S0-BNW-658

Primary Care

A COLLABORATIVE PRACTICE

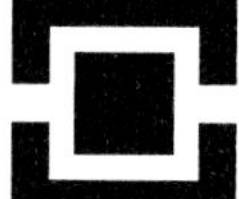

SECOND EDITION

Primary Care

A COLLABORATIVE PRACTICE

Terry Mahan Buttaro, MS, APRN, BC, ANP, GNP, CEN, CCRN
Adult/Gerontologic Nurse Practitioner,
Greenleaf Medical Associates/Lahey Clinic,
Amesbury, Massachusetts;
Beth Israel Deaconess Medical Center (MCCN),
Chelsea, Massachusetts

Patricia Polgar Bailey, MS, MPH, APRN, BC, FNP, CDE
Family Nurse Practitioner,
The Queen's Medical Center;
Clinical Assistant Professor,
University of Hawaii School of Nursing,
Honolulu, Hawaii

JoAnn Trybulski, PhD, APRN, BC, ARNP
Assistant Professor of Clinical Nursing,
University of Miami, School of Nursing,
Miami, Florida

Joanne Sandberg-Cook, MS, APRN, BC, ANP, GNP, CRRN
Adult/Gerontologic Nurse Practitioner,
Dartmouth-Hitchcock Medical Center,
Lebanon, New Hampshire;
Instructor in Medicine,
Dartmouth Medical School,
Hanover, New Hampshire

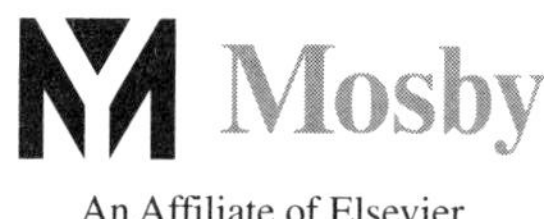

An Affiliate of Elsevier

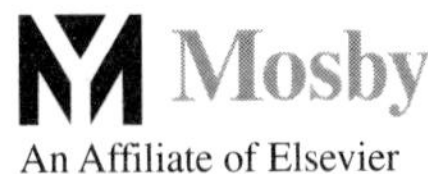

An Affiliate of Elsevier

11830 Westline Industrial Drive
St. Louis, Missouri 63146

PRIMARY CARE: A COLLABORATIVE PRACTICE 0-323-02032-1

NOTICE

Nursing is an ever-changing field. Standard safety precautions must be followed, but as new research and clinical experience broaden our knowledge, changes in treatment and drug therapy may become necessary or appropriate. Readers are advised to check the most current product information provided by the manufacturer of each drug to be administered to verify the recommended dose, the method and duration of administration, and contraindications. It is the responsibility of the licensed prescriber, relying on experience and knowledge of the patient, to determine dosages and the best treatment for each individual patient. Neither the publisher nor the author assumes any liability for any injury and/or damage to persons or property arising from this publication.

The Publisher

Previous edition copyrighted 1999

International Standard Book Number 0-323-02032-1

Acquisitions Editor: Barbara Nelson Cullen
Senior Developmental Editor: Cindi Anderson
Developmental Editor: Stacy Welch
Publishing Services Manager: Deborah L. Vogel
Senior Project Manager: Jodi M. Willard
Design Manager: Bill Drone
Cover and Interior Design: Judy Schmitt

Printed in the United States of America

Last digit is the print number: 9 8 7 6 5 4 3 2

This edition is dedicated to the memory of Dr. Richard Emerine who, for us, embodied our vision for collaborative practice.

Contributors

Murat Anamur, MD
Chief of Oncology Services,
Saints Memorial Medical Center,
Lowell, Massachusetts
Chapters 233, 235

Mary J. Attardo, MSN, RN, C, ANP
Osteoporosis Research and Treatment,
Beth Israel Deaconess Medical Center,
Boston, Massachusetts
Chapter 179

Patricia Polgar Bailey, MS, MPH, APRN, BC, FNP, CDE
Family Nurse Practitioner,
The Queen's Medical Center;
Clinical Assistant Professor,
University of Hawaii School of Nursing,
Honolulu, Hawaii
Chapters 23, 108, 116, 117, 118, 124, 160, 162, 185, 250
Updated Chapters 113, 122, 166, 176, 184

Marie A. Bakitas, ARNP, FAAN
Palliative Care Nurse Practitioner,
Department of Pain Medicine and Palliative Care,
Dartmouth-Hitchcock Medical Center,
Lebanon, New Hampshire
Chapter 12

Claire J. Barrett, RN, MS
Program Director,
Senior Living on Bellingham Hill,
Chelsea, Massachusetts
Chapter 261

Cynthia Erskine Bashaw, MS, RN, CS, FNP
Family Nurse Practitioner,
Department of Internal Medicine,
Pentucket Medical Associates,
Haverhill, Massachusetts
Chapters 17, 127

Rita Beckman-Williams, RNC, MSN
Health Department,
Mount Ida College,
Newton, Massachusetts
Chapter 198

Heather E.T. Bell, MPH, RD, LDN, CHES
Nutrition Consultant,
Smart Cookie Consulting,
Newburyport, Massachusetts
Chapter 14

Martin Jan Bergman, MD, FACR, FACP
Clinical Assistant Professor of Medicine,
Division of Rheumatology,
Medical College of Pennsylvania;
Hanneman University,
Philadelphia, Pennsylvania
Chapter 238

Bonnie L. Bermas, MD
Assistant Professor of Medicine,
Harvard Medical School;
Department of Rheumatology,
Brigham and Women's Hospital,
Boston, Massachusetts
Chapters 240, 243

Wendy L. Biddle, PhD, CFNP
Chief Nurse Practitioner,
Digestive Liver and Disease Specialists,
Norfolk, Virginia
Chapters 148, 149

Rosemary Bill-Fleury, ANP, CDE
Adult Nurse Practitioner,
Department of Internal Medicine,
North Suburban Cardiology,
Stoneham, Massachusetts
Chapter 223

Kathryn Blum, RN, BS, MSN, ANP
Adult Nurse Practitioner,
Newton, Massachusetts
Chapter 225

Maureen B. Boardman, ARNP
Department of Community and Family Medicine,
Dartmouth College,
Hanover, New Hampshire;
Nurse Practitioner,
Dartmouth-Hitchcock Medical Center,
Lebanon, New Hampshire
Chapter 111

Alice Bolton, MS, CS-BC
Private Practice,
Alice Bolton, P.A.,
Sarasota, Florida
Chapters 264, 267

Nancy D. Bolton, RN, MSN, ANP, CCRC
Director of Clinical Research,
Charlottesville Medical Research,
Charlottesville, Virginia
Chapters 146, 156

Karen Borden, MSN, APRN, BC
Nurse Practitioner,
Department of Medical Oncology,
Massachusetts General Hospital,
Boston, Massachusetts
Chapter 254

Marie Elena Botte, MSN, APRN, BC, CDE
Family Nurse Practitioner, Certified Diabetes Educator,
In collaboration with David Richman, MD
Obstetrics and Gynecology,
Malden, Massachusetts;
and with Hayward K. Zwerling, MD
Endocrinology and Internal Medicine,
Lowell, Massachusetts
Chapters 169, 170, 174, 175, 178

David A. Bradshaw, MD, CDR, MC, USN
Head, Pulmonary Division;
Director, Sleep Laboratory,
Naval Medical Center San Diego,
San Diego, California
Chapter 112

Jennifer C. Braimon, MD
Staff Endocrinologist,
Department of Endocrinology,
Lahey Clinic,
Peabody, Massachusetts
Chapter 230

Ann S. Bruner-Welch, AS, PA-C
Physician Assistant,
Multiple Specialties,
Orion Emergency Medical Group,
Santa Rosa, California
Chapters 199, 215, 220

Han Q. Bui, MD
Family Practice,
Naval Hospital Lemoore,
Lemoore Naval Air Station, California
Chapter 248

Terry Mahan Buttaro, MS, APRN, BC, ANP, GNP, CEN, CCRN
Adult/Gerontologic Nurse Practitioner,
Greenleaf Medical Associates/Lahey Clinic,
Amesbury, Massachusetts;
Beth Israel Deaconess Medical Center (MCCN),
Chelsea, Massachusetts
Chapters 3, 25, 28, 30, 31, 32, 42, 115, 116, 125, 143, 154, 162, 226
Updated Chapters 34, 35, 37, 38, 41, 88, 89, 93, 94, 95, 96, 97, 98, 99, 138, 139, 140, 142, 173, 176

Denise T. Bynum, RN, MSN, FNP
Nursing Faculty,
ADN Nursing Division,
Northwest Mississippi Community College,
Senatobia, Mississippi
Chapters 177, 191, 212

Cheryl A. Cahill, RN, PhD
Amelia Peabody Professor of Nursing Research,
MGH Institute of Health Professions,
Boston, Massachusetts
Chapter 2

Cindy D. Campbell, ARNP, ND, CS
Advanced Practice Psychiatric Nurse,
Esprit Professional Services,
Sarasota, Florida
Chapters 266, 267

David R. Campbell, MD
Associate Clinical Professor of Surgery,
Harvard Medical School;
Department of Vascular Surgery,
Beth Israel Deaconess Medical Center,
Boston, Massachusetts
Chapters 135, 137

Virginia Capasso, PhD, APRN, BC
Clinical Nurse Specialist,
Vascular Nursing and Vascular Home Care Program;
Co-Director, Wound Care Center,
Massachusetts General Hospital,
Boston, Massachusetts
Chapters 126, 128

Gretchen Carrougher, MN, RN
Research Coordinator,
Department of Rehabilitation Medicine,
University of Washington Burn Center,
Harborview Medical Center,
Seattle, Washington
Chapter 51

Emily Chandler, RN, CS, MDiv, PhD
Clinical Associate Professor,
Department of Nursing,
Massachusetts General Hospital Institute of Health Professions,
Boston, Massachusetts
Chapter 11

Sharon G. Childs, MS, APRN-BC, CS,CEN, ONC
Adult Nurse Practitioner,
Trauma–Critical Care Clinical Nurse Specialist,
Concentra Medical Center,
Baltimore, Maryland
Chapters 187, 197

Noreen Connolly, RN, CS, MSN
Nurse Educator, Adult Nurse Practitioner,
Caritas St. Elizabeth's Medical Center,
Boston, Massachusetts
Chapter 5

Kathleen M. Craig, RNC, BSN, IBCLC
Lactation Consultant/Birthing Nurse,
Dartmouth-Hitchcock Medical Center,
Lebanon, New Hampshire
Chapter 8

Sandra L. Creamer, RN, CS, PhD, OCN
Oncology/Hematology Nurse Practitioner/ Clinical Specialist,
The Cancer Center,
Saints Memorial Medical Center,
Lowell, Massachusetts
Chapters 233, 235

Susan Cross-Skinner, MSN, RNCS
Adult Nurse Practitioner,
Isham Health Center,
Phillips Academy Andover,
Andover, Massachusetts
Chapter 249

Constance Dahlin, RNCS, MSN, ANP
Nurse Practitioner,
Palliative Care Service,
Massachusetts General Hospital,
Boston, Massachusetts
Chapters 12, 13

Jeffrey B. Dattilo, MD
Assistant Professor of Surgery,
Division of Vascular Surgery,
Vanderbilt University Medical Center;
Attending Surgeon,
Veteran's Administration Hospital,
Nashville, Tennessee
Chapter 128

Eileen M. Deignan, MD
Dermatology Associates of Concord, Inc.,
Concord, Massachusetts
Chapters 45, 48, 49, 51, 52, 53, 58, 59, 60, 69, 70, 73

Sallustio Del Re, MD, FCCP
Teaching Attending,
Departments of Pulmonary and Critical Care,
Atlantic City Medical Center,
Atlantic City, New Jersey
Chapter 110

Karen Dick, PhD, APRN, BC
Assistant Professor and Coordinator,
Adult/Gerontological Nurse Practitioner Program,
University of Massachusetts,
Boston, Massachusetts
Chapters 209, 210

Karin C. Dieselman, MS, RNCS, ANP
Adult Nurse Practitioner,
Department of Occupational Health,
Anna Jaques Hospital,
Newburyport, Massachusetts
Chapters 27, 192

Susan Waldrop Donckers, RN, EdD, CS, FNP
Department of Internal Medicine,
Lewis Gale Clinic,
Salem, Virginia
Chapters 120, 121

Annabel D. Edwards, RN, MSN, ANP
Clinical Nurse Specialist,
Department of Anesthesia—Pain Center,
Massachusetts General Hospital,
Boston, Massachusetts
Chapter 257

Walter Elias, III, MD
Head, Clinical/Business Operations,
Naval Healthcare Support Office San Diego,
San Diego, California
Chapters 33, 47

Kathy J. Fabiszewski, RN, CS, PhD
Assistant Professor,
School of Nursing,
Salem State College,
Salem, Massachusetts;
Nurse Practitioner,
Family Doctors,
Swampscott, Massachusetts
Chapter 203

Julie P. Fago, MD
Associate Professor of Medicine,
Department of Medicine and Geriatrics,
Dartmouth Medical School,
Hanover, New Hampshire
Chapter 202

Jackie S. Fantes, MD
Staff Physician, Family Practice,
Naval Ambulatory Care Center,
Newport, Rhode Island
Chapters 29, 173

Patricia A. Fergus, RN, RRT
Respiratory Therapist,
St. Louis University Hospital,
St. Louis, Missouri
Chapter 21

Michele DuBois Finnell, MS, RNC
Nurse Practitioner,
Department of Rheumatology,
Beth Israel Deaconess Medical Center,
Boston, Massachusetts
Chapter 196

Jane Flanagan, PhD, RNCS
Team Leader,
Pre-Admission Testing Clinic,
Massachusetts General Hospital,
Boston, Massachusetts
Chapter 24

Patricia C. Flanagan, RN, MSN, CS
Clinical Nurse Specialist,
Emergency Department,
Massachusetts General Hospital;
Adjunct Faculty,
MGH Institute of Health Professions,
Boston, Massachusetts
Chapter 130

Diana G. French, PhD, RN, FNP, GNP
Professor,
School of Nursing,
Medical College of Ohio,
Toledo, Ohio
Chapter 193

Michelle E. Freshman, MPH, MSN, RN, CS
Assistant Clinical Care Manager,
Rehabilitation Services,
Newton-Wellesley Hospital,
Newton, Massachusetts
Chapters 224, 246, 247, 251, 252

Elizabeth Friedlander, MS, MEd, ANP/FNP
Clinical Assistant Professor,
Department of Graduate Nursing,
MGH Institute of Health Professions,
Boston, Massachusetts
Chapter 150

Cynthia J. Gantt, RN, PhD, CFNP
Nurse Scientist, Family Nurse Practitioner,
Naval Medical Center San Diego,
San Diego, California
Chapter 171

Denise DeJoseph Gauthier, RN, MS, ACNP
Acute Care Nurse Practitioner,
Department of Cardiology,
Massachusetts General Hospital,
Boston, Massachusetts
Chapter 131

Maryjane B. Giacalone, MS, ANP, ACNP
Department of Cardiology,
Massachusetts General Hospital,
Boston, Massachusetts
Chapter 133

Karen L. Gilbert, MS, ARNP, CNRN
Clinical Coordinator/Nurse Practitioner,
Dartmouth Epilepsy Program,
Department of Neurology,
Dartmouth-Hitchcock Medical Center,
Lebanon, New Hampshire
Chapters 39, 218

Patricia Gillett, RN, MSN, CNS, FNP, ACNP
Family Nurse Practitioner,
First Choice Community Healthcare,
Albuquerque, New Mexico
Chapters 75, 76, 77, 78, 79, 80, 81, 82, 83, 84

Donna M. Glynn, MS, RNCS
Adult Nurse Practitioner,
John Diorio, MD, and Associates,
Compass Medical,
Brockton, Massachusetts
Chapter 156

Kate Goldblum, MSN, RN, CS, CRNO, CFNP
Clinical Nurse Specialist, Ophthalmology,
Nurse Practitioner,
Goldblum Family Eye Care Center,
Albuquerque, New Mexico
Chapters 75, 76, 77, 78, 79, 80, 81, 82, 83, 84

Deanna G. Gordon, PhD, MPH, RN
Professor of Nursing,
School of Nursing,
Capital University,
Bexley, Ohio
Chapter 21

John Joseph Graykoski, BS, PA-C
Physician's Assistant,
Emergency Department,
Sutter Santa Rosa Medical Center,
Santa Rosa, California;
Coppertowers Family Medical Center,
Cloverdale, California
Chapter 208

Marilyn Bleiler Green, MS, RN, CS
Adult Nurse Practitioner,
Granite Medical,
Quincy, Massachusetts
Chapters 18, 160

Brenda L. Hage, MSN, CRNP, CRRN-A
Assistant Professor,
Department of Nursing,
College Misericordia,
Dallas, Pennsylvania
Chapter 15

Susan Harvey, MSN, RN-CS, FNP
Family Nurse Practitioner,
Medical Staff,
Winslow Indian Health Center/Navajo Area,
Winslow, Arizona
Chapters 107, 119

Simon M. Helfgott, MD
Assistant Professor of Medicine,
Harvard Medical School,
Boston, Massachusetts
Chapter 244

Debra Hobbins, MSN, APRN
Associate Chief Nurse,
Clinical Manager, Primary Care,
Veteran's Administration Salt Lake City Health Care System,
Salt Lake City, Utah
Chapters 7, 136, 182

Susan Hoch, MD
Associate Professor,
Department of Medicine,
Drexel University College of Medicine,
Philadelphia, Pennsylvania
Chapters 237, 239

Bonnie Hooper, RN, ANP, MSN, DNC
Nurse Practitioner,
Dermatology Associates,
Encinitas, California
Chapters 48, 73

Eric M. Isselbacher, MD
Assistant Professor of Medicine,
Cardiology Division,
Massachusetts General Hospital;
Harvard Medical School,
Boston, Massachusetts
Chapter 131

David C. Jimerson, MD
Professor of Psychiatry,
Harvard Medical School;
Director of Research,
Department of Psychiatry,
Beth Israel Deaconess Medical Center,
Boston, Massachusetts
Chapter 263

Dorothy Johnson, FNP, DNSc
Department of Rheumatology,
LAC and USC Health Care Network,
Los Angeles, California
Chapters 241, 242

Brenda L. Jordan, MS, APRN, BC
Adult Nurse Practitioner/Gerontologic Clinical Nurse Specialist,
Department of Community and Family Medicine,
Dartmouth-Hitchcock Medical Center,
Lebanon, New Hampshire
Chapter 217

E. Lynne Kelley, MD
Vascular Surgery Fellow,
Department of Vascular Surgery,
Massachusetts General Hospital,
Boston, Massachusetts
Chapter 126

Marianne Kelly, RN, BS
Sleep Disorders Center,
Boston Medical Center,
Boston, Massachusetts
Chapter 16

Philip E. Knapp, MD
Department of Medicine,
Boston University,
Boston, Massachusetts
Chapter 227

Nancy W. Knee, MS, ARNP
Family Practice Nurse Practitioner,
Dartmouth-Hitchcock/Plymouth Pediatrics and Adolescent Medicine,
Plymouth, New Hampshire;
Concord Family Medicine,
Concord, New Hampshire
Chapters 56, 63, 64, 71

Patricia A. Lamb, RN, MN, CNS, CNOR, CRNO
President/Owner,
Ophthalmic Nursing Care of Arizona, Inc.,
Phoenix, Arizona
Chapter 75

Nancy McQueen Le, RNC, MS, GNP, CNRN
Gerontological Nurse Practitioner,
Nova Psychiatric Services,
Quincy, Massachusetts
Chapters 211, 216

Noreen M. Leahy, MS, RN, CS
Nurse Practitioner,
Department of Neuro-Oncology,
Massachusetts General Hospital,
Boston, Massachusetts
Chapters 206, 207, 219

Anne LeMaitre, PT
Director of Rehabilitation,
Department of Rehabilitation,
Port Healthcare Center,
Newburyport, Massachusetts
Chapter 205

Renato Lenzi, MD
Associate Professor,
Gastrointestinal Medical Oncology,
The University of Texas;
M.D. Anderson Cancer Center,
Houston, Texas
Chapter 255

Naaznin Lokhandwala, MD
Endocrinology Fellow,
Department of Endocrinology,
Lahey Clinic,
Burlington, Massachusetts
Chapter 230

Patricia A. Lowry, MS
Acute Care Nurse Practitioner,
Department of Nursing,
Massachusetts General Hospital,
Boston, Massachusetts
Chapter 129

Nancy S. Mahan, MS
Director of Residential Services,
Bay Cove Human Services,
Boston, Massachusetts
Chapters 262, 265

Alan Ona Malabanan, MD, FACE
Clinical Director,
Section of Endocrinology, Diabetes, and Nutrition,
Department of Medicine,
Boston University Medical Center,
Boston, Massachusetts
Chapters 201, 221, 229

Maura Malone, RN, MSN
Clinical Nurse Specialist,
Hematology/Oncology,
Hemophilia and Thrombosis Center,
Dartmouth-Hitchcock Medical Center,
Lebanon, New Hampshire
Chapter 232

Elyse Mandell, MSN, RNCS
Nurse Practitioner,
Hematology Division,
Brigham and Women's Hospital,
Boston, Massachusetts
Chapter 231

Margaret McAllister, RN, PhD, FNP-C, ABRN, BC, FAANP
Associate Professor and Coordinator,
Family Nurse Practitioner Program,
Department of Nursing,
College of Nursing and Health Sciences,
University of Massachusetts—Boston,
Boston, Massachusetts
Chapters 44, 54, 61, 62, 65

Kathleen Golden McAndrew, ARNP, CS, FAAOHN
Executive Director,
University Health Services;
Adjunct Associate Professor,
Department of Nursing,
University of Massachusetts—Boston,
Boston, Massachusetts
Chapter 19

Talli Craig McCormick, MSN, RN-C
Clinical Assistant Professor,
Department of Nursing/Gerontology,
MGH Institute of Health Professions,
Boston, Massachusetts
Chapter 153

Dennis M. McCullough, MD
Chief Clinical Officer,
Department of Community and Family Medicine,
Dartmouth Medical School,
Hanover, New Hampshire
Chapter 222

Claire McGowan, MS, RN, CS, CCRN
Nurse Practitioner,
Pre-Admission Testing Clinic,
Massachusetts General Hospital,
Boston, Massachusetts
Chapter 24

Laurel McKernan, MSN, RN
Clinical Nurse Specialist,
Hematology/Oncology,
Dartmouth-Hitchcock Medical Center,
Lebanon, New Hampshire
Chapter 232

Ruth M. Messer, RN, BSN, OCN
Certified Oncology Nurse,
All Saints Memorial Cancer Center,
Lowell, Massachusetts
Chapter 233

Eran D. Metzger, MD
Instructor of Psychiatry,
Harvard Medical School;
Associate in Psychiatry,
Beth Israel Deaconess Medical Center,
Boston, Massachusetts
Chapter 263

Louise Meyer, MS, ARNP
Nurse Practitioner,
Department of Oncology,
Dartmouth-Hitchcock Medical Center,
Lebanon, New Hampshire
Chapters 145, 151, 155

Cheryl A. Miller, APRN, BC
Geriatric Nurse Practitioner,
Hebrew Rehabilitation Center,
Recuperative Services Unit,
Rosindale, Massachusetts
Chapter 22

Sally-Ann Milne, CRNI, OCN, CEN
Nursing Registry—Outpatient Infusion,
Naples Community Hospital,
Naples, Florida
Chapter 233

Virginia McNally Minichiello, MS, APRN-BC
Adult Nurse Practitioner,
Co-Coordinator, Direct Entry Nursing Program,
Northeastern University,
Boston, Massachusetts
Chapter 196

Catharine Moffett, RN, MSN, FNP
Director,
Student Health Services,
Connecticut College,
New London, Connecticut
Chapter 20

Denise J. Mullaney, MSN, RNCS, ANP, ACNP
Acute Care Nurse Practitioner,
Massachusetts General Hospital,
Boston, Massachusetts
Chapter 133

Debra S. Munsell, MPAS, PA-C
Director, Physician Assistant Student Oncology Program,
Department of Head and Neck Surgical Oncology,
The University of Texas;
M.D. Anderson Cancer Center,
Houston, Texas
Chapters 100, 101, 102, 103, 104, 105, 106

David Patrick Murphy, MD
Fellow, Pulmonary and Critical Care,
Department of Medicine,
Naval Medical Center,
San Diego, California
Chapter 112

Jennifer Neves
Pre-Admission Testing Clinic,
Massachusetts General Hospital,
Boston, Massachusetts
Chapter 24

Kathlyn Nowak, RNC, MS
Nurse Practitioner,
Nutritional Support Services,
Beth Israel Deaconess Medical Center,
Boston, Massachusetts
Chapter 225

Karen Koozer Olson, PhD, FNP-CS
Professor of Nursing,
School of Nursing and Health Sciences,
Texas A & M University—Corpus Christi,
Corpus Christi, Texas
Chapters 85, 86, 90, 91

Daniel W. O'Neill, MD
Assistant Clinical Professor,
Department of Family Medicine,
University of Connecticut School of Medicine,
Farmington, Connecticut
Chapters 50, 66, 214

Marie-Eileen Onieal, PhD (C), MMHS, RNC, PNP, FAANP
Health Policy Coordinator,
Bureau of Health Quality Management,
Massachusetts Department of Public Health,
Boston, Massachusetts
Chapters 186, 195

Maureen O'Hara Padden, MD, MPH
Director of Residency Training,
Naval Hospital Camp Lejuene,
Jacksonville, North Carolina
Chapters 55, 72

Marcia L. Patterson, MSN, RN, NP-C
Advanced Practice Nurse,
Department of Genitourinary Medical Oncology,
The University of Texas;
M.D. Anderson Cancer Center,
Houston, Texas
Chapters 253, 256

Donna Jenell Pease, BSN, MSN
Adult/Geriatric Nurse Practitioner,
Certified Diabetes Educator,
Adult Medicine Clinic,
Tripler Army Medical Center,
Honolulu, Hawaii
Chapter 228

Samara Peña, MD
Fellow in Endocrinology, Diabetes, and Nutrition,
Department of Endocrinology,
Boston Medical Center,
Boston, Massachusetts
Chapter 229

Joanne Marie Petrelli, RN, MSN, CRNP-Adult, LCDR, NC, USN
Department of Internal Medicine,
Naval Medical Center San Diego,
San Diego, California
Chapter 147

Timothy J. Phillips, MD
Family Practice Staff,
Senior Medical Officer,
Branch Clinic,
Yuma, Arizona
Chapter 43

Joyce Powers, RN, MSN, CS, FNP, ACNP
Nurse Practitioner,
Department of Cardiology,
Veteran's Administration,
Albuquerque, New Mexico
Chapters 75, 76, 77, 78, 79, 80, 81, 82, 83, 84

William R. Prebola, Jr., MD, FAAPMR
Private Practice,
Physical and Rehabilitation Medicine,
Northeastern Rehabilitation Associates, PC,
Wilkes-Barre, Pennsylvania
Chapter 15

Judy Ptak, RN, MSN
Infection Control Practitioner,
Dartmouth-Hitchcock Medical Center,
Lebanon, New Hampshire
Chapter 114

Francisco P. Quismorio, Jr., MD
Vice Chief, Professor of Medicine and Pathology,
Division of Rheumatology and Clinical Immunology,
Keck School of Medicine,
University of Southern California,
Los Angeles, California
Chapters 241, 242

Joseph Rampulla, RN, MS, NP, CAS
Nurse Practitioner,
Boston Health Care for the Homeless Program,
Medical Walk-in Unit,
Massachusetts General Hospital,
Boston, Massachusetts
Chapters 259, 268

Roberta N. Regan, MSN, RN
Nurse Practitioner, Evercare,
United Health Care,
Newton, Massachusetts
Chapters 5, 132

Suzanne Mary Rieke, MD
Endocrine Fellow,
Section of Endocrinology, Diabetes and Nutrition,
Boston University School of Medicine,
Boston, Massachusetts
Chapter 221

Robert J. Riggen, MD, MS
Attending Physician,
Emergency Department,
Central Vermont Medical Center,
Berlin, Vermont
Chapter 198

Barbara Jean Roberge, PhD, RN, CS
Geriatric Nurse Practitioner, Nurse Coordinator,
Senior Health Practice—Geriatric Unit,
Massachusetts General Hospital,
Boston, Massachusetts
Chapter 10

JoAnne Sandberg-Cook, MS, APRN, BC, ANP, GNP, CRRN
Adult/Gerontologic Nurse Practitioner,
Dartmouth-Hitchcock Medical Center,
Lebanon, New Hampshire;
Instructor in Medicine,
Dartmouth Medical School,
Hanover, New Hampshire
Chapters 68, 161, 245
Updated Chapters 123, 159, 180, 181

Elizabeth C. Sensenig, MSN, ARNP
Nurse Practitioner,
Clinical Instructor,
Obstetrics and Gynecology,
Department of Reproductive Endocrinology and Infertility,
Dartmouth-Hitchcock Medical Center,
Lebanon, New Hampshire
Chapter 185

Willadene Walker Schmucker, ARNP, MS, MAEd, EdDc
Owner,
The Alternative,
Sarasota, Florida
Chapters 260, 267

Captain Scott W. Shiffer, MSN, FNPC
Family Practice,
U.S. Naval Hospital,
Rota, Spain
Chapters 141, 188

Robert H. Shmerling, MD, FACP
Associate Professor of Medicine,
Harvard Medical School;
Department of Medicine,
Division of Rheumatology,
Beth Israel Deaconess Medical Center,
Boston, Massachusetts
Chapter 236

Cathy J. Sizer, RN, MSN, CPNP
Clinical Instructor,
Department of Graduate Nursing,
Simmons College;
President,
Eastern Massachusetts Chapter,
National Association of Pediatric Nurse Practitioners (NAPNAP),
Boston, Massachusetts
Chapter 6

Sharon R. Smart, MS, RN, CS, FNP
Family Nurse Practitioner,
Greenleaf Medical Associate/Lahey Clinic,
Amesbury, Massachusetts
Chapters 144, 152

LT Clayton M. Smiley, MD
Department of Internal Medicine,
Naval Medical Center San Diego,
San Diego, California
Chapter 109

Chad J. Smith, DO
Family Physician,
Department of Family Medicine,
Naval Hospital Camp Pendleton,
Camp Pendleton, California
Chapters 87, 92

Jean E. Steel, PhD, FAAN
Professor and Chair, Advanced Practice Nursing,
Graduate Program in Nursing,
Massachusetts General Hospital Institute of Health Professions,
Boston, Massachusetts
Chapter 1

Laura Stempkowski, MS, CUNP, AOCN
Nurse Practitioner—Genitourinary Oncology,
Department of Urology,
Dartmouth-Hitchcock Medical Center,
Lebanon, New Hampshire
Chapters 157, 167

Robbyn Takeuchi, MSW
Social Worker,
The Queen Emma Clinics,
The Queen's Medical Center,
Honolulu, Hawaii
Chapters 21, 40

Thomas H. Taylor, MD, MS
Associate Professor of Medicine,
Division of Infectious Diseases,
Dartmouth Medical School,
Hanover, New Hampshire
Chapters 194, 200

Elizabeth Renee Thomas, JD, RN, MSN
Nurse Practitioner,
Department of Interventional Radiology,
Brigham and Women's Hospital,
Boston, Massachusetts
Chapter 176

Debra Toran, MSN, RN, CS
Nurse Practitioner,
Department of Gynecology/Oncology,
Massachusetts General Hospital,
Boston, Massachusetts
Chapter 254

JoAnn Trybulski, PhD, RNCS, APRN, BC
Assistant Professor of Clinical Nursing,
University of Miami, School of Nursing,
Miami, Florida
Chapters 3, 26, 36, 125, 134, 154
Updated Chapter 138

Catherine E. Turner, MSN, FNP-C
CDR, Navy Nurse Corps,
Family Care Clinic,
Halyburton Naval Hospital,
MCAS Cherry Point,
Havelock, North Carolina,
Chapters 57, 67

Susan R. Tussey, MSN, FNP, NP-C
Family Nurse Practitioner,
Family Practice Clinic,
Twentynine Palms Naval Hospital,
Twentynine Palms, California
Chapter 190

Gretchen Van Buren, RN, ARNP
Adult Nurse Practitioner,
General Internal Medicine,
Dartmouth-Hitchcock Medical Center,
Lebanon, New Hampshire
Chapter 213

Janet H. Van Cleave, RN, ACNP-CS, AOCN
Acute Care Nurse Practitioner,
Oncology Care Center,
The Mount Sinai Medical Center,
New York, New York
Chapter 234

Denise A. Vanacore, PhD, CRNP, APRN, BC, CNOR
Coordinator, Adult Nurse Practitioner Program,
Director, Primary Care Health Services,
School of Nursing,
Gwynedd-Mercy College,
Gwynedd Valley, Pennsylvania
Chapters 35, 38, 46, 189

Monika Walczak, MD
Endocrinology Fellow,
Department of Endocrinology,
Lahey Clinic,
Burlington, Massachusetts
Chapter 230

Verra L.N. Wekullo, MD
General Medical Doctor,
University of Nairobi, Kenya;
Third-Year Medical Resident,
Atlantic City Medical Center,
Atlantic City, New Jersey
Chapter 110

Janelle M. West-Koo, MSW, MPA
Social Worker,
The Queen Emma Clinics,
The Queen's Medical Center,
Honolulu, Hawaii
Chapters 21, 40

Carol A. Whelan, MS, CAGS, CS, ANP
Primary Care Division,
Yale University School of Nursing,
New Haven, Connecticut;
Department of Medicine,
Rocky Hill Veteran's Home and Hospital,
Rocky Hill, Connecticut
Chapters 158, 163, 164, 165, 168

Patricia A. White, MS, APRN, BC
Assistant Professor,
Department of Graduate Nursing,
School for Health Studies,
Simmons College,
Boston, Massachusetts
Chapter 4

Cynthia M. Williams, DO, MAEd, CAPT, MC, USN
Assistant Professor,
Department of Family Medicine,
Uniformed Services University of the Health Sciences,
Bethesda, Maryland
Chapters 172, 183

Jane Williams, MSN, RN, FNP, BC
Advanced Practice Nurse,
Department of Genitourinary Medical Oncology,
The University of Texas,
M.D. Anderson Cancer Center,
Houston, Texas
Chapters 253, 256, 258

Barbara Willson, PhD, MSN
Gerontological Nurse Practitioner,
Faculty Emerita,
Massachusetts General Hospital Institute of Health Professions,
Boston, Massachusetts
Chapter 9

Christine M. Wilson, PhD, RN, CS
Assistant Professor,
Graduate Program in Nursing,
Massachusetts General Hospital of Health Professions,
Boston, Massachusetts
Chapter 204

Barbara E. Wolfe, PhD, RN, CS, FAAN
Assistant Professor of Psychiatry,
Harvard Medical School,
Department of Psychiatry,
Beth Israel Deaconess Medical Center,
Boston, Massachusetts
Chapter 263

Mary Young, MSN, ARNP, CS
Adult Nurse Practitioner,
Department of Cardiology,
Kaiser Permanente Medical Clinic,
Wailuku, Hawaii
Chapter 74

Leo R. Zacharski, MD
Professor of Medicine,
Dartmouth Medical School,
Hanover, New Hampshire
Chapter 232

Randall M. Zusman, MD
Associate Professor of Medicine,
Harvard Medical School;
Director, Division of Hypertension and Vascular Medicine,
Cardiac Unit,
Massachusetts General Hospital,
Boston, Massachusetts
Chapter 133

CONTRIBUTORS TO THE FIRST EDITION

James L. Abbruzzese, MD
Detection of Tumor of Unknown Origin

Saralynn H. Allaire, ScD, RN
Rheumatoid Arthritis
Systemic Lupus Erythematosus

Joseph C. Aquilina, MD
Hepatitis

Sheryl M. Barkan, MSN, RN, CS, ANP
Elbow Pain

Joyce S. Billue, EdD, RN, CS, RNP
Bell's Palsy

Beth Blackington, MS, Med, RNCS
Irritable Bowel Syndrome

Susan Browne, MD, FAAP, IBCLC
Lactation

Leslie Burton, RN, MSN, CNN, ANP
Diverticular Disease

Diane L. Carroll, PhD, RN
Heart Failure

Jackie Cassidy, MS, CCC-SP
Dysphagia

Tamera D. Cauthorne-Burnette, RN, MSN, FNP
Dermatitis Medicamentosa
Intertrigo
Nail Disorders
Stasis Dermatitis

Alison B. Christopher, LCSW
Bipolar Disorder

Dorothy S. Cluff, RN, MSN, CFNP
Erectile Dysfunction
Tumors of the Genitourinary Tract
Urinary Calculi

Leslie J. Collins, RN
Unplanned Pregnancy

Inge B. Corless, PhD, RN, FAAN
HIV Infection

Cornelius J. Cornell, MD
Blood Coagulation Disorders

Stephen T. Cruz, MD
Syncope

Maureen Cullen, RN, MS, CCRN, CEN, EMT
Barotrauma and Other Diving Injuries

William L. Daley, MD, MPH
Chest Pain and Coronary Artery Disease

Denise A. DeJoseph, RNCS, ANP
Endocarditis

Thomas G. DiSalvo, MD, MPH
Heart Failure

Linda M. Douville, MS, ARNP
Breast Disorders

Richard J. Dowling, MD
Gastrointestinal Bleeding

Claire Ford Dunbar, ANP-C, MS
Thyroid Disorders

Richard W. Emerine, MD, NPH, FAAFP
Alopecia
Altitude Illness
Screening for Skin Cancer

Mary E. Farrell, PhD(c), RN, CCRN
Sprains, Strains, and Fractures

Annette Gary, RNC, PhD, CNAA, FNP
Testicular Disorders

Denise Ladd Goksel, RN, MSN, MSc, FNP
Abdominal Pain and Infections
Tumors of the Gastrointestinal Tract

Barbara Kingsley Hathaway, C-RNP, ANP, MIH
Hand and Wrist Pain

Judith M. Haywood, ARNP, EdD
Jaundice

Elizabeth Hossan, MD
Basic Principles of Oncology Treatment

Susan Crocker Houde, PhD, RN
Incontinence
Prostate Disorders

Lorraine K. Jacobsohn, RN, MS, CS
Domestic Violence
Sexual Assault

Thomas W. Jenkins, MS, PA-C
Hemoptysis
Sarcoidosis

Vicki Y. Johnson, RN, PhD, CURN
Testicular Disorders

Patricia A. Joyce, RN, MSN, ANP, CS
Lipid Disorders

Nancy Kotzuba, RN, MSN, CS, PNP
Epiglottitis
Peritonsillar Abscess
Pharyngitis and Tonsillitis

Frances J. Lagana, DPM
Diabetes Mellitus

Margaret LaGrange, MSN, RN, CS, ANP
Collaborative Management of the Oncology Patient
Gastrointestinal Symptoms in the Oncology Patient

Laurie Landry, MS, RN, CS
Constipation

Diane Panton Lapsley, MS, RN, CS
Cardiac Arrhythmias
Valvular Heart Disease and Cardiac Murmurs

Eric Larsen, MD
Blood Coagulation Disorders

Dara K. Lee, MD
Cardiac Diagnostic Testing: Noninvasive Assessment of Coronary Artery Disease

Pamela V. Lehmberg, MSN, RN, CS
Genital Human Papillomavirus

Ann H. Lewis, PhD
Cholesteatoma
Impaired Hearing
Inner Ear Disturbances
Tympanic Membrane Perforation

Jane Maffie-Lee, MSN, RN, CS, FNP
Chronic Obstructive Pulmonary Disease

Sheryl A. Martz, MSN, RN, CS, NP-C
Screening for Sexually Transmitted Diseases

Karlwin J. Matthews, MD
Warts

Timothy E. McAlindon, MD, MPM
Rheumatoid Arthritis
Systemic Lupus Erythematosus

Steven T. Meister, MD
Chemical Exposure

Patricia J. Mian, RN, MS, CS
Domestic Violence

Virginia Pender Michel, RN, MSN, ANP
Anorectal Complaints

Katherine B. Mishaw, BSN, MS
Oncology Complications and Paraneoplastic Syndromes

Diane Mitchell, RN, MSN, ANP
Chest Pain (Noncardiac)
Dyspnea
Sleep Apnea

Catherine Morency, MS, RNC
Dementia

Brian S. Morris, MD
Rhinitis

Kathleen L. Neill, RN, CS-ANP, MSN, MA
Chronic Pain

Laura K. Neilley, RN-C, MSN, ANP, GNP
Multiple Sclerosis
Trigeminal Neuralgia

Patrice Kenneally Nicholas, DNSc, RN, ANP
Legal Issues

Cynthia H. Nichols, FNP, RN
Diarrhea

Nancy H. Nicholson, RN, MSN, NP
Vulvar Pruritus and Vulvar Pain

Noreen Heer Nicol, MS, RN, FNP
Fungal Infections

Cheryl A. Ostrowski, MD
Vulvar Dystrophy

Julie A. Patterson, MD
Paget's Disease of the Bone

Alexandra Paul-Simon, PhD, RN
Legal Issues

Lisa Presutto-Curley, RPT
Osteoporosis

Richard D. Quattrone, DO, LT, MC, USN
Cellulitis

Joseph N. Ragan, MD
Cerebrovascular Events
Seizures

Jennifer A. Ramin, MSN, RN, CS
Pap Smear Abnormalities
Pelvic Inflammatory Disease
Vaginitis and Vaginosis

Martha G. Regan-Smith, MD, EdD
Ankylosing Spondylitis and Related Disorders
Polymyalgia Rheumatica and Temporal Arteritis

Jacqueline Rhoads, PhD
Cirrhosis

Catherine Rhuda, RN, MSN, CS
Lymphomas

Thomas P. Rocco, MD
Cardiac Diagnostic Testing: Noninvasive Assessment of Coronary Artery Disease

G.V.R.K. Sharma, MD
Cardiac Arrhythmias

Daniel H. Solomon, MD
Vasculitis

Laura M. Sterling, MD
Poisoning
Thermal Injuries

William S. Strauss, MD
Valvular Heart Disease and Cardiac Murmurs

Tim Stryker, MD
Diabetes Mellitus
Osteoporosis

Paul S. Sullivan, DO
Amyotrophic Lateral Sclerosis
Hepatitis

Stacey A. Swaika, MD
Head Trauma
Hepatitis

Viva Jane Tapper, MSN, ARNP
Parkinson's Disease

Janet E. Tatman, PhD, PA-C
Sleep Disorders

Kathleen Thaney, MS, CRNP-A
Lung Cancer

Deborah M. Thorpe, PhD, RN, CS
Management of Cancer Pain

Cheryle M. Totte, MS, RNC
Osteoarthritis

Eugene G. Tutko, MD
Ocular Emergencies

Peter J. Ungvarski, MS, RN, FAAN, ACRN
HIV Infection

Lynn Valentine, DNSc, FNP, RN
Collaborative Practice

Peggy Vernon, RN, MA, C-PNP
Acne Vulgaris
Contact Dermatitis
Dry Skin
Eczematous Dermatitis (Atopic Dermatitis)
Herpes Zoster (Shingles)
Psoriasis
Scabies
Seborrheic Dermatitis

Joan Domigan Wentz, MSN, RN, CS, ANP
Wound Management

Karen G. Wiberg, MSN, RNC
Obesity

Leila S.L. Williams, DO, LT, USN, MC
Electrical Injuries

Gerri Wittrock-Walton, MS, RN, CS
Pedal Edema

Nancy M. Youngblood, PhD, CRNP, FNP
Chronic Nasal Congestion and Discharge
Epistaxis
Nasal Trauma
Sinusitis
Smell and Taste Disturbances
Tumors and Polyps of the Nose

Reviewers

Christine M. Hatch, MS, RN, CS, FNP
Department of Cardiology and Internal Medicine,
Sea Coast Medical Association,
Newburyport, Massachusetts

Denise G. Max, RN, MSN, APN, C
Capital Health System at Mercer,
Trenton, New Jersey

Richard E. Moon, BSc, MSc, MD, CM, ABIM, ABA, ABPM
Duke University Medical Center,
Department of Anesthesiology,
Durham, North Carolina

Barbara Schaefer, RN, MS, CS-ACNP
Kaiser-Permanente Medical Center,
Department of Neurosurgery,
Anaheim, California

Teri R. Simpson, RN, CS, MSN, FNP, ACNP, CEN, CCRN, CFRN, EMT-P
Metropolitan Hospital,
Grand Rapids, Michigan

Vijay Thadani, MD, PhD
Dartmouth-Hitchcock Medical Center,
Lebanon, New Hampshire

Preface

In the first edition of *Primary Care: A Collaborative Practice*, we recognized that collaboration would be the hallmark for health care delivery in the new millennium. Now that the twenty-first century is underway, we are challenged to articulate *the evidence base for care*. Building the evidence base for practice requires collaboration among researchers and clinicians of multiple disciplines to identify "best practices" and evaluate support for previously unchallenged therapeutic interventions.

This new edition addresses the evolution of thought inherent in any practice discipline. New chapters have been added, and previous chapters have been evaluated and updated with the latest information from an evidence-based perspective. Palliative Care, Presurgical Clearance, Preparticipation Sports Physical, and College Health are among the new chapters of timely interest to primary care providers. The section entitled Weighing the Evidence for Practice represents the essence of our philosophy: primary care practice is collaborative and evolves based on the knowledge created for practice by research. In today's health care environment, primary care providers must be astute consumers of research to deliver the highest quality of care for their patients.

The response to the first edition validated our efforts to provide a multidisciplinary resource for learning and practice. We welcomed comments from practicing clinicians and students and tried in this edition to preserve the balance between a comprehensive and a concise approach to each topic. We have one regret—the loss of one of our key section editors, Dr. Richard Emerine. A source of inspiration for everyone, Rich embodied the spirit of collaboration and encouraged many of the authors who participated in this project. We miss his boundless energy, his mentoring, and gratefully dedicate this edition to him and his memory.

FORMAT

The second edition of *Primary Care: A Collaborative Practice* continues to recognize the increasing complexity of both primary care and the role of the primary care provider. The scope of primary care practice is immense, multifaceted, and in a constant state of evolution. Issues commonly encountered in the delivery of primary care are presented in this text within a framework that encourages comprehensive and cost-effective care. The format of each chapter remains consistent. A health promotion section has been incorporated in many sections to highlight the importance of health teaching and health promotion in the care of patients.

EMERGENCY AND PHYSICIAN REFERRAL ICONS

This text takes a unique approach by recognizing that collaboration among interdisciplinary team members is enhanced when communication is encouraged and the scope of practice of each provider is well defined and understood. This text has clear guidelines for referrals, and icons highlight conditions that require immediate consultation. Experience and skills vary among primary care providers; therefore these icons are organized into the following levels:

The emergency icon represents circumstances concerning specific emergent conditions. Any patient experiencing these signs and symptoms requires immediate emergency department and/or physician referral.

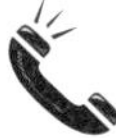

The physician referral icon represents the need for physician consultation for diagnosis or management. The phrase "Physician consultation is indicated" is used for situations in which a physician's consultation is necessary. The phrase "Physician consultation is recommended" is used for situations in which physician consultation may depend on the primary care provider's level of experience.

The reader should be aware that more comprehensive referral or consultation criteria are contained in the text of the chapters that have these special icons. The reader should also realize that the emergency icons might not include all the conditions that need emergency referral. The editors are also aware that experienced providers may not require consultation for all the specified circumstances. State practice regulations may mandate referral under certain circumstances; these regulations supersede any reference to consultation points detailed in this text.

DIAGNOSTICS AND DIFFERENTIAL DIAGNOSIS BOXES

In any patient encounter, critical thinking skills are necessary to construct an appropriate management plan. This text is constructed to assist providers in determining the correct diagnostics and differential diagnoses. Diagnostics boxes list appropriate tests, and Differential Diagnosis boxes list possible differentials. Diagnostics boxes can include up to four categories of testing: (1) **initial** tests (tests that may be performed in the office setting, such as peak flow measurement or pulse oximetry), (2) **laboratory** tests (diagnostic tests performed in a medical laboratory, such as blood hematologies or chemistries), (3) **imaging** tests (radiographic, ultrasound, and nuclear or magnetic resonance studies), and (4) **other** tests (miscellaneous studies that may be necessary in the evaluation of the disorder, such as EEGs or biopsies). Because the clinical presentation differs with each patient, not all diagnostic tests listed may be indicated for each circumstance. An asterisk is placed beside those tests that may be indicated by clinical presentation and physical examination findings. For more detailed information, the reader should refer to the Diagnostics and Differential Diagnosis sections included with each disorder.

MANAGEMENT

The management sections make every attempt to incorporate the contributions that research makes to create an evidence base for practice. Specialty organization guideline recommendations for management, as well as current, ongoing research findings are presented in most chapters where they exist. As with any evolving science, recommendations can be in a state of flux. Management recommendations may change, and new recommendations for practice supersede practices presented in this text. In addition, the reader is directed to check drug indications and dosages in medication product information before administering any medication.

ACKNOWLEDGMENTS

This text represents a collaborative effort. We remain indebted to our contributors, who generously provided their expertise to make this text the resource it is. Their efforts model collaboration, and we remain grateful for their patience with questions and revisions. We must also acknowledge the contributions made by our patients, students, and colleagues. We continue to try to incorporate your suggestions to make this text a useful one for practicing clinicians and students alike.

The support of everyone at Elsevier is greatly appreciated. Still, we are particularly grateful for Jodi Willard, who patiently guided the editing and production process, and for Barbara Cullen, Cindi Anderson, and Stacy Welch, who encouraged and guided us through this second edition.

Finally, our spouses, children, and friends deserve our eternal thanks. They continue to sustain and support us, even when this project has competed with them for our attention.

Terry Mahan Buttaro
JoAnn Trybulski
Patricia Polgar Bailey
Joanne Sandberg-Cook

Contents in Brief

PART 13
Evaluation and Management of Genitourinary Disorders, 675

PART 14
Evaluation and Management of Gynecologic Disorders, 739

PART 15
Evaluation and Management of Musculoskeletal and Arthritic Disorders, 827

PART 16
Evaluation and Management of Neurologic Disorders, 923

PART 17
Evaluation and Management of Endocrine and Metabolic Disorders, 987

PART 18
Evaluation and Management of Hematologic Disorders, 1065

PART 19
Evaluation and Management of Rheumatic and Multisystem Disorders, 1109

UNIT I. RHEUMATIC DISORDERS

UNIT II: MULTISYSTEM DISORDERS

Contents

PART 4
Office Emergencies, 127

PART 5
Evaluation and Management of Skin Disorders, 189

PART 9
Evaluation and Management of Oropharynx Disorders, 337

PART 10
Evaluation and Management of Pulmonary Disorders, 355

PART 11
Evaluation and Management of Cardiovascular Disorders, 445

PART 12
Evaluation and Management of Gastrointestinal Disorders, 573

PART 13
Evaluation and Management of Genitourinary Disorders, 675

PART 14
Evaluation and Management of Gynecologic Disorders, 739

PART 15
Evaluation and Management of Musculoskeletal and Arthritic Disorders, 827

PART 1

Introduction

JOANN TRYBULSKI, Section Editor

CHAPTER 1

Collaborative Practice

Jean E. Steel

During the twentieth century, a major explosion of scientific knowledge significantly impacted health care. New technologies and treatments proliferated. In response to this influx of knowledge and technology was the expansion of professional education, standards, and domains of practice. In addition, the concept of interdisciplinary teams of health care professionals was introduced.

In today's health care environment, patient care concerns are complex and are rarely solved by one profession alone. Meeting these concerns requires that a professional team work together to design, implement, and evaluate patient care. Dialogue among collaborating disciplines is essential to building and maintaining trust during every facet of managing care. The essence of collaborative practice is a collective or a network of professionals that jointly designs, delivers, and evaluates outcomes of care. Patients benefit when more than one discipline focuses attention on planning and managing health care concerns.

A HISTORICAL PERSPECTIVE

In the 1960s the U.S. government began to encourage team training for health care professionals. In 1972 the American Medical Association and the American Nurses Association formed the National Joint Practice Commission (NJPC). The purpose of the NJPC was to describe, research, and refine the value of collaborative practice for nurses and physicians. The NJPC published descriptions of collaborative practices and guidelines for establishing a collaborative practice.[1,2] The NJPC also concluded that joint practice resulted in improved quality of care, increased patient and provider satisfaction, decreased morbidity and mortality, and decreased hospital length of stay.[1]

Since that time, numerous articles and studies have described collaborative practice and have shown multidisciplinary collaboration to be an effective and efficient model of health care delivery.[3-10] Most collaborative practice research has occurred in specialty areas and has linked improved patient outcomes to interdisciplinary collaboration.[11-21] Collaborative practice has provided quality health care services in many settings, but at times it has failed to fulfill its potential.

ELEMENTS OF COLLABORATIVE PRACTICE

Recognition of Patient Needs

The patient is the focus and shapes the elements of collaborative practice. Patient concerns determine the discipline that leads the collaborative care effort. Sometimes medicine or nursing directs the health care team; at other times social service or physical therapy coordinates patient care. The focus of care and attention must be the patient and his or her significant others; therefore leadership of the health care team varies as the patient's needs change.

Trust

Collaborative practice requires respect for each other's knowledge, skill, and clinical decisions. To achieve trust, there must be a broad understanding of the strength and contributions each health care discipline makes to patient care. Each health care professional involved in collaboration should understand the others' assessment of the patient and value the decisions made for this patient.

Recognition of Each Discipline's Contribution

Although state practice laws and professional associations describe responsibility and accountability for practice, these laws, standards, and scopes of practice descriptions may permit several disciplines to provide the same service, thereby increasing access to care. Clearly, health care knowledge and skills are not segregated in a single discipline. Rather, multiple health care disciplines possess common knowledge; in many areas, however, the depth and focus of that knowledge differs. Thus each discipline potentially offers a unique perspective.

Knowledge and understanding of each collaborator's education and experience is vital to the success of collaboration. Educational standards for professional disciplines may appear to be similar, but each has a different emphasis. For example, nurse practitioners value and include health education for patients. Thus, the nurse practitioner curriculum has a strong emphasis on illness prevention and health promotion. The physical therapist examines movement dysfunction and develops and implements exercise interventions to enhance functional outcomes. Both the nurse and the physical therapist are concerned about prevention/promotion and functional outcomes; however, the physical therapist has more extensive education, practice, and experience in these areas.

Members of the collaborating group need to value and acknowledge each other's strengths and challenges. When one provider has a dominant strength, the other members may defer and refer to that expertise.

Another feature of collaborative practice is in the delegation of tasks and responsibilities to other caretakers. Accountability with delegation may vary from situation to situation. State laws also guide accountability in the case of delegation. It is always wise for the professional to determine the line of authority and responsibility when delegating tasks to another professional or lay individual.

Time

Another aspect of collaborative practice centers around the provision of time. Time for discussion and planning of care is essential to ensure that the patient focus remains and that the most appropriate member of the collaborating team directs the effort. Additionally, each professional must believe in the value of collaboration for the patient. Each member of a collaborating team should attend patient care planning meetings to contribute his or her unique expertise. Administrative personnel also need to recognize and support the need for time dedicated to this activity.

CHALLENGES INHERENT IN COLLABORATIVE PRACTICE

In some cases, legal regulation, long-standing traditions, and territorial concerns have hindered the development of collaborative practice among different professions. However, as professional domains of practice have both expanded and contracted in the last few years, there is more evidence of shared activities among professional disciplines. Today nurses are willing and able to initiate care based on professional standards, education, and scope of practice and experience. In collaborative practice, the hierarchy of one professional over another diminishes as each discipline is expected to practice according to its own standards and laws in meeting patient needs.

PROTOCOLS VS. GUIDELINES

In the past, nursing "protocols" listed the step-by-step actions a nurse or nurse practitioner could take in a given situation. Currently, patient care guidelines have become the dominant feature in collaborative practice. These guidelines are designed by a network of health care providers, and they identify suggested treatment options and serve as references for patient care. In this manner, guidelines contribute to the development and expansion of clinical practice.

VALUE OF COLLABORATIVE PRACTICE

The professional literature has reported the benefits of collaborative practice. From the NJPC descriptions of reduced morbidity and mortality, patient and provider satisfaction, and shortened length of stay to many of the current reviews, there is increasing evidence that collaborative practice improves patient care. Outcome research is ongoing and is providing additional information about the value of collaborative practice and is examining the effect of collaborative practice on cost containment and the economics of health care.

The value of outcome research on collaboration can be seen in gerontology nursing practice. Studies in gerontology practice uncovered a need for significant improvement in care as demonstrated by reduced hospitalizations. Consequently, many evaluation and chronic disease management clinics for patients and their families have been developed using collaborative staffing. Subsequent investigations point to a significant reduction in hospitalizations. Other studies have indicated that through collaborative practice, patients have greater comprehension of their condition and its management, fewer broken appointments, fewer hospitalizations, and more efficient use of physician time.[22,23]

CONCLUSION

One of the most significant values of collaboration is the enhancement and expansion of efforts and results. Collaborative research is exponentially productive as it combines resources, expertise, and thinking in the search for truth. Collaborative leadership allows more individuals to participate, and the outcome is from a collective of minds. Collaboration in clinical practice offers improved quality for patients and significant others as professionals share expertise.

The ingredients for successful collaborative practice include a significant and constant degree of trust among members of the team. An understanding of each member's education, expertise, challenges, and scope of practice is essential for successful implementation of collaborative practice. Protected time for planning and evaluating must be allotted within the settings or the delivery of services may be compromised. Continuing research needs to focus on patient care outcomes.

Collaborative practice represents the best response that a group of interdisciplinary medical expert clinicians can offer patients and their families. Collaborative practice efforts are indicators of high quality primary care and should be the goal of every clinician.

REFERENCES

1. National Joint Practice Commission: *Guidelines for establishing joint or collaborative practice in hospitals,* Chicago, 1981, The Commission.
2. Roueche B: *Together: a casebook of joint practices in primary care,* Chicago, 1977, National Joint Practice Commission.
3. Baggs JG, Schmitt MH: Collaboration between nurses and physicians, *Image J Nurs Schol* 20:145-149, 1988.
4. Devereux PM: Does joint practice work? *J Nurs Admin* 11:39-43, 1981.
5. Styles MM: Reflections on collaboration and unification, *Image J Nurs Schol* 16:21-23, 1984.
6. Steel JE: *Issues in collaborative practice,* Orlando, 1986, Grune and Stratton.
7. Prescott PA, Bowen SA: Physician-nurse relationships, *Ann Intern Med* 103:127-133, 1985.
8. Baggs JG, Schmitt MH: Collaboration between nurses and physicians, *Image J Nurs Schol* 20:145-149, 1988.
9. Safriet BJ: Health care dollars and regulatory sense: the role of advanced practice nursing, *Yale J Regul* 9(2):417-488, 1992.
10. Fagin, CMN: Collaboration between nurses and physicians: no longer a choice, *Acad Med* 67:295-303, 1992.
11. Thorne S, Paterson B: Shifting images of chronic illness, *Image J Nurs Sch* 30(2):173-177, 1998.
12. Schaffer J, Wexler LF: Reducing low-density lipoprotein cholesterol levels in an ambulatory care system: results of a multidisciplinary collaborative practice lipid clinic compared with physician-based care, *Arch Intern Med* 155(21):2330-2335, 1995.
13. Grindel CG and others: The practice environment project: a process for outcome evaluation, *J Nurs Admin* 26(5):43-51,1996.
14. Schmitt MH and others: Conceptualizing and measuring outcomes of interdisciplinary team care for a group of long-term, chronically ill, institutionalized patients. In Bachman JE, editor: *Interdisciplinary health care: proceedings of the third annual conference on interdisciplinary team care,* Kalamazoo, Mich, 1981, Center for Human Services, Western Michigan University.
15. Michelson EL: The challenge of nurse-physician collaborative practices: improved patient care provision and outcomes, *Heart Lung* 17:390-391, 1988.
16. Daly BJ, Phelps C, Rudy EB: A nurse-managed special care unit, *J Nurs Admin* 21 (7/8):31-38, 1991.
17. Anvaripour PLK and others: Physician-nurse collegiality in the medical school curriculum, *Mt Sinai J Med* 58(1):91-94, 1991.
18. Baggs JG, Ryan SA: Intensive care unit nurse-physician collaboration and sure satisfaction, *Nurs Econ* 8:386-392, 1990.
19. Evans SA, Carlson R: Nurse/physician collaboration: solving the nursing shortage crisis, *Am J Crit Care* 1(1):25-32, 1992.
20. King ML, Lee JL, Henneman E: A collaborative practice model for critical care, *Am J Crit Care* 2:444-449, 1993.
21. Institute of Medicine: *Primary care: America's health in a new era,* Washington, DC, 1996, National Academy Press.
22. Hankins GD and others: Patient satisfaction with collaborative practice, *Obstet Gynecol* 88(6):1011-1015, 1996.
23. Henneman EA, Lee JL, Cohen JI: Collaboration: a concept analysis, *Adv Nurs* 21:103-109, 1995.

CHAPTER 2

Weighing the Evidence for Clinical Practice

Cheryl A. Cahill

The translation of research findings into clinical practice is an essential element of the clinician's responsibility. However, decisions regarding the sufficiency of evidence to alter usual practices may be difficult to evaluate. This chapter provides clinicians with some guidelines that may be useful in making decisions about evidence-generated changes in care.

Rarely are the results of a single research study sufficient for clinicians to change the usual practice guidelines and standards. Careful evaluation of individual studies to ensure that the study or research question, design, analysis, and conclusions are appropriate is the essential first step. Consistent results from multiple studies are necessary to support changes in practice standards. Because the ultimate purpose of health-related research is to develop and test treatments that prevent illness or restore health, the requisite body of evidence is a clear demonstration of cause-and-effect mechanisms governing the phenomenon of interest. Without an understanding of the mechanisms that regulate the phenomenon of interest, prescriptions and interventions with predictable and consistent outcomes are limited. A systematic investigation is carried out to develop a sufficient understanding of regulatory mechanisms. This investigation begins with identifying the characteristics of the phenomenon and leads to demonstrations of cause-and-effect relationships among variables.

Once cause-and-effect relationships are determined, clinical investigators postulate and test interventions with predictable outcomes. By identifying the level of the question addressed in a single research project, the clinician may determine what is known about the phenomenon of interest and apply that knowledge to clinical practice. This hierarchical view of evidence provides the clinician with a context within which study results may be evaluated for clinical applicability.

LEVEL I RESEARCH QUESTIONS: DESCRIPTION OF CHARACTERISTICS

The progression from description to intervention may be conceptualized as passing through four levels. Determination of the level of the question within this hierarchy is the first step in evaluating the clinical utility of a particular study. The purpose of a Level I question is to describe the pertinent characteristics of the phenomenon of interest. The question usually includes the stem "What is?" For example, "What is the experience of individuals diagnosed with human immunodeficiency virus?"

To answer this question, investigators apply qualitative methods such as structured interviews. Qualitative data may be analyzed with a variety of techniques that guide the investigator to identify ranges of typical responses. Alternatively, investigators may use quantitative methods such as a survey. Analysis of the quantitative data generated in Level I studies includes nonparametric statistics that generate measures of central tendency and dispersion. These measures indicate typical responses by determining the average response (mean, mode, median) and variability of responses (range of responses, standard deviation, other measures of dispersion). The results from this type of study may be used by clinicians to expand the usual assessment parameters but generally do not guide the selection of an intervention or a treatment.

LEVEL II RESEARCH QUESTIONS: RELATIONSHIPS AMONG/BETWEEN VARIABLES

The results of Level I questions provide the basis for Level II questions. Once the fundamental characteristics of a phenomenon have been described, the next logical step is to describe the relationships between and among characteristics or variables. The purpose of Level II questions is to establish associations or differences between variables. Level II questions include the stem "What is the relationship?" or "What are the differences between?" For example, "What is the association between a history of cigarette smoking and the incidence of heart disease in women over 40 years of age?"

Several approaches to this type of question are applicable. For example, investigators may carry out epidemiologic studies in large data sets. This approach has been used to identify the risk factors commonly used to assess patients, to gather specific diagnostic data, and to counsel persons to change behavior. Other studies may be designed to compare the differences in variables between two or more groups. For example, an investigator may measure selected variables in a group of persons with HIV and a group of matched persons without HIV to determine associations between CD4+ counts and fatigue levels. The results of these studies simply describe the associations and differences between the groups and suggest that the differences may be associated with group membership. The data analysis techniques used in Level II studies are measures of association (e.g., correlation coefficients) and differences between and among the research study groups (e.g., t-tests and analysis of variance). The evidence generated with this question level is probably insufficient to demonstrate a mechanistic cause-and-effect relationship between the variables. Demonstrating such a relationship requires more rigorous control of extraneous variables and active manipulation of the independent variable (the variable thought to be the causal variable). The clinician may suggest a change in behavior because of the results of a Level II question, but the results do not guide methods to change those behaviors, nor do they explain how the behavioral change will be effective.

LEVEL III RESEARCH QUESTIONS: CAUSE AND EFFECT

Armed with the results of Level II studies, investigators can design Level III studies. The purpose of Level III studies is to identify the mechanistic relationships among characteristic variables associated with the phenomenon of interest. Level III research questions are more complicated because the investigator has a hypothesis about the nature of the relationships among variables (i.e., which is the causal variable and which is the effect variable). Rather than a research question, the putative relationship tested in the study is often stated as a hypothesis. The format of a hypothesis is a declarative sentence that asserts the relationship: changes in A (the independent variable) cause changes in B (dependent variables). Depending on the amount of preliminary evidence or on the theoretical model proposed by the investigator, the investigator might suggest a directional relationship (e.g., as A increases, B decreases). The design applied to this level of question is either experimental or quasi-experimental.

True Experimental Design

To demonstrate a causal relationship, the investigator must exercise maximum control over the study. A true experiment provides this level of maximum control. A true experiment is characterized by random selection of participants and manipulation of the independent or causal variable. The random selection of subjects ensures that the sample is representative of a population. Several strategies may be used to ensure a representative sample, with each strategy engineered such that each eligible member of the population has an equal chance of being included in the study.

If human subjects are used in a Level III study, considerable care must be taken to control extraneous variables. Extraneous variables are those characteristics of the subject or setting that may influence the behavior of the dependent variable. In addition to random selection of participants, random assignment to the treatment group or the control group provides further control of extraneous variables. For example, if the purpose of the study is to demonstrate that slow and rhythmic breathing by persons with essential hypertension results in lower systolic blood pressure, investigators may send a letter asking for volunteers to all persons being treated at a particular clinic. Because participation in a research study must be voluntary, it is safe to assume that participants "self-select" the study. Willingness to participate in a study may differentiate study participants from the overall population. Therefore random assignment to either the control group or the experimental group adds additional information that may be used to ensure that error was not added by the sampling methods.

Similarly, the investigator may consider other inclusion and exclusion criteria to guide subject recruitment. For example, the investigator may specify that subjects must be following a particular pharmacologic treatment regimen. Because these types of controls increase the complexity of recruitment, the investigator may choose to select persons who are newly diagnosed with hypertension and test them before they begin treatment and again after a specified period of treatment. The study may include a control group of newly diagnosed persons who are monitored in exactly the same way as the experimental group but do not change their respiratory patterns. One way to ensure that environmental stimulation is the same for all subjects is to conduct the experimental sessions in the same laboratory setting. Subjects return at the same time after the initiation of treatment. By contrasting the blood pressure measures of the experimental group with those of the control group, the investigator is able to differentiate the effects of changes in breathing patterns alone from the effects of pharmacologic treatment alone and from the effects of both changes in breathing patterns and pharmacologic treatment (Table 2-1).

Quasi-Experimental Design

In many cases it is not possible to randomly select participants or to randomly assign them to treatment and control groups. For example, if an investigator is interested in the effects of a disease, it would not be possible to assign some subjects to have the disease and others to be free of a disease. In such a case, the disease would be the treatment variable. For example, suppose that an investigator is interested in understanding the pathology of HIV in the immune system. Clearly it would be unethical to randomly assign persons to an experimental group to be infected with HIV. Instead, the investigator monitors persons diagnosed with HIV at baseline and at regular intervals thereafter.

The comparison of baseline data to subsequent observation allows the investigator to characterize the causal relationship between HIV infection and changes in immune parameters. This type of design is referred to as quasi-experimental because there is no random assignment to the experimental condition. Sometimes this type of design is called a repeated measures design, and it is argued that the subject serves as his or her own control. In some ways, this type of design ensures better control of extraneous variables associated with the constitution of individual subjects. However, the investigator should demonstrate with some assurance that every subject is representative of the general population. For example, if the sample lacks diversity of gender, age, and ethnicity, one would wonder to what degree the sample represents the overall population. The application of results can be made only to those individuals represented in the

TABLE 2-1 True Experimental Design

	Baseline	Treatment
Control group	No treatment	Pharmacologic treatment
Experimental group	Rhythmic breathing treatment	Rhythmic breathing treatment *and* Pharmacologic treatment

The purpose of this study is to evaluate the effectiveness of intermittent rhythmic breathing exercises to control hypertension in newly diagnosed persons. During the baseline period, the control group receives no treatment, whereas the experimental group practices the rhythmic breathing treatment. During the treatment period, the control group receives the usual treatment—pharmacologic treatment. The experimental group also receives the usual pharmacologic treatment, because it would be unethical to withhold treatment given the complications of untreated hypertension. A comparison of data from each cell reveals the effects of no treatment, pharmacologic treatment alone, rhythmic breathing treatment alone, and rhythmic breathing with pharmacologic intervention.

sample. In other words, if the sample is not representative of the target population, then the results may not be extrapolated to the population.

Analysis of Level III data test hypothesized relationships between independent and dependent variables. For example, regression techniques generate a mathematical model to predict the change in dependent variables in response to changes in the independent variable. The value of Level III studies to clinicians is that it may provide a degree of confidence in their prediction of outcomes. Clinicians who attempt to anticipate the clinical course of a disease state may use the results of Level III studies. Furthermore, because the results of these studies point to mechanistic associations, standard clinical interventions may be selected to perturb pathology or enhance health.

LEVEL IV RESEARCH QUESTIONS: RANDOMIZED CLINICAL TRIALS

Level IV studies demonstrate the effectiveness of an intervention or treatment. The mechanistic relationships among variables identified by Level III studies support the proposition of the interventions and treatments tested in Level IV questions. The randomized, placebo-controlled, double-blind clinical trial is the gold standard of this type of study because it provides the investigator maximum control of the sources of error inherent human clinical investigations.

Level IV Study Methods

Random Selection/Random Assignment. The random selection of participants for a study is one way to achieve a study sample that is representative of the targeted population. Several methods used by investigators in Level IV studies ensure that all eligible subjects have an equal chance of being included in the study. When the availability of subjects is limited, investigators may conduct the study at a variety of sites. Within each site, all potential subjects are informed of the study and are offered the opportunity to participate. By casting the widest possible net, investigators are ensured of a representative sample.

Random assignment to a treatment group helps to ensure that both groups are comparable. If random assignment is not made, individuals who are significantly better or worse may end up being assigned to one or the other group. For example, if an investigator were free to assign the treatment group, he or she might inadvertently assign those most likely to respond to the new treatment to that group. There might also be a bias toward one treatment over another. A surgeon participating in a randomized clinical trial testing the effectiveness of a lumpectomy in comparison to the usual treatment of mastectomy may prefer to assign young women to the lumpectomy because of the disfigurement associated with mastectomy.

Placebos. Placebos, or sham interventions or treatments, exclude the possibility that changes in patient behavior are due to a desire to please a researcher. The Hawthorne effect must also be acknowledged in any research. The Hawthorne effect produces improvements in performance because subjects are aware they are being observed. Observation of the placebo control group permits investigators to demonstrate effects such as accelerated resolution of symptoms or palliative effects rather than curative effects. For conditions in which an effective treatment exists for the targeted population, those in the placebo group receive the usual treatment rather than a placebo, because in most cases it would be unethical to withhold treatment.

Blinding the Subject and Researcher. Blinding the subject and the researchers and caregivers as to group membership (control group or experimental group) prevents the contamination of results by personal biases. Investigators who are invested in obtaining positive results may be biased in their observations. In the case of pharmaceuticals, only the pharmacist may be aware of which patient is receiving the investigational treatment. Patients who enroll in studies may do so simply because there is no alternate therapy. Hope for a positive effect could bias their reports of effects.

Data Analysis Methods. The aim of data analysis is to demonstrate groupwise differences in treatment effects. Analysis of variance methods or t-tests are most often used, but regression analysis may also be done. The quandary faced by investigators is how to treat the numbers relative to subjects who do not complete a study. Obviously, it is important to know if significantly more subjects died in the treatment group, but what about subjects who withdraw from the study?

One of the important aspects to evaluate in any new treatment is patient preference and a tolerance for side effects. Some have argued that an "intent-to-treat" approach to these data ought to be used. In this approach, subjects who withdraw or die are counted as treatment failures, thus raising the standard for significant results. Consider a case in which 100 subjects are recruited for a study (Table 2-2). Fifty subjects are randomly assigned to the usual treatment, and 50 are assigned to the new treatment. At the end of the study, 10 in each group have died. No subjects withdrew from the usual treatment, but 10 withdrew from the new treatment group. At the end of the study, 20 subjects "got better" with the usual treatment and 20 subjects showed improvement with the new treatment. When calculating success rates, if the number of persons *completing* the study is used as the denominator, the success rate for the usual treatment group is 20 out of 40 (50%) compared to 20 out of 30 (66%) for the new treatment or experimental group. The experimental treatment would appear to be superior. However, if instead the number who *began* the study is used as the denominator, the success rate in the usual treatment group is 20 out of 50 (40%) and in the new treatment group it is 20 out of 50 (40%), which suggests no difference between the groups. Thus with the intent-to-treat approach, one would conclude no difference in success rate between the two treatments and a twofold increase in the failure rate for the new treatment.

ADDITIONAL STUDY PARAMETERS NEEDING EVALUATION

Identification of the level of the question simply informs the clinician of the possible usefulness of the results. The decision to actually modify clinical practices because of the study results must also include some evaluation of the design, subject selection, methods, data analysis scheme and resultant conclusions. Table 2-3 summarizes some of these elements as they

TABLE 2-2 Intent-to-Treat Table

	Usual Treatment			Experimental Treatment		
	N	% Total Intent-to-Treat	% Complete	N	% Total Intent-to-Treat	% Complete
Admitted	50	100	80	50	100	60
Died	10	20	NA	10	20	NA
Withdrew	0	0	NA	10	20	NA
Completed, improved	20	40	50	20	40	66
Completed, did not improve	20	40	50	10	20	33
Total completing	40	80	100	30	60	100

The analysis of data from a clinical trial may be carried out in several ways. Of main concern is how investigators handle participant attrition. The inclusion of participants who begin a study but fail to complete it is referred to as the "intent-to-treat" approach. This table illustrates the difference of results with an intent-to-treat scheme vs. an approach that disregards attrition.

TABLE 2-3 Summary Table

Level of Question	Purpose	Methods	Analysis	Application
I: What is it?	To describe or define a phenomenon of interest To identify pertinent variables or characteristics	Qualitative methods Structured interviews Questionnaires Surveys	Content analysis Ethnography Nonparametric statistics Measures of central tendency	May suggest assessment parameters (Do you experience . . . ?)
II: What is happening here?	To identify relationships between variables—associations and differences	Epidemiologic studies Cross-section studies Correlational studies Studies of groupwise differences	Correlations among variables Differences between variables/groups Mann-Whitney U; analysis of variance; t-test	Suggests avenues of further assessment (If you observe "x", what is the likelihood that "y" will occur?)
III: What is the "nature" of the relationship among variables (cause-and-effect relationship)?	To determine cause-and-effect relationships among variables To explicate mechanisms mediating the phenomenon of interest	Experimental designs Quasi-experimental designs	Analysis of variance Regression analysis	Suggests underlying pathologic conditions that may be treated
IV: What is the therapeutic effect of a proposed intervention? What is the proper "dose" of a treatment to achieve a predictable outcome?	To determine the predictability of a hypothesized outcome at a specific dose in a selected population	Randomized clinical trial	Intent to treat analysis Analysis of variance Regression analysis	Demonstrates the usefulness of a particular treatment for a patient population; with sufficient replication, the clinician may be reasonably sure that the treatment will be effective

relate to the level of the question. Inherent in the progression from description of the phenomenon to clinical trials is an increasing amount of control that the investigator can exert over the conduct of the study. The purpose of the increase in control is to control error. Error is that portion of the measurement that cannot be explained. A simplistic way of describing a statistic is as the ratio between the effect of the experiment and the error.

STATISTICAL ANALYSIS PRINCIPLES

Although it is beyond the scope of this chapter to fully explore statistical methods, it may be helpful to review some basic principles of statistics. The purpose of any statistic is to provide a mathematical measure of the effects of study variables while accounting for error. At the core of statistical analysis is the assumption that variance is normally distributed within a given population. A **population** is defined as all units targeted by the study. A **sample** is defined as that portion of units selected for study that represent the population.

Type I and Type II Errors

One significant source of error in any study is failure of the investigator to include units that represent all characteristics of the population. As discussed previously, one way to avoid this error is to select study participants carefully. A basic element of these strategies is the accrual of a sufficient sample size to ensure that all characteristic elements of the population are included. If a sample is insufficiently representative of a population, the investigator may report false results and may erroneously conclude that the research hypothesis is supported. That is, that the effect of the study may be sufficiently robust to conclude that differences or associations exist between baseline and outcome or between the experimental groups and control groups when in fact there is no difference. This type of error is a Type I error. The investigator also risks what is known as a Type II error, or the failure to detect significant associations or differences when they are present. During the design of a study, the investigator may protect the study from these errors by conducting a power analysis.

Power Analysis

Simply defined, power is an estimate of the probability of detecting significant effects at a given probability of a Type II error. In other words, power is an indication of the confidence one may have that the results are true. In general, research reports discuss power analysis as a way of calculating the sample size needed to adequately represent the target population. In general, the proportional risk of a type II error is set at 0.80. That is, that the investigator estimates that the risk of failure to detect significant results is 2 in 10. If a power analysis has been done, clinicians should be assured that care was taken to ensure that the sample is representative of the target population.

Analysis of Research Study Results

Description of Data and Measures of Central Tendency. A description of the sample and general findings is usually the first step in analyzing the results of a study. Descriptive statistics summarize data. They include measures of central tendency, dispersion, and association. The simplest descriptive statistic may be a graphical representation of the data. A pie chart, bar graph, or line graph is a pictorial representation of the distribution of the data. Measures of central tendency indicate the "typicalness" of the data set. The appropriate measure of central tendency is determined by the way the variable of interest is scaled. The way that the typical representation of gender is categorized as male or female in a sample is by the actual number of participants in each level of the variable or by the value as a proportion of the total. In a case in which the variable of interest may have three or more possible responses, the appropriate measure of central tendency is the mode. The **mode** is the category most frequently selected. For example, suppose the variable of interest was an evaluation of the effectiveness of an educational program for newly diagnosed diabetics. The evaluation tool consists of a list of statements attached to a scale with five possible responses: 1 represents strongly agree; 2, agree; 3, neutral; 4, disagree; and 5, strongly disagree. These responses represent categories with unknown relationships. Therefore the appropriate measure of central tendency for these questions is the mode, or the category with the most responses.

The **median** is an appropriate measure of central tendency for rank order data such as income of participants in a study. Participants are often asked to indicate their annual income by selecting a range of annual incomes. The median is the point on the scale with 50% of the responses below and 50% above. For example, census data generally report the median income in a community or the median price of a home. The appropriate measure of central tendency for discrete data is the **mean**, which is simply the arithmetic mean. For example, a study of the effects of stress on systolic blood pressure might indicate the mean or average baseline systolic blood pressure for the sample.

Standard Deviation. Dispersion is a measure of the variability of the data, or the degree to which data deviate with each other. The range is the difference between the highest score and the lowest score. Standard deviation is a measure of dispersion commonly reported for discrete data. The standard deviation is a summary of the average amount of difference among the data points. A complete description of discrete data would include the mean plus or minus the standard deviation. Assuming that the study group is truly representative of the population, the mean, plus and minus the standard deviation, may represent the "normal" range of responses the clinician may expect to see.

Normal Distribution and Error. If the responses from everyone in a population across the range of possible responses are counted and graphed, the majority of responses fall in the middle, with the rest evenly distributed above and below the middle (Figure 2-1). This sort of distribution is referred to as a normal distribution. Underlying the parametric statistics is the assumption that all responses to an experimental condition are normally distributed. If participants have been truly selected at random from the same population, then the sum of responses should be normally distributed. Individual responses are therefore due to chance. By randomly sampling from a population, the investigator assumes that the sample is representative of the overall population. The distribution of responses of the sample should therefore mirror the distribution of the population. Deviation from a normal distribution model is assumed to be due to error. A well-designed study is engineered to reduce error, and instruments with demonstrated validity and reliability are used. Subject selection is based on clear and reasoned inclusion and exclusion criteria so that only members of the targeted population are included. Data collection protocols are rigorously followed. Despite these best practice methods, however, some error is inevitable.

Statistical Significance (Alpha Values). The purpose of statistical analysis is to estimate the amount of error. Because error is inevitable, the investigator decides before data are collected how much error can be tolerated and still demonstrate significant effects. The amount of tolerable error is defined as the alpha (α) value. The α value is expressed as a decimal representation of the proportional risk for error. An α of 0.05 is interpreted as 5 chances in 100 that an error may occur. Similarly, 0.01 is interpreted as 1 chance in 100. The maximum risk for error is generally set at 0.05.

More rigorous or lower α values are specified to prevent a wrong conclusion that the research has demonstrated positive or significant results. For example, an investigator evaluating a new therapy might decide that the risk of the therapy being ineffective 5 out of 100 times is too high. The α could be set at

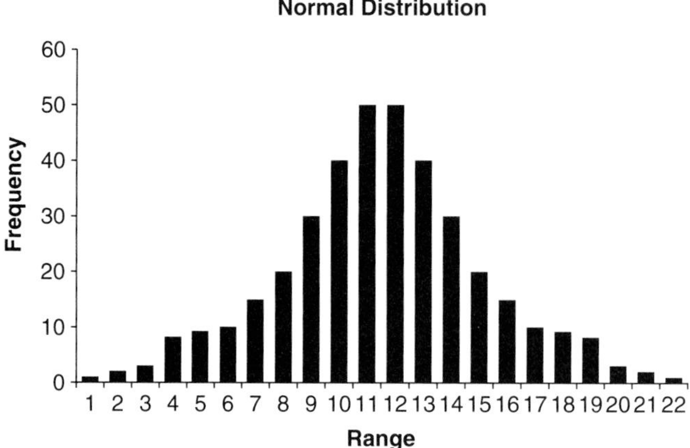

FIGURE 2-1

A graph of a theoretical normal distribution. The x-axis represents all possible responses, and the y-axis is simply the number of responses. This graph demonstrates that the majority of responses cluster in the middle range of possible responses and that the rest are evenly distributed above and below the middle.

0.01, or 1 chance in 100. If that is done, then the results are reported as not significant if statistical analysis demonstrates a p value (the actual proportion of error) of 0.05 at the completion of the study. The clinician may use the strength of the statistical significance to determine the robustness of the effect of the intervention when deciding to change a therapeutic routine. Suppose a study is conducted to compare the usual treatment (drug A) to a new treatment (drug B). The α has been set a priori (beforehand) at 0.05. The reported p values at the end of the study are 0.05, which suggest that the new treatment is better than the old. The clinician must decide whether or not the 5% risk that this conclusion is not true is sufficiently minimal to change the usual prescription.

Statistics of Differences and Associations. Statistics measure associations among variables or differences between variables. During the design of a study, the investigator plans to demonstrate that participants behave in similar or different ways. Association statistics evaluate the similarities among the data. Association statistics compare the distribution of the variables of interest and evaluate whether or not they are consistently similar enough to conclude that they are related. The appropriate association statistic depends on the way the variables are scaled. For example, associations between two categorical variables (the values of the variables are not on a numerical continuum) are evaluated using a goodness-of-fit-statistic, whereas an association between two ranked variables (the values of these variables are in a hierarchical order) are evaluated using a rank order correlation statistic. Associations among continuous data are determined by calculating correlation coefficients. Strong correlations among variables may indicate to clinicians that if one symptom is observed, a second may also be present.

Many times an investigator is interested in discerning the differences among variables or groups. For example, if the purpose of a study is to evaluate the effects of a treatment, the investigator would be interested in demonstrating that a significant difference has occurred. Therefore difference statistics compare the distribution of variables to determine if they are sufficiently different. Because an assumption that all data are normally distributed is central to statistics, difference statistics evaluate the difference between the appropriate measure of central tendency and dispersion to ensure that the distributions are actually independent. In the case of categorical data, differences are determined by the Chi Square statistic. For continuous data, a comparison between two variables are evaluated by a t-test. More than two discrete variables are evaluated with some type of analysis of variance (ANOVA).

The appropriateness of analytic methods is an essential element that the clinician needs to consider when using specific research findings. In general, if the results are consistent across several studies and the analytic methods are similar, the clinician may feel comfortable that the conclusions are correct.

Clinical Significance vs. Statistical Significance. The gold standard for determining the correctness of a research finding is whether or not the statistical analysis yields significant results. However, occasionally an investigator will report the results to be clinically significant despite no statistically significant result. Such an assertion is usually made when the level of significance has approached the 0.05 level. If it is kept in mind that the α is the minimally acceptable risk that a false report is made, then this argument is for increasing that risk. A slightly lower significance is usually the result of small sample sizes. Pragmatically speaking, the time, energy, and resources needed to gather some clinical data may preclude increases in sample sizes. Therefore the clinician must be cautious when considering the usefulness of such data. In these cases, clinicians may be advised to wait for additional studies to be reported before changing their usual practices.

SUMMARY

Clinicians require accurate and precise information in order to deliver safe and effective care. However, the demands of day-to-day practice environments make it difficult to "keep up." The intent of this chapter has been to identify general guidelines useful in evaluating individual studies. The progression of knowledge from description of a phenomenon, disease, or syndrome to effective clinical management requires systematic investigation. Descriptive studies (Level I) characterize the phenomenon of interest and may be used by clinicians to hone their assessment skills. Level II studies aim to detail the essential characteristics of a phenomenon and to demonstrate the relationships among those elements. Clinicians may use these results to guide the diagnosis or recognition of a condition. Level III studies are designed to demonstrate cause-and-effect relationships among variables or elements. Proof of causation may be used by clinicians to treat. Level IV studies test treatments or interventions. Clinicians use the results of these studies to predict the effectiveness of a particular treatment for an individual. This hierarchical conceptualization of scientific progression is an important aspect of evidenced-based practice.

CHAPTER 3

The Provider-Patient Relationship

Terry Mahan Buttaro and JoAnn Trybulski

The purpose of primary care is to encourage wellness, prevent illness, treat chronic disease, and provide palliative care. The majority of primary care visits provide treatment for minor problems or continuing care for chronic diseases. However, the chief complaint is often not the real problem. Each individual has unique health care needs that may be elicited in a caring environment through careful listening.

Textbooks detail the common symptoms of illness and assemble epidemiologic and diagnostic data to permit swift diagnosis and expeditious treatment. However, health care is not a commodity—it is a relationship between the patient and the provider. Historically this has been an intimate partnership based on caring, respect, and trust, but the changing health care environment has wrought widespread changes. For the first time, a sizable number of primary care providers are employees of large corporations. They are now managers responsible for coordinating care and monitoring referrals and prescriptive practices.

In the current health care milieu there is an urgent need for primary care providers to do what they have done so capably for hundreds of years—care for the sick, support their families and friends, and provide education about health. Patients need to feel connected to their provider and know that each infirmity and each anxiety is heard with compassion. Providers must advocate for their patients, ensure quality care, and assist patients in the negotiation of a confusing health care network. All health care disciplines must collaborate to develop plans for care and programs that promote well-being and acknowledge each individual's worth.

All of these functions are components of the provider-patient relationship. In addition, certain provider attributes are important. The first is attentiveness, or the ability to thoughtfully listen and observe. The second is respect for the patient as an individual and for his or her belief system. The third is humility, or that quality of knowing one's strengths and limitations and having the ability to recognize them. The final quality is fortitude, or enduring courage in the face of opposition.

Provider-patient relationships that incorporate the characteristics of respect, trust, and caring will be therapeutic and fruitful. Providers who approach relationships with patients from this perspective will find their effectiveness as a health care provider increased and the quality of their patient interactions enhanced.

Time management has become an essential requirement in medical practice today. The key to efficiency is focus. Distractions must be kept to a minimum; the focus of the provider is the patient. A quiet room is crucial to encourage patients to relate their concerns and anxieties. An accurate clinical picture is imperative and is achieved by obtaining a complete history and understanding the patient's family role, work environment, spirituality, social supports, and psychologic profile.

The history is usually obtained first. The physical examination is based on the patient's complaint, and the history can be obtained after the examination. The history should be reviewed with the patient for clarification. Eating, sleeping, and elimination habits should be discussed. Experience demonstrates that patients return for care until they are satisfied with their management options or until their problem is resolved. If patients are comfortable that their concerns have been addressed, corporate cost containment and time-efficiency goals may be achieved by the elimination of unnecessary tests and visits.

The bond between provider and patient is a confidential, intimate relationship rooted in caring and trust and based on mutual respect. Each touch should inspire confidence. There may be little control over disease progression, but hope and dignity should be sustained. Box 3-1 provides strategies to facilitate interactions between the provider and the patient.

BOX 3-1

STRATEGIES TO ENHANCE PROVIDER-PATIENT INTERACTIONS

- Always introduce yourself and shake hands.
- Allow the patient to remain in street clothes during the initial contact; this may make him or her feel more comfortable.
- Sit at eye level with the patient to facilitate eye contact.
- Begin the encounter by inquiring how you may help the patient.
- Be focused. Distractions must be kept to a minimum.
- Be committed to the patient by listening.
- Do not allow provider prejudices to affect the relationship.
- Allow patient participation in planning therapeutic interventions; this is critical.
- Provide an opportunity for follow-up.
- Close the encounter by asking if the patient has any other concerns.

CHAPTER 4

Ethical Analysis and Decision Making in Primary Care

Patricia A. White

Primary care providers continue to find themselves in clinical situations that involve ethical conflict. Increasing role responsibilities for advanced practice nurses have determined the need for leadership in identifying and managing clinical situations that involve ethical issues and conflicts. These conflicts often result in dilemmas that involve difficult choices for the patient and provider. Current changes in the health care delivery system have created an environment in which ethical dilemmas are more likely to occur. Managed care and the availability of technologic interventions add to the complexity of these dilemmas. In order to advocate for patients in this health care environment, primary care providers need to be well-informed about ethical principles and analysis.

This chapter presents a brief overview of the types of ethical dilemmas faced by primary care providers and the ethical principles involved. Contemporary ethical theories that predominate in the health care delivery environment are also outlined. An approach to analyzing situations that involve ethical dilemmas is provided along with a discussion of ethical principles and how they are used in such analyses. Finally, the role of primary care providers as ethical decision makers is reinforced with suggestions for an advanced role in the practice arena and in the larger health care delivery system.

ETHICAL PRINCIPLES

Ethical dilemmas in clinical situations occur when the perspectives of patients and providers differ regarding the approach to complicated clinical scenarios. Patients and providers often have varied perspectives of the same clinical situation. The values and priorities of patients often differ as they view the dilemmas from their own life histories and current health status. Patients and providers also differ in their adherence to various ethical principles, which are discussed in the following paragraphs.

The major ethical principles include autonomy, beneficence, nonmaleficence, fidelity, justice, and veracity.[1] These principles have been identified as important considerations when ethical dilemmas arise. Autonomy is considered an essential ethical principle because it refers to an individual's right to make decisions about health choices. The legal profession protects the right of all citizens to exert autonomy unless an individual is deemed incompetent by the legal system. Many ethical dilemmas arise in relation to this principle, because a patient's right to decide often conflicts with a family member's or professional's wishes to protect the patient from harm or to prolong his or her life by a surgical procedure. Family members often struggle with a loved one's decision to forgo what might be lifesaving treatment.

The perspectives of patients regarding ethical dilemmas have recently been researched. Pinch and Parsons[2] studied the older population's views about dilemmas regarding end-of-life decisions. They discovered that patients rely heavily on provider input regarding health care decision making. Spielman[3] identifies the ethical dilemmas that arise when caring for older adults with dementia, who often are unable to express their wishes yet need to have their selfhood respected. This much-needed research regarding patients' perspectives is critical for clarifying perspectives that often are not considered when decisions are made. The reliance of patients on provider input as illustrated in this research highlights the care and responsibility inherent in providers' roles as advocates for clients. Vulnerable populations are particularly at risk for not having their views well represented when difficult and life-changing decisions are being made.

Providers bring varied personal views and professional experience, including adherence to their professional codes of ethics. The Code of Ethics of the American Nurses Association requires nurses to consider the consequences of their ethical decisions and ethical principles.[4] Nurses are obligated to demonstrate respect for human dignity and the uniqueness of the individual. The new ANA Code of Ethics (2001) provides additional perspectives for adherence to principles grounded in nursing's long tradition and commitment to ethical practice. This updated Code of Ethics builds on the old code by reiterating the obligation of the nurse to uphold the patient's dignity, worth, and uniqueness. The new Code highlights the need to extend respect for these features of individuals to colleagues, employees, and students, and it emphasizes respect for dignity as a fundamental principle. The Code of Ethics continues to identify the protection of patients as another fundamental value, particularly the protection of patients regarding their right to privacy. It also delineates the responsibility of the nurse to protect patients from the negligent practice of colleagues that is deemed either illegal, incompetent, or unethical. Furthermore, this new Code underscores nurses' obligation to maintain professional competency and contribute to knowledge development through research. Workplace conditions are also addressed in the Code, with an emphasis on identifying a work environment that is conducive to safe practice as an important right of the profession. In addition, the Code accentuates the nurses' responsibility to maintain the integrity of the profession by advocating for the protection of the public from deceptive advertising and false claims from any source. Finally, health promotion is advocated by the Code through nurses' support of public health initiatives and support of policy that positively affects access to care and social change.

Beneficence and Nonmaleficence

Providers also adhere to the ethical principles of beneficence and nonmaleficence when they act on behalf of patients' wishes and try to protect patients from harm. Adherence to these principles is commendable but is sometimes seen as being paternalistic. Concerns also arise in adherence to these principles when a patient makes a decision that may affect his or her safety. Careful identification of the principles involved allows everyone a voice and an opportunity to identify sometimes well intentioned but competing principles.

Ethical Dilemmas

Providers and patients often differ because they may adhere to different principles. Specific examples of ethical dilemmas include providers' concerns about patient safety, which often conflict with patients' perspectives regarding their right to autonomy in decision making about health-related issues. Ethical conflicts also arise when patients and family members disagree about what ought to be done in a particular health care situation.

Providers often experience conflict when environmental constraints such as insurance regulations or practice policies dictate an approach that conflicts with adherence to specific ethical principles. The ethical principle of justice that emphasizes doing the most good for the most people often conflicts with assisting individuals in their access to certain types of care. Managed care regulations often dictate which treatment a patient should receive based on data suggesting that monies might be better spent on providing a preventive approach to more patients. Concerns arise in settings when capitation practices allow only a certain number of visits to specialists when perhaps a patient or provider believes that additional services are warranted.

Clarifying the principles that both the provider and patient consider significant is important when analyzing scenarios that involve ethical dilemmas. The following section identifies the two major traditions in ethical theory in which consideration of ethical principles takes place.

ETHICAL THEORIES

Current tension in ethical thought stems from a belief in persons as rational and individualistic in contrast to a belief that persons exist in relation to others. Waithe[5] describes the historical view of the justice-based and virtue-based traditions that underpin the current tension between the person-centered view and the worldview of individuals as principled and independent. The justice-based, or principle-based, tradition emphasizes the adherence to principles as primary in the analysis of ethical dilemmas. The virtue-based, or care-based, tradition not only emphasizes care and concern for others but also considers the particulars of a clinical situation as primary in the analysis of a case situation.[6]

The polarization of these two traditions has continued to dominate current ethical theory. Fry, Killen, and Robinson[7] speak of the importance of discovering the ways to reconcile these two traditions; the goal is the consideration of ethical principles in relation to the patient's situation. As discussed previously, the consideration of ethical principles in a clinical situation with ethical dilemmas most often needs to consider the contextual features of the patient care situation. Considering the ethical principles involved with this contextual approach can bring the best of both traditions to the consideration of compelling and difficult dilemmas.

ANALYSIS OF EHTICAL DILEMMAS

The analysis of ethical dilemmas requires a thoughtful approach to each case presentation. Veatch and Fry[8] pose four questions that can be used as a guide to analysis. The first question involves distinguishing between moral and nonmoral evaluations and determining who ought to decide the outcome of a clinical scenario. The second question involves the concern about what types of acts are right and requires consideration of the principles involved in the dilemma and how to balance the principles of the parties involved. The third question involves how the rules or principles apply to the specific situation. The application of the principles is a central feature of ethical conflict, because the principles themselves are often competing. How people interpret and view principles is often a concern because some view principles as guides to behavior without regard to context. The fourth stage is the question of what should be done in a particular situation. This stage is the culmination of ethical analysis and should be done only after careful consideration of all perspectives. These stages can be used as a guide to decide if ethical dilemmas and conflict do exist.

PRIMARY CARE PROVIDERS AS ETHICAL DECISION MAKERS

Primary care providers have many leadership opportunities as thoughtful decision makers about the ethical dilemmas that arise in their settings. Using knowledge regarding the nature of ethical dilemmas and analyzing situations as outlined in this chapter will hopefully provide guidelines for this process. Future research needs to consider more carefully the experience of patients involved in ethical dilemmas. There must also be a careful analysis of the types of conflicts and dilemmas as seen from this most important perspective. Research needs to outline the providers' perspective in ethical dilemmas and should determine how environmental factors affect decision making. Particular attention needs to be given to vulnerable populations, whose voice is often not heard when ethical dilemmas arise. Involving patients in decision making and providing a voice for the vulnerable should be at the heart of providers' concerns when ethical dilemmas arise.

As additional research highlights ongoing ethical dilemmas and approaches, advanced practice nurses can continue to bring to their role important reflections regarding ethics. Ethics advisory boards are one way to ensure that a forum exists for providers to discuss and deliberate ethical dilemmas. An interdisciplinary group with community representation can provide an important mechanism to discuss and consider these issues. Clarification of important ethical issues can be a useful outcome of case presentations to advisory boards. Ensuring that a patient has a health care proxy is another way to address patient perspectives and wishes if his or her decision-making capacity becomes impaired.

Patients and primary care providers will benefit from thoughtful ethical analysis and decision making. Clarification of the principles involved for both can contribute to patient well-being and professional satisfaction. Future research will assist in the use of principles within the context of compelling clinical situations. Continued clarification of the perspectives of both providers and patients will also assist primary care providers in their roles as ethical decision makers.

ETHICAL ISSUES IN HUMAN EXPERIMENTATION AND RESEARCH

The history of medical progress is, to a large extent, the history of medical experimentation. Human experimentation and research are based on the philosophy that no patient is ever under any obligation to participate in research.[9] The process of research and human experimentation occurs when the health care provider departs from standard medical practice to obtain new, generalizable knowledge or to test a hypothesis using the scientific method.[9,10]

The ethics of human experimentation and the research process are based on the tenets of the Nuremberg Code, written in 1947 after the trial of Nazi physicians for crimes against humanity. The Nuremberg Code addresses the boundaries of human experimentation on the basis of ten principles. The first principle states that voluntary consent of the human subject is absolutely essential. Implicit in voluntary consent is the requirement that the individual not only has the legal capacity to provide consent but also has sufficient knowledge and comprehension of the choices available in the health care process.

The nine other principles of the Nuremberg Code address facets of the research process, including the benefits of research to society, the study design and its basis on the natural history of a disease, and the avoidance of physical injury and harm, death, or disability during the experimental process. These principles also state that the degree of experimental risk should not exceed the humanitarian importance of the problem, that scientifically qualified persons must conduct the experiment, that the patient may choose to end participation at any time in the research process, and that the researcher must terminate the research process if untoward effects related to the experiment occur.

Within any health care organization, the Institutional Review Board (IRB) is responsible for the review and oversight of proposed research. The role of the IRB is to review research protocols and protect human subjects. Review of informed consent related to any research study is a major function of the IRB. Specific requirements addressed by the IRB in the review relate to minimization of risks, the balance of risks with the anticipated benefits of the research, careful consideration in the selection of human subjects in the study design, and the requirement for obtaining informed consent.

REFERENCES

1. Beauchamp TL, Childress JF: *Principles of biomedical ethics*, ed 4, New York, 1994, Oxford University Press.
2. Pinch WJ, Parsons ME: The ethics of treatment decision making: the elderly patient's perspective, *Geriatr Nurs* 14(6):289-293, 1993.
3. Spielman K: Demented residents' right to refuse treatment, *Clin Excell Nurse Pract* 1(6):376-381, 1997.
4. American Nurses Association: *Code of Ethics with Interpretative Statements*. Kansas City, 2001, The Association.
5. Waithe ME: Twenty three hundred years of women philosophers: toward a gender undifferentiated moral theory. In Brabeck MM, editor: *Who cares? Theory, research and educational implications of the ethic of care*, Westport, Conn, 1989, Praeger.
6. Cooper MC: Principle-oriented ethics and the ethic of care: a creative tension, *Adv Nurs Sci* 14(2):22-31, 1991.
7. Fry ST, Killen AR, Robinson EM: Care based reasoning, caring and the ethic of care: a need for clarity, *J Clin Ethics* 7(1):41-47, 1996.
8. Veatch RM, Fry ST: Four questions of ethics. In Veatch RM, Fry ST, editors: *Case studies in nursing ethics*, Boston, 1995, Jones & Bartlett.
9. Annas GJ: *The rights of patients*, ed 2, Carbondale, Ill, 1989, Southern Illinois University Press.
10. Munson R: *Intervention and reflection: basic issues in medical ethics*, ed 5, New York, 1996, Wadsworth.

CHAPTER 5

Legal Issues

Noreen Connolly and Roberta N. Regan

Rapid changes are continually occurring in the health care field and include the issue of scope of provider practice, as well as access to and the cost and quality of health care. These issues influence the practice of primary care, require focused attention on ethical and legal issues, and demonstrate the importance of a collaborative relationship between medical providers. Areas of concern for the primary care provider include the Patient's Bill of Rights; informed consent; the Patient Self-Determination Act; advance directives; privacy and confidentiality issues; child, elder, and disabled abuse; and malpractice issues.[1]

THE PATIENT'S BILL OF RIGHTS

The Patient's Bill of Rights was adopted in 1973 by the American Hospital Association as a document that views open, honest communication and respect for individual values as essential to the relationship between patients and health care providers. The two basic tenets inherent in the document are (1) respect for the role of the patient in decision making regarding treatment choices and all other aspects of care, and (2) sensitivity to racial, cultural, linguistic, religious, and gender differences, as well as to the needs of persons with disabilities.[1]

The Patient's Bill of Rights provides a foundation for the rights and responsibilities of patients, families, and caregivers, thus offering a health care ethic that respects the role of individuals in decision making. The American Hospital Association encourages health care institutions to tailor this document to their patients by simplifying language and/or providing cultural adaptations when appropriate.

INFORMED CONSENT

Informed consent is a basic element of the provider-patient relationship and involves sharing of information, appropriate interpretation, and deliberation regarding health care decisions. Essential to this process is the presence of trust, commitment to the provider-patient relationship, and adherence to the ethical base for accountability to the patient. In the health care arena, emphasis continues to shift to the importance of this provider-patient relationship. Greater collaboration is required between patients and providers to determine goals and weigh alternative courses of action and approaches to health care. The continued evolution of managed care intensifies the issues surrounding provider-patient relationships.[2]

Informed consent is the responsibility of the primary care provider in all aspects of care, particularly when alternative approaches to the management of a health issue exist. Specifically, the patient has the right to relevant, current, and understandable information concerning diagnosis, treatment, and prognosis and is entitled to request information regarding procedures and/or treatments and their risks, benefits, and alternatives.

BOX 5-1

HOW TO TELL IF A PATIENT IS FIT TO DECIDE TREATMENT

The following questions need to be asked and documented when deciding whether a patient is fit to decide his or her medical treatment[3]:

- What is your medical condition, and what are the treatment options for you?
- What are the benefits if you refuse or accept treatment, and what are the chances the treatment will work for you?
- What will happen if you accept treatment? Reject treatment?

Informed consent requires both information and voluntary participation in health care decision making. Patients must be offered adequate information about their choices whether these choices relate to therapeutic options or to involvement in research. Consent is a voluntary process in which an individual agrees to participate in the plan of care or in research. It is the responsibility of the primary care provider to determine when the patient has an adequate understanding to make informed consent valid (Box 5-1). To be valid, the consent must be voluntary; that is, the patient must be competent and must agree to participate "of his/her own free will."[2]

PATIENT SELF-DETERMINATION ACT AND ADVANCE DIRECTIVES

The Patient Self-Determination Act (PSDA), which was passed in 1991, was designed to empower patients to determine the course of their medical care should incapacitation occur. The PSDA requires all facilities that receive funding from Medicare or Medicaid to provide patients with information concerning the right to create advance directives or to refuse unwanted treatment.[4] Although the PSDA requires these health care facilities to inform patients of their right to record advance directives, it does not stipulate who is responsible for initiating the discussion. The ambiguity regarding primary responsibility may in part account for the low rate of advance directive completion in the United States.[5] Some studies estimate that fewer than one in six Americans create advance directive documents.[5] Another factor is highlighted by the SUPPORT project, which was designed to foster communication between doctors and patients regarding medical care during times of severe illness. In this study, fewer than 50% of the participants were willing to discuss CPR when approached.[6]

There are two principal types of advance directives: (1) the "living will", written statements regarding a patient's wishes for treatment in a variety of hypothetical situations; and (2) a written statement designating a proxy decision maker whose authority is activated in the event of incapacitation. The latter is also known as a health care proxy, health care agent, durable power of attorney for health care, or health care surrogate.[4] Specifically, advance directives provide information regarding the type of treatment an individual wishes to receive in the event that he or she becomes comatose, demented, or unable to communicate during a terminal illness, thus extending autonomy to the last stages of life.[7]

When an advance directive document has not been created and an individual faces a terminal illness without the capacity to make decisions for himself or herself, the principles of medical ethics must be applied as follows: (1) any patient sustaining cardiopulmonary arrest should receive CPR unless compelling reasons exist to indicate that the patient would not want it, (2) a patient has the right to refuse CPR, and (3) CPR should be withheld if initiating this would be considered futile and would serve none of the therapeutic goals as defined by the patient's wishes.[8]

Right to Refuse Treatment

The right to refuse treatment is endorsed by the law as a constitutional right and is protected by the PSDA, which requires that health care organizations offer patients the right to accept or refuse medical treatment. Although the right to refuse treatment is mandated by law for both competent and, in some circumstances, incompetent patients, the right to refuse care can vary across states. Planning health care decisions in advance and establishing open communication between the provider and the patient are essential aspects of the informed consent process.

PRIVACY AND CONFIDENTIALITY

Privacy and confidentiality are essential ethical standards in the practice of primary care. Both the American Medical Association and the American Nurses Association consider confidentiality to be basic to the provision of health care. Patients must trust that all personal and psychologic issues disclosed during communication with a primary care provider will not be disseminated.[9]

In most circumstances, the concept of privileged communication between a patient and his or her provider is protected in the court system, generally barring testimony about patient issues by the provider. In some instances, however, providers may be required to reveal certain information about patients. These circumstances are limited in most states and are permitted only to public health authorities or when criminal or abuse situations arise.[9,10]

CHILD ABUSE

More than three million cases of child abuse are reported each year; 44 out of 1000 children are victims of child abuse. These victims are more likely to use drugs, be arrested, commit suicide, or experience psychiatric disabilities. Victims of sexual abuse are more likely to become prostitutes later in life.[11]

There are different types of child abuse: neglect, physical abuse, and/or sexual abuse. Neglect involves not meeting a child's physical or emotional needs. Parents or caregivers may ignore harmful behavior such as drug or alcohol use, ignore a child's illness, or not feed or clothe the child properly.[11]

Abused children are more likely to live in one-parent homes, have more than four children in a family, and be in a low socioeconomic class. Health care providers must be very careful about looking into all other possible causes for injury. To be falsely accused of child abuse can be traumatic to families.

At the time of injury, health care providers need to obtain a complete history from the child, caretakers with the child, and caretakers at the scene of injury. The child should first be interviewed alone. Health care providers are mandated in every state to report abuse and neglect. Every state provides immunity from potential civil or criminal liability for any health care worker who reports abuse. A child who has been abused should be sent to foster care or admitted to the hospital. There is an increased risk of more abuse and death if the child returns to the abuser.

ELDER ABUSE

In 1998, the annual estimated prevalence of elder abuse in the United States was 3.2%. Since that time, there has been a 94% increase in the number or reported cases, 54% of which are substantiated. The majority of reports are filed by family members (20%), hospital workers (17%), home service providers (9.6%), and doctors, nurses, and clinics (8.4%).[12] Elder abuse is defined by the American Medical Association as "an act or omission which results in harm or threatened harm to the health and welfare of an elderly person."[13] This includes intentional infliction of physical or mental injury, sexual abuse, or the withholding of necessary food, clothing, or medical care to meet the needs of the older adult.[13]

Some of the characteristics associated with an abused older adult include older age, minority status, poor social networks, low income, and functional disability.[12] Functional disability, substance abuse, and cognitive impairment are often present. For many of these reasons, abuse is often difficult to recognize. The older adult may be unable to relate the history due to cognitive impairment, may fear retaliation, or may fear transfer to a nursing home. Signs and symptoms of a mistreated older adult include evidence of head trauma, poor oral hygiene, hematomas, burns, decubiti, welts, bite marks, fractures, weight loss, dehydration, and poor overall hygiene.[13]

When elder abuse is suspected, health care providers should elicit the history of the presenting medical problem, obtain a description of events surrounding the injury, obtain a history of prior injuries, and determine the possible presence of depression. It is important to document the "chain of evidence" with a careful, legible, and thorough collection of physical evidence. When possible, a physical description, laboratory data, and photographs should be obtained to support the claim.[12,13] All health care providers are mandated by law to report suspected elder mistreatment and, when necessary and appropriate, should discuss the situation with the patient and enlist the support of social services.

DISABLED ABUSE

Disability is the inability to care for oneself because of physical, mental, or financial reasons. A disability can be permanent or temporary. The abuse of an individual with a disability can be more difficult to detect than any other abuse. Detection of disabled abuse is complicated by the tendency for disabled persons to delay seeking assistance, because they prefer to remain self-sufficient. When disabled abuse is discovered, the health care provider must report the incidence to the agency governing adult protective services.[14]

MALPRACTICE ISSUES

Almost all malpractice cases result from poor communication and little or no follow-up of patients.[15] Most malpractice suits against nurse practitioners and/or physician assistants include the supervising physician. The supervising physician is liable for reviewing the nurse practitioner or physician assistant's treatment plan.[15]

Malpractice is a deviation from the standard of care compared to what another prudent provider with the same education and skills would do under the same circumstances. The patient must show evidence of four elements to prove malpractice: duty, breach of duty, proximate cause, and damages.[16]

How to Reduce the Risk of Malpractice[17]

1. Quote the patient directly. If patient refuses a test or if you have reviewed with the patient the side effects of a treatment, have him or her sign the chart where the note is written.
2. Have a medical assistant or nurse accompany you to any sensitive examinations. Document that an assistant was with you, and include his or her name.
3. Write your exact thoughts when documenting your differential diagnosis. Do not limit yourself to one differential diagnosis.
4. Document that you discussed the risks and benefits of treatment or refusal of treatment. Document that the patient understands what will happen if treatment is withheld or carried out. Multiple visits may be needed to fully document the patient's understanding of the issue.
5. Dictate in front of the patient, and at the end of dictation ask, "Is this correct?" This helps the patient hear again what is the plan of care.
6. Document that you protected people who are not your patients. For example, if a woman has herpes or a sexually transmitted disease, document that you advised her to tell her sexual contacts so they may receive treatment.
7. Document the goals of care, and document that the patient understands them. For example, "Patient understands he needs to call in 24 hours if abdominal pain is worse or has not improved."
8. When prescribing medications, document that you gave exact instructions on taking the medication and have reviewed the common side effects.

REFERENCES

1. American Hospital Association: *A patient's bill of rights*, Chicago, 1998, The Association.
2. Strumpf NE, Asimos K: Accountability: the covenant between patient and nurse practitioner. In Hickey JV, Ouimette RM, Venegoni SL, editors: *Advance practice nursing: changing roles and clinical applications*, Philadelphia, 1996, JB Lippincott.
3. Tunzi M: Can the patient decide? Evaluating patient capacity in practice, *Am Fam Physician* 64(2):299-306, 2000.
4. Cantor, MD: Learning from the Cruzan decision: the need for advance directives, *JAMA* 265:1751, 1754, 1991.
5. Dexter PR and others: Evidence-based healthcare: a scientific approach to health policy, *Ann Intern Med* 128:102-110, 1998.
6. Covinsky KE: Communication and decision making in seriously ill patients: findings of the SUPPORT project, *J Am Geriatr Soc* 48: S187-193, 2000.
7. Prendergast TJ: Advance care planning: pitfalls, progress, promise. *Crit Care Med* 29:N34-39, 2001.

8. Tilden VP: Ethics perspectives on end-of-life care, *Nurs Outlook* 47:162-167, 1999.
9. Munson R: *Intervention and reflection: basic issues in medical ethics,* ed 5, New York, 1996, Wadsworth.
10. Annas GJ: *The rights of patients,* ed 2, Carbondale, Ill, 1989, Southern Illinois University Press.
11. Jain A: Emergency department evaluation of child abuse, *Emerg Med Clin North Am* 17(3):575-593, 1999.
12. Jogerst GJ and others: Community characteristics associated with elder abuse, *J Am Geriatr Assoc* 48:513-518, 2000.
13. Swagerty DL: Elder mistreatment, *Am Fam Physician* 15:2804-2808, 1999.
14. Birrer R, Singh V, Kumar D: Disability and dementia in the emergency department, *Emerg Med Clin North Am* 17, 505-516.
15. Crane M: A malpractice primer for NPs, *Adv Nurse Pract* 2(23):205-299, 1999.
16. Morrision C: Evolving legal trends affect NPs, *Adv Nurse Pract* 7(5):24, 1999.
17. Teichman P: Documentation for reducing malpractice risk. *Fam Pract Manag* 7(3):29-33, 2000.

PART 2

Primary Care: Adolescence Through Adulthood

JOANN TRYBULSKI, Section Editor

CHAPTER 6

Adolescent Issues

Cathy J. Sizer

Adolescence is the interval in physical, cognitive, emotional, and psychosocial development that occurs between 10 and 21 years of age. Often it is described as a time of intense upheaval for the adolescent and anxiety for the parents. However, these normal developmental changes usually occur without major difficulties.

Successful metamorphosis from adolescence to adulthood involves the attainment of economic and emotional independence from parents, the cultivation of a workable value system, the evolution of a sexual identity, and the development of new and meaningful relationships.[1] Adolescence is also a time when individuals may engage in intentional or unintentional risk behaviors that can lead to significant consequences and complicate their future care.[2] Each year 15,000 to 18,000 adolescents die in accidents.[3] Another 6000 adolescents are homicide victims each year, and approximately 24% of ninth to twelfth graders attempt suicide.[3] These facts mandate increased health promotion, safety awareness, and risk prevention for these young adults. Specific interventions and guidance should be tailored to each adolescent's individual period of development.

Three distinct periods of adolescence characterize the transformation that occurs within this decade of life. Early adolescents (those ages 10 to 14) challenge authority, experience wide mood swings, reject the elements and ideation of childhood, can be argumentative or disobedient, and desire more privacy. There is an intense preoccupation with normal body changes. Anxieties regarding menses or wet dreams and differences in the size of sexual body parts may or may not be expressed. An imaginary judgmental audience may influence behavior and increase insecurities. Peer groups, manifested by close friendships with the same sex along with contact with the opposite sex in groups, substitute for parental influence. These adolescents may express future plans and an emerging value system; although these ideations are initially idealistic, they may change frequently.[4] During this stage, health promotion should focus on the immediate impact of behaviors. Goals include the prevention of cigarette smoking, street drug use, alcohol use, and sexual activity.[5]

Middle adolescents (those ages 15 to 17) are strongly influenced positively and/or negatively by peer groups. Despite this powerful support system, this period is often a lonely one. Family conflict occurs and may escalate as the adolescent strives for independence. Concern about body image decreases, whereas anxiety about attractiveness increases. In addition, the "tired teenager" surfaces, sexual drive heightens, and fad behavior predominates. This is the age of experimentation with sex, drugs, friends, and risk-taking behaviors. However, future goals seem more realistic as the adolescent gains awareness of his or her strengths and limitations. Finally, there is an increased intellectual ability that includes emerging abstract thought, creativity, and contemplation about the future.[4] Health promotion goals continue to include prevention of cigarette smoking, street drug use, alcohol use, and sexual activity, with additional counseling for those engaging in alcohol use or abuse and/or sexual activity, especially unprotected sexual activity.[5]

As they become emancipated from the nuclear family, late adolescents (those ages 18 to 21) begin to assimilate adult roles. At this age adolescents are usually comfortable with their body image, and abstract thinking matures. Peer influence diminishes, and decisions relate more to the individual or to his or her partner. At this age successful adolescents pursue realistic goals, understand the consequences of their behavior, and relate to the family as an adult. They realize their own limitations and mortality and have established a sexual identity as well as an ethical and moral value system.[4] The long-term negative health effects of alcohol abuse, unsafe sex, use/abuse of street drugs, and cigarette smoking should be stressed.[5]

PHYSICAL DEVELOPMENT

Although growth occurs over a continuum, adolescence is marked by a 15% to 18% growth spurt, during which time about 95% of the adult size is reached.[1] Before that growth spurt occurs, other specific pubertal physical changes take place. These changes are regulated by the endocrine feedback systems, including the somatotropic, the adrenal, and the hypothalamic pituitary gonadal axes, as well as by interplay with the thyroid axis. For girls, physical changes usually begin with breast development or breast buds around age 10 years. For boys, testicular enlargement at an average age of 11.5 years marks the initiation of puberty.

The average age for menarche, which follows a growth spurt, is 12.5 years; African-American girls may experience an earlier menarche. Dysmenorrhea is rare, because the first few periods are usually anovulatory. Girls acquire fat during puberty, because a body fat composition of nearly 22% is necessary to maintain regular ovulatory cycles.[6] Girls may have asymmetric breast development in the early stages, as well as extra nipples. Physiologic leukorrhea, which begins several months before menarche, may continue for several years. Puberty for female adolescents is completed with the sculpting of the body that results in the familiar adult shape.

For male adolescents, nocturnal emissions ("wet dreams") begin after testicular and penile growth is underway because dreams become more sexual in nature under the influence of hormones. Male adolescents may have tender or nontender gynecomastia and/or unilateral breast buds, which may be present for about 1 year. Testicular asymmetry is also common. These adolescents may need reassurance that the size of the penis is not an indication of sexual functioning, and they should be made aware that impregnation is a possibility because the testicles are probably capable of producing a few sperm at ejaculation. The remaining male physical developmental changes include voice deepening, auxiliary hair, and facial hair.

Pubertal changes occur in the same sequence for all adolescents. These changes should be tracked with each physical examination using the Sexual Maturation Scale (SMR) or Tanner stages. Often the family history will dictate the timing of puberty, but it is worrisome for boys when testicular enlargement occurs before age 9.5 to 10 years (precocious) or when no changes have occurred by age 13.5 years (delayed). It is equally worrisome for girls when breast buds appear before age of 8 to 8.5 years (precocious) or when no breast buds have appeared by age 13 years (delayed). An easy and inexpensive intervention to evaluate these variations is the bone age radiograph. If the bone age (wrist) is less than the chronologic age but is still appropriate for height, no further diagnostic testing is necessary.

COGNITIVE DEVELOPMENT

Piaget first recognized what is now thought to be the distinguishing feature of adolescent thought: abstract reasoning. By late adolescence, many adolescents can understand and create general principles or formal rules to explain many aspects of human experience. Piaget called this last stage of cognitive development, which is hopefully attained by approximately age 15 years, formal operational thought. However, many adolescents arrive at this cognitive stage later than age 15 years, and some adults never achieve this level of cognition.[7] One of the qualities of adolescence that is most exasperating to parents is the ability of adolescents to reason well in academic subjects but at the same time exhibit illogical thinking about their own lives.[7]

With increasing sophistication and mental agility, an egocentric attitude emerges and peaks at about age 13 years. The belief that they can handle anything and that adults do not understand them can lead adolescents to engage in risk-taking behaviors such as drug use and unprotected sex. As part of this egocentrism, adolescents create the aforementioned judgmental imaginary audience. This same egocentrism sometimes causes adolescents to seek public attention in any way possible.[7] Other aspects of this egocentrism include the "personal fable," or the belief of adolescents that they are special and that the usual laws of nature do not apply to them; "overthinking," or the tendency to make daily circumstances more complicated than necessary; and "apparent hypocrisy," or the belief that rules apply differently to them than to others.[6] An understanding of this as normal development may make communication less difficult and frustrating.

EMOTIONAL DEVELOPMENT

The quest for identity, a major task of adolescence, is accomplished by the development of new goals and the abandonment of childhood aspirations. This ideation is usually positive but can be negative, and it helps explain the apathy, insecurity, or socially unacceptable attributes and behaviors that may occur, such as outrageous hairstyles, hair colors, clothing, drug use, or pregnancy.[7]

Given the ongoing turmoil, conflict, and change that an adolescent experiences, it is no wonder that self-esteem suffers. This can be manifested by depression or suicide. Beginning in seventh grade (a time of overwhelming transition) through the middle to late adolescence periods, many factors contribute to the increasing risk of suicide. Poverty, racial minority status, parental depression, confused sexual identity, rejection by one's own peer group, anger, chronic illness, drug use, adolescent impulsivity, a history of corporal punishment, and divorce are considered potential precipitating factors.[8]

SOCIAL DEVELOPMENT

Successful identity formation in society depends on the support of family and friends. Peer groups buffer the transition between childhood dependency and adult independence and must be respected.[7] These groups identify and define the adolescent. Peer group pressure is positive if it eases the transition to adulthood by decreasing dependence on parents. However, it may also be negative and can lead to experimentation and destructive behaviors.

Given the developmental tasks of adolescence, some parental conflict is inevitable. A consistent and fair parenting style can help alleviate the ongoing conflict. Parents can be influential, especially if family members respect one another and engage in rational discussion. If parents recognize and become more comfortable with the growing autonomy of their adolescent, the difficulties will usually diminish with time.

Community and school are also important influences on development. "Rites of passage" such as bar mitzvahs or bas mitzvahs, achievement awards, "sweet sixteen" parties, driver's licenses, voter registration, and graduation from high school or college foster, focus, celebrate, and further establish the attainment of adult identity.[7]

DEVELOPMENTAL HISTORY

The Guidelines for Adolescent Preventive Services (GAPS) have been developed by the American Medical Association and provide a complete screening history, physical assessment, appropriate testing, and immunization update.[9] Anticipatory guidance for health promotion, safety, and risk issues is also addressed. The focus of these guidelines varies with each stage of adolescence. Therefore modifications based on variations of patient populations are recommended and are acceptable.

THE ADOLESCENT HEALTH VISIT

The initial comprehensive adolescent health visit, with the parent present, begins with an interview to assess the family medical history. Family practices such as household smoking, smoke detector use, and firearm storage are discussed in addition to routine health screening questions.

The presence of the parent at the beginning of the adolescent interview affords the opportunity to observe the relationship between the adolescent and the parent. The adolescent should remain dressed at this stage of the visit. Careful explanation of the changing provider-patient relationship for adolescents and the safeguarding of their privacy is stressed. At this time, parents should be asked about their current concerns or stressors.[10]

The interview continues in privacy with the adolescent. The format of the visit should be explained. Assuring the adolescent of confidentiality is essential. The health history can be organized around the mnemonic *HEADSS FIRST*, which progresses from less threatening topics to potentially more sensitive issues. In this assessment, adolescents are asked about *H*ome, *E*ducation, *A*ctivities, *D*rugs, *S*exual activity, *S*uicide/depression, *F*riends, *I*mage, *R*ecreation, *S*afety issues, and *T*hreats.[2] Affirmative answers to questions concerning the use of street drugs or alcohol can be further explored with two other useful mnemonics: *CAGE* (*C* = "Have you ever felt the need to **cut down** on your use of alcohol or drugs?" *A* = "Have you gotten **annoyed** by someone's criticism of your drug or alcohol use?" *G* = "Do you ever feel **guilty** about your alcohol or drug use?" *E* = "Do you **ever need a drink or drugs in the morning** before school?" Positive screen = Two or more "yes" answers)[11] and *RAFFT* (*R* = "Do you use alcohol or drugs to **relax**, feel better about yourself, or fit in?" *A* = "Do you ever drink or use drugs when you are **alone?**" *F* = "Do any of your close **friends** drink or use drugs?" *F* = "Do any close **family** members have a problem with alcohol or drugs?" *T* = "Have you ever gotten in **trouble** from drinking or taking drugs?" Positive screen = Two or three "yes" answers).[11]

An increased risk for drug use is associated with a family history of alcoholism, parental use of alcohol or drugs, overly permissive or controlling parents, the availability of alcohol or drugs, alcohol- or drug-using friends, school problems, attention deficit–hyperactivity disorder with impulsivity, past physical or sexual abuse, depression or other psychiatric problems, low self-esteem, low religiosity, and/or the need for peer acceptance.[11]

Mental health problems afflict a sizable proportion of adolescents.[12] Unlike adult depression, adolescent depression is not associated with powerlessness or pessimism about the future. Instead, it is directly affected by negative beliefs about self and low parental support. Adolescents tend to mask their depression and exhibit behavioral symptoms such as anger and self-destructive activities. These behaviors are used as a defense mechanism to protect the adolescent from feeling or appearing vulnerable or dependent.[13,14] A referral for immediate psychiatric assessment is indicated if the adolescent has made a suicide plan or has actually attempted suicide. Suicide warning signs are listed in Box 6-1.[15]

The prevalence of violence in society necessitates a violence risk screening (Box 6-2).[13] Affirmative answers to any of the questions in Box 6-2 suggest the need for further intervention. A referral to the appropriate professionals for conflict resolution, anger management, or assertiveness training should be considered. A suspicion of abuse mandates reporting according to the laws in each state.

Sexually active adolescents need counseling concerning the risks of sexual activity and the benefits of delaying future sexual encounters. Particularly, the risks of sexually transmitted diseases (STDs) and HIV infection, as well as the necessity of screening, are discussed. The use and limitations of condoms should be explained. Contraception options are also addressed during this discussion.

The Advisory Committee on Immunization Practice (ACIP) and GAPS recommend a routine comprehensive adolescent visit at age 11 years to lay the groundwork for future annual visits. Immunizations should be reviewed and updated at these annual visits. By 15 years of age, all adolescents should have received three hepatitis B vaccine doses (some states allow a 2-dose schedule, with 10 μg given at each dose and 4 to 6 months between doses), two mumps-measles-rubella (MMR) vaccine doses, four polio vaccine doses, a diphtheria-tetanus (DT) vaccine (if at least 5 years has passed since the previous dose), and Varivax (if there is no reliable history of chickenpox). Routine purified protein derivative (PPD) screenings are not usually performed unless the patient has risk factors for tuberculosis.

A complete gynecologic examination is necessary for sexually active female adolescents, even those younger than age 18 years. These annual preventive visits continue to age 21 years and include appropriate anticipatory guidance and a complete physical examination.[15] When the examination is for a sports physical, it should be sport-specific; at a minimum, the evaluation includes height, weight, blood pressure, visual acuity, cardiovascular assessment, abdominal palpation, testicular and inguinal examination for male adolescents, and a screening orthopedic examination.[16]

Pre-college visits provide an opportune time to update the adolescent's records, including immunization status, and to offer anticipatory guidance regarding sexuality (e.g., contraception, risks and prevention of STDs and HIV, responsible sexual behavior, prevention of sexual assault), cardiovascular health (e.g., nutrition, exercise, smoking), injury prevention (e.g., automobile and campus safety), and mental health (e.g., stress, substance abuse, eating disorders).[16] Patient education should occur at each visit. Box 6-3 lists some available resources.

Good health maintenance habits such as self-examination of the breast or testicles can be discussed during the physical examination. The presence of any abnormal medical conditions should be noted and the adolescent referred to other health professionals as needed. Screenings for preventable and/or treatable conditions (e.g., complete blood count, urinalysis, lipid profile) should be included with each health

BOX 6-1

SUICIDE RISK FACTORS

- Recent loss of a family member
- Social isolation
- Family history of affective disorders
- Interpersonal problems with peers
- Sexual identity concerns
- Abuse/neglect
- Exposure to suicide
- Prior attempts
- Suicidal ideation
- Physical illness or injury
- Intense life stresses
- Poor coping

BOX 6-2

VIOLENCE SCREENING QUESTIONS

- How many fights have you been in during the past year?
- How many of those fights were serious?
- How do you get out of a fight?
- Have you ever been threatened with a weapon?
- Have you ever carried a weapon?
- Does anyone in your family carry a weapon?
- Do your parents physically fight in front of you?
- What is your favorite television show or movie?

BOX 6-3

RESOURCES FOR CARING FOR ADOLESCENTS

American Academy of Child and Adolescent Psychiatry
(800) 333-7636
http://www.aacap.org

American Academy of Pediatrics
PO Box 927
141 Northwest Point Boulevard
Elk Grove Village, IL 60007
(800) 433-9016
http://www.pediatrics.org

American Medical Association
http://www.ama-assn.org (includes resources for parents)

Expect the Best from a Girl
http://www.academic.org (self-esteem website from Mount Holyoke College)

Nutrition and Eating Disorders Hotline
(800) 366-1655

PFLAG—Parents, Families, Friends of Lesbians and Gays
http://www.pflag.org

Suicide Prevention Hotline
(800) 621-4000

Talking to Kids About Tough Issues
http://www.childrennow.org

visit.[9,15,17] Consent for interventions may depend on the individual state regulations regarding emancipation of minors.

Caring for adolescents is challenging. However, the rewards are incalculable because the primary care provider is a privileged witness to the formation of an adult. The potential for the primary care provider to be a positive influence for the emerging adult is immeasurable.

REFERENCES

1. Robinson P: Puberty—am I normal? *Pediatr Ann* 26(2 suppl):S133-S136, 1997.
2. Cavanaugh R: Anticipatory guidance for the adolescent: has it come of age? *Pediatr Rev* 15(12):485-489, 1994.
3. Update: cardiovascular screening for athletes, *Contemp Pediatr* 13(10):16, 1996.
4. Boschere S: Tailor the message to age group, *Pediatr News* 31(7):32, 1997.
5. Burns C and others: *Pediatric primary care,* Philadelphia, 1996, WB Saunders.
6. Greydanus D, editor: *Caring for your adolescent,* New York, 1991, Bantam Books.
7. Nelms B: Suicide—can we help prevent it? *J Pediatr Health Care* 10(3):97-98, 1996.
8. Elster AB, Kuntz NJ, editors: *AMA guidelines for adolescent preventive services (GAPS),* Baltimore, 1994, Williams & Wilkins.
9. Morris G: Tasks of the times, *Contemp Pediatr* 13(6):94-104, 1996.
10. Knight J: Adolescent substance use: screening, assessment, and intervention, *Contemp Pediatr* 14(4):45-72, 1997.
11. Jenkins R, Saxena S: Keeping adolescents healthy, *Contemp Pediatr* 12(6):76-89, 1995.
12. Brown-Jones L, Orr D: Enlisting parents as allies against depression, *Contemp Pediatr* 13(11):67-86, 1996.
13. Morgan IS: Recognizing depression in the adolescent, *MCN* 19:148-155, 1994.
14. Maurer K: Guidelines offer questions to screen for violence, *Pediatr News* 31(2), 1997.
15. Jones CP: ACIP recommends early adolescent health check, *Infect Dis Child,* pp 1-17, Jan 1995.
16. Andrews JS: Making the most of the sports physical, *Contemp Pediatr* 14(3):183-205, 1997.
17. Immunization of adolescents: recommendations of the Advisory Committee on Immunization Practices, the American Academy of Family Physicians, and the American Medical Association, *MMWR* 45(RR-13):10-11, 1996.

CHAPTER 7

Pregnancy

Debra Hobbins

Prenatal care is an important goal of health care systems. Adequate, effective prenatal care is associated with improved birth outcomes.[1-3] There are insufficient data to explain this relationship, however, in part because many studies have evaluated the adequacy of prenatal care by the quantity and early initiation of visits rather than by the specific content of the prenatal care visit.[3-5]

In 1989 the U.S. Public Health Service[6] published specific guidelines for effective routine prenatal care. In 1994, in an effort to define and strengthen prenatal care globally, the World Health Organization (WHO) convened a Working Group to formulate recommendations for prenatal care at the health center level.[7] The U.S. Public Health Service document describes the critical components of each prenatal care visit based on the gestational age of the pregnancy and includes the timing of laboratory tests, examinations, and health promotion activities.[7] Seven essential areas of health behavior advice are recommended for all pregnant women: (1) breastfeeding their infants, (2) reducing or eliminating alcohol, (3) reducing or eliminating smoking, (4) not using illegal drugs, (5) eating the proper foods, (6) taking vitamin and mineral supplements, and (7) gaining an appropriate amount of weight during pregnancy.

Although this chapter may seem to concentrate heavily on the medical or technical aspects of a woman's prenatal care, the impact of the psychosocial aspects of the woman's life and the pregnancy on her emotional well-being and on her relationship with her infant, as well as the implications of childbirth for the family and society, are acknowledged and briefly addressed. There is an association between a woman's social situation, her health, and her use of health services.[8]

Waldenstrom[9] encourages primary care providers to consider different perspectives of childbirth when providing care for childbearing women. From a psychologic viewpoint, childbirth has implications for the woman's identity as a woman, for her maturation into motherhood, and for her relationship with her infant. From a social-psychologic perspective, childbirth has ramifications for the woman's relationships with other people, particularly her partner and parents. From a social point of view, the role of motherhood has implications for all other roles, including professional roles. Childbirth also has economic consequences for the family and society. The birth itself and the procedures surrounding the event are colored by the cultural, ethical, and religious beliefs held by the woman and her family. Therefore social and psychologic support are integral elements of all care provided to pregnant women.[8]

Physician consultation is indicated for many disorders associated with pregnancy. Some patients require emergent evaluation, whereas others require consultation with the appropriate specialist, obstetrician, or primary care provider. Pregnant women with severe hypertension, preeclampsia, or eclampsia; gestational, type 1, or type 2 diabetes; new-onset hyperthyroidism; vaginal bleeding; pyelonephritis; suspected cardiac disease; ectopic pregnancy; or asthma exacerbation may require both physician consultation and hospitalization.

GOALS OF PRENATAL CARE

Ideally, prenatal care includes individualized health education, screening, diagnosis, treatment, and referral.[7] The traditional goals of prenatal care have been to reduce both maternal and fetal morbidity and mortality. The current goals of prenatal care have been broadened to include health promotion for the mother, fetus, and family and have been extended longitudinally through the first year to encompass family development and parenting skills, the reduction of family violence and neglect, injuries, accidents, preventable acute and chronic illnesses, and family planning.[6,10]

BARRIERS TO PRENATAL CARE

Some effort has been made to reduce the traditional barriers to prenatal care in areas such as affordability, transportation, child care, and availability of health care providers. Nonstructural barriers to prenatal care in relation to areas such as attitudes, beliefs, social setting, and culture also exist and may significantly influence a woman's decision about obtaining care, particularly during the first trimester.[11,12] Three cognitive factors are significantly correlated with earlier presentation for prenatal care: (1) the desire for pregnancy, (2) a wish for early confirmation of pregnancy, and (3) an experience of early pregnancy symptoms. The decision to use prenatal care is made within a social, cultural, and historical context that depends on social interpretations.[11]

AMBULATORY PRENATAL CARE

Prenatal care can be effectively and efficiently provided by defining the capabilities and expertise of primary care providers and by ensuring that pregnant women receive risk-appropriate care. All providers must be able to identify a full range of medical and psychosocial risks and refer patients for appropriate care throughout their pregnancy.[13]

Basic prenatal care includes the prenatal care record, physical examination and interpretation of findings, routine laboratory tests, assessment of gestational age and normal progression of pregnancy, ongoing risk identification with consultation/referral mechanisms, psychosocial support, childbirth education, and care coordination. This level of care is safely and appropriately provided by advanced practice nurses (APNs) and physician assistants (PAs) with experience, training, and demonstrated competence, as well as by certified nurse midwives (CNMs).[13] Indeed, based on the evidence in reviews of randomized controlled trials in the Cochrane Pregnancy and Childbirth Database, routinely involving physicians and obstetricians in the care of all women during pregnancy and childbirth is not necessarily uniformly beneficial.[8,14]

Specialty care, which includes additional fetal diagnostic testing and expertise in managing medical and obstetric complications, is generally provided by obstetricians/gynecologists (OB/Gyns). Subspecialty care consisting of advanced fetal diagnoses; medical, surgical, neonatal, and genetic consultation; and management of severe maternal complications is provided by maternal-fetal medicine (MFM) specialists and reproductive geneticists.[15]

Consultation and referral among providers of basic, specialty, and subspecialty levels of prenatal care is instituted on the basis of the patient's circumstances and the expertise of the individual provider. Conditions requiring consultation may be present before conception or may become apparent, arise, or be exacerbated during the pregnancy (Tables 7-1 and 7-2). Follow-up care is determined jointly at the time of consultation, resulting in continued care by collaboration or transfer of care.[13]

CONTENT OF PRENATAL CARE

Although more women are receiving prenatal care, the incidence of low birth weight and preterm labor is increasing, which suggests that a careful evaluation of levels of care and the clinical significance of that care is needed.[16] It has been suggested that the quality of prenatal care, particularly in terms of the patient's receiving all of the recommended health behavior advice, is independent of the quantity of care (number of visits) in predicting improved birth outcomes.[6] It has also been suggested that women who are at greater risk of adverse birth outcomes benefit most from educational health care messages.[3,5] It may be that simply educating patients is of more value in positive perinatal outcomes than measuring, listening to heart tones, and dipping urine.

Diagnosis of Pregnancy

A diagnosis of pregnancy is usually made by a patient's history of missed menses and a positive urine pregnancy test. A home pregnancy test should be confirmed by an office test for urinary human chorionic gonadotropin (hCG) to rule out false-positive or false-negative results.[10]

Estimated Date of Birth

The age of the pregnancy or a clinical estimated date of birth (EDB) or delivery (EDD) should be determined by 20 weeks' gestation, because dating becomes increasingly inaccurate after that time. Accurate dating is important for the management of some pregnancy problems and for the application and interpretation of certain laboratory tests, such as maternal serum alpha-fetoprotein (MSAFP).[13]

Nägele's rule is commonly used to determine the EDB by counting back 3 months from the first day of the last normal menstrual period (LMP) and adding 7 days. For example, if the LMP was April 5, the EDB would be January 12.[17] The duration of a pregnancy is 40 weeks ± 2 weeks. The incidence of pregnancies continuing beyond 42 weeks is 3% to 12%.[18] If there is a size-date discrepancy or if the menstrual dates are uncertain, ultrasound imaging for dating should be performed and is most accurate before 20 weeks' gestation. An ultrasound evaluation is considered consistent with menstrual dates if there is gestational age agreement to within 7 days when the imaging is done at 6 to 11 weeks' gestation, or within 10 days when the imaging is done at 12 to 20 weeks' gestation.[13] The use of routine early ultrasound reduces the incidence of post-term pregnancy, and routine induction of labor at 41 weeks' gestation reduces perinatal mortality with no effect on cesarean birth.[19]

Timing of Visits

Traditionally, prenatal visits are scheduled every 4 weeks from 8 to 28 weeks' gestation, every 2 weeks until 36 weeks' gestation, and weekly thereafter, for a total of 14 visits.[20] A new schedule of fewer visits for healthy, low-risk women, with visits limited to specific purposes during the first 6 months, has also been recommended.[17] The revised schedule consists of visits at 8, 12, 16, 24, 28, 32, 36, 38, and 40 weeks' gestation, for a total of 9 visits. In low-risk women, this new schedule has produced no increases in adverse maternal or perinatal outcomes.[14,20,21] Some suggest, however, that decreasing routine visits may increase urgent clinic visits.[22] Others suggest that because a recommended schedule of visits for high-risk women or women with specific medical conditions has not been established, their needs may be underestimated, whereas adequate use of prenatal care in the total population is overestimated.[23]

Prenatal Visits

A comprehensive summary of recommendations on the diagnostic and educational content of visits is presented in Box 7-1.[24] A version of this summary can be used in clinical practice with dates placed by each item as discussed, ordered, and/or evaluated. It should be noted that the routine early use of ultrasound has been shown to have a trade-off between beneficial and adverse effects.[8]

During pregnancy, only anemia is more common than violence against the woman. Because of the prevalence of violence against women, the increase in violence associated with pregnancy, and the association of pregnancy complications, perinatal morbidity and mortality, and substance abuse with domestic violence, the "abuse screen" item in Box 7-1 should consist of the questions and interventions provided in Boxes 7-2 and 7-3.[13,25]

Although prospective studies have not confirmed an association between hyperthermia and birth defects, animal studies and some human data suggest an association with neural tube defects and impaired brain development. Therefore it is recommended that pregnant women not use a hot tub or sauna with a temperature greater than 38.9° C (102° F) and that exposure be limited to 10 minutes.[18,26]

COMPLICATIONS OF PREGNANCY

Nausea and Vomiting

Nausea and vomiting are the most common symptoms experienced in early pregnancy, with 70% to 85% of women experiencing nausea and 50% experiencing vomiting. A review of randomized controlled trials reveals that vitamin B_6 (pyridoxine) is effective in reducing the severity of nausea; ginger may be of benefit although the evidence is weak. Antiemetics reduce the frequency of nausea, but there is little information available on the effects on fetal outcomes.[27]

TABLE 7-1 Early Pregnancy Indications for Consultation

Indication	Consultant
HEALTH HISTORY/CONDITIONS	
Asthma	
Symptomatic (on medication)	Ob/Gyn
Severe (multiple hospitalizations)	MFM
Autoimmune disease (systemic lupus erythematosus, rheumatoid arthritis, scleroderma, ankylosing spondylitis, Sjögren's syndrome, polymyositis/dermatomyositis)	Ob/Gyn
Cardiac disease	
Cyanotic, prior myocardial infarction, aortic stenosis, primary pulmonary hypertension, Marfan's syndrome, prosthetic valve, American Hospital Association class II or greater	MFM
Other	Ob/Gyn
Diabetes mellitus	
Class A-C	Ob/Gyn
Class D or greater	MFM
Drug/alcohol use	Ob/Gyn
Epilepsy (on medication)	Ob/Gyn
Family history of genetic problems (Down's syndrome, Tay-Sachs disease, cystic fibrosis, Duchenne's muscular dystrophy)	MFM
Hemoglobinopathy (SS-, SC-, S-thalassemia)	MFM
Hypertension	
Chronic with renal or heart disease	MFM
Chronic without renal or heart disease	Ob/Gyn
Phenylketonuria (PKU)	MFM
Prior pulmonary embolus/deep vein thrombosis	Ob/Gyn
Psychiatric illness	Ob/Gyn
Pulmonary disease	
Severe obstructive or restrictive	MFM
Moderate	Ob/Gyn
Renal disease	
Chronic, creatinine $\geq$3 with or without hypertension	MFM
Chronic, other	Ob/Gyn
Requirement for prolonged anticoagulation	MFM
Severe systemic disease	MFM
OBSTETRIC HISTORY/CONDITIONS	
Age $\geq$35 at estimated date of birth	Ob/Gyn
Cesarean birth, prior classical or vertical incision	Ob/Gyn
Incompetent cervix	Ob/Gyn
Prior fetal structural or chromosomal abnormality	MFM
Prior neonatal death	Ob/Gyn
Prior fetal death	Ob/Gyn
Prior preterm birth or preterm premature rupture of membranes (PROM)	Ob/Gyn
Prior low birth weight ($<$2500 g)	Ob/Gyn
Second-trimester pregnancy loss	Ob/Gyn
Uterine leiomyomas or malformation	Ob/Gyn
INITIAL LABORATORY TESTS	
HIV	
Symptomatic or low CD4+count	MFM
Other	Ob/Gyn
CDE (Rh) or other blood group isoimmunization (excluding ABO, Lewis)	MFM
INITIAL EXAMINATION	
Condylomas (extensive, covering vulva/vaginal opening)	Ob/Gyn

Modified from American Academy of Pediatrics, American College of Obstetricians and Gynecologists: *Guidelines for perinatal care,* ed 4, Washington, DC, 1997, The College.
MFM, Maternal fetal medicine.

TABLE 7-2 Ongoing Pregnancy Indications for Consultation

Indication	Consultant
HEALTH HISTORY/CONDITIONS	
Proteinuria (≥2+detected by catheter sample, unexplained by urinary tract infection)	Ob/Gyn
Pyelonephritis	Ob/Gyn
Severe systemic disease affecting pregnancy	MFM
Substance abuse	Ob/Gyn
OBSTETRIC HISTORY/CONDITIONS	
Blood pressure elevation (diastolic ≥90 mm Hg), no proteinuria	Ob/Gyn
Fetal abnormality suspected by ultrasound	
Anencephaly	Ob/Gyn
Other	MFM
Fetal demise	Ob/Gyn
Fetal growth restriction suspected	Ob/Gyn
Gestational age 41 weeks (seen by 42 weeks)	Ob/Gyn
Gestational diabetes mellitus	Ob/Gyn
Herpes, active lesions at 36 weeks	Ob/Gyn
Hydramnios suspected by ultrasound	Ob/Gyn
Hyperemesis persisting beyond first trimester	Ob/Gyn
Multiple gestation	Ob/Gyn
Oligohydramnios suspected by ultrasound	Ob/Gyn
Preterm labor, threatened at <37 weeks	Ob/Gyn
Premature rupture of membranes	Ob/Gyn
Vaginal bleeding ≥14 weeks	Ob/Gyn
LABORATORY/EXAMINATION FINDINGS	
Abnormal MSAFP (low or high)	Ob/Gyn
Abnormal Pap test	Ob/Gyn
Anemia (hematocrit [Hct] <28%, unresponsive to iron therapy)	Ob/Gyn
Condylomas (extensive, covering labia/vaginal opening)	Ob/Gyn
HIV	
Symptomatic or low CD4+ count	MFM
Other	Ob/Gyn
CDE (Rh) or other blood group isoimmunization (excluding ABO, Lewis)	MFM

Modified from American Academy of Pediatrics, American College of Obstetricians and Gynecologists: *Guidelines for perinatal care,* ed 4, 1997, Washington, DC, The College.

Constipation

Constipation is a common problem during pregnancy and is possibly caused by increased levels of circulating progesterone. Bran or wheat fiber increases the frequency of defecation. Stimulant laxatives (bisacodyl, cascara, senna) are more effective than bulk-forming laxatives (psyllium, calcium polycarbophil), but they may cause more side effects.[28]

First-Trimester Bleeding

Approximately 20% to 25% of women experience vaginal spotting or heavier bleeding during the first half of pregnancy; of these women, half will abort. Bleeding may be physiologic and occur around the time of the expected menses. It is caused by cervical lesions or erosion (especially after intercourse) or by cervical polyps.[17] Most women who are threatening to abort will do so no matter what interventions are instituted. Bleeding accompanied by pelvic or back pain requires a cervical and bimanual examination; the prognosis for the pregnancy is poor. Viability may be assessed with transvaginal ultrasound and/or serial quantitative hCG levels, which should increase by at least 65% every 48 hours.[17]

Blood type and Rh type should be determined in cases of threatened, spontaneous, or induced abortion; ectopic gestation; any procedure associated with possible fetal-to-maternal bleeding (e.g., chorionic villus sampling and amniocentesis); and conditions associated with fetal-maternal hemorrhage (e.g., abdominal trauma or abruptio placentae). Women who are unsensitized Rh (D) negative should receive RhoGam within 72 hours. Administration of 300 μg of RhoGam will provide protection in the presence of a fetal-to-maternal bleed of 30 ml. A Kleihauer-Betke test may be used to detect a fetal-maternal hemorrhage greater than 30 ml that would require additional RhoGam.[13]

Second- and Third-Trimester Bleeding

The incidence of second-trimester bleeding is higher than that of third-trimester bleeding and is associated with a perinatal mortality rate of 23% to 32%. Placenta previa, premature placental separation (abruption), molar gestation, and cervical/vaginal lesions are the most common causes of second- and third-trimester bleeding.[18]

The incidence of placenta previa is 1 out of 200 births, occurring in 1 out of 20 grand multiparas, and is associated with an increased risk of congenital abnormalities and intrauterine growth restriction (IUGR). Presentation is typically painless vaginal bleeding at a mean of 32.5 weeks, with blood loss from the first bleed rarely fatal. Ultrasound imaging is the diagnostic technique of choice; vaginal and rectal examinations are not performed. An immediate hospital referral is required.[18,29]

The most common cause of third-trimester bleeding (>80%) is abruptio placentae, which complicates 1 out of 120 pregnancies. The most common clinical correlate of moderate to severe abruption is chronic and/or pregnancy-induced hypertension. Other risk factors are cigarette smoking, cocaine use, and trauma. Abruption is commonly accompanied by uterine pain and tenderness, back pain, and frequent, low-amplitude contractions. An immediate hospital referral is required.[18,29]

Gestational Diabetes

Gestational diabetes is a form of type II diabetes. Women with a history of gestational diabetes have a 30% to 70% risk of developing type II diabetes, the highest risk being for women who had early diagnosis, severe disease, a need for insulin, and impaired glucose tolerance during the postpartum period. Diet therapy is the initial intervention; insulin is added after the diet has failed to control glucose levels.[30] (See Diabetes, p. 28 for the treatment protocol.)

Pregnancy-Induced Hypertension

Pregnancy-induced hypertension (PIH) is hypertension that develops as a consequence of pregnancy and regresses postpartum. PIH complicates 5% of all pregnancies, 20% of nulliparous pregnancies (primarily in adolescents and women over age 35), and 40% of pregnancies in women with chronic renal

BOX 7-1

PRENATAL CARE PROTOCOL: RECOMMENDED DIAGNOSTIC AND EDUCATIONAL COMPONENTS OF VISITS

INITIAL COMPREHENSIVE EVALUATION

History
- Social
- Obstetric
- Medication
- Menstrual
- Health
- Family

Abuse screen

Physical examination (including blood pressure, teeth, height, weight, and pelvic examination)

Laboratory tests
- Cervical cytology
- *Chlamydia trachomatis*
- *Neisseria gonorrhoeae*
- Wet mount (bacterial vaginosis)
- Prenatal labs (CBC, HIV, blood type/Rh, antibody screen, serology, hepatitis B antigen, rubella titer)
- Urine for quantitative culture and protein

Fundal Height (FH)

Fetal heart tones (FHTs)

Education
- Office care/timing of visits
- Danger signs/who to call (vaginal bleeding, swelling of face or fingers, severe or continuous headache, dimness or blurring of vision, abdominal pain, persistent vomiting, chills, or fever ≥38.3° C [101° F], dysuria, escape of fluid from vagina, marked change in frequency or intensity of fetal movements)
- Medication counseling (consider alternative needs for chronic conditions; no ibuprofen, aspirin)
- Alcohol, smoking, illegal drug cessation
- Eating proper foods
- Taking vitamins/minerals
- Weight gain
- Breastfeeding (BF) infant
- Schedule BF class
- Toxoplasmosis awareness (not handling kitty litter, eating well-cooked meat, wearing gloves in garden)
- Morning sickness measures
- Daily fluid intake 2 quart minimum
- Health maintenance practices (e.g., rest, seat belt)

ALL FOLLOW-UP PRENATAL VISITS

Blood pressure, weight, FHTs, FH, urine glucose/protein, fetal movement

8-18 WEEKS

Screening/dating ultrasound

Chorionic villus sampling

Aminocentesis

Education
- Review laboratory results
- Review Pap test results
- Exercise/activity
- Travel
- Discomforts of pregnancy
- Sexuality

16-18 WEEKS

MSAFP

Education
- Prenatal vitamin follow-up
- Financial assistance

26-28 WEEKS

1-hour glucose tolerance

Repeat hemoglobin (Hgb) or hematocrit (Hct)

Repeat antibody test and prophylactic administration
- RhoGam for unsensitized Rh-negative woman

Education
- Fetal movement counts
- Preterm labor signs and symptoms
- Contraception postpartum
- Sign up for classes
- Labor companion(s)
- Alcohol, smoking, illegal drug cessation

Abuse screen

32-36 WEEKS

Testing for sexually transmitted diseases prn

Repeat Hgb or Hct

Presenting part

Education
- Preeclampsia signs and symptoms
- Confirm class attendance
- Left side-lying position
- Push fluids, protein
- Require car seat for infant

36-40 WEEKS

Presenting part/station

GBS culture (35-37 weeks)

Education
- Labor signs and symptoms, when to call
- Labor and delivery procedures
- Labor/birth preferences
- Early labor
- Anesthesia
- Circumcision
- Contraception postpartum
- Breast/bottle feeding
- Discharge planning
- Child care

BOX 7-2

ABUSE SCREEN

These questions may be asked verbally or on a written form. Complete privacy, with only the patient and primary care provider present, is necessary.

1. Have you ever been emotionally or physically abused by your partner or someone important to you?
2. In the year before you were pregnant, were you pushed, shoved, slapped, hit, kicked, or otherwise physically hurt by someone?
3. Since the pregnancy began, have you been pushed, shoved, slapped, hit, kicked, or otherwise physically hurt by someone?
4. In the year before you were pregnant, did anyone force you to have sexual activities?
5. Since the pregnancy began, has anyone forced you to have sexual activities?
6. Are you afraid of your partner or anyone you listed above?

Modified from McFarlane J and others: Safety behaviors of abused women after an intervention during pregnancy, *J Obstet Gynecol Neonatal Nurs* 27(1):64-69, 1998.

BOX 7-3

SAFETY PLAN

Try to do the following:

- Hide money.
- Hide an extra set of house and car keys.
- Establish a code with family and friends.
- Ask a neighbor to call police if violence begins.
- Remove weapons.
- Have available:
  - Social Security numbers (his, yours, children's)
  - Rent and utility receipts
  - Birth certificates (yours and children's)
  - Drivers license (yours and children's)
  - Bank account numbers
  - Insurance policies and numbers
  - Marriage license
  - Valuable jewelry
  - Important phone numbers
- Hide a bag with extra clothing.

Modified from McFarlane J and others: Safety behaviors of abused women after an intervention during pregnancy, *J Obstet Gynecol Neonatal Nurs* 27(1):64-69, 1998.

disease. Other risk factors include a family history of preeclampsia or eclampsia, preexisting hypertensive vascular and autoimmune disease, diabetes, multiple gestation, trisomy 13, hydatidiform mole (earlier than 20 weeks' gestation), and nonimmune or alloimmune fetal hydrops.[17,18]

There are three categories of PIH: (1) hypertension without proteinuria or pathologic edema (edema that is generalized, including the face, hands, and legs); (2) preeclampsia with proteinuria and/or pathologic edema (either mild or severe); and (3) eclampsia with proteinuria and/or pathologic edema, along with convulsions. Transient hypertension develops after the second trimester of pregnancy and is characterized by mild elevations of blood pressure that do not compromise the pregnancy; these mild elevations regress after delivery but may return in subsequent gestations.[17]

Diagnosis of PIH is made when blood pressure is 140/90 mm Hg or greater or rises 30 mm Hg systolic or 15 mm Hg diastolic using Korotkoff's phase V sounds (the disappearance of auscultated sound) as compared with the patient's initial blood pressure reading. Proteinuria, a late sign in PIH associated with an increased risk of poor fetal outcome, is not considered abnormal until it exceeds 300 mg/24 hr. Other clinical indicators may include sudden weight gain and ominous signs such as severe frontal or occipital headache unrelieved by ordinary analgesics, epigastric or right upper quadrant (RUQ) pain, and visual disturbances. Mild preeclampsia is initially managed by rest and observation and requires consultation. Hospitalization is required for severe preeclampsia and eclampsia.[8,17,18]

Gallbladder Disease

The most common type of gallbladder disease, cholelithiasis, is four times more common in women than in men and occurs in approximately 3% to 4% of pregnant women. The majority of these women are asymptomatic. Pregnancy increases the risk of gallstones primarily as a result of incomplete emptying of the gallbladder and the formation of biliary sludge.[17] Rarely, a stone enters the cystic duct, and one of three disorders may occur: biliary colic, acute cholecystitis (accompanied by bacterial infection in 50% to 85% of cases), or obstructive jaundice and pancreatitis. The diagnosis of cholelithiasis is made by ultrasound evaluation of the gallbladder, cystic duct, common bile duct, and liver.[17,31]

Depending on the severity of the disease, patients can usually be managed medically and may require hospitalization for bed rest, nasogastric suctioning, IV hydration, analgesic administration, and broad-spectrum antiinfective coverage. Laboratory tests include a CBC, LFTs, urinalysis, urine culture, serum amylase to exclude pancreatitis, blood cultures in febrile patients, and evaluation of stool color. Surgery for acute gallbladder disease is not common in pregnancy and should be postponed until the postpartum period to avoid the 5% pregnancy loss associated with its performance in the second and third trimesters. More aggressive surgical management is indicated with concomitant biliary pancreatitis. Laparoscopic cholecystectomy has become the treatment of choice.[17,18,31]

MANAGEMENT OF CHRONIC CONDITIONS

Asthma

There is no predictable effect of pregnancy on asthma—one third of patients improve, one third become worse, and one third remain the same. The course of asthma is often similar in subsequent pregnancies. Chronically poor asthma control during pregnancy is associated with PIH, preeclampsia, uterine hemorrhage, increased rate of cesarean birth, preterm birth, IUGR, low birth weight, and congenital malformation.[32]

Women with moderate to severe asthma need to measure and record their daily peak expiratory flow rates (PEFRs) with a portable peak flowmeter at home on rising and 12 hours later. Changes in PEFR values signifying early signs of deterioration often appear before symptoms. PEFR values range from 380 L/min to 550 L/min, with each woman having her own baseline. Adjustments in therapy are made using these measurements. Patients can be symptomatic if they have PEFR variations of 20% or more.

Maintenance therapy for chronic asthma with mild and infrequent symptoms consists of inhaled beta-adrenergic agonists (metaproterenol, albuterol, terbutaline, isoproterenol) as needed, inhaled cromolyn sodium 2 puffs q.i.d., and inhaled corticosteroids for individuals uncontrolled with bronchodilators (beclomethasone 42 μg, 4 puffs b.i.d.). Asthma-associated medications to avoid in pregnancy are alpha-adrenergic compounds other than pseudoephedrine, epinephrine, iodides, sulfonamides (late in pregnancy), tetracyclines, and quinolones.[33,34]

Diabetes

During the first trimester, maternal hyperglycemia and derangements in maternal metabolism may lead to rates of major fetal malformation that are 10% or higher. Maternal glycosylated hemoglobin levels should be checked in the first trimester to assess control during the prior 5 to 6 weeks. MSAFP determinations should be performed at 16 weeks' gestation, comprehensive ultrasound evaluation at 16 to 18 weeks' gestation, and fetal echocardiography at 20 weeks' gestation.[35]

Antepartum care consists of glucose monitoring, insulin therapy, and diet. Capillary glucose monitoring and recording of fasting values (ideal range, 60 to 90 mg/dl) before lunch, dinner, and bedtime (ideal range, 60 to 105 mg/dl), and recording of 2-hour postprandial values at least 1 day per week (<120 mg/dl), is critical. It has been suggested that peak postprandial glucose levels taken 1 hour after beginning a meal are the best predicators of fetal macrosomia.[30] Glycosylated hemoglobin levels should be measured each trimester. Insulin therapy consists of 0.5 units/kg during the first half of pregnancy and 0.7 units/kg during the second half of pregnancy in multiple injections 30 minutes before meals: morning—two thirds of the total dose with two-thirds NPH insulin and one-third regular insulin; and evening—one third of the total dose with one-half NPH insulin and one-half regular insulin. Dietary intake consists of three meals and three snacks totaling 2000 to 2400 kcal/day.[7,35]

Fetal evaluation to prevent demise consists of ongoing maternal assessment of fetal activity beginning at 28 weeks' gestation; nonstress tests (NSTs) weekly at 28 to 30 weeks' gestation and twice weekly at 32 weeks' gestation until birth; evaluation of fetal growth by ultrasound every 4 to 6 weeks; and determination of fetal lung maturity with lecithin-sphingomyelin (L/S) ratio and phosphatidylglycerol (PG) for elective delivery before 39 weeks' gestation.[35]

Thyroid Disease

During pregnancy there is moderate enlargement of the thyroid gland, with increased uptake of radioiodine by the thyroid gland. Total serum thyroxine (T_4) and triiodothyronine (T_3) concentrations rise sharply as early as the second month. Daily T_4 secretion is probably increased, with substantial amounts transferred from the mother to the fetus. Thyroid-binding globulin (TBG) is increased considerably, and thyroid-releasing hormone (TRH) and thyroid-stimulating hormone (TSH) or thyrotropin concentrations are unchanged.[17] Transient lowering of serum TSH is associated with direct stimulation of the maternal thyroid gland by elevated levels of hCG.[36]

Hypothyroidism

Women with untreated hypothyroidism who do become pregnant have a high incidence of preeclampsia and placental abruption, with a correspondingly high number of low-birth-weight and stillborn infants, an increased incidence of fetal distress, and an increased frequency of heart failure. Correction of hypothyroidism can correct these problems. The drug of choice in the treatment of hypothyroidism is levothyroxine. The optimum dose of thyroid hormone is unclear, but the dose should be adjusted so that serum TSH levels are within the normal range. More than 50% of women with hypothyroidism need an increase in thyroid dosage during pregnancy.[17,37]

Hyperthyroidism

Most cases of hyperthyroidism are due to Graves' disease (85%), although nodular goiter and Hashimoto's thyroiditis are occasionally responsible. Early in pregnancy, hydatidiform mole may present with symptoms consistent with thyrotoxicosis. The diagnosis of hyperthyroidism is confirmed by the presence of an increased free thyroxine (FT_4) or free thyroxine index (FT_{4I}), decreased TSH and, in Graves' disease, the presence of TSH receptor antibody (TSHRAb). When the diagnosis is suspected, an endocrinologist should be consulted to assist with diagnosis and management.

Methimazole (10 to 20 mg b.i.d.) or propylthiouracil (100 to 150 mg t.i.d.) are both category D in pregnancy. However, propylthiouracil is usually the preferred treatment because methimazole may be associated with more serious congenital defects. Propylthiouracil should be titrated to the lowest effective dose to minimize the risk for hypothyroidism or goiter in the fetus. Most patients respond to therapy, with an improvement in symptoms and thyroid values within 2 to 4 weeks. When the FT_{4I} improves, the drug dosage is reduced by one half. When the patient is euthyroid, the dosage is further reduced until the total dose is 15 mg of methimazole or 50 mg of propylthiouracil daily. A high titer of TSHRAb (>50%) in the mother at the end of pregnancy is predictive of neonatal hyperthyroidism.[37]

Heart Disease

Pregnancy causes marked changes in the heart. The resting pulse rate increases 10 to 15 beats per minute, and the heart is displaced to the left and upward and is rotated partially on its long axis so the apex is displaced laterally. There is an increase in the cardiac silhouette, and normal pregnant women have some degree of benign pericardial effusion. Heart sounds may also be altered during pregnancy. There may be an exaggerated splitting of the first heart sound with increased loudness of both components; a loud, easily heard third sound; a systolic murmur in 90% of pregnant women (intensified in either inspiration or expiration); a soft diastolic murmur in 20%; and continuous murmurs arising in the breast vasculature in 10%.

Pregnancy produces no changes in the ECG other than slight deviation of the electrical axis to the left.[17]

Cardiac disease should be suspected in women with complaints of dyspnea, chest pain, palpitations or arrhythmia, and cyanosis. Increased attention should be given to women with a history of exercise intolerance, heart murmurs before pregnancy, or rheumatic fever. A general evaluation of heart disease in pregnancy includes a thorough history and physical examination, chest radiographs, ECG, arterial blood gases, and an echocardiogram. If this evaluation suggests cardiac disease, a prompt referral is indicated to classify the type of disorder and evaluate the functional status and reserve in order to counsel the woman regarding the risks to and prognosis for her and her fetus.[17]

ACUTE EPISODIC ILLNESS

The incidence of asymptomatic bacteriuria varies from 2% to 7% depending on parity, race, and socioeconomic status. It is typically present at the first prenatal visit and is diagnosed by the presence of more than 100,000 organisms of a single uropathogen per milliliter in a clean-voided specimen. After an initial negative urine culture, fewer than 1% of women develop a urinary infection during pregnancy. If asymptomatic bacteriuria is not treated, 25% of women will develop an acute symptomatic infection. Renal bacteriuria is present in approximately 50% of cases. Treatment regimens include nitrofurantoin macrocrystals, 100 mg/day for 10 days; or ampicillin, amoxicillin, a cephalosporin, nitrofurantoin, or a sulfonamide for a minimum of 3 days. Prophylactic therapy with 100 mg of nitrofurantoin at bedtime for the duration of the pregnancy is indicated for women with persistent or frequent recurrences of bacteriuria.[17]

Symptoms of cystitis include dysuria, urgency, and frequency, with pyuria, bacteriuria, and hematuria microscopically. More than 90% of infections are limited to the bladder as opposed to asymptomatic bacteriuria with renal involvement. Treatment is the same as for asymptomatic bacteriuria, with the exception that ampicillin, a sulfonamide (cannot be used in the third trimester), nitrofurantoin, or a cephalosporin is given for 10 days.[17]

Upper respiratory tract infections are treated conservatively with rest, hydration, humidification, and medication for the relief of symptoms. Medications include decongestants (pseudoephedrine, 60 mg up to q.i.d., 120-mg sustained-release capsules or tablets b.i.d., or saline nasal spray or drops up to 5 days), antihistamines (chlorpheniramine, 4 mg up to q.i.d. or 8- to 12-mg sustained-release capsules or tablets b.i.d.; or tripelennamine, 25 to 50 mg up to q.i.d. or 100-mg sustained-release capsules or tablets b.i.d.), and cough suppressants (guaifenesin or dextromethorphan, 2 teaspoons q.i.d.). Treatment for sinusitis is with amoxicillin for 3 weeks (if the patient is not allergic to penicillin).[33]

In general, penicillins are safe and lack toxicity for the woman and her fetus; however, there is little experience in pregnancy with the newer penicillins (piperacillin, mezlocillin, and azlocillin), and these should be used only when another, better-studied antibiotic is not effective. There is no evidence of teratogenicity of cephalosporins; the third-generation agents have had limited use in pregnancy. Sulfonamides are not teratogenic but should not be used in a woman with glucose-6-phosphate dehydrogenase (G6PD) deficiency or during the third trimester because of an increased risk of hyperbilirubinemia in the neonate. During the second and third trimesters, tetracyclines can cause a brown discoloration of the teeth, hypoplasia of the enamel, inhibition of bone growth, and other skeletal abnormalities. First-trimester exposure has not been associated with a teratogenic risk. However, tetracycline is considered category D in pregnancy. As an alternate to penicillin, erythromycin is the drug of choice for many diseases in pregnancy. Erythromycin estolate has been associated with reversible hepatotoxicity during pregnancy, but all other forms are recommended. Metronidazole has not been found to increase the incidence of congenital defects or other adverse outcomes of pregnancy for mothers or infants. Because there is some controversy surrounding this drug, deferring therapy until after the first trimester is wise.[38]

HEALTH PROMOTION

As primary prevention continues to gain momentum in the United States, it is likely that the potential for prenatal care to provide a venue for intervention will be recognized. Prenatal care continues to improve some outcomes of pregnancy, whereas other outcomes are seemingly unaffected by prenatal care. It is clear that additional research is needed. Peoples-Sheps[4] asserts that the next decade of prenatal care will be characterized by the following: (1) increasing the recognition and use of components of care that have been shown to be effective; (2) research on psychosocial interventions, preconception care, and the timing of visits; (3) an emphasis on balancing the medical and obstetric components of care with psychosocial components to meet the needs of individual patients; (4) interventions to eliminate smoking during pregnancy; and (5) development and evaluation of more effective ways of delivering services to the poor and to people of color. It may well be that what has been referred to as "enhanced services"—such as Women, Infants, and Children (WIC) services, nutrition counseling, social work services, health education, childbirth education, and violence intervention—are actually the basic services, with the rest (e.g., measuring fundal height and fetal heart tones) may be the "enhanced" or even unnecessary services.[39]

REFERENCES

1. Enkin MW: Effective care in pregnancy and childbirth: the Cochrane Pregnancy and Childbirth Database, *J Perinat Educ* 4(4):23-35, 1995.
2. Haas JS and others: Prenatal hospitalization and compliance with guidelines for prenatal care, *Am J Public Health* 86(6):815-819, 1996.
3. Sable MR, Herman AA: The relationship between prenatal health behavior advice and low birth weight, *Public Health Rep* (112):332-339, 1997.
4. Peoples-Sheps MD: Prenatal care: will the past predict the future? *Women's Health Issues* 6(4):235-236, 1996.
5. Kogan MD and others: Relation of the content of prenatal care to the risk of low birth weight: maternal reports of health behavior advice and initial prenatal care procedures, *JAMA* 271(17):1340-1345, 1994.
6. US Public Health Service: *Caring for our future: the content of prenatal care*, Washington, DC, 1989, US Government Printing Office.
7. Berg CJ: Prenatal care in developing countries: the World Health Organization Technical Working Group on antenatal care, *JAMA* 50(5):182-186, 1995.

8. Enkin MW and others: *A guide to effective care in pregnancy and childbirth,* ed 2, Oxford, 1995, Oxford University Press.
9. Waldenstrom U: Modern maternity care: does safety have to take the meaning out of birth? *Midwifery* 12:165-173, 1996.
10. Byrd J: Content of prenatal care. In Ratcliffe SD, Byrd JE, Sakornbut EL, editors: *Handbook of pregnancy and perinatal care in family practice: science and practice,* Philadelphia, 1996, Hanley & Belfus.
11. Campbell JD, Stanford JB, Ewigman B: The social pregnancy interaction model: conceptualizing cognitive, social, and cultural barriers to prenatal care, *Appl Behav Sci Rev* 4(1):81-97, 1996.
12. Brown SS, editor: *Prenatal care: reaching mothers, reaching infants,* Washington, DC, 1988, National Academy Press.
13. American Academy of Pediatrics, American College of Obstetricians and Gynecologists: *Guidelines for perinatal care,* ed 4, Washington, DC, 1997, The College.
14. Villar J and others: Patterns of routine antenatal care for low-risk pregnancy (Cochrane Review). In *The Cochrane Library, 4,* Oxford, 2001, Update Software.
15. Lockwood CJ: *Autoimmune disease.* In Queenan JT, Hobbins JC, editors: *Protocols for high-risk pregnancies,* ed 3, Cambridge, Mass, 1996, Blackwell Science.
16. Kogan MD and others: The changing pattern of prenatal care utilization in the United States, 1981-1995, using different prenatal care indices, *JAMA* 279:1623-1628, 1998.
17. Cunningham FG and others: *Williams obstetrics,* ed 20, Stamford, Conn, 1997, Appleton & Lange.
18. Scott JR and others: *Danforth's handbook of obstetrics and gynecology,* Philadelphia, 1996, Lippincott-Raven.
19. Crowley P: Interventions for preventing or improving the outcome of delivery at or beyond term (Cochrane Review). In *The Cochrane Library, 4,* Oxford, 2001, Update Software.
20. McDuffie RS and others: Effect of frequency of prenatal care visits on perinatal outcome among low-risk women: a randomized controlled trial, *JAMA* 275(11):847-851, 1996.
21. Binstock MA, Wolde-Tsadik G: Alternative prenatal care: impact of reduced visit frequency, focused visits and continuity of care, *J Reprod Med* 39:1-6, 1994.
22. Ward N, Bayer S, Calhoun B: The impact of alternate prenatal care with reduced frequency of visits in residency teaching program, *Am J Obstet Gynecol* 174(1 pt 2):339, 1996.
23. Alexander GR, Kotelchuck M: Quantifying the adequacy of prenatal care: a comparison of indices, *Public Health Rep* 111:408-418, 1996.
24. Farrington PF, McElligott K, Hobbins-Garbett D: *Prenatal protocol,* unpublished document, Salt Lake City, 1997, Teen Mother and Child Program, University of Utah.
25. McFarlane J and others: Safety behaviors of abused women after an intervention during pregnancy, *J Obstet Gynecol Neonatal Nurs* 27(1):64-69, 1998.
26. Speroff L: Exercise. In Queenan JT, Hobbins JC, editors: *Protocols for high-risk pregnancies,* ed 3, Cambridge, Mass, 1996, Blackwell Science.
27. Jewell D, Young G: Interventions for nausea and vomiting in early pregnancy (Cochrane Review). In *The Cochrane Library, 4,* Oxford, 2001, Update Software.
28. Jewell DJ, Young G: Interventions for treating constipation in pregnancy (Cochrane Review). In *The Cochrane Library, 4,* Oxford, 2001, Update Software.
29. Lockwood CJ: Third trimester bleeding. In Queenan JT, Hobbins JC, editors: *Protocols for high-risk pregnancies,* ed 3, Cambridge, Mass, 1996, Blackwell Science.
30. Jovanovic L: *Diabetes and pregnancy: glucose-mediated macrosomia and the fetus,* 61st Scientific Sessions of the American Diabetes Association, June 23, 2001.
31. Collea JV: Gallbladder. In Queenan JT, Hobbins JC, editors: *Protocols for high-risk pregnancies,* ed 3, Cambridge, Mass, 1996, Blackwell Science.
32. Tan KS, Thomson NC: Asthma in pregnancy, *Am J Med* 109(9):727-733, 2000.
33. Working Group on Asthma and Pregnancy: *Executive summary: management of asthma during pregnancy,* NIH Pub No 93-3279A, Washington, DC, 1993, National Institutes of Health.
34. Kochenour NK: Asthma. In Queenan JT, Hobbins JC, editors: *Protocols for high-risk pregnancies,* ed 3, Cambridge, Mass, 1996, Blackwell Science.
35. Gabbe SG: Diabetes mellitus. In Queenan JT, Hobbins JC, editors: *Protocols for high-risk pregnancies,* ed 3, Cambridge, Mass, 1996, Blackwell Science.
36. Glinoer D: What happens to the normal thyroid during pregnancy? *Thyroid* 9(7):631-635, 1999.
37. Mestman JH: Hypothyroidism. In Queenan JT, Hobbins JC, editors: *Protocols for high-risk pregnancies,* ed 3, Cambridge, Mass, 1996, Blackwell Science.
38. Reece EA and others: *Handbook of medicine of the fetus and mother,* Philadelphia, 1995, JB Lippincott.
39. Mahan CS: Prenatal care indices: how useful? *Public Health Rep* 111:419, 1996.

CHAPTER 8

Lactation

Kathleen M. Craig

Lactation counseling begins during pregnancy with verbal and written health education regarding what to expect in the immediate postpartum period. Expectant mothers should be informed about the benefits of breastfeeding and about the recommendations of the American Academy of Pediatrics that infants be breastfed for the first year of life (and longer if the infant and mother desire).[1] Mothers should know that they can breastfeed even if they are returning to work.

Mothers should be taught to expect to keep their infants close to them in the first 2 weeks as the infant learns to nurse and to plan to sleep when the infant sleeps. Prospective nursing mothers are taught measures to minimize serious breast engorgement and sore nipples, and they are taught that bottles and supplements are avoided during this initial period of lactation. After the infant is born, counseling issues include how to latch on correctly, how to assess milk transfer, and how to assess the adequacy of milk production. The mother is taught that the infant feeds frequently in the first 2 weeks; in general, the infant will begin to space out the feedings after the first 2 weeks. Mothers can be encouraged that mother-infant dyads that make it through the first 2 weeks of breastfeeding generally go on to meet their breastfeeding goals. Community lactation resources for the mother should be provided. The health care provider should refer problems that threaten continued lactation to lactation experts.

DISCHARGE INSTRUCTIONS

Discharge instructions should be clear and in writing. Mothers need to monitor their infants for signs of inadequate milk intake. What constitutes inadequate milk intake for breastfed infants depends on many factors, such as gestational age and size for gestational age. Premature infants may lose more weight, have fewer reserves, and are vulnerable to complications such as low blood sugar. Infants who are large for gestational age or small for gestational age require close monitoring.

It is preferable to teach mothers the expected goals and to teach them to report concerns that the infant may not be meeting these goals rather than teach them the "danger" signs; once the danger signs appear, the infant's condition may be serious. Mothers need to report when their infant is not meeting the standard for a "good" intake, because early intervention is critical. For example, infants are vulnerable to hypernatremic dehydration starvation syndrome and will continue to produce some stool and urine, even when the situation is life threatening.

Therefore discharge instructions center around the appearance of the stool and the optimum feeding and voiding patterns. Infants should feed at least 8 to 12 times per day; after the milk comes in, the stools should be yellow with milk curds. For the first week of life, the number of stools and the number of voids should match the age in days. After this, the infant will develop a personal pattern of elimination that may change again at 1 month of age. Any changes in an infant's established pattern should be evaluated. With an optimum feeding pattern, the infant should latch on securely to the breast and suck and swallow rhythmically and vigorously for at least 10 minutes on each breast. Suckling time at the breast should not be limited.

Mothers should keep a feeding log for the first week, because this is the critical time for lactogenesis. The feeding log should keep track of the number and quality of feeds as well as the number of stools and voids. A feeding log helps the parents to determine at home whether the infant is feeding well. The breasts should soften after feeding, and the infant should be satisfied and may fall asleep after suckling at the second breast.

Mothers are instructed to call the provider if the infant develops jaundice or has difficulty feeding. Infants should be evaluated 2 to 3 days after discharge for hyperbilirubinemia and to assess weight.[2] Infants may lose up to 10% of their birth weight during the first week of life. A supplemental feeding plan should be initiated for infants who lose greater than 10% of their birth weight (Box 8-1).

MANAGEMENT OF BREASTFEEDING PROBLEMS

Breast Engorgement

Breast engorgement may occur on or about the third postpartum day when lactogenesis develops. It can usually be prevented by feeding the infant 8 to 12 times each day in the days leading up to the milk coming in. This may mean waking the infant to nurse. Mothers should keep a feeding log and be taught techniques to awaken a sleepy infant. Mothers should be taught to evaluate the difference between sustained and intermittent suckling. Some women with engorgement may need

BOX 8-1

COMPONENTS OF A PLAN TO IMPROVE BREAST MILK INTAKE

1. Evaluate the breastfeeding technique and correct any problems with sucking technique or positioning.
2. Suggest the appropriate feeding frequency and duration.
3. Use a hospital-grade breast pump with a double-pump setup (pumping both sides at once) to increase breast emptying and stimulation. Use the pumped milk to supplement breastfeedings.
4. Assess adequacy of feeding using pumping volumes and closely following weight gain. If the maternal supply is adequate, weight gain should be at least an ounce a day. If the supply is inadequate and not remediable, supplemental feedings of formula may be required temporarily. Taper them as soon as the supply is increased and weight gain is improved.
5. Slowly taper the pumping sessions after the infant has gained the appropriate weight and is breastfeeding without supplemental measures.
6. If the breastfeeding problem is not improved by improving the sucking technique and supply, contact the referral network for expert help. Continue to maintain contact with the mother and specialists.

to express some milk manually or with a pump to soften the areola enough to allow the infant to latch on. When an engorged breast is not well emptied, the resulting back pressure on the milk glands can result in decreased milk production. If a mother develops sore nipples, the primary care provider or a lactation consultant should be notified.

Infants need to be latched deeply onto engorged breasts to extract the milk. Mothers with engorgement may need to compress their breasts manually to form it for the infant's mouth. Deep latch-on will resolve most nipple problems as well as engorgement. If the engorgement is serious, ice can be applied to the breasts between feeds, and hot packs can be applied before feeds. The mother and infant should receive direct observation of feeding if mother cannot get her infant to latch on. Mother should have a breastfeeding support plan at discharge. This may include visiting nurses, a lactation nurse, or the primary care provider. Obstetric nurses can provide 24-hour phone support to triage concerns and to address early initiation problems.

Latch-On Problems

The infant's inability to suckle effectively is often caused by inappropriate latch-on or attachment. Mothers need to be taught to evaluate the latch and how to present the breast to the infant. Sucking on the nipple tip causes pain and poor let-down. Present the breast to the infant by brushing the nipple slowly on the infant's lower lip to entice him or her to open the mouth wide. The infant must be brought deeply onto the breast so that the chin and nose are touching the breast. Sufficient nipple and areolar tissue must be placed in the infant's mouth so that he or she can strip the milk sinuses. The mother's hand should grasp the breast well behind the areola, compressing and projecting the milk sinuses forward into the front of the breast so that when the infant latches with flanged lips, he or she connects deeply with the milk sinuses to extract colostrum or milk.

Occasionally, the infant's lower jaw needs to be drawn down a bit after latching so that his or her mouth is opened wider as he or she sucks. Every mother-infant pair should have frequent assessment of latch-on during the early postpartum period. This is an opportunity to teach the parents about the infant's unique characteristics and to develop problem-solving techniques. An infant who is consistently dissatisfied after feeding for long periods is not getting enough to eat at the breast and is probably is not latched on correctly. If the mother reports poor feeding after the infant has been discharged, the infant should be brought back to the clinic for evaluation. If the mother is still hospitalized, skilled personnel should work with the mother and infant to improve latch on and colostrum or milk transfer. After milk production has been established, the breasts should soften after feeding, and the infant should be satisfied and may fall asleep after suckling at the second breast.

Let-Down (Milk Ejection) Problems

Let-down, or milk ejection, results from smooth muscle contraction of the myoepithelial cells surrounding the secretory alveoli (glands) of the breast. Oxytocin produced in response to the infant's suckling as well as to the sight, sound, and smell of the infant causes this contraction and the resultant milk flow. Uterine cramping signals early oxytocin production, and the presence of these cramps is a good predictor of ultimate breastfeeding success.[3] The cramping is always worse with second and subsequent infants. Mothers may need analgesics in the early postpartum period to manage the "afterpains." After a few weeks the let-down response can be sensed as a tingling sensation throughout the breasts followed by milk leaking from the nipple. Let-down is inhibited by stress, pain, and alcohol. It can be conditioned through breast massage, thoughts of the infant, and relaxation. It is important for mothers to condition their let-down if they are pumping for premature infants or for a return to work.

Inadequate Milk Production

Inadequate milk production usually results from inadequate suckling and breast emptying. It may also result from inadequate prolactin or, rarely, from inadequate mammary glandular tissue. Prolactin levels measured before and after breastfeeding should show a threefold increase after suckling or pumping. If the problem is the infant, the suckling produces less milk than the pump. If the prolactin level is uniformly low, it suggests an endocrine basis for the low supply. Prolactin levels that respond to stimulation with normal let-down but poor milk supply indicate inadequate glandular tissue. Inadequate glandular tissue can usually be assessed prenatally, with a feeding plan for the infant including close follow-up and early supplementation. Supporting the infant with supplemental feedings while increasing breast stimulation with a breast pump usually improves milk production.

Milk production (galactagogue) stimulators include metoclopramide (10 mg t.i.d. for 1 week and then tapered over 4 days).[4] The mother can use herbal galactogogues such as fenugreek tea, but galactogogues are not consistently reliable. Double pumping in addition to nursing produces the best results for increasing supply.

Low Infant Weight Gain

Low infant weight gain in the first few weeks after birth is a common problem and is usually caused by inappropriate breastfeeding management in the hospital and during the immediate postdischarge period. Infants who have lost 8% or more of their birth weight must be followed to prevent significant problems with breastfeeding. A review of the history may reveal whether feeding frequency, attachment, and let-down are appropriate. Infants who are feeding appropriately should have four or more milk curd stools per day by the fourth day and at least six wet diapers per day. They should be arousable and feeding at least eight times per day for a minimum of 10 minutes of audible sucking and swallowing.

When assessing an infant with inadequate weight gain, providers must observe a breastfeeding session. Strategies to increase success include infant arousal techniques, increased feeding frequency, and breast pumping to increase the milk supply. Sometimes it is necessary to offer the infant supplemental pumped milk or formula to improve sleepiness and weight gain. Ideally, this is done while the infant is feeding at the breast using a supplemental nursing system. Significant infant weight loss or difficult management problems require careful evaluation and follow-up. Consultation with lactation consultants and/or physicians experienced with breastfeeding management and failure to thrive may be necessary.[5]

Cracked Nipples

Cracked nipples are caused by attachment or latch-on problems. When the infant latches on to only the tip of the nipple instead of the areola, the nipple becomes abraded. Treatment includes correcting the latch-on (see Latch-on Problems) and increasing the frequency of the feedings. The duration of suckling may be shortened, but the infant must have active suckling at the breast during each feeding session. Mother should be taught to listen for audible swallowing in the infant. She can remove the infant after the nursing rhythm changes from active deep suckling to leisurely comfort sucking.

Medical-grade lanolin may improve comfort if the nipples are dry and cracked. For severely damaged nipples, hydrogel dressings are useful to maintain a moist wound healing environment. In addition, mothers must avoid overdrying their nipples and should apply warm, moist compresses after feedings to soothe and promote healing. Sometimes the pain of breastfeeding is so severe that pumping or hand expression is required to maintain the supply and prevent engorgement while healing begins. Nipple soreness will resolve after a rest from breastfeeding for 24 hours and with correct latch on. It generally takes 10 days for sore nipples to heal completely. With inadequate improvement, the health care provider must reevaluate the breastfeeding technique and treatment plan; a referral to a lactation specialist may be indicated.[6]

Mastitis

Mastitis, or cellulitis of the interlobular connective tissue of the breast, is often a marker for breastfeeding mismanagement. Mastitis usually presents with fever, generalized malaise, flulike symptoms, local erythema, and breast warmth and tenderness. A combination of unrelieved engorgement and cracked or abraded nipples is often the reason why a plugged milk duct becomes infected. Treatment for mastitis includes the application of warm packs to the breast and frequent breastfeeding or pumping. In addition to these nonpharmacologic interventions, the infection is treated with antibiotics such as amoxicillin/clavulanate, dicloxacillin, or a broad-spectrum cephalosporin to cover a probable staphylococcal or streptococcal infection. The infant's sucking technique and the mother's breastfeeding pattern and support system should also be evaluated. Mastitis can progress to abscess if early intervention is not instituted. Therefore any occurrence of flulike symptoms in a breastfeeding mother mandates an evaluation for mastitis.

Infant Jaundice

Most newborns become mildly jaundiced between the third and fifth days of life. Excessive jaundice in an infant may be a sign of breastfeeding management problems. Other causes of jaundice must be excluded, such as blood group incompatibility, hepatic obstruction, or hepatitis. The latter two causes present as a high direct or conjugated bilirubin level in the infant.

The most common cause of uncomplicated unconjugated hyperbilirubinemia in the first 5 to 10 days of life is infrequent feeding (less than seven sessions per day) and starvation, resulting in an exaggerated physiologic jaundice. This type of jaundice is rare in countries in which breastfeedings on demand are the norm. Frequent feedings result in frequent stools, and bowel movements are the primary excretion route for bilirubin. When feedings and associated stools are infrequent, the bilirubin in the stool is reabsorbed into the bloodstream, which raises the serum bilirubin level and results in clinical jaundice. This is commonly referred to as "no–breast milk" jaundice and is generally associated with less than optimal breastfeeding support. It responds to increased breastfeeding and may require the use of a breast pump to increase the mother's supply. Supplementing with water or formula is counterproductive if breast milk is available. Water and sugar water are not necessary and will not help in the management. Frequent breastfeeding (every 2 to 3 hours) will usually improve the jaundice. Formula supplementation may be required in cases of low milk supply. Every effort should be made to increase the milk supply while protecting the infant from starvation.

Phototherapy may be necessary if jaundice is recognized late and the bilirubin level is above 20 mg/dl. Prematurity, low Apgar scores, and bruising such as in cephalhematoma can be associated with significant early jaundice in breastfeeding infants. True breast milk jaundice usually occurs after 1 to 2 weeks of age (after breastfeeding is well established) and occurs in the setting of appropriate weight gain. True breast milk jaundice may be caused by an inheritable enzymatic defect that inhibits glucuronyl transferase and prevents the conjugation of bilirubin. It results in late-onset, prolonged, unconjugated hyperbilirubinemia. The infant with true breast milk jaundice is typically thriving, gaining weight, and producing four or more milk curd stools per day. A temporary cessation or reduction of breastfeeding for 12 to 24 hours can be tried in severe cases (bilirubin >20 mg/dl). The mother's milk supply should be maintained by pumping while breastfeeding is interrupted. Once the bilirubin level has dropped, breastfeeding can be reestablished. The bilirubin level may raise slightly, but not usually to clinically significant levels.[7]

Weaning

Weaning is a natural process. It is physically and emotionally less painful when it is done gradually and the infant leads the process. As the infant grows, other activities and other foods often replace the need to breastfeed. Weaning can happen as early as 6 to 7 months of age, when solids are introduced, or as late as 2 or 3 years of age.[8] Some mothers and infants choose to breastfeed into the toddler years, and there is no reason to oppose a continuation of this bond. The ethnographic literature suggests that, before the widespread use of artificial infant formulas, children were traditionally nursed for 3 to 4 years. When mothers desire weaning, feedings should be replaced by supplemental milk or formula (depending on the age of the infant), one feeding at a time over a period of a few weeks until all feedings have been replaced. Infants who are less than 1 year of age should receive breast milk or formula. Cow's milk should be withheld until infants are older than 1 year of age. When weaning toddlers, some feedings may be replaced with activities instead of food.

CO-MANAGEMENT ISSUES

Expectant and new mothers should be referred to breastfeeding support groups such as La Leche League, Nursing Mothers' Council, and Women, Infants, and Children (WIC) services. Patients who need additional assistance or specialized help should be referred to breastfeeding or lactation specialists. The Academy of Breastfeeding Medicine, La Leche League Medical Associates, and the International Board of Lactation Consultant Examiners can provide referrals to lactation consultants.[9]

SPECIAL PROBLEMS IN BREASTFEEDING MANAGEMENT

Working Mothers

Mothers who must return to work or school or otherwise be separated from their infants for regular periods of time can usually continue breastfeeding. The milk supply will adjust to the demands. Depending on the mother and the age of the child, the mother may need to pump the breasts two to three times per day to maintain the milk supply and collect it to give to the caregiver for the infant's bottle feedings.

Multiple Births

Mothers of twins or triplets can breastfeed successfully. With proper support and encouragement they can expect to have a sufficient supply. Initially, twins may need to be breastfed separately until they learn how to nurse. After the infants learn how to nurse, they can be breastfed simultaneously. The need for supplemental feedings depends on both the mother's milk supply and the infants' needs.

Breast Pumps

Breast milk can be expressed by hand or by using a breast pump. Hand expression is a learned art that can be taught easily.[10] Many different types of manual and electric pumps are available. Hospital-grade electric pumps are available for rental. Milk should be kept cool after pumping. If refrigerated, it will keep for 48 hours. If frozen at −17.8° C (0° F), it will keep for 6 months. Mothers should be provided with written instructions about milk storage and handling.

REFERENCES

1. American Academy of Pediatrics, Work Group on Breastfeeding: breastfeeding and the use of human milk, *Pediatrics* 100:1035-1039, 1997.
2. Neifert M: Early assessment of the breastfeeding infant, *Contemp Pediatr* 13:142-166, 1996.
3. Newton N: The relation of the milk-ejection reflex to the ability to breastfeed, *Ann NY Acad Sci* 652:484-486, 1992.
4. Errenkranz R, Ackerman B: Metoclopramide effect on faltering milk production by mothers of premature infants, *Pediatrics* 78(4):614-620, 1986.
5. Desmarais L, Browne S: *Breastfeeding and the slow gaining infant: insights and resolutions: lactation consultant educational series,* Garden City Park, NY, 1990, Avery Publishing.
6. Cable B, Stewart M, Davis J: Nipple wound care: a new approach to an old problem, *J Hum Lact* 13(4):313-318, 1997.
7. American Academy of Pediatrics Provisional Committee for Quality Improvement and Subcommittee on Hyperbilirubinemia: practice parameter: management of hyperbilirubinemia in the healthy term newborn, *Pediatrics* 94:558-565, 1994.
8. Stuart-Macadam P, Dettwyler K, editors: *Breastfeeding: biocultural perspectives,* New York, 1995, Walter de Gruyter.
9. Lawrence RA: *Breastfeeding: a guide for the medical profession,* ed 5, St Louis, 1998, Mosby.
10. Marmet C: *Marmet manual expression of breast milk: the Marmet technique,* Pub No 27, Schaumburg, Ill, 1998, La Leche League International.

CHAPTER 9

Aging and Geriatric Issues

Barbara Willson

Those providing primary health care to older adults in the twenty-first century must be responsive to the worldwide demographic shift and be influenced by the findings of gerontologic research. They must also consider current societal attitudes toward aging and the aged.

Demographic predictions for society are that there will be both greater numbers of older adults and increased longevity of the population. The fastest-growing cohort in the late twentieth century was the group identified as "old old" (over age 85 years), and the number of centenarians increased the fastest.[1]

Many individuals reaching the age of 65 years in the coming decades will be robust, with some remaining so until their death. Heart disease, cancer, and cerebrovascular disease continue to be the chief causes of death and disability among older adults. The most common chronic conditions include arthritis, heart disease, hypertension, diabetes, and hearing and vision impairment.[2,3] A demographic imperative exists for the health care system as a result of these data and predictions. Primary care, including health promotion and disease prevention as well as the prevention of disease exacerbation, complications, or disability, must continue in all settings in which older adults live and must be provided by a coordinated team of health care professionals. The goal of primary care of older adults is compression of the period of morbidity to bring improved quality of life until death.

AGEISM

Societal attitudes in the form of ageism are a major barrier to quality health care for older adults. Scientific research dispels many of the myths inherent in ageism, yet it is tenacious, cultural, and universal. Ageism is subtle, and like all prejudices it is based on generalization about members of a group. A recent study of nondiseased older adults extends the understanding of the variations among older adults and of the potential for health and fullness of life in old age. Rowe and Kahn[4] set the stage for this research by proposing a distinction between usual (high risk) and successful (low risk and high function) aging. Gerontologists no longer accept a single pattern or set of signposts for aging (previously termed "normal" aging) but instead describe the diversity within and between each cohort and among individuals. The concept of "normal" aging reflects an internalization of long-standing myths about the aging process that are not easily dispelled.

Robert Butler[5] coined the term *ageism* in 1965 to describe the culturally rooted discomfort with growing older. He observed not only revulsion on the part of young people but also fear of the losses associated with aging. Twenty-five years later Butler[6] noted that ageism continued to prevail, and he predicted that it would not soon disappear. Primary care providers and older adults themselves are influenced by societal ageism.

HALLMARKS OF AGING

In this society, the single most important characteristic of late adulthood is its diversity. The development of biologic and psychosocial aging theories suggests that the nature of individual aging depends more on life experiences than on a universal process or genetic dictate. Environmental conditions and cohort experiences promote many of the observable changes commonly seen with aging. Current research suggests that risk reduction through conscientious primary care is possible with persons aging in the usual manner.[7] Box 9-1 includes selected examples of the findings of gerontologic research that dispel long-held myths about aging.

CHALLENGES IN PRIMARY CARE

The goal of geriatric primary care is to maximize independence and functional status and shorten the morbidity period in the life of each older adult. The challenges in achieving this goal include ageism, a lack of geriatric education, the complexity of illness in older adults, the increasing dependence of older adults, and cost.

Neither older adults nor health care professionals are immune to ageism. Older adults themselves determine when to seek screening or treatment and are known to assume that many symptoms of disease are a result of their advanced age. A common example of this assumption is the reaction to joint pain and stiffness. The use of a variety of analgesics by older adults may promote digestive disturbances and decrease the quality of their nutrition. Inadequately managed pain interrupts sleep and activity. The assessment and guided management of pain avoids unnecessary polypharmacy and interactive complications.

Primary care providers continue to receive minimal education in gerontology and geriatrics, yet research demonstrates that the presentation of disease is often atypical in an aging patient. Treatment must be based on an understanding of the ability of the body to adapt to aging and on an understanding of the effect of aging on pharmacokinetics. Although the human body demonstrates remarkable compensation for aging, stress disrupts this adaptation. The most disturbing stress of the provider-patient interaction is lack of time.

Geriatrics presents special challenges to managed care and cost containment in today's health care system. Effective health care of older adults is best provided by a team that includes the patient (unless he or she is markedly demented), the appropriate

BOX 9-1

FACTS THAT DISPEL MYTHS ABOUT AGING

- Skeletal muscle can be strengthened in very old persons.
- Cardiac output is not automatically diminished with age.
- Aging bodies retain harmony of physiologic functions.
- Unless stress is introduced, age does not destroy the ability to learn.
- Sexual desire and satisfaction are not obliterated by aging.
- The best projector for longevity is the older adult's optimism.
- Basic personality elements continue unless interrupted by advanced dementia.

caregivers, and the leadership of professionals educated in the field of gerontology.

An individual experiencing the usual aging pattern is increasingly vulnerable to multiple health problems and experiences losses that affect stamina, motivation for self-care, and the ability to function effectively. Functional problems affecting the older adult's status and care often include a lack of exercise, constipation, and sleep disturbances. Nonprescription drugs for discomforts and prescriptions from medical specialists often result in a dangerous polypharmacy, which must be recognized to avoid interactions. Reduction of memory and sensory input further complicate the diagnosis and treatment plans. Additional challenges arise from the long-standing use of alcohol and nicotine by the patient as well as from poor nutrition.

Geriatric specialists use the Folstein Mini Mental State Examination (MMSE), the Short Portable Mental Status Questionnaire (SPMSQ), and the Geriatric Evaluation of Mental Status (GEMS) to differentiate short-term memory loss from dementia, to observe the progression of cognitive impairment, and to suggest the etiology of a problem. A detailed history of cognitive change and lifelong habits is a vital element in the differential diagnosis of dementia and often necessitates an interview with an observant family member or friend. Maintaining a record of the patient's baseline mental status and the results of subsequent mental status testing is essential for accurate diagnosis and management.

Tools for the assessment of functional status, including the Barthel Index, the Physical Self-Maintenance Scale (PSMS), and the Katz Index, are also well developed and available and should be used at each patient visit. Function is addressed on two levels: (1) basic, including feeding, bathing, dressing, ambulation, and toileting; and (2) more complex, including cooking, shopping, using the telephone, reading, writing, and managing money. The patient's performance on functional testing can be accomplished quickly in an interview and may explain a failure to respond to medications, a failure to use exercise or diet prescriptions, falls and injuries, and the occurrence of depression or anxiety. A functional and mental status evaluation may lead to a referral to community resources, changes in the patient's living situation, and changes in the treatment plan for chronic health problems.

Screening older adults for disease should be individualized rather than driven by guidelines for all adults. For example, the patient's family and personal history of osteoporosis, cancer, heart disease, dementia, thyroid disease, and diabetes provides important clues to vulnerability as he or she ages. Annual examinations should be comprehensive, are necessarily time-consuming, and when necessary should include responsible family members.

Older adults identify "consistency of provider" when describing what they believe to be high-quality health care.[8] A trusting relationship with one provider ensures greater success when other professionals are included in evaluation and treatment plans. The approach used by a walk-in clinic and by multiprovider groups in which all providers see all patients does not provide the consistency valued by older adults. The relationship of the patient with one provider is particularly important in promoting optimal health and preventing crises. Studies have demonstrated that even very old adults change their behavior based on teaching and counsel—it is never too late. Even more striking are the positive results of strengthening exercise programs in frail and disabled older adults. Not only do they gain strength in the muscles weakened from disuse, but their functional level is dramatically elevated.[9]

Fall prevention is an excellent example of success through the collaborative effort of a multidisciplinary team. Physical and occupational therapists provide appropriate exercise, balance, and gait-training programs and teach patients about environmental hazards. Physicians, nurse practitioners, and physician assistants monitor the treatment of orthostatic hypotension, peripheral vascular disease, and incontinence (a few of the immediate causes of falls). Nutritionists prevent dehydration and anemia through teaching sessions. When falls are prevented, pain, disability, hospitalization, and possibly iatrogenic disaster are also prevented. Falls erode the self-confidence of older adults and intensifies their fear of dependence and loss of control over their lives.

Maintaining the safety of older adults usually involves other family members, whether they are living apart or together. Mental health specialists and community services provide essential caregiver and elder support, and referrals are helpful. Depression is ubiquitous in older adults, often as a result of their ageist thinking, and is contributed to by social isolation; significant losses of relationships, roles, or mobility; and the loss of a sense of wellness.

The primary care of older adults includes a discussion of advance directives and a health care proxy. Ideally, the period of morbidity before death is brief and peaceful, both for efficiency within the health care system and for maximal control over the end of life. A living will or similar document, which describes in detail the wishes of the patient in regard to resuscitation, hospitalization, treatments, and a health proxy, should be part of each patient's health care record.

The challenge for the primary care provider who treats older adults in the twenty-first century is to recognize the individual aging process of each older adult, promote optimal health and functioning, provide care and comfort during illness, and provide for a peaceful death.

REFERENCES

1. Day J: *Population projections of the United States by age, sex, race and Hispanic origin:1995 to 2050,* Current Population Reports (Series P25, No 1130),Washington, DC, 1996, US Government Printing Office.
2. National Center for Health Statistics: *Death rates for 72 selected causes by 10-year age groups, race and sex,* Washington, DC, 1995, US Department of Health and Human Services.
3. Adams P, Marano M: Current estimates from the National Health Interview Survey 1994, *Vital Health Stat* 10(193):83-84, 1995.
4. Rowe J, Kahn T: Successful aging, *Gerontologist* 37(4):433-440, 1997.
5. Butler R: Ageism: another form of bigotry, *Gerontologist* 9(4):243-246, 1969.
6. Butler R: A disease called ageism, *J Am Geriatr Soc* 38(2):178-180, 1990 (editorial).
7. Rowe J, Kahn T: Successful aging, *Gerontologist* 37(4):443-440, 1997.
8. Willson B: *Perceptions of quality home health care among homecare recipients 85 years and older and their providers,* unpublished doctoral dissertation, Ann Arbor, 1994, University of Michigan.
9. Fiatorone M, Evans W: The etiology and reversibility of muscle dysfunction in the aged, *J Gerontol* 48:77-83, 1993.

CHAPTER 10

Management of Common Elder Syndromes

Barbara Jean Roberge

Syndromes are complex, multicausal entities that test the diagnostic powers of the primary care provider. Chaos may reign, but therein lies the challenge in caring for the primary care needs of older individuals. Five common syndromes seen in older adults are discussed in this chapter: polypharmacy, cognitive impairment, dehydration, falls, and failure to thrive. This chapter also contains a definition of an emerging issue in the geriatric literature: domestic violence against older women.

Polypharmacy

DEFINITION/EPIDEMIOLOGY

Polypharmacy is the use of multiple drugs, both prescription and nonprescription. It is a common cause of iatrogenic illness in older adults, who account for 14% of the population but consume 30% of all prescription drugs.[1] For some older adults, drugs consume a high percent of their fixed income.

PATHOPHYSIOLOGY

Drug distribution and clearance are affected by normal age changes, including a reduction in lean body mass and blood flow to the kidney and liver and an increase in body fat. These issues are compounded in frail older adults because, in addition to normal age changes, disease alters the functioning of specific organ systems and affects pharmacokinetics. Drug absorption is not drastically different in healthy older adults. However, because of the increase of achlorhydria with aging, drugs requiring stomach acid for absorption should be avoided. Kidney function declines by approximately one third with aging, and therefore a normal renal function test does not necessarily mean normal renal function.

CLINICAL PRESENTATION

Intrinsic physiology is unalterable; therefore extrinsic factors, namely the type and amount of drug, must be altered. To avoid the negative consequences of polypharmacy, it is important to review all medications with each patient contact and to maintain good communication with consultants. The number of possible adverse reactions and drug interactions is staggering with the addition of just one drug to a multidrug regimen. A drug-related side effect should be considered for any presenting symptom until proven otherwise.

MANAGEMENT

To avoid a negative outcome, patients should be encouraged to order drugs from a pharmacy with computerized drug data. As an educator for both the patient and the primary care provider, the pharmacist plays an important role in preventing poor outcomes.

The drug risk-benefit ratio should be determined when considering the use of a new drug. The recommendations in Table 10-1 should be followed to reduce the risk of drug interactions and adverse reactions. The general principles of drug therapy in geriatrics are first considered, such as the pharmacodynamics of the drug class and common adverse effects experienced by older adults. For example, older adults are more susceptible than younger adults to the anticholinergic effects of drugs. Second, the specific side effect profiles of a drug class and a patient's history of previous adverse effects, morbidity, and general nutritional state are considered. The known or suspected risk is weighted against the presumed benefit of administering the drug. "Start low and go slow" is common advice when prescribing for older adults; however, the heterogeneity of older adults provides a reason to avoid uniform treatment guidelines. An older adult's pain or psychiatric condition may be undertreated because of the primary care provider's fear that a drug may produce adverse effects in all older adults.

Using literature review and expert panel consideration, Knight and Avorn[2] have recently developed twelve quality indicators for appropriate medication use. These indicators are presented in Table 10-2 along with the level of supporting evidence.

Cognitive Impairment

DEFINITION/EPIDEMIOLOGY

The most common and feared cause of a decline in cognition is dementia, and the most prevalent form of dementia is Alzheimer's disease (AD). The cost of treating AD approaches $100 billion annually in the United States. The presence of AD doubles every 5 years after age 65 and approaches 50% by age 85.[3]

PATHOPHYSIOLOGY

Morris has proposed that AD begins with the deposition of beta-amyloid–containing senile plaques (SPs) throughout the neocortex. Plaques exacerbate neurofibrillary tangles and cause

TABLE 10-1 Medication Risk/Benefit Analysis

General Considerations	Specific Considerations
DRUG ISSUES	
Drug class: pharmacokinetic properties of class (e.g., ACE inhibitors affect renal excretion)	Drug class: common side effects (e.g., ACE = hyperkalemia)
PATIENT ISSUES	
Common adverse effects in older adults:	Specific prior problems:
Anticholinergic effects	Renal failure
Constipation/diarrhea	Dehydration
Indigestion	Malnutrition
Delirium	Poor compliance
Dizziness	Drug cost
Depression	
Dermatologic effects	

TABLE 10-2 Quality Indicators: Appropriate Medication Use In Vulnerable Older Adults

Quality Indicator For Vulnerable Older Adults	Supporting Evidence
1. All drugs should have a clearly defined indication documented to avoid indefinite continuation of unnecessary drugs.	No clinical trials, expert panel
2. Drug education may improve adherence and outcomes and alert patient to the side effects.	Meta-analysis review and randomized control trial (RCT)
3. All patient records should contain an up-to-date medication list to eliminate inappropriate duplication and avoid drug interactions.	Cohort study
4. For chronic diseases, document the drug response at a minimum within 6 months of prescribing to provide a basis for continuation.	Expert panel
5. Review the patient's drug regimen at least annually to provide an opportunity for discontinuation and to include new prevention regimens.	Criteria-based literature, one RCT, outcome studies on computer-based retrospective drug-use review (RDUR); RDUR found no change in status, mortality, or morbidity
6. International normalized ratio (INR) should be performed within 4 days of initiating warfarin and at least every 6 weeks. The risk of adverse events is greatest in vulnerable older adults.	Expert panel
7. Electrolytes should be measured within 1 week of initiating thiazide or a loop diuretic and then at a minimum of every year.	No studies of monitoring electrolytes on outcomes; RCT demonstrated the association of hypokalemia with these diuretics; twofold increased risk of ventricular arrhythmias with potassium <3.0 mEq/L
8. Avoid the use of chlorpropamide (Diabinese) because of its prolonged half-life.	473 case-based review plus expert panel
9. Avoid drugs with strong anticholinergic properties that have the potential for adverse effects.	RCTs
10. Barbiturates should not be used if seizure control is not needed because of the potent CNS depressant and addictive properties, the high incidence of drug interactions, and an increased fall risk.	Epidemiologic study of fall rate and barbiturate use
11. Avoid the use of meperidine (Demerol) in vulnerable older adults because of the high risk of delirium.	Case-based study plus RCT comparing meperidine found it no more effective than nonsteroidal antiinflammatory drugs for acute pain
12. Check electrolytes within 1 week of initiating therapy with angiotensin-converting enzyme (ACE) inhibitors because they may cause renal insufficiency and hyperkalemia.	Epidemiologic study plus case-based study; greater risk for developing renal dysfunction immediately after initiating drug, but risk persists for duration of therapy

Modified from Knight E and others: Quality indicators for appropriate medication use in vulnerable elders, *Ann Intern Med* 134(8 pt 2):703-710, 2001.

neuron dysfunction and death, leading to the presentation of symptoms. Brain plaques and tangles noted on autopsy are the hallmark of AD. SP formation is found in asymptomatic individuals at autopsy, but neuronal death is insufficient to cause symptoms. A recent area of intense research interest is in the identification of mild cognitive impairment (MCI). MCI is highly predictive of dementia and is conceptualized as a preclinical stage of dementia.

Cognitive decline is not inevitable with aging. There is great variation in cognition, as there is with all other system functions. Cognition is a factor of education, socioeconomic status, continued social engagement, and wellness. Only modest declines in general intelligence are observed over a lifetime. Tests of simple, relevant tasks show no decline with aging. Daily cognitive functioning, especially with the familiar, does not decline with aging. In fact, older adults demonstrate a larger vocabulary and a greater knowledge of geography and current events than other age-groups. This may be due to greater life experiences. Little research exists on the cognitive abilities of those over age 75. Compared with younger individuals, this group does show a decline in memory, attention, and information processing. However, cognitive, longitudinal studies with the "oldest old" may reveal different results from comparisons of age cohorts.

CLINICAL PRESENTATION

Unlike delirium, dementia is a chronic, irreversible illness with a gradual onset and a steady decline in cognition. Short-term memory loss is the primary symptom in AD along with one or more of the following: disorientation, disturbance in executive functioning (planning, organizing, and abstract thought), problems with activities of daily living, and one of the three *P*s (aphasia, apraxia, and agnosia). Day-night sleep cycles are often reversed, and consciousness and psychomotor changes are not evident until late in the disease. Irritability, withdrawal, and apathy may be exhibited in the early stages of the disease. Psychotic symptoms such as paranoia and agitation are seen later in the disease.

MANAGEMENT

Treatment of AD consists of antioxidants (vitamin E) in high doses, as well as monoamine and cholinesterase inhibitors.[4] The effects of hormone replacement therapy and antiinflammatory

BOX 10-1

COMMON ETIOLOGIES OF DEHYDRATION

INTAKE (FLUID DEPRIVATION)

Environmental Factors
Restricted ambulation
Decreased hearing and/or vision

Increased Metabolic Demands
Infections (resulting in malaise, reduced appetite, and poor intake)

Dysphagia
Poorly fitting dentures
Esophageal lesions
Neurologic disease

Pharmacologic Factors
Narcotics
Sedatives
Neuroleptics
Anticholinergics

Normal Aging Changes
Ineffective water conservation
Decreased thirst drive

Poor Appetite
Fatigue
Constipation
Depression

Fluid Limitations
Preprocedure/preoperatively
To prevent urinary incontinence
Management of heart failure
Management of hyponatremia

OUTPUT (FLUID EXCESS)

Environmental Factors
Hot weather
Alcohol intake

Increased Metabolic Demands
Infections (resulting in tachypnea and sweating)
Diarrhea
Vomiting
Sweating

Endocrine Disorders
Diabetes insipidus
Glycosuria

Pharmacologic Factors
Diuretics
Laxatives

Normal Aging Changes
Ineffective salt conservation

drugs are being studied because epidemiologic studies demonstrate a lower incidence of dementia in individuals who are taking these drugs. Drug treatment has demonstrated a slowing of the disease progression when it is begun in the early to middle stages of the disease, and thus early identification is important.[5]

Dehydration

DEFINITION/EPIDEMIOLOGY

Dehydration is more prevalent in older adults and has a greater likelihood of a negative outcome than in younger adults. It is defined as a state of fluid intake deprivation and/or excess fluid loss. Accompanying electrolyte imbalances may ensue. The most significant electrolyte abnormality is sodium imbalance. Because of this, dehydration is further categorized by the associated relationship between free water and sodium[6]:

- Isotonic dehydration occurs with a balanced loss of water and sodium. An example of this is vomiting and diarrhea, with equal losses of water and electrolytes.
- Hypertonic dehydration, also called hypernatremic dehydration, occurs when water loss is greater than sodium loss. Febrile illnesses and poor fluid intake result in hypertonic dehydration.
- Hypotonic dehydration occurs when sodium loss is greater than water loss, resulting in hyponatremia. The inappropriate use of diuretics causes this type of dehydration.

In older adults, dehydration is often multicausal (Box 10-1). The environmental issues, polypharmacy, and diseases prevalent in older adults predispose this group to dehydration, as do age-related changes in plasma osmolality and thirst.

Dehydration is a common problem in older adults and has a direct and positive effect on increasing rates of morbidity and mortality. For all Medicare beneficiaries age 65 or older (excluding 6% of those beneficiaries in HMOs), 6.7% of the hospitalizations in 1991 (146,960 hospitalizations) had a principal or concomitant diagnosis of dehydration. In the same year, the cost to Medicare for dehydration (not including long-term care cost) was $446 million.[7] Not only is dehydration a common and costly problem, but the consequence to the individual is catastrophic. Almost one half (47%) of older adults hospitalized with a primary diagnosis of dehydration died within 1 year.[7]

PATHOPHYSIOLOGY

Three principal changes in the homeostatic mechanism that controls the volume and osmolality of extracellular fluids occur in older adults. These normal changes result in a reduced adaptability and reserve to deal with system stressors. First the thirst response, which is stimulated by dehydration, is diminished and results in an increased solute-water ratio. Second, decreased renal plasma flow may be responsible for a decline in the ability of the body to concentrate urine. The inability to concentrate urine prevents the body from retaining enough fluid to avert dehydration. Finally, vasopressin release stimulated by low fluid volume is diminished. Therefore the inherent homeostatic mechanism that prevents the sequela of hypovolemia is blunted.[6]

CLINICAL PRESENTATION

The presenting symptoms of dehydration are often vague and nonspecific. These include confusion, lethargy, rapid weight loss, and functional decline. Dehydration is often a feature of failure to thrive. The history should include an assessment of fluid intake, functional status, weight, and cognition. The presence of constipation may indicate a lack of water intake (see Box 10-1).

The physical examination includes a cardiovascular assessment and may reveal an orthostatic drop in blood pressure and a rise in pulse, indicating volume depletion. Temperature may be elevated as a result of dehydration or an inflammatory process. Mucous membranes are often not noticeably dry until severe dehydration is present. Because of changes in skin collagen, poor skin turgor—often used as a sign of dehydration in younger individuals—is unreliable in older adults. The tongue may be swollen and furrowed.

Laboratory data include a review of serum electrolytes, BUN-creatinine ratio, osmolality, hematocrit and hemoglobin, and glucose. A BUN-creatinine ratio of 25:1 or more suggests dehydration. Dehydration is present when the sodium level is greater than 148 mEq/L. However, with isotonic and hypotonic dehydration, serum sodium is normal and low, respectively. Hematocrit is elevated compared to the level of hematocrit when the patient is well hydrated. Respiratory and genitourinary infections are common, and a urinalysis and chest x-ray studies may be appropriate.

Fever, poor fluid intake, iatrogenic drug use, and gastrointestinal fluid losses are the most common causes of dehydration in older adults. Other etiologies of dehydration should be pursued if electrolyte imbalances persist after treatment, with a focus on the endocrine system. However, older adults respond slowly to the treatment of severe electrolyte abnormalities. Hyponatremia, a common and often misdiagnosed clinical finding in older adults, results from an inability to excrete free water. This is due to increased vasopressin release, which causes the kidneys to conserve water and thus increases the ratio of free water to sodium solute. This syndrome is termed the syndrome of inappropriate antidiuretic hormone (SIADH). In SIADH, urine osmolality is greater than 300 mOsm/kg with a low serum sodium level. This high urine osmolality differentiates SIADH from low sodium dehydration. The treatment is limitation of free water, which may then result in dehydration if the patient is not monitored closely.

MANAGEMENT

As described in Table 10-3, management of dehydration is driven by the severity of electrolyte imbalance, the treatment setting, and goals. This distinction is important because all three must be carefully defined before treatment is planned.

The guidelines for oral rehydration have been proposed.[8] In any setting, an oral fluid prescription for a patient should be written with the patient's family in mind; it is important to inform the staff and the family that it is difficult to overhydrate a dehydrated patient with fluids by mouth. Rehydration prescriptions for the first 24 hours include replacement of one half of the fluid deficit plus the ongoing loss and maintenance fluid of at least 1500 ml/day. During the next 2 to 3 days, the remainder of the fluid deficit is replaced and maintenance fluids are given. A simple formula for estimating fluid loss or deficit (based on the fact that 1 L of water weighs 1 kg) has been devised:[5]

$$\text{Preillness weight (kg)} - \text{Current weight (kg)} = \text{Fluid deficit in liters}$$

Because the primary care of older adults occurs in multiple settings, primary care providers may be involved in hypodermoclysis (clysis), the infusion of fluids subcutaneously, or IV fluid administration. A current survey of the geriatric literature suggests that the administration of clysis is gaining in popularity. During this treatment it is best to avoid electrolyte-free or hypertonic solutions because they are poorly absorbed and may precipitate circulatory collapse and death.[9] It should be noted that these recommendations are from poorly designed, older studies using hypertonic solutions that are rarely used today (10% to 25% glucose).

The choice of subcutaneous or IV fluids depends on the serum sodium level and the degree of hypovolemia. If the serum sodium level is normal or low, isotonic saline (0.9%) is infused. If the serum sodium level is high, then a 5% dextrose in one-half normal saline is appropriate after hemodynamic stabilization. If

TABLE 10-3 Dehydration Management

	Low Risk*		High Risk*	
Setting	Treatment	Comfort	Treatment	Comfort
Office practice	OR†	OR	NA	OR
Home	OR/clysis	OR	NA	OR
Nursing home	OR/clysis	OR	Clysis/IV	OR
Hospital	OR	OR	IV	OR

OR, Oral rehydration; *NA,* not applicable.

*Risk is defined by clinical parameters and may include severity of electrolyte imbalance. Though not research based, high risk may be defined as a serum sodium ≥150 mEq/L, an inability to take sufficient fluids by mouth, or co-morbid conditions that increase the risk of complications from rehydration (e.g., congestive heart failure). These definitions of risk are not research based.

†Oral rehydration is used while fluids by mouth are possible.

hypotension, orthostasis, and decreased urine output are present (signaling hemodynamic collapse), the initial IV therapy is rapid infusion of isotonic saline to stabilize these parameters. Hospitalization may be appropriate depending on the treatment goals. After hydration is treated, a return to the premorbid mental status and functional level may take weeks.

Hemodynamic collapse will occur if dehydration is severe and presents as hypotension, orthostasis, and decreased urine output. Overzealous rehydration, or an attempt to replace total water loss within 24 hours, may result in death from cerebral edema.

Education focuses on the prevention of dehydration (Box 10-2). When it occurs, the amounts and types of fluids to ingest are included in the educational plan. Fluids high in sodium (e.g., tomato juice, bouillon, or sports drinks) are appropriate for those with low sodium levels, whereas juice is appropriate for those with high sodium levels. Caffeinated beverages have a mild diuretic effect and should be avoided.

Falls

DEFINITION/EPIDEMIOLOGY

The evaluation and management of an older adult's independence is a priority because functional decline and, specifically, falls are an important morbidity and mortality risk factor. The goal of measuring preclinical functional risk is to permit intervention before the onset of dependence. Falls are a symptom, not a diagnosis.

Falling is an unintentional loss of balance that results in a position change and contact with the ground. The most feared sequela of a fall is a fracture. Quality of life may be severely impacted because of a "fear of falling," with self-imposed isolation and immobility causing a vicious cycle of risk. Fall assessment focuses on known risk factors, including sensory abnormalities and abnormalities of the central and peripheral nervous system, cognition, and mood.[6]

In a community sample, approximately 30% of older adults fall each year. The probability of falling increases with age.[10] In long-term care the annual fall incidence per resident is greater than 50%. Approximately 40% of falls result in minor injuries, and 3% to 5% of falls result in fractures. Falls contribute to 40% of nursing home admissions.[11]

PATHOPHYSIOLOGY

Falls are multifactorial. The majority occur during walking, stepping, or position changes and not during more hazardous activities.[10] Contributing factors are lower extremity weakness, poor balance, orthostatic hypotension, central nervous system disease, cognition and sensory abnormalities, and unsafe environments. The relationship of lower extremity weakness as a marker of preclinical disability has been well demonstrated.[12]

Sensory input from vision, hearing, vestibular function, and proprioception are important in preventing falls. Visual impairment increases as a result of normal age-related changes and the increased prevalence of ocular diseases. Normal age-related changes cause glare intolerance and slower adaptation to the dark than in younger adults. Common ocular diseases include cataracts, glaucoma, conjunctival infections, corneal ulcers, herpes simplex and herpes zoster infections, and macular degeneration.

Presbycusis, or hearing loss associated with normal aging, is initially a result of the loss of hearing high-frequency sounds. Subsequently there is a decrease in the ability to distinguish sounds, especially when background noise is present.

Balance is dependent on sensory cues and vestibular function, both peripheral and central. Disequilibrium and unsteadiness is common in older adults and is related to aging changes and disease in the inner ear as well as to changes in the transmission of signals from the periphery. Acute and chronic changes in mental status, as well as depression, contribute to falls, but the mechanism of action is unclear. Drugs causing sedation, postural hypotension, and electrolyte imbalance have been implicated in the risk for falls. The use of four or more medications increases the risk for falls, regardless of the type of medication.[13]

Normal aging changes in the cardiovascular system blunt the homeostatic mechanisms that maintain adequate organ perfusion and blood pressure control, causing hypotension. Musculoskeletal and joint diseases affect balance and gait, as do loose rugs, cords, and clutter in the home.

CLINICAL PRESENTATION

The clinical presentation of falling is varied. Therefore the health history should focus on previous falls and events surrounding a fall, episodes of syncope, unsteadiness, and dizziness. The mnemonic *DDROPP* (diseases, drugs, recovery, onset, prodrome, and precipitants) helps in remembering the assessment of the event preceding the fall. The assessment should also focus on angina or any history of myocardial infarction, vision and hearing problems, neurologic dysfunction, fractures, cognitive changes, and medications.

Self-reported functional scales quickly supplement the history with information on mobility, self-care abilities, mood, hospitalizations, and nutrition. One of the best-known scales is the Short Form 36 (SF36) along with its condensed version, the Short Form 12 (SF12).[14] It is important to ask questions in reference to current activities. The reply to "How did you get to this appointment?" is immensely informative, as is simply watching how a patient enters the examination room and with whom.

PHYSICAL EXAMINATION

A complete physical examination with a focus on postural vital signs is necessary and should include a cardiovascular and neurologic examination, including Romberg's test with a sternal nudge and a check for nystagmus. Mobility (including gait

BOX 10-2

DEHYDRATION PREVENTION

- Drink six to eight 8-ounce glasses of water/juice daily.
- Take a full glass of water/juice with medications.
- Drink more than usual in hot weather or when you have a fever.
- Keep a fluid intake record for 2 days.
- Poorly fitting dentures will interfere with food and fluid intake.
- People with memory problems need fluid monitoring.

and balance), upper extremity function, cognition, vision, and hearing are also examined. Quick and easy mobility and gait tests are now available and correlate positively with the risk for falls and a decline in self-care ability. With the "get up and go" test,[15] the patient is asked to get up from a chair with his or her arms folded across the chest, walk 10 feet, return to the chair, and sit down using regular footwear and any regular walking aid. The ease of gait, balance, position change, and turning are evaluated. Completion of the task in 20 seconds or less correlates with functional independence; those taking 30 seconds or more are considered functionally dependent.

Lower extremity balance is tested by evaluating the patient standing with the feet side by side, semitandem and tandem, and balancing for 10 seconds. The evaluation of upper extremity strength and coordination is an important marker of frailty. While in a sitting position, the individual is asked to pick up an object off the floor. The Functional Reach Test for balance is completed by asking the individual to reach forward in a parallel plane without taking a step. Individuals with a reach of less than 7 inches are considered very frail and limited in self-care ability.[16] Frailty increases the risk of falls. Patients should be observed by a member of the clinical team while performing the activity associated with the fall.

The initial evaluation should include a CBC (to rule out anemia and infections), electrolytes, BUN, creatinine (to look for dehydration and electrolyte imbalance), serum glucose, and a stool occult blood test. An ECG is indicated, but rhythm disturbances are not a common cause of falls.[17]

If syncope and ECG abnormalities are present, a myocardial infarct is excluded and a careful examination and diagnostic work-up for flow abnormalities is necessary. If the neurologic examination is positive, an MRI will rule out brain infarcts or other abnormalities. The patient with true vertigo is most likely to suffer from inner ear disease. Benign positional vertigo (BPV) is common in older adults. The vertigo of BPV is episodic and is provoked by position changes.

MANAGEMENT

The goal of treatment and education is to alter modifiable risk factors (Box 10-3). Guidelines for fall prevention have been proposed by experts.[18] If lower extremity weakness is present, a referral to a physical therapist for resistance training is recommended. Resistance training benefits even those of advanced age and frailty.[19] If balance is altered, balance training consists of having the patient stand on one foot for 10 seconds and gradually increase the time and frequency. Low-intensity Tai Chi maintenance training has been demonstrated to improve balance.[20] Balance may also be improved by proper footwear and the use of assistive devices. Drug reduction and the avoidance of alcohol are important if hypotension is present. A home safety evaluation or checklist is indicated if trips and falls are prevalent.

Serious complications of falls (e.g., subdural hematoma, cervical fracture) are rare. Because of the high incidence of osteoporosis in older adults, fractures requiring surgical intervention occur with falls, but soft tissue injury is a more common outcome. Consultation should be considered if complications are suspected, particularly if syncope, true vertigo, or abnormal cardiovascular or neurologic findings are present.

BOX 10-3

FALL PREVENTION

- Evaluate the home to eliminate loose cords, clutter, and slippery surfaces.
- Use bathroom and stair rails.
- Change position slowly.
- Treat foot problems and wear well-fitting, low-heeled footwear.
- Light the environment well.
- Exercise to maintain lower leg strength.
- Join a Tai Chi class for balance training.
- Bring all medications, including nonprescriptions, to your health provider.
- Have regular hearing and vision testing.

Failure to Thrive

DEFINITION/EPIDEMIOLOGY

Failure to thrive (FTT) is a syndrome described as a progressive loss of function and general deterioration. The rate of decline exceeds the expected rate as compared with a peer group. It is often initiated by a trigger and follows an at-risk state of frailty.[21] Patients present with weight loss, muscle loss (sarcopenia), and functional decline. Malnutrition is a common problem in nursing homes.

The diagnostic evaluation of FTT seeks to differentiate reversible from irreversible causes. Because of inconsistent definitions of the syndrome, its incidence is unknown. Approximately 15% of hospitalized older adults with FTT die during hospitalization, and 30% of the survivors are discharged to nursing homes.[22]

PATHOPHYSIOLOGY

Normal aging causes a loss of weight and muscle mass and an increase in body fat. Thus only small losses in weight occur with aging. It is hypothesized that changes in body composition are due to age- and disease-related intrinsic and extrinsic causes, such as inactivity.[23] Age-related changes in lean body mass are partially due to changes in growth hormone, estrogen, and androgen secretion. Administering these hormones increases lean body mass but does not necessarily improve functional capacity and strength. Obesity causes insulin resistance, which is not age related. End-stage chronic diseases (e.g., heart failure, pulmonary disease) and malignancy cause weight loss.

CLINICAL PRESENTATION

Patients with FTT may present with any of the following symptoms: weakness, inability to care for self, dizziness, weight and memory loss, and depression. Weight loss in FTT is often gradual. The health history focuses on chronic diseases with signs of organ failure, the presence of gastrointestinal malabsorption, cancer risk factors, infection, thyroid abnormalities, depression, and changes in memory. Nutritional intake and the progression of weight loss are calculated. Adverse reactions to medications, including confusion or anorexia, may be partially responsible for FTT. Any history of smoking and alcohol use, as well as any

BOX 10-4

FAILURE-TO-THRIVE ETIOLOGIES

DISEASE
Organ failure
Metastases
Infection
Stroke
Thyroid disease
Fractures

MEDICATION
Cognitive changes
Anorexia
Dehydration

ENVIRONMENTAL CAUSES
Isolation
Neglect
Poverty

PSYCHIATRIC CAUSES
Depression
Dementia
Psychosis
Delirium

GASTROINTESTINAL CAUSES
Malabsorption
Dysphagia
Dental problems
Diarrhea
Vitamin deficiency

history of transfusions since 1975, is elicited. Reversible causes of FTT are sought (Box 10-4).

PHYSICAL EXAMINATION

A loss of 5% or more of body weight in less than a year requires a search for a reversible cause. A complete physical examination should focus on symptoms, organ failure, infections, and malignancy. However, the physical examination is often benign. A skin, mucous membrane, and eye examination may reveal muscle wasting, ulcerative lesions, and signs of vitamin deficiency, anemia, and dehydration. A complete oral examination, including an evaluation of the dentition and denture fit, is necessary. Tests of swallowing ability and the gag reflex are included in the neurologic examination. A thorough breast examination, a Papanicolaou (Pap) test, and a rectal examination for occult blood loss will evaluate for malignancy. Many older women have not had a vaginal or breast examination for years, if ever; thus it is important to explain the purpose and importance of these examinations. Because of the heterogeneity of older adults, biologic age should not be the only deciding factor in omitting breast and pelvic examinations.

Screening tests should include a CBC, electrolytes, kidney and thyroid studies, fasting blood glucose, liver function tests, calcium levels, urinalysis, and a chest x-ray examination. Additional diagnostics may be indicated and are guided by testing and examination.

Any irreversible cause of FTT, such as malignancy or end-stage organ disease, should be evaluated. The patient and/or family need to be involved in decisions to perform diagnostic testing. Treatment is not always desired by the patient or guardian, and end-of-life support and comfort may be a reasonable approach after the initial evaluation.

A lifelong history of anorexia due to body image concerns has been reported in the literature. Older adults may have lifelong patterns of dieting and anorexia nervosa–like symptoms, which are often overlooked in this population.[24]

MANAGEMENT

Adequate caloric intake and access to food is mandatory. Meals on Wheels and other community support organizations may be necessary if isolation or functional decline is present. Nutritional efforts may improve weight but may not improve clinical outcomes. High-calorie and high-protein supplements are beneficial. A daily multivitamin supplement and 800 IU of vitamin D are beneficial. If decubitus ulcers are present, 220 mg of zinc and 500 mg of vitamin C b.i.d. for 2 weeks (or until healing is complete) can be added until healing is complete. Appetite stimulants are not recommended for reversible causes of weight loss. Depression is treated with an antidepressant.

Creative solutions and their dissemination to prevent malnutrition in nursing home residents have been proposed and include small group dining for dementia patients, the use of volunteers to assist at dinner time, and ethnically appropriate foods.[25] Families need to be included in education and support measures. Often they are the ones to urge patients to seek health care when the patients themselves are reluctant to do so. Patient autonomy must be preserved as long as dementia and depression have been excluded. If irreversible causes of FTT are not found, it may be the natural course of life's end.

Domestic Violence

An important area of emerging research is that of domestic violence (DV) against older women. Research in this area has only recently emerged because the term *domestic violence* usually pertains to younger women. Research on older adults has focused on elder abuse, which usually is rooted in a different definition and focuses on inadequate care of vulnerable populations. DV focuses on physical assault and gender and power issues that may have occurred over a lifetime. The level of research of this emerging issue is at the early stages and has been reported at the case study–qualitative level of research. Phillips[26] informs us that nursing interventions from this emerging literature should consider that wife abuse among older adults exists, that serious physical and emotional harm and death may occur, and that, due to frailty, even low-level violence can cause harm. DV can be associated with lifelong suffering. Finally, DV is a complicated and often hidden issue.[26]

REFERENCES

1. Chrischilles EA and others: Use of medication by persons 65 and over: data from established populations for epidemiologic studies of the elderly, *J Gerontol* 47:M137-144, 1992.
2. Knight E, Avorn J: Quality indicators for appropriate medication use in vulnerable elders, *Ann Intern Med* 134(8 pt 2):703-710, 2001.
3. Morris J: Is Alzheimer's disease inevitable with aging? *J Clin Invest* 104(9):1171-1173, 1999.
4. Sundeland T: Alzheimer's disease: cholinergic therapy and beyond, *Am J Geriatric Psychiatry* 6(2):S56-S63, 1998.
5. Sano M and others: A controlled trial of selegiline, alpha-tocopherol, or both as treatment for Alzheimer's disease, *N Engl J Med* 336(12):1216-1222, 1997.
6. Hazard W and others: *Principles of geriatric medicine and gerontology*, ed 3, New York, 1994, McGraw-Hill.

7. Warren JL and others: The burden and outcomes associated with dehydration among US elderly, 1991, *Am J Public Health* 84(8): 1265-1269, 1994.
8. Hebrew Rehabilitation for the Aged, Morris JN and others, editors: *Quality care in the nursing home,* St Louis, 1997, Mosby.
9. Rochon P and others: A systematic review of the evidence for hypodermoclysis to treat dehydration in older people, *J Gerontol* 52A(3):M169-M175, 1997.
10. Tinetti M, Speechley M, Ginter S: Risk factors for falling among elderly persons living in the community, *N Engl J Med* 319:1701-1707, 1988.
11. Edelberg E: *Falls in the elderly,* Geriatric medicine course, Division on Aging, Boston, 1998, Harvard Medical School.
12. Guralnik J and others: Lower-extremity function in persons over the age of 70 years as a predictor of subsequent disability, *N Engl J Med* 332:556-561, 1995.
13. Nevitt M, Cummings S, Hudes E: Risk factors for injurious falls: a prospective study, *J Gerontol* 46(5):M164-M170, 1991.
14. Ware J, Kosinski M, Keller S: A 12-item short form health survey: construction of scales and preliminary test of reliability and validity, *Med Care* 34:220-233, 1996.
15. Podsiadlo D, Richardson S: The timed "up and go": a test of basic functional mobility for frail elderly persons, *J Am Geriatr Soc* 39: 142-148, 1991.
16. Weiner D and others: Functional reach: a marker of physical frailty, *J Am Geriatr Soc* 40:203-207, 1992.
17. Lipsitz L: An 85-year-old woman with a history of falls, *JAMA* 276:447-453, 1996.
18. Panel on Fall Prevention: Guidelines for the prevention of falls in older persons, *J Am Geriatr Soc* 49:664-672, 2001.
19. Fiatarone MA and others: Exercise training and nutritional supplements for physical frailty in very old people, *N Engl J Med* 330: 1769-1775, 1994.
20. Wolfson L and others: Balance and strength training in older adults: intervention gains and Tai Chi maintenance, *J Am Geriatr Soc* 44: 498-506, 1996.
21. Sarkisian C, Lachs M: Failure to thrive in older adults, *Ann Intern Med* 124:1027-1078, 1996.
22. Berkman B, Foster LW, Campion E: Failure to thrive: paradigm for the frail elder, *Gerontologist* 29:654-659, 1989.
23. Roubenoff R, Harris T: Failure to thrive, sarcopenia, and functional decline in the elderly, *Clin Geriatr Med* 13:613-621, 1997.
24. Miller D and others: Abnormal eating attitudes and body image in older undernourished individuals, *J Am Geriatr Soc* 39:462-466, 1991.
25. Burger and others: *Malnutrition and dehydration in nursing homes: key issues in prevention and treatment,* Pub No 386, Boston, June 2000, The Commonwealth Fund.
26. Phillips LR: Domestic violence and aging women, *Geriatr Nurs* 21(4):188-193, 2000.

CHAPTER 11

Psychosociospiritual Issues

Emily Chandler

Recent discussions surrounding end-of-life issues are often grounded in concerns about pain, loss of control, and quality of life; these problems are far more complex than either legalistic solutions or symptom management would allow.[1] At the root of the fear of patients and their families is the mystery of death itself. A recent Gallup Poll offered revealing answers to the question of what dying patients want. Most reported that they wanted to die at home, be with someone close to them, and have someone pray with them.[2] Hospice and palliative care programs provide what most people wish: managed pain, comfort, quality of life, and a peaceful death. Rather than being a fearful, dreadful experience, dying can be healing, peaceful, and even fulfilling for patients and those closest to them. But the end of life is fraught with crises: physical, psychologic, social, and spiritual. Psychosociospiritual care encompasses all of these phenomena.

The physical aspects of dying are usually more familiar to the primary care provider than the more elusive aspects of the process. Although providing physical comfort and pain management is critical, the elements that cannot be separated from a holistic perspective are equally important. An appreciation for the psychosociospiritual needs that attend the journey of the dying is essential. As beneficial for the caregiver as for the patient, a holistic perspective that attends to whole persons cannot help but strengthen the caregiver's own sense of centeredness in the midst of suffering. A repertoire of psychosociospiritual intervention strategies can address the complex problems of patients in crisis and those who are with them during the process.

IMPACT OF CRISES

Caring for patients and their families at the end of life brings the primary care provider face to face with his or her own experiences of loss. The losses that are lurking and unresolved are those that creep up and surprise us with their tenacity whenever witnessing another's pain. Witnessing and contemplating the unknown, everyone is confronted with feelings of hopelessness and hope, sadness and peace, and fear and trust. A poignant balance is often maintained between these polarized feelings and between the players who, at various points in the process, become the custodians of the feelings. Central to the experience is sorting out which feelings belong to whom.

The primary care provider's own unresolved issues need to be confronted so that any work with patients and families is not blunted by a need to protect the self from being overwhelmed. This is particularly important in the face of compound crises and with the pressure of a caseload filled with too many patients—each of whom need the best the provider can give. Embracing loss and suffering and pain is the starting point for compassionate and trustworthy care that allows others their feelings and experiences without losing hold of the self.

Everyone who deals with crises on a daily basis is at risk for posttraumatic stress disorder (PTSD). Mirroring the fear of patients and the sadness and grief of family members, caregivers who are exposed to stress without adequate means for coping with that stress can become distant and walled off from their feelings. Being overwhelmed with cumulative crises can precipitate the classic symptoms of PTSD: negativism, withdrawal, irritability, blaming, depression, physical complaints, impoverished interpersonal relationships and, the hallmark of PTSD, psychic numbing. When the system cannot bear any more pain, it simply shuts down. Primary care providers who care for terminally ill patients and their families and carry a demanding caseload are at risk for avoiding the patient's and family's sadness in an attempt to prevent the stress from becoming too much. An unwitting unconscious triage is always a possibility: providing care for those patients who are most likely to get well. What is needed to meet patients' needs is a basic knowledge of crisis intervention, a family systems orientation, and familiarity with spiritual care—in short, psychosociospiritual care.

CRISIS INTERVENTION

The vantage point from which the dying process is viewed precipitates widely different perceptions. The circumstances surrounding the death may compound the crisis. Sudden death, violent death, and the death of a child are all situational crises that are superimposed on the developmental crisis of death and dying. Developmental crises and situational crises are always occurring simultaneously within families. However, there is often a recurring pattern in the human response to stress, particularly in regard to universal experiences. Guidelines for responding to those patterns are the crux of well-known crisis intervention strategies.[3] Crisis intervention is no longer the prerogative of mental health practitioners alone; although it may not be specifically named as such, it is continually practiced in primary care.

Increasingly, primary care providers may find themselves to be exactly that: the primary provider of care. The prevalence of home care gives everyone in health care an opportunity to use a diverse array of interventions. One home visit may be worth ten office visits and be far more effective in the long run. With those realities in mind, a model for identifying phases of crises at the end of life and the interventions specific to those phases can aid in the assessment of patients and their families (Table 11-1). The model as proposed is offered as a way of quickly assessing patients' responses to the specific crisis of dying, but it also can prove useful in other contexts.

During the impact phase, which begins with the diagnosis of a terminal illness or the news of the sudden death of a loved one, denial and anger can be most apparent. The patient or family member may be in shock and disbelief, unable to incorporate either information or an emotional response. A steady, caring response of presence is critical at this juncture; the capacity to be fully present with someone in pain sets the stage for an intervention that can be extremely effective, no matter how brief. Being present means staying with the patient, witnessing the grief, listening to the rage, and feeling the stunned reaction that accompanies the news. There is nothing to say. False reassurance is seen as untrustworthy, and an important connection is lost. Small, symbolic gestures say what words cannot; offering tissues and taking them back to discard them is a way of participating in the grief and giving permission to weep. Even offering a glass of water or cup of coffee is a way of attending to the arid reality of the impact phase. Most of all, remaining with patients and their families requires a presence rooted in the certainty of hope and healing that will come in its own time.

The recoil phase typically lasts somewhat longer—hours to days—and is characterized by a need to withdraw from the reality of the event. Patients may avoid scheduled appointments or decide that treatment is unwarranted. They may look to other providers as they search for answers. They may become rejecting, bitter, and angry. It becomes extremely important to initiate overtures at this point, even if one expects to be rebuffed. Patients and families will often remember the overture as helpful long after the event, even though they seemed indifferent at the time help was offered. The recoil phase is one of lonely reality testing as the person tries to come to grips with the enormity of what is happening. The growing awareness of dying and bereavement, as well as the attempt to escape its reality, overshadows everything else.

As the inevitability of the circumstance settles on the family, both the patient and individual family members may experience profound disorganization. This experience may be prolonged, especially if the dying process is slow. Attending to simple activities of daily living, shopping, preparing meals, and caring for children become insurmountable chores. People lock themselves out of cars, forget where they are going, keep appointments they do not have, and can barely keep going. Providing direct, active intervention at this point helps the family carry on in spite of the confusion and exhaustion. Marshaling the forces that have proffered help may be the most important function for the primary caregiver. Most family members are too upset during this phase to organize help for themselves. The opportunity to be part of a holding community of care becomes as much a privilege as it is a responsibility. Brief home visits are particularly appropriate at this point.

TABLE 11-1 Phases of Crises Related to Dying, Death, and Bereavement

Phase	Duration	Intervention
Impact	Minutes to hours	Being present
Recoil	Hours to Week 2	Initiating overtures
Disorganization	Week 3	Actively intervening
Reorganization	Weeks 4-6	Gradually withdrawing
Reemergence	Weeks 6+	Terminating

They give the provider a wealth of information and give the patient and family an opportunity to be in control, in some sense, at home.

The reorganization phase is one of gradual withdrawal for both the patient and the caregiver. There may be instances in which the term *acceptance* is perhaps too strong, but resolve occurs. The patient who is dying and the family or loved one who is grieving come to terms with the reality of what is happening or will happen. It is important to recognize this turn in events and respect the distance that may now be required. The provider needs to learn both how to withdraw and how to invest his or her psychic and spiritual energy in patient situations. Shorter visits, brief telephone calls, and a short note may be helpful. The amount and timing of contact is determined by clinical judgment that considers the dying patient's physical condition and the family's need for support. Premature withdrawal should be avoided; the temptation to retreat before the end can be overwhelming. Being aware of one's own ambivalence about death is critical.

On the other hand, staying too involved to fulfill some unmet personal need betrays the trust the patient has placed in the primary care provider. Patients and families depend on providers to meet their needs as they are able; the patients cannot be expected to meet the needs of the provider. The intensity needed to connect with a dying patient and his or her family can draw the provider into more intimacy than may be healthy. Discussing cases at staff meetings or with peers safeguards against the tendency to care too much. Terminating during the reemergence phase of the process is as necessary for the provider as it is for the family. When such intimate moments as death are shared with families, there is often a pull to stay involved—particularly with loved ones who seem especially alone. Such involvement is not helpful, and it usually promises more than can be given. Saying good-bye is a lesson that the caregiver and the cared for must both learn.

FAMILY SYSTEMS

Every patient comes from a family of origin and from a functional family context, both of which profoundly affect the patient's response to crisis. Anecdotal evidence from clinical practice and clinical research demonstrates that patients who have social and family support fare better than those who do not—regardless of their prognosis.[4] One of the most useful concepts from family systems is the notion of interface, or the overlapping connection points between and among family members. Applying that concept to families in crisis directs the primary care provider toward the relationships that are the most involved and those with the strongest interfaces. Those closest to the patient will become either allies or antagonists in the patient's care depending on how they are approached. A little consideration will prove to be a wise investment of time and energy.

Family stress is mirrored in the patient's response to stress; both need attention. Even family members who have had marginal contact appear along with the crisis of illness—especially terminal illness. Such family members often swoop in when crisis looms and become the focus of attention.[5] Skeletons that have long been dormant tumble out of closets and challenge the family's coping abilities. The intensity of the reactions of family members and significant others is directly related to grief and unresolved relationship issues. Fears, guilt, and grief all come into play and masquerade as anger, rage, and demanding behavior. These reactions can be enormously frustrating—not to mention provoking—for the practitioner whose goal is the patient's care and well-being. A measured response is critical. A referral to a social worker, a mental health clinician, or pastoral care may be appropriate. At the very least, simply acknowledging the existence of those complex emotions and responding with warmth and empathy will lower the anxiety level in the patent's immediate circle.

SPIRITUAL CARE

Spiritual care has historically been a central component of nursing care. Florence Nightingale herself, who was more attracted to mysticism than formal religion, was an early proponent of spiritual care in the service of healing.[6] Confusion, distortion, and numerous interpretations of what spirituality actually is has hampered our understanding and compromised our care. Interest has deepened in the past several years, particularly as the distinction between religion and spirituality becomes more clearly defined and better understood.[7] Research from a variety of fields has focused on spiritual care as a means to ameliorate distress and provide comfort.[8-10] A growing body of data has demonstrated a correlation between spirituality and well-being despite pain and/or disability.[11] The focus on context is a function of professional perspectives. The greatest body of research in medicine has emphasized the impact of religion, or "religious coping,"[12] whereas attention to spiritual care has been a natural concomitant to holistic care in advanced practice. Particularly at the end of life, the capacity to provide spiritual assessment and care is necessary as questions regarding the meaning of life, fear of suffering, fear of death, and the need for forgiveness and reconciliation arise.[13] Simply allowing the patient to explore and name those concerns is often intervention enough.

Giving the spiritual domain its due can present a challenge for those who would not claim to be particularly conversant with the language of the spirit. Although it may be more comfortable for those who are intentional about their own faith journey, spiritual care does not depend on the caregiver's own experience of the spiritual or of faith or religion. In fact, projecting one's own belief systems onto the patient would be inappropriate. What spiritual care does require is an appreciation of mystery and the willingness to be open to the patient's experience.

One clear example of differing perspectives is "nearing death awareness."[14] This term has been suggested for what happens with many patients as death is imminent; it is the sense of setting out on a journey and seeing or speaking to relatives long dead. One might name their experience confusion or disorientation or diagnose it as hypoxia and search for explanations. One might also simply accept that there are phenomena that cannot be explained but simply described. Because the experience of dying is so difficult to articulate, the language used is often symbolic. Listening intently and being attuned to the possible use of metaphor, story, and symbol, one does not only stay in communication with patients but also becomes aware of their peaceful, even joyful experiences.

ACTIVATING HOPE: THE EXPERIENCE OF THE SACRED

The question then becomes the following: "What exactly are we to do for patients when it appears there is nothing to be done?" This is the place for presence and for being rather than for doing. Here is the place for taking full advantage of psychosociospiritual interventions. Most nurses instinctively know that their most meaningful interventions involve the simplest gestures: the touch of a hand, a nod of affirmation, and a look of full and complete attention that exudes presence. There is nothing more powerful and hardly anything more spiritual than touching another soul with one's own. Strategies for intervention that intentionally include spiritual care encourage the patient's own search for meaning and experience of the sacred. Allowing for a spiritual experience that involves the senses—*sensory spirituality*—is a natural access point for nursing.[15]

Patients have a changing sensory function that may constrict their spiritual experience, or experience of the holy, just when their fears may be at their peak. Sensory changes rob patients of positive experiences in their bodies, where the body is often the enemy. Providing a sensory experience that has the potential to invoke a spiritual response is a double benefit. Music is an example of a sensory experience that has extraordinarily soothing effects.[16] "The Chalice of Repose," in Missoula, Montana, trains musicians to play the Celtic harp in the presence of patients and families when death is imminent.[17] They are soothed, and they are calmed; they are enabled to pray without words.

Synesthesia, or the combination of senses (e.g., sight and hearing), can be especially effective in heightening a positive experience.[18] For example, guided imagery can draw on music, voices, images, and color to stimulate a period of helpful relaxation and meditation. Using the arts with patients suffering with chronic pain, or particularly when they are dying, promotes a peaceful environment, can lessen feelings of anxiety and fear and, most important, can facilitate their own sense of the spiritual. That approach is as nourishing to the practitioner as it is to the patient. When one tries to preserve empathy and the capacity to cope simultaneously, recognizing the images, symbols, metaphors, and rituals that activate hope protects one's own reservoir of compassion. What is good for patients is good for us.

Tired bodies and discouraged spirits respond to complementary modalities as a spiritual experience.[19] Relaxation and comfort are easily and quickly attained through the modalities grouped under alternative medicine, such as acupuncture, therapeutic touch, biofeedback, relaxation, Reiki, reflexology, guided imagery, aromatherapy, chiropractic therapy, herbal medicine, and massage.

RESOURCES FOR PSYCHOSOCIOSPIRITUAL CARE

Nursing has lately been getting its own house in order. Rather than depending on chaplains or spiritual counselors, nurses engaged in health ministries and the emerging field of parish nursing are building a treasure trove of resources for spiritual care with patients and families. Referrals to or consultation with those nurses who are articulating new models of spirituality (which may or may not include religious images and rituals) are becoming more available through centers for parish nursing, health ministries, and emerging academic programs. Models of spiritual assessment, especially those tailored for brief intervention, are useful and easily adapted to multiple settings.[20,21] Exploring ways to integrate psychosociospiritual interventions into primary care with patients at the end of life undoubtedly demonstrate the effectiveness of such a model in the care of all patients. Staring death in the face puts life in perspective. Nothing is ever the same again. The world is viewed with a type of wiseheartedness that only the journey into the valley of the deep darkness can provide. Every decision, every priority, every relationship, every wish, and every hope is transformed from that time forward. The provider, too, has become a little more healed and a little more whole in body, mind, and spirit.

REFERENCES

1. Agrawal M, Emanuel EJ: Attending to psychological symptoms and palliative care, *J Clin Oncol* 20(3):624-626, 2002.
2. Gallup G, Jr: *Spiritual beliefs and the dying process,* Princeton, 1997, The George H Gallup International Institute.
3. Augliera DC: *Crisis intervention: theory and methodology,* ed 8, St Louis, 1998, Mosby.
4. Faulkner A: ABCs of palliative care: communication with patients, families, and other professionals, *Br Med J* 16:130-132, 1998.
5. Molloy DW and others: Decision making in the incompetent elderly: the daughter from California syndrome, *J Am Geriatr Soc* 39(4): 396-399, 1991.
6. Macrae J: Nightingale's spiritual philosophy and its significance for modern nursing, *Image J Nurs Schol* 27(1):8-10, 1995.
7. Dyson J, Cobb M, Forman D: The meaning of spirituality: a literature review, *J Adv Nurs* 26(6):1183-1188, 1997.
8. Baldacchino D, Draper P: Spiritual coping strategies: a review of the nursing research literature, *J Adv Nurs* 34(6):833-841, 2001.
9. Hamilton DG: Believing in patients' beliefs: physician attunement to the spiritual dimension as a positive factor in patient healing and health, *Am J Hosp Palliat Care* 15(5):276-279, 1998.
10. Mueller P, Plevak DJ, Rummans TA: Religious involvement, spirituality, and medicine: implications for clinical practice, *Mayo Clin Proc* 76(12):1225-1235, 2001.
11. Chandler E: *Spirituality and well-being in older adults,* unpublished doctoral dissertation, Claremont, Calif, Claremont School Theology.
12. Matthews DA and others: Religious commitment and health status: a review of the research and the implications for family medicine, *Arch Fam Med* 7(2):118-124, 1998.
13. Daaleman T, VandeCreek L: Placing religion and spirituality in end-of-life care, *JAMA* 284(19):2514-2517, 2000.
14. Callanan M, Kelley P: *Final gifts: understanding the special awareness, needs, and communications of the dying,* New York, 1993, Bantam.
15. Chandler E: Spirituality, *Hosp J* 14(3-4):63-74, 1999.
16. Hanser S, Thompson L: Effects of music therapy strategy on depressed older adults, *J Gerontol* 49(6):P265-269, 1994.
17. Schroeder-Sheker T: Music for the dying: a personal account of the new field of music thanatology: history, theories, and clinical narratives, *J Holis Nurs* 12(1):83-99, 1994.
18. Dossey B and others: *Holistic nursing: a handbook for practice,* Gaithersburg, Md, 1995, Aspen.
19. Brown-Saltzman K: Replenishing the spirit by meditative prayer and guided imagery, *Semin Oncol Nurs* 13(4):255-259, 1997.
20. Anandarajah G, Hight E: Spirituality and medical practice: using the HOPE questions as a practical tool for spiritual assessment, *Am Fam Physician* 63(1):81-89, 2001.
21. Highfield MF: Spiritual assessment across the cancer trajectory: methods and reflections, *Semin Oncol Nurs* 13(4):237-241, 1997.

CHAPTER 12

Palliative and End-of-Life Care

Marie A. Bakitas and Constance Dahlin

Almost every medical specialist at some point interacts with patients who are dying. With its dramatic advances in biomedical research and the ability to treat disease and prolong life, however, modern medicine—until recently—has neglected its traditional role of comforting patients and their families when end of life is near."[1]

Entire texts are devoted to birth and obstetric care, yet most medical references barely mention care of the dying patient.[2,3] Unlike the unmistakable signals of impending birth, the objective signs of dying and death are more elusive. Accurately predicting the prognosis is a poorly developed skill in most providers. Some basic strategies for primary care providers may help to improve care for patients with incurable illnesses and their families. This chapter describes the dimensions of palliative and end-of-life care principles that are appropriate for adults with life-threatening illnesses.

How does one know who is dying? A large study of seriously ill patients attempted to answer this question and found that although patients with incurable cancer follow a linear downward path, those dying of chronic cardiopulmonary illness follow a less predictable course.[4] Rather than attempting to determine which patient is "actively" dying, the "surprise" question may be more helpful: "Would you be surprised if this patient died in the next 6 months to a year?"[5] Considering the population in this way can help smooth transitions and lead to an earlier integration of a palliative approach to care.

The key concept is to replace a dichotomous model of cure vs. palliation with one that focuses on palliation in increasing degrees from the time of diagnosis with the life-threatening illness[6] (Figure 12-1). It is appropriate to begin to use a palliative philosophy long before death is imminent but when life-prolonging therapy options have become less effective.[7,8] Primary care providers, focused on continuity of care, are in a unique position to help patient and families understand the concept of palliative care.

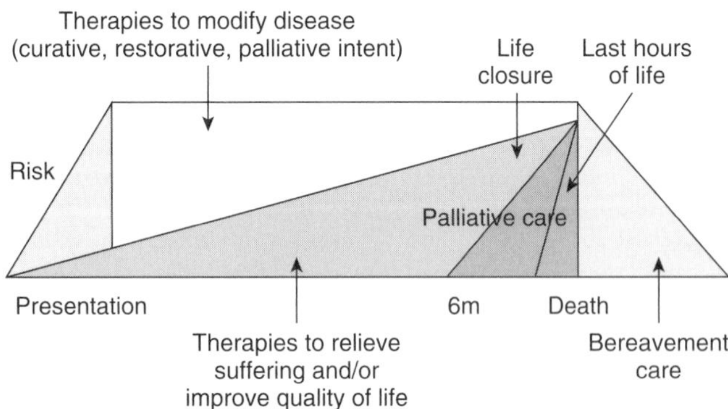

FIGURE 12-1

World Health Organization model. (As modified by Ferris FD: Establishing a palliative care program: rationale. A Center for the Advancement of Palliative Care [CAPC] Management Training Seminar, July 2001, Oakland, Calif. Retrieved December 2001 from the World Wide Web: http//www.capc.org.)

According to the World Health Organization (1990), palliative care is "the active total care of patients whose disease is not responsive to curative treatment. Control of pain and other symptoms and of psychological, social, and spiritual problems is paramount. The goal of palliative care is achievement of the best quality of life for patients and their families."[8] Palliative care affirms life and regards death as a natural and profoundly personal experience for the patient and family. "The goal of palliative care is achieving the best possible quality of life through relief of suffering, control of symptoms, and restoration of functional capacity while remaining sensitive to personal, cultural, and religious values, beliefs and practices."[9]

In a primary care practice, the first step is to understand the patient's preferences, priorities, and wishes about what is important as disease progresses. Advanced care planning includes discussion and documentation of these broad issues as well as the completion of advance directives (see Chapter 5). Most of these standardized forms are written in a defensive tone that indicates the type of care a patient does *not* want. More recently, the "five wishes" approach to advance directives has been promoted.[10] These documents address the type of care a patient *does* want as disease progresses (Table 12-1). If the patient is very near death, giving attention to writing or revising orders that focus on "comfort care" goes a long way in minimizing the procedures that may be "invisible" to the provider but uncomfortable for the patient (e.g., daily weights, lab tests, vital signs).

Because "do not resuscitate" (DNR) orders are generally nonportable, provisions should be made to avoid unwanted care when the patient is at home or in a nursing home. Many states have provisions for "No Code" or DNR orders for patients at home; such provisions allow emergency personnel to provide "comfort care" rather than cardiopulmonary resuscitation if they are called to the home by family members or if patients are brought to an emergency department with a need for symptom control.[11]

In summary, advance care planning is an ongoing process that needs to be revisited whenever a patient's health status or life goals change. To be complete, it should outline the type of care a patient does or does not wish at the end of life, and it should name the proxy decision maker if the patient lacks the capacity to express his or her preferences.

TABLE 12-1 Five Wishes

- The person I want to make care decisions for me when I can't
- The kind of medical treatment I want or don't want
- How comfortable I want to be
- How I want people to treat me
- What I want my loved ones to know

From Five Wishes. An Advanced Directives Document available from The Commission on Aging with Dignity, (888)5WISHES or www.agingwithdignity.org.

Symptom Management in Palliative Care

Holistic symptom care of the patient at the very end of life includes physical, psychologic, social, and spiritual distress of the patient and the family (Figure 12-2).

ANOREXIA/CACHEXIA

Definition

Anorexia is the reduced desire to eat. Because food is the essence of life and often represents love, a loss of interest in food can be very upsetting to the family. Anorexia is characterized by a loss of appetite and a loss of interest in food. Nothing tastes good, or the patient may be too tired or may never get around to eating. Cachexia is a state of general malnutrition marked by weight loss, malnutrition, weakness, and emaciation. It is usually induced by anorexia and is marked by an equal loss of fat, muscle, and bone mineral content. There is often no improvement with nutritional supplements or increased intake.[12]

Pathophysiology

Anorexia is the second most common symptom in patients with cancer, and it is common in patients with HIV. Causes include situational coping, unrelated illnesses, treatment side effects, anxiety, and depression.[13] Physiologic causes include impaired gastric emptying, constipation, pain, medications, oral infections, intracranial disease, and tumor-produced peptides.[14] Progressive anorexia occurs as the patient nears death, and it is a natural part of the dying process.

Clinical Presentation and Physical Examination

The assessment of anorexia is very important and includes the following areas: preferred foods, problems with taste or smell, dry mouth, problems with chewing, bowel assessment, and a social history (including the enjoyment of alcoholic drinks).[13,14]

The physical examination includes an observation of cognition; an oral examination that looks for dryness or lesions, an observation of skin turgor and muscle strength, and an abdominal examination (including a rectal examination). Blood studies may sometimes be appropriate, with particular attention given to nutritional markers that include total lymphocytes, hemoglobin, albumin, and iron.

Management

Education is a cornerstone to care. A loss of appetite is common in dying patients because they cannot tolerate premorbid calorie intake nor do they want to eat. Anorexia usually generates many issues because food as seen as the sustenance and essence of life. Family and friends must be told about the pros and cons of artificial nutrition and hydration.[15,16] In particular, they must be informed about anorexia and cachexia as a natural part of death. IV fluids or feedings via total parenteral nutrition or a nasogastric or gastronomy tube can cause discomfort. The dying patient may experience fluid overload from such strategies because the body is unable to metabolize fluids and proteins in the same way as a "normal, healthy" person. This can result in edema in the arms, legs, and abdomen; incontinence and skin breakdown; as well as pulmonary congestion and ascites causing dyspnea as the abdomen pushes up on the diaphragm.

Realistic goals of nutritional intake (e.g., relief of hunger or thirst, socialization at mealtimes) should be encouraged. The focus should be on giving patients preferred foods that improve their quality of life. Relief from lifelong dietary restrictions (e.g., diabetic, low-salt, or low-cholesterol diets) may be welcomed. Eliminating blood sugar monitoring and evaluating the need for other medications related to diet (e.g., cholesterol-lowering agents) reduces the burden of treatment at this time. An appetite stimulant may be offered if the patient wishes. A progesterone steroid such as megestrol acetate (Megace) 200 to 800 mg/day or dronabinol (Marinol) 2.5 mg PO b.i.d. may be helpful. Medications for depression (e.g., methylphenidate [Ritalin]) or for pain (e.g., dexamethasone [Decadron]) may have the added benefit of helping to increase appetite. A glass of beer, sherry, or wine may stimulate the appetite, particularly if this has been a part of the patient's established routine.

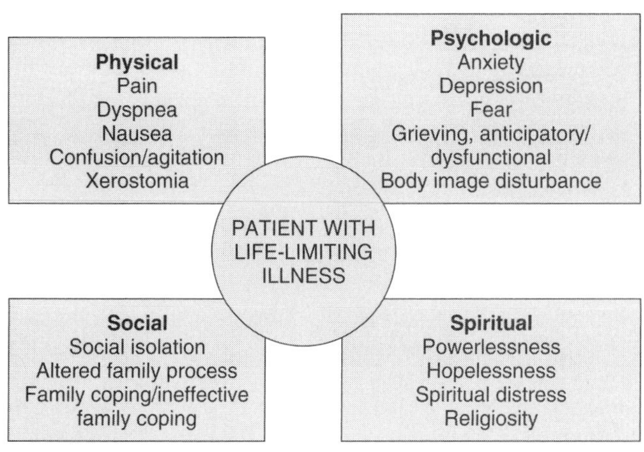

FIGURE 12-2

Symptom model.

ANXIETY/FEAR

Definition

Anxiety is a sense of deep unease. It is related to fear and is characterized by a constellation of signs and symptoms that include insomnia, headache, shortness of breath, weakness, chest pain, palpitations, a sensation of butterflies in the stomach, urinary frequency, pallor, restlessness, tremor, and sweating. The difference between fear and anxiety is that fear has a definable quality.

Pathophysiology

Causes of anxiety at the end of life include situational issues (e.g., financial or family worries, unfinished business, fears, and adjustment to disease) and organic causes (e.g., uncontrolled pain or dyspnea, psychiatric causes, medications, existential distress, altered physiologic status, and a lack of control).[13,14] (See Chapter 260 for a more detailed discussion of the pathophysiology of anxiety.)

Clinical Presentation and Physical Examination

Assessment of anxiety includes a history of the patient's worries and fears. This begins with understanding the patient's knowledge of his or her disease, specifically if there are any fears about dying or death. The patient should be asked about troubling symptoms, previous stressful incidents, and his or her previous coping style with stress and illness. Complaints of tremors, weakness, agitation, limb numbness, or shortness of breath should be noted. The patient may also complain of gastrointestinal upset, palpitations, muscle aches, and sleep disorders.

The physical assessment includes vitals signs, noting a rapid pulse, high blood pressure, or hyperventilation. Generalized signs that include flushing, wheezing, sweating, or tremor may be found on examination. Muscle tightness, nausea, or vomiting can also occur.

Management

Treatment focuses on pharmacologic interventions and on alleviating the specific problem (if possible and if the problem is behavioral). This includes the provision of factual information and the use of psychosocial and spiritual therapists. Pharmacologic interventions include the use of anxiolytics (e.g., benzodiazepines such as lorazepam 0.5 to 2 mg PO/IV/sublingually q 3 to 6 hours or diazepam 2.5 to 10 mg q 3 to 6 hours). Because of expense, the lack of an oral form, and short-term effects, midazolam administered as a continuous infusion should be reserved for use in patients who have intractable symptoms and are unable to swallow.

Alleviation of anxiety may also require relief of a symptom cluster such as the cycle of pain, dyspnea, and anxiety. In such cases it may impossible to separate and treat the "initiating event." The selection of agents that treat multiple symptoms (e.g., morphine, which can relieve pain and dyspnea and provide a calming effect) is often the best approach.

DELIRIUM (TERMINAL AGITATION, TERMINAL DELIRIUM, TERMINAL RESTLESSNESS)

Definition

Delirium is defined as a reversible, sudden, and acute confusional state. It is characterized by sudden changes in mental status, a mental status that waxes and wanes, a reduced attention span, and hyperactivity or hypoactivity.

Pathophysiology

Delirium is common in patients with advanced disease. It may be caused by tumor pressure in the brain; medication side effects, withdrawal, or overdose; uncontrolled pain; metabolic changes; liver or kidney dysfunction; infections; or nutritional deficiencies. More than half of all dying patients experience delirium as they approach death.[17] This may be attributed to the actual dying process or to one of the previously listed causes.

Clinical Presentation and Physical Examination

Delirium often occurs suddenly and may fluctuate during the course of the day. It often worsens in the late afternoon or at night, and the patient's sleep-wake cycle is disturbed. Speech may be incoherent or inappropriate to the situation. The patient may have altered perceptions that manifest as hallucinations or delusions. Disorientation to person, place, date and time, as well as agitation, restlessness, aggressiveness, and/or paranoia are also possible. In addition, he or she may be quite agitated, restless, aggressive, and/or paranoid (see Chapter 209).

A Mini Mental Status Examination (MMSE) is a simple and reliable initial assessment of cognitive function. This test includes orientation to person, place, date, and residence; memory and recall of three objects; attention and calculation; language; response to commands; and ability to copy a design. This assessment can begin to define the degree of disturbance. A thorough neurologic examination may provide further clues to the etiology.

Diagnostics

Diagnostic studies should be undertaken only if the results are likely to change patient management. For example, correcting dehydration, metabolic abnormalities, or hypercalcemia can sometimes reverse delirium, especially if death is not imminent. Other simple blood studies that may reveal easily reversible causes of delirium include glucose levels, kidney function, liver function, and oxygen saturation levels.

Management

First and foremost, educating the family about delirium, its causes (if known or suspected), and its prognosis is critical. If otherwise beneficial medications are the cause, the family needs to help in identifying the patient's priorities for comfort. Older adults are particularly sensitive to medications for pain and symptom control and hence are at high risk for delirium.

Treatment of delirium in a patient in whom death is not imminent includes identifying and treating the reversible causes while keeping the patient in a safe and comfortable environment. The environment should be modified immediately to reduce stimuli, the patient should be reoriented (if possible), and neuroleptics should be administered. If the delirium is a result of opioid or benzodiazepine withdrawal, slowing the tapering process can help. Long-term, high-dose opioids may cause delirium due to the accumulation of metabolites. This is especially common in patients who were previously stable on a particular dose and experience acute dehydration or renal insufficiency. It is usually unrealistic to discontinue opioids in a dying patient. If the current opioid regimen is believed to be the cause of delirium, however, a different opioid in an equianalgesic dose may provide pain relief without delirium. For example, methadone, hydromorphone, and oxycodone may be less deliriogenic than morphine or meperidine. The former agents lack the metabolites that can accumulate and cause delirium.

For the patient who is close to death, the family needs to understand that delirium may signal impending death. This subtlety can be missed. Neuroleptic medications such as haloperidol are the drugs of choice for patients who are delirious in the last few days of life (Table 12-2). These medications may be given to help calm the patient and to ease fear and panic. IV dosing is recommended to initially provide rapid relief and to minimize the extrapyramidal symptoms. Once a dose is established, converting to an equivalent oral dosing regimen (when possible) on a scheduled basis can maintain a calm state. Treatment of delirium using a benzodiazepine alone can result in paradoxical effects and actually worsen the delirium. Hence this often prescribed approach to calm or quiet a delirious patient is discouraged in the dying patient.[18,19]

DEPRESSION

Definition

Depressive disorders are illnesses that affect mood and result in a variety of symptoms, including anhedonia, helplessness, hopelessness, worthlessness, and guilt. Feelings of personal failure are strong.

Diagnosis of depression in a terminally ill patient can be a challenge because the neurovegetative signs that are typically part of the diagnostic criteria of depression are often normally present in most patients with advanced terminal disease. Observing the patient for psychologic and cognitive symptoms of worthlessness, hopelessness, excessive guilt, and suicidal ideation may be more diagnostic. Table 12-3 provides a helpful acronym for diagnosis.[13]

Depression with serious or terminal illness should not be considered "the norm." Although sadness and grief may be anticipated in terminally ill patients, a mood of total despair can lead to suicide, a request for assisted suicide, or other attempts at a "hastened death." The desire for a hastened death is highly linked to depression.[20] Conversely, treating depression in terminally ill patients can allow them to experience pleasure in life, finish the emotional work of saying good-bye, make meaning of their lives, and perform other important activities of life closure.[21]

Clinical Presentation and Physical Examination

The assessment of depression in the terminally ill patient is multifaceted. The appearance of the patient is very important and includes dress and grooming. Affect, speech, and orientation are all factors in the examination. A history with an evaluation of substance abuse and previous depressive or bipolar episodes is critical. Assessment includes mood, affect, and lifestyle changes. A history of sleep disturbances, weight loss, impaired concentration, psychomotor changes, loss of interest in life, feelings of guilt, loss of energy, fatigue, and suicidal thoughts should be noted. It is important to be sensitive to culture and religion during this assessment. Patients must be asked directly about whether they feel depressed, whether they have contemplated taking their own lives, and if they have a plan for doing so (see Chapter 262).

Diagnostics

Diagnostic testing is indicated to exclude other causes of mood disorders. CBC, serum electrolytes, calcium, BUN, creatinine, and TSH are indicated.

Management

Treatment includes pharmacologic and psychotherapeutic modalities. Pharmacologic treatment depends on the prognosis. A psychostimulant or steroid may be the drug of choice if death is likely within 1 month. Methylphenidate is rapid acting and may increase appetite and reduce pain. It can be started at 2.5 to 5 mg/day and increased to 10 to 20 mg/day, given early in the morning, with the same dose repeated at noon to allow the peak effect to wear off by bedtime. Dosing later in the day may cause insomnia. Both psychostimulants and steroids may help to improve multiple common end-of-life symptoms, including depression, appetite, and sedation.

A trial of tricyclic antidepressants (TCAs) or selective serotonin reuptake inhibitors (SSRIs) is appropriate if death is not likely within 1 month. TCAs can help with both neuropathic pain and depression, but the sedating and autonomic properties may cause more side effects. The starting dose for amitriptyline, imipramine, desipramine, or nortriptyline is 10 to 25 mg/day. The dosage can be increased to 25 to 100 mg/day. TCAs should be taken at bedtime because they cause sedation. SSRIs can also be tried. Sertraline is initiated at 12.5 to 25 mg/day with a range up to 50 to 100 mg/day. Fluoxetine is started at 10 mg/day and increased to 20 to 40 mg/day. Paroxetine is started at 10 mg/day. Psychostimulants can be used short term while initiating an SSRI, then weaned as the TCA or SSRI becomes effective.[21]

Some patients benefit from St. John's wort or other herbal remedies. It is important that patients and families understand that herbal remedies are also pharmacologic agents with side effects and adverse effects. Consultation with an herbalist or naturopath may be indicated.

Indications for Referral/Hospitalization

Referrals for the patient and family members to a psychiatrist, psychologist, social worker, pastoral counselor, and/or hospice worker can help in the understanding and management of depression at the end of life. Psychotherapeutic approaches can encourage the patient to talk about past and present experiences as well as the dying experience. Behavioral interventions

TABLE 12-2 Medications Used for Terminal Delirium/Sedation

Generic Name	Approximate Daily Dosage Range	Route
NEUROLEPTICS		
haloperidol	0.5-5 mg q2-12h	PO, IV, SC, IM
chlorpromazine	12.5-50 mg q4-12h	PO, IV, IM
droperidol	0.5-5 mg q12h	PO
BENZODIAZEPINES		
lorazepam	0.5-2.0 mg q1-4h	PO, IV, IM
midazolam	30-100 mg/24h	IV, SC

SC, Subcutaneous; *IM,* intramuscular.

TABLE 12-3 SIGECAPS Mnemonic to Assess Depression

S	Sleep changes (increased or decreased)
I	Interest changes (increased or decreased)
G	Guilt
E	Energy changes (fatigue or loss of energy)
C	Concentration changes (inability to focus)
A	Appetite (decreased or increased)
P	Psychomotor agitation
S	Suicidal thoughts

and cognitive restructuring may also be helpful. A formal psychiatric evaluation may be used to determine the appropriateness of antidepressant medications for patients with co-morbid conditions and for stoic patients who may not be willing to admit depression to their family or primary care provider for fear of causing "disappointment" or appearing weak.

A multidisciplinary approach may be helpful in engaging the patient and acknowledging his or her feelings. Reiteration of the goals of pain and symptom management may provide reassurance and promote feelings of nonabandonment.

DYSPNEA

Definition and Pathophysiology

Dyspnea is a subjective sense of shortness of breath, difficulty breathing, or an uncomfortable awareness of breathing. The patient feels as if he or she is suffocating or choking. This shortness of breath may be accompanied by fear, anxiety, or panic. Dyspnea is common in patients with lung cancer, lung disease, and cardiac disease. Causes include but are not limited to the effects of tumors, the effects of cancer treatment, lung disease, heart disease, infection, muscle weakness, and anxiety.

Clinical Presentation and Physical Examination

A patient's self-report of dyspnea is the most important assessment criteria.[14] The patient may appear short of breath but may deny shortness of breath or vice versa. A 0 to 10 scale can be used, with 0 being no problem and 10 being the worst trouble breathing the patient can imagine. Obtain a history including onset, frequency, and contributing factors.

In addition to subjective reporting, objective examinations include chest auscultation and observations of the patient's breathing and pulse oximetry while at rest, with activity, and in different positions. A chest x-ray examination to check for pneumonia, pleural effusions, or disease progression, or a spiral computed tomography (CT) scan for concern about pulmonary embolism can be helpful. However, these examinations should be performed only if the data would change treatment and the patient is not actively dying.

Management

It is important to consider the prognosis and the patient's values and preferences regarding the treatment of any underlying disease such as infection or progressive cancer. The risks and benefits of the treatment and the potential improvement of the patients symptoms should be considered. If comfort is the goal and the patient is close to death, some simple maneuvers can be helpful. Simply repositioning the patient in upright sitting position may help. Oxygen administration may also be beneficial, with nasal cannulae (and humidification) usually more comfortable than oxygen via a facemask. A fan blowing gently on the face reduces the perception of breathlessness by stimulating the receptors in the cheeks.

Opioids and benzodiazepines can also relieve dyspnea. Morphine is the drug of choice, with a starting dose of 5 to 10 mg PO every 3 to 4 hours in the opioid-naive patient. Doses for older adults can be smaller, starting at 2 to 5 mg PO or subcutaneously every 3 to 4 hours. Oxycodone 5 to 10 mg every 3 to 4 hours may be substituted for older adults or morphine-sensitive patients. Antianxiety agents include lorazepam 0.5 to 2 mg PO every 4 to 6 hours or diazepam 2.5 to 10 mg every 4 to 6 hours. Lorazepam is usually shorter acting than diazepam. The use of nebulized morphine or other nebulized medications (e.g., bronchodilators, steroids for relief of specific symptoms) should be matched to the clinical situation. Many of these interventions lack an evidence base in improving symptoms at the end of life but are perceived by clinicians and patients as beneficial.[14]

At the very end of life, a patient may experience upper airway congestion or a "death rattle." This is usually more distressing to the family than to the patient. Reducing fluid intake, especially IV fluids, can help. This must be done sensitively, and the patient's and family's culture and religion should be considered. If complete discontinuation of an IV is not appropriate, decreasing fluids to a minimum can provide significant relief. Anticholinergic agents may provide some additional relief from this distressing end-stage symptom. These agents include 1.5-mg scopolamine patches (TransDerm Scōp, 1 to 4 patches every 72 hours), hyoscyamine sulfate (Levsin) in drops or pills (0.125 to 0.25 mg every 4 to 6 hours), or glycopyrrolate (Robinul) in either an oral form (1 to 2 mg every 6 hours), injection, or nebulized form. Oral cavity suctioning may help, but secretions will reaccumulate. Deep suctioning is rarely effective and may cause more distress than benefit in the dying person.

DRY MOUTH (XEROSTOMIA)

Definition

Dry mouth, or xerostomia, is the sensation of oral dryness. It is accompanied by decreased salivary secretions and is commonly experienced by patients with advanced progressive disease.[22] It may be difficult to identify the exact underlying cause and contributing factors. However, treatment offers much comfort to patients.

Pathophysiology

Half of all palliative care patients report serious distress from dry mouth, but it may not be prioritized to a high degree by providers. Common causes of dry mouth in terminally ill patients include medication side effects, mouth breathing, oxygen, infection, ulcers, and treatments such as surgery, chemotherapy, and/or radiotherapy.

Clinical Presentation and Physical Examination

Assessment begins with a thorough oral examination that includes inspection for mucosal and buccal dryness and pallor, the presence of a dry fissured tongue or cracked lips, the absence of salivary pooling, and the presence of oral ulcerations, gingivitis, or candidiasis.[22]

Two quick bedside tests are the Cracker Biscuit Test and the Tongue Blade Test. The Cracker Biscuit Test involves giving a patient a dry cracker or biscuit. If he or she cannot eat it, xerostomia is present.[22] The Tongue Blade Test is an extension of the mouth inspection. After inspection is complete, the tongue blade is placed on the tongue. If it sticks, xerostomia is present.[22]

Management

Treatment of xerostomia includes the following steps: treat any underlying infection or disease such as yeast or mucositis; review and, if necessary, alter current medications such as antihistamines or anticholinergics; and stimulate salivary flow using both nonpharmacologic (peppermint water, vitamin C, chewing gum, and mints) and pharmacologic interventions.

Pharmacologic interventions can include pilocarpine 2.5 mg PO t.i.d., slowly titrated up to 10 mg PO t.i.d. Saliva production is greatest after a dose, and the response lasts for approximately 4 hours and varies with severity of xerostomia. Lost secretions are replaced with saliva substitutes, water, and artificial saliva if necessary. An inexpensive spritzer filled with nine parts water and one part fine oil (e.g., grapeseed oil) can be helpful. The teeth should be protected with frequent oral hygiene, and the lips should be lubricated with lip balm. Topical rehydration with water or ice chips is a more subjectively effective remedy to dry mouth and thirst than is IV hydration.[14] Dietary modifications such as the avoidance of spicy or salty foods may help.

NAUSEA/VOMITING

Definition

Vomiting is the expulsion of the contents of the stomach, duodenum, or jejunum through the mouth. Nausea is a feeling of queasiness or a desire to vomit. Nausea manifests itself in a wavelike sensation and can be accompanied by a cold sweat, fast heart rate, or diarrhea.

Pathophysiology

Nausea and vomiting are common at some time during the terminal stage of illness. Causes include delayed stomach emptying, constipation, bowel obstruction, infection, radiotherapy, medications, metabolic disturbances, and increased intracranial pressure.

Clinical Presentation and Physical Examination

Understanding the etiology of nausea and vomiting is critical to facilitate treatment, and therefore a good history is crucial. There should be a review history of nausea, including onset, related factors, and pattern. The presence of peptic ulcer disease, constipation, intracranial pressure, and nausea-inducing medications should be identified. Other important considerations include epigastric pain, pain on swallowing, thirst, hiccups, heartburn, and the last bowel movement.

The physical assessment includes an oral examination, an abdominal examination (with particular emphasis on bowel sounds), a rectal examination, and a neurologic assessment. Studies may include an abdominal x-ray study and, if there is a concern about bowel obstruction, a gastroenterology consultation.

Management

Treatment of nausea and vomiting depends on the etiology. First, the underlying cause is treated if possible. Different classes of antiemetics, alone or in combination, can be administered orally, subcutaneously, intravenously, or via a suppository for symp tomatic relief.[23] Phenothiazines (prochlorperazine, chlorpromazine), butyrophenones (haloperidol), serotonin receptor antagonists (ondansetron, dolasetron), steroids, peristaltic agents (metoclopramide), benzodiazepines (lorazepam), or cannabinoids provide a vast array of choices and combinations.

Nonpharmacologic therapy includes relaxation, distraction, imagery, acupressure, cold therapy, aromatherapy, and music therapy. Diet modifications include eating dry crackers on awakening and eating fewer spicy and greasy foods. Holding or slowing down tube feedings may eliminate nausea induced by bloating. If nausea and vomiting are caused by an obstruction that cannot be relieved, placement of a venting gastrostomy rather than a nasogastric tube may decrease these symptoms, allow the patient the pleasure of eating, and increase patient's overall quality of life.

CONSTIPATION

Definition

Constipation is infrequent rectal emptying (usually defined as less than every 3 days) or physical difficulty in emptying the rectum. This may vary according to patient's usual elimination pattern. Constipation is also characterized by hard or infrequent stools.[24]

Pathophysiology

Constipation is a common problem in terminal care resulting from narcotic therapy, immobility, and decreased fluid and food intake. However, constipation may also be age related, neurologically induced, or associated with colorectal tumors or lesions such a fissures or hemorrhoids.[14,24]

Clinical Presentation and Physical Examination

Assessment of constipation includes a bowel history: day of the last bowel movement, the patient's usual pattern, the use of laxatives or other interventions in an effort to move the bowels, and the current drug regimen with special attention to the narcotic regimen. Physical assessment includes inspection and palpation of the abdomen, bowel sounds, and a rectal examination to check for the presence of stool.

Management

If possible and appropriate, the patient's fluid intake should be increased and a bowel regimen initiated (e.g., senna with stool softener, 1 to 4 tablets q.d. or b.i.d.). An aggressive prophylactic bowel regimen needs to be prescribed concomitantly when opioids are initiated or increased. Lactulose 15 to 30 ml one to three times daily, milk of magnesia 15 to 30 ml twice daily, or citrate of magnesia are alternative stimulants if senna and softener are not adequate. A senna-based tea such as "Smooth Moves Tea" each day is also beneficial. An enema and/or disimpaction may be necessary if there is no stool for several days.[13,14,24] Relief of constipation remains a major comfort measure even toward the very end of life because of its adverse effects on lower abdominal pain, nausea, and restlessness.

BOWEL OBSTRUCTION

Definition

Bowel obstruction is the total or partial occlusion of the bowel lumen and/or the alteration of normal peristaltic motion.[25] It is most likely to occur with advanced abdominal or pelvic cancers such as ovarian, colorectal, and pancreatic cancer. Symptoms can be mild to severe and intermittent or continuous and include distention, intractable nausea and vomiting, and a colicky pain.

Clinical Presentation and Physical Examination

Assessment includes an abdominal examination. Bowel sounds may be normal to absent and hyperactive or hypoactive depending on the location, etiology, and degree of obstruction. Distention will be noted. An abdominal x-ray study and a CT scan will reveal the obstruction.

Management

Treatment depends in part on the patient's prognosis. Acute management is aimed at the immediate relief of symptoms and includes stopping oral intake and inserting a nasogastric tube to alleviate gastric distention. This is the treatment of choice for patients who have a longer prognosis and are able to withstand surgery. Occasionally, endoscopically placed stents can provide relief. Finally, a venting gastrostomy can provide decompression of gas and fluids.[25]

A conservative approach to providing comfort for very ill patients can be accomplished through the use of subcutaneously or intravenously administered agents. Analgesics reduce the pain of abdominal distention. Morphine starting at 1 mg/hr and titrating to the appropriate level to treat the pain is effective. Antiemetics such as Compazine PO or perirectally (PR) or haloperidol 0.5 to 1.5 mg/24 hr can help. Prokinetic agents such as metoclopramide can help in partial obstructions by increasing peristalsis. Antiinflammatories (e.g., corticosteroids) help reduce the inflammatory response and may partially alleviate the obstruction. Dexamethasone 8 to 20 mg/24 hr can reduce inflammatory edema and also help decrease nausea. Somatostatin analogues such as octreotide are thought to inhibit the cascade effect of the glandular secretions and inhibit peristalsis and blood flow to the splanchnic area. Octreotide 300 to 600 mg/24 hr reduces gastrointestinal secretions and motility.

PAIN

Definition

Pain at the end of life is the most feared symptom. It most often occurs when the underlying diagnosis is cancer. However, many other conditions may cause discomfort at the end of life, including arthritis, low back pain, pathologic or compression fractures, pressure sores, and cardiac or other ischemic pain. Patients who continue to follow normal routines and receive unnecessary procedures such as daily weights, laboratory tests, vital signs, and prescribed position changes may also experience unnecessary discomfort. Providing comfort to family members and asking their assessment of patient comfort when the patient cannot communicate is essential to good pain assessment. The following section briefly addresses pain issues specific to end-of-life. (Chapter 13 provides a comprehensive review of many similar principles of chronic pain management.)

Management

Unrelieved pain at the end of life is unnecessary and with few exceptions treatable. Practical issues can be the most challenging, including the loss of oral route for medication administration, a wish to die at home, non–opioid responsive "total pain" or suffering, and a fear that the pain may indicate a hastening death.[26]

Alternatives to oral opioid administration include equianalgesic dosing either rectally (including enteric-coated tablets or suppositories), transdermally, sublingually (via high-concentrate solutions administered to the oral cavity), or subcutaneously (continuously, intermittently, or via a patient-controlled pump).[14] Given these options, there rarely is a need for IV catheters, which can be painful to insert and provide interrupted analgesia when infiltrated. There is no ceiling dose of opioids, and therefore careful increased dosing in response to pain provides an ethically and clinically acceptable approach even if adequate analgesia comes only with sedation.[26]

With the skill and expertise of a hospice home care support, all of the previously mentioned strategies for expert pain relief are available at home or in long-term-care settings.

There is great fear that administering escalating doses of opioids will hasten death. This fear is controversial and difficult to evaluate. Patients who are dying of a terminal illness should continue to receive opioids for pain relief or dyspnea until the time of death. Respirations will ultimately cease. Respiratory depression from opioids is known to occur most often in the opioid-naive person. Careful upwards titration in response to pain rarely causes respiratory depression, because pain is a natural stimulant to the respiratory center. Patients and families as well as nursing staff should be educated about the appropriate use of pain medications for symptom control.[25]

Sedation for Management of Intractable Symptoms in the Dying Patient

The term *terminal sedation* was first applied to the practice of using sedating medications to induce a state of unconsciousness and hence allow a patient to escape physical suffering at the end of life. This language has been changed to eliminate any misunderstanding that the purpose of the sedation is to end the patient's life. More recent terms are *palliative sedation* or *end-of-life sedation*. Sedation is an appropriate treatment of "last resort" in the rare instances in which death is imminent and symptoms such as pain, delirium, dyspnea, and anxiety have become totally refractory to relief. The goal of this sedation is to help calm the patient and alleviate the suffering caused by the unrelieved symptom. An evaluation of the values and beliefs of the acceptability of this approach and the development of a consensus among the patient, family, and providers is critical to ensure the success of this strategy. All those involved in caring for the patient should be involved in the discussion and have their questions answered regarding the proposed treatment modalities and their intended effects.

Settings and Resources for Providing Palliative or End-of-Life Care

Health care systems have evolved to provide episodic, acute, lifesaving care with little emphasis on palliative care until recently. National efforts are now directed at redesigning these systems to adopt a chronic disease model that more easily accommodates patients who wish for less aggressive strategies and expert end-of-life symptom management. Palliative care consultation services and interdisciplinary teams have been developed to bring this expertise back into the mainstream of care. Hundreds of these "specialty" services have developed across the country in hospitals or as an expansion of community hospice services.[27,28] Some are also providing this focus within skilled or extended care and assisted-living facilities. Resources for learning about palliative care approaches and specialists are listed in Box 12-1.

Most Americans express a wish to spend their final days in their own home and surrounded by loved ones. The reality of dying in the United States in the twenty-first century is very different. Up to 50% of people will die in the hospital, and another 25% will die in nursing homes. Only 30% of those dying

BOX 12-1

PALLIATIVE CARE WEB RESOURCES

CENTER TO ADVANCE PALLIATIVE CARE (CAPC)
www.capcmssm.org
Provides technical assistance needed to establish palliative care programs as well as opportunities to network with colleagues in the palliative care community; features CAPC publications, education calendar, and information about advocacy activities.

DYING WELL
www.dyingwell.org
Resources and referral to organizations, websites, and books to empower persons with life-threatening illnesses and their families to live as fully as possible during the dying process. Provides a link to the Missoula Demonstration Project, which demonstrates a community-based approach to end-of-life care.

AMERICA ACADEMY OF HOSPICE AND PALLIATIVE MEDICINE
www.AAHPM.org
A national professional organization dedicated to promoting palliative medicine. Features publications, education, competencies, and certification.

NATIONAL HOSPICE AND PALLIATIVE CARE ORGANIZATION
www.nhpco.org
The National Hospice and Palliative Care Organization is the industry's largest association and leading resource for professionals and volunteers committed to and providing service to patients and their families during end of life.

GROWTH HOUSE: GUIDE TO DEATH, DYING, GRIEF, BEREAVEMENT, AND END-OF-LIFE RESOURCES
www.growthhouse.org
Search engine offers access to the Internet's most comprehensive collection of reviewed resources for end-of-life care.

HOSPICE FOUNDATION OF AMERICA
www.hospicefoundation.org
Provides education and information about death and dying in America.

AMERICANS FOR BETTER CARE OF THE DYING
www.abcd-caring.com
Dedicated to social, professional, and policy reform aimed at improving the care system for patients with serious illness and for their families.

INNOVATIONS IN END-OF-LIFE CARE
www.edc.org/lastacts
On-line journal features peer-reviewed examples of promising practices in end-of-life care. Each bimonthly issue focuses on a different theme.

EDUCATION FOR PHYSICIANS ON END-OF-LIFE (EPEC)
www.epec.net
Educates physicians, through its core curriculum, on essential clinical competencies required to provide quality end-of-life care.

LAST ACTS
www.lastacts.org
A national coalition to improve care and caring near the end-of-life. The goal of the coalition is to bring death-related issues out in the open and help individuals and organizations pursue better ways to care for the dying.

END-OF-LIFE PHYSICIANS EDUCATION RESOURCE CENTER (EPERC)
www.eperc.mcw.edu
Assists physician educators and others in locating high-quality, peer-reviewed training materials. Visitors to the website can search for educational materials indexed by end-of-life care topic areas and educational formats.

ON OUR OWN TERMS: MOYERS ON DYING
www.thirteen.org/onourownterms
Supports the On Our Own Terms outreach campaign with various tools, articles, personal stories, audio and video clips, and interactive opportunities.

will receive hospice services.[29] In the 1997 Institute of Medicine (IOM) report entitled *Approaching Death,* a model of a "good death" was proposed as a target for improvements in the health care system. It stated the following:

"People should be able to expect and achieve a decent and good death—one that is free from avoidable distress and suffering for patients, families and caregivers; in general accord with the patient's and family's wishes; and reasonably consistent with clinical, cultural, and ethical standards."[30]

In truth, palliative care is simply "good" medical care—care that can be provided by any skilled primary care provider, and care that patients and families both want and deserve.

REFERENCES

1. Cassel CK, Foley KM: *Principles for care of patients at the end of life: an emerging consensus among the specialties of medicine.* Milbank Memorial Fund. Retrieved December 2001 from the World Wide Web: http://www.milbank.org/endoflife/index.html.
2. Ferrell BR, Virani R, Grant M: Analysis of end of life content in nursing textbooks, *Oncol Nurs Forum* 26(5):869-876, 1999.
3. Carron AT, Lynn J, Keaney P: End-of-life care in medical textbooks, *Ann Intern Med* 130:82-86, 1999.
4. The SUPPORT Principal Investigators: A controlled trial to improve care for seriously ill hospitalized patients: the study to understand prognoses and preferences for outcomes and risks of treatments (SUPPORT), *JAMA* 274:1591-1598, 1995.
5. Lynn J, Schuster J, Kabcenell A: *Improving care for the end of life: a sourcebook for health care managers and clinicians,* Oxford, 2000, Oxford University Press.
6. Ferris FD: Establishing a palliative care program: rationale. A Center for the Advancement of Palliative Care (CAPC) Management Training Seminar, July 2001, Oakland, Calif. Retrieved December 2001 from the World Wide Web: http://www.capc.org.
7. Foley K, Gelband H, editors: *Improving palliative care for cancer: summary and recommendations,* Institute of Medicine and National Cancer Policy Board, Washington, DC, 2000, National Academy Press.
8. World Health Organization: *Cancer pain relief and palliative care,* Tech Rep No 804, Geneva, 1990, The Organization.
9. Last Act Task Force: Precepts of palliative care, *J Palliative Med* 1(2):109-112. 1998.
10. Five Wishes. An Advanced Directives Document available from The Commission on Aging with Dignity: (888) 5WISHES or http://www.agingwithdignity.org.
11. Commission on Legal Problems of the Elderly, ABA: *Survey of state EMS-DNR laws and protocols, 1999.* Contact http://abaelderly@abanet.org to obtain the full report ($15 fee).
12. Kemp C: Anorexia and cachexia. In Ferrell B, Coyle N, editors: *Oxford textbook of palliative nursing,* Oxford, 2001, Oxford University Press.
13. Dickerson ED and others: *Palliative care pocket consultant.* Oxford, 1999, Oxford International Center for Palliative Care, Academics, Industry, Medicine and Society (AIMS).
14. Waller A, Caroline NL: *Handbook of palliative care in cancer,* ed 2, Boston, 2002, Butterworth-Heinemann.
15. Welk TA: Clinical and ethical consideration of fluid and electrolyte management in the terminally ill client, *J Intraven Nurs* 22(1):43-47, 1999.
16. Kedziera P: Hydration, thirst, nutrition. In Ferrell B, Coyle N, editors: *Oxford textbook of palliative nursing,* Oxford, 2001, Oxford University Press.
17. Block SD: Assessing and managing depression in the terminally ill patient, *Ann Intern Med* 132(3):209-218, 2000.
18. Lawlor PG, Fainsinger RL, Bruera ED: Delirium at the end of life: critical issues in clinical practice and research, *JAMA* 284(19):2427-2429, 2000.
19. Chan D, Brennan N: Delirium: making the diagnosis, improving the prognosis, *Geriatrics* 54(3):28-42, 1999.
20. Quijada E, Billings JA: *Pharmacologic management of delirium: update on newer agents,* January 2002, Fast Facts and Concepts #60, End-of-Life Physician Education Resource Center. Retrieved December 2001 from the World Wide Web: http://www.eperc.mcw.edu.
21. Brietbart W and others: Depression, hopelessness, and desire for hastened death in terminally ill patients with cancer, *JAMA* 284:2907-2911, 2000.
22. Dahlin CD, Goldsmith, TS: Dysphagia, dry mouth, and hiccups. In Ferrell BR, Coyle N, editors: *Oxford textbook of palliative nursing,* Oxford, 2001, Oxford University Press.
23. Letizia M, Shenk J, Jones TD: Intermittent subcutaneous injections for symptom control in hospice care: a retrospective investigation, *Hospice J* 15(2):1-11, 2000.
24. Levy M: Constipation and diarrhea in cancer patients, *Cancer Bull* 43:412-422, 1992.
25. Muir JC: Malignant bowel obstruction. In *Principles and practice of supportive oncology updates,* 2(5):1-7, New Jersey, 1999, Lippincott Williams and Wilkins Healthcare.
26. Wrede-Seaman L: Treatment options to manage pain at end of life, *Am J Hosp Palliat Care* 18(2):89-101, 2001.
27. National Palliative Care Program Directory. Retrieved December 2001 from the World Wide Web (Center for the Advancement of Palliative Care): http://www.capcmssm.org.
28. Beresford L: *Hospital-hospice partnerships in palliative care: creating a continuum of services,* New Jersey, 2001, Robert Wood Johnson Foundation.
29. National Hospice and Palliative Care Organization: *Facts and figures on hospice care in America,* Fax on Request 112. Alexandria, Va, 2001, The Organization.
30. Institute of Medicine: *Approaching death: improving care at the end of life,* Washington, DC, 1997, National Academy Press.

CHAPTER 13

Chronic Pain

Constance Dahlin

DEFINITION/EPIDEMIOLOGY

Although pain is a normal physiologic response that serves as a mechanism against harmful stimulation, chronic pain contributes to morbidity and mortality.[1] It is a poorly understood condition and is therefore undertreated in primary care.[2] Defined as pain that lasts longer than 6 months or persists beyond the expected time of healing, chronic usually encompasses a mechanism separate from that of the original insult.[3] Thus the focus of chronic pain control turns away from repairing damage that may be causing the pain and toward rehabilitation. Rehabilitation focuses on promoting optimal functioning, coping, and quality of life.

Chronic pain can include headaches, low back pain, neck pain, musculoskeletal injury or soft tissue disease, degenerative joint pain, peripheral neuropathy, or neuralgia.[4] Chronic pain is not merely a symptom of disease; it also describes a syndrome that includes depression, alteration in daily activities, and functional and personality changes.[1,3]

Chronic pain is a complex, highly subjective health problem that affects more than 50 million people in the United States.[3] Unlike acute pain, chronic pain serves no protective function. The causes are often multifactorial, and patients' responses are equally varied and individualistic. These patients generally seek a primary care provider at initial presentation for headaches or for abdominal, musculoskeletal, or neurologic pains. Such pains often are the result of work-related stresses or injuries. Low back pain usually is the result of work or automobile accidents.[5] However, pain can also be secondary to other organic disorders, including diabetes, alcoholism, or postherpetic syndromes.

PATHOPHYSIOLOGY

According to Bonica,[3] "chronic pain is caused by a chronic pathologic process in somatic structures or viscera, or by prolonged and sometimes permanent dysfunction of the peripheral and central nervous system or both." Moreover, states Bonica, "the physiologic, affective, and behavioral responses to chronic pain are quite different from those in acute pain."[3]

Pain is a subjective impression that is unique to each patient. Pain is categorized pathophysiologically as either organic or idiopathic (previously referred to as "psychogenic pain"). Organic pain is further delineated as nociceptive or neuropathic.

Nociceptive pain is caused by either direct or threatened injury to tissue and results from the activation of nociceptors, which are peripheral afferent nerve endings that are both sensitive to and transmitters of painful stimuli. Bradykinins, prostaglandins, and other chemical mediators of inflammation found in injured tissue contribute to the pathogenesis of nociceptive pain.[1] Nociceptive pain can manifest as either somatic or visceral pain.

Somatic pain is caused by the activation of nociceptors in the peripheral tissues. Somatic pain is usually described as well localized and is characterized as stabbing, aching, or throbbing. In contrast, visceral pain is usually poorly localized, often is not attributable to the involved organ (i.e., referred pain), and may be described as dull, crampy, or deep. Visceral nociceptive pain can be referred in a dermatomal distribution.

Organic neuropathic pain occurs because of injury to or disease of the nervous system. Neuropathic pain is most often described as burning, shooting, or tingling, and it can follow a dermatomal distribution. Although neuropathic pain may occur spontaneously, evoked pain is the hallmark of neuropathic pain and can be experienced as dysesthesias, altered or abnormal sensations, paresthesia, sensations of electrical shock, hyperalgesia, increased sensitivity to painful stimulation, or allodynia (pain with sensation of ordinarily nonpainful causes, such as cool air or light touch).[1]

Idiopathic, or psychogenic, pain may not demonstrate any clinical evidence of an associated organic etiology but might include additional psychologic elements at the time of clinical presentation. Because the experience of pain is subjective to patients, the reality of their pain is comparable to organic pain and must be treated.

CLINICAL PRESENTATION

The clinical picture of chronic pain is nonspecific and may be noted only in terms of a retrospective review of patient care. Both physical and psychologic perspectives must be considered in a patient with chronic pain. Certain patterns may emerge. First, chronic pain continues for a prolonged period and beyond a "reasonable" healing time for a specific injury. Second, as the autonomic nervous system adapts to the chronicity of the pain, there can be disparity between objective and functional findings because of the lack of signs of heightened sympathetic activity. Therefore the objective physical examination and diagnostic testing may not reveal or provoke a pain response consistent with the patient's subjective description of the pain. However, the patient is adamant that pain exists.

Third, a patient complaining of pain may also present with depression or other psychiatric conditions. The pain as described by the patient may have additional emotional labels such as "cruel," "heartless," or "evil," or a patient may become sadder or more anxious or irritable.[5,6] A diagnosis of chronic pain syndrome may be considered in patients whose continued chronic pain is compounded by psychologic and behavioral changes that lead to functional impairment and emotional distress.[7] Patients with chronic pain may manifest their distress through relationship difficulties, decreased coping abilities, or an inability to work.

Fourth, a pattern of excessive use of the health care system may become apparent as the patient continues to seek various treatment options or additional consultations because of existing pain.[6] Fifth, a history of prolonged or excessive use of opiates, benzodiazepines, or alcohol may exist.[6] Initially these substances may have been taken to promote relaxation and rest, but their excessive use may have become counterproductive to healing. At the same time, the patient may have developed a tolerance to these medications, possibly leading to substance abuse.

PHYSICAL EXAMINATION

Pain is often managed inadequately because of poor clinical assessment. Therefore it is critical that a pain assessment be integrated into the patient's detailed history and physical assessment and continued with each visit. A review of previous diagnostic studies and medical interventions, as well as an assessment of coexisting conditions, is also necessary.[8]

Pain assessment can be aided by the mnemonic device *PQRST:* Provocative-palliative factors, Quality, Region, Severity, Temporal (i.e., time of day, or season in which the pain is more constant or the duration longer). The use of simple pain intensity scales (e.g., 1, no pain; 5, moderate pain; 10, worst possible pain) describes and documents the patient's chronicity and severity of pain; individual pain diaries can also be valuable. A psychiatric assessment including a history of alcohol or other substance use or abuse for pain management should be performed.[2] Signs and symptoms of depression such as fatigue, insomnia, decreased appetite, and decreased activities should be elicited, and the patient's activities of daily living and usual patterns of coping under duress should be reviewed. Finally, it is important to determine how the easing or absence of pain would improve the patient's quality of life.[7]

In addition, it is beneficial to focus not only on the patient's functional disability but also on possible psychologic distress. What is the meaning of pain to the patient, and what are the past experiences of pain? What is the meaning and expression of pain within the patient's culture?

DIAGNOSTICS

No specific diagnostics are indicated, but ECGs, x-ray studies, and laboratory tests such as complete blood count, SMA 20 (sequential multiple analysis of 20 chemical constituents), and a urinalysis should be ordered when appropriate.[9] An electromyogram may also be necessary to localize neurologic pain.

DIFFERENTIAL DIAGNOSES

Etiologies of chronic pain syndromes include trauma to the cervical and lumbar spine, cervical and lumbar disc disease, vascular headaches, arthritis, connective tissue disorders, fibromyalgia, complications from surgical diseases, and neuropathies caused by various viruses, toxins, and diseases.[10]

MANAGEMENT

Many issues may affect the experience of chronic pain, including personal implications of injury, developmental history and past experience of coping, ethnocultural influences, premorbid psychologic health, secondary gain from injury, and environmental influences.[9] Therefore each patient reacts uniquely and has an individual response to pain. It is essential to believe the patient's report of pain.[8] In addition, it is critical to set realistic goals concerning pain control. *Except in rare circumstances,* a patient with a chronic pain syndrome will not be pain free. Thus the most realistic goal is to make the person as comfortable as possible and to encourage the maintenance of optimal mobility and daily functioning.[2] To accomplish this goal, the primary care provider must enter into a partnership with the patient to work together to decrease the pain and increase optimal quality of life.

An individual treatment plan that focuses on both the psychologic and physical components is necessary. Evaluating strategies that have been beneficial in the past may be helpful in developing a manageable strategy for chronic pain. The goal of chronic pain management is not analgesia but rather preserving and maximizing function and enhancing coping skills. In particular, the patient is offered alternative approaches to dealing with the pain, which increases self-promoting behaviors to decrease the negative impact on the quality of life.

Pharmacologic Interventions

Pharmacologic interventions follow the guidelines of the three-step analgesic ladder for pain control as developed by the World Health Organization (WHO) and endorsed by the American Pain Society (APS). Step 1 begins with the use of nonopioids and adjuvants, including nonsteroidal antiinflammatory drugs (NSAIDs), tricyclic antidepressants, selective serotonin reuptake inhibitors (SSRIs), anticonvulsants, or antiarrhythmics.

Although NSAIDS have not been proven to be efficacious in chronic pain, their effectiveness in acute pain is well documented. Thus it is worthwhile to use ibuprofen or naproxen in cases of chronic pain. The new cylcooxygenase-2 (COX-2) class of NSAIDS may relieve pain with fewer side effects.[2]

Tricyclic antidepressants are the initial drugs of choice because both the depressive aspects of chronic pain and the physiologic nerve pain can be treated. Agents include amitriptyline, nortriptyline, imipramine, or desipramine, which can be effective at a starting dose of 25 mg PO at bedtime. (Further consideration must be given to older adults, whose starting dose would be lower.) Failure of one medication in this class does not necessarily indicate that another will fail. Common side effects of this class of medications include dry mouth, constipation, and a feeling of being "hung over." Monitoring blood levels when available can prevent or lessen these side effects.[5]

Second-line medications are anticonvulsants that include phenytoin, carbamazepine, and valproic acid. The anticonvulsants are especially helpful in cases of neuralgia and paresthesia. Initial dosing should be low, such as 50 mg at bedtime for an older adult or 100 mg for a younger patient. Blood levels must be monitored and are kept in the same range as for treating seizures.[5]

The SSRIs, which include fluoxetine, sertraline, and paroxetine, are particularly appropriate for patients who are unresponsive to tricyclics or who have suffered side effects from tricyclics. Side effects of the SSRIs can include rash, urticaria, dizziness, and drowsiness.

Step 2 of the WHO three-step analgesic ladder includes mild opiates such as oxycodone (Percocet), codeine, and acetaminophen/codeine phosphate (Tylenol No. 3), along with adjuvant medications. Side effects include drowsiness and constipation. Tramadol (Ultram) may initiate addiction. This is a concern because tramadol is a synthetic opioid. Patients may not be aware of the potential for the reinitiation of abuse. The newer drug Ultracet (tramadol with acetaminophen) has a similar potential.

Step 3 medication interventions involve opiates. Usually the opiates are considered after other drugs have failed, and they have traditionally been underused because of concerns regarding addiction, tolerance, and side effects such as diversion.[8] Step 3 medications include morphine, fentanyl patches, oxycodone, and hydromorphone. Opiates should be considered only after all other reasonable attempts at analgesia have failed. Meperidine (Demerol) should not be used for chronic pain because the long-acting metabolites can cause central nervous system toxicity, and repetitive injections can cause skin problems. Adjuvant medications such as NSAIDs, tricyclics, SSRIs, anticonvulsants, or antiarrhythmics may be used in combination with the opiates.[8]

Nonpharmacologic Interventions

Patients often use both traditional medicine and alternative therapy. This tandem effect can be very effective, particularly if both the traditional and alternative practitioners work collaboratively. For patients not exposed to alternative therapy, it is important to provide information regarding how such therapies can enhance pain management. The following is a list of nonpharmacologic interventions:

- *Cognitive behavior interventions:* Relaxation, biofeedback, distraction, hypnosis, and support groups. Pain often drains a person's focus and energy. Cognitive behavior interventions can temporarily raise the pain threshold, thereby allowing the patient's attention to be directed toward something other than the pain.
- *Exercise:* Physical therapy, occupational therapy, and exercise programs including hydrotherapy. Exercise can improve general conditioning, thereby improving stamina and endurance. In addition, exercise can promote the production of endorphins, which are the body's natural pain relievers. Stress reduction is a secondary benefit of an exercise program and can assist in overall coping behaviors.
- *Alternative therapies:* Chiropractic treatment, acupuncture, massage therapy, herbal therapies, and homeopathy.
- *Transcutaneous electrical nerve stimulation (TENS):* A process in which a low-voltage electrical pulse is directed through the skin. It is believed to stimulate nerve fibers and interfere with the conduction of painful stimuli.
- *Nerve blocks:* Anesthetic given within a nerve to stop painful conduction.
- *Heat/cold:* Act as counterirritants or reduce muscle spasm.[1,5]

Co-Management with Specialists

Because chronic pain encompasses both physical and psychologic components, pain control is more effective and successful when using a multidisciplinary team approach.[3,5] However, it is crucial for one practitioner to take responsibility for all prescriptions, which allows for a systematic approach to pain medications, permits an adequate trial of medications before change, and ensures avoidance of polypharmacy.

LIFE SPAN CONSIDERATIONS

Chronic pain is rare in a child unless he has undergone a surgical procedure that initiates a response. Usually, chronic pain may begin in young adults precipitated by an accident, incident, or soft tissue injury. It then progresses in middle age and older adults. When onset begins in older adults, it is usually caused by degenerative joint pain.

COMPLICATIONS

Complications can arise with medication misuse or abuse. It is important to monitor a patient's use of NSAIDs for toxicities and the use of opiates because of their potential for abuse. As stated previously, it is important to treat not only the pain, but the psychologic issues that accompany the pain.

INDICATIONS FOR REFERRAL/HOSPITALIZATION

Chronic pain is difficult to manage within one discipline. Consultations with a social worker to assist in the identification of coping mechanisms or with a psychiatric consult to evaluate possible depression may be beneficial. If there is a history of substance abuse, a referral to or consultation with a substance abuse counselor may be helpful.[8] If pain is localized to a specific area, a specialist consultation may be indicated. For example, chronic abdominal pain may require a gastroenterology consultation. Referral to an outpatient pain clinic or pain specialist may also be considered.[11] Some patients require pain management within a specialist program setting, which is appropriate if other pain management interventions have failed. Both inpatient and outpatient pain clinic and rehabilitation programs may be used. Consideration of insurance coverage of these programs and the availability of a program within a reasonable geographic proximity are important.

PATIENT AND FAMILY EDUCATION

Education is the critical core of pain management. Included in patient education are the explanation of the physiology of the affected body system, the pain cycle, and the purpose and side effects of the medications.[7] Education engenders self-assertion and empowers the patient in decisions regarding chronic conditions, possibly ameliorating the lethargy or depression that may be part of the chronic pain syndrome. Education also may provide realistic hope about the pain—that the pain may not be totally eliminated but rather that the quality of life can be improved.

HEALTH PROMOTION

Health promotion activities include good education surrounding activities of daily living. This includes continued participation, distraction, engaging in positive behaviors to avoid a dependency on medications, and the use of various methods in coping with pain.

REFERENCES

1. Garcia J, Altman RD: Chronic pain states: pathophysiology and medical therapy, *Semin Arthritis Rheum* 27(1):1-16, 1997.
2. Khouzam HR: Chronic pain and its management in primary care, *South Med J* 93(10):946-952.
3. Bonica J, editor: General considerations of chronic pain. In *Management of chronic pain,* Philadelphia, 1990, Lea & Febiger.
4. Hitchcock LS, Ferrell BR, McCaffrey M: The experience of chronic nonmalignant pain, *J Pain Symptom Manage* 9(5):312-318, 1994.
5. Nossell M: Chronic nonmalignant pain management. In Salerno E, Willens J, editors: *Pain management handbook: an interdisciplinary approach,* St Louis, 1996, Mosby.
6. Sullivan M, Turner J, Romano J: Chronic pain in primary care: identification and management of psychosocial factors, *J Fam Pract* 32(2):193-199, 1991.

7. Simon JM: Chronic pain syndrome: nursing assessment and intervention, *Rehabil Nurs* 21(1):13-19, 1996.
8. American Pain Society: *Principles of analgesic use in the treatment of acute pain and cancer pain,* ed 4, Skokie, Ill, 1999, The Society.
9. Rodgers C, Thomson T: Pain problems in primary care medical practice. In Tollison CD, Satterwaite JR, Tollison J, editors: *Handbook of pain management,* Baltimore, 1994, Williams & Wilkins.
10. Adams NJ and others: Opioids and the treatment of chronic pain in a primary care sample, *J Pain Symptom Manage* 22(3):791-796, 2001.
11. McCaffrey M, Pasero C: *Pain: clinical manual,* St Louis, 1998, Mosby.

CHAPTER 14

Obesity

Heather E.T. Bell

DEFINITION/EPIDEMIOLOGY

Obesity and overweight are two of the most common conditions addressed by primary care physicians.[1] Classification of obesity and overweight are determined in part by calculating the body mass index (BMI) as a means of estimating body fat:

$$\text{BMI (in kg/m}^2\text{)} = \text{Body weight (in lb) (Height (in in}^2\text{))} \times 704$$

Clinical judgment must be used in interpreting BMI in situations that may affect its accuracy as a reflection of total body fat. These situations include the presence of edema, high muscle mass, wasting of muscle, and individuals with limited stature.[2] Using the above calculation, overweight is defined as a BMI of 25 to 29.9 kg/m^2, and obesity is defined as a BMI of at least 30. It is widely known that obesity is associated with many diseases such as diabetes, hypertension, coronary artery disease, sleep apnea, osteoarthritis, menstrual irregularities, cholelithiasis, cor pulmonale, and various types of cancer.[2] Although obesity in and of itself is not a disease state, its association with major morbidity and mortality is significant, prompting many to redefine obesity as a chronic illness and to treat it as such.

The incidence of obesity varies widely but is becoming more prevalent among developing countries.[3] There is also a familial association resulting from the combination of genetics, shared cultural background, diet, and environment.[4] In the United States, recent studies have shown that more than half of all Americans over age 20 years are overweight, and nearly one fourth are clinically obese.[3] Obesity is insidious, often beginning in childhood and perpetuating with age, but its incidence is not age specific. Many studies have shown an increased risk of morbidity and mortality associated with increasing degrees of body weight, yet experts continue to debate the precise nature of the relationship between weight and health.[3] As for patients, few medical issues are fraught with more anxiety and distress than weight management. It is therefore recommended that providers evaluate individual factors including BMI, waist circumference, disease risk, family history, current health problems, environmental issues, and the patient's orientation to weight management when considering intervention.[3]

PATHOPHYSIOLOGY

Simply put, an overweight state occurs when a positive energy balance is created by an increased energy (caloric) intake that exceeds energy output.[5] If this equation alone were the sole explanation for the nature of obesity, treatment would be rather simple and straightforward and aimed at decreasing caloric intake and increasing energy expenditure. However, multiple factors contribute to the chronic and recurrent nature of obesity. Recent studies of individuals with a wide variance in BMI, in connection with data on their parents, siblings, and spouses, showed that 25% to 40% of the individual differences in body mass or body fat were possibly dependent on genetic factors.[2] In a study of identical and fraternal twins reared apart, however, Stunkard and others[6] found that a 70% variance in BMI was due to genetic influence and only a 30% variance was due to environmental influence.

Considering energy expenditure, the basal metabolic rate (BMR), or the baseline energy that is expended to maintain body functions, can vary widely among individuals and is influenced heavily by heredity, age, gender, and muscle mass. Because of their increased muscle mass, obese individuals have a higher BMR when compared to nonobese individuals. However, there is some evidence to show that obese individuals have unusually low calorie utilization at reduced, more desirable weights. This has led to a theory of individuals having a certain weight "set point." In other words, the body tends to adjust certain regulatory mechanisms to maintain weight at a "set" level, thus preserving homeostasis. Compared to their lean counterparts, obese individuals increase in weight more readily and stabilize at a higher point than desirable and have more difficulty maintaining weight loss.[7]

Increased numbers of fat cells, particularly hypertrophied fat cells, have been observed in obese individuals, particularly those in whom the onset of obesity occurred during early childhood. Some evidence suggests that these individuals plateau in weight when the size of the fat cells is reduced to a critical level with caloric restriction.[7]

Physical activity, both spontaneous (e.g., unconscious fidgeting) and purposeful, varies greatly among individuals. Weight loss resulting from increased physical activity in obese patients may be slow, mainly because their exercise tolerance is low.[8] Therefore weight loss based solely on increased physical activity in these individuals is unrealistic and moreover is likely to promote increased exercise resistance.

Several medications have also been associated with weight gain (Box 14-1), particularly steroids, insulin, and several classes of psychotropic agents.[9]

Finally, other factors contribute to the "energy in equals energy out" equation—mainly socioeconomic, environmental, behavioral, and psychologic factors.[5] Obesity tends to be chronic and recurring, and treatment should be ongoing and lifelong.

BOX 14-1

MEDICATIONS COMMONLY ASSOCIATED WITH WEIGHT GAIN

Corticosteroids
Estrogens
Hormone-replacement therapy
Olanzapine (Zyprexa)
Valproic acid (e.g., Depakote)
Antidepressants
Selective serotonin reuptake inhibitors (SSRIs)
Insulin
Sulfonylureas

From Cummings SM, Pratt JS, Kaplan LM: Evaluation and management of obesity in women. In Carlson K, Eisenstat S, editors: *Primary care of women*, New York, 2001, Mosby.

CLINICAL PRESENTATION

It is important that clinicians be able to both classify a patient's weight and assess the associated disease risk. In general, the greater the degree of obesity, the greater the risk for developing co-morbidities associated with obesity (Box 14-2).

The risk of complications from obesity is related not only to the amount of body fat but also to its distribution. Patients with upper body obesity have an increased independent risk for developing type 2 (non–insulin-dependent) diabetes, hyperinsulinemia, hypertension, hyperlipidemia, and coronary artery disease (CAD) compared with patients with lower body fat distribution, even when the BMI is not markedly increased.[2,5] As a result, measurement of waist circumference is recommended as the most practical method for assessing a patient's abdominal fat content. However, it is unnecessary to measure waist circumference in patients with BMI of 35 kg/m^2 or greater because the measurement will typically be greater than the designated high-risk cut points, and waist measurements lose their predictive power at very high BMIs.[2]

The patient history should include the past medical history, with particular attention given to the existence of associated co-morbidities. The course of the obesity should also be elicited, because obesity that begins in childhood and persists through adulthood suggests a multifactorial cause and genetic predisposition, which may influence the approach to treatment. A history of what the patient has done to lose weight should be obtained, including the use of formalized weight loss programs, diets, and attempts at exercise. This information is helpful in determining what has worked or failed in the past and what might be useful for further treatment. Any history of eating disorders such as anorexia, bulimia, or binge eating disorders should be determined, because a history of these conditions will necessitate a specialized approach to the patient's current

BOX 14-2

CO-MORBIDITIES ASSOCIATED WITH OBESITY

CARDIAC
Coronary artery disease
Cor pulmonale
Hypertension
Congestive heart failure
Pulmonary embolism

RESPIRATORY
Sleep apnea
Hypoventilation
Dyspnea on exertion
Pickwickian syndrome

GASTROINTESTINAL
Cholelithiasis
Diverticulosis
Diverticulitis
Colon cancer
Reflux esophagitis

GENITOURINARY
Amenorrhea
Hypogonadism (men)
Infertility
Urinary incontinence
Breast/uterine cancer (women)

ENDOCRINE
Type II diabetes
Hyperandrogenism (women)
Hypercholesterolemia

MUSCULOSKELETAL
Osteoarthritis
Low back pain

TABLE 14-1 National Heart, Lung, and Blood Institute (NHLBI) Classification of Overweight and Obesity by BMI, Waist Circumference, and Associated Disease Risk

	BMI (kg/m²)	Obesity class	Disease Risk* Relative to Normal Weight and Waist Circumference (Men ≤102 cm [≤ 40 in]; women ≤88 cm [≤35 in])	Disease Risk* Relative to Normal Weight and Waist Circumference (Men >102 cm [>40 in]; women >88 cm [>35 in])
Underweight	<18.5		—	—
Normal	18.5-24.9		—	—
Overweight	25.0-29.9		Increased	High
Obesity	30.0-34.9	I	High	Very high
	35.0-39.9	II	Very high	Very high
Extreme obesity	≥40	III	Extremely high	Extremely high

From National Institutes of Health and National Heart, Lung, and Blood Institute: *Clinical guidelines on the identification, evaluation, and treatment of overweight and obesity in adults: the evidence report,* Washington, DC, 1998, The Institute.
*Disease risk for type 2 diabetes, hypertension, and cardiovascular disease.

weight issues. Finally, the primary care provider should review the patient's motivation for losing weight, if there is one, because much of the success of treatment depends on the patient's commitment to it. Moreover, research in the area of motivational interviewing suggests that clinicians can tailor brief behavior-change messages most effectively when they are cognizant of the patient's motivational status.

PHYSICAL EXAMINATION AND DIAGNOSTICS

The aim of the physical examination should be to assess the patient's overall risk status relative to the degree of obesity as well as the presence and/or degree of existing co-morbid states. Table 14-1 encapsulates the classification guidelines incorporating BMI, waist circumference, and associated disease risk.[2] It is important to note that the defined risk categories denote relative risk, not absolute risk, which is determined by estimates of absolute risk based on the presence of associated disease, target organ damage, or lifestyle risk factors (Table 14-2). Additionally, the following laboratory studies should be considered to rule out causative factors contributing to obesity and co-morbid states: thyroid-stimulating hormone (TSH), fasting glucose and/or HbA_{1c}, fasting cortisol, electrolytes (which may be helpful in diagnosing Cushing's disease), and a fasting lipid profile. Further testing, such as liver and kidney functions, should be considered if gallbladder disease, type 2 diabetes, or nonalcoholic steatohepatitis (NASH)–related cirrhosis is suspected. An ECG, chest x-ray examination, pulmonary function test, and cardiac stress test might be useful if coronary artery disease or cor pulmonale is suspected after examination. Lastly, clinicians should include a sleep study for patients whose neck circumference and sleep history point to obstructive sleep apnea.[9]

DIFFERENTIAL DIAGNOSIS

Care must be taken not to miss the diagnosis of an endocrine disorder, which although rare may in fact be the cause of the obesity (Table 14-3). Although hypothyroidism and Cushing's syndrome are generally correctable, polycystic ovary syndrome (PCOS) does not currently have a specific therapy that improves the associated weight disorder.[9] Eating disorders, particularly bulimia and binge eating disorder, should be considered because patients may have obesity related to the bingeing typical of these diseases.

TABLE 14-2 Identification of Patients at High and Very High Absolute Risk

Conditions Denoting High Absolute Risk*	Conditions Denoting Very High Absolute Risk
Cigarette smoking	Established CAD
Hypertension	History of myocardial infarction
High risk LDL cholesterol	History of angina pectoris (stable or unstable)
Low HDL cholesterol	History of coronary artery surgery
Impaired fasting glucose	History of coronary artery procedures (angioplasty)
Family history of premature CHD	Presence of other atherosclerotic diseases
Male ≥45 years, female ≥55 years (or postmenopausal)	Peripheral arterial disease
	Abdominal aortic aneurysm
	Symptomatic carotid artery disease
	Type 2 diabetes
	Sleep apnea

From National Institutes of Health and National Heart, Lung, and Blood Institute: *Clinical guidelines on the identification, evaluation, and treatment of overweight and obesity in adults: the evidence report,* Washington, DC, 1998, The Institute.
LDL, Low-density lipoprotein; *HDL,* high-density lipoprotein.
*Patients must have three or more of these risk factors to meet the criteria for high absolute risk.

MANAGEMENT

The aim of treatment is to reduce and prevent the occurrence of risks associated with obesity-related co-morbidities. As little as a 5% to 10% reduction in weight has been shown to reduce obesity-related co-morbidities.[2] Because of the chronic, recurrent nature of obesity, the goals of treatment must be reasonable, attainable, and positioned within the context of long-term

TABLE 14-3 Differential Diagnoses to Consider in Obese Patients

Disorder	Clinical Presentation	Diagnostics
Hyperinsulinemia	Use of exogenous insulin Hyperglycemia Use of exogenous steroids, signs of Cushing's disease Polycystic ovary (PCO)	Glucose Insulin levels
Cushing's disease	Moonface Buffalo hump Electrolyte abnormalities Hypertension resistant to medication Tachycardia	Cortisol challenge test Electrolytes Glucose
Polycystic ovary disease	Hirsutism History of oligomenorrhea Infertility	Follicle-stimulating hormone Luteinizing hormone (LH)
Hypothyroidism	Mild obesity Hyporeflexivity Cold intolerance Hair loss Dry skin Amenorrhea Decreased libido	Thyroid-stimulating hormone (TSH) Free T_4
Hypothalamic state (craniopharyngioma)	Delayed sexual development Headache Papilledema Mental deterioration Hypogonadism	CT scan
Growth hormone deficiency (rare)	History of pituitary resection/dysfunction Dwarfism	Growth hormone (GH)

intervention. It is therefore suggested that the clinician and patient gradually establish a weight at which the patient can stay healthy and avoid illness while practicing moderate and balanced food- and exercise-related behaviors. Current guidelines recommend an initial goal of no more than 10% weight loss. Once this weight has been reached and achieved for 1 year, a goal of an additional 10% weight loss, if clinically indicated, can then be suggested. It is also important to note that depending on the clinical needs and motivation of the patient, appropriate goals may also include preventing further acute weight gains or stabilizing weight over the long term—an outcome that is considered particularly significant for patients with a history of weight cycling.[2,9]

Because the state of obesity is multifactorial, treatment should also be multifactorial. For patients with adult-onset obesity who are taking no medications, have no evidence of obesity complications, and for whom weight gain appears to be most strongly related to environmental factors, an appropriate initial intervention would be to develop supportive, realistic, nutrition, and physical activity goals.[9] Such an intervention should promote adequate caloric intake (no fewer than 1000 kcal/day for women, and no less than 1500 kcal/day for men), as well as the inclusion of aerobic activity for cardiovascular development and strength training for the development of lean body mass.[9] The combination of diet and exercise results in much greater weight loss and maintenance than either method alone.[7] Formalized programs in behavior modification, which combine group support with the teaching of more beneficial eating habits (e.g., portion control, recognition of emotional triggers to eating), have been shown to be an important part of adjuvant therapy.[7]

Use of the recommended daily allowance (RDA) Food Guide Pyramid is helpful in teaching patients portion control and the importance of eating a variety of foods. Following the guidelines of the Food Guide Pyramid promotes a high-fiber, low-fat diet, with a limited intake of sweets. In addition, patients should be urged to explore monounsaturated fats such as olive oil, canola oil, and peanuts and to experiment with substituting these for more saturated fats such as animal fats, coconut and palm kernel oils, cocoa butter, and processed hydrogenated items. The primary care provider may believe that certain patients need more specific guidelines for dietary change or more assistance with the emotional aspects of their eating style. Under these circumstances, referral to a dietitian specializing in weight-related medical nutrition therapy is advisable. To prevent treatment failure and/or extreme behaviors with eating and physical activity, it is important to support patients in making small, incremental changes in diet and lifestyle. To encourage patients to continue in their efforts, the goals must be attainable and achievable.

Although physical activity is often promoted as adjunctive therapy in obesity treatment, it may actually be more effective for practitioners to reframe it as being beneficial in its own right. First, beyond the evidence that physical activity increases the likelihood of maintaining weight loss, multiple studies have shown that improved physical fitness reduces the risk of cardiovascular disease and promotes more normalized insulin and blood sugar indices, even if the participants do not experience a significant decrease in BMI.[10,11] Second, reframing physical activity as basic self-care rather than as a means of reshaping the body has been suggested as a more effective means of developing long-term, internal exercise motivation.[12] Lastly, unlinking exercise from weight reduction may assist in the prevention of extreme eating and exercise behaviors, because some researchers have proposed that the pressure to combine diet and exercise to reduce body weight is a significant precipitant in the development of eating disorders.[13]

If there are no medical contraindications to exercise, patients can be encouraged to engage in a regular aerobic exercise program. Recent recommendations state the need to engage in moderate physical activity for a minimum of 30 minutes on most, if not all, days of the week.[5] Patients who are sedentary and deconditioned will need to achieve this level gradually, and very large patients may actually require physical therapy-type exercises to condition their joints and muscles for sustained weight-bearing activity. Examples of moderate-intensity exercise include walking at a brisk pace, swimming, gardening, hiking, low-impact aerobics, and the use of available cardiovascular equipment (e.g., stair climbers, treadmills, and stationary bikes). For more deconditioned patients, practitioners can recommend that they begin by increasing the frequency and duration of activities of daily living such as housecleaning or yard work.[14] Adding weight-resistance training to aerobic exercise increases strength, agility, and endurance. Frequent follow-up visits, perhaps monthly, are helpful in tracking the patient's progress, identifying problem areas that prevent success, and encouraging and supporting the patient's efforts.

Pharmacologic Therapy

Practitioners should be aware that nonprescription drugs are available for weight loss, including chromium, aminophylline cream, Dexatrim, and Acutrim. Patients with bulimia may even resort to using syrup of ipecac as a purgative. However, none of these agents has proven efficacy, and they may have side effects; therefore it is prudent to counsel patients against their use. In general, drug therapy can be appropriate for patients with a BMI of 30 or more without concomitant obesity-related risk factors or diseases or for patients with a BMI of 27 or more with concomitant risk factors or diseases.[2] It is also suggested that pharmacotherapy be reserved for patients who show a proven history of failure to lose and maintain their weight through conventional therapies.[5]

Several medications are currently available for short-term use in a multidisciplinary weight-management intervention. With each, maximal effectiveness is seen in the first year of treatment, and none of these agents have approval of the U.S. Food and Drug Administration (FDA) for use beyond 1 year. Patients who are considering these medications should be informed that these drugs do not replace changes in eating style and physical activity but are potentially useful *additions* to a comprehensive weight management program.[9]

Of the three most common medications currently approved for use, two of them (phentermine and sibutramine [Meridia]) are centrally acting agents that affect the adrenergic and serotonergic synapses and the adrenergic and dopaminergic synapses, respectively, to modestly decrease appetite and enhance resting energy expenditure. Side effects of phentermine and sibutramine may include increased heart rate and blood pressure, and the use of sibutramine is contraindicated in patients with a history of high blood pressure, CAD, congestive heart failure, arrhythmias, or stroke. Patients receiving sibutramine should have their blood pressure monitored regularly. Phentermine may be used for up to 3 months, whereas sibutramine has FDA approval for use up to 1 year. Net weight loss tends to be modest (in the range of 2 to 10 kg) and generally occurs during the early part of therapy.[2,9]

The third medication, orlistat (Xenical), is a pancreatic lipase inhibitor used to decrease dietary fat absorption by blocking up to 30% of the fat consumed in a meal. Adverse effects of orlistat include decreased absorption of fat-soluble vitamins, soft stools and anal leakage (in patients consuming a high-fat meal), and a possible link to breast cancer.[2] Patients taking orlistat should be encouraged to consume meals moderate in fat, as well as a multivitamin supplement, to decrease the possibility of adverse effects. Clinicians should also be alert to the possibility of patients using orlistat as a purgative following a high-fat meal. Orlistat is approved for 1-year use and, as with the medications discussed previously, generally results in modest weight loss.[2]

LIFE SPAN CONSIDERATIONS

Research results on the advisability of weight reduction after the age of 65 years appear to be mixed. Although it is acknowledged that the prevalence of cardiovascular risk factors, functional limitations, and mobility impairments are higher in overweight vs. nonoverweight seniors, there is some question as to whether weight loss will lead to decreased morbidity and mortality. In fact, weight loss at older ages has been associated with increased mortality, although possibly as a result of involuntary weight loss resulting from occult illness.[2] In addition, concerns have been raised about the potential adverse effects of obesity intervention as it affects bone health and dietary adequacy. Weight loss may accelerate bone loss, increasing the risk of osteoporotic fractures, particularly for high-risk groups such as older white women. Restrictions on overall food intake, particularly nutrient-dense, energy-rich foods, could precipitate inadequate intakes of protein and essential vitamins and minerals.[2]

Clinicians considering a weight reduction intervention for an older adult should evaluate the perceived benefits of treatment with respect to quality of life, daily functioning, and risk reduction. They should take steps to select interventions that minimize the possibility of deleterious effects on bone health or general nutrition status.[2]

COMPLICATIONS

As shown in Box 14-1, the associated medical complications of obesity and overweight are many and varied and affect the cardiac, respiratory, gastrointestinal, genitourinary, endocrine, musculoskeletal, and hepatic systems. In addition, obesity and overweight have also been associated with a variety of neoplastic conditions, most notably, reproductive carcinomas.[9]

INDICATIONS FOR REFERRAL/HOSPITALIZATION

Referral to a nutritionist should be considered, particularly when the patient needs more structured information regarding proper diet than the primary care provider can provide or when the patient's emotional and cognitive orientation to eating appears particularly complex.

If a patient's insurance allows or if the patient can afford it, referral to a structured and supervised exercise program may be beneficial. Deconditioned and sedentary patients or patients with chronic obstructive pulmonary disease or other physical limitations would benefit from a supervised program modified to fit their needs. Often these programs are not covered by medical insurance and are an expensive venture. The patient could investigate joining a health club that offers the services of a certified personal training staff that can help the patient develop and follow a specially tailored aerobic fitness program while providing supervision during exercise.

If untreated co-morbidities (e.g., uncontrolled CAD or diabetes) are suspected, the primary care provider should refer the patient to the appropriate subspecialist. If an underlying cause to the obesity is suspected (e.g., hypercortisolism, hyperinsulinemia, or Cushing's disease), the patient should be referred to an endocrinologist.

The primary care provider can consider a referral for surgical intervention for patients with morbid obesity (BMI >40 kg/m^2) and for patients whose BMI is at least 35 with serious co-morbidities (cardiovascular, sleep apnea, uncontrolled type 2 diabetes) and known failure with conventional therapies.[2] Usually either gastroplasty (with vertical bands or adjustable bands) or a gastric bypass (most typically a Roux-en-Y) is performed. Both procedures result in decreased stomach capacity, thereby drastically reducing food consumption, as well as promoting increased satiety. In some cases, mild protein-calorie malabsorption is created.

Follow-up care of patients receiving Roux-en-Y bypass surgery shows that approximately 85% to 90% of these patients achieve a loss of at least 50% of excess body weight, and the addition of intensive postsurgical lifestyle education has been demonstrated to significantly increase the patient success rate at the 5-year point.[9] Associated mortality is less than 1% with these procedures. Major early complications can include wound infection (6%), pneumonia (1.9%), anastomotic leak (1.5%), and thromboembolism (2%). Late complications include incisional hernia (15%), marginal ulcer (6%), transient dumping (15%), and vitamin B_{12} deficiency (25%).[15] A referral for such procedures should be a well thought-out process, with the risk-benefit ratio carefully reviewed with patients. Consultation with a surgeon well experienced in bypass surgery should include appropriate preoperative and postoperative care and education.[5]

PATIENT AND FAMILY EDUCATION

Educating patients in proper diet, exercise, behavior, and lifestyle modifications to promote weight loss and weight maintenance is a cornerstone of conventional therapy. The primary care provider should be familiar with the basic principles of the Food Guide Pyramid, an eating style that promotes variety, balance, and moderation, as well as pleasure. The primary care provider should be comfortable discussing with patients the basics of beginning an aerobic exercise program, keeping in mind that the patient's exercise tolerance is likely to be low, necessitating gradual gains in exercise duration and intensity. Patients should be given information on how to pace themselves by understanding the concept of perceived exertion according to the Borg scale, and how to avoid overexertion and subsequent injury. Goals should be established with patients, particularly regarding the issue of weight loss. The goal should be realistic measures of loss, which can be as modest as $\frac{1}{2}$ to 1 pound per week, or it can also include weight stabilization and prevention of further acute gains. Patients should be reminded that losses of 5% to 10% of total body weight represent significant success, particularly when the losses are maintained.

The information here assumes that the patient is open and receptive to discussing weight status and the possibility of a weight reduction program. More typically, however, patients are ambivalent about the process of weight reduction, and the conversation about weight and health feels awkward and uncomfortable—for both the patient *and* the provider. One study showed that educated, *hospital-employed* women of greater BMI were more likely to state that they delayed medical care because of shame about weight or "because they did not want a lecture regarding their obesity."[16] In addition, the time limits inherent in primary care medicine may make it difficult to have such an intense discussion with as much sensitivity and effectiveness as the provider could wish.

Recent studies of patient education in a primary care setting suggest that use of empathetic communication models such as motivational interviewing are extremely effective at introducing challenging topics in a balanced way that keeps patients engaged. Moreover, these interviews are designed to be brief and focused on the patient's state of motivation, thereby allowing providers to improve patient understanding and patient relations within the constraints of a regular office visit. Table 14-4 matches three possible motivational stages, with the brief content most helpful to the patient in terms of increasing motivation and eventually producing action.[17, 18] It is important for providers to realize that they can be successful with a given interaction, even if the patient leaves the office not yet ready to change his or her behavior. Movement along the motivational continuum *is* success.

The first three stages of change are the points at which provider coaching is most effective. Patients in precontemplation, although likely not open to a prolonged discussion, benefit significantly when providers share their evaluation of health risk status relative to weight, because the patient may be unaware of their clinical risk picture. Similarly, patients in contemplation can use the presentation of the medical benefits of weight management to identify positive outcome expectations if they change their behavior. Lastly, patients in preparation are assisted with successful change when providers offer a clinical perspective on setting appropriate goals for change, as well as offering support with problem solving. In this way, a conversation that could be stressful and demoralizing becomes an opportunity to develop a deeply satisfying relationship between the provider and patient.

TABLE 14-4 Motivational Stages and Processes of Change

Stage of Change	Characteristics	Processes/Techniques
Precontemplation	Patient does not acknowledge a problem; not considering change within the next 6 months.	Establish rapport: validate patient's lack of readiness, acknowledge that the decision belongs to *patient.* Raise patient consciousness of personal risks to health and happiness. Ask about the impact of the problem on significant others.
Contemplation	Patient is ambivalent about change; not considering change within the next month.	Establish rapport: validate lack of readiness, acknowledge that the decision belongs to *patient.* Encourage evaluation of the pros and cons of behavior change. Identify and promote new, positive outcome expectations.
Preparation	Patient is intending to take action within the month, and small steps toward change may have already occurred.	Praise the decision to change. Verify that the patient has the necessary skills for successful change. Identify and assist in problem solving with regard to obstacles. Assist patient in identifying social supports. Encourage small, reasonable "practice" steps.

Data from *Motivating health behavior change: powerful conversations in the exam room,* Courtesy of Steve Taylor, DHSc, St. Anthony Family Medicine Residency Program, Denver CO; and Greene GW and others: Dietary applications of the stages of change model, *J Am Diet Assoc* 99:673-678, 1999.

HEALTH PROMOTION

Modifiable risk factors for overweight and obesity include the patient's eating style, relationship with physical activity, stress management behaviors, and use of certain medications. Primary prevention, which has been called "the most promising therapeutic modality available to combat obesity,"[19] would suggest that providers check in routinely with patients about the quality of their diet, whether they have a consistent exercise practice that they enjoy, and their means of balancing and coping with the increasing demands of work and life. In addition, providers can help with prevention by prescribing alternatives to weight gain-promoting medications whenever possible and exploring instances of significant adult weight gain (>10 pounds).[19]

REFERENCES

1. Yanovski S: A practical approach to treatment of the obese patient, *Arch Fam Med* 2:309-316, 1993.
2. *Clinical guidelines on the identification, evaluation, and treatment of overweight and obesity in adults: the evidence report,* 1998, National Institutes of Health, National Heart, Lung, and Blood Institute.
3. Wickelgren I: Obesity: how big a problem? *Science* 280:1364-1367, 1998.
4. Ravussin E, Swindburn B: Pathophysiology of obesity, *Lancet* 340(8816):404-440,1992.
5. Kushner RF: Office management of the adult obese patient, *Compr Ther* 23(2):116-123, 1997.
6. Stunkard AJ and others: An adoption study of human obesity, *N Engl J Med* 314(4):193-198, 1986.
7. Elliot DL, Goldberg L, Girard DE: Obesity: pathophysiology and practical management, *J Gen Intern Med* 2(3):188-198, 1987.
8. Popovich NG, Wood OB: Drug therapy for obesity: an update, *J Am Pharm Assoc* NS37(1):31-39, 1997.
9. Cummings SM, Pratt JS, Kaplan LM: Evaluation and management of obesity in women. In Carlson K, Eisenstat S, editors: *Primary care of women,* New York, 2001, Mosby.
10. Tremblay A and others: Normalization of the metabolic profile in obese women by exercise and a low fat diet, *Med Sci Sports Exerc* 23(12):1326-1331, 1991.
11. Barnard RJ and others: Role of diet and exercise in the management of hyperinsulinemia and associated atherosclerotic risk factors, *Am J Cardiol* 69:440-444, 1992.
12. Kratina K, King NL, Hayes D: Joyful movement. In *Moving Away From Diets,* Dallas, 1996, Helm Publishing.
13. Epling WF, Pierce WD: Activity based anorexia: a bio-behavioral perspective, *Int J Eating Disord* 7:475-485, 1998.
14. NIDDK Weight Control Information Network: *Active at any size,* Pub No 00-4352, March 2001.
15. Kraal JG: Surgery for obesity, *Clin Perspect Gastroenterol* 298-305, 2001.
16. Olson CL, Schumaker HD, Yawn BP: Overweight women delay medical care, *Arch Fam Med* 3:888-892, 1994.
17. *Motivating health behavior change: powerful conversations in the exam room,* Courtesy of Steve Taylor, DHSc, St. Anthony Family Medicine Residency Program, Denver CO.
18. Greene GW and others: Dietary applications of the stages of change model, *J Am Diet Assoc* 99:673-678, 1999.
19. Rippe JM, Crosley S, Ringer R: Obesity as a chronic disease: modern medical and lifestyle management, *J Am Diet Assoc* 98(10, suppl 2): S9-S15, 1998.

CHAPTER 15

Rehabilitation

Brenda L. Hage and William R. Prebola, Jr.

Approximately 54 million people in the United States—almost one in five Americans—have some type of developmental, physical, or medical disability.[1] The prevalence of disabilities is disproportionately higher among minority populations, rural populations, and those with lower socioeconomic status. These disabling conditions can include physical impairments that affect mobility, vision, speech, swallowing, and/or emotional and mental disability and can limit one or more of the affected individual's activities of daily living (ADLs).[1] Significant efforts must be directed toward increasing the functional status of the disabled. Rehabilitation seeks to assist individuals with restoration of function and maintenance of health and has been described as aiding the individual to reach maximum physical, psychosocial, educational, vocational, and avocational potential consistent with the patient's abilities and limitations.[2]

Rehabilitation uses an interdisciplinary team approach, with a patient- and family-centered plan of care and mutual goal setting in which the patient is an active participant. Several disciplines are involved in the rehabilitative process. A physiatrist, also known as a physical and rehabilitation medicine specialist, is a physician trained in the care of patients with loss of function and usually serves as the leader of the rehabilitation team. Rehabilitation nurses are skilled in caring for patients with disabilities and altered functional ability, and there is a strong emphasis on patient and family education. Advanced practice nurses such as nurse practitioners and clinical nurse specialists provide clinical follow-up care, coordination of care, and staff consultation. Physical therapists focus on gait and mobility issues, and occupational therapists promote self-care abilities used in ADLs. Speech and language therapists assist patients with dysphagia, cognition, and language problems. Dietitians offer consultation regarding nutritional needs. Psychologists provide supportive counseling and diagnostic testing for cognitive problems. Recreational therapists offer patients opportunities to develop and participate in leisure interests. Social workers and case managers coordinate discharge planning. Other health care professionals, such as cognitive therapists, may offer additional services.

The rehabilitation team works together to assist the patient and family. Rehabilitation services may be provided in a variety of settings such as the home, outpatient programs, inpatient rehabilitation units or centers, acute care hospitals, and skilled nursing facilities. The setting is selected on the basis of the patient's underlying function, potential abilities, and individual problems. It is often necessary to use several different settings as the patient moves through the continuum of rehabilitation care.

ASSESSMENT

A comprehensive functional history and assessment are essential to developing the patient's plan of care and measuring patient progress. The key elements of the functional history include the patient's ability to complete ADLs (both currently and before the present illness) and the degree of assistance required. Information regarding the use of wheelchairs, walkers, canes, prosthetics (artificial limbs), orthotics (splints, braces), and any other adaptive equipment, as well as accessibility within the patient's home, is also important.

Indexes of functional assessment include the ability to perform self-care activities (e.g., dressing, bathing, toileting, grooming, hygiene, eating) and mobility (e.g., ambulation, transfers, bed and wheelchair mobility). Social and cognitive functions are also assessed. Some of the many instruments available include the Katz Index of ADL, the Barthel Index, the Kenney Self-Care Evaluation, and the Functional Independence Measure (FIM). The FIM scoring system is the most widely used and consists of 18 functional categories that are further subdivided into mobility, locomotion, self-care, sphincter control, communication, and social cognition.[3] Although sometimes complex and time intensive, the use of FIM scoring or other assessment tools is a valuable means of establishing the patient's baseline functional abilities, measuring treatment outcomes, and facilitating communication with the rehabilitation team. These tools are used at rehabilitation staffing meetings to assist in coordinating the patient's individualized plan of care and in discharge planning. FIM scoring and other assessment measures are also important in fulfilling the documentation requirements of third-party payers, which often require updates showing patients' continued progress for continued rehabilitation eligibility.

PAIN MANAGEMENT

Pharmacologic pain management in rehabilitation is based on many factors, including the patient's age, co-morbid medical problems, medication side effect profile, ease of use, and cost. Nonsteroidal antiinflammatory drugs (NSAIDs) and acetaminophen are helpful for mild to moderate pain. NSAIDs used concomitantly with opioid analgesics allow for lower medication dosages and decrease the incidence of adverse side effects.[4] Chronic, painful conditions such as peripheral neuropathy, lumbar radiculopathy, and fibromyalgia respond well to the analgesic effect of tricyclic antidepressants such as amitriptyline (Elavil) or imipramine (Tofranil), as well as to selective serotonin reuptake inhibitors (SSRIs) such as sertraline (Zoloft) and paroxetine (Paxil). Carbamazepine (Tegretol), divalproex sodium (Depakote), valproic acid (Depakene), and clonazepam (Klonopin) are anticonvulsants that may also be beneficial in relieving the pain associated with neuropathic pain syndromes.[5] Metaxalone (Skelaxin), cyclobenzaprine (Flexeril), or other antispasmodic agents can be prescribed for short-term use to treat pain related to myofascial spasm. Topical agents include lidocaine (Lidoderm) patches and capsaicin cream that are also helpful adjuncts in pain relief.[6]

Chronic, persistent pain associated with reflex sympathetic dystrophy and postherpetic neuralgia may respond well to sympathetic anesthetic blocks, such as a stellate ganglion block.[5] Injections of corticosteroids into joints, the spinal canal (epidural), and the soft tissues are useful in reducing pain and inflammation and may be used in conjunction with other conservative methods.[7] Biofeedback, relaxation techniques, psychologic therapy, and other nonpharmacologic measures of pain relief are also useful adjuncts to pain management.[8]

The use of alternative and complementary health modalities is on the rise. It has been estimated that approximately 15 million adults use herbal products and megavitamins concurrently with prescription medications. Patients often do not disclose the use of these products to their health care provider, thus placing them at risk for untoward adverse drug reactions.[9] The health care practitioner should assess use of herbal and vitamin therapies each time a medication history is obtained. It is imperative that practitioners maintain an open line of communication with patients regarding self-care practices and health beliefs in order to develop an efficacious, acceptable, and safe plan of care.

Some sources suggest that the use of vitamin and herbal therapies may be helpful in the management of chronic pain. Before recommending such therapies, it is important to carefully research the empirical data regarding the use of these alternative and complementary therapies and to evaluate their validity, reliability, and potential for interactions with any prescription medications taken by the patient. As with all therapeutic treatment options, the risk-benefit ratio must be considered.

PHYSICAL MODALITIES

Cryotherapy (cold) can be used to control postoperative pain and, initially, to control pain after musculoskeletal and soft tissue injuries. Chronic problems such as muscle spasm, trigger points, bursitis, and tendinitis also respond well to cold. Hydrotherapy, hot packs, paraffin baths, and ultrasound are all types of therapeutic heat that are useful in pain relief.[8] Transcutaneous electrical nerve stimulation units may benefit patients with postoperative pain and acute pain syndromes. Acupuncture and therapeutic massage have also been shown to be effective in providing pain relief. Interested patients should be referred to a qualified acupuncturist or massage therapist.[10] Prescribing practitioners should be knowledgeable about the various contraindications associated with physical modalities.

THERAPEUTIC EXERCISE

The main goal of therapeutic exercise is mobilization of the patient. The benefits of exercise include preventing or minimizing complications of immobility such as skin breakdown, pneumonia, atrophy, contractures, and deconditioning. Therapeutic exercise should begin when the patient is medically stable. Initially, patients are encouraged to remain out of bed for short periods. Gradually, these periods are increased in length and frequency. A reconditioning program should then be instituted. Isometric and isotonic exercises can be used in conjunction with a gentle strengthening regimen. As the patient's endurance increases, ambulation and transfer training should begin with functional transfers to the wheelchair and commode. With improvement in stamina and mobility, stair training can usually be initiated. The use of exercise bikes and treadmills also aids in improving conditioning and endurance. Later, outdoor ambulation and higher level transfers with a cane, walker, or other assistive device may be tried.

Home evaluations by occupational and physical therapists are useful in identifying equipment needs, environmental and architectural barriers, or other safety hazards within the patient's home. These evaluations, in conjunction with family training sessions, offer additional insights into caregivers' abilities to assist the patient. Patient and family expectations for discharge from the inpatient setting may be unrealistic, and observing the patient function in the home setting may help to create a more realistic picture of abilities.

INDICATIONS FOR REFERRAL/HOSPITALIZATION

A referral to the physiatrist should be considered after any major medical illness or injury that results in severe impairment and disability with profound limitation of function. Patients with multiple concomitant medical problems and chronic pain syndromes with significant limitations should also be referred. Physiatrists are also skilled in electrodiagnostic testing such as electromyography. Patients who require expensive orthotic/prosthetic devices for footdrop or amputation will also benefit from physiatric evaluation. The physiatrist can aid in cost containment by determining whether patients require standardized "off the shelf" equipment vs. customized prescriptions for complex bracing, wheelchair and seating systems, or other appropriate adaptive equipment, thus avoiding unnecessary or inappropriate expenditure of resources.

Early rehabilitation is essential to maximize and maintain the functional abilities of the disabled patient. Individuals with disabilities can enjoy a higher quality of life with an appropriate rehabilitation program.

REFERENCES

1. U.S. Department of Health and Human Services: (Fact Sheet) HHS programs serve Americans with disabilities, Retrieved December 29, 2001 from the World Wide Web: http://www.hhs.gov/news/press/2001pres/01fsdisabilities.html.
2. Stein SA, O'Young B, Young MA: The person, disablement, and the process of rehabilitation. In O'Young B, Young MA, Stein SA, editors: *Physical medicine and rehabilitation secrets*, St Louis, 1996, Mosby.
3. Ottenbacher KJ and others: The reliability of the functional independence measure: a quantitative review, *Arch Phys Rehabil Med* 77(12):1226-1232, 1996.
4. Goddard MJ, Dean BZ, King JC: Basic science, acute pain, and neuropathic pain, *Arch Phys Rehabil Med* 75(5 Spec No):S4-S8, 1994.
5. Dean BZ and others: Therapeutic options in pain management, *Arch Phys Rehabil Med* 75(5 Spec No):S21-S30, 1994.
6. McCaffery M, Pasero C: *Pain: clinical manual*, St Louis, 1999, Mosby.
7. Tan JC: *Practical manual of physical medicine and rehabilitation*, St Louis, 1998, Mosby.
8. Williams FH, Maly BJ: Cancer pain, pelvic pain, and age-related considerations, *Arch Phys Rehabil Med* 75(5 Spec No):S15-S20, 1994.
9. Eisenberg DM: Advising patients who seek alternative medical therapies, *Ann Intern Med* 121:61-69, 1997.
10. Giusto J, Helms JM: Acupuncture. In O'Young B, Young MA, Steins SA, editors: *Physical medicine and rehabilitation secrets*, St Louis, 1996, Mosby.

CHAPTER 16

Sleep Disorders

Marianne Kelly

Disorders of sleep result in an enormous loss of work time, increased employer costs because of accidents, marked social impairment, and even loss of life. Given the rapid development of this field, primary care providers are increasingly obligated to recognize symptoms of sleep disorders to make accurate diagnoses, sound referrals, and successful treatment plans in collaboration with sleep disorders specialists.

In this chapter an overview of normal sleep is presented along with a description of the most common of the 84 currently described disorders of sleep.[1] These disorders are organized according to overarching symptom categories to facilitate improved history-taking skills in primary care providers. Sleep disorders tend to manifest with symptoms of (1) insomnia or poor sleep quality, (2) excessive daytime somnolence, or (3) active sleep behaviors or abnormal physiology-disrupting sleep (parasomnias). These symptom categories may occur alone or in combination, and they serve as a guide to obtaining a detailed history and the ordering of essential diagnostic procedures.

Normal Sleep

DEFINITION/EPIDEMIOLOGY

Sleep is far from a unitary phenomenon. Every night, normal human sleep cycles through three to five stages depending on the patient's age. Sleep stages unfold in a predictable, repeated sequence as a result of the influences of circadian (24-hour) and ultradian (less than 24-hour, often 90-minute) biologic rhythms. This nightly progression is referred to as sleep architecture.

Sleep may be divided into roughly two types: rapid eye movement (REM) sleep and non-REM (NREM) sleep. NREM sleep has four stages or levels of depth that, along with REM sleep, show characteristic EEG patterns. Stage 1 NREM sleep may be little more than a transition into sleep without genuine restorative value; it occupies only a small percentage of the total sleep period. Stage 2 NREM sleep is the workhorse of the system and occupies the greatest portion of the night. Stages 3 and 4 NREM sleep are referred to collectively as delta sleep. Delta sleep is prominent in young children and is the reason they may be difficult to arouse, especially in the first half of the night. Delta sleep may be entirely absent in older adults and, although its restorative value is considerable, may be unnecessary for satisfactory daytime functioning.

REM sleep occupies 15% to 25% of the sleep period in adults and is associated with marked changes in physiology throughout the body, including profound skeletal muscle atonia. This is the stage of sleep in which heart rate, blood pressure, respiration, and autonomic function are considerably less stable. It is also the stage of sleep during which most, but not all, dreaming occurs. REM sleep shows marked sensitivity (suppression) to the effects of medication, particularly antidepressants and other psychoactive drugs, and to anxiety, such as that engendered by the atypical environment of the sleep laboratory.

Normal total sleep time varies considerably with age.[2,3] Although young children require longer sleep times, total sleep time begins to decline by the second decade, remains relatively stable from the third decade through the fifth decade, and falls off more dramatically after age 70. Healthy adults in their 70s may require as little as 4.5 to 5 hours of sleep per night to feel well rested. Judgments about adequate sleep should be made on the basis of a patient's subjective waking sense of well-being, not by a rigid formula.

The circadian rhythms of several neurotransmitters and hormones are strong regulators of sleep-wake cycles. Thus the timing and amount of sleep are influenced by complex interactions between the underlying biologic rhythms and the length of time since the last sleep period. Average human circadian cycles naturally run approximately 25.5 hours but are reset daily to a 24-hour rhythm by a variety of environmental cues, the most important of which is exposure to sunlight. Other circadian cues include work schedules, timing of meals, and social activities.

Normal human sleep is nocturnal; more than 80% of night shift workers can be expected to experience abnormal sleep. These workers tend to get 2 to 4 fewer hours of sleep each night; because of the influence of circadian rhythms, this pattern does not tend to improve over long periods of night work.

Insomnia and Nonrestorative Sleep

DEFINITION/EPIDEMIOLOGY

During any single year, 35% of Americans will report 2 or more weeks of insomnia.[4] Moreover, many patients who are labeled as having insomnia actually have another occult sleep disorders with insomnia as a prominent symptom. With both acute and chronic insomnia, the alternatives to the benzodiazepine hypnotics are effective and should be considered first-line treatments.

Many cases of insomnia may be ultimately diagnosed as either psychophysiologic insomnia (PI) or a circadian rhythm disorder, most commonly delayed sleep phase syndrome (DSPS). Patients with PI complain of difficulty initiating and/or maintaining sleep during a normal sleep period, whereas patients with DSPS have an entrenched propensity for normal sleep quantity and quality at an abnormal time. The pathophysiology of PI (learned anxiety regarding potential inability to sleep coupled with body tension) is manifest in sleep architecture that is abnormally light for the patient's age (i.e., more stage 1 sleep), highly fragmented, and inefficient. The individual with PI spends more time in bed, with greater amounts of wake time needed to achieve increasingly limited total sleep. In contrast, the pathophysiology of DSPS (inability to sleep at normal clock times, with normal sleep occurring late, such as 4 AM to noon) may involve an atypically long circadian cycle that runs considerably longer than a 24-hour day.

Advanced sleep phase syndrome (ASPS) is a less common circadian rhythm disorder, with normal sleep quantity and quality occurring early in the 24-hour day (e.g., 6 PM to 2 AM). It appears to be most common in older adults.

Other common sleep disorders that may result in either insomnia or excessive daytime somnolence (EDS) are restless legs syndrome (RLS) and periodic limb movement disorder (PLMD). These two disorders are often, but not always, found simultaneously in the same patient. The pathophysiology of these disorders involves abnormal sensory (in RLS) or motor (in PLMD) activity in the limbs, most commonly the legs.

CLINICAL PRESENTATION AND DIAGNOSTICS

Polysomnography (PSG) typically contributes little to the diagnosis or treatment of patients with PI or circadian rhythm disorders and therefore should not be the first step in the diagnosis of insomnia. Other primary sleep disorders masquerading as garden variety "insomnia" must first be excluded by a careful history. Detailed information on the timing and amount of sleep is then obtained.

The assessment of insomnia is incomplete without obtaining from the patient a sleep log that covers a minimum of 2 weeks. The log should contain the following information for each night: time of getting into bed, time lights are actually turned out (e.g., after television, reading), estimate of sleep latency (time to begin sleep after lights out), estimate of the number of awakenings and total awake time across the night, time of final awakening, and time of actual arising. These data are essential in treatment planning.

The patient with RLS complains of annoying, "creepy-crawly" sensations in the legs or, less commonly, the arms. These sensations begin when the patient relaxes in bed and attempts to sleep and are relieved only by movement. Less commonly these sensations develop in the evening when the patient sits in a chair. RLS may delay sleep onset by as much as several hours.

With PLMD, the patient may be unaware of the symptom while the bed partner notes rhythmic or periodic leg jerks or twitches occurring every 20 to 60 seconds. The motion typically involves dorsiflexion of the foot at the ankle joint and flexion of the knee. Patients with insomnia may awaken from one of these movements without realizing the cause for the awakening. Conversely, patients with EDS may experience severe and repeated fragmentation of the sleep state secondary to periodic leg movements without any awareness of the sleep disruption.

The night shift worker often complains of short and fragmented daytime sleep and may also complain of dangerous sleepiness during the work shift. These patients are at high risk for accidents and must be evaluated thoroughly and treated aggressively.

MANAGEMENT

Skilled treatment protocols often avoid medication altogether. Behavioral therapies for PI have demonstrated strong success, are remarkably brief, and should be considered before medication, especially in patients with chronic insomnia. Behavioral therapies include sleep restriction therapy, stimulus control, and relaxation training.[5] These therapies are often combined on a case-by-case basis. Training in behavioral therapy for insomnia is available to primary care providers in brief continuing education courses, and a referral to a psychologist familiar with the use of these therapies should be readily available in urban communities.

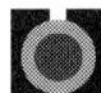

Differential Diagnosis

Insomnia

Psychophysiologic insomnia
Sleep apnea (obstructive or central)
Periodic limb movement disorder and/or restless legs syndrome
Delayed sleep phase syndrome or advanced sleep phase syndrome (circadian rhythm disorders)
Shift work sleep disorder

When medication is deemed necessary for the patient with PI, first-line therapy should often be a low-dose, sedating antidepressant such as trazodone (25 to 50 mg or higher as needed), amitriptyline (10 to 50 mg), or doxepin (10 to 50 mg). The high degree of success achieved with these medications means that habit-forming benzodiazepines can comfortably be considered second-line therapies and used only in selected acute situations.

Bright light therapy has become the treatment of choice for most patients with DSPS and ASPS. The timing and duration of exposure to the lights are critical factors in successful treatment. Improper light levels or duration of exposure may cause retinal or macular damage, and a poorly timed exposure may actually worsen the patient's symptoms. Until this treatment modality achieves greater standardization via large, research-based protocols, it is wise to involve a sleep disorders specialist in the use of bright lights for circadian rhythm disorders. It should be noted that hypnotic medication constitutes ineffective and inappropriate treatment for DSPS and ASPS.

Treatment options for the patient with RLS or PLMD are varied and highly individualized. Several categories of medications may make a contribution, including dopaminergically active compounds (e.g., carbidopa/levodopa, bromocriptine, pergolide), clonazepam, gabapentin, and minor narcotics (e.g., propoxyphene or acetaminophen with codeine). RLS and PLMD are often worsened by antidepressants.

The limited and fragmented daytime sleep of the night shift worker is difficult to treat. Black curtains on the bedroom window to ensure full darkness contribute to remarkable improvement in some patients, no doubt because of modulation of the circadian drive for wakefulness. It is essential that inappropriate social demands on the patient, such as expectations for child care and family errands, be eliminated. A low-dose hypnotic medication may occasionally be required.

PSG is warranted when well-selected treatment protocols for insomnia fail to achieve their expected results. PSG then functions as an important check for RLS, PLMD, or sleep apnea not apparent in the clinical history.

Excessive Daytime Somnolence

DEFINITION/EPIDEMIOLOGY

Considering the known prevalence rates of narcolepsy, other hypersomnias, and sleep apnea, as well as estimates of the prevalence of milder forms of obstructive sleep-disordered breathing, it could be speculated that the overall prevalence of excessive daytime somnolence is as high as 10% of the adult population. Proper evaluation of the patient with EDS requires a careful history and almost always involves PSG.

The pathophysiology of EDS can be thought of as originating from one of two sources. A normal central nervous system (CNS) sleep system may be compromised by physiologic events that repeatedly fragment sleep, such as sleep apnea or PLMD. Alternatively, there may be a CNS deficit that results in a sleep-wake system that is inadequate for maintaining wakefulness and/or overactive in maintaining sleep (e.g., as in narcolepsy).

Narcolepsy is a CNS-based disorder with derangements in components of both REM and NREM sleep. The normal skeletal muscle paralysis of REM sleep may express itself inappropriately during the waking state, resulting in troublesome or dangerous symptoms. Idiopathic CNS hypersomnia also involves CNS sleep system dysfunction, which results in profound EDS. However, with idiopathic CNS hypersomnia, there is no known disease of the REM system, and other symptoms present in narcolepsy are absent. Approximately one third of the cases of idiopathic CNS hypersomnia seem to be genetic; one third may be postviral, and one third are truly idiopathic. Posttraumatic hypersomnia follows closed head injury or other CNS insult.

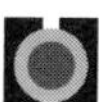

Differential Diagnosis

Excessive Daytime Somnolence

Caused By Sleep-Wake System Deficit
Narcolepsy
Idiopathic CNS hypersomnia
Posttraumatic hypersomnia

Caused By Fragmentation of Sleep
Obstructive or central sleep apnea
Restless legs syndrome
Periodic limb movement disorder

CLINICAL PRESENTATION AND DIAGNOSTICS

Assessment of the patient with EDS usually begins when clinic staff note the patient's unplanned nap in the waiting room. The history includes nodding off involuntarily in a variety of situations including work, noisy family gatherings, conversations and, of most concern, driving. A key piece of history is the frequency of dozing while waiting for traffic lights to change. Information obtained from a family member can be essential to accurate diagnosis, because patients with EDS often deny or minimize the severity of their symptoms. Related complaints include waking up fatigued despite 8 or more hours of unbroken sleep and falling asleep early in the day, such as while reading the morning newspaper.

The history should distinguish among the EDS disorders and must include total sleep time in 24 hours; quantity and duration of nocturnal sleep and daytime naps; presence of snoring and witnessed apneas; awakenings with shortness of breath, choking, or gasping; cataplexy (sudden loss of muscle tone subsequent to strong emotion); restless leg symptoms; active sleep behaviors; a psychiatric history or symptoms; and past and current substance use patterns.

The history of obstructive sleep apnea (OSA) comprises snoring, witnessed apneas, and EDS. The more recently recognized form of sleep-disordered breathing, known as upper airway resistance syndrome (UARS), is a common cause of EDS, impaired daytime functioning, and often vague, depressive symptoms.[6,7] It most commonly involves snoring without apneas, a high degree of sleep fragmentation secondary to snoring and partial airway obstruction, and EDS.

The history of narcolepsy comprises EDS and usually includes most, if not all, of four other symptoms: cataplexy, hypnagogic hallucinations, sleep paralysis, and fragmented, disturbed nocturnal sleep. Cataplexy is thought to be the inappropriate expression of REM atonia during the active waking state, whereas in sleep paralysis the normal atonia of the final REM period of the night may not stop immediately on awakening, which briefly leaves the patient with only eye muscle and diaphragmatic movement. Although the latter two symptoms are naturally terrifying to the patient, there is actually no danger from sleep paralysis because the patient is safely in bed. Hypnagogic hallucinations are dreamlike and often frightening fragments that occur near sleep onset and typically involve patient confusion about whether he or she is awake or asleep.

The history of idiopathic CNS hypersomnia is typically that of unduly long sleep periods (12 hours or more), profound daytime EDS, and none of the other features of narcolepsy.

When the history clearly suggests OSA, a nocturnal PSG may be sufficient for diagnosis. In the absence of a typical OSA history (snoring, witnessed apneas, and EDS), multiple sleep latency testing (MSLT) is warranted and should be ordered in consultation with a sleep disorders specialist, who is responsible for ensuring that the studies most likely to answer the diagnostic questions are performed.

The MSLT is a study of the propensity for daytime sleep. It also is a careful screen for the presence of abnormally occurring REM sleep during daytime naps—an essential sign of narcolepsy. Because of the strong influence of circadian rhythms on the timing and duration of sleep stages, proper scheduling of the PSG and MSLT—with attention to the patient's normal sleep and work routines—may be essential for correct diagnosis, and therefore the role of the sleep specialist cannot be overstated.

Portable equipment for home PSG is available and should be used with caution because great variability exists in the quality of these studies. This service is best provided by a sleep disorders center that can carefully select appropriate patients for either laboratory or home study.

MANAGEMENT

EDS as a result of CNS-based disorders is treated with psychostimulants (e.g., dextroamphetamine, methylphenidate, and pemoline). A non–habit-forming stimulant known as modafinil has been released and offers an option for these patients. Cataplexy is treated by suppressing aspects of REM sleep with an antidepressant, which may in some cases also contribute to a reduction in EDS.

Obstructive sleep apnea and UARS may be treated with nasal continuous positive airway pressure or, in select patients with mild to moderate disease, with a dental appliance designed to increase posterior airway dimensions. Less commonly, appropriate treatment choices may include tracheostomy or, in patients who have undergone a careful preoperative evaluation, maxillofacial surgery.

Parasomnias

DEFINITION/EPIDEMIOLOGY

The parasomnias are a fascinating group of disorders of the arousal process or of specific sleep stages. These disorders result in either abnormal and potentially dangerous behaviors that occur during sleep (e.g., sleepwalking) or abnormal physiology (e.g., REM sleep-related cardiac arrhythmias).[4] Pathophysiology varies greatly across this group. In the case of NREM parasomnias (e.g., sleepwalking, sleep terrors), the mechanism is an abrupt and abnormal arousal from delta sleep. In contrast, REM-sleep parasomnias derive from the loss of normal REM muscle atonia, which results in a patient who "acts out" dreams, often in a highly dangerous fashion. Pathophysiology in nightmares may be physiologic (medication induced or possibly caused by abnormal brainstem mechanisms in the REM-generating system) or psychologic.

CLINICAL PRESENTATION AND DIAGNOSTICS

Patients with parasomnias often experience dangerous or frightening events during sleep. A careful history is helpful in distinguishing NREM parasomnias from REM parasomnias and aids the polysomnographer in planning the most appropriate study. Sleep-related seizures are an important diagnosis that must be excluded on virtually every such patient.

Sleepwalking is a disorder of delta sleep and, because of the circadian propensity for delta sleep in the first half of the night, most commonly occurs within the first 2 to 3 hours of the night. It may involve benign or comical behaviors or may include complex behaviors such as fixing a meal, loading a gun, or driving a car. Sleepwalking is common in childhood and should, at a minimum, be evaluated by PSG if treatment has failed or if dangerous behaviors are occurring. PSG should be routinely included in the workup of adult sleepwalkers.

Sleep-related eating disorders are probably a variant of sleepwalking. Patients with these disorders do little else other than head for the kitchen, where they often fix elaborate meals and occasionally eat inappropriate or uncooked foods. Such patients show no memory for their eating behaviors. There are no associated daytime eating disorder symptoms, such as distorted body image or bingeing/purging.

Patients experiencing sleep terrors, another NREM parasomnia, classically sit bolt upright in bed with a loud scream, may flee from the bed in an apparent panic, and may sustain or cause serious injury. Such patients are typically frightened and disoriented for some time and are difficult to wake to full consciousness. It is often best to gently guide the sleepwalker or suggest that he or she return to bed, without active interference in the behaviors unless injuries are likely. In the morning, patients with NREM parasomnias typically have no memory of their activities.

A total of 30% to 40% of patients with panic disorder experience panic attacks (PAs) at some point in their lifetime that arise out of sleep.[4] These attacks tend to occur during descending stage 2 sleep. Some patients have only sleep-related attacks and never experience a daytime PA.

With REM parasomnias, a patient whose dreams were once benign and nondisturbing now complains of vivid and violent nightmares. There is associated physical activity that often parallels the recalled dream content and may be violent or dangerous. In some cases these patients are diagnosed in the intensive care unit while undergoing treatment for severe injuries sustained during an episode. Bed partners are also at risk for injury.

REM sleep-related cardiac sinus arrest has been described.[1] A high index of suspicion is required to detect cardiac arrhythmias that occur only during sleep and result in vague or nonclassic cardiac symptoms such as choking, shortness of breath, or nausea. A sleep disorders consultation offers the possibility of linking the onset of an arrhythmia to a particular type or stage of sleep. This opens the door to medical options targeted at altering the sleep stage in addition to using specific cardiac drugs.

Proper evaluation of parasomnias, particularly those associated with active or dangerous sleep behaviors, warrants prompt consultation with a sleep disorders specialist. A PSG is required for definitive diagnosis and treatment planning. Home PSG is inappropriate in these cases because the video monitoring available in the laboratory is mandatory for such patients.

MANAGEMENT

Treatment options for the NREM parasomnias include medical, psychologic, and behavioral therapies, which are selected on a case-by-case basis. Sleep terrors may be associated with high levels of anxiety that respond well to psychotherapy. Sleepwalking can be successfully treated with hypnosis and with medication.[8] Clonazepam effectively suppresses delta sleep and should be considered for use in the sleepwalker who demonstrates dangerous behaviors or is unable to sleep in a room on the first floor. Antidepressants seem to be helpful in some patients, but their mechanism of action is unknown. Sleep-related eating disorders have only recently been described and should be managed in collaboration with a sleep disorders specialist. Sleep-related PAs are treated in the same fashion as daytime PAs.

The symptoms of REM parasomnias respond promptly to clonazepam in 90% of cases.[4] Dosing is begun at 0.5 mg at bedtime and is titrated upward as needed, generally to a maximum

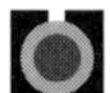

Differential Diagnosis

Parasomnias

NREM sleep
Sleepwalking
Sleep terrors
Sleep-related panic attacks
Sleep-related eating disorders
REM sleep
REM behavior disorders
Nightmares
REM-related cardiac arrhythmias
REM-related painful penile erections

dose of 2 mg at bedtime. Patients who do not respond to clonazepam treatment may respond to carbamazepine, gabapentin, or dopaminergically active compounds.

Behavioral therapies for nightmares show dramatic results.[9] A referral to a psychologist familiar with this treatment is a must for the patient who has impaired daytime functioning because of nightmares.

REFERENCES

1. American Sleep Disorders Association: *International classification of sleep disorders,* Rochester, Minn, 1990, The Association.
2. Williams RL, Karacan I, Hursh CJ: *EEG of human sleep: clinical applications,* New York, 1974, Wiley & Sons.
3. Sheldon S: *Pediatric sleep medicine,* Philadelphia, 1992, WB Saunders.
4. Kryger MH, Roth T, Dement WC: *Principles and practice of sleep medicine,* Philadelphia, 1994, WB Saunders.
5. Morin CM, Culbert JP, Schwartz SM: Nonpharmacological interventions for insomnia: a meta-analysis of treatment efficacy, *Am J Psychiatry* 151:1172-1180, 1994.
6. Guilleminault C and others: A cause of excessive daytime sleepiness: the upper airway resistance syndrome, *Chest* 104:781-787, 1993.
7. Guilleminault C and others: Upper airway sleep-disordered breathing in women, *Ann Intern Med* 122:493-501, 1995.
8. Hurwitz TD and others: A retrospective outcome study and review of hypnosis as treatment of adults with sleepwalking and sleep terror, *J Nerv Ment Dis* 179:228-233, 1991.
9. Krakow B and others: Imagery rehearsal treatment for chronic nightmares, *Behav Res Ther* 7:837-843, 1995.

PART 3

Health Maintenance

JOANN TRYBULSKI, Section Editor

CHAPTER 17

Screening for Cancer

Cynthia Erskine Bashaw

DEFINITION/EPIDEMIOLOGY

Cancer is the second most common cause of death in the United States, accounting for one in every four deaths.[1] Regular screening can result in the detection of certain cancers at earlier stages, when treatment is more likely to be successful. Early detection has been shown to improve survival rates for cancers of the breast, colon, rectum, cervix, prostate, testes, oral cavity, and skin.[2] These screening-accessible cancers account for approximately half of all new cancers.[1] By American Cancer Society (ACS) estimates, the current 81% 5-year survival rate for cancer could be increased to 95% if all Americans participated in regular cancer screenings.[1]

A cancer-related check-up is recommended every 3 years for people 20 to 39 years old and yearly for those 40 years and older.[2] Ideally, this check-up would be incorporated into the periodic health visit. However, many individuals do not schedule routine examinations, and therefore it is incumbent on the health care provider to address cancer-related screening issues during visits for other reasons. A thorough cancer-related check-up includes a complete history to screen for risk factors and early symptoms of disease and a thorough physical examination. Inspection of the skin, oral cavity, breasts, external genitalia, and cervix are essential, as are palpation of the breasts, oral cavity, thyroid, rectum, prostate, testes, ovaries, uterus, and lymph nodes. Health counseling regarding tobacco, sun exposure, diet and nutrition, risk factors, sexual practices, and environmental and occupational exposures should be incorporated into this visit.[2]

More specific guidelines exist for several of the screening-accessible cancers and are outlined in Table 17-1. Screening is defined as a means of accomplishing early detection of disease in asymptomatic people. Screening tests and procedures are usually not diagnostic but serve to sort out persons who are under suspicion for the presence of cancer from those who are not. Screening guidelines are developed in accordance with two requirements: (1) there must be evidence that a test or procedure will detect cancer earlier than if the cancer were detected as a result of the development of symptoms, and (2) there must be evidence that treatment at an earlier stage of the disease will result in an improved outcome.[3]

The following review of current cancer screening recommendations includes a discussion of risk factors for each disorder. Individuals at high risk for a particular disease may require a more aggressive screening approach than is recommended by the existing guidelines that have been developed for the general population.

TABLE 17-1 Summary of American Cancer Society Screening Recommendations

Type of Cancer	Test/Examination	Frequency	Population
Breast	Mammogram	Annually	Women ≥40 years old
	BSE	Monthly	Women ≥20 years old
	Clinical breast examination	Every 3 years	Women 20 to 39 years old
		Annually	Women ≥40 years old
Colorectal	1. FOBT	Annually	Men and women ≥50 years old
	or		
	2. Sigmoidoscopy*	Every 5 years	
	3. Combination of options 1 and 2 (preferred by ACS)		
	or		
	4. Double contrast barium enema*	Every 5 years	
	or		
	5. Colonoscopy*	Every 10 years	
Cervical/pelvic examination and Pap test	All women who are or have been sexually active or who have reached the age of 18 years; after three or more consecutive satisfactory normal annual examinations, the Pap test may be performed less frequently at the discretion of the physician		
Prostate	PSA and DRE	Offer annually with information regarding risks and benefits	Men ≥50 years old with a life expectancy of at least 10 years; begin screening at age 45 years for men at high risk

Source: American Cancer Society's Cancer Facts and Figures—2001.

*A digital rectal examination should be done at the same time as a sigmoidoscopy, colonoscopy, or double-contrast barium enema.

It is recommended that screening guidelines be incorporated into a cancer-related check-up every 3 years for people 20 to 39 years of age and every year for people 40 years of age and older. This check-up should include examinations for cancer of the thyroid, oral cavity, skin, lymph nodes, testes, prostate, and ovaries, as well as health counseling about tobacco, sun exposure, diet and nutrition, risk factors, sexual practices, and occupational exposures.

BREAST CANCER

Breast cancer is the most commonly diagnosed noncutaneous cancer in women and is second only to lung cancer as a cause of cancer deaths in women.[2] It is one of the few cancers for which the benefits of screening, namely mammography, have been unequivocally demonstrated. Tumors of the breast typically metastasize late in the preclinical course or before reaching clinically detectable size. Early detection in the preclinical phase (before metastasis) is possible with mammography, which can detect tumors as small as 1 mm.[4] Large-scale clinical trials have repeatedly shown reductions in breast cancer mortality with regular mammography, and its value as a screening tool is undisputed.[5-8]

Regarding the age range for which regular mammography is appropriate, there is little dispute regarding its value for women between 40 and 70 years of age. The effects can be identified within 10 years after the start of screening for women 40 to 49 years of age and sooner for older women.[8] Meta-analysis examining outcomes from every randomized trial of mammography shows a 25% to 30% reduction in the chance of dying from breast cancer with annual screenings after age 50 years.[7] Data are similar for screening between ages 40 and 50 years.[6-8] There are no data showing a benefit for screening before age 40 years or for performing a baseline mammogram for women in this age range.[7] Although the benefit is less clear and less well studied in women over 70 years, it must be remembered that the annual risk of a 70-year-old being diagnosed with breast cancer is three times that of a 40-year-old and that she has a five times greater annual risk of dying from breast cancer. There are currently no recommendations for stopping mammography at any particular age.[7,8]

ACS guidelines are for annual screening mammography beginning at age 40 years. As cessation of annual screening is not age related but a function of co-morbidity, no age at which screening should be terminated can be specified.[2]

In addition to mammography, a breast self-examination (BSE) is recommended monthly for women 20 years of age and older. A clinical breast examination is recommended every 3 years for women 20 to 39 years of age and annually for those 40 years and older.[2] BSE has not been linked definitively with lowering mortality, but generally women who examine their breasts regularly are familiar with their breasts and are more likely to discover smaller tumors at earlier stages, when more conservative treatment options are possible.[4,7,8] Clinical breast examination is widely used and is particularly important in the 40- to 49-year-old range.[4-6] Some palpable breast cancers are not visible on mammograms, particularly in the dense breasts of younger women.[4,6,8] The ACS's landmark Breast Cancer Detection Demonstration Project found that each screening measure detected cancers not initially found by the others, supporting the rationale for the use of mammography, clinical breast examination, and BSE.[4]

In assessing risk factors for breast cancer, it is important to recognize that approximately 75% of breast cancers occur in women without known risks aside from age and gender.[7] The risk is known to be higher for women who have a personal or family history of breast cancer, biopsy-confirmed atypical hyperplasia, early menarche and/or late menopause, nulliparity or history of first child after age 30, obesity after menopause, recent oral contraceptives or postmenopausal hormone replacement, or excessive alcohol consumption.[1] Possible links to breast density and physical inactivity are under study. Research regarding BRCA-1 and BRCA-2 susceptibility genes is ongoing. General screening of the population for these genes is not recommended.[1] Only 5% of breast cancers are related to these genes.[9] Those at high risk, particularly those with a strong multigenerational family history of breast cancer, may warrant an individualized plan of screening and follow-up monitoring.

COLORECTAL CANCER

Colorectal cancer is the third most common cancer among U.S. men and women.[1] When cancer of this type is confined to the colon-rectum, the 5-year survival rate is 90%. When it spreads to surrounding tissue, the 5-year survival rate falls to 65%.[2] Early detection is therefore critical. It must also be noted that prevention of colorectal cancer can be accomplished by removing colorectal adenomas, which are typically in the form of polyps. These adenomas are precursors to nearly every colorectal cancer and are usually present for several years before their evolution to cancer. With proper screening they are often detected and can be removed before becoming cancerous.[10]

ACS screening guidelines recommend that all men and women have one of the following beginning at age 50 years: (1) annual fecal occult blood test (FOBT), (2) flexible sigmoidoscopy every 5 years, (3) FOBT annually and flexible sigmoidoscopy every 5 years, (4) double-contrast barium enema every 5 years, or (5) colonoscopy every 10 years. It is also recommended that a digital rectal examination (DRE) be performed at the same time as the sigmoidoscopy, barium enema, or colonoscopy.[2] Although there may be benefits to performing the DRE more often for other purposes (e.g., a bimanual pelvic or prostate examination) there is no added benefit in detecting colorectal cancer by DRE more often.[11]

The choice between the recommended options is made on an individual basis with an eye toward enhancing compliance. Low rates of screening for this type of cancer continue, with the ACS reporting that in 1999 only 19.1% of those 50 years and older had undergone FOBT within the preceding year and that only 32.3% had undergone sigmoidoscopy or colonoscopy within the previous 5 years.[2]

The ACS prefers the combination of FOBT annually and sigmoidoscopy every 5 years. Combined testing is better than one or the other alone. FOBT potentially detects blood from lesions anywhere in the colon, including areas that are beyond the reach of the sigmoidoscope, whereas the sigmoidoscopy is superior for detecting lesions in the distal colon and for detecting nonbleeding lesions.[10]

FOBT is accomplished via the collection and testing of six samples from three consecutive stools and has been shown to decrease the risk of death from colon cancer by one third.[10] Because it requires an annual commitment and the inconvenience of eliminating aspirin and nonsteroidal antiinflammatory drugs, red meat, and vitamin C several days before the test, compliance issues are a consideration.

The flexible sigmoidoscopy, when preformed every 5 years, also shows a significant reduction in mortality. Although it allows only for visualization of the distal portion of the colon (because adenomas are often multiple and most typically arise in the lower colon), it identifies 80% of people who have significant neoplasms in the colon.[10] The main drawback is that positive findings must be followed up by a colonoscopy.

The colonoscopy is considered the standard and may be performed at intervals of 10 years. It is the most sensitive test because it allows for direct visualization of the entire colon; however, it is associated with a higher degree of risk than other methods and is more expensive.[10] The double-contrast barium enema is a lower cost alternative and, like the colonoscopy, examines the entire colon. However, it is less effective in detecting small lesions, hence the recommendation of the shorter 5-year interval for screening.[10] Another drawback is that, unlike the colonoscopy, it does not allow for excision of suspicious areas during the same procedure. Both colonoscopy and double-contrast barium enema allow for the elimination of annual FOBT.[2]

The DRE is useful for the identification of masses in the anal canal and lower rectum but has poor sensitivity because of limited reach and is not recommended as sole screening for colorectal cancer. In addition, occult blood testing of stool obtained on the glove should not substitute for the three-stool FOBT protocol because bleeding is often intermittent and not present throughout the whole stool.[10]

Computed tomography colonography and molecular screening of stool DNA are methods being evaluated as potential screening tools. These are not currently ready for widespread clinical application.[10]

Individuals are classified as having an elevated risk of developing colorectal cancer if there is a history of a first-degree relative having developed colon cancer or adenomatous polyps before age 60 years, a history of more than one first-degree relative having been affected at any age, a personal history of adenomatous polyps, a history of inflammatory bowel disease, or a family history of a hereditary colorectal cancer syndrome.[10] People in this category of risk should consult with a gastroenterologist and begin screening earlier and/or undergo screening more often. Other risk factors include age (90% are more than 50 years of age), high-fat/low-fiber diet, and physical inactivity.[1] It is important to recognize, however, that 80% to 85% of all colorectal cancers occur among people with no increased risk except for age.[10]

CERVICAL CANCER

Cervical cancer accounts for 6% of all cancers in women.[12] It has been estimated that 12,900 new cases of cervical cancer would be diagnosed in 2001 and that 4900 women would die of the disease.[1] The tragedy of these figures is that cervical cancer is one of the most successfully treated cancers when detected early. The 5-year survival rate for early invasive cervical cancer is 92%.[2] In addition, cervical cancer has a long lead time and progresses through a series of identifiable, premalignant stages before becoming invasive. Detection of these precancerous changes allows for a variety of treatment options when the disorder is almost certainly curable, thereby decreasing not only mortality from cervical cancer but also its incidence.[6] Early detection of cervical cancer and its precursors depends largely on the Papanicolaou (Pap) test. With increasingly widespread use of this screening tool, deaths from cervical cancer decreased by more than 70% between 1950 and 1995.[13]

Current ACS guidelines recommend an annual Pap test and pelvic examination for women who are or have been sexually active or who have reached the age of 18 years. After three or more consecutive, normal, annual examinations, the Pap test may be performed less frequently at the discretion of the physician.[2] This guideline is consistent with recommendations from other organizations. In general, intervals of up to 3 years are considered acceptable for low-risk women. An upper age limit when such screening ceases to be effective is not known.[6,13] Indeed, the screening recommendations of the National Cancer Institute urge extra effort to reach older women who have not been screened. Of invasive cervical cancers, more than 25% occur in women older than 65 years. In all, 40% to 50% of those who die from cervical cancer are older than 65 years.[13] It should be noted, however, that after a normal Pap test in this age-group, the incidence of abnormal readings during the next 2 years has been shown to be very low; repeat testing within 2 years may not be indicated.[13] Finally, for women who have had a hysterectomy for benign disease, vaginal smears are not necessary or recommended.[13]

In determining an appropriate screening interval for any given woman, a consideration of her individual risk factors is essential. Most important, a causal link has been convincingly established between infection with the human papilloma virus (HPV) and subsequent development of cervical cancer.[6,14-16] HPV is sexually transmitted and is associated with certain sexual behaviors. Among those at risk are women with a history of sexual intercourse before age 16 years.[14] The adolescent cervix is believed to be more susceptible to carcinogenic stimuli because of the active process of squamous metaplasia occurring in the transformation zone during adolescence.[17] Also at risk are those who have had multiple sexual partners or whose partners have had multiple partners. Other risk factors include smoking, HIV infection, poor nutrition, lower socioeconomic status, previously abnormal Pap smear and DES exposure.[2,14]

In general, those with important risk factors should be considered for annual screening. This group includes smokers, those with sexual risk factors, and those with a previously abnormal Pap test. Women who have had a hysterectomy for malignancy and those with a history of DES exposure are at particularly high risk and warrant special consideration and screening at even more frequent intervals.[18]

Extending the interval may be reasonable for women with none of these risk factors. It should be kept in mind, however, that the rate of false-negative Pap smears has been estimated to be 30% or higher.[14,15] More frequent testing provides some measure of protection against missing a diagnosis for an extended period. Considering that a woman's level of risk depends not only on her own behavior but on that of her partner, the number of women who are truly at low risk may be very small.[17]

The advent of liquid-based cytology is promising because it has been shown to increase the sensitivity of detection of high- and low-grade cervical lesions over the conventional Pap test.[13] This type of cell collection is being used ever more widely and may eventually replace the conventional Pap smear. With an eye toward the future, an additional benefit of liquid-based cytology is that it is compatible with screening for HPV. Given the strong association between HPV and cervical cancer, the future may hold recommendations for adjunctive testing for this virus.[6,13]

PROSTATE CANCER

Prostate cancer is the most commonly diagnosed cancer in men, accounting for 29% of new male cancers.[19] It is a disease of aging and is rarely seen in men younger than 50 years of age. Indeed, more than 70% of cases are diagnosed in men older than 65 years, with 70 years the mean age at diagnosis.[19] Another major risk factor is race; the incidence of prostate cancer is 66% higher among African-American men than white men. The mortality rates are also higher.[1,19] Other risk factors include a positive family history and a diet high in animal fat.[1,19]

Considerable controversy exists with regard to screening. Data on screening are limited, and conflicting and professional organizations have not agreed on guidelines.[2] Although both DRE and the prostate-specific antigen (PSA) blood test have shown value for early detection, it is not clear that screening and treatment affect morbidity and mortality.[19] At issue is the concern that some PSA-detected cancers are latent or indolent and unlikely to affect survival. Some men, particularly older men, may well die of other causes before the disease presents itself.[19,20] There is considerable uncertainty about the efficacy of treatment, and sorting out patients for whom there is a clear risk of disease progression has been difficult.[19] In addition, benign prostatic hypertrophy (BPH) and prostatitis yield a high number of false-positives results. Indeed, 25% of men with BPH will have high readings. These men may be subjected to further invasive testing unnecessarily.[19,20]

In acknowledgement of these issues, the ACS specifies in its guidelines that men should be given information about the benefits and limitations of the tests so that an informed choice can be made. The guidelines state that, beginning at age 50 years, men with a life expectancy of at least 10 years should be offered both PSA and DRE annually. Men at high risk (African-American men and men with a first-degree relative who developed prostate cancer at a young age) should be offered screening beginning at age 45 years.[2,10]

TESTICULAR CANCER

It is estimated that 7600 new cases of testicular cancer will be diagnosed in 2001 and that 400 men will die of the disease.[1] Advances in treatment for testicular cancer have reduced mortality by 60% in recent years. The disease occurs most often in white men between 20 and 34 years of age. The most significant factor for developing testicular cancer is cryptorchidism.[21]

Testicular cancer typically presents as a painless lump or hardness of the testicle. Most testicular cancers are first detected by the patient, either unintentionally or by self-examination. Some are discovered on routine physical examination. No studies have been done to determine the effectiveness of testicular self-examination (TSE) or clinical testicular examination in reducing mortality. There is no medical evidence that TSE is any more effective than simple awareness and prompt medical evaluation.[21] The health care provider's main role in the early detection of testicular cancer may be simply fostering an awareness of symptoms among young men and encouraging prompt follow-up evaluation of abnormal findings.[10] It is still recommended that examination of the testicles be included in the routine cancer-related check-up.[2]

OROPHARYNGEAL CANCER

It is estimated that more than 30,000 new cases of oropharyngeal cancer will be diagnosed in 2001.[1] Cancer can affect any part of the oral cavity. Early detection is the key to successful management. Many early changes are either visible or palpable, providing an opportunity during routine examination of the mouth and pharynx to detect this cancer at an early, curable stage. Early lesions have a low propensity to metastasize, and most of these cancers are curable when detected and treated before reaching 2 cm in size.[22]

Signs and symptoms of oropharyngeal cancer include a nonhealing sore, a lump or thickening, or persistent leukoplakia or erythroplakia.[1,22] Particular attention should be directed to high-risk areas in the mouth, which include the floor of the mouth, the ventrolateral aspect of the tongue, and the soft palate complex. The incidence of oral cancer is highest in men and those more than 45 years old. Risk factors include tobacco use and excessive consumption of alcohol.[1,22] Examination of the oral cavity should be incorporated into the cancer screening examination.[2]

SKIN CANCER

Skin cancer is the most common cancer in the United States. The highly curable basal cell and squamous cell cancers are diagnosed in approximately 1 million people each year.[1] Malignant melanoma is far less common yet is responsible for 75% of deaths from skin cancer.[23] Risk factors include a fair complexion, large number of moles, a tendency to freckle, excessive exposure to ultraviolet radiation, a family history of melanoma, a personal or family history of dysplastic nevi, sunburn in childhood, and advancing age.[1,23]

Although data on mass screening of asymptomatic people do not show a reduction in mortality, there is evidence that survival from melanoma is influenced by excision when the tumor is thin.[23] Tumors excised at less that 0.75 mm are lethal in fewer than 5% of cases. By the time they have reached a thickness of 4 mm, they are lethal in more than 50% of cases.[24] There is a prolonged phase of horizontal growth during which the tumor expands horizontally beneath the epidermis before invading the dermis. This phase provides a window of opportunity for early detection and excision before the onset of vertical growth, which carries metastatic potential.[23]

Mortality rates from melanoma rose annually from 1973 to 1990 and have decreased or stabilized since then. It is widely hypothesized that this change may be due to prevention and/or early detection.[23] Although no specific recommendations for screening for skin cancer are supported by research, it is clear that early detection does improve survival. Thus it seems warranted to conduct a careful skin examination during the periodic health visit and to encourage individuals to examine their skin regularly and to report any suspicious lesions. Lesions suspicious for melanoma can be evaluated using the ABCD method. Lesions are examined for A (asymmetry), B (border irregularity), C (color variegation), and D (diameter enlarging to more than 6 mm). Any progressive or sudden change should signal concern.[1]

CONCLUSION

Cancer screening is a vital part of ongoing efforts to decrease cancer mortality. Its success depends on awareness and the use of available screening tools by both patients and caregivers. When integrated into a total approach focusing on healthy lifestyles and disease prevention, it has the potential to increase longevity and enhance quality of life.

REFERENCES

1. American Cancer Society: *Cancer facts and figures 2001,* Retrieved December 2001 from the World Wide Web: www.cancer.org.
2. American Cancer Society: *Cancer prevention and early detection, facts and figures 2001,* Retrieved December 2001 from the World Wide Web: www.cancer.org.
3. National Cancer Institute: *Screening for cancer (pdq): screening/detection for health professionals,* Retrieved December 2001 from the World Wide Web: www.cancernet.nci.nih.gov.
4. Crane R: Breast cancers. In Otto S: *Oncology nursing,* St Louis, 1997, Mosby.
5. Smart CR and others: Twenty-year follow-up of the breast cancers diagnosed during the breast cancer detection demonstration project, *CA Cancer J Clin* 47(3):134-149, 1997.
6. Smith RA and others: American cancer society guidelines for early detection of cancer 2000, *CA Cancer J Clin* 50(1):34-39, 2000, Retrieved December 2001 from the World Wide Web: www.ca-journal.org.
7. Lippman ME: Breast cancer. In Braunwald E and others: *Harrison's principles of internal medicine,* ed 15, New York, 2001, McGraw-Hill.
8. National Cancer Institute: *Screening for breast cancer (pdq), screening/ detection for health professionals,* Retrieved December 2001 from the World Wide Web: www.cancernet.nci.hih.gov.
9. Dixon JM and others: Breast cancer: non-metastatic. In Barton S and others, editors, *Clinical evidence,* ed 5, London, 2001, BMJ Publishing Group.
10. Smith RA *CA Cancer J Clin* 51(1): 2001, Retrieved December 2001 from the World Wide Web: www.ca-journal.org.
11. Herrinton LJ and others: Case-control study of digital-rectal screening in relation to mortality from cancer of the distal rectum, *Am J Epidemiol* 142(9):961-964, 1995.
12. National Cancer Institute: *Cervical cancer (pdq), treatment-health professionals,* Retrieved December 2001 from the World Wide Web: www.cancernet.nci.nih.gov.
13. National Cancer Institute: *Screening for cervical cancer (pdq), screening/detection-health professionals,* Retrieved December 2001 from the World Wide Web: www.cancernet.nci.nih.gov.
14. National Cancer Institute: *Cervical cancer (pdq), prevention-health professionals,* Retrieved December 2001 from the World Wide Web: www.cancernet.nci.nih.gov.
15. Anderson PS, Runowicz CD: Beyond the pap test: new techniques for cervical cancer screening, *Womens Health Primary Care* 4(12): 753-758, 2001.
16. Schiffman MH and others: Epidemiologic evidence showing that human papilloma virus infection causes most cervical intraepithelial neoplasia, *J Natl Cancer Inst* 85(12):958-964, 1993.
17. Savage EW, Parham GP: Cervical dysplasia and cancer. In Hacker NF, Moore JG: *Essentials of obstetrics and gynecology,* Philadelphia, 1992, WB Saunders.
18. Hatcher RA, Trussell J, Stewart F: *Contraceptive technology,* ed 16, New York, 1994, Irvington.
19. National Cancer Institute: *Screening for prostate cancer (pdq), screening/detection-health professionals,* Retrieved December 2001 from the World Wide Web: www.cancernet.nci.nih.gov.
20. National Cancer Institute: *Prostate cancer (pdq), prevention-health professionals, (On-Line),* Retrieved December 2001 from the World Wide Web: www.cancernet.nci.nih.gov.
21. National Cancer Institute: *Testicular cancer (pdq), screening/detection-health professionals,* Retrieved December 2001 from the World Wide Web: www.cancernet.nci.nih.gov.
22. Jackler RK, Kaplan MJ: Ear, nose, and throat. In Tierney LM, McPhee SJ, Papadakis MA: *Current medical diagnosis and treatment 2002,* ed 41,New York, 2002, Lange Medical Books/McGraw- Hill.
23. National Cancer Institute: *Skin cancer (pdq), screening/detection-health professionals,* Retrieved December 2001 from the World Wide Web: www.cancernet.nci.nih.gov.
24. Crosby T, Mason M, Crosby D: Malignant melanoma: non-metastatic. In Barton S and others, editors, *Clinical evidence,* ed 5, London,2001,BMJ Publishing group.

CHAPTER 18

Screening for Sexually Transmitted Diseases

Marilyn Bleiler Green

DEFINITION/EPIDEMIOLOGY

The term *sexually transmitted disease* (*STD*) includes the more than 25 diseases that are spread through sexual contact. Not including HIV, in the United States the most common STDs include chlamydia, gonorrhea, syphilis, genital herpes, human papilloma virus (HPV), and hepatitis B.

Despite efforts designed to promote safe sex practices, STDs, often referred to as the "hidden epidemic,"[1] continue to afflict a large number of people in the United States. The Centers for Disease Control and Prevention (CDC) estimates that more than 65 million people in the United States are currently living with an incurable sexually transmitted disease. An additional 15 million people will become infected each year, and of these about half will develop a lifelong infection. An important statistic is that about one fourth of newly acquired STD infections occur in adolescents.[2]

Efforts to curb and prevent the acquisition and spread of STDs include screening certain higher risk populations. A group is classified as high risk based on age, gender, sexual practices, locale, and other social behaviors or practices that place them at risk to acquire an STD. This chapter reviews the screening recommendation for selected, commonly screened STDs based on recommendations from the CDC and the second[3] and third[4] (in progress) report of the U.S. Preventive Services Task Force (USPSTF).

The goal of screening for disease is early detection of a condition to reduce morbidity and mortality. The value of screening asymptomatic persons must take into consideration the benefits, risks, costs, and effectiveness of screening practices. Effectiveness is determined in part by the characteristics of the screening test, the ease and skill required to perform the test or collect the specimen, and the characteristics of the target population, including age and gender. The USPSTF has developed evidenced-based recommendations for a number of diseases. The CDC is continually revising its recommendation for the prevention, detection, and treatment of STDs. The guidelines in this chapter are based on the recommendations of both groups—the CDC and the USPSTF.

CHLAMYDIA

Chlamydia is an STD caused by an intracellular, parasitic organism *Chlamydia trachomatis*. Currently there are at least 15 recognized serotypes of *C. trachomatis*. Clinical syndromes associated with certain *C. trachomatis* serotypes include nongonococcal urethritis (NGU), mucopurulent cervicitis, pelvic inflammatory disease (PID), lymphogranuloma venereum, acute urethral syndrome in female patients, ocular infections, proctocolitis, epididymitis, and Reiter's syndrome in adults. *C. trachomatis* may be acquired by infants through an infected birth canal, causing pneumonia and conjunctivitis in newborns.[5]

Chlamydia is the most prevalent STD in the United States. Each year, an estimated 3 million new cases of genital infection caused by *C. trachomatis* occur in the United States at a cost of $2.4 billion.[1,2] Chlamydia infection is especially prevalent among adolescents. In the last two decades, genital chlamydial infection has been identified as a major public health problem because of its association with several disease syndromes, including NGU, mucopurulent cervicitis, and PID.[5,6] Up to 40% of women with untreated chlamydia will develop PID, infertility, and tubal pregnancy. Although the disease may be asymptomatic in women, chlamydia causes a painful genital infection in men. Moreover, chlamydia increases the risk for HIV in both men and women. In addition, infants born to women with chlamydia can develop eye infections and pneumonia. In 1999 there were 660,000 reported cases of chlamydia; this is believed to be just the tip of the iceberg, because up to 75% of women and 50% of men with chlamydia may go undiagnosed.[2]

The third USPSTF[4] recommends routine screening for chlamydia in all sexually active women age 25 years and younger and in all women who may be otherwise at risk, whether or not they are pregnant. Evidence suggests that the cost of screening women who are at risk for chlamydia may be less than the cost of treating chlamydia and its complications. Screening patients at greatest risk is more cost-effective than screening all patients. There is no recommendation for or against screening for asymptomatic women ages 26 years and older who are at low risk for infection. There is some evidence that routine screening may be beneficial for all asymptomatic pregnant women ages 25 years or younger and other pregnant women at increased risk for infection.[4] Pregnant women should be screened for chlamydia during their third trimester. There is unclear or insufficient evidence for or against routine screening of asymptomatic men.[7]

Chlamydia organisms, which are obligate and intracellular, are found within urethral, cervical, and rectal epithelial cells, but not in exudate or pus. Because a specimen containing purulent discharge is inadequate for identification of the organism, the cervical os must be cleaned to remove debris and secretions. The DNA probe can be used to test for both chlamydia and gonorrhea. In the future, nucleic acid amplification tests such as PCR and LCR are likely to be considered the standard for diagnosis of STDs, including chlamydia. Regardless of the method used, it is important to closely follow the manufacturer's instructions for specimen collection and transport.[5,8] DNA or RNA amplification tests are more sensitive than culture.

An age of 25 years or younger is the strongest risk factor for chlamydia infection.[4] Other risk factors include having more than one sexual partner, having had an STD in the past, and inconsistent and/or incorrect condom use. The greatest risk for women is not knowing they have chlamydia, because the disease may be asymptomatic but still produce damage.[4]

GONORRHEA

Gonorrhea is a reportable disease caused by the gram-negative diplococcus *Neisseria gonorrhoeae*. It primarily involves mucocutaneous surfaces of the genitourinary tract, pharynx, conjunctiva, and anus. In men it is often characterized by a purulent urethral discharge, whereas in up to 80% of women it is asymptomatic. An estimated 650,000 cases of gonorrhea occur each year in the United States.[2] Populations at risk for gonorrhea include young, sexually active individuals and other individuals who engage in high-risk behaviors such as illegal drug use or prostitution. Recently, researchers have seen indications that gonorrhea may be on the increase among gay and bisexual men. Up to 50% of persons with gonorrhea have a coexistent chlamydial infection.[2]

Laboratory diagnosis of gonorrhea depends on the setting and availability of diagnostic laboratory facilities. Microscopic examination of gram-stained urethral or cervical specimens can detect infection with *N. gonorrhoeae*. The sensitivity of Gram's stain is higher in symptomatic men (90% to 95%) than in asymptomatic men (70%). Gram's stain is less sensitive for cervical infections in women (30% to 65%) and is not useful in diagnosing pharyngeal and rectal infections.[8]

The most sensitive and specific test for detecting gonococcal infection is direct culture from sites of exposure (urethra, endocervix, throat, and rectum). However, other methods are becoming increasingly popular because of the difficulty of handling and storing the culture medium. In women, endocervical canal culture sensitivity is 86% to 96%. Urethral sensitivity is 94% to 98% in symptomatic men and 84% in asymptomatic men.[3,8,9] Male patients should refrain from voiding for at least 2 hours before testing. Female patients should void unless urethral samples are desired.[9]

There is unclear or insufficient evidence to recommend for or against routine screening of asymptomatic high-risk men; however, testing may be indicated on other grounds. In the general population there is some evidence to recommend the exclusion of gonorrhea screening in periodic health examinations in the general population.

There is some evidence to recommend routine screening for gonorrhea for high-risk, asymptomatic women and pregnant women. A test for gonorrhea should be performed during the first prenatal visit for women who are at risk or are living in an area in which the prevalence of gonorrhea is high. A repeat test should be performed during the third trimester for those at continued risk.[7] After delivery, there is clear evidence to recommend routine ophthalmic antibiotic in newborns.[3]

SYPHILIS

Syphilis is a complex systemic STD caused by *Treponema pallidum*. Syphilis has been classified by the CDC into several stages depending on the length of infection. Patients may present with signs and symptoms of primary infection (ulcer or chancre at the infection site; see Color Plate 6), secondary infection (rash, mucocutaneous lesions, and adenopathy), or tertiary infection (cardiac, neurologic, ophthalmic, auditory, or gummatous lesions).[7]

The signs of primary and secondary syphilis may resolve spontaneously even without treatment. The patient then enters the latent stage of the disease, in which there are generally no clinical signs or symptoms of infection and diagnosis is made on the basis of serology. Tertiary syphilis is manifested after a variable period of latency in approximately one third of patients who fail to receive treatment. Late-stage syphilis may occur 10 to 20 years after initial infection. It may present as gummatous disease (rubbery lumps or lesions found in subcutaneous tissue), cardiovascular disease or, in one third of untreated patients, as neurosyphilis. However, neurosyphilis can occur in all stages of syphilis. The diagnosis of neurosyphilis is based on clinical findings and examination of the serum and cerebrospinal fluid.[10]

The latent stage of syphilis is dangerous for pregnant women. Even though she may not have symptoms, a pregnant woman with latent disease can infect her fetus.[10]

Dark field examinations and direct fluorescent antibody tests of lesion exudate or tissue are the definitive methods for diagnosing early syphilis. Serologic nontreponemal tests (e.g., Venereal Disease Research Laboratory [VDRL] or rapid plasma reagin [RPR]) and treponemal tests (e.g., fluorescent treponemal antibody absorbed [FTA-ABS] or microhemagglutination assay for antibody to *T. pallidum* [MHA-TP]) are tests performed to establish a diagnosis. The use of one test alone is not sufficient. A nontreponemal test may be used as the initial screening test. These tests correlate with disease activity and are reported quantitatively. However, false-positive nontreponemal test results are associated with hepatitis, viral pneumonia, pregnancy, infectious mononucleosis, and other viral infections. In addition, chronic false-positive findings are associated with connective tissue diseases such as systemic lupus erythematosus.[10] A treponemal test is used to confirm the diagnosis.[11] Treponemal tests are not used for screening because they remain reactive after the infection is treated.

Both treponemal and nontreponemal tests are used to screen patients with past suspected syphilis infection. Patients treated for early syphilis whose nontreponemal test either shows an increase or fails to show a fourfold decline in *T. pallidum* within 6 months should be retreated. Treponemal tests are used to screen patients for late syphilis when the nontreponemal tests are negative, yet late syphilis is suspected. In later stages of syphilis, antibody titers decline and may be undetectable.

Clear evidence exists to recommend routine screening for syphilis for all pregnant women and all persons at increased risk of infection (commercial sex workers, persons who exchange sex for drugs, those with other STDs including HIV, and contacts of persons with active syphilis).[3] A serologic test for syphilis should be performed on all pregnant women at the first prenatal visit. For those women at high risk, screening should be repeated in the third trimester and again at delivery.[7]

GENITAL HERPES

Herpes simplex virus (HSV) infection is a condition characterized by primary infection of genital or anal lesions with visible, painful, genital, or anal lesions or grouped vesicles at the site of inoculation and regional lymphadenopathy. Recurrent HSV infection is characterized by a normal course of recurring outbreaks of vesicles at the same site.[12]

It is estimated that 16% (approximately 1 in 5) of the U.S. adult population is HSV-2 seropositive.[3,13] In 1999 the estimated prevalence was 19% among the general population between 14 and 49 years old. As many as 1 million people in the United States become infected each year.[2]

Spread of genital herpes is by direct contact because secretions can transmit the virus. Transmissibility is higher with active lesions, but asymptomatic shedding of virus with transmission is also possible. Asymptomatic shedding occurs more often during the first 3 months after primary infection.[13]

Diagnosis of HSV is often a clinical decision based on the patient's history and the morphology of the lesions. The diagnosis is confirmed with a Tzanck test on tissue taken from the base of a lesion or unroofed vesicle.[12,13] Lesions in the process of healing may affect the sensitivity of virologic testing, giving false-negative results.

Routine screening for genital HSV infection is not recommended for asymptomatic persons, including asymptomatic pregnant women. There is unclear or insufficient evidence available at the present time to recommend for or against the examination of pregnant women in labor for signs of active genital HSV lesions, although recommendations to do so may be made on other grounds.[3] Experts have recommended that any serologic testing for herpes simplex should use type-specific assays.[14]

HUMAN PAPILLOMA VIRUS

Human papilloma virus (HPV) is a virus associated with a group of viruses that infect the epithelium of the skin and mucous membranes. There are a number of distinct serotypes of HPV. The infections they cause may be asymptomatic, produce warty lesions, or be associated with a variety of both benign of malignant neoplasia. More than 70 types of HPV are recognized, and distinct types are associated with specific clinical manifestations. Of the 70 types, 30 can infect the genital area. Some cause genital warts or condyloma acuminata. Others may cause subclinical infections that cannot be seen initially. These subclinical infections are more common and can lead to cervical, penile, or anal cancer. On the other hand, genital warts can be treated and cured.[15,16]

It is estimated that 5.5 million people in the United States become infected with HPV each year. Currently, 20 million people in the United States are infected. Women seem to be at higher risk, because persistent cervical infection in women is the single most important risk factor for cervical cancer.[2] Of the oncogenic types of HPV, type 16 accounts for 50% of cervical cancer and high-grade dysplasia. Type 16 (along with types 18, 31, and 45) account for 80% of cervical cancers.[2] According to the CDC, levels of infection with HPV appear to be similar among both men and women.[17] Research indicates that approximately 1% of sexually active adults in the United States have genital warts.[2]

Whereas high-risk types (HPV 16, 18, 31, 33, 35, 39, 45, 51, 52) are associated with low- and high-grade squamous intraepithelial lesions (LSIL and HSIL) and invasive cancer, low-risk types (HPV 6, 11, 42, 43, 44) are primarily associated with genital warts and LSIL. Women with persistent HPV infection, especially high-risk types, are at a greatest risk for developing cervical intraepithelial neoplasia (CIN) and CIN lesions that progress rather than regress. Studies indicate that infection with high-risk and multiple types of HPV and older age are associated with persistent infection.[17]

Genital warts are diagnosed by inspection. They appear as soft, moist, and pink or red swellings. They can be flat, single or multiple, and small or large. Some cluster forming a cauliflower shape. They can appear on the vulva, in or around the anus or vagina, penis, scrotum, groin, or thigh. Incubation varies from weeks (4 to 8) to months.[7,14] Subclinical lesions may be detected with Papanicolaou (Pap) testing, colposcopy, or biopsy or by the application of acetic acid to lesions with light and magnification. Routine use of acetowhitening as a screening test is not recommended. Acetowhitening is not a specific test for HPV infection and therefore can produce false-positive results in populations at low risk for HPV.[7]

A definitive diagnosis of HPV depends on the detection of viral nucleic acid (DNA or RNA) or capsid protein. Pap smear diagnosis of HPV does not always correlate with the detection of HPV DNA in cervical cells. As with mild dysplasia, cell changes attributed to HPV often regress without treatment. Screening for HPV using HPV and RNA tests or acetic acid is not recommended.[7]

HUMAN IMMUNODEFICIENCY VIRUS

HIV was first clinically recognized in 1981 when the CDC noticed increased cases of *Pneumocystis carinii* pneumonia in previously healthy young men.[18,19] The disease soon became recognized in male and female injection drug users. At the same time similar occurrences were being reported in Africans attending European centers for treatment. In 1983, HIV was isolated from a patient and shown to be the causative agent of AIDS. Over the years the case definition of AIDS has undergone several revisions. The etiologic agent of AIDS is HIV, a member of a family of retroviruses and the subfamily of Lentivirinae. Infection with HIV produces a spectrum of diseases that progresses from a clinical latent state or asymptomatic state to AIDS as a late manifestation. The rate of progression is variable. Viral replication is active during all states and increases as the immune system deteriorates. HIV is an RNA virus whose hallmark is the reverse transcription of its RNA to DNA by the enzyme reverse transcriptase. HIV is transmitted by both heterosexual and homosexual contact, by blood and blood products, and by infected mothers to infants either intrapartum, perinatally, or by breast milk.[18,20] HIV is predominantly a sexually transmitted disease. It is characterized by a gradual deterioration of immune functions. During the course of infection crucial immune cells (CD4+, T cells) are disabled and killed and their numbers progressively decline. After a variable period the CD4+ T cell count falls below a critical level and the patient becomes highly susceptible to opportunistic disease.[18,20]

The most common cause of HIV disease throughout the world and in the United States is HIV-1.[7] The prevalence of HIV-2 in the United States is extremely low.[7] Approximately 800,000 to 900,000 persons in the United States are infected with HIV, and approximately 275,000 of these persons might not know they are infected.[20] Early detection of HIV infection is now recognized as a critical component in controlling the spread of HIV infection.[20,21]

Only HIV tests approved by the U.S Food and Drug Administration (FDA) should be used for diagnostic purposes. Several HIV test technologies have been approved by the FDA for diagnostic use in the United States. These tests enable testing of different fluids (i.e., whole blood, serum, plasma, oral fluid, and urine). Informed consent must be obtained before an HIV test is performed.[7] HIV-1 testing consists of initial screening with an electroimmunoassay (EIA) to detect antibodies to HIV-1. Specimens with a nonreactive result from the initial EIA are considered HIV-negative unless new exposure to an infected partner or partner of unknown HIV status has occurred. Specimens with a reactive EIA result are retested in duplicate. If the result of either duplicate test is reactive, the specimen is reported as repeatedly reactive and undergoes confirmatory testing with a more specific supplemental test (e.g., Western blot or, less commonly, an immunofluorescence assay [IFA]). An HIV test should be considered positive only after screening and confirmatory tests are reactive.[20]

A Western blot test may be reported as indeterminate. This may represent the evolving antibody response of a recent infection or may be produced by the presence of nonspecific antibodies. If the indeterminate result was found in a patient who was seronegative for HIV on previous tests, there is concern that this indeterminant result is caused by an new HIV infection. If the result remains indeterminant for 6 months, this probably represents a nonspecific antibody response.

Most infected persons develop a detectable HIV antibody within 3 months of exposure. If the initial negative HIV test was conducted within the first 3 months after exposure, repeat testing should be considered 3 months or longer after the exposure occurred to account for the possibility of a false-negative result. If the follow-up test is nonreactive, it is unlikely that the patient is HIV-positive. However, if the patient was exposed to a known HIV-infected person or if provider or patient concern remains, a second repeat test might be considered 6 months or more from the exposure.[20]

Providers should consider three factors in determining whether to recommend HIV counseling, testing, and referral (CTR) to all patients or to target only selected patients: type of setting, HIV prevalence of the setting, and behavioral and clinical HIV risk of the individual patients in the setting.

Individual risk can be ascertained through risk screening. Under certain circumstances of perinatal transmission, acute occupational exposure, and acute nonoccupational (i.e., high-risk sexual or needle-sharing), exposure providers should recommend HIV CTR regardless of setting prevalence or behavioral or clinical risk.[20]

It is estimated that 120,000 to 160,000 infected women live in the United States. Of these women, 80% are of childbearing age. Approximately 25% of HIV-infected pregnant women who are not treated during pregnancy can transmit HIV to their infants during pregnancy, labor and delivery, or breast-feeding. Effective interventions for HIV-infected pregnant women can protect their infants from acquiring HIV and can prolong the survival and improve the health of these mothers and their children. For these reasons, HIV testing is recommended for all pregnant women. All health care providers should recommend HIV testing to all of their pregnant patients, pointing out the substantial benefit of knowledge of HIV status for the health of women and their infants. HIV screening should be a routine part of prenatal care for all women.[21] Regulations, laws, and policies regarding HIV screening of pregnant women and infants are not standardized throughout all states. Health care workers should be aware of and adhere to the laws and regulations governing their areas of practice related to HIV screening.[21]

Because of recent advances in both antiretroviral and obstetric interventions, pregnant women infected with HIV who know their status prenatally can reduce their risk for transmitting HIV to their infants to 2% or less. Finally, all HIV testing should include counseling, both pretest and posttest.

REFERENCES

1. Institute of Medicine, Committee on Prevention and Control of Sexually Transmitted Diseases: *The hidden epidemic: confronting sexually transmitted diseases,* Washington DC, 1997, National Academy Press.
2. Centers for Disease Control and Prevention: *Tracking the hidden epidemics, trends in STDs in the United States,* Atlanta, 2000, The Centers.
3. US Preventive Services Task Force: *Guide to clinical preventive services,* ed 2, Baltimore, 1996, Williams & Wilkins.
4. Screening for chlamydia infection. What's new from the third USPSTF. AHRQ Pub No APPIP01-0010, Rockville, Md, March 2001, Agency for Healthcare Research and Quality; Retrieved December 2001 from the World Wide Web: http://www.ahrq.gov/clinic/prev/chlamwh.htm.
5. Peeling RW: Chlamydia as pathogens: new species and new issues, emerging infections, *CDC* 2(4):307-319, 1996.
6. Fiumara NJ: *Pictorial guide to sexually transmitted diseases,* New York, 1989, Reed Publishing.
7. Centers for Disease Control and Prevention: 1998 Guidelines for treatment of sexually transmitted diseases, *MMWR* 47(RR-1):1-118, 1998.
8. Test performance characteristics. In *STD/HIV Prevention Training Center of New England: Home study module,* 3-day intensive course, 1997.
9. Sexually transmitted diseases and HIV infection. In US Department of Health and Human Services: *Clinicians' handbook of preventive services: put prevention into practice,* Washington, DC,1994, US Government Printing Office.
10. Larson S, Steiner B, Rudolph A: Laboratory diagnosis and interpretation of tests for syphilis, *Clin Microbiol Rev* 8(1):1-19, 1995.
11. Borgatta L and others: A contemporary approach to curbing STDs, *Patient Care* 30(20):30-42, 1996.
12. Fitzpatrick TB and others: *Color atlas and synopsis of clinical dermatology,* ed 3, New York, 1997, McGraw-Hill.
13. Dorsky D: Herpes simplex virus infections. In *STD/HIV Prevention Training Center of New England: Home study module,* 3-day intensive course, 1997.
14. Division of STD Prevention: Report of an external consultants meeting on prevention of genital herpes, May 5-6, 1998, Retrieved December 2001 from the World Wide Web: http://www.cdc.gov/nchstp/dstd/Reports_Publications/cover.htm.
15. Reichman RC: Human papilloma virus. In Fauci A and others, editors: *Harrison's principles of internal medicine,* New York, 1998, McGraw-Hill.
16. CDC: *Human Papillomavirus: CDC releases first of its kind research,* December 5, 2000. Retrieved December 2001 from the World Wide Web: http://www.cdc.gov/nchstp/dstd/Press_Releases/STDEpidemics2000.htm.
17. Division of STD Prevention. *Prevention of genital HPV infection and sequelae: Report of an external consultants meeting,* U.S. Department of Health and Human Services, Atlanta, 1999, CDC.
18. Fauci AS, Lane HC. Human immunodeficiency virus. In Fauci A and others, editors: *Harrison's principles of internal medicine,* New York, 1998, McGraw-Hill.
19. Wisdom A, Hawkins, DA: *Diagnosis in color, sexually transmitted diseases,* ed 2, London, 1997, Mosby-Wolfe.
20. Centers for Disease Control and Prevention: Revised guidelines for HIV counseling, testing and referral, *MMWR* 50(RR19):1-58, 2001.
21. Centers for Disease Control and Prevention: Revised recommendation for HIV screening of pregnant women, perinatal counseling and guideline consultation, *MMWR* 50(RR19):59-68, 2001.

CHAPTER 19

Principles of Occupational and Environmental Health in Primary Care

Kathleen Golden McAndrew

Occupational and environmental medicine is the application of health care to the worker in relation to the workplace environment. This specialty focuses on injury and illness prevention and worker protection in addition to treatment of work-related injury and illness.

Primary care providers may include occupational health care delivery in their practices. The provider's role in delivering occupational health-related services may vary. Involvement is dependent on the defined scope of service of the practice setting, its proximity to an occupational medicine specialist or program, and the knowledge and interest of the primary care provider.

In addition to treatment and evaluation of workers' compensation injuries, the primary care provider may be involved with work-related injuries and illness through identifying workplace hazards when providing medical evaluations and screenings or during medical assessment and treatment of injured workers. They may also be requested to provide medical information that is needed to assist occupational health professionals with fitness-for-duty or return-to-work issues.

Regardless of the role of the primary health care provider, including an occupational health history as part of the medical history and having an understanding of the risks associated with the job demands of the patient will assist in monitoring and maintaining the health of the working population in each practice. An occupational health history should include at least the following:[1]

- A listing of current and past positions held
- Names of previous employers, years employed, and products manufactured
- A brief description of job duty requirements
- Any current or past exposures to chemical or other hazardous substances

HEALTH PROMOTION

Health promotion is important in maintaining a healthy workplace. The overall health of the worker is an important factor in preventing injury and illness both at home and at work.[2] Many companies encourage and support programs aimed at and resulting in a healthy, productive workforce. A healthy workforce results in reduced risk of work-related injuries, less sick time usage, and improved morale of the employees. To assist with improving the well-being of their employees, many employers offer on-site health promotional programs at the worksite.[2] These offerings may range from on-site exercise programs to health education programs, which include education on smoking cessation, nutrition, exercise, stress reduction, and personal safety. Medical clearance from primary care providers is sometimes requested before employees may participate in programs that involve strenuous physical activity.

Some employers offer periodic screening programs at the worksite. These include blood pressure, weight, blood glucose, cholesterol, and other high-risk factors. Results are used to educate employees on risk reduction through lifestyle changes, as well as a basis for establishing future health promotion programs that target employees' needs. Results of such screening that require evaluation or monitoring are most often referred to the employee's primary care provider.

MEDICAL SCREENINGS

Most employers require a preplacement screening after a job offer. Primary care providers who offer preplacement examinations as part of their practice must understand the purpose and focus of these examinations.

The focus of a preplacement examination is to ensure that the employee is able to perform the essential job functions, with or without accommodation, of the position that he or she has been hired to fill. In addition, the examination serves as baseline data for future screening or work-related injuries, illness, or exposure that may occur throughout employment. Therefore it is essential that the primary care provider be provided with and understands the physical demands and potential for exposure to chemicals or other hazardous substances associated with the job of every patient being screened. The focus of these examinations is specific to the worker's health status and how it relates to the job; the examination is not for diagnostic purposes.

A comprehensive health history is essential to a preplacement examination. It provides a database of both subjective and objective data that encompasses all aspects of the patient's health, including past job duty requirements and any history of exposures.[3]

Components of the preplacement examination should ideally include a job-specific physical examination and appropriate screenings.[4] Job-specific screenings may include spirometry, audiometry, vision screening, a baseline chest x-ray study, various blood studies, and urinalysis. Drug testing or regulatory agency-required testing for certain licenses or certificates might also be provided.

Incidental findings may surface. Although they need to be addressed and plans for follow-up discussed, they should not be addressed as part of the preplacement evaluation or included in the clearance or report to the employer unless they directly affect the employee's ability to perform the job.

After completion of the evaluation, any recommendations, restrictions, abnormal findings, identified special protective measures, or other issues should be discussed with the employee. Any need for periodic monitoring should also be brought to the employee's attention. In addition, the primary care provider should emphasize the need to use appropriate protective equipment and review proper body mechanics as they relate to performing the employee's job duties.

A written recommendation on work fitness should be provided to the employer. The recommendation should be limited to whether the employee is cleared for full work duty or whether any restrictions are recommended. Such restrictions should be specific and described by function. In addition, restrictions should be listed without including the underlying medical reason, because medical information should not be provided to the employer without the employee's written consent.

MEDICAL SURVEILLANCE

Prevention of disease and injuries is the primary purpose of medical surveillance programs and the key focus of occupational health and safety programs.[3,5] Health surveillance is provided to monitor potential exposure to workplace hazards, including biologic, chemical, physical, and ergonomic hazards. Primary care providers need to have a basic understanding of the use of medical surveillance in occupational health settings. To yield optimal results, medical and environmental surveillance results need to be linked. This requires the expertise of experienced occupational medicine or other professionals who are familiar with all components of medical surveillance.[3,4] However, primary care providers may be requested to provide some of the components, such as surveillance examinations, biologic tests, or other health screens, that may be used as part of the overall program monitoring.

The purpose of a surveillance examination is to protect the worker from adverse health effects, evaluate the employee's ability to perform his or her job duties, and meet government surveillance requirements.[6]

Numerous Occupational Safety and Health Association (OSHA) standards require medical surveillance. The nature and frequency of testing are determined by national or state OSHA requirements or by individual employers. The standards are available for each substance (e.g., lead, asbestos), for workers whose job requirements require medical evaluation (e.g., workers requiring respiratory protection, firefighters), or for incidents requiring testing after exposure (e.g., noise exposure, exposure to blood-borne pathogens). Specific requirements are listed in each code and should be referenced before performing evaluations.

DRUG TESTING

Drug and alcohol testing is required of employees who work for companies covered by agencies of the Department of Transportation (DOT) and whose jobs are identified as safety sensitive. In addition, companies or contractors whose federal grants exceed $25,000 are required to establish a drug-free workplace policy that includes drug screening. Individual companies also may choose to implement their own drug-free workplace requirements.[7]

Indications for testing include preplacement screening, random testing, postaccident testing, and testing for reasonable suspicion or "for cause." The most common drugs tested include the panel required by the DOT and other federal agencies. This panel includes marijuana (tetrahydrocannabinol [THC] metabolite), cocaine, amphetamines, opiates, and phencyclidine (PCP). Others may be added by private companies, such as barbiturates, hallucinogens, inhalants, or designer drugs.[7,8] Special panels are sometimes used that include multiple drugs' potential for abuse among specific occupations. Most drug testing programs adopt federal regulations, including their cutoff levels and chain-of-custody procedures required during specimen collection.

Drug screens are normally performed on urine and must be collected by trained staffs that are knowledgeable of the strict federal guidelines. Ethanol (alcohol) testing is done using a Breathalyzer test performed by certified breath alcohol technicians (BATs). Specimens are analyzed by laboratories certified to perform these tests by the Substance Abuse and Mental Health Services Administration (SAMHSA).

Results are sent to a designated medical review officer (MRO). The role of the MRO is to interpret drug screen results and determine whether there is a medical or other explanation for positive results before contacting the employer.

Because strict adherence to guidelines must be followed with every specimen collection, and because facilities must be set up to meet the specifications for collection (e.g., dry bathrooms), most primary care practices defer drug and alcohol testing to occupational medicine programs or to private laboratories that offer drug collection as part of their services.

TREATMENT OF WORK-RELATED INJURIES, ILLNESS, AND EXPOSURES

Workers' compensation is a system that provides medical care, wage replacement benefits and, when necessary, rehabilitation for workers who incur injuries or illness as a result of workplace exposure or activity. With few exceptions for federally administered programs, most are regulated by the individual states.

Many potential hazards in the workplace can cause a work-related injury, illness, or exposure. Some of these injuries may be similar to others or already encountered within a primary care practice. Such hazards include physical hazards of the work environment that may cause injuries (e.g., from objects, falls, noise, heat, or cold). Ergonomics is the cause of a large number of work-related injuries, including back injuries and injuries caused by repetitive motion/cumulative trauma. It is imperative that the work setting be evaluated and altered to lessen the chance of recurrence in these situations.

Exposures may occur when employees work around potentially toxic chemicals or biologic agents. Chemical-related injury, illness, or exposure may occur as a result of normal working conditions or through accidents. These episodes require the primary care provider to have a basic understanding of toxicology. Familiarization with material safety data sheets or access to computerized databases or poison control centers can assist with determining actual exposure and necessary treatment. For biologic exposures, the epidemiology, including mode of transmission, incubation, immunity status of the employee, and appropriate or required follow-up testing, must be known for each exposure. Workers such as health care facility employees, emergency responders, and employees in laboratory and research facilities encounter biologic hazards.

Multiple players are usually involved with workers' compensation cases. The number and type may vary depending on the manner in which each employer is insured. In addition, required forms and regular reports that reflect the employee's status and must be completed within defined time frames. Preauthorization requirements must usually be obtained before referring the patient to specialty, adjunct treatment modalities or when ordering diagnostic tests.

Because there may be different requirements for each employer and within each state, primary care providers who are interested in providing workers' compensation as part of their practice should ensure that they and their support staff have a basic understanding of the system. This can be accomplished by reviewing the applicable state regulations or by attending conferences covering this area.

Regardless of each state's regulations, principles of medical confidentiality regarding work-related injuries and illness limit the information the employer receives regarding the nature of the occupational illness or injury, type of treatment, restrictions and limitations, and the plan for continual care.[4,9]

After each workers' compensation visit, it is advisable and expected that the treating primary care provider notify the case manager or representative of the plan for further medical treatment and the designated work restrictions.[9]

In many situations the injured employee may not be able to perform his or her complete duties while recovering but may be able to perform parts of the job or other tasks. In these cases working with the employer to identify how temporary accommodation of these employees can be provided through modified or light duty is an important part of the treatment plan.[4]

Many companies are mandated or volunteer to develop modified-duty programs. To recommend modified duty, the health care provider must understand the job requirements of each injured employee. It is important that the employer provide this information concerning physical job demands.

When describing limitations or restrictions, it is helpful to describe by function and to qualify and quantify restrictions in as much detail as possible to avoid confusion and to assist the employer in accommodating these restrictions.

REGULATORY AGENCY REQUIREMENTS

In addition to understanding the basics of workers' compensation, primary care providers who choose to address occupational health-related medical issues need to be familiar with other regulations that apply to treatment and screening of employees. Copies of these regulations can be obtained through the respective agency responsible for the regulation, or they can be found on various websites on the Internet.

Occupational Safety and Health Administration

Created by Congress in 1970, OSHA requires each employer to provide "a place of employment, which is free from recognized hazards that are causing or are likely to cause death or serious physical harm to employees."[10] OSHA functions under the Department of Labor. It has the authority to fine or imprison employers who are found to be in violation of its regulations. Although most of OSHA's regulations deal with safety-related concerns, this organization has also issued a number of standards that specify medical evaluations and the testing of employees who may be exposed to certain workplace hazards. Testing is required when exposures meet or exceed a certain level. Other standards require medical clearance before using required protective equipment.

National Institute of Occupational Safety and Health

The National Institute of Occupational Safety and Health (NIOSH) was established under the Occupational Safety and Health Act of 1970 and is part of the U.S. Department of Health and Human Services. Its function is to conduct research and to advise OSHA on issues regarding hazards in the workplace. NIOSH provides educational information helpful to health care providers, employers, and employees.

Americans with Disabilities Act

Congress enacted the Americans with Disabilities Act (ADA) in 1990. It is designed to protect disabled workers from discrimination in the workplace. This act must be considered when offering many occupational health-related evaluations. The ADA requires that an employer make reasonable accommodations in order for the disabled employee to be able to perform those job functions considered essential to the position.[11] In addition, it is also necessary to determine whether disabled employees can perform the job without posing a "direct threat" to the health and safety of themselves or others.[11]

Professional Organizations

Professional organizations such as the American College of Occupational and Environmental Medicine, the American Association of Occupational Health Nurses, and the American Conference of Governmental Industrial Hygienists offer texts, guidelines, and other information that can assist the primary care provider with occupational health-related issues.

REFERENCES

1. Goldman RH: Suspecting occupational disease. In McCunney RJ, editor: *A practical approach to occupational and environmental medicine*, ed 2, Boston, 1994, Little, Brown.
2. Travers P, McDougall C: *Guidelines for an occupational health and safety service*, Atlanta, 1995, American Association of Occupational Health Nurses Publications.
3. Harber P, McCunney RJ, Monosson IH: Medical surveillance. In McCunney RJ, editor: *A practical approach to occupational and environmental medicine*, ed 2, Boston, 1994, Little, Brown.
4. Golden McAndrew K: AAOHN advisory: Nurse practitioners in occupational and environmental health. In the American Association of Occupational Health Nurses Journal. Atlanta, January 1999.
5. Hau ML: Prevention of occupational injuries and illnesses. In Salazar MK, editor: *AAOHN core curriculum for occupational and environmental health nursing*, Philadelphia, 2001, WB Saunders.
6. Burgel B: Direct care in the occupational setting. In Salazar MK, editor: *AAOHN core curriculum for occupational and environmental health nursing*, Philadelphia, 2001, WB Saunders.
7. Golden McAndrew K, McAndrew S: Workplace substance abuse impairment. In the American Association of Occupational Health Nurses Journal. Atlanta, January 2000.
8. Myerson K, Parker-Conrad J: Examples of occupational health and safety programs. In Salazar MK, editor: *AAOHN core curriculum for occupational and environmental health nursing*, Philadelphia, 2001, WB Saunders.
9. McCunney RJ: Occupational medical services. In McCunney RJ, editor: *A practical approach to occupational and environmental medicine*, ed 2, Boston, 1994, Little, Brown.
10. U.S. Department of Labor, Occupational Safety and Health Administration: *General industry OSHA safety and health standards*, 29 CFR 1910, OSHA 2206,Washington, DC, US Government Printing Office.
11. Peterson KW: The Americans with Disabilities Act. In McCunney RJ, editor: *A practical approach to occupational and environmental medicine*, ed 2, Boston, 1994, Little, Brown.

CHAPTER 20

College Health

Catharine Moffett

College or university health services often reflect campus culture and are varied in composition and services. A large university with a medical center can offer a wider variety of providers and specialists than can a small rural college health center. However, one nurse working collaboratively with a local physician at a smaller college might be acquainted with all the students.

The mission of a college or university health service is to provide primary care for the student, promote the well-being of the institution's citizens through health education and illness prevention programs, and contribute ultimately to the academic success of its patients/students.[1] A student health service may also position itself as the student's "interim" primary health care provider, with the understanding that communication with the student's clinician at home will be ongoing.

ROLES OF UNIVERSITY HEALTH CARE PROVIDERS

In college or university health services, the clinician has an ideal opportunity to affect the young adult at a critical time of development. The college years are a transitional stage between the end of adolescence and the beginning of adulthood. The college health care provider can assist in that transition by explaining issues of confidentiality (often a new concept to the student), modeling the practice of partnership between provider and patient in treatment or care decisions, and instructing a student in the sometimes confusing world of health insurance. During this time, the university health care provider can also positively influence the movement from dependent living at home to independent living and from pediatric to adult care.

In addition, health education plays an important role. Some institutions have wellness programs at wellness centers presented in conjunction with the health service. A team composed of university health care provider, health educator, peer educator, and residential life staff, with their various talents and teaching skills, plan and present programs promoting healthier physical, social, and psychologic lifestyles. This collaborative team, with input from other designated individuals, can target the current trends on campus, including risk-taking behavior and drug use, and tailor programs to specific issues and audiences.

TOPICS IN COLLEGE HEALTH

Confidentiality

For some students, receiving health care in the college setting is the first time they are seen without a parent present. If the student is more than 18 years old, he or she is legally able to make a decision relating to health care without parental involvement. Clearly explaining to the student the right to confidentiality can enable more open communication with the provider. Obtaining a student's written permission to discuss a specific illness episode with a parent, professor, or administrator confirms the legal nature of the information in the student's medical chart. On the other hand, parents often need the reassurance that, although their over-18-year-old child may desire privacy regarding visits to the college health center, serious or life-threatening illnesses can and will be made known to parents at the discretion of the professional staff.

If a student is covered on his or her parent's medical insurance plan, confidential information may be inadvertently revealed to the policy holder (parent) as a result of routine billing procedures and documents. When students have the privacy of their own policy, they may be less hesitant in seeking gynecologic care or treatment for contraception and sexually transmitted disease (STD).

Health Care Issues: Female College Students

For some young women, being away from home provides an opportunity for more intimate sexual relationships and the concomitant responsibilities. A first gynecologic visit to the student health service should include enough time for a first pelvic examination (for some), a thorough sexual history, STD education, and contraceptive counseling.

Appointments requested specifically for STD screening or emergency contraception create opportunities for the clinician to explore the college woman's sense of control in a sexual situation, the impact of drug or alcohol use on her decisions, and any sense of guilt or regret connected to her sexual experience. Understanding the student's level of risk-taking behavior enables the clinician to guide the student in contraceptive care, provide a referral to student counseling services, or schedule a follow-up appointment at student health services to continue in the educational/support aspect of her care.

Conflicts pertaining to contraception and religious beliefs or sexual identity and intimacy issues can also be explored during these visits. Other information, such as date rape experience or a history of sexual abuse, may also be revealed and appropriately addressed. Institutions of higher learning are communities in which there are codes of conduct and guidelines for behavior that may be affected by a student's sexual experience. As a supportive member of the community, student health services should have a thorough understanding of the institution's policies and procedures concerning date rape, rape, and sexual harassment. A close working relationship with student counseling services will facilitate appropriate referral and, if necessary, co-management. Unplanned pregnancies can require the collaboration of student health services, student counseling services, and other appropriate counseling services in the community.

College-age women who visit student health services should be observed for evidence of an existing eating disorder or a condition that indicates such a condition. Diagnosis and management of anorexia nervosa or bulimia are addressed elsewhere in this text; however, diagnosis and treatment in the college setting have some unique aspects. Female students are acutely aware of the myth of the "Freshman 15," which purports that freshmen women will gain 15 pounds during their first year on campus.[2] Students with an eating disorder in remission who find college life stressful are prone to regression. Women pressured to compete socially or athletically may respond with disordered eating at college, which can progress to a full eating disorder.

Students living in dorms or sororities and students participating in activities such as athletic teams or dance or theater group may notice fellow students exhibiting behavior indicative of an eating disorder. These students, as well as coaches, professors, or student leaders, should be encouraged to approach student health services to seek advice concerning treatment for a friend or classmate. Whether working alone or in concert with student counseling services, the student health services staff must proceed carefully to protect the individual as well as to reassure the group concerned about the friend or classmate. Depending on the clinical situation, remaining in treatment and meeting established goals in order to remain in college can serve as strong motivating factors for the student with an eating disorder. Unfortunately, the health service is powerless if the student never seeks treatment on her own. Mandated visits have limited value beyond possible diagnosis and can sabotage future treatment.

Health Care Issues: Male College Students

Males 16 to 20 years of age have far fewer health care visits than younger males (11 to 15 years old) or females of their same age cohort.[3] Male college students visit the health center episodically for sick visits or injuries. Therefore there are fewer opportunities for health education or risk-reduction counseling than for college-age women. Efforts to reach this population through outreach programs in dormitories, fraternities, or athletic teams can help bridge this gap.

Young men also present for STI screening. This occasion provides the opportunity to screen for high-risk behaviors including drug and alcohol use, violence, nonrelational sexual activity, and condom use. The STI-screening visit is an excellent opportunity for one-on-one teaching of college men. Because testicular cancer is more prevalent in this age-group, education about testicular cancer and self-examination should be offered to the individual and promoted in wellness efforts. The proper use of condoms can also be taught at an STD screening visit.

Injuries related to violence as a result of male clubs, organizations, or initiation rites may reveal information in conflict with an oath of confidentiality. Understanding the institution's policies about these activities will help guide the clinician's response.

Gay, Lesbian, Bisexual, and Transgender Students

Student health services must initiate outreach to the gay, lesbian, bisexual, and transgender student communities, because these students may be reluctant to have contact with student health services. Student health services can be visible to these communities and understand their special needs by speaking with student gay, lesbian, bisexual, and transgender organizations and requesting feedback on the health service and programs.

Mental Health Issues

As a result of advancements in pharmacologic treatment, increasing numbers of college students have complex psychiatric diagnoses and need various types of on-campus support.[4] Student health services can be involved in medical maintenance, treatment, referral, or co-management of students with mental health needs. The relationship of student health services with student counseling services can vary from a merged, fully integrated center to separate services with shared administration, to completely independent services.

Transfer or coordination of mental health care from home to the college setting can cause various concerns. As with any chronic illness, students may have established a therapeutic relationship with their therapist and now must establish a new relationship with an unfamiliar therapist. Therefore identification and outreach to students who may benefit from counseling services are crucial. Freshmen students with mental health needs can be identified via information on the health form, which should record chronic psychiatric medications. In addition, student health services can serve as a conduit to campus counseling services when the health service is asked by the athletic or dance department to evaluate a student with a potential eating disorder. In addition, the academic or student life department may refer a student with a potential mood, thought, or adjustment disorder. Health service clinicians must be sensitive to the fact that for some, the stigma of seeking mental health services can be a barrier to care, and access through a medical service or for a medically related complaint is more acceptable. Students should be encouraged to sign a release when the referral is made to allow for a collaborative approach to treatment.

Students who are in academic difficulty because of mental health issues may find that student health services or student counseling services can assist in validating a condition that could be interfering with academic performance. Students may request documentation for a medical leave of absence to engage in more intensive therapeutic treatment before returning to campus.

The college years are acutely stressful and accompanied by periods of hopelessness for some students. It is essential that college and university health clinicians maintain a high level of vigilance for suicide risk when assessing all students. Another mental health condition, schizophrenia, has an onset in early adult life and can also present in the college setting (see Chapter 26).

Tobacco/Alcohol

Alcohol use in the college population continues to be a problem despite institutional efforts to curb its use.[5] Secondary effects of binge drinking include sexual assault, violence, property damage, motor vehicle accidents, and death. Among the strategies most often used to curb alcohol consumption are alternative late-night alcohol-free events, peer influence, increased sanctions, student involvement in campus policies, and increased education. Student health services treat both the acute and secondary effects of alcohol intoxication. This encounter affords the opportunity to educate the student in issues connected with alcohol use. In addition, referrals to counseling services, on-campus alcohol education programs, or community alcohol treatment programs may be appropriate.

Tobacco use on the college campus has increased in the past decade; 28% of college smokers begin to smoke regularly at or after age 19 years (when most are already in college).[6] Although most public buildings and most college buildings prohibit smoking, only 27% of the campuses surveyed prohibit smoking in student dormitories.[7]

College or university health clinicians have a role in both policy advocacy for smoking restrictions, as well as in promoting smoking cessation. Tobacco use should be the "fifth vital sign" in student sick visit encounters to initiate the opportunity to discuss smoking cessation. Despite reports from colleges that there is little student demand for formal cessation programs, these programs must remain part of the wellness armamentarium for the student health center.

SCREENINGS AND IMMUNIZATIONS

Evidence of immunity or current immunization to measles, and rubella is usually required for college enrollment. Immunizations or evidence of immunity to hepatitis B, chickenpox, and tetanus are recommended. Prematriculation immunizations are mandated by colleges and universities and by state law. Student health services are responsible for ensuring student compliance with these mandates, including documentation of students who are not immunized because of religious beliefs. The most recent recommendations by the Centers for Disease Control and Prevention Advisory Committee on Immunization Practices, as well as by the American College Health Association, advise students and parents to be educated about the risks of meningococcal disease in the college population and encourage vaccination.[8] Students arriving from tuberculosis-endemic countries within the last 5 years must typically receive tuberculin skin testing before enrollment.[1]

Students studying abroad during college need advice on travel immunizations and information on infectious disease prevention. After students travel to areas where TB is endemic, they should be rescreened for TB.

CULTURAL ISSUES

Cultural competency is crucial to the student health service's success in caring for a diverse student population. Cultural competency is more than cultural awareness (knowledge) and cultural sensitivity (knowledge plus some experience with the culture).[9] Cultural competency encompasses the ability to think about power differentials in relationships and respond with varied skills to establish rapport with diverse individuals.[9] Student health clinicians must be sensitive to voice, body language, and gestures as they communicate with patients. There may be culture-specific meanings for aspects of health care such as pain and reproductive issues in patient populations. University or college health clinicians can expect to experience multiple cultures on their campus and must be leaders in modeling and fostering cultural competency.

RESOURCES

The American College Health Association, a membership representing more than 3200 individuals in 900 institutions of higher education, provides useful standards and guidelines for college health programs and services. Their website can be accessed at www.acha.org.

REFERENCES

1. ACHA Guidelines, Retrieved December 2001 from the World Wide Web www.acha.org.
2. Graham MP, Jones AL: Freshman 15: valid theory or harmful myth? *J Am Coll Health* 50(4):171-173, 2002.
3. Marcell AV and others: Male adolescent use of health care services: where are the boys? *J Adolesc Health* 30:35-43, 2002.
4. *National Survey of Counseling Center Directors,* 2001 International Association of Counseling Services, Alexandria, Va.
5. Wechsler H and others: Trends in college binge drinking during a period of increased prevention efforts, *J Am Coll Health* 50(5):203-217, 2002.
6. Wechsler H and others: Increased level of cigarette use among college students, *JAMA* 280(19):1673-1678, 1998.
7. Wechsler H and others: College smoking policies and smoking cessation programs: results of a survey of college health center directors, *J Am Coll Health* 49(4):1-8, 2001.
8. Advisory Committee on Immunization Practices (ACIP): Meningococcal disease in college students, *MMWR* RR-7, 13-20.
9. ACHA Cultural Competency statement, Retrieved July 10, 2002 from the World Wide Web: www.acha.org.

CHAPTER 21

Lifestyle Assessment

Deanna G. Gordon, Patricia A. Fergus, Janelle M. West-Koo, and Robbyn Takeuchi

Diseases of the industrialized society are often caused by nutritive deficiencies or excesses, inactivity, and ineffective stress management. Nutrition, physical activity, and stress are the dominant lifestyle features that contribute to the three main causes of death in the United States. Heart disease is the major cause of death, followed by cancer and stroke. Mortality rates for 1998, as reported by the National Center for Health Statistics, are 126.6 per 100,000 for heart disease, 123.6 deaths per 100,000 for cancer, and 25.1 per 100,000 for stroke. The rates are adjusted for age.[1]

Healthy People 2010 has incorporated morbidity and mortality data in setting objectives for the nation's health. The document offers a plan to enhance health through health promotion and disease prevention efforts. There are two major goals. The first is to increase life expectancy and quality of life for all, and the second is to eradicate health disparities among the various subgroups of the population. As reported, environmental influences and individual behaviors account for 70% of premature deaths. Two of the major focus areas for healthy lifestyle goals are nutrition/weight management and physical activity/fitness.[2]

INTERCONNECTION AMONG LIFESTYLE COMPONENTS

Lifestyle influences are not mutually exclusive but are interconnected in ways that affect health and well-being. The epidemiology of chronic disease refers to this interconnection as a "web of causation," or multifactorial causation. Nutrition and stress are interrelated in that poor nutritional status may be a stressor. For example, a diet lacking in calcium will likely lead to osteoporosis. Conversely, states of stress may influence eating behaviors. Some individuals consume greater quantities of food when they are under stress, whereas others lose their appetite. Food intake and exercise are linked through metabolic processes. Exercise enhances the effectiveness of metabolic processes, and food is the necessary fuel. Exercise and stress are connected. On one hand, exercise is effective as a means to diffuse the tension associated with stress. Conversely, humans need some stress to perform at peak levels and exercise affords an opportunity to experience positive stress through the exhilaration often experienced after engaging in physical activity.

Overweight and obesity are linked to cardiovascular problems and some forms of cancer. An imbalance in lifestyle influences is associated with a multitude of medical conditions, including type 2 diabetes, sleep apnea, gallbladder disease, hypertension, musculoskeletal injuries, and psychiatric illnesses.

Obesity

The Centers for Disease Control and Prevention has identified a 61% increase in obesity between 1991 and 2000. In 1991, 4 out of 45 states participating in the Behavioral Risk Factor Surveillance System (BRFSS) reported 15% to 19% obesity rates; no state exceeded 20%. In contrast, in 2000 all of the states except Colorado reported rates greater than 15%, with 22 states having rates of at least 20%.

An obesity epidemic exists in the United States.[3] Associated epidemiologic characteristics include age, ethnicity, level of education, and smoking status. The prevalence for obesity exceeds 20% in those between 30 and 70 years of age. Young adults have a rate of 13.5%; older adults, 15.5%. With regard to ethnicity, whites have a rate of 18.5%; blacks, 29.3%; Hispanics, 23.4%; and other races, 12.0%. Those with less than a high school education have a higher prevalence of obesity at 26.1%, whereas high school graduates are at 21.7%. More education is associated with less obesity. In individuals with some college education, 19.5% are obese, whereas those with a college-level or higher education have an obesity rate of 15.2%.[4]

Regrettably, more than half of all Americans are considered overweight.[5] An evidence-based report prepared by a consortium of the National Heart, Lung, and Blood Institute (NHLBI) reported that approximately 97 million adults are overweight or obese. The Expert Panel has defined overweight as a body mass index (BMI) from 25 to 29.9 kg/m^2. Obesity is identified as having a BMI of 30 kg/m^2 or more.[6]

Sedentary Lifestyle

Exacerbating the problem of overweight is the sedentary lifestyle of the majority of Americans. A report of the Surgeon General claims that more than 60% of adults do not meet recommendations for participation in physical activity, with one fourth being not at all active. Moreover, physical inactivity is greater among minorities than among whites. Women are less active than men, and poorer people are less physically active than are those of means.[7]

Stress

The American Institute of Stress, a nonprofit organization, is a clearinghouse for all information related to stress. The Institute touts that stress is the number one health problem in the United States. Research conducted during the past 20 years reveals the impact of stress on health. Health conditions caused by stress affect 43% of adults, and stress-related conditions account for 75% to 95% of visits to primary care providers.[8] Job-related stress is gaining recognition along with the increased incidence of violence in the workplace. Unmanaged stress is linked to hypertension, heart disease, some forms of cancer, gastrointestinal problems, and some emotional health disorders.

LIFESTYLE CHOICES

The effects of lifestyle choices are often readily apparent to the experienced clinician when the patient presents for the physical examination. Clues can be gleaned through observing body size, movement, and affect. The negative effects of poor lifestyle choices are cumulative and usually require a long incubation period before manifestation. Family history may include health conditions that tend to run in the family, such as hypertension and diabetes.

Nutrition

The patient history will provide important clues to lifestyle, including those related to cultural and religious practices that influence food preparation and consumption. Eating habits related to frequency of eating and types of food consumed should be identified. For an individual with weight management problems, the dietary intake of sugar and fats, the inclusion of foods high in fiber content, the amounts of fruits and vegetables, and the amount of food consumed should be evaluated. The consumption of stimulants such as caffeine is important because caffeine may be associated with a pleasant and uplifting feeling for some but may cause irritability and jitteriness in others.

The National Cholesterol Education Program (NCEP) Expert Panel under the auspices of the NHBLI of the National Institutes of Health has established a dietary CAGE questionnaire for practitioners to use in assessing the fat and cholesterol consumption of patients.[9] This instrument is presented in Box 21-1.

Exercise

Physical activity must also be considered as a part of the lifestyle assessment. An insufficient amount has detrimental consequences not only for cardiovascular health and flexibility but also for psychologic well-being. Sedentary patients are unlikely to describe themselves as "energetic"; indeed patients may report becoming easily fatigued. The history should include information about the type and frequency of physical activity. Consequences of the activity as well as any adverse events are important considerations for lifestyle influences on health.

Stress

Stress is a subjective experience and can be detrimental and have profound effects on cardiovascular health. To evaluate the impact of a stressor on a patient and to plan effective interventions, an understanding of the nature of the stressor is important. Attributes of stress should be explored with the patient. What is the source of the stress? Is there a single stressor, or are there multiple stressors? What is the acuity level of the stress? Some stressors are chosen, whereas others present themselves. Is the stress long-standing or newly acquired? Does the patient have prior experience in coping with the particular stressor? How effective are the patient's usual means of managing stress?

Schafer[10] has identified and described behavioral and physical distress symptoms, direct behavioral distress symptoms, and indirect symptoms of stress. Behavioral signs are manifested physically by rigidity and tightness of the body, as is evident with folded or crossed arms or legs. Fists may be clenched to indicate anxiety, or the forehead may be furrowed to signify worry. Direct behavioral distress symptoms reflect internal states and include teeth grinding, irritability, compulsiveness, rapid speech, stuttering, verbal aggression, a withdrawn demeanor, and crying spells. Indirect symptoms encompass addictive and escape behaviors. An elevated level of stress can increase the frequency of unhealthy behaviors. Addictions may be observed in increased smoking, alcohol consumption, the use of drugs to mitigate tension or induce sleep, and excessive consumption of caffeinated products. Common escape modalities are sleeping and television viewing.

Signs of stress may be apparent in self-report of the patient or through distracting mannerisms such as agitation. Questioned about stress in their lives, patients are often forthcoming with evidence and usually can identify their most significant stressors. Stress related to overload is common and is characterized by an urgency about time. Other common sources of stress are interpersonal relationships, relationships within social or work domains, financial worries, and major life changes.

In general, stress is associated with distress. However, happy events and occasions can create a type of stress known as eustress. These events may include a wedding, the birth of a baby, or winning the lottery. The stress accompanies the modifications in behavior required to adapt and adjust to the change. However, the stress associated with the changes accompanying these pleasant events is often not acknowledged.

BOX 21-1

DIETARY CAGE QUESTIONS FOR ASSESSMENT OF INTAKES OF SATURATED FAT AND CHOLESTEROL

C Cheese (and other sources of dairy fats—whole milk, 2% milk, ice cream, cream, whole fat yogurt)
A Animal fats (hamburger, ground meat, frankfurters, bologna, salami, sausage, fried foods, fatty cuts of meat)
G Got it away from home (high-fat meals either purchased and brought home or eaten in restaurants)
E Eat (extra) high-fat commercial products: candy, pastries, pies, doughnuts, cookies

Courtesy US Department of Health and Human Services: *Third Report of the National Cholesterol Education Program on Detection, Evaluation, and Treatment of High Blood Cholesterol in Adults,* Washington, DC, May 2001.

Physical Examination

Assessment of the patient's overall general appearance when he or she is first seen is an important preliminary diagnostic activity. Measurement of vital signs should be taken into account, as well as measures of height and weight. The patient who is well nourished is alert, has good color and smooth skin, stands erect, and is of normal weight for body build and age.[11] A poorly nourished patient is languid with pale, dry skin and poor posture, weighs more or less than normal for body build, and may appear to be high-strung.[11] Ease of movement can be observed to give some indication of body flexibility. Conversely, limited movement may be apparent. A patient under great stress may have signs such as agitation, excessive perspiration, impatience, anxiety, and perhaps even mental dullness.

Recent guidelines from the Obesity Education Initiative (OEI) of the NHLBI[6] recommend the use of surrogate measures to assess body fat. Although technologically sophisticated measures exist, there is evidence that they are expensive and unavailable to many clinicians; therefore BMI and waist circumference should be used. The BMI may be calculated by using the one of the following equations:

$$\text{BMI} = \text{weight (kg)} \times \text{height (m) squared}$$
$$\text{BMI} = \text{weight (lb)} \times 703 \div \text{height (in) squared}$$

The Expert Panel has defined overweight as BMI ranging from 25 to 29.9 kg/m^2 and obesity as a BMI of more than 30 kg/m^2.

In addition, the OEI recommends using waist circumference to measure abdominal fat. A measuring tape is placed on the upper hip bone and at the top of the right iliac crest so it is horizontal and parallel with the floor. The tape measure is extended around the waist in a snug manner but not so as to compress the skin. The measure is made at the end of a normal expiration. For men, a high-risk value is ≥40 inches or ≥102 cm. A measure of >35 inches or >88 cm is considered high risk for females.

The physical examination should include evaluation of cardiovascular fitness, musculature, and flexibility. The heart rate is one indicator of cardiopulmonary fitness. A fit person will have a lower heart rate with greater muscle strength and endurance, plus full range of motion. Patients who are not fit may have dyspnea or chest pain with exertion, be unable to participate in activities for extended periods, have less muscle tone and mass, and have limited range of motion.

Diagnostics

The identification of individuals at risk for health problems is key. The evaluation of blood glucose concentrations will identify those with type 2 diabetes. Lipid profile testing is important to detect individuals at risk for coronary artery disease. Lipoprotein analysis includes the measurement of concentrations of triglycerides, total cholesterol, alpha-lipoproteins (HDLs), beta-lipoproteins (LDLs), and pre–beta-lipoproteins (VLDLs). Epidemiologic investigations suggest that HDL cholesterol is inversely related to coronary disease, with high levels offering protection and lower levels increasing risk.[12] High cholesterol levels may be caused by some drugs such as corticosteroids and by diseases such as hypothyroidism, biliary obstruction, and pancreatic dysfunction.

An at-risk individual over 35 years of age who plans to begin an exercise program should undergo a stress ECG test as a precautionary measure. Younger patients with blood chemistry values and blood pressure readings indicating risk for metabolic or cardiopulmonary disease also need a complete physical examination and stress ECG test.[14] Bone density studies should be conducted on postmenopausal women to ascertain their risk for fracture and as a means to diagnosis osteopenia and osteoporosis.

Lifestyle-Related Medical Problems

Hypertension. Guidelines from the American Heart Association[15] state that a diagnosis of hypertension is based on an average of at least two blood pressure readings taken during two or more office visits after the initial measurement. An optimal reading is <120 mm Hg for systolic blood pressure and <80 mm Hg for diastolic blood pressure. A normal reading is <130 mm Hg for systolic blood pressure and <85 mm Hg for diastolic blood pressure. Patients with blood pressures in these ranges need be checked only once every 2 years. Those with blood pressures in the high-normal category (130 to 139 and 85 to 89 mm Hg for systolic and diastolic, respectively) should be checked every year.

There are three stages of hypertension. In stage 1, the reading ranges between 140 and 159 mm Hg systolic or between 90 and 99 mm Hg diastolic. Patients in this stage should be reevaluated within 2 months. Stage 2 encompasses readings of 160 to 179 mm HG systolic or 100 to 109 mm Hg diastolic. Patients with these values should be seen within 1 month. Stage 3 encompasses readings of ≥180 mm Hg systolic or ≥110 mm Hg diastolic; these patients require immediate evaluation and should be seen again within 1 week as indicated by their clinical situations.

Hyperlipidemia. Cholesterol is a sterol that is synthesized in the liver from fats consumed in the diet and endogenously within body cells.[16] Cholesterol is essential for the production of bile acids, steroids, cell membranes, and sex hormones. Cholesterol enters the bloodstream via lipoproteins, with almost 75% being bound to LDLs.[12] Normally, a value of less than 200 mg/dl is considered an acceptable cholesterol level. Table 21-1 presents the normal ranges of total cholesterol, HDL, and LDL for males and females, allowing for a 10% higher range for African-Americans. The blood triglyceride levels for males and females are presented in Table 21-2.

Diabetes. The concentration of blood glucose will vary depending on the time and contents of the last meal. In general, acceptable glucose levels for whole blood range from 60 to 89 mg/dl for adults under 60 years of age and from 68 to 98 mg/dl for individuals over 60 years of age. The acceptable range for blood serum levels is 70 to 105 mg/dl for adults under 60 years of age and 80 to 115 mg/dl for those greater than 60 years of age.[16]

Metabolic Syndrome. A cluster of risk factors significantly increase the risk for coronary artery disease. In combination the factors increase the risk for coronary heart disease with any level of LDL, according to the NCEP,[9] and the presence of three or more of the risks is sufficient to support a diagnosis of metabolic syndrome (Table 21-3).

Life Span Issues

Adverse health consequences from lifestyle influences have very long incubation periods, ranging up to several decades. It follows that interventions in risk factors at an early age will produce better health outcomes later in life. Risk factors that can be modified are dietary habits, physical activity, and stress management. In addition, methods to intervene in addictions, such as smoking and alcohol consumption, will result in a longer life with more healthy years.

In general, it is not until the middle years of life that problems rooted in earlier patterns of health behaviors begin to arise; these problems include hyperlipidemia and type 2 diabetes, which are presently seen at increasingly early ages. Men are more likely to have coronary problems than are women, although postmenopausal women have risks similar to those of men. The incidence of lung cancer has increased among women, who are more likely to begin smoking at younger ages. Postmenopausal women are at risk for calcium deficiency, which contributes to osteopenia or osteoporosis.

Older persons are particularly susceptible to malnutrition because of decreased physiologic functioning and changes associated with social factors, such as living alone. Suboptimal nutrition is often manifested by osteoporosis, iron deficiency anemia, obesity, and constipation.[19] Because malnutrition in the older patient is difficult to remedy, early detection is imperative.[20]

Older persons often erroneously believe that they have less need for physical activity. In reality, however, moderate to high

TABLE 21-1 Blood Cholesterol

Norm. There is variation in recommended norms in the literature. (*Note:* Range given applies to a healthy population consuming a typical North American diet.)

	Male		Female	
Age	mg/dL	SI Units mmol/L	SI Units mg/dL	mmol/L
TOTAL CHOLESTEROL				
Adults (10% Higher Levels for African-Americans)				
20-24 years	124-218	3.21-5.64	122-216	3.16-5.59
25-29 years	133-244	3.44-6.32	128-222	3.32-5.75
30-34 years	138-254	3.57-6.58	130-230	3.37-5.96
35-39 years	146-270	3.78-6.99	140-242	3.63-6.27
40-44 years	151-268	3.91-6.94	147-252	3.81-6.53
45-49 years	158-276	4.09-7.15	152-265	3.94-6.86
50-54 years	158-277	4.09-7.17	162-285	4.20-7.38
55-59 years	156-276	4.04-7.15	172-300	4.45-7.77
60-64 years	159-276	4.12-7.15	172-297	4.45-7.69
65-69 years	158-274	4.09-7.10	171-303	4.43-7.85
≥70 years	144-265	3.73-6.86	173-280	4.48-7.25
HIGH-DENSITY LIPOPROTEIN CHOLESTEROL (HDL)				
Adult (African-American Levels Approximately 10 mg/dL Higher)				
20-24 years	30-63	0.78-1.63	33-79	0.85-2.04
25-29 years	31-63	0.80-1.63	37-83	0.96-2.15
30-34 years	28-63	0.72-1.63	36-77	0.93-1.99
35-39 years	29-62	0.75-1.60	34-82	0.88-2.12
40-44 years	27-67	0.70-1.73	34-88	0.88-2.28
45-49 years	30-64	0.78-1.66	34-87	0.88-2.25
50-54 years	28-63	0.72-1.63	37-92	0.96-2.38
55-59 years	28-71	0.72-1.84	37-91	0.96-2.35
60-64 years	30-74	0.78-1.91	38-92	0.98-2.38
65-69 years	30-75	0.78-1.94	35-96	0.91-2.48
≥70 years	31-75	0.80-1.94	33-92	0.85-2.38
LOW-DENSITY LIPOPROTEIN CHOLESTEROL (LDL)				
Adult				
20-24 years	66-147	1.71-3.81	57-159	1.48-4.12
25-29 years	70-165	1.81-4.27	71-164	1.84-4.25
30-34 years	78-185	2.02-4.79	70-156	1.81-4.04
35-39 years	81-189	2.10-4.90	75-172	1.94-4.45
40-44 years	87-186	2.25-4.82	74-174	1.92-4.51
45-49 years	97-202	2.51-5.23	79-186	2.05-4.82
50-54 years	89-197	2.31-5.10	88-201	2.28-5.21
55-59 years	88-203	2.28-5.26	89-210	2.31-5.44
60-64 years	83-210	2.15-5.44	100-224	2.59-5.80
65-69 years	98-210	2.54-5.44	92-221	2.38-5.72
≥70 years	88-186	2.28-4.82	96-206	2.49-5.34

Modified from Chernecky C, Berger B, editors: *Laboratory tests and diagnostics procedures,* ed 3, Philadelphia, 2001, WB Saunders.

levels of exercise boost their psychologic functioning, thereby facilitating functional status. In one study, exercise was shown to improve muscle strength, reaction time, and even control over body sway.[21]

COMPONENTS OF A HEALTHY LIFESTYLE

Lifestyle change is difficult, and the course is usually not smooth. There will be setbacks, but it is imperative that the patient begin anew and not be detoured. The therapeutic plan should be as simple as possible because one that is perceived as "too complicated" will become a disincentive.

Lifestyle counseling is essential to primary prevention of disease and disability and will have a positive effect on modifiable risk factors such as hypertension and hyperlipidemia. At the level of primary prevention, health education and counseling regarding nutrition, physical activity, and stress management will produce positive results for the patient.

Nutrition

The American diet has changed substantially during the past few decades. More meals are consumed on the run, away from home and family. Much food is consumed in the form of fast

TABLE 21-2 Triglycerides

		SI Units
SERUM VALUES		
Adult Females		
20-29 years	10-100 mg/dL	0.11-1.13 mmol/L
30-39 years	10-110 mg/dL	0.11-1.24 mmol/L
40-49 years	10-122 mg/dL	0.11-1.38 mmol/L
50-59 years	10-134 mg/dL	0.11-1.51 mmol/L
>59 years	10-147 mg/dL	0.11-1.66 mmol/L
Adult Males		
20-29 years	10-157 mg/dL	0.11-1.77 mmol/L
30-39 years	10-182 mg/dL	0.11-2.05 mmol/L
40-49 years	10-193 mg/dL	0.11-2.18 mmol/L
50-59 years	10-197 mg/dL	0.11-2.22 mmol/L
>59 years	10-199 mg/dL	0.11-2.24 mmol/L
Classification of Triglyceride Levels		
Borderline high	200-400 mg/dL	2.3 mmol/L
High	400-1000 mg/dL	4.5-11.3 mmol/L
Very high	>1000 mg/dL	>11.3 mmol/L

Modified from Chernecky C, Berger B, editors: *Laboratory tests and diagnostics procedures,* ed 3, Philadelphia, 2001, WB Saunders.

TABLE 21-3 Clinical Identification of Metabolic Syndrome

Risk Factor	Defining Level
Abdominal obesity*	Waist Circumference†
Men	>102 cm (>40 in)
Women	>88 cm (>35 in)
Triglycerides	≥150 mg/dL
HDL cholesterol	
Men	<40 mg/dL
Women	<50 mg/dL
Blood pressure	≥130/≥85 mm Hg
Fasting glucose	≥110 mg/dL

Courtesy U.S. Department of Health and Human Services: *Third Report of the National Cholesterol Education Program on Detection, Evaluation, and Treatment of High Blood Cholesterol in Adults,* Washington, DC, May 2001.

*Overweight and obesity are associated with insulin resistance and the metabolic syndrome. However, the presence of abdominal obesity is more highly correlated with the metabolic risk factors than is an elevated body mass index (BMI). Therefore the simple measure of waist circumference is recommended to identify the body weight component of the metabolic syndrome.

†Some male patients can develop multiple metabolic risk factors when the waist circumference is only marginally increased (e.g., 94-102 cm [37-39 in]). Such patients may have a strong genetic contribution to insulin resistance. They should benefit from changes in life habits, similarly to men with categorical increases in waist circumference.

food, which is usually high in fat, calories, and salt. Over time, there is a cumulative effect on the body, with an increase in girth. Early on, the patient needs encouragement to make better food selections. Figure 21-1 depicts the U.S. Department of Agriculture Food Guide Pyramid and can be used as the standard for a healthy diet.

Eating well has several benefits, including providing a sense of vitality, maintaining a better weight, and giving a better overall appearance. Identifying factors that influence food consumption behaviors will enable the primary care provider to adapt health counseling to the patient's unique circumstances. Motives that influence food selection and consumption may relate to culture, habit, or convenience. Cultural practices must be acknowledged and accommodated in health counseling. Habits related to food intake probably require a program of behavioral change. Food consumption behaviors born out of convenience, such as reaching for chips when hunger is felt, may be amendable through health education.

Adequacy of nutritional intake should be ensured. Sufficient intake of daily dietary fiber is often neglected. Fiber in the form of whole-grain foods, fruits, and vegetables is essential to good health and aids in reducing heart disease and cancer. Fiber-rich foods are often neglected because they often require cleaning and preparation. These nutrients are often replaced with prepackaged snack foods. One technique that can be used to avoid convenience foods is to have clean fruits and vegetables prepared in advance and stored so they are ready to eat when a quick snack is desired.

Middle-aged women may be at risk for hypocalcemia resulting from a diet that lacks calcium-rich foods. The ingestion of calcium-enriched orange juice, almonds, spinach, broccoli, kale, turnip greens, milk, cheese, and yogurt should be encouraged. However, caution is advised because overconsumption of calcium may result in hypercalcemia, which is related to the formation of calcium renal calculi.

Caffeine has been classified as a drug because of its effects on the body. Caffeine is used for its stimulating effect, which causes a higher degree of alertness. Excess caffeine, however, can induce caffeinism, which is characterized by headaches, irritability, anxiety, insomnia, and heart palpitations.

Recent studies suggest that moderate intake of caffeine may not have the detrimental consequences once associated with its use. Moderate use is generally considered to be <250 mg per day, or the equivalent of two to three 5-ounce cups of coffee; percolated coffee has 64 to 124 mg of caffeine per 5 ounces, whereas drip-brewed coffee has 110 to 150 mg of caffeine per 5 ounces.[23] Coke has 46 mg of caffeine in a 12-ounce can, and Mountain Dew has 54 mg.[23]

The Vegetarian Diet. Many individuals have chosen to become vegetarians. Reasons for this include political ideologies, concern for excess consumption of saturated fat in beef products, concern over food-borne illnesses associated with meat consumption, and a desire for a healthier lifestyle. Vegetarians should follow the principle of complementation when selecting foods. To ensure that the required amino acids are supplied, complementation combines a grain with legumes or a dairy product (for lactovegetarians). Possible combinations include a peanut butter-and-jelly sandwich, beans and corn, brown bread and baked beans, a flour tortilla and beans, macaroni and cheese, and rice and milk. A major health concern is the adequacy of vitamin B intake because meats are the major source of this nutrient. Because vegetarians may not deliberately plan their meals to incorporate essential nutrients, they should be advised to take a daily multivitamin.

Weight Management. The practice guidelines released by the OEI of the NHLBI[16] advocates that management of overweight

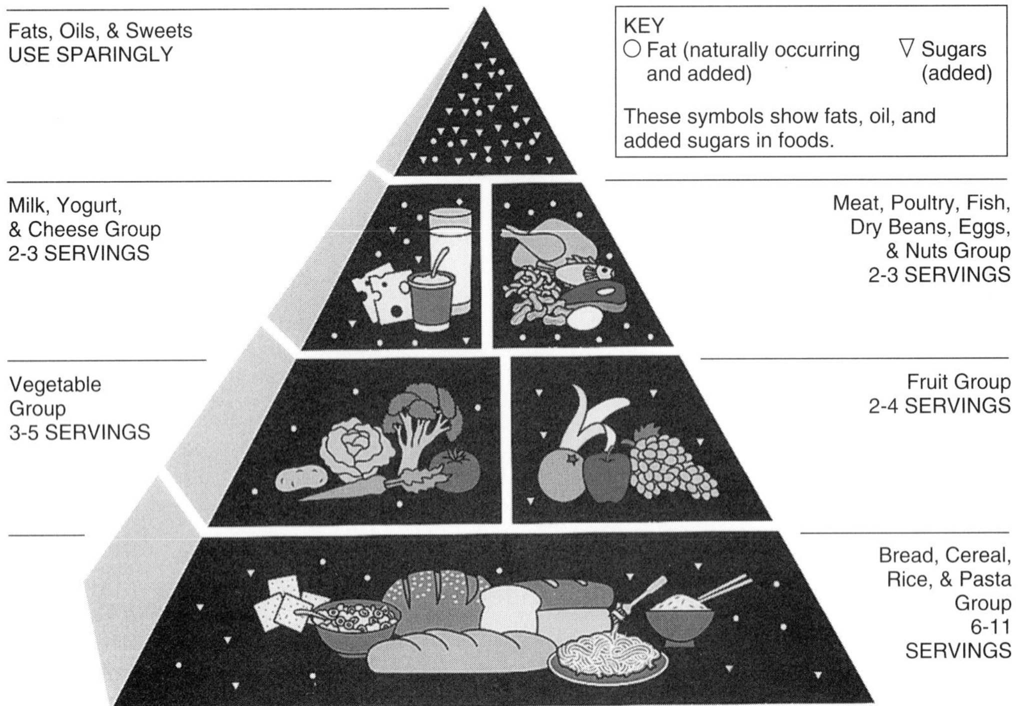

FIGURE 21-1

The Food Guide Pyramid. (Courtesy of U.S. Department of Agriculture and the U.S. Department of Health and Human Services.)

and obesity has many components, including behavioral, dietary, physical, and pharmacologic. The Expert Panel offer several suggestions from a behavioral perspective. The clinician must communicate with the patient in a nonjudgmental manner. The diagnosis of obesity usually comes as no surprise, and the patient may have a long history of frustration and trouble with weight control. In addition, clinicians need to examine their own attitudes toward the condition.

Experts liken obesity to a chronic disease, such as diabetes. Behavioral change is required, and compliance with a long-term regimen of behavioral change is generally poor. Clinicians are advised to build a partnership with the patient, taking into account the patient's weight management goals. Goal setting should be specific yet achievable. A reasonable goal for weight loss can be a reduction of 10% of body weight over a 6-month period. Weight control is not a destination but rather a journey; therefore frequent contact with the health care provider is beneficial to the patient. This can be achieved through frequent monitoring of weight, which has the advantage of being an effective motivator.

Dietary Considerations. According to the OEI practice guidelines,[6] the patient's motivation or inclination toward weight loss is of primary concern. Diet is the cornerstone of a weight management program. According to the recommendations, there are many topics to cover in a patient education program. The patient will need basic instructions on the composition of foods, including information on calorie content, how to read food labels, and what constitutes a serving size. In addition, the patient may need coaching on how to make wise food purchases and techniques for low-calorie food preparation. The patient should understand the value of adequate water intake and the importance of limiting alcohol consumption. Suggested food plans for 1200-calorie and 1600-calorie diets are presented in Tables 21-4 and 21-5, respectively. A guide to food exchanges is presented in Box 21-2.

Exercise

Patients who do not participate in any type of physical activity may have a plethora of excuses. Among the most familiar are lack of time, feeling tired, being too busy, and having a dislike for exercise. Older adults may use their age to justify a lack of physical activity. However, physical activity has been called a "magic bullet" that can ward off heart disease and should be encouraged.

Before encouraging any type of exercise program, the primary care provider must be aware of the patient's existing level of fitness. A patient in mid-life or one who is sedentary and significantly overweight may need medical clearance to begin exercising based on clinical findings in the history and physical examination.

For the sedentary patient, it is extremely important to begin a physical fitness program slowly so that the body can acclimate to the new demands imposed on it. Moreover, a slow start safeguards against injury. An overzealous exercise program is likely to have a negative impact on motivation (i.e., the exercise prescription may serve as a deterrent if it is too rigorous early on). The patient must be committed to carrying out the program. Most individuals are aware of the value of incorporating exercise into their daily schedules, yet many do not follow through. Because exercise requires a personal commitment, individuals need to be deliberate about making time for exercise in their daily lives. Wilbur, Chandler, and Miller[24] investigated women's adherence to a home-based walking program. Frequency of participation

TABLE 21-4 1200-Calorie Diet

	Calories	Fat (grams)	% Fat	Exchange for:
BREAKFAST				
Whole wheat bread, 1 medium slice	70	1.2	15	1 bread/starch
Jelly, regular, 2 tsp	30	0	0	½ fruit
Cereal, shredded wheat, ½ cup	104	1	4	1 bread/starch
Milk, 1%, 1 cup	102	3	23	1 milk
Orange juice, ¾ cup	78	0	0	1½ fruit
Coffee, regular, 1 cup	5	0	0	Free
Breakfast total	**389**	**5.2**	**10**	
LUNCH				
Roast beef sandwich:				
Whole wheat bread, 2 medium slices	139	2.4	15	2 bread/starch
Lean roast beef, unseasoned, 2 oz	60	1.5	23	2 lean protein
Lettuce, 1 leaf	1	0	0	
Tomato, 3 medium slices	10	0	0	1 vegetable
Mayonnaise, low calorie, 1 tsp	15	1.7	96	⅓ fat
Apple, 1 medium	80	0	0	1 fruit
Water, 1 cup	0	0	0	Free
Lunch total	**305**	**5.6**	**16**	
DINNER				
Salmon, 2 ounces edible	103	5	44	2 lean protein
Vegetable oil, 1½ tsp	60	7	100	1½ fat
Baked potato, ¾ medium	100	0	0	1 bread/starch
Margarine, 1 tsp	34	4	100	1 fat
Green beans, seasoned, with margarine, ½ cup	52	2	4	1 vegetable, ½ fat
Carrots, seasoned	35	0	0	1 vegetable
White dinner roll, 1 small	70	2	28	1 bread/starch
Iced tea, unsweetened, 1 cup	0	0	0	Free
Water, 2 cups	0	0	0	Free
Dinner total	**454**	**20**	**39**	
SNACK				
Popcorn, 2½ cups	69	0	0	1 bread/starch
Margarine, ¾ tsp	30	3	100	¾ fat
Total	**1247**	**34-36**	**24-26**	

Modified from National Heart, Lung, and Blood Institute: *The practical guide to the identification, evaluation, and treatment of overweight and obesity in adults,* Bethesda, Md, 2000, NHLBI Information Center.

Traditional American Cuisine—1200 Calories

You can use the exchange list in Box 21-2 to give yourself more choices.

Calories	1,247	Saturated fat, % kcals	7
Total carbohydrate, % kcals	58	Cholesterol, mg	96
Total fat, % kcals	26	Protein, % kcals	19
*Sodium, mg	1,043		

Note: Calories have been rounded.

1200: 100% RDA met for all nutrients except vitamin E 80%, vitamin B_2 96%, vitamin B_6 94%, calcium 68%, iron 63%, and zinc 73%.

*No salt added in recipe preparation or as seasoning. Consume at least 32 ounces of water.

proved to be most problematic; however, once the 24 women began walking, they walked for the prescribed length of time and at the appropriate intensity. Thus patients may need suggestions for scheduling physical activities into their daily routines to ensure frequency of participation in physical activity.

The OEI recommends 30 to 40 minutes of moderate activity 3 to 5 days a week. Good results can be achieved through a program of walking.[6] Table 21-6 provides a suggested plan from the OEI Expert Panel.

Aerobic activity is particularly recommended for cardiac health because it works to strengthen the heart muscle. Aerobic endurance training consists of three phases: the warm-up, aerobics, and the cool down. Warming up for the intensity of aerobic training begins to raise the pulse rate and prepares the muscles and joints. This generally takes 3 to 5 minutes but may take longer in lower temperatures. Often, the warm-up activity is a gentler motion of the same type of physical activity that is part of the aerobic exercise and may involve stretching. The aerobic portion encompasses the dimensions of frequency, intensity, and time (known by the acronym *FIT*). The recommended frequency is three to five times per week, with a day off between workouts being desirable.

TABLE 21-5 1600-Calorie Diet

	Calories	Fat (grams)	% Fat	Exchange for:
BREAKFAST				
Whole wheat bread, 1 medium slice	70	1.2	15.4	1 bread/starch
Jelly, regular, 2 tsp	30	0	0	½ fruit
Cereal, shredded wheat, 1 cup	207	2	8	2 bread/starch
Milk, 1%, 1 cup	102	3	23	1 milk
Orange juice, ¾ cup	78	0	0	1½ fruit
Coffee, regular, 1 cup	5	0	0	Free
Milk, 1%, 1 oz	10	0.3	27	⅛ milk
Breakfast total	**502**	**6.5**	**10**	
LUNCH				
Roast beef sandwich:				
Whole wheat bread, 2 medium slices	139	2.4	15	2 bread/starch
Lean roast beef, unseasoned, 2 oz	60	1.5	23	2 lean protein
American cheese, lowfat and low sodium, 1 slice, ¾ oz	46	1.8	36	1 lean protein
Lettuce, 1 leaf	1	0	0	
Tomato, 3 medium slices	10	0	0	1 vegetable
Mayonnaise, low calorie, 2 tsp	30	3.3	99	⅔ fat
Apple, 1 medium	80	0	0	1 fruit
Water, 1 cup	0	0	0	Free
Lunch total	**366**	**9**	**22**	
DINNER				
Salmon, 3 ounces edible	155	7	40	3 lean protein
Vegetable oil, 1½ tsp	60	7	100	1½ fat
Baked potato, ¾ medium	100	0	0	1 bread/starch
Margarine, 1 tsp	34	4	100	1 fat
Green beans, seasoned, with margarine, ½ cup	52	2	4	1 vegetable, ½ fat
Carrots, seasoned, with margarine, ½ cup	52	2	4	1 vegetable, ½ fat
White dinner roll, 1 medium	80	3	33	1 bread/starch
Ice milk, ½ cup	92	3	28	1 bread/starch, ½ fat
Iced tea, unsweetened, 1 cup	0	0	0	Free
Water, 3 cups	0	0	0	Free
Dinner total	**625**	**28**	**38**	
SNACK				
Popcorn, 2½ cups	69	0	0	1 bread/starch
Margarine, ½ tsp	58	6.5	100	1½ fat
Total	**1613**	**50**	**28**	

Modified from National Heart, Lung, and Blood Institute: *The practical guide to the identification, evaluation, and treatment of overweight and obesity in adults,* Bethesda, Md, 2000, NHLBI Information Center.

Traditional American Cuisine—1600 Calories

You can use the exchange list in Box 21-2 to give yourself more choices.

Calories	1,613	Saturated fat, % kcals	8
Total carbohydrate, % kcals	55	Cholesterol, mg	142
Total fat, % kcals	29	Protein, % kcals	19
*Sodium, mg	1,341		

Note: Calories have been rounded.

1,600: 100% RDA met for all nutrients except vitamin E 99%, iron 73%, and zinc 91%.

*No salt added in recipe preparation or as seasoning. Consume at least 32 ounces of water.

Heart rate is a measure of intensity. The maximum heart rate, calculated by subtracting one's age from 220, represents the heart rate that should not be exceeded during exercise. For example, an individual who is 55 years of age should not have a pulse rate in excess of 165 beats per minute during training. The target heart rate is recommended for maximum effectiveness of aerobic activity and is represented by a range of values between 60% to 80% of the maximum heart rate. Thus the 55-year-old individual is well advised to keep the pulse rate between 99 beats per minute (165 maximum heart rate × 60% = 99) and 132 beats per minute (165 maximum heart rate × 80% = 132). The aerobic portion of activity should be at least 20 minutes long, with the heart beating within the range of the target heart rate. Conditioned individuals may extend their workouts to up to 1 hour.

Any activity that requires rhythmic, continuous movement and the use of the large muscles of the arms and legs may be

BOX 21-2

FOOD EXCHANGE LIST

Within each group, these foods can be exchanged for each other. You can use this list to give yourself more choices.

VEGETABLES

Contain 25 calories and 5 grams of carbohydrate. One serving equals:

- ½ cup cooked vegetables (e.g., carrots, broccoli, zucchini, cabbage)
- 1 cup raw vegetables or salad greens
- ½ cup vegetable juice

If you're hungry, eat more fresh or steamed vegetables.

FAT FREE AND VERY LOW FAT MILK

Contains 90 calories and 12 grams of carbohydrate per serving. One serving equals:

- 8 oz milk, fat free or 1% fat
- ¾ cup yogurt, plain nonfat or lowfat
- 1 cup yogurt, artificially sweetened

VERY LEAN PROTEIN

Choices have 35 calories and 1 gram of fat per serving. One serving equals:

- 1 oz turkey breast or chicken breast, skin removed
- 1 oz fish fillet (flounder, sole, scrod, cod, haddock, halibut)
- 1 oz canned tuna in water
- 1 oz shellfish (clams, lobster, scallop, shrimp)
- ¾ cup cottage cheese, nonfat or lowfat
- 2 each egg whites
- ¼ cup egg substitute
- 1 oz fat-free cheese
- ½ cup beans—cooked (black beans, kidney, chickpeas, or lentils); count as 1 starch/bread and 1 very lean protein

FRUITS

Contain 15 grams of carbohydrates and 60 calories. One serving equals:

- 1 small apple, banana, orange, nectarine
- 1 medium fresh peach
- 1 kiwi
- ½ grapefruit
- ½ mango
- 1 cup fresh berries (strawberries, raspberries, or blueberries)
- 1 cup fresh melon cubes
- ⅛ honeydew melon
- 4 oz unsweetened juice
- 4 tsp jelly or jam

LEAN PROTEIN

Choices have 55 calories and 2 to 3 grams of fat per serving. One serving equals:

- 1 oz chicken—dark meat, skin removed
- 1 oz turkey—dark meat, skin removed
- 1 oz salmon, swordfish, herring, catfish, trout
- 1 oz lean beef (flank steak, London broil, tenderloin, roast beef)*
- 1 oz veal, roast, or lean chop*
- 1 oz lamb, roast, or lean chop*
- 1 oz pork, tenderloin, or fresh ham*
- 1 oz lowfat cheese (3 grams or less of fat per ounce)
- 1 oz lowfat luncheon meats (with 3 grams or less of fat per ounce)
- ¼ cup 4.5% cottage cheese
- 2 medium sardines

***Limit to 1 to 2 times per week.**

MEDIUM FAT PROTEINS

Have 75 calories and 5 grams of fat per serving. One serving equals:

- 1 oz beef (any prime cut), corned beef, ground beef†
- 1 oz pork chop
- 1 oz whole egg (medium)†
- 1 oz mozzarella cheese
- ¼ cup ricotta cheese
- 4 oz tofu (note that this is a heart-healthy choice)

†Choose these very infrequently.

STARCHES

Contain 15 grams of carbohydrate and 80 calories per serving. One serving equals:

- 1 slice bread (white, pumpernickel, whole wheat, rye)
- 2 slices reduced calorie or "lite" bread
- ¼ (1 oz) bagel (varies)
- ½ English muffin
- ½ hamburger bun
- ¾ cup cold cereal
- ⅓ cup rice, brown or white—cooked
- ⅓ cup barley or couscous—cooked
- ⅓ cup legumes (dried beans, peas, or lentils)—cooked
- ½ cup pasta—cooked
- ½ cup bulgur—cooked
- ½ cup corn, sweet potato, or green peas
- 3 oz baked sweet or white potato
- ¾ oz pretzels
- 3 cups popcorn, hot-air popped or microwave (80-percent light)

FATS

Contain 45 calories and 5 grams of fat per serving. One serving equals:

- 1 tsp oil (vegetable, corn, canola, olive, etc.)
- 1 tsp butter
- 1 tsp stick margarine
- 1 tsp mayonnaise
- 1 T reduced fat margarine or mayonnaise
- 1 T salad dressing
- 1 T cream cheese
- 2 T lite cream cheese
- ⅛ avocado
- 8 large black olives
- 10 large stuffed green olives
- 1 slice bacon

Modified from National Heart, Lung, and Blood Institute: *The practical guide to the identification, evaluation, and treatment of overweight and obesity in adults,* Bethesda, Md, 2000, NHLBI Information Center.
Source: Based on the American Dietetic Association Exchange List.

TABLE 21-6 Sample Walking Program

	Warmup	Exercising	Cool Down	Total Time
WEEK 1				
Session A	Walk 5 min	Then walk briskly 5 min	Then walk more slowly 5 min	15 min
Session B	Repeat above pattern			
Session C	Repeat above pattern			
Continue with at least three exercise sessions during each week of the program.				
Week 2	Walk 5 min	Walk briskly 7 min	Walk 5 min	17 min
Week 3	Walk 5 min	Walk briskly 9 min	Walk 5 min	19 min
Week 4	Walk 5 min	Walk briskly 11 min	Walk 5 min	21 min
Week 5	Walk 5 min	Walk briskly 13 min	Walk 5 min	23 min
Week 6	Walk 5 min	Walk briskly 15 min	Walk 5 min	25 min
Week 7	Walk 5 min	Walk briskly 18 min	Walk 5 min	28 min
Week 8	Walk 5 min	Walk briskly 20 min	Walk 5 min	30 min
Week 9	Walk 5 min	Walk briskly 23 min	Walk 5 min	33 min
Week 10	Walk 5 min	Walk briskly 26 min	Walk 5 min	36 min
Week 11	Walk 5 min	Walk briskly 28 min	Walk 5 min	38 min
Week 12	Walk 5 min	Walk briskly 30 min	Walk 5 min	40 min
Week 13 on:				
Gradually increase your brisk walking time to 30 to 60 minutes, three or four times a week. Remember that your goal is to get the benefits you are seeking and enjoy your activity.				

From National Heart, Lung, and Blood Institute: *The practical guide to the identification, evaluation, and treatment of overweight and obesity in adults,* Bethesda, Md, 2000, NHLBI Information Center.

selected. Bicycling, cross-country skiing, and some forms of dancing are examples of aerobic activities. The final component of the workout is the cool down, during which the heart rate gradually returns to normal. Because the muscles are warm, stretching exercises may be incorporated to enhance flexibility.

Resistance training for muscle strength and endurance may be performed before an aerobic activity training or on opposite days. Some individuals lift weights as part of the warm-up. Musculoskeletal training may be achieved through the use of weights or through calisthenics.

The American Heart Association[25] advises that individuals be aware of any sensation of pressure or pain in the mid- or left chest area and/or pallor, cold sweat, sudden light-headedness, or fainting during a workout. If any of these events occur, patients should be instructed to stop exercising and call the primary care provider.

Physical Activity and Chronic Illness

Evidence strongly suggests that physical activity has a significant positive effect on patients with chronic diseases. Sally Fitts, PhD, of the Department of Rehabilitation Medicine at the University of Washington,[26] discovered that stationary bicycling during hemodialysis is beneficial for patients with chronic renal failure and end-stage renal disease. The exercise is not only safe but also increases the efficiency of fluid removal and decreases common problems that accompany dialysis, such as chills, fatigue, and muscle cramping. Fitts cautions that the target heart rate is not a useful measure for patients with end-stage renal disease and instead recommends that the patient's report of perceived exertion be used to determine fitness and intensity.

Patricia Deuster, PhD, MPH, of the Department of Military and Emergency Medicine of the Uniformed Services University of the Health Sciences,[27] affirms that physically active women have a reduced breast cancer risk and that those with osteoporosis, fibromyalgia, or rheumatoid arthritis also benefit from exercise. Osteoporosis, a disease that affects not only postmenopausal women but also female athletes who are amenorrheic, is linked to a low bone mineral density. The condition is averted through impact and weight-bearing exercises. For those with fibromyalgia, cardiovascular conditioning enhances fitness and elevates the pain threshold. Arthritic patients benefit both physically and psychologically. Muscle strength and joint flexibility are improved, and morning stiffness is decreased; psychologically, anxiety and depression are decreased. Exercise regimens that are particularly effective with arthritic patients are water-based exercises and modified dance exercises. Although these preliminary observations hold promise, definitive guidelines must be deferred until the appropriate frequency, intensity, and duration of exercise have been determined.[27]

Stress Management

Behaviors that are beneficial to physiologic wellness, such as engaging in physical activity and a healthy diet, also afford protection against the adverse effects of stress. Excessive stress is harmful because it interferes with the functioning of the immune system, and high levels of stress can impede disease protection.[28] Fortunately, there are many ways to minimize the detrimental consequences, including adequate amounts of sleep, cultivation of interpersonal relationships, relaxation techniques, good time management skills, prayer, a perspective on life, and a sense of humor.

Sleep. Impairment secondary to insufficient sleep is in itself a common health problem that increases the risk for errors in performance and problem solving. Originally, it was believed that sleep was essential to rejuvenate the body physically. Current interest in sleep research is centered on the effect of sleep on the prefrontal cerebral cortex, the part of the brain associated with higher-level thinking abilities. For many, sleep is a low priority and is often sacrificed to make time for other activities. As a consequence, sleep-deprived individuals are more at risk for automobile accidents, anxiety, and depression; are less productive; and are poorer at problem solving. To operate at peak performance, most individuals require from 7 to 8 hours of sleep each day. Some individuals can manage with fewer than 5 hours of sleep, but they represent the exception.

To guarantee adequate time for sleep, time management techniques may be used to deliberately block out the time needed for adequate rest. The sleep schedule should be regular, which means arising at the same time daily. Caffeinated products should be avoided for a minimum of 6 and up to 11 hours before retiring. Sleeping pills and alcohol should be avoided as aids to sleep. A glass of warm milk or a slice of turkey may be helpful because these foods contain the amino acid tryptophan, which is a natural sedative. Daily exercise is also an effective sleep inducer, although it should be avoided before bedtime, when it may have a stimulating effect. Cares and worries should not preoccupy the time before dozing off. Instead, noting concerns and planning courses of action before going to bed may be helpful. Bedtime rituals are also effective for sleep preparation. These may include reading, praying, making preparations for the next day, and bathing.

Interpersonal Relationships. Healthy and satisfying personal relationships are not only rewarding but also buffer some of the stressors in life. Encouraging patients to nurture, maintain, and cherish relationships with family and friends is beneficial. In addition, patients need to have realistic expectations of what to expect from their relationships with others. The quality of relationships takes precedence over quantity; therefore a few good friends confer greater resistance to stress than do many superficial ones.

Relaxation. The relaxation response is an antidote to the physiologic alterations triggered by exposure to a stressor. Blood glucose levels decrease with relaxation, as do the heart rate, respiration rate, and blood pressure. Muscles relax as well. Psychologic advantages may include decreased anxiety and an enhanced ability to cope with fearful situations.

Napping, walking, stroking a pet, participating in a hobby, listening to soothing music, and other activities can elicit the relaxation response. Breathing techniques are also effective for decreasing stress. Deep breathing involves two steps: (1) inhaling through the nose with the intention of inflating the lungs and (2) exhaling through the mouth at a slower rate than inhaling. This is the "cleansing breath" many individuals learn in Lamaze classes. Another technique involves diaphragmatic breathing (i.e., using the diaphragm to regulate respiration). This is sometimes called "belly breathing," which can be observed in the way an infant breathes. The belly is thrust outward as a long, deep breath is taken. Because the relaxation occurs on exhalation, the exhalation should be long and slow.

Time Management. Time is a precious commodity and must be managed wisely. Americans are overextended by the sheer volume of tasks they hope to complete daily. Even youths are beginning to complain of not having enough time in the day—a phenomenon previously reserved for adulthood and its concomitant responsibilities. A common time management technique is to apply an *A, B, C* format to the list of tasks that need to be achieved on a given day. *A* represents what must be achieved during the day, *B* signifies an important task, and *C* means that the activity can wait for another day. The goal is to achieve tasks assigned to the *A* group, make progress on those in the *B* group, and possibly begin the tasks in the *C* group. To ensure successful completion of required and important tasks, individuals should schedule themselves at 75% capacity. Inevitably, tasks, projects, and assignments consume more time than originally allocated. "Underscheduling" will probably convert to a full, rather than overloaded, slate of activities. As the day progresses, it is helpful to ask the question, "What is the best use of my time right now?" Breaks are important and can be used during transition times between activities. A break may be filled with having a meal, engaging in a physical activity (e.g., walking around the block, jumping rope), or calling a friend on the telephone. In the long run, continuously working without a break will diminish productivity and may lead to psychologic burnout.

Prayer. In the aftermath of the events of September 11, 2001, the basic sense of psychologic security was violated in many Americans. Some experienced depression, requiring medication for symptom relief. Others responded by becoming more spiritual and turning to a higher power for assistance in the face of adversity. Overall, those with an active prayer life tend to be more optimistic in their outlooks. Certainly the spiritual domain of health must be acknowledged and faith practices encouraged.

Perspective on Life. Optimists seem to fare better than do pessimists. Patients can be encouraged and supported in their attempts to keep a positive perspective. Care needs to be taken with unduly upset patients or with those who are experiencing a significant personal loss. To coach these individuals in optimism would be to trivialize their needs. These patients could be better served by identifying a source of hope for them.

Humor. A sense of humor serves many purposes. Certainly, it enables one to laugh rather than cry about a situation. Not only does laughter diffuse stress in an individual but, when used appropriately, humor may subdue interpersonal tension in nonamiable social situations.

Safety

Home Safety. Home is regarded as a "safe" haven by many, yet it is the scene for most accidents and injuries. Falls result from navigating cluttered rooms and steps. Kitchen fires can arise from cooking fats and improperly using small appliances. Poisonings occur from chemicals commonly found in household cleaning solutions. In addition, toxic fumes in the form of carbon monoxide or radon may be emitted within homes. Larger appliances, power tools, and electrical cords also pose potential dangers. The use of goggles or safety glasses and ear plugs may be warranted with some types of tools.

Safety at home requires a knowledge of potential sources of trauma and injury. Smoke detectors are recommended for each level of the house. If the smoke detectors are battery powered, batteries should be checked twice a year and replaced as necessary. The schedule should coincide with an event, such as resetting the clock for daylight savings time in April and for standard time in October. Carbon monoxide detectors may be useful for detecting carbon monoxide leaks. Radon, another poisonous gas, can also be detected with a home testing kit. Ventilation systems also need to be checked.

Lighting needs to be assessed for adequacy. In dark homes and in homes with small children or older adults, nightlights may prevent injury from tripping or falling. Floor rugs need to be anchored securely to prevent falls, and stairs should be free of clutter. Slippery floors may also cause household accidents. Electrical cords should not be frayed and should be out of the path of normal daily activity.

Hazardous cleaning supplies need to be stored safely and toxic supplies disposed of properly. Medications should be labeled and kept out of the reach of children. If firearms are kept in the home, extra care needs to be exercised to reduce the risk of injury. Guns should be stored unloaded and be secured under lock and key. Ammunition should be stored away from the firearm, preferably in a locked compartment or container.

The incidence of natural disasters, such as flooding, has increased. Thus it is important for families to have mapped out emergency plans. Important papers and documents, such as birth certificates and Social Security cards for all family members, should be kept in a central place so they are available in the event that household members need to evacuate quickly. Moreover, a supply of any necessary medications should be on hand. A central meeting place should be designated or an extended family member or representative away from the residence should be identified as a communication link should household members become separated in an emergency.

Sports and Vehicular Safety. Seat belts should always be worn. Although some would argue that seat belt use may be responsible for injury or death by trapping an individual in an automobile, this is the rare exception. Most often, seat belts save lives. Drivers need to be alert to the possibility of "road rage," or the expression of impatience and aggression by other drivers. When encountering an individual who may be enraged, it is recommended to avoid eye contact and be alert for opportunities for safety, such as escape routes.

Extra protection should be used to prevent unintentional sports injuries. Mouth guards are advised for those participating in upper body contact sports, such as soccer, basketball, and football. Helmets should be worn for in-line skating, bicycling, riding on a moped or motorcycle, and other activities that present the threat of being forcefully thrown. These include horseback riding and snow skiing. Patients must be advised that additional protective devices such as wrist guards, elbow, and knee protectors prevent traumatic injury with in-line skating.

SMOKING CESSATION

Smoking is the most preventable risk factor for morbidity and mortality in people living in the developed nations of the world.[29] The World Health Organization estimates that tobacco will cause or result in to an annual global rate of 8.4 million deaths by 2020.[29] Nevertheless, the effects of smoking are potentially reversible; smoking represents a treatable condition. Most smokers are aware of the dangers and want to stop but find this very difficult to do.

The causes of smoking are varied; the appeal is different for each smoker. Smoking is pleasurable for some and is a habit for others. Tobacco has more than 4000 components, many of which have biologic activity. Nicotine, a vasoconstrictor, is the most widely known constituent of cigarette smoke. With inhalation of cigarette smoke, nicotine is distributed throughout the body within 10 seconds.[30] At high exposure levels, nicotine is a potentially lethal poison that may cause intoxication in young children who ingest cigarettes. Long-term nicotine exposure affects many organ systems and has been associated with cancer, hypertension, cardiovascular disease, and gastrointestinal and reproductive disorders.

Most smokers use tobacco products regularly because they are addicted to nicotine. Addiction is defined as "compulsive drug seeking and use, even in the face of negative health consequences."[30] Health care providers should remember that approximately 35 million smokers attempt to quit annually but that fewer than 7% of them are able to achieve 1 year of abstinence without help.[30] Cigarettes are very efficient and highly engineered drug delivery systems. Because a typical smoker inhales an average of 10 puffs per cigarette, if that person smokes one pack a day, there will be on average 200 hits a day, which strongly reinforces the habit.[30]

Despite this knowledge, health care professionals may not consistently inquire about a patient's smoking history or counsel patients to stop smoking. One study looked at primary care physicians and found that fewer than half of smokers reported that they even had been advised to quit.[31] Another study found that tobacco was discussed during 633 out of 2963 encounters (21%).[32] Yet the Agency for Health Care Policy and Research (AHCPR) Smoking Cessation Guideline found that just a few minutes of counseling can be an effective mechanism to aid patients in smoking cessation.[33]

Strategies to Help Patients Quit Smoking

In the early 1980s psychologists James Prochaska and Carlo DiClemente sought to understand how people can change behavior, with or without professional intervention. They theorized that patients' willingness to change addictive behavior depended on their state of readiness. There are six distinct phases of change that patients must experience to stop smoking[34] (Table 21-7).

The first stage is *precontemplation,* in which the patient is not considering change. If a patient is not considering change, the primary care provider must be careful not to argue or defend a position on smoking. Arguments are counterproductive, and resistance is a signal to change strategies. Patients should be asked if they smoke and are thinking of quitting. If they say that they smoke and are not thinking of quitting, they should be

TABLE 21-7 Six Processes of Change

Process of Change	Description	Intervention Strategies
Precontemplation	Patient is not considering change.	Raise doubts; increase perception of risks.
Contemplation	Patient shows awareness of a problem.	Evoke reasons to change; list risks of not changing.
Determination	Patient says, "I've got to do something."	Help patient determine steps to take *(if no intervention in this stage, patient may slip back to precontemplation stage).*
Action	Patient stops smoking.	Help patient take steps toward change.
Maintenance	Patient sustains change.	Help patient identify strategies to prevent relapse (self-efficacy important).
Relapse	"Slips" occur.	Help patient to avoid demoralization and discouragement *(sends them back to contemplation).*

Data from DiClimente CC and others: The process of smoking cessation; an analysis of precontemplation and preparation stages of change, *J Consult Clin Psychol* 59:295-304, 1991.

advised to quit and given some literature to read "in case they change their mind." The subject is not pursued at this visit.

The patient may be in denial. Patients who are in denial will disagree with the provider, will express no need for help, and will not accept help if it is offered.[34] Patients who are in denial may perceive further advice as nagging, which may trigger a paradoxical response. If their anxiety levels are increased and they perceive that their freedom is being threatened, they may respond to this threat by increasing smoking.[34]

This does not mean that the provider never brings up the subject again. Patients should be questioned about smoking and offered help at each visit, but the provider's response should be determined by the patient's response. The provider can look for a "teaching moment," raise doubts about smoking, and help the patient increase his or her perception of the risks of smoking. Specific health concerns of the patient (e.g., the number of colds this year) can be pointed out.

Awareness of a problem is the next step toward changing behavior. Once a patient admits there is a problem, he or she is in the *contemplation* stage of change. The provider must "tip the balance" at this point by evoking reasons to change and pointing out the risks of not changing behavior.

When a patient says things such as "I've got to do something," he or she has entered the *determination* stage. The best course of action should be planned together with the patient. This is the crucial point in the "stages of change" model. If there is no intervention at this stage, the patient will return to the precontemplation stage. Any barriers to treatment should be explored and removed if possible. Self-efficacy is an important tool to use for patients to become successful in their goal. The provider should provide the patient information and determine the patient's reaction. Patients should be asked to list the rewards and problems of smoking and identify any past unsuccessful attempts; they should be asked why they thought they did not succeed and what they would do differently this time.

Patients have reached the *action* phase of the model when they have smoked their last cigarette. The patient must have a specific plan by this stage and should have a follow-up visit scheduled so that there is something invested in the smoking cessation attempt.

Maintenance is the phase in which patients must sustain change. The patient needs help identifying strategies to make this a success. The patient needs to be encouraged to find other ways to deal with the urge to smoke, such as taking a walk or doodling, and should be warned of the inherent dangers in thinking of smoking and the importance of substituting alternate behaviors at those times.

Unfortunately, many patients *relapse*. Prochaska found that smokers ordinarily went around the wheel of change three or four times before a stable change was effected.[34] If the patient relapses, it should be pointed out that a coping behavior is learned on each attempt. This can lessen the feeling of failure. Patients should be continually moved toward their goal and counseled to quit.

Smokers should be counseled to quit on every visit. This does not need to be a formal counseling session; a brief talk should suffice. The American Cancer Society advises primary care providers to cover the "four A's"[35]:

- Ask *about smoking at every visit.*
- Advise *patients of the health benefits of quitting smoking (e.g., "As your health care provider, I must advise you to stop smoking now").*
- Assist *the patient in stopping. Identify and remove any barriers to treatment.*
- Arrange *a follow-up visit.*

When patients discover what drives them to smoke, interventions can be designed to help meet those needs. By interviewing the patient to determine specific motivators for smoking, the primary care provider can assist patients in designing a program that is tailored to them (Table 21-8).

Recently, Prochaska conducted a study to determine whether the use of a computer-generated "expert system" would improve outcome rates. Individualized and interactive computer reports were given to patients at 0, 3, and 6 months after randomization. At 24 months, the expert system resulted in 12% sustained abstinence, demonstrating a measurable difference when the message is individualized.[36]

It is important to keep in mind that what we say and how we say it influence how our message is received by the patient. Counseling styles were studied comparing autonomy-supportive and controlling interpersonal styles in brief counseling of smokers. Autonomy-supporting styles, although not directly affecting smoking cessation rates, showed an increase in patient's active involvement in the counseling session. Active

TABLE 21-8 Smoking Motivation and Strategies for Cessation

Motivations for Smoking	Strategies for Cessation
To keep from slowing down; to perk up; to get a lift	Change activity with urge to smoke; stimulate mouth with mouth-wash or brush teeth; avoid fatigue.
Enjoys handling cigarettes; enjoys steps in lighting up; enjoys watching exhaled smoke	Doodle; do crosswords; handle a small object.
Because smoking is pleasant, relaxing; because smoking is pleasurable; to relax	List pleasures of not smoking; contemplate harmful effect of smoking; go to a movie or read to substitute.
When upset; when uncomfortable; when "blue"	Identify what is needed when upset; do deep breathing/relaxation; take up hobby or sport.
Finds it unbearable to run out of cigarettes; very aware of not smoking; feels cravings between cigarettes; most enjoyable cigarette is first of day	Change daily routine to avoid triggers; use nicotine replacement therapy.
Smokes without being aware of it; lights another when one is burning; finds cigarettes in mouth	Throw away all cigarettes, go to places when smoking is prohibited; clean home of all traces of cigarettes.

involvement in turn increases continuous abstinence rates over 30 months.[37]

Modifying the Approach

Patients have different smoking issues that vary by age and gender.[38] The message that the patient is given has greater impact if it is directed toward his or her needs and drives. Women often worry about weight gain after quitting. They should be encouraged to have low-calorie snacks on hand (e.g., carrot sticks) to substitute for handling a cigarette. If medically appropriate, women should also incorporate an exercise program into their quitting plan to increase their metabolic rate and make up for the lowered metabolism that results from the drop in nicotine levels.

Moreover, women who are at different stages of their life need different approaches. A young mother should be warned of the dangers to her born and unborn children. England and others[39] studied the effect of tobacco exposure during pregnancy on the birth weight of term infants. They found that "as third trimester cigarette use increased, birth weight declined sharply but leveled off at more than 8 cigarettes per day . . . women who smoke during pregnancy may need to reduce to low levels of exposure (<8 cigarettes/day) to improve infant birth weight."

Health care providers have an obligation to inform patients that any maternal smoking also increases the danger of fetal death and congenital heart anomalies. Nicotine is contained in breast milk, and infants who breathe environmental tobacco smoke are more prone to otitis media and upper respiratory tract infections. Parents of asthmatic children should be advised to never allow them to be in an environment with tobacco smoke. Infants are at greater risk than older children because their systems are more immature and they are less able independently to escape a smoke environment.

On the other hand, young men may be more interested in the image they convey by smoking. Professional athletes are often shown using smokeless tobacco. Young men should be encouraged to make their own decisions about nicotine use in any form and to not rely on marketing information to make this important health decision.

In addition, adolescents are not convinced of their own mortality; therefore health concerns associated with smoking have a lesser impact on their smoking decisions. Instead, the focus of counseling highlights nicotine's effect on appearance (e.g., yellow teeth and fingers, hair and clothes that smell like smoke, and bad breath). Factors associated with the initiation of adolescent smoking include poor academic performance in middle or high school and prior smoking behavior. Other predictors are a younger age than grade cohorts, an intention to smoke in the following 6 months, and underage drinking. Adolescents who did not start smoking until age 18 and had few friends who smoked were more likely to quit by age 23. This results of this study underscores the importance of early smoking prevention courses and the continuation of these throughout the high school level.[40]

Adults are more receptive to the messages about health concerns with smoking. Counseling should include the effects on blood pressure, the cardiovascular system, and the lungs. The encouragement to stop or refrain from smoking can be individualized according to the patient's personal and family medical history. Patients with high cardiovascular risk factors can be informed of the results of a clinical trial that found that only 8 weeks of smoking reduction resulted in an improvement in fibrinogen levels, WBC counts, and HDL/LDL ratios.[41]

Other smoking effects that have health implications are the effect of smoking on mood and affect. Smoking has been found to have palliative effects on sadness in men as well as palliative effects on anger in both men and women.[42] Therefore patients with depression or anxiety disorders are at particular risk for nicotine addiction. With these patients it may be helpful to augment therapy with an antidepressant, such as bupropion (see p. 105). If the patient has a personal or family history of a psychiatric disorder, nicotine withdrawal may exacerbate symptoms of depression or anxiety. Many of these patients require more extensive psychiatric treatment, behavioral therapy, and support.[43]

Pharmacologic Interventions

Health care providers should remember that pharmacologic adjuncts are most successful when combined with behavior modification strategies or a formalized smoking cessation class. Classes are usually offered at area hospitals or through the American Cancer Society or American Lung Association.

There are basically two types of pharmacologic interventions: one aimed at nicotine replacement and the other aimed at neurochemical mechanisms of the brain pathways. Currently, four medications are available for nicotine replacement therapy (NRT): gum, patches, inhalers, and nasal spray. Nicotine gum is available in 2- or 4-mg dosages. The patient must refrain from smoking while using the gum. With cardiovascular disease patients, nicotine gum should only be used after considering the risk-benefit ratio because nicotine is a potent vasoconstrictor and can precipitate arrhythmias. Other adverse effects include mouth soreness, hiccups, dyspepsia, and jaw ache; these are usually mild and transient.

Generally when commencing NRT, the 2-mg dosage is used initially. Patients using the 2-mg dosage should have a maximum of 30 pieces per day, and patients using the 4-mg dosage should have a maximum of 20 pieces per day.[44] The gum is chewed until a peppery taste emerges and is then held between the cheek and gum. The patient is instructed to chew and hold intermittently for 30 minutes and to avoid eating or drinking anything but water for 15 minutes before; this prevents any interference with buccal absorption.

Nicotine patches are available in varying dosages depending on the manufacturer. Most manufacturers recommend using the higher dosage for the first 4 weeks and then switching to the lower dosages at 2-week intervals. An interval of 8 weeks has been found to be the most effective length of treatment.[45] Light smokers may experience more side effects and may need to begin at a lower dose. The patient must refrain from smoking while using the patch. The same precautions as with the gum apply to patients with cardiovascular disease.

The patch is placed on a relatively hairless location between the neck and waist. Patients should be advised to place the patch on awakening on their quit day. The location should be changed daily. Up to 50% of patients may experience a localized skin reaction, which is usually mild and self-limiting.[44] The reaction can be treated locally with 5% hydrocortisone cream or 0.5% triamcinolone cream if necessary. Rotating patch sites will decrease the likelihood of a skin rash.

Dosing for a nicotine nasal spray begins at 2 to 4 sprays per hour, which may be increased to a maximum of 40 sprays daily. Treatment is recommended to be 8 weeks, followed by a gradual taper over 4 to 6 weeks. Proper technique for dosing with nicotine nasal spray begins by gently blowing the nose, then tilting back the head slightly and spraying the nares. The spray should be aimed toward the center of the nasal opening while avoiding direct spraying of the nasal septum. Sniffing, swallowing, or inhaling the spray should be avoided. Side effects include nasal irritation, blisters or tingling, watery eyes, sneezing, coughing, and change in taste or smell. Additional rarely reported side effects are chest pain, muscle weakness, speech problems, dyspnea, and rash.

Dosing for nicotine inhalers is 6 to 16 cartridges daily. This dose is maintained for 3 months and gradually tapered over the next 3 months. Maximum treatment duration is 6 months. Side effects include headache, mouth/tooth or throat irritation, cough, nasal congestion, change in taste, dyspepsia, and diarrhea. Rarely reported side effects are tachycardia and chest pain.

NRT alone has been proved to double the quit rate of smokers. However, even with this increase, only 10% to 30% of smokers remain continuously abstinent for 1 year.[46] There are two hypotheses for lower success rates. The first is that "no current formulation mimics the extremely rapid, rewarding high arterial nicotine concentrations from inhaled tobacco smoke."[47] The second possible explanation is underdosing of NRT by the user. All standard NRT therapies average half the plasma nicotine concentrations of a heavy smoker. Underdosing is thought to be either from incorrect technique or because the user finds the side effects unpleasant.

Bupropion hydrochloride (Wellbutrin) has been found to be an aid in smoking cessation. Initially marketed and formulated as an antidepressant, the unexpected result was that patients were able to quit smoking. The drug has been remarketed under the name Zyban. The efficacy of bupropion may be explained in part by its effect on the neural uptake of dopamine, prolonging the action of this neurotransmitter. Nicotine, like all addictive drugs, is believed to stimulate increases in the neurotransmitter dopamine. Bupropion should not be prescribed for patients with a seizure disorder, patients with an eating disorder, or patients who are concurrently taking Wellbutrin or any other medication containing bupropion. The dosage may need to be reduced with patients with liver or renal dysfunction. The most common side effect is insomnia. The usual dosage is 150 mg b.i.d. Therapy should begin at 150 mg q.d. for the first 3 days and then be increased to 150 mg b.i.d. Patients may smoke while taking bupropion, and it is recommended that the patient start bupropion 1 to 2 weeks before their intended quit date to allow for stabilization of blood levels.

Individualizing Therapeutic Regimens

Deciding on the most efficacious therapeutic regiment can increase the chances of the successful transition from smoker to ex-smoker. There is only a 20% success rate using one NRT product alone; combining NRT products is another avenue to pursue. Using the patch to keep steady plasma levels (especially overnight) with the addition of faster acting preparations for breakthrough cravings and withdrawal symptoms has been demonstrated to improve quit rates. However, data are not robust and further studies seem warranted.[48]

Studies conducted in the United Kingdom have recommended a four-tiered approach[49]:

1. *Recommendation 1* (for all patients): Systematically record smoking status. This prompts primary caregivers to discuss smoking with all patients.
2. *Recommendation 2* (for motivated light smokers [<10 cigarettes per day]): Give brief advice and refer to formalized smoking cessation program as indicated.
3. *Recommendation 3* (motivated heavy smokers [average >10 cigarettes per day]): Provide NRT and behavioral support (either in-house or local smoking cessation classes).
4. *Recommendation 4* (for motivated heavy smokers [>15 cigarettes per day]): Provide NRT and behavioral support. If unsuccessful, consider adding bupropion and more interventional behavioral support.

Smokers in the relapse phase have been shown to experience less relapse if they remain on bupropion for more than 7 weeks. A clinical trial was performed that included smokers who were prescribed bupropion for 7 weeks. Participants were divided into one group randomized to bupropion for 45 additional weeks and another group randomized to a placebo for 45 weeks. Of the participants who were randomized to bupropion after 7 weeks, 55.1% remained smoke free at week 52 compared with 42.3% of participants in the placebo group. By week 78, the numbers had increased to 47.7% in the bupropion group and 37.7% in the placebo group. However, by week 104, these numbers had leveled off to 41.6% (bupropion) and 40.0% (placebo). This could either reflect a lack of bupropion for 52 weeks or the lack of efficacy of bupropion in long-term smoking abstinence. Interestingly, bupropion was also shown to increase median time to relapse in those smokers who relapsed. Relapse time for smoking was 156 days in the bupropion group vs. 65 days in the placebo group.[50]

Incorporating Smoking Cessation with Primary Care Strategies

Primary providers should remember that it is possible to incorporate basic, brief primary care interventions into a busy practice setting. The five elements of smoking cessation intervention include a strong message to quit smoking, self-help motivational quitting and relapse materials, brief counseling that includes a quit date, use of pharmacologic interventions when indicated, and follow-up support.[51]

Patients may report that they have cut down on the number of packs they smoke per day; while commending their effort, providers should remind these patients that as long as they continue to smoke, carbon monoxide levels will be elevated and mucociliary clearance affected. Patients need to be encouraged that "cold turkey" quitters have the best overall success rates. They should be advised that withdrawal symptoms are short-lived and can be ameliorated by the use of pharmacologic adjuncts. Gradual withdrawal usually makes for more miserable smokers who quickly revert to their previous smoking rate.

A good resource to develop a more structured program can be found in the pamphlet *How to Help Your Patients Stop Smoking,* which is available from the National Institutes of Health in conjunction with the American Cancer Society.[35] Another resource is available at http://www.surgeongeneral.gov/tobacco/default.htm through the Virtual Office of the Surgeon General. It offers a 5-day plan for quitting smoking and tips for the first week. Organizations with materials for smoking cessation include the following:

- American Cancer Society: *phone: (404) 320-3333; website: http://www.cancer.org/*
- American Lung Association: *phone: (212) 315-8700; website: http://www.lungusa.org/*
- Office of Cancer Communications/National Cancer Institute: *phone: (800) 4-CANCER; website: http://cancernet.nci.nhi.gov/*
- Office on Smoking and Health/ Centers for Disease Control and Prevention: *phone: (404) 488-5705; website: http://mentalhealth.about.com/library/h/orgs (search "smoking cessation")*

DOMESTIC VIOLENCE

Definition/Epidemiology

Domestic violence is a significant health care problem with widespread and devastating effects for patients and their children, families, and communities. Approximately 4.8 million intimate partner rapes and physical assaults are perpetrated against women in the United States each year.[52] In the United States, a woman is physically abused by her husband every 12 seconds.[53] In the past, the issue of domestic violence was thought to be a social and judicial concern rather than a health care issue. However, recent research has consistently demonstrated that women seek help in various health care settings and that their health is seriously affected by ongoing abuse. Domestic violence is the leading cause of injury to women between the ages of 15 to 44 in the United States—more than muggings, sexual assaults, and automobile accidents combined.[54] According to the Bureau of Justice statistics (1997), 37% of female patients seen in emergency departments are being abused. Studies in primary care settings have yielded similar results. One Midwestern family practice clinic reported that 23% of female patients were assaulted within the past year; 39% had been assaulted at some time during their life.[55] In one primary care setting, 1 in 7 women reported domestic abuse.[56]

Domestic violence is defined as a pattern of coercive and controlling behavior exercised by one partner over the other. Behaviors can range from economic control, social isolation, and emotional abuse to sexual assault and threats of or actual physical violence. Abusive behavior by the batterer may be sporadic but generally is cyclic and usually escalate in terms of frequency and severity. The majority of victims of domestic violence appear to be women; however, domestic violence occurs in all age, racial, socioeconomic, and sexual orientation groups. The myth that domestic violence occurs in certain populations can result in the error of screening only those believed to be at risk. (Due to the disproportionate representation of women as victims, and for the ease of writing, this chapter may generalize and refer to victims of domestic violence as women.)

Despite the prevalence and significant ramifications of domestic violence on individuals and communities, a variety of barriers to identification and treatment remain. This chapter will further explore these barriers, the basic principles of domestic violence, as well as identify specific techniques for assessment and intervention for the health care professional.

Barriers to Treatment

Power and Control. The relationship dynamics inherent to domestic violence are significant to understanding the barriers patients encounter to obtaining treatment. All abusive relationships are focused on the imbalance of power and control and incorporate the use of specific tactics to maintain this imbalance. It is the perpetrator's desire for increased control over their partner that generates a sense of power over the victim as well as an imbalance of power in the overall relationship. Abusive control and controlling behavior can be exercised in many different ways. Fear is often a powerful deterrent to women seeking appropriate treatment. This includes the use of coercion and threats of physical, psychologic, or economic harm;

intimidation; and physical or sexual violence. Abusive partners attempt to further exert psychologic, emotional, and financial control over their partners through verbal degradation, isolation, and economic abuse. The abuse is often minimized or denied by the perpetrator, and the victim may also be blamed for the abuse, shifting the responsibility for the abusive behavior to the victim. If children are present, they may be used to create guilt or manipulate their victim, or threats to have them taken away or harmed may also be made in a further attempt to control the emotions and reactions of the victim. For female victims, male privilege is commonly used whereby the woman's role in the household is devalued and defined by the male.

Clearly, there are countless tactics by which a perpetrator can exert emotional, physical, and social control over the victim. The more control one partner exercises over the other, the greater sense of power he feels he has in the relationship and over the other individual. Likewise, the less control the victim feels she has in the relationship and with her overall life, the less power she perceives she has, which continues to reinforce this ongoing sense of powerlessness. The more powerless the victim feels, the less likely and able she is to leave the abusive relationship or seek treatment and help.

Cycle of Abuse. Along with the interpersonal dynamics between the abuser and the victim, the evolving dynamics of the relationship itself are also important factors to consider while exploring barriers to treatment. The dynamics of abusive relationships are often a part of a systematic pattern of dominance and control characterized as occurring in a cycle; each turn of the cycle perpetuates the dynamics of the ongoing violence and controlling behavior.[52] The first stage of the cycle often represents the baseline of the relationship without any acute issues at hand. Slowly, the relationship may enter a tension-building phase in which stress level and tension are raised, ultimately leading to an explosive event. This may be characterized by a verbal argument and may also result in physical or sexual abuse. After this explosion, the tension and stress that had been building previously are expelled and a false sense of calm returns to the relationship. Often after an explosive event, the relationship goes through a phase commonly referred to as the "honeymoon period." During this time, the abuser often appears more loving and sensitive toward his partner, perhaps in some respect atoning for the recent abusive episode. The relationship at this time may even appear to have improved, which often serves as reinforcement to the victim that her partner is changing and that the abuse will end. Unfortunately, the cycle repeats itself over time with some modifications. As this cycle of abuse self-perpetuates over time, it appears that the length of the "honeymoon period" shortens with each turn of this cycle, thereby increasing the frequency and severity of these abusive episodes.

Barriers to Identification

Despite the high prevalence of domestic violence, abuse is often not identified, and an opportunity to intervene and offer resources and follow-up is missed. The reason for this is twofold and can be attributed to the patient's reluctance to disclose this information and the issues presented by the health care provider.

Patient Barriers. Aside from the interpersonal and relationship dynamics that often hinder access to treatment, other factors also contribute to the difficulty in identifying abuse. Patients may be reluctant to disclose information due to shame or embarrassment or feel that it is culturally inappropriate to discuss information with others regarding their intimate relationships. Previous negative or unhelpful experiences with past disclosure of abuse sometimes result in patients having reservations about repeating this experience. This negative experience may include not being asked by the provider despite the patient's attempts to raise the issue themselves or not being asked in a caring or empathic manner. The victim's impaired insight or awareness into her abusive situation may also present a barrier to identification; these ongoing patterns of abusive power and control may seem "normal" to victims, thereby decreasing their ability to recognize the lethality of their situations.

Provider Barriers. In addition, health care providers unfortunately create their own barriers to identification. The greatest barrier to the identification of abuse is often self-imposed by providers by simply not asking about abuse. Primary care providers may be unaware of the prevalence of abuse or have inadequate understanding about domestic violence. This includes having misconceptions about abuse risks, settings, and lethality, thereby resulting in missed opportunities for screening. These false stereotypes may also result in practitioners thinking that abuse does not occur within the population they serve, and they may be concerned about offending their patients by asking.

Providers may also feel a sense of powerlessness to address the problem and may therefore feel ill-equipped to deal with the situation and provide adequate intervention. However, the results of one study clearly indicated that health care providers can be effective in helping victims of domestic violence and were rated almost as highly as counselors and support groups.[57] The magnitude of the problem may also overwhelm the provider, who feels that he or she lacks the time or the resources to address the situation. However, findings suggest that providers can improve their ability to respond to these situations by educating themselves and their patients about domestic violence and familiarizing themselves with local resources available to provide support for these patients.[57]

Clinical Presentation

Domestic violence is a primary reason for admission into emergency departments for women in the United States.[57] Therefore a history of recent visits to the emergency department for repeated physical injuries may indicate that the patient is in a violent domestic situation. Likewise, repeated office visits for either physical injuries or complaints may suggest that abuse is occurring. The National Violence Against Women Survey (2000) found that physical and/or sexual violence resulted in more than 320,000 outpatient visits annually.[52] A patient who has been battered may show obvious signs of abuse, or the symptoms may be more obscure. In general, clinical indicators of domestic violence may be categorized into physical complaints, psychosocial indicators, or a combination of the two.

Physical Complaints. Injuries to the head and neck are the most common injuries in domestic abuse situations, followed by upper extremity, breast, back, and buttock injury.[58] In a large domestic violence study conducted in a primary care setting, researchers found that frequent or serious bruises or cuts, sprains, broken bones, and various pains (e.g., chest, stomach, pelvic, and genital) were associated with high levels of abuse.[59] Some of the less obvious signs and symptoms include a loss of appetite, eating binges and self-induced vomiting, vaginal discharge, diarrhea or constipation, fainting, difficulty passing urine, hyperventilation, and headaches. Other indicators of domestic violence include injuries in various stages of healing, repeated office visits, delayed treatment for an injury, reluctance to talk about an injury, or explanations that are inconsistent with the type of injury.[60]

Sexual assault can occur with physical and/or emotional abuse, or it can be the only form of abuse in the relationship. Intimate partner sexual assault includes any forced sex acts that occur within the context of any intimate relationship and may include the use of objects, rape, or uncomfortable or embarrassing sexual experiences.[61] Studies in San Francisco and Boston revealed that 8% to 10% of participants were victims of intimate partner rape.[52] Men who sexually abuse their partners are particularly dangerous, which means that women are at greater risk in terms of lethality.[62] Although approximately one third of women injured in their most recent incident of intimate partner rape seek medical treatment, only one fifth of the incidents are reported to the police.[52] This disparity supports the critical role health care providers have in identifying domestic violence and offering support and resources to their patients. Evidence of sexual assault should automatically prompt further exploration by providers. This form of violence can result in problems such as pelvic inflammatory disease, sexually transmitted diseases (STDs), HIV/AIDS, vaginal/anal tearing, urinary tract infections, dysmenorrhea, unexplained vaginal bleeding, or pelvic pain.[58] The male partner may exert control over his partner by not using a condom, thereby increasing her risk for STDs and unintended pregnancy.

Physical abuse during pregnancy poses a significant health risk for mother and fetus; therefore assessment for abuse during pregnancy should be part of routine prenatal care.[59] For some relationships, domestic violence may begin when a woman becomes pregnant; if domestic violence is already present, it may escalate during pregnancy.[63] Research indicates that one in six women are battered during pregnancy. Possible complications of domestic violence during pregnancy include low birth weight and miscarriage. Both of these symptoms could result from abdominal trauma, inadequate prenatal care, suboptimal weight gain, an unhealthy diet, and/or severe stress.[64] The stress from abuse may increase the likelihood that the pregnant woman would smoke or abuse substances, which would be another cause for low birth weight.[64] Because pregnancy may be the only time healthy women come in frequent contact with health care providers, this is an opportune time to ask about domestic violence.[60]

Psychosocial Indicators. In addition to physical injuries and complaints, patients may experience a variety of psychosocial problems. A recent study supports the need for better understanding of the effects of nonphysical forms of abuse. Women may be treated for symptoms of depression or anxiety without assessing for domestic violence; treatment may be ineffective if these symptoms are taken out of context of the abuse.[57] Psychologically, the patient can experience a complex traumatic stress response, which includes the symptoms of posttraumatic stress disorder (e.g., intrusive thoughts, nightmares, disassociated flashbacks, psychic numbness, hypervigilance, and exaggerated startle response).[65] Depression, anxiety, and their related symptoms are often commonly experienced by victims; these include anhedonia, difficulty concentrating, changes in sleep and eating patters, depressed mood, somatization, decreased self-esteem, and suicidal ideations. There may be an alteration in affect (predominantly depressed or restricted), alteration in perceptions of the perpetrator (seeing the abuser as omnipotent), and an alteration in the sense of self (disappearance of self and increased feelings of self-blame).[64] This complex traumatic response can be immobilizing and prevent the victim from escaping the abusive relationship or seeking help.

Universal Screening. All patients seen in primary care settings should be routinely screened for domestic violence. Because many patients are reluctant to disclose that they are being abused the first time that the subject is raised, they may be more likely to disclose information after they have developed some level of trust with the provider. Therefore screening should not be limited to the first visit and providers should continue to screen at subsequent visits.

Framing the Question. Privacy and confidentiality are essential when screening or interviewing a patient about domestic violence. The patient's partner or a third party should never be informed that the patient is being screened for domestic violence because this may place the patient and provider at risk for retaliation. Providers should use their own style of communication to introduce the subject and convey the need for screening due to the seriousness and prevalence of domestic violence. It may be helpful to normalize the process for patients using statements such as, "Since domestic violence is so prevalent, I have started screening all of my patients." It is usually most beneficial to use direct questions when screening,[66] such as the following:

- Have you ever been hit, slapped, kicked, or otherwise physically hurt by someone? If yes, by whom?
- Have you ever been threatened, controlled, or forced to do things you did not want to do? If yes, by whom?
- Are you afraid of your partner or anyone else?

The presentation of the provider when screening a patient can negatively influence the patient's willingness to disclose her victimization. If the provider is not comfortable with the subject matter and the screening process, it is advisable to have an appropriate staff member screen patients. It is essential that the provider is not only aware of how to appropriately interview patients to screen for domestic violence but also how to respond to them when the screening has been completed. It is recommended that the provider compile a list of resources and related brochures and have them available to aid in the education of the patient regarding domestic violence.

Patient Denies Abuse. If the patient denies abuse, the provider should document in the patient's chart that the screening was completed. If the patient presents with injuries that are inconsistent with her explanation as to how they occurred and denies abuse, document in the patient's chart that the "injury is inconsistent with explanation." There is generally no therapeutic benefit of challenging the patient's explanation. Consider the need to report to appropriate authorities if the patient is a minor or a dependent adult. It is recommended that the provider be acquainted with the mandatory reporting laws in the state in which he or she practices because there is a great deal of variation from state to state. Even when a patient denies abuse and is well known to the provider, the patient should be rescreened at subsequent visits. Providers should continue to convey to the patient that they are available to assist, if needed.

Patient Discloses Abuse. When a patient discloses that she is being abused, the provider can use the opportunity to convey concern, to educate, and to provide information on available resources. The patient should be assured that she is not at fault for the battering, regardless of what she may or may not have done. Efforts to verify patient's report with her partner or other family members should not be attempted. The primary focus should be on the patient's safety and providing her with appropriate referrals. It is important to remember that victims of domestic violence will present in many different ways. Even if the victim does not cry or appear distraught when disclosing incidences of abuse or violence, it does not mean that she has not been victimized.

Management

Clinical Intervention. The health care provider can assist the patient who admits to being a victim of domestic violence by assessing and treating medical problems, educating about the dynamics of domestic violence, discussing safety issues, and providing referrals.

It is important to address the patient's urgent and nonurgent health care needs at the time of the visit, time permitting. Some victims of domestic violence may have difficulty returning to the health care provider's office for follow-up. Patients who report domestic violence and who are not ready to leave the abusive relationship may benefit from education and services targeting the prevention of unintended pregnancy. When treating the patient's illness or injuries, the provider should take caution to not prescribe any medication that may impair the patient's judgment or ability to respond, because this would place the patient at increased risk for further harm. If necessary, refer to a specialist for additional health care needs.

Documentation of the patient's visit is very important and may be needed for legal proceedings. The patient's account of domestic violence should be documented in the medical record using the patient's own words, when possible. It is advisable to avoid using the term "alleges." An appropriate substitute is "patient reports" or "patient states." Caution should be used when documenting the patient's demeanor. Because the patient's medical record may be used in legal proceedings, accuracy is important. Documentation should also indicate when and how the patient sustained the injuries. It should include the identity of the person who caused the injury. It is important that the health care provider stick to his or her area of expertise. Documented inferences that are out of the provider's area of expertise may create legal difficulties for a patient who pursues legal action against the abuser.[67] Documentation should include a detailed description of the injuries as well as a body map to identify the location of injuries. Care should be taken to not attempt to place a date on when injuries occurred based on the appearance of the injuries; instead document objective data, such as color and size of bruises. Dating injuries can create complications with legal proceedings.

If available, offer to take photographs of the patient's injuries. The patient's written consent is required before having pictures taken, and all pictures must be labeled with the patient's name and medical record number. When appropriate, it is recommended that an object of standard size be placed into the picture and near the injury to illustrate size (e.g., a tape measure or a coin). This will aid in providing an accurate perspective of the injuries should they be needed for review at a later date. The patient may need the photographs as evidence of the assault for legal purposes. Care should be taken to preserve the patient's dignity while photography is taking place, and the patient should not be asked to remove more clothing than is necessary. Some of the photographs of the injuries should include the patient's face, when possible, to protect against a possible dispute of the identity of person photographed.[67]

If a patient was recently sexually assaulted, the provider should consider referring the patient to an emergency department that has a program to assist victims of sexual assault before commencing with a physical examination. They can assist with securing evidence that may be lost during a regular physical examination. This should be encouraged even if the patient is not considering notifying law enforcement at the time of disclosure of sexual assault. There are time restrictions on these types of services; therefore the local hospital should be contacted for service guidelines.

Psychosocial Intervention. Repeated abuse can have a monumental psychologic impact on the victim. Care should be taken to discuss the patient's psychologic well-being. Patients may experience feelings of intense fear and helplessness. Some victims may develop posttraumatic stress disorder.[68] Victims of chronic abuse should be screened for suicidal and homicidal ideations because they may feel there is no way out of the abusive relationship other than death. If appropriate, the patient should be referred for crisis intervention. Referrals to individual counseling and support groups specific to domestic violence are also appropriate. However, couples counseling is highly discouraged due to the potential for further harm to the patient. Information should be given to the patient that indicates how to access emergency shelters and financial and legal assistance.

Children who are exposed to family violence should be referred to age-appropriate counseling. Many organizations that provide services to adult victims of domestic violence have age-appropriate services for children. Patients who have children should be encouraged to have their children examined by a pediatrician for assessment of their physical and psychological well-being. Many people often mistakenly think that if a child was not physically assaulted, he or she is not in need of services. Children who are exposed to violence are at significant risk for using violence themselves, becoming delinquent, experiencing school and behavioral problems, and having serious and possible life-long mental health problems.[69]

Safety Assessment and Planning. On identification and discussion of the domestic violence, the health care provider should perform a thorough assessment and discuss a safety plan. Information on the history of the violence should be obtained; it should include when the violence first occurred, types of incidents, whether weapons were used, and the frequency of assaults. This will assist in determining whether the violence is escalating, as well as aid in raising the victim's awareness of the progression of violence. The presence of weapons in the home increases the potential lethality of the situation. Patients need to make their own decisions about their safety and whether they should leave the abusive relationship. Violence will often escalate when the victim attempts to leave; as a result, patients should be advised to take extra precautions to protect their safety when leaving a relationship.

If the patient is in immediate danger while in the clinical setting, the appropriate security services should be contacted immediately. The health care provider should not attempt to mediate between the victim and her partner.

The safety plan should consider various scenarios that the patient may find herself in and need to escape from. It may include having the patient develop a code with someone she trusts who lives in the home or next door; this code would indicate that patient needs help and that the police should be notified. Details should be discussed regarding where the patient would go if the home is not safe. Patients should be encouraged to use domestic violence shelters to protect their safety. They should be discouraged from going to the homes of family or friends, where the abuser is likely to be able to locate them.

The patient should be encouraged to compile important documents such as birth certificates and photo identification, as well as an address book, checkbook, bank cards, medical cards, Social Security cards, chronic medication, and clothing. The patient's safety is of the ultimate importance and if compiling documents places her at greater risk, she should not be encouraged to do so. Providers should help patients in identifying people and agencies that are able to assist. A follow-up appointment, as appropriate, should be scheduled before the patient leaves. Furthermore, the health care provider should inquire about whether the patient can be contacted through the mail or on the telephone. The provider's good intention of calling the patient later to inquire about her well-being may actually further jeopardize her safety.

A determination of the success of an intervention should not hinge on whether the patient leaves the abusive relationship. A successful intervention is one in which the provider has acknowledged and validated the situation and offered the appropriate referrals. The patient may decide at a later date to seek services based on the groundwork that was laid at a previous visit.

REFERENCES

1. National Center for Health Statistics: *Fast stats A to Z: death/mortality.* Retrieved August 12, 2002, from the World Wide Web: http://www.cdc.gov/nchs/fastats/death.htm.
2. U.S. Department of Health and Human Services: *Healthy People 2010,* ed 2, *with understanding and improving health and objectives for improving health,* 2 vols, Washington, DC, 2000, U.S. Government Printing Office.
3. Centers for Disease Control and Prevention/National Center for Chronic Disease Prevention and Health Promotion: *Nutrition and physical activity obesity trends. prevalence of obesity among U.S. adults, region and state: Behavioral Risk Factor Surveillance System (1991-2000); self-reported data.* Retrieved August 12, 2002, from the World Wide Web: http://www.cdc.gov/nccdphp/dnpa/obesity/trend/prev_reg.htm.
4. Centers for Disease Control and Prevention/National Center for Chronic Disease Prevention and Health Promotion: *Nutrition and physical activity obesity trends. prevalence of obesity among U.S. adults, by characteristics: Behavioral Risk Factor Surveillance System (1991-2000); self-reported data.* Retrieved August 12, 2002, from the World Wide Web: http://www.cdc.gov/nccdphp/dnpa/obesity/trend/prev_char.htm.
5. National Center for Chronic Disease Prevention and Health Promotion: *Nutrition and Physical Activity. Center for Disease Control and Prevention. Obesity Trends. U.S. Obesity Trends 1985 to 2000.* Retrieved August 12, 2002, from the World Wide Web: http://www.cdc.gov/nccdphp/dnpa/obesity/trend/maps/index.htm.
6. National Heart, Lung, and Blood Institute: *The practical guide to the identification, evaluation, and treatment of overweight and obesity in adults,* Bethesda, Md, 2000, NHLBI Information Center.
7. Centers for Disease Control and Prevention/National Center for Chronic Disease Prevention and Health Promotion: *Physical activity of health: a report of the surgeon general—adults.* Retrieved August 12, 2002, from the World Wide Web: http://www.cdc.gov/nccdphp/sgr/adults.htm.
8. The American Institute of Stress: *America's #1 health problem: why is there more stress today?* Retrieved August 12, 2002, from the World Wide Web: http://www.stress.org/problem.htm.
9. U.S. Department of Health and Human Services: *Third report of the National Cholesterol Education Program on Detection, Evaluation, and Treatment of High Blood Cholesterol in Adults,* Washington, DC, 2001, U.S. Government Printing Office.
10. Schafer W: *Stress management for wellness,* Austin, Tex, 1996, Holt, Rinehart & Winston.
11. Stanhope M, Knollmueler RN: *Public and community health nurse's consultant: a health promotion guide,* St Louis, 1997, Mosby.
12. Pagana K, Pagana T: *Mosby's diagnostic and laboratory test reference,* ed 5, St Louis, 1999, Mosby.
13. Reference deleted in galleys.
14. Maud PJ, Foster C: *Physiological assessment of human fitness,* Champaign, Ill, 1995, Human Kinetics.
15. American Heart Association, Inc: *Blood pressure levels.* Retrieved August 12, 2002, from the World Wide Web: http://216.185.112.5/presenter.jhtml?identifier=4450.
16. Chernecky C, Berger B, eds: *Laboratory tests and diagnostic procedures,* ed 3, Philadelphia, 2001, WB Saunders.
17. Reference deleted in galleys.
18. Reference deleted in galleys.
19. Fisher C: Nutrition and quality of life, *Can Nurs Home* 4(1), 1993.
20. Guigoz Y, Vellas B, Garry PJ: Assessing the nutritional status of the elderly: the mini nutritional assessment as part of the geriatric evaluation, *Nutr Rev* 54(1 pt 2):559-565, 1996.
21. Lord S, Castell S: Effect of exercise on balance, strength and reaction time in older people, *Arch Phys Med Rehabil* 75(6):648-652, 1994.
22. Reference deleted in galleys.
23. Payne WA, Hahn DB: *Understanding your health,* ed 4, St Louis, 1995, Mosby.
24. Wilbur J, Chandler P, Miller A: Measuring adherence to a women's walking program, *West J Nurs Res* 23(1):8-32, 2001.

25. American Heart Association: *Exercise and your heart: a guide to physical activity,* Dallas, Tex, 1993, The Association.
26. Fitts SS: Physical benefits and challenges of exercise for people with chronic renal disease, *J Renal Nutr* 7(3):123-128, 1997.
27. Deuster PA: Exercise in the prevention and treatment of chronic disorders, *Women's Health Issues* 6(6):320-331, 1996.
28. Lego S: Women and stress, *Imprint* 43(2):57-60, 1996.
29. Vainio H and others: Smoking cessation in cancer prevention, *Toxicology* 166(1-2):47-52, 2001.
30. National Institute on Drug Abuse: *NIDH research report series: nicotine addiction,* NIH Publication No. 01-4342.
31. Park E and others: The development of a decisional balance measure of physician smoking cessation interventions, *Prev Med* 33(4):261-267, 2001.
32. Ellerbeck EF and others: Direct observation of smoking cessation activities in primary care practice, *J Fam Pract* 50(8):688-693, 2001.
33. Amar S and others: The efficacy of a doctor-patient appointment in a primary care setting dedicated to preventative medicine, *Harefuah* 140(8):689-693, 2001.
34. DiClimente CC and others: The process of smoking cessation; an analysis of precontemplation and preparation stages of change, *J Consult Clin Psychol* 59:295-304, 1991.
35. Glynn TJ, Manley M: *How to help your patients stop smoking: a National Cancer Center Institute manual for physicians,* NIH Publication No. 95-3064, Washington, DC, 1995, National Cancer Institute.
36. Prochaska JO and others: Evaluating a population-based recruitment approach and a stage-based expert system intervention for smoking cessation, *Addict Beh* 26(4):583-602, 2001.
37. Williams GC, Deci EL: Activating patients for smoking cessation through physician autonomy support, *Med Care* 39(8):813-823, 2001.
38. Goring S, Arnold J: *Health promotion handbook,* St Louis, 1998, Mosby.
39. England LJ and others: Effects of smoking reduction during pregnancy on the birth weight of term infants, *Am J Epidemiol* 154(8):694-701, 2001.
40. Ellickson PL and others: Predictors of late-onset smoking and cessation over 10 years, *J Adolesc Health* 29(2):101-108, 2001.
41. Eliasson B and others: Effects of smoking reduction and cessation on cardiovascular risk factors, *Nicotine Tob Res* 3(3):249-255, 2001.
42. Delfino RJ and others: Temporal analysis of the relationship of smoking behavior and urges to mood states in men versus women, *Nicotine Tob Res* 3(3):245-248, 2001.
43. Ziedonis D, Brady K: Dual diagnosis in primary care: detecting and treating both the addiction and mental illness, *Med Clin North Am* 81:1017-1036, 1997.
44. Hodgson BB, Kizior RJ: *Nursing drug handbook,* Philadelphia, 2002, WB Saunders.
45. Silagy C and others: Nicotine replacement therapy for smoking cessation, *Cochran Database Syst Rev* (3):CD000146, 2000.
46. Wagena EJ, Huibers MJ, van Schayck CP: Therapies for smoking cessation (antidepressants, nicotine-replacement and counseling) and implications for the treatment of patients with chronic obstructive pulmonary disease, *Ned Tijdsch Geneash* 145(31):1492-1496, 2001.
47. Stapleton J: Commentary: progress on nicotine replacement therapy for smokers, *BMJ* 318(7179):289, 1999.
48. Sweeney CT and others: Combination nicotine replacement therapy for smoking cessation: rationale, efficacy and tolerability, *CNS Drugs* 15(6):453-467, 2001.
49. Coleman T: Smoking cessation: integrating recent advances into clinical practice, *Thorax* 56:579-582, 2001.
50. Hays JT and others: Sustained-release bupropion for pharmacological relapse prevention after smoking cessation: a randomized, controlled trial, *Ann Intern Med* 135(6):423-433, 2001.
51. Goring S Arnold J: *Health promotion handbook,* St Louis, 1998, Mosby.
52. *Findings from the National Violence against Women Survey, July 2000.* © 2002 Family Education Network. Retrieved August 12, 2002, from the World Wide Web: http://www.infoplease.com/ipa/A0875303.html.
53. Bureau of Justice Statistics: *Report to the nation on crime and justice. The data,* Washington, DC, 1983, Office of Justice Programs, U.S. Department of Justice.
54. Stark E, Flitcraft A: Violence against intimates: an epidemic review. In Van Hassett VB and others, editors: *Handbook of family violence,* New York, 1988, Plenum Press.
55. Hamburger K, Saunders DG, Hovey M: Prevalence of domestic violence in community practice and rate of physician inquiry, *Fam Med* 24:283-287, 1992.
56. Freund K, Blackhall L: Detection of domestic violence in a primary care setting, *Clin Res* 38:736A-738A, 1990.
57. Gordon J: *Helping survivors of domestic violence,* New York, 1998, Garland Publishing, Inc.
58. Eisenstat SA: Domestic violence. In Carlson K, Eisenstat SA, editors: *Primary care of women,* St Louis, 1995, Mosby.
59. McCauley J and others: The "battering syndrome": prevalence and clinical characteristics of domestic violence in primary care internal medicine, *Ann Intern Med* 123(10):737-746, 1995.
60. Alpert EJ: Violence in intimate relationships and the practicing internist: new "disease" or new agenda? *Ann Intern Med* 123(10):774-781, 1995.
61. Campbell JC, Alford P: The dark consequences of marital rape, *Am J Nurs* 89(7):946-949, 1989.
62. Council of Scientific Affairs, American Medical Association: Violence against women: relevance for medical practitioners, *JAMA* 267(23):3184-3189, 1992.
63. McFarlane J and others: Assessing for abuse during pregnancy, *JAMA* 267(33):3176-3178, 1992.
64. Campbell JC, Lewandowski LA: Mental and physical health effects of intimate partner violence on women and children, *Psychiatr Clin North Am* 20(2):353-374, 1997.
65. Herman J: *Trauma and recovery,* New York, 1994, Basic Books.
66. Feldhaus KM and others: Accuracy of three brief screening questions for detecting violence in the emergency department, *JAMA* 277(17):1357-1361, 1997.
67. Schornstein S: *Domestic violence and health care: what every professional needs to know,* Thousand Oaks, Calif, 1997, Sage Publications, Inc.
68. Kubany E and others: PTSD among women survivors of domestic violence in Hawaii, *Hawaii Med J* 55:164-165, 1996.
69. Walker L: *The battered woman syndrome,* New York, 2000, Springer Publishing Company, Inc.

CHAPTER 22

Immunizations

Cheryl A. Miller

Vaccine-preventable infectious diseases, such as influenza and pneumococcal pneumonia, continue to be leading causes of significant medical costs, morbidity, and mortality.[1] Immunization rates have improved in some populations, but poor access to health care and inadequate public education continue to have an impact on immunization rates. Most of the vaccine-preventable diseases in the United States occur in the adult population. Adults and young adults are often unaware of the need for adult immunizations. Many adolescents also do not receive the recommended immunizations.

One of the goals of *Healthy People 2010* is to prevent disease, disability, and death from vaccine-preventable illnesses. Progress has been made as the schedules for vaccination have been clarified. Inactivated vaccines can be given simultaneously at different injection sites. A live attenuated vaccine (e.g., mumps or measles vaccine) can be given simultaneously with an inactive vaccine (e.g., influenza vaccine) if separate injection sites are used. Combination vaccines are also helpful in decreasing the number of injections required.[1-4]

Health care providers in all settings, including schools, colleges, outpatient clinics, workplaces, and emergency departments, should take advantage of the opportunities to discuss immunization history, including past and present illnesses, age, employment, family history, and risk factors. This history should also include allergies and prior allergic or untoward reactions. Women of childbearing age should be questioned about the possibility of pregnancy, because certain vaccines are contraindicated during pregnancy. Adolescents should have their immunization history updated at age 11 or 12 years.[2-5] Patients are educated about the potential side effects of each vaccine and should be encouraged to keep a record of their vaccination history. As with any injected medication, observation for approximately 15 minutes is recommended because of the danger of anaphylaxis. Immunosuppressed patients (e.g., patients with HIV infection or leukemia, or patients receiving chemotherapy or steroids) should not be given live vaccines because this may lead to disseminated disease. Table 22-1 provides information, including dosages and side effects, on the currently recommended vaccines.[6,7] Other information regarding immunizations can be obtained by calling the Centers for Disease Control and Prevention Hotline (800-232-2522) or by accessing the website (http://www.immunize.org/express).

REFERENCES

1. U.S. Department of Health and Human Services: *Healthy People 2010*, ed 2, Washington, DC, 2000, Government Printing Office.
2. LoBuono C: Steps to improve immunization rates, *Patient Care* 34(9):93-111, 2000.
3. Schaffer S and others: Adolescent immunization practices: a national survey of U.S. physicians, *Arch Pediatr Adolesc Med* 155(5):566-571.
4. Reid K, Grizzard T, Poland G: Adult immunizations: recommendations for practice, *Mayo Clin Proc* 74(4):377-384, 1999.
5. Selekman J: Recommended immunization schedule: 2001, *Pediatr Nurs* 27(3):303, 2001.
6. National Coalition for Adult Immunization: *Adult immunization schedule (September, 2001)*. Retrieved November 9, 2001, from the World Wide Web: http://www.nfid.org/ncai/schedules/adults.
7. Waldrop J: Childhood vaccination update: a new weapon against pneumococcal bacteria, *Adv Nurse Pract* 9(2):34-40, 2001.

TABLE 22-1 Quick Reference for Routine Immunizations

Vaccine Antigen Dose and Route	Routine Administration Schedule*	Precautions†‡ Contraindications	Adverse Reactions	Serious Adverse Reactions	Education Indications
DTP					
Diphtheria-tetanus-pertussis§ Child: 0.5 ml IM Adult: see Td D—Toxoid T—Toxoid P—Bacteria	2, 4, 6, 12-15 months Booster: 4-6 years (Contains aluminum) Administer deep IM; avoid compressing plunger when withdrawing needle to prevent leakage into subcutaneous fat. 6 months should elapse between third and fourth dose.	Neurologic disorder with progressive developmental delay or changed neurologic findings Neurologic condition predisposing to seizures or neuro deterioration 7 years or older Serious adverse reactions to previous immunization	Local pain, erythema Fussiness Fever <104.9° F Sleepiness Painless lump at injection site that may last several weeks	Once for every 100-1000 doses: Fever >104.9° F within 48 hours Persistent, inconsolable cry for >3 hours or high-pitched cephalic cry within 48 hours of dose Once for every 1750 doses: Convulsions, facial neurologic signs, alteration in consciousness Collapse or shocklike state Very rarely: Anaphylaxis Coma	A warm compress to injection site if red, swollen. Report serious adverse reactions to health care provider. Acetaminophen for fever. Adverse effects may last 12-24 hours.
DTaP	Consider fourth and fifth doses only for children ≥15 months.				
DT					
Diphtheria-tetanus (pediatric) 0.5 ml IM	Only used if child had serious reaction to DTP; "D" (larger dose of diphtheria) is not given to children ≥7 years		Local pain at injection site		

Modified from Osguthorpe MC, Morgan EP: An immunization update for primary health care providers, *Nurse Pract* 20(6):52-65, 1995.

*Recommended schedules differ for infants and children who do not begin immunizations at usual time or who are behind schedule. See specific guidelines from American Academy of Pediatrics or Advisory Committee on Immunization Practices, USDHHS/CDC.

†No immunization should be given to a client who is moderately or severely ill.

‡Pregnancy is a precaution with any immunization. Special cases must be considered on an individual basis.

§DTP/Hib combination vaccines are available. See specific guidelines from Advisory Committee on Immunization Practices, USDHHS/CDC, and American Academy of Pediatrics.

continued

TABLE 22-1 Quick Reference for Routine Immunizations—cont'd

Vaccine Antigen Dose and Route	Routine Administration Schedule*	Precautions†‡ Contraindications	Adverse Reactions	Serious Adverse Reactions	Education Indications
Td					
(Tetanus diphtheria) Child: 14-16 years Adult: 0.5 ml IM	Unvaccinated children ≥7 years Children 14-16 years and q 10 years Adults: booster q 10 years All adults (18-65) who did not complete a primary series in childhood Dose 1 Dose 2—at least 6 weeks later Dose 3—6-12 months after second dose	History of neurologic reaction or severe hypersensitivity (anaphylaxis or generalized urticaria)	Local reactions (induration and erythema) Arthus-type hypersensitivity—severe local reaction, fever, and malaise may occur if tetanus boosters given too often.	Very rarely: Serious allergic reaction Deep, aching pain and muscle wasting in upper arm 2 days to 4 weeks after the injection and may last months	Td is recommended for persons seeking medical attention for clean, minor wounds if more than 10 years since last dose. Td is recommended for deep puncture wounds if more than 5 years since last dose.
POLIOMYELITIS VACCINES					
(OPV no longer recommended in United States) IPV killed virus Dosage: 0.5 ml SQ	2, 4, 6 months (dosage may be given through 18 months) Booster: 4-6 years Can be substituted for some or all doses of OPV	Altered immunity in recipient or household HIV-positive Larger dose corticosteroid ≥18 years Allergic reaction to neomycin or streptomycin	Local pain at injection site	1 case for every $1\frac{1}{2}$ million after first dose 1 case for every 30 million later doses Paralytic polio in recipient or close contact (more common in adults) Anaphylaxis	Virus can be shed in stool for 4-6 weeks—need for good handwashing and proper disposal of diapers. IPV is recommended for previously unvaccinated adults—travelers to areas where wild poliovirus is endemic and epidemic.
MMR					
Measles, mumps, rubella Live virus Mix with diluent and give contents of single-dose vial SC. Measles, mumps, and rubella vaccines may be administered separately (see insert recommendations).	12-15 months Booster: either at 4-6 years or at 11-12 years Adults: 1 dose MMR, unless contraindicated, if not immunized as a child (ACIP recommends a second dose of MMR for certain high-risk individuals: those entering post–high school educational settings, persons in health care settings with direct patient care contact, travelers to areas with endemic measles.)	Severe allergy to eggs or neomycin Altered immunity in recipient Serum immune globulin, whole blood, or blood products within past 3 months Large dose corticosteroid Pregnancy contraindicated for 3 months after rubella immunization (use contraception).	Mild burning sensation at injection site Measles Fever starting 5-12 days after vaccination Rash Mumps Swelling of salivary glands Fever Rubella Joint pain/swelling 1-3 weeks after immunization, lasting 1 day to 3 weeks—more common among older, not previously immunized clients	Very rarely: Serious allergic reaction Anaphylaxis Postvaccination encephalitis Coma Residual seizure disorder Low number of platelets—usually temporary	All adults born in 1957 or later should receive 1 dose of measles/mumps vaccine unless there is laboratory evidence of immunity. Rubella vaccine is recommended for adults (especially women) without proof of vaccination or laboratory immunity. There is no evidence that revaccination with MMR in persons with natural or acquired immunity, to any of or all of the three diseases, causes increased risk. Measles vaccine may suppress tuberculin activity for 4-6 weeks.

Hib					
0.5 ml IM DTP/Hib combination vaccines are available. See specific guidelines from AAP and ACIP and review package insert information. After the primary infant Hib conjugate vaccine series is completed, any other licensed Hib conjugate vaccines may be used for 12-15 months booster dose.	2, 4, 6 months (Children who received PRP-OMP at 2 and 4 months do not require a dose at 6 months.) Booster: 12-15 months	≥5 years of age (Unimmunized children ≥5 years with chronic disease that is associated with *Hemophilus influenzae* should receive 1 dose.) Previous anaphylactic reaction to diphtheria toxoid if using HbOC (HibTITER) or PRP-D (Pro-HIBIT). These vaccines contain small amounts of diphtheria toxoid.	Local pain at injection site Mild fever		Protects child against some illnesses caused by *H. influenzae* (e.g., *H. influenzae* meningitis, pneumonia)
HEPATITIS B					
Recombinant antigen Infants: 0.25 ml IM (The dose for infants born to HBsAG-positive mothers is 0.5 ml IM. These infants are also given hepatitis B immune globulin [HBIG] at birth.) Child <11 years: 0.25 ml IM Child 11-19 years: 0.5 ml IM Adult ≥20 years: 1 ml IM Recombivax HB dialysis formulation is recommended for adult predialysis and dialysis patients (see package insert).	Infants: series of 3 doses Option 1: at birth, 1-2 months, 6-18 months Option 2: 1-2 months, 4 months, 6-18 months Infants born to HBsAg-positive mothers should receive hepatitis B immunoprophylaxis before hospital discharge. 7 years-adult: series of 3 doses—at first visit, then 2 months later, then 6 months after second dose	Hypersensitivity to yeast If symptoms of sensitivity occur after an injection, do not give additional immunizations.	Local pain, erythema, swelling Fatigue, weakness, headache Fever (≥100° F), malaise	Anaphylaxis	3-dose regimen provides a protective level against hepatitis B viral infection. Hepatitis B can cause cirrhosis and cancer of the liver. Duration of protection is generally 7 years. Vaccination is recommended for following at-risk groups: 1. Health care and public safety personnel 2. Employees of chronic care facilities 3. Subpopulations with a known high incidence of disease—Alaskan Eskimos, Indochinese, Haitian, and sub-Saharan refugees 4. Illicit injectable drug users 5. Prisoners 6. Morticians 7. Persons who have heterosexual activity with multiple partners, persons who repeatedly contract STDs, homosexually active males, prostitutes 8. Patients who frequently require blood transfusions or clotting factor concentrates 9. Household contacts of HBV carriers 10. Military personnel and travelers to areas with high endemic levels

Modified from Osguthorpe MC, Morgan EP: An immunization update for primary health care providers, *Nurse Pract* 20(6):52-65, 1995.

*Recommended schedules differ for infants and children who do not begin immunizations at usual time or who are behind schedule. See specific guidelines from American Academy of Pediatrics or Advisory Committee on Immunization Practices, USDHHS/CDC.

†No immunization should be given to a client who is moderately or severely ill.

‡Pregnancy is a precaution with any immunization. Special cases must be considered on an individual basis.

§DTP/Hib combination vaccines are available. See specific guidelines from Advisory Committee on Immunization Practices, USDHHS/CDC, and American Academy of Pediatrics.

continued

TABLE 22-1 Quick Reference for Routine Immunizations—cont'd

Vaccine Antigen Dose and Route	Routine Administration Schedule*	Precautions†‡ Contraindications	Adverse Reactions	Serious Adverse Reactions	Education Indications
INFLUENZA					
(Subviron or split virus) Children: 1 or 2 doses (Children <9 years who are receiving influenza vaccine for the first time should be given 2 doses, at least 1 month apart.) 6-35 months: 0.25 ml IM of split virus at least 1 month apart in AL thigh 3-9 years: 1 or 2 doses of 0.5 ml IM of split virus in AL thigh or deltoid ≥9 years: 1 dose of 0.5 ml IM deltoid Adult: 0.5 ml IM deltoid	Annually in the fall	History of allergy to eggs History of serious reaction to influenza vaccine Pregnancy—postpone immunization to second or third trimester.	Soreness at the injection site Myalgia, fever, flulike symptoms		CDC targets the following high-risk groups: 1. Persons >65 years old 2. Residents of nursing homes or other chronic care facilities 3. Adults and children with chronic disorders of pulmonary or cardiovascular system (e.g., asthma, bronchopulmonary dysplasia) 4. Persons who require regular medical follow-up or hospitalization during previous year because of chronic metabolic diseases (e.g., diabetes, renal dysfunction), hemoglobinopathies, or immunosuppressants (e.g., HIV, AIDS, or immunosuppression) because of medications 5. Family members, health care providers, and employees and volunteers who are potentially capable of transmitting influenza to high-risk patients
PNEUMOCOCCAL POLYSACCHARIDE VACCINE					
(23 valent) Inactivated antigen (Killed vaccine) Child: 0.5 ml IM or SC Adults: 0.5 ml IM or SC (Persons who received the 14-valent vaccine should not be reimmunized unless they are very high risk.)	Adults ≥65 years 1 dose: revaccination recommended only for those at highest risk ≥6 years after first dose. Children: 1 dose at ages 2, 4, and 6 months, with a booster dose at 12-15 months Age 24 months or greater: give 1 or 2 doses at least 6-8 weeks apart	Safety in pregnancy has not been evaluated.	Localized pain and erythema at the injection site Low-grade fever for 24 hours		CDC targets the following high-risk groups: 1. Adults ≥65 years old 2. Children or adults with chronic cardiac or respiratory illnesses or at risk for respiratory illness 3. Immunocompromised children/adults (e.g., splenic dysfunction, HIV, AIDS, sickle cell disease) 4. Revaccination should be considered ≥6 years after the first dose for those at highest risk of fatal pneumococcal disease or rapid decline in antibody levels.

VARICELLA <12 months: not recommended 12 months-12 years: 0.5 ml SC >12 years: First dose of 0.5 ml SC, then a repeat dose in 4-8 weeks (same for adults who have never received this immunization)		Anaphylactic allergy to gelatin or neomycin Pregnancy Immunocompromised patients Acute febrile illness Blood dyscrasias, leukemia, lymphoma Active, untreated TB Defer vaccination for 5 months after blood transfusions or administration of immune globulin or VZIG Avoid use of salicylates for 6 weeks after vaccination	Mild local pain at injection site Rare: mild varicella-like illness with a few fever vesicles	Anaphylaxis	Offer to high risk groups with no history of varicella illness: teachers of young children, day care workers, health care workers.

Modified from Osguthorpe MC, Morgan EP: An immunization update for primary health care providers, *Nurse Pract* 20(6):52-65, 1995.

*Recommended schedules differ for infants and children who do not begin immunizations at usual time or who are behind schedule. See specific guidelines from American Academy of Pediatrics or Advisory Committee on Immunization Practices, USDHHS/CDC.

†No immunization should be given to a client who is moderately or severely ill.

‡Pregnancy is a precaution with any immunization. Special cases must be considered on an individual basis.

§DTP/Hib combination vaccines are available. See specific guidelines from Advisory Committee on Immunization Practices, USDHHS/CDC, and American Academy of Pediatrics.

CHAPTER 23

Travel Medicine

Patricia Polgar Bailey

Every year millions of Americans travel overseas for business and pleasure; within the next two decades, the number of international travelers is expected to double.[1] In addition to the increased numbers of travelers, destinations once considered remote and unreachable are often visited by tourists. As a result, many travelers are at an increased risk of infectious and tropical disease. Although approximately 1300 persons die each year while traveling abroad, most travel-related deaths are caused by cardiovascular events and accidents. Only 1% of deaths are caused by infection.[2] Cardiac infarctions are the single greatest cause of deaths; most of these occur in older travelers who have a preexisting history of cardiac disease. Most deaths in travelers under the age of 55 are due to accidents, of which the majority could be prevented.[2]

The risk of acquiring an infectious illness or a tropical illness is dependent on the country visited, length of stay, present health status, risk behaviors, and preventive measures taken before departure. Nevertheless, the risk of acquiring many of the common travel-related illnesses, including hepatitis A, typhoid, malaria, and yellow fever, can be greatly minimized with a combination of education, immunizations, and chemoprophylaxis.

Primary care providers are often asked for recommendations about travel-related health issues. Travelers often receive conflicting information from family, friends, and the media. Therefore it is paramount that primary care providers be knowledgeable about these issues or at least know where to refer patients for up-to-date information. Primary care providers need to review the travel itinerary of prospective travelers, determine their risk for disease exposure, administer the required or recommended immunizations, and prescribe pharmacotherapy for disease prevention or for the treatment of episodic illness that can occur while traveling. In addition, travelers may need to be seen or referred to specialists for travel-related illnesses acquired while traveling.

Unfortunately, health conditions throughout the world change frequently and it is often difficult, if not impossible, to provide complete and up-to-date health information in one reference. Nevertheless, it is the primary care provider's responsibility to educate patients about travel-related health issues, determine their risk for disease exposure, administer immunizations and prescribe medications to protect them from travel-related illness or refer them to readily available resources (including computer programs and Internet access), facilitate the data acquisition for safe travel, and provide information about travel-related illnesses (Box 23-1). This information simplifies pretravel health screenings, helps determine what immunizations are required or recommended, and provides guidance regarding chemoprophylaxis for malaria, treatment of episodic illnesses (particularly traveler's diarrhea), water purification, traveling precautions, and medical care abroad.

PRETRAVEL PREPARATION

Adequate preparation and knowledge are advised for all travelers. Health care insurance may not provide coverage for travelers outside the United States. Medicare, for example, will not provide coverage for illness or accidents occurring outside the United States, including Canada.[2] Thus all travelers should be encouraged to closely examine their health care policies. If provisions for foreign travel are not included, it is generally possible to obtain an inexpensive, short-term policy to cover episodic needs that can occur while traveling. Travelers with serious preexisting medical conditions should consider purchasing evacuation insurance.[3]

Travelers with chronic health conditions should carry a written summary of their health problems, a list of current medications, and a copy of a recent ECG if available. A list of additional recommended travel documentation is included in Box 23-2. Medical identification bracelets are also recommended. Travelers who use inhalers (which may arouse suspicion), require needles or syringes (e.g., for insulin administration), or use controlled substances may find it worthwhile to carry a letter from their physician certifying their diagnosis and treatment in case of customs or security questions.[3] Travelers should take an adequate supply of regularly used medication. The medications should be kept in clearly labeled bottles, with the possible exception of medication to treat HIV and related illnesses.

Guidebooks and other travel publications provide invaluable information about the climate, culture and customs, economics and politics of countries throughout the world. In addition, several websites offer current weather and three-day forecasts for hundreds of cities around the world.

IMMUNIZATIONS

Although routine immunizations should be updated, travel immunizations, including hepatitis viruses A and B, typhoid fever, polio, meningococcal meningitis, yellow fever, Japanese encephalitis, and rabies, may be required or recommended depending on the destination, length of stay, current disease outbreaks, prior destinations, and other factors. Immunizations requirements should be reviewed at least 8 weeks before travel commences to ensure adequate time for antibody response as well as sufficient time to complete vaccine series such as Japanese encephalitis and rabies.

Specific guidelines for recommended and required immunizations are available in two publications from the Centers for Disease Control and Prevention (CDC): *Health Information for International Travel* (The Yellow Book), which is updated biannually, and "Summary of Health Information for International Travel (The Blue Sheet), which is updated weekly. These resources can also be accessed from the CDC website (http://www.cdc.gov), and information can also be obtained from the CDC automated International Traveler's Voice Information Service (404-332-4559), local health departments, and numerous other travel resources (Box 23-1).

Overseas travelers may need some vaccines not readily available in many primary care offices. For example, the yellow fever vaccine can be obtained only in offices officially licensed to administer the vaccine. In addition, many physicians in the

BOX 23-1

TRAVEL RESOURCES

Centers for Disease Control and Prevention (CDC)
(404) 639-3311
Website: http://www.cdc.gov
CDC Division of Vector-Borne Diseases
(970) 221-6400
CDC Health Information for International Travel (Yellow Book)
Superintendent of Documents
PO Box 371954
U.S. Government Printing Office
Washington, DC 20402
Website: http://www.cdc.gov/travel/yellowbk.htm
CDC International Travelers' Hot Line
(Clinical information for health care providers)
(404) 332-4559
Website: http://www.cdc.gov/travel/travel.html
CDC National Immunization Program Voice Information System
(800) CDC-HOT-SHOT
CDC Public Inquiries
(404) 639-3534
CDC Summary of Health Information for International Travel
(Blue Sheet document number 220022)
Fax: (404) 332-4565
HIV Testing Requirements for Entry into Foreign Countries
Website: http://www.travel.state.gov/HIVtestingreqs.html
International Association for Medical Assistance to Travelers
417 Center Street
Lewistown, NY 14092
(716) 754-4883
International Certificate of Vaccination
Superintendent of Documents
PO Box 371954
U.S. Government Printing Office
Washington, DC 20402
(Uniform stamp from local state government is necessary for validation of International Certificate of Vaccination when yellow fever vaccination is required.)
Malaria Hot Line
(404) 488-4046 or (404) 639-2888
Travel Medicine Advisor
American Health Consultants, Inc.
PO Box 740056
Atlanta, GA 30374
(800) 688-2421
Travel Medicine, Inc.
351 Pleasant Street
Northampton, MA 01060
(800) TRAVMED
e-mail: travel@travmed.com
Website: http://www.travmed.com
University of Washington Medical Center
Travel Medicine Service Audio Library
(206) 548-4888
Website: http://www.weber.u.washington.edu/~travmed/
U.S. Department of State Consular Affairs Automated Fax Service
(Information sheets regarding foreign embassy addresses and phone numbers, entry requirements, traveler advisories, and medical facilities)
U.S. Department of State Overseas Citizens Services and Consular Affairs Automated Voice Service
(Provides information for Americans abroad with financial, health, or legal questions)
(202) 647-5225
Website: http://www.travel.state.gov
U.S. Department of State Overseas Citizen's Emergency Center
(202) 647-5226
World Wide Web Travel Information page
Website: http://www.cdc.gov/travel/travel.html

United States are unfamiliar with tropical diseases such as malaria. Furthermore, because the health status and travel plans of each individual are unique, pretravel advice and appropriate recommendations may be more readily determined by health care providers specializing in travel medicine or in travel clinics. Travel medicine specialists and travel clinics are available in each state to provide the necessary information, documentation, risk assessment, immunizations, and recommendations needed for safe travel throughout the world. Some of these clinics have health care providers who offer a broader range of services, including the diagnosis and treatment of tropical and infectious diseases. Several Internet websites offer a list of travel clinics, including Travel Medicine Inc. (http://www.travmed.com), Shoreland's Travel Health Online (http://www.tripprep.com), International Society of Travel Medicine (http://www.istm.org), and American Society of Tropical Medicine and Hygiene (ASTMH) Directory of Travel Clinics and Consulting Physicians (http://www.astmh.org/clinics/clinindex.html).

MEDICATIONS AND PRESCRIPTIONS

Malaria

The need for prophylactic medications should be based on a traveler's itinerary. Malaria threatens nearly 40% of the world's population, and at least 100 countries are considered areas of malaria risk. However, most cases of malaria can be prevented. Avoiding malaria depends on knowledge of malaria-endemic areas, protection against mosquito bites (e.g., clothing, mosquito netting, DEET-containing insect repellants), and taking a prophylactic medication. In addition, travelers should be educated about the symptoms of malaria so that they can seek medical treatment should such symptoms occur.

BOX 23-2

TRAVEL DOCUMENTATION

- Passport and visa information
- Green card if applicable
- Birth certificate and photo ID
- Yellow fever and/or cholera vaccination requirements (International Certificate of Vaccination)
- Immunizations (All routine immunizations should be updated, but some immunizations may be advised based on disease patterns throughout the world. All immunizations should be recorded and signed by physician or designee in the "Traveler's International Certificate of Vaccination" or traveler's medical diary.
- HIV testing requirements for entry into foreign countries
- Tuberculosis testing requirements
- International driver's permit
- Physician's letter for prescription medications, syringes, HIV status (with copy of test result), exemption from vaccines with reason for exemption, and traveler's specific health needs
- Notarized parental consent—if traveling with children
- Physicians or hospitals abroad to contact for obtaining care, if needed

International travelers who take medications for chronic conditions should be advised to carry two supplies of these medications: one in their carry-on bag and one in their checked luggage.

Food and Water Precautions and Traveler's Diarrhea

Although not as serious as malaria, diarrhea is by far the most common medical problem among travelers to underdeveloped and tropical countries. However, diarrhea is not a disease but rather a symptom of an intestinal infection that is most commonly caused by contaminated food and water. Intestinal infections can be cause by bacteria, parasites, and viruses, although the most common cause of traveler's diarrhea is the bacterium *Escherichia coli*. Other causes of watery bacteria include *Salmonella, Campylobacter,* and *Vibrio* bacteria. Approximately 10% of cases of watery diarrhea are causes by intestinal viruses.[2] In contrast to watery diarrhea, bloody diarrhea suggests dysentery, which is caused by both bacteria (*Shigella, Campylobacter jejuni, Yersinia*) and sometimes parasites (*E. histolytica*). Other causes of bloody diarrhea include amebiasis, cryptosporidiosis, schistomiasis, and cyclosporidiasis. Only about 2% of travelers develop chronic diarrhea, which is usually caused by a parasite known as *Giardia*.

Because most travelers' diarrhea is caused by bacteria, antibiotics (particularly the fluoroquinolones [quinolone]) are especially helpful in its treatment. In general, one or two doses of a quinolone is sufficient to treat travelers' diarrhea, although in some cases longer treatment is warranted (i.e., a 5- to 7-day course may be indicated for a case of *Shigella*).[2] The benefit of broad-spectrum antibiotics is that they can be used effectively to treat some other episodic illnesses experienced while traveling, such as urinary tract infections, bronchitis, and uncomplicated skin infections.

Drugs other than antibiotics, such as Pepto-Bismol (bismuth subsalicylate) and loperamide, can be used to treat diarrhea. Both of these medications reduce the number of unformed stools and, in some cases, the duration of illness. There has been concern that these and other antimotility drugs may actually prolong the illness by interfering with the body's natural "flushing mechanism"; this has not been observed in most cases of travel-related watery diarrhea. However, antimotility drugs are not recommended in cases of bloody diarrhea and/or with a temperature of ≥101° F.[2]

Education about proper food and water precautions is imperative. Travelers should be advised to eat only cooked food and peeled fruits and vegetables and to drink only bottled beverages. Cooked foods should be served hot. Milk and milk products that have not been pasteurized should be avoided. Beverages made from boiled or hot water, such as tea and coffee, are generally safe. However, ice should be avoided. Travelers should be suspicious of locally bottled water, which may have been filled with local tap water, and of uncapped bottled water. Looks can be deceiving; clear wilderness stream and lake water can be contaminated with *Giardia* or *Campylobacter.* The adage "boil it, cook it, peel it, or forget it" is helpful to pass on to travelers. Travelers should avoid buying food from street vendors and from eating in establishments that appear to be unclean or have dirty restrooms.

Medications to prevent and treat motion and altitude sickness are helpful. The travel itinerary as well as the traveler's medical history can help guide the choice of appropriate medication. A back-up pair of eyeglasses or contact lenses is also recommended.

AIR TRAVEL RISKS

Air travel of more than 6 hours' duration increases the risk of deep vein thrombosis and peripheral edema. To minimize this risk, travelers should be encouraged to get up, walk, and stretch during flights. On most flights cabin pressure is maintained at a level equivalent to that of altitudes of 8000 feet or lower, which does result in some reduction in available oxygen. As a result, travelers with chronic pulmonary or cardiac disease can require supplemental oxygen. Travelers should wait at least 3 weeks after a myocardial infarction to fly and should be aware that supplemental oxygen may be needed for up to 4 months after the event.[1]

Air travel during pregnancy is usually safe but should be avoided after the eighth month. Pregnant women should be encouraged to walk around at least every 2 hours to avoid deep vein thrombosis.

Travelers with diabetes must monitor their serum glucose levels closely as changes in time zone and diet and exercise routines can cause significant changes even in those with good control. Travelers with recently diagnosed and unstable diabetes should be advised to wait until glycemic control is stabilized before traveling. Stuart Rose's[2] *International Travel Health Guide* includes protocols for adjusting insulin dosages across multiple time zones based on the direction and duration of travel.

SAFE TRAVEL

All travelers should be aware of safety risks while traveling and take appropriate measures to mitigate those risks. Crime is a problem in most parts of the world, and travelers should take precautions to avoid being robbed. Valuables should be kept in a hotel safe if available. Travelers should refrain from wearing expensive jewelry, should minimize the amount of cash carried, use Travelers' Checks or the equivalent, and dress modestly and inconspicuously.

The leading cause of health problems while traveling is motor vehicle accidents. Seatbelts should be worn and general motor vehicle safety precautions implemented at all times. In addition, travelers should be advised to plan trips in advance and to review directions before departure if they will not be traveling as part of a tour. Travelers should know how to protect themselves and receive help in case of a crime or emergency as well as where to obtain medical care while in a foreign country.

SUMMARY

As international travel becomes increasingly common, primary care providers need to have at least a basic knowledge about travel medicine and to have referral options for travelers requiring additional services. All travelers should know about required and recommended immunizations as well as the need for malaria prophylaxis. In addition, an understanding of appropriate food and water precautions and the treatment of traveler's diarrhea is also necessary. General and country-specific travel education should include information about jet lag, motion and altitude sickness, protection against insect bites, sources of medical care, and a country's culture and customs.

REFERENCES

1. Aerospace Medical Association, Air Transport Medicine Committee: Medical guidelines for air travel, *Aviat Space Environ Med* 667(10 suppl):B1-B16, 1996.
2. Rose SR: *International travel health guide,* Northampton, MA, 1999, Travel Medicine, Inc.
3. Bratton RL: Advising patients about international travel: what they can do to protect their health and safety, *Postgrad Med* 106(1):57-64, 1999.

Presurgical Clearance

Jane Flanagan, Jennifer Neves, and Claire McGowan

As the type and number of outpatient surgical procedures have multiplied, the need for presurgical medical evaluation to ascertain an individual patient's medical readiness to undergo surgery has increased exponentially. The patient's primary care team or a medical team from a presurgical clinic affiliated with either the surgeon or the hospital where the surgery is scheduled may perform the presurgical clearance examination.

TYPES OF PATIENTS NEEDING PRESURGICAL CLEARANCE

The types of adult patients needing presurgical clearance can vary greatly by age, medical condition, and diagnosis. They can be young and healthy with a minor athletic injury, older and requiring a surgical procedure with several co-morbidities present such as cardiac and pulmonary disease, or surgical oncology patients who may have a poor prognosis but are otherwise healthy. The one common characteristic shared by all these patients is that they are considered elective, non-emergent admissions. It is this characteristic that serves as a basis for classifying these patients from an anesthesia-risk perspective.

COMPONENTS OF PRESURGICAL CLEARANCE

All patients presenting for presurgical clearance are considered outpatients. They can come from home, rehabilitation centers, nursing facilities, or other extended care environments, and the intent is that they will return to that environment after clearance. Presurgical clearance can occur 1 to 30 days before surgery and, ideally, will be scheduled so that all necessary consults can be conducted and reviewed by the appropriate providers. For example, the health care provider performing the presurgical clearance decides that pulmonary function tests are warranted in a patient with asthma who will be undergoing elective hip replacement. The provider must allow for enough time to schedule this test and review the results with the anesthesia team, who will then determine the appropriate anesthesia plan for the patient.

History

A general review of systems, including smoking history, drug and alcohol use and or abuse, intake of herbal remedies and vitamins, medication or latex allergies, recent blood transfusions, pregnancy (full-term or incomplete), recent history of chemotherapy or radiation therapy, and a personal or family history of problems with anesthesia or bleeding should be obtained. Additionally, in-depth information about medical conditions such as cardiac disease, respiratory disease, diabetes, gastrointestinal problems, and psychiatric issues are all pertinent to the presurgical medical history.

Physical Examination

The physical examination focuses on the presenting surgical problem and probable type of anesthesia. The general examination should include generalized appearance and baseline vital signs that include oxygen saturation, height, and weight. The airway, dentition, and range of motion of the head and neck should also be evaluated. Abnormalities should be noted in the appearance of neck veins, presence of bruits, and the auscultation of heart, lungs, and abdomen. An additional examination that includes the presence of abdominal masses, genitourinary or rectal problems, peripheral pulses, and cranial nerves may be warranted depending on the reason for surgery, medical history, and anesthetic plan.

For example, a 32-year-old healthy man presents with a herniated lumbar disk. The physical examination should include all of the preceding tests because this patient may present with neurologic or peripheral vascular changes or may experience them during the postoperative period. In addition, sexual, urinary, and bowel function could be a presenting symptom associated with his back problem or may develop in the postoperative period as an untoward result of the surgery.

Diagnostics

Diagnostic testing for presurgical clearance is variable and depends on several factors: (1) presenting diagnosis, (2) patient age, (3) co-morbidities, and (4) type of anesthetic agent planned. Much of what was considered necessary preoperative testing in the past has been reviewed by collaborating staff, and guidelines in many presurgical clinics have been developed to be consistent with research in this area.[1] The guidelines used in one presurgical clinic are outlined in Table 24-1.

Collaborative Management of Patient Co-Morbidities

Ideally, patients who present for presurgical clearance will have good primary care and will have underlying medical conditions well managed on presentation. There are two instances in which the provider performing the presurgical clearance must address the management of co-morbid disease processes: (1) when a patient does not have appropriate primary care, and (2) when a patient does have good primary care but needs further testing as a result of the anesthesia plan and co-morbid diseases.

For instances in which the patient does not have a primary care provider, the presurgical clearance provider determines if any primary care issues must be addressed in the preoperative period. If there are none, then the patient progresses through presurgical clearance but is educated about the importance of primary care. If the patient requires primary care before surgery, the surgeon is contacted and the patient is referred to a primary care provider before undergoing the surgical procedure.

At other times a patient has been well managed by a primary care provider but the primary care provider is unsure what diagnostic tests may be needed before surgery. In these instances the provider performing the presurgical clearance makes recommendations for further extensive testing and refers the patient to the primary care provider. For example, a patient who has a history of well-managed angina but has not had a recent stress test and is scheduled for a total hip replacement with a general anesthetic would need a stress test before surgery. This may be arranged in collaboration with the primary care provider, or the patient may be referred back to the primary care provider, who then orders the test and sends the results to the presurgical clinic. Other tests that may be

TABLE 24-1 Tests for Presurgical Clearance

Test	When Performed
Chest x-ray study	Patient is over age 60 years, has a smoking history of >20 pack-years, has a history of cardiovascular or pulmonary diseases or is having a thoracic procedure, or has malignant disease
ECG	Patient is above a certain age (males >45 years, females >55 years) or has a history or symptoms of cardiac disease, diabetes, morbid obesity, significant pulmonary disease, cocaine abuse
Complete blood count	Patient is over age 60 years; has a history of pulmonary, cardiovascular, or renal disease; has a smoking history >20 pack-years; has a history of radiation therapy or chemotherapy; has a history of bleeding disorder; or presents with symptoms of infectious process (increased temperature and cough)
Coagulation studies	Patient is presently undergoing coagulation therapy, has a history of alcohol abuse or hepatic disease or a family or personal history of easy bruising or bleeding disorders or malignant disease, or is undergoing procedures with associated blood loss or postoperative coagulation therapy
Pregnancy test	Patient is a woman of childbearing age (except a woman who has had an oophorectomy)
Electrolytes	Patient is on dialysis; is diabetic or has hypertension, heart disease, or other disease process; or is on medication that may cause alteration in electrolytes
Liver function tests	Patient has a history of alcohol abuse, hepatitis, or known hepatic disease
Urinalysis or urine culture and sensitivity	Patient is undergoing urologic procedure, is receiving a prosthetic device, or has a history of frequent urinary tract infections
Albumin	Patient is malnourished or has a history of alcohol abuse or hepatic or malignant disease

required because of the anesthesia plan include echocardiograms in patients with known valve disease or pulmonary function tests in patients with chronic obstructive pulmonary disease (COPD).

Medication and Fasting Recommendations

Medication and fasting requirements are other management issues addressed by the provider performing the presurgical clearance. All herbal medications and vitamin E should be stopped 2 weeks before surgery. All medications used to control conditions such as hypertension, heart disease, eye problems, anxiety, pain, and COPD should be continued and taken on the morning of surgery.

Oral diabetic agents should not be taken the morning of surgery except for metformin (Glucophage), which should be stopped 3 days before surgery. In general, patients taking insulin are instructed to take half their usual dose of longer-acting agent and are instructed to withhold shorter-acting insulin. This plan may require a referral to the endocrinologist for confirmation or more tailored management.[2]

Recommendations for fasting guidelines vary among hospitals. It is generally accepted, however, that all patients can have clear fluids until 5 hours before surgery, except for patients who have gastroesophageal reflux (GERD) or for those having surgery that requires them to be in a prone position; such patients need to fast from both food and fluids for 8 hours before surgery. In addition, the presence of upper gastrointestinal disease (including GERD) may predispose a patient to aspiration of stomach contents during intubation. To diminish the risk of aspiration, these patients should take an H_2-receptor antagonist the night before and on the morning of surgery.[3]

Review of Surgical Complications

Complications related to anesthesia are multiple and range from major and life threatening (rare) to more benign and easily resolved (more common). Complications vary by anesthetic type, with co-morbid conditions adding to the risk. For general anesthesia, complications can range from nausea, vomiting, sore throat, and fatigue to stroke, myocardial infarction, allergic reaction, and death. For spinal or other regional anesthesia, complications can include headache, nerve damage, infection, and limb loss. All potential complications are reviewed before surgery to stratify risk and minimize perioperative morbidity and mortality. Given the seriousness of the potential risks, the complications are again addressed by the anesthetist who is providing care on the day of surgery before obtaining consent.

Patient and Family Education

Patient and family education is related to the surgical and anesthesia plan of care. After the patient has been assessed and with the patient's permission, the family can be included in preoperative and postoperative teaching. Expectations regarding the patient's care on discharge either to home or another facility can also be discussed. Teaching the anesthesia plan of care is also completed in the presurgical setting and includes possible complications and effects of anesthesia as well as intraoperative and postoperative pain management.

Health Promotion

Many patients who present for presurgical clearance have lifestyle issues that may promote or exacerbate disease processes. This encounter presents an excellent opportunity to address these issues. For example, a patient who smokes can be encouraged to quit smoking during the preoperative period, and appropriate referrals to smoking cessation programs can be made. Assessment and teaching around other issues such as alcohol or drug abuse, stress management, exercise, home safety, and domestic violence are also addressed in this setting. A patient may or may not be ready to make the appropriate alterations in lifestyle; thus it requires skillful assessment to determine the timing of such teaching.

PRESURGICAL CLINICS

Before the late 1980s, patients were admitted to the hospital for a minimum of 1 day before surgery for presurgical clearance. At this time they were screened and assessed by a surgical team that included anesthesiologists, surgeons, and nurses. They would also complete presurgical preparations and tests. The improvement of surgical and anesthesia techniques led to a reduced need for extensive testing and preparation. Concurrently, patients were expressing a desire to be in their own home with family or other loved ones the night before surgery, and there was an increasing demand to implement cost containment measures by health care organizations.[4,5]

As a result, hospitals throughout the United States created presurgical clearance clinics by the late 1980s in an effort to provide patients and their families with the same level of preparation that they had received previously.[2] Initially these clinics were established to prepare patients undergoing minor surgeries, but with increasing demands on hospitals to save costs and continued improvements in surgical technologies, there was a greater push to prepare a larger variety and a more acute population of patients. These clinics have been one reason that the length of stay for surgical procedures has decreased nationwide. For example, in the 1980s the average length of stay for major joint repair was 4 weeks, which often included 1 or 2 preoperative days. Between 1995 and 1997, the average length of stay for major joint repair was 4 days.[6]

It has also been reported that the numbers of surgeries has been increasing. In one Massachusetts hospital the number of people having surgery requiring a hospital stay increased from 21,000 to 22,000 between 1999 and 2000, with 90% of these surgical patients being admitted on the same day of surgery.[7]

COLLABORATIVE PRACTICE IN PRESURGICAL CLINICS

Midlevel providers in presurgical clinics collaborate with the anesthesiologists who will be providing the anesthetic as well as with primary care providers and surgeons regarding the plan of care. In conjunction with primary care providers and surgeons, these APNs (advanced practice nurses) or PAs (physician assistants) make referrals to cardiologists and other specialists if needed to determine the safest anesthesia plans. In presurgical clinics, midlevel providers and anesthesiologists review the results of these tests and discuss with surgeons the proposed anesthesia plans. These midlevel providers then communicate the proposed plans to the primary care providers.

Theoretically, patients presenting in presurgical clinics should have their general health managed in the primary care setting. In some cases, however, this does not occur. If this is the case, it is an excellent opportunity to review the importance of good primary care and to make a referral to a primary care physician in a location that will be convenient for the patient.

REFERENCES

1. Everett L, Kallar S: Pre-surgical evaluation and laboratory testing. In Twersky R, editor: *The ambulatory anesthesia handbook*, St Louis, 1995, Mosby.
2. Cygan R, Waitzkin H, Hsaio R: When to stop and restart medications in the perioperative period, *J Intern Med* 11:29, 1993.
3. Moyers JR, Vincent CM: Preoperative medication. In Barash PG, Cullen BF, Stoelting RK, editors: *Clinical anesthesia*, Philadelphia, 2001, Williams & Wilkins.
4. DeFazio-Quinn DM: Ambulatory surgery: an evolution, *Nurs Clin North Am* 32:377-386, 1997.
5. Jones D, Coakley A, Flanagan J: Nursing diagnosis at 24 and 72 hours following same day surgery with general anesthesia. In Rantz M, LeMore P, editors: *Proceedings of the Thirteenth North American Nursing Diagnosis*, Glendale, Calif, 1999, CNAHL Information Systems.
6. Lagoe R, Arnold K, Noetscher C: Benchmarking hospital lengths of stay using histograms. *Nurs Economics* 17:75-92, 1999.
7. Kowalczyk L: Elective surgeries soar. In *The Boston Globe* 258:A1, B4, 2000.

CHAPTER 25

Preparticipation Sports Physical

Terry Mahan Buttaro

Primary care providers are often asked to do preparticipation examinations (PPEs) for student athletes. Most states require these examinations for both junior and high school athletes. Physicians experienced in sports medicine recommend that student athletes have a preparticipation physical for middle school, junior high school, high school, and college athletics.[1] The American Heart Association recommends cardiovascular preparticipation screening and a history and physical examination for all athletes participating in high school and college sports and prefers that a physician perform the examination.[2] Some states allow nurse practitioners and physician assistants to perform sports physicals, and others do not.[2]

Historically, the primary goal for these examinations has been to identify adolescent athletes at risk for a cardiovascular event. It is also necessary that other medical problems be identified and treated before the student is cleared to participate in any athletics. Determining the overall health of the athlete, providing counseling, and strengthening the provider-patient relationship are other objectives. The importance of the sports participation physical examination cannot be understated. The examiner must be skilled and have sufficient experience in performing both the cardiovascular and musculoskeletal examination to identify any condition that would prohibit participation in the chosen sport.

Although some PPEs have been performed in the school in the past, it is preferable to perform the examination in the office so that adequate time can be spent ascertaining the student's and family's health history and performing the examination. If possible, the examination should be performed at least 6 weeks before the beginning of the sports season. It is also important that a parent accompany the student to the examination to fully establish the family history and cardiovascular risk factors. It is often helpful to have the student and parent complete and sign a preparticipation health history form before the examination. *It is essential that the provider review the form with the student and parent and specifically question the parent and student about each item on the health history form.*

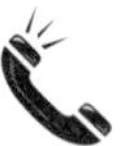

Physician consultation is recommended for preparticipation sports physical.

HISTORY

Allergies, current and past medications, and the personal and family history should be carefully assessed. Answers to the following questions should be determined before the examination commences.

1. Medical history, including the following:
   - Allergic or untoward reactions to exercise, medications, pollens, foods, and stinging insects (the specific nature of the reaction should also be determined)
   - Current medications, including vitamins or herbal supplements, prescribed or over-the-counter medications, and nutritional supplements
   - Habits such as smoking, caffeine, alcohol or drug use
   - Immunization history: tetanus, hepatitis, chickenpox, and MMR (measles, mumps, rubella)
   - Previous surgeries (particularly orthopedic, genital, kidney, or eye surgeries)
   - Previous hospitalizations
   - Loss of an organ such as eye, kidney, or testicle
2. Present or past illness, including the following:
   - Recent viral illness such as mononucleosis or myocarditis
   - Recent weight loss or gain
   - Previous sports restriction
   - History of heat-related illness
   - Skin reactions (hives, rashes, infections)
   - Head injury, neck injury, loss of consciousness, fainting, concussion, headaches, seizures
   - Visual problems such as blurred vision or a history of detached retina; does the patient wear glasses or contacts?
   - History of heart surgery, hypertrophic cardiomyopathy, or coronary artery abnormalities; history of chest pain or palpitations (heart racing or skipped heart beats) with or after exercise; history of hypertension; history of weakness or dizziness with or after exercise; history of murmur or syncope
   - Breathing problems such as wheezing, coughing, or trouble breathing with or after exercise; history of asthma
   - History of musculoskeletal injury such as fracture or dislocation; neck injury or pain; shoulder injury or pain; back injury or pain; elbow, hand, or finger injury or pain; knee, ankle, foot, or toe injury or pain

     History of use of special equipment for sports-related activities

     History of numbness or tingling in the upper or lower extremities

     History of eating disorder, excessive fatigability, diabetes, bleeding problems, anemia, hepatitis, mononucleosis

     History of stress, anxiety, or depression

     Menstrual history: menarche, last menstrual period, frequency of menses (number of menstrual periods in the past year)
3. Family history, including the following:
   - History of premature or sudden death, long QT syndrome, Wolfe-Parkinson-White syndrome, arrhythmias, hypertrophic cardiomyopathy, or Marfan's syndrome
   - Family history of coronary artery disease

PHYSICAL EXAMINATION

The physical examination should be focused and thorough to determine the presence of an acute infection or any impairment that would prohibit participation in the selected sport. General appearance, posture, overall health, and height, weight, and percentage of body fat should be determined. It is vital that congenital deformities such as arachnodactyly (Marfan's syndrome) be noted. Additional components of the physical examination should include the following:

1. Visual acuity with Snellen chart: corrected visual acuity should be 20/40 or better
2. Vital signs
3. Blood pressure and heart rate at rest, 3 minutes after exercise, and again 6 minutes after exercise
4. Skin evaluation for signs of fungal, candida, or other infection
5. Head, eyes, ears, nose, and throat (HEENT) evaluation to determine infectious processes and evaluate any lymphadenopathy
6. Cardiovascular examination
   - The heart sounds must be assessed in the supine, standing, and squatting position. Special emphasis is necessary to determine the presence of any murmurs or arrhythmias. Arrhythmias, extra heart sounds (S_3, S_4), a new murmur, a diastolic murmur, a systolic murmur grade 3/6 or higher, a systolic murmur that increases in intensity with the Valsalva maneuver, or a mitral valve click accompanied by a murmur requires further evaluation before clearance for sports participation can be given.
   - Radial and femoral pulses should be symmetric to exclude coarctation of the aorta.
   - Blood pressure must be compared to age-adjusted tables. Elevated blood pressure requires treatment and must be within the accepted range before medical clearance is given. The use of beta blockers and/or diuretics may prohibit athletic participation in some states.[1]
7. Pulmonary examination: lung sounds should be assessed anteriorly and posteriorly
8. Abdominal examination: organomegaly requires further evaluation*
9. Genitourinary examination
   - The testes must be descended.
   - The presence of inguinal hernias must be determined.
10. Musculoskeletal examination
    - Is there neck pain on examination or with range of motion (ROM)?*
    - With the patient standing, the back should be evaluated for scoliosis, flexibility, and pain with ROM.*
    - All extremities and joints, including the shoulders/arms, elbow/forearm, wrist/hand, hip/thigh, knee, leg/ankle, foot, and acromioclavicular joint, must be evaluated for flexibility, symmetry, tenderness, and ROM. Resisted shoulder shrug and resisted flexion

*Any pain or deficit requires further evaluation before medical clearance is given for sports participation.

and extension must be determined.* Asymmetry or pain with ROM requires further evaluation.
- The physical signs of Marfan's syndrome should be excluded.
- Can the patient "duck walk" at least 4 steps?
- Can the patient hop on each foot several times?

11. Neuromuscular examination
    - Cranial and sensory nerves
    - Deep tendon reflexes
    - Cerebellar function

DIAGNOSTICS

Diagnostics are not usually necessary, although some states can require urinalysis to determine the presence of protein or sugar in the urine. Other diagnostics such as ECG, exercise stress test, or echocardiogram are necessary if the history and physical examination suggests any cardiac abnormalities. Hemoglobin and hematocrit should be determined as necessary in female athletes.

MEDICAL CLEARANCE

Physician consultation/referral is indicated and medical clearance deferred if there is a history of detached retina, posttraumatic convulsive disorder, or the absence of an eye, kidney, or testicle (these conditions usually prohibit participation in any contact sport). Appropriate consultation/referral is also indicated if the student is unable to perform duck walk maneuvers or if there is evidence of diminished visual acuity, hypertension, an acute systemic infection, cardiac abnormalities, neurologic deficit, neck pain or history of cervical stenosis, shoulder asymmetry, joint tenderness or pain with ROM. Medical clearance is deferred pending specialist evaluation. Patients with significant lymphadenopathy, abdominal organomegaly, uncontrolled diabetes or asthma, obesity, and eating disorders also require further evaluation before medical clearance can be provided. Students with controlled asthma, diabetes, or other chronic illness can participate in sports but must have careful medical management.

PATIENT AND FAMILY EDUCATION

Students, parents, and coaches can exert considerable pressure on the primary care provider to provide medical clearance for the athlete. However, the primary care provider's fundamental responsibility is to protect the student from harm. Any concerns elicited during the history or physical examination must be carefully explained to both the parent and student. It is important that both the parent and student understand that medical clearance cannot be given until the results of diagnostic testing and/or specialist evaluation are known. The parent and student should also understand that a preparticipation sports physical examination has limitations and cannot completely eliminate the risks inherent in any athletic activity.

REFERENCES

1. Hergenroeder AC: *The preparticipation sports physical in children and adolescents.* Retrieved from the World Wide Web August 20, 2002: http://www.uptodate.com.
2. Lyznicki JM and others: Cardiovascular screening of student athletes, *Am Fam Physician* 62(4):765-774, 2000.

PART 4

Office Emergencies

TERRY MAHAN BUTTARO, Section Editor

CHAPTER 26

Acute Bronchospasm

JoAnn Trybulski

DEFINITION/EPIDEMIOLOGY

Bronchospasm, or constriction of the bronchioles, occurs in conjunction with multiple entities. Bronchospasm may develop in a patient as a reaction to medication administered in the office, or the patient may already have bronchospasm when he or she comes to the office for an examination.

Clinical conditions that are associated with bronchospasm include anaphylactic reactions to medications or other allergens, congestive heart failure, pulmonary embolism, asthma, chronic obstructive pulmonary disease, lower respiratory tract infection, mechanical airway obstruction by anatomic changes or tumor, and vocal cord dysfunction.[1] The actual incidence of bronchospasm is difficult to determine because many cases are intermittent and the conditions that cause bronchospasm are multiple.

Immediate emergency department referral/physician consultation is indicated for patients in acute respiratory distress.

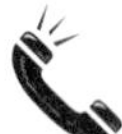

Physician consultation is indicated for patients with an Sao_2 of less than 92% on room air and failure to improve with nebulizer treatment given three times or epinephrine injection administered three times to a peak flow of greater than 80% of predicted.

PATHOPHYSIOLOGY

Bronchospasm results when hyperreactivity of the airways, caused by inflammatory substances, produces airway bronchoconstriction, edema, and obstruction. The bronchospasm may be intermittent and resolve without treatment, or the obstruction may progress to respiratory arrest, with its potential for death.

CLINICAL PRESENTATION

Patient presentations can vary from mild anxiety to acute respiratory distress. Most often, wheezing, coughing, and dyspnea are present. A repetitive, spasmodic cough may be the only sign of bronchospasm. The inability of the patient to speak a full sentence without pausing to breathe indicates severe bronchospasm. The psychologic states of patients vary according to their previous experience with this condition and the severity of symptoms. Patients with a history of asthma may have experienced bronchospasm quite frequently and may have even come to accept this as a usual daily pattern, whereas patients who experience their first episode or a severe episode may understandably be quite anxious.

PHYSICAL EXAMINATION

Vital signs may show tachypnea, tachycardia, and a normal or slightly elevated blood pressure. Hypotension occurs in an allergic reaction with anaphylaxis. The presence of pulsus paradoxus of greater than 25 mm Hg is a uniform indicator of severe respiratory compromise.[2]

Skin color may be normal, flushed, or pale. The presence of pruritus or a rash is a diagnostic aid with an allergic etiology.

The use of accessory muscles is noted as a sign of more severe bronchospasm. Wheezing may be audible or present with auscultation on inspiration and/or expiration. The finding of a silent chest indicates severe spasm and is an ominous sign. With audible wheezing, the trachea should be auscultated to discern whether these sounds are indicative of laryngospasm or partial airway obstruction with a foreign body.

DIAGNOSTICS

Peak flow measurements will be reduced from the patient's normal or from what is considered normal for age and height. Pulse oximetry values below 90% in adults indicate more severe bronchospasm. Arterial blood gas (ABG) analysis is best performed in an emergency department.

Chest radiographs may delineate the cause of bronchospasm. With asthma or allergy, the chest radiograph can be normal or show hyperinflation.

DIFFERENTIAL DIAGNOSIS

Potentially fatal conditions require immediate exclusion. The presence of an urticarial rash with decreasing blood pressure is a sign of anaphylaxis, necessitating immediate treatment with supplemental oxygen via nasal cannula or mask and diphenhydramine (Benadryl) 25 to 50 mg IV or epinephrine 0.3 mg SC depending on the patient's condition and cardiac status.

Cardiac failure may present as bronchospasm in the setting of known cardiac disease. Clinical presentation with paroxysmal nocturnal dyspnea, distended neck veins, or pedal edema confirms the diagnosis. Vascular redistribution or pleural effusion may be seen on chest radiographs. Obtaining chest radiographic studies should not delay treatment for cardiac failure.

Bronchospasm with acute dyspnea may herald impending respiratory failure in patients with chronic lung disease. Other causes of respiratory failure include depressed respiratory drive, pneumonia, atelectasis, asthma, airway obstruction, pulmonary edema, pulmonary hemorrhage, pulmonary contusion, and adult respiratory distress syndrome (ARDS). The history and clinical presentation indicate the origin of the respiratory failure.

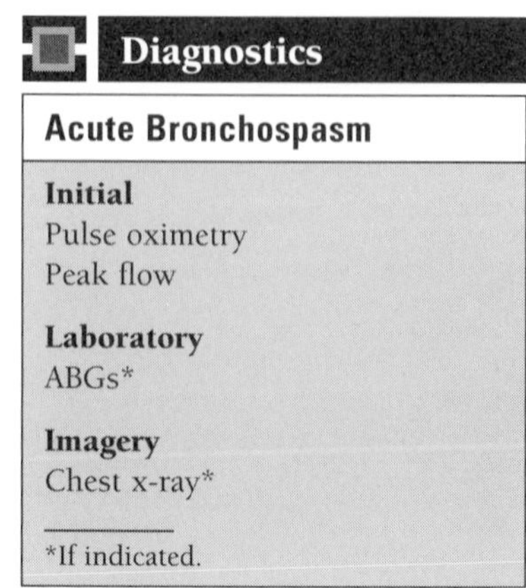

Diagnostics

Acute Bronchospasm

Initial
Pulse oximetry
Peak flow

Laboratory
ABGs*

Imagery
Chest x-ray*

*If indicated.

Pulmonary embolization should be suspected when bronchospasm occurs in a patient at risk for a pulmonary embolus. These patients include those who smoke and those with signs of vascular thrombosis, a history of atrial fibrillation, or a history of oral contraceptive use.

Recurrent bronchospasm or a poor response to bronchodilation medication indicates the need for reassessment and thorough evaluation for mechanical airway obstruction caused by anatomic changes or tumor, as well as vocal cord dysfunction, a missed case of heart failure, or pulmonary embolus.

INITIAL STABILIZATION AND MANAGEMENT

Acute bronchospasm occurring in the setting of lower respiratory tract infection, asthma, or chronic obstructive pulmonary disease is initially managed by supplemental oxygen via nasal cannula or mask and inhalation of a beta agonist via a metered-dose inhaler (MDI) or nebulizer. Treatment via an MDI consists of 2 to 4 puffs of albuterol every 20 minutes; up to three treatments may be given to reverse bronchospasm as long as tachycardia does not increase or palpitations are not precipitated by the treatments.[1] As an alternative, nebulizer treatment with 0.25 to 0.50 ml of a 0.5% solution of albuterol diluted to 3 to 5 ml with saline may be used; this treatment may also be given every 20 minutes for up to three treatments.[3] Ipratropium bromide 0.5 mg may be added to the nebulizer solution with saline and given every 6 hours to augment and prolong bronchodilation.

Worsening respiratory status, increased respiratory difficulty, decreasing pulse oximetry values, and failure to respond to beta agonist therapy indicate impending respiratory failure. The primary care provider should be prepared to support respiration via intubation and mechanical ventilation while transferring the patient to the nearest emergency facility for other therapeutic modalities. Inhalation of an oxygen-helium mixture has shown some benefit in severe cases of bronchoconstriction. Use of a parenteral steroid (60 to 80 mg of methylprednisone IV) needs to be considered, but objective improvement in airway functioning may not occur for 6 to 12 hours after administration.[2] Once acute bronchospasm is resolved, the use of oral prednisone starting at 60 mg daily and tapered over 2 weeks is generally prescribed to reduce inflammation. Recent studies point to the efficacy of using magnesium sulfate IV as an adjunct to treat acute bronchospasm.[4] Doses for magnesium sulfate IV reported in a meta-analysis ranged from 10 to 25 mg/kg with infusion over 20 minutes.[4]

Differential Diagnosis

Acute Bronchospasm	
Anaphylaxis	Pulmonary embolism
Congestive heart failure	Tremor
Respiratory failure	Vocal cord dysfunction

DISPOSITION AND REFERRAL

The primary care provider should be acquainted with the capabilities of the local emergency medical services system and have in place a plan for the emergency transport of patients. Patients who fail to respond to treatment or who do not improve with initial therapy should be transported to an emergency treatment facility.

PREVENTION AND PATIENT EDUCATION

The primary care provider needs to be prepared to manage acute bronchospasm in the office setting and must have a plan for emergency medical services system support. Equipment and supplies needed in initial patient management include, at a minimum, oxygen, peak flow meters (disposable or capable of being decontaminated), beta agonist inhalers (albuterol), and epinephrine. If an emergency department is not readily available, additional recommended supplies include IV access capability, parenteral steroids, anticholinergic medication (ipratropium), intubation equipment, and a hand-held nebulizer. Increasingly, medical offices have access to pulmonary function testing machines and pulse oximetry. Office personnel who triage telephone calls and make appointments should receive guidelines for which patients to reroute to the emergency department via ambulance.

Patients with known asthma need to have a management plan devised that includes parameters for seeking medical evaluation. These patients also require extensive education regarding their medication regimens, care and use of inhalers, and how to measure and use peak flow measurements.

REFERENCES

1. Richmond E: Asthma diagnosis and management, *Clin Rev* 7(8):76-112, 1997.
2. Abou-Shala N, MacIntyre N: Emergent management of acute asthma, *Med Clin North Am* 80(4):677-699, 1996.
3. Murphy JL, editor: *Nurse practitioner's prescribing reference,* New York, 1997, Prescribing Reference.
4. Alter HJ, Koepsell TD, Hilty WM: Intravenous magnesium as an adjuvant in acute bronchospasm: a meta-analysis, *Ann Emerg Med* 36(3):191-197, 2000.

CHAPTER 27

Altitude Illness

Karin C. Dieselman

DEFINITION/EPIDEMIOLOGY

Altitude illness is a syndrome complex of mild to severe symptoms that results from rapid ascent into an hypoxic environment, especially in nonacclimatized people. This syndrome complex is manifested as acute mountain sickness (AMS), high-altitude pulmonary edema (HAPE), and high-altitude cerebral edema (HACE). AMS, HAPE, and HACE are separate clinical syndromes with a continuum of mild to severe symptoms. This complex of symptoms can cause coagulation abnormalities, focal neurologic deficits, syncope, peripheral edema, retinopathy, pharyngitis, bronchitis, immune suppression, and flatus expulsion.

More than 300 million people worldwide inhabit high-altitude regions, with 50% living above 2400 m (8000 feet).[1] In the United States more than 40 million people travel above 2400 m (8000 feet) annually.[2,3]

AMS occurs within the first 24 hours of a rapid ascent to 2000 m (6600 feet) or higher and is seen in 33% of climbers.[2] This syndrome develops in nearly three out of four climbers to 4500 m (15,000 feet). The incidence at 2220 m (7200 feet) and 2700 m (9000 feet) is 17% and 40%, respectively. AMS occurs in 40% of trekkers in Nepal on the path to Mount Everest; this number increases to 70% during ascent to the top.[4] Two thirds of the climbers of Mount Rainer and 25% of travelers to Colorado ski resorts experience AMS.[1]

Men and women are equally susceptible to AMS; children and individuals with preexisting diseases (e.g., arteriosclerotic cardiovascular disease [ASCVD], chronic obstructive pulmonary disease [COPD], congestive heart failure [CHF], sickle cell anemia) are more susceptible. HAPE is less common, occurring in 1% to 2% of those who rapidly ascend to 3000 m (10,000 feet).[2] HAPE is more common in climbers and skiers who have not acclimatized. With HAPE, 20 deaths worldwide are reported annually, with men having a preponderance of 87% over women.[3]

Immediate emergency department referral/physician consultation is indicated for patients with altitude illness.

PATHOPHYSIOLOGY

AMS results in a decrease of oxygen delivery to the tissues at the alveolar level. At 1500 m (5000 feet), PaO_2 as measured with arterial blood gas sampling is 80 mm Hg; at 2250 m (7500 feet), 70 mm Hg; and at 4500 m (15,000 feet), 50 mm Hg. Hypoxia ensues, which stimulates changes in the lungs, heart, brain, and kidneys.

The pulmonary effects of AMS include hyperventilation and increased tidal volume, which lead to a decrease in PCO_2 or a respiratory alkalosis. Pulmonary circulation constricts, resulting in an increased pressure that leads to pulmonary edema. Hypoxia stimulates the hypoxic ventilatory response (HVR) of the peripheral chemoreceptors in the carotid bodies. The inhibition of central chemoreceptors results in a decrease in minute ventilation. This interaction controls respiratory rate and heart rate and is indirectly responsible for the renal control of bicarbonate. In AMS, the hypobaric hypoxia is the underlying cause. Although the exact sequence of events is unclear, an increase in aldosterone and antidiuretic hormone (ADH) levels and renin-angiotensin secretion interaction results in fluid overload, which leads to cerebral and pulmonary edema.

In HAPE, pulmonary hypertension is present as a result of the hypoxia. Pulmonary wedge pressures and left ventricular function are not affected. Theories include overperfusion (fluid leakage into alveoli), pulmonary venous obstruction, and capillary permeability.[3] With HACE, there is alteration in the blood-brain barrier and increased cerebral blood flow, which leads to cerebral edema.

CLINICAL PRESENTATION

As stated previously, AMS, HAPE, and HACE are separate clinical syndromes that fall on a continuum of mild to increasingly severe symptoms (Table 27-1). AMS manifests within 6 hours of arrival or even after 1 day or longer and is similar to an alcoholic hangover. The headache is bifrontal and worsens when bending over or performing the Valsalva's maneuver. The gastrointestinal and constitutional symptoms are outlined in Table 27-2. There is irritability, a worsening headache, emesis, and dyspnea. In its most severe form, AMS can lead to HAPE, HACE, and coma within 12 hours.

As noted in Table 27-2, HAPE manifests between 6 hours and 4 days after arrival to altitude. Many of the symptoms appear nocturnally as a result of arterial desaturation during sleep. Symptoms can be mild (dyspnea on exertion, dry cough), moderate (weakness, fatigue with walking, raspy cough, headache), or severe (dyspnea at rest, productive cough, orthopnea, stupor, or coma). The progression of the cough from dry to wet and mental status changes indicate a worsening condition. Coma and death occur quickly if left untreated.

HACE, the advanced stage of AMS, is characterized by a worsening of the AMS symptoms listed in Table 27-2. Visual problems, papilledema, paralysis, and seizures characterize progressive neurologic involvement.[2]

PHYSICAL EXAMINATION

The physical findings for altitude illness vary and depend on the severity of the condition; see Table 27-2 for a comparison. With mild AMS, the findings are nonspecific. Fluid retention is the hallmark.

In HAPE, the physical findings vary with the severity of the illness. Hackett and Rabold[4] classify this severity as follows: mild HAPE reveals a normal heart rate, a normal respiratory rate, dusky nail beds and, possibly, pulmonary rales. Moderate HAPE reveals a normal heart rate, a respiratory rate of 16 to 30, cyanotic nail beds, rales, and ataxia. Severe HAPE includes tachycardia (>110 beats per minute), a respiratory rate of greater than 30, facial and nail bed cyanosis, and ataxia.

TABLE 27-1 Altitude-Related Findings

	High Altitude	Very High Altitude	Extreme Altitude
Elevation (in meters)	1500-3500	3500-5500	>5500
Elevation (in feet)	4900-11,500	11,500-18,000	>18,000
Pa_{O_2}	>90%	<90%	<70-90
Impairment of O_2 transport	None	Yes	Yes
Severity	Mild	Moderate to severe	Severe and life threatening
Findings	↓ Exercise performance ↑ Respiratory rate	Mild/moderate hypoxemia	Severe hypoxemia Death without O_2

TABLE 27-2 Altitude Illness

Onset	Symptoms	Physical Examination	Management	Prevention
ACUTE MOUNTAIN SICKNESS				
1-6 hours to several days Rapid	Headache Anorexia Cough Nausea Emesis Weakness Insomnia	Increased heart rate, decreased blood pressure	Descend ≥500 m, or stop, rest, acclimatize Acetazolamide 125 to 250 mg PO, emetics, and analgesics	Ascend slowly. Avoid strenuous exertion and rapid accent >2750 m. Consider acetazolamide 1 day before and 2 days after ascent to high altitude. Spend night at intermediate altitude.
Moderately severe AMS			O_2 1 to 2 L, dexamethasone 4 mg PO/IM q 6 hours until symptoms resolve	
HIGH-ALTITUDE PULMONARY EDEMA				
6 hours to 4 days	Fatigue Irritability Shortness of breath Cough Confusion Hemoptysis Nocturnal illness	Increased heart and respiratory rates Decreased blood pressure Cyanosis Frothy sputum Oliguria Mental status changes Rales Ataxia	Immediate descent Portable hyperbaric chamber or O_2 4 to 6 L, then 2 to 4 L Nifedipine 10 mg × 1, then 30 mg extended release q 12 hours initially, then 4 mg q 6 hours Dexamethasone if neurodeterioration	Ascend slowly. Avoid overexertion. Consider nifedipine 20 to 30 mg ER q 12 hours in persons with prior episode.
HIGH-ALTITUDE CEREBRAL EDEMA				
Hours to days	Nausea Emesis Irritability Severe headache Insomnia Ataxia Irrationality	Decreased loss of consciousness Cranial nerve palsies Seizures Coma Rales	O_2 2 to 4 L Descend as soon as possible Hyperbaric chamber Dexamethasone 8 mg PO/IM/IV initially, then 4 mg PO q 6 hours Acetazolamide if descent delayed	Ascend slowly at graded rate. Avoid overexertion. *Consider acetazolamide 125 to 250 mg 1 day before and 2 days after at high altitude.

Modified from Hackett PH, Roach RC: High altitude illness, *N Engl J Med* 345(2):107-113, 2001.
AMS, Acute mountain sickness; *HAPE,* high-altitude pulmonary edema; *HACE,* high-altitude cerebral edema.
*For persons with repeated episodes.

The progressive neurologic signs of HACE are listed in Table 27-2. Focal neurologic findings are a result of increased intracranial pressure and include the third and sixth cranial nerve palsies, papilledema, and pulmonary rales.

DIAGNOSTICS

The clinical presentation and physical findings indicate the diagnosis. Pulse oximetry, arterial blood gases (ABGs), and chest x-ray studies confirm the severity of the presentation of AMS. Pulse oximetry values vary depending on the severity of AMS. Normal values are greater than 90% in adults and greater than 94% in infants and children. The chest x-ray study will be normal in patients with AMS, but with HAPE/HACE there is a patchy bilateral interstitial edema.[5]

DIFFERENTIAL DIAGNOSIS

Unlike a viral illness, a patient with uncomplicated AMS does not present with fever or myalgia. Hangover, exhaustion, and dehydration may be difficult to differentiate. A history of alcohol intake, recent vigorous activity, and other reasons for lack of water intake may assist the practitioner. Hypothermia and the use of sedatives may slow the mental processes and cause ataxia.[1] With HAPE, patients with preexisting cardiac (ASCVD), hematologic (sickle cell anemia), and pulmonary (COPD) diseases need to be differentiated through the history, physical examination, chest x-ray study, and ECG. HACE may mimic transient ischemic attacks (TIAs) or cerebrovascular accidents (CVAs). Brain tumors present similarly.

INITIAL STABILIZATION AND MANAGEMENT

Preventive measures and early recognition by the patients and timely intervention by the practitioner result in timely and effective management (Box 27-1). In all cases, the ascent should be stopped and a descent should be initiated. General measures on presentation include a complete medical history, physical examination, and pulse oximetry.

AMS, the most common of the syndromes, rapidly improves over 24 to 48 hours when acclimatization occurs. Simple measures ameliorate the symptoms; a descent of 150 to 300 m (500 to 1000 feet) will help for sleep disturbances. More severe symptoms require acetazolamide 250 mg b.i.d. (5 mg/kg/day in divided doses), supplemental oxygen 1 to 2 L/min, prochlorperazine (Compazine) 5 to 10 mg IM t.i.d. p.r.n. for nausea, dexamethasone 4 mg every 6 hours, and/or diuretics (furosemide [Lasix] 20 to 40 mg every 12 hours). Hyperbaric bags reduce altitude sickness and diminish symptoms in 1 to 2 hours.[1,3,5,6]

HAPE usually resolves with an immediate descent of 300 m (1000 feet). Severe cases should initially be managed as AMS is managed, but management should also include urgent treatment with nifedipine 10 mg PO. Nifedipine ER 30 mg PO should be continued every 12 to 24 hours.[2,5,6] Oxygen 4 to 6 L/min is also indicated until improvement is noted; the flow rate can then be decreased to 2 to 4 L/min to conserve the supply. The use of diuretics has had mixed results and may in fact worsen symptoms.[2,3] Despite therapy, the overall mortality rate is 11% for those who descended and 44% for those who did not.[2]

Diagnostics

Altitude Illness

Initial
Pulse oximetry

Laboratory
ABGs

Imaging
Chest x-ray

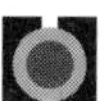

Differential Diagnosis

Altitude Illness

Acute Mountain Sickness (AMS)
Viral illness or bacterial infection
Hangover
Dehydration
Exhaustion
Hypoglycemia
Hyponatremia
Hypothermia
Sedatives, alcohol, or other medications
Transient ischemic attack or cerebrovascular accident
Psychosis
Brain tumor
Carbon monoxide poisoning
Seizure
Migraine

High-Altitude Pulmonary Edema (HAPE)
Transient ischemic attack or cerebrovascular accident
Brain tumor
Sickle cell anemia
Chronic obstructive pulmonary disease
Cardiac disease/congestive heart failure
Brain tumors
Asthma
Bronchitis
Pneumonia
Pulmonary edema
Pulmonary embolus

High-Altitude Cerebral Edema (HACE)
Transient ischemic attack or cerebrovascular accident
Brain tumor

BOX 27-1

TREATMENT OF ALTITUDE ILLNESS

ACUTE MOUNTAIN SICKNESS
Analgesics, descent, avoidance of alcohol, benzodiazepines
Use of acetazolamide, prochlorperazine (Compazine), oxygen, dexamethasone, hyperbaric bag, diuretics (if indicated)

HIGH-ALTITUDE PULMONARY EDEMA
Immediate descent, rest, evacuation (if not improved)
Nifedipine, oxygen, hyperbaric bag

HIGH-ALTITUDE CEREBRAL EDEMA
Immediate descent and evacuation
Dexamethasone, hyperbaric bag, BCLS, ACLS, seizure control (if indicated)

HACE requires emergent evacuation. Treatment may include oxygen 2 to 4 L/min and dexamethasone 8 mg PO, IM, or IV followed by 4 mg every 6 hours.[5] Acetazolamide can be administered if descent is delayed. Supportive measures may include basic life support (BLS), advanced cardiac life support (ACLS), and seizure control. Hyperventilation in patients who are intubated can decrease intracerebral pressure.

DISPOSITION AND REFERRAL

Patients with AMS that does not improve should be evacuated; hospital admission for more intensive treatment monitoring is essential. HAPE and HACE require immediate descent and urgent treatment.

PREVENTION AND PATIENT EDUCATION

AMS is best prevented with acclimatization and the avoidance of alcohol, strenuous activity, or abrupt ascents.[2,4-6] Acetazolamide 125 to 250 mg b.i.d. for 24 to 48 hours before ascent is helpful, especially for those with a history of AMS or abrupt ascent without acclimatization. This treatment is continued for 2 days and stopped unless symptoms recur.[4,5] Nifedipine 20 mg t.i.d. 24 hours before ascent may help prevent HAPE. Spending one night at 1500 to 2000 m (5000 to 6600 feet) before ascent and sleeping at altitudes below 2500 m (8200 feet) will be beneficial. Gradually ascending 300 m/day, avoiding abrupt ascents to more than 3000 m (10,000 feet), and allowing 2 nights for each 800- to 1000-m (2666- to 3333-ft) altitude gain may prevent AMS. For altitude climbing, Zafren and Honigman[1] recommend the maintenance rule, "climb high, sleep low." Patients who have experienced HAPE have a recurrence rate of 66%.[6]

REFERENCES

1. Zafren K, Honigman B: High-altitude medicine, *Emerg Med Clin North Am* 15(1):191-222, 1997.
2. Braun R, Krishel S: Environmental emergencies, *Emerg Med Clin North Am* 15(2):451-476, 1997.
3. Hultgren HN: High-altitude pulmonary edema: current concepts, *Annu Rev Med* 47:267-284, 1996.
4. Hackett PH, Rabold M: High altitude medical problems. In Tintinalli JE, Ruiz E, Krome RL, editors: *Emergency medicine: a comprehensive study guide*, New York, 1996, McGraw-Hill.
5. Hackett PH, Roach RC: High altitude illness, *N Engl J Med* 345(2): 107-113, 2001.
6. Harris MD and others: High-altitude medicine, *Am Fam Physician* 57(8):1907-1914, 1998.

CHAPTER 28

Anaphylaxis

Terry Mahan Buttaro

Immediate emergency department referral/physician consultation is indicated for patients with angioedema, respiratory distress, and vascular collapse.

DEFINITION/EPIDEMIOLOGY

Anaphylaxis is a systemic, life-threatening allergic reaction characterized by urticaria, pruritus, angioedema (Color Plate 8), gastrointestinal symptoms, respiratory distress, and cardiovascular collapse. Anaphylactic reactions are commonly underreported, and the exact number of individuals affected by this disorder is uncertain. However, it is estimated that more than 40 million people are at risk for anaphylaxis and that this disorder causes approximately 500 to 1000 deaths in the United States each year.[1] Although individuals may respond differently, anaphylactic reactions usually occur within seconds to minutes after sensitization to a specific antigen. The response is typically immediate, but reactions can occur several hours after the exposure. To prevent death, prompt recognition and treatment are essential. Antibiotics are commonly associated with anaphylaxis, but latex, other medications, foods, additives, hymenoptera stings, venoms, chemicals, exercise, and cold urticaria can also cause anaphylaxis (Box 28-1). Often the cause is idiopathic.

PATHOPHYSIOLOGY

An immunoglobulin E (IgE)-mediated response, anaphylaxis is a profound, immediate allergic reaction with life-threatening bronchospasm, hypoxemia, and hypotension. A similar presentation occurs in an anaphylactoid reaction, a non–antigen, non–antibody-mediated response.[2] Both reactions are caused by mediators from basophils and mast cells, which precipitate the release of histamines, causing increased capillary permeability, vasodilation, and bronchospasms. Urticaria and pruritus are a result of mild allergic reactions, whereas facial angioedema (well-defined subcutaneous edema), respiratory distress, and vascular collapse indicate a severe reaction.

CLINICAL PRESENTATION

Within seconds of exposure to the offending agent, the individual may experience a variety of symptoms, including weakness, pruritus, urticaria, nausea, vomiting, abdominal cramping, diarrhea, incontinence, throat tightness, stridor, a "lump" in the throat, hoarseness, wheezing, angioedema, and/or chest tightness. The reaction is fairly immediate and occurs within 1 to 45 minutes after exposure to the allergen. A careful history is important to elicit information about previous exposure to offending agents, onset of symptoms, other illnesses, medications, and allergies.

BOX 28-1

COMMON ALLERGENS ASSOCIATED WITH ANAPHYLAXIS

- Allergen extracts: pollen and nonpollen extracts
- Antiserums
- Blood products
- Dyes (fluorescein, radiographic contrast media)
- Environmental allergens (dust, mold, grasses, trees, animals)
- Enzymes
- Exercise
- Foods
    - Additives such as monosodium glutamate (MSG)
    - Beans (including soybeans)
    - Chocolate
    - Cottonseed oil
    - Eggs
    - Grains
    - Mango
    - Milk
    - Nuts (especially peanuts)
    - Seafood (particularly shellfish)
    - Sesame and sunflower seeds
    - Spices: mustard
    - Strawberries
    - Wheat, buckwheat
- Hormones (insulin, progesterone, vasopressin)
- Hymenoptera stings (bees, wasps, yellow jackets, hornets, imported fire ants)
- Idiopathic
- Intravenous colloids: dextran
- Medications
    - Anesthetics
    - Angiotensin-converting enzyme inhibitors
    - Antibiotics, particularly penicillins, cephalosporins
    - Antineoplastic compounds
    - Aspirin
    - Corticosteroids
    - Insulin
    - Lidocaine
    - Muscle relaxants
    - Nitrofurantoin
    - Nonsteroidal antiinflammatory drugs
    - Opiates
    - Procaine
    - Vaccines
    - Vitamins: thiamine, folic acid
- Mite-contaminated food ingestion
- Occupational chemicals and proteins
    - Ethylene oxide
    - Latex
    - Rubber products
- Venom

PHYSICAL EXAMINATION

Physical examination reveals characteristic pruritic, urticarial eruptions. Facial angioedema may be significant and associated with vocal changes, stridor, or wheezing, indicating the need for intubation and immediate transfer to the nearest emergency facility. Tearing, rhinorrhea, pallor, cyanosis, confusion, restlessness, anxiety, tachycardia, bronchospasm, arrhythmias, hypoxia, accessory muscle use, distant heart and lung sounds, and hypotension may also be present. Airway obstruction and cardiopulmonary arrest may occur within minutes to hours after allergen exposure.

DIAGNOSTICS

The ECG may reveal ST-segment elevation, hyperacute or inverted T waves, arrhythmias, or asystole. Arterial blood gas analysis, if available, is indicated. A chest x-ray examination also may be appropriate.

DIFFERENTIAL DIAGNOSIS

The presentation and history are usually sufficient to accurately diagnose an anaphylactic reaction, although acute bronchospasm, upper airway obstruction, and pulmonary edema should be considered in the differential diagnosis. However, these disorders do not cause urticaria or angioedema and are not usually associated with gastrointestinal symptoms. Identification of the offending antigen, if possible, will aid in the prevention of future reactions.

INITIAL STABILIZATION AND MANAGEMENT

Immediate subcutaneous epinephrine is widely accepted to stimulate vasoconstriction and bronchial smooth muscle relaxation as well as to reduce capillary permeability. Individuals with mild reactions, normal blood pressure, and adequate respiratory exchange may be managed with subcutaneous epinephrine 0.2 to 0.5 ml of a 1:1000 solution (children, 0.1 ml/kg up to 0.3 ml). More serious reactions may require repeat dosing at 20-minute intervals. Diphenhydramine 50 to 100 mg PO with mild symptoms or IM/IV with more severe symptoms will help alleviate urticaria and angioedema. Aminophylline 0.25 to 0.5 g IV may be indicated for bronchospasm. Although not effective immediately, the

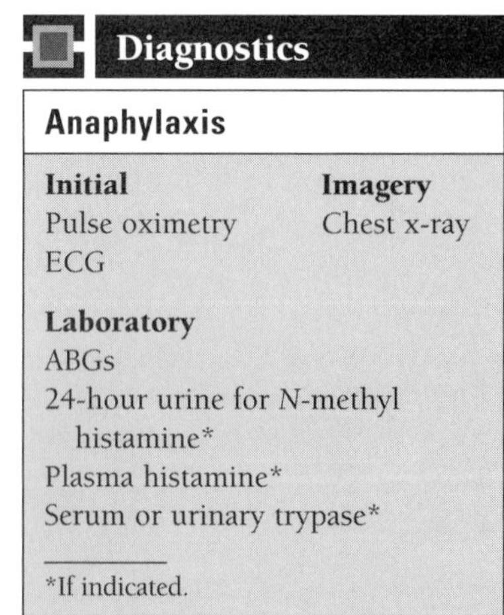

Diagnostics

Anaphylaxis

Initial
Pulse oximetry
ECG

Imagery
Chest x-ray

Laboratory
ABGs
24-hour urine for N-methyl histamine*
Plasma histamine*
Serum or urinary trypase*

*If indicated.

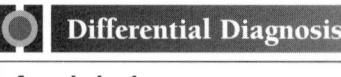

Differential Diagnosis

Anaphylaxis

Bronchospasm
Upper airway obstruction
Pulmonary edema

use of corticosteroids should be discussed with the physician to prevent recurrent anaphylaxis.

In critical anaphylaxis, subcutaneous epinephrine may not be effective. Epinephrine 0.5 to 1.0 ml of a 1:10,000 solution slow IV push at 5- to 10-minute intervals; isotonic fluid replacement (0.9% normal saline); high-flow oxygen; continuous monitoring of airway, breathing, and circulation (ABCs); and rapid transport to an emergency facility are immediately indicated. Physician consultation is essential because epinephrine can cause myocardial ischemia, arrhythmias, seizures, and severe systolic hypertension.

Sublingual or endotracheal epinephrine can be given in life-threatening situations if IV access is unobtainable. IV aminophylline, diphenhydramine, H_2-blockers, vasopressors, and steroids may also be considered in consultation with the physician. Physician consultation is also indicated for patients undergoing beta blocker therapy who may be resistant to epinephrine and require glucagon 1 mg IV.[2]

If the reaction has occurred in response to an insect bite, the area should be carefully examined and the stinger, if present, should be removed (see Chapter 29). The area should be carefully cleaned and cool packs should be applied to the area.

DISPOSITION AND REFERRAL

The patient should be immediately transferred to an emergency facility if initial stabilization and treatment are not effective. All patients require continued observation in the emergency department or hospital for several hours or overnight because anaphylaxis may recur after initial stabilization.

PREVENTION

The prevention of future anaphylactic reactions is the primary goal. Patients identified as being allergic to aspirin should understand the importance of avoiding all aspirin and nonsteroidal antiinflammatory drug–containing products. Any allergens must be forever avoided, and consultation with an allergist is recommended. Radioallergosorbent (RAST) and skin testing may be recommended to determine the cause of the reaction, although skin testing should not be conducted within 6 weeks of any anaphylactic event. With all allergy testing, there is the potential risk of precipitating a fatal anaphylactic reaction.

For reactions associated with venom stings, a referral for desensitization is strongly recommended. The importance of wearing shoes outdoors and avoiding perfumes and bright clothing should be stressed. Beta blocker therapy may be contraindicated for patients with a history of hymenoptera stings.

Patients with a food allergy must be particularly attentive, because fatal reactions in this population are not uncommon.[3] The importance of reading labels carefully and always carrying an epinephrine pen should be frequently reiterated and emphasized.

PATIENT AND FAMILY EDUCATION

Individuals who have experienced an anaphylactic reaction should wear a medical alert bracelet. Patients, families, and coworkers should be instructed in the use of a home epinephrine kit, which should contain a premeasured, disposable syringe of 1:1000 epinephrine and an antihistamine tablet. The importance of having immediate access to the kit at all times, of urgently administering epinephrine and antihistamine, and of calling 911 immediately if wheezing, breathing difficulties, or facial, lip, or tongue swelling occurs should be emphasized and understood by the individual and family members. Patients should be reminded to replace the medication in the home epinephrine kit yearly.

In addition, a trained health care provider should teach patients, teachers, and caregivers how to use the epinephrine autoinjector pen.[4]

REFERENCES

1. Neugut AI, Ghotek AT, Miller RL: Anaphylaxis in the United States: an investigation into its epidemiology, *Arch Intern Med* 161(1):15-21, 2001.
2. O'Dowd L, Zweiman B: Anaphylaxis. Retrieved from the World Wide Web May 23, 2002: http://www.uptodate.
3. Bock SA, Munoz-Furlong A, Sampson HA: Fatalities due to anaphylactic reactions to foods, *J Allergy Clin Immunol* 107(1):191-193, 2001.
4. Grouhi M and others: Anaphylaxis and epinephrine auto-injector training: who will teach the teachers? *J Allergy Clin Immunol* 104(1): 190-193, 1999.

CHAPTER 29

Bites and Stings

Jackie S. Fantes

Insect Bites and Stings

DEFINITION/EPIDEMIOLOGY

There are more species of insects in existence than any other form of multicellular life. Insects that bite and infest include mosquitoes, flies, bedbugs, kissing bugs, fleas, lice, blister beetles, centipedes, millipedes, scabies, chiggers, and ticks. Stinging insects include vespids, bees, and ants. The medical importance of insects is that they bite, sting, and envenomate; are vectors for infectious pathogens; and cause hypersensitivity reactions. Insect bites and stings can cause toxic reactions that range from local and mild to life threatening.[1]

Immediate emergency department referral/physician consultation is indicated for anaphylaxis and suspected black widow or brown recluse spider bites.

PATHOPHYSIOLOGY AND CLINICAL PRESENTATION

Although many insect bites and stings are simply a nuisance, some patients can have severe skin or systemic reactions. Vespids (yellow jackets, hornets, and wasps), bees (honeybees and bumblebees), and ants inject venom with a stinger. The sting results in immunoglobulin E (IgE)-mediated systemic reactions that cause the release of mediators (histamines, the slow-reacting substance of anaphylaxis [SRS-A], and eosinophil chemotactic factors of anaphylaxis [ECF-A])[2] from mast cells and culminating in local inflammation involving many cell types and numerous mechanisms.[3]

These stings induce local, toxic, systemic, and delayed reactions. A local reaction consists of erythema, edema, and pruritus at the sting site. A toxic reaction presents as gastrointestinal distress, light-headedness, syncope, headache, fever, drowsiness, muscle spasms, edema, and, occasionally, seizures. A systemic reaction is anaphylaxis, which initially presents as itchy eyes, facial flushing, generalized urticaria, and dry cough. Anaphylaxis can quickly intensify to respiratory distress, and it may deteriorate to respiratory or cardiovascular failure. A delayed reaction can occur 10 to 14 days after the sting and cause fever, malaise, headache, urticaria, lymphadenopathy, and polyarthritis.[2] Table 29-1 describes the pathophysiology and clinical presentation of other insect bites and stings.[1]

PHYSICAL EXAMINATION

The initial assessment of bites and stings should determine any compromise in airway, breathing, and circulation (i.e., evidence of anaphylaxis). A thorough examination of the bite or sting and surrounding area should be made to determine the extent of envenomation and any associated infection.

DIAGNOSTICS

Adults with systemic allergic reactions should be considered for venom immunotherapy, which is successful in virtually all patients. The diagnosis of insect sting allergy can be made on the basis of a history of anaphylaxis with a sting, positive skin tests, or radioallergosorbent tests (RASTs).[3] Otherwise, no specific laboratory evaluation is required unless indicated by the clinical course.

DIFFERENTIAL DIAGNOSIS

The diagnosis of all insect bites and stings is made by obtaining a careful history. It is helpful if the patient brings in the insect. Insect bites are commonly confused with contact dermatitis and viral exanthemas. Flea bites may resemble varicella. Bullous impetigo and burns may resemble reactions to blister beetles. Because of such similarities, a history of exposure may be the only diagnostic clue.[4]

INITIAL STABILIZATION AND MANAGEMENT

The management of all insect bites and stings begins with local wound care to include removal of the stinger and the use of ice packs, antihistamines (H_1- and H_2-blockers) for itching, topical steroids for inflammation, topical or systemic antibiotics for secondary infection, and nonsteroidal antiinflammatory drugs to relieve discomfort.[4] Any evidence of a systemic reaction must be treated as anaphylaxis.

Management also includes eradication of the insect. For flea infestation it is necessary to vacuum thoroughly; wash the rugs, pets, and beds; and use an insecticide. Lice and scabies are eradicated by applying 1% lindane lotion or shampoo (Kwell, Scabene) on two consecutive nights. Permethrin (NIX, Elimite) is another effective scabies treatment. Ticks are removed either with forceps—grasping the tick close to the mouth, flipping the tick so the backside is closest to skin, and pulling—or by suffocating the tick with mineral oil, nail polish, petrolatum, or chloroform. After removing the tick, the bite area must be explored for retained mouth parts.[4]

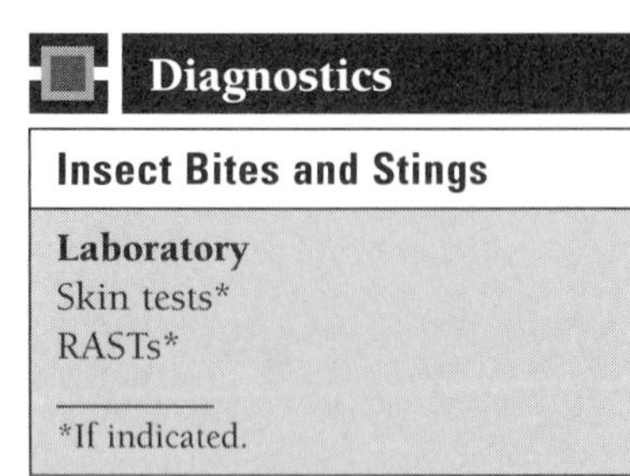

Diagnostics

Insect Bites and Stings

Laboratory
Skin tests*
RASTs*

*If indicated.

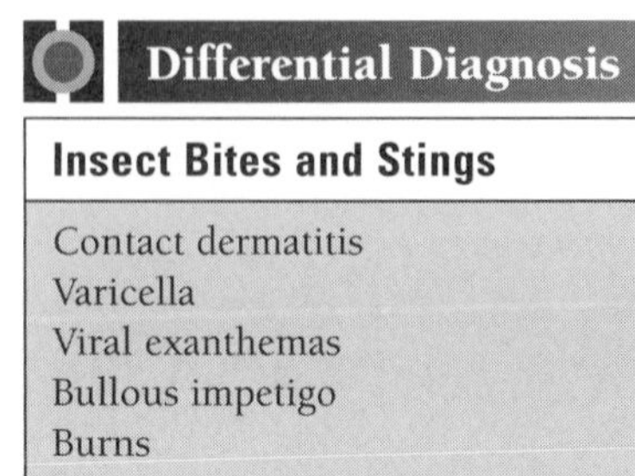

Differential Diagnosis

Insect Bites and Stings

Contact dermatitis
Varicella
Viral exanthemas
Bullous impetigo
Burns

DISPOSITION AND REFERRAL

Systemic reactions to bites and stings may be life threatening. Thus any systemic or anaphylactic reaction requires a referral to the emergency department for definitive management and possible hospitalization.

PREVENTION AND PATIENT EDUCATION

Preventive management against bites and stings includes avoidance and protective clothing. Repellents can be used and include diethyltoluamide

TABLE 29-1 Summary of Insect Bites and Stings

Insect	Clinical Presentation	Pathophysiology
Wasps, bees, ants, hornets, yellow jackets	Local reaction Toxic reaction Systemic reaction Delayed reaction	Inject venom with stinger
Fire ants	Papule progressing to sterile pustule in 6-24 hours	Inject venom with stinger
Mosquitoes, flies	Pruritic, painful papule Secondary infection common	Inject salivary material
Bed bugs, kissing bugs	Clustered, erythematous, pruritic nodules	Painlessly suck blood
Fleas	Pruritic grouped welts, papules, vesicles Secondary infection common	Deposit saliva in bite
Lice	Pruritus Nits in scalp, body, or pubic hair	Deposit saliva in bite
Blister beetles	Large blisters	Release hemolymph
Centipedes	Pain and itching with local necrosis	Inject venom with fangs
Millipedes	Brown-stained area with blistering	Excrete toxic chemicals
Scabies	Burrow lesion with pruritus Secondary infection common	Burrow in epidermis
Chiggers	Pruritic papules or vesicles Secondary infection common	Release digestive substances in bite
Ticks	Pruritic papule with tick present Secondary infection common	Attach to victim with painless bite

(DEET), dimethyl phthalate, dimethyl carbate, ethyl hexanediol, butopyronoxyl (Indalone), benzyl benzoate, and Skin-So-Soft bath oil (Avon).[5] Any person with a history of anaphylaxis from wasp or bee stings should be given medical warning tags and epinephrine injector kits.[2]

Spider Bites

DEFINITION/EPIDEMIOLOGY

There are more than 30,000 species of spiders worldwide, of which 50 are medically important to humans.[2] In the United States, the bites of only two spiders cause problems: brown recluse spiders and black widow spiders.[6] The brown recluse spider is a six-eyed nocturnal spider that avoids people. It is yellow, brown, or black with thin legs that are five times the body length; the entire spider is approximately the size of a quarter. It has a violin-shaped marking on its back. The brown recluse spider is found in warm, dry areas such as abandoned buildings, woodpiles, and cellars.[2]

The female black widow spider is the most venomous of all spiders and has a body size of approximately 1.5 cm and a leg span of 4 to 5 cm.[2] Despite the name "black" widow, these spiders may be black, brown, tan, or variegated.[6] The classic orange-red, hourglass-shaped marking is actually found on only one species *(Latrodectus mactans)* and may be merely an indistinct yellow or orange spot. The male spider is only one third the size of the female; his bite cannot penetrate human skin. Black widow spiders are aggressive and tend to live in basements, woodpiles, and garages.[2]

PATHOPHYSIOLOGY AND CLINICAL PRESENTATION

The venom of the brown recluse spider is chemotactic, which results in endothelial injury and subsequent thrombosis.[6] It is a neurotoxin that causes the release of acetylcholine and norepinephrine at the neurosynaptic junction.[2] The bite of the brown recluse spider is almost painless and most commonly presents as a mild, erythematous lesion that may become firm and then heal over several days to weeks. The bite can also be more severe, causing erythema, blistering, and a bluish discoloration within 24 hours and possibly becoming necrotic within 3 to 4 days. The lesions can vary in size from 1 to 30 cm and take 6 weeks to 4 months to heal. The victim may have a systemic response and experience fevers, chills, nausea, vomiting, myalgias, arthralgias, petechiae, hemolysis, or seizures within 24 to 48 hours of the bite. Severe systemic manifestations can lead to hemoglobinuria, renal failure, disseminated intravascular coagulation, and death.[2]

The bite of the black widow spider is mildly to moderately painful, with erythema, swelling, and muscle cramps beginning at the site within 30 minutes to 12 hours. The muscle cramping progresses to large muscle groups and the abdomen and can mimic peritonitis. The muscle pain can subside over a few hours but can flare over 2 to 3 days, with muscle weakness and intermittent spasms persisting for weeks to months. Hypertension can be a serious complication. Anxiety or confusion can also occur. Severe envenomation may lead to shock, coma, or respiratory failure secondary to muscle paralysis.[6]

PHYSICAL EXAMINATION

The physical examination of the patient should be complete. The primary survey should determine any compromise of the airway, breathing, or circulation (i.e., evidence of anaphylaxis). A thorough examination of the bite and surrounding area is then necessary to determine the extent of envenomation and any associated infection.

DIAGNOSTICS

If a brown recluse spider bite is suspected, CBC, BUN, electrolytes, blood sugar, creatinine, coagulation profile, and urinalysis (for hemoglobinuria) tests should be ordered. There are no specific laboratory tests indicated for a suspected black widow spider bite.[2] However, CBC, urinalysis, BUN, creatinine, glucose, electrolytes, and an acute abdominal series may be indicated because the presentation may mimic an acute abdomen.

DIFFERENTIAL DIAGNOSIS

Brown recluse and black widow spider bites should be included in the differential diagnosis of any spider bite. However, the diagnosis of either of these spider bites can be difficult, especially in the absence of the actual spider. The unusual presentation of acute abdominal pain requires that all causes of acute abdomen be considered in the differential diagnosis.

INITIAL STABILIZATION AND MANAGEMENT

The bite of the brown recluse spider requires no medications, and currently no antivenom is available. Tetanus prophylaxis and supportive measures should be provided. Antibiotics are indicated only if infection is suspected. Pain relief may be required in some cases. Daily wound care is important for those with necrotic lesions, and surgery may be required for necrotic lesions larger than 2 cm.[2]

The initial therapy for black widow spider bites is basic supportive care—airway, breathing, and circulation. Local wound care and tetanus prophylaxis should always be provided. Narcotic analgesics, benzodiazepines, and calcium gluconate are all effective means of pain relief and muscle relaxation. Antivenom is indicated only for a severe bite because of the risk of anaphylaxis and serum sickness.[6]

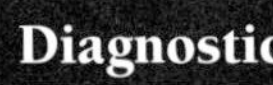

Diagnostics

Spider Bites

Laboratory (Brown Recluse)
CBC and differential
Serum electrolytes
BUN
Serum glucose
Creatinine
Coagulation profile
Urinalysis

Laboratory (Black Widow—to distinguish bite from acute abdomen)
CBC and differential
Serum electrolytes
BUN
Creatinine
Serum glucose
Urinalysis

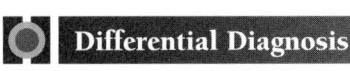

Differential Diagnosis

Spider Bites

All spider bites
All causes of acute abdominal pain

The wolf spiders, of which the tarantula is the most common, cause bites the equivalent of a wasp sting without necrosis. These bites usually require only supportive care.[4]

DISPOSITION AND REFERRAL

Adults and children with evidence of significant systemic reactions should be referred for hospitalization and close observation. Patients with black widow spider bites that require antivenom should always be referred to the emergency department and/or for hospital admission.

PREVENTION AND PATIENT EDUCATION

Everyone in endemic areas should be taught to recognize the brown recluse spider and avoid its habitats. Clothing, bed linens, attics, closets, and woodpiles should be examined closely in endemic areas because the spider is aggressive only if forced into contact with the substrate.[7]

Black widow spiders are more commonly found in their webs at night. Therefore the webs should be cleaned cautiously at night and the spider mechanically destroyed. Professional exterminators are indicated for heavy infestations. Everyone in endemic areas should be taught to recognize the black widow spider. Protective sleeves and gloves are recommended in handling wood and brush in infested areas.[7]

Reptile Bites and Scorpion Stings

In the United States, the venomous snakes include the pit vipers and coral snakes. Pit vipers include rattlesnakes, copperheads, cottonmouths (water moccasins), and bushmasters. Each year approximately 5000 snakebites are reported to poison control centers in the United States, but only one third to one half of these are caused by venomous snakes. The most severe envenomations tend to occur with rattlesnakes. Of the venomous snake bites, 20% result in no envenomation and 40% result in only mild envenomation.[8]

Other reptiles to consider are Gila monsters, which are slow-moving lizards in the deserts of the southwestern United States. Medically significant scorpion stings also occur in the southwestern United States from the bark scorpion[6] (so named because it often lives under the bark of trees).[9]

PATHOPHYSIOLOGY

The venom of the pit viper is a complex mixture of cytotoxic, hemotoxic, and neurotoxic enzymes that cause local tissue injury, systemic vascular damage, hemolysis, fibrinolysis, and neuromuscular dysfunction.[2] Coral snake venom is neurotoxic.[2] Gila monster venom is as toxic as rattlesnake venom, but Gila monsters lack the apparatus to effectively inject it; they have short, grooved teeth and therefore require a prolonged bite for envenomation.[2] Scorpion venom is primarily neurotoxic and is composed of proteins and polypeptides that activate sodium channels to produce a hyperadrenergic state.[9]

CLINICAL PRESENTATION

For the bites in which there is no envenomation, the only clinical finding is the puncture wound. The clinical picture of patients who are envenomated depends on several factors: amount of venom introduced, anatomic location of the bite, size and age of the patient, and patient's overall state of health. The bites are classified by the degree of envenomation: none, minimal, moderate, or severe. The presentation of no envenomation is minimal pain and no significant swelling. Minimal envenomation presents as local swelling of less than 15 cm from the bite wound and no systemic manifestations. Moderate envenomation has local swelling of 15 to 30 cm with systemic signs and symptoms. Severe envenomation has local swelling of more than 30 cm with severe systemic signs and symptoms, including coagulation abnormalities.[8]

Coral snake bites resemble scratch marks and are somewhat painful. Patients present with neurologic symptoms such as tremors, salivation, dysarthria, diplopia, dysphagia, dyspnea, and seizures. These symptoms, which are usually delayed up to 1 to 6 hours, may progress to respiratory muscle paralysis and death.[8] In most cases the bite of the Gila monster causes only local pain and swelling that worsens over several hours and subsides over the next several hours. Only occasionally will a systemic reaction occur, with weakness, light-headedness, paresthesias, diaphoresis, or hypertension.[2] Scorpion stings may present as mild symptoms with only local pain and/or paresthesias, or they may progress to somatic or cranial nerve dysfunction. Motor nerve effects include roving eye movements, fasciculations, and dysphagia, as well as the autonomic effects of tachycardia and excessive secretions.[9]

PHYSICAL EXAMINATION

The physical examination of the patient should be complete. First, any compromise of the airway, breathing, or circulation (i.e., anaphylaxis) should be determined. This is followed by a thorough examination of the bite and surrounding area to determine the extent of envenomation.

DIAGNOSTICS

Several corroborating laboratory studies are needed, including CBC, coagulation studies, fibrinogen, electrolytes, BUN, creatinine, and urinalysis. A type and crossmatch for blood, an arterial blood gas (ABG) analysis, and an ECG are needed if the envenomation is severe.[8]

Diagnostics

Reptile Bites and Scorpion Stings

Laboratory	
CBC and differential	BUN
Coagulation studies	Creatinine
Fibrinogen	Urinalysis
Serum electrolytes	

DIFFERENTIAL DIAGNOSIS

The diagnosis is made on the basis of a history of a snakebite or scorpion bite, with a clinical presentation consistent with envenomation. It is helpful if the victim can identify the snake or scorpion with use of a picture.

INITIAL STABILIZATION AND MANAGEMENT

First aid measures must be instituted first, but all patients bitten by venomous snakes or scorpions must be taken to a health care facility. First aid measures include retreating beyond striking range, remaining calm, immobilizing the extremity involved, keeping physical activity minimal, wiping the bite site, identifying the snake if it can be done safely, and closely observing the patient's respiratory status. Incision of the wound, suction of the wound, and tourniquets are not recommended. In the prehospital or office setting, management includes providing advanced cardiac life support as appropriate, immobilizing the limb, establishing IV access, and administering oxygen. The wound should be cleaned and tetanus prophylaxis administered.[9]

The major determinant of the required therapy is the degree of envenomation, with the mainstay of therapy for moderate to severe venomous snakebites being antivenom.[8] For Gila monsters, local wound care is probably sufficient and must include the removal of any teeth in the wound; no antivenom is available.[2] For scorpion bites, management is supportive with analgesics and wound care; there is antivenom for severe bites, but it is available only in Arizona and is rarely used.[9]

DISPOSITION AND REFERRAL

Because the clinical symptoms can be delayed, all bites by venomous snakes and scorpions need to be observed for a minimum of 8 hours. The patient must be in an emergency department or hospital setting in which antivenom is available. For snakebites, consultation with a physician or poison control center familiar with envenomation is always recommended.[8]

PREVENTION AND PATIENT EDUCATION

Knowledge of reptile habits and habitats can help prevent envenomation. Anyone who may come in contact with these reptiles should be educated on their habits.

REFERENCES

1. Schlossberg D: Arthropods and leeches. In Cecil RL, Goldman L, Bennett JC, editors: *Cecil textbook of medicine*, Philadelphia, 2000, WB Saunders.
2. Salluzzo RI: Insect and spider bites. In Tintinalli JE, editor: *Emergency medicine: a comprehensive study guide*, New York, 1996, McGraw-Hill.
3. Lichtenstein L: Insect sting allergy. In Cecil RL, Goldman L, Bennett JC, editors: *Cecil textbook of medicine*, Philadelphia, 2000, WB Saunders.
4. Nichols CG: Insect bites and infestations. In Harwood-Nuss AL, editor: *The clinical practice of emergency medicine*, Philadelphia, 1996, Lippincott-Raven.
5. Elston DM: Bugs and bites, *Dela Med J* 68(9):445-450, 1996.
6. Gateley A, McKinney P: Arthropod envenomation. In Noble J, editor: *Textbook of primary care medicine*, ed 3, St Louis, 2001, Mosby.
7. Allen C: Arachnid envenomations, *Emerg Med Clin North Am* 10(2):269-298, 1992.
8. Adam R, Sullivan J: Venomous snake bites. In Cecil RL, Goldman L, Bennett JC, editors: *Cecil textbook of medicine*, Philadelphia, 2000, WB Saunders.
9. Walter F, Bilden E, Gibly R: Environmental emergencies, *Crit Care Clin* 15(2):353-386, 1999.

CHAPTER 30

Bradycardia

Terry Mahan Buttaro

DEFINITION/EPIDEMIOLOGY

Absolute bradycardia is defined as a heart rate of less than 60 beats per minute. Athletes, older adults, and other individuals may have normally slow heart rates, and bradycardia may not be pathologic during sleep or after the Valsalva maneuver or other vagal stimulation. Relative bradycardia occurs when the heart is unable to respond as expected to traumatic or hypovolemic hypotension.[1] Although the heart rate in relative bradycardia can be greater than 60 beats per minute, medications or sinoatrial (SA) node dysfunction can repress the heart rate.

Medications, cardiac disease, hypothyroidism, hypothermia, hypoxemia, acidemia, and other disease states can also produce bradycardia. Asymptomatic bradycardia does not require urgent intervention. However, careful monitoring and therapy are indicated if the bradycardia causes symptoms or is related to type II second-degree (Mobitz II) or third-degree atrioventricular (AV) block.[2]

Immediate emergency department referral/physician consultation is indicated for patients with symptomatic bradycardia, Mobitz II, or third-degree heart block.

PATHOPHYSIOLOGY

Bradycardia may result from sinus node dysfunction or AV block. Sinus node dysfunction can be a result of increased vagal tone, as seen in athletes or conditioned young people or in older adults as the result of underlying disease processes, medications, or toxicity. AV block is also associated with various disease processes, including myocardial infarction, coronary artery spasm, digitalis toxicity, cardiac mesotheliomas, and infectious processes. Medications, particularly beta blockers and calcium channel blockers, may induce either sinus node or AV dysfunction.

CLINICAL PRESENTATION

Some symptoms may be nonspecific, but dizziness, fatigue, and syncope are complaints commonly identified with bradycardia. Nausea, vomiting, and confusion have also been correlated with bradycardia. Any bradyarrhythmia associated with chest pain, shortness of breath, exercise intolerance, decreased level of consciousness, hypotension, congestive heart failure, or myocardial infarction is considered a prearrest condition.

PHYSICAL EXAMINATION

Although associated symptoms will often guide the physical examination, a focused history and physical examination are necessary. The patient's level of responsiveness and vital signs (including temperature, blood pressure, pulse, respiratory rate, and oxygen saturation) are significant and should be continually reassessed. Hypotension, ventricular arrhythmias, and pulmonary congestion are serious signs indicating the need to identify the cardiac rhythm and institute rapid appropriate treatment.

DIAGNOSTICS

An ECG is necessary for rhythm analysis and appropriate management. Further diagnostics are guided by the history and physical examination but can include drug levels, electrolytes, glucose, BUN, creatinine, CBC, creatine kinase (CK)-MB, troponin T or I, thyroid studies, and chest x-ray studies.

DIFFERENTIAL DIAGNOSIS

Determination of the bradyarrhythmia and associated pathology is essential for treatment (see Chapter 127). Common causes include medications, infections, vasovagal syncope, myocardial infarction, digitalis toxicity, sick sinus syndrome, bradycardia-tachycardia syndrome, hypothyroidism, and other disease states.

INITIAL STABILIZATION AND MANAGEMENT

Current American Heart Association guidelines are based on evidence that has been categorized into five recommendation classes.[3] Advanced cardiac life support (ACLS) guidelines advise differentiating the symptoms caused by the bradycardia from those not related to the slow rate. No intervention is necessary if the patient is stable and asymptomatic. However, continuous patient observation and continuous monitoring of oxygen saturation, vital signs, oxygen administration, IV access, and 12-lead ECG are vital. Identification of cardiac rhythm is essential. Patients with suspected myocardial infarction should be treated according to the acute coronary syndrome algorithm with oxygen, aspirin (if not aspirin allergic—162 to 325 mg chewed), nitroglycerin, and morphine (Figure 30-1).

Symptomatic patients with worsening clinical symptoms or prearrest conditions related to the bradycardia may require urgent intervention before a definitive underlying condition is identified. Atropine 0.5 to 1 mg IV push every 3 to 5 minutes (total dose

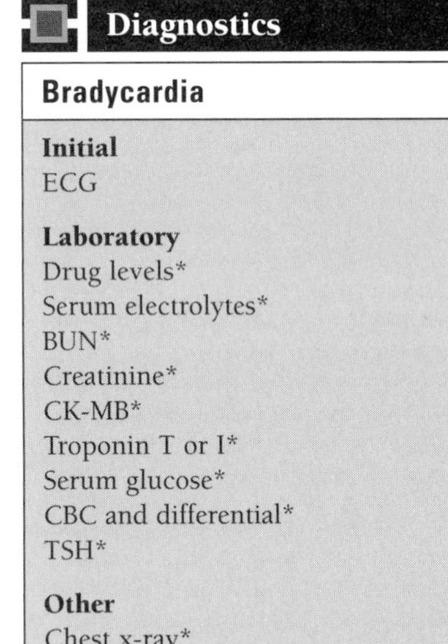

Diagnostics

Bradycardia

Initial
ECG

Laboratory
Drug levels*
Serum electrolytes*
BUN*
Creatinine*
CK-MB*
Troponin T or I*
Serum glucose*
CBC and differential*
TSH*

Other
Chest x-ray*

*If indicated.

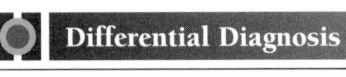

Bradycardia

Medication induced
Infection
Vasovagal syncope
Myocardial infarction
Digitalis toxicity
Sick sinus syndrome
Hypothyroidism
Bradycardia/tachycardia syndrome

PREHOSPITAL	EMERGENCY DEPARTMENT
Initial Assessment (Goal: Targeted Clinical Exam and 12-Lead ECG Within 10 Minutes)	
• Obtain a brief, targeted history/physical exam (determine age, gender; signs/symptoms, pain presentation, including location of pain, duration, quality, relation to effort, time of symptom onset, Hx CAD, CAD risk factors present?) Hx of Viagra use? • Assess vital signs, determine oxygen saturation If previous consistent with possible or definite ACS: • Use checklist (yes-no), focus on eligibility for reperfusion therapy, evaluate contraindications to aspirin and heparin • Establish IV access, ECG monitoring • Administer aspirin 162 to 325 mg (chewed) if no reason for exclusion • Obtain 12-lead ECG (machine interpretation or transmission of ECG to physician) • Draw blood for initial serum cardiac marker levels (to lab on arrival in Emergency Department) Consider triage to facility capable of angiography and revascularization if any of the following are present: • Signs of shock • Pulmonary edema (rales > halfway up) • Heart rate ≥100 beats/min and SBP ≤100 mm Hg	RN triage for rapid care • Targeted history: determine age, gender, signs/symptoms, pain presentation, including location of pain, duration, quality, relation to effort, time of symptom onset; Hx CAD, CAD risk factors present? Hx of Viagra use? • Assess vital signs, determine oxygen saturation • Establish IV access, ECG monitoring • Obtain 12-lead ECG (present to physician for review) Physician evaluation If previous consistent with possible or definite ACS: • Obtain brief, targeted history/physical exam • Evaluate eligibility for reperfusion therapy + contraindications to aspirin and heparin • Administer aspirin 162 to 325 mg (chewed) if no reason for exclusion • Administer nitroglycerin as indicated • Evaluate 12-lead ECG: Categorize patient into one of three groups: ST-elevation or new or presumably new LBBB, ST-depression/ transient ST-segment/T wave changes, normal or nondiagnostic ECG • Obtain serial ECGs in patients with Hx suggesting MI and nondiagnostic ECG • Obtain baseline serum cardiac marker levels (CK-MB, Troponin T or I, myoglobin) • Obtain lab specimens (CBC, lipid profile, electrolytes, coagulation studies) • Obtain portable chest x-ray film • Evaluate results

Routine Measures

- Oxygen 4 L/min by nasal cannula for first 2 to 3 hours (Class IIa)
- Oxygen 4 L/min by cannula, titrate if pulmonary congestion, SaO_2 <90% (Class I)
- Aspirin 162 to 325 mg chewed (if hypersensitivity exists, ticlopidine); may administer via rectal suppository (325 mg) if nausea, vomiting, upper GI disorder present
- Nitroglycerin SL or spray (ensure IV access, SBP >90 mm Hg, HR >50 beats/min, no RV infarction)
- Morphine 2 to 4 mg IV if pain not relieved with nitroglycerin; may repeat every 5 minutes (ensure SBP >90 mm Hg)

Routine Measures: Oxygen, Aspirin, Nitroglycerin, Morphine (MONA)

Studies suggest that oxygen administration may limit ischemic myocardial injury and reduce ST-segment elevation in patients with MI.

1. Oxygen
   a. Give at 4 L/min
   b. Overt pulmonary congestion, arterial oxygen desaturation (SaO_2 <90%) (Class I)
   c. Routine administration to all patients with uncomplicated MI during the first 2 to 3 hours (Class IIa)

FIGURE 30-1

Initial assessment and general treatment of the patient with an acute coronary syndrome. (From Aehlert B: *ACLS quick review study guide*, ed 2, St Louis, 2000, Mosby.)

continued

2. Aspirin
   a. Administer 162 to 325 mg (chewed); may be administered via rectal suppository (325 mg) if nausea, vomiting, upper GI disorder present
   b. Other antiplatelet agents such as dipyridamole, ticlopidine, or clopidogrel may be substituted if true aspirin allergy is present or if patient is unresponsive to aspirin
3. Nitroglycerin
   a. Pain relief is a priority
      (1) Benefits: Decreases anxiety and pain, may decrease BP and heart rate, decreases myocardial oxygen demand, decreases risk of arrhythmias
      (2) Possible complications: hypotension
   b. Therapy
      (1) Nitroglycerin SL or spray
         (a) Ensure IV access, systolic BP >90 mm Hg
         (b) Avoid nitroglycerin administration in the presence of marked bradycardia (<50 beats/min) and in patients with suspected right ventricular infarction. "Patients with right ventricular infarction are especially dependent on adequate right ventricular preload to maintain cardiac output and can experience profound hypotension during administration of nitrates."
         (c) Avoid nitroglycerin administration if patient has used Viagra within past 24 hours
         (d) Avoid long-acting oral nitrate preparations in the early management of acute MI
      (2) Morphine 2 to 4 mg IV (if discomfort is not relieved with nitroglycerin)—may repeat every 5 minutes (ensure SBP >90 mm Hg) titrated to pain relief
         (a) Respiratory depression secondary to morphine administration is unusual with acute MI; however, if it occurs it can be treated with IV naloxone

MONA

MONA is an acronym that may be used to recall medications used in the management of acute coronary syndromes (although not in the order they are administered).

M = morphine
O = oxygen
N = nitroglycerin
A = aspirin

FIGURE 30-1, cont'd

For legend, see previous page.

0.03 mg/kg), may be given in emergent clinical situations[4] (Figure 30-2). However, atropine can induce cardiac ischemia, precipitate ventricular tachycardia or fibrillation, and be deleterious in the presence of Mobitz type II second-degree heart block or third-degree heart block associated with wide-complex ventricular escape beats.[1]

Transcutaneous pacing (TCP) is an appropriate intervention for symptomatic bradycardia and is considered to be a Class I intervention (definitely recommended) by the American Heart Association[3] (see Figure 30-2). Although often not available, these pacers are currently obtainable with some defibrillator/monitors. However, this treatment may be uncomfortable and is not always successful.

If available, IV dopamine or epinephrine can be used to treat critical bradycardia. A dopamine infusion of 5 to 10 μg/kg/min can improve cardiac output and increase blood pressure, although an epinephrine infusion of 1 to 2 μg/min may be indicated in extremely urgent situations.[3] IV isoproterenol infusion (Isuprel) 2 to 10 μg/min, now infrequently used to treat bradycardia, can be helpful in low doses (Class IIb) but is considered harmful in higher doses and should be used with caution (Class III).[2]

DISPOSITION AND REFERRAL

Patients experiencing signs and symptoms related to bradyarrhythmias require constant reassessment and definitive management in an emergency department. Immediate transfer to an emergency center is required.

PREVENTION

Prevention, when possible, may avert complications or serious injury. Patients who complain of syncope, fatigue, or other symptoms that may be related to bradycardia require diagnostic correlation. A permanent pacemaker may be indicated for bradycardia associated with sinus node dysfunction.

PATIENT AND FAMILY EDUCATION

Patients should understand the importance of calling their health care provider if they experience syncope, light-headedness, or a slow heart rate that hinders activities. In addition,

Basic Life Support

Perform Primary ABCD Survey
(Correct critical problems IMMEDIATELY as they are identified)
Assess responsiveness, **A**irway, **B**reathing, **C**irculation,
ensure availability of monitor/**D**efibrillator

↓

Advanced Life Support

Perform Secondary ABCD Survey
Administer oxygen, establish IV access, attach cardiac monitor,
administer fluids as needed (O2, IV, monitor, fluids)

↓

Assess vital signs, attach pulse oximeter, and monitor blood pressure
Obtain and review 12-lead ECG, portable chest x-ray film
Perform a focused history and physical exam

↓

Identify the Patient's Cardiac Rhythm

↓

Is the patient experiencing serious signs and symptoms because of the bradycardia?

SIGNS	SYMPTOMS
Low blood pressure, shock, pulmonary congestion, congestive heart failure, angina, acute MI, ventricular ectopy	Chest pain, weakness, fatigue, dizziness, lightheadedness, shortness of breath, exercise intolerance, decreased level of responsiveness

- If no serious signs and symptoms, observe
- If serious signs and symptoms are present, further intervention depends on the cardiac rhythm identified

Is the QRS narrow or wide?

NARROW QRS BRADYCARDIA

- **Sinus bradycardia**
- **Junctional rhythm**
- **Second-degree AV block, type I**
- **Third-degree (complete) AV block**

- **Atropine 0.5 to 1.0 mg IV:** May repeat every 3 to 5 min to a total dose of 2.5 mg (0.03 to 0.04 mg/kg). Total cumulative dose should not exceed 2.5 mg over 2.5 hours
- **Transcutaneous pacemaker (TCP):** Pacing should not be delayed while waiting for IV access or for atropine to take effect.
- **Dopamine infusion:** 5 to 20 mcg/kg/min
- **Epinephrine infusion:** 2 to 10 mcg/min
- **Isoproterenol infusion:** 2 to 10 mcg/min (low doses)

WIDE QRS BRADYCARDIA

- **Second-degree AV block, type II**
- **Third-degree (complete) AV block**
- **Ventricular escape (idioventricular) rhythm**

- **Transcutaneous pacemaker:** As an interim device until transvenous pacing can be accomplished
- **Dopamine infusion:** 5 to 20 mcg/kg/min
- **Epinephrine infusion:** 2 to 10 mcg/min
- **Isoproterenol infusion:** 2 to 10 mcg/min (low doses)

FIGURE 30-2

Symptomatic bradycardia. (From Aehlert B: *ACLS quick review study guide*, ed 2, St Louis, 2000, Mosby.)

patients and caregivers should know how to activate the emergency medical system (911) if these symptoms occur with chest discomfort or shortness of breath.

Careful explanation and supportive therapy will enhance patient and family understanding. These measures will also help allay the anxiety inherent in an emergent situation. Medication regimens, if associated with the bradyarrhythmias, should be reviewed to prevent misinterpretation.

REFERENCES

1. Demetriades D and others: Relative bradycardia in patients with traumatic hypotension, *J Trauma* 45(3):534-539, 1998.
2. American Heart Association: *ACLS provider's manual*, Dallas, 2001, The Association.
3. American Heart Association: *2000 Handbook of emergency cardiovascular care for healthcare providers*, Dallas, 2000, The Association.
4. Aehlert B: *ACLS quick review study guide*, ed 2, St Louis, 2000, Mosby.

CHAPTER 31

Cardiac Arrest

Terry Mahan Buttaro

DEFINITION/EPIDEMIOLOGY

More than 300,000 cardiac arrests occur in the United States each year.[1] Nearly one third of the victims die, usually within the first hour, the result of the abrupt cessation of normal heart rhythm. Cardiac arrest was previously considered to be the result of malignant ventricular arrhythmias or ventricular fibrillation (VF). More recent studies have revealed that asystole and pulseless electrical activity are also common causes of cardiac arrest and that these victims also benefit from CPR and aggressive advanced cardiac life support (ACLS) management.[2]

Fortunately, cardiac arrest patients are usually seen in the emergency department. However, some patients present to their primary care provider with prearrest conditions; these conditions should be quickly identified to facilitate emergency care. If cardiac arrest does occur, resuscitative efforts should be initiated immediately. Trained personnel should begin basic cardiac life support (BCLS) to maintain airway, breathing, and circulation (ABCs) until advanced cardiac life support (ACLS) is available[3,4] (Table 31-1). Preplanning requires that each member of the office team have a specified role if a cardiac arrest occurs and that providers be trained in BLS and ACLS.

Immediate emergency department referral/physician consultation is indicated for cardiac arrest.

PATHOPHYSIOLOGY

Cardiac arrest may result from either cardiac causes or extraneous circumstances. The net effect is the cessation of cardiac rhythm and the resultant tissue hypoxia and acidosis. Biologic death will occur if resuscitative measures are not instituted immediately.

CLINICAL PRESENTATION

There may be no warning that an acute event is about to occur. Presentation can include the classic midsternal, crushing, "vise-like" chest pressure with radiation to the arm, neck, or jaw and the accompanying diaphoresis, or it may consist of vague, nonspecific symptoms that include chest tightness, discomfort, nausea, shortness of breath, palpitations, light-headedness, or syncope. A recent history of angina, fatigue, and other nonspecific complaints are also reported. A medical history of smoking, hypertension, elevated cholesterol level, diabetes, and a sedentary lifestyle and family history of coronary artery disease (CAD) are significant risk factors for cardiac arrest; therefore obtaining this information is beneficial. If information cannot be elicited from the patient, family members or others should

TABLE 31-1 Primary ABCD Survey

ASSESS RESPONSIVENESS
If responsive, ask patient questions to determine adequacy of airway and breathing
If unresponsive, call for help (9-1-1 "Phone first"), call for defibrillator
Continue Primary ABCD Survey

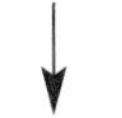

AIRWAY
Open the airway
If the airway is open, evaluate breathing
If the airway if not open, assess for sounds of airway compromise and look in the mouth for blood, broken teeth, loose dentures, gastric contents, and foreign objects
Clear the airway and insert an airway adjunct as needed to maintain an open airway

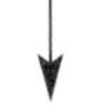

BREATHING
Look, listen, and feel for breathing
If the patient is responsive and breathing is adequate, evaluate circulation
If the unresponsive patient is breathing adequately, place in recovery position if no signs of trauma
If breathing is difficult and the rate is too slow or too fast, provide positive-pressure ventilation with 100% oxygen
If breathing is absent, insert an airway adjunct (if not previously done) and provide positive-pressure ventilation with a pocket mask or bag-valve-mask and 100% oxygen
Deliver two slow breaths and ensure the patient's chest rises with each breath
Administer oxygen as soon as it is available
Continue Primary ABCD Survey

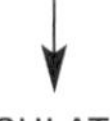

CIRCULATION
Assess for the presence of a pulse
If the patient is unresponsive, assess the carotid pulse on the side of the patient's neck nearest you
If the patient is responsive, assess the radial pulse. If a pulse is present, quickly estimate the rate and determine the quality of the pulse (e.g., fast/slow, regular/irregular, weak/strong), then perform the Secondary ABCD Survey
If there is no pulse, begin chest compressions until an AED or monitor/defibrillator is available

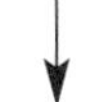

DEFIBRILLATION
Attach AED or monitor/defibrillator when available
If cardiac rhythm is pulseless VT or VF:
Defibrillate up to 3 times in rapid succession, pausing only to analyze/verify rhythm ("serial shocks")
Defibrillate with 200 J, 200 to 300 J, 360 J, or equivalent biphasic energy as necessary
If cardiac rhythm is not VT/VF, perform Secondary ABCD Survey

From Aehlert B: *ACLS quick review study guide,* ed 2, St Louis, 2000, Mosby.

be questioned to determine the patient's medical history and specific details of the circumstances surrounding the event.

PHYSICAL EXAMINATION

Assessing unresponsiveness in a calm but efficient manner is critical in the initial management of cardiac arrest. If there is no evidence of trauma, the American Heart Association (AHA) recommends gently shaking the victim and shouting, "Are you okay? Are you okay?" If unresponsiveness is confirmed in an adult patient, it is necessary to immediately call 911 to activate the emergency medical services (EMS) system to enable rapid procurement of an automated external defibrillator (AED) or a conventional defibrillator.[5]

If a second person is available to activate the EMS system, the provider should be positioned on the left at the victim's head to adequately perform the primary survey. The primary survey consists of opening and inspecting the airway with the head tilt–chin lift or jaw thrust maneuver, assessing breathlessness, verifying an obstructed airway with two slow breaths ($1\frac{1}{2}$ to 2 seconds per breath), confirming pulselessness or other signs of circulation (movement, coughing, or breathing) for no more than 10 seconds, and providing positive pressure ventilations (preferably oxygenated) and chest compressions according to the standards established by the AHA. There is *limited evidence* suggesting the benefit of a precordial thump in the witnessed arrest of a pulseless patient when an AED or a conventional defibrillator is unavailable. However, the AHA considers the precordial thump to be an acceptable intervention for health care providers if a defibrillator or AED is not available.[5] As soon as an AED or a conventional defibrillator is available, the leads should be attached to the victim, the rhythm assessed and, if appropriate, the victim defibrillated according to AHA standards[4] (see Table 31-1).

Continual assessment of airway, breathing, circulation, and the need for defibrillation (ABCD) is ongoing. Heart rate, blood pressure, oxygen saturation, and the effectiveness of intubation, CPR, and defibrillation should be reassessed at frequent intervals.

DIAGNOSTICS

An ECG, defibrillator monitor, or AED is needed to determine cardiac rhythm, which indicates the necessity of defibrillation and appropriate ACLS intervention. Serum electrolytes, drug levels, and cardiac enzymes are required for more definitive diagnosis but may be deferred to emergency department management.

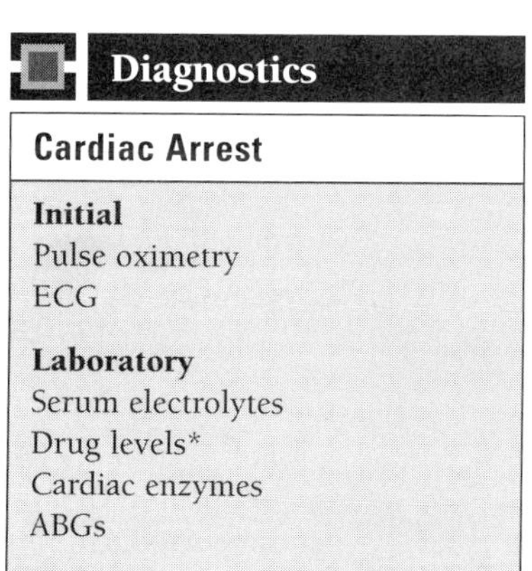
Diagnostics

Cardiac Arrest

Initial
Pulse oximetry
ECG

Laboratory
Serum electrolytes
Drug levels*
Cardiac enzymes
ABGs

*If indicated.

DIFFERENTIAL DIAGNOSIS

Sudden cardiac death is often associated with VF. Other emergency situations associated with cardiac arrest include significant but nonlethal arrhythmias, hypotension, shock, pulmonary edema, pulmonary embolus, toxicologic cardiac emergencies, metabolic imbalance, near-drowning, hypothermia, cardiac tamponade, tension pneumothorax, electric shock, and lightning strike. It is important to consider, determine, and treat reversible causes of the arrest.

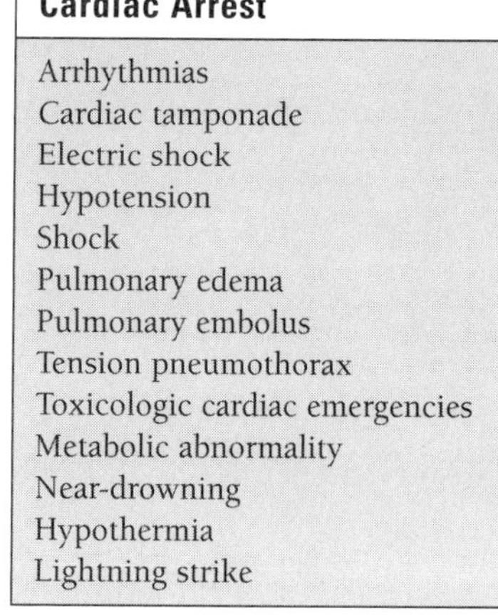
Differential Diagnosis

Cardiac Arrest

Arrhythmias
Cardiac tamponade
Electric shock
Hypotension
Shock
Pulmonary edema
Pulmonary embolus
Tension pneumothorax
Toxicologic cardiac emergencies
Metabolic abnormality
Near-drowning
Hypothermia
Lightning strike

INITIAL STABILIZATION AND MANAGEMENT

Management should follow the guidelines of the AHA[4] (Tables 31-1 and 31-2). If the patient's collapse may have caused trauma, the head, neck, and spine must be maintained in a straight line to stabilize the cervical spine. After activation of the EMS system, the patient should be positioned on a flat, firm surface, and BLS should be initiated. The cause of the cardiac arrest should be considered throughout the resuscitative effort to facilitate appropriate interventions and promote successful resuscitation.

Because most victims of cardiac arrest are in VF, the AHA still considers early defibrillation the most effective treatment for adult victims of cardiac arrest[4] (Table 31-3). There is *evidence suggesting the benefit* of early CPR and defibrillation; approximately 85% to 90% of cardiac arrest victims will respond to early CPR and the three initial defibrillation stacked

TABLE 31-2 Secondary ABCD Survey

(ADVANCED) AIRWAY
Reassess the effectiveness of initial airway maneuvers and interventions
Perform endotracheal intubation, if needed

↓

BREATHING
Assess ventilation
Confirm endotracheal tube placement (or other airway device) by at least two methods
Provide positive-pressure ventilation
Evaluate effectiveness of ventilations

↓

CIRCULATION
Establish peripheral intravenous (IV) access
Attach ECG
Administer medications appropriate for cardiac rhythm/clinical situation

↓

DIFFERENTIAL DIAGNOSIS
Consider possible cause(s) of the arrest, rhythm, situation

From Aehlert B: *ACLS quick review study guide,* ed 2, St Louis, 2000, Mosby.

TABLE 31-3 Pulseless Ventricular Tachycardia (VT)/Ventricular Fibrillation (VF)

Basic Life Support

PERFORM PRIMARY ABCD SURVEY
(Correct critical problems IMMEDIATELY as they are identified)
Assess responsiveness
Call for help/call for defibrillator
Airway—open the airway
Breathing—deliver two slow breaths, administer oxygen as soon as it is available
Circulation—perform chest compressions
Ensure availability of monitor/**D**efibrillator
On arrival of AED/monitor/defibrillator, evaluate cardiac rhythm

If PEA or asystole, continue CPR and go to appropriate algorithm.
If pulseless VT/VF, shock up to three times (200 J, 200 to 300 J, 360 J, or equivalent Biphasic energy).

Reevaluate cardiac rhythm

- If persistent or recurrent pulseless VT/VF, continue CPR and perform secondary ABCD Survey
- If PEA or asystole, continue CPR and go to appropriate algorithm

If return of spontaneous circulation (ROSC):
- Assess vital signs
- Maintain open airway
- Provide ventilation
- Administer medications appropriate for rhythm, blood pressure, and heart rate

Advanced Life Support

PERFORM SECONDARY ABCD SURVEY
(ADVANCED) *A*IRWAY
Reassess effectiveness of initial airway maneuvers and interventions
Perform invasive airway management

*B*REATHING
Confirm ET tube placement (or other airway device) by at least two methods
Provide positive-pressure ventilation/Evaluate effectiveness of ventilations
Secure airway device in place with commercial tube holder (preferred) or tape

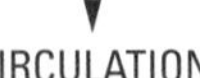

*C*IRCULATION
Establish IV access and administer appropriate medications

*D*IFFERENTIAL DIAGNOSIS
Search for and treat reversible causes

Pattern becomes CPR-drug-shock or CPR-drug-shock-shock-shock

Epinephrine (Class Indeterminate) 1 mg (1:10,000 solution) IV every 3 to 5 min
(ET dose 2 to 2.5 mg diluted in 10-mL normal saline or distilled water)

or

Vasopressin (Class IIb) 40 U IV bolus (administer only once)
(If no response to vasopressin, may resume epinephrine after 10 to 20 min; epi dose 1 mg every 3 to 5 min)

Defibrillate with 360 J (or equivalent Biphasic energy) within 30 to 60 sec

Consider antiarrhythmics (avoid use of multiple antiarrhythmics because of potential proarrhythmic effects)
- **Amiodarone** (Class IIb): Initial bolus: 300 mg IV bolus diluted in 20 to 30 mL of NS or D_5W. Consider repeat dose (150 mg IV bolus) in 3 to 5 min. If defibrillation successful, follow with 1 mg/min IV infusion for 6 hours (mix 900 mg in 500 ml NS), then decrease infusion rate to 0.5 mg/min IV infusion for 18 hours. Maximum daily dose 2.0 g IV/24 hours
- **Lidocaine** (Class Indeterminate): 1 to 1.5 mg/kg IV bolus, consider repeat dose (0.5 to 0.75 mg/kg) in 5 min; maximum IV bolus dose 3 mg/kg. (The 1.5 mg/kg dose is recommended in cardiac arrest.) Endotracheal dose: 2 to 4 mg/kg. A single dose of 1.5 mg/kg is acceptable in cardiac arrest
- **Magnesium** (Class IIb if hypomagnesemia present): 1 to 2 g IV (2 to 4 ml of a 50% solution) diluted in 10 ml of D_5W if Torsades de Pointes or hypomagnesemia
- **Procainamide** (Class IIb for recurrent pulseless VT/VF; Class Indeterminate for persistent pulseless VT/VF): 20 mg/min; maximum total dose 17 mg/kg
- Consider **sodium bicarbonate** 1 mEq/kg

From Aehlert B: *ACLS quick review study guide,* ed 2, St Louis, 2000, Mosby.

TABLE 31-4 Asystole

Basic Life Support

PERFORM PRIMARY ABCD SURVEY
(Correct critical problems IMMEDIATELY as they are identified)
Assess responsiveness
Call for help/call for defibrillator
Airway—open the airway
Breathing—deliver two slow breaths, administer oxygen as soon as it is available
Circulation—perform chest compressions
Ensure availability of monitor/**D**efibrillator
On arrival of AED/monitor/defibrillator, perform secondary ABCD Survey if rhythm is NOT pulseless VT/VF

Scene Survey—Documentation or other evidence of Do Not Attempt Resuscitation (DNAR)?
Obvious signs of death? If yes, do not start/attempt resuscitation

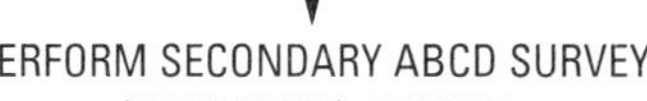

Advanced Life Support

PERFORM SECONDARY ABCD SURVEY
(ADVANCED) *A*IRWAY
Reassess effectiveness of initial airway maneuvers and interventions
Perform invasive airway management

*B*REATHING
Assess ventilation
Confirm ET tube placement (or other airway device) by at least two methods
Provide positive-pressure ventilation/evaluate effectiveness of ventilations
Secure airway device in place with commercial tube holder (preferred) or tape

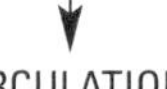

*C*IRCULATION
Confirm presence of asystole
(Check lead/cable connections, ensure power to monitor is on, correct lead is selected, gain turned up, confirm asystole in second lead)
Establish IV access and administer appropriate medications

*D*IFFERENTIAL DIAGNOSIS
Search for and treat reversible causes ***(PATCH-4-MD)***

Consider immediate transcutaneous pacing

Epinephrine 1 mg (1:10,000 solution) IV every 3 to 5 min
(ET dose 2 to 2.5 mg diluted in 10 ml normal saline or distilled water)

Atropine 1 mg IV every 3 to 5 min to maximum 0.04 mg/kg (Class IIb)
(ET dose 2 to 3 mg diluted in 10 ml normal saline or distilled water)

Consider sodium bicarbonate 1 mEq/kg:
- Known preexisting hyperkalemia (Class I)
- Cyclic antidepressant overdose (IIa)
- To alkalinize urine in aspirin or other drug overdoses (IIa)
- Patient that has been intubated + long arrest interval (IIb)
- On return of spontaneous circulation if long arrest interval (IIb)

Consider termination of efforts:
- Evaluate the quality of the resuscitation attempt
- Evaluate the resuscitation for atypical clinical features (e.g., hypothermia, reversible therapeutic or illicit drug use)
- Does support for cease-effort protocols exist?

Possible causes of asystole: **PATCH-4-MD**

Pulmonary embolism
Acidosis
Tension pneumothorax
Cardiac tamponade
Hypovolemia
Hypoxia
Heat/cold (hypo-/hyperthermia)
Hypo-/hyperkalemia (and other electrolytes)
Myocardial infarction
Drug overdose/accidents (cyclic antidepressants, calcium channel blockers, beta-blockers, digitalis)

From Aehlert B: *ACLS quick review study guide,* ed 2, St Louis, 2000, Mosby.

TABLE 31-5 Pulseless Electrical Activity (PEA)

Basic Life Support

PERFORM PRIMARY ABCD SURVEY
(Correct critical problems IMMEDIATELY as they are identified)
Assess responsiveness
Call for help/call for defibrillator
Airway—open the airway
Breathing—deliver two slow breaths, administer oxygen as soon as it is available
Circulation—perform chest compressions
Ensure availability of monitor/**D**efibrillator
On arrival of AED/monitor/defibrillator, perform secondary ABCD Survey if rhythm is NOT pulseless VT/VF

Advanced Life Support

PERFORM SECONDARY ABCD SURVEY
(ADVANCED) *A*IRWAY
Reassess effectiveness of initial airway maneuvers and interventions
Perform invasive airway management

*B*REATHING
Assess ventilation
Confirm ET tube placement (or other airway device) by at least two methods
Provide positive-pressure ventilation/evaluate effectiveness of ventilations
Secure airway device in place with commercial tube holder (preferred) or tape

*C*IRCULATION
Establish IV access
Assess blood flow with Doppler
(If blood flow detected with Doppler, treat using hypotension/shock algorithm)
Administer appropriate medications

*D*IFFERENTIAL DIAGNOSIS
Search for and treat reversible causes ***(PATCH-4-MD)***
(Fast narrow-QRS—consider hypovolemia, tamponade, pulmonary embolism, tension pneumothorax; slow wide QRS—consider cyclic antidepressant overdose, calcium channel blocker, beta-blocker, or digitalis toxicity)

Possible causes of PEA:
PATCH-4-MD

Pulmonary embolism
Acidosis
Tension pneumothorax
Cardiac tamponade
Hypovolemia (most common cause)
Hypoxia
Heat/cold (hypo-/hyperthermia)
Hypo-/hyperkalemia (and other electrolytes)
Myocardial infarction
Drug overdose/accidents (cyclic antidepressants, calcium channel blockers, beta-blockers, digitalis)

Epinephrine 1 mg (1:10,000 solution) IV every 3 to 5 min
(ET dose 2 to 2.5 mg diluted in 10 ml normal saline or distilled water)

If the rate is slow, atropine 1 mg IV every 3 to 5 min to max 0.04 mg/kg (Class IIb)
(ET dose 2 to 3 mg diluted in 10 ml normal saline or distilled water)

Consider sodium bicarbonate 1 mEq/kg:
- Known preexisting hyperkalemia (Class I)
- Cyclic antidepressant overdose (IIa)
- To alkalinize urine in aspirin or other drug overdoses (IIa)
- Patient that has been intubated + long arrest interval (IIb)
- On return of spontaneous circulation if long arrest interval (IIb)

Consider termination of efforts

From Aehlert B: *ACLS quick review study guide,* ed 2, St Louis, 2000, Mosby.

shocks.[6] Therefore defibrillation with a biphasic defibrillator, a conventional defibrillator, or an AED should occur as soon as the defibrillator is available. Defibrillation with a conventional defibrillator consists of three shocks: first at 200 J, then at 200 to 300 J, and again at 360 J, if necessary. The pulse should be checked after the third defibrillation.

If circulation is not restored with the initial stacked shocks, it is important to continue CPR and to determine the cardiac rhythm. Further treatment should follow ACLS guidelines[4] (Tables 31-3, 31-4, and 31-5).

COMPLICATIONS

Death will ensue rapidly if CPR, defibrillation, and treatment are not immediately initiated; few victims will survive if CPR is not started within 4 minutes. Those who do survive cardiac arrest may sustain central nervous system injury, hemodynamic instability, and arrhythmias.

DISPOSITION AND REFERRAL

Circulation has been restored if a pulse is present. Airway, breathing, and circulation should be supported and the patient transported to the nearest emergency department. Emergency department personnel should be advised of pertinent medical information.

PREVENTION

Primary prevention of cardiac arrest is the ultimate goal. Patients with dyspnea, light-headedness, angina, palpitations, or fatigue should be evaluated for underlying CAD. The identification of risk factors for CAD and the appropriate interventions are indicated to decrease the number of sudden cardiac deaths. In addition, community programs enhance the understanding of coronary disease, reinforce early management of chest pain, and promote early access to the EMS system.

Training in CPR and emergency cardiac care is essential for any health care provider. Caregivers of patients with CAD should also be trained in BLS and understand the warning signs associated with sudden cardiac death.

If the cardiac arrest was the result of sustained ventricular tachycardia (VT), the victim will need therapy to reduce the chance of future events. An automated implantable cardioverter/defibrillator or cardiac surgery may be appropriate. Antiarrhythmic pharmacologic therapy may not be useful for the prevention of ventricular arrhythmias and in fact may be proarrhythmic.[7] There is clear evidence, however, that amiodarone is superior to other antiarrhythmic agents, and current ACLS guidelines recommend amiodarone for shock-refractory VT/VF, stable monomorphic and polymorphic VT, and wide-complex tachycardia in stable patients.[8] Research continues on the use of beta blockers and other medications, as well as invasive therapies to prevent episodes of ventricular arrhythmias.

PATIENT AND FAMILY EDUCATION

Patients and caregivers should be aware that chest discomfort that increases in intensity or is associated with sweating, palpitations, irregular heartbeat, shortness of breath, light-headedness, nausea or vomiting, loss of consciousness, or discomfort that radiates to the jaw, neck, or arm necessitates calling 911 or other emergency service immediately. It is important to explain that presentation can be atypical, particularly in women, diabetic persons, or older adults. Everyone should be encouraged to learn BLS, but families who have loved ones with CAD should know how to perform CPR. In addition, patients with risk factors for CAD should constantly be encouraged to make lifestyle changes to reduce the risk of cardiac arrest.

REFERENCES

1. Thel MC, O'Connor CM: Cardiopulmonary resuscitation: historical perspective to recent investigations, *Am Heart J* 137(1):39-48, 1999.
2. Stratton SJ, Niemann JT: Outcome from out-of-hospital arrest caused by nonventricular arrhythmias: contribution of successful resuscitation to overall survivorship supports the current practice of initiating out-of-hospital ACLS, *Ann Emerg Med* 32(4):448-453, 1998.
3. Cobb LA and others: Influence of cardiopulmonary resuscitation prior to defibrillation in patients with out-of-hospital ventricular fibrillation, *JAMA* 281(13):1182-1188, 1999.
4. Aehlert B: *ACLS: quick review study guide*, ed 2, St Louis, 2000, Mosby.
5. American Heart Association: *2000 Handbook of emergency cardiovascular care for healthcare providers*, Dallas, 2000, The Association.
6. American Heart Association: *ACLS provider's manual*, Dallas, 2001, The Association.
7. Reiffel JA: Prolonging survival by reducing arrhythmic death: pharmacologic therapy of ventricular tachycardia and fibrillation, *Am J Cardiol* 80(8A):45G-55G, 1997.
8. Kudenchuk P and others: Amiodarone for resuscitation after out-of-hospital cardiac arrest due to ventricular fibrillation, *N Engl J Med* 341(12):871-878, 1999.

CHAPTER 32
Cerebrovascular Accident

Terry Mahan Buttaro

DEFINITION/EPIDEMIOLOGY

Strokes (cerebrovascular accidents [CVAs]) are responsible for the deaths of approximately 160,000 Americans each year and represent the third leading cause of death in this country.[1,2] An additional 750,000 Americans survive the neurologic insult associated with a stroke but may have profound deficits.[1] Strokes are the most common cause of adult disability in the United States.[1]

Nearly 85% of strokes are classified as ischemic; the remaining are the result of subarachnoid or intracerebral hemorrhage.[2] Impairment may be mild or severe depending on the type of stroke, location, size, and neurologic recovery. Because strokes are caused by ischemia or hemorrhage, identification of the type of stroke is essential. Eligibility for treatment of ischemic stroke with fibrinolytic (thrombolytic) therapy requires that patients with a clinical diagnosis of stroke and evident neurologic deficit have a baseline computed tomography (CT) scan performed to exclude intracranial hemorrhage. Fibrinolytic therapy in patients with intracerebral hemorrhage is absolutely contraindicated. Patients diagnosed with ischemic stroke and without contraindications for fibrinolytic therapy should receive treatment within 3 hours of symptom onset.[3] *Timely evaluation and transport to an emergency facility equipped to treat stroke patients within 60 minutes of symptom onset are critical if the serious neurologic sequelae associated with ischemic or hemorrhagic strokes are to be limited.*

Hypertension has been associated with both ischemic and hemorrhagic strokes and is the most significant risk factor.[3] Other risk factors include age, gender, race/ethnicity, heredity, prior personal history of stroke or transient ischemic attacks (TIAs), nicotine abuse, diabetes, elevated blood cholesterol level, increased RBC count, heart disease, sickle cell anemia, obesity, sedentary lifestyle, and the presence of a carotid bruit. Congestive heart failure and coronary artery disease, particularly atrial fibrillation, significantly increase the risk of thromboembolic stroke. Pregnancy, cancer, cocaine use, and protein S and C deficiencies have also been identified as risk factors for stroke.

Immediate emergency department referral/ physician consultation is indicated for victims of a CVA, or "brain attack."

PATHOPHYSIOLOGY

Most strokes are ischemic in nature, are the result of a cerebral embolism or cerebral thrombosis, and are categorized by vascular distribution or anatomic location. Embolic strokes occur precipitously and result from migrating clots that develop in another part of the body and then travel to the brain. Thrombotic strokes develop in the brain itself, often have a fluctuating course, and may be preceded by a series of small strokes or TIAs. Transient arterial occlusions are responsible for the reversible focal symptoms of a TIA. The characteristics of strokes and TIAs are similar, although TIAs persist for several minutes or hours and then resolve. The resolution of these symptoms results in a negative neurologic examination, and the diagnosis of a TIA may be based on the history. However, many patients with a TIA subsequently experience a complete stroke, often within 30 days; therefore TIAs should be managed aggressively.[2]

Strokes are usually classified by the affected anatomic location or artery.[2] The signs and symptoms suggest the affected artery and the involved areas of the brain (Table 32-1). Anterior circulation strokes involve the cerebral hemispheres and are associated with the carotid artery, whereas posterior circulation strokes are associated with the vertebrobasilar artery. Lacunar strokes are thrombotic strokes that affect the small arteries deep within the white matter of the brain.

Subarachnoid hemorrhage and intracerebral hemorrhage are the causes of hemorrhagic strokes. A ruptured aneurysm is the most common cause of subarachnoid hemorrhage and is associated with a sudden, severe, relentless headache and significant mortality rate. Intracerebral hemorrhage results when a blood vessel in the brain ruptures and bleeds.

CLINICAL PRESENTATION

Determination and documentation of symptom onset from the patient, family, or witnesses are critical because fibrinolytic therapy for an acute ischemic stroke should be administered within 3 hours of symptom onset. Warning signs of stroke may be fleeting or mild in a TIA but can last as long as 24 hours. However, any sudden focal neurologic deficit or alteration in consciousness or cognitive ability should prompt consideration that a stroke has occurred. Characteristics customarily associated with a stroke include a fall; facial paralysis; vertigo; language, visual, or gait disturbances; and unilateral numbness, weakness, or clumsiness. These symptoms may be prominent in both ischemic and hemorrhagic strokes, although headache, nausea, vomiting, neck pain, light/sound intolerance, and decreased consciousness suggest a hemorrhagic stroke. Seizures, particularly in older adults, also suggest the possibility that a stroke has occurred.[2]

History is essential to differentiate a stroke from other disorders with similar presentations (i.e., hypoglycemia, syncope, seizure, migraine, infection, or drug overdose). A previous history of hypertension, coronary artery disease, diabetes, and CVA or TIA should be established and the patient's activity before the event determined. Eliciting allergies and the names of current medications (particularly antihypertensive agents, aspirin, anticoagulants, amphetamines, oral contraceptives or hormone replacement therapy, and diabetic medications) is essential. Over-the-counter medications or street drug use, as well as medical, psychiatric, and head trauma history, is also very important. In addition, any contraindication to thrombolytic therapy should be determined (Box 32-1).

PHYSICAL EXAMINATION

The initial assessment should ensure that airway, breathing, and circulation (ABCs) are intact. The airway status, level of consciousness, focal neurologic assessment, and vital signs

TABLE 32-1 Clinical Manifestations of Stroke

Affected Artery	Structures Supplied by Affected Vessel	Signs and Symptoms of Occlusion
Anterior cerebral	Supplies medial surfaces and upper portions of frontal and parietal lobes and medial surface of hemisphere	Emotional lability Confusion Weakness, numbness on affected side Paralysis of contralateral foot and leg Impaired mobility, with sensation greater in lower extremities than in upper Urinary incontinence Loss of coordination Personality changes Impaired sensory function
Middle cerebral Most commonly occluded vessel in stroke Largest branch of the internal carotid artery	Supplies a portion of the frontal lobe and lateral surface of the temporal and parietal lobes, including the primary motor and sensory areas of the face, throat, hand and arm and, in the dominant hemisphere, the areas for speech	Alterations in communication, cognition, mobility, and sensation, including: Aphasia Dysphasia Reading difficulty (dyslexia) Inability to write (dysgraphia) Visual field deficits Contralateral sensory deficit Contralateral hemiparesis (more severe in the face and hand than in the leg) Altered level of responsiveness
Posterior cerebral	Supplies medial and inferior temporal lobes, medial occipital lobe, thalamus, posterior hypothalamus, visual receptive area	Hemiplegia Receptive aphasia Sensory impairment Dyslexia Coma Visual field deficits Cortical blindness from ischemia
Internal carotid	Supplies the cerebral hemispheres and diencephalon	Headaches Altered level of responsiveness Bruits over the carotid artery Profound aphasia Ptosis Weakness, paralysis, numbness, sensory changes, and visual deficits (e.g., blurring) on the affected side Unilateral blindness
Vertebral or basilar	Supplies the brainstem and cerebellum	Incomplete occlusion Transient ischemic attacks Unilateral and bilateral weakness of extremities Visual deficits on affected side (e.g., diplopia, color blindness, lack of depth perception) Nausea, vertigo, tinnitus Headache Dysarthria Numbness Dysphagia "Locked-in" syndrome—no movement except eyelids; sensation and consciousness preserved Complete occlusion or hemorrhage Coma Decerebrate rigidity Respiratory and circulatory abnormalities

BOX 32-1

CONTRAINDICATIONS TO THROMBOLYTIC THERAPY

- Minor stroke symptoms or rapidly resolving stroke symptoms
- Presence of intracranial bleeding on non–contrast-enhanced CT or high suspicion for subarachnoid hemorrhage
- History of internal bleeding within past 3 weeks (21 days)
- History of serious head trauma, intracranial surgery, or stroke within past 3 months
- History of serious trauma or major surgery within past 2 weeks (14 days)
- History of lumbar puncture within past week (7 days)
- History recent arterial puncture at noncompressible site
- History of intracranial hemorrhage, arteriovenous malformation, or aneurysm
- History of recent myocardial infarction
- History of known bleeding diathesis, platelet count $<100{,}000/mm^3$, heparin administration within past 48 hours and partial thromboplastin time greater than normal, or recent anticoagulant use (warfarin) with prothrombin time >15 seconds
- Witnessed seizure during stroke onset
- Consistently elevated systolic blood pressure >185 mm Hg or diastolic blood pressure of >110 mm Hg

Modified from American Heart Association: Exclusion criteria for fibrinolytic therapy checklist for ischemic stroke. In *ACLS provider manual,* Dallas, 2001, The Association.

BOX 32-2

CINCINNATI PREHOSPITAL STROKE SCALE

1. If any one of the following signs is abnormal, stroke probability = 72%
2. *Facial droop/weakness:* Ask patient to "Show me your teeth" or "Smile for me"
   a. *Normal:* Both sides of face move equally well
   b. *Abnormal:* One side of face does not move at all
3. *Motor weakness (arm drift):* With eyes closed, ask patient to extend arms out in front of him or her 90 degrees (if sitting) or 45 degrees (if supine)
   a. *Normal:* Both arms move the same *or* both arms do not move at all
   b. *Abnormal:* One arm either does not move *or* one arm drifts down compared to the other
   c. Drift is scored if the arm falls before 10 seconds
4. *Aphasia (speech):* Ask patient to say "You can't teach an old dog new tricks," "The sky is blue in Cincinnati," or similar phrase
   a. *Normal:* Phrase is repeated clearly and correctly
   b. *Abnormal:* Words are slurred (dysarthria) or abnormal (aphasia), or patient is mute

From Aehlert B: *ACLS quick review study guide,* ed 2, St Louis, 2000, Mosby.

(including temperature and blood pressure measurement in both upper arms) should be promptly and continuously assessed. The blood pressure may be elevated on an acute basis, and fever can be present in an acute stroke as well as with infection.

In addition, examination should include an inspection for tongue or buccal mucosa lacerations, evidence of incontinence, and evidence of trauma, which may indicate seizure activity.[3] Evidence of facial droop, arm drift, aphasia, unilateral weakness, or slurred or inappropriate speech is strongly suggestive of a stroke and mandates immediate transport by ambulance to the emergency department or stroke center. The Glasgow Coma Scale score helps to establish the patient's level of consciousness, and the Cincinnati Prehospital Stroke Scale[3] (Box 32-2) assists in determining the probability of a stroke.

Other components of the physical examination include skin evaluation for evidence of trauma from a fall (particularly head trauma), purpura, cholesterol, or ecchymosis; eye examination to determine reactivity, equality, and pupil size; funduscopic examination for papilledema or cholesterol emboli; carotid artery examination for pulses and bruits; cardiac evaluation for arrhythmias or murmur; and examination of the lower extremities for a deep vein thrombosis. However, this examination should not delay the immediate transfer of the patient to an emergency department or stroke center.

DIAGNOSTICS

Patients with suspected stroke should be promptly transferred to a stroke center where clinical diagnosis is confirmed with a spiral CT scan or non–contrast-enhanced cranial CT scan.

Diagnostics

Cerebrovascular Accident†

Initial	Imaging
Spiral CT scan or noncontrast cranial CT scan	Chest x-ray
ECG	Lateral cervical spine x-ray*
Laboratory	**Other**
Serum electrolytes	Lumbar puncture*
Serum glucose	CT angiography*
BUN Creatinine	ECG
CBC and differential	Chest x-ray
Coagulation studies	
Drug/alcohol levels*	
Toxic screen*	
Type and crossmatch	
Serum hCG*	

*If indicated.
†All tests should be conducted at a stroke center.

Current recommendations advise that the CT scan be obtained within 25 minutes and interpreted within 45 minutes of arrival at the stroke center. CT angiography, when available, provides further information and options for recanalization and intraarterial thrombolysis. Fibrinolytic therapy should not be administered until hemorrhagic stroke has been excluded.[2,3]

On admission to the stroke center, CBC, erythrocyte sedimentation rate, serum glucose, electrolytes, BUN, creatinine, LFTs, toxicology screen, coagulation studies (prothrombin time

[PT], partial thromboplastin time [PTT], platelet count, and international normalized ratio [INR]), and type and crossmatch should be obtained. Serum beta-hCG is indicated for all women of childbearing age. An ECG to exclude arrhythmias and a chest x-ray examination are also indicated to aid diagnosis. Lateral cervical spine x-ray studies and lumbar puncture may be advised to exclude other problems if clinically indicated. However, lumbar puncture should not be performed until subarachnoid hemorrhage is excluded by CT scan.

DIFFERENTIAL DIAGNOSIS

Coexisting illness or prior neurologic impairment may make diagnosis enigmatic, although any sudden onset of neurologic dysfunction is strongly indicative of a stroke. Hyperglycemia and hypoglycemia should be also considered, particularly in the presence of diabetes. Drug, alcohol, or other toxins; trauma; seizure; hyponatremia; syncope; thrombotic thrombocytopenic purpura; meningitis or encephalitis; aneurysm; intracranial tumor; subdural or epidural hematoma; metabolic or hypertensive encephalopathy; and migraine may also cause focal neurologic changes or altered consciousness.

INITIAL STABILIZATION AND MANAGEMENT

Management should model the American Heart Association guidelines for suspected stroke patients. Assessment of the ABCs is essential because airway obstruction, aspiration, and poor ventilation are concerns. Pulse oximetry, administration of oxygen (if necessary), airway and seizure management, and treatment of documented hypoglycemia are crucial. IV access with isotonic fluid only is recommended, although bolus administration of IV fluid is not indicated unless hypotension is present. A neurologic examination should be performed within 10 minutes of arrival in the emergency department or stroke center.

Poststroke hypertension is not uncommon. Treatment is not usually recommended before hospitalization[2] and is usually customary only in a hypertensive emergency, acute myocardial infarction, aortic dissection, hypertensive encephalopathy, or severe left ventricular failure. However, if systolic blood pressure is greater than 220 mm Hg or diastolic blood pressure is greater than 120 mm Hg, the American Heart Association recommends treatment with labetalol 10 to 20 mg IV or nitroglycerin paste.[3] Patients with blood pressure greater than 185/110 mm Hg should not receive fibrinolytic therapy until the blood pressure is reduced below this level.[3]

Seizures should be controlled and the patient protected from injury. Lorazepam 1 to 4 mg IV over 10 minutes is indicated for seizures initially. Phenytoin may be subsequently administered for longer-acting seizure control. A loading dose of phenytoin 1 g IV is indicated in new-onset seizures; administration in adults should not exceed 50 mg/min.

Differential Diagnosis

Cerebrovascular Accident
Hyperglycemia/hypoglycemia
Trauma
Seizure
Syncope
Meningitis
Encephalitis
Aneurysm
Intracranial tumor
Subdural/epidural hematoma
Metabolic or hypertensive encephalopathy
Migraine
Drug/alcohol/toxin induced
Thrombotic thrombocytopenia purpura

DISPOSITION AND REFERRAL

Immediate transport by emergency medical services (EMS) personnel to an emergency care center equipped to provide CT scanning and stroke therapy is indicated for all suspected stroke victims. Neurosurgical consultation is recommended if acute hemorrhage is suspected.

PREVENTION AND PATIENT AND FAMILY EDUCATION

Controllable risk factors for stroke should be addressed with all patients and families. Increased awareness of the dangers of smoking, alcohol, a sedentary lifestyle, and obesity are continuing public health concerns. Lifestyle and medical interventions for hypertension, hypercholesterolemia, diabetes, and other controllable risk factors require continued assessment for optimal benefit. Patients with a history of TIAs require a careful explanation that symptoms usually resolve in 24 hours, that neurologic defects are not permanent, and that there is an increased risk for stroke. Thus an appropriate evaluation of carotid bruits and cardiac risk factors for stroke is necessary. Oral anticoagulation or aspirin is usually prescribed if atrial fibrillation is present. In addition, health care providers have a responsibility to heighten public awareness of stroke symptoms, potential stroke therapies, and the need for prompt medical evaluation and treatment of stroke.

REFERENCES

1. National Stroke Association: Retrieved May 19, 2002 from the World Wide Web: http://www.stroke.org/brain_stat.cfm.
2. Aehlert B: *ACLS quick review study guide,* ed 2, St Louis, 2001, Mosby.
3. American Heart Association: *ACLS provider manual,* Dallas, 2001, The Association.

CHAPTER 33

Chemical Exposure

Walter Elias, III

DEFINITION/EPIDEMIOLOGY

Harmful chemicals are found in every aspect of life, particularly the home and workplace. Common household chemicals that are dangerous include shoe polishes, cosmetics, over-the-counter and prescription medications, alcohols (isopropyl alcohol, methanol, and ethanol), detergents, cleaning products (especially chlorine, ammonia, or lye-containing cleaners), rodent and insect poisons, common yard chemicals, and paints and paint products.

Chemicals abound in the workplace, and many of these cause irritation or toxicity if exposed to the human body. The Occupational Safety and Health Administration (OSHA) requires that all employers and employees be advised of chemical hazards by means of a Hazards Communication Program, which includes having a Material Safety Data Sheet (MSDS) for each chemical used in the workplace. The employer must ensure that MSDSs are readily accessible to employees during each work shift when they are in the work area.[1] MSDSs are fact sheets provided by chemical manufacturers that list chemical, physical, and health hazard data for a particular substance. Health hazard data include routes of entry, acute and chronic effects, signs and symptoms of exposure, and emergency and first aid procedures.[2] For safety reasons and because federal law requires accurate labeling on chemical containers, it is wise to avoid the unnecessary transfer of potentially dangerous chemicals into any other containers. If transfer to another container is necessary, OSHA labeling requirements must be followed.[1]

More than 1.8 million poisonings were reported to poison control centers in the United States in 1992; 90% of these poisonings occurred in the home, and 60% involved children younger than 6 years of age.[3] Poisoning was the third leading cause of unintentional injury or death in 1998, resulting in 10,255 deaths.[4] These statistics demonstrate the importance of taking preventive measures against accidental chemical exposures. Prevention is best achieved by keeping medications and cleaners out of the sight and reach of children[4] and by keeping the materials clearly labeled.[1] Essential first aid materials for poisoning and the telephone number of the poison control center should also be readily available.

Immediate emergency department referral, physician consultation, and contact with a poison control center are indicated for chemical exposure.

PATHOPHYSIOLOGY

The pathophysiologic and systemic effects of a chemical exposure are dependent on the characteristics and effects of the substance, the degree and route of exposure, and patient comorbidities.

CLINICAL PRESENTATION

For poisoning, the history should address the "Five Ws": *who*—the patient's age, weight, sex, and relationship to others present; *what*—the name and dosage of substance, co-ingestants, and amount ingested; *when*—the time and date of ingestion; *where*—both the route of poisoning and the geographic location in which the poisoning occurred, and *why*—whether the ingestion was intentional or unintentional, plus associated details. A detailed past medical history should be obtained, including previous poisonings, medical conditions, and concurrent medications that might affect the patient's response to and the metabolism or elimination of ingestants, psychiatric history, and history of substance abuse. Particular attention should be given to eliciting a history of alcoholism and renal or hepatic disease.[5]

The patient who has had a toxic exposure may be affected in many different ways. The presentation of chemical exposures can range from a viral, respiratory-like syndrome to severe burns or coma.[6] With children, there often is physical evidence (e.g., a smell of cleaning products, pill or plant fragments, nonfood stains, open bottles or containers), which can be more suggestive than the symptoms themselves.[3] Adults commonly know the type of exposure unless they are incapacitated by it, in which case witnesses can usually identify the exposure. If the exposure is occupational, the chemical may be readily identifiable. Reviewing MSDSs for pertinent information after an occupational exposure may be helpful.

The following paragraphs describe a few common presentations of chemical exposure related to specific classes of chemicals. *Anticholinergics* include prescription medications such as dimenhydrinate, diphenhydramine, astemizole, loratadine, meclizine, promethazine, tricyclic antidepressants, and household and wild plants such as mandrake, jimsonweed ("loco weed"), and nightshades. Anticholinergics cause a syndrome that is best remembered by the mnemonic "hot as Hades, blind as a bat, red as a beet, dry as a bone, mad as a hatter," which describes the syndrome of hyperthermia; mydriasis; flushed skin; dry mucous membranes, urinary retention, and decreased bowel motility; and hallucinations or frank psychosis, respectively.[7]

Alkalis are found in numerous household cleaning products, batteries, and other substances and cause irritation to the oral mucosa, esophagus, and stomach. This irritation ranges from mild to extremely severe. Both acids and alkalis cause extensive tissue damage to mucous membranes and the gastric system. The alkalis, however, are associated with a much more serious prognosis because they tend to penetrate tissues more deeply and rapidly than do the acids, particularly if the eye is involved.[7]

Hydrocarbons are the basis of many chemicals commonly used in industry and are found in garages and sheds. These substances cause a host of reactions that include coughing, vomiting, a chemical odor to the breath and, in severe exposure, unconsciousness and coma.

PHYSICAL EXAMINATION

The initial physical examination for chemical exposure must be rapid and focused. Airway, breathing, and circulation (ABCs) must be supported and cardiac function monitored.

Vital signs and cardiac function should be frequently reassessed, and a possible deterioration in the patient's status should be anticipated. The examination must focus on systems to help determine clues to the chemical exposure (i.e., pupils, skin, mucous membranes, etc.) and adjuvant diagnostic laboratory studies.

DIAGNOSTICS AND DIFFERENTIAL DIAGNOSIS

Useful diagnostic studies in the evaluation of a chemical exposure include CBC, an electrolyte panel to calculate the anion gap, and LFTs. If an inhalation injury is suspected, arterial blood gas (ABG) studies are indicated to assess ventilation or perfusion problems related to the possible exposure. Other diagnostics should be ordered as the history warrants; examples include methemoglobin level for possible carbon monoxide toxicity or blood/serum measurements of specific chemicals such as lead, arsenic, or mercury.

The differential diagnosis is dependent on the type, length, and route of exposure as well as on the patient's presenting signs and symptoms. Etiologies not related to the exposure (e.g., head trauma in a patient with altered mental status) and co-morbidities should be considered in the differential diagnosis. The poison control center and appropriate texts should be consulted for specific recommendations.

INITIAL STABILIZATION AND MANAGEMENT

The initial objective in the treatment of any chemical exposure or poisoning is to first protect and/or establish an airway and breathing and to ensure adequate circulation. Once the ABCs have been established, it is very important to consult the nearest poison control center. Poison control center personnel are able to help identify the chemical and guide appropriate treatment. The poison control telephone number is region specific, and *every primary care provider should be aware of the location of the telephone number to the regional poison control center.*

For ingestions, therapy depends on the material ingested. It is essential to check toxicologic clinical guidelines for specific recommendations based on the substance. Possible therapeutic modalities can include gastrointestinal decontamination via gastric lavage or with activated charcoal. Gastric lavage is accomplished by inserting an orogastric tube through the mouth to the stomach and then instilling and withdrawing warmed water or normal saline using a syringe. Gastric lavage is acceptable for some ingestions, such as for a patient who has ingested a potentially life-threatening amount of poison, and the procedure can be undertaken within 60 minutes of ingestion.[8] Because the act of lavage often initiates vomiting in the victim, adequate airway protection must always be ensured. Syrup of ipecac should not be administered routinely in the management of poisoned patients.[8] It should not be administered to a patient who has a decreased level or impending loss of consciousness or who has ingested a corrosive substance or hydrocarbon with high aspiration potential.[8] However, it may be useful for the telephone management of childhood ingestion in non–high-risk patients when the patient cannot reach medical care within 1 hour.[5]

Activated charcoal 1 to 2 g/kg is the mainstay of gastrointestinal decontamination. The charcoal adsorbs ingested substances due to its high surface area, thereby reducing absorption by the gastrointestinal tract. However, it is not helpful for caustic acids and alkalis, alcohols, lithium, or heavy metals.[5] Activated charcoal may be given with any diluent (e.g., water, magnesium citrate, sorbitol) mixed at 240 ml/30 g of charcoal. Magnesium citrate and sorbitol can enhance gastric motility and provide a decrease in the body's absorption of the toxin.[5] Cathartics should not be administered to children younger than 1 year of age.[9]

Specific toxins have specific antidotes. The poison control center is the single best source to quickly determine these antidotes. Table 33-1 can be used as a supplementary guide until the poison control center can be reached.

Most skin exposure to chemicals must be treated immediately with copious irrigation with water (i.e., "dilution is the solution to pollution"). Removal of saturated clothing and vigorous showering off of the chemical with large quantities of water are essential to prevent further damage to the patient. Exposed areas should be irrigated for a minimum of 15 to 30 minutes. This minimizes the amount of time that the offending agent is in direct contact with the skin, thus limiting the amount of damage caused by the chemical agent.

Diagnostics

Chemical Exposure

Initial
Pulse oximetry, if inhalation exposure

Laboratory
CBC and differential
Serum electrolytes
BUN
Creatinine
Serum glucose
Anion gap
LFTs
ABGs, if inhalation exposure
Methemoglobin for carbon monoxide (CO)
Serum lead, arsenic, mercury or other specific chemical tests*

Imagery
Chest x-ray may be indicated for inhalation exposure

*If indicated.

DISPOSITION AND REFERRAL

Once a patient has been initially stabilized, he or she should be referred for definitive care. If the exposure has been minimal, follow-up with the primary care provider may be all that is necessary. Severe intoxication may warrant admission to the intensive care unit. Hospital admission should be considered if the extent of exposure is unknown or if the patient has had a significant exposure; this is especially true for older adults and the very young.

PREVENTION AND PATIENT EDUCATION

Toxic and chemical exposure can be easily prevented by correctly labeling, storing, and locking up potentially harmful agents and by using appropriate protective measures such as wearing appropriate personal protective equipment. MSDSs are available online at http://www.ilpi.com/msds. The telephone number for the poison control center should be posted on every home and business telephone for ready access if required.

TABLE 33-1 Common Chemical Exposures and Initial Management

Toxin	Symptom/Physical Examination	Initial Stabilization	Management
Acids (toilet cleaner, drain cleaner, hydrochloric acid, sulfuric acid, battery acid)	Burns of oral mucosal, drooling, odynophagia, abdominal pain	Airway maintenance, circulatory support; sucralfate 1 g PO may decrease symptoms but not complications	Copious washing of mouth with cold water; do not induce vomiting, lavage, or administer charcoal
Alkalis	Caustic—burns	Dilution with water	Do not induce vomiting or lavage; large amounts of water/milk ingestion only
Anticholinergics	Flushing of skin, blurred vision/mydriasis, tacky mucous membranes, hypoactive bowel sounds	Physostigmine	0.5-2.0 mg IV/IM over 2 minutes, q 30-60 min p.r.n.
Carbon monoxide	Headache, cherry red lips, altered consciousness, coma	Oxygen	100%, hyperbaric oxygen if available
Ethylene glycol	Cough, dizziness, headache, abdominal pain, dullness, nausea, unconsciousness, vomiting	Ethanol	10 ml/kg of a 10% ethanol solution in D_5W over 30 minutes followed by 1.5 ml/kg/hr of a 10% ethanol solution to maintain blood alcohol level (BAL) of 100-150 mg/dl
Isopropyl alcohol	Ethyl alcohol–like (ETOH-like) effects (altered consciousness, stupor, slurred speech)	Lavage with charcoal	Do not induce emesis; lavage indicated if performed within 30 minutes of ingestion
	Dizziness, gastroenteritis, stupor to coma, incoordination	Emesis, gastric lavage, correction of electrolyte alterations	Nasogastric (NG) or orogastric tube with lavage; may require dialysis
Methanol	Cough, dizziness, headache, nausea, dry skin, redness	Ethanol	See ethylene glycol
Petroleum products	Vomiting, chest/abdominal pain, cough, dyspnea, fever, arrhythmias, seizures, altered level of consciousness	Prompt gastric lavage, O_2, respiratory support, and airway management	Gastric emptying initiated by ipecac in the alert patient (one time only); intubation and lavage in the unconscious or stuporous patient; activated charcoal is controversial; support of respiration and metabolic parameters

REFERENCES

1. Occupational Safety Health Administration: OSHA regulations. Standards—29 CFR. Hazards communication—1900. Available at http://www.osha.gov.
2. Occupational Safety Health Administration: Appendix III material safety data sheet. Available at http://www.osha.gov.
3. Rakel RE: *Saunder's manual of medical practice.* Philadelphia, 1996, WB Saunders.
4. National Safety Council: Report on injuries in America, 2001. Retrieved January 6, 2002 from the World Wide Web: http://www.nsc.org/library/rept2000.htm.
5. Larsen LC, Cummings DM: Oral poisonings: guidelines for initial evaluation and treatment, *Am Fam Phys* 57(1):85-92, 1998.
6. Verdon ME: Common clinical presentations of occupational respiratory disorders, *Am Fam Phys* 52(3):939-946, 1995.
7. Tintinalli JE, Ruiz E, Krome RL: *Emergency medicine: a comprehensive study guide,* ed 4, New York, 1996, McGraw-Hill.
8. Krenzelok EP, McGuigan M, Lheur P: Position statement: ipecac syrup. American Academy of Clinical Toxicology; European Association of Poisons Centres and Clinical Toxicologists, *J Toxicol Clin Toxicol* 35(7):699-709, 1997.
9. Hay WW and others: *Current pediatric diagnosis and treatment,* ed 13, Stanford, Conn, 1997, Appleton & Lange.

CHAPTER 34

Electrical Injuries

Updated by Terry Mahan Buttaro

DEFINITION/EPIDEMIOLOGY

Injuries from an electrical accident can be minor or can cause severe damage, electrocution, or death from cardiopulmonary arrest. In the United States, more than 100,000 people are killed each year in electrical accidents. Although the actual number of accidental and environmental electrical injuries is uncertain, the second leading cause of death in the workplace is electrical injury.[1] Lightning is the most common lethal natural phenomenon, causing approximately 90 deaths yearly.[2,3] From 20% to 30% of persons struck by lightning die; 70% of the survivors have permanent sequelae. Electrical injuries caused by low-voltage current account for 60% to 70% of reported electrical injury and are responsible for nearly half of deaths from electrical shock and 1% of accidental deaths in the home.[2] The majority of household electrocutions involve 110- or 220-V current and are usually due to failure to ground tools or appliances or the use of hair dryers or other electrical devices near water. Contact with low- and high-voltage electric current is responsible for a significant number of injuries in children.[4] The most common cause of electrical injury in children under age 6 years is oral contact with electrical cords or wall sockets and the placement of conductive bodies in wall sockets. Adolescent boys 11 to 18 years of age often sustain high-voltage injuries.[4]

Immediate emergency department referral/physician consultation is indicated for patients with electrical injuries.

PATHOPHYSIOLOGY

Electrical injuries result from the direct effects of current and from the conversion of electrical energy into thermal energy as current passes through body tissues. Factors that determine the severity and distribution of injury include the type of current, voltage, amperage, tissue resistance, surface contacted, pathway of current, duration of contact, and other associated trauma. Alternating current (AC), the more common cause of electrical injuries, is more dangerous than direct current (DC) because it can produce tetanic skeletal muscle contractions and prevent the victim from releasing the hold from the energized source, thus increasing current delivery to the victim. AC voltage at 25 to 300 Hz and 25 to 220 V is the common household current level and can easily cause ventricular fibrillation if the pathway of the current includes the heart. Low-voltage contact, although potentially lethal, does not result in the magnitude of tissue necrosis seen with high-voltage injury. The voltage in a lightning strike is in the range of 10 million to 2 billion V, but the duration of a lightning strike is short.

Heat generation is responsible for most of the burns seen with electrical injuries. Heat damage is proportional to tissue resistance. Tissues with high fluid and electrolyte content conduct electrical current better than others. Listed in decreasing order of magnitude of tissue necrosis are nerves, blood vessels, muscle, skin, tendon, fat, and bone. Nerve tissue has the least resistance to direct flow and therefore is more easily damaged.[5] Electrical current passing through the head or crossing the thorax is more likely to cause respiratory arrest or ventricular fibrillation than current passing through the leg. Skin, the initial barrier to current flow, is an effective insulator to deeper tissues. As current flows from the contact point, tissue with the least electrical resistance sustains the greatest current density and destructive injury. The most severe cutaneous and deep injuries are adjacent to contact sites, and the damage decreases with increasing distance from damage points.

CLINICAL PRESENTATION

The spectrum of electrical injury ranges from a transient unpleasant sensation to instantaneous death. Cardiopulmonary arrest is the primary cause of immediate fatalities from electrical injury and is common in patients with high-voltage electrical and lightning injury. Respiratory paralysis, burns, fractures, ruptured tympanic membrane, hyphema, vitreous hemorrhage, and injuries to the spinal cord, peripheral nervous system, and vascular systems are not uncommon.[1,6] Oliguria or anuria from deep tissue damage and rhabdomyolysis can cause acute renal failure.[6] Visible myoglobinuria indicates massive acute muscle necrosis and impending renal failure. Disseminated intravascular coagulation can result from massive trauma.[6] Neurologic deficits are sometimes evident immediately after the current exposure. However, complications such as reflex sympathetic dystrophy and motor neuron disease may not become apparent for days to months after the electrical trauma.[6,7] Long bone fracture often occurs with falls, and fractures (particularly of the vertebral column) can result from tetanic muscle contraction at the time of electrocution.[8] Cataracts can form up to 2 years after such injury. Direct injury to internal organs is uncommon.

PHYSICAL EXAMINATION

When evaluating a victim with an electrical injury, the primary care provider should always completely undress the patient to determine entry and exit wounds as well as associated injuries. Patients should be assessed for associated cranial, spinal, or other trauma, and the neck should initially be treated as being unstable, particularly with DC injuries. Arrhythmic conduction disturbances and infarct patterns can be present on the ECG. Cardiopulmonary presentations vary, and most patients lack the characteristic chest discomfort indicative of myocardial ischemia. Transient, mild paresthesias and complete and irreversible impairment of sensory or motor function, or both, can be present in patients with electrical injuries. Absent pulses, decreased peripheral perfusion, and impaired neurologic function are also seen in patients with acute vascular complications from electrical trauma.

Injuries consistent with findings of blunt trauma to the head, spinal cord, musculoskeletal, intrathoracic, and intraabdominal areas can be present in patients who were thrown from the energized current source, had forceful tetanic muscle contractions associated with AC injuries, or fell after losing consciousness and muscle control. Skin wounds are typically leathery or charred areas of full-thickness skin loss. The patient with lightning injury may have linear, punctate, feathery burns that often are referred to as "Lichtenberg's flowers." The entry and exit sites are usually depressed, giving the appearance that current exploded the tissue. Underlying injury to a major muscle compartment is accompanied by edema formation. Circulatory integrity is best judged with Doppler ultrasound of distal pulses.

DIAGNOSTICS

Initial studies include CBC, electrolytes, glucose, BUN, creatinine, coagulation profile, arterial blood gas (ABG) analysis, a creatinine phosphokinase (CK) level, a creatine kinase-muscle/brain (CK-MB) fraction, and a myoglobin level.[9] A 12-lead ECG and continuous cardiac monitoring are necessary for all patients with electrical injury. Fetal monitoring is necessary if the victim is pregnant.[10] Patients with suspected spinal injuries should receive cervical spine radiographs. Other x-ray studies are indicated to exclude fracture if localized edema and pain are present.[8] Consideration of other diagnostic studies should be coordinated with the consulting specialists.

DIFFERENTIAL DIAGNOSIS

The diagnosis of electrical injury may be unclear, particularly in unwitnessed cases in which the victim is confused, amnesic, or unconscious or in instances in which external signs of injury are absent. In these cases, several conditions should be considered as part of the differential diagnosis: cardiopulmonary arrest, arrhythmias, peripheral neuropathies, seizures, and nonelectrical trauma. Circumstances surrounding the electrical injuries should also be sought to determine the possible mechanism of the injury. Precipitating factors such as intoxication, suicidal intention, or foul play should be considered.

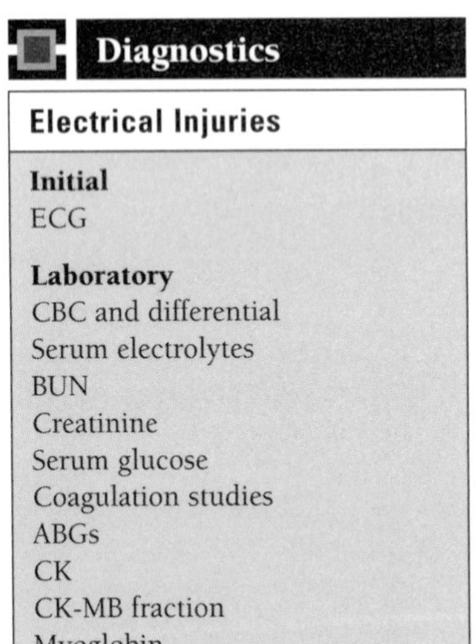

Diagnostics

Electrical Injuries

Initial
ECG

Laboratory
CBC and differential
Serum electrolytes
BUN
Creatinine
Serum glucose
Coagulation studies
ABGs
CK
CK-MB fraction
Myoglobin

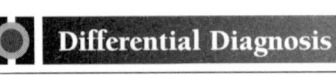

Differential Diagnosis

Electrical Injuries

Cardiopulmonary arrest
Arrhythmias
Peripheral neuropathies
Seizures
Nonelectrical trauma

INITIAL STABILIZATION AND MANAGEMENT

Immediate priorities for patients include the airway, breathing, and circulation (ABCs) taught in basic life support (BLS) and advanced cardiac life support (ACLS) classes. The cervical spine should be immobilized and the airway should be secured while supporting respiration, with adequate oxygenation and stabilization of circulation if required. CPR must be initiated, and the emergency medical services (EMS) system should be activated if necessary. Intravascular volume is replenished with lactated Ringer's or normal saline solution with a bolus of 10 to 20 ml/kg to maintain urine output at approximately 1 ml/kg/hr. Myoglobinuria is treated by alkalinizing the urine by adding sodium bicarbonate to the IV fluids (i.e., 44 to 50 mEq of bicarbonate to 1 L of lactated Ringer's or normal saline solution).[11]

Wound care involves treating both cutaneous and deep soft tissue injuries with a saline dressing. Consultation with a surgeon should be considered to evaluate the need for formal wound exploration and/or debridement. Tetanus prophylaxis should be updated. Prophylactic antibiotics have not been shown to decrease episodes of infection and usually are not indicated. Management of other complications resulting from electrical trauma generally follows standard emergency therapy.

DISPOSITION AND REFERRAL

Prompt specialty consultation is required in addition to the liberal involvement of surgical specialists. All patients who have lost consciousness or sustained cardiac or respiratory arrest, as well as those with ischemic chest pain, myoglobinuria, or significant burn wounds, should be hospitalized. A referral to a burn center is often necessary for electrical burns because considerable injury to deeper neurovascular and musculoskeletal structures may not be obvious until several days after the injury.

PREVENTION AND PATIENT AND FAMILY EDUCATION

All discharged patients should have reliable home support. Patients should be advised to return immediately to their primary care provider if any symptoms occur. A specific follow-up should be arranged with a primary care provider familiar with electrical injuries, and patients should receive careful explanation of the injury and recuperative process. Open sockets and outlets must be covered with "childproof" devices, and children must be watched carefully. Plug-in electrical appliances should be kept away from the bathtub. Community education programs, particularly at school and at work, are necessary to help prevent accidents. Safety standards in industry and in the community must be constantly updated and enforced.[12]

REFERENCES

1. Pinto DS, Clardy P: *Environmental electrical injuries*. Retrieved July 31, 2002 from the World Wide Web: http://www.uptodate.com.
2. Rakel R: *Textbook of family practice*, ed 5, Philadelphia, 1995, WB Saunders.
3. Lightning associated deaths: United States, *MMWR* 47(19):391-394, 1998.
4. Rai J and others: Electrical injuries: a 30-year review, *J Trauma* 46(5):933-936, 1999.
5. Tintinalli J, Ruiz E, Krone R: *Emergency medicine*, New York, 1996, McGraw-Hill.
6. Fish RM: Electrical injuries, part 2: specific injuries, *J Emerg Med* 18(1):27-34, 2000.
7. Jafari H and others: Motor neuron disease is a potential complication of lightning or electrical shock, *J Neurol Neurosurg Psychiatr* 71(2):265-267, 2001.
8. Hostetler MA, Davis CO: Galeazzi fracture resulting from electrical shock, *Pediatr Emerg Care* 16(4):258-259, 2000.

9. Schwartz GR: *Principles and practice of emergency medicine*, Philadelphia, 1992, Lea & Febiger.
10. Fish RM: Electrical injuries, part 3: cardiac monitoring indications, the pregnant patient, and lightning, *J Emerg Med* 18(2):181-187, 2000.
11. Bennett J, Plum F: *Cecil textbook of medicine*, Philadelphia, 1996, WB Saunders.
12. Rosen P and others: *Emergency medicine: concepts and clinical practice*, ed 4, St Louis, 1998, Mosby.

CHAPTER 35

Head Trauma

Denise A. Vanacore; Updated by Terry Mahan Buttaro

DEFINITION/EPIDEMIOLOGY

Each year more than 50,000 people die from traumatic brain injury (TBI).[1] Most of these deaths are related to motor vehicle accidents, violence, or falls. Other causes include sports injuries and bicycle accidents. In children, bicycle accidents account for an estimated 140,000 head injuries each year.[1] Head injuries from falls occur most often in children younger than 2 years of age and in persons older than 65 years of age, whereas motor vehicle accidents are the leading cause of brain injury in persons ages 5 to 64 years.[1,2] Approximately 11% of falls are fatal, usually from TBI.[1] Older patients are particularly vulnerable and can sustain a subdural hematoma even when the head injury is not associated with loss of consciousness.[3]

The National Center for Injury Prevention and Control reports that 5.3 million Americans have a TBI-related disability.[1] Brain injury can be mild or severe enough to dramatically affect a patient's intellectual and physical capacity, as well as their psychologic, social, and economic well-being. Loss of consciousness is one of the most significant indicators of brain injury. The severity of damage can be described by an injury-rating system such as the Glasgow Coma Scale (GCS) score (Box 35-1). The GCS assesses eye opening responses, motor responses, and verbal responses. A number is assigned for the level of functioning attained in each category and then totaled.

BOX 35-1

GLASGOW COMA SCALE

Sign	*Score*
EYE OPENING	
Spontaneous	4
To verbal command	3
To pain	2
No response	1
BEST MOTOR RESPONSE	
Obeys verbal commands	6
Localizes pain	5
Movement or withdrawal to pain	4
Flexion response to pain (decorticate)	3
Extension response to pain (decerebrate)	2
No response	1
BEST VERBAL RESPONSE	
Alert and oriented	5
Converses but confused/disoriented	4
Nonsensical/inappropriate words	3
Nonspecific sounds	2
No response	1

A normal patient has a score of 15, whereas a patient who is brain dead has a score of 3. Minor head trauma is defined as an initial GCS of 13 to 15 and a period of unconsciousness of less than 20 minutes. Moderate head injury refers to an initial GCS score of 9 to 12 with or without loss of consciousness. Severe head trauma is defined as an initial GCS of less than 8 or a comatose state for 6 hours or more.[4]

Immediate emergency department referral/physician consultation is indicated for head trauma with alteration in level of consciousness, paralysis, paresthesia, rhinorrhea, raccoon's sign (ecchymosis beneath both eyes), Battle's sign, otorrhea, and hemotympanum.

PATHOPHYSIOLOGY

Head trauma can consist of soft tissue injury or skull fracture, or both. Brain injury from trauma can occur in two stages: primary and secondary. Primary injury is sustained as a direct result of the initial insult and may result from lacerations or contusions of the brain or from direct disruption of brain tissue by the shearing of axons. Secondary injury may occur as a result of increased intracranial pressure (ICP), cerebral hypoxia, or decreased cerebral blood flow. This may cause further neuronal damage, which can compromise an already injured brain. The cranial vault is a fixed space that contains the brain, cerebrospinal fluid (CSF), and blood. Because the skull limits intracranial volume, neurologic damage after head injury can be directly related to cerebral edema that causes increased ICP, which in turn decreases cerebral blood flow and causes cerebral ischemia.

CLINICAL PRESENTATION

It is important to establish the mechanism of the trauma, the stability or progression of the patient's symptoms, the patient's prior condition, and the patient's significant medical history. The cause of the injury should be determined: Was it accidental or intentional?[2] Changes in mentation and level of consciousness should be noted and elicited from witnesses. A history of amnesia for the traumatic event often indicates altered consciousness. It is also necessary to ascertain consciousness before the head injury to determine other pathologic conditions such as stroke, myocardial infarction, or respiratory distress. Additional causes of altered mental status, such as hypoglycemia, drug overdose, hyperthermia, or arrhythmias, must also be investigated. Alcohol intoxication can mask the signs and symptoms of a head injury; therefore it is important to determine if alcohol was involved. The history should also elicit complaints of headache, nausea, vomiting, unsteady gait, visual changes, tinnitus, difficulty concentrating, and emotional lability.

PHYSICAL EXAMINATION

The patient with head trauma can fluctuate from being awake and alert to being comatose and in respiratory distress. The initial evaluation should follow the standard protocol developed for all trauma patients. The patient's airway, breathing, and circulation (ABCs) and cervical spine must be evaluated and stabilized. The initial observation should assess the patient's level of consciousness, vital signs, and determination of GCS score. A quick but thorough neurologic examination is necessary to assess brain injury, focal deficits, and patient stability. The neurologic examination should include pupillary response, extraocular motion, Romberg's test, gait, finger to nose, memory, and concentration. The skull must also be examined for the presence of fractures, penetrating injuries, lacerations, or CSF drainage. It is also important to perform repeated neurologic examinations to determine if the patient is stable, improving, or deteriorating. However, a normal neurologic examination does not eliminate the possibility of brain injury.

DIAGNOSTICS

Because patients with head injury can have an associated cervical spine fracture, an x-ray examination of the cervical spine is necessary. A nonenhanced computed tomography (CT) scan is indicated for patients with a depressed or deteriorating level of consciousness, skull fracture, neurologic deficit, open head wound, penetrating head injury, or amnesia or if there is a high risk of intracranial injury. Repeat CT scans may be necessary if neurologic deficits develop. Laboratory studies should include CBC, electrolytes, serum glucose, urinalysis, arterial blood gases (ABGs), coagulation panel, blood alcohol level and, if indicated, a drug screen. Blood for type and crossmatch should be sent immediately. Further examinations may be indicated in cases of severe trauma.

DIFFERENTIAL DIAGNOSIS

The differential diagnosis must include skull fracture, concussion, cerebral contusion, epidural hematoma, subdural hematoma, subarachnoid bleed, cerebral edema, and penetrating injuries. *Cerebral concussion* is defined as the loss of consciousness without significant anatomic damage to the brain. The severity of the injury is quantified by the duration of amnesia—the length of amnesia before impact (antegrade amnesia) plus the length of amnesia after impact (retrograde amnesia). It is usually helpful to determine the time interval between the first thing and the last thing remembered. Cerebral contusions usually occur on the undersurface of the poles of the frontal lobes or on the poles of

Diagnostics

Head Trauma

Initial
Pulse oximetry

Laboratory
CBC and differential*
Serum electrolytes*
Serum glucose*
Urinalysis*
ABGs*
Coagulation panel*
Blood alcohol/drug level*

Imaging
CT scan
X-ray of spine

*If indicated.

Differential Diagnosis

Head Trauma

Skull fracture/concussion/contusion
Epidural/subdural hematoma
Subarachnoid bleed
Cerebral edema
Penetrating injuries

the temporal lobes. The patient is typically awake and alert after the initial injury, but increasing ICP, a decreased level of consciousness, and focal neurologic deficits may develop as the contusion mass increases in size.

INITIAL STABILIZATION AND MANAGEMENT

The main priority in the patient with head injury is the same as that for all trauma patients—management of the ABCs and cervical spine. Once that is achieved, the principal goal is to assess the primary injury and to rapidly recognize a surgically correctable lesion. CT scans are not indicated for patients with minor head trauma or a GCS score of 15 or more. Patients without loss of consciousness, amnesia, focal neurologic deficits, or depressed skull fracture do not require a CT scan. These patients may be discharged home if observation is available and instructions are given on proper patient evaluation. Minor head injuries (loss of consciousness for less than 5 minutes, amnesia, a GCS score of 12 to 14, impaired alertness, or depressed skull fracture) require a diagnostic CT scan.

Health care providers must always be aware of the "talk and deteriorate" syndrome. Patients with this syndrome utter recognizable words after the head injury and then deteriorate to a severe, brain-injured condition within 48 hours. The most common neurologic findings are altered mental status and focal hemispheric deficits. Early and appropriate use of CT scanning is helpful in detecting significant intracranial lesions before clinical neurologic deterioration occurs.

DISPOSITION AND REFERRAL

The patient may be discharged home with proper instructions if the CT scan is normal and if a family member or friend can provide close observation for 24 hours. If no one is available to monitor the patient or if there is evidence of a pathologic condition, the patient should be admitted to the hospital for observation. A patient who has had more than 5 minutes of unconsciousness, posttraumatic seizures, a GCS score of 12 to 14, focal neurologic deficits, a lesion on the CT scan, or a moderate head injury (a GCS score of 9 to 12) should be hospitalized, stabilized, and closely observed for any neurologic deterioration; a neurosurgical evaluation is also indicated. Patients with severe head trauma (a GCS score of 8 or less, penetrating skull injuries, or compound skull fractures) should be evaluated at the nearest hospital and have a neurosurgical evaluation.

PREVENTION AND PATIENT EDUCATION

Specific instructions must be provided to those who will be observing the patient who is discharged home. The patient should remain in the care of a competent caregiver and rest in a quiet environment for the first 24 hours after discharge. The first 24 hours after the injury are the most important. The patient should return for treatment if any of the following develop: drowsiness or difficulty awakening (the patient should be awakened every 2 hours during sleep), continuous nausea, vomiting more than twice, seizures/convulsions, visual disturbances or pupillary changes, new-onset weakness or an inability to move body parts, severe headache, confusion, personality changes, unusual restlessness, difficulty breathing, dizziness, or difficulty walking.[4] Aspirin (and medications that contain aspirin), alcohol, and narcotics should not be taken for 1 week after the injury.

Patients should also be informed about the posttraumatic or postconcussion syndrome, which is not life threatening but may disable a patient for weeks to months. Symptoms may include headache, tinnitus, memory loss, dizziness, giddiness, poor concentration, emotional lability, irritability, nervousness, disturbed sleep, fatigue, and decreased libido. Symptoms last for 2 to 6 weeks in most cases but can be present for 1 to 2 years. Treatment consists of rest, reassurance, and analgesics. It is also extremely important that patients return to work as soon as possible, even if a reduced workload is necessary.

Patients must be educated regarding safety issues such as the proper use of bicycle helmets, seatbelts, and car seats for infants and children. Safety issues in the home should also be reviewed (e.g., staircases, gates, throw rugs, and lighting) in an attempt to reduce falls in children and older adults.

REFERENCES

1. National Center for Injury Prevention and Control. Retrieved May 30, 2002 from the World Wide Web: http://www.cdc.gov.
2. Caviness AC: Skull fractures in children. Retrieved May 30, 2002 from the World Wide Web: http://www.uptodate.com.
3. Evans RW: Geriatric headache, *Ann Long-Term Care* 10(5):28-35, 2002.
4. Logan P: *Principles of practice for the acute care nurse practitioner*, Stamford, Conn, 1999, Appleton & Lange.

CHAPTER 36

Hypotension

JoAnn Trybulski

DEFINITION/EPIDEMIOLOGY

Hypotension, or low blood pressure, is a relative term, and its evaluation in the office setting presents a challenge. Whatever the absolute blood pressure measurement or cause, primary care providers must be prepared to manage hypotension in the ambulatory setting.

In those patients accustomed to elevated pressures, a sudden decrease to 110 mm Hg systolic may cause symptoms. On the other hand, some patients may routinely have a systolic blood pressure in the 90s and be asymptomatic. Clinical conditions may also produce symptomatic low blood pressure. Postural hypotension is low blood pressure that results from assumption of the upright position and has been found in epidemiologic surveys to affect from 5% to 20% of patients over 65 years of age.[1] Another form of hypotension, postprandial hypotension, occurs after meals. The causes of symptomatic hypotension are multiple, and the morbidity ranges from the transient symptoms of vasovagal episodes to life-threatening conditions such as hemorrhage, pulmonary embolus, myocardial failure, myocardial infarction, or arrhythmia.

Immediate emergency department referral/ physician consultation is indicated for unstable, hemodynamically compromised patients.

PATHOPHYSIOLOGY

When blood pressure is decreased, one explanation may be visualized as an alteration in one of the three basic components necessary for the maintenance of blood pressure. The first component is the state of contraction of the muscles in the vessel walls themselves. Some physiologic, endocrine states or autonomic nervous system dysfunction may cause abnormal relaxation of the muscles in the vessel walls, sequestering blood and causing a decrease in blood pressure. The second component is the intravascular volume. When fluid is depleted through bleeding, vomiting, or diarrhea, this decrease in intravascular volume produces a low blood pressure. The final component is the state of the cardiac muscle. Any failure in critical pumping function of the heart produces decreased pressure in the vascular system.

The pathophysiologic mechanisms for postural hypotension involve autonomic failure or volume depletion. Autonomic failure represents a dysfunction of the postganglionic sympathetic nerves in which these neurons fail to release appropriate amounts of norepinephrine, producing impaired vasoconstriction, thus reducing intravascular volume and producing hypotension.[1] Autonomic failure is produced by some medications (e.g., antihypertensives, vasodilators, nitrates, calcium channel blockers, antidepressants, opiates, alcohol) or as a result of neurologic conditions such as reflex syncope (e.g., carotid sinus hypersensitivity, micturition syncope, defecation syncope), postural orthostatic tachycardia syndrome, degenerative neurologic diseases, and some peripheral neuropathy syndromes.[1] Decreased baroreceptor sensitivity is the pathophysiologic mechanism for the often observed, milder form of postural hypotension seen in older persons.[1]

The mechanism of postprandial hypotension is poorly understood. Normally, there is meal-induced pooling of blood in the splanchnic circulation, with resulting sympathetic nervous system activation as compensatory mechanism. A default in this sympathetic compensation produces a decrease in cardiac output and systemic vascular resistance, resulting in hypotension.[1] Other factors implicated include vasodilation produced by postprandial insulin release or gastrointestinal peptides that have vasoactive effects.[1]

Symptomatic hypotension produces low perfusion of all body tissues. Vital organs such as the kidneys, brain, and heart are particularly at risk in hypoperfusion states. Hypoperfusion of the kidneys precipitates failure. With inadequate oxygen supplied to the brain, function and consciousness are impaired. Moreover, hypoperfusion of cardiac muscle carries the risk of myocardial ischemia.[2]

CLINICAL PRESENTATION

Most patients with hypotension complain of being dizzy or light-headed. Some may relate that their symptoms occur only when they sit or stand. Patients exhibiting a vasovagal response also describe a sensation of impending syncope. Tachycardia is produced as a compensatory attempt to maintain blood pressure. The existence of associated signs and symptoms such as vomiting, chest pain, diaphoresis, urticaria, dyspnea, hematochezia, or palpitations provides important clues concerning the etiology of the hypotension.

PHYSICAL EXAMINATION

Pulse and blood pressure are measured in the lying, sitting, and standing positions if patient response allows it. A low blood pressure, absolute or in comparison with the patient's normal pressure, when the patient is lying down confirms the diagnosis, particularly if the decrease is associated with dizziness, light-headedness, or tachycardia.

DIAGNOSTICS

A 20 mm Hg decrease in systolic blood pressure, a 10 mm Hg decrease in diastolic blood pressure, or symptoms of dizziness or light-headedness when the patient changes position from lying to standing confirm the diagnosis of postural or orthostatic hypotension.[3] Failure to increase the pulse with the decrease in blood pressure is indicative of cardiac disorder or autonomic dysfunction.[3] However, young patients may maintain their systolic blood pressure and exhibit an increased pulse with a position change in conjunction with symptoms of cerebral hypoperfusion (fatigue, light-headedness, exercise intolerance, or cognitive impairment); this represents the syndrome of postural autonomic tachycardia.[1]

Additional physical examination and diagnostic tests, including an ECG, electrolytes, glucose, BUN, creatinine, chest x-ray examination, computed tomography (CT) or lung scan, and endocrine studies, are obtained to confirm or eliminate conditions as the cause of hypotension, based on the patient's presentation. In addition, a thorough medication history is obtained and a side effect profile for each drug is reviewed because many hypertension medications, psychotropics, or muscle relaxants have hypotension as a potential side effect.

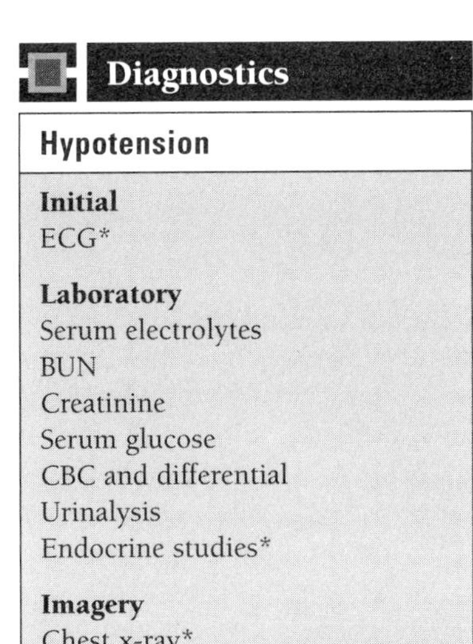

Diagnostics

Hypotension

Initial
ECG*

Laboratory
Serum electrolytes
BUN
Creatinine
Serum glucose
CBC and differential
Urinalysis
Endocrine studies*

Imagery
Chest x-ray*
CT scan

*If indicated.

DIFFERENTIAL DIAGNOSIS

See the Differential Diagnosis box for possible causes of hypotension.

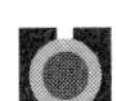

Differential Diagnosis

Hypotension

Hypovolemia
Vasovagal response
Myocardial disease
Heart failure
Active bleeding
Pulmonary embolus
Arrhythmia
Diabetic neuropathy
Malnutrition
Adrenal insufficiency
Drug-induced condition
Organic dementia
Anaphylaxis
Heat exhaustion
Autonomic dysfunction

INITIAL STABILIZATION AND MANAGEMENT

The patient with hypotension initially should be placed in a recumbent position. Supplemental oxygen is essential for those patients in whom bleeding, myocardial infarction or failure, arrhythmia, or pulmonary embolus is suspected or for any patient with breathing difficulty. If hypovolemia is suspected, a fluid challenge of 250 to 500 ml of normal saline solution is administered intravenously, and its effect on the blood pressure is assessed.[4]

The suspected etiology of the hypotension guides further diagnostic evaluation and management. Nonpharmacologic interventions for postural hypotension include arising slowly; avoiding coughing, straining, or walking in hot weather; raising the head of the bed 10 to 20 degrees for sleep; using custom-fitted elastic stockings (although these may not be tolerated by patients with motor dysfunction or neuropathies); exercising; increasing water intake; and crossing the legs to stand.[5] Postprandial hypertension treatment recommendations include a reduction in carbohydrate intake, avoiding large meals, limiting alcohol ingestion, and reducing activity immediately after eating.[5]

Pharmacologic therapy is instituted in conjunction with physician consultation. Medications that are used include fludrocortisone as a first-line agent for orthostatic hypotension; second-line agents are sympathomimetics such as milodrine.[5] Supplementary agents such as nonsteroidal antiinflammatory drugs, caffeine, and erythropoietin are used in conjunction with first- or second-line medications.[5] There are a variety of third-line agents and investigational medications.

DISPOSITION AND REFERRAL

Patients with hypotension as a result of dehydration may be hydrated on an outpatient basis. Patients with poor response to a fluid challenge may need rapid transport to an emergency facility for further diagnosis, consultation, and treatment.

PREVENTION AND PATIENT EDUCATION

Patients taking medication who have orthostatic hypotension as a side effect are taught to change position or to arise from sitting slowly. Maintaining adequate fluid intake while in a hot environment, and when vomiting or diarrhea occurs, is essential to avoid hypovolemia from dehydration. Patients at risk for dehydration (or their caregivers) are instructed to report any signs of dehydration (e.g., dry mucous membranes, lightheadedness, altered mentation, or diminished urine output) to the primary care provider.

REFERENCES

1. Kaufman H, Kaplan NM, Freeman R: Mechanisms and causes of orthostatic and postprandial hypotension, *Up to Date*. Retrieved January 18, 2001 from the World Wide Web: http://www.uptodate.com
2. Beique F, Ramsey V: Cardiopulmonary circulation in the critically ill. In Garrard C, Foex P, Westaby S, editors: *Principles and practices of critical care*, New York, 1997, Oxford University Press.
3. Reilly BM, editor: *Practice strategies in outpatient medicine*, ed 2, Philadelphia, 1991, WB Saunders.
4. Iseke RJ: Heat related illnesses. In Noble J, editor: *Textbook of primary care medicine*, ed 3, St Louis, 1996, Mosby.
5. Kaufman H, Freeman R, Kaplan NM: Treatment of orthostatic and postprandial hypotension, *Up to Date*. Retrieved February 18, 2001 from the World Wide Web: http://www.uptodate.com

CHAPTER 37

Ocular Emergencies

Updated by Terry Mahan Buttaro

Severe trauma, ocular burns, and orbital cellulitis are serious eye conditions in which a delay in definitive care potentiates permanent damage. "Red eye" is the most common ocular concern seen in primary care and may be related to a variety of inflammatory and infectious diseases (see Table 75-1).[1] A number of other entities cause acute vision loss and require urgent diagnosis and treatment if vision is to be preserved (Table 37-1).

Immediate emergency department/ophthalmology referral is indicated for orbital fracture, severe trauma, penetrating eye injury, rust ring, acute-angle glaucoma, retinal detachment, hyphema, hyperactive bacterial conjunctivitis, endophthalmitis, uveitis, herpetic keratitis, central artery occlusion peripheral ulcer, and vitreous hemorrhage.

Trauma, Eyelid Laceration, Foreign Bodies, and Corneal Abrasion

DEFINITION/EPIDEMIOLOGY

Eye injuries from foreign bodies may involve dirt or debris, high-speed tools, tree branches, or exploding fragments. Trauma may be blunt or penetrating and result in orbit fracture with nerve entrapment, hyphema, eyelid laceration, globe rupture, or corneal abrasion. Corneal abrasions are superficial lesions that result from trauma, foreign bodies, or exposure to ultraviolet (UV) light.[2]

CLINICAL PRESENTATION AND PHYSICAL EXAMINATION

Patients often can describe the circumstances surrounding the injury. The pertinent history should include the use of contact lenses, immunization status, medications, allergies, history of glaucoma, previous eye injuries, and mechanism of injury. Pain, photophobia, and constant tearing are common with corneal abrasions or foreign bodies. Diplopia or blurred, cloudy, or reduced vision is often identified with trauma.

Whether simple or complex, eye trauma requires a careful examination of the entire eye (including funduscopic examination) to exclude serious injury. The initial inspection should assess location, degree of enophthalmus or exophthalmus, visual acuity or two-point discrimination, and pupillary light response. The presence of lacerations, penetrating or perforating wounds, edema, foreign bodies, hemorrhage or blood in the anterior chamber (hyphema), tearing, scleral injection, rust ring, and visual fields should be determined. Extraocular movements are indicated to exclude muscle/nerve entrapment. Eyelid inversion is necessary to inspect for foreign bodies that may have lodged beneath the lids. Palpation of the orbital bones is essential in suspected orbital trauma. *If globe rupture or overt trauma is considered, a no-touch examination is indicated to prevent further damage.* Testing should be deferred and the eye shielded.

DIAGNOSTICS AND DIFFERENTIAL DIAGNOSIS

Cobalt blue light or a slit lamp examination with fluorescein stain may reveal corneal abrasions. X-ray examinations or computed tomography (CT) scans are necessary for suspected fractures or penetrating foreign bodies. The differential diagnosis includes foreign bodies, corneal abrasion or ulceration, orbit fracture, globe rupture, hyphema, and detached retina. Intraocular disease, blood dyscrasia, and trauma should be considered for hyphema.

INITIAL STABILIZATION AND MANAGEMENT

Bleeding must be stabilized; overt eye trauma requires eye shielding. A tetanus booster is necessary. Tetracaine 0.5% or another optical topical analgesic may be necessary during the examination but should not be prescribed for pain. Using a slit lamp or magnifying glass, foreign bodies embedded superficially in the cornea may be removed with a 25-gauge needle by practitioners skilled in the procedure. Normal saline irrigation may be indicated to flush superficial dirt or debris (see Chapter 33). A moistened cotton applicator may also be used to swab superficial foreign bodies. Treatment of abrasions consists of providing pain relief with cycloplegic medications and nonsteroidal antiinflammatory drugs, preventing infections with topical antibiotics, and promoting reepithelialization. Recent studies have questioned the efficacy of eye patching.[2] Patching is no longer required for small (<5-mm) and noncentral lesions; patching should never be used to treat corneal abrasions from contact lenses because increased pseudomonal infections have occurred in these cases.

DISPOSITION AND REFERRAL

Patients with suspected orbit fracture, globe rupture, hyphema, retinal detachment, eyelid laceration, or rust ring require immediate ophthalmology referral. For corneal abrasions or foreign bodies, patients should have follow-up in 24 hours to document healing. If the abrasion is healing, the eye patch can be removed at this time, and antibiotics should be continued for 7 to 14 days. An ophthalmology consult is indicated if the abrasion has not healed in 24 hours.

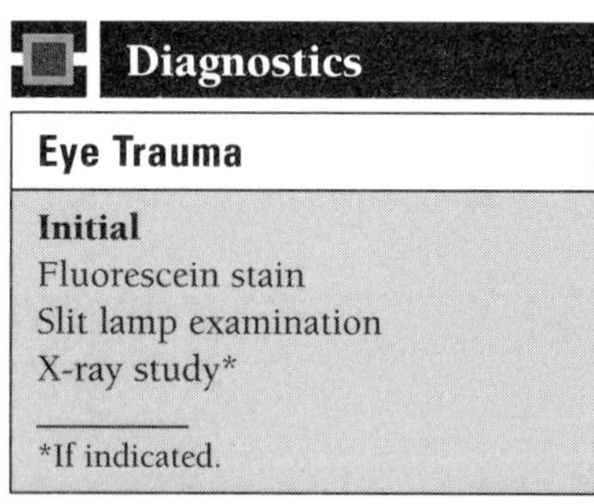

Diagnostics

Eye Trauma

Initial
Fluorescein stain
Slit lamp examination
X-ray study*

*If indicated.

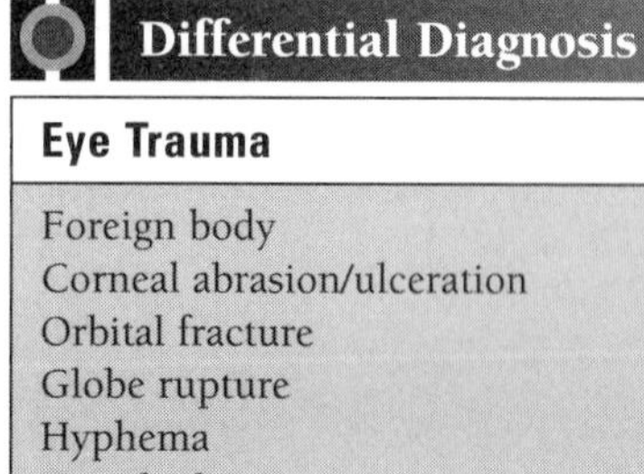

Differential Diagnosis

Eye Trauma

Foreign body
Corneal abrasion/ulceration
Orbital fracture
Globe rupture
Hyphema
Detached retina

TABLE 37-1 Acute Vision Loss Treatment Guidelines

Entity	Clinical Presentation	Physical Examination	Management
Hyphema	History of blunt trauma; variable vision decrements; no pain	Minute to obvious blood in anterior chamber; pupil reacts poorly; retina obscure	Urgent ophthalmology referral
Vitreous hemorrhage	Painless; sudden shower of floaters; etiologies include retinal tear, hypertension, vein occlusion	Vision variable; possibly no red reflex; retina obscured	Urgent telephone consultation/referral to ophthalmology for possible hospital admission and vitrectomy
Hemianopsia (differential diagnoses: stroke, migraine, hysteria)	Blindness in ½ visual field of one/both eyes Hysteria: C/O tubular/tunnel vision	Visual field abnormalities Hysteria: Vision testing variable; no discernible abnormalities	Suspected stroke: Physician consultation and urgent transfer to stroke center/emergency department All patients with hemianopsia require MD evaluation
Retinal hemorrhage	Variable, painless vision loss associated with trauma, hypertensive crisis, systemic disease, local ocular conditions	Decreased visual acuity	Physician consultation indicated for evaluation because treatment is based on cause Emergency department transfer may be indicated for hypertensive emergency
Central artery occlusion/ central vein occlusion	Vein: Sudden, variable vision loss Artery: More complete vision loss Systemic factors: emboli, high blood pressure, diabetes, blood disorders, reduced perfusion	Vein: Dilated tortuous veins, retinal and macular edema, multiple diffuse hemorrhages Artery: Pale retina/optic disc, boxcar retinal veins	Urgent ophthalmology referral Permanent vision loss may occur in 1 hour in central artery occlusion Evaluate for embolic source if arterial Consider giant cell arteritis in older adults
Retinal detachment	Sudden, painless, unilateral vision loss or hazy/smoky change in visual acuity; past medical history may reveal recent cataract surgery	Unilateral visual decrement; visibly detached retina	Urgent ophthalmology referral Permanent central vision loss may occur in 24-48 hours if macula is involved
Retrobulbar neuritis	Pain with eye movement; multiple causes, may be unilateral/bilateral; unilateral retrobulbar neuritis may indicate multiple sclerosis	Central scotoma; optic head nonhyperemic	Ophthalmology referral within 24-48 hours
Optic neuritis	May have pain with eye movement; multiple systemic causes, including neurologic, systemic, and environmental chemical exposure	Large vein congestion, central scotoma, hyperemic optic nerve head, blurred disc margins, sluggish pupillary reflex	Ophthalmology referral within 24-48 hours
Acute-angle glaucoma	See Table 75-1		Urgent ophthalmology referral
Endophthalmitis/uveitis	See Table 75-1		Urgent ophthalmology referral

PREVENTION AND PATIENT EDUCATION

See Prevention and Patient Education under Ocular Burns.

Ocular Burns

DEFINITION/EPIDEMIOLOGY

Ocular burns may be caused by an acidic (battery acid) or alkaline (lye) agent or vapor, as well as by UV light. The deep penetration of alkaline exposures typically causes more damage.

CLINICAL PRESENTATION AND PHYSICAL EXAMINATION

Eye exposures to chemicals usually cause significant eye pain and may cause light sensitivity. UV radiation can produce a painful actinic keratitis after exposure to arc welding, high-voltage short circuits, tanning lights, and reflection from snow. Vision loss is dependent on the type and length of exposure.

DIAGNOSTICS AND DIFFERENTIAL DIAGNOSIS

Funduscopic examination, fluorescein stain, and a slit lamp evaluation are essential diagnostic tools. The nature of the exposure (acidic vs. alkaline) must also be determined.

INITIAL STABILIZATION AND MANAGEMENT

Immediate copious normal saline irrigation for a minimum of 20 to 30 minutes is indicated for chemical burns to the eye. Topical anesthetics (tetracaine hydrochloride, 1 to 2 drops of a 0.5% solution) and lid retractors are advantageous for irrigation, particularly with severe blepharospasm. Lid retraction with irrigation is important after exposure to alkaline agents because residual particles can cause progressive damage. Litmus paper is used to monitor pH; irrigation is continued until

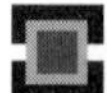

Diagnostics

Ocular Burns
Initial Fluorescein stain Slit lamp examination

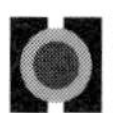

Differential Diagnosis

Ocular Burns
Acidic burns Alkaline burns

the pH is 7.4.[3] Oral analgesics, cycloplegic medications, and topical antibiotics are used to prevent pain and secondary infection.

Treatment for exposure to UV light, tanning lights, or welders' arcs includes a lubricating ointment, oral analgesics, and eye patching. Topical anesthetics may be used once for the examination but should not be prescribed for pain.

DISPOSITION AND REFERRAL

Hospitalization and an ophthalmologic consultation are indicated, because complications can be extensive. Alkalis are associated with increased ocular pressure from scleral contraction and damage to the trabecular meshwork. Other complications include angle-closure glaucoma, scarring, and keratitis sicca.

PREVENTION AND PATIENT EDUCATION

Intense eye pain and a sudden visual disturbance are both important symptoms that should not be ignored. All individuals should be reminded to wear safety glasses when playing racket sports or working with chemicals or tools. The importance of avoiding bright sunlight and the need to wear sunglasses that block UV light should also be stressed.

First aid measures should include a careful explanation and demonstration of how to flush the eyes at home. After flushing, follow-up is recommended if (1) pain persists, (2) a whitening or redness of the eye is noted, or (3) there is a change in visual acuity. It is important that patients receive careful instruction regarding the use of eye medications. In addition, patients should be reminded to not operate heavy equipment or drive while wearing the eye patch.

REFERENCES

1. Hara J: The red eye: diagnosis and treatment, *Am Fam Physician* 54(8):2423-2428, 1996.
2. Torok P: Corneal abrasions: diagnosis and management, *Am Fam Physician* 53(8):2521-2531, 1996.
3. Edlich RF and others: Chemical injuries. In Marx JA and others, editors: *Rosen's emergency medicine: concepts and clinical practice*, ed 5, St Louis, 2002, Mosby.

CHAPTER 38

Poisoning

Denise A. Vanacore; Updated by Terry Mahan Buttaro

DEFINITION/EPIDEMIOLOGY

Although poisonings are most commonly associated with ingestion, toxic effects can also be caused by injection, inhalation, or absorption through skin or mucous membranes. The effects of the poisoning are not always initially obvious, but the toxic substances can subsequently affect various organ systems. The American Association of Poison Control Centers (AAPCC) reports more than 2 million poisonings annually, although accidental and intentional ingestions of toxic substances are not always reported. In 2000, there were 2.2 million reported poison exposures in the United States; 920 deaths occurred as a result of these exposures.[1] Poisoning remains one of the leading causes of death in the United States and in 2000 was the primary cause of death in the home.[2] More than 50% of poisonings occur in children less than 6 years of age.[1] Fortunately, the AAPCC is available 24 hours a day (800-222-1222) to provide treatment information regarding toxicologic substances.[1,3]

Immediate emergency department referral/physician consultation is indicated for victims of poisoning. The goal is to treat the immediate event as quickly as possible.

PATHOPHYSIOLOGY

Pathophysiology depends on the poisonous substance as well as on the route and duration of exposure. The patient's underlying physical condition and initial first aid measures will also affect the impact of the toxin.

CLINICAL PRESENTATION

Specific signs and symptoms sometimes enable medical personnel to identify the type of poisoning. A thorough history and physical examination also can aid in identifying the substance. Often, however, these details are not readily available because of the patient's mental status and physical condition. Identification of the toxin, time and amount of exposure, and cause (accidental/intentional) are important details that sometimes can be elicited from family, friends, or witnesses, or can be determined by examination of the patient's clothes, valuables, or objects noted at the scene of the exposure. In addition, some toxins cause a characteristic group of symptoms called *toxidromes* (a constellation of signs/symptoms related to a particular toxic substance), which can alert the practitioner to the presence of a particular substance (Table 38-1).

PHYSICAL EXAMINATION

The physical examination should assess mental status and vital signs, and determine the presence of any toxidromes. A focused but complete examination of the cardiovascular, respiratory, and

TABLE 38-1 Symptoms and Substances

Symptom	Toxic Substance
Hallucinations	Atropine, cocaine, phencyclidine, LSD
Seizures	Strychnine, anticholinergics, isoniazid, theophylline, nortriptyline
Increased vital signs	Sympathomimetics, anticholinergics
Mydriasis	Anticholinergics, sympathomimetics
Miosis	Organophosphates, narcotics, bromide, acetone, clonidine, heroin
Nonreactive pupils	Anticholinergics
Horizontal nystagmus	Alcohol, lithium, carbamazepine, solvents, memprobamate, quinine, primidone
Decreased respirations	Opiates, organophosphates, barbiturates, beta blockers, benzodiazepines, alcohol, clonidine
Bradycardia	Opiates, organophosphates, barbiturates, beta blockers, benzodiazepines, alcohol, clonidine
Decreased temperature	Opiates, organophosphates, barbiturates, beta blockers, benzodiazepines, alcohol, clonidine
Periorbital edema	Fish poisoning
Abdominal cramps, nausea/vomiting, diarrhea	Fish poisoning, corrosive materials (lye, iodine), cocaine
Tachycardia	Cyclic antidepressants, strychnine, cocaine

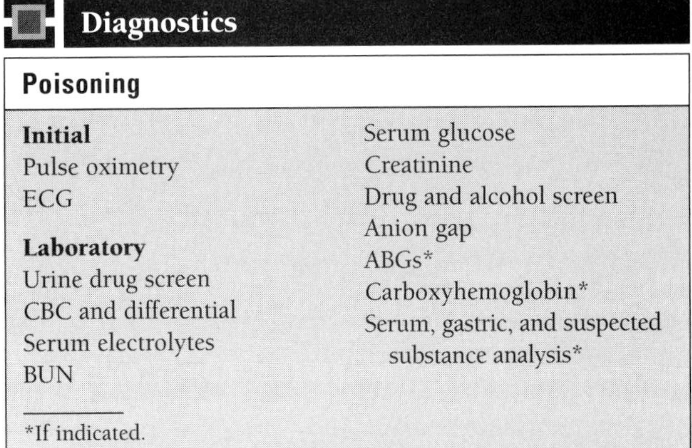

Diagnostics

Poisoning

Initial
Pulse oximetry
ECG

Laboratory
Urine drug screen
CBC and differential
Serum electrolytes
BUN
Serum glucose
Creatinine
Drug and alcohol screen
Anion gap
ABGs*
Carboxyhemoglobin*
Serum, gastric, and suspected substance analysis*

*If indicated.

Differential Diagnosis

Poisoning

Trauma
Metabolic abnormality
Neurologic injury
Alcohol
Medications
Illicit substances
Iron
Plants
Food
Insecticides
Carbon monoxide
Heavy metals
Cyanide
Inhalation
Petroleum distillates
Transient ischemic attack (TIA)
Gastrointestinal disorders

neurologic systems is essential. The toxicologic substance and type of poisoning will dictate the need for additional evaluation (e.g., skin, gastrointestinal [GI]).

Many substances can cause changes in mental status that range from agitation or delirium to coma. Some characteristic signs and symptoms may suggest a particular substance. Atropine, cocaine, phencyclidine, and LSD may cause hallucinations. Strychnine can cause seizures in an otherwise alert patient. Other drugs that are known to cause seizures include anticholinergics, isoniazid, and theophylline. Sympathomimetics and anticholinergics cause increased vital sign values. A below-normal temperature, respiratory rate, and heart rate may be a result of opiates, organophosphates, barbiturates, beta blockers, benzodiazepines, alcohol, or clonidine. Anticholinergic and sympathomimetic substances can cause mydriasis, whereas organophosphates, narcotics, bromide, acetone, clonidine, and nicotine may cause miosis. Cocaine does not interfere with reactivity of the pupils, but anticholinergics cause nonreactive pupils. Nystagmus can be caused by a variety of substances. Alcohols, lithium, carbamazepine, solvents, meprobamate, quinine, and primidone may cause horizontal nystagmus. Sometimes characteristic odors emanate from patients and may give clues to aid in identification.

DIAGNOSTICS

In addition to vital signs and physical findings, laboratory values can be an important aspect of the diagnostic evaluation and aid in management. Diagnostic tests should be dictated by the toxicologic exposure. Some substances, including alcohol, aspirin, acetaminophen, illicit drugs, iron, lead, mercury, carboxyhemoglobin, and ethylene glycol, can be measured directly. In addition, many psychopharmacologic substances, including lithium hydroxide, divalproex sodium (Depakote), carbamazepine (Tegretol), oxcarbazepine (Trileptal), gabapentin (Neurontin), and nortriptyline (Pamelor), can be calculated. Assessment of arterial blood gases, the anion gap, the osmolar gap, and the oxygen saturation gap may provide additional information.

Other laboratory studies are helpful in assessing end-organ involvement and should include electrolytes, glucose, blood urea nitrogen, creatinine, and liver function tests. Urine screens may be indicated if cocaine, opiates, or marijuana are suspected. A pregnancy test should be obtained, if indicated. An electrocardiogram is necessary with specific poisons and in some instances will need repeated assessment.[4] Further evaluation should be directed if abnormalities such as acidosis or hypoxia are discovered.

DIFFERENTIAL DIAGNOSIS

Initial diagnostic determination and treatment are usually based on the history and physical examination. If the patient is confused or comatose, all potential causes for the change in mental status should be considered. Laboratory analysis and the patient's response to therapeutic intervention provide additional diagnostic information. The differential diagnosis should include trauma, metabolic abnormality, neurologic injury, alcohol, medications, illicit substances, cleaning agents, plants, insecticides, food, trauma, carbon monoxide, heavy metals, cyanide, inhalation, and petroleum distillate poisoning. If GI symptoms are present, the differential diagnosis should include any possible GI disorders.

INITIAL STABILIZATION AND MANAGEMENT

Regardless of the poison, the initial assessment of the poisoned patient requires attention to airway, breathing, and circulation. Oxygen and continuous airway maintenance are critical. IV access is also necessary. If the patient is comatose, a standard cocktail of glucose 25 to 50 g IV, thiamine 100 mg IV, and naloxone 2 to 4 mg IV has been recommended in the past, and the benefits of this regimen seem to outweigh the potential risks.[5,6] *Ambulance transport to the nearest emergency department is vital.* When the specific substance is known, the local poison control center should be contacted to provide specific management and treatment recommendations.[1] Further management should be directed to reverse the known side effects (i.e., ingestion poisonings require GI decontamination with activated charcoal, 25 to 100 g by mouth or via nasogastric tube to prevent absorption of toxic substances).

Considering the large number of substances that could potentially act as toxins, a relatively small number of antidotes are available. Some commonly used antidotes include *N*-acetylcysteine, flumazenil, and naloxone. *N*-acetylcysteine is administered at an initial dose of 140 mg/kg by a standard protocol based on a nomogram to determine the necessity of treatment for acetaminophen overdoses. Flumazenil administered intravenously in 0.2-mg doses every minute to a maximum of 1 to 3 mg reverses the effects of benzodiazepine but could be detrimental if given to patients with mixed substance overdose, alcohol, or seizure history.[7] Naloxone is an opiate antagonist and is given in doses of 0.4 to 0.8 mg IV for adults to a maximum of 8 to 22 mg and in doses of 0.01 mg/kg IV for children.[4,8] More detailed listings that include antidotes for other substances are available.[4,6]

DISPOSITION AND REFERRAL

Immediate transfer or referral to an emergency department is recommended. Most patients who are treated for poisoning require a minimum observation period, if not hospitalization.

PREVENTION AND PATIENT EDUCATION

Education about the prevention of accidents and injuries is of utmost importance. To prevent exposures to potentially harmful substances, patients must understand the risks of inappropriate contact with medications and other household items. Information regarding the toxic effects of specific substances and the safe usage, storage, and handling of potential toxins at home and in the workplace is always useful and is an important reminder for us all. For patients with children, reminders about childproofing the home (particularly the importance of locking medications and cleaning agents in a childproof cabinet) can potentially prevent accidental exposures.

REFERENCES

1. Centers for Disease Control. Retrieved May 31, 2002 from the World Wide Web: http://www.cdc.gov/ncipc/factsheets/poiz.htn.
2. National Safety Council. Injury Facts. Retrieved May 31, 2002 from the World Wide Web: http://www.nsc.org.
3. American Association of Poison Control Centers (AAPCC). Retrieved June 4, 2002 from the World Wide Web: http://www.aapcc.org.
4. Bone R: Approach to the poisoned patient, *Dis Mon* 42(9):511-607, 1996.
5. Kirk M, Pace S: Pearls, pitfalls, and updates in toxicology, *Emerg Med Clin North Am* 15(2):427-429, 1997.
6. Tintinalli JE, Ruiz E, Krome RL: *Emergency medicine*, ed 4, San Francisco, 1996, McGraw-Hill.
7. Mazda R: Poisoning and drug toxicity. In Logan P, editor: *Principles and practice for the acute care nurse practitioner*, Stamford CT, 1999, Appleton & Lange.
8. Hodgson BB, Kizior RJ: *Saunders nursing drug handbook*, Philadelphia, 2002, WB Saunders.

CHAPTER 39

Seizures in an Emergency Setting

Karen L. Gilbert

DEFINITION/EPIDEMIOLOGY

A seizure is a neurologic event characterized by excessive, paroxysmal firing of neurons in the brain, which typically produces a transient disturbance in brain function. A single seizure may result from discrete, temporary abnormalities such as a high fever in small children, hyperventilation, or alcohol withdrawal. A first seizure may present itself in the form of status epilepticus (SE). SE is defined as more than 30 minutes of continuous seizure activity, or two or more seizures without recovery of baseline consciousness between attacks.

Single seizures are not by themselves indicative of epilepsy. Epilepsy is a disease characterized by recurrent seizures or chronic susceptibility to seizures. The International League Against Epilepsy has divided seizures into three classes:

1. *Generalized.* Both cerebral hemispheres are involved (includes absence, myoclonic, clonic, tonic, tonic-clonic, and atonic seizures).
2. *Partial.* Only one cerebral hemisphere is involved. Partial seizures are further divided into simple partial seizures (which do not result in impaired consciousness) and complex partial seizures (which do impair consciousness).
3. *Unclassified.* These seizures defy classification because of inadequate or incomplete data.

In the United States approximately 2.5 million people—1% of the population—have epilepsy.[1] An estimated 5% of the U.S. population will experience a seizure during their lifetime.[2] Incidence rates are highest in childhood, plateau between the ages of 15 and 65 years of age, and rise again among older adults.

Immediate emergency department referral and physician consultation are indicated for SE or new-onset seizures.

PATHOPHYSIOLOGY

Seizures are symptoms of an underlying problem; they are not a disease in themselves. Any internal or external phenomenon that alters the structure of the brain or its biochemical environment may be a cause of seizures. Most seizures (60%) are idiopathic—there is no discrete identifiable cause, and the seizures are probably primarily genetic in origin.[1] They often emerge in early childhood and are uncommon in the older adult population. The remaining 40% of seizures may be caused by an acute active process (e.g., central nervous system [CNS] infection, tumors, toxins, drugs) or by a more remote event such as congenital CNS disorders, encephalopathy from asphyxia or hypoxia, or stroke.[3] In an emergency setting, symptomatic seizures may be provoked by an acute medical or neurologic illness. Etiologies may include febrile illnesses, metabolic encephalopathy, drug or alcohol withdrawal, encephalitis, or meningitis. In these cases, treatment of the underlying cause is as important as the treatment of seizures.

CLINICAL PRESENTATION

Because many seizures result in alterations in consciousness or amnesia, a reliable eyewitness description of the event is important in establishing a diagnosis. The patient may remember experiencing prodromal symptoms such as a headache or an aura (e.g., queasy epigastric discomfort, fearful feeling, déjà vu) before the seizure. Other factors important to the history are systemic illness, drug use or abuse, pregnancy, head trauma, focal weakness, family history of seizure disorder, risk factors for HIV or other infection, and specific circumstances surrounding the seizure. Detailed questioning of the patient with seizures may elicit a history of nocturnal enuresis, unexplained bruises, aching muscles, shoulder dislocations, tongue biting during sleep, unexplained blood on the pillow, or a sudden decline in work or school performance.[2]

The clinical presentation varies according to the type and location of seizure. For example, a patient having a simple partial seizure does not lose consciousness and is aware of the seizure manifestations, which may be a jerking of an extremity, a sensory distortion, an emotion, or an indescribable feeling. In a complex partial seizure, the patient may stare vacantly into space, fail to respond to others, and perform meaningless, stereotypic, and repetitive movements. A tonic-clonic, or grand mal, seizure is the easiest to recognize. These seizures are characterized by a predictable progression from tonic stiffening of the limbs (which usually lasts from 30 to 60 seconds) to clonic convulsions of the body (which last 1 to 2 minutes). After the seizure ends, the patient may be lethargic and sleepy for several hours or more.

PHYSICAL EXAMINATION

A careful physical and neurologic examination should be performed, with attention given to vital signs, evidence of systemic illness or drug abuse, focal neurologic deficits, heart murmurs, arrhythmias, and bruits. Except in the course of the seizure itself, the physical examination is usually normal in the majority of patients with epilepsy.

DIAGNOSTICS

A reliable eyewitness account of the event is crucial for establishing a diagnosis. Routine laboratory tests are usually not useful in evaluating a first seizure in an otherwise well patient. However, a CBC may be helpful in determining whether the patient has an infection. Glucose, electrolytes, calcium, magnesium, phosphorus, BUN, creatinine, and liver function tests may be helpful in ruling out a metabolic cause. In addition, a serum prolactin level drawn within 15 to 30 minutes of the event may be useful in differentiating a true seizure from a pseudoseizure.[3] The prolactin level may be elevated after a true seizure but is normal after a psychogenic nonepileptic seizure.

Neuroimaging (head computed tomography [CT] scan or magnetic resonance imaging [MRI]) is usually done to determine

Diagnostics

Seizures

Laboratory	Anticonvulsant drug levels*
CBC and differential	ABGs*
Serum electrolytes	**Imaging**
BUN	CT scan or MRI (if first seizure)
Creatinine	
Serum glucose	
LFTs	**Other**
Drug/alcohol screen	EEG*
Urinalysis	

*If indicated.

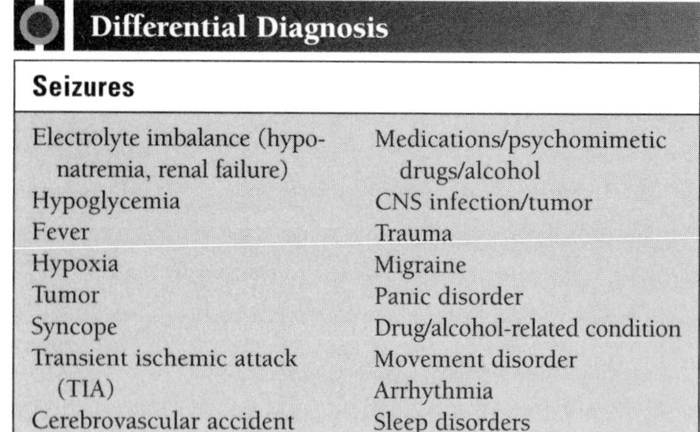

Differential Diagnosis

Seizures

Electrolyte imbalance (hyponatremia, renal failure)	Medications/psychomimetic drugs/alcohol
Hypoglycemia	CNS infection/tumor
Fever	Trauma
Hypoxia	Migraine
Tumor	Panic disorder
Syncope	Drug/alcohol-related condition
Transient ischemic attack (TIA)	Movement disorder
	Arrhythmia
Cerebrovascular accident (CVA)	Sleep disorders
	Idiopathic

the presence of a structural lesion (tumor, aneurysm, intracranial bleeding) as a cause for the seizure. An MRI is superior to a CT scan, but CT scans are more commonly available in the emergency department evaluation of a first seizure.[3] An EEG provides useful and highly specific data—an abnormal EEG is highly predictive of seizure recurrence. However, a normal EEG does not exclude epilepsy or the presence of a structural lesion.[3]

Video/EEG monitoring may be helpful for cases in which the history, eyewitness description, clinical examination, neuroimaging, and EEG fail to yield a diagnosis. Other special diagnostic procedures include positron emission tomography, single photon emission computed tomography, and magnetoencephalographic recording of brain activity; however, these tests are not available on an emergency basis. For patients in SE, a battery of laboratory tests is usually performed: CBC, electrolytes, glucose, magnesium, calcium, BUN, creatinine, liver function tests, coagulation studies (prothrombin time/partial thromboplastin time), alcohol level, toxicology screen, anticonvulsant drug levels, urinalysis, and a pregnancy test. These should be done concurrently with stabilization of the patient. Examination of the cerebrospinal fluid is required if meningitis or encephalitis is suspected. Viral encephalitis should be treated empirically with acyclovir until the results of diagnostic studies for herpes virus are available. Similarly, suspected bacterial meningitis should be treated with appropriate antibiotics until culture results are available.

DIFFERENTIAL DIAGNOSIS

Events that may be mistaken for seizures are numerous and include syncope, transient ischemic attack, migraine, hypoglycemia, movement disorders, psychogenic pseudoseizures, cardiac arrhythmias, hypotension and hypoperfusion, sleep disorders, paroxysmal vertigo, breath-holding spells in children, and panic disorder.

INITIAL STABILIZATION AND MANAGEMENT

In the acute setting, most seizures resolve spontaneously within a few minutes and require no specific treatment apart from close observation to ensure that patients do not harm themselves. However, SE is a medical emergency that requires simultaneous medical stabilization (airway, breathing, circulation, and medications to control the seizures) and a search for the underlying cause. The Epilepsy Foundation of America's Working Group on Status Epilepticus defines SE as a continuous seizure lasting 30 minutes or more, or two consecutive seizures in a row without mental clearing.[4] Efforts have been made recently to change the definition from 30 minutes of continuous seizure activity to 10 minutes. This is based on the duration of seizure activity that may produce permanent injury. Generalized convulsive SE (GCSE) is a medical emergency that can lead to transient or permanent brain damage.

Early treatment is a key factor in the outcome and prognosis. Initial management should include maintaining homeostasis and respiratory support. If seizures persist beyond 30 minutes, a vicious circle of maladaptive physiologic responses occurs.[5] SE may be complicated by hypotension, hypertension, hyperthermia, hypoglycemia, hypoxemia, acidosis, arrhythmias, rhabdomyolysis, pulmonary edema, fractures, and dislocations.

Mortality and morbidity rates have been related to the etiology of SE and time from onset to treatment. In patients with known epilepsy, half of the hospital-reported cases of GCSE have been associated with subtherapeutic antiepileptic drug (AED) levels.[6] This is usually due to patients not taking their medication as prescribed. Other common causes of SE are meningitis, head trauma, eclampsia, and progressive neurologic and neurodegenerative disorders.[4] In a study by the Veterans Affairs Status Epilepticus Cooperative Study Group comparing four treatments (lorazepam, phenytoin, phenobarbital, and diazepam) for GCSE, lorazepam was more likely than phenytoin to be successful when used as the initial treatment.[7] Recommendations for treating acute episodes of SE are listed in Table 39-1. The following conditions warrant consideration for admission: SE, incomplete recovery or prolonged postictal state, illness suspected that requires treatment, drug or alcohol withdrawal, febrile illness (adult), expanding mass lesion, history of recent head trauma, or focal signs on examination.[3] Depending on a number of variables, including the potential for seizure recurrence, first seizures are generally not treated with AEDs. Only about 30% of persons who have a single unprovoked generalized tonic-clonic seizure have a second one whether or not they are treated with medications.[8] Medication

TABLE 39-1 Recommended Emergency Treatment and Timetable for Status Epilepticus

Time (min)	Action
0-5	Diagnose status epilepticus Give oxygen by nasal cannula/mask; consider intubation if indicated. Establish an IV; obtain blood samples for glucose, serum chemistry, hematology screen, toxicology and antiepileptic drug levels.
6-9	If hypoglycemia is established or blood glucose unknown, administer glucose: Adults: give thiamine 100 mg followed by 50 ml of 50% glucose IV Children: 2 ml/kg of 25% glucose
10-20	Administer either 0.1 g/kg of lorazepam at 2 mg/min *or* 0.2 mg/kg of diazepam at 5 mg/min by IV (if diazepam used, also give phenytoin in follow-up treatment).
21-60	If SE persists, administer 15-20 mg/kg of phenytoin no faster than 50 mg/min in adults and 1 mg/kg per min in children by IV. Monitor ECG and blood pressure.*
>60	If status does not stop after 20 mg/kg of phenytoin, give 20 mg/kg of phenobarbital IV at 100 mg/min. If status persists, obtain anesthesia consult for possible pentobarbital coma.

Modified from Treatment of convulsive status epilepticus: recommendations of the Epilepsy Foundation of America's Working Group on Status Epilepticus, *JAMA* 270(7):856, 1993.
*In most centers, fosphenytoin is replacing phenytoin. It is dosed in phenytoin equivalents and can be dosed twice as fast as phenytoin. It also causes less damage if it infiltrates.

may delay recurrence or somewhat reduce its likelihood. Factors that should be considered in the decision to treat or not to treat a first seizure include the following:

- The type of seizure that occurred (complex partial seizures are more likely to be recurrent than generalized tonic-clonic ones)
- Environment and occupation (i.e., dangerous work environment such as construction)
- Results of imaging studies and EEG; if either is abnormal, it would be prudent to treat, because a recurrence is more likely

The decision to treat carries with it a change in the patient's lifestyle, driving and occupational restrictions, social stigma, and the costs and side effects of medications. The risk-benefit ratio may not justify use of AEDs in this setting. A consultation with a neurologist is helpful in deciding on whether or not to treat.

If AED therapy is indicated, a number of factors should be considered: the patient's age, seizure type, daily activities, social and economic ramifications, and medication side effect profile. The goal should be the restoration of a normal life, with complete control of seizures through the use of a single drug and minimization of side effects. Success, however, does not always mean 100% seizure control. Failure is defined as inadequate seizure control and/or unacceptable side effects.[1]

Well-established AEDs that are considered first-line therapy include carbamazepine, phenytoin, valproic acid, phenobarbital, and primidone. Newer, less well-established AEDs include felbamate, fosphenytoin, gabapentin, lamotrigine, tiagabine, zonisamide, levetiracetam, and topiramate. Each of these drugs has its own unique profile regarding indications, risks, side effects, complications, and required laboratory monitoring (see Chapter 218). The primary care provider can initiate the use of antiepileptic medications. If acceptable seizure control cannot be achieved with a single drug, referral should be made to a neurologist. Other reasons for referral include focal neurologic findings on physical examination, a CNS lesion seen on CT or MRI, a change in habitual seizure patterns, or the patient's desire for pregnancy.[3] If seizures remain refractory to medical management (up to 20% of the epilepsy population), the patient should be evaluated by an epileptologist to determine whether surgery—localization and resection of the epileptogenic focus—is feasible.[9]

DISPOSITION AND REFERRAL

From the emergency setting, the patient should be referred to a primary care provider and/or neurologist. The primary care provider and neurologist are a team. Collaboration in decision making is essential. It is important to have clear communication between primary care providers and specialists to maintain consistency of care. Medication changes should be communicated to all providers to avoid confusion and medication errors. Older adults and patients with multiple medical problems require closer coordination among providers.

PREVENTION AND PATIENT EDUCATION

Epilepsy does not affect life span so much as lifestyle. The life span of the average patient with well-controlled epilepsy is identical to that of persons without epilepsy. Patients with acute symptomatic seizures are at risk for increased morbidity and mortality from their underlying disease processes (e.g., CNS infection, stroke, trauma). SE, as previously noted, also confers a higher morbidity and mortality. Even during a brief seizure, a patient (particularly an older adult) may suffer an injury from falling. The AEDs have side effects that range from minor to severe and life threatening.

Driving and operating dangerous machinery are obviously hazardous to patients whose seizures are not well controlled. Patients undergoing a seizure evaluation should be advised not to drive or operate potentially dangerous machinery until the evaluation has been completed and the risk of recurrence has been determined. Some states have specific laws mandating that physicians report persons with seizures to the state division of motor vehicles; in other states the patient is responsible for reporting. The physician or other practitioner should carefully document his or her discussion with the patient regarding increased driving risks and the patient's as well as the physician's responsibility to conform to the laws of the state.

Patients must be educated regarding the side effects of their medications and the interactions with other medications, including birth control pills. Potential factors initiating seizures (e.g., flashing lights, sleep deprivation, stress) should be reviewed with the patient. The importance of the medication regimen in the control of seizures should be emphasized along with the caveat that the regimen may fail.

Family planning should be discussed thoroughly with women of childbearing age. Patients planning a pregnancy should be referred to a neurologist. Most pregnancies in women with epilepsy are routine, and the children are delivered healthy. However, the risk of congenital fetal anomalies in mothers with epilepsy is two to three times that of the general population, irrespective of medical treatment. Both seizures and AEDs can adversely affect the developing fetus.[10] Patients need to be aware that oral and injectable contraceptives and levonorgestrel (Norplant) have a higher failure rate in women taking antiepileptic medications.

REFERENCES

1. Booss J: *Management of epilepsy: federal practitioner supplement*, Birmingham, Ala, 1995, Department of Veterans Affairs, Birmingham Regional Medical Education Center.
2. Brodie MJ, Dichter MA: Antiepileptic drugs: review article, *N Engl J Med* 334(3):168-173, 1996.
3. Moore-Sledge CM: Evaluation and management of first seizures in adults, *Am Fam Physician* 56(4):1113-1120, 1997.
4. Working Group on Status Epilepticus: Treatment of status epilepticus, *JAMA* 270:854-859, 1992.
5. Gilbert K: An algorithm for diagnosis and treatment of status epilepticus in adults, *J Neurosci Nurs* 31(1):27-36, 1999.
6. Ramsay E: Treatment of status epilepticus, *Epilepsia* 34(suppl.1): 71-81, 1993.
7. Treiman D and others: A comparison of four treatments for generalized convulsive status epileptics, *N Engl J Med* 339(12): 792-798, 1998.
8. Freeman J, Pedley T: Indications for treatment. In Engel J Jr, Pedley T, editors: *Epilepsy: a comprehensive textbook*, Philadelphia, 1997, Lippincott-Raven.
9. Engel J: Surgery for seizures: review article, *N Engl J Med* 334(10): 647-652, 1996.
10. Liporace JD: Women's issues in epilepsy, *Postgrad Med* 10(1):102-118, 1997.

CHAPTER 40

Sexual Assault

Janelle M. West-Koo and Robbyn Takeuchi

DEFINITION/EPIDEMIOLOGY

The terms *sexual assault* and *rape* are often used interchangeably, although there are clear differences between them. Rape is a legal term and not a medical diagnosis. The legal definition of rape may vary among states, but the common components of the definition include a lack of consent, a threat or use of force, and penetration of a bodily orifice.[1] Sexual assault has a much broader definition. It is defined as any sexual act that is forced or coerced without the consent of the victim.[2] Rape and sexual assault are not sexually motivated acts; rather, they are motivated by rage, aggression, and the determination to dominate another human being.

According to recent statistics, the rate of sexual assault is increasing.[3] In 1999, 89,107 rapes were reported to the police in the United States.[4] Statistics from the National Crime Victimization Survey (NCVS) within the United States revealed that 141,000 completed rapes and 60,000 attempted rapes occurred in 1999, for a total of 201,000 rape cases.[5] Further surveys indicate that 1 out of 6 women in the United States experience either a completed or attempted rape at some point in their lifetime.[3] Rapes are about 10 times higher for women than men, although men are less likely to report the occurrence. (For the purposes of this chapter, the term "she" will be used, although this information can also apply to men who have been victims of sexual assault.) As previously discussed, it is important to consider the differences between the terms *rape* and *sexual assault*, as these statistics account for only reported rape cases and do not indicate the incidence of sexual assault, which has a much broader scope.

There are no known risk factors for becoming a victim of sexual assault. In fact, anyone can be a victim regardless of age, race, gender, or socioeconomic status. However, sexual assault victims are predominately female, and the perpetrators are almost always heterosexual males. Female victims are more likely to be assaulted by someone they know, rather than a stranger.[3] Sexual assault can also occur in the context of any intimate partner relationship. This includes marital, nonmarital, gay, lesbian, or past relationships. However, this type of sexual assault is often recurring and is one of the symptoms of a larger domestic violence problem that needs to be addressed. Consequences for this type of ongoing, sexual violence by an intimate partner are severe and require ongoing monitoring and attention by the primary care provider. (See Chapter 21 for further information regarding evaluation and management.)

CLINICAL PRESENTATION

The physical presentation of the sexual assault victim in the clinic setting is immensely varied. Some patients may report a chief complaint of sexual assault to their primary care provider, whereas others may not mention that a sexual assault has occurred. Likewise, the presentation of psychologic effects of trauma also varies among victims. Some patients may choose to disclose that a sexual assault occurred if asked by a trusted primary care provider. However, other patients may still deny that violence occurred despite the evidence of trauma and inquiry. Whatever the reasons for the patient's denial, this still must be respected, and all the primary care provider may be able to do is offer support. It is not up to the practitioner to determine whether sexual assault occurred; that must be left for the court to decide. Rather, it is often helpful for the primary care provider to let the patient know that sexual assault is, unfortunately, a common experience, and that it is a problem that the provider may be able to assist with. This may help to leave the door open should the patient decide in the future to disclose what happened.

There are specific circumstances, however, in which providers are mandated to report the sexual assault to the proper authorities. Any sexual assault perpetrated against a victim who is under 18 years of age or against any adult who is physically dependent or cognitively impaired must be reported to the local Child Protective or Adult Protective Agency. Health care providers are mandated to report any suspicion of sexual assault in these populations, regardless of whether the patient reports that sexual assault has occurred. Although it is not the responsibility of the provider to prove that the violence occurred, it is his or her responsibility to act on the clinical evidence presented. As laws may vary among states, providers should become familiar with the laws within their area.

INITIAL STABILIZATION AND MANAGEMENT/PHYSICAL EXAMINATION

If the patient does disclose that he or she was sexually assaulted, the provider should further explore whether the patient desires to pursue legal action. The provider should defer a physical examination and refer the patient to the emergency department if the sexual assault occurred within the last 5 days and if the patient desires to pursue legal actions. A referral to the emergency department will ensure that the appropriate measures are taken to collect evidence and comply with standardized protocol, which are integral to support the patient's desire for legal pursuits. Further, the emergency department will also be able to provide patients with comprehensive and compassionate services, including crisis intervention, rape counseling, and referrals to appropriate community agencies. The primary care provider can prepare the patient for what to expect in the emergency department. It is not important that the provider request specific information about the assault, because this information will be gathered in the emergency department. Retelling the story can be more traumatizing for the patient. Rather, providers can attentively listen to and document what the patient desires to express. The primary care provider should carefully note emotional responses (e.g., crying, restlessness, anxious behavior, shaking, withdrawal), as this would be useful in court as an adjunct to the emergency department records.

If the patient does not desire to pursue legal action, or if more than 5 days have passed since the assault, medical care can be managed in the office setting. The provider needs to obtain a detailed history and perform a physical and gynecologic examination. Possible gynecologic injuries include vaginal or anal tearing, rectal bleeding, bruising, or soreness. Other physical symptoms associated with trauma include gastrointestinal irritability, dysmenorrhea, pelvic pain, and urinary tract infection. (For specific treatment considerations, see chapters that address the specific injury, infection, and medical disorder.)

Potential consequences of sexual assault further include the risk for pregnancy, sexually transmitted diseases (STDs), and HIV/AIDS. If it has been more than 72 hours since the sexual assault, it is not feasible to offer pregnancy or STD prophylactics. A pregnancy test should be completed, with appropriate counseling pending the results. The patient should be tested for STDs (gonorrhea and chlamydia are the most prevalent), and standard treatment should be followed if the results are positive. The patient may express fears about having contracted HIV/AIDS; however, testing cannot be done until 3 to 6 months after the assault because of the length of time required for seroconversion to occur. If the appropriate time has passed, patients should have pretest and posttest education and counseling. Education should include risks of acquiring the infection, potential transmission of the virus, and instruction about safe sex practices at least until testing is complete, or longer if the results are positive.

Clearly, appropriate referrals need to be made for any symptoms, illnesses, or injuries whose treatment is beyond the scope of the office setting. Patients may also commonly report psychosomatic complaints, including fatigue and tension headaches, with or without the report of sexual assault. These symptoms may need further exploration through a psychosocial assessment.

PSYCHOSOCIAL ASSESSMENT

When a patient reports that she has been a victim of sexual assault, and it has been determined that she will be treated in the primary care setting, it is important to assess more than the patient's physical well-being. Patients may seek care soon after the assault or after an extended period of time. The patient's account of the assault will aid the provider in understanding the patient's experience and what type of services the patient may benefit from.

Patients who seek care shortly after the assault may display a range of emotions. Some may appear frightened, shocked, or angry. Regardless of their presentation, they are in need of understanding and support. The patient's emotional presentation is not indicative of the level of trauma that has been experienced. A review of the patient's home environment and support system is appropriate. Because of a stigma that some victims of sexual assault, it is sometimes difficult for them to inform significant people in their life about their victimization. Some fear that their intimate partner or parent may seek physical revenge against the perpetrator when the perpetrator is known to them. As a result, they may be reluctant or unwilling to disclose information in an effort to protect their partner or parent from potential legal problems. Unfortunately, some patients are afraid to inform someone about the assault because they feel that no one will believe them or that they are to blame for the assault. This is especially true if the patient consumed alcohol or drugs before the assault or if they felt they were dressed in provocative attire. This may result in the patient not receiving in-depth support.

Patients can be assisted with identifying people in their lives who they are able to disclose the assault to and who are able to provide them with support. They may also benefit from a discussion on the various ways that they can talk with their family or partner about the assault. The patient may experience a high degree of fear over the potential for further harm and may be afraid to be alone or return home. Patients must be assisted in finding the means to appropriately address their fears.

Patients who initially seek care after a length of time after the assault may be prompted to do so because of physical complaints such as STDs or pregnancy, as well as psychologic difficulties. Some patients may experience symptoms of psychologic distress that are consistent with posttraumatic stress disorder (PTSD). One study revealed that almost one third of rape victims develop PTSD at some point in their lifetime after a rape; this rate is six times higher than the rate for women who have not been raped.[4]

Reactions of people who have been sexually assaulted will vary depending on a variety of factors, including age, gender, and circumstances surrounding the assault. Regardless of when the patient seeks care after a sexual assault, it is important for the provider to gain an accurate understanding of the patient's concerns, level of functioning, and support system before an appropriate treatment plan can be developed. The primary care provider's comfort level with the subject matter may affect the patient's willingness to disclose information that will provide insight into the patient's needs. The provider is in a pivotal role to aid the patient in identifying the need for additional services, including mental health services.

DOCUMENTATION

Accurate and precise documentation of the patient's physical and emotional signs and symptoms of sexual assault serves to corroborate the patient's testimony in court. It is essential that health care providers use medical rather than legal terminology. For example, calling the assault the "alleged rape" should be avoided; rather, it should be described as the "reported sexual assault." Likewise, the word *patient* should be used rather than *victim*. Further consideration regarding the connotation of words is essential. *Penetration* is a better word than *intercourse*, as the latter may sound as though the act was consensual. If the patient does not wish to have a certain part of the examination completed, it should not be documented as "refused," as this makes the patient sound uncooperative; rather, one should write the patient "declined" the examination. Using the patient's own words in quotations whenever possible works best to capture the description of the incident and is extremely helpful in court. One should avoid writing "no weapons used" but should describe exactly what happened, because there may have been verbal or implied threats. It is also important to be wary of avoiding medical jargon that leaves room for misinterpretation. If the patient appears calm and collected, it is better to document that than to say "no apparent distress." Documenting unnecessary history that is not related to the chief complaint (e.g., psychiatric history, substance abuse history) could be used in court to discredit the patient's testimony.

SPECIFIC POPULATIONS

Male Patients

Although male victims are in the minority of the sexual assault victims, it is critical that they be treated the same as female patients with the exception of the gynecologic examination. Male victims may experience rectal or penile trauma, bleeding or discharge, infection, or trauma to the mouth and pharynx. The patient may receive frontal injuries from being in a prone position during the assault. Men are usually assaulted by other men. For a multitude of reasons, men are less likely to seek services after being sexually assaulted. It is common for them to experience physical and emotional reactions similar to those of women who are assaulted. Men may also feel that they are less of a man, may experience shame about not being able to defend themselves, and may be confused about their sexuality. If the assailant was a woman, the patient may feel particularly weak or inferior. As with all victims of sexual assault, it is important for the patient to receive mental health services.

Older Adults

Older patients are particularly vulnerable because of age-related illness and overall decrease in physical strength. They may sustain more overall injuries and specifically more genital injuries. Older women are less likely to report being sexually assaulted; they may feel extreme embarrassment, humiliation, and shame because they were raised during a time when issues related to sex were not discussed. Some patients may be concerned that reporting the assault will result in a loss of their independence.

Adolescents

Adolescents are also at increased risk for victimization. Studies indicate that young women are at a greater likelihood of experiencing violence. The National Survey of Adolescents found that 13% of female adolescents had experienced sexual violence at some point in their lives.[4] They also have a tendency not to seek services for a variety of reasons. Some may feel responsible for the assault, or they may be concerned that their parents will find out or that they will be further victimized if they disclose information. Adolescence can be a difficult period for patients as a result of developmental and social changes and of patients' attempts to define themselves as they mature. Being sexually assaulted may create a multitude of problems for an adolescent including difficulty establishing trust and the development of psychiatric symptoms. Adolescents should be referred to age-appropriate mental health services.

Immigrants

In general, many immigrants have difficulty accessing care because of their limited resources, language barriers, and a lack of awareness regarding how to access services; however, there are additional concerns with respect to receiving services for sexual assault. Some patients may be afraid to report the sexual assault to authorities because of concern that it may have a negative impact on their immigration status, especially if the patient is an undocumented alien. They may also not understand that it is illegal for them to be assaulted, and they have the right to report the crime. Another significant factor for immigrants in accessing services to address sexual assault is their cultural beliefs. Some may feel that it is inappropriate for them to discuss intimate matters with a professional, although they may not have the means or methods to address their issues within a cultural context. It is important for the health care provider to be aware of cultural factors when providing care, to modify their treatment to the extent that they are able, and to ensure that the patient is aware of his or her rights and the availability of services.

DISPOSITION AND REFERRAL

Under certain circumstances, the victim of sexual assault may be treated in a primary care setting; however, it is preferable that the patient be treated in a specially equipped emergency department by trained staff if the examination occurs within several days of the assault. Because different facilities operate under different guidelines, it is imperative that the primary care provider be aware of the guidelines for the facilities in their area so that appropriate referrals can be made. The patient should always be referred to mental health services that are specific to addressing issues surrounding sexual assault. If the patient is treated in the primary care setting, an assessment must be made to determine their physical, mental health, and legal needs, as well as the patient's level of functioning and willingness to pursue additional services. The primary care provider should use his or her influence to encourage patients to accept additional services as deemed appropriate based on the provider's assessment.

PREVENTION AND PATIENT EDUCATION

Sexual assault occurs in a variety of settings and may victimize people of all ages, races, religions, and socioeconomic backgrounds. There are various tips that patients can be given to protect their general safety; however, there is no known prevention for sexual assault. The primary care provider should educate the patient about the dynamics of sexual assault, including the fact that it is an act of violence, and encourage the patient to seek mental health services.

REFERENCES

1. U.S. Department of Justice, Bureau of Justice Statistics: *Selected findings: violence against women: estimates from the redesigned survey,* Rockville, Md, 1995, National Crime Justice Reference Services.
2. Massachusetts Department of Public Health in Collaboration with the Massachusetts Coalition Against Sexual Assault: *Supporting survivors of sexual assault,* ed 1, Boston, 1997, The Department.
3. Macguire K, Pastore AL: *1994 Sourcebook of criminal justice statistics,* Washington, DC, 1995, US Department of Justice, Bureau of Justice Statistics.
4. Hodgson J, Kelley D: *Sexual violence: policies practices, and challenges in the United States and Canada,* Westport, Conn, 2002, Praeger.
5. Bureau of Justice Statistics 2000: *Criminal victimization, 1999.* Washington, DC, 2000, U.S. Department of Justice, Bureau of Justice Statistics.

CHAPTER 41

Syncope

Updated by Terry Mahan Buttaro

DEFINITION/EPIDEMIOLOGY

Syncope is defined as a temporary loss of consciousness and postural tone that is followed by spontaneous recovery and does not require resuscitation. Presyncope or near-syncope is a sensation of light-headedness or faintness in which the patient senses that true syncope may be imminent but complete loss of consciousness never occurs.

The incidence of syncope in the general population is not known. The closest estimates come from the Framingham study, in which approximately 3% of individuals experienced at least one syncopal episode over a 26-year period.[1,2] Among those who experienced syncope, the incidence of recurrence was approximately 30%.[1-4] It can be assumed that those who practice medicine long enough will eventually encounter a case of syncope or presyncope. Each year, cases of syncope can account for up to 600,000 visits to the emergency department.[5]

Immediate emergency department referral/physician consultation is indicated for syncope in a patient with a family history of sudden death or for syncope associated with exercise, chest pain, congestive heart failure (CHF), palpitations, acute hemorrhage, transient ischemic attacks, seizure, or an abnormal ECG or chest x-ray study. Patients with syncope and a past medical history of anatomic heart disease or previous surgical repair of a cardiac lesion also require emergency department referral/physician consultation.

PATHOPHYSIOLOGY

Syncope is a symptom of an underlying process (Box 41-1). There are two main pathophysiologic mechanisms by which syncope may occur. The first is through the deprivation of nutrients to the brain. In most cases this deprivation results from decreased blood flow to the brain secondary to hypovolemia, cardiac outflow obstruction, cardiac arrhythmias, or neurovascular etiologies. The second underlying mechanism is deprivation of oxygen delivery to the brain, which may be seen with hypoxia or anemia. True syncope needs to be distinguished from seizure disorders or other conditions that might result in altered levels of consciousness, such as iatrogenic syncope from medication therapy, drug or alcohol intoxication, concussions, amnesia, or metabolic causes such as hypoglycemia. It is important to note that seizurelike activity may be present with syncope; this is secondary to generalized cerebral hypoxia.

Cardiac causes need to be diagnosed early in the evaluation because these etiologies are associated with a 1-year mortality rate of 20% to 30% and an increased incidence of sudden death.[6,7]

BOX 41-1

CAUSES OF SYNCOPE

CARDIAC

Mechanical/Obstructive Pprocesses

Cardiac valvular diseases
Atrial myxoma
Hypertrophic/obstructive cardiomyopathy
Pulmonary hypertension
Pulmonary embolism
Pericardial disease
Cardiac tamponade
Myocardial infarction/ischemia

Arrhythmias

Sick sinus syndrome
Atrioventricular conduction disturbances
Supraventricular/ventricular tachycardia
Prolonged QT syndrome
Pacemaker malfunction

NEUROLOGIC

Reflex/Neuromediated

Vasovagal (common faint)
Situational (postmicturition, cough, swallow, defecation)
Carotid sinus hypersensitivity (primarily found in older adults)

Cerebrovascular

Vertebrovascular transient ischemic attack

MISCELLANEOUS

Hypoglycemia
Psychiatric disease (panic disorder, hysteria, depression)
Hypovolemia (especially in older patients who are taking antihypertensive medications)

The cardiac causes consist of two major categories: (1) mechanical or ventricular outflow obstructive processes, and (2) arrhythmia. Possible mechanical or obstructive processes responsible for syncope include cardiac valvular disease, atrial myxoma, hypertrophic or obstructive cardiomyopathy, pulmonary hypertension, pulmonary embolism, pericardial disease/tamponade, acute myocardial infarction/ischemia, and possible prosthetic valve malfunction. Possible rhythm disturbances include sick sinus syndrome, atrioventricular conduction disturbances, supraventricular and ventricular tachycardias, long QT syndrome, and pacemaker system malfunction.

Neurovascular etiologies of syncope may be classified into reflex or neuromediated causes and cerebrovascular causes. Among the reflex or neuromediated causes of syncope are vasovagal causes (also known as the common faint), situational causes (including postmicturition, cough, swallowing, defecation), and carotid sinus syncope (often associated with tight collars, shaving, head turning, and older adults). These neuromediated causes of syncope are thought to result from a poorly understood neural pathway in which neural signals sent from the medulla result in a vasodilatory response with venous pooling and cardioinhibition that results in bradycardia. In carotid sinus syncope and postmicturition syncope, the trigger sites are thought to be peripheral receptors that respond to mechanical stimuli. The main cerebrovascular type of syncope centers around the vertebrobasilar arteries through which the brainstem is perfused. The main causes of this type of syncope are transient ischemic attack, compression (i.e., cervical rib) of the vertebrobasilar circulation, and subclavian steal.

Several miscellaneous causes of syncope are not easily classified into any of the previously mentioned categories. Hypoglycemia is a possible metabolic case of syncope and is usually found in individuals with diabetes who have taken too much of a particular hypoglycemic agent. Hyperventilation is another possible cause. Several psychiatric causes, including depression, hysteria, and panic attacks, may subsequently result in hyperventilation, which can result in hypocarbia and cerebral vasoconstriction compounded by possible peripheral vasodilation. In approximately 38% to 50% of cases, no definitive etiology is found despite thorough evaluations.[8,9]

CLINICAL PRESENTATION

The history of present illness is essential to helping the primary care provider determine if a particular case should be treated on an outpatient or inpatient basis. The history needs to include a detailed account of the syncopal episode. In many cases a witness is needed to determine the specific details of the event. It should be established what the patient was doing before the syncopal episode and whether there were any preceding symptoms. A history of urinating, defecating, swallowing, coughing, shaving, turning the head, neck pressure, or pain before syncope is consistent with some form of neurally mediated syncope. Fainting just before a stressful event is consistent with vasovagal syncope. If the patient is able to relate the presyncopal or syncopal episode to a change from a horizontal to a vertical position, the episode may be a result of hypovolemia or orthostatic hypotension. Numbness and tingling in the face and hands suggest hyperventilation.

The patient may have felt some nausea, diaphoresis, or warmth just before losing consciousness. The presence of an aura, such as a peculiar smell, might be a clue to the presence of an underlying seizure disorder. Differentiating between a seizure and postsyncope, seizurelike activity can be difficult. A possible underlying cardiac etiology needs to be considered if the syncopal episode was sudden and without warning. The sudden onset of syncope is consistent with an arrhythmia, whereas the onset of syncope with exertion may be associated with a mechanical or obstructive process. The presence of chest pain, palpitations, syncope with exertion, and a positive family history of coronary artery disease also necessitates excluding a cardiac cause.[10]

How the patient acted while unconscious is important. Most syncopal events are brief; patients often recover once they are in the horizontal position, which allows the resumption of blood flow to the brain. The presence of seizure activity, urinary incontinence, fecal incontinence, and tongue biting may be of help in differentiating a seizure from true syncope. Postictal symptoms during the recovery phase are more consistent with seizure.

Certain medications may be the underlying or contributing cause. Antihypertensive medications may aggravate orthostatic symptoms, especially in older adults. Antiarrhythmic drugs may have proarrhythmic side effects. It is important to know if the patient is being treated for a seizure disorder, any psychiatric disorders, or diabetes and if the patient has been taking medications as prescribed.

A thorough review of the patient's past medical history is also necessary. The social history should include alcohol use, any possible illicit drug use, and the patient's occupation. In patients suspected of having an underlying cardiac problem, the presence of any cardiac risk factors for coronary artery disease should be determined. Risk factors include male gender, a family history of premature coronary artery disease, hypercholesterolemia, hypertension, smoking, and diabetes.

PHYSICAL EXAMINATION

After establishing that the patient is stable, the initial physical evaluation needs to focus on the cardiovascular system. Auscultation may reveal murmurs, gross rhythm disturbances, or extra heart sounds such as S_3 or S_4. The lungs should be auscultated for rales or crackles, which might indicate the presence of CHF possibly secondary to an acute myocardial infarction or pulmonary disease. Other signs of CHF include the presence of jugular venous distention, hepatojugular reflux, and edema.

Orthostatic blood pressures (also known as *tilts*) should be measured to determine the presence of hypovolemia. These measurements are obtained by having the patient lie in the supine position for at least 5 minutes and then measuring the blood pressure and pulse. The blood pressure and pulse are checked while the patient is sitting up and then while standing. A drop in systolic pressure by at least 20 mm Hg or an increase in the pulse rate by at least 20 beats per minute when assuming a more upright position is considered a positive test.

Hypersensitive carotid sinus baroreceptors may be another underlying cause of syncope. If there are no carotid bruits, this baroreceptor response may be tested by a specialist. In this test, the patient is supine, IV access is established, and atropine is available, if needed. The patient's heart rhythm is observed on a cardiac monitor while carotid sinus pressure is applied. The monitor is checked for the presence of asystole for at least 3 seconds. The blood pressure should be measured to determine if the systolic blood pressure dropped at least 50 mm Hg.[10] Obviously this test should be reserved for a more controlled setting in which possible deleterious consequences can be reversed. A complete neurologic examination, including a funduscopic examination, should also be performed on these patients. A rectal examination will help determine if gastrointestinal bleeding is present.

DIAGNOSTICS

Initial laboratory testing should include electrolytes, blood urea nitrogen, creatinine, glucose, and hematocrit. A chest x-ray study will help reveal any significant cardiac etiologies that may

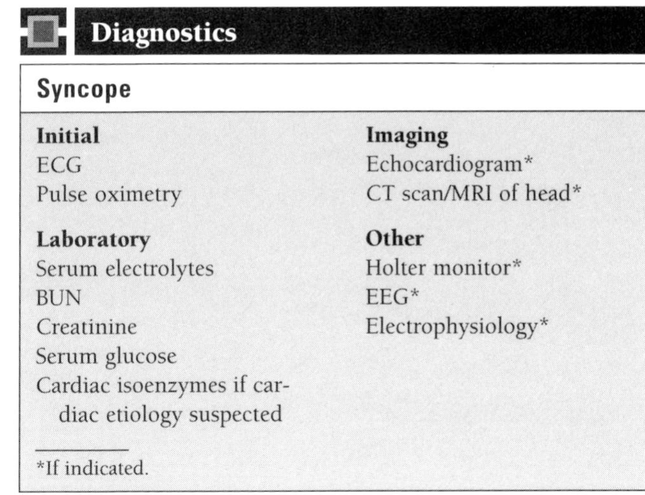

Diagnostics

Syncope

Initial	**Imaging**
ECG	Echocardiogram*
Pulse oximetry	CT scan/MRI of head*
Laboratory	**Other**
Serum electrolytes	Holter monitor*
BUN	EEG*
Creatinine	Electrophysiology*
Serum glucose	
Cardiac isoenzymes if cardiac etiology suspected	

*If indicated.

result in CHF. Cardiomegaly is considered to be a heart shadow that takes up more than half of the chest cavity on the posteroanterior view. An ECG should be performed to help detect the presence of any possible arrhythmias. Cardiac enzymes should be drawn if the patient possesses several cardiac risk factors with a history of chest pain or if there are physical findings consistent with CHF. If a cardiac obstructive cause is suspected, an echocardiogram may be indicated. A pregnancy test should be performed on all female patients of childbearing age.[10]

DIFFERENTIAL DIAGNOSIS

The differential diagnosis of syncope includes vasovagal syncope, orthostatic hypotension, seizure disorder, alcohol abuse, cardiovascular disease with obstruction, cardiac arrhythmias, transient ischemic attack, concussion, hypovolemia, hypoglycemia, anemia, or hypoxia. In addition, syncope may be related to medication therapy or an anxiety attack.

INITIAL STABILIZATION AND MANAGEMENT

During a witnessed event, the patient should be placed in a supine position. Tight clothing should be loosened and the patient's head turned to the side. If the history and diagnostic testing indicates that an initial episode of syncope was not secondary to a cardiac etiology, therapy can be directed at the underlying disorder. If the patient is unstable, the appropriate advanced cardiac life support and advanced trauma life support protocols need to be followed.

DISPOSITION AND REFERRAL

In the case of neuromediated syncope, and especially with recurring episodes, the patient should be referred to a neurologist for possible tilt-table testing and treatment, possibly with fludrocortisone, desmopressin, or pressor agents.[11] Cases of syncope with possible underlying cardiac etiologies need to be referred to an accepting physician as soon as possible for further evaluation. Patients who may possibly have new-onset seizure disorder need to be referred for possible admission. Older patients deserve a thorough history to determine if some other problem in their home environment is preventing them from staying hydrated or taking their medications properly. These patients may need the help of a social worker or health benefits advisor.

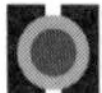

Differential Diagnosis

Syncope
Seizure
Alcohol abuse
Concussion
Drug-induced or medication-related condition
Anemia
Metabolic etiology (hypoglycemia)
Cardiac arrhythmia
Vasovagal reaction
Pregnancy

All patients need to understand the importance of adequate hydration and need to avoid circumstances that might precipitate syncope. They should be told to return to the clinic if the syncope becomes recurrent. Depending on the suspected underlying etiology, a referral to either a neurologist or cardiologist is appropriate at this time.

PREVENTION AND PATIENT EDUCATION

Patients and families should have careful explanation regarding the cause of the syncopal event. In the case of vasovagal, carotid sinus, and situational syncope, patients need to be made aware of the particular behaviors, activities, or circumstances that might result in syncopal episodes, and they should be given adequate avoidance strategies. Prevention of orthostatic changes necessitates that patients learn to rise slowly from the bed or chair, exercising the leg muscles before standing. Although syncope is often not recurrent, patients with syncope should be advised not to operate motorized equipment until the etiology of the event is determined and treated.[12,13]

REFERENCES

1. Benditt DG, Lurie KG, Fabian WH: Clinical approach to diagnosis of syncope: an overview, *Cardiol Clin* 15(2):165-176, 1997.
2. Savage DD and others: Epidemiologic features of isolated syncope: the Framingham study, *Stroke* 16:626-629, 1985.
3. Bass EB and others: Long-term prognosis of patients undergoing electrophysiologic studies for syncope of unknown origin, *Am J Cardiol* 62:1186-1191, 1988.
4. Kapoor WN and others: A prospective evaluation and follow-up of patients with syncope, *N Engl J Med* 309:197-204, 1983.
5. Junaid A, Dubinsky IL: Establishing an approach to syncope in the emergency department, *J Emerg Med* 15(5):593-599, 1997.
6. Kapoor WN: Evaluation and outcome of patients with syncope, *Medicine* 69(3):160-175, 1990.
7. Silverstein MD and others: Patients with syncope admitted to medical intensive care units, *JAMA* 248(10):1185-1189, 1982.
8. Linzer M and others: Diagnosing syncope. Part 2: Unexplained syncope, *Ann Intern Med* 127(1):76-86, 1997.
9. Kapoor WN: Evaluation and management of the patient with syncope, *JAMA* 268(18):2553-2560, 1992.
10. Linzer M and others: Diagnosing syncope. Part 1: Value of history, physical examination, and electrocardiography, *Ann Intern Med* 126(12):989-996, 1997.
11. Kaufmann H: Syncope: a neurologist viewpoint, *Cardiol Clin* 15(2):177-194, 1997.
12. Bhatia A and others: Driving safety among patients with neurocardiogenic syncope, *Pacing Clin Electrophysiol* 22:1576, 1999.
13. LI H and others: Potential risk of vasovagal syncope for motor vehicle driving, *Am J Cardiol* 85:184, 2000.

CHAPTER 42

Tachycardia

Terry Mahan Buttaro

DEFINITION/EPIDEMIOLOGY

Tachycardia is described as a heart rate exceeding 100 beats per minute. Normal sinus tachycardia will not usually require medical intervention, but other tachyarrhythmias can result in hemodynamic compromise and warrant urgent treatment. A rapid assessment of airway, breathing, and circulation, as well as a complete history, physical examination, and 12-lead ECG, are indicated.

Asymptomatic individuals with tachycardia can have stable cardiac rhythms that do not require emergent treatment. Fever, nicotine, exercise, stimulants, medications, and anxiety can precipitate normal sinus tachycardia. Pregnancy, coronary heart disease, congestive heart failure, valvular heart disease, pulmonary embolus, pericardial disease, valvular disorders, ischemia, metabolic and electrolyte abnormalities, medications, toxins, infection, and volume depletion should be considered as possible precipitants identified with atrial and ventricular arrhythmias, as well as tachycardia.[1]

Emergency department referral/physician consultation is indicated for new-onset atrial fibrillation, atrial flutter, ventricular tachycardia (VT), or supraventricular tachycardia (SVT).

PATHOPHYSIOLOGY

The pathology of tachycardia is varied. Sinus tachycardia is a normal physiologic response and should not be considered pathologic. Atrial fibrillation and flutter, the narrow-complex tachycardias (ectopic atrial tachycardia, multifocal atrial tachycardia, junctional tachycardia, and paroxysmal SVT tachycardia), the stable wide-complex tachycardias of unknown type, and monomorphic/polymorphic ventricular tachycardia are tachyarrhythmias that can cause hemodynamic instability (see Chapter 127). In narrow-complex tachycardia, such as paroxysmal tachycardia, the heart rate increases suddenly and rapidly, then decreases suddenly. The attack may last seconds or days, during which time the ventricular rate is rapid, regular, and usually between 150 and 225 beats per minute. This pathology is most likely related to an aberrant reentry involving the arteriovenous (AV) node, although an obscure bypass tract near the AV node may cause the aberrant conduction (as in Wolfe-Parkinson-White syndrome).

Atrial fibrillation and atrial flutter are rhythm disturbances characterized by rapid atrial stimulation and varied ventricular response. In flutter this can be a fleeting phenomenon. In fibrillation it can be related to stress. However, atrial arrhythmias are commonly related to varied disease states. These include coronary heart disease, rheumatic fever, mitral stenosis, thyrotoxicosis, infection, metabolic abnormalities, pulmonary embolism, and chronic lung disease.

Diagnostics

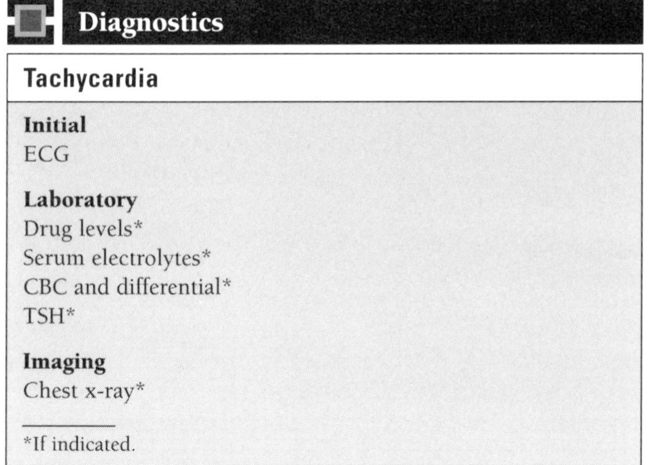

Tachycardia

Initial
ECG

Laboratory
Drug levels*
Serum electrolytes*
CBC and differential*
TSH*

Imaging
Chest x-ray*

*If indicated.

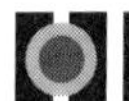

Differential Diagnosis

Tachycardia	
Drug induced	Hypotension
Hyperthyroidism	Hypoxia
Acute myocardial infarction	Hypovolemia
Congestive heart failure	Infection
Pulmonary embolus	Electrolyte disturbance

Whether monomorphic or polymorphic, VT is a rhythm disturbance that arises in the ventricles. The arrhythmia is life threatening if the patient is pulseless, but the patient can be hemodynamically stabile when VT is associated with a pulse.

CLINICAL PRESENTATION

Some tachyarrhythmias are well tolerated, but anxiety, restlessness, shortness of breath, weakness, fatigue, dizziness, and palpitations are common presenting symptoms.[2] Any tachycardia associated with acute myocardial infarction, an alteration in consciousness, chest pressure, hypotension/shock, shortness of breath, dyspnea on exertion, congestive heart failure, or dizziness requires emergency care.

PHYSICAL EXAMINATION

Because tachycardia can precipitate hemodynamic instability, an assessment of vital signs (including temperature, blood pressure, heart rate, respirations, and oxygen saturation) should be continuous. A heart rate greater than 150 beats per minute can cause serious signs and symptoms, but a careful history will help determine whether an underlying pathologic condition is causing the tachycardia and will facilitate appropriate treatment. The physical examination should be focused and exact. This will help establish whether the patient is stable or unstable and whether the tachycardia has precipitated serious signs and symptoms.

DIAGNOSTICS

Continuous assessment, cardiac monitoring, and a 12-lead ECG are necessary to identify the tachyarrhythmia and any deterioration in the patient's condition. A chest x-ray study and laboratory studies, including drug levels, electrolytes, a complete blood count, and thyroid studies, may also be indicated.

DIFFERENTIAL DIAGNOSIS

Atrial fibrillation, atrial flutter, narrow-complex tachycardias, stable wide-complex tachycardia of uncertain type, and ventricular tachycardia are tachyarrhythmias with potentially serious consequences. Emergency Cardiovascular Care Guidelines 2000 recommends classifying patients as stable or unstable, identifying whether serious signs and symptoms are present, and determining whether the arrhythmia has caused these signs and symptoms.[3] Identification of the tachycardia and its related pathology is essential for appropriate treatment (Figures 42-1 to 42-6). To prevent inappropriate therapy, the patient's condition and the etiology of the tachycardia should be carefully considered before treatment is initiated. Medications, pregnancy, hyperthyroidism, acute myocardial infarction, congestive heart failure, pulmonary embolus, hypotension, hypoxia, hypovolemia, infection, electrolyte abnormalities, and other disorders may precipitate a rapid heart rate and its resultant symptoms. Treatment of the specific disorder may result in resolution of the tachycardia.

INITIAL STABILIZATION AND MANAGEMENT

Oxygen administration, IV access, a 12-lead ECG, and continuous monitoring of the patient's oxygen saturation and vital signs are critical. In addition, suction, intubation, and defibrillation equipment should be readily available.

Advanced Cardiac Life Support (ACLS) Guidelines 2000 does not recommend treatment for tachycardia if chest pressure, acute myocardial infarction, change in mental status, hypotension, shortness of breath, congestive heart failure, or other signs and symptoms indicating instability are not present. Identification of the tachycardia is critical for appropriate treatment. However, immediate cardioversion is indicated if the patient is unstable because of the tachycardia (Figures 42-1 to 42-6). Urgent cardioversion is rarely necessary when the heart rate is less than 150 beats per minute.[3] Specific medications can also be used to treat specific tachyarrhythmias if the patient is stable (see Figures 42-1 to 42-6).[4] The choice of medications or cardioversion may also depend on the immediate availability of a defibrillator.

DISPOSITION AND REFERRAL

Ideally, symptomatic patients with tachycardia should be stabilized with initial management. Immediate transfer by ambulance to an emergency department is indicated for patients requiring continued assessment and management.

PREVENTION AND PATIENT EDUCATION

Tachyarrhythmias often recur. Careful explanation of the specific disorder and recognition of untoward symptoms are an important part of patient education. Because electrolyte disturbances and medications can precipitate some tachyarrhythmias, it is important that primary care providers consider and review medication therapies regularly. Amiodarone, sotalol, or other antiarrhythmic medications; implantable cardioversion/defibrillators; pacemakers; or ablation therapy may be indicated for the prevention of recurrent symptomatic tachycardia.[5,6]

Perform Primary ABCD Survey (Basic Life Support)
(Correct critical problems IMMEDIATELY as they are identified)
Assess responsiveness, **A**irway, **B**reathing, **C**irculation,
ensure availability of monitor/**D**efibrillator

↓

Perform Secondary ABCD Survey (Advanced Life Support)
Administer oxygen, establish IV access, attach cardiac monitor, administer fluids as needed (O_2, IV, monitor, fluids)
Assess vital signs, attach pulse oximeter, and monitor blood pressure
Obtain and review 12-lead ECG, portable chest x-ray film
Perform a focused history and physical exam

↓

Is the patient stable or unstable?
Is the patient experiencing serious signs and symptoms because of the tachycardia?

↓

Attempt to identify patient's cardiac rhythm using:

- 12-lead ECG, clinical information
- Vagal maneuvers
- Adenosine 6 mg rapid IV bolus over 1 to 3 sec. If needed, administer adenosine 12 mg rapid IV bolus over 1 to 3 sec after 1 to 2 min. May repeat 12 mg dose in 1 to 2 min if needed. Follow each dose immediately with 20 ml IV flush of NS. Use of adenosine is relatively contraindicated in patients with asthma. Decrease dose in patients on dipyridamole (Persantine) or carbamazepine (Tegretol); consider increasing dose in patients taking theophylline or caffeine-containing preparations

↓

Identify the Patient's Cardiac Rhythm

↓

Junctional Tachycardia		**Paroxysmal Supraventricular Tachycardia (PSVT) (Includes AVNRT or AVRT)**		**Ectopic Atrial Tachycardia, Multifocal Atrial Tachycardia (MAT)**	
Stable Patient		Stable Patient		Stable Patient	
Normal Cardiac Function	**Impaired Cardiac Function***	**Normal Cardiac Function**	**Impaired Cardiac Function***	**Normal Cardiac Function**	**Impaired Cardiac Function***
Amiodarone (IIb) **or** Beta blocker (Indeterminate) or Ca^{++} channel blocker (Indeterminate)	Amiodarone (IIb)	*Priority order:* Ca^{++} channel blocker (Class I) Beta blocker (Class I) Digoxin (IIb) Sync cardioversion	*Priority order:* Sync cardioversion Digoxin (IIb) Amiodarone (IIb) Diltiazem (IIb)	Ca^{++} channel blocker (IIb) **or** Beta blocker (IIb) **or** Amiodarone (IIb) **or** Flecainide (IIb) or Propafenone (IIb) **or** Digoxin (Indeterminate) **Cardioversion ineffective**	Amiodarone (IIb) **or** Diltiazem (IIb) **or** Digoxin (Indeterminate) **Cardioversion ineffective**

UNSTABLE PATIENT
If hemodynamically unstable PSVT, perform synchronized cardioversion: 50 J, 100 J, 200 J, 300 J, 360 J (or equivalent Biphasic energy)

*Impaired cardiac function = Ejection fraction <40% or CHF.

Medication Dosing

Amiodarone—150 mg IV over 10 min, followed by an infusion of 1 mg/min for 6 hours and then a maintenance infusion of 0.5 mg/min. Repeat supplementary infusions of 150 mg as necessary for recurrent or resistant arrhythmias. Maximum total daily dose 2.0 g.
Beta blockers—*Esmolol:* 0.5 mg/kg over 1 min, followed by a maintenance infusion at 50 mcg/kg/min for 4 min. If inadequate response, administer a second bolus of 0.5 mg/kg over 1 min and increase maintenance infusion to 100 mcg/kg/min. The bolus dose (0.5 mg/kg) and titration of the maintenance infusion (addition of 50 mcg/kg/min) can be repeated every 4 min to a maximum infusion of 300 mcg/kg/min. *Metoprolol:* 5 mg slow IV push over 5 min × 3 as needed to a total dose of 15 mg over 15 min.
Calcium channel blockers: *Diltiazem*—0.25 mg/kg over 2 min (e.g., 15 to 20 mg). If ineffective, 0.35 mg/kg over 2 min (e.g., 20 to 25 mg) in 15 min. Maintenance infusion 5 to 15 mg/hr, titrated to heart rate if chemical conversion successful. Calcium chloride (2 to 4 mg/kg) may be given **slow** IV push if borderline hypotension exists before diltiazem administration. *Verapamil*—2.5 to 5.0 mg slow IV push over 2 min. May repeat with 5 to 10 mg in 15 to 30 min. Maximum dose 20 mg.
Digoxin—Loading dose 10 to 15 mcg/kg lean body weight.
Flecainide, propafenone—IV form not currently approved for use in the United States.

FIGURE 42-1

Narrow QRS tachycardia. (From Aehlert B: *ACLS quick review study guide*, ed 2, St Louis, 2000, Mosby.)

Perform Primary ABCD Survey (Basic Life Support)
(Correct critical problems IMMEDIATELY as they are identified)
Assess responsiveness, **A**irway, **B**reathing, **C**irculation, ensure availability of monitor/**D**efibrillator

↓

Perform Secondary ABCD Survey (Advanced Life Support)
Administer oxygen, establish IV access, attach cardiac monitor, administer fluids as needed (O_2, IV, monitor, fluids)
Assess vital signs, attach pulse oximeter, and monitor blood pressure
Obtain and review 12-lead ECG, portable chest x-ray film, perform a focused history and physical exam

↓

Is the patient stable or unstable?
Is the patient's cardiac function normal or impaired?
Is the patient experiencing serious signs and symptoms because of the tachycardia?
Attempt to identify patient's cardiac rhythm using 12-lead ECG, clinical information
Is Wolff-Parkinson-White syndrome (WPW) present? If yes, see WPW algorithm
Has atrial fibrillation/atrial flutter been present for more or less than 48 hours?

↓

STABLE PATIENT

Normal Cardiac Function		Impaired Cardiac Function*	
Onset <48 hours	**Onset >48 hours**	**Onset <48 hours**	**Onset >48 hours**
Control Rate	**Control Rate**	**Control Rate**	**Control Rate**
Calcium channel blocker (Class I) **or** Beta blocker (Class I) **or** Digoxin (IIb)	Calcium channel blocker (Class I) **or** Beta blocker (Class I) **or** Digoxin (IIb)	Diltiazem (IIb) **or** Amiodarone (IIb) **or** Digoxin (IIb)	Diltiazem (IIb) **or** Amiodarone (IIb) **or** Digoxin (IIb)
Convert Rhythm	**Convert Rhythm**	**Convert Rhythm**	**Convert Rhythm**
Cardioversion **or** Amiodarone (IIa) **or** Procainamide (IIa) **or** Ibutilide (IIa) **or** Flecainide (IIa) **or** Propafenone (IIa)	Delayed cardioversion **or** Early cardioversion	Cardioversion **or** amiodarone (IIb)	Delayed cardioversion **or** Early cardioversion

Delayed cardioversion: Anticoagulation therapy for 3 weeks before cardioversion, for at least 48 hours in conjunction with cardioversion, and for at least 4 weeks after successful cardioversion. **Early cardioversion:** IV heparin immediately, transesophageal echocardiography (TEE) to rule out atrial thrombus, cardioversion within 24 hr, anticoagulation × 4 wks

Unstable Patient

If hemodynamically unstable, perform synchronized cardioversion: Atrial fibrillation: 100 J, 200 J, 300 J, 360 J, or equivalent Biphasic energy. Atrial flutter: 50 J, 100 J, 200 J, 300 J, 360 J, or equivalent Biphasic energy

Medication Dosing

Amiodarone—150 mg IV bolus over 10 min followed by an infusion of 1 mg/min for 6 hours and then a maintenance infusion of 0.5 mg/min. Repeat supplementary infusions of 150 mg as necessary for recurrent or resistant arrhythmias. Maximum total daily dose 2.0 g.
Beta blockers—*Esmolol:* 0.5 mg/kg over 1 min followed by a maintenance infusion at 50 mcg/kg/min for 4 min. If inadequate response, administer a second bolus of 0.5 mg/kg over 1 min and increase maintenance infusion to 100 mcg/kg/min. The bolus dose (0.5 mg/kg) and titration of the maintenance infusion (addition of 50 mcg/kg/min) can be repeated every 4 min to a maximum infusion of 300 mcg/kg/min. *Metoprolol:* 5 mg slow IV push over 5 min × 3 as needed to a total dose of 15 mg over 15 min. *Propranolol:* 0.1 mg/kg slow IV push divided in 3 equal doses at 2 to 3 min intervals. Do not exceed 1 mg/min. Repeat after 2 min, if necessary. *Atenolol:* 5 mg slow IV (over 5 min). Wait 10 min, then give second dose of 5 mg slow IV (over 5 min).
Calcium channel blockers: *Diltiazem*—0.25 mg/kg over 2 min (e.g., 15 to 20 mg). If ineffective, 0.35 mg/kg over 2 min (e.g., 20 to 25 mg) in 15 min. Maintenance infusion 5 to 15 mg/hr, titrated to heart rate if chemical conversion successful. Calcium chloride (2 to 4 mg/kg) may be given **slow** IV push if borderline hypotension exists before diltiazem administration. *Verapamil*—2.5 to 5.0 mg slow IV push over 2 min. May repeat with 5 to 10 mg in 15 to 30 min. Maximum dose 20 mg.
Ibutilide—Adults ≥60 kg: 1 mg (10 ml) over 10 min. May repeat × 1 in 10 min. Adults <60 kg: 0.01 mg/kg IV over 10 min.
Procainamide:—100 mg over 5 min (20 mg/min). Maximum total dose 17 mg/kg. Maintenance infusion 1 to 4 mg/min.
Flecainide, propafenone—IV form not currently approved for use in the United States.
Sotalol—1 to 1.5 mg/kg IV slowly at a rate of 10 mg/min.

*Impaired cardiac function = Ejection fraction <40% or CHF.

FIGURE 42-2

Atrial fibrillation/atrial flutter algorithm. (From Aehlert B: *ACLS quick review study guide*, ed 2, St Louis, 2000, Mosby.)

Perform Primary ABCD Survey (Basic Life Support)
(Correct critical problems IMMEDIATELY as they are identified)
Assess responsiveness, **A**irway, **B**reathing, **C**irculation, ensure availability of monitor/**D**efibrillator

↓

Perform Secondary ABCD Survey (Advanced Life Support)
Administer oxygen, establish IV access, attach cardiac monitor, administer fluids as needed (O_2, IV, monitor, fluids)
Assess vital signs, attach pulse oximeter, and monitor blood pressure
Obtain and review 12-lead ECG, portable chest x-ray film, perform a focused history and physical exam

↓

Is the patient stable or unstable?
Is the patient experiencing serious signs and symptoms because of the tachycardia?
Is the patient's cardiac function normal or impaired?
Attempt to identify patient's cardiac rhythm using 12-lead ECG, clinical information
Is Wolff-Parkinson-White syndrome (WPW) present? (e.g., young patient, HR >300, ECG: short PR interval, wide QRS, delta wave)
Has WPW been present for more or less than 48 hours?

↓

Normal Cardiac Function		**Impaired Cardiac Function***	
Onset <48 hours	**Onset >48 hours**	**Onset <48 hours**	**Onset >48 hours**
Control Rate	**Control Rate**	**Control Rate**	**Control Rate**
Cardioversion **or** Amiodarone (IIb) **or** Procainamide (IIb) **or** Flecainide (IIb) **or** Propafenone (IIb) **or** Sotalol (IIb)	Use antiarrhythmics with extreme caution because of embolic risk	Cardioversion **or** Amiodarone (IIb)	Use antiarrhythmics with extreme caution because of embolic risk
Convert Rhythm	**Convert Rhythm**	**Convert Rhythm**	**Convert Rhythm**
Cardioversion **or** Amiodarone (IIb) **or** Procainamide (IIb) **or** Flecainide (IIb) **or** Propafenone (IIb) **or** Sotalol (IIb)	Delayed cardioversion **or** Early cardioversion	Cardioversion	Delayed cardioversion **or** Early cardioversion

Delayed cardioversion: Anticoagulation therapy for 3 weeks before cardioversion for at least 48 hours in conjunction with cardioversion and for at least 4 weeks after successful cardioversion. **Early cardioversion:** IV heparin immediately, transesophageal echocardiography (TEE) to rule out atrial thrombus, cardioversion within 24 hr, anticoagulation × 4 weeks

Medication Dosing

Amiodarone—150 mg IV bolus over 10 min followed by an infusion of 1 mg/min for 6 hours and then a maintenance infusion of 0.5 mg/min. Repeat supplementary infusions of 150 mg as necessary for recurrent or resistant arrhythmias. Maximum total daily dose 2.0 g.
Procainamide—100 mg over 5 min (20 mg/min). Maximum total dose 17 mg/kg. Maintenance infusion 1 to 4 mg/min.
Flecainide, propafenone—IV form not currently approved for use in the United States.
Sotalol—1 to 1.5 mg/kg IV slowly at a rate of 10 mg/min.

*Impaired cardiac function = Ejection fraction <40% or CHF.

FIGURE 42-3

Wolff-Parkinson-White (WPW) syndrome algorithm. (From Aehlert B: *ACLS quick review study guide*, ed 2, St Louis, 2000, Mosby.)

Perform Primary ABCD Survey (Basic Life Support)
(Correct critical problems IMMEDIATELY as they are identified)
Assess responsiveness, **A**irway, **B**reathing, **C**irculation, ensure availability of monitor/**D**efibrillator

↓

Perform Secondary ABCD Survey (Advanced Life Support)
Administer oxygen, establish IV access, attach cardiac monitor, administer fluids as needed (O_2, IV, monitor, fluids)
Assess vital signs, attach pulse oximeter, and monitor blood pressure
Obtain and review 12-lead ECG, portable chest x-ray film, perform a focused history and physical exam

↓

Is the patient stable or unstable?
Is the patient experiencing serious signs and symptoms because of the tachycardia?
Determine if the rhythm is monomorphic or polymorphic VT and determine patient's QT interval

↓

Stable Patient

Normal Cardiac Function	Impaired Cardiac Function*

May proceed directly to synchronized cardioversion or use **one** of the following:

Normal Cardiac Function	Impaired Cardiac Function*
• Procainamide (IIa)	• Amiodarone (IIb)
• Sotalol (IIa)	• Lidocaine (Indeterminate)
• Amiodarone (IIb)	
• Lidocaine (IIb)	

↓

If medication therapy ineffective, perform synchronized cardioversion

Unstable VT with a Pulse

If hemodynamically unstable, sync 100 J, 200 J, 300 J, and 360 J (or equivalent Biphasic energy)
If hypotensive (systolic BP <90), unresponsive, or if severe pulmonary edema exists, defibrillate with same energy

Medication Dosing

Amiodarone: 150 mg IV bolus over 10 min. If chemical conversion successful, follow with IV infusion of 1 mg/min for 6 hours and then a maintenance infusion of 0.5 mg/min. Repeat supplementary infusions of 150 mg as necessary for recurrent or resistant arrhythmias. Maximum total daily dose 2.0 g.
Lidocaine: 1 to 1.5 mg/kg initial dose. Repeat dose is half the initial dose every 5 to 10 min. Maximum total dose 3 mg/kg. If chemical conversion successful, maintenance infusion 1 to 4 mg/min. If impaired cardiac function, dose = 0.5-0.75 mg/kg IV push. May repeat every 5 to 10 min. Maximum total dose 3 mg/kg. If chemical conversion successful, maintenance infusion 1 to 4 mg/min.
Procainamide: 100 mg over 5 min (20 mg/min). Maximum total dose 17 mg/kg. If chemical conversion successful, maintenance infusion 1 to 4 mg/min.
Sotalol: 1 to 1.5 mg/kg IV slowly at a rate of 10 mg/min.

*Impaired cardiac function = Ejection fraction <40% or CHF.

FIGURE 42-4

Sustained monomorphic ventricular tachycardia. (From Aehlert B: *ACLS quick review study guide*, ed 2, St Louis, 2000, Mosby.)

Perform Primary ABCD Survey (Basic Life Support)
(Correct critical problems IMMEDIATELY as they are identified)
Assess responsiveness, **A**irway, **B**reathing, **C**irculation, ensure availability of monitor/**D**efibrillator

↓

Perform Secondary ABCD Survey (Advanced Life Support)
Administer oxygen, establish IV access, attach cardiac monitor, administer fluids as needed (O_2, IV, monitor, fluids)
Assess vital signs, attach pulse oximeter, and monitor blood pressure
Obtain and review 12-lead ECG, portable chest x-ray film, perform a focused history and physical exam

↓

Is the patient stable or unstable?
Is the patient experiencing serious signs and symptoms because of the tachycardia?
Determine if the rhythm is monomorphic or polymorphic VT and determine patient's QT interval

↓

Polymorphic VT Normal QT interval		**Polymorphic VT** **Prolonged QT interval** (Suggests torsades de pointes)	
Stable Patient			
Normal Cardiac Function	**Impaired Cardiac Function***	**Normal Cardiac Function**	**Impaired Cardiac Function***
Treat ischemia if present Correct electrolyte abnormalities May proceed directly to electrical therapy or use **one** of the following: Amiodarone (IIb) Lidocaine (IIb) Procainamide (IIb) Sotalol (IIb) Beta blockers (Indeterminate)	May proceed directly to electrical therapy or use **one** of the following: Amiodarone (IIb) Lidocaine (Indeterminate)	DC meds that prolong QT Correct electrolyte abnormalities May proceed directly to electrical therapy or use **one** of the following: Magnesium (Indeterminate) Overdrive pacing with or without beta blocker (Indeterminate) Isoproterenol (Indeterminate) Phenytoin (Indeterminate) Lidocaine (Indeterminate)	May proceed directly to electrical therapy or use **one** of the following: Amiodarone (IIb) Lidocaine (Indeterminate)
If medication therapy ineffective, use electrical therapy			
Unstable Patient			
Sustained (>30 sec or causing hemodynamic collapse) polymorphic VT should be treated with an unsynchronized shock, using an initial energy of 200 J; if unsuccessful, a second shock of 200 to 300 J should be given and, if necessary, a third shock of 360 J			
Medication Dosing			

Amiodarone—150 mg IV bolus over 10 min. If chemical conversion successful, follow with IV infusion of 1 mg/min for 6 hours and then a maintenance infusion of 0.5 mg/min. Repeat supplementary infusions of 150 mg as necessary for recurrent or resistant arrhythmias. Maximum total daily dose 2.0 g.

Beta blockers—*Esmolol:* 0.5 mg/kg over 1 min followed by a maintenance infusion at 50 mcg/kg/min for 4 min. If inadequate response, administer a second bolus of 0.5 mg/kg over 1 min and increase maintenance infusion to 100 mcg/kg/min. The bolus dose (0.5 mg/kg) and titration of the maintenance infusion (addition of 50 mcg/kg/min) can be repeated every 4 min to a maximum infusion of 300 mcg/kg/min. *Metoprolol:* 5 mg slow IV push over 5 min × 3 as needed to a total dose of 15 mg over 15 min. *Atenolol:* 5 mg slow IV (over 5 min). Wait 10 min then give second dose of 5 mg slow IV (over 5 min).

Isoproterenol—Can be used as a temporizing measure until overdrive pacing can be instituted if no evidence of coronary artery disease, ischemic syndromes, or other contraindications. 2 to 10 mcg/min. Mix 1 mg in 500 ml NS or D_5W.

Lidocaine—1 to 1.5 mg/kg initial dose. Repeat dose is half the initial dose every 5 to 10 min. Maximum total dose 3 mg/kg. If chemical conversion successful, maintenance infusion 1 to 4 mg/min. If impaired cardiac function, dose = 0.5 to 0.75 mg/kg IV push. May repeat every 5 to 10 min. Maximum total dose 3 mg/kg. If chemical conversion successful, maintenance infusion 1 to 4 mg/min.

Magnesium—Loading dose of 1 to 2 g mixed in 50 to 100 ml over 5 to 60 min IV. If chemical conversion successful, follow with 0.5 to 1.0 g/hr IV infusion.

Phenytoin—250 mg IV at a rate of 25 to 50 mg/min in NS using a central vein.

Procainamide—100 mg over 5 min (20 mg/min). Maximum total dose 17 mg/kg. If chemical conversion successful, maintenance infusion 1 to 4 mg/min.

Sotalol—1 to 1.5 mg/kg IV slowly at a rate of 10 mg/min.

*Impaired cardiac function = Ejection fraction <40% or CHF.

FIGURE 42-5

Polymorphic ventricular tachycardia. (From Aehlert B: *ACLS quick review study guide*, ed 2, St Louis, 2000, Mosby.)

Perform Primary ABCD Survey (Basic Life Support)
(Correct critical problems IMMEDIATELY as they are identified)
Assess responsiveness, **A**irway, **B**reathing, **C**irculation, ensure availability of monitor/**D**efibrillator

↓

Perform Secondary ABCD Survey (Advanced Life Support)
Administer oxygen, establish IV access, attach cardiac monitor
Administer fluids as needed (O_2, IV, monitor, fluids)
Assess vital signs, attach pulse oximeter, and monitor blood pressure
Obtain and review 12-lead ECG, portable chest x-ray film, perform a focused history and physical exam

↓

Is the patient stable or unstable?
Is the patient experiencing serious signs and symptoms because of the tachycardia?

Use 12-lead ECG/clinical information to help clarify rhythm diagnosis

↓

Rhythm confirmed as SVT Go to narrow-QRS tachycardia algorithm	**Wide-Complex Tachycardia of Unknown Origin Stable Patient**	**Rhythm confirmed as VT Go to VT algorithm**

Normal Cardiac Function	**Impaired Cardiac Function***
Sync cardioversion **or** Procainamide (IIb) **or** Amiodarone (IIb)	Sync cardioversion **or** Amiodarone (IIb)

↓

If medication therapy ineffective, perform synchronized cardioversion

Unstable Patient

If hemodynamically unstable, sync 100 J, 200 J, 300 J, and 360 J, or equivalent Biphasic energy. If hypotensive (systolic BP <90), unresponsive, or if severe pulmonary edema exists, defibrillate with same energy

Medication Dosing

Amiodarone—150 mg IV bolus over 10 min. If chemical conversion successful, follow with IV infusion of 1 mg/min for 6 hours and then a maintenance infusion of 0.5 mg/min. Repeat supplementary infusions of 150 mg as necessary for recurrent or resistant arrhythmias. Maximum total daily dose 2.0 g.

Procainamide: 100 mg over 5 min (20 mg/min). Maximum total dose 17 mg/kg. If chemical conversion successful, maintenance infusion 1 to 4 mg/min.

*Impaired cardiac function = Ejection fraction <40% or CHF.

FIGURE 42-6

Wide QRS tachycardia of unknown origin. (From Aehlert B: *ACLS quick review study guide*, ed 2, St Louis, 2000, Mosby.)

REFERENCES

1. Shotan A and others: Incidence of arrhythmias in normal pregnancy and relation to palpitations, dizziness, and syncope, *Am J Cardiol* 79(8):1061-1064, 1997.
2. Wood KA, Drew BJ, Scheinman MM: Frequency of disabling symptoms in supraventricular tachycardia, *Am J Cardiol* 79(2):145-149, 1997.
3. American Heart Association: *2000 handbook of emergency cardiovascular care for healthcare providers*, Dallas, 2000, The Association.
4. Aehlert B: *ACLS quick review study guide*, St Louis, 2000, Mosby.
5. Singh BN: Controlling cardiac arrhythmias: an overview with historical perspective, *Am J Cardiol* 80(8A):4G-15G, 1997.
6. Stevenson WG and others: Ablation therapy for cardiac arrhythmias, *Am J Cardiol* 80(8A):56G-66G, 1997.

CHAPTER 43

Thermal Injuries

Timothy J. Phillips

Extremes of environmental conditions often contribute to the development of heat- and cold-related injuries, including hyperthermia and hypothermia. A history of increased physical activity in the heat or prolonged exposure to cold temperatures may suggest thermal injury, but conditions such as alcohol or drug ingestion, trauma, psychiatric conditions, or medical conditions should also be considered.

Immediate emergency department referral/physician consultation is indicated for hypothermia or heatstroke/heat exhaustion.

Heat-Related Injuries

DEFINITION/EPIDEMIOLOGY

Heat stress and heat cramps are milder forms of heat-related injuries, whereas heatstroke and heat exhaustion are more severe. Heat injuries are differentiated not by specific temperature ranges but by symptoms and systemic changes that develop as body temperature increases.

Some cases are too mild to be diagnosed, and some cases do not get reported. Therefore it is difficult to estimate with accuracy the number of heat-related injuries. However, one report has listed 84 fatal heatstroke injuries among football players from 1955 to 1990.[1]

PATHOPHYSIOLOGY

Heat-related injuries occur when the metabolic demands of exercise raise the temperature of the body or when environmental heat stress is maximal. In warm environments, evaporation of sweat from the skin is the most important mechanism of heat dissipation.[2] Under certain conditions, however, an inadequate transfer of heat occurs and body temperature increases. Heat exhaustion is associated with a combination of conditions, including dehydration, loss of the normal electrolyte balance, and respiratory alkalosis caused by exercise. Heatstroke caused by failure of the normal thermoregulatory mechanisms is believed to be related to dehydration complicated by a compensatory vasoconstriction of the peripheral vasculature.

CLINICAL PRESENTATION

Patients with heat stress usually exhibit mild changes in mental status and may also complain of dizziness and fatigue. Heat cramps are characterized by muscle spasms that may be accompanied by weakness, fatigue, nausea, and vomiting. More severe forms of heat injury, including heat exhaustion and heatstroke, are differentiated by worsening mental status changes. Heat exhaustion may be accompanied by a variety of symptoms that include but are not limited to nausea, vomiting, fatigue, irritability, headache, syncope, dyspnea, weakness, and increased sweating. Heatstroke may be characterized by vomiting, diarrhea, coma, seizures, and mental status changes.

PHYSICAL EXAMINATION

The spectrum of physical findings and presenting symptoms reflects the severity of the injury. Blood pressure and heart rate typically are elevated in patients presenting with heat stress. Heart rate, blood pressure, and body temperature may be normal when heat cramps are present. In heat exhaustion, orthostatic vital signs and mental status changes may also be present, and core body temperature is typically less than 39° C (102.2° F). In addition to a core body temperature greater than 39° C (102.2° F), symptoms of heatstroke may include decreased blood pressure and mental status changes.

DIAGNOSTICS

Because the liver, kidneys, muscles, and coagulation systems are most susceptible to heat injury, laboratory assessment should include electrolytes, glucose, BUN, creatinine, liver function tests (LFTs), creatinine phosphokinase, and coagulation studies. A urinalysis should be obtained to assess kidney involvement. A variety of ECG changes may be observed. It is important to monitor patients with heatstroke for rhabdomyolysis, acute renal failure, and disseminated intravascular coagulation, which are well-known complications. Note that hepatic damage (elevated LFTs) is a consistent feature of heatstroke, and therefore an absence of this casts doubt on the diagnosis.[2]

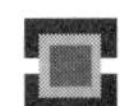

Diagnostics

Heat-Related Injuries

Initial
ECG

Laboratory
Serum electrolytes
BUN
Creatinine
CPK
Serum glucose
LFTs
Coagulation studies (PT/PTT)
Urinalysis
CBC and differential

DIFFERENTIAL DIAGNOSIS

It is essential to recognize the seriousness of heat-related injuries. Heat stress, heat cramps, heat syncope, heatstroke, and heat exhaustion must be differentiated to ensure proper treatment. Presentation of the more emergent heat-related injuries may mimic other conditions, including systemic infections, dehydration, seizures, metabolic or neurologic abnormalities, cardiac arrhythmias, myocardial infarction, and cocaine overdose. These should be considered if the patient does not respond to cooling measures.

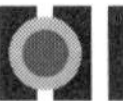

Differential Diagnosis

Heat-Related Injuries

Heat stress/cramps/stroke/exhaustion/syncope
Systemic infection
Dehydration
Seizures
Metabolic/neurologic abnormality
Cardiac arrhythmias
Myocardial infarction
Cocaine overdose

INITIAL STABILIZATION AND MANAGEMENT

The degree of hyperthermia affects treatment. However, all patients with hyperthermia should be treated with rest, hydration, and cooling regardless of severity. Either oral or IV hydration can be used for minor heat cramps, but heat exhaustion requires IV hydration with either normal saline or lactated Ringer's solution at 250 ml/hr.[3]

Heatstroke needs to be identified and treated immediately. Because outcome and resultant damage are related to the duration of hyperthermia, the core body temperature should be lowered quickly to 38° C (100.4° F). Simple, quick cooling measures include immersing the patient in ice water, covering the patient with an ice water cooling blanket, fanning, and placing ice packs in the groin, axilla, and neck area. IV hydration should be started immediately, but rapid delivery of excessive fluids should be avoided. If other symptoms develop, specific therapy may be necessary for patients with coma, renal failure, coagulopathies, or acid-base abnormalities.

DISPOSITION AND REFERRAL

All patients with heat injuries should be assessed rapidly and treated initially with hydration, cooling measures, and rest. The level of treatment available at the treatment facility should dictate the necessity for referral. Transfer to the appropriate facility should be arranged for patients requiring hospitalization or critical care.

PREVENTION AND PATIENT EDUCATION

Prevention of heat-related injuries includes physical conditioning and acclimatization. Daily exposure for 100 minutes a day results in near-maximal acclimatization in 7 to 14 days.[2] Patients should also understand the importance of drinking extra fluids during hot weather or if working or exercising in the heat because individuals do not voluntarily drink as much as they lose, replacing only two thirds of the fluids lost.[2]

Cold-Related Injuries

DEFINITION/EPIDEMIOLOGY

Hypothermia is caused by decreased core body temperature. Unlike hyperthermia, it is categorized by specific ranges of core body temperatures. Frostbite injury results from exposure to cold temperatures and causes irreversible tissue damage.

From 1979 to 1995 hypothermia was the underlying cause of 12,368 deaths in the United States.[4] Frostbite, which usually affects the feet, occurs most commonly in adults between 30 and 49 years of age.[5]

PATHOPHYSIOLOGY

As core body temperature decreases, cardiac output, blood pressure, and heart rate initially increase, then decrease. An initial increase in respiratory rate is followed by a decrease in rate. The oxyhemoglobin dissociation curve is shifted to the left, with a subsequent decrease in oxygen delivery. This combination of decreased metabolic functioning leads to abnormalities in the functional capabilities of the pulmonary, cardiac, and central nervous systems.[3] When frostbite occurs, the tissue is damaged by the progressive effects of freezing, decreased oxygen, and the release of inflammatory factors into the tissue.

CLINICAL PRESENTATION

Mild hypothermia corresponds to a core body temperature of 32° to 35° C (89.6° to 95.0° F). Moderate hypothermia develops if cooling continues until the core body temperature reaches 28° to 32° C (82.4° to 89.6° F). Severe hypothermia results if the core body temperature decreases to less than 28° C (82.4° F).[6] Frostbite may have a varying degree of symptoms depending on the degree of local tissue injury; however, numbness is the most common presenting symptom 75% of the time.[7]

PHYSICAL EXAMINATION

In addition to the specific core temperature noted in patients with hypothermia, certain common symptoms are associated with each level of hypothermia. Symptoms associated with mild hypothermia often include shivering, tachycardia, tachypnea, and diuresis. Changes in skin color, balance, and memory may also be present in some cases. Shivering decreases and mental status changes are noticeable with a further decrease of temperature to moderate hypothermia. With severe hypothermia, the loss of reflexes, stupor or coma, and fixed, dilated pupils may be observed. Characteristic ECG changes depend on temperature. Above 35° C (95.0° F), sinus tachycardia is most common. Between 35° and 32° C (95.0° and 89.6° F), sinus bradycardia commonly occurs. Below 32° C (89.6° F), characteristic J waves may be seen. At 30° C (86.0° F), atrial arrhythmias are usual, whereas at 28° C (82.4° F), ventricular arrhythmias are more common. Asystole occurs at temperatures less than 20° C (68° F).[8]

Superficial frostbite is characterized by decreased sensation and erythema surrounding a central white area with or without blisters. Deep frostbite is characterized by hemorrhagic blisters or necrosis with tissue loss.[5]

DIAGNOSTICS

Patients with hypothermia require cardiac monitoring and close observation for arrhythmias. Rectal temperature, preferably obtained with a continuous rectal probe, and vital signs are indicated. CBC, glucose, BUN, creatinine, serum electrolytes, coagulation studies (PT/PTT), cardiac isoenzymes, and arterial blood gases (ABGs) are also necessary.

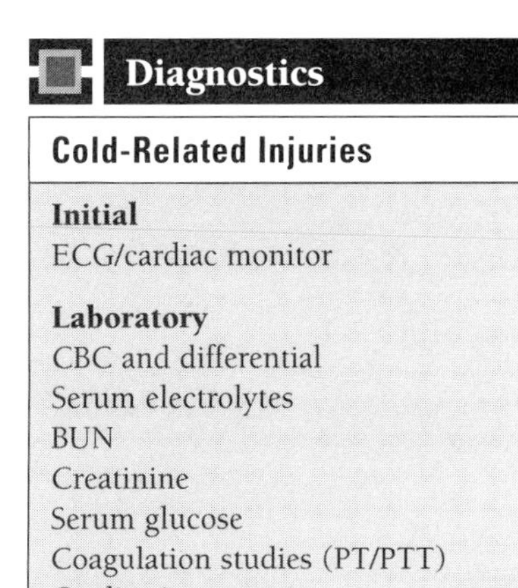

Diagnostics

Cold-Related Injuries

Initial
ECG/cardiac monitor

Laboratory
CBC and differential
Serum electrolytes
BUN
Creatinine
Serum glucose
Coagulation studies (PT/PTT)
Cardiac isoenzymes
ABGs

DIFFERENTIAL DIAGNOSIS

Although the symptoms associated with hypothermia can be associated with other conditions, the core body temperature will indicate hypothermia. Further differentials should include the specific differences between mild, moderate, and severe hypothermia, as well as

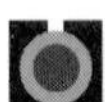

Differential Diagnosis

Cold-Related Injuries
Mild/moderate/severe hypothermia Superficial/deep frostbite

the difference between superficial and deep frostbite. This information will guide rewarming and treatment.

INITIAL STABILIZATION AND MANAGEMENT

Cold injuries require rewarming, and the method of rewarming is based on the clinical circumstances and availability of resources.[8] Regardless of the degree of cold injury, all patients with hypothermia should immediately have all cold or wet clothing removed and be covered with warm and dry blankets to prevent further heat loss. In addition, patients with moderate or severe hypothermia should be handled gently to prevent arrhythmias such as ventricular fibrillation. The care of patients in cardiac arrest necessitates rewarming because "death cannot be pronounced until the patient is warm and dead."[9]

Passive external rewarming includes placing these patients in a warm environment and covering them with warm, dry blankets. Active external rewarming includes warmed blankets, hot packs, warm bodies, or forced air rewarming.[8] Core rewarming includes perfusion of the body with warm IV fluids, administration of heated and humidified oxygen, and a body cavity lavage with warm fluids. Hemodialysis and extracorporeal circulation are also considerations for rewarming.

Hypothermia precautions are also applicable to patients with frostbite. The injured part should be rewarmed as soon as possible with water between 37° and 40° C (98.6° and 104° F). Ibuprofen should be given at a dose of 12 mg/kg/day to decrease the effects of inflammation. Tetanus immunization status should be updated, and penicillin is recommended at a dose of 500,000 units every 6 hours during the first 72 hours of treatment.[5] One precaution to follow is to not rewarm an affected extremity if there is a chance of refreeze before definitive treatment, as thaw/freeze/thaw creates tremendous tissue damage.

DISPOSITION AND REFERRAL

For mild symptoms that are resolved after rewarming, patients can be discharged. Other patients should be evaluated for hospitalization.[3] All patients with frostbite that exceeds the minimal symptoms should be hospitalized.

PREVENTION AND PATIENT EDUCATION

Hypothermia is preventable, yet nearly 700 people die each year from cold-related injuries.[10] Prevention of these injuries requires education regarding proper clothing and shelter. Layering of clothes to protect against extreme temperatures should also be advised. In addition, patients and families should understand that massaging the affected areas is contraindicated and that cold sensitivity is a common sequela of hypothermic injury. Use the motto of "comfortably cool" in cold environments to prevent sweating, because sweating can lead to hypothermia and frostbite later.

REFERENCES

1. Tom PA, Garmel GM, Auerbach PS: *Environment-dependent sports emergencies, Med Clin North Am* 78(2):305-325, 1994.
2. Yarbrough B, Vicario S: Heat illness, 1997-2009. In Marx JA and others, editors: *Rosen's emergency medicine: concepts and clinical practice,* ed 5, St Louis, 2002, Mosby.
3. Tintinalli JE, Ruiz E, Krome RL, editors: *Emergency medicine,* ed 4, San Francisco, 1996, McGraw-Hill.
4. Lee-Chiong TL, Stilt JT: Accidental hypothermia: when thermoregulation is overwhelmed, *Postgrad Med* 99(1):77-80, 83-84, 87-88, 1996.
5. Reamy BV: Frostbite: review and current concepts, *J Am Board Fam Pract* 11(1):34-40, 1998.
6. Gentilello LM: Advances in the management of hypothermia, *Surg Clin North Am* 75(2):243-256, 1995.
7. Danzl DF: Frostbite, 1972-1978. In Marx JA and others, editors: *Rosen's emergency medicine: concepts and clinical practice,* ed 5, St Louis, 2002, Mosby.
8. Hanania NA, Zimmerman JL: Accidental hypothermia, *Crit Care Clin* 15(2):235-249, 1999.
9. Braun R, Krishel S: Environmental emergencies, *Emerg Med Clin North Am* 15(2):451-476, 1997.
10. Hypothermia-related deaths: Utah, 2000 and United States, 1979-1998, *MMWR* 51(4):76-78, 2002.

PART 5

Evaluation and Management of Skin Disorders

JOANN TRYBULSKI, Section Editor

CHAPTER 44

Examination of the Skin and Approach to Diagnosing Skin Disorders

Margaret McAllister

DEFINITION/EPIDEMIOLOGY

Skin problems occur in more than 25% of the general population and are the presenting complaint in 10% of primary care patients.[1] A large number of skin diseases present in similar ways. Factors such as age, ethnic and genetic makeup, risk factors, body habitus, skin surface, and self-care practices may confound a diagnosis. An underlying systemic pathologic condition may also contribute to the difficulty of making a definitive diagnosis of skin lesions.

OVERVIEW OF SKIN FUNCTION, ANATOMY, AND STRUCTURES

The primary functions of the skin include protection of the underlying body structures from the ingress of microorganisms, control of body heat and elimination of body waste through perspiration, and prevention of injury to core body structures. The skin protects the body from infectious agents; protects against loss of body heat through conduction, convection, and radiation; and provides a first-line defense against mechanical, chemical, and thermal injury. Glands in the dermal layer of the skin secrete a substance that lubricates the body surface and assists with a variety of body functions. The peripheral sense receptors contained in the skin alert the body to pain, temperature changes, pressure, and touch.

The skin is composed of three layers: the epidermis, the dermis, and the hypodermis (or subcutis). The outer epidermal (or cuticle) layer is avascular and is divided into an outer horny layer (the stratum corneum) and an underlying horny layer (the stratum mucosum). The stratum corneum consists of keratinocytes—cells that originate in the basal cell layer of the epidermis and migrate upward to the stratum corneum and slough off as dead cells called squames. As long as the outer horny layer is intact, normal skin bacteria are prevented from invading deeper skin and gaining access to the bloodstream. The lower layer of the epidermis contains the Langerhans' cells, which function as antigen-presenting cells that migrate to the lymph nodes and play an important role in the allergic skin response. Melanocytes found in the basal layer of the epidermis constitute the body's principal protection against ultraviolet (UV) radiation.[1]

The second layer of the skin, the dermis—also termed the cutis, corneum, or true skin—holds the epidermis in place. The dermis is composed of an outer papillary layer and an inner reticular layer that contains connective tissue and the blood supply, as well as lymphatic vessels, peripheral nerves, elastic tissue, and a reservoir of water and electrolytes. The dermal appendages are contained within the reticular layer and include the eccrine sweat glands that control body temperature via evaporation, the sebum-producing sebaceous glands that lubricate the stratum corneum through openings in the skin (called pores), hair follicles, and the nail bed. Other appendages include apocrine glands attached to hair shafts located in the axillary, perianal, and genital areas. These glands respond to the increased hormone levels associated with puberty, adolescence, and young adulthood and decrease their activity with normal aging. A variation of the apocrine gland is the cerumen-producing glands lining the external auditory canal. The oily substance, cerumen, protects the skin lining the ear canal from bacterial invasion.

A third layer of the skin, the hypodermis, or subcutis, functions to store fat and insulate the body from extremes in temperature and provide a cushion against injury. It also contributes to the skin's mobility over underlying body parts.

CHANGES IN THE SKIN ASSOCIATED WITH AGING

Both structural and functional changes occur in the skin during the aging process. These changes include a decrease in the number of Langerhans' cells; a variation in the size, shape, and staining of the keratinocytes; a decrease in the thickness of the dermis; and a loss of elastic tissue. There is a decrease in the number of sweat glands, hair follicles, and specialized nerve endings, as well as decreased vascularity and increased fragility of existing capillaries. Functional changes in the skin include a decreased inflammatory response, increased time for wound healing, thinning of the skin resulting in increased fragility and risk of injury, decreased sweat capacity, and increased dryness secondary to less sebum production.[2,3]

ASSESSMENT

Formulating a differential diagnosis for skin lesions is based on in-depth knowledge of various common skin disorders and their characteristic physical properties, including location and shape. In addition, knowledge of the associated history typical of common rashes is essential. Variations in color, texture, and continuity of a patient's skin may be a normal genetic or ethnic variant, an indicator of local skin pathology, or an indicator of an underlying systemic disease process. Proper assessment forms the basis for an appropriate plan of care and patient education for self-care of acute and chronic skin lesions, as well as the prevention of recurrence. Assessment begins with a careful history and physical examination. Additional investigative techniques, such as Wood's light examination, laboratory data, or microscopic skin scraping examination, may be necessary to ensure a definitive diagnosis.

Health History

Subjective components of a dermatologic history include the patient or caregiver's history of the onset and progression of the rash, associated symptoms, past history of any skin disorder, medication history, social history, occupational history, and dietary practices. The primary care provider inquires about self-care practices such as homeopathic remedies, lotions, soaps, any change in laundry products, new clothing or fabrics, rubber glove use, cosmetics, sunbathing, tanning salons, and the humidity of the patient's typical ambient environment. In addition, a family or self-history of skin disorders, allergy, atopy, asthma, or eczema in childhood is reviewed.

BOX 44-1

PRIMARY LESIONS

Macules are localized changes in the skin color. They are flat and nonpalpable, but they may be scaly. Examples include freckles, lentigines (or "age spots"), actinic lentigines on sun-exposed areas, large macules of melasma seen in pregnancy, and the hypopigmented macular lesions of vitiligo and pityriasis alba. Oblique lighting may assist in determining if a macule is flat or raised, suggesting a papule.

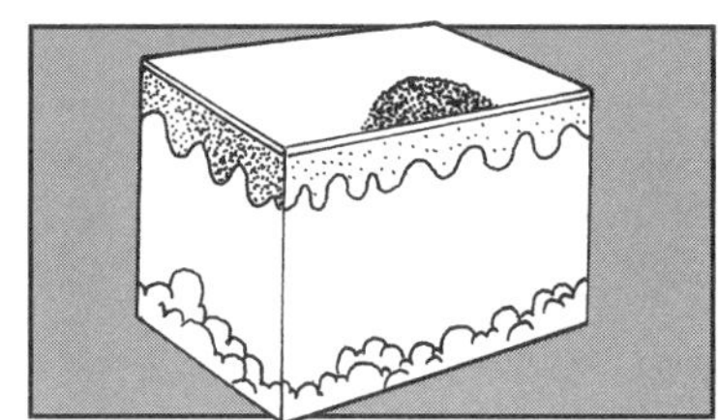

Papules can be solid or fluid-filled lesions that are elevated and are less than 5 mm in diameter. The size and shape of a papule can vary from pointed to flat-topped lesions. Examples of papules include atopic eczema or a viral exanthema that is a combined macular-papular rash.

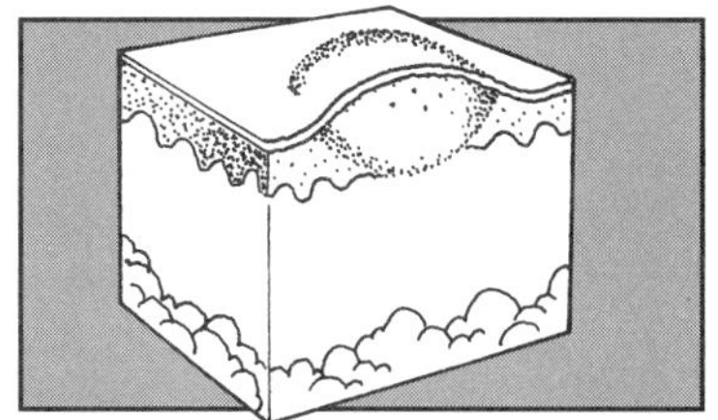

Nodules are both solid and elevated above the surface of the skin but usually originate deeper in skin layers. Nodules measure greater than 5 mm in diameter. Palpation assists in determining the depth of a nodule. If the skin slides over the nodule, it is beneath the dermis and in the subcutaneous layer. If the skin moves with the lesion, then it is located in the dermis. A hemanginoma, a basal cell carcinoma, or melanoma may be termed a nodule.

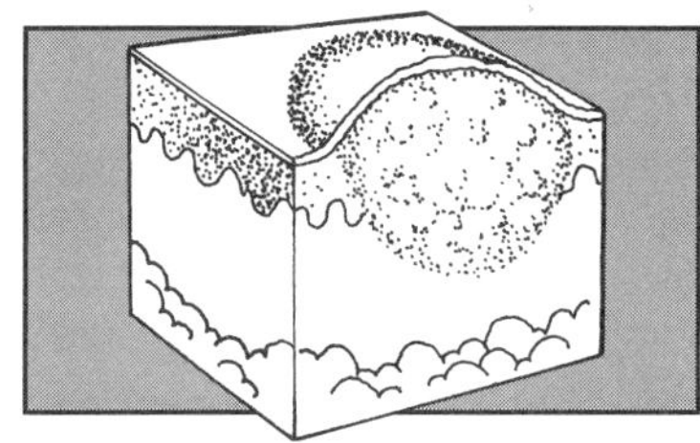

Plaques are elevated lesions that are larger than 5 mm in diameter. Like papules, they may take on a variety of shapes. A plaque is often a close grouping of multiple papules, such as is seen in seborrheic dermatitis, tinea corporis, tinea versicolor, or psoriasis.

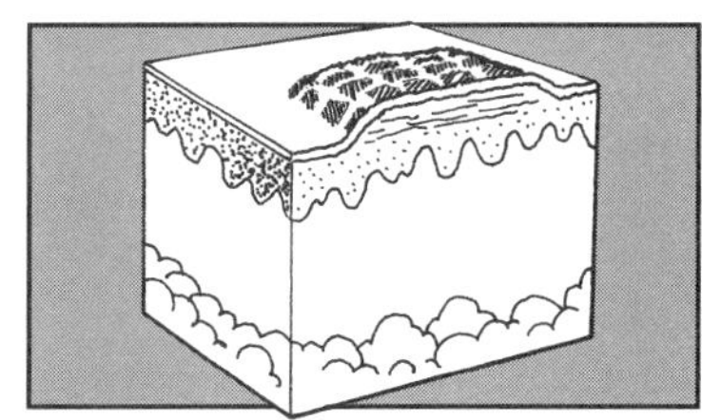

Vesicles and *bullae* are well-circumscribed, fluid-filled areas under the superficial layers of the skin. A vesicle can measure 5 mm in diameter. The covering over the vesicle is a thin layer of epithelium that is easily punctured. An example is the vesicle of herpes simplex or impetigo. Bullae are accumulations of fluid under the superficial layers of the skin that measure greater than 5 mm in diameter. Burns of the second degree constitute bullae, as do large impetigo lesions and the lesions of a fixed drug eruption.

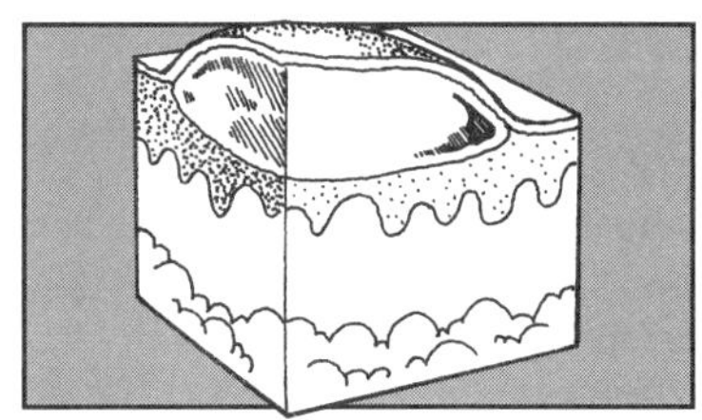

Wheals are an accumulation of fluid within the dermal layer of the skin that forms an edematous plaque. Wheals are localized edema of the skin, and they may appear in a variety of sizes and shapes. The color depends on the amount of fluid in the wheal. Examples of wheals include hives and angioedema.

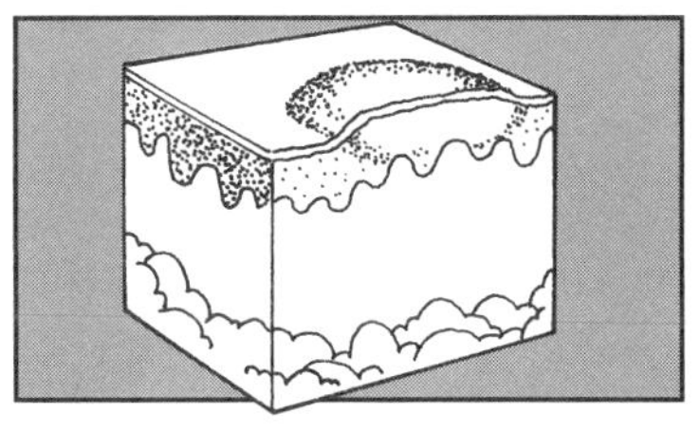

Pustules are abscessed lesions filled with pus. Furuncles and acne lesions are pustular and often respond to antibiotic and local therapy.

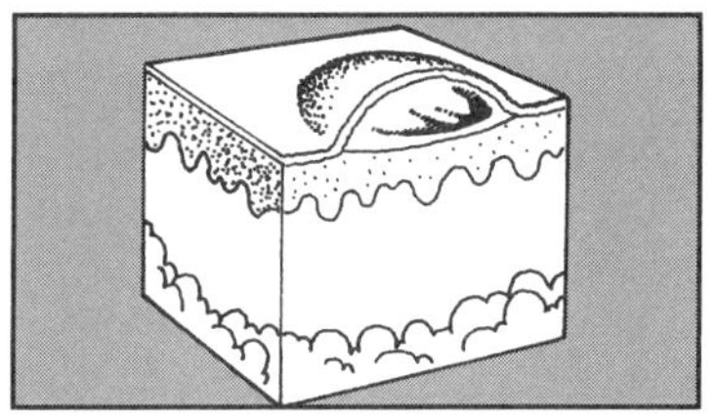

BOX 44-2

SECONDARY LESIONS

Secondary lesions are changes that occur in primary lesions as a result of environmental factors, self-care practices (such as scratching), inflammation of surrounding tissues, healing and scar formation, infection, and the use of topical medications, such as steroids.

Scales are dried, thin, platelike lesions of cornified epithelium. These lesions are partially attached, partially separated from the epidermis, and commonly associated with exfoliative skin conditions. Scales are commonly seen with psoriasis or seborrheic dermatitis.

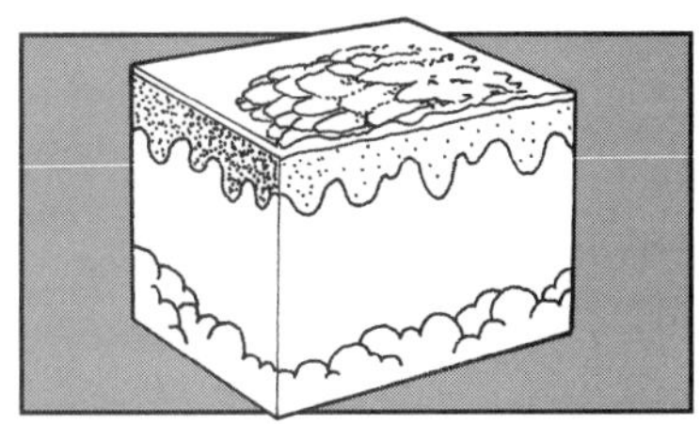

Crusts are hard, dried exudates that occur on the surface of ruptured vesicles or pustules. Crusted lesions and vesicles on an erythematous base are often seen in perioral herpes simplex or in herpes zoster.

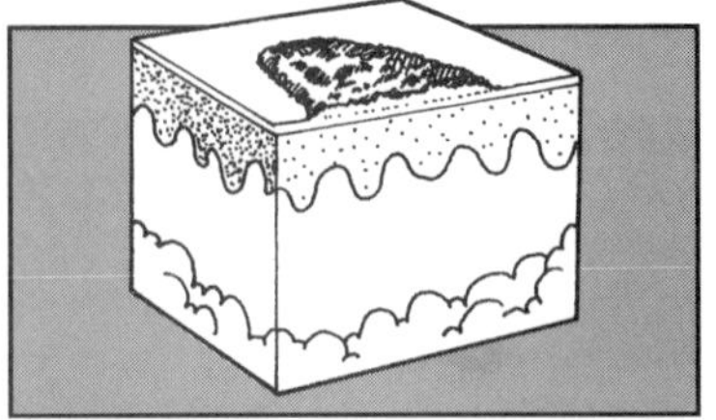

Erosions are skin injuries that may result from rubbing or shearing. This type of lesion is moist and may also result from a ruptured vesicular or pustular lesion.

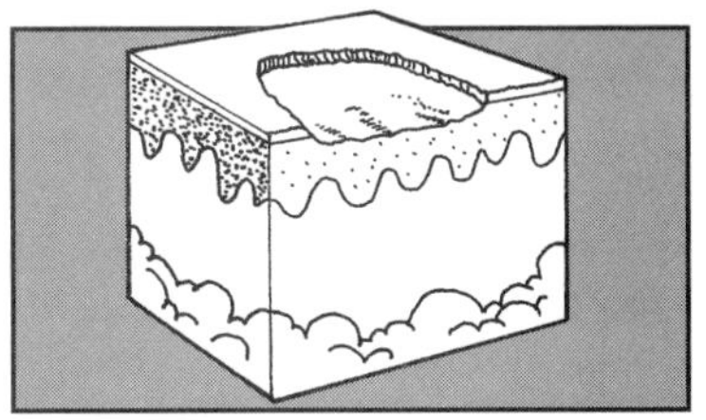

Fissures are slivered lesions that extend from the epidermis into the dermis. Fissures may occur from trauma but are also associated with inflexible, dried skin that cracks when stretched.

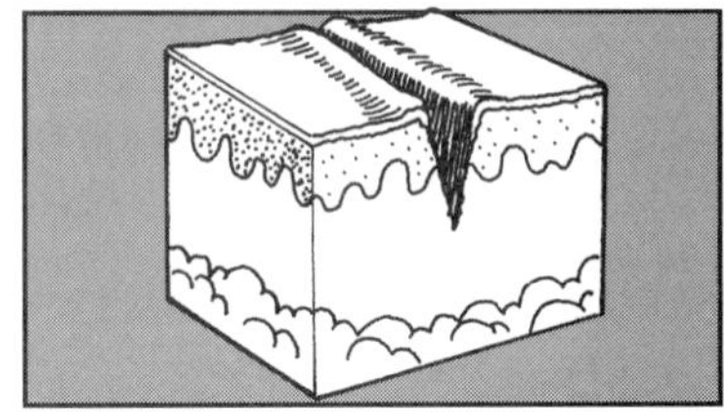

Atrophy is used to describe lesions that are inelastic and have lost characteristic rhomboid lines. In discoid lupus erythematosus, the lesions commonly seen on the scalp, face, arms, and torso have central atrophy but may have accompanying erythematous borders, scales, and telangiectasia.

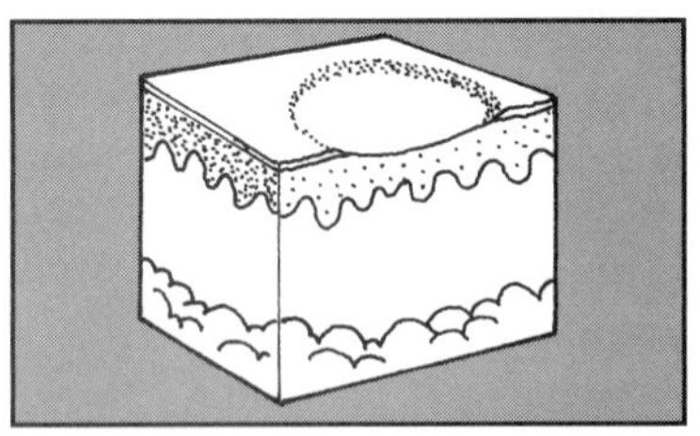

Ulcers are concave lesions with a sunken appearance. The result of trauma and/or poor circulation, ulcers extend from the epidermis into the dermis.

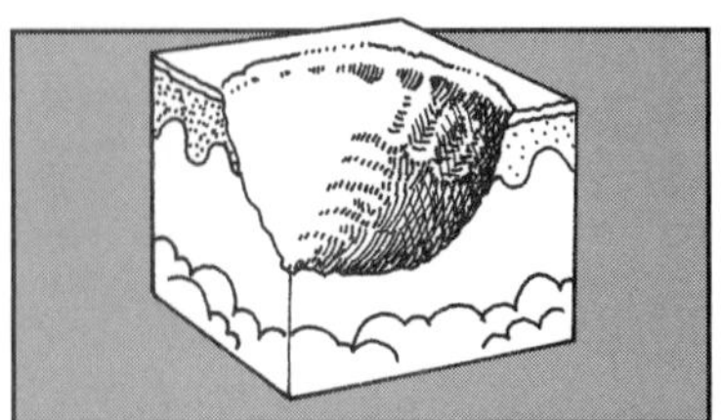

Scars are fibrous lesions that result from trauma to the skin. The appearance depends on the etiology of the injury, but new scars are generally hyperpigmented. As the lesion ages, the scar will fade and become hypopigmented.

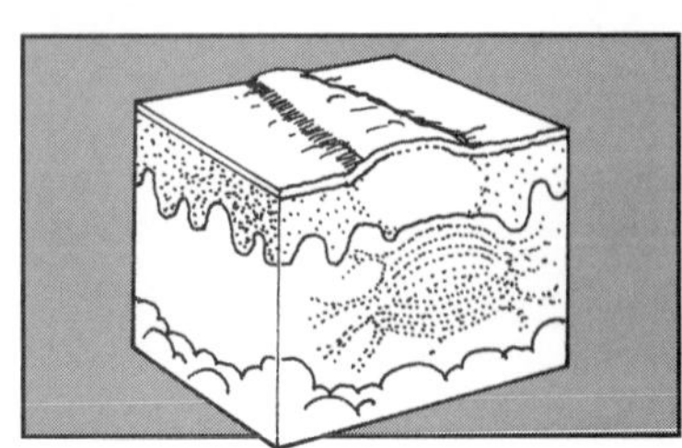

BOX 44-3

SKIN EXAMINATION TECHNIQUES

Diascopy can be performed using a flat microscope slide or other clear instrument, such as a magnifying glass. Blanching of blue to red lesions followed by a gradual refilling indicates blood in the capillaries; absence of blanching indicates blood leaching outside of the capillaries, such as in petechiae.

Gram's stain of exudates from lesions is helpful in distinguishing the etiology as either a gram-positive or gram-negative organism.

The *Tzanck test* with Wright's or Giemsa's stain can uncover multinucleated giant cells that are typical of herpes simplex or varicella zoster virus. The top of the vesicle must be removed in order to obtain fresh fluid from the base of the lesion.

A *10% to 30% potassium hydroxide (KOH) stain* determines the presence of hyphae and spores consistent with candidiasis or uncovers the spaghetti-and-meatball appearance of tinea versicolor, caused by the skin fungus *Pityrosporum orbiculare* or *Pityrosporum ovale*.[5] Attempts should be made to obtain scrapings from the top of a lesion or from the advancing edge of a lesion. The skin lesion is aligned vertical to the microscopic slide, and a gentle scraping of the lesion with the side of a slide or a scalpel loosens skin debris collected on the slide below. KOH is applied directly to the scale debris, a coverslip is placed over the skin scraping, or the KOH is applied alongside the edge of the coverslip. KOH then gravitates to cover the specimen by capillary action. The specimen is then set under the microscope for examination, first using ×10 power and then proceeding to ×40 power for finer detail. The examiner must be sure to close the condenser diaphragm and turn the condenser down to enhance the detail of hyphae that are embedded in the scaly debris.[6]

Culture for herpesvirus, streptococcus, staphylococcus, or *Pseudomonas* organisms requires removal of the outer crust or cuticle of the lesion to obtain fluid for culturing. The fluid at the base of the lesion is most likely to be positive for the contributing organisms and free of contamination from the skin surface. A special viral culture-collecting device must be used in accordance with laboratory specifications. Bacterial cultures for streptococcus and staphylococcus organisms can be collected with a regular throat culture–collecting swab. *Candida* organisms can be grown on Sabouraud's agar in a 2- to 6-day period, whereas dermatophytes will take up to 2 to 4 weeks to grow on the same agar. The organisms of tinea versicolor will grow only on special media.[6]

In *scabies preparation* a superficial skin shaving from a skinfold area is obtained from the top of a burrow and examined under oil immersion. Oil or potassium hydroxide solution should be placed on the lesion first. With a scalpel the top is shaved off of the lesion, and the debris is placed on a microscopic slide. Additional oil and a coverslip are added, and the specimen is examined under ×10 magnification.[7] The presence of adult mites, eggs, or feces in the burrows is sufficient for a diagnosis of scabies.

Physical Examination

A hand-held magnifying lens (5× to 10×) is an important adjunct to the objective examination of skin lesions. Magnification affords the examiner the advantage of determining if the lesion is a disruption in the horny outer layer of the skin and can reveal changes in pigmentation throughout the lesion, such as in a melanoma. Regular or irregular contours in the borders of lesions can also be determined. The addition of oil to the skin further enhances the translucency of the horny outer layer of the stratum corneum and permits better visualization of skin fissures and the presence of hair follicles in the lesions, as well as pores.[4] The presence of scaling and inflammation can also be determined. A listing of primary and secondary lesions is provided in Boxes 44-1 and 44-2.

Access to a freestanding light that can be adjusted to provide direct or oblique lighting is a necessary adjunct. Darkening the ambient lighting allows for greater illumination and contrast of the involved lesion. Overillumination, however, may wash out important details of a lesion. Direct lighting with an intense penlight or the ophthalmoscope head with a halogen light permits visualization of closed vesicles or pustules and differentiation of fluid or cystic masses.

Another form of lighting is the Wood's light, or black light, which emits long wavelengths above 365 nm of UV rays through a Wood's filter made of nickel oxide and silica, thus rendering the UV rays harmless to the skin. The advantage of this lighting method is that skin diseases such as tinea versicolor fluoresce a white to yellow color; erythrasma, a scaly skin condition caused by *Corynebacterium minutissimum*, fluoresces a bright coral red color under the Wood's light.[5] Even small amounts of decreased melanin, such as vitiligo, are accentuated under the Wood's light and appear stark white. *Pseudomonas* infections appear yellow-green.[4]

Palpation of skin lesions provides information on the extent of the lesion below the skin surface, its consistency, its exact size, and the presence of associated pain. Certain lesions, such as dermatofibromas, indent with lateral palpation; this distinguishing characteristic is known as Fitzpatrick's sign. Dermatographism is a phenomenon that arises when the skin of a person with urticaria is lightly rubbed with a pointed object, such as the back of a fingernail. Histamine is released under the skin surface, and the skin becomes raised and red, depicting the exact configuration inflicted by the pointed object.

Diagnosis involves a close evaluation of the lesion's distribution or location, configuration, borders, size, shape, color, and surface characteristics or appearance. Documentation includes a description of the lesion's size, color, shape, surface characteristics, distribution, and configuration.

A discussion of skin examination techniques is provided in Box 44-3.

REFERENCES

1. Greenberger N, Hinthorn DR: *History taking and physical examination: essentials and correlates*, St Louis, 1993, Mosby.

2. Goldsmith L, Lazarus GS, Tharp MD: *Adult and pediatric dermatology: a color guide to diagnosis and treatment*, Philadelphia, 1997, FA Davis.
3. Ebersol P, Hess P: *Towards healthy aging: human needs and nursing responses*, ed 5, St Louis, 1998, Mosby.
4. *Merck manual of geriatrics*, ed 2, Whitehouse Station, NJ, 1995, Merck.
5. Habif TP: *Clinical dermatology: a color guide to diagnosis and therapy*, ed 3, St Louis, 1996, Mosby.
6. Reves JT, Maibach HI: *Clinical dermatology illustrated: a regional approach*, ed 3, Philadelphia, 1998, FA Davis.
7. Fitzpatrick TB and others: *Color atlas and synopsis of clinical dermatology*, ed 3, New York, 1997, McGraw-Hill.

CHAPTER 45

Surgical Office Procedures

Eileen M. Deignan

As an external organ, the skin is accessible for diagnostic biopsies and therapeutic procedures. In the changing health care environment, more patients are seeing nondermatologists for skin problems. In fact, more nondermatologists than dermatologists receive visits for malignant skin tumors.[1,2] The diagnosis of malignant skin tumors by clinical examination and lesion biopsy is an important skill for a primary care provider.

Skin biopsies are fundamental techniques in the diagnosis and management of neoplastic skin disease. With practice, they can be performed safely and with minimal scarring. However, these technical skills cannot substitute for clinical knowledge. Before performing a biopsy, the primary care provider should always consider the diagnostic possibilities of the neoplasm, select the optimal biopsy site and technique, and determine if referral to a more experienced colleague is necessary. Inflammatory lesions that require a biopsy for diagnosis are probably best treated by a dermatologist.

INDICATIONS FOR BIOPSY

All suspicious neoplastic lesions should be biopsied. It is a greater error not to biopsy a suspicious lesion than to biopsy benign lesions too often. In a study of the ability of primary care residents to diagnose and manage possibly cancerous lesions, 33% did not recommend a skin biopsy in cases in which it was appropriate.[3] In many cases an excisional biopsy also serves as the treatment for some precancerous and malignant lesions.

A lesion that clinically appears to be an atypical nevus or malignant melanoma should be completely removed to the level of the subcutaneous fat with a punch or elliptical excision.[4] The thickness of a melanoma is the single most important criterion for predicting survival of nonmetastatic melanoma.[5] In the event that the lesion is indeed a malignant melanoma, it is important that it be removed to the level of the subcutaneous fat so that its depth can be measured accurately. If a partial-thickness biopsy is performed on a melanoma, the true thickness of the lesion cannot be adequately evaluated.

BIOPSY REFERRAL

Patients with bleeding disorders, hematologic malignancies, and conditions that require anticoagulation therapy are more likely to develop complications from biopsies. Additionally, lower leg biopsies of patients with diabetes or vascular disease may be complicated by delayed wound healing. Thus these individuals should be referred to a dermatologist or surgeon for biopsy. If careful attention is given to hemostasis, patients who are taking aspirin can undergo biopsies in the primary care provider's office.

Certain anatomic locations are more difficult to biopsy safely. The scalp, for example, is a particularly vascular area, and biopsies in this site often bleed profusely. The palms of the hands, soles of the feet, and lateral aspects of the fingers are also challenging areas to biopsy because of the underlying neurovasculature and fascia. Overall, the face is a cosmetically sensitive area; technically, the eyelids and nose are particularly challenging areas to biopsy. Patients requiring biopsies in any of these areas should be referred to an experienced dermatologist or surgeon.

SITE SELECTION

The goal of a biopsy is to obtain a specimen representative of the lesion. Small, suspicious lesions can be removed entirely with a punch or shave biopsy. For a larger lesion, often just a part is removed. In such cases, the area that is thickest or has the most abnormal color should be sampled. These areas will be most likely to have a specific pathologic condition.

The punch biopsy should not be used to sample part of a melanocytic lesion. The sampled area may not include the most worrisome part of the lesion, and the result could be falsely reassuring. Melanocytic lesions are best approached with an excisional biopsy, in which the entire lesion is removed for histologic analysis.

TECHNIQUE CHOICE

Punch Biopsy

A punch biopsy is used to sample a lesion that appears to extend below the epidermis. As a diagnostic procedure, it is useful both to identify the disease process and to ascertain the depth of the process. For instance, the entire thickness of the epidermis should be sampled to diagnose a squamous cell carcinoma. If only part of the epidermis is sampled, neither the thickness of the epidermal abnormality nor the degree of invasion can be assessed. As a result, an actinic keratosis cannot be distinguished from a squamous cell carcinoma in situ or from an invasive squamous cell carcinoma (Table 45-1).

A punch biopsy is performed with a cylindrical instrument called a "punch." These instruments have a sharp circular edge to bore out a cylindrical piece of tissue and are manufactured in diameters from 2 to 10 mm. The 2-mm punch should be reserved for very small lesions or cosmetically sensitive areas. It may not provide enough tissue for adequate analysis of most lesions. Depending on the location on the body, punches larger than 6 mm can have a cosmetic complication when the wound is repaired. The standing cutaneous horns ("dog ears") at the ends of a large oval wound closure can result in an unsightly scar. Instead of using a large punch, the primary care provider should consider removing the lesion with an elliptic excision, thereby eliminating the standing cutaneous horns.

Shave (Parallel Plane) Biopsy

The shave biopsy is best for lesions that are elevated above the level of the epidermis or have a disease confined to the epidermis. Examples include superficial basal cell carcinoma, seborrheic keratosis, verruca vulgaris, and pyogenic granuloma (see Table 45-1). Because it is more superficial, a shave biopsy site usually heals more rapidly and with less scarring than a punch biopsy.

Scissor Excision

The scissor excision is useful for removing small exophytic or pedunculated growths such as acrochordons (skin tags), filiform warts, and polypoid nevi (see Table 45-1). A scissor excision that does not remove a significant amount of epidermis does not result in scarring because of the superficial nature of the wound.

PREPARATION

The rationale for the biopsy and the wound care involved should be outlined for the patient, and informed consent should be obtained. The major complications of biopsies and scissor excisions are bleeding, infection, allergic contact dermatitis, and scarring. These possibilities should be stated for every patient before starting the procedure.

Shave biopsies leave a round or oval-shaped, depressed, and hypopigmented or hyperpigmented scar. Ideally, a sutured punch biopsy leaves a linear scar. A site left to close by secondary intention heals with a round, depressed scar.

The primary care provider should inquire about the patient's tendency to form hypertrophic scars or keloids, which tend to occur on the deltoids and the chest. If a lesion on the chest or deltoid is to be biopsied, the patient should be counseled that a hypertrophic or keloid-type scar may form, even if there is no history of abnormal scarring.

Before the procedure, patients should be asked about medical conditions and medications that can predispose them to bleeding. Any sensitivities to the items used to care for the biopsy wound, such as antibiotic ointment or adhesive tape, should be ascertained. Immunosuppressive diseases or medications that could predispose the patient to infection or delay wound healing should be noted, and the patient should be advised.

TABLE 45-1 Optimal Techniques for Biopsying Common Lesions

Lesion	Punch	Shave	Scissor	Ellipse
Suspicious pigmented lesion	Yes*	No	No	Yes
Basal cell carcinoma	Yes	Yes	No	Yes
Squamous cell carcinoma	Yes	No	No	Yes
Verruca vulgaris	No	Yes	Yes	No
Seborrheic keratosis	No	Yes	No	No
Pyogenic granuloma	No	Yes	Yes	No

*If lesion is small enough to be excised by punch.

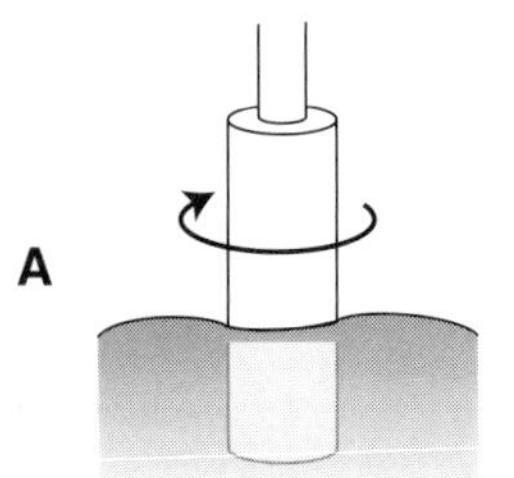

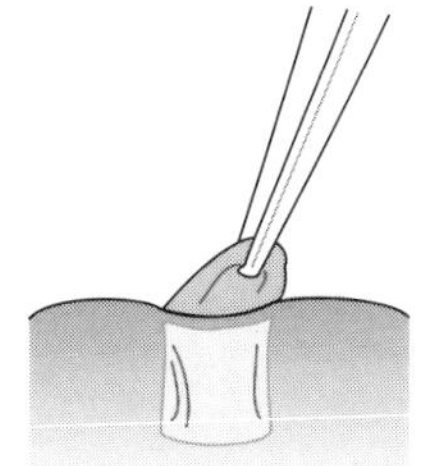

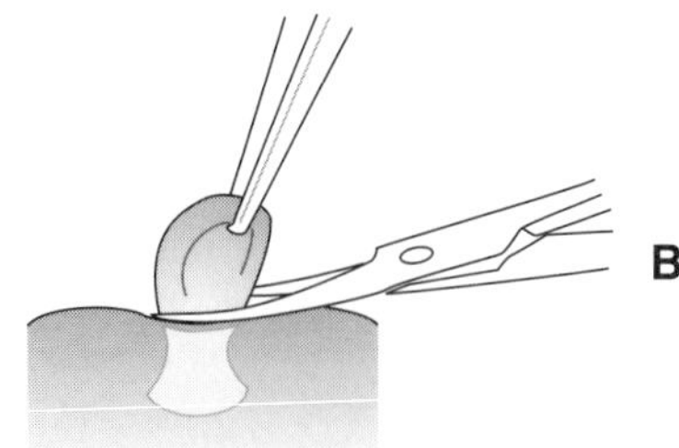

FIGURE 45-1

A, Punch biopsy. **B**, Scissor excision. (From Edmunds MW, Mayhew MS: *Procedures for primary care practitioners*, ed 2, St Louis, 2002, Mosby.)

THE BIOPSY PROCEDURE

Shave biopsies, punch biopsies, and scissor excisions are clean but not sterile procedures. Practitioners should wear gloves and eye protection, but masks and gowns are not necessary. A fenestrated drape will provide a clean field.

Materials

It may be helpful to assemble biopsy materials in one location. A complete set includes marking pens, alcohol pads, 1% or 2% lidocaine with and without epinephrine, 20-gauge (for drawing up) and 30-gauge (for injecting) needles, 3-ml syringes, gauze pads, fenestrated drapes, a selection of disposable punches, #15 blades, toothed forceps, scissors, needle drivers, 4-0, 5-0, and 6-0 nylon suture, antibiotic ointment (bacitracin or mupirocin, not triple antibiotic with neomycin), and adhesive bandages.

Anesthetic

The lesion should be marked with an indelible pen, because the lesion may disappear after the injection of a local anesthetic—a result of the vasoconstrictive effect of lidocaine. The area is cleaned with alcohol, and 0.2 to 0.5 ml of 1% to 2% lidocaine with 1:100,000 epinephrine is infused. The lesion is raised by infusing anesthetic into and under the lesion; this facilitates the shave biopsy. Epinephrine causes local vasoconstriction, which decreases bleeding and prolongs the duration of anesthesia. Maximum vasoconstriction is achieved in 15 to 20 minutes. Lidocaine without epinephrine is used if the area to be biopsied is the tip of the nose, the finger, the toe, or the penis. The vasoconstrictive effect of epinephrine in these distal areas, which have limited blood supply, could result in necrosis.

Punch Biopsy

The skin is stabilized with the thumb and forefinger of one hand and is pulled perpendicular to the relaxed skin tension lines. The punch is held perpendicular to the skin and rotated into the skin with a firm, constant, circular motion (Figure 45-1). The punch is advanced until the tissue "gives" as the punch advances into the subcutaneous fat. The punch should be advanced cautiously in thin areas such as the fingers or face. The punch is removed, and either side of the wound is pressed gently. The core of tissue is grasped gently with the forceps and elevated out of the wound to expose the base. Care should be taken not to crush the specimen with the forceps. Scissors are used to sever the base of the sample from the underlying fat. The specimen is placed immediately in 10% neutral buffered formalin.

Because of normal skin tension, the defect created by the biopsy will be oval. The defect is closed with monofilament nylon suture using a simple interrupted suture. One or two sutures should be sufficient. In general, 4-0 or 5-0 sutures can be used on the trunk and extremities; the finer 6-0 suture should be used for the face. Care should be taken while suturing to approximate and evert the wound edges for optimal healing.[5] The goal of suturing a punch biopsy is twofold: (1) hemostasis, and (2) improving the cosmetic result. Suturing requires more expertise and time, but the end result is often noticeably better than a wound that has been closed with Steri-Strips or allowed to heal by secondary intention.

Shave Biopsy

With a shave biopsy, the area should be prepared and anesthetized in the same way as for a punch biopsy. The lesion is stabilized between the thumb and forefinger. A #15 blade is held parallel to the surface of the skin and stroked smoothly under the lesion, avoiding a sawing motion. To avoid creating a deep wound, strict attention should be given to keeping the blade parallel to the skin (Figure 45-2). The sample is grasped gently with forceps and placed immediately in 10% formaldehyde.

Holding pressure on the wound for 5 minutes can usually control the small vessel bleeding created by the sampling. If needed, the field is blotted dry, and a cotton-tipped swab soaked in a chemical hemostatic agent (e.g., 20% aluminum chloride in absolute alcohol) is rolled across the field several times. Ferric subsulfate (Monsel's solution) and silver nitrate are also useful as hemostatic agents but should be avoided with cutaneous procedures. They are more corrosive than aluminum chloride and can tattoo the skin.

Scissor Excision

Because the pain of administering an anesthetic is often greater than the excision itself, very small lesions do not require an anesthetic. The lesion is held up with forceps and snipped at the base (see Figure 45-1). Aluminum chloride can be used for hemostasis. A bandage usually is not necessary.

WOUND CARE

The biopsy site will heal faster in a moist, occluded environment. Therefore the wound is dressed with an antibiotic ointment and an adhesive bandage. The patient should be instructed to leave the dressing in place for 12 to 24 hours. Thereafter the area is washed once a day with soap and water and covered again with an antibiotic ointment and adhesive bandage. Suture sites should be cleaned and dressed in this manner until the sutures are removed. Shave biopsy wounds, which heal by secondary intention, should reepithelialize in 7 to 10 days. After reepithelialization, no special care is needed in the area.

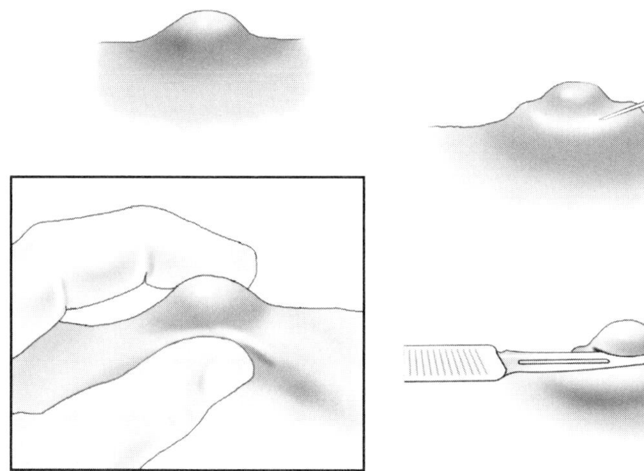

FIGURE 45-2

Shave biopsy. (From Edmunds MW, Mayhew MS: *Procedures for primary care practitioners*, ed 2, St Louis, 2002, Mosby.)

The timing of the biopsy suture removal is important for the cosmetic result. Sutures should be left in place long enough to prevent the wound from stretching or dehiscing but not so long that suture marks ("railroad tracks") remain at the wound edge. As a general rule, sutures in areas not under tension (e.g., the face) should be removed in 5 to 7 days. Sutures in areas that are under tension (e.g., the trunk and extremities) should be left in place for 10 to 14 days.[6]

COMPLICATIONS

Infection, bleeding, scarring, and allergic reactions are the most common complications of biopsies. If a patient notes oozing of blood from the wound, he or she should place direct pressure on the site for 20 minutes. This intervention should be adequate to control small vessel bleeding. Immediate evaluation is essential if the wound continues to bleed. The sutures should be removed and the wound explored for a bleeding vessel.

Postbiopsy bacterial infections are usually caused by *Staphylococcus aureus* or group A streptococcus species.[7] Any purulent drainage should be cultured, and oral or topical antibiotic therapy should be considered. Biopsies on the hands and feet or in intertriginous areas such as the groin and axillae can become infected with *Candida* organisms. These infections usually respond well to topical antifungals.[8]

If erythema and pruritus develop around the wound site, a contact allergy to the antibiotic cream or dressing should be considered. The neomycin in triple antibiotic cream is a notorious cause of contact allergy at biopsy sites. The alleged offending agent should be discontinued. Petroleum jelly is substituted if the reaction appears to be to the antibiotic ointment. A gauze pad held in place by paper tape is usually well tolerated by patients who react to adhesive bandages. Very exuberant reactions that vesiculate may require a short course of low-potency topical cortisone.[9]

DOCUMENTATION

Careful documentation is the responsibility of the provider who performs the biopsy. The age, gender, and pertinent history of the patient (e.g., duration of lesion, skin cancer risk factors, previous malignancies) are indicated on the pathology requisition sheet. A brief clinical description and the clinical diagnosis or differential diagnosis of the biopsied lesion should be provided for the pathologist.

The procedure is documented in the patient's chart. Along with the description and clinical diagnosis or differential diagnosis, the location of the lesion should be carefully described or drawn. It is particularly critical to identify the location of the lesion when a shave excision is performed. Otherwise, it may be difficult to locate the lesions should they require further treatment, because the scar may not be apparent after the wound has healed. Indications for the biopsy, informed consent, procedure, specimen disposition, dressing, wound care instructions, and follow-up plans should also be documented.

REFERENCES

1. Alguire PC, Mathes BM: Skin biopsy techniques for the internist, *J Gen Intern Med* 13(1):46-54, 1998.
2. Stern RS, Gardocki GJ: Office-based care of dermatologic disease, *J Am Acad Dermatol* 14(2 pt 1):286-93, 1986.
3. Gerbert B and others: Primary care physicians as gatekeepers in managed care. Primary care physicians' and dermatologists' skills at secondary prevention of skin cancer, *Arch Dermatol* 132(9):1030-1038, 1996.
4. Bolognia JL: Biopsy techniques for pigmented lesions, *Dermatol Surg*, 26(1);89-90, 2000.
5. Balch CM and others: Tumor thickness guide to surgical management of clinical stage I melanoma patients, *Cancer* 43(3):883-888, 1979.
6. Moy RL, Waldman B, Hein DW: A review of sutures and suturing techniques, *J Dermatol Surg Oncol* 18(9):785-795, 1992.
7. Haas AF, Grekin RC: Practical thoughts on antibiotic prophylaxis, *Arch Dermatol* 134(7):872-873, 1998.
8. Haas AF, Grekin RC: Antibiotic prophylaxis in dermatologic surgery, *J Am Acad Dermatol* 32(2 pt 1):155-176, quiz 177-180, 1995.
9. Gette MT, Marks Jr JG, Maloney ME: Frequency of postoperative allergic contact dermatitis to topical antibiotics, *Arch Dermatol* 128(3):365-367, 1992.

CHAPTER 46

Principles of Dermatologic Therapy

Denise A. Vanacore

DEFINITION/EPIDEMIOLOGY

The critical first step in treating any dermatologic condition is accurate diagnosis. Other important components are the type of lesion to be treated, the medication, the vehicle of the active medication, and the method used to apply the medication.

In dermatologic therapy the type of lesion guides therapy. Moist, weeping lesions are treated with Burow's solution to hasten drying while providing soothing relief. In dry dermatitis, therapeutic agents incorporated into creams or ointments help to increase moisture in the skin and provide relief from pruritus.

SKIN STRUCTURE

The skin is the largest organ of the body. The primary function of the skin is to provide a barrier to substances from passage into the body. Three main layers form this barrier.[1] The stratum corneum is the most superficial layer and consists of enucleated keratinocytes, which are filled with keratin and an interfilamentous matrix. The epidermis is the middle layer and consists of stratified squamous epithelium. The innermost layer is the dermis, which contains connective tissue.

The thickness and permeability of the stratum corneum vary on different areas of the body. When the stratum corneum is irritated and inflamed, the protective skin barrier is interrupted. These characteristics have clinical implications for dermatologic therapy, because they affect drug absorption.

MEDICATIONS

Variables to Consider When Prescribing

Several variables affect the pharmacologic response when dermatologic agents are applied to the skin.[2] The first variable is the regional variation in drug penetration, which is based on the thickness of the stratum corneum. There is an inverse relationship between the thickness of the stratum corneum and drug concentration. In areas such as the face, scalp, and scrotum, the stratum corneum is more permeable than others. In addition, there is increased permeability when the skin is inflamed. In addition, the concentration of the dermatologic medication affects its absorption in the skin. Finally, because the principal transport mechanism is passive diffusion, increasing the concentration gradient increases absorption.

Dermatologic Vehicles

The base in which the active medication is delivered (the vehicle) affects the ability of the drug to permeate the skin. The vehicle may also provide important therapeutic effects to the skin, such as hydration. Drug absorption may be enhanced up to 10 times with the application of occlusive dressings.

The most common vehicles are combinations of powders, oils, and liquids in varying proportions. Powders aid in absorbing moisture, decrease friction, and help to cover wide areas. Oils provide an emollient function and, because of their occlusive properties, often enhance drug absorption. Liquids provide a cooling, soothing sensation by evaporation while helping exudative lesions to dry. Some common pharmacotherapeutic preparations are described in Table 46-1.[3]

Ointments. Ointments consist mainly of water suspended in oil and are an excellent lubricant. Goldstein and Goldstein[3] stated that ointments are generally the most potent vehicles because of their increased occlusive effect; however, they are not useful in hairy areas, and the greasiness of the product is not aesthetically acceptable to many patients. Ointments are best for dry, lichenified lesions because of the effects of lubrication and heat retention through decreased transepidermal water loss.

Creams. Creams are less potent than ointments, stronger than lotions, and consist of a semisolid emulsion of oil in water. Creams are a cosmetically appealing vehicle that can be washed off with water. They are used on nonhairy areas such as the palms of the hands and soles of the feet.[3]

Lotions. Lotions consist of a powder-in-water preparation and are a less potent vehicle.[3] Indications for the use of lotions include moist areas, dermatoses, pruritus, hairy areas, or large treatment areas. Lotions are commonly used to provide a cooling effect on the skin.

Solutions. Solutions consist of water in combination with various medications or substances. When used as bath soaks, solutions provide coolness and aid in drying exudative lesions.[3] Solutions are best for open or closed dressings, for infected dermatoses, or in hairy areas.

Gel. A gel is an oil-in-water, semisolid emulsion with alcohol in the base; it is transparent and colorless and liquefies on contact with the skin. Gels are an excellent vehicle for use on hairy body areas, and they combine the best therapeutic advantages of ointments with the best cosmetic advantages of creams.[3]

The optimal vehicle selections for specific body sites are listed in Table 46-2. With variations in skin thickness, body hair, and type of lesion, it is important to choose the most appropriate vehicle.

Topical Corticosteroids

Some of the most useful topical agents for treating a variety of dermatologic conditions are corticosteroids. The major effects of corticosteroids are the reduction of inflammatory response, vasoconstriction, and a decrease in collagen synthesis.[3] They are available in several classes based on potency (Table 46-3), and they come in a variety of strengths and vehicles (Table 46-4).

Topical corticosteroids are exceptionally useful in treating various dermatologic diseases, but they are not without potential adverse effects. The higher the potency and the more prolonged the use, the higher the chance of developing adverse effects. Collagen synthesis is affected, which results in striae and tissue atrophy. These effects may be reversible when the drug is discontinued. Visible distended capillaries (telangiectasia) and purpura

TABLE 46-1 Topical Pharmacotherapeutic Preparations

Category	Examples	Special Considerations
Lotions	Calamine, Valisone, lindane	Cools and dries as it evaporates; useful for treating moist or pruritic skin
Creams	Nivea, Purpose, most topical corticosteroids, antifungal agents	Helps retain water; cosmetically appealing; useful in high-humidity environments; easily washed off
Gels	Benzoyl peroxide, Erygel, Topicort, Lidex	Becomes liquid on contact; cosmetically appealing; avoid on acutely inflamed skin because alcohol base may cause stinging
Ointments	Petrolatum, Aquaphor, Eucerin, most topical corticosteroids	Helps retain water, hydrating; avoid use in exudative, infected lesions; may be greasy; complications include folliculitis, maceration, and miliaria
Emulsions	Cetaphil, Unibase	Water-in-oil preparations that are less occlusive than ointments
Pastes	Zinc oxide paste	Less greasy than ointments, with some drying action; good as protective barrier
Wet dressings		
Open	Apply 6-8 layers of gauze or a handkerchief, soaking wet, for 15 min 3 times daily	Antiinflammatory action and vasoconstriction aid in decreased edema and crust removal; evaporation and cooling offer relief of pruritus
Closed	Same as for open, with plastic cover	Retains heat and causes maceration
Bath soaks	Aveeno, Alpha-Keri	Temperature should be lukewarm, not hot; limit to 20-30 min; oils may make tub slippery
Powder	Zeasorb, Micatin, Tinactin	Promotes drying; increases surface area; decreases maceration and moisture; avoid in open wounds
Fixed	Unna's boot (zinc oxide gelatin boot)	Proper application will aid in decreasing edema; leave the dressing in place for 1 week, then remove by soaking in warm water

From Goldstein B, Goldstein A: *Practical dermatology,* ed 2, Philadelphia, 1997, Mosby.

TABLE 46-2 Optimal Vehicle Selection for Specific Body Sites

Vehicle	Smooth, Nonhairy Skin, Thick, Hyperkeratotic Lesions	Hairy Areas	Palms, Soles	Infected Areas	Between Skin Folds; Moist, Macerated Lesions
Ointment	+++		+++		
Cream	++	+	++	+	++
Lotion		++		++	++
Solution		+++		+++	++
Gel		++		+	+
Spray: little clinical usefulness					

Modified from Goldstein B, Goldstein A: *Practical dermatology,* ed 2, Philadelphia, 1997, Mosby.
+, Infrequently used vehicle; ++, acceptable vehicle; +++, preferred vehicle.

TABLE 46-3 Classes of Topical Corticosteroids

Class	Potency	Considerations	Examples	Indications
I	Ultra high	Consult MD	0.05% betamethasone dipropionate 0.05% clobetasol propionate	Severe inflammatory dermatoses unresponsive to standard treatment Two-week use restriction; never use on the face or groin
II	Very high	Consult MD	0.05-0.25% desoximetasone 0.2% fluocinolone acetonide 0.5% triamcinolone acetonide	Severe inflammatory dermatoses (e.g., psoriasis, severe atopic dermatitis, or severe contact dermatitis)
III	High	Use with caution	0.025% betamethasone benzoate 0.025% fluocinolone acetonide 0.1% triamcinolone acetonide	Moderate cutaneous dermatoses
IV	Intermediate	Use with caution	0.025% triamcinolone acetonide 0.01% fluocinolone acetonide	Moderate cutaneous dermatoses
V	Low		2.5% hydrocortisone 0.2% betamethasone	Mild cutaneous dermatoses
VI	Very low		0.25-1.0% hydrocortisone (i.e., OTC strengths)	Very mild, self-limiting dermatoses

Modified from Goldstein B, Goldstein A: *Practical dermatology,* ed 2, St Louis, 1997, Mosby.

TABLE 46-4 Topical Corticosteroid Potency, Strongest (Class I) to Weakest (Class VI)

Brand Name	Generic Name	Preparation	Size
CLASS I (ULTRA HIGH)	*Unresponsive severe inflammatory dermatoses*		
Cordran tape 4 μ/sq cm^2	Flurandrenolide	Tape	2 × 3 in, 24 × 3 in, 80 × 3 in
Diprolene 0.05%	Betamethasone dipropionate*	Cream, ointment, gel	15, 45 g
		Lotion	30, 60 ml
Diprolene AF 0.05%	Betamethasone dipropionate	Cream	15, 45 g
Psorcon 0.05%	Diflorasone diacetate	Cream, ointment	15, 30, 45, 60 g
Temovate E 0.05%	Clobetasol propionate*	Cream, ointment	15, 30, 45 g
		Lotion	25, 50 ml
		Gel	15, 30, 60 g
		Emollient cream	15, 30, 60 g
Ultravate 0.05%	Halobetasol propionate	Cream, ointment	15, 50 g
CLASS II (VERY HIGH)	*Severe inflammatory dermatoses*		
Aristocort 0.5%	Triamcinolone acetonide*	Cream, ointment	15, 240 g
Cyclocort 0.1%	Amcinonide	Cream, ointment	15, 30, 60 g
		Lotion	20, 60 ml
Diprosone 0.05%	Betamethasone dipropionate*	Cream, ointment	15, 45 g
		Aerosol	85 g
		Lotion	30, 60 ml
Florone 0.05%	Diflorasone diacetate	Cream, ointment	15, 30, 60 g
Halog 0.1%	Halcinonide	Cream, ointment	15, 30, 60, 240 g
		Solution	20, 60 ml
Lidex 0.05%	Fluocinonide*	Cream, ointment	15, 30, 60, 120 g
		Solution	20, 60 ml
		Gel	15, 30, 60, 120 g
		Solution	60 ml
Lidex E 0.05%	Fluocinonide	Cream	15, 30, 60, 120 g
Kenalog 0.05%	Triamcinolone acetonide*	Cream, ointment	20 g
Maxiflor 0.05%	Diflorasone diacetate	Cream	30, 60 g
		Ointment	15, 30, 60 g
Topicort 0.25%	Desoximetasone*	Cream	15, 60, 120 g
		Ointment	15, 60 g
		Gel 0.05%	15, 60 g
CLASS III (HIGH)	*Moderate cutaneous dermatoses*		
Aristocort 0.1%	Triamcinolone acetonide*	Cream, ointment	15, 60, 240, 2520 g
Aristocort A 0.1%	Triamcinolone acetonide*	Cream	15, 60, 240 g
		Ointment	15, 60 g
Cutivate 0.05%	Fluticasone propionate	Cream	15, 30, 60 g
0.005%		Ointment	15, 30, 60 g
Dermatop 0.1%	Prednicarbate	Cream	15, 60 g
Elocon 0.1%	Mometasone furoate	Cream, ointment	15, 45 g
		Lotion	30, 60 ml
Kenalog 0.1%	Triamcinolone acetonide*	Cream	15, 60, 80, 240, 2520 g
		Ointment	15, 60, 80, 240 g
		Lotion	15, 60 ml
Synalar 0.025%	Fluocinolone acetonide*	Cream, ointment	15, 30, 60, 425 g
		Solution 0.01%	20, 60 ml
Synemol 0.025%	Fluocinolone acetonide*	Cream	15, 30, 60 g
Valisone 0.1%	Betamethasone valerate*	Cream	15, 45, 110, 430 g
		Ointment	15, 45 g
		Lotion	20, 60 ml
		Powder	5, 10 g

From Goldstein B, Goldstein A: *Practical dermatology,* ed 2, St Louis, 1997, Mosby.

*Available generically, but may not be so predictably effective. In most cases, however, it is much less expensive.

TABLE 46-4 Topical Corticosteroid Potency, Strongest (Class I) to Weakest (Class VI)—cont'd

Brand Name	Generic Name	Preparation	Size
CLASS IV (INTERMEDIATE)	*Moderate cutaneous dermatoses*		
Aristocort 0.025%	Triamcinolone acetonide*	Cream	15, 60, 2520 g
Kenalog 0.025%	Triamcinolone acetonide*	Cream	15, 80, 240, 2520 g
		Lotion	60 ml
		Ointment	15, 80, 240 g
Locoid 0.1%	Hydrocortisone butyrate	Cream, ointment	15, 45 g
		Solution	30, 60 ml
Valisone 0.01%	Betamethasone valerate*	Cream	15, 60 g
Westcort 0.2%	Hydrocortisone valerate	Cream	15, 45, 60 g
		Ointment	15, 45, 60 g
CLASS V (LOW)	*Mild cutaneous dermatoses*		
Aclovate 0.05%	Alclometasone dipropionate	Cream, ointment	15, 45, 60 g
Derma-Smoothe/FS 0.01%	Fluocinolone acetonide	Oil	120 ml
DesOwen 0.05%	Desonide*	Cream	15, 60, 90 g
		Ointment	15, 60 g
		Lotion	60, 120 ml
FS Shampoo 0.01%	Fluocinolone acetonide	Shampoo	180 ml
Synalar 0.01%	Fluocinolone acetonide*	Cream	15, 30, 60, 425 g
		Solution	20, 60 ml
Tridesilon 0.05%	Desonide*	Cream, ointment	15, 60 g
CLASS VI (VERY LOW)	*Very mild, self-limiting dermatoses*		
Hytone 1%	Hydrocortisone*	Cream, ointment	30, 120 g
		Liquid	45, 75, 120 ml
		Lotion	120 ml
		Roll-on stick	14 g
Hytone 2.5%	Hydrocortisone*	Cream	30, 60 g
		Ointment	30 g
		Lotion	60 ml
Pramosone 1%	Hydrocortisone with pramoxine HCl 1%	Cream	30, 60 g
		Ointment	30 g
		Lotion	60, 240 ml
Pramosone 2.5%	Hydrocortisone with pramoxine HCl 1%	Cream	30 g
		Ointment	30 g
		Lotion	60, 120 ml

TABLE 46-5 Amount of Topical Medication to Dispense for Adult Use*

	b.i.d./1 wk	t.i.d./2 wk	b.i.d./4 wk
Face and neck	15 g	45 g	60 g
Trunk	60 g	180 g	240 g
One arm	15 g	45 g	60 g
One leg	30 g	90 g	120 g
Hands and feet	15 g	45 g	60 g
Body	180 g	0.75-1 kg	1.25-2 kg

From Goldstein B, Goldstein A: *Practical dermatology*, ed 2, St Louis, 1997, Mosby.
*For children, use one third to one half these amounts.

may result from a thinning of the epidermis. Classes I to IV should never be used on the face or the genitals. The primary care provider should use caution when prescribing classes I, II, and III and should consider consultation with a physician.

When corticosteroids are used with occlusive dressings, there is an increase in drug penetration in the skin and an increase in the potential adverse reactions. Learning a few drugs in each class will benefit the primary care provider when prescribing topical corticosteroids.

PATIENT AND FAMILY EDUCATION

The first guideline of dermatologic therapy is to keep the treatment as simple as possible. Primary care providers should prescribe enough medication to complete therapy. The amount of topical medication to dispense for adult use is listed in Table 46-5.

Application procedures should be written out, and the patient should fully understand the instructions. Important information to review with the patient includes whether to moisten the skin first, how much topical medication to apply, where to apply it, and whether the area can be occluded by a dressing. Patients should be instructed not to apply the dermatologic medication to areas other than where instructed. In addition, patients should be aware of possible adverse reactions and should know when to call the office and return for follow-up evaluation.

REFERENCES

1. DiPiro J and others: *Pharmacotherapy: a pathophysiologic approach*, Stamford, Conn, 1997, Appleton & Lange.
2. Katzung B: *Basic and clinical pharmacology*, Stamford, Conn, 1998, Appleton & Lange.
3. Goldstein B, Goldstein A: *Practical dermatology*, ed 2, St Louis, 1997, Mosby.

CHAPTER 47

Screening for Skin Cancer

Walter Elias, III

DEFINITION/EPIDEMIOLOGY

Although early detection and treatment of skin cancer can improve patient outcomes, evidence is insufficient to recommend for or against routine screening for skin cancer using a total-body skin examination for its early detection.[1] Nevertheless, the purpose of skin cancer screening is to educate both the patient and the practitioner to be able to identify the characteristic changes associated with skin cancer. These cancers include nonmelanomatous skin cancers (NMSCs) (e.g., basal cell carcinoma [BCC], squamous cell carcinoma [SCC]) and melanomatous (malignant melanoma [MM]) skin cancers.

It is known that 1 in 6 Americans develops skin cancer at some point.[2] Approximately 1.3 million cases of BCC or SCC are diagnosed each year. Between 1973 and 1995, the incidence of MM increased from 5.7 per 100,000 to 13.3 per 100,000.[1] Approximately 47,700 cases of MM were diagnosed in the year 2000. An estimated 9600 persons died of skin cancer in 2000, with 7700 dying of MM, and 1900 dying of other skin cancers.[3] In contrast to NMSC, which typically affects older adults, the frequency of MM peaks between 20 and 45 years of age.

The rising incidence of skin cancer over the past several decades may be primarily attributed to increased sun exposure associated with societal and lifestyle shifts in the U.S. population and to depletion of the protective ozone layer.[2] Acute sunburns place the patient at increased risk. Second-degree burns before age 18 can double the incidence of NMSC and greatly increase the risk for MM.[4] Fair-skinned men and women older than 65 years, patients with atypical moles, and those with more than 50 nevi constitute known groups at substantially increased risk for developing melanoma.[2]

PATHOPHYSIOLOGY

Repeated and unprotected exposure to ultraviolet light causes photoaging of the skin over time. Normal skin aging begins by age 30 to 35 years and is characterized by thinning, atrophy, decreased elasticity, and fragility that leads to wrinkling. Skin that is photoaged from sun damage may be coarse with yellow discoloration (solar elastosis), irregularly pigmented, rough, or atrophic with deep wrinkling. Reactive hyperplasia of melanocytes results in persistent hyperpigmentation and hypopigmentation of the hands, forearms, legs, chest, and back. Chronic exposure disrupts the maturation of the outer layer of the epidermis, resulting in scaling, roughness, seborrheic keratoses, actinic keratoses, and NMSCs[4-6]; heavy sun exposure is also a risk factor for MM.[1]

CLINICAL PRESENTATION

Clinicians and patients can reliably measure some risk factors for melanoma. Patients presenting for routine physical examinations should be queried concerning any changes in the appearance or size of skin lesions as listed in Table 47-1. Questions about the patient's use of sunscreens, repeated sun exposure without protection, tendency to burn, outdoor employment, or family history of melanoma are beneficial to estimate the risk for NMSC or MM.[2,5]

PHYSICAL EXAMINATION

The most commonly advocated screening test for skin cancer is a complete and thorough total-body skin examination. With the patient disrobed, the examiner must systematically inspect the entire skin surface, including the nails and the soles of the feet.[1] Detection of a suspicious skin lesion such as a basal cell carcinoma warrants biopsy or referral (Color Plate 1). NMSC lesions such as BCC may vary from a normal flesh-colored lesion to a slightly pigmented lesion (see Color Plate 1). These are characterized by a raised, shiny appearance, often with pearly borders. An SCC lesion is a roughened, scaling area that does not heal and readily bleeds when scraped (Color Plate 3). Keratinization of these can lead to a heaped-up appearance that flakes. MM is characterized by a lesion that is best described as the ABCDEs of MM (Color Plates 4 and 5).[1,2] These include *A*symmetry (of the entire lesion), *B*order (irregularities), *C*olor (variability within the lesion from a brown to black discoloration), *D*iameter (size greater than 6 mm), and *E*levation (recently raised). Additional symptoms suspicious for skin cancer include nonhealing skin areas, ulceration, bleeding, and weeping sores. In African-Americans, Asian-Americans, and dark-skinned individuals, abnormal lesions of the nails, hands, or feet should also be evaluated, because these are common sites for melanomas in these populations (see Color Plate 5).

DIAGNOSTICS

Skin biopsy is the "gold standard" of diagnosis and is best performed by an experienced practitioner. A shave or punch biopsy technique is appropriate for diagnostic evaluation of suspected NMSC (see Chapter 45). Excisional biopsy (total removal) of suspicious MM lesions should be followed with a wider excision if MM is diagnosed.

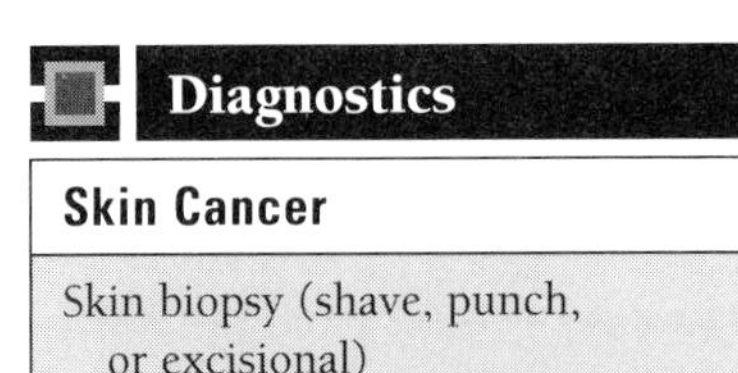
Diagnostics

Skin Cancer

Skin biopsy (shave, punch, or excisional)

DIFFERENTIAL DIAGNOSIS

Screening for skin cancer includes the evaluation of skin for all atypical-appearing lesions. Skin cancers may range from a seborrheic keratosis (Color Plate 2) to a premalignant solar (actinic) keratosis to a BCC, SCC,

Differential Diagnosis

Skin Cancer

Actinic keratoses
Basal cell carcinoma
Squamous cell carcinoma
Malignant melanoma
Dysplastic nevi

TABLE 47-1 Signs Suggesting Malignancy in Pigmented Lesions

Sign	Implication
CHANGE IN COLOR	
Sudden darkening; brown, black	Increased number of tumor cells, the density of which varies within the lesion, creating irregular pigmentation
Spread of color into previously normal skin	Tumor cells migrating through epidermis at various speeds and in different directions (horizontal growth phase)
Red	Vasodilation and inflammation
White	Areas of regression or inflammation
Blue	Pigment deep in dermis, sign of increasing depth of tumor
CHANGE IN CHARACTERISTICS OF BORDER	
Irregular outline	Malignant cells migrating horizontally at different rates
Satellite pigmentation	Cells migrating beyond confines of primary tumor
Development of depigmented halo	Destruction of melanocytes by possible immunologic reaction and inflammation
CHANGES IN SURFACE CHARACTERISTICS	
Scaliness	
Erosion	
Oozing	
Crusting	
Bleeding	
Ulceration	
Elevation	
Loss of normal skin lines	
DEVELOPMENT OF SYMPTOMS	
Pruritus	
Tenderness	
Pain	

From Habif TP: *Clinical dermatology: a color guide to diagnosis and therapy,* ed 3, St Louis, 1996, Mosby.

or MM. An actinic keratosis is a persistent or recurrent reddened and roughened area that scales or crusts. These lesions are effectively treated with liquid nitrogen using a freeze-thaw technique to obtain a 1- to 3-mm rim of freeze, which allows appropriately slow thawing over 20 to 40 seconds.[6]

MANAGEMENT

BCC is treated with electrodesiccation and curettage. Definitive treatment of SCC is total excision. An experienced dermatologist or surgeon is best equipped to treat an MM lesion with a wide excision. If an NMSC or MM is recognized early by the patient or practitioner, surgical cure is close to 100%.

Co-Management with Specialists

An annual skin examination of sun-exposed areas is recommended for patients with the diagnosis of BCC or SCC. A family physician or dermatologist can accomplish this. A total annual skin examination by an experienced family physician or dermatologist is recommended for patients diagnosed with MM lesions.

COMPLICATIONS AND LIFE SPAN CONSIDERATIONS

Despite the tendency of NMSC lesions to be slow growing, failure to diagnose them can result in disfigurement. There is indirect evidence that the shift to earlier tumor stages of melanoma found with screening may be associated with better clinical outcomes.[1] The survival rate at 5 years is inversely proportional to the depth of the MM at the time of diagnosis—the deeper the lesion at diagnosis, the lower the survival rate at 5 years. There are minimal risks from total-body skin examination; however, the examination may be embarrassing to some patients and could result in unnecessary treatment as a result of misdiagnosis or detection of lesions that might not have caused clinical consequences but were biopsied.[1]

INDICATIONS FOR REFERRAL/HOSPITALIZATION

The identification of atypical-appearing skin lesions warrants referral or a biopsy. If the biopsy reveals an NMSC or MM, a trained family physician, dermatologist, or surgeon should provide the definitive treatment.

PATIENT EDUCATION AND HEALTH PROMOTION

Knowing that damage to the skin caused by the sun is additive may help patients take precautions against sun exposure and thereby reduce their risk; 80% of lifetime sun exposure is obtained before 18 years of age.[1] Precautions include avoiding the sun, wearing protective clothing, and using sunscreens to prevent solar damage to the skin, both for young children and adults. Prevention of sunburns, which carry a high risk of malignant transformation over time, is paramount. Education of patients at higher risk is crucial. (See the Clinical Presentation section for factors that place patients at higher risk.) The incidence of melanoma doubled between 1973 and 1995.

Sun exposure for longer than 15 minutes requires protection with a sunscreen that has a sun protection factor (SPF) of at least 15. Sunscreens should be applied before sun exposure and reapplied every 2 hours or after swimming. It is important for patients to know they should seek medical attention for nonhealing sores (sores usually heal with 4 to 6 weeks) or for any lesion that changes in size, shape, texture, or color. Early identification of atypical-appearing skin lesions results in timely referral and effective treatment.

REFERENCES

1. *Screening for skin cancer: recommendations and rationale.* U.S. Preventive Services Task Force. Article originally in *Am J Prev Med* 2001, 20(3S): 44-6. Agency for Healthcare Research and Quality, Rockville, MD. Retrieved Dec 5, 2001 from the World Wide Web: http://www.ahrq.gov/clinic/ajpmsuppl/skcarr.htm.
2. Jerant AF, Johnson JT, Sheridan CD, Caffrey TJ: Early detection and treatment of skin cancer, *Am Fam Physician* 62(2):357-368, 2000.
3. American Cancer Society. Prevention and early detection. Retrieved Sept 21, 2000 from the World Wide Web: http://www.cancer.ort/statistics/cff2000/selected_toc.html.
4. Kaminester LH: Current concepts: photoprotection, *Arch Fam Med* 5:289-295, 1996.
5. Cockerell CJ, Howell JB, Balch CM: Think melanoma, *South Med J* 86(12):1325-1333, 1993.
6. Habif TP: *Clinical dermatology: a color guide to diagnosis and therapy,* ed 3, St Louis, 1996, Mosby.

CHAPTER 48

Acne Vulgaris

Eileen M. Deignan and Bonnie Hooper

DEFINITION/EPIDEMIOLOGY

Acne vulgaris is the most common dermatologic disorder seen in the United States. It is first observed in the pediatric age-group and can last well into the adult years. Although it is usually not a serious medical problem, acne should never be dismissed as a minor condition that will eventually be outgrown. The psychologic effects of prolonged acne and scars can be devastating. Advances in acne treatment enable management of this disease in many cases.

Acne vulgaris is a disorder of the pilosebaceous follicles. Its most prominent appearance during adolescence ("the peak of life") results in its name, which is attributed to the Greek and Latin words *akme* and *acme,* meaning "prime of life."

Early lesions of acne develop in 40% of children 8 to 10 years old, and 85% of all adolescents develop some form of acne. Of adults in their thirties and forties, 10% continue to experience active lesions, and 6% to 10% of adults in their fifties have varying degrees of this disorder.[1,2] There appears to be a familial tendency toward acne, and it is more common in males than in females.

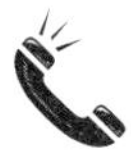

A dermatologic referral is indicated for isotretinoin (Accutane) therapy.

PATHOPHYSIOLOGY

The production of sebum appears to be directly related to androgenic stimulation. Before and during puberty, hormonal stimulation increases the production of the sebaceous glands in the pilosebaceous follicles. Abnormally adherent keratinocytes cause plugging of the pilosebaceous follicles, which contributes to the formation of the primary lesion (the comedone). Comedones include the open comedone (blackhead) and the closed comedone (whitehead). The open comedone is an obstruction at the follicular mouth, which is filled with plugs of stratum corneum cells. The black color is a result of compacted follicular cells, not dirt.[2] Closed comedones are a result of cystic swelling of the follicular duct below the epidermis. The microscopic opening of the closed comedone keeps its contents from escaping. These closed comedones are the precursors of inflammatory papules and pustules (Color Plate 9). Inflammatory reactions to sebum, fatty acids, and *Propionibacterium acnes* cause chemotactic factors and proinflammatory cytokines to be produced.[1,2] Inflammatory material around the comedone creates inflammatory papules and pustules.

Deeper lesions that develop in the lower portion of the follicle become nodulocystic lesions. Inflammatory acne may result in scars, most commonly from self-inflicted trauma from scratching and squeezing the lesions. These scars tend to be small pits. Rupture of cystic acne lesions also results in scar formation without any manipulation of the lesions. Another aftereffect of acne is that keloids can form, especially over the sternum. Especially in darker skin patients, inflammatory lesions often resolve with postinflammatory hyperpigmentation. Patients can be reassured that this "staining" is not scarring and usually clears spontaneously after several months.[3]

CLINICAL PRESENTATION/PHYSICAL EXAMINATION

The duration of acne, past treatments, the use of products, medical abnormalities, menstrual history, and all medications should be included in the patient's history. It is important to document how long previous treatments were used and any side effects. One frustrating fact of acne therapy is that most treatments require 6 to 12 weeks to take effect. If a therapy has been used for less than 6 to 12 weeks, it may not have been given an adequate trial.

In the history, it must be considered that seasonal and hormonal factors affect acne flares. More severe lesions occur during the winter months because acne is an inflammatory condition that responds to ultraviolet light; there is less sunlight during the winter. In addition, female patients typically report premenstrual acne flares.

A careful history should include an inquiry about exposure to cosmetic and hair styling products. Cosmetic acne can result from oil-based cosmetics, lotions, and hair products. It is usually worse in the areas in contact with the cosmetic. Similarly, pomade acne is seen on the forehead and neck as the result of oily lotions and creams used to style the hair.

Mechanical acne can result from friction from headbands, hats, helmets, chin straps, collars, and tight bras, and patients should be queried about this. Typically this presentation demonstrates acneform lesions in the area where these devices contact the body, whereas other locations are spared. Acne excoriee is a subtype of acne in which the primary lesions have been scratched. Patients with acne excoriee are encouraged to stop manipulating or scratching these lesions as an important part of successful therapy for this acne condition.[4]

A medication history is essential in evaluating acne, because certain medications can induce or aggravate acne (Box 48-1).[2,3]

BOX 48-1

DRUGS THAT INDUCE OR AGGRAVATE ACNE

- Androgens
- Adrenocorticotropic hormone (ACTH)
- Bromides
- Glucocorticoids
- Oral and fluorinated topical corticosteroids
- Hydantoins
- Iodides
- Isoniazid
- Lithium
- Phenobarbital
- Phenytoin
- Rifampin
- Trimethadione

In some cases of drug-induced acne, such as steroid-induced acne, the lesions are monomorphous. Typically, drug-induced acne has a rapid onset and may involve the usual acne areas as well as unusual areas such as the postauricular area, upper arms, lower back, abdomen, and legs.

A physical examination documents the type, location, and extent of acne lesions. The highest concentration of sebaceous glands occurs on the face, chest, back, and shoulders. Patients may present with a variety of lesions, including comedones, papules, pustules, and nodules. Surprisingly, the skin of a patient with acne will not necessarily be oily.

DIAGNOSTICS/DIFFERENTIAL DIAGNOSIS

Acne is diagnosed by physical examination. Laboratory blood testing is necessary only if adrenal or gonadal dysfunction is a possible cause. Other conditions may be misdiagnosed as acne. These include milia, rosacea (Color Plate 10), the adenoma sebaceum lesions of tuberous sclerosis, nevus comedonicus, miliaria of the newborn, flat warts, and molluscum contagiosum.

MANAGEMENT

Therapy should be individualized according to the degree and severity of acne. Goals of treatment include (1) normalizing keratinization of the follicular epithelium, (2) decreasing sebum production, (3) reducing *P. acnes*, proliferation, (4) reducing inflammation, and (5) minimizing scarring.

Mild cleansers and cleansing bars are helpful to remove sebum from the surface of the skin. They do not alter sebum production. Harsh soaps, astringents, "buff puffs," and grainy washes should be avoided because they may dry the skin or aggravate inflammatory lesions. Moisturizers, makeup, and hair products should be water based.

Excessive desquamation of the follicular epithelium, together with excess sebum production, contributes to comedone formation. Topical medications (keratolytics) that affect this process are tretinoin (Retin A), adapalene (Differin), tazarotene (Tazorac), azelaic acid (Azelex), and salicylic acid. These agents are applied to clean skin once daily, usually before bedtime. Side effects include erythema, dryness, and sun sensitivity. Systemic isotretinoin (Accutane) also decreases comedogenesis.

Several topical agents are available to decrease *P. acnes* proliferation and inhibit the production of inflammatory mediators. These agents include erythromycin, clindamycin, metronidazole, sulfonamide, azelaic acid, and benzoyl peroxide. There are also combination products with benzoyl peroxide combined with erythromycin or clindamycin. These are usually applied once or twice a day after cleansing. Although these agents may be used alone, they also work synergistically with keratolytics.

Diagnostics

Acne Vulgaris

Laboratory
Adrenal/gonadal testing*

*If indicated.

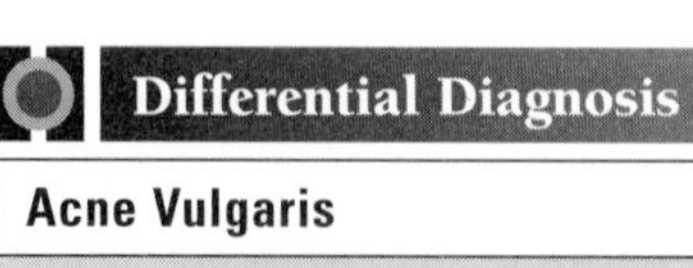

Differential Diagnosis

Acne Vulgaris

Tuberous sclerosis
Nevus comedonicus
Flat warts
Molluscum contagiosum

Oral antibiotics are effective for inflammatory acne by decreasing *P. acnes* and by reducing the concentration of free fatty acids, thereby inhibiting comedogenesis. Treatment for a minimum of 4 to 6 weeks is necessary to show improvement and may continue for several months. The most commonly used oral antibiotics include erythromycin, tetracycline, doxycycline, and minocycline. Less commonly used antibiotics include clindamycin, trimethoprim-sulfamethoxazole, azithromycin, cephalexin, ampicillin, and amoxicillin. Most patients require long-term treatment or intermittent courses of oral antibiotics until remission occurs.

Systemic medications that cause sebaceous gland suppression include estrogen and spironolactone. They act by suppressing the androgenic stimulation of sebum production and may be beneficial to female patients with acne. The most effective estrogen dose is at least 50 µg of ethinyl estradiol per day. Most combination oral contraceptives contain 35 µg or less of ethinyl estradiol. Fortunately, these doses of estrogens can be effective in acne suppression when combined with a nonandrogenic progestin such as norgestimate or desogestrel. Spironolactone is an antiandrogen that also reduces sebum production. Combination oral contraceptives and spironolactone are contraindicated in pregnant and lactating women and in the presence of thromboembolic disorders, renal impairment, and hyperkalemia.

Isotretinoin (Accutane) is restricted for the treatment of recalcitrant nodulocystic acne that has been unresponsive to standard therapies.[5] Its use is best managed by a dermatologist or dermatology nurse practitioner. It is thought to inhibit sebum production, decrease follicular obstruction, and have an antiinflammatory effect. Careful monthly monitoring of CBC, triglycerides, and hepatic function, as well as human chorionic gonadotropin (hCG) in female patients is required. Isotretinoin is teratogenic in humans, and contraceptive measures should be taken. Sexually active women of childbearing years must take effective birth control measures and be monitored for pregnancy monthly. Treatment usually lasts for 4 to 6 months. Approximately 60% of patients who complete a course of isotretinoin therapy will experience a long-term remission. Of the other 40%, some require further courses of isotretinoin, but some will have acne that is controllable with simpler forms of acne therapy.

Contrary to popular wisdom, acne does not appear to be related to certain foods. Therefore dietary restrictions are not indicated.

LIFE SPAN CONSIDERATIONS

Rosacea

Sometimes called acne rosacea (see Color Plate 10), this condition is rare in children and occurs most often between 30 and 50 years of age. It often coexists with acne vulgaris and may closely mimic it. The hallmark or distinction, however, is that comedones do not occur in rosacea. Rosacea may arise de novo or may follow acne, sometimes by years. Occasionally rosacea is confused with perioral dermatitis, which is much more common in the younger population.

MANAGEMENT

Neutral soaps are recommended. Plexion cleanser (sodium sulfacetamide 10% and sulfur 5%) has helped to reduce both erythema and papules. Makeup does not need to be avoided. Topical steroids may cause acneform eruptions and/or rebound flushing, although they may help with stinging and burning.

Persistent erythema and edema is difficult to treat but may be improved with lasers, particularly the Intense Pulsed Light system. Transient flushing, especially of the central face, is also difficult to treat. Avoidance of trigger factors (e.g., alcohol, hot fluids, spicy foods) is essential. Papules and pustules are best treated with antibiotics. Both topical and oral antibiotics help to disrupt the link between flushing and papules.

Treatment usually begins with metronidazole 0.75% gel, cream, or lotion applied b.i.d. Topical antibiotics (e.g., erythromycin gel) may also be effective. Oral antibiotics may be tried for cases in which control is inadequate. Tetracycline 250 to 500 mg PO b.i.d. or minocycline 50 to 100 mg PO q.d. is the usual first line of therapy and should be continued for 2 to 3 months or until clearance occurs. Maintenance doses of tetracycline 250 mg to 500 mg q.d. or minocycline 50 mg to 100 mg q.d. may continue indefinitely as needed for control. Accutane may be used in recalcitrant or severe cases and is effective in low doses (0.1 mg/kg to 0.2 mg/kg body weight per day). Telangiectasis, often the result of constant flushing, responds readily to Intense Pulsed Light (laser) treatments. Granuloma formation (rhinophyma) may last for years with periods of exacerbation and remission. Surgical intervention is the most effective treatment modality. Depending on severity, antidepressants may be a helpful adjunct in managing the psychosocial sequelae.

COMPLICATIONS

Acne-related facial scarring is the most obvious complication. A more common complication is hyperpigmentation, or staining, at the site of inflammatory lesions. Complications can also result from therapy. Serious side effects are associated with some systemic therapies, particularly isotretinoin, which is not only teratogenic but may also cause hypertriglyceridemia, thrombocytopenia, and hepatic dysfunction. In addition, serious social and psychologic effects are also associated with severe acne.

The most serious medical complication of rosacea is the ocular form in which rosacea keratitis may develop, with resultant corneal ulcers. If this complication is suspected, the patient should be referred to an ophthalmologist. Most complications of rosacea center on the psychosocial aspects. Cosmetic disfigurement with the resultant depression and defensiveness about one's appearance may develop. The patient may be perceived as an alcoholic because of the enlarged flushed nose and cheeks. In an effort to avoid trigger factors, patients may not participate in common social practices such as drinking wine and hot liquids (coffee, tea) and eating spicy foods. Occasionally, they feel compelled to stay indoors to avoid sun and heat.

INDICATIONS FOR REFERRAL/HOSPITALIZATION

All patients with recalcitrant or severe nodulocystic acne should be referred to a dermatologist for treatment. Issues related to depression and self-esteem should be referred to a mental health professional.

PATIENT AND FAMILY EDUCATION

Acne management and treatment takes weeks to months before improvement is appreciated. Patience and understanding of the prescribed treatment regimen are crucial. Phone contact and periodic office visits will help evaluate improvement and compliance. This type of support is often important for this frustrating and often long-term or recurrent disorder. Patients with rosacea can contact the National Rosacea Society at http://www.rosacea.org for more information.

HEALTH PROMOTION

Patients are encouraged to wash their skin; in particular, their face should be washed twice a day. An awareness that non–water-based cosmetic and hair products may cause acne is an important fact to remember. Patients may have jobs that require them to wear protective headgear and should be encouraged to maintain a careful face cleansing routine to minimize the occurrence of mechanical acne.

REFERENCES

1. Hurwitz S: *Clinical pediatric dermatology*, ed 2, Philadelphia, 1993, WB Saunders.
2. Weston WL, Lane AT, Morrelli JG: *Color textbook of pediatric dermatology*, ed 2, St Louis, 1996, Mosby.
3. Dershewitz RA: *Ambulatory pediatric care*, ed 2, Philadelphia, 1993, JB Lippincott.
4. Fox J: *Primary health care of children*, St Louis, 1997, Mosby.
5. Leyden JJ: Therapy for acne vulgaris, *N Engl J Med* 336(16):1156-1162, 1997.

CHAPTER 49

Alopecia

Eileen M. Deignan

DEFINITION/EPIDEMIOLOGY

Alopecia is a term used to describe abnormal hair loss. There are multiple causes of hair loss ranging from unusual congenital hair abnormalities to the commonly observed alopecia from androgenetic or pattern hair loss.

Hair loss is a disturbing and highly emotional issue for many patients. The evaluation of the patient with alopecia involves a carefully elicited history, a physical examination, and sometimes laboratory studies or a biopsy of the scalp. The treatment of alopecia depends on the cause.

PATHOPHYSIOLOGY

Alopecia (except for congenital alopecia) can be divided into two types: scarring and nonscarring alopecia. The nonscarring alopecias, in which the hair follicles are still present, are usually a result of an abnormality of the hair cycle. The scarring alopecias, in which the hair follicles are absent or fibrosed, are usually the result of an intensely inflammatory process of the scalp such as discoid lupus or kerion formation from tinea capitis.

A person is born with the 100,000 or so hair follicles that he or she will have throughout life.[1] Each hair follicle goes through a highly programmed cycle over and over again throughout its life cycle.[2] The cycle of hair growth involves three phases: anagen, catagen, and telogen. The anagen (growth) phase varies depending on the location of the follicle on the body. It is the longest on the scalp (producing long hairs) and much shorter on the eyebrows (producing short hairs). During the catagen phase, the hair involutes. This is the shortest of the three stages. During the telogen phase, the mature hair is shed. Most people lose 50 to 150 scalp hairs per day.

Three common types of hair loss are a result of anagen phase disturbance: androgenetic alopecia, anagen effluvium, and alopecia areata. Androgenetic alopecia, the most common type of hair loss, is seen as the hereditary thinning of hair in susceptible men and women. Patterned thinning of the hair begins in men and women as early as their teens. Fifty percent of men and women have some androgenetic alopecia by age 50.[1] This condition results from the sensitivity of hair on certain portions of the scalp to androgens. Testosterone, an androgen, is converted to dihydrotestosterone (DHT) peripherally. DHT binds to receptors on scalp hair follicles, causing a series of events that leads to the shortening of the anagen or growth part of the cycle. As a result, hair follicles that previously produced thick, pigmented, and terminal hairs now make thin, vellus hairs. This process is called miniaturization and produces the thinning hair seen in androgenetic alopecia or pattern hair loss.

Anagen effluvium is used to describe the alopecia from the diffuse, rapid, and dramatic loss of anagen hairs. The most common cause is chemotherapy. Chemotherapeutic agents prevent the rapid division of the hair matrix cells. Hair production stops, and the hairs that are already present become frail, break off, and are shed. Normal hair production resumes when the antineoplastic medication is stopped.[2]

Alopecia areata is an autoimmune condition that results in well-demarcated areas of alopecia on the scalp or body. The condition is fairly common, affecting about 2% of the United States population.[1] In alopecia areata, there is an idiopathic inflammatory response around the hair bulb at the base of the hair. The inflammation forces the hair out of the anagen (growth) phase and into the telogen (shedding) stage. Spontaneous remission is common.

The transient shedding of telogen phase hairs is termed telogen effluvium. In this condition, the hair prematurely enters the telogen (shedding) phase. Multiple factors, including high fever, certain medications, endocrine abnormalities, anemia, childbirth, and malnutrition can cause the hair to prematurely enter this stage.[1] The alopecia from telogen effluvium usually begins 4 to 6 weeks after any of these circumstances occur and can persist for several months.

CLINICAL PRESENTATION

The history is a critical part of the evaluation of a person with alopecia. The clinician should inquire about the duration and rapidity of the hair loss. Long and insidious hair loss is more indicative of androgenetic alopecia. It is important to ask if the patient has had this type of hair loss before. Alopecia areata is often recurrent. The clinician should also inquire about acute and chronic illnesses and current and past medications. An acute illness such as a high fever can trigger a telogen effluvium, as can hyperthyroidism or hypothyroidism. A family history of hair loss may represent a clue for androgenetic alopecia, a hereditary disorder. It is important to inquire about associated symptoms. The presence of scalp itching, pain, or flaking point to an inflammation of the scalp from psoriasis or contact dermatitis from hair dye. These conditions inflame the scalp and cause hair breakage with resultant alopecia. In addition, symptoms of scalp itching and flaking can indicate tinea capitis, a fungal infection of the scalp that produces alopecia because the hairs are weakened by the infection.

PHYSICAL EXAMINATION

The physical examination begins with an evaluation of the pattern of hair loss. Androgenetic alopecia in males usually presents as recession of the hair line at the temples and thinning in the frontal areas and the vertex. Women with androgenetic alopecia usually have diffuse thinning that is most pronounced in the frontal and parietal areas. A rim of hair along the frontal hairline is usually preserved.

Alopecia areata usually presents as well-demarcated patches of hair loss. Singular, "exclamation point" hairs are sometimes visible. These "exclamation point" hairs are normal distally but are thinned proximal to the scalp. The scalp is not inflamed in alopecia areata. In addition, the eyebrows and eyelashes may be affected. Men may experience alopecia areata in the beard area. When the whole scalp is affected, the process is called alopecia totalis. If the whole body is involved, the process is called alopecia universalis.

Anagen effluvium tends to lead to a diffuse loss of hair as does telogen effluvium. Scarring of the scalp suggests an inflammatory process such as lupus or lichen planopilaris. Scaling on the scalp may suggest psoriasis or tinea capitis. Patch hair loss with regrowing hairs of multiple lengths suggests trichotillomania, a condition in which the patient pulls or twists the hair.

DIAGNOSTICS

Findings from the history and physical examination guide diagnostic testing. If there is scaling on the scalp that is suggestive of tinea capitis, then several hairs or a scalp scraping is examined after preparation with potassium hydroxide (KOH). The presence of hyphae in the KOH preparation confirms the presence of a fungal etiology for the alopecia.

Diagnostics

Alopecia

Laboratory
KOH preparation
TSH
CBC
Serum glucose
Ferritin level*
VDRL*
DHEA-5*
Testosterone level*

*If indicated.

A hair pull test, in which a few dozen hairs are grasped firmly at the base and pulled, can help determine a telogen or anagen effluvium. The hair bulb from these pulled hairs is examined for abnormalities with a magnifying glass or under the microscope.

If telogen effluvium is suspected and there is no obvious cause, an underlying illness should be considered. Patients need an evaluation for hypothyroidism or hyperthyroidism. Iron deficiency anemia should be evaluated with hemoglobin, serum iron, iron-binding capacity, and ferritin tests.

A hormonal evaluation of a woman with androgenetic alopecia is not necessary unless she has other signs of a hormonal imbalance such as irregular menses, infertility, hirsutism, cystic acne, virilization, or galactorrhea.[1] In these women, evaluation for alopecia may include testosterone or DHEA-5 levels in addition to the other hormonal tests indicated by their symptoms.

Secondary syphilis is a cause of patchy alopecia. Patients suspected of having secondary syphilis should have a VDRL test performed. Finally, a scalp biopsy is sometimes helpful when the cause of the alopecia is not clear.

DIFFERENTIAL DIAGNOSIS

The differential diagnosis of hair loss is somewhat large. Table 49-1 can be used to differentiate among these conditions. The cause can usually be isolated with a careful history, physical examination, and some diagnostic tests.

MANAGEMENT

When an external factor is found with anagen or telogen effluvium, the key to the management of alopecia is removal of this causative factor. Anagen effluvium as a result of chemotherapy

Differential Diagnosis

Alopecia

Generalized Hair Loss
Telogen effluvium
- Acute blood loss
- Childbirth
- Inadequate protein intake
- High fever
- Medications (heparin, propranolol, vitamin A, warfarin, propylthiouracil, isotretinoin, lithium, beta blockers, amphetamines, etretinate)
- Stress
- Metabolic abnormalities (hypothyroidism, hyperthyroidism, diabetes)
- Severe illness
- Anemia

Anagen effluvium
- Cancer therapy (chemotherapy, radiation)
- Poisoning (arsenic, thallium)

Generalized patchy
- Secondary syphilis

Localized Hair Loss
Androgenic alopecia (male or female pattern)
Alopecia areata
- Atopic dermatitis
- Anemia
- Diabetes
- Pregnancy
- Thyroid disease
- Infection
- Stress
- Tick bite
- Lupus erythematosis
- Myasthenia gravis
- Vitiligo
- Hirsutism

Scarring alopecia
- Developmental defects (aplasia cutis)
- Physical injury (burns, pressure)
- Infection (bacterial [folliculitis, furuncle], fungal [karion], viral [herpes zoster])
- Neoplasms (metastatic cancer, sclerosing basal cell)
- Lupus
- Lichen planus

Cicatricial pemphigoid
- Scleroderma

Traction alopecia
Trichotillomania

TABLE 49-1 Diagnosis of Alopecia

Disease	Duration (years)	Scalp	Pattern	Pull Test
Alopecia areata	<1	Normal	Patchy + ! hairs*	+/−
Tinea capitis	<1	Scale, crust	Patchy	Hair breakage
Trichotillomania	>1	Normal to scarring	Patchy with stubble	−
Telogen effluvium	<1	Normal	Diffuse	↑ telogen
Androgenetic alopecia	>1	Normal	Pattern baldness	−
Systemic disease	<1	Normal	Diffuse	Normal/↑ telogen
Hair breakage	<1	Normal	Patchy	Age appropriate

**! hairs,* Short, stubby, straight, "exclamation point–like" hairs.

will reverse when the medication is stopped and the hair matrix is allowed to mature again. Telogen effluvium will also reverse when the causative factor or event is over or corrected and the hair cycle is allowed to return to normal.

Currently, androgenetic alopecia is most often medically treated with two medications: minoxidil and finasteride. Minoxidil is the only medication approved by the Food and Drug Administration for use by women. It is applied twice a day to the dry scalp. The side effects of the medication include dryness and irritation of the scalp. Hypertrichosis occurs in 3% to 5% of women. This effect diminishes after a year of therapy.

Finasteride is an oral medication. It works by blocking the peripheral conversion of testosterone to dihydrotestosterone (DHT). DHT is the hormone responsible for causing the miniaturization of hairs in androgenetic alopecia. The medication is taken daily and is safe and well tolerated. Both minoxidil and finasteride should be used for 8 to 12 months to determine if they are effective.[2]

Many cases of alopecia areata resolve spontaneously; however, several treatment options are available. Therapies include topical and intralesional corticosteroids. Anthralin, an immunomodulating agent, and minoxidil are two topical agents that can be effective treatments. Topical immunotherapy, or contact sensitization, is an effective therapy but is not widely available.

COMPLICATIONS

Some types of hair loss are the result of systemic illness. Complications can result from these illnesses. In addition, complications can occur as a result of the psychologic effects that patients may experience with the loss of their hair.

INDICATIONS FOR REFERRAL/HOSPITALIZATION

Alopecia without a timely response to standard management options or cases in which the cause is unclear requires consultation with a dermatologist. Patients should also be referred to a dermatologist or surgeon for consideration of hair transplantation. Patients with suspected trichotillomania may benefit from a mental health referral.

PATIENT AND FAMILY EDUCATION

Patients with androgenetic alopecia may be reassured to know that this is a common disorder. They should be reminded there are no restrictions on types of grooming products that they use. In addition, the frequency of hair washing will not affect the hair loss process.[1]

Patients with alopecia areata should know that spontaneous remissions and recurrences are common. They should also know that vitiligo, atopy (eczema, asthma, and hayfever), and thyroid disease are more common in people with alopecia areata.[3]

REFERENCES

1. Price VH: Treatment of hair loss, *N Engl J Med* 341(13):964-973, 1999.
2. Paus R, Costarelis G: The biology of hair follicles, *N Engl J Med* 341(7):491-497, 1999.
3. Arnold HL, Odom RM, James WD: *Andrews' diseases of the skin: clinical dermatology,* ed 8, Philadelphia, 1990, WB Saunders.

CHAPTER 50

Animal and Human Bites

Daniel W. O'Neill

DEFINITION/EPIDEMIOLOGY

Half of all Americans will be bitten by an animal or another human in their lifetime, with an incidence of about 5 million each year. Most of these bites are minor, but there is a significant risk of injury and infection. One million people seek medical attention annually, with an estimated health care cost of $30 million a year. Dog bites account for 80% to 90% of those bites that require medical care, most commonly affect the extremities, are seen more often in children and young adults, and occur most commonly when the animal is provoked. Dog bites have the lowest incidence of wound infection (2% to 20%), but serious trauma can occur, especially with the increasingly common larger-breed dogs. Cat bites are the second most common type of mammalian bite, with an incidence of 400,000 per year. The infection rate is much higher (from 30% to 80%), probably as a result of the deep puncture wounds from the animal's sharp teeth.

Human bites account for 3% to 23% of bite wounds, usually result from overly aggressive behavior, and have overall infection rates from 10% to 50%.[1] Bites not located on the hand have an infection rate similar to that of routine lacerations, but the clenched fist injury, or "fight bite," has a much higher complication rate because of the high penetrating force causing local tissue destruction and potentially osteomyelitis, tendonitis, and septic arthritis.

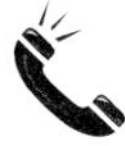

Physician consultation is indicated for suspected rabid animal bites, facial or extensive bites, tendon, bone or joint involvement, or significant infectious complications.

PATHOPHYSIOLOGY

The morbidity associated with mammalian bites is mostly related to tissue injury or, more commonly, polymicrobial infections near the bite site. The risk factors for infection are listed in Box 50-1. The most common aerobic bacteria in animal bites are *Pasteurella, Streptococcus, Staphylococcus,* and *Corynebacterium* species. *Eikenella corrodens* is another important pathogen. *Bacteroides, Actinomyces,* and *Fusobacterium* species are common anaerobic isolates and may produce beta lactamase. A rare but serious bacterial infection caused by *Capnocytophaga canimorsus* causes overwhelming sepsis, disseminated intravascular coagulation, and a 25% mortality rate in patients with predisposing conditions such as asplenia, liver disease, or immunosuppressive therapy.[1] Other pathogens that can rarely be transmitted through animal bites are those that cause tularemia, leptospirosis, cat scratch disease, rat-bite fever, tetanus, plague, sporotrichosis, blastomycosis, and rabies, which is uniformly fatal if not prevented.

BOX 50-1

RISK FACTORS FOR BITE WOUND INFECTION

- Location on the hand or foot
- Puncture wounds
- Crush injuries
- Treatment delay >12 hours
- Failure to irrigate and debride wound during initial management
- Age >50 years
- Asplenia
- Immunocompromised state
- Alcoholism
- Diabetes mellitus
- Preexisting edema at the bite site
- Peripheral vascular disease

Human bites are also polymicrobial, with similar pathogens; however, there are some important differences. *Pasturella* and *Capnocytophaga* species are not transmitted through humans. The anaerobes and many of the *Staphylococcus aureus* isolates produce beta lactamase. *E. corrodens* is present in 25% of clenched-fist injuries, is often resistant to certain antibiotics, and can lead to a serious indolent infection. Rare organisms from humans include herpes simplex 1 and 2, hepatitis B and C, and *Mycobacterium tuberculosis*. HIV has a biologic possibility of transmission through a bite wound, but there remains little evidence for this.[2]

CLINICAL PRESENTATION

A bite history must include the location and time of the bite, the breed and behavior of the animal, the domestication and rabies vaccine status of animal, whether or not the animal was provoked, drug allergies, current immunization status for tetanus and rabies, alcohol use, current medications, and past medical history with an emphasis on immunocompetence, history of splenectomy, chronic edema, or liver disease. Patients may be unwilling to admit to human bite wounds, particularly in a clenched-fist injury.

PHYSICAL EXAMINATION

Physical examination should document the location, extent, and depth of the wounds; type of wound (puncture, scratch, tear or avulsion); and tenderness and other signs of infection (e.g., erythema, streaking, fluctuation, adenopathy, purulent discharge). There should be careful testing for involvement of underlying tendons, joints, and nerves and for signs of compartment syndrome.

DIAGNOSTICS

Aerobic and anaerobic wound cultures should be obtained from all *infected* wounds before treatment. There is no benefit in culturing fresh bite wounds. Blood cultures and CBC are indicated if there are signs of

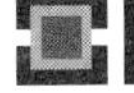

Diagnostics

Animal and Human Bites

Laboratory

Aerobic and anaerobic cultures of infected wounds

Imaging

X-rays for any bone or joint involvement or foreign body

systemic infection. Radiographs are necessary if there is possible bone or joint involvement or if a foreign body is present.

DIFFERENTIAL DIAGNOSIS

None.

MANAGEMENT

After assessing for and treating life-threatening injuries, the wound should first be irrigated with copious amounts of sterile saline solution. Devitalized tissue and foreign bodies are cautiously debrided. Primary closure of bite wounds is controversial. There are data to support primary closure in low-risk dog bites after appropriate wound care and in both old and new facial human bite wounds.[1,3,4] It is generally accepted that most cat and human bites, deep puncture wounds, clinically infected wounds, wounds over 24 hours old, and bites to the hand should be left open because of the high risk of infection.[1] Some wounds can be closed by secondary intention in 1 to 3 days. Aggressive drainage, irrigation, and wound packing are necessary if there is an established wound infection after cultures are obtained. The wound area should be immobilized and elevated for 2 to 3 days. Close outpatient follow-up monitoring is recommended to track complications or treatment failures.

Antibiotic prophylaxis in fresh bite wounds with low risk of infection is controversial. Most authorities recommend empiric antibiotic prophylaxis for 3 to 5 days in the following high risk cases: moderate to severe wounds associated with crush injuries or edema; location on the hand, head, face, or foot; involvement of bone, tendon, joint, or vascular structures; patients with a history of liver disease, splenectomy, or immunocompromise; deep puncture wounds that have been unable to be irrigated; and most cat and human bites.

Infected bites require 10 to 14 days of targeted antibiotic therapy. The selection of antibiotics is based on knowledge of the most common organisms encountered and on susceptibility testing of cultured organisms from infected wounds. Erythromycin, clindamycin, dicloxacillin, and first-generation cephalosporins are not efficacious because of the resistance of *Pasturella* species. Amoxicillin covers *Pasturella* species but is not recommended alone because of the beta lactamase production of *E. corrodens, S. aureus,* and *Bacteroides fragilis* (in human bites). Empiric therapy with amoxicillin/clavulanic acid (500 to 850 mg b.i.d.) or cefuroxime (500 mg b.i.d.) are the most effective, with relative risk reductions of 0.56.[5] In patients who are allergic to penicillin, doxycycline (100 mg b.i.d.) or the combination of trimethoprim/sulfamethoxazole or a fluoroquinolone plus clindamycin can be used. Macrolides should be reserved for pregnant patients allergic to beta-lactams.[6]

Tetanus toxoid (0.5 ml IM) must be administered to those who have not had a tetanus and diphtheria toxoid (Td) booster within the past 10 years. Some authorities recommend tetanus toxoid in infected or extensive wounds if 5 years or more have elapsed. Patients who have not completed a full primary series of three injections or whose vaccination status is unknown will require tetanus immune globulin (250 to 500 U IM) with the first of three monthly doses of tetanus toxoid.[7]

Rabies is a dreaded complication of animal bites. The decision to provide postexposure antirabies treatment should include the following considerations based on the guidelines of the Centers for Disease Control and Prevention.[8] The type of exposure is the first consideration, such as a bite or close contact of an open wound with the saliva of a potentially infected animal. Species such as bats, raccoons, skunks, and foxes are the most commonly infected in the United States, but in other countries dogs and cats are predominant carriers. Most rodents, such as squirrels, hamsters, guinea pigs, gerbils, rats, and mice are rarely infected. The exception is woodchucks. Reports of aggressive, unprovoked, or bizarre animal behavior raise the suspicion of rabies. The city or state health department should be contacted for reporting, recommendations, and assistance if there is any question about the risk.*

The wound must be immediately washed with soap and water or povidone-iodine solution, which significantly lowers transmission rates, and every effort must be made with the help of public health authorities to make a decision regarding quarantine (isolation and observation) or sacrifice of the biting animal for pathologic brain examination. If it is clearly indicated or recommended, and if the patient has not received the primary series of human diploid cell rabies vaccine (HDCV), the patient should receive passive immunization with human rabies immunoglobulin (HRIG) 20 to 40 IU/kg, with half the dose injected around the wound and half given intramuscularly (gluteal).[8] In addition, active immunization with HDCV 1 ml IM (deltoid) on days 0, 3, 7, 14, and 28, is indicated.[9] Individuals with a preexposure HDCV vaccination history should receive a HDCV booster on days 0 and 3 but do not require HRIG.[8]

COMPLICATIONS

Infection is the most serious complication resulting in cellulitis, tenosynovitis, septic arthritis, osteomyelitis, and even death from sepsis. Patients with human bite and clenched fist injuries are particularly at risk for these complications. Other potential complications include hemorrhage, disfigurement, and decreased motor function. Hepatitis B or other systemic disease from human bites is an additional concern.

INDICATIONS FOR REFERRAL/HOSPITALIZATION

Although most bite wounds can be handled on an outpatient basis, there are a few indications for hospitalization (1% to 2% of patients) and referral. Patients with systemic manifestations of infection (fever and chills); severe cellulitis; suspicion of noncompliance; infected bites refractory to oral or outpatient therapy; involvement of a joint, nerve, bone, or tendon (orthopedic referral); underlying illness such as poorly controlled diabetes, peripheral vascular disease, or an immunocompromised state (infectious disease referral); significant hand bites (hand surgery referral); extensive wounds requiring reconstructive surgery (plastic surgery referral); and head injuries (otolaryngologic or neurosurgery referral) should be considered for hospitalization.[1]

PATIENT EDUCATION AND HEALTH PROMOTION

All patients should be encouraged not to provoke domestic animals or handle wild animals, especially raccoons, skunks, foxes, and bats. A rabies vaccine for pets (both dogs and cats)

*For good sources of patient education on rabies, go to http://www.intrepid.net/~twila/rabies.htm. For clinical guidelines on rabies, go to http://www.cdc.gov/ncidod/dvrd/rabies/professional/professi.htm.

is mandatory in the United States but not in many foreign countries, including Mexico. Nervousness, aggressiveness, excessive drooling or foaming at the mouth, or fearlessness should raise the suspicion of rabid animals and prompt notification of the animal warden or health authorities.

Preexposure immunization with HDCV should be considered for high-risk groups such as animal handlers, veterinarians, certain laboratory workers, and persons living in or visiting countries with a significant rabies risk. The regimen would be 1 ml IM on days 0, 7, and 21 and a booster every 2 years.[8]

Td boosters should be given every 10 years routinely in all patients. Instructions to clean all bite wounds and seek medical care immediately should be given, especially for "fight bites" to the hand.

REFERENCES

1. Griego RD and others: Dog, cat and human bites: a review, *J Am Acad Dermatol* 33:1019-1029, 1995.
2. Richman KM, Rickman LS: The potential for transmission of HIV through human bites, *J Acquir Immune Defic Synd* 6(4):402-406, 1993.
3. Ruskin RD and others: Treatment of mammalian bite wounds of the maxillofacial region, *J Oral Maxillofac Surg* 51:174-176, 1993.
4. Donkor P, Bankas DO: A study of primary closure of human bite injuries to the face, *J Oral Maxillofac Surg* 55(5):479-481, 1997.
5. Fleisher GR: The management of bite wounds, *N Engl J Med* 340(2):138-140, 1999.
6. Goldstein EJC: Outpatient management of dog and cat bite wounds, *Fam Pract Recertification* 22(2):67-86, 2000.
7. Kelleher AT, Gordon SM: Management of bite wounds and infection in primary care, *Cleve Clin J Med* 64(3):137-141, 1997.
8. Advisory Committee on Immunization Practices: Human rabies prevention—United States, 1999, *MMWR* 48(RR-1):1-52, 1999.
9. Baevsky RH, Bartfield JM: Human rabies: a review, *Am J Emerg Med* 11:279-286, 1993.

CHAPTER 51

Burns, Minor

Eileen M. Deignan and Gretchen Carrougher

DEFINITION/EPIDEMIOLOGY

The skin is the largest organ of the body and functions as an excellent barrier against external injury. A burn can disturb this barrier function. A burn may be sustained from electrical, thermal, or chemical agents. Thermal burns constitute a large majority of these injuries, and a relatively small percentage are chemical burns.[1]

In the United States, approximately 2 million patients present with burn injuries each year. Of these burns, 80% are minor and can be managed on an outpatient basis.[2]

Immediate emergency department referral/physician consultation is indicated for burns that cause respiratory injury (inhalation or facial burns); burns of the hands, feet, genitals, or perianal area; full-thickness burns >2% of the total body surface area (TBSA); minor burns >10% TBSA in patients older than 50 years of age; or patients 10 to 50 years of age with burns of >15% TBSA.

PATHOPHYSIOLOGY

The temperature or heat content of the burning agent and the duration of exposure determine the extent of burn injury. A burn wound is best described by the zones of injury. Typically, three zones exist, with the innermost zone (zone of coagulation) representing the most damaged area. Cellular death and thrombosis of the blood vessels occur in this zone. The area of tissue adjacent to this zone is the zone of stasis, where blood flow is compromised. This zone may quickly progress to ischemia, or it may return to normal depending on several factors related to resuscitation. The outermost zone is the zone of hyperemia. This zone has received minimal damage, is characterized by increased blood flow, and will fully recover.[3]

A burn wound is defined by the size and depth of the wound. The size of the burn is quantified by the percentage of the TBSA burned. This percentage can be estimated in several ways. A very quick method acknowledges that the back of the patient's hand is approximately 1% of the patient's TBSA. Therefore the percentage of TBSA burned is the number of "hands" equal to the size of the burn.[3] Another method is the "rule of nines," which is illustrated in Figure 51-1.

The depth of a burn is described by the depth of skin injured and is either first, second, or third degree. First-degree (superficial) burns involve only the epidermis. Second-degree (partial-thickness) burns involve the dermis. Third-degree burns are full-thickness burns that extend to the subcutaneous fat. The hallmark of the third-degree burn is that the burn site is insensate.[3]

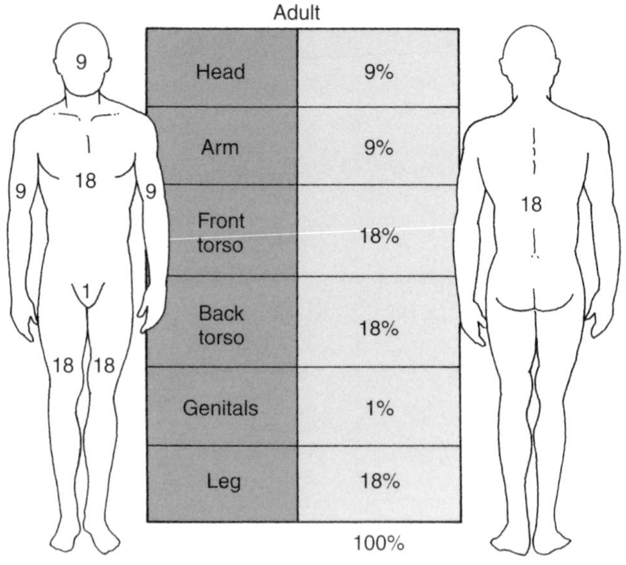

FIGURE 51-1

"Rule of nines" burn chart.

CLINICAL PRESENTATION

The primary care provider must obtain a full history of the mechanism of injury. The type of thermal or chemical exposure, the duration of exposure, and the time since the injury are important details. This history will help determine any risk for associated traumatic, pulmonary, or ocular injury. A preexisting illness will affect the prognosis and disposition.[4]

PHYSICAL EXAMINATION

The physical examination of the burn victim should be methodic and thorough. Airway, breathing, and circulation should be assessed first. A circumferential burn in a limb may compromise circulation in the involved appendage. The depth, extent (percentage of TBSA burned), and location of the burn must be accurately determined and recorded. The examination should also include a search for any associated injuries.[4]

DIAGNOSTICS

The skin is a barrier, and infection and metabolic abnormalities can result when this barrier is disrupted. Simple thermal burns do not require diagnostic testing. For more serious injuries, CBC, glucose, electrolytes, BUN, creatinine, urinalysis, and tissue cultures may be necessary. A chest x-ray study is indicated for a suspected inhalation injury.

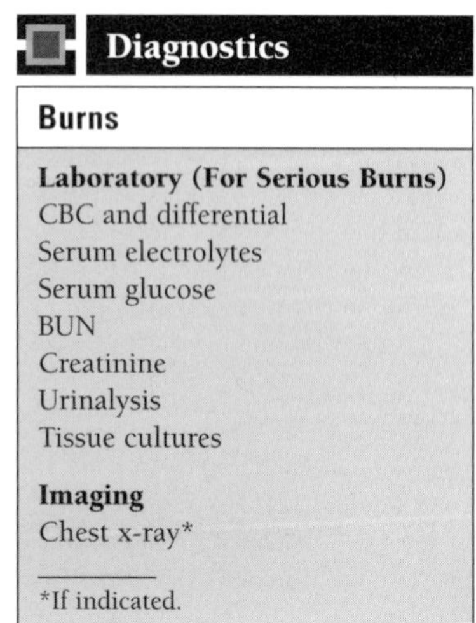

Diagnostics

Burns

Laboratory (For Serious Burns)
CBC and differential
Serum electrolytes
Serum glucose
BUN
Creatinine
Urinalysis
Tissue cultures

Imaging
Chest x-ray*

*If indicated.

DIFFERENTIAL DIAGNOSIS

The differential diagnosis is determined primarily by history. Certain skin conditions (e.g., staph scalded skin syndrome, toxic epidermal necrolysis) can resemble a generalized burn.

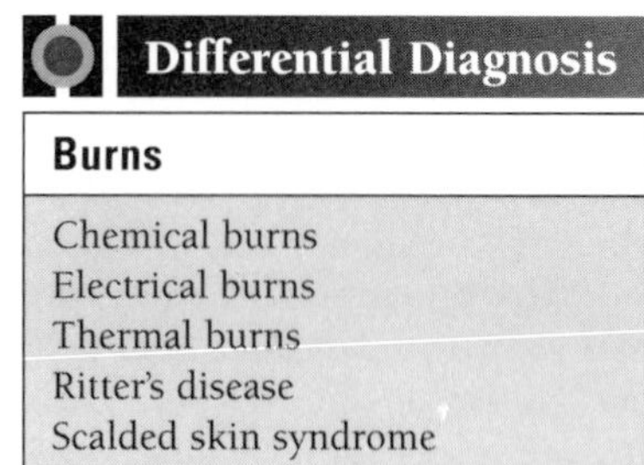

Differential Diagnosis

Burns

Chemical burns
Electrical burns
Thermal burns
Ritter's disease
Scalded skin syndrome

MANAGEMENT

Management of the patient with burns depends on the classification of the burn. The severity, extent, and location of the burn guide the decisions for treatment. The American Burn Association classifies burns as major, moderate, and minor. Low-risk patients are those between 10 and 50 years of age. High-risk patients are those under 10 years of age and over 50 years of age. Poor-risk patients are those with underlying medical conditions such as heart disease, diabetes, or pulmonary problems. Minor burns involve <15% of TBSA in the 10- to 50-year age-group or <10% of TBSA in patients under 10 years of age or over 50 years of age. Minor full-thickness burns are <2% of TBSA in all age-groups.

Minor burns also have no other associated injuries and can be managed in the office or outpatient setting.[3] If the burn was caused by a chemical agent, the initial therapy is to remove the offending chemical and garments and begin aggressive irrigation. Otherwise, thermal and chemical burn management is similar.[1]

Minor burns are painful, and treatment should begin with analgesics. Ibuprofen, with its antiprostaglandin properties, is a good antiinflammatory and analgesic medication. Narcotic agents such as codeine are also appropriate analgesics. The burn wound needs to be cleaned with mild soap and water or saline; blisters should be debrided. Tetanus prophylaxis should be given as indicated.

Finally, a dressing must be applied. There are several ways to dress minor burns. The burn is usually covered with a thin layer of antimicrobial cream or ointment. The most common topical therapy used is silver sulfadiazine cream (Silvadene), but it cannot be used in patients with sulfa allergy. It should be used cautiously on the face, because the silver in the cream may be deposited in the skin, causing tattooing or staining. Bacitracin ointment is a good alternative. The wound should be washed and redressed twice daily. The dressing needs to be removed twice daily, the wound thoroughly washed, an antibiotic cream or ointment reapplied, and a new dressing applied. This regimen should continue for 7 to 10 days until the wound is healed. A burned extremity may require splinting and elevation.[3,4,5]

Some burns may require open dressings in which a topical agent is applied without a dressing. The most common sites for open dressings are the face, neck, and perineum. The wound should be thoroughly washed 2 to 3 times a day and the topical agent reapplied.[4]

Alternative burn dressings include synthetic dressings such as DuoDerm, Opsite, Epigard, Epi-Lock, Biobrane, or Tegaderm. These biosynthetic dressings are applied to the fresh, clean, moist burn and are sized to approximate the outline of the burn with a slight amount of tension to achieve maximum adherence. These dressings are left in place until the wound heals (approximately 1 to 2 weeks). The dressing can be trimmed away as it spontaneously separates from the wound. Excessive fluid collection under the dressing must be aspirated, or the dressing should be changed. An outer dry dressing needs to be applied and changed daily.[3,4]

COMPLICATIONS

Complications of minor burns typically include local infection and inflammation. Treatment may include the need for antibiotic therapy and/or a change in topical therapy. Serious complications are rare.

INDICATIONS FOR REFERRAL/HOSPITALIZATION

Any burn injury larger than the American Burn Association's criteria for minor burns should be referred to the nearest emergency department for further evaluation and hospitalization as necessary. Burns that may result in functional or cosmetic impairment, have an associated injury, or involve high-risk patients require a referral for emergency evaluation.

PATIENT AND FAMILY EDUCATION

All burn patients should be seen in 24 hours for a wound check and for assessment of the depth and extent of the burn. Patients should be given clear discharge instructions that explain wound care. They also should be alerted for any signs and symptoms of infection or vascular compromise. If an extremity is involved, it should be elevated. Pain medications may be required. If pain medicine is prescribed, an explanation of how to use the analgesic and of the potential side effects is also necessary.

HEALTH PROMOTION

Home and work safety is the cornerstone of burn prevention. Manufacturer recommendations for protective equipment such as gloves, protective eyewear, and ventilation with certain household cleaning products and at the worksite can prevent chemical and inhalation burns. To prevent electrical burns, the electrical current must be turned off before attempting any electrical repairs, electric outlets should have covers, and frayed electrical cords should be repaired or the fixture discarded. Lowering hot water temperatures will reduce the risk of scald injuries. Loose clothing should be restricted when cooking or when around open flames. Everyone should be familiar with the stop, drop, and roll technique if their clothes catch fire.

REFERENCES

1. Griglak MJ: Thermal injury, *Emerg Med Clin North Am* 10(2):369-383, 1992.
2. Schwartz LR: Thermal burns. In Tintinalli JE, editor: *Emergency medicine: a comprehensive study guide*, ed 4, St Louis, 1996, McGraw-Hill.
3. Jordan BS, Harrington DT: Management of the burn wound, *Nurs Clin North Am* 32(2):251-273, 1997.
4. Martin ML, Harchelroad FP: Chemical burns. In Tintinalli JE, editor: *Emergency medicine: a comprehensive study guide*, ed 4, St. Louis, 1996, McGraw-Hill.
5. Monafo WW: Initial management of burns, *N Eng J Med* 335(21): 1581-1586, 1996.

CHAPTER 52

Cellulitis

Eileen M. Deignan

DEFINITION/EPIDEMIOLOGY

Cellulitis is an acute skin infection that rapidly spreads and extends deeply from the dermis to the subcutaneous tissue. Cellulitis may progress to a more severe soft tissue infection.[1] The clinical presentation is characterized by erythema, induration, and pain.

Staphylococcus aureus and group A beta-hemolytic streptococci are the most common causative agents in this cutaneous process in adults. *Haemophilus influenzae* type B cellulitis is found more commonly in children less than 3 years old.[2,3] Non-group A streptococcus is seen more commonly in patients with underlying abnormalities of the lymphatic system, such as lymphedema. In addition to the more common organisms, adults with co-morbid diseases such as diabetes mellitus or immunodeficiency may be infected with *Acinetobacter, Clostridium septicum, Enterobacter, Escherichia coli, H. influenzae, Pasteurella multocida, Proteus mirabilis, Pseudomonas aeruginosa,* and group B streptococcus.[2,4,5]

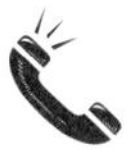

Physician consultation is indicated for patients with periorbital or orbital cellulitis, extensive cellulitis, and cellulitic infections that do not respond to antibiotic therapy within 24 to 48 hours.

PATHOPHYSIOLOGY

Cellulitis most often occurs after a break in the skin such as a laceration, ulceration, chronic dermatoses, or surgical wound. It may, however, develop after trauma to the skin or arise in apparently normal-appearing skin. The lower extremity is the most commonly affected site, but cellulitis may occur anywhere on the body. Areas of the body that have venous or lymphatic compromise from previous cellulitis, radiation treatments, or lymph node resection are more susceptible to recurrent cellulitis.[2]

CLINICAL PRESENTATION AND PHYSICAL EXAMINATION

The classic signs of cellulitis are erythema, induration, and pain. The borders of the infected area are usually sharply defined and may be slightly elevated. Blisters, abscesses, erosions, and necrosis may develop in the area of cellulitis. These signs may be accompanied by systemic symptoms, such as malaise, fever, and chills (Color Plate 11). The site of entry of the bacteria may be evident as breaks in the skin or ulcerations. Regional lymph nodes may be enlarged and tender.

Erysipelas is a superficial form of cellulitis that involves the lymphatic system. Erysipelas is characterized by a sharply demarcated, indurated border and lymphangitic "streaking" toward a regional lymph node. Typical areas involved include the lower legs, face, and ears. Facial erysipelas may follow a streptococcal infection of the upper respiratory tract.[6]

DIAGNOSTICS

The diagnosis of cellulitis is made primarily through the recognition of its distinctive clinical features (erythema, induration, and pain). Because the culture yield of aspirates and biopsy specimens is low, isolation of the etiologic agent is usually not attempted in healthy adults.[6,7] In adults with underlying disease, however, the results of cultures may be more helpful in selecting an appropriate antibiotic. The site most productive for needle aspirate for cultures has been found to be halfway between the leading edge and the center of the cellulitis.[8] Draining wounds or abscesses have a much higher culture yield and should be performed.[8] Draining abscesses also allows for more affective penetration of antibiotics into the infected area.

Patients with cellulitis typically have a mild leukocytosis and an elevated erythrocyte sedimentation rate (ESR). However, routine use of a complete blood count, ESR, and blood cultures is unwarranted in otherwise young, healthy adults.

DIFFERENTIAL DIAGNOSIS

The differential diagnosis of cellulitis includes erysipelas, stasis dermatitis, deep vein thrombosis, contact dermatitis, urticaria, erythema nodosum, erythema migrans, and early herpes zoster.[9] More severe, life-threatening infections such as necrotizing fasciitis, staphylococcal scalded skin syndrome, and toxic epidermal necrolysis must also be differentiated early from cellulitis. Cellulitis may also be superimposed on concurrent skin disease such as stasis dermatitis.

MANAGEMENT

In healthy adults, uncomplicated cases of cellulitis should be treated with antibiotics effective against staphylococcus and streptococcus, the presumptive etiologic agents.[6] A penicillinase-resistant penicillin such as dicloxacillin (500 mg PO q.i.d.), or a cephalosporin such as cephalexin (250 mg PO q.i.d.) for 7 to 10 days is appropriate. Erythromycin (250 to 500 PO q.i.d.) is appropriate for those with a penicillin allergy. For more extensive but relatively uncomplicated infections, patients may receive an initial dose of a parenteral antibiotic such as cefazolin 1 g or ceftriaxone 1 g before leaving the office, followed by a full course of oral antibiotics. For patients with more severe symptoms (e.g., fever) or with underlying medical conditions that warrant closer monitoring, a once-daily dose of a long-acting parenteral antibiotic such as ceftriaxone 1 to 2 g or cefazolin with probenecid may be given until a good response is observed.[10] The patient may then be switched to an oral antibiotic to complete a total of 7 to 10 days of treatment. Initially, close follow-up monitoring of the patient is indicated to be sure the infection is responding to the antibiotic regimen.

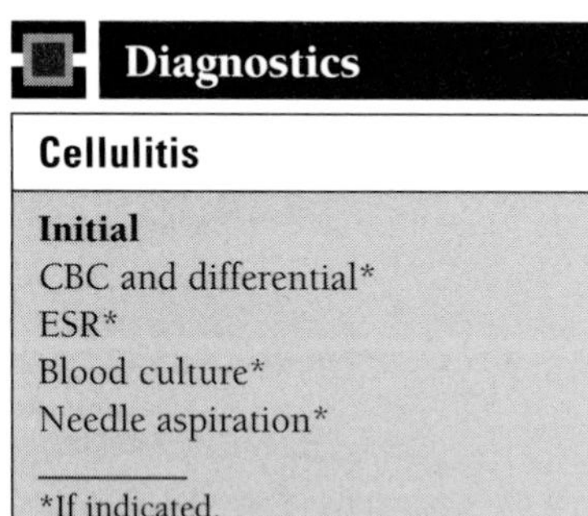

Diagnostics

Cellulitis

Initial
CBC and differential*
ESR*
Blood culture*
Needle aspiration*

*If indicated.

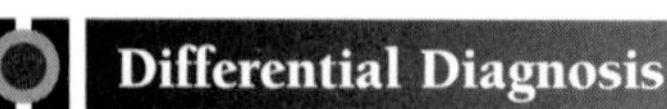

Differential Diagnosis

Cellulitis

Erysipelas
Atopic dermatitis
Folliculitis
Necrotizing fasciitis
Scalded skin syndrome
Toxic epidermal necrolysis

In addition to rest, nonpharmacologic therapies such as the application of moist heat and elevation of the affected region should be advocated in all cases of cellulitis. In patients with abscess formation, incision and drainage are required.

COMPLICATIONS AND INDICATIONS FOR REFERRAL/HOSPITALIZATION

In severe cellulitic infections or in patients who are unresponsive to previously mentioned therapies, referral for IV antibiotics is appropriate. Periorbital cellulitis is typically a result of a sinusitis, upper respiratory tract infection, or eye trauma and is more common in children. Symptoms typically include erythema and edema of the eyelid, conjunctivitis, and chemosis (conjunctival edema). This condition is treated with warm soaks and aggressive antibiotic therapy as previously mentioned.

Far more uncommon is orbital cellulitis, in which there is exophthalmos, orbital pain, restricted eye movement, chemosis, and occasionally visual disturbances. This is an emergency and must be treated as such. Often the infection stems from an ethmoid or maxillary sinusitis and should be evaluated by a computed tomography (CT) scan. Complications may include blindness, diplopia, brain abscess, and meningitis if the infection is not aggressively treated. IV antibiotics are indicated for all patients, with ceftriaxone 1 to 2 g IV every 12 to 24 hours being effective against most etiologic agents. Referral to an otolaryngologist is recommended for closer evaluation.

Soft tissue infections of the hands must be carefully evaluated to determine whether tendon sheaths, joint spaces, or muscle spaces are involved. Necrotizing soft tissue infections are a surgical emergency. The condition starts with redness and painful swelling of the deep tissues. A black eschar rapidly develops with necrosis of the underlying tissues. If necrotizing fasciitis, necrotizing cellulitis, or myonecrosis is suspected, immediate referral is indicated for prompt surgical debridement and IV antibiotics.[9,11]

Patients with diabetes mellitus need to be followed closely, particularly when cellulitis involves the feet or hands. As a result of decreased circulation in the extremities from microvascular compromise, persons with diabetes are at a greater risk for developing ulcerations and osteomyelitis. Radiographs of the affected extremity are indicated to evaluate for bony involvement or the presence of air in the soft tissues.[11] Uncomplicated cases of nonulcerative cellulitis in patients with diabetes can be treated with amoxicillin-clavulanate or quinolones. These antibiotics are chosen because they cover gram-negative organisms and anaerobes that may infect patients with diabetes.[11,12] Ciprofloxacin 750 mg PO b.i.d. plus clindamycin 300 mg PO q.i.d. or metronidazole 500 mg PO q.i.d. may be used for mild cases of infected diabetic ulcers. More severe ulcerative infections or cases of osteomyelitis require IV antibiotics and referral to a surgeon for debridement.

PATIENT AND FAMILY EDUCATION

Prevention of skin infections can be enhanced by cleaning all skin wounds through thorough washing and/or irrigation and covering wounds with dressings. Patients with diabetes should be encouraged to make a visual inspection of their feet on a daily basis to evaluate for pressure wounds and breaks in the skin. Underlying dermatoses such as tinea pedis, stasis dermatitis, and lymphedema should be treated aggressively, particularly in patients with diabetes, so the skin does not become a portal of entry for bacteria.

REFERENCES

1. Lewis RT: Soft tissue infections, *World J Surg* 22(2):146-151, 1998.
2. Carroll JA: Common bacterial pyodermas: taking aim against the most likely pathogens, *Postgrad Med* 100(3):311-322, 1996.
3. Howe PM, Fajardo JE, Orcutt MA: Etiologic diagnosis of cellulitis: comparison of aspirates obtained from the leading edge and the point of maximal inflammation, *Pediatr Infect Dis J* 6:685-686, 1987.
4. Boddour LM, Bisno AL: Non-group A beta-hemolytic streptococcal cellulitis, *Am J Med* 79:155-159, 1985.
5. Kieflhofner MA, Brown B, Dall L: Influence of underlying disease process on the utility of cellulitis needle aspirates, *Arch Intern Med* 148:2451-2452, 1988.
6. Brogan TV, Nizet V, Waldhausen JH: Streptococcal skin infections, *N Engl J Med* 334(4):240-245, 1996.
7. Sachs MK: Cutaneous cellulitis, *Arch Dermatol* 127:493-496, 1991.
8. Epperly TD: The value of needle aspirate in the management of cellulitis, *J Fam Pract* 23(4):337-340, 1986.
9. Fitzpatrick TB: *Color atlas and synopsis of clinical dermatology: common and serious diseases*, ed 3, New York, 1997, McGraw-Hill.
10. Brown G and others: Ceftriaxone versus cefazolin with probenecid for severe skin and soft tissue infections, *J Emerg Med* 14(5):547-551, 1996.
11. Elliot DC, Kufera JA, Myers RA: Necrotizing soft tissue infections: risk factors for mortality and strategies for management, *Ann Surg* 224(5):672-683, 1996.
12. Wood MJ, Logan MN: Ciprofloxacin for soft tissue infections, *J Antimicrob Chemother* 18(suppl D):159-164, 1986.

CHAPTER 53

Contact Dermatitis

Eileen M. Deignan

DEFINITION/EPIDEMIOLOGY

Contact dermatitis is an acute or chronic inflammatory reaction that results from a substance coming in contact with the skin. Common substances that create irritant dermatitis include acne preparations, harsh soaps, detergents, solvents, alkalis, and acids. Occlusion and sweating also contribute to irritant dermatitis.[1]

Allergic contact dermatitis is the result of a delayed-type hypersensitivity reaction to an allergen. Common causes of allergic contact dermatitis include poison ivy and poison oak, nickel, latex, rubber, and para-aminobenzoic acid (Table 53-1).[2,3]

Chemical substances cause another type of contact dermatitis when they irritate skin. The resultant irritation is called irritant or nonallergic contact dermatitis.

PATHOPHYSIOLOGY

Irritant contact dermatitis results from prolonged exposure to an irritant that penetrates the epidermal barrier. The pathophysiology of allergic contact dermatitis differs. With the initial irritant exposure in cases of allergic contact dermatitis, epidermal Langerhans' cells absorb the irritant, or antigen. These specialized dendritic cells then present the antigen in the form of MCH class II molecules to lymphocytic T-cells. The T-cells then proliferate and enter the circulation. A second exposure to the antigen elicits activation of the T-lymphocytes to release inflammatory mediators, causing the skin reaction.[1-3]

CLINICAL PRESENTATION AND PHYSICAL EXAMINATION

A pruritic rash is a common presenting symptom with both irritant and allergic contact dermatitis. The rash of irritant contact dermatitis is sharply limited to the area of exposure. This dermatitis develops within a few hours of contact with the offending agent. Involved areas are initially erythematous and may develop vesicles, erosions, or crusting.

Allergic contact dermatitis also is usually sharply demarcated to the site of exposure, but there can also be spreading of the dermatitis to areas that were not exposed. In some cases, the eruption may become generalized. These lesions follow a similar pattern with initial erythema. Papules, vesicles, erosions and crusts may develop[4] (Color Plate 12).

DIAGNOSTICS AND DIFFERENTIAL DIAGNOSIS

Irritant contact dermatitis may resemble atopic dermatitis or nummular dermatitis. The diagnosis of contact dermatitis is made when the location and pattern of the rash are consistent with the exposure history. Localization to the soles of the feet suggests a reaction to the insole of the shoe. Dermatitis around the neck suggests a reaction to a piece of jewelry. Impetigo, candidal infections, and dermatophyte infections may be confused with allergic contact dermatitis. A careful history or irritant

TABLE 53-1 Contact Dermatitis: Distribution Diagnosis

Location	Material
Scalp and ears	Shampoo, hair dyes, topical medicines, metal earrings, eye glasses
Eyelid	Nail polish (transferred by rubbing), cosmetics, contact lens solution, metal eyelash curlers
Face	Airborne allergens (poison ivy from burning leaves, ragweed), cosmetics, sunscreens, acne medications (e.g., benzoyl peroxide), aftershave lotion
Neck	Necklaces, airborne allergens (ragweed), perfumes, aftershave lotion
Trunk	Topical medication, sunscreens, poison ivy, plants (phototoxic reactions), clothing, undergarments (e.g., spandex bra, elastic waistband), metal belt buckles
Axillae	Deodorant (axillary vault), clothing (axillary folds)
Arms	Same as hand; watch and watchband
Hands	Soaps and detergents, foods, poison ivy, industrial solvents and oils, cement, metal (pots, rings), topical medications, rubber gloves in surgeons
Genitals	Poison ivy (transferred by hand), rubber condoms
Anal region	Hemorrhoid preparations (benzocaine, Nupercaine), Mycolog cream
Lower legs	Topical medication (benzocaine, lanolin, neomycin), dye in socks
Feet	Shoes (rubber or leather), cement spilling into boots

From Habif TP: *Clinical dermatology*, ed 3, St Louis, 1996, Mosby.

exposure may confirm the correct diagnosis. Cultures and potassium hydroxide preparation can screen for infectious or fungal etiologies. Patch testing can sometimes help identify a contact allergen.

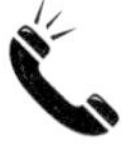

Physician consultation is recommended for oral steroid use.

MANAGEMENT

Treatments for both irritant and allergic contact dermatitis involve avoidance of the offending agents. Gentle cleansing with mild soaps and cleansing creams followed by lubrication of the skin and application of high potency topical glucocorticoid creams two to three times a day will clear irritant dermatitis. If the involvement of allergic contact dermatitis is extensive, the eruption may best be treated with oral glucocorticosteroids in consultation with a physician. The course of prednisone should start at about 1 mg/kg. The dose should be tapered off over 2 weeks.[4] A short course of oral steroids in the form of dose packs does not maintain the antiinflammatory effects adequately, and rebound is common.[2,3] If the lesions are vesicular and weepy, Domeboro compresses two or three times a day for 1 or 2 days will help dry the lesions. Antihistamines can be used to help control the itching.

COMPLICATIONS

The most common complication of acute contact dermatitis is a superimposed bacterial infection. This may be treated with topical or systemic antibiotic depending on the severity of involvement. If correctly treated, patients usually recover without serious sequelae.

Diagnostics

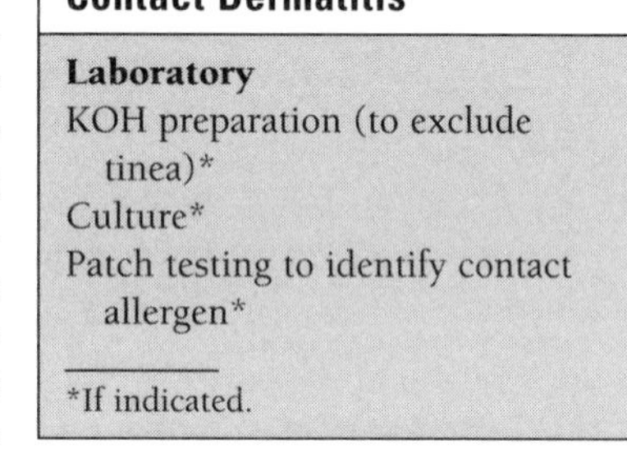

Contact Dermatitis

Laboratory
KOH preparation (to exclude tinea)*
Culture*
Patch testing to identify contact allergen*

*If indicated.

INDICATIONS FOR REFERRAL/ HOSPITALIZATION

Referral to a dermatologist or dermatology nurse practitioner may be indicated for contact dermatitis. Specialty consultation is appropriate for widespread or recalcitrant contact dermatitis or when the exact diagnosis remains elusive.

Differential Diagnosis

Contact Dermatitis

Atopic dermatitis
Dyshidrotic eczema
Bacterial infections
Candidal infections
Phytophotodermatitis

PATIENT AND FAMILY EDUCATION

Patient education to avoid the offending antigen is crucial. Patients should understand the importance of continuing treatments for 2 to 3 weeks to prevent rebound. They should also be educated about proper application of steroid creams and their potential side effects. With oral corticosteroid use, patients must be told that the medications should be taken with food and only as prescribed, and they must be educated concerning the medications' potential side effects. In addition, patients must be able to recognize the signs and symptoms of infection.

REFERENCES

1. Dershewitz RA: *Ambulatory pediatric care*, ed 2, Philadelphia, 1993, JB Lippincott.

2. Arndt K: *Manual of dermatologic therapeutics*, ed 5, Boston, 1995, Little, Brown.
3. Weston WL, Lane AT, Morrelli JG: *Color textbook of pediatric dermatology*, ed 2, St Louis, 1996, Mosby.
4. Fitzpatrick TB: *Color atlas and synopsis of clinical dermatology: common and serious diseases*, ed 3, New York, 1997, McGraw-Hill.

CHAPTER 54

Corns and Calluses

Margaret McAllister

DEFINITION/EPIDEMIOLOGY

Corns and calluses are a painful reaction to pressure or friction on the underlying dermis covering the digital and plantar surfaces of the feet. Areas of excessive pressure or friction lead to hyperkeratotic, thickened skin that forms a padded area of protection for underlying skin structures. Corns, also termed helomas, are of two types: soft (heloma molle) and hard (heloma durum). Calluses (tylomas), although unsightly, are less bothersome than corns and are generally a reaction to friction on the metatarsal heads or other bony prominences and may be a response to body weight distribution.[1,2] Calluses are not well circumscribed and lack a central core that is found in corns.

PATHOPHYSIOLOGY

Soft corns stem from hyperkeratotic development in response to excessive pressure or friction. A soft corn is a spongy hyperkeratosis in the interdigital areas of the toes. The pain associated with soft corns is often extreme because the inflammation excites pressure on the nerve receptors in the dermis. Pressure on the skin over the heads and bases of the condyles of the metatarsals and phalanges results from extrinsic factors (including an improperly fitting toebox, short shoes, or shoes with stiff soles) or from intrinsic factors such as arthritic changes, fractures, or congenital foot deformity. Both intrinsic and extrinsic factors contribute to the development of a compensatory response of the foot and toes. Downward pressure on the metatarsal heads and contracture of the phalanges set the stage for friction and pressure, leading to corn and callus formation. Both produce pain because the conical-shaped keratin points into the dermis, thereby stimulating painful sensory nerve endings.[2] Pain is triggered by development of an underlying bursitis or adventitious bursa that acts as a buffer of protection for the underlying bone.[2]

CLINICAL PRESENTATION

Corns generally produce problems when symptoms interfere with the performance of daily activities. It is important to obtain a good occupational history and to inspect the style and fit of the patient's customary shoe. An inability to move the toes in the toebox or wearing pointed-toe or high-heeled shoes is often reported. Self-treatment by cutting or using over-the-counter plasters to remove the outer horny layer of tissue is common. Occasionally, soft corns present with evidence of maceration, inflammation, oozing, and severe pain. Secondary infections of interdigital soft corns are common and are painful.

PHYSICAL EXAMINATION

Corns appear as well-circumscribed, translucent formations of keratin derived from the stratum corneum of the epidermis. Corns and calluses are located in areas of mechanical trauma.

The dorsolateral aspect of the fifth toe or the dorsal surface of the distal interphalangeal joints of the second, third, and fourth toes are the areas most commonly affected by pressure. Seed corns are small, localized lesions anywhere on the plantar surface; hard corns are located over bony prominences; soft corns occur between the toes, most often in the fourth web space; and "pump bumps" appear in adolescents as thickened soft tissue at the posterior aspect of the calcaneus secondary to wearing shoes that are too short.[3]

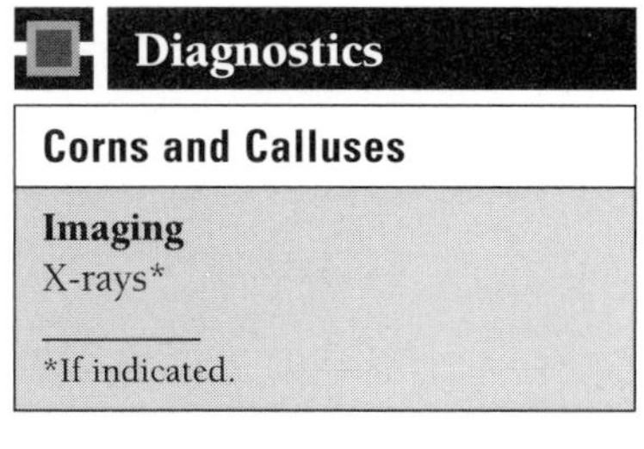
Diagnostics

Corns and Calluses

Imaging
X-rays*

*If indicated.

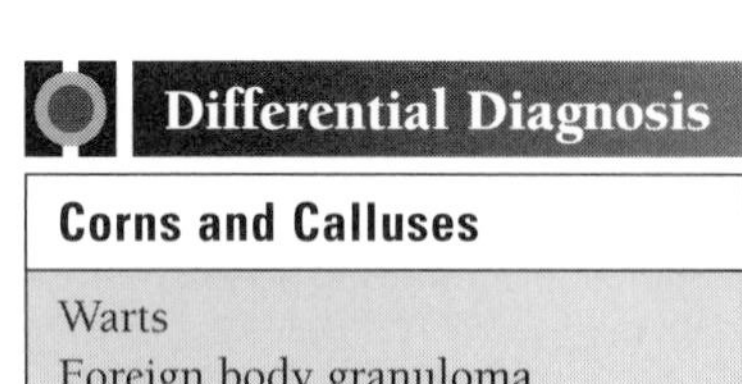
Differential Diagnosis

Corns and Calluses

Warts
Foreign body granuloma
Porokeratosis plantaris discreta

DIAGNOSTICS AND DIFFERENTIAL DIAGNOSIS

Inspection and examination are the only diagnostics generally indicated. Hard corns are distinguished from warts by their slow onset, location over bony prominences, and painful response to direct pressure. Other factors include the lack of punctate bleeding when the corn is pared with a surgical scalpel, as well as evidence of furrowed skin lines on magnification, which are not present in warts.[4] In some instances radiographs of the bony structures of the feet may be necessary to determine the intrinsic etiology of corn and callus formation, such as arthritis, bony prominences, condylar projections, and malunion of an old fracture.[4,5]

MANAGEMENT

Caustic solutions should not be used in the management of either corns or calluses. Principles of treatment include the following: (1) provide pain relief, (2) discover and correct the etiology for increased mechanical stress, (3) recommend appropriate footwear and orthotic devices, and (4) recommend surgery if conservative approaches fail.[5] Patients should be advised to wear shoes with extra depth to increase room for their toes. All corns and calluses can be scraped and pared by the primary care provider in the office using a scalpel with a #15 blade. Padding may prove helpful in the form of toe crests and metatarsal pads that redistribute weight from the metatarsal head to the pad. Toe crests work well for patients with painful hammertoes but must be worn in conjunction with shoes with a sufficiently wide toebox. Other, more recent advances include a variety of shoe pads.*

Soft corn infections can be treated by twice-daily warm soaks and the application of a topical antibiotic, such as mupirocin, that is effective against gram-positive organisms. If signs of cellulitis are present, additional oral medication should be started in the form of penicillinase-resistant penicillin, a first-generation cephalosporin, or erythromycin. After healing, the patient should be instructed to wear lamb's wool between the longer and shorter toes that is thick enough to prevent pain when the toes are juxtaposed. The patient should be instructed to wear open-toe shoes if possible and to purchase shoes that promote proper foot alignment and provide room for movement of the toes in the toebox.

Treatment for calluses includes regular sanding with a pumice stone after softening the callus in warm water. Proper footwear, as well as posture and body habitus, are further considerations in managing calluses.

Co-Management with Specialists

Patients should be referred to a podiatrist and/or orthopedic surgeon who specializes in the care of feet if conservative treatments fail to relieve pressure and restore foot health. Patients with arthritis or hip deformities, those who bear weight only on one foot, and those who use assistive devices for ambulation are at greater risk for severe corns and calluses that do not respond to conservative treatment, because intrinsic factors are the underlying cause of the mechanical stress. These individuals are also more likely to develop painful hammertoes. Surgical remodeling of the toes can be achieved to provide the patient with marked relief from painful pressure spots and enhances quality of life. Custom shoes are also a helpful adjunct.

LIFE SPAN CONSIDERATIONS

Adolescents and young adults are more likely to wear shoes that fit improperly to be fashionable or to make their feet look smaller. Foot inspection during annual physical examinations should focus on early detection of corns, calluses, and bunions that result from short, tight-fitting footwear. Women have a greater incidence of corns, calluses, bunions, and foot deformities than do men. Patients over 65 years of age have more foot problems than the general population.[5] Older adults are at increased risk for foot infections secondary to corns and callus formation, poor circulation, and poor-fitting shoes. Foot assessment should be included in the comprehensive physical examination as a means to evaluate foot health and provide necessary preventive education. Working men and women who stand for long hours on the job are at greater risk for foot problems. Efforts should be made to assess their feet frequently and determine the adequacy of shoe fit for comfort and prevention of pressure points.

COMPLICATIONS

Secondary infections often occur in soft corns. Other complications are primarily in the form of irritation, self-inflicted injury from paring down the corns, and chemical burns from the use of caustic over-the-counter keratolytic solutions.

INDICATIONS FOR REFERRAL/HOSPITALIZATION

Hospitalization is generally not warranted unless serious infection or surgery is indicated for corns that fail to respond to conservative treatment. Diabetic patients with infected corns may require IV antibiotic treatment. Other indications for referral include custom fitting for orthotic shoes.[5] Patients with severe foot deformity who are unable to purchase commercially available shoes that do not put pressure on the feet and toes may benefit from custom-fit shoes, which are expensive

*Available from Hapad. Samples and a catalog can be obtained by calling (800) 544-2723.

but are worth the investment for comfort and freedom from pressure-induced pain. Custom-fit shoes promote optimal balance and assist in the prevention of falls.

PATIENT AND FAMILY EDUCATION

Education focuses on prevention and treatment with properly fitting footwear that allows for sufficient toe space and an even distribution of body weight over the plantar surface of the foot.[5] Shoes should provide a shock-absorbing quality that absorbs rather than creates pressure and friction. Gait and body habitus are other considerations.

REFERENCES

1. DeGown RL, Brown DD: *DeGown's diagnostic examination*, ed 7, New York, 2000, McGraw Hill.
2. Robbins JM: Recognizing, treating, and preventing common foot problems, *Cleve Clin J Med* 67(1):45-56, 2000.
3. Silfverskklold JP: Common foot problems, *Postgrad Med* 89(5): 183-188, 1991.
4. Singh D, Bentley G, Trevino SG: Fortnightly review: callosities, corns, and calluses, *Br Med J* 312(7403):1403-1406, 1996.
5. Brainard BJ: Managing corns and plantar calluses, *Phys Sports Med* 19(12):61-66, 1991.

CHAPTER 55

Cutaneous Herpes

Maureen O'Hara Padden

DEFINITION/EPIDEMIOLOGY

Cutaneous infections caused by the herpes simplex virus (HSV) can be of two serologic types: HSV-1 and HSV-2. HSV-1 is responsible for 90% of oral lesions, whereas the predominance of genital lesions is associated with HSV-2 (Color Plate 13). However, either virus can cause infection at each site. Oral HSV-1 infection recurs more than oral HSV-2 infection and, likewise, genital HSV-2 infection recurs more often than genital HSV-1 infection.[1] The reason for this is not understood. Clinically, the lesions produced by each strain of the virus are indistinguishable.

There is a high prevalence of HSV-1 and HSV-2 throughout the world. Infection with the virus shows no seasonal variation. Approximately 100 million individuals are infected with HSV-1, and 40 to 60 million are infected with HSV-2.[2] One third to one half of infected individuals lack clinical manifestations of infection.[3] Asymptomatic individuals can shed the virus in the absence of symptoms. In fact, transmission has been shown to occur most often in the setting of asymptomatic virus shedding. HSV shedding has been shown to be three times higher in genital secretions sampled between, rather than during, clinical recurrences.[4] Seroprevalence increases with age and with the number of sexual partners. Recent data suggest that 21.9% of persons age 12 years or older living in the United States have serologic evidence of infection with HSV-2—a 30% increase since the 1970s. It is more common among females, less-educated individuals, cocaine users, and African-Americans and Mexican-Americans.[5]

PATHOPHYSIOLOGY

Transmission of HSV occurs by direct contact with active lesions or with secretions containing the virus. HSV-1 and HSV-2 share approximately 50% of their DNA, and therefore infection with one form affords some protection against the other.[6] HSV can invade the mucous membranes or any cutaneous site where there is skin disruption. The virus attaches itself to epithelial cells, enters, and replicates, exploiting cellular components. Once infected, cells die and release clear fluid, causing the formation of vesicles and fusing to form multinucleated giant cells. During the infection process, the virus gains access to and infects regional, sensory, or autonomic nerves. The virus travels via the nerve axon to the ganglion, where it establishes a latent infection. Subsequently, the virus can reactivate and travel down the axon, where it causes a recurrent infection in the cutaneous area innervated by the affected root.

CLINICAL PRESENTATION

There are three distinct phases of HSV infection: primary, latent, and recurrent infection. Lesions of the primary infection typically appear 2 to 12 days after inoculation, with a mean of 4 days.[1] Virus excretion in primary mucocutaneous infections can persist for up to 23 days. The occurrence of lesions may be preceded by a prodrome of burning or tenderness at the site of subsequent eruption. Multiple painful vesicles then appear at the site of infection and may be accompanied by tender lymphadenopathy in regional nodes. Fever, dysuria, vaginal discharge, or malaise may accompany the primary infection. Ulceration subsequently occurs, and lesions crust over and heal in immunocompetent patients within 2 to 3 weeks.

During the latent phase the virus remains dormant in the ganglion of the nerve that serves the affected dermatome. The recurrent phase is characterized by virus reactivation and the reappearance of lesions in the dermatome affected during the primary infection. The outbreak may not occur at exactly the same site. Reactivation of the virus can be caused by local or systemic stimuli such as immunodeficiency, trauma, fever, menses, ultraviolet light, and sexual intercourse. Although stress has been considered to be a trigger of HSV recurrence, recent evidence suggests that this may not be the case.[7] The primary infection may last for 2 to 6 weeks, whereas recurrent infections are shorter (4 to 6 days) and are less severe, with markedly fewer lesions.

PHYSICAL EXAMINATION

The lesions of HSV infection are very distinct. Grouped vesicles on an erythematous base appear on the lips, facial area, throat, or genital area (see Color Plate 13). The fluid contained in the vesicles turns cloudy and the vesicles rupture, leaving an erosion that subsequently crusts over. Regional lymphadenopathy may be associated with primary or recurrent infections but is more common with primary infections. The various stages of lesions can often make diagnosis challenging.

DIAGNOSTICS

A diagnosis of HSV infection can be made clinically with a thorough history and physical examination. However, laboratory confirmation should be considered in patients who present with a newly diagnosed primary infection. In addition, it is important to elicit any history of HSV infection, HIV infection, or pregnancy. The "gold standard" for the diagnosis of cutaneous herpes simplex infections remains viral culture. Viral cultures can take 4 to 5 days with a sensitivity of 70% to 80%. Diagnosis may also be made using fluid obtained from a freshly unroofed vesicle for Tzanck preparation or by using a direct fluorescence antibody (DFA) test. Both tests have lower sensitivity rates than culture. Viral cultures are most likely to be positive when fresh, moist lesions exist; however, the DFA test may still be positive in crusted, healing lesions.[8]

Serologic testing is available but often does not differentiate HSV-1 from HSV-2 and may only reveal previous exposure. In fact, in one study, fewer than 10% of individuals who were HSV-2 seropositive reported a history of genital herpes.[5] Antigen detection tests are also of limited usefulness in primary infections, because antibody development may be delayed.[6,9] Polymerase chain reaction (PCR) tests are extremely sensitive and specific but are expensive and are not indicated for mucocutaneous infections. PCR is most useful in the assessment of patients with suspected HSV encephalitis.[8]

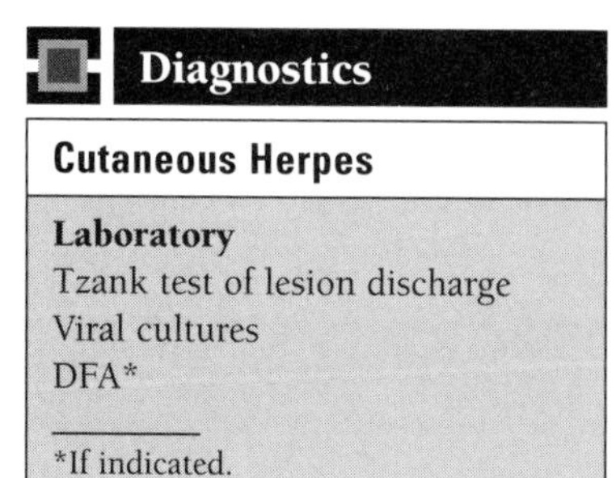

Diagnostics

Cutaneous Herpes

Laboratory
Tzank test of lesion discharge
Viral cultures
DFA*

*If indicated.

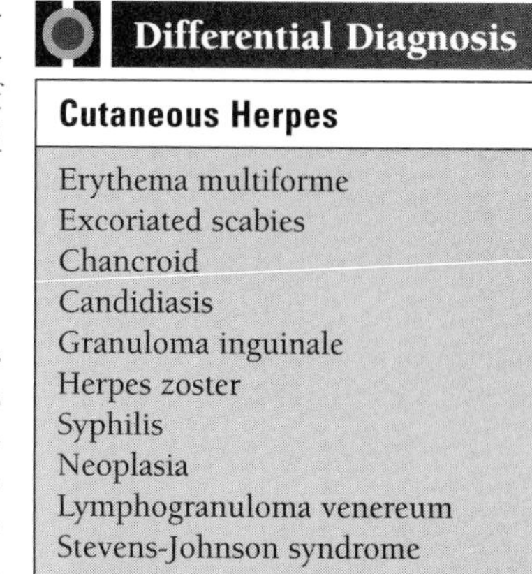

Differential Diagnosis

Cutaneous Herpes

Erythema multiforme
Excoriated scabies
Chancroid
Candidiasis
Granuloma inguinale
Herpes zoster
Syphilis
Neoplasia
Lymphogranuloma venereum
Stevens-Johnson syndrome
Trauma
Ulcerative balanitis

DIFFERENTIAL DIAGNOSIS

The differential diagnosis of HSV infections is varied. Erythema multiforme, excoriated scabies, chancroid, candidiasis, granuloma inguinale, herpes zoster, syphilis, neoplasia, lymphogranuloma venereum, Stevens-Johnson syndrome, mechanical ulceration secondary to trauma, and ulcerative balanitis should be considered.

MANAGEMENT

Acyclovir remains the treatment of choice for most HSV infections (Table 55-1). Two newer precursor drugs, valacyclovir (which is converted to acyclovir) and famciclovir (which is converted to penciclovir) have been licensed for use and have been shown to have better bioavailability than acyclovir or penciclovir. However, they are considerably more expensive. Their clinical benefit is similar, and no evidence exists that one is better than the others. Their usefulness lies in the convenience of the dosing schedule, which may be important in patients with poor compliance. From a cost-benefit perspective, acyclovir is probably most useful in the management of herpes simplex infections, because it is now available in generic form.[10]

TABLE 55-1 Dosing Schedule Summary for Mucocutaneous Herpes Simplex Infections

Drug	Dosage
INITIAL EPISODE	
Acyclovir	200 mg PO 5 times daily for 7-10 days 5 mg/kg IV q 8 hr for 5-7 days 400 mg PO t.i.d. for 7-10 days
Valacyclovir	1 g PO b.i.d. for 7-10 days
Famciclovir	250 mg PO t.i.d. for 5-10 days
RECURRENT EPISODES	
Acyclovir	400 mg PO b.i.d. for 5 days
Acyclovir "stat"	400 mg PO once at onset of prodrome*
Valacyclovir	500 mg PO b.i.d. for 5 days
Famciclovir	125-250 mg PO b.i.d. for 5 days
SUPPRESSION	
Acyclovir	400 mg PO b.i.d.
Valacyclovir	500 mg or 1000 mg PO q.d.
Famciclovir	250 mg PO b.i.d.

*Recurrent orolabial HSV, limited evidence.

Oral Gingivostomatitis

Evidence exists that oral acyclovir suspension (given for 7 days at a dose of 15 mg/kg per dose five times a day to children afflicted with herpetic gingivostomatitis) significantly shortens duration of oral lesions and reduces eating and drinking difficulties.

Primary Herpes Labialis

Evidence exists that initial orolabial infection with HSV should be treated with acyclovir 200 mg PO five times daily for 7 to 10 days.[11,12] Topical acyclovir has little efficacy and should not be used to treat mucocutaneous HSV infections.[13,14] However, the U.S. Food and Drug Administration (FDA) has approved penciclovir cream, applied every 2 hours (while awake) for 4 days, for treatment of herpes labialis. Limited evidence exists that penciclovir cream is useful in treating recurrent herpes labialis with reduced pain and faster healing of lesions.[15]

Recurrent Herpes Labialis

Evidence of the benefit of treatment is unclear for recurrent herpes labialis. Only severe cases of recurrent herpes labialis should be treated. Recurrent outbreaks can be treated with the following acyclovir regimens: (1) 200 mg PO five times daily, (2) 400 mg PO t.i.d., or (3) 800 mg PO b.i.d. until lesions are crusted or for approximately 5 days.[11] Limited evidence exists regarding the benefit of a single "stat" dose of 800 mg acyclovir at the onset of prodrome to prevent recurrent outbreaks of HSV in some patients.[16]

Primary Genital Herpes

Evidence exists for benefit of treatment of primary genital herpes with either IV or oral acyclovir.[12] Patients may be treated with one of the following regimens: (1) 200 mg PO five times daily for 7 to 10 days, (2) 5 mg/kg IV every 8 hours for 5 to 7 days or (3) 400 mg PO t.i.d. for 7 to 10 days.[1] Valacyclovir and famciclovir may also be used, but there is no evidence to suggest they are any more effective clinically, and they cost considerably more. They do offer the benefit of easier dosing with valacyclovir given daily and famciclovir given three times daily. This may be important if compliance or ease of dosage schedule is an important consideration. When given, the following dosing regimens may be used: (1) valacyclovir 1 g PO b.i.d. for 7 to 10 days, or (2) famciclovir 250 mg PO t.i.d. for 5 to 10 days.[1]

Recurrent Genital Herpes

Limited evidence exists for benefit of treatment of recurrent genital herpes labialis with acyclovir, famciclovir, or valacyclovir when started within 24 hours of onset.[17-20] However, medication only shortens the duration of lesions by 1 to 2 days, and there is no change in time to recurrence of infection. When given, the following regimens may be used: (1) acyclovir 400 mg PO b.i.d. for 5 days, (2) valacyclovir 500 mg PO b.i.d. for 5 days, or (3) famciclovir 125 to 250 mg PO b.i.d. for 5 days.[1]

Suppression of Frequent Recurrences

Evidence exists for benefit of suppression in patients with frequently recurring HSV infections (>6 per year) with acyclovir, famciclovir, or valacyclovir.[3,21-24] Patients may be treated with one of the following long-term suppressive therapy regimens: (1) acyclovir 400 mg PO b.i.d., (2) famciclovir 250 mg PO b.i.d., or (3) valacyclovir 500 to 1000 mg PO q.d.[1] This reduces the number of recurrences and the frequency of asymptomatic shedding. It is important to understand that famciclovir and valacyclovir are no more effective for treating recurrent HSV infections than acyclovir.[22,23] Because of their cost, valacyclovir and famciclovir find greatest usefulness where compliance or convenience of dosing is an issue. The FDA has approved suppressive therapy with acyclovir for 12 months, although studies extending treatment to 5 years show no cumulative toxicity.[21] Patients with frequent orolabial HSV infection can be treated with similar regimens.

LIFE SPAN CONSIDERATIONS

Patients should understand that infection with HSV is lifelong and that there is no cure. There is currently no vaccination available.[3] In most individuals the frequency and severity of attacks diminish with time.

COMPLICATIONS

Complications of HSV are rare and typically occur in women with primary infections. Possible complications include aseptic meningitis, urinary retention, cutaneous dissemination, bacterial superinfection, erythema multiforme, and spontaneous abortion. A cesarean section is indicated if the mother has active herpes lesions at or around the time of delivery.

INDICATIONS FOR REFERRAL/HOSPITALIZATION

Patients for whom a diagnosis of HSV is in question, who have superimposed HIV infection, who are on long-term suppressive therapy, or who fail to respond to routine therapy should be referred to a physician or specialist. Pregnant women also represent a special population and should be referred for evaluation by their obstetrician or family physician immediately.

Patients requiring large amounts of pain medication or patients who have severe disseminated infections, severe superimposed bacterial infections, an inability to void, or an inability to take anything by mouth should be considered for hospitalization.

PATIENT AND FAMILY EDUCATION

Patients must be made aware of their ability to transmit HSV even when they have no apparent lesions. The use of condoms should be encouraged. The risk of neonatal transmission during pregnancy must be explained to both male and female patients. Patients should be encouraged to use lip balm with sunscreen when exposed to ultraviolet light to avoid precipitation of an outbreak.

Patients may experience shame or depression because of their infection with HSV and should be referred to the National Herpes Hotline at (919) 361-8488 for available resources.

HEALTH PROMOTION

Patients can reduce their risk of acquiring genital herpes by limiting their lifetime number of sexual partners, by using condoms, and through education regarding transmission and shedding. In that manner, they can choose to avoid high-risk situations. The risk of orolabial herpes infection can also be reduced by limiting sexual partners and by avoiding direct contact with individuals with cold sores. Patients with orolabial and genital herpes must be counseled not to excoriate or rub the herpes lesions because of the risk for autoinoculation of other parts of the body.

REFERENCES

1. Whitley RJ: Herpes simplex virus infections, *Lancet* 357:1513-1518, 2001.
2. Whitley RJ: Prospects for vaccination against herpes simplex virus, *Pediatr Ann* 22(12):726-732, 1993.
3. Spruance SL and others: A large scale placebo-controlled, dose-ranging trial of perioral Valacyclovir for episodic treatment of recurrent herpes genitalis: Valacyclovir HSV Study Group, *Arch Intern Med* 156(15):1729-1735, 1996.
4. Wald A and others: Virologic characteristics of subclinical and symptomatic genital herpes infections, *N Engl J Med* 333:770-775, 1995.
5. Fleming DT and others: Herpes simplex virus type 2 in the United States, 1976 to 1994, *N Engl J Med* 337:1105-1111, 1997.
6. Annunziato PW and others: Herpes simplex virus infections, *Pediatr Rev* 17(12):415-423, 1996.
7. Green J and others: Psychological factors in recurrent genital herpes. *Genitourin Med* 73:253-258, 1997.
8. Erlich KS: Management of herpes simplex and varicella-zoster virus infections, *West J Med* 166(3):211-215, 1997.
9. Leflore S and others: A risk-benefit evaluation of acyclovir for the treatment and prophylaxis of herpes simplex virus infections. *Drug Saf* 23(2):131-142, 2000.
10. Clark JL and others: Management of genital herpes, *Am Fam Physician* 51:175-182, 187-188, 1995.
11. Centers for Disease Control and Prevention: 1993 sexually transmitted diseases treatment guidelines, *MMWR* 42:22-26, 1993.
12. Whitley RJ: Acyclovir: a decade later, *N Engl J Med* 327:782-789, 1992.
13. Review: Topical acyclovir is of limited or no benefit to patients with recurrent herpes labialis, *ACP Journal Club* 15: 6, 1991.
14. Worrall G: Topical acyclovir for recurrent herpes labialis in primary care, *Can Fam Physician* 37:92-98, 1991.
15. Spruance SL: Penciclovir cream for the treatment of herpes simplex labialis, *JAMA* 277(17):1374-1379, 1997.
16. Shelley WB and others: "Stat" single dose of acyclovir for prevention of herpes simplex, *Cutis* 57(6):453, 1996.
17. Reichman RC and others: Treatment of recurrent genital herpes simplex infections with oral acyclovir: a controlled trial, *JAMA* 251: 2103-2107, 1984.
18. Famciclovir reduced lesion healing time in recurrent genital herpes, *ACP Journal Club* 125:69, 1996.
19. Diaz-Mitoma and others: Oral famciclovir for the suppression of recurrent genital herpes: a randomized controlled trial, *JAMA* 280: 887-892, 1998.
20. Patel R and others: Valacyclovir for the suppression of recurrent genital HSV infection: a placebo controlled study of once daily therapy. International Valacyclovir HSV Study Group, *Genitourin Med* 73(2): 105-109, 1997.
21. Wald A and others: Suppression of subclinical shedding of herpes simplex virus type II with acyclovir, *Ann Intern Med* 124:8-15, 1996.
22. Chosidow O and others. Famciclovir vs. acyclovir in immunocompetent patients with recurrent genital herpes infections: a parallel-groups, randomized, double blind clinical trial, *Br J Dermatol* 144(4):818-824, 2001.
23. Tyring SK and others. A randomized, placebo-controlled comparison of oral valacyclovir and acyclovir in immunocompetent patients with recurrent genital herpes infections: The Valacyclovir International Study Group, *Arch Dermatol* 134(2):185-191, 1998.
24. Mertz GJ and others: Oral famciclovir for suppression of recurrent genital herpes simplex virus infection in women, *Arch Intern Med* 157:343-349, 1997.

CHAPTER 56

Dermatitis Medicamentosa

Nancy W. Knee

DEFINITION/EPIDEMIOLOGY

Dermatitis medicamentosa (drug eruption) is an eruption of the skin or mucous membranes that can occur up to 2 weeks after drug administration. These eruptions imitate almost all of the morphologies in dermatology, including exanthemas, urticaria, photosensitivity, fixed-drug reactions, palpable purpura, bullae, alopecia, onycholysis, acral erythema, lichenoid and acneiform lesions, toxic epidermal necrolysis, and erythema multiforme syndrome. Drug reactions may occur at any age, are more common in women, and are the most common form of drug sensitivity reactions.[1]

Immediate emergency department referral/ physician consultation is indicated for anaphylaxis, severe erythema multiforme, or Stevens-Johnson syndrome.

PATHOPHYSIOLOGY

Drug eruptions are hypersensitivity manifestations of immunologic or nonimmunologic mechanisms stimulated by oral, topical, or parenteral drug administration.[2] Immunologic responses occur when specific antibodies or specifically sensitized lymphocytes to a drug develop during the sensitization period, which may be 4 or 5 days after initial exposure. Subsequent exposure to the drug results in a reaction that may occur within minutes, hours, or days.

Nonimmunologic responses, the most common, may be caused by accumulation of a drug, pharmacologic action of a drug, genetic factors, reaction of the drug with ultraviolet light, irritancy of topical solutions, and unknown factors.[2,3] Hypersensitivity reactions to antibacterial agents (mostly penicillin), protease inhibitors (PIs) are examples of the latter, involving maculopapular rashes and/or urticaria.[2]

Protease inhibitors may cause acute generalized exanthematous pustulosis (AGEP). AGEP presents with onset of acute clinical symptoms, including fever higher than 38° C (100.4° F) and widespread exfoliative dermatitis following a pustular, morbilliform eruption that heals with discontinuation of the PI.[4]

CLINICAL PRESENTATION

Patients may present with a variety of skin reactions (Table 56-1). The most common is a confluent, maculopapular rash that may be pruritic (Color Plate 14). Onset can occur 7 to 10 days after starting the drug but may not occur until the course of medication is finished. The rash may last 1 to 2 weeks and then fades.[2] The rash may also be urticarial or a fixed-drug reaction that occurs in the same area each time the drug is taken.

TABLE 56-1 Skin Reactions

Dermatologic Types	Causative Agents	Manifestations
Exanthemas	Cillins, sulfonamides, barbiturates	Bright red scarlatiniform lesions, usually on trunk
Urticaria	Cillins, salicylates, erythromycin, carbamazepine	Typical, well-defined wheals on hands, feet, lips, generalized
Photosensitivity	Phenothiazines, tetracyclines, sulfonamides, artificial sweeteners	Dermatitis or gray-blue hyperpigmented areas on skin exposed to sun
Fixed-drug reactions	Phenolphthalein, tetracycline, sulfonamides	Dusky red or purple lesions that reappear in same area with repeated drug exposure
Purpura	Chlorothiazide, meprobamate, anticoagulants	Nonblanching purple lesions, usually generalized and on lower extremities
Bullae	Cillins, barbiturates, iodines, sulfonamides	Symmetric, erythematous, edematous, bullous lesions
Lichenoid lesions	Antimalarials, gold, thiazides, chlorpromazine	Angular papules that turn into scaly patches
Acneiform lesions	Corticosteroids, iodines, bromides, hydantoins	Acnelike but no comedones and with sudden onset
Toxic epidermal necrolysis	Barbiturates, hydantoins, cillins, sulfonamides	Areas of loosened, easily detached epidermis with a scalded appearance
Erythema multiforme	Cillins, barbiturates, sulfonamides	Vary from small vesicles or ulcers to widespread bullous lesions (Stevens-Johnson syndrome)

PHYSICAL EXAMINATION

Careful skin examination is indicated. The category of lesions and distribution should be noted. Further examination of the head, eyes, ears, nose, throat, and cardiopulmonary status may be necessary to exclude viral exanthema or anaphylaxis, a more severe, systemic reaction.

DIAGNOSTICS

No laboratory tests are available that can establish the diagnosis, although occasionally a CBC may reveal eosin-ophilia. Skin tests can evaluate sensitivity to penicillin. Diagnosis is dependent on a thorough drug history, including known allergies or hypersensitivities to all oral, topical, parental, over-the-counter, prescription, vitamin and "natural" preparations and duration of symptoms.[5]

DIFFERENTIAL DIAGNOSIS

Other dermatologic processes must be excluded. These include urticaria, purpura, photosensitivity, bullous impetigo, contact or irritant dermatitis, acne vulgaris, rosacea, scarlet fever, staphylococcal infections, secondary syphilis, and viral rashes (e.g., herpes simplex mycoplasma).[5] Usually the sudden onset and symmetric nature of the eruptions (except in cases of topical administration of the offending product) establish the diagnosis as dermatitis medicamentosa. For example, urticaria-related drug reactions present as transient wheals in the skin caused by acute dermal edema. The more sudden and explosive the appearance of the urticaria, the more likely that a potent, life-threatening anaphylaxis may occur. Immediate discontinuation of the drug is imperative. Urticaria lesions are distinguished from erythema multiforme by the former's pruritic nature and will often "move" over 1 to 2 hours. Erythema multiforme lesions are not pruritic, are often painful, and may last 1 to 4 weeks.[5] Readministration of the pharmacologic preparation will confirm sensitivity; however, this may be life threatening, especially in immunologic responses.

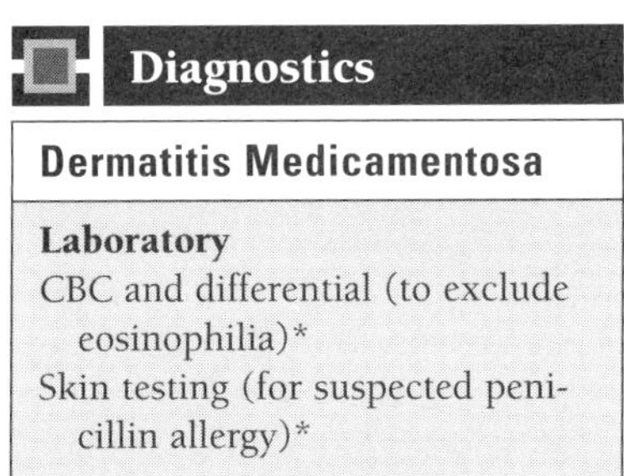
Diagnostics

Dermatitis Medicamentosa

Laboratory
CBC and differential (to exclude eosinophilia)*
Skin testing (for suspected penicillin allergy)*

*If indicated.

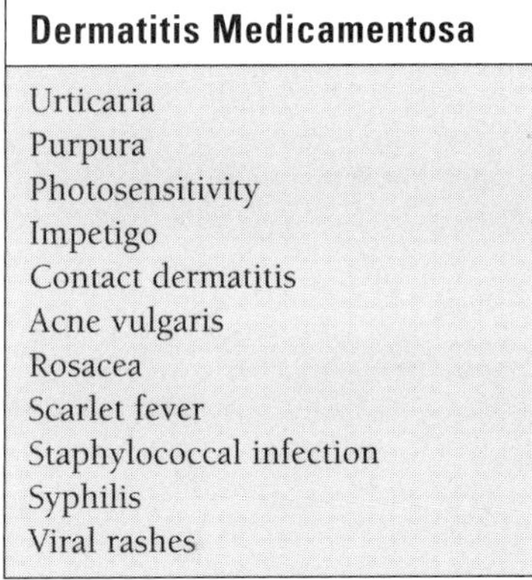
Differential Diagnosis

Dermatitis Medicamentosa

Urticaria
Purpura
Photosensitivity
Impetigo
Contact dermatitis
Acne vulgaris
Rosacea
Scarlet fever
Staphylococcal infection
Syphilis
Viral rashes

MANAGEMENT

Identification of the offending preparation and its removal will usually resolve the drug reaction, although the course of the reaction may progress for several days until the preparation is eliminated from the body.

Symptomatic treatment is advised. Cool compresses and tepid baths may be soothing. For nonacute eruptions with dry, scaly, nonpruritic lesions, cooling lotions (e.g., Sarna Anti-Itch) may be applied.[2] Topical corticosteroid ointment can be administered to a small area for more pruritic eruptions. If effective, the preparation may be applied to the entire eruption four times per day.[3] Oral antihistamines should also be administered to manage pruritus. For refractory cases oral corticosteroids may prove beneficial. For severe reactions, including those with anaphylaxis, epinephrine 1:1000 (0.2 ml SC) should be administered. Antihistamines should be used adjunctively.

COMPLICATIONS

Anaphylaxis is a potential life-threatening complication of reexposure to the offending preparation, especially in immunologic responses. Immunologic responses vary and may progress to Stevens-Johnson syndrome (epidermis peels off in sheets), erythema multiforme (eruption of symmetric erythematous and edematous lesions of the skin or mucous membranes), myocarditis (inflammation of the myocardium), or other life-threatening conditions.

INDICATIONS FOR REFERRAL/HOSPITALIZATION

Patients with erythema multiforme, Stevens-Johnson syndrome, or anaphylaxis require immediate referral. Any patient who does not experience a resolution of symptoms in a timely manner should be referred for confirmation of the diagnosis and additional consultation.

PATIENT AND FAMILY EDUCATION/HEALTH PROMOTION

Patients should be encouraged to wear medical alert bracelets or devices that list medication allergies. Home anaphylaxis or epinephrine kits should be prescribed, and both the patient and family should be instructed in their use. The patient's record should be flagged to alert other health care providers of the allergy, and all patients, including children, should be encouraged to tell providers about the allergy before any antibiotics or other medications are prescribed.

REFERENCES

1. Fitzpatrick T and others: *Color atlas and synopsis of clinical dermatology,* ed 2, New York, 1991, McGraw-Hill.
2. Habif T and others: *Skin disorders: diagnosis and treatment,* St Louis, 2001, Mosby
3. Berkow R: *The Merck manual,* ed 16, Rahway, NJ, 1992, Merck Research Laboratories.
4. Ward HA, Russo GG, Shrum J: Cutaneous manifestations of antiretroviral therapy, *J Am Acad Dermatol* 6:2, 2002.
5. Hebert AA, Ralston JP: Cutaneous reactions to anticonvulsant medications, *J Clin Psychiatry* 62(suppl 14):22-26, 2001.

CHAPTER 57

Dry Skin

Catherine E. Turner

DEFINITION/EPIDEMIOLOGY

Dry skin is literally skin that lacks moisture or water. It is often characterized as rough or xerotic. Dry skin is common in dry climates and during the winter months and it is especially prevalent in older adults.

PATHOPHYSIOLOGY

Environments in which the humidity is below 30% cause dehydration of the stratum corneum layer of the skin. Cold air and heat in buildings, cars, and homes also contribute to skin dehydration, especially during the winter months.

Repeated exposure to solvents and soaps removes lipids from the skin. Natural skin oils are removed, and their protective nature is lost. Loss of water, lipids and/or proteins alters the overall skin integrity and its ability to perform its protective functions.[1]

CLINICAL PRESENTATION AND PHYSICAL EXAMINATION

Many individuals report having dry skin most of their lives, whereas others state that the problem developed with aging. Some report skin changes with the seasons or after an illness. In general, the dryness presents as a rough patch that itches. Pruritis is worse on the lower extremities. This area has less fat and muscle mass and less ability to replace the lipid layer elements. The hands and face are also common sites because of exposure to wind/air and handwashing. If moisture is not replaced, the skin becomes rough and occasionally loses its suppleness. It often becomes cracked and fissured.[2] Erythema craquelé, an uneven diamond pattern with erythema at the edges, can develop (Color Plate 15).

DIAGNOSTICS AND DIFFERENTIAL DIAGNOSIS

Dry skin is a visual diagnosis. The differential diagnosis includes all other forms of dermatitis, including eczema, ichthyosis vulgaris, and scabies.[2,3] Secondary skin changes occurring as a result of scratching can complicate the appearance of the skin, making accurate diagnosis difficult.

MANAGEMENT

Xerotic skin is dry because of a lack of water. Treatment with lubricants and water-in-oil emulsions two to three times daily will restore moisture. Patients should be advised to take "short" baths with water that is not hot. For infants and even some older adults, foregoing the bath and spot washing the axilla and groin can help to minimize moisture loss. When toweling, the skin should be patted dry. Oils can be added to the skin immediately after toweling or just before rinsing. If applied before rinsing, the oil helps prevent the loss of moisture caused by rinsing and drying. If applied immediately after rinsing, the oils help prevent further loss of moisture and should be applied within 2 to 3 minutes of drying. Caution is advised, because using oils can make the skin "slippery." Infants can be at risk for being dropped, and all patients could be at risk for falls—a particular concern in older adults.

Differential Diagnosis
Dry Skin
Eczema
Ichthyosis vulgaris
Scabies

Antihistamines are often used to minimize scratching. Caution is advised, because the sedative effects of traditional antihistamines are potentially problematic. In older patients, interactions of the antihistamines with other medications or other disease entities are also a consideration (e.g., urinary retention secondary to benign prostatic hypertrophy may be exacerbated in older males). Creams and lotions containing the chemicals menthol and phenol can often help in the relief of pruritis[1] and, based on patient situation and severity, may be tried before systemic oral therapy. Dry skin treated early with moisturizers and emollients will help prevent secondary lesions resulting from scratching and irritation.

COMPLICATIONS

Although complications are uncommon, they do occur. Infections and even cellulitis have occurred as a result of scratching. Other complications are generally secondary to treatment. Local reactions to perfumes in moisturizers can occur, as well as atrophy from long-term use of topical steroids.

INDICATIONS FOR REFERRAL/HOSPITALIZATION

A dermatology referral and hospitalization are not usually indicated. A referral to dermatologist is warranted if the diagnosis is unclear.

PATIENT EDUCATION AND HEALTH PROMOTION

Patients with dry skin should understand the importance of keeping the room temperature comfortably low or as close to 68° F as possible to help prevent the skin from drying. Humidifiers can help put moisture back in the air and are advisable for many patients. Chronic use of humidifiers includes education on periodic cleaning with vinegar to keep impurities to a minimum. Bath water should be warm but not hot. Moisturizers should be applied just before rinsing or immediately after drying. Their use should include caution for slippage to prevent falls or injuries. Mild soaps or cleansers should be used sparingly. Low to medium potency topical corticosteroid ointments provide rapid relief for associated eczematous changes but should be discontinued when symptoms have resolved. The patient should be cautioned against scratching, because scratching leads to complications and exacerbates the irritated skin. Overall long-term management from year to year in appropriate patients can help prevent dry skin. The use of good skin care programs that can be modified seasonally can help to control and prevent dry skin and/or its complications.

Travel increases during the winter and holiday months. Because air travel can significantly pull moisture from the air and lead to drying of the skin, patients should be instructed to keep well hydrated and use moisturizers as necessary. In addition, patients susceptible to dry skin should be cautioned to avoid extended use of high settings on car heaters, because these cause a loss of moisture from skin surfaces.

Patients should stay well hydrated. Soups and stews help replace water in the diet and are good sources of nutrients during the winter months. Older adults should be cautioned to limit their sodium consumption, but the need for adequate hydration both externally and internally is important. Vitamins can be added to the daily regimen for patients who are not already taking a multivitamin or whose nutritional balance is of concern. This will help promote good skin integrity via overall nutritional health. It is important to encourage the basics: adequate nutrition, exercise, and rest. Medications added as needed will help prevent dry skin problems.

REFERENCES

1. Habif T: *Skin disease: diagnosis and treatment*, St Louis, 2001, Mosby.
2. Arndt K: *Manual of dermatologic therapeutics*, ed 5, Boston, 1995, Little, Brown.
3. Weston WL, Lane AT, Morrelli JG: *Color textbook of pediatric dermatology*, ed 2, St Louis, 1996, Mosby.

CHAPTER 58

Eczematous Dermatitis (Atopic Dermatitis)

Eileen M. Deignan

DEFINITION/EPIDEMIOLOGY

Eczematous dermatitis, or atopic dermatitis (AD), is a chronic disorder characterized by exacerbations and remissions of dry, itchy red skin. It is associated with an increased incidence of asthma, hay fever, or allergies. Patients with a tendency toward the development of these three conditions are called *atopics*. Many atopic patients also have a family history of atopy. From 30% to 80% of atopic patients experience eczematous flares throughout life.[1] AD is often called "the itch that rashes." Patients initially are bothered by itching, scratch an area, and then develop a rash at the site of scratching. Factors that aggravate atopic dermatitis include dry skin, sweating, heat, and dry environments. Topical agents (e.g., harsh soaps and detergents) and wool also intensify AD. In addition, AD can be exacerbated by infections, stress, and allergies.

PATHOPHYSIOLOGY

Although the primary cause of AD remains unknown, patients with AD have elevated serum immunoglobulin E (IgE) levels and altered cell-mediated immunity. However, despite the correlation between elevated IgE levels and the severity of AD, not all patients with elevated IgE levels experience AD.[2]

CLINICAL PRESENTATION AND PHYSICAL EXAMINATION

AD is characterized by pruritic, erythematous, dry patches of skin, often with scale. Linear excoriations may be seen as a secondary change (Color Plate 16). The borders of eczematous lesions are not initially well defined. Crusting and oozing are common. Thickened skin with well-defined skin markings (lichenification) may develop in longer-standing lesions as the result of scratching. In adults, eczema or atopic dermatitis may be generalized with a tendency to develop lesions on the face, neck, flexural folds, wrists, and dorsa of the feet.

DIAGNOSTICS AND DIFFERENTIAL DIAGNOSIS

AD is a clinical diagnosis that is based on a careful history and presentation. Seborrheic dermatitis can be differentiated from AD by its presentation and distribution. Seborrheic dermatitis typically presents as nonpruritic, yellow, waxy plaques on the face, postauricular area, and scalp. Psoriasis is characterized by well-demarcated, intensely erythematous plaques with characteristic, overlying silvery scale. Areas of trauma such as the scalp, elbows, and knees are commonly involved.

Scabies typically presents as a poorly defined pruritic eruption, often with linear burrows in the web spaces of the fingers. The breasts and genital areas are also often involved. The condition is commonly complicated by eczematous changes from scratching and rubbing. The diagnosis is confirmed by scraping a burrow and microscopically identifying mites, eggs, or fecal material in the scraped material.

Molluscum contagiosum lesions are small, dome-shaped papules with central umbilication. They are not easily confused with AD, but patients with molluscum often develop dermatitis in the area of molluscum lesions. In AD, dozens to hundreds of molluscum contagiosum lesions are sometimes seen, usually around the eyes, axillae, and proximal extremities.[3]

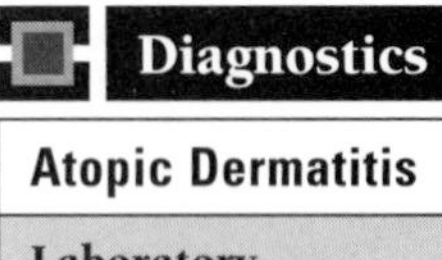

Diagnostics

Atopic Dermatitis

Laboratory
KOH preparation (to exclude other disorders)

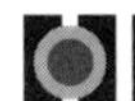

Differential Diagnosis

Atopic Dermatitis

Seborrheic dermatitis
Psoriasis
Scabies
Molluscum contagiosum
Tinea

Tinea (or superficial fungal infection) lesions have a sharply demarcated border with scale at the edge and central clearing. They are usually limited in number and sometimes form an arciform array. A scraping of the border of the lesion and treatment of the removed sample with potassium hydroxide (KOH) reveal hyphae on microscopic evaluation.

MANAGEMENT

Patient education is the cornerstone of AD treatment. The patient must learn to avoid rubbing and scratching the involved areas, because this only exacerbates the condition. With AD, it is said that "one scratch is too much and a thousand scratches is not enough." Therefore the goals of treatment are management of pruritus to prevent scratching and rubbing and skin hydration to prevent the primary disease.

Antihistamines can control itching, allay anxiety, and induce sleep. Diphenhydramine and hydroxyzine are the drugs of choice, although nonsedating antihistamines may be preferred for daytime use.

Hydration through bathing in an oatmeal powder bath of tepid water can be soothing during an acute flare of AD. The bathing should be immediately followed by the application of a bland emollient such as hydrated petrolatum.

Topical corticosteroid ointments are usually necessary to alleviate inflammation during an acute flare. These medications are applied to the erythematous areas two or three times per day. As the flare subsides, alternating the corticosteroids with lubricants will lessen the risks of prolonged steroid use.[2] Topical corticosteroids should be discontinued when the inflammation has subsided, whereas the use of lubricants and emollients should be continued.

People with AD should be aware of the drying affect of soaps. Mild soaps can be used to wash the body folds and genital area but should be avoided on other body parts.

Secondary bacterial infections should be treated with appropriate topical and systemic antibiotics. Systemic corticosteroids are seldom used in the treatment of AD and should be reserved for extreme cases that are not controlled with topical treatments. Phototherapy with ultraviolet B (UVB) light and photochemotherapy with psoralen plus ultraviolet A (PUVA) light may be helpful in patients in whom standard therapies have failed.

The immunosuppressant topical FK506, or tacrolimus, is a relatively new agent for the treatment of AD.[4] It is available in an ointment base in 0.03% and 0.1% concentrations. The ointment is applied twice daily to the skin. It can be used both for eczema flares and intermittently for maintenance that is nonresponsive to other therapies. The medication is generally well tolerated except that many patients experience transient stinging with the first few applications of the medication.

COMPLICATIONS

Secondary bacterial infections are common from chronic excoriations. Group A beta-hemolytic streptococci and staphylococci are the most common bacterial organisms. Bacterial secondary infection should be considered, cultured for, and treated in patents with purulent or weepy lesions and in cases of AD that are slow to respond to standard therapies.

Patients with AD have a higher incidence of herpes simplex virus, molluscum contagiosum, and warts. These infections can be more frequent and widespread in patients with AD. Increases in cutaneous viral infections are related to defective cell-mediated immunity in the skin as well as to the use of topical steroids.

A particularly serious viral complication of AD is eczema herpeticum. A patient with this condition has an underlying skin disorder (usually AD) and develops a widespread eruption of vesicles and erosions. A Giemsa-stained scraping of the base of a vesicle will reveal multinucleated giant cells. Eczema herpeticum should be treated with oral antiviral medications.

INDICATIONS FOR REFERRAL/HOSPITALIZATION

Failure to respond to topical treatments requires referral to a dermatologist or dermatology nurse practitioner for management. An eruption that is recalcitrant to treatment may resemble AD but actually be another disorder. For example, bullous pemphigoid and cutaneous T-cell lymphoma can sometimes resemble AD in their early stages.

In addition, evaluation and management by an allergist or allergy nurse practitioner may be needed for optimal care in a patient with known allergies or with suspicions for an allergic role in the disease.

Hospitalization may be required for intensive topical or systemic treatments. Hospitalization is also indicated for patients who are unresponsive to outpatient therapies.

PATIENT AND FAMILY EDUCATION

Patients should understand that there is no cure for AD. Weeks or months of control will be followed by sudden exacerbations. Patients should understand the proper use of antihistamines to control itching, as well the continuous use of lubricants and emollients to moisturize the skin. Careful education on proper bathing and moisturizing is very important, as is an understanding of the proper use of baths and lubricants to decrease the need for topical corticosteroids. Identification of aggravating factors such as stress, infections, weather change, dry skin, and contact sensitivity will aid in management.

REFERENCES

1. Arndt K: *Manual of dermatologic therapeutics,* ed 5, Boston, 1995, Little, Brown.
2. Hannifin J: *Dermatologic therapy,* vol 1, Copenhagen, 1996, Munksgaard.
3. Weston WL, Lane AT, Morrelli JG: *Color textbook of pediatric dermatology,* ed 2, St Louis, 1996, Mosby.
4. Odom RB, James WD, Berger TG: *Andrew's diseases of the skin,* ed 9, Philadelphia, 2000, WB Saunders.

CHAPTER 59

Fungal Infections (Superficial)

Eileen M. Deignan

Superficial fungal infections are common problems. These fungal infections can cause a primary or secondary infection of the skin that may be difficult to accurately diagnose. Greater exposure to fungal pathogens is occurring in the healthy and fitness-minded population, in debilitated patients using systemic antibiotics, and in patients who are immunocompromised.

Dermatophyte Infections

DEFINITION/EPIDEMIOLOGY

A dermatophyte is a fungus that invades and proliferates within the nonviable keratinized tissues—the stratum corneum of the skin, hair, and nails. Three of the most common pathologic dermatophytes are *Trichophyton, Microsporum,* and *Epidermophyton.* The infections produced by dermatophytes are known as tinea, dermatophytosis, or ringworm. *Tinea* is derived from the Latin word for "worm" and was probably chosen because of the common presence of a migrating, circular pattern with the infection.[1]

PATHOPHYSIOLOGY

Fungal infections are usually transmitted through close contact with an infected person or animal. Indirect contact with fomites (infected towels, clothing) may also cause dermatophyte infections.

CLINICAL PRESENTATION AND PHYSICAL EXAMINATION

Tinea infections are transmitted by direct contact with organisms in the environment, animals, or other people. They are characterized and named according to their location. Tinea capitis (head/scalp) can present as patchy, scaly, nonscarring areas of hair loss (Color Plate 17). Depending on the infectious organism, the lesions may become inflamed, boggy, and pustular. Tinea corporis (body) appears on skin as erythematous plaques and papules in an annular or arciform pattern. Lesions often have slightly elevated orders with central clearing (Color Plate 18). Tinea cruris (jock itch) appears on the groin and upper inner thigh and extends to the gluteal folds as erythematous scaling patches with raised borders. The scrotum is often spared. Tinea pedis (athlete's foot) can occur as interdigital scaling, maceration, and fissuring (Color Plate 19). It can also present as a mild erythematous scaling eruption that involves the sole and sides of the foot (moccasin distribution). Tinea manus (hand) is often a dry, scaly eruption of the palms, with sharply marginated plaques on the dorsum of the hands. The feet are often also involved. Tinea unguium (nail), also called onychomycosis, most commonly presents as the distal subungual type. The infection begins in the distal nail bed and spreads to infect the nail plate, causing the nail to appear thickened and yellowed, with subungual keratinacious debris. Onychomycosis appears on lateral nail margins as a yellow discoloration. Increased nail thickness and distortion usually occur over time.

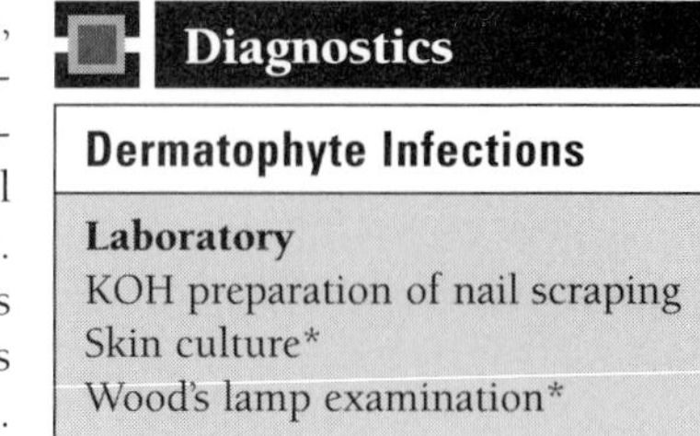

Diagnostics

Dermatophyte Infections
Laboratory
KOH preparation of nail scraping
Skin culture*
Wood's lamp examination*

*If indicated.

Differential Diagnosis

Dermatophyte Infections
Dermatitis
Figurate erythemas
Granulomatous dermatoses
Papulosquamous eruptions
Psoriasis
Skin cancer
Tinea
Urticaria

DIAGNOSTICS

The diagnosis of all fungal infections is based on clinical features and simple diagnostic procedures. The potassium hydroxide (KOH) microscopy preparation is a valuable, cost-effective tool that provides rapid confirmation of many types of fungal infections.[2] The key to a reliable KOH preparation includes properly obtaining an adequate specimen by scraping the active, leading border of a lesion. A #15 blade should be used to collect the scrapings on a glass slide. A 10% to 20% solution of KOH is placed directly on the collected scale, a coverslip is applied, the sample is gently heated, and a microscopic examination is performed. A negative KOH result does not always exclude dermatophyte infections. Fungal culture can be helpful to detect infection in the absence of a positive KOH result. Dermatophytes usually take a few weeks to grow in culture. Examination with long-wave ultraviolet light (Wood's lamp) is helpful for screening for tinea capitis caused by certain fungal species. *Trichophyton tonsurans,* the most common cause of tinea capitis in the United States, however, does not fluoresce.[3]

DIFFERENTIAL DIAGNOSIS

See the Differential Diagnosis box.

MANAGEMENT

The treatment of tinea infections consists of removing the infecting organisms. Acute exudative lesions are treated with wet dressings. Topical antifungal solutions and creams reduce superficial scaling and organisms; keratolytic agents remove thick scales on the hands and feet, which allows these agents to work better. Several topical applications are available to treat tinea corporis: oxiconazole nitrate (Oxistat), clotrimazole (Lotrimin), econazole nitrate (Spectazole), ketoconazole (Nizoral), ciclopirox olamine (Loprox), or topical terbinafine HCl (Lamisil) (Table 59-1). Treatment is usually continued 1 week past clearing to discourage recurrence; however, a recurrence of tinea infections is common depending on the source.

Systemic antifungal medications are used for widespread tinea or infections that involve the nails or scalp. A long-standing treatment for tinea capitis is griseofulvin for 2 to 4 months,

TABLE 59-1 Examples of Cream Topical Treatment

	Recommended Application to Affected Areas	Indicated for		
		Tinea (Pedis, Cruris, Corporis) (T)	Candidiasis (C)	Tinea Versicolor (TV)
Imidazoles				
Clotrimazole (Lotrimin)	Twice daily	X	X	X
Econazole (Spectazole)	Once daily for T and TV; twice daily for C	X	X	X
Miconazole (Monistat-Derm)	Twice daily for T and C; once daily for TV	X	X	X
Ketoconazole (Nizoral)	Once daily	X	X	X
Oxiconazole (Oxistat)	Once or twice daily	X		
Ciclopirox (Loprox)	Twice daily	X	X	X
Nystatin (Mycostatin)	Twice daily		X	
Terbinafine (Lamisil)	Twice daily	X		

GENERAL CONSIDERATIONS

Clinical improvement may be seen fairly soon after initiating treatment. Twice-daily applications, when indicated, should be done morning and evening. In general, all infections should be treated for 2 weeks to reduce the possibility of recurrence. Tinea pedis may require 6 weeks or more of treatment.

or 2 weeks after negative KOH or culture results are obtained. Griseofulvin needs to be taken with high-fat food for complete absorption. Newer antifungal agents such as terbinafine are effective with only 2 to 4 weeks of therapy.[4] The use of oral medications requires careful dosing and monitoring for potential side effects. Treatment should not be considered complete until a follow-up negative fungal culture is obtained.[3]

Onychomycosis may be treated with oral terbinafine (Lamisil) or with oral itraconazole (Sporanox). The oral dose of terbinafine is 250 mg daily—6 weeks for fingernail onychomycosis and 12 weeks for toenail involvement.[5-7] Terbinafine is not recommended if there is a history of renal or liver dysfunction. Monitoring of liver function is required every 6 weeks or if the patient experiences nausea, anorexia, or fatigue during therapy. Neutropenia has been reported as a side effect of terbinafine therapy; therefore a CBC should be performed every 6 weeks or if there are symptoms suggestive of neutropenia.[7]

Oral itraconazole is prescribed at 200 mg twice daily for 1 week of each month—for 3 months for toenail involvement and for 2 months for fingernail involvement.[7] Liver function should be assessed before beginning therapy and after 6 weeks of therapy. Itraconazole affects the cytochrome P450 enzyme system and has several important drug interactions that require individual assessment before initiating therapy.[8]

Topical therapy for onychomycosis is relatively ineffective. Neither the oral nor the topical form of either medication is recommended for pregnant or nursing women. Unfortunately, the recurrence of onychomycosis is high, even with compliant therapy.

COMPLICATIONS

An uncommon complication of tinea capitis is the formation of a kerion, a boggy, exudative area on the scalp. It is a hypersensitivity reaction to the fungus. Kerion formations (tinea capitis) may result in permanent hair loss and scarring.[4] Fungal infections can also be complicated by bacterial superinfections. Other complications are associated with side effects and drug interactions with oral antifungal medications.

INDICATIONS FOR REFERRAL/HOSPITALIZATION

Dermatophyte infections usually respond at least partially to treatment. Severe infections or infections that do not respond to treatment require a referral to a dermatologist. A referral to a dermatologist or dermatology nurse practitioner is recommended for treatment with oral antifungal medications.

PATIENT AND FAMILY EDUCATION

See the Patient and Family Education section under Candidiasis, p. 232.

Candidiasis

PATHOPHYSIOLOGY

Candida albicans, a yeast, can normally be found on mucous membranes, in the gastrointestinal tract, in the vagina, and on the skin (Color Plate 20). *Candida* is usually an opportunistic organism. It is able to behave as a pathogen usually only in the presence of immune modulation or in intertriginous areas. Predisposing factors to *Candida* infection include pregnancy; the use of birth control pills, antibiotics, or corticosteroids; malnutrition; diabetes and other endocrine diseases; or immunosuppressed conditions. A local environment that is warm, moist, macerated, and/or occluded favors the growth of this organism.

CLINICAL PRESENTATION AND PHYSICAL EXAMINATION

The clinical appearance of candidiasis depends on its location. Candidiasis of the mucous membranes is called "thrush." Thrush appears as white or gray membranous plaques that are adherent to the buccal. If the plaques are scraped away, the base is macerated and brightly erythematous. The lesions can extend down the esophagus and to the lips and corners of the mouth. Perleche, or angular cheilitis, is a fissuring and maceration of the corners of the mouth. The common causes of perleche include candidal infection, bacterial infection, and irritant dermatitis.

Common sites of skin infection with *Candida* are axillary, gluteal, perianal, and interdigital folds (see Color Plate 20). These intertriginous candidiasis lesions are usually pink or red moist patches bordered by a thin collarette of scale. They are sometimes surrounded by characteristic "satellite" pustules. Vaginal thrush causes intense itching and often a "cheesy" vaginal discharge. Candidal paronychia, or nail fold infection, is an inflammation of the nail fold. There is rounding and lifting of the nail fold, sometimes with a pus discharge. The nail can overtimes become thickened and discolored. Untreated severe candidiasis in any location has the potential to cause fungal septicemia in an immunocompromised patient.

DIAGNOSTICS

The diagnosis of candidiasis is based on clinical appearance, microscopic evaluation with a KOH preparation to look for budding yeast with or without hyphae, and/or a fungal culture. *C. albicans* grows readily on fungal media within 48 to 72 hours.

DIFFERENTIAL DIAGNOSIS

The differential diagnosis is dependent on the affected area.

MANAGEMENT

The treatment of candidiasis is aimed at eliminating both the predisposing factors and the organism. A variety of agents—powders, vaginal douches, oral suspensions, creams, and tablets—are commonly used for the treatment of candidal infections (see Table 59-1). Superficial infections should usually be treated with topical therapy. If the infection is so widespread that the use of topical agents is impractical or too expensive, oral fluconazole (Diflucan) or oral ketoconazole (Nizoral) is appropriate.

COMPLICATIONS

The most serious complication of candidiasis is fungal septicemia, which may be seen in immunocompromised, hospitalized patients. Candidal esophagitis is a potential complication of antibiotic therapy or may be noted in patients who are severely immunocompromised, particularly patients with AIDS.

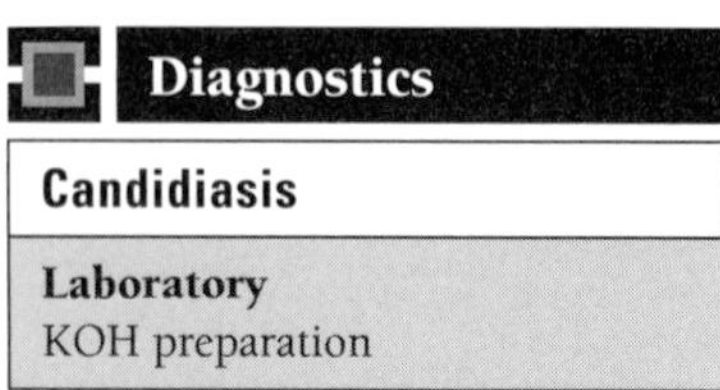

Diagnostics

Candidiasis
Laboratory KOH preparation

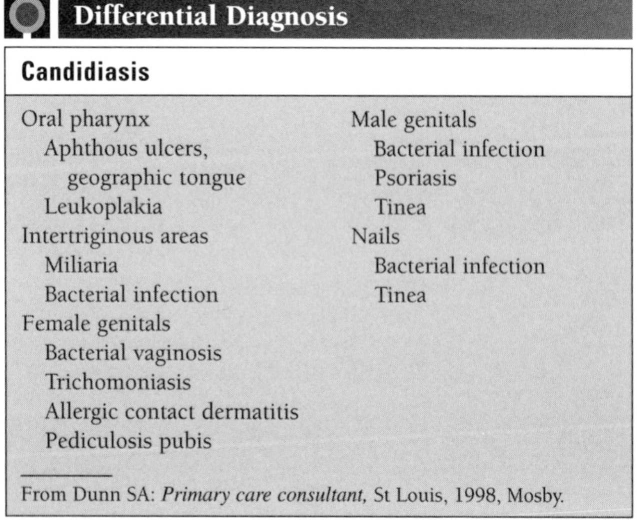

Differential Diagnosis

Candidiasis	
Oral pharynx	Male genitals
Aphthous ulcers, geographic tongue	Bacterial infection
Leukoplakia	Psoriasis
Intertriginous areas	Tinea
Miliaria	Nails
Bacterial infection	Bacterial infection
Female genitals	Tinea
Bacterial vaginosis	
Trichomoniasis	
Allergic contact dermatitis	
Pediculosis pubis	

From Dunn SA: *Primary care consultant,* St Louis, 1998, Mosby.

INDICATIONS FOR REFERRAL/HOSPITALIZATION

Treatment is usually effective and a referral is not indicated. The differential diagnosis of *Candida* infection is large, however. Therefore infections recalcitrant to treatment require a physician or dermatology referral to look for other etiologies for the eruption. Patients with yeast septicemia or other systemic manifestations or infection also require a physician consultation.

PATIENT AND FAMILY EDUCATION

Methods for reducing environmental factors that encourage heat, moisture, maceration, and trauma should be emphasized: drying thoroughly after bathing (especially in the axillae and toe webs and between and under the breasts), wearing absorbent materials such as cotton underwear and socks, changing socks frequently and avoiding constrictive clothing, not wearing the same shoes each day, and wearing sandals in warm weather.

During active infections or in the hope of preventing recurrence, a simple talc powder or antifungal powder (tolnaftate [Zeasorb AF]) should be applied to intertriginous or interdigital areas twice daily. With the reintroduction of many powders that contain cornstarch, it is extremely important to inform patients who are prone to fungal infections to avoid cornstarch-containing products because this substance encourages fungus growth.

Patients using oral steroid inhalers should understand the importance of rinsing the oral cavity after using these inhalers. Although there is no clearly documented benefit, some clinicians recommend that their patients eat yogurt daily while on antibiotic therapy to help prevent vaginal or oral yeast infections.

Tinea Versicolor

DEFINITION/EPIDEMIOLOGY

Tinea versicolor is a chronic, asymptomatic, and superficial fungal infection. This skin manifestation is common in young adults.

PATHOPHYSIOLOGY

The causative organism of tinea versicolor is *Malassezia furfur. Pityrosporum orbiculare* is the yeast form of the organism. The fungus is found on normal skin, and the infection is due to a change in the host's resistance to this organism. Tinea versicolor causes lesions in some individuals during periods of high heat and humidity. Thus the condition is more prevalent during the summer and in hot, humid regions. Exposure to sunlight often initiates an episode.

CLINICAL PRESENTATION AND PHYSICAL EXAMINATION

Lesions vary in color and are either white or light pink in the hypopigmented version, or tan or brown in the hyperpigmented version. They are slightly scaly and are round or oval coalescing papules and plaques. The usual sites for these lesions are the sternal region; the sides of the chest, abdomen, or back; the pubis; and the intertriginous areas. Hypopigmented lesions are more noticeable in darkly pigmented skin. Patients should be reassured that repigmentation will occur after treatment and with exposure to natural sunlight. However, this process can take several months.

DIAGNOSTICS

Diagnosis is by KOH examination, which reveals numerous short, straight hyphae and clusters of round, budding yeast; this configuration is commonly referred to as "spaghetti and meatballs." A KOH examination may be falsely negative if the patient has just showered.

DIFFERENTIAL DIAGNOSIS

Vitiligo, pityriasis alba, pityriasis rosea, and small plaque parapsoriasis should be considered in the differential diagnosis. Lesions may resemble seborrheic dermatitis, but tinea versicolor most commonly affects the trunk, neck, and upper extremities, whereas seborrheic dermatitis affects hairy body areas. Although uncommon, secondary syphilis should be considered in the differential diagnosis.

MANAGEMENT

Common antifungal creams, such as the imidazoles, are useful in treating tinea versicolor (see Table 59-1). Medication is applied to the entire torso during active infections to eliminate inapparent lesions. Oral antifungal agents can also be used. Topical shampoos and/or suspensions containing selenium sulfide or pyrithione zinc are also very effective in treatment or prophylaxis. Shampoos are applied to affected areas, allowed to dry, and rinsed away after remaining in place approximately 10 minutes. This treatment is repeated for 7 to 14 consecutive days during active infections, followed by periodic use of these shampoos or soaps if the patient is prone to frequent infections. Specific instructions should be reviewed with every product or drug.

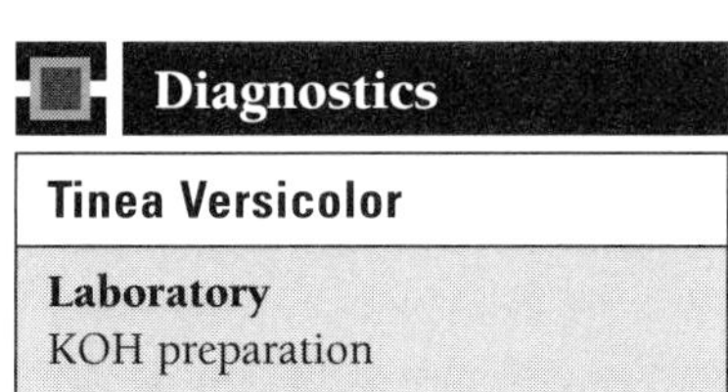

Diagnostics

Tinea Versicolor

Laboratory
KOH preparation

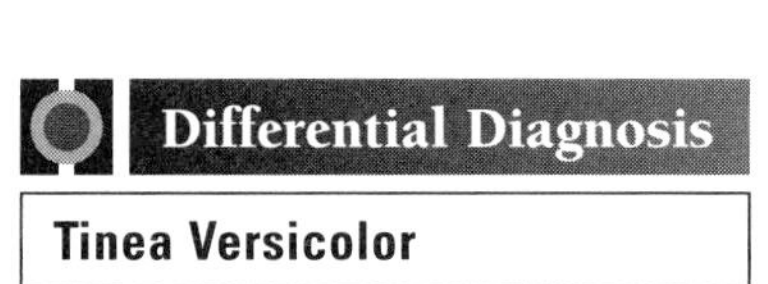

Differential Diagnosis

Tinea Versicolor

Pityriasis alba
Pityriasis rosea
Vitiligo
Seborrheic dermatitis
Secondary syphilis

COMPLICATIONS

Complications are unusual. Some patients may develop *Pityrosporum folliculitis,* although this disorder usually resolves with topical therapy.

INDICATIONS FOR REFERRAL/HOSPITALIZATION

A referral is not usually necessary. Rashes recalcitrant to treatment require a dermatology referral to reconsider the diagnosis.

PATIENT AND FAMILY EDUCATION

Patients should understand that tinea versicolor commonly recurs but is not a serious disorder. The regular use of any selenium sulfide shampoo for 10 minutes each day for a week followed by consistent weekly treatments will often prevent recurrences.

REFERENCES

1. Nicol NH, Huether SE: Alteration on the integument in children. In McCance J, Huether SE, editors: *Pathophysiology: the biologic basics for disease in adults and children,* ed 3, St Louis, 1998, Mosby.
2. Nicol NH, Black JM: Assessment of clients with integumentary disorders. In Black JM, Matassarin-Jacobs E, editors: *Medical-surgical nursing: clinical management for continuity of care,* ed 5, Philadelphia, 1997, WB Saunders.
3. Bradley BJ and others: Tinea capitis today: what nurses need to know about identifying and managing fungal infections of the scalp in the school setting, *J Sch Nurs* (suppl):1-16, 1996.
4. Odom RB, James WD, Berger TG: *Andrews' diseases of the skin: clinical terminology,* ed 9, Philadelphia, 2000, WB Saunders.
5. Nicol NH, Black JM: Nursing care of clients with integumentary disorders. In Black JM, Matassarin-Jacobs E, editors: *Medical-surgical nursing: clinical management for continuity of care,* ed 5, Philadelphia, 1997, WB Saunders.
6. Elewski B, Weil M: Dermatophytes and superficial fungi. In Sams WM, Lynch P, editors: *Principles and practices of dermatologic therapy,* ed 2, New York, 1996, Churchill Livingstone.
7. *Physicians Desk Reference,* Montvale, NJ, 1998, Medical Economics.
8. Murphy JL: *Nurse practitioner's prescribing reference,* New York, 1998, Prescribing Reference.

CHAPTER 60

Herpes Zoster (Shingles)

Eileen M. Deignan

DEFINITION/EPIDEMIOLOGY

Herpes zoster (shingles) is caused by the varicella zoster virus. This is the same virus that causes chickenpox. After primary varicella infection (chickenpox) or vaccination, the virus lies dormant in the sensory root ganglion cells. The zoster eruption results from reactivation of the latent varicella infection in the dorsal root or cranial nerve ganglion cells.[1] The cause of reactivation is not known, but zoster is more common in older adults and immunosuppressed persons. Lesions appear over several days and last up to 7 weeks. The eruption can be quite painful and can result in significant residual pain, which is called *postherpetic neuralgia.*

Although zoster is self-limiting and common in adults, there are circumstances in which consultation is recommended.

Ophthalmologic consultation is indicated for ocular involvement.
Physician consultation is recommended for lesions that cross dermatomes or for cheek or nose involvement.

PATHOPHYSIOLOGY

After initial varicella infection, the virus is dormant in the dorsal root ganglia. The causes of reactivation are not clear but may result from stress, trauma, reexposure to varicella, radiation therapy, or immunosuppressive therapy. Once reactivated, the virus replicates and travels down the sensory nerve into the skin.[2]

CLINICAL PRESENTATION AND PHYSICAL EXAMINATION

Zoster classically presents as a unilateral eruption within a dermatome. It is common to have some lesions in the dermatome above and below the one primarily affected. The eruption is often preceded by pain in the affected dermatome. Because there is no accompanying eruption, the pain is sometimes mistaken for angina pectoris, sciatica, or early glaucoma. The eruption initially consists of erythematous papules and then, over the course of hours, develops into vesicles (Color Plate 21). New lesions may continue to develop over the course of several days. Healing time varies, ranging from 1 to 7 weeks. Low-grade fever and lymphadenopathy may be present. The most common areas of involvement are the thoracic, cranial (especially the trigeminal nerve), and lumbar nerves.[3]

DIAGNOSTICS

Diagnosis is based on the clinical presentation of an eruption in a dermatomal distribution. Patients may develop several lesions outside of the primarily affected dermatome. Disseminated herpes zoster is a generalized eruption of lesions along with the typical segmental distribution.

A Tzanck test is a rapid way to confirm the diagnosis of zoster in the provider's office. Direct fluorescent antibody test is another rapid test that is available at some hospitals. Both tests are preferred over a viral culture because they are more rapid and often more sensitive.

DIFFERENTIAL DIAGNOSIS

The pain associated with zoster can precede the eruption by 4 or 5 days. Depending on the distribution, the pain may mimic angina, renal colic, or pleuritic pain. Once the eruption is present, the cause of the pain is more obvious. Varicella is seldom confused with zoster because of the distribution of lesions. Herpes simplex infection can sometimes mimic zoster. A direct fluorescence antibody test or viral culture will differentiate the two. Coxsackievirus (hand-foot-and-mouth disease) is generally limited to the acral areas.

MANAGEMENT

The treatment of uncomplicated herpes zoster is symptomatic treatment of lesions and prevention of secondary infection. Analgesic agents may be administered if necessary. Topical moist compresses and agents, such as calamine or ethyl chloride spray, are soothing and will help dry vesicles. Antiviral therapy is an important part of zoster therapy. When started within the first few days of the eruption, it reduces zoster-associated pain. Antiviral treatment also is associated with faster healing of lesions. Acyclovir is effective in both localized and disseminated herpes zoster. If treatment with acyclovir is started within 48 hours of onset, it can shorten the course and may reduce postherpetic neuralgia.

Acyclovir is dosed at 800 mg five times daily for 7 to 10 days. The newer antiviral agents valacyclovir and famciclovir are at least as affective as acyclovir, and perhaps more so because they achieve higher blood levels of medication. They are more expensive, however. In addition, they should be used with caution in patients with renal impairment. The use of antihistamines is helpful to reduce pruritus.[1,2]

Diagnostics

Herpes Zoster
Laboratory
Tzanck test (of lesion discharge)*
Antibody titer*
Direct fluorescent antibody test

*If indicated.

COMPLICATIONS

Postherpetic neuralgia is the most common complication of zoster. Older adults tend to have more persistent pain after the zoster lesions have healed.[4] Postherpetic neuralgia is often difficult to control; some patients benefit from ibuprofen therapy. Other therapies include topical lidocaine preparations and topical capsaicin.

There is some evidence that older adults

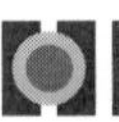

Differential Diagnosis

Herpes Zoster
Varicella
Hand-foot-and-mouth disease
Rickettsialpox
Dermatitis herpetiformis

who are at risk for significant acute zoster-associated pain may benefit from concurrent antiviral and systemic corticosteroid treatment during the acute infection.

Herpes zoster on the tip of the nose, around the eyes, and on the forehead requires immediate ophthalmologic examination. These findings signal possible involvement of the branch of the trigenimal nerve that innervates the cornea, which may cause ulceration on the cornea and result in permanent damage. Motor paralysis and facial palsy (Ramsay Hunt syndrome) may follow herpes zoster. Immunosuppressed individuals may develop dissemination, pneumonia, hepatitis, meningoencephalitis, and purpura fulminans.[1,2,5]

INDICATIONS FOR REFERRAL/HOSPITALIZATION

In ophthalmic zoster, ocular complications occur in approximately 50% of cases. Immediate referral to an ophthalmologist is indicated. Patients with generalized disseminated zoster should be evaluated for malignancy, immunodeficiency, or AIDS.[2] Hospitalization is often necessary in patients with disseminated herpes zoster.

PATIENT AND FAMILY EDUCATION

Lesions of herpes zoster may contain varicella zoster virus, enabling transmission to susceptible individuals. Herpes zoster itself is not transmissible; therefore although care should be taken to avoid exposure to susceptible or immunosuppressed contacts, patients with herpes zoster may continue to work and attend school.

Care should be taken to educate patients should be about the time course of zoster lesions and associated pain. They should also be given instructions about topical lesion care and pain relief.

REFERENCES

1. Arndt K: *Manual of dermatologic therapeutics*, ed 5, Boston, 1995, Little, Brown.
2. Hurwitz S: *Clinical pediatric dermatology*, ed 2, Philadelphia, 1993, WB Saunders.
3. Gilden DH and others: Neurologic complications of the reactivation of varicella-zoster virus, *N Engl J Med* 342:635, 2000.
4. Sershewitz RA: *Ambulatory pediatric care*, ed 2, Philadelphia, 1993, JB Lippincott.
5. Odom RB, James WD, Berger TG: *Andrew's diseases of the skin*, ed 9, Philadelphia, 2000, WB Saunders.

CHAPTER 61

Hidradenitis Suppurativa (Acne Inversa)

Margaret McAllister

DEFINITION/EPIDEMIOLOGY

Hidradenitis suppurativa, now also referred to as acne inversa, has long been considered a disease of the apocrine glands. Recent histopathologic research indicates that the primary lesion is infundibulofolliculitis with secondary infection of apocrine glands.[1,2] The disease is characterized by abscesses, draining sinus tracts, and comedomes. The prevalence of hidradenitis is greater in females, with genitofemoral lesions being most common; axillary lesions are found equally in males and females, and anogenital lesions are found more commonly in males.[3-5] All ethnic groups are affected, with African American populations having a more severe form of the disease.[4] A hereditary predisposition has been noted in females, with a mother-daughter transmission being most common,[4] and a familial autosomal dominant tendency exists.[1]

PATHOPHYSIOLOGY

The exact cause of hidradenitis is not known and is controversial. Theories of causation include keratin plugging of the apocrine ducts or a primary failure of the apocrine glands to drain effectively. An association with immunosuppression is cited in the literature.[2,6] With keratin plugging, the apocrine duct and hair follicle are occluded by keratin, which causes increased ductal pressure and inflammation. Bacteria cause the ducts to rupture and, with extension of infection, lead to cysts, sinus tracks, and fistula formation. Acne inversa is proposed as a more appropriate name for this disease.[2] In a study of 41 patients with active hidradenitis suppurativa, bacteria isolated in 49% (20 out of 41) of abscess lesions included *Staphylococcus aureus, Streptococcus milleri, Staphylococcus epidermidis,* and *Staphylococcus hominis.*[7] Other organisms implicated include *Escherichia coli, Proteus mirabilis, Pseudomonas aeruginosa,* and gram-negative organisms.[3,6]

CLINICAL PRESENTATION

The hallmarks of hidradenitis suppurativa are single or multiple areas of swelling, pain, and erythema accompanied by acute abscess formation. The active phase of the disease is proceeded by the appearance of double or triple black comedones on the affected skin surface. The condition often progresses to a chronic state of pain, sepsis, sinus tract and fistula formation, purulent discharge, and keloids. Disfiguring scar formation marks long-standing hidradenitis. Patients usually give a history of multiple episodes of repeat abscesses that have been drained and treated with antibiotic medications over a period of years. Unlike acne, the disease is unrelenting and often progressive, leaving hypertrophic scars that form a basketweave configuration accented by marked erythema beneath the breast and in the axilla, suprapubic, groin, and anogenital regions. Sinus tracks form under the skin in which connecting, inflamed, and plugged glands drain into each other and trap bacteria. Patients are concerned about the cause of the problem and may fear they have a malignant disease. Predisposing factors include obesity, a history of acne, and obstruction of the apocrine ducts.[4]

PHYSICAL EXAMINATION

The lesions are palpated to determine their readiness for incision and drainage. The axilla, groin, perianal region, buttocks, chest, inframammary area, and back are examined to determine the involvement and extent of the disease.

DIAGNOSTICS

The initial diagnosis is based on clinical observation. Lesions that are actively discharging are cultured, and sensitivity tests are performed. A skin biopsy is performed for patients with stubborn cases or suspicious lesions. Laboratory tests may be needed to exclude other, more serious underlying diseases.

DIFFERENTIAL DIAGNOSIS

The differential diagnosis for hidradenitis suppurativa includes bacterial folliculitis, furunculosis, scrofuloderma, granuloma inguinale, lymphogranuloma venereum, and squamous cell carcinoma.[8-10]

MANAGEMENT

There are a variety of treatment measures, including topical, oral, and surgical interventions.

Fluctuant abscesses in which the skin has become thin and the underlying mass is soft can be surgically incised and drained in the primary care provider's office. Local anesthesia with 1% to 2% lidocaine with or without epinephrine is provided through a 30-gauge needle and a 1- to 3-ml syringe. The sting of lidocaine can be buffered by preparing a mixture of 1 ml of $NaHCO_3$ with 9 ml of lidocaine. A pointed, lance-shaped #11 surgical blade is recommended for incision. The blade is inserted parallel to the skin lines, cutting across the thin area of skin and creating an opening through which purulent material can drain. Pressure is applied to the surrounding tissue to facilitate drainage. A curette drawn back and forth through the abscess will loosen adhesions and aid in the removal of necrotic material. A semiocclusive sterile dressing with a thin film of topical bacitracin should then be applied. Care must be taken to cleanse the area daily with soap and water; the dressing is reapplied for 3 to 5 days.

Smaller nodules can be injected with triamcinolone acetonide 3 to 5 mg/ml diluted with lidocaine and followed by a course of oral antibiotics. Larger cysts can be injected with triamcinolone 3 to 5 mg/ml directly into the wall of the lesion and later incised. Low-grade inflammation is responsive to oral antibiotics, but long-term treatment is necessary before clinical remission is evident. Erythromycin 250 to 500 mg four times daily, tetracycline 250 to 500 mg four times daily, or minocycline 100 mg twice daily should be considered. Erythromycin 500 mg four times daily may be effective in a large adult during periods of active inflammation.[6] Topical isotretinoin cream 0.05% may be efficacious in relieving keratin plugging of the apocrine glands.[6] Isotretinoin 1 mg/kg daily for 20 weeks may be tried under co-management with a physician in the early stages of the disease or as an adjunct to surgical intervention.[4,6] Because of the teratogenic effects of this medication, all women must be screened for pregnancy before taking isotretinoin and protected against pregnancy while taking the medication. For severe pain and inflammation, a tapering dose of 70 mg of prednisone over a 14-day period is prescribed.

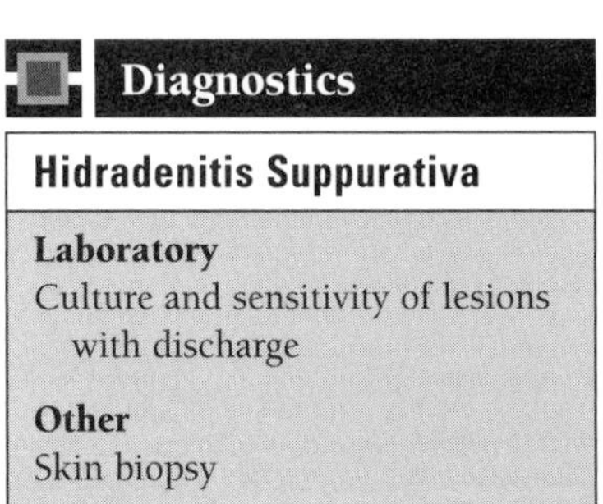

Diagnostics

Hidradenitis Suppurativa

Laboratory
Culture and sensitivity of lesions with discharge

Other
Skin biopsy

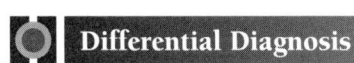

Differential Diagnosis

Hidradenitis Suppurativa

Bacterial folliculitis
Bacterial furunculosis
Scrofuloderma
Granuloma inguinale
Lymphogranuloma venereum
Squamous cell carcinoma

Co-Management with Specialists

A referral to a dermatologist is recommended for patients with hidradenitis that is recalcitrant to traditional oral therapy or for patients with recurrent lesions after incision and drainage. Patients treated with oral isotretinoin 1 mg/kg daily for 20 weeks may be co-managed with the nurse practitioner or physician assistant for the purposes of determining treatment response and monitoring for side effects.

LIFE SPAN CONSIDERATIONS

The onset of hidradenitis suppurativa is usually between the second and fifth decades, with onset as early as puberty in some individuals.[8] Many cases of hidradenitis disappear after patients reach 35 years of age.

COMPLICATIONS

The primary care provider should be aware of the impact of body image changes on patients with this disease, especially young adolescents. As with any chronic illness, an assessment for clinical depression and threats to self-esteem should be included as part of the ongoing care. Complications other than chronicity are rare, but fistulas from the groin area to the urethra and bladder have been reported.[4] Cases of reactive arthritis have been identified in the literature.[11] Vigilant follow-up is necessary to exclude patients who fail to respond to treatment. Cases of anogenital squamous cell carcinoma have been diagnosed in patients with long-term hidradenitis.[9,10] Other complications are related to the treatment regimen. Patients taking large doses of erythromycin may experience damage to their auditory nerve and deafness.

INDICATIONS FOR REFERRAL/HOSPITALIZATION

Surgical excision is recommended for patients with chronic, recurrent hidradenitis suppurativa that involves the sinus tracts and fibrotic scarring. Complete excision of the involved glands and skin grafting may be necessary. Carbon dioxide laser treatments can be performed by a qualified dermatologist skilled in this technique. If surgery requires extensive surgical resection and reconstruction of the female genitalia, the services of a gynecologic oncologist may be required.[5]

PATIENT AND FAMILY EDUCATION

Patient education should include careful explanation that a clear cause for the disease is not known. A complete explanation of the hypothetical causes of the disease process should be provided. The average length of time for abscesses to heal is 6.9 days. Patients should be assured that neither antiperspirants nor shaving nor other underarm deodorants or depilatories are implicated as a cause. Topical isotretinoin may cause skin irritation, and caution should be exercised to avoid excessive use. Sun sensitivity with the use of isotretinoin should be stressed, and appropriate protective clothing should be worn while in the sun. Patients should be educated on the side effects of the prescribed antibiotics, including photosensitivity. Patients taking erythromycin must be advised to avoid the concurrent ingestion of terfenadine, astemizole, and ketoconazole.

REFERENCES

1. Jansen I, Altmeyer P, Piewig GJ: Acne inversa (alias hidradenitis suppurativa), *Eur Acad Dermatol Venereol* 5:532, 2001.
2. Boer J, Weltevreden EF: Hidradenitis suppurativa or acne inversa: a clinicopathological study of early lesions, *Br J Dermatol* 135:721, 1996.
3. Jemec GB, Heidenheim M, Nielsen NH: Prevalence of hidradenitis suppurativa in Denmark, *Ugeskr Laeger* 160:847, 1998.
4. Fitzpatrick TB and others: *Color atlas and synopsis of clinical dermatology,* ed 4, New York, 2000, McGraw-Hill.
5. Goldberg JM, Buchler DA, Dibbell DG: Advanced hidradenitis suppurativa presenting with bilateral vulvar masses, *Gynecol Oncol* 60: 494, 1996.
6. Habif TP: *Clinical dermatology,* ed 3, St Louis, 1996, Mosby.
7. Jemec GB and others: The bacteriology of hidradenitis suppurativa, *Dermatology* 193:203, 1996.
8. Barker R, Burton JR, Zieve PD: *Ambulatory care medicine,* ed 5, Baltimore, 1998, Williams & Wilkins.
9. Li M, Hunt MJ, Commens CA: Hidradenitis suppurativa, Dowling Degos disease and perianal squamous cell carcinoma, *Australas J Dermatol* 38:209, 1997.
10. Gur E and others: Squamous cell carcinoma in perineal inflammatory disease, *Ann Plast Surg* 38:653, 1997.
11. Bhalla R, Sequeira W: Arthritis associated with hidradenitis suppurativa, *Ann Rheum Dis* 53:64, 1994.

CHAPTER 62

Hyperhidrosis

Margaret McAllister

DEFINITION/EPIDEMIOLOGY

Hyperhidrosis is a condition of excessive sweating marked by sweaty palms, excessive axillary sweating, and sweaty feet. Most cases are idiopathic or primary in nature and only rarely indicate underlying secondary pathology because the sweating in hyperhidrosis is localized to defined body areas.[1-3]

PATHOPHYSIOLOGY

Perspiration is one of the body's mechanisms for thermal regulation, as well as fluid and electrolyte balance. The center for body temperature regulation is located in the hypothalamus. Cooling perspiration is under hypothalamic control, whereas emotional perspiration is under cerebral control.

Hyperhidrosis is primarily a dysfunction or hyperfunction of eccrine sweat glands. These eccrine glands are commonly found throughout the body, with the largest concentration located in the palms of the hands, soles of the feet, and axillae.[4] Secretions from these eccrine glands function to cool the body through sweat evaporation from the skin. The eccrine glands are innervated by the sympathetic nervous system with regulation by acetylcholine, a cholinergic neurotransmitter, rather than norepinephrine.[5] With axillary hyperhidrosis there is usually overactivity of the thoracic sympathetic ganglion. In addition, the axillary apocrine sweat glands may be involved with axillary hyperhidrosis. Apocrine glands are found primarily in the axillary and anogenital areas, are activated at puberty, and are responsive to adrenergic sympathetic stimulation caused by emotional stressors.[4]

CLINICAL PRESENTATION

The presentation of primary hyperhidrosis is excessive sweating unrelated to ambient heat or humidity. Areas most commonly affected include the palms, soles, and axillae, but the condition may involve any body surface or take on a unilateral distribution. Concern over the social consequences of this disorder (and its resulting body odor) and embarrassment may create a barrier to intimate relationships or affect the patient's choice of occupation. When the soles of the feet are involved, widespread fungal infections of the skin and nails are accompanied by foot odor. More generalized body sweating is associated with an underlying condition, whereas localized sweating confined to the palms, soles, and axillae is more often a response to anxiety or heat or is idiopathic. Episodic sweating may be associated with hypoglycemia. A history of medications, including oral hypoglycemic agents and selective serotonin reuptake inhibitors (SSRIs), and alcohol intake is an important consideration.

PHYSICAL EXAMINATION

Based on the history and presenting complaint, attempts should be made to locate evidence of any underlying disease process. A complete history and physical assessment is done, searching for signs and symptoms of systemic disorders such as infections, malignancies, acromegaly, hyperthyroidism, diabetes, collagen vascular disease, pheochromocytoma, and sarcoidosis.

In assessing the patient with generalized sweating, the examiner should look for miliaria rubia, an abnormal blocking of the sweat ducts. In this condition, sweat is trapped in the stratum corneum, creating tiny, pinpoint, clear papules that with pressure rupture the sweat ducts, creating an erythematous macular papular rash. Other associated presentations include dyshidrotic eczema; this is a simple eczema promoted by the retention of sweat in the stratum corneum.

DIAGNOSTICS

Thyroid and fasting blood sugar studies are indicated to exclude thyroid disease and diabetes. If night sweats are present, a purified protein derivative (PPD) test is necessary to exclude tuberculosis. For perimenopausal women with hyperhidrosis, tests for follicle-stimulating hormone (FSH) and luteinizing hormone (LH) are recommended to document menopause and to provide patient reassurance. SSRIs may provoke night sweats. A different SSRI should be considered before changing drug classes.

DIFFERENTIAL DIAGNOSIS

The most common cause of excessive perspiration is a sympathetic mediated response to stress. A careful history and examination will indicate the necessity to exclude hyperthyroidism with an ultrasensitive test for thyroid-stimulating hormone (TSH) and thyroxin (T_4).

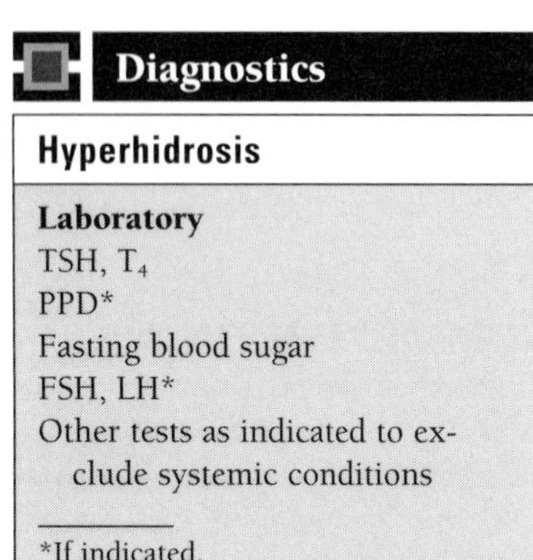

Diagnostics

Hyperhidrosis

Laboratory
TSH, T_4
PPD*
Fasting blood sugar
FSH, LH*
Other tests as indicated to exclude systemic conditions

*If indicated.

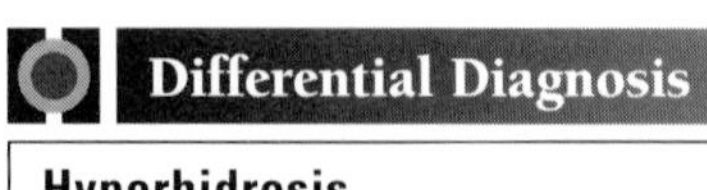

Differential Diagnosis

Hyperhidrosis

Hyperthyroidism
Infection
Malignancy
Tuberculosis
Diabetes mellitus
Pheochromocytoma
Alcoholism
Central nervous system diseases
Autonomic peripheral neuropathy
Other hormonal imbalances

A patient symptom diary of provoking factors, responses to foods, body temperature, and amount and location of perspiration provides a helpful adjunct in determining the cause of sweating. If infection or malignancy is suspected, a thorough evaluation is mandated. A tuberculin skin test should be performed for those with complaints of night sweats. A fasting blood sugar study is performed to exclude diabetes mellitus. In women with variations in the length and amount of menses, a search for accompanying symptoms of vasomotor hot flashes and objective evidence of ovarian failure is necessary. Symptoms of sweating and flushing accompanied by marked hypertension require an evaluation for pheochromocytoma. Evidence of central nervous system disease or autonomic peripheral neuropathy warrants referral to a neurologist. Other causes of generalized sweating include infections, malignancies, hormonal imbalances, alcoholism, and some medications.[1]

MANAGEMENT

Topical applications of 20% alcoholic solution of aluminum chloride hexahydrate (Drysol) can be effective in decreasing excessive perspiration on the hands, soles of the feet, and axillae. These treatments provide for chemodenervation of the eccrine sweat glands.[6] A less potent solution of 6.25% aluminum chloride (Xerac) can be prescribed for patients who have more sensitive skin. The perspiring area is coated lightly with the solution and allowed to dry. An occlusive wrap is then applied (or vinyl gloves can be worn on the hands), and the solution is left on for 8 hours, followed by a complete soap-and-water wash of the affected areas. Applications are repeated every 2 to 3 days as tolerated. With satisfactory dryness, maintenance requires a once-weekly application.[2,3]

Liposuction of the axillary sweat glands has been effective,[7,8] as has surgical excision of axillary tissue.[9] Persistent primary palmar hyperhydrosis has shown a positive response to thoracic endoscopic surgery. Bilateral interruption of the upper dorsal sympathetic chain of D2 and D3 can provide a cure for primary hyperhydrosis.[10]

Co-Management with Specialists

Consultation with a dermatologist may be useful for patients who are refractory to topical treatments. A number of other remedies may be attempted by the dermatologist, including iontophoresis, in which an electrical current may be used to obstruct the sweat ducts.[3,11,12] Botulinum toxin has been found to be an effective modality for hyperhidrosis affecting the axillae and palms and for gustatory sweating.[13] Liposuction has shown to be effective for axillary hyperhydrosis.[7,8] Consideration of these other and treatments warrants consultation with an appropriate specialist. Sweating associated with anxiety or panic attacks warrants co-management with a mental health specialist or neuropsychiatrist.

COMPLICATIONS

Patients with hyperhidrosis may experience difficulty functioning in social or occupational situations as a result of this disorder. The latter may significantly affect a patient's quality of life. Other complications are rare, although patients with sensitive skin may develop reactions to the topical solutions prescribed for treatment. In most instances, decreasing the concentration of the solution will decrease skin irritation. Patients who undergo sympathectomy may experience compensatory sweating.

INDICATIONS FOR REFERRAL/HOSPITALIZATION

Evidence of an underlying medical condition leading to secondary hyperhidrosis, such as pheochromocytoma, warrants referral. Primary hyperhidrosis refractory to topical treatments is referred for evaluation to a surgeon experienced in thoracoscopic sympathicolysis,[10] liposuction,[7,8] or axillary dissection.[9] Patients with excessive perspiration associated with anxiety or panic disorders can benefit from a program of mental health counseling.

PATIENT AND FAMILY EDUCATION

Education is critical to assist patients with coping and understanding this socially stigmatizing condition. A complete explanation of the etiology of primary hyperhidrosis and an explanation regarding sympathetic overactivity are provided. Patients need assurance that a search for an underlying pathologic reason for the disorder has been conducted. Results of laboratory tests must be provided. Support in the form of education for family members and significant others is an important aspect of comprehensive care. Good personal hygiene is encouraged with axillary sweating. Both open-toe and canvas shoes with cotton socks promote evaporation of foot perspiration while decreasing foot odor and preventing fungal infections of the feet. Occupational environments should be well ventilated and include air conditioning.

REFERENCES

1. Rzany B, Spinner DM: Interventions for localised sweating, *The Cochrane database of systemic reviews.* Retrieved March 4, 2002, from the World Wide Web: http://gateway1.ovid.com/ovidweb.cgi.
2. Rakel RE: *Textbook of family practice,* ed 5, Philadelphia, 1997, WB Saunders.
3. Rassner G: *Atlas of dermatology,* ed 3, Philadelphia, 1994, Lea & Febiger.
4. Baker DJ, Heymann WR: Eccrine glands and apocrine glands, *Am Acad Dermatol.* Retrieved March 4, 2002, from the World Wide Web: http://www.aad.org/education/eccrine.htm.
5. Collin J, Whatling P: Treating hyperhidrosis: surgery and botulinum toxin are treatments of choice in severe cases, *Br Med J* 320: 1221, 2000.
6. Benohanian A and others: Localized hyperhidrosis treated with aluminum chloride in a salicylic acid gel base, *Int J Dermatol* 37: 701, 1998.
7. Christ JE: The application of suction assisted lipectomy for the problem of axillary hyperhidrosis, *Surg Gynecol Obstet* 169:457, 1989.
8. Payne CMER: Liposuction for axillary hyperhidrosis, *Clin Exp Dermatol* 23:9, 1998.
9. Atkins JL, Butler PEM: Treating hyperhidrosis, *Br Med J* 321:702, 2000.
10. Drott C, Claes G: Hyperhidrosis treated by thoracoscopic sympathecotomy, *Cardiovasc Surg* 4:788, 1996.
11. Shen JL, Lin GS, Li WM: A new strategy of iontophoresis for hyperhidrosis, *J Am Acad Dermatol* 22:239, 1990.
12. Murphy R, Harrington CI: Iontophoresis should be tried before other treatments, *Br Med J* 321:702, 2000.
13. Odderson IR: Hyperhidrosis treated by botulinum A exotoxin, *Dermatol Surg* 24:1237, 1998.

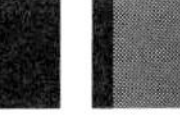

CHAPTER 63

Intertrigo

Nancy W. Knee

DEFINITION/EPIDEMIOLOGY

Intertrigo is a superficial mycotic infection that occurs between juxtaposed moist skin surfaces. Common sites include the inframammary folds, inner thighs, and axillary and perianal areas. Sweat retention, moisture, warmth, alterations in systemic immunity, systemic antibiotic therapy, and overgrowth of resident microorganisms are related factors.

Patients are susceptible to intertrigo at any age. Infants with thrush or a diaper rash, women with vulvovaginitis, men with balanitis, individuals infected with HIV, and prolonged steroid users are particularly susceptible.[1] Other predisposing conditions and factors include psoriasis, eczema, diabetes, obesity, pregnancy, oral contraceptive use, and chemotherapy.[2]

PATHOPHYSIOLOGY

Intertrigo is caused by *Candida albicans.* This yeastlike fungus is normally found in the mouth, vagina, and gastrointestinal tract. Skin breakdown results from the release of toxins on the integumentary surface that subsequently cause irritation and result in maceration of cutaneous tissue.[3]

CLINICAL PRESENTATION AND PHYSICAL EXAMINATION

Intertrigo presents as red, moist, and glistening plaques/patches or moist, red papules and pustules. The borders are well defined, and the patches erode the epidermis, resulting in scaling.

DIAGNOSTICS

A potassium hydroxide (KOH) wet mount or gram-stained specimen with scrapings from the lesion is performed. A KOH preparation that is positive for pseudohyphae and budding spores confirms the diagnosis. Bacterial superinfection may be identified by culture.[2]

DIFFERENTIAL DIAGNOSIS

For intertriginous areas, the differential diagnosis should include tinea, miliaria, psoriasis, seborrheic dermatitis, eczema, erythrazma, bacterial folliculitis, and contact dermatitis. Genital rashes may be caused by pediculosis pubis.[2] In females, bacterial vaginosis or trichomoniasis must be considered in the differential diagnosis.

MANAGEMENT

The site of the infection must be considered when selecting a medication. Topical nystatin, imidazole, or allylamine creams and powders may be applied three or four

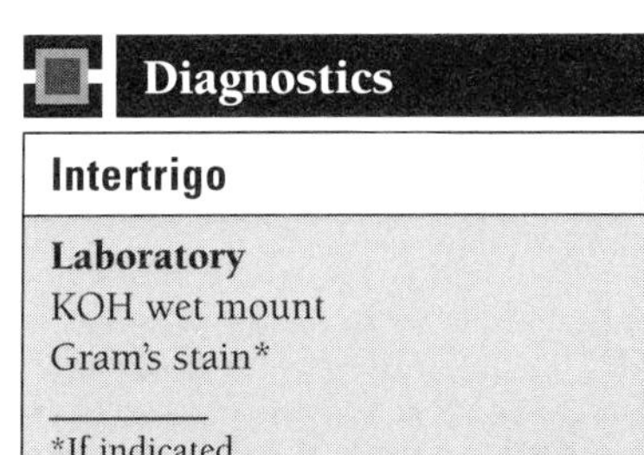

Diagnostics

Intertrigo

Laboratory
KOH wet mount
Gram's stain*

*If indicated.

times daily for 7 to 14 days. Treatment should be continued several days after the skin clears. If antiinflammatory or antipruritic properties are needed, equal amounts of a low-strength hydrocortisone cream are added to the antifungal creams.[1] If the infection is recalcitrant or recurrent, nystatin oral suspension 100,000 units/ml, 5 ml swished and swallowed q.i.d. for 7 days, is indicated.[4] Oral ketoconazole can be effective, but the risk of hepatic toxicity must be considered and monitored. The infected area should be treated with a compress of cool water or Burow's solution applied for 20 minutes several times a day until the skin remains dry.[2] The affected area should be air-dried frequently, and loose cotton clothing should be worn. An absorbent powder, not necessarily medicated, such as Zeasorb, acting as a dry lubricant, may be applied after the inflammation subsides.[2]

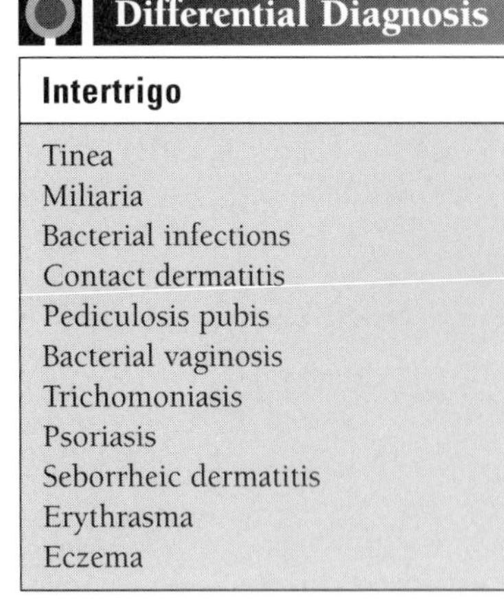
Differential Diagnosis

Intertrigo

Tinea
Miliaria
Bacterial infections
Contact dermatitis
Pediculosis pubis
Bacterial vaginosis
Trichomoniasis
Psoriasis
Seborrheic dermatitis
Erythrasma
Eczema

LIFE SPAN CONSIDERATIONS

New parents should be counseled about the possibility of candidal rashes in the diaper area of infants. Women of childbearing age should be informed of the risk of these infections while taking oral contraceptives and during pregnancy.

COMPLICATIONS

A secondary bacterial infection may develop from scratching or other vehicles that may also affect skin integrity. Patients with frequent candidal infections should be evaluated for HIV, diabetes mellitus, or other immunocompromised states.

INDICATIONS FOR REFERRAL/HOSPITALIZATION

Any patient who does not experience a resolution of symptoms of intertrigo within 2 weeks should be referred for additional consultation and confirmation of diagnosis. Immunocompromised patients require consultation with the appropriate specialist.

PATIENT AND FAMILY EDUCATION/HEALTH PROMOTION

Assistance with weight reduction may be indicated for patients with intertrigo. Affected areas need to be exposed to light and air several times daily. A hair dryer set on cool can be effective for drying inframammary areas. Once the affected epidermis has healed, patients should be encouraged to keep prone areas clean and dry. Cornstarch- and talc-containing powders should be avoided. Wearing clean cotton underwear and avoiding tight clothing may also be beneficial in reducing reoccurrence rates.

REFERENCES

1. Fitzpatrick T and others: *Color atlas and synopsis of clinical dermatology,* ed 2, New York, 1991, McGraw-Hill.
2. Habif T: *Skin disorders: diagnosis and treatment,* St Louis, 2001, Mosby.
3. Porth C: *Pathophysiology: concepts of altered health states,* ed 2, Philadelphia, 1986, JB Lippincott.
4. Berkow R: *The Merck manual,* ed 16, Rahway, NJ, 1992, Merck Research Laboratories.

CHAPTER 64

Nail Disorders

Nancy W. Knee

Immediate emergency department-surgical referral is indicated for paronychial infection of the tendon sheath.

Herpetic Whitlow

DEFINITION/EPIDEMIOLOGY

Herpetic whitlow is an infection of the area between the fascial planes of the distal finger, usually surrounding the nail. This infection is most often seen in children with gingivomatitis, in women with genital herpes, and in nurses.[1]

PATHOPHYSIOLOGY

The infecting pathogen is herpes simplex virus. The inoculation with the initial virus is often obscure. The virus remains dormant in the nerve ganglia; secondary eruptions may be related to stress, certain foods, sun exposure, and unknown precipitants.

CLINICAL PRESENTATION

Herpetiform vesicles or blisters erupt on the distal phalanx, sometimes after a short prodromal period of tingling or pruritus in the area of the eruption. Painful vesicles can be singular or coalescent, resemble a group of warts or a bacterial infection, and persist for 8 to 12 days; lesions then begin to dry, forming crusted fissures.[1] The course of the eruptions can persist for 21 days until resolution; healing may take longer in areas that remain moist. Persistent eruptions may cause scarring and atrophy.[2] In addition to the vesicles, the fingertip may be edematous, erythematous streaking may be evident on the forearm, and the axillary lymph nodes may become enlarged.[3]

PHYSICAL EXAMINATION

The nails should be inspected for shape, configuration, texture, and herpetiform vesicles. Axillary and epitrochlear nodes should be examined for lymphadenopathy.

DIAGNOSTICS AND DIFFERENTIAL DIAGNOSIS

Visualization of multinucleated giant cells using the Tzanck test confirms the diagnosis.[4] If the Tzanck test is negative, a herpes simplex culture should be obtained. The differential diagnosis should include a bacterial or candidal infection, such as paronychia.

MANAGEMENT

Although no conclusive evidence supports the use of antiviral therapy, valacyclovir (Valtrex) may be given at 1 g b.i.d. for 10 days for initial episodes and 500 mg b.i.d. for 5 days for recurrent episodes. Chronic cases of herpetic whitlow may be treated with valacyclovir 500 mg to 1 g daily for up to 1 year. Creatinine clearance should be checked and the dose adjusted according to the creatinine clearance values if abnormal. L-Lysine is ineffective.[1] Cool water compresses can be used to decrease erythema and debride crusts, thus promoting healing.[1] Analgesia such as ibuprofen 800 mg t.i.d. may be administered for pain control; however, vesicular pain may require barbiturate analgesia.[4]

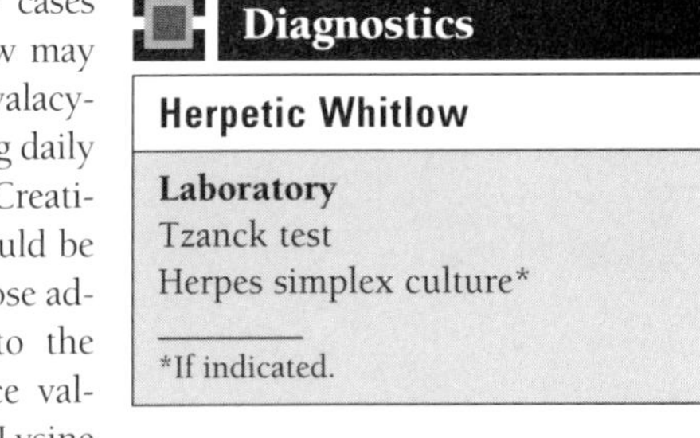

Diagnostics

Herpetic Whitlow

Laboratory
Tzanck test
Herpes simplex culture*

*If indicated.

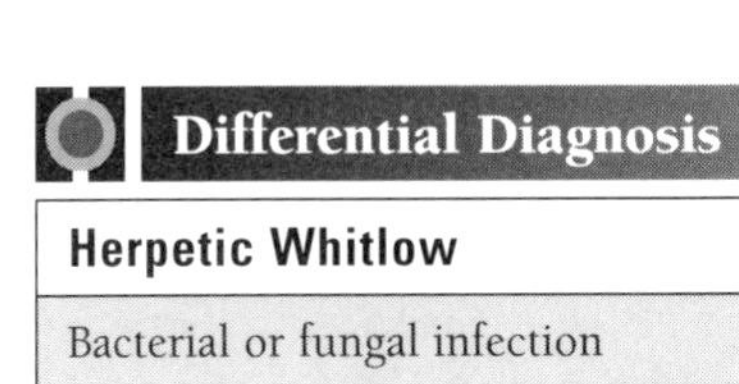

Differential Diagnosis

Herpetic Whitlow

Bacterial or fungal infection

COMPLICATIONS

Secondary bacterial infection in conjunction with the viral syndrome is possible. However, there is little evidence that this is a concern.

INDICATIONS FOR REFERRAL/HOSPITALIZATION

Physician referral is necessary if the virus is recalcitrant to treatment after 3 weeks. Hospitalization should not be required.

PATIENT AND FAMILY EDUCATION/HEALTH PROMOTION

Patients will require education regarding medication administration. Valacyclovir should be administered within 48 hours of the first prodromal signs. Patients should be advised to keep their infected digit(s) away from their mouth and eyes to prevent inoculation of these surfaces with the virus. If patients work in occupations in which they could infect other persons (e.g., nurse, manicurist), they should be advised to wear gloves when working. Signs and symptoms of infection should be carefully explained, and the patient should be encouraged to call if complications develop.

Paronychial Infections

DEFINITION/EPIDEMIOLOGY

Paronychial infections manifest as acute or chronic inflammation of the periungual tissues with an underlying bacterial or fungal infection. The microorganism can penetrate the periungual tissues through a split in the epidermis from trauma, a hangnail, irritation, or chronic exposure to water or irritants.[2]

Paronychial infections may be seen more often in women than in men; this may be related to manicures or the application of acrylic nails. Postmenopausal women may be at greater risk for chronic, candidal, paronychial infections because of diminished estrogen levels. An antiretroviral, indinavir, is also associated with paronychias because of interference with the alteration of retinoid metabolism.[5] Patients who work with chemicals are more at risk for infections because of the irritant nature of these substances, as well as the risk of trauma.

PATHOPHYSIOLOGY

The causative organisms include *Pseudomonas, Proteus, Streptococcus, Staphylococcus,* and *Candida albicans.*[2,4,6] The periungual tissues are inoculated via trauma, inert vehicles such as water, or soluble chemicals. Usually the infection follows the nail margin, or the infection may penetrate under the nail.

CLINICAL PRESENTATION AND PHYSICAL EXAMINATION

The nail folds, nail, and even digits are often described as throbbing. The nail may display distal onycholysis, discoloration, distortion, and ridging. Erythema and edema around the nail folds can be present. Force applied to the affected area releases purulent, often foul-smelling discharge.[4] Pyogenic granuloma-like lesions and granulation tissue are seen in the nail sulci in paronychias associated with indinavir.[5]

DIAGNOSTICS AND DIFFERENTIAL DIAGNOSIS

Potassium hydroxide (KOH) preparation will determine the presence of pseudohyphae and spores, which indicate candidal infection. Exudate can be cultured to determine the pathogen and to guide treatment.

The differential diagnosis includes herpetic whitlow and onychomycosis. However, paronychial infection is usually readily recognized.

MANAGEMENT

Treatment for acute infection includes hot compresses four times per day and systemic antibiotics if the pathogen is bacterial. Antibiotic therapy consists of a 7- to 10-day regimen of penicillin 25 to 50 mg/kg/day in divided doses every 6 to 8 hours, cephalexin 25 to 50 mg/kg/day in divided doses every 6 to 8 hours, or erythromycin 40 mg/kg/day in divided doses every 6 hours.[7] Ibuprofen or acetaminophen is used for analgesia. Any area with an accumulation of purulent secretions should be excised and drained, and then cleansed with half-strength iodine twice per day.

If *Candida* organisms are present, the affected area requires treatment with an antifungal lotion such as ciclopirox, miconazole, or ketoconazole cream three times per day for 2 weeks.[2] The nail should be trimmed back to the juncture of the nail plate and nail bed. For chronic candidal infections, it is important to keep the hands dry and free of moisture. The patient should be treated with oral nystatin 500,000 U q.i.d. for 2 weeks because the likely source of infection is the mouth.

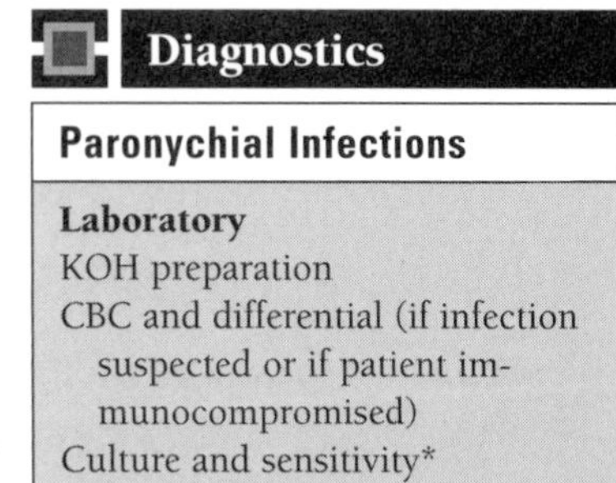

Diagnostics

Paronychial Infections

Laboratory
KOH preparation
CBC and differential (if infection suspected or if patient immunocompromised)
Culture and sensitivity*

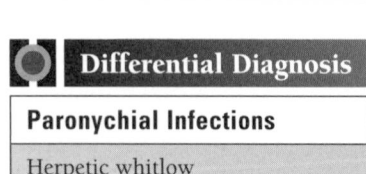

*If indicated.

Differential Diagnosis

Paronychial Infections

Herpetic whitlow
Onychomycosis

COMPLICATIONS

If untreated, the paronychial infection can invade deep into the digit, infecting the tendon and tendon sheaths. Infection along the tendon sheath requires immediate surgical intervention. Chronic mucocutaneous candidiasis can cause hyperkeratosis of the entire nail plate. These chronically infected nails can become distorted and may require excision.

INDICATIONS FOR REFERRAL/HOSPITALIZATION

Physician referral is necessary if the infection continues after 2 weeks of treatment. Suspected infection of the tendons or tendon sheaths requires immediate referral to a physician or surgeon. Hospitalization may be required for surgical intervention.

PATIENT AND FAMILY EDUCATION/HEALTH PROMOTION

It is imperative that patients understand the importance of keeping hands and nails as clean and dry as possible. Patient education should address the causative factors. Patients who have manicures or who wear acrylic nails should be advised to rest their nails and hands for 1 week every month.[4] The patients who deal with caustic chemicals and irritants are advised to wear protective gloves. The hands should be gloved when washing dishes or clothing by hand. Keeping the nail trimmed and dry will help prevent further infections.

Onychomycosis and Tinea Unguium

DEFINITION/EPIDEMIOLOGY

The terms *onychomycosis* and *tinea unguium* are often used interchangeably; however, onychomycosis is any infection of the nails caused by a fungus, and tinea unguium, or ringworm, of the nail is defined as a dermatophyte infection of the nail plate. These infections cause thickening, roughness, and splitting of the nail, resulting in dystrophy of the nail and onycholysis. The distal component of the nail subsequently separates and then falls off.[2] Often ringworm of the toenails is seen in patients with long-standing tinea pedis. Both varieties are very common in advancing age as a result of a reduction in blood flow.[4] "Trauma prediposes to infection; they are life-long, there is no spontaneous remission."[1]

PATHOPHYSIOLOGY

The most common pathogens associated with tinea unguium are *Trichophyton rubrum* (most common in the general population and in patients with HIV), *Trichophyton mentagrophytes, Trichophyton interdigitale, Trichophyton unguium,* and *Epidermophyton floccosum.*[8] Onychomycosis due to nondermatophytes is associated with *Candida* organisms.[4] Multiple organisms may be present in a single nail.[1]

CLINICAL PRESENTATION

Table 64-1 describes the physical presentation of nail dystrophies.

TABLE 64-1 Nail Dystrophies

Nail Disorder	Clinical Presentation	Manifestations
Distal/lateral subungual onychomycosis	White to brownish yellow discoloration of nail	Subungual hyperkeratosis; separation of nail plate and nail bed
White superficial onychomycosis	White, sharply outlined area on nail plate; nail surface rough and friable	Common in fingernails and toenails of HIV-infected patients
Proximal subungual onychomycosis (rare)	Whitish brown area on proximal aspect of nail plate	None
Candidal infections	Thickening of nail plate	Nail eventually disintegrates

PHYSICAL EXAMINATION

Careful examination of the toes and fingers is essential. The color may be white or yellowed, and the texture powdery or thickened. Noting the condition of the subungual nail bed, that is, the degree of elevation and separation of nail from nail bed, and surrounding tissue is important to determine the presence of concurrent bacterial infection.

DIAGNOSTICS

Confirmation of the diagnosis is made via microscopic examination of nail scrapings with a potassium hydroxide (KOH) preparation or culture of nail debris.[9] It is essential to determine the invading organism as a dermatophyte or *Candida* for appropriate treatment. Histologic tests and acid-Schiff staining are reliable for an accurate diagnosis to identify organisms susceptible to specific therapeutic agents.[1]

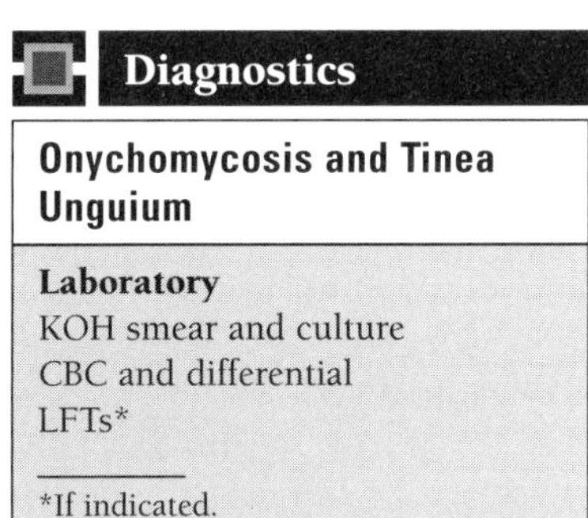

Diagnostics

Onychomycosis and Tinea Unguium

Laboratory
KOH smear and culture
CBC and differential
LFTs*

*If indicated.

DIFFERENTIAL DIAGNOSIS

Conditions that must be excluded include psoriasis, eczema, trauma, lichen planus, and onychogryposis, onycholysis, and leukonychia.[1] Psoriasis is often mistaken for dermatophyte and fungal infections, but the two may coexist (Color Plate 22).[1]

Differential Diagnosis

Onychomycosis and Tinea Unguium

Psoriasis
Eczema
Trauma
Lichen planus
Onychogryposis
Herpetic whitlow
Subungual malignant melanoma
Peripheral vascular disease
Pityriasis
Medications
Trophic changes
Black nail paronychia
Darier's disease
Endocrine disorders

MANAGEMENT

Fingernail onychomycosis may be treated with terbinafine (Lamisil) 250 mg daily for 6 weeks, when the infected nail bed is debrided. An alternative is itraconazole (Sporanox) 200 mg daily for 6 weeks or pulse dosing 200 mg b.i.d. for 1 week on and then 3 weeks off; repeated two or three times for fingernails.[1] Fingernails respond better than do toenails, although recurrence rates are very high, especially in older persons, who may not respond to pharmacotherapy.[4] Renal, liver, and hematopoietic function tests should be obtained before initiating therapy, and periodically thereafter. Patients with liver, renal, and hematopoietic dysfunction may not be candidates for therapy with Lamisil or itraconazole; consultation is advised for these patients. Toenail onychomycosis should be treated with terbinafine 250 mg/day for 12 weeks or pulse dosing of itraconazole 200 mg b.i.d. for 1 week on and 3 weeks off, repeated three or four times.[1] LFTs should be obtained before initiating therapy and at 6 weeks into therapy.[1] Multiple drug interactions exist with itraconazole. Consistent, prolonged application of a topical antifungal agent after clinical response to an oral agent may prevent nail reinfection. Removing the infected nail affords better cure rates and longer remissions.[1]

COMPLICATIONS

Chronic dermatophytosis and infection result in hyperkeratosis. The nail plate separates from the nail bed, resulting in total dystrophic onychomycosis whereby the nail bed disappears, leaving behind a keratinized nail bed.[8]

INDICATIONS FOR REFERRAL/HOSPITALIZATION

Patients with poor liver function or liver disease require referral to a physician before the initiation of therapy. The liver toxicity from the systemic preparations used in the treatment of these infections may preclude treatment. Discussion with the physician regarding newer forms of "pulse therapy" or short-term therapy is also a consideration for referral.

PATIENT AND FAMILY EDUCATION/HEALTH PROMOTION

In many cases, nails do not become clear in 12 weeks. Patients should be assured that the medication remains in the nail plate for months and will continue to kill fungus.[1] These infections can be recalcitrant to treatment, and treatment can take months or even years for complete resolution of the pathogens. Patient education should be targeted toward causative factors. It is imperative that patients keep their hands and nails as dry as possible. Footwear should be evaluated annually for size and suitability. Education concerning medication administration and instruction regarding signs of liver toxicity should be reviewed.

REFERENCES

1. Habif T and others: *Skin disease: diagnosis and treatment,* St Louis, 2001, Mosby.
2. Berkow R: *The Merck manual,* ed 16, Rahway, NJ, 1992, Merck Research Laboratories.
3. Cauthorne-Burnette T, Estes ME: *Clinical companion for health assessment and physical examination,* Albany, NY, 1998, Delmar.
4. Fitzpatrick T and others: *Color atlas and synopsis of clinical dermatology,* ed 2, New York, 1991, McGraw-Hill.
5. Ward HA, Russo GG, Shrum J: Cutaneous manifestations of antiretroviral therapy, *J Am Acad Dermatol* 46:284, 2002.
6. Murphy L: *Nurse practitioners' prescribing reference,* New York, 1998, Prescribing References.
7. White G: *Levene's color atlas of dermatology,* ed 2, London, 1997, Mosby-Wolfe.
8. Fenstermacher K, Hudson B: *Practice guidelines for family nurse practitioners,* Philadelphia, 1997, WB Saunders.
9. Mir A: *Atlas of clinical diagnosis,* Philadelphia, 1995, WB Saunders.

CHAPTER 65

Pigmentation Changes (Vitiligo)

Margaret McAllister

DEFINITION/EPIDEMIOLOGY

Vitiligo is a skin disorder characterized by either a lifelong or a rapid disappearance of pigment-producing melanocytes in the epidermis and hair follicles. Lack of melanin leads to the appearance of progressive, symmetrically patterned, milky-white macules that merge to form larger depigmented areas. The macules give a variegated appearance to the skin that is similar to the white patches on a Holstein calf—hence the origin of the word from the Greek word *vitelius,* which means "calf." The disease is psychologically troublesome, particularly in dark-skinned individuals such as African-American and Indian populations, in which the variegated appearance to the skin is most striking and socially stigmatizing. The disease manifests itself in two forms: type A, a nondermatomal distribution, and type B, a segmental or dermatomal distribution (zosteriform) characterized by rapid spread.

Vitiligo is seen in 1% to 2% of the general population, without regard to race, ethnic origin, or gender. The condition has an inherited tendency, with 30% of cases reporting a family history of vitiligo in parents, offspring, or siblings.[1] Although familial cases of vitiligo have been associated with autoimmune endocrine disorders, a definitive genetic locus has not yet been reported.[2] Disease onset occurs between 10 and 30 years of age, with 50% of the cases occurring before age 20 and fewer cases reported in infancy and old age.[1,3,4]

PATHOPHYSIOLOGY

The cause of vitiligo is not known. Except for the absence of melanocytes, skin function is normal. There is a progressive destruction of pigment-producing cells at the border of the dermis and epidermis. The nonsegmental (nondermatomal) variety of vitiligo is associated with a small risk of autoimmune-related disorders, such as type 1 diabetes mellitus and thyroid disease.[5]

Several theories exist to explain the phenomenon of vitiligo. The autoimmune theory proposes that there is a destruction of the cutaneous melanocytes with loss of the melanin-producing pigment. Histologic examination indicates that lymphocytes build up within the dermis and are involved in the destruction of the melanocytes. Coexisting diseases such as alopecia areata, autoimmune thyroid disorders, Addison's disease, atrophic gastritis, pernicious anemia, and type 1 diabetes underscore the relationship of dermatomal vitiligo to autoimmunity. Serum autoimmune antibodies against melanocytes, thyroid and adrenal tissue, islet cells, gastric parietal cells, and intrinsic factors have been demonstrated.

A second explanation, the neurogenic theory, supposes that a toxic substance is released by the peripheral nerve endings and interferes with the production of melanin. A third theory

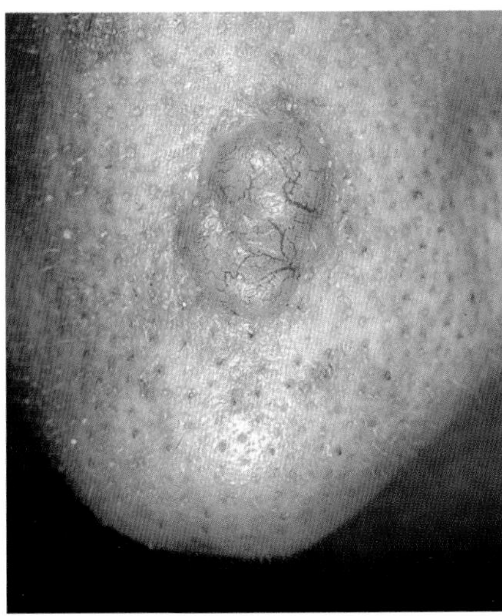

1

Nodular basal cell carcinoma. (From Habif TP and others: *Skin disease: diagnosis and treatment,* St Louis, 2001, Mosby.)

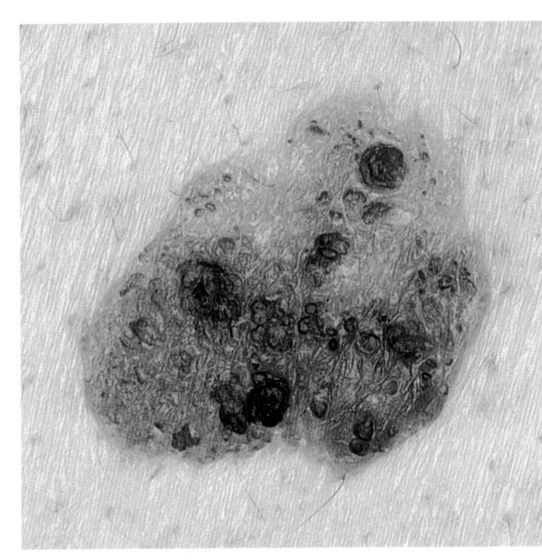

2

Seborrheic keratosis (mimicking melanoma). (From Habif TP and others: *Skin disease: diagnosis and treatment,* St Louis, 2001, Mosby.)

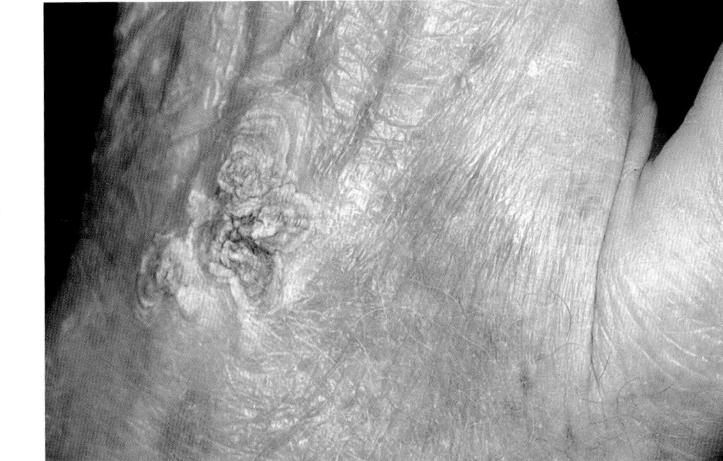

3

Squamous cell cancer. (From Habif TP and others: *Skin disease: diagnosis and treatment,* St Louis, 2001, Mosby.)

4

Superficial spreading melanoma. (From Habif TP and others: *Skin disease: diagnosis and treatment,* St Louis, 2001, Mosby.)

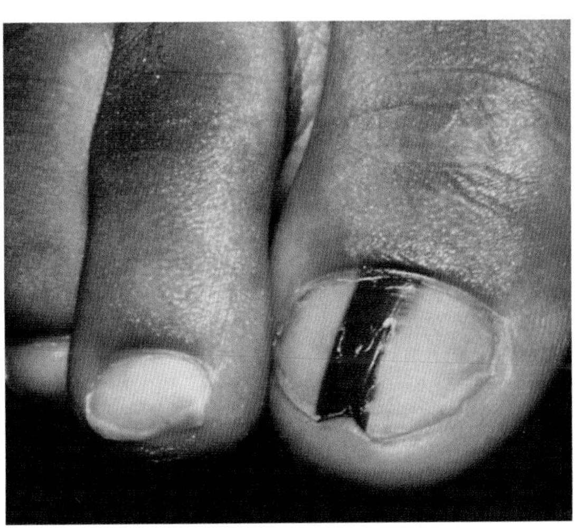

5

Acral-lentiginous melanoma. It occurs most often on hands, feet, or nail beds of dark-skinned individuals. Very common in African Americans and Asian Americans. (From Habif TP and others: *Skin disease: diagnosis and treatment,* St Louis, 2001, Mosby.)

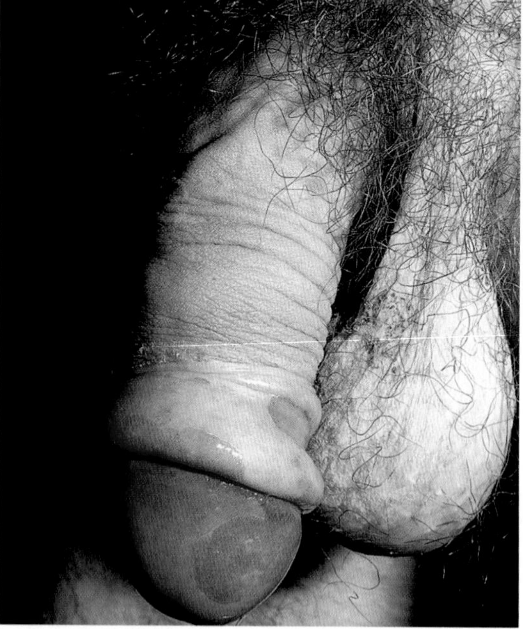

6

Multiple syphilitic chancres. (From Fisher BK, Margesson LJ: *Genital skin disorders: diagnosis and treatment,* St Louis, 1998, Mosby.)

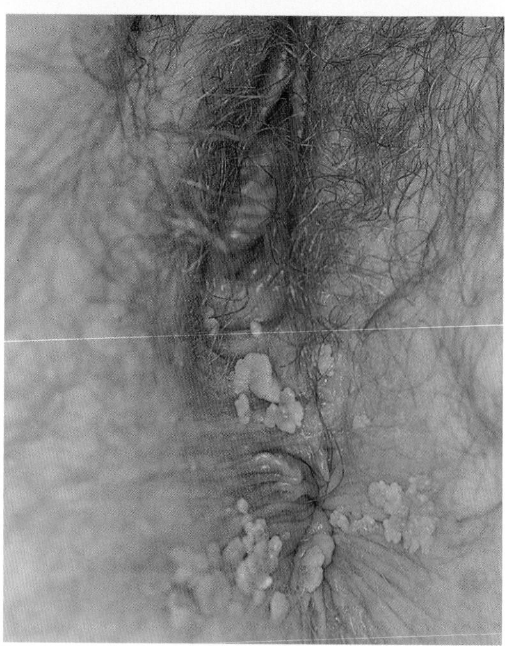

7

Multiple condylomata in the perineum and perianal area. (From Fisher BK, Margesson LJ: *Genital skin disorders: diagnosis and treatment,* St Louis, 1998, Mosby.)

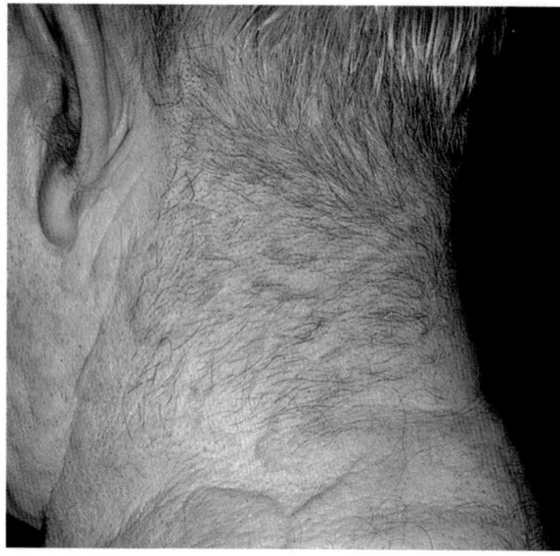

8

Angioedema affects the face, lips, palms, soles, or a portion of an extremity. It may become confluent and cover wide areas. The color is uniform. Hives vary in color. (From Habif TP and others: *Skin disease: diagnosis and treatment,* St Louis, 2001, Mosby.)

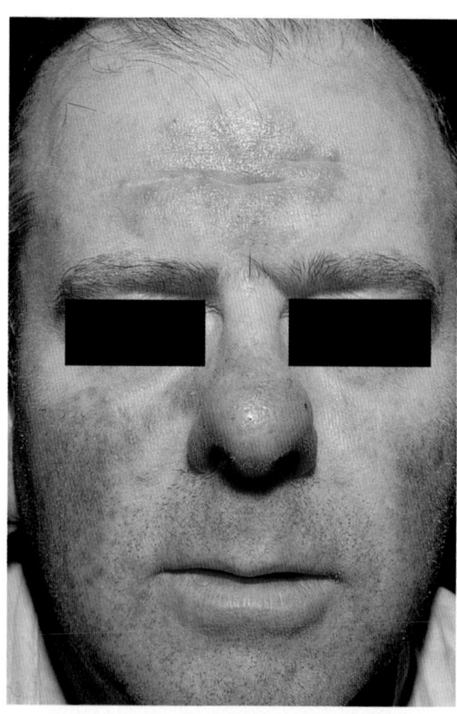

10

Rosacea. (From Habif TP and others: *Skin disease: diagnosis and treatment,* St Louis, 2001, Mosby.)

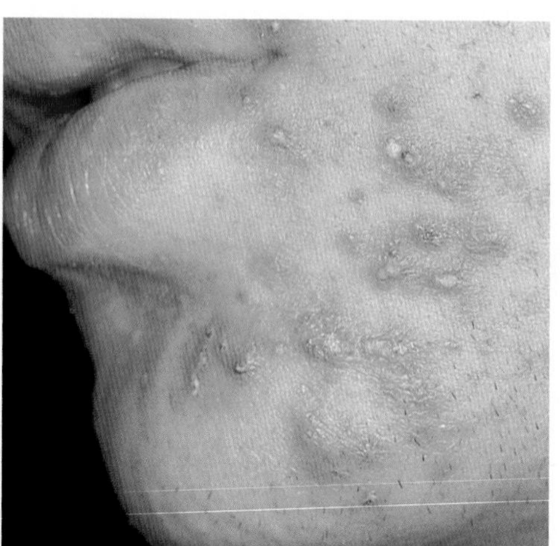

9

Pustular acne. (From Habif TP and others: *Skin disease: diagnosis and treatment,* St Louis, 2001, Mosby.)

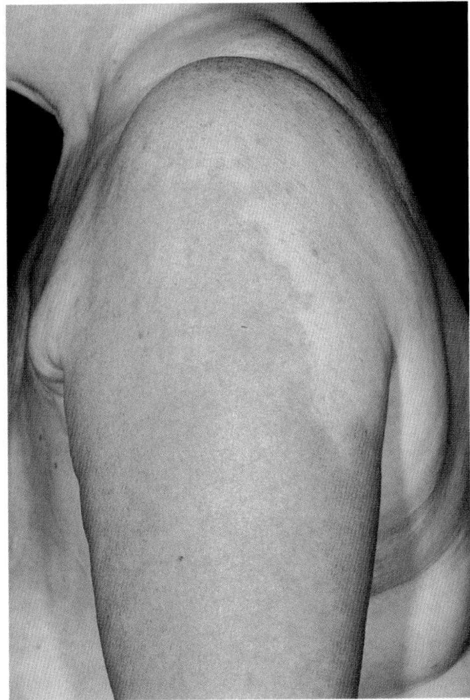

11

Cellulitis. (From Habif TP: *Clinical dermatology: a color guide to diagnosis and therapy,* ed 3, St Louis, 1996, Mosby.)

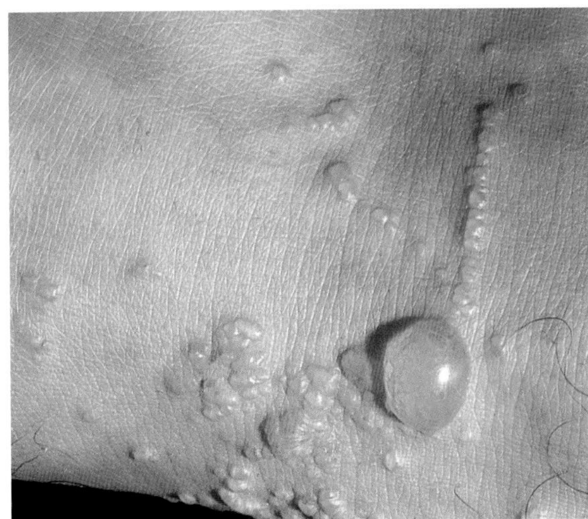

12

Rhus dermatitis (poison ivy). (From Habif TP and others: *Skin disease: diagnosis and treatment,* St Louis, 2001, Mosby.)

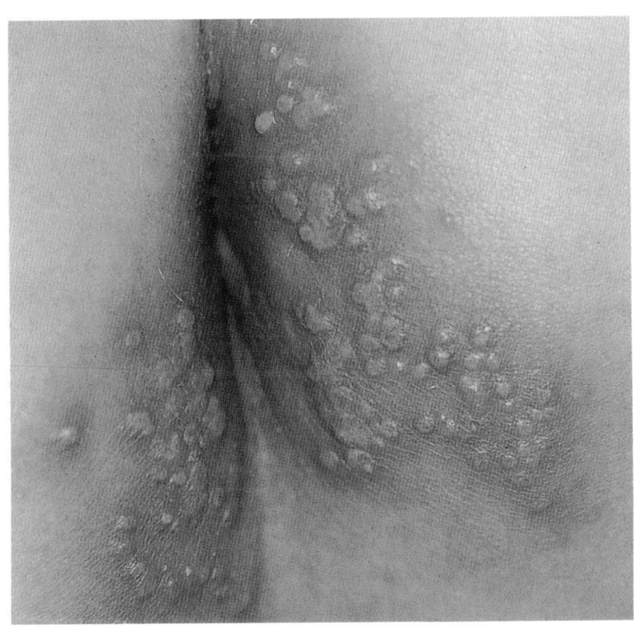

13

Herpes simplex. Primary herpes simplex on the perineum and buttocks with groups of vesicles on a red base. (From Fisher BK, Margesson LJ: *Genital skin disorders: diagnosis and treatment,* St Louis, 1998, Mosby.)

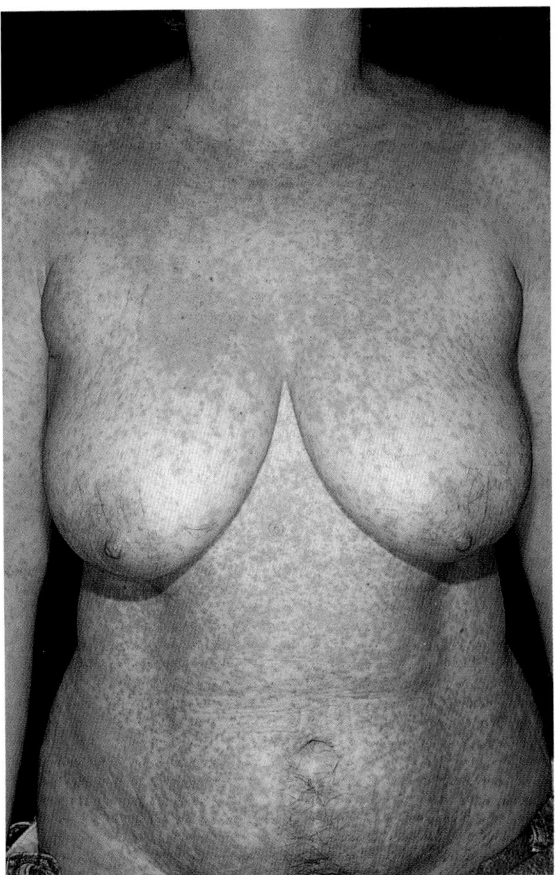

14

Cutaneous drug reaction. (From Habif TP and others: *Skin disease: diagnosis and treatment,* St Louis, 2001, Mosby.)

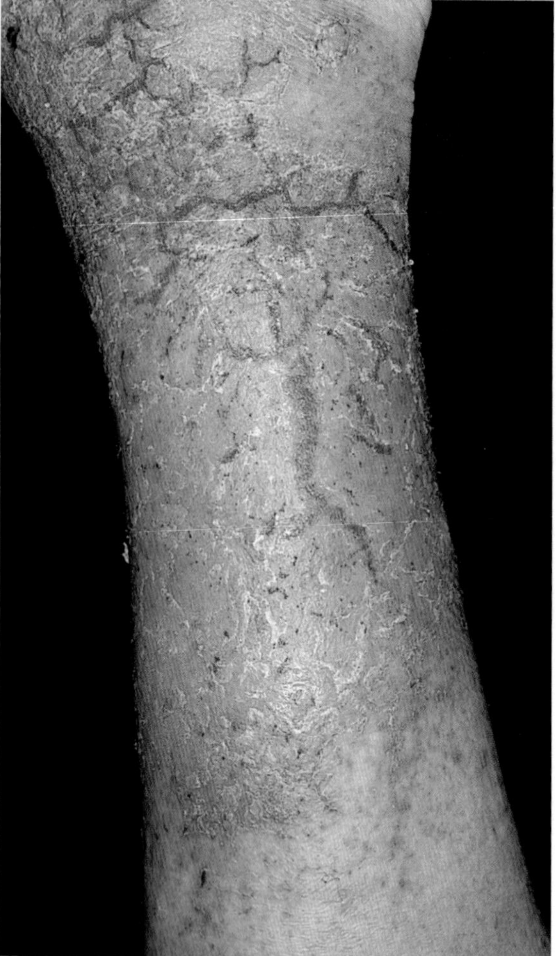

15

Asteatotic eczema. (From Habif TP and others: *Skin disease: diagnosis and treatment,* St Louis, 2001, Mosby.)

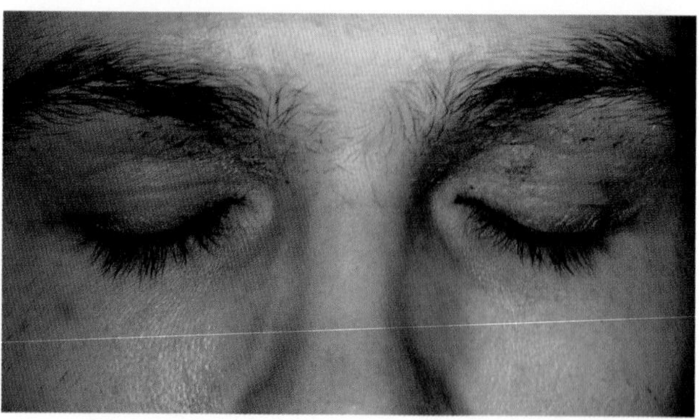

16

Atopic dermatitis. (From Habif TP and others: *Skin disease: diagnosis and treatment,* St Louis, 2001, Mosby.)

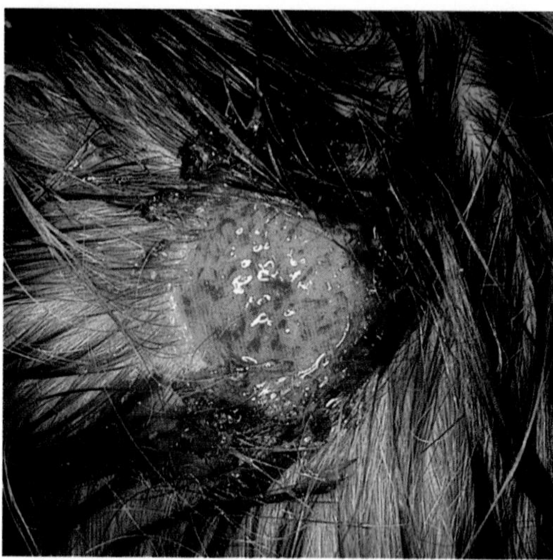

17

Tinea capitis. (From Habif TP and others: *Skin disease: diagnosis and treatment,* St Louis, 2001, Mosby.)

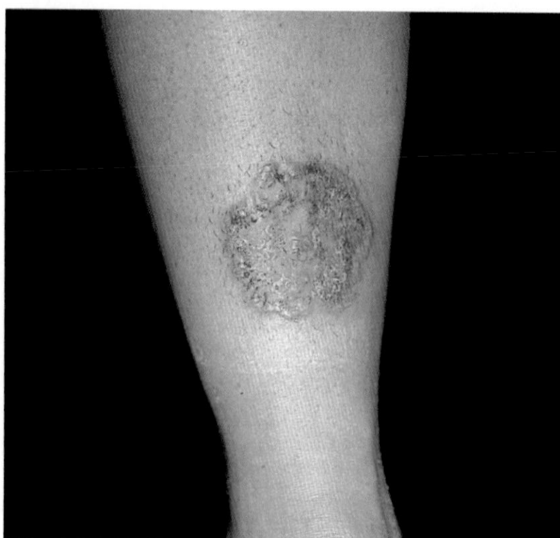

18

Tinea corporis (ringworm of the body). (From Habif TP and others: *Skin disease: diagnosis and treatment,* St Louis, 2001, Mosby.)

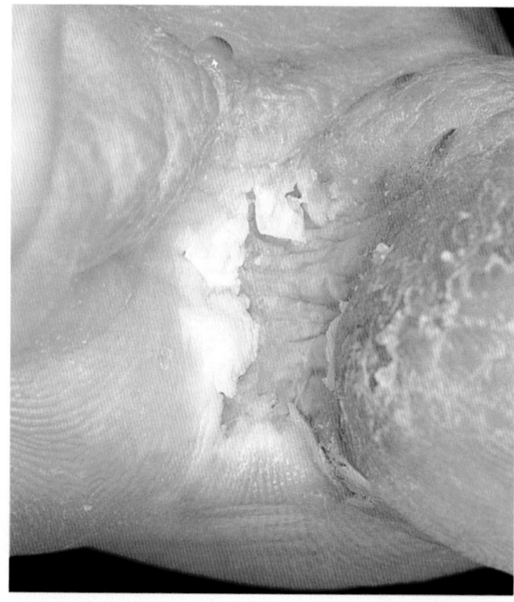

19

Interdigital tinea pedis (toe web infection). (From Habif TP and others: *Skin disease: diagnosis and treatment,* St Louis, 2001, Mosby.)

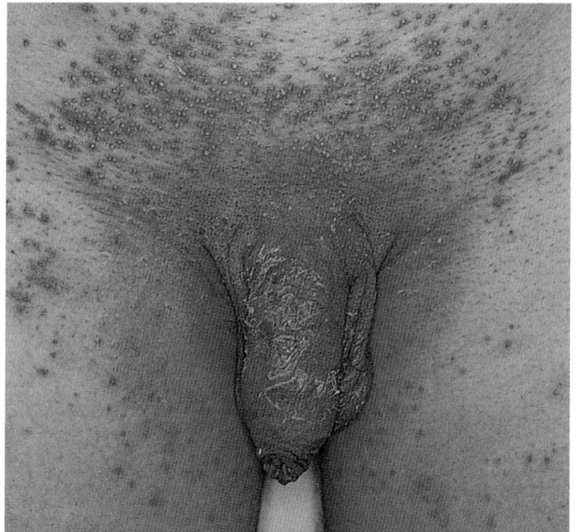

20

Moniliasis (candidiasis). (From Fisher BK, Margesson LJ: *Genital skin disorders: diagnosis and treatment,* St Louis, 1998, Mosby.)

21

Ophthalmic zoster. (From Habif TP and others: *Skin disease: diagnosis and treatment,* St Louis, 2001, Mosby.)

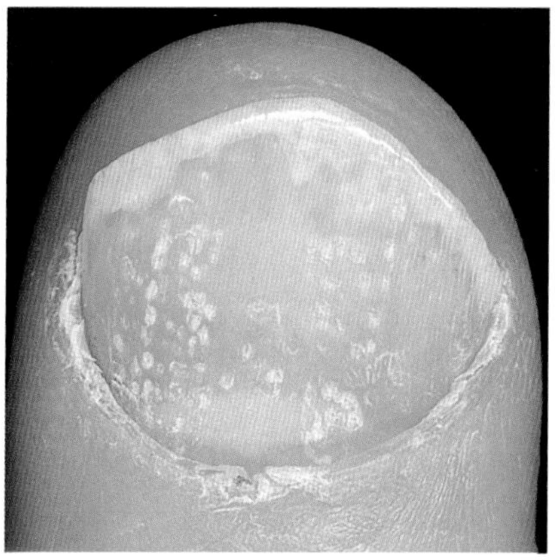

22

Psoriasis of nails. (From Habif TP and others: *Skin disease: diagnosis and treatment,* St Louis, 2001, Mosby.)

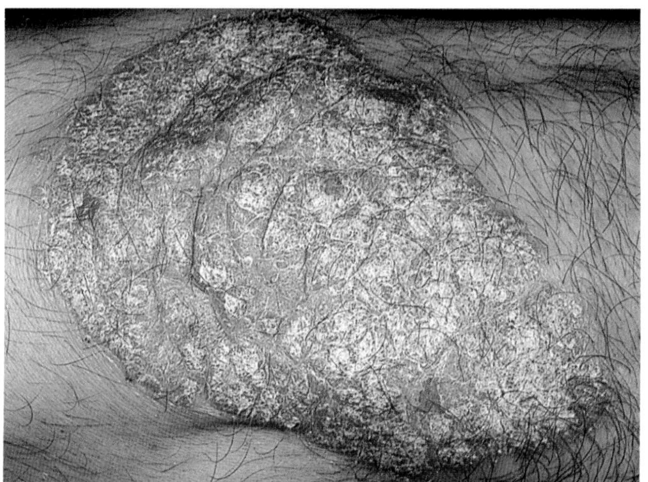

23

Psoriasis. Thick, red plaques have a sharply defined border and an adherent silvery scale. (From Habif TP and others: *Skin disease: diagnosis and treatment,* St Louis, 2001, Mosby.)

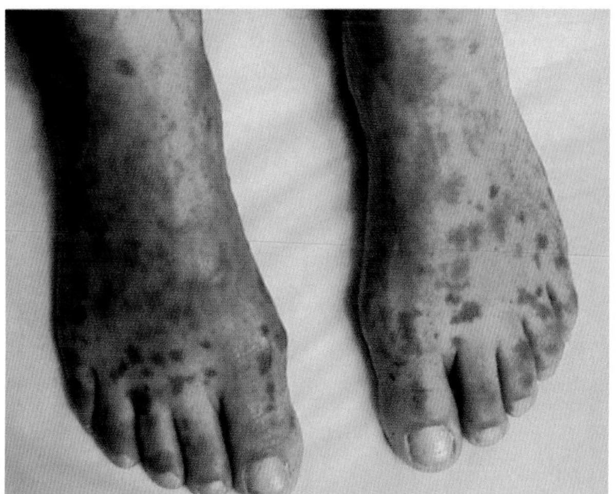

24

Palpable purpura. (Reprinted from the *Clinical Slide Collection on the Rheumatic Diseases,* © 1991, 1995. Used by permission of the American College of Rheumatology.)

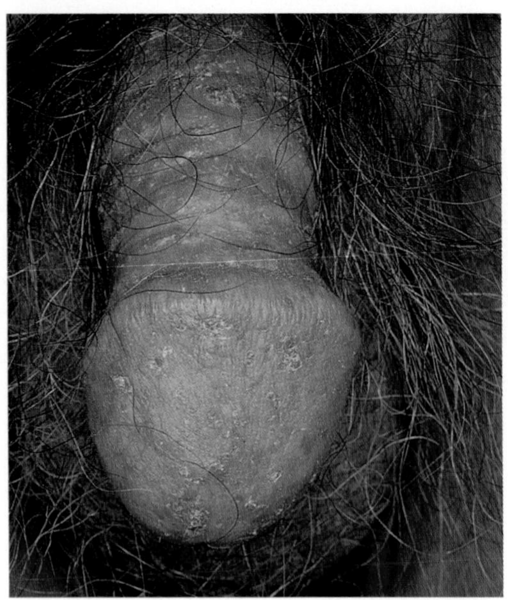

25

Scabies. (From Fisher BK, Margesson LJ: *Genital skin disorders: diagnosis and treatment,* St Louis, 1998, Mosby.)

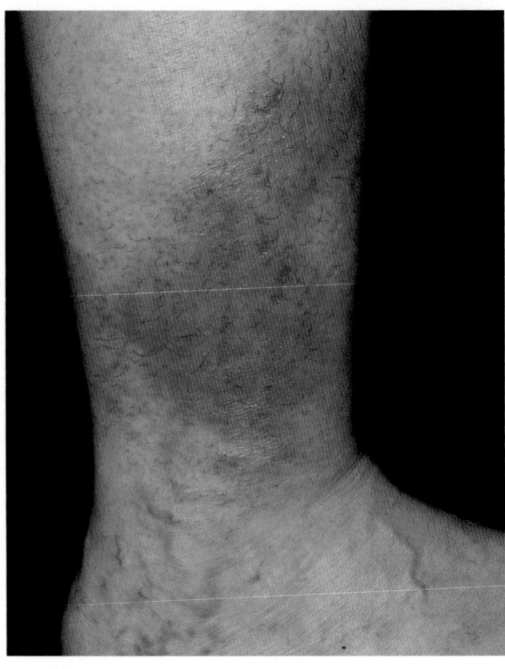

26

Stasis dermatitis in early stage with erythema and erosions. (From Habif TP: *Clinical dermatology: a color guide to diagnosis and therapy,* ed 3, St Louis, 1996, Mosby.)

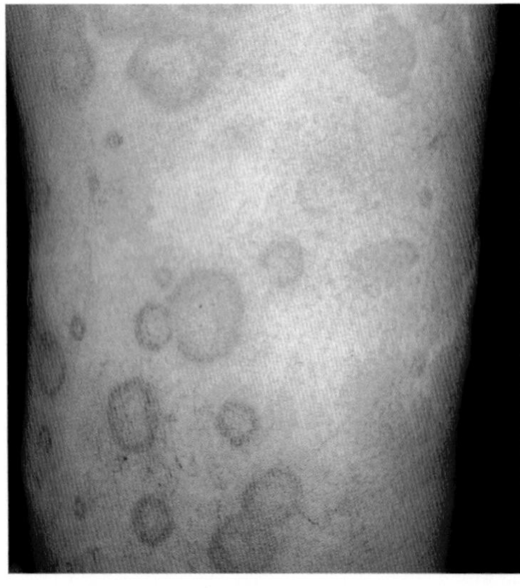

27

Urticaria. (From Habif TP and others: *Skin disease: diagnosis and treatment,* St Louis, 2001, Mosby.)

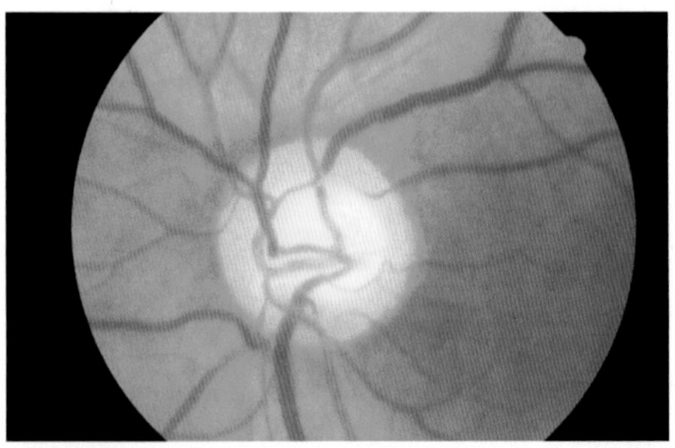

28

Glaucoma with cupping. (Courtesy Buddy Crofton, CRA, COT.)

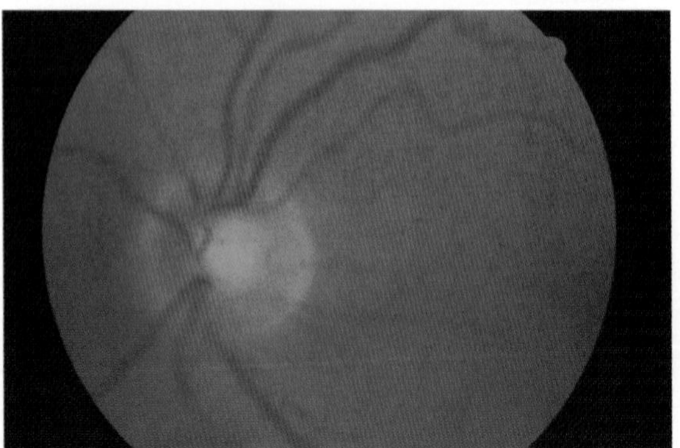

29

Glaucoma without cupping. (Courtesy Buddy Crofton, CRA, COT.)

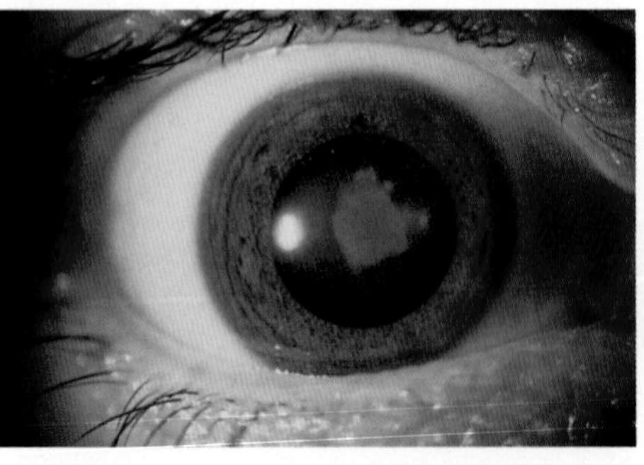

30

Cataracts (dilated pupil). (Courtesy Buddy Crofton, CRA, COT.)

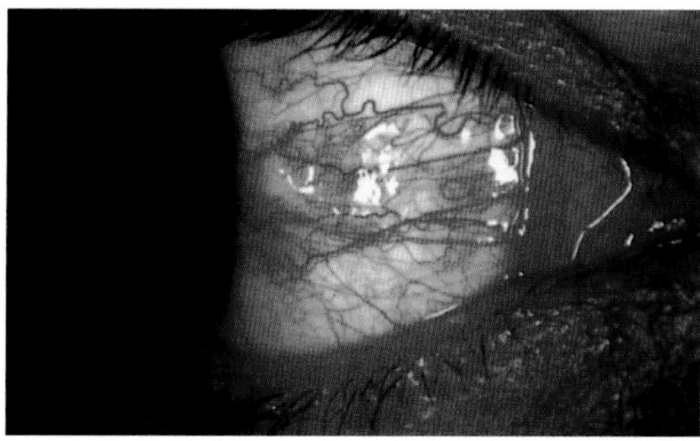

31

Pingueculum. (Courtesy Buddy Crofton, CRA, COT.)

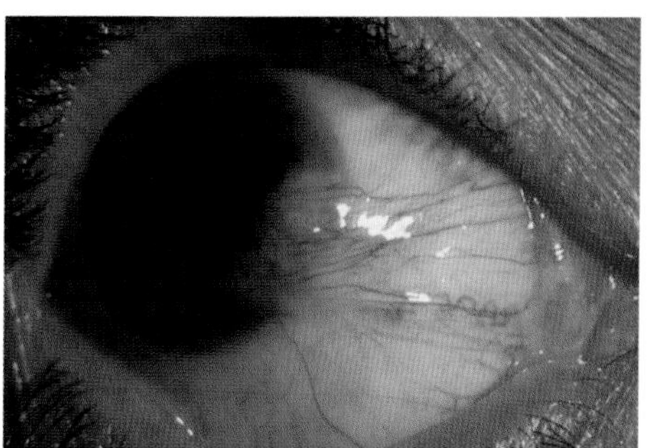

32

Pterygium. (Courtesy Buddy Crofton, CRA, COT.)

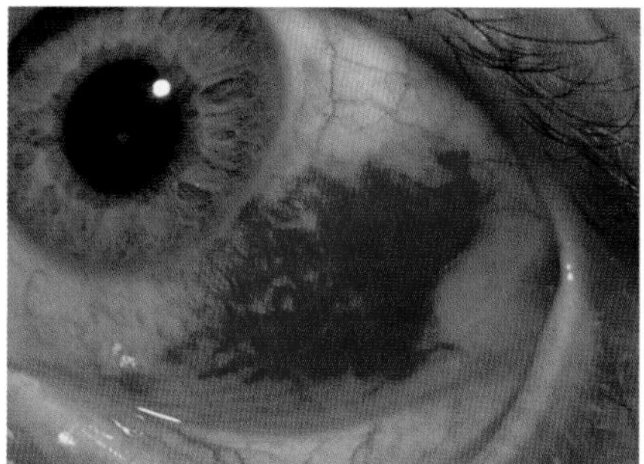

33

Subconjunctival hemorrhage. (Courtesy Buddy Crofton, CRA, COT.)

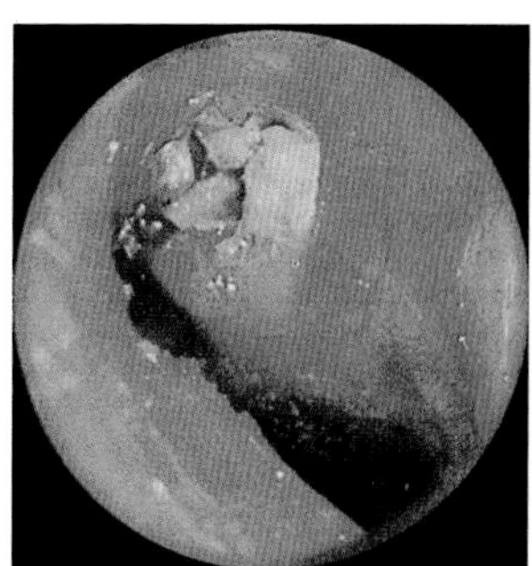

34

Cholesteatoma. (From Malasanos L and others: *Health assessment,* ed 3, St Louis, 1986, Mosby; courtesy Richard A Buckingham, MD, University of Illinois—Chicago.)

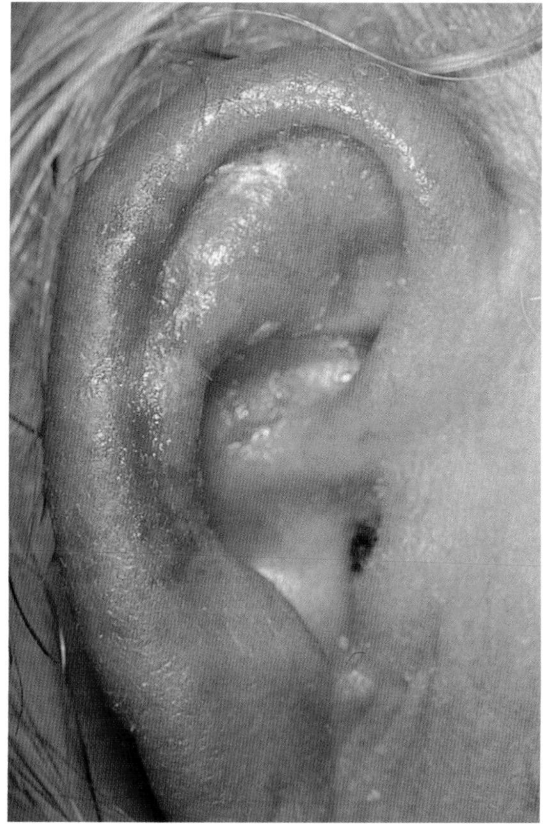

35

Malignant otitis externa. (From Habif TP and others: *Skin disease: diagnosis and treatment,* St Louis, 2001, Mosby.)

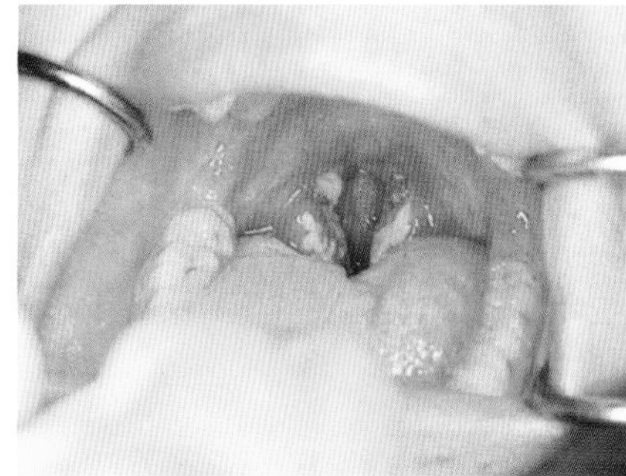

36

Pharyngitis/tonsillitis. (From Barkauskas VH and others: *Health and physical assessment,* ed 2, St Louis, 1998, Mosby.)

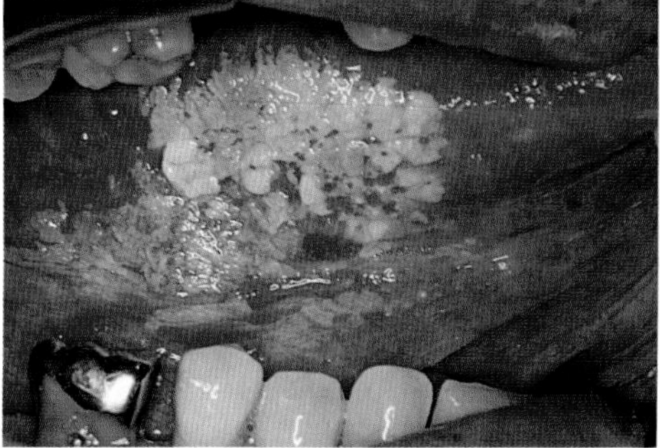

37

Leukoplakia on the ventrolateral aspect of the tongue. (From Eisen D, Lynch DP: *The mouth: diagnosis and treatment,* St Louis, 1998, Mosby.)

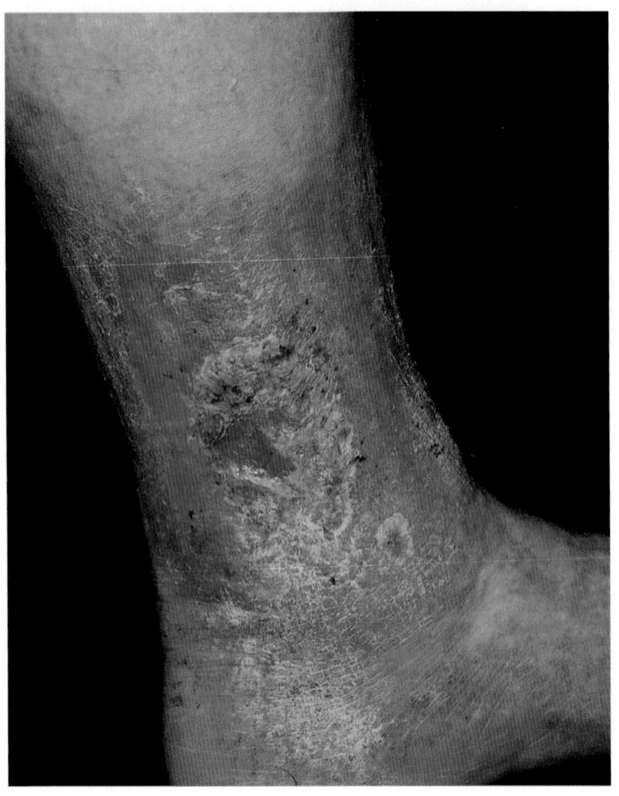

38

Venous leg ulcers. (From Habif TP and others: *Skin disease: diagnosis and treatment,* St Louis, 2001, Mosby.)

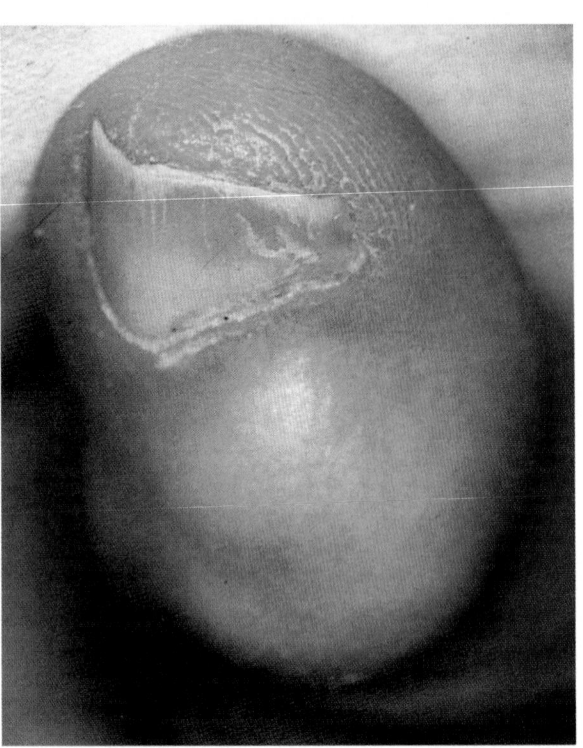

39

Gout with tophus. (From Baran R and others: *Color atlas of the hair, scalp, and nails,* St Louis, 1991, Mosby.)

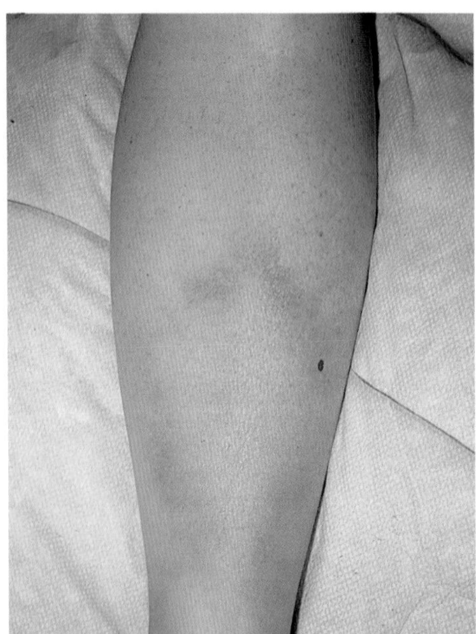

40

Lyme disease. (From Habif TP and others: *Skin disease: diagnosis and treatment,* St Louis, 2001, Mosby.)

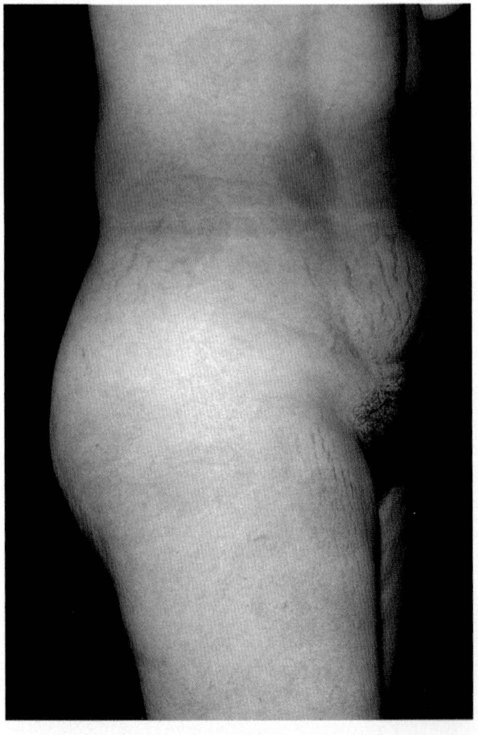

41

Lyme disease. (From Habif TP and others: *Skin disease: diagnosis and treatment,* St Louis, 2001, Mosby.)

suggests there is a defect in the natural protective mechanism of melanin synthesis by melanocytes. Toxic substances accumulate during normal melanin production and later precipitate the destruction of the melanocytes.[1] The variation in presentation and progression of the two types of vitiligo indicates that the underlying pathologic condition for the two forms of disease may be distinctly different.

CLINICAL PRESENTATION

Vitiligo is characterized by a progressive and invasive hypopigmentation of the skin that is found on sun-exposed areas and extensor surfaces of the upper body. Most patients have no other clinical findings.[3] There is a likely family predisposition, and onset may follow an injury to the skin such as a burn, bruise, or contusion (Koebner's phenomenon). In fair-skinned individuals, the disease may go undetected until summer, when the sun-exposed areas tan and the melanin-free areas appear as contrasting chalky-white areas.

PHYSICAL EXAMINATION

The extensor surfaces may have been traumatized previously; depigmentation first appears here in a symmetric fashion typical of the more common nondermatomal variety. The segmental variety is more often seen in children and follows a dermatomal distribution that progresses more rapidly. The dermatomal variety is not likely to be associated with autoimmune disorders or Koebner's phenomenon.[3] The border is not sharply demarcated but instead exhibits a tricolored, uneven appearance.[6] Box 65-1 indicates the usual presentation of the hypopigmented lesions of vitiligo.

Vitiligo can be best described as a white, flat macule within the epidermis that varies in size from 5 mm to 5 cm with a convex outer edge. In the common nonsegmental variety, the lesion presents in a symmetric distribution on the body parts. Macules may eventually merge to cover the entire body in a condition termed *vitiligo universalis*. Variations of the lesion include smaller lesions mixed with larger ones and the appearance of elevated, erythematous, pruritic lesions known as *inflammatory vitiligo*. The segmental variety occurs in a band-type distribution on one side of the body.

DIAGNOSTICS

The clinical presentation and physical examination are generally sufficient to make a diagnosis. In some instances (lighter-skinned individuals and in areas under the arms and genital regions), a Wood's light examination is necessary to make the diagnosis. A Wood's light will illuminate depigmented areas as chalky white. A skin scraping for a potassium hydroxide (KOH) examination fails to demonstrate hyphae or spores consistent with tinea versicolor, another common depigmenting lesion. Although not usually necessary, a skin biopsy will show an absence of melanocytes and melanin in the epidermis.

Vitiligo patients show an increased frequency of autoimmune disorders such as thyroid disease, insulin-dependent diabetes, and pernicious anemia.[7] The patient should be assessed for signs and symptoms of thyroid disease; a screening for thyroid-stimulating hormone (TSH) and thyroxine (T_4) is recommended. However, the treatment of thyroid disease has no impact on the progression of vitiligo.[1] A fasting blood glucose is included in the initial diagnostic evaluation. A CBC with indices is performed to detect the presence of macrocytosis followed by an evaluation for vitamin B_{12} deficiency if indicated.

BOX 65-1

HYPOPIGMENTED VITILIGO LESIONS

Bony surfaces—Back of hands and fingers, elbows and knees
Body orifices—Around the eyes, mouth, and nose
Body folds—Armpits and groins
Other areas—Legs, wrists, nipples, and genitals
Hair—Area within the affected patch may become white

Diagnostics

Vitiligo

Laboratory
Wood's lamp examination
KOH preparation
TSH, T_4
Fasting blood sugar
CBC and differential
B_{12}

Other
Skin biopsy*

*If indicated.

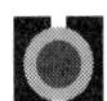

Differential Diagnosis

Vitiligo

Albinism
Piebaldism
Tuberous sclerosis
Nevus anemicus
Chemical leukoderma
Tinea versicolor
Leprosy
Pityriasis alba
Lichen sclerosis
Psoriasis
Eczema

DIFFERENTIAL DIAGNOSIS

Early or atypical lesions often require the exclusion of other hypopigmented disorders, including albinism, piebaldism, tuberous sclerosis, nevus anemicus, tinea, pityriasis alba, and lichen sclerosis. Some of these disorders are associated with patchy depigmentation with inflammation and scaling or atrophy induration.

MANAGEMENT

Care of the patient with vitiligo involves the use of sunscreens (SPF 15 to 30) to protect the nonpigmented skin from burning and to reduce the tanning of melanin-producing areas of the skin. Extensive sunburn can produce a response similar to Koebner's phenomenon and extend the depigmentation process. Cosmetic cover-ups assist the patient with management of the psychologic aspects of the disease and improve body image and self-coping mechanisms. A variety of cosmetic substances are commercially available and are marketed under the names of Covermark (Lydia O'Leary) and Dermablend (Flori Roberts). These products can be customized to match individual skin tones. Although these products do not come off in water, they do rub off and therefore may not sustain long periods of wear. Tanning creams containing dihydroxyacetone may be applied to induce the tanning of affected areas; these substances can be used for eyelids. Some patients desire no treatment aside from cosmetics and prefer to allow the disease to progress until all body parts are depigmented. However, it is difficult to judge how long this will take, which limits the usefulness of this approach in the treatment regimen.

After coexistent autoimmune disorders have been excluded, patients with vitiligo are generally referred to a dermatologist for treatment options. Therapy is directed toward either repigmentation therapy of the affected areas or depigmentation therapy of the unaffected areas. Repigmentation involving the use of high- to mid-potency steroid creams applied twice a day to the affected areas is usually the first approach. Patients must be monitored every 2 months for evidence of skin atrophy.

Recently occurring lesions and those of the facial and genital areas are the most responsive to topical steroid treatment.[3,6] A response to treatment is indicated by the development of follicular pigmented spots that widen with time and persist. Areas with minimal hair follicles are slower to repigment.

Efforts are in progress to develop guidelines in the management of vitiligo. Meta-analysis of studies using class 3 corticosteroids and narrow-band ultraviolet B (UVB) have shown these methods to be effective and safe for localized and generalized vitiligo, respectively.[8] However, steroid treatment failure is seen in nearly 20% of cases; failure is likely if no response is seen by the end of 2 months.[6] At this time, the patient should be referred back to the specialist for further evaluation and for treatment with psoralens plus ultraviolet light of the A wavelength (PUVA), either topical or systemic. PUVA treatments should be performed by a qualified specialist. Close monitoring of the patient for response to treatment is necessary. Prevention of eye exposure to UV light must be strictly enforced by ensuring that the patient wears glasses that filter all UV light. Up to 2 years of treatment may be necessary before repigmentation occurs.[6] Another technique is chemical depigmentation to produce an artificially induced vitiligo universalis if more than 50% to 80% of the body is affected. This technique involves the application of a monobenzone 20% cream twice daily. The application produces an irreversible depigmentation that takes up to 2 to 3 months to begin.[1] The primary care provider can monitor this treatment regimen if prescribed by the specialist. Patients are generally very pleased with the outcome of this treatment.

Laser therapy is an option for those trained in the use of this technique; XTRAC is the first U.S. Food and Drug Administration (FDA)-approved laser treatment for vitiligo.[9]

COMPLICATIONS

Treatment with steroids may involve atrophy and striae formation, which increases the risk for easy bruising and infection. Steroid-induced glaucoma and cataracts are complications of steroid application around the eyes. Complications of PUVA treatment include a phototoxic reaction and ocular damage if appropriate UV protective sunglasses are not used. Consultation with the specialist is necessary if evidence of skin atrophy, adrenal axis suppression, or steroid-induced glaucoma presents.

INDICATIONS FOR REFERRAL/HOSPITALIZATION

Once therapy has been instituted by a dermatologist, primary care providers can assist with monitoring therapy, with a dermatology consultation for treatment questions. After coexistent autoimmune disorders have been excluded, patients with vitiligo are referred to a dermatologist for treatment options. The primary care provider monitors the therapy, with a dermatology consultation for treatment questions. The involvement of eye pigment mandates a referral to an ophthalmologist for evaluation. A referral for mental health counseling may be indicated because this disorder can be psychologically stressful.

PATIENT AND FAMILY EDUCATION

Education includes teaching patients about the nature of the pigment changes and the lack of exact scientific knowledge concerning the true cause of the disease. Patients should be taught that the treatment response includes repigmentation that occurs first in areas with residual melanocytes. Vitiligo with late-life onset or long-standing lesions is less likely to respond to treatment. Risk factors associated with topical steroids include easy bruising, infection, and decreased vision. Patients are taught to observe their skin closely for the development of suspicious skin lesions suggestive of melanoma. The rule of fingertip units should be adhered to in prescribing and monitoring patients on topical steroids. One fingertip unit weighs 0.5 g and is the amount expressed from a tube applied to the fingertip. One half of a fingertip unit will cover the dorsum of the hand, and 2.5 fingertip units will cover the face. For lesions affecting the face, a 30-g tube should last for 10 days.[3] Patients should avoid using more steroid cream than directed and should avoid applying steroids around the eyes and moist genital areas, where thin skin enhances systemic absorption. Patients should avoid sunlight for 48 hours after each PUVA treatment.

Assessment of the patient's psychologic response to vitiligo includes body image adjustment, use of cosmetic coverings, and knowledge concerning the noncontagious nature of vitiligo. Family members should be included in the office visit for support and explanation concerning the benign nature of the disorder and the expected response to treatment. Instruction concerning the use of sunscreens to protect depigmented areas is critical.

REFERENCES

1. Habif TP: *Clinical dermatology*, ed 3, St Louis, 1996, Mosby.
2. de la Fuente-Fernandez R: Mutations in GTP-cyclohydrolase I gene and vitiligo (research letters), *Lancet* 350:640, 1997.
3. Schwartz RA, Janniger CK: Vitiligo, *Cutis* 60:239, 1997.
4. Hann SK, Chun WH, Park YK: Clinical characteristics of progressive vitiligo, *Int J Dermatol* 36:353, 1997.
5. Fitzpatrick TB and others: *Color atlas and synopsis of clinical dermatology*, ed 3, New York, 1997, McGraw-Hill.
6. Reeves JT, Maibach HI: *Clinical dermatology illustrated: a regional approach*, ed 3, Philadelphia, 1998, FA Davis.
7. You-Min Y, Hong-Yong K: A study on the frequency of the autoimmune disorder in vitiligo patients, *Ann Dermatol* 13:218, 2001.
8. American Medical Association: The development of guidelines for the treatment of vitiligo, *Arch Fam Med* 9:954, 2000.
9. Psoriasis: revolutionary new laser treatment reaches patients, *Med Devices Surg Technol Week* October 21:30, 2001. Retrieved August 12, 2002, from the World Wide Web: http://www.newsrx.com.

CHAPTER 66

Pruritus

Daniel W. O'Neill

DEFINITION/EPIDEMIOLOGY

Pruritus is a sensation that leads to a desire to scratch. It is a common symptom that can be found in many dermatologic and systemic illnesses.

PATHOPHYSIOLOGY

Pruritus is characterized by the activation of a network of free nerve endings situated at the dermoepidermal junction by local mediators such as histamine and/or numerous other peptides and proteases.[1] These impulses are carried by unmyelinated C fibers to the central nervous system, where the impulses are modulated by opioid peptides. Prostaglandins in the skin lower the threshold for itching. The exact pathophysiologic mechanisms leading to itching in systemic disease is ill defined. Scratching leads to symptomatic relief by temporarily destroying the nerve endings or stimulating pain fibers, but this often leads to the release of more mediators and the scratch-itch cycle, in which one scratch is too many and a million are not enough.

CLINICAL PRESENTATION AND PHYSICAL EXAMINATION

Dermatologic disorders can present with characteristic primary skin lesions; therefore after obtaining a basic history of the present illness, a total skin examination is necessary to first identify or exclude dermatologic disorders.[1] Often the secondary skin lesions, such as excoriations (scratches), secondary infections (e.g., impetigo), hyperkeratotic skin changes, and lichenification (thickening, which indicates chronicity), obscure the primary lesion. If a diagnosis is not evident on initial examination, then a thorough history should include diurnal rhythms, character, severity, distribution, exacerbating and alleviating factors, and previous treatments. The history should also include medication use, alcohol use, past medical history, exposures (e.g., to people who are scratching, pets, soaps, detergents, dry air, chemicals), and a complete review of systems. A complete physical examination with emphasis on evaluation for organomegaly and adenopathy is then performed.

DIAGNOSTICS

If no etiology is found, screening laboratory examinations include a CBC with differential, serum glucose, aspartate and alanine transaminase, alkaline phosphatase, bilirubin, BUN, creatinine, thyroid panel, urinalysis, and chest radiograph. If indicated, a skin biopsy can be sent for pathologic examination (mycosis fungoides), immunofluorescence (pemphigoid and dermatitis herpetiformis), or special staining (mastocytosis). Serum ferritin, protein and immunoelectrophoresis, stool for ova and parasites, or other studies may also be indicated. Occasionally it is necessary to perform repeated evaluations in

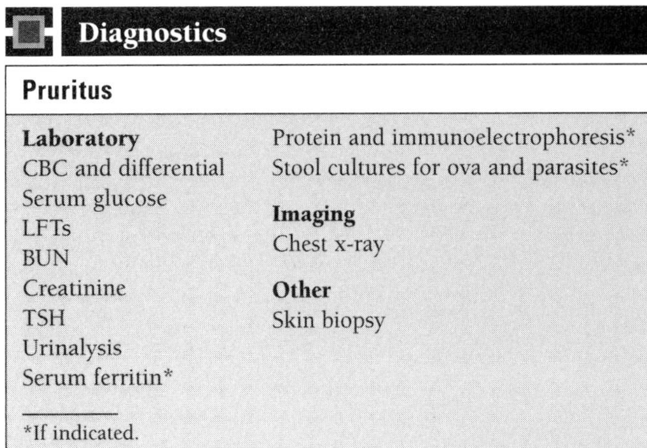

Diagnostics

Pruritus

Laboratory	Protein and immunoelectrophoresis*
CBC and differential	Stool cultures for ova and parasites*
Serum glucose	**Imaging**
LFTs	Chest x-ray
BUN	
Creatinine	**Other**
TSH	Skin biopsy
Urinalysis	
Serum ferritin*	

*If indicated.

follow-up or to refer the patient for dermatologic or psychiatric evaluation.

DIFFERENTIAL DIAGNOSIS

Dermatologic disorders with pruritus as a predominant symptom are common. Some of these disorders are covered in detail in other chapters, and each has its own etiology, clinical presentation, and treatment considerations. Pruritus without diagnostic skin lesions that persists longer than 2 weeks and is undiagnosed after 2 weeks of evaluation is called *pruritus of undetermined origin* (PUO) and may indicate a systemic disorder. Other causes and types of pruritus have been described but are quite rare.[1] Medications are also an important cause of pruritus.

MANAGEMENT

The success of treatment for pruritus depends on identification of the underlying dermatologic or systemic cause. In addition to appropriate treatment, pruritus will require interventions to alleviate this annoying symptom, although often not completely. Disrupting the scratch-itch cycle by alleviating pruritus is a mainstay of therapy for dermatitis. Medications that cause pruritus should be stopped. Taking steps to avoid irritants (e.g., wool or misguided topical therapy), reducing stress, and keeping the nails trimmed should be pursued. Cooling of the skin by the use of light clothing, air-conditioning, or frequent application of cool wet compresses, cooling lotions such as calamine, or aqueous creams is useful. Phenol, menthol, and camphor have been used. A tepid bath before retiring can alleviate pruritus long enough for the patient to fall asleep. Decreased bathing frequency and emollients are effective for any condition in which dry skin (xerosis) is present. Pramoxine hydrochloride (often combined with other topical agents) and 5% doxepin cream, a topical tricyclic antidepressant, have proved effective in several trials.[2] Topical and oral corticosteroids should be reserved only for cases of cutaneous inflammation. Topical antihistamines and anesthetics are sensitizers and therefore should be discouraged. Capsaicin works for localized pruritus.[3]

Oral therapy consists of H_1 antagonists such as diphenhydramine (25 to 50 mg every 6 hours), chlorpheniramine (4 mg every 4 to 6 hours), or hydroxyzine (25 to 50 mg every 4 to 6 hours), which can be beneficial, especially at bedtime. Sedative

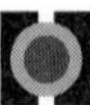

Differential Diagnosis

Pruritus

Pruritic Dermatologic Disorders

- Inflammatory disorders
  - Xerosis (asteatotic eczema)
  - Atopic dermatitis (eczema, the "itch that rashes")
  - Nummular eczema
  - Dyshydrotic eczema
  - Lichen simplex chronicus
  - Contact dermatitis (chemical or allergic)
  - Urticaria and dermatographism
  - Lichen planus
  - Psoriasis
  - Aquagenic pruritus
  - Rhus dermatitis (poison ivy and poison oak)
  - Miliaria
  - Nodular prurigo
  - Bullous and prebullous pemphigoid
  - Dermatitis herpetiformis
  - Pruritic urticarial papules and plaques of pregnancy
  - Polymorphic light eruption (and other photosensitive reactions)
- Infectious disorders
  - Viral exanthema (e.g., varicella)
  - Dermatophytes
  - Folliculitis (hot tubs)
  - Impetigo
- Infestations
  - Scabies
  - Pediculosis
  - Sea bather's eruption (jelly fish larvae)
  - Insect bites (e.g., fleas, mites, bedbugs)
  - Parasitic infections (e.g., onchocerciasis, echinococcosis, schistosomiasis)
- Neoplastic disorders
  - Mycosis fungoides
  - Mastocytosis
- Environmental disorders
  - Sunburn
  - Fiberglass dermatitis
  - Pernio/chilblains
  - Winter itch (dry ambient environment, excessive bathing)
  - Other (wool, hairs, fabric softeners, brighteners, other chemicals)
  - Aquagenic pruritus (histamine mediated, lasts 1 hour after exposure to water)

Systemic Disorders Associated with Pruritus

- Metabolic and endocrine disorders
  - Diabetes mellitus (anogenital pruritus more common)
  - Postmenopausal estrogen withdrawal (anogenital and generalized)
  - Adrenal insufficiency
  - Carcinoid syndrome
  - Hypothyroidism (secondary to dry skin in myxedema)
  - Hyperthyroidism (secondary to elevated skin temperature)
- Hematologic disorders
  - Polycythemia vera (typically water induced or "bath itch")
  - Iron deficiency anemia
  - Paraproteinemia
  - Waldenström's macroglobulinemia
- Malignant neoplasms
  - Lymphoma (Hodgkin's) and leukemia
  - Abdominal visceral carcinoma
  - CNS tumors
  - Multiple myeloma
  - Mycosis fungoides
- Hepatobiliary disorders
  - Primary biliary cirrhosis (from bile salts and associated substances)
  - Biliary obstruction (cholestasis)
  - Cholestasis of pregnancy
- Renal disorders
  - Chronic renal failure (80% of patients on hemodialysis, can be from secondary hyperparathyroidism)
- Parasitic infestations
  - Hookworm, onchocerciasis, ascariasis, trichinosis
- Infections
  - HIV (pruritus can be the primary presentation)
- Psychologic states
  - Delusions of parasitosis
  - Neurotic excoriations (can be extensive)
  - Psychogenic pruritus (anxiety induced)

Medications That Cause Pruritis

- Opiates and derivatives
- Aspirin
- Quinidine
- Phenothiazines*
- Tolbutamide*
- Erythromycin estolate*
- Hormones* (e.g., anabolic steroids, estrogens, progestins, testosterone)
- Vitamin B complex
- Psoralen plus ultraviolet A light (PUVA)
- Antimalarials
- Subclinical sensitivity to any drug

*Via cholestasis.

side effects are common, which may explain their therapeutic benefit. Nonsedating antihistamines have yielded inconsistent results in clinical trials but are better tolerated during the day.[4] The oral tricyclic antidepressant doxepin (25 mg every night up to 300 mg daily [in divided doses]) is a potent H_1 and H_2 receptor blocker that has anxiolytic effects. Amitriptyline (25 mg at night up to 150 mg daily [in divided doses]) is a less favorable alternative. Opiate antagonists such as naltrexone have been used for various causes of pruritus with success but are in general not first-line agents.[5] Oral activated charcoal is a safe, effective therapy for uremic pruritus.[6] Cholestyramine (4 g once to three times daily) is effective for pruritus caused by cholestasis, but it can have untoward gastrointestinal side effects and should be taken with vitamin K and multivitamin supplements. Colestipol works similarly but is better tolerated. In refractory cases of cholestatic pruritus, ursodiol, phenobarbital, and rifampin have been used with good results.[3] Patients with liver disease should have diets high in polyunsaturated fatty acids. Danazol is effective therapy for myeloproliferative disorders and other systemic disorders.[7] Cyproheptadine (4 mg t.i.d.) and aspirin have both been shown to help patients with pruritis from polycythemia vera. Ultraviolet B (UVB), sunlight, and topical clobetasol are all efficacious in pruritus associated with HIV disease.[3]

COMPLICATIONS

Secondary skin lesions from scratching and secondary infections are common. Other complications include an undiagnosed underlying systemic illness or untoward side effects from drug therapy.

INDICATIONS FOR REFERRAL/HOSPITALIZATION

Consultation with a dermatologist should be considered for intractable cases of pruritus or when the etiology remains unknown after the preliminary evaluation and follow-up. UVB phototherapy is very effective for uremic pruritus (i.e., those receiving dialysis). Psoralen plus ultraviolet A (PUVA), intralesional corticosteroid therapy, or other methods may be used. Other approaches include the use of acupuncture, transcutaneous electrical stimulation, mechanical vibratory stimulation, or referral to a pain relief clinic. Psychotherapeutic interventions have been shown to be beneficial in some patients.[8] If a systemic disorder is discovered, referral to an endocrinologist, hematologist, oncologist, gastroenterologist, nephrologist, psychiatrist, or other subspecialist may be in order.

PATIENT AND FAMILY EDUCATION/HEALTH PROMOTION

Lifestyle interventions to alleviate pruritus require a concerted effort at patient education to identify factors that provoke or worsen itching. Avoiding dry skin through the use of humidifiers, limited bathing, mild soaps, and emollients is critical. Elimination of wool and other clothing irritants, stress reduction measures, and instructions on medication side effects are also very helpful in the management of pruritus.

REFERENCES

1. Bernhard JD: Pruritus: pathophysiology and clinical aspects. In Moschella SL, Hurley HJ, editors: *Dermatology,* ed 3, Philadelphia, 1992, WB Saunders.
2. Millikan LE: Treating pruritus: what's new in safe relief of symptoms? *Postgrad Med* 99:173, 1996.
3. Rupp JF, Kaplan DL: Pruritis: causes-cures, parts 1, 2, and 3, *Consultant* November:3157, 1999; December:3367, 1999; February:321, 2000.
4. Behrendt H, Ring J: Histamine, antihistamines and atopic eczema, *Clin Exp Allergy* 20(suppl 4):25, 1990.
5. Wolfhagan FH and others: Oral naltrexone treatment for cholestatic pruritus: a double blind, placebo-controlled study, *Gastroenterology* 113:1264, 1997.
6. Giovannetti S and others: Oral activated charcoal in patients with uremic pruritus, *Nephron* 70:193, 1995.
7. Kolodny L and others: Danazol relieves refractory pruritus associated with myeloproliferative disorders and other diseases, *Am J Hematol* 51:112, 1996.
8. Kimyai-Asadi A, Usman A: The role of psychological stress in skin disease, *J Cutan Med Surg* 5:140, 2001.

CHAPTER 67

Psoriasis

Catherine E. Turner

DEFINITION/EPIDEMIOLOGY

Psoriasis is a papulosquamous eruption characterized by well-circumscribed erythematous macular and papular lesions with loosely adherent silvery white scale. It is a chronic, unpredictable disorder that is characterized by remissions and exacerbations throughout the life span. First episodes often appear in young adulthood, but they can appear later in life as well. Stress, anxiety, and illness often precede flares. Strep pharyngitis (sore throat) and some drug therapies (beta blockers, antimalarial agents, systemic steroids)[1,2] may precipitate or exacerbate an outbreak. Time lost from school and work, as well as the emotional and financial constraints on families, mandates cost-effective and convenient treatments. Symptoms can be treated but as yet there is no cure. Remissions are common and can last for short periods or years, although in some persons treatment can be refractory.[3]

The etiology is unknown, and the course is unpredictable. Although most patients experience localized plaques, extensive involvement may develop and cause the patient and family great social, psychologic, and economic distress.

From 1% to 3% of the population is affected by psoriasis, with 25% to 45% beginning after age 10.[4] Psoriasis is slightly more prevalent in women.[5] Congenital psoriasis is rare. It does seem to be passed genetically and thus a familial tendency can increase risk, although many individuals cannot recall family members who had the disease.

PATHOPHYSIOLOGY

The pathogenesis of psoriasis is unclear. The epidermis is thickened in psoriatic patients. The normal cell transit time of 20 to 28 days is shortened. Transit time from basal skin layer to the surface is 3 to 4 days. Scaly papules and plaques form and collect on the surface in well-demarcated lesions. The lesions have an erythematous base with silvery white plaques that are adherent. The dermis is highly vascular, and tiny bleeding points are revealed if the scales are removed (Auspitz's sign).[2]

CLINICAL PRESENTATION AND PHYSICAL EXAMINATION

Psoriasis is a clinical diagnosis based on the characteristic silvery white scales (Color Plate 23). Common sites include the elbows, knees, scalp, genitalia, and intergluteal cleft. In contrast to adult psoriasis, childhood psoriasis often involves the face. Many patients exhibit nail dystrophies (see Color Plate 22), including pitting, yellowing of the distal portion, separation of the nail plate (onycholysis), and thickening of the entire nail (hyperkeratosis).

Cutaneous trauma can induce psoriasis 1 to 3 weeks after injury. This isomorphic response, also known as Koebner's phenomenon, occurs in a linear fashion along the lines of a scratch, abrasion, sunburn, or pressure.

Discrete scaly plaques that begin on the trunk and spread to the extremities, sparing the palms and soles, are indicative of guttate psoriasis. The word *guttate* is derived from the Latin word *gyttata,* meaning "drop." Guttate psoriasis presents after a streptococcal infection and is most common in adolescents. These patients are likely to develop psoriasis vulgaris later in life (common, plaque-like psoriasis).

Erythroderma and pustular psoriasis are more serious forms of the disease. They are most common in patients older than 50 years and may be precipitated by infection and recent use of systemic steroids. Erythrodermic forms generally appear over a large portion of the body and can be precipitated by various treatments themselves. (It can occur after treatment with systemic steroids, emotional stress, other toxic medication, or a severe illness.)

Although most psoriatic lesions are asymptomatic, itching is variable. However, picking and scratching the lesions can produce Koebner's response, and the lesions worsen. Skinfold lesions tend to itch more than do common plaque-type lesions. The vulva is a common site for intense itching, or "inverse psoriasis."[3]

In psoriatic arthritis, one or several joints are involved. Although rare in children, it is recognized with increasing frequency in patients younger than 16 years. It is most common in female patients, with the peak onset at age 9 to 12 years. The clinical presentation is similar to that of any inflammatory arthritis.[4,6] The rheumatoid factor is negative, and the distal interphalangeal joints are common sites for arthralgias.[2]

DIAGNOSTICS

The presence of silvery scales on red, erythematous plaques is characteristic; therefore the diagnosis is based on presentation.

DIFFERENTIAL DIAGNOSIS

In children the plaques of psoriasis are thinner and less scaly than in those adults with psoriasis and are often confused with seborrhea and fungal infections. Seborrhea on the scalp tends to be patchy, red, and a bit more oily in appearance. Psoriasis is more plaque-like with thick scales. Psoriasis generally appears on extensor surfaces, whereas atopic dermatitis is found on most flexor surfaces. Lichen planus papules have more of a purple hue, and patients exhibit Wickham's striae (lacy reticular crisscrossed whitish lines) on many lesions. Flat warts do not have scale on the surface. Guttate psoriasis is often confused with pityriasis rosea, but it lacks the characteristic herald patch, and the scale is thicker and more diffuse in psoriasis. Changes in the nails are often confused with onychomycosis. Culturing for the presence of fungus will help establish the diagnosis. Yellow discoloration is common in both fungal and psoriatic changes, as is nail separation. The nails in psoriasis are not well formed as debris collects underneath, again due to rapid shedding of the skin layers. This debris leads to failure in the integrity of the nail and the onycholysis.

MANAGEMENT

Good control can be achieved but requires meticulous and consistent home care. Therapy is aimed at reducing epidermal proliferation and decreasing inflammation. Topical corticosteroids produce rapid resolution of plaques. Moderate- to high-potency topical glucocorticosteroids applied two or three times per day produce maximal benefit in 2 to 3 weeks. This is less messy than some treatments and can reduce pruritus. Tolerance can occur, and atrophy can occur with continued use over time. Occlusion with moist wraps can hasten the therapy on large or thick plaques. Thin layers of Duoderm alone can be placed and left for 5 to 7 days. Some providers prefer to start here, thinking initial corticosteroid use can make later use of other modalities recalcitrant.[2]

Differential Diagnosis

Psoriasis
Lichen planus
Flat warts
Pityriasis rosea
Rheumatoid arthritis
Nail fungus
Seborrheic dermatitis
Atopic dermatitis
Lichen planus
Flat warts
Pityriasis rosea
Fungal infections (in nails)

Intralesional injections with a corticosteroid suspension produce satisfactory results after one or two injections; this treatment requires a dermatology referral. Limitation of this therapy is atrophy and obvious discomfort from injections.

Phototherapy in the form of ultraviolet B (UVB) light therapy and psoralen plus ultraviolet A light (PUVA) is highly effective for recalcitrant psoriasis. Therapy in the structured environment of a dermatologist's office is of more therapeutic value than sunbathing. Care must be taken to avoid sunburn and resultant Koebner's phenomenon. Long-term therapy is often required, and skin should be monitored for changes. Skin cancer risk increases, especially in fair individuals, and patients should be advised to shield the eyes to prevent cataract risk with any phototherapy modality.

Scalp psoriasis requires softening and removing the scales. A combination of 3% salicylic acid in mineral oil, glycerin, or olive oil, or a mixture of phenol and sodium chloride, should be massaged into the scalp and left on for several hours or overnight. An appropriate tar shampoo should then be used. Daily use of this therapy will remove the scale and allow penetration of a corticosteroid lotion to reduce inflammation.[7]

Coal tar preparations are an effective treatment and were a mainstay of therapy for many years. Newer preparations are more pleasant but are considered only moderately effective. Tar preparations can cause folliculitis and stain the skin and clothing. Their use has largely been replaced by topical corticosteroids. Anthralin can be irritating if not thoroughly washed off the skin, stains the skin and clothing, and is difficult to apply.

Newer topical vitamin D (Dovonex) and retinoid (Tazorac) preparations, applied once daily, may be equally effective as topical corticosteroid treatments and can be used in combination with steroid and phototherapy treatments. These topical treatments reduce cell proliferation and induce remissions.

Oral retinoids (Tegison, Soriatane) are useful for pustular and erythrodermic psoriasis. However, their side effects are similar to those of isotretoin and should be used with caution in women of childbearing age because they are teratogenic. In addition, their effects on growing bones limit their use in children.

Methotrexate is an antimetabolite that is highly effective in treating severe, recalcitrant psoriasis and psoriatic arthritis. Its side effects include mucous membrane ulcers, lowered platelet and leukocyte counts, elevated liver enzyme levels, and gastrointestinal disturbances. It should be reserved for patients unresponsive to other therapies and for those with psoriatic arthritis.[8] Methotrexate and retinoid therapy should be co-managed with a dermatologist.

Cyclosporin is efficacious but is also limited in use because of its potential nephrotoxicity. Relapse is also common once therapy is stopped. Patients who require cyclosporin therapy should be managed by a dermatologist.

Combination therapy with topical agents, oral agents, and phototherapy is common. Even in patients maintained on topical treatments alone, it is useful to use multiple agents simultaneously for their synergistic effects. If more than 20% to 30% of the body is involved, generally the phototherapies and more systemic treatments are required. For smaller flares or chronicity, early treatment with combination therapies centered around topical treatments can manage the disease and minimize risk.

Guttate psoriasis should be treated with oral antibiotics to eliminate the streptococcal infection, in addition to topical preparations to reduce the scale and inflammation. Antistreptolysin levels should be monitored and elevations treated until remission.

Oral steroids should be used with caution because they can induce a pustular flare. They may be useful in controlling persistent erythroderma but are not indicated in the treatment of psoriasis.

COMPLICATIONS

Complications are usually related to infection. Scratching can introduce bacteria from beneath fingernails into lesions. Guttate psoriasis, erythrodermic psoriasis, and pustular psoriasis are also potential complications. Both erythrodermic psoriasis and pustular psoriasis are rare, but serious sequelae, including congestive heart failure and sepsis, are potential hazards. Other complications are generally secondary to treatment; these can include atrophy of skin with corticosteroid use, the risk with phototherapy of skin cancer and cataracts if the eyes are not protected, and the side effects of strong antimetabolites or retinoids to the metabolic profiles.

INDICATIONS FOR REFERRAL/HOSPITALIZATION

A patient with recalcitrant or unresponsive psoriasis should be referred to a dermatologist for management with phototherapy and for management with oral therapies. If dermatology referral is not possible, an internist may be appropriate for oral therapy. Referral to a rheumatologist or internist for patients with psoriatic arthritis is advised.

PATIENT AND FAMILY EDUCATION/HEALTH PROMOTION

It is crucial for the patient and family to understand the chronic nature of psoriasis, as well as the genetic and environmental factors. Adherence to the prescribed regimen is necessary for effective treatment, but this requires meticulous and consistent home care.

Patients should understand the use of moisturizers and lubricants to maintain control. Education regarding treatment modalities and emotional support for families, as well as patients, is an important part of treatment. Patients may contact the National Psoriasis Foundation (NPF) (http://www.psoriasis.org/), a not-for-profit organization dedicated to research, education, and support.

REFERENCES

1. Lehne R: *Pharmacology for nursing care,* ed 2, Philadelphia, 1994, WB Saunders.
2. Habif T: *Clinical dermatology: a color guide to diagnosis and therapy,* ed 3, St Louis, 1996, Mosby.
3. Tierney LM, McPhee SJ, Papadakis MA: *Current: Medical diagnosis and treatment 1997,* ed 36, Stamford, CT, 1997, Appleton & Lange.
4. Vernon P: The heartbreak of psoriasis: no laughing matter, *J Pediatr Health Care* 11:32, 1997.
5. National Psoriasis Foundation. Retrieved August 12, 2002, from the World Wide Web: http://www.psoriasis.org.
6. Hurwitz S: *Clinical pediatric dermatology,* ed 2, Philadelphia, 1993, WB Saunders.
7. Arndt K: *Manual of dermatologic therapeutics,* ed 5, Boston, 1995, Little, Brown.
8. Weston WL, Lane AT, Morrelli JG: *Color textbook of pediatric dermatology,* ed 2, St Louis, 1996, Mosby.

CHAPTER 68

Purpura

Joanne Sandberg-Cook

DEFINITION/EPIDEMIOLOGY

Purpura is a hemorrhaging into the skin. The size of the bleeding vessel determines the size of the lesion, which in turn may provide clues to the etiology. Petechiae are lesions less than 3 mm in diameter; these indicate capillary bleeding. Lesions ranging from 3 mm to 1 cm are often referred to as purpura. Lesions larger than 1 cm are referred to as *ecchymoses.* All show a predilection for the limbs. Purpura is divided into two groups: inflammatory (palpable) and noninflammatory. Noninflammatory purpura is further divided into hemostatic defects, nonpalpable purpura, and nonhemostatic defects (vascular purpuras).[1]

PATHOPHYSIOLOGY

Purpura is characterized by an extravasation of red blood cells into the dermis from small cutaneous vessels. Hemosiderin or hematoidin may be present if the purpura is chronic; this causes a characteristic red or brown discoloration. Purpura may be oval or round or irregularly outlined; it may be flat or raised (palpable) as a result of edema or induration.

Palpable purpura consists of raised, erythematous lesions that do not blanch when the skin is pressed with a glass slide. Dilated superficial capillaries, in which the blood remains confined within the vessels, do blanch when pressed, thereby distinguishing it from true purpura.

Extravasation of blood from the vessel depends on the integrity of the blood vessel, which in turn depends on the strength of the vessel, the transmural pressure gradient that drives blood out of the vessel, and the competence of the mechanism that combats the basal level of vascular trauma.[1]

CLINICAL PRESENTATION

Because purpura is a symptom of many systemic diseases, these lesions seldom present without other symptoms. A review of systems should include an inquiry into other bleeding sites, abnormally heavy menstrual bleeding, trauma, recent infection (including sexually transmitted diseases), exposure to ticks or a tick bite, and recent travel to areas where Rocky Mountain spotted fever or Lyme disease is endemic or epidemic. A complete medication history (including over-the-counter medications and allergies) should be taken. Any history of autoimmune disease or other serious illnesses such as leukemia or lymphoma should be noted. Recent complaints of fever, chills, arthralgias, and myalgias should also be determined.

PHYSICAL EXAMINATION

The skin is the focus of the physical examination. The size, location, and shape of the lesions should be documented. Bullae and ulcerations can develop within any lesion larger than petechiae.[2] Lesions should be palpated for swelling (palpable purpura) or flatness against the skin. Palpable purpura is generally associated with inflammation of the vessel (Color Plate 24) (see

Chapter 244). A glass slide pressed against the lesion determines whether it is blanchable, thereby differentiating it from erythema or dilated superficial capillaries.[1] Excoriation may imply pruritus.

The remainder of the general examination includes an oral examination to look for lesions of the gums or tongue and a joint examination to look for swelling, inflammation, or deformities that would suggest connective tissue disease. Fever, nuchal rigidity, organomegaly, or a new heart murmur may imply serious systemic disease or infection.

Observations of weight, nutritional status, or skin turgor may suggest nutritional deficiencies. Evidence of trauma (healing bruises, fractures) may indicate ongoing trauma as an etiology.

DIAGNOSTICS

Laboratory studies help differentiate between inflammatory and noninflammatory purpura. (Inflammatory purpura [vasculitis] is discussed in Chapter 244.) A CBC with a platelet count (not an estimate) is most helpful. An erythrocyte sedimentation rate (ESR) can be beneficial in excluding an inflammatory cause. A bleeding time, platelet count, prothrombin time (PT), partial thromboplastin time (PTT), and an international normalization ratio (INR) will determine the presence of coagulopathies. BUN, creatinine, and LFTs are necessary to exclude organ disease. Immune studies to exclude autoimmune diseases such as lupus, rheumatoid arthritis, cryoglobulinemias, or scleroderma may be indicated depending on other physical findings and symptoms.

DIFFERENTIAL DIAGNOSIS

The differential diagnosis of purpura is extensive. Inflammatory and noninflammatory causes of purpura should be differentiated. Inflammatory purpura is most often palpable and is associated with the vasculitides. These syndromes can be life threatening and require prompt treatment in conjunction with a specialist (see Chapter 244). Causes of noninflammatory purpura include serious infectious diseases, medication hypersensitivity, trauma, vascular disorders, and bleeding disorders.

Systemic infections such as HIV/AIDS, cytomegalovirus, hepatitis virus B and C, herpes zoster, Lyme disease (see Chapter 238), Rocky Mountain spotted fever, meningitis, syphilis, and gonococcemia have been associated with purpura.[2] Subacute bacterial endocarditis may present with fever, petechial skin rash, and a new heart murmur.

Noninfectious presentations are often related to medications, including the long-term use of oral steroids and fluorinated topical steroids. Drug-induced vasculitis is the most common cause of palpable purpura and can occur at any time during the course of the medication. These allergic reactions to medication may be associated with fever, arthralgia, and urticaria.[2] The most common causative agents are antibiotics, sulfonamides, thiazide diuretics, phenytoin, and allopurinol. Nonsteroidal antiinflammatory medications, including aspirin, can also cause petechial skin rashes.[4] Hypersensitivity syndromes, including allergic reactions to medications, can cause petechial skin rashes. Heparin, low-molecular-weight heparin, and warfarin (Coumadin) can cause bleeding, which can result in purpura.

Trauma to blood vessels presents as classic bruising, often involving the extremities, feet, hands (in the case of repetitive pounding), or face. The lesions associated with child abuse may involve bruising from pinching or grabbing or palpebral

Diagnostics

Purpura

Laboratory
- CBC and differential
- BUN
- Creatinine
- LFTs
- Platelet count
- ESR
- Bleeding time
- PT/PTT
- INR
- Rheumatoid factor*
- Antinuclear antibodies*
- Antineutrophil cytoplasmic antibody (ANCA)*

Other
- Skin biopsy

*If indicated.

Differential Diagnosis

Purpura

Inflammatory
- Palpable
  - Vasculitis
  - Cryoglobulinemia

Noninflammatory
- Hemostatic defects
  - Platelet abnormalities
  - Coagulation abnormalities
- Nonpalpable purpuras
  - Increased pressure
    - Venous stasis
  - Decreased vessel integrity
    - Senile purpura
    - Steroid excess
    - Vitamin C deficiency
    - Hormonal
  - Trauma
    - Physical injury
    - Solar injury
  - Infectious
    - Bacterial (meningococcemia)
    - Viral
    - Rickettsial (Lyme disease, Rocky Mountain spotted fever)
- Embolic
  - Atheroembolic
    - Cholesterol
- Neoplastic
  - Leukemia
  - Lymphoma
- Allergic
  - Medications
  - Contact
- Thrombotic
  - Disseminated intravascular coagulation
  - Purpura fulminans
  - Antiphospholipid syndrome
  - Idiopathic thrombotic thrombocytopenia purpura (ITTP)

conjunctivae resulting from strangulation or smothering.[1] Senile purpura presents as large ecchymoses on the extensor surfaces of the arms and hands of (usually) an older adult. Such lesions occur as a result of the skin thinning associated with age, sun damage, or prolonged steroid use in combination with minor trauma or shearing.[3] Laboratory studies are normal, and the patient should be reassured that the lesions are benign.

A variety of syndromes associated with vascular diseases can cause purpura. Atheroemboli secondary to cholesterol can cause petechiae, purpura, nodules, ulceration, and occlusion leading to gangrene. Fat emboli that occur 2 to 3 days after severe trauma can present with petechiae of the upper extremity, thorax, and conjunctivae.[1] Disseminated intravascular coagulation (DIC) demonstrates both thrombotic and hemorrhagic features. Purpura fulminans is a rare complication of DIC and results in hemorrhagic necrosis of the skin.[4]

Idiopathic thrombotic thrombocytopenia purpura (ITTP) is a syndrome of platelet aggregation in the microcirculation producing ischemia in the various organs. There is an association with von Willebrand factor.[5] Hemolytic anemia, thrombocytopenia, neurologic symptoms, renal disease, and fever can all be seen with this extremely serious syndrome.[5]

Petechiae and ecchymoses are quite common.[3] Stasis dermatitis presents with petechiae caused by capillary injury. This results from chronic venous stasis because of valve incompetence. Later stages of chronic venous stasis are associated with an accumulation of hemosiderin, resulting in the characteristic brown discoloration of the lower extremities.[4]

Miscellaneous causes of purpura include hemorrhagic gingivitis or stomatitis related to vitamin C deficiency (scurvy). Young women occasionally tend to bruise easily because of hormonal changes. A tendency toward early stroke, multiple miscarriages, and/or thrombocytopenia may be associated with the presence of antiphospholipid antibodies, sometimes known as lupus anticoagulant. HIV/AIDS and carcinomas, including lymphomas and leukemias, can produce petechial or purpuric lesions.[2] Finally, defects in clotting factors or platelet abnormalities, including the quantity and quality of platelets, can lead to cutaneous bleeding (see Chapter 232).

MANAGEMENT

Treatment of purpura is directed toward the etiology. Patients with disorders of platelet count or function should be referred to a hematologist for possible bone marrow biopsy. Patients with palpable purpura should be advised that an extensive evaluation, including a skin biopsy, may be indicated. A referral to appropriate specialists, usually a hematologist or rheumatologist, is indicated.

Patients with stasis dermatitis may benefit from the application of 1% hydrocortisone cream to help with the associated pruritus. A reassurance that the lesions are benign is needed for young women who bruise easily because of hormonal changes and for older patients with senile purpura.

LIFE SPAN CONSIDERATIONS

Purpura associated with hormonal change is most often seen in young women. Senile purpura is primarily a disease of older adults but can result from chronic steroid use. Antiphospholipid antibodies are most commonly found in women of childbearing years, but men and older women can also be affected. The vasculitides are most often seen in middle-aged patients, with several notable exceptions.

COMPLICATIONS

Complications of the skin lesions themselves include the formation of bullae, skin breakdown, and ulcer formation. Ulcers are slow to heal and can involve a large area. Necrosis of the skin, especially the fingertips, can be a complication of vascular lesions.

INDICATIONS FOR REFERRAL/HOSPITALIZATION

Any patient with fever and a petechial skin rash should be hospitalized to exclude or evaluate life-threatening infection, systemic vasculitis, or neoplasm. This is especially necessary if the patient has a connective tissue disease such as lupus or rheumatoid arthritis, has a malignancy, or has been exposed to meningitis. Patients with acute bleeding disorders may require hospitalization to control bleeding and for transfusion. All patients with palpable purpura should be referred to a hematologist or rheumatologist for evaluation and treatment recommendations.

PATIENT AND FAMILY EDUCATION/HEALTH PROMOTION

Medications that may contribute to bleeding should be avoided unless the patient is advised to continue as part of a treatment plan. Patients with stasis should be advised to avoid tight-fitting garments and prolonged standing. Chronic use of steroid creams or ointments should be discouraged because it leads to skin thinning and increased susceptibility to minor trauma.

REFERENCES

1. Beutler E and others: *William's hematology,* ed 5, New York, 1995, McGraw-Hill.
2. Braverman IM: *Skin signs of systemic disease,* ed 3, 1998, WB Saunders.
3. Soter N: Vasculitis in primary care dermatology. In Arndt K and others, editors: Philadelphia, 1997, WB Saunders.
4. Weedon D: *Skin pathology,* New York, 1997, Churchill Livingstone.
5. Moake J, Chow T: Thrombotic thrombocytopenic purpura: understanding a disease no longer rare, *Am J Med Sci* 316:105, 1998.

CHAPTER 69

Scabies

Eileen M. Deignan

DEFINITION/EPIDEMIOLOGY

Scabies is an infection caused by infestation of the *Sarcoptes scabiei* mite. It can affect people of all ages and is more common in crowded living conditions and institutional facilities.

PATHOPHYSIOLOGY

The scabies mite is not visible to the unaided eye. The female mite is responsible for the infestations. The mite is oval in shape and has four pairs of legs. It burrows into the stratum corneum and lays up to 38 eggs for 1 to 2 months before dying. The eggs hatch in approximately 1 week and reach maturity in 3 weeks, starting a new cycle.[1] The intense pruritus experienced with scabies infestation is a hypersensitivity reaction to the mites. It usually begins 2 to 4 weeks after infection in a person who is not previously sensitized. Pruritus may begin within a day of reinfestation in a previously sensitized person. Scabies is usually acquired through close personal contact, although the mite can survive off the human host for up to 3 days.

CLINICAL PRESENTATION AND PHYSICAL EXAMINATION

The clinical presentation of scabies is variable. Most commonly there are minimal findings in the setting of intractable pruritus. The skin lesions of scabies can be classified into two categories: lesions at the site of infestation and lesions secondary to hypersensitivity to the mite. Intraepidermal burrows are linear or serpiginous ridges that are produced by the infesting female mite. Common sites of burrows are the interdigital spaces of the hands, flexures of the wrists and arms, genitals, feet, buttocks, and axillae (Color Plate 25). A hypersensitivity reaction to the mites can be manifested as urticaria, eczematous dermatitis, and scabetic nodules. Excoriations, lichen simplex chronicus, and secondary infection may result from scratching.

DIAGNOSTICS

The classic burrow, a straight or S-shaped ridge 5 to 20 mm long, is present less than 20% of the time. Definitive confirmation is made with a scabies prep. A drop of mineral oil is placed on a burrow, and the lesion is scraped with a #15 blade. The sample is viewed under a microscope and examined for mites, eggs, or feces.[2] There are usually only a few scabies mites on an infected patient. As a result, several areas may need to be sampled to get a positive result.

DIFFERENTIAL DIAGNOSIS

Scabies may easily be mistaken for other skin disorders. The differential diagnosis should include contact dermatitis, asteatotic dermatitis, insect bites, animal scabies, seborrheic dermatitis, and psoriasis.

MANAGEMENT

Topical application of 5% permethrin cream (Elimite) is the treatment of choice. The cream should be applied from the neck down, giving attention to the interdigital webs, axilla, umbilicus, gluteal cleft, genitals, and areas under the nails. Because scabies can infest the hairline of older adults, the product is massaged into the skin from head to toe in these patients. The medication should be left on for 8 to 12 hours and then washed off.[3,4] This product can be safely used again in 1 week because it is rapidly metabolized.[3,4]

Diagnostics

Scabies

Laboratory
Microscopic examination for mites or eggs

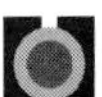

Differential Diagnosis

Scabies

Atopic dermatitis
Insect bites
Pediculosis
Pityriasis rosea
Animal scabies
Seborrheic dermatitis
Syphilis
Contact dermatitis
Psoriasis

An important change in treatment guidelines is that lindane (Kwell) is no longer recommended for the treatment of scabies. Absorption of lindane is 10 times higher than permethrin. There have been reports of seizures with repeated exposure.

Persistent pruritic papules and eczematous manifestations may result from both infestation and treatment. Lubrication and topical corticosteroids are used to treat the inflammation, and antihistamines are used to treat the pruritus. A secondary infection may result from scratching. Pustules, impetigo, and ecthyma should be treated with appropriate antibiotics.

Ivermectin is an antihelminthic medication that is useful for treatment of scabies. It is effective and relatively easy to use because it is administered orally. Because ivermectin is an oral medication that does not need to be absorbed by the skin, it is useful for patients with crusted scabies. The dose of ivermectin is 200 μg/kg. The average adult dose is 12 to 18 mg, administered as a single, one-time dose.[5]

COMPLICATIONS

Superinfection is a potential complication. Acute glomerulonephritis has been associated with streptococcal superinfection. Serious toxicity has been associated with lindane treatment. Thus treatment with lindane should be used cautiously, particularly with children.

INDICATIONS FOR REFERRAL/HOSPITALIZATION

Elimite (permethrin) is not approved by U.S. Food and Drug Administration for use in infants less than 2 months old. Whether permethrin is secreted in human milk is not known. Deaths have been associated with the use of ivermectin for scabies in older adults. Therefore this medication should be used with caution. Consultation with the physician or specialist is recommended if scabies is identified in these patients before a specific medication is chosen.[5-7]

PATIENT AND FAMILY EDUCATION

All household contacts should be identified and treated. All clothing and bedding must be washed in hot water and dried on the hot cycle, and stuffed sofas and chairs should be vacuumed. Materials that cannot be washed should be placed in a plastic bag for 1 week. Patients should be given written and verbal instructions. Recalcitrant infestation or persistent pruritus requires physician consultation.

REFERENCES

1. Weston WL, Lane AT, Morrelli JG: *Color textbook of pediatric dermatology,* ed 2, St Louis, 1996, Mosby.
2. Arndt K: *Manual of dermatologic therapeutics,* ed 5, Boston, 1995, Little, Brown.
3. Hurwitz S: *Clinical pediatric dermatology,* ed 2, Philadelphia, 1993, WB Saunders.
4. Fox J: *Primary health care of children,* St Louis, 1997, Mosby.
5. Chouela E and others: Diagnosis and treatment of scabies: a practical guide, *Am J Clin Dermatol* 3(1):9-18, 2002.
6. *Nurse practitioners' prescribing reference:* vol. 5, number 2, New York, 1998, Prescribing Reference.
7. Wilson BA, Shannon MT, Stang CC: *Nurses drug guide,* Norwalk, Conn, 1995, Appleton & Lange.

CHAPTER 70

Seborrheic Dermatitis

Eileen M. Deignan

DEFINITION/EPIDEMIOLOGY

Seborrheic dermatitis is a chronic, common dermatosis. It is characterized by greasy, slightly erythematous scaling that occurs in areas with the highest concentration of sweat glands or sebaceous glands, including the scalp, face, postauricular, and intertriginous areas.[1]

PATHOPHYSIOLOGY

The cause of seborrheic dermatitis is unknown. Although an inflammatory reaction to *Pityrosporum orbiculare* has been postulated, it is possible that seborrheic dermatitis may be caused by yeast secondary to prolonged retention of sebum on the skin.[2,3]

CLINICAL PRESENTATION AND PHYSICAL EXAMINATION

Seborrheic dermatitis is seen in both young and old patients. In infants, the most common presentation is yellow or brown scaling lesions on the scalp, and is called "cradle cap." In adolescents and adults, another common presentation is dry, flaky scales on the scalp. This disorder is known as dandruff.

On the face and auricular area, seborrheic dermatitis presents as greasy, erythematous, sharply marginated plaques. Polycyclic plaques are commonly seen on the sternal area. In the axillae and groins, the eruption presents as more confluent plaques with a fine scale and less well-defined borders. This disorder may persist throughout life and may be worse during adolescence. Lesions are usually asymptomatic, although occasionally pruritus is present.[4]

DIAGNOSTICS AND DIFFERENTIAL DIAGNOSIS

The differential diagnosis is broad. More common diseases that can resemble seborrheic dermatitis include psoriasis, impetigo, dermatophytosis, tinea versicolor, intertriginous candidiasis, otitis externa, blepharitis, and systemic lupus erythematosus. Dermatophytosis, candidiasis, fungal otitis externa, and tinea versicolor can be differentiated from seborrhea with a potassium hydroxide scraping positive for hyphae. Psoriasis is often difficult to distinguish from seborrheic dermatitis. History and characteristic findings of psoriasis such as nail changes and lesions on the extensor surfaces help to differentiate the two diseases.

Less common diseases that can resemble seborrheic dermatitis include Langerhans' cell histiocytosis, acrodermatitis enteropathica, pemphigus foliaceous, and glucagonoma syndrome. If these disorders are considered, there should be consultation with a dermatologist.[2,5]

MANAGEMENT

Treatment depends on the location and severity of the disorder. In some cases, patients who wash their hair only every week or less often will clear with more frequent washing. Antiseborrheic shampoos used three or four times a week will decrease

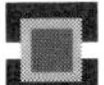

Diagnostics

Seborrheic Dermatitis

Initial
KOH wet preparation

Other
Skin biopsy*

*If indicated.

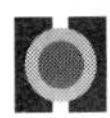

Differential Diagnosis

Seborrheic Dermatitis

Dandruff
Scabies
Tinea
Contact dermatitis
Psoriasis
Pemphigus
Impetigo
Dermatophytosis
Candida
Langerhans cell histiocytosis
Acrodermatitis enteropathica
Pemphigus foliaceous
Glucagonoma syndrome

eruptions or clear up the condition some cases. Some patients may require a topical steroid in the form of a lotion applied once a day after washing with an antiseborrheic shampoo. The topical steroid should be discontinued when the dermatitis improves. Mineral oil preparation massaged into the scalp and left to sit overnight on the scalp will loosen the scales in the more severe, psoriasis form of scalp seborrheic dermatitis.[4]

There are several options for therapy on the face. A simple solution is to use the lather of an antiseborrheic shampoo to wash the face on a daily basis. If this intervention does not help, a mild topical steroid can be used daily until the eruption clears. The shampoo should be continued for maintenance. Similar therapies can be used for eruptions on the chest and in intertriginous areas. Secondary bacterial or candidal infections should be treated with antibiotic and antifungal agents.

COMPLICATIONS

Secondary candidal infections and bacterial infections may occur, especially around the eyes and in intertriginous areas. These should be treated with appropriate antifungal medications and antibiotics. Periorificial dermatitis is a papular eruption that can occur around the eyes, nose, and mouth as a result of topical steroid overuse on the face. If this eruption occurs, topical steroids should be tapered off.

INDICATIONS FOR REFERRAL/HOSPITALIZATION

Patients with unresponsive seborrheic dermatitis should be referred to a dermatologist for further workup. As indicated previously, several dermatoses can resemble seborrheic dermatitis but will not respond to the same therapies.

PATIENT AND FAMILY EDUCATION

Seborrheic dermatitis is chronic and recurrent. Proper use of antiseborrheic preparations several days per week will usually control the disorder.

REFERENCES

1. Hurwitz S: *Clinical pediatric dermatology*, ed 2, Philadelphia, 1993, WB Saunders.
2. Dershewitz RA: *Ambulatory pediatric care*, ed 2, Philadelphia, 1993, JB Lippincott.
3. Arndt K: *Manual of dermatologic therapeutics*, ed 5, Boston, 1995, Little, Brown.
4. Odom RB, James WD, Berger TG: *Andrew's diseases of the skin*, ed 9, Philadelphia, 2000, WB Saunders
5. Weston WL, Lane AT, Morrelli JG: *Color textbook of pediatric dermatology*, ed 2, St Louis, 1996, Mosby.

CHAPTER 71

Stasis Dermatitis

Nancy W. Knee

DEFINITION/EPIDEMIOLOGY

Stasis dermatitis is a persistent inflammation or chronic dermatitis of the skin of the lower extremities. The condition is usually associated with chronic venous insufficiency, and ulceration is a potential complication.[1] The condition is most often seen in persons over 50 years of age and is more common in women than in men. Obesity is an associated factor, and relapses are common.[2]

PATHOPHYSIOLOGY

Stasis dermatitis is a recalcitrant condition related to venous incompetence associated with valve destruction. Valve leaflets become constricted and are unable to prevent venous regurgitation. This condition results in ischemia of the vasculature, skin, and supporting structures in the subcutaneous and dermis layers.[3] Perivascular fibrin deposits and small vessel vasoconstriction may be contributing factors.[4]

CLINICAL PRESENTATION AND PHYSICAL EXAMINATION

The hallmark sign of stasis dermatitis is bronzing (hemosiderin staining) of the affected skin. The eruption can be unilateral or bilateral and is initially localized to the ankle (Color Plate 26). Edema, a common manifestation, progresses from distal to proximal, and varicose veins are often present.[5] The condition is often insidious; full manifestation of the signs and symptoms may take months. Patients may present with mild pruritus, xerosis, a scaly and erythematous rash, cutaneous atrophy, and bulla formation. The skin may be cyanotic when the extremity is in a dependent position. Secondary bacterial infection (usually staphylococcal) ensues, and painful ulceration eventually occurs.[4] Often there is a past history of deep vein thrombosis.

DIAGNOSTICS

Doppler ultrasound and a venogram are used to diagnose venous insufficiency. Ulcers should be cultured for bacterial infection if indicated.

DIFFERENTIAL DIAGNOSIS

Other etiologies of ulceration should be considered. These include arterial insufficiency, carcinoma, sickle cell anemia, necrobiosis lipoidica, and pyoderma gangrenosum, and contact dermatitis (i.e., neomycin).[2]

MANAGEMENT

Therapeutics are based on the extent and acuity of the medical condition. The leg should be elevated above the heart for 30 minutes of rest at least four times a day to promote venous return and diminish or prevent edema. The patient should be fitted for graduated compression hose, and topical emollients should be applied daily. Maintenance of optimal skin integrity includes avoidance of trauma (including hot water in showers or baths). Mild soaps (e.g., Dove, Neutrogena) and adequate fluid intake should be encouraged. Systemic antibiotics are necessary for any cellulitis. Irritants such as lanolin, wool, and alcohol should be avoided.[4] Occasionally topical corticosteroids are indicated for pruritic, nonulcerated areas. A midpotency steroid can be used for a short time, with gradual reduction to a low-potency steroid cream. However, steroids should not be used if there are any signs of infection.

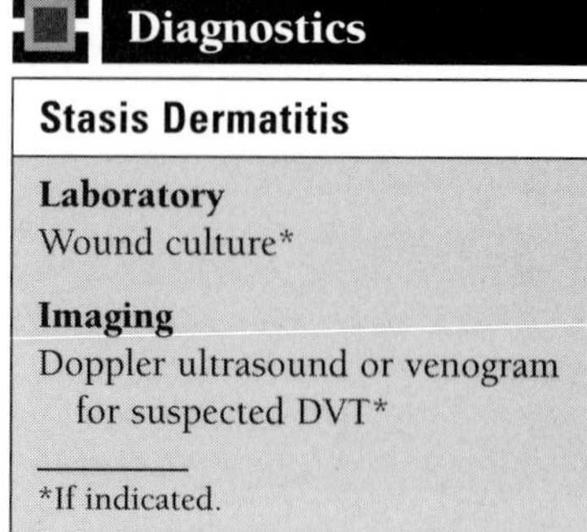

Diagnostics

Stasis Dermatitis

Laboratory
Wound culture*

Imaging
Doppler ultrasound or venogram for suspected DVT*

*If indicated.

Differential Diagnosis

Stasis Dermatitis

Arterial insufficiency
Carcinoma
Sickle cell anemia
Necrobiosis lipoidica
Pyoderma gangrenosum
Contact dermatitis

In the ulcerative phase, wet-to-dry normal saline dressings should be applied two to four times per day. Silver sulfadiazine may be applied between wet-to-dry dressings provided there is no known sulfa allergy.[1] Cultures should be obtained to guide management if there is infection. The wound should be kept free of necrosis. In some instances Dakin Solution #1 may be indicated, but consultation with a wound care specialist is recommended before instituting anything other than normal saline wet-to-dry dressing.[1] Early trials of Daflon, a venotropic drug, 500 mg b.i.d. have demonstrated a significant effect in reducing edema, healing venous leg ulcers, and reducing inflammation.[5] In select instances (e.g., small ulcerative areas that do not inhibit ambulation), a zinc gelatin bandage, Unna's paste boot, or absorptive dressing such as calcium alginate under a compression bandage may be used.[4] These devices should be changed every 2 to 3 days initially, then once or twice a week when the edema diminishes and the ulcer begins to heal.[4] Elevation and compression bandages should be used in conjunction with these therapies.

COMPLICATIONS

Ulceration or cellulitis may progress to osteomyelitis or pyoderma gangrenosum. Either of these conditions can cause significant morbidity and may even be fatal in compromised hosts.

INDICATIONS FOR REFERRAL/HOSPITALIZATION

Ulcerations that are recalcitrant to therapy or that penetrate past the dermis layer require referral to a general surgeon or plastic surgeon for partial-thickness grafting and/or recommended ulcer treatments.

Hospitalization is indicated for patients who require surgical intervention, lack the ability to perform medical therapies at home, or have infections that require IV antibiotics.

PATIENT AND FAMILY EDUCATION/HEALTH PROMOTION

Patients need to receive instruction and often closely monitored assistance regarding the application of compression hose, topical medications, colloid paste, or special dressing applications. The appropriate use, side effects, interactions, and contraindications of antibiotics should be carefully explained. Patients with chronic stasis dermatitis need to understand the importance of keeping the legs elevated as much as possible. The need for good nutrition, supplemental vitamins when indicated, and weight reduction should be encouraged.

REFERENCES

1. Fitzpatrick T and others: *Color atlas and synopsis of clinical dermatology,* ed 2, New York, 1991, McGraw-Hill.
2. Habif T and others: *Skin disorders: diagnosis and treatment,* St Louis, 2001, Mosby.
3. Berkow R: *The Merck manual,* ed 16, Rahway, NJ, 1992, Merck Research Laboratories.
4. Fenstermacher K, Hudson B: *Practice guidelines for family nurse practitioners,* Philadelphia, 1997, WB Saunders.
5. Ramelet AA: Clinical benefits of Daflon 500 mg in the most severe stages of chronic venous insufficiency, *Angiology* 52(suppl 1):S49-S50, 2001.

CHAPTER 72

Urticaria

Maureen O'Hara Padden

DEFINITION/EPIDEMIOLOGY

Urticaria, also referred to as hives, is caused by a vascular reaction that occurs in the upper dermis of the skin. It is characterized by the development of wheals on the body surface (Color Plate 27). Acute urticaria is defined as episodes of hives lasting less than 6 weeks. Conversely, chronic urticaria is defined as hives persisting for more than 6 weeks. Physical urticaria is a distinct form of urticaria caused by exposure to physical triggers such as mechanical, thermal, water, or cold. The hives associated with physical urticaria typically fade within an hour, except in the case of pressure urticaria, in which the hives take longer to develop and subsequently take longer to fade. In some cases, there is an association between thyroid autoimmunity and urticaria.[1] Historically, it had been believed that urticaria could be associated with an underlying malignancy such as lymphoma, leukemia, or colon cancer. Recent limited evidence suggests that such an association may not really exist.[2] It has been suggested that an association between *Helicobacter pylori* and urticaria exists, and this particular question is currently the subject of much investigation.

Urticaria is a common disorder and is estimated to affect 10% to 20% of the population at some time during their life.[3] In most cases it is relatively mild in presentation, albeit frustrating for the patient. In other cases, however, it represents part of a continuum that includes anaphylaxis and can be life threatening. Two thirds of all cases occur between the 20 and 40 years of age, and there appears to be no racial predilection.[4] *Acute* urticaria is more common in young adults, children, and atopic individuals. This form of urticaria is most often due to exposure to food allergens, food additives, medications, or radiocontrast media. *Chronic* urticaria is more common in middle-aged women, occurs twice as often in women as in men, and does not show the same predilection for individuals with atopy[4]; 75% of all cases are idiopathic. Only 50% of cases of chronic urticaria remit within a year, and up to 40% of cases lasting longer than 6 months persist for 10 years or more.[5]

Immediate emergency department referral/physician consultation is necessary for patients with angioedema, respiratory failure, or hemodynamic compromise.

PATHOPHYSIOLOGY

Urticaria is an immediate hypersensitivity reaction that occurs after exposure to an allergen or antigen. Mast cells located in the loose connective tissue of the skin release histamine in response to the exposure. Histamine binds to H_1-receptors, leading to dilation of capillaries and vascular permeability. Arteriolar dilation leads to flaring around the lesions, and extravasation of fluid from the leaky capillaries leads to wheals. The histamine that is released causes the pruritus.[6] The superficial itchy swellings in the skin caused by extravasation of fluid from leaky capillaries are referred to as wheals. Deeper swellings of the skin and alimentary tract can occur in some cases; these swellings tend to be more painful than pruritic and are consistent with angioedema.

Mast cells can also be activated by the immunoglobulin E (IgE) antibodies stimulated by foods, drugs, insect stings, latex, or animals. Alternatively, activation can occur directly by drugs, including opiates or radiocontrast media given to the patient. Other cell mediators such as complement and neuropeptides (substance P) may be involved. Rarely, chronic urticaria may be caused by IgG autoantibodies directed against the IgE receptor.[5]

CLINICAL PRESENTATION

Patients presenting with urticaria initially note pruritus followed by the development of hives. Lesions appear in crops that last for 2 to 3 hours and then disappear, only to flare up elsewhere later. They generally fade in less than 24 hours, leaving no trace. Episodes can occur as often as daily and in chronic urticaria can last for up to 2 years.

Important history can be simplified into the six *I*s: *i*nfections, *i*ngestants (food), *i*njectants (drugs), *i*nsect stings, *i*nhalants (pollen), and *i*nternal disease. Latex allergy is an increasing cause of urticaria. Other historical factors to be elicited are exposure to heat, fever, cold, exercise, change in menses, and emotional stress. In more severe cases of urticaria, the patient may experience angioedema and complain of difficulty breathing.

PHYSICAL EXAMINATION

Physical examination reveals edematous pink or red wheals surrounded by a bright red flare. The center of the lesions may be clear or, rarely, may develop bullae. Lesions typically appear on the torso but may occur anywhere on the body. The patient with physical urticaria caused by exposure to some physical stimulus may show what is referred to as dermatographism on examination. Dermatographism is the development of a wheal-and-flare reaction when the skin is stroked with a pen or other physical stimulus. In severe cases of urticaria with angioedema, there may be swelling of the face or oropharynx and deeper swelling in the dermis.

DIAGNOSTICS

Laboratory tests are generally of little value unless the history or examination suggests that they are needed. In fact, most cases of urticaria require no laboratory investigation, especially if mild disease is responding to therapy. They may be helpful in cases of chronic urticaria where physical causative agents have been excluded. Typical laboratory workup would include a complete blood count, white blood cell differential, and erythrocyte sedimentation rate. Urinalysis, hepatitis panel, thyroid panel, thyroid antimicrosomal antibody, antinuclear antibody, rheumatoid factor, serum complement C3 and C4, cryoglobulin, serum IgE and IgM, chest radiograph, and sinus series are less likely to be needed but may be ordered when indicated by history, physical examination, or consultation with a specialist. A skin biopsy may be done to assess for vasculitis if the sedimentation rate is increased or if hives are accompanied by arthralgia or burning sensation in the skin. Specific allergy or provocative tests may prove useful in certain patients (e.g., atopic individuals with severe urticaria) to establish sensitivity to certain foods that should be avoided.

DIFFERENTIAL DIAGNOSIS

The following should be considered in the differential diagnosis: insect bites, vasculitis, pityriasis rosea, syphilis, bullous pemphigoid, systemic lupus erythematosus, urticaria pigmentosa, drug eruptions, and erythema multiforme.

MANAGEMENT

Identification of the responsible exposure and elimination would be ideal. However, most cases of urticaria are idiopathic, and providers must often turn to pharmacologic therapy. Evidence exists for the benefit of treatment of acute and chronic urticaria with H_1-receptor antagonists, H_2-receptor antagonists, tricyclic antidepressants, leukotriene receptor antagonists and, in some cases, steroids (Table 72-1).

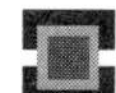
Diagnostics

Urticaria

Laboratory*
CBC and differential†
ESR†
Urinalysis†
LFTs†
TSH†
Thyroid antimicrosomal antibodies†
Antinuclear antibodies†
Rheumatoid factor†
Serum complement C_3 and C_4†
Cryoglobulin†
Serum IgE†
Serum IgM†
Hepatitis†

Imaging
Chest x-ray†

*If no physical causes present.
†If indicated.

Differential Diagnosis

Urticaria

Insect bites
Vasculitis
Pityriasis rosea
Syphilis
Erythema multiforme
Bullous pemphigoid
Systemic lupus erythematous
Urticaria pigmentosa
Drug eruptions
Erythema multiforme

Although older antihistamines such as Benadryl and Atarax were used commonly in the past, they have largely been replaced by newer, nonsedating H_1-blockers such as loratadine (Claritin), cetirizine (Zyrtec), and fexofenadine (Allegra). There is evidence for clinical benefit when these medications are used at higher doses.[7] Their efficacy combined with reduced sedation and anticholinergic side effects have made them first-line therapy in the treatment of urticaria. Because higher doses of the H_1-blockers are often needed to treat the symptoms of urticaria—doses that in most individuals would lead to significant sedation with the older H_1-blockers—the newer nonsedating H_1 blockers have found favor.[8] However, the addition of a sedating antihistamine (e.g., chlorpheniramine 4 to 12 mg or hydroxyzine 10 to 50 mg) at bedtime to the regimen of a patient already taking a nonsedating

TABLE 72-1 Medications Used in Management of Urticaria and Angioedema

Medications	Dosage
H_1-RECEPTOR ANTAGONISTS	
Cetirizine HCl (Zyrtec)	Adults: 10-20 mg/day (tablet)
Loratadine (Claritin)	Adults: 10 mg/day (tablet)
Fexofenadine (Allegra)	Adults; 120 mg/day (capsules/tablets)
H_2-RECEPTOR ANTAGONISTS	
Cimetidine (Tagamet)	300 mg q.i.d. (tablet, liquid)
Ranitidine HCl (Zantac)	150 mg PO b.i.d. (tablet, capsule, liquid, injection)
TRICYCLIC ANTIDEPRESSANTS	
Amitriptyline HCl (Elavil)	10-100 mg PO q.d. (tablet)
Doxepin (Sinequan)	10-100 mg PO q.d. (capsule, oral concentrate)
LEUKOTRIENE RECEPTOR ANTAGONISTS	
Montelukast sodium (Singulair)	Adults: 10 mg/day (tablet)
Zafirlukast (Accolate)	Adults: 20 mg PO b.i.d. (tablet)

H_1-blocker may help the patient sleep better. There is little evidence, however, that such an addition adds much to H_1-receptor blockade.

Evidence exists for clinical benefit when an H_2-blocker is added to an H_1-blocker in the case of urticaria that is refractory to H_1-blockade. An H_2-blocker such as cimetidine (Tagamet 300 mg PO q.i.d.) or ranitidine (Zantac 150 mg PO b.i.d.) can be added.[9] An H_2-blocker should be used only in conjunction with an H_1-blocker, because the evidence that exists pertains to the benefit of H_2-blockers in cases of chronic urticaria that is refractory to treatment with H_1-blockers alone.[10-12] Evidence also exists for the benefit of treatment of refractory chronic urticaria with the tricyclic antidepressants.[13,14] Doxepin is the most potent H_1-blocker in the class and when used should be started at 25 mg PO h.s. and titrated to effect with a maximum dosage of 100 mg PO h.s. Alternatively, amitriptyline (Elavil) may be used at the same dosing interval of 10 to 100 mg PO h.s.

Limited evidence exists for a clinical benefit to treatment of refractory chronic urticaria with the calcium channel blocker nifedipine in addition to antihistamines in dosages of 10 mg PO b.i.d. to 20 mg PO t.i.d.[15] Recent limited evidence also suggests that the leukotriene inhibitors may be useful in some patients with chronic refractory urticaria.[16] Evidence exists for benefit of treatment of acute urticaria with oral corticosteroids such as prednisolone at a dose of 50 mg/day for 3 days.[7] Long-term oral corticosteroids should not typically be used in chronic urticaria but may be used in select refractory cases under specialty consultation.[7]

Remember that cases of acute urticaria typically last no more than 5 to 7 days. Chronic urticaria is different. Individuals affected by chronic urticaria must seek to modify their lifestyle to avoid the irritant(s) that trigger the symptoms. Patients with a history of severe urticaria and/or angioedema should carry an epinephrine autoinjector for emergency use. Epinephrine 1:1000 (0.3 ml SC) may be used in addition to the H_1-blocker if the patient exhibits any signs of angioedema or if urticaria is severe. A short course of oral corticosteroids may also be considered in the case of angioedema that affects the mouth.

LIFE SPAN CONSIDERATIONS

Patients must learn to avoid triggers, because urticaria can plague them throughout their life. Patients predisposed to severe urticaria, anaphylaxis, or angioedema should be educated in crisis management, including the use of subcutaneous epinephrine to avoid unnecessary morbidity or mortality.

COMPLICATIONS

Pruritus may lead to scratching, excoriation, and secondary infection. The most severe complication is angioedema or anaphylaxis accompanying the urticaria, which can lead to airway obstruction and/or cardiopulmonary arrest.

Immediate emergency department referral/physician consultation is necessary for patients with angioedema, respiratory failure, or hemodynamic compromise. Patients should be hospitalized if they require intubation or are at risk for airway compromise, severe anaphylaxis, or shock.

INDICATIONS FOR REFERRAL/HOSPITALIZATION

Patients should be referred to a physician or specialist for further evaluation when the diagnosis is in question, when an underlying systemic disease is suspected or found, and when routine medical therapy is not effective.

PATIENT AND FAMILY EDUCATION

Patients should be educated on the natural course and history of the disease. Surveillance should be conducted to identify triggers of the disorder. Patients and their family should be educated regarding signs and symptoms of anaphylaxis and angioedema and should understand the importance of avoiding known precipitants. If patients have a history of anaphylaxis or angioedema, they should be provided with an injectable epinephrine preparation such as an EpiPen for emergency use. Both patient and family members should be educated on its use.

REFERENCES

1. Leznoff A, Sussman GL: Syndrome of idiopathic chronic urticaria and angioedema with thyroid autoimmunity: a study in 90 patients, *J Allergy Clin Immunol* 84(1):66-71, 1989.
2. Lindelof B and others: Chronic urticaria and cancer: an epidemiological study of 1155 patients, *Br J Dermatol* 123:453-456, 1990.

3. Mahmood T: Physical urticarias, *Am Fam Physician* 49(6):1411-1414, 1994.
4. Mahmood T: Urticaria, *Am Fam Physician* 51(4):811-816, 1995.
5. Greaves M: Chronic urticaria, *N Engl J Med* 332(26):1767-1772, 1995.
6. Sveum R: Urticaria: the diagnostic challenge of hives, *Postgrad Med* 100(2):77-84, 1996.
7. Grattan C, Powell S, Humphreys F: Management and diagnostic guidelines for urticaria and angioedema, *Br J Dermatol.* 144(4): 708-714, 2001.
8. Goldsmith P, Dowd PM: The new H_1 antihistamines: treatment of urticaria and other clinical problems, *Dermatol Clin* 11(1):87-95, 1993.
9. Juhlin D and others: Drug therapy for chronic urticaria, *Clin Rev Allergy* 10:349-369, 1992.
10. Singh G: H_2 blockers in chronic urticaria, *Int J Dermatol* 23(9): 627-628, 1984.
11. Harvey RP, Schocket AL: The effect of H_1 and H_2 blockade on cutaneous histamine response in man, *J Allergy Clin Immunol* 65(2): 136-139, 1980.
12. Phanuphak P, Schocket AL, Kohler PF: Treatment of idiopathic urticaria with combined H_1 and H_2 blockers, *Clin Allergy* 8(5):429-433, 1978.
13. Rao KS and others: Duration of the suppressive effect of tricyclic antidepressants on histamine-induced wheal and flare reactions in human skin, *J Allergy Clin Immunol* 82(5 pt 1):752-757, 1988.
14. Gupta M and others: Antidepressant drugs in dermatology: an update, *Arch Dermatol* 123:647-652, 1987.
15. Bressler RB and others: Therapy of chronic idiopathic urticaria with nifedipine: a demonstration of beneficial effect in a double-blind, placebo controlled crossover trial, *J Allergy Clin Immunol* 83:756-763, 1989.
16. Nettis E and others: Comparison of montelukast and fexofenadine for chronic idiopathic urticaria, *Arch Dermatol* 137(1):99-100, 2001.

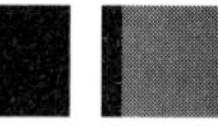

CHAPTER 73

Warts

Eileen M. Deignan and Bonnie Hooper

DEFINITION/EPIDEMIOLOGY

Verruca, or warts, are benign epidermal neoplasms. They are caused by various types of human papillomavirus (HPV), which are characterized as double-stranded DNA viruses that are members of the family Papovaviridae. Approximately 70 types of HPV have been identified on the basis of their DNA homology.[1-3] Although these genotypes can invade any anatomic site of the body, typically each has a predilection for a preferred body area. For example, HPV-1 and HPV-4 are usually identified in plantar, planus, and common warts. Several HPV types are associated with an increased risk for developing genital cancers. A strong association has been established between infection by HPV types 16, 18, 31, 33, 35, 45, 51, 52, and 56 and the subsequent development of cervical cancer.

The prevalence of warts in the general population has not been studied. Patients in the first and second decades of their lives bear a greater rate of occurrence.[4] HPV infection is estimated to occur in approximately 10% of children and young adults, with peak incidence in those 12 to 16 years of age.[2] There is a decreased incidence of warts in African-Americans and older adults.[2,5]

Individuals with decreased cellular immunity are particularly susceptible to HPV infection. In these patients verruca can be rather extensive in terms of lesion size and area of involvement. Individuals previously infected with warts have three times the risk for reinfection.[5]

Certain environmental and occupational factors also increase the risk for developing verruca. Periungual warts are much more common in butchers and in patients whose hands are exposed to chronic wet conditions, including chronic nail biters. Hyperhidrosis increases the chance for developing plantar warts.[6]

PATHOPHYSIOLOGY

Infection always originates from persons who harbor the host-specific HPV. It is postulated that infection occurs through breaks in the skin as a result of close contact with infected persons or their desquamated keratinocytes.[7] Once the virus gains access, it uses the host cell resources to coordinate its own gene expression and replicate. Although viral particles are found in the basal layer of infected tissue, replication occurs only in upper-level, differentiated epithelial cells. Autoinoculation can occur at sites of cutaneous trauma. Vertical transmission from infected mothers to their offspring (i.e., by ascending infection and passage through an infected birth canal) is a well-documented source of anogenital and laryngeal infection in infants.

Infection depends on the number of viral particles, the extent of contact, and the cellular immunity of the host. Even though the virus confines itself to the epidermis, it generally spreads laterally for a considerable distance beyond the line that demarcates the wart from the normal skin. HPV may be actively replicating or may lie in a dormant, or latent, state. Lesions recur when the host's cell-mediated immunity can no longer hold the virus in check. Incubation periods range from 1 to 8 months.

CLINICAL PRESENTATION AND PHYSICAL EXAMINATION

HPV infection is usually asymptomatic. When it does result in clinical changes, it becomes manifest with several different morphologic characteristics. Verruca vulgaris, or common warts, are skin-colored hyperkeratotic papules that occur most often on the backs of the hands and on the knees and periungual areas. Filiform warts are a variant and are distinguished by their fine, fingerlike projections. They usually occur on the face and occasionally may be tender. Verruca plana, or flat warts, mainly affect children. They are commonly seen on the face and extremities in crops of 1- to 2-mm papules that are smooth, flat, and skin-colored to brown. Verruca plantaris, or plantar warts, are skin-colored papules or plaques on plantar pressure points. They are often studded with black pinpoints that represent thrombosed capillaries. These warts may be extremely tender and preclude weight bearing. The depth of plantar warts makes their treatment long and complicated.[6,7] Condyloma acuminata, or anogenital warts, are sexually transmitted and range from unobtrusive, small, skin-colored papules to large, cauliflower-like growths (Color Plate 7). Warts have also been described on the oral and nasal mucous membranes, conjunctivae, larynx, and cervix.

DIAGNOSTICS AND DIFFERENTIAL DIAGNOSIS

To date there are no cultures, vaccines, antiviral therapies, or widely accessible serologic tests that can lead to a definitive diagnosis of or treatment for HPV. Diagnosis is confirmed clinically by debriding the thickened hypertrophic epidermis with a scalpel or curette until the thrombosed capillary tips that rise perpendicular to the surface cause a speckled "seeds" appearance in the dermis.[4] The absence of skin lines within the lesion is considered a key diagnostic indicator. The differential diagnosis of verruca includes keratoma, callus, lichen planus, squamous cell carcinoma, molluscum contagiosum, and foreign body.

MANAGEMENT

Most warts are benign and asymptomatic and generally regress spontaneously over time. A total of 50% of all warts involute spontaneously by the end of 12 months, and 66% to 70% disappear within 24 months.[5,8] According to a task force of the American Academy of Dermatology's Committee on Guidelines of Care, indications for treatment include (1) the patient's desire for therapy; (2) the presence of pain, bleeding, itching, or burning; (3) lesions that are disabling or disfiguring; (4) large numbers or size of lesions; (5) prevention of spreading to unblemished skin; and (6) an immunocompromised state.[8]

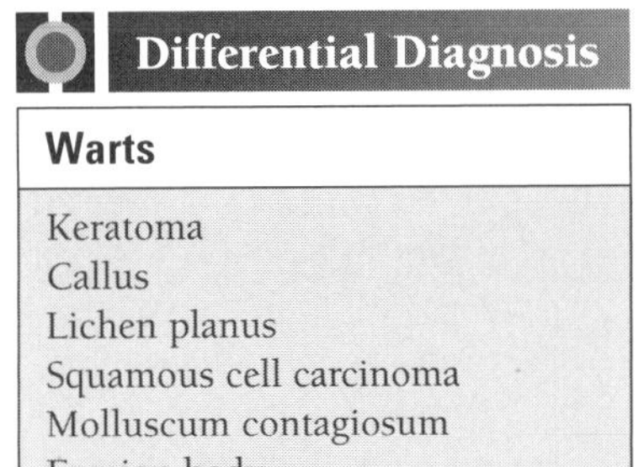
Differential Diagnosis

Warts

Keratoma
Callus
Lichen planus
Squamous cell carcinoma
Molluscum contagiosum
Foreign body

Therapies are directed toward destruction of the lesions and include chemical destruction, cryotherapy, electrodesiccation, and laser ablation. Chemical destruction is with a liquid agent or transdermal patches. Liquid preparations of salicylic acid, lactic acid, and dichloroacetic or trichloroacetic acid are used on common, flat, periungual, and plantar verruca. Application once or twice a day along with paring or filing of the lesion has resulted in cure rates that exceed 60%.[8] A petroleum-based substance can be applied on the surrounding skin to protect it from chemical burn. Treatment may take up to 12 weeks. Cantharidin, applied every 2 to 3 weeks, presents another option.[1,2] Daily use of topical tretinoin (Retin-A) has been advocated for flat warts. Podophyllum resin has a potential for systemic absorption, and serious adverse gastrointestinal and nervous system effects have been reported from this absorption.[1,5] Therefore podophyllum resin needs to be washed from the skin 1 to 4 hours after application, and it should never be used with patients who are pregnant.

Cryotherapy with liquid nitrogen, ether, or nitrous oxide is commonly used to treat verruca. This therapy causes a stinging or burning sensation with application, produces minimal scarring, and allows for rapid healing. Treatment may be needed every other week to every third week until resolution. Nerve damage can occur if treatment is too vigorous in areas where the nerves are superficial, such as the lateral phalanges. Cryotherapy used in combination with topical acids may produce a synergistic effect.[5]

Treatment with pulsed dye or other vascular laser destroys the blood supply to the wart, thereby increasing nourishment to the virus and enhancing resolution. A temporary bruise will result at the treatment site.

More aggressive surgical techniques are available if topical agents and cryotherapy fail. Excision, curettage, and electrocautery increase the risk of scarring, and there is no evidence of improved success.[1,2,7] Administration of an anesthetic may cause a viral tract, which can potentially result in reinfection.

COMPLICATIONS

Plantar warts can be particularly painful and, if left untreated, may result in altered activity, abnormal gait, or foot deformities. Infections are rare, but autoinoculation from one area to another is common.

Genital warts (condyloma acuminata) are transmitted sexually and can be transmitted from mother to infant during childbirth. For both males and females, there is an increased risk of genital and rectal carcinoma.

INDICATIONS FOR REFERRAL/HOSPITALIZATION

A referral to a dermatologist or podiatric surgeon is advised if all of the common techniques have failed or if the lesion is too large. Therapies include the use of intralesional bleomycin or interferon injections, laser ablation, poison ivy extract, and radiologic treatment.[5,6] Cure rates with these more advanced techniques are not reported to be much higher than the modalities used so commonly in the past.

Several unconventional therapies may also be helpful adjuncts. Cimetidine (Tagamet) 25 to 40 mg/kg/day in three or four divided doses has been reported as benign and successful in approximately 80% of patients within 2 to 3 months.[9,10] Success rates appear higher in children, although this treatment method remains somewhat controversial and more recently has fallen out of favor. Hyperthermia water bath treatments may be an effective alternative in treating recalcitrant or extensive verruca.[1,8,10] For this form of therapy to be effective, a temperature range of 45° to 48° C (113° to 118.4° F) needs to be maintained for at least 30 minutes per treatment session.[10]

PATIENT AND FAMILY EDUCATION

Patients and families should understand that most warts are benign, viral lesions that can spread from person to person (particularly in showers, locker rooms, or other public places) and may resolve spontaneously, although sometimes only after many years. Education should include self-treatment options as well as the side effects of all medications. Specific instructions (soaking and paring the wart before application of medicines) should be given regarding the proper use of over-the-counter treatments to enhance efficacy.

REFERENCES

1. Ordoukhanian E, Lane AT: Warts and molluscum contagiosum: beware of treatments worse than the disease, *Postgrad Med* 101(2): 223-235, 1997.
2. Siegfried EC: Warts on children: an approach to therapy, *Pediatr Ann* 25(2):79-90, 1996.
3. Frasier LD: Human papillomavirus infections in children, *Pediatr Ann* 23(7):354-360, 1994.
4. Esterowitz D and others: Plantar warts in the athlete, *Am J Emerg Med* 13(4):441-443, 1995.
5. Kimble-Haas S: Primary care treatment approach to nongenital verruca, *Nurse Pract* 21(10):29-36, 1996.
6. Glover MG: Plantar warts, *Foot Ankle* 11(3):172-178, 1990.
7. Bolton RA: Nongenital warts: classification and treatment options, *Am Fam Physician* 43(6):2049-2056, 1991.
8. Landow K: Nongenital warts: when is treatment warranted? *Postgrad Med* 99(3):245-249, 1996.
9. Glass AT, Solomon BA: Cimetidine therapy for recalcitrant warts in adults, *Arch Dermatol* 132:680-682, 1996.
10. Kang S, Fitzpatrick TB: Debilitating verruca vulgaris in a patient infected with the human immunodeficiency virus: dramatic improvement with hyperthermia therapy, *Arch Dermatol* 130(3):294-296, 1994.

CHAPTER 74

Wound Management

Mary Young

DEFINITION/EPIDEMIOLOGY

Tissue trauma accounts for significant morbidity and financial concern, with the cost of wound care estimated to be greater than $2 billion in the United States each year.[1-3] The incidence and prevalence of acute and chronic wounds vary with populations, geographic and demographic status, and general medical conditions. Acute wounds consist of lacerations, abrasions, avulsions, crush injuries, puncture wounds, insect or mammalian bites, traumatic or surgical wounds, burns, and skin tears. Chronic wounds consist of pressure ulcers, venous and arterial ulcers, diabetic foot ulcers, and nonhealing surgical or traumatic wounds. Pressure ulcers affect 1.5 to 3 million Americans at any given time. In all, 60% to 90% occur in older adults, with 66% of older adults with hip fractures developing pressure ulcers; 15% to 25% of persons admitted to long-term care facilities reportedly have a pressure ulcer. Acute care incidence is 2.7% to 29.5%, with prevalence at 3.5% to 29.5%.[4-11] Venous ulcers are present in 3.5% of persons over age 65 years; the recurrence rate is more than 70% as a result of chronic venous insufficiency. Arterial ulcers occur in a large percentage of patients with peripheral vascular disease. These ulcers are particularly difficult to heal as a result of poor perfusion, and revascularization is often needed to promote reperfusion and the hope of healing the ulcer. Diabetic foot ulcers occur in approximately 15% of the more than 16 million people with diabetes. Ulcers precede amputation 85% of the time, with the cost of treatment exceeding $28,000 for the first 2 years after diagnosis.[12-17]

Surgical wounds are often treated in the outpatient setting secondary to rising costs of acute care management and reimbursement concerns. Wound infection and dehiscence preclude wound healing by secondary intention, with the primary care provider and home health care nurse managing these difficult-to-heal wounds.[3] A broad understanding of wound healing physiology and general management principles will assist the provider in facilitating maximum wound repair.

Immediate referral to a specialist is indicated for deep lacerations, especially when a fracture or tendon injury is suspected.
Immediate referral to a hand specialist is indicated for hand injuries.
Immediate referral to a plastic surgeon is indicated for facial and hand wounds because of the high priority in minimizing scarring and ensuring a return to normal motor function.[2]

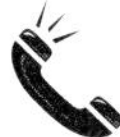

Physician consultation is indicated for deep puncture wounds of the foot, hand, chest, abdomen, and head.

Physician consultation is indicated for wounds requiring large amounts of debridement and wounds with continuous bleeding.

PATHOPHYSIOLOGY

Wound healing begins at the time of injury and proceeds over several months through the stages of inflammation, proliferation, and remodeling. Inflammation, which begins at the time of injury, is an essential first step in wound healing to provide local vasospasm and initiation of the clotting process. Neutrophils, oxygen, and nutrients are transported to the wound site, and proliferation begins. In this phase, epithelial cells migrate over the surface of the wound, collagen synthesis begins, and the wound begins to contract. Remodeling occurs over the next several months, with layering of collagen providing further contraction and tensile strength.[16,17]

Wound healing is affected by many internal and external factors. Internal factors include age, preexisting co-morbidities (i.e., diabetes mellitus, cardiovascular disease, autoimmune disorders), perfusion, oxygenation, nutrition, hydration, and some medications (especially steroids, immune suppressants, and chemotherapeutic drugs). External factors include pressure, friction, shear, moisture, contamination with bacteria, debris or necrotic tissue, and the wound environment (pH, moisture).[18-20]

Stages of wound healing may be interrupted by changes in the internal and external wound healing factors. Two common examples are the occurrence of anemia during wound healing, which slows the healing response as a result of decreased oxygenation, and pressure exerted over the site, which decreases perfusion and prolongs or delays wound healing.

Classification of wounds is unique to wound type, and reference to established classification systems is recommended. Wounds involving only the epidermal layer are classified as superficial or partial thickness. Examples include simple lacerations, skin tears, first-degree burns, abrasions, and shallow ulcerations. These wounds usually heal easily within 2 to 6 days and require the least intervention.

Full-thickness wounds involve the epidermis and dermis and may extend through subcutaneous tissue into muscle and bone. Examples include deep lacerations, second- and third-degree burns, various types of ulcers, and surgical or traumatic wounds.

Pressure ulcers may be partial or full thickness and are staged 1 through 4 according to the guidelines of the Agency for Health Care Research and Quality (formerly the Agency for Health Care Policy and Research) (Box 74-1). Burns are classified as first, second, or third degree and require a unique approach. A referral is indicated when the burn is full thickness and/or occurs on the face, feet, hands, or perineum[20] (Box 74-2). Skin tears are a common occurrence in frail older adults, often occurring during routine daily activities such as washing and dressing. The shearing and friction forces against frail skin cause the tear, separating the epidermis from the dermis (partial thickness) or the dermis from underlying structures (full thickness).[21-23] The Payne-Martin Classification System for grading tears is easy to use and is helpful in documentation[23] (Box 74-3). Diabetic foot ulcers and arterial and venous ulcers are determined by etiology and are usually full thickness. Several classification systems have emerged; Table 74-1 displays the University of Texas system for staging diabetic foot ulcers.

Surgical wounds heal by primary, secondary, or tertiary intention. Primary intention implies that the wound edges are approximated and sutured, stapled, taped, or glued. Secondary intention implies that the wound edges are not approximated, usually because of failed primary intention (dehiscence) or infection. Secondary intention healing is prolonged and results in significant scarring. Delayed primary intention, or tertiary

BOX 74-1

PRESSURE ULCER STAGING; AHCPR GUIDELINES

Stage I: Nonblanchable erythema of intact skin; the heralding lesion of skin ulceration.
Stage II: Partial-thickness skin loss involving epidermis and/or dermis. The ulcer is superficial and presents clinically as an abrasion, blister, or shallow crater.
Stage III: Full-thickness skin loss involving damage or necrosis of subcutaneous tissue that may extend down to, but not through, underlying fascia. The ulcer presents clinically as a deep crater with or without undermining of adjacent tissue.
Stage IV: Full-thickness skin loss with extensive destruction, tissue necrosis, or damage to muscle, bone, or supporting structures (e.g., tendon or joint capsule). Note: Undermining and sinus tracts may also be associated with Stage IV pressure ulcers.

From Agency for Health Care Policy and Research: *Clinical practice guidelines: pressure ulcers in adults: prediction and prevention,* Rockville, Md, 1994, US Department of Health and Human Services, Public Health Service, Agency for Health Care Policy and Research.

BOX 74-2

BURNS CLASSIFICATION

First degree: Superficial, involving only the epidermis. The skin appears dry and erythematous, without blisters, and is sensitive. The classic example is sunburn. Healing occurs in 5 to 10 days.
Second degree: Partial thickness, involving the epidermis and dermis. The skin appears pink, wet, mottled, and with blisters. The site is very painful, such as after a burn from boiling water. Healing occurs in 10 days to 2 weeks.
Third degree: Full thickness, involving the epidermis and dermis, extending into subcutaneous tissue. The wound appears pale white, cherry red, or black. The tissue is very dry and often has necrotic areas to debride. This type of wound is anesthetic. Direct flames, electricity, or chemicals are common causative agents. Skin grafting is often required.

Modified from Wysocki A: Wound care management, *Nurs Clin North Am* 34(4):791, 1999.

intention, refers to wounds that were not initially closed (usually because of infection, contamination, or wound stress) and are closed after some secondary intention healing has occurred.

CLINICAL PRESENTATION

Any break in skin integrity in the immunocompromised or diabetic patient warrants timely and complete evaluation. Early evaluation and intervention in this population of patients may prevent complications of healing, including infection.

Acute wounds are most often caused by accidental injury and result in lacerations, abrasions, burns, bites, and puncture wounds. Patients with co-morbidities, especially diabetes mellitus and peripheral vascular disease, may present with lower extremity ulcers related to neuropathy and poor perfusion. Patients with decreased functioning resulting from brain injury, neurologic disease, or spinal cord injury often present with pressure ulcers. Prevention, early identification, and appropriate management are of primary importance to prevent costly and irreversible tissue damage, especially in the medically compromised patient.

The patient's medication history is important to evaluate and guides management decisions. Immunosuppressive drugs, including chemotherapy and steroids, adversely affect wound healing by interrupting the inflammatory process, an important first step in mounting a healing response. Critical factors to elicit include the patient's age, allergies, employment, nutritional status, drug/alcohol use, smoking history, and immune status, including the last tetanus booster.

Moreover, conditions that adversely affect wound healing include diabetes mellitus, autoimmune disorders, malnutrition, positive smoking history, chronic respiratory disease, and peripheral vascular disease; these affect management plans.[17,18]

BOX 74-3

PAYNE-MARTIN CLASSIFICATION SYSTEM FOR SKIN TEARS

CATEGORY I

Skin tears without tissue loss

Linear type; epidermis and dermis have been pulled apart

Flap type; epidermal flap completely covers the dermis to within 1 mm of wound margin

CATEGORY II

Skin tears with partial tissue loss

Scant tissue loss; 25% or less of flap is lost

Moderate to large tissue loss; more than 25% of epidermal flap is lost

CATEGORY III

Skin tear with complete tissue loss

Epidermal flap is absent

Modified from Baranoski S: Skin tears: the enemy of frail skin, *Adv Skin Wound Care* 13(3 pt 1):123-126, 2000.

PHYSICAL EXAMINATION

Assessment of the wound must follow a thorough history. The nature and timing of the wound, along with the patient's medical history, determine management strategies. Wound location, type, depth, previous treatments, and surrounding tissue assessment guide treatment decisions.

In addition to a thorough wound evaluation (including noting tunneling, the presence and odor of exudate, and the appearance of all tissue in and around wound bed), a focused physical examination is important. In lower extremity wounds, determining perfusion by pulse assessment, and noninvasive diagnostic testing if necessary, are required. The absence or presence of peripheral perfusion and associated changes of edema, tissue color and warmth, and neurovascular status are essential to determine.[16]

Wounds that are healing or have the potential to heal will demonstrate pink or red tissue and the absence of excessive exudate, infection, and debris. The size of the wound, measured weekly, should slowly decrease. Healing wounds are pink, robust, and bumpy (granulation tissue), with pink/red healing edges that demonstrate migration by contact with the wound bed. Tissue is not healing if it is pale, nonblanchable, flat, and has raised hard edges.

DIAGNOSTICS

X-ray studies may be necessary in acute injuries to determine bone or tendon involvement. Separation, fracture, or dislocation usually requires referral to a specialist. Compound fractures, especially in hand injuries, require diligent management and antibiotic administration.

Noninvasive vascular studies are useful to determine arterial flow in patients with lower extremity ulceration. Bone scans or an MRI is helpful in diagnosing osteomyelitis; a bone biopsy is sometimes necessary for definitive diagnosis.[12]

CBCs are useful in detecting anemia, which can slow wound healing progression by decreasing perfusion and

TABLE 74-1 Diabetic Foot Ulcer Grades; University of Texas Classification System

	0	1	2	3
A	Preulcerative or postulcerative lesion completely epithelialized	Superficial, not involving tendon, joint capsule or bone	Penetrating to tendon or joint capsule	Penetrating to tendon or joint capsule
B	With infection	With infection	With infection	With infection
C	With ischemia	With ischemia	With ischemia	With ischemia
D	With infection and ischemia	With infection and ischemia	With infection and ischemia	With infection and ischemia

Modified from University of Texas Classification System in Diabetic Foot Exam, pp 12-13.
Retrieved February 11, 2002 from the World Wide Web: http://sh-aux.lsumc.edu/cme/diabetic-foot-exam.

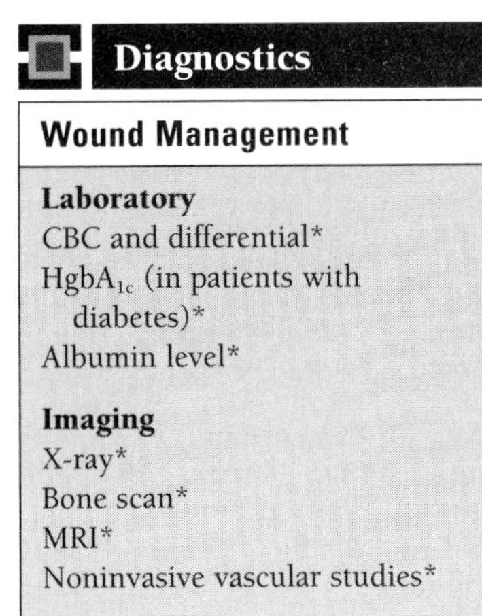

Diagnostics

Wound Management

Laboratory
CBC and differential*
$HgbA_{1c}$ (in patients with diabetes)*
Albumin level*

Imaging
X-ray*
Bone scan*
MRI*
Noninvasive vascular studies*

*If indicated.

oxygenation. A slightly elevated WBC count may be indicative of the inflammatory response, whereas a WBC count that continues to rise may indicate an infection. Immunosuppressive disorders delay wound healing, and may be first detected on CBC. A total lymphocyte count less than 1500 cells/ml^3, coupled with an albumin of less than 3.5 g/dl, is indicative of malnutrition, which delays wound healing. Patients with diabetes who have a hemoglobin A_{1C} of greater than 8 are at increased risk of failed wound healing as a result of hyperglycemia.[12-14]

DIFFERENTIAL DIAGNOSIS

The nature and location of the wound determine diagnosis as well as treatment. Acute wounds are determined by the nature of injury. Diagnosis and treatment of chronic wounds are determined by patient history, the presence of medical conditions, and the location and appearance of the wound.

Ulcers are chronic wounds that have several different underlying medical conditions as etiologies. The diagnosis of the underlying etiology is essential, because treatment of this condition affects ulcer recurrence rates. Most pressure ulcers occur over bony prominences, with 95% occurring over the sacrum, greater trochanter, ischial tuberosity, heel, or lateral malleolus.[16] The location of venous ulcers is typically on the medial lower leg, above the medial malleolus. The wound is often large with irregular wound edges; the wound bed appears beefy red and granular, with moderate to heavy exudate. Associated skin changes include a brawny texture, edema, and hyperpigmentation. Venous ulcers are not usually painful.[15] Arterial ulcers occur most often over the pretibial area, tips of the toes, or over the lateral malleolus; they are painful, flat, and dry and have well-demarcated edges. The limb is traditionally thin, cool, pale or hyperemic, hairless, and shiny as a result of decreased perfusion. Diabetic foot ulcers appear most commonly on the plantar surface of the foot, often at the head of the first metatarsal joint of the great toe. They are often painless secondary to neuropathy, and they have dry, pale edges and wound bed and a black eschar cover.[16]

Thermal wounds are the most common type of burn, with more than 2 million occurrences each year. A total of 80% of these burns are handled in the outpatient setting; burn center referral is based on the American Burn Association's criteria for burn center referral.[20]

MANAGEMENT

The use of universal precautions is essential in wound assessment and treatment. The first step—establishing the type and nature of injury—guides wound management decisions. Referral to a specialist is indicated for deep lacerations, especially when a fracture or tendon injury is suspected. Facial and hand wounds are also best managed by specialists because of the high priority in minimizing scarring and ensuring a return to normal motor function. Regardless of wound type, practicing the principles of wound healing will guide management. Ensuring wound bed moisture, nutrition, perfusion, pH balance, freedom from infection and debris, and protection are imperative. Management of co-morbid conditions and reduction of risk factors, including careful blood glucose monitoring and control, smoking cessation, correction of malnutrition, and enhancing perfusion are important strategies. Ensuring adequate protein intake and essential vitamins and minerals, especially vitamin C and zinc, may also enhance wound healing.[16,17]

Acute Wounds

Lacerations, Abrasions, Avulsions, Crush Injuries, Bites, Puncture Wounds, Other Traumatic or Surgical Wounds. The primary management of all acute wounds is to control major hemorrhage, protect the patient and the wound, and promote comfort. After examining the wound, cleaning and debriding it are essential to remove dirt, debris, and foreign bodies. All traumatic wounds are considered contaminated and should be irrigated with normal saline solution (0.9%). The best method of irrigation is attaching a syringe and 22-gauge angiocatheter to a liter of normal saline via IV tubing. This allows for extensive irrigation under pressure (5 to 15 psi is recommended), which is most effective for cleansing. (Use of a piston or bulb syringe alone does not generate enough pressure for adequate irrigation.) Sharp debridement of nonviable or necrotic tissue and complete hemostasis further decrease the risk for infection.

Decisions about wound closure depend on the wound type, location, depth, and tension of the wound edges. A wound with smooth edges that is not grossly contaminated (e.g., a laceration from a knife or razor) may be closed by approximating the wound edges and applying wound adhesive, Steri-Strips, or suturing with appropriate material. Staples are an efficient closure medium but are usually used when closure must be quick and the wound is not located in an area where scarring is of concern. Wounds easily closed include small lacerations not over a joint; wounds with clean, even edges approximated without inversion or eversion; and lacerations not in areas with redundant tissue. Suturing guidelines are reviewed in Table 74-2. Abrasions, avulsions, crush injuries, bites, and puncture wounds are not usually closed. Tissue approximation, when appropriate, and the application of an antibiotic ointment covered by a sterile nonadherent dressing is standard practice. Keeping the wound out of water, observing for signs and symptoms of infection, and changing the dressing according to principles will aid wound healing.[18,19]

A dressing is applied after wound exploration, irrigation, cleansing, debridement, and closure (when appropriate). Dressings serve the purposes of protection, drainage absorption, insulation, maintenance of moisture and cleanliness, and gaseous exchange. They should be easily removed without traumatizing tissue and are often multilayered. No single dressing may afford all of these properties, and several hundred wound care products are available to choose from.[24-28]

TABLE 74-2 Recommendations for Suturing

Location	Suggested Suture Size	Suggested Suture Removal
Scalp	Superficial closure: 4-5; deep closure: 4	6-7 days
Trunk	Superficial closure: 4-5; deep closure: 3-4	6-8 days
Arms	Superficial closure: 4-5; deep closure: 3-4	Extensor surfaces: 10-14 days; all others: 7-10 days
Legs	Superficial closure: 4-5; deep closure: 3-4	Same as for arms
Hands: referral indicated, although simple lacerations may be repaired	Superficial closure: 5-6; deep closure: 4	Palms: 7-10 days; extensor surfaces: 10-14 days
Feet (soles): referral indicated for tendon or nerve injury	Superficial or deep closure: 3-4	7-14 days
Facial (including eyelids, lips, ears): pressure dressing; referral indicated		3-5 days
Penis/scrotum: referral indicated		
Dog bites: bites over 6 hours old and puncture wounds should not be sutured; consultation suggested for wounds less than 6 hours old		
Cat bites: puncture wounds should not be sutured		
Human bites: wounds should not be sutured		

Selection of dressing is based on function, availability, cost, and comfort. The external layer is protective; several types of bulky gauze are available to choose from for this layer. Dressings may be secured with tape, stockinet, binders, or straps. Being mindful of decreasing tissue trauma can guide the choice of dressing security. For example, wounds that are large and highly exudative and require frequent changes should be secured with a binder, stockinet, or Montgomery straps. This will decrease skin tearing and trauma from frequent tape removal.

The second layer should be highly absorptive and usually is thick cotton gauze. The primary layer protects the wound edges wound bed; it should not adhere to the wound and should be easily removed. Examples include xeroform, Adaptic, and transparent dressings.

Tetanus immunization should be reviewed in all patients after any type of tissue trauma. Tetanus and diphtheria toxoid and tetanus immune globulin should be administered if immunization is unknown or if the patient has received fewer than three lifetime doses. Immunization with tetanus-diphtheria toxoid is recommended for all patients with tetanus-prone wounds (including all contaminated wounds) if the previous immunization was more than 5 years ago[18] (Table 74-3 and Box 74-4).

Antibiotic prophylaxis with Augmentin 875/125 is recommended for all cat bite wounds because 80% become infected. Early prophylaxis (within 12 hours of the bite) is recommended for human and dog bite wounds, although the risk of infection is less. Clindamycin is an appropriate antibiotic for patients who are allergic to penicillin. Traumatic nonbite wounds should be treated prophylactically with cefazolin 1 g IV initially, followed by oral antibiotics. Contaminated wounds must be treated systematically (Table 74-4). Other wounds that require antibiotics are listed in Box 74-5.

Skin Tears. Skin tears should be gently cleansed with normal saline and patted dry or left to air dry; the skin should be as

TABLE 74-3 Tetanus Immunization*

	Unknown Primary Immunization or Fewer Than Three Doses	Three or More Doses
Tetanus-prone wounds	Tetanus and diphtheria toxoid (Td) and tetanus immune globulin (TIG)	Td if >5 years since booster
Non–tetanus-prone wounds	Td	Td if >10 years since booster

From ACIP: General recommendations on immunization, *MMWR* 51(RR-2), 1-35, 2002.
***Dosages (for age 7 years or older):** Td, 0.5 ml IM; TIG, 250 U IM.

BOX 74-4

TETANUS-PRONE VS. NON–TETANUS-PRONE WOUNDS

TETANUS-PRONE WOUNDS

Puncture wounds
Crush injuries
Wounds over 6 hours old
Stellate wounds
Wounds greater than 1 cm long
Wounds with devitalized tissue
Obviously contaminated wounds

NON–TETANUS-PRONE WOUNDS

Wounds less than 6 hours old
Wounds with clean margins
Wounds without devitalized tissue
Wounds without organic contamination
Wounds with clearly defined edges

TABLE 74-4 Suggested Systemic Antibiotics for Contaminated Wounds

	Primary Antibiotics	Alternate Antibiotics
Afebrile wounds	Ampicillin/clavulanate First-generation cephalosporin	Erythromycin Clarithromycin Azithromycin Clindamycin
Febrile wounds with sepsis	Ampicillin/sulbactam Ticarcillin/clavulanate Piperacillin-tazobactam Imipenem cilastatin Meropenem	Penicillin-resistant synthetic penicillins *and* Antipseudomonal aminoglycosoids *and* Clindamycin

Modified from Gilbert DN, Moellering RC, Jr, Sande MA: *The Sanford guide to antimicrobial therapy,* Hyde Park, Vt, 2001, Antimicrobial Therapy.

BOX 74-5

WOUNDS THAT REQUIRE ANTIBIOTIC THERAPY

- Wounds more than 8 hours old
- Crushing injuries
- Grossly contaminated wounds
- Fingertip avulsions with bone exposed
- Open fractures
- Tendon or joint involvement
- Mammalian bites
- Paronychia with pus
- Wounds in felons
- Wounds in immunocompromised patients
- Wounds in patients with diabetes

closely approximated as possible. Steri-Strips may be useful in holding the wound edges together, especially in a grade 2 or 3 tear. A dressing that requires infrequent changes while supplying moisture to the wound bed is recommended for treatment. A transparent dressing left in place 5 to 7 days is a good choice. Otherwise, a hydrogel or impregnated gauze such as xeroform may also be selected. Removal of any dressing from a skin tear must be done carefully to avoid interrupting the delicate tissue adherence.[22,23]

Burns. Immediate treatment includes moving the patient away from the source of heat, removing jewelry or metal (which may continue to conduct heat), and applying cool compresses to decrease skin temperature. All burns should be cleansed with normal saline and gauze initially; necrotic tissue should be sharply debrided, and a topical antimicrobial cream or ointment should be applied. Ideally, the product should penetrate eschar, not interfere with healing, be minimally absorbed and nontoxic, and provide wide spectrum antibiotic coverage. Silvadene is the most common choice. Bactroban can be used for patients who are allergic to sulfa. Application twice a day, with normal saline cleansing at each dressing change, is recommended. Excessive use can lead to a secondary infection of *Pseudomonas aeruginosa* or *Enterobacter cloacae*, and therefore its use should be limited to 14 to 21 days. Chemical burns should be emergently treated with rapid and copious irrigation with normal saline or water, then treated as described previously.[2]

Chronic Wounds

The principles of wound management guide treatment decisions, regardless of wound type. However, chronic wounds command specific intervention based on etiology. The Wound Care Product Selection Algorithm (Figure 74-1) can guide the selection of a dressing based on the appearance of the wound. The use of cytotoxic products, including Betadine, hydrogen peroxide, Dakin solution, and other bacteriostatic products previously thought to be beneficial, is not currently recommended. Antibiotic creams and ointments, including Silvadene, are appropriate for short periods of time in infected wounds and are prescribed for only 14 to 21 days. Normal saline 0.9% is the cleansing, irrigating, and wound packing product of choice in most wounds because it is isotonic, available, and inexpensive.

Pressure Ulcers. Pressure ulcers are treated by removing pressure and avoiding friction, shear, and moisture. The ulcers are cleaned twice daily with normal saline irrigation or a surfactant cleanser if fecal or urine contamination is a concern. Wound care products are selected to ensure protection, absorption of exudates, and gentle debridement. Stage 4 ulcers must be packed with a moist product, such as saline impregnated gauze or a hydrogel; highly exudative wounds benefit from calcium alginate products. Stage 1 or 2 ulcers that are not infected may be treated with a hydrocolloid dressing, which may be left in place 5 to 7 days.

Venous Ulcers. Treatment of venous ulcers involves reducing edema with leg elevation, compression stockings, or graded compression devices. Unna's boot has been a useful dressing for many years; it provides compression and cannot be easily removed by the patient. However, it is not absorptive and therefore becomes less effective as the limb compresses over time.[15] Absorptive dressings (e.g., calcium alginate) combined with decompression are more effective in venous ulcer care.

Arterial Ulcers. With arterial ulcers, perfusion is promoted by avoiding compressive stockings or dressings and by encouraging dependent limb position most of the time. Four-inch wooden blocks placed under the head of the bed promote dependence while sleeping. Providing warmth to the lower extremities with cotton stockings and protecting from injury with well-fitting shoes can aid in prevention. Arterial ulcers should be gently cleansed with normal saline, and moisture may be provided with topical creams, hydrogels, or hydrocolloids. Saline dressings may macerate the surrounding tissue and are difficult to maintain. Unna's boot is inappropriate in the care of arterial ulcers because it dries an already dry wound bed and provides compression in a poorly perfused limb.

Diabetic Foot Ulcers. The high incidence and recurrence rate makes diabetic foot ulcers a common issue in diabetes care. Management of blood glucose is an essential component for foot ulcer prevention and healing. Additionally, specific ulcer management techniques include debridement to a clean ulcer

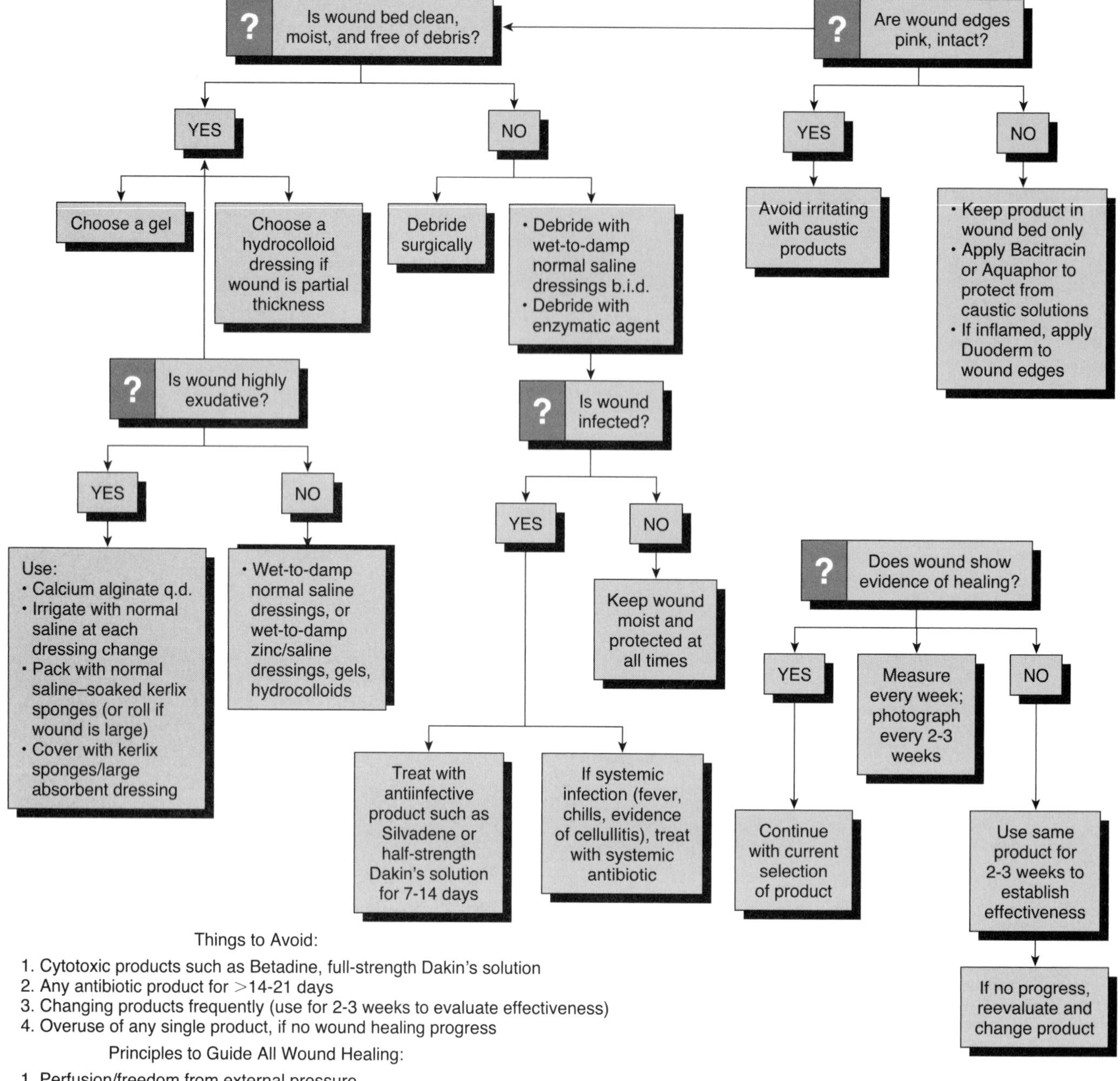

FIGURE 74-1

Algorithm for wound care product selection.

base, treatment of any infection in the ulcer, consideration of modalities to promote wound healing, and the use of accommodative pressure-reducing devices such as custom-molded shoes or shoe inserts to off-load ulcer sites.

Debridement can be accomplished by surgical, mechanical, or autolytic methods. Surgical debridement is used to remove hyperkeratotic or necrotic tissue and should cause only minimal healthy tissue trauma and bleeding. Mechanical debridement involves the use of high-pressure water sprays. Whirlpool treatments are not recommended by some sources, because these treatments have a risk for skin burning and maceration in a patient population where there is impaired healing mechanisms (the diabetic population).[29,30] In the office setting, a 30-ml syringe with an 18-gauge needle can be used for mechanical debridement. Autolytic debridement with film and hydrocolloid dressings allow leukocytes on the ulcer surface to degrade and release lysosomal enzymes that break down protein and mucopolysaccharide components of ulcer eschar;

however, dressings that retain moisture are contraindicated in the presence of infection.[29]

Once the ulcer is debrided, prevention of infection is imperative to reduce risk of amputation; however, detection of infection is often difficult secondary to neuropathy and decreased inflammatory response. Dressings must be changed frequently, at least every 24 hours, and the ulcer is continually assessed for infection. Prolonged hyperglycemia may be the first indication of infection. Systemic antibiotics and assessing for osteomyelitis are essential to prevent amputation.[12-14]

Currently, limited evidence exists for the benefit for other treatment modalities such as cultured human dermis, hyperbaric oxygen therapy, total contact casting, and tissue growth factors.[30] This is an area where there is emerging data; however, some of these treatment modalities have had limited investigation because of their high cost. Graftskin, a bilayered skin substitute, has been used as a healing adjunct for full-thickness ulcers that do not have tendon, muscle, joint capsule, or bone exposure and have not responded to conventional therapy.[29]

Once ulcers are healed, patients require close, continuous monitoring to minimize recurrences. Pressure-relieving modalities (see Health Promotion, p. 272) may be used. Patients should be monitored daily, weekly, biweekly, and finally at 2-month intervals until stabile and then at least at 6-month intervals.[29]

Nonhealing Surgical or Traumatic Wounds. Wounds healing by secondary intention are often large and highly exudative. Wound packing with a hydrogel or calcium alginate to absorb exudate is often effective. The use of new technologic advances to enhance healing, such as vacuum-assisted closure (VAC), has promoted wound healing in large, open wounds.[31]

Adjunctive therapies are useful in chronic wounds; hyperbaric oxygen therapy is being used in treating diabetic foot ulcers with moderate success.[26] VAC, developed by Kinetics Concepts, Inc., is useful to promote healing in chronic, moist, stage 3 or 4 pressure ulcers, as well as nonhealing surgical wounds and some lower extremity ulcers. Ultrasound, topical oxygen, and E-STIM may also be beneficial in certain wounds.[17,24-26,32]

Documentation must include the nature of the injury, wound type, location, size in centimeters, (length, width, depth), integrity of supporting structures (bone, wound, vasculature), and appearance of all exposed and surrounding tissue. A picture of the wound is most helpful, as is a drawing that demonstrates shape and where measurements were taken.[31] Depth is assessed with a sterile Q-tip placed into the deepest part of the wound, then measured (Box 74-6).

BOX 74-6

DOCUMENTATION OF WOUNDS

- Wound
  - Location
  - Length
  - Depth
  - Edges
- Presence of foreign bodies
- Accompanying injuries
  - Fractures
  - Dislocations
  - Tendon or ligament injuries
  - Neurologic and cardiovascular findings
- Diagnostic findings, radiologic conclusions
- Treatments
- Possible scar formation
- Follow-up

LIFE SPAN CONSIDERATIONS

Impaired skin integrity is common in older adults as a result of age-related skin changes, immobility, malnutrition, incontinence, immunocompromise, polypharmacy, sensory deficits, and co-morbidities. Thinning of the epidermis, dermis, and subcutaneous tissue coupled with decreased tensile strength and elasticity and poor epidermal-dermal adhesion, contribute to easy skin tears, pressure ulcers, and lower extremity ulcers.[18,22]

In addition, wound healing time is prolonged in older adults because of decreased oxygenation and perfusion and a decreased inflammatory response. Although the same principles of wound management apply in all populations, special diligence is recommended in caring for older adults. Consideration of the diminished ability to provide self-care and travel easily to and from medical facilities should prompt the provider to select appropriate dressings and to consider a referral to home health agencies for wound evaluation and care in the patient's setting. The risk of delayed wound healing contributes to infection, pain, and a decreased quality of life in patients who may already be compromised.[17,18]

COMPLICATIONS

Complications of wound healing include infection, dehiscence, delayed wound healing, extensive scarring, and sepsis. Serious infection of the face or hands and cellulitis that has not responded to oral antibiotic treatment require IV antibiotics and/or hospitalization.

INDICATIONS FOR REFERRAL/HOSPITALIZATION

The location and nature of the wound, injury to bone, vasculature or tendons, and the experience of the primary care provider guide referral decisions. Fractures, deep tissue, vascular or organ damage, facial and hand injuries, and/or severely contaminated wounds require referral to a specialist. Large, open wounds or deep puncture wounds most likely require surgical intervention. Facial or hand wounds that are infected may require hospitalization and IV antibiotics. Chronic wounds such as ulcers may be best managed by referral to a wound care specialist and as part of an interdisciplinary team.

PATIENT AND FAMILY EDUCATION

Signs and symptoms of wound infection should be reviewed with the patient and family both verbally and in writing. Infection of the wound can greatly affect outcome and may impede wound healing and return of function. Demonstrating wound dressing techniques with the patient and family and observing a return demonstration when possible are helpful in ascertaining patient understanding. A patient teaching pamphlet or videotape with specific directions for wound cleansing and care reinforces teaching.

Reevaluation and follow-up evaluation for suture removal should be scheduled before discharge. Sutures are removed according to the location of the wound and the type of suture used. Referral for visiting nurses may be important for dressing changes, support in managing medications (especially antibiotics), and wound evaluation in the home. Follow-up monitoring of most wounds should occur within 7 to 10 days.

HEALTH PROMOTION

The cost of wound care in all populations exceeds $2 billion annually in the United States. Prevention of lower extremity ulcers in patients with diabetes mellitus and peripheral vascular disease will prevent amputations, decrease the cost of multiple hospitalizations, and improve overall quality of life. Diligent foot care in patients with diabetic and peripheral vascular disease patient can prevent unnecessary amputations, thus improving and prolonging lives. The use of pressure-relieving interventions such as callus removal, padded hosiery to reduce callus buildup, extra depth shoes, and insoles to redistribute foot pressure have demonstrated some benefit in ulcer prevention.

The following health promotion behaviors are strategic interventions in the prevention of traumatic wounds: teaching safety in the home, promoting gun control, working to decrease violence, encouraging automobile safety including seat belt use, and ensuring child safety practices. These practices should be part of health care encounters for patients in multiple sites.

REFERENCES

1. Bryant R: *Acute and chronic wounds: nursing management*, St Louis, 2000, Mosby.
2. Hughes P: Wounds and wound management. In Sheehy S and others: *Manual of clinical trauma care*, ed 3, St Louis, 1999, Mosby.
3. Kravitz, M: Outpatient wound care, *Crit Care Nurs Clin North Am* 8(2): 217-223, 1996.
4. Bostrom J and others: Preventing skin breakdown: nursing practices, costs and outcomes, *Applied Nurs Res* 9(4):184-188, 1996.
5. Kemp M, Krouskop T: Pressure ulcers: reducing incidence and severity by managing pressure, *J Gerontol Nurs* 20:27-34, 1994.
6. Bergman-Evans B, Cuddigan J, Bergstrom N: Clinical practice guidelines: prediction and prevention of pressure ulcers, *J Gerontol Nurs* 20:19-26, 1994.
7. Olson B and others: Pressure ulcer incidence in an acute care setting, *J Wound Ostomy Care Nurs* 23(1):15-22, 1996.
8. Evans J and others: Pressure ulcers: prevention and management, *Symposium on Geriatrics, Part II*, Mayo Foundation 789-799. 1995.
9. Cassidy S: Pressure ulcers: prevention and treatment, *J Care Manag* 2(3suppl):1-10, 1996.
10. Bergstrom N and others: *Treatment of pressure ulcers, clinical practice guidelines No 15, Agency for Health Care Policy and Research*, Rockville, Md, 1994, US Department of Health and Human Services, Public Health Service, Agency for Health Care Policy and Research.
11. Harrison M and others: Practice guidelines for the prediction and prevention of pressure ulcers: evaluating the incidence, *Applied Nurs Res* 9(1):9-17, 1996.
12. Mulder G: Evaluating and managing the diabetic foot: an overview, *Adv Skin Wound Care* 13(1):33-36, 2000.
13. American Diabetes Association: Consensus development conference on diabetic foot wound care, *Diabetes Care* 22:1354-1360, 1999.
14. Halpin-Landry J, Goldsmith S: Feet first: diabetes care, *Am J Nurs* 99(2):26-34, 1999.
15. Hess C: Management of the patient with a venous ulcer, *Adv Skin Wound Care* 13(2):79-83, 2000.
16. Bates-Jenson B: Chronic wound assessment, *Nurs Clin North Am* 34(4):799-839, 1999.
17. Krasner D, Sibbald R: Nursing management of chronic wounds, *Nurs Clin North Am* 34(4):935-943. 1999.
18. Boynton P, Jaworski D, Paustian C: Meeting the challenges of healing chronic wounds in older adults, *Nurs Clin North Am* 34(4):921-932. 1999.
19. Nayduch D: Trauma wound management, *Nurs Clin North Am* 34 (4):896-906,1999.
20. Gordon M, Goodwin C: Initial assessment, management and stabilization of burns, *Nurs Clin North Am* 32 (2):237-249, 1999.
21. Wipke-Tevis D and others: Prevalence, incidence, management, and predictors of venous ulcers in the long-term-care population using the MDS, *Adv Skin Wound Care* 13(5):218-214, 2000.
22. Davidson M: Impaired skin integrity in elderly patients, *Med Surg Nurs Q* 1(3):87-97, 1993.
23. Baranoski S: Skin tears: the enemy of frail skin, *Adv Skin Wound Care* 13(3 Pt 1):123-126, 2000.
24. Krasner D: Wound care products, *Ostomy Wound Manage* 33:47-60, 1991.
25. Fowler E and others: Wound care 1999, *Home Healthcare Nurse* 17 (7):437-444, 1999.
26. Boykin J: The nitric oxide connection: hyperbaric oxygen therapy, becaplermin, and diabetic ulcer management, *Adv Skin Wound Care* 13:169-174, 2000.
27. Ovington L: Wound care products: how to choose, *Home Healthcare Nurse* 19(4):224-232, 2001.
28. Ladin D: Understanding dressings, *Clin Plastic Surg* 25(3):433-441, 1998.
29. Brill LR, Stone JA: New treatments for lower extremity ulcers, *Patient Care Nurse Pract* 4(120):9-20, 2001.
30. NHS Center for Reviews and Dissemination: A systematic review of foot ulcers in patients with type 2 diabetes mellitus II: treatment, Database of Abstract and Reviews of Effectiveness, 1(10). Retrieved August 2001 from the World Wide Web: http://gateway1.ovid.com/ovidweb.cgi.
31. Argenta L, Morykwas M: Vacuum-assisted closure: a new method for wound control and treatment: clinical experience, *Ann Plastic Surg* 38 (6):563-577, 1997.
32. Louis D: Photographing pressure ulcers to enhance documentation, *Decubitus* 5(7):38-45, 1992.

PART 6

Evaluation and Management of Eye Disorders

TERRY MAHAN BUTTARO, Section Editor

CHAPTER 75

Evaluation of the Eyes

Kate Goldblum, Patricia Gillett, Patricia A. Lamb, and Joyce Powers

Ocular assessment may focus on ocular health promotion, preventive vision care, or an episodic problem. Prevention includes regular eye examinations (especially after age 40 years) and the need for protective eyewear in sports, at work, and around hazardous materials. Early detection of ocular disorders, as well as patient education about ocular symptoms requiring immediate evaluation, is also an integral component of ocular health promotion. Episodic ocular problems require rapid examination. Visual acuity in each eye (noting any differences in visual acuity between the two eyes or from previous measurements), ocular alignment and mobility, pupillary equality and reaction to light, gross visual fields, and the status of the optic discs should all be assessed.

Evaluation of the eyes may also provide further evidence of systemic disorders. Patients with diabetes or hypertension may have ocular fundus changes. Some neurologic disorders may also present as abnormalities on ocular examination. A thorough assessment can help identify patients with common vision-threatening problems such as cataracts, glaucoma, diabetic retinopathy, and age-related macular degeneration. Once identified, patients with these problems should be referred for appropriate evaluation and treatment.

Immediate ophthalmology/emergency department referral is indicated for patients with sudden-onset vision loss not associated with an obvious disorder.

HISTORY

History of Present Illness

Careful documentation of the symptoms is crucial for diagnosis. It is important to consider the following elements in evaluating and documenting the symptom(s): location; severity; circumstances surrounding the onset; quality or character; aggravating, alleviating, or associated factors; duration; frequency; timing; and impact on activities of daily living. Identification of current or prior use of eye medications, documentation of any history of ocular symptoms, and identification of any recent systemic illnesses, such as upper respiratory tract symptoms, are also important.

Past Medical History

A complete list of systemic and ocular medications helps identify disorders commonly associated with ocular manifestations such as diabetes and hypertension and may avoid adverse effects such as systemic beta-blocker potentiation by ophthalmic beta agonists. In addition, many systemic medications may induce blurred vision or dry eye symptoms. Identification of drug allergies and sensitivities is always important. The ocular history should include glasses or contact lens wear, previous ocular injuries or surgeries, and patching or poor vision in childhood. A history of previous intraocular surgery is important information in evaluating an abnormally shaped pupil. Knowing that patching occurred in childhood may be useful information in evaluating a difference between the right and left visual acuity in an adult.

Family History

The presence of any of the following should be included in the ocular family history: glaucoma, diabetes, cataracts, macular degeneration, retinitis pigmentosa, retinoblastoma, keratoconus, color blindness, nystagmus, albinism, choroideremia, and corneal dystrophies. The most significant medical conditions with ocular manifestations include diabetes, hypertension, hyperthyroidism, vascular disorders, migraine headache, von Recklinghausen's disease, Marfan syndrome, sickle cell anemia, and arthritis.[1]

Social History

A general assessment of employment and leisure activities may identify concerns related to environmental hazards and the potential for ocular injury or trauma. This information is useful for patient education related to ocular injury prevention and the use of protective eyewear. Assessment of contact lens wear and hygiene practices may identify other ocular risks.

OCULAR EXAMINATION

Vision Screening

Screening for visual impairment is an important function in primary health care. Routine screening for amblyopia and strabismus in children during the preschool period and routine visual acuity testing in older adults are recommended.[2,3] Although routine vision screening of other age-groups and routine ophthalmoscopic assessment in older adults is not supported by evidence in the literature, screening my be justified on other grounds.[4]

Visual Acuity Testing

The importance of measuring visual acuity in each eye before any further assessment, manipulation, or treatment cannot be overemphasized. It is imperative to assess and document visual acuity in each eye separately. This is important not only from a clinical standpoint but also from a medicolegal perspective, particularly in any situation involving ocular trauma. Visual acuity assessment and documentation provide evidence of the patient's visual acuity before diagnostic evaluation. This documentation provides an important clinical baseline and precludes subsequent allegations that vision loss was related to the examination technique or subsequent treatment.

Evaluation of both near and far vision in each eye separately, assessment with and without glasses, and avoidance of the pinhole effect obtained with squinting are important in determining visual acuity. Results may vary as a result of motivation, attention, intelligence, and environmental variants. Visual acuity is determined by the smallest object that can be clearly seen and distinguished. Results of clinical visual acuity testing indicate foveal function, assuming the remainder of the visual system is normal.

The most common method of measuring visual acuity is a *Snellen chart* placed 20 feet from the patient, with results recorded as a fraction (e.g., 20/20 or 20/80). A measure of 20/80 means the person tested identifies letters at 20 feet that a person with average vision could identify at 80 feet. The individual with average vision sees 20/20. A modified chart with pictures, numbers, or tumbling Es is useful for illiterate or younger patients. The *Allen figure chart* is commonly used for this purpose. Allen figures are pictures of easily recognized objects used in place of letters or the tumbling E to quantify visual acuity in those unable to read letters on a Snellen chart or who are confused about the tumbling E chart. The Allen figure chart is useful to determine visual acuity in preschoolers, mentally handicapped older children or adults, and illiterate adults.

If the patient cannot identify the largest letter or object on the chart, the next level of visual acuity testing involves *counting fingers* at a certain distance. If the longest distance at which the patient can count fingers is 3 feet, the visual acuity is recorded as "CF at 3 feet." If the patient is unable to count fingers at any distance, the next measure is *hand movement,* again recorded as the longest distance that the patient can see the hand move (e.g., "HM at 6 inches"). If hand movement is not visible at any distance, the examiner uses a bright penlight to determine whether the patient has *light perception*. If the patient can see the light, the visual acuity is recorded as "LP." If not, "NLP" (no light perception) is recorded.

A *Jaeger chart* is used to measure near vision. The card is placed at 12 to 14 inches, and results are recorded as the smallest line read (e.g., J_1 or J_{10}). J_1 is the level of near vision equivalent to 20/20 at distance and is equivalent in size to 4-point type. J_5 is 8-point type and J_{10} is 14-point type. Standard newspaper print is 8-point type.

Children who see better with one eye than the other should be referred to an ophthalmologist for evaluation for amblyopia.[5] If amblyopia is not treated before age 10 to 12 years, previously treatable amblyopia becomes a permanent vision loss.

Pupil Evaluation

The pupil should be evaluated for dilation and constriction functions, equality, size, and shape. Pupillary response to light is either direct or consensual. Normal pupils are round and equal and react to light directly and consensually. A pupil that appears abnormal on examination may be indicative of acute glaucoma, iatrogenic dilation, iritis, drug effects, congenital iris abnormalities; acquired iris abnormalities from trauma or prior surgery; or neurologic abnormalities. Anisocoria (unequal pupil size) is a normal finding in approximately 20% of the population.[6]

Extraocular Muscle Function

Extraocular muscle examination evaluates the movement of the six extraocular muscles innervated by three cranial nerves: CN III, CN IV, and CN VI. *Hirschberg's test* uses the corneal light reflex as a simple, practical evaluation of muscle balance. A light source is held midway between the patient's two eyes at a distance of 10 to 12 inches. The light is directed at the pupils as the patient looks straight ahead, and the light reflex is examined to determine if it is reflected symmetrically in each pupil. In the normal person both reflexes will be symmetric. If one eye is not straight, the light reflexes will be asymmetric when compared. Evaluation of the cardinal gaze positions is a further assessment of extraocular muscle function and is done by asking the patient to follow an object in each of the nine cardinal gaze positions.

The *cover/uncover test* also evaluates muscle function. One eye is occluded while the patient fixates on some object in primary gaze. The eye under the cover should be observed for movement as the occluder is removed. The second eye should be covered and the process repeated. There should be no movement in the uncovered eye. If the eye under the occluder deviates after the occluder is removed (while the opposite eye fixates), it is an indication that extraocular muscle function is compromised. This may occur as a result of abnormal innervation related to diabetic neuropathy or stroke. Abnormal extraocular muscle function may also result from a mechanical restriction such as in thyroid myopathy, muscle entrapment occurring secondary to orbital fractions, or an orbital neoplasm.

Visual Field Evaluation

The confrontation visual field examination evaluates visual function of the peripheral retina and identifies large visual field losses, which are usually accompanied by some functional impairment. Each eye should be tested separately, with the nontested eye covered and the patient's visual field compared with the examiner's visual field. Reasons for defects include advanced glaucoma, stroke, neoplasm, or retinal detachment. Visual field assessment is dependent on subjective patient replies. The results should be reproducible.

External Examination

The eyebrows, eyelids, eyelashes, and orbital rim should be inspected and palpated. The cornea, conjunctiva, iris, pupil, and anterior chamber should be inspected. The normal bulbar conjunctiva is translucent, moist, and membranous with rich vasculature. The cornea is a clear and avascular structure; the sclera is white. Anterior chamber depth can be assessed by shining a light obliquely across the eye. If the iris is abnormally close to the posterior corneal surface, the oblique light will not reach the opposite side of the eye. The irides are normally the same color. The symmetry of all structures should be noted. The eyelashes should be evenly distributed and curve outward. Normal lid margins are against the globe; lacrimal ducts are patent and without discharge. The skin should be intact and without redness, discharge, or lesions.

Intraocular Pressure Evaluation

Intraocular pressure can be measured in the primary care setting using a Schiøtz tonometer. If a Schiøtz tonometer is not available, a gross estimation of intraocular pressure can be obtained by lightly palpating the globe through the closed upper lids. This method can be especially useful in evaluating acute glaucoma, which usually is unilateral. In these patients, a distinct difference in firmness between the involved eye and the uninvolved eye may be appreciated. An enlarged cup-disc ratio may be an indication that the patient has had a long period of elevated intraocular pressure (Color Plates 28 and 29).

Ophthalmoscopic Examination

Of all organs, the eye is most accessible to direct examination. The direct ophthalmoscope provides a magnified, upright image of the retinal structures. The ocular lens should be clear and centered behind the iris. The vitreous should be translucent and can normally contain floaters visible by ophthalmoscopic examination. If all of the ocular media are clear, the retina should appear as a red reflex. The retina and optic disc should be examined. To facilitate a thorough retinal examination, the ophthalmoscope should be held stable at the pupil, and the patient should look in all four directions. The entry of the optic nerve into the globe forms the physiologic cup, which should be visible. The normal cup-disc ratio is less than 0.5. The macula lies 2 disc diameters from the optic nerve and somewhat superior to it. The macula is avascular and should be examined last because it is the most sensitive part of the retina.

SIGNS AND SYMPTOMS OF OCULAR DISEASE

Red Eye

Red eye is one of the most common ocular complaints in the primary care setting. Often the underlying disorder is self-limiting with minimal visual consequences, but it is important to recognize serious, vision-threatening conditions. The term *red eye* denotes hyperemia of the conjunctiva or sclera. It is sometimes used to denote redness of the adnexal structures or periocular area.

The most common cause of red eye is *conjunctivitis*, which may be allergic, bacterial, or viral. Patients may also present with a red eye from *episcleritis* or *scleritis*. These are inflammatory conditions, although scleritis may have a microbial etiology very rarely. Episcleritis is almost always self-limiting and rarely requires topical antiinflammatory therapy. Scleritis is a more serious condition that can be vision-threatening and is often related to an underlying autoimmune disorder. Patients with possible scleritis should be referred to an ophthalmologist.

The uveal tract of the eye consists of the iris, ciliary body, and choroid. Any or all of these structures may become inflamed, causing a red eye. *Iritis* is an inflammation of the anterior uveal structure, the iris. *Uveitis* is an inflammation that also involves the posterior uveal structures. These inflammatory conditions are often associated with systemic disorders, many with an autoimmune component. Patients with iritis or uveitis should be referred to an ophthalmologist. These and other ocular disorders that must be considered in the differential diagnosis of a patient presenting with red eye are presented in Table 75-1.

Accurate diagnosis is critical in determining the appropriate therapy for red eye. For example, treating bacterial conjunctivitis with steroids may exacerbate the infection, and steroid use with a corneal abrasion or ulcer may lead to corneal melting and serious visual consequences. Conversely, treating a herpetic keratitis with an antibiotic may delay appropriate therapy and lead to potentially serious consequences. Many ocular disorders can be difficult to accurately diagnose without a slit lamp. The

TABLE 75-1 Red Eye: Differential Diagnosis and Management Guidelines

Disorder	Signs and Symptoms	Pain	Management
DISORDERS ASSOCIATED WITH OCULAR ADNEXA REDNESS			
Blepharitis	Ocular burning; eyelid margins red with scaling or crusting	Yes	Warm compresses; daily lid scrubs; erythromycin or bacitracin ophthalmic ointment for anterior blepharitis; see Chapter 77
Cellulitis			
Orbital	Vision may or may not be affected; localized tenderness, erythema, edema; fever; proptosis	Yes	Referral to ophthalmology for hospitalization, IV antibiotics; see Chapter 82
Periorbital	Vision usually not affected; localized tenderness, erythema, edema; fever may or may not be present	Yes	Systemic, broad-spectrum antibiotic; office follow-up visit in 12 to 24 hours; see Chapter 82
Dacryocystitis	Chronic tearing; eyelash crusting; localized tenderness; circumscribed erythema, edema in the inferior medial canthal area; may be able to express purulent material from the nasolacrimal duct	Yes	Warm compresses; gentle massage; topical and/or systemic antibiotics; see Chapter 81
Eyelid lesions			
Chalazion	Nontender in chronic lesions; localized erythema, edema of eyelid(s)	No	Warm compresses; daily lid scrubs; lid massage; see Chapter 77
Hordeolum	Localized tenderness, erythema, edema of eyelid(s); internal lesions point to external or internal eyelid surface; external lesions point to eyelid margin	Yes	Warm compresses; lid scrubs for recurrent lesions; topical antibiotics; see Chapter 77
Soft tissue hemorrhage	Localized tenderness may or may not be present; erythema, ecchymosis, edema of affected area	±	Cold compresses; if orbital floor fracture suspected, tomograms or CT scan; see Chapter 31

CT, computed tomography.

TABLE 75-1 Red Eye: Differential Diagnosis and Management Guidelines—cont'd

Disorder	Signs and Symptoms	Pain	Management
DISORDERS ASSOCIATED WITH OCULAR SURFACE REDNESS			
Angle-closure glaucoma	Severe pain; nausea, vomiting; halos around lights; photophobia; cornea may be cloudy with variable decrease in vision; conjunctival hyperemia; pupil middilated and fixed; firm globe; shallow anterior chamber	Yes	Refer emergently to ophthalmology; consider pilocarpine 2% 1 gtt q 15 min and/or acetazolamide 250-500 mg PO stat
Chemical exposure	Pain; conjunctival hyperemia, chemosis; corneal haze; decreased visual acuity	Yes	Immediate copious irrigation essential; refer emergently to ophthalmology; see Chapter 37
Conjunctivitis			
Allergic	Pruritus; conjunctival hyperemia, chemosis; watery or stringy discharge	No	Avoiding allergens; cold compresses; topical and/or systemic medication; see Chapter 78
Bacterial	Photophobia with blepharospasm; mucopurulent discharge with eyelash mattering; edema, hyperemia; preauricular adenopathy only with hyperacute disorder	±	Topical antibiotic drops; systemic antibiotics necessary for gonococcal or chlamydial etiology; see Chapter 78
Viral	Acute onset often associated with systemic illness; photophobia or foreign body sensation; preauricular adenopathy; hyperemia; chemosis; watery discharge; classic dendritic corneal lesion present with herpes simplex; periocular lesions present with herpes zoster ophthalmicus	±	Supportive treatment, including cool compresses, topical artificial tears; referral to ophthalmology for herpetic conjunctivitis; see Chapter 78
Corneal foreign body, abrasion or ulcer	Foreign body sensation with intense pain; photophobia; conjunctival hyperemia; may have decreased visual acuity; ulcers usually present as white or opaque corneal lesion; immediate prior history of trauma usually precedes abrasion but not erosion	Yes	Topical antibiotics (for prophylaxis) and systemic pain relievers in abrasions and after foreign body removal; no patching generally, *never* with ulcers or contact lens–related problems; urgent referral to ophthalmology for erosions, emergent referral for ulcers; see Chapter 79
Dry eye	Sandy, gritty, foreign body sensation; burning; pruritus; conjunctival hyperemia; decreased visual acuity		Topical artificial tears; lubricating ointments at night; warm compresses; gentle eyelid massage; evaluation for systemic disorders; see Chapter 80
Episcleritis/scleritis	Mild to severe pain; circumscribed erythema of affected sclera; vision unaffected	Yes	Episcleritis usually self-limiting; with possible scleritis, refer to ophthalmology; see Chapter 75
Hyphema	Microscopic or visible blood layering in anterior chamber usually after blunt trauma; often associated with other ocular symptoms	Yes	Refer urgently to ophthalmology; see Chapter 37
Iritis/uveitis	Pain; photophobia; conjunctival hyperemia; pupil constriction; may have epiphora but no mucopurulent discharge	Yes	Refer urgently to ophthalmology; see Chapter 75
Keratitis	Pain, photophobia; conjunctival hyperemia; corneal cloudiness with stromal involvement	Yes	Refer urgently to ophthalmology; see Chapter 75
Pinguecula and pterygium	Ocular irritation or pain when inflamed; dry eye symptoms; fleshy lesion medial on conjunctiva; with pterygium, lesion extends onto cornea	Yes	Ocular lubricants; topical NSAIDs; with pterygium, refer routinely to ophthalmology; see Chapter 83
Subconjunctival hemorrhage	No subjective symptoms; bright red spot of blood visible under overlying conjunctiva; remainder of conjunctiva remains white	No	Reassurance; no treatment necessary; see Chapter 84

primary care provider should not hesitate to refer patients to an ophthalmologist for cases in which treatment does not produce the expected result or in which the diagnosis remains obscure.

Vision Loss and Other Visual Disturbances

Visual disturbances can include decreased central or peripheral vision, *metamorphopsia* (distorted images), *photopsia* (light flashes), or *vitreous opacities* (floaters). It is critical to assess the vision of each eye individually. For the patient who normally wears corrective lenses, the visual acuity should be checked with glasses in place. If the glasses are unavailable, getting a pinhole acuity will approximate a corrected acuity. If reduced visual acuity disappears with corrective lenses or pinhole testing, a refractive error is most likely. It is also imperative to obtain a detailed history of the onset, duration, and other characteristics of symptoms. Visual loss may be unilateral or bilateral, may be transient or permanent, may occur suddenly or gradually, and may involve central or peripheral vision. Complaints of decreased peripheral vision are not common in the primary care setting because patients usually perceive only significant scotomas. "Sudden" vision loss must be distinguished from "suddenly noticed." A gradual vision loss in one eye may be "suddenly" noticed when the better eye is inadvertently occluded by a hand or some other object. Table 75-2 lists common causes of vision loss.

Amaurosis fugax is a transient, periodic visual loss. This condition may result from ophthalmic artery spasms in occlusive diseases of the internal carotid artery or from abnormalities of the aortic arch, both of which require referral for a cardiovascular evaluation. Amaurosis fugax may also result from temporal arteritis, which usually appears with accompanying tenderness or pain. These patients should be referred to an ophthalmologist for definitive diagnosis and management to prevent permanent vision loss. Transient visual loss, photopsia, floaters, photophobia, metamorphopsia, or scintillating scotomas may accompany migraine headaches. Ocular symptoms common in migraines can occur without an associated headache. Unless the patient has a clear past history of ocular migraine, these patients should be referred to an ophthalmologist to rule out other potential problems such as retinal or vitreal detachment.

TABLE 75-2 Vision Loss: Differential Diagnosis

Sudden	Gradual
UNILATERAL VISION LOSS	
Acute angle-closure glaucoma	Amblyopia
Central retinal vessel occlusion	Cataracts
Hyphema or other trauma	Corneal opacities
Iritis/uveitis	Iritis/uveitis
Optic neuritis	Macular degeneration
Temporal arteritis	Vitreous opacities
Retinal hemorrhage	
Retinal detachment	
BILATERAL VISION LOSS	
Hyphema or other trauma	Cataracts
Meningitis	Glaucoma
Migraine	Macular degeneration
Retinal hemorrhage	Pituitary tumor
Retrobulbar neuritis	
Stroke	

Metamorphopsia is commonly seen with macular degeneration. Any patient reporting new-onset visual distortion or a change in previously noted metamorphopsia should be referred to an ophthalmologist because effective treatments are available for certain types of age-related macular degeneration.[7,8]

Photopsia (flashes or flickers of light) may result from a retinal problem or cortical stimulation. Photopsia from retinal problems may be another indication of an impending or actual retinal tear or detachment, or a posterior vitreous detachment with retinal traction. Cortically induced photopsia may indicate migraine headache or occipital epilepsy.[9] Retinal detachment may also produce a persistent symptom described as a "curtain," "shadow," or "veil" falling over part of the visual field.

The vitreous is a thick, gellike structure that degenerates and liquefies with aging. When this occurs, aggregates form *vitreous floaters*, which are perceived by the patient as gray or black shapes floating within the visual field. Depending on the size and number, floaters may be simply annoying or may cause visual disability. They are often absorbed. If floaters occur suddenly or increase in frequency or quantity, urgent referral to an ophthalmologist is necessary. These symptoms may indicate the presence of a posterior vitreous detachment, primary vitreous hemorrhage, retinal tear, or retinal detachment.

Ocular and Periocular Pain

Ocular or periocular pain can include any discomfort in or around the eye and may be described as burning, aching, throbbing, boring, stabbing, or irritating, as with a foreign body sensation. Any condition that stimulates the numerous pain receptors present in the eyelids, cornea, conjunctiva, and uveal tract will cause ocular or periocular pain. Any inflammatory disorder of the conjunctiva, superficial layers of the cornea, or uveal tract can cause ocular irritation, burning, discomfort, or frank pain. Symptoms may be related to exposure to environmental irritants such as tobacco smoke or chemical fumes. Pain may also be referred from adjacent structures innervated by the ophthalmic division of cranial nerve V. Noninflammatory conditions affecting the optic nerve, retina, or vitreous do not usually result in pain.

Pain may occur coincidentally with other ocular symptoms, including decreased visual acuity, photophobia, ocular discharge, eyelid edema or erythema, ptosis, proptosis, or corneal cloudiness. Important history includes the following:

- Decrease in visual acuity
- Suddenness of onset
- Associated symptoms (including systemic symptoms such as nausea or vomiting)
- Contact lens use
- Exposure to ultraviolet light (such as outdoor activities or arc welding)
- Neurologic or systemic disorders
- Trauma

A complete ocular assessment should be performed in any patient with ocular pain. It is also important to examine the structures of the head and neck in any patient with a history of trauma. However, the eye should *never* be manipulated if there is any possibility of laceration or rupture of the ocular tissues. A shallow anterior chamber or abnormally shaped pupil may indicate a loss of aqueous humor secondary to a penetrating injury. Acute glaucoma should be excluded by measuring the intraocular pressure with a Schiøtz tonometer or palpating the globes and comparing the affected eye with the unaffected eye. Patients with a painful eye from acute glaucoma usually have associated redness, nausea, and vomiting. The cornea and conjunctiva may be assessed to identify abrasions or ulcers by applying fluorescein dye and examining the external eye under fluorescent light. Applying a topical anesthetic such as proparacaine hydrochloride 0.5% (Ophthaine) or tetracaine hydrochloride 0.5% (Pontocaine) will help differentiate the superficial pain caused by corneal surface disorders from pain resulting from problems with the deeper structures.

It may be useful to approach the differential diagnosis of ocular pain by grouping possible causes according to accompanying symptoms. This approach is summarized in Table 75-3.

Other Ocular Signs and Symptoms

Chemosis is edema of the bulbar conjunctiva. The conjunctiva becomes balloonlike and translucent in appearance around the corneal limbus, making the cornea appear sunken. The most common cause is an allergic reaction. The history of onset and recent activities should help with diagnosis.

Epiphora is excessive tearing. Causes include obstruction of the normal tear drainage system and excessive production of tears caused by irritation or inflammation. Although persistent tearing of one or both eyes in an infant is a cardinal sign of congenital glaucoma, this is a rare condition. Tearing in infants is most often due to congenital nasolacrimal duct obstruction. The patient should be referred to an ophthalmologist when no underlying cause is apparent or if the epiphora worsens.

Ocular discharge may be clear, watery, purulent or mucopurulent, stringy, or ropy. The differential diagnosis of an ocular disorder may be aided by observing the nature of abnormal ocular secretions. Pus in the conjunctival sac causes the eyelashes to stick together and is most common in mucopurulent conjunctivitis. A profuse watery discharge with a burning or gritty sensation and pain may be present in viral conjunctivitis. Pruritus associated with a discharge varying from a watery to a stringy, mucuslike consistency may indicate allergic conjunctivitis.

Photophobia may occur for no known reason. However, almost any condition resulting in ocular irritation or inflammation may cause photophobia. Conditions to consider include iritis or uveitis, conjunctivitis, conjunctival or corneal foreign bodies, corneal abrasion, keratitis, congenital glaucoma in infants, and acute glaucoma in adults. Photophobia may also result from exposure keratitis. This condition occurs most commonly in arc welders, swimmers, or skiers who do not use lenses for protection from excessive direct or reflected ultraviolet light exposure.

Pruritus is the most common complaint in allergic conditions, including allergic conjunctivitis. The symptom is usually bilateral and may be seasonal with associated hay fever symptoms. Unilateral pruritus associated with erythema and chemosis may be iatrogenic or caused by an allergic reaction to topical ophthalmic preparations or, commonly, the preservative in the preparation. Patients with severe dry eye or a chemical injury may also experience pruritus.

REFERENCES

1. Goldblum K: Nursing assessment. In Lamb P, Goldblum K, editors: *Core curriculum for ophthalmic nursing*, ed 2, Dubuque, Iowa, 2002, Kendall/Hunt Publishing.
2. Capriolo J and others: *Comprehensive adult medical eye evaluation*, San Francisco, 2000, American Academy of Ophthalmology.
3. Bateman JB and others: *Pediatric eye evaluations*, San Francisco, 1997, American Academy of Ophthalmology.
4. US Preventive Services Task Force: *Guide to clinical preventive services*, ed 3, Baltimore, 2000-2002, Williams & Wilkins.
5. American Academy of Pediatrics Committee on Practice and Ambulatory Medicine, Section on Ophthalmology: Eye examination and vision screening in infants, children, and young adults (RE9625), *Pediatrics* 98(1):153-157, 1996; http://www.aap.org/policy/01461.html.
6. Newman SA and others: *Basic and clinical science course: neuro-ophthalmology*, San Francisco, 2001, The Foundation of the American Academy of Ophthalmology.
7. Age-Related Eye Disease Study Research Group: A randomized, placebo-controlled clinical trial of high-dose supplementation with vitamins C and E, beta-carotene, and zinc for age-related macular degeneration and vision loss, *Arch Ophthalmol* 119(10):1417-1436, 2001.
8. Wormald R and others: Photodynamic therapy for neovascular age-related macular degeneration, Cochrane Review. In *The Cochrane Library* Issue 4, 2001, Oxford, Update Software.
9. Trobe JD: *The physician's guide to eye care*, San Francisco, 1998, American Academy of Ophthalmology.

TABLE 75-3 Symptoms Associated with Ocular Pain and Possible Causes

Associated Symptom	Possible Causes
Photophobia	Acute glaucoma, migraine, corneal trauma, keratoconjunctivitis, iritis, uveitis, scleritis
Nausea and vomiting	Acute glaucoma, endophthalmitis
Itching	Chemical injury, severe dry eye, allergy
Pain on eye movement	Orbital pseudotumor, myositis, posterior scleritis, optic neuritis, trauma, orbital cellulitis
Foreign body sensation	Corneal ulcer or abrasion, conjunctivitis, overexposure to ultraviolet light, entropion, trichiasis, conjunctival or eyelid lesion (rule out actual corneal or conjunctival foreign body)

CHAPTER 76

Cataracts

Kate Goldblum, Patricia Gillett, and Joyce Powers

DEFINITION/EPIDEMIOLOGY

A cataract is an opacity in the crystalline lens of the eye. Although not all cataracts significantly affect visual acuity, they are a common cause of decreased visual acuity and the leading cause of preventable blindness in the United States for individuals over age 40 years.[1] Most cataracts occur in the aging population and can significantly affect the quality of life in older adults. Almost everyone will develop a cataract if he or she lives long enough. Between ages 65 and 74 years, 14% of men and 24% of women have visually significant cataracts. After age 75 years, these figures increase to 39% and 46%, respectively. The incidence of cataracts is higher in patients with diabetes. Age-related cataracts are usually bilateral but may develop at different rates. Congenital cataracts occur in approximately 1 in 2000 live births.[2] Congenital cataracts are an urgent ophthalmic problem because of the rapid development of amblyopia in the neonate.

PATHOPHYSIOLOGY

Cataracts form when altered metabolic processes affect the structure of the lens fiber. These changes are associated with aging, diabetes, trauma, heavy smoking, corticosteroid use, electrical shock, and exposure to ultraviolet light.

CLINICAL PRESENTATION

Initially the patient may complain of visual problems such as blurry vision or a "film" that obscures vision. The patient may also complain of glare from any source of bright light or altered color perception. Occasionally, a significant unilateral cataract will appear to cause a "sudden" loss of vision. The vision loss is not actually sudden; the patient notices it suddenly when the nonaffected eye becomes obscured in some way. The history may include a gradual decrease in vision. Significant cataracts may cause a loss in the ability to continue usual leisure activities or to perform activities of daily living.

PHYSICAL EXAMINATION

The external ocular structures and the pupillary aperture should be examined. The red reflex may be dull. With an advanced cataract, the pupil will appear opaque because of the mature cataractous lens behind the iris (Color Plate 30). Ophthalmoscopic examination may reveal lens opacities and obscured retinal vasculature.

DIAGNOSTICS

None indicated.

DIFFERENTIAL DIAGNOSIS

The differential diagnosis includes any cause of decreased visual acuity, including macular degeneration and diabetic retinopathy. With advanced cataracts, the completely opaque lens may resemble an intraocular tumor that obscures the pupillary aperture.

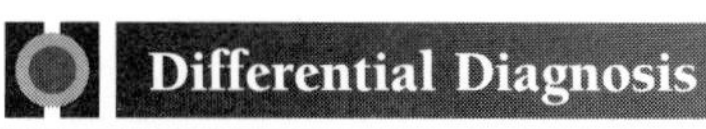

Cataracts
Macular degeneration
Diabetic retinopathy
Intraocular tumor
Retinal detachment
Scarring from previous trauma or irradiation

MANAGEMENT

A regular ophthalmic examination and changes in eyeglasses will temporarily improve the patient's ability to see as the cataract develops. Other mediating measures include using increased magnification and increased lighting to improve functional ability. It may be acceptable for the patient to make lifestyle modifications (e.g., ceasing nighttime driving), at least temporarily. The best clinical evidence to date supports that surgery will improve quality of life and is indicated when visual needs exceed the level of vision allowed by the cataract.[1]

LIFE SPAN CONSIDERATIONS

Congenital cataracts or cataracts that develop in children ages 10 years or younger must be urgently managed because of the certain risk of amblyopia. The morbidity attached to the extensive incidence of cataracts in older adults warrants referral for surgery even in individuals with multiple co-morbidities. Advances in cataract surgery and management, including topical anesthesia, small incision surgery, and intraocular lenses, reduce the risks and hasten postoperative visual rehabilitation, making this surgery appropriate even for very old patients.[3] Older patients with no deficits other than poor vision are 2.5 times more likely to experience a decline in functional ability than are patients with normal vision.[1]

COMPLICATIONS

Usually the only complication associated with cataracts is decreased visual acuity. In rare instances a cataract may cause phacolytic glaucoma or anterior uveitis and require immediate surgery. Mature cataractous lenses are more likely to dislocate. Mature cataracts may cause complete blindness, but surgery can still provide a good visual outcome.

INDICATIONS FOR REFERRAL/HOSPITALIZATION

The patient should be referred to an ophthalmologist when visual acuity is reduced to a level that does not meet the patient's visual needs. The level at which this occurs varies from person to person.

PATIENT AND FAMILY EDUCATION

Larger-print materials, the use of magnifying devices, and increased lighting may allow adequate vision during the early phase of cataract development. Patients should be informed that cataracts are progressive and irreversible but that surgical removal is safe and effective. Surgery is elective. Patients should be advised that only they can determine when their vision no longer meets their visual needs.

HEALTH PROMOTION

Patients should avoid known risk factors such as heavy smoking, ultraviolet radiation, and alcohol consumption. Other risk factors over which patients may have some control include diabetes, corticosteroid use, electrical shock, and trauma.[4]

REFERENCES

1. Masket S and others: *Preferred practice patterns: cataract in the adult eye,* San Francisco, 2001, American Academy of Ophthalmology.
2. Johns KJ and others: *Basic and clinical science course: lens and cataract,* San Francisco, 2001, Foundation of the American Academy of Ophthalmology.
3. Lundstrom M, Steneve U, Thorburn W: Cataract surgery in the very elderly, *J Cataract Refract Surg* 26:408-414, 2000.
4. Goldblum K: Lens disorders. In Lamb P, Goldblum K, editors: *Core curriculum for ophthalmic nursing,* ed 2, Dubuque, Iowa, 2002, Kendall/Hunt Publishing.

CHAPTER 77

Chalazion, Hordeolum, and Blepharitis

Kate Goldblum, Patricia Gillett, and Joyce Powers

DEFINITION/EPIDEMIOLOGY

Chalazia and hordeola are both inflammatory processes involving the glandular tissues of the eyelid, usually the upper eyelid. A hordeolum is also called a stye. An external hordeolum is an infection of the glands of Moll or Zeis, whereas an internal hordeolum is an infection of the meibomian gland. A chalazion also involves the meibomian gland but is a granulomatous inflammatory lesion rather than an infectious process. Although an acute infection of the meibomian gland is actually an internal hordeolum, it is sometimes referred to as an *acute chalazion.* These inflammatory lesions are often associated with blepharitis, an inflammatory condition of the eyelid margins. Blepharitis may be acute or chronic and is often categorized as *anterior* or *posterior* depending on the anatomic structures involved.[1] Anterior blepharitis involves the anterior lid margin surrounding the eyelashes and may extend to the posterior lid margin, conjunctiva, and cornea. When associated with *Staphylococcus aureus* infection, 80% of patients with the condition are women, probably related to use of contaminated eye makeup. Posterior blepharitis involves abnormal function of the meibomian glands, either hyperactive secretion or obstruction of the gland. These conditions are among the most common ocular disorders seen in primary care.[2]

PATHOPHYSIOLOGY

The glandular structures involved in a chalazion or hordeolum become obstructed, leading to an inflammatory process. In the case of a hordeolum, a gland of Moll or Zeis becomes acutely inflamed and infected. The most commonly associated organism is *S. aureus*. In contrast, a chalazion involves a chronically inflamed meibomian gland without accompanying infection. Anterior blepharitis is most commonly associated with *S. aureus* infection but is also associated with other organisms. It may also involve abnormal sebaceous gland secretory function and is then termed *seborrheic blepharitis.* Excessive meibomian oil secretions or solidification of the oil with resulting blockage of the gland results in posterior blepharitis.

CLINICAL PRESENTATION

A chalazion or hordeolum may present with a localized erythematous swelling. A hordeolum is often tender to palpation, whereas chronic chalazia are normally nontender. There is usually no visual disturbance unless lid swelling is excessive. Larger lesions may press on the corneal surface and induce astigmatism, decreasing vision. An internal hordeolum typically points either externally to the skin or internally to the conjunctival surface. An external hordeolum is more superficial and points to the lid margin. A chalazion is usually located in the mid tarsus away from the lid margin and is usually a

TABLE 77-1 Clinical Presentation of Blepharitis

	Crusting	Erythema/Edema	Loss of Eyelashes
Anterior	Hard	Yes	Yes
Anterior Seborrheic	Oily	Yes	Rare
Posterior	+/−	Yes	No

chronic lesion that presents with or without acute inflammatory signs.

All forms of blepharitis may present with crusting and an erythematous lid margin. Alteration of the tear film layer may induce symptoms of dry eye (Table 77-1).

PHYSICAL EXAMINATION

The ocular adnexa, especially the lid margins, should be carefully inspected. Adequate lighting and some magnification are particularly helpful during this assessment. With blepharitis, the lid margins may be reddened and scaly. The lid should be palpated for swelling and masses, and the eyelid should be everted to examine the tarsal conjunctival surface for pointing. This maneuver may be difficult when the lid is swollen and painful. The sclera and conjunctiva should be inspected for erythema, edema, or exudate. Hordeola and chalazia may be initially indistinguishable. However, the initial acute manifestations of a chalazion will resolve within a few days, leaving a painless, slowly growing lid mass.

DIAGNOSTICS

None indicated.

DIFFERENTIAL DIAGNOSIS

Patients with multiple or recurrent chalazia or hordeola may have underlying diabetes mellitus. Benign or malignant tumors must be considered in patients with recurrent or atypical lesions. In addition to chalazia, hordeola, and blepharitis, the differential diagnosis for eyelid disorders includes cellulitis or abscess of the eyelid and acute dacryocystitis.[3]

MANAGEMENT

Frequent application of warm, moist compresses to a hordeolum will often hasten the process of pointing and draining. If associated with a specific eyelash, pulling the lash will also hasten draining. Topical antibiotics may be helpful and should be used four times daily and continued for 1 week. Topical antibiotics include neomycin/polymyxin B/gramicidin (Neosporin ophthalmic solution) or tobramycin 0.3% (Tobrex ophthalmic solution). The more broad-spectrum topical antibiotics such as ofloxacin 0.3% (Ocuflox ophthalmic solution) or ciprofloxacin (Ciloxan ophthalmic solution) should be avoided unless the hordeolum recurs frequently or does not respond to other therapy. Ointments can be messy and blur the vision, and many patients prefer drops for these reasons. Recurrent lesions require daily lid margin scrubs and topical antibiotics. Although commercial products for lid scrubs are available, an inexpensive and effective alternative is diluted baby shampoo (see Patient and Family Education). Patients with chronic or recurrent lesions may be co-managed with the ophthalmologist. Chronic chalazia may require steroid injection. If this is not effective, lesions must be surgically incised and removed by an ophthalmologist. Lid scrubs are also indicated for blepharitis management. Therapy for anterior blepharitis includes topical antibiotics. Table 77-2 summarizes the specific management of hordeola, chalazia, and the different forms of blepharitis.

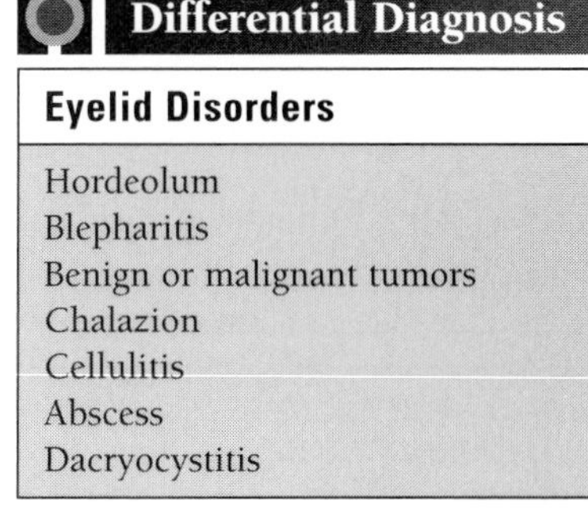
Differential Diagnosis

Eyelid Disorders

Hordeolum
Blepharitis
Benign or malignant tumors
Chalazion
Cellulitis
Abscess
Dacryocystitis

LIFE SPAN CONSIDERATIONS

Hordeola are more common in children and adolescents and may occur in groups of lesions because individuals in these age-groups tend to rub their eyelids and spread the infection. In contrast, chalazia are more common in adults.[4] In children, a large lesion causing astigmatism or obstructing the visual axis may induce amblyopia. Younger children can develop significant amblyopia within weeks. Anterior blepharitis is more common in younger patients, and posterior blepharitis is more common in older patients.[5]

COMPLICATIONS

If left untreated, these lesions may progress to eyelid or periorbital cellulitis and require systemic antibiotics. Large lesions may induce astigmatism or mechanically restrict the visual field, but this is rare. Chronic blepharitis may result in scarring and the loss of protective eyelashes.

INDICATIONS FOR REFERRAL/HOSPITALIZATION

Complicated cases may require referral to an ophthalmologist. Patients with recurrent or atypical lesions, lesions unresponsive to therapy, or unexplained vision loss should also be referred to an ophthalmologist. Blepharitis that does not respond to conservative management should be referred to an ophthalmologist for further evaluation and management, including possible systemic antibiotic therapy.

PATIENT AND FAMILY EDUCATION

Patients need instructions regarding good hygienic practices and daily lid scrubs. An inexpensive alternative to commercially available products for lid scrubs is 1 part baby shampoo diluted in 1 part water. The patient should be instructed to dip a clean, cotton-tipped swab in the solution and gently scrub the lid margins. A separate swab should be used for each eyelid. After the scrub, the patient should thoroughly rinse the area and pat it dry. Although it is an expensive recommendation, the patient with a hordeolum or blepharitis associated with *S. aureus* infection should be instructed to discard all eye and face makeup, opened contact lens solutions, and used contact lens cases because of the risk of reinfection from contamination.

HEALTH PROMOTION

Good lid hygiene to control chronic blepharitis and prevent the recurrence of chalazia and hordeola is the primary consideration in health promotion.

TABLE 77-2 Management of Lid Disorders

	Compresses	Antibiotic	Steroid	Other
HORDEOLUM				
Internal: Zeis or Moll gland infection *External:* meibomian gland infection (sometimes referred to as "acute chalazion")	Frequent warm, moist compresses to hasten pointing and drainage	Topically to prevent secondary infection from drainage; continue for 1 week; systemic doxycycline for recurrent lesions	None	Lid scrubs, especially if lesions recurrent; discard opened eye makeup to avoid reinfection
CHALAZION				
Meibomian gland *inflammation* (acute *infection* is more properly termed external hordeolum)	Frequent warm, moist compresses to liquefy glandular secretions	Not indicated	Intralesional injection may be effective in resolving lesion	Lid massage to help express impacted secretions; lid scrubs useful if associated with blepharitis
BLEPHARITIS				
Anterior	Daily or more frequent warm, moist compresses to help loosen crusts	Topical ophthalmic erythromycin or bacitracin ointment	None	Lid scrubs at least daily or more often to help remove crusts
Anterior seborrheic	Daily or more frequent warm, moist compresses to help loosen crusts	None	Occasional topical steroid if inflammation prominent	Lid scrubs at least daily or more often to help remove oily secretions
Posterior	Daily or more frequent warm, moist compresses to help liquefy secretions	None	None	Lid scrubs at least daily or more often to help remove oily secretions

REFERENCES

1. Cioffi GA: *The Devers manual: ophthalmology for the health care professional*, Baltimore, 1997, Williams & Wilkins.
2. Bajart AM: Lid inflammations. In Albert DM, Jakobiec FA, editors: *Principles and practice of ophthalmology*, ed 2, 2000, WB Saunders.
3. Robinson D, Kidd P, Rogers KM, editors: *Primary care across the lifespan*, St Louis, 2000, Mosby.
4. Wilson ME and others: *Basic and clinical science course: pediatric ophthalmology and strabismus*, San Francisco, 2001, The Foundation of the American Academy of Ophthalmology.
5. Wilhelmus KR and others: *Basic and clinical science course: external disease and cornea*, San Francisco, 2001, The Foundation of the American Academy of Ophthalmology.

CHAPTER 78

Conjunctivitis

Kate Goldblum, Patricia Gillett, and Joyce Powers

DEFINITION/EPIDEMIOLOGY

Conjunctivitis is an inflammation or infection of the conjunctiva. Only the bulbar conjunctiva covering the sclera may be involved, or the inflammation may also involve the tarsal conjunctiva that lines the inside of the eyelids. The cornea may become involved with more severe inflammatory or infectious responses, in which case the condition is termed *keratoconjunctivitis*.

Conjunctivitis is a common ocular condition and can occur in all age-groups. Allergic conjunctivitis occurs seasonally or after ocular contact with sensitizing substances, such as occurs in contact lens wearers who develop sensitivities to their lenses or the solutions used to care for them. Allergic conditions, which usually begin in childhood or adolescence, are more common in patients with a positive family history of allergy. These conditions are more common in males.[1] Bacterial conjunctivitis is much less common than other types; viral conjunctivitis is the most common cause of an acute red eye.[2] Adenoviruses cause most cases of conjunctivitis and keratoconjunctivitis, including epidemic keratoconjunctivitis, which is highly contagious and is often spread via public swimming pools. Gonococcal and chlamydial infections are more likely to occur in the neonate or in patients at risk for sexually transmitted diseases. Chlamydial conjunctivitis, also called *inclusion conjunctivitis,* is becoming more common in the United States as a result of sexual spread of the causative organism.[3] The chlamydial organism may also be transferred from the mother's birth canal to infants during delivery. Toxic conjunctivitis occurs with exposure to noxious agents such as chlorinated water in swimming pools, hair sprays, other aerosol agents, and strong chemical fumes.

PATHOPHYSIOLOGY

Allergic conjunctivitis is an immunologically mediated response to a wide variety of allergens. Another noninfectious mechanism is a toxic response to various agents such as crab lice or to the benzalkonium chloride preservative in many topical medications. Bacterial conjunctivitis results from a variety of infectious organisms, including *Staphylococcus aureus, Streptococcus* species, *Haemophilus influenzae, Neisseria gonorrhoeae, Proteus* species, and *Klebsiella pneumoniae.* Viral conjunctivitis commonly involves the adenoviruses, herpes simplex virus, and herpes zoster virus.

CLINICAL PRESENTATION

A variety of symptoms may be present depending on the cause and severity of the conjunctivitis. The most common sign of conjunctivitis is conjunctival hyperemia. Allergic conjunctivitis often causes generalized hyperemia, mild to severe itching, and an ocular discharge that may be clear and watery or stringy and mucoid. There may also be mild to severe chemosis. Severe edema may cause the cornea to appear sunken in the boggy conjunctiva. Vision is usually unaffected or mildly affected if there is significant tearing. Antecedent history of atopy is helpful in diagnosing allergic conjunctivitis.

Viral conjunctivitis has an acute onset and may be unilateral or bilateral with a watery discharge and preauricular or submandibular adenitis. It may be associated with fever and pharyngitis, especially in children. Viral conjunctivitis is usually self-limiting but may take weeks to completely resolve. Photophobia or a foreign body sensation may be present. Herpes simplex conjunctivitis presents with a classic dendritic corneal lesion visible with fluorescein staining. Herpes zoster dermatitis may also involve the ocular structures, including the conjunctiva. Although variably reliable, the presence of a lesion on the tip of the nose, called Hutchinson's sign, is an indication of ocular involvement.[4]

In contrast, the only bacterial conjunctivitis that causes preauricular adenitis is the hyperacute purulent conjunctivitis caused by the *Neisseria* species, primarily *N. gonorrhoeae* or, less commonly, *N. meningitidis.*[5] Bacterial conjunctivitis has an acute onset and is not associated with systemic illness. Hyperemia, chemosis, photophobia with blepharospasm, and tearing may be present. Symptoms often begin in one eye and then involve the second eye. The patient may report that the eye may be "stuck shut" with mucopurulent drainage on awakening. If a mucopurulent discharge is present in association with preauricular adenitis, a careful history should be obtained to determine whether there is an increased risk for other sexually transmitted disease because chlamydia is found in up to one third of all patients with gonococcal conjunctivitis.[6]

PHYSICAL EXAMINATION

Although the history is the most helpful factor in making the correct diagnosis, the examination may provide additional clues or help exclude other causes of the patient's symptoms. The pupils should be observed for symmetry and response to light, and the eyelids should be examined for erythema, swelling, or hyperemia. The upper lids should be everted and the tarsal conjunctival surface checked for a cobblestone appearance, which indicates an allergic response. The possible presence of conjunctival foreign bodies should be evaluated using magnification. The sclera and conjunctiva should be observed for redness, edema, or discharge. The cornea should be evaluated for clarity. Herpetic lesions, foreign bodies, and ulcers should be excluded using magnification and an ultraviolet light source after fluorescein staining. The preauricular and submandibular glands should be palpated for the presence of lymphadenopathy.

DIAGNOSTICS

Patients with conjunctivitis should have corneal fluorescein staining to identify any possible corneal surface pathology that may cause similar symptoms. Cultures are generally not necessary in the primary care setting. Exceptions include neonates with mucopurulent discharge, as well as adolescents and adults at risk for sexually transmitted diseases. In such cases the discharge must be

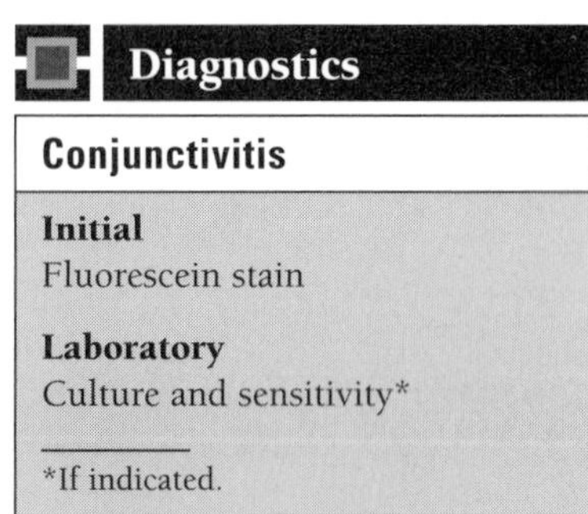
Diagnostics

Conjunctivitis

Initial
Fluorescein stain

Laboratory
Culture and sensitivity*

*If indicated.

cultured to determine whether the conjunctivitis is of gonococcal or chlamydial origin.[7]

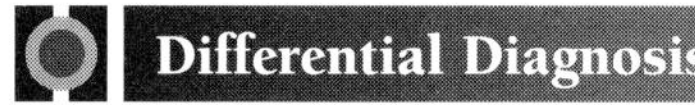

Conjunctivitis

Nasolacrimal obstruction
Acute anterior uveitis
Acute glaucoma
Blepharitis
Corneal abrasions or ulcers
Corneal or conjunctival foreign bodies

DIFFERENTIAL DIAGNOSIS

Other causes of a red eye include nasolacrimal duct obstruction, acute anterior uveitis, acute glaucoma, blepharitis, corneal abrasions or ulcers, and corneal or conjunctival foreign bodies. Further causes of a red eye are listed in Table 75-1.

MANAGEMENT

Topical decongestant/antihistamine combinations such as naphazoline hydrochloride 0.025%/pheniramine maleate 0.3% (Naphcon-A) or naphazoline/antazoline (Vasocon-A) and the newer selective antihistamines levocabastine hydrochloride 0.05% (Livostin) and emedastine 0.05% (Emadine) are effective for relieving the symptoms of allergic conjunctivitis. Nonsteroidal antiinflammatory agents such as ketorolac (Acular) or diclofenac (Voltaren) and the mast cell stabilizers lodoxamide tromethamine 0.1% (Alomide) or cromolyn sodium 4% (Crolom) can be helpful in allergic conjunctivitis. Severe allergic conjunctivitis may require topical steroid therapy, but such therapy can cause increased intraocular pressure (IOP) in susceptible patients and therefore should not be used unless the IOP can be checked periodically. Systemic antihistamines or other antiallergy agents may be helpful. Cold compresses may relieve itching and edema.

Although acute bacterial conjunctivitis is often self-limiting, topical antibiotics may hasten resolution.[8] Topical antibiotic drops such as sulfacetamide 10% (Bleph-10, Isopto Cetamide, or Sodium Sulamyd) or tobramycin (Tobrex) are effective in treating most uncomplicated cases of bacterial conjunctivitis. Chlamydial and gonococcal conjunctivitis must be treated with topical and systemic antibiotic therapy. The primary care provider may manage the systemic antimicrobial therapy for gonococcal and chlamydial conjunctivitis. The ophthalmologist manages the ocular therapy and monitors the patient's progress.

Systemic penicillin and doxycycline therapy are the respective treatments of choice for gonococcal and chlamydial infections. Gentamycin 3 mg/ml (Garamycin Ophthalmic, Genoptic S.O.P., or Gentacidin), ofloxacin 0.3% (Ocuflox), or norfloxacin (Chibroxin) ophthalmic drops may be used for gonococcal conjunctivitis. Tetracycline ophthalmic ointment (Terak) may be used for chlamydial conjunctivitis.

Viral conjunctivitis is usually self-limiting. Cool compresses may provide some symptomatic relief. Antiinfectives, steroids, and topical vasoconstrictors should not be used. Conjunctivitis of herpetic etiology should be referred to an ophthalmologist for antiviral therapy.

LIFE SPAN CONSIDERATIONS

Conjunctivitis can occur in all age-groups. During the first month of life, conjunctivitis is called *ophthalmia neonatorum.* Hyperacute purulent bacterial conjunctivitis is most common in neonates, adolescents, and adults because of its association with the *Neisseria* species and requires culture for confirmation. Viral conjunctivitis is more likely to be associated with fever and pharyngitis in children.

COMPLICATIONS

Severe allergic conjunctivitis can progress to vernal conjunctivitis and lead to corneal ulceration. Bacterial conjunctivitis can also involve the cornea, leading to keratitis and possibly ulceration. Infected corneal ulcers may result in intraocular infection and loss of the eye. Severe viral conjunctivitis may cause extensive scarring and cicatricial complications.

INDICATIONS FOR REFERRAL/HOSPITALIZATION

Neonates with conjunctivitis should be referred to an ophthalmologist. All patients with suspected bacterial conjunctivitis should be referred to an ophthalmologist if the condition is unresponsive to antimicrobial therapy or if there is suspected corneal involvement. An ophthalmic referral is also necessary for complaints of significant ocular pain or decreased visual acuity. Steroid therapy for severe viral conjunctivitis is controversial and should be initiated by an ophthalmologist, as should treatment for herpetic viral keratoconjunctivitis.

PATIENT AND FAMILY EDUCATION

Patients should be instructed to use the prescribed medication for allergic conjunctivitis during the acute allergic periods and to avoid rubbing the eyes to prevent further irritation. Comfort measures such as cold compresses can be helpful. Patients should be warned to avoid the offending allergen whenever possible. Appropriate hygienic measures to prevent transmission to others are imperative with contagious conjunctivitis. Frequent and thorough handwashing is necessary for the patient and all close contacts. Patients should be advised not to share linens with others and to limit public contact during the acute phase when drainage occurs. In any case of infectious conjunctivitis, patients should be instructed to discard all opened eye makeup and to replace their contact lenses, cases, and opened solutions.

HEALTH PROMOTION

Eye makeup, ocular medications, and contact lens solutions and cases should not be shared with other individuals. They should also be replaced regularly to avoid possible ocular infections from contaminated items. Patients need to be informed that sexually transmitted diseases can infect the ocular structures through oral-genital contact.

REFERENCES

1. Abelson MB, Udell IJ: Allergic and toxic reactions. In Albert DM, Jacobiec FA, editors: *Principles and practice of ophthalmology,* ed 2, Philadelphia, 2000, WB Saunders.
2. Trobe JD: *The physician's guide to eyecare,* San Francisco, 1997, American Academy of Ophthalmology.
3. Isada CM, Meisler DM: Gonococcal ocular disease. In Fraunfelder FT, Roy FH, Randall J, editors: *Current ocular therapy,* ed 5, Philadelphia, 2000, WB Saunders.
4. Pavan-Langston D: Viral disease of the cornea and external eye. In Albert DM, Jacobiec FA, editors: *Principles and practice of ophthalmology,* ed 2, Philadelphia, 2000, WB Saunders.

5. Foulks GN, Gordon JS, Kowalski RP: Bacterial infections of the conjunctiva and cornea. In Albert DM, Jacobiec FA, eds: *Principles and practice of ophthalmology,* ed 2, Philadelphia, 2000, WB Saunders.
6. Wilhelmus KR and others: *Basic and clinical science course: external disease and cornea,* San Francisco, 2001, The Foundation of the American Academy of Ophthalmology.
7. Dawson CR: Inclusion conjunctivitis. In Fraunfelder FT, Roy FH, Randall J, editors: *Current ocular therapy,* ed 5, Philadelphia, 2000, WB Saunders.
8. Wormald R and others: Antibiotics versus placebo for acute bacterial conjunctivitis (Cochrane Review). In *The Cochrane Library* Issue 4, 2001, Oxford, Update Software.

CHAPTER 79

Corneal Surface Defects and Ocular Surface Foreign Bodies

Kate Goldblum, Patricia Gillett, and Joyce Powers

DEFINITION/EPIDEMIOLOGY

The corneal surface may be disrupted by an abrasion, erosion, ulcer, or foreign body. An abrasion is a partial or complete defect in the epithelial layer of cells after some traumatic event or overexposure to ultraviolet (UV) light. An erosion is also a partial or complete defect in the epithelium but is not associated with trauma immediately preceding the symptoms. A corneal ulcer involves the underlying stromal layer in addition to the epithelial defect. This may or may not be infected. Ocular foreign bodies may be any foreign matter that becomes lodged in the corneal or conjunctival tissues. Abrasions resulting from trauma may occur in any age-group. Foreign bodies are a common source of ocular injuries seen in primary care or emergency departments. Certain workers, such as mechanics, woodworkers, and other construction workers, have an increased risk of corneal abrasions or ocular foreign bodies if they do not use appropriate protective eyewear. Contact lens wearers are at increased risk for corneal abrasions. Extended contact lens wear increases the risk of corneal ulcers approximately sixfold over that of daily contact lens wear.[1] Erosions occur in patients with a history of prior corneal abrasion.

Immediate ophthalmology referral is indicated for all corneal ulcers and for all ocular foreign bodies that are penetrating, obviously impacted, associated with rust ring, or not readily removed by irrigation.
Immediate ophthalmology referral is indicated for ocular herpes simplex and ocular herpes zoster.

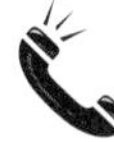

Urgent ophthalmology referral is indicated for suspected corneal erosions.
Urgent ophthalmology referral is indicated for corneal abrasions not resolved in 24 hours and for corneal lesions that are dendritic or punctate.

PATHOPHYSIOLOGY

An abrasion of the corneal epithelium may be caused by chemical or mechanical debridement resulting from trauma or UV radiation exposure. Corneal erosions occur if an abrasion disrupts Bowman's membrane. Decreased evaporation during sleep results in the formation of a fluid layer above the incompletely healed Bowman's membrane, below the epithelium.

This allows repeated sloughing of the overlying epithelium when the patient awakes and opens the lid, removing the loose epithelial cells. Epithelial defects, whether abrasions or erosions, may allow bacterial, viral, or fungal organisms to invade the corneal stroma, resulting in an ulcer. Sterile corneal ulcers may also occur.

CLINICAL PRESENTATION

Because the cornea is highly innervated, any disruption in the corneal surface causes intense pain. Similar pain may be caused by a *foreign body* under the upper eyelid that rubs the corneal surface with each blink. Small disruptions in the corneal surface may initially produce a sandy or gritty sensation. With more extensive involvement, intense pain, ocular redness, tearing, photophobia, and often a foreign body sensation are present. A *corneal ulcer* usually appears as a white or opaque lesion. A clear history of trauma or excessive UV exposure usually precedes a *corneal abrasion*. The history may include contact lens wear or any recent ocular irritation that may have caused vigorous eye rubbing resulting in an abrasion. In contrast, there may not be a clear history of exposure to an *ocular foreign body* when one is present. *Corneal erosions* are not immediately preceded by trauma. Careful questioning may elicit a history of prior corneal abrasion. There may or may not be decreased visual acuity depending on the extent and location of the pathology.

PHYSICAL EXAMINATION

The upper lid of the involved eye should be everted and the tarsal conjunctival surface examined under magnification for the presence of foreign bodies. The cornea should be examined after the instillation of fluorescein. Corneal defects will stain and fluoresce when exposed to UV light, as will defects caused by foreign bodies. The conjunctiva should be examined for erythema and edema. The corneal surface should be evaluated, checking clarity and looking for areas of opacity or surface irregularity. An oblique light source can be used to assess anterior chamber depth and to identify hypopyon (pus in the anterior chamber). A perforated corneal ulcer or a penetrating foreign body may cause a flat anterior chamber, which is evident when the chamber is compared with the fellow eye.

DIAGNOSTICS

A corneal ulcer is an ophthalmic emergency, especially in the presence of hypopyon. Immediate culture and institution of antimicrobial therapy after an ophthalmology consult may be necessary in some settings in which an ophthalmologist is not immediately available.

DIFFERENTIAL DIAGNOSIS

The differential diagnosis includes corneal laceration, conjunctivitis, herpetic and other forms of keratitis, blepharitis, dacryocystitis, inflamed pingueculum or pterygium, and early hordeolum or chalazion.

MANAGEMENT

Minor corneal abrasions can be managed in the primary care setting. An antibiotic ointment such as tobramycin (Tobrex), gentamycin (Garamycin, Gentacidin, or Genoptic), or erythromycin (Ilotycin) is applied. Patching does not hasten healing time, lessen pain, or decrease reports of blurred vision. In addition, compliance with the medication regimen is improved when the patient's eye is not patched.[2] A pain reliever should be prescribed and the patient reexamined every 24 hours until the lesion is completely healed. Preparations with a steroid component should not be used because the steroid can slow healing and encourage bacterial growth. All patients with apparent erosions should be urgently referred, and patients with corneal ulcer should be emergently referred to an ophthalmologist for evaluation and further therapy. If there is any delay in referral of a corneal ulcer, the lesion should be cultured, and broad-spectrum topical antibiotic drops should be started and given every 30 minutes until seen by the ophthalmologist.[3] Ciprofloxacin ophthalmic solution (Ciloxan) is a broad-spectrum antibacterial agent effective against *Pseudomonas aeruginosa*. The patient's tetanus immunization status should be determined.

Superficial corneal and conjunctival foreign bodies can be safely removed in the primary care setting. After application of a topical anesthetic, a moist, cotton-tipped applicator may be used to remove the foreign body. If the foreign body is superficially embedded, a 25-gauge needle may be necessary for removal if the provider is skilled in this procedure and has adequate magnification. Topical antibiotic therapy should be prescribed prophylactically. Clinical studies do not show any benefit in patching the eye in these patients. In any case, *a firm patch should not be applied nor any medications instilled if there is any possibility or suspicion of a penetrating injury.* In addition, any patient with a contact lens–associated abrasion or ulcer should never be patched.

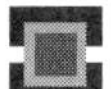

Diagnostics

Corneal Surface Defects and Foreign Bodies

Initial (Corneal Ulcer)
Fluorescein scan

Laboratory (Corneal Ulcer)
Culture and sensitivity (if immediate ophthalmology consultation not available)

Initial (Foreign Body)
Fluorescein stain

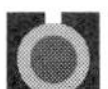

Differential Diagnosis

Corneal Surface Defects and Foreign Bodies

Conjunctivitis
Keratitis
Blepharitis
Dacryocystitis
Inflamed pinguecula or pterygium
Hordeolum (early)
Chalazion (early)
Corneal lacerations

LIFE SPAN CONSIDERATIONS

Infants and children may not be cooperative, which makes careful examination and removal of foreign bodies too difficult in the primary care setting. These patients should be urgently referred to an ophthalmologist. The majority of eye injuries occur in the second and third decades of life. In children, many injuries are sports related and most occur between the ages of 11 and 15 years.[4]

COMPLICATIONS

Corneal abrasions usually heal without complications but may result in a secondary bacterial keratitis. Corneal erosions and ulcers may cause corneal scarring with vision loss. Corneal ulcers may also result in endophthalmitis, an extensive ocular infection. Subsequent phthisis bulbi (wasting of the globe) and complete blindness may occur. Metallic foreign bodies produce a rust ring that must be completely removed using a slit lamp biomicroscope to prevent chronic problems. Cataract formation is common after any penetrating injury or ulcer.

INDICATIONS FOR REFERRAL/HOSPITALIZATION

Referral to an ophthalmologist is necessary if a corneal abrasion (1) has not significantly improved within 24 hours, (2) has not completely resolved in 48 to 72 hours, or (3) shows any signs of infection. All patients with corneal ulcers should be emergently referred. Hospitalization may be required for IV antibiotic therapy. Any deeply embedded or centrally located corneal foreign body also requires referral to an ophthalmologist, as do metallic foreign bodies. All chemical injuries and any suspicion of ocular penetration require emergent referral to an ophthalmologist.

PATIENT AND FAMILY EDUCATION

It is imperative to instruct the patient to remove contact lenses immediately if there is any redness, ocular irritation, pain, or decrease in vision. Patients should be advised not to resume contact lens wear until 24 to 48 hours after a superficial abrasion has healed. Culture and subsequent disposal are necessary for all lens supplies and solutions if a corneal ulcer is present. Patients should dispose of any opened cosmetics because of the risk for contamination. Patients should be informed that corneal abrasions or surface defects that remain after foreign body removal can cause significant discomfort for 12 to 24 hours. They should be encouraged to use appropriate pain medications. Patients should be instructed to return before the scheduled follow-up examination if there is any purulent drainage, increased pain or redness, or decreased vision.

HEALTH PROMOTION

The use of proper protective eyewear is imperative during many work and leisure activities to prevent ocular injury. Information regarding such use should be obtained on all patients in the primary care setting, and patients should be encouraged to use appropriate protection.

REFERENCES

1. Wilhelmus KR and others: *Basic and clinical science course: external disease and cornea*, San Francisco, 2001, The Foundation of the American Academy of Ophthalmology.
2. Kaiser PJ: A comparison of pressure patching versus no patching for corneal abrasions due to trauma or foreign body removal: Corneal Abrasion Patching Study Group, *Ophthalmology* 102(12):1936-1942, 1995.
3. Foulks GN, Gordon JS, Kowalski RP: Bacterial infections of the conjunctiva and cornea. In Albert DM, Jacobiec FA, editors: *Principles and practice of ophthalmology*, ed 2, Philadelphia, 2000, WB Saunders.
4. Mason GA: Traumatic disorders. In Lamb P, Goldblum K, editors: *Core curriculum for ophthalmic nursing*, ed 2, Dubuque, Iowa, 2002, Kendall/Hunt Publishing.

CHAPTER 80

Dry Eye Syndrome

Kate Goldblum, Patricia Gillett, and Joyce Powers

DEFINITION/EPIDEMIOLOGY

Dry eye is a condition in which the ocular surface becomes desiccated. It affects the tarsal and bulbar conjunctivae and the cornea. The severity of the condition ranges from mild to severe, with more serious involvement resulting in extensive ocular surface changes. The term *keratoconjunctivitis sicca* is often used interchangeably with dry eye. Dry eye occurs in the majority of patients with Sjögren's syndrome, a combination of dry eyes and dry mouth often linked with conditions mediated by the autoimmune system.[1]

Dry eye is relatively common, affecting up to 15% of adults.[2] It is more common among females and older adults. Older adults are more likely to develop symptoms of dry eye as a result of the physiologic changes that accompany aging. Children with true dry eye are more likely to have a congenital cause.

Dry eye is commonly associated with autoimmune diseases and other systemic disorders such as multiple sclerosis, lymphoma, and human immunodeficiency virus.[2] Many medications may contribute to dry eye, including diuretics, antihistamines, tricyclics, atropine, isotretinoin, and many anticholinergics. Environmental factors such as low humidity and wind also play a role.

PATHOPHYSIOLOGY

Dry eye may be caused by inadequate tear production, increased tear evaporation, abnormal tear composition, or abnormal tear spreading. It can also result from lacrimal gland dysfunction, mucin deficiency, environmental factors, lipid abnormalities, or inadequate tear film spread resulting from abnormal eyelid function or anatomic surface abnormalities.[3] Dry eye is a common problem in patients with abnormal lid function due to Bell's palsy.

CLINICAL PRESENTATION

Redness, contact lens intolerance, visual blurring, and symptoms of ocular irritation such as burning, itching, scratchiness, foreign body sensation, or "sand in the eye" may be the initial manifestations of dry eye. Symptoms worsen when environmental factors exacerbate tear evaporation or increase ocular irritation. Warmth, low humidity, fans, and secondhand smoke contribute to the symptoms. The bulbar conjunctiva may become erythematous and the periorbital skin may become dry and irritated if the patient rubs the eye in an effort to alleviate the symptoms. Conversely, excessive tearing may be the initial complaint if the tear film lacks adequate mucin or lipid. Important history includes exposure to environmental factors that contribute to dryness, medications, previous injury, and the presence of symptoms that suggest autoimmune disease.

PHYSICAL EXAMINATION

Careful external examination of the ocular surface and adnexa will identify conditions such as inadequate lid function or anatomic abnormalities that prevent normal tear distribution. Evaluation of the skin and joints is important to identify a systemic etiology for dry eyes.

DIAGNOSTICS

Many diagnostic modalities exist to evaluate dry eye. Schirmer tear testing can be done in the primary care setting. This test measures tear production using filter paper with or without prior instillation of a topical anesthetic. Without topical anesthesia, the normal eye will usually produce enough tears to wet the filter paper to at least 10 mm within 5 minutes.

DIFFERENTIAL DIAGNOSIS

Other causes of ocular irritation that may mimic the symptoms of dry eye include environmental irritants and ocular infection. Frequent use of preserved topical preparations may also cause or exacerbate ocular irritation.

MANAGEMENT

Treating or controlling the underlying cause of dry eye is the basis of therapy. Topical therapy with ocular lubricants is often effective in alleviating symptoms. Artificial tears containing methylcellulose or polyvinyl alcohol (Celluvisc, OcuCoat, HypoTears) are usually the most effective. However, there is great variation among individuals, and the patient should be encouraged to try several different preparations. Lubricating ointments may be helpful before sleeping, especially with incomplete eyelid closure, but they are not appropriate for use during waking hours. Using preservative-free, unit-dose preparations helps prevent iatrogenic allergic responses, which greatly exacerbate the problem. Warm compresses and gentle eyelid massage may also be helpful. Systemic disorders associated with dry eye may require consultation and co-management with multiple specialists.

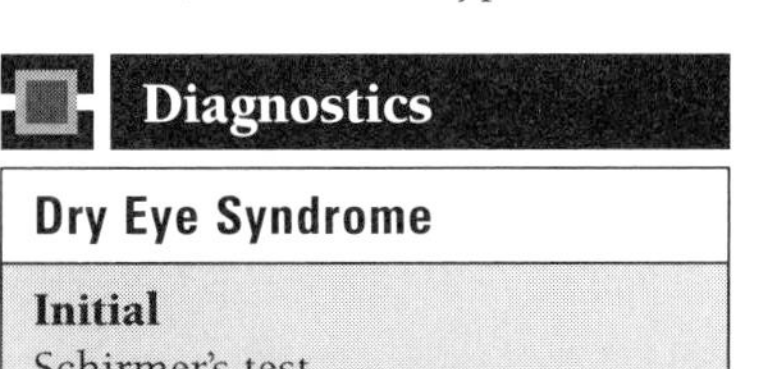

Diagnostics

Dry Eye Syndrome
Initial Schirmer's test

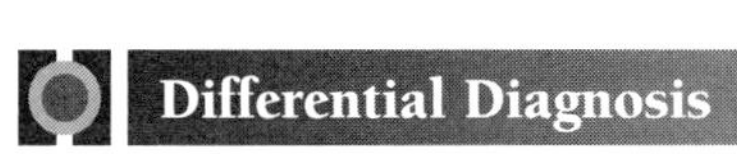

Differential Diagnosis

Dry Eye Syndrome
Ocular irritants (particularly preserved topical preparations) Environmental irritants Ocular infection

LIFE SPAN CONSIDERATIONS

Dry eye is more common in older patients.[4]

COMPLICATIONS

Severe dry eye can result in corneal ulceration and extensive corneal scarring with subsequent visual disability. Conjunctival scarring with adhesions may also occur.

INDICATIONS FOR REFERRAL/HOSPITALIZATION

Ocular lubricants and environmental control may not adequately relieve symptoms. In these situations, referral to an ophthalmologist for additional therapy such as lacrimal plugs is appropriate.

PATIENT AND FAMILY EDUCATION

Patients should be taught the importance of good handwashing before instilling ocular medications as well as the risks of sharing medications. They should also be taught appropriate technique for eyelid massage and warm compresses.

HEALTH PROMOTION

Dry eye syndrome is a chronic condition. Knowledge of the environmental factors that exacerbate the condition and how to avoid or ameliorate those conditions is essential. Frequent or excessive use of preserved topical preparations may worsen symptoms and should be avoided.

REFERENCES

1. Strochschein M: Systemic disorders. In Lamb P, Goldblum K, editors: *Core curriculum for ophthalmic nursing*, ed 2, Dubuque, Iowa, 2002, Kendall/Hunt Publishing.
2. Wilhelmus KR and others: *Basic and clinical science course: external disease and cornea*, San Francisco, 2001, The Foundation of the American Academy of Ophthalmology.
3. Goroll AH, May LA, Mulley AG: *Primary care medicine: office evaluation and management of the adult patient*, ed 3, Philadelphia, 1995, JB Lippincott.
4. Hogan RN: The eye in aging. In Albert DM, Jacobiec FA, editors: *Principles and practice of ophthalmology*, ed 2, Philadelphia, 2000, WB Saunders.

CHAPTER 81

Nasolacrimal Duct Obstruction and Dacryocystitis

Kate Goldblum, Patricia Gillett, and Joyce Powers

DEFINITION/EPIDEMIOLOGY

Nasolacrimal duct obstruction (NLDO), also called dacryostenosis, is a congenital, acute, or chronic blockage that may be partial or complete. Abnormal duct patency and the resulting disruption of normal drainage may lead to dacryocystitis, an inflammation of the lacrimal sac. Approximately 6% of newborn infants have congenital dacryostenosis.[1]

PATHOPHYSIOLOGY

Congenital NLDO is usually caused by a mucosal membrane over the distal end of the duct.[2] Obstruction that is not congenital may result from involutional stenosis, trauma, neoplasia, or anatomic obstructions such as a deviated septum, polyps, or hypertrophied inferior turbinates. Chronic dacryocystitis may lead to scar tissue formation and NLDO in adult patients.

CLINICAL PRESENTATION

Infants with congenital dacryostenosis usually have chronic tearing or mucopurulent discharge and eyelash crusting. These symptoms usually appear within the first few weeks of life but occasionally occur later in early infancy. Adults often have similar symptoms, although the etiology differs. Inadequate tear drainage results in an accumulation of tears in the palpebral fissure with eventual overflow down the cheeks. Mucopurulent discharge from the punctum may be present.

PHYSICAL EXAMINATION

The ocular adnexa and surface structures should be carefully examined for signs of inflammation, although the eye itself is not usually red unless there is an associated conjunctivitis. Palpation is an important part of the examination to assess for edema or tenderness. Pressing on the lacrimal sac may express discharge from the nasolacrimal punctum on the involved side. Fever and leukocytosis may be present in acute dacryocystitis.

DIAGNOSTICS

Diagnostics are usually not necessary. However, if purulent discharge is present, culture and sensitivity may be indicated, particularly in recalcitrant infections. A CBC may be indicated if fever is present.

DIFFERENTIAL DIAGNOSIS

Tearing and ocular irritation may also indicate the presence of conjunctivitis, blepharitis, glaucoma, corneal abrasion, or a corneal foreign body. Mechanical obstruction should be considered, and the presence of a tumor, other neoplastic growth, or foreign body should be excluded. Dacryocystitis may be confused with or a cause of preseptal cellulitis.[3]

MANAGEMENT

Diagnostics

Nasolacrimal Duct Obstruction and Dacryocystitis

Laboratory
Culture and sensitivity (if discharge is present)
CBC and differential (if fever is present)

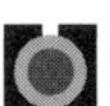

Differential Diagnosis

Nasolacrimal Duct Obstruction and Dacryocystitis

Dacryocystitis
Conjunctivitis
Blepharitis
Glaucoma
Corneal abrasion
Corneal foreign body
Tumor
Foreign body
Preseptal cellulitis

Because congenital NLDO clears spontaneously in most infants, the only treatment usually necessary is gentle daily massage over the lacrimal sac to promote drainage and encourage opening of the obstructing nasolacrimal duct membrane. Warm compresses over the involved eye will help loosen crusting on the eyelashes and may be most necessary after the infant awakens. Topical antibiotics may be prescribed for associated conjunctivitis or excessive mucopurulent drainage caused by *Streptococcus pneumoniae, Staphylococcus* organisms, *Pseudomonas* organisms, and *Haemophilus influenzae* (primarily in children). Infants with acute dacryocystitis should also receive systemic antibiotic therapy. Treatment for dacryocystitis in adults with an acute or chronic obstruction includes hot compresses and topical or systemic antibiotics. Antibiotic choice is based on Gram's stain. Topical antibiotics include neomycin/polymyxin B/gramicidin (Neosporin ophthalmic solution) or ofloxacin 0.3% (Ocuflox ophthalmic solution), 1 drop every 1 to 6 hours. Systemic therapy may include a first-generation cephalosporin such as cephalexin (Keflex) or erythromycin (Erythrocin), 500 mg every 12 hours. In the absence of mucopurulent drainage, prolonged use of topical antibiotics is not necessary in infants or adults.

Infants with congenital NLDO should be co-managed with a pediatric ophthalmologist if complications occur. Conservative management with massage and warm compresses is appropriate up to 12 months of age if no complications occur. Beyond age 12 months, NLD probing is indicated.

LIFE SPAN CONSIDERATIONS

There is frequent spontaneous clearing of congenital NLDO in infants. By 6 months of age, approximately 50% to 90% of cases have spontaneously resolved. Beyond 12 months of age, spontaneous resolution becomes much less likely, and there is an increased possibility of permanent consequences. Conversely, definitive treatment to relieve the obstruction is often necessary in adults.

COMPLICATIONS

NLDO usually precedes dacryocystitis, which can progress to abscess formation. The use of systemic antibiotics is necessary for abscess formation, ineffective topical antibiotic therapy, or recurrent dacryocystitis.

INDICATIONS FOR REFERRAL/HOSPITALIZATION

After initial antibiotic therapy, adults with acute dacryocystitis should be referred to an ophthalmologist because the infection is secondary to obstruction and likely to recur without definitive treatment. The presence of dacryocystitis or abscess with systemic signs of fever, malaise, or leukocytosis may require hospitalization for IV antibiotic therapy.

PATIENT AND FAMILY EDUCATION

The parents or patient should receive instructions on warm compress application, nasolacrimal duct massage, and instillation of topical antibiotics. Patients should be told that antibiotics treat the infection but do not cure the obstruction. To avoid the unnecessary delay of definitive treatment when it is indicated, parents should be aware that NLD probing may be done in the ophthalmologist's office and does not require the use of a general anesthetic.

HEALTH PROMOTION

Immunizations should be encouraged to avoid potential complications of dacryocystitis resulting from *H. influenzae*.[4]

REFERENCES

1. Uphold CR, Graham MV: *Clinical guidelines in child health,* ed 2, Gainesville, Fla, 1999, Barmarrae Books.
2. Boger WP: Congenital nasolacrimal duct obstruction. In Albert DM, Jacobiec FA, editors: *Principles and practice of ophthalmology,* ed 2, Philadelphia, 2000, WB Saunders.
3. Fraioli AJ: Conjunctivitis and orbital cellulitis in childhood. In Albert DM, Jacobiec FA, editors: *Principles and practice of ophthalmology,* ed 2, Philadelphia, 2000, WB Saunders.
4. Wilson ME and others: *Basic and clinical science course: pediatric ophthalmology and strabismus,* San Francisco, 2001, The Foundation of the American Academy of Ophthalmology.

CHAPTER 82

Orbital and Periorbital Cellulitis

Kate Goldblum, Patricia Gillett, and Joyce Powers

DEFINITION/EPIDEMIOLOGY

The orbital septum is a connective tissue structure that separates the anterior third of the orbit from the posterior two thirds. Orbital and periorbital cellulitis are bacterial infections involving the tissues of these areas. Periorbital cellulitis, also called preseptal cellulitis, involves the tissues anterior to the orbital septum; orbital cellulitis, also called postseptal cellulitis, involves the posterior tissues.

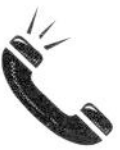

Ophthalmology consultation is recommended for periorbital cellulitis.
Ophthalmology referral is indicated for orbital cellulitis.

PATHOPHYSIOLOGY

The most common bacteria responsible for orbital and periorbital infections include *Staphylococcus aureus,* group A streptococcus, *Streptococcus pneumoniae,* and *Haemophilus influenzae.* Fungal infection should also be suspected, especially in immunocompromised patients. The mechanism of infection in orbital and periorbital cellulitis may involve the spread of infection from superficial lid infections, insect bites or other local trauma, respiratory infections, middle-ear infections, dental infections, or bacteremia.[1] However, it is most commonly secondary to sinusitis.

CLINICAL PRESENTATION

The initial signs and symptoms of periorbital or orbital cellulitis may include a history of trauma or insect bite to the periocular tissues. The most common signs and symptoms of periorbital cellulitis include erythema, warmth, and tenderness. Fever may or may not be present, and the eye is usually white with good mobility and vision. There may be pain with ocular movement. Orbital cellulitis usually presents with similar signs and symptoms with the addition of proptosis, decreased ocular motility, fever, and leukocytosis. Vision and the pupillary response may or may not be decreased. Unilateral involvement is the most common presentation. All signs may be present in either periorbital or orbital cellulitis, but proptosis, restriction of eye movement, ocular redness, and decreased visual acuity are more suggestive of orbital cellulitis.

PHYSICAL EXAMINATION

The ocular tissues and adnexa should be carefully examined and palpated for erythema, warmth, edema, tenderness, drainage, restriction of extraocular muscle action, and proptosis. Evaluating the cranial nerves (CNs) involved in extraocular muscle movements (CNs III, IV, and VI) and assessing corneal sensitivity to identify potential involvement of CN V is important. The eye should be examined carefully for any sign of injury that may provide clues regarding the etiology of the infection. The patient should be assessed for temperature elevation and other signs of systemic toxicity.

DIAGNOSTICS

A complete blood count with differential should be obtained. Any drainage should be cultured and blood cultures obtained if the signs and symptoms suggest a possible orbital cellulitis. In young children, blood cultures should be obtained in any case of cellulitis associated with fever.

DIFFERENTIAL DIAGNOSIS

Any disorder causing unilateral proptosis should be included in the differential diagnosis. Conjunctivitis with periocular tissue involvement, hordeolum, chalazion, dacryocystitis, or dacryoadenitis should be considered. Other considerations include pyoderma, insect bites, orbital tumor, pseudotumor, Graves' disease, and severe allergies.

MANAGEMENT

Periorbital cellulitis requires systemic, broad-spectrum antibiotic therapy. Follow-up evaluation in the office within 12 to 24 hours to monitor for signs of progression or lack of response to antibiotic therapy is important. Appropriate adult oral therapy for periorbital cellulitis includes cefuroxime (Ceftin) 250-500 mg PO b.i.d. Pediatric patients are prescribed 20 mg/kg/day. Patients with significant systemic symptoms, periorbital cellulitis that fails to respond to oral antibiotics, or possible orbital cellulitis should be referred to an ophthalmologist for hospitalization and an IV antibiotic such as cefuroxime (Zinacef) 1.5 g IV every 8 hours. These patients should be monitored closely during the first 24 to 48 hours of hospitalization for lack of improvement or deterioration in condition.

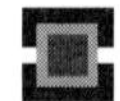

Diagnostics

Orbital and Periorbital Cellulitis

Laboratory
CBC and differential
Culture and sensitivity
Blood culture (particularly in children)

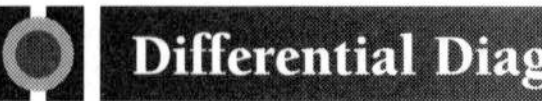

Orbital and Periorbital Cellulitis

Conjunctivitis
Hordeolum
Chalazion
Dacryocystitis
Dacryoadenitis
Pyoderma
Insect bite
Orbital tumor
Graves' disease
Severe allergies

LIFE SPAN CONSIDERATIONS

A primary concern in periorbital and orbital cellulitis is the age of the patient. Neither orbital nor periorbital cellulitis is common over the age of 20 years. Children under the age of 5 years are more likely to have periorbital rather than orbital cellulitis.[2] After age 5 years, orbital cellulitis is more common. Any cellulitis in children under 5 years of age is potentially more serious. *H. influenzae* type B is potentially life threatening in young children because it can lead to meningitis. This possibility should be a special concern in unvaccinated children.

COMPLICATIONS

Orbital cellulitis is a potentially fatal condition.[3] The possible complications of periorbital and orbital cellulitis can pose significant risk to the patient and include (1) meningitis; (2) cavernous sinus thrombosis; (3) central retinal artery or vein thrombosis; (4) retinal ischemia resulting from increased intraocular pressure; (5) subperiosteal, orbital, epidural, subdural, or brain abscess; (6) optic nerve involvement with subsequent blindness; (7) involvement with paresis of CNs III, IV, V, and VI; and (8) fungal orbital cellulitis in immunosuppressed and diabetic patients.

INDICATIONS FOR REFERRAL/HOSPITALIZATION

Patients with decreased visual acuity, systemic symptoms, or neurologic signs should be referred to an ophthalmologist. Patients with periorbital cellulitis that does not improve within 24 hours when treated with oral antibiotics should also be referred to an ophthalmologist. Patients with orbital cellulitis require hospitalization for initiation of IV antibiotics and other supportive therapy as indicated.

PATIENT AND FAMILY EDUCATION

When oral antibiotic therapy is prescribed, patients should be instructed to return before their scheduled follow-up visit (in 12 to 24 hours) if their symptoms increase in severity. They should also be reminded to complete the full course of antibiotic therapy and to return before the end of therapy if signs and symptoms do not continue to improve or if there is any worsening of the condition. Patients and families should be informed that fever, lethargy, and irritability are signs of possible sepsis or meningitis.

HEALTH PROMOTION

H. influenzae vaccination should be promoted in all children.

REFERENCES

1. Durboraw CE, Stasior GO, Hrohel GB: Orbital cellulitis and abscess. In Fraunfelder FT, Roy FH, Randall J, editors: *Current ocular therapy*, ed 5 Philadelphia, 2000, WB Saunders.
2. Fraioli AJ: Conjunctivitis and orbital cellulitis in childhood. In Albert DM, Jakobiec FA, editors: *Clinical practice: principles and practice of ophthalmology*, ed 2, Philadelphia, 2000, WB Saunders.
3. Westfall CT, Baker AS, Shore JW: Infectious processes of the orbit. In Albert DM, Jakobiec FA, editors: *Principles and practice of ophthalmology*, ed 2, Philadelphia, 2000, WB Saunders.

CHAPTER 83

Pingueculum and Pterygium

Kate Goldblum, Patricia Gillett, and Joyce Powers

DEFINITION/EPIDEMIOLOGY

Pinguecula and pterygia are degenerative lesions of the conjunctiva.[1] Pinguecula are often considered precursors of pterygia.[2] A pingueculum is confined to the bulbar conjunctiva, whereas a pterygium eventually extends onto the cornea, usually from the nasal aspect. These lesions occur most often in patients with a long history of outdoor activity.

PATHOPHYSIOLOGY

Pinguecula and pterygia result from epithelial hyperplasia secondary to degenerative changes. Chronic exposure to sunlight and other environmental irritants, such as wind, induce these changes.[3]

CLINICAL PRESENTATION

A pingueculum is characterized by an elevated, yellowish growth, almost always in the nasal aspect of the palpebral conjunctiva (Color Plate 31). When inflamed, the lesion is usually erythematous. Inflamed lesions produce mild to moderate ocular discomfort. Elevated lesions disrupt normal tear film distribution, resulting in symptoms of dry eye. A pterygium is characterized by a vascularized lesion that usually extends from the conjunctiva of the nasal palpebral fissure onto the nasal cornea (Color Plate 32). If the pterygium extends into the visual axis, vision loss occurs. Pterygia may also become inflamed and produce ocular discomfort. Contact lens wearers may experience discomfort and problems sooner.

PHYSICAL EXAMINATION

The ocular surface should be examined carefully, preferably under lighted magnification, looking for signs of inflammation such as edema and injection. Whether the lesion extends past the corneoscleral junction onto the cornea is important in determining the significance of the lesion.

DIAGNOSTICS

The discomfort from a pterygium or pingueculum may mimic that of a corneal abrasion or erosion. If there is any question that a corneal lesion is present, fluorescein should be applied and the cornea carefully examined under fluorescent lighting.

DIFFERENTIAL DIAGNOSIS

Any ocular irritation may cause similar symptoms. The differential diagnosis includes episcleritis, scleritis, conjunctivitis, conjunctival dermoid, and corneal abrasion or erosion.

MANAGEMENT

Topical ophthalmic lubricants constitute initial therapy. Topical antiinflammatory agents such as ketorolac (Acular) and diclofenac (Voltaren) are useful in managing the mild inflammation of a pingueculum. More severely inflamed pinguecula may require topical steroid therapy. It is important to determine the intraocular pressure (IOP) before instituting topical steroids because they can raise the IOP. Some newer topical steroid preparations have less tendency to raise IOP than do many of the older topical steroids. Rimexolone (Vexol) or loteprednol (Alrex) ophthalmic solution 1 drop q.i.d. is less likely to cause a rise in IOP than is a steroid preparation such as prednisolone (Pred-Forte). These medications should not be continued for longer than 1 week. It is also important to rule out the presence of corneal surface defects before prescribing topical steroids. In the primary care setting it is more difficult to exclude corneal ulcer or abrasion, but it is imperative to do so. If topical steroids are required, it is most appropriate to refer the patient to an ophthalmologist. Pinguecula may often be managed in the primary care setting, but co-management with an ophthalmologist is necessary if there are frequent or severe episodes of inflammation. An acutely inflamed pterygium may also require steroid therapy. Any lesion that begins to encroach on the cornea should be referred to an ophthalmologist for surgical evaluation.

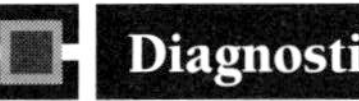

Diagnostics

Pingueculum and Pterygium
Initial
Fluorescein stain*

*If indicated.

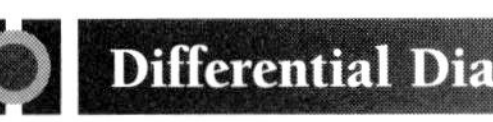

Differential Diagnosis

Pingueculum and Pterygium
Episcleritis
Scleritis
Conjunctivitis
Conjunctival dermoid
Corneal abrasion or erosion

LIFE SPAN CONSIDERATIONS

Because of the degenerative nature of pinguecula and pterygia, they do not occur in children, but they often occur in older adults who live in sunny or windy climates.

COMPLICATIONS

A pingueculum may evolve to a pterygium. As a pterygium extends onto the cornea and into the visual axis, it affects visual acuity. Surgical excision is necessary before this occurs, to avoid postoperative scarring in the central cornea with subsequent loss of visual acuity.

INDICATIONS FOR REFERRAL/HOSPITALIZATION

Patients with inflamed pinguecula that do not respond to short-term topical antiinflammatory therapy should be referred to an ophthalmologist. All patients with pterygia approaching the corneoscleral border should be nonurgently referred for evaluation regarding the timing of surgical intervention. If topical steroid therapy is considered, physician consultation is recommended.

PATIENT AND FAMILY EDUCATION

Patients should be cautioned to not use over-the-counter vasoconstrictors for relief of redness. They may increase irritation and, if overused, can cause rebound conjunctival congestion.

HEALTH PROMOTION

The avoidance of excessive exposure to ultraviolet light and dry, windy environments may lessen the incidence of pterygia and pinguecula. Sunglasses with adequate blocking of ultraviolet A (UVA) and ultraviolet B (UVB) light should be recommended to all patients to help prevent these lesions.

REFERENCES

1. Wilhelmus KR and others: *Basic and clinical science course: external disease and cornea,* San Francisco, 2001, The Foundation of the American Academy of Ophthalmology.
2. Farah S and others: Tumors of the cornea and conjunctiva. In Albert DM, Jakobiec FA, editors: *Principles and practice of ophthalmology,* ed 2, Chapter 75 [CD ROM], 2000, WB Saunders.
3. Grossniklaus HE and others: *Basic and clinical science course: Ophthalmic pathology and intraocular tumors,* San Francisco, 2001, The Foundation of the American Academy of Ophthalmology.

CHAPTER 84

Subconjunctival Hemorrhage

Kate Goldblum, Patricia Gillett, and Joyce Powers

DEFINITION/EPIDEMIOLOGY

A subconjunctival hemorrhage is an area of bleeding under the conjunctiva. These bright red lesions can occur at any age.

PATHOPHYSIOLOGY

A subconjunctival hemorrhage occurs when a break in a conjunctival blood vessel results in blood leaking into the subconjunctival space. They are usually benign lesions caused by a Valsalva maneuver such as sneezing, coughing, or vomiting. They can also be caused by rubbing the eye or by other minor or major trauma to the eye. They can be associated with hypertension, severe conjunctival inflammation, or any systemic condition that increases the risk of bleeding.[1] They can also occur spontaneously.

CLINICAL PRESENTATION

A subconjunctival hemorrhage presents with a bright red spot of blood visible under the overlying conjunctiva (Color Plate 33). The rest of the conjunctiva remains white. The lesion can be small or involve the entire bulbar conjunctiva. There usually is no pain, itching, or decrease in visual acuity. The history may include rubbing the eye or a recent sudden Valsalva maneuver from vomiting, coughing, or sneezing. With a severe hemorrhage, the conjunctiva may be edematous from the underlying hematoma, making the cornea appear sunken.

PHYSICAL EXAMINATION

The external ocular structures and the ocular surface should be carefully examined for edema, tenderness, discharge, symmetry, and signs of external trauma. The pupillary symmetry and function should be evaluated, and the ocular fundus examined for signs of hemorrhage. The patient's blood pressure should be measured.

DIAGNOSTICS

Diagnostic testing is not indicated because the physical examination will confirm the diagnosis. However, diagnostic tests may be indicated if hypertension or other systemic disorders are suspected. If the hemorrhage is associated with a history of trauma, x-ray studies (plain films), ultrasonography, CT, or MRI may be indicated to rule out other occult trauma.

DIFFERENTIAL DIAGNOSIS

It is important to determine that subconjunctival hemorrhage is not associated with other complaints and that the history is negative other than for a Valsalva maneuver such as coughing, sneezing, or rubbing the eye. This information may be difficult to elicit. Acute, mucopurulent conjunctivitis may be associated with a subconjunctival hemorrhage.[2] Subconjunctival hemorrhage must also be differentiated from other common causes of red eye, but in general this is easy to do because there typically are no associated symptoms with subconjunctival hemorrhage. It is important to consider the more serious systemic disorders that may increase the risk of spontaneous bleeding. A full diagnostic evaluation is not necessary, but a careful history that focuses on the possibility of hypertension and the potential causes of increased bleeding risk is appropriate. In addition, patients with an atypical presentation may have conjunctival Kaposi's sarcoma and should be evaluated for occult human immunodeficiency virus (HIV).[3]

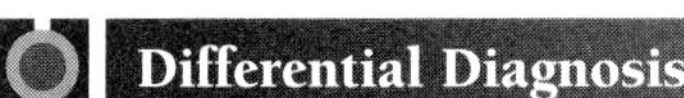

Subconjunctival Hemorrhage
Conjunctivitis
All causes of red eye
Trauma
Hypertension
Bleeding disorders
Kaposi's sarcoma

MANAGEMENT

No treatment is necessary for a subconjunctival hemorrhage. The use of topical decongestants such as naphazoline HCl 0.025%/pheniramine maleate 0.3% (Naphcon-A) or naphazoline HCl 0.05%/antazoline phosphate 0.5% (Vasocon-A) may relieve some redness but may not significantly reduce the time required for the hemorrhage to resorb.

LIFE SPAN CONSIDERATIONS

In the pediatric population it may be difficult to elicit a good history. The possibility of trauma, including child abuse, should be carefully considered.[4] In older patients, the risk of an underlying disease process that predisposes the patient to bleeding should be assessed.

COMPLICATIONS

Complications are uncommon; however, if trauma is a possibility, there may be a retinal hemorrhage or other obvious or occult ocular pathology present. Because such injuries are potentially serious, the patient should be assessed for further injury and referred to an ophthalmologist if necessary.[5]

INDICATIONS FOR REFERRAL/HOSPITALIZATION

A retinal hemorrhage on funduscopic examination may indicate hypertension or possible trauma. Ocular trauma with retinal hemorrhage necessitates an ophthalmic referral. If there is no history of ocular trauma in the presence of subconjunctival and retinal hemorrhages, a referral to a physician may be indicated to determine the underlying cause of the bleeding. In addition, patients with any associated ocular symptoms should be referred to an ophthalmologist.

PATIENT AND FAMILY EDUCATION

It is important to provide reassurance that a subconjunctival hemorrhage, although unsightly, is not serious. Treatment to alleviate the redness of the hemorrhage is neither necessary nor effective.

HEALTH PROMOTION

Subconjunctival hemorrhages do not usually recur unless there is an underlying systemic problem. If patients do present with a recurrent hemorrhage, they should be instructed not to rub their eyes and to avoid strenuous Valsalva maneuvers.

REFERENCES

1. Wilhelmus KR and others: *Basic and clinical science course: external disease and cornea*, San Francisco, 2001, The Foundation of the American Academy of Ophthalmology.
2. Foulks GN, Gordon JS, Kowalski RP: Bacterial infections of the conjunctiva and cornea. In Albert DM, Jakobiec FA, editors: *Principles and practice of ophthalmology*, ed 2, Chapter 68 [CD ROM], 2000, WB Saunders.
3. McMullen WW, D'Amico DJ: AIDS and its ophthalmic manifestations. In Albert DM, Jakobiec FA, editors: *Principles and practice of ophthalmology*, ed 2, Chapter 348 [CD ROM], 2000, WB Saunders.
4. Wilson ME and others: *Basic and clinical science course: pediatric ophthalmology and strabismus*, San Francisco, 2001, The Foundation of the American Academy of Ophthalmology.
5. Mead MD, Colby KA: Evaluation and initial management of patients with ocular and adnexal trauma. In Albert DM, Jakobiec FA, editors: *Principles and practice of ophthalmology*, ed 2, Chapter 371 [CD ROM], 2000, WB Saunders.

PART 7

Evaluation and Management of Ear Disorders

TERRY MAHAN BUTTARO, Section Editor

CHAPTER 85

Auricular Disorders

Karen Koozer Olson

DEFINITION/ETIOLOGY

Auricular disorders are those conditions that affect the external ear. The incidence and prevalence of the individual condition vary. The auricular disorder may be a secondary issue or may be discovered during the physical examination. Auricular disorders may be benign conditions associated with other disease processes, may be related to cultural practices such as body piercing, or may be a symptom of a serious illness that requires immediate referral and treatment.

Certain disease processes are associated with specific abnormalities of the auricle. Patients with Addison's disease may have calcification of the cartilage. The nodules of Hansen's disease may appear on the earlobe and present as multiple nodules on the ear and face. Patients with chronic arthritis may have hard nodules develop in the auricle. These rheumatoid nodules are usually accompanied by similar nodules on the hands, elbows, knees, or heels. Tophi are painless, hard or gritty, and irregular uric acid crystal deposits in the auricle. They form in relation to years of high uric acid levels. Pressure on these deposits may result in the expulsion of a white crystalline substance. A hematoma of the auricle occurs in response to blood disorders or trauma and presents as a tender, blue doughy mass that, if not drained, results in a deformity commonly referred to as "cauliflower ear."[1]

Common problems associated with piercing of the earlobes and the helix are local infection and tears from the pierced site. *Keloids,* which are firm masses of scar tissue that are not cosmetically acceptable but are otherwise benign, may also occur at the pierced site. Keloids occur more often in dark-skinned people.

Chondrodermatitis helicis is a chronic inflamed lesion, usually on the helix or anthelix, that most often affects older men. It is painful and may have crusting. A biopsy examination distinguishes it from carcinoma. Two types of skin cancer may be found on the auricle. Basal cell carcinoma is the most common form of skin cancer and the least deadly. It is a slow-growing cancer that is often found in areas exposed to the sun, such as the top of the auricle. This type of disorder is found in older persons, in fair-skinned patients, and in patients who have a history of sun exposure. The lesion appears as a shiny, irregular painless area. This form of cancer rarely metastasizes.

Squamous cell carcinoma (SCC) is also usually found in fair-skinned patients and in patients with a history of sun exposure. The typical lesion has a raised, crusted border around a center ulcer. SCC is a more serious form of skin cancer. It metastasizes to regional lymph nodes and can cause death. Skin cancer is probably the most common significant auricular disorder seen in primary care.

Malignant otitis externa is a severe form of otitis externa. It presents with a severely swollen, erythematous, and tender auricle. It can lead to a life-threatening infection of the head and face. It is most likely to occur in patients with diabetes and in those who have compromised immune systems. The causative organism is usually *Pseudomonas aeruginosa.*

PATHOPHYSIOLOGY

The auricle is the external ear structure that is composed chiefly of cartilage covered by skin. It is firm and elastic. It is divided into three parts: the top portion is the helix, the midsection is the anthelix, and the lower portion is the lobe. The function of the outer ear is to aid in receiving sound waves from the environment.

CLINICAL PRESENTATION

Often the patient is being seen for a general examination or follow-up. The complaint related to an auricular disorder is usually a minor issue. For tears and infection, the patient may present with a specific episode of trauma and/or an erythematous, tender earlobe. Malignant otitis externa may present as sequelae to an infection or a respiratory illness and most often occurs in immunosuppressed or diabetic patients.

PHYSICAL EXAMINATION

The parameters of the auricular disorder should be noted; these include the onset, duration, and intensity of any symptoms. Any medications, treatments, or remedies that have been used on the auricle or systemically should also be documented, as well as all related symptoms and past history of treatments and outcomes. A complete inspection and palpation of the auricle form the basis for evaluation. The examination should be modified to the individual findings. The normal ears are placed level with the eyes. The ears of neonates are usually flat; however, in older infants this may indicate persistent side lying. Protruding ears should be examined to exclude edema from insect bites or infection. Normal earlobes are similar in size and placement and should move freely and painlessly. Infected pierced earlobes will be warm, tender, and erythematous and may have exudate. The lobes of older patients may be more prominent and/or pendulous. Dry or scaly skin of the external ear may indicate psoriasis or seborrhea. The external ear may also have skin breakdowns or erosions from prolonged pressure from eyeglasses or oxygen tubing. Cancerous or precancerous lesions are most often found on the top of the auricle. They may appear as shiny, irregular painless lesions (basal cell) or as raised crusted lesions around a center ulcer (squamous cell).

DIAGNOSTICS

The diagnostic tests are dependent on the underlying disease process. A biopsy should be performed on any small, crusted, ulcerated or indurated lesion that does not heal properly. If the biopsy findings are positive, a complete cancer screening should be ordered. Rheumatoid arthritis profiles should

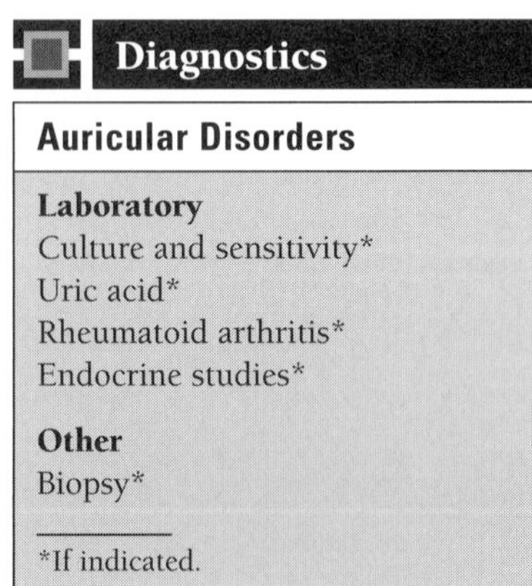

Diagnostics

Auricular Disorders

Laboratory
Culture and sensitivity*
Uric acid*
Rheumatoid arthritis*
Endocrine studies*

Other
Biopsy*

*If indicated.

be obtained in patients with rheumatoid nodules. If tophi are present, a uric acid chemistry profile is indicated. Calcification nodules related to Addison's disease indicate the need for endocrine studies.

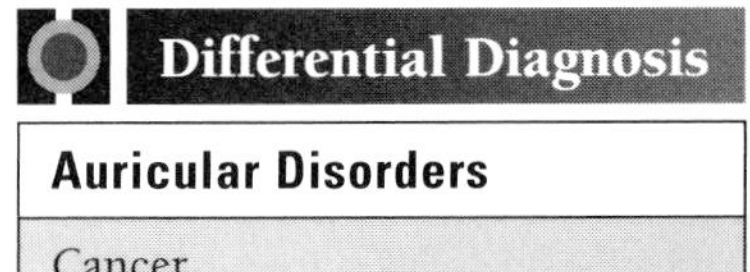

Auricular Disorders

Cancer
Rheumatoid arthritis
Gout
Addison's disease
Infection

DIFFERENTIAL DIAGNOSIS

The differential diagnosis includes all of the diagnoses mentioned earlier.

MANAGEMENT

Infections of the earlobe that are a result of piercing can be treated with topical alcohol and antibiotic ointment or systemic antibiotic treatment such as ceftriaxone or cephalexin. Mild infections can be treated with cephalexin or dicloxacillin 500 mg PO q.i.d. for 7 to 10 days. Erythromycin is appropriate for penicillin-allergic patients. More severe infections should be treated with ceftriaxone 1 g IM or IV daily for ≥1 day, depending on the severity of the infection. Oral antibiotic therapy should then be prescribed as previously noted. Most patients with malignant otitis externa require immediate referral to a physician or an otolaryngologist, admission to a hospital, and aggressive antimicrobial therapy. Patients with very early disease may be treated with Cipro (ciprofloxacin) 500 to 750 mg PO b.i.d. for 7 to 10 days with very frequent follow-up.[2] A biopsy should be performed on any chronically inflamed lesion to ascertain whether it is malignant. An auricular hematoma should be drained using sterile technique and treated with topical antibiotic ointment or systemic antibiotics, depending on the extent of the wound.

LIFE SPAN CONSIDERATIONS

Life span considerations are related to the specific disease disorders. Complications from piercing are more likely in the young. Skin cancers are most likely to occur in middle-aged and older patients.

COMPLICATIONS

Complications are unusual but do occur. Trauma, if untreated, may result in painful nodules or a distorted "cauliflower ear." Painless pinnal nodules may be a complication of Addison's disease, and any painless nodule may represent a carcinoma. Infections, if untreated, may spread systemically. Recurring pinnal infections should prompt concern for relapsing polychondritis, a degenerative cartilage disease that can cause tinnitus or deafness.

INDICATIONS FOR REFERRAL/HOSPITALIZATION

Patients with torn earlobes are usually referred to a plastic surgeon for repair. A biopsy should be performed on any cancerous or suspicious lesion. Malignant otitis externa requires immediate referral to a physician or hospital admission.

PATIENT AND FAMILY EDUCATION

Understanding the importance of sunscreen protection for the ears is essential. In addition, the signs of skin cancer—asymmetry, borders (irregular, ragged, notched, or blurred), color (irregular), and diameter (the lesion is >¼ inch or growing)—should be carefully explained.[3,4] The importance of how to clean and care for the external ear canal and the auricle should be stressed. When selecting ear-piercing facilities, patients should look for facilities that employ licensed personnel and are inspected or approved by public health authorities. In addition, wearing heavy earrings or earrings that dangle around small children or in circumstances where the earring might be torn from the ear should be discouraged.

HEALTH PROMOTION

Health promotion is primarily related to the specific disease. Sun screens and protective clothing are the best choice for the prevention of skin cancer.

REFERENCES

1. DeGowin R: *DeGowin and DeGowin's diagnostic examination*, ed 6, New York, 1994, McGraw-Hill.
2. Gilbert D, Moellering R, Sande M: *The Stanford guide to antimicrobial therapy*, ed 31, Hyde Park, VT, 2001, Antimicrobial Therapy, Inc.
3. American Cancer Society: *Facts on skin cancer*, Atlanta, GA, 1988, The Society.
4. American Cancer Society: *All about skin cancer*, Atlanta, GA, 2001, The Society. Retrieved August 12, 2002, from the World Wide Web: http://www.cancer.org/eprise/main/docroot/CRI/CRI_2x?sitearea=LR.

CHAPTER 86

Cerumen Impaction

Karen Koozer Olson

DEFINITION/ETIOLOGY

Cerumen impaction is a common problem that occurs when increased amounts of hard cerumen either partially or completely occlude the external ear canal. Cerumen can become dry and immobile and occlude the canal for a variety of reasons. Dirt and other debris in the ear can contribute to the impaction. Cotton-tipped swabs used to clean the ear can push this material back into the canal; fibers from the swabs often complicate the situation.

PATHOPHYSIOLOGY

Cerumen is a soft, yellow, waxy, protective substance that is secreted by glands in the external ear canal. It is part of the mechanism used to protect the ear canal and tympanic membrane (TM) from dirt and debris. Excessive cerumen production, a narrow ear canal, or obstruction may predispose a patient to impaction.

CLINICAL PRESENTATION

Patients with cerumen impaction typically complain of unilateral fullness or hearing loss. Itching, discomfort, tinnitus, and dizziness are also common complaints.

PHYSICAL EXAMINATION

The outer ear should be inspected for size, shape, color, and placement; the lobe, helix, and preauricular and postauricular lymph nodes should be bilaterally palpated. The body temperature and lymph nodes are usually normal. The normal ear should be inspected by having the patient tip his or her head toward the opposite shoulder. In adults, the pinna is pulled gently up and backward; for young children and infants, the ear is pulled downward. The largest speculum that will fit into the ear canal is gently inserted. Cerumen impaction may prevent the speculum from being fully inserted. The impaction will appear as a light-yellow to dark-brown mass that prevents or partially blocks visualization of the TM. Blood in the external ear canal appears as bright red to black and may be liquid or a solid mass. Sanguineous drainage often appears as honey-colored fluid.

DIAGNOSTICS

No diagnostics are indicated.

DIFFERENTIAL DIAGNOSIS

The primary differential diagnosis is a foreign body in the external ear canal.

MANAGEMENT

If a ruptured TM is not suspected and there is no history of tympanostomy tubes or recent ear surgery, removal of the impaction is appropriate. If possible, a commercial wax softener or 2 or 3 drops of baby oil or mineral oil should be inserted in the affected ear daily for 3 to 5 days before removal is attempted. Removal with a cerumen spoon or curette is appropriate if direct visualization is available and the cerumen is in the lateral third of the external ear canal. If the cerumen is deeper in the canal, a tepid water irrigation with a WaterPik, the Welch Allyn Ear Wash System, or a regular syringe is required. A ceruminolytic agent instilled in the canal for 15 to 20 minutes before the lavage will soften the cerumen and aid in removal. Liquid docusate sodium has also been used successfully to soften cerumen.[1] These agents should not be used if infection or perforation is suspected. The auricle should be straightened as much as possible and the irrigant directed upward in the canal. The canal should be irrigated until clear unless the patient experiences pain or dizziness.

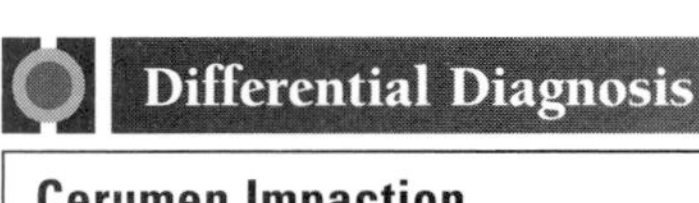

Cerumen Impaction
Foreign body

Instillation of Cortisporin Otic solution (hydrocortisone/neomycin sulfate/polymyxin B sulfate) (4 drops q.i.d. for 7 to 10 days) or 2 or 3 drops of a 2:3 mixture of white vinegar/rubbing alcohol in the canal every day for 2 to 3 days after the procedure will reduce the risk of otitis externa.[2] Whenever cerumen impaction is noted in one ear, the other ear should be examined for ceruminosis.

LIFE SPAN CONSIDERATIONS

In older adults, the glands that produce cerumen may become less productive, which can result in cerumen that is drier and more likely to collect in the canal and become impacted. Adults who work in noisy industries and are required to wear hearing protection may have an increased risk for cerumen impaction. Hearing aids and earplugs inserted into the external auditory canal can push the cerumen into the canal and predispose the patient to cerumen impaction.

COMPLICATIONS

Cerumen accumulation can also decrease auditory acuity and cause pressure on and perforation of the TM. Removal of cerumen that has adhered to the wall of the external ear canal may leave an abraded or irritated area that can develop into otitis externa. Hearing loss and injury to the TM are other potential complications.

INDICATIONS FOR REFERRAL/HOSPITALIZATION

Patients with suspected perforation, tympanostomy tubes, or recent ear surgery should be referred to an otolaryngologist, as should patients who experience acute pain, dizziness, hearing loss, or damage to the external ear canal or TM during the ear lavage.

PATIENT AND FAMILY EDUCATION

Patients should be cautioned about the use of cotton-tipped swabs to clean the ear canal. The use of these swabs can push the cerumen farther into the ear, and fibers from the swab can help to hold the cerumen in a mass. Soft cloths and soap and water should be used to clean the auricle. The external ear canal does not require cleaning. Patients must understand the importance of a medical evaluation if pain or discharge is noted.

HEALTH PROMOTION

Commercial ceruminolytics or baby oil, one or two drops in the ear canal once or twice a week, will help prevent cerumen from becoming hard and imbedded. Patients who wear hearing aids are more at risk for the development of ceruminosis and, if possible, should not wear the hearing aid while sleeping.

REFERENCES

1. Singer AJ, Sauris E, Viccellio AW: Ceruminolytic effects of docusate sodium: a randomized controlled trial, *Ann Emerg Med* 36:228, 2000.
2. Gilbert D, Moellering R, Merle S: *The Stanford guide to antimicrobial therapy*, ed 31, Hyde Park, VT, 2001, Antimicrobial Therapy.

CHAPTER 87

Cholesteatoma

Chad J. Smith

DEFINITION/EPIDEMIOLOGY

A *cholesteatoma* is an invasive growth of keratin-producing squamous epithelial cells typically found within the middle ear or mastoid air spaces.

PATHOPHYSIOLOGY

Based on their etiology, cholesteatomas may be broadly categorized as congenital or acquired. Congenital cholesteatomas occur as nests of embryonic squamous epithelial cells in an ear without a history of tympanic membrane (TM) perforation or chronic infections.[1] Acquired cholesteatomas occur as squamous epithelial cells enter the middle ear after perforation or prolonged chronic negative pressure with a retraction pocket in the TM (Color Plate 34). Over time this tumor enlarges, producing proteolytic enzymes that cause destruction of the ossicles and erosion of inner ear structures, mastoid bone, and other cranial contents.[2] Chronic otitis media, drainage, mastoiditis, and disseminated infection may coexist.

CLINICAL PRESENTATION

Although congenital cholesteatomas are often asymptomatic, acquired lesions have a history of recurring ear infections and drainage or TM retractions due to eustachian tube dysfunction. Impaired hearing may be the first sign of middle ear destruction from a cholesteatoma.

PHYSICAL EXAMINATION

A complete otologic examination with attention to the ear canal, TM, and mastoid regions may reveal a white mass behind or perforating through the TM. Drainage indicates infection.

DIAGNOSTICS AND DIFFERENTIAL DIAGNOSIS

An audiogram can reveal conductive hearing loss. A CT scan aids in the diagnosis and determination of the extent of tumor involvement. The differential diagnosis should include all causes of conductive hearing loss.

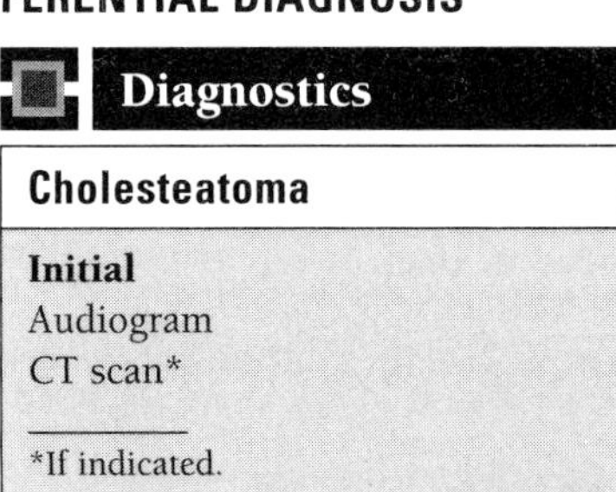

Diagnostics

Cholesteatoma

Initial
Audiogram
CT scan*

*If indicated.

MANAGEMENT

Cholesteatomas require surgical excision. Concurrent suppurative otitis media requires systemic antibiotic therapy and removal of debris from the canal.

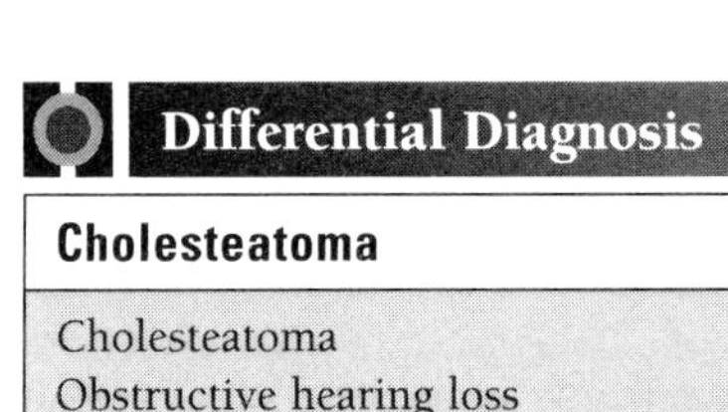

Differential Diagnosis

Cholesteatoma

Cholesteatoma
Obstructive hearing loss
Eardrum disorders
Otosclerosis

COMPLICATIONS

Complications include deafness, mastoiditis, and disseminated infection.

INDICATIONS FOR REFERRAL/HOSPITALIZATION

All patients with a cholesteatoma must be evaluated and managed by an otolaryngologist. Surgical excision is the primary treatment. Even after appropriate surgical treatment, recurrence rates may be as high as 50%.[1]

PATIENT AND FAMILY EDUCATION

Patient education should include information about this condition and its association with chronic ear infections and TM perforations. The importance of documenting complete healing after TM perforations is stressed.

REFERENCES

1. Thompson JW: Cholesteatomas, *Pediatr Rev* 20(4):134-136, 1999.
2. Seidman MD, Simpson GT, Khan MJ: Common problems of the ear. In Noble J, editor: *Textbook of primary care medicine,* ed 3, St Louis, 2001, Mosby.

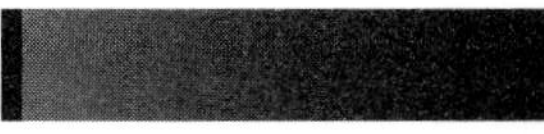

CHAPTER 88

Impaired Hearing

Updated by Terry Mahan Buttaro

DEFINITION/EPIDEMIOLOGY

Impaired hearing is a defect in the proper identification of external sound. Impaired hearing affects both communication ability and personal safety and can also be a socially isolating experience. The prevalence of hearing loss increases with advancing age; it is a common condition for many aging adults. Hearing loss may go undetected for many years but can be greatly improved with both traditional and new interventions for hearing restoration. Conductive loss is more amenable to treatment than is sensorineural loss.

Immediate otolaryngologist/neurologist referral is indicated for patients with abrupt hearing loss.

PATHOPHYSIOLOGY

Hearing loss occurs as the result of dysfunction in the mechanical conduction of external sound (conductive), in the sensorineural structures and pathways to the brain (sensorineural), or from a combination of the two (mixed).[1] In conductive hearing loss, any component of the anatomic structures of the external or middle ear can be involved. In the external ear such factors include impacted cerumen, infection with edema, cholesteatoma tumors, overgrowth of the bony wall, tumors, congenital atresia, and fibrotic stenosis from recurrent infection. Perforation, scar tissue, negative pressure for eustachian tube dysfunction, or any condition that impairs the mobility of the tympanic membrane (TM) can impair hearing sensitivity. Causes of conductive loss from middle ear disease include acute otitis media, chronic serous otitis, and TM disorders. *Otosclerosis,* which is fusion of the stapes over the oval window, is a common cause of hearing loss in aging adults. It is a genetically inherited condition in 10% of the population; if significant, it is amenable to surgical intervention. Other conditions that interfere with the mechanical transmission of sound in the middle ear are trauma that damages the ossicles, congenital malformations, and cholesteatomas.

Sensorineural hearing loss is caused by disorders of the cochlea and the retrocochlear region, including the auditory nerve and its connection in the brainstem. Noise trauma is a principal cause of cochlear damage. Persistent or repeated exposure to excessive noise causes stress to the structures of the hair cells in the cochlea. High frequencies are affected initially, and then all frequencies are affected. A loud, explosive noise may cause temporary damage to these structures. *Presbycusis* is a gradual degeneration within the cochlea that accompanies aging. There may also be degeneration of the mechanical structures and the central auditory connections. This condition is symmetric, irreversible, progressive, and may have a hereditary component; high frequencies are most commonly affected. Ototoxicity needs to be considered with sensorineural hearing loss. The prime suspects in ototoxicity include antineoplastics, salicylates, aminoglycosides, furosemide, and quinine-related drugs. Sensorineural hearing loss may be caused by viral or bacterial infection.

Retrocochlear hearing loss involves the auditory nerve, brainstem, or central nervous system (CNS). Causes of this type of hearing loss include the sequelae of CNS infection (meningitis) or cerebrovascular injury, demyelinating diseases or neoplasms, multiple sclerosis, and syphilis.

Mixed hearing loss combines elements of both conductive and sensorineural loss. Common causes of this loss include injury to the ear, infection, and congenital disorders.

CLINICAL PRESENTATION

Most people experience some degree of hearing loss over time, although hearing loss is often so gradual that many people are unaware of their hearing deficit. Other patients may complain of abrupt hearing loss or diminished hearing accompanied by headache, earache, tinnitus, or vertigo. Important information to determine is family history of hearing loss, occupational history, the onset of the hearing loss, whether the loss was precipitated by trauma or infection, and whether there is associated isolation, behavioral change, or depression.

PHYSICAL EXAMINATION

A complete examination of the head, neck, and throat and an evaluation of cranial nerves and the auditory and vestibular system are essential. The pinna and external auditory canal should be inspected for malformations, lesions, exudates, and obstruction. Examination of the TM should ensure TM mobility (via pneumoscopy) and determine whether effusion, infection, perforation, or cholesteatoma is present. The Weber and Rinne tests help differentiate conductive and sensorineural hearing loss. A screening audiogram is also necessary.

DIAGNOSTICS

A audiogram in a soundproof environment is recommended if hearing is impaired. The qualities of sound tested are loudness of tone (measured in decibels [dB]) and the frequency or pitch of the tone (measured in Hertz [cycles] per second). The threshold of normal hearing is 0 to 20 dB. Patients who begin to hear sound at 40 dB have difficulty hearing faint or distant speech and require favorable seating. At 55 dB, patients understand normal speech at 3 to 5 feet; at 90 dB, patients hear a loud voice at a 1-foot distance from the ear.[1] Brainstem auditory evoked response and neuroimaging studies may be useful in diagnosing tumors and traumatic injuries.[2] A rapid plasma reagin (RPR) or Venereal Disease Research Laboratory (VDRL) test (to exclude syphilis) and a CT scan (if a tumor is suspected) may also be indicated.

DIFFERENTIAL DIAGNOSIS

The differential diagnosis for conductive loss includes cholesteatoma, otosclerosis, or any disorder of the external or middle ear. Sensorineural hearing loss can be inherited or result from neurologic disorders, metabolic abnormalities, autoimmune diseases, or noise- or medication-induced presbycusis. The sensorineural hearing loss associated with labyrinthitis is usually accompanied by vertigo. Hearing loss in Meniere's disease fluctuates and usually presents after other symptoms, such as vertigo and tinnitus. Other possibilities include congenital disorders or a fistula that involves leakage of perilymphatic fluid after trauma. Hearing loss from retrocochlear diseases may result from infection, stroke, intracranial bleeding, concussion, demyelinating or other degenerative diseases, and neoplasms such as vestibular schwannoma, congenital keratoma, meningioma, and primary intracranial malignancy or metastasis.[1]

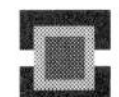

Diagnostics

Impaired Hearing

Initial
Audiogram

Laboratory
CBC and differential (if anemia or infection is suspected)*
VDRL or RPR (to rule out syphilis)*
ESR, antinuclear antibodies (ANA), rheumatoid factor (RF) (if autoimmune cause is suspected)
TSH (if hypothyroid or hyperthyroid disorder is suspected)

Imaging
CT scan/MRI (if tumor is suspected)*

*If indicated.

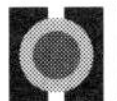

Differential Diagnosis

Impaired Hearing

Conductive Hearing Loss
Congenital atresia of the external auditory canal
Cholesteatoma
Foreign body
Impacted cerumen
Infection (otitis media, otitis externa)
Otosclerosis
Psoriasis or other dermatologic disease
Trauma to external auditory canal
Tumor
Tympanic membrane perforation

Sensorineural Hearing Loss
Acoustic neuroma
Autoimmune hearing loss: polyarteritis nodosa, relapsing polychondritis, rheumatoid arthritis, systemic lupus erythematosus, Wegener's granulomatosis
Barotrauma
Congenital/hereditary
Infection: meningitis, viruses
Meniere's disease
Metabolic abnormality: anemia, diabetes
Neurologic disorder: multiple sclerosis, cerebrovascular accident, transient ischemic accident, Arnold-Chiari malformations, syphilis
Ototoxic medications
Paget's disease
Presbycusis
Trauma

MANAGEMENT/CO-MANAGEMENT WITH SPECIALISTS

Conductive hearing loss associated with cerumen impaction or infection usually responds to impaction removal and antibiotic therapy. Otolaryngology referral is indicated for patients with hearing deficit associated with trauma, congenital hearing loss, tumors, obstructions of the external auditory canal, nonhealing TM rupture, and otoslerosis. Tumors and obstructions of the external auditory canal must be surgically excised. Treatment for otosclerosis requires stapedectomy or sound amplification, whereas TM perforation may heal spontaneously or require a surgical patch or graft. Presbycusis and some other hearing impediments can be treated with hearing aids.

COMPLICATIONS

Impaired hearing may lead to social isolation, economic hardship, and accidents. Missed diagnoses may result in deafness.

INDICATIONS FOR REFERRAL/HOSPITALIZATION

Referral to an otolaryngologist is appropriate when the diagnosis is unclear, when preliminary assessment is a serious condition, or when surgical intervention is an option. Referral to an audiologist is always appropriate for definitive testing. Abrupt hearing loss is cause for immediate referral to an appropriate specialist, usually an otolaryngologist or a neurologist.

PATIENT AND FAMILY EDUCATION

Patients should be aware that a sudden hearing loss, difficulty understanding what other people are saying, or a constant ringing in the ear requires further evaluation. They should receive a careful explanation about their particular type of hearing loss, as well as how medications, such as aspirin, nonsteroidal antiinflammatory drugs, antibiotics, and diuretics, can cause hearing loss. Information about referral resources and options for management should also be presented to patients and their families. For patients considering hearing aids, careful explanation about the types of hearing devices available, their cost, and the fact that hearing loss cannot be completely restored is important to prevent any misunderstandings. Family members who live with a hearing impaired person should understand the importance of decreasing background noise, facing the person when speaking so that the face and mouth are visible, and involving the hearing impaired person in conversations.

HEALTH PROMOTION

Ototoxic medications should be monitored or, if possible, eliminated. After age 50, hearing should be checked at the annual physical examination. Ears should also be checked yearly for cerumenosis and, if necessary, irrigated. Employees at risk for hearing loss from trauma or prolonged and elevated noise exposure are mandated by the Occupational Safety and Health Administration to limit their exposure and to wear protective equipment. Earplugs or protective equipment to prevent home, occupational, and recreational noise exposure should be encouraged to prevent any hearing loss.

REFERENCES

1. Seidman MD, Simpson GT, Khan MJ: *Common problems of the ear.* In Nobel J, editor: *Primary care medicine,* St Louis, 1996, Mosby.
2. Weller KA: *Impaired hearing.* In Rakel RE, editor: *Saunders' manual of medical practice,* Philadelphia, 1996, WB Saunders.

CHAPTER 89

Inner Ear Disturbances

Updated by Terry Mahan Buttaro

Patients often present to the office or emergency department with a complaint of lightheadedness, dizziness, unsteadiness, or disequilibrium. Often the description is vague, but it is essential to have the patient explain what he or she is experiencing to differentiate between dizziness and vertigo. Inner ear disturbances can be associated with both *vertigo,* the abnormal perception of movement, and *dizziness,* the feeling of rotary movement. A complete physical examination including orthostatic vital signs, cranial nerve evaluation, and assessment of gait and balance is essential to help exclude pathologic disorders.

Labyrinthitis

DEFINITION/EPIDEMIOLOGY

Labyrinthitis is a usually short-lived disorder of the inner ear characterized by the sudden onset of vertigo. This sensation of abnormal movement is often described by patients as a feeling of unsteadiness, whirling, spinning, or dizziness. Labyrinthitis commonly occurs after an upper respiratory infection or an acute inflammation of the inner ear. Vertigo is often extreme, and patients are unable to sit or stand without losing their balance or vomiting.[1] Falls are common.

Vestibular neuronitis causes similar symptoms and is associated with a viral infection. However, hearing is not affected in vestibular neuronitis.

PATHOPHYSIOLOGY

Labyrinthitis is usually caused by an irritation of the inner ear from a middle ear or an upper respiratory infection; viral infection is the most common cause.[2] Bacterial labyrinthitis is more serious and may be a complication of otitis media or meningitis.[2] Labyrinthitis may also be caused by irritation from serous products associated with otitis media or by vasculitis, medications, head injury, and tumors.[2]

CLINICAL PRESENTATION

Patients with labyrinthitis complain of severe, vertigo, nausea, and vomiting aggravated by head movement. Tinnitus and hearing loss can be present. The most severe symptoms of vertigo usually subside within 48 to 72 hours, but they can last 4 to 5 days. Although most episodes resolve spontaneously, vertigo may reoccur for weeks or months when the head is turned suddenly.[1]

The history should include current medication use, history of head trauma, and the duration, episodic nature, and severity of the vertigo. Past medical history and recent infection, particularly in the respiratory tract, should be elicited. Precipitating or provoking factors including cough, sneeze, or change in head position, and associated symptoms should be ascertained to help determine the cause of the vertigo.

PHYSICAL EXAMINATION

A thorough ear, nose, and throat examination and a careful neurologic evaluation are recommended. Screening hearing examination, plus labyrinthine tests for positional nystagmus, past pointing, and balance (Romberg), should be included. Spontaneous nystagmus, horizontal or rotary, is almost always present, has fast phases, and is directed in the opposite direction from the affected ear. An abnormal neurologic examination suggests a more serious etiology.

DIAGNOSTICS

More definitive examinations to test hearing and to assess vertigo may be warranted. A CBC to assess the presence of infection may be beneficial. If a tumor is suspected, MRI or a CT scan is indicated.

DIFFERENTIAL DIAGNOSIS

Additional causes of vertigo including other causes of peripheral and central vertigo must be considered. Benign positional vertigo is associated with changes in head position, especially when the patient is recumbent. Vestibular neuronitis is characterized by unilateral vestibular dysfunction without hearing loss. Meniere's disease is associated with vertigo that recurs over months and years. Central causes of vertigo, such as vascular disorders or tumors, are less common, have a more gradual onset, and usually have milder symptoms.[2] Multiple sclerosis, post-concussion syndrome, and medication-induced labyrinthitis can also cause similar symptoms.

MANAGEMENT

Patients are encouraged to lie in a side-lying position with the affected ear uppermost because bed rest provides the best relief from symptoms. Activity can be increased as tolerated. Medications to control vertigo include meclizine 12.5 to 50 mg PO every 6 hours or diphenhydramine (Benadryl) 25 to 50 mg PO every 6 hours.[2] Sedatives, such as diazepam 2.5 mg PO t.i.d., and antiemetics, such as promethazine 25 to 50 mg PO every 6 hours, can also help control the symptoms.

To avoid dehydration and to maintain adequate nutrition, the frequent ingestion of small amounts of bland liquids and foods should be encouraged. Antibiotics are

Diagnostics

Labyrinthitis

Laboratory
CBC and differential*

Imaging
MRI or CT scan*

*If indicated.

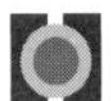

Differential Diagnosis

Labyrinthitis

Benign positional vertigo
Postpositional vertigo
Vestibular neuronitis
Meniere's disease
Vascular disorders
Tumors
Demyelinating disease (multiple sclerosis)
Medication induced
Inflammation (syphilis, vasculitis, otitis media)
Endocrine disorders
Postocclusion syndrome

appropriate if there is associated bacterial infection. There is no evidence to support treatment with systemic corticosteroids.[3]

LIFE SPAN CONSIDERATIONS

Medications for labyrinthitis can cause drowsiness and sedation. In older adults, lower doses of medications (i.e., 12.5 mg meclizine) should be considered to control sedation.

COMPLICATIONS

Sensorineural hearing loss can occur after inflammation of the inner ear. Suppurative otitis media, meningitis, or mastoiditis may be associated with labyrinthitis.[3]

INDICATIONS FOR REFERRAL/HOSPITALIZATION

Consultation with an otolaryngologist is indicated when the diagnosis is unclear, if the bacterial infection is severe, or if symptoms do not resolve within 4 to 6 weeks. Associated suppurative otitis media, meningitis, or mastoiditis also necessitates referral. Severe dehydration indicates a need for IV rehydration and possible hospitalization.

PATIENT AND FAMILY EDUCATION

The provision of information about the disorder and reassurances will be helpful to patients and families. The importance of slowly changing positions should be discussed. In addition, adequate hydration and safety should be stressed. Patients, particularly older adults, may require assistance with activities of daily living (ADLs) and/or a walker or cane during the acute phase of the illness. Driving and operating heavy equipment should be avoided while on sedatives and/or antihistamines.

Because the disorder usually resolves within 4 to 6 weeks, patients should understand the importance of notifying the primary care provider if the symptoms continue or increase in severity. Follow-up evaluation should be scheduled to reassess the patient and ensure the vertigo is resolving.

Meniere's Disease

DEFINITION/EPIDEMIOLOGY

Meniere's disease is a chronic condition of the inner ear characterized by recurrent vertigo and hearing loss that can affect the quality of life and functional capacity. It is a complex of four symptoms that may or may not occur simultaneously: dizziness described as spinning vertigo, low-frequency sensorineural hearing loss, tinnitus, and a feeling of fullness in the affected ear. It is estimated that Meniere's disease affects 150 out of 100,000 people, with men and women affected equally.[4] Most patients acquire the disease after the fifth decade of life, although it is common from age 20 through 50; 30% of cases have bilateral involvement.[5,6]

PATHOPHYSIOLOGY

Meniere's disease involves excess fluid and pressure in the labyrinth of the inner ear that episodically distends the structures of the labyrinth and damages the vestibular and cochlear hair cells. There is no known cause, although allergies, metabolic disorders, vascular anomalies, viruses, syphilitic infections, and trauma are suspected.[6]

CLINICAL PRESENTATION

Early in the disease process, patients have intermittent attacks of vertigo that last from minutes to hours, often associated with nausea and vomiting. These episodes are commonly accompanied by pressure in the ear, low-pitched tinnitus fluctuating in intensity, and hearing loss, usually in one ear. There can be long periods of remission. During later stages, the attacks of vertigo may occur quite often, and the hearing loss is constant.

PHYSICAL EXAMINATION

Diagnosis is primarily based on symptom analysis, but it is necessary that Meniere's disease be differentiated from other causes of vertigo. A thorough head and neck examination to exclude acute otitis media or other infectious process and a comprehensive neurologic examination are important. On physical examination, the Weber's test will lateralize to the unaffected ear, and in the Rinne test, air conduction will be greater than bone conduction. Spontaneous nystagmus occurs during attacks and may not be present between attacks.[2]

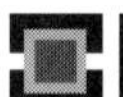

Diagnostics

Meniere's Disease

Initial
Audiogram

Laboratory
TSH
FTA-ABS
Lipid profile
Serum electrolytes

Imaging
MRI with gadolinium enhancement (to rule out neuroma)

Other
Electrocochleography*

*If indicated.

DIAGNOSTICS

Diagnosis is usually established by history. However, serologic testing (lipid profile, serum electrolyte levels, thyroid function tests, and FTA-ABS [to exclude syphilis infection] and other diagnostic evaluations can include a neurootologic examination, audiogram, vestibular evaluation with caloric testing, MRI with gadolinium enhancement, and electrocochleography.[5,6]

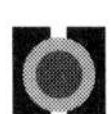

Differential Diagnosis

Meniere's Disease

Paroxysmal positional vertigo
Viral labyrinthitis
Vestibular neuronitis
Vertebrobasilar insufficiency
Atherosclerosis
Acoustic neuroma
Migraine
Head trauma
Thyroid dysfunction
Anemia
Arrhythmias
Hypoglycemia
Muscular sclerosis
Brain tumor
Cerebral infarcts
Cogan's syndrome
Mondini dysplasia
Drug toxicity

DIFFERENTIAL DIAGNOSIS

Meniere's disease is in large part diagnosed by excluding other disorders and is classified as idiopathic. Meniere's disease can present with only hearing loss or vertigo, both symptoms of many disorders. If vertigo is the only presenting symptom, the differential diagnosis includes drug toxicity, benign paroxysmal positional vertigo, viral labyrinthitis, vestibular neuronitis, vertebrobasilar insufficiency, atherosclerosis, acoustic neuroma, migraine headache, and head trauma. Other causes include Cogan's syndrome, Mondini dysplasia, thyroid dysfunction, anemia, arrhythmias, hypoglycemia, and central nervous system (CNS) disorders, such as muscular sclerosis, brain tumor, and cerebral infarcts.[5,6]

MANAGEMENT/CO-MANAGEMENT WITH SPECIALISTS

If Meniere's disease is suspected, patients should be referred to the otolaryngologist for testing and management. The treatment can be difficult. The goals of therapy include managing the episodes of vertigo and arresting the disease process. Bed rest may be the most valuable recommendation during an acute episode. Limiting the intake of caffeine, alcohol, tobacco, and dietary sodium is also often suggested, although there are no studies that confirm the benefit of these recommendations.[7]

Betahistine hydrochloride and diuretic therapy can reduce the severity of the attacks, but clear evidence of benefit still must be explored.[8] Diuretics such as triamterene/hydrochlorothiazide (Dyazide or Maxzide) or a carbonic anhydrase inhibitor such as acetazolamide (Diamox) can be used in acute episodes. In addition, benzodiazepines such as lorazepam (Ativan) or diazepam (Valium) for short-term use and antihistamines such as meclizine (Antivert) can be beneficial. Promethazine (Phenergan) or prochlorperazine (Compazine) can help manage the nausea and vomiting for some patients. Tricyclic antidepressants may be helpful for resistant cases. There are no studies to suggest that herbal medications, vitamin therapies, or vestibular rehabilitation are helpful.[7]

In severe cases, chemical labyrinthectomy with intracochlear gentamicin or surgical procedures such as labyrinthectomy, vestibular neurectomy, or decompression of the endolymphatic sac have been considered. These treatments are controversial, but these interventions can provide relief for patients with unrelenting symptoms.[6]

LIFE SPAN CONSIDERATIONS

Although Meniere's syndrome is more commonly diagnosed in middle-aged adults, older adults and children can also be afflicted.[5,6] The disorder can be particularly difficult to treat in pregnancy because medications are toxic to the fetus.

COMPLICATIONS

Hearing loss may be permanent. Injury from falls is a possible complication.

INDICATIONS FOR REFERRAL/HOSPITALIZATION

Referral to an otolaryngologist or a neuro-otologist is indicated for diagnostic evaluation and management. Hospitalization is rarely indicated unless the patient becomes dehydrated or injured as a result of a fall. Hospitalization is necessary for surgical intervention.

PATIENT AND FAMILY EDUCATION

Patient information should include information about the disease pathology, expected course, and treatment choices. Reassurance will help to allay anxiety. Specific recommendations include the avoidance of ototoxic drugs and noise exposure as well as the maintaining adequate nutrition and hydration.[6] Patient safety during acute episodes of vertigo and the sedative side effects of prescribed medications should be emphasized.

Tinnitus

DEFINITION/EPIDEMIOLOGY

Tinnitus is usually a chronic, benign, but annoying ringing in one or both ears that can be constant or intermittent. It can, however, herald a more serious disorder. It is often accompanied by high-frequency sensorineural hearing loss. Tinnitus can either accompany or cause anxiety and depression and can affect the patient's quality of life. There are a wide range of causes, including presbycusis, toxins, noise trauma, acoustic neuroma, vascular abnormalities, and neuromuscular conditions, complicating both diagnosis and treatment. Most patients adjust to the condition by refocusing attention. Those with a more disabling form of the condition require referral for diagnosis and management, which can include hearing aids, sound masking, counseling, alternative therapies, drugs, or surgery.

Tinnitus is also a subjective symptom of perceived sound—ringing, buzzing, hissing, high-pitched screeching, whistling, or other noise that seems to be coming from the ears. Rarely, tinnitus can be an objective, real sound audible to the examiner. It is estimated that as many as 50 million Americans have the condition. Tinnitus worsens with age, affecting about 10% of aging adults. A significant number of patients (approximately 12 million) seek medical assistance or are disabled by tinnitus.[9]

PATHOPHYSIOLOGY

Tinnitus results from many causes, including ototoxins, otosclerosis with aging, excessive noise exposure, intracranial pressure, eustachian tube dysfunction, whiplash injury, temporal mandibular dysfunction, uncontrolled hypertension, hyperlipidemia, or hypothyroidism. Either conductive or sensorineural hearing loss accompanies tinnitus. High-frequency loss is more common than the low-frequency hearing loss associated with Meniere's disease.[9] It is estimated that 90% of cases of tinnitus have an otologic origin. Tinnitus can also occur with conditions such as chronic otitis, allergy, excess cerumen, perforation of the tympanic membrane, fluid in the middle ear, multiple sclerosis, anemia, migraine headache, tumor, or head injury.[10,11] It can be aggravated by anxiety or depression.[10] It is believed that both auditory and nonauditory factors contribute to the problem.[12] The cause may be the result of either peripheral or central auditory pathology. Current research is under way into the role of the central auditory system, the way in which the brain responds to sound and the absence of sound, and the links between the auditory nervous system and the brain. Objective tinnitus may be related to a vascular condition such as carotid artery stenosis, a neuromuscular condition, an intracranial or a head/neck tumor, or a structural defect in the ear.[10]

CLINICAL PRESENTATION

Patients with tinnitus have varying degrees of symptomatology and levels of debilitation, depending on the type and level of perceived sound. There is usually some degree of hearing loss.

Tinnitus can interfere with the patient's social, emotional, and health status. Persons with tinnitus can experience emotional or psychologic problems, such as depression, insomnia, and decreased concentration.[9,10]

PHYSICAL EXAMINATION

A thorough evaluation for tinnitus consists of a comprehensive history and physical examination to determine whether tinnitus is caused by metabolic, systemic, or infectious disease or an inflammatory condition.[10] The history should include onset, duration, frequency, characteristics, and location of the sound. The description of the sound is very important because a rushing, pulsating, or humming sound associated with positional changes indicates pulsatile tinnitus, which can indicate tumor, increased intracranial pressure, or vascular abnormalities.

If the tinnitus is associated with hearing loss, any dizziness, vertigo, ear pressure, pain, or discharge should be noted. In addition, any allergy history, previous ear disease or injury, past noise exposure, medications, family history of hearing disorders, and ingestion of caffeine, chocolate, and soda drinks should be ascertained.[10]

The physical examination should include a complete ear, nose, throat, head, and neck examination, including auscultation of the head (preauricular areas, temples, orbits, mastoids) and neck (jugular veins) for bruits, as well as evaluation of the temporal mandibular joint for clicking. Blood pressure, hearing tests, cardiac assessment, and a complete neurologic (including cranial nerves) examination are also indicated.[9,10] There are usually no specific physical findings in most patients.

DIAGNOSTICS

A tinnitus handicap questionnaire is available to measure the degree of severity of tinnitus.[10] All patients with tinnitus should receive a complete audiologic evaluation, including bone and air conduction, which will determine a symmetric high-frequency sensorineural hearing loss if the cochlea is involved. The hearing test can also reveal asymmetric results that suggest retrocochlear tinnitus associated with CNS conditions or tumors. Laboratory testing should include a CBC, lipid levels, erythrocyte sedimentation rate (ESR), serum electrolytes, serum glucose, BUN, creatinine, and thyroid function.[10] If indicated, additional diagnostics include auditory evoked potential (AEP), auditory brainstem response test (ABR), electronystagmography (ENG), and MRI and/or CT scan. Further diagnostic evaluation of dizziness, vertigo, or nystagmus may also be necessary.[12]

DIFFERENTIAL DIAGNOSIS

The differential diagnosis should include those conditions that distinguish benign tinnitus from tinnitus caused by serious pathology. Excessive noise exposure and presbycusis are common causes of hearing loss and tinnitus. Medications, such as aspirin, can cause permanent or reversible tinnitus. Tinnitus of short duration is often caused by an acute process such as otitis, labyrinthitis, or noise exposure. Vascular disorders can cause pulsatile tinnitus and require in-depth evaluation by an otolaryngologist or a neurologist. Spasm in the muscles of the ear or palate can be heard as an intermittent tapping sound. An acoustic neuroma is usually associated with unilateral tinnitus. Meniere's disease is characterized by fluctuating tinnitus, hearing loss, or vertigo. Tinnitus accompanied by vertigo, facial nerve dysfunction, and symptoms of a transient ischemic attack (TIA) or cerebrovascular accident (CVA) signal CNS disorders.[9]

Diagnostics

Tinnitus

Initial
Audiology evaluation

Laboratory
CBC and differential
Serum glucose
Serum electrolytes
BUN
Creatinine
TSH
ESR
Lipid profile*

Imaging
MRI or CT scan*

Other
AEP*
ENG*
ABR test*

*If indicated.

Differential Diagnosis

Tinnitus

Noise exposure
Medication induced
Otitis
Labyrinthitis
Vascular disorders
Acoustic neuroma
TIA/CVA
CNS disorders
Meniere's disease

MANAGEMENT

Intermittent tinnitus is not usually considered serious, but unilateral tinnitus has been associated with an acoustic tumor and therefore consultation with the primary care physician is indicated to determine the need for MRI and/or CT scanning. Pulsatile tinnitus is also considered a serious symptom and necessitates evaluation by an otolaryngologist or a neurologist.

All ototoxic medications and excessive noise exposure need to be eliminated. The use of nicotine and caffeine has been discouraged, although there is no clear evidence that supports these recommendations.[13] Obvious local pathologic conditions should be treated (e.g., cerumen removal or administration of antibiotics for infection).

Most patients with mild to moderate tinnitus adjust to the condition, and although it is annoying, they do not find it debilitating. Patient education and reassurance are often all that can be offered. Other patients, with more severe tinnitus, find the condition disabling. Although there are options for treatment, the lack of a known cause makes tinnitus difficult to treat. If a sensorineural hearing loss is associated, referral for the application of other treatment modalities, such as hearing aids, sound masking, or behavioral counseling, may be indicated.[10] If no hearing loss is present, sound maskers alone, such as electronic noise-generating devices, mood tapes, or radio static, can diminish the intrusiveness of tinnitus.

Alternative therapies, including vitamins, herbal remedies, biofeedback, acupuncture, and magnetic and hypnotherapy, have not been proved to be effective.[14] The benefit of psychotherapy is unclear, but antidepressants, such as nortriptyline, have proved somewhat helpful if depression or anxiety accompanies tinnitus. However, results are varied in patients without associated anxiety or depression.[9,10]

Patients with symptoms that interfere with the quality of life or are debilitating require referral to an otolaryngologist for evaluation and therapy. A principal goal of behavioral therapy is to induce and facilitate habituation to the tinnitus signal. This habituation is achieved through counseling and with low-level broadband noise produced by wearable generators and environmental sound. With this approach, the patient still perceives the tinnitus when focusing on it but otherwise is unaware of the sound and is less annoyed.

COMPLICATIONS

There are no complications associated with chronic, benign tinnitus. Missed diagnosis of tinnitus that is caused by serious, underlying pathology may lead to untreated disease and major complications.

INDICATIONS FOR REFERRAL/HOSPITALIZATION

Consultation with the primary care physician is necessary when referral to an otolaryngologist or a neurologist is indicated. If there is a suspicion that the tinnitus is not benign or if pulsatile or unilateral tinnitus is present, the patient should be seen by the appropriate specialist.

PATIENT AND FAMILY EDUCATION

Information on the causes of tinnitus and hearing loss increases understanding for most patients. A discussion of treatment options and resources for treatment is beneficial. Reassurance about the benign and common experiences of tinnitus is also helpful. Resources about tinnitus can be obtained from the American Tinnitus Association.*

*PO Box 5, Portland, OR 97207.

REFERENCES

1. Plum F, Posner JB: Dizziness and vertigo. In Andreoli T et al, editors: *Cecil's essentials of medicine,* Philadelphia, 1997, WB Saunders.
2. Pepper RM: Dizziness. In Rakel RE, editor: *Saunders' manual of medical practice,* Philadelphia, 1996, WB Saunders.
3. Seidman MD, Simpson GT, Khan MJ: Common problems of the ear. In Noble J, editor: *Textbook of primary care medicine,* St Louis, 1996, Mosby.
4. Schessel DA, Minor B, Nedzelski J: Meniere's disease and other peripheral vestibular disorders. In Cummings CW, editor: *Otolaryngology head and neck surgery,* St Louis, 1998, Mosby.
5. Knox GW, McPherson A: Meniere's disease: differential diagnosis and treatment, *Am Fam Physician* 55:1193, 1997.
6. Nelson SL: Meniere's disease. In Rakel RE, editor: *Saunders' manual of medical practice,* Philadelphia, 1996, WB Saunders.
7. James A, Thorp M: Meniere's disease. In Barton S and others, editors: *Clinical evidence,* London, 2001, BMJ Publishing.
8. Van de Claes J, Heyning PH: A review of medical treatment for Meniere's disease, *Acta Otolaryngol* 544(Suppl):34, 2000.
9. Cullen PT: Tinnitus. In Rakel RE, editor: *Saunders' manual of medical practice,* Philadelphia, 1996, WB Saunders.
10. Ciocon JO and others: Tinnitus: a stepwise workup to quiet the noise within, *Geriatrics* 50:18, 1995.
11. Seidman MD, Jacobson GP: Update on tinnitus, *Otolaryngol Clin North Am* 29:455, 1996.
12. Jastreboff PJ, Gray WC, Gold SL: Neurophysiological approach to tinnitus patients, *Am J Otolaryngol* 17:236, 1996.
13. Dobie RA: A review of randomized clinical trials in tinnitus, *Laryngoscope* 109:1209, 1999.
14. Waddell A, Canter R: Tinnitus. In Barton S and others, editors: *Clinical evidence,* London, 2001, BMJ Publishing.

CHAPTER 90

Otitis Externa

Karen Koozer Olson

DEFINITION/EPIDEMIOLOGY

Otitis externa is commonly referred to as *earache* and is a superficial inflammation or infection of the external ear that usually presents with unilateral pain in the external auditory canal.

Immediate physician/otolaryngology consultation is indicated for patients with malignant otitis externa (Color Plate 35).

PATHOPHYSIOLOGY

The superficial inflammatory process of the external auditory canal may have multiple precipitants, including cerumen impaction, trauma related to vigorous cleaning of the canal with cotton-tipped swabs, swimming in pools that are not properly maintained, or swimming in lakes, rivers, and oceans. The most common causative organisms are *Staphylococcus aureus, Pseudomonas, Candida,* and *Aspergillus* sp.[1-4]

CLINICAL PRESENTATION

The usual presentation of otitis externa is unilateral pain in the ear canal. A feeling of fullness or itching may accompany the pain. Tenderness of the tragus may also be present, as may be mild lymphadenopathy and a low-grade fever.

PHYSICAL EXAMINATION

The physical examination may reveal a normal temperature and normal lymph nodes, but pain and tenderness are evident with palpation of the tragus and inspection of the external ear canal. The external ear canal may be erythematous and edematous. The tympanic membrane may be poorly visualized because of cerumen and/or edema and exudate in the auditory canal. Unilateral hearing deficits may be evident if the canal is markedly swollen or impacted with cerumen.

DIAGNOSTICS

Diagnostic testing is often unnecessary. However, a culture of canal drainage with antibiotic sensitivities is indicated for severe external otitis or for malignant otitis externa. The erythrocyte sedimentation rate (ESR) may be elevated in malignant otitis externa. A CT scan or MRI is indicated if osteomyelitis of the temporal bone is suspected in patients with malignant otitis externa.

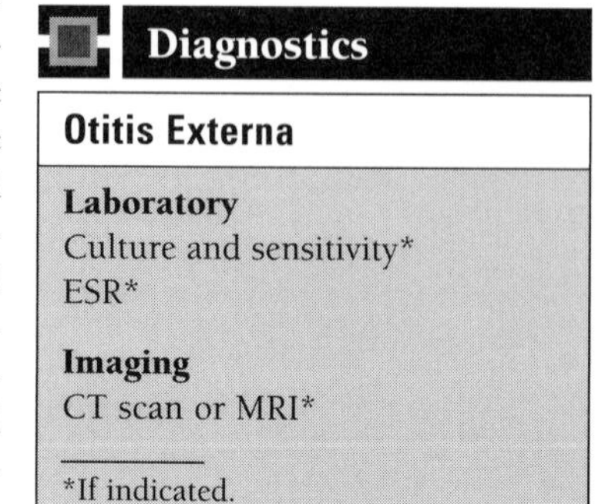

Diagnostics

Otitis Externa

Laboratory
Culture and sensitivity*
ESR*

Imaging
CT scan or MRI*

*If indicated.

DIFFERENTIAL DIAGNOSIS

The most common differential diagnoses are cerumen impaction and the presence of a foreign body in the external ear canal.

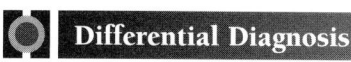

Differential Diagnosis

Otitis Externa

Cerumen impaction
Foreign body
Malignant otitis externa

MANAGEMENT

Management of otitis externa is dependent on the complaint and the causative factors. Over-the-counter nonsteroidal antiinflammatory drugs and complete cleaning and drying of the canal may be all that are necessary for mild inflammatory processes. *Staphylococcal* infections, which are characterized by yellow, crusty exudate, can be treated topically with an antibiotic/hydrocortisone compound (e.g., Cortisporin otic suspension [hydrocortisone/neomycin sulfate/bacitracin zinc/polymyxin B sulfate] 4 drops t.i.d. or q.i.d. for 7 days in the external canal).[2] For acute disease, dicloxacillin 500 mg PO q.i.d. can be used for 7 to 10 days.[2] The insertion of a wick into the affected ear may enhance healing in particularly edematous and inflamed canals. *Pseudomonas* infections, which are often accompanied by a greenish exudate, also are treated with topical agents such as Cortisporin. A fine, white material on the affected skin may be indicative of fungal infections and is best treated with clotrimazole (Lotrimin) 1% 2 drops t.i.d. into the affected ear.[2]

LIFE SPAN CONSIDERATIONS

Otitis externa is most common in young people and in swimmers; the incidence increases during the summer.

COMPLICATIONS

Complications of otitis externa are very rare but include malignant otitis externa. This condition is usually caused by *Pseudomonas aeruginosa* and is most commonly seen in patients who have diabetes or are immunocompromised. It is associated with severe pain, necrosis, and osteomyelitis.

INDICATIONS FOR REFERRAL/HOSPITALIZATION

Patients with suspected malignant otitis externa should be referred to an otolaryngologist or admitted to the hospital. Very early disease can be treated with Cipro (ciprofloxacin) 500 to 750 mg PO b.i.d. for 7 to 10 days with frequent follow-up.[2] In general, an erythematous, edematous, and tender auricle is indicative of virulent involvement of the deeper structures, which can progress to a life-threatening infection of the face and head. This condition requires immediate physician consultation and possible hospitalization for aggressive antimicrobial therapy. Patients who have diabetes or are immunocompromised may also require a referral for specialized care. Patients with severe otitis externa and frequent recurrences should be referred to an ear, nose, and throat specialist.

PATIENT AND FAMILY EDUCATION

Patients need to be educated about medication management, the use of earplugs when swimming, and avoidance of the use of cotton-tipped swabs in the external ear. The importance of immediate follow-up if there is increased pain or increasing signs of infection should be stressed.

HEALTH PROMOTION

Swimmers should use earplugs, as well as a mixture of 1:2 white vinegar/rubbing alcohol drops in each ear after swimming.[2]

REFERENCES

1. Bates B, Bickley L, Hoekelman B: *Physical examination and history taking*, ed 6, Philadelphia, 1995, JB Lippincott.
2. Gilbert D, Moellering R, Merle S: *The Stanford guide to antimicrobial therapy*, ed 31, Hyde Park, VT, 2001, Antimicrobial Therapy.
3. Uphold C, Graham M: *Clinical guidelines in family practice*, ed 3, Gainesville, FL, 1998, Barmarrae Books.
4. Ferri F: *Ferri's clinical advisor: instant diagnosis and treatment*, St Louis, 2001, Mosby.

CHAPTER 91

Otitis Media

Karen Koozer Olson

DEFINITION/EPIDEMIOLOGY

Otitis media is an inflammatory or infective process of the middle ear that may be bacterial, fungal, or viral in origin and is most often associated with upper respiratory tract infections or allergies. Acute otitis media has a rapid onset and short duration. Otitis media with effusion describes an inflammation/infection of the middle ear with an accompanying accumulation of serous fluid that can last up to 3 weeks. Subacute otitis media is a middle ear effusion that lasts from 3 weeks to 3 months. If the effusion has persisted for >3 months, it is classified as chronic otitis with effusion. Recurrent otitis media is an inflammation/infection of the middle ear that occurs frequently (three or more episodes in 6 months) but resolves between episodes.

PATHOPHYSIOLOGY

Otitis media is a dysfunction of the eustachian tube. The actual etiology is unknown, but it may be sequelae of upper respiratory tract infections or allergies that result in edema of the eustachian tube. Antecedent events are possibly infections or allergies that cause edema or congestion of the middle ear. Narrow eustachian tubes may predispose patients to episodes of otitis media. Exposure to cigarette smoke acts in several ways to increase the individual's risk for otitis media. Smokers are at higher risk for upper respiratory tract infections, plus the smoke may decrease the mucociliary functioning in the eustachian tube. When middle ear secretions accumulate in the eustachian tube, the opportunity for pathogen growth also increases. The most common pathogens are bacterial and viral. The most common bacterial causative agents are *Streptococcus pneumoniae* and *Haemophilus influenzae*. Chronic serous otitis is often associated with adenoidal hypertrophy, allergies, a deviated nasal septum, and the sequelae of upper respiratory tract infections and purulent otitis media.[1,2]

CLINICAL PRESENTATION

Clinical findings are related to the etiology. If the otitis media is related to allergic rhinitis, the clinical presentation will be significantly different than it would be if it were related to an upper respiratory tract infection. The patient with acute otitis media presents with a painful ear and probably has other symptoms of illness, including warm, tender, and enlarged postauricular and cervical lymph nodes; rhinorrhea; vomiting; diarrhea; and fever. Patients with chronic otitis media or serous otitis may be asymptomatic or have mild pain. Vertigo, hearing loss, mild stuffiness, and a fullness or popping sensation in the ear are additional complaints.

PHYSICAL EXAMINATION

A past history of ear infections, upper respiratory tract infections, allergies, smoke exposure, and any treatments and their effectiveness should be elicited. The development of the current illness, including the onset and duration of symptoms, the presence of ear pain or drainage, fever, irritability, hearing loss, tinnitus, or dizziness, should be noted. Associated symptoms, such as headache, nasal congestion, sore throat, or mouth pain, require investigation. Activities that involve barometric pressure changes, such as scuba diving and flying, may affect ear equilibrium. Temperature and vital signs may be within normal range, or the temperature may be elevated. The mouth, eyes, and nose examination may also be normal or may show signs and symptoms of upper respiratory tract infection. The frontal and maxillary sinuses are often tender on palpation and do not transilluminate. Mild to significant lymphadenopathy may be present. The tympanic membrane (TM) may be slightly erythematous or significantly inflamed and bulging. Bubbles seen behind the membrane indicate effusion.

The color of the TM may range from gray to red. Erythema of the TM is an inconclusive finding and may be related to crying or fever. In otitis media with effusion, the TM is dull gray and may be injected. Fluid levels may be visible behind the membrane. A very white TM may be the result of scarring from previous infections or of pus behind the eardrum. Discharge in the canal suggests perforation. Purulent discharge in the ear canal may be cultured and used as a basis for antibiotic selection. Bullae between the TM layers is most often associated with *Mycoplasma pneumoniae*. In chronic serous otitis, the TM may appear retracted with a diffuse light reflex. It has limited movement and bubbles, or a fluid line may be seen behind the membrane.[1,2]

In acute otitis media, the TM is red and bulging with obscure landmarks. Acute otitis media is often characterized by a throbbing, painful earache. Often there is fever. Hearing is usually impaired, and the patient may have nausea or dizziness. The TM is bright red and bulging. The disease is usually accompanied by cold or influenza symptoms. In serous otitis media, there may be fullness and impaired hearing. Fluid levels or air bubbles may be seen behind the TM.

DIAGNOSTICS

Diagnosis is normally based on the otoscopic examination. Weber's test and the Rinne test may be indicated to determine whether conduction and sensorineural hearing have been affected. Allergy testing should be considered in patients who have recurrent or chronic otitis symptoms and a history of allergies and/or allergic rhinitis. A sinus x-ray study or a CT scan of the sinuses may also be indicated with patients who have recurrent or chronic otitis media.

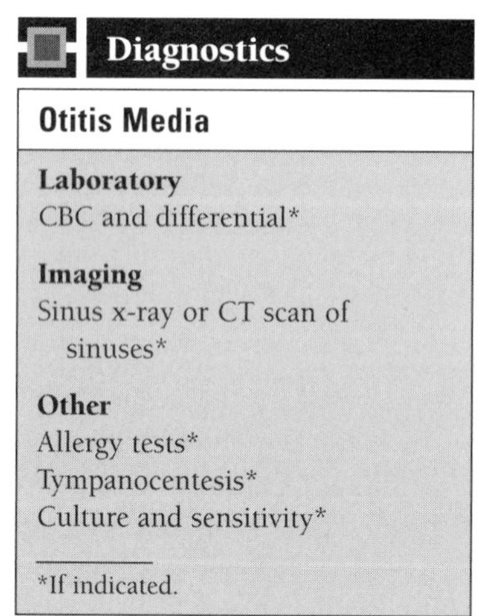
Diagnostics

Otitis Media

Laboratory
CBC and differential*

Imaging
Sinus x-ray or CT scan of sinuses*

Other
Allergy tests*
Tympanocentesis*
Culture and sensitivity*

*If indicated.

Immune status should be considered in patients with atypical otitis media or those who do not respond to therapy. Tympanocentesis may be indicated for recurrent otitis media to identify causative organisms. A CBC with differential should be ordered in immunocompromised patients.

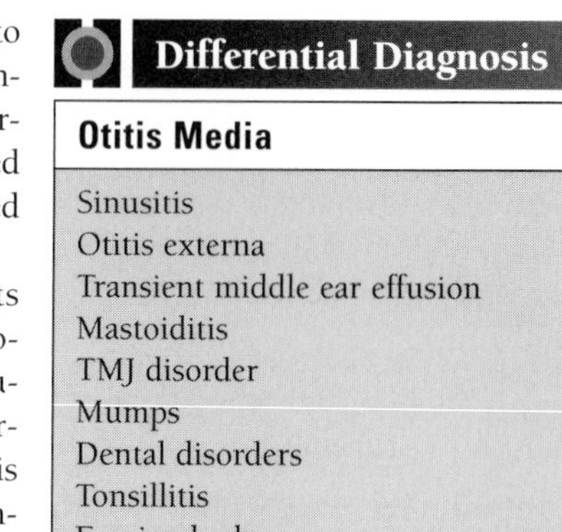
Differential Diagnosis

Otitis Media

Sinusitis
Otitis externa
Transient middle ear effusion
Mastoiditis
TMJ disorder
Mumps
Dental disorders
Tonsillitis
Foreign body
Head or ear trauma

Several other tests are available for diagnosis. The use of the pneumatic otoscope to determine whether the TM is mobile is the most commonly used technique. Acoustic reflectometry, which is the use of sound waves to determine TM mobility, is rarely used.

DIFFERENTIAL DIAGNOSIS

Otitis externa, transient middle ear effusion related to barometric changes, mastoiditis, temporomandibular joint (TMJ) disorder, mumps, dental disorders, and tonsillitis should be considered. In addition, ear pain can result from a foreign body either in the nose or in the ear (more likely in young children) or from head or ear trauma.

MANAGEMENT

The management of bacterial otitis media has traditionally relied on the use of antibiotics (Table 91-1). However, many cases of otitis media can be treated symptomatically with acetaminophen or ibuprofen.[3] One third of all cases of otitis media have no bacterial component, and up to 80% of all cases resolve without antimicrobial treatment.[2,3] Antibiotic therapy should be determined on an individual basis and is dependent on the history and presentation.

Amoxicillin continues to be the antibiotic of choice for the initial treatment of otitis media. It is relatively easy to use, inexpensive, and effective. Increasingly, however, a significant number of organisms, usually those that produce beta-lactamase, are amoxicillin resistant. If initial therapy is not successful, a medication effective against these organisms, such as amoxicillin/clavulanic acid, should be considered. Other antibiotics commonly used are sulfonamides, cephalosporins, and macrolides.[1-3]

Prophylactic antibiotic use for the treatment and prevention of chronic or recurrent otitis media is still being debated. Prophylaxis is recommended after the occurrence of three or more otitis episodes in 6 months and is usually given for 3 months during the high-incidence winter and early spring months. The patient should be evaluated every 4 weeks. The prophylactic treatment for patients who are not allergic to penicillin is amoxicillin 20 mg/kg at h.s.[3] The use of acetaminophen or ibuprofen for fever and discomfort is also recommended. The treatment of viral otitis media is symptomatic. Acetaminophen or ibuprofen is recommended for fever and discomfort. The use of antihistamines and decongestants has not been shown to be effective. However, they may be effective in the prevention of otitis media related to allergic rhinitis. Nasal sprays are recommended for symptomatic relief of otitis media with effusions or relief of serous otitis. The recommendation for adults

TABLE 91-1 Antibiotic Recommendations for Acute Otitis Media (Bacterial)

Antibiotic	Adult Dosage	Pediatric Dosage
Amoxicillin	250 to 500 mg t.i.d. × 10 days	40 mg/kg/day in 3 divided doses × 10 days
Trimethoprim/sulfamethoxazole (Septra DS)	1 tablet b.i.d. × 10 days	1 ml/kg/day in divided doses q 12 hr × 10 days
Erythromycin	333 to 500 mg t.i.d. × 7 to 10 days	30 to 50 mg/kg/day in divided doses t.i.d. × 7 to 10 days
Amoxicillin/clavulanic acid (Augmentin)	250 to 500 mg t.i.d. × 10 days	40 mg/kg/day in 3 divided doses × 10 days
Cefaclor	500 mg t.i.d. × 10 days	40 mg/kg/day in 3 divided doses × 10 days

is internasal cromolyn sodium (NasalCrom) 1 spray in each nostril four to six times daily or beclomethasone dipropionate (Beconase AQ) 1 or 2 sprays in each nostril b.i.d.[2,3] Nonpharmacologic treatment for recurrent or chronic otitis media with effusion includes the use of myringotomy with tubes.

LIFE SPAN CONSIDERATIONS

Acute otitis media is primarily a disease of young children. In adults it most often occurs in smokers and in adults who are exposed to second-hand smoke

COMPLICATIONS

Usually no long-term complications are evident. The most common short-term consequence is decreased conductive hearing loss. This may be a barrier to learning and may contribute to language development delays, especially if the problem is chronic and occurs in the preschool and early school-aged child. Eardrum perforation represents common sequelae of both acute otitis media and chronic otitis media with effusion. Hearing loss, perforation of the eardrum, cholesteatoma, acute mastoiditis, meningitis, and epidermal abscess are less common complications of otitis media.

INDICATIONS FOR REFERRAL/HOSPITALIZATION

The patient with chronic or acute otitis media that does not respond to therapy in 2 to 3 days should be switched to an alternative therapy. If there is no response to the alternative therapy, then referral to a physician or otolaryngologist is necessary. In addition, patients with chronic or recurrent otitis media warrant physician consultation.

PATIENT AND FAMILY EDUCATION

The risk of otitis media can be decreased by not smoking and by minimizing exposure to smoke. Smoking cessation should be encouraged (see Chapter 21). Otitis media is not contagious. However, patients may require careful explanation about symptomatic rather than antibiotic treatment of otitis media.

HEALTH PROMOTION

The best health promotion for patients to prevent otitis media is cessation of smoking and exposure to second-hand smoke.

REFERENCES

1. Uphold C, Graham M: *Clinical guidelines in family practice*, ed 3, Gainesville, FF, 1998, Barmarrae Books.
2. Ferri F: *Ferris clinical advisor: Instant diagnosis and treatment*, Philadelphia, 2001, Mosby.
3. Gilbert D, Moellering R, Merle S: *The Stanford Guide to antimicrobial therapy*, ed 31, Hyde Park, VT, 2001, Antimicrobial Therapy.

CHAPTER 92

Tympanic Membrane Perforation

Chad J. Smith

DEFINITION/EPIDEMIOLOGY

Tympanic membrane (TM) perforation is an opening in the otherwise intact membrane that, as a mechanical component of hearing, separates the external from the middle ear. TM perforation results from a variety of causes and is a cause of conductive hearing loss. These perforations usually heal spontaneously and rarely require surgical intervention.

PATHOPHYSIOLOGY

Perforation can be caused by a variety of traumatic, infectious, and neoplastic processes. The TM can be lacerated or perforated by foreign objects in the external canal. Barotrauma, physical trauma, or a fracture of the temporal skull can tear or perforate the TM. Occasionally the TM perforates with the pressure and inflammation of acute otitis media. Perforations often precede the development of a cholesteatoma.[1]

CLINICAL PRESENTATION AND PHYSICAL EXAMINATION

TM perforations are usually discovered at the time of trauma or during the evaluation for middle ear infection. Perforation may also be observed in association with a cholesteatoma. Most patients with traumatic perforation experience pain and some degree of hearing loss. A thorough ear examination and an evaluation of hearing status should be included in the initial assessment.

DIAGNOSTICS AND DIFFERENTIAL DIAGNOSIS

After the perforation has healed, an audiogram is helpful in evaluating the presence or extent of hearing impairment. The differential includes all causes of perforation, including trauma, infection, and neoplasm.

MANAGEMENT

Most TM perforations heal spontaneously unless they become secondarily infected or are very large. Patients should keep water out of the ear until the perforation has healed. Antibiotic drops and/or systemic antibiotics are often necessary when infection is evident.

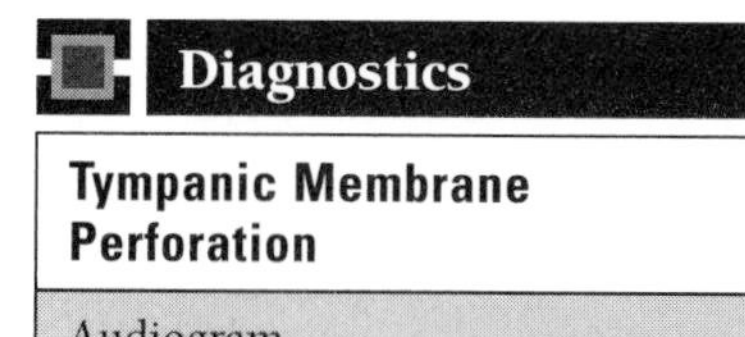

Tympanic Membrane Perforation

Audiogram

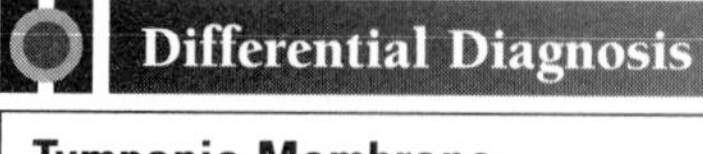

Tympanic Membrane Perforation

Barotrauma
Trauma
Infection
Neoplasm

COMPLICATIONS AND INDICATIONS FOR REFERRAL/ HOSPITALIZATION

A middle ear infection, cholesteatoma, and impaired hearing are potential complications of a TM perforation. A referral to an otolaryngologist is appropriate for large perforations or for those that do not show evidence of timely healing.

PATIENT AND FAMILY EDUCATION

Patient education should include measures to protect the TM while it heals. Patients should not permit water to enter the ear until healing has occurred, and they should be encouraged to return for follow-up. The etiology of the perforation should be determined so that repeat perforations are avoided. Special emphasis on the importance of not inserting objects (e.g., cotton-tipped applicators) into the external ear canal is also necessary.

REFERENCE

1. Seidman MD, Simpson GT, Khan MJ: Common problems of the ear. In Noble J, editor: *Textbook of primary care medicine*, ed 3, St Louis, 2001, Mosby.

PART 8

Evaluation and Management of Nose Disorders

TERRY MAHAN BUTTARO, Section Editor

CHAPTER 93

Chronic Nasal Congestion and Discharge

Updated by Terry Mahan Buttaro

DEFINITION/EPIDEMIOLOGY

It is estimated that 15% to 20% of the population experiences chronic or recurrent nasal congestion during their lifetime.[1] In fact, some people may experience chronic nasal congestion most of the time. These people may seek constant treatment because chronic nasal congestion has a profound effect on the quality of life. Lives are affected by constant discomfort and/or coughing, absenteeism from work, inability to participate in leisure activities, and the expense of treating the problem. Often the primary care provider must be able to distinguish between the symptoms that indicate allergic rhinitis and those of an obstruction, inflammation, or vasomotor instability. Management of the condition can be achieved through the proper use of allergy testing and the effective use of antihistamines, decongestants, and topical corticosteroids.

PATHOPHYSIOLOGY

The pathology of chronic nasal congestion and discharge depends on the specific disease process that is causing the signs and symptoms. Acute nasal congestion is usually related to the common cold. Chronic rhinitis can be related to allergic and nonallergic rhinitis, medications, mechanical obstruction, pregnancy, hypothyroidism, and chronic inflammatory disease or to syphilis, rhinosclerosis, rhinosporidiosis, leishmaniasis, blastomycosis, histoplasmosis, and leprosy. The latter diseases are conditions that present with granuloma formation and destruction of soft tissue, cartilage, and bone.

CLINICAL PRESENTATION

The clinical presentation of chronic nasal congestion and discharge depends on the specific disease process that is causing the signs and symptoms. The most common causes include colds, medications, mechanical obstruction, chronic inflammatory disease, atrophic rhinitis, and hormonal etiologies. Other causes such as syphilis, rhinosporidiosis, leishmaniasis, blastomycosis, and histoplasmosis should also be considered. The clinical presentations of these diseases are found in Box 93-1.

PHYSICAL EXAMINATION

The patient should be asked to blow the nose with one side occluded to identify obstruction and then repeat with the other side. The nasal mucous membranes are inspected for erythema, pallor, atrophy, edema, crusting, and discharge. Any abnormalities, such as polyps, erosions, and septal deviations or perforations, should be noted. The vestibules should be inspected with a penlight while the patient's head is tipped back. A nasal speculum should be used for the examination to allow better visualization of the nasal cavity. The speculum blades should be inserted gently about ½ inch into the nostril. Control of the

BOX 93-1

COMMON CAUSES OF CHRONIC NASAL CONGESTION AND DISCHARGE

SYPHILIS

Secondary syphilis occurs about 6 to 8 weeks after exposure and the primary infection
Characterized by a skin rash (macular, papular, or follicular), which often involves the palms and soles; this may last 2 to 6 weeks
Erosions of the mucous membranes may occur
Flulike symptoms: headache, generalized arthralgia, and malaise

RHINOSPORIDIOSIS

Pedunculated polyps on mucous membranes
Polyps may be on mucosa of the nose, larynx, eyes, penis, vagina, and sometimes skin

LEISHMANIASIS

Localized cutaneous ulcers on the face
Single or multiple, sharply demarcated, granulomatous, autoinoculable lesions of the face and mucous membranes

BLASTOMYCOSIS

Signs and symptoms of bronchopneumonia
A dry, hacking cough
Chest pain, fever
Nasal discharge

HISTOPLASMOSIS

Nasal, oral ulcerations
Lymphadenopathy, hepatomegaly, splenomegaly

DRUGS

Nasal congestion
Nasal mucosa erythema
Atrophy of septal mucosa
Septal perforation

HORMONAL ETIOLOGIES FOR CHRONIC NASAL CONGESTION

Nasal congestion
Nasal obstruction

MECHANICAL OBSTRUCTION

Visualization of polyps, tumor, deviated septum, or foreign body
Unilateral obstruction, mild discomfort, and sneezing
Unilateral purulent nasal discharge

CHRONIC INFLAMMATORY DISEASE

Nasal ulceration
Nasal obstruction

ATROPHIC RHINITIS

Atrophic and sclerotic mucous membrane
Abnormal patency of the nares
Crust formation
Foul odor

speculum can be increased by resting the index finger on the side of the patient's nose and steadying the patient's head with the nondominant hand. The blades should be opened gently to avoid pressure to the sensitive areas of the nose.

Inspection may be hampered by nasal congestion. In that case it may be necessary to shrink the nasal membranes with a topical vasoconstrictor (e.g., phenylephrine hydrochloride). When the medication is being instilled, the patient is asked to say "e" and to hold the sound. The technique occludes the upper airway and prevents the medication from running into the pharynx.[2]

DIAGNOSTICS

Selection of laboratory studies depends on the differential diagnosis and suspected disease process. Antigen challenge testing may be helpful in determining whether the symptoms are related to allergic or nonallergic disease. In vivo and in vitro testing methods are used for antigen challenge testing.

In vitro testing for allergen-specific immunoglobulin E (IgE) is the test of choice for the detection of allergen-specific IgE. The test involves skin testing for environmental allergens (dusts, molds, animal dander, and pollens). The testing is performed by introducing these potential allergens into the skin with needle pricks.

Because a false-negative finding may result, antihistamines should not be taken for 12 to 24 hours before the testing. The size of the wheal and flare correlates well with the level of allergen-specific IgE.

DIFFERENTIAL DIAGNOSIS

Syphilis

In acquired syphilis, *Treponema palladium* enters the body through the mucous membranes anywhere in the body. Although this is classified as a sexually transmitted disease, structures of the mouth and nose can become infected. During the secondary stage of the disease, which immediately follows the primary stage, *T. pallidum* invades the skin and mucous membranes. It can mimic several skin disorders and cause erosions of the mucous membranes, including the nose.

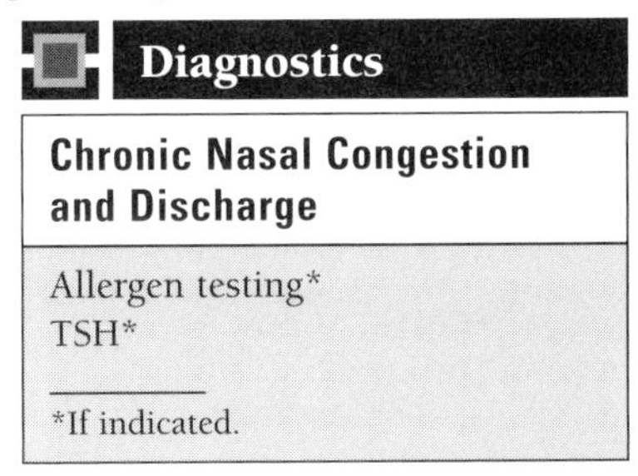

Diagnostics

Chronic Nasal Congestion and Discharge

Allergen testing*
TSH*

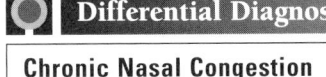

*If indicated.

Differential Diagnosis

Chronic Nasal Congestion and Discharge

- Syphilis
- Rhinosporidiosis
- Leishmaniasis
- Blastomycosis
- Histoplasmosis
- Medications, including street drugs (cocaine)
- Hormonal etiologies
- Mechanical obstruction
- Chronic inflammatory disease
- Atrophic rhinitis

Rhinosporidiosis

Rhinosporidiosis is characterized by large, friable, sessile, or pedunculated polyps on the mucous membranes of the nose, eyes, larynx, penis, and vagina. It is apparently contracted by swimming in stagnant water and occurs mostly in boys and men from India and Ceylon. Spores can be found in biopsy material.

Leishmaniasis

Leishmaniasis is a disease caused by parasitic flagellate protozoa that are transmitted by the bite of a female sandfly. The lesions present as ulcers principally involving mucous membranes of the nasopharyngeal and nasal cavity. Secondary infection producing nasal discharge may be the first sign of the infection. The infection is found in large part in people from developing countries.

Blastomycosis

An infectious disease caused by a fungus, blastomycosis primarily involves the lungs but can be spread (rarely) hematogenously to the oral and nasal mucosa. Initially the disease presents with papulopustules; it progresses to a large lesion with an abruptly sloping, purplish red, abscess-studded border. Discharge may occur, particularly if a secondary infection is present. Diagnosis is by made with a culture.

Histoplasmosis

Histoplasmosis is a fungal infection characterized by a primary pulmonary lesion with ulcerations of the oropharynx. The disseminated form is a defining disease for AIDS. Infection develops after the inhalation of dust that contains fungal spores. The majority of people who become infected live in the midwestern section of North America. The disease is diagnosed by culture.

Medications and Street Drugs

When nasal decongestants (e.g., oxymetazoline, phenylpropanolamine, pseudoephedrine) are overused, there may be a worsening of symptoms. After more than 3 days of continuous use, response to these agents becomes blunted (tachyphylaxis). Once the response to these medications has changed, the patient is likely to increase the number of times that the medication is used to obtain a therapeutic response. Cessation of the medication at this point may result in rebound nasal congestion. The congestion is believed to be a result of reflex vasodilatation. The nasal mucosa appears to be erythematous.

Cocaine abuse is becoming a more common cause of nasal congestion in primary care. Nasal snorting of cocaine results in nasal congestion and discharge. Cocaine is a potent sympathomimetic, and the reaction of the nasal passages is similar to that of nasal decongestant abuse. Recurrent nasal use of cocaine causes the nasal septal mucosa to become ischemic. This leads to tissue atrophy and telltale septal perforation.[1]

Hormonal Changes

The hormonal changes that occur during pregnancy and in hypothyroidism may cause the turbinate to become pale and edematous, leading to nasal congestion. Hypothyroidism may be subclinical except for nasal obstruction. The edema of the turbinates may be related histologically to the pathology found in myxedema, which is a result of an alteration in the composition of the tissues. The connective fibers of certain structures become separated by an increased amount of protein and mucopolysaccharides. This complex binds to water, producing edema.[3] With pregnancy, the congestion is related to the fluid retention that normally occurs.

Mechanical Obstruction

Congestion, discharge, and recurrent episodes of sinusitis that are unilateral are the classic signs of mechanical obstruction. The obstruction can be due to a tumor, polyp, deviated septum, or foreign body in the nose. Neoplasms are rare, and polyps generally occur in association with allergic and vasomotor rhinitis, chronic sinusitis, aspirin-induced asthma, cystic fibrosis, and drug abuse.

Chronic Inflammatory Disease

Midline granuloma is a rare illness of unknown etiology. The predominant sign of this disease is the development of ulceration that causes destruction of the upper respiratory tract. The ulceration may cause destruction of nasal structures. The presenting signs and symptoms include nasal stuffiness, crusting, and granulations. When this condition is found in patients older than 50 years, there may be a history of allergic rhinitis.

Atrophic Rhinitis

Atrophic rhinitis is characterized by an atrophic and sclerotic mucous membrane, abnormal patency of the nasal cavities, crust formation, and foul odor. The etiology is unknown, and the disease appears primarily in women.

The nasal turbinates are dry and atrophic, with crusts and fetid green nasal drainage, which is most likely a secondary infection. Anosmia is a common result of the disease process, as are frequent nosebleeds.

MANAGEMENT AND INDICATIONS FOR REFERRAL/HOSPITALIZATION

Syphilis

Penicillin (penicillin G benzathine 2.4 million U IM) is the treatment of choice for primary, secondary, and early latent syphilis (<1 year's duration).[4] Patients who are allergic to penicillin may be treated with doxycycline 100 mg PO b.i.d. for 15 days or tetracycline 500 mg PO q.i.d. for 15 days.[4] Pregnant women who are allergic to penicillin can be treated with erythromycin 500 mg PO, q.i.d. for 14 days.[4] Neurosyphilis or late latent syphilis requires a lumbar puncture and longer treatment regimens.

Rhinosporidiosis

This disease is rarely fatal unless the airway or other vital organs are compromised. However, the patient is at risk of the development of secondary infections, which may be fatal. Complete excision of the early lesions is curative and is the treatment of choice for this disease.

Leishmaniasis

Healing occurs spontaneously in 2 to 18 months, leaving a depressed scar. Secondary infections must be treated with antibiotic/antiprotozoal agents. Patients who are suspected of having this disease should be referred to an infectious disease specialist. If the ulcers do not spontaneously resolve, treatment with sodium antimony glutonate, pentamidine, or amphotericin B is indicated.[5]

Blastomycosis

If untreated, blastomycosis is progressively fatal. Treatment should follow the guidelines of the Infectious Disease Society of America (IDSA), although amphotericin B is usually effective.[6] Referral to a specialist in infectious diseases is indicated. Improvement begins in 1 week.

Histoplasmosis

The primary form of histoplasmosis is benign; however, it can be fatal in patients with AIDS. Referral to an infectious disease specialist is indicated. Treatment is based on IDSA guidelines, but both amphotericin B or itraconazole have been used effectively.[7]

Medications

When topical decongestants have been abused, the rebound nasal congestion will resolve 2 to 3 weeks after the medication is stopped. If cocaine has been abused, the septum will slowly heal once the drug is stopped.

Hormonal Changes

Nasal symptoms resolve with the correction of the hypothyroidism. The hormonal changes associated with pregnancy resolve after delivery.

Mechanical Obstruction

The nasal passages must be carefully cleared with suction. Care must be used to not push the object farther into the nose. Topical decongestants can shrink mucous membranes so that the object can be more easily visualized. One side of the nose can be occluded, and the patient is asked to blow forcefully. If this does not remove the object, an alligator forceps may be used to remove it. If the primary care provider is unable to remove the object, referral to an emergency department or otolaryngologist is necessary.

Chronic Inflammatory Disease

The patient should be referred to an otolaryngologist for treatment.

Atrophic Rhinitis

The goals of treatment are reduction of crusting and the cessation of odor. Topical antibiotics, such as bacitracin, can be used, or topical or other estrogens and vitamins A and D may be effective.

COMPLICATIONS

Complications are dependent on the etiology; ulcerations, infection, and septal perforation may occur if the underlying disorder is undetected.

PATIENT AND FAMILY EDUCATION

The patient and family should understand the importance of treatment recommendations. The patient should also be aware of the signs and symptoms of complications and/or recurring disease and know what to do if these signs and symptoms occur. Follow-up should be stressed.

HEALTH PROMOTION

Prevention of diseases such as syphilis, blastomycosis, and other protozoal or fungal infections will thwart the development of chronic nasal congestion. All patients should be educated about the dangers of decongestant abuse, cocaine, and exposure to chronic irritants and allergens.

REFERENCES

1. Goroll AH, May LA, Mulley AG: *Primary care medicine*, ed 3, Philadelphia, 1995, JB Lippincott.
2. Black J, Matassarin-Jacobs E: *Medical-surgical nursing: clinical management for continuity of care*, ed 5, Philadelphia, 1997, WB Saunders.
3. McCance K, Huether S: *Pathophysiology: the biological basis for disease in adults and children*, ed 3, St Louis, 1998, Mosby.
4. Hicks CB, Sparling PF: *Early syphilissxxxz Retrieved June 15, 2002*, from the World Wide Web: http://www.UpToDate.com.
5. Leder K, Weller PF: *Treatment and prevention of leishmaniasis*. Retrieved June 15, 2002, from the World Wide Web: http://www.UpToDate.com.
6. Chapman SW: *Treatment of blastomycosis*. Retrieved June 15, 2002, from the World Wide Web: http://www.UpToDate.com.
7. Wheat J: *Diagnosis and treatment of pulmonary histoplasmosis*. Retrieved June 15, 2002, from the World Wide Web: http://www.UpToDate.com.

CHAPTER 94

Epistaxis

Updated by Terry Mahan Buttaro

DEFINITION/EPIDEMIOLOGY

Epistaxis is a common problem experienced by most people at some point during their lifetime. Most episodes of epistaxis are benign, but some require emergency treatment and hospitalization.[1] Some individuals are more prone to nosebleeds because of the fragile mucous membranes that cover Kiesselbach's plexus and other surfaces that cover the anterior septum. Predisposing factors include nasal trauma, rhinitis, drying of the nasal mucosa from low humidity, deviation of the nasal septum, alcohol use, and antiplatelet medications.

PATHOPHYSIOLOGY

Epistaxis (nosebleed) may result from irritation, trauma, infection, or tumors. It can also be the result of systemic disease (e.g., hypertension, blood clotting disorders), systemic treatment (e.g., chemotherapy, anticoagulants), or nasal trauma (e.g., nose picking, foreign bodies, forceful nose blowing). Bleeding can occur anteriorly or posteriorly. Most nosebleeds occur within Kiesselbach's plexus, a vascular plexus on the anterior nasal septum, and are associated with irritated mucosal membranes or trauma.[2] This plexus is particularly vulnerable and easily injured. Posterior nosebleeds occur within the posterior branches of the sphenopalatine artery, are idiopathic or associated with vascular disease, and can be difficult to control.[3]

CLINICAL PRESENTATION

Patients with epistaxis will present with scant to copious amounts of blood emerging from the nares. Depending on the amount of bleeding, small clots may also emerge. Patients may report that the bleeding began spontaneously or that nasal trauma preceded the bleeding. A thorough history and elicitation of prescription or over-the-counter medication use, both oral and intranasal, are important to establish the cause of the bleeding and institute treatment.

PHYSICAL EXAMINATION

Vital signs and airway safety should first be determined and the patient should be instructed to sit up straight, tilt the head forward, and apply firm, continuous pressure to the affected nostril. If the epistaxis is the result of trauma, the nose should be checked for fractures. An internal examination may be deferred until the blood flow has subsided, but if the bleeding does not readily subside, the nose should be examined with a nasal speculum. Good illumination and suction are necessary to locate the bleeding site. Topical 4% cocaine applied either as a spray or on a cotton strip serves both as an anesthetic and as a vasoconstricting agent. If this preparation is not available, a topical agent decongestant (e.g., oxymetazoline) can be used in conjunction with a topical anesthetic (e.g., tetracaine) to examine the nose.[4]

DIAGNOSTICS

It is important to consider any underlying condition that may have caused the epistaxis. Laboratory assessment of bleeding parameters may be necessary to exclude underlying disease, especially if the bleeding recurs without a clinical explanation. A CBC should be obtained if severe bleeding has occurred; prothrombin time (PT)/international normalized ratio (INR) should be obtained if the patient is taking an anticoagulant.

DIFFERENTIAL DIAGNOSIS

Sudden epistaxis demands conscientious consideration. Although nasal trauma is the most common cause of nasal bleeding, it is critical to recognize other conditions that may result in bleeding from the nose. Other causes of recurrent epistaxis, such as hereditary hemorrhagic telangiectasia (Osler-Weber-Rendu disease) or tumor, should be considered.

MANAGEMENT

Most cases of epistaxis can be successfully treated with the application of direct pressure to the anterior portion of the nose for a minimum of 10 minutes. This technique is often successful because the most common source of epistaxis is the anterior part of the septum, where Kiesselbach's plexus is located. The patient should also be encouraged to sit in an upright position, because venous pressure is reduced in this position. The patient should also lean forward to decrease the swallowing of blood. Depending on the amount of bleeding, short-acting topical nasal decongestants (e.g., phenylephrine, 0.125% to 1% solution, 1 or 2 sprays), which act as vasoconstrictors, may help to stop the blood flow. If the bleeding area is noted anteriorly, the area can be dried and cauterized with a silver nitrate stick.[3]

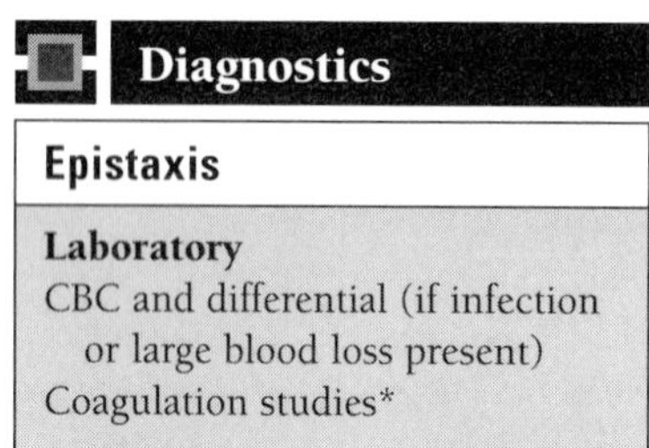

Diagnostics

Epistaxis

Laboratory
CBC and differential (if infection or large blood loss present)
Coagulation studies*

*If indicated.

If the bleeding site does not respond to direct pressure or cautery with the silver nitrate stick, *nasal packing with a nasal tampon or iodoform gauze must be placed by a practitioner skilled in this procedure.* The tampon or packing should be lubricated with petroleum jelly or bacitracin. Once in place, the pack is not removed for 48 to 72 hours.[3,5] If the bleeding continues, the opposite nostril should be packed in a similar fashion. Continued bleeding suggests there is a posterior rather than an anterior bleed and requires specialist consultation and possible hospitalization. Twice-daily oral amoxicillin-clavulanate (875 mg/125 mg) or trimethoprim-sulfamethoxazole (double strength) is usually prescribed while the packing is in place.[3]

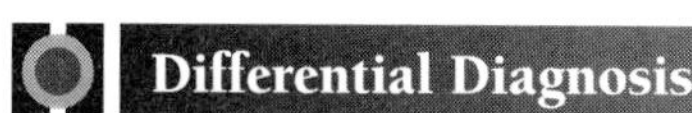

Differential Diagnosis

Epistaxis

Allergies
Colds or other infectious processes
Low humidity
Medications (aspirin, nonsteroidal antiinflammatory drugs, warfarin)
High altitude
Trauma
Coagulation defect
Hypertension
Neoplasm
Septal perforation
Vascular abnormality
Osler-Weber-Rendu syndrome

COMPLICATIONS

Complications are rare, because most nosebleeds are easily controlled. However, respiratory function can be compromised and patients may become hypotensive if bleeding is severe. Other complications are usually related to treatment and include abscess formation, septal perforation, or sinus infection. Toxic shock syndrome has also been reported as a complication of nasal packing.[3]

INDICATIONS FOR REFERRAL/HOSPITALIZATION

Occasionally a site of bleeding is inaccessible to direct control, or attempts to directly control the bleeding may be unsuccessful. In such cases, anterior and posterior nasal packing may be required. When the packing is in place in the posterior pharynx, the choana (posterior nares) are occluded so that an anterior pack can be placed. The packing should be done in an operating room or specialist's office, because it is uncomfortable and the patient may become hypoxic.

Surgical intervention may be necessary if medical measures are not sufficient to eliminate epistaxis. Internal maxillary or ethmoid artery ligation may be required to control nasal bleeding.[6] This technique is certainly necessary when the bleeding becomes life threatening and other treatments have failed. The surgery is usually performed after posterior packing has failed to stop the bleeding.

PATIENT AND FAMILY EDUCATION/HEALTH PROMOTION

After the bleeding has stopped, the patient is advised to avoid vigorous exercise and aspirin-containing medications for several days. The patient and family should also understand the importance of calling the primary care provider if the bleeding recurs (particularly while packing is in place) and recognize the necessity of follow-up evaluation within 48 to 72 hours to ensure healing of the lesion.

Avoidance of tobacco and hot, spicy foods is also advisable because they may cause vasodilation. Avoidance of nasal trauma, including digital self-trauma, is an obvious necessity. Lubrication of the mucous membranes with petroleum jelly or bacitracin ointment may reduce nasal discomfort and reduce the need to manipulate the nasal passages. Home humidification may also prevent the nasal irritation that results from a dry environment. Patients should also understand how to treat nosebleeds at home by providing firm pressure to the nostrils for 10 to 30 minutes.

REFERENCES

1. Tomkinson A and others: Patterns of hospital attendance with epistaxis, *Rhinology* (35):129, 1997.
2. Alvi A, Joyner-Triplett N: Acute epistaxis: how to spot the source and stop the flow, *Postgrad Med* 99:83, 1996.
3. Alter H: Approach to the patient with epistaxis. Retrieved March 21, 2002 from the World Wide Web: http://www.uptodate.com.

4. Jackler R, Kaplan M: Ear, nose, and throat. In Tierney L, McPhee S, Papadakis M, editors: *Current medical diagnosis and treatment*, Stamford, Conn, 1997, Appleton & Lange.
5. Jassen W: Treatment for emphysema: an overview of lung volume reduction surgery, *Perspect Respir Nurs* 7(1):1-5, 1996.
6. Black J, Matassarin-Jacobs E: *Medical-surgical nursing: clinical management for continuity of care*, ed 5, Philadelphia, 1997, WB Saunders.

CHAPTER 95

Nasal Trauma

Updated by Terry Mahan Buttaro

DEFINITION/EPIDEMIOLOGY

Nasal fractures are the most common trauma to the nose. The nasal bones are fractured more often than are other facial bones, and the nasal pyramid is the most commonly fractured bone in the body. Fractures of the nose may also include the ascending processes of the maxilla and the septum. Open nasal fractures are rare.[1] Nasal trauma, even if minor, can also cause septal hematomas.

Immediate emergency department/neurologic referral is indicated for nasal trauma associated with leaking cerebrospinal fluid or a suspected dural tear.

PATHOPHYSIOLOGY

Nasal trauma is the result of a severe blow to the face. In adults, most facial blows are related to automobile accidents and sports injuries. However, falls and abuse are also associated with nasal and orbital trauma.

CLINICAL PRESENTATION

The mechanism of injury, past medical history, allergies, and current medications should be discerned. Diplopia, visual changes, facial numbness, and other associated symptoms must also be determined. If the injury is recent, bleeding, which results from torn mucous membranes, can be profuse. Soft tissue swelling also develops promptly, may obscure the break, and can cause nasal obstruction. If the injury is older, edema may still be present and hematomas or ecchymosis visible.

PHYSICAL EXAMINATION

Inspection should determine the presence of periorbital ecchymosis, edema, abrasions/lacerations, epistaxis, cerebral spinal fluid leakage (blood-tinged liquid), as well as trauma to the teeth, neck, chest, and obvious deformity. Respiratory and cervical spine stability, as well as vital signs, should be determined. Mouth breathing suggests the presence of a septal hematoma.

The dorsum (bridge) of the nose should be gently palpated for deformity, instability, crepitus, and point tenderness. It is also important to assess for a palpable step-off of the infraorbital rim, as this is an indication of a zygomatic complex fracture. Stability of the teeth and palate should also be evaluated. Intranasal examination is necessary to exclude septal hematoma, which appears as a widening of the anterior septum, visible just posterior to the columella. Septal fracture, displacement/deviation, hematoma, or laceration should be noted.[2] However, internal examination may be deferred until the blood flow has subsided. Epistaxis is almost always present when there has been trauma, and bleeding is a sign that the nose has been fractured.

DIAGNOSTICS

The diagnosis of nasal trauma begins with a history of a blow to the nose, usually with concurrent epistaxis. The classic signs and symptoms are tenderness, crepitation, or movement of nasal bones on palpation of the nose. Septal hematoma may be found on visual inspection. An x-ray examination may confirm the physical examination and identify any additional facial fractures. However, x-ray studies of the nasal bones seldom provide additional information and are not recommended unless there is suspicion of extensive trauma that extends beyond a simple nasal fracture. CT scan is necessary if cerebral spinal fluid leakage is noted or if more complex facial fractures are considered.

DIFFERENTIAL DIAGNOSIS

The differential diagnosis of nasal trauma is based on the force of the trauma. Frontal sinus fractures result from trauma to the forehead and because of the location may present as a nasal fracture. Brisk hemorrhage from the nasal cavity accompanies these fractures. Fractures of the posterior wall of the frontal sinus may cause dural tears and leakage of cerebrospinal fluid into the nasal cavity. Common injuries that should be included in the differential diagnosis include septal hematomas, other facial fractures, and orbital fractures.

MANAGEMENT

Initial treatment consists of cool, local pressure to the affected area(s) to decrease edema and bleeding. A nasal fracture without deformity or septal hematoma may be treated with analgesia alone. Acetaminophen (Tylenol) with codeine or its equivalent is usually adequate. A simple laterally displaced fracture can be manually reduced. The patient should be given a topical intranasal anesthesia with codeine before reduction is attempted by a practitioner skilled in this procedure. The anesthetic is applied by inserting cotton pledgets that have been rolled into cylindric shapes into the nasal cavities. The pledgets are inserted with nasal forceps into the upper and lower nasal cavities and are left in place for 15 minutes. Topical anesthesia may be more effective if it is given with a local injected anesthetic. Nasal fracture reduction in children should be performed with the patient under general anesthesia.

A simple, laterally displaced fracture can be reduced by exerting thumb pressure on the nose in the direction opposite that of the initial fracture force. If the fracture has been reduced or if it is nondisplaced, otolaryngologic consultation within 3 days is indicated. Consultation is also recommended for suspected septal hematoma.

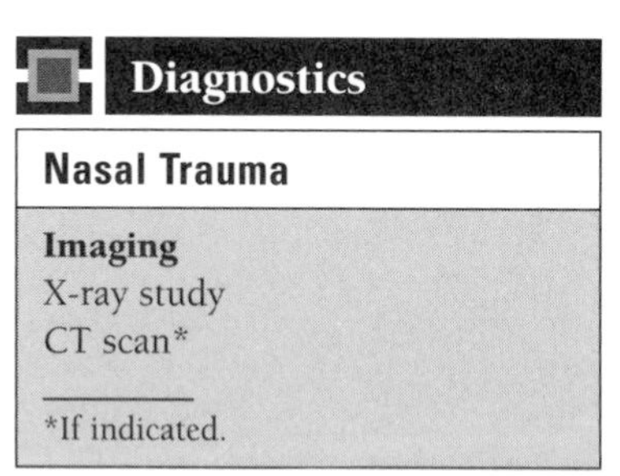

Diagnostics

Nasal Trauma

Imaging
X-ray study
CT scan*

*If indicated.

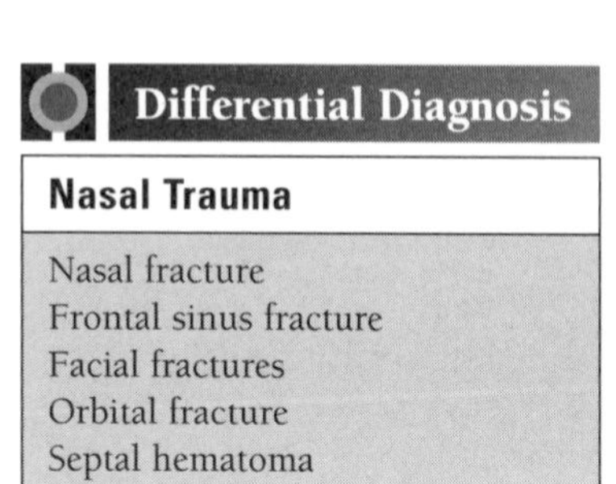

Differential Diagnosis

Nasal Trauma

Nasal fracture
Frontal sinus fracture
Facial fractures
Orbital fracture
Septal hematoma

COMPLICATIONS

Septal hematomas may develop and can occlude the airway. Nasal trauma may result in a nasal hematoma that separates the septal cartilage from the adherent mucoperichondrium, which supplies the septum with nutrition.[1] A subperichondrial hematoma that remains untreated can result in the loss of nasal cartilage because the mucoperichondrium cannot reattach to the septum. Therefore the blood supply is lost and the septum becomes necrotic. The loss of nasal cartilage results in a saddle nose deformity. Failure to treat a hematoma may easily cause it to become infected. *Staphylococcus aureus* is the most likely organism involved because of its prevalence in the nose and on the skin.

Deviations of the nasal septum are often a complication of nasal trauma. The deviation may cause varying degrees of nasal obstruction and predispose the patient to sinusitis and epistaxis. This is a result of the loss of natural defenses such as the nasal cilia. Septal ulcers and perforations may occur after repeated trauma and even constant nose picking.

INDICATIONS FOR REFERRAL/HOSPITALIZATION

If airflow obstruction develops in the nasal passages or if obvious deformity is present when the swelling subsides, consultation with an otolaryngologist within 3 to 5 days is warranted. Ideally, nasal fractures with deformity but no associated soft tissue swelling should be reduced immediately before edema develops. If edema develops, reduction should be delayed until the edema subsides, usually in 3 to 5 days. Reduction should not be delayed beyond 10 to 14 days. Any suspicion of leaking cerebrospinal fluid or a suspected dural tear mandates immediate neurosurgical referral.

PATIENT AND FAMILY EDUCATION

The patient should understand the signs and symptoms of complications and whom to call if problems develop. In particular, the patient should return for evaluation if the pain becomes intense, if the bleeding is profuse, and if nasal discharge becomes purulent, with a foul odor. If packing has been placed, the patient should understand the importance of not removing the packing, that the primary care provider will remove it. The patient should avoid any nose touching or picking, increase the amount of humidified air at home, and increase fluid intake. The dressings should not get wet, and swimming is not allowed until the dressings are removed and the primary care provider gives permission to do so. Antihistamine use and smoking are contraindicated during the recovery period.

REFERENCES

1. Crumley R: Maxillofacial and neck trauma. In Saunders C, Ho M, editors: *Current emergency diagnosis and treatment*, Stamford, Conn, 1992, Appleton & Lange.
2. Jackler R, Kaplan M: Ear, nose and throat. In Tierney L, McPhee S, Papadakis M, editors: *Current medical diagnosis and treatment*, Stamford, Conn, 1997, Appleton & Lange.

CHAPTER 96

Rhinitis

Updated by Terry Mahan Buttaro

Allergic Rhinitis

DEFINITION/EPIDEMIOLOGY

Allergic rhinitis is an atopic process characterized by sneezing, rhinorrhea, nasal congestion, pruritus of the nose and eyes, popping of the ears, throat clearing, and coughing. It is caused by an immunoglobulin E (IgE)-mediated hypersensitivity response to foreign allergens and can affect any age-group. The hallmark of this condition is the temporal correlation of symptoms with exposure to allergens. The most common allergens are pollens, weeds, trees, animal dander, dust mites, foods, insects, and mold spores.

The prevalence of allergic rhinitis varies by location and depends on the type and quantity of airborne allergens. It has been estimated that more than 20 million Americans are affected by allergic rhinitis, making it second only to dental care as a reason for office visits.[1] Each year allergic rhinitis results in more than 30 million office visits, and it is the leading cause of restricted activity and loss of productivity at work, at home, and in schools.[2] Pharmacologic agents and surgical interventions to treat the symptoms are estimated to cost billions of dollars annually.[3]

PATHOPHYSIOLOGY

Symptoms of allergic rhinitis do not begin with primary exposure to the antigen. Instead, the initial exposure leads to antigen processing by helper T-cells. With subsequent exposure to allergens, antibody production of B-cells is stimulated, and the mast cells ultimately become coated with IgE antibodies. With repeated exposures, antibody cross-linking results in mast cell degranulation and the release of various mediators. These products, which include histamines and bradykinins, are responsible for the classic itching, sneezing, and rhinorrhea.

CLINICAL PRESENTATION

Allergic rhinitis should be suspected with seasonal or recurrent sneezing, disturbances of taste or smell, nasal congestion, dry mouth, postnasal discharge, and complaints of fatigue. Nasal discharge is thin and clear and there can be nasal obstruction and facial discomfort. Watery, itchy, and puffy eyes commonly occur, but fever and chills are unusual. Typically, there is a personal or family history of asthma, eczema, or other atopic disease.

A detailed environmental exposure history is essential. Dust mites, animal dander, and indoor allergens should be suspected when winter symptoms predominate, because heating systems disseminate dust particles and aggravate symptoms during the winter months. Patients with seasonal symptoms are typically allergic to outdoor allergens such as pollen or ragweed. Symptoms that occur during late spring and early summer are generally triggered by grass pollens, whereas symptoms during late summer and early fall tend to be linked to weed pollens. Tree pollens tend to be associated with symptoms in late winter or early spring. These generalizations vary with geographic changes and daily fluctuations in allergen counts.

Because symptoms related to allergic rhinitis cause itching in the nose and throughout the upper respiratory tract, the pattern of symptoms is important. When is the patient asymptomatic? What medications has the patient been using? Where and when do symptoms occur? Is there associated itching and, if so, where?

The exact anatomic location of congestion should also be determined. Anatomic obstructions tend to cause unilateral nostril blockage, whereas nasal polyps generally cause bilateral obstruction.

PHYSICAL EXAMINATION

The physical examination can be performed with either a nasal speculum or an otoscope with an attached speculum. The classic boggy, swollen nasal turbinates with pale, bluish mucosa are often associated with bleeding, mucus, crusting, and other signs of inflammation. Common findings also include enlarged tonsils, the "allergic salute," a crease across the nose from manipulating the tip of the nose, and conjunctival irritation.[4]

DIAGNOSTICS

The diagnosis of allergic rhinitis is generally based on the patient's history. However, nasal cytology (Wright's stain) can determine the presence of neutrophils or eosinophils and determine if the symptoms are related to allergic rhinitis or infection. Further diagnostic tests are typically performed by an allergist. The scratch test or patch tests are used to test for skin response to suspected allergens. Radioallergosorbent tests (RASTs) determine serum levels of allergen-specific IgE titers. Skin testing is less expensive and more sensitive and is therefore the preferred diagnostic.[5] However, RASTs are more specific and can be used in patients with dermatographism or equivocal skin tests or in patients who cannot discontinue antihistamines.[5]

DIFFERENTIAL DIAGNOSIS

Although many cases of rhinitis are allergic in nature, other causes need to be considered, including vasomotor rhinitis and rhinitis medicamentosa. An infectious source is common and tends to be associated with fever, purulent sinus drainage, and other signs of infectious sinusitis. Causes of noninfectious rhinitis include aspirin sensitivity, anatomic blockage (nasal polyp, deviated nasal septum), hypothyroidism, and pregnancy. The use of reserpine, methyldopa, nonsteroidal antiinflammatory drugs (NSAIDs), and beta blockers has also been associated with rhinitis.[6]

MANAGEMENT

Environmental Control

The most important way to control allergic rhinitis is through environmental control. Because the patient is typically allergic to several allergens, control of the indoor and

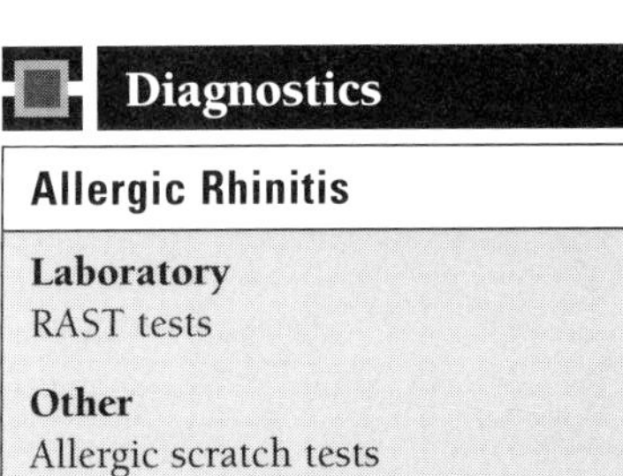

Diagnostics

Allergic Rhinitis

Laboratory
RAST tests

Other
Allergic scratch tests

Differential Diagnosis

Allergic Rhinitis

Allergic	Endocrine
Seasonal	Hypothyroidism
Perennial	Pregnancy
Infectious	Iatrogenic
Viral	Rhinitis medicamentosa
Bacterial	Aspirin
Anatomic	Methyldopa
Nasal polyps	Estrogen
Deviated septum	Reserpine
Neoplasm	Oral contraceptives
Adenoidal hypertrophy	Beta blockers
Immunologic	Vasomotor
AIDS	
Primary ciliary dyskinesia	
Cystic fibrosis	
Humoral deficiencies	

outdoor environment is crucial.[6] Nonspecific irritants (e.g., smoke) and indirect contact (e.g., secondary contact of animal dander) can cause symptoms that are indistinguishable from those of allergies.[1] Although techniques to control environmental allergens are arduous, time consuming, and sometimes expensive, they are often essential for symptom control. In general, it tends to be the time commitment involved, not the costs, that makes environmental control difficult for patients.

If the allergen is outdoors, minimizing both direct and indirect exposures is recommended. Long-sleeved clothing and a mask may also be necessary to minimize direct contact. However, often it is the indirect contact—when the allergen is brought into the house—that proves to be most bothersome. Keeping the windows closed and bathing and changing clothes immediately after entering the home should minimize exposures.

Often an indoor allergen is the cause of complaints. House dust contains the waste products of dust mites that live in furniture, carpets, bedding, and mattresses. Stuffed animals are a significant problem for some patients. Pets, particularly cats and dogs, are also a major cause of allergic symptoms. Removing the pet is not an effective means of environmental control because many people are not willing to give up their animal. Effective strategies include keeping the pet out of the bedroom at all times, keeping the pet outdoors as much as possible, washing the pet and pet bedding weekly, ventilating the home frequently to promote air exchange, having a friend or family member who is not allergic clean regularly with a high efficiency particulate air (HEPA) or double bag vacuum, and minimizing carpeting, drapes, and upholstered furniture. If carpets cannot be removed, an acaricide powder can be used every other month to kill dust mites.[5] Carpeting should be made of synthetic and short-napped fibers. Rugs should be washable; all loose or old rugs should be removed. Curtains (which should be cotton and, preferably, washable) and furniture should be cleaned and wiped regularly; dust-catching Venetian blinds should be avoided.

Other recommendations include keeping closet doors shut; covering machine-washable polyester pillows and mattresses with allergy-free and zippered plastic covers; wet dusting; washing stuffed animals, sheets, and comforters in hot water (>130° F) at least weekly; removing house plants and books; trimming bushes from the house; cleaning central heating and air-conditioning units; cleaning walls; using mold inhibitors when painting; reducing mold growth and humidity; and using a frost-free refrigerator. Although the efficacy of HEPA filters is unclear, HEPA furnace filters and room cleaners may also decrease allergen exposure.

In a closed environment, the quality of the air has a significant impact on symptoms. Studies have suggested that sleeping in an allergy-free bedroom can be beneficial to symptom relief.[1] Smoking should not be allowed in the home. Humidification between 30% and 40% is optimal during the winter. High humidity can lead to mold growth, and therefore dehumidifying in the summer months is crucial. Any heating, humidifying, or air-conditioning device that depends on the delivery of forced air must have an effective air filter. There are two types of effective air filtration devices: (1) electrostatic filters, which depend on electrostatic precipitation of particulate matter as it is drawn through a charged field by a blower; and (2) HEPA filters, which depend on trapping particulate matter in a specially treated cellulose high efficiency particulate air filter.[6] Electrostatic filters require that the particle trapping device be washed, whereas HEPA filters often require that accessory filters be replaced on a regular basis. The accessory filters are needed to trap larger particles that would otherwise impair the efficiency of the unit. Keeping these units clean and free of dust should be a priority.

The provider-patient relationship is crucial in the control of environmental exposures. Recommendations should be reasonable and made with compassion and clarity. If possible, a visit to the home and workplace will help determine which recommendations may be most beneficial.

Medications

Pharmacologic interventions are appropriate if strict environmental control has not worked sufficiently, but they should be used only when allergies significantly affect quality of life. Because pharmacologic agents may be used for extended periods, the safety, side-effect profile, and cost-effectiveness of each agent must be considered carefully.

In the past, antihistamines were typically the first line of therapy for allergic rhinitis. However, a more recent meta-analysis of randomized, controlled trials revealed that antihistamines did not control symptoms as well as intranasal corticosteroids.[7] Nasally applied steroids alleviate nasal symptoms with fewer side effects and can be as effective for obstructive symptoms as the antihistamines and decongestants combined.[4] Formulations are equally effective and include beclomethasone, budesonide, flunisolide, fluticasone, and triamcinolone. Both aqueous and nonaqueous formulations are available. Patients with a dry, irritated nose tend to prefer the aqueous formulations, whereas those with naturally lubricated nasal passages tend to prefer the nonaqueous preparations.[4] Most nasal inhalers (except dexamethasone) can be safely used at the recommended dosage without concerns about systemic absorption. Once symptoms have been alleviated, the lowest dose that keeps the patient symptom free is recommended.

Burning, stinging, or epistaxis is occasionally reported with the use of nasal steroids, particularly in winter months. These problems are minimized by using proper technique, applying a small amount of petroleum jelly to the nasal vestibules before using the nasal spray, and also by using a saline spray. Septal perforation is a rare complication; in fact, signs of atrophy of the mucosa are not commonly seen. Any such effects can be minimized by aiming the spray toward the lateral side of the nose and away from the septum. Patients over 60 years of age should be screened by an ophthalmologist before using nasal steroids, because reports have linked usage to open-angle glaucoma and cataracts in older adults.[4] The spray should be used regularly, but nasal steroids can take days or weeks to work. Antihistamine-decongestant combinations, although more effective if used before the exposure, can have more short-term benefits than steroid sprays. For patients with severe nasal obstruction, a short course of oral steroids can also be effective, although a combination of nasal steroids and antihistamines is safer.

Antihistamines directly minimize the allergic symptoms of rhinorrhea, itching, sneezing, conjunctival erythema, and tearing by blocking the effects of histamines. These symptoms are mainly related to the early allergic response and antihistamines are more effective if given before allergen exposure.[8] Antihistamines are much less effective at dealing with the late allergic response of nasal congestion.

The original first-generation antihistamines are available over the counter and are quite effective. However, they tend to be sedating and are not always practical for daytime use. Studies have shown an increased number of injuries and motor vehicle-related deaths when sedating antihistamines have been taken.[9,10] Therefore first-generation antihistamines are best used at bedtime. Chlorpheniramine, diphenhydramine, and hydroxyzine are available in liquid form and reach peak levels in approximately 2 hours.[11] Diphenhydramine is particularly effective because its half-life is approximately 3.5 hours; however, caution should be used with older adults.

The sedating effect of the antihistamines varies by medication and is less problematic with the second-generation agents. Regimens that involve using a nonsedating, second-generation antihistamine in the morning and a sedating antihistamine before sleep have been useful for many patients.

The second-generation antihistamines are effective throughout the allergic cycle and do not produce significant sedation. They are indicated if sedation is experienced with first-generation antihistamines, if benign prostatic hyperplasia is present, if narrow-angle glaucoma has been diagnosed, or if anticholinergic side effects are a problem.[12] Although more expensive than the first-generation agents, the improved quality of life and work performance allowed by the second-generation antihistamines can dramatically offset the cost. Second-generation antihistamines include astemizole (which can increase the appetite and cause weight gain), terfenadine, loratadine, cetirizine, acrivastine, fexofenadine, and levocabastine. Concerns regarding the arrhythmogenic potential of terfenadine have caused the Food and Drug Administration to remove it from the market in 1999.

Astemizole and terfenadine can cause cardiovascular effects (torsades de pointes, ventricular tachycardia, ventricular fibrillation) when used at higher than recommended doses or when taken in conjunction with erythromycin, clarithromycin, ketoconazole, itraconazole, or other medications that limit metabolism.[10] This effect results from common metabolism by the CYP3A4 isoenzyme of the cytochrome P-450 hepatic enzyme system. Other agents, such as loratadine and cetirizine, have not precipitated cardiovascular arrhythmias. Although loratadine is metabolized by the CYP3A4 isoenzyme, it has a second, alternate pathway that uses the CYP2D6 isoenzyme; this alternate pathway can be activated if the primary pathway becomes overloaded. Thus increased drug levels do not occur with loratadine.

Although second-generation antihistamines are extremely effective, they tend not to alleviate nasal congestion. Therefore combination formulations with decongestants, such as Allegra-D or Claritin-D, have become useful. Unfortunately, the decongestant component can cause sleeplessness, tachycardia, tremors, and other side effects. Antihistamines and decongestants are contraindicated for patients with hypertension, prostate enlargement, or narrow-angle glaucoma.

Other intranasal agents that can be helpful in controlling allergic rhinitis include azelastine (Astelin), cromolyn, and ipratropium bromide. Astelin is an antihistamine spray, but is expensive and can cause an unpleasant taste if not used correctly. Intranasal cromolyn affects the inhibition of mast cell degranulation; thus it affects local cytokine release. If taken regularly, cromolyn can prevent early- and late-phase allergy responses.[1] Unlike intranasal steroids, cromolyn is much less effective against nasal congestion; however, it is quite therapeutic for symptoms of sneezing, rhinorrhea, and itching.[4] The major problem is the dosing, which is four times daily. Nevertheless, its safety profile makes it an appealing choice for some patients.[4]

Intranasal ipratropium bromide, an anticholinergic agent, may also be effective for rhinorrhea and sneezing but is less useful for nasal congestion.[13,14] It is the treatment of choice for gustatory and skier's rhinitis and is often used to treat symptoms of the common cold.[4] It is generally safe and well tolerated. The most common drug-related problems are dryness and epistaxis.

Relief of nasal symptoms can also be achieved through the combined use of antihistamines and decongestants, topical nasal cromolyn, or topical nasal steroids.[4] For some patients, thick mucus secretions are a problem. Saline nasal sprays and high-dose guaifenesin can be helpful in thinning the thick discharge and improving symptoms.[4] Allergic rhinitis should not be treated with prolonged oral corticosteroid therapy; however, in some instances, short-term oral therapy may be beneficial.

Co-Management with Specialists

Immunotherapy is a long-term treatment for allergic rhinitis. Although it is beneficial for 9 out of 10 patients with seasonal allergic rhinitis caused by grass and ragweed, the effectiveness of immunotherapy is limited for other types of allergic rhinitis.[6] It may be effective if occupational exposures cannot be avoided and is generally considered when symptoms are present for more than 6 months, if symptoms are not relieved by environmental control and pharmacologic agents, and when the cost of immunotherapy is less than that of pharmacologic therapy. Injections are given every week in progressively increasing doses until a maintenance dose is achieved; after that, injections are given monthly.[15] Immunotherapy is not recommended for patients on beta-blocker therapy.

There is a risk of immediate and delayed reactions with immunotherapy. Generalized reactions tend to occur within 20 to 30 minutes, but more systemic reactions can be delayed. Although the risk of a severe reaction is small, the response can be fatal. Therefore patients should wait in the office for 30 minutes after the injection and carry an EpiPen if appropriate. The proper resuscitative equipment should be accessible if immunotherapy is offered and a physician should be readily available.

COMPLICATIONS

Complications of allergic rhinitis are rare but potentially serious. Sleep apnea can be a problem in untreated rhinitis.[16] Thus, treatment with medications and strict environmental control can be beneficial.

INDICATIONS FOR REFERRAL/HOSPITALIZATION

Older adults with new-onset rhinitis may need a physician evaluation to exclude anatomic obstruction. However, most patients with new-onset rhinitis have been recently exposed to a new and offending agent and can be managed effectively without a referral. Some patients require a referral to an otolaryngologist. Any patient who presents with new nasal complaints of congestion should have a nasal examination to assess for anatomic problems. Although nasopharyngeal neoplasms are rare, nasal polyps are common and often require surgical intervention. These patients can also have aspirin sensitivity and allergic asthma. A deviated septum can also produce symptoms that mimic classic rhinitis.

A second careful review of the patient's history, medication use, exposure to cigarette smoke and perfumes, and occupational exposures is indicated before making any referral. In addition, a home visit and review of inhaler technique are invaluable. Medications and medical problems that may be contributing to the symptoms should be investigated.[6] T-cell deficiencies (e.g., acquired immunodeficiency syndrome), cystic fibrosis, hypothyroidism, and humoral deficiencies should be considered. A referral to an allergist is indicated if the signs and symptoms continue and anatomic problems have been excluded.

Allergic rhinitis rarely requires hospitalization. Rare circumstances include anaphylaxis, a life-threatening hypersensitivity immune response, or the need for a surgical procedure (e.g., nasal polypectomy). Hospitalization is typically required for treatment and continued observation.

PATIENT AND FAMILY EDUCATION

Once the environmental allergens have been identified, recommendations can be made and a therapeutic regimen agreed on. Education is crucial in the management of allergic rhinitis. A dramatic improvement in symptoms is often noted when patients become experts on the triggers that activate symptoms. Therefore an allergy diary is often useful. Reducing exposure to dust mites, animal dander, molds, cockroaches, pollens, smoke, and other irritants is essential. Patients should also understand how to use nasal inhalers correctly and the importance of using inhalers regularly to promote their effectiveness. The side effect profile of these medications as well as over-the-counter and prescription antihistamines and decongestants should also be discussed.

Idiopathic or Vasomotor Rhinitis

DEFINITION/EPIDEMIOLOGY

Vasomotor rhinitis, which is now known as idiopathic rhinitis, is an important, often overlooked, nonallergic, noninfectious cause of perennial nasal congestion and rhinorrhea. Idiopathic rhinitis is not associated with itchiness of the eyes and nose or sneezing. It occurs in response to environmental triggers that can include cold air, strong smells, irritants, changes in weather, some medications (angiotensin-converting enzyme inhibitors, beta blockers), stress, exercise, or certain foods.[11] In contrast to the symptoms of allergic rhinitis, which tend to be seasonal and periodic, vasomotor symptoms tend to be year-round and chronic. Idiopathic rhinitis tends to affect both genders equally. Information on this disorder is scant and treatment is limited.[11]

PATHOPHYSIOLOGY

Symptoms of idiopathic rhinitis are provoked by environmental stimuli. Poorly understood, idiopathic rhinitis may be an abnormality of autonomic control of the vascular and glandular systems of the nose.[11] It has been postulated that the cause of vasomotor rhinitis involves an abnormal balance that favors parasympathetic control over sympathetic control of the nasal mucosa.[11] The underlying cause of this imbalance is unknown.

CLINICAL PRESENTATION

With idiopathic rhinitis, patients often report perennial nasal congestion but little discharge. There are few, if any, symptoms on arising, but nasal congestion can begin shortly after getting out of bed. Exposure to cold bedrooms or bathrooms is often reported. Stress, odors, spicy foods, sunlight, and other environmental exposures are often cited as causes. These irritants appear to be nonspecific triggers for exaggerated physiologic responses.

One characteristic that distinguishes vasomotor rhinitis from allergic rhinitis is that itching, sneezing, and other irritative symptoms tend to occur with allergic rhinitis, whereas obstructive symptoms tend to occur with vasomotor rhinitis.[11] Tearing and itching of the eyes and sneezing are common in allergic rhinitis but are uncommon with vasomotor rhinitis. Sneezing can occur at times with vasomotor rhinitis, but this usually occurs in response to temperature changes.

PHYSICAL EXAMINATION

The physical appearance of the nasal mucosa often differs in allergic rhinitis and vasomotor rhinitis. Nasal polyps are often present in patients with allergic rhinitis (especially those with aspirin sensitivity); the presence of such polyps excludes a diagnosis of vasomotor rhinitis.[11] Moreover, the nasal mucosa is typically pale in allergic rhinitis but is often erythematous in vasomotor rhinitis.

DIAGNOSTICS/DIFFERENTIAL DIAGNOSIS

Idiopathic rhinitis can be difficult to distinguish from allergic rhinitis. Although there is no definitive test, certain diagnostic tests can be useful. The appearance of nasal eosinophils is common in allergic rhinitis but is rarely seen with vasomotor rhinitis.[11] Skin testing is often positive in allergic rhinitis but not in vasomotor rhinitis.[11] In patients with vasomotor rhinitis, there is little correlation between positive skin tests and exposure history.[11] A positive skin test to a seasonal allergen in a patient with perennial symptoms is not clinically significant. Medication side effects, hypothyroidism, pregnancy, rhinitis medicamentosa, allergic rhinitis, aspirin sensitivity, infections, and nasal obstructions should also be considered in patients with symptoms of vasomotor rhinitis.

MANAGEMENT

Unlike allergic rhinitis, idiopathic rhinitis does not usually respond to antihistamines. Oral decongestants are often effective and are best used around the clock.[6] Intranasal steroids can also be effective. As with allergic rhinitis, environmental avoidance is the best treatment; immunotherapy is often not effective. Idiopathic rhinitis is chronic, and avoidance of stimuli is important. Smoking, using perfumes or colognes, and eating spicy foods should be discouraged. Autonomic denervation of the nasal mucosa has been attempted, and some success has been achieved.[11] Otolaryngologists can also perform cryosurgery of the inferior turbinates, which can be helpful.[11]

COMPLICATIONS

Although little information is available on the long-term complications of idiopathic rhinitis, chronic problems can occur. Patients can suffer from sleep deprivation and a poor quality of life.

INDICATIONS FOR REFERRAL/HOSPITALIZATION

Most patients can be managed effectively. A referral may be indicated if the diagnosis remains elusive, if treatments have not been effective, or if anatomic causes are being considered.

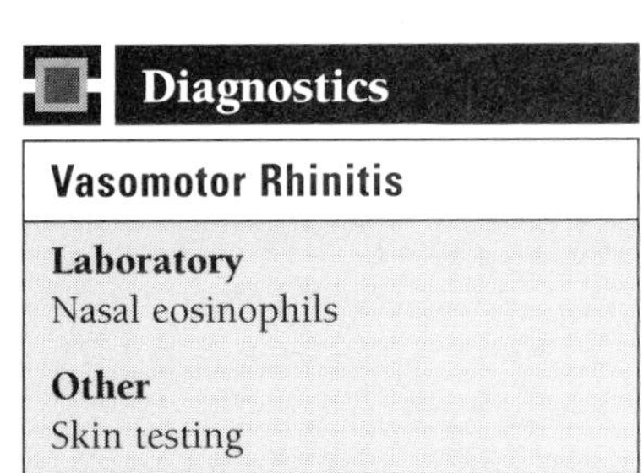

Diagnostics

Vasomotor Rhinitis

Laboratory
Nasal eosinophils

Other
Skin testing

PATIENT AND FAMILY EDUCATION

It is important for the patient to understand that idiopathic rhinitis is a chronic condition and that the effectiveness of symptomatic treatment is limited. A detailed environmental history and minimization of potential exposures is most beneficial. Many of the measures that are effective for patients with allergic rhinitis will be effective in patients with vasomotor rhinitis. Regular use of topical decongestants should be avoided because of the potential for developing a tolerance to these agents.

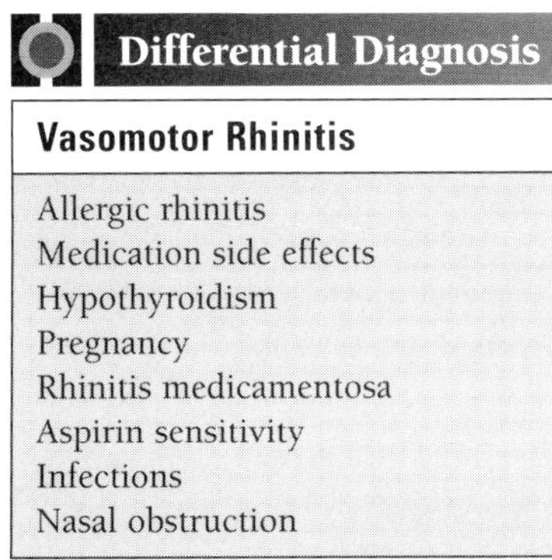

Differential Diagnosis

Vasomotor Rhinitis

Allergic rhinitis
Medication side effects
Hypothyroidism
Pregnancy
Rhinitis medicamentosa
Aspirin sensitivity
Infections
Nasal obstruction

Other Causes of Rhinitis

INFECTIOUS

Upper respiratory infections typically are associated with rhinitis. A coexistent infection is present, and relatively prompt relief of symptoms occurs with resolution of the infection. Purulent discharge is common but not always present.

ANATOMIC

Anatomic causes of rhinitis include a deviated nasal septum, nasal polyps, and nasal tumors. In particular, neoplasms should be suspected in older adults. The most common cause of anatomic problems is nasal polyps, which can cause impressive obstructive symptoms. These are often found incidentally in patients with asthma who also have aspirin sensitivity. Symptoms can be perennial and difficult to differentiate from allergic rhinitis or vasomotor rhinitis. Treatment options include intranasal steroids or surgery.

RHINITIS MEDICAMENTOSA

Symptoms of nasal congestion may result from the chronic administration of sympatholytic drugs, NSAIDs, or topical decongestants. This most commonly develops with tolerance to topical decongestants. After approximately 1 or 2 weeks of using topical decongestants, the nasal mucosa suffers rebound engorgement through increased blood flow. Although these symptoms tend to continue for days or weeks, discontinuation of the offending drug is curative. A 1- to 2-week course of nasal steroids or, rarely, systemic steroids can be helpful during the withdrawal period.

PHARMACOLOGIC

Various medications, including beta blockers, estrogen, and oral contraceptives, can mimic symptoms of allergic rhinitis. Treatment involves discontinuation of the medication.

OTHER MEDICAL CAUSES

Pregnancy and hypothyroidism are common causes of rhinitis. Other causes include cocaine use and atrophic changes. Treatment is directed at the underlying medical problem.

REFERENCES

1. Georgitis JW, Kaiser HB, Kaliner M: Allergic rhinitis: taming the troubled nose, *Patient Care* 31:51-60, 1997.
2. Kopke RD, Jackson RL: Rhinitis. In Bailey BJ, editor: *Head and neck surgery: otolaryngology*, Philadelphia, 1993, JB Lippincott.
3. Wood RP, Jafek BW, Eberhard R: Nasal obstruction. In Bailey BJ, editor: *Head and neck surgery: otolaryngology*, Philadelphia, 1993, JB Lippincott.
4. Ferguson BJ: Allergic rhinitis: options for pharmacotherapy and immunotherapy, *Postgrad Med* 101(5):117-131, 1997.
5. Ferguson BJ: Allergic rhinitis: recognizing signs, symptoms, and triggering allergens, *Postgrad Med* 101(5):110-116, 1997.

6. Martin D, Valentin MD: Allergies and related conditions. In Barker LR, Burton JR, Zieve PD, editors: *Principles of ambulatory medicine*, ed 4, Baltimore, 1995, Williams & Wilkins.
7. Weiner JW, Abramson MJ, Puy RM: Intranasal corticosteroids versus oral H-1 receptor antagonists in allergic rhinitis: systematic review of randomized controlled trials, *Br Med J* 314:1624, 1998.
8. Kause HF: Therapeutic advances in the management of allergic rhinitis and urticaria, *Otolaryngol Head Neck Surg* 111:364-372, 1994.
9. Gilmore TM and others: Occupational injuries and medication use, *Am J Ind Med* 30:234-239, 1996.
10. Corren J and others: Emerging trends in the management of allergic respiratory disorders, *Clin Cour* 16(1):1-7, 1997.
11. Stewart TW: Vasomotor rhinitis: neglected cause of nasal congestion, *Postgrad Med* 67(1):171-177, 1980.
12. Bousquet J and others: Assessment of quality of life in patients with perennial allergic rhinitis with the French version of the SF-36 Health Status Questionnaire, *J Allergy Clin Immunol* 94(2 pt 1):182-188, 1994.
13. Kaiser HB and others: Long-term treatment of perennial allergic rhinitis with ipratropium bromide nasal spray 0.06%, *J Allergy Clin Immunol* 95:1128-1132, 1995.
14. Georgitis JW: Nasal atropine sulfate: efficacy and safety of 0.050 percent and 0.075 percent solutions for severe rhinorrhea, *Arch Otolaryngol Head Neck Surg* 124:916, 1999.
15. Varney VA and others: Usefulness of immunotherapy in patients with severe summer hay fever uncontrolled with antiallergic drugs, *Br Med J* 302:265-269, 1991.
16. McNicholas WT and others: Obstructive apneas during sleep in patients with seasonal allergic rhinitis, *Am Rev Respir Dis* 126(4): 625-628, 1982.

WEBSITES

Allergy, Asthma, and Immunology Online: http://allergy.mcg.edu/home.html/
American Academy of Allergy, Asthma, and Immunology: http://www.aaaai.org/
American Rhinologic Society: http://www.american-rhinologic.org/
National Institute of Allergy and Infectious Diseases (NIAID): http://www.niaid.nih.gov

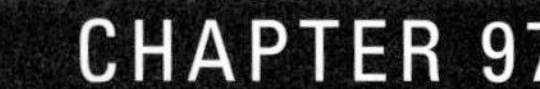

Sinusitis

Updated by Terry Mahan Buttaro

DEFINITION/EPIDEMIOLOGY

Sinusitis can be defined as an inflammation of the mucosal surface of the paranasal sinuses. There are numerous subclassifications, but the most useful definitions include acute and chronic sinusitis. Acute sinusitis resolves with treatment within 2 to 3 weeks, whereas chronic sinusitis continues over an extended period of time. This is an important distinction, as treatment of chronic sinusitis is more complicated than treatment of acute sinusitis.

Acute sinusitis is an inflammatory process in the paranasal sinuses caused by viral, bacterial, and fungal infections or allergic reactions. The most common cause of acute sinusitis is a bacterial infection caused by *Streptococcus pneumoniae, Haemophilus influenzae,* or staphylococci and is usually precipitated by an acute viral respiratory tract infection. Less common pathogens are *Chlamydia pneumoniae, Streptococcus pyogenes,* viruses, and fungi. The symptoms of acute sinusitis are often confused with an upper respiratory tract infection. The presenting signs and symptoms include nasal congestion, purulent nasal discharge, and a headache that becomes more intense when the patient bends forward. Fever, fatigue, and other constitutional symptoms are common. The onset is abrupt, with infection in one or more paranasal sinuses. The benefit of antibiotic therapy in decreasing the symptoms and duration of illness has been documented.[1]

Chronic sinusitis occurs with episodes of prolonged sinus infection that resist treatment or with recurrent acute infections that are inadequately treated and never resolve. The presentation of this disease is the frequent exacerbations of sinus infections that are caused by gram-negative rod or anaerobic microorganisms. In about 25% of cases chronic maxillary sinusitis is secondary to dental infection. The importance of the identification of an anaerobic infection is that this is an infection that can result in an anaerobic brain abscess that is hematologically spread from the sinuses. Gram-negative bacilli may cause sinusitis in patients who are intubated through the nose or who have a nasogastric tube placed in the nose. It is the trauma and the obstruction caused by these tubes that lead to a sinus infection.

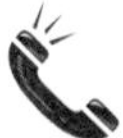

Physician consultation is recommended when there is evidence of periorbital cellulitis, high fever, or acute focal pain.

PATHOPHYSIOLOGY

Most sinus disease involves the maxillary and anterior ethmoidal sinuses. The maxillary sinus is the largest of the paranasal sinuses, and its ostium into the nose is superiorly placed, thereby failing to take advantage of gravity. These anatomic characteristics cause it to be the most commonly infected sinus. In community acquired sinusitis, the sinus may fill with fluid during a viral infection, such as the flu or common cold, and because the fluid is unable to drain, it becomes a good medium for bacterial growth. Bacterial sinusitis is most often a complication of a viral rhinosinusitis, but is also associated with allergies, dental infection, or fluid introduced into the sinuses by diving and swimming. Sinusitis may also develop when fluid is trapped in the sinuses by anatomic abnormalities such as a deviated septum, adenoidal hypertrophy, neoplasms, or a foreign body. Patients with cystic fibrosis have thick mucosa that is not easily expelled by the normal mucociliary clearance mechanism and are at increased risk for sinusitis.

As the infection develops, the sinuses become inflamed; sensations of pain and pressure become intense and are the common symptoms of a sinus infection. Pain may be referred to the upper incisor and canine teeth via the branches of the trigeminal nerve, which traverse the floor of the sinus.

Chronic sinusitis is thought to result from an acute sinus infection that has not completely resolved with antibiotic treatment because the sinuses have not drained completely. Patients with chronic sinusitis may have an anatomic abnormality that inhibits normal mucus clearance and thus may not be able to completely recover from a sinus infection.

CLINICAL PRESENTATION

Acute sinusitis is characterized by nasal congestion, pain, fever, and a yellow or green nasal discharge. Sensations of pain that may be present in the teeth and forehead are worse in the morning and when the patient bends forward from the waist. Acute frontal sinusitis usually causes pain and tenderness of the forehead. This pain can be elicited by palpation of the orbital roof just below the medial end of the eyebrow. Palpation here is more accurate than percussion of the supraorbital area.[2] An infection in the frontal sinuses produces pain and tenderness in the lower portion of the forehead and purulent drainage from the middle meatus of the nasal turbinates. Maxillary sinus infections produce pain and tenderness over the cheek area and may also cause erythema over the upper, lateral aspect of the check. The anterior ethmoid cells drain through the middle meatus, and the posterior cells drain through the superior meatus. Sphenoid sinusitis is rare but may cause pain behind the eyes or at the vertex, as well as facial pain. These sinuses drain through the superior meatus.

The common cold and allergic and vasomotor rhinitis are common antecedents to an acute sinus infection. A sore throat is common and may develop from the postnasal drip that is present with sinus infections. The drainage down the back of the throat may cause the sensation of material in the back of the pharynx, a need to swallow frequently to clear the throat, and a persistent cough when the patient is in a prone position. Gastrointestinal symptoms result from the swallowing of mucus.

Symptoms of chronic sinusitis may vary but typically will involve one or more symptoms of acute sinusitis. Nasal congestion, discharge, and a cough that lasts for more than 30 days are common. Severe pain and headache are not usually present in chronic sinusitis. The pain that is present is usually a dull ache or pressure across the forehead and/or midface. Nasal drainage may be thick and green or yellow. A constant postnasal drip and chronic cough are present. Chronic sinusitis is thought to be one of the primary causes of reactive airway disease. Worsening of asthma is not unusual and may be a result of the sinobronchial reflex, mouth breathing, and postnasal drip containing inflammatory chemicals from the sinuses.[3] The patient with chronic sinusitis may also experience an increase in allergic symptoms, including nocturnal asthma, allergic rhinitis, and eczema.[3] When a patient is in a prone position, sinusitis symptoms worsen, especially at night.

PHYSICAL EXAMINATION

The presence of fever and vital signs should first be determined. Then evaluation of the nasal tract for nasal turbinate edema and erythema, as well as discharge in the nasal cavity and in the area of the turbinates, is necessary. The patency of both nares should be determined, and the nose inspected for septal deviation and polyps; however, examining the nose with a nasal speculum is often inadequate in evaluating sinusitis. Transillumination of the sinuses may provide helpful information. If the sinuses can be transilluminated, they are not likely to contain fluid; inability to transilluminate the sinuses suggests the presence of fluid in the sinuses. However, this test must be done with care, as improper technique can result in a false reading. Examination of the eyes, noting periorbital swelling and the presence of allergic shiners (dark circles under the eyes) and erythema, should precede percussion of the frontal and maxillary sinuses for tenderness—all of which indicate that a sinus infection is present. The pharynx should be examined for postnasal drip, erythema, and lymphoid hypertrophy. Because otitis media commonly occurs with sinusitis, otic examination is extremely important. The sinuses drain into the nasopharynx, and bacteria found in this discharge are easily transported to the eustachian tube, where they ascend to the middle ear, creating a middle ear infection.

The teeth should be examined for caries, and the gingivae should be examined for inflammation. Approximately 5% to 10% of patients with maxillary sinus infections have dental root infection; therefore the maxillary teeth should be tapped to determine if the teeth are infected.[1]

DIAGNOSTICS

Acute sinusitis can be diagnosed empirically from the history and physical examination. Sinus x-ray studies may be indicated for refractory cases. However, with the advent of CT scanning, sinus x-ray studies are obtained infrequently. If they are done, anteroposterior, lateral, and occipitomental views are ordered to provide the information needed for diagnosis. CT and MRI are necessary if the diagnosis is difficult and more information is required. These tests are highly sensitive, but any upper respiratory infection can cause the CT scan to appear abnormal.[4]

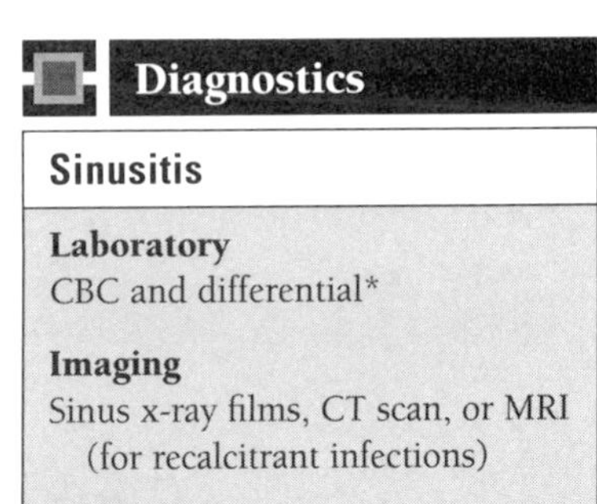
Diagnostics

Sinusitis

Laboratory
CBC and differential*

Imaging
Sinus x-ray films, CT scan, or MRI (for recalcitrant infections)

*If indicated.

DIFFERENTIAL DIAGNOSIS

Other possible explanations for facial pain include dental abscess, trigeminal neuralgia, optic neuritis, viral rhinosinusitis, and migraine headache. Chronic rhinitis may occur in syphilis, rhinosporidiosis, leishmaniasis, blastomycosis, and histoplasmosis. These are all conditions characterized by granuloma formation and destruction of soft tissue, cartilage, and bone. Mechanical obstruction and atrophic rhinitis can also present with the same symptoms as chronic sinusitis and should be included in the differential diagnosis.

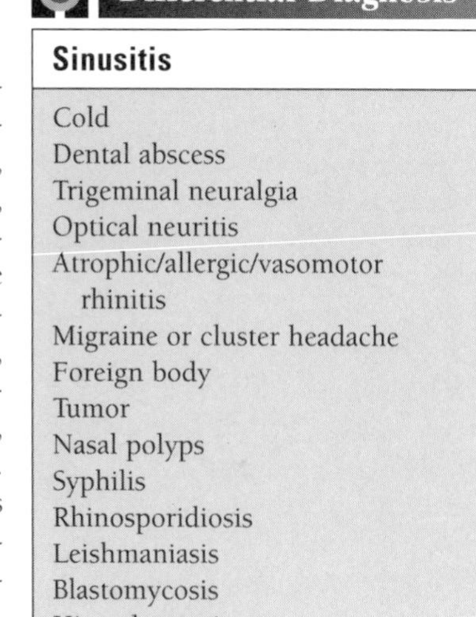
Differential Diagnosis

Sinusitis

Cold
Dental abscess
Trigeminal neuralgia
Optical neuritis
Atrophic/allergic/vasomotor rhinitis
Migraine or cluster headache
Foreign body
Tumor
Nasal polyps
Syphilis
Rhinosporidiosis
Leishmaniasis
Blastomycosis
Histoplasmosis

Dental Abscess

A dental abscess is an infection beside a tooth, usually near the root. The symptoms are localized or may radiate to the sinuses. An abscess is a collection of purulent material and is evidenced by inflammation, with fluctuation and pointing. Constitutional symptoms may be present. Fever, with chills and sweating, may progress to septicemia. If the abscess has been present for a long time, anemia may be present.

Trigeminal Neuralgia

Trigeminal neuralgia is degeneration of pressure on the trigeminal nerve, resulting in severe pain in and around that nerve. The pain is stabbing and radiates from the angle of the jaw along the branches of the nerve. Pain in the first branch presents as lightning-like sensations along the eye and back over the forehead; it resembles the pain of a sinus infection.

Optic Neuritis

Optic neuritis is an inflammation that causes hyperesthesia, paresthesia, dysesthesia, or paralysis. The pain that results from optic neuritis can resemble the pain of sinusitis.

Viral Rhinosinusitis

The common cold often involves the paranasal sinuses. The common cold is an acute, afebrile infection of the respiratory tract, with inflammation of the upper airway, including the nose, parasinuses, throat, larynx, and often both bronchi.

Migraine Headache

A paroxysmal disorder characterized by recurrent attacks of headache, migraine can occur with or without associated visual and gastrointestinal disorders. The mechanism is thought to be related to episodic reductions in systemic serotonin concentrations, which in turn lead to the observed vasomotor changes. There may or may not be an aura. The pain begins after the aura subsides and may be unilateral or generalized. Migraine headaches often resemble the headaches that are present with a sinus infection.

MANAGEMENT

Treatment of the rhinorrhea, sneezing, and coughing associated with viral rhinosinusitis consists of a first-generation antihistamine, nonsteroidal antiinflammatory drug (NSAID), and decongestant or cough suppressant.[5] Antibiotics are not recommended for viral rhinosinusitis in healthy adults.[6] If symptoms continue for more than a week or are accompanied by *unilateral* facial pain and purulent nasal secretions, antibiotic therapy and decongestants are recommended, as there is evidence that antibiotics are beneficial.[5-7] Amoxicillin 250 to 500 mg PO t.i.d. for 10 to 14 days is the drug of choice for the treatment of acute sinusitis in patients who are not allergic to penicillin.[2,7] Alternatives include trimethoprim-sulfamethoxazole 160 mg/800 mg (Bactrim DS 1 tablet b.i.d.), amoxicillin-clavulanate (Augmentin 250 to 500 mg t.i.d.), or ciprofloxacin (Cipro 250 to 750 mg b.i.d.). Patients who do not respond to the initial antibiotic treatment can be given a different antibiotic for a longer period or referred to an otolaryngologist.

Topical therapy to reduce obstruction and mucosa inflammation is helpful in reducing the symptoms associated with sinusitis. Saline solutions may be used to liquefy secretions. Decongestants such as oxymetazoline (Neo-Synephrine) may decrease nasal congestion and edema, promoting drainage. Nasal steroid preparations such as flunisolide (Nasalide 2 puffs in each nostril b.i.d.) are beneficial in decreasing nasal congestion and in the long-term management of rhinitis. Intranasal steroids in acute and chronic sinusitis have not been extensively studied, but symptomatic relief was documented in one study.[8]

Oral decongestants can decrease nasal congestion and facilitate drainage. Pseudoephedrine (Sudafed 30 to 120 mg b.i.d.; maximum adult dosage of 240 mg/day) is a major component of most oral decongestants and can be purchased over the counter.

COMPLICATIONS

In the antibiotic era it has become uncommon for sinusitis to become life threatening. However, a chronic infection may interfere with the quality of life, as chronic sinusitis can continue for extended periods, possibly for years. The cost in time, pain, expense, and emotional stress is significant. Chronic sinusitis is also associated with asthma and may be a cause of chronic asthma.

Osteomyelitis of the frontal bone is a potential complication. If osteomyelitis develops, fever, pain, and edema over the involved bone will be present. The edema is called Pott's puffy tumor.[9]

An orbital infection is also a possible complication of sinus infection because the orbit is surrounded on three sides by the paranasal sinuses. This complication occurs more often when the ethmoid sinuses are infected and the bacteria can extend through the lamina papyracea. The orbital infection may cause so much edema that the patient has difficulty with vision. Visual loss can also be a result of pressure on the optic nerve, which can cause a permanent loss of vision. In addition, if the optic nerve becomes infected, the infection can spread to the intracranial vault. Intracranial suppuration can develop, creating a brain abscess or meningitis. Patients with this condition are usually acutely ill and have an elevated temperature, severe headache, and symptoms of increased intracranial pressure.

Invasive fungal sinusitis is a rare, but potentially fatal complication of chronic sinusitis in patients with a co-morbid immunologic disorder such as malignancy, human immunodeficiency virus infection, diabetes, or drug-induced neutropenia.[10] Prompt recognition of the serious signs and symptoms (fever, facial pain, epistaxis, and cognitive or visual changes in an immunocompromised patient) associated with invasive fungal sinusitis is essential to prevent proliferation of the infection.[10] Invasive fungal sinusitis should not be confused with allergic fungal sinusitis, a benign but unremitting sinus infection more common in young people with asthma.[10]

INDICATIONS FOR REFERRAL/HOSPITALIZATION

The patient who is not symptom free after the second treatment with antibiotics should be referred to an otolaryngologist and/or allergist. If the patient has allergies, immunotherapy as indicated by skin testing may be necessary for patients with chronic recurrent sinusitis. Surgery may be indicated when the symptoms of sinusitis do not respond to medical therapy, if chronic pain is present, or if recurrent reactive airway disease develops. Endoscopic transnasal surgery has become more common and involves irrigation and suctioning of the sinuses. External approaches, such as the Caldwell-Luc operation, provide better visualization but can have severe complications such as optic nerve damage blindness. In addition, the bone may be perforated and meningitis may result.[11]

Immediate physician consultation is indicated for immunocompromised patients with suspected fungal sinusitis. Hospitalization for IV therapy with amphotericin B and surgical consultation for biopsy or debridement are imperative.[10]

Scuba divers with chronic sinusitis can experience sinus barotraumas. Usually, this condition is not serious, but these patients can be at risk for neurologic compromise. For this reason, scuba divers with chronic sinusitis should be evaluated by an otolaryngologist.[12]

PATIENT AND FAMILY EDUCATION/HEALTH PROMOTION

Patients should be aware that although the symptoms of an upper respiratory infection and sinusitis are similar, antibiotic therapy is not beneficial in viral rhinosinusitis.[13] However, upper respiratory infections that increase in severity, do not resolve after 7 to 10 days, and are accompanied by symptoms suggestive of bacterial sinusitis do require treatment. The patient treated for sinusitis should be instructed to return for further evaluation if the symptoms have not improved in 48 to 72 hours. In addition, the patient must be able to recognize complications such as periorbital swelling and know to contact the primary care provider immediately.

Patients with upper respiratory infections should understand the importance of blowing the nose gently to prevent the introduction of nasal fluid into the sinuses.[6] The patient should also know the signs and symptoms of viral respiratory infections and how to manage them with first-generation antihistamines, NSAIDs and, if indicated, a decongestant or cough suppressant so that sinusitis can be controlled or at least treated early in the disease.[6]

If allergic rhinitis is a precursor to sinusitis, environmental control should be stressed. Humidified air and increased fluid intake are important to relieve nasal discomfort and liquefy secretions. Warm, moist air in the form of steam inhalation or warm compresses may relieve the feeling of pressure and headache, and any activity that might introduce fluid into the sinuses, such as swimming or diving, should be avoided.

Smoking cessation is also strongly encouraged.

REFERENCES

1. DeFerranti SD and others: Are amoxicillin and folate inhibitors as effective as other antibiotics for acute sinusitis? A meta-analysis, *Br Med J* 317:632-637, 1998.
2. Jackler R, Kaplan M: Ear, nose and throat. In Tierney L, McPhee S, Papadakis M, editors: *Current medical diagnosis and treatment*, Stamford, Conn, 1997, Appleton & Lange.
3. Ticenor W: Sinusitis for physicians, 1997, Retrieved January 1997 from the World Wide Web: http://www.wtichenorpol.net.
4. Gwaltney JM Jr and others: Computerized tomographic study of the common cold, *N Engl J Med* 330:25, 1994.
5. Gwaltney JM: Acute sinusitis. Retrieved February 2002 from the World Wide Web: http://www.uptodate.com.
6. Hickner JM and others: Principles of appropriate antibiotic use for acute rhinosinusitis in adults: background, *Ann Internal Med* 134(6):498-505, 2001.
7. Glasziou P, DelMar C: Upper respiratory tract infection, *Clin Evidence* 6:1200-1207, 2001.
8. Meltzer EO and others: Added relief in the treatment of acute recurrent sinusitis with adjunctive mometasone furoate nasal spray. The Nasonex Sinusitis Group, *J Allergy Clin Immunol* 106:630-637, 2000.
9. Goroll AH, May LA, Mulley AG: *Primary care medicine*, ed 3, Philadelphia, 1995, JB Lippincott.
10. Cox GM, Perfect acute sinusitis. Retrieved February 2002 from the World Wide Web: http://www.uptodateonline.
11. Katz P: Wegener's granulomatosis. In Hurst J, editor: *Medicine for the practicing physician*, ed 4, Stamford, Conn, 1996, Appleton & Lange.
12. Parell GJ, Becker GD: Neurologic consequences of scuba diving with chronic sinusitis, *Laryngoscope* 110(8):1358-60, 2000.
13. Gonzales R and others: Principles of appropriate antibiotic use for treatment of acute respiratory tract infections in adults: background, specific aims, and methods, *Ann Emerg Med* 37(6):690-697, 2001.

CHAPTER 98
Smell and Taste Disturbances

Updated by Terry Mahan Buttaro

DEFINITION/EPIDEMIOLOGY

Disorders of smell and taste can be seriously debilitating to patients and are often diagnostic dilemmas for primary care providers. Olfactory dysfunction can be described as the loss of the sense of smell (anosmia), smell distortion (parosmia or dysosmia), or the diminished sense of smell (hyposmia). These dysfunctions can result from aging, tobacco, toxins, medications, endocrine disorders, nasal inflammation, infection, malnutrition, head or facial trauma, Parkinson's disease, Alzheimer's disease, CNS disturbances, or varied other conditions.

Taste disorders include diminished taste (hypogeusia), unpleasant taste (aliageusia or phantogeusia), and any persistent taste (dysgeusia). Ageusia or absent taste does occur, but is less common. Taste disorders are often related to olfactory dysfunction, but can also be associated with anesthesia, malignancies, head and neck irradiation, surgical procedures, kidney or gastric dysfunction, metabolic or hepatic disorders, or psychiatric disturbances.

PATHOPHYSIOLOGY

During the process of smelling, odorant molecules are taken in through the nose; these molecules must pass through the nasal cavity to reach the cribriform area and become soluble in the mucus that lies over the dendrites of the olfactory receptor cells.[1] The inability of odorant molecules to reach the receptor cells of the olfactory nerve (cranial nerve I) is the most common cause of olfactory dysfunction. Therefore anosmia or hyposmia can by caused by any disease process that prevents the odorant molecules from reaching these receptor cells, including polyps, septal deformities, rhinitis, and nasal tumors. The olfactory dysfunction can also be associated with epithelial cell changes and can be either transient or permanent depending on the cause of the dysfunction. Approximately 20% of the dysfunction is idiopathic, usually developing after a viral illness.[1] An absent, diminished, or distorted smell or taste can also be a sign of an endocrine disorder.

Any condition that causes the nasal mucus to be diminished, such as a drying of the nasal mucosa, can impair taste. Other conditions that can impair taste include heavy smoking, Sjögren's syndrome, radiation therapy of the head and neck, or peeling of the skin on the tongue. Ageusia also may result from disease of the chorda tympani or the gustatory fibers. Overuse of condiments and certain drugs can take away the sense of taste. Lesions involving sensory pathways to the taste centers of the brain, or diseases of the taste centers of the brain itself, can also interfere with the sense of taste.

CLINICAL PRESENTATION

Problems with taste and smell may or may not be associated with symptoms related to disorders that cause ageusia and anosmia. Most often, the presenting complaint is loss of taste or smell after an upper respiratory infection. In young adults the loss of smell often results from head trauma. If a patient has lost or experienced a decrease in the sense of smell, a thorough evaluation for intranasal and intracranial disease is required. A complete medical, occupational, smoking, and medication history is essential to diagnosis. Onset of symptoms (gradual versus acute) and associated symptoms should also be determined.

PHYSICAL EXAMINATION

The examination should confirm the patient's subjective complaint. Assessment for the loss of taste and smell focuses on the cranial nerves (CNs) that provide information about taste and smell. The olfactory nerve (CN I) is a sensory nerve. Testing of this nerve begins with asking the patient to identify odors that are nonirritating and aromatic, such as coffee, isopropyl alcohol, and toothpaste. After testing CN I, the nasopharynx should be inspected for abnormalities (e.g., polyps), crusting, amount of mucus present, and any signs of upper respiratory problems. The pharyngeal examination should determine presence of lesions, inflammation, or exudate.

The glossopharyngeal nerve (CN IX) is a mixed sensory/motor nerve. The sensory portion controls the taste sensation for the posterior third of the tongue. CN IX is tested along with the facial nerve (CN VII), which also is a mixed sensory/motor nerve. The sensory part of CN VII controls taste sensation for the anterior two thirds of the tongue. Each side of the tongue should be tested with sweet, salty, sour, and bitter flavors. The tongue should be protruded while the patient is identifying the taste, and the mouth should be rinsed before testing the other side. This process should be repeated with the posterior portion of the tongue.

After determining if the complaint is related to olfactory or taste dysfunction, a more comprehensive examination is necessary. Weight, vital signs, plus a conscientious ear, nose, throat, and neurologic evaluation are indicated.

DIAGNOSTICS

Assessment of odor and taste identification is an essential component of diagnostic testing for the loss of taste and smell. Both the University of Pennsylvania Smell Identification Test (UPSIT) and the Threshold, Discrimination, Identification Test (TDIT) can be used in the primary care setting and can help assess smell disorders.[2] If these tests are unavailable, the patient should be referred to a specialist for specific assessment of smell and taste dysfunction. Laboratory testing should include complete blood test, electrolytes, BUN, creatinine, LFTs, thyroid-stimulating hormone, antinuclear antibodies, and erythrocyte sedimentation rate. If Sjögren's syndrome is suspected antibodies to Ro/SSA and LA/SSB should be included.[2] An enhanced CT scan of the head or MRI may also be indicated to exclude neoplasms and unsuspected fractures of the floor of the cranial fossae. Further testing should be based on clinical presentation and physical findings.

DIFFERENTIAL DIAGNOSIS

The differential diagnosis for the loss of taste or smell includes disease processes that can affect the upper respiratory tract. The most common conditions are allergic and bacterial rhinitis, viral infections, head trauma, sinusitis, nasal polyps, and benign neoplasms. Anosmia can also be congenital or related to a meningioma, glioma, dementia, or aneurysm. Depression can be a cause of dysosmia. Aging, olfactory dysfunction, infection, radiation therapy, medications, malnutrition, Sjögren's syndrome, gastroesophageal reflux, endocrine disorders, trauma, cancer, and cancer therapy should be considered in the differential diagnosis of taste disorders.[3]

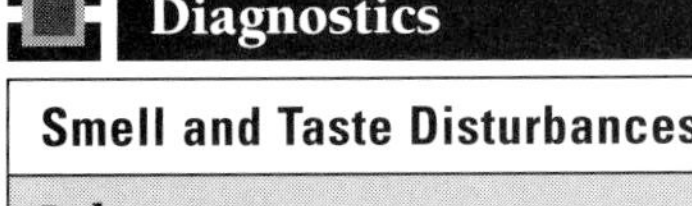

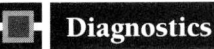

Smell and Taste Disturbances

Laboratory
CBC and differential
Electrolytes
Creatinine
LFTs
TSH
Antinuclear antibodies
Erythrocyte sedimentation rate
Ro/SSA and LA/SSB*

Imaging
CT scan or MRI

*If indicated.

MANAGEMENT AND INDICATIONS FOR REFERRAL/ HOSPITALIZATION

The cause of a disrupted sense of taste or smell should be identified. It is particularly important to distinguish between olfactory and taste disturbance. Treatment of rhinitis, sinusitis, infection, gastroesophageal reflux disease (GERD), or anemia may restore the lost function. The diet should be reviewed and the overuse of condiments eliminated. If possible, medications that may be associated with this disorder should be discontinued or changed. Zinc therapy has been effective for some patients with taste disorders associated with head and neck cancer, malnutrition, and some other disorders, but the benefit of zinc and vitamin therapy for the treatment of smell and taste disorders is unclear.[2,4,5]

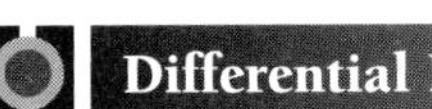

Smell and Taste Disturbances

Viral infection
Allergic/bacterial sinusitis
Nasal polyps
Benign neoplasms/tumors
Sjögren's syndrome
Endocrine disturbances
Trauma
Medications
Irradiation
Degenerative disorder
Sinusitis
GERD
Cancer
Malnutrition
Depression

If such measures are unsuccessful, the patient should be referred to an otolaryngologist for a comprehensive nose and throat examination. If smell and taste testing cannot be performed in the primary care setting, the patient should be referred to a specialist for diagnostic evaluation. Suspected central nervous system disorders or conditions that cause destruction of the neuroepithelium or its central pathway require referral to a neurologist. Patients whose symptoms are related to allergies may benefit from consultation with an allergist, whereas those with dental disorders require referral to a dentist.

COMPLICATIONS

Complications of smell and taste disorders include a permanent loss of smell or taste. The loss of taste and smell can indicate a serious problem such as a brain tumor or degenerative nerve disease. The loss of these senses profoundly affects quality of life and depression is a potential problem.[6] Patients may lose their appetite and lose weight. Olfactory dysfunction can also compromise safety

PATIENT AND FAMILY EDUCATION AND HEALTH PROMOTION

If the sensory loss is permanent, the patient should be instructed about using spices to season food. Patients who have lost the sense of smell should be counseled about smoke detectors and the use of electrical rather than gas appliances. The importance of continued personal hygiene and the avoidance of aggressively strong colognes should also be discussed.

REFERENCES

1. Hellerman D: Arthritis and musculoskeletal disorders. In Saunders C, Ho M, editors: *Current emergency diagnosis and treatment,* Stamford, Conn, 1997, Appleton & Lange.
2. Mann NM, Lafreniere D: Evaluation of taste and smell disorders. Retrieved February, 2002, from the World Wide Web: http://www.uptodate.com.
3. Johnson FM: Alterations in taste sensation: a case presentation of a patient with end-stage pancreatic cancer, *Cancer Nurs* 24(2):149-55, 2001.
4. Henkin RI and others: Efficacy of exogenous oral zinc in treatment of patients with carbonic anhydrase VI deficiency, *Am J Med Sci* 318(6):392-405, 1999.
5. Ripamonti C and others: A randomized, controlled clinical trial to evaluate the effects of zinc sulfate on cancer patients with taste alterations caused by head and neck irradiation, *Cancer* 82(10):1938-1945, 1998.
6. Miwa T and others: Impact of olfactory impairment on quality of life and disability, *Arch Otolaryngol Head Neck Surg* 127(5):497-503, 2001.

CHAPTER 99

Tumors and Polyps of the Nose

Updated by Terry Mahan Buttaro

Nasal Tumors and Polyps

DEFINITION/EPIDEMIOLOGY

Primary sites for malignant tumors can occur in the nose, nasopharynx, and paranasal sinuses. The broad spectrum of malignant lesions that occur in the nose and paranasal sinuses include carcinomas, lymphomas, sarcomas, and melanomas. The most common, however, is squamous cell carcinoma.

The most common type of benign tumor is an inverted papilloma, which arises from the common wall between the nose and maxillary sinuses. A highly vascular benign tumor, the juvenile angiofibroma, is common in adolescent males, bleeds easily, and can cause nasal obstruction. These tumors are nonmalignant, but they can cause considerable problems as they spread through the nasopharynx.[1]

Nasal polyps represent an inflammatory disorder of the nose and paranasal sinuses that can result in chronic nasal obstruction and a diminished sense of smell. The etiology of these pale, edematous masses is unknown, but the lesions are commonly seen in patients with allergic rhinitis, which predisposes polyp formation, as well as in acute and chronic infections. The presence of polyps in children may indicate the possibility of cystic fibrosis.

PATHOPHYSIOLOGY

The pathophysiology of benign and malignant tumors of the nasopharynx is varied and makes diagnosis difficult. However, a basic understanding of the different pathologies can assist in diagnosis. Squamous cell carcinomas arise from the malpighian cells (the stratum germinativum and stratum spinosum layer) of the epithelium. This cancer develops in normal skin, in preexisting actinic keratosis, or in a patch of leukoplakia. The incidence is higher in men and is associated with smoking and heavy alcohol consumption. The inverted cell papillomas develop from the squamous cells in which the epithelium is invaginated into the vascular connective tissue stroma. They are invasive and behave in a locally malignant manner. Juvenile angiofibromas are vascular and may actually hemorrhage. They also act in a locally malignant manner. They spread from the nasopharynx to the nasal cavity, the sphenoid, and the parasinuses and may extend extradurally. Nasal polyps form at the site of massive dependent edema in the lamina propria of the mucous membrane, usually around the ostia of the maxillary sinuses.

CLINICAL PRESENTATION

Malignant tumors can occur in the nose, nasopharynx, and paranasal sinuses. Generally, these malignancies remain asymptomatic until late in their course. Early symptoms are nonspecific, mimicking those of rhinitis or sinusitis. Unilateral nasal obstruction and discharge accompanied by pain, recurrent hemorrhage, headache, or visual or olfactory changes suggest the presence of cancer. For this reason, any patient with unilateral or persistent nasal symptoms requires thorough evaluation.

Benign nasal tumors are associated with nasal obstruction, discharge, or facial swelling. These tumors can bleed easily and cause recurrent epistaxis. The tumor is usually easily visualized because of its growth and spread.

Symptoms of nasal polyps include nasal obstruction, hyposmia or anosmia, recurrent sinusitis, headache, and postnasal drip. In some patients, nasal polyps are accompanied by intrinsic asthma and intolerance to acetylsalicylic acid.[1] A developing polyp is teardrop shaped; when mature, it resembles a peeled seedless grape.

PHYSICAL EXAMINATION

A complete examination of the head and nasopharynx is essential. The vestibules should be inspected with a penlight while the patient's head is tipped back. Each naris should be examined, checking for erythema, edema, discharge, bleeding, or tumor. Further examination includes pharyngeal inspection and determination of lymph node involvement.

DIAGNOSTICS

Diagnostic testing for benign tumors and nasal polyps can include sinus x-ray studies for information about fluid levels and bone involvement, but CT scan or MRI is usually indicated if tumor is suspected. Endoscopic evaluation and biopsy are necessary for definitive diagnosis and treatment of suspected tumors. Complete blood studies are necessary to determine the presence of anemia or other hematologic disease.

DIFFERENTIAL DIAGNOSIS

The differential diagnosis for tumors and polyps includes mucoceles, granulomas without systemic involvement, and Wegener's granulomatosis, a systemic vasculitis of unknown etiology, associated with granulomatous changes. Wegener's granulomatosis is associated with glomerulonephritis, as well as granulomatous lesions in the upper and lower respiratory tract. Other organ systems can also be affected.

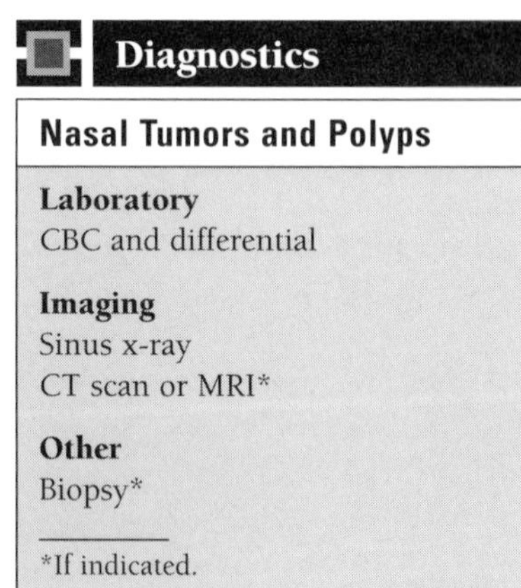

Diagnostics

Nasal Tumors and Polyps

Laboratory
CBC and differential

Imaging
Sinus x-ray
CT scan or MRI*

Other
Biopsy*

*If indicated.

MANAGEMENT AND INDICATIONS FOR REFERRAL/HOSPITALIZATION

The successful treatment of small polyps involves the use of nasal steroid sprays. A short course of oral corticosteroid (e.g.,

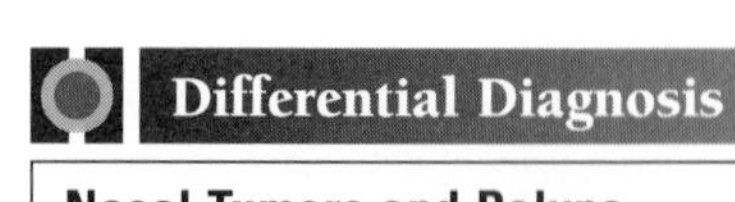

Differential Diagnosis

Nasal Tumors and Polyps

Benign/malignant polyps
Wegener's granulomatosis

prednisone, 6-day course of twenty-one 5-mg tablets: 30 mg on the first day and tapering by 5 mg each day) may also be therapeutic. When medical management is unsuccessful, evaluation by an otorhinolaryngologist is necessary. Polyps often will require surgical removal. Benign and malignant tumors should be surgically excised; benign tumors can be removed endoscopically, but malignant tumors require a large surgical excision. If the tumor is malignant, chemotherapy and/or radiation therapy may be indicated. Patients with suspected Wegener's granulomatosis require specialist referral.

COMPLICATIONS

Complications of benign tumors and polyps include chronic nasal obstruction and/or olfactory dysfunction. Patients may have frequent recurrence of the tumors or polyps, requiring frequent need for surgical procedures. A cancerous tumor may be terminal despite extensive therapy.

PATIENT AND FAMILY EDUCATION

Patients with benign or malignant tumors need to understand the importance of therapy. The patient should be aware of the signs and symptoms of complications or disease recurrence and the importance of continued follow-up monitoring.

Wegener's Granulomatosis

DEFINITION/EPIDEMIOLOGY

Wegener's granulomatosis is a vasculitis characterized by glomerulonephritis plus granulomas of the nose and lung. The most destructive lesions of bone, cartilage, and soft tissue of the nose and paranasal sinuses are ultimately found on biopsy to be malignant neoplasms, such as lymphomas or carcinomas. The etiology of this rare disorder is unknown. Without treatment Wegener's granulomatosis is invariably fatal; most patients survive less than a year after diagnosis.[2] However, the prognosis is good if the disease is diagnosed and treated early. The disease usually occurs in those older than 40 years, with equal frequency in men and women. The skin, eyes, heart, and gastrointestinal, nervous, and musculoskeletal systems can also be affected.

PATHOPHYSIOLOGY

A necrotizing vasculitis associated with autoimmunity, Wegener's granulomatosis is one of the many autoimmune diseases that occur when the immune system reacts against self-antigens and destroys host tissue. The body has a hypersensitive response; inflammation results and causes the destruction of healthy tissue. In this disease the probable self-antigen is unknown. The hypersensitivity results in chronic inflammation and causes the formation of a granuloma, a dense infiltration of lymphocytes and macrophages. If the macrophages cannot protect the body against tissue damage, the body attempts to wall off the infected site and a granuloma is formed.[3] In the vasculitis of Wegener's granulomatosis, immune complex is deposited in the blood vessel walls. Complement is activated, resulting in direct cellular injury and a decrease in the circulating levels of the complement components.[4] Once the process begins, the disorder usually develops over 4 to 12 months.[2]

CLINICAL PRESENTATION

Most patients with this condition present with respiratory tract symptoms such as nasal congestion, nasal ulcerations, rhinitis, sinusitis, otitis media, otorrhea, hearing loss, gingival hypertrophy, cough, dyspnea, or hemoptysis.[2] Fever, weakness, malaise, weight loss, conjunctivitis, rashes or skin lesions, and polyarthralgias are other common complaints. The lungs are affected in 40% of newly diagnosed patients.[2] As the disease progresses, the percentage of lung involvement progresses, eventually reaching 80%, but patients with pulmonary involvement can be asymptomatic.[2] Renal disease is rarely apparent on initial presentation, although hematuria, red blood cell casts, and impaired renal function suggest renal involvement.[5]

PHYSICAL EXAMINATION

Physical findings may be absent initially despite numerous subjective complaints. If physical signs are present, they are usually associated with the upper respiratory airway and include nasal congestion and crusting, rhinorrhea, ulceration of the nasal septum, and epistaxis. The destruction of the nasal septum that results in saddle nose deformity, a characteristic sign of Wegener's granulomatosis, occurs late in the disease process. Infrequently there may be erosions through the skin that cover the nose and sinuses.[5] If there is pulmonary involvement, localized rales, rhonchi, and wheezing can be heard during auscultation. Other physical findings include unilateral proptosis, red eye, otitis media, symmetric polyarticular arthritis, and purpura.

DIAGNOSTICS

Routine laboratory studies add little to the diagnosis of Wegener's granulomatosis. Most patients will have normocytic, normochromic anemia; leukocytosis; thrombocytosis; and elevated erythrocyte sedimentation rate. A urinalysis, plus BUN and creatinine, should be obtained to assess renal involvement.

A chest x-ray study is necessary to determine the presence of infiltrates, nodules, masses, and cavities, as well as sarcoidosis, tumor, or infection. Sinus x-ray studies may also be indicated to determine if sinusitis or sinus destruction is present.

Most patients with Wegener's granulomatosis test positive for circulating antineutrophil cytoplasmic antibodies (cANCA), which are commonly found in this disorder.[2] Although a positive cANCA suggests Wegener's granulomatosis, tissue biopsy of a suspicious lesion confirms diagnosis. Lung biopsy is preferred, although other sites can be used. The biopsy site depends on the severity of the illness,

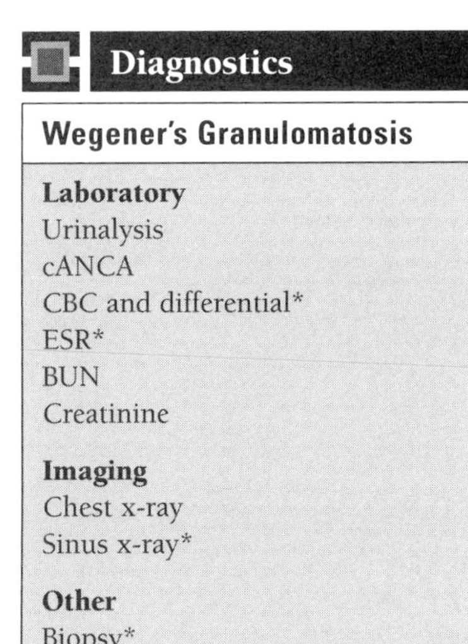

Diagnostics

Wegener's Granulomatosis

Laboratory
Urinalysis
cANCA
CBC and differential*
ESR*
BUN
Creatinine

Imaging
Chest x-ray
Sinus x-ray*

Other
Biopsy*

*If indicated.

the risks of the surgical procedure, and the organ system involved.

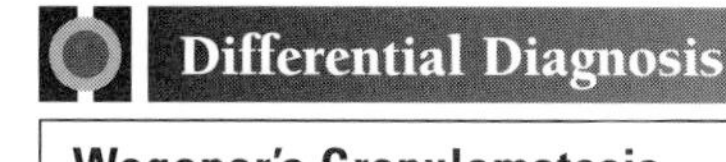

Wegener's Granulomatosis

Goodpasture's syndrome
Churg-Strauss vasculitis
Systemic lupus erythematosus
Vasculitic disorders
Rheumatic disorders

DIFFERENTIAL DIAGNOSIS

The differential diagnosis for Wegener's granulomatosis includes other pulmonary-renal syndromes such as Goodpasture's syndrome, Churg-Strauss vasculitis, and systemic lupus erythematosus. Other vasculitides and rheumatic disorders should also be considered.

MANAGEMENT AND INDICATIONS FOR REFERRAL/HOSPITALIZATION

A patient suspected of having Wegener's granulomatosis should be referred to a specialist as soon as the disease is suspected. In general, most patients will be hospitalized for diagnosis and the initiation of treatment. Currently, it is recommended that Wegener's granulomatosis be treated with immunosuppressive cytotoxic drugs such as cyclophosphamide (Cytoxan).[5] In most patients, therapy is started at a dose of 1 to 2 mg/kg per day PO as a single dose. A response to this drug occurs within 2 weeks, and remission can be induced in up to 75% of patients[2]; however, most patients have relapses of the disease. Prednisone 1 mg/kg per day reduces the vascular edema and is given concurrently. After 2 or 3 weeks, the steroids are slowly reduced to a maintenance dose and in some cases may be discontinued after 4 months.[6] The cyclophosphamide is given for at least 1 full year and then is reduced by 25 mg every 2 to 3 months.[5] Treatment may differ for patients who have more critical pulmonary or kidney involvement and, in some instances, other drug regimens may be indicated.[6]

The most serious side effect of cyclophosphamide is leukopenia; therefore the blood count needs to be checked on a routine basis. It is recommended that patients with Wegener's granulomatosis who are being treated with cyclophosphamide drink 1 to 2 quarts of liquid per day and empty the bladder frequently because of the risk of bladder cancer from the medication.

COMPLICATIONS

The complication for this disease is the inability to create a remission. If the patient does not receive early treatment, the disease is generally fatal. Once proteinuria or hematuria develops, progression to renal failure can be rapid.[2] Morbidity may result from the disease or be related to toxicity from the treatment.

Pneumocystis carinii pneumonia is a potential treatment complication necessitating prophylactic therapy with trimethoprim-sulfamethoxazole.[6]

PATIENT AND FAMILY EDUCATION

Patients need to understand the necessity of adherence to therapy and the need for frequent follow-up evaluation. Medication and side effects must be explained and understood. These patients should also be able to recognize the signs of renal, pulmonary, and other complications. In particular, they should be alert to the recurrence of nasal discharge, sinusitis, fever, and pulmonary changes.

REFERENCES

1. Jackler R, Kaplan M: Ear, nose and throat. In Tierney L, McPhee S, Papadakis M, editors: *Current medical diagnosis and treatment 1997*, Stamford, Conn, 1997, Appleton & Lange.
2. Hellermann D: Arthritis and musculoskeletal disorders. In Saunders C, Ho M, editors: *Current emergency diagnosis and treatment*, Stamford, Conn, 1997, Appleton & Lange.
3. McCance K, Huether S: *Pathophysiology: the biological basis for disease in adults and children*, ed 3, St Louis, 1998, Mosby.
4. Puett D, Sergent B: Vasculitis. In Noble J, editor: *Textbook of primary care medicine*, ed 2, St Louis, 1996, Mosby.
5. Katz P: Wegener's granulomatosis. In Hurst J, editor: *Medicine for the practicing physician*, ed 4, Stamford, Conn, 1996, Appleton & Lange.
6. Rose BD and others: Treatment of Wegener's granulomatosis and microscopic polyangiitis. Retrieved October 2002 from the World Wide Web: http://www.uptodate.com.

PART 9

Evaluation and Management of Oropharynx Disorders

JOANN TRYBULSKI, Section Editor

CHAPTER 100

Dental Abscess

Debra S. Munsell

DEFINITION/EPIDEMIOLOGY

Infection of the periapical tissue is commonly known as a dental abscess. These infections are often encountered in the general population and may resolve spontaneously.[1] However, they can cause chronic infections or life-threatening complications.

PATHOPHYSIOLOGY

Poor dental hygiene is a cause of dental abscesses. These abscesses arise as a result of infection by normal oral flora in a carious tooth or as a result of traumatized gingival mucosa.[1] Dental abscesses begin with necrosis of the tooth pulp, leading to bacterial invasion of the pulp chamber and deeper tissues. Deep cavities (caries) cause necrosis by initiating vasodilation and edema, which lead to pressure and pain in the rigid walls of the tooth. This pressure cuts off the circulation to the pulp, and the infection can invade the surrounding bone.

Multiple organisms are usually found in abscesses, sometimes as many as 5 to 10. Initially, aerobic bacteria invade the necrotic pulp and create a hypoxic climate that favors the growth of anaerobic bacteria.

CLINICAL PRESENTATION

Abscesses usually occur in the setting of carious teeth or poor dental hygiene and cause pain, localized edema, and purulent discharge from the affected site. The tooth may be partially elevated out of the socket. The pain responds poorly to analgesic agents. If the abscess is minor, systemic signs may not be evident. More advanced infections may by associated with fever and lymphadenitis.

PHYSICAL EXAMINATION

Inspection of the gingiva surrounding the area of pain will reveal edema and erythema of the soft tissues, and possibly a purulent discharge from a draining sinus tract. If progression of the infection has occurred beyond the local area, orbital cellulitis, retropharyngeal space involvement, fascial plane invasion, or cavernous sinus thrombosis can occur.

DIAGNOSTICS

Physical examination remains the standard of diagnosis for a dental or periapical abscess. Routine radiologic screening is not recommended, as thickening of the periodontal membrane is the only finding visible before abscess formation, and abscesses develop rapidly. Chronic abscesses may reveal a radiolucent area at the tooth apex. A CBC may be indicated if cellulitis is suspected. Other diagnostics are dependent on complications.

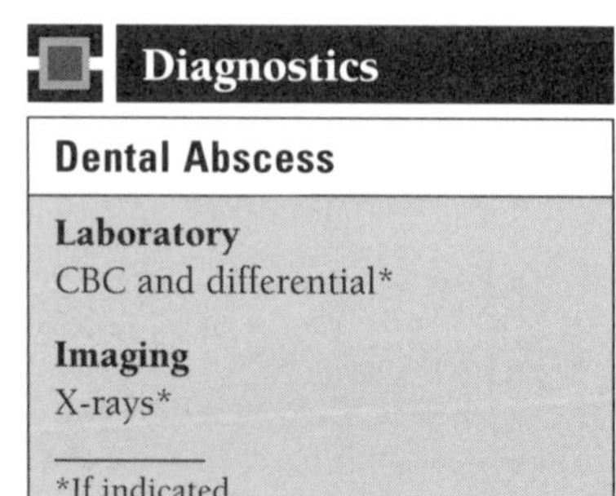

Diagnostics

Dental Abscess

Laboratory
CBC and differential*

Imaging
X-rays*

*If indicated.

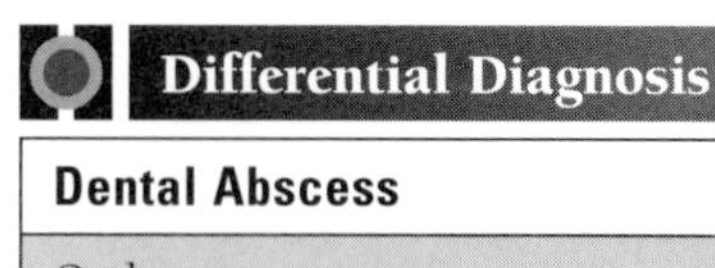

Differential Diagnosis

Dental Abscess

Oral cancer

DIFFERENTIAL DIAGNOSIS

All oral lesions must be evaluated for potential malignancy. If there is doubt about the lesion, a biopsy is necessary to exclude malignant disease, especially in populations predisposed to oral cavity cancer.

MANAGEMENT

Management of a periapical abscess is primarily surgical. Dental extraction allows for the release of pressure and drainage of the abscess. Alternatively, many abscessed teeth are candidates for root canal therapy. Antibiotic coverage for both aerobic and anaerobic bacteria enhances infection resolution. Oral antibiotic therapy includes the following antibiotics: penicillin, clindamycin, and metronidazole. Metronidazole may be used in combination with penicillin but not alone. Amoxicillin with clavulanic acid is an alternative to penicillin. For those patients who cannot take these antibiotics, erythromycin, cephalexin, sulfa, quinolone, and tetracycline are not as effective but may be used. If indicated, parenteral antibiotic therapy with penicillin, clindamycin, and metronidazole should be used. Cefazolin and cefoxitin are less effective. Gentamycin, chloramphenicol, tobramycin, amikacin, or any third-generation cephalosporins are not recommended because they fail to provide adequate protection, have adverse complications (chloramphenicol), are very expensive, or are more broad spectrum than necessary.[1]

Empiric therapy is usually indicated. Culture of the purulent discharge can result in a more specific bacterial diagnosis, and appropriate therapy can then be implemented. Analgesic therapy is instituted as an adjunct to antibiotic and surgical treatment.

COMPLICATIONS

Complications arising from dental abscesses can range from minor to life threatening. Minor complications include the need for antibiotic therapy and/or dental extraction or endodontic work (i.e., root canal). Major complications can include orbital cellulitis, fascial plane infections, osteomyelitis, cavernous sinus thrombosis, and bacteremia with sepsis.[1] Up to 30% of deep neck space infections may be caused by dental abscesses.[1] In addition, the life-threatening complication of Ludwig's angina is a possibility. This infection of the deep mandibular space presents with trismus, drooling, induration of the tongue and submandibular area, tachypnea, and dyspnea. Airway compromise can occur.

INDICATIONS FOR REFERRAL/HOSPITALIZATION

Dental abscesses are co-managed with dentists or endodontists to ensure adequate resolution of the initial infection, prevent complications, and institute preventive treatment. When signs and symptoms of bacteremia, orbital cellulitis, cavernous sinus thrombosis, or fascial plane involvement are present, prompt hospitalization and team management with a dentist or endodontist and an infectious disease consultant are indicated. Other indications for hospitalization include edema and erythema of the eyelids, exophthalmos, and conjunctival edema. Deep neck space infection is also an indication for hospitalization.

PATIENT AND FAMILY EDUCATION/HEALTH PROMOTION

Early and proper dental care prevents most dental infections. Daily brushing, flossing, and appropriate dental hygiene are stressed. Early care of carious teeth can prevent future dental infections. Older adults and those with valvular disorders are strongly encouraged to practice good dental hygiene with early repair of carious teeth and prompt treatment of abscesses to prevent complications. The role of dental and gingival infection in myocardial infarction is an area of investigation.

REFERENCES

1. Cummings CW and others: *Otolaryngology-head and neck surgery*, ed 3, St Louis, 1998, Mosby.

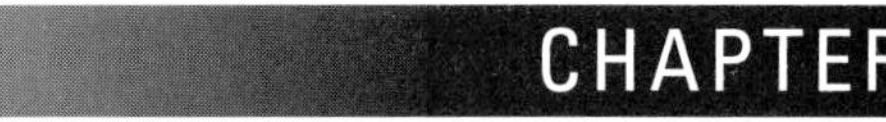

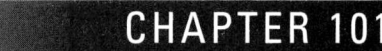

CHAPTER 101

Diseases of the Salivary Glands

Debra S. Munsell

DEFINITION/EPIDEMIOLOGY

The salivary glands comprise the paired parotid glands, the submandibular and sublingual glands, and the numerous minor salivary glands found in the upper aerodigestive tract. Diseases that affect the salivary glands are divided into neoplastic and nonneoplastic categories. The nonneoplastic category is further divided into infectious and noninfectious origins; neoplastic diseases can be either benign or malignant. Acute suppurative sialadenitis is covered in Chapter 104.

Salivary gland infections can be found in all age ranges and populations. Malignant neoplasms that involve the salivary glands account for approximately 5% of all head and neck tumors, not including skin cancers. The distribution of salivary tumors among men and women is virtually equal, with 1.2 per 100,000 for men and 0.7 per 100,000 for women. Warthin's tumor, a benign neoplasm, is more common in men than women. Salivary tumors in older adults most commonly affect the parotid glands. Several studies have identified an increased incidence of breast cancer in patients who have had mucoepidermoid carcinoma of the salivary glands, and an increase in minor salivary gland adenocarcinoma has been associated with occupational exposure to furniture, woodworking, and boot and shoe manufacturing.[1]

PATHOPHYSIOLOGY

Several disease entities are considered in the category of noninfectious salivary gland disease, including recurrent parotitis, sialolithiasis (salivary gland stones), branchial cleft anomalies, Sjögren's syndrome, xerostomia, ptyalism, sialosis, and the benign epithelial lesion of Godwin. Sialectasis, either acquired or congenital, can lead to recurrent parotitis. This dilation of the gland can be produced either by stone formation or strictures. Sialolithiasis, which mainly affects the submandibular glands, refers to the formation of stones or calculi in the glands. These stones are predominantly hydroxyapatite, and there may be more than one.[1] First branchial cleft anomalies also affect the salivary glands, primarily the paired parotid glands. Sinus tracts and cysts associated with these anomalies can affect the facial nerve.

Sjögren's syndrome is an autoimmune disorder that affects the salivary glands. On pathologic evaluation, a lymphocytic infiltrate with acinar atrophy, ductal epithelial hyperplasia, and metaplasia can be found. Benign lymphoepithelial lesion of Godwin is an inflammatory condition often found in association with human immunodeficiency virus (HIV) infection. It can be confused pathologically with malignant lymphoma, metastatic carcinoma, sarcoidosis, or chronic sialoadenitis.[2]

Xerostomia is a term used to describe a dry mouth. Several diseases, as well as radiation therapy and drug therapy, can cause these symptoms. The production of excess saliva is called ptyalism; drug treatments and other medical conditions are the underlying causes. *Sialosis* is a term used to refer to bilaterally recurring salivary gland edema. Acinar cell hypertrophy, interstitial edema, and striated duct atrophy may be present on pathologic examination. Metabolic disorders such as diabetes, alcoholism, and various vitamin deficiencies can also initiate enlargement of the salivary gland. Certain drugs, including the phenothiazines, thioureas, and iodine, can cause salivary gland enlargement as a result of their cholinergic effects.

Infectious diseases that affect the salivary glands include parotitis, viral infections, syphilis, HIV, and granulomatous diseases. Granulomatous diseases include tuberculosis, sarcoidosis, and actinomycosis.

Neoplastic changes also affect the salivary glands; 80% of salivary gland tumors involve the paired parotid glands.[3] Benign tumors that involve the salivary glands include pleomorphic adenoma, monomorphic adenoma, Warthin's tumor, and oncocytoma.

Malignant tumors of the salivary glands are more likely to be found in the minor salivary glands.[1] Parotid malignant tumors account for approximately one third of the malignant tumors of the salivary glands. These malignancies include mucoepidermoid carcinomas, acinic cell carcinomas, adenocarcinomas, and adenoid cystic, malignant mixed, and squamous cell carcinomas.[1] Mucoepidermoid carcinomas are the most common cancers of the major salivary glands and are most commonly seen in the parotid gland.[4]

CLINICAL PRESENTATION

The noninfectious entities that cause enlargement of the salivary gland usually present as a painless swelling of the salivary gland. One exception is sialolithiasis, or stones in the gland, which is evidenced by painful edema of the affected gland and increased symptoms with meals. Sjögren's syndrome, associated with connective tissue diseases such as rheumatoid arthritis, polyarteritis nodosa, and systemic lupus erythematosus, presents with the classic xerostomia, abnormal taste, keratoconjunctivitis sicca, dry tongue, and intermittent unilateral or bilateral swelling of the salivary gland. Bilateral salivary gland cysts characterize the benign lymphoepithelial lesion of Godwin, whereas a lack of saliva or excess salivary gland production is associated with xerostomia and ptyalism. Infectious diseases of the salivary glands usually cause a rapid onset of colicky pain with meals, edema, indurations of the affected gland, malaise, and chills.[2]

Benign and malignant processes of the salivary gland present as painless, unilateral masses. They may be cystic in nature, such as with Warthin's tumor. A prior history of radiation may be elicited. A small number of patients may complain of pain, and a few may present with facial nerve paralysis or palsy.[1] Squamous cell carcinoma and malignant mixed tumors have a history of rapid growth and may present with facial pain and fixation of underlying structures. The salivary glands may also be the sites of metastatic spread of other malignancies of the head and neck, most commonly squamous cell carcinoma and malignant melanoma, with the primary sites above the clavicles.[4] Primary malignant lymphomas have been reported but are rare.

PHYSICAL EXAMINATION

Nonneoplastic, noninfectious diseases of the salivary glands involve unilateral or bilateral swelling of the affected gland. In the case of sialolithiasis, a stone may be palpated in the corresponding duct. With Sjögren's syndrome, xerostomia and keratoconjunctivitis accompany unilateral or bilateral swelling of the salivary gland. Bilateral cystic masses may be palpated with a benign lymphoepithelial lesion of Godwin. Sialosis presents as a bilateral, recurrent swelling of the affected glands.

Infectious diseases of the salivary gland will demonstrate inflammation, edema, and bilateral or unilateral involvement of the gland. Purulent discharge is present in acute bacterial infections. With a localized parotid abscess, pitting edema may be found. In viral infections such as mumps parotitis, a bilaterally and painfully enlarged gland and difficulty in opening the jaws may be encountered.

Neoplastic diseases are usually distinguished by painless, firm masses that may be fast or slow growing. Late presentation produces paralysis of the facial nerve, fixation of underlying structures and, possibly, skin involvement.

DIAGNOSTICS

Evaluation of salivary gland disease relies heavily on the patient's history and physical examination. A culture of purulent discharge from the affected duct may be performed if infectious entities are suspected. Fine-needle aspiration of the affected gland may be beneficial in diagnosing infectious agents, such as bacterial and granulomatous diseases. Systemic evaluation of serum may be indicated to establish a diagnosis of HIV infection, mycobacterial disease, toxoplasmosis, and tularemia.[2] Skin testing may be useful in the diagnosis of tuberculosis and cat-scratch disease.

Viral titers may be done if viral infectious etiologies are suspected. Antibodies to the S and V antigen greater than 1:192 are expected. A CT scan or ultrasonographic evaluations of the glands may be used if neoplastic disease is suspected. Sialography in conjunction with plain-tissue films is used to diagnose sialolithiasis.

DIFFERENTIAL DIAGNOSIS

The differential diagnosis of noninfectious, nonneoplastic salivary gland disease includes drug therapy, sialolithiasis, branchial cleft anomalies, Sjögren's syndrome, xerostomia, ptyalism, and metabolic disorders such as diabetes. Infectious etiologies that can affect the salivary gland are numerous and include HIV infection; viral infections such as mumps, paramyxovirus, and Epstein-Barr virus; bacterial

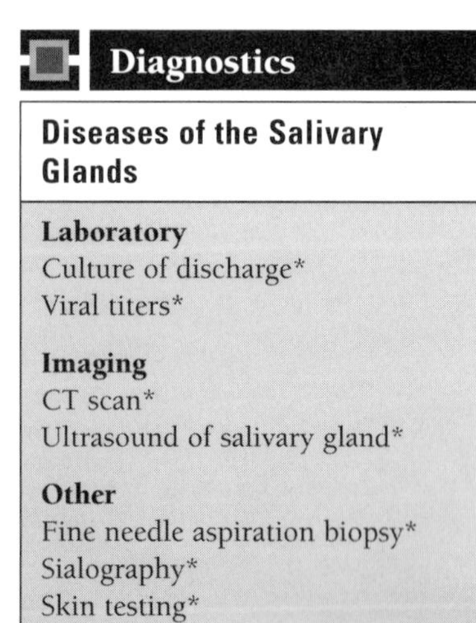
Diagnostics

Diseases of the Salivary Glands

Laboratory
Culture of discharge*
Viral titers*

Imaging
CT scan*
Ultrasound of salivary gland*

Other
Fine needle aspiration biopsy*
Sialography*
Skin testing*

*If indicated.

infections, including *Staphylococcus aureus* and *Streptococcus* organisms, tuberculosis, tularemia, actinomycosis, and cat-scratch disease; and parasitic diseases such as toxoplasmosis.[2]

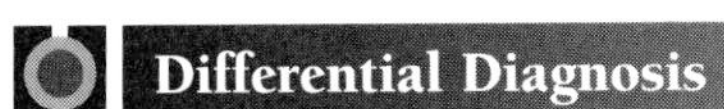

Diseases of the Salivary Glands

Infections (bacterial, viral, granulomatous, parasitic)
Drug therapy
Branchial cleft anomalies
Sjögren's syndrome
Benign/malignant tumors
Sialolithiasis
Xerostoma
Ptyalism
Metabolic disorders (diabetes)

Neoplastic involvement of the salivary glands includes both benign and malignant disease. Included in the differential for benign lesions are pleomorphic adenoma, Warthin's tumor, monomorphic adenoma, and oncocytoma. Malignant tumors that can affect the salivary glands include mucoepidermoid carcinoma, acinic cell carcinoma, adenocarcinoma, adenoid cystic carcinoma, malignant mixed tumors, and squamous cell carcinoma. The salivary glands can also be the site of metastatic disease to the head and neck. Included in these metastatic tumors are malignant melanoma, squamous cell carcinoma, and lymphoma. Primary malignant lymphoma of the salivary glands has been reported but is rare.[1]

MANAGEMENT

Management of many noninfectious diseases of the salivary gland is conservative. Recurrent parotitis may be treated with surgical removal of the affected gland if the patient remains symptomatic. Sialolithiasis can be managed with warm compresses, analgesics, and sialagogues. Sialagogues are agents that stimulate the production and flow of saliva, such as lemon balls and chewing gum. Fluid and electrolyte replacement should be addressed. Surgical removal of the offending stone may be required. Branchial cleft anomalies are treated with surgical excision. Sjögren's syndrome is treated symptomatically with local and systemic therapy to address the xerostomia and xerophthalmia. Ptyalism may require surgical intervention.

Management of infectious diseases of the salivary glands depends on the etiology of the disease. Management of acute suppurative parotitis is discussed in Chapter 104. Viral infection of the salivary glands, most commonly caused by the mumps paramyxovirus, requires conservative therapy that consists of adequate hydration, rest and, possibly, diet modification. Hospitalization and consultation with infectious disease specialists may be necessary if infection progresses to involve other organs or structures. Infections that are suspected to be HIV infection should be evaluated by an HIV specialist; surgical intervention should be undertaken to evaluate appropriately for possible lymphoma, which has been associated with HIV salivary gland enlargement. Granulomatous infection of the salivary glands should be treated with the appropriate agents. Tubercular infections and nontubercular mycobacterial infections may require surgical removal because these infections may not respond to traditional therapies. Mild actinomycosis can be treated with penicillin VK 500 to 1000 mg PO q.i.d. for two months.[5] Clindamycin or erythromycin can be substituted if the patient is allergic to penicillin.[5] Cat-scratch disease can be treated symptomatically, without antibiotic therapy. Toxoplasmosis infections can be treated with combination therapy that consists of pyrimethamine and trisulfapyrimidines, although in most cases this regimen is reserved for those with systemic disease and for those who are immunocompromised or pregnant.[2] Parenteral antibiotics, such as the aminoglycosides streptomycin or gentamycin, can be used for tularemia. Tetracycline has also been used for tularemia, but with mixed results.

Suspected benign or malignant salivary gland masses are managed surgically. With surgery of the parotid gland, preservation of the facial nerve is critical unless the nerve is already nonfunctional or has tumor involvement. A superficial parotidectomy is the surgical procedure of choice. Some surgeons propose that both the deep and superficial lobes of the parotid gland be treated with a total parotidectomy. Tumors of the minor salivary glands are treated with surgical excision. The extent of the procedure is dictated by the tumor site and the disease. Radiation therapy as a primary treatment modality is no longer recommended, although postoperative radiation therapy may be necessary for certain tissue types.[1] Neck dissection performed at the time of the surgical procedure may be indicated for tumors larger than 4 cm, cancers that originate in the submandibular gland, and primary squamous cell carcinoma. If there is undifferentiated carcinoma and high-grade mucoepidermoid carcinoma, a neck dissection should also be performed at the time of the initial surgery.

LIFE SPAN CONSIDERATIONS

Older adults are at high risk for all types of salivary gland tumors. Sjögren's syndrome has a higher incidence in postmenopausal women because of the increased incidence of connective tissue disorders in this population.

COMPLICATIONS

Complications of diseases of the salivary glands include recurrent bouts of salivary gland swelling, pain, and stone formation, which necessitates surgical intervention. Xerostomia produces serious dental caries because of the lack of saliva. Infectious etiologies of salivary gland disease have a potential for sepsis. Encephalitis, meningitis, and cochleitis are serious consequences of mumps paramyxovirus infection. Bacterial infections and granulomatous diseases can be serious in patients who are immunocompromised.

Benign tumors of the salivary gland rarely cause complications unless they are neglected and invade the facial nerve, underlying structures, or overlying skin. The recurrence rate is low for tumors excised appropriately and properly. However, malignant tumors of the salivary glands can be difficult to treat. Tumors such as adenoid cystic carcinoma, squamous cell carcinoma, and adenocarcinoma may metastasize to other local and regional sites. To ensure a good outcome, it is important to initiate appropriate surgical consultation if a tumor is suspected.

INDICATIONS FOR REFERRAL/HOSPITALIZATION

Primary care providers may manage many infectious and noninfectious diseases that affect the salivary glands. A team of qualified practitioners should manage acute suppurative parotitis (sialoadenitis). Suspected benign and malignant masses should be referred to an appropriate head and neck surgeon for proper diagnosis and treatment. Sialolithiasis requires consultation with an otolaryngologist. Hospitalization may be required to manage the underlying condition causing salivary enlargement or to manage complications.

PATIENT AND FAMILY EDUCATION

Patients should be encouraged to examine themselves for signs and symptoms of salivary gland disease. Painful or painless swelling of the salivary glands, xerostomia, ptyalism, and purulent discharge from salivary gland ducts are important conditions to investigate.

HEALTH PROMOTION

Important topics for health promotion include adequate hydration, good oral hygiene, and immunizations. In addition, it is important that the patient be taught to avoid risk factors such as radiation exposure and exposure to animals that may be vectors of disease.

REFERENCES

1. Lee KJ: *Essential otolaryngology: head and neck surgery,* ed 6, Norwalk, Conn, 1995, Appleton & Lange.
2. Cummings CW and others: *Otolaryngology: head and neck surgery,* ed 3, St Louis, 1998, Mosby.
3. Tierney LM Jr, McRhee SJ, Papadakis MA: *Current medical diagnosis and treatment,* ed 37, Stamford, Conn, 1998, Appleton & Lange.
4. Myers E, Suen J: *Cancer of the head and neck,* ed 3, Philadelphia, 1996, WB Saunders.
5. Sharkawy AA, Chow AW: Cervicofacial actinomycosis. Retrieved October 17, 2002 from the World Wide Web: http://www.uptodate.com.

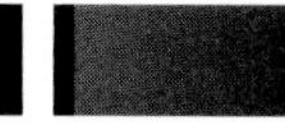

CHAPTER 102

Epiglottitis

Debra S. Munsell

DEFINITION/EPIDEMIOLOGY

Epiglottitis (supraglottitis) is an inflammation of the epiglottis and the surrounding structures. The inflammation is typically caused by a bacterial infection and less commonly occurs as a result of a viral illness or caustic and thermal injury to the epiglottis. Epiglottitis is a rare but serious life-threatening condition.

From the 1950s to the early 1990s epiglottitis typically was associated more often with children than with adults.[1] However, with the advent of vaccination for *Haemophilus* sp., a dramatic decline in childhood epiglottitis has been noted. Epiglottitis is presently more common in the adult population than in children. In 1980 the ratio of children to adults with epiglottitis was 2.6:1; by 1993 it had declined to 0.4:1.[2] The state of Rhode Island reported a decline in the incidence of epiglottitis in children from 38 cases between 1975 and 1977 to a single case between 1990 and 1992; however, in the adult population epiglottitis increased from 17 cases between 1975 and 1977 to 69 cases between 1990 and 1992.[3] Incidence is now decreasing in all age-groups, possibly as a result of a general decrease of *Haemophilus influenzae* type B (HIB) disease in the general population. Other pathogens associated with this disease include group A, B, and C *Streptococcus; Streptococcus pneumoniae; Klebsiella pneumoniae; Candida albicans; Staphylococcus aureus; Haemophilus parainfluenzae; Neisseria meningitidis;* varicella zoster; and various other viral pathogens.[4]

Male predominance has been reported with epiglottitis; however, male-female ratios have varied. The average age of adults with epiglottitis varies from 42 years to that age plus or minus 18.5 years.[5] One study noted an increase in cases during the summer months; however, most experts agree that there is not a predictable seasonal occurrence of epiglottitis.[6]

Epiglottitis among adults may follow an unpredictable clinical course, ranging from relatively benign disease to rapidly progressive disease with acute airway obstruction and possibly death.[5] The mortality rate for children is now less than 1%, but the mortality rate for the adult population is in the range of 6% to 7%.[1]

Delay in diagnosis is associated with a 9% to 18% mortality rate.[4]

Immediate emergency department referral/ physician consultation is indicated for patients with suspected epiglottitis.

PATHOPHYSIOLOGY

Epiglottitis can be caused by a variety of microorganisms. Two of the most common offending organisms are HIB and beta-hemolytic streptococcus. In patients with underlying disease, *Aspergillus, Klebsiella,* and *Candida* organisms have been identified.

A viral etiology has been postulated for some cases of adult epiglottitis, especially the milder cases.[7] Also, herpes simplex has been positively identified in adult epiglottitis.

CLINICAL PRESENTATION

Patients with epiglottitis present with severe sore throat, dysphagia, odynophagia, fever, and shortness of breath. Other complaints include the inability to swallow their own secretions, neck tenderness, lymphadenopathy, cough, drooling, stridor, respiratory distress, and hoarseness. The onset and duration of symptoms before the patient's initial contact with the primary care provider vary. Depending on the severity of symptoms, patients may seek treatment after having symptoms for less than 8 hours, or they may have had them for more than 4 days.

PHYSICAL EXAMINATION

Patients with epiglottitis may or may not have fever and a toxic appearance, depending on the severity of the infection. Physical findings by indirect laryngoscopy reveal an erythematous, edematous epiglottis with a narrow glottic opening. Depending on the severity of respiratory distress, posturing in the upright "sniff" position with drooling may be noted. Substernal and supraclavicular retractions, tachycardia, tachypnea, and inspiratory stridor may be noted. With severe respiratory distress, changes in mental status, anxiety, pallor, cyanosis, and other signs of hypoxia may be present.

Precautions during the physical examination are required. If epiglottitis is suspected, the pharynx should not be examined. Any inspection of the oral cavity requires that emergency airway management equipment be immediately available in case of laryngospasm.

DIAGNOSTICS

A definitive diagnosis of epiglottitis is made by indirect laryngoscopy with a flexible fiberoptic scope or a laryngeal mirror. Indirect laryngoscopy is considered a safe diagnostic tool in the adult population but not in children.

A lateral neck film may be useful but may not be diagnostic in the adult population. Findings on the lateral neck film suggestive of epiglottitis include a swollen epiglottis presenting like a "thumbprint" sign. Because they have a fairly low sensitivity (true positives) rate, lateral neck films are not a true diagnostic tool.

A CBC often reveals leukocytosis with a shift to the left. Blood cultures may be obtained to exclude septicemia. A culture of the epiglottis is helpful in identifying the offending organism. Arterial blood gasses may also be indicated.

DIFFERENTIAL DIAGNOSIS

Other conditions should be considered in the differential diagnosis. These include Ludwig's angina, retropharyngeal and peritonsillar infections, tumor, trauma to the larynx, allergic drug reactions, and angioneurotic edema. Signs and symptoms of Ludwig's angina, retropharyngeal abscess, and peritonsillar cellulitis or abscess are somewhat similar to those of epiglottitis, as all present with an infectious process. Ludwig's angina is an infection, or cellulitis, of the floor of the mouth, often involving the submental, sublingual, and/or submandibular spaces. Ludwig's angina typically results from a dental infection and can be easily diagnosed by CT scan. Retropharyngeal abscess can also be identified by CT scan and can be excluded by negative findings on physical examination. Peritonsillar cellulitis or abscess can be excluded by negative physical examination findings.

A tumor, trauma to the larynx, allergic drug reaction, or angioneurotic edema may present with signs similar to those of epiglottitis. A tumor or trauma to the larynx may cause sore throat, hoarseness, dysphagia, and respiratory distress; however, infectious findings are negative. Allergic drug reaction or angioneurotic edema typically present with respiratory distress and dermatologic findings.

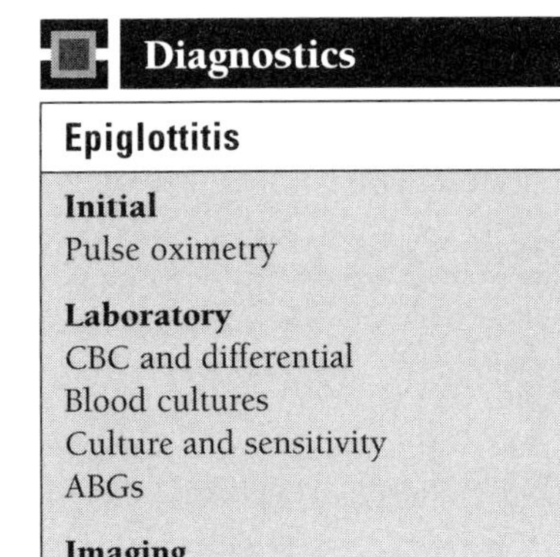

Diagnostics

Epiglottitis

Initial
Pulse oximetry

Laboratory
CBC and differential
Blood cultures
Culture and sensitivity
ABGs

Imaging
Lateral neck x-ray

Other
Indirect laryngoscopy

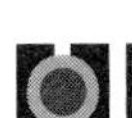

Differential Diagnosis

Epiglottitis

Ludwig's angina
Retropharyngeal and peritonsillar infections
Tumor
Trauma
Allergic reaction
Angioneurotic edema

MANAGEMENT

Patients should be allowed to sit upright in a quiet environment with humidified oxygen. Treatment of epiglottitis consists of close observation for airway management, antibiotics, and, in some cases, steroids. The patient should be hospitalized in an intensive care unit for aggressive airway monitoring. Isolation is sometimes recommended for the first 24 hours after the initiation of antibiotic therapy. Patients with an increased risk of airway obstruction (those with respiratory distress, tachycardia, tachypnea, or an increased white blood cell count) may require an artificial airway by intubation or tracheotomy. Continuous oxygen therapy and monitoring of oxygen saturation are necessary.

IV antibiotics should be initiated as soon as possible. In the past the usual treatment for epiglottitis was ampicillin and chloramphenicol; however, because of ampicillin-resistant *H. influenzae,* it is no longer recommended. Chloramphenicol is not often used because of the increased risk of aplastic anemia. A second- or third-generation cephalosporin (e.g., ceftriaxone IV or cefotaxime), ampicillin/sulbactam, or trovafloxacin are the current recommended medications for treatment.[8] Although many experts advocate the use of steroids, it is not a universal standard of treatment. Controlled trials that prove any benefit from steroids are not available.

The use of rifampin as a prophylaxis against infection in close contacts is sometimes recommended. There have been cases of transmission of *Haemophilus* infection from children to adults and adults to children.[1]

LIFE SPAN CONSIDERATIONS

With the changes in the age of those affected by HIB infection, careful evaluation of all age-groups is suggested. A suspicion of epiglottitis should prompt an immediate referral to an emergency department capable of airway support.

COMPLICATIONS

Epiglottitis is a serious and potentially fatal condition. Death from airway obstruction may result. Other potentially fatal complications include septicemia and meningitis, resulting from the spread of infection.

INDICATIONS FOR REFERRAL/HOSPITALIZATION

All cases of epiglottitis or suspected epiglottitis require immediate referral. Hospitalization is necessary for close observation of the airway and initiation of appropriate antibiotic therapy.

PATIENT AND FAMILY EDUCATION

Explanation of all procedures is necessary to allay patient and family anxiety. The importance of the medical regimen should be stressed to enhance adherence. When steroids are prescribed, information on steroids and tapering of doses must be reviewed.

HEALTH PROMOTION

Health promotion should include an age-appropriate immunization status review. Cases of thermal inhalation injuries resulting in epiglottitis have been documented in crack cocaine users. Caustic ingestions, foreign bodies, and other thermal inhalations have also resulted in signs and symptoms of epiglottitis.[8]

REFERENCES

1. Carey MJ: Epiglottitis in adults, *Am J Emerg Med* 14(4):421-424, 1996.
2. Frantz TD, Rasgon BM: Acute epiglottitis: changing epidemiological patterns, *Otolaryngol Head Neck Surg* 109:457-460, 1993.
3. Park KW, Darvish A, Lowenstein E: Airway management for adult patients with acute epiglottitis, *Anesthesiology* 88:254-261, 1988.
4. Fairbanks DNF: *Pocket guide to antimicrobial therapy in otolaryngology-head and neck surgery*, ed 10, Alexandria, Va, 2001, The American Academy of Otolaryngology-Head and Neck Surgery Foundation.
5. Hebert PC and others: Adult epiglottitis in a Canadian setting, *Laryngoscope* 108:64-69, 1998.
6. Kass EG and others: Acute epiglottitis in the adult: experience with a seasonal presentation, *Laryngoscope* 103:841-844, 1993.
7. Shapiro J, Eavey RD, Baker AS: Adult supraglottitis: a prospective analysis, *JAMA* 259:563-567, 1988.
8. Felter R: Pediatrics, Epiglottitis, *eMedicine Journal*, June 5 2001, Volume 2, Number 6; http://www.emedicine.com.

CHAPTER 103

Oral Infections

Debra S. Munsell

DEFINITION/EPIDEMIOLOGY

Aphthous ulcers, stomatitis, and thrush *(Candida)* infections are often encountered in primary care practice. Mechanical irritation, drug reactions, trauma, nutritional deficiencies, stress, and infection (bacterial, viral, or fungal) irritate and inflame the sensitive oral mucosa. These conditions may be localized to the oral mucosa or associated with systemic disease. Therefore it is important to accurately diagnose and appropriately care for these lesions.

Aphthous ulcers (canker sores) are defined as shallow, painful, and often recurrent lesions of the oral mucosa. They typically affect adolescents and young adults, with more females than males affected. Patients with known ulcerative colitis, Crohn's disease, or gluten-sensitive enteropathy are also affected. *Stomatitis* is a general term that refers to the inflammation of the soft tissues of the oral cavity. Chemical or heat injuries may initiate stomatitis; aspirin may cause an ulcerative lesion when used as a topical anesthetic on the oral mucosa. Burns sustained from hot food or liquids may also cause mucosal irritations. Certain food substances, chewing gum, oral mouth rinses, and dental products may induce painful lesions. Cinnamon flavoring has been implicated as a common culprit.[1]

Thrush, or candidal infection of the oral mucosa, is caused by the overgrowth of *Candida albicans,* bacteria that are normally found in the flora of the gastrointestinal tract. Immunocompromised hosts; patients with diabetes, ulcerative colitis, Crohn's disease, gluten sensitivity, vitamin deficiencies, or poor oral hygiene; patients who wear dentures; and others with poor general health are susceptible to oral mucosal lesions. These lesions may occur from infancy through maturity and can be a recurrent source of irritation.

PATHOPHYSIOLOGY

Aphthous ulcers (recurrent aphthous ulceration, canker sores) are a common presenting problem for all age-groups. Although the exact etiology of these ulcers is not readily known, it is thought that cell-mediated hypersensitivity to the oral mucosa may be the cause. Other proposed etiologic factors include stress; deficiencies of vitamin B_{12}, folic acid, or iron; microbial agents; and hypersensitivity states (gluten-sensitive enteropathy). Generalized stomatitis may be caused by poor oral hygiene, ill-fitting dentures, nicotine abuse, mechanical trauma, chemical trauma from caustic substances, or hot foods. Thrush more typically occurs with underlying diabetes or with immunocompromised states. Parenteral antibiotic or steroid use has been implicated as a precursor to oral candidiasis.

CLINICAL PRESENTATION

Aphthous ulcers are painful, shallow ulcerations of the oral mucosa and occur as solitary or multiple lesions. They are not typically found on the anterior hard palate or gingiva, and they may be recurrent. Ranging in size from 2 mm to many centimeters, aphthous ulcers may have a gray-yellow, pseudomembranous base surrounded by erythema. Fever and lymphadenopathy are not usually present.

There are three categories of aphthous ulcers. Minor aphthous ulcers are generally the most common and range in size from 2 to 10 mm; healing occurs over 10 to 14 days. Many people attribute these minor ulcers to stress, trauma, or even menses. Major aphthous ulcers may present as painful lesions that are 2 to 3 cm in diameter and are often in a state of cyclical eruption. Scarring is associated with these lesions. The third category is the herpetiform ulceration, which often is mistaken for lesions of the herpes simplex virus. These lesions are small (2 to 3 mm), are widely scattered or closely grouped, and may be recurrent. Viral cultures of these lesions are negative.

Stomatitis may be attributed to many different causes, most commonly denture irritation, poor oral hygiene, and nicotine abuse. Typically, stomatitis caused by denture irritation presents as irritation of the soft tissue associated with denture contact. It is erythematous and painful. *Candida* infections (thrush) usually appear as white, cottage cheeselike lesions that can be easily removed with a swab. The underlying tissue may bleed after manipulation.

PHYSICAL EXAMINATION

An aphthous ulceration can occur as a solitary lesion or multiple lesions. The usual presentation is a 2- to 10-mm, ulcerative mucosal lesion that has a white-yellow central fibrinous pseudomembrane.[1]

Stomatitis lesions caused by poor oral hygiene and denture wearing are found underlying the denture or appliance, and they are erythematous and painful. Secondary candidiasis may also be associated with denture stomatitis.[2] Stomatitis from chemical or thermal injury presents with a painful, sloughing, whitish mucosal surface, or the lesions may be erythematous with a white keratotic surface. Nicotinic stomatitis presents as multiple, 1- to 2-mm papules on a background of white mucosa. The hard palate and anterior soft palate are most often involved, and the papules have erythematous centers.

DIAGNOSTICS

Aphthous ulcerations, as well as lesions of nicotinic and traumatic stomatitis, are diagnosed by clinical presentation and physical examination. *Candida* infections can also be diagnosed from the physical examination and presentation, but a microscopic examination of oral scrapings will reveal the classic findings of hyphae. Cultures on a mycologic medium (Sabouraud's dextrose agar, Pagano-Levin) may be obtained for confirmation.

DIFFERENTIAL DIAGNOSIS

Carcinoma of the oral cavity should be suspected with oral erosive lesions that are slow to heal or with thickened white patches that adhere to the oral mucosa. Alcohol or tobacco use increases the risk for oral cancers.

Although similar in appearance to aphthous ulcers, herpetic lesions are usually found only on the oral mucosa attached to bony structures. Additional etiologies of mucosa ulceration that are indicative of systemic disease include acute necrotizing ulcerative gingivitis (Vincent's gingivitis), bullous pemphigoid, Behçet's syndrome, Crohn's disease, immune dysfunction, and hand-foot-and-mouth disease.

In acute necrotizing ulcerative gingivitis (ANUG), multiple ulcerative lesions occur with illness or stress and are associated with fetid odor, metallic taste, excessive salivation, and friable gingiva. In its most severe form, ANUG requires systemic antibiotic therapy to prevent septic sequelae, particularly with patients who are immunocompromised.

Bullous pemphigoid is a cutaneous disorder in which lesions commence as fixed urticarial plaques followed by clear bullae that appear on both normal and urticarial areas. This chronic eruption primarily affects flexor surfaces but may be generalized. The lesions occur in crops and transiently affect the oral mucosa.

Behçet's syndrome produces ulcerative lesions on oral and genital areas, with associated symptoms of uveitis and arthritis. Involvement of the central nervous system is less common; the ocular effects of Behçet's syndrome include retinal vasculitis and necrosis. Loss of vision can occur, even with aggressive treatment.

The lesions of Crohn's disease affect the mucosal surfaces of the gastrointestinal tract, including the oral cavity. Careful evaluation for gastrointestinal symptoms is recommended when oral lesions are extensive or recurrent. Extensive or recurrent involvement of oral lesions necessitates investigation of immune status and a screening for diabetes or other systemic disorders.

Hand-foot-and-mouth syndrome less commonly affects the buttocks and proximal extremities. This viral syndrome produces a mild, self-limiting illness. Inquiry concerning the sudden onset of gastrointestinal systems is helpful when clear vesicular lesions that ulcerate are found in the mouth and on the hands and feet.

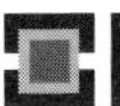

Diagnostics

Oral Infections

Initial
KOH preparation or Tzanck test*

Laboratory
CBC and differential*
Serum glucose*
B_{12}/folate*

*If indicated.

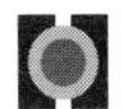

Differential Diagnosis

Oral Infections

Aphthous ulcers
Mechanical/chemical/thermal injury
Drug reactions
Nutritional deficiencies
Infectious etiologies (bacterial, viral, fungal)
Carcinoma
Systemic disease (diabetes, Crohn's, Behçet's, acute necrotizing ulcerative gingivitis, hand-foot-and-mouth)
Immune dysfunction

MANAGEMENT

Aphthous stomatitis can be a vexing problem because recurrence is common. Treatment is directed at symptomatic relief. Methods of symptomatic relief with unclear benefit include the application of topical steroids (e.g., triamcinolone in Orabase, a dental paste) or a steroid mouth rinse with betamethasone syrup.[1]

Current treatments that have likely benefit to reduce the severity and duration of episodes, but not likely to affect recurrence rates include (1) Gly-Oxide rinse (carbamic peroxide) or Kaopectate and diphenhydramine (Benadryl) mixed in equal measures and applied to the irritated surfaces as a mouth rinse six times a day; and (2) avoidance of irritating, acidic, hot, or spicy foods. Other treatments with likely benefit are varied mouth rinse preparations. Viscous lidocaine is also used as a rinse, but careful observation is needed because this treatment may affect the swallowing and gag reflexes. Amlexanox oral paste, ¼ inch paste four times daily after oral care, is also indicated.[3] Several preparations or "mouthwash" recipes have been developed to assist in the relief of patients suffering from aphthous stomatitis.[4] One such compounded suspension consists of 30 ml diphenhydramine elixir and 60 ml Mylanta, taken as a 5-ml swish and swallow three times daily and at bedtime.[3] Another compound is 60 ml Maalox and 4 g sucralfate used in the same manner.[3] Other treatments include the combination of diphenhydramine liquid, dexamethasone, nystatin suspension, and tetracycline (from capsules), swished and swallowed 1 teaspoon six times a day (after and in-between meals and at bedtime). Advice from a pharmacist should be obtained concerning this formulation. Acemannan oral gel or rinse p.r.n. can be used to sooth irritated tissue. For use in children and for those in whom tetracycline is prohibited, amoxicillin/clavulanate can be substituted for the tetracycline.[5] However, severe eruptions may respond only to systemic steroids.

Nicotinic stomatitis can be treated by cessation of tobacco abuse. Denture stomatitis can be treated with thorough daily dental hygiene and removal of dentures at night. Secondary *Candida* infections, if suspected, should be treated appropriately. Trauma and chemical or thermal burns should be treated symptomatically with analgesics and baking soda-salt water rinses. If the offending agent is known, it should be avoided.

Candida infections may be treated in several ways because antifungal agents are now supplied in many forms. A nystatin oral suspension, 100,000 units/ml is a commonly used therapy; 5 ml of the suspension is swished and swallowed four times a day until 48 hours after the lesions have resolved. Lozenges of nystatin may also be prescribed. For patients with dentures, nystatin powder is applied to the dentures three to four times daily. Oral clotrimazole or nystatin troches are also widely prescribed. Antifungal creams may be applied under dental appliances. Some infections may respond only to systemic therapy with fluconazole 100 mg/day for 14 days.[2] In patients with diabetes, maintaining proper glucose levels is an important therapeutic component.

COMPLICATIONS

Aphthous stomatitis is usually a short-lived entity; there are few, if any, complications. Denture stomatitis and nicotine stomatitis are not thought to cause serious complications and are not associated with further development of oral carcinomas. *Candida* infections of the oral cavity can be managed without complication in most instances. However, care should be taken to identify patients who may be immunocompromised or nutritionally at risk to adequately assess their needs.

INDICATIONS FOR REFERRAL/HOSPITALIZATION

Aphthous stomatitis, dental and nicotinic stomatitis, and routine *Candida* infections rarely require referral. A physician or subspecialist in infectious diseases should be consulted if questions arise concerning possible carcinoma or if the patient is immunocompromised. Patients with routine eruptions are not candidates for hospitalization, but severely immunocompromised patients or patients with diabetes may need hospitalization for treatment of the underlying disease.

PATIENT EDUCATION/HEALTH PROMOTION

Aphthous stomatitis is usually a recurrent eruption. Treatment of the underlying causes, if known, may alleviate future outbreaks. Crohn's disease; ulcerative colitis; stresses; deficiencies of vitamin B_{12}, iron, and folic acid; and estrogen sensitivity have been implicated in outbreaks. Avoidance of irritating food, beverages, and chemicals may alleviate some of the symptoms and decrease the number of recurrences. Proper oral hygiene and good denture care prevent most problems with denture-related stomatitis. Avoidance of excessively heated food and drink will prevent thermal stomatitis. *Candida* infections can be anticipated in patients who are taking long courses of steroids and antibiotics; treatment for these patients should be started as soon as symptoms occur. Patients who are known to be immunocompromised should be monitored regularly for the signs and symptoms of developing *Candida* infections and treated accordingly. Patients with diabetes should be taught proper glycemic control measures and routine surveillance of skin and mucosal surfaces.

REFERENCES

1. Cummings CW and others: *Otolaryngology: head and neck surgery,* ed 3, St Louis, 1998, Mosby.
2. Rakel RE: *Conn's current therapy,* Philadelphia, 1998, WB Saunders.
3. *Tarascon pocket pharmacopoeia,* Loma Linda, Calif, 2001, Tarascon Publishing.
4. *MDACC 2001/2002 pharmacy formulary and therapeutic index, division of pharmacy,* Hudson, Ohio, 2001, Lexi-Comp, Inc.
5. Fairbanks DNF: *Pocket guide to antimicrobial therapy in otolaryngology: head and neck surgery,* ed 10, Alexandria, Va, 2001, American Academy of Otolaryngology—Head and Neck Surgery Foundation.

CHAPTER 104

Parotitis

Debra S. Munsell

DEFINITION/EPIDEMIOLOGY

An inflammatory reaction of the parotid gland, parotitis may be caused by bacterial, viral, fungal, or mycobacterial invasion. The most common infection is viral mumps. Parotitis is often encountered in the sixth to seventh decade of life in an equal male-female ratio.[1] This condition is also referred to as acute suppurative sialadenitis, surgical parotitis or surgical mumps, postoperative parotitis, or secondary parotitis.[1] Chronic illness, an immunocompromised host, recent surgical procedure, and hypovolemia are common precipitating factors.[1] Intrinsic factors such as medications (anticholinergics) and extrinsic factors such as radiation therapy may also precipitate a reaction. It is important to note that salivary gland enlargement can be the initial manifestation of human immunodeficiency virus (HIV) infection.[1]

PATHOPHYSIOLOGY

Multiple factors can contribute to the development of parotitis. Most commonly the infection begins with retrograde migration of oral cavity flora via Stensen's duct. Stasis of saliva, ductal obstruction, decreased stimulation (anorexia), decreased mastication, and poor oral hygiene contribute to retrograde migration.[2] Chronically ill patients, recent surgical candidates, and those with acute or chronic hypovolemia (hemorrhage, diarrhea, emesis) exhibit factors that lead to stasis and retrograde migration. In addition, parotid salivary secretions are an inferior bacteriostatic medium and may also augment inflammatory reactions.

CLINICAL PRESENTATION

The usual presentation consists of a rapid onset of localized pain, edema, and induration of the infected gland.[2] Systemic symptoms may include fever, chills, and malaise.[1] Viral inflammatory reactions most often present with edema (usually bilateral) and pain, which is exacerbated by mastication. Low-grade fever, arthralgias, malaise, and headache may also be present. Although parotitis may sometimes be referred to as "surgical mumps," it is not related to the viral syndrome mumps, which is caused by the mumps paramyxovirus. Surgical mumps refers to the similar appearance of glandular swelling seen in mumps and parotitis. Infection with the HIV virus may produce bilaterally enlarged, painless parotid glands that gradually produce smaller amounts of saliva, resulting in complaints of xerostomia.[1]

PHYSICAL EXAMINATION

Bimanual palpation of the gland with attention to Stensen's duct should be performed. In parotitis, palpation of the gland elicits a suppurative discharge from Stensen's duct.[2] Bilateral edema is suggestive of viral infection, and a clear discharge is found on palpation of the duct. Suppurative discharge should be cultured. If the process has been present for several days, fluctuance of suppurative sialadenitis may not be palpable because of the anatomic septations in the parotid.[2]

DIAGNOSTICS

The diagnosis of parotitis is based on the clinical presentation and physical examination. A CBC with differential may reveal a leukocytosis with neutrophilia in suppurative etiologies.[1] Appropriate cultures and sensitivities should be obtained, and fungal and mycobacterial studies should be requested when indicated. Radiographs or oblique soft tissue films are obtained if obstruction caused by calculus is suspected.

DIFFERENTIAL DIAGNOSIS

The differential diagnosis of parotitis should include bacterial, viral, mycobacterial, or fungal infections. Cytomegalovirus, coxsackievirus and Epstein-Barr virus have all been identified as agents of infection. Mechanical or extrinsic factors such as radiotherapy or drug-induced parotitis should also be included in the differential diagnosis. In addition, anticholinergic medications can initiate parotitis. Such medications include antiparkinsonian agents, atropine, dicyclomine hydrochloride, glycopyrrolate, scopolamine, and hyoscyamine sulfate.

MANAGEMENT

Nonsurgical treatments include parenteral antibiotics such as beta lactamase-resistant penicillins or cephalosporins. Recommended antibiotic therapy includes amoxicillin with clavulanic acid, and clindamycin. Cefoxitin and nafcillin are suggested for refractory disease[3] (Box 104-1). Fluid and electrolyte replacement is necessary.[1] Attention to proper oral hygiene and the use of sialagogues, such as lemon balls and chewing gum, are also recommended. Sialagogues are agents that stimulate the production and flow of saliva. There is a questionable role for the use of steroids. Analgesics and local heat for relief of pain are beneficial. External/bimanual massage (from distal to proximal) of the duct is also recommended.[1] Surgical drainage is appropriate if the infection is refractory for more than 3 or 4 days. A CT scan or ultrasound examination of the parotid and neck is indicated if abscess formation has occurred after 3 or 4 days while the patient is taking aggressive parenteral antibiotics. Because of the usually debilitated states of patients predisposed to

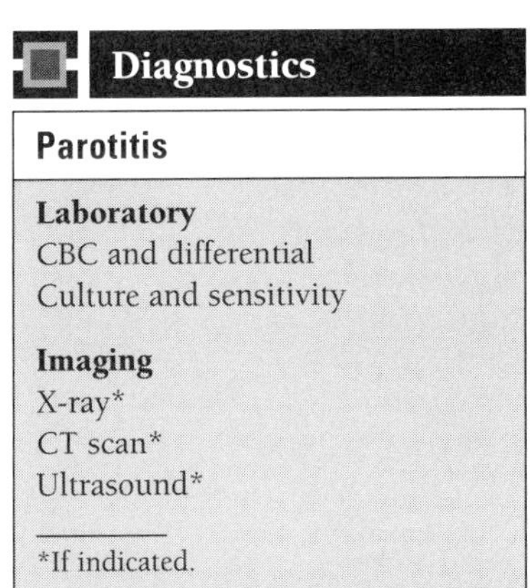

Diagnostics

Parotitis

Laboratory
CBC and differential
Culture and sensitivity

Imaging
X-ray*
CT scan*
Ultrasound*

*If indicated.

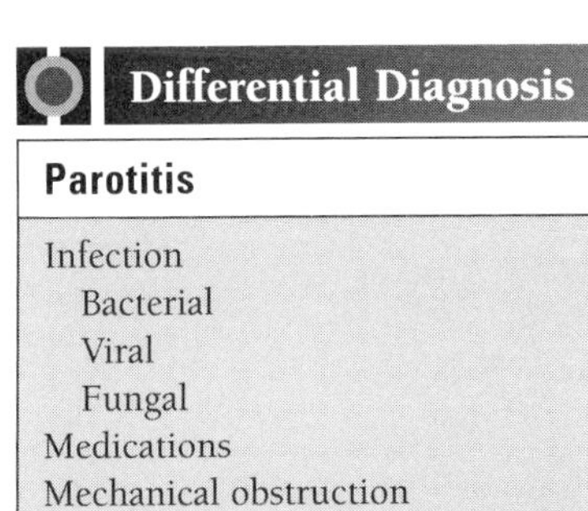

Differential Diagnosis

Parotitis

Infection
- Bacterial
- Viral
- Fungal

Medications
Mechanical obstruction

BOX 104-1

ANTIBIOTICS RECOMMENDED IN THE TREATMENT OF BACTERIAL PAROTITIS

- Amoxicillin with clavulanic acid (Augmentin)
- Ampicillin with sulbactam (Unasyn IV)
- Antistaphylococcal penicillin
- Clindamycin
- Cephalexin
- Cefoxitin
- Nafcillin
- Vancomycin IV and metronidazole

parotitis, a poor prognosis is associated with postoperative patients who develop parotitis. A 20% mortality rate is associated with the development of this infection.[1]

COMPLICATIONS

Complications include abscess formation and the need for surgical drainage. The discomfort associated with this disorder may prevent the patient from eating and drinking, increasing the risk of hypovolemia and further compromising the patient.

INDICATIONS FOR REFERRAL/HOSPITALIZATION

Consultation with an otolaryngologist-head and neck surgeon is recommended. Patients who develop parotitis often require hospitalization for fluid replacement, careful monitoring, and IV antibiotics.

PATIENT AND FAMILY EDUCATION/HEALTH PROMOTION

Preoperative attention to hydration and overall health status should be addressed if the patient is not a candidate for emergent surgery. After diagnosis, attention to hydration, parenteral antibiotics, oral hygiene, and sialagogue use should be addressed. Patients should be instructed in proper oral hygiene, which includes brushing and flossing the teeth and proper care of dentures and dental appliances. The side effects of medications should be discussed with the patient to determine if medication is causing decreased salivary secretions.

REFERENCES

1. Cummings CW and others: *Otolaryngology-head and neck surgery,* ed 3, St Louis, 1998, Mosby.
2. DeWeese DD: *Otolaryngology-head and neck surgery,* ed 7, St Louis, 1988, Mosby.
3. Way L: *Current surgical diagnosis and treatment,* ed 10, Norwalk, Conn, 1994, Appleton & Lange.

CHAPTER 105

Peritonsillar Abscess

Debra S. Munsell

DEFINITION/EPIDEMIOLOGY

A peritonsillar abscess (PTA) is an accumulation of pus located within the peritonsillar tissue. The abscess usually occurs in patients with a history of recurrent, chronic, or improperly treated tonsillitis. PTA may also develop in patients properly treated with penicillin. In such cases the abscess results from penicillin-resistant strains of bacteria.

Peritonsillar cellulitis and abscess formation are common occurrences in young adults.[1] The incidence rate for PTA is approximately 30 per 100,000 person-years, or approximately 45,000 cases annually in the United States and Puerto Rico.[2] The relatively high incidence of PTAs reported raises the possibility that the decreasing rate of tonsillectomies might be increasing the risk for developing PTAs.[2]

Patients with a history of chronic tonsillitis are at risk for developing a peritonsillar abscess. The recurrence of peritonsillar abscess is reported to be variable—from 0% to 23%.[2] The risk of recurrence is higher if the patient is less than 30 years of age.

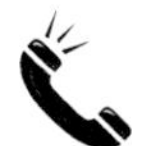

Physician consultation is recommended for peritonsillar abscess.

PATHOPHYSIOLOGY

PTAs, which occur at either the superior or inferior tonsillar poles, are caused by microorganisms that invade the tissue. Studies of tonsillitis have shown a high incidence of anaerobic organisms (principally bacteroids) and aerobic bacteria; group A beta-hemolytic streptococci (GABS) are commonly involved.[1] Beta-lactamase production by anaerobes and some staphylococci result in ineffective treatment of pharyngitis, which can potentially precipitate a PTA.

The abscess formation results from the body's attempt to localize the infection. Erythema and swelling of the peritonsillar region result from increased blood supply and the collection of pus. The pus consists of cells, bacteria, and necrotic tissue.

CLINICAL PRESENTATION

Typically the presentation consists of fever, often 38.8° C (102° F) or higher, chills, fatigue, malaise, foul breath, and severe odynophagia. The patient may appear acutely ill and often complains of pain radiating to the ear of the affected side. Trismus (spasms of the masticatory muscles) is often noted. Drooling is typically present because of the inability to handle secretions. A "hot potato" voice is commonly noted.

PHYSICAL EXAMINATION

With a superior pole PTA there is marked edema and erythema of the peritonsillar tissue and soft palate; this tissue is often fluctuant. Inferior pole PTA is difficult to diagnose, and radiologic assistance in the form of a CT scan with contrast is warranted.[1] The findings are almost always unilateral, with the tonsil typically displaced downward and medially. The uvula is often edematous and displaced to the opposite side.[3] With an inferior pole PTA, the physical findings may not be as prominent or may be absent. Other findings include tender cervical adenopathy and signs of dehydration.

DIAGNOSTICS

Superior pole PTAs are easily diagnosed on the basis of physical findings. Inferior pole PTA is an unusual disorder and is suspected when severe unilateral odynophagia is extremely inconsistent with the physical findings.[3] A CT scan with contrast will confirm abscess formation.

A CBC often reveals leukocytosis. A Monospot test may be performed to exclude infectious mononucleosis. Aspiration of the abscess for culture by an otolaryngologist typically reveals both aerobic and anaerobic bacteria.

DIFFERENTIAL DIAGNOSIS

When considering a diagnosis of peritonsillar abscess, it is imperative to exclude other conditions that present with similar signs and symptoms. These conditions include infectious mononucleosis, tumors, cervical adenitis, epiglottitis, retropharyngeal abscesses, aneurysms of the internal carotid artery, and dental, salivary, or mastoid infections.

Infectious mononucleosis can be excluded on the basis of clinical presentation, physical examination, and serologic findings. With mononucleosis, headache, malaise, fatigue, and anorexia are typically present before the sore throat. A tumor in the peritonsillar region is eliminated from diagnostic consideration by a lack of the physical findings usually present in an infectious process. A CT scan and, possibly, a biopsy are indicated if a tumor is suspected.

The signs and symptoms of PTAs are similar to epiglottitis, which is a potentially fatal condition if not diagnosed. Epiglottitis is less likely when there is peritonsillar swelling with preserved ability to swallow and no stridor auscultated over the larynx on physical examination. Indirect visualization of the epiglottis is a reliable method in the adult and may be necessary to exclude epiglottitis as a cause of symptoms.

Diagnostics

Peritonsillar Abscess

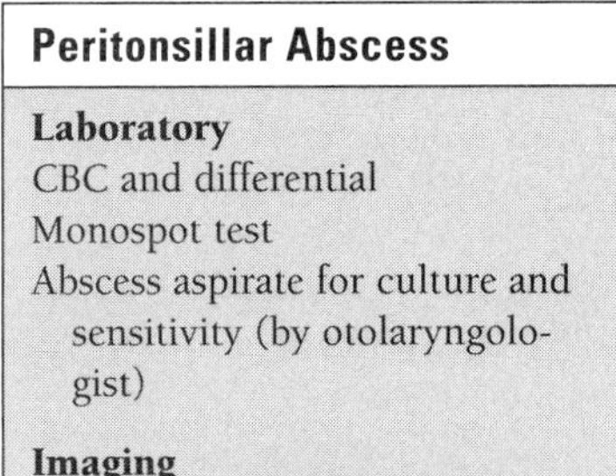

Laboratory
CBC and differential
Monospot test
Abscess aspirate for culture and sensitivity (by otolaryngologist)

Imaging
CT scan (for inferior pole peritonsillar abscess)*

*If indicated.

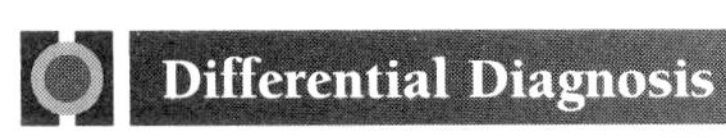

Differential Diagnosis

Peritonsillar Abscess

Infectious mononucleosis
Tumors
Cervical adenitis
Epiglottitis
Retropharyngeal abscess
Aneurysm of internal carotid artery
Dental/salivary/mastoid infection

Cervical adenitis and retropharyngeal abscesses may be similar in their presentation. Both conditions reveal an ill or toxic patient, with signs of infection and neck pain. A retropharyngeal abscess can be identified with a CT scan. Dental, salivary, and mastoid infections can be excluded by observing the physical appearance of the oropharynx. Dental and salivary infections are more localized to the floor of the mouth, and mastoid infections are localized behind the affected ear. An absence of infectious signs and symptoms helps distinguish an aneurysm of the internal carotid artery from other causes. If an aneurysm of the internal carotid artery is suspected, an MRI or ultrasound is necessary.

MANAGEMENT

Oral antibiotic therapy is not sufficient for effective treatment of a PTA. Surgical intervention is required with needle aspiration, incision and drainage, or tonsillectomy. The majority of PTAs can be treated effectively with needle aspiration, antibiotics, and pain medication.[4] A tonsillectomy may be indicated in certain situations; it is very rare to develop a PTA after tonsillectomy. Tonsillectomy is indicated for PTA associated with a history of chronic or recurrent tonsillitis or for the case of the unusual presentation of the abscess.[1] Optimum hydration of the patient must be maintained, either orally or IV.

LIFE SPAN CONSIDERATIONS

Although peritonsillar abscess is an entity of the young, a high index of suspicion must be kept in all age-groups. Early detection and treatment can prevent a life-threatening complication.

COMPLICATIONS

Serious and potentially fatal complications may result from a PTA. The abscess can result in airway obstruction from spread of the infection. Rupture of the abscess with aspiration of the infected material can cause severe and serious sequelae. If untreated, the infection may spread to involve the superior constrictor muscle, other deep spaces of the neck, and the mediastinum.[4] Necrosis of the muscle may result.

Other complications of PTA include thrombophlebitis, chronic peritonsillar abscess, glottic edema, epiglottitis, septicemia, endocarditis, myocarditis, and hemorrhage. Poststreptococcal complications such as rheumatic fever and glomerulonephritis may result if the infected material consists of GABS. Thrombosis of the internal jugular vein (Lemierre syndrome) is a rare sequelae, usually the result of infection with *Fusobacterium necrophorum*. IV antibiotic therapy and surgical treatment of the abscess are required. Ligation or excision of the internal jugular vein is mandatory if septic emboli are noted. Anticoagulation therapy is a controversial issue for this syndrome.[1]

INDICATIONS FOR REFERRAL/HOSPITALIZATION

After diagnosis of a PTA has been made, patients should be referred immediately to an otolaryngologist for an evaluation concerning surgical intervention and antibiotic therapy. Hospitalization may not be necessary, although the patient is usually hospitalized after aspiration and started on IV antibiotics.

Patients may be discharged in 24 hours or less if symptoms subside and the abscess does not reappear. Otolaryngologists prefer cephalexin or another first-generation cephalosporin, with or without metronidazole because of penicillin-resistant microorganisms. Alternative therapy includes the use of cefuroxime (with or without metronidazole), clindamycin, trovafloxacin or, if mononucleosis has been excluded, amoxicillin/clavulanate.[5] A follow-up visit with an otolaryngologist is necessary if tonsillectomy is indicated.

PATIENT AND FAMILY EDUCATION

Education concerning PTA as a complication of tonsillitis is important. PTA can recur, and therefore the signs and symptoms should be described. These include fever, chills, malaise, odynophagia, ear pain, inability to open the mouth, dysphagia, drooling, and a "hot potato" (hoarse) voice. Information regarding the possible side effects of antibiotic therapy should be discussed. These side effects may include nausea, vomiting, diarrhea, abdominal pain, lethargy, vaginitis, or a secondary yeast infection. Signs and symptoms of an allergic reaction, including urticaria, shortness of breath, wheezing, or tightness in the chest, indicate the necessity for immediate emergency treatment.

Patients should be informed that penicillin can decrease the effectiveness of oral contraceptives; therefore a back-up method of contraception is advised for the entire pill cycle in which antibiotic use occurs. In addition, penicillin is best absorbed on an empty stomach.

HEALTH PROMOTION

Patients with histories of recurrent tonsillitis, chronic tonsillitis, and inadequately treated tonsillitis should be monitored closely for signs of peritonsillar abscess. Consultation with an otolaryngologist is a must for these patients. Stress must be placed on emphasizing that the patient complete any antimicrobial therapy regimen in order to minimize the development of resistant strains of bacteria.

REFERENCES

1. Shah UK: Tonsillitis and peritonsillar abscess, *eMedicine Journal* 2(7), 2001; http://www.emedicine.com.
2. Herzon FS: Peritonsillar abscess: incidence, current management practices, and a proposal for treatment guidelines, *Laryngoscope* 105(8 pt 3 suppl 74):1-17, 1995.
3. Licamelli GR, Grillone GA: Inferior pole peritonsillar abscess, *Otolaryngol Head Neck Surg* 118:95-99, 1998.
4. Millan SB, Cumming WA: Supraglottic airway infections, *Prim Care* 23(4):741-758, 1996.
5. Fairbanks DNF: *Pocket guide to antimicrobial therapy in otolaryngology-head and neck surgery,* Alexandria, Va, 2001, The American Academy of Otolaryngology—Head and Neck Surgery Foundation.

CHAPTER 106

Pharyngitis and Tonsillitis

Debra S. Munsell

DEFINITION/EPIDEMIOLOGY

Pharyngitis is a condition that encompasses infection or irritation of the pharynx and tonsils.[1] A common illness affecting both children and adults, pharyngitis is a common reason for people to seek health care.[2] Pharyngitis can present as an acute illness or a chronic condition. The causes are numerous and include both infectious and noninfectious agents.

Noninfectious causes of pharyngitis include referred pain, allergies, trauma from foreign bodies or burns, cancer, chemotherapy, radiation, psychosomatic illness, and irritation. Irritation of the pharynx may result from dust, smoke, dryness, or toxins, either inhaled or swallowed.

Infectious agents responsible for pharyngitis include viruses, bacteria, and, uncommonly, fungi or parasites. Viral infection is the most common cause of pharyngitis in all age-groups and can occur during any season.[3] The most common viruses, responsible for 6% to 20% of all cases, are the rhinovirus and adenovirus.[1] Other responsible agents include the Epstein-Barr virus, which causes mononucleosis, herpes simplex virus, influenza virus, parainfluenza virus, and cytomegalovirus.

The most common cause of bacterial infection is *Streptococcus pyogenes. S. pyogenes* includes groups A, C, and G beta-hemolytic streptococcus. Group A beta-hemolytic streptococcus (GABHS) is important to identify, as it is responsible for acute rheumatic fever (ARF) and glomerulonephritis. GABHS typically peaks in the late winter and early spring, but it can be seen year-round. Group C disease is more common among college students and adolescents. Community-wide and food-borne causes of pharyngitis have been connected to group G organisms.[1] Other offending agents include *Mycoplasma, Arcanobacterium haemolyticus, Chlamydia, Neisseria, Corynebacterium,* and anaerobic bacteria.

Tonsillitis and pharyngitis are similar in clinical presentation, physical findings, diagnosis, and management (Color Plate 36). Tonsillitis is an acute or chronic inflammation of the tonsils and usually results from GABHS infection, although it may be caused by other bacteria or viruses. Tonsillitis may not be a concern unless the patient is symptomatic.

Immediate emergency department referral/physician consultation is indicated for pharyngeal abscess.

PATHOPHYSIOLOGY

The normal flora of the oral pharynx region consists of various and numerous microorganisms. These microorganisms are not harmful unless the immune system is weakened, resulting in increased susceptibility to illness. Pharyngitis/tonsillitis develops from an exposure to a viral or bacterial agent, although some people can harbor or be colonized with pathogenic bacteria and remain free of infection.

Of debate recently has been the possibility of family pets acting as reservoirs for group A streptococcal infection. At this point there is no credible evidence that supports the idea of pets as reservoirs or that pets contribute to familial spread.[4]

CLINICAL PRESENTATION

The clinical presentation of pharyngitis/tonsillitis is varied depending on the offending agent. Noninfectious pharyngitis presents somewhat differently from infectious pharyngitis. Typically, with noninfectious pharyngitis the patient will report a sore throat and dryness, and if environmental allergens are the cause, symptoms will often include rhinorrhea, watery eyes, and a postnasal drip. Patients receiving radiation or chemotherapy may present with complaints of pain, dryness, and dysphagia. Oropharyngeal moniliasis (thrush) may be present in these patients secondary to the immunosuppression.

The infectious causes of pharyngitis/tonsillitis are bacterial and viral. The presentation of symptoms can be quite similar. Viral causes are more common, and typically patients will report the sudden onset of a sore throat, fever, malaise, cough, headache, myalgias, and fatigue. Patients may also report rhinitis, conjunctivitis (adenovirus), congestion, and a cough with sputum production.

One of the most common causes of bacterial pharyngitis/tonsillitis is GABHS. Patients may report a sudden onset of sore throat, painful swallowing, fever, chills, headache, nausea, vomiting, and abdominal pain.[1] With bacterial pharyngitis, rhinitis, conjunctivitis, and myalgias are not typically present.

Other bacterial causes should be investigated if indicated, as *Neisseria gonorrheae* and *Chlamydia* organisms can cause pharyngitis. Often these patients will report a mild throat discomfort in addition to urethritis or vaginitis.

PHYSICAL EXAMINATION

In viral pharyngitis, findings include mild erythema with little or no pharyngeal exudate, although the pharynx may appear swollen, boggy, or pale.[5] Painful or tender lymphadenopathy is not typically present. Infectious mononucleosis typically produces pharyngeal erythema, tonsillar hypertrophy, white to grayish green exudate, petechiae at the junction of the hard and soft palate, and posterior cervical adenopathy. Hepatomegaly and splenomegaly may be identified in less than 50% of patients. Jaundice may be present, but that is unusual.[3]

In GABHS infection, the physical examination reveals marked erythema of the throat and tonsils; patchy, discrete, white or yellowish exudate; uvular edema; and tender anterior cervical adenopathy (see Color Plate 36). Pressure on the tonsillar pillars may produce purulent drainage. The uvula may also be edematous, and fever greater than 38.3° C (101° F) is typical. Occasionally GABHS may present with an erythematous, persistent sore throat with little fever and no exudate.

DIAGNOSTICS

Although it is sometimes difficult to differentiate between viral and bacterial pharyngitis/tonsillitis, clinical presentation may indicate the diagnosis. No specific diagnostic test exists for viral pharyngitis.[3]

Diagnostic studies used to detect GABHS include a throat culture, rapid antigen detection test (RADT), and sometimes an antistreptolysin titer (ASO). The ASO titer is not used during initial diagnostic screening but is obtained to identify or confirm a diagnosis of GABHS weeks to months after the infection. The RADT is often used because it is rapid and convenient. However, the RADT is less sensitive (true positives) than a throat culture. If the diagnosis of GABHS is suspected and the RADT is negative, a throat culture is performed for confirmation. A CBC often reveals leukocytosis with GABHS.

DIFFERENTIAL DIAGNOSIS

The presence of an inflamed pharynx requires further investigation. The differential diagnosis should include infectious mononucleosis, allergies, thrush, peritonsillar cellulitis or abscess, pharyngeal abscess, epiglottitis, and upper respiratory tract infection.

Infectious mononucleosis differs from pharyngitis or tonsillitis in clinical presentation, physical examination, and serologic findings. This diagnosis is seen more commonly in adolescents and young adults.[5] These patients usually present with headache, malaise, fatigue, and anorexia before the sore throat occurs. Hepatosplenomegaly may be noted during the physical examination. A CBC often reveals leukocytosis with atypical lymphocytes. A positive Monospot test reveals heterophil antibodies. The Monospot test is highly specific and sensitive, but it may take 1 to 2 weeks to produce a positive result. Therefore an initial false-negative finding may occur. Associated symptoms of teary, watery discharge from the eyes; pruritus; rhinitis; postnasal drip; pale, boggy nasal mucosa; and an erythematous pharynx with mucus are commonly seen with seasonal allergies. Thrush, a white, thick, cheeselike material that can be scraped off, is identified with a positive potassium hydroxide test result. Peritonsillar cellulitis differs from pharyngitis by the physical examination and the absence of pus on aspiration. Peritonsillar abscess can be diagnosed by presenting signs and symptoms and the aspiration of pus. Tonsillitis may be present with pharyngitis.

Although presenting signs and symptoms are similar to viral pharyngitis, an upper respiratory tract infection usually is distinguished by cough, congestion, rhinitis, sneezing, injected conjunctiva, erythematous

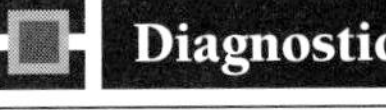

Diagnostics

Pharyngitis and Tonsillitis

Laboratory
Throat culture or RADT
CBC and differential*

*If indicated.

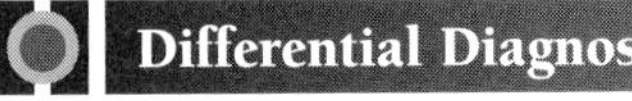

Differential Diagnosis

Pharyngitis and Tonsillitis

Infectious mononucleosis
Allergies
Thrush
Peritonsillar cellulitis/abscess
Epiglottitis
Upper respiratory tract infection
Diphtheria
Trauma
Cancer
Chemotherapy
Radiation
Irritation
Viral/bacterial/fungal etiologies

and edematous nasal mucosa, and an erythematous pharynx. Epiglottitis must be excluded by radiographic imaging or direct laryngoscopy once it is suspected; typically, however, patients with epiglottitis cannot effectively swallow even their own saliva.

Severe exudative pharyngitis/tonsillitis is usually present in mononucleosis. A thick, gray membrane over the tonsils and pharynx is indicative of diphtheria. Leukoplakia, a white patch, is a premalignant change that may arise anywhere on the oral mucosa (Color Plate 37). If it is suspected, a thorough history is warranted. If the lesion remains for more than 2 weeks, a biopsy is indicated.

MANAGEMENT

Treatment of viral pharyngitis includes rest, fluids, humidification, voice rest, and warm saline gargles to ease the discomfort. Acetaminophen or ibuprofen should be used for fever and general discomfort. Topical anesthetic sprays and throat lozenges are of benefit; however, they may produce further irritation in a small number of individuals.

Antibiotic therapy (penicillin V 250 mg q.i.d. for 10 days) is indicated in GABHS to prevent complications. A one-time dose of benzathine penicillin, 1.2 million units IM, has also been proven effective. Penicillin is often prescribed because of the low cost, safety, and efficacy. Amoxicillin 250 mg t.i.d. to q.i.d. or 500 mg b.i.d. for 10 days is also appropriate. Erythromycin 250 mg q.i.d. for 10 days is indicated for patients with penicillin allergy.

A first- or second-generation cephalosporin is effective initially or for recurrent disease. There is a small chance, however, of cephalosporin allergy if the patient is allergic to penicillin. Clindamycin and amoxicillin/clavulanate have been proven effective in recurrent episodes of GABHS. One of the newer macrolides, azithromycin, offers the convenience of once-a-day dosing for 5 days and has been proven effective, but it is expensive. The supportive measures described with viral pharyngitis also apply to GABHS pharyngitis/tonsillitis.

Treatment for non-group A streptococci is given for symptomatic relief, as the organisms are not linked to serious sequelae and do not produce a major antibody response.[1] Penicillin or erythromycin is effective, but the duration of treatment remains unclear.

Management of chronic pharyngitis/tonsillitis with GABHS infection may require tonsillectomy, although tonsillectomy is not done as often as in the past. Current recommendations suggest six or seven documented episodes of GABHS within 1 year, five episodes a year for 2 consecutive years, or three episodes a year for 3 years before tonsillectomy is warranted.

LIFE SPAN CONSIDERATIONS

More than 40 million visits annually occur for pharyngitis in the adult population. More prescriptions are written for treatment of pharyngitis than any other respiratory infection, including pneumonia and otitis.[6] Reflux laryngitis is another cause for pharyngitis. Clearly, pharyngitis is an entity the affects all age-groups and populations. Significant amounts of health care dollars are spent annually in the treatment of this problem. A comprehensive head and neck examination and history are required to accurately assess the situation and prescribe appropriate treatment. Pharyngitis that lasts more than 2 weeks in an adult smoker should be considered a cancer until proven otherwise. Prompt and proper diagnosis of patients who truly have *S. pyogenes* infections can have a significant effect on the morbidity of the disease.[7]

COMPLICATIONS

Peritonsillar cellulitis or abscess, retropharyngeal abscess, scarlet fever, ARF, and poststreptococcal glomerulonephritis may result if GABHS infections are untreated. Unfortunately, glomerulonephritis may result even with proper treatment. ARF can be prevented by prompt antibiotic therapy for the prescribed length of time.

Complications from chronic tonsillitis include upper airway obstruction, sleep apnea, and sleep disturbances.

INDICATIONS FOR REFERRAL/HOSPITALIZATION

An evaluation by an otolaryngologist should be sought for recurrent GABHS infections or for complications that may result from pharyngitis. In addition, potential airway obstruction from pharyngitis or abscess requires immediate referral to an otolaryngologist and hospitalization. Peritonsillar abscess and retropharyngeal abscess require hospitalization for observation and IV antibiotics. Abscesses usually require incision and drainage. Patients with ARF and poststreptococcal glomerulonephritis may require hospitalization depending on symptoms. Patients diagnosed with ARF will require antibiotic prophylaxis, although debate exists regarding the duration of prophylaxis.

PATIENT AND FAMILY EDUCATION

Education is extremely important, and adherence to antibiotic therapy must be stressed. Patients should understand that they are infectious until 24 hours after the start of antibiotic therapy and that a full course of antibiotics is needed to prevent reinfection or complications.

Education stresses adherence to prescribed therapy to ensure eradication of organisms. Possible side effects of antibiotic therapy, including allergic reaction, nausea, vomiting, diarrhea, abdominal pain, lethargy, vaginitis, and secondary yeast infection, should be explained. Signs and symptoms of an allergic reaction, urticaria (hives), shortness of breath, wheezing, or tightness in the chest mandate immediate medical attention. Furthermore, since penicillin can decrease the effectiveness of oral contraceptives, additional contraception is recommended for the entire pill cycle in which the antibiotics are used. All patients with GABHS should be instructed to call the primary care provider if symptoms escalate or if respiratory distress or difficulty swallowing develops. In general, patients should start to feel better 24 to 48 hours after the start of antibiotic therapy. Patients should be encouraged to use a new toothbrush 48 hours after antibiotic therapy is started to decrease the possibility of a recurrent infection. The old toothbrush should be discarded.

Education for the patient with viral pharyngitis is important. Supportive measures should be encouraged. Patients can expect symptom resolution of the pharyngitis over a 1- to 3-week period. Antibiotics are inappropriate in viral infections, but patients and families may require considerable teaching to understand the importance of avoiding antibiotic therapy when appropriate.

HEALTH PROMOTION

Health promotion involving pharyngitis covers many areas. Proper oral hygiene should be addressed with all age-groups at all visits. Education regarding the misuse of antibiotic therapy for viral entities should also be stressed. Of importance is teaching patients, families, and health care workers the importance and need for appropriate hand-washing technique. Limiting exposure to individuals with pharyngitis must also be included in patient teaching. Evaluation for age-appropriate immunization status should be stressed.

REFERENCES

1. Middleton DB: Pharyngitis, *Prim Care* 23(4):719-739, 1996.
2. Centor R, Meier F: Sore throat. In Dornbrand L, Hoole A, Pickard CG, editors: *Manual of clinical problems in adult ambulatory care,* Boston, 1992, Little, Brown.
3. Ruppert SD: Differential diagnosis of common causes of pediatric pharyngitis, *Nurse Pract* 21:38-48, 1996.
4. Bisno AL: Diagnosis and management of group A streptococcal pharyngitis: a practice guideline, *Clin Infect Dis* 25:574-583, 1997.
5. Seller R: *Differential diagnosis of common complaints,* Philadelphia, 1993, WB Saunders.
6. Muller C: *Pharyngitis: Grand Rounds presentation.* University of Texas—Galveston, April 2001.
7. Stephenson KN: Acute and chronic pharyngitis across the lifespan, *Lippincotts Primary Care Prac,* Sep-Oct 4, 2000.

PART 10

Evaluation and Management of Pulmonary Disorders

PATRICIA POLGAR BAILEY, Section Editor

CHAPTER 107

Acute Bronchitis

Susan Harvey

DEFINITION/EPIDEMIOLOGY

Acute bronchitis is an acute inflammation of the tracheobronchial tree and is associated with a generalized upper respiratory tract infection. The diagnosis is usually made in the winter months, when other upper respiratory tract infections occur with frequency.

Each year approximately 12 million episodes occur in individuals 18 years and older in the United States.[1] In more than 90% of cases of acute bronchitis, the etiology is associated with common cold viruses such as rhinovirus and coronavirus, as well as with more invasive viruses such as influenza and adenovirus.[2,3] Less common nonviral causes of acute bronchitis include *Bordetella pertussis, Mycoplasma pneumoniae*, and *Chlamydia pneumoniae* (which is different from the *Chlamydia trachomatis* that causes pneumonia in neonates). Despite the evidence that viruses play a significant role in the cause of acute bronchitis, primary care providers still commonly prescribe antibiotics. In one study more than 31% of the total number of antibiotic prescriptions written were for acute bronchitis.[2] This statistic is alarming considering that in 1980 most isolates of *Streptococcus pneumoniae* were sensitive to penicillin, whereas currently there is approximately a 25% to 30% resistance to the drug.[3] Inappropriate antibiotic use has likely contributed to this increasing microbial resistance.

PATHOPHYSIOLOGY

Acute bronchitis causes edematous changes in the mucous membrane of the tracheobronchial tree and an increase in secretions. Destruction of the bronchial epithelium and loss of cilia function is usually minimal with the common cold viruses but may be more extensive with *M. pneumoniae* and influenza viruses. Cigarette smoking and chemical irritants increase the severity of the infection. Current literature suggests that people who suffer from recurrent attacks of acute bronchitis may have mild asthma.[4] This has lead to more research investigating the role of bronchodilators in the treatment of acute bronchitis.[3,4]

CLINICAL PRESENTATION AND PHYSICAL EXAMINATION

A cough with or without sputum production is the most common symptom reported with acute bronchitis. It begins early in the course of the upper respiratory tract infection. The sputum may be clear at the onset of the infection and become mucoid. The cough may also produce a burning substernal pain with inspiration. Nasal and pharyngeal symptoms subside after 3 to 4 days, but the cough usually remains prominent and progressive. The patient may also have a low-grade fever. Wheezes, rhonchi, and coarse rales may be present on physical examination. Community-acquired pneumonia should be suspected if the patient's history includes dyspnea, high fever, tachycardia, evidence of consolidation on examination, or the presence of symptoms for 2 or more weeks.

Acute bronchitis is easy to identify in children, but adults usually do not present with all of the classic signs. Infection with *B. pertussis* should also be suspected in adults who have a paroxysmal cough, especially when accompanied by whooping or vomiting. Although infection with *B. pertussis* is not life threatening in adults, it is important that it be diagnosed because of the complications it can cause in older adults or in infants who have not been vaccinated against the disease.

DIAGNOSTICS

No diagnostic tests are necessary for acute bronchitis. Routine sputum cultures are useless in the diagnosis because the nasopharyngeal area is colonized with bacterial flora. However, nasopharyngeal cultures should be obtained if *B. pertussis* or the influenza virus is suspected.

A chest radiograph may be useful if the history and physical examination suggest the possibility of community-acquired pneumonia. A heightened suspicion of community-acquired pneumonia is reasonable in older adults because they may present with more subtle symptoms of lower respiratory tract infection.

DIFFERENTIAL DIAGNOSIS

Acute bronchitis is often viral in origin. The most important differential diagnosis is community-acquired pneumonia, which is usually bacterial and requires antimicrobial therapy. Other differential diagnoses include rhinitis, sinusitis, foreign body aspiration, tuberculosis, tumors, and other chronic lung diseases.

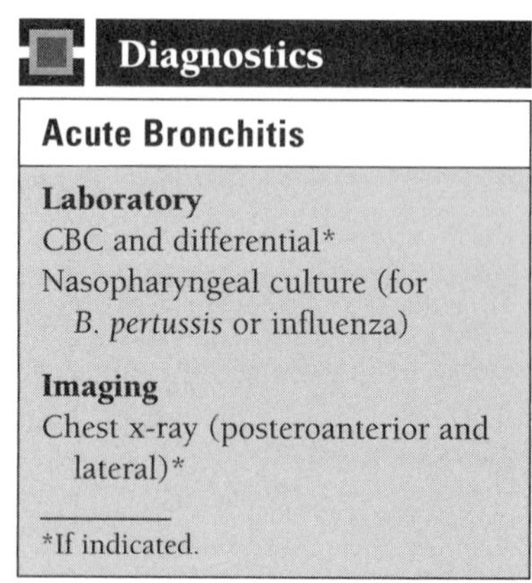
Diagnostics

Acute Bronchitis

Laboratory
CBC and differential*
Nasopharyngeal culture (for *B. pertussis* or influenza)

Imaging
Chest x-ray (posteroanterior and lateral)*

*If indicated.

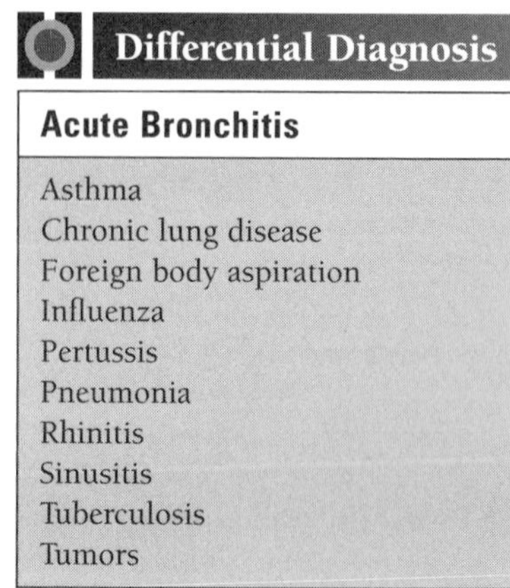
Differential Diagnosis

Acute Bronchitis

Asthma
Chronic lung disease
Foreign body aspiration
Influenza
Pertussis
Pneumonia
Rhinitis
Sinusitis
Tuberculosis
Tumors

MANAGEMENT

The mainstay of treatment in acute bronchitis is directed toward symptom reduction. Because most causes of acute bronchitis are viral, antibiotics are generally not warranted. Decreasing the cough with dextromethorphan cough preparation (30 mg/5 ml, 1 to 2 teaspoons PO every 4 hours as needed; maximum of 4 doses per day) is reasonable. Codeine may be useful at bedtime if the cough is severe. Antipyretics, bed rest, and increasing fluid consumption to thin the secretions are also beneficial treatments. The role of beta-adrenergic bronchodilators is emerging as a more attractive option, especially in patients with wheezes or rhonchi.[3,4]

Reassurance and education are probably the most important modalities for treatment of acute bronchitis. With the rapid emergence of antibiotic-resistant strains of bacteria, it is prudent to withhold the use of antibiotics in stable, otherwise healthy adults.[5,6] Patients should be treated with antimicrobial agents if *C. pneumoniae* or *B. pertussis* is suspected. *C. pneumoniae* should be treated with a tetracycline, such as doxycycline 100 mg b.i.d. for 7 to 10 days or a macrolide such as erythromycin 250 mg q.i.d., 333 mg t.i.d., or 500 mg b.i.d. for 10 days. *B. pertussis* should be treated with a 10-day course of erythromycin. Amantadine 200 mg daily in 1 to 2 divided doses is used if influenza A virus is suspected but only if fewer than 48 hours have passed since onset of the illness.[4] Older adults should receive a reduced dosage (100 mg/day) because of the increased risk of renal dysfunction associated with this medication.

COMPLICATIONS

Although acute bronchitis is often viral and self-limiting, complications do occur. The development of a chronic cough, usually the result of postbronchitic reactive airway disease, can cause discomfort and sleep loss. Pneumonia results from bacterial superinfection and can cause dyspnea, chest pain, and anxiety in addition to other symptoms. Acute respiratory failure, although uncommon, is a potential sequelae. Patients with chronic bronchitis are more susceptible to superinfection and can develop exercise intolerance and hypoxia.

INDICATIONS FOR REFERRAL/HOSPITALIZATION

Acute bronchitis that does not respond to symptomatic treatment and lingers longer than 2 weeks may require physician referral. Patients with progressive dyspnea, oxygen saturation <90%, and signs of sepsis require hospitalization for IV therapy, enhanced pulmonary therapy, and IV antibiotics.

PATIENT AND FAMILY EDUCATION

Patients should be counseled about smoking cessation and the need to avoid air pollutants and irritants. An appropriate face mask can be helpful if work involves chemicals, dust, or other irritants. Rest, increased fluids, and breathing moist air from a clean humidifier or warm shower should be encouraged. In addition, patients should be encouraged to call their primary care provider if the symptoms continue or increase in severity.

Additional patient education information can be obtained from The American Lung Association, 1740 Broadway, New York, NY 10019 ([800] 586-4872; http://www.lungusa.org).

REFERENCES

1. Gonzales R, Sande M: Uncomplicated acute bronchitis, *Ann Intern Med* 133(12):981-991, 2000.
2. Stone S and others: Antibiotic prescribing for patients with colds, upper respiratory tract infections, and bronchitis: a national study of hospital based emergency departments, *Ann Emerg Med* 36(4):320-327, 2000.
3. Gonzales R and others: Special report: CDC principles of judicious antibiotic use, *Ann Emerg Med* 37(6):720-727, 2001.
4. Snow V and others: Principles of appropriate antibiotic use for treatment of acute bronchitis in adults, *Ann Intern Med* 134:518-520, 2001.
5. Gonzales R and others: Decreasing antibiotic use in ambulatory practice, *JAMA* 281(16):1512-1519, 1999.
6. Gwaltney J: Acute bronchitis. In Mandell G, Bennett J, Dolin R, editors: *Mandell, Douglas, and Bennett's Principles and practice of infectious diseases,* ed 5, Philadelphia, 2000, Churchill Livingstone.

CHAPTER 108

Asthma

Patricia Polgar Bailey

DEFINITION/EPIDEMIOLOGY

Asthma is a chronic inflammatory disorder of the airways characterized by increased responsiveness of the tracheobronchial tree to various stimuli, resulting in episodic reversible narrowing and inflammation of the airways.[1,2] In susceptible individuals this bronchial inflammation causes recurrent episodes of wheezing, shortness of breath, chest tightness, and cough. These episodes are usually associated with widespread but variable airflow obstruction that is often reversible either spontaneously or with treatment. The inflammation also causes an associated increase in the existing bronchial hyperresponsiveness to a variety of stimuli.[3,4] This definition of asthma, specifically the concept of asthma as a chronic and inflammatory process, represents a change in the previous understanding of the disease and has important implications for its management.

Asthma is the most common chronic respiratory disorder among all age-groups, with a reported prevalence of 5% to 10%, which represents an increase of 75% since 1980. In the United States, asthma affects 14 to 15 million persons and is responsible for more than 5000 deaths annually; 30% to 40% of those affected by asthma are less than 18 years old. The mortality rate for asthma increased 118% from 1970 to 1995.[5] Every year, more than 10 million school days and more than 3 million work days are missed because of asthma. Asthma is the sixth most common reason for visits in ambulatory settings, and two thirds of patients with asthma obtain their care from a primary care provider.[1,2,6-8] Nonetheless, asthma is still responsible for a disproportionate and increasing number of emergency department visits (>1.5 million) and hospitalizations (>500,000) during recent years.[9]

High mortality rates are associated with high rates of hospitalization in impoverished urban areas. Asthma hospitalization rates have been highest among African-Americans (19% higher incidence), women, and children; death rates have been consistently disproportionately higher among African-Americans, especially those between 15 and 24 years of age.[4] Although prevalence is higher among racial and ethnic minorities, a more valid relationship may exist between socioeconomic status and increased asthma prevalence, morbidity, and mortality than between race and asthma prevalence. Asthma mortality has also been associated with poverty, urban living conditions, exposure to oxidant pollutants, and passive smoking.[7,10] Allergic asthmatic children exposed to high levels of indoor allergens, such as those associated with cockroaches, rodents, and mold, have more severe and more frequent episodes of asthma.[11]

Occupational asthma is currently the most common occupational ailment. Widespread exposure in the workplace environment to airborne dusts, gases, vapors, or fumes contributes to both the development of asthma and the worsening of asthma for those already afflicted. Lost work productivity is estimated at $1033 per person with asthma, or $4.4 billion for all workers afflicted with asthma.[12]

The financial impact of asthma is considerable. At least 1% of all U.S. health care costs are spent on asthma. Direct and indirect asthma-related costs were estimated to be $11.3 billion in 1998, with emergency department visits and hospitalizations responsible for the majority of the cost.[3] Most of those hospitalized or seen in the emergency department had been there before, reflecting the fact that inadequate health behaviors result in increased costs.[1,2,13]

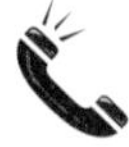

Physician consultation is indicated for patients with Sa_{O_2} <90% on room air, peak flow <70%, and failure to improve with nebulizer treatment ×3 or epinephrine injection ×3.

PATHOPHYSIOLOGY

It is now believed that the primary event in asthma is airway inflammation and that airway hyperresponsiveness and airflow obstruction are secondary and symptomatic features of the disease. Underlying airway inflammation, which involves cellular infiltration, edema, nerve irritation, and vasodilation, results in constriction of airway smooth muscle, increased mucus production, and airway hyperresponsiveness. Atopy, which is the genetic tendency for developing immunoglobulin E (IgE)-mediated hypersensitivity reactions in response to environmental antigens and allergens, is considered to be one of the strongest predisposing factors for the development of asthma. Certain stimuli induce asthma by causing or increasing airway inflammation, whereas other stimuli provoke bronchoconstriction in individuals who already have asthma or airway hyperresponsiveness. Inducers, stimuli that are known to increase inflammation, include inhaled allergens, low–molecular-weight sensitizers, viral or mycoplasmal respiratory infections, and high concentrations of noxious gases. Stimuli that "trigger" or cause bronchoconstriction include exercise, cold air, laughter, emotional upset, and inhaled irritants. Triggers of sudden severe bronchoconstriction include acetylsalicylic acid/nonsteroidal antiinflammatory drugs, beta-adrenergic blockers, food allergens, certain food additives, stings, bites, injections (e.g., allergy shots), and inhaled allergens.[14]

These stimuli set the stage for a cascade of cellular activation, which includes subsequent cytokine release and neurologic excitation. Certain cellular processes act to limit the antigenic response, including mast cell activation through cytokines and infiltration by inflammatory cells, including neutrophils, eosinophils, and lymphocytes. The inflammatory cells are also the source of mediators, which induce bronchoconstriction, excess mucus production, airway edema, and further inflammatory cell influx, all of which lead to bronchial obstruction. The late-phase reaction, which generally occurs 3 to 8 hours after antigen exposure, is the result of new cellular infiltration and activation. Nocturnal and early morning bronchospasm, which occurs with relative frequency in persons with asthma, may be related to circadian variations in cortisol and epinephrine levels, vagal tone, and inflammatory mediators.[15]

One common, often overlooked, exacerbating factor of asthma is esophageal reflux of gastric contents. The incidence of gastroesophageal reflux in adults with asthma has been reported to range between 34% and 89%.[16,17] Gastroesophageal reflux may worsen asthma by inducing a reflex response to esophageal acid exposure, resulting in bronchoconstriction, or by increasing airway hyperreactivity. In addition, aspiration of refluxed material may induce or worsen asthma symptoms. Based on shared vagal innervation of the esophagus and bronchial tree, esophageal acid may induce a reflex bronchoconstriction.[15]

CLINICAL PRESENTATION

The clinical hallmarks of asthma include episodic wheezing associated with dyspnea, cough, and sputum production. Between episodes, symptoms may improve or completely resolve. Symptoms vary from mild to severe, with varying effects on activity. An increased index of suspicion for asthma is essential when respiratory symptoms, including cough, wheeze, shortness of breath, chest tightness, or soreness, persist or recur often.[13,18]

Although wheezing is probably the symptom most typically associated with asthma, the most common symptom of asthma, and often the most troublesome, is cough. However, cough is also the third most common presenting symptom in the ambulatory setting, with a corresponding long list of potential causes. Cough is the only asthma symptom 7% to 57% of the time; this type of asthma is referred to as cough-variant asthma. Cough is often treated symptomatically, which can easily result in a delayed or missed diagnosis of asthma. A diagnosis of asthma should be considered in the differential diagnosis of all patients with a cough, as it is such a common cause. Most persons with cough do not have associated variable airflow obstruction; if obstruction is present and reversible with bronchodilator medication, the diagnosis of asthma is confirmed.[19]

In addition to chronic cough, there are several common clinical presentations of asthma. An acute asthmatic episode is characterized by airway obstruction, which manifests as symptoms of breathlessness and anxiety, often accompanied by wheezing and sometimes cough. These symptoms may resolve within several hours if treatment is given or within 1 to 3 days, even without specific intervention, or they may progress to more severe airway obstruction and respiratory compromise if no therapy is provided. Between acute asthmatic episodes, airflow is normal and symptoms are absent. Several specific conditions are associated with acute asthma exacerbations.

Exercise-induced asthma refers to the development of airway obstruction in an individual after the cessation of exercise, even after brief periods of exercise. Symptoms usually begin 5 to 10 minutes after the completion of exercise and resolve within 1 to 4 hours. Certain forms of exercise, including skiing, ice hockey, and running in the cold, more commonly precipitate airway obstruction; other forms of exercise, such as swimming, less commonly precipitate airway obstruction, most likely because of the warmer and more humid air being inspired. Cold or dry air often predisposes an asthmatic individual to airway obstruction, such as occurs, for example, when a dry, air-conditioned environment (such as an indoor mall) is entered from the warmer, more humid outside air. Common allergens that precipitate asthma include cat allergen (dander), house dust mite allergen, cockroach allergen, and tree and grass pollen. Viral illnesses can also induce airway obstruction in asthmatic individuals; symptoms may persist for weeks to months if therapy is not initiated. Occupational exposures are a common cause of asthma triggers; early responses may occur within several hours; however, late responses may not occur for 8 to 12 hours after exposure. Often occupation-induced asthma symptoms may persist long after the individual has left the workplace; an important consideration is the development of the differential diagnosis. Approximately 1% to 10% of individuals with moderate to severe asthma have aspirin-induced asthma, which is characterized by symptoms of moderately severe airway obstruction, rhinorrhea, sneezing, tearing, dermal changes, and in some cases gastrointestinal symptoms (nausea, vomiting, cramping) when exposed to aspirin or other prostaglandin (H synthase type I) inhibitors. The onset of aspirin-induced asthma occurs most often during the twenties and thirties. The diagnosis of aspirin-induced asthma is important for two reasons: drugs should be avoided, as they may induce life-threatening asthma attacks, and effective treatment is available specifically for this type of asthma.[2]

Acute severe asthma, although not pathologically distinct from acute asthma, represents a more severe and prolonged form of the illness. Acute severe asthma is often characterized by unremitting asthma symptoms (including shortness of breath, diminished exercise tolerance, and wheezing) for weeks with less than optimal response to therapy. Often asthmatic individuals develop prolonged severe asthma by inappropriately self-medicating with beta$_2$-adrenergic agonist inhalers for weeks before seeking medical attention, at which point the risk of respiratory collapse and asphyxia may be great.[2]

Chronic stable asthma refers to asthma that is characterized by episodes of airway obstruction and airway symptoms. Although multiple asthma episodes may occur during a period of several months, most are of moderate severity and respond promptly to therapy. Asthma symptoms and exacerbations can generally be controlled through chronic medication use.[2]

Sample questions for the diagnosis and initial assessment of asthma have been developed by the National Institutes of Health (NIH), National Asthma and Education Prevention Program (NAEPP) (Box 108-1). In addition to an assessment of symptoms, an individual's family history is helpful when a diagnosis of asthma is being considered. Often persons with asthma have a family history of asthma or atopy. Also, family members are often able to identify specific exposures or circumstances that precipitate the patient's symptoms.[18]

PHYSICAL EXAMINATION

The physical examination of the individual with asthma or suspected asthma can be divided into four objectives: (1) diagnosis and differential diagnosis, (2) assessment of asthma severity, (3) identification of adverse effects of medications, and (4) identification of concomitant medical problems. A complete physical examination is necessary if assessment of respiratory exertion or compromise is needed, to identify or evaluate coexisting medical conditions, or if the presentation is complex.[19]

The diagnosis of asthma is based on the history, physical examination, and certain diagnostic tests, particularly spirometry. The physical examination, although an essential part of the evaluation, may correlate poorly with objective measures of airway obstruction, such as pulmonary function tests (PFTs). In the asymptomatic patient the physical examination may be

BOX 108-1

COMPONENTS OF THE PRACTITIONER'S FOLLOW-UP ASSESSMENT: SAMPLE ROUTINE CLINICAL ASSESSMENT QUESTIONS*

MONITORING SIGNS AND SYMPTOMS

(Global assessment) Has your asthma been better or worse since your last visit?

(Recent assessment) In the past 2 weeks, how many days have you:

- Had problems with coughing, wheezing, shortness of breath, or chest tightness during the day?
- Awakened at night from sleep because of coughing or other asthma symptoms?
- Awakened in the morning with asthma symptoms that did not improve within 15 minutes of inhaling a short-acting inhaled $beta_2$ agonist?
- Had symptoms while exercising or playing?

MONITORING PULMONARY FUNCTION

Lung function

What is the highest and lowest your peak flow has been since your last visit?

Has your peak flow dropped below ___ L/min (80% of personal best) since your last visit?

What did you do when this occurred?

Peak flow monitoring technique

Please show me how you measure your peak flow.

When do you usually measure your peak flow?

MONITORING QUALITY OF LIFE/FUNCTIONAL STATUS

Since your last visit, how many days has your asthma caused you to:

- Miss work or school?
- Reduce your activities?
- (For caregivers) Change your activity because of your child's asthma?

Have you had any unscheduled or emergency department visits or hospital stays?

MONITORING EXACERBATION HISTORY

Since your last visit, have you had any episodes/times when your asthma symptoms were a lot worse than usual?

- If yes—What do you think caused the symptoms to get worse?
- If yes—What did you do to control the symptoms?

MONITORING PHARMACOTHERAPY

Medications

What medications are you taking?

How often do you take each medication? How much do you take each time?

Have you missed or stopped taking any regular doses of your medications for any reason?

Have you had trouble filling your prescriptions?

How many puffs of your short-acting inhaled $beta_2$ agonist (quick-relief medicine) do you use per day?

How many __________ (name short-acting inhaled $beta_2$ agonist) inhalers (or pumps) have you been through in the past month?

Have you tried any other medicines or remedies?

MONITORING PHARMACOTHERAPY

Side effects

Has your asthma medicine caused you any problems?

- Shakiness, nervousness, bad taste, sore throat, cough, upset stomach

Inhaler technique

Please show me how you use your inhaler.

MONITORING PATIENT-PROVIDER COMMUNICATION AND PATIENT SATISFACTION

What questions have you had about your asthma daily self-management plan and action plan?

What problems have you had following your daily self-management plan? Your action plan?

Has anything prevented you from getting the treatment you need for your asthma from me or anyone else?

Have the costs of your asthma treatment interfered with your ability to get asthma care?

How can we improve your asthma care?

Let's review some important information:

- When should you increase your medications? Which medication(s)?
- When should you call me [your doctor or nurse practitioner]? Do you know the after-hours phone number?"
- If you can't reach me, what emergency department would you go to?

From National Institutes of Health, National Heart, Lung, and Blood Institute: *Highlights of the Expert Panel Report 2: guidelines for the diagnosis and management of asthma,* NIH pub no 97-4051A, Washington DC, 1997, US Department of Health and Human Services.

*These questions are examples and do not represent a standardized assessment instrument. The validity and reliability of these questions have not been assessed.

entirely normal. Nonetheless, assessing the severity of asthma and airway obstruction is the most important objective in evaluating a person with asthma. Wheezing may be detectable or elicited during forced expiration. In general, mild bronchospasm is associated with expiratory wheezing. As obstruction becomes more significant, wheezing is heard during both the inspiratory phase and the expiratory phase, with a prolongation of the latter. With profound obstruction, wheezing may be heard only during the inspiratory phase or may be entirely absent. With severe obstruction the intensity of the breath sounds diminish. As obstruction increases, accessory muscles of respiration are used; as the obstruction becomes more significant, there may be evidence of hyperinflation with a low diaphragm and an increased anteroposterior diameter. Another rough measure of the degree of obstruction is pulsus paradoxus. An inspiratory decline in systolic blood pressure of greater than 10 mm Hg is abnormal, and one greater than 20 mm Hg generally reflects profound obstruction. However, this measure is crude and should not substitute for more direct measures of the degree of obstruction, such as spirometry.[13]

TABLE 108-1 Classifying Severity of Asthma Exacerbations*

	Mild	Moderate	Severe	Respiratory Arrest Imminent
SYMPTOMS				
Breathless	While walking	While talking (infant: softer, shorter cry; difficulty feeding)	While at rest (infant: stops feeding)	
	Can lie down	Prefers sitting	Sits upright	
Talks in	Sentences	Phrases	Words	
Alertness	May be agitated	Usually agitated	Usually agitated	Drowsy or confused
SIGNS				
Respiratory rate	Increased	Increased	Often >30/min	
		Guide to rates of breathing in awake children *Age* — *Normal rate* <2 months — <60/min 2-12 months — <50/min 1-5 years — <40/min 6-8 years — <30/min		
Use of accessory muscles; suprasternal retractions	Usually not	Commonly	Usually	Paradoxical thoracoabdominal movement
Wheeze	Moderate, often only end-expiratory	Loud; throughout exhalation	Usually loud; throughout inhalation and exhalation	Absence of wheeze
Pulse per minute	<100	100-120	>120	Bradycardia
		Guide to normal pulse rates in children *Age* — *Normal rate* 2-12 months — <160/min 1-2 years — <120/min 2-8 years — <110/min		
Pulsus paradoxus	Absent <10 mm Hg	May be present 10-25 mm Hg	Often present >25 mm Hg (adult) 20-40 mm Hg (child)	Absence suggests respiratory muscle fatigue
FUNCTIONAL ASSESSMENT				
PEF (% predicted or % personal best)	80%	Approximately 50%-80%	<50% predicted or personal best or response lasts <2 hours	
Pao_2 (on air)	Normal (test not usually necessary)	>60 mm Hg (test not usually necessary)	<60 mm Hg: possible cyanosis	
and/or				
Pco_2	<42 mm Hg (test not usually necessary)	<42 mm Hg (test not usually necessary)	≥42 mm Hg: possible respiratory failure	
Sao_2% (on air) at sea level	>95% (test not usually necessary)	91%-95%	<91%	
	Hypercapnia (hypoventilation) develops more readily in young children than in adults and adolescents.			

From National Institutes of Health, National Heart, Lung, and Blood Institute: *Highlights of the Expert Panel Report 2: guidelines for the diagnosis and management of asthma*, NIH pub no 97-4051A, Washington DC, 1997, US Department of Health and Human Services.

***Notes:**
- The presence of several parameters, but not necessarily all, indicates the general classification of the exacerbation.
- Many of these parameters have not been systemically studied, so they serve only as general guides.

Severe asthma exacerbations are characterized by labored respirations, diaphoresis, anxiety, and breathlessness (inability to finish a complete sentence). A respiratory rate of 30 breaths per minute or more and a heart rate of 120 beats per minute or more suggest severe bronchospasm. Other signs and symptoms that often herald impending respiratory failure include agitation, confusion, somnolence, and cyanosis. Unilateral loss of breath sounds may reflect mucus plugging and secondary atelectasis, but pneumothorax must also be considered in this situation.[13] However, even a careful physical examination provides only a crude estimate of airway obstruction, and significant airway obstruction is possible even when the physical examination is entirely normal. Assessment of respiratory status is best accomplished through measurement of lung function with spirometry or peak flow meters.[20] The National Heart, Lung and Blood Institute (NHLBI) system of classifying the severity of asthma exacerbations is presented in Table 108-1.

The physical examination is also important in identifying adverse effects of asthma medications. Side effects of $beta_2$-adrenergic medications and theophylline include tachycardia and tremors. Inhaled corticosteroids can cause oral thrush and dysphonia. Adverse effects of oral (systemic) corticosteroids include central adiposity, hypertension, ecchymoses, cataracts, kyphosis, muscle weakness, and alterations in mental status.[20]

Coexisting medical problems can be conceptualized in two ways. There are certain co-morbid conditions that are commonly associated with asthma, such as nasal polyps, allergic rhinitis, sinusitis, and eczema. In addition, there are coexisting medical problems that may be unrelated to asthma, but their identification and management have important implications for asthma therapy and control. Such possible co-morbidities include glaucoma, hypertension, gastroesophageal reflux, diabetes mellitus, arthritis, and/or a history of current malignancies.[20]

DIAGNOSTICS

A diagnosis of asthma is based on three components: (1) demonstration of episodic symptoms of airflow obstruction (e.g., wheeze, cough, shortness of breath), (2) evidence that airflow obstruction is at least partially reversible, and (3) exclusion of other conditions from the differential diagnosis.[4,20] A thorough history and physical examination are essential to making the diagnosis of asthma. Physical findings can be helpful in identifying significant obstruction as it occurs, but at best provide only a crude estimate of the degree of obstruction. However, significant obstruction may not be manifested as an abnormal physical finding; in addition, findings are likely to be completely normal between episodes. In fact, reduced expiratory flow rates ([FEV_1]) and increased airway resistance may not be recognized as dyspnea until a 30% to 40% decline in FEV_1 has occurred.[13] Thus objective measures of pulmonary function, such as spirometry and peak flow meters, are essential in establishing the diagnosis of asthma, as well as in assessing the severity of asthma. Spirometry is now recommended (1) at the time of initial assessment to confirm the diagnosis of asthma, (2) after treatment is initiated and symptoms and peak expiratory flow (PEF) have been stabilized, and (3) at least every 1 to 2 years.[4]

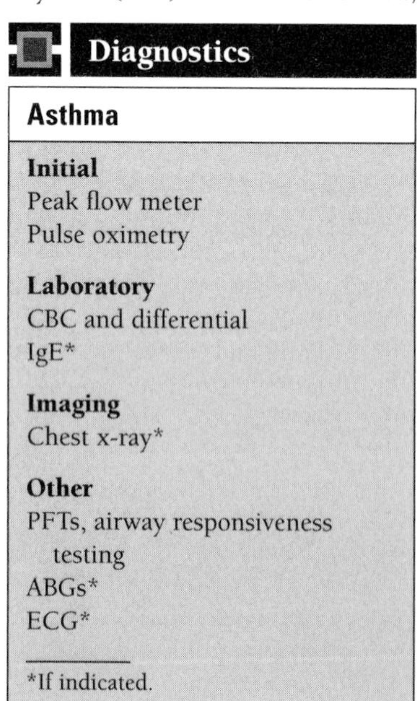
Diagnostics

Asthma

Initial
Peak flow meter
Pulse oximetry

Laboratory
CBC and differential
IgE*

Imaging
Chest x-ray*

Other
PFTs, airway responsiveness testing
ABGs*
ECG*

*If indicated.

Although spirometry provides many measures, the most useful for evaluating asthma include the peak expiratory flow rate (PEFR), the FEV_1, the maximum mid-expiratory flow rate (MMEFR), and the forced vital capacity (FVC). Results are compared with expected values, derived from a population of healthy, nonsmoking adults, and are expressed as a percentage of the expected value.

Decreased rates of airflow throughout the vital capacity are the most common pulmonary function abnormality in mild asthma as reflected by abnormalities in the PEFR, the FEV_1, and the MMEFR (forced expiratory flow [FEF_{25-75}]). During bronchospasm, spirometry reveals obstruction with a decrease in FEV_1 and decreased MMEFR. The FEV_1 to FVC is also reduced. As obstruction increases, an increased residual volume and functional residual are noted. One of the diagnostic hallmarks of asthma is reversal of obstruction after the administration of a bronchodilator, which corresponds both with clinical improvement and with improved spirometric values. In addition to helping establish the diagnosis of asthma, spirometry helps assess the adequacy of therapy, the need for further therapy and evaluation during emergencies, or the need for hospital admission. The severity of asthma attacks must be assessed by accurate and reproducible measures of airflow. Health care providers tend to underestimate the degree of airway obstruction in individuals with acute asthma, and knowledge of a person's pulmonary function has potentially important implications for treatment. For this reason, the NAEPP guidelines recommend the use of pulmonary function testing as part of the assessment and monitoring during the treatment of acute asthma.[21] During a severe asthma attack, recording of the entire spirogram may be difficult, but the FEV_1 can still be measured. As the asthma attack resolves, both the PEFR and the FEV_1 increase, whereas the MMEFR usually remains significantly diminished.[2]

Other laboratory tests that may be used to diagnose asthma or be included as part of the evaluation include airway responsiveness testing, arterial blood and other serum analysis, radiography, an electrocardiogram (ECG), and sputum cultures. Airway responsiveness testing measures the bronchoconstrictor response elicited by a standard stimulus. The FEV_1 is measured after inhalation of an aerosol containing graded amounts of a bronchoconstrictor agonist. The most common bronchoconstrictors used are methacholine and histamine.[2]

Individuals with asthma often have atopy, which is often reflected in blood eosinophilia as high as 4% to 8%. In addition, IgE serum levels are also often elevated. In fact, epidemiologic studies indicate that asthma is unusual in individuals with low IgE levels.[2]

Generally, the chest radiographs of individuals with asthma are normal. Therefore chest radiography is not indicated in the routine evaluation of patients with asthma unless physical examination findings are suggestive of infectious illness or respiratory complications such as pneumomediastinum and pneumothorax. If an asthma exacerbation is severe enough to warrant hospital admission, a chest x-ray film should be taken. The x-ray film may show hyperinflation (indicated by diaphragmatic depression) and abnormally translucent lung fields.[2]

Between asthma attacks, in the absence of respiratory infection, the sputum is usually clear. During an asthma attack, even in the absence of infection, the sputum may be yellow to green. This does not necessarily indicate infection; the color change may be from eosinophil peroxidase. Sputum cultures are generally not obtained unless there is suspicion of an acute infectious respiratory infection.[2]

An ECG is not part of the routine evaluation of a patient with asthma. If it is obtained during an asthma exacerbation, an ECG in the absence of cardiac disease is usually significant only for sinus tachycardia. In severe attacks, right axis deviation, right bundle branch block, cor pulmonale, or even ST-T wave abnormalities may occur. If these abnormalities resolve as the asthma attack abates, no further cardiac evaluation is necessary. ECG findings should be monitored during asthma attacks for individuals with significant cardiac disease to monitor for myocardial infarction, which can result from attack-induced stress.[13]

DIFFERENTIAL DIAGNOSIS

The medical conditions most likely to be confused with asthma involve the upper respiratory system (e.g., croup, vocal cord dysfunction) and lower respiratory system (e.g., pneumonia, chronic obstructive pulmonary disease [COPD]), the cardiovascular system (e.g., valvular disease and cardiomyopathy), and the gastrointestinal system (e.g., gastroesophageal reflux disease [GERD]).[20]

Not all wheezing is due to asthma, and other causes should be excluded before a diagnosis of asthma is made. Spirometry can be used to help differentiate asthma from other possible conditions in the differential diagnosis. An FEV_1 of 80% of predicted or less with a reduced FEV_1/FVC ratio that normalizes or significantly improves with bronchodilator therapy raises the suspicion of asthma. Other causes of wheezing and upper airway obstruction include tracheomalacia, tracheal or bronchial masses, and laryngeal (vocal cord) dysfunction. The presence of stridor or focal wheezing on physical examination and with flow limitation on a flow volume loop are characteristic of tracheomalacia and tracheobronchial masses. Laryngeal dysfunction is caused by abnormal apposition of the vocal cords during the respiratory cycle and can generally be treated effectively by speech therapy. Laryngeal dysfunction is often initially misdiagnosed as asthma and often inappropriately treated with high-dose systemic steroids. Laryngoscopy is needed to confirm laryngeal dysfunction.[13]

Persons with COPD, including emphysema and chronic bronchitis, may have acute episodes of airway obstruction and wheezing, especially during exacerbations of their disease. COPD is often accompanied by a history of smoking, less response to bronchodilator therapy, and irreversible PFT changes over time. In addition, COPD may be distinguished from asthma by signs of hyperinflation, such as diminished breath sounds, decreased heart sounds, and a flattened diaphragm. Chest wall deformities are suggestive of restrictive lung diseases. Dullness to percussion may indicate the presence of pneumonia or a pleural effusion. Foreign body aspiration should be considered if lateralizing wheezes are heard.[13,20]

Alpha$_1$-antitrypsin (AAT) deficiency is an inherited disorder, caused by an inborn error in the liver's production of AAT, which is the dominant protease in the lung and which protects alveoli from the destructive effects of serine proteases. AAT deficiency causes a syndrome of abnormalities including neonatal jaundice, airflow obstruction, premature emphysema, and cirrhosis of the liver.[22,23] The primary respiratory effect of AAT deficiency is degradation of the protein elastin, a protein that is essential for the elastic recoil required for pulmonary expiratory function. As a result, chronic persistent airflow obstruction develops. AAT deficiency is a well-established cause of panacinar emphysema, but its role in the pathophysiology of asthma is less well understood. The prevalence of AAT deficiency is about 0.01% to 0.02% in those with emphysema; the prevalence of AAT deficiency among patients with asthma is not known.[22] Individuals with AAT deficiency often have symptoms similar to those of bronchial asthma; pulmonary function may be normal, especially among those who do not smoke. Hence, a diagnosis of AAT deficiency is often missed or delayed. However, bronchopulmonary infections are common in persons with AAT deficiency, and their family history almost always includes lung disease. Asthmatic patients with AAT generally have more severe disease and often respond less to bronchodilators than do those without the disorder. Primary care providers should have a high level of suspicion for AAT deficiency in young persons whose symptoms do not respond to appropriate asthma therapy, especially in the absence of smoking. Diagnosis of AAT deficiency is based on AAT serum levels but may also involve other diagnostic measurements, including pulmonary function testing, chest radiography, serum electrophoresis, and genotyping. Although there are some similarities in the management of AAT deficiency, there are also important differences; diagnosis of AAT has critical implications for an individual's prognosis and quality of life.[23]

Differential Diagnosis

Asthma	
Acute bronchiolitis (infectious, chemical)	Chronic obstructive pulmonary disease (chronic bronchitis or emphysema)
Airway obstruction by masses	Cystic fibrosis
Central thoracic tumors	Endobronchial sarcoid
Metastatic cancer	Eosinophilia pneumonia
Primary lung tumors	Foreign body aspiration
Substernal thyroid tumors	Interstitial fibrosis
Alpha$_1$-antitrysin deficiency	Pleural effusion
Aspiration (foreign body)	Pulmonary emboli
Bronchiolitis obliterans organizing pneumonia	Systemic mastocytosis
Bronchial stenosis	Systemic vasculitis (polyarteritis nodosa)
Carcinoid syndrome	Tracheomalacia
Cardiac failure	

MANAGEMENT

Although the role of inflammation in the pathogenesis of asthma was recognized in the earlier 1991 NHLBI guidelines on asthma management, asthma is now defined as a chronic inflammatory disease of the airways.[24] This new understanding of asthma pathology also suggests that much of asthma care will be provided by individuals and their families outside of and away from health care institutions and practitioners. In addition, inflammation is now understood to be one of the preeminent problems in asthma, which has shifted the focus of treatment from symptomatic to preventive therapy, including the need for antiinflammatory medications, environmental controls, and patient education.[12] The NAEPP of the NHLBI has identified six goals of asthma treatment (Box 108-2).

The NHLBI Expert Panel for the Diagnosis and Management of Asthma has developed a classification system of asthma severity based on the frequency and severity of symptoms.

Characteristics of each of these categories are presented in Table 108-2. According to the guidelines, individuals should be assigned to the most severe asthma category in which any characteristic occurs. The major change from previous classification systems is the division of asthmatic patients into those with and those without mild persistent symptoms. This distinction has important clinical implications because, in general, the only persons not requiring antiinflammatory medications are those with intermittent symptoms.

Asthma pharmacotherapy is determined by the severity of the disease, and a summary of disease classification and corresponding recommended medications is found in Table 108-3. The most effective medications for long-term control of asthma continue to be those with antiinflammatory effects, including the inhaled corticosteroids, mast-cell stabilizers such as cromolyn, long-acting $beta_2$-adrenergic agonists, and the leukotriene modifiers. These medications are referred to in the Expert Panel Report (EPR) 2 as long-term–control medications to emphasize their role in achieving and maintaining control of persistent asthma (Tables 108-4 and 108-5). Relief of exacerbations and control of acute symptoms are achieved through the use of "quick-relief medications," chief among them being the short-acting $beta_2$-adrenergic agonists, but also including anticholinergic and systemic glucocorticoids (Table 108-6). The new EPR guidelines also emphasize a stepwise management approach in which therapies should be initiated at higher levels (steps, not dosages) to establish control as quickly as possible. After control has been achieved, therapy should be tapered for long-term management.[25] Despite the fact that the approach to asthma therapy has been recommended by the NHLBI since 1991, studies indicate that there remains an overreliance on

BOX 108-2

GOALS OF ASTHMA TREATMENT

- Prevent chronic and troublesome symptoms (e.g., coughing or breathlessness in the night, in the early morning, or after exertion).
- Maintain (near) "normal" pulmonary function.
- Maintain normal activity levels (including exercise and other physical activity).
- Prevent recurrent exacerbations of asthma and minimize the need for emergency department visits or hospitalizations.
- Provide optimal pharmacotherapy with minimal or no adverse effects.
- Meet patients' and families' expectation of and satisfaction with asthma care.

From National Institutes of Health, National Heart, Lung and Blood Institute: *1997 Guidelines for the diagnosis and management of asthma: highlights of the Expert Panel Report 2*, Pub No 97-4051A, Washington DC, 1997, US Government Printing Office.

TABLE 108-2 Stepwise Approach for Managing Asthma in Adults and Children Over 5 Years of Age

GOALS OF ASTHMA TREATMENT

- Prevent chronic and troublesome symptoms (e.g., coughing or breathlessness in the night, in the early morning, or after exertion)
- Maintain (near) "normal" pulmonary function
- Maintain normal activity levels (including exercise and other physical activity)
- Prevent recurrent exacerbations of asthma and minimize the need for emergency department visits or hospitalizations
- Provide optimal pharmacotherapy with minimal or no adverse effects
- Meet patients' and families' expectation of and satisfaction with asthma care

CLASSIFICATION OF SEVERITY: CLINICAL FEATURES BEFORE TREATMENT*

	Symptoms†	Nighttime Symptoms	Lung Function
STEP 4 Severe persistent	Continual symptoms Limited physical activity Frequent exacerbations	Frequent	FEV_1 or PEF ≤60% predicted PEF variability >30%
STEP 3 Moderate persistent	Daily symptoms Daily use of inhaled short-acting $beta_2$ agonist Exacerbations affect activity Exacerbations ≥2 times per week; may last days	>1 time per week	FEV_1 or PEF >61% ≤80% predicted PEF variability >30%
STEP 2 Mild persistent	Symptoms >2 times per week but <1 time per day Exacerbations may affect activity	>2 times per month	FEV_1 or PEF ≥80% predicted PEF variability 20%-30%
STEP 1 Mild intermittent	Symptoms ≤2 times per week Asymptomatic and normal PEF between exacerbations Exacerbations brief (from a few hours to a few days); intensity may vary	≤2 times per month	FEV_1 or PEF ≥80% predicted PEF variability <20%

From National Institutes of Health, National Heart, Lung, and Blood Institute: *Highlights of the Expert Panel Report 2: guidelines for the diagnosis and management of asthma*, NIH pub no 97-4051A, Washington DC, 1997, US Department of Health and Human Services.

*The presence of one of the features of severity is sufficient to place a patient in that category. An individual should be assigned to the most severe grade in which any feature occurs. The characteristics noted in this table are general and may overlap because asthma is highly variable. Furthermore, an individual's classification may change over time.

†Patients at any level of severity can have mild, moderate, or severe exacerbations. Some patients with intermittent asthma experience severe and life-threatening exacerbations separated by long periods of normal lung function and no symptoms.

TABLE 108-3 Stepwise Approach for Managing Asthma in Adults and Children Over 5 Years of Age Treatment

	Long-Term Control	Quick Relief	Education
Preferred treatments are in bold print.			
STEP 4 Severe persistent	*Daily medication:* **Antiinflammatory: inhaled corticosteroid (high dose)** *and* Long-acting bronchodilator: either long-acting inhaled beta$_2$ agonist, sustained-release theophylline, or long-acting beta$_2$-agonist tablets *and* Corticosteroid tablets or syrup long term (2 mg/kg/day, generally do not exceed 60 mg/day).	Short-acting bronchodilator: **inhaled beta$_2$ agonists** as needed for symptoms. Intensity of treatment will depend on severity of exacerbation. Use of short-acting inhaled beta$_2$ agonists on a daily basis or increasing use indicates the need for additional long-term–control therapy.	*Steps 2 and 3 actions plus:* Refer to individual education/counseling.
STEP 3 Moderate persistent	*Daily medication:* Either **Antiinflammatory: inhaled corticosteroid (medium dose)** *or* Inhaled corticosteroids (low-medium dose) and add a long-acting bronchodilator, especially for nighttime symptoms: either **long-acting inhaled beta$_2$ agonist,** sustained-release theophylline, or long-acting beta$_2$-agonist tablets. If needed Antiinflammatory: inhaled corticosteroids (medium-high dose) *and* Long-acting bronchodilator, especially for nighttime symptoms; either **long-acting inhaled beta$_2$ agonist,** sustained-release theophylline, or long-acting beta$_2$-agonist tablets.	Short-acting bronchodilator: **inhaled beta$_2$ agonists** as needed for symptoms. Intensity of treatment will depend on severity of exacerbation. Use of short-acting inhaled beta$_2$ agonists on a daily basis or increasing use indicates the need for additional long-term–control therapy.	*Step 1 actions plus:* Teach self-monitoring. Refer to group education if available. Review and update self-management plan.
STEP 2 Mild persistent	*Daily medication:* **Antiinflammatory:** either **inhaled corticosteroid** (low doses) or **cromolyn or nedocromil** (children usually begin with a trial of cromolyn or nedocromil). Sustained-release theophylline to serum concentration of 5-15 μg/mL is an alternative. Zafirlukast or zileuton may also be considered for patients ≥12 years of age, although their position in therapy is not fully established.	Short-acting bronchodilator: **inhaled beta$_2$ agonists** as needed for symptoms. Intensity of treatment will depend on severity of exacerbation. Use of short-acting inhaled beta$_2$ agonists on a daily basis or increasing use indicates the need for additional long-term–control therapy.	*Step 1 actions plus:* Teach self-monitoring. Refer to group education if available. Review and update self-management plan.

From National Institutes of Health, National Heart, Lung, and Blood Institute: *Highlights of the Expert Panel Report 2: guidelines for the diagnosis and management of asthma,* NIH pub no 97-4051A, Washington DC, 1997, US Department of Health and Human Services.

Notes:

- The stepwise approach presents general guidelines to assist clinical decision making; it is not intended to be a specific prescription. Asthma is highly variable; clinicians should tailor specific medication plans to the needs and circumstances of individual patients.
- Gain control as quickly as possible, then decrease treatment to the least medication necessary to maintain control. Gaining control may be accomplished either by starting treatment at the step most appropriate to the initial severity of the condition or by starting at a higher level of therapy (e.g., a course of systemic corticosteroids or higher dose of inhaled corticosteroids).
- A rescue course of systemic corticosteroid may be needed at any time and at any step.
- Some patients with intermittent asthma experience severe and life-threatening exacerbations separated by long periods of normal lung function and no symptoms. This may be especially common with exacerbations provoked by respiratory infections. A short course of systemic corticosteroids is recommended.
- At each step, patients should control their environment to avoid or control factors that make their asthma worse (e.g., allergens, irritants); this requires specific diagnosis and education.

continued

TABLE 108-3 Stepwise Approach for Managing Asthma in Adults and Children Over 5 Years of Age Treatment—cont'd

	Long-Term Control	Quick Relief	Education
STEP 1 Mild intermittent	No daily medication needed.	Short-acting bronchodilator: **inhaled $beta_2$ agonists** as needed for symptoms. Intensity of treatment will depend on severity of exacerbation. Use of short-acting inhaled $beta_2$ agonists more than 2 times a week may indicate the need to initiate long-term–control therapy.	Teach basic facts about asthma. Teach inhaler/spacer/holding chamber technique. Discuss roles of medications. Develop self-management plan. Develop action plan for when and how to take rescue actions. Discuss appropriate environmental control measures to avoid exposure to known allergens and irritants.
↓Step down Review treatment every 1 to 6 months; a gradual stepwise reduction in treatment may be possible.		**↑Step up** If control is not maintained, consider step up. First, review patient medication technique, adherence, and environmental control (avoidance of allergens or other factors that contribute to asthma severity).	

From National Institutes of Health, National Heart, Lung, and Blood Institute: *Highlights of the Expert Panel Report 2: guidelines for the diagnosis and management of asthma,* NIH pub no 97-4051A, Washington DC, 1997, US Department of Health and Human Services.

TABLE 108-4 Long-Term–Control Medications

Name/Products	Indications/Mechanisms	Potential Adverse Effects	Therapeutic Issues
CORTICOSTEROIDS (GLUCOCORTICOIDS)			
Inhaled Beclomethasone dipropionate Budesonide Flunisolide Fluticasone propionate Triamcinolone acetonide	***Indications*** Long-term prevention of symptoms; suppression, control, and reversal of inflammation. Reduce need for oral corticosteroids. ***Mechanisms*** **Antiinflammatory.** Block late reaction to allergen and reduce airway hyperresponsiveness. Inhibit cytokine production, adhesion protein activation, and inflammatory cell migration and activation. Reverse $beta_2$ receptor down-regulation, inhibit microvascular leakage.	Cough, dysphonia, oral thrush (candidiasis). In high doses systemic effects may occur, although studies are not conclusive and clinical significance of these effects has not been established (e.g., adrenal suppression, osteoporosis, growth suppression, skin thinning, and easy bruising.)	Spacer/holding chamber devices decrease local side effects and systemic absorption. Preparations are not absolutely interchangeable on a microgram or per-puff basis. New delivery devices may provide greater delivery to airways, which may affect dose. The risks of uncontrolled asthma should be weighed against the limited risks of inhaled corticosteroids. Dexamethasone is not included because it is highly absorbed and has long-term suppressive side effects.
Systemic Methylprednisolone Prednisolone Prednisone	***Indications*** For short-term (3-10 days) "burst": to gain prompt control of inadequately controlled persistent asthma. For long-term prevention of symptoms in severe persistent asthma: suppression, control, and reversal of inflammation. ***Mechanisms*** Same as inhaled.	Short-term use: reversible abnormalities in glucose metabolism, increased appetite, fluid retention, weight gain, mood alteration, hypertension, peptic ulcer and, rarely, aseptic necrosis of femur. Long-term use: adrenal axis suppression, skin thinning, hypertension, diabetes, Cushing's syndrome, cataracts, muscle weakness, and—in rare instances—impaired immune function. Consideration should be given to coexisting conditions that could be worsened by systemic corticosteroids, such as herpes virus infections, varicella, tuberculosis, hypertension, peptic ulcer, and *Strongyloides.*	Use at lowest effective dose. For long-term use, alternate-day AM dosing produces least toxicity. If daily doses are required, one study shows improved efficacy with no increase in adrenal suppression when administered at 3 PM rather than in the morning.

From National Institutes of Health, National Heart, Lung, and Blood Institute: *Highlights of the Expert Panel Report 2: guidelines for the diagnosis and management of asthma,* NIH pub no 97-4051A, Washington DC, 1997, US Department of Health and Human Services.

TABLE 108-4 Long-Term–Control Medications—cont'd

Name/Products	Indications/Mechanisms	Potential Adverse Effects	Therapeutic Issues
CROMOLYN SODIUM AND NEDOCROMIL			
Cromolyn Nedocromil	***Indications*** Long-term prevention of symptoms; may modify inflammation. Preventive treatment before exposure to exercise or known allergen. ***Mechanisms*** **Antiinflammatory.** Block early and late reaction to allergen. Interfere with chloride channel function. Stabilize mast cell membranes and inhibit activation and release of mediators from eosinophils and epithelial cells. Inhibit acute response to exercise, cold dry air, and sulfur dioxide.	15%-20% of patients complain of an unpleasant taste from nedocromil.	Therapeutic response often occurs within 2 weeks, but a 4- to 6-week trial may be needed to determine maximum benefit. Dose of cromolyn MDI (1 mg/puff) may be inadequate to affect airway hyperresponsiveness. Nebulizer delivery (20 mg/ampule) may be preferred for some patients. Safety is the primary advantage of these agents.
LONG-ACTING BETA$_2$ AGONISTS			
Inhaled Salmeterol	***Indications*** Long-term prevention of symptoms, especially nocturnal symptoms, *added to antiinflammatory therapy.* Prevention of exercise-induced bronchospasm. **Not to be used to treat acute symptoms or exacerbations.** ***Mechanisms*** **Bronchodilation.** Smooth muscle relaxation following adenylate cyclase activation and increase in cyclic AMP producing functional antagonism of bronchoconstriction. In vitro, inhibit mast cell mediator release, decrease vascular permeability, and increase mucociliary clearance. Compared to short-acting inhaled beta$_2$ agonist, salmeterol (but not formoterol) has slower onset of action (15-30 minutes) but a longer duration (>12 hours).	Tachycardia, skeletal muscle tremor, hypokalemia, prolongation of QT$_c$ interval in overdose. A diminished bronchoprotective effect may occur within 1 week of chronic therapy. The clinical significance has not been established.	**Not to be used to treat acute symptoms or exacerbations.** Clinical significance of potentially developing tolerance is uncertain because studies show symptom control and bronchodilation are maintained. Should not be used in place of antiinflammatory therapy. May provide more effective symptom control when added to standard doses of inhaled corticosteroid compared to increasing the corticosteroid dosage.
Oral Albuterol, sustained release			Inhaled long-acting beta$_2$ agonists are preferred because they are longer acting and have fewer side effects than oral sustained-release agents.
METHYLXANTHINES			
Theophylline, sustained-release tablets and capsules	***Indications*** Long-term control and prevention of symptoms, especially nocturnal symptoms. ***Mechanisms*** **Bronchodilation.** Smooth muscle relaxation from phosphodiesterase inhibition and possibly adenosine antagonism. May affect eosinophilic infiltration into bronchial mucosa as well as decrease T-lymphocyte numbers in epithelium. Increases diaphragm contractility and mucociliary clearance.	Dose-related acute toxicities include tachycardia, nausea and vomiting, tachyarrhythmias (SVT), central nervous system stimulation, headache, seizures, hematemesis, hyperglycemia, and hypokalemia. Adverse effects at usual therapeutic doses include insomnia, gastric upset, aggravation of ulcer or reflux, increase in hyperactivity in some children, difficulty in urination in older males with prostatism.	Maintain steady-state serum concentrations between 5 and 15 μg/ml. Routine serum concentration monitoring is essential due to significant toxicities, narrow therapeutic range, and interindividual differences in metabolic clearance. Absorption and metabolism may be affected by numerous factors, which can produce significant changes in steady-state serum theophylline concentrations. Not generally recommended for exacerbations. There is minimal evidence for added benefit to optimal doses of inhaled beta$_2$ agonists. Serum concentration monitoring is mandatory.

continued

TABLE 108-4 Long-Term–Control Medications—cont'd

Name/Products	Indications/Mechanisms	Potential Adverse Effects	Therapeutic Issues
LEUKOTRIENE MODIFIERS			
Zafirlukast tablets	***Indications*** Long-term control and prevention of symptoms in mild persistent asthma for patients ≥12 years of age. ***Mechanisms*** **Leukotriene receptor antagonist.** Selective competitive inhibitor of LTD4 and LTE4 receptors.	No specific adverse effects to date. As with any new drug, there is the possibility of rare hypersensitivity or idiosyncratic reactions that cannot usually be detected in initial premarketing trials. One reported case of reversible hepatitis and hyperbilirubinemia; high concentrations may develop in patients with liver impairment.	Administration with meals decreases bioavailability; take at least 1 hour before or 2 hours after meals. Inhibits the metabolism of warfarin and increases prothrombin time; it is a competitive inhibitor of the CYP2C9 hepatic microsomal isozymes. (It has not affected the elimination of terfenadine, theophylline, or ethinyl estradiol drugs metabolized by the CYP3A4 isozymes.)
Zileuton tablets	***Indications*** Long-term control and prevention of symptoms in mild persistent asthma for patients ≥12 years of age. ***Mechanisms*** **5-lipoxygenase inhibitor.**	Elevation of liver enzymes has been reported. Limited case reports of reversible hepatitis and hyperbilirubinemia.	Zileuton is a microsomal CYP3A4 enzyme inhibitor that can inhibit the metabolism of terfenadine, warfarin, and theophylline. Doses of these drugs should be monitored accordingly. Monitor hepatic enzymes (ALT).
Montelukast tablets	***Indications*** Prophylaxis and treatment of asthma; not recommended for children <2 years of age ***Mechanisms*** Same as zafirlukast	Adults: Headache, fatigue, fever, GI upset Children: flu/cold symptoms, eye or leg pain, thirst	Not for primary treatment of acute attack; not for monotherapy in exercise-induced bronchospasm Caution when withdrawing from oral steroids Pregnancy category B, nursing mothers Monitor with drugs that induce CYP450 (e.g., rifampin, phenobarbital)

From National Institutes of Health, National Heart, Lung, and Blood Institute: *Highlights of the Expert Panel Report 2: guidelines for the diagnosis and management of asthma,* NIH pub no 97-4051A, Washington DC, 1997, US Department of Health and Human Services.

TABLE 108-5 Usual Dosages for Long-Term–Control Medications

Medication	Dosage Form	Adult Dose	Child Dose	Comments
SYSTEMIC CORTICOSTEROIDS				
Methylprednisolone	2, 4, 8, 16, 32 mg tablets	7.5-60 mg daily in a single dose or q.i.d. as needed for control Short-course "burst": 40-60 mg per day as single or 2 divided doses for 3-10 days	0.25-2 mg/kg daily in single dose or q.i.d. as needed for control Short course "burst": 1-2 mg/kg/day, maximum 60 mg/day, for 3-10 days	For long-term treatment of severe persistent asthma, administer single dose in AM either daily or on alternate days (alternate-day therapy may produce less adrenal suppression). If daily doses are required, one study suggests improved efficacy and no increase in adrenal suppression when administered at 3:00 PM. Short courses or "bursts" are effective for establishing control when initiating therapy or during a period of gradual deterioration. The burst should be continued until patient achieves 80% PEF personal best or symptoms resolve. This usually requires 3-10 days but may require longer. There is no evidence that tapering the dose following improvement prevents relapse.
Prednisolone	5 mg tablets, 5 mg/ml, 15 mg/ml solution			
Prednisone	1, 2.5, 5, 10, 20, 25 mg tablets, 5 mg/ml solution			
CROMOLYN AND NEDOCROMIL				
Cromolyn	MDI 1 mg/puff Nebulizer solution 20 mg/ampule	2-4 puffs t.i.d./q.i.d. 1 ampule t.i.d./q.i.d.	1-2 puffs t.i.d./q.i.d. 1 ampule t.i.d./q.i.d.	1 dose before exercise or allergen exposure provides effective prophylaxis for 1-2 hours.
Nedocromil	MDI 1.75 mg/puff	2-4 puffs b.i.d./q.i.d.	1-2 puffs t.i.d./q.i.d.	See cromolyn above.

From National Institutes of Health, National Heart, Lung, and Blood Institute: *Highlights of the Expert Panel Report 2: guidelines for the diagnosis and management of asthma,* NIH pub no 97-4051A, Washington DC, 1997, US Department of Health and Human Services.

TABLE 108-5 Usual Dosages for Long-Term–Control Medications—cont'd

Medication	Dosage Form	Adult Dose	Child Dose	Comments
LONG-ACTING $BETA_2$ AGONISTS				
	Inhaled			
Salmeterol	MDI 21 μg/puff, 60 or 120 puffs	2 puffs q 12 hr	1-2 puffs q 12 hr	May use 1 dose nightly for symptoms.
	DPI 50 μg/blister	1 blister q 12 hr	1 blister q 12 hr	Should not be used as a rescue inhaler for symptom relief or for exacerbations.
	Tablet			
Sustained-release albuterol	4 mg tablet	4 mg q 12 hr	0.3-0.6 mg/kg/day, not to exceed 8 mg/day	
METHYLXANTHINES				
Theophylline (numerous manufactures)	Liquids Sustained-release tablets and capsules	Starting dose 10 mg/kg/day up to 300 mg maximum; usual maximum 800 mg/day	Starting dose: 10 mg/kg/day; usual maximum: ≥1 year of age: 16 mg/kg/day <1 year: 0.2 × (age in weeks) + 5 = mg/kg/day	Adjust dosage to achieve serum concentration of 5-15 μg/ml at steady state (at least 48 hours on same dosage). Due to wide interpatient variability in theophylline metabolic clearance, **routine serum theophylline level monitoring is important.** See below for factors that can affect levels.
LEUKOTRIENE MODIFIERS				
Zafirlukast	20 mg tablet	40 mg daily (1 tablet b.i.d.)		For zafirlukast, administration with meals decreases bioavailability; take at least 1 hour before or 2 hours after meals.
Zileuton	300 mg tablet 600 mg tablet	2400 mg daily (two 300 mg tablets or one 600 mg tablet, q.i.d.)		For zileuton, monitor hepatic enzymes (ALT).

TABLE 108-6 Quick-Relief Medications

Name/Products	Indications/Mechanisms	Potential Adverse Effects	Therapeutic Issues
SHORT-ACTING INHALED $BETA_2$ AGONISTS			
Albuterol Bitolterol Pirbuterol Terbutaline	***Indications*** Relief of acute symptoms; quick-relief medication. Preventive treatment before exercise for exercise-induced bronchospasm. ***Mechanisms*** **Bronchodilation.** Smooth muscle relaxation following adenylate cyclase activation and increase in cyclic AMP producing functional antagonism of bronchoconstriction.	Tachycardia, skeletal muscle tremor, hypokalemia, increased lactic acid, headache, hyperglycemia. Inhaled route, in general, causes few systemic adverse effects. Patients with preexisting cardiovascular disease, especially older adults, may have adverse cardiovascular reactions with inhaled therapy.	Drugs of choice for acute bronchospasm. Inhaled route has faster onset, fewer adverse effects, and is more effective than systemic route. The less $beta_2$-selective agents (isoproterenol, metaproterenol, isoetharine, and epinephrine) are not recommended due to their potential for excessive cardiac stimulation, especially in high doses. Albuterol liquid is not recommended. For patients with mild intermittent asthma who are not taking antiinflammatory medication, regularly scheduled daily use neither harms nor benefits asthma control. Regularly scheduled daily use is not generally recommended. Increasing use or lack of expected effect indicates inadequate asthma control. >1 canister a month (e.g., albuterol—200 puffs per canister) may indicate overreliance on this drug; ≥2 canisters in 1 month poses additional adverse risks. For patients frequently using a $beta_2$ agonist, antiinflammatory medication should be initiated or intensified.

From National Institutes of Health, National Heart, Lung, and Blood Institute: *Highlights of the Expert Panel Report 2: guidelines for the diagnosis and management of asthma,* NIH pub no 97-4051A, Washington DC, 1997, US Department of Health and Human Services.

continued

TABLE 108-6 Quick-Relief Medications—cont'd

Name/Products	Indications/Mechanisms	Potential Adverse Effects	Therapeutic Issues
ANTICHOLINERGICS			
Ipratropium bromide	***Indications*** Relief of acute bronchospasm (see Therapeutic Issues column). ***Mechanisms*** **Bronchodilation.** Competitive inhibition of muscarinic cholinergic receptors. Reduces intrinsic vagal tone to the airways. May block reflex bronchoconstriction secondary to irritants or to reflux esophagitis. May decrease mucous gland secretions.	Drying of mouth and respiratory secretions, increased wheezing in some individuals, blurred vision if sprayed in eyes.	Reverses only cholinergically mediated bronchospasm; does not modify reaction to antigen. Does not block exercise-induced bronchospasm. May provide additive effects to $beta_2$ agonist but has slower onset of action. Is an alternative for patients with intolerance to $beta_2$ agonists. Treatment of choice for bronchospasm due to beta-blocker medication.
CORTICOSTEROIDS			
Systemic Methylprednisolone Prednisolone Prednisone	***Indications*** For moderate-to-severe exacerbations to prevent the progression of exacerbation, reverse inflammation, speed recovery, and reduce rate of relapse. ***Mechanisms*** **Antiinflammatory.**	Short-term use: reversible abnormalities in glucose metabolism, increased appetite, fluid retention, weight gain, mood alteration, hypertension, peptic ulcer and, rarely, aseptic necrosis of femur. Consideration should be given to coexisting conditions that could be worsened by systemic corticosteroids, such as herpes virus infections, varicella, tuberculosis, hypertension, peptic ulcer, and *Strongyloides*.	Short-term therapy should continue until patient achieves 80% PEF personal best or symptoms resolve. This usually requires 3-10 days but may require longer. There is no evidence that tapering the dose following improvement prevents relapse.

short-acting bronchodilators and underuse of antiinflammatory medications on the part of both practitioners and persons with asthma. This suggests that the underlying pathophysiology of asthma and its implications for therapy are still not widely understood. As emphasized in the EPR stepwise approach, all patients except those with mild, intermittent asthma benefit from maintenance antiinflammatory medication. The use of antiinflammatory medications for maintenance (long-term control) of mild to moderate asthma results in fewer asthma exacerbations, fewer emergency department visits, decreased cost of care, fewer school or work days missed, and an improved quality of life.[18]

An integral component of asthma management is the treatment of coexisting diseases, including rhinitis, sinusitis, and GERD. Intranasal glucocorticoids may be helpful in the management of chronic rhinitis, whereas antibiotics are indicated for bacterial sinus infections. Annual influenza vaccine is recommended for all persons with persistent asthma. For persons with GERD, acid suppressive therapy may decrease asthma symptoms. Individuals with GERD often do not describe symptoms suggestive of GERD; approximately 25% to 30% of patients with asthma have clinically silent reflux.[26]

Given the known role of environmental triggers in the pathophysiology of asthma, it is essential that environmental interventions be implemented along with clinical approaches in the management of asthma. Interventions at the household level must include efforts to eliminate cockroaches, rodents, and mold. Individual efforts to sustain pest-free environments, especially in apartment complexes, will be effective only if efforts at the building, neighborhood, and city level are in place to bolster those efforts.

Medications

Long-Term Control Medications

Corticosteroids. Corticosteroids are the most potent and effective antiinflammatory medications available for the treatment of moderate to severe asthma. Although the mechanism of action is not completely understood, they have been shown to reduce the synthesis of inflammatory mediators and to inhibit late responses to allergen (those occurring several hours after allergen exposure). Their ability to inhibit a wide variety of inflammatory responses probably accounts for their effectiveness in many types of asthma. Inhaled corticosteroids are the most effective long-term therapy for persistent asthma and are recommended for every individual with persistent asthma symptoms. Inhaled corticosteroids are generally well tolerated in low to moderate doses and have fewer side effects for a given level of therapeutic effect. There is no consensus on the specific type or dose of inhaled steroid to be used. In general, dosage begins with 2 to 4 puffs per day and is increased based on the individual's response. Each of the inhaled steroids has its own maximum number of doses per day.

High-potency inhaled corticosteroids, budesonide (Pulmicort) and fluticasone (Flovent), provide the same therapeutic effect as other inhaled corticosteroids but in fewer puffs. Both drugs come in preparations of different potencies; therefore with the higher-potency inhalers, fewer puffs are necessary to deliver the same dose as compared with other types of steroid inhalers.

The major side effect of inhaled steroids is oral thrush, which can be prevented by good oral hygiene and the use of aerosol spacers during delivery. The safety of long-term therapy with high-dose inhaled steroids has not been well established, and their use may be associated with untoward side effects, including adrenal suppression, bone loss, skin bruising, glaucoma, behavioral abnormalities, and the possibility of inhibited growth in children. It is still unknown whether the use of high-potency steroids increases the risk of adrenal suppression and other systemic side effects.[2,18,24]

Systemic corticosteroids are used in the management of asthma symptoms not responding to standard treatment. In general, a steroid "pulse" with initial doses of prednisone of 40 to 60 mg/day and tapered to zero over the ensuing 1 to 2 weeks is prescribed. If symptoms reexacerbate during this period, the dose is increased and the taper restarted. For persons not responding to a prednisone taper or with life-threatening symptoms, in-hospital treatment is necessary and IV methylprednisolone is often used.[2] Untoward side effects of systemic corticosteroids include hypothalamic adrenal axis suppression, electrolyte imbalances, myopathy, osteoporosis, peptic ulcer, dermal atrophy, carbohydrate intolerance, increased intracranial pressure, and psychiatric disturbances.

Cromolyn and Nedocromil. Cromolyn sodium (Intal) and nedocromil sodium (Tilade) are antiinflammatory agents whose specific mechanism of action is not yet well understood. Both are used in the prophylaxis of mild to moderate asthma, rather than for the treatment of acute symptoms. Both of these agents are more useful when exposure to an identifiable exposure triggers symptoms, such as exercise, cold air, or animal dander. These agents may be useful prophylactically when a known asthma trigger cannot be avoided. In such situations they may be good alternatives to inhaled steroids because they have a better safety and side effect profile. Both agents tend to be more useful in the pediatric population than in the adult population. In addition, if it is effective in controlling symptoms, nedocromil may be preferred to corticosteroid therapy during pregnancy for safety reasons. Nedocromil may also be particularly helpful in persons whose primary asthma symptom is cough. Nedocromil is the more potent of the two agents and has the advantage of twice-daily dosing. It is not well tolerated in up to 12% of patients because of a perceived bitter taste or throat irritation.

Xanthine Derivatives. Xanthine derivatives, such as theophylline, are used for long-term asthma management and sustained relief of symptoms. Theophylline and aminophylline have a long history of use in asthma and have been traditionally considered to be bronchodilators of moderate potency. Recent evidence suggests they may have other beneficial effects in asthma, including an inotropic effect on the diaphragm and antiinflammatory activity. One of the major difficulties with using theophylline is its relatively narrow therapeutic index and the potentially significant variations in plasma levels, both in a single individual and within a population over time. A number of drugs affect the metabolism of theophylline, and careful monitoring of serum levels during treatment is recommended (Table 108-7). Acceptable therapeutic plasma levels are between 10 and 20 μg/ml, although clinical improvement has been noted at "subtherapeutic levels." Higher plasma levels are associated with gastrointestinal, cardiac, and central nervous system toxicity, including such symptoms as headache, nausea, vomiting, diarrhea, cardiac arrhythmias, and seizures.[2]

The use of theophylline in asthma management has declined with the availability of other maintenance medications that have fewer side effects and do not require monitoring of serum levels. Nonetheless, theophylline may be useful in certain situations (e.g., as an additional agent to inhaled corticosteroids when better long-term control is still needed).

Leukotriene Modifiers. Two of the newest medications for asthma include the antileukotriene agents zafirlukast (Accolate) and zileuton (Zyflo). These antiinflammatory agents target a single group of inflammatory mediators; they interfere with the effects of leukotrienes by either blocking the leukotriene receptor or reducing the activity of enzymes required for leukotriene synthesis. As inflammatory mediators, leukotrienes increase endothelial permeability, which increases airway edema and mucus secretion, further increasing airway obstruction. In addition, the leukotrienes directly potentiate bronchoconstriction mediated by leukotriene receptors on bronchial smooth muscle.[18] In persons with persistent asthma the leukotriene modifiers have been shown to increase persistent bronchodilation, reduce asthma symptoms, including nocturnal asthma symptoms, reduce medication use, and decrease the need for prednisone quick-relief therapy.[2] Both drugs can increase prothrombin times in persons receiving anticoagulant therapy; prothrombin times should be monitored more closely in these cases.

Zafirlukast and montelukast are oral leukotriene-receptor antagonists, which prevent the binding of leukotrienes at receptor sites. Zafirlukast has a relatively rapid onset of action, and its effects are additive with beta-adrenergic bronchodilators. It has been shown to be helpful in reducing cold air-, exercise-, and allergen-induced bronchoconstriction and nocturnal asthma symptoms. In clinical trials the most common side effects included headache, gastritis, pharyngitis, and rhinitis, although these symptoms occurred with the same frequency in placebo groups. Zafirlukast should be taken on an empty stomach. The other leukotriene-receptor antagonist, montelukast, is also rapidly absorbed after oral administration, with peak plasma levels achieved in 2.5 to 4 hours, depending on the dose. Montelukast is to be used in conjunction with other asthma therapies for the prophylaxis and chronic treatment of asthma. It should not be used as monotherapy for the treatment

TABLE 108-7 Factors Affecting Serum Theophylline Concentrations*

Factor	Decreases Theophylline Concentrations	Increases Theophylline Concentrations	Recommended Action
Food	↓ Or delays absorption of some sustained-release theophylline (SRT) products	↑ Rate of absorption (fatty foods) products	Select theophylline preparation that is not affected by food.
Diet	↑ Metabolism (high protein)	↓ Metabolism (high carbohydrate)	Inform patients that major changes in diet are not recommended while taking theophylline.
Systemic, febrile viral illness (e.g., influenza)		↓ Metabolism	Decrease theophylline dose according to serum concentration level. Decrease dose by 50% if serum concentration measurement is not available.
Hypoxia, cor pulmonale, and decompensated congestive heart failure, cirrhosis		↓ Metabolism	Decrease dose according to serum concentration level.
Age	↑ Metabolism (1 to 9 years)	↓ Metabolism (<6 months, older adults)	Adjust dose according to serum concentration level.
Phenobarbital, phenytoin, carbamazepine	↑ Metabolism		Increase dose according to serum concentration level.
Cimetidine		↓ Metabolism	Use alternative H_2 blocker (e.g., famotidine or ranitidine).
Macrolides: TAO, erythromycin, clarithromycin		↓ Metabolism	Use alternative antibiotic or adjust theophylline dose.
Quinolones: ciprofloxacin, enoxacin		↓ Metabolism	Use alternative antibiotic or adjust theophylline dose. Circumvent with ofloxacin if quinolone therapy is required.
Rifampin	↑ Metabolism		Increase dose according to serum concentration level.
Ticlopidine		↓ Metabolism	Decrease dose according to serum concentration level.
Smoking	↑ Metabolism		Advise patient to stop smoking; increase dose according to serum concentration level.

From National Institutes of Health, National Heart, Lung and Blood Institute: *Highlights of the Expert Panel Report 2: guidelines for the diagnosis and management of asthma,* NIH pub no 97-4051A, Washington DC, 1997, US Department of Health and Human Services.
*This list is not all inclusive; for discussion of other factors, see package inserts.

and management of exercise-induced bronchospasm and should also not be used for the treatment of acute asthma attacks. In clinical trials, the most common adverse side effects were similar to those associated with zafirlukast. In addition, in rare cases montelukast therapy has been associated with systemic eosinophilia, although a causal relationship has not been established.[27]

Zileuton is an oral leukotriene synthesis inhibitor with similar effects in clinical trials to the leukotriene receptor antagonists. Zileuton can be taken without regard to meals. In clinical trials zileuton therapy was associated with elevated liver enzyme levels in some subjects. For this reason, it is recommended that liver enzyme levels be obtained at baseline and monitored at regular intervals throughout the first year and periodically thereafter for persons receiving zileuton therapy. Its use is contraindicated in persons with active liver disease or with abnormal liver function tests. Zileuton also increases serum levels of theophylline, and in persons receiving concurrent theophylline therapy the dosage generally needs to be reduced by approximately 50%.[24] Several other antileukotriene agents are currently in clinical trials and are likely to receive Food and Drug Administration approval in the near future.

Because antileukotriene agents have only recently been approved for use in asthma management and because they are less potent than corticosteroids, specific guidelines for their use in asthma therapy have not yet been developed. Their use is recommended for the treatment of chronic persistent asthma. They may be helpful in reducing the quantity of inhaled or oral corticosteroids needed to control symptoms, which would be especially helpful for persons who experience troubling corticosteroid side effects. In addition, they may be effective alternatives to long-acting bronchodilators, such as salmeterol and theophylline. They may also be helpful for persons with aspirin-induced asthma, as they offer some protection against a variety of environmental substances that often produce cross-reactions in persons with aspirin sensitivities.[24]

Long-Acting Beta$_2$-Adrenergic Agonists. Salmeterol (Serevent) is currently the only long-acting bronchodilator, with an onset of action within 1 to 2 hours of administration and a duration of

10 to 14 hours. Because of its slow onset of action, salmeterol should never be used as a quick-relief medication for short-term relief of acute symptoms. The best use for long-acting beta$_2$-adrenergic agonists has not yet been determined. Salmeterol has been used effectively in controlling nocturnal asthma symptoms. In addition, salmeterol may be effective in controlling anticipated exercise-induced asthma and may mitigate the need to use short-acting bronchodilators before each activity. When salmeterol is prescribed, patients need to be specifically instructed not to use this drug for relief of acute bronchospasm.[2,24]

Quick-Relief Medications

Short-Acting Beta$_2$-Adrenergic Agonists. Short-acting beta$_2$-adrenergic agonists (bronchodilators) act as bronchodilators by relaxing airway smooth muscle that has become constricted as a result of stimuli in the environment (Table 108-8). Short-acting bronchodilators may also provide effective prophylaxis against anticipated asthma triggers, including exercise, cold air, and certain allergens. Short-acting beta$_2$-adrenergic agonists usually provide rapid relief of symptoms, but they do not affect the underlying inflammation associated with asthma. Short-acting beta agonists are not approved as maintenance medications because their use does not improve long-term asthma control. An increase in the use of bronchodilator therapy indicates worsening asthma; in fact, the need for more than 2 puffs once or twice daily of bronchodilator (quick-relief) medication or the use of more than 1 canister per month is generally an indication that a person's asthma is inadequately controlled.[28] In such cases the asthma management plan should be reviewed, and antiinflammatory medication should probably be added to the therapy, or if it is already being used, prescribed at an increased dose.[18] Short-acting beta$_2$-adrenergic agonists are available in inhaled (metered-dose inhaler [MDI] or nebulizer), oral, and intravenous preparations. All beta$_2$-adrenergic agonists used routinely for asthma therapy have an onset of action in 10 to 15 minutes and a duration of effect of 4 to 6 hours. Side effects of the short-acting bronchodilators include tachycardia, hypertension, tremors, nervousness, headache, dizziness, hyperactivity, insomnia, nausea, and muscle cramps.

Because these medications are generally administered by MDI, it is important that inhaler technique be reviewed on a regular basis. When bronchodilators do not promptly and completely resolve symptoms of bronchoconstriction, systemic glucocorticoid therapy is indicated for suppression and reversal of underlying airway inflammation.[25]

Anticholinergic Agents. Anticholinergic agents such as ipratropium bromide (Atrovent) are sometimes useful in reversing bronchoconstriction. Bronchial smooth muscle receptors, innervated by the vagus nerve, respond to acetylcholine, which induces bronchoconstriction. Anticholinergic agents have been shown to have a bronchodilator effect in persons with mild to moderate asthma, but the effect is generally not as significant as that of the short-acting beta$_2$-adrenergic agents. They may be used as alternatives for symptomatic relief for those who have difficulty tolerating the side effects of the beta$_2$-adrenergic bronchodilators.

Monitoring Therapy and Asthma Severity

Asthma management guidelines stress the importance of assessment of pulmonary function using PEFR meters rather than basing assessment on the individual's perception of dyspnea (POD). Studies have shown that in 60% of individuals there is no correlation between POD and simultaneous peak flow measurements and that the majority of individuals have a blunted POD (i.e., an underestimation of respiratory compromise) resulting in undertreatment of asthma, a delay in treatment changes and may even predispose individuals to fatal asthma attacks.[29] Therefore it is recommended that all individuals with moderate to severe asthma learn how to monitor their PEF and have a flow meter at home. PEF monitoring during exacerbations should be encouraged for all those with moderate to severe, persistent asthma, and PEF should guide management. In addition, long-term daily peak flow monitoring is recommended for individuals with moderate to severe asthma to help maintain control of symptoms; however, if long-term monitoring is not done, periodic short-term monitoring is recommended for evaluating responses to therapy or assessing the effect of environmental exposures. All individuals with asthma who experience periodic severe asthma exacerbations may benefit from peak flow monitoring.[4]

Peak flow monitoring helps individuals follow the course of their disease, predict exacerbations, identify triggers, and assess their response to treatment.[18] PEF values, specifically the individual's *personal best* PEF, should be used as the basis for an action plan. An individual's personal best PEF can be estimated after a 2- to 3-week period during which the PEF is recorded at least once a day in the early afternoon. Additional measurements should be made after beta$_2$-adrenergic inhalers are used for symptomatic relief. The personal best is usually achieved in the early afternoon after maximal effect of any therapy has stabilized or resolved the symptoms. The personal best should be reassessed periodically to account for progression of disease. A PEF value that is significantly higher than all the other measurements should be interpreted with caution; rather than reflecting a personal best, an outlying value may be due to spitting or coughing into the peak flow meter.[4]

A zone system similar to a traffic light has been successfully used to help individuals interpret their symptoms and PEFR results. The use of this system is particularly helpful for asthmatic patients who are unable to recognize the severity of their asthma based on symptoms, which is estimated to be the case for more than 50% of patients. In addition, many studies have shown that asthma symptoms correlate poorly with the level of airway obstruction as determined by spirometry (FEV_1 and PEF). After treatment, subjective improvement in asthma symptoms may occur without a corresponding improvement in the degree of airway obstruction. For this reason, current guidelines recommend that airway obstruction be measured objectively when assessing patients with chronic asthma.[30]

The zone system is made up of green, yellow, and red zones (or lights if the traffic light analogy is used). The green zone (or light) corresponds to a PEF measurement that is ≥80% of an individual's personal best or optimal control. For individuals with very irritable airways who decompensate quickly, the cutoff may be adjusted to 90%.[12] A measurement in the green zone reflects

TABLE 108-8 Usual Dosages for Quick-Relief Medications

Medication	Dosage Form	Adult Dose	Child Dose	Comments
SHORT-ACTING INHALED $BETA_2$ AGONISTS				
	MDIs			
Albuterol	90 μg/puff, 200 puffs	2 puffs 5 minutes before exercise	1-2 puffs 5 minutes before exercise	An increasing use or lack of expected effect indicates diminished control of asthma. Not generally recommended for long-term treatment. Regular use on a daily basis indicates the need for additional long-term control therapy. Differences in potency exist so that all products are essentially equipotent on a per puff basis. May double usual dose for mild exacerbations. Nonselective agents (i.e., epinephrine, isoproterenol, metaproterenol) are not recommended due to their potential for excessive cardiac stimulation, especially at high doses.
Albuterol HFA	90 μg/puff, 200 puffs	2 puffs t.i.d.-q.i.d.	2 puffs t.i.d.-q.i.d.	
Bitolterol	370 μg/puff, 300 puffs			
Pirbuterol	200 μg/puff, 400 puffs			
Terbutaline	200 μg/puff, 300 puffs			
	DPIs			
Albuterol Rotahaler	200 μg/capsule	1-2 capsules q 4-6 hr as needed and before exercise	1 capsule q 4-6 hr as needed and before exercise	
	Nebulizer solution			
Albuterol	5 mg/ml (0.5%)	1.25-5 mg (0.25-1 ml) in 2-3 ml of saline q 4-8 hr	0.05 mg/kg (minimum 1.25 mg, maximum 2.5 mg) in 2-3 ml of saline q 4-6 hr	May mix with cromolyn or ipratropium nebulizer solutions. May double dose for mild exacerbations.
Bitolterol	2 mg/ml (0.2%)	0.5-3.5 mg (0.25-1 ml) in 2-3 ml of saline q 4-8 hr	Not established	May not mix with other nebulizer solutions.
ANTICHOLINERGICS				
	MDIs			
Ipratropium	18 μg/puff, 200 puffs	2-3 puffs q 6 hr	1-2 puffs q 6 hr	Evidence is lacking for producing added benefit to $beta_2$ agonists in long-term asthma therapy.
	Nebulizer solution			
	0.25 mg/ml (0.025%)	0.25-0.5 mg q 6 hr	0.25 mg q 6 hr	
SYSTEMIC CORTICOSTEROIDS				
Methylprednisolone	2, 4, 8, 16, 32 mg tablets	Short course "burst": 40-60 mg/day as single or 2 divided doses for 3-10 days	Short course "burst": 1-2 mg/kg/day, maximum 60 mg/day, for 3-10 days	Short courses or "bursts" are effective for establishing control when initiating therapy or during a period of gradual deterioration. The burst should be continued until the patient achieves 80% PEF personal best or symptoms resolve. This usually requires 3-10 days but may require longer. There is no evidence that tapering the dose following improvement prevents relapse.
Prednisolone	5 mg tablets, 5 mg/ml, 15 mg/ml solution			
Prednisone	1, 2.5, 5, 10, 20, 25 mg tablets; 5 mg/ml solution			

From National Institutes of Health, National Heart, Lung, and Blood Institute: *Highlights of the Expert Panel Report 2: guidelines for the diagnosis and management of asthma,* NIH pub no 97-4051A, Washington DC, 1997, US Department of Health and Human Services.

good asthma control and that it is *safe* to proceed. The yellow zone (or light) means *caution* and refers to a PEF measurement that is within 50% to 80% of the individual's personal best or optimal control. Some guidelines use a range of 60% to 80% for the yellow zone; the more conservative value of 60% promotes earlier intervention as the patient's condition begins to deteriorate. Symptoms that interfere with daily activities may be present; typical symptoms include cough, wheeze, chest tightness, shortness of breath, and nocturnal awakening. A measurement in the yellow zone indicates the need for a temporary increase in medication dose or frequency. The specific medication change is tailored for each individual and may include increased bronchodilator therapy, increased or added corticosteroid therapy, and a short course of oral corticosteroids. In many ways, the yellow zone is the key to the entire asthma action plan (AAP), as a measurement in this zone reflects worsening airway obstruction, which will usually continue to worsen if action is not taken. The written AAP should identify at what point the next level of provider should be contacted; in general, individuals should be instructed to contact their primary care provider for mild to moderate symptoms that do not respond to treatment or for PEFs that remain within the yellow zone (50% to 60% of personal best). A PEF value or symptoms in the red zone mean *danger* and indicate the need for emergency treatment. A reduction in the PEF >50% (or 40%) and dyspnea are the general criteria for the red zone. Other associated symptoms may include inability to blow into the peak flow meter, accessory respiratory muscle use, difficulty walking or talking because of asthma, and cyanosis. Immediate use of inhaled rescue bronchodilator therapy and initiating or increasing oral corticosteroid therapy are necessary. If the PEFR does not improve after emergency treatment, the individual should be instructed to call 911 (or an emergency number) or proceed to the emergency department (or to his or her primary care provider). The AAP should clearly state in the red zone portion when patients need to seek emergency care.[12,18] The NAEPP has developed a self-management program for asthma exacerbations that is based on the zone system (Figure 108-1).

It has been well established that improving asthma adherence can lead to better control. Despite growing awareness of the importance of asthma education, however, adherence to asthma treatment, including medications, the use of peak flow meters, and avoidance of environmental irritants, is still poor. The provider-patient relationship is central to improving adherence; all specific strategies aimed at improving adherence (such as simplifying medication regimens, AAPs) must be developed in a therapeutic, trusting provider-patient relationship to be effective.[31] Studies have shown that asthma therapy based on influencing behavior and self-management of acute exacerbations results in improved control and decreased asthma morbidity.[12,32,33]

Current practice guidelines recommend follow-up visits at 1- to 6-month intervals, depending on the severity of asthma and the degree of control. Persons with mild asthma who, for example, experience occasional exacerbations only after exercise may need only an annual visit for asthma or have it addressed as part of an annual examination. On the other hand, persons with moderate to severe asthma with frequent exacerbations may need monthly visits to review PEFR readings and assess the effectiveness of medications.[28]

Co-Management with Specialists

The current NIH guidelines state that all patients who have had an asthma-related hospitalization (and thus, by definition, have chronic severe asthma) be evaluated by an asthma specialist. In addition, general reasons for consultation with a specialist include poorly controlled asthma, asthma that is unresponsive to appropriate therapy, the desire to obtain a second opinion, and periodic patient evaluation. Specific reasons for specialist consultation may include classification of asthma type and severity, interpretation of PFT results, assessment of possible occupational asthma, allergy skin testing, and advice about pharmacotherapy.[34] Evidence of poorly controlled asthma, including frequent missed days of work or school, dissatisfaction with the quality of life, and frequent emergency department visits and hospitalizations, may reflect lack of recognition of the disease severity by the patient or primary care provider or treatment plans that are too simplistic. In such cases, referral to an asthma specialist is warranted and will likely improve control and the quality of life and decrease asthma-related morbidity and mortality.

LIFE SPAN CONSIDERATIONS

The preparation for pregnancy in women with asthma, if possible, should begin well in advance to achieve good asthma control before and during the pregnancy. In about equal proportions of women, the control of asthma will improve, worsen, or remain unchanged during pregnancy. Just as with any individual, unmanaged asthma in a pregnant woman may result in emergency department visits, hospitalizations, respiratory failure, and even death. In addition, poorly managed asthma has also been associated with certain complications of pregnancy, including an increased incidence of preeclampsia, eclampsia, low birth weight, premature delivery, and infant mortality.[35] Given the potential for and possible consequences of asthma complications during pregnancy, it is vitally important that pulmonary function (minimally peak flow monitoring) be monitored throughout pregnancy. Because a 20% drop in peak flow often precedes the onset of symptoms, pregnant women need to be able to recognize when they fall 80% below their baseline. In addition, an appreciation of ability to improve or lack of improvement is essential so that appropriate prompt treatment can be initiated.

The basic management of asthma during pregnancy is similar to that in nonpregnant individuals. In an effort to minimize the need for medications, environmental and lifestyle controls assume an even more important role. No asthma therapy has been proved to be absolutely safe during pregnancy. For women who require only beta$_2$-adrenergic agonists, metaproterenol is usually the drug of choice. For women requiring antiinflammatory medication, the use of beclomethasone or cromolyn is considered relatively safe. During more severe exacerbations of asthma, tapered regimens of oral prednisone are used, as the risks of anoxia to the fetus outweigh the possible risks of oral corticosteroid therapy.[13,15]

There has been a steady increase in the prevalence of asthma from adolescence to old age. Asthma tends to be less well recognized among older adults, as symptoms are often attributed to other respiratory ailments such as COPD, congestive heart failure, pulmonary aspiration, pulmonary embolism, and bronchogenic carcinoma. However, the tools usually used to diagnose asthma are still helpful in ruling out the differential diagnoses in this population. If the clinical picture is indistinguishable from either COPD or asthma, it is often useful to consider age of onset; asthmatics have generally experienced symptoms at an earlier age as well as having had a clearer history during their younger years.[36,37]

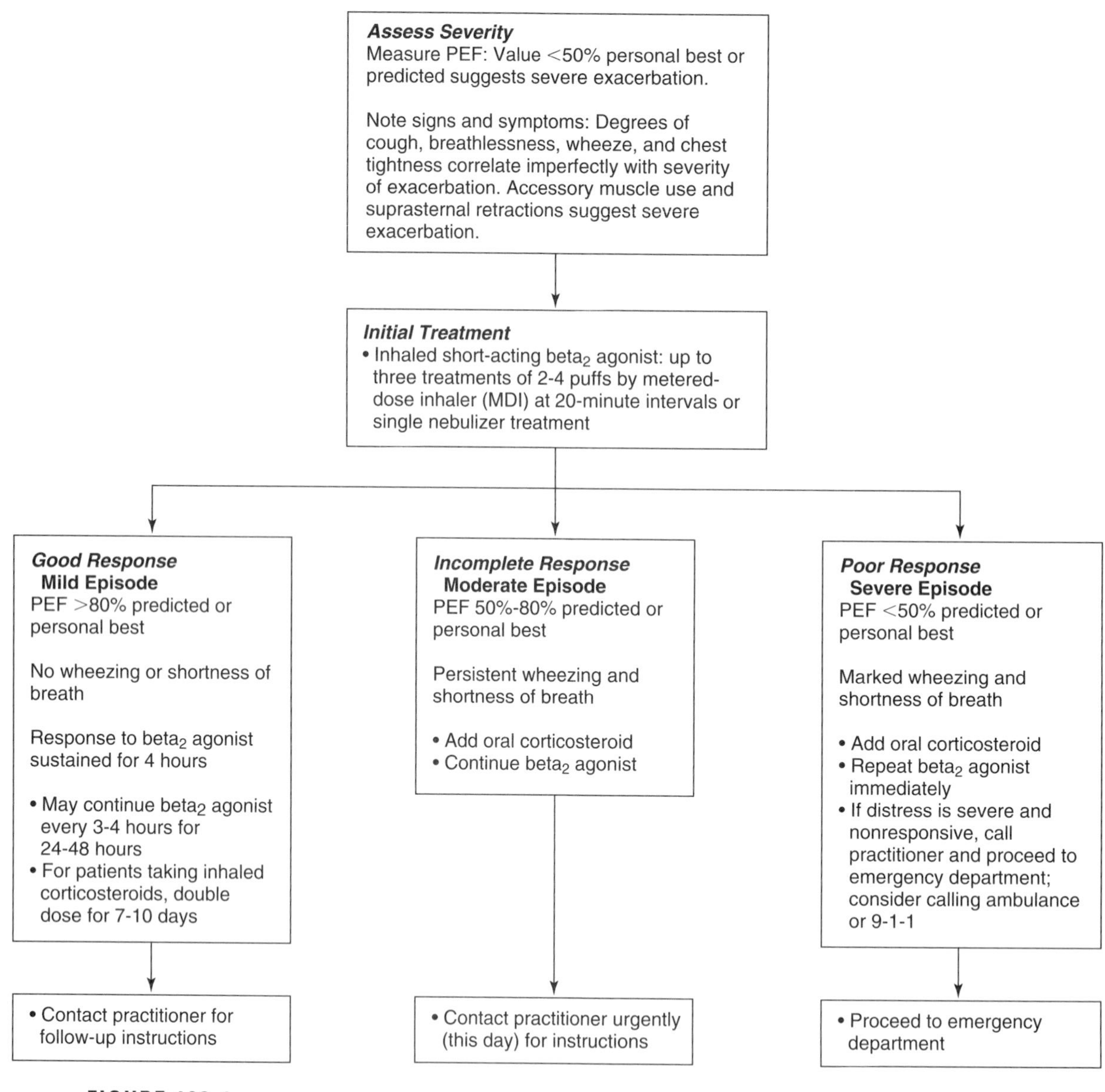

FIGURE 108-1

Management of asthma exacerbations: home treatment. (From National Institutes of Health, National Heart, Lung, and Blood Institute: *1997 Guidelines for the diagnosis and management of asthma: highlights of the Expert Panel Report 2,* Pub No 97-4051A, Washington DC, 1997, US Government Printing Office.)

In addition, subjective awareness and perception of symptoms tend to be poorer among older adults. For these reasons, asthma remains underdiagnosed and suboptimally treated in this population.[30] In older adults, chronic bronchitis may coexist with asthma, which may affect management. Asthma medications may aggravate coexisting medical conditions, such as cardiac disease and osteoporosis; adjustments in the pharmacotherapy may need to be made. Certain drugs commonly used in older people, including aspirin and beta blockers, may adversely affect asthma. Finally, older adults may have particular difficulty with inhaler administration; their technique should be carefully reviewed, and devices such as spacers may be especially helpful in improving drug delivery in this population. Overall, asthma tends to be associated with poor overall health and a greater handicap in mobility, despite adjustment for living conditions, depression, cognition, visual or auditory impairment, and joint pain.[36]

Nonetheless appropriate care in older individuals is achievable. Most adverse reactions to asthma drugs may require dose adjustment but are generally not significant to warrant discontinuation of the drug. The use of large volume spacers improves the inhalation technique, and most older individuals prefer using this device compared to using the MDI alone.[36]

COMPLICATIONS

Complications of asthma include status asthmaticus and fatal asthma. Status asthmaticus is present when symptoms do not improve or remit with initial treatment of an acute exacerbation.

During status asthmaticus, despite maximum therapy, respiratory failure may develop.[13] Signs and symptoms indicative of respiratory failure include paradoxical thoracoabdominal movement, absence of wheeze, bradycardia, and a deterioration in mental status. If an exacerbation is severe enough that respiratory failure seems possible, intubation should be performed sooner rather than later.[25]

The increasing rates of asthma morbidity and mortality are very disturbing. The reasons for these increasing rates are unclear; however, certain risk factors for fatal asthma have been identified. Co-morbidity (such as from cardiovascular disease or COPD) and serious psychiatric disease or psychosocial problems increase the risk of fatal or near-fatal asthma. Difficulty perceiving airflow obstruction or its severity and a history of sudden severe exacerbations also increase the risk of fatal asthma. However, a period of 2 to 7 days of worsening asthma symptoms rather than a sudden deterioration often precedes hospitalizations, providing a window of opportunity to implement more aggressive therapy in an effort to prevent fatal or near-fatal events. Additional risk factors include hospitalization or emergency care for asthma within the past month, prior asthma-related ICU care, three or more emergency department visits or two or more hospitalizations for asthma during the past year, and prior intubation for asthma. Other risk factors include current use or withdrawal from systemic glucocorticoids and the use of three or more canisters of inhaled short-acting beta$_2$-adrenergic agonists per month. Urban residence, low socioeconomic status, and illicit drug use also increase the risk for fatal asthma.[4,7,38] These risk factors affirm the need for interventions designed to prevent and control asthma, as well as therapy that includes the self-management of asthma symptoms during periods of exacerbations, especially for those at high risk.

Research has demonstrated that in comparison with other patient groups, adults with asthma who have lower socioeconomic status and less education are likely to receive care that has less continuity and is less intensive after hospital or emergency department discharge. In addition, a minority of these patients tend to have AAPs or adequate communication with their primary care providers during the acute stages of the exacerbation. In addition, those most at risk for fatal asthma are more likely to depend primarily on the emergency department for management of exacerbations. In other words, those individuals who are at highest risk for complications of asthma are likely to receive the type of care that increases rather than mitigates the risk of future complications.[6,7,38-40]

INDICATIONS FOR REFERRAL/HOSPITALIZATION

Referral to an asthma specialist for consultation or co-management is recommended if there are any difficulties achieving or maintaining control of asthma or if step 3 or 4 care is required. Hospitalizations should be considered for all individuals whose symptoms do not improve or remit with initial aggressive treatment of the acute exacerbation. The NHLBI's guidelines for the management of asthma exacerbations in the emergency department and hospital are included in Figure 108-2.

PATIENT EDUCATION

Patient education is both one of the most important and one of the most challenging aspects of asthma management. Asthma is a chronic disease and, like other chronic diseases, requires ongoing maintenance and prevention. Asthma that is treated only episodically when exacerbations occur will result in symptomatic relief at best. To achieve the other goals of asthma treatment (such as preventing symptoms, maintaining near-normal pulmonary function, minimizing the adverse effects of pharmacotherapy, and minimizing the need for emergency department visits and hospitalizations), patients and their families need to be well educated about the disease, its basis, and their role in monitoring symptoms and preventing exacerbations. Table 108-9 includes a summary of asthma education to be included as part of patient care visits.

Every individual with asthma should participate with their primary care provider in setting up an individualized written asthma management plan, or AAP, that includes their own asthma triggers, a detailed description of relevant environmental control measures, instructions on the role and use of medications and delivery devices (e.g., spacers, nebulizers), monitoring techniques (e.g., PEFR meters), and instructions on how to tailor therapy to deal with changing symptoms. Proper inhaler technique is described in Box 108-3. Patients should be taught how to recognize symptom patterns, interpret PEFR results, and increase treatment during exacerbations of asthma.[12,18] An AAP should be developed for each individual based on signs and symptoms and/or PEFR, with instructions on how and when to change pharmacotherapy and when to contact the primary care provider. Emphasis should be placed on the long-term control medications (anti-inflammatory medications) used to achieve and maintain control of persistent asthma and quick-relief medications (bronchodilators) used to treat acute symptoms and exacerbations.[4] In addition to allowing for the early recognition of symptoms and earlier initiation of treatment, which can minimize the severity of exacerbations, AAPs also increase confidence, security, and ability for self-control in individuals with asthma and their families.[12]

Patients with asthma should have a copy of their AAP at home, work, and school, with all medications available at each location. In addition, they should be reminded and encouraged to plan ahead for vacations—to have an AAP with them and know emergency department locations and phone numbers.[12]

BOX 108-3

PROPER METERED-DOSE INHALER TECHNIQUE WITH AND WITHOUT A SPACER

1. Remove cap, hold inhaler upright, and shake inhaler well.
2. Tilting your head back slightly, exhale slowly and fully.
3. Place mouthpiece between lips or open mouth widely and hold inhaler 1 to 2 inches from mouth.
4. Press down on inhaler once as you start to inhale slowly and deeply.
5. Continue to inhale slowly and deeply as long as you can.
6. Hold breath for 10 seconds (at least 4 seconds).
7. Exhale slowly through nose or pursed lips.
8. Repeat puffs as prescribed, waiting at least 1 minute between puffs.

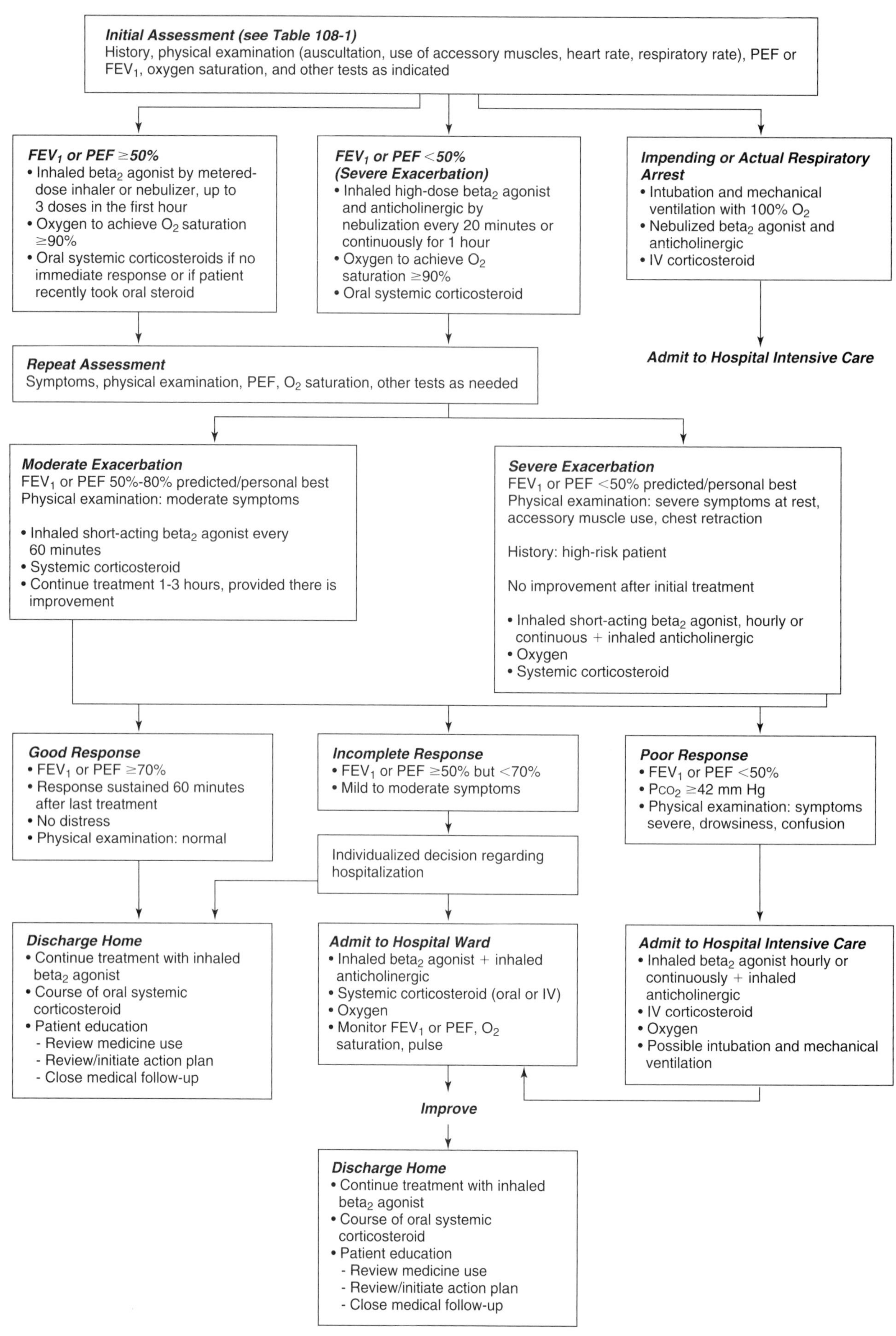

FIGURE 108-2

Management of asthma exacerbations: emergency department and hospital-based care. (From National Institutes of Health, National Heart, Lung, and Blood Institute: *1997 Guidelines for the diagnosis and management of asthma: highlights of the Expert Panel Report 2,* Pub No 97-4051A, Washington DC, 1997, US Government Printing Office.)

TABLE 108-9 Delivery of Asthma Education by Clinicians During Patient Care Visits

Assessment Questions	Information	Skills
RECOMMENDATIONS FOR INITIAL VISIT		
Focus on: • Concerns • Quality of life • Expectations • Goals of treatment	Teach in simple language.	Teach and demonstrate.
"What worries you most about your asthma?" "What do you want to accomplish at this visit?" "What do you want to be able to do that you can't do now because of your asthma?" "What do you expect from treatment?" "What medicines have you tried?" "What other questions do you have for me today?"	What is asthma? A chronic lung disease. The airways are very sensitive. They become inflamed and narrow; breathing becomes difficult. Asthma treatments: two types of medicines are needed: • Long-term control: medications that prevent symptoms, often by reducing inflammation • Quick relief: short-acting bronchodilator relaxes muscles around airways Bring all medications to every appointment. When to seek medical advise. Provide appropriate telephone number.	Inhaler and spacer/holding chamber use. Check performance. Self-monitoring skills that are tied to an action plan: • Recognize intensity and frequency of asthma symptoms • Review the signs of deterioration and the need to reevaluate therapy: Walking at night with asthma Increased medication use Decreased activity tolerance Use of a simple, written self-management plan and action plan
RECOMMENDATIONS FOR FIRST FOLLOW-UP VISIT (2 TO 4 WEEKS OR SOONER AS NEEDED)		
Focus on: • Concerns • Quality of life • Expectations • Goals of treatment	Teach or review in simple language.	Teach or review and demonstrate.
Ask relevant questions from previous visit and also ask: "What medications are you taking?" "How and when are you taking them?" "What problems have you had using your medications?" "Please show me how you use your inhaled medications."	Use of two types of medications. Remind patient to bring all medications and the peak flow meter to every appointment for review. Self-evaluation of progress in asthma control using symptoms and peak flow as a guide.	Use of a daily self-management plan. Review and adjust as needed. Use of an action plan. Review and adjust as needed. Peak flow monitoring and daily diary recording. Correct inhaler and spacer/holding chamber technique.
RECOMMENDATIONS FOR SECOND FOLLOW-UP VISIT		
Focus on: • Expectations of visit • Goals of treatment • Medications • Quality of life	Teach or review in simple language.	Teach or review and demonstrate.
Ask relevant questions from previous visits and also ask: "Have you noticed anything in your home, work, or school that makes your asthma worse?" "Describe for me how you know when to call your doctor or go to the hospital for asthma care." "What questions do you have about the action plan? Can we make it easier?" "Are your medications causing you any problems?"	Relevant environmental control/avoidance strategies: • How to identify home, work, or school exposures that can cause or worsen asthma • How to control house-dust mites, animal exposures if applicable • How to avoid cigarette smoke (active and passive) Review all medications. Review and interpret peak flow measures and symptom scores from daily diary.	Inhaler/spacer/holding chamber technique. Peak flow technique. Use of daily self-management plan. Review and adjust as needed. Use of the action plan. Confirm that patient knows what to do if asthma gets worse.

From National Institutes of Health, National Heart, Lung, and Blood Institute: *Highlights of the Expert Panel Report 2: guidelines for the diagnosis and management of asthma,* NIH pub no 97-4051A, Washington DC, 1997, US Department of Health and Human Services.

continued

TABLE 108-9 Delivery of Asthma Education by Clinicians During Patient Care Visits—cont'd

Assessment Questions	Information	Skills
RECOMMENDATIONS FOR SUBSEQUENT VISITS		
Focus on: • Expectation of visit • Goals of treatment • Medications • Quality of life	Teach or review in simple language.	Teach or review and demonstrate.
Ask relevant questions from previous visits and also ask: "How have you tried to control things that make your asthma worse?" "Please show me how you use your inhaled medication."	Review and reinforce all: • Educational messages • Environmental control strategies at home, work, or school • Medications Review and interpret from diary: • Peak flow • Symptom scores	Inhaler/spacer/holding chamber technique. Peak flow technique. Use of daily self-management plan. Review and adjust as needed. Use of the action plan. Confirm that patient knows what to do if asthma gets worse. Periodically review and adjust the written action plan.

From National Institutes of Health, National Heart, Lung, and Blood Institute: *Highlights of the Expert Panel Report 2: guidelines for the diagnosis and management of asthma,* NIH pub no 97-4051A, Washington DC, 1997, US Department of Health and Human Services.

Persons with asthma and other household members need to be educated about the role of environmental triggers of asthma and efforts that they can take to reduce environmental hazards with the home and surrounding areas. Often cleaning crews require specialized training and equipment to decrease allergen levels in the environments they are servicing.

REFERENCES

1. Bailey R and others: Impact of clinical pathways and practice guidelines on the management of acute exacerbations of bronchial asthma, *Chest* 113(1):28-33, 1998.
2. Drazen JM: Bronchial asthma. In Baum GL and others, editors: *Textbook of pulmonary diseases,* ed 6, Philadelphia, 1998, Lippincott-Raven.
3. National Heart, Lung and Blood Institute: *Global initiative for asthma,* NIH Pub No 95-3659, Washington, DC, 1995, US Government Printing Office.
4. National Institutes of Health, National Heart, Lung and Blood Institute: *1997 Guidelines for the diagnosis and management of asthma: highlights of the Expert Panel Report 2,* Pub No 97-4051A, Washington, DC, 1997, US Government Printing Office.
5. National Heart, Lung, and Blood Institute Data fact sheet: *Asthma statistics.* NIH, U.S. Department of Health and Human Services, Bethesda, Md, 1999 (January), NHLBI.
6. Hanania NA and others: Factors associated with emergency department dependence of patients with asthma, *Chest* 111(2):290-295, 1997.
7. Hartert TV and others: Inadequate outpatient medical therapy for patients with asthma admitted to two urban hospitals, *Am J Med* 100(4):386-394, 1996.
8. Vollmer VM and others: Specialty differences in the management of asthma, *Arch Intern Med* 157(11):1201-1208, 1997.
9. Castro M and others: Risk factors for asthma morbidity and mortality in a large metropolitan city, *J Asthma* 38(8):625-635, 2001.
10. Lang DM, Sherman MS, Polansky M: Guidelines and realities of asthma management: the Philadelphia story, *Arch Intern Med* 157(11):1193-2000, 1997.
11. Kinney PL and others: On the front lines: an environmental asthma intervention in New York City, *Am J Public Health* 92(1):24-26, 2002.
12. Flaum M, Lung CL, Tinkelman D: Take control of high-cost asthma, *J Asthma* 34(1):5-14, 1997.
13. Bigby TD: Asthma: clinical presentation and diagnosis. In Bordow RA, Moser KM, editors: *Manual of clinical problems in pulmonary medicine,* Boston, 1996, Little, Brown.
14. Varner AE, Busse WW: Inflammation in asthma: why it's so important, *J Respir Dis* 17(7):605-616, 1996.
15. Kleerup EC, Tashkin DP: Outpatient treatment of asthma, *West J Med* 163(1):49-63, 1995.
16. Harding SM, Richter JE: Gastroesophageal reflux disease and asthma, *Semin Gastrointest Dis* 3:139-150, 1992.
17. Harding SM and others: Asthma and gastroesophageal reflux: acid suppressive therapy improves asthma outcome, *Am J Med* 100(4): 395-405, 1996.
18. Keenan JM: Asthma management: the case for aiming at control rather than merely relief, *Postgrad Med* 103(3):53-69, 1998.
19. Irwin RS and others: Managing cough as a defense mechanism and as a symptom: a consensus panel report of the American College of Chest Physicians, *Chest* 114(2 suppl):113S-181S, 1998.
20. Li JTC, Sheeler RD: The asthma physical exam: what's valuable, what's not? *J Respir Dis* 17(9):735-738, 1996.
21. Emerman CL, Cydulka RK: Effect of pulmonary function testing on the management of acute asthma, *Arch Intern Med* 155(20):2225-2228, 1995.
22. Blank CA, Brantly M: Clinical features and molecular characteristics of alpha$_1$-antitrypsin deficiency, *Ann Allergy Asthma Immunol* 72(2): 105-120, 1994.
23. Pina JS, Horan MP: Alpha$_1$-antitrypsin deficiency and asthma: the continuing search for the relationship, *Postgrad Med* 101(4):305, 1997.
24. Fish JE and others: Asthma care: new treatment strategies, new expectations, *Patient Care* 31(16):82-100, 1997.
25. Richman E: Asthma diagnosis and management: new severity classifications and therapy alternatives, *Clin Rev* 7(8):76-112, 1997.
26. Simpson WG: Gastroesophageal reflux disease and asthma: diagnosis and management, *Arch Intern Med* 155(8):798-803, 1995.
27. *Drug facts and comparisons 2003: pocket version,* St Louis, 2002, Facts and Comparisons.
28. Li JTC, Sheeler RD: Getting the most out of a 15 minute asthma visit, *J Respir Dis* 18(2):135-141, 1997.
29. Magadle R and others: The risk of hospitalization and near fatal and fatal asthma in relation to the perception of dyspnea, *Chest* 121(2): 329-333, 2002.

30. Teeter JG, Bleecker ER: Relationship between airway obstruction and respiratory symptoms in adult asthmatics, *Chest* 113(2):272-277, 1998.
31. Bender B, Milgram H, Rand C: Nonadherence in asthmatic patients: is there a solution to the problem? *J Allergy Asthma Immunol* 79(3): 177-185, 1997.
32. Taitel MS and others: A self-management program for adult asthma. II. Cost-benefit analysis, *J Allergy Clin Immunol* 95(3):672-676, 1995.
33. Kotses H and others: A self-management program for adult asthma. I. Development and evaluation, *J Allergy Clin Immunol* 95(2):529-540, 1995.
34. Li JTC, Sheeler RD: Asthma specialty consultation: a two-way street, *J Respir Dis* 18(11):953-990, 1997.
35. Murdock MP: Asthma in pregnancy, *J Perinatal Neonatal Nurs* 14(4):27-36, 2002.
36. Quadrelli SA and others: Features of asthma in the elderly, *J Asthma* 38(5):377-389, 2001.
37. Parameswaran K and others: Asthma in the elderly: underperceived, underdiagnosed and undertreated: a community survey, *Respir Med* 92(3):573-577, 1998.
38. Turner MO and others: Risk factors for near fatal asthma: a case-control study in hospitalized patients with asthma, *Am J Respir Crit Care Med* 157(6 pt 1):1804-1809, 1998.
39. Haas JS and others: The impact of socioeconomic status on the intensity of ambulatory treatment and health outcomes after hospital discharge for adults with asthma, *J Gen Intern Med* 9(3):121-126, 1994.
40. Gottlieb DJ, Beiser AS, O'Connor GT: Poverty, race, and medication use are correlates of asthma hospitalization rates: a small area analysis in Boston, *Chest* 108(1):28-35, 1995.

CHAPTER 109

Chest Pain (Noncardiac)

Clayton M. Smiley

DEFINITION/EPIDEMIOLOGY

Noncardiac chest pain is a recurrent substernal chest pressure or other chest discomfort believed to be unrelated to the heart after a reasonable cardiac evaluation. Its reported long-term mortality rate is excellent at 10 years.[1] Nevertheless, symptoms of chest pain are frightening to patients and can be associated with significant morbidity. Ockene and others[2] surveyed patients who had chest pain but normal coronary arteries at cardiac catheterization and found that despite reassurance, 47% limited their activity, 51% were unable to work, and 57% still believed they had heart disease after a mean follow-up period of 16 months.

Patients commonly present with chest pain in the primary care setting. The etiology of these patients' symptoms can be life threatening, but more often are the result of benign causes. One report detailed that 67% of chest pain diagnoses in primary care patients were due to musculoskeletal, gastrointestinal (GI), psychiatric, or pulmonary disorders. Only 16% were secondary to cardiac causes of all types, and another 16% were idiopathic.[3] The correct diagnosis is most often obtained with a detailed history, supporting physical examination findings, and an ECG and/or chest x-ray study if indicated. Ruling out cardiac causes of chest pain or other noncardiac life-threatening conditions is an essential first step. The evaluation of cardiac chest pain is discussed separately.

Immediate emergency department referral/physician consultation is indicated for hemodynamic instability or suspected pulmonary embolism, pneumothorax, esophageal rupture, or aortic dissection.

PATHOPHYSIOLOGY

The sympathetic chain, vagus, and phrenic nerves are responsible for carrying pain impulses in the thoracic cage. All of the structures in the chest, including the chest wall, esophagus, lungs, heart, and diaphragm have overlapping innervation. Thus, pain from different organs, including those in the abdomen that abut the diaphragm (liver, spleen, stomach) may have similar referral patterns. In addition, patients may have a difficult time localizing pain from deep structures, whereas diseases involving more superficial structures such as the chest wall or pleura are more easily localized. Because there is no sensory innervation in the lung parenchyma, disease involving the alveoli or interstitium does not cause chest pain unless the pulmonary vasculature, bronchi, or pleura are involved.[4]

CLINICAL PRESENTATION

The history is crucial in determining the differential diagnosis and appropriate management in individuals presenting with chest pain. Careful questioning usually clarifies the cause. Some examples of questions are listed in Box 109-1. The following descriptions should be pursued when questioning the patient:

- *Quality.* Myocardial ischemia is more often a pressure that is vicelike or constricting. Sharp, stabbing, knifelike pain suggests a noncardiac cause.
- *Location.* Pain that localizes to a small area of the chest suggests pleural or chest wall involvement.
- *Intensity.* Aortic dissection, pneumothorax, or pulmonary embolism pain has an abrupt onset with the greatest intensity at the beginning. Ischemic chest pain is more gradual, and psychogenic causes of chest pain have a more vague onset.
- *Duration.* If the chest pain lasts only seconds, or has been constant for weeks, it is not cardiac.
- *Aggravation.* Symptoms related to eating such as dysphagia, odynophagia, and/or heartburn are more suggestive of esophageal chest pain, whereas exercise that worsens the chest pain is more classic for cardiac ischemia. Position changes, deep breathing, or cough points to a musculoskeletal or pleural disorder.
- *Alleviation.* Repeated palliation with antacids and food likely points to a GI source. Esophageal and cardiac causes are both made better with sublingual nitroglycerin.[5]

The patient's description of his or her symptoms should be viewed in the context of any history of cardiac, pulmonary, psychiatric, or musculoskeletal diseases. A thorough review of current medications may also contribute to the decision-making process.

PHYSICAL EXAMINATION

Examination of a patient with chest pain begins with an assessment of his or her general appearance and vital signs. The general appearance suggests the severity and possibly the seriousness of the symptoms. Abnormalities in the vital signs point to an infectious, pulmonary, cardiac, or malignant process. Hemodynamic instability should prompt immediate referral to the emergency department. The majority of patients with noncardiac chest pain should have normal vital signs.

BOX 109-1

SAMPLE QUESTIONS FOR PATIENTS PRESENTING WITH CHEST PAIN

- Where is the pain?
- How long have you had the pain?
- Do you have recurrent episodes of pain?
- How long does each episode last?
- What makes the pain better? Worse? (Breathing? Lying flat? Moving your arms, neck?)
- How would you describe the pain? (Burning? Crushing? Throbbing? Stabbing? Knife-like?)
- When does the pain occur? (With exertion? After eating? When moving your arms?)
- Is the pain associated with shortness of breath? (Cough? Palpitations? Nausea/vomiting? Fever? Leg pain? Coughing up blood?)

Modified from Swartz MB, editor: The heart. In *Textbook of physical diagnosis: history and examination,* Philadelphia, 1994, WB Saunders.

A general inspection of the chest may reveal a skin rash such as the unilateral rash of herpes zoster in a thoracic dermatome. Evidence of trauma either confirms the history or possibly indicates domestic violence, which the patient did not discuss.

The neck examination should focus on the presence of lymphadenopathy in the cervical chains or supraclavicular fossa. Elevation of the neck veins indicates volume overload and possible heart failure. Tracheal deviation points to a possible pneumothorax.

Palpation of the chest and range of motion of the upper body may cause chest pain in the presence of costochondritis, musculoskeletal disease, a rib fracture, or trauma. Dullness to percussion over a portion of the posterior chest indicates the presence of either a pleural effusion or a consolidative pulmonary process such as pneumonia.

Auscultation of the lungs may elicit asymmetric breath sounds, a pleural friction rub, wheezing, crackles, or absent or decreased breath sounds, all of which should prompt additional investigation with a chest x-ray study. The cardiac examination should evaluate for the presence of murmurs, extra heart sounds (S_3 or S_4), or friction rubs.

Examination of the abdomen may reveal tenderness in the epigastric area, or right or left upper quadrants causing irritation of the diaphragm and resultant referred chest pain.

Finally, it should be remembered that many patients with noncardiac chest pain have a completely normal physical examination.

DIAGNOSTICS

The diagnostic testing options for chest pain are often limited in the primary care setting. If the patient's chest pain is considered cardiac in origin, a 12-lead ECG may demonstrate characteristic abnormalities. Although a normal ECG reduces the likelihood of an acute coronary syndrome by 70% to 90%, however, it does not completely rule it out. The ECG should be interpreted in the context of the patient's history and risk factors for heart disease.[6]

The chest x-ray study is a useful diagnostic took for detecting cardiac and pulmonary abnormalities. Pulse oximeters should be available to determine the oxygen saturation. Occasionally, other studies may be needed such as an arterial blood gas or a complete blood count with differential. In most cases, however, a detailed history, physical examination, and possibly an ECG and/or chest x-ray study should give enough information to form a hypothesis regarding the etiology of the symptoms.

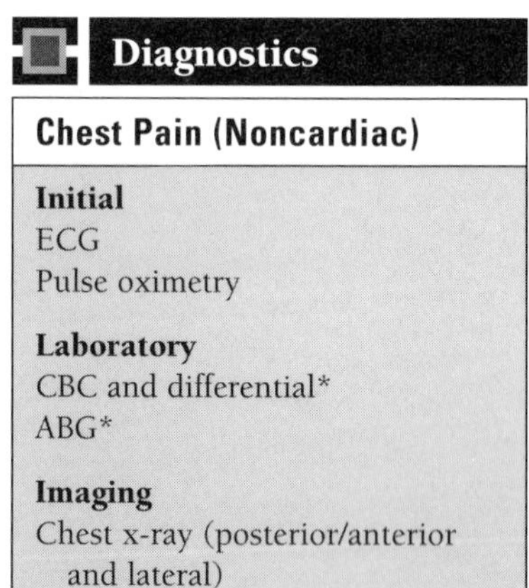
Diagnostics

Chest Pain (Noncardiac)

Initial
ECG
Pulse oximetry

Laboratory
CBC and differential*
ABG*

Imaging
Chest x-ray (posterior/anterior and lateral)

*If indicated.

DIFFERENTIAL DIAGNOSIS

The most common causes of noncardiac chest pain in the primary care setting are due to musculoskeletal, gastrointestinal, psychiatric, and pulmonary disease.[3]

Musculoskeletal chest pain is often nagging and persistent, lasting anywhere from hours to weeks. Patients complain of superficial chest pain localized in a small area. The symptoms are aggravated by position, deep breathing, turning, or arm movement. Causes of musculoskeletal chest wall pain include costochondritis, routine muscle strains, rheumatologic diseases such as rheumatoid arthritis, ankylosing spondylitis, fibromyalgia, and other nonrheumatologic diseases such as neoplasms or fractures.

Esophageal chest pain may result from reflux disease, rupture of the esophagus (Boerhaave's syndrome), or pill-induced esophagitis. Symptoms highly suggestive of an esophageal disorder, specifically reflux disease, include dysphagia, odynophagia, regurgitation, and heartburn.[7] The classic history for Boerhaave's syndrome is profound diffuse chest pain following severe retching and vomiting. Recent use of prescriptions such as doxycycline, nonsteroidal antiinflammatory drugs (NSAIDs), or alendronate might suggest pill-induced esophagitis.

Psychiatric diseases may underlie symptoms of chest pain in many primary care patients. In one study, patients with noncardiac chest pain and no abnormalities on upper endoscopy or other explanation for their symptoms had a higher prevalence of panic disorder, obsessive-compulsive disorder, and major depressive episodes.[8] These patients tend to be younger and female and have atypical symptoms and other diagnosed psychiatric illnesses.

Finally, the lungs may cause chest pain if the vasculature, parenchyma, or pleural tissue is affected. Pulmonary embolism (PE) is a common and often missed diagnosis. According to a landmark study, 97% of patients with a PE had dyspnea, pleuritic chest pain, or cough.[9] These symptoms are obviously nonspecific and require a high degree of clinical suspicion with special attention to known risk factors of PE such as immobilization, history of previous venous thromboembolism, recent surgery, pregnancy, or malignancy. Another diagnosis that should be considered in patients with the sudden onset of sharp, stabbing chest pain is pneumothorax. Patients with primary pneumothorax are typically young tall males who smoke and have no history of lung disease.[4] Secondary spontaneous pneumothoraces occur in patients with cystic fibrosis, chronic obstructive pulmonary disease, and human immunodeficiency virus in patients with *Pneumocystis* pneumonia. Patients who have community acquired pneumonia as the underlying cause of their chest pain are usually easily diagnosed based on the cough, fever, sputum production, and findings on physical examination and chest x-ray study.

Differential Diagnosis

Chest Pain (Noncardiac)

Pulmonary	**Musculoskeletal**
Bronchitis	Arthritis
Malignancy	Costochondritis
Pleurisy	Herpes zoster
Pneumonia	Rib fractures
Pneumothorax	
Pulmonary embolism	**Gastrointestinal**
	Esophageal hyperalgesia
Cardiac	Reflux disease
Angina pectoris	Referred gallbladder, pancreatic, hepatic, or splenic pain
Dissecting aortic aneurysm	
Hypertrophic cardiomyopathy	Esophageal spasm
Myocardial infarction	
Pericarditis	**Psychiatric**
Valvular heart disease	Major depression
	Panic disorder
	Generalized anxiety disorder

MANAGEMENT

Management of patients with chest pain depends on the etiology of the disease process (Figure 109-1). Exclusion of coronary artery disease or other life-threatening noncardiac causes of chest pain is an essential first step.

Musculoskeletal chest pain therapy includes the use of NSAIDs, rest, heat, or ice. For those patients who cannot tolerate traditional NSAIDs (older patients, those with a history of ulcer disease or previous GI bleeding), selective COX-2 inhibitors (celecoxib 100 to 200 mg daily or b.i.d. or rofecoxib 12.5 to 50 mg daily) may be indicated. Scheduled Tylenol 650 mg q 4-6 hours may also be helpful in these patients.

When the clinical picture suggests an esophageal source, an empiric trial with twice daily proton pump inhibitors (pantoprazole 40 mg b.i.d., omeprazole 20 mg b.i.d., lansoprazole 30 mg b.i.d., rabeprazole 20 mg b.i.d.) has been shown to be safe, cost-effective, and diagnostically accurate.[10] Therapy may be given for up to 8 weeks.[11] If the symptoms resolve, maintenance therapy with daily proton pump inhibitors (PPIs) should then follow. If no resolution occurs, a referral to a gastroenterologist for 24-hour ambulatory pH monitoring and additional workup is appropriate.

Psychiatric disease as a cause for noncardiac chest pain is common; however, it should always be a diagnosis of exclusion. If a diagnosis of panic disorder, depression, or generalized anxiety disorder is suspected, selective serotonin reuptake inhibitors (SSRIs) are effective. One study even demonstrated a benefit of reducing noncardiac chest pain by 50% in those patients who did not meet DSM-IV criteria for panic disorder, major depressive disorder, or generalized anxiety disorder but did not otherwise have an explanation for their symptoms.[12] In addition, patients with these diagnoses have been shown to benefit from enrollment in cognitive behavioral therapy.[13]

If a pulmonary disorder is suspected, and the chest x-ray findings confirm suspicion, treatment will be self-evident. In the case of pneumonia first-line treatment is with antibiotics such as doxycycline 100 mg b.i.d., a macrolide (clarithromycin 500 mg b.i.d. or azithromycin 500 mg on day 1 then 250 mg on days 2-5), or one of the fluoroquinolones with enhanced activity against *Streptococcus pneumoniae* (ciprofloxacin 750 mg b.i.d., levofloxacin 500 mg q.d., sparfloxacin 400 mg for 1 day then 200 mg q.d., gatifloxacin 400 mg q.d., moxifloxacin 400 mg q.d.) for 10 to 14 days.[14] A follow-up chest x-ray study should be done 6 to 8 weeks after treatment in all patients over the age of 50 years to document resolution of the infiltrate and to assess for an underlying cause of the process such as a malignancy or another structural defect.

Patients with a pneumothorax or suspected pulmonary embolism should be triaged to the emergency department. An

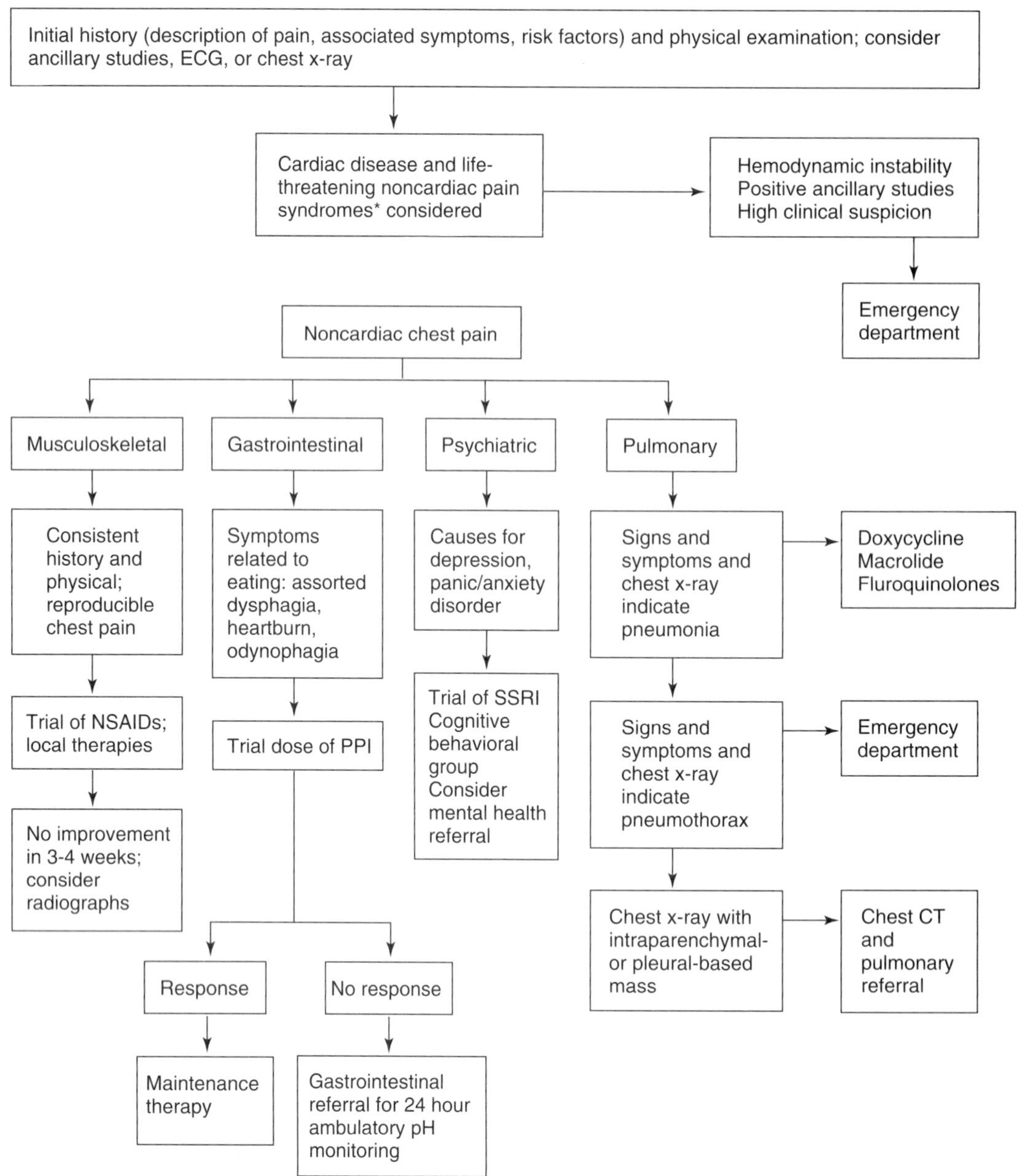

FIGURE 109-1

Approach to the patient with noncardiac chest pain. (Modified from Fang J and others: *Am J Gastroenterol* 96: 958-968, 2001.)

intraparenchymal or pleural-based mass causing chest pain deserves additional workup with a chest CT, pain management with analgesics, and a referral to a pulmonologist.

LIFE SPAN CONSIDERATIONS

After cardiac and life-threatening noncardiac conditions are excluded, the age of the patient is often an important factor in determining the diagnosis. Younger patients' chest pain is generally caused by more benign underlying conditions, whereas older patients with more risk factors and co-morbid conditions should be approached with caution. Regardless of the patient's age, cardiac and life-threatening noncardiac conditions should be ruled out first.

COMPLICATIONS

Pulmonary embolism can be life threatening if diagnosis and treatment are delayed. Thus clinical suspicion of pulmonary embolism is important in all patients who present with respiratory or cardiac complaints. A pneumothorax can develop into a tension pneumothorax if it is not treated appropriately. With a tension pneumothorax, there is a mediastinal and tracheal shift to the contralateral side that causes hypotension and an increase in respiratory distress. This condition can be rapidly fatal if not diagnosed and treated. Pneumonia can proceed to respiratory failure even in young and otherwise healthy patients. Esophageal perforation leads to mediastinitis. Finally, acute aortic dissection can lead to cardiac valvular insufficiency, rapid hemodynamic collapse, and death if not addressed promptly.

INDICATIONS FOR REFERRAL/HOSPITALIZATION

In patients with suspected reflux causing chest pain, nonresponse to high-dose PPI therapy should prompt a referral to a gastroenterologist. A pulmonologist should be consulted for any mass on chest x-ray film and in patients with recurring or nonresolving pneumonia, because these conditions may indicate an underlying malignancy or immune deficiency.

Emergency department referral/physician consultation is necessary when a cardiac origin of chest pain or a life-threatening noncardiac cause cannot be excluded.

PATIENT AND FAMILY EDUCATION

Noncardiac chest pain can be a diagnosis with significant morbidity.[2] Ensuring that patients are well informed about their diagnosis, its natural history, and possible complications improves the probability of a positive outcome.

Patient education should emphasize how to recognize cardiac, pulmonary, or musculoskeletal chest pain and what to do when it occurs, including when to call 911. If the patient smokes, counseling on the importance of tobacco cessation should be done at every visit. If any medications are prescribed, instructions should incorporate the correct administration of the drugs as well as their possible side effects.

REFERENCES

1. Chambers JBC: Chest pain with normal coronary anatomy: a review of natural history and possible etiologic factors, *Progr Cardiov Dis* 33:161-184, 1990.
2. Ockene I and others: Unexplained chest pain in patients with normal coronary arteriograms: a follow-up of functional status, *N Engl J Med* 303:1249-1252, 1980.
3. Klinkman BS and others: Episodes of care for chest pain: a preliminary report from MIRNEJ: Michigan Research Network, *J Fam Pract* 38:345-352, 1994.
4. White P and others: Common pulmonary problems: cough, hemoptysis, dyspnea, chest pain, and the abnormal chest x-ray. In Barker LR, Burton JR, Zieve PD, editors: *Principles of ambulatory medicine*, Baltimore, 1999, Williams & Wilkins.
5. Fang I and others: A critical approach to non-cardiac chest pain: pathophysiology, diagnosis, and treatment, *Am J Gastroenterol* 96: 958-968, 2001.
6. Panju AA and others: Is this patient having a myocardial infarction? *JAMA* 280:1256-1263, 1998.
7. Alban-Davies H and others: Angina-like esophageal pain: differentiation from cardiac pain from history, *J Clin Gastroenterol* 29:392-397, 1994.
8. Ho K and others: Noncardiac, nonesophageal chest pain: the relevance of psychological factors 43:105-110, 1998.
9. The PIOPED Investigators: Value of the ventilation/perfusion scan in acute pulmonary embolism. Results of the prospective investigation of pulmonary embolism diagnosis (PIOPED), *JAMA* 263: 2753-2759, 1990.
10. Ofman JJ and others: The cost-effectiveness of the omeprazole test in patients with non-cardiac chest pain, *Am J Med* 107:219-227, 1999.
11. Castell DO and others: The acid suppression test for unexplained chest pain, *Gastroenterology* 115:222-224, 1998.
12. Varia I and others: Randomized trial of sertraline in patients with unexplained chest pain of non-cardiac origin, *Am Heart J* 140:367-372, 2000.
13. van Peski-Oosterbaan AS and others: Cognitive-behavioral therapy for non-cardiac chest pain: a randomized trial, *Am J Med* 106:424-429, 1999.
14. Bartlett JG and others: Practice guidelines for management of community acquired pneumonia in adults, *Clin Infect Dis* 31:640-653, 2000.

CHAPTER 110

Chronic Cough

Sallustio Del Re and Vera Wekullo

DEFINITION/EPIDEMIOLOGY

Cough, an important reflex action and respiratory defense mechanism, is designed to prevent the aspiration of foreign material into the lower respiratory tract and to clear excessive secretions, fluids, or foreign matter from the airway.[1,2] Although cough has a protective role, excessive and chronic cough can result in numerous complications, including anxiety, fatigue, insomnia, myalgia, dysphonia, perspiration, and urinary incontinence. In addition, chronic cough may also be a symptom of underlying disease. For these reasons, a persistent chronic cough is a cause for concern for both the patient and primary care provider. Most coughs are acute and self-limiting, but a cough that persists for more than 3 weeks and has failed initial treatment is defined as chronic and should be investigated. Overall, cough is the fifth most common symptom for which medical care is sought, accounting for 30 million visits annually[3] and costing more than $1 billion each year in both prescribed and over-the-counter medications.[4] It is a common complaint of patients with smoking-related pulmonary disease, along with dyspnea and chest pain, but it also has an incidence of 20% among nonsmoking adults.[4,6]

Although most smokers have a cough, they do not generally seek medical attention for the cough in particular. In adults, chronic cough is most often (up to 94% of the time) the result of five disorders, including postnasal drip syndrome, asthma, gastroesophageal reflux disorder (GERD), chronic bronchitis (primarily from cigarette smoking), and bronchiectasis. Chronic cough in immunocompetent, nonsmoking adults who have normal chest x-ray examinations and do not take angiotensin-converting enzyme (ACE) inhibitors can be attributed to postnasal drip, asthma, GERD, or a combination of these problems. Chronic cough has been shown to be simultaneously due to multiple causes in a majority of cases. In addition, cough due to multiple causes has been the result of three diseases up to 42% of the time.[1,3]

An understanding of the anatomic, physiologic, and pathophysiologic aspects of cough is important for diagnosis and appropriate treatment. The systematic, diagnostic protocol uses the anatomic characteristics of the cough reflex and enervation as a guide to finding the etiology of the cough (Box 110-1).

PATHOPHYSIOLOGY

When a neural receptor along the respiratory tree is stimulated, an afferent signal is transmitted to the "cough center" of the brain, which is located in the medulla. From this center via a complex reflex arc, the impulse is passed down the efferent pathway to the expiratory musculature.

The receptors of the afferent limb can be found anywhere along the respiratory tree. These include the vagus from the ears, larynx, trachea, bronchi, pleurae and gastrointestinal tract; the trigeminal from the nose and the sinuses; the glossopharyngeal from the pharynx; and the phrenic from the diaphragm.

BOX 110-1

CHARACTERISTICS OF CHRONIC COUGH

- When did the cough start?
- Is it severe at night or during the day?
- Is it productive or dry?
- What characteristic does the sputum have?

The efferent limb consists primarily of the phrenic and spinal nerves. After the stimulus reaches the cough center, the cough begins with a deep inspiration to approximately 50% of the vital capacity. This allows for maximum expiratory flow by increasing the lung elastic recoil and by decreasing airway frictional resistance. During this phase the glottis opens widely to allow rapid entry of large amounts of air into the lung. The glottis rapidly closes and the abdominal and intercostal muscles contract, increasing the intrapleural pressures to 100 to 200 mm Hg. In a fraction of a second, the glottis reopens, causing an explosive release of air. During this phase the tracheobronchial tree narrows, resulting in forces sufficient enough to strip mucus off the walls, creating sputum.

CLINICAL PRESENTATION

Studies have shown that a careful and detailed history will provide the diagnosis in 80% of all cases of cough.[3,7-9] Careful consideration of the various characteristics of cough may aid diagnosis (Figure 110-1). A cough that lasts for 3 consecutive months for more than 2 consecutive years is indicative of chronic bronchitis. A sudden onset of cough when a patient is in supine position with an associated sour taste in the mouth suggests esophageal reflux. A cough associated with constant throat clearing and thick mucus production, especially on rising from bed, is consistent with postnasal drip and sinusitis. Intermittent productive cough associated with wheezing is most probably asthma. A cough associated with rhinorrhea and/or sneezing may be a viral syndrome or the common cold. If it recurs annually at the same time of year, allergic rhinitis is possible. A loud hacking cough during the daytime that is nonproductive, leads to exhaustion, and is associated with emotional stress may suggest psychogenic cough. In addition, some authors have attributed certain sputum characteristics to a particular disease process (Box 110-2). Evaluation of these attributes may also aid in diagnosis.

PHYSICAL EXAMINATION

The physical examination has been reported to be diagnostic in 60% of cases.[9,10] Obvious findings include the following:

- Pharyngeal erythema with or without cobblestoning of the mucosa and purulent secretions, as seen in sinusitis, postnasal drip, or allergic disease
- Diffuse inspiratory crackles characteristic of pulmonary edema or fibrosis
- Expiratory wheezes as in asthma or chronic obstructive pulmonary disease
- Occasional hair rubbing against the eardrum or cerumen impaction in the canal

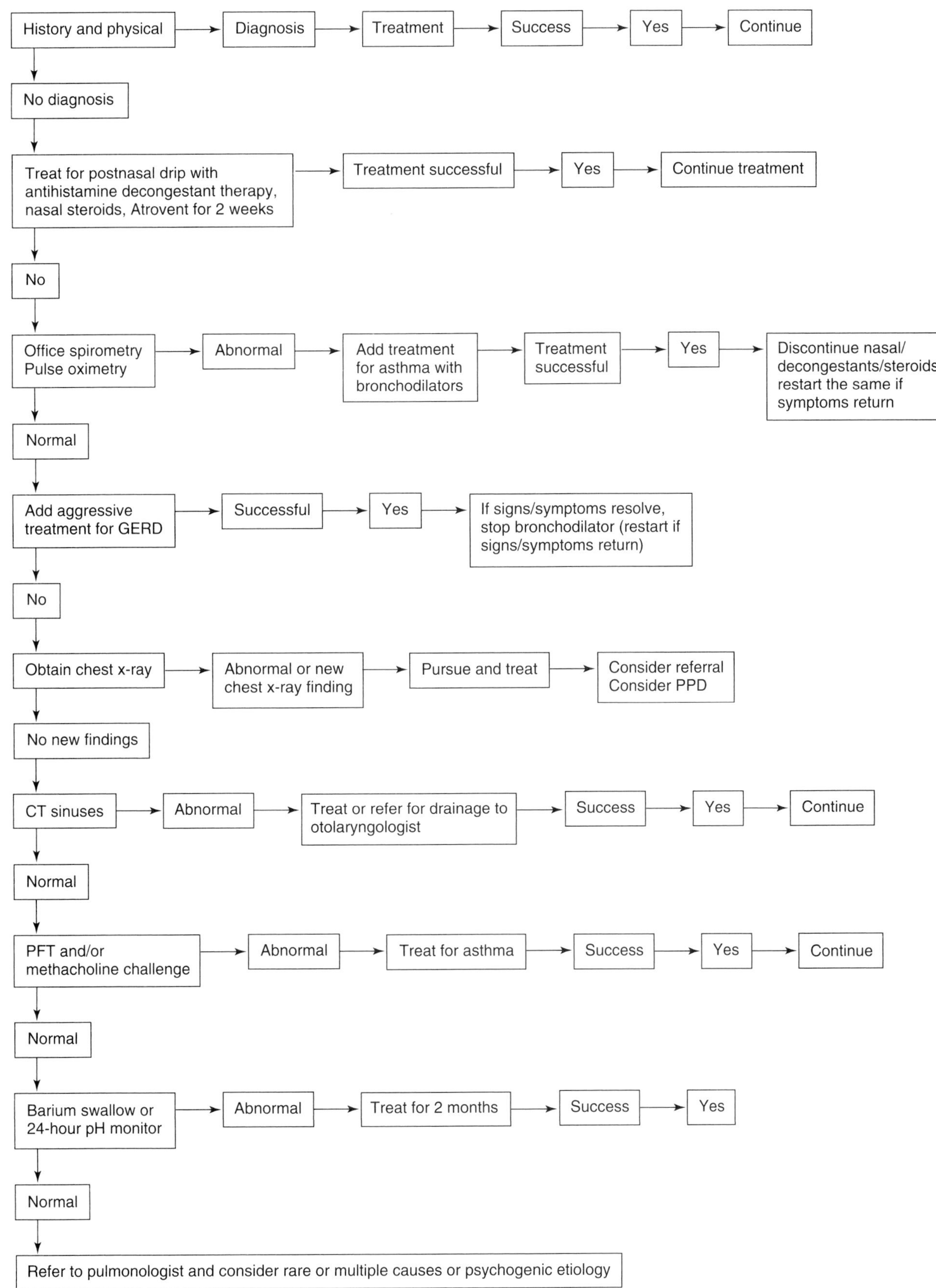

FIGURE 110-1

Diagnostic chronic cough protocol.

BOX 110-2

SPUTUM CHARACTERISTICS OF VARIOUS PULMONARY DISORDERS

- Hemoptysis: bronchogenic cancer, pulmonary embolus, tuberculosis
- Yellow/green, purulent; bronchitis
- Pink frothy: pulmonary edema
- Fetid purulent: anaerobic infections
- Rust colored: pneumococcal pneumonia
- Foam, serous, mucopurulent layers: bronchiectasis

If the history and physical examination cannot establish the cause of the cough, an x-ray study is necessary. However an x-ray finding is diagnostic in only 2% to 4% of cases.[3,10]

DIAGNOSTICS

X-ray examination will reveal the presence of a lung mass or parenchymal abnormalities, such as sarcoidosis, fibrosis, emphysema, and congestive heart failure. A bronchoscopy should be planned only for a specific diagnosis. However if chest x-ray findings are negative, especially for a mass, a bronchoscopy is diagnostic in only 2% to 5% of patients with a cough.[10] If the diagnosis is still not found, routine pulmonary function tests (PFTs) are indicated, and if these are negative a methacholine challenge test is necessary.

At this point, up to 70% of the coughs will have been diagnosed. If the cause is still undetermined, however, a gastrointestinal evaluation with a barium swallow and a 24-hour pH esophageal monitoring should be considered. Further diagnostic tests include a CT scan of the sinuses or otolaryngologic evaluation. Approximately 98% of patients should now have a definitive diagnosis.[6,10] The remaining 2% will most likely have a psychogenic cough, or the cause will be undetermined. Up to 25% to 50% of patients will have multiple causes.[11]

DIFFERENTIAL DIAGNOSIS

The causes of cough are plentiful and diverse. Postnasal drip syndrome is believed to be the most common cause of chronic cough. In general, it occurs after viral upper respiratory tract infections. Other causes of postnasal drip syndrome include perennial rhinitis (e.g., rhinitis due to seasonal allergens), irritants, drugs, vasomotor responses, and chronic sinusitis.[1]

Diagnostics

Chronic Cough

Imaging
Chest x-ray study*
Barium swallow*
Sinus CT*

Other
Bronchoscopy*
PFTs*
Purified protein derivative*
Methacholine challenge test*
24-hour esophageal pH monitoring*

*If indicated.

Differential Diagnosis

Chronic Cough (Adults)

Most Common	Rare
Postnasal drip	Tracheobronchial collapse
Asthma	Lung cancer
Chronic bronchitis	Tuberculosis
GERD	Occupational/environment induced
Less Common	Interstitial lung disease
Bronchiectasis	Hyperthyroidism
Medications	Retrosternal goiter
Cardiac disease	Carcinoid tumor
Postinfectious cough syndrome	Retained suture
Sarcoidosis	Hodgkin's disease
Foreign body aspiration	Zenker's diverticulum
Postradiation pneumonitis	Habit cough
Psychogenic	
Ear canal irritation	
Gastrointestinal disturbances	

Differential Diagnosis

Chronic Cough (Children)

Most Common
Asthma
Upper and lower respiratory infections
GERD

Less Common
Congenital anomalies
Heart disease
Foreign bodies
Aspiration
Environmental

Early asthma may present as chronic cough, and bronchial asthma is the second most common cause of chronic cough. The cough may precede audible wheezes and is the only presenting symptom in up to 57% of asthma cases (cough variant asthma). Given the high and increasing prevalence of asthma, it should always be considered as a possible cause of chronic cough. The degree and reversibility of obstruction is most accurately assessed by spirometry, which measures forced expiratory volume in 1 second (FEV_1). An FEV_1 that is less than 80% of predicted value and is strongly responsive to inhaled $beta_2$ agonist bronchodilators (an increase of at least 12% in the measured FEV_1) is strongly suggestive of asthma.[1]

If the PFT results are normal, an attempt to induce bronchospasm using bronchoconstrictor such as methacholine should be tried. This is known as the methacholine challenge test and is diagnostic in 25% of patients.[12] A nebulized solution of methacholine is administered in a stepwise fashion, incrementally increasing the dose and repeating the spirometry after each dose. A 20% drop in FEV_1 from baseline is considered a positive result.[3] Other substances used as bronchoconstrictors include histamine, cold air exposure, and ultrasonic water mists.

Chronic bronchitis, most often caused by smoking, accounts for between 5% and 12% of patients with chronic cough.[3,7,9,11] Spirometry reveals an airflow obstruction that does not significantly respond to inhaled bronchodilators (or improvement in FEV_1 >12%). Smoking cessation is the most effective therapeutic intervention, because the majority of patients will have resolution of cough or improvement within 8 weeks. Unfortunately, the cough of persistent smokers is usually resistant to most, if not all, forms of therapeutic interventions.

Bronchiectasis, another major airway disease, may also cause chronic cough. Responsible for only 4% of coughs, bronchiectasis is an enlargement of the peripheral airways that in the worst cases may give the lungs a "Swiss cheese" appearance on anatomic section.[3,7,9] Diagnosis is dependent on the history and recurrent episodes of purulent sputum, which, when left standing in a cup, may separate into three layers: frothy top, serous middle, and purulent bottom. The most efficient diagnostic modality is a high-resolution CT scan with characteristic finding of "tram tracking, saccules, and signet rings."

Gastroesophageal reflux accounts for 10% to 20% of all chronic coughs.[3,4] This cough can occur at any age, although the average is 67.2 years. It occurs slightly more in women. Most patients refer to concurrent abdominal complaints, such as dyspepsia or heartburn, although it is not unusual for patients to have no symptoms at all. The reflux material does not necessarily need to be aspirated or even reach the glottis to cause cough or bronchospasm. Studies commonly used for diagnosis include a barium swallow, esophagoscopy, manometry, and pH probe monitoring.

Postinfectious cough syndrome constitutes between 10% and 20% of all cough complaints in the primary care setting.[11] It occurs after an upper respiratory tract infection and may cause a cough for 8 weeks or more. Most cases start with a viral syndrome; thus antibiotics are ineffective. Most coughs respond well to cough suppressants; some will require inhaled steroids or a short course of oral prednisone. In nonsmokers some success has been reported with inhaled ipratropium bromide (Atrovent). Medication-induced cough affects 10% of patients receiving angiotensin-converting enzyme (ACE) inhibitors.[11,13] The mechanism is poorly understood and may affect patients early in the course of therapy or after several months or years. Cough usually resolves within 2 to 4 weeks of stopping the medication. All ACE inhibitors should then be avoided, and patients should be started on a different class of antihypertensives or an angiotensin II receptor blocker.

In adults of all ages and in children older than 1 year of age, postnasal drip syndrome, asthma, and GERD are the three most common causes of chronic cough. More often than not, chronic cough is a result of multiple causes.[1,3] Cardiac disease, particularly left ventricular failure, interstitial lung disease, bronchogenic carcinoma, sarcoidosis, foreign body aspiration, postradiation pneumonitis, and *metastatic* lung carcinoma, may all have a cough as the sole presenting symptom. (Although many primary care providers are concerned about missing lung carcinoma, isolated chronic cough is a rare presentation of lung cancer.[15]) Other rare causes of cough include esophageal diverticulitis, stomach ulcer, pericardial effusion, and ear canal irritation.

The literature suggests that psychogenic cough is generally a loud, barking cough that is associated with high stress and typically does not occur at night. However, a cough that is not psychogenic can also be barking or honking, and most persons with chronic cough usually do not wake up during the night once they have fallen asleep. Because a psychogenic cough has no distinguishing features or diagnostic tests, it should remain a diagnosis of exclusion after all other possibilities have been excluded.[3] In 0.5% of cases the course will be undetermined.[3,11] Infectious causes such as pertussis and tuberculosis are reemerging and need to be considered as important differentials of chronic cough.

MANAGEMENT

Therapy is either antitussive (to prevent, control, or eliminate cough) or protussive (to make cough more effective and productive). Antitussive cough is indicated when the cough serves no useful purpose such as clearing the airway and can be specific or nonspecific. Specific treatment is directed at the mechanism directly responsible such as smoking cessation. Nonspecific therapy is directed at the symptom and is meant to control the cough where specific therapy has failed or is not possible (e.g., inoperable lung cancer). Protussive treatment is indicated for patients for whom coughing serves a useful function, as with cystic fibrosis.[16]

Specific therapy is encouraged for the causative agent if a definitive diagnosis is found. Empiric therapy is appropriate when there is a reasonable suspicion of a specific diagnosis. Asthmatic patients should be treated with inhaled $beta_2$ agonists, inhaled corticosteroids, or inhaled nonsteroidal antiinflammatory medications such as cromolyn sodium or nedocromil sodium, and occasionally oral steroids.

Postnasal drip caused by sinusitis is treated with oral decongestants, nasal steroids, and possibly, but not necessarily, antibiotics. When postnasal drip is related to allergic or nonallergic rhinitis, an H_1-antihistamine is an appropriate alternative to antibiotic therapy. Antibiotics are indicated when there is purulent nasal drainage and sinus tenderness.

Chronic bronchitis is best treated with smoking cessation, an ipratropium bromide inhaler, and a $beta_2$ agonist inhaler. When purulent sputum is present, a 7- to 10-day course of antibiotics is indicated.

Management of GERD involves a trial of antireflux therapy. A combination of a proton pump inhibitor and a prokinetic agent relieves the GERD-associated cough in most cases. However, it may take 6 months before the full benefit of therapy is realized. In addition, preventive measures such as weight reduction, smoking cessation, a diet low in acidic foods, and the raising of the head of the bed may help reduce the tone of the lower esophageal sphincter, thus mitigating symptoms.[1]

Demulcents are agents high in sugar content and are believed to coat the sensory receptors in the upper airways. They also promote swallowing, which may help suppress the cough reflex. Expectorants such as guaifenesin are believed to change the consistency of the sputum, thus making it easier to expectorate.

Opiates increase the latency threshold of the cough center. Codeine, oxycodone, and nonopiate dextromethorphan are standard therapy for severe nonproductive coughs. All are CNS depressants and except for dextromethorphan are very addicting. Local anesthetics such as nebulized lidocaine are extremely effective and directly suppress the sensory nerve; however, these agents are difficult to administer.

COMPLICATIONS

Patients often develop costochondritis or hemoptysis as a result of strenuous coughing. Although usually not serious, these developments can be quite frightening for patients and families. Other complications include rib fractures, ruptures, emphysematous blebs, cough, syncope, wheezing, dyspnea, and sleep interruption.

INDICATIONS FOR REFERRAL/HOSPITALIZATION

All patients with coughs that do not respond to or resolve with treatment require physician consultation. Those patients with coughs related to cardiac disease, carcinoma, foreign body aspiration, or other suspected pathology require referral to the appropriate specialist with documentation of diagnostic evaluation, treatment, and treatment evaluation. Hospitalization may be indicated for wheezing and hypoxia as well as for bronchoscopy or other therapeutic interventions (Box 110-3).

PATIENT AND FAMILY EDUCATION

Cough is a major concern for patients that usually requires medical attention. Diagnostic studies are rarely needed, and a systematic and logical approach generally affords relief for the vast majority of patients. Patients and families need to understand, however, that many coughs are viral in origin and that coughs may last 4 to 8 weeks. Careful explanation of the prescribed therapy, the need to use antibiotics only when indicated, and the signs and symptoms of serious cough-related illness should be carefully explained.

BOX 110-3

INDICATIONS FOR REFERRAL

COMPLICATED COUGH WITH ANY OF THE FOLLOWING

Cardiac causes
Carcinoma: primary or metastatic
Chronic aspiration (e.g., in patients with history of cerebrovascular accident)
Foreign body in ear requiring evaluation
Sinusitis requiring drainage

ABNORMAL TESTS REQUIRING SPECIALIST INTERVENTION

GERD requiring 24-hour pH monitoring
Any suspicion of allergy requiring bronchoprovocation testing
Occupational exposure requiring legal intervention
Suspicion of sarcoid, carcinoma, bronchiectasis, carcinoid, Zenker's diverticulum requiring bronchoscopy
Retrosternal goiter requiring surgery
Chronic obstructive pulmonary disease patients requiring home-oxygen supplementation
Chest x-ray film suggestive of empyema

DANGER SIGNALS INDICATING COMPLICATED COUGH

Hemoptysis
Weight loss

Further testing or evaluation is indicated before concluding that the cough is psychogenic, a habitual cough, or a smoker's cough.

REFERENCES

1. D'Urzo A, Jugovic P: Chronic cough: three most common causes, *Canad Fam Physician* 48: 1311-1316, 2002.
2. Duffy NC, Angus R: Casebook: chronic cough, *The Practitioner* 246: 84-96, 2002.
3. Irwin RS and others: Managing cough as a defense mechanism and as a symptom. A consensus panel report of the American College of Chest Physicians, *Chest* 114(2 Suppl):133S-181S, 1998.
4. Irwin RS, Curley FJ, Freanch CL: Chronic cough: the spectrum and frequency of causes, key components of the diagnostic evaluation, and outcomes of specific therapy, *Am Rev Respir Dis* 141:640-647, 1990.
5. Reference deleted in galleys.
6. Irwin RS, Madison M: Anatomical diagnostic protocol in evaluating chronic cough with specific reference to gastroesophageal reflux disease, *Am J Med* 108(4A): 126S-130S, 2000.
7. Irwin RS, CurJey FJ: The treatment of cough, *Chest* 99:1477-1484, 1991.
8. Wartak JF, Sproule BJ, King EG: Differentiating causes of cough: an algorithmic approach, *J Respir Dis* 10:77-94, 1989.
9. Pratter MR and others: An algorithmic approach to chronic cough, *Ann Intern Med* 11:977-983, 1993.
10. Poe RH and others: Chronic persistent cough: experience in diagnosis and outcome using anatomical diagnostic protocol, *Chest* 95:723-728, 1989.
11. Poe RH, Israel R: Evaluating and managing that nagging chronic cough, *J Respir Dis* 11:297-313, 1990.
12. Boyards MC: Why is this patient still coughing? *J Respir Dis* 19:199, 1998.
13. Faller EW, Jackson DM: Physiology and treatment of cough, *Thorax* 45:425-430, 1990.
14. Reference deleted in galleys.
15. Irwin RS, Madison JM: Symptom research on chronic cough: A historical perspective, *Ann Intern Med* 134: 809-814, 2001.
16. Lawler WR: An office approach to the diagnosis of chronic cough, *Am Fam Physician* 58(9):2015-2022, 1998.
17. Rose VL: American College of Chest Physicians issues a consensus statement on the management of cough, *Am Fam Physician* 59(3): 697-699, 1999.

CHAPTER 111

Chronic Obstructive Pulmonary Disease

Maureen B. Boardman

DEFINITION/EPIDEMIOLOGY

Chronic obstructive pulmonary disease (COPD) refers to a cluster of disorders of the bronchi, the conducting airways, and the lung parenchyma. It includes chronic bronchitis and emphysema. Asthma can also be included within the general category of COPD because it shares the same pathophysiologic common denominator: slowing of the expiratory flow rate. The terms *chronic obstructive airway disease* (COAD), *chronic obstructive lung disease* (COLD), *chronic airflow or airway obstruction* (CAO), and *chronic airflow limitation* (CAL) all refer to the same disorder.

Chronic bronchitis is defined clinically as a chronic, persistent cough and/or sputum production for 3 consecutive months each year for 2 consecutive years, with periodic acute exacerbations during which the symptoms worsen.[1] The pathologic features include inflammation of the cells lining the bronchial wall, hyperplasia of the mucous glands, and narrowing of the small airways.[2]

Emphysema is the permanent and abnormal enlargement of any part of the airspaces distal to the terminal bronchioles. Emphysema also involves destruction of the alveolar walls without fibrosis.[2]

Asthma is inflammation of the small airways. Signs and symptoms include hyperactive airways with productive cough, exertional dyspnea, and airflow obstruction, all of which usually reverse with appropriate medication.[3] Asthma can result in progressive airflow obstruction that over time becomes less and less reversible and resembles the obstruction seen in patients with chronic bronchitis and emphysema. Although asthma and COPD are generally considered separate diseases, patients with COPD can have a mix of emphysema, chronic bronchitis, and/or asthma that ranges from a "pure" emphysematous picture to a mixture of all three.

COPD is the fourth most common cause of death in the United States. According to Social Security Disability statistics, it is second only to coronary heart disease in causing disability. According to the American Lung Association, the mortality rate of COPD has been increasing steadily over the past 20 years; during this same time period the mortality rates of many other chronic diseases have been in decline.[4,5] Together, all three components of this disease—chronic bronchitis, emphysema, and asthmatic bronchitis—affect more than 16 million people in the United States. It is likely that at least the same number of people have minimal or no symptoms and go undiagnosed, making the true prevalence of this disease probably as high as 30 to 35 million cases.[6]

COPD is predominantly a smoker's disease that clusters in families and worsens with age. A hereditary pattern caused by alpha$_1$-antitrypsin deficiency contributes to the "pure" emphysematous forms of this disease.

The risks for COPD include genetic, behavioral, socioeconomic, and environmental factors (Box 111-1). Cigarette smoke and an occupation that involves regular exposure to a dusty environment are the two major external factors. Because smoking cessation slows the decline in the expiratory airflow, it is clear that smoking is a powerful factor in determining outcome.[7] When the disease is far advanced, however, degeneration of lung function will probably continue, even with smoking cessation. COPD is more common among individuals who are poor or undereducated. Cigarette smoking is also more common in these groups, but indigent populations still have worse lung function even when adjusted for smoking status. Other contributing factors include crowded living conditions with exposure to frequent viral infections, poorly ventilated homes, inadequate nutrition, exposure to passive cigarette smoke, and suboptimal care for childhood respiratory infections. It is possible that high levels or air pollution contribute to the development of chronic lung disease, but this has not been proven definitively.[8]

Morbidity and mortality rates from COPD are higher in Caucasians than in African-Americans.[7] Mortality has always been higher in men than in women. However, data from the last 3 decades have demonstrated a gender shift in the number of smoking-related COPD cases being diagnosed each year. By the mid 1990s more women than men were hospitalized for COPD exacerbations, and whereas the mortality rate for men from COPD has remained stable, the mortality rate for women has increased.[9] Because of the long latency period between smoking exposure and the development of clinical disease, deaths from this disease continue to increase despite the declining smoking rates in the United States.[10]

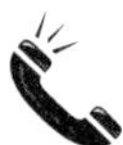

Physician consultation is recommended for the initial diagnosis and management of patients with a significant change in condition or a failure to improve with prescribed therapies.

PATHOPHYSIOLOGY

The etiology of chronic bronchitis is not well understood, but chronic infection and airway hyperreactivity play important roles. The inflammatory process continues unabated even after withdrawing prolonged exposure to bronchial irritants such a smoke, dust, and fumes. Airway edema, airway wall thickening, excess mucus production, and loss of ciliary function result. Airflow is

BOX 111-1

RISK FACTORS FOR DEVELOPING CHRONIC OBSTRUCTIVE PULMONARY DISEASE

- Cigarette smoking
- Airway hyperreactivity
- Childhood respiratory infections
- Occupational exposures
- Age
- Air pollution
- Passive exposure to smoke
- Poor nutrition
- Low socioeconomic status
- Crowded living conditions
- Family members with COPD
- Alpha$_1$-antitrypsin deficiency

obstructed during both inspiration and expiration. Widespread bronchial narrowing with mucus plugging produces hypoxemia because of the mismatching of ventilation and perfusion. Hypercarbia results from the lack of ventilation. Chronic hypoxia and hypercarbia increase pulmonary arterial resistance and may lead to the development of pulmonary hypertension and, eventually, cor pulmonale. A sudden worsening of symptoms in severe chronic bronchitis can precipitate acute right heart failure. Chronic bronchitis causes much less parenchymal damage than emphysema; therefore diffusing capacity, lung volumes, and compliance of lung tissue are not greatly altered.[2]

Enlargement of air spaces in emphysema is the result of alveolar wall destruction. This process is not completely understood but probably results from increased numbers of activated neutrophils that produce elastases—enzymes that destroy the elastin elements in the alveolar walls. Neutrophil-derived elastase is one of a group of destructive proteases contained in alveolar tissue. Usually a small amount of neutrophil elastase is inactivated by antielastases (also known as antiproteases), which are found in the serum and lung lining layer. The prime antielastases, which is present in the largest quantities, is alpha$_1$-antitrypsin.

Even though they account for fewer than 3% of cases, patients with a hereditary deficiency of alpha$_1$-antitrypsin have less inhibition of elastase and a much higher risk of developing emphysema.[2] The primary role of alpha$_1$-antitrypsin is to inhibit the function of several proteases, most notably human neutrophil elastase. Human neutrophil elastase degrades the protein elastin, which is key to the elastic recoil mechanism necessary for the lung's expiratory function. The lack of alpha$_1$-antitrypsin can lead to panacinar emphysema. Because the alveoli have lost their recoil mechanism, the driving force during respiration decreases and causes a chronic persistent airflow obstruction. In addition to inhibiting proteases, alpha$_1$-antitrypsin inhibits the function of lymphocytes, macrophages, and neutrophils.[11] Patients with a hereditary deficiency of alpha$_1$-antitrypsin have less inhibition of elastase and a much higher risk of developing emphysema.

Cigarette smoking also increases elastase activity by causing an influx of elastase-rich neutrophils into the alveoli and by causing the oxidative inactivation of antitrypsin. These processes result in a 30-fold increase in the risk of COPD.

Regardless of the mechanism, the end result of COPD is the destruction of alveolar architecture and the capillary bed lying within the alveolar wall. Initially, the reduction in size of the vascular bed parallels the fall in alveolar surface area. Ventilation still roughly matches perfusion, and significant hypoxemia does not ensue. As the disease progresses, the elastic recoil of the airways is lost, and the poorly supported noncartilaginous airways collapse during expiration. Expiratory flow rates fall as a result, causing decreased airflow. Because this airflow obstruction is not uniform throughout the lung, there is uneven distribution of ventilation and blood perfusion. This uneven distribution causes arterial hypoxemia (decreased PaO_2); decreased ventilation causes hypercarbia (increased $PaCO_2$).

CLINICAL PRESENTATION

A thorough patient history, physical examination, and diagnostic testing are necessary for diagnosis. The most common presenting complaint is dyspnea on exertion. This symptom develops late in the course of this disease, when irreversible changes may have already occurred.

COPD must be considered as a diagnosis in every patient who smokes, even in the absence of respiratory symptoms. Discussing smoking habits at every visit is an important strategy in the prevention of irreversible disease. Documentation should include onset of smoking, the average number of packs per day, and whether there have been any successful cessation attempts. Information about other respiratory symptoms, such as cough, sputum production, and exertional dyspnea, should be elicited and quantified.

The important medical history includes any recurrent or prolonged respiratory tract infections that have required antibiotic treatment. A childhood history of frequent respiratory tract infections and bronchitis and any history of asthma, recurrent sinus infections, or nasal polyps should be documented because such conditions are common in patients with COPD.

The family history, including allergies, tuberculosis, cystic fibrosis, COPD, and other chronic lung conditions, should be elicited. A detailed occupational history with special attention to exposure to noxious inhalants is essential.[7]

PHYSICAL EXAMINATION

Early in the disease process the physical examination is often normal. Even without the findings of advanced COPD, it is impossible to exclude the diagnosis in the person at risk. In fact, in a large autopsy series, only one out of eight cases of emphysema had been diagnosed clinically.[12] In the late stages of COPD, the general physical findings include those resulting from hyperinflation. Inspection of the skin may show tobacco stains on the fingers and, occasionally, clubbing of the fingernails. Chest inspection reveals an increase in the anteroposterior diameter, an increase in the intercostal spaces and, in severe cases, abnormal retraction of the interspaces during inspiration. With inspiration there is diminished movement of the rib cage and increased movement of the abdominal wall. Abdominal and sternocleidomastoid muscles may be well developed but accompanied by diminished muscle mass in the thighs and legs. A forward-sitting posture with both hands on the knees to fix the shoulders, thereby permitting more effective use of the accessory cervical muscles, may be noted. Pursed-lip breathing with prolonged expirations is also characteristic of COPD.[13,14]

There is increased resonance on chest percussion. The diaphragm seems low and moves poorly with deep inspiration and expiration. Diminished transmission of breath sounds on auscultation is the most reliable finding; this indicates chronic airflow limitation. Early inspiratory crackles are commonly found. Wheezing may be elicited with forced expiration, but the presence of wheezing is more often found in reversible bronchospasm.[13]

Lung disease causes hypertrophy of the right ventricle of the heart, resulting in cor pulmonale. Therefore, chronic cor pulmonale may be present in the advanced stage of COPD. The physical examination may reveal neck vein distention, peripheral edema, and hepatomegaly from an elevated right atrial pressure. Pulmonary hypertension and distention of the right ventricle cause a pronounced cardiac impulse in the epigastrium.

DIAGNOSTICS

Early detection of COPD is important for decreasing the associated morbidity and mortality. COPD can result in the loss of 40% to 50% of lung capacity before any problems are noticed.[10] During the presymptomatic period, laboratory measurements show airflow obstruction and can detect disease. A simple office maneuver may help to determine if further testing is needed. After a maximal inspiration, the patient exhales as forcefully as possible through the mouth. The practitioner auscultates the trachea over the upper sternum and measures the time between the first and last sound of forced expiration (forced expiratory time [FET]). An FET of 6 seconds or more is considered abnormal and suggests significant airflow obstruction.[15] An FET of fewer than 3 seconds makes significant airflow obstruction unlikely.

A prolonged FET should be confirmed with spirometric testing. The American Thoracic Society recommends providing screening spirometry in the office. Mild degrees of emphysema probably result in hyperinflation even before airflow abnormalities are present.[16] Spirometry should be performed at least once in every smoker over the age of 40 years and in anyone who has cough, shortness of breath, or wheezing. Forced vital capacity (FVC), forced expiratory volume in 1 second (FEV_1), and the ratio of the two (FEV_1/FVC) are the primary spirometric measurements used for diagnosis.[7] Both FVC and residual volume increase with mild COPD (Box 111-2). Even slight decreases in FEV_1 or increases in FVC can lower the ratio below the normal 70% to 75%. The FEV_1-FVC ratio correlates with the early loss of ventilatory function and the early emergence of symptomatic COPD.[10] The severity of airflow obstruction is also reflected in the FEV_1. Repeating these tests after patients use an inhaled bronchodilator may help identify a bronchospastic element of the disease. If the FVC or FEV_1 improves by 12% or more, bronchospasm is present.[7] Even if flow rates do not respond to bronchodilators during the testing, some benefit may still be obtained from prolonged use.[13,17]

A posteroanterior and lateral chest x-ray study is useful for both the diagnosis of COPD and detection of its complications, such as pneumonia, pulmonary hypertension, and pneumothorax. The diagnosis of emphysema can be made if two or more of the following findings are present on the x-ray film: flattening of the diaphragm and blunting of the costophrenic angle on the posteroanterior view, enlargement of the retrosternal space on the lateral view, flattening or concavity of the diaphragmatic contour on the lateral view, or irregularity of lung field lucency.[7]

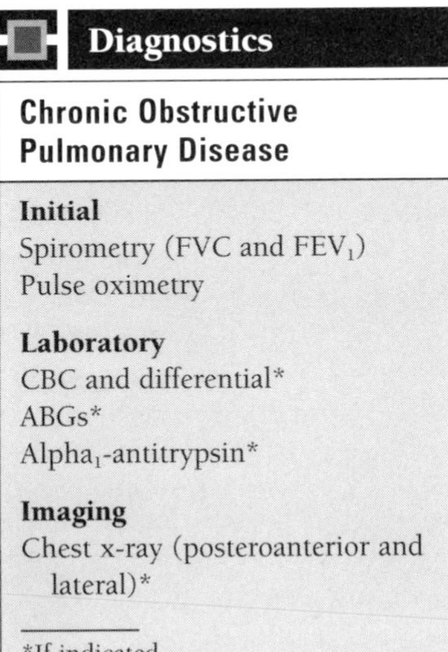

Diagnostics

Chronic Obstructive Pulmonary Disease

Initial
Spirometry (FVC and FEV_1)
Pulse oximetry

Laboratory
CBC and differential*
ABGs*
$Alpha_1$-antitrypsin*

Imaging
Chest x-ray (posteroanterior and lateral)*

*If indicated.

BOX 111-2

SPIROMETRY FINDINGS IN MILD OR EARLY CHRONIC OBSTRUCTIVE PULMONARY DISEASE

FVC > predicted
FEV_1 < predicted
FEV_1/FVC ratio will be < 70%

Pulse oximetry to estimate oxygen saturation can be helpful, but blood gas measurements are necessary to assess and manage patients during exacerbations and when oxygen therapy is indicated. The baseline measurement of blood gases is especially important when severe chronic bronchitis is present because it allows for a comparison with gases obtained during acute exacerbation.[7]

Elevations of hematocrit and hemoglobin provide a measure of the severity of hypoxemia. Phlebotomy may become necessary if the elevation is severe. An ECG can indicate the severity of the lung disease as well as the presence of cor pulmonale. Significant findings include sinus tachycardia, multifocal atrial tachycardia, signs of right atrial enlargement (peaked P waves in leads II, III, and aV_F), signs of right ventricular hypertrophy (a tall R wave in lead V_1 and a deep S wave in lead V_6), and right axis deviation.[7] Sputum is not routinely examined, but its inspection can help differentiate between a pulmonary infection and an exacerbation of reactive airways. Detection of neutrophils or eosinophils in the sputum help determine whether antibiotic or corticosteroid therapy is indicated. Measurement of the $alpha_1$-antitrypsin levels is indicated if the patient has a strong family history of premature emphysema or $alpha_1$-antitrypsin deficiency.[7]

DIFFERENTIAL DIAGNOSIS

Distinguishing COPD from other causes of chronic cough or dyspnea is important for initial diagnosis and in acute exacerbations. A chronic cough could simply be secondary to chronic sinusitis or chronic rhinitis from allergies or postinfectious states. Gastroesophageal reflux, neoplasms, tuberculosis, interstitial lung diseases, and heart diseases (e.g., mitral stenosis or those causing chronic pulmonary edema) may cause chronic cough. Chronic coughs may also result from drugs such as angiotensin-converting enzyme inhibitors, beta blockers, and amiodarone.

Disease that cause chronic dyspnea include COPD, chronic bronchitis, emphysema, cystic fibrosis, and asthma. Less common entities include diffuse interstitial lung disease, pulmonary vascular disease (including recurrent pulmonary emboli, pulmonary hypertension, and arteriovenous malformation), and malignancies (including bronchogenic carcinoma and pulmonary metastatic disease). Phrenic nerve dysfunction or neuromuscular diseases can cause respiratory muscle weakness. Chest wall abnormalities, especially kyphoscoliosis, will cause chronic dyspnea. There are also nonpulmonary causes for dyspnea, including anemia, obesity, ascites, metabolic acidosis, hyperthyroidism, congenital heart disease, and abnormal hemoglobinopathies.

MANAGEMENT

Certain therapeutic interventions for symptomatic COPD improve survival, and some improve symptoms. In the presence of hypoxemia, smoking cessation and oxygen therapy improve survival. Interventions that improve symptoms include pharmacotherapy, education, exercise, psychologic support, nutrition, and surgery.

The goals of treatment are to reverse or reduce airflow obstruction, control cough and secretions, prevent and eliminate infection, and control complications, including polycythemia, hypoxemia, and right heart failure. It is important to relieve underlying depression and anxiety, maximize exercise tolerance, and educate patients about avoiding aggravating factors such as bronchial irritants.[18]

Smoking cessation is the single-most important intervention to reduce the rapid decline of lung function.[19] Patients may be more inclined to stop smoking if they understand that smoking cessation is critical to preventing premature loss of lung function.

Home oxygen is used in later stages of COPD because, unlike some pharmacotherapeutics, it improves survival in hypoxemic COPD. In fact, survival is related to the number of hours of supplemental oxygen used per day.[20] In one study, survival rates improved somewhat in patients who received oxygen 12 to 15 hours per day but improved most in those who received it 19 to 24 hours per day.[21] Other benefits of long-term oxygen include reduction in polycythemia, reduced pulmonary artery pressures, reduced dyspnea, and improvement in neuropsychiatric testing. Another benefit may be the reduction of nocturnal arrhythmias, but it is unclear whether this translates into reduced mortality.

The Medicare criteria for 24-hour supplemental oxygen (Box 111-3) are PaO_2 of 55 mm Hg or less or an O_2 saturation of 88% or less while breathing room air. Patients with cor pulmonale or erythrocytosis (hematocrit greater than 55%) and a PaO_2 of 56 to 59 mm Hg or an SaO_2 of 89% also qualify.[18] Patients with exercise-induced desaturation below 85% should use oxygen during exercise to reduce dyspnea and prevent hypoxemia. In the presence of daytime hypoxemia (a PaO_2 less than 55 mm Hg), a hematocrit greater than 50% to 55%, morning headaches, daytime sleepiness, and poor exercise tolerance are indications of oxygen desaturation during sleep.[22] Monitoring of oxygen saturation during the night may be indicated for these patients because sleep can cause hypoventilation and nocturnal hypoxemia. Oxygen therapy at night will reduce the incidence of nocturnal hypoxemia.[18]

Differential Diagnosis

Chronic Obstructive Pulmonary Disease

Chronic Cough
Chronic sinusitis
Chronic rhinitis
Gastroesophageal reflux
Neoplasm
Asthma
Tuberculosis
Interstitial lung disease
Congenital heart disease
Cardiac disease (mitral stenosis, congestive heart failure)
Medications (angiotensin-converting enzyme inhibitors, beta blockers, amiodarone)

Dyspnea
Asthma
Cystic fibrosis
Interstitial lung disease
Pulmonary embolism
Pulmonary hypertension
Arteriovenous malformation
Other pulmonary vascular diseases
Phrenic nerve dysfunction
Neuromuscular disease
Kyphoscoliosis or chest wall abnormalities
Malignancy
Anemia
Obesity
Ascites
Metabolic acidosis
Hyperthyroidism
Congenital heart disease
Abnormal hemoglobinopathies
Hereditary emphysema (alpha$_1$-antitrypsin)

Pharmacotherapy

Pharmacotherapy will not alter the progression of COPD but can relieve symptoms and improve exercise tolerance (Table 111-1). Inhaled bronchodilators relieve bronchospasm; methylxanthine therapy further enhances bronchodilation, albeit within a narrow therapeutic window; and corticosteroids reduce inflammation. Antibiotics will not treat exacerbations of COPD unless these exacerbations are precipitated by infections. Even though few patients with COPD actually have alpha$_1$-antitrypsin deficiency and the long-term efficacy of replacement therapy is unclear, its identification and treatment are important. Diuretics may also be useful in patients with cor pulmonale.

Bronchodilators include beta$_2$-adrenergic agonists and anticholinergics. Ipratropium bromide is a more effective first choice in patients with nonasthmatic COPD but is less effective than beta$_2$-adrenergic agonists in patients with asthmatic COPD. In general, ipratropium bromide is considered the first drug of choice unless symptoms are intermittent, in which case a beta$_2$-adrenergic agonist should be the first choice.[19,21]

Anticholinergic Therapy. Anticholinergic therapy is usually more clinically effective for COPD than for asthma.[3] Stimulation of the cholinergic nerves to the bronchial smooth muscle causes bronchoconstriction. Decreased cholinergic stimulation lessens bronchoconstriction. The cholinergic receptors are plentiful in the proximal airways, and these are the ones that

BOX 111-3

CRITERIA FOR 24-HOUR SUPPLEMENTAL OXYGEN

PaO_2 of 55 mm Hg or less, or an O_2 saturation of 88% or less while breathing room air

PaO_2 of 56-59 mm Hg or an O_2 saturation of 89% or less with evidence of pulmonary hypertension, cor pulmonale, or erythrocytosis

TABLE 111-1 Pharmacologic Agents for COPD Therapy

Agent	Recommended Dose Range	Notes
ANTICHOLINERGIC		
Ipratropium bromide metered dose inhaler (MDI), 18 μg/inhalation	2-4 puffs, 4-6 times per day	Poorly absorbed systemically; few side effects; should be used regularly, not p.r.n.
Also as solution for nebulization, 500 μg in 2.5 ml	3-4 times per day, separate doses by 6-8 hours	Precautions with narrow-angle glaucoma, prostatic hypertrophy, and bladder neck obstructions
$BETA_2$-ADRENERGIC AGONISTS		
Albuterol sulfate MDI, 90 μg/inhalation	1-2 puffs, q 4-6 hr	Use on a p.r.n. basis is better than a fixed-use schedule No more than 12 inhalations daily
Also as solution for nebulization, 0.5 ml of 0.5% solution	3-4 times per day	Relatively short-acting drug; excessive use should be avoided Caution with cardiac disease, hyperthyroidism, diabetes, seizure disorders
Bitolterol mesylate MDI, 370 μg/inhalation	2 puffs at 1- to 3-minute intervals followed by a third puff if needed, q 8 hr Maximum dose: 3 puffs, q 6 hr or 2 puffs, q 4 hr	Same as albuterol
Also as solution for nebulization, 2 mg/ml; dilute to 2-4 ml	2-4 times per day, 4 hours apart	
Metaproterenol sulfate MDI, 650 μg/inhalation	2-3 puffs, q 3-4 hr	Same as albuterol
Also as solution for nebulization, 5.0% solution	0.2-0.3 ml of 5.0% solution in 2.5 ml of normal saline, 3-4 times per day	
Pirbuterol acetate MDI, 200 μg/inhalation	2 puffs, q 4-6 hr	Same as albuterol
Terbutaline sulfate MDI, 200 μg/inhalation	2 puffs, q 4-6 hr	Same as albuterol
Salmeterol xinafoate MDI, 21 μg/inhalation	2 puffs, q 12 hr Maximum is 2 doses/day	Same as albuterol Not for treatment of acute attacks May be helpful for nocturnal symptoms in COPD because it is a long-acting preparation
METHYLXANTHINE		
Theophylline		
Immediate-release tablets	10 mg/kg/day in 4 divided doses	Follow serum levels to regulate dose between 8 and 13 mg/day; reduce dose in patients with liver disease, cardiac disease, or seizures
Sustained-release tablets	10 mg/kg/day in 1-3 doses	Check for drug-drug interactions
ORAL CORTICOSTEROIDS		
Methylprednisolone	40-48 mg/day in divided doses for 3-4 days	Used to treat acute exacerbations
Prednisone	3- to 4-week tapering course: Begin with 40-60 mg; taper by 10 mg q 4-5 days, ending with 4 or 5 days of 5 mg/day	Used to treat acute exacerbations
	2- to 3-week trial of steroids: 20-40 mg/day	Used for patients not responding to optimal doses of other drugs Steroid therapy is associated with many side effects—osteoporosis, cataracts, hypertension, diabetes, peptic ulcers, psychic disorders, aseptic necrosis of hip, masking of infections, increased appetite, weight gain, and cushingoid effects This form of steroid should be replaced with inhaled form as soon as possible

continued

TABLE 111-1 Pharmacologic Agents for COPD Therapy—cont'd

Agent	Recommended Dose Range	Notes
INHALED CORTICOSTEROIDS		
Beclomethasone diproprionate MDI, 42 μg/inhalation	2 puffs, 3-4 times per day or 4 puffs, 2 times per day; maximum 20 puffs/day	Patients should be taught that inhaled corticosteroids are not bronchodilators These must be used regularly to be effective; mouth should be rinsed after use Hoarseness, dry mouth, oral fungal infections are side effects
Flunisolide MDI, 250 μg/inhalation	2 puffs, 2 times per day Maximum 8 puffs/day	Same as beclomethasone diproprionate
Triamcinolone acetonide MDI, 100 μg/inhalation	2 puffs, 3-4 times per day or 4 puffs, 2 times per day; maximum 16 puffs/day	Same as beclomethasone diproprionate
Fluticasone/salmeterol	100, 250, 500 μg/50μg per inhalation 1 inhalation q 12 hr	Dry-powder inhaler Same as beclomethasone diproprionate
Budesonide	200 μg/inhalation 1-2 inhalations b.i.d.	Dry-powder inhaler Same as beclomethasone diproprionate
Fluticasone propionate	Metered dose inhaler 44, 110, or 220 μg/puff; initial: 88 μg b.i.d., maximum: 440 μg b.i.d. 2-4 puffs b.i.d.	Same as beclomethasone diproprionate
MUCOACTIVE AGENTS		
Iodinated glycerol	60 mg, 4 times per day	Prolonged use can lead to hypothyroidism
Supersaturated potassium iodide solution (SSKI)	0.03-0.06 ml, 3 times per day	Patients need 7-10 days of treatment before therapeutic effect occurs Prolonged use can lead to hypothyroidism Most side effects are gastrointestinal

influence COPD. Adrenergic receptors are more plentiful in the distal airways, which play a larger role in asthma.

For persistent dyspnea and cough, anticholinergic treatment may be more effective than beta$_2$-adrenergic agonists.[20] The effects of anticholinergics are slower in onset but are more prolonged and intense, making them more useful for patients with sustained symptoms. The current preparation, ipratropium bromide, has virtually no side effects because it is poorly absorbed systemically. The usual dose is 2 to 4 inhalations four to six times daily, with a recommended maximum of 12 inhalations daily. This medication should be used on a regular, not p.r.n., basis. Newer products with a longer duration of action are being developed and should be on the market in the near future.[3,18,20,23]

Beta$_2$-Adrenergic Agonist Therapy. Beta$_2$-adrenergic agonists (bronchodilators) cause bronchial smooth muscle dilation and can also improve mucocilliary clearance. The major side effects include tachycardia and tremor from stimulation of beta$_1$ receptors in muscle. Unfortunately, recommended doses of these agents have been based on studies of patients with moderate, stable asthma. These dosages may not be appropriate for patients with COPD. As the severity of bronchospasm increase, the efficacy of beta$_2$-adrenergic agonists decreases.

Some studies demonstrate that p.r.n. use of beta$_2$-adrenergic agonists is superior to a fixed-use schedule.[24] Most agents in this class have a 4- to 6-hour duration. The dosage should not exceed 4 to 12 inhalations per day for the shorter-acting preparations (albuterol, pirbuterol acetate, metaproterenol sulfate, isoetharine, and terbutaline) or twice daily for the longer-acting preparations (salmeterol xinafoate). The longer-acting inhaled preparations or the oral form of these medications may be more helpful in patients with nocturnal symptoms. Toxicity and drug-drug interactions must be avoided in older adults, especially in the presence of coexisting heart disease.

Methylxanthine Therapy. Theophylline is considered a third-line agent because its bronchodilatory effect is limited and its therapeutic range is narrow. Placebo-controlled studies have shown a significant positive effect of theophylline on spirometry, respiratory muscle strength, and resting blood gases. Other studies have shown the theophylline, in combination with bronchodilators, improves the subjective sensation of dyspnea and enhances quality of life.[25-27] Theophylline improves cardiac output, reduces pulmonary vascular resistance, and may have antiinflammatory effects. It may be used in patients who have not responded well to the first-line agents. Monitoring serum levels is important to determine the dosage needed to keep the level of theophylline between 8 and 13 mg/dl. If levels rise, the risk of toxicity increases with little therapeutic gain. Theophylline is not recommended for patients receiving H_2-receptor blockers or fluoroquinolone or macrolide antibiotics, because there is a likelihood of reduced theophylline clearance and a risk of toxicity.

Corticosteroids. Although recent studies suggest that oral corticosteroids may significantly improve airflow and gas exchange with acute exacerbations of COPD, their role remains uncertain.[28,29] Complications, especially in older adults, make long-term therapy with oral corticosteroids problematic. These complications include skin damage, cataracts, diabetes, obesity, peptic ulcer disease, osteoporosis, and secondary infection. Oral steroids can be used to treat acute exacerbations. A 3- to 4-week tapering course of prednisone may be helpful. A dose of 40 to 60 mg of prednisone should be initiated and tapered by 10 mg ever 4 or 5 days, ending with 4 or 5 days of 5 mg/day. Rebound bronchospasm can occur with faster tapers.

For patients who do not respond to optimum doses of other drugs, it is reasonable to try prednisone in doses of 20 to 40 mg/day. This trial of steroids should last 2 to 3 weeks. A 20% to 30% increase in FEV_1 must be demonstrated to justify continued use of oral steroids. Twice the lowest daily dose that maintains improvement should be prescribed on an every-other-day regimen to minimize side effects. If patients are taking long-term corticosteroids, other measures to improve symptoms of COPD should be considered. Lung volume reduction surgery or lung transplantation are two possible options.

The use of inhaled corticosteroids in the treatment of COPD remains controversial. Results of five large-scale, double-blind, placebo-controlled, randomized trials published since 1998 failed to show an improvement in lung function long term as measured by FEV_1.[30] However, three of these studies did show a significant reduction in the number or severity of the exacerbations in patients using inhaled corticosteroids in comparison with placebos.[30]

The World Health Organization's Global Initiative for Chronic Obstructive Lung Disease, or Gold Guidelines, suggest that inhaled corticosteroid use is appropriate for patients with COPD who have shown a documented spirometric response and symptomatic improvement with these medications, or who have severe disease.

Thus there is a place for inhaled corticosteroids in the stepwise approach to the treatment of symptomatic COPD. The FEV_1 should be rechecked after 3 to 4 months of therapy with inhaled corticosteroids. If the FEV_1 improves or stays the same, the same dosage should be continued. If the FEV_1 declines, discontinuation of the inhaled steroid should be considered. The side effects of inhaled corticosteroids are minimal. Oral candidiasis can be minimized by rinsing the mouth with water or mouthwash after every use or by using a spacer.[3]

Mucoactive Agents. Some patients with COPD form increased quantities of abnormal mucus. Increasing hydration by the IV route, aerosolized route, or oral route does not decrease the thickness of secretions. Iodinated glycerol 60 mg PO q.i.d. may be helpful. Another option for patients who have trouble coughing up thick, tenacious sputum is supersaturated potassium iodide solution 0.03 to 0.06 ml PO t.i.d. Patients may need to take this medication for 7 to 10 days before a therapeutic effect occurs.

Antibiotics. Viruses are probably responsible for at least half of the exacerbations of COPD. Antibiotics have no value in the prevention or treatment of exacerbations of COPD unless there is evidence of a bacterial infection. Although antibiotics do reduce the severity and duration of these types of exacerbations, treatment is usually empiric because cultures of sputum are not cost-effective.[31] In a bacterial infection the most common pathogens include *Streptococcus pneumoniae, Haemophilus influenzae, Chlamydia pneumoniae,* and *Moraxella catarrhalis.*[3,20,31]

The mainstay antibiotics are broad-spectrum oral agents that the patient can keep at home to use at the first sign of an acute exacerbation. Typical choices are amoxicillin, ampicillin, cefaclor, doxycycline, and trimethoprim-sulfamethoxazole. Newer, more expensive antibiotics that extend the spectrum of coverage can be used for second-line therapy and include cefpodoxime, azithromycin, clarithromycin, levofloxacin, gatifloxacin, and moxifloxacin. Changing from a first- to a second-line antibiotic is necessary if symptoms do not improve within 2 days, especially if persistent fever or purulent sputum is present.[31]

Pulmonary Rehabilitation

Pulmonary rehabilitation has now become the treatment of choice for patients with COPD.[32,33] Pulmonary rehabilitation is a multidiscipline-team approach to care. It is designed to be highly individualized to meet the needs of each patient. The team makeup may vary from program to program but usually consists of a physician, a respiratory therapist, an exercise therapist and/or a physical therapist, an occupational therapist, psychosocial staff, and a dietitian/nutritionist. Pulmonary rehabilitation programs are an excellent source of support. Instruction on nutrition, exercise, upper body weight training, breathing techniques, and guidance with maximizing energy reserves are critical components of any rehabilitation program.

Exercise Training

Formal exercise programs are another component of pulmonary rehabilitation.[32-35] Programs emphasize lower extremity training, upper extremity training, and strength training. Most pulmonary rehabilitation exercise programs consist of 20- to 30-minute sessions three times a week for 6 to 8 weeks.[32] Participants are also taught breathing strategies such as pursed-lip breathing and controlled coughing as methods to improve patients' ability to perform activities of daily living.

Immunizations

A yearly immunization with the influenza vaccine is essential to decrease morbidity and mortality from influenza epidemics. Patients with COPD are at high risk for pneumococcal pneumonia and should receive the currently available polyvalent pneumococcal vaccine.[3,31]

Psychologic Support

Patients with COPD may feel anxious, depressed, and fatigued. Counseling is recommended for patients exhibiting signs and symptoms of major depression. Many of these problems improve when patients become involved in a pulmonary rehabilitative program. There is evidence that 15 to 20 rehabilitation sessions including exercise, isolated physical therapy, and breathing techniques are more effective in reducing anxiety than a similar number of counseling sessions. Sometimes an antidepressant is beneficial. Issues about sexuality should be discussed because most patients will not raise this sensitive issue themselves. If necessary, sexual counseling may be initiated.[20]

Nutrition

COPD often precipitates weight loss because the increased work of breathing can double resting energy expenditures. This, along with decreased physical activity, tends to diminish fat and muscle stores. Weight loss is also aggravated by disease exacerbations or anorexia from medications or emotional issues. Severe dyspnea, coughing, and sputum production can interfere with eating. Caloric intake may need to be increased to 45 kcal/kg/day. Patients should be encouraged to eat frequent, small meals instead of a large meal; large meals cause abdominal distention, which impairs diaphragmatic function. Vitamin supplementation and commercially prepared drinks are convenient, easily digested, and high in protein, calories, and vitamins. Consultation with a registered dietitian is often necessary to plan for adequate nutrition.[18]

Surgery

Two types of surgery may be beneficial for some patients with COPD: lung volume reduction surgery and lung transplantation. The proposed benefit of lung volume reduction surgery is improved elastic recoil and diaphragmatic function, which is accomplished by reducing the volume of the lung and thereby decreasing hyperinflation.[6] Most patients will not benefit from lung volume reduction surgery, and optimal candidates have not been defined. Therefore before any patient is considered for this surgery, all other conventional therapies must be exhausted without significant improvement in the patient's quality of life.

End-stage COPD is the most common indication for single-lung transplantation. This surgery has become an accepted therapy for end-stage COPD. However, as with volume reduction surgery, optimal candidates have not been defined. Survival statistics vary significantly among centers. Costs associated with lung transplantation are very high, and donor availability is limited.[3]

COMPLICATIONS

Complications may be related to the disease or associated with treatment. Drug effects should always be considered if there is a change in clinical condition. Long-term corticosteroids increase the risk for compression fractures because of accelerated osteoporosis. Some complications can be prevented by keeping the corticosteroid dose as low as possible, encouraging calcium supplementation, replacing estrogen in women (if appropriate), and prescribing etidronate or alendronate treatment for patients unable to reduce their prednisone dose to less than 20 mg every other day.[7]

Theophylline toxicity should be considered in the presence of gastrointestinal symptoms, tremors, headache, or tachycardia. Other medications may affect the metabolism of theophylline. Corticosteroid or diuretic therapy may be responsible for hyperglycemia, hypokalemia, or azotemia.

Depression or marked anxiety often accompanies COPD. Patients with stable COPD tolerate antidepressant therapy, but most often depression improves when airflow obstruction improves; antiinflammatory therapy needs to be maximized during acute infections. Atypical mycobacterial disease should always be considered if chest radiographs show cavitary apical disease. Purified protein derivative (PPD) testing and a sputum examination for acid-fast bacilli are indicated.[7]

Fungal infections are important in the differential diagnosis of certain infiltrates in patients with COPD. Histoplasmosis is endemic in the Ohio and Mississippi River valleys. In the southwestern United States, coccidioidomycosis is endemic and can reach epidemic proportions after a dust storm. Aspergillus is a fungus that can be particularly dangerous in patients with COPD. Consultation is recommended before initiating specific antifungal therapy.[7]

Three other complications occur as a result of the disease process: sleep disorders, acute respiratory failure, and cor pulmonale. Although not always recognized, nocturnal oxygen desaturation in patients with COPD is fairly common. It is not usually caused by sleep apnea but by ventilation-perfusion abnormalities and short-term hypoventilation during REM (rapid eye movement) sleep. Patients who are not obese rarely develop coexisting upper airway obstruction. In some individuals who are obese, however, there is an added obstructive component to the usual mechanisms of transient hypoxemia. Sleep-related hypoxemia is suggested by an increased hematocrit in a patient who complains of morning headaches and daytime somnolence. Often the patient's significant other complains of intense snoring. Overnight home monitoring with pulse oximetry establishes the diagnosis. It is appropriate to prescribe home oxygen for nocturnal use if home monitoring with a pulse oximeter identifies an oxygen saturation of <88% and if symptoms of headache, fatigue, and poor exercise tolerance are present. Continuous positive airway pressure (CPAP) via a well-fitting nasal mask is helpful for patients with an obstructive component. If nocturnal oxygen desaturation is suspected, a referral should be made to a pulmonologist or sleep disorders specialist.[7]

Acute respiratory failure is the most severe complication of COPD. Acute worsening of arterial blood gases necessitates consultation and possible hospitalization.

Cor pulmonale is a severe complication of COPD and is an indication for consultation. Its pathologic definition is right ventricular enlargement, hypertrophy, or dilation secondary to lung disease.[7] Peripheral edema, elevation of the neck veins, and a congested liver reflect right-sided heart failure. In the presence of a significant degree of COPD and an elevated hematocrit with hypoxemia, the diagnosis of cor pulmonale as a complication of COPD can be made without further expensive tests other than an ECG. Standard therapy for cor pulmonale is to treat the underlying airflow obstruction and improve oxygenation. Restriction of salt intake to 2 g/day and a 24-hour diuretic can benefit mild heart failure. If decompensation continues, the addition of supplemental oxygen is indicated to achieve arterial oxygen saturation in the 90% to 95% range 24 hours a day. Hematocrit or hemoglobin levels should be monitored at 4- to 8-week intervals. If the patient is adequately oxygenated, the elevated hematocrit will resolve within that period. Persistent erythrocytosis reflects insufficient oxygen administration or the presence of desaturation during sleep despite the oxygen. A sleep study at this point may help to determine if additional therapy, such as CPAP, is needed during the night.

INDICATIONS FOR REFERRAL/HOSPITALIZATION

Consultation is appropriate when (1) the disease progresses and the need for oral corticosteroids is evident, (2) presentation includes escalation of symptoms and fever, (3) hospitalization is indicated, (4) continuous or nocturnal oxygen is required, and (5) there is evidence of right-sided heart failure and cor pulmonale is present. Murray and Petty[7] outlined 12 indications for consultation with a pulmonary specialist:

1. Particularly severe disease, including persistent dyspnea with activities of daily living despite therapy and frequent recurrent exacerbations
2. Evaluation for and maintenance of oxygen therapy, including consideration of nocturnal oxygen therapy or transtracheal oxygen therapy
3. Inability to successfully taper the patient from systemic corticosteroids
4. Preoperative assessment for thoracic surgery or other surgery, which places the patient at high risk for pulmonary complications
5. Failure to respond after two courses of antibiotics for an acute exacerbation
6. Consideration of long-term intermittent or continuous antibiotic therapy
7. Persistent pulmonary infiltrate(s) on chest radiograph with no response to a course of antibiotics
8. Evaluation of sleep disturbances, including obstructive sleep apnea
9. Management of severe acute respiratory failure, especially if mechanical ventilation is a consideration
10. Cor pulmonale with clinical right-sided heart failure that is unresponsive to usual therapy
11. Consideration of new techniques in lung volume reduction surgery
12. Consideration of alpha_1-antitrypsin augmentation therapy

Hospitalization is based on the severity of the underlying respiratory dysfunction, progression of symptoms, new or worsening cor pulmonale, or the existence of other co-morbidities. Hypoxemia and hypercapnia are probably increasing if a patient does not respond adequately to treatment or is confused or unable to walk, eat, or sleep without aid. Hospitalization is warranted in these cases.

Some patients require admission to a specialized respiratory care unit. Issues that require admission include (1) severe dyspnea that does not respond to initial emergency therapy; (2) confusion, lethargy, or respiratory muscle fatigue characterized by paradoxic diaphragmatic motion; (3) persistent or worsening hypoxemia despite supplemental oxygen, or severe or worsening acidosis; and (4) the need for assisted mechanical ventilation.[18]

PATIENT AND FAMILY EDUCATION

Education is a cornerstone of pulmonary rehabilitation. Patients need to understand that COPD refers to emphysema and chronic bronchitis, because these two diseases often occur together. Patients can better recognize and treat the symptoms of COPD if they understand the nature of the disease and the implications of treatment. The importance of medication, oxygen therapy, smoking cessation, nutrition, exercise, breathing techniques to minimize dyspnea, and health promotion should be stressed.

Patients with COPD who travel are at some risk; therefore it is important that patients and families understand the necessary precautions. Although commercial air travel is safe for most patients with COPD, flying exposes them to hypobaric hypoxia because aircraft are not routinely pressurized at sea level. The goal is to maintain the patient's PaO_2 above 50 mm Hg during the flight. Oxygen delivered by nasal cannula to 2 to 3 L/min will replace the inspired oxygen partial pressure lost at 8000 feet compared with sea level. Lesser amounts of oxygen are sufficient for most patients. Patients who are accustomed to receiving continuous oxygen therapy at home usually require an additional 1 to 2 L/min during air travel. Patients cannot take their own supply of oxygen on board; they must use oxygen supplied by the airline and make arrangements for oxygen at their destination. The Federal Aviation Administration requires a physician's statement of need before a patient can receive continuous oxygen during a flight.

REFERENCES

1. Celli BR and others: The challenge of COPD: step by step through the workup, *Patient Care* 31(2):21-52, 1997.
2. Celli BR: Pathophysiology of chronic obstructive pulmonary disease, *Chest Surg Clin North Am* 5(4):623-633, 1995.
3. Boyars MC: COPD: a step-care approach when FEV_1 is deteriorating, *Consultant* 37(6):1673-1687, 1997.
4. Hunter MH, Kim DE: COPD: management of acute exacerbations and chronic stable disease, *Am Fam Physician* 64(4):603-612, 2001.
5. American Lung Association: *Trends in chronic bronchitis and emphysema: morbidity and mortality,* New York, 2001, Epidemiology and Statistics Unit.
6. Petty TL: A new national strategy for COPD, *J Respir Dis* 18(4): 365-369, 1997.
7. Petty TL: *Frontline treatment of COPD,* ed 2, Denver, 2000, Snowdrift Pulmonary Foundation.
8. Bates DV, Sizto R: The Ontario air pollution study: identification of the causative agent, *Environ Health Perspect* 79:69-72, 1989.
9. Closing the gender gap: women and COPD, *J COPD Management* 2(4):16-19, 2001.
10. Pina JS, Horan MP: Alpha_1-antitrypsin deficiency and asthma, *Postgrad Med* 101(4):153-168, 1997.
11. Goroll AH: Management of chronic obstructive pulmonary disease. In Coroll AH, May LA, Mulley AG, editors: *Primary care medicine: office evaluation and management of the adult patient,* ed 3, Philadelphia, 1995, JB Lippincott.
12. Bates B: *A guide to physical examination and history taking,* ed 5, Philadelphia, 1991, JB Lippincott.
13. Badgett RG and others: Can moderate chronic obstructive pulmonary disease be diagnosed by historical and physical findings alone? *Am J Med* 94(2):188-196, 1993.
14. Lal S, Ferguson AD, Campbell EJM: Forced expiratory time: a simple test for airway obstruction, *Br Med J* 1:814-817, 1964.
15. Petty TL, Silvers GW, Stanford RE: Mild emphysema is associated with reduced elastic recoil and increased lung size but not with airflow limitation, *Am Rev Respir Dis* 136(4):867-871, 1987.
16. American Thoracic Society: Lung function testing, selection of reference values, and interpretation strategies, *Am Rev Respir Dis* 144: 1202-1208, 1991.
17. Celli BR and others: The challenge of COPD: therapeutic strategies that work, *Patient Care* 31(5):101-118, 1997.
18. Anthonisen NR and others: Effects of smoking intervention and the use of an inhaled anticholinergic bronchodilator on the rate of decline in FEV_1: the lung health study, *JAMA* 272:1497-1505, 1994.
19. Celli BR: Current thoughts regarding treatment of chronic obstructive pulmonary disease, *Med Clin North Am* 80(3):589-609, 1996.
20. Gross NJ: COPD management: options for patients with severe disease, *J Respir Dis* 17(6):494-501, 1996.
21. Celli BR and others: The challenge of COPD: managing the special problems of chronic lung disease, *Patient Care* 31(7):87-98, 1997.

22. Petty TL: Developments in the early recognition and treatment of COPD, *Hosp Med* 32(8):13-20, 1996.
23. van Schayck CP and others: Bronchodilator treatment in moderate asthma or chronic bronchitis: continuous or on demand? A randomized study, *Br Med J* 303:1426-1431, 1991.
24. Mahler DA and others: Sustained-release theophylline reduces dyspnea in non-reversible obstructive airway disease, *Am Rev Respir Dis* 131:22-25, 1985.
25. McKay SE and others: Value of theophylline in the treatment of patients handicapped by chronic obstructive pulmonary disease, *Thorax* 48:227-232, 1993.
26. Pulmonary Rehabilitation Research NIH Workshop Summary: *Am Rev Respir Dis* 49:825-830, 1994.
27. Callahan CM, Dittus RS, Katz BP: Oral Corticosteroid therapy for patients with stable chronic obstructive pulmonary disease: a meta-analysis, *Ann Intern Med* 114:216-223, 1991.
28. Thompson WH and others: Controlled trial of oral prednisone in outpatients with acute COPD exacerbation, *Am J Respir Crit Care Med* 154:407-412, 1996.
29. Kertjens HAM and others: A comparison of bronchodilator therapy with and without inhaled corticosteroids therapy for obstructive airway disease, *N Engl J Med* 327:1413-1419, 1992.
30. The debate over inhaled corticosteroid use in COPD, *J COPD Management* 2(5):13-16, 2001.
31. Lacasse Y and others: Meta-analysis of respiratory rehabilitation in chronic obstructive pulmonary disease, *Lancet* 348:1115-1119, 1996.
32. Kharestan A: The role of pulmonary rehabilitation in the treatment of COPD patients, *J COPD Management* 2(4):10-15, 2001.
33. Celli BR: Pulmonary rehabilitation for COPD: a practical approach for improving ventilatory conditioning, *Postgrad Med* 103:159-160, 167-168, 173-176, 1998.
34. Casaburi R: Exercise training in chronic obstructive pulmonary disease, In Casaburi R, Petty TL, editors: *Principles and practice of pulmonary rehabilitation,* Philadelphia, 1994, WB Saunders.
35. Cooper CB: Exercise in chronic pulmonary disease: aerobic exercise prescription, *Med Sci Sports Exerc* 33(July Suppl):5671-5679, 2001.

CHAPTER 112

Dyspnea

David Patrick Murphy and David A. Bradshaw

DEFINITION/EPIDEMIOLOGY

Dyspnea is the word medical practitioners use when patients complain of breathing difficulty. The complex nature of this symptom prompted an American Thoracic Society consensus panel to define dyspnea as "... a term used to characterize a subjective experience of breathing discomfort that consists of qualitatively distinct sensations that vary in intensity. The experience derives from interactions among multiple physiologic, psychologic, social, and environmental factors, and may induce secondary physiologic and behavioral responses."[1] Although breathlessness is expected after vigorous exercise, dyspnea is a cardinal manifestation of cardiopulmonary disease that warrants appropriate evaluation and treatment.

PATHOPHYSIOLOGY

The mechanisms responsible for the sensations we identify as dyspnea are complex and vary by disease. Conceptually, it has been suggested that dyspnea occurs whenever sensory input from receptors in the airways, lung, and chest wall does not match up with respiratory drive.[2] These sensory receptors may respond to chemicals, stretch, irritation, or passive distention. For example, there appears to be a dissociation between sensory input and motor output in conditions that impose a mechanical load on the respiratory system by either decreasing compliance of the lung (e.g., pneumonia, pulmonary edema, fibrosis) and/or chest wall (e.g., kyphoscoliosis, rib fractures, circumferential thorax burns) or inhibiting airflow (e.g., asthma, chronic bronchitis, emphysema).[3] In addition, neuromuscular weakness or fatigue may cause dyspnea symptoms because or the inability of weakened muscles to generate an expected level of ventilation. Hypoxemia and hypercapnia (carbon dioxide retention) stimulate chemoreceptors that may cause dyspnea through increased respiratory motor drive. Somewhat surprisingly, there is a poor correlation between dyspnea and blood gas abnormalities. Dyspneic patients are often perplexed to learn that they have adequate oxygen saturation or when supplemental oxygen administration does not relieve symptoms. Finally, it is important to understand that the perception of dyspnea varies greatly among patients and is influenced by various psychologic, social, and environmental factors.

CLINICAL PRESENTATION

Dyspnea is a common complaint. The following dimensions are useful in elucidating the disease process that causes dyspnea: quality, timing, intensity, associated symptoms, and environmental exposures.

Quality

The descriptors patients use to describe dyspnea sensations may be diagnostically useful.[4-7] For example, patients with asthma tend to complain of "chest tightness" or "constriction."

Diseases associated with an increased mechanical load (either resulting from decreased compliance or increased airway resistance) are often associated with feelings of excessive "work" or "effort." Patients with an increased drive to breathe (e.g., resulting from hypoxemia or hypercapnia) experience air hunger and they may complain that they "can't get enough air in." Most pulmonary diseases probably activate multiple dyspnea mechanisms leading to a composite of sensations that defy easy classification.

Timing

Although it is often impossible to pinpoint the precise onset of dyspnea, it is important to distinguish between acute and chronic symptoms. Sudden onset of dyspnea often heralds serious cardiopulmonary disease that requires immediate evaluation and treatment (e.g., pulmonary embolism, pneumothorax, myocardial infarction). Relative stability, intermittent exacerbations, or progressive debilitating symptoms may characterize chronic dyspnea. Patients with increasing symptoms or intermittent exacerbations should be carefully reevaluated for worsening disease or a new problem.

Intensity

Dyspnea severity is difficult to quantify, and therefore activity limitation is commonly used as a surrogate marker. Dyspnea is almost always first noticed with physical exertion and may progress to symptoms at rest. The degree of activity necessary to elicit symptoms may be quantified by asking questions such as, "how many flights of stairs" or "how far can you walk on level ground?" One commonly used scale for classifying the severity of dyspnea was proposed and published by the Medical Research Council (Table 112-1).

Associated Symptoms

In addition to dyspnea, chest pain, cough, hemoptysis, and wheezing are cardinal symptoms of pulmonary disease. Chest pain is one manifestation of ischemic heart disease, but may also result from pneumothorax, pulmonary embolism, or rib trauma. Hemoptysis is a very distressing symptom that may accompany dyspnea. Expectorated blood can originate from the nose, airways, or lung parenchyma. Cough is an exceedingly common symptom of acute and chronic pulmonary disease. Persistent cough is most often caused by postnasal drip, gastroesophageal reflux, or asthma. Wheezing signifies airway diseases such as asthma and chronic obstructive pulmonary disease (COPD), or focal obstruction by tumor or aspirated foreign body. Patients who present with fever, chills, or night sweats should be evaluated for acute or chronic lung infections including pneumonia, tuberculosis, and chronic bronchiectasis.

TABLE 112-1 Dyspnea Scale

Grade	Degree	Defining Clinical Characteristics
0	None	Not troubled with breathlessness except with strenuous exercise
1	Slight	Troubled by shortness of breath when hurrying on level ground or walking up a slight hill
2	Moderate	Walks more slowly than people of the same age when on level ground because of breathlessness or has to stop for breath when walking at own pace on level ground.
3	Severe	Stops for breath after walking about 100 yards or after a few minutes on level ground
4	Very severe	Too breathless to leave the house or breathless when dressing or undressing

Exposures

The lungs are uniquely susceptible to various environmental hazards including air pollution, dust, and smoke. A careful history of current and past tobacco use is essential in the evaluation of tobacco-related diseases such as asthma, chronic bronchitis, emphysema, spontaneous pneumothorax secondary to bullous disease, ischemic heart disease, respiratory bronchiolitis, and eosinophilic granuloma. In addition, many medications, as well as therapeutic radiation, are known to damage the lungs.

PHYSICAL EXAMINATION

The physical examination begins with careful assessment of the patient's vital signs. Normal respiratory rate in adults ranges from 12 to 20, and a rapid or labored breathing pattern is often, but not always, evident in dyspneic patients. Many practitioners consider pulse oximetry a "vital sign," as it usually provides a reliable measure of arterial oxygen saturation. A normal oxygen saturation level, however, does not rule out carbon dioxide retention and ventilatory insufficiency (carbon dioxide levels must be directly measured with an arterial blood gas sample). Expiratory peak flow measurement may also be included in the initial assessment of patients with known airways disease or when wheezing is detected.

Breathing pattern and body position provide important clues to disease severity. The acutely dyspneic patient often sits upright and leans forward to optimize breathing mechanics. The inability to speak in full sentences and accessory respiratory muscle use indicate increased work of breathing. Patients with COPD often adopt a characteristic "pursed-lip" appearance. Shallow, rapid breathing or panting is characteristic interstitial lung diseases. The skin may be diaphoretic and the patient may appear anxious. Bluish discoloration of the skin and mucous membranes (cyanosis) results from increased amounts of deoxygenated hemoglobin. Central cyanosis, detected in the tongue and mucous membranes, is a more reliable indicator of oxygenation than peripheral cyanosis, which can also result from intense vasoconstriction of vessels in the extremities. Mental status may be depressed by either severe hypoxemia or hypercapnia. Digital or finger clubbing is an important finding often attributed to various lung diseases, but it is also seen in other disorders such as in inflammatory bowel disease and congenital heart disease.

The lung examination includes careful inspection of the thorax and abdomen. Chest wall deformities may limit lung expansion and contribute to dyspnea. Normally the chest and abdomen move symmetrically or "in phase." When the chest rises and the abdomen falls, the pattern of breathing is said to be "paradoxical" and indicates diaphragmatic weakness or fatigue. Palpation of the chest wall is useful in assessing tracheal position, symmetry of chest movement, areas of tenderness, and crepitus (subcutaneous air from pneumothorax or pneumomediastinum). Airless lung transmits sounds more efficiently than air-filled lung and is the basis for auscultatory consolidative findings including bronchial breath sounds, egophony (E to A changes), and whisper pectoriloquy. The classic example of a disease that causes lung consolidation is pneumonia, although any process that fills (pus, water, blood. protein, cells) or collapses alveoli yields these findings. Abnormal or "adventitious" lung sounds are distinguished by whether they are continuous (high pitched = wheezing, low pitched = rhonchi) or discontinuous (crackles). Wheezing signifies bronchoconstriction or airway obstruction from secretions, tumor, or foreign body. Crackles are heard in a number of disease processes including congestive heart failure and interstitial lung disease. Pleural friction rubs are grating sounds that may occur in inspiration and/or expiration as inflamed pleural surfaces rub against each other.

A detailed discussion of the cardiac examination is beyond the scope of this chapter, but is an important component of the evaluation of dyspneic patients. The pulse should be carefully analyzed for rate and rhythm. Atrial fibrillation is a common arrhythmia that can usually be diagnosed at the bedside by its "irregularly irregular" character. Left ventricular dysfunction and valvular heart disease also lend themselves to bedside diagnosis through palpation and auscultation. The extremities should also be assessed for pulse and edema.

In summary, the physical examination is an essential part of the workup of dyspneic patients and should be used to help direct the diagnostic evaluation. Studies suggest that the absence of specific physical examination findings is of greater diagnostic utility than positive findings in patients with chronic dyspnea. For example, interstitial lung disease and congestive heart failure are unlikely causes of dyspnea in a patient without crackles on lung examination.

DIAGNOSTICS

After a thorough history and physical examination are completed, further diagnostic studies may be necessary. A plain chest radiograph is helpful in elucidating many causes of dyspnea. Radiographic findings of hyperinflation, flattened hemidiaphragms, increased anterior clear space, and bulla support a diagnosis of chronic obstructive lung disease. Parenchymal infiltrates occur in many different disease processes but, in the context of an acute infectious syndrome, implies pneumonia. Congestive heart failure is recognized by cephalization of vessels, Kerley's B lines, and an enlarged cardiac silhouette. Frank pulmonary edema presents with bilateral perihilar air-space filling ("bat wing" appearance) and pleural effusions. Pneumothorax and pleural effusion are generally easily detected on a plain chest radiograph, although small effusions may require decubitus views for confirmation. The chest radiograph is usually normal or reveals only subtle abnormalities in asthma and pulmonary embolism.

Spirometry is essential to the diagnosis and management of asthma and COPD. A decrease in the ratio of forced expiratory volume in 1 second to forced vital capacity (FEV_1/FVC) is the spirometric hallmark of obstruction. Bronchoprovocation testing with either methacholine or exercise may be necessary to diagnose asthma in patients with normal baseline spirometry. Proportionately reduced FEV_1 and FVC suggest restriction (a useful pneumonic for restrictive lung processes is "PAINT" *p*leural disease, *a*lveolar filling process, *i*nterstitial lung disease, *n*euromuscular disease, or *t*horacic cage abnormalities) that should be confirmed with lung volume measurements. Diaphragmatic and respiratory muscle weakness may be detected with maximal inspiratory pressure and maximal expiratory pressure maneuvers, although these tests are neither sensitive nor specific.

The workup for pulmonary thromboembolic disease can be complicated and is often driven by the availability and expertise of local medical resources. An appropriate evaluation may initially include a ventilation/perfusion scan or CT angiogram. Symptomatic lower extremity clots (the source for most pulmonary emboli) are usually detected by ultrasound. Pulmonary angiography remains the "gold standard" for the diagnosis of pulmonary embolism.

Cardiac rhythm disturbances and hypertrophy may be noted on routine ECG, although intermittent arrhythmias may be detected only by long-term monitoring (e.g., telemetry, Holter, or event monitoring). Echocardiography is extremely useful in assessing left ventricular function, cardiac valve status, pericardial effusions, and, in some cases, pulmonary hypertension.

Other routine studies with utility in the evaluation of patients with dyspnea include hemoglobin level to exclude anemia and thyroid function tests to exclude hyperthyroidism. More sophisticated testing such as formal cardiopulmonary exercise testing and cardiac catheterization obviously require referral to specialists.

DIFFERENTIAL DIAGNOSIS

Dyspnea is most commonly caused by cardiopulmonary disease, although anemia, neuromuscular weakness, gastroesophageal reflux, deconditioning, and psychogenic causes must be considered. The most common causes of acute dyspnea are asthma, bronchitis, pneumothorax, pneumonia, pulmonary embolism, chest trauma with rib fractures or pulmonary contusions, ischemic heart failure, psychogenic causes, and acute blood loss. The majority of patients with

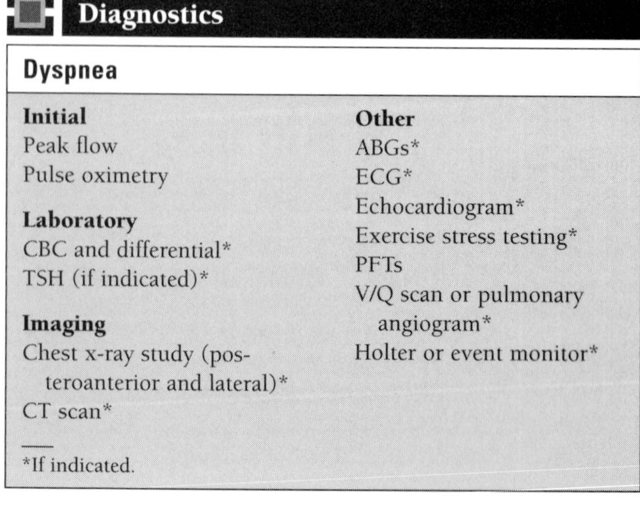

Diagnostics

Dyspnea

Initial
Peak flow
Pulse oximetry

Laboratory
CBC and differential*
TSH (if indicated)*

Imaging
Chest x-ray study (posteroanterior and lateral)*
CT scan*

Other
ABGs*
ECG*
Echocardiogram*
Exercise stress testing*
PFTs
V/Q scan or pulmonary angiogram*
Holter or event monitor*

*If indicated.

long-standing dyspnea have one of four etiologies: asthma, COPD, interstitial lung disease, or cardiomyopathy.[3]

MANAGEMENT

The treatment of dyspnea entails treatment of the underlying disease process and symptomatic relief. Supplemental oxygen should be administered initially to all acutely dyspneic patients and to chronically dyspneic patients who are hypoxemic. The standard Medicare criteria for supplemental oxygen are as follows: PaO_2 at rest of <55 mm Hg or oxygen saturation <89%. Patients with a PaO_2 of 56 to 59 mm Hg warrant supplemental oxygen if they have underlying congestive heart failure or pulmonary hypertension. These criteria are based on two large studies that demonstrated improved survival in hypoxemic COPD patients treated with supplemental oxygen.[8,9] Patients who desaturate during sleep or exercise also qualify for supplemental oxygen, although the data supporting these indications are not as strong. Administration of supplemental oxygen may worsen CO_2 retention in some patients with COPD. These patients require assessment with an arterial blood gas to ensure adequate carbon dioxide elimination. Energy conservation strategies (e.g., slow walking pace; periodically using resting positions, such as leaning forward while sitting in a chair, avoiding fatigue; and spacing chores at times when feeling good) and specific breathing techniques are often effective in patients with obstructive lung disease. Patients with difficulty mobilizing secretions (e.g., chronic bronchitis, bronchiectasis, cystic fibrosis) benefit from chest physiotherapy and airway clearance adjuncts such as the flutter device or vest airway clearance system. Anxiolytics and narcotics are sometimes effective in relieving dyspnea, but must be used cautiously due to inherent respiratory depressant properties.

Formal pulmonary rehabilitation programs effectively incorporate dyspnea management therapies with nutrition and exercise. These programs have been shown to improve quality of life and may reduce unscheduled medical visits.[10-12]

Differential Diagnosis

Dyspnea

Acute	Chronic
Acute blood loss	Anemia
Airway obstruction	Asthma
Asthma	Cardiomyopathy
Bronchitis	Chronic obstructive pulmonary disease
Carbon monoxide poisoning	Congestive heart failure
Congestive heart failure/pulmonary edema	Cystic fibrosis
Foreign body aspiration	Gastroesophageal reflux disease
Ischemic heart disease	Interstitial pulmonary fibrosis
Neuromuscular weakness	Ischemic heart disease
Pleural effusion	Obesity
Pneumonia	Pectus excavatum
Pneumothorax	Pleural effusion
Psychogenic	Pulmonary hypertension
Pulmonary contusions	Sarcoidosis
Pulmonary emboli	Severe kyphoscoliosis
Trauma (rib fractures or pulmonary contusions)	Spondylitis

COMPLICATIONS

Dyspnea limits activity and alters lifestyle. The consequences of uncontrolled dyspnea symptoms may include anxiety, depression, loss of job, and social isolation. Physical deconditioning results from decreased exercise and leads to a downward spiral of ever-decreasing activity.

INDICATIONS FOR REFERRAL/HOSPITALIZATION

Patients with chronic dyspnea should be referred to a pulmonary specialist when the etiology is not obvious from the history, physical examination, and screening studies including complete blood count, chest radiograph, and spirometry. An echocardiogram and treadmill stress test may help differentiate between cardiac and pulmonary disease before the consultation.

The decision to hospitalize a patient depends initially on identifying the likely cause of respiratory distress. Conditions that need to be readily identified and mandate hospital admission include pulmonary embolism and myocardial infarction. Criteria for hospitalization of patients with other conditions such as pneumothorax, asthma, and COPD depend on the severity of the illness, response to treatment, and presence of co-morbid conditions.

PATIENT AND FAMILY EDUCATION

Patients with chronic dyspnea need to be taught techniques that control symptoms and to recognize warning signs that signal need for medical assistance. Pulmonary rehabilitation programs provide intense education for patients with severe pulmonary disease, but are expensive and not always available. All patients who use inhaled bronchodilators and corticosteroids should be regularly instructed in proper inhaler techniques. Asthmatic patients may benefit from home peak-flow monitoring to detect worsening airflow obstruction, which offers an opportunity for early intervention. Smoking cessation is critical in the management of any cardiopulmonary disease and clinicians play a pivotal role in educating their patients regarding the adverse effects of tobacco use and strategies to stop smoking.

REFERENCES

1. Meek PM and others: Dyspnea: mechanisms. Assessment, and management. A consensus statement, *Am J Respir Crit Care Med* 159: 321-340, 1999.
2. Schwartzstein RM and others: Breathlessness induced by dissociation between ventilation and chemical drive, *Am Rev Respir Dis* 139: 1231-1237, 1989.
3. Pratter MR and others: Cause and evaluation of chronic dyspnea in a pulmonary disease clinic, *Arch Intern Med* 149:2277, 1989.
4. Harver A and others: Descriptor of breathlessness in healthy individuals. Distinct and separable constructs, *Chest* 118:679-690, 2000.
5. Moy ML and others: Quality of dyspnea in bronchoconstriction differs from external resistive loads, *Am J Respir Crit Care Med* 162:451-455, 2000.
6. O'Donnell DE, Chau LK, Webb KA: Qualtitative aspects of exertional dyspnea in patients with interstitial lung disease, *J Appl Physiol* 84(6):2000-2009,1998.
7. Mahler DA and others: Descriptor of breathlessness in cardiorespiratory diseases, *Am Respir Crit Care Med* 154:1357-1363, 1996.

8. Nocturnal Oxygen Therapy Trial Group: Continuous or nocturnal oxygen therapy in hypoxemic chronic obstructive lung disease: a clinical trial, *Ann Intern Med* 93:391-398, 1980.
9. Medical Research Council Working Party: Long-term domiciliary oxygen therapy in chronic hypoxic cor pulmonale complicating chronic bronchitis and emphysema, *Lancet* 1:681-686, 1981.
10. Fishman AP: Pulmonary rehabilitation research. NIH workshop summary, *Am Rev Respir Dis* 149:825-833, 1994.
11. Ries AL: Position paper of the American Association of Cardiovascular and Pulmonary Rehabilitation: scientific basis of pulmonary rehabilitation, *J Cardiopulm Rehabil* 10:418-441, 1990.
12. Pulmonary rehabilitation. Joint ACCP/AACVPR evidence-based guidelines, *Chest* 112:1363-1396, 1997.

CHAPTER 113

Hemoptysis

Updated by Patricia Polgar Bailey

DEFINITION/EPIDEMIOLOGY

Hemoptysis refers to the expectoration of blood or blood-stained sputum from a site in the tracheobronchial tree, lung parenchyma, or pulmonary circulation. It can range from a small amount of blood-streaked sputum, which is commonly seen in bronchitis, to a massive hemorrhage that rapidly causes death by asphyxiation. Massive hemoptysis is uncommon but requires immediate attention because the reported mortality rate is 38% or higher.[1] Even slight bleeding may signify a serious condition, such as bronchogenic carcinoma or tuberculosis.

More than 100 causes of hemoptysis have been reported, but only a few of these are responsible for the majority of cases.[2,3] Infection is the most common cause of hemoptysis worldwide. In the Western world, hemoptysis is often related to neoplasms and acute bronchitis.

PATHOPHYSIOLOGY

For hemoptysis to occur, there must be some communication between the airways and the blood vessels of the lungs. The lungs receive blood from two relatively independent circulations: pulmonary and bronchial. The pulmonary circulation is characterized by lower pressures and higher volumes and is supplied with mixed venous blood via the pulmonary arteries. In contrast, the bronchial circulation supplies oxygenated blood in a high-pressure, low-volume circuit.

The bronchial arteries can become enlarged and more numerous in association with a variety of inflammatory or neoplastic diseases. Chronic inflammation, often associated with infectious processes, can lead to destruction of the connective tissue of blood vessels or result in erosion through the vessel wall. Angiographic studies have revealed that hemoptysis typically originates from the bronchial arteries. This is presumably related to the connection of these arteries to the proliferative nests of small vessels often found in areas of inflammation and tumors.

CLINICAL PRESENTATION

It is common for patients to confuse hemoptysis with hematemesis or epistaxis. Blood from the airways is usually bright red, alkaline, and frothy because of the presence of surfactant. Blood originating in the gastrointestinal tract is usually dark red and acidic and may be intermixed with food particles.

It is important to carefully determine the chronology and volume of hemoptysis. Quantifying blood loss may be difficult in patients who are clinically stable because they are often anxious. Urgent evaluation and possible hospitalization are indicated if more than 50 ml of blood has been expectorated in the previous 24 hours. For smaller amounts of blood loss, a thorough diagnostic evaluation can be initiated in the office of the primary care provider.

A long history of small-volume, recurrent hemoptysis with little or no sputum production indicates a process such as bronchogenic carcinoma, bronchial adenoma, or vascular malformation. A history of chronic sputum production suggests an infectious etiology such as bronchitis, bronchiectasis, lung abscess, or tuberculosis. Hemoptysis associated with bacterial pneumonia is suggested by an acute onset of fever, sputum production, and, commonly, pleuritic chest pain. Hemoptysis is commonly a late symptom of bronchogenic carcinoma and is preceded by a chronic cough, fatigue, and constitutional symptoms. Abrupt hemoptysis associated with cigarette smoking is often seen with bronchitis and/or bronchogenic carcinoma.

PHYSICAL EXAMINATION

The presence of a fever is indicative of infection. A thorough examination of the ears, nose, and throat can detect upper airway sources of bleeding, such as laryngeal carcinoma lesions. The presence of stridor or findings suggestive of chronic obstructive pulmonary disease, congestive heart failure, or pneumonia can be determined by auscultation of the chest.

Localized wheezing may indicate a local obstruction, foreign body, or bronchogenic carcinoma. A pleural friction rub may be the only sign of pulmonary infarction associated with a pulmonary embolism. Isolated crackles are nonspecific for the location of the primary disease because they may represent an inflammatory reaction to blood aspirated from another site.

Digital clubbing is suggestive of chronic lung disease, such as bronchiectasis or malignancy. Cardiac examination may help determine the presence of mitral stenosis. Localized adenopathy, especially a supraclavicular node, may be indicative of a lung malignancy. A bleeding disorder is suggested by the presence of petechiae or ecchymoses.

DIAGNOSTICS

The most important routine study for evaluating hemoptysis is chest radiography. Comparing the chest x-ray film with an earlier one is valuable in determining whether the lung process is acute or chronic. Important diagnostic findings include an air-fluid level of a lung abscess, the "crescent sign" of a mycetoma, a nodule that suggests a neoplasm, evidence of volume loss, or consolidation distal to an airway obstruction. Although the value of a CT scan of the chest in patients with a nondiagnostic chest x-ray film is uncertain, the CT scan remains a sensitive diagnostic test when used alone.[1]

Sputum studies may reveal a specific infectious agent or occasionally may provide a cytologic diagnosis. A routine Gram's stain, culture and sensitivities, acid-fast stains, and cytologic studies are recommended. Other routine laboratory tests should be tailored to the clinical situation.

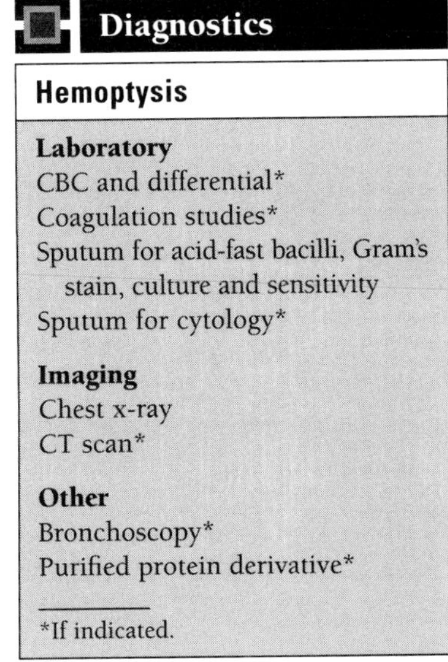

Diagnostics

Hemoptysis

Laboratory
CBC and differential*
Coagulation studies*
Sputum for acid-fast bacilli, Gram's stain, culture and sensitivity
Sputum for cytology*

Imaging
Chest x-ray
CT scan*

Other
Bronchoscopy*
Purified protein derivative*

*If indicated.

Differential Diagnosis

Hemoptysis

Bronchitis*	Congestive heart failure*
Bronchogenic carcinoma	Mitral valve prolapse
Tuberculosis*	Metastatic tumor
Bronchiectasis*	Bronchopulmonary sequestration
Mycetoma	Endobronchial foreign body
Lung abscess*	Bleeding diathesis
Lung cancer*	Wegener's granulomatosis
Bronchial adenoma	Trauma
Foreign body	Fungal infection
Pneumonia*	Parasitic infection
Pulmonary embolism*	Medication (amiodarone)
Arteriovenous malformation	
Goodpasture's syndrome	

*Common causes.

Fiberoptic bronchoscopy has become the most valuable diagnostic tool in evaluating hemoptysis. This procedure allows direct visualization of the airways and localization of the bleeding source. Biopsy and lavage samples from the airways and alveolar spaces can be sent for cytologic and microbial studies. This procedure is relatively safe, is well tolerated, and can be performed on an outpatient basis. The proper timing for fiberoptic bronchoscopy is somewhat controversial. Most thoracic specialists prefer to perform bronchoscopy earlier in the course of hemoptysis. However, some specialists advocate delaying bronchoscopy until the hemoptysis has subsided because it is possible that the procedure will induce coughing and increase bleeding.

DIFFERENTIAL DIAGNOSIS

Despite a thorough evaluation, many patients who present with hemoptysis do not receive a specific diagnosis. The differential diagnosis is extensive, but common causes include infection, bronchiectasis, and lung cancer.[1-5] Less commonly, trauma, a foreign body, or medications may be associated with hemoptysis.

MANAGEMENT

Patients with massive hemoptysis require rapid and decisive care. The immediate goal is to prevent asphyxiation, and therefore airway control should be ensured as rapidly as possible. To protect the unaffected lung, insertion of a double-lumen endotracheal tube that allows selective and individual ventilation and suctioning of each lung is usually indicated. Bleeding can be contained by introducing a special balloon-tipped catheter through a bronchoscope and inflating the balloon in the bronchus where the bleeding arises.[6] If the bleeding site is known, patients should be directed to lie with the bleeding side down to prevent blood from draining into the noninvolved lung.

The availability of typed and cross-matched blood is a necessity. Other temporizing measures include an endobronchial iced saline lavage and the application of fibrinogen-thrombin through the bronchoscope. If there is no response to these measures or if the condition worsens, two major modes of therapy are available: surgical resection of the bleeding site and angiographic embolization.

Cough suppressants such as codeine and hydrocodone are often used in patients with hemoptysis. Antibiotics are indicated if the cause of hemoptysis is believed to be a bacterial infection.

COMPLICATIONS

Patients with hemoptysis resulting from noninfectious causes are at risk for frequent recurrences. The most obvious complication of massive hemoptysis is asphyxiation, which accounts for the majority of deaths from hemoptysis.

INDICATIONS FOR REFERRAL/HOSPITALIZATION

Patients with hemoptysis are often referred to a pulmonary specialist for diagnostic evaluation unless their symptoms suggest infection and the hemoptysis responds to antibiotics. Hospitalization is rarely necessary unless hemoptysis is greater than 50 to 100 ml in 24 hours or there is significant respiratory compromise.

PATIENT AND FAMILY EDUCATION

Education about hemoptysis should include information about the diagnostic evaluation. It is important that the patient be taught the importance of adhering to the prescribed treatment. The rate of recurrence in patients who smoke is likely to be high because common causes such as bronchitis and bronchogenic carcinoma are often related to smoking. Therefore it is imperative that patients be encouraged to quit smoking. Because hemoptysis can be particularly disconcerting, emotional support for the patient and family is especially important.

REFERENCES

1. Hershberg B and others: Hemoptysis: etiology, evaluation, and outcome in tertiary referral hospital, *Chest* 112(2):440-444, 1997.
2. Mroz BJ and others: Hemoptysis as the presenting symptom in bronchiolitis obliterans organizing pneumonia, *Chest* 111(6):1775-1776, 1997.
3. Nelson JE, Forman M: Hemoptysis in HIV-infected patients, *Chest* 110(3):737-743, 1996.
4. Goldstein I and others: Very early onset of acute amiodarone pulmonary toxicity presenting with hemoptysis, *Chest* 111(5):1446-1447, 1997.
5. Lick SD, Conti VR: Automatic internal cardioverter-defibrillator patch erosion into the upper airway presenting as a cavitary lesion, *Chest* 112(4):1144-1146, 1997.
6. Freitage L: Development of a new balloon catheter for management of hemoptysis with bronchofiberscopes, *Chest* 103:593, 1993.

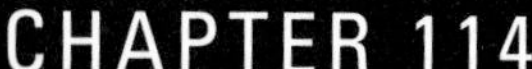

CHAPTER 114

Influenza

Judy Ptak

DEFINITION/EPIDEMIOLOGY

Influenza is an acute infection of the respiratory tract caused by influenza virus type A or B. It is usually a self-limited disease that occurs in outbreaks, primarily during the winter months in temperate climates, and may occur year round in the tropics. Influenza is highly contagious and occurs in all age-groups. It tends to occur in outbreaks that can rapidly affect 10% to 40% of the population.[1]

PATHOPHYSIOLOGY

Influenza is transmitted from person to person via respiratory secretions that contain virus. These respiratory secretions are spread in the form of droplets that are produced when a person talks, coughs, or sneezes. Virus is detectable and may be shed in respiratory secretions up to 24 hours before the onset of symptoms.

Once virus reaches the epithelium cells of the respiratory tract it penetrates the cells and begins replication. This viral replication leads to cell death and release of large amounts of virus that can infect adjacent cells. This quickly causes desquamation of the ciliated epithelium. Onset of the acute symptoms coincides with this desquamation.[1]

CLINICAL PRESENTATION

After an incubation period of 1 to 2 days there is an abrupt onset of symptoms. These symptoms include fever, chills, headache, malaise, myalgia, and loss of appetite. Respiratory symptoms are also present but are usually overshadowed by the severity of the systemic symptoms. Respiratory symptoms include dry cough, nasal congestion and clear discharge, and sore throat. The cough is usually the most prominent of these respiratory symptoms.

The patient's temperature rises rapidly after onset, peaking at 37.7° to 40.0° C (100° to 104° F) in about 12 hours. The fever typically begins to decline on the second or third day and may last as long as 4 to 8 days. Systemic symptoms become less prominent as the fever decreases. A convalescent phase of 1 to 2 weeks follows the acute febrile stage. Cough, malaise, and fatigue, often extreme, are often seen during the convalescent phase.

Some patients have mild illness that resembles the common cold. Older adults, people with underlying chronic diseases, and women in the third trimester of pregnancy may experience a rapidly worsening course of influenza.

PHYSICAL EXAMINATION

Uncomplicated cases of influenza have minimal physical findings. At the onset of symptoms the patient's face is often flushed and the eyes may be watery and red. The skin may be hot and moist. Cervical lymph nodes may be enlarged and tender. The pharynx is usually unremarkable and the chest examination is usually normal.[2]

DIAGNOSTICS

Virus can be isolated from nose and throat specimens such as nasal swabs or washings, sputum, and throat swabs. Virus can be detected in cell cultures in 2 to 7 days. There are several techniques to detect the presence of viral antigens in nose and throat specimens that yield results rapidly, ranging from 1 hour to 24 to 48 hours. These rapid tests may not be as sensitive as cell culture, however, and they may be most useful in the management of individual patients at high risk for serious complications from influenza, who may benefit most from appropriate antiviral treatment. These rapid diagnostic tests for influenza may also be helpful in institutional settings where prophylaxis for other residents is indicated.[3]

Infection with influenza virus can also be confirmed by showing at least a fourfold rise in antibody titer in convalescent serum taken 10 to 20 days after an acute serum sample.

Clinical diagnosis in the setting of a confirmed influenza outbreak is very accurate.

DIFFERENTIAL DIAGNOSIS

On an individual basis in the absence of a known outbreak of influenza, it may be difficult to distinguish a case of the flu from many of the other respiratory viruses such as the common cold and respiratory syncytial virus. Other things to consider are *Mycoplasma pneumoniae,* bacterial pneumonia, and severe streptococcal pharyngitis.

MANAGEMENT

Treatment of influenza is primarily symptomatic. Patients should rest as much as possible. They should maintain an adequate fluid intake. Antipyretics and analgesics can be used to control fever and relieve headache and myalgia.

In the United States four antiviral medications are currently approved for treatment of influenza: amantadine (Symmetrel), rimantadine (Flumadine), zanamivir (Relenza), and oseltamivir (Tamiflu). Amantadine and rimantadine are approved for chemoprophylaxis and treatment of influenza A. Zanamivir and oseltamivir may be used for treatment of uncomplicated influenza. Oseltamivir may also be used for chemoprophylaxis of influenza. When used as treatment for influenza, these drugs must be started within 48 hours of the onset of symptoms and can reduce the severity of the symptoms and the duration of symptoms by about 1 day.[4] Recommendations for the treatment and prophylaxis of influenza with antiviral drugs are listed in Boxes 114-1 and 114-2.

BOX 114-1

RECOMMENDATIONS FOR TREATMENT OF INFLUENZA WITH ANTIVIRAL DRUGS

- All people at risk for complications in whom influenza develops
- People with severe influenza
- Consider for people with influenza who wish to shorten the duration of their illness

From Prevention and Control of Influenza. Recommendations of the Advisory Committee on Immunization Practices (ACIP), *MMWR* 50(RR04); 1-46, 2001.

LIFE SPAN CONSIDERATIONS

Influenza can cause mortality in any age-group; however, mortality is highest in older people. In the United States, about 20,000 people die each year from influenza or its complications. People 65 years old or older account for more than 90% of these deaths. In a large retrospective study of women between 15 and 64 years old, Neuzil and colleagues[5] found a significant increase in acute cardiopulmonary hospitalizations and deaths during influenza season.

COMPLICATIONS

The primary complications of influenza are pulmonary. The most notable pulmonary complications are primary influenza pneumonia, which is rare, or secondary bacterial pneumonia. Other pulmonary complications include croup in children and exacerbation of chronic pulmonary disease. CNS complications such as Guillain-Barré syndrome and encephalitis rarely occur after influenza infection. The association with influenza infection and Reye's syndrome in children prompted the recommendation that aspirin be avoided when treating children with influenza. Other complications that have been associated with influenza infection are myositis, which is seen primarily in children, and toxic shock syndrome.

INDICATIONS FOR REFERRAL/HOSPITALIZATION

Patients who do not begin to gradually improve a few days after the onset of symptoms should be reevaluated and referred as appropriate. Hospitalization may be indicated for patients with underlying chronic conditions that are complicated by the added stress of influenza infection. Anyone who is rapidly getting worse should be considered for hospitalization.

PATIENT AND FAMILY EDUCATION

Patients and their families should be educated about the need to get the influenza vaccine on a yearly basis. Basic personnel hygiene measures such as good hand washing may help to reduce the risk of acquiring influenza.

HEALTH PROMOTION

The influenza vaccine is the primary method of preventing influenza infection. People at risk for complications from influenza infection should be encouraged to receive the influenza vaccine, as well as people who are likely to transmit influenza to those at high risk for complications. The vaccine should be

BOX 114-2

RECOMMENDATIONS FOR PROPHYLAXIS OF INFLUENZA WITH ANTIVIRAL DRUGS

- Persons at high risk who have not been vaccinated
- Persons at high risk who are vaccinated after influenza activity has begun
- Unvaccinated household members of persons at high risk
- Unvaccinated persons who provide care to those at high risk
- Persons who have immune deficiency

From Prevention and Control of Influenza. Recommendations of the Advisory Committee on Immunization Practices (ACIP), *MMWR* 50(RR04); 1-46, 2001.

BOX 114-3

RECOMMENDATIONS FOR USE OF INFLUENZA VACCINE

- People 50 years or older
- Residents of long-term-care facilities
- Adults and children with chronic pulmonary or cardiovascular disease (including asthma)
- Adults and children requiring care for chronic metabolic disease, renal dysfunction, hemoglobinopathy, or immunosuppression (including HIV)
- Children (6 months to 18 years) receiving long-term aspirin therapy
- Women who will be in the second or third trimester of pregnancy during the influenza season (usually December through March)
- People who can transmit influenza to those at high risk
  - Health care personnel
  - Employees of long-term-care facilities
  - Employees of residences for people at high risk
- Providers of home care to people at high risk
  - Household members (including children) of people at high risk
- Groups to consider for vaccination
  - People at high risk traveling to locations where influenza may be circulating
  - People providing essential community services
  - Students and others in institutional settings
  - Any person who wishes to reduce the risk of infection with influenza

From Prevention and Control of Influenza. Recommendations of the Advisory Committee on Immunization Practices (ACIP), *MMWR* 50(RR04); 1-46, 2001.

given each year at least 2 weeks before the expected start of the influenza season. In the temperate climates mid October to the start of the flu season is the preferred time to vaccinate people. The vaccine that is presently available in the United States contains three inactivated strains of influenza virus, two influenza subtypes and one influenza B type. On an annual basis the U.S. Food and Drug Administration determines the influenza strains to be included in the next year's vaccine based on which viruses are most likely to cause epidemics in the coming winter.[6] A live attenuated influenza virus vaccine given via intranasal spray is currently being developed. Recommendations for the use of influenza vaccines are listed in Box 114-3.

REFERENCES

1. Mandell G and others: *Principles and practice of infectious diseases*, ed 5, Philadelphia, 2000, WB Saunders.
2. Fauci A and others: *Harrison's principles of internal medicine*, ed 14, New York, 1998, McGraw-Hill.
3. Coonrad JD: Influenza: will new diagnostic tests and antiviral drugs make a difference? *Chest* 119(6):1630-1632, 2001.
4. Advisory Committee on Immunization Practices: Prevention and control of influenza, *MMWR* 50(RR04):1-46, 2001.
5. Neuzil KM and others: Influenza-associated morbidity and mortality in young and middle-aged women, *JAMA* 281(10):901-907, 1999.
6. Couch RB: Prevention and treatment of influenza, *N Engl J Med* 343(24):1778-1787, 2000.

CHAPTER 115

Lung Cancer

Kathleen Thaney and Terry Mahan Buttaro

DEFINITION/EPIDEMIOLOGY

Throughout the world lung cancer continues to be the leading cause of cancer-related deaths, and in the United States more than 154,000 people are expected to die from lung cancer in 2002.[1] More women now die of lung cancer than of breast cancer and in this country lung cancer causes more deaths than breast, colorectal, and prostate cancer combined.[1] African-American men and women have a higher incidence of cancer in general and lung cancer specifically than do Caucasian men and women. Risk factors for lung cancer include (1) tobacco abuse, (2) low socioeconomic status, (3) less education, (4) occupational exposure to additional carcinogens (e.g., asbestos), (5) genetic predisposition, and (6) concurrent excessive alcohol intake, poor diet, and stress. The need to promote prevention, early detection, and treatment in this population is urgent, yet often this is the same population that finds it difficult to access health care.

Recent research in lung cancer has focused not only on developing new and more effective treatment strategies, but also on early identification of malignant transformation, genetic markers, early chemoprevention, and tobacco cessation strategies. Early identification of high-risk individuals, appropriate interventional studies, and implementation of prevention strategies are essential to reduce the number of new cases. Unfortunately, screening for lung cancer in the United States is not currently recommended. Two randomized trials, the Mayo Lung Project and the Czechoslovakia Lung Cancer Screening Study, did not show a reduction in lung cancer mortality even though screening did detect a higher number of cancers. In Japan, however, smokers are screened with sputum cytology and radiography and the 5-year survival rates seem to have improved substantially (from 33.7% to 58.4%).[2] The National Cancer Institute is currently investigating the utility of chest x-ray studies for lung cancer screening in the National Cancer Institute PLCO (prostate, lung, colorectal, and ovarian) Cancer Screening Trial, and some studies suggest that screening with spiral CT scanning and sputum cytology will identify early tumors and improve survival.[2] Newer nonradiographic technologies (i.e., molecular sputum analysis for tumor markers) are also being investigated.[3] In the interim it is essential that primary care providers are mindful of the risk factors associated with lung cancer and have a heightened awareness of the symptoms related to this highly lethal cancer.

PATHOPHYSIOLOGY

Of the lung cancers in the United States, 80% to 90% are directly related to tobacco abuse, whether active or passive. The major determinant is the number of cigarettes actively smoked or the amount of passively inhaled smoke, not the amount of tar in each cigarette. There is a fourfold increase in the risk of developing lung cancer when a person increases cigarette intake from

BOX 115-1

WORLD HEALTH ORGANIZATION HISTOLOGIC CLASSIFICATION OF EPITHELIAL CANCER OF LUNG

I. Benign
II. Dysplasia and carcinoma in situ
III. Malignant
   A. Squamous cell (epidermoid) and spindle (squamous) carcinoma
   B. Small cell carcinoma
      1. Oat cell
      2. Intermediate cell
      3. Combined oat cell
   C. Adenocarcinoma
      1. Acinar
      2. Papillary
      3. Bronchoalveolar
      4. Mucus secreting
   D. Large cell carcinoma
      1. Giant cell
      2. Clear cell

From Kreyburg L and others: *Histological typing of lung tumours*, ed 2, Geneva, 1981, World Health Organization.

one half pack to one pack of cigarettes per day. Other factors that lead to increased risk of lung cancer are (1) asbestos exposure, (2) radon exposure, (3) previous lung or upper respiratory tract cancer, (4) genetic predisposition, and (5) air pollution.[4] Lung cancer cells may have 10 or more acquired genetic lesions, most commonly mutations in *ras* oncogenes; amplification, rearrangement, or transcriptional activation of the *myc* family genes; or overexpression or deletions involving chromosomes.[5] Loss of 3_p and 9_p are the earliest events detectable even in hyperplastic bronchial epithelium p53 abnormalities, and *ras* mutations are usually found only in invasive cancers.

There is no apparent threshold in the dose-response relation between the degree of smoking and the incidence of lung cancer. As a result, the potential of smoke in the environment of nonsmokers to produce lung cancer has become an important issue. Smoke inhaled by nonsmokers has a chemical composition similar to that inhaled by smokers. One small study supported the hypothesis that nonsmokers exposed to environmental smoke metabolized a carcinogenic substance associated with lung cancer.[6] Approximately 10,000 cases of lung cancer are diagnosed each year in nonsmokers; more than 20% of these cases are attributed to environmental secondhand smoke.[7]

Lung cancer is divided into two major categories: (1) non–small cell lung cancer (NSCLC), which includes squamous cell, adenocarcinoma, and large cell carcinoma and (2) small cell lung cancer (SCLC). The World Health Organization classification is accepted worldwide (Box 115-1). Of the four major types, epidermoid (squamous) cell cancers account for 20% to 30% of lung cancer cases; adenocarcinoma, including bronchoalveolar adenocarcinoma, accounts for 30% to 40% of cases; large cell cancer accounts for 10% of cases; and small cell (oat cell) cancer accounts for 20% of cases.[1] The histology of the cancer (small cell vs. non–small cell) is a major determinant of the treatment approach. Small cell cancer is usually disseminated at the time of diagnosis, whereas non–small cell cancer may be localized. Epidermoid and small cell carcinomas correlate with significant tobacco smoke exposure. They usually present as central masses, whereas adenocarcinomas present as peripheral nodules or masses. The rate of adenocarcinoma presentations is increasing, especially in nonsmoking women. With the exception of T1 N0 tumors, it appears that adenocarcinomas have a poorer prognosis for stage than squamous cell cancers.[2] However, the 5-year survival rate for all types of lung cancer in the United States has been less than 15% for 30 years.[2]

BOX 115-2

SIGNS AND SYMPTOMS OF LUNG CANCER DEPENDING ON LOCATION OF TUMOR

I. Local effect on airway—cough, hemoptysis, dyspnea, wheeze, stridor, pneumonitis, abscess, chest pain. Regional tumor impingement on extrapulmonary mediastinal structures—tracheal destruction, laryngeal nerve paralysis (hoarseness), dysphasia, plural effusion, superior vena cava obstruction
II. Metastatic manifestations—seizures (brain), bone pain, liver metastases, spinal cord compression
III. Paraneoplastic—syndrome of inappropriate antidiuretic hormone, hypercalcemia, Cushing's syndrome, hypertrophic pulmonary osteoarthropathy
IV. Systemic symptoms—anorexia, weight loss, fatigue, weakness

CLINICAL PRESENTATION

Approximately 10% of all lung cancers present asymptomatically[1]; thus a careful history to determine previous asbestos or carcinogenic exposure, tobacco use, or second-hand smoke exposure is an essential component of the yearly physical examination. Signs and symptoms depend on the location of the primary tumor, presence of regional spread, and presence of metastasis (Box 115-2). Symptoms may be classified according to the (1) effect on the major airway, (2) impingement of the tumor on extrapulmonary mediastinal structures, (3) presence of paraneoplastic syndromes (most often seen in oat-cell cancers), (4) effect of distant metastases, and (5) presence or absence of systemic symptoms (e.g., weight loss). The principal symptom of lung cancer is chronic cough, which is also widespread in chronic cigarette smokers. A persistent cough or change in cough warrants a chest x-ray study and possibly further follow-up evaluation. Other clinical manifestations of lung cancer include dyspnea, dysphagia, anorexia, weight loss, wheezing, frequent bouts of pneumonia or respiratory tract infections, hemoptysis, hoarseness, chest pain, fatigue, and upper extremity pain and/or edema.

PHYSICAL EXAMINATION AND DIAGNOSTICS

The physical examination of a patient with risk factors or symptoms suspicious for lung cancer should be comprehensive. The presence of masses (i.e., nasopharyngeal, thyroid, breast, abdominal, prostate, rectum), lymphadenopathy, as well as signs of infection or malignancy should be determined.

Diagnostics

Lung Cancer

Laboratory
CBC and differential
Electrolytes
Glucose
BUN
Creatinine
LFTs
Sputum cytology
Purified protein derivative

Imaging
Chest x-ray study
CT scan of chest and abdomen
Bone scan*
Positron emission tomography scan*

Other
Bronchoscopy
Mediastinoscopy
ECG

*If indicated.

To design appropriate treatment, certain diagnostic tests are performed to stage the patient's disease. Staging of NSCLC refers to defining the (1) size of the tumor, (2) absence or presence of regional spread, (3) presence of metastases, and (4) presence of paraneoplastic syndrome with or without systemic symptoms.

General staging procedures and diagnostic staging include (1) a complete and thorough physical examination and laboratory studies that include a CBC, electrolytes, LFTs, and ECG; (2) a chest x-ray film that shows a definable mass; (3) a CT or positron emission tomography scan (more sensitive and specific than CT) of the chest to determine mediastinal involvement; (4) an abdominal CT scan to evaluate the liver and adrenal glands (the adrenal glands are common sites of metastasis and are often asymptomatic); (5) sputum cytology; (6) bronchoscopy; (7) mediastinoscopy; (8) bone scan (controversial at present); and (9) other scans as appropriate if distant metastasis is suspected.

Tissue diagnosis is essential for staging the patient. Pretreatment prognostic factors include the size of the tumor, tumor histology, performance status of the patient, and presence or absence of weight loss.[7]

On completion of the diagnostic evaluation, the patient is staged according to tumor size (T), presence or absence of regional lymph node involvement (N), and presence or absence of metastasis (M) (Table 115-1).

The primary tumor is divided into four categories (T1 to T4), depending on size, site, and local involvement. Lymph node spread is subdivided into bronchopulmonary (N1), ipsilateral mediastinal (N2), and contralateral or supraclavicular disease (N3), and according to whether metastatic spread is present or absent.[5] Patients are then classified as having stage I, II, III, or IV cancer.

DIFFERENTIAL DIAGNOSIS

Cough, dyspnea, hemoptysis, and wheezing are associated with a number of lung conditions. When weight loss, cachexia, and anorexia are also present, serious illness is easily suspected. More moderate symptoms, however, should not be overlooked, as early identification of lung cancer may enable long-term survival. Although patients with lung cancer may be asymptomatic, chronic cough, dyspnea, hemoptysis, wheezing, and other pulmonary symptoms necessitate investigation for infection, tumor, or other pulmonary disorder.

TABLE 115-1 International TNM Staging System for Lung Cancer

Stage	TNM Descriptions	5-Year Survival (%)
I	T1-2 N0 M0	60-80
II	T1-2 N1 M0	25-50
IIIA	T3 N0-1 M0	25-40
	T1-3 N2 M0	10-30
IIIB	Any T4 or N3 M0	<5
IV	Any M1	<5

PRIMARY TUMOR (T)	
T1	Tumor
T2	Tumor >3 cm in diameter or with associated atelectasis-obstructive pneumonitis extending to hilar region
T3	Tumor with direct extension into chest wall (including superior sulcus tumors), diaphragm, mediastinal pleura, or pericardium
T4	Tumor invading mediastinum (heart, great vessels, trachea, esophagus, vertebral body, or carina) or with presence of a malignant pleural effusion
REGIONAL LYMPH NODES (N)	
N0	No node involvement
N1	Metastasis to lymph nodes in peribronchial and/or ipsilateral hilar region
N2	Metastasis to ipsilateral mediastinal or subcarinal lymph nodes
T3	Metastasis to contralateral mediastinal or hilar nodes, or any scalene or supraclavicular nodes
DISTANT METASTASES	
M0	No known metastasis
M1	Distant metastasis present with site specified (e.g., brain)

Modified from DeVita VT: *Cancer: principles and practice of oncology,* ed 5, Philadelphia, 1997, JB Lippincott. Data from the *AJCC manual for staging,* ed 5, Philadelphia, 1997, JB Lippincott.

Differential Diagnosis

Lung Cancer

Infection	Small cell carcinoma
Interstitial pulmonary fibrosis	Adenocarcinoma
	Large cell carcinoma
Metastatic cancer	Mesothelioma
Granuloma	Tuberculosis
Squamous cell carcinoma	Benign tumor

MANAGEMENT

Treatment can include surgery, radiotherapy, and/or chemotherapy and can be curative or palliative. A number of factors including type of tumor, stage of the disease, patient age, and functional status determine appropriate interventions for each patient.

Surgery

In NSCLC, when the tumor is limited to a hemithorax and can be totally encompassed by excision, surgery provides the best chance for cure.[8] In stage I and stage II disease, when the tumor has not extended past the bronchopulmonary lymph nodes, excision is almost always possible. There is controversy over treatment of stage IIIA disease, especially if ipsilateral lymph nodes are involved. N2 disease has a poorer prognosis than stage IIIA disease with only a T3 tumor. Newer approaches to treatment of stages IIIA and IIIB disease involve pretreatment with neoadjuvant chemotherapy followed by surgical excision. Stage IV disease is not appropriate for surgical intervention, as it is disseminated at the time of diagnosis. Chemotherapy or palliative therapy is the primary management modality for stage IV disease.

Small cell carcinoma is always considered disseminated, and chemotherapy (usually with multiple chemotherapeutic agents) is the initial intervention. Chemotherapy is also being combined with radiation therapy for some patients. Surgical resection combined with chemotherapy is used for a single pulmonary nodule. Palliative surgery can also be valuable to preserve airway function for patients with obstructive tumor.

Radiotherapy

Radiotherapy in NSCLC has experienced significant changes in a short time with respect to evolution of appropriate patient selection, radiobiologic principles, technical innovation, and the use and integration of chemotherapy and surgery. Factors such as the quality of life during and after therapy, cost of treatment, and management of side effects and toxicities must be considered in today's health care environment.[8] Only one third of patients with NSCLC present without mediastinal nodal metastasis. In these cases the goal of radiation therapy is to eradicate tumor in the lymph nodes. This is usually done after curative surgery. In more advanced stages radiotherapy is considered palliative and is now commonly combined with adjuvant chemotherapy.

Chemotherapy

Chemotherapy can be considered standard therapy for advanced stages III and IV NSCLC and is the primary modality in the treatment of SCLC. In locoregionally advanced stages IIIA and IIIB cancer, chemotherapy is used as a component of multimodality treatment.[9] Therapy is now given with curative intent, and it is hoped that integration of chemotherapy will not only increase median survival time, but in some instances will also render curative therapy. It has become common acceptable practice in stage III NSCLC to use several courses of neoadjuvant therapy before surgery.[8] Active drugs in NSCLC include combinations of carboplatin and paclitaxel, of cisplatin and vincristine, or of cisplatin plus etoposide. Continuous research is scrutinizing the effect of varied combinations of these and newer chemotherapeutic agents.

Dose-limiting factors include neutropenia, anemia, and thrombocytopenia. However, the addition of colony-stimulating factors has made possible the administration of higher doses and better response rates. Successful chemotherapy depends on the age and performance status of the patient, and the presence or absence of other serious medical illnesses. Box 115-3 provides an outline for treatment according to stage.

BOX 115-3

SUMMARY OF TREATMENT APPROACH TO PATIENTS WITH LUNG CANCER

NON–SMALL CELL LUNG CANCER

Resectable (stages I, II, IIIa, and selected T3 N2 lesions)

- Surgery
- Radiotherapy for "nonoperable" patients
- Postoperative radiotherapy for N2 disease

Nonresectable (N2 and M1)

- Confined to chest: high-dose chest radiotherapy (RT), if possible, plus chemotherapy (CT); consider neoadjuvant CT followed by surgery
- Extrathoracic: RT to symptomatic local sites; CT for patients with good performance status and evaluable lesions)

SMALL CELL LUNG CANCER

Limited stage (good performance status)

- CT plus chest RT

Extensive stage (good performance status)

- CT

Complete tumor responders (all stages)

- Prophylactic cranial RT

Patients with poor performance status (all stages)

- Modified-dose CT
- Palliative RT

ALL PATIENTS

RT for brain metastases, spinal cord compression, weight-bearing lytic bony lesions, symptomatic local lesions (nerve paralyses, obstructive airway, hemoptysis in non–small cell lung cancer and in small cell cancer not responding to CT

Appropriate diagnosis and treatment of other medical problems and supportive care during CT

Encouragement to stop smoking

From Wilson JD and others: *Harrison's principles of internal medicine*, ed 14, New York, 1998, McGraw-Hill.

COMPLICATIONS

Complications are myriad and may be related to the cancer or treatment. Medications and particularly chemoradiotherapeutics may have significant side effects, including increased mortality. Metastatic disease, coagulation and thrombotic disorders, anemia, paraneoplastic syndromes, and superior vena cava syndrome are among the many complications that require prompt identification and treatment.

INDICATIONS FOR REFERRAL/HOSPITALIZATION

Diagnostic evaluation and clinical staging are initiated by the primary care provider. However, medical management of lung cancer is best provided by experienced oncologists. With the exception of early stage I and II disease (which involves primarily a surgical referral), lung cancer requires multidisciplinary collaboration among surgical, medical, and radiation oncologists. The role of the primary care provider includes coordination of care among specialties, close supervision of other medical conditions, and supportive interventions. Hospitalization for surgical excision of the tumor is obvious. Hospitalization may also be appropriate if complications from radiation, chemotherapy, or the cancer itself occur.

PATIENT AND FAMILY EDUCATION

Continuous patient education about the dangers of smoking is essential. Primary care providers must continually encourage patients to stop smoking and advise family members to avoid second-hand smoke.

When a diagnosis of cancer is made, patients and families require careful explanation of the disease, staging, treatment, and side effects. Pain management, bowel protocols, and observation for complications require continuous reinforcement and support.

REFERENCES

1. Strauss GM: Overview and clinical manifestations of lung cancer. Retrieved September 5, 2002 from the World Wide Web: http://www.uptodateonline.com.
2. Petty TL: Early screening for lung cancer: weighing in on the controversy, *Consultant* 41(7):957-961, 2001.
3. Mandel J, Weinberger SE: Screening for lung cancer. Retrieved September 5, 2002 from the World Wide Web: http://www.uptodateonline.com.
4. Pope CA III and others: Lung cancer, cardiopulmonary mortality, and long-term exposure to fine particulate air pollution, *JAMA* 287: 1132-1141, 2002.
5. Fauci AS and others, editors: Summary of treatment approaches to lung cancer. In *Harrison's principles of internal medicine,* ed 14, New York, 1998, McGraw-Hill.
6. Hecht SS and others: A tobacco-specific carcinogen in the urine of men exposed to cigarette smoke, *N Engl J Med* 329(21): 1543-1546, 1993.
7. Samet J: Passive smoking. Retrieved October 25, 2002 from the World Wide Web: http://www.uptodateonline.com.
8. Minna J and others: Cancer of the lung. In DeVita V, Hellerman S, Rosenberg S: *Cancer: principles and practice of oncology,* ed 5, Philadelphia, 1997, Lippincott-Raven.
9. Idhe DC: Chemotherapy of lung cancer, *N Engl J Med* 327(20): 1434-1441, 1992.

CHAPTER 116

Occupational Respiratory Disease

Patricia Polgar Bailey and Terry Mahan Buttaro

DEFINITION/EPIDEMIOLOGY

Occupational respiratory disease results from work-related exposures to inhaled dusts, powders, solvents, gases, or fumes that adversely affect the upper and lower respiratory tract. Occupational respiratory diseases have been recorded since ancient history. Egyptian pictographs and the writings of Hippocrates document the role of occupational exposures in lung disease. Because many exposures do not result in acute symptoms, workers may be unaware that they have been exposed to potentially hazardous materials. The challenge for primary care providers, especially those unfamiliar with occupational medicine, is to maintain a high index of suspicion that a symptom or cluster of symptoms may have a connection with a patient's job or work history. It is important to remember that work-related exposures do occur in occupations other than the obvious.[1]

Although the true scope of occupational lung disease is difficult to quantify, it is well recognized that a small percentage of chronic occupational respiratory disease is correctly associated with work-related exposures. Asthma is the most common type of occupational pulmonary disease in the industrialized world; an estimated 2% to 15% of all adult asthma cases are work related. Occupational asthma may be related to specific antigens in the workplace (i.e., flour or latex) or to chemical irritants (i.e., ammonia, chlorine, sulfur dioxide).[2] Interstitial pulmonary fibrosis, which results from workplace exposure to asbestos and silica, persists throughout the world despite knowledge regarding the potential hazards of these substances and effective means for prevention. Silicosis mortality rates have been estimated to be as high as 7.36 per 100,000 men in some industrialized countries.[3] Approximately 65,000 men in the United States have asbestosis; it is estimated that occupational asbestos exposure will contribute to 19,000 cases of mesothelioma and 55,000 cases of lung cancer by 2009. In the United States, 85,000 cotton mill workers are permanently or partially disabled as a result of exposure to cotton dust. As many as 30% of coal miners (both active and retired) have coal workers' pneumonoconiosis.[4] The prevalence of latex hypersensitivity, including latex-induced asthma, is as high as 14% among some groups of health care workers.[5] Despite these significant statistics, the number of affected individuals captured in any occupational surveillance system remains a gross underestimate because the majority of cases are undiagnosed or are not attributed to workplace exposures.[3]

PATHOPHYSIOLOGY

Inhaled noxious exposures affect the respiratory tract in several ways. Direct irritation results in increased mucus production; cough and airway hyperreactivity, which may cause bronchospasm; chest tightness or pain; dyspnea; pneumonitis; or pulmonary edema. The full effect of certain irritants may not be realized until 12 to 24 hours after the exposure. Small particles (≤ 5 μm) may remain in the lung to induce a fibrotic or granulomatous response. A latency period of 15 to 20 years between exposure and onset of clinical disease often obscures the causal relationship, which makes the diagnosis of occupational lung disease more difficult. Hypersensitivity and abnormal functioning of the immune system may contribute to the development of certain occupational respiratory diseases, including asthma, hypersensitivity pneumonitis, asbestosis, and chronic beryllium disease. The presence of certain host factors, such as cigarette smoking and the home environment (e.g., proximity to sources of pollutants), plays a role in the development of work-related lung disease. For example, cigarette smoking and asbestos exposure have a synergistic effect on the risk for lung cancer that is greater than the risk of either of these two exposures alone.[2,4]

Occupational respiratory diseases include obstructive airway diseases (asthma, byssinosis), interstitial lung disease (coal worker's pneumonoconiosis, asbestosis, silicosis, acute and chronic beryllium disease, hypersensitivity pneumonitis), industrial bronchitis, cancer, and noncardiogenic pulmonary edema. Asthma, one of the most common types of occupational respiratory disease, has been associated with at least 250 specific workplace exposures. In comparison to many other occupational illnesses, asthma produces more persistent, even permanent, effects.[6] Byssinosis is another obstructive airway disease; it is associated with exposure to cotton, hemp, and flax processing and is characterized by shortness of breath and chest tightness. Prolonged exposures can cause irreversible byssinosis, which is associated with fixed airway obstruction. Cigarette smoking significantly increases the risk of irreversible byssinosis.[7]

Many occupational toxins contribute to the development of interstitial lung disease, including coal dust, asbestos, silica, and beryllium. The occurrence and extent of disease often depend on the level and chronicity of the exposure. Depending on the specific disease, fibrosis of the lung parenchyma, pleural thickening, and the formation of pleural plaques contribute to respiratory failure and increase the risk for the subsequent development of lung cancer and mesothelioma.

Bronchitis is a common manifestation of airway irritation and inflammation that is associated with many occupational exposures, including irritant gases, welding fumes, and coal dust. *Chronic bronchitis* is defined as the presence of cough and sputum on most days for ≥ 3 months per year and for ≥ 2 consecutive years.

Occupational exposures are associated with different types of pleuropulmonary malignancies—including laryngeal, bronchogenic, and oat cell carcinomas—as well as with mesothelioma, a tumor of the pleura and peritoneum.

Certain groups of health care professionals are at increased risk for the development of occupational respiratory problems as a result of their exposure to specific pathogens and toxins. Occupational asthma resulting from latex allergy (as well as latex-related dermatitis and life-threatening anaphylaxis) is becoming an increasing problem among health care workers. Establishing a diagnosis of latex-related asthma is essential to avoid permanent respiratory compromise. With the resurgence of tuberculosis (TB) in this decade, increasing numbers of health care workers have become infected with TB. The risk for infection is compounded by the fact that there is a convergence of immunocompromised individuals in various types of settings staffed by health care workers, including long-term care facilities, hospitals, homeless shelters, correctional facilities, and drug treatment centers. Since 1990 there have been a number of TB outbreaks in these settings, resulting in approximately 300 cases of TB. These outbreaks were characterized by transmission of both isoniazid-resistant TB and, in many cases, multidrug-resistant TB.[8]

CLINICAL PRESENTATION

Obtaining a thorough history from patients, including environmental and occupational exposures, smoking habits, and a careful review of respiratory symptoms, is important. The review of symptoms should include questions about onset of symptoms, rhinitis, conjunctivitis, cough, sputum production, wheezing, dyspnea, chest tightness or pain, history of allergies, asthma, and respiratory infections.[2] In addition, it is important to elicit the temporal relationship of symptoms to time spent at work. For example, an improvement of symptoms during periods away from work or an intensification during periods at work might suggest an occupational exposure.

To accurately diagnose and manage occupational disease, primary care providers must familiarize themselves with their patients' social and occupational environments. However, much more is involved than simply knowing an individual's work history. Detailed information about the jobs performed (including an outline of a typical workday), work habits, materials used (dyes, solvents, dusts, powders, fumes, acids, alkalis, gases, metals), and the use of protective equipment must be elicited. All workers should be asked about any safety or health concerns they might have. For many practitioners, some investigation and research are necessary before an accurate assessment of exposures is possible.

Exposures to noxious substances can cause various types of reactions in both the upper and lower respiratory tract. Acute symptoms of upper respiratory tract irritation include nasal and paranasal sinus irritation, sinus congestion, frontal headaches, rhinorrhea, and, occasionally, epistaxis. A dry cough and hoarseness may indicate pharyngeal and laryngeal inflammation, respectively. Mid–respiratory tract irritation and inflammation often result in bronchospasm, of which asthma is an example. Acute irritation of the deep respiratory tract causes pulmonary edema and pneumonitis.

Chronic respiratory exposures can result in various permanent pulmonary reactions. Chronic bronchitis is one of the most common pulmonary responses to long-term occupational exposures and results from excessive mucus production in the bronchi. Toxic workplace exposures that can cause chronic bronchitis include mineral dusts and fumes (e.g., from coal, fibrous glass, asbestos, metal, and oils), organic dusts (e.g., from cotton, grains, and wood), gases (e.g., ozone and nitrous oxide), plastic compounds (isocyanates), acids, and smoke. Fibrosis or pneumonoconiosis (localized and nodular) is usually due to small particles of inorganic dust and produces symptoms that initially include a nonproductive cough and shortness of breath; in the later stages there is a productive cough, distant breath sounds, and right-sided heart failure. Pleural plaques and diffuse pleural thickening are manifestations of asbestos exposures. Emphysema-related changes, which include destruction of alveolar walls and air trapping, results from chronic exposures to coal dust or cadmium. The formation of pulmonary granulomas is a less common response to inhaled work-related exposures but can occur from chronic exposure to metal dust.[7]

PHYSICAL EXAMINATION

Many workplace exposures do not cause acute respiratory symptoms, and therefore the physical examination may be entirely normal. This is the one reason why occupational exposures are often not considered in the differential diagnosis and why the magnitude of occupational respiratory disease is grossly underestimated. However, it is important to always consider occupational asthma when an adult suddenly develops asthma.[2] The physical examination is most helpful when the results are abnormal because a normal physical examination does not negate the possibility of work-related respiratory disease. In fact, once an occupational exposure results in obvious acute symptoms, the disease may have already progressed to the point that symptomatic relief, rather than a cure, is all that is possible.

A thorough physical examination with special attention to the respiratory system is necessary. Auscultation can provide helpful diagnostic clues. Fine basilar crackles and a pleural friction rub are more common in certain interstitial lung diseases such as asbestosis. Wheezes, especially in association with a temporal relationship to work exposures, may raise the suspicion of asthma. Digital clubbing in a worker with a history of asbestos exposure might raise the suspicion of asbestosis, especially if other manifestations of the disease have already become apparent.

A cardiac examination is important; ventricular failure may reflect underlying lung disease; left ventricular failure may present as dyspnea, and right ventricular failure may denote severe and advanced lung disease.[7] In addition to assessing the respiratory and cardiac systems, a complete physical examination is necessary to identify signs that may be manifestations of chronic or acute occupational exposures and may provide clues to the etiology of the specific respiratory syndrome being evaluated.

DIAGNOSTICS

Important diagnostic tests include a chest radiograph and pulmonary function tests (PFTs). A chest x-ray examination can help identify early evidence and progression of parenchymal and pleural disease, including opacities, calcifications, and pleural thickening. In addition to a standard reading, chest x-ray studies should be interpreted according to the International Labor Organization (ILO) nomenclature and classification system. The ILO system provides a standardized set of comparison radiographs that can be used to classify x-ray films at one point in time or to follow an individual or group for changes over time.[7] Although chest x-ray studies do reveal evidence of abnormalities, they do not provide information about the degree of disability or impairment, nor do they provide an accurate assessment of lung function. For example, the chest x-ray film of an individual with severe obstructive lung disease might appear relatively normal.

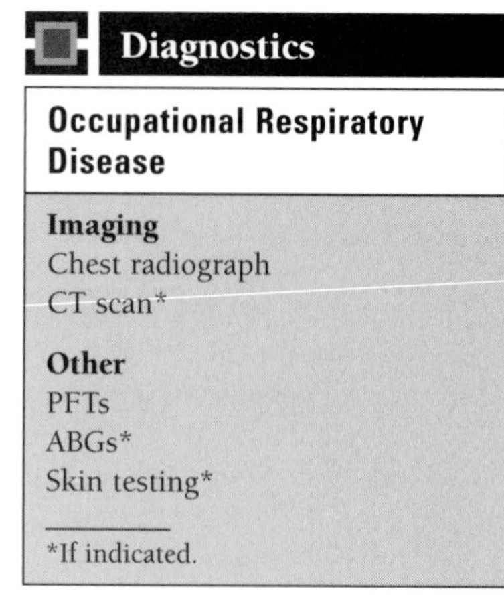

Diagnostics

Occupational Respiratory Disease

Imaging
Chest radiograph
CT scan*

Other
PFTs
ABGs*
Skin testing*

*If indicated.

PFTs are used to assess lung function. They are of value in determining the type and extent of lung disease, following the progression of disease for changes in severity or response to therapy, and fulfilling legal and compensatory purposes. The basic tests of ventilatory function can be performed with a spirometer, which can provide an accurate assessment of the relationship between chronic respiratory symptoms and diminished ventilatory capacity.[9] Although spirometry provides many measures, the most useful for evaluating work-related respiratory disease include forced vital capacity (FVC), forced expiratory volume in the first second of a forced vital capacity maneuver (FEV_1), and the ratio of these two measurements (FEV_1/FVC). FVC refers to the maximal volume of air that is exhaled after a maximal inspiration. FEV_1 is an estimate of the flow rate and is obtained by measuring the volume exhaled during the first second. Results are compared with expected values—which are derived from a healthy population of nonsmoking adults—and are expressed as a percentage of the expected value.[7]

Obstructive diseases such as asthma involve an obstruction in airflow without a reduction in lung volume. Therefore measurements of FVC remain within 80% to 120% of the population standard and are considered normal. However, measurements of both FEV_1 and FEV_1/FVC are decreased in asthma and other obstructive diseases. In contrast, restrictive disease, including silicosis, asbestosis, and coal worker's pneumoconiosis, are characterized by reductions in both FEV_1 and FVC, resulting a normal or greater ratio of FEV_1/FVC. Mixed pulmonary conditions may also be present; this occurs when cigarette smoking or multiple environmental exposures coexist with a given occupational exposure and may confuse the results of the PFTs. Nonetheless, PFTs are a useful instrument for considering the general characteristics of work-related lung disease. The response to bronchodilator inhalation is another method for differentiating between obstructive and restrictive airway disease.[7]

Additional PFTs include the measurement of residual volume (RV), pulmonary diffusion lung capacity (DL), arterial blood gases (PaO_2, PCO_2, and pH), and exercise testing. Pulmonary compliance measures the distensibility of the lungs, which is reduced when lungs stiffen.

Skin testing can be helpful in identifying specific antigens, such as flour.[2] A diagnosis of occupational asthma is a strong consideration if skin testing is positive and the patient has been having bronchospasms.

DIFFERENTIAL DIAGNOSIS

Primary care providers play a pivotal role in identifying occupational lung diseases and differentiating them from non–work-related respiratory disorders. More often than not, correctly diagnosed respiratory symptoms are incorrectly attributed to factors other than work because most primary care providers are unfamiliar with their patients' jobs or job-related exposures.

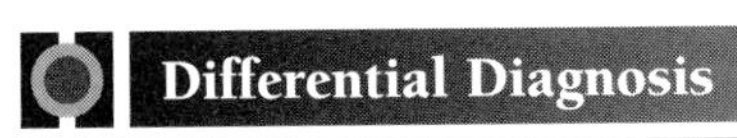

Occupational Respiratory Disease

- Asthma
- Bronchitis
- Chronic obstructive pulmonary disease
- Emphysema
- Fibrosis
- Asbestosis
- Respiratory tract irritants
- Pulmonary granuloma
- Noncardiogenic pulmonary edema
- Neoplasm

Most of the symptoms related to occupational respiratory toxins are the same or similar to those associated with other respiratory illnesses, whether or not they are work related. Exploration of the work connection when obtaining patient histories, performing examinations, and evaluating symptoms is essential in the development of the differential diagnosis.[1]

MANAGEMENT

The management of occupational respiratory diseases is a multifaceted process and should include general guidelines and specific instructions for modifying hazardous work conditions. Important steps include elimination of the exposure source, referral to a specialist, early diagnosis, effective treatment, and Worker's Compensation (if indicated).[9] It is useful to distinguish between exposures that cause acute symptoms, those that may produce irreversible symptoms after prolonged exposure, and those that produce disease that is manifest only after a long latency period. Workers whose exposures produce airway changes that are acute or reversible once the exposure has been removed benefit the most from environmental controls (e.g., an exhaust system), alteration of work practices (e.g., wetting asbestos before removing it), and substitution of a nonhazardous substance for a hazardous one. Other preventive measures that benefit workers to a lesser extent include education regarding specific work hazards, use of personal protective equipment, administrative measures (e.g., job rotation), and screening for early detection of disease.

The management of occupational respiratory disease depends on the specific respiratory illness treated. It is essential that the patient be removed from the exposure as promptly as possible after symptoms have developed. For many occupational respiratory diseases, the most important prognostic determinant is the length of exposure before diagnosis. The principles of managing occupational symptomatic asthma are the same as for nonoccupational asthma.[6] Treatment modalities specific to the disease and close monitoring of symptoms and lung function must be maintained for every individual with an occupational respiratory disease.

LIFE SPAN CONSIDERATIONS

Certain occupational respiratory toxins affect both the female and male reproductive processes, compromising the health of both the workers and their children. Information about pregnant women's work activities and those of their partner (including work done at home) and all related exposures should be obtained as part of the perinatal history. Although performed by more women in American society than in any other, household work is often forgotten as a source of potential respiratory toxins. Products used routinely in the home—including scouring powders, chlorine bleaches, furniture polish, drain cleaners, furniture or paint strippers containing organic solvents, glues, paints, epoxies, and pesticides—are all potential hazards, especially when used in a small or poorly ventilated area.[10]

Another important life span consideration related to occupational respiratory disease involves latency and older adults. Many occupational respiratory diseases are characterized by long asymptomatic periods from the time of exposure to clinical evidence of disease. The manifestation of certain cancers may not appear for 10 to 20 years or even longer after an occupational exposure. The screening of workers at risk for certain diseases such as cancer must take into consideration such latency issues. In addition, the differential diagnosis for a constellation of signs and symptoms must reflect occupational exposure that may have occurred many years before.

COMPLICATIONS

Complications of occupational respiratory disease depend on the specific disease process. TB or a fungal infection is a complication peculiar to silica pneumonoconiosis. The increased risk of mortality associated with certain chronic respiratory exposures is now well recognized. For example, asbestos-related pleural thickening can cause respiratory failure. Multiple occupational exposures, including those to arsenic, chromium, vinyl chloride monomer, asbestos, and radiation, have been causally identified with respiratory tract cancers.

INDICATIONS FOR REFERRAL/HOSPITALIZATION

Most primary care providers are unfamiliar with occupational medicine. Patients should be referred to an occupational medicine specialist if a diagnosis is not clear or if symptoms are unresponsive to treatment. Chronic work-related respiratory tract illnesses are often best managed by an occupational medicine or pulmonary specialist. This includes the management of many respiratory diseases resulting from chronic exposures (e.g., asbestosis or byssinosis) but may also include the management of acute problems such as silicosis-related TB.

PATIENT AND FAMILY EDUCATION

Education must include an explanation of diagnostic tests and the specific treatment modalities being considered and used. The specifics will depend on the specific respiratory disease involved. Occupational medicine is at its best preventive health care. Patients need to be educated about the relationship of their symptoms to workplace exposures, the consequences of continued exposures, and their rights and responsibilities as employees. Employers are required by law to maintain Material Safety Data Sheets (MSDSs), which describe toxic substances, their proper handling, and the symptoms that may arise from contact with them. However, many workers are unaware of the existence of MSDSs and need to be encouraged to read those that are relevant to their jobs. Education needs to include information about the importance of personal protective equipment and workplace hygiene. A list of resources, such as those offered through the Occupational Safety and Health Administration (OSHA) and the National Institute of Occupational Safety and Health (NIOSH), should be made available to the patient.

REFERENCES

1. Chester TJ and others: Caution: work can be hazardous to health, *Patient Care*, Feb 1996.
2. Chan-Yeung M, Malo J-L: *Overview of occupational asthma*. Retrieved September 6, 2002, from the World Wide Web: http://www.uptodateonline.com.
3. Wagner GR: Asbestosis and silicosis, *Lancet* 349:1311, 1997.
4. Oliver CL, Stoeckle JD: Prevention and evaluation of occupational respiratory disease. In Goroll AH, May LA, Mulley AG, editors: *Primary care medicine: office evaluation and management of the adult patient*, Philadelphia, 1995, JB Lippincott.
5. Burton AD: Latex allergy in health care workers, *Occup Med* 12:609, 1997.
6. Bardana EJ, Harber P, Lockey JE: Occupational asthma: breathing easier on the job, *Patient Care*, Feb 1996.
7. Wegman DH, Christiani DC: Respiratory disorders. In Levy BS, Wegman DH, editors: *Occupational health: recognizing and preventing work-related disease*, ed 2, Boston, 1988, Little, Brown.
8. McDiarmid MA: Tuberculosis in the health care industry, *Occup Med* 12:767, 1997.
9. Kahan E, Weingarten MA, Appelbaum T: Attitudes of primary care physicians to the management of asthma and their perception of its relationship to patients' work, *Isr J Med Sci* 32:757, 1996.
10. Quinn MM, Woskie SR: Women and work. In Levy BS, Wegman DH, editors: *Occupational health: recognizing and preventing work-related disease*, ed 2, Boston, 1988, Little, Brown.

CHAPTER 117

Pleural Effusions

Patricia Polgar Bailey

DEFINITION/EPIDEMIOLOGY

A pleural effusion is an abnormal amount of fluid within the pleural space. The pleural space is an area approximately 10 to 20 μm in width that is situated between the mesothelium of the parietal and visceral pleura. The parietal pleura lines the chest cavity, covering the chest wall, diaphragm, and mediastinum. The parietal pleura contains sensory nerves, and its blood supply comes from the systemic circulation and hence has hydrostatic pressure. The visceral pleura covers the entire surface of both lungs and contains no pain fibers. Its blood flow is supplied by branches of the pulmonary circulation. The parietal and visceral pleurae are continuous at the hilum, where they are penetrated by both the pulmonary and bronchial vessels.[1,2] Pleural fluid is normally produced in quantities just sufficient to lubricate the parietal and visceral surfaces. This small amount of fluid is constantly replenished and reabsorbed; absorption is principally via the lymphatic system.

The pleural space is referred to as one of the body's "potential spaces," referring to the fact that there is normally only a very small amount of fluid volume within this space. Approximately 0.1 ml/kg of fluid is normally contained within the pleural space unless some disease process or trauma has caused fluid or solid tissue to collect there. A volume greater than 7 to 14 ml is abnormal.[3,4]

Pleural effusions are a common manifestation of many pulmonary and systemic diseases, most notably congestive heart failure (CHF), because of the elevation of pulmonary venous pressure. Approximately 25% to 30% of persons referred to a pulmonologist have evidence of pleural disease.[4]

PATHOPHYSIOLOGY

An increased amount of fluid (an *effusion*) accumulates in the pleural space whenever the rate of fluid formation exceeds the rate of fluid absorption. There are numerous conditions that may lead to pleural effusions, including viral and bacterial infections, neoplasms, thromboemboli, cardiovascular dysfunction, and immunologic dysfunction (Box 117-1). Mechanisms that contribute to increased pleural fluid accumulation include (1) an increase in microvascular pressure (e.g., CHF), (2) a decrease in plasma osmotic pressure (e.g., hypoalbuminemia), (3) an increase in the permeability of microcirculation (e.g., pneumonia), (4) a decrease in pleural pressure (e.g., atelectasis), (5) impaired lymphatic drainage from pleural spaces (e.g., malignant effusions), and (6) movement of fluid across the diaphragm from the peritoneal cavity (e.g., inflammation from acute pancreatitis).[1] Malignant pleural effusions are a common problem encountered in persons with advanced cancer. Breast, lung, and ovarian carcinomas and lymphoma account for more than 75% of all malignant pleural effusions.[5]

Pleural effusions are often categorized as transudates and exudates. Exudative pleural effusions result primarily from pleural

BOX 117-1

POTENTIAL CAUSES OF PLEURAL EFFUSIONS

Congestive heart failure (most common cause)
Pneumonia
Malignancy (carcinoma, lymphoma, mesothelioma, leukemia)
Pulmonary embolism
Atelectasis
Tuberculosis
Infectious parasitic and fungal diseases
Cirrhosis
Hepatic and splenic abscesses
Nephrotic syndrome
Rheumatoid arthritis
Systemic lupus erythematous and other connective tissue diseases
Sarcoidosis
Drug-induced effusions
Benign asbestos-related effusions
Pancreatitic disease
Intraabdominal abscesses
Peritoneal dialysis
Radiation therapy
Viral illness, including AIDS
Endocrine dysfunction
Esophageal perforation

and lung inflammation (e.g., pneumonia) or impaired lymphatic drainage of the pleural space (e.g., malignancy). In fact, a variety of disease mechanisms, including infection, malignancy, immunologic and lymphatic abnormalities, and iatrogenic factors, can cause exudates. Transudates are produced by imbalances in hydrostatic and oncotic pressures in the chest. CHF, as well as disease processes that cause movement of fluid from the peritoneal space (e.g., cirrhosis) or retroperitoneal space, can cause transudates. Transudative pleural effusions have a lower specific gravity and lower concentrations of protein and lactic dehydrogenase compared with exudative effusions.[1]

CLINICAL PRESENTATION

Persons with pleural effusions often present asymptomatically. However, when symptoms do occur, the most common presenting complaints include pleuritic chest pain, dyspnea, and nonproductive cough.[4] Pleuritic pain is associated with inflammation of the parietal pleura and is caused by irritation of its sensory fibers.[1] This pain is often sharp, unilateral, and localized to the affected area, although it may also be experienced in the lower chest and ipsilateral shoulder or referred to the abdomen. Exacerbating factors include deep inspiration, cough, or other movement of the upper body. Malignant tumors involving the parietal pleura generally cause steady, dull pain compared with the sharp, intermittent pain associated with an acute inflammatory process. Pleural effusions cause compression of adjacent lung tissue and reduce the amount of possible lung expansion, which may result in varying degrees of dyspnea, depending on the size and functional status of the underlying lung and the rate of fluid accumulation. However, dyspnea does not necessarily correlate with blood oxygen levels or the size of the pleural effusion but rather seems to be related to the increased thoracic cage size, which affects respiratory muscle function. Malignant pleural effusions in particular are often characterized by complaints of dyspnea that seem out of proportion to the size of the effusion.[6] The nonproductive cough is most likely due to lung compression and bronchial irritation.[4]

A thorough history is important. Information about the presence of fever, cough, sputum production, dyspnea, or abdominal pain should be elicited. Past medical history, including systemic and chronic illnesses, previous surgeries, prior exposures (such as to tuberculosis and asbestos), and previous alcohol abuse, is important.

PHYSICAL EXAMINATION

Several findings on physical examination are suggestive of a pleural effusion; however, the clinical manifestations of the effusion may be overshadowed by the underlying disease process.[7] Common physical examination findings include decreased or absent breath sounds over the effusion, decreased respiratory excursion, dullness to percussion, reduced tactile fremitus, and decreased bronchial breath sounds, sometimes with egobronchophony (E-to-A change) at the upper fluid borders. Pleural inflammation is often accompanied by a friction rub that is transitory and that generally disappears as fluid accumulates in the pleural space. Small effusions (<500 ml) may be associated with minimal or no findings. In situations where effusions are greater (>1500 ml) or pulmonary compromise is more substantial, the use of accessory muscles of respiration, inspiratory lag, cyanosis, bulging intercostal margins, mediastinal shift, and jugular vein distention may be evident. In addition to assessing the respiratory status, a complete physical examination is necessary to identify signs that may be manifestations of systemic or acute illness and suggest the etiology of the effusion. For example, nonthoracic signs such as pedal edema, jugular venous distention, and an S_3 gallop might suggest CHF.[7]

DIAGNOSTICS

Once a pleural effusion is suspected, chest x-ray films should be obtained to confirm its presence and to look for other abnormalities that might be helpful in determining its etiology. Normal amounts of fluid are not visible on chest radiographs. Chest x-ray films may fail to detect smaller effusions (<100 ml). Those effusions that are detected (usually >100 ml) appear as blunting and medial displacement of the sharp costophrenic angle, pleural-based densities, infiltrates, hilar adenopathy, or signs of CHF. A subpulmonic effusion is suspected if the diaphragm is elevated. Chest radiographs do not attain 100% sensitivity until pleural effusions are >500 ml.[8]

Smaller effusions should be confirmed by ultrasonography, which will detect effusions of 5 to 50 ml and are 100% sensitive for effusions of >100 ml.[4,8] In addition to their use in detecting smaller effusions, ultrasound examinations are used to guide diagnostic thoracentesis, which has resulted in improved yield and decreased complication rates for thoracentesis.

Once a pleural effusion has been discovered, identification of the disease process, procedure, or drug that caused the effusion is essential. Diagnostic evaluation relies heavily on examination of pleural fluid obtained by thoracentesis. In experienced hands, thoracentesis can be performed safely at the bedside and can be used to diagnose the cause of pleural effusions in 75% of cases.[1] Although a definitive diagnosis, such as the finding of malignant cells, can be established in only 25% of cases, relevant information (from fluid analyses, including cellular counts, chemistry profiles, cultures, and stains) that is useful for clinical decision making and for excluding certain causes of a pleural effusion is obtained in an additional 15% to 20% of cases.[4] In certain situations where the clinical diagnosis and cause of the effusion are relatively secure and the clinical course is uncomplicated (e.g., uncomplicated CHF, small effusions after thoracic or abdominal surgery, and postpartum effusion), therapy may be initiated and a thoracentesis performed only if the response to therapy is inadequate. However, whenever the cause of a pleural effusion is unclear, a diagnostic thoracentesis is generally warranted.[8]

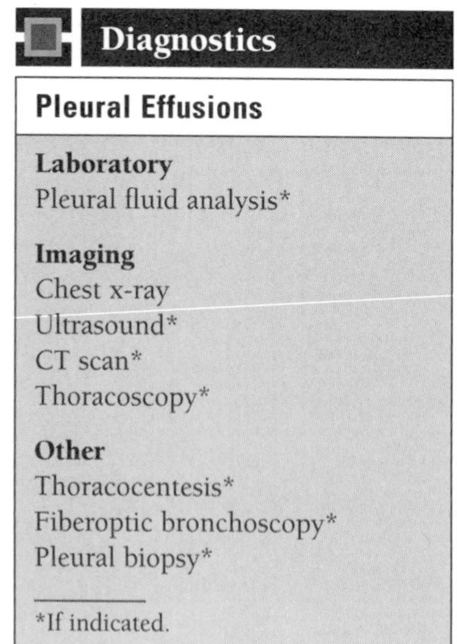
Diagnostics

Pleural Effusions

Laboratory
Pleural fluid analysis*

Imaging
Chest x-ray
Ultrasound*
CT scan*
Thoracoscopy*

Other
Thoracocentesis*
Fiberoptic bronchoscopy*
Pleural biopsy*

*If indicated.

There are no absolute contraindications to thoracentesis. However, relative contraindications include a bleeding diathesis, anticoagulation, a small volume of pleural fluid, mechanical ventilation, inability of the patient to cooperate, and cutaneous disease such as herpes zoster infection at the needle entry site.[1,7] The complication rate of thoracentesis is approximately 20% and includes pneumothorax, cough, and, rarely, bleeding, empyema, and spleen or liver puncture.[4]

Other tests needed to establish a definitive diagnosis may include a CT scan of the chest, thoracoscopy, fiberoptic bronchoscopy, and pleural biopsy. A chest CT scan is not obtained initially to confirm the presence of a pleural effusion; it is most useful after thoracentesis for further evaluation of suspected parenchymal or pleural abnormalities. Bronchoscopy and thoracoscopy are useful in the evaluation of exudative effusions whose etiology is still unclear. Open pleural biopsy is required when other procedures have failed to provide a diagnosis.[4,8]

DIFFERENTIAL DIAGNOSIS

A number of diseases can cause symptoms similar to those characteristic of pleural effusions, including pneumothorax, pulmonary embolism, CHF, neoplasms, trauma, and tuberculosis. Once the presence of a pleural effusion has been established, the differential diagnosis is based on the presence of transudative and exudative effusions, although a number of conditions can cause both. The presence of a transudative pleural effusion is generally associated with a systemic condition rather than a pleural disease. An exudate usually suggests a pathologic condition that specifically involves the pleural space. Pleural fluid characterized by high erythrocyte counts (>100,000/ml) is most often seen in cases of trauma, malignancy, and pulmonary embolism. Other laboratory evaluations, such as a pleural fluid eosinophil count, glucose concentration, and pH, can be used to help distinguish between the potential causes of the effusion.

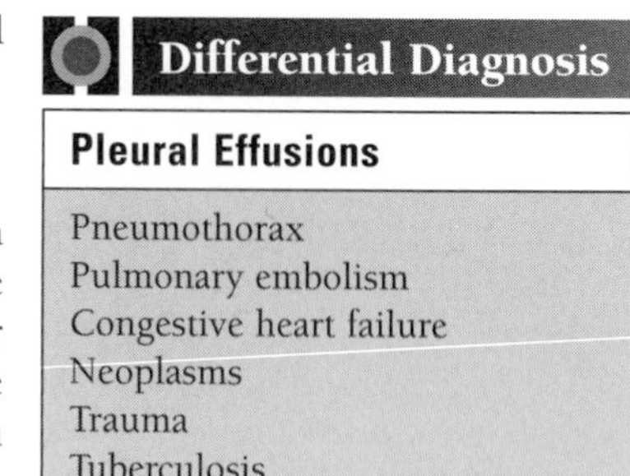
Differential Diagnosis

Pleural Effusions

Pneumothorax
Pulmonary embolism
Congestive heart failure
Neoplasms
Trauma
Tuberculosis

MANAGEMENT

Management is based on treating the cause of the effusion, and a number of specialists may be needed, depending on the cause. In addition, symptomatic treatment is aimed at making the patient more comfortable, beginning when the evaluation is initiated and while the underlying cause is being treated. When an effusion is large, the removal of only 300 to 500 ml through thoracentesis may result in a marked decrease in dyspnea. Indomethacin is often used successfully to treat pleuritic pain and does not suppress respirations as do narcotics. Malignant pleural effusions, especially in the face of advanced disease, are generally very difficult to treat, and management is often focused on providing comfort measures. Some effusions are caused by viral infections and most often resolve without medical intervention.

COMPLICATIONS

Complications depend on the cause and extent of the effusion, accompanying respiratory or systemic compromise, comorbidity, and the treatment modalities available. Malignant pleural effusions are a major cause of morbidity in cancer patients with advanced disease. Treatment is usually palliative, although treatment of the primary malignancy and temporizing symptomatic relief (e.g., repeated thoracentesis for recurrent effusions) may be helpful.

INDICATIONS FOR REFERRAL/HOSPITALIZATION

The evaluation and treatment of a pleural effusion depend on the underlying disease process, degree of respiratory distress, and other contributory factors, such as coexistent health problems. Persons without evidence of respiratory compromise can often be assessed and treated on an outpatient basis. Those with substantial respiratory compromise should be admitted to the hospital for further evaluation and treatment. Referral to a specialist is necessary to establish a definitive diagnosis and management plan.

PATIENT AND FAMILY EDUCATION

Education will vary, depending on the cause of the pleural effusion. In all cases teaching must include an explanation of the diagnostic tests, such as thoracentesis. In addition, education should focus on relieving uncomfortable symptoms, such as dyspnea. Because multiple specialists are often involved in the evaluation of a pleural effusion, the primary care provider's role in coordinating care and keeping the patient well informed and at the focus of decision making is essential.

REFERENCES

1. Sahn SA: Pleural anatomy, physiology, and diagnostic procedures. In Baum GL and others, editors: *Textbook of pulmonary diseases*, ed 6, Philadelphia, 1998, Lippincott-Raven.

2. Celli BR: Diseases of the chest wall. In Bennette C, Plum F, editors: *Cecil textbook of medicine*, ed 20, Philadelphia, 1996, WB Saunders.
3. Pronchik DJ, Sexton J: Emergency department presentation of an unusual pleural effusion, *Am J Emerg Med* 16:163, 1998.
4. Holm K, Antony VB: Pleural effusions: when to suspect, how to proceed, *J Respir Dis* 16:906, 1995.
5. Patz EF: Malignant pleural effusions: recent advances and ambulatory sclerotherapy, *Chest* 113(1 suppl):74S, 1998.
6. Light RW: Disorders of the pleura, mediastinum, and diaphragm. In Fauci AS and others, editors: *Harrison's principles of internal medicine*, ed 14, New York, 1998, McGraw-Hill.
7. Moser K: Pleural effusion. In Bordow RA, Moser KM, editors: *Manual of clinical problems in pulmonary medicine*, ed 4, 1996, Little, Brown.
8. Barterr T, Akers SM, Pratter MR: The evaluation of pleural effusion, *Chest* 106:1209, 1994.

CHAPTER 118

Pleurisy

Patricia Polgar Bailey

DEFINITION/EPIDEMIOLOGY

Pleurisy is chest pain caused by stimulation of the pain fibers in the parietal pleura and is associated with inflammation of the pleural lining. The pain is usually described as sharp or stabbing and is generally exacerbated by deep breathing, coughing, or sneezing. Pleuritic pain is usually experienced over the lower portion of the chest. Pleural involvement is characteristic of numerous localized and systemic disease processes.[1,2]

PATHOPHYSIOLOGY

Pleurisy is caused by *pleuritis* (inflammation of the pleural lining) with or without pleural effusion. The pleural layers are highly permeable and in close contact with microcirculation, which makes them very responsive to local or systemic immunologic or inflammatory processes.[2] The most common causes of pleuritis include viral, bacterial, or tuberculosis infections, as well as pulmonary infarction or connective tissue diseases such as lupus erythematosus.[1] Trauma to the chest wall is a less common cause of pleurisy.

Pleurisy is rarely caused by malignant processes; malignant tumors that involve the pleura generally cause a steady, dull pain compared with the sharp, stabbing, intermittent pain associated with pleural inflammation. Certain drugs, including nitrofurantoin, methysergide, methotrexate, and procarbazine, have been associated with pleurisy.[3]

CLINICAL PRESENTATION

A thorough history is instrumental in determining the differential diagnosis for any type of chest pain. Pain on breathing (which may be minimal to severe depending on the degree of inflammation) and a stabbing or shooting chest pain are characteristics of pleurisy. Milder pleurisy may be described as a "stitch in the side." Pleuritic pain is generally made worse by breathing, coughing, sneezing, or talking. Often the most comfortable position for the patient is lying on the affected side, which limits expansion of the chest wall.[3]

PHYSICAL EXAMINATION

Pleuritic pain is usually located directly over the site of inflammation, and tenderness is increased with deep palpation. Rapid and shallow breathing may be associated symptoms, with limited chest wall expansion on the affected side. Percussion over the affected area may be dull if there is underlying consolidation or pleural effusion. Increased or diminished fremitus may also denote the presence or absence of consolidation. A pleural friction rub, which varies in intensity from a faint scratching sound to a loud creak, confirms the diagnosis of pleurisy. However, the absence of a pleural friction rub does not negate the presence of pleurisy because the presence of pleural fluid may mitigate or even nullify the rub.

A pleural friction rub may be heard during both phases of respiration but is often most pronounced at or near the end of inspiration. It disappears when patients hold their breath. A pleural friction rub may be localized or heard over a wider area and is generally most audible over the lateral and posterior regions of the inferior thorax. It is rarely heard over the upper thorax and lung apices because of the limited movement of the lung in these areas compared with the lung bases. In general, a rub is heard only if the person takes a deep breath; a rub, even if present, is not audible during splinting or shallow breathing. Crackles can sometimes sound similar to a rub, but a cough usually diminishes crackles and has no effect on a rub. A sound similar to a pleural friction rub can be produced by sliding a stethoscope over the skin; firm pressure of the stethoscope on the skin should eliminate this "false rub" and intensify the sound of a real friction rub if present.[3]

DIAGNOSTICS

Several laboratory tests, although themselves not diagnostic of pleurisy, may help elucidate the underlying cause. An elevated leukocyte count with a shift to the left suggests a bacterial infection such as pneumonia, an esophageal rupture, or the presence of an abscess. Leukopenia may reflect a viral process or lupus erythematosus. A chest x-ray examination may help diagnose bacterial pneumonia, pneumothorax, an esophageal rupture, or problems below the diaphragm such as a subphrenic abscess or effusion. Thoracentesis and pleural fluid analysis can help identify the underlying cause once the existence of a pleural effusion has been established (see Chapter 117). If the cause of the pleurisy is still unclear, other studies, including a CT scan of the chest, a ventilation-perfusion scan, a pleural biopsy, and/or esophageal contrast studies, may be indicated.

DIFFERENTIAL DIAGNOSIS

Problems that originate in other chest wall structures can produce pain similar to pleurisy and include pneumothorax, rib fractures, costochondritis, vertebral fractures, and nerve root pain from herpes zoster infection. The presence of a pleural friction rub confirms the pleuritis, but a patient history, physical examination, and pertinent diagnostic tests are still necessary to determine the most likely differential diagnosis.

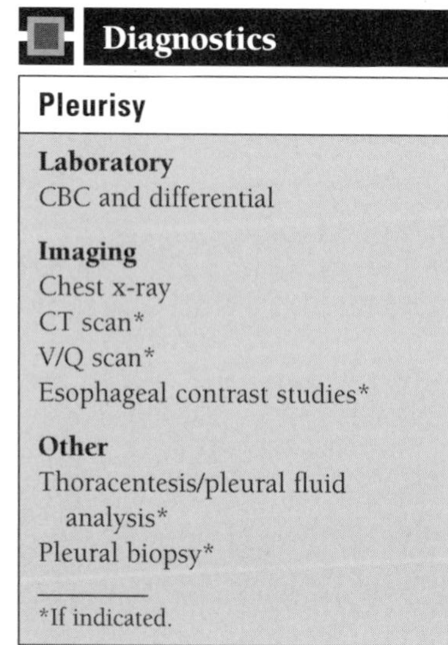

Diagnostics

Pleurisy

Laboratory
CBC and differential

Imaging
Chest x-ray
CT scan*
V/Q scan*
Esophageal contrast studies*

Other
Thoracentesis/pleural fluid analysis*
Pleural biopsy*

*If indicated.

Differential Diagnosis

Pleurisy

Pulmonary hypertension	Cervical spine disease
Pulmonary embolism	Musculoskeletal pain
Tracheitis	Pancreatitis
Pneumothorax	Gallbladder disease
Pleurodynia	Subphrenic abscess
Pneumonia	Peptic ulcer disease
Myocardial infarction	Esophageal disorder
Angina	Tumor neuritis
Pericarditis	Myositis
Rib fracture	Aneurysm
Costochondritis	Thoracic outlet syndrome
Metastatic bone pain	Herpes zoster

Pleural effusion is a finding commonly associated with pleurisy and may be helpful in determining the diagnosis. Viral infections, rheumatic disease, and sarcoidosis often cause pleurisy in the absence of a pleural effusion. In contrast, pneumonia, mycobacterium tuberculosis, lupus pleuritis, and postcardiac injury syndrome are generally associated with pleural effusions.[2,3]

The patient's history may be helpful in narrowing the differential diagnosis. For example, a recent leg fracture with casting raises the possibility of a pulmonary embolism. Occupational asbestos exposure might suggest asbestos pleurisy. A history of lupus erythematosus or sarcoidosis increases the suspicion of systemic connective tissue disease as the underlying cause of the pleurisy.[3]

Many types of pain experienced in the chest area are not pleuritic. Cardiac chest pain is often central and diffuse and is described as a pressing or squeezing rather than a sharp and intermittent pain. Cardiac pain (angina, acute myocardial infarction, dissecting aortic aneurysm) often radiates to the neck, jaw, or arms and worsens with exertion, which is not characteristic of pleurisy. Pericardial pain can be similar in character to pleuritic pain but is usually felt on the anterior side of the chest and back and is exacerbated by lying down. Chronic chest pain is not usually a result of parenchymal lung disease because the lung and visceral pleura are not innervated by pain fibers.

MANAGEMENT

The management of pleurisy is based on treatment of the underlying disease. Co-management with a specialist is necessary for all except the most benign causes of pleural inflammation. Drainage of the pleural space may be indicated if a pleural effusion is present (see Chapter 117). Certain systemic causes of inflammation, such as lupus erythematosus, respond well to corticosteroids. Nonsteroidal antiinflammatory drugs are used to provide symptomatic pain relief. Malignant diseases rarely cause pleurisy, and pleurisy generally resolves with appropriate and prompt treatment.[3]

COMPLICATIONS

The extent and complications of pleural inflammation depend on the underlying disease process. Some causes are self-limiting and have no chronic sequelae or complications. When the inflammation is chronic or if pleural repair processes cause fibrosis, an inelastic membrane ("pleural peel") may form around the lung. This membrane causes lung entrapment and impairs respiratory function.[2]

INDICATIONS FOR REFERRAL/HOSPITALIZATION

A referral is often necessary to determine or treat the underlying cause of the pleurisy. The requisite evaluation and management depend on the cause of the inflammation. Patients without evidence of respiratory compromise or acute illness can often be evaluated and treated on an outpatient basis. Patients with more significant respiratory compromise or highly contagious disease (e.g., active pulmonary tuberculosis) may need to be hospitalized for further evaluation and treatment.

PATIENT AND FAMILY EDUCATION

Patient education varies depending on the cause of the pleurisy. Teaching must include an explanation of and rationale for all diagnostic tests. Education should also focus on symptomatic relief. As in all cases in which multiple practitioners may be involved, the role of the primary care provider is important in coordinating care and in keeping the patient well informed and at the focus of decision making.

REFERENCES

1. Ball WC: Approach to the patient with pulmonary disease. In Stobo JD and others, editors: *Principles and practice of medicine,* ed 23, Stamford, Conn, 1996, Appleton & Lange.
2. Kroegel C, Antony VB: Immunobiology of pleural inflammation: potential implications for pathogenesis, diagnosis, and therapy, *Eur Respir J* 10:2411, 1997.
3. Sahn SA, Heffner JE: Approach to the patient with pleural disease. In Kelley WN and others, editors: *Textbook of internal medicine,* ed 3, Philadelphia, 1997, Lippincott-Raven.

CHAPTER 119

Pneumonia

Susan Harvey

DEFINITION/EPIDEMIOLOGY

Pneumonia is an infection of the lower respiratory tract that is usually accompanied by cough, fever, malaise, and chest x-ray abnormalities. Sputum production, pleurisy, dyspnea, chills, hypoxia, and hemoptysis may be present in some individuals with pneumonia, depending on the causative organism. In most cases diagnosis of the disease is made by the presence of symptoms; however, identification of the etiologic agent is usually not necessary. Although the list of organisms causing pneumonia is long and increasing, most pneumonias are caused by relatively few organisms. In primary care practice, two of the most important issues are awareness of the most common infectious pathogens and their treatment, and decisions regarding the appropriateness of outpatient treatment.

The successful treatment of pneumonia depends on the correct empiric antibiotic selection and knowledge of its proven effectiveness in vivo. A working knowledge of the organisms that most commonly infect different age-groups and the habits or characteristics that put an individual at risk for specific etiologic agents is essential. The most common cause of bacterial pneumonia is *Streptococcus pneumoniae.*[1] It is estimated that 20% to 60% cases of pneumonia are caused by *S. pneumoniae.* Gram-negative organisms include *Haemophilus influenzae, Klebsiella pneumoniae,* and *Moraxella catarrhalis. M. catarrhalis* and *K. pneumoniae* infections are more commonly diagnosed when there is coexistent alcoholism. *Staphylococcus aureus* and *H. influenzae* infections often occur after a primary influenza infection. *M. catarrhalis,* a gram-negative organism not thought to be pathogenic, is most commonly found in those with chronic lung conditions such as chronic obstructive pulmonary disease (COPD). It is also found in those with other underlying chronic lung conditions such as malignancy, with steroid use, and with diabetes.[2]

Another organism responsible for pneumonia is *Legionella pneumophila.* This organism was first implicated in 1976 after 182 people became ill in Philadelphia while attending an American Legion convention. The organism is a gram-negative bacillus that survives in water and soil. Contamination with the organism is acquired through inhalation of aerosolized droplets, thus making air-conditioning ventilating systems an obvious reservoir.

Finally, the atypical and nonbacterial organisms responsible for pneumonia include *Mycoplasma pneumoniae, Chlamydia pneumoniae* (the Taiwan acute respiratory disease [TWAR] strain), and multiple viruses. Mycoplasma organisms lack cell walls and cannot be stained and visualized by conventional methods. Infection with this organism causes a disease that is usually found in younger individuals and follows a milder course. Chlamydial infection also presents as a mild infection spread from person to person by aerosolized droplet secretions.

Pneumonia remains one of the leading causes of morbidity and mortality in the United States, especially in older adults and in those with underlying chronic disease. Specifically, pneumonia of any etiology is the sixth leading cause of death in the United States. It is estimated that there are 4 million episodes of pneumonia diagnosed in the United States every year, with a total of >30 million days of disability.[3] These are surprising statistics given the advent of broad-spectrum antibiotics, a multivalent *Pneumococcus* vaccine, and very sophisticated hospital care.

Clues to the specific cause of the pneumonia can be found in the patient's history. The community-acquired pneumonias include most of the organisms found in Table 119-1 except for the enteric gram-negative bacilli, *Pseudomonas* organisms, and staphylococci, which are often found in patients who are hospitalized or live in nursing homes.

The incidence of some causes of pneumonia is linked to the season of the year and the geographic area. Influenza illness in the winter increases the prevalence of secondary *S. pneumoniae*, *S. aureus*, and *H. influenzae* pneumonias. *H. influenzae* is known to have a short incubation period and moves through communities rather quickly. Mycoplasmal infection usually moves through communities slowly because of a longer incubation period and lower communicability. *Legionella* organisms have been known to infect a large number of people simultaneously by infecting many within a group from a single reservoir.

PATHOPHYSIOLOGY

The lungs are usually a sterile environment maintained by a host of natural defenses. The airways act as a filtration and humidification system of inspired air. Epithelial cells line the entire respiratory tract and contain cilia that constantly beat upward toward the pharynx. This action is a physical means of elimination of foreign material. Also, an intact gag reflex prevents the entry of particles, mucus, and food debris. Finally, the immune system is responsible for defense mechanisms, such as the action of phagocytes, macrophages, neutrophils, complement, and immunoglobulins, to retard advancement of pathogenic organisms that do gain access to this normally sterile environment.

In the healthy adult, the above-mentioned host mechanisms prevent disease much of the time. However, there are a number of mechanisms that, when present, allow for pathogens to gain entry into the lungs, such as an altered level of conscious from stroke, seizure, anesthesia, alcohol abuse, intoxication, and the sleep state. Epiglottic closure may be compromised in these situations and allow normal oral flora to gain entry.

Certain other conditions may predispose an individual to recurrent pneumonias; these include individuals with compromised immune function, cystic fibrosis, esophageal abnormalities, bronchial obstruction, and bronchiectasis.

TABLE 119-1 Epidemiologic Characteristics Related to Specific Pathogens

Characteristics	Pathogen(s)
Alcoholism	Oral anaerobes *Streptococcus pneumoniae* Gram-negative bacilli
COPD/tobacco use	*Haemophilus influenzae* *Streptococcus pneumoniae* *Moraxella catarrhalis*
Nursing home resident	*S. pneumoniae* Gram-negative bacilli *H. influenzae* *Staphylococcus aureus*
Poor dental hygiene	Oral anaerobes
Recent exposure to plumbing/water	*Legionella* organisms
Exposure to birds	*Chlamydia psittaci* Histoplasmosis
HIV infection	*Pneumocystis carinii* *S. pneumoniae* *H. influenzae* *Mycobacterium tuberculosis*
Exposure to excreta of wild rodents	Sin nombre virus (Hantavirus pulmonary syndrome)

Reprinted with permission from File TM and others: Community acquired pneumonia, *Postgrad Med 99*(1):102, 1996. ©1996 McGraw-Hill.

CLINICAL PRESENTATION/PHYSICAL EXAMINATION

The clinical presentation of pneumonia includes a history of fever, malaise, and cough with or without sputum production. The patient may also complain of hemoptysis, dyspnea, and pleuritic chest symptoms. The history alone does not distinguish between bacterial, viral, and atypical pneumonia syndromes. Chest auscultation may reveal rales that do not clear with a cough, which may be found in both bacterial and atypical pneumonia. Consolidation, including dullness to percussion, bronchial breath sounds, and egobronchophony (E-to-A changes), is found more commonly in the bacterial pneumonia syndromes. Chest radiographs are highly variable and may be normal in the early course of the disease. In addition, chest x-ray films of patients with viral and mycoplasmal pneumonia may show large infiltrates with minimal outward symptoms. Older adults may show none of the classic signs of pneumonia but may have a history of sudden alteration in mental status, such as confusion, lethargy, stupor, or coma.

Bacterial Pneumonia Syndromes

Gram-Positive Bacteria. *S. pneumoniae* is the leading cause of pneumonia in any adult age-group with or without co-morbid conditions.[1-4] Pneumococcal pneumonia that is associated with bacteremia has a 20% mortality rate.[5] Those at risk for this condition characteristically have some chronic condition, such as diabetes, COPD, asplenia, advanced age, cigarette smoking, congestive heart failure, dementia, alcoholism, or immunosuppression. From 20% to 60% percent of all hospitalized patients are infected with pneumococci.[1]

The history may include an abrupt onset of high fever with shaking chills; cough with productive, purulent sputum; and possibly pleuritic-type chest pains. Physical examination may reveal signs of consolidation (egobronchophony, increased fremitus, dullness to percussion, rales, and rhonchi) and chest x-ray films that reveal single or multiple lobar consolidation. Sputum analysis by Gram's stain indicates gram-positive diplococci in pairs and short chains and large numbers of polymorphonuclear leukocytes.

S. aureus, although rarely a cause of community-acquired pneumonia, must be considered, especially after a primary influenza infection, in older adults and in those with diabetes. From 2% to 10% of acute community-acquired pneumonias are due to staphylococci.[5] Suppurative conditions, including empyema, lung abscess, and pneumothorax, are common complications. Seeding to distant sites, such as bones, joints, liver, endocardium, and the meninges, may also occur.

Group A streptococci rarely cause community-acquired pneumonia but have been found in epidemics among close groups that live together, such as military units. Symptoms may be similar to those of *S. pneumoniae*, and Gram's stain reveals clumped spherical cocci, similar in appearance to a bunch of grapes.

Gram-Negative Bacteria. *H. influenzae*, another etiologic agent of community-acquired pneumonia, is a small gram-negative rod with a polysaccharide capsule. There are six serotypes, of which type b is the most severe and invasive (causing meningitis and sepsis). Some strains of *H. influenzae* are nonencapsulated and therefore cannot be typed. These are also capable of causing disease, but usually the disease is noninvasive and therefore less severe. It is these nontypeable strains of *H. influenzae* that are usually found in acute bronchitis. Pneumonia caused by *H. influenzae* is usually caused by an encapsulated strain. Older adults and those with underlying chronic lung conditions are most susceptible to this bacteria.[6,7]

The history usually includes an abrupt onset of fever, shaking chills, and cough with purulent sputum. The patient may describe pleuritic chest pain, and physical examination reveals signs of consolidation. A bronchopneumonia pattern is seen on the chest x-ray film.

Aerobic gram-negative bacilli rarely colonize the upper airway in healthy individuals but are often found in people with an underlying disease such as alcoholism and in those who reside in health care facilities or nursing homes. Aspiration of the organisms is thought to be the mode of infection. *Pseudomonas* organisms, *Klebsiella pneumoniae*, and *Escherichia coli* may also become pulmonary pathogens. Studies show that the mortality rate of gram-negative pneumonia collectively may be 35% to 60%. Therefore a history of recent hospitalization or nursing home residency should heighten suspicion for a gram-negative pathogenesis. Polymicrobial infection is especially seen in older adults, and increased colonization of gram-negative bacilli of the upper airway is related to recent antimicrobial use, decreased activity, diabetes, and alcohol use.

Moraxella (Branhamella) catarrhalis is a beta lactamase–producing gram-negative aerobic *Diplococcus* that was recently identified as a common pathogen found in individuals with COPD.[1,2] Often in patients with COPD, it is the only organism isolated from the lower respiratory tract. Other chronic conditions, such as alcoholism, steroid use, diabetes, and malignancy, increase the risk of *M. catarrhalis* infection. The highest incidence of this infection tends to be in the winter months.

Atypical Pneumonia Syndromes

Atypical pneumonia syndromes largely refer to pneumonias caused by nonbacterial organisms and by bacterial organisms that do not share the expected characteristics of most bacteria. *M. pneumoniae* is the most common offending organism in the majority of cases of pneumonia in those under 40 years of age.[2] It has a predominance in older children and young adults. This "atypical" pneumonia syndrome is characterized by a prodrome of fever, headache, myalgias, and dry cough. These individuals usually appear less ill than do those with bacterial pneumonia. Symptoms may last up to 6 weeks and include a dry, hacking cough that may require a narcotic cough suppressant. Because of the long incubation period, mycoplasmal infection may spread slowly among family members. It should be viewed as a systemic disease with a pulmonary component.

The physical examination usually reveals fine rales with no signs of lung consolidation. A cutaneous manifestation may be present in the form of maculopapular eruptions. Rarely, examination of the tympanic membranes shows evidence of bullous myringitis, which can be very painful. Chest x-ray films reveal patchy alveolar densities or nonhomogeneous segmental infiltrates. The WBC count may be normal or only slightly elevated. Full recovery is expected with no residual effects in a previously healthy individual. However, the disease can be severe in those with sickle cell anemia, in older adults, and in those with immunosuppression.

C. pneumoniae (TWAR strain) is the etiologic agent for a common atypical pneumonia syndrome in younger individuals. Outbreaks occur in groups such as military units and on college campuses among younger adults. Symptoms are very similar to those of mycoplasmal infection. Clinical presentation may include laryngitis, a hoarse voice, and nonexudative pharyngitis, in addition to the symptoms described above for mycoplasmal infection. Laryngitis is not present in any other atypical pneumonia syndrome. Chest x-ray films may show patchy consolidation, interstitial infiltrates, and/or funnel-shaped lesions. The WBC count is also usually normal.

Multiple viruses, including adenoviruses, respiratory syncytial virus, and parainfluenza virus, may also cause pneumonia. Predilection for infection in children is most common. Cytomegalovirus and *Pneumocystis carinii* may be the cause of pneumonia in the immunocompromised host. Recently, infection with hantavirus has been recognized in the southwestern part of the United States. Fever, myalgias, and respiratory distress resembling acute respiratory distress syndrome (ARDS) are present.[1]

Legionnaire's Disease

Infection with *Legionella pneumophila* was only recently identified as a pulmonary pathogen. Symptoms include dry cough, fever with a temperature between 38.3° and 38.9° C (101° and 102° F), altered mental status, relative bradycardia, headache, and gastrointestinal symptoms, including diarrhea.

Legionnaire's disease is caused by a gram-negative bacillus that is considered an atypical organism because it does not respond to the beta lactam antibiotics as do other gram-negative organisms. Suspicion for infection with *Legionella* organisms should be high, especially in older adults and in those with chronic underlying disease who are most at risk for death. Chest x-ray films reveal rapid progression of asymmetric infiltrates without signs of consolidation. Serum titer levels for *Legionella* organisms can be obtained but are most often negative early in the disease. To be diagnostic, the titer must be greater than 1:256. Treatment with tetracycline and the macrolide antibiotics is recommended.

DIAGNOSTICS

Chest Radiography

The results of chest x-ray films are most valuable when considered in the context of the history and physical examination. Not every case of pneumonia needs to be confirmed with a chest x-ray film, especially if the patient is young, is without co-morbid disease, and is expected to recover in a timely manner. However, a chest x-ray film can help to differentiate between conditions that mimic pneumonia, such as pneumocystic disease and tuberculosis. Posteroanterior and lateral chest x-ray films confirm pneumonia when new infiltrates are found on the films. However, a chest x-ray film that is negative does not exclude the diagnosis of pneumonia. Dehydration and neutropenia may result in false-negative findings. Comparison of the current chest x-ray film with old radiographs is always important to assess for current changes. Bacterial patterns on the chest x-ray film include lobar consolidation, cavitation, and large pleural effusions.

Sputum Analysis

Analysis of the sputum can be very helpful in identifying an etiologic agent in pneumonia. Culture and Gram's stain are excellent methods of identifying the pathologic agent when needed. A good sputum sample comes from the bronchial tree; it is not the same as saliva from the mouth. Although not usually available during the clinic visit, sputum produced on awakening in the morning is typically a good sample because of the strong reflex to cough when rising to an upright position. Sputum that contains <10 squamous epithelial cells and <25 neutrophils is considered an adequate sample. The patient is encouraged to rinse the mouth with water several times before trying to produce a sample. Inhalation of a warmed 3% to 10% saline solution may help the patient to provide an adequate sample.

Fiberoptic bronchoscopy, lung biopsy, and examination of the pleural fluid are invasive diagnostic techniques implemented in the hospital environment when the diagnosis is not clear or an etiologic agent needs to be ascertained. These are not used in the outpatient setting and therefore are not usually useful in the initial attempt to diagnose pneumonia.

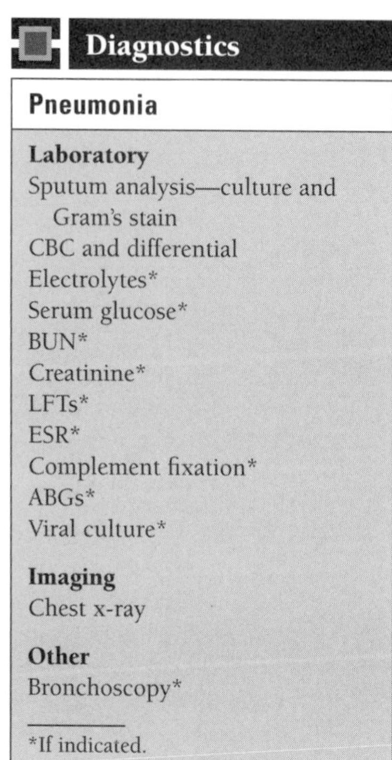

Diagnostics

Pneumonia

Laboratory
Sputum analysis—culture and Gram's stain
CBC and differential
Electrolytes*
Serum glucose*
BUN*
Creatinine*
LFTs*
ESR*
Complement fixation*
ABGs*
Viral culture*

Imaging
Chest x-ray

Other
Bronchoscopy*

*If indicated.

Other Tests

Multiple serologic and antigen studies are available in an attempt to identify the pathogen(s) responsible for the pneumonia. These are not routinely used in the outpatient setting. However, if bacterial pneumonia is suspected, blood cultures should be obtained and can be very valuable. When positive, blood cultures provide definitive proof of the offending organism. Even after extensive diagnostic testing has been completed, many times the pathogen remains unidentified.

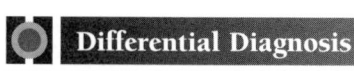

Differential Diagnosis

Pneumonia

Streptococcus pneumoniae
Mycoplasma pneumoniae
Respiratory viruses (including cytomegalovirus and hantavirus)
Chlamydia pneumoniae (TWAR strain)
Haemophilus influenzae
Legionella pneumophila
Staphylococcus aureus
Mycobacterium tuberculosis
Endemic fungi
Aerobic gram-negative bacilli (e.g., *Pseudomonas aeruginosa*)
Anaerobic infections
Polymicrobial infections
Pulmonary embolus
Congestive heart failure
Pulmonary tumors
Inflammatory lung diseases
Acute and chronic bronchitis

DIFFERENTIAL DIAGNOSIS

Multiple organisms must be considered in the differential diagnosis of pneumonia, as well as syndromes that can mimic symptoms of the disease. These may include pulmonary emboli, congestive heart failure, pulmonary tumors, and some inflammatory lung diseases.

MANAGEMENT

Resistance patterns to all antibiotics are an increasing problem that is now more evident and widespread than at any other time in medical history. Careful, prudent use of antibiotics is absolutely necessary to curb this growing problem. The routine practice of trying to cover for all pathogens, especially gram-negative organisms, should be avoided; this only leads to increased resistance patterns. Initiation of antibiotic treatment in patients with community-acquired pneumonia is empirically determined because the history and physical examination will not determine a specific cause for the disease.[8-11] Despite the use of sputum culture, Gram's stain, and chest x-ray studies, the practitioner can accurately identify the causative organism only 40% to 70% of the time. Therefore the patient's age, the competency of the host immune system, underlying chronic conditions, patterns of resistance in the community, and knowledge of the most likely pathogen(s) must be considered to accurately determine empiric antimicrobial therapy.

Recommendations for initial empiric antimicrobial therapy in the outpatient setting vary.[1,4] The recommendations for treatment of community-acquired pneumonia are taken from the most recent guidelines and recommendations published by the American Thoracic Society in 2001.[1] Since the last publication of these recommendations in 1993, there has been a shift from age-groups and co-morbid conditions to the most likely pathogens combined with modifying factors (Table 119-2) and/or cardiopulmonary disease (Tables 119-3 to 119-6). Group I includes outpatients without cardiopulmonary disease and without modifying factors. Modifying factors include human immunodeficiency virus infection (HIV), presence of risk factors for infection with drug-resistant *Pneumococcus*, presence of risk factors for gram-negative infection (including nursing home residence), and risk factors for *Pseudomonas aeruginosa*. Group II includes

TABLE 119-2 Modifying Factors That Increase the Risk of Infection with Specific Pathogens

Penicillin-resistant and drug-resistant pneumococci
- Age >65 years
- Beta-lactam therapy within the past 3 months
- Alcoholism
- Immune-suppressive illness (including therapy with corticosteroids)
- Multiple medical co-morbidities
- Exposure to a child in a day care center

Enteric gram-negatives
- Residence in a nursing home
- Underlying cardiopulmonary disease
- Multiple medical co-morbidities
- Recent antibiotic therapy

Pseudomonas aeruginosa
- Structural lung disease (bronchiectasis)
- Corticosteroid therapy (>10 mg of prednisone per day)
- Broad-spectrum antibiotic therapy for >7 days in the past month
- Malnutrition

From American Thoracic Society: Guidelines for the management of adults with community-acquired pneumonia: diagnosis, assessment of severity, antimicrobial therapy and prevention. *Am J Respir Crit Care Med* 163:1730-1754, 2001.

TABLE 119-3 Group I: Outpatients, No Cardiopulmonary Disease, No Modifying Factors*†

Organisms	Therapy
Streptococcus pneumoniae *Mycoplasma pneumoniae* *Chlamydia pneumoniae* (alone or as mixed infection) *Haemophilus influenzae* Respiratory viruses Miscellaneous *Legionella* spp. *Mycobacterium tuberculosis* Endemic fungi	Advanced-generation macrolide: azithromycin or clarithromycin‡ *or* Doxycycline§

From American Thoracic Society: Guidelines for the management of adults with community-acquired pneumonia: diagnosis, assessment of severity, antimicrobial therapy, and prevention, *Am J Respir Crit Care Med* 163:1730-1754, 2001.
* Excludes patients at risk for HIV.
† In roughly 50%-90% of the cases no etiology was identified.
‡ Erythromycin is not active against *H. influenzae,* and the advanced generation macrolides azithromycin and clarithromycin are better tolerated.
§ Many isolates of *S. pneumoniae* are resistant to tetracycline, and it should be used only if the patient is allergic to or intolerant of macrolides.

outpatients with cardiopulmonary disease (congestive heart failure or COPD) and/or other modifying factors (risk factors for drug-resistant *S. pneumoniae* or gram-negative bacteria). Group III includes inpatients, not in the intensive care unit, and group IV includes inpatients admitted to the intensive care unit.[1]

Most of the time monotherapy is adequate treatment for outpatients with pneumonia but without co-mordid illness or modifying factors. Traditionally erythromycin was the most widely recommended antibiotic for this group of individuals. The most common pathogens in this group include *S. pneumoniae, M. pneumoniae,* respiratory viruses, *C. pneumoniae,* and *H. influenzae*. Other identified pathogens, including *Legionella* organisms, *S. pneumoniae, M. tuberculosis,* and endemic fungi, cause pneumonia to a lesser extent. The macrolide antibiotics, including erythromycin, azithromycin, and clarithromycin, are commonly used to treat this group. The American Thoracic Society (ATS) recommends an advanced-generation macrolide such as azithromycin or clarithromycin; both of these cover the expected organisms infecting group I. The ATS reports that the use of macrolides or doxycycline constitutes level III evidence, which includes case studies and expert opinion. The studies include in vitro antibiotic susceptibility. Erythromycin was dropped as a recommendation due to its lack of activity against *H. influenzae,* which often infects cigarette smokers. However, it remains a reasonable choice if cost or availability is a factor and the patient is not likely to be infected with *H. influenzae*.

TABLE 119-4 Group II: Outpatient, with Cardiopulmonary Disease, and/or Other Modifying Factors*†

Organisms	Therapy‡
Streptococcus pneumoniae (including DRSP) *Mycoplasma pneumoniae* *Chlamydia pneumoniae* Mixed infection (bacteria plus atypical pathogen or virus) *Haemophilus influenzae* Enteric gram-negatives Respiratory viruses Miscellaneous *Moraxella catarrhalis, Legionella* spp., aspiration (anaerobes), *Mycobacterium tuberculosis,* endemic fungi	Beta-lactam (oral cefpodoxime, cefuroxime, high-dose amoxicillin, amoxicillin/clavulanate; or parenteral ceftriaxone followed by oral cefpodoxime) *plus* Macrolide or doxycycline§ *or* Antipneumococcal fluoroquinolone (used alone)

From American Thoracic Society: Guidelines for the management of adults with community-acquired pneumonia: diagnosis, assessment of severity, antimicrobial therapy, and prevention, *Am J Respir Crit Care Med* 163:1730-1754, 2001.
* Excludes patients at risk for HIV.
† In roughly 50%-90% of the cases no etiology was identified.
‡ In no particular order.
§ High-dose amoxicillin is 1 g every 8 h; if a macrolide is used, erythromycin does not provide coverage of *H. influenzae,* and thus when amoxicillin is used, the addition of doxycycline or of an advanced-generation macrolide is required to provide adequate coverage of *H. influenzae.*

Doxycycline, a second antibiotic choice, offers predictable coverage against the atypical pathogens and *H. influenzae.* However, doxycycline is less likely to cover drug-resistant *S. pneumoniae,* which is an unlikely pathogen in this group. Doxycycline is inexpensive, offers twice-daily dosing, and has few gastrointestinal side effects.

Group II includes outpatients with cardiopulmonary diseases (congestive heart failure and COPD) or risk factors for drug-resistant *S. pneumoniae,* which include age greater than 65 and nursing home residence. The pathogens are changed but *Pneumococcus* remains the most likely cause of pneumonia for this group, especially *Pneumococcus* that is resistant to penicillin. Other organisms include *E. coli, Klebsiella* spp., and *P. aeruginosa.* Aspiration with anaerobes should be considered if there is poor dentition, neurologic illness, or impaired consciousness.

TABLE 119-5 Group III: Inpatients, Not in ICU*†

Organisms	Therapy‡
CARDIOPULMONARY DISEASE AND/OR MODIFYING FACTORS (INCLUDING BEING FROM A NURSING HOME)	
Streptococcus pneumoniae (including DRSP) *Haemophilus influenzae* *Mycoplasma pneumoniae* *Chlamydia pneumoniae* Mixed infection (bacteria plus atypical pathogen) Enteric gram-negatives Aspiration (anaerobes) Viruses *Legionella* spp. Miscellaneous *Mycobacterium tuberculosis,* endemic fungi, *Pneumocystis carinii*	Intravenous beta-lactam§ (cefotaxime, ceftriaxone, ampicillin/sulbactam, high-dose ampicillin) *plus* Intravenous or oral macrolide or doxycycline ‖ *or* Intravenous antipneumococcal fluoroquinolone alone
NO CARDIOPULMONARY DISEASE, NO MODIFYING FACTORS	
S. pneumoniae *H. influenzae* *M. pneumoniae* *C. pneumoniae* Mixed infection (bacteria plus atypical pathogen) Viruses *Legionella* spp. Miscellaneous *M. tuberculosis,* endemic fungi, *P. carinii*	Intravenous azithromycin alone If macrolide allergic or intolerant: Doxycycline and a beta-lactam *or* Monotherapy with an antipneumococcal fluoroquinolone

From American Thoracic Society: Guidelines for the management of adults with community-acquired pneumonia: diagnosis, assessment of severity, antimicrobial therapy, and prevention, *Am J Respir Crit Care Med* 163:1730-1754, 2001.
* Excludes patients at risk for HIV.
† In roughly one-third to one-half of the cases no etiology was identified.
‡ In no particular order.
§ Antipseudomonal agents such as cefepime, piperacillin/tazobactam, imipenem, and meropenem are generally active against DRSP, but not recommended for routine use in this population that does not have risk factors for *P. aeruginosa.*
‖ Use of doxycycline or an advanced-generation macrolide (azithromycin or clarithromycin) will provide adequate coverage if the selected beta-lactam is susceptible to bacterial beta-lactamases.

TABLE 119-6 Group IV: ICU-Admitted Patients*†

Organisms	Therapy‡§
NO RISKS FOR *PSEUDOMONAS AERUGINOSA*	
Streptococcus pneumoniae (including DRSP) *Legionella* spp. *Haemophilus influenzae* Enteric gram-negative bacilli *Staphylococcus aureus* *Mycoplasma pneumoniae* Respiratory viruses Miscellaneous *Chlamydia pneumoniae, Mycobacterium tuberculosis,* endemic fungi	Intravenous beta-lactam (cefotaxime, ceftriaxone)‖ *plus either* Intravenous macrolide (azithromycin) *or* Intravenous fluoroquinolone
RISKS FOR *PSEUDOMONAS AERUGINOSA*‖	
All of the above pathogens plus *P. aeruginosa*	Selected intravenous antipseudomonal beta-lactam (cefepime, imipenem, meropenem, piperacillin/tazobactam)# *plus* intravenous antipseudomonal quinolone (ciprofloxacin) *or* Selected intravenous antipseudomonal beta-lactam (cefepime, imipenem, meropenem, piperacillin/tazobactam)# *plus* intravenous aminoglycoside *plus either* intravenous macrolide (azithromycin) *or* intravenous nonpseudomonal fluoroquinolone

From American Thoracic Society: Guidelines for the management of adults with community-acquired pneumonia: diagnosis, assessment of severity, antimicrobial therapy, and prevention, *Am J Respir Crit Care Med* 163:1730-1754, 2001.
* Excludes patients at risk for HIV.
† In roughly one-third to one-half of the cases no etiology was identified.
‡ In no particular order.
§ Combination therapy required.
‖ Antipseudomonal agents such as cefepime, piperacillin/tazobactam, imipenem, and meropenem are generally active against DRSP and other likely pathogens in this population but are not recommended for routine use unless the patient has risk factors for *P. aeruginosa.*
If beta-lactam allergic, replace the listed beta-lactam with aztreonam and combine with an aminoglycoside and an antipneumococcal fluoroquinolone as listed.

Recommended initial therapy includes beta lactam drugs (penicillins and cephalosporins) as outlined in Table 119-4, with the addition of a macrolide or doxycycline. Second-line therapy could be monotherapy with an antipneumococcal fluoroquinolone; these include levofloxacin, moxifloxacin, and gatifloxacin. These recommendations from the ATS constitute level II evidence, which is supported by well-designed, controlled trials without randomization (including cohort, patient series, and case control studies).[1] Groups III and IV are not discussed here but are included to complete the recommendations by the ATS. A treatment algorithm is provided (Figure 119-1).

The choice of antibiotic therapy depends on careful consideration of the cost, especially with second- and third-generation cephalosporins, the consequences of failing to respond to initial outpatient treatment, the need for hospitalization, and the social situation of the patient. Additional concerns include the likelihood of adherence to the treatment regimen, the existence of a supportive home environment, access to emergency department care if needed, the presence of an involved individual to identify significant changes in this illness should they occur, and the opportunity for follow-up in 24 to 48 hours.

The duration of therapy is usually 7 to 14 days, depending on the severity of the illness, co-morbid illness, and resolution of the illness. The long half-life of azithromycin allows for a shorter duration of therapy, usually 5 days. In the immunocompromised

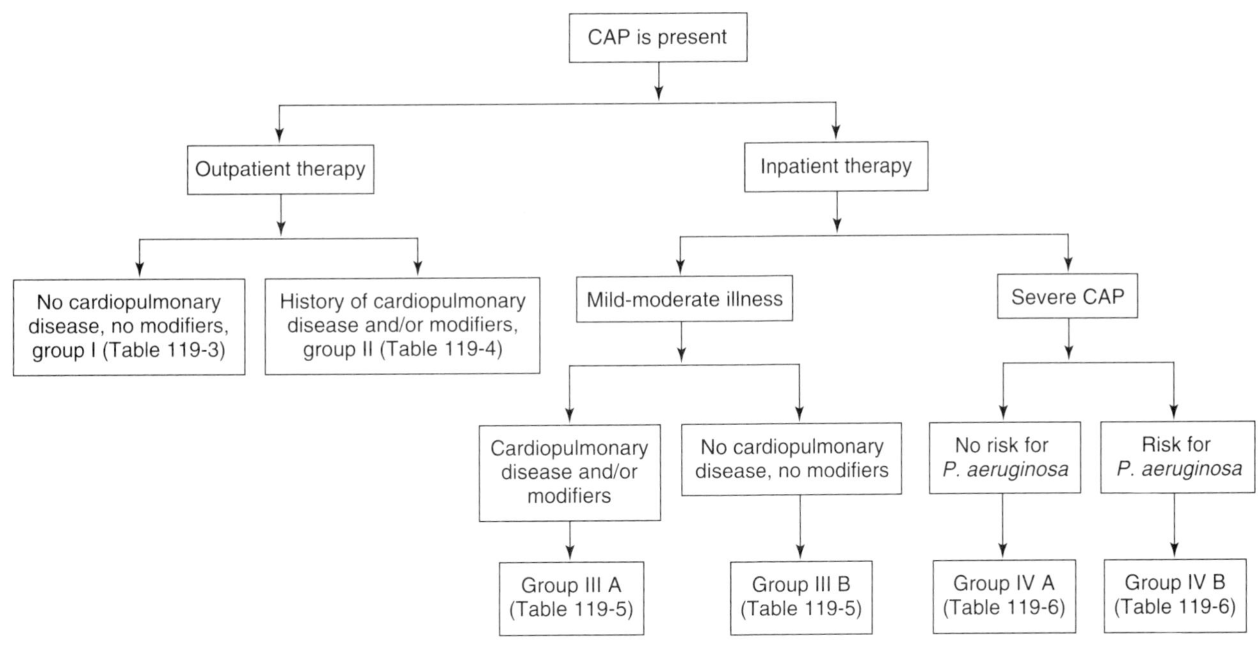

FIGURE 119-1

Treatment algorithm for pneumonia. *CAP,* Community acquired pneumonia. (From American Thoracic Society: Guidelines for the management of adults with community-acquired pneumonia: diagnosis, assessment of severity, antimicrobial therapy and prevention, *Am J Respir Crit Care Med* 163:1730-1754, 2001.)

patient, in general 50% additional time is needed for antibiotic therapy. Suspected mycoplasmal or chlamydial pneumonia requires 10 to 14 days. Infection with *Legionella* organisms, which takes the longest to resolve of all the community-acquired pneumonias, requires ≥14 days of antibiotic therapy.[1,3,4,6]

Older adults and those with coexisting illness are at increased risk of developing more virulent pneumonia, have longer healing times, need more supportive treatment, and require closer follow-up, especially with delayed resolution of pneumonia. Younger individuals without co-morbid disease who are infected with pneumonia usually respond quicker and have fewer complications.

With the increased prevalence of HIV/acquired immune deficiency syndrome (AIDS), the suspicion of compromised immune function must be considered when there is delayed resolution of pneumonia or when a young individual seems to be more ill than would be expected with preserved immune function. A common cause of pneumonia in the patient with AIDS is *P. carinii,* which should be suspected despite the use of prophylactic antibiotic treatment before the onset of symptoms. Other common pathogens must also be considered, such as *S. pneumoniae, H. influenzae,* cytomegalovirus, and *M. tuberculosis,* as well as other pathogens.

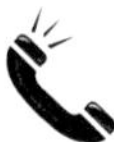

Physician consultation is recommended for patients with oxygen saturation of <90% on room air, rigors, change in mental status, extremely abnormal vital signs, or co-morbid disease (e.g., diabetes, HIV, cancer, or COPD).

COMPLICATIONS

With minimal diagnostic testing and empiric antibiotic treatment, most patients will improve and show resolution of pneumonia. In most cases improvement is seen within 48 to 72 hours after initiation of antibiotics. Pneumonia that fails to resolve shows little clinical improvement after 4 weeks of therapy. Fever, cough, sputum production, and shortness of breath may still be present. Chest x-ray films also do not show improvement within this time frame.

When there is poor response to therapy, possibly either the initial antibiotic choice was not correct, there was poor adherence to the oral antibiotic therapy, or the diagnosis of pneumonia was not accurate. Considerations should include the possibility of opportunistic fungal infections, *P. carinii,* tuberculosis, bronchogenic carcinoma, Wegener's granulomatosis, bronchiolitis obliterans with organizing pneumonia (BOOP), and congestive heart failure. A diagnostic bronchoscopy, CT scan, and transthoracic needle aspiration may be warranted to exclude these. If the diagnosis is still undetermined and there is no resolution, an open lung biopsy may be considered, and consultation with a pulmonologist is clearly warranted. Other complications of pneumonia include abscess, empyema, pulmonary vascular congestion, and pulmonary embolism.

INDICATIONS FOR REFERRAL/HOSPITALIZATION

Delayed resolution of pneumonia and inpatient treatment generally require consultation. Pneumonia is the leading cause of death due to an infectious agent and, overall, is the sixth leading cause of death in the United States. Therefore it is imperative to recognize patients who are not candidates for outpatient therapy. Indications for hospital admission are discussed in a similar fashion throughout the literature. Certain clinical criteria observed in the patient warrant hospitalization (Box 119-1). However, clinical judgment of the primary care provider always supersedes written recommendations.

PATIENT AND FAMILY EDUCATION

Once the diagnosis of pneumonia has been made, patient education should include directions for use of the antibiotic and information on potential untoward effects of the drug. Follow-up instructions, depending on the clinical situation, may include 24-hour telephone contact or follow-up in the office after 24 to 48 hours. This will improve adherence to the prescribed therapy, provide an opportunity to address side effects of drug therapy, and allow progress to be monitored. The need for hospitalization should be assessed throughout the course of the illness. Education should include instructions to drink plenty of fluids and instructions on use of an antipyretic to control fever and myalgias when needed. Use of cough medicines should be avoided because the cough reflex and sputum expectoration enhance removal of thick secretions. However, in the event of a constant, nonproductive cough, as found especially with mycoplasmal infection, a narcotic such as codeine at night allows for more restorative sleep.

HEALTH PROMOTION

Patients at risk for pneumonia should receive the pneumonia vaccination and should also be encouraged to receive a flu shot each year. Avoiding smoke and contact with persons who have a respiratory infection also decreases the risk of pneumonia. Daily exercise and eating healthy foods high in vitamins, nutrients, and fiber should also be encouraged.

BOX 119-1

INDICATIONS FOR HOSPITALIZATION

- Severe abnormality in vital signs:
  - Heart rate >125 beats per minute
  - Systolic blood pressure <90 mm Hg
  - Respiratory rate >30 breaths per minute
- Altered mental status
- Oxygen saturation by pulse oximetry <90% on room air
- Suppurative pneumonia-related infection (empyema, septic arthritis, meningitis, endocarditis)
- Severe electrolyte imbalance or metabolic abnormality not known to be chronic:
  - Sodium <130 mEq/L
  - Hematocrit <30%
  - Absolute neutrophil count <1000/mm^3 or WBC count <5000
  - BUN >50 mg/dl
  - Creatinine >2.5 mg/dl
- Acute coexistent medical condition requiring hospital admission that is independent of pneumonia
- Failure to respond to outpatient treatment within 48-72 hours

From Niederman MS and others: Guidelines for the initial management of adults with community-acquired pneumonia: diagnosis, assessment of severity, and initial antimicrobial therapy, *Am Rev Respir Dis* 148(5):1418-1426, 1993.

REFERENCES

1. American Thoracic Society: Guidelines for the management of adults with community-acquired pneumonia: diagnosis, assessment of severity, antimicrobial therapy and prevention, *Am J Respir Crit Care Med* 163:1730-1754, 2001.
2. Donowitz G, Mandell G: Acute pneumonia. In Mandell G, Bennett J, Dolin R, editors: *Principles and practice of infectious disease*, ed 5, New York, 1995, Churchill Livingstone.
3. Mandell L: Antibiotic therapy for community-acquired pneumonia, *Clin Chest* Med 20(3):589-598, 1999.
4. Bartlett J and others: Guidelines from the Infectious Disease Society of America: practice guidelines for the management of community-acquired pneumonia in adults, *Clin Infect Dis* 31:347-382, 2000.
5. Lieberman D: Atypical pathogens in community acquired pneumonia, *Clin Chest Med* 20(3):489-498, 1999.
6. Cunha B, Segreti J, Yaamauchi T: Community-acquired pneumonia: new bugs, new drugs, *Patient Care* 30(5):142-162, 1996.
7. Cunha B: Community-acquired pneumonia, *Med Clin North Am* 84(1):43-77, 2001.
8. Farber M: Managing community-acquired pneumonia, *Postgrad Med* 105(4):106-114, 1999.
9. Heffelfinger J and others: Management of community-acquired pneumonia in the era of pneumococcal resistance, *Arch Intern Med* 160:1399-1408, 2000.
10. Holten KB, Onusko EM: Appropriate prescribing of oral beta-lactam antibiotics, *Am Fam Physician* 62(3):611-620, 2000.
11. Gonzales R and others: Special report: CDC principles of judicious antibiotic use, *Ann Emerg Med* 37(6):690-702, 720-727, 2001.

WEBSITE RESOURCES

Alliance for the Prudent Use of Antibiotics. http://www.healthsci.tufts.edu/apua/apua.html

American Society for Microbiology. Retrieved August 12, 2002 from the World Wide Web: http://www.asm.org.

American Thoracic Society: Guidelines for the Management of Adults with Community Acquired-Pneumonia. Retrieved August 12, 2002 from the World Wide Web: http://www.thoracic.org.

Centers for Disease Control and Prevention: Active Bacterial Core Surveillance of the Emerging Infections Program Network. Retrieved August 12, 2002 from the World Wide Web: http://www.cdc.gov/ncidod/eid/vol7no1/schuchat.htm

Antmicrobial Resistance: Prevention Tools. Retrieved August 12, 2002 from the World Wide Web: http://www.cdc.gov/drugresistance/technical/prevention_tools.htm.

National Center for Infectious Diseases: A Public Health Action Plan to Combat Resistance. Retrieved August 12, 2002 from the World Wide Web: http://www.cdc.gov/drugresistance/.

FDA Center for Drug Evaluation and Research. Retrieved August 12, 2002 from the World Wide Web: http://www.fda.gov/cder/.

Infectious Disease Society of America: Practice Guidelines. Retrieved August 12, 2002 from the World Wide Web: http://www.idsociety.org/pg/toc/htm.

Johns Hopkins Division of Infectious Diseases Antibiotic Guide. Retrieved August 12, 2002 from the World Wide Web: http://www.hopkins-abxguide.org/.

CHAPTER 120

Pneumothorax

Susan Waldrop Donckers

DEFINITION/EPIDEMIOLOGY

Pneumothorax is defined as an accumulation of air in the pleural space. It is caused by a variety of conditions, including disease processes and trauma. The most common cause of primary spontaneous pneumothorax (PSP) is spontaneous rupture of subpleural blebs at the apex of the lungs in tall, thin, healthy men 30 to 40 years of age.[1] More than 90% of patients with PSP are smokers or ex-smokers. The incidence of spontaneous pneumothorax is 7.4 per 100,000 men and 1.2 per 100,000 women, for a total of 20,000 cases per year.[2] Secondary or complicated pneumothorax occurs in middle-aged adults and results from systemic lupus erythematosus, sarcoidosis, emphysema, asthma, cystic fibrosis, and other pulmonary diseases.[1-4] Both penetrating and nonpenetrating trauma can cause pneumothorax and may occur at any age. There also are numerous iatrogenic causes, including the insertion of central lines or barotrauma related to surgery or resuscitation efforts. There are reports in the literature of pneumothorax in pregnancy, labor, and the postpartum period. Approximately one half of pregnant women have a previous respiratory infection, asthma, or previous pneumothorax. The Valsalva maneuver that occurs with vomiting and in the second stage of labor may cause the rupture of unrecognized blebs.[5] The Valsalva maneuver to augment the "high" in those smoking marijuana or using cocaine has also been associated with the development of a pneumothorax as well as from needle sticks from "main lining" into neck veins. Several studies have described a familial incidence of PSP.[2]

Immediate emergency department referral/physician consultation is indicated for patients with respiratory compromise.

PATHOPHYSIOLOGY

The loss of negative pressure when air enters the pleural space causes the lung or a portion of it to collapse. Air in the pleural space may occur spontaneously or may be caused by trauma, a ruptured bleb, or gas generated by microorganisms in empyema.

CLINICAL PRESENTATION

Although some patients with pneumothorax may be asymptomatic, the most common complaint is an acute onset of dyspnea, pain, and cough. The pain is sharp and is exacerbated by any type of movement. The pertinent history should include current medications; allergies; history of strenuous exercise, smoking, or trauma; and other medical conditions.

PHYSICAL EXAMINATION

The physical findings depend on the size and nature of the pneumothorax. A tension or large pneumothorax is a medical emergency. Acute respiratory distress, diaphoresis, tachycardia, hypoxemia, tachypnea, tracheal deviation, cyanosis, neck vein distention, extreme anxiety, and impending cardiopulmonary arrest are unmistakable.[6] A smaller pneumothorax may cause dyspnea and discomfort, or the patient may be asymptomatic. Asymmetric chest excursion, absent breath sounds, and decreased tactile fremitus and hyperresonance on the affected side may be evident but depend on the size of the pneumothorax.

DIAGNOSTICS

Pulse oximetry should be determined. Chest x-ray studies, including anteroposterior and lateral views, are required. Expiratory or lateral decubitus films may be necessary to verify a small pneumothorax. A CT scan may be helpful in some cases.[5] Arterial blood gases, if available, should be obtained. Thoracoscopy also may be indicated.[3]

DIFFERENTIAL DIAGNOSIS

Dyspnea and chest pain are identified with a large number of clinical problems. A history of lung diseases (e.g., emphysema, cancer, or a rare condition such as Marfan's syndrome) is important to note. Many pneumothoraces occur as a result of trauma, and therefore rib fractures, contusions, costochondral separation, and muscle strains need to be excluded. Other differential diagnoses to consider include pulmonary embolism, myocardial infarction, dissecting aortic aneurysm, pleurisy, pericarditis, and costochondritis.

MANAGEMENT

A tension pneumothorax requires immediate intervention. To prevent fatality, a 16-gauge or larger-bore needle should be inserted into the pleural space at the midclavicular line of the second intercostal space on the affected side. Air is released immediately, but the needle must be left in place until a chest tube can be inserted.

No treatment is needed if the pneumothorax is small (<20% of the hemithorax) and the patient is asymptomatic. Spontaneous resolution occurs in 7 to 14 days.[7] Chest tube placement is vital in patients with symptoms; these patients should be referred for emergency care. The chest tube is left in place until the leak seals, which is usually 2 to 4 days. Ventilatory support is indicated in some cases.[1] Patients used to require a long hospital stay for pneumothorax

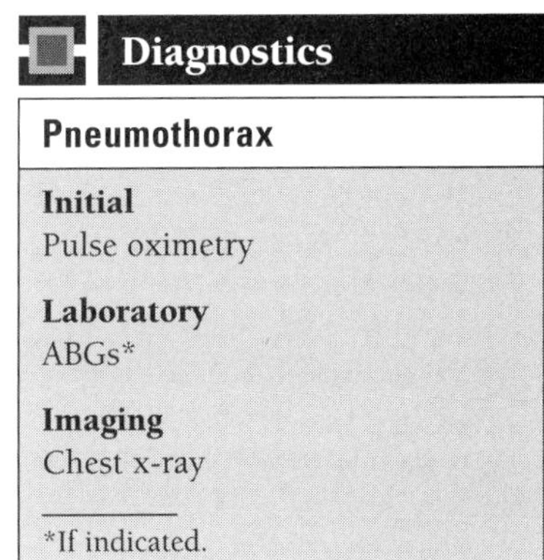

Diagnostics

Pneumothorax

Initial
Pulse oximetry

Laboratory
ABGs*

Imaging
Chest x-ray

*If indicated.

Differential Diagnosis

Pneumothorax

Lung disease
Trauma—blunt (contusion) or penetrating (fractured ribs)
Pulmonary embolism
Myocardial infarction
Pericarditis
Pleurisy
Muscle strain/costochondritis
Dissecting aortic aneurysm
Diaphragmatic hernia

treated with an indwelling chest tube. However, patients with chest tubes have recently been successfully managed on an outpatient basis. Options to prevent recurrences include the instillation of chemical agents such as talc, doxycycline, tetracycline, or minocycline through a chest tube or thorascope; laser therapy; pleural abrasion; or thoracotomy.[1]

LIFE SPAN CONSIDERATIONS

The frequency of reoccurrence is as high as 30%,[2] of which the complications may be more severe if there is concomitant respiratory or cardiac disease, especially chronic diseases that worsen with age. Efforts should be made to minimize and treat all possible exacerbating and complicating factors.

COMPLICATIONS

A large pneumothorax causes cardiac and ventilatory compromise, which may result in death. Numerous complications can arise from chest tube placement, including pulmonary edema, lung infarction, infection, trauma, bleeding, and subcutaneous emphysema.

INDICATIONS FOR REFERRAL/HOSPITALIZATION

A patient with a large pneumothorax requires hospitalization for chest tube placement and resolution. A pulmonologist may be consulted if the patient has underlying lung disease.

PATIENT AND FAMILY EDUCATION

Patient education should center on information regarding the cause, prevention, and treatment of a pneumothorax. Patients will also need education regarding the care of chest tubes. If genetic testing is performed, patients and families will need specific information and support.

Smoking cessation is an important educational issue with any lung problem and is an issue for patients with a pneumothorax, whatever the cause. If the patient has frequent, spontaneous recurrences, education regarding the importance of emergency care is necessary. Patients need to be cautioned against scuba diving and traveling to high altitudes.

HEALTH PROMOTION

Health promotion is aimed primarily at the elimination of smoking in those at risk and the prevention of trauma.

REFERENCES

1. Baum GL and others: Diseases of the pleura and pleural space. In Baum GL and others, editors: *Textbook of pulmonary diseases*, ed 6, Philadelphia, 1998, Lippincott-Raven.
2. Fraser RS and others: Pneumothorax. In Fraser RS and others: *Diagnosis of diseases of the chest*, ed 4, vol 4, Philadelphia, 1998, WB Saunders.
3. Baumann MH and others: Management of spontaneous pneumothorax: an American College of Chest Physicians Delphi consensus statement, *Chest* 119(25):590-600, 2001.
4. Sood N and others: Outcomes of intensive care unit care in adults with cystic fibrosis, *Am J Respir Crit Care Med* 163:335-338, 2001.
5. Wallach SL: Spontaneous pneumothorax, *N Engl J Med* 343(4):300-301, 2000.
6. Golden PA: Thoracic trauma, *Orthop Nurse* 19(5):37-46, 2000.
7. Richardson C, Baldwin D: Diagnosing acute shortness of breath in adult patients, *Practitioner* 244(5):478-482, 2000.

CHAPTER 121

Pulmonary Hypertension

Susan Waldrop Donckers

DEFINITION/EPIDEMIOLOGY

Pulmonary hypertension occurs when the pulmonary arterial pressure is inappropriately high for a given level of blood flow through the lungs.[1] The clinical definition is a pulmonary artery pressure of more than 25 mg Hg at rest or more than 30 mg Hg with exercise.[1,2]

Primary pulmonary hypertension (PPH) is a clinical syndrome of pulmonary hypertension that progresses rapidly to right ventricular failure and death.[1,2] The incidence of this process is small: 1 to 2 persons per 1 million worldwide.[2] PPH is generally considered to be a disease of younger people, with the greatest incidence between the ages of 20 and 45. PPH has been reported in older adults but is difficult to diagnosis because of the increased incidence of heart or lung diseases. In the PPH Patient Registry, the ratio of women to men is 7:1, regardless of age at diagnosis.[1]

A variety of factors have been associated with this progressive and usually fatal disease, including genetic predisposition, endothelial cell dysfunction, hypoxia, abnormalities in vasomotor control, thrombotic obliteration of vascular lumen, and vascular remodeling through cell proliferation and matrix production.[1-6] Reports describe the mean survival time of this complex process as less than 4 years.[7] Persons at risk for PPH include those with human immunodeficiency virus (HIV) infection, persons with a history of taking fenfluramine, persons with portal hypertension, and persons with a history of cocaine or IV drug abuse.[2] PPH is distinct from secondary pulmonary hypertension (SPH); in PPH no disease that causes a chronic increase in pulmonary artery pressure is clearly detectable.[2] SPH occurs as a complication of other disorders such as chronic bronchitis or chronic obstructive pulmonary disease (COPD).

PATHOPHYSIOLOGY

A number of different conditions cause pulmonary hypertension; however, basically pulmonary hypertension develops when flow or resistance to flow across the pulmonary vascular bed increases. Cardiac output increases three to fivefold during exercise, and the increased pulmonary blood flow raises the pulmonary artery (PA) pressure. In a healthy person the vasculature accommodates the increase in flow through the distention of vessels. The increase in flow during exercise is also temporary. However, with certain clinical conditions such as an atrial or a ventricular septal defect (ASD or VSD, respectively), the increase in flow is sustained, which leads to a thickening of the vessels. With the increase in blood flow and resistance, the pulmonary pressure rises.

Increases in blood viscosity and decreased vessel radius also increase vascular resistance. Causes include vessel destruction as in COPD, pulmonary fibrosis, resection, or pulmonary embolus.[8]

The most common cause of increased pulmonary vascular resistance associated with chronic respiratory disease is hypoxia, which causes vasoconstriction, thickening of the vascular media (remodeling), and polycythemia.[8] The mechanisms responsible for hypoxic pulmonary vasoconstriction remain undefined, even after years of intensive study.[8] The etiology of sustained pulmonary hypertension is multifactorial, regardless of the original insult.[1] The variety of pathologic changes has given rise to a variety of treatment modalities.[6-8]

CLINICAL PRESENTATION

Patients are generally asymptomatic until the condition becomes severe. Sixty percent of patients present with dyspnea. Other associated symptoms include fatigue, angina, syncope, cough, hemoptysis, Raynaud's phenomenon, edema, and decreased exercise tolerance. Symptoms are insidious, and the average time for the onset of symptoms and diagnosis is 2 years.[1]

PHYSICAL EXAMINATION

Physical findings initially may be subtle. Findings include a loud second heart sound (pulmonic component), decreased carotid pulse, evidence of right ventricular dilation (lifts or heaves), a murmur of tricuspid regurgitation, or pulmonic insufficiency. Signs of right ventricular failure with jugular vein distention, a loud S3 on inspiration, cor pulmonale, increased liver size, ascites, and edema are signs of advanced disease. Lung fields are generally clear.

DIAGNOSTICS

A variety of noninvasive and invasive studies are necessary to evaluate pulmonary hypertension. ECG changes include signs of right ventricular hypertrophy (an S wave in lead I and a Q wave and an inverted T wave in lead III may be the first changes; however, when seen, the condition is usually advanced). ECG changes suggestive of pulmonary embolism are the same as those in right ventricular hypertrophy and occur acutely. Chronic right ventricular pressure results in right-axis deviation and an R wave–to S–wave ratio of >1 in V_1.[1]

Chest x-ray examination may reveal pulmonary arteries that are increased in size. Although hypoxemia is a common finding, pulmonary function tests may demonstrate normal or only minimally restrictive elements. Arterial blood gases (ABGs), ventilation-perfusion (V/Q) studies (to rule out an embolus), Doppler studies, and echocardiography are helpful, as are radionuclear diagnostics and/or CT or MRI. A typical blood gas study will show hypoxia and respiratory alkalosis. In certain cases an open lung biopsy may be necessary to exclude interstitial lung disease.[1] Exercise studies may also be useful to evaluate response to treatment.[5] Pulmonary capillary wedge pressures are calculated during cardiac catheterization and are necessary for a definitive diagnosis. Serologic studies to screen for connective tissue diseases may also be indicated.[1]

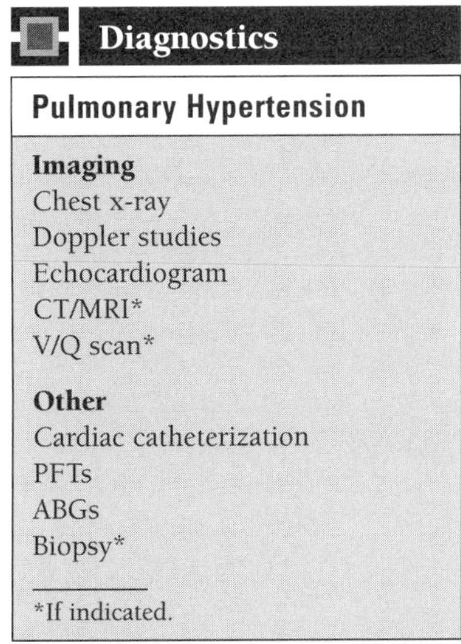

Diagnostics

Pulmonary Hypertension

Imaging
Chest x-ray
Doppler studies
Echocardiogram
CT/MRI*
V/Q scan*

Other
Cardiac catheterization
PFTs
ABGs
Biopsy*

*If indicated.

Differential Diagnosis

Pulmonary Hypertension

Restrictive lung disease	Pulmonary artery stenosis
Obstructive lung disease	Pulmonary venous hypertension
Granulomatous lung disease	Thromboembolic disease
Chronic liver disease	Parasitic infection
Congenital heart disease	IV drug use
Valvular heart disease	Connective tissue disease
Myocardial heart disease	

DIFFERENTIAL DIAGNOSIS

It is important to identify the underlying problem to ensure proper treatment. The differential diagnosis includes restrictive, obstructive, and granulomatous lung disease; chronic liver disease; congenital, valvular, and myocardial heart disease; pulmonary artery stenosis; pulmonary venous hypertension; and thromboembolic disease. Other etiologies to be considered include parasitic infection and IV drug use.

MANAGEMENT

Recognition of the disease process is important for appropriate cardiac or pulmonary referral, particularly if an acute event such as pulmonary embolus is suspected. Oxygen therapy, correction of acid-base balances, bronchodilation, treatment for emboli or mitral stenosis, antibiotics for infection, treatment for obstructive sleep apnea, and measures to improve left ventricular failure are all recommended.[1,4,8] In PPH, anticoagulation and high-dose calcium channel blockers (nifedipine 30 to 240 mg/day) may lower pulmonary resistance.[1,2,6-8] Recent studies have shown that long-term therapy with IV epoprostenol (prostacyclin) and sildenafil lowers pulmonary resistance, improves symptoms measurably, increases exercise capacity, and improves hemodynamic values.[2,6-8] Epoprostenol has antithrombic properties and is a potent vasodilator for both systemic and pulmonary arteries.[7,8] For some patients, a lung transplant may be an option.[7,8]

COMPLICATIONS

Complications of pulmonary hypertension include the development of right and eventually left ventricular hypertrophy and death. Other complications include arrhythmias, both bradycardia and tachycardia, acute pulmonary embolism, pulmonary hemorrhage, and pneumonia. Only 34% of patients survive more than 5 years.[1] Hospitalization may be necessary for medication adjustment, monitoring, and imaging.

INDICATIONS FOR REFERRAL/HOSPITALIZATION

Because accurate diagnosis is crucial, referral to an appropriate specialist is recommended. Imaging, cardiac catheterization, pulmonary function testing, medication recommendations, and lung transplantation all require specialist referral.

PATIENT AND FAMILY EDUCATION

Patients with pulmonary hypertension often require a tremendous amount of support from primary care providers. Careful explanation of the disease process and the need for moderation during activity is very important because exercise may increase pulmonary vascular resistance and hypoxia. The side effects and adverse reactions of all medications should be carefully explained and understood by both patients and families.[2]

For patients with end-stage pulmonary hypertension, lung transplantation may be an option, although the waiting list for organ transplants is often long. Transplantation criteria are dependent on age, past medical history, and the overall condition of the patient at the time of transplantation. The risk management and complications of transplantation should be thoroughly explained.[8]

The incidence of familial PPH is 6% of the 187 cases of PPH in the National Institutes of Health registry.[3] Although this is an uncommon form of pulmonary hypertension, families will need education and support if a genetic workup if chosen.

HEALTH PROMOTION

PPH is an uncommon disease process, occurring in approximately 1 to 2 per 1 million persons worldwide. The exact mechanisms of the disease are still undergoing study; however, the clinical course is deadly. Until recently patients and families had little hope for remission of this progressive disease.[2] Because secondary pulmonary hypertension occurs as a complication of other disorders, such as COPD, sleep apnea, sickle cell crisis, connective tissue diseases, cardiac diseases, thromboembolism, and others, these are the disease processes that must be monitored for the onset of complications. Lung diseases are the most common causes of pulmonary hypertension, so the prevention of lung disease is a major challenge[2]; one of the major preventive measures for eliminating lung disease would be the prevention of smoking.

REFERENCES

1. Rounds S, Cutaia MV: Pulmonary hypertension: pathophysiology and clinical disorders. In Baum GL and others, editors: *Textbook of pulmonary medicine*, ed 6, Philadelphia, 1998, Lippincott-Raven.
2. Cheever KH and others: Epoprostenol therapy for primary pulmonary hypertension, *Crit Care Nurse* 19(4):20-27, 1999.
3. Loscalzo J: Genetic clues to the cause of primary pulmonary hypertension, *N Engl J Med* 345(5):367-368, 2001.
4. Kessler R and others: The obesity-hypoventilation syndrome revisited, *Chest* 120(2):369-376, 2001.
5. Sun XG and others: Exercise pathophysiology in patients with primary pulmonary hypertension, *Circulation* 24(104):429-435, 2001.
6. Zhao L and others: Sildenafil inhibits hypoxia-induced pulmonary hypertension, *Circulation* 104(4):424-428, 2001.
7. Rich S: Medical treatment of pulmonary hypertension: a bridge to transplantation? *Am J Cardiol* 75:63A-66A, 1995.
8. Russo-Magno PM, Hill NS: New approaches to pulmonary hypertension, *Hosp Pract* 36(3):29-32, 37-40, 2001.

Sarcoidosis

Updated by Patricia Polgar Bailey

DEFINITION/EPIDEMIOLOGY

Sarcoidosis is a multisystem, granulomatous disease of unknown origin that commonly affects young and middle-aged adults. It involves the lungs and intrathoracic lymph nodes in more than 90% of affected patients, but it may essentially affect any organ. Other commonly involved sites include the skin, eyes, liver, spleen, myocardium, central nervous system, kidney, and bone. More than 80% of patients are between 20 and 45 years of age; the disease is rare in children and older adults. The incidence may vary with geographic location. In Europe, the United Kingdom, Japan, and North America, incidence rates of 10 to 20 per 100,000 population have been cited. Sarcoidosis appears to be rare in Africa and in Central and South America. No clear genetic basis has been established for sarcoidosis, but genetic factors may modulate its evolution and expression.[1] Sarcoidosis is approximately eight times more common in African-Americans and is slightly more common in females; sporadic cases have been described in families.

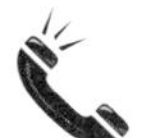

Physician consultation is indicated for all suspected cases of sarcoidosis.

PATHOPHYSIOLOGY

The characteristic pathologic feature of sarcoidosis is the noncaseating granuloma. The collection of macrophages that compose the granuloma does not show evidence of frank necrosis or caseation, as would be seen with tuberculosis or histoplasmosis.

The initial cutaneous anergy observed in sarcoidosis seems to be caused by the nonavailability of lymphocytes. Lymphopenia is a prominent feature. The helper-suppressor T-cell ratio is reduced in the peripheral blood but increased at the site of granulomatous inflammation. The helper T-lymphocytes fight the inflammation and leave inadequate numbers in the peripheral blood to elicit a cutaneous reaction. Although the initial antigen is unknown, the alveolitis begins the accumulation of helper T-lymphocyte (CD4) cells and macrophages. It is believed that activated macrophages may be responsible for the eventual development of fibrosis in some patients with sarcoidosis.

In the lung, granulomatous inflammation and fibrosis result in ventilation-perfusion imbalance and widening of the alveolar-arterial oxygen gradient. In the early stages, PaO_2 may be within the normal range at rest but decreases with exertion.

CLINICAL PRESENTATION AND PHYSICAL EXAMINATION

Sarcoidosis may affect almost any organ system and may appear in acute, subacute, or chronic form. Sarcoidosis typically presents asymptomatically with an abnormal chest radiograph.[2]

Approximately one third of patients with this disorder have nonspecific features—fever, fatigue, anorexia, weight loss, and, occasionally, chills and night sweats. The symptoms and related organ involvement consistent with sarcoidosis are found in Table 122-1. Involvement of the upper airways and posterior pharynx may result in upper airway obstruction with worsening symptoms of dyspnea. Hoarseness and nasal obstruction may occur as a result of vocal cord and nasal mucosa granulomas (polyps). Hemoptysis is rarely seen; when present, it suggests the presence of mycetoma.

It is unusual to detect adventitious lung sounds on auscultation. Wheezing is occasionally audible in patients with advanced disease. Digital clubbing and hemoptysis are rare. Dyspnea, dry cough, and chest pain occur commonly. Chest pain can be severe and difficult to distinguish from cardiac chest pain.[3]

Joint pain without deformity is present in 25% to 90% of patients with sarcoidosis. Ocular lesion are often seen, especially uveitis. Clinical involvement of the central nervous system is unusual, but cranial nerve involvement can be seen. Asymptomatic granulomas can occur in any part of the female reproductive system, including the breast. Skin lesions that are seen include erythema nodosum and lupus pernio.[3]

DIAGNOSTICS

Chest radiographs are abnormal in more than 90% of patients.[4] In general, one of the following patterns is demonstrated: (1) bilateral hilar lymphadenopathy (50% to 80% of cases), (2) parenchymal interstitial infiltrates (25% to 50%) with a predilection for upper- and mid-lung field distribution, and (3) both lymphadenopathy and interstitial disease. Bilateral hilar lymphadenopathy (BHL) is often the lesion that suggests the diagnosis of sarcoidosis.

Unless lymphadenopathy is present, the appearance of the chest radiograph may be indistinguishable from other interstitial lung disorders. Typically, radiographic lesions are bilateral and are distributed relatively symmetrically; asymmetric involvement is occasionally seen.

TABLE 122-1 Clinical Features of Sarcoidosis

Organ System	Symptoms or Presentation
Pulmonary	Dyspnea, cough, wheezing, chest pain
Upper airway	Dyspnea, nasal congestion, hoarseness, stridor, polyps
Dermatologic	Nodules, papules, plaques
Ocular	Photophobia, tearing, pain, decreased visual acuity, lacrimal gland enlargement, uveitis
Rheumatologic	Polyarthropathy, monoarthropathy, myopathy
Neurologic	Headache, hearing loss, paresthesias, seizures, cranial nerve palsy
Cardiologic	Syncope, dyspnea, arrhythmias, congestive heart failure, cardiac tamponade
Gastrointestinal	Dysphagia, abdominal pain, jaundice, hepatomegaly
Hematologic	Lymph node enlargement, hypersplenism
Renal	Kidney failure, calculi

Staging systems based on the appearance of the chest radiograph have been in widespread use since 1957. The consensus now favors the following classification[3]:

- Stage 0: Normal chest radiograph
- Stage 1: Bilateral hilar lymphadenopathy (BHL)
- Stage 2: BHL with pulmonary infiltrates
- Stage 3: Pulmonary infiltrates without BHL
- Stage 4: Pulmonary fibrosis

CT and high-resolution computed tomography (HRCT) of the chest are superior to a conventional chest x-ray study in defining the extent of parenchymal abnormalities in sarcoidosis. HRCT can help differentiate between reversible (mostly inflammatory) changes and irreversible (presumably fibrotic) alterations.

Hypergammaglobulinemia is seen in more than 30% of cases of sarcoidosis. Even when the serum gamma globulin level is not high in the active phase, it is often higher than during regression of sarcoidosis. The level of serum angiotensin-converting enzyme (ACE) is elevated in approximately 60% of patients with sarcoidosis; this level may be useful in following the course of the disease. Anemia occurs in 4% to 20% of patients.[3] Hypercalcemia and hypercalciuria occasionally occur secondary to increased gastrointestinal absorption, abnormal vitamin D metabolism, and increased calcitriol production by sarcoid granulomas. Skin testing often reveals cutaneous anergy.

Pulmonary function tests (PFTs) may be normal or may reveal a restrictive pattern. Radionuclide scanning reveals high uptake of gallium-67 in pulmonary lesions of sarcoidosis. However, ^{67}Ga is also taken up by the lungs in patients with a large number of other diseases; therefore a high level of ^{67}Ga is not specific for sarcoidosis.

It is often reassuring to have a tissue diagnosis, and there are many techniques for this. The most specific location to biopsy for diagnosis is the lung. Bronchoscopy with transbronchial biopsies are positive in 50% to 60% of patients who do not have radiographic evidence of parenchymal disease. This positivity increases to 85% to 90% when there are radiographic abnormalities. A bronchoalveolar lavage performed at the time of fiberoptic bronchoscopy retrieves inflammatory and immune effector cells from the lower respiratory tract that

Diagnostics

Sarcoidosis

Laboratory
- CBC and differential
- Electrolytes
- Glucose
- BUN
- Creatinine
- Calcium
- Phosphorus
- LFTs
- Erythrocyte sedimentation rate
- Serum gamma globulin
- Serum ACE

Imaging
- Chest x-ray
- CT scan

Other
- PFTs
- Bronchoscopy
- Purified protein derivative

can also be diagnostic. Biopsies can also be taken from other organ systems suspected to involve sarcoid (conjunctivae, skin, lymph nodes).

DIFFERENTIAL DIAGNOSIS

Many conditions can present with dyspnea, diffuse pulmonary infiltration, and granulomas. Hypersensitivity pneumonitis, asbestosis, silicosis, drug effects, bacterial or fungal infections, and malignancies should all be considered.

MANAGEMENT

Hospitalization is rarely needed during the diagnostic or treatment phases of sarcoidosis. No treatment is recommended for asymptomatic patients with stage 1 sarcoidosis. Those with fever or joint pains often respond to nonsteroidal antiinflammatory drugs (NSAIDs). Low-dose prednisone 15 to 20 mg/day may occasionally be needed to control symptoms that do not respond to NSAIDs. If symptoms of dyspnea or a cough develop, airway obstruction may be present, and corticosteroid therapy is advisable. In some cases inhaled corticosteroids may be effective.[2]

Patients with stage 2 disease who are symptomatic are treated with corticosteroids. Only observation is suggested for patients who are asymptomatic and have only mild impairment of lung function; treatment is needed for individuals who have progressive impairment of lung function. Patients with stage 3 or 4 sarcoidosis almost always require treatment with corticosteroids or another type of immunosuppressive treatment, but this is often unsatisfying. Lung transplantation may eventually be required in some of these patients.

Sarcoidosis is very sensitive to corticosteroids. Typical regimens consist of a single daily dose of 20 to 40 mg of prednisone, which is gradually tapered over 6 months.[3] Some patients require a maintenance dose of prednisone of approximately 10 to 15 mg/day, whereas others remain off prednisone indefinitely or for extended periods.

Methotrexate and azathioprine are other treatment options for patients who either develop severe side effects or do not respond to prednisone.[3,5] The use of these agents is clearly valuable for selected patients, but there are no controlled studies of indications for use or efficacy. These agents along with antimalarial agents, including chloroquine and hydroxychloroquine, are also often used as the initial drug of choice in the treatment of chronic skin lesions from sarcoidosis. More studies are required before recommending these drugs as part of the routine therapy for sarcoidosis.

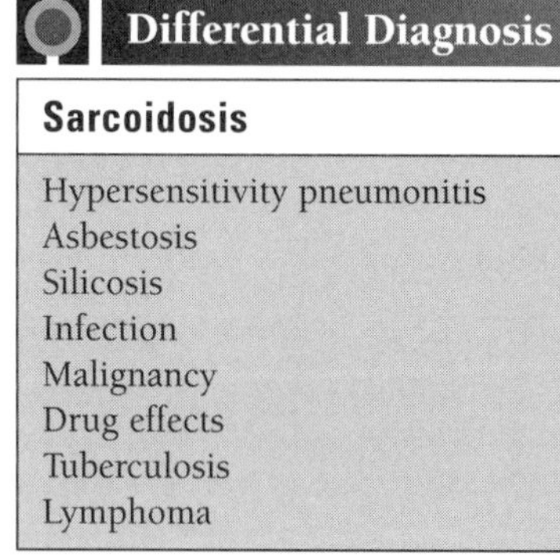

Differential Diagnosis

Sarcoidosis

Hypersensitivity pneumonitis
Asbestosis
Silicosis
Infection
Malignancy
Drug effects
Tuberculosis
Lymphoma

LIFE SPAN CONSIDERATIONS

Sarcoidosis does not affect pregnancy but may flare after delivery. Sarcoidosis in children younger than age 15 showed the same organ distribution as in adults. The prognosis for children seems better than that for adults.[3]

COMPLICATIONS

Most complications of sarcoidosis occur as a result of corticosteroid therapy and include osteoporosis, hyperglycemia, and gastric ulcers. Relapses are common and are determined by the reappearance of clinical signs and symptoms, chest radiograph abnormalities, and an elevated ACE level. In this situation, a return to a previously high maintenance dose is sufficient to control recurrence.

INDICATIONS FOR REFERRAL/HOSPITALIZATION

Sarcoidosis is a serious multisystem disease that requires physician consultation. Lung biopsies are usually necessary for diagnosis and require referral to a pulmonary specialist. If other biopsies are indicated, the appropriate specialist should be consulted. Therapy during the acute and chronic phases should be directed by the physician or specialist to ensure proper treatment. Hospitalization may be necessary for severe dyspnea and hypoxia or for severe cardiac dysfunction.

PATIENT AND FAMILY EDUCATION

The nature of the disease, including its varied presentation, must be carefully explained to patients. Medications, if indicated, and their side effects need to be discussed. It is very important that patients understand the risk for worsening lung impairment or other organ damage if compliance with therapy is poor. It is important that patients be familiar with the clinical signs suggestive of possible recurrence of sarcoidosis.

REFERENCES

1. Sharma OP, Badr A: Sarcoidosis: diagnosis, staging, and role of newer diagnostic modalities, *Clin Pulm Med* 1(1):18, 1994.
2. Sharma OP: Pulmonary sarcoidosis and corticosteroids, *Am Rev Respir Dis* 147(6 pt 1):1598-1600, 1993.
3. American Thoracic Society: Statement on sarcoidosis, *Am J Respir Crit Care Med* 160:736-755, 1999.
4. Lynch JP III, Strieter RM: Sarcoidosis. In Lichetenstein LM, Fauci AS, editors: *Current therapy in allergy, immunology, and rheumatology*, Philadelphia, 1992, BC Decker.
5. Lower EE, Baughman RP: Two years of methotrexate therapy in sarcoidosis: efficacy and toxicity, *Sarcoidosis* 11(suppl 1):331, 1994.

CHAPTER 123

Sleep Apnea

Updated by Joanne Sandberg-Cook

DEFINITION/EPIDEMIOLOGY

Sleep apnea is a serious disorder with potentially life-threatening complications. It is often characterized by collapse of the upper airway while sleeping, resulting in breathing cessation. Apneic periods lasting at least 10 seconds and as long as 2 to 3 minutes may be experienced. Sleep apnea is diagnosed when apneic periods occur five or more times per hour and the patient has daytime hypersomnolence.[1]

There are two predominant forms of this disturbance. Central sleep apnea (CSA) occurs with poor ventilatory drive and results in an absence of airflow. Obstructive sleep apnea (OSA), the more common form, occurs with intermittent closure of the upper airway.[2] This results in decreased or absent airflow despite persistent ventilatory effort.[3] Mixed apnea is a combination of both CSA and OSA.

Sleep apnea affects the quality of life. Fatigue, excessive sleepiness, morning headaches, memory and judgment problems, irritability, and difficulty concentrating are often reported.[4,5] These symptoms may result in depression.[6] In addition, several studies indicate that daytime hypersomnolence resulting from OSA increases the risk for automobile and work-related accidents.[5-8] It has been estimated that the loss of productivity in the United States is more than $20 billion annually.[7]

Sleep apnea is considered a common condition among adults. CSA is rare and occurs most often in infants or individuals over age 65.[9] This may be a result of a major cerebral disease, brainstem or spinal disorder, or cardiovascular disease. OSA is considered a common cause of breathing difficulties. A prevalence of sleep apnea in 2% of women and 4% of men has been reported.[1] Risk factors for OSA include male gender, obesity, older age, and craniofacial anomalies.[4-6] More recently, menopausal status and ethnic origin have been found to put people at risk for sleep apnea.[2] African-Americans develop this condition more often and at a younger age than do whites.[2]

PATHOPHYSIOLOGY

The signs and symptoms of OSA are attributed to the narrowing and collapse of the upper airway. This usually occurs at the oropharynx, but it can occur anywhere from the soft palate to above the epiglottis. Relaxation of the upper airway muscles and partial airway obstruction result in loud snoring. With complete obstruction, breathing stops for a period of 10 seconds to more than 1 minute.[6] A struggle to breathe and severe hypoxia occur during this period. A brief arousal with loud snoring follows after the airway is reopened. A short period of hyperventilation rapidly corrects the hypoxemia. As the number of apneic events increases, the severity of symptoms and their sequelae intensify.

CLINICAL PRESENTATION

Snoring is one of the most common symptoms associated with OSA. Patients are often unaware of this problem or its severity; thus it is beneficial to interview the patient's bed partner to determine the pattern of snoring and breathing.[4] Intermittent loud snoring with periods of silence longer than 10 seconds may indicate sleep apnea. Patients with CSA do not complain about snoring but often are concerned about insomnia, morning fatigue, and daytime hypersomnolence.

Another major indicator for OSA is daytime hypersomnolence. This may be assessed using the Epworth Sleepiness Scale.[9] With this tool, the tendency to fall asleep is correlated with a variety of daytime activities (Box 123-1). Occasionally this assessment tool may not portray an accurate degree of sleepiness. Some patients may deny that they have this difficulty; therefore confirmation with family members is often helpful.

Patients with OSA may report a variety of other complaints, including nocturnal arousals with or without choking spells, nocturnal diaphoresis, abnormal motor activity during sleep, enuresis, gastroesophageal reflux, headaches, chest pain, diminished libido, impotence, loss of memory and concentration, personality changes, and depression.[1,3-5] Pertinent history should include smoking, caffeine, and alcohol habits; current medications; and co-morbid illnesses.

PHYSICAL EXAMINATION

The physical examination is often unremarkable. Positive findings periodically reveal obesity and a short, thickened neck. A neck circumference of more than 43 cm for men or more than 40 cm for women is a positive finding in some patients with OSA.[5] Reddened pharyngeal mucosa with a thick, soft palate and marked tonsillar hypertrophy are other indicators of this condition.[10] Patients with acromegaly or neurologic or cardiac disorders will demonstrate abnormal changes associated with these disorders.

DIAGNOSTICS

Methods for OSA screening continue to be controversial. Polysomnography is often considered the primary diagnostic test to establish a definitive diagnosis. Measurements obtained include sleep staging, airflow, ventilatory effort, arterial oxygen saturation, ECG, body position, and limb movements.[1] This requires an overnight stay in a sleep laboratory, where a sleep technician is constantly available to monitor the study and may be able to initiate treatment with nasal continuous positive airway pressure (CPAP) during the first night of study.

Home monitors are available for determining airflow, ventilatory effort, heart rate, oxygen saturation, and sleep parameters. The benefits of home monitoring include increased comfort and decreased costs. However, because home monitoring is done without the assistance of a technician to monitor equipment, data may be less accurate than that generated in a sleep laboratory. If home monitoring results are negative, a full sleep study in a sleep laboratory should be conducted. Disadvantages arise with equipment difficulties and lack of monitoring sensitivity and specificity. The severity of symptoms should determine the priority for how OSA is diagnosed.

DIFFERENTIAL DIAGNOSIS

Daytime hypersomnolence and snoring can occur for a variety of reasons. The most common causes of daytime hypersomnolence are insufficient sleep and insomnia. A decrease in daily caffeine consumption may also cause this symptom. Narcolepsy, restless leg syndrome, idiopathic hypersomnolence, use of alcohol or sedatives, endocrine disorders (hypothyroidism, Addison's disease, hypothalamic disease), chronic obstructive pulmonary disease (COPD), congestive heart failure (CHF), asthma, gastroesophageal reflux disease (GERD), and panic attacks are possible etiologies to consider.[4] Narrowed upper airways may cause the patient to snore. This may result from nasal deviation or polyps, tonsillar hypertrophy, acromegaly, micrognathia, Shy-Drager syndrome, or myotonic dystrophy.[11]

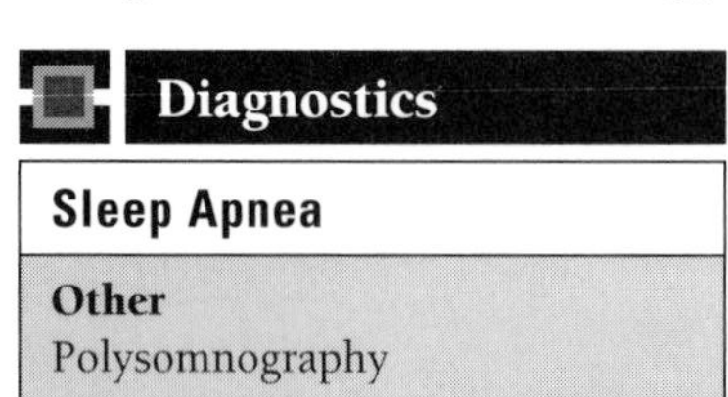
Diagnostics

Sleep Apnea

Other
Polysomnography

Differential Diagnosis

Sleep Apnea

Asthma	Restless leg syndrome
Chronic obstructive pulmonary disease	Idiopathic hypersomnolence
Congestive heart failure	Alcohol
Gastroesophageal reflux disease	Sedatives
Hypersomnolence caused by	Endocrine disorders
Decreased caffeine consumption	Hypothyroidism
Insomnia	Addison's disease
Insufficient sleep	Hypothalamic disease
Panic attacks	Nasal polyps or deviation
Narcolepsy	Tonsillar hypertrophy
	Acromegaly
	Micrognathia

MANAGEMENT

Treatment should be individualized to the symptoms, especially when daytime hypersomnolence presents. The severity of the sleep disorder should not be the only factor considered when determining patient management.

Behavioral approaches may be considered for some patients with OSA. Weight loss (diet and exercise), elimination of alcohol in the evening, and avoidance of the supine position in bed may be beneficial.[1,4,7,8]

For moderate to severe cases of OSA, nasal CPAP is the preferred treatment. A mask is fitted over the nose, and tubing from the mask is connected to a machine that forces air through the nasal passages. This restores unobstructed breathing by maintaining the patency of narrowed, collapsible upper airways. The initial pressure level is usually set at 4 to 5 cm H_2O. This may be titrated up to 20 cm H_2O, if necessary, to restore regular breathing. Absolute contraindications to CPAP include floppy epiglottis and skull fracture.[8] A bilevel positive airway pressure (BiPAP) unit, in which inspiratory and expiratory pressures vary, may allow for better comfort, especially for those unable to tolerate higher CPAPs.[12]

Strategies to increase patient adherence with this intervention are important considerations. Careful mask fit and pressure adjustments increase comfort. Decongestants are beneficial for nasal congestion. Adding moisture to the forced air will provide humidity and decrease mucosal membrane dryness.

Pharmacologic therapy occasionally provides more restful sleep, especially if patients are having trouble adjusting to nasal CPAP. A trial of low-dose benzodiazepines, such as lorazepam 0.5 mg h.s. or low-dose selective serotonin reuptake inhibitors (SSRIs) may improve sleep quality. Protriptyline 5 to

BOX 123-1

EPWORTH SLEEPINESS SCALE

Name ______________________ Age ______
Date ______________________ Sex ______

How likely are you to doze off or fall asleep in the following situations, in contrast to feeling just tired? This refers to your usual way of life in recent times. Even if you have not done some of these things recently, try to work out how they would have affected you.

Use the following scale to choose the most appropriate number for each situation:

0 = Would never doze
1 = Slight chance of dozing
2 = Moderate chance of dozing
3 = High chance of dozing

SITUATION	CHANCE OF DOZING
Sitting and reading	______
Watching TV	______
Sitting inactive in a public place (e.g., a theater or a meeting)	______
As a passenger in a car for an hour without a break	______
Lying down to rest in the afternoon when circumstances permit	______
Sitting and talking to someone	______
Sitting quietly after a lunch without alcohol	______
In a car, while stopped for a few minutes in traffic	______
	Total ______

From Johns MW: A new method for measuring daytime sleepiness: the Epworth Sleepiness Scale, *Sleep* 14:540-545, 1991.

10 mg h.s. may also act as a mild appetite suppressant and assist with weight reduction.[4,10] Evaluation of the effectiveness of the medication, along with the potential side effects of dry mouth and constipation, should be assessed.

Oral/dental devices are often considered, especially for patients with abnormal facial structures or patients who do not tolerate nasal CPAP. When directly compared with CPAP, oral appliances are preferred and therefore should be considered in those who have refused CPAP or for whom CPAP has failed.[12] Mandibular advancement devices move the jaw forward, which enlarges the retroglossal air space and reduces upper airway resistance.[5]

Uvulopalatopharyngoplasty (UPPP), which is the resection of redundant pharyngeal tissue, is considered only after medical treatment fails.[1,5,6] Unfortunately, the success rate, as measured in the number of apneic episodes per hour, is <50%.[12] For severe OSA, tracheostomy allows adequate oxygenation and sleep comfort.

Central apnea is sometimes treated with nasal CPAP. This may prevent hypoxia and bradyarrhythmias. Patients with significant lung disease often benefit from oxygen supplementation.

LIFE SPAN CONSIDERATIONS

Adenotonsillar hypertrophy accounts for most cases of sleep apnea in children and can lead to poor school performance. In older adults, relaxation of the pharyngeal musculature is thought to contribute to increased incidence. However, a survivor effect might exist in very old adults, with many middle-aged patients not surviving to old age.[12] More reports of an increased incidence of sleep apnea in postmenopausal women are emerging.[12]

COMPLICATIONS

Cardiovascular and pulmonary complications are potential consequences of OSA. Apnea-induced hypoxia results in systemic vasoconstriction, causing increased blood pressure. Hypertension has been reported in 50% to 60% of patients with OSA.[6,12] Arrhythmias, myocardial ischemia, and myocardial infarction are possible in patients with OSA and coronary heart disease.[1] OSA markedly aggravates left ventricular failure in patients with underlying heart disease.[4] Pulmonary hypertension and, in severe cases, cor pulmonale may result from severe OSA. OSA can also exacerbate other medical conditions, which can lead to a premature death. Complications can also include automobile and work-related accidents that result from daytime hypersomnolence.

INDICATIONS FOR REFERRAL/HOSPITALIZATION

Because complications are a concern, a supervising physician is often consulted to assist with the management of patients with OSA. A referral to a sleep specialist is usually indicated before a formal sleep study is conducted. The study should be analyzed, and recommendations made by the consultant. An otolaryngologic consultation is necessary if surgery is being considered to correct upper airway anatomy.

There is a substantial mortality and morbidity risk for patients with OSA. Critically ill patients may have cardiopulmonary failure and require intensive care. Pulmonary hypertension, right ventricular failure, polycythemia, and chronic hypercapnia and hypoxemia may develop in a large percentage of patients with this disorder[1,5,6]; this is often referred to as the pickwickian syndrome. With increased respiratory difficulties, hospitalization is often required.

PATIENT AND FAMILY EDUCATION

A discussion of how sleep apnea occurs, including anatomy of the upper airway, may increase the patient's understanding of this disorder and enhance adherence to treatment. Lifestyle changes, including diet and exercise for weight loss, are important topics for the practitioner to review. Substances known to potentially aggravate sleep should be avoided, including alcohol and muscle relaxants. If sedatives are prescribed, the potential side effects should be reviewed, and patients should understand when to contact the primary care provider. Patients should also understand that sleeping on the side rather than on the back might be beneficial. Sleep practice issues should be discussed. These include having a consistent sleep time, reserving the bed for sleep and sexual intercourse, and minimizing noise, light, and temperature extremes.[10] Patients should also be advised about the possible hazards of driving. Education of the patient and bed partner about the benefits of treatment and proper use of nasal CPAP is essential.

REFERENCES

1. Young T and others: The occurrence of sleep disordered breathing among middle-aged adults, *N Engl J Med* 328:1230-1235, 1993.
2. Malhotra A, White DP. Obstructive sleep apnea, *Lancet* 360: 237-245, 2002.
3. Chaska B and others: Sleep apnea: is your patient at risk? National Heart, Lung and Blood Institute Working Group on Sleep Apnea, *Am Fam Physician* 53(1):247-253, 1996.
4. Man GC: Obstructive sleep apnea: diagnosis and treatment, *Med Clin North Am* 80(4):803-820, 1996.
5. Stradling JR: *Respiratory problems during sleep,* Priory Lodge Education Limited, Version 1.0, April 1997, Oxford, England.
6. Noureddine SN: Sleep apnea: a challenge in critical care, *Heart Lung* 25(1):37-44, 1996.
7. Riley RW and others: Obstructive sleep apnea: trends in therapy, *West J Med* 162:143-148, 1995.
8. Baumel MJ, Maislin G, Pack AI: Population and occupational screening for obstructive sleep apnea: are we there yet? *Am J Respir Crit Care Med* 155:9-14, 1997.
9. Johns MW: A new method for measuring daytime sleepiness: the Epworth Sleepiness Scale, *Sleep* 14:540-545, 1991.
10. Neubauer DN, Smith PL, Early CJ: Sleep disorders. In Barker LR, Burton JR, Zieve PD, editors: *Principles of ambulatory medicine,* ed 4, Baltimore, 1995, Williams & Wilkins.
11. Polo O and others: Management of obstructive sleep apnoea/hypopnoea syndrome, *Lancet* 344:656-660, 1994.
12. Lavie P, Here P, Hoffstein V : Obstructive sleep apnoea syndrome as a risk factor for hypertension: population study, *Br Med J* 320:479-482, 2000.

CHAPTER 124

Tuberculosis

Patricia Polgar Bailey

DEFINITION/EPIDEMIOLOGY

Tuberculosis (TB) is an airborne infectious disease caused by *Mycobacterium tuberculosis*, an "acid-fast" aerobic bacterium that is capable of remaining alive outside the host for a relatively long time. In the United States, the vast majority of TB cases are caused by *M. tuberculosis*, also referred to as the *tubercle bacillus*. However, several closely related mycobacteria can cause disease in humans, including *M. bovis*, the cause of TB in cattle; *M. avium*, one of the causes of TB in birds; and *M. africanum*. TB caused by these organisms was relatively rare in the United States until they were identified as the cause of opportunistic infections in patients infected with human immunodeficiency virus (HIV). *M. microti*, another mycobacterium, does not cause TB in humans.[1]

TB has reemerged as one of the most pressing public health problems in the United States and throughout the world. In 1993, the World Health Organization (WHO) declared TB to be a "global health emergency," and a 1995 report identified it as the leading single-infection killer of adults. Approximately 90 million new cases will have occurred worldwide during the 1990s, with approximately 95% of those cases occurring in developing countries, particularly sub-Saharan Africa and Southeast Asia.[2]

During the mid-twentieth century the United States benefited from relatively successful control of TB. From 1953 to 1985, the reported cases of TB in the United States dropped from 84,000 cases to 22,000 cases. Since 1985 that decline has reversed; by 1993 there had been a 14% increase in TB cases.[1] In some U.S. cities, including New York, Miami, and Los Angeles, the incidence of TB has more than doubled during this time period.[2] Historically, TB in the United States has been a disease that affects primarily older adults; increasingly, younger adults and children are being affected. Minority populations are disproportionately affected by TB, with more than two thirds of reported TB cases occurring among nonwhite racial and ethnic groups.[3]

Many factors have contributed to the increased incidence of TB, including the HIV epidemic and higher rates of poverty, homelessness, incarceration, and drug use. An increasing number of immigrants, many of whom live in crowded housing and have inadequate health care, and an increased number of residents in long-term care facilities have also contributed to this public health problem. Deterioration in the health care infrastructure and reductions in TB outreach programs, which historically improved compliance with treatment regimens, have also contributed to the resurgence of TB.

In addition to the increasing incidence of TB, a serious concern is the recent emergence of drug-resistant strains. In 1991 in New York City (one of the U.S. cities with the highest incidence of TB), 33% of TB cases were resistant to at least one antitubercular drug, and 19% were resistant to both isoniazid (INH) and rifampin (RIF)—the two most effective drugs for the treatment of TB. Multidrug resistance to TB significantly increases the cost and duration of treatment while decreasing the efficacy of therapy.[4]

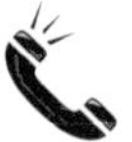

Physician consultation is recommended for any patient suspected of having pulmonary or extrapulmonary TB.

PATHOPHYSIOLOGY

TB is spread primarily through direct infection (person-to-person), but it can also be spread indirectly via the airborne transmission of the tubercle bacilli, which can remain suspended in the air for several hours. Transmission, which may occur if these bacilli-laden sputum droplets (each containing one to three organisms) are inhaled, depends on three factors: the infectiousness of the person with TB, the environment in which the exposure occurred, and the duration of exposure.[1] Although theoretically one organism implanted in the alveolus can initiate this process, 5 to 200 organisms are usually required.[5] Most of the larger inhaled particles become lodged in the upper respiratory tract, where infection is unlikely to take place. Infection begins if the droplet nuclei reach the alveolar macrophage and multiplication of the tubercle bacilli is initiated. A small number of mycobacteria spread through the lymph system to regional lymph nodes and via the bloodstream to more distant tissues and organs, including areas in which TB is more likely to develop, such as the apices of the lung, the kidneys, the brain, and the bone. Eighty-five percent of all TB cases involve the lungs; other common sites include the pleura, central nervous system (CNS), lymphatic system, genitourinary system, and bones and joints. TB can also become disseminated and then is referred to as *miliary TB*.

There are two distinct epidemiologic patterns of TB disease. Reactivation, or postprimary, disease is the most common clinical form of TB. Most symptomatic cases of TB arise in persons with a history of TB infection who were inadequately treated or were not treated. The second epidemiologic profile is referred to as primary infection, which does not usually present as a symptomatic infection except in persons infected with HIV. More than 90% of persons with primary infection are entirely asymptomatic, and infection with TB is identified only by a positive reaction to a tuberculin skin test.

Certain medical conditions increase the risk that TB infection will progress to active disease. The risk may be three times greater (as with coexistent diabetes mellitus) to 100 times greater (as with HIV infection) for persons who have these conditions compared with those who do not.[1] Medical conditions that increase the risk of active TB are listed in Box 124-1.

CLINICAL PRESENTATION

Persons who have been infected with *M. tuberculosis* but do not have active disease are completely asymptomatic. There is no evidence of infection, and there is no clinical or radiographic evidence of TB.

Symptoms of pulmonary TB (the most common site) include fatigue, anorexia, weight loss, night sweats, cough, chest

BOX 124-1

CONDITIONS THAT INCREASE THE RISK OF ACTIVE TUBERCULOSIS

- HIV infection
- Recent infection with *M. tuberculosis* (within the past 2 years)
- Chest radiograph findings suggestive of previous TB (in a person who receives inadequate or no treatment)
- Diabetes mellitus
- Silicosis
- Substance abuse (notably drug injection)
- Prolonged corticosteroid therapy
- Other immunosuppressive therapy
- Cancer of the head and neck
- Hematologic and reticuloendothelial diseases (e.g., leukemia and Hodgkin's disease)
- End-stage renal disease
- Intestinal bypass or gastrectomy surgery
- Chronic malabsorption syndrome
- Low body weight (≥10% below the ideal)

pain, hemoptysis, irregular menses, and a low-grade fever. Symptoms in adults are often subtle and may appear in conjunction with or simulate other illness and therefore are often not associated with TB. However, one third of persons with pulmonary TB are asymptomatic on initial presentation.[1,2]

Approximately 15% of cases of TB are extrapulmonary, with common sites including the bones and joints, genitourinary system, the lymphatic system, and the CNS. The symptoms of extrapulmonary TB depend on the site affected. TB of the spine often causes back pain, whereas TB of the genitourinary system may result in hematuria or persistent dysuria.

PHYSICAL EXAMINATION

A complete physical examination is an essential part of the evaluation but cannot be used alone to confirm or exclude the presence of TB. Even if the physical examination is entirely negative, it can provide useful information about the patient's overall condition. Certain findings, although not diagnostic of TB, may be suggestive of the diagnosis. Rales in the upper posterior portion of the chest, evidence of pleural effusion, lymphadenopathy, weight loss, and fever may increase the suspicion for TB. Confirmation of TB is based on the diagnostic evaluation presented in the next section.

DIAGNOSTICS

Screening is the first step in the diagnostic evaluation of TB and is performed to identify infected patients at high risk for TB who would benefit from preventive therapy as well as patients with TB who need treatment. Because the vast majority of patients infected with TB are asymptomatic, primary care providers should administer the tuberculin skin test to all high-risk persons as part of their routine evaluation. Persons with any of the medical conditions listed in Box 124-1 should be screened annually unless there is prior documentation of a positive tuberculin skin test.[6] Other high-risk groups include close contacts of a person with infectious disease; foreign-born persons from areas in which TB is common (e.g., Asia, Africa, and Latin America); the medically underserved and low-income populations, including high-risk racial and ethnic groups (e.g., Asians and Pacific Islanders, African-Americans, Latinos, and Native Americans); residents of long-term care facilities (e.g., correctional facilities and nursing homes); and other groups identified as having a disproportionate prevalence of TB, including migrant farm workers and homeless persons. Routine institutional screening is also recommended for health care workers and the staff of long-term institutional facilities who may have occupational exposures to TB or who would pose a risk to large numbers of susceptible persons if they developed active disease (e.g., staff member of an acquired immune deficiency syndrome [AIDS] hospice).[1]

Diagnostics

Tuberculosis

Initial
PPD (Note: Patients with a previous history of a positive PPD should not undergo this test again.)

Laboratory
Sputum culture for acid-fact bacilli × 3*

Imaging
Chest x-ray*

*If indicated.

The standard and preferred method of screening for TB infection is the Mantoux tuberculin skin test, which is administered by the injection of 5 tuberculin units (0.1 ml) of purified protein derivative (PPD) intradermally into either the volar or dorsal surface of the forearm. The injection should be made with a disposable tuberculin syringe with the needle bevel pointing upward. The injection should produce a discrete, pale elevation of the skin (a wheal) that is 6 to 10 mm in diameter and disappears within several hours. If a wheal is not produced, the injection was probably too deep and will likely result in a false-negative reading. In the absence of a wheal, the skin test should be repeated. The amount of induration, rather than the erythema, is measured. All reactions should be recorded in millimeters of induration, even those classified as negative. If no induration is found, "0 mm" should be recorded.

The skin test is read within 48 to 72 hours. If the patient fails to show up for a scheduled reading within 72 hours, a positive reaction may still be measurable up to 1 week. However, all negative responses not documented within 72 hours should be repeated.[1] The criteria for determining whether a skin test is significant depend on a patient's risk for developing disease or ability to mount a reaction to the PPD. The criteria for a positive PPD test are listed in Box 124-2. Once a patient has had a positive tuberculin skin test, no subsequent tuberculin skin testing should be performed.

A variety of factors can cause a false-negative tuberculin skin test, including the recipient's age, the simultaneous administration of a live vaccine, concomitant infections, metabolic deficiencies, underlying disease, and improper placement or storage of the PPD. Live vaccinations such as the measles, mumps, rubella (MMR) vaccine and the oral poliovirus vaccine may cause a false-negative response for up to 2 months after immunization. However, results of the PPD skin test performed simultaneously with inoculation of these vaccines are unaffected.[6] Other potential causes of false-negative test results are listed in Box 124-3.

Because there are many potential causes of a false-negative tuberculin test, the absence of a positive reaction does not exclude TB disease or infection. Anergy, which is a decreased or absent, delayed-type hypersensitivity response, can be caused by severe or febrile illness, miliary or pulmonary disease, and most of the factors listed in Box 124-3. Of all patients with TB, 10% to 25% have negative reactions to the tuberculin skin test. Approximately one third of patients with HIV infection and more than 60% of patients with AIDS have skin test reactions of <5 mm, even though they have been infected with *M. tuberculosis*.[1]

Differentiating between a negative skin test reaction due to noninfection and a negative test due to anergy is made possible by the simultaneous administration of the Mantoux test and at least one other delayed-type hypersensitivity antigen. One of several antigens to which most adult patients have been exposed, such as tetanus toxoid, mumps, or the *Candida* species, is administered in the same way as the Mantoux test. A reaction of ≥3 mm to any of the antigens, including PPD, excludes anergy. Persons who have a positive reaction to the tuberculin should be regarded as having been infected with *M. tuberculosis*, regardless of their reaction to the antigen testing. The results of the anergy test should be recorded in millimeters of induration, similar to the PPD reading. If the person is determined to be anergic, the probability of disease or infection should be assessed on the basis of risk factors and presentation. In the absence of findings consistent with active disease, anergic individuals with a high risk of exposure should be considered for preventive therapy. Low CD4 T-lymphocyte counts (≤200/μL) have been closely correlated with anergy, but anergy can also occur in persons with relatively high CD4 counts. Similarly, reactivity to the tuberculin skin test and control antigens may be present at very low CD4 levels; therefore TB screening should be performed unless anergy has been previously documented.[1]

False-negative reactions can result from a decreased or waning delayed-type hypersensitivity reaction over time, especially among older adults who may have been infected years before being screened for TB. Although previously infected with TB, their hypersensitivity to the PPD antigen has been blunted over time. Although they may not respond to the initial skin test, the skin test may stimulate or "boost" their ability to react to the tuberculin on a subsequent test. Therefore skin testing is repeated in 1 to 3 weeks. A positive reaction to the second test probably represents a boosted reaction rather than a reaction to new infection. On the basis of this two-step testing, the patient should be classified as previously infected, and management should proceed accordingly.[1] Guidelines for interpreting the results of a two-step tuberculin skin testing are included in Box 124-4.

Many foreign countries vaccinate against TB using the bacille Calmette-Guérin (BCG) vaccine. Sensitivity to tuberculin varies significantly among persons who have received the BCG vacci-

BOX 124-2

CRITERIA FOR A POSITIVE TUBERCULIN SKIN TEST

INDURATION ≥5 MM

Persons with HIV infection
Household or close contacts of persons with TB infection
Persons with fibrotic lesions or evidence of old, healed TB on chest x-ray studies
Patients who are immunosuppressed

INDURATION ≥10 MM

Foreign-born persons from countries with high TB prevalence
Medically underserved, low-income populations, including high-risk minority populations
Homeless persons
Prisoners
Alcoholics
IV drug users
Persons with other medical factors known to increase the risk of TB, including the following:

- Silicosis
- Diabetes
- Immunosuppressive or steroid therapy
- Chronic obstructive pulmonary disease
- Hematologic and reticuloendothelial disease
- End-stage renal disease
- Intestinal bypass
- Postgastrectomy
- Carcinomas of the oropharynx and upper gastrointestinal tract
- Persons ≥10% below ideal body weight

Health care workers
Persons with prior bacille Calmette-Guérin vaccination

INDURATION ≥15 MM

Persons at low risk for TB

BOX 124-3

POTENTIAL CAUSES OF FALSE-NEGATIVE TUBERCULIN TEST REACTIONS

- Age (>45 years, newborns)
- Immunosuppression (e.g., corticosteroids, chemotherapy, or other agents)
- Systemic viral, fungal, and bacterial infections
- Live virus vaccinations (e.g., measles, mumps, rubella, trivalent oral poliovirus vaccine)
- Malnutrition/cachexia or nutritional derangement (e.g., severe protein deficiency, zinc deficiency)
- Chronic renal failure
- Hematologic/lymphoreticular disorders (e.g., Hodgkin's lymphoma)
- Sarcoidosis
- Stress (e.g., burns, postoperative status, mental illness)
- Jejunoileal bypass surgery
- Alcoholism
- Mechanical (injection too deep, inexperienced reader)
- Improper storage (exposure to light or heat)

Modified from American Thoracic Society: Diagnostic standards and classification of tuberculosis, *Am Rev Respir Dis* 142(3):725-735, 1990.

nation; this variance depends in part on the strain of BCG used and the person vaccinated. A history of BCG vaccination often confuses the diagnostic picture because there is no reliable way to determine whether a reaction to the tuberculin skin test is due to the BCG vaccine or to infection with *M. tuberculosis*. Nevertheless, a prior history of BCG vaccination is not considered a contraindication to PPD tuberculin skin testing. A reaction to the tuberculin skin test is probably a result of infection with *M. tuberculosis* rather than the BCG vaccine if the induration is large, if significant time has elapsed since BCG vaccination, if the person has had a recent exposure to someone with infectious TB, if there is a family history of TB, if the person comes from an area in which TB is endemic, or if the chest x-ray study shows evidence of previous TB infection. Patients who have received the BCG vaccine should be screened, evaluated, and managed in a manner similar to those who have not been vaccinated with BCG.[1,6]

Persons with a positive tuberculin skin test should have an anteroposterior chest x-ray study to exclude active pulmonary TB and to detect the presence of fibrotic lesions, which may suggest an old TB infection or silicosis. Once these conditions have been excluded, no subsequent chest radiographs are indicated unless the person is symptomatic. In addition, anergic persons who have symptoms consistent with TB or have risk factors for TB should have a chest x-ray examination. Abnormalities in the apical and posterior segments of the upper lobe or in the superior segments of the lower lobe are those most often seen with pulmonary TB. Infiltrates without cavities and mediastinal or hilar lymphadenopathy may also be seen. HIV infection and other immunocompromising illnesses may result in unusual chest x-ray findings. Chest x-ray findings may be suggestive of TB but are never diagnostic. Nevertheless, they may be used to exclude the possibility of pulmonary TB.[1]

Persons suspected of having pulmonary or laryngeal TB should have at least three sputum cultures performed to detect the presence of acid-fast bacilli (AFB). A positive smear is strongly suggestive but not diagnostic of TB because the AFB on a smear may be due to mycobacterium other than *M. tuberculosis*. It is also possible for those with TB to have negative AFB smears. Species of mycobacterium are identified using a variety of methods, including nucleic acid probes, liquid chromatography, and polymerase chain reactions (PCRs). The diagnosis is confirmed by a positive culture of *M. tuberculosis* complex, *M. avium*, or *M. intracellulare*. The mycobacterium isolates are then tested for drug susceptibility. Drug susceptibility is important to ensure appropriate treatment and should be repeated within 2 months if there has not been an adequate response to treatment.

BOX 124-4

CRITERIA FOR INTERPRETATION OF TWO-STEP TUBERCULIN SKIN TESTING

- If the first test is positive, consider the person infected.
- If the first test is negative, give second test 1 to 3 weeks later.
- If the second test is positive, consider the person infected. If the second test is negative, consider the person uninfected.

Modified from the Centers for Disease Control and Prevention, *Core curriculum on tuberculosis: what the clinician should know*, ed 3, Atlanta, 1994, US Department of Health and Human Services.

DIFFERENTIAL DIAGNOSIS

The differential diagnosis of TB varies depending on the type of TB and the site of involvement. The signs and symptoms associated with pulmonary TB are consistent with other respiratory illnesses such as pneumonia, acute bronchitis, or carcinoma. Extrapulmonary TB can occur in any organ; therefore persistent signs and symptoms in any organ should lead to a consideration of TB.

MANAGEMENT

The management of TB depends entirely on the current clinical classification system of disease, which is based on the pathogenesis of the disease and the diagnostic results. The classification system is described in Table 124-1.

Class 0 and class 1 TB require no treatment. Patients with class 1 TB should have another tuberculin skin test performed within several months given the history of known exposure to TB.

Patients with class 2 TB have been infected

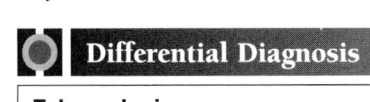

Tuberculosis

Pneumonia
Acute bronchitis
Carcinoma

TABLE 124-1 Clinical Classification System for Tuberculosis

Class	Type	Description
0	No TB exposure Not infected	No history of exposure Negative reaction to tuberculin skin test
1	TB exposure No evidence of infection	History of exposure Negative reaction to tuberculin skin test
2	TB infection No disease	Positive reaction to tuberculin skin test Negative bacteriologic studies (if done) No clinical or radiographic evidence of TB
3	Current TB disease	*M. tuberculosis* cultured (if done) *or* Positive reaction to tuberculin skin test *and* Clinical or radiographic evidence of current disease
4	Previous TB disease	History of episode(s) of TB *or* Abnormal but stable radiographic findings Positive reaction to the tuberculin skin test Negative bacteriologic studies (if done) *and* No clinical or radiographic evidence of current disease
5	TB suspected	Diagnosis pending

From Centers for Disease Control and Prevention: *Core curriculum on tuberculosis: what the clinician should know*, ed 3, Atlanta, 1994, US Department of Health and Human Services.

with TB but do not have any evidence of disease. The main purpose of preventive therapy is to decrease the risk that latent TB infection will progress to clinically active TB disease. INH is most commonly used for preventive therapy and is highly effective when taken as prescribed. INH is bactericidal, relatively nontoxic, inexpensive, and easily administered. The degree of protection conferred by INH varies depending on the percentage of mycobacterium eradicated. INH has been shown to reduce the incidence of disease by 54% to 90%; the primary reason for this variation in efficacy appears to be the actual amount of INH taken during the year it was prescribed.

INH remains less widely prescribed in the United States than it should be. Some studies have shown that fewer than one third of patients at risk for TB are screened with the tuberculin skin test; of those with class 2 TB, only 5% of those eligible for preventive therapy were offered it by their health care provider.[3] Preventive therapy should be considered for persons younger than 35 who have tuberculin skin tests of ≥10 mm who have any risk factors for TB. Patients younger than 35 with no known risk factors should be evaluated for preventive therapy if their reaction to the tuberculin skin test was ≥15 mm. Unless otherwise indicated, INH preventive therapy should be offered to individuals with class 2 TB (tuberculin positive), regardless of their history of BCG vaccination.

The major side effect of INH is hepatitis. Other problems associated with INH include peripheral neuropathy, gastrointestinal upset, and mild CNS effects. From 10% to 20% of patients started on INH develop mild abnormalities of liver function, which often resolve even if INH therapy is continued. INH should be discontinued if any of the liver function tests (LFTs) reach three to five times the upper limit of normal.[7] The risk for INH-induced hepatitis increases directly with increasing age; therefore INH is recommended for patients older than 35 only if they are at high risk for the development of TB. Baseline and monthly LFTs and a monthly clinical evaluation should be performed for all persons undergoing INH therapy.[6] High-priority candidates for TB preventive therapy, regardless of age, are listed in Box 124-5. Alcohol consumption has also been identified as a contributing risk factor in the development of INH-induced hepatitis. Other drugs that increase the risk of INH-induced hepatitis include acetaminophen, phenytoin (Dilantin), steroids, methimazole (Tapazole), estropipate (Ogen, Ortho-Est), and metoclopramide (Reglan, Maxolon). INH administration increases the serum levels of certain drugs, including phenytoin, theophylline, carbamazepine (Tegretol), benzodiazepines, and anticoagulants. During INH administration the serum levels of these drugs should be monitored more closely. Drugs that decrease the serum concentration of INH include antacids, corticosteroids, and laxatives.

Peripheral neuropathy is associated with the administration of INH and most likely results from interference with pyridoxine absorption. It is recommended that pyridoxine (10 to 50 mg/day) be administered in conjunction with INH to patients who have medical problems where neuropathy is already common, such as diabetes, uremia, alcoholism, and malnutrition. In addition, pyridoxine should be administered to pregnant women and to patients with a seizure disorder who are undergoing INH therapy.

BOX 124-5

HIGH-PRIORITY CANDIDATES FOR TUBERCULOSIS-PREVENTIVE THERAPY

Preventive therapy should be recommended for the following persons with a positive skin test, regardless of age (criterion for a positive reaction in millimeters of induration is listed in parentheses):

- Persons with known or suspected HIV infection, including persons who inject drugs whose HIV status is unknown (≥5 mm)
- Close contacts of persons with infectious clinically active TB (≥5 mm)
- Persons who have chest x-ray findings suggestive of previous TB and who have received inadequate or no treatment (≥5 mm)
- Persons who inject drugs and are known to be HIV negative (≥10 mm)
- Recent tuberculin skin test converters (≥10-mm increase within a <2-year period for those <35 years of age; ≥15-mm increase for those >35 years of age)
- Persons with medical conditions that increase the risk of TB, such as diabetes mellitus, prolonged corticosteroid therapy, immunosuppressive therapy, some hematologic and reticuloendothelial diseases, IV drug use, end-stage renal disease, and clinical situations associated with rapid weight loss (≥10 mm)

The usual preventive therapy regimen is INH 300 mg/day for 6 to 12 months; the duration of therapy depends on the risk factors for TB and the associated co-morbidity. Six months of therapy has been shown to confer a high degree of protection (approximately 69%) if the medication is taken as prescribed. Twelve months of therapy reduces the risk by more than 90% if the entire course of therapy is completed. Patients infected with HIV should receive 12 months of therapy.[1]

For persons with a positive tuberculin skin test and evidence of silicosis or old fibrotic lesions without evidence of clinically active disease, alternative regimens include 4 months of INH and RIF or 12 months of INH. For persons who have had close contact with individuals with INH-resistant TB, preventive therapy with RIF for ≥6 months should be considered. RIF preventive therapy can also be considered for patients who are INH intolerant.[1]

RIF is bactericidal, relatively nontoxic, and easily administered. The most common side effect of RIF is gastrointestinal upset. Other adverse reactions include rashes, hepatitis, and, rarely, thrombocytopenia and cholestatic jaundice. RIF is a cytochrome P450 (hepatic microsomal enzyme) inducer that may increase the clearance of drugs metabolized by the liver, including oral hypoglycemic agents, glucocorticoids, estrogens, Coumadin (warfarin) derivatives, methadone, theophylline, antiarrhythmic agents (quinidine, verapamil, mexiletine), anticonvulsants, ketoconazole, and cyclosporin. By interfering with estrogen metabolism, RIF may also interfere with the effectiveness of oral contraceptives.[7]

Treatment of class 3 or clinically active TB requires multidrug therapy. The development of the specific drug regimen should be done in consultation with a specialist familiar with the management of TB. Four drugs are included in the initial regimen: INH, RIF, pyrazinamide (PZA), and ethambutol (EMB) or streptomycin (SM); the purpose is to prevent the development of multidrug-resistant TB. Once the drug susceptibility results are known, the regimen is adjusted. If susceptibility to INH and RIF is demonstrated, administration of these two drugs is continued after the initial 2 months of multidrug therapy. Three-drug therapy (INH, RIF, PZA) is sometimes used as initial therapy if drug resistance is unlikely.[1]

The most important side effect of PZA is hepatotoxicity. However, the risk for liver injury does not seem to increase when this drug is coadministered with INH and RIF. Other adverse effects include hyperuricemia (acute gout is uncommon), arthralgias, skin rashes, and gastrointestinal side effects. Salicylates are often effective in relieving PZA-related arthralgias.[7] Baseline and monthly LFTs and monthly uric acid levels should be obtained for patients taking PZA.

The most common adverse reactions to EMB are optic neuritis, decreased visual acuity, and the loss of red-green perception. These side effects appear to be dose related and are more common in patients with renal failure, probably as a result of decreased clearance of the drug. All patients taking this drug should receive monthly red-green discrimination and visual acuity testing. Ototoxicity is the most common serious side effect of SM, often resulting in vertigo or hearing loss. Nephrotoxicity occurs less commonly, but both of these adverse effects are more common in patients who are older than 60 or who have renal damage.

"Second-line" antitubercular drugs, such as para-aminosalicylic acid, ethionamide, and cycloserine, tend to be less effective and more toxic than the "first-line" drugs previously discussed. They are generally used only in cases of drug-resistant TB or atypical mycobacterial infections. Research on newer antitubercular drugs continues to be of importance, especially in this era of emerging drug resistance.

The antitubercular drug regimens used to treat extrapulmonary TB are similar to those used to treat pulmonary TB. Additional therapies such as corticosteroid therapy or surgery may be required depending on the site of TB infection. The type of follow-up and bacteriologic evaluation required is determined by the site of infection.

The diagnosis of nonclinically active TB (class 4 TB) is defined by a history of previous episodes of TB or stable radiographic findings in a patient with a positive tuberculin skin test. Sputum cultures, if obtained, are negative; there is no radiographic evidence of clinically active disease. Patients with class 4 TB may be treated in several ways depending on TB risk factors and the coexisting medical conditions. Some patients may have completed a course of preventive therapy, and some may be receiving preventive therapy; for others, preventive therapy may not be indicated. Current, clinically active TB must be excluded before a patient can be classified as class 4.

Patients are categorized as having class 5 TB while the evaluation for TB is still being done and the diagnosis of TB is pending. Patients remain in this class until all diagnostic studies have been performed but should not remain in this class for more than 3 months. If clinically active TB is strongly suspected, patients are started on multidrug therapy while the evaluation is still pending. If a diagnosis of clinically active TB (class 3) is confirmed, multidrug therapy is continued. If TB disease is excluded, the drug regimen is altered accordingly. For example, if a diagnosis is changed to infectious (class 2) TB, preventive therapy is continued if indicated. If active TB is highly possible, it is imperative to start multidrug therapy initially and alter the regimen accordingly, because progressing from single-drug therapy (e.g., INH) to multidrug therapy once a diagnosis of active disease is confirmed increases the risk of spreading the disease and of the development of drug-resistant TB.

One of the most significant problems associated with TB control is adherence to antitubercular regimens. Approximately 25% of patients receiving TB treatment do not complete their prescribed regimen within 12 months.[1] Directly observed therapy (DOT) is one way to ensure medication compliance. With DOT, a health care provider or other designated person directly observes the patient taking each dose of TB medication. DOT is routinely implemented in many areas, such as homeless shelters and institutional settings. Antitubercular regimens can often be prescribed to be taken two or three times weekly, making DOT less burdensome. DOT has been shown to be cost-effective when such intermittent regimens are used.[1]

The law in every state requires that a diagnosis of TB be reported to the local health department. All drug susceptibility test results should be forwarded to the health department. Reporting TB is important for source and contact identification, epidemiologic surveillance, and the provision of resources for case management.

Co-Management with Specialists

Consultation with a specialist is required for the management of all patients requiring multidrug therapy, those with active clinical disease (class 3), and those for whom the evaluation is pending (class 5 TB). In addition, consultation is indicated for patients with evidence of TB infection (class 2) and coexistent medical conditions, especially those that alter immune responsiveness, which may increase the risk of development of clinically active disease.

LIFE SPAN CONSIDERATIONS

Pregnant women should receive tuberculin skin testing unless otherwise indicated. Women with evidence of TB infection (class 2) should be considered for INH preventive therapy using the standard criteria. INH therapy is generally initiated 3 months after delivery, although the drug is not contraindicated in pregnancy. Pregnant women with clinically active TB (class 3) must receive adequate therapy as soon as TB is suspected. Untreated TB presents a much greater danger to a woman and her fetus than does treatment of the disease. The preferred initial drug regimen includes INH, RIF, and EMB. These drugs do cross the placenta but have no demonstrated teratogenic side effects. A woman on antitubercular therapy should not be discouraged from breastfeeding; although small concentrations of the drug are found in breast milk, they do not cause toxicity in newborns. SM is contraindicated during pregnancy, and PZA is not routinely used because its effects on the fetus are still unknown.[1,7]

Older adults receiving antitubercular therapy must be monitored more closely for drug side effects. Many of the adverse reactions increase with advancing age and decreased renal function.

COMPLICATIONS

Complications of TB can result from the disease process itself or can be secondary to drug therapy. The death rate of untreated pulmonary TB is approximately 60%, with a median time until death of 2½ years. Patients with miliary or disseminated TB often become ill before radiographic changes are apparent or a diagnosis of TB has been made. Without treatment, the prognosis for miliary TB is poor. However, miliary TB responds to the same drug regimens used to treat other forms of TB.

Persons taking antitubercular drugs need to be monitored closely for side effects and drug toxicities. Baseline laboratory evaluations and monthly examinations are indicated for most of the drugs used to treat TB.

INDICATIONS FOR REFERRAL/HOSPITALIZATION

Most patients with clinically active pulmonary TB should be considered for hospitalization during the first couple of weeks of therapy. After 2 weeks of multidrug therapy, the infectiousness of these patients is reduced significantly and they are no longer a threat to public health. Patients with extrapulmonary TB are generally much less infectious and can generally be managed as outpatients.

Persons with multidrug-resistant TB should be referred to an infectious disease specialist or a pulmonologist with expertise in the treatment of TB. Immunocompromised patients with active TB or any patients with disseminated disease should also be referred.

PATIENT AND FAMILY EDUCATION

Patient education is critical to controlling the resurgence of TB. The public must be educated about the role of TB screening and the need to identify persons infected with TB before active disease develops so they can benefit from preventive therapy. The importance of medication adherence must be carefully explained to patients receiving INH or multidrug therapy. Untreated TB can lead to reactivation of the disease in the future, progression of the disease, continued spread of the disease, and the development of drug resistance. In addition, the potential drug side effects must be carefully discussed, and patients should be instructed to contact their primary care provider as soon as any signs or symptoms associated with drug toxicity develop.

REFERENCES

1. Centers for Disease Control and Prevention, *Core curriculum on tuberculosis: what the clinician should know,* ed 3, Atlanta, 1994, US Department of Health and Human Services.
2. Comstock GW, Reichman LB, Starke JR: Can we control TB this time? *Patient Care* 1995.
3. American Thoracic Society: Control of tuberculosis in the United States, *Am Rev Respir Dis* 146(6):1623-1633, 1992.
4. Centers for Disease Control and Prevention, Recommendations of the Advisory Council for the Elimination of Tuberculosis: Initial therapy for tuberculosis in the era of multidrug resistance, *MMWR* 42(RR-7): 1-8, 1993.
5. Danneburg AM: Immune mechanisms in the pathogenesis of pulmonary tuberculosis, *Rev Infect Dis* 11(suppl 2):S369-S378, 1989.
6. McColloster P, Neff NE: Outpatient management of tuberculosis, *Am Fam Physician* 53(5):1579-1594, 1996.
7. American Thoracic Society: Treatment of tuberculosis and tuberculosis infection in adults and children, *Am J Respir Crit Care Med* 149(5):1359-1374, 1994.

PART 11

Evaluation and Management of Cardiovascular Disorders

JOANN TRYBULSKI, Section Editor

CHAPTER 125

Cardiac Diagnostic Testing: Noninvasive Assessment of Coronary Artery Disease

JoAnn Trybulski and Terry Mahan Buttaro

DEFINITION/EPIDEMIOLOGY

The accurate noninvasive assessment of the presence and severity of coronary artery disease (CAD) remains a major cause of concern with clinical practitioners. The current standard for noninvasive evaluation of CAD in patients presenting with chest pain or in patients with known CAD presenting for risk stratification is the exercise ECG, also called the *exercise tolerance test* (ETT). However, the exercise ECG has significant limitations in many patients, including those in whom the resting ECG is abnormal (Table 125-1) and those who are unable to exercise to an aerobic workload adequate to exclude provocable ischemia.

As a consequence of these and other limitations, it has become common to interface an imaging modality, such as myocardial perfusion imaging (MPI) or cardiac ultrasound, with the exercise ECG in an effort to improve the sensitivity and specificity of noninvasive CAD detection and therefore improve the ability to predict the presence of coronary heart disease.

PATHOPHYSIOLOGY

To understand the application of exercise testing in patients with CAD, it is helpful to understand oxygen delivery to the myocardium. Unlike most other circulatory beds in the body, the coronary circulation allows for maximal oxygen extraction from the blood when the body is at rest. Increases in oxygen demand obligate an increase in myocardial blood flow. The healthy coronary circulation can increase flow approximately five times above the baseline level. The fundamental pathophysiology in CAD is a limitation of the ability of the coronary circulation to vasodilate appropriately. As a result, the ability to increase flow in the face of increased myocardial oxygen demand is limited.

In an ETT, patients are asked to perform incremental exercises. This results in positive chronotropic (rate) and inotropic (strength of contraction) stimulation of the cardiovascular system, which increases myocardial oxygen demand. The normal hemodynamic response to these stimuli is an increase in absolute coronary blood flow. However, this ability is reduced in the presence of CAD, which leads to an imbalance between oxygen supply and demand and results in myocardial ischemia.

EXERCISE TOLERANCE TEST

The standard first-line approach to provocative testing for CAD is the ETT, during which the patient (attached to a 12-lead ECG) is monitored continuously during graded exercise. The ECG response of normal hearts is maintenance of an "isoelectric" ST segment during exercise and recovery. By standard criteria, a positive test for CAD is defined by the development of horizontal or downsloping ST-segment depression of >1 mm measured 80 msec after the J point of the QRS complex (the junction between the QRS complex and the ST segment). ECG changes such as upsloping ST-segment depression or isolated T-wave changes have not demonstrated predictive value.

Because the interpretation of the test is based primarily on the development of characteristic ischemic ST-segment and T-wave changes, it is not surprising that resting ECG abnormalities can lead to a reduction in test sensitivity and specificity. The specificity of the routine ETT is reduced if the patient has had a prior myocardial infarction (MI) because this produces persistent ST-segment and T-wave abnormalities.

A number of other factors can interfere with the sensitivity of the exercise test in detecting CAD. Because an increase in coronary blood flow is related to an increasing heart rate, it is clear that the sensitivity of the test is effort dependent. The standard is the peak heart rate achieved during exercise. Specifically, a test will be considered negative for CAD only if the patient exercises to at least 85% of the age-predicted maximum heart rate without evidence of inducible ischemia (maximum heart rate = ~[220 − age]). If the patient fails to achieve this "target" heart rate, the test should be considered nondiagnostic, or insufficient to exclude ischemia. On the other hand, if there is evidence of ischemia (typical angina, ischemic ST changes) before the patient's target heart rate is reached, the test is considered strongly predictive of significant CAD. A second important predictor of more advanced CAD is exercise-induced hypotension (i.e., a fall in systolic blood pressure of at least 20 mm Hg at any point during exercise).

Medications such as beta blockers can attenuate the heart rate, making the rest of the exercise test less diagnostic. The decision to discontinue beta blockers 1 to 2 days before testing is influenced by the purpose of the exercise test. For ETTs ordered to detect angina, it is recommended that the cardiologist be consulted about withholding the medication before performing the test. ETTs performed to assess effectiveness of pharmacologic therapy require normal daily medication regimens. Imaging studies may be useful in patients who undergo a stress test during beta-blocker therapy.

Another potential contributor to the lack of sensitivity of the ETT is derived from the limitations of the surface ECG related to the spatial distribution of the electrical abnormalities that occur in ischemia. This concept may be better understood if the ECG is considered as an imaging tool that examines the forces of cardiac depolarization and repolarization. To detect ischemia, the repolarization phase of the cardiac cycle—the ST segment and T wave—is examined for abnormalities. ST-segment and T-wave changes in the surface ECG are related to both the extent and the severity of myocardial ischemia. As might be expected, the ETT is more sensitive for the detection of severe disease. Detection of ischemia that is confined to the posterior and/or lateral segments of the left ventricle can be more difficult.

Additional insight into the limitations of routine exercise testing has been provided by observations made in the invasive laboratory. In the setting of myocardial ischemia (produced by balloon inflation during coronary angioplasty), the events described in the following sections have been shown to occur sequentially.

TABLE 125-1 Exercise Testing Comparisons

Test	Benefits	Limitations
Treadmill exercise	Assess ischemia, functional capacity, prognosis Equipment widely available Accuracy established in different populations	Sensitivity lower Poor specificity with: females, resting ECG ST-T abnormalities, digoxin, LBBB, pacemakers No accuracy for site localization or extent of MI
Exercise myocardial perfusion imaging	Reproducible results Improved sensitivity and specificity over treadmill alone More accurately determines extent of CAD and prognosis Assess myocardial viability	Increased cost Requires longer testing times Modest radiation exposure Specificity depends on laboratory and image reading Artifacts due to soft tissue (breast), diaphragm signal attenuation Requires additional equipment/personnel Low specificity with LBBB
Thallium	More extensive validation for detecting viable myocardium with rest-redistribution technique Assessment of pulmonary uptake	
Sestamibi	Superior image with female or obese patients Measures left ventricular function	
Exercise radionuclide angiography	Well validated to identify patients with severe disease Risk stratification after MI Good images with obese or COPD patients Accurate information about ejection fractions	Limited availability and high expense Uses bicycle, not treadmill exercise Inaccurate when heart rate is irregular Reduced specificity with: females, abnormal resting left ventricular function
Exercise echocardiography	Sensitivity and specificity comparable with exercise nuclear imaging Provides information on presence/extent of CAD Results immediately available Portable Less test time, lower cost than nuclear imaging Assesses multiple parameters: global/regional ventricular function, chamber size, wall thickness, valve function Accurate for diagnosis of CAD with resting ECG abnormalities, LBBB Detects left anterior descending coronary artery and multivessel disease	Interpretation nonstandardized and subjective Difficult to interpret with resting wall motion abnormalities Images may be nondiagnostic due to poor image quality Prognostic potential uncertain due to a limited number of studies
Pharmacologic stress with dipyridamole or adenosine	Accurate assessments in patients unable to exercise Useful for preoperative risk assessment in patients with claudication or musculoskeletal limitations Relatively safe in selected patients (side effects rapidly reversible by ending infusion or administering aminophylline) More accurate to diagnose CAD with LBBB than perfusion imaging	Cannot assess functional capacity ECG abnormalities less likely to occur than with exercise Contraindicated with: hypotension, sick sinus syndrome, high-grade heart block, hyperreactive airways, with oral dipyridamole therapy Must discontinue theophylline-containing medications for 72 hours and caffeine for 24 hours before testing Serial testing cannot be used to assess therapy Dipyridamole may induce ischemia in 45% patients with severe CAD Specificity is reduced with right ventricular pacemakers
Dobutamine echocardiography	Accurate CAD assessments in patients unable to exercise Relatively safe in selected patients (side effects rapidly reversible by terminating infusion or administering a beta blocker) Detects threshold of myocardial ischemia Assesses myocardial viability More accurate to diagnose CAD with LBBB than perfusion imaging Establishes prognosis for LBBB, in absence of previous MI	Cannot assess functional capacity ECG abnormalities less likely to occur than with exercise Needs good echocardiographic windows Difficult with obese or COPD patients Requires extensive experience to read Labor intensive Can precipitate dangerous ventricular arrhythmias, especially with severe CAD, poor left ventricular function Contraindicated with aortic aneurysm

Data from Weiner DA: Advantages and limitations of different exercise testing modalities, *UpToDate*. Retrieved January 9, 2002, from the World Wide Web: http://www.uptodate.com.
COPD, Chronic obstructive pulmonary disease; *LBBB,* left bundle branch block.

Ischemic Cascade

Ischemic cascade can be described as follows:

Ischemia → decreased left ventricular compliance → abnormal regional wall motion → ECG changes → chest pain

The ST-segment and T-wave changes that are central to demonstrate ischemia on the ECG occur relatively late in the ischemic cascade. It has been demonstrated that these events resolve in reverse order.

Imaging Adjuncts to the Exercise Tolerance Test

The various imaging modalities that can be used as adjuncts to the graded exercise test can be viewed in the context of the "ischemic cascade." Myocardial perfusion imaging (MPI) is designed to detect the spatial distribution of myocardial blood flow (i.e., to define the regional heterogeneity of flow that characterizes regional ischemia). Cardiac ultrasound (two-dimensional echocardiography [2DE]) is designed to detect the abnormalities in regional wall motion that develop as a consequence of regional myocardial ischemia.

Examining the limitations of routine exercise testing from a historical perspective yields interesting information. The limitations detailed previously were clinically acceptable when the exercise study was performed principally as a binary diagnostic test (to determine whether CAD was present or absent) in patients presenting with chest pain. The limited sensitivity of this test in a subgroup of patients with minimal CAD did not produce significant consequences. However, even with patients with minimal CAD, the use of the ETT did not yield significant answers about CAD status, primarily because these patients have a cardiovascular event rate of only 1% to 2% per year.

With the advent of effective coronary revascularization surgery, the ETT has assumed additional predictive clinical relevance. It is clear that powerful predictors of outcomes reside in clinical data and in ETT results independent of the ST-segment response, such as the hemodynamic response and the aerobic work capacity as reflected by exercise duration.

In contrast, the more recent expansion of interventional therapies to affect coronary revascularization has resulted in an important shift in the data that practitioners seek from provocative testing. For example, in patients with stable coronary syndromes, the judicious application of percutaneous transluminal coronary angioplasty (PTCA) requires that both the presence and territorial distribution of ischemia be defined. Further, in patients who have sustained prior myocardial injury, decisions regarding revascularization require a definition of ischemia both within and remote from the site of injury, as well as tissue viability within the zone of infarction.

It should also be emphasized that the usefulness of these adjunctive imaging modalities depends in part on the prevalence of disease in the patient population being studied. In general, these adjunctive modalities are most useful in patient populations with an intermediate pretest clinical probability of disease.

In the evaluation of patients presenting with stable chest pain syndromes and normal surface ECGs, the conventional ETT typically provides adequate clinical information for diagnostic purposes. Similarly, in patients with known CAD and stable coronary syndromes, the ETT is typically adequate as a means of observing disease progression for purposes of prognostication and timing of revascularization procedures. However, with respect to the delineation of damaged myocardial regions and residual myocardial viability in zones of prior injury, it has become clear that adjunctive radiopharmaceutical and/or cardiac ultrasound imaging substantially improves test sensitivity and specificity (Box 125-1).

When considering ETT, primary care providers should be aware that there are relative contraindications for ETT. For these patients, consultation with a cardiologist is recommended. The following clinical alterations are relative contradictions to ETT: uncontrolled hypertension; significant ventricular arrhythmias; uncontrolled severe congestive heart failure; severe valvular heart disease consistent with aortic stenosis, mitral stenosis, or idiopathic hypertrophic subaortic stenosis; atrial fibrillation with an uncontrolled ventricular response; and a recent MI or unstable angina (may select modified testing 6 to 7 days after MI).

MYOCARDIAL PERFUSION IMAGING

Thallium-201 and Technetium-99m Sestamibi

At the present, thallium-201 chloride and technetium Tc-99m sestamibi are the radiopharmaceutical agents used for the detection of CAD in MPI. The distinctive properties of these two agents are well recognized. They appear comparable for CAD detection in patients with stable coronary syndromes: a number of sources have documented the clinical efficacy of sestamibi with thallium-201 chloride.[1-4]

Sestamibi imaging provides the capacity to "simultaneously" define left ventricular systolic function and myocardial perfusion. This offers a means to assess the impact of reperfusion therapies in patients presenting with acute coronary syndromes.

The minimal redistribution of sestamibi, when combined with its protracted myocardial clearance (half-life of approximately 5 hours), is well suited to the imaging of patients presenting with acute coronary syndromes. Unlike thallium-based perfusion imaging, sestamibi image acquisition can be performed up to several hours after tracer injection. This allows for appropriate treatment and triage of patients presenting with acute MI and unstable angina; the image acquired after such treatment will represent the status of myocardial perfusion at the time of tracer injection. Tracer injection can be repeated at a later time to assess myocardial salvage/residual viability in

BOX 125-1

INDICATIONS FOR COUPLING NUCLEAR OR ULTRASOUND IMAGING TO THE STANDARD EXERCISE TOLERANCE TEST

- Left ventricular hypertrophy with ST-segment and T-wave abnormalities on resting ECG.
- Abnormal baseline ST-segment and T-wave abnormalities on resting ECG for any reason
- Recent MI, particularly with persistent rest ST-segment abnormalities
- Clinical use of digoxin
- Wolff-Parkinson-White syndrome
- Bundle branch block
- Ventricular pacemaker

infarct patients or to define the presence, extent, and territorial distribution of ischemia in patients with unstable angina.

Researchers have found that sestamibi images performed in the emergency department may be useful in identifying low-versus high-risk patient presenting with suspected myocardial ischemia. Furthermore, although MPI with thallium-201 chloride is typically coupled to exercise or pharmacologic stress, a number of reports have demonstrated that rest-redistribution imaging may provide valuable information in patients with unstable coronary syndromes—who are not suitable candidates for stress studies.

Because the diagnosis of perfusion defects requires the detection of decreased flow in one region relative to another, there will be occasional instances of false-negative scans in patients with severe three-vessel or left main coronary disease. These "balanced" flow disturbances (i.e., a decrease in coronary flow in more than two geographic territories) should be suspected in patients in whom clinical suspicion of severe CAD is high but the MPI reveals uniform tracer uptake.

EXERCISE ECHOCARDIOGRAPHY

The practice of exercise echocardiography has expanded dramatically in recent years. Current data suggest that adjunctive echocardiographic imaging enhances the sensitivity and specificity of CAD detection to an extent comparable to that provided by nuclear techniques. The 2DE evidence for ischemia includes an abnormal left ventricular ejection fraction (LVEF) response to exercise and/or the development of regional wall motion abnormalities.

As previously demonstrated in thallium imaging, the sensitivity of the 2DE technique for CAD detection is enhanced in patient subsets with multivessel CAD and/or prior MI. In addition, the sensitivity of exercise echocardiography is decreased in patients with resting wall motion abnormalities. In practical terms, patients in whom adequate ultrasound imaging views cannot be obtained (often including obese patients or those with severe emphysematous lung disease) should be considered for alternate imaging modalities.

COMPARISON OF MYOCARDIAL PERFUSION IMAGING WITH TWO-DIMENSIONAL ECHOCARDIOGRAPHY

In summary, the available literature indicates that exercise 2DE with Doppler Flow Study is comparable to MPI for the detection of CAD. However, there are relative strengths of the respective modalities that merit comment. First, there is a greater accumulation of literature for MPI with respect to prognostication in patients with CAD. In addition, it appears that MPI may be preferable to 2DE for the recognition of incremental ischemia in myocardial regions characterized by abnormalities of resting wall motion. Further, quantification of myocardial perfusion data has been more extensively validated than comparable quantification of cardiac ultrasound; the latter technique has been limited by the technical difficulties attendant to endocardial border recognition. The majority of studies with exercise 2DE have been limited to qualitative visual assessment; it is also clear that the early 2DE data were acquired in patient groups with a relatively high incidence of significant CAD. Finally, MPI (e.g., rest-redistribution thallium-201 chloride scintigraphy and rest-injected technetium Tc-99m sestamibi) is more amenable to the detection of ischemia in patients with unstable coronary syndromes in whom exercise is contraindicated. Serial rest 2DE images acquired in patients with unstable coronary syndromes may occasionally be useful if new or more extensive wall motion abnormalities can be detected during recurrent ischemia.

In contrast, 2DE offers access to the incremental information regarding left ventricular contractile performance that is analogous to that provided by exercise radionuclide ventriculography. LVEF response to exercise provides important prognostic information in patients with CAD; such information is available only inferentially by myocardial perfusion scintigraphy (i.e., pulmonary thallium uptake). Finally, with respect to viability assessment, it is to be emphasized that the detection of preserved contractile function in myocardial segments supplied by diseased coronary arteries is essential.

THREE-DIMENSIONAL/DOPPLER FLOW ECHOCARDIOGRAPHY

Three-dimensional (3D) echocardiographic techniques are currently available that use MRI as well as computer-assisted 3D acquisition systems for 2DE. However, the cost of the 3D technology is higher. Three-dimensional technology is still in the process of development, so current evidence-based guideline evaluations center on 2DE with Doppler flow study.[5]

Current investigations of 3D technology involve electron beam CT (EBCT). This emerging 3D technology performs a heart scan at a rapid rate, thus "freezing" cardiac motion. Coronary artery calcification is analyzed and a total calcium score for a patient's coronary arteries is calculated based on the areas of calcification and the maximum CT calcium density.[6] With significant CAD (>50% stenosis), only 2.5% of coronary segments have no detectable calcium on EBCT.[6]

Doppler flow studies are used to localize and quantify obstructions in the cardiovascular system. Primarily, the addition of Doppler flow study to an echocardiogram enhances the ability to evaluate prosthetic valve function, detect and evaluate the blood shunting from a septal defect, and gauge the severity of valvular stenosis or regurgitation.[5]

PHARMACOLOGIC STRESS TESTING

The clinical usefulness of adjunctive imaging modalities has been expanded by the coupling of such techniques to "pharmacologic" stress, an important advantage in patients who are unable to perform conventional treadmill or ergometer exercises. At the present, the pharmacologic agents used are coronary vasodilators (e.g., dipyridamole [Persantine] and adenosine) or inotropic/chronotropic drugs (e.g., dobutamine).

The vasodilator drugs are applied to assess the effective coronary flow reserve (i.e., the ratio of maximal flow to basal flow). Because the extraction of tracer is proportional to blood flow, the coupling of vasodilators with MPI allows for the detection of regional flow disturbances. These regional perfusion abnormalities can be characterized as reversible (normal uptake at baseline, with decreased uptake after vasodilator) or fixed (indicative of prior infarction). The fact that vasodilators do not induce ischemia but simply unmask regional variations in flow reserve means that the ECG portion of the test will very rarely demonstrate ischemic changes. However, on rare occasions ECG changes may be observed, and up to 20% of patients may experience angina. Ischemia may be caused by "coronary steal." The effects of dipyridamole can be reversed by IV aminophylline, and the effects of adenosine and dobutamine can be reversed by discontinuation of the infusion.

Another approach is to induce cardiac ischemia using a beta agonist such as dobutamine, which is applied in gradually increased doses until the goal heart rate is achieved (the provocation of ischemic chest pain or ST-segment changes may also lead to termination of the test). Dobutamine increases cardiac work, initially via an inotropic effect; a normal cardiac response to dobutamine is an increase in global left ventricular contractility. The chronotropic effects of this agent become apparent at higher infusion rates (20 to 50 μg/kg/min). Most commonly, inducible ischemia occurs at these higher infusion rates.

As previously described, the development of regional wall motion abnormalities is often an early manifestation of ischemia. For this reason, dobutamine is most commonly coupled with 2DE (which is performed after each increase in dose) to determine regional abnormalities in left ventricular function or decreases in LVEF. The onset of new regional hypokinesis in a previously normally contracting segment is highly predictive of the presence of CAD in the artery supplying the dysfunctional segment. Alternatively, MPI can be coupled with dobutamine in patients with poor echocardiographic windows. The accuracies of dobutamine echocardiography and dobutamine MPI are comparable.

In a study by Sawada and others,[7] dobutamine echocardiography was shown to have comparable usefulness in patients with baseline normal wall motion (89% sensitivity and 85% specificity); however, the sensitivity was somewhat lower in patients with abnormal resting wall motion (81% sensitivity and 86% specificity). In another study, adenosine had similar sensitivity (86%) to dipyridamole when coupled with nuclear imaging but lower specificity (specificity 71% and accuracy 80%).[8] The poor performance of adenosine echocardiography (sensitivity 58%, specificity 87%, and accuracy 69%) underscores the importance of coupling vasodilators with perfusion imaging rather than with cardiac ultrasound, which requires the induction of ischemia to produce regional contractile dysfunction.

Another study found the sensitivity of dobutamine stress 2DE to be comparable to that of dobutamine single-photon emission CT (SPECT) (85% versus 80%, respectively); the specificity of the two techniques was also comparable (82% versus 74%, respectively), as were the predictive values.[8]

In summary, on the basis of these data, the following conclusions can be drawn:

- Vasodilator stress echocardiography is less sensitive for the detection of CAD than similar stress tests coupled with perfusion scintigraphy.
- Vasodilator stress echocardiography is less sensitive than exercise or dobutamine 2DE for disease detection.
- Vasodilator perfusion scintigraphy compares favorably with exercise/dobutamine scintigraphy or exercise/dobutamine 2DE with respect to CAD detection.

CONCLUSION

The recognized limitations of the exercise ECG have resulted in the development of adjunctive, noninvasive imaging tests to evaluate patients with CAD. In particular, modalities that assess the contractile performance of the left ventricle, as well as those that evaluate the status of regional myocardial perfusion, have gained widespread application. Cardiac ultrasound and MPI are of comparable usefulness in detecting CAD. The data with respect to prognostication are most extensive for MPI techniques, but ultrasound-based prognostication data are accumulating.

Both functional studies and perfusion imaging have demonstrated clear usefulness in addressing the complex question of myocardial viability. These testing modalities are used to assess the presence of functional heart muscle in patients with ischemic heart disease and regional contractile dysfunction.

Although it is often inferred that ultrasound-based techniques and MPI techniques are competitive, it is clear that these modalities may in fact be complementary in the evaluation of selected patients with CAD. Recently, the American College of Cardiology (ACC)/American Heart Association (AHA) Task Force on Practice Guidelines suggested that exercise MPI or exercise echocardiography may be used as the initial test for diagnosis in patients with chronic stable angina who are able to exercise.[9] In addition, The ACC/AHA Committee on Clinical Application of Echocardiography recognizes that an exercise or a pharmacologic stress echocardiogram can be used to evaluate the presence or extent of ischemia where there is an underlying ECG abnormality that affects ECG interpretation (i.e., prior ischemia, left bundle branch block, Wolff-Parkinson-White syndrome).[5] There is conflicting evidence whether echocardiography techniques are preferable when there are no resting ECG abnormalities.[5]

REFERENCES

1. Wackers FJ and others: Technetium-99m hexakis 2-methoxyisobutyl isonitrile: human biodistribution, dosimetry, safety, and preliminary comparison to thallium-201 for myocardial perfusion imaging, *J Nucl Med* 30(3):301-311, 1989.
2. Maisey MN and others: European multicenter comparison of thallium-201 and technetium-99m methoxy isobutyl isonitrile in ischemic heart disease, *Eur J Nucl Med* 16:869, 1990.
3. Kiat H and others: Comparison of technetium 99m methoxy isobutyl isonitrile and thallium 201 for evaluation of coronary artery disease by planar and tomographic methods, *Am Heart J* 117(1):1-11, 1989.
4. Henkin RE and others: ACR appropriateness criteria for chronic chest pain, without evidence of myocardial ischemia/infarction, *Radiology* June (suppl):85-88, 2000.
5. Cheitlin and others: ACC/AHA guidelines for the clinical application of echocardiography, *Circulation* 95(6):1686-1744, 1997. Retrieved February 2, 2002, from the World Wide Web: http://www.acc.org. clinical/guidelines/ech/ec1A.htm.
6. Laudon DA and others: Use of electron beam computed tomography in the evaluation of chest pain patients in the emergency department, *Ann Emerg Med* 33(1):15-21, 1999.
7. Sawada SG and others: Echocardiographic detection of coronary artery disease during dobutamine infusion, *Circulation* 83(5): 1605-1614, 1991.
8. Marwick T and others: Selection of the optimal nonexercise stress for the evaluation of ischemic regional myocardial dysfunction and malperfusion: comparison of dobutamine and adenosine using echocardiography and 99mTc-MIBI single photon emission computed tomography, *Circulation* 87(2):345-354, 1993.
9. Gibbons RJ and others: Guidelines for the management of patients with chronic stabile angina, *J Am Coll Cardiol* 33(7):2092-2197, 1999.

CHAPTER 126

Abdominal Aortic Aneurysm

Virginia Capasso and E. Lynne Kelley

DEFINITION/EPIDEMIOLOGY

Abdominal aortic aneurysm (AAA) is a progressive localized dilation of the abdominal aorta. With an AAA, the diameter of the suspicious area exceeds the normal diameter by 50% (1.5 times).[1] AAA develops in about 3% to 4% of adults older than 65 years.[2] Since the 1970s, the Western world has seen a dramatic rise in the incidence of aneurysms that remains valid even when better screening and access to health care is taken into effect.[3] Thus at least 1 million Americans have a clinically recognized AAA.

AAA is an important clinical diagnosis because it is associated with considerable risk of rupture and death as the aneurysm enlarges to a diameter of ≥5 cm.[4] In 1991, 16,696 deaths in the United States were attributed to aortic aneurysms; aneurysms involving the infrarenal abdominal aorta accounted for 52% of deaths.[5] Between 1979 and 1990, the death rates from AAA decreased slightly among white males while they increased slightly for black males and white females. Overall, the rates were higher for whites than for blacks and for males than for females.

Risk factors for AAA include atherosclerotic vascular disease, white race, male gender, advanced age, hypertension, smoking, chronic obstructive pulmonary disease (COPD), history of hernias, family history of AAA, and presence of other aneurysms.[6] Despite extensive investigation, the link between COPD and AAA remains elusive. Recent evidence suggests that the high prevalence of AAA in patients with COPD may be related to medications (oral steroids) and coexisting diseases, rather than a common pathway of pathogenesis involving plasma elastase or alpha$_1$-antitrypsin deficiency.[7] Another recent study suggests an association between AAA and elevated homocysteine plasma levels.[8] Homocysteine levels have been shown to be higher in patients with AAA than in control subjects without AAA. In addition, aneurysmal size has been shown to be larger in patients with hyperhomocysteinemia than in those with normohomocysteinemia. However, this may be explained by the increased prevalence of hyperhomocysteinemia in patients with atherosclerosis independent of the presence of an aneurysm.

The proposed etiologies of AAA include atherosclerosis, inflammation, mycotic infection, inheritable connective tissue disorders (Marfan's syndrome, type IV Erlos-Danlos), and trauma. Traditionally, atherosclerosis has been considered the most common cause of AAA. However, aneurysm formation is associated with atherosclerosis in only 25% of cases.

PATHOPHYSIOLOGY

AAA is a disease of the medial wall layer of the aorta. It is characterized by degeneration of the extracellular matrix proteins and the presence of an inflammatory cell infiltrate composed predominantly of T-cells. Degradation of the cell wall proteins in the medial layer occurs as a result of complex interactions between genetic factors, inflammatory cytokines, matrix metalloproteinases (MMPs), tissue inhibitors of MMPs (TIMPs), and others. The consequences include dissolution and fragmentation of collagen and elastin, leading to expansion of the vessel wall.[9] When the aortic wall tension exceeds the tensile strength of the wall collagen and the wall can no longer withstand the repetitive force of systolic contraction, the aneurysm ruptures.

CLINICAL PRESENTATION

Although an AAA may cause symptoms as a result of the pressure on surrounding structures, about 75% are asymptomatic at initial diagnosis.[10] Asymptomatic AAAs are generally detected during an incidental radiologic or surgical procedure. Alternatively, in thin patients, a supine abdominal examination may readily show a pulsatile abdominal mass. Inflammatory AAAs may present with chronic abdominal pain or back pain and, sometimes, ureteral obstruction.[4] Other clinical symptoms may result from embolization or rupture of the aneurysm.

Thromboembolic phenomena may herald the presence of an AAA. Microembolic infarcts in the lower extremity of a patient with easily palpable pedal pulses may suggest either abdominal or popliteal aneurysm. Embolization of mural thrombus from an abdominal aneurysm may present with acute limb ischemia due to femoral or popliteal occlusion.[10]

The classic diagnostic triad of hypovolemic shock, pulsatile abdominal mass, and abdominal or back pain is encountered in only a minority of patients with a ruptured AAA. Ruptured AAAs should be suspected in any patient who presents with hypotension and atypical abdominal or back pain symptoms. In a patient with a history of aneurysm or pulsatile mass, the presence of abdominal pain must be considered to represent a rapidly expanding or ruptured aneurysm and must be treated accordingly. In the community setting, the death rate from ruptured AAA is almost 90% because 80% die before reaching the hospital and about 50% die during surgery to repair the rupture.

PHYSICAL EXAMINATION

Palpation of the abdomen for AAA is one of the few physical examination maneuvers that is an evidence-based recommendation in the periodic health examination of older men.[11] To detect AAA on physical examination, the patient is positioned supine with knees flexed to relax the abdominal wall. The examiner places the palm of the hand over the epigastrium to detect a transmitted pulsation. The examiner then places both hands on the abdomen with palms down and an index finger on either side of the pulsating area to measure the aortic width. An AAA is suspected when the aorta is judged to be at least 3.0 cm in maximum diameter.

Unfortunately, abdominal palpation has only moderate overall sensitivity for detecting AAA (68%).[11] The sensitivity of abdominal palpation increases with AAA diameter, from 61% for AAA of 3.0 to 3.9 cm, to 69% for AAA of 4.0 to 4.9 cm, and to 82% for AAA of ≥5.0 cm. The sensitivity of abdominal palpation also increases (91%) when the abdominal girth is <100 cm (40-inch waistline). When the girth is ≥100 cm and the aorta is palpable, the sensitivity is less (82%). Overall, when the girth is <100 cm and the AAA is ≥5.0 cm, abdominal palpation is highly sensitive (100%) for detecting AAA.

DIAGNOSTICS

Currently, ultrasound is the imaging study ordered most often for screening and initial confirmation of an aneurysm. This modality can provide a reasonably accurate measurement of initial size and be used for serial follow-up evaluation.[12] The most accurate measurement of size by ultrasound is the anteroposterior diameter. (The transverse measurement may be larger due to distortion of the aorta.) High-resolution ultrasound allows the visualization of important anatomic markers, including the origin of the superior mesenteric artery, left renal vein indicating the level adjacent to the renal arteries, and the iliac arteries. Ultrasound also allows visualization of the "halo effect" of an inflammatory aneurysm. Duplex ultrasound illuminates aortoiliac occlusive disease.

CT with intravenous contrast is the most widely used imaging technique before aortic aneurysm repair. It permits the detection of inflammatory aneurysms, aneurysmal leakage, and penetrating aortic ulcers. It also delineates venous anomalies, periaortic lymphadenopathy, and horseshoe kidneys.[12]

The era of endoluminal repair of AAA necessitates selection of the proper endograft according to precise measurement of the size and length of both the proximal neck of the aneurysm and the common iliac arteries. This is best achieved by helical or spiral CT scanning, which allows the creation of three-dimensional images that can be rotated for viewing in any projection. This technique requires breath-holding for 30 seconds. It also requires the administration of contrast medium (120 to 150 ml), which may be detrimental in patients with renal insufficiency.

Standard contrast aortography is the simplest method to define the presence of significant associated renal, visceral, or iliofemoral occlusive disease. Although no longer routinely recommended for all patients with AAA, selective indications for preoperative aortography include suspicion of suprarenal extension, suspected visceral or renal artery disease, iliofemoral occlusive disease, horseshoe kidney, prior aortic or colonic surgery, and unusual aneurysms (e.g., mycotic, aortocaval fistula).[13]

MRI and magnetic resonance angiography (MRA) are alternative approaches to aortography.[12] Gadolinium-enhanced MRA images provide clear delineation of the renal and visceral vessels as well as occlusive disease of the iliofemoral vessels. In many centers, MRA has become the imaging study of choice for patients with renal insufficiency.

MRI and MRA have limitations. The limitations include inability to use on patients with pacemakers or other metallic hardware that would affect the magnetic field. In addition, for certain patients, claustrophobia or unstable medical conditions would preclude their being in the tube during the necessary acquisition time. In addition, MRA has not yet been validated as a method of sizing for endovascular aneurysm repair.

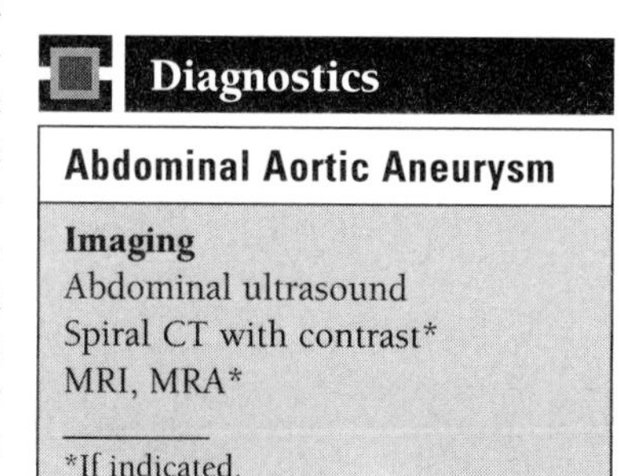

Diagnostics

Abdominal Aortic Aneurysm

Imaging
Abdominal ultrasound
Spiral CT with contrast*
MRI, MRA*

*If indicated.

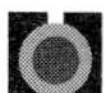

Differential Diagnosis

Abdominal Aortic Aneurysm	
Nephrolithiasis	Appendicitis
Myocardial infarction	Pyelonephritis
Esophageal rupture	Ischemic bowel
Perforated gastric ulcer	Back strain
Pancreatitis	Arthritis
Bowel obstruction	Neoplasm
Cholelithiasis	Other causes of abdominal pain
Diverticulitis	Other causes of back pain
Gastrointestinal bleed	

DIFFERENTIAL DIAGNOSIS

The differential diagnoses for AAA include conditions associated with abdominal pain or back pain. These conditions include nephro-lithiasis, myocardial infarction, esophageal rupture, perforated gastric ulcer, pancreatitis, bowel obstruction, cholelithiasis, diverticulitis, gastrointestinal bleed, appendicitis, pyelonephritis, ischemic bowel, back strain, arthritis, or neoplasm.[14] CT is the most readily available method to rule out alternate causes of abdominal pain.

MANAGEMENT

The goal of AAA management is to prevent aneurysmal rupture while minimizing surgical risk. Thus the size of the aneurysm is the critical factor in deciding the timing of elective AAA repair. A fair amount of controversy persists about the best timing and method of AAA repair (operative or endoluminal) with consideration of preoperative risk factors and postoperative complications.

The majority of aneurysms expand slowly at a rate of 0.2 to 0.3 cm/yr, or 10% of the diameter.[15] However, the risk of rupture increases significantly when an AAA exceeds 5 cm in diameter. This was shown in a recent population-based study in which the estimated risk of rupture based on the latest ultrasound study was 0% per year for an aneurysm less than 4 cm, 1% per year for an aneurysm 4.0 to 4.9 cm, 11% per year for an aneurysm 5.0 to 5.9 cm, and 25% for aneurysms greater than 6 cm.[16]

Recent data from the United Kingdom Small Aneurysm Trial[17] and the Veterans Administration Aneurysm Detection and Management Trial (ADAM)[18] help to guide decision making about the timing of surgical repair of small AAA (4.0 to 5.0 cm) versus surveillance with serial ultrasound examinations. These studies concluded that unless the aneurysm exceeds 5.5 cm, there is no long-term survival advantage of early surgery over serial ultrasonographic surveillance at 6-month intervals. Elective repair is appropriately indicated for healthy patients with AAA measuring 5.0 to 6.0 cm.[4]

Preoperative Cardiac Risk Stratification

Several large surveys have demonstrated that coronary artery disease is the most important underlying medical illness contributing to morbidity and mortality among individuals who undergo major vascular surgery, regardless of the type of peripheral vascular surgery, particularly when they are 70 years of age or older.[19-22] The American College of Cardiology (ACC) and the American Heart Association (AHA) developed guidelines to aid in cardiac risk stratification before noncardiac surgery.[23]

According to the ACC/AHA guidelines,[23] aortic and other vascular procedures are considered high risk. Therefore patients should proceed to surgery without further cardiac evaluation only when they have no clinical predictors or minor clinical predictors (advanced age, abnormal ECG, cardiac rhythm other than sinus, low functional capacity, history of stroke, uncontrolled hypertension) with moderate or excellent functional capacity (≥4 METS, that is, activities such as doing light housework like dusting and washing dishes or climbing a flight of stairs or a hill).[24,25] Preoperative noninvasive testing (pharmacologic stress testing) is indicated when patients are undergoing high-risk vascular surgery and they have two or more intermediate predictors of clinical risk (mild angina pectoris, prior myocardial infarction, compensated or prior congestive heart failure, diabetes mellitus, renal insufficiency) and poor functional capacity (≤4 METS). The results of noninvasive testing are then used to plan further perioperative management. This includes intensified medical therapy, cardiac catheterization, coronary revascularization, or, potentially, cancellation or delay of noncardiac surgery.

Other medical conditions may increase the mortality rate of aneurysm repair by twofold or threefold. They include chronic renal failure (serum creatinine level, >3 mg/dl, or hemodialysis), COPD (forced expiratory volume >1 L), and liver cirrhosis with portal hypertension. These conditions increase the mortality rate from 3% to 5% to 8% to 10%.[4]

Open Surgical Repair

Open surgical repair of an AAA is usually approached through a midline or a left flank retroperitoneal incision. Overall, these two approaches are generally interchangeable in the treatment of infrarenal aneurysm, although specific indications for the transperitoneal approach include right renal graft, right iliac artery aneurysm, prior left colectomy, and aneurysmal neck that turns to the right. Indications for the retroperitoneal approach include multiple prior laparotomies or abdominal surgeries, selected abdominal stoma, horseshoe kidney, inflammatory aneurysms, obesity, and juxtarenal and suprarenal aortic aneurysms.[26]

During open surgical repair of an AAA, the aneurysm is exposed and normal segments of the proximal and distal aorta are cross-clamped. The aneurysm is incised. Lumbar arteries, which backbleed into the aneurysm, are oversewn. A prosthetic graft is positioned in the aorta, extending from a segment of normal aorta above the aneurysm to a segment of normal aorta below the aneurysm. If the aneurysm extends to the iliac arteries, a bifurcated prosthetic graft is used. The distal ends of the bifurcated limbs extend into the iliac or femoral arteries. The wall of the aneurysm is closed over the newly placed graft. The posterior peritoneum, and then the abdomen, is closed in the standard manner.

A number of advancements contributed to improved outcomes of open surgical repair. These include autotransfusion, balanced general and epidural anesthesia, and improved pain management with continuous epidural analgesia in the postoperative setting.

Today, most patients undergoing surgical repair of an AAA have their preoperative workups done as outpatients. After restricting their dietary intake and managing their bowel evacuation at home on the day before surgery, these patients are admitted for same-day surgery. The surgery lasts between 2 to 4 hours. Patients undergoing infrarenal AAA repair typically stay in the intensive care unit for 1 night. They are transferred to the general care unit on postoperative day 1, when they get out of bed to the chair or ambulate. If the graft extends down to the femoral vessels, they are kept at bed rest until postoperative day 2. Also on postoperative day 2, the diet of patients who undergo AAA through a retroperitoneal approach is advanced to clear liquids and then diet as tolerated. If the operation is performed through a transperitoneal approach, return of bowel function may take a few days longer. Discharge to home with skilled nursing visits is projected for postoperative day 5, although it ranges from day 5 to day 7. Home nursing care focuses on the incision, pain management, appetite and food intake, bowel function, and progression of activity.

Endovascular Stent Grafts

In 1991, Parodi and others[27] reported the deployment of the first stent graft for the repair of AAA. A growing number of studies have documented the efficacy and generally satisfactory early results for a variety of transluminally placed endovascular grafts.[28-31]

Endoluminal AAA repair is associated with reduced length of hospital stay and decreased recovery time, accounting for its appeal to patients and physicians, as well as an upsurge of enthusiasm for the development and use of such devices.[32]

Endoluminal repair of AAA is achieved through exclusion of the aneurysm from the circulation by means of a prosthetic graft that is inserted from a remote site to the desired intraluminal location, under radiologic guidance, and then secured by an expandable stent attachment system. The devices may be commercially manufactured or custom made. They may consist of a bifurcated graft or a tube graft with a single limb (aortouniiliac). In addition, a modular product allows the creation of a variable bifurcated graft through the deployment and attachment of a contralateral limb and extensions. Also, if it is necessary to exclude the contralateral iliac artery but restore flow to the contralateral extremity, an aortouniiliac device has been combined with a standard operative femorofemoral bypass graft. When only tube grafts were available, endoluminal repair was possible for <10% of patients, but this rate has increased to <50% with the availability of bifurcated grafts and aortouniiliac grafts.[33]

The initial successful deployment of a stent graft has been reported in 95% to 97% of cases.[34] In most cases, the procedure time is now less than 2 hours. Most procedures are performed under epidural anesthesia combined with conscious sedation. Only very infrequently does an endovascular patient require an intensive care unit stay. Patients are sent home after CT confirmation of graft placement and the absence of a leak at the attachment sites for the graft. The average length of hospital stay is now approximately 2.4 days, with more than 85% of patients being discharged on their first or second postoperative day.[32]

The first routine follow-up visit with the vascular surgeon occurs 1 month after hospital discharge, at which time another

CT scan is obtained to reaffirm the position of the graft, presence or absence of any leak, and evidence of sac shrinkage. Thereafter, CT scans are obtained every 6 months for several years. If the aneurysm and the prosthesis remain stable, the frequency of follow-up can be decreased to annual visits.

Patients report a return to a sense of preoperative health status in 11 days after endoluminal repair versus 47 days after open surgical repair.[32] However, as discussed later, long-term data about device durability and frequent endoleaks (leaks around the endovascular graft) preclude a universal shift from open surgical repair to endoluminal repair.

Ruptured AAAs present a unique challenge to endovascular repair. Because the first indication of their presence is often the back pain and hypotension associated with acute enlargement and rupture, the primary goal is patient stabilization. This is accomplished by gaining control of the rupture and preventing further hemorrhage. Once the patient is stabilized, repair of the aorta can be accomplished.

For elective repairs, grafts typically are chosen based on a series of measurements and often using three-dimensional reconstructions of CT scans and/or angiograms. The process can take several days, which is a luxury that is not available with an acute rupture. However, with increasing surgical experience and the availability of a range of graft sizes at hand, this less-invasive method of repair has been applied with some degree of success.[35-37] Clearly, as the technology improves, this method of repair will play a wider role in the repair of ruptured AAAs. We hope the dismal 90% mortality rate for ruptured AAA will improve.

LIFE SPAN CONSIDERATIONS

In general, AAA is considered a disease of older, white men. However, AAA repair is often performed on young patients (≤50 years). Aneurysms are more commonly symptomatic in younger patients, although perioperative mortality and morbidity rates are not significantly different for young patients compared with older patients (≥65 years) with degenerative (atherosclerotic) AAAs.[38]

COMPLICATIONS

Complications vary for surgical repair and endoluminal repair of AAAs. Mortality rates and short- and long-term graft complications are compared for the two techniques.

In most large series, the 30-day mortality rate for surgical repair is 3% to 5%.[6] Early surgical complications of arterial thrombosis, anastomotic rupture or bleeding, peripheral emboli, and limb loss are rare at centers with experience (1% to 3%). In a recent 36-year population-based study of late graft complications, the 1-, 3-, and 5-year rates of survival free of graft complications were 97%, 95%, and 93%, respectively.[39] Further, the incidence of long-term complications is very low but includes anastomotic pseudoaneurysm (3%), graft thrombosis (2%), aortoenteric fistula (1.6%), graft infection (1.3%), anastomotic hemorrhage (1.3%), colonic ischemia (0.7%), and atheroembolism (0.3%).

The 30-day mortality rates for stent graft repairs are similar (3%) to those for standard surgical repair. However, for patients at high risk, mortality rates have been as high as 10% to 13%. The most common early complications include groin hematoma (6% to 7%), arterial thrombosis (2% to 3%), iliac artery rupture (1% to 1.5%), and thromboemboli (1% to 2%).

Although long-term follow-up is limited, the most common long-term problem is endoleak. An endoleak involves persistent filling of the aneurysm from either an anastomotic site or collateral blood vessels, most commonly caused by persistent bleeding from lumbar or inferior mesenteric artery branches in the AAA sac. Endoleaks occur in about one third of cases. Endoleaks close spontaneously in more than 50% of cases by 6 to 12 months after the procedure. Secondary catheter-based reinterventions are required to close an additional 10%. Surgical intervention has been required to treat 2% to 3% of long-term leaks. Aneurysm rupture occurs in 1% of patients within 1 to 2 years. Other common late complications include severe graft kinking (2%), graft migration (2%), and graft thrombosis (3%).

INDICATIONS FOR REFERRAL/HOSPITALIZATION

Patients with an AAA of ≥4.0 cm should be referred to a vascular surgeon. Recent evidence suggests that outcomes for open repair of intact AAA are better at large, urban institutions.[40] Therefore referral to a center with a vascular service experienced in treating AAAs is indicated with elective repairs. Using ultrasound examination, the vascular surgeon monitors expansion of aneurysms of ≤4.5 cm every year and every 6 months for patients with aneurysms of ≥4.5 cm. Although elective repair is usually considered when the AAA enlarges into the range of 5 to 6 cm, repair of smaller aneurysms may occur if the patient cannot commit to the surveillance program. Rapid expansion beyond 10% of the diameter per year is also an indication for surgical repair. Finally, repair may be delayed until the diameter is ≥6 cm in poor-risk patients.

If the aneurysm enlarges and is being considered for repair, a thin-slice CT scan may be performed for evaluation for stent graft placement. However, indications for stent grafting versus standard surgical repair have not yet been fully elucidated. Because the long-term outcomes of stent grafts are unknown, stent grafts are often reserved for older patients with limited life expectancy or for patients with other significant medical comorbidity for open surgical repair.

PATIENT EDUCATION

During the period of surveillance of small aneurysms, patient education addresses modification of risk factors such as hypertension, smoking, and diabetes to slow AAA expansion; protocols for surveillance; options for elective treatment; indications for emergent evaluation; and surveillance of first-degree relatives. During the periprocedural phase, patient education focuses on the trajectory of care, including length of hospital stay, and postdischarge recovery, including of the care of the incision or catheterization site, resuming usual activities of daily living (ADLs), and long-term monitoring of graft patency and prevention or detection of subsequent aneurysms.

Hypertension and cigarette smoking are critical risk factors for expansion of AAA. Although beta blockade with propranolol has not demonstrated a significant difference in the rate of expansion of small AAA or the need for surgery, treatment with beta blockers continues because of its effect on reducing coronary events.[41,42] Smoking cessation is likely to occur in only 15% to 25% of smokers.

The frequency of surveillance varies depending on the size of the aneurysm at the most recent ultrasonographic study. Patients must commit to serial ultrasonographic examinations or consider early repair of a small aneurysm with the inherent risks and benefits of open surgical or endovascular repair.

Physicians and surgeons should describe both the standard open surgical procedure and endovascular stent graft procedure. The explanation should include early and late results of both types of procedures to inform the patient and assist in decision making.

After the detection of AAA, patients should be counseled to report the new-onset symptoms of aneurysmal enlargement, such as abdominal or back pain, to their vascular surgeon. Symptoms of impending rupture, requiring immediate emergency care, include severe abdominal, flank, or back pain unrelieved by position change. The abdominal pain may be characterized as deep, boring, or tearing. Low back pain may be dull, radiating to the legs, similar to musculoskeletal pain. The flank pain may radiate to the groin and be associated with hematuria.

Strong evidence suggests a genetic predisposition to AAA.[43,44] Approximately 20% of patients with AAA will have a first-degree relative with AAA, suggesting the importance of annual ultrasonographic screening after age 50 in these family members. This is most applicable to male siblings, who appear to be at highest risk.

REFERENCES

1. Johnston KW and others: Suggested methods for reporting on arterial aneurysms, *J Vasc Surg* 13:452-458, 1991.
2. Hallett JW: Abdominal aortic aneurysm: natural history and treatment, *Heart Dis Stroke* 1:303-308, 1992.
3. Greenhalgh RM, Mannick JA, editors: *The care and management of aneurysms,* London, 1990, WB Saunders.
4. Hallett J: Management of abdominal aortic aneurysms, *Mayo Clin Proc* 75:395-399, 2000.
5. Gillum RF: Epidemiology of aortic aneurysm in the United States, *J Clin Epidemiol* 48:1289-1298, 1995.
6. Zarins C and others: AneuRx stent graft versus open surgical repair of abdominal aortic aneurysms: multi-center prospective clinical trial, *J Vasc Surg* 29:292-308, 1999.
7. Lindholt JS and others: Natural history of abdominal aortic aneurysm with and without coexisting chronic obstructive pulmonary disease, *J Vasc Surg* 28:226-233, 1998.
8. Brunelli T and others: High prevalence of mild hyperhomocysteinemia in patients with abdominal aortic aneurysm, *J Vasc Surg* 32:531-536, 2000.
9. Marian AJ: On genetics, inflammation, and abdominal aortic aneurysms: can single nucleotide polymorphisms predict the outcome? *Circulation* 1103:2222, 2001.
10. Thompson MM, Bell PR: ABC of arterial and venous disease. Arterial aneurysms, *Br Med J* 320:1193-1196, 2000.
11. Fink HA and others: The accuracy of physical examination to detect abdominal aortic aneurysm, *Arch Intern Med* 160:833-836, 2000.
12. Hallett JW: What imaging studies does the surgeon really need before abdominal aortic aneurysm repair? In Abbott WM, editor: *Proceedings of current issues in vascular surgery,* Boston, 1999, Division of Vascular Surgery.
13. Vignati JJ and others: The role of preoperative imaging studies in the evaluation of asymptomatic and symptomatic abdominal aortic aneurysms. In Perler BA, Becker GJ, editors: *Vascular intervention: a clinical approach,* New York, 1997, Theime.
14. Ketterling M: Abdominal aortic aneurysm. Patients at peril, *Clin Rev* 11:59-64, 2001.
15. Cronenwett JL and others: Variables that affect the expansion rate and outcomes of small abdominal aortic aneurysms, *J Vasc Surg* 11: 260-269, 1996
16. Reed WW and others: Learning from the last ultrasound: a population-based study of patients with abdominal aortic aneurysm, *Arch Intern Med* 157:2064-2068, 1997.
17. UK Small Aneurysm Trial Participants: Mortality results for randomized controlled trial of early elective surgery or ultrasonographic surveillance for small abdominal aortic aneurysms, *Lancet* 352: 1649-1655, 1998.
18. Lederle FA and others: Design of abdominal aortic aneurysm detection and management (ADAM) study, *J Vasc Surg* 20:296-303, 1994.
19. Plecha FR and others: The early results of vascular surgery in patients 75 years of age and older: an analysis of 3259 cases, *J Vasc Surg* 2:769-774, 1985.
20. Goldman L: Cardiac risks and complications of non-cardiac surgery, *Ann Intern Med* 98:504-513, 1983.
21. Ashton CM and others: The incidence of perioperative myocardial infarction in men undergoing noncardiac surgery, *Ann Intern Med* 118:504-510, 1993.
22. Roger VL and others: Influence of coronary artery disease on morbidity and mortality after abdominal aortic aneurysmectomy: a population-based study. 1971-1978, *J Am Coll Cardiol* 14:1245-1252, 1989.
23. Eagle KA and others: ACC/AHA guideline update for perioperative cardiovascular evaluation for noncardiac surgery: a report of the American College of Cardiologists/American Heart Association Task Force on Practice Guidelines (Committee to Update 1996 Guidelines on Preoperative Cardiovascular Evaluation for Noncardiac Surgery), 2002, American College of Cardiology Website. Retrieved August 12, 2002, from the World Wide Web: http:/www.acc.org/clinical/guidelines/perio/dirIndex.htm.
24. Hlatky MA and others: A brief self-administered questionnaire to determine functional capacity (the Duke Activity Status Index), *Am J Cardiol* 64:651-654, 1989.
25. Fletcher GF and others: Exercise standards. A statement for healthcare professional from the American Heart Association Writing Group, *Circulation* 91:580-615, 1995.
26. Cambria RP and others: Transperitoneal versus retroperitoneal approach for aortic reconstruction: a randomized prospective study, *J Vasc Surg* 11:314-325, 1990.
27. Parodi JC and others: Transfemoral intraluminal graft implantation for abdominal aortic aneurysms, *Ann Vasc Surg* 5:491-499, 1991.
28. Marin and others: Initial experience with transluminally placed endovascular grafts for treatment of complex vascular lesions, *Ann Surg* 222:449-469, 1995.
29. Edwards WH and others: Endovascular grafting of abdominal aortic aneurysms: a preliminary study, *Ann Surg* 223:568-575, 1996.
30. Moore WS and others: Transfemoral endovascular repair of abdominal aortic aneurysm: results of the North American EVT phase I trial, *J Vasc Surg* 23:543-553, 1996.
31. Chuter TAM and others: Clinical experience with a bifurcated endovascular graft for abdominal aortic aneurysm repair, *J Vasc Surg* 24:655-666, 1996.
32. Brewster DC: How well does endovascular AAA repair work? seven-year MGH experience. In Abbott WM, editor: *Proceedings of vascular and endovascular surgery,* Boston, 2001, Division of Vascular Surgery.
33. Brewster DC and others: Initial experience with endovascular aneurysm repair: comparison of early results with outcome of conventional open repair, *J Vasc Surg* 27:992-1005, 1998.
34. May J and others: Endovascular treatment of infrarenal abdominal aortic aneurysms, *Ann Vasc Surg* 12:391-395, 1998.
35. Ohki T, Veith FJ: Endovascular grafts and other image-guided catheter-based adjuncts to improve the treatment of ruptured aortoiliac aneurysms, *Ann Surg* 232:466-479, 2000.

36. Yusuf SW and others: Emergency endovascular repair of leaking aortic aneurysm, *Lancet* 344:1645, 1994.
37. Greenberg RK and others: An endoluminal method of hemorrhage control and repair of ruptured abdominal aortic aneurysms, *J Endovasc Ther* 7:1-7, 2000.
38. Cherr G and others: Survival of young patients after abdominal aortic aneurysm repair, *J Vasc Surg* 35:94-99, 2002.
39. Hallett JW and others: Graft-related complications after abdominal aortic aneurysm repair: reassurance from a 36-year population-based experience, *J Vasc Surg* 25:277-284, 1997.
40. Huber TS and others: Experience in the United States with abdominal aortic aneurysm repair, *J Vasc Surg* 33:304-311, 2001.
41. Gadowski GR and others: Abdominal aortic aneurysm expansion rate: effect of size and beta-adrenergic blockade, *J Vasc Surg* 19:727-731, 1994.
42. Poldermans D and others: The effect of bisoprolol on perioperative mortality and myocardial infarction in high risk patients undergoing vascular surgery, *N Engl J Med* 341:1789-1794, 1999.
43. Johansen K, Koepsell T: Familial tendency for abdominal aortic aneurysms, *JAMA* 256:1934-1936, 1986.
44. Tilson MD, Dang C: Generalized arteriomegaly. A possible predisposition to the formation of abdominal aortic aneurysms, *Arch Surg* 116:1030-1032, 1981.

CHAPTER 127

Cardiac Arrhythmias

Cynthia Erskine Bashaw

Cardiac arrhythmias vary widely in type and causality and occur in both the presence and absence of cardiac disease. They also vary in severity from trivial to life threatening. Classification is commonly accomplished by dividing the arrhythmias into two major subsets: tachyarrhythmias, or those producing heart rates of greater than 100 beats per minute, and bradyarrhythmias, or those producing heart rates below 60 beats per minute. Arrhythmias may arise from conductive tissue anywhere within the atria, atrioventricular (AV) junction, or ventricles and are often further classified according to their place of origin. Symptoms, however, are more closely related to the ventricular rate and to the severity of underlying heart disease than to the origin of the arrhythmia.[1]

Emergency department referral/physician consultation is indicated for patients with life-threatening arrhythmias.

Physician consultation is indicated for new-onset rhythm disturbances and for arrhythmias associated with chest pain, syncope, dizziness, or treatment failure.

Tachyarrhythmias

DEFINITION/EPIDEMIOLOGY

Approximately 60% of all cardiac arrhythmias arise in or involve the atria.[2] Atrial fibrillation is the most common sustained arrhythmia encountered in clinical practice.[3] It occurs in 12% of patients over the age of 75 and in 30% of those over the age of 80.[4,5] Ventricular tachyarrhythmias, especially in the setting of serious, underlying organic cardiac disease, may predispose the patient to sudden death and increase mortality rates.[6,7] Sudden cardiac death claims more than 300,000 lives annually in the United States and accounts for 50% of cardiac deaths.[8] In the majority of cases it is caused by ventricular fibrillation preceded by ventricular tachycardia (VT).[8,9] Risk factors for sudden death include ischemia, hypertrophic or dilated cardiomyopathy, and valvular or congenital heart disease.[7] Nonsustained VT develops in up to 10% of individuals after an acute myocardial infarction (MI).[7]

PATHOPHYSIOLOGY

The three major mechanisms responsible for most tachyarrhythmias are reentry, abnormal or enhanced automaticity, and triggered activity.[1,10] Reentry accounts for 80% to 90% of tachyarrhythmias and results from changes in the transmembrane potential of cardiac cells, which serve to alter the conduction pathways and refractoriness of cell membranes.[11]

Reentry

The mechanism for reentry involves the existence of two conduction pathways with nonhomogeneous refractory periods. They are connected both proximally and distally by conductive tissue, thereby creating a potential electrical circuit. Most typically, reentry is initiated into this system by a premature beat. The premature impulse, on finding one pathway still in its refractory period, travels along the pathway, with the shorter refractory period arriving at the distal portion of the circuit just as the other pathway becomes nonrefractory. The impulse is then conducted in retrograde fashion back to the proximal portion of the loop, finding the original pathway again ready to conduct. In this manner a circus movement is established whereby a single impulse is repeatedly conducted around the reentrant circuit.[1,10,11] The impulse escapes the loop at some point within each lap and depolarizes the rest of the myocardium, thereby creating a tachyarrhythmia.[10]

Abnormal or Enhanced Automaticity

Automaticity, or the ability to depolarize spontaneously, is a property common to all cardiac cells. Normally the automatic discharge of the sinus node proceeds at a rate faster than that of the remaining cardiac tissue, thereby establishing an orderly sequence of cardiac depolarization. However, a variety of factors, including ischemia, hypoxia, electrolyte imbalances, and drug effects, may enhance the automaticity of an ectopic focus, allowing it to depolarize more rapidly than the sinus node. Repeated discharge of an ectopic focus in excess of the sinus node results in a tachyarrhythmia.[1]

Triggered Activity

Triggered activity arises as a result of afterdepolarizations, or oscillations of membrane potential that attend or follow the action potential. When these oscillations depolarize the cell to threshold potential, they cause action potentials that result in extrasystoles and tachycardia.[12] Triggered activity is thought to be the mechanism underlying the tachyarrhythmias associated with digoxin toxicity.[12,13] It may also be induced by antiarrhythmic agents and electrolyte imbalances.[12] Torsades de pointes (polymorphic VT associated with long QT intervals) is thought to be a triggered arrhythmia.[13]

CLINICAL PRESENTATION

Tachyarrhythmias may be entirely asymptomatic. Symptoms, when they do occur, are in large part related to the ventricular rate, the extent of underlying heart disease, ventricular function, and associated precipitating factors. Palpitations are the most common symptom caused by tachyarrhythmias. In patients with paroxysmal attacks, palpitations are usually regular and start and terminate abruptly. In patients with atrial fibrillation, palpitations are typically irregular and may be more sustained.[1] Extrasystoles may also cause palpitations or an awareness of isolated extra beats. The pause that follows an extrasystole may be experienced as an actual cessation of the heartbeat.[14] Other causes of palpitations include thyrotoxicosis, hypovolemia, regurgitant valvular disease, anemia, hypoglycemia, pheochromocytoma, fever, and drugs (particularly digitalis, tricyclic antidepressants [TCAs], and antiarrhythmic agents).[14] Palpitations may be a manifestation of an episode of acute anxiety.[9,14] Palpitations also commonly accompany the hot flashes of menopause.[15] Pertinent history includes the use of alcohol, tobacco, caffeine, sympathomimetics (commonly found in over-the-counter cold medicines), cocaine, theophylline, and thyroid medication because any of these may cause tachycardia and palpitations.[14] Any history of underlying heart disease and/or previous rhythm disturbance and its treatment is also relevant.

Because tachyarrhythmias tend to shorten diastole, ventricular filling is compromised, causing a drop in blood pressure, cardiac output, and coronary perfusion. Resultant symptoms may include light-headedness, dizziness, syncope, fatigue, shortness of breath, and chest pain.[16-18]

A serious tachyarrhythmia may result in hemodynamic decompensation, causing hypotension, chest pain, heart failure, change in level of consciousness, or even sudden cardiac death. It is important to assess both the arrhythmia and its tolerance by the patient to determine the degree of urgency and the appropriate setting for intervention.

PHYSICAL EXAMINATION

The general appearance of the patient, particularly color, perspiration, respiratory effort, and manifestations of anxiety, is important in evaluation of an arrhythmia. Indicators of the patient's hydration status, including skin turgor, status of mucous membranes, and orthostatic vital signs, are also relevant because dehydration and hypovolemia may cause a reflex tachycardia. Blood pressure, pulse, temperature, and assessment of the patient's mental status should accompany the initial assessment. Tachycardia with hypotension is indicative of cardiovascular compromise, requiring prompt intervention.

The chest is inspected and/or palpated for parasternal lifts, heaves, and thrills. Auscultation of the heart for rate, rhythm, and the presence of murmurs, clicks, or extra heart sounds is essential. A benign systolic ejection murmur may accompany a tachycardia, whereas a murmur of any type may be associated with an underlying valve disorder. An S3 sound may warn of impending heart failure and is a significant finding. The irregularly irregular rhythm that is the hallmark of atrial fibrillation may also be the result of multiple extrasystoles, whereas a regular tachycardia is more often associated with sinus tachycardia and other forms of supraventricular tachycardia (SVT). Alterations in pulse volume and irregularity may accompany ventricular ectopic beats, depending on the timing and force of ventricular contractions.

Assessment of the neck veins may provide information regarding atrial activity. An intermittent a wave may be observed. The a wave is absent with atrial fibrillation as atrial systole is lost. A more prominent a wave than v wave may be observed with 2:1 AV block. Cannon a waves, or forceful, irregular expansions in the jugular pulse, may occur with AV dissociation as the atria contract against closed AV valves, causing a reflux of blood to the jugular veins.[12]

As part of the assessment, the examiner auscultates the lungs for rales, wheezes, or rhonchi and inspects the legs for edema. These may be present with associated cardiac failure as an indication that the rhythm is poorly tolerated by the patient.

Other important findings include exophthalmos, an enlarged or nodular thyroid gland, or skin and hair changes commonly associated with hyperthyroidism.

DIAGNOSTICS

12-Lead Electrocardiogram

The 12-lead ECG is indicated for initial evaluation of a suspected arrhythmia. This diagnostic tool has the notable limitation of providing only a brief view of the heart's electrical activity. Although sustained rhythms may easily be captured, paroxysmal rhythms may be elusive. However, even when the rate and rhythm are normal, the resting ECG may yield valuable information about the etiology of an arrhythmia such as ventricular hypertrophy, MI, ischemia, drug effects, or electrolyte imbalance.[9] Indications of conduction abnormalities may also be present and include the widened QRS that accompanies intraventricular conduction delay; the shortened PR interval that accompanies preexcitation syndromes, such as Wolff-Parkinson-White (WPW); or the prolonged QT interval that may accompany idiopathic long QT syndrome or drug effects.[1,9,12] When abnormal rhythms are captured on the 12-lead ECG, the examiner needs to obtain a rhythm strip by allowing the tracing to continue for several minutes to fully evaluate the rhythm. With tachyarrhythmias, minor depressions of the ST segment and inversion of the T wave are commonly rate related and may be mistaken for indications of coronary disease.[14] These changes can be reevaluated once the rate is controlled.

Holter Monitoring

Continuous ambulatory ECG (Holter monitoring) is a useful option for evaluating a suspected arrhythmia when symptoms are paroxysmal in nature. Use of this portable device allows continuous recording of the heart's activity over a 24-hour period. The patient keeps a diary of activities and symptoms that can later be correlated with the tracing. For the patient with infrequent symptoms, intermittent ambulatory ECG (event recording) may be more appropriate because the device can be worn for a long period of time and is dormant until activated by the user at the onset of symptoms.[1,11]

Diagnostics

Tachyarrhythmias

Initial	**Imaging**
ECG	Echocardiography (if left ventricular dysfunction or valve disease is suspected)
Pulse oximetry	
Laboratory	**Other**
Hemoglobin/hematocrit	Event monitor
Serum electrolytes	Holter monitor
TSH	Provocative testing
Blood glucose	Valsalva's maneuver*
Digoxin level*	Carotid sinus massage*
Drug levels*	

*If indicated.

Provocative Testing/Electrophysiologic Studies

Provocative testing (e.g., the exercise ECG) may be helpful when the history suggests an arrhythmia in association with a specific activity. It is used for provocation of arrhythmias caused by ischemia or increased sympathetic activity.[1] Rhythms that put the patient at high risk for adverse events (very rapid SVT, WPW syndrome, complex ventricular ectopy, and VT) warrant referral to a specialist for electrophysiologic studies to properly identify and treat the problematic rhythm. Electrophysiologic studies may also be indicated for investigating palpitations and syncope when noninvasive techniques have failed to definitively identify the problem.[1]

Signal-Averaged Electrocardiogram

The signal-averaged ECG may also identify patients at risk for tachyarrhythmias. This technique permits identification of low-voltage signals by means of high-gain amplification of the ECG. Low-amplitude deflections at the end of the QRS complex indicate a heightened risk of ventricular tachyarrhythmias. Their presence has been used for prognostic assessment after MI, but this technique is rarely used today because of the advent and availability of electrophysiologic studies.[1]

Carotid Sinus Massage/Valsalva's Maneuver

The use of carotid sinus massage and the Valsalva maneuver may help to differentiate one rhythm from another and are important diagnostic and therapeutic tools. Diagnostically, carotid sinus massage and Valsalva maneuvers may cause transient AV block; this results in slowing of the ventricular response, enabling identification of the underlying rhythm. Therapeutically, these techniques may terminate rhythms for which the AV node is part of the reentry circuit, such as in AV nodal reentry tachycardia.[12]

Other Diagnostics

Diagnostics, when appropriate, might include a hemoglobin level to determine the presence of anemia, electrolytes to exclude hypokalemia and other electrolyte disturbances, a thyroid-stimulating hormone (TSH) level if hyperthyroidism is suspected, a blood glucose determination if hypoglycemia is suspected, and a drug level for patients being treated with digoxin or other medications that might cause arrhythmia. Echocardiography may be indicated when hypertrophy or valvular disease is suspected as an associated condition.

DIFFERENTIAL DIAGNOSIS

Narrow QRS Tachycardia

Any rhythm with a QRS of 0.12 second or less is termed supraventricular, having originated at or above the AV node. The rhythms in the following paragraphs are included in this group and are described as they appear on the ECG.

Sinus Tachycardia

In sinus tachycardia there is a P wave preceding each QRS in a consistent 1:1 relationship. The rhythm is regular, the P waves are identical, the QRS complexes are normal and narrow, and the PR and QRS intervals are within normal ranges. The rate is over 100 beats per minute (Figure 127-1).

Premature Atrial Contractions

Premature atrial contractions (PACs) do not, in and of themselves, constitute a tachyarrhythmia but are important in that they may initiate a tachyarrhythmia in the susceptible heart. Also, if they are numerous, they may cause the patient to complain of palpitations or a skipped or extra beat.[14] They are typically identified on the ECG within a prevailing sinus rhythm, which would be completely regular were it not for the premature beats. The PAC is a normal-looking beat in every way except that it occurs prematurely. Because its origin is outside the sinus node, the P wave, although normal, may appear different from the P waves of the prevailing rhythm. Because it is premature, the P wave may be buried or appear as a notch in the previous T wave. The PR interval may differ slightly from that of the prevailing rhythm, although it remains within the normal range. Because the beat depolarizes the sinus node, there is typically a partially compensatory pause before the next sinus beat (Figure 127-2).

Differential Diagnosis

Tachyarrhythmias

Narrow Complex	Wide Complex
Sinus tachycardia	Supraventricular tachycardia with aberrancy
Multifocal atrial tachycardia	Ventricular tachycardia
Paroxysmal atrial tachycardia	Ventricular fibrillation
AV nodal reentry tachycardia	
AV reciprocating tachycardia	
Atrial flutter	
Atrial fibrillation	
Premature atrial contractions	
Premature junctional contractions	

Premature Junctional Contractions

Premature junctional contractions (PJCs) are another cause of irregularity in the heart rhythm. Also known as ectopic atrial contractions, PJCs are premature beats that originate in the AV node. They do not constitute a tachyarrhythmia but, like PACs, may initiate one in the susceptible heart. Because the impulse is carried to the ventricles along normal pathways, the resultant QRS is narrow and appears similar to the QRS complexes of the sinus rhythm. There may be retrograde conduction to the atria, yielding a P wave that can occur before, during, or after the QRS. If the P wave occurs before the QRS complex, the PR interval is less than 0.12 second. When a P wave is visible, it is typically negative in leads II, III, and aVF.[12]

Multifocal Atrial Tachycardia

In multifocal atrial tachycardia, the heart rate is usually 100 to 130 beats per minute, and the rhythm is irregular. The P waves have three or more different morphologies. The PP interval and the PR interval will be variable. This rhythm is usually seen in older patients with pulmonary, cardiovascular, or metabolic disturbances.

Paroxysmal Supraventricular Tachycardia

Paroxysmal supraventricular tachycardia (PSVT) is a rapid (rate of 140 to 240 beats per minute), generally regular rhythm that is typically initiated by a single beat and starts and stops abruptly. P waves may differ slightly in morphology compared with the sinus rhythm. The QRS is most typically narrow. P and QRS waves may exist in a 1:1 relationship, or variable AV block may alter this relationship. If the rate is very fast, P

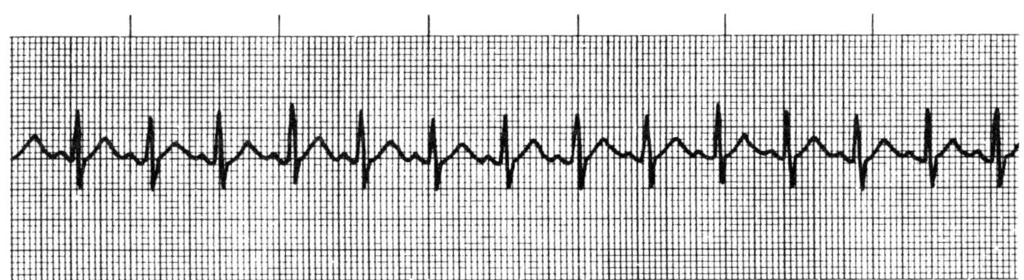

FIGURE 127-1

Sinus tachycardia. (From Andreoli KG and others: *Comprehensive cardiac care*, ed 2, St Louis, 1971, Mosby.)

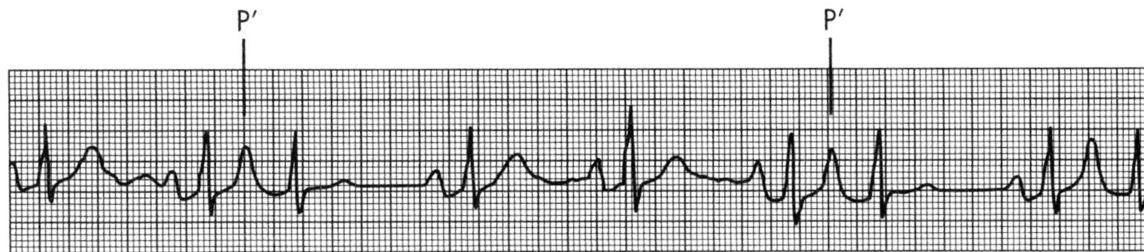

FIGURE 127-2

Premature atrial complexes hidden in T waves (lead II). (From Conover MB: *Understanding electrocardiography*, ed 7, St Louis, 1996, Mosby.)

waves may be buried in the previous beat. Paroxysmal atrial tachycardia (PAT), particularly PAT with block, is often associated with digoxin toxicity.[12]

Atrioventricular Nodal Reentry Tachycardia

In AV nodal reentry tachycardia (AVNRT), the most common mechanism for PSVT, there are dual pathways within the AV node that are responsible for the circus conduction. P waves, when they are visible, exist in a 1:1 relationship with the QRS. Often, in very fast rhythms, they are buried within the QRS and either are not visible or are seen as a distortion at the end of the QRS complex. This distortion appears as a pseudo-S wave in leads II, III, and aVF and/or a pseudo-r′ wave in lead V_1.[12,19] The rate is usually 140 to 180 beats per minute and regular. The QRS is narrow and morphologically similar to that of the sinus rhythm. It is typically paroxysmal in nature and will terminate with the Valsalva maneuver or carotid sinus massage.

Atrioventricular Reentry Tachycardia

With AV reentry tachycardia (AVNT), the reentry is because of an accessory pathway between the atria and ventricles that bypasses the AV node. This mechanism is responsible for preexcitation syndromes such as Lown-Ganong-Levine syndrome and WPW syndrome. Typically there is a short PR interval. The QRS may be normal or wide. In WPW a delta wave, which is a slurred upstroke at the beginning of the QRS, may be seen. In orthodromic tachycardia, the impulse is conducted first down the AV pathway and then back up via the accessory pathway. A narrow QRS results. In antidromic tachycardia the impulse conducts first down the accessory pathway and then back up through the AV pathway. The result is a wide QRS. Reentrant rhythms conducted in this manner tend to be very fast because of the shorter refractory period of the accessory pathway.[9]

Atrial Flutter

In atrial flutter the atrial rate ranges from 250 to 350 beats per minute, producing a sawtooth appearance of the P waves. The atrial rate of 300 beats per minute usually has a 2:1 conduction to the ventricle, producing a QRS rate of 150 beats per minute.

Atrial Fibrillation

Atrial fibrillation has the normal P wave replaced by fibrillatory f waves, producing a wavy baseline. The atrial rate is estimated to be between 350 and 650 beats per minute. There is an irregularly irregular ventricular response because the AV node will allow only a fraction of the atrial impulses to reach the ventricle (Figure 127-3).

Wide QRS Tachycardia

A QRS that is greater than 0.12 second may be SVT with aberrancy (a wide QRS produced by a refractory block of one of the bundle branches as the rapid impulses from the atria attempt to depolarize the ventricles), VT, or ventricular fibrillation. Differentiation between VT and SVT with aberrant conduction is often challenging but critical because treatment approaches differ significantly depending on the origin of the arrhythmia. A combination of leads is superior to one lead in making this differentiation.[20]

Supraventricular Tachycardia

In SVT with aberrancy, the QRS is greater than 0.12 second wide but typically not greater than 0.14 second. Often a triphasic RSR′ right bundle branch pattern is seen in lead V_1. Because of the fast ventricular rate, the P wave may be buried in the previous beat or may present as a peaked or notched T wave in the previous beat. Carotid sinus massage may slow (and hence yield a 1:1 relationship of the P to the QRS) or even terminate the tachycardia.

Ventricular Tachycardia

VT is defined as three or more consecutive ventricular ectopic beats. The rhythm may be sustained or nonsustained, lasting more than or less than 30 seconds, respectively. The QRS width is greater than 0.12 second and often is greater than 0.14 second. It is usually fairly regular with a rate between 100 and 300 beats per minute. The most reliable criterion for correctly diagnosing VT is AV dissociation. P waves may be seen as distortions at different points in the ECG cycle. These are independent P waves that bear no relationship to the QRS. Other indicators that favor a diagnosis of VT over SVT are a QRS greater than 0.14 second; extreme right-axis deviation between (180 and −90); concordance of the QRS pattern in all precordial leads (i.e., all positive or all negative deflections), particularly when concordance is negative; and a wide QRS pattern inconsistent with typical right or left bundle branch patterns.[12,13] This rhythm will not respond to carotid sinus massage (Figure 127-4).

Torsades de Pointes

The QRS morphology of VT may be uniform (monomorphic VT) or variable (polymorphic VT). A specific type of VT, torsades de pointes, deserves mention because the pharmacologic treatment for this disorder differs markedly from standard treatment for VT. Torsades de pointes is characterized by polymorphic QRS complexes that change in amplitude and cycle length.

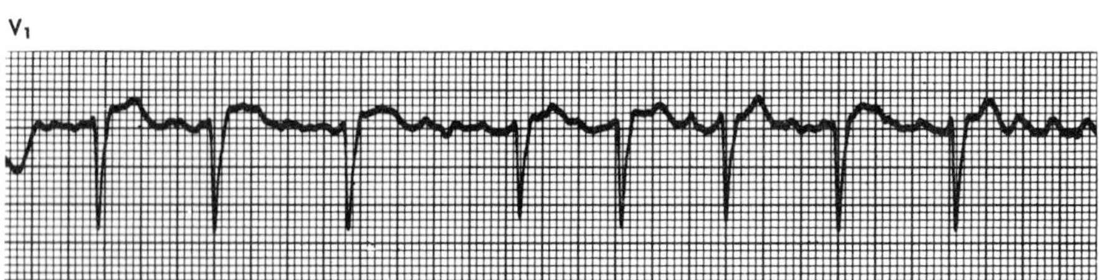

FIGURE 127-3

Atrial fibrillation. (From Conover MB: *Cardiac arrhythmias: exercises in pattern interpretations*, St Louis, 1974, Mosby.)

It is associated with QT prolongation, which may be idiopathic or related to drug effects (antiarrhythmic agents of class Ia, IIc, and III; TCAs; and phenothiazines) or electrolyte imbalances (particularly hypokalemia or hypomagnesemia).[12,13]

Ventricular Fibrillation

Ventricular fibrillation is a rapid, disorganized electrical activity within the ventricles with no discrete QRS complexes. The heart is unable to contract, and the patient is in cardiac arrest.

Premature Ventricular Contractions

Premature ventricular contractions (PVCs) are extra premature beats that originate in the ventricle. They are characterized by wide (>0.12 second), bizarre QRS complexes that interrupt the prevailing rhythm. The P wave is typically absent, and the beat is most often followed by a full compensatory pause (the distance from the QRS preceding the PVC to the QRS that follows it is equal to twice the RR interval of the prevailing sinus rhythm). Typically, the T wave deflection is in opposition to that of the QRS complex.[11] Their description is included here because of their association with ventricular tachyarrhythmias (Figure 127-5).

MANAGEMENT

Antiarrhythmic drugs have limited efficacy and a high propensity to produce serious side effects, including life-threatening arrhythmias. Results of clinical trials, such as the Cardiac Arrhythmia Suppression Trials (CAST I and CAST II), which demonstrated an increase in mortality in all treatment groups (patients with asymptomatic ventricular dysfunction after acute MI treated with encainide, flecainide, or moricizine) compared with a placebo group, have emphasized the need to critically analyze the need for antiarrhythmia therapy.[21] The concept of proarrhythmia, or antiarrhythmic agents inducing the very arrhythmias they are used to suppress, has radically altered antiarrhythmic therapy. The two general conditions for which antiarrhythmic therapy is appropriate are a potentially life-threatening arrhythmia and an arrhythmia that is significantly symptomatic.[9,10] The treatment of serious, recurrent, or potentially life-threatening arrhythmias generally requires referral to a cardiologist for aggressive management, possibly involving guided drug therapy based on electrophysiologic study results or electrical (implantable cardioverter-defibrillators [ICDs]) or surgical (ablation) intervention.[1,10]

With these general principles in mind, the following discussion reviews general approaches to each arrhythmia. Pharmacologic agents are further outlined in Table 127-1.

For patients with atrial tachyarrhythmias who are hemodynamically unstable, immediate synchronized cardioversion may be recommended. Cardioversion is successful in 85% to 90% of cases.[4,16,18] Acute management may also be accomplished with the IV administration of adenosine, calcium channel blockers, or beta blockers.[9]

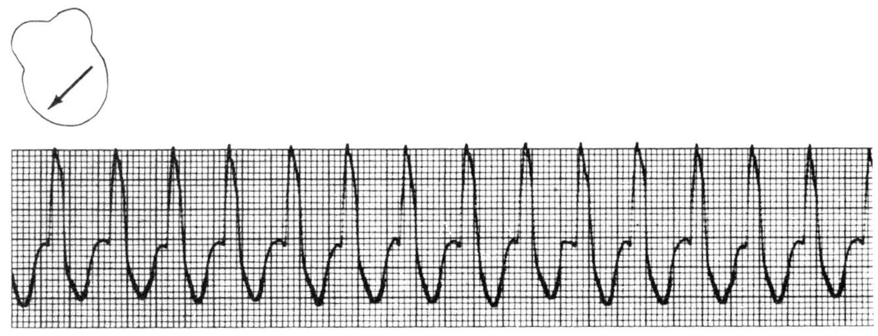

FIGURE 127-4

Ventricular tachycardia. (From Conover MB: *Understanding electrocardiography*, ed 5, St Louis, 1988, Mosby.)

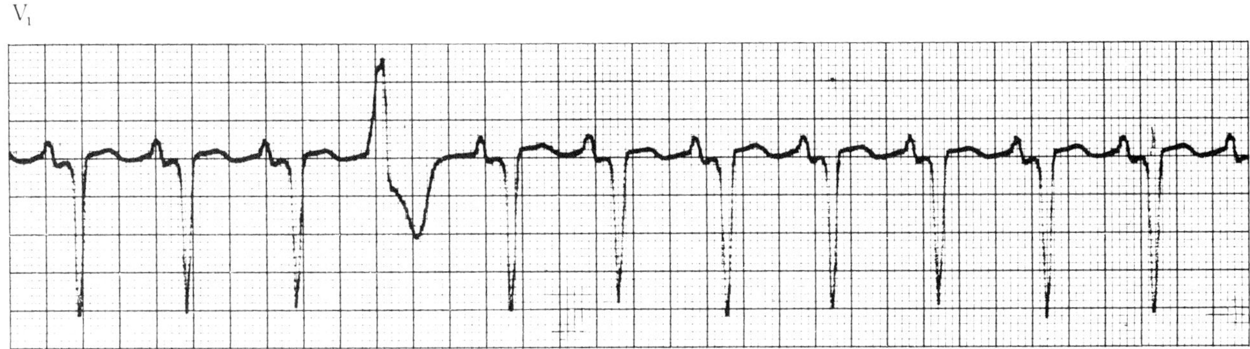

FIGURE 127-5

Premature ventricular contractions. (From Conover MB: *Pocket guide to electrocardiography*, ed 3, St Louis, 1994, Mosby.)

TABLE 127-1 Pharmacologic Arrhythmia Management

Agent	Dose	Cautions
CLASS I AGENTS*		
IA		
Procainamide	IV: 20 mg/min; maximum: 15 mg/kg PO: 750-1250 mg q 6 hr	GI upset, hypotension, widening of QRS, lupuslike syndrome, anorexia, rash, proarrhythmia
Quinidine	IV: 6-10 mg/kg; rate of 0.4-0.5 mg/kg/min PO: 200-400 mg q 6 hr	GI upset, diarrhea, cinchonism, fever, rash, proarrhythmia, anorexia, tinnitus, increased digoxin and warfarin levels
IB		
Lidocaine	IV: 1-1.5 mg/kg; total: 3 mg/kg	Drowsiness, paresthesia, muscle twitching, lack of orientation, convulsions
IC		
Flecainide	PO: 100-200 mg q 12 hr	Proarrhythmia, decreased left ventricular function, dizziness, visual disturbances, dyspnea, headache, nausea, fatigue, palpitation, chest pain, tremor, constipation; to be avoided in AV block or left ventricular dysfunction
Propafenone	PO: 150-300 mg q 8-12 hr	Proarrhythmia, unusual taste, dizziness, AV block, intraventricular conduction defect, constipation, headache, diplopia, fatigue; to be avoided in severe congestive heart failure (CHF), AV block, or chronic obstructive pulmonary disease (COPD)
CLASS II AGENTS†		
Esmolol	IV: 500 μg/kg/min over 5-min load; 50-200 μg/Kg/min infusion	Nausea, vomiting, diarrhea, fatigue, weakness, CHF, hallucinations, insomnia, gait disturbance, mental status change, conduction abnormality, exacerbation of asthma; all beta blockers to be avoided in bronchospasm, CHF, and hypotension
Metoprolol	IV: 5 mg IV push q 5 min up to 15 mg PO: 50-450 mg/day in divided doses	
Propranolol	IV: 2 mg IV push; maximum: 0.1 mg/kg PO: 20-160 mg q 6 hr	
CLASS III AGENTS‡		
Sotalol	PO: 80-320 mg q 12 hr	Prolongation of QT, proarrhythmia, nausea, vomiting, dry mouth, diarrhea, retroperitoneal fibrosis, depression, fatigue, impotence, headache, bradycardia, AV block
d-Sotalol	PO: 100-400 mg q 12 hr	
Amiodarone	IV: 150 mg over 10- to 30-min load; 1 mg/min × 6 hr; 0.5 mg/min up to 1 g/day PO: 800-1600 mg/day for 3-14 days; 100-400 mg/day maintenance	Corneal microdeposits, photosensitivity, liver/lung toxicity, hypothyroidism, pulmonary fibrosis, proarrhythmia, AV block, increase in warfarin or digoxin levels, skin discoloration, prolonged elimination (half-life: 60 days)
Ibutilide	IV: 1 mg over 10 min, repeat ×1 in 10 min; 0.01 mg/kg for patient <60 kg	Proarrhythmia, AV block, bradycardia, nausea, headache
Bretylium	IV: 5-10 mg/kg up to 30 mg; infuse 1-2 mg/min	Hypotension, nausea, vomiting, bradycardia, initial catecholamine release with increase in heart rate/blood pressure
CLASS IV AGENTS§		
Verapamil	IV: 0.075-0.15 mg/kg over 2 min PO: 120-480 mg/day	Contraindicated in WPW, sick sinus syndrome, excess beta blocker, procainamide, quinidine, or digoxin
Diltiazem	IV: 0.25-0.35 mg/kg over 2 min; 5-15 mg/hr constant × 24 hours PO: 120-480 mg/day	CHF, hypotension, nausea, edema, fatigue, conduction abnormalities, pain at injection site
MISCELLANEOUS AGENTS		
Adenosine	IV: 6- to 12-mg bolus	Facial flushing, dyspnea, chest pain, nausea, headache, light-headedness, bronchospasm
Digoxin	IV: 0.5-1 mg/24 hr in divided doses PO: 0.125-0.375 mg/day	Interactions with other agents (requiring reduction of digoxin), anorexia, nausea, vomiting, diarrhea, constipation, visual disturbances, psychiatric disturbances, all types of arrhythmias
Magnesium	IV: 1- to 2-g load over 1-2 min; 0.5-1 g/hr infusion	AV block, hypotension, flushing, sweating, depressed reflexes, respiratory paralysis, diarrhea
Epinephrine	IV: 1 mg every 3-5 min; 0.1 mg/kg for high dose	Ischemia with increased ventricular ectopy
Atropine	IV: 0.5-1 mg every 5 min; maximum: 0.04 mg/kg	Tachycardia, delirium, flushed/hot skin, ataxia, blurred vision, ischemia

*Depress automaticity, increase refractoriness, and inhibit sodium channels.
†Beta-blocking effects.
‡Prolong the action potential and interfere with potassium-dependent repolarizing currents.
§Block inward calcium channels of SA and AV node.

Sinus Tachycardia

Sinus tachycardia is treated by removal or treatment of the underlying cause (e.g., fever, hypovolemia, hyperthyroidism, anxiety). Elimination of tobacco, alcohol, caffeine, or sympathomimetics (such as those found in over-the-counter cold medications and nose drops) may result in a return to normal heart rate.[12] Patients with inappropriate sinus tachycardia may be considered for radiofrequency ablation.[9]

PACs do not usually require treatment, but the cause may be investigated, particularly when the patient is aware of and bothered by them. In normal individuals PACs may be a result of various stimuli, including tobacco, alcohol, and caffeine. Their occurrence may diminish or disappear when these stimuli are withdrawn. PACs are also associated with ischemia, hypokalemia and hypomagnesemia, hypoxia, and myocardial stretch in early congestive heart failure. Correction of the underlying cause may halt the PACs.[12]

PJCs are not usually treated. If they initiate a tachyarrhythmia, treatment is directed toward controlling that rhythm.[12]

Multifocal Atrial Tachycardia

Multifocal atrial tachycardia occurs primarily in older patients with co-morbid disease. Sixty percent of these patients have significant pulmonary disease.[12,22] The diagnosis often occurs in the setting of congestive heart failure, exacerbation of the underlying pulmonary condition, or electrolyte imbalance. As with sinus tachycardia, therapy is directed at correcting the precipitating factor (e.g., improving oxygenation, correcting electrolyte imbalance).[12]

Paroxysmal Supraventricular Tachycardia

Most cases of PSVT are reentrant and amenable to radiofrequency ablation when symptoms are significant and recurrent. Ablation is most often preferable to antiarrhythmic agents because of safety and tolerability concerns.[9] Pharmacologically, narrow-complex PSVT is treated by slowing AV conduction with digoxin, calcium channel blockers, or beta blockers and/or by suppressing atrial automaticity with class Ia, Ic, or III antiarrhythmic agents. An important cause of PAT is digoxin toxicity. A patient taking digoxin who has PAT should be assumed to be digoxin toxic until it has been proved otherwise.[12]

Wide-complex PSVT must be managed with care in conjunction with a cardiologist. Radiofrequency ablation is the treatment of choice. If pharmacologic management is instituted, care must be exercised because agents that increase the refractoriness of the AV node (digoxin, calcium channel blockers, and beta blockers), when used alone, may decrease the refractoriness of the accessory pathway and have the potential to cause a faster ventricular rate. Class Ia, Ic, and III agents are preferred because they increase the refractoriness of the bypass tract. In long-term therapy, these agents are sometimes used in combination with agents that increase the refractoriness of the AV node.

Atrial Fibrillation/Atrial Flutter

Management of the patient with atrial fibrillation/atrial flutter may be challenging because the best approach is often not clear and treatment must be highly individualized. The three therapeutic goals are rate control, restoration and maintenance of sinus rhythm, and prevention of thromboembolism. The risks and benefits of each treatment must be considered for each patient.[3]

Because atrial fibrillation and atrial flutter are often related to an underlying disease process, treatment of these arrhythmias must include a search for a cause. Common causes include rheumatic heart disease, mitral valve disease, hypertension (particularly with left ventricular hypertrophy), coronary heart disease, cardiomyopathy, hyperthyroidism, acute alcohol intoxication or withdrawal, stimulant ingestion (caffeine, amphetamines, theophylline), and acute pulmonary disease.[3,10]

A major decision to be made in treating atrial fibrillation is whether to attempt to restore and maintain sinus rhythm or to opt merely for ventricular rate control. Reasons for opting for restoration and maintenance of sinus rhythm include symptom relief, prevention of embolism, and prevention of cardiomyopathy. Cardioversion can be accomplished via either electrical or pharmacologic means. Direct current (DC) cardioversion is more effective but carries with it the need for sedation or anesthesia. Pharmacologic cardioversion is most effective when initiated within 7 days after the onset of atrial fibrillation. Side effects and proarrhythmia are concerns. Flecainide, ibutilide, propafenone, amiodarone, and quinidine are the drugs of choice. Procainamide, sotalol, and digoxin may also be used. Both electrical and pharmacologic cardioversion carry the risk of thromboembolism.[3] When the rhythm has been sustained for longer than 48 hours, anticoagulation for 3 weeks before and 4 weeks after elective cardioversion is necessary.[16,18,23] A transesophageal echocardiogram may also be obtained before cardioversion to exclude the presence of atrial thrombus.[9]

Without continuous antiarrhythmic therapy, 80% of patients who attain sinus rhythm relapse within 1 year after cardioversion and 50% relapse even when treated with antiarrhythmic drugs.[3,9,10] Unfortunately, the medications used to maintain sinus rhythm in the setting of atrial fibrillation are proarrhythmic and introduce an element of risk to pharmacologic intervention, particularly when there is underlying heart disease. One major consideration in determining treatment is the patient's tolerance of the lost atrial contraction that accompanies atrial fibrillation. Loss of AV synchrony and the irregularity of the ventricular rhythm both contribute to a decline in cardiac output that has been estimated to be about 15%.[3] Although patients without serious underlying disease may be able to tolerate this reduction without difficulty, a patient with limited cardiac reserve may decompensate quickly. The presence of mitral stenosis, restrictive or hypertrophic cardiomyopathy, pericardial disease, or ventricular hypertrophy increases the likelihood of hemodynamic deterioration with the onset of atrial fibrillation.[3] When the loss of atrial contraction is not as critical and the patient is hemodynamically stable, the decision is less obvious. Neither conversion to and maintenance of sinus rhythm nor rate control is clearly superior.[3] Information should be provided regarding the relative efficacy and potential side effects of antiarrhythmic agents. The duration of atrial fibrillation is an important determinant of success: the longer a patient experiences atrial fibrillation, the lower are the odds of maintaining sinus rhythm. The odds are very low, for instance, after 3 months of atrial fibrillation.[10]

Drugs that are used in the maintenance of sinus rhythm include those from class 1a (e.g., procainamide, quinidine), 1c (e.g., flecainide, propafenone), and III (e.g., sotalol, amiodarone).[3]

Rate control is easier to achieve and is an acceptable goal in hemodynamically stable patients. Digoxin, beta blockers, and calcium channel blockers are the drugs of choice. Amiodarone may also be used.[3]

Patients with preexcitation syndromes who have episodic atrial fibrillation or flutter require electrophysiologic testing because they are at risk for sudden death. Radiofrequency ablation is recommended.

Thromboembolism is a major complication of recurrent or persistent atrial fibrillation. One third of these patients eventually experience strokes, of which 75% are thought to be embolic.[3] Anticoagulation greatly reduces this risk. Anticoagulation, when indicated, is accomplished with warfarin to maintain the international normalized ratio (INR) between 2 and 3 (see Chapter 232). For those who cannot take anticoagulants, aspirin 325 mg/day is an acceptable but less effective alternative.[3] Anticoagulation in low-risk patients, those younger than 60 years of age without heart disease, is generally not indicated. For those younger than 60 with heart disease but no other thromboembolic risks and for those 60 years old or older with no heart disease or other thromboembolic risk, anticoagulation may be accomplished with aspirin as mentioned. For all others, warfarin is preferred if not contraindicated because of other factors.[3]

Finally, those with problematic or refractory atrial fibrillation may be candidates for nonpharmacologic approaches, including the surgical MAZE procedure, which has been shown to be useful in controlling the tachyarrhythmia that occurs with atrial fibrillation.[3,24]

Premature Ventricular Contractions

PVCs occur in both normal and diseased hearts. In the normal heart PVCs are of no prognostic significance, and in the absence of severe symptomatology they require no treatment. However, complex ventricular ectopy (defined as >0 PVCs/min over 24 hours or nonsustained VT) is rare in the normal heart, and the appearance of such should provoke an evaluation for underlying cardiac disease. The patient with cardiac disease (previous MI or depressed left ventricular ejection fraction) and complex ectopy is at increased risk for sudden death. However, antiarrhythmic therapy, although it may reduce the ectopy, has not been shown to decrease mortality; in the CAST studies, it was actually shown to increase the risk of sudden cardiac death.[10] When treatment is instituted, beta blockers are the drugs of choice.

Ventricular Tachycardia

Clinical management of nonsustained VT first includes identification and management of any underlying cause (e.g., digoxin toxicity, electrolyte imbalance, hypoxia, ischemia). In the absence of symptoms and underlying heart disease, treatment is rarely indicated. Patients with previous MI, structural heart disease, and low ejection fractions who have nonsustained VT, however, are at particularly high risk for adverse events, including sudden death. Beta blockers reduce these risks. Referral for electrophysiologic testing should be considered for this group, as well as for those with severe symptomatology.[10]

Sustained VT is typically an emergent situation requiring care at an acute care facility. Synchronized cardioversion with 100 to 360 J is indicated for VT with hemodynamic compromise. Immediate defibrillation for ventricular fibrillation or VT without a pulse is required to prevent immediate death.[25] Therapy to prevent recurrent sustained VT may include either pharmacologic management or ICDs. Those with significant left ventricular dysfunction are at particularly high risk for sudden death. Current evidence suggests that these patients are best managed with ICDs. For those with normal left ventricular function, a combination of amiodarone and a beta blocker may be used.[9] Radiofrequency ablation is appropriate for those with reentrant VT.

COMPLICATIONS, INDICATIONS FOR REFERRAL/HOSPITALIZATION, PATIENT AND FAMILY EDUCATION

See Complications, Indications for Referral/Hospitalization, and Patient and Family Education under Bradyarrhythmias.

Bradyarrhythmias

DEFINITION/EPIDEMIOLOGY

Bradyarrhythmias may result from abnormalities in conduction between the sinus node and atrium, within the AV node, and in the intraventricular conduction pathways.[26] Sinus node dysfunction is most often found in older adults as an isolated phenomenon resulting from idiopathic fibrosis.[1,26] Interruption of blood supply to the sinus node from myocardial ischemia or infiltration of the structure as a result of collagen vascular disease, sarcoid, tumors, or amyloid will cause disruption of sinus node discharge. Sinus bradycardia may occur with hypothyroidism, advanced liver disease, hypothermia, or severe hypoxia and in patients taking calcium channel blockers or beta blockers. It may also occur normally in highly trained athletes.[26]

Idiopathic fibrosis is a major cause of AV block, particularly in older adults.[1] Diseases that can influence AV conduction include MI, coronary spasm, myocarditis, rheumatic fever, mononucleosis, Lyme disease, sarcoidosis, amyloidosis, and neoplasms. Drugs such as digitalis, beta blockers, calcium channel blockers, and quinidine may also cause AV nodal conduction disturbances.[26]

Bundle branch block (BBB) may occur in the presence or absence of structural heart disease. It may be congenital or acquired, chronic or intermittent. It is often rate related and may be seen only when the heart exceeds some critical rate. Left bundle branch block (LBBB) is often a marker for ischemic heart disease, long-standing hypertension, severe aortic valve disease, or cardiomyopathy.[27]

PATHOPHYSIOLOGY

The sinus node is the cardiac conduction tissue with the highest intrinsic firing rate. It is the pacemaker of the normal heart. When sinus node discharge is suppressed or blocked by drugs or disease, bradycardia may result. The pacemaker function may be assumed by "escape" foci in the atrial tissue, the AV node, the His-Purkinje tissue, or the ventricular myocardium.

Because the intrinsic rates of these areas are slower than in the sinoatrial (SA) node, bradycardia may result.[1]

Conduction Blocks

Conduction blocks can also occur in the AV node or the His-Purkinje system. When the impulse is merely delayed, as with first-degree AV block or BBB, the heart rate may be unaffected. However, with higher degrees of block, a significant bradycardia may occur. In second-degree AV block, impulse conduction through the AV node is intermittently blocked. An adequate ventricular rate may or may not be maintained. In third-degree, or complete, heart block, there is complete failure of AV conduction, and continuing ventricular activity depends on the emergence of an escape rhythm. Depending on where the escape rhythm originates, an adequate heart rate may or may not be maintained. The higher the level in the conduction system at which the block occurs, the faster is the escape rhythm. A block within the AV node, for instance, may result in an escape rhythm fast enough to prevent syncope. If both bundle branches are blocked, the ventricular escape rhythm may be too slow to maintain an adequate cardiac output, and syncope and death may result.[1]

CLINICAL PRESENTATION

Symptoms accompanying bradycardia are largely dependent on the ventricular rate relative to metabolic demand and on the presence of underlying cardiac disease. Those with limited cardiac reserve would obviously tolerate a slow rate less well than would those with normal hearts. The American Heart Association recognizes two types of bradycardia: absolute and relative. Absolute bradycardia refers to any heart rate below 60 beats per minute. Relative bradycardia refers to a heart rate that is too slow to maintain normal blood pressure or cardiac output even if the rate is greater than 60 beats per minute.[28]

Bradycardia may be asymptomatic and may be an incidental finding on a routine ECG. In such cases it is most likely that the needs of the body are being met despite the slow heart rate. Such a finding may indicate occult disease or may merely represent the nonpathologic, physiologic sinus bradycardia that occurs in highly trained athletes. Symptomatic bradycardia is defined as a documented bradyarrhythmia that is directly responsible for the development of frank syncope or near-syncope, transient dizziness, or light-headedness and confusional states resulting from cerebral hypoperfusion attributable to a slow ventricular rate.[29] Other symptoms include fatigue, exercise intolerance, and frank congestive heart failure. These symptoms may occur at rest or with exertion.[29]

Relevant aspects of the history include a careful review of all medications, as well as the presence of any underlying cardiac disease. It is important to discern whether the symptoms occur at rest or with exertion and whether there are any outstanding aggravating or alleviating factors. A vagal mechanism for bradycardia may be implicated, for instance, if the symptoms occur only with straining, such as with vomiting or moving the bowels.

PHYSICAL EXAMINATION

As with tachyarrhythmias, the focus of the physical examination for the patient with a suspected bradyarrhythmia is a thorough cardiopulmonary examination. Blood pressure and heart rate and rhythm are crucial, as are careful cardiac auscultation and respiratory assessment. Any murmurs or extra heart sounds are relevant, as are any signs of impending cardiac failure (rales, S3, jugular vein distention, peripheral edema, or respiratory effort). Signs of congestive heart failure might indicate cardiovascular compromise as a result of the bradycardia.

When the presenting complaint is syncope, near-syncope, dizziness, or altered level of consciousness, a neurologic examination is necessary to explore the possibility of noncardiac causes. Orthostatic vital signs are also important to exclude orthostatic hypotension as a cause of syncope.

Finally, palpitations may be the presenting complaint when the bradyarrhythmia is a manifestation of sick sinus syndrome. This syndrome is often characterized by recurrent SVTs alternating with bradycardia (often called "tachy-brady syndrome"). The long pauses that often follow the termination of tachycardia may also cause symptoms, including syncope, dizziness, or confusion. Persistent bradycardia, sinus arrest, or SA exit block may also accompany sick sinus syndrome, with symptomatology similar to that of other forms of bradycardia.[9]

DIAGNOSTICS

Electrocardiography

As in any arrhythmia, the ECG is vital to accurate diagnosis. Ambulatory ECG (Holter monitoring, event recording) plays a special role in the diagnosis of bradyarrhythmias in that definite correlation of symptoms with a bradyarrhythmia is a requirement to fulfill the criteria of symptomatic bradycardia. Decisions about the need for a pacemaker are necessarily influenced by the presence or absence of symptoms that are directly attributable to bradycardia.[29] Ambulatory monitoring allows for this definitive correlation.

Provocative Testing

Provocative testing in the form of a tilt test may elicit bradyarrhythmias related to position change, such as malignant vasovagal syndrome, which is evidenced by exaggerated vagal response to emotional or painful stimuli. Carotid sinus massage during simultaneous ECG recording is useful for provoking symptomatic bradycardia in the carotid sinus syndrome, a disorder in which bradycardia occurs in response to carotid sinus hypersensitivity.[1]

Diagnostics

Bradyarrhythmias

Initial	Imaging
ECG	Echocardiography (if left ventricular dysfunction or valve disease is suspected)
Pulse oximetry	
Laboratory	**Other**
Hemoglobin/hematocrit	Event monitor
Serum electrolytes	Holter monitor
TSH	Provocative testing
Blood glucose	
Digoxin level*	
Drug levels*	

*If indicated.

Other Diagnostics

Other tests may be necessary to exclude other causes of bradycardia. These include serum electrolytes to exclude hyperkalemia and other electrolyte imbalances, a digoxin level for patients being treated with digoxin, and a TSH level to exclude hypothyroidism.

DIFFERENTIAL DIAGNOSIS

Sinus Bradycardia

In sinus bradycardia, the sinus node fires at a rate less than 60 beats per minute with a 1:1 relationship between each P wave and QRS complex. PR and QRS intervals are within normal range.

Sinoatrial Exit Block

SA exit block is the sudden cessation of sinus rhythm that results in long pauses. These pauses usually occur in a fixed pattern.

Atrioventricular Nodal Block

AV nodal block, in which conduction is delayed or blocked completely at the level of the AV node, may be transient, intermittent, or permanent. The block is termed first, second, or third degree, depending on the ability of the AV node to allow conduction of P waves to the ventricle. In first-degree AV block, the PR interval is greater than 0.20 second, but every P wave is conducted to the ventricle, resulting in a related QRS complex. First-degree block may occur in the presence or absence of bradycardia.

Second Degree, Type I. In second-degree, Mobitz type I AV block, there is progressive prolongation of the PR interval until a P wave is not conducted to the ventricle. The atrium/ventricle conduction ratio is usually 3:2 or 4:3, and a typical "group beating" of complexes occurs. This rhythm is also called Wenckebach's block (Figure 127-6).

Second Degree, Type II. In second-degree, Mobitz type II AV block, there is a constant PR interval until a P wave is simply not conducted (not followed by a QRS). This type of block is less common and more severe than Mobitz type I block and has a higher propensity to progress to complete heart block (Figure 127-7).

Third-Degree AV Block. In third-degree (complete) AV block, none of the atrial impulses are conducted to the ventricle. The P waves have no relationship to the QRS waves (AV dissociation). Typically, the pacemaker function is picked up by an escape focus, resulting in either a junctional or ventricular escape rhythm. Because these escape foci have lower intrinsic rates than the sinus node, a bradycardia may result. A junctional escape rhythm is characterized by a slow rate (40 to 60 beats per minute) with QRS complexes of normal width, which are not related to P waves (P waves may be absent or may occur but bear no relationship to the QRS complexes whatsoever). A ventricular escape rhythm typically produces a bradycardia of less than 40 beats per minute and is characterized by wide QRS complexes (>0.12 second) that are not connected to P waves.

Differential Diagnosis

Bradyarrhythmias

Sinus bradycardia	Bundle branch block
Sinoatrial exit block	Right bundle branch block
AV nodal block	Left bundle branch block
First-degree AV block	Left posterior hemiblock
Second-degree AV block	Left anterior hemiblock
Mobitz type I	
Mobitz type II	
Third-degree (complete) AV block	

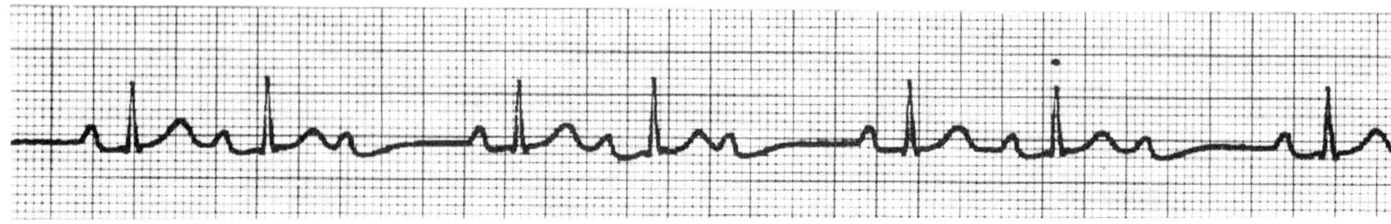

FIGURE 127-6

Second-degree AV block, Mobitz type I. (From Conover MB: *Understanding electrocardiography,* ed 7, St Louis, 1996, Mosby.)

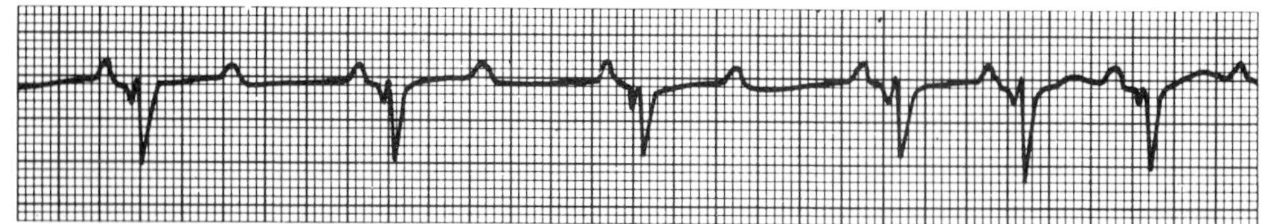

FIGURE 127-7

Second-degree AV block, Mobitz type II. (From Conover MB: *Cardiac arrhythmias: exercises in pattern interpretations,* St Louis, 1974, Mosby.)

Bundle Branch Blocks

Once impulses pass across the AV node, conduction occurs rapidly to all sections of the ventricular muscle by way of the right and left bundle branches. In BBB, conduction is disrupted down one or both of these branches, resulting in distortion and prolongation of the QRS complex. A QRS duration of 0.10 to 0.11 second results from incomplete BBB, whereas a QRS duration of 0.12 second or longer results from complete BBB. When conduction down the right bundle is blocked (right bundle branch block [RBBB]), the left bundle will conduct to the ventricle first. The ECG shows a small R wave, followed by an S wave and then a final R′ in lead V_1, whereas V_6 will show a deep, slurred S wave after initially normal Q and R waves. When conduction down the left bundle is blocked (LBBB), the right bundle will conduct to the ventricle first. The ECG shows a broad, slurred S wave in lead V_1 and an R′ in lead V_6.

Hemiblocks

The left bundle divides into the left anterior fascicle and the left posterior fascicle. When conduction is impaired in only one of the fascicles, a hemiblock occurs. A right-axis deviation will be noticed on the ECG with left posterior hemiblock, and a left-axis deviation will occur with left anterior hemiblock.

MANAGEMENT

Emergent treatment of the patient with a bradyarrhythmia who is hemodynamically compromised involves the administration of IV atropine. However, atropine must be used with extreme caution in the setting of suspected MI because it may worsen ischemia or result in tachyarrhythmias.[28]

In the primary care setting, management of the patient with a bradyarrhythmia who is hemodynamically stable involves discerning whether the rhythm has a reversible or an irreversible cause. Many drugs may cause bradyarrhythmias. Withdrawal of the offending drug may be all that is required for restoration of an adequate ventricular rate. Correction of electrolyte imbalances, in particular hyperkalemia, may also result in resolution of the problem.

In general, patients with symptomatic bradycardia should be referred to a cardiologist unless a reversible cause can be identified and corrected. Patients with asymptomatic bradycardia may or may not require further intervention; this is determined in large part by the type of block, as described in the following paragraphs.

Sinus Bradycardia

Sinus bradycardia is treated only if the patient is symptomatic (e.g., light-headedness or syncope occurs in the setting of a decrease in heart rate). Withdrawal of drugs that produce an increase in vagal tone (i.e., Tensilon or digitalis) or that decrease sympathetic tone (e.g., beta blockers, calcium channel blockers, amiodarone, or reserpine) may result in an increase in sinus node activity. A drug such as atropine, which blocks vagal tone, will increase the heart rate. A permanent pacemaker may be necessary for patients with chronic, symptomatic bradycardia.

Sinoatrial Exit Block

SA exit block is managed by removing the offending cause. Medications (e.g., quinidine, procainamide, or digitalis), ischemia, or excessive vagal tone may all induce this arrhythmia. In the absence of a reversible cause, the rhythm is managed as a sinus bradycardia, and treatment is not indicated unless the pauses are symptomatic.[12]

Heart Blocks

Heart block is treated by first correcting any underlying causes. First-degree AV block may be corrected by removing agents such as digitalis, beta blockers, calcium channel blockers, or class III agents (sotalol, amiodarone) or by treating hyperkalemia or ischemia after an MI. A pacemaker is generally not indicated. As with first-degree block, second-degree AV block is usually alleviated by correcting the underlying cause. Atropine may be given to increase the atrial rate, and a temporary or permanent pacemaker may be necessary. Virtually all patients with third-degree AV block will require a permanent pacemaker unless the block is likely to be temporary (e.g., acute MI, drug effects).[1] The rhythm may be treated emergently with atropine, epinephrine, or isoproterenol. The sudden development of a BBB requires treatment of the underlying cause, but a temporary pacemaker may be necessary in the presence of an MI.

LIFE SPAN CONSIDERATIONS

Older patients have the highest incidence of arrhythmias, as well as other co-morbid conditions.[4] Renal, hepatic, and cardiovascular disease will greatly affect left ventricular function, tolerance of the arrhythmia, and the ability for clearance of antiarrhythmic agents. Interactions with other agents must also be considered when treating an older patient for arrhythmias. Prescribing an agent such as amiodarone to a patient who is already taking warfarin or digoxin will, for example, increase the plasma levels of these drugs.

COMPLICATIONS

The most important determinants of mortality from an arrhythmia are the degree and nature of left ventricular dysfunction.[6] Sudden cardiac death is a real and present danger with complex ventricular arrhythmias, particularly in the setting of underlying cardiac disease. Exacerbation of cardiac ischemia/infarction or heart failure may also occur with tachyarrhythmias or bradyarrhythmias. Reduction in cardiac output will result in decreased perfusion to other vital organs (e.g., brain, kidney). The risk of thromboembolism and stroke with atrial fibrillation has been previously discussed, as have the proarrhythmic effects of many of the antiarrhythmic agents. Lethal proarrhythmias occur in 1% to 2% of patients receiving antiarrhythmic therapy.[5,16,22,30]

INDICATIONS FOR REFERRAL/HOSPITALIZATION

Obviously, any arrhythmia that produces hemodynamic decompensation (loss of pulse, blood pressure, syncope, chest pain) requires immediate hospitalization. Referral to an electrophysiologist is required if treatment for the arrhythmia will require nonpharmacologic agents, such as a pacemaker, catheter ablation, or ICD implantation. Electrophysiologic studies are required for guided pharmacologic therapy in the treatment of complex, potentially life-threatening arrhythmias. Electrophysiologic testing is also necessary if the patient is refractory to standard drug therapy or if the drug therapy itself produces life-threatening proarrhythmia.

PATIENT AND FAMILY EDUCATION

First, the nature of any particular arrhythmia should be explained. When the arrhythmia is harmless, this information may serve to alleviate unnecessary fears and alterations in lifestyle. When a potentially serious arrhythmia does exist, a frank discussion of the problem and treatment options may serve to enhance understanding and guide the decision-making process.

Discussion regarding the avoidance of any potential stimuli (e.g., alcohol, caffeine, cocaine, cigarettes) is important. Recommendations concerning steps to follow when the arrhythmia occurs should include a plan that addresses where and when to seek treatment. Careful medication teaching, including proper scheduling of doses, potential side effects, and interactions with over-the-counter medications, is essential.

For those who have a permanent pacemaker or automatic implantable cardioverter-defibrillator (AICD), there is a review of special precautions. The manufacturer is often able to provide excellent educational materials specific to any particular device.

Finally, the importance of involving family and significant others in teaching cannot be overemphasized. Depending on the nature of an arrhythmia, an individual may be rendered incapable of intervening on his or her behalf during an acute event. Family or others who are able to act in a timely and appropriate fashion may influence the outcome and survival of the affected individual. The families of patients with arrhythmias should learn cardiopulmonary resuscitation and develop an emergency plan.

REFERENCES

1. Timmis AD, Nathan AW, Sullivan ID: *Essential cardiology,* ed 3, Malden, Mass, 1997, Blackwell Science.
2. Mandel WJ: *Cardiac arrhythmias: their mechanisms, diagnosis, and management,* Philadelphia, 1987, JB Lippincott.
3. Fuster V and others: *ACC/AHA/ESC guidelines for the management of patients with atrial fibrillation 2001.* Retrieved August 12, 2002, from the World Wide Web: http://www.acc.org/clinical/guidelines/atrial_fib/af_index.htm.
4. Kayser SR: Antiarrhythmic drug therapy, III: atrial fibrillation, *Prog Cardiovasc Nurs* 11:35-43, 1996.
5. Antman EM and others: Therapy of refractory symptomatic atrial fibrillation and atrial flutter: a staged approach with new antiarrhythmic drugs, *J Am Coll Cardiol* 15:698-707, 1990.
6. Singh B: Controlling cardiac arrhythmias: an overview with an historical perspective, *Am J Cardiol* 80(8A):4G-14G, 1997.
7. Banerji S, Kayser SR: Antiarrhythmic drug therapy, IV: ventricular arrhythmias, *Prog Cardiovasc Nurs* 12:32-36, 1997.
8. Myerburg RJ, Castellanos A: Cardiovascular collapse, cardiac arrest, and sudden death. In Brunwald E and others, editors: *Harrison's principles of internal medicine,* ed 15, New York, 2001, McGraw-Hill.
9. Massie BM, Amidon TA: Heart. In Tierney LM, McPhee SJ, Papadakis MA, editors: *Current medical diagnosis and treatment,* ed 41, New York, 2001, Lange Medical Books/McGraw-Hill.
10. Fogoros RN: *Antiarrhythmic drugs,* Malden, Mass, 1997, Blackwell Science.
11. Canobbio MM: *Cardiovascular disorders,* St Louis, 1990, Mosby.
12. Conover MB: *Understanding electrocardiography,* ed 8, St Louis, 2003, Mosby.
13. Josephson ME, Zimetbaum P: The tachyarrhythmias. In Brunwald E and others, editors: *Harrison's principles of internal medicine,* ed 15, New York, 2001, McGraw-Hill.
14. Lee TH: Chest discomfort and palpitation. In Isselbacher KJ and others, editors: *Harrison's principles of internal medicine,* ed 15, New York, 2001, McGraw-Hill.
15. Hacker NF, Moore JG: *Essentials of obstetrics and gynecology,* ed 2, Philadelphia, 1992, WB Saunders.
16. Sopher SM, Camm AJ: Atrial fibrillation: maintenance of sinus rhythm versus rate control, *Am J Cardiol* 77:24A-37A, 1996.
17. Ukani ZA, Ezekowitz MD: Contemporary management of atrial fibrillation, *Med Clin North Am* 79:1135-1149, 1995.
18. Morley J and others: Atrial fibrillation, anticoagulation, and stroke, *Am J Cardiol* 77:38A-44A, 1996.
19. Ching TT and others: A new electrocardiographic algorithm using retrograde p waves for differentiating atrioventricular node reentrant tachycardia from atrioventricular reciprocating tachycardia mediated by concealed accessory pathway, *J Am Coll Cardiol* 29:394-402, 1997.
20. Kellen JC and others: The Cardiac Arrhythmia Suppression Trial: implications for nursing practice, *Am J Crit Care* 5:19-25, 1996.
21. Kayser SR: Antiarrhythmic drug therapy, I: general principles of drug selection, *Prog Cardiovasc Nurs* 11:33-37, 1996.
22. Kastor JA: Multifocal atrial tachycardia, *N Engl J Med* 322:1713-1717, 1990.
23. Schlicht JR and others: Physician practices regarding anticoagulation and cardioversion of atrial fibrillation, *Arch Intern Med* 156:290-294, 1996.
24. Stevenson WG and others: Ablation therapy for cardiac arrhythmias, *Am J Cardiol* 80:56G-66G, 1997.
25. American Heart Association: *Advanced life support,* Dallas, Tex, 1997, The Association.
26. Josephson ME: The bradyarrhythmias: disorders of sinus node function and AV conduction disturbances. In Brunwald E and others, editors: *Harrison's principles of internal medicine,* ed 15, New York, 2001, McGraw-Hill.
27. Goldberger AL: Electrocardiography. In Brunwald E and others, editors: *Harrison's principles of internal medicine,* ed 15, New York, 2001, McGraw-Hill.
28. Hayes DD: Bradycardia: keeping the current flowing, *Nursing* 27:50-55, 1997.
29. Gregoratos G and others: *ACC/AHA guidelines for implantation of cardiac pacemakers and antiarrhythmia devices,* Aug 1998. Retrieved August 12, 2002, from the World Wide Web: http://www.americanheart.org/scientific/statements/.
30. Campbell RW: Atrial fibrillation: steering a management course between thromboembolism and proarrhythmic risk, *Eur Heart J* 16(suppl G):28-31, 1995.

CHAPTER 128

Carotid Artery Disease

Virginia Capasso and Jeffery Dattilo

DEFINITION/EPIDEMIOLOGY

Stroke is the third leading cause of death in the United States. Each year about 600,000 people experience a new or recurrent stroke; about 500,000 of these are first attacks and 200,000 people die.[1] The vast majority of these strokes are ischemic strokes. Ischemic strokes result from oxygen deprivation to the brain as a result of partial or complete occlusion of an artery. Atherosclerosis of the larger extracranial and intracranial vessels, such as the carotid or middle cerebral arteries (MCAs), is implicated in most ischemic strokes.[2] Estimates of ischemic strokes from extracranial carotid lesions range from 15% to 52%.[3] Atherosclerotic carotid artery stenosis (CS) is the most common cause of stroke in young adults.[4]

The annual rate of primary vascular events sustained by persons with >50% occlusion of a carotid artery is more than twice that for individuals with <50% CS (11% versus 4.2%).[5] The annual rate of stroke and vascular death is almost 3 times higher among individuals with >50% stenosis (5.5%) than among persons with <50% stenosis (1.9%). The yearly rate of ipsilateral stroke with 50% to 79% stenosis is low (1.4%). When stenosis exceeds 80%, the yearly rate of unheralded ischemic stroke at least triples to 4.2%[5] and may rise as high as 10.4%.[6]

In general, the risk factors for CS are the same as for atherosclerotic cardiovascular disease. High systolic blood pressure, high cholesterol levels, and smoking have been specifically linked to an increased risk of CS in older adults.[7] When compared with individuals 60 years of age or older, younger adults (50 years of age or younger) undergoing carotid endarterectomy (CEA) for CS are significantly more likely to have a history of smoking, hypertension, and premature coronary artery disease and lower levels of high-density lipoprotein (HDL) cholesterol.[4]

Elevated levels of plasma homocysteine may be another important risk factor for CS. Among individuals 55 to 74 years of age, hyperhomocysteinemia has been associated with thickening of the common carotid intima-media lining.[8] However, one study failed to demonstrate a strong genetic link between carotid artery abnormalities and homocysteine levels in first-degree relatives of young adults with hyperhomocysteinemia.[9] Furthermore, current investigation in animal models found that normalization of plasma homocysteine levels does not restore normal vascular function.[10]

PATHOPHYSIOLOGY

Atherosclerotic CS initially involves infiltration of lipids into the intima of the carotid artery. The fatty streak eventually develops into an atherosclerotic plaque. The carotid bifurcation seems to be particularly susceptible to plaque formation. Although the exact reason is unclear, it is probably related to unique hemodynamic characteristics at the carotid bifurcation. Blood flow to the brain can be reduced or interrupted by severe narrowing or occlusion of the internal carotid artery. In addition, turbulence may actually damage the atherosclerotic plaque, resulting in the loss of intimal continuity or ulceration. Platelets and fibrin aggregate on the roughened intimal surface, and there is subsequent thrombosis. Fragments of a fractured plaque or thrombus may embolize to smaller distal arteries. Interruption of cerebral blood flow and cerebral infarction are the potential life-threatening sequelae.[11]

CLINICAL PRESENTATION

Patients with CS may be asymptomatic or symptomatic. Patients with severe CS may be asymptomatic if the circle of Willis is competent and adequately perfuses the territory of the middle cerebral artery (MCA). With patients who are asymptomatic, a bruit may be detected on routine physical examination.

Patients with symptomatic CS may present with one of three primary vascular events: (1) transient ischemic attack (TIA), (2) reversible ischemic neurologic deficit, and (3) stroke.

A TIA is a brief episode of neurologic deficit that lasts between 30 minutes and 24 hours. It is followed by complete functional recovery without any residual deficit. TIA is the most important omen of impending stroke, with one third of patients having a stroke within 5 years of the first occurrence of TIA.

A reversible ischemic neurologic event is a neurologic deficit that lasts longer than 24 hours. It leaves no residual signs or symptoms after days to weeks. However, it is considered a completed stroke with minimal residual deficit.

A stroke-in-evolution develops for a period of hours to days. Most thrombotic strokes have a gradual progression of manifestations up to 72 hours after infarct. This progression correlates with the degree of edema caused by the inflammatory process. A completed stroke is characterized by a neurologic deficit that remains unchanged for 2 to 3 days.

Symptoms derived from carotid artery occlusion, which develop gradually or in a stepwise pattern, include monocular blindness (amaurosis fugax), contralateral hemiparesis, and contralateral hemianesthesia. Global aphasia is present when the dominant hemisphere is involved. When the nondominant hemisphere is affected, the patient exhibits neglect of the opposite side of the body.

PHYSICAL EXAMINATION

The physical examination should include a complete cardiovascular and neurologic examination. Important components of the cardiovascular examination include palpation and auscultation of all bilateral peripheral pulses for bruits, as well as blood pressures in bilateral upper extremities in the lying and sitting position. The neurologic examination should include an examination of mental status, cranial nerves (including funduscopic examination), and motor and sensory function.

Although a carotid bruit is routinely listed as a clinical indicator of CS, it has been shown to be a poor predictor of moderate to severe CS.[12] Other predictors of CS include certain blood pressure characteristics. In a study of 187 older adults with isolated systolic hypertension, an elevated systolic blood pressure and increased pulse pressure were significant predictors of CS.[13] In addition, an increased pulse pressure and decreased diastolic blood pressure were independent risk markers for CS. The characteristic changes in blood pressure reflect compensation for reduced blood flow through the narrowed arterial lumen. Thus when diastolic blood pressure drops, the pulse pressure widens as peripheral vascular resistance decreases to dilate the arterial lumen in the presence of worsening arterial occlusive disease.

DIAGNOSTICS

Duplex ultrasound is now the primary diagnostic tool for CS. Studies have demonstrated a high agreement between duplex ultrasound and arteriography in the detection of >45% stenosis in the carotid artery.[14] It also has been shown that the operative plan is rarely changed by adding arteriography to diagnostic duplex ultrasonography that already suggests the need for CEA. Therefore the cost of care may be reduced more than $2000 by eliminating arteriography from the diagnostic evaluation.

DIFFERENTIAL DIAGNOSIS

The differential diagnosis of carotid artery disease depends on the presentation. In the presence of a carotid bruit, a negative duplex ultrasound necessitates further diagnostic evaluation. An echocardiogram will detect an intracardiac source of a murmur (e.g., valvular incompetency or septal defect) that is transmitted to the neck. An arteriogram of the aortic arch will demonstrate stenosis of extracranial vessels that are inaccessible to physical examination or noninvasive vascular testing.

MANAGEMENT

Management of asymptomatic and symptomatic CS is based on guidelines developed from recent randomized trials. The detection of a carotid bruit, development of transient ischemia, or a Duplex ultrasound that reveals 60% or more occlusion of the internal carotid artery (ICA) indicates the need for referral to a specialist (surgeon or neurologist). Carotid endarterectomy (CEA) is the "gold standard" for the treatment of symptomatic and asymptomatic patients with severe CS. Recently, carotid angioplasty and stenting have been advocated as an alternative to surgical treatment with CEA.

Carotid Endarterectomy

In 1998, the American Heart Association updated its guidelines for CEA.[1] Recommendations vary according to the presence or absence of symptoms and the degree of stenosis (Figure 128-1). CEA is recommended for asymptomatic individuals, with low surgical risk (<3%) and life expectancy of more than 5 years, who have a stenotic lesion that reduces the diameter of the outflow tract by 60% or more.[15] Among symptomatic patients, CEA is beneficial for those who have had TIA or mild cerebrovascular accident (CVA) within the previous 6 months. It is also indicated for symptomatic patients with 70% stenosis or more.

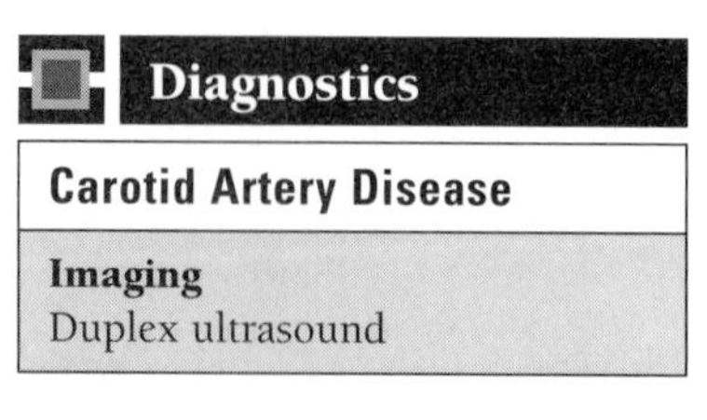
Diagnostics

Carotid Artery Disease

Imaging
Duplex ultrasound

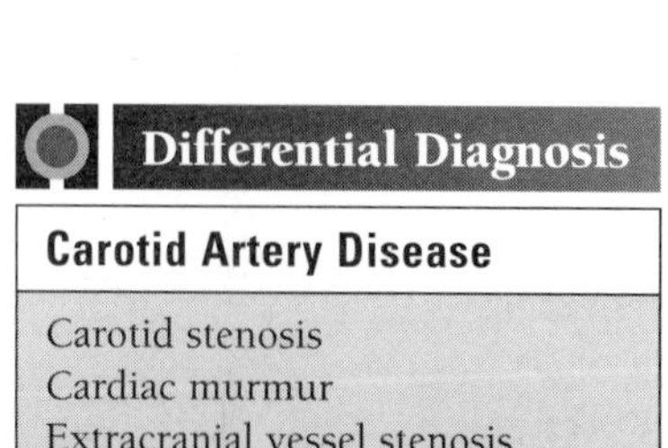
Differential Diagnosis

Carotid Artery Disease

Carotid stenosis
Cardiac murmur
Extracranial vessel stenosis

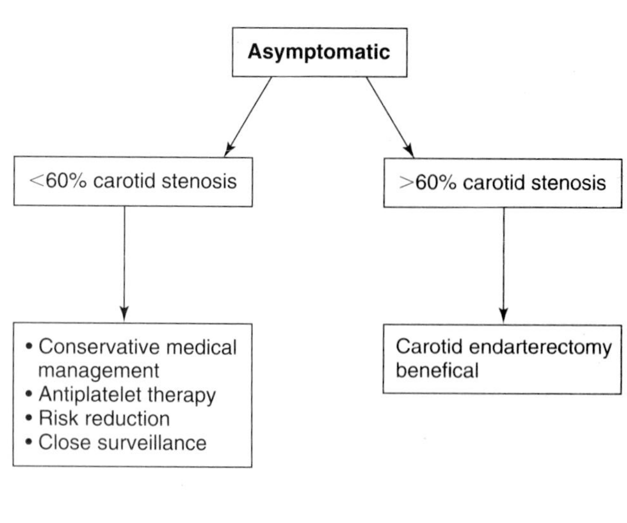

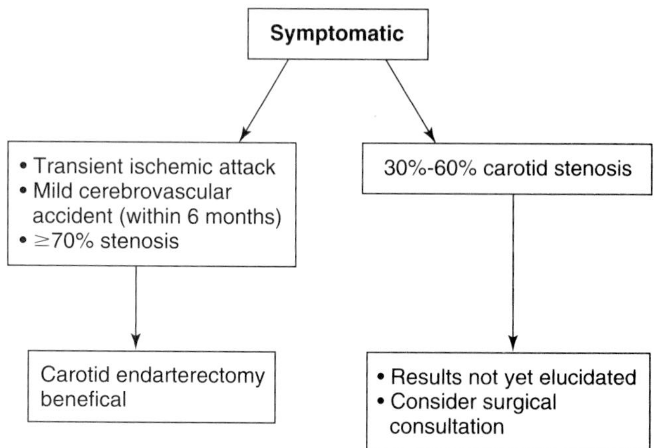

FIGURE 128-1

Guidelines for carotid endarterectomy. (Modified from Datillo JB: Peripheral vascular disease. In Hess ML, editor: *Heart disease in primary care*, Philadelphia, 1999, Williams & Wilkins.)

However, the usual practice is watchful waiting for patients with less than 60% stenosis. During this period, a duplex ultrasound is repeated every 6 months, and anticoagulants (aspirin, ticlopidine, warfarin) are prescribed for stroke prophylaxis. The dosage of aspirin, which inhibits thrombosis through its antiplatelet effect, usually ranges from 81 to 325 mg/day. The American Heart Association[12] recommends 325 mg/day as an initial dosage for stroke prevention. The effective dose of ticlopidine, which may be prescribed for individuals who cannot tolerate aspirin or who continue to have cerebral ischemic events while taking aspirin, is 250 mg/day. Because ticlopidine may cause serious neutropenia, the blood neutrophil count should be monitored during the first 3 months of therapy. Balloon angioplasty and carotid artery stenting may also be considered, although further research and evaluation of the efficacy of these procedures are necessary.

Temporary anticoagulation with warfarin may be beneficial for the occasional patient who has recurrent TIAs while taking aspirin or ticlopidine. The initial approach is to anticoagulate to a prothrombin time (PT) of 1.5 to 1.8 times the control value or to an INR (international normalized ratio) of 2.5 to 3.5. If cerebral ischemic events do not recur after 3 months, anticoagulation is reduced to an INR of 2.0 to 3.0. In the absence of ischemic cerebral events, warfarin may be discontinued after an additional 3 months, and antiplatelet agents may be resumed.[13] New medications are being developed for stroke prophylaxis.

Stroke prevention also includes the reduction of risk factors. The reduction of isolated systolic hypertension in people more than 60 years of age decreases the incidence of stroke by 36%.[16] Smoking cessation promptly reduces the risk of stroke by an amount proportional to the number of cigarettes smoked. The recent Scandinavian Simvastatin Survival Study (4S) reported a 30% reduction in fatal and nonfatal strokes in patients taking simvastatin; other studies of statin drugs used ultrasound and found a slowing of the progression of carotid atherosclerosis.[17-19] Although heavy alcohol use is associated with an excessive risk of stroke, moderate use may serve a protective role by raising HDL cholesterol, thereby reducing the risk of atherosclerotic cardiovascular disease and consequent ischemic stroke. The role of postmenopausal estrogen replacement in stroke replacement remains uncertain.[20]

Carotid Angioplasty/Stenting

In 1998, the American Heart Association published guidelines for carotid angioplasty and stenting.[21] The guidelines include (1) carotid restenosis after CEA with hyperplastic lesions within 3 years, (2) anatomically high lesions that would require extraordinary surgical manipulations, (3) radiation-induced stenosis, and (4) high-risk surgical patients. The recommendations were derived from the current lack of clinical evidence to suggest that angioplasty and stenting have results comparable to those of CEA in preventing stroke. Currently, there are randomized studies under way to investigate and compare CEA and angioplasty/stenting, including the Carotid Revascularization Endarterectomy versus Stent Trial (CREST). Until these results are available, carotid angioplasty and stenting should be reserved for patients in randomized trials and the subset of high-risk patients.

LIFE SPAN CONSIDERATIONS

According to the National Heart, Lung, and Blood Institute's Framingham Heart Study, 28% of people who experience a stroke are less than 65 years of age.[1] For people more than 55 years of age, the incidence of stroke more than doubles in each successive decade. The chance of having a stroke before age 70 is 1:20 for both sexes.

In individuals younger than 45 years of age, CEA has been shown to be a safe procedure, with postoperative mortality, CVAs, and cardiac complications of less than 2%.[21] The 10-year disease-free interval may exceed 75%. However, when compared with groups of older patients undergoing CEA, the 10-year survival rate is lowest for patients younger than 45 years of age. The poor life expectancy is attributed to complications of atherosclerosis.

COMPLICATIONS

Complications of CEA include stroke (1% to 3%), hypertension (19% to 25%), hypotension (5% to 30%), myocardial infarction (0.8% to 3%), bleeding (<1%), and cranial nerve injury (16%).[22] Most strokes (60%) are evident on awakening from the anesthetic. Thrombotic strokes often occur 2 to 3 hours after surgery; embolic strokes, up to 2 days after surgery; and cerebral hemorrhages, 1 to 3 days after surgery. Hypertension, which may result from carotid sinus injury or increased baroreceptor activity, usually occurs 1 to 6 hours after surgery and may require the administration of IV antihypertensive medications. Hypotension, which occurs within 1.5 hours of surgery and may persist for 15 hours after surgery, may require low-dose phenylephrine infusion and, subsequently, precautions for orthostatic changes during mobilization of the patient.

Expanding hematomas in the neck pose a risk of respiratory compromise and require exploration. The most common cranial nerve injuries involve cranial nerve (CN) X (8%), CN XII (5% to 8%), and CN VII (2%). Injury to the recurrent laryngeal branch of the vagus nerve (CN X) causes hoarseness and ineffective cough, whereas injury to the superior laryngeal branch of the vagus nerve causes minor swallowing difficulty and an easily fatigued voice. Deviation of the tongue to the ipsilateral side provides evidence of injury to the hypoglossal nerve (CN XII). Drooping of the lip on the ipsilateral side and an inability to smile reflects injury to the marginal mandibular branch of the facial nerve (CN VII). Cranial nerve deficits are usually minor and transient, resolving in 4 to 6 weeks.

INDICATIONS FOR REFERRAL/HOSPITALIZATION

All patients with suspected carotid artery disease resulting in ischemia should be referred for assessment regardless of whether a bruit is present. In most centers, patients are referred to vascular surgeons for CEA because surgical therapy with CEA is considered superior to medical therapy alone for the treatment of severe CS (>70%).[23-26]

CEA involves surgical atherectomy with or without a vein patch at the site of arteriotomy. CEA restores ipsilateral arterial blood flow in the common carotid artery (CCA), ICA, and MCA, which renders cerebral blood flow less dependent on collateral flow through the basilar artery.[22]

Preoperative evaluation includes cardiac risk assessment for silent myocardial ischemia. Identification of positive predictive factors of perioperative cardiac events (advanced age, previous myocardial infarction, and ventricular ectopic activity) indicate a need for exercise stress testing or pharmacologic nonstress testing. Unfortunately, most patients with peripheral arterial disease have intermittent claudication, which prevents adequate exercise stress testing. Silent ischemia is more effectively demonstrated by reversible defects on dipyridamole (Persantine)-thallium or dobutamine-atropine scans. Extensive coronary disease necessitates coronary arteriography and intervention. When indicated, CEA and coronary artery bypass grafting (CABG) may be performed sequentially during a single procedure. The most appropriate management of patients at moderate risk for perioperative events is less clear. The addition of beta blockers to the therapeutic regimen is the only therapy shown to prevent perioperative myocardial infarction.

CEA should be performed in a center with low rates of morbidity and mortality (<6%). Most patients undergoing elective CEA are admitted to the hospital on the morning of the procedure. Intake of all food and fluid is restricted after 12:00 AM.

A general anesthetic agent is administered to most patients. A regional anesthetic agent may be used for high-risk patients, especially those with chronic respiratory diseases. The operative time is between 1 and 2 hours for an uncomplicated case. Patients are extubated and awake at the end of the procedure. They are transferred to the postanesthesia care unit (PACU) for 2 to 4 hours of observation before transfer to the general care unit. Infusion of IV fluid is discontinued in the PACU. The IV infusion of low-molecular-weight dextran-40 (Rheomacrodex) for antiplatelet effect continues until the morning of postoperative day (POD) 1. Oral fluids may be started in the PACU, and the diet is advanced after transfer to the general care unit.

Most patients complain of only minor incisional discomfort, which is adequately managed with oral oxycodone with acetaminophen or acetaminophen alone. Other minor complaints include a sore throat (usually related to endotracheal intubation) and numbness of the ear and neck (related to nerve trauma by surgical retraction). In some centers, discharge occurs in the afternoon or evening of POD 1. Labile blood pressure during the postoperative period necessitates reevaluation of the patient's antihypertensive regimen before discharge; this is necessary to prevent syncopal episodes related to hypotension. In some institutions, the treatment plan includes two home visits for blood pressure monitoring. The visits correspond with periods of high risk for bleeding resulting from reperfusion (POD 2 or 3 and POD 5 or 6).

PATIENT AND FAMILY EDUCATION

Patient education focuses on preventing the complications of CEA and secondary prevention of recurrent CS. The importance of adhering to the antihypertensive regimen in preventing hyperfusion syndrome and stroke is emphasized, as is the need for the patient to report transient loss of consciousness, severe headache, and transient or persistent neurologic deficit.[20]

Secondary prevention of recurrent CS is directed at reducing risk factors. Because cigarette smoking is a risk factor for restenosis, efforts are directed at smoking cessation.[27] Elevated serum cholesterol levels may contribute to CS, and therefore patients who have undergone CEA should be counseled and treated according to the guidelines of the Expert Panel on Detection, Evaluation, and Treatment of High Blood Cholesterol in Adults.[28] Heavy alcohol use is discouraged.

REFERENCES

1. American Heart Association: *2002 heart & stroke statistical update*, Dallas, Tex, 2001, The Association.
2. Weber CE: Stroke: brain attack, time to react, *AACN Clin Issues* 6: 562-575, 1995.
3. Whittemore AD: Carotid endarterectomy for acute stroke. In Abbott WM, editor: *Proceedings of current issues in vascular surgery*, Boston, 1997, Massachusetts General Hospital, Division of Vascular Surgery.
4. Levy PJ and others: Carotid endarterectomy in adults 50 years of age and younger: a retrospective comparative study, *J Vasc Surg* 25: 326-331, 1997.
5. Mackey AE and others: Outcome of asymptomatic patients with carotid disease: asymptomatic cervical bruit study group, *Neurology* 48:896-903, 1997.
6. Rockman CB and others: Natural history and management of the asymptomatic, moderately stenotic internal carotid artery, *J Vasc Surg* 25:423-431, 1997.
7. Wilson PW and others: Cumulative effects of high cholesterol levels, high blood pressure and cigarette smoking on carotid stenosis, *N Engl J Med* 337:516-522, 1997.
8. Bots ML and others: Homocysteine, atherosclerosis and prevalent cardiovascular disease in the elderly: the Rotterdam Study, *J Intern Med* 242:339-347, 1997.
9. DeJong SC and others: High prevalence of hyperhomocysteinemia and asymptomatic vascular disease in siblings of young patients with vascular disease and hyperhomocysteinemia, *Arterioscler Thromb Vasc Biol* 17:2655-2662, 1997.
10. Lentz SR and others: Consequences of hyperhomocysteinemia on vascular function in atherosclerotic monkeys, *Arterioscler Thromb Vasc Biol* 17:2930-2934, 1997.
11. Mumma CM: Nursing role in management of stroke patient. In Lewis SM, Collier IC, Heitkemper MM, editors: *Medical-surgical nursing*, ed 4, St Louis, 1996, Mosby.
12. American Heart Association: *Guidelines for the management of patients with acute ischemic stroke*, Dallas, Tex, 1994, The Association.
13. Bruno A: Ischemic stroke. Part 2: optimal treatment and prevention, *Geriatrics* 48:37-54, 1993.
14. Ballard JL and others: Cost-effective evaluation and treatment for carotid disease, *Arch Surg* 132:268-271, 1997.
16. SHEP Cooperative Research Group: Prevention of stroke by antihypertensive drug treatment in older persons with isolated systolic hypertension: final results of the Systolic Hypertension in Elderly Program (SHEP), *JAMA* 265:3255-3264, 1991.
17. Randomized trial of cholesterol lowering in 4444 patients with coronary heart disease: the Scandinavian Simvastatin Survival Study (4S), *Lancet* 344:1383-1389, 1994.
18. Furberg CD and others: Effect of lovastatin on early carotid atherosclerosis and cardiovascular events, *Circulation* 90:1679-1687, 1994.
19. Crouse JR and others: Pravastatin, lipids and atherosclerosis in the carotid arteries (PLAC-II), *Am J Cardiol* 75:455-459, 1995.
20. Biller J and others: Guidelines for carotid endarterectomy: a statement for healthcare professionals from a special writing group of the Stroke Council, American Heart Association, *Stroke* 29:554-562, 1998.
21. Bettmann MA and others: Carotid stenting and angioplasty: a statement for healthcare professionals from the Councils of Cardiovascular Radiology, Stroke, Cardiothoracic and Vascular Surgery, Epidemiology and Prevention, and Clinical Cardiology, American Heart Association, *Stroke*, 29:336-338, 1998.
22. Mingoli A and others: Carotid endarterectomy in young adults: is it a worthwhile procedure? *J Vasc Surg* 25:464-470, 1997.
23. Blankensteijn JD and others: Flow volume changes in the major cerebral arteries before and after carotid endarterectomy: an MR angiography study, *Eur J Endovasc Surg* 14:446-450, 1997.
24. Mayberg MR and others: Carotid endarterectomy and prevention of cerebral ischemia in symptomatic carotid stenosis, *JAMA* 266: 3289-3294, 1991.
25. Warlow CP: Symptomatic patients: the European Carotid Surgery Trial (ECST), *J Mal Vasc* 18:198-201, 1993.
26. Biller J and others: Guidelines for carotid endarterectomy: a statement for healthcare professionals from a special writing group of the Stroke Council, American Heart Association, *Circulation*, 97:501-509, 1998.
27. Morganstern LB and others: The risks and benefits of carotid endarterectomy in patients with near occlusion of the carotid artery: North American Symptomatic Carotid Endarterectomy Trial (NASCET) Group, *Neurology* 48:911-915, 1997.
28. O'Brien MS, Ricotta JJ: Postoperative treatment of patients undergoing carotid endarterectomy, *J Vasc Surg* 12:1-5, 1994.

CHAPTER 129

Chest Pain and Coronary Artery Disease

Patricia A. Lowry

DEFINITION/EPIDEMIOLOGY

Coronary heart disease remains the primary cause of death for both men and women in the United States. Each year 1.1 million Americans suffer a myocardial infarction (MI) mostly as a result of coronary thrombosis. Approximately 466,000 of these heart attacks are fatal. Nearly 220,000 people will die before ever reaching a hospital, primarily as a result of ventricular arrhythmias.[1] The majority of deaths among patients who do reach the hospital are attributable to left ventricular failure and cardiogenic shock within 96 hours after infarction.

Early reperfusion treatment of patients with an acute MI improves left ventricular systolic function and survival; therefore every effort must be made to minimize hospital delay. Although time is critical in the treatment of MI, patient delay, not transport or system inadequacy, has proved to be the biggest obstacle to obtaining timely medical treatment. Studies have shown that only one out of five patients arrive at the hospital during that "golden hour," the time frame during which they would obtain the greatest benefits from reperfusion therapy. Many reasons exist for hospital delays including the patient's lack of knowledge regarding heart attack symptoms. In random phone surveys 90% could identify chest pressure as a symptom of a heart attack, 67% could identify arm pain, 50% knew that shortness of breath could be related, and only 21% were aware that sweating could be a symptom. Overall the average patient interviewed could identify only 2 of the 11 heart attack symptoms.[2]

Immediate emergency department referral/physician consultation is indicated for patients with suspected MI.

Risk Factors for Coronary Artery Disease

It is currently believed that it is coronary artery plaque composition and morphology, not the degree of plaque stenosis, that determines the risk of cardiovascular events. Modification of controllable cardiac risk factors has been shown to decrease the frequency of cardiovascular morbidity and mortality.

Historically, risk factors have been subdivided into factors that are nonmodifiable, such as gender, age, and family history, and factors that are modifiable, such as smoking cessation, cholesterol levels, diabetes mellitus, and hypertension. It is now known that some cardiac risk factors are more predictive of coronary artery events than others.

Pasternak and others[3] have developed an evidence-based system whereby known and potential coronary risk factors have been placed into a hierarchy based on four factors:

- Risk factors for which there is a strong causal relationship to coronary artery disease (CAD) and for which interventions have been *proved* to reduce the incidence of CAD events (cigarette smoking, low-density lipoprotein [LDL] cholesterol, dietary factors, hypertension, thrombogenic factors)
- Risk factors that strongly suggest a causal relationship to CAD and for which interventions are *likely,* based on current pathophysiologic understanding and on epidemiologic and clinical trial evidence, to reduce the incidence of CAD events (diabetes, physical inactivity, high-density lipoprotein [HDL] cholesterol, obesity, postmenopausal status)
- Risk factors that are clearly associated with an increased CAD risk and for which modifications *might* lower the incidence of CAD events (psychosocial factors such as stress and depression, triglycerides, Lp(a) lipoprotein, homocysteine, oxidative stress)
- Risk factors associated with increased risk but that cannot be modified or whose modifications would be *unlikely* to change the incidence of CAD events (age, gender, family history) (Table 129-1)

In addition to these risk factors, information is beginning to emerge that shows a relationship between sleep apnea and the development of coronary ischemia. Sleep apnea syndrome, irrespective of the type (obstructive, central, or mixed), leads to cessation of airflow and a fall in oxygen saturation. When the oxygen saturation drops, often to profoundly low levels during sleep, disturbance in cardiac rhythm and elevation in pulmonary arterial pressure may occur as a consequence of hypoxia-induced pulmonary hypertension. Similar physiologic disturbances of hypoxia occur in the coronary arterial circulation. In

TABLE 129-1 AHA/ACC Secondary Prevention for Patients with Coronary Artery Disease

Risk Factors	Goal
Smoking	Complete cessation
Blood pressure control	<140/90 mm Hg <135/85 mm Hg if heart failure or renal insufficiency
Lipids	LDL <100 as goal <7% saturated fat diet <20 mg/day cholesterol Triglycerides <200 as goal
Physical activity	30 minutes 3-4 days/week minimum 30 min/day optimal
Weight management	Body mass index (BMI) of 18.5-24.9 kg/m^2
Diabetes mellitus	Hemoglobin A_{1C} <7% is advised
Medications	
ASA	75 to 325 mg PO daily; if ASA is contraindicated use of clopidogrel or warfarin
Beta blockers	Implemented within first 24 hours
ACE inhibitors	Implemented within first 24 hours

From AHA/ACC Guidelines for preventing heart attack and death in patients with atherosclerotic cardiovascular disease, *Circulation* 104:1577-1579, 2001.

the presence of critical coronary stenosis, hypoxia-induced coronary vasoconstriction as a result of impaired endothelial function may lead to coronary ischemia. The treatment of choice depends on the type of sleep apnea syndrome.

PATHOPHYSIOLOGY

Chronic Stable Angina

Chronic stable angina is precipitated by exertion and relieved by rest. A reduction in myocardial oxygen supply or increases in myocardial oxygen demand are the determinants of coronary ischemia. Although the pathology for unstable angina and the pathology for chronic stable angina both result from atherosclerotic lesions in the coronary arteries, the pathophysiology of each varies.

Under normal circumstances an increase in myocardial oxygen demand is balanced by an increase in myocardial oxygen supply. The three most important factors that determine myocardial oxygen demand are heart rate, systemic blood pressure (peripheral vascular resistance), and left ventricular wall tension. The heart rate and the systolic blood pressure exert independent influence on myocardial oxygen requirements, because both determine myocardial workload (heart rate × systolic blood pressure = myocardial workload). Therefore activities (e.g., exercise, hurrying, lifting) and increased metabolic demands (e.g., with fever, anemia, thyrotoxicosis) that increase the workload of the heart in the presence of a fixed and limited oxygen supply will increase myocardial oxygen requirements and thus precipitate ischemia and angina.

The coronary arteries exhibit changes in vascular tone (vasomotion). These changes play a significant role in the development of coronary ischemia. The endothelial lining is the innermost layer of the coronary artery. It is a monolayer, exocrine organ that actively participates in homeostasis and regulation of vascular tone by producing, secreting, and responding to a number of vasoactive substances, including prostacyclin, thrombin, histamine, serotonin, adenosine, endothelium-derived relaxing factor (EDRF), endothelin, and cholinergic agonists. Under normal circumstances the endothelium responds to vasoactive stimuli, such as mental stress, cold, and catecholamines, by releasing EDRF to maintain vasodilation.[4-6] In the presence of atherosclerosis, however, the endothelial function is impaired; hence the vasoconstrictive response is unopposed, leading to constriction at the site of atherosclerosis and adjacent areas. This results in a decrease in myocardial blood flow and induces coronary ischemia.

Silent Myocardial Ischemia

It has been recognized that asymptomatic occurrences of ischemia are more common than symptomatic episodes in patients with exertional anginal symptoms. Silent myocardial ischemia occurs when there is objective evidence of ischemia in the absence of symptoms. Since the advent of continuous ambulatory ECG monitoring, many patients with typical stable angina have been found to have frequent episodes of asymptomatic ischemia.

The full clinical implications of silent ischemia are not well understood, but several longitudinal studies have shown an increased incidence of ischemia, MI, and sudden death in asymptomatic patients with positive exercise stress test results. In addition, patients with asymptomatic ischemia who have had an MI are at greater risk for a second coronary event. Ischemia can occur with or without evidence of increased myocardial oxygen demand (increased product of heart rate and blood pressure).

The pathogenesis of silent myocardial ischemia is not well understood, although several hypotheses exist. It has been suggested that some individuals have a higher endorphin level than others, which may play a role in the perception of pain. In addition, some patients have a higher ischemic pain threshold, as well as more tolerance to cold-induced ischemia. Finally, autonomic dysfunction, particularly in patients with diabetes, is thought to contribute to silent ischemia.

Microvascular Angina

The diagnosis of microvascular angina (syndrome X) is suspected when (1) there is a convincing history of anginal chest pain with or without documented reversible ischemic ECG changes, (2) angiography fails to demonstrate obstruction or spasm of a major coronary artery, and (3) other conditions have been excluded from the differential diagnosis.

The etiology of microvascular angina is still not fully understood, although studies have demonstrated that some patients with this syndrome have an abnormal vasodilating response of their small or resistance vessels (diminished coronary reserve). Still other patients may have a low pain threshold or other noncardiac causes of pain.

Variant Angina (Coronary Artery Spasm, Prinzmetal's Angina)

In variant angina, coronary artery spasm should be suspected on the basis of the patient's history. Spasm can occur in any coronary artery; however, the right coronary artery, and to a lesser extent the left anterior descending artery, are more commonly affected. The spasm tends to be focal and reproducible at the same location. However, diffuse single-vessel coronary artery spasm may occur. Multivessel spasm is extremely rare; when it occurs, it is associated with intractable ventricular tachycardia. The etiology of coronary artery spasm is abnormal endothelial cell function. This is especially true when injury to the endothelium results in decreased concentration of EDRF.

Unstable Angina and Non–ST-Segment Elevation Myocardial Infarction

The pathophysiology of acute MI has been controversial since Hippocrates first postulated that heart disease could cause sudden death. The causes of MI can be divided into those that decrease myocardial oxygen supply and those that increase myocardial oxygen demand. Atherosclerotic plaque results in a reduction of coronary blood flow, thereby reducing oxygen supply. These plaques reduce the cross-sectional area of coronary artery lumen, thus reducing coronary perfusion pressure. When a critical stenosis develops, coronary blood flow is adequate at rest but cannot increase to meet metabolic demands during exertion. The subendocardium blood reserve becomes much more limited than that of the subepicardium; therefore ischemia and infarction occur first in the subendocardial layer. When the infarction is limited to the subendocardial layer, the term non-ST elevation MI or non-Q wave MI is applied.

The development of a vulnerable coronary artery lesion is multifactorial and is dependent on the biochemical and physical properties of that lesion. Unstable angina/non-ST-segment MI is most commonly due to coronary artery narrowing caused by a nonocclusive thrombus that has developed from a ruptured atherosclerotic plaque. According to one theory, coronary atherosclerosis is initiated by oxidized LDLs, which are toxic to the endothelium of the coronary artery. Such toxicity initiates an inflammatory response, which stimulates chemotactic factors for circulating monocytes. Monocytes enter the vessel wall, transform into tissue macrophages, and ingest oxidized LDLs. Over time, lipid-filled macrophages (foam cells) die, creating an extracellular lipid pool with eventual formation of a fibrous cap. Proteolytic enzymes produced by activated macrophages erode the fibrous cap, producing areas that are fragile and prone to rupture. Increases in shear stress and vasomotor changes placed on this vulnerable lesion make it highly likely to rupture. Therefore the role of the inflammatory response as a trigger for plaque rupture cannot be overemphasized. Evidence is beginning to focus on the role of bacterial and viral infections and their effects on existing atheromatous lesions, making them more vulnerable and unstable with a predisposition to rupture and thrombose.

When plaque rupture occurs, the size of the resultant thrombus, whether a small mural or an occlusive thrombus, will depend on several factors, including the amount of thrombogenic substrate that is exposed, the amount of local blood flow disturbances, and the actual thrombotic propensity of the vessel.

Therefore lesion disruption is a dynamic process that may lead to transient vessel occlusion and ischemia by a labile thrombus, resulting in unstable angina. These thrombotic occlusions often resolve spontaneously; however, they can recur within hours or days. In other cases formation of a fixed thrombus and a more chronic occlusion may occur, resulting in acute MI.

Coronary artery narrowing of less than 80% generally does not induce development of collateral vessels. For this reason, smaller plaques that rupture are more likely to cause a significant clinical event during thrombotic occlusion of the vessel as a result of the absence of protective collateral flow.

Acute ST-Segment Elevation Myocardial Infarction

The pathophysiology of an acute ST elevation MI has been controversial since Hippocrates first postulated that heart disease could cause sudden death. The causes of MI can be divided into those that decrease myocardial oxygen supply and those that increase myocardial oxygen demand. Atherosclerotic plaque results in a reduction of coronary blood flow, thereby reducing oxygen supply. These plaques reduce the cross-sectional area of coronary artery lumen, thus reducing coronary perfusion pressure. When a critical stenosis develops, coronary blood flow is adequate at rest but cannot increase to meet metabolic demands during exertion. The subendocardium blood reserve becomes much more limited than that of the subepicardium; therefore ischemia and infarction occur first in the subendocardial layer. When the infarction is limited to the subendocardial layer, the term non-ST elevation MI or non–Q-wave MI is applied.

In most cases MI occurs when an atherosclerotic plaque ruptures, which serves as a nidus for thrombus formation with resultant coronary artery occlusion. The atherosclerotic plaque most likely to rupture is the nonocclusive plaque, which may rupture several times before producing MI. On each rupture, blood, fibrin, and platelet aggregates accumulate into the plaque, forming intraintimal or intraplaque thrombus and resulting in an increase in plaque size, intraplaque pressure, and increased obstruction of the coronary lumen. When such a plaque ruptures, fissures, or ulcerates, MI and/or sudden death may occur. Plaque rupture with resulting thrombus formation is the common physiologic mechanism underlying unstable angina, MI, and sudden death. The amount of myocardial injury sustained is directly related to several factors. These factors include the amount of thrombus present, the ability of the intrinsic lytic system to promote lysis, the impact of local vasoconstrictor substances on impeding blood flow, whether the vessel affected is partially or totally occluded, the presence or absence of collateral vessels and the quantity of blood they supply to the affected area, and the amount of myocardium supplied by the affected vessel.

The platelet is not only the smallest cell, it is also the most active in thrombus formation. The platelet consists of membranes, tubules, granules, and receptors. During activation the resting platelet undergoes a dramatic change that induces platelet-platelet interaction or aggregates. Such platelet aggregates play an important role in acute coronary syndromes and MI. In several autopsy studies of patients who died of unstable angina, MI, and sudden cardiac death, platelet aggregation, fibrin, and microthrombi were common findings. Because platelets are important in the pathophysiology of acute ischemic syndrome and MI, inhibiting platelet activation should be beneficial in reducing and preventing acute coronary syndromes.

CLINICAL PRESENTATION

Chronic Stable Angina

The patient with chronic stable angina demonstrates characteristic symptoms that occur with predictable frequency, severity, duration, and provocation. These symptoms occur with exertion, are relieved by rest or no more than one nitroglycerin, and generally last for only 1 to 3 minutes. Chronic stable angina remains constant unless an acceleration of the disease process intervenes. The clinical presentation can best be evaluated by a detailed history of anginal quality, location, radiation, severity, duration, and precipitating and relieving factors. Associative factors such as dyspnea, diaphoresis, nausea, vomiting, eructations, diarrhea, and fatigue should also be evaluated (Box 129-1).

William Heberden first defined the peculiar discomfort of myocardial ischemia as angina pectoris, which translated means a "strangling in the chest." The majority of patients do not refer to their anginal symptoms as pain; thus questioning related to "chest pain" may prove misleading, and the diagnosis of angina pectoris may be missed. Discomfort originating from the chest may arise from many structures, including the skin, subcutaneous tissue, bone, muscle, vascular structures, nerves, pleura, lungs, pericardium, heart, esophagus, or gastrointestinal viscera.

Adjectives used to describe the *quality* of angina can be variable and are often conveyed as a pressure, heaviness, aching, constriction, tightness, squeezing, numbness, or burning sensation. Patients may demonstrate a clenched fist over the sternal area (Levine's sign) to further elucidate this feeling. The *location* of discomfort is predominantly behind the midsternum (retrosternal) or just to the left of the sternum, the area of which should be approximately the size of a clenched fist. If the patient is able to localize the area of discomfort as being no larger than a fingertip, the etiology is seldom related to myocardial ischemia, and other causes should be considered. Myocardial ischemia can also encompass the territory between the epigastrium and the lower jaw, lower teeth, and hard palate, with sensations of tightness or constriction in the throat area.

Radiation symptoms are not uncommon and are related to involvement of the C8 to T4 spinal ganglia. These ganglia receive impulses from the heart, as well as from peripheral dermatomes, which are transmitted to the spinal cord via afferent nerve fibers. When myocardial ischemia occurs, the sharing of these ganglia can produce discomfort to the other dermatomal areas. Therefore stimulation of the dermatomes affecting the brachial plexus can result in discomfort or numbness anywhere along the medial surface of the left arm, including the fourth and fifth digits. Isolated wrist discomfort has also been reported. The right arm and lateral surfaces can be affected, although with less frequency.

Stimulation of the cervical plexus can result in suprascapular and intrascapular discomfort. Precipitating factors, including increased exertion, coitus, or emotion, tend to induce myocardial ischemia by increasing circulating catecholamine levels. This increases the metabolic oxygen needs of the heart in the setting of a limited oxygen supply, thereby producing anginal symptoms. Eating a large meal may precipitate discomfort, as can increased metabolic demands from fever, chills, thyrotoxicosis, anemia, hypoglycemia, exposure to cold air, and the nicotine from cigarette smoking.

Relief of stable anginal symptoms generally occurs within 1 to 3 minutes after the discontinuation of activity and/or with rest. When angina is related to emotional upheaval, it may take longer to decrease catecholamine levels, and anginal symptoms may persist for a longer period. Nitroglycerin administration will usually provide relief within 5 minutes and is a useful diagnostic tool. When symptoms persist for longer than 20 minutes, the patient should no longer be considered to be having chronic stable angina and should be instructed to seek prompt medical attention.

Although cessation of activity generally produces relief of pain, it has been noted that some patients who develop angina with walking are able to continue walking, with eventual alleviation of the angina. These patients are able to "walk through" the anginal event. There are several proposed hypotheses for the relief of angina during exercise. These include (1) dilation of functioning collateral blood vessels during exercise, (2) relief of coronary arterial spasm, and (3) vasodilation of systemic blood vessels with a corresponding decline in systemic arterial blood pressure and heart rate, which in turn reduces myocardial oxygen demand.

The Canadian Cardiovascular Society Classification (CCSC) is a useful tool to determine the exercise tolerance of patients with stable angina pectoris and to determine the degree of disability that anginal symptoms are imposing on the patient (Box 129-2).

Anginal Equivalents

For reasons that continue to remain unclear, myocardial ischemia can be experienced as dyspnea and/or fatigue rather than actual chest pressure. Symptoms of dyspnea are generally noted to be stable when they occur with moderate exertion and unstable when they occur with minimal exertion or when they begin to awaken the patient during the night. The etiology of stable symptoms is related to increased myocardial demand, and the etiology of unstable symptoms is related to decreased myocardial supply. The dyspnea produced is due to myocardial ischemia resulting in diastolic dysfunction, which produces increased left-sided filling pressures. Fatigue often follows an activity and resolves within several minutes. The etiology is related to left ventricular dysfunction resulting in decreased cardiac output.

BOX 129-1

HISTORY QUESTIONS FOR THE PATIENT WITH ANGINA

Chest pain information
- Precipitating factors (exertion, meals, stress, cold)
- Quality (pressure, squeezing, burning, stabbing)
- Radiation (shoulders, arm, wrist, neck, jaw, back)
- Relief measures (rest, nitroglycerin [hallmark], food)
- Severity (1-10 scale)
- Timing (activity, bedtime, meals, history of occurrence, duration)

Associative factors
- Dyspnea
  - Provoked by activity (chest pain first or dyspnea)
  - Orthopnea (how many pillows)
  - Paroxysmal nocturnal dyspnea (how soon after retiring to bed)
- Diaphoresis
- Gastrointestinal complaints (nausea, vomiting, diarrhea)
- Fatigue

Presence of cardiac risk factors
Current medication profile

BOX 129-2

CANADIAN CARDIOVASCULAR SOCIETY CLASSIFICATION

Class I—Prolonged exertion evokes angina, without limits to normal activity.
Chest II—Walking >2 blocks evokes angina, with slight limits to normal activity.
Class III—Walking <2 blocks evokes angina, with marked limits to normal activity.
Class IV—Minimal activity or rest evokes angina, with severe restrictions to activity.

Microvascular Angina

The clinical presentation of microvascular angina is similar to that of classic angina, although atypical features are common, including rest pain, prolonged pain, and pain that is less responsive to nitroglycerin. Although there is no apparent gender difference in the perception of angina, the syndrome of microvascular angina is found predominantly in women.

Variant Angina

The sine qua non of variant angina pectoris is a history of spontaneous or unprovoked episodes of typical angina. Discomfort occurs predominantly at rest and is usually not provoked by exertion. Patients sometimes note that beta-blockers exacerbate symptoms. The differential diagnosis on presentation should be unstable angina until it is proven otherwise.

Unstable Angina and Non–ST-Segment Elevation Myocardial Infarction

Diagnosis of unstable angina and non–ST-segment elevation MI depends predominately on a detailed patient history. The five most important factors from the initial history that enhance the likelihood of the patient experiencing an episode of ischemia are (1) the nature of symptoms, (2) prior history of CAD, (3) age greater than 75 years, (4) male sex, and (5) number of risk factors present for CAD. In addition, several factors may suggest an acceleration of the patient's chronic anginal symptoms to an unstable or non–ST-segment elevation MI. These factors may include the anginal event occurring with less provocation or at rest, a prolongation of the anginal symptoms, an increase in the severity of symptoms, or newly associated findings with the chest discomfort. Physical examination finding of pulmonary edema, a new or worsening mitral regurgitation murmur, an S3, hypotension, bradycardia and/or tachycardia suggest the patient to be at high risk. A 12-lead ECG, preferably with and without chest pain, should also be obtained (Box 129-3).[7] It is particularly important to assess the duration of anginal events and whether rest pain has been present to determine the patient's short-term risk of complications. Patients who present with prolonged chest pressure or an anginal equivalent lasting longer than 20 minutes or in a crescendo pattern, coupled with ST-segment depression or T-wave inversion on the ECG, have a higher likelihood of suffering a non–ST-segment elevation MI as a result of an unstable anginal event.[8] This is important, because patients who develop a non-ST-segment elevation MI have a 70% higher risk of death and an 8.5% higher potential for reinfarction than those with unstable angina alone.

BOX 129-3

UNSTABLE ANGINA PRESENTATIONS

- Angina while at rest within 1 week of presentation
- New-onset angina of Canadian Cardiovascular Society Classification (CCSC)
- CCSC class III or IV within 2 months of presentation
- Angina increasing to at least CCSC III or IV
- Variant angina
- Non–Q-wave myocardial infarction
- Post-myocardial infarction angina (>24 hours)

Data from US Department of Health and Human Services, Agency for Health Care Policy and Research: Diagnosing and managing unstable angina, *Clin Pract Guide* 2-18, 1994.

Acute ST-Segment Elevation Myocardial Infarction

Classically, acute MI is diagnosed as a constellation of symptoms. Chest pain described as pressure, heaviness, squeezing, crushing, and aching is often associated with nausea, vomiting, diaphoresis, and/or dyspnea. Generally, the pain involves the sternum and/or epigastrium, and in many cases it may radiate to the arm, elbow, jaw, or neck. Any combination of these symptoms may occur in an individual patient. An unusual presentation may be cranial pain, which is usually different from a classic headache syndrome. Epigastrium pain secondary to acute MI may be misdiagnosed as indigestion, and referred pain to the shoulder on deep inspiration may be misdiagnosed as being splenic in nature. In the older patient MI may present as a sudden onset of dyspnea, weakness, loss of consciousness, and/or confusion. Although chest discomfort may be the most common presenting symptom, it may be atypical or absent in some patients with acute coronary syndrome (silent acute MI). In addition, the chest discomfort of MI may be similar to etiologies of chest wall pain.

PHYSICAL EXAMINATION

Inspection of the chest may reveal the point of maximal impulse (PMI) to be downward or laterally displaced, suggestive of cardiomegaly, perhaps from hypertension. The PMI may also have a rocking quality, perhaps related to a left ventricular aneurysm from a previous MI. The thorax should be inspected to determine the presence of any rashes or vesicles, which may suggest a herpetic etiology. Inspection of the neck veins should be performed to assess the jugular venous pulse for any elevation. The contour of the internal jugular waveforms should also be noted. A funduscopic examination may reflect hypertension or diabetic retinopathy. Xanthomas or an early arcus senilis may be indicative of elevated cholesterol levels. The peripheral circulation should be assessed for any vascular lesions indicative of arterial or venous disease.

Palpation during cardiac assessment is confined to assessing the upstroke of the carotid artery pulse and the PMI of the cardiac apex. The carotid upstroke should be brisk, yet not hyperdynamic. A prolonged carotid upstroke may be indicative of aortic stenosis as ventricular emptying becomes delayed when ejected across a significantly stenotic valve. Conversely, a brisk carotid upstroke may be indicative of aortic regurgitation.

The PMI should be confined to the fifth intercostal space at the midclavicular line. With any downward or lateral displacement of the PMI, cardiomegaly should be considered. In a follow-up inspection, palpation of the PMI should confirm any aneurysmal formation.

Auscultation of the chest may reveal a ventricular gallop (S_3) produced just after the second heart sound, which may be either physiologic or pathologic in nature. A physiologic S_3 may be heard in children and adults up to 35 to 40 years old. It may also be noted in women during their third trimester of pregnancy. A pathologic S_3 may be related to decreased myocardial contractility and is suggestive of congestive heart failure caused by volume overload of the ventricles. This may be related to either mitral or tricuspid regurgitation.

An atrial gallop (S_4) may be noted just before the first heart sound and is produced by an increased resistance to ventricular filling caused by ventricular stiffness after atrial contraction. Left ventricular etiologies of an S_4 include cardiomyopathy, hypertension, MI, and aortic stenosis. Right ventricular etiologies include pulmonary hypertension and pulmonary stenosis. An S_4 may also be noted in trained athletes.

A holosystolic murmur audible at the apex during an episode of chest pain is most likely consistent with mitral regurgitation. It is often secondary to papillary muscle dysfunction as a result of left ventricular ischemia. A ventricular septal defect (VSD) post-MI should also be considered and further evaluated with echocardiography.

Inflammation around the pericardium may produce a pericardial friction rub, which generally has one systolic and two diastolic components. The systolic component is produced when the ventricles contract in systole, whereas the diastolic components are produced in early and late diastole. The early diastolic component occurs as a result of rapid, passive ventricular filling, whereas the late diastolic component occurs with atrial contraction. The sound produced is very high and of a scratching/grating quality.

Adventitious breath sounds suggest heart failure. Their occurrence and the presence of any vascular bruits, indicating further vascular disease, should prompt further evaluation.

The physical examination is generally normal when the patient is not having episodes of variant angina; however, during episodes the patient may develop hypertension and tachycardia in response to the pain. In addition, the patient may have associated diaphoresis, nausea, and radiation of pain to the arm. Auscultation of the chest during an episode may reveal a gallop or transient systolic murmur originating from the mitral valve.

Approximately 90% of the diagnosis of an acute coronary event is made from the patient's history. The physical examination findings will support this diagnosis and help determine if the patient is in congestive heart failure or is manifesting evidence of a cardiac arrhythmia. The patient will understandably be anxious and on occasion will be diaphoretic. Generally, the pulse rate and blood pressure may be normal; however, with an extensive area of MI, the patient may have a compensatory tachycardia and be hypotensive (Box 129-4).

BOX 129-4

CARDIAC PHYSICAL ASSESSMENT

INSPECTION

PMI—displaced downward and laterally, aneurysmal
Skin and extremities—color, edema, xanthomas, lesions
Neck veins—elevated jugular venous distention, contour of internal jugular pulse
Thorax—rashes, zoster
Funduscopic examination—evaluate for risk factors: diabetes mellitus, elevated cholesterol

PALPATION

Carotid upstroke—may be prolonged with aortic stenosis
PMI—may be diffuse with cardiac enlargement

AUSCULTATION

Ventricular gallop (S_3)—heart failure
Atrial gallop (S_4)—hypertension, MI; due to resistance of ventricular filling
Systolic mitral regurgitation murmur consistent with an ischemic papillary muscle
Pericardial friction rub—inflammation around the pericardial sac; may have one systolic and two diastolic components
Adventitious breath sounds
Carotid bruits—other vascular location

DIAGNOSTICS

Chronic Stable Angina

Electrocardiogram. In chronic stable angina the ECG can be useful to detect cardiac ischemia during actual episodes of angina. During this period, ST-segment depressions with symmetric T-wave inversions in the affected leads may be noted. During pain-free intervals, however, the ECG will revert to normal limits. Other possible changes include evidence of a prior MI, left ventricular hypertrophy, and repolarization abnormalities.

Exercise Tolerance Testing (Stress Testing). It has been estimated that in 1994 more than two thirds of treadmill testing was performed in the practitioner's office, with 33% of the testing being performed by noncardiologists. It is important, therefore, to understand the indications, contraindications, and interpretation of exercise stress testing results.

Because of the nondiagnostic potential of the ECG in patients with intermittent episodes of chest pain, all patients who are suspected of having coronary ischemia should undergo an exercise tolerance test within 72 hours of presentation of symptoms. Stress testing is performed for diagnostic, prognostic, and management purposes. Prognostically, the exercise tolerance test is directly related to a 4- to 5-year survival. Individuals who have stable exertional angina without left main CAD carry a 4% mortality rate annually. Patients with hypertension or a prior MI carry a worse prognosis. In addition, patients unable to complete the second stage of a Bruce protocol because of ST-segment depression have more than a 50% likelihood of progression of coronary heart disease in the succeeding 4 years. Those who develop ischemia after moderate exercise have less than a 50% likelihood of progression of disease in the next 4 years, and patients with ischemia only after strenuous exercise have less than a 20% likelihood of progression of disease in the next 4 years.[9]

When ordering stress testing consideration should be given as to whether imaging is indicated. For those patients with uninterpretable resting ECGs resulting from the following conditions, imaging either with thallium or sestamibi should be added: (1) preexisting 1-mm ST segment depressions, (2) left ventricular hypertrophy with strain, (3) left bundle branch block, (4) digoxin therapy, (5) ventricular pacing, or (6) patients with Wolfe-Parkinson-White syndrome.

The most commonly used definition for a positive exercise tolerance test result is the development of ECG changes consistent with ischemia. This ECG finding is a 1-mm or greater horizontal or down-sloping ST-segment depression or ST-segment elevation that persists for at least 60 to 80 msec after the end of the QRS complex.

The ST-segment changes on a stress test are indicative of viable cardiac muscle being supplied by a narrowed coronary artery. The time frame in which symptoms or ECG changes appear should be noted, as should the hemodynamic response. Stress testing should not be performed in individuals with exacerbation of congestive heart failure, uncontrolled cardiac arrhythmias, severe hypertension, unstable angina, an acute evolving MI, or critical aortic stenosis.

Coronary Angiography. The primary purpose of coronary angiography is to define the anatomy of the coronary arteries. Coronary angiography is presently the only method available for defining the coronary vasculature. MRI and electron beam CT continue to be investigational tools in defining the coronary anatomy. Coronary angiography is used not only in diagnosis of CAD, but also in directing therapeutic interventions. It is important to note that coronary angiography does not provide information about the functional significance of a given coronary lesion, nor does it provide information regarding the patient's functional status and symptoms. Therefore coronary angiography in the setting of chronic stable angina should be reserved for those patients in whom the diagnosis is in doubt, those who have failed to respond to medical therapy, and those in whom an intervention is being contemplated. In patients with chronic stable angina, coronary angiography should be preceded by an exercise stress test with or without imaging as deemed appropriate. Angiography should not be performed in all patients with a diagnosis of CAD. Studies have shown that patients with good exercise tolerance and whose CAD is easily controlled by medications will not benefit from an interventional procedure and for that reason do not require a coronary angiography.

Variant Angina

Electrocardiogram. Transient ST-segment elevation on a 12-lead ECG during an episode of variant angina is essential to make the diagnosis. ECG changes are usually observed in the leads related to the ventricular areas supplied by the affected vessels. On occasion, ECG changes may be dramatic but resolve readily with the use of sublingual nitroglycerin or nifedipine.

Echocardiogram. An echocardiogram obtained during a period of variant angina may reveal segmental wall motion abnormality, depending on the severity of the spasm and duration of the episode.

Exercise Tolerance Testing. An exercise tolerance test should be performed to exclude atherosclerotic disease. Most patients with noncritical CAD who have variant angina have a negative exercise tolerance test result.

Coronary Angiography. Patients with unprovoked chest discomfort at rest that is typical of angina may have variant angina. An exercise tolerance test should be the initial testing modality. On occasion, this test may be negative for ischemia, even though the patient is still experiencing chest discomfort. At that time, patients may undergo coronary arteriography to evaluate further for CAD. If variant angina is indeed suspected, all vasoactive medications should be discontinued at least 24 hours before coronary arteriography or any other provocative testing. Provocation of spasm with acetylcholine has been used to induce endothelial cell vasoreactivity. However this practice has fallen out of vogue because of the potential to induce global spasm and hence lethal cardiac arrhythmias. Therefore diagnosis of variant angina is generally made from a patient history revealing nonexertional events that often are nocturnal.

Unstable Angina/Non–ST Elevation Myocardial Infarction

Electrocardiogram. The 12-lead ECG continues to be the principal diagnostic tool in the differentiation of an unstable anginal/non-ST elevation MI event. During an episode of anginal discomfort, the ECG findings depend on several factors including the location of the involved vessel, amount of myocardium involved, duration of ischemia, and transient nature of the pathophysiologic process. During an episode of ischemia, the electrical properties of the myocardial cells within and surrounding the area of ischemia are altered, producing changes on the surface ECG.

ST-segment depression, along with symmetrically inverted T waves, is generally present within minutes during an acute ischemic event. According to guidelines of the Agency for Health Care Policy and Research (AHCPR), ST depressions more than 1 mm indicate a high likelihood of an unstable anginal event, whereas ST depressions of 0.5 to 1 mm indicate an intermediate likelihood. These changes generally return to baseline once the ischemic event is resolved. As a rule, Q waves do not develop, and there is no distinct change in the R wave. Persistence of ST-segment depression for longer than 48 hours usually differentiates an unstable anginal event from a non-ST elevation MI. It should be emphasized that an absence of ST-segment or T-wave changes does not exclude the possibility of myocardial ischemia. In particular, ischemia affecting the left circumflex territory is not always demonstrated on the ECG.

Exercise Tolerance Testing. A standard low level exercise stress test is considered the most reasonable test in patients able to exercise who have a resting ECG that is notable for ST segment changes. Those patients with an ECG pattern that would interfere with test interpretation should have imaging performed.

Laboratory Data. Laboratory blood work for the patient with a potential unstable anginal pattern should consist of hemoglobin and hematocrit levels to exclude anemia as a precipitating factor. Measurements of sodium, potassium, chloride, carbon dioxide, BUN, and creatinine should be obtained, along with a urinalysis. A fasting blood glucose level should be obtained, as well as a fasting cholesterol profile, to identify potential coronary risk factors. Thyroid functions should be considered to exclude hyperthyroidism or hypothyroidism. Magnesium levels should be considered for repletion purposes. Cardiac markers (creatine phosphokinase [CPK], CPK-MB and troponin levels) should be obtained to determine an unstable ischemic event from a non-ST elevation MI (Table 129-2).[10] C-reactive proteins may also be drawn to determine the presence of an inflammatory response, which is gaining enhanced recognition as a precursor to plaque rupture.

Echocardiography. The echocardiogram is helpful during an acute ischemic event in several ways. Most important, it assists in detecting the location and extent of regional and/or global left ventricular dysfunction. Second, it assists in risk stratification before discharge, and, finally, it is helpful for future evaluation of the remodeling and healing process. The ECG detects ischemia by evaluating the motion and thickening of the left ventricular walls. This becomes particularly helpful when the patient has chest pressure and nondiagnostic ECG findings.

Although there are many techniques to assess ventricular wall motion, the method most commonly used is the two-dimensional echocardiogram with M-mode. In acute coronary ischemia the two-dimensional ECG with M-mode may demonstrate abnormal wall motion of the ischemic section, which occurs almost immediately. Wall motion abnormalities, however, can be influenced by any abnormalities in the adjacent muscle to which it is attached. Perhaps a more specific finding for ischemic cardiac muscle would be the inability of the affected myocardial muscle to thicken during systolic contraction. The nonischemic, or normal, region reveals normal motion and thickening toward the left ventricular cavity during systole. The M-mode echocardiogram is ideal for measuring wall thickness and chamber dimensions, whereas color Doppler is used in conjunction with the M-mode to assess a regurgitant lesion.

Acute Myocardial Infarction

Electrocardiogram. ST elevations are generally representative of myocardial injury but may also be seen with left ventricular hypertrophy, hypertrophic cardiomyopathy, Prinzmetal's angina, pericarditis, hyperkalemia, early polarization, and left bundle branch block. In addition, ST-segment and T-wave changes may be seen in a variety of disease processes, including infiltrative myocardial disease (neoplasm, sarcoidosis, amyloidosis, hemochromatosis), chest deformities, muscular dystrophy, electrolyte abnormalities, cerebrovascular accidents, pharmacologic treatments (digoxin, tricyclics), hyperventilation, and anxiety. Therefore it is the history and presenting symptoms that remain the basis for the diagnosis of an acute or chronic coronary syndrome.

TABLE 129-2 Cardiac Markers

Cardiac Marker	Rises	Peaks	Normalizes
CPK-MB isoforms	3-12 hours	24 hours	48-72 hours
Myoglobin	1-3 hours	6 hours	24 hours
Troponin T and I	3-12 hours	3-4 hours	14 days

The initial ECG presentation during an acute MI may demonstrate "hyperacute T-wave changes," which are demonstrated by their tall, peaked shape (Figure 129-1). Within minutes to an hour after the acute event, the ST segment becomes elevated in the leads reflecting the area of myocardium involved. Within hours to days, the T waves usually become inverted and Q waves may develop (Figure 129-2). Pathologic Q waves generally represent a Q-wave or transmural MI. A Q wave is best defined by a width of greater than 0.04 seconds and a height at least one-third of the associated R wave, provided that the R wave exceeds 5 mm in height. Within 1 week the ST segment returns to baseline unless a left ventricular aneurysm develops. In this case ST-segment elevation will persist. It may take up to 1 or more months for the T wave to return to positivity. The occurrence of pericarditis after MI will be reflected by ST-segment elevation in all leads except aV_F and V_1, which will show ST-segment depression with a convex rather than concave curvature.

Reciprocal changes may be evident in the leads opposite the area of infarction, as opposed to those recorded by the leads facing the infarct zone. Reciprocal changes are evidenced by an abnormal Q wave being replaced by an abnormal R wave, an ST-segment elevation being replaced by an ST-segment depression, and deep, symmetric negative T waves being replaced by tall, symmetric positive T waves.

In many healthy individuals some degree of ST-segment elevation, especially in the precordial leads (V_2 to V_5) may be noted on the routine ECG. In most people the degree of elevation is minimal; however, it can vary from 1 to 4 mm in height. This phenomenon has been attributed to early ventricular repolarization. It can be differentiated from the ST-segment elevation of an acute MI by the following: an upward concavity of the ST segment, an elevated takeoff of the ST segment at the J point (the junction of the end of the QRS complex and the beginning of the ST segment), and a distinct notching or slurring on the downstroke of the R wave.

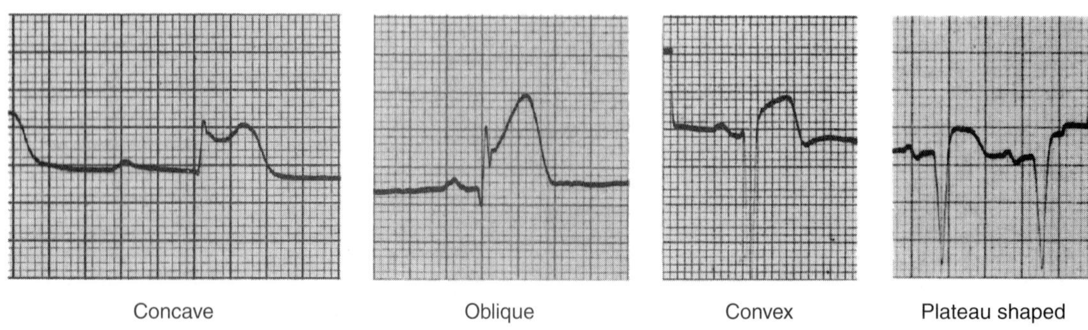

FIGURE 129-1

ST-segment elevations in acute MI. (From Conover MB: *Understanding electrocardiography,* ed 7, St Louis, 1996, Mosby.)

Although the 12-lead ECG is useful in localizing the region of myocardial ischemia, it is limited in both the sensitivity and the specificity needed to distinguish the culprit coronary artery (Box 129-5 and Figures 129-3 to 129-5).

Laboratory Data. For almost 30 years the creatine kinase (CK) and the creatine kinase MB (CPK-MB) have been used to detect myocardial cell injury. They were found to be moderately sensitive and specific. Recently the American College of Cardiology has recommended the use of myocardial markers such as the troponins and myoglobin. Troponin I and T are presently the new "gold standard" because of their high sensitivity and specificity. Like CPK-MBs, cardiac troponins become elevated within 3 to 4 hours. Troponin levels continue to be released for up to 11 days (7- to 14-day range) after a cardiac event. Thus it is more diagnostic of predicting the occurrence of an acute coronary event as well as serving as a late cardiac marker. Myoglobin is found exclusively in both cardiac and

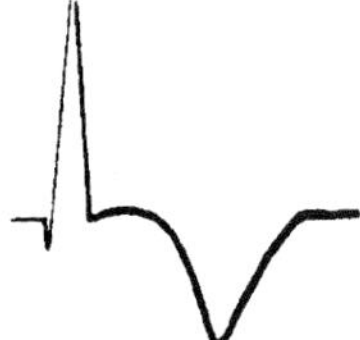

FIGURE 129-2

Typical coved ST segment and inverted T-wave of evolving MI. (From Conover MB: *Understanding electrocardiography*, ed 7, St Louis, 1996, Mosby.)

BOX 129-5

TWELVE-LEAD ECG AND MYOCARDIAL INFARCTION TERRITORY

Lead	*Territory*
II, III, aV_F	Inferior wall
II, III, aV_F, V_5, V_6	Inferoapical wall
I, aV_L, V_5, V_6	Inferolateral wall
V_1-V_4	Anterior wall
I, aV_L, V_1-V_6	Anterolateral wall
V_1-V_3	Anteroseptal wall ST-segment elevations
V_5-V_6	Apical wall
I, aV_L, V_5-V_6	Lateral wall
V_1-V_3	Posterior wall ST-segment depressions; tall, upright R wave
V_1-V_2	Septal wall ST-segment elevations

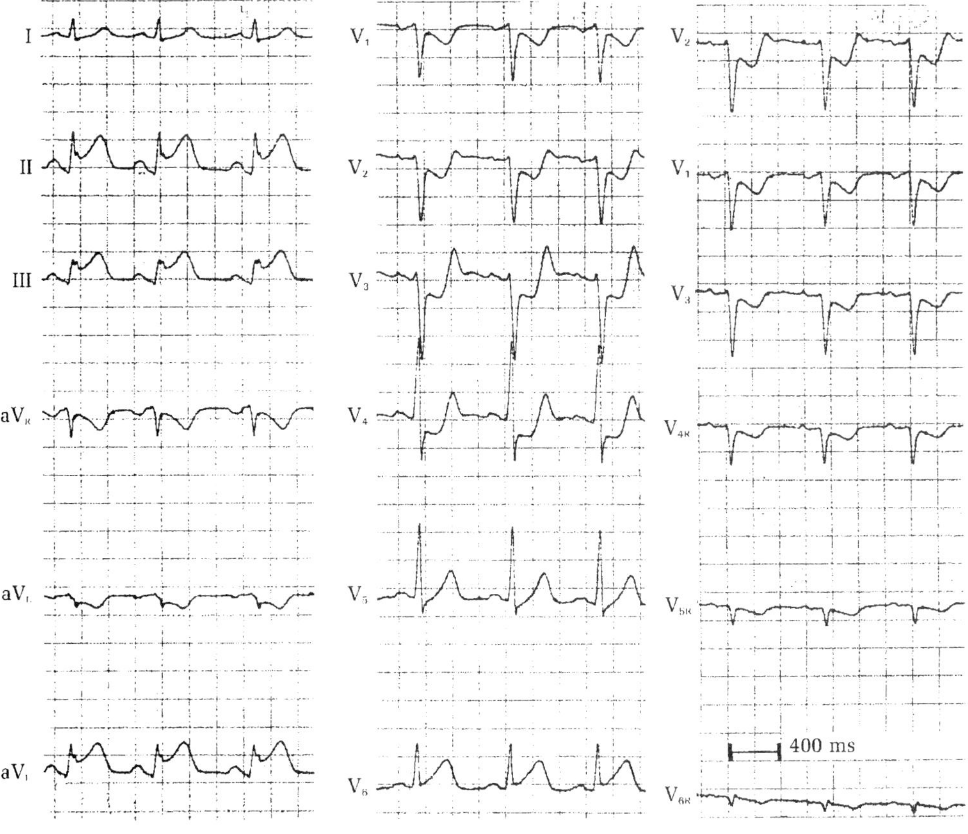

FIGURE 129-3

Acute inferior MI caused by circumflex artery occlusion. Diagnosis was determined by the negative T wave in lead V_{4R} and the fact that the ST segment is higher in lead II than in lead III.(From Wellens HJJ, Conover MB: *The ECG in emergency decision making*, Philadelphia, 1991, WB Saunders.)

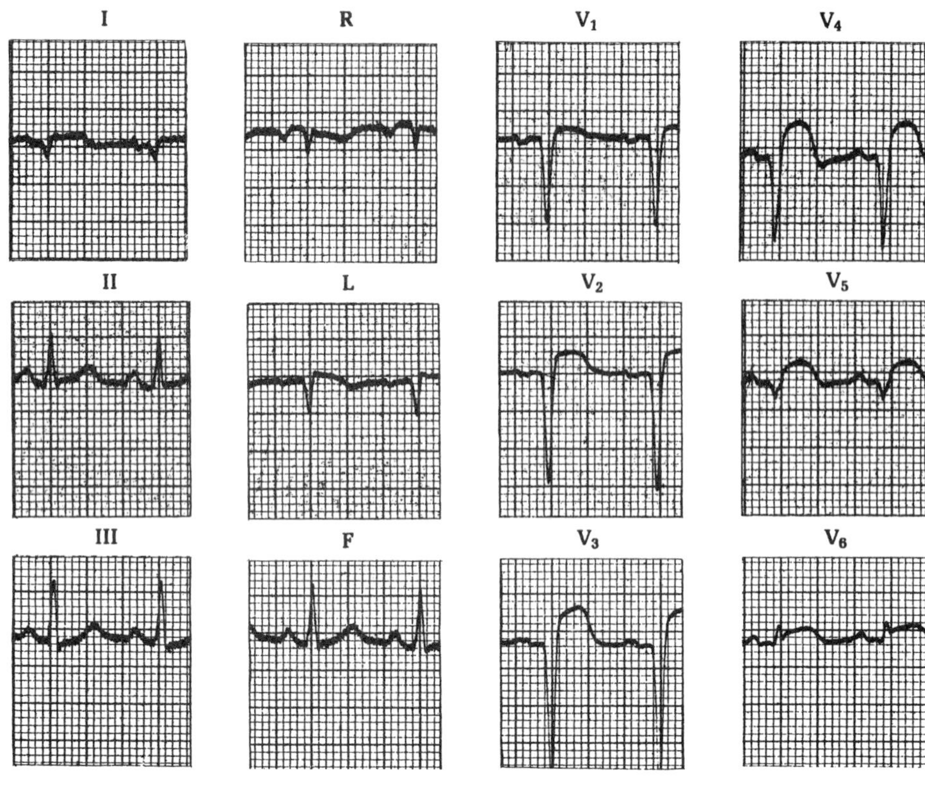

FIGURE 129-4

Anterolateral MI. Diagnosis was made by the loss of the R-wave progression from lead V1 to lead V6 and the ST-segment elevation in those leads. (From Conover MB: *Understanding electrocardiography,* ed 7, St Louis, 1996, Mosby.)

skeletal striated muscle. It is released within 1 to 3 hours after a myocyte cell injury, which currently makes it the earliest marker of cell injury. Unfortunately, myoglobin lacks the cardiac specificity of the troponins. This can lead to false-positive results as a result of skeletal, renal, or other cardiac issues. Additionally, a mild leukocytosis of approximately 15,000/mm^3 may persist for up to 1 week.

When patients present with an acute MI caused by a known thrombotic lesion, there may be reason to suspect that they carry with them the additional burden of a hypercoagulable state. Therefore it may prove prudent to obtain a hypercoagulable panel for these patients.

Stress Testing. Myocardial perfusion imaging with thallium-201 or sestamibi, although very sensitive for the diagnosis of MI, cannot distinguish acute infarction from chronic scarring. Stress testing post-MI is often performed to determine any future ischemic events and to provide an exercise prescription for cardiac rehabilitation.

Echocardiogram. Two-dimensional echocardiography can be of value in identifying wall motion abnormalities; estimating left ventricular ejection fraction; assessing for pericardial effusion, ventricular aneurysm, and left ventricular thrombus, and for collaborating clinical and physical diagnosis of right ventricular infarction. Doppler echocardiography is useful in the detection of valvular regurgitant lesions, as well as ventricular and atrial septal defects. Echocardiography obtained early in the course of an evolving MI is helpful in diagnosis and can aid in the decision-making process. In addition, the echocardiogram can provide prognostic information regarding left ventricular function and identify patients who may be at risk for developing complications. Therefore serial echocardiograms are beneficial for future comparison.

DIFFERENTIAL DIAGNOSIS

The primary focus in the ambulatory care setting is to differentiate cardiac from noncardiac chest pain. Four chest pain syndromes have a particularly high mortality rate and therefore need to be expediently detected, diagnosed, and managed. These conditions include aortic dissection, MI, pulmonary embolus, and a spontaneous pneumothorax. Conditions included in the differential diagnosis that have a lower mortality rate include gastrointestinal, pulmonary, valvular, inflammatory, integumentary, and psychologic disturbances (Table 129-3).

MANAGEMENT

Chronic Stable Angina

Treatment of chronic stable angina involves many modalities. As this is a chronic disease, however, it is important to have a good provider-patient relationship and a means of objectively evaluating specific therapeutic interventions. Such an objective measure of evaluation and classification is the previously noted classification of the CCSC.

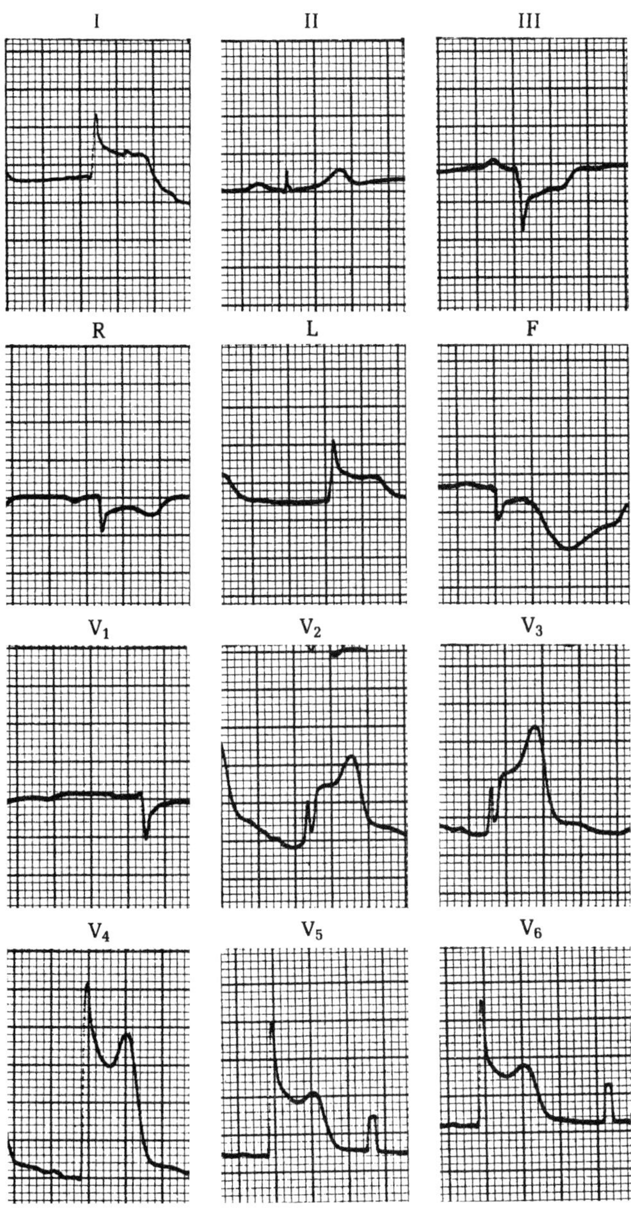

FIGURE 129-5

ECG showing massive anterolateral MI. ST elevation is evident in all superior leads. (From Conover MB: *Understanding electrocardiography*, ed 7, St Louis, 1996, Mosby.)

Patients should undergo baseline stress testing to determine their cardiac risk potential. Medication regimen should include acetylsalicylic acid (ASA), beta blockers, lipid-lowering agents based on a fasting cholesterol profile, and nitrates as needed. Risk factor modification is paramount to decrease the potential for disease progression.

Patients should be cautioned about specific anginal triggers, such as isometric exercise and walking in cold air. Lifting a heavy load or performing arm exercise (isometric exercise) may precipitate anginal symptoms because of an increase in myocardial oxygen demand. Walking in cold air may induce coronary vasoconstriction. It is advisable therefore to educate patients to cover their nose and mouth with a scarf when walking in cold air. Patients should be aware that sexual activity could precipitate angina and that this anginal trigger is not position related. Finally, patients should be encouraged to exercise, as exercise appears to result in an eventual reduction in coronary blood flow for a given workload. As previously noted, patients should be aware of the "walk-through phenomenon," which is the relief of anginal symptoms during exercise as exercise activity continues.

Silent Myocardial Ischemia

There have been few studies to evaluate whether pharmacologic intervention for silent myocardial ischemia has the same effect as seen in patients who manifest symptoms of angina pectoris. It appears that the same principles apply and that all three classes of antianginal drugs may be beneficial. The use of aspirin in patients with asymptomatic ischemia after MI has been shown to reduce coronary events. Because vasoconstriction is thought to be a significant pathophysiologic component of this condition, a calcium channel blocker is recommended as first-line therapy. Beta blockers may also be used. Management of patients with asymptomatic myocardial ischemia must be individualized. Treatment interventions should be based on the following: (1) the degree of positivity of the exercise stress test, with particular attention to the stage at which ECG evidence of ischemia appears, (2) the magnitude and number of perfusion defects seen on thallium or sestamibi scintigraphy, (3) the ECG localization of ischemia, and (4) the change in left ventricular function documented on radionuclide ventriculography or echocardiography. Coronary arteriography is recommended in patients with evidence of severe ischemia on noninvasive testing. Asymptomatic patients with silent ischemia and significant left main CAD or three-vessel CAD and impaired left ventricular function are appropriate candidates for coronary artery bypass surgery. In the ACIP study (Asymptomatic Cardiac Ischemic Pilot Study), coronary revascularization significantly reduced the duration of silent ischemia and hospital readmissions over a 1-year period when compared with medical strategies.[11] Patients with silent myocardial ischemia require close follow-up monitoring with noninvasive testing to determine changes in left ventricular function and the time required for positivity of the exercise test, which indicates ischemia.

Microvascular Angina

Many patients with microvascular angina respond to beta blockers, calcium channel blockers, and nitrates; however, a large number of patients continue to have pain. The natural history of the disorder is variable. Many patients have resolution of symptoms with time but may have periods of exacerbation. Even in patients with persistent symptoms, there does not appear to be a risk for MI or sudden death. Patient reassurance is an important part of therapy.

Variant Angina

Acute treatment of the chest pain episode is generally sublingual nitroglycerin. Calcium channel blockers are the long-term treatment of choice for this condition. In most cases a single agent is sufficient, but in resistant cases combination therapy with a dihydropyridine calcium channel blocker such as nifedipine or amlodipine (Norvasc) coupled with a non-dihydropyridine such

TABLE 129-3 Differential Diagnosis: Chest Pain

	Symptoms	Physical Examination Findings
INTEGUMENTARY		
Herpes zoster	Prodrome symptoms of chest pressure Tingling, tenderness, and pain along involved dermatome(s)	Grouped vesicles along erythematous base
CHEST WALL DISCOMFORT		
Costochondritis	Anterior chest pain, sharply localized	Reproducible by pressure on costochondral junction
LUNGS		
Pneumonia	Pain occurs when inflammatory process extends to pleura, resulting in chest pain that worsens with inspiration Fever, chills, cough, sputum production, dyspnea	Crackles or rales and/or decreased breath sounds over affected area Bronchial breath sounds with dense consolidation, increased fremitus, and egophony (E to A changes) Dullness to percussion
Pneumothorax	Sudden-onset, severe unilateral chest pain, generally pleuritic in nature Dyspnea	Diminished breath sounds on affected side Mediastinal emphysema may be present
Pneumothorax/tension	Same as pneumothorax, yet with substernal chest pressure with throat tightness	Same as pneumothorax, yet hypotension may be present Tracheal and mediastinal shift
Pulmonary embolus	Dyspnea Chest pain secondary to pulmonary infarction or inflammatory response (pleuritic)	Decreased breath sounds in affected area Hypotension with massive pulmonary embolus as a result of low cardiac output Hemoptysis, tachycardia, and hypoxia
Pulmonary hypertension	Mimics symptoms of ischemic chest pain Dyspnea	Prominent parasternal lift at lower left sternal border or xiphoid Pulmonic/tricuspid or mitral regurgitation murmur(s) S_4 may be audible
HEART		
Aortic stenosis	Easy fatigability, dyspnea on exertion, syncope or near-syncope, anterior chest pressure	Systolic murmur best heard over right base Delayed carotid upstrokes
Aortic dissections	Sudden onset of severe tearing, stabbing pain over anterior chest (proximal dissection) or interscapular/abdominal region (distal dissection) Diaphoresis, nausea, vomiting, near-syncope	Hypertension in 50% of patients Pulses are diminished or absent Neurologic symptoms (decreased cerebral/spinal cord perfusion) Aortic regurgitation murmur may be present as a result of aortic root dissection
Mitral valve prolapse	Sharp left anterior chest pain generally occurs in response to stress or emotional events Chest discomfort may last seconds to days Palpitations and dyspnea	Mitral valve click may be noted in systole at left lower sternal border
Pericarditis	Anterior chest pain that may radiate to shoulder area if diaphragmatic surface of pericardium is involved Chest pain is sharp; increases with inspiration or supine positioning (pleuritic) and lessens with forward positioning	Fever with bacterial or viral etiology Friction rub may or may not be present
GASTROINTESTINAL SYMPTOMS		
Reflux (gastroesophageal reflux disease)	Substernal burning, may radiate to neck, occurs 30 to 60 minutes after eating	
Acute cholecystitis	Right upper quadrant pain/epigastric pain Nausea, vomiting, and anorexia	Right upper quadrant tenderness + Murphy's sign Fever may be present
PAIN DISORDERS	Intense anxiety that may last for several days May note avoidance behavior because of inability to seek a safe refuge during an attack period Chest pain that is atypical Hypertension may be noted	

as diltiazem or verapamil is useful. Continuous nitrate therapy is not recommended because of problems with tolerance, but targeted nitrates may be helpful in patients with a predictable pattern of pain. Beta blockers are contraindicated.

The natural history of spasm is one of periods of symptomatic exacerbation followed by periods of relative quiescence. Once a patient who is receiving therapy has been without symptoms for 6 to 12 months, medication withdrawal can be attempted. Patients with spasm without significant fixed coronary stenoses are not candidates for mechanical intervention.

Unstable Angina and Non–ST Elevation Myocardial Infarction

Early risk stratification should be performed to determine the likelihood of an acute cardiac ischemic event from a non-ST elevation MI. The immediate management of this patient population consists of a detailed patient history, physical examination, 12-lead ECG, and cardiac markers. From this information the health care provider can generally classify the patient with chest pain to one of four categories: a noncardiac etiology, a stable anginal etiology, a possible acute coronary artery syndrome, or a patient with a definite coronary artery syndrome.

Patients who present at low risk for adverse cardiac outcomes may be managed on an outpatient basis. These patients present with new-onset or worsening anginal symptoms yet have not had a severe, prolonged, or at-rest event within the past 2 weeks. Their ECG is normal or unchanged during an episode of chest discomfort and cardiac markers are within normal limits. Low-risk patients should be immediately started on aspirin therapy, 160 to 325 mg, unless contraindicated, along with daily beta-blocker therapy and sublingual nitroglycerin as needed. Identifiable precipitating clinical circumstances should be uncovered, as should any secondary etiologies (e.g., fever, anemia, hypotension, cardiomyopathy, aortic stenosis, thyrotoxicosis, or recent stressful events). Symptoms of unstable angina may resolve once the precipitating event is treated.

Low-risk patients should be seen for follow-up evaluation within a 72-hour period, at which time symptoms should be reevaluated for any further instability. Early exercise tolerance testing should also be performed. Patients should be educated regarding cardiac risk factors and aggressive plans for risk factor modification.

Patients presenting in the intermediate- or high-risk category should be hospitalized for careful monitoring, risk stratification, and management. If the symptoms of acute coronary syndrome are identified in the office setting, immediate referral to an emergency department should be undertaken. The patient should be given sublingual nitroglycerin and chewable aspirin immediately. If chewable aspirin is not available, a regular aspirin tablet should be crushed and given to the patient. Once in the emergency department setting, beta-blocker therapy should be considered if presenting hemodynamic profile permits, with the dose titrated to a heart rate of 50 to 60 beats per minute. Heparin should be given in a bolus of 80 units/kg of body weight and infused at 14 units/kg. The dosage is then titrated to achieve an activated partial thromboplastin time of 1.5 to 2.0 times the control. Low-molecular-weight heparin may also be considered in lieu of heparin therapy. A platelet GPIIb/IIIa receptor antagonist should be added to patients with continuing ischemia or with other high risk features and to patients for whom a percutaneous coronary intervention is planned.

Acute ST-Elevation Myocardial Infarction

Treatment goals for the patient with an acute MI are to restore blood supply to cardiac muscle, to relieve pain, and to decrease the incidence of complications (such as heart failure, myocardial rupture, valvular dysfunction, as well as fatal and nonfatal arrhythmias). Prevention of recurrent ischemia and infarction as well as efforts to decrease mortality should also be undertaken.

With these goals in mind, patients with an acute evolving ST elevation MI should be admitted to a specialized coronary unit, where continuous cardiac rhythm and hemodynamic monitoring can take place. Patients with a suspected MI who are considered low risk for arrhythmias and hemodynamic compromise may be admitted to a telemetry unit where continuous arrhythmia monitoring is available.

The mortality rate of patients with an ST elevation MI is higher than for those with a non-ST elevation MI in the early phases of the acute event. However, recurrent infarction in the late hospital period is much higher in patients with a non-ST elevation MI. When reinfarction occurs, it is associated with a high mortality rate. Thus the difference in long-term prognosis between an ST elevation MI and a non-ST elevation MI is not statistically significant.

Management of an acute ST elevation MI has changed considerably in the past several years. The major area of interest has been the use of thrombolytic therapy, antiplatelet agents, and angioplasty to reestablish coronary artery patency and limit infarct size. The most crucial aspect of management is aimed at preserving the myocardium and reestablishment of coronary flow within a critical time frame. Studies indicate that maximum benefit is achieved from lytic therapy when it is initiated within 1 to 3 hours after the onset of symptoms. Modest benefit is attained when therapy is instituted 3 to 6 hours after the onset of infarction, and some benefit is possible when therapy is given up to 12 hours after the onset of infarction if chest pain is ongoing and ST-segment elevation is apparent in ECG leads that do not demonstrate new Q waves. General contraindications to lytic therapy include recent surgery or head trauma, active internal bleeding, suspected aortic dissection, pregnancy, diabetic hemorrhagic retinopathy, severe hypertension, and a history of cerebrovascular accident or previous allergic reaction to the thrombolytic agent. Hemorrhagic stroke is the most common complication. The rate increases with advancing age. Patients above age 70 years have strokes at twice the rate of younger patients; however, several studies have shown that these groups of patients benefit from lytic therapy. Decisions about thrombolytic therapy must be made on a case-by-case basis in these patients.

Thrombus and platelet aggregation play an important role in the pathogenesis of acute MI. The use of heparin and aspirin to impede the process is indicated. Both heparin and aspirin have been shown to reduce the risk of fatal and nonfatal MI. Unless contraindicated, aspirin (325 mg daily) should be given to all patients. This should be started immediately by having the patient chew an aspirin and should be continued indefinitely.

Clopidogrel should be administered to all patients unable to take aspirin because of a hypersensitivity reaction. Heparin is generally administered by weight adjustment to keep the partial thromboplastin time 1.5 to 2 times normal. A GP IIb/IIIa receptor antagonist should be administered to patients with continuing ischemia, a planned coronary intervention, or other high-risk features.

Nitroglycerin paste or infusion is used if patients continue to have ongoing ischemia. Nitroglycerin reduces systemic vascular resistance and pulmonary capillary wedge pressure and increases collateral coronary blood flow to the subendocardium, thereby protecting ischemic myocardium. When nitroglycerin is administered, an adequate coronary perfusion pressure should be maintained. (IV nitroglycerin 10 μg/min initial dose and up to 300 μg/min for the first 24 to 48 hours is usually administered.)

The early use of IV beta blockers for patients with increased heart rates in the absence of contraindications (e.g., severe congestive heart failure, hypotension, bradycardia, atrioventricular [AV] block) has been shown to reduce myocardial oxygen demand, infarct size, and ventricular fibrillation. In addition, beneficial effects of long-term beta blockers, without intrinsic sympathomimetic activity, have been well documented in large-scale trials, which have demonstrated reduction in mortality, reinfarction, and sudden death. Caution must be taken when administering beta blockers because of their occasional unpredictable hemodynamic effects. Metoprolol (Lopressor 5 mg every 5 minutes for a total of 15 mg IV) is the most commonly used beta blockers at this time. For patients who tolerate the IV dosing, oral dosing should be initiated 15 minutes after the last IV dose at 25 to 50 mg every 6 hours for 48 hours. During this time the patient should periodically be assessed for bradycardia and heart block on cardiac monitor as well as for physical examination findings of bronchospasm. If patients continue to tolerate this dosing regimen they can be placed on 50- to 100-mg PO b.i.d.

The use of angiotensin-converting enzyme (ACE) inhibitors has improved the mortality rate as well as the prevention of heart failure and recurrent MI in patients with left ventricular function of 40% or less. If possible, ACE inhibitors should be started once the patient is hemodynamically stable. Renal issues should also be considered when starting ACE inhibitor therapy; renal artery stenosis is a contraindication to this therapy.

Calcium channel blockers have been shown to be effective in acute and chronic stable angina, but there have been conflicting reports about their use for the patient with an acute MI. It is currently recommended that short-acting calcium antagonists not be used for patients with angina. Patients with continued post-MI ischemia caused by coronary vasospasm might benefit from a calcium channel blocker. Diltiazem, in both long- and short-term studies, has been beneficial (prevention of reinfarction and reduction in mortality) after non-Q wave MI in patients who do not have congestive heart failure.

Arrhythmia prevention studies have failed to demonstrate any survival advantage for patients given prophylactic antiarrhythmic therapy after admission to a monitored unit. Arrhythmias should be promptly diagnosed and treated to prevent further deterioration related to increased myocardial oxygen demands, decreased cardiac output, or electrical instability. The routine use of lidocaine is not recommended.

Pain relief is best remedied by enhancing coronary blood flow or by decreasing myocardial oxygen demand. With ongoing chest pain, morphine sulfate may be administered to decrease myocardial preload because of its vasodilatory effects. It should be noted that as a narcotic, morphine may mask ischemic chest pain; thus the patient may be having ongoing ischemia, but become too sedate to communicate ongoing ischemic symptoms. Morphine may be dosed in 2-mg increments, with many patients requiring up to a total of 15 to 20 mg. Caution must be used in older patients and those with chronic obstructive pulmonary disease (COPD).

Pharmacologic Therapy for Coronary Artery Disease

Aspirin. Aspirin is effective in the treatment of CAD because of its effects on platelets and vasculature endothelial cells. In platelets aspirin *irreversibly* inhibits the synthesis of cyclooxygenase, preventing the formation of thromboxane A_2, which is responsible for platelet aggregation. In vascular endothelial cells aspirin *temporarily* inhibits the synthesis of cyclooxygenase, which inhibits prostacyclin production and platelet aggregation. The clinical benefits of aspirin have been demonstrated at doses of 75 to 325 mg daily. Although aspirin in doses of 75 mg has been demonstrated to inhibit platelet aggregation, its effectiveness on endothelial prostaglandin inhibition has yet to be determined. Therefore aspirin in doses of less than 162 mg daily for the treatment of CAD cannot be recommended at this time.

Aspirin reaches appreciable plasma levels within 20 minutes and results in platelet inhibition within 60 minutes.[11] The antiplatelet effect of aspirin lasts for the 10-day life of the platelet; however, 10% of circulating platelets are replaced on a daily basis. Normal hemostasis can be achieved with only 20% of aspirin-free platelets. This becomes an important consideration in the timing of aspirin withdrawal for elective surgical procedures.

The U.S. Physicians Health Study evaluated 22,071 male physicians receiving alternate-day doses of 325 mg of aspirin and found a 44% reduction in risk of first MI.[12] Findings for overall cardiovascular mortality were inconclusive because of an inadequate number of events. It should be noted that although this study was encouraging, additional data on primary prevention are needed to assess the risk-benefit ratio of aspirin in a healthy population. Clinical judgment should be used for patients at risk for MI until further evidence becomes available.

Aspirin therapy has been proved to benefit patients in the acute phase of an evolving MI and should be routinely administered with an initial loading dose of 162 mg PO unless an anaphylactic aspirin allergy is known.[13] Enteric-coated tablets should be chewed or crushed for more rapid absorption.

The most convincing evidence of the efficacy of using aspirin therapy in an acute evolving MI came from the Second International Study of Infarct Survival.[14] In this trial 17,187 patients presented within 24 hours of symptoms and were randomly assigned to receive aspirin (162 mg daily) or a placebo. After 5 weeks, patients who received aspirin therapy had a 23% reduction in mortality and a 49% reduction in nonfatal reinfarction when compared with the placebo group. In addition, there was no increase in gastrointestinal bleeding in the aspirin-treated group. For those patients with unstable angina, or in those evolving an acute MI and are unable to take aspirin due to a hypersensitivity reaction, clopidogrel should be administered.

Beta Blockers. Beta blockers have become the mainstay of therapy for patients with CAD. Beta blockers decrease myocardial oxygen consumption by decreasing the heart rate at rest and with exercise, by lowering the blood pressure, and by reducing myocardial contractility, thereby eliciting a negative inotropic effect. In contrast, these agents are not useful for vasospastic angina and may worsen the condition. Beta blockers have been shown to reduce total mortality, the rate of nonfatal infarction, cardiovascular mortality, and sudden cardiac death. In addition, they have been shown in some studies to reduce infarct size.

Beta blockers can be classified according to their relative cardioselectivity and lipid solubility. Beta blockers may be "nonselective" (have an affinity for both $beta_1$- and $beta_2$-receptors) or "selective" (have an affinity for $beta_1$-receptors). $Beta_1$-receptors are located in the myocardium, with small amounts of $beta_2$-receptors in the atrium. $Beta_2$-receptors are primarily located in the bronchioles, peripheral vascular smooth muscles, and other specialized sites, such as pancreatic islet cells. Thus blockade of $beta_2$-receptors may lead to bronchoconstriction/bronchospasm and peripheral vascular constriction, resulting in claudication. In addition, the mechanism whereby insulin-induced hypoglycemia is countered by stimulation of the liver to mobilize liver glycogen is $beta_2$-receptor dependent. Thus blockade of $beta_2$-receptors in a patient with diabetes may lead to an inappropriate response to hypoglycemia. This is important, as patients with CAD and one of the following—asthma, COPD, diabetes, or intermittent claudication—may benefit from a low dose of $beta_1$-selective agents administered with caution. However, as one increases the dose of such agents, selectivity is lost, and both types of receptors become blocked (Box 129-6).

BOX 129-6

BETA BLOCKER AGENTS

NONSELECTIVE $BETA_1$ AND $BETA_2$ BLOCKERS
Propranolol (Inderal)
Timolol (Blocadren)
Nadolol (Corgard)
Sotalol (Sotacar,* Betapace)
Penbutolol (Levatol)

NONSELECTIVE/VASODILATORY
Carteolol (Cartrol)
Labetalol (Trandate/Normodyne)
Pindolol (Visken)

CARDIOSELECTIVE—$BETA_1$ RECEPTORS ONLY
Acebutolol (Sectral)
Atenolol (Tenormin)
Metoprolol (Lopressor/Betaloc,* Toprol XL)

*Canada-only drugs.

Side effects of beta blockers include fatigue, impotence, cold extremities, bronchospasm, worsening claudication, bradycardia, and cardiac conduction disturbances. CNS side effects are based on the lipid solubility property of the agent. Agents that are lipid soluble readily cross the blood-brain barrier and are more likely to cause insomnia, depression, and nightmares; this may be seen in any patient but is commonly observed in older adults. Patients should be cautioned that sudden discontinuation of beta-blocker therapy may precipitate anginal symptoms or lead to MI as a result of rebound tachycardia. Although much has been written about the beta-blocker withdrawal syndrome, the incidence is quite low. However, in discontinuing the drug, one should be prudent and taper the drug over several days. Some beta blockers have the capacity to stimulate either one or both $beta_1$- and $beta_2$-receptors, hence the term *intrinsic sympathomimetic activity,* as seen with pindolol. This property limits the efficacy of treating patients with angina because at higher doses the heart rate is not decreased and may even be increased. These agents may be beneficial in patients who have symptomatic sinus bradycardia when treated with other beta blockers. The major effect of beta blockers with sympathomimetic activity is lowering of blood pressure. Labetalol possesses both beta- and alpha-blocking actions. This drug can be used to treat patients with angina, as well as patients with significant hypertension.

Nitrates. Nitrates are recommended for the treatment of stable and unstable angina, as well as in the management of an acute MI. The clinical effectiveness of nitrates is in their ability to promote vascular smooth muscle relaxation, resulting in arteriolar and venous dilation. In smaller doses nitrates dilate the venous system, which causes peripheral pooling and decreased venous return to the heart (preload). This reduction in preload decreases the left ventricular size, ventricular filling pressures, and myocardial wall tension. In larger doses, nitrates dilate the arterial vasculature, lowering systemic blood pressure (afterload) and thereby decreasing the resistance to ventricular ejection, making it easier for the heart to contract. This overall reduction in left ventricular workload decreases myocardial oxygen consumption. The arteriolar dilating effect, however, may produce a reflex tachycardia, thereby increasing myocardial oxygen consumption. This effect may be attenuated by concurrent use of beta blockade. In addition, the combination of nitrates with calcium channel blockers should be undertaken cautiously, as postural hypotension may be a problem.

Coronary vasodilation is induced through the exogenous production of nitric oxide from nitrate metabolism, which is now known to be EDRF. In the coronary circulation, damage to the endothelial layer from atherosclerosis results in decreased availability of EDRF and hence a decreased vasodilatory response. Nitrates are endothelium-independent vasodilators and therefore do not require a functioning endothelium to deliver a vasodilating response. Nitrate administration results in the endogenous production of nitric oxide, which replaces the vasodilating effects of EDRF and promotes coronary vessel vasodilation.

Presently the three nitrate preparations available for use in the United States are nitroglycerin, isosorbide dinitrate (ISDN), and isosorbide mononitrate (ISMN) (Table 129-4).

TABLE 129-4 Nitrate Preparations*

Preparation	Brand Name	Starting Dose	Maximum Dose	Onset of Action	Duration of Action
SUBLINGUAL					
Nitroglycerin	Nitrostat	0.4 mg (1 tablet)	3 tablets in 15 minutes	1 minute	<30 minutes
SUBMUCOSAL					
Nitroglycerin	Nitrolingual	0.4 mg (metered spray)	3 sprays in 15 minutes	1 minute	<30 minutes
ORAL					
ISDN	Isordil, Sorbitrate	20 mg q 4-6 hr	60-80 mg q 4 hr	60-90 minutes	4-6 hours
ISDN-SR	Dilatrate-SR	40 mg q 12 hr	80 mg b.i.d. or t.i.d.		
ISMN	Ismo, Monoket	20 mg in AM and 20 mg 7 hours later			
ISMN-SR	Imdur	30-60 mg q day	120-240 mg q day		
TOPICAL					
Ointment (2%)	Nitro-Bid, Nitrol	0.5 inches q 4-6 hr	4-5 inches q 3-4 hr	30-60 minutes	3-6 hours
Patch	Transderm-Nitro, Nitro-Dur, Nitrodisc, Deponit	5 mg/24 hr (0.1 to 0.4 mg/hr)	2-3 patches of 15 mg in 24 hours	30 minutes	24 hours

*Dosing for nitrate preparations should include a dose-free interval each day to prevent refractory tolerance.

Sublingual nitroglycerin tablets in doses of 0.4 μg are most useful for acute anginal events because of the rapid course of action of sublingual nitroglycerin. Sublingual nitroglycerin is also recommended for prophylactic use before the patient engages in a physical activity or a stressful event that has historically precipitated an anginal event. Sublingual nitroglycerin works within 3 to 5 minutes; however, antiischemic effects last for less than 30 minutes. Because of its short duration of action, sublingual nitroglycerin should be combined with oral nitrates for sustained effectiveness. Patients should be taught to take one nitroglycerin tablet over a 5-minute period for a total of three tablets in a 15-minute period. Nitroglycerin is taken while the patient is in a seated position to decrease preload by maximizing blood flow to the dilated peripheral circulation. If no relief is obtained after three nitroglycerin tablets, the patient should be transported by ambulance to the nearest medical facility. Nitroglycerin tablets retain their potency for up to 6 months after the bottle has been opened. Patients should be encouraged to keep nitroglycerin tablets in their amber-colored glass bottle, protected from moisture and extremes of temperature and light.

Nitroglycerin spray is particularly useful for patients with visual or neurologic impairments who may have difficulty handling a small tablet. The spray is delivered in a metered dose of 0.4 μg and should be applied to the surface of the tongue. Patients should be reminded not to inhale the spray. Each canister contains approximately 200 doses, and the canister will maintain its potency for up to 3 years.

Oral nitroglycerin is the nitrate of choice in the ambulatory population and can be taken as either ISDN or ISMN. ISDN is extensively metabolized in the liver, where over half of it is converted to ISMN. Because of this bypass effect, ISDN is not effective for the treatment of angina or in enhancing exercise capacity in doses of less than 20 mg q 4 hours. In 1991 the U.S. Food and Drug Administration approved ISMN, which does not undergo hepatic degradation, so that 100% of it is available after oral dosing. The main advantage of the ISMNs is that they can be administered once or twice daily, as compared with the need to administer ISDNs three to four times per day. The main disadvantage is the cost. ISMN preparations cost several times more than the generic ISDN, and this needs to be considered in prescribing practices. Aside from these two factors, there is no distinct advantage in using one of these preparations over the other.

Topical nitroglycerin is absorbed through the skin and can be administered either through a 2% ointment or through premeasured skin patches in doses of 5, 10, 15, or 20 mg daily. The advantage of nitroglycerin ointment over other methods of administration is that the ointment can be removed promptly if any side effects develop. However, its disadvantages seem to outweigh its advantages in the ambulatory population. The ointment is messy to apply, can soil clothing, is seldom dosed consistently each time, and may produce a localized skin rash. The nitroglycerin patch produces a more controlled dosing and is generally favored over the ointment by most patients. Although initially topical nitroglycerin is very effective, long-term usage can lead to nitrate tolerance and thus a decreased therapeutic effect. It is therefore recommended that topical nitroglycerin be removed from the skin for 8 hours daily.

Nitrate tolerance results from plasma nitrate levels sustained from continued nitrate administration. Nitrate tolerance is important to identify because it leads to a reduction in antiischemic benefits. The etiology of nitrate tolerance is a complex, multifactorial phenomenon, and the mechanism has remained elusive. However, the theory that is commonly associated with nitrate tolerance involves vascular depletion of sulfhydryl groups. The metabolism of nitrates requires the use of sulfhydryl to form intracellular nitric oxide from nitrates. This is the active molecule that stimulates guanylate cyclase to produce vasodilation. Continuous use of nitrates produces excess nitric oxide formation, thus depleting sulfhydryl groups. A sulfhydryl donor such as acetylcysteine has been used in experiments to counteract nitrate tolerance.

To avoid the effects of nitrate tolerance dosing, intervals free of nitrates must occur. For oral ISDN administration, a three-times-per-day dosing schedule (8 AM, 1 PM, and 6 PM) rather than a four-times-per-day schedule should be prescribed. With sustained-release ISDN administration, dosing at 8 AM and 2 PM would support nitrate-free intervals in the evening. Topical nitrates should be removed for 8 to 12 hours daily. This dosing schedule provides periods during the evening hours whereby the patient is without antiischemic therapy. For this reason, combined with the reflex tachycardia often seen with vasodilation in response to nitrate therapy, combination therapy with beta blockers or calcium channel blockers is recommended.

Calcium Channel Blockers. Calcium channel blockers are used in the treatment of hypertension and angina pectoris. They selectively inhibit the influx of calcium into the calcium-L channel in both smooth muscle and myocardial cells. All have a peripheral arteriolar and coronary vasodilating effect and a negative inotropic effect, although the latter is modest in the case of nifedipine. Two distinct classes of calcium channel antagonists have emerged on the basis of molecular structure: (1) the dihydropyridines (DHPs), related to nifedipine, and (2) the non-DHPs, related to verapamil (papaverine derivative) and diltiazem (benzothiazepine derivative).

The DHPs are more vascular selective; thus their dominant effect is peripheral and coronary vasodilation. They have minimal or no effect on the sinus and AV nodes. The rapid vasodilatory effects of these agents may lead to reflex tachycardia, exacerbation of congestive heart failure, and stimulation of the renin-angiotensin system. These undesirable effects are more common among the short-acting DHPs, and as such should be avoided in the patient with an acute MI. Since the advent of truly long-acting agents (nifedipine XL, amlodipine, felodipine), there have been fewer side effects. In the PRAISE Trial, amlodipine had no detrimental effect on patients with ischemic class II or III congestive heart failure.[15] The non-DHPs, which are less vascular selective than the DHPs, predominantly inhibit nodal tissue (decrease sinus rate) and myocardial contraction. These agents should be used with caution in patients taking beta blockers and in patients with left ventricular dysfunction. They may be safely used in appropriately selected patients without sinus node or AV node disease. Calcium antagonists have the ability to prevent coronary vasoconstriction. In general, verapamil or diltiazem is preferred over nifedipine and other DHPs for monotherapy, as agents in the latter group have the potential to cause a reflex tachycardia (Box 129-7).

BOX 129-7

CALCIUM CHANNEL BLOCKERS

DIHYDROPYRIDINES

Amlodipine (Norvasc)
Isradipine (DynaCirc)
Felodipine (Plendil)
Nicardipine (Cardene)
Nifedipine (Procardia/Adalat)
Nisoldipine (Sular)

NONDIHYDROPYRIDINES

Diphenylalkylamines derivative
Verapamil (Calan, Covera HS, Isoptin, Verelan)
Benzothiazepines derivative
Diltiazem (Cardizem, Dilacor, Tiazac)

Angiotensin-Converting Enzyme Inhibitors. The conical shape of the heart is designed for optimal efficiency in performance and energy utilization. MI induces alteration in the contour of the heart, leading to decreased left ventricular performance and increased energy requirement for a given workload. Preserving the contour of the heart after MI is essential for effective left ventricular performance and prevention of the development of left-sided heart failure. The consequences of poor left ventricular performance result in an increased 5-year mortality ranging from 26% to 75%.[16]

It is clear that stimulation of the renin-angiotensin-aldosterone system plays an important pathophysiologic role in the development of congestive heart failure and poor left ventricular performance. ACE inhibitors can therefore inhibit or counteract the adverse hemodynamic and neurohumoral effects (increased preload, afterload, heart rate, sympathetic tone, catecholamines, and renin-angiotensin system activity) contributed by the system.

Several large trials have shown that administration of ACE inhibitors shortly after acute MI, once the patient is hemodynamically stable, has prevented the development of heart failure in patients with left ventricular dysfunction but without clinical heart failure.[17-19] In addition, ACE inhibitors reduced long-term mortality in patients with and without clinical evidence of heart failure through their ability to reverse the major hemodynamic and neurohumoral abnormalities associated with poor left ventricular performance.[20]

Anticoagulation. The use of anticoagulation with aspirin and heparin has significantly reduced the short-term risk of thromboembolic complications during an acute MI. However, the continuing use of a low-molecular-weight heparin beyond 1 week has not been shown to be effective in further risk reduction.[20] There continues to exist a significant percentage of patients with acute coronary syndrome who experience major vascular events either during or within the first few months after their hospital stay. One alternative oral therapy to minimize cardiac complications is the use of the thienopyridine derivatives, the most promising of which is clopidogrel (Plavix). This medication, in doses of 75 mg daily in addition to aspirin therapy, was shown in the CURE Trial to significantly decrease the incidence of nonfatal MI, strokes, and in-hospital refractory ischemia or severe ischemic episodes as well as heart failure events for up to 6 months.[21]

Left Ventricular Thrombus. The use of two-dimensional echocardiography to evaluate left ventricular function has been of great value in identifying ventricular mural thrombi. Thrombi are more common in patients with a large rather than small area of MI. Thrombi are often observed in the left ventricle, particularly in the apex, where aneurysm and pseudoaneurysm commonly form. On rare occasions, with extensive infarction, thrombus may be observed in the right ventricular apex.

Warfarin (Coumadin) therapy is indicated in patients with a mural thrombus, especially in cases where the thrombus is mobile, has an irregular surface, and is protruding. Warfarin therapy is generally initiated for 3 to 6 months, after which time echocardiographic evaluation to assess the presence or absence of mural thrombus is performed. If the thrombus persists after warfarin therapy, it does not necessarily indicate continued embolic potential unless there is evidence of mobility. In addition, warfarin therapy is indicated in patients with severe left ventricular dysfunction and an ejection fraction of less than 20%.

The Coumadin Aspirin Reinfarction Study (CARS)[22] was prematurely discontinued, because there was no difference between the combined therapy of warfarin plus aspirin and aspirin or warfarin alone.[22] This was a double-blind trial; however, there was difficulty in achieving an international normalized ratio (INR) of 1.5 or greater.

Cholesterol-Lowering Agents. An estimated 99,500,000 American adults have total blood cholesterol levels of 200 mg/dl or greater. Numerous clinical trials have demonstrated that elevated low-density lipoproteins (LDLs) are a major risk factor for CAD. Likewise, recent clinical trials have found that reductions in LDLs have reduced the risk of overall mortality, coronary mortality, major coronary events, coronary artery procedures, and strokes. Therefore an LDL cholesterol of less than 100 ml/dl is optimal. A cholesterol profile should be obtained on hospital admission or within 24 hours thereafter. LDL cholesterol levels begin to decline in the first few hours after an event and may remain low for many weeks. Two major modalities of LDL-lowering therapy are therapeutic lifestyle changes (weight reduction, increased physical activity, and dietary reductions in saturated fats and cholesterol intake) and medication therapy. The drug of choice is usually a statin; however, a bile acid sequestrant or nicotinic acid may be used. After 12 weeks of drug therapy, the response to therapy can be reassessed. If the patient's goal has yet to be achieved, a more intensive drug therapy along with careful lifestyle analysis for compliance should be undertaken. Should the patient still have difficulty in achieving his or her goal, the patient should be referred to a specialist. Once the LDL goal has been achieved the patient may be monitored every 4 to 6 months. Liver function tests and CPK levels should be periodically evaluated to detect any evidence of liver abnormalities or myositis.

Interventional Management of Coronary Artery Disease

Diagnostic Catheterization. In the United States an estimated 1,291,000 inpatient cardiac catheterizations and 472,000 outpatient catheterizations are performed annually. The goal of the cardiac catheterization procedure is to provide detailed structural information to assess patient prognosis and to select an appropriate management strategy. According to AHCPR guidelines, patients considered for cardiac catheterization over ongoing medical therapy include those patients who (1) have recurrent symptoms that are not controlled with medical therapy; (2) are stratified into a high-risk group on noninvasive testing; (3) opt for early invasive strategy; (4) had prior angioplasty, bypass surgery, or MI; and (5) have significant congestive heart failure and/or impaired left ventricular function and angina pectoris.

Percutaneous Coronary Intervention. Percutaneous transluminal coronary angioplasty (PTCA) is a cardiac catheterization technique designed to decrease coronary artery obstruction, thus improving coronary blood flow. Since the inception of PTCA, its clinical and anatomic indications have expanded from the treatment of proximal single-vessel disease to multivessel disease and acute coronary syndromes. Although the use of PTCA has broadened, the mortality and emergency bypass rates have remained less than 1%. The low mortality rate can be attributed to improvement in medical therapy (clopidogrel, glycoprotein IIb/IIIa receptor blockers) and new adjunctive devices such as stents, atherectomy, and rotablation.

The general indications for PTCA and adjunctive therapy are due to the following high-risk indicators: (1) patients with recurrent angina/ischemia at rest or with low level activities, (2) recurrent angina/ischemia with congestive heart failure symptoms, (3) high-risk findings on noninvasive stress testing, (4) depressed left ventricular systolic function of less than 40% on noninvasive studies, (5) hemodynamic instability, (6) sustained ventricular tachycardia, (7) percutaneous coronary intervention within the last 6 months, and (8) a prior history of coronary artery bypass graft (CABG) surgery. PTCA is contraindicated for significant left main CAD when the left main coronary artery is not protected by previous CABG.

No differences have been noted in the complication rates of death, MI, emergency need for CABG, abrupt vessel closure, or hemorrhage when comparing the early invasive treatment group to the noninvasive treatment group.[23] Stent restenosis occurs at a rate of approximately 20%, generally between 3 and 6 months as a result of fibrocellular intimal hyperplasia. After PTCA, coronary artery stenting and rotablation procedures patients are generally discharged the next morning, with a follow-up cardiology appointment within 1 to 2 weeks. Medication therapy consists of aspirin (325 mg daily), beta-blocker therapy, cholesterol-lowering therapy as indicated, and nitroglycerin if needed. Clopidogrel (Plavix), an antiplatelet medication, is prescribed daily for a minimum of 4 weeks in doses of 75 mg for those patients with stent placement. With the advent of these antiplatelet agents, the incidence of early stent thrombus has decreased to less than 1%. Subacute intracoronary stent thrombosis generally occurs 5 days after stent implantation, whereas endothelium restenosis generally occurs around the tenth to twelfth week. After any PCI, patients must be educated to seek immediate attention if anginal symptoms should recur, indicating a potential vessel re-stenosis.

Coronary Artery Bypass Surgery. CABG is one of the most commonly performed surgical procedures in the United States. In 1997 an estimated 607,000 of these procedures were performed on 366,000 patients. The indication for CABG is to improve the overall quality of life. Approximately 90% of patients have their symptoms relieved initially, with 70% of patients remaining free of symptoms at 1 to 3 years. When cardiac symptoms redevelop, they are generally associated with bypass graft occlusion. Overall, the occlusion rate for saphenous vein grafts is greater than that for left internal mammary artery grafts.

Because surgical treatment of ischemic heart disease is palliative, reoperative CABG is now common. The treatment of choice—reoperative coronary artery bypass, cardiology intervention, or medical therapy—depends on the patient's symptoms, medical history, coronary anatomy, and left ventricular function.

LIFE SPAN CONSIDERATIONS

Recently, the gender differences between men and women with respect to coronary anatomy, clinical presentation, and treatment modalities have been under investigation. The clinical presentation of women often does not typify the midsternal chest tightness with shoulder and arm radiation that men often experience. Instead, women may present with indigestion as their only symptom. Because the mortality rate from an MI is 44% in women compared to 27% in men, it is important that gender bias be eliminated from the clinical decision making and that the nuances of CAD in women be acknowledged.[24]

The diagnosis of CAD in women has also proven difficult because of false-positive exercise tolerance testing in women. The ECG response to such testing in women has been shown to elicit an abnormal ischemic response in up to 67% of those tested, despite normal coronary arteries. Speculation into this area suggests women's lower hematocrit levels and higher circulating estrogen levels as plausible culprits. In an effort to provide greater test sensitivity and specificity, radionuclide testing may be performed. Despite the increased accuracy this testing provides, there is still a significant number of false-positive results mainly as a result of breast attenuation artifact, which may produce septal and anterior wall defects. Stress echocardiography may prove to be a more accurate method of noninvasive CAD testing in women.

COMPLICATIONS

The complications of ischemic heart disease and MI are potentially life threatening. Recurrent ischemia and reinfarction can increase the area of nonfunctioning myocardial tissue, creating mechanical complications such as papillary muscle rupture, ventricular aneurysm, or ventricular septal defect. Rhythm and conduction disturbances may arise without premonitory signs. Chest pain and anxiety associated with cardiac disease can produce hypertension, increasing afterload and oxygen demand. Heart failure, hypotension, and shock impair systemic perfusion and cardiac function.

INDICATIONS FOR REFERRAL/HOSPITALIZATION

The patient whose condition is complicated by multiple co-morbid diseases (e.g., diabetes mellitus, hypertension, heart failure, hyperlipidemia, and peripheral vascular disease) should be referred to a cardiologist. Patients with chronic stable angina who develop a change in anginal pattern should also be referred to a specialist. In addition, all patients with a documented history of coronary ischemic syndrome should be co-managed with a cardiologist. The patient's symptoms and co-morbid diseases should determine the frequency of visits to the specialist.

It is well established that deaths occurring from acute MI occur within the first hour of onset. Therefore the importance of symptom education of an MI, and rapid transport and early admission to a hospital cannot be overemphasized.

Ischemic CAD represents a spectrum of coronary insufficiency ranging from chronic stable angina, unstable angina, or non–Q-wave MI (subendomyocardial infarction) to transmural MI. Hospitalization is based on specific criteria.

Patients who are having unstable angina pectoris, defined as new-onset angina (angina occurring within 1 month), angina occurring at rest and with minimal exertion, or crescendo angina, should be admitted to the hospital. All patients who are suspected of, or are having, an acute MI should be hospitalized.

PATIENT AND FAMILY EDUCATION

Considerations for patients with CAD include careful management of co-morbid illnesses, along with a thorough understanding of their disease process and prescribed medical regimen. Women who are candidates for hormone replacement therapy should be offered information about the risks and benefits of estrogen or hormone replacement therapy after menopause.

Patients need to be educated about CAD and heart attack warning signs. Anginal symptoms are often present days to weeks before the onset of an acute MI. Therefore education to assist patients to recognize cardiac symptoms and an early action plan should be undertaken. The National Institutes of Health suggests the use of a "TIME method." This method places emphasis on *t*alking with your patients about their risk of a heart attack, how to recognize symptoms and an action step plan. Next to *i*nvestigate their feelings about MI, and to *m*ake an action plan. Lastly the provider should *e*valuate the patient's understanding regarding the discussed recommendations and delay risks.

Both patients and families should understand the importance of calling 911 or an ambulance if the symptoms of a heart attack occur or are not relieved with sublingual nitroglycerin. These symptoms include chest pressure or discomfort; pain radiating to the arm, neck, or jaw; diaphoresis; nausea and/or vomiting; shortness of breath; dizziness; rapid or irregular pulse; and loss of consciousness. All families who have a family member with CAD should be encouraged to learn CPR.

HEALTH PROMOTION

Despite growing evidence from clinical trials establishing that risk factor modification can decrease coronary artery morbidity and mortality, the majority of patients still are not being treated. A "Get with the Guidelines Program" has been developed by the American Heart Association to ensure patients are being discharged on appropriate medications and risk factor counseling. These guidelines focus on smoking cessation, lipid lowering, ACEI use, beta blocker therapy, hypertension management, weight and exercise management, diabetes management, atrial fibrillation management, ASA or other antithrombotic medication, and alcohol and drug abuse management.

REFERENCES

1. American Heart Association: *2001 heart and stroke statistical update*, Dallas, Texas, 2001, AHA.
2. Goff D and others: Knowledge of heart attack symptoms in a population survey in the United States: the REACT trial, *Arch Intern Med* 158:2329-2338, 1998.
3. Pasternak R and others: 27th Bethesda Conference: Matching the intensity of risk factor management with the hazard for coronary disease

events, Task force 3: spectrum of risk factors for coronary heart disease, *J Am Coll Cardiol* 27(5):978-990, 1996.
4. Yeung AC and others: The effect of atherosclerosis on the vasomotor response of coronary arteries to mental stress, *N Engl J Med* 325: 1551-1556, 1991.
5. Nabel EG and others: Dilation of normal and constriction of atherosclerotic coronary arteries caused by the cold pressor test, *Circulation* 77:43-52, 1988.
6. Vita JA and others: The coronary vasomotor response to acetylcholine relates to risk factors for coronary artery disease, *Circulation* 81: 491-497, 1990.
7. Braunwald E and others: ACC/AHA guidelines for the management of patients with unstable angina and non-ST-segment elevation myocardial infarction: a report of the American College of Cardiology/American Heart Association Task Force on Practice Guidelines (Committee on the Management of Patients with Unstable Angina), *Circulation* 102:1193-1209, 2000.
8. Cannon C et al: Predictors of non–q-wave MI in patients with acute ischemic syndrome: an analysis from the thrombolysis in myocardial ischemia (TIMI) III trials, *Am J Cardiol* 75:977-981, 1995.
9. Ellestad MH: *Stress testing principles and practice,* Philadelphia, 1975, FA Davis.
10. Puleo P and others: Use of a rapid assay of subforms of creatine kinase MB to diagnose or rule out acute myocardial infarction, *N Engl J Med* 331:561-566, 1994.
11. Hirsh J and others: Aspirin and other platelet active drugs: the relationship between dose, effectiveness, and side effects, *Chest* 102(suppl): 327S-336S, 1992.
12. Steering Committee of the Physicians' Health Study Research Group: Final report on the aspirin component of the ongoing Physicians' Health Study, *N Engl J Med* 321:129-135, 1989.
13. Harpaz D and others: Effect of aspirin on mortality in women with symptomatic or silent myocardial ischemia, *Am J Cardiol* 78:1215-1219, 1996.
14. ISIS-2 (Second International Study of Infarct Survival) Collaborative Group: Randomized trial of intravenous streptokinase, oral aspirin, both, or neither among 17,197 cases of suspected acute myocardial infarction: ISIS-2, *Lancet* 2:349-360, 1988.
15. Packer M and others: Prospective randomized amlodipine survival evaluation trial (PRAISE), *N Engl J Med* 335:1107-1114, 1996.
16. Cowie MA: The epidemiology of heart failure, *Eur Heart J* 18:208-225, 1997.
17. The SOLVD Investigators: Effects of enalapril on mortality and the development of heart failure in asymptomatic patients with reduced left ventricular ejection fractions, *N Engl J Med* 327:685-691, 1992.
18. McKelvie R, Benedict, C, Yusuf, S: Prevention of congestive heart failure and management of asymptomatic left ventricular dysfunction, *Br Med J* 318:1400-1402, 1999.
19. CONSENSUS Trial Study Group: Effects of enalapril on mortality in severe congestive heart failure: results of the Cooperative North Scandinavian Enalapril Survival Study (CONSENSUS), *N Engl J Med* 316:1429-1435, 1987.
20. Fragmin and Fast Revascularization during Instability in Coronary Artery Disease (FRISC II) Investigators: Long-term low molecular-mass heparin in unstable coronary artery disease: FRISC II prospective randomized multicentre study, *Lancet* 354:701-707, 1999.
21. The Clopidogrel in Unstable Angina to Prevent Recurrent Events Trial Investigators: Effects of clopidogrel in addition to aspirin in patients with acute coronary syndromes without ST-segment elevations, *N Engl J Med* 345:494-503, 2001.
22. Coumadin Aspirin Reinfarction Study (CARS) Investigators: Randomized double-blind trial of fixed low-dose warfarin with aspirin after myocardial infarction, *Lancet* 350:389-396, 1997.
23. Bowden W and others for the VANQWISH Trial Investigators: Outcomes in patients with acute non-q-wave myocardial infarction randomly assigned to an invasive as compared with a conservative management strategy, *N Engl J Med* 338:1785-1792, 1998.
24. McGrath D: Coronary artery disease in women, *Am J Nurse Pract* 2(6):7-23, 1998.

CHAPTER 130

Outpatient Management of Deep Venous Thrombosis

Patricia C. Flanagan

DEFINITION/EPIDEMIOLOGY

Deep venous thrombosis (DVT) occurs when blood flow is partially or completely obstructed by a thrombus in a deep vein, potentially posing complications ranging from regional tissue damage to fatal pulmonary embolism. The incidence of DVT is widely variable, with estimates ranging from 43 to 145 per 100,000 annually in the United States.[1]

DVT most commonly occurs in the lower extremity, involving the iliac, femoral, or popliteal veins. Thrombi in the proximal venous system, particularly above the level of the knee, pose a greater risk of embolization than those in calf veins. The axillary and subclavian veins of the upper extremity can also be affected by DVT.

Risk factors, potential complications, diagnostic evaluation, and therapeutic modalities are essentially the same for DVT in upper or lower extremities. Risk factors for DVT include surgery, trauma, immobilization, malignancy, extremity paralysis, anesthesia, insertion of a central venous catheter or pacemaker, postpartum state, estrogen use, family history of DVT, previous history of DVT, recent hospitalization, recent air travel, inherited blood disorders (Box 130-1), and advancing age.[2]

Early detection and treatment can significantly reduce the risk of complications, particularly life-threatening pulmonary embolisms. Management of DVT is increasingly occurring in the primary care setting and selected patients may be managed in subacute units or as outpatients. Outpatient management is possible because the development of rapidly effective, readily controllable anticoagulation therapy with low-molecular-weight heparin.

PATHOPHYSIOLOGY

Although the specific etiology of DVT is unclear, at least two of the three indicators that compose Virchow's triangle are usually present: venous stasis abnormality of the intimal layer of the vascular wall, and altered blood coagulation.[3] Venous stasis can occur in association with chronic illness, obesity, immobilization (as in casting, long airplane or car journeys, or bed rest), and lower extremity trauma. Injury to the venous intima can result from direct trauma, inflammation resulting from medication administration, or vascular disease. Upper extremity DVT is associated with indwelling central venous catheters and repetitive motion of the extremity resulting in vessel inflammation. Hypercoagulability may occur when anticoagulant medications are abruptly discontinued, or may be due to inherited deficiencies of naturally occurring anticoagulants such as antithrombin III, protein C, or protein S fibrinogen abnormalities, or antibodies to phospholipids.

Whatever the course, DVT develops from platelet aggregation at the wall of a deep vein. Resulting propagation of the blood clot may partially or completely occlude the vessel, causing decreased venous circulation and extremity swelling below the level of the clot.

Thrombus formation may also occur in the superficial veins, typically in the setting of varicose veins. Superficial thrombi pose far less risk of embolization because of a tendency to spontaneously dissolve.

BOX 130-1

BLOOD DYSCRASIA RISK FACTORS FOR DEEP VENOUS THROMBOSIS

- Antithrombin III deficiency
- Protein C deficiency
- Protein S deficiency
- Activated protein C resistance
- Antiphospholipid antibody syndrome
- Polycythemia vera
- Erythrocytosis
- Factor V Leiden mutation
- Mutation G20210A in prothrombin gene

CLINICAL PRESENTATION

The most common presenting complaint is unilateral swelling, accompanied by pain in the affected extremity. For some patients, the first indication of DVT will be the complication of pulmonary embolization from the DVT. These patients present with shortness of breath and chest pain.

Obtaining a thorough patient history is crucial in order to identify pertinent risk factors such as recent surgery or injury, phlebitis, malignancy, immobilization or inactivity, and medication history. A family history to determine the presence of episodes of thrombosis or any blood coagulation disorders is an essential part of assessment for DVT.

PHYSICAL EXAMINATION

The signs of DVT are often subtle and nonspecific. Physical examination of the affected extremity may reveal tenderness, swelling, warmth, and erythema. With suspected lower extremity DVT, the circumference of the affected leg should be measured 10 cm below the tibial tuberosity and the measurement compared with the opposite extremity.

Prominent varicosities or dilated superficial veins may be present and it may be possible to palpate a cordlike vein. Alternatively, complete obstruction of the vasculature may occur and present with prominent superficial veins and cyanosis below the level of the clot. Homan's sign (calf pain in dorsiflexion of the foot) is an unreliable indicator of DVT.

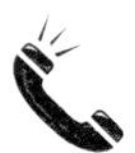

Physician consultation is indicated for all patients suspected of DVT.

DIAGNOSTICS

Diagnostic testing is nearly always indicated in the work up for suspected DVT because of the difficulty of determining the presence of DVT based on clinical presentation, patient history, and physical examination. A method for managing the diagnosis of DVT can be based on a classification system developed by Anderson and associates[4] for use in the emergency department setting. This classification can be used to group patients into a high, medium, and low pretest probability for DVT, and this grouping is used to guide diagnostic testing (Box 130-2). With this system, low probability patients can have DVT excluded by a negative duplex ultrasound (DU) with follow-up evaluation indicated. Those with moderate or high probability can have serial ultrasounds the next day and then serially if the ultrasound is negative.[5] Alternatively, medium- to high-risk patients can undergo anticoagulation and have either a repeat DU (medium probability) or immediate venography (high probability) if the initial DU is negative.[4] (Clinicians should note that noninvasive tests like DU may not be accurate and can yield false-negative results in the setting of previous DVT or congestive heart failure).[5] In these cases, patients should have venography (phlebography.)[5] Other testing may be indicated by continuing symptoms, or when the suspicion of DVT remains high.

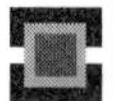
Diagnostics

Deep Venous Thrombosis

Imaging
Duplex venous ultrasound
Impedance plethysmography (more sensitive for thrombi in the proximal venous system or do not fully obstruct blood flow)
Contrast venography
MRI (for proximal DVT)

Laboratory
Laboratory tests for hypercoagulability*

*If indicated.

BOX 130-2

GUIDE FOR PRETEST PROBABILITY OF LOWER EXTREMITY DEEP VENOUS THROMBOSIS

Score 1 point for each of the following findings:
- Presence of cancer (current active or palliative treatment or treatment in last 6 months)
- Recent immobilization of lower extremity, presence of paralysis or paresis
- Tenderness localized to deep vein system distribution
- Swelling of entire leg
- Affected calf measurement > or = 3 cm larger than nonaffected calf
- Affected leg with pitting edema (nonaffected leg has no pitting edema)
- Presence of dilated superficial veins near affected area (nonvaricose)

Subtract 2 points from score:
- There could be as likely probability for an alternative diagnosis

Total the result:
- High probability > or = 3 points total
- Medium probability 1 or 2 points total
- Low probability 0 or less total

Modified from Anderson DR and others: Thrombosis in the emergency department: use of a clinical diagnosis model to safely avoid the need for urgent radiological investigation, *Arch Intern Med* 159(5):477-482, 1999.

There are two noninvasive tests for DVT. The first, duplex venous ultrasound (DU), is a common noninvasive study that involves imaging the deep veins. Duplex venous ultrasonography involves imaging the deep veins in order to visualize the thrombus and identify abnormalities of blood flow in the affected area. Failure of the vein to collapse when pressure is applied during ultrasonography is highly suggestive of underlying thrombosis. DU is less sensitive for clots confined to the calf than for those extending to the proximal venous system, so a series of studies may be necessary to identify propagation of the thrombus.

Another noninvasive test, impedance plethysmography, detects changes in blood flow using a thigh blood pressure cuff. Plethysmography is generally more sensitive for determining the presence of thrombi in the proximal venous system than for those in the distal venous system and thrombi that do not fully obstruct blood flow.

Contrast venography is more sensitive and specific than DU and is used when clinical presentation, history, and physical examination findings are highly suggestive of DVT, but initial noninvasive studies are negative. This invasive diagnostic test involves injecting dye into a foot vein and monitoring blood flow for defects characteristic of thrombus. However, venography is uncomfortable and poses risks because of its invasive nature and the potential for an adverse reaction to the injected contrast medium. The procedure itself may cause thrombosis.

Measurement of blood levels of d-dimer, a fibrin degradation product, has been used in the workup of DVT and pulmonary embolism, but is generally considered insensitive and nonspecific for definitive diagnosis. In particular, with cancer patients, one study found that a negative d-dimer test result does not reliably exclude DVT, as the negative predictive values of the d-dimer test is significantly lower in patients with cancer.[6] Studies have indicated that a negative d-dimer level in the setting of negative ultrasonography may be sufficient to eliminate the need for further noninvasive studies.[5]

MRI can be useful for detecting proximal DVT. Specifically, thrombi in the vena cava or pelvic veins can be visualized with MRI.

If noninvasive studies are positive, primary care practitioners may opt to proceed with anticoagulation therapy without pursuing contrast venography. Although noninvasive studies are less likely to initially detect DVT in the calf veins, it is crucial to ensure that calf thrombi do not propagate to the popliteal vein, where the risk of embolization is greater. Thus an initially negative noninvasive study in the setting of a high degree of clinical suspicion indicates the need for repeat imaging. Observation alone may be a reasonable strategy if noninvasive studies are negative, clinical presentation and physical examination are unimpressive, and patient history is noncontributory.

Consideration of a hypercoagulable state should be given in patients with documented DVT who are less than 60 years old and have no known risk factors for DVT. Assays to evaluate hypercoagulability may be performed (see Chapter 232). However, the timing of these tests is crucial, because heparin or warfarin may affect these measurements.

DIFFERENTIAL DIAGNOSIS

Differential diagnoses that should be considered include cellulitis, musculoskeletal injury, ruptured Baker's cyst, and peripheral edema from other causes such as congestive heart failure or lymphatic obstruction.

MANAGEMENT

Inpatient Management

DVT can be managed in the inpatient setting with IV unfractionated heparin to stabilize the existing thrombus and oral anticoagulation with warfarin to prevent the formation of new thrombi. Anticoagulation in the hospital setting typically involves administration of IV heparin for about 1 week, with concurrent administration of warfarin, which takes about 5 days to reach therapeutic blood levels after initial dosing. The goal of therapy is to prevent propagation of the clot and prevent new thrombi from forming. Heparin and warfarin will not lyse existing clots, but will promote fibrinolysis. The most common side effect of heparin is hemorrhage.

Outpatient or Subacute Management

Development of low-molecular-weight heparin now offers an alternative of home therapy for patients who are stable, specifically those with DVT in the calf veins, without significant risk for pulmonary embolism or other complications, and who are able to actively participate in the treatment plan.[7] Evidence supports the benefit of treating these selected patients for DVT out of the hospital.[8-11] Home therapy is contraindicated if the patient is medically unstable or pregnant, or has a history of recent trauma or surgery, renal insufficiency, iliac thrombus, or heparin-induced thrombocytopenia.

One method of outpatient treatment for patients weighing between 50 and 115 kg is to start anticoagulation with dalteparin 100 units/kg (round to nearest 500 U) SC every 12 hours (maximum of 9000 U every 12 hours) for 5 days.[5] Warfarin (Coumadin) is begun on day 2, dosing based on the prothrombin time/international normalized ratio (PT/INR) measurement. The PT/INR is measured daily to adjust the warfarin dosage. On day 5, platelets are also measured and the dalteparin may be discontinued after day 5 if the PT INR is >2 for 2 days (INR goal is 2 to 3).[5] The patient is on bed rest for 2 days with no exertional activity until the condition stabilizes. Patients are monitored daily for vital signs (pulse, blood pressure, respiration), size of pulmonary embolus, increased leg pain, and swelling. An alternative regimen includes admission for 24 hours for initial anticoagulation with heparin.[5]

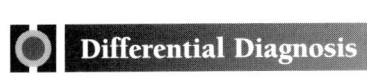

Deep Venous Thrombosis

Cellulitis
Musculoskeletal injury
Ruptured Baker's cyst
Peripheral edema from other causes (e.g., congestive heart failure, lymphatic obstruction)

Adjunct Treatment

Treatment strategies for all patients with DVT should include elevation and compression of the affected extremity to promote venous return. Patients should be instructed to avoid sitting for extended periods. Elastic compression stockings, either calf or thigh-high (depending on location of the clot) should be worn when ambulating.

Deep Venous Thrombosis Prophylaxis

Low-molecular-weight heparins are approved for DVT prophylaxis and are more expensive than unfractionated heparin; however, they have a more predictable response, a longer half-life, and greater bioavailability than unfractionated heparin. They also cause less bleeding than heparin and are associated with a lower incidence of heparin-induced thrombocytopenia.[3,12] These drugs, ardeparin, dalteparin, danaparoid, and enoxaparin, also are administered for 5 to 7 days in conjunction with the initiation of warfarin therapy. All are approved for DVT prophylaxis, some in specific settings, and danaparoid is also approved for DVT treatment.

Warfarin therapy is generally initiated with 10 mg q.d. and adjusted based on evaluation of the PT/INR. Goal INR is between 2.0 and 3.0 to maintain the desired therapeutic anticoagulation effect while incurring the least risk of hemorrhage. With patients treated in the hospital for DVT, PT/INR is measured daily in the hospital setting, every few days in the outpatient setting until the goal INR is reached, and monthly thereafter.

Duration of oral anticoagulation therapy is determined by causative factors typically up to 6 weeks when associated with short-term immobilization or surgery, 3 months for other causes, and indefinitely in the setting of persisting risk factors.

Recurrent Deep Venous Thrombosis

If anticoagulation is contraindicated for any reason, or if DVT recurs despite adequate anticoagulation, placement of an inferior vena cava filter may be indicated. Thrombolytic therapy is usually reserved for extensive DVT occurring in the iliac or femoral system as a result of the higher risk of embolization of thrombi in these locations and the drug's increased potential for causing hemorrhage.

Superficial vein thrombosis does not require anticoagulation therapy. A reasonable management strategy includes nonsteroidal antiinflammatory drug therapy, extremity elevation, and the application of moist heat therapy.

LIFE SPAN CONSIDERATIONS

Anticoagulation is initiated with caution in the older adults. This group has a greater likelihood of co-morbidities and polypharmacy, and potentially increased risk of sustaining injury from falling.

Women of childbearing age should be advised about the potential risks and benefits of anticoagulation. Careful consideration should be given to the prevention of pregnancy during anticoagulation therapy, because the safety of low-molecular-weight heparin during pregnancy has not been established, and warfarin is contraindicated in pregnancy.

COMPLICATIONS

The most lethal complication of DVT is pulmonary embolism, which causes an estimated 200,000 deaths annually in the United States. Pulmonary embolism occurs when a thrombus breaks apart and a resulting embolus lodges in one of the pulmonary arteries. Signs and symptoms include acute-onset shortness of breath, chest pain, anxiety, tachycardia, and hypoxemia. A significant obstruction can be rapidly fatal and presents with the signs and symptoms of complete circulatory collapse.

Other complications of DVT include chronic venous insufficiency and the development of postphlebitic syndrome, which is characterized by venous valvular incompetence and chronic edema.

INDICATIONS FOR REFERRAL/HOSPITALIZATION

Low-molecular-weight heparin therapy may be appropriate for certain stable patients, specifically those with DVT in the calf veins, with limited risk factors for pulmonary embolism and no other contributing problems. A short observational hospital admission may be indicated for medically complicated patients, those with co-morbidities, or those who are not able to adequately manage home anticoagulation therapy for any reason.

Visiting nursing services may be required in certain circumstances when anticoagulation therapy is indicated. Older adults and those requiring assistance with the activities of daily living may be overwhelmed by the need for accurate dosing and medication administration. A home safety evaluation may be in order to identify injury risks in the dwelling.

PATIENT AND FAMILY EDUCATION

The patient who is placed on anticoagulant therapy should be educated about the adverse side effects of low-molecular-weight heparins and warfarin, and should be encouraged to immediately report signs or symptoms of unusual bleeding. Avoiding injury is important, so the patient should refrain from contact sports and other potentially injurious activities. Signs and symptoms of pulmonary embolization (chest pain/pressure, breathing difficulty, rapid pulse) should be taught. If these signs and symptoms occur, the emergency plan should be reviewed and individualized for each patient based on the availability of emergency response in the patient's area.

The patient should avoid excessive consumption or pattern change in the intake of foods that are rich in vitamin K, which interferes with warfarin synthesis. These foods include green leafy vegetables such as spinach, cabbage, and broccoli; beans; cheeses; cauliflower; avocado; turnips; rice; milk; pork; and fish.

Multiple drugs interact with warfarin to produce an enhanced or reduced response. New medications should be initiated only after carefully considering potential adverse interactions. The patient should be instructed to refrain from using over-the-counter, supplemental, or herbal remedies without consulting their primary care provider.

HEALTH PROMOTION

Prevention of recurrent DVT development should be addressed by discussing lifestyle changes including weight loss, the benefits of a daily walk, and the importance of elevating the legs when sitting. Additionally, the patient should be instructed to avoid sitting or standing for a prolonged period, and to wear elastic stockings to help promote venous return. Particularly, the importance of frequent position changes and the risk for DVT when riding in cars or airplanes should be reviewed. Patients over 60 years of age and those with other DVT risk factors should be encouraged to wear compression stockings when flying.

REFERENCES

1. Silverstein MD and others: Trends in the incidence of deep vein thrombosis and pulmonary embolism: a 25-year population-based study, *Arch Intern Med* 158:585-593, 1998.
2. Heit JA and others: Risk factors for deep vein thrombosis and pulmonary embolism: a population-based case-control study, *Arch Intern Med* 160:809-815, 2000.
3. Weismantel D: Treatment of the patient with deep vein thrombosis, *J Fam Pract* 50:249-256, 2001.
4. Anderson DR and others: Thrombosis in the emergency department: use of a clinical diagnosis model to safely avoid the need for urgent radiological investigation, *Arch Intern Med* 159(5):477-482, 1999.
5. Barry MJ: Diagnosis and treatment of deep venous thrombosis: physician's guide. In MGH clinical pathways, primary care operations improvement, Retrieved August 30, 2001 from the World Wide Web: http://www.mdguide_files/physicians_guide.htm.
6. Lee AY and others: Clinical utility of a rapid whole blood d-dimer assay in patients with cancer who present with suspected acute deep vein thrombosis, *Ann Intern Med* 131(6):417-423, 1999.
7. Harrison L and others: Assessment of outpatient treatment of deep-vein thrombosis with low-molecular-weight heparin, *Arch Intern Med* 158:2001-2003, 1998.
8. Boccalon H and others: Clinical outcome and cost of hospital vs home treatment of proximal deep vein thrombosis with a low-molecular-weight heparin: the Vascular Midi-Pyrenees study, *Arch Intern Med* 160(12):1769-1773, 2000.
9. O'Shaughnessy D, Miles J, Wimperis J: Patients with deep-vein thrombosis can be safely treated as out-patients [In Process Citation], *QJM* 93(10):663-667, 2000.
10. Grau E and others: Home treatment of deep venous thrombosis with low molecular weight heparin: long-term incidence of recurrent venous thromboembolism, *Am J Hematol* 67(1):10-14, 2001.
11. Dunn AS and others: Outpatient treatment of deep venous thrombosis in diverse inner-city patients, *Am J Med* 110(6):458-462, 2001.
12. Kearon C, Gent M: Heparin therapy for deep vein thrombosis: from hospital to home, *Am J Med* 110:501-502, 2001.

CHAPTER 131

Endocarditis

Denise DeJoseph Gauthier and Eric M. Isselbacher

DEFINITION/EPIDEMIOLOGY

The clinical characteristics and bacteriologic evidence associated with infective endocarditis were recognized before the advent of antimicrobial therapy to combat the offending organisms. Before the discovery of antibiotics, endocarditis was a progressive and eventually fatal disorder. Despite diagnostic advancements and the availability of newer antimicrobial agents, infective endocarditis still carries a significant morbidity rate and can be life threatening. Although the overall incidence of infective endocarditis is relatively low, certain populations are at a higher risk. Primary prevention in these high-risk groups is of critical importance.[1-5]

Infective endocarditis refers to a microbial infection within the heart. These vegetations most often involve the heart valves, but they can occur on the intraventricular septum or mural endocardium. The majority of cases of endocarditis are the result of a bacterial infection; a few cases result from fungal organisms. Rarely, endocarditis may be the result of a rickettsial, spirochete, or chlamydial infection.[1-5]

Historically, endocarditis has been classified as acute or subacute according to its clinical course. Although classifications based on acuity are helpful, a more descriptive system has been introduced and is of greater therapeutic and prognostic value. Because the incidence of acute rheumatic heart disease is on the decline in developed countries, patients with mitral valve prolapse, prosthetic valve replacements, congenital abnormalities, or degenerative valve disease, as well as users of IV drugs, now account for the majority of patients diagnosed with endocarditis. Therefore endocarditis is presently classified according to the underlying valve anatomy together with the infectious etiology (e.g., native valve viridans streptococcal endocarditis).[3-5]

Native Valve Endocarditis

The majority of patients with native valve endocarditis who do not use IV drugs have a predisposing cardiac lesion. In the majority of cases, the underlying cardiac lesion is mitral valve prolapse.[3-5] The overall incidence of native valve endocarditis in non-IV drug users is 3 times higher in men than in women. The patients at highest risk are men with a systolic murmur of mitral regurgitation, especially those over 45 years of age.[2,4]

Endocarditis associated with rheumatic heart lesions is on the decline but still accounts for 30% of cases. Patients in this group tend to be middle-aged or older, and the mitral valve is most often involved. Lesions associated with congenital heart disease are the underlying cause in 10% to 20% of patients. Advances in the management of these structural abnormalities, including septal defects and patent ductus arteriosus, have significantly reduced the number of individuals at risk.[1,3]

Calcific degeneration of the valves is a predisposing factor in older adults. Previous endocarditis itself is a predisposing factor because of the valvular damage that results from the infection.[3] However, infective endocarditis can occur on valves that are morphologically normal; in recent years there has been an increasing number of patients with no detectable predisposing cardiac lesion.[1,4]

Streptococcal species account for 50% to 70% of native valve endocarditis in non-IV drug users.[1,3] Viridans streptococci are normal inhabitants of the oropharynx and account for more than half of all streptococcal endocardial infections. Organisms in this group include *S. sanguis, S. salivarius, S. mutans*, and *S. mitis*. Viridans streptococci usually infect abnormal valves and are typically highly sensitive to penicillin.[1,4,6]

S. bovis, a group D *Streptococcus*, is the causative organism in a small percentage of cases, but it is more common in individuals over 60 years of age and is strongly associated with a malignant or premalignant gastrointestinal lesions. Therefore patients with *S. bovis* endocarditis should be evaluated for an undetected gastrointestinal malignancy. *S. bovis* is a virulent microorganism, associated with significant valvular damage and resultant hemodynamic compromise, as well as a high risk of embolism. Although the microorganism is highly sensitive to penicillin, valvular destruction and persistent large vegetations are indications for surgical intervention.[3,6-8]

Group A beta-hemolytic and group B streptococci account for fewer than 5% of cases; these organisms are capable of attacking normal valves, leading to rapid destruction and embolization of vegetative matter. Group B streptococci are normal flora of the gastrointestinal tract, oropharynx, vagina, and urethra. Co-morbid conditions associated with endocardial infection by these organisms include diabetes mellitus, carcinoma, osteomyelitis, malignancy, and hepatic failure. Penicillin alone may not be bactericidal; an aminoglycoside antibiotic may be necessary.[2,3,6]

Enterococci are indigenous to the gastrointestinal tract and urethra and are responsible for 10% of native valve endocarditis in non-IV drug users. *Enterococci faecalis, E. faecium*, and *E. durans* can attack normal or abnormal valves. Enterococcal endocarditis is usually seen in older men and young women who have a recent history of genitourinary surgery, trauma, or malignancy. Although rare, this condition may also occur in women who have undergone an abortion, a pregnancy, or a cesarean delivery. Enterococcal organisms are resistant to penicillin alone, and therefore an aminoglycoside is necessary to achieve eradication. The treatment of enterococcal endocarditis has become further complicated by beta-lactamase-producing and aminoglycoside-resistant strains.[3,4,6]

Staphylococci are responsible for 20% to 25% of cases of native valve endocarditis, with most of these cases due to *S. aureus* (coagulase-positive *Staphylococcus*). The majority of endocardial infections involving IV drug users can be attributed to this microorganism. *S. aureus* endocarditis is characterized by the rapid destruction of the involved valve with multiple metastatic abscesses; this often results in heart failure or death within days. Coagulase-negative species, such as *S. epidermidis*, are uncommon pathogens in native valve endocarditis but are commonly associated with prosthetic valve involvement. Staphylococcal species are highly resistant to penicillin because of their ability to produce beta-lactamase.[1,3,4,6]

Other potential pathogens in native valve endocarditis include the gram-negative organisms in the HACEK group

(*Haemophilus, Actinobacillus, Cardiobacterium, Eikenella,* and *Kingella*), which are components of the oropharyngeal flora. These organisms account for approximately 5% to 10% of cases in non–IV drug users. Although the clinical course is typically subacute, these organisms are capable of producing large vegetations with a high risk of embolization. Unfortunately, the HACEK organisms are quite difficult to isolate from blood, which makes their diagnosis challenging.[2-4,6]

Fungal organisms are rarely responsible for native valve endocarditis in non–IV drug users. However, *Candida* and *Aspergillus* organisms can cause endocarditis in patients with IV catheters, especially if patients are immunocompromised or are receiving broad-spectrum antimicrobial therapy. The course is subacute, but the prognosis is poor because of the relative ineffectiveness of current antifungal medications. Fungal infections result in large, friable vegetations that often embolize; therefore early surgical intervention is indicated.[3,4,9]

Prosthetic Valve Endocarditis

The overall risk of endocarditis in patients with prosthetic valves ranges between 1% and 4%, with the highest incidence within the first 12 months after surgery. The risk is increased 5% in patients who undergo valve replacement during active infection.[1,3,5,10-12] Although native valve endocarditis in non–IV drug users most often involves the mitral valve, there is no significant difference in infection rates between prosthetic aortic and prosthetic mitral valves. There also appears to be no significant long-term difference between bioprosthetic and mechanical implants. However, mechanical valves have a higher incidence of early prosthetic valve endocarditis (PVE). Other factors associated with an increased infection risk include advanced age, antecedent native valve infection, and a longer cardiopulmonary bypass time. Gender does not appear to alter the risks associated with mitral valve replacements.[5,11,12]

PVE is categorized as "early" when symptoms occur within 60 days of surgery or "late" when they occur after 1 year. The clinical presentation, microbiology, and morbidity and mortality rates differ. Early PVE is the result of perioperative seeding; it occurs either intraoperatively through direct contamination of the surgical field or postoperatively through contamination of central lines, pacemaker wires, or other indwelling sources. Despite prophylactic antibiotic therapy, the majority of early infections are the result of staphylococcal species, most commonly *S. epidermis* followed by *S. aureus*. Other pathogens include gram-negative bacilli, fungi (especially *Candida*), streptococci, enterococci, and diphtheroids.[5,12]

Late PVE occurs after the new valve has endothelialized. The source of the infection is not related to the surgical procedure but may result from a transient bacteremia as a consequence of a dental, gastrointestinal, or genitourinary procedure, often in the setting of inadequate prophylaxis. The microbial isolates are similar to those seen in native valve endocarditis. Viridans streptococci account for the majority of cases that occur more than 1 or 2 years after implantation. Other streptococcal species, enterococci, staphylococci, gram-negative bacilli, fungi, and diphtheroids are more often involved within the first 18 months after surgery.[3,12]

Infections associated with early PVE usually result in rapid valvular dysfunction and destruction of the integrity of the suture line, thus heralding an acute and rapidly deteriorating course with a high mortality rate. Because late PVE is often caused by less virulent organisms, it often has a subacute course. However, if the offending organism is virulent, late PVE may also present as an acute, fulminant infection.[12]

Endocarditis in Intravenous Drug Users

Those who develop endocarditis associated with IV drug use tend to be younger (with a mean age in the 30s) and are most often male. The actual risk of infection among IV drug users is variable depending on the drugs injected, their method of preparation, and frequency of use. In this population, infection involving the tricuspid valve is most common. Right-sided endocarditis is otherwise rare; therefore IV drug use should be suspected when this type of endocarditis is discovered. Involvement of the aortic valve alone or mitral valve alone is seen in a small number of patients, whereas even fewer have a combination of left- and right-sided endocarditis. The majority of IV drug users who develop infective endocarditis have structurally normal valves before the infection; a significant minority, approximately 20%, have an underlying cardiac lesion from congenital disease or previous endocardial infection.[3,5]

Skin flora is the most common source of pathogenic microorganisms in users of IV drugs; contaminated drugs and drug paraphernalia are also bacterial sources. *S. aureus* is the most common offending organism; it is isolated in 60% of total cases and in 80% of cases involving the tricuspid valve. Various streptococcal and enterococcal species account for approximately 20% of total cases; gram-negative bacilli, particularly *Pseudomonas* and *Serratia* organisms, are responsible for an additional 10% of infections. Fungi, most often *Candida* organisms, are isolated only 5% of the time. More than one organism is isolated in approximately 5% of individuals.[1]

The majority of patients with right-sided endocarditis are noted to have pneumonia or septic pulmonary emboli as a result of direct embolization. These patients appear ill, with high fevers and shaking chills. Patients with a clinical syndrome consistent with tricuspid valve endocarditis should also be evaluated for a potential extracardiac source of the endovascular infection, such as septic thrombophlebitis. The overall mortality rate for right-sided endocarditis is approximately 10%.[1,5]

Endocarditis in Pregnancy

Endocarditis is a potentially serious complication of pregnancy; fortunately, it is uncommon. The overall incidence of endocarditis associated with pregnancy is declining as a result of a decreasing incidence of rheumatic heart disease, improvements in the management of complications during pregnancy and the postpartum period, and the legalization and standardization of abortion. Underlying cardiac lesions (which are present in the majority of women affected) and the use of illicit IV drugs are predisposing factors to endocarditis.[13,14]

Although dental procedures have been the most common means of bacterial entry, puerperal bacteremia can occur after a vaginal or cesarean delivery. Premature labor, prolonged rupture of the membrane, prolonged labor, or manual removal of the placenta may be predisposing factors. If these occur in the setting of an underlying cardiac lesion, the risk is substantial, and prophylactic antibiotics should be administered.[13,14]

PATHOPHYSIOLOGY

The development of endocarditis depends on the invasion of the bloodstream by a pathogen capable of attaching to an endothelial surface. The normal endothelium is not conducive to bacterial deposition. A high-velocity jet stream, a narrow valvular orifice, and a flow from a high- to a low-pressure chamber are hemodynamic features that predispose to endocarditis. This forceful flow denudes the endothelium and allows for platelet and fibrin deposition. This layering of platelets and fibrin creates a nonbacterial sterile vegetation, which in turn provides an ideal medium for bacterial adherence and growth. Virulent microorganisms, especially the staphylococcal species, are capable of attaching to even normal endothelium.[1,3,4]

Microorganisms attach just distal to the narrowed orifice of a turbulent jet, such as on the atrial surface of the mitral leaflets in mitral regurgitation or on the ventricular surface of the aortic cusps in the setting of aortic insufficiency. After colonization of the endothelial surface, bacteria begin the replication process. Further platelet and fibrin deposition over the bacteria provides insulation from phagocytic cellular defenses, which allows the microorganisms to thrive and form vegetations. Proliferation of the microorganism leads to local valvular destruction, tissue invasion, and possible embolization of the vegetative material.[1-4]

Morphologic characteristics of the vegetations depend on the offending organism and the duration of the infection. Lesions range from small, flat, or granular deposits to large, pedunculated, and friable formations. During the course of effective antimicrobial therapy, leukocytes and fibroblasts penetrate vegetations. This healing process results in fibrosis, occasionally with calcification, and eventual reendothelialization of the valvular surface.[11,15]

The signs and symptoms of infective endocarditis vary according to the causative organism and the degree of systemic involvement. Valvular infection can result in the disruption of valvular integrity, including perforation of a valve leaflet, rupture of chordae tendineae or papillary muscles, or leaflet prolapse. Penetration of bacteria into the adjacent myocardium can result in myocardial or perivalvular abscesses, which may result in conduction system disturbances and heart block. Further penetration of infection may produce fistulas between cardiac chambers. Large vegetations associated with fungal or *Haemophilus* infections can cause obstruction of the valvular orifice. Even after a bacterial cure has been achieved, fibrosis of the valve leaflets can result in hemodynamically significant valvular stenosis or regurgitation.[1,5,16]

Embolization of vegetative matter is not uncommon and most often involves the renal, splenic, coronary, or cerebral circulation. Myocardial infarction can be the result of embolization of the vegetative material down the coronary arteries. Pulmonary embolism is a complication associated with right-sided endocarditis in IV drug users or patients with fungal infections. Embolization of septic material can lead to abscess formation. Mycotic aneurysms occur as a direct result of septic invasion into the arterial wall or septic embolization, which weakens the vessel wall and predisposes it to rupture.[4,17,18]

Persistent bacteremia triggers an immune complex response of both the humoral and cell-mediated immune systems. As seen in many chronic infections, a generalized hypergammaglobulinemia develops. Immune complexes containing IgG, IgM, and IgA and complement are deposited along the glomerular basement membrane of the kidney, precipitating glomerulonephritis. Peripheral manifestations of arthritic discomforts and cutaneous vasculitis may also be attributed to deposition of immune complexes in the joints and mucocutaneous vessels.[1,4,5]

CLINICAL PRESENTATION AND PHYSICAL EXAMINATION

The onset of symptoms usually occurs within days to weeks of the introduction of the microorganisms, but the symptoms may initially be nonspecific. Early symptoms of infection involving a less virulent organism such as viridans streptococci include generalized fatigue, malaise, night sweats, chills, and mild weight loss. A highly pathogenic organism such as *S. aureus* may present with an abrupt onset that prompts the patient to seek early medical attention. The virility of the invading microorganism dictates the pace and severity of the disease course.[2,19]

Fever is present in the majority of patients but may be absent in older adults, immunocompromised hosts, or patients previously treated with antibiotics. The degree of fever is dependent on the causative microorganism; high-grade fevers are primarily associated with virulent infections.[1,2,4,5] The majority of patients become afebrile within 72 hours of initiating the appropriate antibiotic therapy. Persistent fever suggests an ineffective antimicrobial regimen or a myocardial or distant (metastatic) abscess formation.[16]

Heart murmurs are detectable in the majority of patients but may be absent early in the course or in patients with right-sided endocarditis. A new murmur of regurgitation or a true change in an existing murmur suggests an acute process and often heralds the development of congestive heart failure. The diagnosis of infective endocarditis must be entertained in any patient with a heart murmur and fever of unknown etiology.[1,2,4]

Splenomegaly was commonly associated with endocarditis before the advent of antibiotic therapy, but it is now a rare finding.[1] Petechiae may be noted on the conjunctivae, palate, buccal mucosa, and extremities and are associated with a long-term infection. Splinter hemorrhages are linear, subungual hemorrhages that may appear in infective endocarditis. Both petechiae and splinter hemorrhages may represent embolic phenomena or vasculitis. Although sometimes seen in patients with infective endocarditis, they may also appear with other disease processes.[1,2,4,5]

Janeway's lesions and Osler's nodes are cutaneous lesions associated with endocarditis. Janeway's lesions are nontender, hemorrhagic macules (1 to 4 mm) on the palms of the hands and soles of the feet and are the result of septic embolization. Osler's nodes are painful nodules on the finger and toe pads that last hours to days. They have also been noted on the forearms, ears, and dorsa of the feet. Their pathogenesis is uncertain, but they are thought to be related to microembolization and subsequent inflammation or immune complex mediation. Osler's nodes are an uncommon finding and may also be associated with other disease processes.[1,2,4,5]

Roth's spots are retinal hemorrhages with a pale center located near the optic disc. They are an uncommon finding and can be associated with infective endocarditis as well as hematologic and connective tissue disorders.[1] Other ocular manifestations that have been documented include amaurosis fugax and painful blurring of vision.[2]

Evidence of neurologic involvement may be seen in approximately 20% to 40% of patients with infective endocarditis. Major embolization of the middle cerebral artery, the most commonly involved territory, manifests as hemiplegia. Mycotic aneurysms are a potentially life-threatening complication that occurs in 1% of patients, but they are most often associated with infections involving less virulent pathogens. They typically occur early in the course of the disease but can occur months or even years after a bacteriologic cure has been achieved. A severe unrelenting headache, transient neurologic changes, or signs of cranial nerve involvement suggest the possibility of an intracranial mycotic aneurysm. Brain abscesses, purulent meningitis, arteritis, transient ischemic attacks, embolic strokes, cranial nerve palsy, intracerebral bleeding, subarachnoid hemorrhage, and encephalomalacia have also been reported.[2,4,20]

Congestive heart failure is a serious complication and is the primary cause of death in patients with infective endocarditis. It may be secondary to valvular destruction, coronary embolization resulting in myocardial infarction, myocarditis, or myocardial abscess formation. Early recognition of cardiac decompensation and intensive intervention are critical. Failure of antimicrobial therapy or the development of refractory congestive heart failure is an indication for surgical intervention. Intracardiac complications requiring surgical intervention include valvular dehiscence, ruptured chordae tendineae, perforation of valve leaflets, and the formation of an aneurysm or abscess. In these situations, surgical intervention may be lifesaving; therefore the presence of an active infection is not considered a surgical contraindication. Surgical intervention is also indicated in patients infected with brucella or fungi and those with recurrent emboli, early prosthetic valve endocarditis, or late prosthetic valve endocarditis secondary to *S. aureus*.[9]

Renal involvement is another serious complication of infective endocarditis. Renal insufficiency is often the result of glomerulonephritis secondary to immune complex deposition on the glomerular basement membrane. It may also occur secondary to septic embolization, leading to renal infarction or abscess formation.[1]

Metastatic infections such as pyogenic meningitis, pyelonephritis, splenic abscesses, and osteomyelitis are most often noted in patients with *S. aureus* endocarditis. Metastatic infections are rarely seen in endocarditis involving less virulent microorganisms. Metastatic infections increase the risk of a relapse of infective endocarditis.[4]

Complaints of arthralgias and myalgias are common. Arthralgias tend to involve the proximal joints and lower extremities and may be monoarticular. Myalgias, often localized to the thigh or calf, are commonly unilateral and have no radicular pattern. These discomforts are often described at the time of presentation and may in part be a manifestation of elevated circulating immune complexes.[2,4]

Pulmonary embolism is most often associated with tricuspid valve endocarditis among IV drug users. It may also occur in patients with indwelling central venous catheters or in patients with left-sided endocarditis who have left-to-right shunting from a septal defect.[1,2]

DIAGNOSTICS

To establish the diagnosis of infective endocarditis, an effort should be made to isolate the pathogenic microorganisms from the blood. Three sets of blood cultures should be obtained from different venipuncture sites with samples drawn at least 30 to 60 minutes apart before initiating antimicrobial therapy. Cultures can be obtained at any time; a febrile state at the time of culture is not critical. There also is no particular advantage to drawing the culture from arterial blood rather than from venous blood.[2,5,21,22]

The first consideration when interpreting positive blood culture data is whether the bacteremia is sustained or transient. Intravascular infections such as endocarditis produce a sustained bacteremia, which is defined as the presence of the same microorganism in the blood for at least 1 hour. In contrast, transient bacteremia clears within 30 minutes or less. Consequently, only one blood culture in the series is likely to be positive in transient bacteremia, whereas all cultures are likely to be positive with sustained bacteremia. A single positive blood culture is most consistent with transient bacteremia (or contamination) but is not diagnostic for endocarditis.[22]

The next consideration is whether the identified pathogen is one typically associated with an intravascular infection or is more likely a result of another source of infection. Salmonellae, brucellae, and enteric gram-negative bacteria can produce sustained bacteremia yet are rarely pathogens in endocarditis. Organisms such as viridans streptococci and coagulase-negative staphylococci are common pathogenic organisms in endocarditis.

Other abnormal laboratory findings commonly found in infective endocarditis include a normochromic, normocytic anemia, especially in infections of longer duration. The WBC count is usually within normal limits in less virulent infections, perhaps with a slight shift to the left. A marked leukocytosis with a shift to the left is a common finding in endocarditis caused by a virulent microorganism. The erythrocyte sedimentation rate is elevated, except in patients with cardiac or renal failure. A positive rheumatoid factor can be detected in half of the patients who have a duration of infection greater than 3 to 6 weeks. Circulating immune complexes are present in most patients; these levels decline as the infection is effectively treated. The serum complement level is usually decreased, especially in patients with glomerulonephritis.[1,2,5] The urinalysis result is most often abnormal, with proteinuria, microscopic hematuria, or pyuria. Serum creatinine may be elevated and reflects the degree of renal involvement secondary to glomerulonephritis or renovascular embolization.[1]

Echocardiography plays an important role in the evaluation of suspected or documented endocarditis. Vegetations appear as abnormal sessile or pedunculated echogenic masses

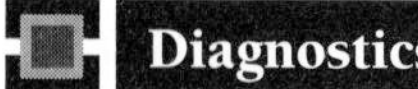

Diagnostics

Endocarditis

Laboratory
CBC and differential
ESR
Rheumatoid factor
Serum complement
Creatinine
Urinalysis
Blood cultures × 3 (30 minutes apart)

Imaging
Transthoracic echocardiogram

attached to valve leaflets. Unfortunately, vegetations of less than 5 mm can be difficult to identify with transthoracic echocardiography; the sensitivity of this technique for native valve endocarditis is therefore only about 60%. With its greater resolution, transesophageal echocardiography can identify lesions as small as 2 to 3 mm and therefore has sensitivity as high as 90% to 100%.[18,23]

Identifying vegetations in the presence of a prosthetic valve is more difficult because the prosthesis causes acoustic shadowing of parts of the ultrasound image; in this setting, the sensitivity of transthoracic echocardiography falls to approximately 20%.[24] Transesophageal echocardiography is capable of imaging prosthetic valves reliably, especially those in the mitral position; its sensitivity for vegetations in this setting falls only slightly to 86% to 94%.[25] Consequently, transesophageal echocardiography is preferred for evaluating suspected endocarditis in patients with valve prostheses.[18]

In addition to documenting the presence of vegetations in patients with endocarditis, echocardiography provides additional data of prognostic importance. First, the size, location, and mobility of vegetations as determined by echocardiography may be useful predictors of subsequent embolism. Second, echocardiography reliably identifies leaflet damage or associated valvular regurgitation that arises as a consequence of endocarditis. Finally, echocardiography can detect evidence of local invasion by an aggressive infection—such as an abscess or a fistula formation—that may be an indication for surgical repair.[11,15]

Clinical information, including the presenting signs and symptoms, findings on physical examination, laboratory and blood culture data, and echocardiographic findings, must be considered collectively by the practitioner when a diagnosis of infective endocarditis is considered. To help guide the diagnosis systematically, the new Duke criteria (Box 131-1) have become widely accepted.[26,27]

DIFFERENTIAL DIAGNOSIS

The diagnosis of infective endocarditis must be considered in any patient with a cardiac murmur and a fever of unknown cause. The diagnosis should also be entertained in any febrile IV drug user, any patient with a prosthetic valve who is febrile or has evidence of valvular dysfunction, or any young person with a cerebrovascular accident.[1] The definitive diagnosis of endocarditis requires (1) the isolation of a pathogenic organism from the blood or embolic material or (2) the demonstration of endocardial vegetations on echocardiography or at the time of surgery or autopsy.[24]

Other conditions can mimic the signs and symptoms of infective endocarditis, which makes a definitive diagnosis difficult at the time of initial presentation. A comprehensive diagnostic evaluation will usually yield an accurate diagnosis in a timely manner. Disease processes such as acute rheumatic fever, atrial myxoma, lymphoma, systemic lupus erythematosus, tuberculosis, thrombotic thrombocytopenia purpura, connective tissue disorders, sickle cell disease, and nonbacterial thrombotic endocarditis can produce a similar constellation of symptoms.[2,16]

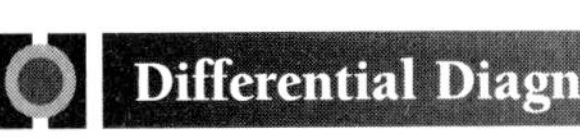

Endocarditis

Acute rheumatic fever
Atrial myxoma
Systemic lupus erythematosus
Thrombotic thrombocytopenia purpura
Connective tissue disorders
Sickle cell disease
Nonbacterial thrombotic endocarditis

BOX 131-1

DUKE CRITERIA FOR THE DIAGNOSIS OF INFECTIVE ENDOCARDITIS

MAJOR CRITERIA

1. Positive blood cultures
2. Evidence of endocardial involvement
   a. Echocardiogram demonstrating vegetation, abscess, or new prosthetic valve dehiscence
   or
   b. New valvular regurgitation

MINOR CRITERIA

1. *Predisposition:* Preexisting heart conditions
2. Fever: 38° C (100.4° F) or higher
3. *Vascular phenomena:* Arterial emboli, septic pulmonary emboli, mycotic aneurysms, intracranial hemorrhage, conjunctival hemorrhage, Janeway lesions
4. *Immune phenomena:* Nephritis, Osler's nodes, Roth's spots, positive rheumatoid factor
5. *Echocardiographic:* Consistent with diagnosis but not meeting major criteria
6. *Microbiologic:* Positive blood cultures that do not meet major criteria, *or* serologic evidence of active infection with a microorganism consistent with endocarditis

DEFINITE INFECTIVE ENDOCARDITIS

1. Pathologic criteria
   a. *Microorganisms:* Documented by culture or histologic examination of vegetation, embolic material, or intracardiac abscess
   b. *Pathologic:* Presence of vegetation or intracardiac abscess, histologic confirmation of active endocarditis
   c. *Clinical criteria:* 2 major criteria, *or* 1 major and 3 minor criteria, *or* 5 minor criteria

POSSIBLE INFECTIVE ENDOCARDITIS

Presentation and findings that are consistent with diagnosis but fall short of *definite* criteria (but not *rejected*)

INFECTIVE ENDOCARDITIS REJECTED

1. Firm alternate diagnosis established *or*
2. Resolution of symptoms after 4 days or fewer of antibiotic therapy
3. No pathologic evidence at surgery or autopsy after 4 days or fewer of antibiotic therapy

Modified from Durak DT and others: Duke Endocarditis Service: new criteria for diagnosis of infective endocarditis: utilization of specific echocardiographic findings, *Am J Med* 96:200-209, 1995; and Dajani AS and others: Prevention of bacterial endocarditis: recommendations by the American Heart Association, *JAMA* 277:1794-1801, 1997.

It is important to note that blood cultures obtained before the initiation of antimicrobial therapy will be positive in more than 95% of patients with infective endocarditis.[5] Therefore negative culture data should prompt further investigation into other possible causes of the fever and symptoms. If there is clinical suspicion of infective endocarditis in a patient with negative blood cultures, intensive efforts should be undertaken to identify fastidious microorganisms; these include prolonged incubation periods, culturing on special mediums, and serologic assessment. Microorganisms including *Coxiella burnetti* (Q fever), *Chlamydia* sp., *Tropheryma whipplei*, and *Bartonella* sp. are difficult to isolate. Pathogens may potentially be isolated from embolized material or excised valve tissue.[5,21]

MANAGEMENT

The identification of the infecting organism and the institution of high-dose bactericidal therapy are the cornerstones of treatment. Parenteral administration of antibiotics is preferred to ensure predictably high serum levels. Throughout the prolonged course of treatment, ongoing assessment of the patient's response to therapy, as well as vigilance for the development of potential complications, is crucial. Clinical improvement with reduction of fever is usually seen within 1 week of appropriate antimicrobial therapy. Blood cultures should be rechecked and should become negative after several days of effective pharmacologic treatment. Persistent fevers should raise the suspicion of an intracardiac abscess, metastatic foci of infection, or inadequate antimicrobial therapy.[2,5,16]

The selection of antimicrobial agents and the duration of therapy vary depending on the microorganism isolated and the duration of infection. Infective endocarditis caused by highly penicillin-sensitive viridans streptococci can often be cured within 2 weeks with a dual regimen of penicillin and an aminoglycoside. Intracardiac prostheses or infections of longer duration (which produce large vegetations) require a prolonged antibiotic course to achieve a successful cure. Tables 131-1 to 131-6 summarize the current treatment recommendations formulated by a consensus group of the American Heart Association.[27] Although these recommendations do not include all subgroups or potential pathogens, they do provide treatment regimens for the most commonly encountered cases of infective endocarditis.[6]

Co-Management with Specialists

Infective endocarditis is a potentially life-threatening infection and should be managed collaboratively with a cardiologist. Any patient presenting with fever and symptoms consistent with

TABLE 131-1 Suggested Antibiotic Regimens for Native Valve Endocarditis due to Penicillin-Sensitive Viridans Streptococci and *Streptococcus bovis*

Antibiotic	Dosage* and Route	Duration	Comments
Penicillin G *or*	12-18 million units/24 hr, either continuously or in 6 equal doses	4 weeks	Preferred in most patients over 65 years of age and in patients with impaired renal or cranial nerve VIII function.
Ceftriaxone	2 g/day IV/IM	4 weeks	
Penicillin G *with*	12-18 million units/24 hr IV, either continuously or in 6 equal doses	2 weeks	Gentamicin dosing based on ideal body weight, not actual body weight.
Gentamicin	1 mg/kg IV/IM q 8 hr	2 weeks	
Vancomycin	30 mg/kg/24 hr IV in 2 divided doses, not to exceed 2 g/24 hr unless serum levels monitored	4 weeks	Recommended for patients allergic to penicillins or other beta-lactams.

Modified from American Heart Association, Dallas, 2002, The Association.
*Dosages recommended are for adults with normal renal function.
Desirable peak serum gentamicin level (1 hour after infusion) is approximately 3 μg/ml.
Desirable peak serum vancomycin level (1 hour after infusion) is 30-45 μg/ml, for twice-daily dosing.

TABLE 131-2 Regimens for Native Valve Endocarditis due to Strains of Viridans Streptococci and *Streptococcus bovis* Relatively Resistant to Penicillin G

Antibiotic	Dosage* and Route	Duration	Comments
Penicillin G *with*	18 million units/24 hr IV, either continuously or in six equal doses	4 weeks	Cefazolin or other first-generation cephalosporin may be used in patients whose penicillin hypersensitivity is not of the immediate type.†
Gentamicin	1 mg/kg IM or IV q 8 hr	2 weeks	
Vancomycin	30 mg/kg/24 hr in 2 equal doses, not to exceed 2 g/24 hr unless serum levels monitored	4 weeks	Vancomycin is recommended for patients allergic to beta-lactams.

Modified from American Heart Association, Dallas, 2002, The Association.
*Dosages recommended for adults with normal renal function. For special dosing considerations for gentamicin and vancomycin, see the footnotes in Table 131-1.
†Cephalosporins should not be used in patients with immediate-type sensitivity reactions to penicillins (urticaria, angioedema, anaphylaxis).

TABLE 131-3 Standard Regimen for Enterococcal Endocarditis*

Antibiotic	Dosage† and Route	Duration	Comments
Penicillin G *with*	18-30 million units/24 hr, either continuously or in 6 equal doses	4-6 weeks	4 weeks if symptoms <3 months; 6 weeks if symptoms >3 months.
Gentamicin‡	1 mg/kg IM or IV q 8 hr	4-6 weeks	
Ampicillin *with*	12 g/24 hr, continuously or in 6 equal doses	4-6 weeks	Duration as recommended above.
Gentamicin‡	1 mg/kg IM or IV q 8 hr	4-6 weeks	
Vancomycin‡ *with*	30 mg/kg/24 hr IV in 2 equal doses, not to exceed 2 g/24 hr unless serum levels monitored	4-6 weeks	Vancomycin is recommended for patients allergic to beta-lactams; cephalosporins are not an alternative if penicillin allergic.
Gentamicin‡	1 mg/kg IM or IV q 8 hr	4-6 weeks	

Modified from American Heart Association, Dallas, 2002, The Association.
*All enterococcal endocarditis must be tested for antimicrobial susceptibility. This table is only for gentamicin- or vancomycin-susceptible organisms.
†Dosages recommended are for adults with normal renal function.
‡For special dosing considerations for gentamicin and vancomycin, see the footnotes in Table 131-1.

TABLE 131-4 Regimens for Staphylococcus Endocarditis in the Absence of Prosthetic Material

Antibiotic	Dosage* and Route	Duration	Comments
Nafcillin or oxacillin *with optional*	2 g IV q 4 hr	4-6 weeks	Benefit of additional aminoglycoside is unclear.
Gentamicin†	1 mg/kg IM or IV q 8 hr	3-5 days	
If allergic to beta-lactams:			
Cefazolin or another first-generation cephalosporins *with optional*	2 g IV q 8 hr	4-6 weeks	Avoid cephalosporins in patients with a hypersensitivity to penicillin.
Gentamicin†	1 mg/kg IM or IV q 8 hr	3-5 days	
Vancomycin	30 mg/kg/24 hr IV in 2 equal doses, not to exceed 2 g/24 hr unless serum levels monitored	4-6 weeks	Recommended for patients with penicillin allergy or methicillin-resistant staphylococci.

Modified from American Heart Association, Dallas, 2002, The Association.
*Dosages recommended are for adults with normal renal function.
†For special dosing considerations for gentamicin and vancomycin, see the footnotes in Table 131-1.

TABLE 131-5 Regimens for Endocarditis due to HACEK Microorganisms*

Antibiotic	Dosage† and Route	Duration	Comments
Ceftriaxone	2 g daily IV or IM	4 weeks	Cefotaxime or other third-generation cephalosporin may be substituted
Ampicillin *with*	12 g/24 hr IV, either continuously or in 6 equal doses	4 weeks	Ampicillin should not be used if organism produces beta-lactam
Gentamicin‡	1 mg/kg IM or IV q 8 hr	4 weeks	

Modified from American Heart Association, Dallas, 2002, The Association.
*HACEK microorganisms include *Haemophilus parainfluenzae, Haemophilus aphrophilus, Actinobacillus actinomycetemcomitans, Cardiobacterium hominis, Eikenella corrodens, and Kingella kingae.*
†Dosages recommended are for adults with normal renal function.
‡For special dosing considerations for gentamicin, see the footnotes in Table 131-1.

TABLE 131-6 Regimens for Staphylococcal Endocarditis in the Presence of Prosthetic Material

Antibiotic	Dosage* and Route	Duration	Comments
Vancomycin† *with*	30 mg/kg/24 hr IV in 2 to 4 equal doses, not to exceed 2 g/24 hr unless serum levels monitored	≥6 weeks	Regimen for methicillin-resistant staphylococci
Rifampin† *and with*	300 mg PO q 8 hr	≥6 weeks	Rifampin increases warfarin sodium requirements for antithrombotic therapy
Gentamicin‡	1 mg/kg IM or IV q 8 hr	2 weeks	
Nafcillin or oxacillin *with*	2 g IV q 4 hr	≥6 weeks	Regimen for methicillin-susceptible staphylococci
Rifampin *and with*	300 mg PO q 8 hr	≥6 weeks	
Gentamicin‡	1 mg/kg IM or IV	2 weeks	First-generation cephalosporin or vancomycin should be used in patients allergic to beta-lactams§

Modified from American Heart Association, Dallas, 2002, The Association.
*Dosage recommendations are for adults with normal renal function.
†Rifampin plays a crucial role in the eradication of staphylococci in the setting of prosthetic material.
‡For special for gentamicin and vancomycin, see the footnotes in Table 131-1.
§Cephalosporins should be avoided in patients with an immediate-type hypersensitivity to penicillin.

endocarditis should be hospitalized for immediate evaluation. Hemodynamic deterioration can be sudden, and intravenous antibiotic therapy should be initiated immediately after blood culture results have been obtained.

Cardiac surgery with replacement of the infected valve often becomes necessary in the treatment of patients who develop complications of infective endocarditis, most commonly as the result of a virulent pathogen. Surgery is indicated in the setting of refractory congestive heart failure secondary to valvular dysfunction. Cardiac surgery is required for patients with prosthetic valve endocarditis who show evidence of prosthetic instability or dehiscence. If the patient does not respond to appropriate and adequate antibiotic therapy, with the persistence of positive blood cultures, surgery may be necessary to eradicate the infection. Finally, the presence of an invasive infection that results in a perivalvular abscess or fistula often requires surgery to debride the necrotic tissue, repair the anatomic damage, and replace the infected valve. Infective endocarditis as a result of brucella or fungal infections can rarely be treated with antimicrobial therapy; therefore surgery is indicated in such cases.[5,9]

LIFE SPAN CONSIDERATIONS

Because infective endocarditis is associated with significant morbidity and mortality, primary prevention for patients at risk is critical. The cardiac conditions believed to predispose patients to infective endocarditis are listed in Box 131-2. Identification and education of patients at risk are essential and are the responsibility of all providers. The current recommendations of the American Heart Association for endocarditis prophylaxis are summarized in Box 131-3 and Tables 131-7 and 131-8. Prophylaxis is most effective when administered before the procedure. Recent data have demonstrated that adequate antibiotic blood levels are maintained for several hours after the initial dose; therefore single-dose therapy is now recommended.[25]

These guidelines are general. Practitioners must use their own clinical judgment in specific cases. For example, special consideration is required for patients with rheumatic heart disease who are receiving chronic penicillin therapy for the prevention of recurrent episodes of rheumatic fever. In this setting, oropharyngeal organisms may have become resistant to penicillin. Consequently, before the procedure patients should receive prophylaxis with another appropriate antibiotic, such as clindamycin. One exception is rheumatic prophylaxis with monthly injections of benzathine penicillin. This regimen does not usually result in penicillin resistance, and therefore penicillin prophylaxis may be used safely.[25]

COMPLICATIONS

The acute complications associated with infective endocarditis are numerous, may involve all major organ systems, and are potentially life threatening. Cardiac complications are often the result of direct pathogen invasion, whereas metastatic complications result from septic embolization or immune complex deposition.

Another concern is the possibility of a relapse. After completion of the antibiotic course, blood cultures should be checked once or twice during the first 2 months. Relapses usually occur within the first few months, and blood cultures may become positive before clinical manifestation. Patients with a relapse in native valve endocarditis often respond to further antimicrobial treatment, but surgical intervention should be considered for patients with prosthetic valves or persistent enterococcal endocarditis.[5]

Occasionally it is impossible to completely eradicate the microorganism with antimicrobial therapy, and surgery may not be an option because of the high operative risk associated with co-morbid conditions. In this case, chronic suppressive therapy may help prevent the manifestations and complications of endocarditis.

INDICATIONS FOR REFERRAL/HOSPITALIZATION

A diagnosis of infective endocarditis must be considered in any patient with a murmur and fever of unknown cause. This diagnosis must be considered in IV drug users or in patients with prosthetic valves who have a fever of unknown origin.

BOX 131-2

ENDOCARDITIS RISK FACTORS

ENDOCARDITIS PROPHYLAXIS RECOMMENDED

High Risk

Prosthetic valves—mechanical bioprostheses and homografts
Prior episode of infective endocarditis
Complex congenital heart disease (e.g., single ventricle, transposition of the great vessels, tetralogy of Fallot)
Surgically constructed pulmonary shunts

Moderate Risk

Congenital cardiac defects
Acquired valvular dysfunction (e.g., rheumatic heart disease)
Hypertrophic cardiomyopathy
Mitral valve prolapse with regurgitation and/or thickening of leaflets

ENDOCARDITIS PROPHYLAXIS NOT RECOMMENDED

Negligible Risk (no greater than the general population)

Isolated secundum atrial septal defects
Surgically repaired atrial or ventricular septal defects or patent ductus arteriosus (without residua after 6 months)
Previous coronary artery bypass graft surgery
Mitral valve prolapse without regurgitation
Physiologic, functional, or innocent heart murmurs
Previous Kawasaki syndrome without valvular dysfunction
Previous rheumatic fever without valvular dysfunction
Cardiac pacemakers or implanted defibrillators

Modified from Dajani AS and others: Prevention of bacterial endocarditis: recommendations by the American Heart Association, *JAMA* 277:1794-1801. 1997.

BOX 131-3

PROCEDURES AND ENDOCARDITIS PROPHYLAXIS

ENDOCARDITIS PROPHYLAXIS RECOMMENDED*

Dental Procedures

Prophylactic cleaning
Dental extractions or implant placement
Periodontal procedures
Root canal
Placement of subgingival antibiotic fibers
Initial placement of orthodontic bands but not brackets

RESPIRATORY TRACT PROCEDURES

Tonsillectomy/adenoidectomy
Rigid bronchoscopy
Surgical procedures involving respiratory mucosa

GASTROINTESTIONAL PROCEDURES†

Sclerotherapy for varices
Esophageal dilation
Endoscopic retrograde cholangiography with biliary obstruction
Biliary tract surgery
Surgery involving intestional mucosa

GENITOURINARY PROCEDURES

Cystoscopy
Urethral dilation
Prostate surgery

ENDOCARDITIS PROPHYLAXIS NOT RECOMMENDED

Dental Procedures

Restorative dentistry, including fillings
Local anesthetic injections (nonintraligamentary)
Postoperative suture removal
Orthodontic adjustment
Fluoride treatment and dental radiographs

Respiratory Tract Procedures

Endotracheal intubation
Flexible bronchoscopy with or without biopsy‡

Gastrointestinal Procedures

Transesophageal echocardiogram‡
Endoscopy with or without biopsy‡

Genitourinary Procedures

Vaginal hysterectomy‡
Vaginal delivery‡
Cesarean section
Involving noninfected tissue

- Urethral catheterization
- Dilation and curettage
- Therapeutic abortion
- Sterilization procedures
- Insertion and removal of intrauterine devices

Other Procedures

Cardiac catheterization, including angioplasty and intracoronary stent placement
Implantation of cardiac pacemakers and defibrillators
Incision or biopsy of surgically scrubbed skin
Circumcision

Modified from Dajani AS and others: Prevention of bacterial endocarditis: recommendations by the American Heart Association, *JAMA* 277:1794-1801. 1997.
*Prophylaxis recommended for patients with high- and moderate-risk cardiac conditions.
†Prophylaxis recommended for high-risk patients; optional for moderate-risk patients.
‡Prophylaxis optional for high-risk patients.

TABLE 131-7 Antibiotic Prophylaxis for Dental, Oral, Respiratory Tract, or Esophageal Procedures

	Antibiotic	Dosage* and Route
Standard prophylaxis	Amoxicillin PO	*Adults:* 2 g *Children:* 50 mg/kg 1 hour before procedure
Inability to take oral medication	Ampicillin IM or IV	*Adults:* 2 g *Children:* 50 mg/kg Within 30 minutes before procedure
Allergy to penicillin	Clindamycin PO *Or* Cephalexin† or cefadroxil† PO *Or* Azithromycin PO *Or* Clarithromycin PO	*Adults:* 600 mg *Children:* 20 mg/kg 1 hour before procedure *Adults:* 2 g *Children:* 50 mg/kg 1 hour before procedure *Adults:* 500 mg *Children:* 15 mg/kg 1 hour before procedure
Allergy to penicillin and inability to take oral medication	Clindamycin IV *Or* Cefazolin† IM or IV	*Adults:* 600 mg *Children:* 20 mg/kg Within 30 minutes of procedure *Adults:* 1 g *Children:* 25 mg/kg Within 30 minutes of procedure

Modified from Dajani AS and others: Prevention of bacterial endocarditis: recommendations by the American Heart Association, *JAMA* 277:1794-1801, 1997.
*Total children's dose not to exceed adult dose.
†Cephalosporins should not be used in patients with hypersensitivity reactions to penicillins.

Immediate consultation and hospitalization are warranted if the history, symptoms, and clinical findings raise a suspicion of infective endocarditis.

A diagnostic evaluation, including blood cultures and echocardiography, must be performed. After obtaining blood cultures, the early initiation of an IV antibiotic regimen is vital in minimizing the risks of valvular destruction and the metastatic complications associated with pathogenic invasion.

The availability of a wide assortment of infusion pumps and percutaneous central catheters has made home therapy an acceptable, cost-effective option for certain patients. Outpatient therapy may be considered for completing the prolonged antibiotic course only for patients who have demonstrated a response to treatment (negative blood cultures and afebrile state), are hemodynamically stable, are without complications such as congestive heart failure or embolic events, are reliable (non–IV drug users), and will comply with regular follow-up.[28]

PATIENT EDUCATION/HEALTH PROMOTION

Education of patients and family members is crucial. The etiology and treatment of endocarditis, as well as the diagnostic tests, should be carefully explained. Patients should understand the importance of preventive therapy and current prophylaxis recommendations. Patients treated for infective endocarditis should understand the risk of relapse and the importance of obtaining follow-up diagnostics and contacting the primary care provider if there are any signs of illness.

REFERENCES

1. Bansal RC: Infective endocarditis, *Med Clin North Am* 79:1205-1240, 1995.

TABLE 131-8 Antibiotic Prophylaxis for Genitourinary and Gastrointestinal Procedures*

	Antibiotic	Dosage and Route§
High-risk patients	Ampicillin *plus* gentamicin†	*Adults:* Ampicillin 2 g IV/IM plus gentamicin† 1.5 mg/kg IV within 30 minutes of procedure; then ampicillin 1 g IV/IM or amoxicillin 1 g PO 6 hours later *Children‡:* Ampicillin 50 mg/kg IV/IM plus gentamicin 1.5 mg/kg within 30 minutes of procedure; then ampicillin 25 mg/kg IV/IM or amoxicillin 25 mg/kg PO 6 hours later
High-risk patients allergic to penicillin	Vancomycin *plus* gentamicin†	*Adults:* Vancomycin 1 g IV over 1-2 hours plus gentamicin 1.5 mg/kg IV/IM; complete infusion/injection within 30 minutes of procedure *Children:* Vancomycin 20 mg/kg IV over 1-2 hours plus gentamicin 1.5 mg/kg IV/IM; complete within 30 minutes of procedure
Moderate-risk patients	Amoxicillin *or* ampicillin	*Adults:* Amoxicillin 2 g PO 1 hour before procedure, or ampicillin 2 g IV/IM within 30 minutes of procedure *Children:* Amoxicillin 50 mg/kg PO 1 hour before procedure, or ampicillin 50 mg/kg IV/IM within 30 minutes of procedure
Moderate-risk patients allergic to penicillin	Vancomycin	*Adults:* Vancomycin 1 g IV *Children:* Vancomycin 20 mg/kg IV Infusions given over 1-2 hours to be completed within 30 minutes of procedure

Modified from Dajani AS and others: Prevention of bacterial endocarditis: recommendations by the American Heart Association, *JAMA* 277:1794-1801, 1997.
*Excludes esophageal procedures.
†Gentamicin dose not to exceed 120 mg.
‡Total children's dose not to exceed adult dose.
§No second dose of vancomycin or gentamicin is recommended.

2. Cunha BA, Gill V, Lazar JM: Acute infective endocarditis: diagnostic and therapeutic approach, *Infect Dis Clin North Am* 10:811-834, 1996.
3. Korzeniowski OM, Chowdhury MH: Endocarditis of natural and prosthetic valves: Treatment and prophylaxis. In Schlossberg D, editor: *Current therapy of infectious disease*, ed 2, St Louis, 2001, Mosby.
4. Wilson WR, Barasch E: Infective endocarditis. In Willerson JT, Cohn JN, editors: *Cardiovascular medicine*, ed 2, Philadelphia, 2000, Churchill Livingstone.
5. Mylonakis E, Claderwood SB: Medical progress: infective endocarditis in adults, *N Engl J Med* 345:1318-1330, 2001.
6. Wilson WR and others: Antibiotic treatment of infective endocarditis due to streptococci, enterococci, staphylococci, and HACEK microorganisms, *JAMA* 274:1706-1713, 1995.
7. Kupferwasser HD and others: Clinical and morphological characteristics in Streptococcus bovis endocarditis: a comparison with other causative microorganisms in 177 cases, *Heart* 80:276-280, 1998.
8. Pergola V and others: Comparison of clinical and echocardiographic characteristics of Streptococcus bovis endocarditis with that caused by other pathogens, *Am J Cardiol* 88:871-875, 2001.
9. Guerra JM and others: Long term results of mechanical prosthesis for treatment of active infective endocarditis, *Heart* 86:63-68, 2001.
10. Gordon SM and others: Early onset prosthetic valve endocarditis: the Cleveland Clinic experience 1992-1997, *Ann Thorac Surg* 69:1388-1392, 2000.
11. DiSalvo G and others: Echocardiography predicts embolic events in infective endocarditis, *J Am Coll Cardiol* 37:1069-1076, 2001.
12. Piper C and others: Prosthetic valve endocarditis, *Heart* 85:590-593, 2001.
13. Mueller SD, Willerson JT: Pregnancy and the heart. In Willerson JT, Cohn JN, editors: *Cardiovascular medicine*, ed 2, Philadelphia, 2000, Churchill Livingstone.
14. Mendelson MA, Lang RM: Pregnancy and cardiovascular disease. In Barron WM, Limdheimer MD, editors: *Medical disorders during pregnancy*, ed 3, St Louis, 2000, Mosby.
15. Vuille C and others: Natural history of vegetations during successful medical treatment of endocarditis, *Am Heart J* 128:1200-1209, 1994.
16. Meine TJ and others: Cardiac conduction abnormalities in endocarditis defined by the Duke criteria, *Am Heart J* 142:280-285, 2001.
17. Oakley CM, Hall RJC: Endocarditis: problems—patients being treated for endocarditis and not doing well, *Heart* 85:470-474, 2001.
18. Bayer AS and others: Diagnosis and management of endocarditis and its complications, *Circulation* 98:2936-2948, 1998.
19. Netzer RO-M and others: Infective endocarditis: clinical spectrum, presentation and outcome. An analysis of 212 cases 1980-1995, *Heart* 84:25-30, 2000.
20. Heiro M and others: Neurologic manifestations of infective endocarditis: a 17-year experience in a teaching hospital in Finland, *Arch Intern Med* 160:2781-2787, 2000.
21. Eykyn SJ: Endocarditis: basics, *Heart* 86:476-480, 2001.
22. Shulman ST, Phair JP: Infective endocarditis. In Shulma ST and others, editors: *The biologic and clinical basis of infectious diseases*, ed 5, Philadelphia, 1997, WB Saunders.
23. Lindner JR and others: Diagnostic value of echocardiography in suspected endocarditis: an evaluation based on the pretest probability of disease, *Circulation* 93:730-736, 1996.
24. Durack DT and others: New criteria for diagnosis of infective endocarditis: utilization of specific echocardiographic findings: Duke Endocarditis Service, *Am J Med* 96:200-209, 1994.
25. Andrews MM, von Reyn CF: Patient selection criteria and management guidelines for outpatient parenteral antibiotic therapy for native valve endocarditis, *Clinical Infectious Disease* 33:203-209, 2001.
26. Durak DT, Lukes AS, Bright DK: Duke Endocarditis Service: new criteria for diagnosis of infective endocarditis: utilization of specific echocardiographic findings, *Am J Med* 96:200-209, 1995.
27. Dajani AS and others: Prevention of bacterial endocarditis: recommendations by the American Heart Association, *JAMA* 277:1794-1801, 1997.

CHAPTER 132

Heart Failure

Roberta N. Regan

DEFINITION/EPIDEMIOLOGY

Heart failure is the final pathophysiologic state in the progression of most cardiovascular disorders. Packer[1] defines heart failure as a complex clinical syndrome characterized by abnormalities of left ventricular function and neurohormonal regulation accompanied by effort intolerance, fluid retention, and reduced longevity. The spectrum of clinical presentation is wide, ranging from mild, effort-related signs and symptoms caused by fluid retention to life-threatening arrhythmias and cardiogenic shock.

The etiology of heart failure can be divided into three broad categories: (1) anatomic or functional abnormalities of the coronary vessels, myocardium, or cardiac valves; (2) biochemical and physiologic abnormalities that increase the myocardial workload or reduce myocardial oxygen delivery, thus impairing myocardial contraction; and (3) extracardiac factors that cause excessive demand on the cardiovascular system.[2] Treatment requires identification of the specific etiology or etiologies and exacerbating factors for appropriate management and amelioration of precipitating factors.

With the widespread use of objective measures of myocardial function, such as echocardiography, it has become clear that there is a surprising variability in the degree of ventricular dysfunction despite a similar degree of clinical symptomatology. Left ventricular systolic dysfunction, present in the majority of patients with heart failure, is usually associated with symptoms when the left ventricular ejection fraction falls to less than 35%. Recent studies, including the V-HeFT II trial[3] and the SOLVD trial,[4] have shown that coronary artery disease is the most common etiology of systolic dysfunction. At least 15% to 30% of patients with classic symptoms of heart failure have normal or minimally subnormal left ventricular ejection fractions. Most of these patients have primary left ventricular diastolic dysfunction. In this disorder left ventricular filling pressures are high, and during exercise there is a decreased stroke volume response.[5] The most common etiology of heart failure resulting from primary diastolic dysfunction is hypertension.

Hypertension and valvular heart disease were considered the most common etiologies for heart failure 30 to 50 years ago. Today, in order of prevalence, the most common causes of heart failure are coronary artery disease, hypertension, alcohol, and idiopathic dilated cardiomyopathy. Most forms of chronic heart disease predispose the patient to heart failure over time, especially those disease processes that have the common pathophysiologic feature of left ventricular hypertrophy (Box 132-1).

Heart failure is a leading cause of morbidity and mortality and represents a major public health problem in the United States. It is the only cardiovascular condition that is increasing in incidence in the United States. An estimated 4.6 million Americans carry the diagnosis of heart failure, and an estimated 400,000

BOX 132-1

ETIOLOGIES OF HEART FAILURE

CARDIOVASCULAR DISEASE

Ischemic heart disease
Toxic cardiomyopathy (e.g., alcohol, chemotherapeutic agents)
Idiopathic cardiomyopathies
- Dilated
- Hypertrophic
- Restricted

Hypertension
Valvular heart disease
Pericardial disease
Congenital defects
Chronic tachycardia

NONCARDIAC DISEASE

Endocrine/metabolic disorders (contractility not usually impaired; rather, metabolic demands are in excess of normal cardiac output; volume overload of the left ventricle)
Thyrotoxicosis
Anemia
Pregnancy
Fever, systemic infection
Ateriovenous fistulas
Vitamin B_1 deficiency (beri-beri)

CONNECTIVE TISSUE DISEASES

Systemic lupus erythematosus
Polymyositis
Progressive systemic sclerosis (scleroderma)

PULMONARY DISEASES

Cor pulmonale secondary to chronic obstructive pulmonary disease
Pulmonary hypertension

From Moser DK, Cardin S: Heart failure. In Clochesy JM and others, editors: *Critical care nursing*, ed 2, Philadelphia, 1996, WB Saunders.

new cases are identified each year. An estimated $20 billion was spent on care of patients with heart failure in 1999 alone.[6] Approximately 50% of persons with heart failure are symptomatic and over 65 years of age.[7]

The Framingham Heart Study enrolled more than 5000 people free of cardiac disease in a prospective observational study in the late 1940s. The study's data showed an increased incidence of heart failure with advancing age, with the incidence of heart failure doubling with each decade of life, especially in those who have a diagnosis of hypertension. There is a slightly higher incidence in men because of their greater vulnerability to coronary artery disease.[8] A total of 10% of Americans over 70 years old have been diagnosed with heart failure.[9]

In 1990 in the United States there were 722,000 hospital admissions for heart failure, four times the number reported in 1971, validating the increasing prevalence of heart failure as the population ages. Hospitalizations for heart failure are increasing most rapidly in the over 65 year age-group.[1,10] In all, 60% of patients with heart failure carry a diagnosis of another serious, noncardiac co-morbid illness. In one study, subjects had a mean of three chronic conditions in addition to heart failure, with diabetes, chronic obstructive pulmonary disease (COPD), and anemia being the most common.[11] Because the prevalence of heart failure is expected to double in the twenty-first century, ambulatory and home care services for heart failure will have to increase.

A significant cause of mortality, heart failure has a 5-year survival rate of 25% in men and 38% in women. Thus heart failure is a more lethal condition than certain cancers.[12] Heart failure mortality increases with age, and the mortality rate is 50% higher in African-Americans than in Caucasians and one third higher in men. The annual number of deaths directly from heart failure has increased from 10,000 in 1968 to 42,000 in 1993, with another 219,000 deaths related to this condition.[13]

Physician consultation is indicated for new onset of heart failure in a patient with no previous history of cardiac disease.
Physician consultation is recommended for patients with deterioration of previously stable congestive heart failure.

PATHOPHYSIOLOGY

Heart failure is in many ways a prototypical disorder of cardiovascular aging. Age-related cardiac changes combine with the high prevalence of cardiovascular disease in older adults in the United States, so that heart failure has become increasingly prevalent.[14] The etiology of heart failure can be multifactorial, resulting from ischemic heart disease, hypertension, cardiomyopathy, or hyperthyroidism. In this complex physiologic state, there is either a decline in the ability of the heart to pump enough blood at a sufficient rate to sustain body physiologic functions, or the existence of elevated ventricular filling pressures. Thus, in general, there are two distinct mechanisms for heart failure: (1) systolic dysfunction with impaired ventricular contractility and (2) diastolic dysfunction with increased ventricular stiffness and/or reduced ventricular compliance.[15]

With diastolic dysfunction, the key problem is increased ventricular stiffness and reduced compliance, thus producing a rise in cardiac pressures during diastolic filling and the inability of the left ventricle to relax and accommodate a sufficient amount of oxygenated blood returning from the lungs. Left ventricular distensibility is reduced during part of or throughout the whole of diastole, and filling pressures must increase to maintain a constant ventricular volume. This condition in the left ventricle results in an increase in cardiac filling pressures during both rest and exercise, failure of the normal rise in cardiac output during exertion, and, occasionally, a reduction in cardiac output at rest. The heart attempts to compensate for this impaired distensibility through the "booster" effect of augmented atrial contraction. The most common causes of diastolic dysfunction are hypertension, ischemia resulting from coronary artery disease, aortic stenosis, and infiltrative or restrictive myocardial diseases.

Systolic dysfunction remains the most common type of heart failure with a decrease in both the ejection fraction and cardiac output. In systolic dysfunction the three determinants of ventricular function—preload, contractility, and afterload—are usually all altered. Preload is the degree of myocardial fiber stretch at the end of ventricular filling. When the heart ejects subnormally, there is an increased volume of blood left in the ventricular chambers (increased left ventricular end-systolic volume). This excess volume leads to distention of the ventricles and increased interventricular pressure at the onset of diastole. Filling must then occur at higher pressures during diastole. At small increases of volume/pressure, nonfailing myocardial fibers have the intrinsic property of increasing their force of contraction in an attempt to "revert" the subsequent volume/pressure conditions of both heart ejection and filling back to normal. This intrinsic property also enables the heart to maintain the cardiac output during states of pressure or volume overload.[2] However, in the failing heart, the failing myocardial fibers are both excessively overloaded and stretched beyond lengths commensurate with the normal reflex-increased force of contraction. Cardiac output eventually falls, precipitating symptoms and signs of either inadequate cardiac output or systemic or pulmonary congestion.

The ventricular dysfunction in heart failure is accompanied by a decrease in myocardial contractility, or force of contraction. This decline in contractility produces a reduction in ejection fraction and often stroke volume and cardiac output. Contractile force can be improved with the administration of positive inotropic agents, such as digoxin, and beta agonists, such as catecholamines. Physiologic states such as hypoxia and acidosis cause a reduction in contractility, as can both beta blockers and calcium channel blockers.

Afterload is the amount of left ventricular wall tension that develops during systole to eject blood. It is determined by both the size of the ventricular chamber (since wall tension must increase as the radius of the ventricle increases according to Laplace's law) and the dynamic vascular resistance against which the heart contracts. Systolic blood pressure reasonably approximates afterload and is a clinically important indicator of myocardial load. Because afterload determines the ease or speed of ventricular contraction, the ejection fraction is a function of afterload. The ejection fraction is an afterload-dependent measure of contractility. The ejection fraction of a normal heart with normal contractility may, in fact, fall if the afterload is extremely high. Thus it is important to consider the severity of the elevation of afterload before deciding that contractility as measured by the afterload-dependent ejection fraction is truly abnormal. One must remember that each determinant of ventricular function is interrelated and may potentially contribute to ventricular systolic dysfunction. Eventually, ventricular dysfunction is evidenced by a decline in stroke volume and cardiac output.

Several systemic compensatory mechanisms exist for the body to compensate for the reduction in cardiac output. Early on, these compensatory mechanisms serve to increase cardiac output and tissue perfusion. In the long run, however, they lead to further cardiac injury and further decompensation.

Compensatory Mechanisms

Several interrelated compensatory mechanisms attempt to maintain normal ventricular contractility, ventricular pressures, cardiac output, and blood pressure. The three primary compensatory mechanisms include (1) increased sympathetic adrenergic activity with a resultant increase in circulating neurohormones, (2) neuroendocrine activation of the renin-angiotensin-aldosterone system, and (3) ventricular remodeling. To appreciate the mechanisms of heart failure, one must remember that these same three compensatory mechanisms are responsible for the deterioration of cardiac function as time passes.

Sympathetic Adrenergic Activity. Abnormalities of the baroreceptors and cardiac reflexes have been documented in heart failure.[16] Normally, stimulation of the baroreceptor reflex results in activation of the parasympathetic nervous system and an inhibition of the sympathetic nervous system, so that heart rate and systemic vascular resistance are reduced. The opposite occurs when the baroreceptors are inhibited in response to a reduction in blood pressure. In heart failure the baroreceptors are inhibited by the reduction in cardiac output and the activation of the sympathetic nervous system. As heart failure progresses, the baroreceptor function is depressed further, leading to even greater sympathetic over activity despite intense vasoconstriction and volume retention.

In heart failure, the reduction in cardiac output leads to tissue hypoperfusion and direct activation of the sympathetic nervous system. In turn, the activated sympathetic adrenergic system stimulates release of catecholamines from the cardiac adrenergic nerves and the adrenal medulla. Release of catecholamines causes not only direct stimulation of contractility and heart rate, but also vasoconstriction in less metabolically active organs (e.g., skin, kidneys) and also, venoconstriction. The resultant venoconstriction increases preload by the increase in venous return. Catecholamines also affect the cardiac cells, producing an increased myocardial oxygen demand, hypertrophy of the cells themselves, and tissue necrosis. Over time, these cardiac myocyte effects can increase heart failure.

Moreover, as a result of sympathetic activation, plasma norepinephrine levels are elevated. The degree of plasma norepinephrine elevation correlates with the severity of heart failure, and are predictive of mortality in heart failure. In addition, exposure of the myocardial beta receptors to high levels of circulating catecholamines produces a decrease in both the number of beta-adrenergic receptors and their responsiveness to catecholamine stimulation. This elevation of circulating catecholamines and the sustained stimulation of the sympathetic nervous system can produce arrhythmias.

Neuroendocrine Activation. There are two additional vasoconstrictor systems that act as compensatory mechanisms and therefore are affected with heart failure: the renin-angiotensin-aldosterone system and arginine vasopressin. The renin-angiotensin-aldosterone system is activated as a result of a decline in blood pressure in the renal juxtaglomerular cells, which causes the release of increased renin, an enzyme. In fact, the degree of renin activity in plasma is related to the severity of heart failure. Renin acts on angiotensinogen, the plasma protein produced by the liver, to form angiotensin I. Angiotensin I is in turn converted into angiotensin II, a potent vasoconstrictor, through the action of angiotensin-converting enzyme (ACE), which is localized primarily in the lungs. This potent vasoconstrictor, angiotensin II, constricts the renal arterioles, thereby potentiating its own release. Other actions of angiotensin II are the stimulation of the thirst center, the release of aldosterone from the adrenal glands, and the trigger for the additional release of norepinephrine. In turn, aldosterone release promotes intravascular volume expansion by helping sodium and water retention and stimulating potassium excretion. These multiple, synergistic mechanisms eventually place the failing myocardium at more risk by increasing preload and afterload, promoting electrolyte imbalance, and increasing the risk for ischemia and arrhythmias.

The other vasoconstrictor system involves arginine vasopressin, a substance released from the posterior pituitary gland. Of note, the serum levels of arginine vasopressin are proportional to the severity of the heart failure, as this substance is not released in all heart failure patients.[17]

In addition to the renin-angiotension-aldosterone system and arginine vasopression, there are also, endothelium-derived factors, such as endothelin, that contribute to the vasoconstriction seen in heart failure. At the present time, however, the significance of these endothelium-derived factors are less clear.[18]

During the course of neuroendocrine activity in heart failure, several vasodilators are also activated and serve as counterregulatory systems. In response to the increased atrial stretch that occurs during heart failure, atrial natriuretic factor, a peptide, is released into the circulation from atrial myocytes. This hormone attenuates the vasoconstrictor effects of the other constrictor hormones, inhibits the renin-angiotensin system, reduces aldosterone release, and suppresses the release of norepinephrine.[19] Other vasodilators, such as prostaglandins, bradykinin, kallidin, and dopamine, are also released, but these may be overwhelmed by the potent vasoconstrictor systems activated in heart failure.

Ventricular Remodeling. Yet another compensatory response to heart failure is ongoing remodeling of ventricular three-dimensional morphology. Both myocardial hypertrophy and dilation occur in varying degrees, depending on the etiology of the heart failure. Dilation is an increase in the ventricular end-diastolic volume and represents an early compensatory response in volume overload in an attempt to increase contractility. In dilation, each individual myocyte lays down additional sarcomeres in series. Dilation preserves stroke volume and maintains cardiac output, but it also causes significantly increased wall stress. In turn, increased wall stress increases myocardial oxygen demand, a deleterious condition if significant coronary artery disease is present. Also, excessive wall stress may lead to myocyte loss and fibrosis of cardiac tissue.

Moreover, the condition of ventricular hypertrophy is a direct result of attempts to compensate for the increase in wall stress. Ventricular hypertrophy is the increase in the number of sarcomeres within each myocyte of ventricular heart muscle; these abnormal, large cells cannot contract as efficiently. Initially, myocardial hypertrophy distributes the greater degree of wall stress to a greater myocardial mass and thus "normalizes" the increased load per myocyte. Hypertrophy also increases the force of the ventricular contraction. Ultimately, however, ventricular remodeling in heart failure progresses to the point that it can no longer offer any compensatory advantage, especially when loading conditions remain abnormal or when myocardial disease causes myocyte loss.[19]

At the onset of heart failure, all the compensatory mechanisms described are beneficial; however, over time, these compensatory mechanisms may themselves exacerbate heart failure. The fluid retention intended to enhance contractile force can cause pulmonary and systemic congestion. Arterial vasoconstriction can cause impaired tissue perfusion and increased afterload. Myocardial hypertrophy and the sympathetic activity can increase myocardial oxygen consumption. The result of all of these responses is an increase in myocardial burden and an escalation in the degree of heart failure.

CLINICAL PRESENTATION AND PHYSICAL EXAMINATION

There is no single symptom, sign, or laboratory test that can definitively diagnose heart failure. Therefore prudent clinical judgment and an understanding of the pathophysiology of heart failure are critical to evaluating the significance of an individual patient's presenting signs and symptoms, in conjunction with their past medical history. The New York Heart Association (NYHA) functional classification is typically used to classify a patient's status; this classification expresses the relationship between the onset of symptoms (fatigue, dyspnea, palpitations, angina) and the degree of physical exertion (Box 132-2).

The American College of Cardiology (ACC) and American Heart Association (AHA) have devised a new classification system to complement, not replace, the NYHA. This new classification system grades patients in Stages A-D.[20] Stage A designates patients at risk for development of failure: patients with hypertension, diabetes, coronary artery disease, myocarditis, use of cardiotoxic medications, or a family history of cardiomyopathy, but without symptoms of failure or evidence of structural heart damage. Stage B includes those patients with structural heart disease (previous MI, left ventricular systolic dysfunction, asymptomatic valvular disease) but without symptoms of failure. Stage C encompasses those patients with

BOX 132-2

NEW YORK HEART ASSOCIATION FUNCTIONAL CLASSIFICATION

Class I—No limitations. Ordinary physical activity does not cause undue fatigue, dyspnea, or palpitations.

Class II—Slight limitation of physical activity. Such patients are comfortable at rest. Ordinary physical activity results in fatigue, palpitations, dyspnea, or angina.

Class III—Marked limitation of physical activity. Although patients are comfortable at rest, less than ordinary activity will lead to symptoms.

Class IV—Inability to carry on any physical activity without discomfort. Symptoms of congestive heart failure are present even at rest. With any physical activity, increased discomfort is experienced.

From the American Heart Association: *Nomenclature and criteria for the diagnosis of diseases of the heart and great vessels*, ed 9, Dallas, 1994, The Association.

known structural heart disease and prior or current symptoms of failure. The final stage, Stage D, is reserved for patients with refractory heart failure requiring specialized interventions: patients with marked symptoms at rest, on maximum medication therapy, or recurrent hospitalizations for failure.[20]

Dyspnea and Fatigue

Dyspnea and fatigue are the cardinal presenting symptoms of heart failure. The principal difference between exertional dyspnea in normal subjects and in the patient with heart failure is the degree of activity necessary to induce the symptom. Increasing heart failure is usually heralded by a change in the severity of dyspnea. Therefore it is necessary for the practitioner to ascertain whether there is a change in the extent of the exertion that actually causes the dyspnea. As the ventricular dysfunction advances, there is a progressive decline in the intensity of the exertion needed to cause symptoms. Interestingly, for sedentary patients with heart failure, there may be a total absence of dyspnea.[21]

Fatigue that is seen with heart failure is a direct result of the generalized hypoxia of body tissues from the decrease in cardiac output and the resultant decrease in oxygen saturation of the blood. This results in easy fatigability, weakness, and dizziness. In addition, the loss of potassium induced by the increased levels of aldosterone can also cause muscle weakness. To compound this muscle weakness, there is an alteration of the normal vascular response to exercise. Adequate vasodilation fails to occur during exercise, thereby reducing blood flow to the muscle and causing further muscle deconditioning. Recent studies have provided strong evidence that muscle deconditioning plays a more important role in fatigue than previously recognized.[21,22]

Orthopnea and Paroxysmal Nocturnal Dyspnea

Orthopnea is a common finding with heart failure. Orthopnea is shortness of breath occurring in the supine position and is typically relieved in part by the upright or sitting position. Although interstitial and alveolar pulmonary congestion are most likely present at all times, when a person is in an upright position, fluid in the lungs gravitates to the bases, making breathing somewhat easier. Paroxysmal nocturnal dyspnea is the onset of acute breathlessness at night. The exact etiology for this symptom is unknown but is believed to be related to increased reabsorption of fluid from the periphery in the recumbent position, which leads to left ventricular overload, increasing the symptoms of failure.

Bronchospasm and Wheezing

In some patients, heart failure may cause reflex bronchospasm and wheezing. This condition, called cardiac asthma, results from pulmonary interstitial or alveolar edema present with congestive heart failure.[23] Typically, with cardiac asthma, there is a nonproductive cough, especially with the patient in the recumbent position.

Crackles

Other adventitious lung sounds, crackles, may be heard on auscultation secondary to pulmonary fluid transudation; however, crackles are not always present with heart failure. In new-onset or acute escalation of heart failure, crackles are commonly present. When crackles are heard in early failure, they are at the lung bases because of the effects of gravity. In chronic heart failure, increased pulmonary fluid transudation may be accommodated by an increase in lymphatic drainage, so that the interstitial spaces and alveoli remain relatively dry and crackles may be absent.

Hemoptysis and Dysphagia

With more advanced heart failure, hemoptysis and dysphagia can be seen. Hemoptysis may result from bronchial vein bleeding resulting from venous distention, and dysphagia can occur as a result of esophageal compression from distention of the left atrium.

Pulmonary Edema

Perhaps the most dramatic clinical presentation of heart failure is failure causing acute pulmonary edema. This potentially life-threatening complication manifests as severe dyspnea, diaphoresis, and anxiety, with shallow, rapid breathing and, in a number of cases, pink, frothy sputum. Elevated blood pressure is common with pulmonary edema, probably because of an outpouring of endogenous catecholamines. Sinus tachycardia is also a component, although this finding may be absent in patients taking beta blockers, calcium channel blockers, or antiarrhythmic medications, all of which blunt heart rate response.

Abnormal Cardiac Examination Findings

Abnormalities in the cardiac examination are the presence of extra heart sounds, gallops (S_3, S_4) or murmurs, and the lateral displacement and abnormalities of the apical impulse. S_4 is the sound caused by the overdistention of the ventricles produced during late diastole as the stiffened ventricles expand further to accommodate the final diastolic filling volume of blood injected from the atria by atrial contraction (atrial kick). The presence of an S_3 indicates early diastolic rapid, turbulent left ventricular filling and is often evident when left ventricular systolic dysfunction is the mechanism of heart failure. These gallop sounds, S_4 and S_3, are best heard with the patient in the left lateral position. The presence of a loud S_4 gallop in the absence of an S_3 gallop suggests early failure or the presence of predominantly diastolic dysfunction, such as results from hypertensive heart disease, or hypertrophic or restrictive cardiomyopathy.

The location and character of the left ventricular apical impulse can provide important information regarding the mechanism of the heart failure. Displacement of the palpable apical impulse away from the midclavicular line toward the anterior axillary line indicates left ventricular enlargement. Furthermore, the palpable apical impulse should be a quick tap, narrow in distribution, not more than 1 to 2 cm in diameter. An impulse that is palpable with the palm of the hand, lasts longer, or is forceful indicates increased cardiac output or ventricular hypertrophy.

In addition, with increased cardiac volume or overload, a palpable impulse may be elicited with the palm of the hand placed on the sternum. This finding is a right ventricular tap or heave, indicating right ventricular enlargement and volume overload.

In all patients with heart failure, a careful auscultatory examination is important to exclude acute or chronic valvular disease and other structural heart disease. A vigilant search for regurgitant or stenotic aortic and mitral valve murmurs is essential, as these conditions are an important, yet potentially reversible, cause of heart failure. In severe aortic stenosis the small-volume, but high-velocity, turbulent jet of blood flowing across the valve during systole creates a loud and harsh systolic murmur. In acute severe aortic or mitral regurgitation, however, the large-volume, less turbulent jet of blood creates a softer murmur.

Jugular Venous Pressure, Hepatomegaly, and Peripheral Edema

The jugular veins provide a useful index of right atrial pressure and, thus, a guide to the presence of volume overload that can manifest as peripheral edema. Normal jugular venous pressure can be assessed by noting the upper limit of visible pulse undulation in the internal jugular veins with the patient supine and his or her head elevated at a 45-degree angle. With normal pressure, the upper level of jugular vein undulation is approximately 4 cm or less above the sternal angle. Ideally, the internal jugular vein is inspected, but as the external jugular venous system is more easily identified, it can also be used. The external jugular vein is compressed in the supraclavicular fossa, and as the examiner's finger strips the vein cephalad, blood rises in the more proximal portion of the vein; the height of this blood volume above the patient's clavicles reflects the central venous pressure. The height of the venous column normally falls during inspiration as a result of the accompanying decrease in intrathoracic pressure.

In patients with mild heart failure the jugular venous pressure may be normal at rest but rises quickly to abnormal levels with compression of the right upper quadrant, a sign known as the hepatojugular reflex. This sign is assessed by having the patient lie supine and semirecumbent at a 45-degree angle. Pressure with the examiner's hand is exerted on the patient's right upper quadrant and the jugular veins are observed for distention. This maneuver causes a sudden increase in venous return causes right ventricular end-diastolic and right atrial pressures to rise and remain elevated, which can be detected as jugular venous distention.

With heart failure, hepatomegaly, or liver enlargement, may be present and liver tenderness may be noted on abdominal palpation because of the stretching of the hepatic capsule. With chronic heart failure, however, liver tenderness is reduced, although liver enlargement persists. This enlargement of the liver is responsible for the anorexia, abdominal fullness, and/or nausea reported by patients with heart failure.

Although peripheral edema can be a common manifestation of heart failure, it does not correlate well with the level of systemic venous pressure and should not be used to estimate the degree of failure. In chronic heart failure, fluid volume may be already sufficiently expanded to cause edema in the presence of only slight elevations of systemic venous pressure.[24] Peripheral edema, usually symmetric, is pitting, generally occurs in the dependent portions of the body, and is greatest at the end of the day. In advanced heart failure, generalized body edema, including ascites and anasarca, may be present.

Nocturia

Nocturia occurs as a result of nocturnal diuresis. This nocturnal diuresis lessens the degree of fluid retention. Nocturnal diuresis with nocturia results from fluid resorption and redistribution in the supine position, as well as a reduction in renal vasoconstriction that occurs at rest.

Altered Hemodynamics

As previously discussed, the major determinants of cardiac output are stroke volume and heart rate. Heart rate is altered by activation baroreceptors found in the carotid arteries by means of a complex feedback mechanism. Zucker[16] has identified abnormalities in these baroreceptors in patients with heart failure that causes the abnormal activation of the sympathetic nervous system, the renin-angiotensin-aldosterone system, and vasopressin release and by the activation of these systems prevents an increase in heart rate in response to a reduction in pressure. In advanced heart failure, however, sympathetic activation overwhelms the compensatory neurohormonal response and results in a resting tachycardia

DIAGNOSTICS

The majority of patients with heart failure present with ventricular systolic dysfunction with a variable degree of diastolic dysfunction; however, a subset of patients have predominantly diastolic dysfunction. Because the clinical management of these two disease processes differs, a thorough diagnostic evaluation is critical. Table 132-1 reviews the history, physical examination, and diagnostic testing differences between systolic and diastolic dysfunction. The diagnostic evaluation should be limited to those studies necessary to (1) determine the type of ventricular dysfunction, primarily systolic or diastolic; (2) uncover correctable etiologies; (3) determine the prognosis; and (4) guide treatment.[25]

Chest X-Ray Examination

The size and shape of the cardiac silhouette, as well as the presence of interstitial and alveolar edema determine radiologic evidence of heart failure. A common chest x-ray study finding in heart failure is cardiomegaly, with a cardiothoracic (size of heart to width of chest) ratio that is increased more than 50%. Normally, in the upright position, pulmonary blood flow is greater to the lung bases than to the apexes. This is evidenced on the plain chest x-ray film when the caliber of the vessels, particularly the veins, of the lower lung

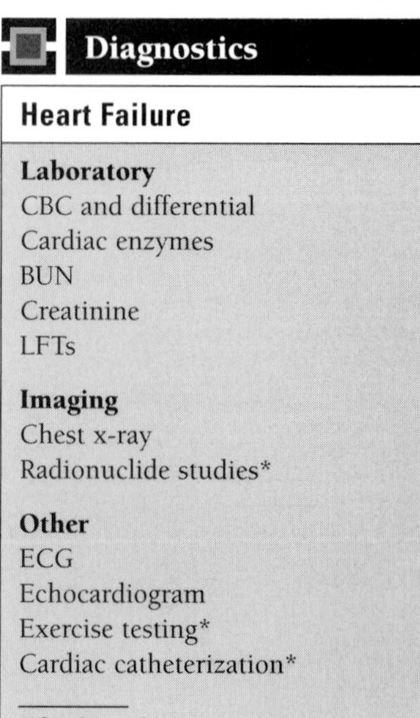
Diagnostics

Heart Failure

Laboratory
CBC and differential
Cardiac enzymes
BUN
Creatinine
LFTs

Imaging
Chest x-ray
Radionuclide studies*

Other
ECG
Echocardiogram
Exercise testing*
Cardiac catheterization*

*If indicated.

TABLE 132-1 Systolic vs. Diastolic Dysfunction in Heart Failure: Differences in History, Physical Examination, and Diagnostic Tests*

Parameter	Systolic	Diastolic
HISTORY		
Coronary artery disease	++++	+
Hypertension	++	++++
Diabetes	+++	+
Valvular heart disease	++++	−
Paroxysmal dyspnea	++	+++
PHYSICAL EXAMINATION		
Cardiomegaly	+++	+
Soft heart sounds	++++	+
S_3 gallop	+++	+
S_4 gallop	+	+++
Hypertension	++	++++
Mitral regurgitation	+++	+
Rales	++	++
Edema	+++	+
Jugular venous distention	+++	+
CHEST X-RAY EXAMINATION		
Cardiomegaly	+++	+
Pulmonary congestion	+++	+++
ELECTROCARDIOGRAM		
Low voltage	+++	−
Left ventricular hypertrophy	++	++++
Q waves	++	+
ECHOCARDIOGRAM		
Low ejection fraction	++++	−
Left ventricular dilation	++	−
Left ventricular hypertrophy	++	++++

From Young JB: Assessment of heart failure. In Colucci WS, editor: Heart failure: cardiac function and dysfunction. In Braunwald E, editor: *Atlas of heart disease,* vol 4, Philadelphia, 1995, Current Medicine.

*Plus signs indicate "suggestive" (the number reflects relative weight). Minus signs indicate "not very suggestive."

zones is compared with the caliber of the vessels of the upper lung zones. Patients with heart failure have a redistribution of pulmonary blood flow to the upper zones, so that the caliber of the upper zone vessels becomes equal to or greater than the caliber of lower zone vessels. This redistribution occurs because interstitial edema is more severe in lower lung fields as a result of gravity. The microvasculature is consequently compressed, and blood flow is shunted upward.

Another radiologic indicator of heart failure, interstitial pulmonary edema, occurs when the left atrial pressure is elevated above 20 mm Hg. The radiologic pattern of interstitial edema consists of varying combinations of septal, perivascular, and subpleural edema. Septal edema is manifested by Kerley's B lines, which are short, nonbranching lines seen at the periphery of the lower lung fields, extending to and perpendicular to the pleural surface. Perivascular edema is manifested both as central (hilar) haze and as loss of definition of lower zone vessels. Subpleural edema is indicated by a sharp pleural margin associated with a poorly defined density extending into the underlying lung. Interstitial edema may also be seen as peribronchial "cuffing" when airways are viewed in cross section.

Alveolar edema, a third radiologic finding indicative of heart failure, occurs when the left atrial pressure is elevated above 30 mm Hg. This appears on the chest x-ray film as frank pulmonary opacification. The distribution of alveolar edema may be a typical central "bat wing" pattern, may be diffuse, or may be asymmetric, even unilateral. Opacification seen with alveolar edema is usually homogeneous but occasionally may be patchy, even mimicking pneumonia.

When left atrial pressure rises acutely, as in myocardial infarction, clinicians should remember that there may be a lag of several hours before the appearance of radiologic pulmonary edema. In these patients crackles that suggest acute pulmonary edema are usually heard despite an unimpressive radiographic appearance. Conversely, when the left atrial pressure is rapidly lowered with therapy and crackles disappear, the edema may continue to be present on the chest x-ray film for several hours.

Echocardiography and Radionuclide Ventriculography

Measurement of ventricular performance is a critical step in the diagnostic evaluation. The combined use of history, physical examination, chest x-ray examination, and the ECG cannot be relied on to distinguish among major etiologies of heart failure. The use of echocardiography or radionuclide ventriculography can substantially improve the accuracy of differentiating between systolic and diastolic dysfunction as compared with clinical evaluation alone.[26]

The value of echocardiography cannot be overestimated in the diagnostic evaluation of known or suspected heart failure. It currently represents the single most effective tool in widespread clinical use for the assessment of heart failure.[27]

Approximately 70% of patients with heart failure have left ventricular systolic dysfunction, defined as a left ventricular ejection fraction less than 40%.[21,27] Two-dimensional Doppler echocardiography provides information regarding biventricular systolic performance, wall thickness, and chamber dimensions. Segmental or regional wall motion abnormalities, chamber enlargement, and valvular disease can also be detected and quantified by echocardiography. Diastolic dysfunction can often be detected as well. Doppler echocardiography allows for the characterization of abnormal left ventricular filling in diastole. With significant diastolic dysfunction, this presents as increased velocity, reduced volume, and delayed timing on the Doppler echocardiogram. The Advisory Council to Improve Outcomes Nationwide in Heart Failure and the ACC and AHA guidelines both recognize echocardiography as the preferred diagnostic tool for evaluating the cause of heart failure in patients.[21,27]

Radionuclide angiography is more accurate than echocardiography in the measurement of ejection fraction. In combination with exercise and a myocardial perfusion imaging agent (such as thallium or sestamibi), exercise radionuclide myocardial scintigraphy is a sensitive and specific diagnostic tool in the assessment of suspected or known coronary artery disease. The usefulness of radionuclide angiography as a diagnostic tool is limited by the inability to characterize valvular abnormalities, cardiac chamber volumes, wall thickness, and estimation of intracardiac pressures.[21]

Exercise Testing

The exercise test, or stress test, provides important data on exercise and functional capacity, as well as prognostic information. Measurement of peak oxygen consumption during cardiopulmonary exercise testing is likely the single best predictor of survival in patients with advanced heart failure and currently determines the appropriateness and timing of heart transplantation.[26] Serial exercise testing with quantification of the workload achieved is helpful in determining the response to medical therapy. Exercise testing also permits the identification of suspected exercise-induced arrhythmias.

The use of submaximal exercise testing, such as the 6-minute walk test, is a viable option for those who do not have access to equipment to measure respiratory gases. The 6-minute walk test is a 100-foot self-paced walk during which the subject is asked to cover as much ground as possible.[28] The 6-minute walk test correlates well with peak oxygen consumption and predicts short-term survival in patients with advanced heart failure. Univariate and multivariate analysis found that the distance ambulated during the test was the strongest predictor of peak oxygen consumption and was equivalent to left ventricular ejection fraction in predicting mortality and hospital readmissions for heart failure.[29-31]

Cardiac Catheterization/Endomyocardial Biopsy

Clinical information gleaned from cardiac catheterization and measurement of hemodynamics is invaluable in patients with heart failure who have advanced symptoms or suboptimal response to medical therapy. Catheterization provides valuable information about the origin of congestive vs. low-output symptoms through direct measurement of filling pressure and cardiac output, and permits the direct measurement of systemic vascular resistance. Hemodynamic measurement provides an assessment of valvular dysfunction and identifies the presence of intracardiac shunts. From a therapeutic perspective, hemodynamic assessment can guide medical therapy in refractory cases, determine the need for circulatory support, and provide data for identifying the timing for valvular surgery.[32]

In addition, cardiac catheterization remains the best procedure for evaluation of diastolic dysfunction properties because ventricular filling pressures can be measured directly. Although catheterization may not be beneficial for all heart failure patients, cardiac catheterization should be considered in patients with acute or acutely decompensated chronic heart failure not responding to treatment. Cardiac catheterization should also be considered in patients with angina or other signs of ischemia not responding to appropriate treatment.[21,27]

It has been established that during exercise radionuclide myocardial imaging, many patients with significant left ventricular dysfunction and dilation irrespective of cause have a positive myocardial redistribution study suggestive of coronary artery disease. Coronary artery angiography performed during cardiac catheterization is often necessary to diagnose the presence, extent, and severity of an existing coronary artery disease. Furthermore, cardiac catheterization and coronary angiography are used with radionuclide imaging to assess viability of revascularization strategies for patients with ischemic cardiomyopathy.

Conversely, the role of right ventricular endomyocardial biopsy in the diagnostic evaluation is controversial. Biopsy is usually performed only in cases with a clear-cut acute symptomatic onset (within 6 months), with compelling clinical suspicion of infiltrative cardiomyopathy (such as amyloidosis, sarcoidosis, or metastatic cancer), or with suspected Adriamycin cardiotoxicity.

Cardiac Magnetic Resonance Imaging

MRI is used to measure cardiac volumes, wall thickness, and left ventricular mass. Cardiac MRI also quantifies myocardial perfusion and function and detects pericardium thickening and degree of myocardial necrosis. Currently, use of MRI is not widespread and is recommended only if other imaging techniques are not diagnostically satisfactory.[27]

DIFFERENTIAL DIAGNOSIS

A variety of cardiac, pulmonary, and systemic disease states have dyspnea as a typical symptom and can be confused with heart failure on the basis of this symptom. Therefore systematic evaluation of dyspnea is critically important to properly diagnose the underlying disease. The common disease processes leading to dyspnea can be broadly characterized as abnormalities in gas exchange, pulmonary circulation, respiratory mechanics, or cardiac function. Ferrin and Tino[33] identified four categories for use in making a differential diagnosis of dyspnea: (1) pulmonary causes (airway, parenchyma, pleura, chest wall, and vasculature), (2) cardiac causes (pericardial, myocardial, valvular, coronary arteries), (3) neuromuscular dysfunction, and (4) anxiety disorders.

Chronic Pulmonary Conditions

The dyspnea of heart failure might be confused with chronic pulmonary conditions (Figure 132-1). The most common adult disorders of COPD, chronic bronchitis, asthma, exacerbated cystic fibrosis, and lung cancer are coincidentally seen in the same age range at risk for heart failure; however, these pulmonary conditions have physical examination findings that help distinguish them from heart failure. COPD represents a spectrum of disease severity and pathophysiology and is a common co-morbidity in patients with heart failure. In patients with underlying COPD and heart failure, it is often challenging to distinguish the dyspnea of pulmonary origin from the dyspnea of cardiac origin. Chronic dyspnea caused by COPD is often exacerbated by bending over forward (e.g., while putting on one's shoes), whereas dyspnea caused by heart failure is usually not aggravated by this. This simple maneuver may aid in the discernment of the origin of a patient's dyspnea.

Orthopnea (worsening dyspnea when the patient assumes a recumbent position) and paroxysmal nocturnal dyspnea (sudden waking from sleep with marked dyspnea) may result from either COPD or heart failure. These entities may be difficult to identify on the basis

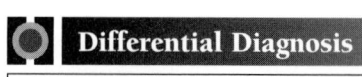

Heart Failure

Pulmonary causes
Cardiac causes
Neuromuscular dysfunction
Anxiety disorders

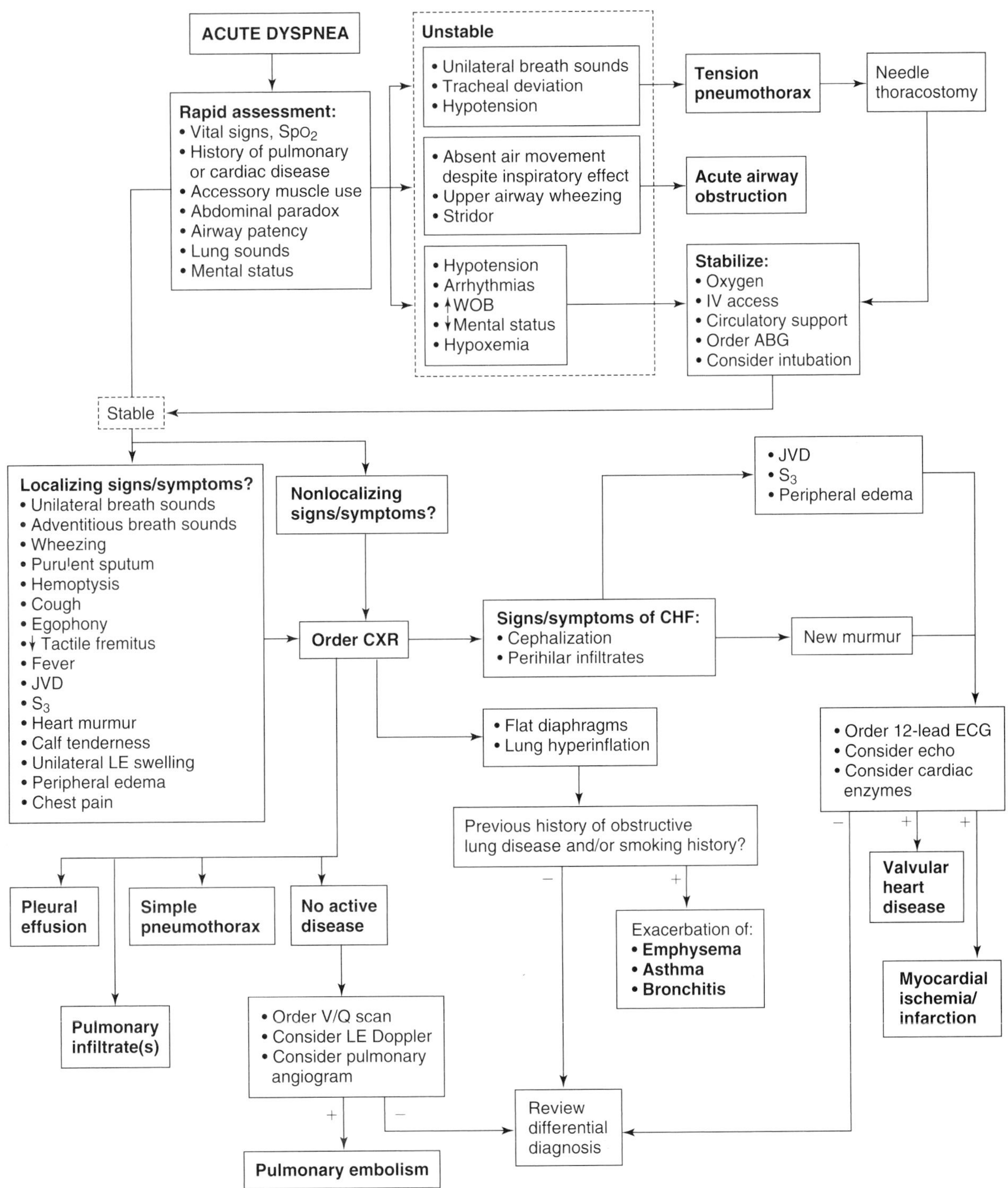

FIGURE 132-1

Acute dyspnea algorithm. *Spo_2*, Peripheral saturation of oxygen; ↑, increase; ↓, decrease; *WOB*, work of breathing; *IV*, intravenous, *ABG*, arterial blood gas; *JVD*, jugular venous distention; *S_3*, third heart sound; *LE*, lower extremity; *CXR*, chest radiograph; *CHF*, congestive heart failure; +, present, −, absent; *V/Q*, ventilation/perfusion ratio; *echo*, echocardiogram. (From Ferrin M, Tino G: Acute dyspnea, *AACN Clin Issues* 8(3):398-410, 1997.)

of symptom analysis; past medical history, risk for heart failure, and cardiac examination findings (S_3, S_4, jugular venous distention) in combination with other symptoms such as increased fatigue may help elucidate the cause as heart failure.

Asthma and Upper Respiratory Infection

In clinical practice, new-onset heart failure is often mistaken for asthma or an upper respiratory infection (URI) because dyspnea is predominant symptom. However, the duration of the dyspnea can be a clue to distinguish new-onset heart failure from asthma or URI. The asthmatic patient is usually free of chronic dyspnea but experiences episodic dyspnea, with prominent inspiratory and expiratory wheezing. Because pulmonary edema can trigger bronchospasm and wheezing, an acute asthma attack may mimic acute pulmonary edema, but usually airflow limitation and wheezing are more marked in acute asthma, and also the cardiac examination is notable for the lack of an enlarged apical impulse or an S_3 gallop.

Airway Obstruction

Aspiration with associated airway obstruction may produce acute dyspnea that can be mistaken for that of heart failure, as can the acute dyspnea associated with pneumonia or pneumothorax. However, a careful consideration of the entire clinical picture, with attention to the pulmonary examination indicating consolidation or absent breath sounds, helps the clinician distinguish heart failure from these pulmonary etiologies of dyspnea.

Pleural Effusions

Pleural effusions produce dyspnea of a more chronic nature that can be confused with heart failure. Dyspnea associated with effusions is usually gradual in onset and is nonexertional.[31] To further complicate this picture, clinicians must recall that pleural effusions may result from chronic heart failure, as well as from other systemic conditions. Pleural effusions produce dyspnea through compression of underlying lung parenchyma and reduction in ventilated lung volume. Diminished breath sounds, dullness to percussion, and diminished tactile fremitus are noted on physical examination.

Pleural effusions are primarily transudative or exudative, both of which can be an aid to distinguish among the etiologies. Differentiation between transudative and exudative is made on the basis of the protein content and lactate dehydrogenase levels in the pleural fluid as compared with those levels in the serum. In all, 70% of transudative effusions are caused by heart failure because of abnormally high pleural capillary pressures. Transudative effusions can also result from liver failure, chronic renal failure, or hypoalbuminemia; however, these produce specific laboratory findings that can distinguish them from effusions caused by heart failure. Protein-enriched exudative effusions are primarily seen in malignancy, infection, and collagen vascular diseases.

Pulmonary Effusions

Pulmonary embolism may present with acute dyspnea and therefore be confused with heart failure. Symptoms of pulmonary embolism may be subtle and range from none, to mild dyspnea with pleuritic chest pain, to cardiac arrest. The most common etiology of a pulmonary embolus, however, is a lower extremity deep vein thrombosis, which can cause unilateral leg pain and swelling that can suggest embolus as a cause for chest pain and dyspnea. In pulmonary embolus, arterial blood gas analysis may show hypoxemia; however, the best diagnostic test to identify a pulmonary embolus is the ventilation-perfusion scan that exhibits ventilation-perfusion mismatch.

Neuromuscular Disorders

Neuromuscular disorders, such as myasthenia gravis and Guillain-Barré syndrome, can be differentiated from heart failure because the dyspnea from neuromuscular causes originate from respiratory muscle weakness and other neurologic findings distinguish them from heart failure as well.

Anxiety

Finally, anxiety as the sole cause of dyspnea is uncommon and is always a diagnosis of exclusion. Clinicians must remember that anxiety is common with dyspnea of any cause, adds to the perceived severity, and prolongs the duration of the dyspnea.

MANAGEMENT

Chronic or acute heart failure requires sufficient diagnostic testing to determine the specific etiology or cause. Coronary artery disease, valvular heart disease, and pericardial disease may be surgically treatable, mandating appropriate diagnostic studies. Once a specific diagnosis has been made, the first task in the treatment of heart failure is to treat specific reversible etiologies. Once reversible etiologies are treated, management of the residual heart failure can be initiated. Heart failure caused by diastolic dysfunction must be differentiated from that caused by systolic dysfunction, as treatment options differ.

In general, the primary objectives in treatment of heart failure are fourfold: (1) prevention of further myocardial injury, (2) prevention of recurrence of clinical failure (congestive or low output), (3) relief of symptoms and signs, and (4) improvement in prognosis.[26] Correct selection and application of pharmacologic therapy require an understanding of the patient's pathophysiology and a careful history and physical examination.

The ACC/AHA classification stages represent a framework for management of left heart failure. In Stage A patients (risk, no symptoms, no structural abnormality), clear benefit exists for control of systolic and diastolic hypertension. Selected studies support treatment of lipid disorders, ACE inhibitor use in patients with diabetes and other cardiovascular risk factors, and control of tachycardic ventricular rates.[20] Benefits are unclear and are the result of expert consensus opinion for periodic evaluation for signs and symptoms of heart failure, smoking cessation, dietary salt reduction, nutritional supplements, avoidance of illicit drug use, limitation of alcohol consumption, or regular exercise.[20]

For Stage B patients (those with structural heart disease, previous MI, left ventricular systolic dysfunction, asymptomatic valvular disease but without symptoms of failure), clear evidence exists for ACE inhibition and beta blockade, irrespective of the ejection fraction.[20] Evidence is unclear and is the result of consensus opinion for ACE inhibition or beta blockade for patients with reduced ejection fraction, valve replacement for hemodynamically significant stenosis or regurgitation, digoxin for patients with systolic dysfunction in sinus rhythm, or the recommendations made for Stage A patients.[20]

Management for Stage C patients (with known structural heart disease and with prior or current symptoms of failure) includes the health promotion measures previously mentioned in conjunction with daily weights, limitation of exercise during periods of acute decompensation, and close monitoring for decompensation. In these patients, nonadherence to medication and dietary regimens can rapidly precipitate deterioration. Pharmacologic therapy in Stage C typically involves four classes of medications: a diuretic, an ACE inhibitor, a beta blocker, and digitalis.[20]

In Stage C patients, there are additional interventions that have demonstrated value in selected patients. These include the use of aldosterone antagonists, angiotension-receptor blockers, hydralazine, isosorbide dinitrate, and exercise training. Further interventions not currently recommended but under investigation include vasopeptidase inhibitors, endothelin antagonists, and cytokine antagonists. The value of synchronized biventricular pacing, external counterpulsation, and respiratory support techniques are being explored for patients with heart failure.[20]

Stage D patients with refractory heart failure require meticulous control of fluid balance. Clear evidence exits for benefit with both ACE inhibitors and beta blockers. It is important to recognize, however, that the increased role of neurohormonal factors in compensation of severe heart failure can place Stage D patients at risk for hypotension and renal insufficiency with ACE inhibition, as well as increased risk for increasing failure with beta blockade. Thus these agents should be used in small doses and with caution in these patients. Stage D patients are candidates for specialized interventions such as circulatory support measures, cardiac transplantation, and left ventricular assist devices.[20]

Pharmacologic Therapy Overview

Therapy for heart failure can be subdivided by pathophysiology (systolic vs. diastolic dysfunction) and by the level of symptomatic presentation defined by the NYHA classification. The NYHA subgroups are class I/II, without significant symptoms; class II/III, with mild to moderate signs and symptoms of clinical heart failure; and class III/IV, with persistent signs of disabling heart failure. Box 132-3 identifies the appropriate class of pharmacologic agents for each subgroup. Another way to view the overall management of systolic dysfunction (ejection fraction <40%) is based on the volume status. With no evidence of fluid excess, therapy with an ACE inhibitor (vasodilator) is begun. Once the ACE dosage is stabilized, a beta blocker is added. A diuretic and/or digoxin can be added to manage new or persistent symptoms. With patients who have a fluid overload as evidenced by edema, pulmonary rales, or jugular venous distention, therapy is initiated with a diuretic and an ACE inhibitor. When the patients are stabilized on these medications, digoxin may be added to reduce symptoms and increase exercise tolerance. Once the fluid overload is resolved, a beta-blocking agent may be added for persistent symptoms. Of course, a patient's renal status and other co-morbid conditions may impact decisions regarding therapy.

BOX 132-3

TARGETING OF PHARMACOLOGIC THERAPY FOR LEFT VENTRICULAR DYSFUNCTION BY SUBGROUP

NYHA CLASS I/II
Prophylactic use of ACE inhibitors

NYHA CLASS II/III
Combination therapy: digoxin, diuretics, vasodilators, ACE inhibitors

NYHA CLASS III/IV
Combination therapy plus inotropic agents, transplantation

NYHA, New York Heart Association.

Vasodilators. Vasodilators reverse several of the characteristic physiologic compensatory mechanisms that accompany the development of heart failure. Vasodilators affect peripheral vasculature tone and have beneficial lowering effects on preload and afterload. Predominant venous vasodilators (such as nitroglycerin) increase venous compliance and redistribute blood volume to the venous capacitance vessels, thereby reducing ventricular filling volume and pressure. Predominant arterial vasodilators (such as ACE inhibitors) decrease arteriolar resistance, which reduces impedance to the left ventricular outflow, resulting in augmentation of the cardiac output and stroke volume. Vasodilators are an appropriate therapy for both systolic and diastolic dysfunction.

ACE Inhibitors. ACE inhibitors are the cornerstone of chronic management of symptomatic heart failure. The role of the ACE inhibitor emerged from the recognition that neurohormonal activation contributes to the pathogenesis of heart failure. By suppressing the production of angiotensin II, a potent vasoconstrictor, ACE inhibitors decrease systemic and pulmonary vascular resistance by preventing the release of aldosterone and norepinephrine while elevating the levels of the vasodilator hormone bradykinin.

ACE inhibitors should be considered a priority in all patients with left ventricular systolic dysfunction, unless absolutely contraindicated.[32] The following are potential contraindications: (1) history of compelling intolerance or adverse reaction to these agents, (2) serum potassium level greater than 5.5 mEq/L, or (3) symptomatic hypotension. Care should be used in patients who have a serum creatinine level greater than 3 mg/dl.[26] With the exception of these contraindications, ACE inhibitors should be used in all patients with left ventricular dysfunction and a left ventricular ejection fraction less than 40%, regardless of the level of symptoms.[33] ACE inhibitors have been shown to significantly reduce mortality, improve functional status, and reduce hospital admissions in patients with mild, moderate, and severe heart failure and left ventricular systolic dysfunction.[5,27,32-34] Concerns regarding side effects have been cited as a reason for the low usage of ACE inhibitors.[26] The average reduction in blood pressure and the abnormal alteration in serum chemistry values were quite small in the SOLVD trial, with only 2.2% of patients achieving a symptomatic reduction in blood pressure.[4] These results indicate that patients who begin ACE inhibitors should have their blood pressure, renal function, and serum potassium level monitored within 1 week. Maximum daily doses should be attempted in all patients (captopril 50 mg t.i.d., enalapril 20 mg b.i.d., lisinopril 40 mg q.d.). In patients with hypotension, hyperkalemia, and/or renal dysfunction, a test dose should be given initially (captopril 6.25 mg or enalapril 2.5 mg) in the office, and incremental dose escalation tried cautiously. Despite the clear demonstration of benefits and nominal number of potential side effects, the EPICAL Study[35] notes continued underutilization of these drugs in daily practice.

Angiotensin-Receptor Blocker Agents. Angiotension-receptor blocking agents are the newer medications that act directly on the angiotensin-renin-aldosterone system. These agents modify the effects of angiotensin II, the substance that promotes vasoconstriction, abnormal cell growth, and the release of aldosterone. All of these responses, which are detrimental in heart failure, are mediated through the angiotensin I (AT1) receptor. Although ACE inhibitors decrease the conversion of angiotensin I to angiotensin II and prevent the breakdown of bradykinin, these agents do not completely suppress angiotensin II, which is formed by way of alternate pathways. Angiotensin-receptor blocker agents are selective for the AT1 receptor and thereby complete the process by interfering with the action of angiotensin II at the receptor level, shunting the angiotensin II to the AT2 receptor, which mediates vasodilation and decreased cell growth.[36] Recent evidence suggests that angiotensin receptor binder (ARBs) may delay nephropathy in type 2 diabetes.[37]

Losartan, irbesartan, valsartan, and candesartan are currently available in a variety of dosages, which should be titrated with respect to blood pressure and laboratory monitoring when used alone or in conjunction with an ACE inhibitor.

Both the ELITE I and ELITE II trials compared losartan and captopril, revealing no significant difference in performance. The latter trial, however, revealed losartan to be better tolerated in terms of side effects. It has been suggested that the addition of an ARB to an ACE inhibitor will provide more complete blockade of angiotensin II production, preventing more of the deleterious effects on the myocardium and the periphery.[34,38]

Additional Options for Patients Unable to Tolerate ACE Inhibitors. AHCPR guidelines state that hydralazine combined with isosorbide dinitrate (Isordil) or isosorbide mononitrate (Imdur) is an appropriate alternative for patients who are unable to tolerate ACE inhibitors.[34]

Hydralazine is a direct arteriolar vasodilator, and isosorbide dinitrate is a venodilator. The combination of these agents results in an increase in cardiac output secondary to decreased impedance to ventricular ejection and decreased preload. The combination of hydralazine and isosorbide dinitrate improves survival and exercise tolerance in patients with heart failure.[4,39] These were the first medications to show improved survival in heart failure, but are currently not specifically recommended.[34] Side effects have been a significant problem in clinical trials, with 18% to 33% of patients discontinuing these medications because of headache, palpitations, and nasal congestion. Isosorbide dinitrate should generally be initiated at a dose of 10 mg t.i.d. and increased weekly to 40 mg t.i.d. as tolerated. Hydralazine should be initiated at a dose of 10 to 25 mg t.i.d. and increased weekly to 75 to 100 mg t.i.d. as tolerated. Therapy for hypotensive patients and those with severe heart failure should be initiated at lower doses. Three-times-per-day dosing is recommended to enhance compliance because there is poorer compliance and identified nitrate tolerance at four-times-per-day dosing.

BOX 132-4

FACTORS CONTRIBUTING TO EXCESS SODIUM AND WATER RETENTION IN HEART FAILURE

- Decreased cardiac output
- Decreased glomerular filtration rate secondary to reduced renal blood flow
- Redistribution of intrarenal blood flow to salt-conserving medulla
- Increased renal sympathetic nerve activity
- Increased arginine vasopressin (antidiuretic hormone) levels
- Activation of the renin-angiotensin-aldosterone system

From Moser DK, Cardin S: Heart failure. In Clochesy JM and others, editors: *Critical care nursing*, ed 2, Philadelphia, 1996, WB Saunders.

Diuretics. Unlike ACE inhibitors, diuretics have not yet been shown to reduce mortality overall in patients with heart failure. No large controlled clinical trial has been conducted with regard to diuretics and heart failure; however, diuretics are important agents to relieve the signs and symptoms of systemic and pulmonary congestion caused by volume overload in heart failure. Many factors contribute to the sodium and water retention that causes volume overload in heart failure (Box 132-4). Diuretics promote sodium and fluid excretion, thus relieving both the symptoms (dyspnea, orthopnea, and paroxysmal nocturnal dyspnea) and the accompanying signs (crackles, S_3, jugular venous distention, hepatic engorgement, peripheral edema, and ascites) of volume overload.

Initial therapy with a thiazide diuretic is appropriate in mild heart failure. A loop diuretic, which is more potent, should be used with severe heart failure, renal insufficiency, or persistent edema.[26] If congestion does not resolve with a thiazide diuretic, a loop diuretic should be initiated to replace the thiazide diuretic. Symptoms of severe heart failure or significant renal dysfunction usually always require a loop diuretic agent. Loop diuretics are associated with acute and chronic distal tubular compensation and may be combined with a thiazide, thereby increasing diuretic potency by minimizing distal tubular compensation.[32] Diuretic dosing is summarized in Table 132-2. The standing dose of diuretic is dependent on the patient's body size, age, estimated glomerular filtration rate, renal function, amount of edema, and compliance with a low-sodium and fluid-restricted diet.

Intravascular volume depletion following diuretic administration reduces preload but has little effect on afterload. Excessive depletion of intravascular volume may actually increase afterload by causing reflex sympathetic stimulation and subsequent release of vasoconstrictors such as norepinephrine,

TABLE 132-2 Diuretics Used in the Treatment of Chronic Heart Failure

Drug	Initial Dose (mg)	Recommended Maximum Dose (mg)	Potential Adverse Reactions
THIAZIDE DIURETICS			
Hydrochlorothiazide	25 q day	50 q day	Postural hypotension, hypokalemia, hyperuricemia
Chlorthalidone	25 q day	50 q day	
LOOP DIURETICS			
Furosemide	10-40 q day	240 b.i.d.	Same as thiazide diuretics
Bumetanide	0.5-1 q day	10 q day	
POTASSIUM-SPARING DIURETICS			
Spironolactone	25 q day	100 b.i.d.	Hyperkalemia (especially if given with ACE inhibitors), gynecomastia, rash
Triamterene	50 q day	100 b.i.d.	
Amiloride	5 q day	10 b.i.d.	
THIAZIDE-RELATED DIURETICS			
Metolazone	2.5 as single dose initially	20 q day	Same as with thiazide diuretics

From Konstam M and others: *Heart failure: evaluation and care of patients with left-ventricular systolic dysfunction,* Clinical Practice Guideline No 11, AHCPR Pub No 94-0612, 1994, Rockville, Md, US Department of Health and Human Services, Public Health Service, Agency for Health Care Policy and Research.

epinephrine, renin, and angiotensin. Increased afterload may reduce cardiac output and lead to orthostatic hypotension, causing further activation of already-augmented vasoconstrictive mechanisms. These diuretic-induced stimulatory effects on the renin-angiotensin-aldosterone system can be blocked to some extent by the concomitant administration of an ACE inhibitor.[40] Potent diuretics can cause serious electrolyte abnormalities such as hypokalemia and hypomagnesemia that require periodic measurement of serum potassium and magnesium. In instances of significant potassium wasting, potassium-sparing diuretics such as triamterene may be useful.

With disease progression the use of intermittent IV diuretics to overcome the significant neurohormonal responses that are antecedent to the increase in sodium and fluid retention may be necessary. A state of relative diuretic resistance is common in advanced heart failure or in long-term diuretic therapy.

Metolazone, a potent oral thiazide-like agent, can be added to loop diuretics in such instances. Metolazone is usually effective with reduced renal function. Although the thiazide diuretics alone are usually ineffective in severe heart failure, the combination of a thiazide diuretic with a loop diuretic may be able to promote diuresis in refractory heart failure.

Recently the RALES trial (Randomized Aldactone Survival Study) suggested a benefit in the addition of spironolactone in those patients who present with the following criteria: (1) symptoms of dyspnea at rest currently or within the last 6 months, or (2) those characterized as having "severe" or NYHA Class IV heart failure.[32] This potassium-sparing diuretic and aldosterone antagonist is often helpful to promote diuresis in patients taking high doses of loop diuretics and metolazone and has been shown to decrease both mortality and hospitalization rates in these patients. The blockade of aldosterone receptors by spironolactone substantially reduced the risk of morbidity and death and improved symptoms as measured by NYHA class.[40] Such diuretics promote hyperkalemia, however, and their use must be carefully monitored. Also, to date, there have been no trials to assess the safety or efficacy in patients with less severe heart failure.[32]

Digoxin. The cardiac glycosides, such as digoxin, have been used to treat heart failure for more than 200 years, but controversy still surrounds their use in heart failure.[41] Digoxin improves physical functioning and symptoms in patients with systolic dysfunction, but the addition of digoxin to diuretics and ACE inhibitors has not been clearly shown to reduce mortality.[32,42,43] There are three current recommendations for the use of digoxin in heart failure: (1) patients who have atrial fibrillation in conjunction with heart failure, (2) patients who have dyspnea at rest or a recent history of dyspnea at rest, and (3) those who remain symptomatic despite adequate dosages of diuretics, ACE inhibitors, and beta blockers.[32] In addition, the Digitalis Investigation Group trial revealed a trend toward excess mortality resulting from myocardial infarction and sudden death in those who likely had ischemic heart disease as the underlying etiology of heart failure.[43]

Digoxin acts as a positive inotropic agent by increasing intracellular calcium in myocytes by altering calcium-sodium exchange (see Positive Inotropic Agents, p. 521, for further discussion). The increase in intracellular calcium available to actin-myosin filaments results in an increased contractile state of myocytes.[42] In addition, digoxin may resensitize baroreceptors that have been suppressed by increased neurohormonal sympathetic activity. Current evidence suggests that digoxin is an appropriate addition to ACE inhibitors and diuretics for the treatment of systolic dysfunction. Digoxin is not indicated in patients with primary diastolic dysfunction and preserved systolic function.[26,42] Loading doses of digoxin are not necessary in heart failure. In the presence of normal renal function, the typical daily dose of 0.25 mg can be initiated. In patients with abnormal renal function, conduction defects, and small body size, as well as in older patients, digoxin dosing should be started at 0.125 mg daily and titrated on the basis of serum digoxin levels. There are numerous interactions with digoxin and other drugs, particularly amiodarone, quinidine, procainamide, diltiazem, verapamil, antibiotics, and anticholinergic agents. Patients taking these other agents should also be dosed with digoxin 0.125 mg daily.

There are no data to support regular measurement of serum digoxin levels. As a clinical rule of thumb, however, digoxin levels should be obtained when (1) heart failure worsens, (2) renal function deteriorates, (3) medications are added that affect digoxin levels, or (4) digoxin toxicity is suspected (Box 132-5). An adequately digitalized patient will have a serum digoxin concentration of 0.7 to 1.4 ng/ml; most patients with digoxin toxicity have elevated serum digoxin levels. Hypokalemia, hypomagnesemia, and hypercalcemia exacerbate digoxin toxicity.

Beta Blockers. One of the most important mechanisms responsible for progression of heart failure is activation of the sympathetic nervous system. This observation led to the hypothesis that drugs that interfere with the actions of the sympathetic nervous system (e.g., beta blockers) may be beneficial in heart failure.[45] In several studies to date, beta blockers in carefully selected patients with heart failure have been shown to improve ventricular function, hemodynamics, functional status, and exercise tolerance, as well as reduce heart failure exacerbations.[46-51] In three published trials, as well as the COPERNICUS Study (October 2002), treatment with carvedilol, metoprolol, or bisoprolol reduced mortality by at least 34% in patients with heart failure.[32] Beta-adrenergic blocking agents exert their actions by occupying beta-adrenergic receptor sites, which results in the inability of the beta agonists to exert their effects. Beta blockers reduce heart rate and thereby reduce myocardial oxygen consumption, inhibit the release of renin, and decrease the activation of the renin-angiotensin system. Beta-adrenergic blockade is not recommended in those with heart failure who have bradycardia, significant heart block, moderate to severe COPD, or brittle insulin-dependent diabetes. Beta blockers are currently recommended for all patients with NHYA Class II or III systolic heart failure, except for those with dyspnea at rest or any symptoms of dyspnea at rest within the previous 6 months. The benefits are especially well described for those patients with a history of myocardial infarction and most patients with left ventricular dysfunction.[32]

Adjunctive Therapy

Anticoagulants. Many practitioners opt to anticoagulate patients with advanced systolic dysfunction (left ventricular ejection fraction <30% to 35%) because of the potential risk of systemic embolization. Review of a number of clinical trials has found that the risk is much lower than ordinarily thought and data to date remain limited and controversial.[27,32,52] Further evidence suggests that the risks associated with anticoagulation may outweigh potential benefits in many patients with heart failure. Current recommendations are to avoid routine anticoagulation except in patients with heart failure who have a risk of embolization that is higher than baseline. Characteristics that place patients at a higher than baseline risk of cardiac thromboembolism include left ventricular ejection fraction <30% to 35%, paroxysmal or chronic atrial fibrillation, or significant mitral regurgitation. There is no evidence to support use of anticoagulation in patients with sinus rhythm, even if a history of a previous vascular event exists or evidence of an intracardiac thrombus.[27]

Anticoagulation with warfarin with a target international normalized ratio (INR) of 2 to 3, along with close monitoring, is recommended. Close monitoring is especially important if right-sided heart failure and hepatic congestion worsen. Patients and their families need to understand the signs and symptoms of excess anticoagulation, as well as the need to take the appropriate dose of anticoagulant and to have blood work completed at the prescribed times.[26]

BOX 132-5

SIGNS OF DIGOXIN TOXICITY

- New arrhythmias
- Anorexia
- Nausea
- Confusion
- Visual disturbances

Antiarrhythmics. Between 35% and 50% of deaths resulting from heart failure are sudden and caused by presumed malignant tachyarrhythmias.[53] This observation has led to intense interest in the use of antiarrhythmic pharmacologic therapy and devices to reduce the risk of sudden arrhythmic cardiac death in patients with heart failure. Given the widespread availability of implantable cardioverter-defibrillators (ICDs) in particular, management of ventricular arrhythmias in patients with heart failure is rapidly evolving.

Frequent premature ventricular contractions (PVCs) and nonsustained ventricular tachycardia are common in heart failure as a result of elevated ventricular wall stress, focal myocardial fibrosis, electrolyte imbalances, effects of pharmacologic agents, high levels of circulating catecholamines, and myocardial ischemia. As the severity of heart failure progresses, nonsustained ventricular tachycardia is a nearly ubiquitous finding on Holter or telemetry monitoring. Although the presence of nonsustained ventricular tachycardia is a marker of a poorer prognosis, it is not necessarily a marker of a greater risk of sudden cardiac death.[54] There is no evidence to date that the suppression of asymptomatic PVCs or nonsustained ventricular tachycardia by antiarrhythmics is beneficial in patients with heart failure; however, there are a number of adverse factors associated with the use of antiarrhythmic agents in patients with heart failure. Class I agents are considered to be proarrhythmic on the ventricular level, whereas Class II agents have been associated with sudden death in heart failure.[27,44] On the basis of these facts, the routine use of antiarrhythmics in patients with heart failure who have brief, asymptomatic episodes of nonsustained ventricular tachycardia is not recommended.

Amiodarone. Two interventions that hold promise for patients with symptomatic or malignant arrhythmias and heart failure are amiodarone and the ICD. Amiodarone is effective against most supraventricular and ventricular arrhythmias and may restore sinus rhythm in patients with heart failure and atrial fibrillation. Amiodarone is the only antiarrhythmic drug without clinically significant negative inotropic effects. Data to date, however, do not show an improvement in overall mortality. In addition, potential side effects include hyperthyroidism or hypothyroidism, hepatitis, neuropathy, and pulmonary fibrosis. Careful monitoring is required with the use of amiodarone, and routine administration is not recommended in patients with heart failure.[27]

Implantable Cardioverter-Defibrillators. ICDs reliably detect and terminate malignant ventricular arrhythmias. In patients with reduced ejection fraction, prior myocardial infarction, and inducible ventricular tachycardia, ICDs prevent sudden cardiac death. The role of ICDs in patients with reduced ejection fraction and prior myocardial and nonischemic cardiomyopathy is under investigation. As the cost, ease of implantation, and safety of ICDs improve, ICDs will likely be implanted more often in patients with significant depression of systolic function.

Positive Inotropic Agents

Positive inotropic agents increase the force of myocardial contraction. Despite the development of the newer generations of effective vasodilators, there is an ongoing search for a safe and efficacious orally administered positive inotropic agent. The long-term use of oral inotropic agents in clinical studies has been hampered by their risk of precipitating serious ventricular arrhythmias and increasing the risk of sudden cardiac death. To date, nearly every long-term orally administered inotropic agent has led to an increase in mortality from sudden cardiac death in patients with heart failure. There is as yet no safe, available oral inotropic agent other than digoxin. A recently studied promising agent, vesnarinone, a drug with complex pharmacologic effects, including positive inotropy, improved functional capacity and the quality of life but led to decreased survival, likely because of sudden cardiac death.[55]

Long-term use of parenteral positive inotropic agents such as phosphodiesterase inhibitors (milrinone, amrinone, enoximone) and beta-adrenergic agonists (dobutamine) has resulted in improved symptoms but increased rates of sudden cardiac death when patients receive therapy at home.[56,57] At present, the use of continuous or intermittent parenteral positive inotropic agents is largely palliative in patients with end-stage heart failure. Such agents can be helpful, however, for patients with refractory volume overload or threatened end-organ dysfunction. Dobutamine directly stimulates beta-adrenergic receptors of the heart, leading to an increase in heart rate and contractile force. The self-limited institution of an IV inotropic agent such as dobutamine can transiently improve systolic function, palliate low-output states, and improve end-organ dysfunction. Renal performance can also be improved with low-dose dopamine, which stimulates renal dopaminergic receptors, leading to renal vasodilation.[26] At higher doses dopamine may be deleterious by increasing myocardial oxygen demand and afterload. Because both dopamine and dobutamine at higher doses may cause vasoconstriction, the potent vasodilator nitroprusside may be necessary to counteract this vasoconstrictor effect.

These results underscore the importance of factors other than myocardial contractility in determining the outcome of heart failure. To date, improvements in contractility have not led to improved outcomes. Continual pharmacologic modulation of myocardial preload and afterload, as well as pharmacologic inhibition of progressive myocyte hypertrophy and myocardial chamber dilation, are likely to be of more importance.

Nonpharmacologic Therapy

The modern approach to the management of chronic heart failure is directed primarily at manipulating myocardial preload and afterload. Although pharmacologic therapy is the mainstay of treatment for patients with heart failure, several nonpharmacologic interventions are important and useful adjuncts to overall management.

Diet. Reduced-sodium diets have been recommended for the management of heart failure, although there have as yet been no clinical studies to evaluate a specific sodium restriction. Volpe and others[58] found that patients with mild heart failure exhibited impaired sodium excretion when given a high-sodium diet as compared with normal subjects. In addition, patients with heart failure did not have an increase in atrial natriuretic factor in response to the oral sodium load, whereas the normal subjects had an increase in atrial natriuretic factor by 40%. These findings underscore the susceptibility of sodium retention in patients with mild heart failure and indirectly support the usefulness of sodium restriction.

Diets restricted to 2 g of sodium are somewhat unpalatable for most patients, and the added cost of low-sodium foods makes adherence to them a challenge. However, patients with severe heart failure should try to adhere to a 2-g sodium diet whenever possible. Patients with mild to moderate heart failure should be advised to follow a 3-g sodium diet, which is a more reasonable and realistic goal for most patients and their families. This diet can be attained by avoiding foods with high sodium content, removing the salt shaker from the table, and not cooking with salt. Patients with heart failure require specific dietary instructions and guidelines on how to read the labels on all food packages. Involvement of family members who prepare the foods cannot be underestimated; these persons need to be included in all dietary education.

Alcohol consumption should be infrequent and modest. Alcohol should be completely prohibited in any patient with known or suspected alcohol-induced cardiomyopathy.[26]

Sudden increases in sodium intake in patients with well-compensated but relatively severe heart failure can lead to acute decompensation. Holidays and seasonal festivities are particularly problematic because of the alteration in food preparation, increased daily activity levels, and increase in emotional stressors during these times. Ethnic foods prepared during holiday seasons are often high in sodium. Careful selection and alterations in holiday eating patterns need to be discussed with patients and their families, and alternative food choices offered. Dietary referral may be beneficial.

Activity. Until recently, reduced activity, including occasional periods of bed rest, were considered a standard part of management for patients with heart failure. Bed rest is thought to promote diuresis in the short term, but in the long term the negative effects of bed rest likely outweigh its benefits.

The clinical benefits that occur as a result of exercise training result from the salutary effects of exercise on skeletal muscle rather than substantial improvements in myocardial function. Both bicycle ergometry and arm ergometry have been used for training programs, and improvements in patients who exercise at home have been noted.

Studies have demonstrated improvements in exercise tolerance and patient symptoms with varying modes, intensities, durations, and frequencies of exercise.[58,59] Therefore guidelines regarding exercise for patients with heart failure are not clear at present. It is necessary to adapt recommendations regarding exercise to the current health status of the patient. Box 132-6 lists the relative criteria for initiating or increasing an exercise training program.

For most patients a regular walking program may be the most effective and functional mode of exercise. Most patients should begin with frequent, short walks and progress to less frequent, longer walks. Progression is based on individual prescriptions with adequate rest periods. Because dyspnea is the most common complaint, the level of perceived dyspnea is an acceptable method to define exercise intensity. Patients should exercise to a level that produces a moderate degree of dyspnea, with a rating of 3 on a scale of 1 to 10.

BOX 132-6

EXERCISE TRAINING GUIDELINES FOR PATIENTS WITH HEART FAILURE

I. **Relative criteria for the initiation of an aerobic exercise training program**
   A. Compensated heart failure
      1. Ability to speak without signs or symptoms of dyspnea (able to speak comfortably with a respiratory rate of <30 breaths per minute)
      2. Less then moderate fatigue
      3. Crackles (rales) present in more than half of the lungs
      4. Resting heart rate of <120 beats per minute
      5. Cardiac index of ≥1.8 L/min/m^2 (for invasively monitored patients)
      6. Central venous pressure of <12 mm Hg (for invasively monitored patients)

II. **Relative criteria indicating a need to modify or terminate exercise training**
   A. Marked dyspnea or fatigue
   B. Respiratory rate >40 breaths per minute during exercise
   C. Development of an S_3 heart sound or pulmonary crackles
   D. Increase in pulmonary crackles
   E. Increase in the sound of the second component of the second heart sound (P_2)
   F. Poor pulse pressure (<10 mm Hg difference between the systolic and diastolic blood pressure)
   G. Decrease in heart rate or blood pressure of >10 beats per minute or 10 mm Hg, respectively, during continuous (steady state) or progressive (increasing workload) exercise
   H. Increased supraventricular or ventricular ectopy
   I. Increase of >10 mm Hg in the mean pulmonary artery pressure (for invasively monitored patients)
   J. Increase or decrease of >6 mm Hg in the central venous pressure (for invasively monitored patients)
   K. Diaphoresis, pallor, or confusion

Modified from Cahalin L: Exercise training guidelines for patients with congestive heart failure, *Phys Ther* 76:516-533, 1997.

Surgical Therapy

Mechanical Circulatory Support. For hospitalized patients with heart failure who have severe symptoms despite maximal medical therapy, including parenteral inotropic agents, mechanical circulatory support with intraaortic balloon pumps (IABPs), and ventricular assist devices (VADs), may provide a lifesaving bridge to cardiac transplantation. Intraaortic balloon counterpulsation unloads the left ventricle and increases coronary artery perfusion. Myocardial ischemia is ameliorated, and left ventricular performance improves. The intraaortic balloon is positioned in the descending aorta, and it is inflated and deflated in synchrony with the mechanical events of the cardiac cycle. The usual role of the IABP in patients with heart failure is supportive while the patient is waiting for emergent cardiac transplantation. VADs (e.g., external centrifugal pumps, extracorporeal membrane oxygenation systems, pulsatile short-term pumps, internal mechanical assist devices) were originally designed to support the left ventricle. Current VADs may also be used to support the right ventricle. Unlike the IABP, VADs completely unload either the right or left ventricle. The indication for VAD is cardiogenic shock refractory to conventional pharmacologic therapy and to IABP.[60]

Currently, the mean duration of mechanical circulatory support before transplantation is 50 days.[61] For this reason, considerable effort is made to support patients with portable left VADs outside of the hospital. For portable VADs, the assist device pump or energy converter is implanted surgically, and the control or power source is worn externally. The control units and batteries are lighter (8 pounds) than those in the past and allow patients to be ambulatory.[62] Patients in whom a VAD has been implanted and who go on to transplantation have a long-term survival similar to that of patients who undergo routine transplantation.

Cardiac Transplantation. Cardiac transplantation is a reasonable therapeutic option for end-stage heart failure. For patients with severe symptoms and diminished life expectancy, cardiac transplantation may offer the only hope of improved quality of life and survival. After transplantation, survival is 85% at 1 year and 70% at 5 years.[63] In patients with severe symptoms almost refractory to medical therapy, the quality of life is clearly better for those who undergo cardiac transplantation.[23] Unfortunately, cardiac transplantation is an option for relatively few patients because of the limited supply of donor hearts. An estimated 20,000 patients per year could benefit from cardiac transplantation, but only 2000 donor hearts are available per year.[64] Careful and expert medical management in selected patients may provide acceptable outcomes when cardiac transplantation is unavailable because of the shortage of donor hearts.

Management of Diastolic Dysfunction

Diastolic dysfunction, or impairment of ventricular relaxation, is present in 20% to 40% patients with heart failure.[20] The origin of diastolic dysfunction can be structural as a result of a cardiomyopathy, age-related changes in conjunction with hypertension, or can remain elusive.[20] Diagnosis of diastolic dysfunction is made on the basis of the existence of signs and symptoms of heart failure with the absence of valvular abnormalities and normal left ventricular ejection fraction.[20]

Medical management of patients with diastolic dysfunction includes control of blood pressure, reduction in central blood volume (preload), and prevention of tachycardia and myocardial ischemia.[20] Unclear evidence exits for benefit in treatment for isolated diastolic dysfunction with ACE inhibitors, digoxin, beta blockers, calcium channel blockers, or ARBs; however, many patients with diastolic dysfunction require these medications for treatment of their other medical conditions.[20] Recommendations for the use of antiarrhythmics and anticoagulation are similar to those previously discussed with systolic dysfunction.[20]

COMPLICATIONS

Arrhythmias

Studies have demonstrated a high prevalence of ventricular and atrial arrhythmias in patients with heart failure. Atrial fibrillation occurs in at least 20% of patients with heart failure and is associated with increased mortality.[65] Patients with rapid atrial fibrillation require rate control with either digoxin, a beta blocker, or in some cases a calcium channel blocker. At least one attempt at chemical or electrical cardioversion should be undertaken in most patients with heart failure and atrial fibrillation. Uncontrolled or new-onset atrial fibrillation can worsen heart failure or lead to acute decompensation. It is always prudent to try to convert new-onset atrial fibrillation to normal sinus rhythm. This often requires several weeks of anticoagulation and initiation of closely supervised antiarrhythmic therapy.

Low-dose amiodarone is an increasingly attractive option as an atrial stabilizing agent in patients with symptoms refractory to other agents. In rare instances catheter ablation may be necessary to prevent uncontrolled, rapid ventricular rates,[24] especially in patients with hypertrophic cardiomyopathy or severe left ventricular failure.

Ventricular arrhythmias are present in nearly all patients with heart failure. Asymptomatic ventricular arrhythmias should not be treated. Because all antiarrhythmic agents can produce negative inotropic effects or proarrhythmia in patients with heart failure, initiation of therapy should occur in a hospital setting.

Metabolism

Long-standing severe heart failure may lead to anorexia as a result of hepatic and intestinal congestion. Occasionally there is impaired intestinal absorption of fat and protein.[66] The patient with heart failure may have an increase in total metabolism from an augmentation of myocardial oxygen consumption, excessive work of breathing, low-grade fevers, and elevated levels of tumor necrosis factor, a cytokine produced by monocytes.[67] The combination of reduced caloric intake and higher metabolism leads to a reduction in tissue mass that is often masked by the increase in fluid retention.

In heart failure, caloric malnutrition may be related to anorexia and early satiety, fat malabsorption may be due to congestion or altered hepatic management of lipids, and protein malnutrition may be related to changes in the bowel from elevated lymphatic production as a result of elevated systemic venous pressure. Medical therapy with vasodilators and diuretics tailored to normalize intracardiac pressures may decrease the prevalence of malnutrition in patients with heart failure.[66]

Vitamin supplements may be advisable for water-soluble vitamin loss associated with diuresis and problems with intestinal absorption of the fat-soluble vitamins. Frequent small snacks may also assist patients in meeting their caloric intake, and excessive fluid intake should be avoided.

INDICATIONS FOR REFERRAL/HOSPITALIZATION

Patients with heart failure may benefit from cardiology consultation when symptoms appear to be refractory to the standard therapies of vasodilators, diuretics, ACE inhibitors, and digoxin. The onset of arrhythmias, coronary ischemia, and/or myocardial infarction should prompt consultation as well. Cardiac transplantation may be considered for young patients failing to respond to maximal medical therapy.

Even with pharmacologic advances in heart failure management, the hospital readmission rate among older patients is between 29% and 47%.[68] This high readmission rate is related to inadequate symptom management by the patient, nonadherence to complex pharmacologic schedules and dietary regimens, social isolation, and the natural illness trajectory.[68]

Thus there has been increasing interest in developing disease management guidelines and strategies. Seven management strategies identified by a cardiology advisory board were (1) heart failure clinics, (2) home health advanced practice nurses, (3) community-based case managers, (4) patient telemanagement, (5) cardiac rehabilitation, (6) emergency department observation units, and (7) heart failure subacute care.[69] Heart failure clinics have provided a mechanism for patients to be seen in a clinic for physical assessment, medication instruction, dietary education, and exercise training.

For patients with heart failure who are unable to attend clinic sessions, the home health advanced practice nurse may be an appropriate referral. The advanced practice nurse with expertise in heart failure can see the patient at home three times per week for assessment of weight, vital signs, heart and lung sounds, and signs of peripheral edema. During the home visit the advanced practice nurse can continue patient teaching regarding medications, diet, and activity and develop a plan with the patient and family regarding emergency care and when to call the primary care provider.

The use of telemedicine technology as a tool in disease management is expanding rapidly to meet the needs of patients in integrated health care delivery systems. A number of innovative attempts at telemedicine with patients with heart failure are underway and may be potential alternatives for management of these patients in their home.[70,71] Specifically, patients with heart failure are using telephone and computer technology to transmit data on vital signs, symptoms, and weight to a central repository where the health care providers can review trends.

Indications for hospitalization include suspicion of new-onset heart failure for diagnostic evaluation, clinical or ECG evidence of acute myocardial ischemia, pulmonary edema or severe respiratory distress, oxygen saturation below 90%, severe medical complications (e.g., pneumonia, renal failure), anasarca, symptomatic hypotension or syncope, heart failure refractory to treatment with a maximal program, and the need to evaluate home support for safe management in the community.[26]

In addition, hospitalization may be necessary for IV administration of diuretics such as metolazone to reduce intestinal edema, and for the institution of IV dobutamine or renal-dose dopamine to increase renal blood flow.[26]

PATIENT AND FAMILY EDUCATION

Many of the important concepts for managing heart failure have been discussed in previous sections of this chapter. Patients and their families can take an active role in the management of this disorder if there is understanding of the condition and its treatments. Support for weight reduction and smoking cessation, if applicable, may be helpful. Reinforcement of the importance of restricting salt, reducing stress, taking medications (and reporting side effects), and balancing rest with exercise is also of benefit. All patients should be weighed daily or every other day and should call the primary care provider if they have a weight gain of more than 2 pounds in 2 days.

HEALTH PROMOTION

Prevention of congestive heart failure is linked to prevention of ischemic heart disease. Accordingly, all patients should be screened for heart disease risk and encouraged to reduce their risk by a healthy lifestyle, including normalization of weight, low-fat diet, smoke exposure avoidance, and exercise. Interventions to screen for heart disease risk include a family history, blood pressure measurement, lipid screen, and blood glucose or hemoglobin A1C to screen for diabetes. Patients should be encouraged to seek medical attention promptly for any heart attack signs/symptoms, unexplained fatigue, or dyspnea. Good control of blood pressure and diabetes is an essential component of prevention of congestive heart failure. Other cardiovascular diseases need close monitoring with timely intervention for any condition change.

REFERENCES

1. Packer M: Survival of patients with chronic heart failure and its potential modification by drug therapy. In Cohn JN, editor: *Drug treatment of heart failure*, ed 2, Secaucus, NJ, 1998, ATC International.
2. Braunwald E, Colucci WS, Grossman W: Aspects of heart failure: high-output failure: pulmonary edema. In Braunwald E, editor: *Heart disease*, ed 5, Philadelphia, 1997, WB Saunders.
3. Cohn JN and others: A comparison of enalapril with hydralazine-isosorbide dinitrate in the treatment of chronic congestive heart failure, *N Engl J Med* 325:303-310, 1991.
4. The SOLVD Investigators: Effect of enalapril on survival in patients with reduced left ventricular ejection fractions and congestive heart failure, *N Engl J Med* 325:293-302, 1991.
5. Bonow RO, Udelson JE: Left ventricular diastolic dysfunction as a cause of congestive heart failure, *Ann Intern Med* 117:502-510, 1992.
6. Senni M and others: Outcomes research review, *J Am Coll Cardiol* 33:164-170, 1999.
7. Kannel WB: Need and prospects for prevention of cardiac failure, *Eur J Clin Pharmacol* 49:S3-S9, 1996.
8. Kannel WB, Belanger AJ: Epidemiology of heart failure, *Am Heart J* 121:951-957, 1991.
9. Schocken DD, Arrieta MI, Leaverton PE: Prevalence and mortality rate of congestive heart failure in the United States, *J Am Coll Cardiol* 20:301-306, 1992.
10. Kannel WM, Ho K, Thom T: The changing epidemiologic features of cardiac failure, *Br Heart J* 72 (suppl 2):S3-S9, 1994.
11. Friedman MM: Older adults' symptoms and their duration before hospitalization for heart failure, *Heart Lung* 26:169-176, 1997.
12. Ho KK and others: The epidemiology of heart failure: the Framingham study, *J Am Coll Cardiol* 22(suppl A):6A-13A, 1993.
13. National Heart, Lung and Blood Institute: *National Institutes of Health data fact sheet*, Bethesda, Md, 1996, US Department of Health and Human Services, Public Health Service.
14. Rich MW: Epidemiology, pathophysiology, and etiology of congestive heart failure in older adults, *J Am Geriatr Soc* 45:968-974, 1997.
15. Goldsmith SR, Dick C: Differentiating systolic from diastolic heart failure: pathophysiologic and therapeutic considerations, *Am J Med* 95:645-655, 1993.
16. Zucker IH: Baro and cardiac reflex abnormalities in chronic heart failure. In Zucker IH, Gilmore JP, editors: *Reflex control of the circulation*, Boca Raton, Fla, 1991, CRC Press.
17. Benedict CR and others: Relation of neurohormonal activation to clinical variables and degree of left ventricular dysfunction: a report from the Registry of Studies of Left Ventricular Dysfunction, *J Am Coll Cardiol* 23:1410-1420, 1994.
18. Katz SD and others: Impaired endothelium-mediated vasodilatation in the peripheral vasculature of patients with congestive heart failure, *J Am Coll Cardiol* 19:918-925, 1992.
19. Opie LH: *The heart: physiology and metabolism*, New York, 1991, Raven Press.
20. ACC/AHA Committee: ACC/AHA guidelines for the evaluation and management of chronic heart failure in the adult, *Circulation* 104:2996-3007, 2001.
21. Wagoner A: Congestive heart failure and the role of two-dimensional Doppler echocardiography: a primer for cardiac sonographers, *J Am Soc Echocardiogr* 13:157-163, 2000.
22. Wilson JR, Mancini DM: Factors contributing to the exercise limitation of heart failure, *Circulation* 22(suppl A):93A-98A, 1993.
23. Manning HL, Schwartzstein RM: Mechanism of disease: pathophysiology of dyspnea, *N Engl J Med* 333:1547-1553, 1995.
24. Stevenson LW, Perloff JK: The limited reliability of physical signs for estimating hemodynamics in chronic heart failure, *JAMA* 261:884-888, 1989.
25. Guidelines for the evaluation and management of heart failure: report of the American College of Cardiology/American Heart Association Task Force on Practice Guidelines, *J Am Coll Cardiol* 26:1376-1398, 1995.
26. Konstam MA and others: *Heart failure: evaluation and care of patients with left-ventricular systolic dysfunction, Clinical Practice Guideline No 11*, AHCPR Pub No 94-0612, Rockville, MD, 1994, US Department of Health and Human Services, Public Health Service, Agency for Health Care Policy and Research.
27. Remme WJ: Guidelines for the diagnosis and treatment of congestive heart failure, *Eur Heart J* 22:1527-1560, 2001.
28. Griffin BP and others: Incremental prognostic value of exercise hemodynamic variables in chronic congestive heart failure secondary to coronary artery disease or to dilated cardiomyopathy, *Am J Cardiol* 67:848-853, 1991.
29. Guyatt GH and others: How should we measure function in patients with chronic heart and lung disease? *J Chronic Dis* 38:517-524, 1985.

30. Cahalin LP and others: The six-minute walk test predicts peak oxygen uptake and survival in advanced heart failure, *Chest* 110:325-332, 1996.
31. Bittner V and others: Prediction of mortality and morbidity with a 6-minute walk test in patients with left ventricular dysfunction, *JAMA* 270:1702-1707, 1993.
32. Chavey W and others: Cardiovascular medicine update: guideline for the management of heart failure caused by systolic dysfunction: Part II treatment, *Am Fam Physician* 64:6, 2001.
33. Ferrin MS, Tino G: Acute dyspnea, *AACN Clin Issues* 8:398-410, 1997.
34. CONSENSUS Trial Study Group: Effects of enalapril on mortality in severe congestive heart failure, *N Engl J Med* 316:1429-1335, 1987.
35. Echemann M: Determinants of angiotensin-converting enzyme inhibitor prescription in severe heart failure with left ventricular systolic dysfunction: the EPICAL study, *Am Heart J* 139:624-631, 2000.
36. Miller AB: Angiotensin receptor blockers and aldosterone antagonists in congestive heart failure, *Cardiol Clin* 19:195-202, 2001.
37. ADA: Standards of medical care for patients with diabetes mellitus, *Diabetes Care* 25(Suppl):33-49, 2002.
38. Carson PE: Rationale for the use of combination angiotensin-converting enzyme inhibitor/angiotensin II receptor blocker therapy in heart failure, *Am Heart J* 140:361-366, 2000.
39. SOLVD Investigators: Effects of enalapril on mortality and the development of heart failure in asymptomatic patients with reduced left-ventricular ejection fraction, *N Engl J Med* 327:685-691, 1992.
40. Pitt B and others: The effect of spironolactone on morbidity and mortality in patients with severe heart failure, *N Engl J Med* 341:709-716, 1999.
41. Cohn JM and others: Effects of vasodilator therapy on mortality in chronic heart failure: results of the Veterans Administration Cooperative Study, *N Engl J Med* 314:1547-1552, 1986.
42. The Captopril-Digoxin Multicenter Research Group: Comparative effects of therapy with captopril and digoxin in patients with mild to moderate heart failure, *JAMA* 259:539-544, 1988.
43. Kelly RA, Smith TW: Digoxin in heart failure: implications of recent trials, *J Am Coll Cardiol* 22(suppl A):107A-112A, 1993.
44. Cleland J and others: What is the optimal medical management of ischemic heart failure? *Prog Cardiovasc Dis* 43:101-103, 2001.
45. Packer M and others: Withdrawal of digoxin from patients with chronic heart failure treated with angiotensin-converting enzyme inhibitors, *N Engl J Med* 329:1-7, 1993.
46. Dibianco R and others: A comparison of oral milrinone, digoxin, and their combination in the treatment of patients with chronic heart failure, *N Engl J Med* 320:677-683, 1989.
47. Jaeschle R, Oxman AD, Guyatt GH: To what extent do congestive heart failure patients in sinus rhythm benefit from digoxin therapy? A systematic overview and meta-analysis, *Am J Med* 88:279-286, 1990.
48. Colucci WS and others: Carvedilol inhibits clinical progression in patients with mild heart failure, *Circulation* 94:2800-2806, 1996.
49. Bristow MR: Pathophysiologic and pharmacologic rationales for clinical management of chronic heart failure with beta-blocking agents, *Am J Cardiol* 71:12C-22C, 1993.
50. Eichhorn EJ, Hjalmarson A: Beta-blocker treatment for chronic heart failure, *Circulation* 90:2153-2156, 1994.
51. CIBIS Investigators and Committees: A randomized trial of beta-blockade in heart failure: the Canadian Insufficiency Bisprolol Study (CIBIS), *Circulation* 90:1765-1773, 1994.
52. Australia/New Zealand Heart Failure Research Collaborative Group: Randomised, placebo-controlled trial of carvedilol in patients with congestive heart failure due to ischaemic heart disease, *Lancet* 349:375-380, 1997.
53. Cohn JN and others: Thromboembolism in left ventricular dysfunction, *Circulation* 86:I-252, 1992.
54. Podrid PJ, Fogel RI, Fuchs TT: Ventricular arrhythmias in congestive failure, *Am J Cardiol* 69:82G-98G, 1992.
55. Cleland JCF and others: Clinical, haemodynamic and anti-arrhythmic effects of long-term treatment with amiodarone on patients in heart failure, *Br Heart J* 57:436-445, 1987.
56. Feldman AM and others: Effects of vesnarinone on morbidity and mortality in patients with heart failure, *N Engl J Med* 329:149-155, 1993.
57. Packer M and others: Effect of oral milrinone on mortality in severe chronic heart failure, *N Engl J Med* 325:1468-1475, 1991.
58. Volpe M and others: Abnormalities of sodium handling and of cardiovascular adaptations during high salt diet in patients with mild heart failure, *Circulation* 88(pt 1):1620-1627, 1993.
59. Coats AJS and others: Effects of physical training in chronic heart failure, *Lancet* 335:63-66, 1990.
60. Mancini DM and others: Benefits of selective respiratory muscle training on exercise capacity in patients with chronic congestive heart failure, *Circulation* 91:320-329, 1995.
61. Vargo RL: Bridging to transplant: mechanical support for heart failure, *Crit Care Nurs Clin North Am* 5:649-659, 1993.
62. Mehta SM and others: Combined registry for the clinical use of mechanical ventricular assist pump and the total artificial heart in conjunction with heart transplantation: sixth official report, 1994, *J Heart Lung Transplant* 14:585-593, 1995.
63. Moroney DA, Powers K: Outpatient use of left ventricular assist devices: nursing, technical, and educational considerations, *Am J Crit Care* 6:355-362, 1997.
64. Hosenpud JD and others: The registry of the International Society for Heart and Lung Transplantation: Fourteenth official report, 1997, *J Heart Lung Transplant* 16:691-712, 1997.
65. Evans RW: The economics of heart transplantation, *Circulation* 75: 63-75, 1987.
66. Carson M and others: The influence of atrial fibrillation on prognosis in mild to moderate heart failure, *Circulation* 87(6 suppl):VI102-VI110, 1993.
67. Berkowitz D, Croll MN, Likoff W: Malabsorption as a complication of congestive heart failure, *Am J Cardiol* 11:43-47, 1963.
68. Carr JG and others: Prevalence and hemodynamic correlates of malnutrition in severe congestive heart failure secondary to ischemic or idiopathic dilated cardiomyopathy, *Am J Cardiol* 63:709-713, 1989.
69. Vinson JM and others: Early readmission of elderly patients with heart failure, *J Am Geriatr Soc* 38:1290-1295, 1990.
70. Cardiology Preeminence Roundtable: *Beyond four walls: cost effective management of chronic congestive heart failure,* Washington DC, 1994, Advisory Board Co.
71. Williams RE and others: Telemanagement of congestive heart failure: results of daily weights and symptom tracking, *J Am Coll Cardiol* 29:247A, 1997.

CHAPTER 133

Hypertension

Maryjane B. Giacalone, Denise J. Mullaney, and Randall M. Zusman

DEFINITION/EPIDEMIOLOGY

In 1972 the National Heart, Lung, and Blood Institute initiated a campaign to improve public awareness of the need for treatment of hypertension.[1] The campaign has been successful in improving awareness and increasing treatment, but adequate control of hypertension (as measured by a systolic blood pressure under 140 mm Hg or a diastolic blood pressure less than 90 mm Hg) has not progressed to the same extent.[2,3]

In all, 20% of Americans, or approximately 50 million people, have hypertension.[3] Hypertension is a risk factor for coronary artery disease (CAD), heart failure, stroke, peripheral arterial disease, kidney disease, and retinopathy and therefore represents a significant public health threat. When hypertension is combined with other risk factors, its effect on the development of CAD is profound, contributing approximately 35% of the risk.[4-6]

In 1998, hypertension was directly responsible for 44,435 deaths (males 41.5%, females 58.5%) in the United States.[7] Research has shown that small gains in the control of hypertension can result in health improvements. Data extrapolated from the INTERSALT study have shown that an overall drop of 2 mm Hg in the distribution of blood pressure would result in a 6% annual reduction in stroke, a 4% reduction in CAD, and a 3% reduction in all-cause mortality.[8] The most recent data available reveal that although 68.4% of Americans are aware of their high blood pressure, only 53.6% are undergoing treatment, with only 27.4% having adequate blood pressure control.[9]

Blood pressure is that force in arterial structures created by an interplay of flow, volume, and constriction. High blood pressure, or hypertension, has been defined by determining the levels of blood pressure that cause target organ damage, morbidity, and mortality as arterial flow is delivered. It is known that 95% of all hypertension is primary or essential hypertension and has no known cause. The remaining 5% is termed *secondary hypertension* and is directly attributable to structural, circulatory, or chemical abnormalities. Published in 1997, the Sixth Report of the Joint National Committee on Prevention, Detection, Evaluation, and Treatment of High Blood Pressure (JNC VI) provides classifications for blood pressure values (Table 133-1) based on risk.[9] Since that time, the improved outcomes for diabetics with lower blood pressure values in the Hypertension Optimal Treatment (HOT) study[10] has prompted interest in modifying the JNC VI classifications to recommend a lower target blood pressure of 130/80 for diabetics.

Incidence and Prevalence

Both systolic and diastolic blood pressures rise throughout childhood and early and middle adulthood; each is an independent predictor of cardiovascular disease whether occurring alone or concurrently in individuals under the age of 50 years.[5,6] The rate of rise in diastolic blood pressure tends to level off or drop slightly in approximately the fifth decade of life. The resulting widened pulse pressure becomes equally as important in predicting cardiovascular risk.[11] Systolic blood pressure continues to rise with advancing age, making isolated systolic hypertension more prevalent in the older adult. Three million individuals over 60 years of age have isolated systolic hypertension.[12] More than half of individuals between ages 65 and 74 years and more than three fourths of those 75 years and over have hypertension.[13]

TABLE 133-1 Blood Pressure Classification

Category	Systolic (mm Hg)		Diastolic (mm Hg)
Optimal	<120	*and*	<80
Normal	<130	*and*	<85
High-normal	130-139	*and*	85-80
Hypertension			
Stage 1	140-159	*or*	90-99
Stage 2	160-179	*or*	100-109
Stage 3	≥180	*or*	≥110

From National Institutes of Health: *The Sixth Report of the Joint National Committee on Prevention, Detection, Evaluation, and Treatment of High Blood Pressure,* NIH pub no 98-4080, Bethesda, Md, November 1997, The Institute.

There is a higher prevalence of hypertension among men until the fifth and sixth decade of life. After menopause, women have a higher incidence of this condition; by age 65, women have a higher overall prevalence of hypertension.[7,14-16]

In general, people of lower socioeconomic means and lower educational levels have a higher prevalence of hypertension. In these groups, poor diet, stress, and poor access to health care may play a role in the development of high blood pressure.[5]

African-Americans have higher rates of hypertension than Caucasians. The baseline blood pressure in African-American children is higher than in Caucasian children and rises at a faster rate, producing higher rates of hypertension at younger ages. African-Americans have a higher incidence of cardiovascular, stroke, and renal complications and have a higher mortality rate related to hypertension than do people of other ethnic backgrounds.[3,7,17-19] Enhanced renal sodium resorption occurs in 57% of African-Americans as compared with 27% in other groups. This salt sensitivity—along with a generally poorer economic base, diet, and access to health care—contribute to the problem of high blood pressure among African-Americans.

Risk Factors

Obesity, a higher dietary intake of fat, a sodium intake in excess of sodium need, physical inactivity, and excessive alcohol intake are characteristics associated with Western culture and the development of hypertension.[5,8,19-21]

Generally, the risk for hypertension is significant for both systolic and diastolic measurements and tends to increase as blood pressure increases. Prevention, detection, and treatment of hypertension should be public health priorities. The development of hypertension is probably multifactorial and therefore necessitates a coordinated, thoughtful, and individualized approach to diagnosis and treatment.

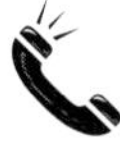

Physician consultation is indicated for patients with pregnancy-induced hypertension, a systolic blood pressure greater than 180 mm Hg, a diastolic blood pressure greater than 110 mm Hg, or signs of cardiovascular, renal, or retinopathic complications.

PATHOPHYSIOLOGY

Blood pressure is the product of cardiac output (heart rate, myocardial contractility, and circulating volume and its impact on myocardial stretch) and peripheral resistance (vascular constriction and compliance). Anything that affects any part of this equation can affect blood pressure. In a properly functioning system, feedback loops maintain homeostasis.

Primary Hypertension

Sympathetic Nervous System. An increased heart rate can be caused by stimulation of the sympathetic nervous system in response to hypovolemia (baroreceptor response) or to physical or psychologic stressors (fever, anger, anxiety, exercise). An increased heart rate leads to an increase in cardiac output. The increase in blood pressure that follows is a normal response in these situations and is usually self-limiting because the heart rate response is caused by catecholamines or reduced by the parasympathetic response. Chronic stress may be an environmental factor that leads to the development of hypertension.

Excessive myocardial contractility (hyperkinesis) may also be the result of neurohormonal stimulation and has been hypothesized as a cause of mild hypertension, primarily in young adults. It has also been hypothesized as a cause of myocardial hypertrophy leading to hypertension, but there is no clear evidence to support this view. Hypertrophy is associated with hypertension but is usually considered a compensatory buildup of myocardial myofibrils to overcome high peripheral pressures.[22]

Sodium Balance and Salt Sensitivity. For years sodium has played a controversial role in the pathogenesis of hypertension. Sodium's primary effect on blood pressure is related to excess circulating volume, but it may also affect contractility and vascular resistance.[22] A controversial and well-publicized meta-analysis of the role of sodium in the development of hypertension concluded that there is insufficient evidence to warrant sodium restriction as a preventive measure.[23] However, many other authorities claim that most of the trials in this study were short-term and that an excessive sodium intake over many years can play a role in the development of hypertension.[24]

Hypertension associated with salt sensitivity has been postulated to be caused by (1) an inability to normally excrete sodium via the kidneys (either through an upward shift in the arterial pressure required for sodium excretion or through a decrease in renal mass or filtration surface), resulting in an effectively increased circulating volume and a slight excess of total body sodium despite pressure natriuresis; (2) a resetting of the pressure-natriuresis curve, requiring higher blood pressures to maintain normal sodium and water balance; (3) abnormal electrolyte transport, resulting in disturbances in the cytosolic sodium/calcium balance and increased vasoconstriction; or (4) low renin levels, reduced numbers of nephrons, and modified sympathetic nervous system activity.[25-31]

Epidemiologic studies generally support a link between higher salt intakes and the prevalence of hypertension.[8] Less well defined, however, is whether lowering salt intake, alone or in combination with antihypertensive medications, can prevent hypertension or universally lower blood pressure in individuals with hypertension.[26] Studies support some element of salt sensitivity among certain individuals, but there is no simple test to determine this sensitivity.[31] Some salt sensitivity has been linked to defects of the angiotensinogen gene.[32] Age, African-American heritage, diabetes, low renin levels, and nonmodulating hypertension often predict salt sensitivity.

Renin-Angiotensin System. Renin is an enzyme produced and released by the juxtaglomerular apparatus of the kidney in response to sensation of a low-flow state (reduced renal perfusion pressure or low circulating intravascular volume), sympathetic nervous system stimulation and/or catecholamine release, and hypokalemia. Once released, renin acts on angiotensinogen to create angiotensin I. In the pulmonary circulation, angiotensin-converting enzymes change angiotensin I to angiotensin II, a potent vasoconstrictor that over time and with prolonged production causes arterial stiffening and hypertrophy. Angiotensin II also causes aldosterone stimulation, which enhances sodium and water reabsorption from the renal tubules and effectively increases circulating volume. The resulting higher blood pressure should provide feedback to maintain homeostatic responses.

Feedback loops may not work properly in some individuals, allowing for higher circulating levels of renin and thus a higher blood pressure. Unabated renin production may be related to undetectable arteriolar disease or ischemia that affects some nephrons. Renin levels are low in approximately 30% of individuals with hypertension, normal in 60%, and high in 10%.[32] One hypothesis suggests that individuals with high renin levels have hypertension related to vasoconstriction, whereas those with low renin levels have hypertension attributable to increased circulating volume and may be more responsive to diuretic therapy.[33]

Vascular Hypertrophy. In addition to the effect of angiotensin II, vascular hypertrophy may result from growth-enhancing substances such as excessive levels of insulin, catecholamines, natriuretic hormone, and growth hormone.[21] Studies are being conducted on certain paracrine factors—particularly endothelins, which cause vasoconstriction and vascular hypertrophy, and the opposing endothelium-derived relaxing factor (EDRF), also known as nitric oxide.[34,35]

Obesity. There is a direct correlation between increasing weight and increasing blood pressure. Obesity, especially central obesity, has been linked to hypertension and cardiovascular mortality. Several theories have been advanced to explain the association between obesity and hypertension. One theory states that an increased sympathetic nervous system output results in activation of the renin-angiotensin-aldosterone system, thereby promoting sodium and water retention, increased circulating volume, increased cardiac output without increased peripheral resistance, and cardiac alterations. Other theories include those of metabolic

TABLE 133-2 Secondary Hypertension

	Clues			
	History and Physical	Screening	Diagnostic Testing	Treatment
CONDITION: ENDOGENOUS				
Renovascular condition (RAS)	Age <30 (fibromuscular) or >50 (atherosclerotic) History of atherosclerosis or risk factors Family history of RAS Abdominal bruits	Urinalysis Creatinine	Captopril flow scan Renal magnetic resonance arteriogram Renal arteriogram	Control hypertension: beta blockers Avoid ACEIs Angioplasty Bypass surgery
Pheochromocytoma	5 *Hs* (hypertension, hyperhydrosis, hypermetabolism, hyperglycemia, headache) Hypertension after anesthetics, tricyclics Family history of endocrine disorders Hypertension after abdominal palpation Labile hypertension	Spot urine vanillylmandelic acid (VMA) 24-hour urine VMA and metanephrines	Spot urine VMA 24-hour urine VMA and metanephrines Plasma catecholamines (clonidine suppression test) CT scan of abdomen and pelvis Scintigraphy/MIBG imaging (to check for extrarenal and malignant masses)	Control hypertension: alpha blocker followed by beta blocker, or alpha/beta blocker Surgery
Hyperaldosteronism	Weakness Headache Fatigue Hypertension Hypokalemia	Unprovoked hypokalemia	Aldosterone levels before and after saline challenge Renin levels 24-hour urinary aldosterone 17 hydroxycorticosteroids CT scan of abdomen and pelvis Adrenal scintigraphy (if CT scan is negative) Adrenal vein catheterization (if CT scan and scintigraphy are negative)	If adrenal tumor: surgery If bilateral hyperplasia: potassium-sparing diuretics
Coarctation of the aorta	Young age Arm blood pressure > leg blood pressure Possible claudication Fatigue Late systolic murmur Apical heave	Chest x-ray	Echocardiogram Chest CT scan Aortogram	Surgery Angioplasty Stent
Thyroid disorder	Weight change Fatigue Metabolic change Temperature intolerance Edema Change in bowel habits Thyromegaly	Thyroid-stimulating hormone Weakness Muscle spasms Unprovoked hypokalemia	Triiodothyronine Thyroxine Thyroid-binding hormone	Treat underlying disorder Control hypertension in interim

anomalies, specifically hyperinsulinemia and insulin resistance.[30,35] Approximately 25% to 30% of Americans are obese. Results from the Framingham Heart Study indicate that obesity accounts for 78% of hypertension in men and 65% of hypertension in women.[4] Some of the benefits of weight loss are decreased insulin levels, improved insulin sensitivity, and decreased plasma norepinephrine levels. Other benefits not yet proven are decreased renin production and improved blood flow associated with a reduction in intracellular calcium levels.

Hypertension and obesity, glucose intolerance, or hyperlipidemia often occur together and greatly raise the risk for developing atherosclerotic cardiovascular disease.[4] Research studies in central obesity, hyperglycemia, hyperinsulinemia, and insulin resistance have not yet shown that insulin-resistance syndromes have a pathogenic role in high blood pressure.

Other Dietary Influences. There are insufficient data to support recommendations regarding calcium, potassium, magnesium, or protein changes in the diet.[9] The Dietary Approaches to Stop Hypertension (DASH) study showed that blood pressure is decreased in response to a universally recommended diet that contains generous servings of fruits,

TABLE 133-2 Secondary Hypertension—cont'd

	Clues			
	History and Physical	Screening	Diagnostic Testing	Treatment
Renal parenchymal disease Polycystic kidney disease Glomerulonephritis Diabetic nephropathy Chronic renal failure Obstruction	Edema Nocturia Diabetes History of urinary tract infections (UTIs) Pruritus Family history of polycystic kidney disease	Urinalysis Creatinine	24-hour urine: protein, creatinine, creatinine clearance Renal ultrasound IV pyelogram Diabetes testing	Depends on specific cause; control volume intake, diuretics, and additional medical therapy; ACEI if diabetic (otherwise use with caution), control glycemia, relieve obstruction
Cushing's syndrome	Hirsutism Edema Buffalo hump Moon facies Truncal obesity Red/purple striae	24-hour urine: free cortisol	Dexamethasone suppression test Pituitary MRI CT scan of thorax/abdomen	Surgery Control of hypertension
Other: Anxiety Pregnancy Sleep apnea				
CONDITION: EXOGENOUS				
Alcohol Cocaine	History of use			Cessation of substance
NSAIDs	History of arthritis			Alternative treatment if necessary
Steroids	History of steroid-dependent conditions			
Sympathomimetics (over-the-counter cold remedies)	History of recent URI			
Weight control remedies				
Erythropoietin				
MAO inhibitors				

vegetables, and low-fat dairy products with reduced saturated and total fat.[36]

Alcohol Intake. Excessive alcohol consumption is associated with hypertension and should be suspected in individuals who have been resistant to treatment. Alcohol may raise blood pressure by causing increases in sympathetic nervous system activity, activation of the renin-angiotensin system, and/or decreases in peripheral vascular tone and impairment of baroreceptor effectiveness.[30,35,37] Marked increases in blood pressure may occur with acute alcohol withdrawal but are unrelated to mechanisms of chronic hypertension. Overall reduction of alcohol intake results in a lowered blood pressure in hypertensive, heavy drinkers. Decreases in blood pressure are slow with alcohol restriction and peak in approximately 4 to 6 weeks.[38]

Exercise/Activity. Acute exercise can raise blood pressure in individuals with normotension and hypertension. The blood pressure rise is most dramatic and serious in those with uncontrolled hypertension. However, regular exercise can be beneficial if the person can adhere to an established exercise routine. The Centers for Disease Control and Prevention recommends regular exercise as an aid in lowering blood pressure. Regular isometric exercise has been shown to prevent the development of hypertension.[39] Regular aerobic exercise has been shown to reduce the incidence of cardiovascular events.[40]

Secondary Hypertension

Secondary hypertension can be ascribed to renal artery stenosis, pheochromocytoma, hyperaldosteronism, coarctation of the aorta, Cushing's syndrome, sleep apnea, thyroid disease, alcohol, and the use of steroids, oral contraceptives (hormone replacement therapy is an infrequent cause), or nonsteroidal antiinflammatory drugs (NSAIDs) (Table 133-2). Although secondary causes account for approximately 5% of all hypertension etiologies, it is important to keep in mind that 5% translates to more than 2.5 million cases.

Renal Artery Stenosis. Renal artery stenosis (RAS) results in hypertension when there is a 70% to 80% blockage of a renal artery,[41] resulting in activation of the renin-angiotensin system.[42] Two different mechanisms have been shown to cause renal artery stenosis. In individuals less than 30 years old, fibrodysplasia or fibromuscular dysplasia causes tight fibrous bands that alternate with normal or thin tissue along the renal artery, usually the medial portion. Fibrodysplasia affects more women than men. After age 50 years, atherosclerosis is the more likely cause of RAS and usually presents in the proximal artery, extending from aortic plaque.[41-44] Hypertension from RAS can coexist with essential hypertension. Angioplasty is the preferred treatment for fibrodysplastic RAS. Atherosclerotic RAS may also be treated with angioplasty if the lesion is not ostial, but there is a 40% restenosis rate; angioplasty can be repeated. Surgical bypass of the renal artery is another option as long as the individual is healthy enough to undergo surgery.[44]

Pheochromocytoma. Pheochromocytoma is a catecholamine-producing tumor of the adrenal glands and is responsible for 0.1% to 1% of all cases of hypertension.[41,42,44] A small percentage of these tumors are malignant.[43] Hypertension seen with pheochromocytoma is constant in 50% of cases and labile in the other 50%.[43] Approximately 50% of cases include the "5 Hs": hypertension, headache, hyperhidrosis, hypermetabolic state, and hyperglycemia. Bilateral headache, hyperhidrosis, and palpitations occur in 95% of the cases.[41]

Primary Hyperaldosteronism. Primary hyperaldosteronism is seen in fewer than 0.5% of all cases of hypertension and is more common in women. Adrenal adenoma accounts for 70% of all cases and is correctable by surgery. The other 30% result from bilateral adrenal hyperplasia, which must be managed medically. Primary hyperaldosteronism is suspected in patients with unprovoked hypokalemia.[41-43]

Coarctation of the Aorta. Coarctation of the aorta (a localized stricture of the aorta) is usually found in youth. It is typified by hypertension in the presence of claudication, delayed femoral pulses, decreased blood pressure in the lower extremities, and notching of ribs on chest x-ray films.[43,44] It is surgically correctable.

Cushing's Syndrome. It is known that 80% of individuals with Cushing's syndrome have hypertension.[41] Cushing's syndrome is caused by hypersecretion of glucocorticoids by the adrenal cortex. This hypersecretion results from an adrenal tumor or overstimulation by the anterior pituitary.

Use of Certain Medications. The use of oral corticosteroids and anabolic steroids may also result in hypertension. NSAIDs have been associated with hypertension, with indomethacin and naproxen having the greatest effect on blood pressure.[45]

Obstructive Sleep Apnea. Obstructive sleep apnea, which affects 2% to 4% of the population,[46] is associated with hypertension and is thought to result from a hypoxia-driven sympathetic nervous system discharge.[47] Early studies show improvement in blood pressure with mechanical ventilation and avoidance of the supine position during sleep.[46] It may be more common in individuals with heart failure, end-stage renal disease, or central obesity.

Renal Parenchymal Disease. Renal parenchymal disease is associated with the development of hypertension and is also considered a result of hypertension. Renal insufficiency is apparent when creatinine levels rise higher than 1.5 mg/dl and the glomerular filtration rate falls to less than 50 ml/min. Renal parenchymal disease encompasses glomerular diseases (e.g., chronic renal failure, systemic lupus erythematosus, nephritis, diabetic nephropathy, glomerulonephritis, renal vasculitis), and interstitial diseases (e.g., polycystic kidney disease, chronic interstitial nephritis).[41]

The pathophysiology of renal parenchymal disease and hypertension likely involves factors that impair sodium excretion and lead to increased circulating volume. Over time, an increase in peripheral vascular resistance, which perpetuates blood pressure elevation, may result from changes in cytosolic electrolytes, heightened vascular reactivity, and proliferation of the smooth muscle cells. Increased activity of the renin-angiotensin system, which is more common in end-stage renal disease but is present in some cases of milder renal insufficiency, raises peripheral resistance by direct vasoconstriction and by increasing total available sodium.[48,49] Endothelins and the effects of reduced renal clearance of EDRF inhibitors are potential areas for study and possible future treatment.

CLINICAL PRESENTATION

Because most patients with hypertension are asymptomatic, the importance of screening cannot be overemphasized. Symptoms of high blood pressure usually occur only after the physical consequences of organ damage arise. Stroke, renal dysfunction, retinopathy, aortic dissection, and the sequelae of left ventricular hypertrophy are potential presenting conditions that result from long-standing undiagnosed hypertension. Secondary causes of hypertension are more likely to present with early symptoms reflective of the underlying etiology, such as diabetic nephropathy and Cushing's syndrome. The Joint National Committee on Detection, Evaluation, and Treatment of High Blood Pressure[9] therefore recommends that health care providers measure blood pressure at each patient visit.

After obtaining an initial history and physical examination, a follow-up evaluation should be scheduled on the basis of the systolic and diastolic blood pressure values obtained, the presence of concomitant cardiovascular risk factors, and evidence of end-organ dysfunction resulting from hypertension. On the basis of blood pressure alone, a systolic pressure greater than or equal to 180 mm Hg and/or a diastolic pressure greater than or equal to 110 mm Hg necessitates an evaluation within 1 week (Table 133-3) or immediate intervention if the patient exhibits signs of cardiac, cerebral, vascular, and/or renal complications.

The medical history, physical examination, and laboratory data obtained from a patient with high blood pressure should focus on eliciting the presence of cardiovascular risk factors, dysfunction of target organs, and evidence of possible secondary causes of hypertension.[9]

Cardiac risk factors are assessed in the medical history. The health risks associated with hypertension are compounded by tobacco use, hyperlipidemia, left ventricular hypertrophy, glucose intolerance, and a positive family history.[50] In addition, a complete cardiovascular, cerebrovascular, renovascular, endocrine, and family history are documented.

Any recent surgical, psychologic, social, environmental, or traumatic stress should be elicited. Such events may precipitate a temporary elevation in blood pressure or suggest a secondary cause of hypertension. For example, pheochromocytoma can adversely affect hemodynamic stability during surgery.

All over-the-counter and prescribed medications (both currently or formerly used by the patient) should be listed, including nicotine, herbal treatments, steroids, oral contraceptives, NSAIDs, sedatives, sympathomimetics, amphetamines, cyclosporine, erythropoietin, tricyclic antidepressants, monoamine oxidase inhibitors, and alpha- and beta-adrenergic agonists. The dosage, frequency, and duration of medications should be documented. A dietary assessment of sodium, cholesterol, fat, and alcohol intake must also be obtained.

Clues for potential secondary causes of hypertension, such as sleep apnea (loud snoring, erratic sleep, daytime somnolence), pheochromocytoma (severe headaches, diaphoresis, palpitations), aldosteronism (muscle cramps, weakness, polyuria, polydipsia, nocturia, rhabdomyolysis, paresthesias), mineralocorticoid alteration (licorice intake, chewing tobacco, and oral steroid use), and renovascular (hematuria) should be elicited.

Symptoms indicative of target organ damage must be sought. These symptoms can be neurovascular (transient weakness or blindness, loss of visual acuity, severe headache, confusion, lethargy, seizures), vascular (coarctation, impotence, claudication), cardiovascular (chest pain, dyspnea, palpitations, syncope), and renal (oliguria, hematuria, dysuria).

PHYSICAL EXAMINATION

Accurate assessment of blood pressure is crucial. The JNC VI and the American Heart Association recommend that, to get an accurate reading, patients abstain from caffeine and nicotine for 30 minutes before measurement of blood pressure.[51,52] In addition, a cuff of the appropriate size (the bladder of the cuff should encompass 80% to 100% of arm circumference) is applied 1 cm above the antecubital fossa. The patient's arm is positioned with support and is horizontal to the fourth intercostal space; the sphygmomanometer must be at the practitioner's eye level. The systolic value is the level at which the first Korotkoff sound appears; the diastolic value is the level at which sound disappears. Blood pressure and heart rate are measured in each arm while the patient is supine or seated with feet on the floor; these measurements are repeated after the patient has been standing for 2 minutes.[53,54]

Height and weight are recorded and guide weight management decisions. Other components of the physical examination gather evidence of end-organ impairment and secondary etiologies for hypertension.

Sustained hypertension produces a vascular effect. Retinal changes include arteriolar narrowing, arteriovenous nicking, exudates, hemorrhages, and, in severe cases, papilledema. The carotid arteries and aorta may have bruits, and impaired cerebral circulation may manifest as deficits on neurologic testing. Evidence of cardiac dysfunction (e.g., adventitious lung sounds, cardiac gallops, or displaced apical pulse) or left ventricular enlargement indicates complications of hypertension and impacts treatment decisions. Pulse changes (diminished or absent) and skin changes (thinning, loss of extremity hair) point to peripheral circulatory impairment.

Hypertension produced as a result of other processes affects multiple organ systems. Striae, neurofibroma, or pruritic areas are important to note. Radial-femoral pulse delays and differences in blood pressure between arms or between arms and legs require further evaluation. Renal artery bruits or enlarged kidneys are evidence of kidney involvement. Thyroid findings of enlargement, bruits, or nodules necessitate additional testing.

DIAGNOSTICS

Because multiple factors may transiently increase or decrease blood pressure values, a diagnosis of hypertension is based on measurements obtained during at least three office visits.[9] Anxiety, sympathomimetic decongestants, oral contraceptives, nicotine, caffeine, and appetite suppressants are some of the more common causes of increased blood pressure.[51,52] Fluid loss and bed rest can decrease blood pressure.[55]

Routine evaluation of hypertension includes urinalysis, CBC, serum potassium, BUN, serum creatinine, fasting blood

TABLE 133-3 Follow-Up Blood Pressure Measurement

Initial Blood Pressure Reading		
Systolic (mm Hg)	**Diastolic (mm Hg)**	**Follow-Up Recommended**
<130	<85	Recheck in 2 years
130-130	85-80	Recheck in 1 year
140-159	90-99	Confirm within 2 months
160-179	100-109	Evaluate or refer to source of care within 1 month
≥180	≥110	Evaluate or refer to source of care immediately depending on clinical situation

From National Institutes of Health: *The Sixth Report of the Joint National Committee on Prevention, Detection, Evaluation, and Treatment of High Blood Pressure,* NIH pub no 98-4080, Bethesda, Md, November 1997, The Institute.

Diagnostics

Hypertension

Laboratory	Imaging
Urinalysis	Chest x-ray*
CBC and differential	Abdominal ultrasound*
Serum glucose	Renal angiogram*
Serum electrolytes	**Other**
BUN	ECG
Creatinine	Echocardiogram*
Fasting lipid profile	
Calcium	
Phosphorus	
Uric acid	
TSH*	
24-hour urine cortisol (if Cushing's syndrome is suspected)	
24-hour creatinine, catecholamines, and metanephrines (if pheochromocytoma is suspected)	

*If indicated.

glucose, plasma lipoproteins, serum uric acid, and calcium. An ECG is obtained to assess evidence of ischemic heart disease or left ventricular hypertrophy (Figure 133-1). Left ventricular hypertrophy by ECG is manifested by a large S wave in V_1 and a large R wave in V_5. These two deflections will add up to more than 35 mm.[56]

DIFFERENTIAL DIAGNOSIS

The initial evaluation of a patient with hypertension should exclude the possibility of secondary hypertension. Diagnosis and treatment of an underlying secondary etiology may ultimately resolve the hypertension. The more commonly noted secondary causes of hypertension, their symptoms, and diagnostic testing can be found in Table 133-2.

Among the differential diagnoses is "white coat hypertension," which is an elevated blood pressure related to the anticipation or anxiety of visiting a health care provider. When white coat hypertension is suspected, home blood pressure monitoring or ambulatory blood pressure monitoring may be beneficial. Some cases of white coat hypertension are thought to be predictive of high blood pressure; in such cases patients may benefit from nonpharmacologic primary prevention techniques.[9]

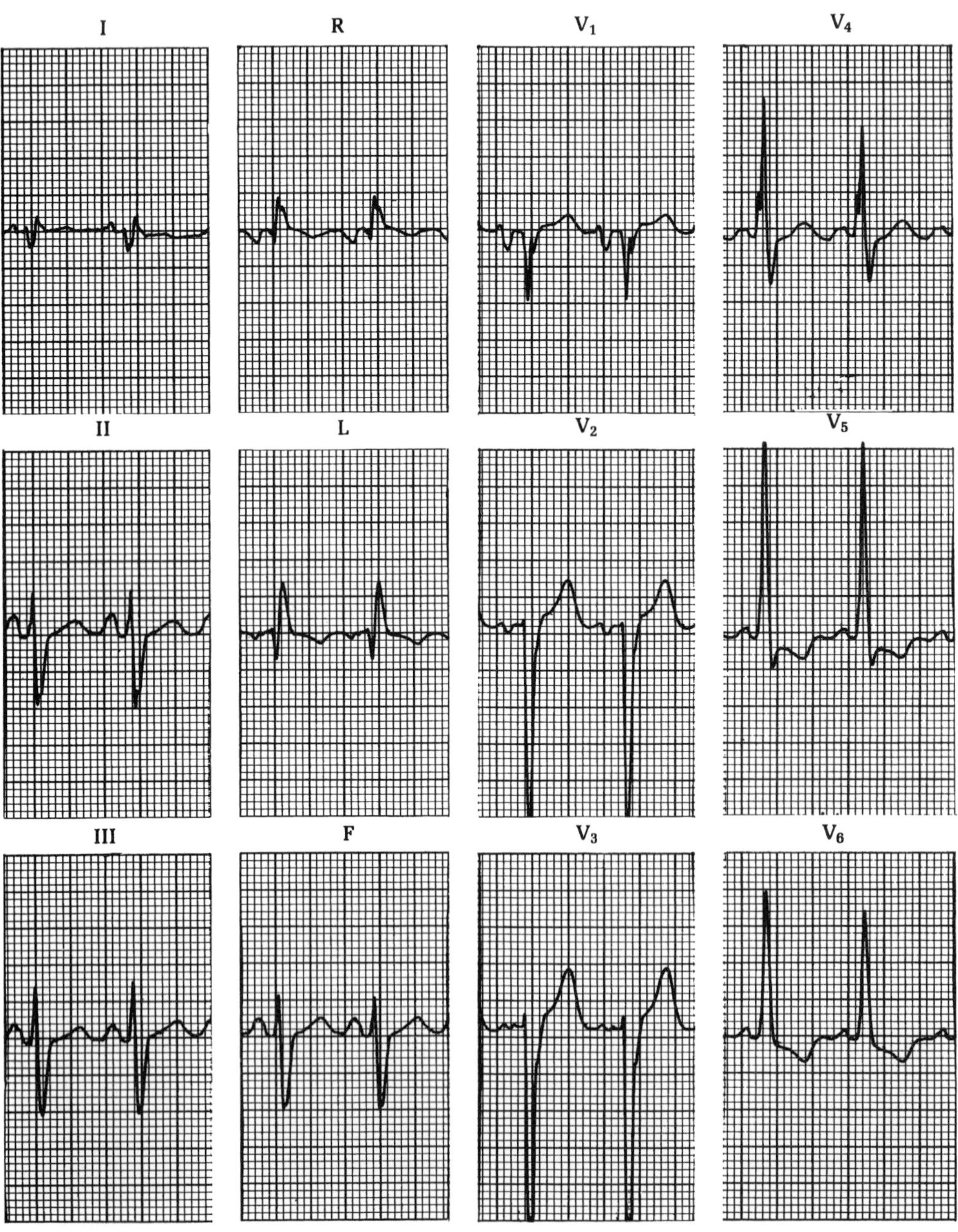

FIGURE 133-1

Left ventricular hypertrophy and strain with left atrial enlargement. (From Conover MB: *Understanding electrocardiography,* ed 7, St Louis, 1996, Mosby.)

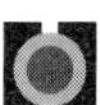 Differential Diagnosis

Hypertension

Primary hypertension
Secondary hypertension
- Pheochromocytoma
- Cushing's syndrome
- Renal vascular disease
- Medications (see Table 133-2)
- Coarctation of the aorta
- Hypercalcemia
- Primary aldosteronism
- Alcohol
- Acromegaly
- Sleep apnea

MANAGEMENT

JNC VI[9] recommends using a risk stratification strategy for treatment on the basis of blood pressure, the presence of cardiac risk factors, and target organ damage (Table 133-4). This approach ensures that those at highest risk will receive aggressive treatment. For primary prevention and treatment, all individuals should adhere to nonpharmacologic recommendations such as weight reduction, salt restriction, moderation of alcohol intake, exercise, and smoking cessation. Primary prevention is especially important because the risk of heart disease with hypertension is much greater than the risk reduction provided by secondary prevention of hypertension.[57]

Nonpharmacologic Therapy

Nonpharmacologic therapy is the initial management technique attempted with borderline hypertension and is an adjunct for both primary prevention of hypertension and pharmacologic therapy. Lifestyle interventions form the cornerstone of nonpharmacologic therapy.

Weight Reduction. A 10-lb weight reduction has been shown to result in a lowered blood pressure; when necessary, a weight loss of more than 10 pounds improves the results further.[38,58] Weight reduction is indicated if the patient is more than 110% of ideal body weight.

Ideal body weight can be roughly calculated as 110 pounds for the first 5 feet of height plus 6 pounds for each inch over 5 feet (males), or 110 pounds for the first 5 feet of height plus 5 pounds for each inch over 5 feet (women). A typical daily caloric intake is estimated through a 24-hour diet recall by the patient. Calories may be reduced by 500 kcal/day to achieve a modest 1 lb/week weight reduction. Strategies for successful weight reduction include an emphasis on short-term weight reduction goals, avoidance of terms with negative connotations (e.g., "diet"), and follow-up visits for encouragement regarding reaching goals and maintaining healthy eating practices.

Salt Restriction and Healthy Eating Habits. Evidence in the DASH study has shown that a diet rich in fruits, whole grains and vegetables and low in red meats, saturated fat, cholesterol and sugar-containing drinks lowered blood pressure.[36] In general, salt restriction has been shown to lower blood pressure among all blood pressure levels, but especially in individuals who are salt sensitive.[29,30,38]

A subset of the DASH study looked at three levels of sodium intake, finding that the lower the salt intake, the lower the blood pressure, especially among African-Americans. These blood-pressure lowering effects were in addition to those achieved with the overall healthier eating patterns in the DASH diet.[59] Maintaining a low-sodium diet can be difficult and is often marked by recidivism. Weight reduction may lead to decreased salt sensitivity, thereby obviating the need for salt restriction.[29]

Other Lifestyle Modifications. Additional important lifestyle recommendations involve exercise, limitation of alcohol use, stress management, and smoking cessation. Specific exercise recommendations and guidelines for alcohol use are found in Chapter 21 (Lifestyle Assessment) and under Patient Education. Strategies for smoking cessation are found in Chapter 21 (Lifestyle Assessment)

Pharmacologic Therapy

The decision to start pharmacologic therapy should be individualized for each patient. The elements that factor into this decision include level of blood pressure; the presence of cardiac risk factors (hyperlipidemia, tobacco use, family history, diabetes, premature menopause without hormone replacement therapy); and the presence, severity, and acuity of target organ damage (heart, blood vessels, brain, and kidney) as described in Table 133-5.

There are many different categories of antihypertensives: diuretics, beta blockers, angiotensin-converting enzyme (ACE) inhibitors, angiotensin receptor blockers (ARB), calcium channel blockers, and alpha blockers. New antihypertensive drugs are currently under investigation. Each of the drugs in each of these categories has been shown to reach a certain level of efficacy in

TABLE 133-4 Risk Stratification and Treatment of Hypertension

Blood Pressure Stages (mm Hg)	Risk Group A (No Risk Factors; No TOD/CCD)	Risk Group B (At Least One Risk Factor, Not Including Diabetes; No TOD/CCD)	Risk Group C (TOD/CCD and/or Diabetes, With or Without Other Risk Factors)
High-Normal (130-139/85-89)	Lifestyle modification	Lifestyle modification	Lifestyle modification and drug therapy
Stage 1 (140-159/90-99)	Lifestyle modification (up to 12 months)	Lifestyle modification (up to 6 months)	Lifestyle modification and drug therapy
Stages 2 and 3 (≥160/≥100)	Drug therapy and lifestyle modification	Drug therapy and lifestyle modification	Drug therapy and lifestyle modification

Modified from National Institutes of Health: *The Sixth Report of the National Committee on Prevention, Detection, Evaluation, and Treatment of High Blood Pressure,* NIH pub no 98-4080, November 1997, The Institute.
TOD/CCD, Target organ damage/clinical cardiovascular disease.

TABLE 133-5 Hypertensive Medications

Medication	Dosage	Compelling Indications	Effect on Coexisting Conditions: Favorable	Effect on Coexisting Conditions: Unfavorable
DIURETICS		Heart failure; Isolated systolic hypertension in older patients	Type 2 diabetes (low dose); osteoporosis (thiazides)	Types 1 and 2 diabetes (high dose); gout; renal insufficiency
Thiazide				
Chlorthalidone	12.5-50 mg/day			
Hydrochlorothiazide	12.5-50 mg/day			
Indapamide	1.25-5 mg/day			
Metolazone	2.5-10 mg/day			
Loop				
Bumetanide	0.5-4 mg divided b.i.d./t.i.d.			
Ethacrynic acid	25-100 mg divided b.i.d./t.i.d.			
Furosemide	40-240 mg divided b.i.d./t.i.d.			
Potassium-Sparing				
Amiloride	5-10 mg/day			
Spironolactone	25-100 mg/day			
Triamterene	25-100 mg/day			
ALPHA BLOCKERS			Hyperlipidemia; benign prostatic hypertrophy	
Doxazosin	1-16 mg/day			
Prazosin	2-30 mg divided b.i.d./t.i.d.			
Terazosin	1-20 mg/day			
BETA BLOCKERS		MI (nonintrinsic sympathomimetic activity)	Angina; atrial tachycardia and atrial fibrillation; essential tremor; Migraine (noncardioselective); hyperthyroidism; preoperative hypertension	Bronchospasm; depression; diabetes types 1 and 2; hyperlipidemia; atrioventricular heart block; peripheral vascular disease
Acebutolol	200-800 mg/day			
Atenolol	25-100 mg/day-b.i.d.			
Betaxolol	5-20 mg/day			
Metoprolol tartrate	50-300 mg b.i.d.			
Metoprolol succinate	50-300 mg/day			
Nadolol	40-320 mg/day			
Pindolol	10-60 mg/day			
Propranolol	40-480 mg divided			
Timolol maleate	20-60 mg b.i.d.			
ALPHA/BETA BLOCKERS			Heart failure (carvedilol)	Liver disease (labetalol)
Carvedilol	12.5-50 mg b.i.d.			
Labetalol	200-1200 mg/b.i.d.			

From National Institutes of Health: *The Sixth Report of the Joint National Committee on Prevention, Detection, Evaluation, and Treatment of High Blood Pressure,* NIH pub no 98-4080, Bethesda, Md, November 1997, The Institute.

Efficacy		Side Effects		
Increase	Decrease	Caution With	Short-Term Use	Possible
Combination diuretics with different sites of action	Steroids; NSAIDs; resin-binding drugs	Lithium (increased levels); potassium-sparing and ACEIs may cause hyperkalemia	Increases cholesterol, blood glucose	Hyponatremia, hypokalemia (except in potassium-sparing), hypomagnesemia, hyperuricemia, hypercalcemia, hyperglycemia, sexual dysfunction
				Decreased clearance of verapamil with prazosin
Concomitant use of hepatically metabolized beta blockers; cimetidine; quinidine; food	NSAIDs; rifampin; Phenobarbital; inducers of hepatic metabolism	Severe heart failure; asthma, bronchospastic COPD; diabetes (decreased hypoglycemic awareness); heart block; hypertriglyceridemia (associated with nonintrinsic sypathomimetic activity)		Bradycardia; fatigue; impaired circulation in extremities; sexual dysfunction; depression
				Postural hypotension; bronchospasm

continued

TABLE 133-5 Hypertensive Medications—cont'd

Medication	Dosage	Compelling Indications	Effect on Coexisting Conditions	
			Favorable	Unfavorable
CALCIUM CHANNEL BLOCKERS		Isolated systolic hypertension (long-acting dihydropyridine)	Angina; cyclosporine-induced hypertension; diabetes type 1 and 2; nondihydropyridine: atrial tachycardia, atrial fibrillation, and migraine headache	Heart failure (except amlodipine) and types 2- and 3-degree AV block (nondihydropyridine)
Dihydropyridines				
Amlodipine	2.5-10 mg/day			
Felodipine	2.5-10 mg/day			
Isradipine	5-20 mg/day			
Nicardipine	30-60 mg b.i.d. (long-acting only)			
Nifedipine (long-acting only)	30-120 mg/day			
Nondihydropyridines (Long-Acting Only)				
Diltiazem	120-360 mg*			
Verapamil	90-480 mg*			
ANGIOTENSIN-CONVERTING ENZYME INHIBITORS		Heart failure; diabetes type I; MI with systolic dysfunction	Diabetes type I; renal insufficiency (with creatinine <3 mg/dl)	Kidneys in renal artery stenosis; pregnancy
Captopril	25-100 mg divided b.i.d. or q.i.d.			
Enalapril	5-40 mg/day or b.i.d.			
Lisinopril	5-40 mg/day			
Quinapril				
ANGIOTENSIN II BLOCKERS				
Losartan	25-100 mg/day or b.i.d.			
Valsartan	80-320 mg/day			
Irbesartan	150-300 mg/day			
Candesartan	8-32 mg divided q.d.-b.i.d.			
VASODILATORS			Heart failure (with hydralazine along with nitrates when ACEIs cannot be prescribed)	
Hydralazine	50-300 mg/day			
Minoxidil	5-100 mg/day			

*Frequency depends on formulation.

Efficacy		Side Effects		
Increase	Decrease	Caution With	Short-Term Use	Possible
Cimetidine or ranitidine with CCBs hepatically metabolized	Rifampin; Phenobarbital; inducers of metabolism			**Dihydropyridines only:** Lower extremity edema, flushing, headache **L-channel nondihydropyridines only:** Conduction defects, heart failure, lower lithium levels (with verapamil); increased levels of quinidine, digoxin, sulfonylureas, and theophylline (competitive hepatic metabolism) with nondihydropyridines
With chlorpromazine	NSAIDs; antacids; food may decrease some absorption	Potassium-sparing diuretics **Contraindicated in pregnancy**		Cough; angioedema (rare); hyperkalemia; leukopenia; increased lithium levels
				Angioedema (isolated); hyperkalemia; less cough than with ACEIs
		MAO inhibitors		Edema/fluid retention; tachycardia; lupus syndrome (hydralazine) hirsutism (minoxidil)

lowering blood pressure and therefore has been approved by the U.S. Food and Drug Administration (FDA). Diuretics and beta blockers have the advantage of being the most studied and have been proven effective in preventing stroke and reducing the risk of coronary disease. For this reason, they were recommended by the Joint National Commission on Hypertension as first-line pharmacologic treatments for uncomplicated hypertension in 1993 and, with some caveats, in 1997.[9] Certain individuals have concomitant conditions that include specific indications for drugs other than diuretics or beta blockers. These patients should be started on the pharmacologic therapy most appropriate for their needs.[9]

In general, it is recommended to start with the lowest dose possible. Lower doses are associated with fewer side effects and are better tolerated so patients more readily adhere to a drug regimen. For better antihypertensive effects where needed, the dosage of an individual drug can be increased, or another drug (in a small dosage) can be added. There are fixed combination drugs on the market for such treatment; they are popular because they are often effective, have a low side-effect profile, and are often less expensive than two separate pills.[60-62] If necessary (because of untoward effects or poor blood pressure control), another antihypertensive medication can be substituted.

Diuretics. Diuretics have been a mainstay of antihypertensive therapy and include thiazides, loops, and potassium-sparing diuretics. Because of their natriuretic nature, diuretics are especially effective in patients whose hypertension is typified by low sodium excretion and high circulating volume. Thiazide diuretics are the preferred choice for initial therapy because of their potency and their long duration of action.[9] African-Americans, older adults, and obese individuals often benefit from thiazides.[17]

Mainly reserved for hypertension that is resistant to treatment or for patients with renal disease, loop diuretics may be substituted when the glomerular filtration rate reaches approximately 60% or when the serum creatinine is greater than 1.7 (150 μmol/L). Patients cannot be classified as "resistant" to treatment unless they remain hypertensive after a diuretic has been added to the regimen.[62]

By preventing some exchange of sodium for potassium in the distal tubule, potassium-sparing diuretics (i.e., triamterene or spironolactone) are useful in combination with other diuretics to prevent hypokalemia. By using a combination therapy such as hydrochlorothiazide with spironolactone, lower doses of each drug may produce better antihypertensive effects with better patient tolerance.

Patients should be followed for efficacy of blood pressure control or for problems with side effects, cost, or adherence. Laboratory testing for glucose, potassium, lipid levels, and renal function should be performed several times during the first year of therapy to detect any possible adverse effect.

Problems with hypokalemia can be prevented and/or combated by advising a higher intake of potassium-rich fruits and vegetables,[21] such as bananas, greens, spinach, baked potatoes, and orange juice. Hypokalemia can also be controlled by adding a potassium supplement or adding an ACE inhibitor to antihypertensive therapy, if indicated. A potassium supplement should not be added to an ACE inhibitor unless the practitioner is certain that hypokalemia still exists; the potassium should be carefully checked at close intervals after the initiation of such therapy.

Beta Blockers. Along with diuretics, beta blockers have been recommended by the JNC V as first-line therapy and by the JNC VI as first-line therapy for uncomplicated hypertension.[9,53] Many beta blockers are now available with many different classifications: cardioselective vs. nonselective, with intrinsic sympathomimetic activity vs. without intrinsic sympathomimetic activity, lipophilic vs. hydrophilic, and combined alpha and beta blockers (Box 133-1). Beta blockers are inexpensive, well tolerated, and cardioprotective after myocardial infarction and improve outcomes in patients with heart failure.[63-67] Beta blockers are sometimes used for stage fright or for patients with hypertension and concomitant anxiety. A relative contraindication exists for individuals with diabetes and hyperlipidemia and for patients with peripheral vascular disease who have ischemia at rest.[63,64] Because beta blockers may produce bronchoconstriction, they are contraindicated in asthma and in other conditions with a bronchospastic component. Recent studies also suggest that beta blockers, when used as monotherapy in older adults, may not be effective.[68,69]

Angiotensin-Converting Enzyme Inhibitors. ACE inhibitors interrupt the conversion of angiotensin I to angiotensin II and are effective antihypertensive agents. Treatment with an ACE inhibitor improves triglyceride levels and insulin sensitivity and has a neutral or beneficial effect on other lipids and glucose levels in patients with diabetes.[70,71] ACE inhibitors are renoprotective and there is documented improved survival rates in patients with congestive heart failure and regression of left ventricular hypertrophy.[70-73]

The JNC VI recommends ACE inhibitor treatment of hypertension after first-line treatment unless special circumstances exist, such as patients with diabetes or heart failure with systolic dysfunction. ACE inhibitor therapy is also recommended for a minimum of 6 weeks after acute anterior myocardial infarction with ST-segment elevation to prevent remodeling and indefinitely with echocardiographic evidence of left ventricular systolic dysfunction (ejection fraction <40%) with or without symptoms.[65]

ACE inhibitors are contraindicated in pregnancy and are relatively contraindicated in hyperkalemia and with creatinine levels more than 3.0 mg/dl. Laboratory testing for serum potassium and creatinine is indicated 48 hours after initiation of therapy and weekly for several weeks.

BOX 133-1

BETA BLOCKERS

Nonselective: propranolol, nadolol, sotalol, timolol, oxprenolol
Cardioselective: atenolol, metoprolol, acebutolol
Intrinsic sympathomimetic activity: oxprenolol, celiprolol, pindolol, acebutolol
Lipid-soluble: propranolol, metoprolol, pindolol
Lipid-insoluble: atenolol, sotalol, nadolol
Alpha/beta: labetalol, carvedilol

Angiotensin Receptor Blockers. ARBs received FDA approval for treatment of hypertension in 1995. These agents have a similar antihypertensive effect as ACE inhibitors. Definite evidence shows they are beneficial in patients with heart failure[74] when patients are unable to take ACE inhibitors and they have had proven renoprotective benefits similar to ACE inhibitors in patients with type 2 diabetes.[75-78] These findings primarily occurred after JNC VI, but the strength of the data would support the use of ARBs as first-line therapy for people with type 2 diabetes and hypertension. Like ACE inhibitors, ARBs are contraindicated in pregnancy.

Calcium Channel Blockers. Calcium channel blockers perform by blocking calcium within cells, primarily the vascular and cardiac muscle cells. The calcium channel blockers consist of the dihydropyridines (nifedipine and amlodipine) and the nondihydropyridines (verapamil and diltiazem).

Calcium channel blockers are efficacious and well tolerated and have a relatively low side-effect profile and a high adherence rate in comparison to other therapies.[78] They are metabolically neutral, which makes them advantageous for patients with diabetes or hyperlipidemia.[79] They are also effective antianginal medications.[80]

Unfortunately, short-acting calcium channel blockers, especially nifedipine, have been associated with a greater risk of cardiovascular death.[81] This effect has not been seen with long-acting preparations of calcium channel blockers.[82] However, there are other disadvantages. With the exception of amlodipine, calcium channel blockers may worsen heart failure and in general are contraindicated in patients with systolic dysfunction (ejection fraction <40%). In some patients, the dihydropyridines have been associated with leg edema unresponsive to diuretic therapy. There have also been concerns that calcium channel blockers may be associated with an increased risk of cancer. This may be related to slowed calcium influx and delayed apoptosis, although there are insufficient data to support this theory.

Calcium channel blockers can be used as first-line therapy in patients with hypertension and concomitant angina, although long-acting formulations are preferred. Nondihydropyridines should be avoided in patients with sick sinus syndrome or bradycardia (heart rate <55 beats per minute) at rest. Caution is advised if these drugs are being combined with digoxin or a beta blocker.

Alpha-Adrenergic Blockers. Alpha-adrenergic blockers have some favorable effects, which prompted the JNC VI to recommend them in certain circumstances.[9] The doxazosin arm of the ALLHAT study,[83] conducted after JNC VI was published, was discontinued prematurely because of higher rates of cardiovascular events and hospitalizations for heart failure among patients on doxazosin. Thus there is evidence that despite its positive effect on benign prostatic hypertrophy (BPH) and on lipids, doxazosin and alpha-adrenergic blockers in general should not be used as first-line pharmacologic treatment in hypertension. There have been no studies that have looked at alpha-adrenergic blockers as an added therapy. Therefore, although some sources recommend alpha-adrenergic blockers as additional therapy for patients with significant hyperlipidemia, severe hypertension, and hypertension related to renal disease may also benefit, there is no comparative data to support their use.[84]

Vasodilators (Minoxidil, Hydralazine). The direct vasodilators are recommended as second- or third-line medications for hypertension and are best used in combinations that control untoward effects such as edema or flushing.[9] Hydralazine is the most commonly used of these drugs and is most useful when used in combination with a diuretic to reduce compensatory volume expansion and with beta blockers to blunt the catecholamine response.[80] Hydralazine and nitrates can be used together in patients with hypertension and heart failure who do not tolerate ACE inhibitors or ARB.[85] Hydralazine requires three or four times a day dosing, so adherence may be a problem for many patients. In high doses hydralazine may cause a lupuslike reaction. Minoxidil is not recommended in women because of the possibility of facial hirsutism.

Monitoring

Follow-up strategy depends on the initial blood pressure (see Table 133-3). If blood pressure is not in good control, therapy can be advanced. If previously well-controlled blood pressure has risen, several areas should be explored. Poor adherence to the medical regimen because of a difficult dosage schedule, side effects, cost, or lack of understanding may be the cause. The patient history and physical examination should focus on possible secondary causes of hypertension. New conditions, such as renal parenchymal disease or renal artery stenosis, can elevate a previously controlled blood pressure. Other causes may include new over-the-counter or mail-order herbal treatments, the use of NSAIDs, or excessive alcohol intake.[41,43]

Co-Management with Specialists

Patients with concomitant diseases that are affected by or can cause hypertension may require collaborative management by a specialist in that field. An endocrinology consultation may be indicated for patients with diabetes. Nephrologists can provide collaborative care to patients with renal disease, and cardiologists can provide care to those with active CAD.

LIFE SPAN CONSIDERATIONS

In general, systolic blood pressure rises with age, whereas diastolic blood pressure reaches a peak around 60 years of age and then begins to decrease mildly. Isolated systolic hypertension is especially a problem for patients over age 60 years, and is thought to result from aging, stiffening, and lack of compliance of the arteries. Isolated systolic hypertension responds well to most antihypertensive medications and especially to diuretics and calcium channel blockers. Advancing age does not preclude nonpharmacologic therapy. In fact, trials in older patients have shown beneficial outcomes in terms of stroke and total mortality in the treatment of systolic hypertension[14] and diastolic hypertension.[86] In this population, pharmacologic therapy may require gentle initiation and advancement to prevent excessive drops in blood pressure or orthostatic hypotension, which can result in falls.[87-89] Blood pressure goals are the same with older persons, however, and progress toward those goals has been associated with improved/preserved cognitive function.[90]

Secondary hypertension should be considered when hypertension develops before the age of 30 years (i.e., coarctation of the aorta or fibromuscular renal artery stenosis) or after the age of 55 (i.e., atherosclerotic renal artery stenosis). Hypertension during pregnancy (preeclampsia) is beyond the scope of this discussion.

COMPLICATIONS

Long-term complications of hypertension include left ventricular hypertrophy, heart failure, CAD, myocardial infarction, sudden death, aortic dissection, cerebrovascular disease, proteinuria, renal insufficiency, atherosclerotic conditions, retinopathy,[91,92] and hypertensive urgencies and emergencies.[93,94] Complications can result from long-term uncontrolled hypertension that assails target organs over time or from sudden surges of acute hypertension that result, for example, from acute glomerulonephritis or cocaine ingestion. A decline in cognitive functioning[95] and a higher incidence of dementia and Alzheimer's disease[96] have been associated with hypertension in older individuals.

Hypertensive Crises

Hypertensive emergencies are relatively rare events. Earlier and more pervasive diagnosis and treatment have reduced the incidence of malignant hypertension from untreated high blood pressure and has reduced mortality rates. A hypertensive crisis is present when blood pressure is high enough to threaten target organs acutely. JNC VI[9] differentiates between hypertensive emergencies and hypertensive urgencies as follows:

Hypertensive Emergency Characteristics	*Hypertensive Urgency Characteristics*
Hypertensive encephalopathy	Upper levels stage 3 hypertension
Intracranial hemorrhage	Hypertension with optic disc edema
Unstable angina pectoris	Progressive target organ complications
Acute myocardial infarction	Severe perioperative hypertension
Pulmonary edema	
Dissecting aortic aneurysm	
Eclampsia	

The initial assessment of hypertensive crises should be aimed at two primary goals: (1) determining a threat to the most commonly affected target organs: fundi, brain, heart, and kidneys; and (2) finding a cause. Kaplan[97] noted that, because various diagnostic options may be contaminated by drugs, blood, and urine, samples should be collected quickly before treatment but without delaying it:

Drug	*Interferes With*
Labetalol	Catecholamine assays (alpha blocker)
Diuretics/potassium	Primary aldosteronism evaluation
Renin-suppressing drugs	Renovascular evaluation

Oral antihypertensive therapy is usually indicated for hypertensive urgencies. It may be advisable to coordinate the treatment of the cause (e.g., relief of pain in a postoperative patient) with the adjustment or initiation of the oral medication. Observation of the patient for several hours after treatment to determine safety and efficacy is recommended.

Hypertensive emergencies require admission to an intensive care unit and parenteral treatment (Table 133-6). The goal of treatment should be to reduce blood pressure slowly over a few hours, because rapid lowering of blood pressure can produce a shock effect in target organs. The brain maintains cerebral perfusion pressure by autoregulation, which balances perfusion via cerebral vasoconstriction or vasodilation in response to rises and falls in blood pressure. Normal autoregulation is easily maintained with blood pressure ranges of 70/40 mm Hg to 190/130 mm Hg (allowing for some individual variation). However, the autoregulation curve skews to the right and upward in patients with chronic hypertension. If blood pressure exceeds the limits of autoregulation or if blood pressure is dropped precipitously, signs of cerebral hypoperfusion may be present.

Initially, patients with severe hypertension may appear with headache, dizziness, altered consciousness (lethargy, slowed mentation, confusion, agitation), and nausea.[98] Other target organs may produce profound symptoms in response to severe hypertension; pulmonary edema may occur in the setting of diastolic heart failure from excessively high afterload (peripheral resistance); retinal hemorrhage may occur. The physical examination, especially the retinal examination, should focus on target organ damage. Groups III and IV Keith-Wagener-Barker funduscopic changes may be the only or the initial sign of rapid deterioration with severe hypertension. Other possible changes may include blood pressure variation resulting from coarctation or aortic dissection, ECG changes and chest pain consistent with unstable angina or myocardial infarction, and hematuria resulting from renal decompensation.

TABLE 133-6 Parenteral Medications for Severe Hypertension

Drug (Type)	Duration	Cautions and Comments
Nitroprusside (vasodilator)	1-10 minutes	Most rapid; use arterial monitoring; raises intracranial pressure
Nitroglycerin (vasodilator)	Minutes	Good for heart failure, coronary artery disease (CAD); tolerance may develop
Labetalol (alpha/beta blocker)	3-6 hours	Avoid in asthma; caution in heart failure
Esmolol (beta blocker)	<30 minutes	Avoid in heart failure and asthma
Nicardipine (calcium channel blocker)	3-6 hours	Prevents cerebral vasospasm; may cause ischemia
Furosemide (diuretic)	4 hours	Use with vasodilators
Hydralazine (diuretic)	>1 hour	Indicated for eclampsia; avoid in CAD, dissection
Fenoldopam (peripheral vasodilator and diuretic)	15 minutes	Contraindicated in glaucoma; may cause reflex tachycardia

JNC VI[9] recommends initially reducing blood pressure by no more than 25% in the first 2 hours; the goal over the next 2 to 6 hours is 160/100 mm Hg. The rate of fall should be gradual. Effort should be made to control the pressure and avoid precipitous drops. For this reason, the prior practice of using sublingual, short-acting nifedipine is contraindicated.[9] Particular caution should be exercised with older adults, in patients with chronic hypertension, in patients who might have hypovolemia (diuretic use, recent loss of appetite, vomiting, or diarrhea), or in patients who are taking vasoactive medications. In patients of all ages, overly aggressive therapy has been associated with adverse outcomes such as blindness, coma, and death.[93] The necessity of preventing permanent cerebral damage must be carefully achieved while lowering blood pressure enough to protect vital organs in circumstances such as acute heart failure, threatened myocardial infarction, or acute aortic dissection.

INDICATIONS FOR REFERRAL/HOSPITALIZATION

A physician consultation is necessary when hypertension is resistant to therapy and when secondary causes attributable to lifestyle considerations or habits have been excluded. Certain secondary causes may be best diagnosed and managed collaboratively. A referral may also be wise in patients with stage 3 hypertension before treatment is initiated.

Referral to a hypertension specialist is recommended when so-called "triple therapy" (three antihypertensive drugs, including a diuretic) has failed. A patient who has known secondary hypertension caused by renal artery stenosis should be referred to a hypertension specialist and a vascular radiologist or surgeon. Primary aldosteronism may require specialized input from an endocrinologist.

Patients who have severe hypertension may require immediate treatment, consultation, referral and, possibly, hospitalization. Both the level of the blood pressure elevation and the presence of accompanying signs or symptoms of acute damage will dictate the next level of care.

Hospitalization is recommended for those with stage 3 hypertension, a diastolic blood pressure greater than or equal to 130 mm Hg, and grade 3 or 4 retinopathy (exudates and hemorrhage).[9,87,91,92] Although retinopathy may be the first presenting sign, target organ symptoms should be rapidly assessed. Neurologic symptoms include altered mental status, dizziness, blurred vision or loss of vision, focal neurologic deficits, and gastrointestinal symptoms. Cardiac symptoms include chest pain (or an anginal equivalent) and/or dyspnea accompanied by ECG changes, rales, and an S_3 on physical examination, and possibly heart failure on chest x-ray study. Vascular symptoms may include tearing or burning chest pain or interscapular pain, with a variation in bilateral arm or leg blood pressure measurements, decreased pulses in lower extremities, or a widened mediastinum on the chest x-ray film. Renal signs may include oliguria, hematuria, proteinuria, or red cell casts by urinalysis.

PATIENT AND FAMILY EDUCATION

Topics that must be addressed include dietary instructions, exercise recommendations, risk factor modification, lifestyle issues, and the side effects associated with the medication prescribed. Patient comprehension is increased when handouts are given as references after the office visit.

General dietary recommendations include four servings of fruit, four servings of vegetables, and three servings of low-fat dairy products [DASH trial][36]; reduction of cholesterol (<300 mg/day), saturated fat (<10% of total calories), and total fat (<30% of total calories)[American Heart Association]; control of blood sugar; and moderate alcohol intake (no more than 2 ounces 100 proof liquor, 8 ounces wine, or 34 ounces beer daily; half this amount for individuals smaller than the average male). Total alcohol cessation may be necessary when hypertension is resistant to treatment.

Salt intake should be restricted to a maximum of 2.4 g/day. The DASH study[59] showed that the lower the salt intake, the lower the blood pressure. As noted previously, adherence may be difficult for many patients at extremely low levels.

Measures that help with salt restriction include avoiding adding salt to food, cooking with herbs, using fresh fruits and vegetables instead of canned, choosing fresh meats instead of deli or processed meats (e.g., bacon, sausage), and avoiding obviously salty foods (e.g., potato chips, pretzels, salted nuts). According to guidelines of the FDA and the United States Department of Agriculture, healthy foods are those containing less than 360 mg sodium per serving. Labels showing sodium-free (5 mg/serving), very-low-sodium (<36 mg/serving), or low-sodium antacids (<141 mg/serving) should be selected.

Exercise recommendations are geared around provision of a specific exercise prescription (see Physical Activity, Chapter 21), with consideration of screening for CAD by physician consultation and/or stress testing in males over 40 years of age and females over 50 years of age.[99] The goal should be an established routine of exercise that is enjoyable and maintains interest with consistent progression of activity. Factors that need emphasis include adequate hydration, stretching, and warm-up and cool-down periods with more strenuous exercise.

Self-monitoring of blood pressure is a reasonable goal. If the patient agrees, family members should be provided with information concerning therapeutic recommendations. Individual knowledge concerning optimum level of blood pressure, factors affecting blood pressure, the necessity of treatment for control rather than cure of blood pressure, dosing, mechanism, monitoring required, side effects of medications, and dangers of quick weight loss programs is crucial. Involvement of patients in the decision-making process, exploration of feelings concerning treatment regimens, exit interviews, and making regular follow-up visits help the patient to achieve therapeutic goals.

HEALTH PROMOTION

Health promotion involves risk factor modification that is directed toward cardiovascular disease and diabetes. Reduction to normal weight, smoking cessation, control of lipid levels, glycemic control, and stress management are key components of risk factor modification.

REFERENCES

1. National Heart, Lung, and Blood Institute: Scientific advances: under pressure: hypertension. Retrieved August 11, 1997 from the World Wide Web: www.nhlbi.nih.gov/personal/condonv/t1/html/hyper.htm.

2. Burt VL and others: Trends in the prevalence, awareness, treatment, and control of hypertension in the adult US population: data from the health examination surveys, 1960-1991, *Hypertension* 26(1):60-69, 1995.
3. Burt VL and others: Prevalence of hypertension in the US adult population: results from the Third National Health and Nutrition Examination Survey, 1988-1991, *Hypertension* 25(3):305-313, 1995.
4. Kannel WB: Blood pressure as a cardiovascular risk factor, *JAMA* 275(24):1571-1576, 1996.
5. Whelton PK: Epidemiology of hypertension, *Lancet* 344:101-106, 1994.
6. Mortality after 16 years for participants randomized to the Multiple Risk Factor Intervention Trial, *Circulation* 94(5):946-951, 1996.
7. American Heart Association: Biostatistical Fact Sheet. Retrieved January 29, 2002 from the World Wide Web: www.americanheart.org/presenter.jhtml?identifier=695.
8. Stamler R: Implications of the INTERSALT study, *Hypertension* 17(suppl I):116-120, 1991.
9. National Heart, Lung, and Blood Institute: *The sixth report of the Joint National Committee on Prevention, Detection, Evaluation, and Treatment of High Blood Pressure*, NIH Pub No 98-4080, Bethesda, Md November 1997, US Department of Health and Human Services. Web site: www.nhlbi.nih.gov/nhlbi/nhlbi.htm.
10. Hansson L and others: Effects of intensive blood-pressure lowering and low-dose aspirin in patients with hypertension, *Lancet* 351:1755-1762, 1998.
11. Millar JA and others: Pulse pressure as a risk factor for cardiovascular events in the MRC Mild Hypertension Trial, *J Hypertens* 17:1065-1072, 1999.
12. Curb JD and others: Effect of diuretic-based antihypertensive treatment on cardiovascular disease risk in older diabetic patients with isolated systolic hypertension: systolic hypertension in the elderly program cooperative research group, *JAMA* 276(23):1886-1892, 1996.
13. National Center for Health Statistics: *Health, United States, 1995*, Hyattsville, Md, 1996, Public Health Service.
14. Materson BJ and others: Single-drug therapy for hypertension in men: a comparison of six antihypertensive agents with placebo, The Department of Veterans Affairs Cooperative Study Group on Antihypertensive Agents, *N Engl J Med* 328(13):914-921, 1993.
15. Materson BJ, Reda DJ, Cushman WC: Department of Veterans Affairs single-drug therapy of hypertension study: revised figures and new data, Department of Veterans Affairs Cooperative Study Group on Antihypertensive Agents, *Am J Hypertens* 8(2):189-192, 1995.
16. Dannenberg AL, Garrison RJ, Kannel WB: Incidence of hypertension in the Framingham Study, *Am J Public Health* 78(6):676-679, 1988.
17. SHEP Cooperative Research Group: Prevention of stroke by antihypertensive drug treatment in older persons with isolated systolic hypertension: final results of the systolic hypertension in the elderly program, *JAMA* 265(24):3255-3264, 1991.
18. Kaplan NM: Ethnic aspects of hypertension, *Lancet* 344:450-452, 1994.
19. Kaplan N: Primary hypertension: pathogenesis. In *Clinical hypertension*, ed 6, Baltimore, 1994, Williams & Wilkins.
20. Kaplan NM: Alcohol and hypertension, *Lancet* 345:1588-1589, 1995.
21. Ashida T and others: Effects of dietary salt on sodium-calcium exchange and ATP-driven calcium pump in arterial smooth muscle of Dahl rats, *J Hypertens* 10(11):1335-1341, 1992.
22. Midgley JP and others: Effect of reduced dietary sodium on blood pressure: a meta-analysis of randomized controlled trials, *JAMA* 275(20):1490-1597, 1996.
23. Campese VM and others: Pressor reactivity to norepinephrine and angiotensin in salt-sensitive hypertensive patients, *Hypertension* 21: 301-307, 1993.
24. Kaplan NM: Primary hypertension: from pathophysiology to prevention, *Arch Intern Med* 156:1919-1920, 1996.
25. Cowley AW, Roman RJ: The role of the kidney in hypertension, *JAMA* 275(20):1581-1589, 1996.
26. Navar LG: The kidney in blood pressure regulation and development of hypertension, *Med Clin North Am* 81(5):1165-1198, 1997.
27. Frohlich ED: Current clinical pathophysiologic considerations in essential hypertension, *Med Clin North Am* 81(5):1113-1129, 1997.
28. Pecker MS: Salt sensitivity in hypertensive patients: pathogenesis, identification, and treatment. In Laragh JH, Brenner BM, editors: *Hypertension: pathophysiology, diagnosis, and management*, ed 2, New York, 1995, Raven Press.
29. Reisin E: Nonpharmacologic approaches to hypertension: weight, sodium, alcohol, exercise, and tobacco considerations, *Med Clin North Am* 81(6):1289-1303, 1997.
30. Sullivan JM: Salt sensitivity: definition, conception, methodology, and long-term issues, *Hypertension* 17(suppl I):I61-I68, 1991.
31. Oparil S, Calhoun DA: High blood pressure. In Dale DC, Federman DD, editors: *Scientific American medicine*, New York, 1997, Scientific American.
32. Massie BM: Systemic hypertension. In Tierney LM, McPhee SJ, Papadakis MA, editors: *Current medical diagnosis and treatment*, ed 36, Stamford, Conn, 1997, Appleton & Lange.
33. Mann SJ, Blumenfeld JD, Laragh JH: Issues, goals, and guidelines for choosing first-line and combination antihypertensive drug therapy. In Laragh JH, Brenner BM, editors: *Hypertension: pathophysiology, diagnosis and management*, ed 2, New York, 1995, Raven Press.
34. Forte P and others: Basal nitric oxide synthesis in essential hypertension, *Lancet* 349:837-842, 1997.
35. Haffner ST and others: Metabolic precursors of hypertension: the San Antonio heart study, *Arch Intern Med* 156:1994-2001, 1996.
36. Conlin PR and others: The effect of dietary patterns on blood pressure control in hypertensive patients: results from the Dietary Approaches to Stop Hypertension (DASH) trial, *Am J Hypertens* 13(9):949-955, 2000.
37. Ramsey LE and others: Non-pharmacological therapy of hypertension, *Br Med Bull* 50(2):494-508, 1994.
38. Alderman MH: Non-pharmacological treatment of hypertension, *Lancet* 344:307-311, 1994.
39. Blair SN et al: Physical fitness and incidence of hypertension in healthy normotensive men and women, *JAMA* 252:487-490, 1984.
40. Paffenbarger RS Jr and others: The association of changes in physical activity level and other lifestyle characteristics with mortality among men, *N Engl J Med* 328:538-545, 1993.
41. Adcock BB, Ireland RB Jr: Secondary hypertension: a practical diagnostic approach, *Am Fam Physician* 55(4):1263-1270, 1997.
42. Dustan HP: Renal arterial disease and hypertension, *Med Clin North Am* 81(5):1199-1212, 1997.
43. Ram CVS: Secondary hypertension: workup and correction, *Hosp Pract* 29(4):137-150, 1994.
44. Schamess A, Bernik T, Tenner S: Refractory hypertension due to Conn's syndrome, *Postgrad Med* 95(4):199-203, 1994.
45. Pope JE, Anderson JJ, Felson DT: A meta-analysis of the effects of nonsteroidal anti-inflammatory drugs on blood pressure, *Arch Intern Med* 153:477-484, 1993.
46. Berger M et al: Avoiding the supine position during sleep lowers 24-hour blood pressure in obstructive sleep apnea (OSA) patients, *J Hum Hypertens* 11(10):657-664, 1997.
47. Guilleminault C, Robinson A: Sleep-disordered breathing and hypertension: past lessons, future directions, *Sleep* 20(9):806-811, 1997.
48. Preston RA, Singer I, Epstein M: Renal parenchymal hypertension: current concepts of pathogenesis and management, *Arch Intern Med* 156:602-611, 1996.
49. National High Blood Pressure Education Program Working Group: 1995 Update of the Working group reports on chronic renal failure and renovascular hypertension, *Arch Intern Med* 156:1938-1947, 1996.
50. McCarron D: High blood pressure. In Dale DC, Federman DD, editors: *Scientific American medicine*, New York, 1995, Scientific American.
51. Pentel P: Toxicity of over-the-counter stimulants, *JAMA* 252(14): 1898-1903, 1984.
52. Freestone S, Ramsay LE: Pressor effect of coffee and cigarette smoking in hypertensive patients, *Clin Sci* 63:403, 1982.
53. The Fifth Report of the Joint National Committee on Detection, Evaluation, and Treatment of High Blood Pressure (JNC V): 1993, *Arch Intern Med* 153:154-182, 1993.

54. Frohlich ED, Grim C, Labarthe DR: Recommendations for human blood pressure determination by sphygmomanometers: report of a special task force appointed by the Steering Committee, AHA, *Hypertension* 11:209A-222A, 1988.
55. Hossman V, Fitzgerald GA, Dollery CT: Influence of hospitalization and placebo therapy on blood pressure and sympathetic function in essential hypertension, *Hypertension* 3:113, 1981.
56. Dubin D: *Rapid interpretation of EKGs*, ed 4, 1994, Imago.
57. Stamler J, Stamler R, Neaton JD: Blood pressure, systolic and diastolic, and cardiovascular risks: US population data, *Arch Intern Med* 153:598-615, 1993.
58. American Heart Association Subcommittee of Nutritionists: American Heart Association guidelines for weight management programs for healthy adults, *Heart Dis Stroke* 3(4):221-228, 1994.
59. Sacks FM and others: Effects on blood pressure of reduced dietary sodium and the dietary approaches to stop hypertension (DASH) diet, *N Engl J Med* 34(1):3-10.
60. Kaplan NM: Implications for cost-effectiveness: combination therapy for systemic hypertension, *Am J Cardiol* 76:595-597, 1995.
61. Epstein M, Bakris G: Newer approaches to antihypertensive therapy: use of fixed dose combination therapy, *Arch Intern Med* 156:1969-1978, 1996.
62. Kaplan NM, Gifford RW: Choice of initial therapy for hypertension, *JAMA* 275(20):1577-1580, 1996.
63. Lyons D, Petrie JC, Reid JL: Drug treatment: present and future, *Br Med Bull* 50(2):472-493, 1994.
64. Rutherford JD, Braunwald E: Chronic ischemic heart disease. In Braunwald E, editor: *Heart disease: a textbook of cardiovascular medicine*, ed 4, Philadelphia, 1992, WB Saunders.
65. ACC/AHA Task Force on Practice Guidelines: ACC/AHA guidelines for the management of patients with acute myocardial infarction: a report of the American College of Cardiology/American Heart Association Task Force on Practice Guidelines (Committee on Management of Acute Myocardial Infarction), *Circulation* 28:1328, 1996.
66. Effect of metoprolol CR/XL in chronic heart failure: metoprolol CR/XL randomized intervention trial in congestive heart failure(MERIT-HF), *Lancet* 353: (9169):2001-2007, 1999.
67. Packer M and others (US Carvedilol Heart Failure Study Group): The effect of carvedilol on morbidity and mortality in patients with chronic heart failure, *N Engl J Med* 334(21):1349-1355, 1996.
68. Messerli FH, Grossman E, Goldbourt U: Are beta-blockers efficacious as first-line therapy for hypertension in the elderly? *JAMA* 279:1903-1907, 1998.
69. Staessen JA and others: Randomised double-blind comparison of placebo and active treatment for older patients with isolated systolic hypertension: the Systolic Hypertension in Europe (Syst-Eur) Trial Investigators, *Lancet* 350:757-764, 1997.
70. Gifford RW: Antihypertensive therapy: angiotensin-converting enzyme inhibitors, angiotensin II receptor antagonists, and calcium antagonists, *Med Clin North Am* 81(6):1319-1333, 1997.
71. Consensus statement: Treatment of hypertension in diabetes, *Diabetes Care* 19(suppl 1): S107-S113, 1996.
72. The EUCLID study group: Randomised placebo-controlled trial of lisinopril in normotensive patients with insulin-dependent diabetes and normoalbuminuria or microalbuminuria, *Lancet* 349:1787-1791, 1997.
73. The SOLVD Investigators: Effect of enalapril on survival in patients with reduced left ventricular ejection fractions and congestive heart failure, *N Engl J Med* 325:293-302, 1991.
74. Cohn JN and others: A randomized trial of the angiotensin-receptor blocker valsartan in chronic heart failure, *N Engl J Med* 345(23): 1667-1675, 2001.
75. BM Brenner and others: Effects of losartan on renal and cardiovascular outcomes in patients with type 2 diabetes and nephropathy, *N Engl J Med* 345:861-869, 2001.
76. EJ Lewis and others: Renoprotective effect of the angiotensin-receptor antagonist irbesartan in patients with nephropathy due to type 2 diabetes, *N Engl J Med* 345:851-860, 2001.
77. Parving HH and others: The effect of irbesartan on the development of diabetic nephropathy in patients with type 2 diabetes, *N Engl J Med* 435:870-878, 2001.
78. Epstein M: The calcium antagonist controversy: the emerging importance of drug formulation as a determinant of risk, *Am J Cardiol* 79(10A):9-19, 1997.
79. Sowers JR: Effects of calcium antagonists on insulin sensitivity and other metabolic parameters, *Am J Cardiol* 79(10A):24-28, 1997.
80. Frishman WH: Use of calcium antagonists in patients with ischemic heart disease and systemic hypertension, *Am J Cardiol* 79(10A):37-38, 1997.
81. Psaty BM and others: The risk of myocardial infarction associated with antihypertensive drug therapies, *JAMA* 274(8):620-625, 1995.
82. Alderman MH: Effect of long-acting and short-acting calcium antagonists on cardiovascular outcomes in hypertensive patients, *Lancet* 349:594-598, 1997.
83. ALLHAT Collaborative Research Group: Major cardiovascular events in hypertensive patients randomized to doxazosin vs chlorthalidone in the antihypertensive and lipid-lowering treatment to prevent heart attack trial (ALLHAT), *JAMA* 283:1967-1975, 2000.
84. Kaplan NM: Systemic hypertension: therapy. In Braunwald E, editor: *Heart disease: a textbook of cardiovascular medicine*, ed 4, Philadelphia, 1992, WB Saunders.
85. Cohn J and others: A comparison of enalapril with hydralazine-isosorbide dinitrate in the treatment of chronic congestive heart failure, *N Engl J Med* 325:303-310, 1991.
86. Dahlof B and others: Morbidity and mortality in the Swedish Trial in Old Patients with Hypertension (STOP-Hypertension), *Lancet* 338:1281-1285, 1991.
87. Glynn RJ and others: Use of antihypertensive drugs and trends in blood pressure in the elderly, *Arch Intern Med* 155:1855-1860, 1995.
88. Kaplan NM: Hypertension in the elderly, *Annu Rev Med* 45:27-35, 1995.
89. Sadowski AV, Redeker NS: The hypertensive elder: a review for the primary care provider, *Nurse Pract* 21(5):99-118, 1996.
90. Forette F and others: Prevention of dementia in randomized double-blind controlled Systolic Hypertension in Europe (Syst-Eur) trial, *Lancet* 352:1347-1351, 1998.
91. Chobanian AV, Alexander W: Exacerbation of atherosclerosis by hypertension, *Arch Intern Med* 156:1952-1956, 1996.
92. Arnett DK and others: Hypertension and subclinical carotid artery atherosclerosis in blacks and whites: the Atherosclerosis Risk in Communities Study, *Arch Intern Med* 156:1983-1989, 1996.
93. Thach AM, Schultz PJ: Nonemergent hypertension, *Emerg Med Clin North Am* 13(4):1009-1035, 1995.
94. Psaty BM and others: Health outcomes associated with antihypertensive therapies used as first-line agents: a systematic review and meta-analysis, *JAMA* 277(9):739-745, 1997.
95. Elias MF and others: Untreated blood pressure level is inversely related to cognitive functioning: The Framingham Study, *Am J Epidemiol* 138(6):353-364, 1993.
96. Skoog I and others: 15-year longitudinal study of blood pressure and dementia, *Lancet* 347:1141-1145, 1996.
97. Kaplan NM: Management of hypertensive emergencies, *Lancet* 344:1335-1338, 1994.
98. Murphy C: Hypertensive emergencies, *Emerg Med Clin North Am* 13(4):973-1006, 1995.
99. ACC/AHA Guidelines for exercise testing: executive summary, *Circulation* 96:345-354, 1997.

CHAPTER 134

Myocarditis

JoAnn Trybulski

DEFINITION/EPIDEMIOLOGY

Myocarditis, or inflammation of the myocardium, affects the myocardial cell, interstitium, or vascular components singularly or in combination, producing varied symptoms of variable duration.[1] The presentation of myocarditis may be subacute with minor symptoms that resolve spontaneously or acute with severe, even life-threatening symptoms; moreover, symptoms may persist for extended time in a chronic form of the illness.[1]

Myocardial inflammation is caused by a myriad of viruses, including human immunodeficiency virus; in addition, fungi, rickettsiae, bacteria, spirochetes, protozoans, helminthes, medications, chemicals, systemic and metabolic disorders, pregnancy, radiation, physical agents (the most common is alcohol), hypersensitivity, or autoimmune reactions are precipitants (Box 134-1).[1,2] The incidence varies; epidemic outbreaks and clustering in families have been observed.[2]

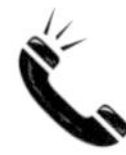

Physician consultation is indicated for patients with suspected myocarditis.

PATHOPHYSIOLOGY

The origin of myocarditis can be multifactorial. Current explanations of pathogenesis center on two mechanisms: infectious and autoimmune or hypersensitivity. In infectious myocarditis the replication of the pathogen in myocardial tissue can damage myocardial cells by tissue toxins, which initiates a cellular and humoral immunologic response.[1,2] A maladaptive response produces myocardial damage by means of sensitized and hyperreactive T lymphocytes, resulting in autoimmune reactions of varying degrees and duration.[2] Factors that affect the immunologic response and cause the maladaptive response are toxic effects of the pathogen or substance on myocardial tissue in combination with host factors such as familial predisposition, peripartum state, hypoxia, exercise, nutritional status, ethanol intake, ionizing radiation, and exposure to temperature extremes.[3] The autoimmune response may be triggered by an infectious agent as explained previously or initiated as a reaction to a substance or condition. The common pathway seems to be the existence of cytokines, which are present in any T-cell–mediated response.[3]

Recovery can be complete and without any damage, or the clinical course can be marked by progression to heart failure. Myocarditis has been found to be a precursor of cardiomyopathy, which may present years after the initial inflammation.[4]

Three stages characterize viral myocarditis; each stage has different pathophysiology and manifestations. In phase 1, the viral phase, the virus enters the myocytes and trigger an immune response. This immune response modulates further replication of the virus but also enhances additional viral entry that may continue immune activation; this secondary immune response is predominant in the pathogenesis of mycocarditis.[5] Phase 2 includes triggering of an autoimmune response via T-cell activation, cytokine activation, and CD4 cell activation that produces autoreactive antibodies. The activated products destroy the virus-containing cells, in this case the myocytes, reducing the number of functional heart muscle cells.[5] This destruction of heart muscle cells over time produces dilated cardiomyopathy and represents the third phase of viral myocarditis. In one trial, patients with a more aggressive early immune response had a less severe course, whereas those with high levels of circulating CD2+ T-cells, indicating a greater late immune response and activation capable of mediating an autoimmune type of response, had an increased incidence of dilated cardiomyopathy and poorer survival statistics.[6]

CLINICAL PRESENTATION

Presenting symptoms range from asymptomatic, with diagnosis an incidental finding on autopsy, to cardiomyopathy with end-stage heart failure. Brief cardiac inflammation is quite common with viral infections and may account for the transient weakness and transient exertional tachycardia early in viral illnesses.[1]

These symptoms resolve after several days. Reports of continued fatigue, coupled with tachycardia associated with minimal exertion or palpitations, should prompt investigation for myocarditis. Patients often recount accelerated pulse or palpitations in response to stimulants such as caffeine or alcohol and to even mildly exciting or stressful situations such as watching a sporting event or movie or reading a tense book passage. The clinical presentation may be characterized by various degrees of heart failure. Fever may be present,[2] as well as symptoms commonly found in the condition causing the myocarditis.

Acute chest pain mimicking myocardial infarction or the coexistence of pericarditis can occur with myocarditis.[1] Signs and symptoms of pulmonary and systemic embolism can coexist as a complication.[1] Regrettably, sudden death secondary to arrhythmia or heart block or failure can be the initial presentation.[1,3]

PHYSICAL EXAMINATION

Tachycardia, either resting, with minimal exertion, or out of proportion to any fever, is a prominent feature.[1,3] Ectopy is often detected. Because the presentation of myocarditis ranges from asymptomatic to overt heart failure, the physical examination finding will reflect this spectrum. Some infectious agents such as the coxsackievirus also affect the pericardium, producing pericardial pain, audible friction rub, or pleural effusion.[7]

Signs of heart failure vary with its severity. In myocarditis accompanied by heart failure, an S_3 and/or S_4 may be detected by cardiac auscultation. Milder cases may show only vascular redistribution of flow to upper lobes on chest x-ray film and no abnormal cardiac examination findings, whereas in more severe cases gallops, murmurs, peripheral edema, and an abnormal chest x-ray film showing an enlarged heart may be present.[1]

BOX 134-1

COMMON CAUSES OF MYOCARDITIS

INFECTIOUS
Rickettsia (typhus, Q fever, Rocky Mountain spotted fever)
Diphtheria
Gonococcal
Typhoid fever
Salmonella
Streptococci
Tuberculosis
Menigococci
Brucellosis
Clostridia
Staphylococci
Psittacosis
Mycoplasma pneumoniae
Melioidosis
Syphillis
Leptospirosis
Borelliosis
Lyme disease
Fungal (e.g., aspergillosis, candidiasis, coccidioidomycosis)
Helminthic disease (e.g., trichinosis)
Protozoal disease

VIRAL
Coxsackie virus
Echovirus
HIV
Cytomegalovirus
Poliomyelitis
Mononucleosis
Hepatitis
Rubeola
Varicella
Respiratory syncytial virus
Herpes simplex virus
Arbovirus
Adenovirus
Yellow fever
Rabies

SYSTEMIC CONDITIONS
Pregnancy
Kawasaki disease
Collagen-vascular disorders (e.g., lupus)
Infiltrative disorders (e.g., sarcoidosis)
Hypereosinophilia
Wegener's granulomatosis
Thyrotoxicosis

DRUGS/SUBSTANCES
Hypersensitivity reactions
Insect/snake bites
Acetozolamide
Alcohol
p-Aminosalicylic acid
Amphetamines
Amphotericin B
Antimony
Arsenic
Barbiturates
Caffeine
Carbamazepine
Carbon monoxide
Catecholamines
Chloramphenicol
Cocaine
Diphenylhydatoin
Diphtheria or tetanus toxoid
Diuretics
5-Fluorouracil
Heavy metals
Horse serum
Immunosuppressives
Indomethacin
Isoniazid
Lithium
Penicillins
Phenothiazines
Phenylbutazone
Quinidine
Rapeseed oil
Smallpox vaccine
Streptomycin
Sulfonamides
Sulfonylureas
Theophylline
Tetracycline

Modified from Rodenheffer R, Gersh B: Dilated cardiomyopathies and the mycarditides. In Guilani ER and others, editors: *The Mayo Clinic practice of cardiology,* St Louis, 1996, Mosby.

DIAGNOSTICS

Because myocarditis has varied presentations, the diagnosis is made either by clinical signs and symptoms or by pathologic cell biopsy criteria; these are neither uniformly sensitive or specific.[8] Uniformly accepted diagnostic criteria are lacking.[9]

Initial laboratory evaluation includes CBC, cardiac enzymes, evaluation of renal and liver function, and appropriate titers, including viral or Lyme. In addition, other tests are indicated to elicit the suspected cause of myocardial inflammation as necessary.

A chest x-ray study is obtained; as mentioned previously, results are consistent with the degree of heart failure present. The ECG can be normal or reveal ST segment and T-wave abnormalities. These abnormalities may vary and the ECG may revert to normal on recovery.[2]

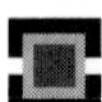

Diagnostics

Myocarditis

Initial
Pulse oximetry*
Monitoring for palpitations

Laboratory
CBC and differential
Cardiac enzymes
BUN
Creatinine
LFTs
Disease titers

Imaging
Chest x-ray
MRI*

Other
Myocardial biopsy*
Echocardiogram
Electrocardiogram
Holter or event monitoring

*If indicated.

Atrial and/or ventricular arrhythmias with or without atrioventricular conduction blocks occur.[1] Consideration for 24-hour cardiac monitoring is helpful when palpitations are reported to assess their clinical implications. An echocardiogram detects valvular, wall motion, and left ventricular output abnormalities.

If pulse oximetry is available in the office setting, it can be a useful modality to assist with diagnosis in mildly symptomatic cases with questionable tachycardia. The pulse oximeter is attached, and resting pulse rate and oxygen saturation in arterial blood (SaO_2) are recorded. The patient can then be asked to perform the maneuver that precipitates the tachycardia, such as walking a certain distance or climbing a flight of stairs, while pulse rates and SaO_2 are recorded. Tachycardia and mild desaturation have been observed. Of course, any findings of heart failure or reports of symptomatic palpitations or chest discomfort eliminate this as a recommended diagnostic aid.

The patient's clinical status and potential for deterioration in condition determine whether the initial evaluation is done as outpatient or in the monitored hospital setting. Patients with severe cases of myocarditis are evaluated for myocardial biopsy to determine the diagnosis and to assess therapeutic response.[1] However, the rate of positive biopsy ranges from 5% to 60% in patients with a clinical diagnosis of myocarditis.[4] The low correlation of histologic evidence with clinical findings may be because of the difficulty of pathologists to apply the Dallas Criteria as accepted pathologic proof of myocarditis.[4] The Dallas Criteria consider evidence of myocyte damage to be the presence of inflammatory infiltrate, T-cell lymphocytes only, with potential for disagreement on the minimum number of T-cells needed to meet criteria for diagnosis.[4] These criteria, established in 1984, exclude other evidence of inflammation such as cytokines, B-cells, adhesion molecules, activated macrophages, and expressions of class II major histocompatibility antigens.[4]

The difficulty in establishing uniformly applicable diagnostic criteria may stem from the failure to define cellular markers or cell pathology indicative of myocarditis; or perhaps the multiple etiologies produce distinctly different clinical presentations.[6] Also, the infiltrative process of myocarditis may be transient, confounding biopsy results.[7]

Measurement for elevation in serum troponin I, a serum marker associated with cardiac injury that persists for up to 14 days, is under investigation as a diagnostic aid.[8] Nuclear imaging modalities such as antimyosin immunoscintigraphy have been used by cardiologists.[9] Therefore decisions about the specific diagnostic testing that a patient requires are made in consultation with cardiology.

DIFFERENTIAL DIAGNOSIS

Other causes for arrhythmia, heart failure, and poor exercise tolerance, including coronary artery, pulmonary, or valvular heart disease, must be excluded. Particularly, the existence of cardiomyopathy needs to be disproved. Cardiomyopathy is cardiac muscle disease, classified as dilated, hypertrophic, or restrictive.[1,10] If cardiomyopathy is suspected, appropriate testing to exclude reversible etiologies and tests evaluating cardiac function are required. Reversible causes of cardiomyopathy include metabolic and infiltrative diseases (i.e., hemochromatosis, amyloidosis, sarcoidosis, or glycogen storage disease), metabolic disorders (i.e., thyroid disease, acromegaly, Cushing's disease, or pheochromocytoma), toxic effects (i.e., alcohol, cocaine, antineoplastic agents, or amphetamines), radiation effects, nutritional deficiencies (i.e., thiamine or hypophosphatemia), collagen disorders, rheumatic fever, rheumatoid arthritis, neuromuscular disorders, septic shock, or transplant rejection.[1,9] An interesting cause of cardiomyopathy is Chagas' disease, a parasitic infection found predominately in Central and South America, which may present with cardiomyopathy years after the initial infection.

MANAGEMENT

Supportive therapy with bed rest; quiet environment; and restriction of smoking, alcohol, and caffeine is indicated for all patients. The decision to hospitalize is determined by the patient's clinical status, the etiology of the myocarditis, and the presence of arrhythmias or heart failure. Some patients with mild viral myocarditis and no heart failure or life-threatening arrhythmias may be managed as outpatients.

There is controversy over the role of prednisone alone or in combination with immunosuppressive agents in the treatment of myocarditis.[4,6] Therefore management of a patient with myocarditis is best achieved in consultation with a cardiologist. With infectious myocarditis, suppression of the early immune response with nonsteroidal antiinflammatory agents has shown increased viral replication and inflammation, producing more cardiac injury.[3] Therefore use of nonsteroidal agents should be restricted during the acute phase of the viral disease. Immunosuppression may be recommended in cases of biopsy-proven myocarditis, those patients not responding to conventional therapy, before transplantation, and in patients with giant-cell myocarditis (severe symptoms with rapid disease progression).[11]

With viral myocarditis, an assessment of the phase of the disease is helpful, as recommendations have the potential to increase damage when the nonsteroidal agents are used at an incorrect stage of the disease. In phase 1, the viral replication phase, antiviral therapies are considered less

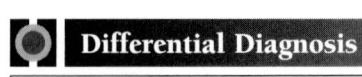

Differential Diagnosis

Myocarditis

Cardiomyopathy
Valvular heart disease
Pulmonary heart disease
Coronary heart disease
Arrhythmia etiologies

helpful, as viral replication precedes development of the cardiac manifestations that characterize the condition, unless the specific viral agent has been identified or when there is a know viral epidemic.[5] Immunosuppressive therapies are typically avoided at this stage. Because studies have yielded inconsistent results with immunosuppressive therapies, only well-studied immunosuppressive drugs should be used and their use confined to well-defined stage 2 patients.[5] One study points to the benefit of immunosuppressive therapy in patients with inflammatory dilated cardiomyopathy and active immune damage as demonstrated by the presence of human leukocyte antigen with myocardial biopsy.[12] The use of high-dose intravenous immunoglobulin for acute viral myocarditis is an area of ongoing investigation.[13]

Antiarrhythmic medications are used to suppress life-threatening arrhythmias.[2] Cardiac failure is managed with conventional heart failure regimens including angiotensin-converting enzyme inhibitors, diuretics, salt restriction, digitalis, beta blockers, vasodilators, aldosterone antagonists, and other modalities as determined by the patient's status.[14] Temporary or permanent pacing is indicated for symptomatic heart block.[2] Ventricular assist devices are currently being investigated. In one case report a ventricular assist device was used successfully for short-term use (20 days) with refractory ventricular fibrillation that was time limited.[15] Cardiac transplantation may be indicated in severe, irreversible cases. All management decisions are made with cardiology consultation.

LIFE SPAN CONSIDERATIONS

Young adults who present with chest pain and ECG changes suggestive of acute myocardial infarction should be investigated for nonrheumatic poststreptococcal myocarditis.[16] Myocarditis, leading to dilated cardiomyopathy, can be a complication of pregnancy, presenting in the last month or the first months after delivery.[2]

COMPLICATIONS

Sudden death from heart block, failure, or arrhythmia may occur.[1,3] Thromboembolic episodes can occur. Cardiomyopathy may ensue or occur years after apparent recovery.[3] Also, patients are at risk for continued cardiac symptoms in the chronic form of myocarditis.[1]

INDICATIONS FOR REFERRAL/HOSPITALIZATION

Physician consultation is indicated during the initial evaluation and management and with follow-up evaluation of all patients with myocarditis. All patients suspected of myocarditis should have cardiology consultation to assist with their diagnosis and management and, if necessary, myocardial care biopsy.

All patients with myocarditis associated with heart failure or the potential for life-threatening arrhythmias should be hospitalized. In other patients the severity of the condition causing the myocarditis in association with the clinical status determines whether hospitalization is warranted.

PATIENT AND FAMILY EDUCATION

Patients with altered cardiac function are understandably anxious about their condition. A careful, sensitive explanation about the cause for the condition, rationale for testing, and realistic appraisal of their clinical status is vital for all patients with myocarditis.

Because stress has been found to cause tachycardia and palpitations in these patients, the importance of avoiding stimulating situations and substances such as caffeine, alcohol, chocolate, and cold medications should be emphasized. Rest with avoidance of any physical exercise, even housework or driving, is indicated in the acute phase. If patients are managed at home, family members should also be informed regarding the importance of observing these restrictions.

Teaching about any medication is essential, as is reviewing the signs and symptoms that prompt immediate attention (i.e., fatigue, dyspnea, weight gain, swollen ankles, chest pain, mentation difficulty, unilateral leg pain, dizziness, or light-headedness in conjunction with palpitations). Patients should be instructed to "listen to their body" as they recover and resume activity gradually, while monitoring for elevated pulse rate and palpitations as indicators that an activity is still not tolerated. Frequent rest periods are indicated during the recovery period.

Work restrictions may be necessary for an extended period, even with mild cases. Patients should be seen regularly for support and guidance during the sometimes lengthy convalescent period. The importance of yearly vaccination against influenza is stressed with these patients. Continued support and explanations of the recovery process for family members are mandatory.

Anecdotally a mild, transient recurrence of palpitations and exertional tachycardia with subsequent infection has been observed. Patients recently recovered from myocarditis can be reassured about this occurrence, providing there are no symptomatic palpitations or signs of heart failure. However, it is not known if this is a variant of or a marker for a chronic form of the disease.

All patients with a history of myocarditis should be assessed periodically for signs and symptoms of cardiomyopathy (i.e., dyspnea, exercise intolerance, and cardiac enlargement). The role of alcohol in the development of cardiomyopathy should be explained.

REFERENCES

1. Shah PM: Cardiomyopathies. In Stein JH, editor: *Internal medicine*, ed 5, St Louis, 1998, Mosby.
2. Rodenheffer R, Gersh B: Dilated cardiomyopathies and the myocarditides. In Guiliani ER et al, editors: *The Mayo Clinic practice of cardiology*, St Louis, 1996, Mosby.
3. Roddenheffer R, Gersh BJ, Kennel AJ: Myocarditis, dilated cardiomyopathy, and specific myocardial disease. In Guiliani ER et al, editors: *Cardiology: fundamentals and practice*, St Louis, 1991, Mosby.
4. McKenna WJ, Davies MJ: Editorial on immunosuppressive therapy for myocarditis, *N Engl J Med* 333(5):312, 1995.
5. Liu PP, Mason JW: Advances in the understanding of myocarditis, *Circulation* 104(9):1076-1082, 2001.
6. Mason JW and others: A clinical trial of immunosuppressive therapy for myocarditis, *N Engl J Med* 333(5):269-275, 1995.
7. Abelmann WH: Myocarditis. In Hurst JW, editor: *Medicine for the practicing physician*, Stamford, Conn, 1996, Appleton & Lange.
8. Smith SC and others: Elevations of cardiac troponin I associated with myocarditis, *Circulation* 95(1):163, 1997.
9. Khaw BA, Narula J: Non-invasive detection of myocyte necrosis in myocarditis and dilated cardiomyopathy with radiolabelled antimyosin, *Eur Heart J* 16(suppl O):119-123, 1995.

10. Baughmann KL, Kasper EK, Hershkowitz A: Myocardial and pericardial disease. In Noble J, editor: *Primary care medicine*, ed 2, St Louis, 1996, Mosby.
11. Caforio AL, McKenna WJ: Recognition and optimum management of myocarditis, *Drugs* 52(4):515-525, 1996.
12. Wojcincz R and others: Randomized, placebo-controlled study for immunosuppressive treatment of inflammatory dilated cardiomyopathy: two year follow-up results, *Circulation* 104:39-45, 2001.
13. Tedeschi A and others: High-dose intravenous immunoglobulin in the treatment of acute myocarditis: a case report and review of the literature, *J Intern Med* 251(2):169-175, 2002.
14. Parrillo JE: Inflammatory cardiomyopathy (myocarditis): which patients should be treated with anti-inflammatory therapy? *Circulation* 104(1):4, 2001.
15. McGovern PC and others: Successful explantation of a ventricular assist device following fulminant influenza type A-associated myocarditis, *J Heart Lung Transplant* 21(2):290-293, 2002.
16. Gill MV, Klein NC, Cunha BA: Non-rheumatic poststreptococcal myocarditis, *Heart Lung* 24(2):425, 1995.

CHAPTER 135

Peripheral Arterial Insufficiency

David R. Campbell

Peripheral arterial insufficiency is the condition that results when there is insufficient blood flow to the extremities. It is much more likely to occur in the lower extremities, although the increasing use of catheter interventions has made upper extremity problems more common. If the symptoms have been present for weeks or months, the condition is defined as chronic. If the symptoms develop over hours or days, it is referred to as acute.

Immediate physician/vascular surgeon referral is indicated for suspected arterial occlusion or dissecting aneurysm.

Chronic Arterial Insufficiency

DEFINITION/EPIDEMIOLOGY

Chronic arterial insufficiency is one disease that has increasing prevalence as the population ages. As the major cause is atherosclerosis, the risk factors for chronic arterial insufficiency are the same as those for coronary artery disease. Diabetes, hypertension, hyperlipidemia, and tobacco intake are all independent risk factors. Smokers are twice as likely to develop claudication.[1] Vascular disease is one of the most common complications of diabetes. Genetic factors have also long been recognized as being important, and recently an increased level of homocysteine has been shown to be associated with premature atherosclerosis.[2] Even in younger patients, premature atherosclerosis is the most common cause of chronic arterial insufficiency, although rare causes include entrapment syndromes and adventitial cystic disease of the popliteal artery.

Numerous studies have confirmed that most patients with obstructive arterial disease have underlying coronary artery disease or diabetes and have on average a 10-year shorter life span.[1] The amputation rate is about 1% per year. However, the amputation rate is much higher in patients with diabetes and in active smokers.[1]

PATHOPHYSIOLOGY

The atherosclerotic plaque causing leg ischemia is identical to that seen in coronary artery disease and carotid disease. It is an intimal lesion that may affect any of the vessels of the lower extremity. The blockage may build up slowly, allowing collateral vessels to develop and thereby minimizing symptoms. Alternatively, intraplaque hemorrhage and thrombosis may lead to sudden expansion and acute symptomatology. The infrarenal aorta and iliac arteries are known as the inflow arteries, whereas the femoral popliteal and tibial vessels are the outflow vessels. Obstruction of the aortoiliac and femoral arteries is often seen in smokers, whereas tibial artery disease is much more common in patients with diabetes.

CLINICAL PRESENTATION

The classic symptom of peripheral arterial insufficiency is claudication. Claudication a tightening or cramping pain usually in the calf muscles that is precipitated with exercise and is relieved with rest. With exercise there is an increased demand for blood that cannot be met. Subsequently lactic acid and other metabolites build up in the muscle, causing discomfort. The severity is assessed by how far a patient can walk before pain ensues. Although the distance may be reduced by an incline, cold weather, or a recent meal, it generally tends to be fairly consistent. Pain is always relieved immediately by stopping the activity and never occurs when the patient is at rest. Sometimes the thigh or buttock muscles are affected first. This is indicative of iliac artery obstruction (Leriche's syndrome). As the obstruction becomes more severe, the patient may develop pain at rest because circulation to the feet is impaired. Characteristically, the patient will go to bed and be awakened after a couple of hours by pain in the toes that is only relieved by gravity (e.g., getting out of bed or hanging the feet over the side of the bed). The patient may resort to sleeping in a chair to avoid the pain. Eventually, there is not enough blood to sustain viability, and gangrene ensues, usually beginning in the toes or heels. Ischemic rest pain is consistent; it occurs every night, unlike the intermittent leg cramps seen so often in older adults, which are not related to arterial insufficiency.

PHYSICAL EXAMINATION

On physical examination, muscle wasting, loss of hair, and reduced temperature in the affected limb may be noted. Careful pulse examination is very important. Absent femoral pulses suggest inflow disease, whereas the absence of popliteal pulses implies isolated tibial disease. One physical sign that can be helpful in the diagnosis of peripheral vascular disease is the presence of dependent rubor. If the ischemic leg is elevated for 30 seconds, it becomes pale, as blood is unable to travel uphill. This renders the tissue ischemic, and the capillaries vasodilate. If the leg is then made dependent, blood travels down to those dilated capillaries, and a deep red color ensues. The longer the rubor takes to develop, the worse the ischemia. A careful history and physical examination will allow for a good assessment of the functional severity of the obstruction and the likely location.

DIAGNOSTICS

The most useful tool in assessing peripheral arterial insufficiency in the office is a portable Doppler instrument and a sphygmomanometer cuff. By using these tools, it is possible to compare the systolic pressure at the brachial artery with that in the dorsalis pedis and posterior tibial arteries. This measurement is expressed as the ankle brachial index (ABI) and should be greater than the one in the normal extremity. An ABI of 0.75 to 0.5 is consistent with claudication, and an ABI below 0.5 is consistent with rest pain or gangrene.

Patients with mild claudication may have palpable pulses at rest but lose them with exercise. This is best demonstrated in the vascular laboratory with an exercise noninvasive study. During this test, the patient is placed on a treadmill and ABIs are measured at rest, while exercising, and on recovery.

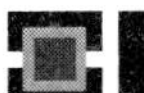

Diagnostics

Chronic Arterial Insufficiency

Initial
Doppler ankle/arm indexes

Laboratory
Serum glucose and lipid profile

Imaging
Doppler flow studies

Other
Treadmill testing
Plethysmography
Arteriography

Sometimes related medical conditions, such as obesity or peripheral edema, make it impossible to assess the pulse status. In these situations the pocket Doppler instrument may be invaluable. A normal pulse is triphasic but becomes increasingly monophasic with proximal obstruction. With practice it is relatively simple to distinguish these pulses. If there are good triphasic pulses by Doppler ultrasonography in the feet, there is unlikely to be significant ischemia. If the vascular status is unclear with physical examination, patients should be referred to the vascular laboratory for formal evaluation. Evaluation will provide the ABIs, the level at which the pulse becomes monophasic, and the pulse volume recording (a plethysmographic test that records the volume of the extremity with each heartbeat). The forefoot tracing is helpful for the vascular surgeon to determine whether there is enough circulation to heal a foot lesion. This is particularly important in patients with diabetes, in whom ABIs are often inaccurate.

Other tests are available but are used less often except in research protocols. Chief among these is the measurement of transcutaneous oxygen, which reflects the metabolic state of the target tissues. Unfortunately, variants such as ambient temperature make this test impractical as a routine test. Instead of a treadmill test, it is possible to use reactive hyperemia obtained after inflating a pressure cuff to suprasystolic pressure to produce vasodilation; however, this is somewhat uncomfortable and has not become routinely available.

DIFFERENTIAL DIAGNOSIS

The presence of peripheral neuropathy in diabetes makes the diagnosis of peripheral insufficiency quite difficult. Damage to the peripheral nerves may mask the symptoms of arterial insufficiency. Thus if patients have no feeling in their legs, they may simply complain that their legs get tired of walking. Without sensation, there may be no rest pain, and patients may present with painless gangrene. Other conditions that should be considered include cauda equina syndrome, Buerger's disease, leg cramps, or musculoskeletal disorders.

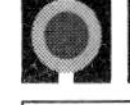

Differential Diagnosis

Chronic Arterial Insufficiency

Acute peripheral arterial occlusion
Peripheral neuropathy
Cauda equina syndrome
Buerger's disease
Musculoskeletal condition
Leg cramps

Cauda Equina Syndrome

Spinal stenosis causing pressure on the nerve roots may result in symptoms of claudication from the hip downward, which can easily be confused with Leriche's syndrome. This is becoming increasingly common as the population ages and progressive degenerative joint disease becomes more prevalent. The correct diagnosis can be made by ordering noninvasive exercise studies. In cauda equina syndrome there will be no pressure drop when the patient exercises on a treadmill.

Buerger's Disease

Buerger's disease is an inflammatory occlusive disease involving primarily the medium and smaller arteries of both the upper and lower extremities. Although uncommon in the United States, it is seen more often in the Middle and Far East and appears to be directly related to the effects of smoking. Patients manifest the signs and symptoms of chronic arterial insufficiency, but apart from smoking have no other risk factors for atherosclerosis. Bypass surgery is rarely indicated because disease is more distal, but patients will experience remission if exposure to nicotine is avoided.

MANAGEMENT

Management of chronic arterial insufficiency depends on the severity of the symptoms. If the patient has stable claudication and is managing without much difficulty, then it is reasonable to treat the patient conservatively. Patients with mild, recent-onset claudication are quite likely to improve with conservative measures alone. These include lifestyle modifications as indicated, particularly tobacco cessation. Studies comparing exercise with angioplasty have shown that a daily exercise program involving walking to the point of pain as often as possible is as effective as angioplasty in providing relief of symptoms.[3] Because the ABI does not change, it is believed that this effect is produced by training the muscles rather than producing increased flow to the foot. Hypertension, hyperlipidemia, and diabetes must be treated aggressively.

Because these patients are at high risk for coronary artery disease, it is prudent to start them on a daily aspirin dosage as well. The literature on the role of aspirin, dipyridamole, and ticlopidine in peripheral vascular disease is extensive and quite confusing.[4] There is much disagreement as to whether aspirin confers benefit either preoperatively or postoperatively in patients with peripheral vascular disease. There is agreement, however, that low-dose aspirin (81 to 650 mg/day) reduces the incidence and mortality of subsequent myocardial infarction in patients over 50 years old. It makes sense therefore to initiate low-dose aspirin for all patients with peripheral vascular disease provided that there are no contraindications. There has never been a study demonstrating a benefit to adding dipyridamole to that regimen. Ticlopidine, another antiplatelet agent, is at least as effective as aspirin, but it is expensive and has significant side effects. Clopidogrel (Plavix) is also more effective than aspirin and safer than ticlopidine, but it, too, is expensive and its role, if any, in the management of peripheral vascular disease remains to be determined.

Pentoxifylline (Trental) has been shown to increase the distance that 30% of patients with claudication can walk, although the effect has been small. Recent trials of cilostazol (Pletal), a phosphodiesterase III inhibitor, have demonstrated significant improvement over both placebo and pentoxifylline in distance walked without symptoms for patients with claudication.[5] The main contraindication for cilostazol is a history of congestive heart failure. It is safe to say that neither of these drugs has had the impact on the management of claudication as hoped.

COMPLICATIONS

Lower extremity ulcers may result from neuropathy, arterial insufficiency, infection, or a combination of these (see Box 137-1). Infection such as cellulitis or ulcers with extensive involvement may result in osteomyelitis. The presence of infection can also disturb blood glucose control, complicating diabetes management.

Associated with peripheral neuropathy is the development of calcification of the arteries. This is not related to the atherosclerotic lesion, which is an intimal lesion, but it does render the vessels relatively incompressible. This means that the ABI may be artifactually elevated and less helpful in assessing the degree of ischemia. In these cases the pulse volume recording can be particularly helpful.

A total of 30% of patients with neuropathy also have an autonomic neuropathy, which is sometimes called an autosympathectomy. This condition results in diversion of blood from the nutrient vessels to the skin, making the skin unnaturally warm. Thus it is possible to see a diabetic patient with a minor skin lesion but with no symptoms and a warm foot that is critically ischemic. Failure to recognize this may result in further loss of tissue.

Diabetic Foot Ulcer

Diabetic neuropathy is a polyneuropathy and has a motor component. The paralysis of the intrinsic muscles results in clawing of the foot, and the patient tends to develop traumatic lesions over the metatarsal heads and on the tops of the toes. Healing may be impaired by relative arterial insufficiency.

Any infection requires treatment with appropriate debridement and antibiotics. Also, bed rest is indicated to minimize damage that may go undetected if neuropathy is present. If the ulcer is superficial, it can be treated on an outpatient basis, with non–weight bearing, dressing care, and a first-generation cephalosporin. If the ulcer is deep or there is a significant cellulitis, hospitalization is advised and broad-spectrum antibiotics instituted. Failure to heal with treatment suggests arterial insufficiency and merits referral to a vascular surgeon for possible arteriography (see Chapter 74).

INDICATIONS FOR REFERRAL/HOSPITALIZATION

If patients present with severe claudication, rest pain, or gangrene, they should be referred promptly to a vascular surgeon for further evaluation. Once the extent of the severe ischemia has been identified, arteriography is indicated to demonstrate the extent and location of the obstruction. Treatment may involve angioplasty and stent placement or surgery. Magnetic resonance arteriography (MRA) may be used in preference to standard arteriography in patients with abnormal renal function. MRA is also helpful in demonstrating arteries in the lower leg not seen on standard arteriography. In general, neither arteriography nor MRA should be ordered without vascular surgical consultation. Once the location and extent of the blockage have been identified, the surgeon and radiologist can collaborate to determine the appropriate therapy. More extensive and more distal disease is more likely to require bypass either with prosthetic material or with the patient's own saphenous vein.

Diabetic patients with neuropathy or arterial insufficiency require regular podiatry consultation. The podiatrist will determine the frequency of visits based on callus development. With appropriate shoes and care of calluses and nails, many patients with ischemia can avoid problems for long periods. Regular podiatry visits enable early recognition of potential problems and ensure expeditious referral and treatment.

Patients with superficial ulcers who do not improve with bed rest and treatment require referral to a vascular surgeon. More extensive ulcers require immediate vascular consultation.

PATIENT AND FAMILY EDUCATION

All patients should be advised to follow a low-fat diet, exercise regularly, and avoid all tobacco products. Patients over age 50 years without contraindications should understand the importance of low-dose daily aspirin. Patients with diabetes, particularly if neuropathy is present, should be instructed to visually inspect their feet daily and seek professional help for any foot lesion. Many patients with diabetes are terrified of amputation and should be reassured that with good podiatric care and immediate attention to any problem, amputation can usually be avoided. All patients with arterial insufficiency should have their toenails cut by a podiatrist. In addition, the patient should be given instructions about general foot protection measures, including properly fitting shoes, avoiding synthetic materials in shoes that do not "breathe," and always wearing shoes or slippers. Direct contact with very hot or very cold substances or surfaces must be avoided. It is imperative to seek immediate medical evaluation for prolonged pain, sudden color changes, or a numb feeling in the extremities.

Acute Arterial Insufficiency

DEFINITION/EPIDEMIOLOGY

Acute arterial insufficiency is the sudden onset of the symptoms of ischemia. The incidence of acute arterial occlusion seems to be increasing.[6] This increase is partly related to better diagnosis and recognition, but also to the fact that patients with advanced heart disease are living longer and undergoing more invasive procedures. It is critical to make the diagnosis expeditiously to avoid loss of limb or life.

PATHOPHYSIOLOGY

Acute ischemia may result from an embolus from another source in a distal vessel. The most common source of an embolus is the heart. This may be the clot that forms on the ventricular wall after a myocardial infarction or a clot from the atrium in patients with atrial fibrillation. Rarely, a tumor in the heart such as atrial myxoma may break off and travel to the peripheral vessels.

Acute thrombosis of preexisting atherosclerotic lesions is the other major cause of acute ischemia. This type may be less severe than acute ischemia secondary to embolization, as collateral circulation has had time to develop. Aneurysms of the abdominal aorta or popliteal artery may cause acute ischemia secondary to acute thrombosis of the aneurysm. Once the embolus becomes lodged, the arteries and veins distal to the occlusion become spasmatic. After a few hours, vasodilation occurs, and the thrombus begins to organize. At this point the ischemia becomes irreversible. It is generally accepted that if acute occlusion of the limb occurs and there is no collateral circulation, necrosis will begin after 6 hours unless the ischemia is relieved.

CLINICAL PRESENTATION

Classically, the patient will present with a history of sudden onset of pain in an extremity. A history of recent myocardial infarction or atrial fibrillation and the presence of normal circulation in the other limb suggests an embolus as the source. A previous history of peripheral vascular disease suggests acute thrombosis as the cause.

PHYSICAL EXAMINATION

On examination the limb is usually pale and pulseless with absent or diminished capillary refill. If there is loss of sensation or immobility of the foot, tissue loss is imminent. These signs and symptoms are often referred to as the five Ps: *P*ain, *P*allor, *P*ulselessness, *P*aresthesias, and *P*aralysis. Untreated, the limb becomes edematous, mottled, and eventually gangrenous. The sudden onset of pain with signs of acute ischemia and mottling from the waist down suggests acute aortic occlusion and demands immediate diagnosis and treatment if the patient is to survive.

DIAGNOSTICS

Diagnosis is generally based on the clinical presentation and examination. Doppler studies are necessary to determine the presence or absence of arterial pulses. Arteriography may be indicated in some circumstances.

DIFFERENTIAL DIAGNOSIS

The patient history will usually suggest whether the ischemia is related to an embolus or thrombus.

The most common error is to misdiagnose acute ischemia as an acute neurologic event. The consequent delay in treatment can result in limb loss or, in the case of acute aortic occlusion, death. Careful pulse examination at the time of presentation will avoid this problem. Other causes of acute arterial insufficiency or arterial occlusion include blue toe syndrome and aneurysms.

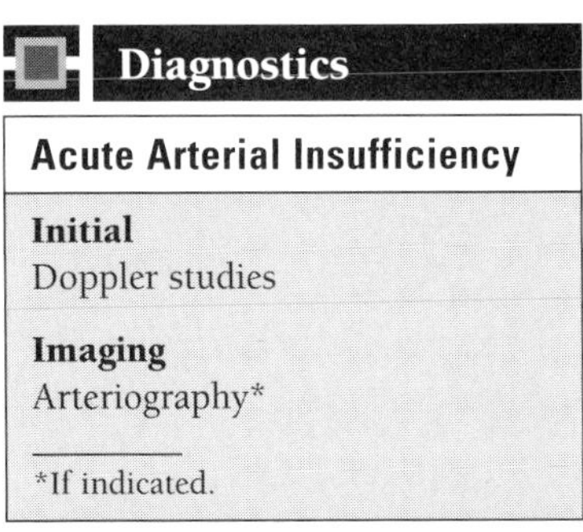

Diagnostics

Acute Arterial Insufficiency

Initial
Doppler studies

Imaging
Arteriography*

*If indicated.

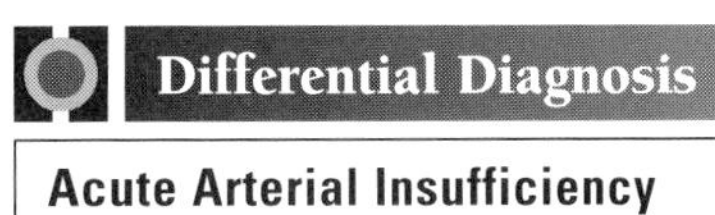

Differential Diagnosis

Acute Arterial Insufficiency

Ruptured aneurysm
Thrombotic event
Embolic event
Neurologic event

Blue Toe Syndrome

Bluish discoloration or localized gangrene of the feet without evidence of ischemia, infection, or peripheral neuropathy is known as blue toe syndrome. Blue toe syndrome results from microemboli from the heart, aorta, or peripheral arteries that are small enough to lodge in the capillaries. These emboli may be small thrombi from the heart or from an aortic or popliteal aneurysm. They may also be cholesterol emboli or atheroemboli from atherosclerotic plaques in the aorta, iliac arteries, or femoral arteries.

When blue toe syndrome is suspected, careful physical examination for the presence of an abdominal or popliteal aneurysm is mandatory. If there is no evidence of ischemia, infection, or peripheral neuropathy, a cardiac echocardiogram and abdominal ultrasound study should be obtained. If these are negative for a clot or abdominal aneurysm, antiplatelet therapy is begun and the patient is monitored closely. Consultation with a vascular surgeon is appropriate at this point. Usually, the lesion will improve over the next few weeks, but if it does not, or if emboli recur, a transesophageal echocardiogram and an aortogram of the thoracic aorta to the femoral arteries are indicated. If a localized lesion is discovered, it can be addressed, although diffuse atherosclerosis of the suprarenal aorta is often the source. In these cases recurrent embolization often leads to chronic renal failure, as well as distal gangrene. Ligation of the iliac arteries with axillobifemoral bypass and preparation for dialysis are the current available therapies.

Aneurysm

An aneurysm is a localized enlargement of an artery that causes symptoms by expansion, rupture, or thrombosis. A true aneurysm is said to be present when the wall of the aneurysm is an arterial wall. If the wall is compressed connective tissue, however, then the rupture is a contained rupture, or false aneurysm.

Infrarenal aortic aneurysms are a common cause of death secondary to rupture. Often they are asymptomatic, although they may cause an acute onset of back or abdominal pain. If a pulsatile abdominal mass is discovered on physical examination, further evaluation with either abdominal ultrasound or a CT scan is indicated. If the presence of an aneurysm is confirmed, referral to a vascular surgeon is indicated. Femoral or popliteal aneurysms are less common but may be detected on physical examination and usually cause symptoms by expansion and thrombosis. They are often associated with aortic aneurysms, and an abdominal ultrasound should also be obtained if either of these is detected.

Patients with aneurysms should be advised that this condition is often congenital and that any blood relatives over age 50 years should probably have an abdominal ultrasound.

MANAGEMENT

As soon as the diagnosis of acute arterial occlusion is made, a bolus of intravenous heparin (5000 units) should be given to prevent a clot from forming distal to the occlusion. Hospitalization and prompt referral to a vascular surgeon for evaluation with treatment are essential. Ideally, treatment, whether surgical or thrombolytic therapy, should be instituted within 6 hours of the occlusion.

COMPLICATIONS

Complications are less dependent on the effect of the acute occlusion than on the cause. Thus patients with an embolus at the time of a massive myocardial infarction will do poorly in comparison with those whose clot is from atrial fibrillation. Studies show a mortality rate with arterial occlusion of 22% to 39% and an amputation rate of 11% to 17%, respectively.[6,7]

INDICATIONS FOR REFERRAL/HOSPITALIZATION

Immediate evaluation by a vascular surgeon is imperative. Acute arterial occlusion is an emergency in which treatment delay can impair limb viability or threaten life.

PATIENT AND FAMILY EDUCATION

Review of the signs and symptoms for acute arterial occlusion at regular intervals is indicated. For other educational points for review, see the Patient Education section under Chronic Arterial Insufficiency, p. 551.

REFERENCES

1. Coffman JD: Peripheral vascular disease. In Noble J, editor: *Textbook of primary care medicine*, ed 2, St Louis, 1996, Mosby.
2. Molgaard J and others: Hyperhomocystinaemia: an independent risk factor for intermittent claudication, *J Intern Med* 231:273-279, 1992.
3. Perkins JM and others: Exercise training versus angioplasty for stable claudication: long and medium term results of a prospective randomized trial, *Eur J Vasc Endovasc Surg* 11(4):409-413, 1996.
4. Humphrey PW, Silver D: Antithrombotic therapy. In Rutherford, editor: *Vascular surgery*, Philadelphia, 1995, WB Saunders.
5. Dawson DL and others: A comparison of cilostazol and pentoxifylline for treating intermittent claudication, *Am J Med* 109(7):523-530, 2000.
6. Brewster DC: Acute peripheral arterial occlusion, *Cardiol Clin* 9(3): 497-513, 1991.
7. Baxter-Smith D and others: Peripheral arterial embolism: a 20-year review, *J Cardiovasc Surg* 29(4):453-457, 1988.

CHAPTER 136

Peripheral Edema

Debra Hobbins

DEFINITION/EPIDEMIOLOGY

Pedal/lower extremity edema can be a symptom of a potentially serious disease. Early detection of the underlying disease process enables early treatment and prevents more serious complications. Pedal edema may be ignored or missed completely because it is slow to develop; patients often will not complain until their shoes no longer fit.

Edema is caused by excess interstitial fluid in the tissues and is described as trace (barely detectable) to 4+ pitting.[1] A weight gain of 4 to 5 pounds usually precedes the visible signs of edema. Severe edema can cause tissues to be rocklike. Obstruction of the lymph flow in an extremity causes lymphedema.

The implications of peripheral edema depend on a patient's health status and/or disease state. It can be an expected finding in a normal pregnancy as a result of the increase in total body water and increased peripheral venous pressure. It may also be a side effect of certain medications, such as calcium channel blockers or steroids. However, disease states such as venous and/or arterial insufficiency, congestive heart failure, renal failure, and cirrhosis account for the majority of cases of peripheral edema.[2,3]

PATHOPHYSIOLOGY

The amount of fluid in the interstitial space depends on several parameters: capillary pressure and permeability, the interstitial and osmotic pressure that results from plasma colloids, lymphatic circulation, and total extracellular fluid. A change in any of these factors causes increased interstitial volume with resultant edema. Because of the effects of gravity, interstitial fluid tends to be first noted in the peripheral system; for example, an individual who remains predominately in the supine position will first accumulate interstitial fluid in the sacral area.

The peripheral edema that results from congestive heart failure is produced by an elevation in venous pressure and capillary pressure. The resulting systemic venous congestion produces peripheral edema. Congestive heart failure also predisposes an individual to venous stasis. Venous stasis results from incompetent valves or a weakness in the venous walls themselves, causing dilation and valve failure with resultant reflux. Venous valves can also degenerate as a result of genetic factors, resolving thrombi, or advancing age.

With venous thrombi, obstruction of venous outflow causes an increase in pressure. As a result, fluid is pushed through the capillary membranes into the tissue space, which leads to edema.

The peripheral edema associated with cirrhosis or hypoalbuminemia results from decreased albumin. A decrease in plasma protein or an increase in the protein content of the interstitial fluid decreases oncotic pressure and results in fluid accumulation.

Electrolyte imbalance also plays a role in the development of peripheral edema. Edema is one of the most common manifestations of sodium excess. Whenever there is abnormal retention of salt in the body, water is also retained. The kidneys assume the major role in sodium balance. Reducing salt intake results in hypotonicity of the plasma with an increased loss of water via the kidneys. Many diuretics act directly on the kidney tubules to prevent sodium reabsorption.

Peripheral edema also results from lymphedema, which may be caused when there is interference with the drainage of lymph from any part of the body. The function of the lymphatic vessels is to return to the bloodstream the water, protein, and products of cellular metabolism that cannot be reabsorbed by blood capillaries. The lymphatic channels drain the interstitial fluid. Blockage of the lymphatic system may be the result of an infection, malignant process, surgical procedure, or radiation therapy.

CLINICAL PRESENTATION

The presence of edema does not necessarily mandate urgent treatment. A systematic approach is recommended to determine the underlying disease process. The patient may present with unilateral or bilateral swelling of the foot or leg. The color of the affected area may range from normal to pink, red, or brown. Pain and respiratory difficulties may or may not be present.

PHYSICAL EXAMINATION

Obtaining the past medical and current medication histories is critical. In addition, these are important factors related to the history of a patient with peripheral edema: location of the edema; unilateral or bilateral nature; history of acute trauma; any alteration in the fitting of clothing or shoes; the presence of a cough, progressive shortness of breath, or nocturnal dyspnea; and a report of the urine volume, color, and frequency.

During the physical examination, it is important to note the extent and severity of the edema, the color and temperature of the skin, and the presence of any breakdown or lesions. Also, the presence of any gait difficulty should be determined. The patient's current weight should be compared with previously recorded weights. During the cardiovascular examination, the presence of new gallops, murmurs, or jugular venous distention should be assessed. The presence of ascites in the abdomen or rales on pulmonary auscultation should be determined, as these can indicate increased fluid volume.

DIAGNOSTICS

A careful history and physical examination are helpful in determining the necessary screening tests searching for the etiology of the peripheral edema. In unilateral edema with acute onset and pain, a lower extremity ultrasound is obtained to exclude deep vein thrombosis. The ultrasound should be repeated in cases of persistent unilateral painful edema. A urinalysis is obtained to check for protein. Serum electrolytes, BUN, creatinine, total protein, albumin, and globulin may elicit the cause of the edema. With more generalized edema, LFTs, and a thyroid-stimulating hormone level are necessary. The presence of pelvic lymphadenopathy and peripheral edema necessitates an evaluation for a pelvic mass with appropriate radiographs, a CT scan, or an MRI of the abdomen and pelvis. Vascular or arterial studies are indicated if the lower extremities also show brawny skin color changes or symptoms suggesting venous or arterial insufficiency.

DIFFERENTIAL DIAGNOSIS

When there is evidence of lower extremity edema, the differential diagnosis ranges from idiopathic edema, stasis secondary to long periods of immobility and excessive sodium intake, the Charcot foot of diabetes, to serious entities such as renal failure, cirrhosis, pulmonary hypertension, human immunodeficiency virus, or congestive heart failure.[4,5] Certain medications (e.g., calcium channel blockers, intrathecal opiate infusions) may also cause peripheral edema.[6] A drug history is necessary to prevent unnecessary diagnostic testing or inappropriate treatment. A history of phlebitis is important to note; postphlebitic syndrome is characterized by a chronically swollen limb and in some individuals can appear after 10 to 20 years because of incompetent veins.[7]

MANAGEMENT

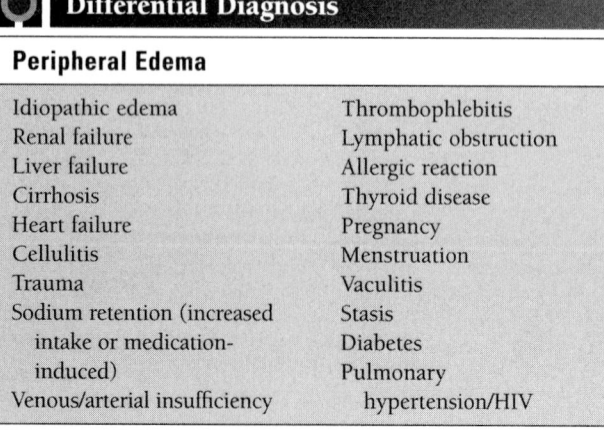

Management of peripheral edema is dictated by the underlying cause. Restriction of sodium and elevation of the affected extremities are helpful strategies; the use of support or compression stockings is a beneficial adjunct. These interventions may be all that is necessary when the edema is due to increased hydrostatic or decreased osmotic pressure. If the edema is a side effect of a drug, the medication may need to be changed, or a diuretic may need to be added to the regimen. When the underlying cause is cardiac failure, renal failure, or cirrhosis, treatment depends on the severity of the disease and the systems affected.

Co-Management with Specialists

In most cases the primary care provider can manage the patient with peripheral edema. If there is significant renal or cardiac disease, there must be careful and ongoing communication regarding the choice of therapy and the understanding of changes to the medication regimen. Home care nurses are a valuable resource for patients with more complicated conditions. Diuresis can often be accomplished at home with a record of daily weights, determination of postural vital signs, and respiratory and cardiac assessment by the home care nurse in conjunction with monitoring of electrolytes and kidney function tests.

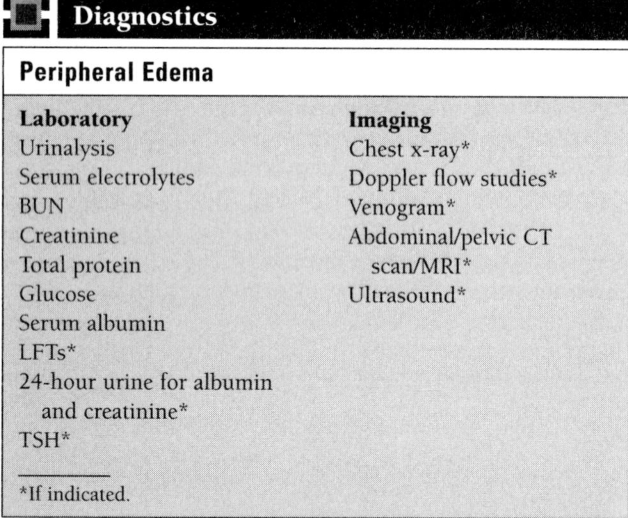

Diagnostics

Peripheral Edema

Laboratory	Imaging
Urinalysis	Chest x-ray*
Serum electrolytes	Doppler flow studies*
BUN	Venogram*
Creatinine	Abdominal/pelvic CT scan/MRI*
Total protein	Ultrasound*
Glucose	
Serum albumin	
LFTs*	
24-hour urine for albumin and creatinine*	
TSH*	

*If indicated.

Differential Diagnosis

Peripheral Edema

Idiopathic edema	Thrombophlebitis
Renal failure	Lymphatic obstruction
Liver failure	Allergic reaction
Cirrhosis	Thyroid disease
Heart failure	Pregnancy
Cellulitis	Menstruation
Trauma	Vaculitis
Sodium retention (increased intake or medication-induced)	Stasis
Venous/arterial insufficiency	Diabetes
	Pulmonary hypertension/HIV

COMPLICATIONS

Complications of peripheral edema result from a failure to recognize the early warning signs and a delay in diagnosing a pathologic condition. Deep vein thrombosis can lead to embolization and life-threatening risks. Persistent peripheral edema may lead to tissue breakdown and resultant cellulitis.

INDICATIONS FOR REFERRAL/HOSPITALIZATION

Consultation with the appropriate specialist is appropriate for edema that results from cardiac, renal, or liver disease. The patient with significant venous insufficiency and persistent stasis ulcers may benefit from a vascular surgery consultation to discuss treatment options. Hospitalization and heparinization may be recommended for deep vein thrombosis. However, low-molecular-weight heparin (Lovenox) may enable a shorter hospital stay and closely monitored outpatient management for some patients.[8] Severe cellulitis often requires hospitalization.[8,9] In other circumstances hospitalization is recommended if the underlying pathologic condition (e.g., congestive heart failure) needs stabilization.

PATIENT AND FAMILY EDUCATION

The patient should understand the significant symptoms (e.g., increased weight in edema) that may indicate a deteriorating medical condition. The importance of good foot care, properly fitting footwear, rest, and elevation of the affected extremity is also important. Patients should understand the importance of reporting any change in the appearance or sensation of the foot. The type of footwear can be observed during the office visit, and recommendations can be made if there is a problem. It is wise to ask the patient periodically if there has been a recent change in shoe size.

REFERENCES

1. Degowin E and others: *Bedside diagnostic exam,* New York, 1981, Macmillan.
2. Dornbrand L, Hoole A, Picard C: *Manual of clinical problems in adult ambulatory care,* Boston, 1992, Little, Brown.

3. Treiman GS and others: Factors influencing ulcer healing in patients with combined arterial and venous insufficiency, *J Vasc Surg* 33(6):1158-1164, 2001.
4. Sommer TC, Lee TH: Charcot foot: the diagnostic dilemma, *Am Fam Physician* 64(9):1591-1598, 2001.
5. Mehta NJ and others: HIV-related pulmonary hypertension: analytic review of 131 cases, *Chest* 118(4):1133-1141, 2000.
6. Aldrete JA, Couto da Silva JM: Leg edema from intrathecal opiate infusions, *Eur J Pain* 4(4):361-365, 2000.
7. Noble J and others: *Textbook of primary care medicine*, St Louis, 1996, Mosby.
8. Levine M and others: A comparison of low-molecular-weight heparin administered primarily at home with unfractionated heparin administered in the hospital for proximal deep-vein thrombosis, *N Engl J Med* 334(11):677-681, 1996.
9. Koopman MMW and others: Treatment of venous thrombosis with intravenous unfractionated heparin administered in the hospital as compared with subcutaneous low-molecular-weight heparin administered at home: The Tasman Study Group, *N Engl J Med* 334(11):682-687, 1996.

CHAPTER 137

Peripheral Venous Insufficiency

David R. Campbell

Peripheral venous insufficiency occurs whenever there is obstruction to venous return in the superficial or deep veins of the upper or lower extremities. Important venous insufficiency clinical syndromes include deep vein thrombosis, venous stasis, varicose veins, stasis dermatitis, and leg ulceration.

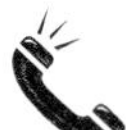

Physician consultation is indicated for all patients with deep vein thrombosis as documented by Doppler ultrasound.

Deep Venous Thrombosis of the Lower Extremity

DEFINITION/EPIDEMIOLOGY

Deep venous thrombosis (DVT) is the development of a blood clot in the deep veins of the lower or, occasionally, the upper extremity. A DVT may include the iliac veins and the vena cava and is characterized by a relatively loose thrombotic attachment to the vein wall until the healing process starts.

Although the term *phlebitis* is often used to describe DVT, it should in fact be reserved for superficial phlebitis. Superficial phlebitis is an inflammation of the affected superficial veins as a result of local trauma, venous stasis, or infection; chemical injury may result from an IV injection. Because the clot is part of an inflammatory process that involves the vessel wall, there is no risk of pulmonary embolism unless the process extends to involve the deep system.

PATHOPHYSIOLOGY

The deep veins of the lower extremity are the main conduit by which the legs are emptied of blood. Blood travels back to the heart as a result of compression of the deep veins by leg muscles. Valves in the vein prevent reflux back down the vein because of gravity. Blood runs from the superficial system to the deep veins through perforator veins, which are also protected from reflux by the presence of valves. Any condition that produces stasis or hypercoagulability is likely to result in the formation of clots in the deep veins.[1] A major risk factor is surgery, particularly gynecologic operations or orthopedic procedures on the hip and knee. Bed rest produces stasis and may result in DVT. Long airplane or car rides are also risk factors.[2] Patients who have a tendency for hypercoagulation, particularly patients with malignancy, may present with DVT. A lesser but definite risk factor for DVT is use of oral estrogen preparations, contraceptive pills, or hormone replacement therapy, and these should be considered in patients with other risk factors.[2]

A clot may form in any part of the deep venous system and may either propagate or remain localized. It may cause symptoms in two ways. First, there is a local effect in obstruction of blood flow, which rarely is so significant that it results in venous gangrene. Second, the clot may become detached and migrate to the lungs, forming an embolus. This is a common cause of death in at-risk patients.

CLINICAL PRESENTATION AND PHYSICAL EXAMINATION

A history of previous DVT, prolonged inactivity, estrogen use (oral contraceptive or hormone replacement therapy), or recent surgery or trauma should be obtained from the patient. The classic signs of DVT are leg edema and calf tenderness. Calf pain on dorsiflexion of the foot is known as Homans' sign. All of these signs are relatively nonspecific; up to 50% of patients with DVT have no symptoms at all. Together, extensive thrombosis and extreme leg swelling have in the past been known as phlegmasia alba dolens.

The history and examination for superficial phlebitis differ from that for DVT. The patient may have a localized area of edema, erythema, and tenderness over a superficial vein, with increased temperature in the surrounding skin.

DIAGNOSTICS

The diagnosis of superficial phlebitis is based on the clinical findings; diagnostic tests are not usually indicated. If a DVT is suspected on the basis of clinical signs or risk factors, the diagnosis can be made simply by duplex ultrasound of the legs.[3] Test results should document clot visualization, normal blood flow, compressibility of the veins, augmentation of flow with respiration, or reflux in the deep and superficial systems. The most common sites for DVT are the femoral veins; in this situation the duplex ultrasound is as accurate as venography. Isolated tibial or iliac vein thrombosis may be more difficult to diagnose; venography or magnetic resonance venography may be indicated if there is a high index of suspicion. Appropriate testing for malignancy, connective tissue disorders, or inherited autocoagulation deficiencies may be necessary. The need for further investigation is guided by the clinical presentation, past medical history, and family history.

Diagnostics

Peripheral Venous Insufficiency

DEEP VEIN THROMBOSIS
Imaging
Duplex ultrasound*
Venography/magnetic resonance venography*

Laboratory
Protein C, Protein S
Antithrombin III
Antiphospholipid antibodies
Factor V Leiden

CHRONIC VENOUS STASIS
None indicated

VARICOSE VEINS
Imaging
Duplex scan

VENOUS STASIS ULCERATION
Initial
Doppler ultrasound

*If indicated.

DIFFERENTIAL DIAGNOSIS

It is not possible to diagnose DVT accurately on the basis of clinical presentation or physical examination alone. Other differential diagnoses that should be considered are superficial phlebitis, cellulitis, ruptured Baker's cyst, strained muscle, or a malignant neoplasm that is compromising the veins.

The possibility of an underlying malignancy or the existence of a connective tissue disorder must also be considered. Inherited deficiencies of protein C, protein S, or antithrombin III are important (albeit less common) causes, particularly in recurrent cases or in patients with a family history of DVT.

MANAGEMENT

Management of superficial vein phlebitis consists of elevation of the leg and compression with an Ace bandage. Nonsteroidal antiinflammatory drugs and antibiotics are also indicated. It is important to note that superficial phlebitis may coexist with DVT.

Management of DVT requires that heparin be initiated immediately to prevent a pulmonary embolism. Traditionally this has meant admission to the hospital for systemic heparinization. Typically a bolus of 5000 U is given, followed by a continuous infusion at 800 to 1400 units/hr (80 units/kg heparin bolus followed by an infusion of 18 units/kg) to maintain a partial thromboplastin time (PTT) that is twice the normal rate. The PTT should be checked after 6 hours. The heparin infusion should be continued until the PTT has been in the therapeutic range for a minimum of 2 consecutive days. Warfarin (Coumadin) is started within the first 24 hours, and the patient is discharged once the international normalized ratio is between 2 and 3.[4] The regimen of warfarin is usually continued for 3 to 6 months.

Low-molecular-weight heparin (e.g., enoxaparin) given by subcutaneous injection has been shown in studies to be safe for at-home treatment of uncomplicated DVT.[5] These studies show the same or a lower incidence of complications when compared with standard heparin. Because enoxaparin has a long half-life, it can be given twice a day subcutaneously; its predictable anticoagulant response obviates the need for PTT monitoring. As it becomes more widely used, this type of therapy is expected to reduce the cost of treating DVT.

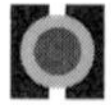

Differential Diagnosis

Peripheral Venous Insufficiency

Deep Vein Thrombosis
Superficial phlebitis
Cellulitis
Ruptured Baker's cyst
Strained muscle
Malignant neoplasm

Chronic Venous Stasis
Heart failure
Malnutrition
Lymphatic obstruction

Varicose Veins
Venous/arterial insufficiency
Peripheral neuritis
Arthritis

Venous Stasis Ulceration
Venous stasis ulceration
Ischemic ulceration
Neuropathic ulceration

LIFE SPAN CONSIDERATIONS

DVT that is diagnosed during pregnancy should be managed on an individual basis after consultation with a vascular surgeon and the patient's obstetrician.[6] Heparin is generally safe during pregnancy and can be given to pregnant women to treat DVT. The use of warfarin (Coumadin) is contraindicated during pregnancy. Any woman of childbearing age who is taking this medication should be advised of the risks of pregnancy. The introduction of enoxaparin has made the management of these patients much simpler.

A number of measures have been shown to be effective for DVT prophylaxis in patients undergoing surgery. Cuffs that provide intermittent leg pressure to reduce stasis are combined with subcutaneous heparin until the patient is mobile. Low-molecular-weight heparin has been approved for very-high-risk procedures (e.g., hip replacement) and is now being used instead of perioperative warfarin. Subcutaneous heparin twice a day is usually sufficient for medical patients who have been prescribed bed rest.

COMPLICATIONS

Pulmonary embolism is one of the major causes of postoperative morbidity and mortality.[7] In high-risk patients the key to prevention is appropriate surveillance for DVT with the duplex scan. Pulmonary embolism usually occurs within 2 weeks of DVT. After this time, the clot is sufficiently organized to make detachment unlikely. Symptoms of a pulmonary embolus include the sudden onset of pleuritic chest pain and shortness of breath. The patient is noted to be hypoxic yet has a relatively normal chest x-ray film. Evidence of a clot in the leg by duplex scan combined with a positive lung scan is sufficient for diagnosis. A pulmonary arteriogram is indicated if the duplex scan is negative or if the lung scan is equivocal. Increasingly the lung scan and pulmonary angiography are being replaced by CT angiography, which is less invasive. If the patient's condition is critical, thrombolytic therapy can be started through the catheter used for the pulmonary arteriogram.

Postphlebitic syndrome is a chronic condition that may develop as a sequela to DVT. DVT can produce chronic changes in veins with loss of valve competence, and it is a cause of chronic venous stasis.[8]

All patients receiving heparin should have their platelet count checked every few days; a sudden drop in the count may be indicative of heparin-induced thrombocytopenia. If this occurs or if the patient has a known allergy to heparin, treatment with low-molecular-weight dextran should be used instead. Prophylactic placement of a vena cava filter to prevent pulmonary embolism should be considered if other medical conditions prevent the use of anticoagulation therapy.[9]

INDICATIONS FOR REFERRAL/HOSPITALIZATION

A documented DVT in any patient requires a physician consultation, during which time the need for hospitalization and IV heparin vs. outpatient treatment with low-molecular-weight heparin can be determined. Vascular consultation is necessary for patients who may require placement of a vena cava filter.[10] If the inflammatory process continues despite treatment, excision may occasionally be indicated; in such cases a vascular consult should be sought.

PATIENT AND FAMILY EDUCATION

Other options for birth control should be discussed with patients, particularly those who smoke. High-risk patients should understand the risks associated with long plane and automobile journeys. They should also be advised to wear support stockings and to take an aspirin every day while traveling. Low-dose aspirin (81 to 365 mg) has been shown conclusively to reduce the incidence and mortality of myocardial infarction in patients over 50 years old; it may be recommended in patients at risk for DVT who travel long distances. Adequate fluid intake, frequent rest breaks to stretch and exercise the legs, and passive intermittent contraction of the calf muscles enhance blood flow to the lower extremities during prolonged, confined travel conditions.

Anticoagulant therapy should be carefully explained to patients. The importance of routine laboratory testing to monitor therapy should be stressed. Patients should understand the importance of contacting the primary care provider if abnormal bleeding occurs.

HEALTH PROMOTION

See Chapter 130.

Chronic Venous Stasis

DEFINITION/EPIDEMIOLOGY

Chronic venous stasis results from increased pressure in the deep veins. This condition produces edema, varicose veins, chronic skin changes, and ulceration.

PATHOPHYSIOLOGY

Human beings are relatively poorly adapted to walking on two legs for extended periods. The distribution of blood to the feet is accomplished by the heart in concert with gravity, but it is only the muscle pump and fragile venous valves that return the blood to the heart. Prolonged standing and a tall stature increase hydrostatic pressure on the valves. During pregnancy the hormone relaxin, which allows the pelvis to stretch, also causes the veins to distend and the valves to become incompetent. Resolution of this condition after pregnancy is often incomplete, resulting in increased venous stasis. Obesity and age-associated loss of tissue turgor are also factors that produce venous stasis.

Increased pressure may also result from proximal venous obstruction secondary to an old DVT or more commonly from reflux secondary to valvular incompetence. Valvular incompetence may result after recanalization after a DVT, or it may be primary in nature.

Even if the valves of the perforator and saphenous veins remain competent, deep venous hypertension does affect the foot and ankle. The foot tends to swell, particularly if the patient stands much of the day. The point of maximum pressure is the ankle, and the skin becomes thickened and may react to the pressure with an eczematous reaction known as stasis eczema.

Consequently, blood cells in the tiny venules break down under high pressure; hemosiderin is deposited under the skin to produce a characteristic brown staining that progresses with time.

CLINICAL PRESENTATION AND PHYSICAL EXAMINATION

The clinical appearance of chronic venous stasis varies depending on whether the superficial or deeper veins are affected. Chronic edema and skin discoloration on the legs and ankles may be present. Varicose veins, ulceration, and even cellulitis may result.

DIAGNOSTICS AND DIFFERENTIAL DIAGNOSIS

Diagnostic tests are unnecessary because the diagnosis is based on the clinical history and physical findings. The physical findings also guide the diagnosis. However, the peripheral edema associated with chronic venous stasis may also be caused by other disease entities. Medications, congestive heart failure, lymphatic obstruction, and malnutrition may all be associated with lower extremity edema (see the Diagnostics and Differential Diagnosis boxes on p. 556.

MANAGEMENT

Compression stockings and periodic leg elevation are the most important methods for controlling chronic venous insufficiency and preventing skin ulcers. Careful monitoring is important when venous ulcers occur. Normal saline wet-to-dry dressings or topical antibiotic therapies are indicated. Ulcer infections should be treated with the appropriate antibiotic.

COMPLICATIONS

Venous ulcers are the most common complication of chronic venous stasis. A superimposed infection and cellulitis are additional concerns. Severe edema may result in decreased mobility and an increased risk for falls or DVT.

INDICATIONS FOR REFERRAL/HOSPITALIZATION

Venous ulcers or peripheral edema that does not respond to conventional therapies may require a referral to the appropriate specialist. Severe ulcers with extensive tissue loss may require evaluation by a plastic surgeon for possible grafting. Most patients can be successfully managed with careful outpatient follow-up visits. However, hospitalization may be indicated for severe edema, infection, or surgical valvuloplasty.

PATIENT AND FAMILY EDUCATION

The most effective treatment for leg swelling and stasis dermatitis is the use of support stockings.[11] Severe stasis eczema may require the use of 0.5% hydrocortisone cream in combination with compression. The hydrocortisone cream should be discontinued once the condition has resolved.

Varicose Veins

PATHOPHYSIOLOGY

Varicose veins are caused by pathologic distention and proliferation of the superficial veins. Varicose veins include primary and secondary varicose veins as well as spider veins.

Primary varicose veins are usually familial. There is no previous history of DVT, and the varicosities are usually exacerbated by pregnancy. Progressive dilation of the superficial veins may be local or more extensive. Primary varicose veins result from incompetent perforators, which produce local varicosities, or from incompetence of the saphenous vein valves, which produces more generalized varicosities. Secondary varicose veins result from a previous DVT. Most commonly these are caused by incompetent valves following recanalization. When the deep venous system is totally occluded, these varicose veins may represent the main venous drainage from the leg; in this instance removal of the veins would be harmful. Telangiectasia or spider veins may result from increased pressure in the superficial veins. It is not clear why this condition is more predominant in some patients.

CLINICAL PRESENTATION AND PHYSICAL EXAMINATION

The pooling of blood in large varicose veins tends to produce symptoms of heaviness and discomfort in the legs while standing. Large varicose veins are unsightly and may produce severe anxiety and cause major lifestyle changes. Trauma to a varicose veins may result in severe bleeding, particularly in older adults, as their skin may be atrophic and thereby provides less protection.

DIAGNOSTICS AND DIFFERENTIAL DIAGNOSIS

Diagnosis is based on inspection of the lower extremities when the patient is standing. Further differential consideration is usually unnecessary. The only important test indicated for varicose veins is the duplex scan to determine whether the deep system is patent and whether there is saphenofemoral reflux. Individual incompetent perforators in the leg may also be identified. If varicosities are not present, venous and arterial insufficiency, peripheral neuritis, and arthritis should be considered (see the Diagnostics and Differential Diagnosis boxes on p. 556).

MANAGEMENT

Asymptomatic varicose veins do not require treatment. There is no effective way to reduce venous pressure in the lower legs except with support stockings.

COMPLICATIONS

Occasionally a superficial varicosity will rupture and significant bleeding may be noted. Topical compression and elevation of the extremity usually control the bleeding. Skin ulcerations are an additional complication of varicose veins.

INDICATIONS FOR REFERRAL/HOSPITALIZATION

Referral to a vascular surgeon is indicated if support stockings are not effective in controlling symptoms or are poorly tolerated by the patient.

Treatment by a specialist may involve removal of the varicose veins or, alternatively, injection or laser treatment. Large veins are more appropriately removed in outpatient surgery, whereas smaller veins can be injected. Spider veins can be treated by either injection or laser treatment. Recent reports of obliteration of the long saphenous vein using a catheter and a radiofrequency generator may reduce the morbidity of saphenectomy.[12]

PATIENT AND FAMILY EDUCATION

It is important to inform patients that none of the treatments for varicose veins eradicate the problem of high venous pressure. Therefore recurrence is the rule rather than the exception. This knowledge may affect a patient's decision to proceed with surgery. Patients should also understand that compression stockings and periodic leg elevation are beneficial.

Venous Stasis Ulceration

DEFINITION/EPIDEMIOLOGY

Venous stasis ulceration is the most severe complication of postphlebitic syndrome and rarely occurs without a history of preceding DVT. With the introduction of heparin and the prompt diagnosis and treatment of DVT, venous stasis ulceration is now much less common.

PATHOPHYSIOLOGY

A number of factors contribute to venous ulceration. At first, peripheral edema increases as a result of incompetent valves in the venous system. This edema leads to capillary distention and the leakage of fluid and other substances into the surrounding tissue. If there is trauma to the skin of the affected extremity, oxygen and essential nutrients for healing are prevented from reaching the injured area. As a result, a superficial, irregularly shaped ulceration occurs. These ulcers can continue to erode, and cellulitis and superimposed infection can occur.

CLINICAL PRESENTATION AND PHYSICAL EXAMINATION

The patient with venous stasis ulceration typically presents with an ulcer above the medial malleolus, and there are usually other signs of venous stasis (Color Plate 38). The ulcers have a distinctive presentation that permits differentiation from ischemic or diabetic ulcers (Box 137-1). At the time of presentation, the wound may be secondarily infected. Pulses may not be palpable because of local swelling or coexistent ischemia.

DIAGNOSTICS AND DIFFERENTIAL DIAGNOSIS

Diagnostic tests are usually unnecessary. A portal Doppler can be used to assess pulses if they are not readily palpable. The differential diagnosis should encompass all peripheral ulcers (see the Diagnostics and Differential Diagnosis boxes on p. 556).

MANAGEMENT

Management of venous stasis ulceration consists of bed rest. A wet-to-dry dressing may be tried; however, the ulcer should be debrided as indicated and oral antibiotics started, guided by aerobic and anaerobic cultures results whenever possible. A nonstick dressing may be less painful once the ulcer is clean. This treatment is accompanied by compression with an Ace wrap.

Compliance can be a real problem for many patients; some centers combat this by using a rigid dressing such as the Unna's paste boot, which provides compression and a dressing that needs to be changed only once a week. The Unna's paste boot should not be used if there is peripheral arterial disease. A referral is sometimes indicated for refractory cases.

BOX 137-1

CHARACTERISTICS OF LEG ULCERS BY ETIOLOGY*

VENOUS STASIS
Occur around ankle, particularly medial side
History of previous phlebitis
Signs of venous stasis
Painful when secondarily infected
Improved by elevation

ISCHEMIC
Occur at tips of extremities or heel
History of claudication common
Very painful, but much worse on elevation
Absent pulses on physical examination
Secondary infection likely to spread very quickly

NEUROPATHIC (DIABETIC)
Occur at pressure points
Painless but coexistent neuritic pain may be confusing
Often present after secondary infection

*More than one etiology may be involved.

COMPLICATIONS

Superimposed infection is a constant concern with venous stasis ulceration. Osteomyelitis is a potential hazard for ulcers that become infected.

INDICATIONS FOR REFERRAL/HOSPITALIZATION

A surgical referral is indicated if the ulcer fails to heal with the simple measures outlined previously. If the ulcer is clearly deteriorating, hospitalization may be required.

PATIENT AND FAMILY EDUCATION

Patient education is extremely important in preventing the recurrence of this condition. Patients must understand the need to maintain compression and to be fitted with appropriate support stockings. In cases of severe edema, an external pneumatic compression stocking may be necessary to reduce swelling at the end of the day.

Many patients fail to wear their prescribed support stockings because the wrong stockings are provided. In general, knee-high stockings are much better tolerated than any tight support that crosses the knee. The main exceptions are pregnant women and women with varicose veins in the thigh, who may find support pantyhose comfortable. When ordering stockings the key factor is pressure (Table 137-1). The thick or fine-knit quality of the stockings affects only durability and patient acceptance.

TABLE 137-1 Recommendations for Support Stockings

Pressure (mm Hg)	Recommendations
0-10	Normal socks
10-20	Over-the-counter support stockings Recommended for individuals who are on their feet all day and for prophylaxis for DVT when traveling
30-40	Lowest pressure therapeutic stocking Good for individuals who are looking for more pressure than over-the-counter stockings or who cannot tolerate the higher pressures
30-40	Standard pressure for therapeutic stockings Patients should be instructed to shower in the evening so these stockings can be put on before getting out of bed; otherwise many patients, particularly older adults, will have trouble putting them on
40-50	Should be prescribed only for patients who do not get enough compression with 30-40 mm Hg Almost impossible to get on!

REFERENCES

1. Nordstrom M and others: A prospective study of the incidence of deep-vein thrombosis within a defined urban population, *Intern Med* 232(2):155-160, 1992.
2. Lapostolle F and others: Severe pulmonary embolism associated with air travel, *N Engl J Med* 345(11):779-783, 2001.
3. Venous thrombotic disease and combined oral contraceptives: results of international multicentre case-control study: World Health Organization Collaborative Study of Cardiovascular Disease and Steroid Hormone Contraception, *Lancet* 346(8990):1575-1582, 1995.
4. Masuda EM, Kistner RL: Prospective comparison of duplex scanning and descending venography in the assessment of venous insufficiency, *Am J Surg* 164(3):254-259, 1992.
5. Schulman S and others: A comparison of six weeks with six months of oral anticoagulant therapy after a first episode of venous thromboembolism: Duration of Anticoagulation Trial Study Group, *N Engl J Med* 332(25):1661-1665, 1995.
6. Hirsh J et al: Low molecular weight heparins in the treatment of patients with acute venous thromboembolism, *Thromb Haemost* 74: 360-363, 1995.
7. Ginsberg JS and others: Venous thrombosis during pregnancy: leg and trimester of presentation, *Thromb Haemost* 67:519-520, 1992.
8. Quinn DA and others: A prospective investigation of pulmonary embolism in women and men, *JAMA* 268:1689-1696, 1992.
9. Franzeck UK and others: Prospective 12-year follow-up of clinical and hemodynamic sequelae after deep vein thrombosis in low-risk patients, *Circulation* 93(11):74-79, 1996.
10. Alexander JJ, Yuhas JP, Piotrowski JJ: Is the increasing use of prophylactic IVC filters justified? *Am J Surg* 168(2):102-106, 1994.
11. Abu-Own A and others: Microangiopathy of the skin and the effect of leg compression in patients with chronic venous insufficiency, *J Vasc Surg* 19:1074-1083, 1994.
12. Pichot O and others: Role of duplex imaging in endovenous obliteration for primary venous insufficiency, *J Endovasc Ther* 7(6):452-459, 2000.

CHAPTER 138

Valvular Heart Disease and Cardiac Murmurs

Updated by Terry Mahan Buttaro and JoAnn Trybulski

When a murmur is heard for the first time, it is important to determine whether it represents a pathologic condition and what type of condition it may represent. The generation of the sounds called murmurs is the same whether the cause is benign or due to severe pathology and therefore is impossible to differentiate on the basis of the sound alone. What distinguishes benign from pathologic murmurs is often the associated physical findings or symptoms (Table 138-1). Some patients will require referral for diagnostic testing, whereas the clinical assessment of others will suggest that diagnostic testing is unnecessary.

A murmur is the relatively lengthy series of sounds produced by the turbulent flow of blood. Under normal conditions, blood flow is uniform or laminar within the vessel or chamber and is therefore free of audible vibration. When flow velocity is excessively high, or when normal flow occurs across an obstruction, turbulence and its resultant audible vibration occur. In a classic article on auscultation of the heart, Leatham[1] noted that all murmurs were related to three factors: (1) high rates of flow through a normal or abnormal valve; (2) forward flow through a constricted or irregular valve or into a dilated vessel; or (3) backward flow through a regurgitant valve, septal defect, or patent ductus arteriosus.

Murmurs may be characterized by a number of factors: location, intensity, pitch, radiation, and timing. Of these, timing is the most important factor. Timing delineates the critical division between systolic and diastolic murmurs, as well as the relationship to the heart sounds (S_1 and S_2; e.g., ending well before, right at, or continuing through S_2). As the heart rate increases, diastole shortens, and systole and diastole approach similar intervals. When this occurs, differentiating between S_1 (beginning of systole) and S_2 (beginning of diastole) on the basis of cadence alone becomes difficult. Palpation of the carotid pulse while simultaneously auscultating the heart at the base will easily permit the listener to focus in and time S_1 (the onset of systole), which will occur slightly before the onset of the carotid pulse rise. Although the two components of S_2 (aortic, or A_2, and pulmonic, or P_2) are almost superimposed at end-expiration, with inspiration P_2 splits later, creating an easily audible gap. This will be best appreciated over the upper left sternal border. A systolic murmur that ends at or before A_2 will be a left-sided murmur (e.g., aortic stenosis [AS] or mitral regurgitation [MR]), whereas one that extends beyond A_2 will be emanating from the right side of the heart (i.e., pulmonic stenosis or tricuspid regurgitation).

Intensity, or loudness, which is related to the velocity of blood flow, describes how audible the murmur is. However, loudness does not equate with the severity of the underlying problem. Some of the loudest murmurs are due to a small muscular ventricular septal defect (VSD) in an adolescent, which is destined to

TABLE 138-1 Murmurs*

Diagnosis	Characteristic	Location/Radiation	Physical Examination Findings	Effect of Valsalva's Maneuver	ECG Findings	Chest X-Ray Findings
COMMON SYSTOLIC MURMURS						
Aortic stenosis	Harsh, cresendo-decresendo	Right sternal border; radiation to neck	Delayed carotid upstroke; narrowed pulse pressure; systolic thrill at second right intercostal space	Decreases murmur	Left atrial enlargement; left axis deviation; atrioventricular conduction delay; left ventricular hypertrophy	Aortic valve calcification; left ventricular hypertrophy
Mitral regurgitation	Holocystolic blowing*	Apex; radiation to axilla	Laterally displaced, hyperdynamic apical impulse; brisk carotid upstroke	No change	Left ventricular hypertrophy	Left ventricular enlargement
Mitral valve prolapse	Mid to late systolic; occasionally honking; may have midsystolic click; click and murmur can be intermittent	Lower left sternal border	May have scoliosis or pectus excavatum in connective tissue disorder	Murmur and/or click may move to later systole or disappear	Usually within normal limits; occasionally flat or inverted T in leads II, III, aV_F	Skeletal abnormalities, if present
Tricuspid regurgitation	Early, mid, late, or pansystolic	Lower left sternal border; radiation to right sternal border	Sustained precordial lift	Decreases murmur	Right atrial hypertrophy; right axis deviation	Usually normal
Hypertrophic cardiomyopathy	Peaks midsystole	Left sternal border	Murmur decreases with change from standing to squatting; S_4 gallop may be present	Increases murmur	Left atrial enlargement; increased voltage; may have LVH	May have slight cardiac enlargement
Benign or innocent*	Early systolic; crescendo-decrescendo; changes intensity with rate	Variant	No underlying systemic findings; no findings of cardiac enlargement or failure; murmur disappears with breath holding	Murmur disappears	Normal ECG	Normal findings
Ventricular septal defect	Holosystolic; louder in midsystole	Left sternal border; radiation to right sternal border	May have systolic thrill at lower left sternal border	Increases murmur	May have left atrial and ventricular enlargement	
COMMON DIASTOLIC MURMURS						
Aortic regurgitation	Loud, blowing, high pitched	Lower left sternal border	Widened pulse pressure; abrupt rise and fall in carotid upstroke	Increases murmur	Left ventricular hypertrophy; sinus tachycardia	Left ventricular hypertrophy; aortic valve calcification; ascending aortic dilation
Mitral stenosis	Low-pitched, diastolic rumble (mid)	Apex, left lateral position	Opening snap	No change or increases murmur	Left atrial enlargement; right axis deviation	Left atrial enlargement; calcified mitral valve
Tricuspid stenosis	Decrescendo, low pitched	Fourth or fifth left intercostals space	Absent right ventricular impulse; diastolic thrill; lower left intercostal border may have opening snap at fourth left intercostal space	Decreases murmur	Height of p wave in lead II >2.5 mm; PR shortened; right atrial hypertrophy	Right atrial and vena cava shadows

*Assurance of whether a murmur is benign or innocent cannot be determined with 100% accuracy.

close spontaneously. Murmurs are graded 1 (barely audible), 2 (faint but clearly heard), 3 (easily heard but without being able to palpate the vibrations on the chest wall), 4 (heard with a palpable thrill), 5 (heard with the stethoscope only partially in contact with the chest wall with a palpable thrill), or 6 (heard without a stethoscope with a palpable thrill). The location where a murmur is best heard is also generally noted (e.g., at the upper right sternal border [second intercostal space], upper left sternal border, lower left sternal border, or apical areas) of the chest wall. These terms have largely superseded the earlier descriptors of aortic, pulmonic, tricuspid, and mitral locations because of the variable radiation or transmission of the sounds.

Systolic murmurs are classified into two general types: ejection type (midsystolic) and regurgitant type (holosystolic). In the ejection type of murmur there is a period of time between S_1 (closure of the mitral and tricuspid valves) and the onset of the murmur. During this time the ventricle is generating pressure (isovolumetric contraction) to overcome the pressure in the great vessels (aorta and pulmonary artery) and open the aortic and pulmonic valves. The murmur builds in intensity as velocity increases, followed by a decrease in intensity, which occurs well before S_2 (closure of the aortic and pulmonic valves). Thus the murmur is diamond shaped, or crescendo-decrescendo. This murmur occurs with left ventricular outflow obstrùction whether the obstruction is from rheumatic or calcific AS, idiopathic hypertrophic subaortic stenosis (IHSS), or pneumonic stenosis. Most murmurs are of this type.

In contrast are the murmurs resulting from flow from a high-pressure chamber to a low-pressure chamber, which occurs in incompetent valves (mitral or tricuspid regurgitation) or with a VSD. As soon as pressure starts to develop, flow occurs throughout systole (holosystolic flow). The pressure gradient and therefore the intensity of the murmur is largely unchanged throughout systole. Such murmurs are described as plateau shaped. The murmurs of chronic tricuspid regurgitation or MR are the epitomes of the holosystolic murmur. However, when a significant gradient or differential of pressure does not exist between chambers, the murmurs will be truncated. Thus the murmur of acute severe MR may occur only during early systole because of rapid equalization of left atrial pressure with left ventricular pressure. Similarly, the classic murmur of a VSD, which may ordinarily be indistinguishable from that of chronic MR, may be truncated or even totally absent in the face of pulmonary hypertension (Eisenmenger's complex). The murmur of mitral valve prolapse is classically late systolic, often after a midsystolic click. Variation in intensity of the murmur with respiration is strongly associated with right-sided (pulmonic or tricuspid valve) abnormalities.[2]

Diastolic murmurs are related to regurgitation across either the aortic or the pulmonic valve, or to filling rumbles caused by flow across a normal (in exaggerated flow states) or obstructed mitral or tricuspid valve. Listening for the high-pitched diastolic murmur of aortic insufficiency or pulmonic insufficiency (regurgitation) is difficult and may require proper positioning of the patient. These murmurs are loudest early in diastole, when there is a large pressure gradient between the aorta and the left ventricle; they then fall in intensity as the pressure gradient falls, producing a decrescendo pattern of sound. They are best heard with the patient sitting, leaning forward, and exhaling—all of which minimize the distance from the stethoscope to the heart. The diaphragm of the stethoscope should be used because of the high-frequency response of the murmur.

The etiology of the murmur cannot be discerned by the character of the murmur; however, it is generally acknowledged that aortic insufficiency murmurs heard best at the upper right sternal border are more likely related to dilation of the aortic root, in contrast to murmurs caused by damage to the aortic valve themselves. If the aortic insufficiency is acute and severe, the duration of the murmur may be truncated as a result of the rapid and premature equalization of pressures between the left ventricle and the aorta. Pulmonic insufficiency is usually found in the setting of pulmonary hypertension with dilation of the pulmonic artery and produces the Graham Steell's murmur, which by clinical examination is almost indistinguishable from the murmur of aortic insufficiency. Low-pitched rumbles in diastole are caused by forward flow across a stenotic mitral or tricuspid valve. Such low-pitched murmurs are best appreciated using the bell of the stethoscope at the apical area with the patient lying slightly on the left side. Because the filling of the ventricles occurs primarily in early diastole (the rapid filling phase) and at the end of diastole (from atrial contraction), the murmur is loudest during these times. Therefore patients with atrial fibrillation will lack the presystolic accentuation of their diastolic rumbles, as they have no atrial contraction.

The duration of the murmur correlates with the severity of the obstruction. However, the severity of the obstruction does not correlate with the intensity or loudness of the murmur. Less severe stenosis will result in a shorter gradient across the stenotic valve, and a shorter murmur will result; more severe stenosis will result in a longer gradient across the stenotic valve, and a longer murmur (to the end of diastole) will result. Hyperdynamic states, such as anemia or fever, or the presence of atrial or ventricular septal defects producing shunting of blood from one chamber to the other during diastole, may produce murmurs in mid-diastole. Left atrial myxomas may obstruct flow across the mitral valve during diastole, producing a similar rumble, but one that is associated with a "tumor plop," instead of an opening snap.

Continuous murmurs begin in systole and extend at least partway into diastole. The classic continuous murmur is exemplified by the murmur associated with a patent ductus arteriosus. Intracardiac shunting between a high-pressure system (aorta) and a low-pressure system (pulmonary artery) exists throughout the cardiac cycle and may be heard in the region just beneath the left clavicle. Fistulas or localized arterial obstructions may also produce continuous murmurs. In addition, continuous murmurs are often the findings associated with benign high-flow states. A continuous murmur, known as a venous hum and heard in the neck, is commonly noted in children and adolescents. It may be abolished by compression of the jugular vein. Similarly, women in the late stages of pregnancy, or shortly postpartum in lactating women, may develop a continuous "mammary shuffle" over the breast that may be obliterated with firm pressure.

A group of murmurs that are not due to any pathologic obstruction to flow are termed innocent, benign, or functional.

As noted previously, the acoustic-mechanical phenomena that create benign or innocent murmurs are the same as those that create pathologic conditions. The differentiation is based on the lack of other findings (e.g., abnormal carotid or peripheral pulses, associated symptoms). Several clues may help distinguish innocent murmurs from pathologic ones.[3] Murmurs that are due to an increased cardiac output (e.g., as a result of fever, thyrotoxicosis, anemia) may be termed functional because they are caused by excess flow across the outflow tract. Many older adults have decreased mobility of the aortic valves as a result of fibrosis and calcification (aortic sclerosis), which distorts the flow, without producing a significant gradient across the valve. Other older patients may have outflow murmurs that are due to ejection of blood into a kinked, tortuous aorta. A number of adolescents and young adults have ejection murmurs that mimic the flow murmur across the pulmonic valve as a result of an atrial septal defect. These patients have a narrowed anteroposterior chest dimension that is due to either a decreased curvature of the spine (straight back syndrome) or pectus excavatum.[3]

Aortic Stenosis

DEFINITION/EPIDEMIOLOGY

Based purely on clinical findings, it is more difficult to assess the degree of severity of AS than it is to assess any other valvular abnormality. Valvular AS may be caused by rheumatic damage, congenital abnormality (bicuspid aortic valve), or degeneration caused by the aging process—calcific AS of older adults.[4] Over the past three decades, with the successful treatment of streptococcal pharyngitis, the etiology has shifted away from rheumatic to calcific. All share the fact that over 20 to 30 years the repetitive mechanical trauma of the blood against the valve results in fibrosis, calcification, and eventually stenosis.

PATHOPHYSIOLOGY

Any reduction of the normal aortic valve orifice of approximately 3 cm^2 will cause obstruction to the flow of blood from the left ventricle into the aorta during ventricular systole. A systolic pressure gradient develops between the left ventricle and the aorta. Left ventricular pressure rises, increasing systolic wall stress. The left ventricle hypertrophies as a compensatory mechanism to maintain an adequate cardiac output. Valvular stenosis is generally considered to be significant when the valve area is reduced to 25% of normal. Therefore hemodynamically significant AS would be an aortic valve area <0.75 cm^2 in an adult, which is associated with a gradient of >50 mm Hg. A large pressure gradient across the aortic valve may be sustained for many years without a reduction in contractile function, with left ventricular dilation generally a very late manifestation. Persistent pressure overload to the left ventricle may eventually lead to left ventricular dilation, left atrial enlargement, and pulmonary hypertension.

CLINICAL PRESENTATION

Chest pain, syncope, and dyspnea are the classic symptoms associated with severe AS. With chronic AS there generally is a long latent period before the development of symptoms. Once symptoms develop, however, the progression to end-stage disease or death is precipitous, averaging 2 to 5 years.[5] Calcific AS has now become more predominant than rheumatic aortic stensosis,[6] and as a result the mean age of presentation is now in the sixties. Angina and syncope become manifest while the left ventricular function remains preserved; dyspnea indicates congestive heart failure (CHF) and left ventricular dysfunction.[6] Exertional angina occurs in about two thirds of patients with severe AS and may be due to coronary atherosclerosis or to the markedly increased myocardial oxygen demand. This may occur even in the presence of normal coronary arteries.[7,8] Although uncommon, patients with severe AS have suffered sudden death, usually in association with exertion, and although the mechanism remains uncertain, a common hypothesis is an abnormal baroreceptor response, the Bezold-Jarisch reflex.[9] Dizziness or frank syncope occurs in 15% to 30% of patients and has been attributed to an abrupt fall in systemic vascular resistance in the presence of a fixed cardiac output, abrupt failure of the overloaded left ventricle during effort, or arrhythmia.[10] Left ventricular failure eventually occurs with symptoms of fatigue, cough, progressive dyspnea on exertion, orthopnea, and paroxysmal nocturnal dyspnea. If the problem is unrelieved, death is likely within 2 years in patients with heart failure, 3 years in those with syncope, and 5 years in those with angina.[11]

PHYSICAL EXAMINATION

No physical finding can reliably assess the severity of obstruction. Classically the carotid pulse has a slow rise with delayed peak and small volume (pulsus parvus and pulsus tardus). A notch or shudder in the upstroke (anacrotic notch) may be appreciated. The average examiner, however, is unable to distinguish a slow-rising pulse from a normal one.[12] Auscultation reveals a harsh crescendo-decrescendo systolic election murmur that begins after the first heart sound. The murmur of AS is loudest at the second right sternal edge and radiates to the left lateral sternal border and carotids. A thrill is often present. The murmur may become softer, or even inaudible, in patients with end-stage AS. Paradoxic splitting of the second heart sound (S_2) occurs as a result of delay in closure of the aortic valve. In severe stenosis the A_2 is often inaudible; therefore no splitting of S_2 is appreciated. An additional early systolic ejection sound or click may be heard, more commonly in younger patients with congenital or bicuspid AS. Left ventricular hypertrophy (LVH) produces a sustained thrust or heave of the apical impulse. Displacement of the apical impulse downward and to the left occurs after left ventricular failure develops and the ventricle dilates.

DIAGNOSTICS

The single most important fact concerning laboratory tests in patients with AS is that with the exception of echocardiography, normal findings (e.g., lack of LVH or normal chest x-ray findings) do not exclude severe disease. The ECG demonstrates normal sinus rhythm with signs of LVH. Atrial fibrillation usually represents either end-stage disease with left ventricular decompensation or other associated disease. Conduction abnormalities, such as first-degree atrioventricular block, bundle branch block, and intraventricular conduction disturbances, are fairly common. The chest x-ray film may demonstrate rounding or prominence of the left ventricle as a result of concentric hypertrophy of the left ventricle, poststenotic dilation of the aorta, and calcification of the valve cusps, or the chest x-ray findings may be completely normal.

In contrast, a technically satisfactory, well-performed two-dimensional echocardiogram has the ability to exclude significant obstruction of the aortic valve. The Doppler portion of the examination is able to provide an assessment of the outflow gradient that closely approximates that obtained by cardiac catheterization. By combining Doppler ultrasonography and the echocardiogram, reasonable calculation of the aortic valve area may be made. Thickened, calcified, and immobile leaflets are readily noted by transthoracic two-dimensional echocardiography. The echocardiogram also demonstrates poststenotic dilation of the aorta and left ventricular wall thickening. Dilation of the left ventricle and/or reduced contractility (ejection fraction) occurs with myocardial failure. Equally important, additional valvular abnormalities (e.g., mitral regurgitation or stenosis) are apparent, as are the findings of IHSS.

Cardiac catheterization can determine the severity of obstruction by recording the gradient across the valve and by calculation of the valve area. Additional functional assessment of the left ventricle is possible. In the current era these findings often serve to confirm those obtained by Doppler echocardiography. In adults the major indication for cardiac catheterization is to delineate the coronary anatomy. Even in patients without angina, approximately 50% will have significant coronary obstructions[7] (see the Diagnostics box on p. 570).

DIFFERENTIAL DIAGNOSIS

The major condition in the differential diagnosis for a systolic ejection murmur without valvular disease is the functional or innocent murmur (i.e., flow murmur without disease). The absence of symptoms or other physical abnormalities will generally lead to this diagnosis. In the adult the major pathologic state that must be differentiated is IHSS or hypertrophic stenosis. These patients may have similar symptomatology; however, the carotid upstroke is very brisk, with at times two distinct humps (the bispheriens pulse). The primary distinguishing characteristic is the response of the murmur to maneuvers that increase or decrease the dynamic obstruction. Thus standing or the strain phase of the Valsalva maneuver decreases venous return, resulting in a smaller left ventricular outflow tract and an increase in the murmur intensity.

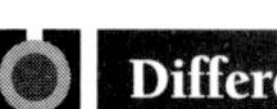

Differential Diagnosis

Systolic Murmurs

Ejection Murmurs
Aortic stenosis
Idiopathic hypertrophic subaortic stenosis
Pulmonary stenosis

Regurgitant Murmurs
Mitral regurgitation or insufficiency
Tricuspid regurgitation or insufficiency
Ventricular septal defect

Late Systolic Murmurs
Mitral valve prolapse

Continuous Murmurs
Patent ductus arteriosus
Benign (innocent)
Mammary shuffle

MANAGEMENT

Management of the patient with symptomatic AS is almost entirely surgical. Medications cannot increase the forward flow across a critically stenosed valve. Indeed, treatment of the symptomatic patient with high-grade AS is fraught with difficulties. Nitrates may decrease systemic vascular resistance and perfusion pressure. Calcium channel blockers and beta blockers may decrease left ventricular function and precipitate heart failure. Diuretics may result in hypovolemia and underperfusion similar to that with nitrates. Thus each must be used with great caution. Digoxin may provide some benefit to a patient with AS who is symptomatic with evidence of left ventricular dysfunction. Medical therapy for the asymptomatic patient with AS consists of antibiotic prophylaxis for the prevention of infective endocarditis. Strenuous physical exertion should be avoided only in patients with high-grade lesions.

Co-Management with Specialists

Co-management with a specialist is reasonable for patients with AS to obtain a Doppler echocardiogram every 2 years for mild disease and annually for more severe disease. Patients with significant obstruction and modest symptoms, or those who are asymptomatic yet have severe obstruction, may require a Doppler echocardiogram every 6 months.

LIFE SPAN CONSIDERATIONS

Once patients with AS become symptomatic with angina or syncope, the average survival time is 2 to 3 years. Patients with CHF demonstrate an average survival time of 1.5 to 2 years.[5]

COMPLICATIONS

The initial symptoms associated with AS are generally angina and syncope/presyncope, as well as dyspnea and frank CHF, which, in the patient with solely AS, are manifestations of a failing left ventricle. Atrial fibrillation occurs in less than 10% of patients with AS, and its occurrence should raise the possibility of concomitant mitral valve disease. If it occurs, prompt cardioversion is often required, as loss of atrial contraction may markedly impair left ventricular performance as a result of the markedly noncompliant left ventricle. Systematic calcium embolization to the retinal artery may result in partial visual loss and may be an additional indication for prompt surgical repair.[13]

INDICATIONS FOR REFERRAL/HOSPITALIZATION AND PATIENT EDUCATION

See Indications for Referral/Hospitalization and Patient Education under Mitral Stenosis, p. 571.

Aortic Insufficiency

DEFINITION/EPIDEMIOLOGY

Aortic regurgitation occurs when the aortic valve fails to close completely, allowing blood to flow back into the left ventricle during ventricular diastole. This process may be either chronic or acute. It may occur as a result of involvement of the leaflets themselves or as a result of distortion of the aortic root. Pathologic processes that affect the aortic valve, leading to chronic aortic regurgitation, are inflammation (e.g., resulting from rheumatic fever, syphilis, rheumatoid arthritis), structural processes (e.g., unicuspid, bicuspid, aneurysm), disruptive processes (e.g., trauma, infective endocarditis, dissection), congenital conditions, or stress from hypertension, whereas acute aortic regurgitation most commonly occurs as a result of infective endocarditis, with dissecting aortic aneurysm and acute chest trauma being less common causes.

PATHOPHYSIOLOGY

Aortic regurgitation, or aortic insufficiency (AI), produces a volume overload to the left ventricle during diastole. The volume of blood regurgitated into the left ventricle determines whether the volume overload is mild, moderate, or severe. Regurgitant volume is determined by (1) the area of the regurgitant valve orifice, (2) the diastolic pressure gradient between the aorta and the left ventricle, and (3) the duration of diastole.[5] In chronic AI the left ventricle dilates, compensating with a gradual increase in end-diastolic volume. Initially, forward output is maintained as normal, and the ventricle may not ever have increased end-diastolic pressure, but wall stress is dramatically elevated. In acute aortic regurgitation there is no time for this adaptation to occur, and a dramatic increase in left ventricular end-diastolic pressure occurs with only minor increases in end-diastolic volume.

CLINICAL PRESENTATION AND PHYSICAL EXAMINATION

Patients with chronic aortic regurgitation may be asymptomatic for decades. When symptoms do occur, the patient usually complains of symptoms of CHF, especially dyspnea and fatigue. Patients may also complain of angina in the absence of significant coronary artery disease. Patients with acute aortic regurgitation present with symptoms of severe left-sided failure (dyspnea at rest, orthopnea, paroxysmal nocturnal dyspnea, fatigue, exhaustion) that have occurred suddenly. Symptoms of low forward cardiac output (fatigue and exhaustion) are overshadowed by symptoms of pulmonary congestion in patients with acute AI.

A number of physical findings differ between acute and chronic AI. In chronic AI the rate of rise of the peripheral pulse is rapid with quick collapse (Corrigan's, or water-hammer, pulse) as a result of the forceful ejection of blood in early systole and regurgitation during early diastole. The carotid pulse is often bisferious. Arterial blood pressure usually demonstrates a low diastolic pressure (Korotkoff sounds may even be zero) with a normal systolic blood pressure, thus causing a widened pulse pressure in a patient with moderate or severe chronic AI. Patients with acute AI usually demonstrate a carotid arterial pulse with a sharp rise to a single, rapidly collapsing peak without a widened pulse pressure. A pulsus alternans may be present in acute severe AI, but it is unusual in patients with chronic AI. With chronic AI the apical impulse is displaced to the left and downward and is hyperdynamic. Auscultation of the patient with AI often reveals an S_3. The diastolic murmur of chronic regurgitation is usually high pitched and blowing, with the duration correlating best with the severity of the insufficiency. In acute AI the murmur may be very short or even absent. A rumbling mid or late diastolic murmur, the Austin Flint murmur, may be heard at the apex in the presence of at least moderate insufficiency. This represents functional mitral stenosis (MS) of the mitral valve from the torrential regurgitant flow produced by the AI impinging on the anterior mitral valve leaflet. A loud systolic ejection murmur is common in both acute and chronic AI, even in the absence of valve stenosis.

DIAGNOSTICS

The characteristic findings on the ECG for a patient with chronic AI is LVH, especially in the precordial leads. Conduction disturbances may occur with aortic regurgitation secondary to inflammatory processes. In acute severe AI the ECG is usually normal except for sinus tachycardia, without evidence of LVH.

As the severity of chronic aortic regurgitation increases, the left ventricular contour enlarges, producing a boot-shaped heart silhouette on the chest x-ray film. The aortic knob and ascending aorta become prominent with moderate to severe chronic AI. Patients with acute AI do not demonstrate cardiac enlargement but will exhibit increased venous redistribution to the upper lobes because of pulmonary venous and capillary hypertension secondary to an increased left ventricular end-diastolic pressure and left atrial pressure.

Echocardiography combined with color Doppler imaging has become the primary diagnostic tool for assessment of AI. Evidence of mild AI may be detected on Doppler imaging long before it is audible on auscultation. Transthoracic two-dimensional echocardiography may help to identify possible etiologies for the regurgitation by documenting flail or prolapsing leaflets, a dilated aortic root, or evidence of vegetation. The greatest impact, however, is the ability of Doppler echocardiography to assess the severity of the regurgitation and assist in determining the optimal time for valve replacement, especially in the asymptomatic patient. Color Doppler imaging has been investigated for the ability to "quantify" the degree of regurgitation; however, not surprisingly, only a relative, "qualitative" assessment is possible, because the amount of regurgitation is dependent not only on the "size of the hole," but also on both the upstream and downstream pressures. However, echocardiography is able to quantify the ventricular dimensions and ventricular function (ejection fraction) well. Evidence of reduction in systolic function or marked and/or progressive ventricular dilation is an indication for surgery. Patients with a left ventricular end-systolic dimension >55 mm have been found to have an increased risk of operative death or subsequent death from CHF[14] (see the Diagnostics box on p. 570).

DIFFERENTIAL DIAGNOSIS

The murmur of AI is an early diastolic murmur that must be differentiated from other early diastolic murmurs (pulmonary regurgitation and VSD). Most early diastolic murmurs are related to either pulmonary or aortic regurgitation. However, an early diastolic flow murmur can also sometimes be heard in patients with a VSD and a large left-to-right shunt.

MANAGEMENT

Medical therapy for chronic aortic regurgitation consists of antibiotic prophylaxis. Once left ventricular failure develops, digitalis glycosides, diuretics, and vasodilators are necessary to

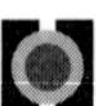

Differential Diagnosis

Diastolic Murmurs

Early Diastole
Aortic insufficiency
Pulmonary insufficiency
Ventricular septal defect

Mid to Late Diastole
Mitral stenosis
Tricuspid stenosis
Austin Flint murmur

improve left ventricular function and to reduce the aortic regurgitant fraction. Hydralazine and other vasodilators have been found to be useful in the asymptomatic or minimally symptomatic patient for reducing ventricular volumes, improving ejection fraction, and potentially delaying the need for surgery.[15,16] The primary therapy for an incompetent valve, however, remains valve replacement. The critical issue is the timing of surgery. Surgery is advocated for symptomatic patients who have confirmed moderate to severe chronic AI or who have impaired or progressively worsening left ventricular function. Surgery is usually not indicated for asymptomatic patients with severe chronic AI who have good exercise tolerance and normal left ventricular function. The natural history of such patients has been excellent.[17] However, recent emphasis has been placed on distinguishing the patient with mild symptoms (New York Heart Association [NYHA] functional class II) from the truly asymptomatic patient, with strong consideration for early operation for the former.[18] Although the need for surgery at the onset of symptoms or ventricular dysfunction has been emphasized, even the patient with a grossly impaired left ventricular performance or severe symptoms may experience marked improvement in ventricular function and symptoms[19] and therefore should be considered as a candidate for valve replacement.

Co-Management with Specialists

Co-management with a specialist is considered when the patient with AI becomes symptomatic. Patients may live for years or decades with AI before the development of symptoms. However, as with AS, once symptoms develop, progressive deterioration will occur over the subsequent few years unless surgical intervention occurs.

COMPLICATIONS

Other than progressive ventricular dysfunction and development of symptoms, the major complication is infective endocarditis. Patients who are nearing the time for consideration of valve replacement should undergo dental consultation.

INDICATIONS FOR REFERRAL/HOSPITALIZATION AND PATIENT EDUCATION

See Indications for Referral/Hospitalization and Patient Education under Mitral Stenosis, p. 571.

Mitral Regurgitation

DEFINITION/EPIDEMIOLOGY

Mitral insufficiency, or mitral regurgitation, may result from a disturbance of any of the functional components of the mitral valve or its supporting structures, which include the valve leaflets, papillary muscle, mitral valve annulus, chordae tendineae, or left ventricle itself. Rheumatic heart disease was generally the most common cause of chronic MR; however, with the reduction in the incidence of rheumatic fever, other causes such as ischemic heart disease and mitral valve prolapse have become the most common etiologies. Additional causes of MR, either acute or chronic, include isolated rupture of the chordae tendineae, papillary muscle dysfunction, and infective endocarditis. Dilation of the left ventricle from any cause is likely to cause the mitral leaflets to fail to coapt. Acute regurgitation may occur as a result of spontaneous rupture of the chordae tendineae, blunt chest trauma, or necrotic disruption of a papillary muscle as a sequela of a myocardial infarction.

PATHOPHYSIOLOGY

The burden placed on the heart as a result of MR is independent on the amount of reflux and the ventricular and atrial ability to compensate. During systole the left ventricle will be simultaneously ejecting blood forward through the aortic valve or backward across an incompetent valve into the left atrium. The volume of mitral regurgitant flow in either chronic or acute MR therefore depends on the size of the regurgitant orifice and on the pressure gradient between the left ventricle and the left atrium. The latter will be affected by the balance between the ease of regurgitation into the "low-pressure sump" of the left atrium and the flow out to the aorta. Regurgitant flow will be decreased by any agent that decreases left ventricular size (such as diuretics) or shifts the balance toward forward output (such as afterload-reducing vasodilators). In contrast, regurgitation is increased by any factor that enlarges the left ventricle, depresses myocardial function, or increases resistance to forward flow (such as hypertension or AS). With chronic MR the increased volume of blood ejected back into the left atrium causes stretching and thinning of the atrial wall. The large, thin-walled atrium accommodates the large volume of blood ejected into it during ventricular systole. Although the pressure in the left atrium and pulmonary capillaries and veins will be elevated during systole, the left atrial pressure decreases to near normal during ventricular diastole. The left ventricle dilates and becomes hypertrophied in response to the increased volume from the left atrium, so that a sufficient cardiac output is maintained. Initially the additional volume to be ejected by the ventricle (increased preload) results in enhanced emptying. Therefore the ejection fraction will be increased. "Normal" ejection fraction or other measures of cardiac systolic performance actually are likely to represent significantly abnormal ventricular function. Pulmonary hypertension rarely develops in the patient who has developed MR gradually over time.

In contrast, patients with acute MR develop a rapid increase in left atrial pressure as a result of the sudden volume overload into a normal, nondilated left atrium and ventricle. This results in sudden increased left ventricular end-diastolic, left atrial, and pulmonary venous pressure, producing interstitial edema that leads to pulmonary edema. Pulmonary hypertension may develop.

CLINICAL PRESENTATION

The patient with MR may remain asymptomatic for decades. Patients generally complain of fatigue and, later in the course of the disease, dyspnea on exertion. The former is a result of reduced forward cardiac output, whereas the latter occurs with the onset of left ventricular dysfunction. The severity of symptoms, as well as clinical outcome, of chronic MR depends not only on the degree of regurgitation, but also on associated additional valvular abnormalities, the presence of underlying ventricular dysfunction, and concomitant coronary artery disease. Palpitations are often noted, even in the patient without evidence of atrial fibrillation. Symptoms of CHF appear late in the course of chronic MR as a result of the gradual increase in volume overload. By the time symptoms appear, the degree of ventricular dysfunction may have progressed to such an extent as to be irreversible.

Those who develop acute MR have an abrupt onset of symptoms resulting from the sudden overload of the left atrium. A patient with rupture of a few chordae from subacute bacterial endocarditis or trauma usually complains of easy fatigue, dyspnea, pedal edema, and occasionally intermittent chest pain. A patient with a complete rupture of a papillary muscle generally has severe hypotension and florid pulmonary edema. With MR, palpation of the carotid pulse will generally demonstrate a rapidly rising pulse. The apical impulse is hyperkinetic and displaces downward and to the left. Auscultation of the patient with chronic MR reveals a soft S_1. A loud P_2 or an extenuated pulmonic component of S_2 suggests the presence of pulmonary hypertension. An audible S_3 is present when there is hemodynamically significant MR, and in combined MS and regurgitation, S_3 is indicative of predominant regurgitation. The hallmark murmur of MR is the pansystolic, blowing murmur best heard at the apex and radiating to the axilla or back. The murmur may radiate to other locations such as the back or sternum if papillary muscle dysfunction or partial rupture of supporting structures is present. Maneuvers that decrease left ventricular volume by decreasing impedance to left ventricular outflow or venous return (such as sudden standing or inhalation of amyl nitrite) will result in a decreased murmur, as will more chronically decreasing ventricular volume with diuresis. Increasing the impedance to left ventricular ejection (ask the patient to squeeze both fists in a handgrip) will increase regurgitation and thereby the intensity of the murmur.

DIAGNOSTICS

The ECG in chronic MR usually demonstrates normal sinus rhythm with left atrial hypertrophy in the early stage and atrial fibrillation later on. If the MR is secondary to underlying ventricular dysfunction and dilation, evidence of LVH is generally noted on the ECG. The chest x-ray film demonstrates an increase in both left ventricular and left atrial size.

Doppler echocardiography detects the high-velocity jet of regurgitant flow back into the left atrium. It permits sensitive detection of regurgitation of even a mild degree. Although the ability to "quantify" the degree of the regurgitation remains imprecise, the technique permits the more important prediction of clinical outcomes. The severity can be roughly estimated by the distance the jet goes into the atrium. Chronic MR usually produces a volume overload pattern and a large left atrium. Structural abnormalities such as flail leaflets, endocarditic vegetation, and thickened, rheumatic chordae can be detected by echocardiography. Determination of the end-systolic volume of the ventricle has proved to be a more reliable predictor of clinical prognosis.[20] Patients with dimensions >50 mm had poor outcomes after surgery, in contrast to those with end-systolic diameters <40 mm (see the Diagnostics box on p. 570).

DIFFERENTIAL DIAGNOSIS

The murmur of MR or mitral insufficiency is a holosystolic murmur. Other holosystolic murmurs include the murmur of tricuspid regurgitation and VSD. On rare occasions the murmur of patent ductus arteriosus can be a holosystolic murmur also. Often, if the patient is tachycardic, these murmurs are difficult to distinguish from long systolic ejection murmurs. Because holosystolic murmurs are pathologic murmurs, differentiation is essential (see the Differential Diagnosis box on p. 564).

MANAGEMENT

All patients with chronic MR, even those who are asymptomatic, should receive antibiotic prophylaxis before any dental or surgical procedure. If atrial fibrillation develops, digitalis glycosides are given to control the ventricular rate. Other agents such as calcium channel blockers or beta blockers may be less tolerated, given their potential to exacerbate the degree of regurgitation as a result of their negative contractile potential. Anticoagulation should be strongly considered to prevent systemic emboli. Dietary sodium restriction and diuretics will be useful for symptomatic patients. Agents that reduce afterload (hydralazine or converting enzyme inhibitors) will increase forward flow of blood and thereby improve symptoms, reverse hemodynamic alterations, and even delay the necessity for surgical intervention.[21] Recent investigations suggest the benefit of angiotensin receptor blocker therapy for the patient intolerant of angiotensin-converting enzyme inhibitors.[22]

Co-Management with Specialists

Co-management with a specialist should be considered once the patient with MR becomes symptomatic and surgery is considered. Surgical therapy is aimed at improving symptoms, relieving severe pulmonary hypertension, and decreasing left ventricular volume and mass. The Veterans Administration Cooperative Study has recommended surgery for significant MR or MS/MR before left ventricular election fraction is decreased to below 0.5, the end-systolic volume index is increased to above 101 ml/m^2, or pulmonary hypertension develops, because left ventricular size and systolic function will likely be normal postoperatively and survival and functional class will be enhanced.[23] Other investigators have recommended using an ejection fraction cutoff of 60% as being indicative of significant ventricular dysfunction.[24] Patients with marked left ventricular dysfunction may remain symptomatic even after surgical treatment. Such patients may show a decrease in ejection fraction and an increase in end-systolic volume immediately after surgery as the abolition of MR removes their "low-pressure sump," essentially increasing the afterload that the ventricle faces. These patients may require vasodilator treatment in the immediate postoperative period and in fact may be difficult to wean off bypass. Such patients may benefit by only partial repair of the valve, leaving some regurgitation.

Surgical techniques used to treat MR are valve repair/reconstruction and valve replacement. Valve repair/reconstruction repairs the disrupted functional component of the valve. Mitral valve repair retains the tethering effect of chordal attachments, which may prevent postoperative dilation of the left ventricle, and decreases the chance of left ventricular dysfunction, which occurs after mitral valve replacement. A significant increase in exercise ejection fraction and stroke volume after mitral valve replacement has been found in patients in whom the chordae and papillary muscles were preserved.[25]

LIFE SPAN CONSIDERATIONS

Life span considerations for patients with MR will depend on the degree of symptoms and the status of the left ventricular function. Patients with MR may remain asymptomatic for decades, with only a small percentage progressing to more severe MR requiring surgery.[26] Patients commonly may tolerate even significant MR for decades without development of symptoms.

COMPLICATIONS

Atrial fibrillation affects approximately 75% of patients with MR and is related to the size of the left atrium. Other complications include systemic embolization (generally in the presence of atrial fibrillation) and bacterial endocarditis.

INDICATIONS FOR REFERRAL/HOSPITALIZATION AND PATIENT EDUCATION

See Consideration for Referral/Hospitalization and Patient Education under Mitral Stenosis, p. 571).

Mitral Valve Prolapse

DEFINITION/EPIDEMIOLOGY

A unique subset of patients with MR are those with mitral valve prolapse (MVP). Although the regurgitation is usually mild and often free of associated papillary muscle dysfunction, MVP appears to occur more often in patients with small ventricles resulting from thoracic deformities, such as the straight back syndrome or pectus excavatum. The syndrome seems to be most prevalent in young women between 20 and 40 years old, although it has been detected in males of all ages, with men over the age of 45 years at increased risk of developing complications of severe MR and endocarditis.[27]

PATHOPHYSIOLOGY

MVP is typically described as the posterior displacement or prolapse of one or both (more commonly the posterior) leaflets of the mitral valve into the left atrium during systole. This billowing back of the leaflet places stress on the chordae tendineae and papillary muscles, which may be the cause of the nonischemic chest discomfort. The myxomatous degeneration may, over time, result in thickened and redundant valves. As the valvular dysfunction progresses, insufficient coaptation will result in MR. The connective tissue changes may extend into the mitral annulus, enhancing the tendency for MR, and into the chordae tendineae, potentially resulting in sudden chordal rupture.

CLINICAL PRESENTATION

Most persons with MVP are asymptomatic. When symptoms do occur, the patient usually complains of chest discomfort, palpitations, mild dyspnea, fatigue, and anxiety. These symptoms are similar to those reported in the panic disorder syndrome. Both disorders may be a result of automatic dysfunction.[28] The chest symptoms, along with the tremendous frequency of this disorder in the general population, mandate familiarity with its presentation. Although as many as 17% of healthy females may have auscultatory findings suggestive of this syndrome, a more valid estimate, relying on appropriate echocardiographic criteria, would place the frequency at 4% to 6%, or affecting more than 10 million males and females in the United States.[29,30]

MVP should probably be thought of as a continuum from the exaggeration of the normal, slight billowing of the mitral valve into the left atrium during systole, to a fully "floppy" valve, and finally to variable degrees of MR when the floppy, redundant leaflets no longer are able to coapt. At times the regurgitation may become severe, often as a result of the rupture of the chordae tendineae. Most commonly, the disorder exists by itself, generally in association with a characteristic pathologic myxomatous degeneration of the mitral valve. There appears to be a strong hereditary predisposition to the condition, although it may be associated with other conditions, some rare (e.g., Ehlers-Danlos syndrome) and others common (e.g., atrial septal defect). MVP has been noted in patients with coronary artery disease. The ischemic discomfort is usually described as brief attacks of severe, piercing pain localized to the apex. Palpitations are common and may result from a variety of arrhythmias.

Most cases of MVP are diagnosed on routine physical examination. Auscultation of the patient with MVP reveals a midsystolic click. This is a snapping extra heart sound heard best at the lower left sternal border or at the apex, and it may be only intermittently appreciated. The presence of an apical systolic murmur varies with the degree of MR. This systolic murmur is usually a late systolic–crescendo type that can be loud and musical. Maneuvers that decrease the left ventricular volume, such as standing, will both move the click earlier in systole and make the murmur longer. Holosystolic murmurs are usually an indication of pronounced MVP resulting in a more severe form of MR.

DIAGNOSTICS

Patients with MVP, most commonly those who are symptomatic, may demonstrate inverted T waves and nonspecific ST-segment changes in the inferior and left precordial leads of the ECG. These changes may be a manifestation of the ischemia to the papillary muscles resulting from the strain placed on these muscles by the prolapsed valve leaflets. Stress ECGs and thallium-201 or sestamibi exercise scans should be used when there is a need to differentiate MVP from coronary artery disease. This is especially important when the patient with suspected MVP complains of chest discomfort.

Supraventricular tachycardia is not uncommon in MVP. Other ventricular and supraventricular arrhythmias, as well as conduction disturbances, may also occur. There seems to be a slightly increased incidence of sudden death, presumably as a result of ventricular fibrillation, although this finding has not been firmly established.

Echocardiography, specifically two-dimensional echocardiography, is regarded by some as the single best technique to define this disorder. The echocardiogram shows the posterior mitral valve leaflet or both leaflets bowing or bulging back into the left atrium during systole. Such displacement, noted solely on the four-chamber view, is now recognized as a normal finding.

Patients with thickened and redundant mitral valves form a higher-risk subgroup for subsequent complications.[30] Other echocardiographic findings include MR and flail leaflets in patients with ruptured chordae (see the Diagnostics box on p. 570).

DIFFERENTIAL DIAGNOSIS

The murmur of MVP is a late systolic murmur and is characterized by a midsystolic click. This click heralds the onset of the murmur. Because it is a murmur of mitral insufficiency, it should be differentiated from the holosystolic murmur of mitral insufficiency (see the Differential Diagnosis box on p. 564).

MANAGEMENT

Most persons with MVP are asymptomatic and require no intervention other than periodic clinical and echocardiographic follow-up evaluation every 3 to 5 years. Asymptomatic patients need reassurance that the condition is benign and usually uncomplicated, and that the prognosis is good. If a systolic murmur is present, however, the patient with MVP, even if asymptomatic, requires more frequent monitoring. Those with holosystolic murmurs are more likely to have more MR and require the same approach as noted for MR. However, even in the face of severe MR, many patients will continue to do well.[26]

Antibiotic prophylaxis, although controversial, appears reasonable for MVP with evidence of MR. Patients with a history of palpitations or prolonged QT intervals should have 24-hour ambulatory monitoring. Beta-blocker therapy is often useful for palpitations and/or nonischemic chest pain. Patients with syncope or near-syncope should be referred for more complete arrhythmia evaluation.

Co-Management with Specialists

Co-management with a specialist and life span considerations for MVP are related to the severity of the MR and are the same as previously described for MR. Surgical treatment of MVP is necessary when the MR has been progressive and severe. Mitral reconstruction with ring annuloplasty has been successful.

COMPLICATIONS

In addition to chordal rupture and progressive MR, endocarditis and sudden death have been associated with this disorder[31]; however, their incidence remains uncertain. Most reviews conclude that endocarditis and sudden death are rare. All of the complications are more common in older men or those with MVP and thickened leaflets.[27,30]

INDICATIONS FOR REFERRAL/HOSPITALIZATION AND PATIENT EDUCATION

See Indications for Referral/Hospitalization and Patient and Family Education under Mitral Stenosis, p. 571).

Mitral Stenosis

DEFINITION/EPIDEMIOLOGY

MS is almost always caused by rheumatic heart disease. Thus with the marked reduction of rheumatic carditis over the last four decades, the occurrence of MS has lessened. Less common causes of obstruction across the mitral valve that prevents normal emptying of the left atrium into the left ventricle during diastole include congenital stenoses, masses such as vegetation, clots or benign tumors (atrial myxomas), and profound calcification of the mitral annulus. Damage to the mitral valve from rheumatic fever will cause the commissures of the leaflets themselves to fuse, the leaflets to thicken and fibrose, and the chordae to thicken and shorten, resulting in a thickened, scarred valve that is funnel shaped with a "fish mouth" appearance.

PATHOPHYSIOLOGY

The central pathophysiologic feature of MS is obstruction across the mitral valve during diastole. This results in a pressure gradient between the left atrium and the left ventricle. The increased left atrial pressure is transmitted to the pulmonary veins and capillaries, and eventually to the pulmonary arteries and right side of the heart. The normal mitral valve area is 4 to 6 cm^2. There is usually no detectable pressure gradient across the normal mitral valve, even when flow is increased with exercise. As the valve area is reduced, the gradient across the valve increases. When the valve area is reduced to 25% of normal, hemodynamically significant stenosis is present. Critical MS occurs when the mitral valve opening is reduced to 1 cm^2. With this degree of obstruction, the mean gradient, even at rest, is likely to be >20 mm Hg throughout diastole. With a further rise to 25 to 30 mm Hg, the left atrial pressure will exceed plasma oncotic pressure, and episodes of orthopnea and/or paroxysmal nocturnal dyspnea will develop. Chronic elevation of left atrial pressure produces a passive pressure load on the pulmonary vessel and causes hypertrophy and hyperplasia. In addition, there is a reactive vasoconstrictive aspect. Pulmonary hypertension may develop, which over time may produce right ventricular hypertrophy. In long-standing, severe MS, pulmonary hypertension may approach or exceed systemic levels.

A major advance in the ability to assess valvular obstruction was the derivation by Gorlin of a hydraulic formula for calculation of the cardiac valve area. An understanding of this formula is helpful to better understand the factors that result in increases in this gradient. This equation describes the relationship between the size of the opening (valve area) and how it relates to the flow rate across the valve and the pressure drop (gradient) across the valve. Thus for any given valve area, an increase in flow volume (cardiac output) results in an increase in gradient. The "rate" aspect relates to the time available to get the blood across the valve (diastolic filling period). Increases in blood flow (resulting from hypervolemia or pregnancy) will increase the gradient. More dramatic is the effect of heart rate. As diastole, not systole, shortens with an increase in heart rate, fever or exercise may significantly elevate the gradient, especially because the gradient increases as a square of the increase in flow rate (i.e., a doubling of the heart rate will quadruple the gradient). Thus patients with mild to moderate MS who were previously asymptomatic may develop florid heart failure with the development of atrial fibrillation (which generally has a rapid ventricular response on initial occurrence).

CLINICAL PRESENTATION

The principal symptom of MS is dyspnea, which is graded according to the NYHA classification. Patients with asymptomatic MS are graded as functional class I. Patients with dyspnea that occurs with greater than ordinary exertion are graded as class

II; patients with dyspnea that occurs with only mild exertion (less than ordinary activity) are class III; and those with dyspnea on minimal exertion, with episodes of orthopnea, paroxysmal nocturnal dyspnea, or pulmonary edema are class IV. Fatigue is also common with MS and in some cases may be more severe than dyspnea. If atrial fibrillation develops, patients may also complain of palpitations. Hemoptysis may occur as a result of pulmonary hypertension and in rare instances may be massive. Hoarseness (Ortner's syndrome) may develop from compression of the left recurrent laryngeal nerve by a dilated left atrium. A small number of patients complain of angina-like chest pain, which may be due to concomitant coronary artery disease, pulmonary embolus, or pulmonary hypertension. Thromboembolism may be the presenting symptom in some patients.

Auscultation will typically reveal a loud S_1, an accentuated pulmonic component of S_2 (P_2) if pulmonary hypertension is present, and an opening snap heard with the diaphragm of the stethoscope. This snap is caused by the snapping of the thickened mitral valve as it reaches the end of its maximal excursion during early diastole. This must be distinguished from an S_3 gallop sound, which is lower in pitch and occurs later in diastole (typically 0.12 seconds after S_2) than the opening snap, which occurs 0.04 to 0.10 seconds after S_2. The classic diastolic rumble of MS is heard with the bell of the stethoscope near the apex. It begins shortly after the opening snap and may have a presystolic accentuation in patients who are still in normal sinus rhythm. The murmur may be difficult to appreciate in the early stages of MS and can be better appreciated by listening with the patient in the left lateral decubitus position or by increasing the flow by having the patient perform mild exercise. As the severity of MS increases and valve leaflets become markedly calcified, the S_1 sound will decrease in intensity while the diagnostic rumble progresses to a pandiastolic murmur.

DIAGNOSTICS

The characteristic findings on the ECG are evidence of left atrial enlargement (widened, notched P wave in lead II with pronounced terminal negativity in V_1) in patients still in normal sinus rhythm and evidence of right axis deviation of the QRS or right ventricular hypertrophy. Atrial fibrillation is common. Chest x-ray examination may reveal a straightening of the left heart border or "double density" in the midportion of the cardiac silhouette, both of which are manifestations of left atrial enlargement. With chronic pulmonary hypertension the pulmonary vessels become prominent, and flow redistributes fluid in the upper lobes. Chronic accumulation of transudated fluid in the interstitial spaces of the lungs and lymphatic engorgement result in linear shadows perpendicular to the pleura, which are known as Kerley's B lines.

Diagnostics

Murmurs

Initial
ECG

Imaging
Chest x-ray

Other
Stress ECG*
Thallium ECG*
Sestamibi exercise scan*
Echocardiogram (including two-dimensional and Doppler)*
Cardiac catheterization*

*If indicated.

Probably no cardiac lesion has been so closely aligned with echocardiography as MS. Echocardiography has largely superseded cardiac catheterization as a means of quantifying the magnitude of the gradient, valve area, determining the presence of additional valvular lesions, and assessing ventricular function. Coronary arteriography still may be required in adults to exclude coronary artery disease. The M-mode echocardiogram is able to demonstrate the characteristic motion of the mitral valve, which resembles a square wave. In MS the anterior and posterior leaflets demonstrate "concordant" movement (both leaflets moving in concert anteriorly during diastole) as opposed to the normal "discordant" movement (leaflets moving in opposite directions). Two-dimensional echocardiography demonstrates the reduced excursion of the valve, with "doming" of the valve during diastole, and permits accurate assessment of the valve area by planimetry of the valve on the cross-sectional, or short-axis, view. In addition, dense echoes suggest calcification of the valve, which, along with assessment of the pliability, permits judgment as to the feasibility of commissurotomy vs. valve replacement.[32] Two-dimensional echocardiography will also assess the size of the left atrium, as well as identify other causes for mitral obstruction, such as atrial myxoma. Doppler study not only documents the presence of regurgitation, but also permits another accurate method for estimating valve area, by means of either the "pressure–half-time" technique or the continuity equation. In the presence of tricuspid regurgitation, some degree of which is almost always present, estimation of pulmonary pressure can be made.

DIFFERENTIAL DIAGNOSIS

The murmur of MS is classified as a mid to late diastolic murmur. Other mid to late diastolic murmurs that should be considered in the differential diagnosis include an atrial presystolic murmur, the Austin Flint murmur, and the murmur of tricuspid stenosis. (See the Differential Diagnosis box on p. 566.)

MANAGEMENT

Treatment of the underlying obstructive lesion of MS is an operative procedure. Medical therapy aims to prevent recurrent episodes of rheumatic fever, systemic embolism, and treatment of atrial fibrillation. All patients with MS must receive penicillin prophylaxis for infections, surgery, or any instrumentation procedure. Patients who have had one episode of rheumatic fever are at risk for a second episode. Recurrent episodes of rheumatic fever are dramatically lessened with secondary prophylaxis against streptococcal infections. Anemia or infections should be promptly treated because they increase the heart rate and therefore the gradient. Similarly, occupations that demand strenuous physical exertion should be avoided by patients with more than mild MS. Patients who are symptomatic should be treated with oral diuretics and sodium restriction.

Patients with MS who have atrial fibrillation should be treated with digoxin, beta blockers, and/or calcium channel blockers to slow the ventricular rate. Electrical cardioversion may be attempted in patients with mild MS and new-onset atrial fibrillation. Anticoagulation is required for 3 weeks before cardioversion to prevent emboli during conversion from atrial fibrillation to normal sinus rhythm. After cardioversion to normal sinus rhythm, antiarrhythmic therapy to maintain normal sinus rhythm may be indicated. The rate of successful cardioversion is low in patients who have been symptomatic for several years and who have a left atrium larger than 5 cm as documented by echocardiography; however, a single attempt is often worthwhile.

Anticoagulant therapy can help prevent venous thrombosis and pulmonary embolism and can reduce the frequency of systemic embolism in patients with MS who have experienced previous embolic episodes.[33] No benefit of anticoagulation has been shown for patients in normal sinus rhythm without a prior history of embolism. However, anticoagulation may be reasonable to consider for those patients found to have moderate MS by echocardiogram or those with symptoms, as the occurrence of systemic embolization is well recognized in these patients.

The primary determinant for surgical consideration is the degree of symptoms. Patients in NYHA class II to III would be considered surgical candidates. The onset of atrial fibrillation intensifies symptomatology and, even if the patient is successfully cardioverted, the atrial fibrillation is a harbinger of impending need for intervention. Arterial thromboembolism increases the need for surgery. Two surgical approaches are used: commissurotomy, either open (under direct visualization) or closed (using a dilator), and valve replacement. The former is by necessity palliative, reducing the degree of obstruction, and is most successful in patients without huge atria or significant regurgitation calcification. Otherwise, patients require valve replacement. An alternative in selected cases is balloon mitral valvuloplasty. This technique has been demonstrated to be superior to closed commissurotomy and equivalent to open commissurotomy.[34] Given the lower costs and avoidance of open heart surgery, the balloon procedure should be considered the treatment of choice for pliable, stenotic valves. Suitable patients almost always would be considered earlier in their symptomatic natural history than they would be if full replacement were required.

Co-Management with Specialists and Life Span Considerations

Co-management with a specialist is necessary when cardioversion, surgery, or balloon valvuloplasty is being considered. Life span considerations include the need for anticoagulation to prevent emboli in atrial fibrillation and antibiotic therapy to prevent bacterial endocarditis.

COMPLICATIONS

Patients with MS are at risk for thromboembolization. An additional complication is severe pulmonary hypertension. The clinical course of these patients must be differentiated from that of patients with congenital heart disease. It is well recognized that the unfortunate patient with pulmonary hypertension due to congenital heart disease (Eisenmenger's syndrome) has a very poor result after surgery. Initially it was believed that patients with mitral valve disease and marked pulmonary hypertension shared the same fate. However, a number of studies have demonstrated that although they do have an increased operative mortality when compared with patients who are less severely affected, these patients demonstrate a striking and rapid improvement in pulmonary pressures.[35] For this reason, no such patient should be considered as not being a surgical candidate.

INDICATIONS FOR REFERRAL/HOSPITALIZATION

Any patient with valvular heart disease will require cardiology referral and hospitalization for cardiac catheterization, balloon angioplasty, or surgical intervention when necessary. Patients with acute bacterial endocarditis will require IV antibiotics. Hospitalization may also be required for the management of complications such as heart failure or pulmonary edema.

PATIENT AND FAMILY EDUCATION

Patients with valvular disorders, whether from a stenotic valve or regurgitant valve, will require basic knowledge of their condition to prevent complications. The medication regimen should be explained and its importance reinforced at every visit. Because antibiotic prophylaxis is required before any instrumentation procedure, this should also be explained and its importance reinforced periodically (see Chapter 131).

REFERENCES

1. Leatham A: Auscultation of the heart, *Lancet* 703-708, 757-766, 1958.
2. Lembo NJ and others: Bedside diagnosis of systolic murmurs, *N Engl J Med* 318:1572-1578, 1988.
3. Castle RF: The innocent heart murmur, *J Colorado Med Soc* 69:45-48, 1972.
4. Rackley CE and others: Aortic valve disease. In Hurst JW and others, editors: *The heart*, New York, 1990, McGraw-Hill.
5. Alpert JS: Chronic aortic regurgitation. In Dalen JE, Alpert JS, editors: *Valvular heart disease*, Boston, 1986, Little, Brown.
6. O'Rourke RA, Walsh RA: Recognition and treatment of acute aortic regurgitation, *J Intens Care Med* 1:33-46, 1986.
7. Julius BK and others: Angina pectoris in patients with aortic stenosis and normal coronary arteries: mechanisms and pathophysiologic concepts, *Circulation* 95:892-898, 1997.
8. Gould KL: Why angina pectoris in aortic stenosis, *Circulation* 95: 790-792, 1997.
9. Mark A: The Bezold-Jarisch reflex revisited: clinical implications of inhibitory reflexes originating in the heart, *J Am Coll Cardiol* 1(1): 90-102, 1983.
10. Seltzer A: Changing aspects of the natural history of valvular aortic stenosis, *N Engl J Med* 317:91-98, 1987.
11. Ross J, Braunwald E: Aortic stenosis circulation, 38(1 suppl):V61-V67, 1968.
12. Spodick DH and others: Rate of rise of the carotid pulse, *Am J Cardiol* 49(1):159-162, 1982.
13. Brockmeir LB and others: Calcium emboli to the retinal artery in calcific aortic stenosis, *Am Heart J* 101:32-37, 1981.
14. Henry WL and others: Observations on the optimal time for operative intervention for aortic regurgitation. I. Evaluation of the results of aortic valve replacement in symptomatic patients, *Circulation* 61:471-483, 1980.
15. Greenberg B and others: Long-term vasodilator therapy of chronic aortic insufficiency, *Circulation* 789:92-103, 1988.
16. Scognamiglio R and others: Nifedipine in asymptomatic patients with severe aortic regurgitation and normal left ventricular function, *N Engl J Med* 331:689-694, 1994.
17. Bonow RO and others: The natural history of asymptomatic patients with aortic regurgitation and normal left ventricular function, *Circulation* 68(3):509-517, 1983.
18. Klodas E and others: Optimizing timing of surgical correction in patients with severe aortic regurgitation: role of symptoms. *J Am Coll Cardiol* 130:746-752, 1997.

19. Stone PH and others: Determinants of prognosis of patients with aortic regurgitation who undergo aortic valve replacement, *J Am Coll Cardiol* 3(5):1118-1126, 1984.
20. Wisebaugh T and others: Prediction of outcome after valve replacement for rheumatic mitral regurgitation in the era of chordal preservation, *Circulation* 89:191-197, 1994.
21. Greenberg B and others: Beneficial effects of hydralazine in severe mitral regurgitation, *Circulation* 58:273-278, 1978.
22. Dujardin KS and others: A prospective trial on the effects of losartan on the degree of mitral regurgitation, *Circulation* 94:I-468, 1997.
23. Crawford M and others: Determinants of survival and left ventricular performance after mitral valve replacement, *Circulation* 81:1173-1181, 1990.
24. Enriquez-Sarano M and others: Echocardiographic prediction of survival after surgical correction of organic mitral regurgitation, *Circulation* 90:830-837, 1994.
25. David T and others: Mitral valve replacement for mitral regurgitation with and without preservation of chordae tendineae, *J Thorac Cardiovasc Surg* 88:718-725, 1984.
26. Rosen SE and others: The natural history of asymptomatic patients with severe mitral regurgitation secondary to mitral valve prolapse and normal right and left ventricular performance, *Am J Cardiol* 74: 374-380, 1994.
27. Devereux RB, Kramer-Fox R, Kligfield P: Mitral valve prolapse: causes, clinical manifestations, and management, *Ann Intern Med* 111: 305-317, 1989.
28. Weissman NJ and others: Contrasting patterns of autonomic dysfunction in patients with mitral valve prolapse and panic attacks, *Am J Med* 82:880-888, 1987.
29. Markiewicz W and others: Mitral valve prolapse in one hundred presumably healthy young females, *Circulation* 53:464-473, 1976.
30. Marks AR and others: Identification of high risk and low risk subgroups of patients with mitral valve prolapse, *N Engl J Med* 320: 1031-1036, 1989.
31. Mills P and others: Long term prognosis of mitral valve prolapse, *N Engl J Med* 297:13-18, 1977.
32. Wilkins GT and others: Percutaneous mitral valvotomy: an analysis of echocardiographic variables related to outcome and the mechanism of dilatation, *Br Heart J* 60:299-308, 1988.
33. Siegel R and others: Effects of anticoagulation on recurrent systemic emboli in mitral stenosis, *Am J Cardiol* 60:1191-1192, 1987.
34. Farhat MB and others: Percutaneous balloon vs surgical closed and open mitral commissurotomy, *Circulation* 97:245-250, 1998.
35. Braunwald E and others: Effects of mitral valve replacement on the pulmonary vascular dynamic of patients with pulmonary hypertension, *N Engl J Med* 273:509-514, 1965.

PART 12

Evaluation and Management of Gastrointestinal Disorders

TERRY MAHAN BUTTARO, Section Editor

CHAPTER 139

Abdominal Pain and Infections

Updated by Terry Mahan Buttaro

DEFINITION/EPIDEMIOLOGY

Abdominal pain represents one of the most common, yet challenging complaints in primary care. Chronic pain that is intermittent or constant may be organic or functional. Severe abdominal pain for longer than 6 hours in a previously well patient usually indicates a condition requiring surgical intervention.[1]

The patient's description of the pain often suggests the pathologic condition. With ulceration, pain is often described as burning or gnawing. Hollow tube obstruction (bowel, biliary tree, ureters) has an intermittent colicky or wavelike quality, whereas the pain of peritoneal irritation is steady and increases with coughing, palpation, or movement. With metabolic disturbances or altered bowel motility, the pain may be crampy, and the distribution can be localized or generalized. Vascular insufficiency is evidenced by a crampy discomfort or pain that occurs primarily in the midabdominal region but is related to meals (abdominal angina). Thrombosis produces a more progressive and severe pain. The pain associated with distention of an encapsulated structure (liver, kidney, spleen, ovary) is constant and aching. Nerve irritation can be severe and has a dermatome distribution. A dissecting aneurysm usually produces pain that is described as "tearing."[1]

The location of pain may also suggest the source of the patient's discomfort. Pain localized to the right upper abdominal quadrant generally emanates from the chest cavity, liver, gallbladder, stomach, bowel, or right kidney or ureter. The most common diagnoses of pain in this area are cholecystitis and leaking duodenal ulcer.[1] Left upper quadrant pain is usually associated with the heart or chest cavity, spleen, stomach, pancreas (especially acute pancreatitis), left kidney, or ureter.[1] The source of left lower abdominal pain can include the bowel, left ureter, or pelvis and is most commonly associated with diverticulitis.[1] Right lower quadrant pain is associated with the appendix, bowel, right ureter, or pelvis, with the most common diagnosis being appendicitis. Cholecystitis or peptic ulcer perforation also must be considered.[1] Pain that migrates across several quadrants is typically associated with the bowel, whereas abdominal wall pain from trauma or inflammation can occur in any quadrant.

Abdominal pain can be subtle and the diagnosis obscure, particularly in older adults. The older patient is less likely to mount a fever or pain response than is a young patient but is more likely to present with lethargy or mental status changes. In women of childbearing age, it is imperative to exclude the possibility of ectopic pregnancy, even in women with a history of tubal ligation.

With acute abdominal pain, an accurate diagnosis is highly dependent on history, physical examination, and appropriate laboratory and radiologic procedures. Diseases that may cause acute abdominal pain include appendicitis, cholecystitis, diverticulitis, small bowel obstruction, perforated peptic ulcer, peritonitis, ruptured ectopic pregnancy, and ruptured abdominal aortic aneurysm. It is important that all women of childbearing age with abdominal pain have a serum beta-hCG to exclude pregnancy. (Cholecystitis, diverticulitis, and ectopic pregnancy are discussed in Chapters 141, 145, and 175.) It is also essential to remember that acute diseases of the chest—including myocardial infarction, congestive heart failure, pulmonary infarction, and pneumonia—may mimic primary diseases of the abdomen.

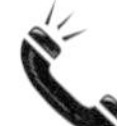

Physician consultation is indicated for suspected gastrointestinal bleeding, bowel obstruction, postural vital sign changes, abnormal findings, jaundice, a positive pregnancy test, severely localized or unilateral lower abdominal pain, or a history of trauma.

Appendicitis

DEFINITION/EPIDEMIOLOGY

Acute appendicitis is an inflammatory disease of the wall of the appendix that may result in perforation with subsequent peritonitis. Acute appendicitis is a common reason for emergency surgery, and the diagnosis is based on the history and physical examination.

PATHOPHYSIOLOGY

Acute appendicitis is classified as simple, gangrenous, or perforated on the basis of operative findings. In simple appendicitis the appendix is viable and intact. Gangrenous appendicitis is characterized by necrosis of the appendiceal wall. Perforated appendicitis refers to disruption of the appendix. Acute appendicitis is thought to be secondary to obstruction of its orifice, with secondary bacterial infection.[2,3] Sixty percent of patients with appendicitis demonstrate lymphoid hyperplasia on pathologic examination. Lymphoid hyperplasia occurs most commonly after periods of dehydration and viral infection and is most common in the young. This may account for the increased incidence of appendicitis in younger populations.[4] One third of patients demonstrate a mechanical obstruction with solid fecal material.[2,5] Other causes of luminal obstruction include tumors, parasites, foreign bodies, and bacterial or viral agents.[2,3,5]

When the appendiceal lumen becomes obstructed, the mucosa continues to secrete fluid until the intraluminal pressure exceeds venous pressure. At this point, the appendix becomes hypoxic, the mucosa ulcerates, and bacteria invade the wall. Infection causes additional swelling and ischemia due to thrombosis of small intramural vessels. Gangrene and perforation usually develop in 24 to 36 hours. Perforation leads to a release of the luminal contents into the peritoneal cavity.

CLINICAL PRESENTATION

The most reliable historical feature in the diagnosis of acute appendicitis is the sequence of symptoms. The classic sequence of symptoms is pain at some site in the abdomen, anorexia, nausea, or vomiting; these symptoms are followed by pain over the appendix and fever. Not all patients will have every symptom; however, when they occur in any other order, the diagnosis of appendicitis should be questioned.

Pain is the initial symptom of appendicitis and begins in the epigastrium or periumbilical area. However, abdominal pain may be diffuse or localized in the right lower quadrant from the onset. The initial pain is described as colicky and not severe, but it reaches its peak in approximately 4 hours. The pain gradually subsides but reappears in the right lower quadrant, progressing to a severe ache that is exacerbated by movement. The practitioner should recognize that the exact location of pain may be variable due to the variable location of the diseased appendix: ascending, iliac, or pelvic.[1] The most valuable physical finding is localized tenderness.

PHYSICAL EXAMINATION

The diagnosis of acute appendicitis requires a careful history and a thorough physical examination. The physical examination usually reveals a low-grade fever. Abdominal tenderness is elicited by asking the patient to cough. The patient can usually localize the painful spot with one finger. By systematically palpating the abdomen with one finger, the practitioner confirms localized tenderness, usually in the right lower quadrant between the umbilicus and the anterosuperior iliac spine (McBurney's point). There may be signs of peritoneal irritation, including guarding, rebound tenderness, and obturator and psoas signs. The psoas sign is elicited by asking the supine patient to raise the straightened right leg against resistance by the practitioner. The obturator sign is elicited by passive rotation of the right leg with the patient supine and the right hip and knee flexed. A rectal examination may reveal tenderness or a mass.

DIAGNOSTICS

Most agree that the diagnosis of acute appendicitis is suggested by the history and physical examination. In fact, the rate of normal or perforated appendices at surgery has not changed since the addition of ultrasound or CT to the evaluation of suspected appendicitis, underscoring the importance of careful a clinical history and physical examination.[6] The primary care provider should immediately refer a patient with suspected appendicitis for surgical consultation. Laboratory data in support of appendicitis include a WBC count that ranges from 10,000 to 16,000 cells/μl. A serum beta human chorionic gonadotropin (beta-hCG) level should be performed in women of childbearing age to assist in excluding a ruptured ectopic pregnancy. In a recent prospective study, rebound tenderness, guarding, WBC count, and C-reactive protein levels were independent predictors of appendicitis.[7]

Diagnostics

Appendicitis

Laboratory
CBC and differential
hCG*
Urinalysis

Imaging
Barium enema x-ray*
Ultrasound*
CT scan*

Other
Laparoscopy/laparotomy*

*If indicated.

Imaging studies are not required in most cases of suspected appendicitis. However, imaging modalities may be necessary if the presentation is atypical or in patients at the extremes of age. Plain abdominal radiographs show nonspecific signs and are no longer recommended. Barium enema x-ray studies are safe and are thought to exclude a diagnosis of appendicitis if the appendix fills with barium. However, failure of the appendix to fill with barium does not necessarily indicate acute appendicitis; therefore other imaging modalities are generally used.

Ultrasonographic evidence of appendicitis includes appendiceal wall thickening, luminal distention, and lack of compressibility.[8] Its usefulness is strictly limited by operator-dependent skill and interpretation. If the ultrasound is negative, clinical findings of acute appendicitis require intervention by laparoscopy or laparotomy. A CT scan is not usually justified in routine acute appendicitis unless the ultrasound is found to be normal or reliable ultrasound is not available.[4] CT is reliable in differentiating a periappendiceal phlegmon from an abscess.[3,9]

DIFFERENTIAL DIAGNOSIS

Other conditions that may mimic acute appendicitis include gastroenteritis, mesenteric lymphadenitis, acute salpingitis, mittelschmerz, ruptured ectopic pregnancy, ureteral colic, Meckel's diverticulitis, sigmoid diverticulitis, perforated peptic ulcer, cholecystitis, intestinal obstruction, cecal diverticulitis, and perforated colonic carcinoma. Basilar pneumonia may also be confused with appendicitis.

MANAGEMENT

With appendicitis, a prompt appendectomy, preferably within 24 hours of symptom onset, is essential to prevent perforation and peritonitis.[1] Little preparation for surgery is required, but fluid and electrolyte repletion is necessary. Older patients should be evaluated and treated for systemic disease. Perioperative systemic antibiotics such as metronidazole and ceftizoxime have been shown to prevent wound infection in simple appendicitis.[3] If the appendix is perforated, triple antibiotic therapy with ampicillin, gentamicin, and clindamycin or monotherapy with a second-generation cephalosporin such as cefotetan is essential, as is fluid resuscitation with crystalloids followed by prompt appendectomy.[3,9] Surgery for an appendiceal abscess may spread a localized

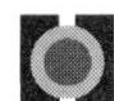

Differential Diagnosis

Appendicitis

Gastroenteritis
Mesenteric lymphadenitis
Acute salpingitis
Mittelschmerz
Ruptured ectopic pregnancy
Ureteral colic
Meckel's diverticulitis
Sigmoid diverticulitis
Perforated peptic ulcer
Cholecystitis
Intestinal obstruction
Cecal diverticulitis
Perforated colonic carcinoma
Basilar pneumonia
Pyelonephritis
Intestinal obstruction
Ureteral calculus
Salpingitis/pelvic inflammatory disease
Ruptured corpus luteum cyst
Endometriosis
Regional enteritis/Crohn's disease

infection to other parts of the peritoneal cavity; therefore percutaneous CT-guided drainage of an abscess is used to allow the acute inflammation to resolve before proceeding with elective appendectomy in 6 weeks to 3 months.[3]

COMPLICATIONS

Complications of appendicitis include gangrene, perforation with peritonitis, and abscess formation. Pylephlebitis, which is septic thrombophlebitis of the portal venous system, should be suspected in any patient with appendicitis who has shaking chills. Septicemia, urinary retention and infection, small bowel obstruction, and mesenteric thrombophlebitis may also occur. The most common complication from appendectomy is wound infection, but pneumonia, intraperitoneal abscesses, enterocutaneous fistulas, wound or inguinal hernias, or minor bleeding can also occur.[5]

INDICATIONS FOR REFERRAL/HOSPITALIZATION

Immediate surgical referral or a transfer to the emergency department is indicated for suspected appendicitis or other acute abdominal pain. Hospitalization is indicated for monitoring and surgical care, if necessary.

PATIENT AND FAMILY EDUCATION

Abdominal pain may be a sign of serious illness or may be related to a chronic disorder. Patients should understand that localized abdominal pain or pain that increases in severity warrants discussion with the primary care provider. Patients must also understand that abdominal pain accompanied by fever, chills, severe vomiting or diarrhea, significant rectal bleeding, black and tarry stools, weakness, or dizziness requires a visit to their primary care provider. Families of older patients should understand that pain perception may be diminished; the associated delay in presentation results in more than 30% of older adults with appendicitis having perforation at presentation.[4] In older adults, any of the previously listed symptoms, even if unaccompanied by abdominal pain, should be evaluated by a medical professional.

Small Bowel Obstruction

DEFINITION/EPIDEMIOLOGY

Small bowel obstruction is a mechanical occlusion of the bowel lumen or a paralysis of intestinal musculature that results in fluid and gas accumulation proximal to the obstruction. It is essential to recognize bowel obstruction because it can cause vascular compromise, bowel ischemia, and peritonitis. Adhesions, hernias, and tumors are the most common causes of small bowel obstruction. Other conditions, such as abscesses, inflammatory bowel disease, volvulus, intussusception, and radiation enteritis, can also be responsible.

PATHOPHYSIOLOGY

In a bowel obstruction, distention results in decreased absorption and increased secretions, which causes further distention and fluid and electrolyte imbalances. Bacterial proliferation may occur as a result of stasis. Distention increases the risk of bowel perforation and diffuse peritonitis. Mechanical obstruction of the bowel lumen may occur from polypoid tumors, intussusception, volvulus, gallstone ileus, impacted feces, or bezoar formation. Intussusception, often recognized as an abdominal mass on examination with a history of acute symptom onset, occurs when a bowel segment telescopes into the adjacent bowel, resulting in symptoms of intermittent bowel obstruction. Volvulus results from abnormal twisting of a bowel segment along its mesenteric axis. Intrinsic and extrinsic lesions of the bowel that may cause obstruction include congenital, neoplastic, and inflammatory lesions.[5]

CLINICAL PRESENTATION

Bowel obstruction presents with intermittent and crampy abdominal pain, vomiting, obstipation, abdominal distention, and fever. The pain is usually relieved by vomiting, intestinal tube decompression, or the passage of intestinal contents through a partial obstruction. Pain that progresses in severity, localizes, or becomes constant demonstrates progression to a strangulated obstruction; this condition requires urgent surgery. Particular attention should be placed on prior history of abdominal or pelvic operations, which would predispose to adhesions as a cause of obstruction.

PHYSICAL EXAMINATION

Tachycardia and hypotension tend to be late symptoms and may be present depending on the degree of hypovolemia that results from persistent vomiting or from toxemia caused by intestinal gangrene.[5,10] The physical examination also reveals a distended abdomen, with diffuse midabdominal tenderness to palpation. Peristaltic rushes and a high-pitched tinkling may be auscultated over the abdomen. Rectal and sigmoidoscopic examinations may reveal stool, masses, or tenderness, and occult blood suggests carcinoma, intussusception, or bowel ischemia.[10] Particular attention needs to be placed on examination of potential hernial orifices, especially the area of the femoral ring because of its small opening and potential for bowel strangulation.[1]

DIAGNOSTICS

The radiographic evaluation should include upright and supine x-ray films of the abdomen and the upright chest. The upright abdominal film identifies a distended bowel proximal to the obstruction in addition to air-fluid levels. It may show free air if perforation has occurred. The supine radiograph may distinguish between ileus and obstruction. With an ileus, the radiograph will show distended loops in both the large and small bowel; with an obstruction, the segment proximal to the obstruction is distended, and the distal bowel loops are decreased in caliber.[10] Ileus most commonly occurs after trauma, significant operative procedure, or high-dose or frequent narcotic use. The patient should also be evaluated for intraperitoneal masses, ascites, gallstones, renal calculi, foreign bodies, and gas within the bowel wall, portal venous system, or biliary tree.[10] Contrast radiography (e.g., an upper gastrointestinal study, small bowel study, and barium enema) can be helpful in intermittent or suspected partial small bowel obstruction. Recent studies suggest that CT scanning after the administration of oral and IV contrast media may be the technique of choice in locating and identifying intestinal obstruction in the nonacute setting.[11]

Laboratory data usually reflect a progressively increasing WBC count. A serum beta-hCG should be performed to exclude pregnancy in women of childbearing age.

DIFFERENTIAL DIAGNOSIS

The differential diagnosis of small bowel obstruction includes gastroenteritis, paralytic ileus, intestinal perforation, ischemic colitis, idiopathic inflammatory bowel disease, mesenteric thrombosis, and retroperitoneal hemorrhage. Addison's disease, poisoning, diabetes mellitus, and tertiary syphilis may also mimic small bowel obstruction.

MANAGEMENT

Immediate hospitalization is required for the treatment of suspected bowel obstruction, and consultation with a surgeon is essential. Initial management of bowel obstruction includes restriction of all oral intakes, IV fluid therapy, electrolyte and acid-base correction, optimization of cardiopulmonary and renal function, and nasogastric decompression. Urgent laparotomy is required if there is no response to supportive care or if there is advanced illness, ischemia, or perforation.[5,10] Otherwise, patients can be observed with serial physical examinations and radiographs. Antibiotic therapy usually has no role except as an adjunct to surgery.

COMPLICATIONS

A bowel obstruction may progress to bowel ischemia. Signs of an ischemic bowel include fever, severe and continuous pain, hematemesis, shock, gas in the bowel wall or portal vein, abdominal free air, peritoneal signs, and acidosis.[5]

INDICATIONS FOR REFERRAL/HOSPITALIZATION AND PATIENT AND FAMILY EDUCATION

See Indications for Referral/Hospitalization and Patient and Family Education under Appendicitis, p. 576.

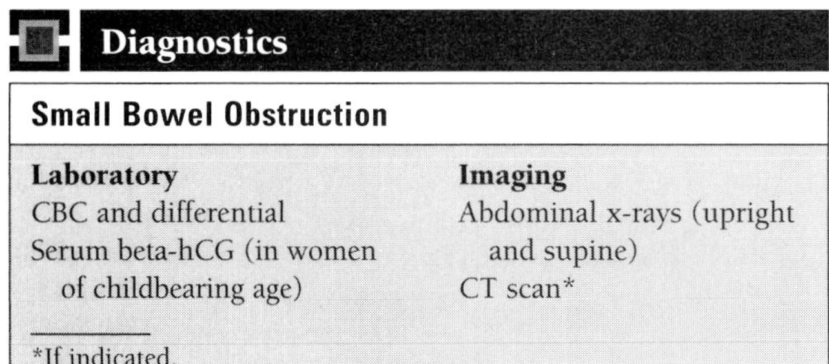

Diagnostics

Small Bowel Obstruction

Laboratory	Imaging
CBC and differential	Abdominal x-rays (upright and supine)
Serum beta-hCG (in women of childbearing age)	CT scan*

*If indicated.

Differential Diagnosis

Small Bowel Obstruction

Gastroenteritis	Retroperitoneal hemorrhage
Paralytic ileus	Addison's disease
Intestinal perforation	Poisoning
Ischemic colitis	Diabetes mellitus
Idiopathic inflammatory bowel disease	Tertiary syphilis
Mesenteric thrombosis	Neoplasm

Perforated Peptic Ulcer

DEFINITION/EPIDEMIOLOGY

Peptic ulcer perforation is a life-threatening complication of peptic ulcer disease and is more common with duodenal ulcers than with gastric ulcers. Perforation may lead to a free perforation into the peritoneal cavity or perforation of an adjacent organ such as the pancreas, with resulting peritonitis or pancreatitis. Factors that predispose a patient to peptic ulcers are *Helicobacter pylori* infections, nonsteroidal antiinflammatory drugs (NSAIDs), tobacco abuse, and hypersecretory states such as Zöllinger-Ellison syndrome.[12] The overall mortality rate for perforated gastric ulcers is approximately 10%.[2,12]

PATHOPHYSIOLOGY

Peptic ulcer perforations can be classified as (1) those in which the luminal contents freely escape into the peritoneal cavity and (2) those in which the penetration is sealed by surrounding structures of peritoneum.[2] Because the anterior walls of the stomach and duodenum are not defended by contiguous tissue, ulcers in these locations are more likely to be complicated by free perforation, which leads to generalized peritonitis and the accumulation of air in the abdominal cavity.[2] Posterior gastric ulcers perforate into the lesser peritoneal sac, where the inflammatory reaction may be contained and form an intraabdominal abscess. Ulcers may also penetrate into the pancreas, liver, or greater omentum and cause intractable symptoms.

CLINICAL PRESENTATION

The most common presentation of a perforated peptic ulcer is the abrupt onset of severe abdominal pain followed rapidly by peritoneal signs. Pain begins in the epigastrium and spreads rapidly throughout the abdomen with frequent early radiation of pain to the scapular areas. The abruptness, severity, and rapid progression of symptoms lead the patient to seek prompt medical attention. Clinically, patients often demonstrate signs of improvement such as decreased pain and vomiting 6 to 12 hours after perforation. However, peritoneal signs remain and the clinical improvement does not last long. By about 12 hours, the patient appears seriously ill, usually grunting with shallow respirations and the knees drawn up to the chest.

PHYSICAL EXAMINATION

Upper abdominal tenderness is accompanied by board-like rigidity of the abdomen. If it has been less than 24 hours since the perforation, a low-grade fever and tachycardia are often present, but hypotension is unusual.[9] Continued spilling of gastric and intestinal contents into the peritoneum causes chemical peritonitis and subsequent hypovolemia with the development of progressive hypotension and fever. Bowel sounds are absent in most cases.

DIAGNOSTICS

Perforation is suggested by the history and physical examination. The suspected diagnosis is confirmed by the detection of pneumoperitoneum on upright abdominal or chest x-ray films. If a pneumoperitoneum is absent, a water-soluble contrast examination may be used to demonstrate perforation.[9] A left lateral decubitus radiograph usually demonstrates air over the liver. When the diagnosis is suspected and the x-ray studies are negative, the diagnosis may be confirmed by endoscopy.[12] A serum beta-hCG level should be performed in women of childbearing age to assist in excluding ectopic pregnancy. Laboratory tests include a peripheral WBC count that shows mild leukocytosis as well as elevated amylase levels in the serum and peritoneal fluid.[13]

DIFFERENTIAL DIAGNOSIS

The differential diagnoses of a perforated peptic ulcer include acute pancreatitis, acute cholecystitis, perforated acute appendicitis, colonic diverticulitis, intestinal obstruction, ruptured ectopic pregnancy, and postemetic esophageal rupture. Myocardial infarction may also mimic a perforated peptic ulcer.

MANAGEMENT

Immediate hospitalization and consultation with a surgeon are essential. Treatment of a perforate peptic ulcer is surgical in 95% of patients.[14] Management includes IV fluid resuscitation, correction of electrolyte abnormalities, and continuous nasogastric suction.[15] IV broad-spectrum antibiotics, such as ampicillin-sulbactam and gentamicin, are also required.[12] Blood transfusions may also be necessary in the presence of hemorrhage. Early suspicion, recognition, and surgical repair are the keys to survival and decreased morbidity.

COMPLICATIONS

Fifty percent of patients with a perforated peptic ulcer die of hemorrhage.[2] Peptic ulcer penetration into the pancreas, gastrohepatic omentum, biliary tract, liver, greater omentum, and colon may occur.[12] Surgical complications include recurrent ulcer, dumping syndrome, and vitamin deficiency.[13]

INDICATIONS FOR REFERRAL/HOSPITALIZATION AND PATIENT AND FAMILY EDUCATION

See Indications for Referral/Hospitalization and Patient and Family Education under Appendicitis, p. 576.

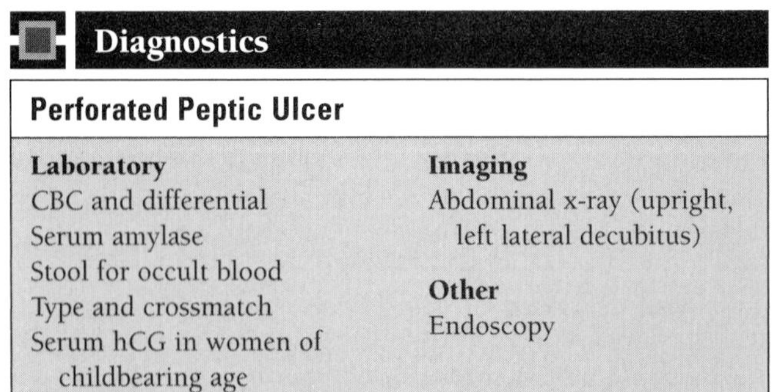

Diagnostics

Perforated Peptic Ulcer

Laboratory	Imaging
CBC and differential	Abdominal x-ray (upright, left lateral decubitus)
Serum amylase	
Stool for occult blood	**Other**
Type and crossmatch	Endoscopy
Serum hCG in women of childbearing age	

Differential Diagnosis

Perforated Peptic Ulcer

Acute pancreatitis	Myocardial infarction
Acute cholecystitis	Intestinal obstruction
Perforated appendix	Perforated colon
Colonic diverticulitis	

Peritonitis

DEFINITION/EPIDEMIOLOGY

Primary spontaneous bacterial peritonitis refers to a peritoneal infection in the absence of a clear precipitating factor such as a perforated viscus. The most common cause of spontaneous bacterial peritonitis in adults is cirrhosis complicated by portal hypertension and ascites.[2] Secondary peritonitis refers to spillage of gastrointestinal or genitourinary microorganisms into the peritoneal space. Secondary peritonitis is most commonly a result of appendicitis, diverticulitis, cholecystitis, penetrating wounds of the bowel, or perforation of a gastric or duodenal ulcer.[16] In these instances, a secondary infection may occur as either generalized peritonitis or localized abscesses.[16]

PATHOPHYSIOLOGY

Primary peritonitis is thought to result from a hematogenous and lymphogenous spread of bacteria through an intact gut wall from the intestinal lumen. The gut wall is thought to be more permeable to bacterial translocation because of wall edema from portal hypertension. In patients with cirrhosis, microorganisms removed from circulation by the liver may not be properly phagocytized by impaired liver macrophages and thus contaminate hepatic lymph and pass into the ascitic fluid. Portosystemic shunting also diminishes hepatic clearance of microorganisms, which perpetuates bacteremia and increases the potential for ascitic fluid infection.[16] Enteric microorganisms account for the majority of pathogens in patients with cirrhosis. *Escherichia coli* is the most commonly identified pathogen, followed by *Streptococcal pneumoniae, Klebsiella pneumoniae,* and other streptococcal species, including enterococci. Other organisms responsible for primary peritonitis may include *Neisseria gonorrhoeae, Chlamydia trachomatis, Mycobacterium tuberculosis,* and *Coccidioides immitis. Bacteroides fragilis* and *E. coli* are most commonly found when gastrointestinal perforation is the precipitating event.[16] Primary bacterial peritonitis is almost exclusively monomicrobial, and if multiple organisms are identified the diagnosis should be questioned and other sources for infection sought, such as perforated viscus.[17]

CLINICAL PRESENTATION

In patients with cirrhosis, a temperature of greater than 37.7° C (100° F) may be the only manifestation of peritoneal infection.[16] Additional complaints include diffuse abdominal pain, tenderness, nausea, vomiting, and diarrhea.

PHYSICAL EXAMINATION

With peritonitis, the physical examination may reveal diffuse abdominal tenderness, decreased bowel sounds, rebound tenderness, and guarding. Fever, tachycardia, and hypotension may also be present. Rectal examination may reveal tenderness if abscesses occur near this area.

DIAGNOSTICS

The diagnosis of peritonitis should be suspected on the basis of fever, abdominal pain and tenderness, and leukocytosis. Initially, a CBC and electrolytes may be obtained in the primary care setting. Suspected peritonitis, especially that accompanied by decreasing bowel sounds, increasing tenderness, and the development of rebound tenderness, warrants a laparotomy to confirm the diagnosis. Hospitalization and consultation with an internist, a gastroenterologist, and a surgeon are therefore required.

Patients with cirrhosis and spontaneous bacterial peritonitis should be diagnosed on the basis of the clinical setting, presence of ascites, and ascitic fluid analysis, not a laparotomy.[18] Patients with ascites should undergo paracentesis in the hospital setting with peritoneal fluid analysis for cell count, differential, protein concentration, and a Gram's stain and culture.[16] The diagnosis of primary bacterial peritonitis requires more than 250 to 500 WBCs in the ascitic fluid, with more than 50% of them being polymorphonuclear neutrophils.[17] More than 500 WBCs/μl indicates possible perforated viscus.[17] The ascitic fluid analysis will typically show a low protein concentration, pH of less than 7.35, and a lactate concentration of greater than 25 mg/dl.[16] In primary bacterial peritonitis, 30% to 50% of ascites fluid cultures are negative.[17] When a suspected intraabdominal abscess is present, CT or ultrasound-guided aspiration is standard practice.[16]

DIFFERENTIAL DIAGNOSIS

Diseases that may mimic peritonitis include pancreatitis, appendicitis, diverticulitis, gastroenteritis, salpingitis, and ischemic colitis. Secondary causes of peritonitis should also be considered, including perforated duodenal ulcer, perforated gastric ulcer, small bowel infarction or perforation, appendicitis, large bowel perforation, and cholecystitis with or without perforation or pericholecystic abscess.

Diagnostics

Peritonitis

Laboratory	Other
CBC and differential	Laparotomy/endoscopy*
Serum electrolytes	Biopsy*
Bun, creatinine	CT scan
Ascitic fluid analysis*	Ultrasound guided aspiration
Serum hCG in women of childbearing age	

*If indicated.

Differential Diagnosis

Peritonitis

Pancreatitis	Appendicitis
Appendicitis	Cholecystitis
Diverticulitis	Ruptured ectopic pregnancy
Gastroenteritis	Acute granulomatous peritonitis
Salpingitis	Chylous ascites
Ischemic colitis	Mesenteric lipodystrophy
Perforated duodenal ulcer	
Perforated gastric ulcer	
Small or large bowel perforation	

MANAGMENT

With primary bacterial peritonitis, the peritoneal fluid Gram's stain is often negative; therefore antibiotic therapy is usually empiric and is based on the most likely pathogens.[16] Cefotaxime 1 to 2 g IV every 6-8 hours or cefotaxime 500 to 1000 mg IV every 12 hours are proven treatments.[19] Third-generation cephalosporin antibiotics and the combination of ampicillin and an aminoglycoside have also proved to be effective.[16,20] Alternative antibiotic therapies include broad-spectrum penicillins, carbapenems, and beta-lactam antibiotics combined with beta-lactamase inhibitors.[16] Usual duration for therapy ranges from 3 to 7 days, but a recent meta-analysis of therapies has not shown a particular antibiotic or length of treatment to be most beneficial.[19,21] Antimicrobial therapy should be continued for cases in which peritoneal cultures are sterile but there is a strong suspicion of primary bacterial peritonitis.[16] Clinical improvement and a decline in the ascitic fluid leukocyte count (<250) should occur after 24 to 48 hours of antimicrobial therapy; a failure to respond to therapy should prompt suspicion for other pathologic conditions. Preventive treatment in patients with cirrhotic ascites is recommended to reduce the incidence of spontaneous bacterial peritonitis. Oral norfloxacin 400 mg/day, ciprofloxacin once weekly, or double-strength trimethoprim-sulfamethoxazole administered daily for 5 days each week has been shown to reduce the incidence of peritonitis in these patients.[16,19,22] This reduction in rate of primary peritonitis does not change the mortality rate for cirrhotics, which is related to their underlying hepatic dysfunction.[17] Treatment of secondary peritonitis includes the use of appropriate antimicrobial therapy and surgical management as necessary.

COMPLICATIONS

Primary peritonitis is an ominous sign in the cirrhotic patient. After the first episode, only one third of patients will survive 1 year, and of these, one half will have a recurrence of peritonitis with a mortality rate of 50%.[23] These patients also have a very high rate of umbilical and other abdominal wall hernias that can eventually lead to strangulation of contents and secondary peritonitis.

Nosocomial infections are common among patients with intraabdominal infections. Invasion by *Pseudomonas, Serratia, Enterobacter, Enterococcus, Staphylococcus,* and *Candida* spp. organisms may occur in the treatment setting.[13] Multiorgan failure occurs as a result of sepsis from intraabdominal infections and is the major cause of death in patients with intraabdominal infection.[24]

INDICATIONS FOR REFERRAL/HOSPITALIZATION AND PATIENT AND FAMILY EDUCATION

See Indications for Referral/Hospitalization and Patient and Family Education under Appendicitis, p. 576.

Ruptured Aortic Aneurysm

DEFINITION/EPIDEMIOLOGY

An abdominal aortic aneurysm (AAA) is an abnormal dilation of the abdominal aorta that may rupture and cause exsanguination into the peritoneum. Fifty percent of patients with a ruptured AAA die before reaching a treatment facility, and 24% of those who do reach a facility die before reaching an operating room for attempted repair.[25] Most AAAs are atherosclerotic in origin; the remainder are caused by trauma, vasculitis, syphilis, or other infections.[26] Risk factors for AAA include atherosclerosis, hypertension, peripheral vascular disease, smoking (8:1 increased risk), male gender (4:1 increased risk), and advancing age.[4,27] AAA is a relatively common condition (30 to 66/1000 persons) and is increasing as the population ages.[25]

PATHOPHYSIOLOGY

The pathogenesis of most dissecting AAAs is atherosclerosis; the common underlying defect is vessel wall weakness secondary to a loss of elastin and collagen tissue in the aorta. The focal loss of elastic and muscle fibers in the media leads to cystic spaces filled with a metachromatic myxoid material. Weakening and replacement of elastin and collagen over time lead to increased aneurysm diameter and length. The initial event triggering the medial dissection is controversial, but more than 95% of cases show a transverse tear in the intima and internal media, and many postulate that a spontaneous laceration of the intima allows blood from the lumen to enter and dissect the media.[28] Alternatively, it has been postulated that a hemorrhage from the vasa vasorum into the media (which has been weakened by cystic medial necrosis) initiates stress on the intima, which leads to the intimal tear.[28]

CLINICAL PRESENTATION

A patient may present with a throbbing, aching back pain that can precede actual rupture. Conversely, a patient may present days after a contained rupture.[1] In the majority, however, the rupture of an AAA is accompanied by the sudden onset of severe abdominal pain that may be confined to the flank, low back, or groin with radiation to the back that brings them in urgently. Symptoms occur in this distribution because most AAAs rupture posterolaterally into the retroperitoneum.[25] Pain may worsen in the recumbent position and is relieved by sitting up or leaning forward. Faintness and syncope may occur as a result of blood loss and gradually worsen until shock finally supervenes.[9] It is not uncommon for a patient with a ruptured AAA to present with a chief complaint of angina due to unrecognized blood loss that may actually delay full evaluation and definitive treatment.[1]

PHYSICAL EXAMINATION

During dissection, a pulsatile, painful mass can be palpated in the abdomen between the xiphoid process and the umbilicus. In AAAs, the pulsations are felt directly over the mass and displace the examining fingers laterally. An aortic bruit may be present. Peripheral pulses may be unequal or absent but can be normal. Profound shock may rapidly ensue as a result of intraperitoneal leakage of blood.

DIAGNOSTICS

Additional diagnostic tests are not required if a ruptured AAA is suspected. The patient should be hospitalized immediately, with resuscitation and therapy in the operating room. If the diagnosis of rupture is in doubt and time allows, a CT scan is the standard for evaluation of an AAA because it can determine the extent of the aneurysmal process. Angiography is used preoperatively in elective repairs to demonstrate aortic and vascular anatomy and renal vessel involvement. An ultrasound can be a helpful screening tool in the early stages of the disease process or in the questionable emergency department patient. Abdominal plain x-ray films may show a soft-tissue mass in the region of the abdominal aorta. A chest radiograph should also be obtained to evaluate the thoracic aorta. Laboratory tests should include a CBC, type and cross-match, electrolytes, and renal function tests.

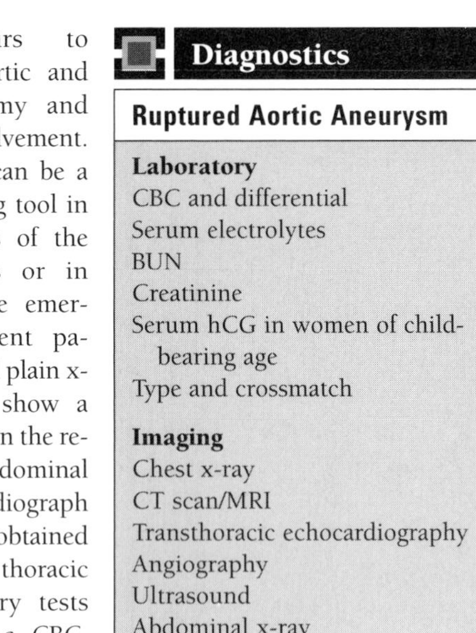

Diagnostics

Ruptured Aortic Aneurysm

Laboratory
CBC and differential
Serum electrolytes
BUN
Creatinine
Serum hCG in women of child-bearing age
Type and crossmatch

Imaging
Chest x-ray
CT scan/MRI
Transthoracic echocardiography
Angiography
Ultrasound
Abdominal x-ray

Other
ECG

DIFFERENTIAL DIAGNOSIS

The most common misdiagnosis of ruptured AAA is myocardial infarction.[9] Other diseases or conditions that may mimic AAA include a perforated peptic ulcer, diverticulitis, appendicitis, peritonitis, acute pancreatitis, pyelonephritis, renal colic, renal infarct, and mesenteric ischemia.[27]

MANAGEMENT

When a rupture is strongly suspected, IV fluids should be initiated with no less than two large-bore peripheral IV sites; the patient should be cross-matched for blood, and an immediate laparotomy should be performed. Surgical excision of the aneurysm and prosthetic graft placement within the aneurysmal sac are urgently required.[26,27] The postoperative mortality rate is approximately 50%.[9]

COMPLICATIONS

Postoperative complications of ruptured AAA repair include colon infarction, sepsis, congestive heart failure, myocardial infarction, arrhythmias, liver dysfunction, renal failure, respiratory failure, pneumonia, and lower extremity ischemia.

INDICATIONS FOR REFERRAL/HOSPITALIZATION AND PATIENT AND FAMILY EDUCATION

See Indications for Referral/Hospitalization and Patient and Family Education under Appendicitis, p. 576.

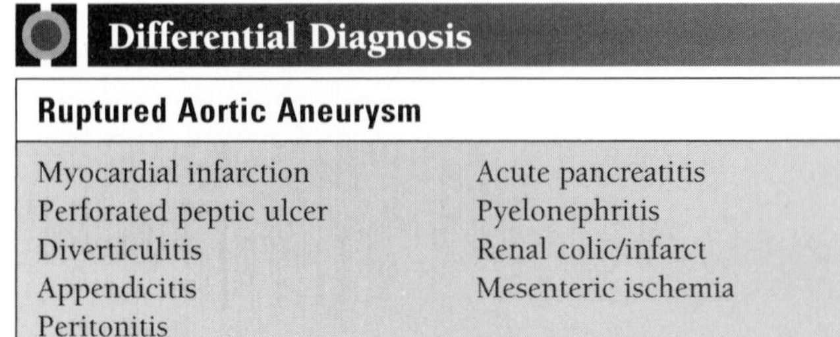

Differential Diagnosis

Ruptured Aortic Aneurysm

Myocardial infarction	Acute pancreatitis
Perforated peptic ulcer	Pyelonephritis
Diverticulitis	Renal colic/infarct
Appendicitis	Mesenteric ischemia
Peritonitis	

REFERENCES

1. Silen W: *Cope's early diagnosis of the acute abdomen,* ed 19, New York, 1996, Oxford University Press.
2. Rubin E, Farber JL: The gastrointestinal tract. In Rubin E, Farber JL, editors: *Pathology,* ed 2, Philadelphia, 1994, JB Lippincott.
3. Schrock TR: Acute appendicitis. In Sleisenger MH, Fordtran J, editors: *Gastrointestinal disease,* ed 5, Philadelphia, WB Saunders.
4. Liu CD, McFadden DW: Acute abdomen and appendix. In Greenfield LJ and others, editors: *Surgery scientific principles and practice,* ed 2, Philadelphia, 1997, Lippincott-Raven.
5. Blackbourne LH: Small intestine and appendicitis. In Blackbourne LH, editor: *Surgical recall,* Baltimore, 1994, Williams and Wilkins.
6. Flum DR and others: Has misdiagnosis of appendicitis decreased over time? a population-based analysis, *JAMA* 286:1748-1753, 2001.
7. Andersson RE and others: Diagnostic value of disease history, clinical presentation, and inflammatory parameters of appendicitis, *World J Surg* 23:133-140, 2001.
8. Karp SJ, Morris J, Soybel D: Small intestine and appendicitis. In Marino BS, editor: *Blueprints in surgery,* Malden, 1998, Blackwell Science.
9. Mulholland MW: Approach to the patient with acute abdomen. In Yamada T, editor: *Textbook of gastroenterology,* ed 2, Philadelphia, 1995, JB Lippincott.
10. Schuffler MD, Sinanan MN: Intestinal obstruction and pseudo-obstruction. In Sleisenger MH, Fordtran JS, editors: *Gastrointestinal disease: pathophysiology, diagnosis, management,* ed 5, Philadelphia, 1993, WB Saunders.
11. Quigley EM, Hasler WL, Parkman HP: AGA technical review on nausea and vomiting, *Gastroenterology* 120:263-286, 2001.
12. Graham DE: Ulcer complications and their nonoperative treatment. In Sleisenger MH, Fordtran JS, editors: *Gastrointestinal disease: pathophysiology, diagnosis, management,* ed 5, Philadelphia, 1993, WB Saunders.
13. Blackbourne LH: Upper GI bleeding. In Blackbourne LH, editor: *Surgical recall,* Baltimore, 1994, Williams and Wilkins.
14. Lowe RC, Wolfe MM: Acid-peptic disorders, gastritis, and helicobacter pylori. In Noble J, editor: *Textbook of primary care medicine,* ed 3, St Louis, 2001, Mosby.
15. Karp SJ, Morris J, Soybel D: Gallbladder. In Marino BS, editor: *Blueprints in surgery,* Malden, Mass, 1998, Blackwell Science.
16. Johnson CC, Baldessarre J, Levison ME: Peritonitis: update on pathophysiology, clinical manifestations, and management, *Clin Infect Dis* 24:1035-1045, 1997.
17. Lucey MR: Diseases of the peritoneum, mesentery, and omentum. In Goldman L, editor: *Cecil textbook of medicine,* ed 21, Philadelphia, 2000, WB Saunders.
18. Runyon BA: Surgical peritonitis and other diseases of the peritoneum, mesentery, omentum, and diaphragm. In Sleisenger MH, Fordtran JS, editors: *Gastrointestinal disease: pathophysiology, diagnosis, management,* ed 5, Philadelphia, 1993, WB Saunders.
19. Friedman SL: Alcoholic liver disease, cirrhosis, and its major sequelae. In Goldman L, editor: *Cecil textbook of medicine,* ed 21, Philadelphia, 2000, WB Saunders.
20. Guss DA: Disorders of the liver, biliary tract, and pancreas. In Rosen P, editor: *Emergency medicine: concepts and clinical practice,* ed 4, St. Louis, 1998, Mosby.
21. Soares-Weiser K, Brezis M, Leibovici L: Antibiotics for spontaneous bacterial peritonitis in cirrhotics, *Cochrane Database Syst Rev* (3):CD002232, 2001.
22. Singh N and others: Trimethoprim-sulfamethoxazole for the prevention of spontaneous bacterial peritonitis in cirrhosis: a randomized trial, *Ann Intern Med* 122:595-598, 1995.
23. Garcia-Tsao G: The diagnosis of bacterial peritonitis: comparison of pH, lactate concentration, and leukocyte count, *Hepatology* 5:91, 1985.
24. Gorbach SL: Intraabdominal infections, *Clin Infect Dis* 17:961-965, 1993.
25. Brandt LJ, Boley SJ: Ischemic and vascular lesions of the bowel. In Sleisenger MH, Fordtran JS, editors: *Gastrointestinal disease: pathophysiology, diagnosis, management,* ed 5, Philadelphia, 1993, WB Saunders.
26. Blackbourne LH: Vascular surgery. In Blackbourne LH, editor: *Surgical recall,* Baltimore, 1994, Williams and Wilkins.
27. Goldstone J: Abdominal aortic aneurysms. In Greenfield LJ and others, editors: *Surgery scientific principles and practice,* ed 2, Philadelphia, 1997, Lippincott-Raven.
28. Rubin E, Farber JL: Blood vessels. In Rubin E, Farber JL, editors: *Pathology,* ed 2, Philadelphia, 1994, JB Lippincott.

CHAPTER 140

Anorectal Complaints

Updated by Terry Mahan Buttaro

Anorectal complaints often encountered in the primary care setting include hemorrhoids, anal fissure, pruritus ani, and anorectal abscess and fistula. However, other anorectal conditions such as a polyp, condyloma accuminata, malignancy, or a dermatologic disorder should be considered because these disorders often cause similar symptoms. A careful history and thorough physical examination are vital in making a correct diagnosis.

Hemorrhoids

DEFINITION/EPIDEMIOLOGY

Hemorrhoids are masses of vascular tissue that, along with connective and muscular tissue, form a cushion in the submucosal layer of the anal canal. One of their functions is to help maintain closure of the anus. They are part of normal human anatomy, and therefore symptomatic hemorrhoids can potentially develop in all adults. External hemorrhoids lie below the dentate line and are covered with squamous epithelium. Internal hemorrhoids are located above the dentate line and are covered by columnar epithelium.[1]

PATHOPHYSIOLOGY

The exact cause of hemorrhoids is not completely understood. It is thought that when these vascular cushions enlarge or prolapse as a result of increased pressure applied to the pelvic floor from straining, prolonged standing, or lifting, external or internal hemorrhoids develop.[2]

CLINICAL PRESENTATION

The most common presenting symptoms of hemorrhoids are bleeding, pruritus, protrusion, and pain. Internal hemorrhoids are usually associated with intermittent, painless, bright red rectal bleeding that occurs after defecation. The blood may be seen on the toilet paper, in the toilet water, or sometimes on the outside of the stool. Blood mixed in with the stool or dark-colored blood often indicates more proximal disease. Internal hemorrhoids can be divided into four categories on the basis of severity: first-degree hemorrhoids may bulge but do not prolapse through the anal orifice; second-degree hemorrhoids prolapse during defecation but reduce spontaneously; third-degree hemorrhoids prolapse with defecation and require manual reinsertion; and fourth-degree hemorrhoids protrude permanently.[2,3] External hemorrhoids are less likely to bleed and are often asymptomatic unless thrombosis develops. The patient can present with anal irritation, pruritus, or a palpable nodule. Symptoms of a thrombosed external hemorrhoid include edema and moderate to severe pain.

PHYSICAL EXAMINATION

The entire perineum and perianal area should be inspected in a position that is comfortable for the patient (knee-chest, lithotomy, or left lateral prone). External hemorrhoids can be visualized around the anal orifice as the patient bears down, whereas internal hemorrhoids are best visualized using an anoscope as the patient bears down. An internal hemorrhoid is not palpable on rectal examination unless the hemorrhoid is thrombosed. Inflamed external hemorrhoids are erythematous and sensitive, whereas a thrombosed external hemorrhoid appears as a dark, bluish nodule on one side of the anus and is tender to palpation.[4]

DIAGNOSTICS

If the history reveals heavy, prolonged bleeding, a CBC should be obtained to exclude anemia. To screen for bleeding from a more proximal site in the colon, the adult patient should be given stool cards for serial fecal occult blood testing once all hemorrhoidal bleeding has resolved. However, any patient who complains of rectal bleeding should undergo flexible sigmoidoscopy or colonoscopy to exclude malignancy.[5]

DIFFERENTIAL DIAGNOSIS

The differential diagnosis includes other anorectal conditions that can cause pain, bleeding, or protrusion. Examples are rectal prolapse, anal skin tags, hypertrophied anal papillae, rectal polyps or cancer, anal fissure, anal papillitis, inflammatory bowel disease, and condyloma or other sexually transmitted disease.

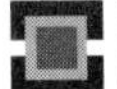

Diagnostics

Hemorrhoids

Laboratory
Serial fecal occult blood testing
CBC and differential*

Other
Flexible sigmoidoscopy*
Colonoscopy*

*If indicated.

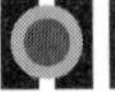

Differential Diagnosis

Hemorrhoids

Rectal prolapse
Anal skin tags
Anal fissure
Hypertrophied anal papillae
Rectal polyps
Anal papillitis
Inflammatory bowel disease
Condyloma acuminatum

MANAGEMENT

Although currently under revision, guidelines for the treatment of hemorrhoids have been published by The American Society of Colon and Rectal Surgeons.[6] The treatment of hemorrhoids is based on the degree of the patient's symptoms. Most cases of hemorrhoids can be managed conservatively, and some patients will require little or no treatment. A high-fiber diet and increased fluid intake are almost always recommended. Fiber absorbs water and helps soften the stool, thus preventing constipation and straining. Bulk-forming agents and stool softeners are sometimes used in addition to diet therapy to keep stools soft. In one study, psyllium was effective in controlling hemorrhoidal bleeding.[7] Topical hydrocortisone creams, suppositories, or foams (Table 140-1), frequent warm water sitz baths, and analgesics can help reduce inflammation and promote patient comfort.

If a thrombosed external hemorrhoid is identified within 48 hours of onset, it can be evacuated by first infiltrating a local anesthetic into the base of the hemorrhoid. An elliptical incision is then made into the thrombus and the clot is expressed. Relief is immediate. This procedure can usually be carried out in the clinic setting by a primary care provider. Care includes a gauze pad applied to the site for 12 hours, followed by a sitz bath to remove the bandage and cleanse the area. Continued daily sitz baths and a mini-pad to protect clothing are recommended for several more days. If a thrombosed external hemorrhoid has been present for more than 48 hours or is not too painful, conservative measures, including mild analgesics, sitz baths, and topical anesthetic ointments, can be used.[4,7]

A more conservative treatment for acute thrombosed external hemorrhoids with topical nifedipine was proved to be helpful in one study.[8] A topical preparation of 0.5% nitroglycerin ointment can be applied topically to the thrombosed hemorrhoid.

Patients with continued symptoms can require more aggressive therapy. Rubber band ligation, laser coagulation, sclerotherapy, bipolar diathermy coagulation, cryosurgery, or hemorrhoidectomy may be necessary to alleviate symptoms.

LIFE SPAN CONSIDERATIONS

Symptomatic hemorrhoids are a common disease entity. Although they can occur at any age in both sexes, they are more common with advancing age. The prevalence in the United States has been estimated to be as high as 50% of adults over the age of 50.[9]

COMPLICATIONS

Fourth-degree hemorrhoids are at risk for strangulation because they are irreducible. Strangulated hemorrhoids can become gangrenous, requiring immediate surgical intervention.[10]

Rubber band ligation has been associated with increased pain, infection, and sepsis. Hemorrhoidectomy has been associated with urinary tract infections, urinary retention, fecal impaction, delayed hemorrhage, and, rarely, infection.[7]

INDICATIONS FOR REFERRAL/HOSPITALIZATION

If conservative measures fail, patients should be referred to a gastroenterologist for infrared photocoagulation, electrocoagulation, or rubber banding before surgical hemorrhoidectomy is suggested. Surgery is the treatment of choice for fourth-degree hemorrhoids, most third-degree hemorrhoids, strangulated hemorrhoids, or hemorrhoids that have not responded to other therapies.[10] Flexible sigmoidoscopy or colonoscopy should be performed on all patients with rectal bleeding to exclude a more proximal lesion, which could exist in addition to hemorrhoids.[11]

PATIENT AND FAMILY EDUCATION

Patients should be instructed on how to increase dietary fiber and in the correct use of topical antiinflammatory agents. They should be taught preventive measures, including increased fluid intake, keeping the stool soft, avoiding straining during bowel movements, regular exercise to help promote regular bowel movements, and keeping the anal area clean and dry. The importance of follow-up needs to be stressed if symptoms do not resolve with conservative measures.

Anal Fissure

DEFINITION/EPIDEMIOLOGY

An anal fissure is a painful linear crack or tear in the lining of the anal canal. A fissure present for less than 6 weeks is considered acute, whereas fissures present for longer than 6 weeks are qualified as chronic.

PATHOPHYSIOLOGY

Anal fissures are sometimes seen in patients with Crohn's disease, tuberculosis, or leukemia.[12] However, most anal fissures are caused by trauma to the anal canal from passage of a large, hard stool. Other causes include frequent diarrhea, which can result in a chemical burn from severe alkalinity, and anal stenosis, which may predispose the patient to fissure formation. An

TABLE 140-1 Topical Anorectal Antiinflammatory Preparations*

Preparation	Actions	How Supplied	Usual Dosage and Administration
ProctoCream-HC 2.5% (hydrocortisone acetate) Anusol-HC 2.5% (hydrocortisone)	Antiinflammatory and antipruritic	Creams	Apply to affected area two to four times per day, depending on severity of condition
Analpram-HC 1%/1% and 2.5%/1% (hydrocortisone acetate/pramoxine)	Antiinflammatory and antipruritic, topical anesthetic		
Anusol-HC suppositories (hydrocortisone acetate)	Antiinflammatory and antipruritic	Suppositories	One suppository in rectum in morning and one at night for 2 weeks
ProctoFoam-HC (hydrocortisone acetate/pramoxine)	Antiinflammatory and antipruritic, topical anesthetic	Aerosol container and anal applicator	Apply to affected area nightly for 2 weeks; may be used up to three or four times a day

*Topical anal preparations containing hydrocortisone should not be used continuously for more than 2 weeks to avoid skin atrophy.

acute fissure often resolves without intervention. However, a chronic ulcer surrounded by scar tissue may develop if the underlying sphincter goes into involuntary spasm, leading to diminished blood flow to the area.[2]

CLINICAL PRESENTATION

Many patients will seek treatment with the thought that they have hemorrhoids. Classic symptoms of an anal fissure are severe rectal pain during and after bowel movements and small amounts of bright red rectal bleeding seen on the toilet paper. Some patients will avoid having a bowel movement because of the pain and thus produce even harder stools, which exacerbates the problem.[13]

PHYSICAL EXAMINATION

Because of the severe pain associated with an anal fissure, the physical examination should be done gently and with reassurance. The fissure is most easily visualized by spreading the buttocks to expose the anus. Ninety percent of fissures will be located at the posterior midline, and the remainder are situated in the anterior midline. A fissure located in a more lateral position usually indicates another underlying disease.[4,10] If the fissure is chronic, the examination may reveal a hypertrophied anal papilla proximal to the fissure and a sentinel pile or skin tag distal to the fissure at the anal verge.[10] These findings are indicative of repetitive inflammation and healing with resultant formation of scar tissue and can lead to anal stenosis. If the fissure is extremely painful, digital rectal and anoscopic examination may be deferred. If the fissure is touched with a cotton-tipped applicator, the symptoms will often be reproduced, helping to confirm the diagnosis.

DIAGNOSTICS

There are no routine laboratory abnormalities.

DIFFERENTIAL DIAGNOSIS

Chronic anal fissures are often misdiagnosed as hemorrhoids because of the presence of a sentinel tag. The practitioner should keep in mind that pain during bowel movements is not symptomatic of hemorrhoidal disease.[2] Sometimes a large hypertrophied anal papilla can be mistaken for a polyp on digital rectal examination. Inflammatory bowel disease, carcinoma of the anus, syphilis, and other sexually transmitted diseases are also included in the differential diagnosis.

MANAGEMENT

Increased fiber and sitz baths are a proven effective treatment for anal fissures.[12] Other therapies include the use of stool softeners, as well as cream, suppositories, or foam containing antiinflammatory agents (see Table 140-1). Topical anesthetic gel (lidocaine [Xylocaine] 2% jelly) applied before bowel movements can be helpful to reduce pain and spasm. There is some evidence that suggests that by increasing blood flow and decreasing sphincter pressure, topical 0.2% glyceryl trinitrate ointment expedites healing.[12,14] Botulinum toxin injection also has been shown to be effective for healing.[12,14] However, the studies involving nitroglycerin cream and botulinum injections were small, and fissures did recur in some patients.[14]

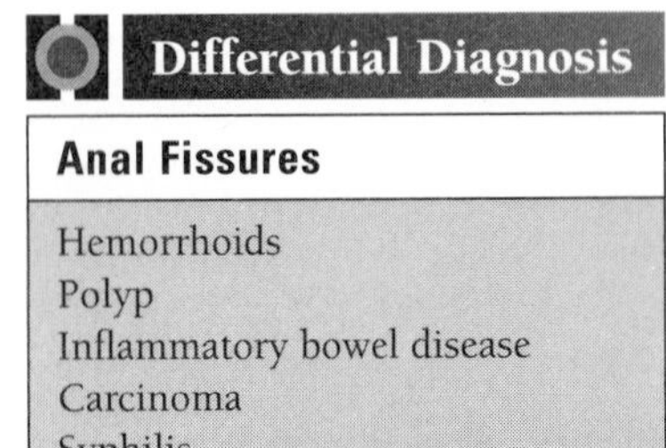

Differential Diagnosis

Anal Fissures

Hemorrhoids
Polyp
Inflammatory bowel disease
Carcinoma
Syphilis

LIFE SPAN CONSIDERATIONS

Anal fissures are commonly seen in young and middle-aged adults but can occur at any age.[9] Both sexes seem to be equally affected. Although very common, the exact incidence of this disease is unknown.[13]

COMPLICATIONS AND INDICATIONS FOR REFERRAL/HOSPITALIZATION

Patients with chronic or recurrent fissures that do not respond to conservative therapy should be referred for surgery. Lateral subcutaneous internal sphincterotomy reduces internal sphincter tone, allowing the fissure to heal. This surgery is sometimes combined with excision and repair of the entire ulcer complex.[2] Complications of this procedure can include poor wound healing and rectal incontinence but are usually avoided.[13]

PATIENT AND FAMILY EDUCATION

Patients need to be informed that healing can take up to 6 weeks with conservative measures. They should be advised to return for follow-up if symptoms do not resolve or if they become recurrent. Prevention includes keeping the stools soft with a high-fiber diet and adequate fluid intake and the avoidance of straining during bowel movements.

If topical nitroglycerin is prescribed, patients should understand how to use the preparation and be able to recognize the side effects associated with all nitrates. Nitrates are contraindicated in patients using sildenafil citrate.

Pruritus Ani

DEFINITION/EPIDEMIOLOGY

Pruritus ani or itching of the anus and perianal skin is a fairly common condition, affecting up to 5% of the population.[13] Although the true prevalence of this disorder is unknown, men are affected four times more often than women.[13,15]

PATHOPHYSIOLOGY

There are many different causes of pruritus ani. In many patients the condition has no identified cause. However, a recent study suggests that varied dermatologic conditions can cause the persistent itching that plagues some patients.[16] Pruritus ani can also be related to improper hygiene habits or to the ingestion of certain foods or beverages. Common offenders include coffee, tea, soda, alcohol, tomatoes, citrus fruits, and chocolate.[3,7] These foods possibly affect the function of the internal anal sphincter, permitting the fecal soilage associated with pruritus ani.[15]

CLINICAL PRESENTATION

The patient often complains of an uncontrollable urge to scratch the anus. The symptoms tend to be worse at night or after a bowel movement. Sometimes the itching will involve the perianal area, buttocks, and vulva or scrotum. Scratching provides only transient relief and can lead to an itch-scratch cycle that results in exacerbation of the condition.

PHYSICAL EXAMINATION

Diagnosis is made by a careful history and physical examination. The anus should be thoroughly inspected for obvious anorectal, infectious, or dermatologic disease. A digital rectal examination is also indicated. If the pruritus is chronic, the perianal skin may appear moist, excoriated, and macerated.

DIAGNOSTICS

Cultures may be useful if an infectious etiology is suspected. If the pruritus is primarily nocturnal, cellophane tape can be applied to the perianal skin in the early morning. The tape is then placed on a glass slide and examined under a microscope for the presence of pinworm eggs. If a dermatologic disease is believed to be the cause, a biopsy sample obtained by a dermatologist can help to confirm the diagnosis.

DIFFERENTIAL DIAGNOSIS

Psoriasis, malignancy, candidal infection, hidradenitis suppurativa, parasitic infection, sexual transmitted diseases, and anal fissures should be considered in the differential. See the Differential Diagnosis box.

MANAGEMENT

Any identified infectious or dermatologic disease should be treated. Once other pathologic causes of pruritus ani have been excluded, the patient's hygiene and dietary habits should be addressed. The anal area should be kept clean and dry, and overvigorous wiping or scratching should be avoided. Perfumed toilet paper, soaps, and hygiene products should not be used. A 1% hydrocortisone cream can be used initially but should be discontinued after 2 weeks to avoid skin atrophy.[10] Nonmedicated talcum powder or a barrier cream such as zinc oxide can also be helpful.[15] Dietary restrictions of possible offending foods should be tried. A psyllium product can be used to bulk the stool in an attempt to prevent fecal soilage if loose stools are a problem.[15] Medications and foods that cause loose stools should be avoided if at all possible. If severe nocturnal itching is a problem, an antihistamine with antipruritic properties, such as hydroxyzine (Atarax), can help the patient sleep and assist in breaking the itch-scratch cycle. Relief of symptoms usually occurs in 4 to 6 weeks.[13]

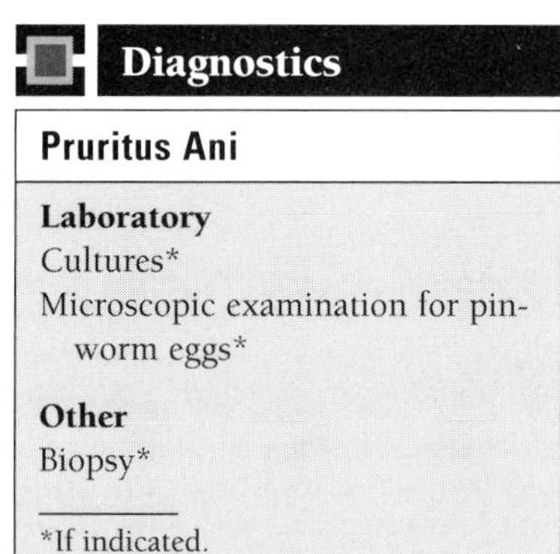

Diagnostics

Pruritus Ani

Laboratory
Cultures*
Microscopic examination for pinworm eggs*

Other
Biopsy*

*If indicated.

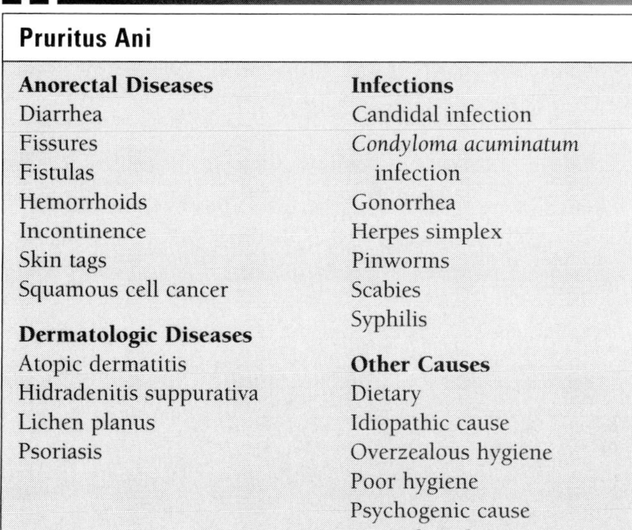

Differential Diagnosis

Pruritus Ani

Anorectal Diseases	**Infections**
Diarrhea	Candidal infection
Fissures	*Condyloma acuminatum* infection
Fistulas	Gonorrhea
Hemorrhoids	Herpes simplex
Incontinence	Pinworms
Skin tags	Scabies
Squamous cell cancer	Syphilis
Dermatologic Diseases	**Other Causes**
Atopic dermatitis	Dietary
Hidradenitis suppurativa	Idiopathic cause
Lichen planus	Overzealous hygiene
Psoriasis	Poor hygiene
	Psychogenic cause
	Warmth and moisture

LIFE SPAN CONSIDERATIONS

Pruritus ani is most common in the fourth, fifth, and sixth decades; however, this disorder can occur at any age.[13]

COMPLICATIONS

Scratching associated with pruritus ani can cause excoriations. These can become infected and require antibiotic therapy. Vaginal infections are also potential complications. Pruritus ani related to pinworm infestation can be easily spread to others, and reinfection is common.

INDICATIONS FOR REFERRAL/HOSPITALIZATION

Referral to a specialist is rarely indicated for pruritus ani. If a dermatologic disease is suspected but not clearly identified, the patient should be referred to a dermatologist for further evaluation.[16] Suspicious lesions require biopsy, and any signs or symptoms suggesting bowel pathology require colonoscopy to exclude malignancy. If medical treatment has failed, referral to a gastroenterologist is indicated.[15]

PATIENT AND FAMILY EDUCATION

The patient should be educated about the possible etiology of this condition. To help identify offending foods, the patient can be taught an elimination diet. The patient should be instructed about proper anal hygiene habits and to avoid scratching the area.

Anorectal Abscess or Fistula

DEFINITION/EPIDEMIOLOGY

An anorectal abscess is an infection that occurs from obstruction of the duct of a perianal gland in the intersphincteric space. An anorectal fistula is the drainage of an abscess through an abnormal communication to the perianal skin. An abscess is the acute manifestation of an infection, and a fistula is the chronic manifestation.[2,10] The incidence is higher in men than in women, with the most common ages being the third and fourth decades of life.[10]

PATHOPHYSIOLOGY

The most common cause of anorectal abscesses and fistulas is bacterial infection of the anal glands. These glands may become infected if obstruction with resulting stasis occurs from trauma, hard stools, foreign bodies, or diarrhea. Another common cause of anorectal abscesses or fistulas is Crohn's disease.[4,10]

CLINICAL PRESENTATION

Symptoms of an abscess include acute pain and swelling. The pain increases with movement, sitting, or bowel movements. Malaise and fever may also be present. The most common complaint of patients with an anorectal fistula is a persistent purulent drainage. The patient may give a history consistent with a prior anorectal abscess.[10]

PHYSICAL EXAMINATION

Inspection of the perineum may reveal erythema, heat, swelling, and tenderness. If the abscess is located higher in the anorectum, the perineum may be unrevealing, and the abscess may manifest as localized tenderness on rectal examination. On anoscopy, pus may be seen exuding from an opening into the anal canal. A fistula may present with pus oozing from a sinus or opening in the perineal skin. Inguinal lymph nodes may be enlarged.[1]

DIAGNOSTICS

A CBC may reveal leukocytosis. With recurrent fistulas, a small bowel follow-through, colonoscopy, or barium enema may be indicated to exclude Crohn's disease.

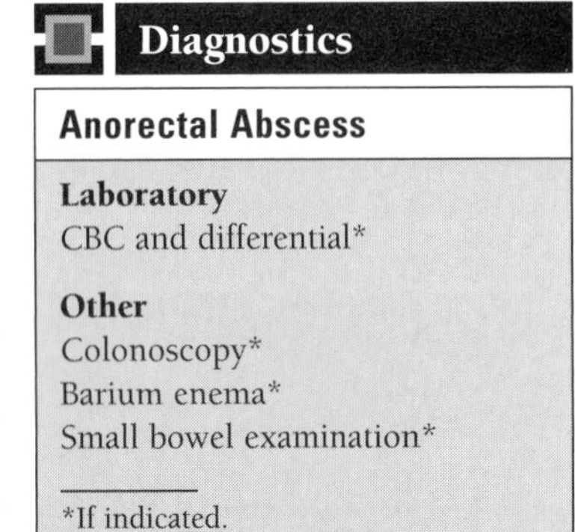

Diagnostics

Anorectal Abscess

Laboratory
CBC and differential*

Other
Colonoscopy*
Barium enema*
Small bowel examination*

*If indicated.

DIFFERENTIAL DIAGNOSIS

With recurrent fistulas, Crohn's disease should be considered. Also included in the differential diagnosis is pilonidal sinus, hidradenitis suppurativa, anorectal malignancy, actinomycosis, sexually transmitted diseases, and lymphoma.[1,10]

Differential Diagnosis

Anorectal Abscess

Crohn's disease
Pilonidal sinus
Hidradenitis suppurativa
Carcinoma
Actinomycosis
Sexually transmitted diseases

MANAGEMENT, COMPLICATIONS, AND INDICATIONS FOR REFERRAL/HOSPITALIZATION

The treatment of an anorectal abscess or fistula is always surgical. Because the risk of sepsis is potentially fatal, medical management by itself is never indicated. When an anorectal abscess or a fistula is suspected, antibiotics should be started. Surgery involves drainage of the abscess and fistulotomy if indicated.[2,10] The major complication of surgery for an abscess or a fistula is incontinence.[2]

PATIENT AND FAMILY EDUCATION

After surgery, the patient should be instructed to keep the stools soft with bulk-forming agents, a high-fiber diet, and stool softeners. Warm sitz baths can help with hygiene, promote healing, and provide comfort until healing is complete. The importance of follow-up visits to inspect the wound for proper healing should be emphasized.

REFERENCES

1. Fierst SM: Fissure in ano; hemorrhoids. In Hurst JW, editor: *Medicine for the practicing physician,* ed 4, Stamford, Conn, 1996, Appleton & Lange.
2. Kodner IJ: Differential diagnosis and management of benign anorectal diseases, *Gastrointest Dis Today* 5:8-16, 1996.
3. Henley CE: Diseases of the rectum and anus. In Taylor RB, editor: *Family medicine: principles and practice,* ed 4, New York, 1994, Springer-Verlag.
4. Spiro HM: *Clinical gastroenterology,* ed 4, New York, 1993, McGraw-Hill.
5. Bleday R, Breen E: *Treatment of hemorrhoids.* Retrieved August 4, 2002, from the World Wide Web: http://www.uptodate.com.
6. The American Society of Colon and Rectal Surgeons. Retrieved August 12, 2002, from the World Wide Web: http://www.fascrs.org/ascrs-parameters.html.
7. Bassford T: Treatment of common anorectal disorders, *Pract Ther* 45:1787-1994, 1992.
8. Perotti P and others: Conservative treatment of acute thrombosed external hemorrhoids with topical nifedipine, *Dis Colon Rectum* 44:405-409, 2001.
9. Goligher JC: *Surgery of the anus, rectum and colon,* ed 5, London, 1984, Bailliere Tindall.
10. Barnett JL, Raper SE: Anorectal diseases. In Yamada T, editor: *Textbook of gastroenterology,* ed 2, Philadelphia, 1995, JB Lippincott.
11. Schussman LC, Lutz LJ: Outpatient management of hemorrhoids, *Prim Care* 13:527-540, 1986.
12. Breen E, Bleday R: Anal fissures. Retrieved August 4, 2002, from the World Wide Web: http://www.uptodate.com.
13. Mazier WP: Hemorrhoids, fissures, and pruritus ani, *Surg Clin North Am* 74:1277-1292, 1994.
14. Jones M, Scholefield J: Anal fissures, *Clin Evidence* 6:330-335, 2001.
15. Bonis PAL and others: Approach to the patient with anal pruritus. Retrieved August 4, 2002, from the World Wide Web: http://www.uptodate.com.
16. Dasan S and others: Treatment of persistent pruritus ani in a combined colorectal and dermatological clinic, *Br J Surg* 86:1337-1340, 1999.

CHAPTER 141

Cholelithiasis and Cholecystitis

Scott W. Shiffer

DEFINITION/EPIDEMIOLOGY

Cholelithiasis and cholecystitis are worldwide disorders that result from inflammatory, infectious, neoplastic, metabolic, and congenital conditions. Gallbladder disease affects all cultures and is prevalent in most Western countries. From 20 to 25 million Americans have cholelithiasis, and each year more than half of patients with newly diagnosed gallstone disease undergo a cholecystectomy.[1] In the United States, Native Americans have a very high incidence of gallstones compared with other groups.[2] The highest incidence of acute cholecystitis is in adults aged 30 to 80 years; women have approximately twice the incidence of gallstones as men. Unfortunately, older men seem to be at risk for the development of acalculous cholecystitis, an uncommon condition that is being seen with increasing frequency.[3] Risk factors include age, ethnicity (Scandinavians and Pima Indians seem to have an increased incidence), family history, gender, medications, obesity, rapid weight loss, and hyperalimentation, as well as co-morbid disorders such as diabetes, Crohn's disease, alcoholic and biliary cirrhosis, and hyperparathyroidism (Table 141-1).[4]

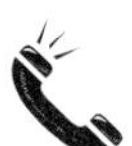

Physician consultation is indicated for acute cholecystitis.

PATHOPHYSIOLOGY

Gallstones are formed from bile constituent crystals and are divided into three primary types of stones: cholesterol, pigmented, and mixed.

Cholesterol gallstones occur as a result of several conditions. First, a supersaturation of cholesterol in the bile must be present. Second, a "snowball" effect via nucleation of filamentous, helical, or tubular forms of nonhydrated cholesterol crystals must occur because there is either an excess of pronucleating factors or a lack of antinucleating factors.[5] Third, biliary sludge accumulates as a result of delayed gallbladder emptying and stasis. Pregnancy and very low calorie diets leading to rapid weight loss are also associated with biliary sludge formation and lithogenesis.[6] Biliary proteins and lipids may act as cofactors in the cholesterol crystallization process, and there appears to be a link between an iron-deficient diet and cholesterol crystal formation.

Pigment gallstones result from excess unconjugated, insoluable bilirubin that precipitates into bilirubin crystals. This mechanism also can form the basis for a mixed-type of stone associated with alcoholic liver disease and chronic hemolysis.[6] Black-pigmented gallstones remain in the gallbladder. Brown-pigmented gallstones and cholesterol stones can be found in the gallbladder, intrahepatic ducts, cystic duct, and common bile duct.

Small gallstones pass uneventfully through the common bile duct and do not cause distress. Larger stones may cause obstruction of the cystic or common bile duct, causing increased pressure to the ductal system that results in pain, nausea, and vomiting as a result of the contractile spasms of the smooth muscle. Because of the blockage, bile is prevented from entering the duodenum, reducing the ability of the body to digest fat. The undigested fat passes from the small intestine into the large intestine, where bacteria convert the excess undigested fat into fatty acid derivatives. The fatty acid derivatives alter water absorption from the colon, which results in diarrhea and excess fluid loss. The obstruction also prevents bile secretion into the small intestine, resulting in jaundice.[2]

The gallbladder becomes inflamed as a result of various processes, including continued blockage of the cystic or common bile duct. This inflammation causes the release of prostaglandins and other chemicals that further inflame

TABLE 141-1 Risk Factors for Gallstone Formation

	Risk Factor
*A*ge	Increasing age*
*B*ody habitus	Obesity, rapid weight loss
*C*hildbearing	Pregnancy
*D*rugs	Fibric acid derivatives (or fibrates), contraceptive steroids, postmenopausal estrogens, progesterone, octreotide (Sandostatin), ceftriaxone (Rocephin)
*E*thnicity	Pima Indians, Scandinavians
*F*amily	Maternal family history of gallstones
*G*ender	Females
*H*yperalimentation	Total parenteral nutrition,† fasting
*I*leal and other metabolic diseases	Ileal disease (Crohn's disease), resection or bypass,* high triglycerides, diabetes mellitus, chronic hemolysis,* alcoholic cirrhosis,* biliary infection,* primary biliary cirrhosis, duodenal diverticula,* truncal vagotomy, hyperparathyroidism, low level of high-density lipoprotein cholesterol

From Ahmed A, Cheung RC, Keefe EB: Management of gallstones and their complications, *Am Fam Physician* 61(6):1673-1680, 1687-1688, 2000.
*Risk factors for pigment gallstone formation.
†Risk factor for cholesterol and pigment gallstone formation.

gallbladder tissue. In 75% of cases, bacterial infections contribute to the inflammatory response in acute cholecystitis.[7] The most common bacteria involved in biliary tract infections are *Escherichia coli, Klebsiella* sp., and enterococci.[8] Gangrene of the gallbladder and possible perforation can result if the process is not stopped.

Cholecystitis can also occur in the absence of stones; this condition is labeled acute or chronic *acalculous cholecystitis.* Acalculous cholecystitis is classified as acute if the duration of symptoms is less than 1 month and as chronic if the symptoms have been present longer than 3 months. The pathophysiology of this condition is poorly understood. The inflammatory process is similar to cholecystitis except that gallstones are not present. A common cause of chronic acalculous cholecystitis is biliary dyskinesia. Risk factors associated with acute acalculous cholecystitis are outlined in Box 141-1.

CLINICAL PRESENTATION

Symptoms do not appear in 60% to 80% of patients with gallstones.[9] However, patients with chronic cholecystitis often describe a recurrent, mild to moderate, right upper quadrant and epigastric abdominal pain accompanied by nausea and vomiting. The pain may radiate to the region of the posterior right shoulder/scapula and is often associated with eating fatty foods.

Classically, symptomatic cholelithiasis presents as biliary colic with intermittent or steady, right upper quadrant abdominal pain that radiates to the right posterior shoulder within an hour of eating any type of large meal.[10] The pain may be constant or intermittent and tapering, sometimes without complete relief. It is described as mild to severe and lasts from 1 to 6 hours. The biliary colic is accompanied by nausea and vomiting. There can be a history of these episodes, which increase in frequency.

Acute cholecystitis develops in a manner similar to symptomatic cholelithiasis, but biliary colic lasts longer than 6 hours. There usually is a past history of intermittent colic consistent with chronic cholecystitis, and there may be anorexia, fever, and chills in addition to the nausea and vomiting observed in symptomatic cholelithiasis. As the gallbladder becomes progressively inflamed, the pain in the right upper quadrant becomes sharp. Charcot's triad of right upper quadrant abdominal pain, fever, and jaundice can be observed if a stone is lodged in the common bile duct.

Traditionally, patients with acute acalculous cholecystitis are critically ill and require hospitalization. Presentation includes generalized complaints, fever, nausea, vomiting, and loss of appetite. Often there is no significant past medical history, although surgery, trauma, burns, and other disorders have been associated with acalculous cholecystitis. This condition should be considered in all patients who present with right upper quadrant pain in the absence of gallstones.[11]

BOX 141-1

RISK FACTORS ASSOCIATED WITH ACUTE ACALCULOUS CHOLECYSTITIS

- Coronary artery disease
- Previous myocardial infarction
- Diabetes
- Peripheral/cerebral vascular disease
- Polyarteritis nodosa
- Prolonged labor
- Prolonged fasting
- Immediate postoperative period
- Hyperalimentation
- Dehydration
- Fibrosis of the gallbladder
- Obstruction of the biliary or pancreatic ducts
- Thrombosis of the cystic artery
- Critical illnesses (e.g., bone marrow transplant)
- Severe illnesses
    - Trauma
    - Burns
    - Sepsis
- Major diseases
    - AIDS
    - Leptospirosis

PHYSICAL EXAMINATION

Depending on the severity of the condition, the physical examination in symptomatic cholelithiasis and chronic cholecystitis may be unremarkable. Right upper quadrant abdominal pain may be accompanied by tenderness. The diagnosis is based on the history, the exclusion of other disorders, and the results of the gallbladder ultrasound.

With acute cholecystitis, there may be moderate distress from systemic toxicity, including tachycardia and fever. The right upper quadrant abdominal pain is associated with tenderness and muscle guarding or rigidity. The gallbladder is not commonly palpable, but a distended tender gallbladder confirms the suspected diagnosis. Hypoactive bowel sounds and a positive Murphy's sign (an inability to take a deep breath during palpation beneath the right costal margin) may be noted. Dehydration is not uncommon. Jaundice is present in approximately 20% of patients and is the result of long-standing biliary obstruction or chronic hemolysis.[12]

The physical findings in acalculous cholecystitis are similar to those found in symptomatic gallstones. Right upper quadrant pain, vomiting, fever, jaundice, and a positive Murphy's sign are present.

DIAGNOSTICS

Laboratory testing should be individualized, but a CBC, urinalysis, liver function tests, and serum pancreatic enzymes are usually indicated (Table 141-2). A test for human chorionic gonadotropin (hCG) is essential in women of childbearing age, if potentially teratogenic clinical imaging studies are considered. An ECG is necessary if cardiac risk factors are present or if cardiac involvement is suspected.

Plain abdominal radiographs will demonstrate biliary air, marked hepatomegaly, and, in some cases, gallstones. A chest x-ray study will exclude right lower lobe pneumonia. Ultrasound is the most practical imaging study for evaluating the gallbladder and is considered accurate at least 95% of the time.[10] Pregnancy is not a contraindication for ultrasound examination.[13]

If further studies are required, scintigraphic imaging should follow ultrasonography. Biliary scintigraphy is the most accurate and specific test for diagnosing acute cholecystitis.

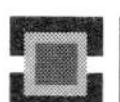

Diagnostics

Cholelithiasis and Cholecystitis

Laboratory
CBC and differential
LFTs (bilirubin, alkaline phosphate)

Imaging
Ultrasound
Biliary scintigraphy

Other
Endoscopic retrograde cholangiopancreatogram (ERCP)*

*If indicated.

DIFFERENTIAL DIAGNOSIS

There are an extensive number of differential diagnoses for cholecystitis. See the Differential Diagnosis box for a list of the more common differential diagnoses.

Differential Diagnosis

Cholelithiasis and Cholecystitis

Neoplasm	Pneumonia (right lower lobe)
Hepatitis or hepatic abscess	Pleuritis
Pancreatitis	Pyelonephritis
Gastritis	Myocardial ischemia or infarction
Peptic ulcer disease	Diverticulitis
Irritable bowel syndrome	Herpes zoster
Appendicitis	Renal colic
Fitz-Hugh–Curtis syndrome	
Pelvic inflammatory disease	

MANAGEMENT

In general, asymptomatic gallstones do not require surgical intervention. However, there is a 20% chance of the development of symptoms, and prophylactic cholecystectomy is sometimes recommended.[14] Asymptomatic patients in the following groups could be considered for a laparoscopic cholecystectomy[1]:

- Certain women of childbearing age
- Young children
- Patients with very large gallstones
- Certain patients with diabetes (should be discussed with the primary care physician or general surgeon)

The initial management of symptomatic gallbladder disease begins with isotonic IV rehydration, correction of electrolyte abnormalities and, possibly, antibiotic therapy. Oral hydration is contraindicated during this time. Antispasmodic and antiemetic medications are used for uncomplicated cholelithiasis. In addition to an antiemetic, a nasogastric tube should be used for protracted vomiting to decompress the stomach. Pain should be managed with parenteral analgesics.[14] Meperidine is usually used because it causes less spasm of the sphincter of Oddi compared with other narcotics. An injectable nonsteroidal antiinflammatory prostaglandin inhibitor (ketorolac tromethamine) is also an effective pain reliever in nonbacterial gallbladder distention.[2]

With uncomplicated symptomatic cholelithiasis, discharge is appropriate once the condition has stabilized and oral hydration is maintained. Surgical consultation before discharge is advised. Acute cholecystitis should be suspected if the symptoms do not resolve within 4 to 6 hours; in this case, timely surgical referral is essential.

Co-Management with Specialists

Medical dissolution, biliary lithotripsy, or surgical intervention requires further consultation to ensure optimal health care. Patients with diabetes and asymptomatic disease should have a consultation with a gastroenterologist or surgeon to determine whether further management is required.

After initial patient stabilization, treatment options for uncomplicated symptomatic cholelithiasis include medical dissolution therapy (oral or direct gallbladder irrigation), biliary lithotripsy, cholecystostomy (as an alternative surgical procedure), and open or laparoscopic cholecystectomy. Medical

TABLE 141-2 Expected Laboratory Values in Biliary Tract Disease

	Serum Laboratory Tests						
	WBC	Bilirubin	Alkaline Phosphate	Aspartate Aminotransferase	Alanine Aminotransferase	Amylase	Lipase
Chronic cholecystitis	Normal	Normal	Normal	Normal	Normal	Normal	Normal
Symptomatic cholelithiasis	Normal	Normal or slight rise	Normal or slight rise	Normal	Normal	†	†
Acute cholecystitis	Normal or rise	Rise in 45% of patients	Rise in 23% of patients	Rise in 40% of patients	Normal	Rise in 13% of patients†	Normal
Acute acalculous cholecystitis	Rise	Slight rise	Slight rise	Slight rise	Slight rise	Normal	Normal
Chronic acalculous cholecystitis	Normal	Normal	Normal	Normal	Normal	Normal	Normal
Choledocholith	Rise	Rise	Rise	Rise*	Rise*	Rise†	Rise†

*A rise in the transaminases is associated with prolonged obstruction leading to hepatocellular destruction.
†A rise in the serum amylase and lipase is associated with pancreatitis secondary to ampulla of Vater stone obstruction.

dissolution therapy of gallstones is attractive to patients who are poor surgical candidates or those who refuse surgery.[14]

The oral bile acid (chenodeoxycholic or ursodeoxycholic acid) method attempts to reduce the ability of the body to create gallstones by limiting cholesterol saturation in the bile. This method is best for patients who have cholesterol stones smaller than 2 cm and have a functioning gallbladder. This therapy usually requires at least 9 months to become effective; stones recur in 50% of patients within 5 years when the treatment is stopped. The high cost of the medication may be a deterrent for this type of medical management.[10] Pending an improved long-term success rate, these drugs are best reserved for patients who may not be safe surgical candidates.

A second medical dissolution regimen involves direct gallbladder irrigation with ether-type solvents. This method dissolves small stones in approximately 2 to 4 hours. Unfortunately, stone recurrence is not unusual.

Biliary lithotripsy can be considered in 20% to 25% of patients presenting with gallstones and is relatively safe. Energy waves are generated through a water bath and into the soft tissue and are transmitted into the stone. The relatively painless shock waves fracture the stones into smaller pieces that are then passed into the small intestine. The criteria for biliary lithotripsy are quite specific; in addition, it is an expensive therapy, and gallstone recurrence is reported at 50% by 5 years.[15]

Cholecystostomy is an alternative surgical procedure to open or laparoscopic cholecystectomy and is used if there is too much inflammation or if the patient is too ill for cholecystectomy. Either operatively or percutaneously, stones and bile are removed via the gallbladder fundus, and a tube is placed as an external drain.

An open cholecystectomy requires a subcostal surgical incision on the right side. The skin is separated with retractors, and the gallbladder is isolated from the liver. The cystic duct and cystic artery are ligated, and the diseased gallbladder is removed. This open surgical approach is necessary when there are relative contraindications for the laparoscopic method; these contradictions include coagulopathy, cirrhosis, portal hypertension, pregnancy, peritonitis, severe cardiopulmonary disease, and prior surgical adhesions.

Because of its safety, convenience, reduced postoperative pain, and shorter hospitalization (outpatient surgery at some facilities), laparoscopic cholecystectomy is the standard treatment for symptomatic gallbladder disease. Choledocholithiasis, or stones in the common bile duct, can also be managed through the laparoscopic approach, although in some instances this will be too difficult to manage safely. Some laparoscopic approaches will require a conversion to the open cholecystectomy procedure—5% of patients undergoing treatment for chronic cholecystitis and 25% of patients with acute cholecystitis.[10]

In addition to the initial treatment of gallstone disease, perioperative antibiotics may be indicated. Bacteria associated with acute cholecystitis include *E. coli, Klebsiella pneumoniae, Clostridium welchii, Clostridium perfringens,* and *Streptococcus faecalis.* A third-generation cephalosporin antibiotic is appropriate for cases in which there is no sepsis. Obvious infection is better managed with ampicillin, gentamicin, and clindamycin or the equivalent.

When acalculous cholecystitis is recognized, an antibiotic regimen sensitive to gram-negative organisms is the first step to treating the infection. Surgical drainage or removal of the gallbladder is considered the definitive treatment. Laparoscopic cholecystectomy may be chosen to treat the condition. Ultrasound-guided percutaneous cholecystostomy under a local anesthetic agent is an excellent alternative and has a very low mortality rate. Although symptoms of chronic acalculous cholecystitis and gallbladder dysfunction are relieved with cholecystectomy, caution is advised for this type of management pending further trials. Either a cholecystectomy or a cholecystostomy is required depending on the severity of the illness. Cholecystostomy is the treatment of choice if severe disease is present or there is extensive inflammation.[7]

COMPLICATIONS

Potential organ damage depends on the location of the gallstone obstruction in the biliary system. Patients with recurrent pain have twice the complication rate as patients without symptoms, and patients with symptomatic gallstones have a 70% chance of developing complications over their lifetime.[14] The most common complication is choledocholithiasis. In general, symptomatic gallstones require surgical intervention. If left untreated, potential complications of the disease include a pus-filled gallbladder, which can lead to perforation. Local perforation can occur within 1 week after the onset of acute cholecystitis and can lead to the formation of a pericholecystic abscess. There is a 25% mortality rate if a free perforation into the abdominal cavity occurs.[12] Should a large gallstone pass into the intestinal lumen, a small bowel obstruction is possible; this is called a *gallstone ileus.* Three times more common in men and associated with diabetes, gas-forming bacteria (*Clostridium* and coliform organisms) can lead to an emphysematous cholecystitis that further leads to gallbladder perforation.[12] The gallbladder may become gangrenous when extensive inflammation causes necrosis and thrombosis of the cystic artery. Stones lodged in the ampulla of Vater can cause gallstone pancreatitis. The porcelain gallbladder, an uncommon condition associated with cancer, is observed on plain radiographs. The porcelain appearance of the gallbladder rim is caused by calcification of the gallbladder.

The complication rate of gallstone disease varies and depends on the procedure chosen to manage the disease, the size of the gallstone, the age of the patient, and co-morbid issues. The complication and mortality rates of laparoscopic cholecystectomy and open cholecystectomy are listed in Table 141-3.

INDICATIONS FOR REFERRAL/HOSPITALIZATION

Asymptomatic cholelithiasis does not require referral for surgical management except as previously discussed. Symptomatic gallstones or evidence of acalculous disease supported by ultrasound or oral cholecystogram requires further medical and/or surgical consultation for management and maintenance.

Acute cholecystitis requires hospitalization for IV antibiotics and fluid therapy. Nearly three fourths of patients who are medically managed have complete remission of their symptoms within 2 to 7 days of hospitalization.[6]

The postoperative course after a cholecystectomy varies according to whether the surgeon used the laparoscopic or the

TABLE 141-3 Complication Rate of Gallstone Disease

	Complication Rate (%)	Mortality Rate (%)
Open cholecystectomy	7.7	0.03 (<65 years) 0.5 (>65 years)
Laparoscopic cholecystectomy	1.9	0.08

open approach. Some patients who have undergone a laparoscopic cholecystectomy may return to unrestricted activity approximately 8 days after surgery.[16,17] Patients who have undergone an open cholecystectomy may return to unrestricted activities approximately 35 days after surgery.[16,17] Patients diagnosed with acalculous cholecystitis are admitted to the hospital for the surgical procedure. If a percutaneous catheter placement is used to drain the gallbladder (cholecystostomy), the catheter remains in place for at least 7 days.

PATIENT AND FAMILY EDUCATION

Patients who are obese should be counseled about the increased risk of gallstone formation. Patients should understand the importance of lifestyle dietary changes. Although some risk factors have been implicated and not clearly demonstrated for cholelithiasis, it may be wise for patients to avoid excessive caffeine and alcohol intake and prolonged fasting. Although birth control pills may increase the possibility of gallstone disease during the first years of use, the clinical impact is not sufficient to avoid use because pregnancy has the same physiologic effect and the low-dose oral contraceptives in current use are less likely to affect gallbladder disease.[18] Patients with known gallstones should not be started on clofibrate, an antilipemic agent, because it is associated with a significantly higher incidence of cholelithiasis. An increase in the relative risk of stone formation is associated with thiazides; if possible, dosages should be reduced or the medication discontinued.

If gallstones are incidentally noted on x-ray, ultrasound, or other clinical imaging studies of the abdomen, reassurance that asymptomatic stones do not require surgery is needed. Patients presenting with symptomatic gallbladder disease need an explanation of laboratory and imaging tests, referral, and management.

Many patients who are anticipating laparoscopic cholecystectomies underrate or have unrealistic expectations about postoperative pain and activity. Preparatory guidance in this area may be efficacious to ensure a more realistic postoperative course. Older patients can expect to spend additional time in the hospital after a cholecystectomy.

REFERENCES

1. Vander AJ, Sherman JH, Luciano DS: Pathophysiology of the gastrointestinal tract. In Vander AJ, Sherman JH, Luciano DS, editors: *Human physiology*, ed 6, New York, 1994, McGraw-Hill.
2. Aufderheide TP, Brady WJ: Cholecystitis and biliary colic. In Tintinalli JE, Ruiz E, Krome RL, editors: *Emergency medicine*, New York, 1996, McGraw-Hill.
3. Chung SC: Acute acalculous cholecystitis: a reminder that this condition may appear in a primary care practice, *Postgrad Med* 98(3): 199-204, 1995.
4. Ahmed A, Cheung RC, Keefe EB: Management of gallstones and their complications, *Am Fam Physician* 61(6):1673-1680, 1687-1688, 2000.
5. Portincasa P, Van Erpecum KJ, Vanberge-Henegouen GP: Cholesterol crystallization in bile, *Gut* 41(2):138-141, 1997.
6. Greenberger NJ, Isselbacher KJ: Diseases of the gallbladder and bile ducts. In Fauci AS and others, editors: *Harrison's principles of internal medicine*, New York, 1998, McGraw-Hill.
7. Neal DD, Moritz MJ, Jarrell BE: Liver, portal hypertension, and biliary tract. In Jarrell BE, Carabasi RA III, editors: *Surgery*, ed 3, Baltimore, 1996, Williams & Wilkins.
8. Garrison RN and others: Surgical infections. In Lawrence PF, Bell RM, Dayton MT, editors: *Essentials of general surgery*, ed 2, Baltimore, 1992, Williams & Wilkins.
9. Malet PF, Soloway RD: Diseases of the gallbladder and bile ducts. In Wyngaarden JB, Smith LH, Bennett JC, editors: *Cecil textbook of medicine*, Philadelphia, 1992, WB Saunders.
10. Giurgiu DI, Roslyn JJ: Treatment of gallstones in the 1990s, *Prim Care* 23(3):497-513, 1996.
11. Pinto KM: Acalculous cholecystitis: a case report, *Nurse Pract* 21(10):120-122, 1996.
12. DiMarino AJ: Gastrointestinal diseases. In Myers AR, editor: *Medicine*, ed 2, Philadelphia, 1994, Harwal.
13. Yates MR, Baron TH: Pregnancy and liver disease, *Clin Liver Dis* 3(1):131-146, 1999.
14. Dayton MT and others: The biliary tract. In Lawrence PF, Bell RM, Dayton MT, editors: *Essentials of general surgery*, ed 2, Baltimore, 1992, Williams & Wilkins.
15. Schwesinger WH, Diehl AK: Changing indications for laparoscopic cholecystectomy: stones without symptoms and symptoms without stones, *Surg Clin North Am* 76(3):493-504, 1996.
16. Soper NJ and others: Comparison of early postoperative results for laparoscopic versus standard open cholecystectomy, *Surg Gynecol Obstet* 174(2):114-118, 1992.
17. Jatzko GR and others: Multivariate comparison of complications after laparoscopic cholecystectomy and open cholecystectomy, *Ann Surg* 221(4):381-386, 1995.
18. Grimes DA, editor: Benign gallbladder disease: newer data suggest little or no excess risk with oral contraceptive use, *Contraception Rep* 8(5), 1997.

CHAPTER 142

Cirrhosis

Updated by Terry Mahan Buttaro

DEFINITION/EPIDEMIOLOGY

Cirrhosis is a serious, irreversible disease caused by exposure to persistent toxins that cause hepatocellular injury and compromise liver function. Alcohol and various drugs, including acetaminophen, amiodarone, chemotherapeutic agents, antibiotics, and carbon tetrachloride, are the most common toxins associated with cirrhosis. The cause can be idiopathic, but primary and secondary biliary cirrhosis; viruses; infections such as hepatitis B, C, and D; hemochromatosis; autoimmune hepatitis; and other disorders also play a role in the development of cirrhosis (Box 142-1).

Cirrhosis is often classified by the underlying pathology, but another common classification of cirrhosis is based on histologic findings. There are three types of cirrhosis: micronodular, macronodular, and mixed form.[1] Micronodular cirrhosis, often associated with ethanol and drug abuse, occurs when there is repeated presence of an offending agent that prevents the regeneration of normal tissue. As a result, the regenerating tissue produces small nodules that have limited functional abilities. Macronodular cirrhosis is often seen in hepatocellular carcinoma and is distinguished by larger nodules (2 to 3 cm in diameter) that may contain their own blood supply. The larger nodules resemble scar tissue and have limited functional abilities. Mixed-form cirrhosis consists of both macronodules and micronodules. This class or variety of cirrhosis has mixed characteristics, and the patient's liver functions are also varied.[1]

The prognosis of cirrhosis depends on the etiology and classification of the disease.[2] If the cirrhosis is related to alcohol or hepatotoxic drugs, the major factor that determines survival is the patient's ability to stop drinking alcohol or taking hepatotoxic drugs. Progression of the disease can be halted if this occurs.

Child's classification is a functional tool that assesses the patient's nutritional and hepatic status (Table 142-1).[3] It is a fairly reliable prognostic indicator for patients with cirrhosis and end-stage liver disease. This classification demonstrates that patients with a combination of an albumin concentration of less than 3 g/dl, a serum bilirubin concentration of more than 3 g/dl, severe ascites, encephalopathy, and generalized wasting have a 50% operative mortality rate.[3] In established cases of cirrhosis with severe hepatic dysfunction, only 50% survive 2 years and 35% survive 5 years.[3]

BOX 142-1

DISEASES CAUSING CIRRHOSIS

- Metabolic disease (diabetes mellitus)
- Wilson's disease
- Hemochromatosis
- Antitrypsin deficiency
- Cardiac failure (congestive heart failure, myocardial infarction, valvular heart disease)
- Biliary tract obstruction
  - Primary obstruction (calculi)
  - Secondary obstruction (tumor)
- Venoocclusive disease (Budd-Chiari syndrome)
- Autoimmune disease (lupus erythematosus)

PATHOPHYSIOLOGY

Hepatocellular injury occurs when the liver is continually exposed to toxins or diseases that produce toxemia, inflammation, ischemia, and necrosis of the hepatic tissue. The persistent inflammation and necrosis stimulate hepatocellular regeneration, causing the development of fibrous (scar) tissue such as collagen by fibroblasts. As the regeneration process progresses, rigid nodules form, distorting the normal surrounding hepatic tissue. This deformation produces increased resistance to normal blood circulation, decreased blood flow, and even obstruction of normal portal venous flow resulting in decreased liver functional abilities.[4] Portal hypertension results when increased hydrostatic pressure within the portal venous circulation develops as a result of inflammation and obstruction of blood flow. As cirrhosis progresses, the pressure in the portal circulation rises, increasing resistance to portal venous flow. Collateral circulation develops to bypass areas of obstruction and maintain adequate blood flow.[4] The collateral path to portal circulation occurs in many areas, most commonly the peritoneum, retroperitoneum, and thoracic cavities. Collateral circulation can also occur in the rectum, esophagus, and gastric areas. These collateral vessels contain varicosities and appear as dilated convoluted veins with limited flexibility.[5] As a result, they are susceptible to spontaneous rupture and hemorrhage and result in significant morbidity and mortality.[6]

CLINICAL PRESENTATION

The onset of symptoms can be insidious, and patients with cirrhosis can be asymptomatic. In primary biliary cirrhosis (PBC), fatigue is reportedly the most common symptom.[7] Fatigue is also one of the most common complaints in hereditary hemochromotosis.[8] Other complaints associated with cirrhosis are nonspecific and include weakness, malaise, pruritus, and weight loss. As the patient's condition weakens, anorexia is present and is often associated with nausea and vomiting. Hematemesis can

TABLE 142-1 Child's Criteria for Hepatic Functional Reserve

	A (Minimal)	B (Moderate)	C (Advanced)
Serum bilirubin	<2 mg/dl	2-3 mg/dl	>3 mg/dl
Serum albumin	>3.5 g/dl	3-3.5 g/dl	<3 g/dl
Ascites	None	Easily controlled	Poorly controlled
Neurologic disorders	None	Minimal	Advanced coma
Nutrition	Excellent	Good	Poor (wasting)

From Child CG III, Turcotte J: The liver and portal hypertension. In Dunphy JE, editor: *Major problems in clinical surgery*, Philadelphia, 1964, WB Saunders.

also be a common presenting complaint. Abdominal pain, if present, is related to ascites and the stretching of the muscles around the enlarged liver. Chest pain caused by cardiomegaly has also been reported.[9] Menstrual abnormalities, impotence, and sterility are other complaints.[9] Neuropsychiatric symptoms such as difficulty concentrating, irritability, and confusion are associated with liver function failure.[10]

PHYSICAL EXAMINATION

A careful history, particularly a personal history of alcohol, toxic drug, or substance use and a specific review of the patient's social and work history, can identify high-risk behaviors such as IV drug use or a homosexual lifestyle. Occupations such as those in health care increase a person's susceptibility to hepatic disease. A history of recent blood transfusion or residence in an area of high hepatitis virus incidence also can suggest the diagnosis of cirrhosis.

Bruising, hematemesis, melena, and hematochezia associated with clotting dysfunction may be the presenting signs of cirrhosis. Low-grade fever, anorexia, jaundice, or right upper quadrant pain can be present. The liver may be nodular, firm, enlarged, or shrunken (seen in late stages of cirrhosis), and the spleen may be enlarged. A fluid wave and increased abdominal girth will be evident if ascites are present.[11] The presence of high pressures in the portal circulation often leads to the development of rectal varices as well as esophageal varices. As a result of the fluid shifts, peripheral edema is found in the feet, legs, and hands.[10] Lethargy and coma occur in the later stages of cirrhosis.

Asterixis, or liver flap, can be elicited with severe cases of liver failure. Other physical signs associated with cirrhosis include spider angiomas on the face, chest, and abdomen; palmar erythema; gynecomastia in men; and changes in body hair distribution in women.

DIAGNOSTICS

Hypoalbuminemia, elevated serum protein, hyperbilirubinemia, and elevated liver enzymes all indicate hepatocellular inflammation or injury. Additional diagnostics depend on patient presentation, but it is essential to determine the exact cause of the cirrhosis in newly diagnosed patients with cirrhosis. Thus initial serology workups should screen for antimitochondrial antibodies (a marker of primary biliary cirrhosis [PBC] that distinguishes PBC from secondary biliary cirrhosis), antinuclear antibodies, anti–smooth muscle antibodies, antibodies to hepatitis C, hepatitis B surface antigen, and antibodies to hepatitis B core antigen and surface antigen. Fasting serum ferritin, transferrin saturation, and total iron-binding capacity should be obtained to exclude hereditary hemochromatosis.[8] If the transferrin saturation is significantly elevated (>45%), genetic testing (C282Y and H63D) for hereditary hemochromatosis is indicated.[8] Other suggested serology workups include serum protein electrophoresis and, if Wilson's disease is a consideration (patient <50 years old), serum ceruloplasmin.

Other abnormalities in laboratory results are common. Pancytopenia, anemia, thrombocytopenia, abnormal clotting mechanisms, and prolongation of prothrombin time all contribute to an increased potential for gastrointestinal bleeding.[12] Hyponatremia can indicate advanced illness, but other electrolyte abnormalities and renal insufficiency are also common.

Diagnostics

Cirrhosis

Laboratory
- CBC and differential
- Serum electrolytes
- Serum glucose
- BUN
- Creatinine
- Serum protein
- Albumin
- Globulin
- LFTs
- Bilirubin
- Alpha-fetoprotein*
- Antimitochondrial antibodies
- Anti–smooth muscle antibodies
- Hepatitis screen
- Fasting serum ferritin
- Transferrin saturation
- Total iron-binding capacity
- C282Y*
- H63D*
- Serum protein electrophoresis*
- Serum ceruloplasmin*

Imaging
- Ultrasound
- CT scan
- Doppler studies

Other
- Liver biopsy
- Esophagogastroscopy

*If indicated.

Ultrasound or CT scan can be used to confirm liver size, assess portal circulation, and determine the presence of occult ascites or tumor.[6,13] Doppler studies can evaluate patency of hepatic, splenic, and portal veins, whereas upper endoscopy establishes the presence of esophageal and/or gastric varices. However, liver biopsy, which may be contraindicated if coagulopathies, are present is the preferred diagnostic test to confirm cirrhosis and determine the etiology of the liver dysfunction.[14] Abdominal paracentesis and abdominal fluid analysis (to determine bacterial peritonitis or peritoneal carcinomatosis) are indicated in the presence of ascites.[11]

DIFFERENTIAL DIAGNOSIS

Hepatocellular injury has varied causes, but it can be idiopathic. PBC is a chronic, progressive cholestatic disease of unknown etiology, although one recent study suggests environmental factors may play a role.[15] The nonsuppurative, granulomatous inflammatory destruction of the small interlobular bile ducts associated with PCB occurs within the liver and results in the development of cholestasis, liver failure, and cirrhosis.[13]

Secondary biliary cirrhosis occurs when the

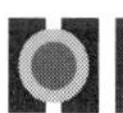

Differential Diagnosis

Cirrhosis

- Primary biliary cirrhosis
- Secondary biliary cirrhosis
  - Cardiac failure
  - Hemochromomatosis
  - Wilson's disease
  - Uremia
  - Nephrotic syndrome
  - Metabolic disorders
  - Pericarditis
  - Blood dyscrasias
  - Biliary disease
  - Hepatitis
  - Thrombosis
  - Tumor
  - $Alpha_1$-antitrypsin deficiency
  - Nonalcoholic steatohepatitis
  - Primary sclerosing cholangitis
  - Parasitic infection
  - Pancreatitis
  - Common bile duct obstruction

disease is related to extrahepatic disease, as seen with cardiac failure, hemochromatosis, or Wilson's disease.[13] Patients aged 40 years or younger with neuropsychiatric symptoms should be evaluated for Wilson's disease. Uremia, nephrotic syndrome, metabolic disorders, pericarditis, various blood dyscrasias, biliary disease, and hepatitis are conditions that impair liver function and mimic cirrhosis.[14] Thrombosis that is the result of cardiac or hematologic manifestations can obstruct blood flow and significantly alter liver function. The presence of a tumor (hepatocellular carcinoma or metastatic tumors) can be detected by imaging and suspected on the basis of an elevated serum alpha-fetoprotein concentration. The diagnosis of emphysema accompanied by liver dysfunction, especially in younger patients, suggests possible alpha$_1$-antitrypsin deficiency.[12] The presence of diabetes and endocrine disturbances in an older patient suggests hemochromatosis.[12] Nonalcoholic steatohepatitis (NASH), primary sclerosing cholangitis, or a parasitic infection such as *Schistosoma mansoni* should also be considered as a possible cause of hepatocellular injury.[16]

MANAGEMENT

Cirrhosis is an irreversible disease process; however, careful management and early treatment of complications can improve survival.[16] Thus the main focus of treatment involves the prevention of further liver dysfunction and the treatment of complications. Reversible causes of cirrhosis such as alcohol or hepatotoxic medications must be eliminated (Box 142-2) because the continued use will result in a limited life expectancy.[17] The treatment of primary biliary cirrhosis is primarily palliative, although transplantation may be beneficial in severe cases. Patients who have ongoing viral hepatitis B or C infection can have increased life expectancy with antiviral therapy, whereas those with autoimmune hepatitis benefit from corticosteroid therapy.

Patients with portal hypertension require careful monitoring for complications such as ascites and varices. Paracentesis or the placement of a peritoneovenous shunt will help with fluid redistribution if a 2000 mg/day sodium diet, fluid restriction, and diuretic therapy are not successful[18] (Box 142-3). Management of varices entails confirming the presence and location of varices. Although numerous drugs are currently being studied, only nonselective beta-adrenergic blockers (e.g., propranolol and nadolol) have shown clear benefit in decreasing the risk of hemorrhage and death in patients who have large varices but have not yet had a variceal bleed.[19] Both of these medications seem to provide some protection in preventing subsequent bleeding. Somatostatin infusions for acute variceal bleeding seem to be effective and are associated with improved survival.[20] Bleeding varices can also be treated by

BOX 142-2

HEPATOTOXIC DRUGS AND SUBSTANCES

ENVIRONMENTAL TOXINS
Arsenic
Fluorine
Trichloroethylene
Copper
Vinyl chloride
Toluene

DRUGS
Isoniazid
Folic acid analogues
Sodium valproate
Quinolone antibiotics
Acetaminophen
L-Asparaginase
Purine antimetabolites
Heavy metal chemotherapeutics
Phenothiazines
Ketoconazole
Cytidine analogues
Anthracenediones
Megadose vitamin E

DRUGS—cont'd
NSAIDs
Iron salts
Gold sodium thiomalate
Tetracycline
Testosterone and derivatives
Thioxanthenes
Aspirin (high dose: >2 g/day)
Nitrofurantoin
Interleukins
Inhaled anesthetics
Retinoic acid and derivatives
Estrogen antagonist/agonists
Alkylating agents
Hetastarch
Flutamide, goserelin
Griseofulvin
Clozapine
Butyrophenones
Methyldopa
Dantrolene

BOX 142-3

MANAGEMENT OF ASCITES

DIETARY MANAGEMENT
Sodium restriction to 2 g/day
Dietary consultation
Protein restriction to 50 g/day

FLUID MANAGEMENT
Restriction to 1500 ml when there is marked hyponatremia
Consider referral for large-volume paracentesis (5-6 L)—admit for procedure

PHARMACOLOGIC MANAGEMENT
When sodium levels remain high, begin spironolactone 100 mg/day in divided doses
Check sodium levels in 1 week, and if natriuresis and diuresis do not occur, increase daily dose to 100 mg every 4-5 days to a maximum of 400 mg/day
Adjust diuretic doses so that no more than 0.5 kg (1 pound) of fluid is lost per day
If patient has ascites and peripheral edema, no more than 1 kg of fluid loss is acceptable
Decrease dosage of diuretics by 50% if patient has signs and symptoms of hypovolemia

LABORATORY TESTS
Monitor weight, potassium, BUN, and creatinine every week or more often if patient's condition warrants it

balloon tamponade, injection sclerotherapy, endoscopic variceal band ligation, transjugular interhepatic portosystemic stent shunts (TIPS), portosystemic shunts, and/or peri-esophageal devascularization procedures[6,19-22] (Box 142-4).

Endoscopic sclerotherapy and endoscopic band ligation have both been associated with improved survival.[6]

Neurotoxin development is associated with severe liver disease and causes the cognitive defects of hepatic encephalopathy.[6] Numerous factors, including infections, medications, gastrointestinal bleeding, and constipation, have been linked to the development of hepatic encephalopathy. The serum ammonia (NH_3) level may or may not be elevated. Oral lactulose 30 to 45 ml PO t.i.d. or q.i.d. to produce two or three daily soft stools helps treat and prevent hepatic encephalopathy, but the underlying cause should also be corrected.[6] If the patient develops diarrhea, the dosage should be decreased to prevent fluid and electrolyte imbalance.[6]

Attention to each patient's nutritional status is necessary to ensure correction of iron deficiency, electrolyte balance, and protein-calorie malnutrition. The primary care provider and nutritionist can design a patient-centered plan that will focus on consumption of foods that meet the patient's physical and emotional needs. Multivitamin supplementation each day is also advised. Patients with Wernicke's encephalopathy will also require thiamin supplementation.

The use of herbal medications has been studied, but these medications have not proved to be beneficial and, in some instances, may even be harmful.[19]

Co-Management with Specialists

Management of the patient with cirrhosis is complex and requires coordinated efforts by specialists. For patients with drug or alcohol abuse, the first priority is to assist the patient in eliminating the agent from use. Drug and alcohol treatment programs can help both the patient and the family. Collaboration with mental health specialists provides information about the patient's progress with alcohol or drug abuse and determines safe medication choices for patients if pharmacologic support for detoxification is needed.

The availability of social services is helpful in acquiring financial, physical, or psychologic assistance; attaining therapeutic home aids and home health nursing care; recommending support groups; or arranging transportation. If long-term care is needed, the social worker can provide information about available facilities that will meet the patient's and family's needs.

Endoscopic evaluation by the gastroenterologist is recommended to assess the presence of varices when cirrhosis is diagnosed and if variceal bleeding is suspected. Surgical consultation may also be indicated for surgical decompression of the portal system.

COMPLICATIONS

Ascites is often associated with cirrhosis and is produced by an imbalance between the formation and distribution of peritoneal fluid. Spontaneous bacterial peritonitis is a serious infection and a potential consequence of ascites. A recent study has shown an increased incidence of gram-positive cocci in bacterial peritonitis and an increased resistance to quinolone therapy.[23]

Endocrine abnormalities are common, and diabetes is often associated with cirrhosis, particularly when related to alcohol or hemochromatosis. Other complications associated with cirrhosis include hepatocellular carcinoma, portal hypertension, gastrointestinal bleeding, hepatorenal syndrome, pulmonary hypertension, hypoxemia, hepatic hydrothorax, coagulopathies, and splenomegaly or splenic hemorrhage.[24-26] Some patients can be severely immunocompromised and at risk for infection.

When hepatocellular damage is extensive, hepatic failure results. Hepatic encephalopathy, a neuropsychiatric syndrome typified by mental status changes and asterixis, is caused by high ammonia levels and rising toxic waste products (end products of metabolism). Hepatic encephalopathy can be chronic or acute and is often associated with gastrointestinal bleeding, increased dietary protein, fluid and electrolyte disorders, medications, or infection. Early recognition, correction of the underlying precipitant, careful monitoring, and treatment with lactulose or other medications to control ammonia production are essential[6] (Box 142-5).

INDICATIONS FOR REFERRAL/HOSPITALIZATION

Primary care providers manage most patients with cirrhosis and monitor for complications. Prompt consultation and hospitalization are indicated for gastrointestinal bleeding, encephalopathy,

BOX 142-4

PREVENTION OF GASTROINTESTINAL BLEEDING

- Administer a beta blocker (propranolol 80 mg/day) for prophylaxis in patients at an increased risk for bleeding (because of ascites, encephalopathy, confirmed presence of varices).
- Consider consultation with a gastroenterologist for patients to have sclerotherapy and shunt procedures for prevention of recurrent variceal bleeding
- Monitor prothrombin time and platelet count. Although patients can have severe alterations in PT/PTT, bleeding may not occur, and treatment is not indicated. To make sure that a vitamin K deficiency is not contributing to the alterations in PT/PTT, consider administering 10-25 mg of vitamin K for 1 to several days to be sure that the liver is synthesizing to its capacity.

BOX 142-5

HEPATIC FAILURE MANAGEMENT

1. Further restrict protein intake to 20-30 g/day.
2. Consult dietitian to make sure patient's intake of amino acids is adequate.
3. Monitor mental status—check asterixis by using a five-point star or signature testing.
4. Monitor ammonia levels.
5. Consider oral lactulose 15-30 ml q 4-6 hr, with subsequent adjustments in dosage to allow two to three soft stools per day. Consider adding oral neomycin 1 g b.i.d., or metronidazole 250 mg if lactulose does not decrease ammonia levels.

BOX 142-6

PATIENT AND FAMILY EDUCATION

1. Eliminate use of alcohol and any hepatotoxic drugs.
2. Maintain strict dietary discipline.
   Sodium restriction to 2 g/day
   Protein restriction to 50 g/day
   Consult dietitian when in doubt about any phase of the diet
3. Follow exercise plan.
   Consult with physical therapy to determine plan for patient.
4. Participate in support group activities.
   Alcoholics Anonymous
   Al-Anon
5. Watch for signs of peripheral edema—call office for weight gain greater than 2 pounds/day.
6. Instruct patient's family to report any changes in patient's sensorium, posture/gait.

increasing azotemia, peritoneal irritation, or unexplained fever.[26] Consultation with a gastroenterologist is indicated for ascites unresponsive to fluid and sodium restriction, diuresis, large-volume paracentesis (5 to 6 L), or gastrointestinal bleeding from varices. Patients with intractable ascites, variceal bleeding, progressive encephalopathy, Wilson's disease, end-stage liver disease, or hemochromatosis and candidates for liver transplantation are managed by a gastroenterologist. Consultation with a nephrologist is indicated for patients with oliguria, anuria, or azotemia.[9]

PATIENT AND FAMILY EDUCATION

The patient and family should understand the benefit of the treatment plan. Dietary discipline, avoidance of hepatotoxic drugs (including nonsteroidal antiinflammatory drugs [NSAIDs]), and support group activities are ways to achieve a successful outcome (Box 142-6).

The patient and family should also be aware of the importance of reducing the risk of gastrointestinal bleeding, recognizing the signs of variceal bleeding, and taking the appropriate course of action if bleeding occurs.

Many patients with cirrhosis may be depressed. However, the use of antidepressant drugs is not usually indicated because of the high risk of oversedation and toxicity.[27] Consultation with a psychopharmacologist could assist in the design of a treatment regimen that could help the patient through this depression. Signs and complications of depression, as well as indications for immediate intervention, should be reviewed with the patient and family.

REFERENCES

1. Tobias M: Cirrhosis. In *Of the GI system and the liver*, Philadelphia, 1995, JB Lippincott.
2. Kaplan MM: Survival in asymptomatic primary biliary cirrhosis: not as good as previously reported? *Gastroenterology* 21:1707-1709, 1990.
3. Freidman L: Liver, biliary tract and pancreas. In Tierney LM Jr, McPhee SJ, Papadakis MA, editors: *Current medical diagnosis and treatment*, ed 36, Stamford, Conn, 1997, Appleton & Lange.
4. Kowdley KV: Update on therapy for hepatobiliary disease, *Nurse Pract* 7:78-86, 1996.
5. Groszman RJ: Complications of portal HTN: esophogastric varices and ascites, *Gastroenterol North Am* 21:22-27, 1992.
6. Yamada T and others: Cirrhosis, portal hypertension, and end-stage liver disease. In Yamada T, Alpers DH, Powell DW, editors: *Handbook of gastroenterology*, New York, 1998, Lippincott Williams & Wilkins.
7. Prince MI and others: Validation of a fatigue impact score in primary biliary cirrhosis: towards a standard for clinical and trial use, *J Hepatol* 32:368-373, 2000.
8. Perlman BL: Hereditary hemochromatosis: early detection of a common yet elusive disease, *Consultant* 42:237-250, 2002.
9. Butler RW: Managing the complications of cirrhosis, *Am J Nurs* 94: 46-49, 1994.
10. Gerschwin ME: Newer concepts relating to the pathogenesis of primary biliary cirrhosis. In Sorrell MF, editor: *Common liver problems: an update on practice and science*, Postgraduate course of the American Association for the Study of Liver Disease, Thorofare, NJ, 1990, Charles Slack.
11. Gershwin ME, Mackay IR: New knowledge in primary biliary cirrhosis, *Hosp Pract* 30:29-81, 1995
12. Portis R and others: HELLP syndrome: pathophysiology and anesthetic considerations, *AANA J* 65:37-47, 1997.
13. Tucker H: Primary biliary cirrhosis: current diagnosis and treatment, *Soc Gastroenterol Nurses* 15:70-76, 1992.
14. Covington H: Nursing care of patients with alcoholic liver disease, *Crit Care Nurse* 13:47-59, 1993.
15. Prince MI and others: The geographical distribution of primary biliary cirrhosis in a well-defined cohort, *Hepatology* 34:1083-1088, 2001.
16. Trotter FJ, Brenner DA: Current and prospective therapies for hepatic fibrosis, *Comprehens Ther* 21:303-318, 1995.
17. Elcheroth J and others: Role of surgical therapy in management of intractable ascites, *World J Surg* 18:240-245, 1994.
18. Such J, Runyon BA: Cirrhosis: diagnosis and initial therapy. Retrieved August 2001 from the World Wide Web: http:// www.uptodate.com.
19. Terblanche J and others: Long-term management of variceal bleeding: the place of varix injection and ligation, *World J Surg* 18:185-192, 1994.
20. Moitinho E and others: Multicenter randomized controlled trial comparing different schedules of somatostatin in the treatment of acute variceal bleeding, *J Hepatol* 35:712-718, 2001.
21. Mudge C: Hepatorenal syndrome, *AACN Clin Issues Crit Care Nurs* 3(3):614-632, 1992.
22. Pomier–Layrargues G and others: Transjugular intrahepatic portosystemic shunt (TIPS) versus endoscopic variceal ligation in the prevention of variceal bleeding in patients with cirrhosis: a random trial, *Gut* 48:390-396, 2001.
23. Fernandez J and others: Bacterial infections in cirrhosis: epidemiological changes with invasive procedures and norfloxacin prophylaxis, *Hepatology* 35:140-148, 2002.
24. Benvegnu L and others: Evidence for an association between the aetiology of cirrhosis and pattern of hepatocellular carcinoma development, *Gut* 48:110-115, 2001.
25. Arroyo V, Gines P, Planas R: Treatment of ascites in cirrhosis: diuretics, peritoneovenous shunt and large-volume paracentesis, *Gastroenterol Clin North Am* 21:237-255, 1992.
26. Kuper H and others: The risk of liver and bile duct cancer in patients with chronic viral hepatitis, alcoholism, or cirrhosis, *Hepatology* 34 (4 Pt 1):714-718, 2001.
27. DiPiro J: *Pharmacotherapy: a pathophysiological approach*, ed 3, Stamford, Conn, 1996, Appleton & Lange.

CHAPTER 143

Constipation

Terry Mahan Buttaro

DEFINITION/EPIDEMIOLOGY

Constipation is the most commonly occurring gastrointestinal complaint; it affects 10% of the general population, with an estimated $725 million expended on laxatives every year.[1,2] Although this disorder does affect the pediatric population, it is a common complaint among older adults and appears to be more prevalent in women, resulting in at least 2.5 million visits annually.[3-6] The increased incidence in older adults is related to diminished vitality, decreased activity, and the consequences of many illnesses and medications[3,4] (Box 143-1). Although not usually considered life threatening, constipation can be disconcerting and disabling and has been associated with impaction and ileus.[2,3] For this reason, all patients in the primary care setting should be queried about their bowel habits.

Constipation is usually defined as a decrease in the frequency of bowel movements. However, two of the following symptoms must have been present for at least 12 weeks in the past year to fulfill the Rome II criteria for constipation: fewer than two bowel movements per week or the passage of hard or lumpy stools; a sensation of straining, a feeling of incomplete evacuation, and/or anorectal obstruction; and manual maneuvers to aid defecation in more than 25% of defecations.[6,7] Less than three stools per week is usually considered abnormal. Soft, easily passed stools are not indicative of constipation. A true clinical diagnosis is the finding of a large amount of feces in the rectal ampulla on digital examination and/or excessive feces in the colon, rectum, or both on the abdominal radiograph.

PATHOPHYSIOLOGY

The primary function of the large intestine is to store and concentrate fecal material before defecation. If the fecal contents remain in the large intestine for long periods, almost all water is absorbed, resulting in hard stools. Normal colonic motility depends on the integrity of the central nervous system, autonomic nervous system, gut wall innervation and receptors, circular smooth muscle, gastrointestinal neurotransmitters, and hormones. Healthy adults have normal gut transit time; total gut transit time is prolonged in patients with constipation.

Disordered colonic transit and pelvic floor or anorectal dysfunction (a failure to adequately empty the rectal contents) are the two primary causes of constipation.[8] Secondary causes include ignoring the urge to defecate, inadequate fiber or fluid intake, hypothyroidism, medications, diabetes, pregnancy, irritable bowel syndrome, hypokalemia, hypercalcemia, psychologic disturbances, neurologic disorders, and anatomic lesions such as fistulas, hemorrhoids, rectocele, abscesses, or neoplasms. Parasitic infections such as *Ascaris lumbricoides* (an intestinal nematode) have been identified with intestinal obstruction and should be considered in patients who travel to or live in endemic areas of the United States.[9]

BOX 143-1

MEDICATIONS ASSOCIATED WITH CONSTIPATION

- Amantidine
- Amitriptyline
- Antacids
- Anticholinergics
- Antihistamines
- Calcium channel blockers
- Calcium supplements
- Diuretics
- Iron supplements
- Narcotics
- NSAIDs

CLINICAL PRESENTATION

Constipation is a subjective complaint and varies from one individual to another. Patients may complain of constipation and describe a feeling of nausea, bloating, cramping, and difficulty passing stools. The patient history should include the change in bowel pattern, number of stools per day/week, last bowel movement, need to strain during defecation, feeling of incomplete evacuation, impaction, fecal incontinence, diarrhea, abdominal pain, and presence of blood or pain with defecation.[10,11] In addition, a past history of associated illnesses, a 24-hour dietary and fluid review, a complete medication review (including laxative and over-the-counter medication use), and any related symptoms should also be elicited.

PHYSICAL EXAMINATION

Although it is not uncommon to have normal findings, the physical examination is performed to exclude or verify the symptom of constipation. Orthostatic hypotension and/or tachycardia implies dehydration; weight loss suggests anorexia or carcinoma. The oral examination may suggest poor dentition, ill-fitting dentures, lesions, or dehydration. Abdominal scars indicate a surgical history. Peristalsis and bowel sounds may be increased or decreased, suggesting a threatened obstruction or ileus. There may be increased dullness over areas of stool, and masses may be palpated. Rebound tenderness suggests a peritoneal inflammation. A gynecologic examination may demonstrate a rectocele. A rectal examination and anoscopy should determine sphincter tone, pain, lesions, rectal prolapse, impaction, hemorrhoids, or fissures. The neurologic examination may elicit autonomic dysfunction.

DIAGNOSTICS

Diagnostics exclude underlying pathologic conditions and metabolic disturbances. A recent change in bowel habits or the presence of abdominal pain or rectal bleeding mandates an evaluation for an obstructing neoplasm with colonoscopy or a barium enema. Abdominal x-ray studies are indicated in the presence of abdominal discomfort, nausea, and/or vomiting to exclude obstruction, ileus, or volvulus. Abdominal radiographs or an abdominal ultrasound, plus a stool culture, are also indicated if ascariasis is suspected.[9] A urinalysis and culture may reveal chronic cystitis, which may be related to constipation. A stool sample for occult blood, thyroid-stimulating hormone (TSH), CBC, and chemistry profile, specifically calcium, potassium, and blood glucose, should also be obtained. Colonic transport, anorectal manometry, electromyelography, and other studies may be indicated for constipation that does not respond to therapeutic intervention.[12]

DIFFERENTIAL DIAGNOSIS

It is critical to recognize the pathologic conditions that may first present as constipation. Colorectal carcinoma, ovarian cancer, hypothyroidism, ileus, parasitic infection, rectal fissure, hypokalemia, hypercalcemia, obstruction, and irritable bowel syndrome with alternating constipation and diarrhea must be considered.

MANAGEMENT

Prevention and management of constipation are dependent on both the underlying cause and the individual patient. Volvulus and obstruction require immediate surgical evaluation. Ileus and pseudo-obstruction can be medically managed with nasogastric suction and IV fluid.

Once a pathologic or life-threatening condition has been excluded, patients should be encouraged to keep a stool diary (noting frequency of stooling and associated symptoms) to both substantiate the constipation and aid in determining the effectiveness of intervention.[13] Although there is limited evidence specifying the correct management for constipation, the initial approach should include management of secondary causes, dietary measures, increased fluids to 1.5 to 2 L/day, periodic exercise, and bowel training.[3,14] An increase in fiber to 20 to 40 g/day over a period of weeks is appropriate. Often five prunes per day or 2 tablespoons of bran with meals followed with at least 8 ounces of liquid is adequate. If a patient is unable to consume the required diet, fiber supplements such as Fiberall or Fibercon combined with increased fluids are recommended. Initiating a moderate exercise program may help to increase peristalsis, although exercise has not been proved to be an effective therapy. Patients should also be encouraged to develop regular bowel habits by allowing enough time for satisfactory bowel elimination and by attempting to defecate during a specific time period each day. Because the gastrocolic response is stimulated by eating, the patient should be encouraged to toilet 30 minutes after eating a meal.

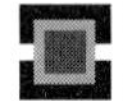 **Diagnostics**

Constipation

Laboratory
Urinalysis*
Stool for occult blood
TSH
CBC and differential
Chemistry profile (including calcium, potassium, serum glucose)
Stool culture*

Imaging
Abdominal radiographs (KUB—flat plate and upright)*
Abdominal ultrasound*

Other
Barium enema*
Colonoscopy or flexible sigmoidoscopy*
Anorectal manometry*
Electromyelogram*
Colonic transport studies*

*If indicated.

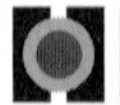 **Differential Diagnosis**

Constipation

Carcinoma
Ovarian cancer
Hypothyroidism
Ileus
Parasitic infection
Rectal fissure
Electrolyte disturbance
Obstruction
Irritable bowel syndrome

Pharmacologic treatment is appropriate if there is no response to conservative measures. Although there is no evidence to suggest that fiber is superior to laxatives, bulking agents such as psyllium or methylcellulose are suitable initially.[15] Metamucil or Citrucel 5 ml (1 tsp) q.d. to t.i.d. is administered in 240 ml of water. Docusate sodium may be added to soften the stool if bulk-forming agents are ineffective.

If straining is still present, a laxative is indicated. There is no clear evidence to recommend any particular laxative, although some laxatives can have significant side effects. The use of a stimulant laxative (senna or bisacodyl) every 3 days is acceptable, the chronic use of castor oil, senna, cascara, or bisacodyl has been associated with intestinal mucosal damage and electrolyte abnormalities; therefore these medications should be avoided, if possible. Milk of magnesia is readily available and inexpensive, but it should be used judiciously in patients with a history of congestive heart failure or renal insufficiency to avoid fluid and electrolyte abnormalities.[6] Other osmotic laxatives such as lactulose or MiraLax (polyethylene glycol) are relatively safe alternatives (provided liquid intake is adequate) and can be titrated to produce a daily bowel movement.[16] Although not contraindicated, lactulose should be used cautiously in patients with diabetes. The use of mineral oil has been associated with vitamin deficiency and therefore is not recommended.

A suppository, Fleet's enema, or tap water enema may also be used. Other medications, including colchicine, are currently under investigation for the treatment of constipation, but more studies are necessary to establish safety and efficacy.

Patients with constipation related to pelvic floor dysfunction or neurologic injury may benefit from biofeedback training if a center that is equipped to provide electromyogram-guided biofeedback is available.[17,18] Surgical evaluation is necessary for patients with rectal prolapse and for those who require surgical intervention.[18] The phases of constipation management are listed in Box 143-2.

COMPLICATIONS

Complications of constipation include the development of an ileus, megacolon, hernia, hemorrhoids, fecal impaction, or rectal or uterine prolapse. Laxative dependency is an added consequence.

INDICATIONS FOR REFERRAL/HOSPITALIZATION

Nausea, vomiting, fever, and abdominal pain may indicate the presence of an ileus and must be managed accordingly. Treatment is usually supportive and requires physician consultation when hospitalization is necessary to provide parenteral fluids and pain management. Referral to a gastroenterologist is indicated if a pathologic condition is suspected or if therapies are unsuccessful.

BOX 143-2

CONSTIPATION MANAGEMENT

PHASE 1

Lifestyle changes

1. Exercise regularly.
2. Develop regular bowel habits.

Dietary changes

1. Increase dietary fiber to 20-40 g/day (prunes, bran, beans, broccoli, spinach, carrots, corn, potato, apple, and pears with skin).
2. Decrease fats, particularly cheese.
3. Increase fluids to 1.5-2 L/day.

PHASE 2

1. Bulk-forming laxatives: methylcellulose (Citrucel) or psyllium (Metamucil), 1 teaspoon to 1 tablespoon one to three times daily in 240 ml water; or calcium polycarbophil (FiberCon), 2 tablets with 8 ounces of water one to four times daily, followed by a second glass of water; fluid intake should be increased

PHASE 3

1. Stool softeners

   Dioctyl sodium sulfosuccinate: 100 mg PO t.i.d. followed by 8 ounces of water

PHASE 4

1. Saline laxatives

   Lactulose: 30-45 ml PO up to q.i.d., or 1 tablespoon every hour until bowel movement

   Milk of magnesia: 30 ml PO p.r.n. h.s.

   Magnesium citrate: 30 ml PO p.r.n. h.s.

   Miralax: 17 g in 8 oz water p.r.n. q.d.*

   Fleet enema: one enema per rectum

PHASE 5

1. Stimulant laxatives

   Bisacodyl: 5-15 mg PO q.d. p.r.n.

   Senna (Senokot): 2 tablets PO p.r.n. h.s.

   Bisacodyl (Dulcolax) suppository: 1 per rectum q 3 days p.r.n.

PHASE 6

1. Severely constipated patients may require both oral laxatives and enemas or a suppository to alleviate constipation.

*Avoid prolonged use.

PATIENT AND FAMILY EDUCATION AND HEALTH PROMOTION

It is imperative that lifestyle changes be reinforced to establish consistent bowel habits. Patients should not delay in responding to the call to defecate and should be encouraged to sit on the toilet, with feet placed on a stool, at the same time each day for approximately 10 minutes; this should occur preferably after meals and/or the ingestion of a warm liquid to stimulate the gastrocolic reflex. The promotion of a low-fat, high-fiber diet and a minimum of 2 L of fluid/day are essential. However, dietary fiber should be gradually introduced to avoid severe cramping and bloating. It is very important that patients receive a careful explanation of medication side effects and understand the importance of avoiding laxatives when pregnant or unless necessary. Patients should also contact the primary care provider for any change in bowel habits or if the constipation is associated with fever, bleeding, weight loss, and abdominal pain.

REFERENCES

1. Sweeney M: Constipation: diagnosis and treatment, *Home Care Prov* 2(5):250-255, 1997.
2. Norton C: The causes and nursing management of constipation, *Br J Nurs* 5(20):1252-1258, 1996.
3. Abyad A, Mourad F: Constipation: common sense care of the older patient, *Geriatrics* 51(12):28-34, 1996.
4. Talley NJ and others: Constipation in an elderly community: a study of prevalence and potential risk factors, *Am J Gastroenterol* 91(1): 19-25, 1996.
5. Harari D and others: Bowel habit in relation to age and gender: findings from the National Health Interview Survey and clinical implications, *Arch Intern Med* 156(3):315-320, 1996.
6. Robson K, Lembo T: Management of constipation in geriatric patients, *Long-Term Care Interface* 2(10):54-58, 2001.
7. Thompson WG and others: Functional bowel disorders and functional abdominal pain, *Gut* 45(suppl 2):43-47, 1999.
8. Ashraf W and others: An examination of the reliability of reported stool frequency in the diagnosis of idiopathic constipation, *Am J Gastroenterol* 91(1):26-32, 1996.
9. Pfeifer J, Agachan F, Wexner SD: Surgery for constipation: a review, *Dis Colon Rectum* 39(4):444-460, 1996.
10. Wasadikar PP, Kulkarni AB: Intestinal obstruction due to ascariasis, *Br J Surg* 84(3):410-412, 1997.
11. Agachan F and others: A constipation scoring system to simplify evaluation and management of constipated patients, *Dis Colon Rectum* 39(6):681-685, 1996.
12. Koch A and others: Symptoms in chronic constipation, *Dis Colon Rectum* 40(8):902-906, 1997.
13. Bassotti G and others: Upper gastrointestinal motor activity in patients with slow-transit constipation: further evidence for an enteric neuropathy, *Dig Dis Sci* 41(10):1999-2005, 1996.
14. Ashraf W and others: Constipation in Parkinson's disease: objective assessment and response to psyllium, *Move Dis* 12(6):946-951, 1997.
15. Benton JM and others: Changing bowel hygiene practice successfully: a program to reduce laxative use in a chronic care hospital, *Geriatr Nurs* 18(1):12-17, 1997.
16. Tramonte SM and others: The treatment of chronic constipation in adults: a systemic review, *J Gen Intern Med* 12(1):15-24, 1997.
17. Clausen MR, Mortensen PB: Lactulose, disaccharides and colonic flora: clinical consequences, *Drugs* 53(6):930-942, 1997.
18. Ko CY and others: Biofeedback is effective therapy for fecal incontinence and constipation, *Arch Surg* 132(8):829-833, 1997.

CHAPTER 144

Diarrhea

Sharon R. Smart

DEFINITION/EPIDEMIOLOGY

Diarrhea is defined as an increased liquidity and frequency of stools. Acute diarrhea usually has an abrupt onset and lasts less than 1 week, although some cases of acute diarrhea may last up to 2 weeks. Most cases of acute diarrhea are infectious and occur within hours of exposure. A variety of symptoms with varying degrees of severity, including abdominal cramping, fever, chills, nausea, and vomiting, often occur with acute diarrhea, but the patient is rarely seriously ill unless there is a high fever, protracted vomiting, or severe dehydration. Most cases are self-limiting, require no medical treatment, and resolve spontaneously within several days. Medications, particularly chemotherapeutic agents, fecal impaction, and enteral feedings can also cause acute diarrhea.

Chronic diarrhea lasts longer than 2 or 3 weeks, can be intermittent or continuous, and is classified as inflammatory, osmotic, secretory, factitious, or related to altered intestinal motility (irritable bowel syndrome). Occasionally, chronic diarrhea is the end result of an acute diarrheal infection.

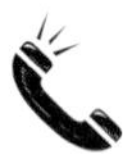

Physician consultation is indicated if diarrhea is accompanied by high fever, abdominal pain, dehydration, or bloody stools.

PATHOPHYSIOLOGY

Pathogens such as viruses, bacteria, or parasites can cause diarrhea. Viruses usually occur on a year-round basis but peak in the winter months. Bacterial illnesses are more common in the summer or early fall. Infectious diarrhea, the most common type of diarrhea, is spread by food or water contamination, person-to-person contact, the fecal-oral route, or animals.[1] Noninfectious causes of diarrhea include organic disorders and irritable bowel syndrome or other functional disorders.[2,3]

Diarrhea can be caused by laxative abuse or (1) an osmotic mechanism that is altered by a large amount of poorly absorbed ingested solutes that produce an osmotic pressure on the intestinal mucosa (e.g., lactose intolerance or laxative overuse), (2) an abnormal ion transport that results in a hypersecretory diarrhea in which there is diffuse mucosal disease of the small intestine (e.g., celiac sprue or enteric infections), (3) deranged or enhanced motility with an increase of fluid throughout the gut (e.g., chronic diseases or malignancy), or (4) an exudation of blood and pus on or in the intestinal mucosa, resulting in an impairment of the absorption of water and electrolytes (e.g., dysentery or ulcerative colitis). Any of these mechanisms can cause a disturbance of the normal flow and transport of intestinal fluids, resulting in an increased intestinal intraluminal fluid load that cannot be properly absorbed. Eventually the consistency of the stool is affected, becoming loose and liquid. If the integrity of the intestinal mucosa has been affected, as in bacterial invasion, rectal bleeding and fecal leukocytosis occur.[2-4]

CLINICAL PRESENTATION

The history will be the most helpful in determining the etiology of the diarrheal illness and should include a description of the alterations in normal day-to-day bowel habits, as well as duration of the illness and the frequency and liquidity of the stools. This information will assist in differentiating between acute and chronic diarrhea and determine the aggressiveness of the diagnostic evaluation and/or need for immediate referral.

The history should include associated symptoms such as nausea, vomiting, and abdominal pain or cramping, as well as any episodes of fever or chills (indicating dehydration or an inflammatory infection). Other pertinent information includes increased thirst; oliguria; dizziness; tenesmus; rectal discomfort; presence of bloody, mucoid, or purulent exudates in stools, weight loss (gradual or acute); previous or current diagnosed medical conditions, such as diabetes, thyroid disease, or malignancies; and associated bowel symptoms, including alternating patterns of constipation and diarrhea; nocturnal diarrhea; and any history of hemorrhoids. All current medications, over-the-counter and prescription, including antibiotic treatment within the past 3 months, should be reviewed. A detailed dietary history, including any nutritional or dietary supplement or diet aides, is also necessary because sugar-free products contain sorbitol or mannitol, which are poorly absorbed and may cause diarrhea. A social history should include any recent travel to areas with poor sanitation and water systems (i.e., to assess for infection with enterotoxigenic *Escherichia coli, Shigella* organisms, or giardiasis), alcohol or substance use or abuse, type of residence (i.e., urban versus rural), type of employment (e.g., workers in day care centers or nurseries, prisons, nursing homes; food handlers), and stress-related issues. Sexual practices should be explored because sexually active homosexual persons are at risk for enteric infections.

Family history should include any recent diarrhea illnesses in family members. Food poisoning should be suspected if others, either family members or close cohorts, have similar symptoms. Specific inquiry should be made as to whether there has been any consumption of raw milk or meats. Common causes of food poisoning include *Staphylococcus aureus, Clostridium perfringens,* and *Bacillus cereus.*[1,3]

PHYSICAL EXAMINATION

A complete examination should include weight and temperature, as well as orthostatic vital signs (blood pressure and heart rate while lying, sitting, and standing) to assess volume status. The skin should be examined, noting color, turgor, rashes, or joint inflammation (Reiter's syndrome). The head and neck should be assessed for evidence of conjunctivitis (suggesting Reiter's syndrome), dehydration, infection, thyromegaly, or lymphadenopathy. A cardiovascular examination is indicated to determine the patient's response to the illness and to exclude the cardiovascular complications associated with some illnesses. Particular emphasis during the abdominal examination is necessary to determine abdominal distention, peristalsis, masses, organomegaly, tenderness, rigidity, rebound, guarding, fecal impaction, or bleeding. In a female patient with lower abdominal symptoms, a pelvic examination is imperative. In an older patient, exclusion of fecal impaction is essential.[3]

DIAGNOSTICS

Acute diarrhea in an afebrile individual is usually a self-limiting illness, even with coexistent nausea or vomiting. Diagnostic evaluation is not usually indicated because this type of diarrheal illness is usually viral and is considered benign. Some bacteria have a noninflammatory effect on the intestinal mucosa, and symptoms will usually resolve within 1 week without treatment. Further evaluation is not necessary, and a diagnosis is rarely documented.

In an immunocompromised patient or patient with fever, abdominal pain, dehydration, protracted nausea and vomiting, diarrhea lasting longer than 1 week, and/or the presence of blood in the stool, diagnostic testing should be more aggressive. A CBC, serum electrolytes, BUN, creatinine, and stool evaluation for occult blood and fecal leukocytes are necessary. Normally there are no fecal leukocytes or polymorphonuclear cells in the stool, but fecal leukocytes are present in inflammatory diarrhea and are associated with *Campylobacter, Shigella,* or *Salmonella* organisms; *Clostridium difficile;* and enterohemorrhagic *E. coli.* If fecal leukocytes are present, the stool should be further evaluated for ova and parasites, and a stool culture obtained. If infection with *C. difficile* is suspected, a stool sample for both culture and *C. difficile* toxin is necessary.

If a small bowel obstruction or stool impaction with overflow incontinence (commonly seen in older adults) is suspected, plain x-ray films (kidney-ureter-bladder [KUB] and upright) of the abdomen are necessary. Other diagnostics to consider include imaging (CT scan if acute diverticulitis is suspected) or colonoscopy, if the diarrhea continues despite appropriate treatment.

If diarrhea continues after 2 weeks with no coexisting factors, a consideration may be lactose intolerance. No diagnostics are necessary other than a trial of abstinence from foods or liquids that contain lactose. However, if the lactose-free diet trial fails to solve symptoms, bacterial causes, such as giardiasis or infection with *Entamoeba* organisms or other pathogens, should be considered.

DIFFERENTIAL DIAGNOSIS

Infectious diarrhea can be classified into inflammatory and noninflammatory causes. The inflammatory pathogens usually affect the integrity of the lower intestinal mucosa, and presentation usually includes fever and bloody stools. Noninflammatory infectious pathogens usually affect the upper gastrointestinal tract (Box 144-1). Fever may or may not be present, but bloody diarrhea is not a common presenting symptom. Other causes of diarrhea that should be considered include medications, toxins, human immunodeficiency virus (HIV) infection, malignancy, acute diverticulitis, Crohn's disease, and ulcerative colitis.

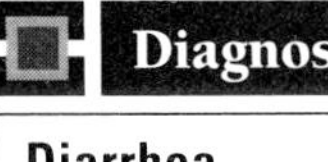

Diagnostics

Diarrhea

Laboratory
- CBC and differential*
- Serum electrolytes
- Serum glucose
- BUN
- Creatinine*
- Stool for occult blood and fecal leukocytes*
- Stool for ova and parasites, culture for *Clostridium difficile**

*If indicated.

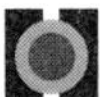

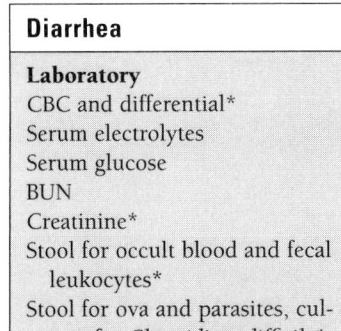

Differential Diagnosis

Diarrhea

Acute Diarrhea*	Chronic Diarrhea
Amebiasis (usually associated with travel)	AIDS
Staphylococcus aureus (associated with contaminated food)	Colitis
Campylobacter organisms	Crohn's disease
Giardia lambia (associated with contaminated water)	Diet related diarrhea (lactose intolerant)
Salmonella organisms (associated with contaminated food)	Impaction
Shigella organisms	Irritable bowel
Toxigenic *Escherichia* coli (traveler's diarrhea)	Medication-related diarrhea
Viral infection	

*Diarrhea lasting <2 weeks.

MANAGEMENT

Because diarrhea is usually self-limiting, treatment measures should be directed toward symptomatic relief, comfort measures, rest, and rehydration to prevent further dehydration. IV hydration is indicated for severe dehydration or for young, old, or immunocompromised patients. Oral fluid replacement initiated in the office is advised to manage a mild, uncomplicated illness. Sports drinks can be used in healthy adults to prevent dehydration. However, these preparations should be used cautiously in the pediatric population because the hypertonic solutions have a high carbohydrate and low electrolyte content, which can intensify the diarrhea.

If the patient shows evidence of mild dehydration and is not vomiting, a hypo-osmolar solution containing glucose and electrolytes is advised to prevent future increased intestinal intraluminal fluid overload. Commercial preparations include Pedialyte or Rehydralyte; however, the American College of Gastroenterology recommends homemade solutions that are consumed alternately (Box 144-2). A cereal-based rehydrating solution, Ricelyte, which contains more calories than the glucose-based solution, may be used to decrease stool volume and the duration of diarrhea. If Ricelyte or another similar commercial product is not available, a preparation can be made with the following ingredients: 1 to 2 cups of rice cereal, 4 cups of water (boil if traveling), and $\frac{1}{2}$ teaspoon of salt. If abdominal cramping is an associated symptom, fasting for a brief period of 8 to 12 hours and applying moist heat to the abdomen as a comfort measure may help.[5]

Solid food products should be reintroduced as symptoms resolve and stools become more formed. Dietary restrictions are

BOX 144-1

CAUSES OF DIARRHEA

INFECTIOUS DIARRHEA	NONINFECTIOUS DIARRHEA
Noninflammatory Type	Drugs
Viruses	Laxatives
Rotavirus	Antibiotics
Norwalk-like virus	Antiarrhythmic agents
Bacteria	Diuretics
Enterotoxigenic *Escherichia coli*	Lactose intolerance
Clostridium perfringens	Toxins
Staphylococcus aureus	Heavy metals
Bacillus cereus	Insecticides
Vibrio cholerae	Endocrine disorders
Parasites	Thyroid disease
Giardia lamblia	Diabetes
Cryptosporidium organisms	Irritable bowel syndrome
Inflammatory Type	Inflammatory bowel disease
Bacteria	Crohn's disease
Campylobacter jejuni	Malignancies
Shigella organisms	HIV disease
Enterohemorrhagic *E. coli*	Tropical sprue
Clostridium difficile	Celiac sprue
Vibrio parahaemolyticus	Scleroderma
Salmonella organisms	Short bowel syndrome
Parasites	Whipple's disease
Entamoeba histolytica	

BOX 144-2

HOMEMADE ORAL REHYDRATING SOLUTIONS

8 oz orange or apple juice
½ tsp honey or corn syrup
Pinch of salt
Followed by
8 oz clear water
¼ tsp baking soda
or
4½ cups water
¼ tsp salt substitute (with potassium)
½ tsp baking soda
½ tsp salt
2-3 tbsp sugar, honey, or corn syrup

necessary only if the patient cannot tolerate certain food products. If lactose intolerance does occur, with symptoms of bloating and gas, dairy products should be avoided. If symptoms of lactose intolerance persist, irritable bowel syndrome, food allergies, or even giardiasis should be considered. Other food products that may aggravate symptoms are caffeine, sugar-free products that contain sorbitol, and foods high in fiber.

Medications for symptomatic relief of nausea and vomiting, abdominal cramping, and diarrhea are used to facilitate the improvement of stool formation and are generally used in older children and otherwise healthy adults. Absorbents such as kaolin-pectin preparations (Kaopectate; 4 tablespoons every 4 hours) and antispasmodic/anticholinergic/sedatives such as Donnatal (atropine sulfate/scopolamine hydrobromide/hyoscyamine sulfate/phenobarbital; 1 or 2 tablets t.i.d.) are used to decrease abdominal cramping. Antisecretory agents, which have an anti-inflammatory effect and include bismuth subsalicylate (Pepto-Bismol; 2 to 4 tablespoons every 30 minutes, not to exceed 8 doses/24 hr or 1 or 2 tablets every 4 to 6 hours), are commonly used if there is vomiting and abdominal cramping.[1,6] However, these products may cause aspirin toxicity and should be used cautiously. Patients taking warfarin should be cautioned as well because anticoagulation will be affected. Bismuth subsalicylate is not recommended in the HIV-positive or immunocompromised patient since encephalopathy is possible. The concomitant use of bismuth subsalicylate with antibiotics should be avoided because of the decreased effectiveness of the antibiotics.[6]

Because the diarrhea is a clearance mechanism to eliminate toxins in the gastrointestinal tract, the use of antimotility agents, which inhibit intestinal motility, should be avoided, particularly in the presence of bloody diarrhea or fecal leukocytosis. Diarrhea caused by an inflammatory pathogen, such as *Salmonella* or *Shigella* organisms, has been documented to worsen with the use of antimotility agents.

Antimotility agents that are commonly used in noninflammatory diarrhea include loperamide (Imodium; 4-mg caplets: 2 caplets initially, then 1 after each loose stool, not to exceed 16 mg/24 hr), diphenoxylate hydrochloride/atropine sulfate (Lomotil [2.5 mg/tablet]; 2 tablespoons or 2 tablets every 4 to 6 hours), or tincture of opium (10 mg/ml; 0.3 to 0.6 ml PO every 6 hours p.r.n.). Loperamide is preferred in children, pregnant women, and immunocompromised patients. If nausea is the main complaint, treatment with promethazine (Phenergan), prochlorperazine (Compazine), or another antiemetic is recommended.[6]

Empiric treatment with antibiotics should be considered in the presence of fecal leukocytes without a confirmed positive stool culture, with occult blood, and/or if the patient has fever with profuse, watery diarrhea because the most likely cause of the infection is *Salmonella, Shigella,* or *Campylobacter* organisms. Ciprofloxacin (500 mg b.i.d. for 3 days) or norfloxacin (400 mg b.i.d. for 3 days) can be started until the stool culture results are verified, but they should not be used in children or pregnant or lactating women. If the diarrhea has persisted for longer than 2 weeks and if infection with *Giardia* organisms is suspected, metronidazole (250 mg q.i.d. for 7 days) can be initiated.[5,6]

Vomiting is usually the predominant symptom in a viral illness. Infection with rotavirus usually lasts approximately 24 hours but can last 4 to 8 days. This is the most common virus seen in infants and young children. Norwalk and Norwalk-like viruses most often affect older children and adults and are associated with contaminated food or water. Both are transmitted fecal-orally. Oral rehydration therapy and antiemetics or bismuth subsalicylate are commonly used to decrease vomiting and abdominal cramping.[6,7]

Enterotoxigenic *E. coli* infection, or traveler's diarrhea, starts within 24 to 72 hours of incubation and lasts 3 to 6 days. The diarrhea is accompanied by fever and vomiting. Treatment includes oral rehydration and antimotility agents. Antibiotics are not usually necessary; however, they are sometimes used to shorten the course of the illness. These include trimethoprim/sulfamethoxazole (Bactrim DS) (160/800 mg b.i.d.), doxycycline (100 mg b.i.d.), or ciprofloxacin (500 b.i.d.), each administered for 3 to 5 days. Prophylactic antibiotic therapy is not recommended in healthy travelers. The preparation most often recommended is bismuth subsalicylate.[6,8]

Infection with *C. perfringens* is caused by a toxin found in contaminated meat, poultry, or legumes. The incubation period is within 8 to 14 hours. Diarrhea with abdominal cramping usually lasting 24 hours is the most common complaint. *S. aureus* food poisoning has a rapid onset of action, usually within 2 to 6 hours, and lasts up to 10 to 12 hours. Nausea and vomiting often occur. This illness commonly occurs in group outbreaks.

B. cereus is an organism that causes food poisoning and is associated with contaminated fried rice. The illness becomes evident within 6 hours of exposure. Presenting symptoms include diarrhea, abdominal cramping, nausea, and vomiting. Oral rehydration therapy and antimotility or antisecretory agents are used.[1,2,9]

Infection with *V. cholerae* is common in South or Central America, Asia, or Africa, but it has also been documented in Texas and Louisiana. The incubation period is usually 12 to 24 hours, and symptoms include nausea, vomiting, and profuse, watery diarrhea. Treatment includes fluids and antibiotic therapy. Commonly prescribed medications include tetracycline or doxycycline. An alternative treatment is ciprofloxacin (30 mg/kg, not to exceed 1 g, as a single dose) for adults and erythromycin (40 mg/kg t.i.d. for 3 days) for children.[2,8,9]

Parasitic diarrheal illnesses are not usually seen in the United States. However, worldwide they are a significant cause of serious illness and even death. Travelers, immigrants, homosexual males, and institutionalized individuals are at risk. Giardiasis is the most common parasite in the United States and is often seen in hikers and/or campers. Giardiasis occurs with person-to-person contact and with water and food contamination. The illness is mild to severe, occurring 1 to 3 weeks after contact with or ingestion of the cysts. The illness often has a prolonged course. Explosive watery diarrhea is present, but other symptoms, such as epigastric abdominal pain, belching, bloating, flatus, and nausea and vomiting, can be prominent. Diarrhea can resolve within 1 week; however, flatus and belching can persist. The presence of fever or bloody stools is uncommon. The medication commonly prescribed is metronidazole (250 mg t.i.d. to q.i.d. for 7 days). This treatment will resolve the illness in the majority of cases. Other medications used are furazolidone (Furoxone) and quinacrine.[2,6,8]

Another common parasite found in contaminated water that causes noninflammatory diarrhea is *Cryptosporidium*. The individual ingests oocysts and often is asymptomatic unless immunocompromised. Common symptoms include profuse, watery diarrhea with fever, nausea, vomiting, and anorexia that typically lasts 1 to 2 weeks. There is no effective treatment except for supportive measures with antidiarrheal agents and fluid replacement. Occasionally paromomycin (500 to 750 mg q.i.d. for 14 to 28 days followed by 500 mg indefinitely) is used to alleviate some of the severe symptoms. Azithromycin (2.4 g on day 1, followed by 1.2 g/day for 27 days, then 600 mg/day indefinitely) can also be used.[6]

Inflammatory bacterial diarrheal illnesses are not always treated with antibiotics, particularly in mild illness states. If the individual has debilitating symptoms, most likely antibiotics will be used along with supportive measures.

Campylobacter jejuni is the leading cause of foodborne diarrheal illness in the United States. Illness is usually mild and self-limiting, with fever, nausea, and abdominal cramping 2 to 6 days after exposure to contaminated undercooked meat or nonpasteurized products or animal contact. Most patients have spontaneous resolution of symptoms without antibiotic treatment. However, in a prolonged illness (lasting up to 2 weeks), treatment with antibiotics is initiated, such as ciprofloxacin (500 mg b.i.d. for 7 to 10 days), erythromycin (250 to 500 mg q.i.d. for 5 to 7 days), or tetracycline (250 mg q.i.d. for 5 to 7 days).[2,8]

Shigella, a foodborne pathogen, includes several strains; however, the most common in the Untied States is *Shigella sonnei*, which is transmitted via person-to-person, usually among household contacts. The most commonly affected individuals are children and homosexual males. Diarrhea ranges from mild to severe, is usually seen within 1 to 7 days of incubation, and lasts for 4 to 7 days. Fever and abdominal cramping may also be present. Treatment includes oral rehydration therapy and antibiotics. Trimethoprim/sulfamethoxazole (Bactrim DS) (160/800 mg b.i.d.) or ampicillin (500 mg q.i.d.) for 5 to 10 days has been commonly used. However, there has been documentation of increasing resistance to these drugs; thus ciprofloxacin (500 mg b.i.d. for 3 to 7 days) or a single dose of tetracycline can also be used.[1,2,6]

Enterohemorrhagic *E. coli*, which is often foodborne, causes bloody diarrhea. Antibiotics have not been found to be of benefit to patients and are not recommended.[2,6] Hydration therapy is advised in this illness.

Infection with *C. difficile*, or pseudomembranous colitis, is caused by an enterotoxin or a cytotoxin that alters the patient's normal intestinal flora after antibiotic therapy. *C. difficile*–induced diarrhea can occur up to 3 months after the medication has been taken. The illness may completely resolve after discontinuation of the offending medication. If antibiotics are used, the treatment of choice is metronidazole (250 to 500 mg q.i.d. in adults). Vancomycin (125 to 500 mg in adults) can be used if the patient cannot tolerate or does not respond to metronidazole, but it is considerably more expensive. If diarrhea persists despite treatment, cholestyramine (4 g/day) with or without lactobacilli (1 to 2 g q.i.d.), combined with vancomycin (125 mg q.o.d.) for 3 to 4 weeks, may be tried. Antimotility agents should be avoided.[1,2,10,11]

Infection with *Vibrio parahaemolyticus* is associated with the ingestion of uncooked seafood. Symptoms occur within 4 hours to 4 days after ingestion. Watery diarrhea is accompanied by abdominal cramps, nausea, vomiting, fever, and chills. Usually oral hydration therapy is advised, However, in severe cases; tetracycline (500 mg q.i.d. for 5 to 7 days) is also prescribed.[2,6]

Infection with *Salmonella* organisms is transmitted through the ingestion of contaminated food, particularly eggs and poultry, improperly washed fruits and vegetables, or water. Pet turtles have also been implicated in the transmission. Clinical illness is mild and lasts 1 to 2 weeks. Fever may or may not be present.

Antibiotic treatment is required only for persistent symptoms. Commonly prescribed medications include trimethoprim/sulfamethoxazole (Bactrim DS) (160/800 mg b.i.d.) or ciprofloxacin (500 mg b.i.d.), with each administered for 7 to 14 days. *Salmonella* organisms can invade any organ and even cause sepsis in a prolonged illness. The mortality rate is high, particularly in the immunocompromised patient.[1,2,6]

Entamoeba histolytica infection, or amebiasis, is a parasitic illness that causes death worldwide. It commonly occurs in the tropics, Mexico, Central and South America, India, Asia, and Africa. Those individuals at risk are travelers, immigrants, sexual contacts, and institutionalized patients. Illness occurs 2 to 6 weeks after the ingestion of cysts from contaminated water and food or from person-to-person contact. The illness may initially be mild with gradually increasing severity of symptoms. The patient may have 10 to 12 liquid stools per day with blood and mucus in the stool, malaise, weight loss, and diffuse abdominal pain. Hepatomegaly is rarely seen; however, close observation is indicated if this occurs because hepatic abscess can occur. Hospitalization is common for these individuals. Medication treatment includes metronidazole (750 mg t.i.d. for 7 to 10 days), followed by iodoquinol (650 mg t.i.d. for 20 days), diloxanide furoate (500 mg t.i.d. for 10 days [obtained from the Centers for Disease Control and Prevention]), or paromomycin (500 mg t.i.d. for 10 days).[1,2,6]

COMPLICATIONS

Complications of diarrhea usually result from dehydration; therefore regardless of the cause, attention should be directed toward fluid and electrolyte replacement. Hypocalcemia, hypomagnesemia, and hypokalemia are common in persistent diarrhea. Continuous diarrhea can require hospitalization for fluid and electrolyte replacement if the patient is unable to maintain hydration with oral fluid replacement. Sepsis and cardiovascular collapse are potential complications, and infants, older adults, and immunosuppressed patients are more susceptible to these complications. Refractory diarrhea is usually a symptom of a more serious illness and requires diagnostic evaluation and immediate physician consultation.

INDICATIONS FOR REFERRAL/HOSPITALIZATION

If dehydration is severe and/or protracted vomiting is present, IV fluids should be initiated. If symptoms of the illness persist beyond 3 weeks despite treatment measures, chronic lactose intolerance, giardiasis, malignancies, and disease states such as diabetes, thyrotoxicosis, lupus, HIV infection, or irritable bowel syndrome should be considered. Physician consultation is imperative in these cases.

PATIENT AND FAMILY EDUCATION

Listed here are some general recommendations that should be discussed with the patient[5,6]:

- Practice good handwashing after each bowel movement to lessen the possibility of spread to other family members.
- Drink frequent, small sips of fluids (water, tea, boullion, flat cola, flat ginger ale, or sports drink) to avoid dehydration.
- Avoid foods and let your stomach rest for the first 12 hours or until you begin to feel better. Gradually add small amounts of food (i.e., crackers, toast, rice, bananas), but avoid those that will aggravate symptoms (i.e., dairy products, caffeine, high-fat or high-fiber foods, carbonated beverages, sugar-free products, and alcohol).
- It is better to avoid antidiarrheal products because most cases of diarrhea are self-limiting.
- Rest.
- If symptoms persist or are accompanied by mental confusion, fever with a temperature of more than 38.3° C (101° F), chills, vomiting, weakness (especially muscle weakness), dizziness, dry mouth, extreme thirst, little or no urine output, severe abdominal discomfort, blurred vision, or black or bloody stools, immediately notify the health care provider.
- Some medications, particularly Pepto-Bismol, will cause stools to appear black.
- Children or food handlers should remain at home until the diarrhea resolves.

HEALTH PROMOTION/ILLNESS PREVENTION

Prevention of diarrhea should be the primary goal. Important information to convey to patients includes the following:

- When traveling, especially out of the country, drink and brush teeth with bottled water and eat only peeled fruits and vegetables. Never drink untreated water.
- Avoid high-risk foods, such as raw seafood, raw eggs, nonpasteurized dairy products, and undercooked poultry and beef.
- Avoid raw or undercooked meats. Avoid foods that have sat out at room temperature for more than 2 hours, particularly foods not refrigerated or heated in buffets or food stands.
- Handwashing remains the best preventive measure. Always wash hands after handling chicken or other raw meats. Wash cutting boards frequently (plastic cutting boards that can be washed in a dishwasher are preferable).
- Defrost meats in the microwave (as directed) or refrigerator.
- Cook foods to the proper temperature. Use a meat thermometer to check temperatures of roasts, chicken, and hamburger.

REFERENCES

1. Bitterman RA: Acute gastroenteritis and constipation. In Rosen P, editor: *Emergency medicine: concepts and clinical practice*, ed 4, St Louis, 1998, Mosby.
2. Fauce A, editor: Infectious diarrhea. In Braunwald E and others, editors: *Harrison's principles of internal medicine*, ed 14, New York, 1998, McGraw-Hill.
3. Fine KO: Diarrhea. In Sleisenger MH, editor: *Gastrointestinal and liver disease*, vol 1, ed 6, Philadelphia, 1998, WB Saunders.
4. Powell DW: Approach to the patient with diarrhea. In Kelly WN, editor: *Textbook of internal medicine*, vol 1, Philadelphia, 1997, Lippincott-Raven.
5. Mawhorter SD: Travel medicine for the primary care physician, *Cleve Clin J Med* 64(9):483-492, 1997.
6. Dupont HL and the Practice Parameters Committee of the American College of Gastroenterology: Guidelines on acute infectious diarrhea in adults, *Am J Gastroenterol* 92(11):1962-1975, 1997.

7. Keith ML: Continuing Education Forum: pediatric diarrhea, *J Am Acad Nurse Pract* 9(12):577-579, 1997.
8. Hamer DH, Gorbach SL: Infectious diarrhea and bacterial good poisoning. In Sleisenger MH, editor: *Gastrointestinal and liver disease,* vol 2, ed 6, Philadelphia, 1998, WB Saunders.
9. Cole M: Acute diarrhea. In Rakel RE, editor: *Saunders' manual of medical practice,* Philadelphia, 1996, WB Saunders.
10. Bartlett JD: Pseudomembranous enterocolitis and antibiotic-associated colitis. In Sleisenger MH, editor: *Gastrointestinal and liver disease,* ed 6, Philadelphia, 1998, WB Saunders.
11. Afghani B, Stutman HR: Toxin-related diarrhea, *Pediatr Ann* 23(10):549-555, 1994.

CHAPTER 145

Diverticular Disease

Louise Meyer

Diverticular disease is a common disorder of the colon occurring more often as life expectancy increases and as dietary practices include more refined foods. The disease manifests itself in a variety of clinical spectrums and can present in three different clinical patterns: (1) diverticulosis or uncomplicated diverticular disease, the asymptomatic or symptomatic presence of noninflamed multiple colonic diverticula; (2) diverticulitis or complicated diverticular disease associated with inflammation in one or more of the diverticula, with possible resultant perforation leading to abscess or fistula formation; and (3) hemorrhage, another complication of diverticular disease, often associated with a right-sided diverticulum or diverticula.

Diverticulosis

DEFINITION/EPIDEMIOLOGY

Diverticulosis derives its name from the basic unit of diverticular disease, the diverticulum, which is an outpouching of mucosa through the colon wall. The occurrence of a single diverticulum is uncommon; hence the term *diverticulosis* is used to describe the condition of numerous diverticulum, or diverticula, in the colon. This term is an anatomic descriptor. Clinically, diverticulosis is an uncomplicated, asymptomatic or symptomatic disease without inflammation or bleeding.

The prevalence of colonic diverticulosis varies greatly in different geographic areas of the world. It is most common in the Western hemisphere and is rare in Africa, Asia, and many parts of South America. This disease is considered a deficiency disease of twentieth century Western civilization. Its emergence parallels a change in dietary habits that occurred during the industrial revolution of the 1850s, including the mechanical milling of crude cereal grain and wheat flour and the resultant loss of the nonabsorbable fiber content. Coincidentally, at this time, there was also an increased consumption of white flour, refined sugar, conserves, and meat.[1] Studies from less industrialized regions (e.g., Africa and Asia) document prevalence rates of diverticulosis of less than 0.2%.[1] The worldwide prevalence of diverticular disease is not truly known, but in the United States and other developed countries its prevalence approaches 10%.[2]

In addition to geographic distribution, age is another important variable and is the key risk factor. Diverticulosis is rare before age 40 years, but occurs in later years, with an estimated incidence of 50% to 65% by age 80.[3-6]

PATHOPHYSIOLOGY

Colonic diverticula are defects of the large colon, especially the sigmoid, that develop with advancing age. They are saclike herniations of the mucosa through the muscularis propria and are actually pseudodiverticula because they do not contain the muscle layer.

The pathophysiologic changes common to all cases of diverticulosis of the colon are not entirely clear. Herniation of the muscular layer of the colon is the result of two factors: (1) an increased pressure gradient between the colonic lumen and the serosa, and (2) areas of relative weakness in the colonic wall.[7]

One commonly accepted hypothesis of diverticula formation is that low-fiber diets decrease the amount of intraluminal bulk in the colon causing muscular hypertrophy as the colon tries to move the fecal matter along.[1] Lack of fecal bulk is thought to produce uncoordinated and irregular colonic peristalsis, which creates sacculations in the colon wall. There is increased pressure within these sacs, which results in diverticular outpouchings. These sacs occur at weak points, or natural breaks, in the muscle layer of the colon where the nutrient vessels, the vasa recta, pass through the muscularis propria into the submucosa. In addition, the colon wall, which is covered by connective tissue, loses its flexibility and tensile strength with age. A weakened bowel wall develops and may predispose an individual to formation of diverticula.

Therefore increasing fiber intake will reduce the incidence of diverticular disease.[8] This hypothesis is supported by another study in which vegetarians living in England had a 12% incidence of diverticular disease as compared to a 33% incidence among nonvegetarians who ingested half of the mean daily intake of dietary fiber.[9]

In terms of size and distribution, diverticula range from 1 to 2 mm to giant diverticula. In Western societies, diverticula occur predominantly in the sigmoid colon. In Asians who have adopted a Western diet, right-sided diverticula are more common.[10]

CLINICAL PRESENTATION

Patients with uncomplicated colonic diverticula, or diverticulosis, are often asymptomatic and rarely seek medical attention; at least 80% to 85% of these individuals never present with a clinical problem.[11] Symptomless diverticula are often noted when the colon is studied for another reason via a barium enema, colonoscopy, CT scan, or ultrasound.

By contrast, symptomatic patients may complain of irregular defecation, intermittent abdominal pain, bloating, or excessive flatulence. In general, there is a change in stool caliber, with descriptors that can range from flattened or ribbonlike to hard pellets. Associated complaints can include urinary dysfunction, nausea and vomiting, and heartburn. Older individuals often relate recurrent bouts of steady or crampy pain (mostly in the left lower quadrant) in combination with constipation or alternating periods of diarrhea and constipation. They may also have abdominal distention that is relieved with the passage of flatus or stool. These symptoms can often mimic irritable bowel syndrome except that they are experienced at an older age.

Those who present with right-sided pain tend to be younger and their pain is easily mistaken for appendicitis.[6]

PHYSICAL EXAMINATION

For patients with uncomplicated symptoms, the physical examination (both a pelvic and rectal examination) is usually normal. However, physical findings can reveal mild, left lower quadrant tenderness with a thickened palpable sigmoid and descending colon. Rectal bleeding is uncommon.

DIAGNOSTICS

A CBC and urinalysis should be obtained. Screening laboratory values should be normal in uncomplicated diverticulosis. A stool for occult blood is necessary because diverticulosis is not known to cause occult rectal bleeding. Plain abdominal x-ray films will be normal and are unnecessary. Rigid sigmoidoscopy usually cannot be performed beyond the rectosigmoid junction and for this reason is not particularly useful. The diagnosis of diverticulosis is most often established with a barium enema examination; this method is the best for determining the extent and severity of the disease. Although it is often used as a diagnostic tool, a colonoscopy is best used to assess the large bowel for a coexisting pathologic condition rather than for an actual diagnosis of diverticular disease.

DIFFERENTIAL DIAGNOSIS

The hallmark of symptomatic diverticulosis is colicky abdominal pain in the absence of an inflammatory process. The cause of this pain is not fully understood but possibly is related to spasms in the sigmoid colon or an element of obstruction related to the spasms. This clinical entity must be differentiated from diverticulitis and any disease that causes abnormal intestinal motility.

The challenge is not so much in making the diagnosis as it is in distinguishing patients who have symptomatic diverticular disease from those who have diverticula plus other lesions that may be responsible for the symptoms. Irritable bowel syndrome and colorectal cancer should be considered in the differential.

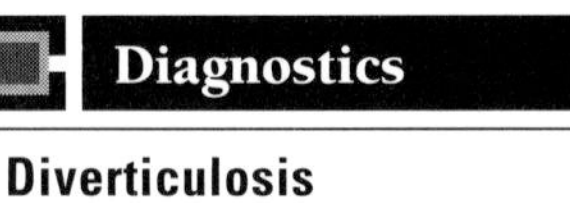

Diverticulosis

Laboratory
CBC and differential
Urinalysis
Stool for occult blood

Imaging
Barium enema

Other
Colonoscopy*

*If indicated.

MANAGEMENT

Fiber is essential for normal intestinal function. Pioneering studies in the 1960s and 1970s revealed the relationship between colonic

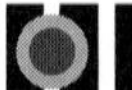

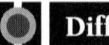

Differential Diagnosis

Diverticulosis

Diverticulitis	Infectious colitis
Irritable bowel disease	Radiation-induced colitis
Cancer	Gynecologic inflammatory or neoplastic diseases
Cystitis	Vascular ectasia
Appendicitis	Ectopic pregnancy
Inflammatory bowel disease	Anorectal disease
Crohn's disease	Small or large bowel obstruction
Peritonitis	
Chronic ulcerative colitis	
Ischemic colitis	

diverticulosis and low consumption of dietary fiber.[1,9] Earlier studies revealed that increased dietary fiber can provide symptomatic relief in patients with painful diverticulosis or recurrent diverticulitis.[12-14] A diet that includes 35 g of fiber may bring about significant change. In the United States adults consume approximately 11 to 23 g of fiber per day—half of the 27 to 40 g of daily fiber recommended by the World Health Organization and less than the 20 to 35 g proposed by the American Dietetic Association.[15,16]

Increased fiber intake can be achieved through the consumption of whole grains and cereals, fruits, vegetables, and legumes. These foods should be introduced gradually over a period of weeks to months to avoid excessive bloating and flatulence. Bran, a concentrated form of fiber, can be used as an adjunct to fiber consumption but should not be a replacement for other high-fiber foods. Some patients may need 2 g of bran three times a day to provide the bulk; it should be soaked or mixed in mediums such as hot cereal, applesauce, juice, or milk.

Fiber can also be given through commercially available high-fiber supplements or bulk formers such as psyllium hydrophilic mucilloid, methylcellulose, and calcium polycarbophil. These products work similarly to bran and must be taken with several glasses of fluid to be effective. They produce a softer, more frequent stool.

Current literature does not support the elimination of certain dietary foodstuffs in the management of diverticulosis. Nonetheless, the following foods are generally avoided: popcorn, corn, nuts, and seeds.

Anticholinergic and antispasmotic agents have been used without substantiated evidence of their effectiveness. They may be used to relieve spasms. Care should be taken to avoid constipation. Surgical resection for pain relief, in the absence of documented inflammatory complications, is associated with a high rate of symptom recurrence and is therefore not recommended.[11]

LIFE SPAN CONSIDERATIONS

Diverticular disease is usually observed in adults older than 40 years and incidence increases with age. Younger adults, however, can develop diverticular disease as well as associated complications such as diverticulitis and diverticular bleeding.

COMPLICATIONS

The majority of patients with diverticular disease have an uncomplicated course. However, several older studies have shown that 10% to 25% of individuals develop diverticulitis, with 5% eventually experiencing massive bleeding from a diverticulum.[3,17]

INDICATIONS FOR REFERRAL/HOSPITALIZATION

Uncomplicated diverticular disease can be managed in the primary care setting. Questionable radiographic findings on any barium studies necessitate a referral to a gastroenterologist for further evaluation. Patients with rectal bleeding need further evaluation, and a referral and/or consultation are indicated.

Although the primary care provider assumes responsibility for patient education, a referral to a dietitian may be considered and may be beneficial for patients with recurrent, painful disease.

PATIENT AND FAMILY EDUCATION/HEALTH PROMOTION

Patients' diet and symptoms should be reviewed at every session for prevention and health promotion. All patients need to be instructed about a nutritionally well-balanced diet that includes whole grain breads and cereals as well as fresh fruits and vegetables to attain the benefits of both types of fiber (see Figure 21-1).[16] The goal of 30 g of fiber per day requires the consumption of five fruits and vegetables (15 g), four high-fiber starches (8 g), and one high-fiber cereal (7 g).

It is important that patients be advised to increase their fiber intake gradually to prevent flatulence and abdominal discomfort. Patients can often tolerate 5- to 10-g increments every few weeks on the basis of symptoms. Bloating or flatulence resulting from bran intake usually resolves with continued use. If patients are taking pharmaceutical fiber supplements, it is especially important that they increase their fluid intake to at least eight 8-ounce glasses of fluid per day.

Diverticulitis

DEFINITION/EPIDEMIOLOGY

Diverticulitis, or complicated diverticular disease, is the most common complication of diverticulosis. An inflammatory condition that involves one or more colonic diverticula, diverticulitis is almost always symptomatic. Diverticulosis must be present before there can be an attack of diverticulitis.

The possibility of experiencing diverticulitis increases with the longer duration of diverticular disease and with increasing age. In one study approximately one fifth, or 20%, of all patients with radiologic evidence of diverticulosis developed diverticulitis in the sixth decade; this fraction increased to one third by the ninth decade.[3] A recent study by Marinella and Mustafa[18] observed that, although rare, diverticulitis can occur in patients less than 35 years old.

PATHOPHYSIOLOGY

The inflammation associated with diverticulitis is thought to result from the stagnation of fecal material in a single diverticulum. This produces a fecalith that leads to pressure necrosis of the mucosa and subsequent inflammation.[19] This inflammatory process progresses and either a microperforation or a macroperforation ensues. A small perforation is easily contained by the pericolic tissues and becomes a localized phlegmon. A larger perforation may result in a walled-off pericolic abscess whose erosion may produce fistulas into adjacent structures such as the urinary bladder, vagina, small bowel, or anterior abdominal wall. If there is free perforation in the abdominal cavity, fecal peritonitis may occur.

CLINICAL PRESENTATION

The diagnosis of diverticulitis is often clinical, especially in a patient with known diverticula. Most patients with infection or localized inflammation have mild to moderate, colicky to steady, aching abdominal pain usually present in the left lower quadrant (93% to 100%) accompanied by fever (57% to 100%) and leukocytosis (69% to 83%).[2] Constipation or loose stools may or may not be present. There may be nausea and vomiting. Hematochezia is uncommon in diverticulitis and is more suggestive of other diagnoses. In some instances the patient presents with complications of diverticulitis, such as recurrent urinary tract infections or feculent vaginal discharge resulting from fistulization. In other cases, a patient may exhibit few or no symptoms and therefore does not seek medical attention for several days. Older patients or patients who are immunocompromised may have minimal abdominal pain, no fever, and a relatively benign physical examination, but still be septic.

PHYSICAL EXAMINATION

The physical examination of patients with diverticulitis may reveal mild distention. Bowel sounds are hyperactive if there is obstruction but are otherwise normal. Generally there is tenderness in the suprapubic region or over the involved colonic segment (often found in the left lower quadrant). A mass may or may not be palpated. Pain in the right lower quadrant can be mistaken for acute appendicitis. There can be involuntary guarding and percussion tenderness localized in this area indicating localized peritoneal inflammation. Patients who experience generalized abdominal pain and abdominal wall rigidity could have a perforated viscus. A rectal examination may reveal some tenderness in the pelvis, and occasionally a mass is palpated anteriorly. Stools are not usually positive for occult blood, but hematochezia is possible. In female patients, a pelvic examination is a necessary component of the physical examination. Fever can be present, but a past study found that 14% of patients were afebrile at presentation.[20]

DIAGNOSTICS

Initial laboratory studies may not be useful in determining a diagnosis of diverticulitis. Although a CBC is usually obtained, leukocytosis is not a requisite symptom of this condition. Urinalysis may reveal white blood cells if the inflammatory process is adjacent to the bladder or ureter. The presence of bacteria in the urine sample consistent with urinary infection is suggestive of a fistula.

Supine and upright plain x-ray films can be obtained to assess the presence of an ileus, a small or large bowel obstruction, or free abdominal air, which indicates perforation. A CT scan of the abdomen and pelvis has been used increasingly to evaluate patients with diverticulitis. It is the test of choice if diverticular complications are suspected because it gives a more accurate estimate of the degree of inflammation than do other studies.[21,22] Some authorities suggest that not all patients with acute diverticulitis require a CT scan for successful management, but recommend that it be performed under the following conditions: a questionable diagnosis, a suspected abscess or fistula, inadequate clinical improvement with medical treatment, as a diagnostic for patients who are immunocompromised (e.g., steroid dependent) where clinical evaluation is not a reliable indicator of the patient's condition, or an unusual clinical situation such as right-sided diverticulitis.[11] A barium enema is not recommended with acute diverticulitis because of the risk of barium peritonitis.

Additional tests include ultrasound, flexible sigmoidoscopy, and colonoscopy. Ultrasonography is used to reveal extracolic fluid collections and to guide percutaneous drainage of pelvic and paracolic abscesses; however, they are more operator dependent than CT scans. Patients may not be able to tolerate the external pressure and imaging is limited in an obese patient.[6] Flexible sigmoidoscopy is often used during an episode of suspected diverticulitis. Its main usefulness arises in the event of colonic obstruction to differentiate an obstructing carcinoma from an obstructing diverticular mass. Colonoscopy is useful after the inflammatory process subsides.

Diagnostics

Diverticulitis

Laboratory
CBC and differential
Stool for occult blood
Urinalysis

Imaging
Angiography (if patient is bleeding)
CT scan*
Ultrasound*

Other
Colonoscopy*
Flexible sigmoidoscopy*

*If indicated.

DIFFERENTIAL DIAGNOSIS

Diverticulosis is sometimes associated with marked local tenderness and a palpable sigmoid loop and therefore may be mistaken for diverticulitis; however, fever and leukocytosis are generally absent with diverticulosis. Other differential diagnoses include acute appendicitis, peritonitis, cystitis, neoplasm, inflammatory bowel disease, ischemic colitis, radiation colitis, infectious colitis, small bowel obstruction, and gynecologic disorders such as pelvic inflammatory disease, endometriosis, ovarian cysts, and ectopic pregnancy.

MANAGEMENT

The clinical spectrum of acute diverticulitis is diverse. Spontaneous resolution is common for many patients with low-grade fever, mild leukocytosis, and minimal abdominal tenderness. These patients do not require hospitalization. Treatment generally consists of clear liquids, limiting physical activity, and prescribing oral antibiotics such as trimethoprim/sulfamethoxazole (Bactrim DS) 160 mg/800 mg b.i.d. or ciprofloxacin 500 mg b.i.d. plus metronidazole 500 mg t.i.d. for 7 to 14 days.[6,23,24] If fever and leukocytosis are absent, the patient may have only painful diverticular disease and not diverticulitis; for this condition antibiotics are withheld. The duration of treatment is determined by clinical response and generally is discontinued when symptoms have resolved and the patient is afebrile. Pain medication is discouraged; symptomatic relief may be achieved with warm packs. Nonopiate analgesics may be used if necessary.

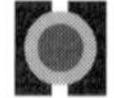

Differential Diagnosis

Diverticulitis

Diverticulosis	Radiation colitis
Acute appendicitis	Infectious colitis
Peritonitis	Small bowel obstruction
Cystitis	Pelvic inflammatory disease
Neoplasm	Endometriosis
Inflammatory bowel disease	Ovarian cysts
Ischemic colitis	Ectopic pregnancy

Immediately after an attack of diverticulitis, a short-term low-fiber diet that consists of 15 g or less of dietary fiber is prescribed to reduce the volume of fecal material in the lower bowel and to prevent irritation to the colon. When the patient is asymptomatic, a gradual modification to a diet high in fiber (and free of seeds) may help to reduce pressure inside the colon, thus reducing the chances of future attacks.[15] A colonoscopy is recommended after symptoms resolve to exclude carcinoma.[6]

At the opposite end of this spectrum are patients acutely ill with systemic peritonitis, sepsis, and hypovolemia. Any patient with a temperature of 38.5° C (101.3° F) or above and with marked tenderness, signs of localized peritonitis, intestinal obstruction, or a suspected intraabdominal or pelvic abscess must be admitted to the hospital. Hospitalization is also recommended for diabetic or immunosuppressed patients, older adults, and patients with chronic renal failure in whom diverticulitis is suspected in the absence of the previously listed criteria. Hospital management includes assessment of fluid status and intravenous replacement, nasogastric suction if there is an obstruction or ileus, blood cultures, and broad-spectrum intravenous antibiotics that cover gram-negative anaerobes and gram-negative aerobes. Antibiotic selection might include metronidazole (anaerobic gram-negative bacilli) 750 to 1000 mg IV every 12 hours (15 mg/kg loading dose, then 7.5 mg/kg every 6 hours), plus an aminoglycoside such as gentamycin (aerobic gram-negative bacilli) 1.0 mg/kg IV every 8 hours (maximum dose 5 mg/kg/day in divided doses in life-threatening situations).[21,25] Treatment time depends on symptom resolution and is usually maintained for 7 to 10 days. Variations of these treatments are based on patient needs. Only meperidine should be used for pain management. Morphine increases colonic spasm and may accentuate hypersegmentation.[6]

Further evaluation and management depend on patients assessment and response to initial treatment. If fever, abdominal signs, and leukocytosis have mostly resolved and bowel function has returned with the passage of flatus, a liquid diet can be started and slowly advanced to a low-fiber diet. When the patient is asymptomatic, a high-fiber diet can be gradually introduced. The patient is discharged with a regimen of oral antibiotics such as metronidazole 500 mg t.i.d. for 7 to 10 days. Studies such as a barium enema or colonoscopy should be performed 4 to 6 weeks after hospital discharge.

A CT scan is required if the patient fails to improve after 2 to 4 days of medical treatment, if there is doubt about the diagnosis, or if a pelvic or abdominal abscess, fistula, or obstruction needs to be excluded. Occasionally, a peridiverticular abscess of more than 5 cm can be drained by CT as long as the patient has adequate antibiotic coverage.[6]

Because most patients with uncomplicated diverticulitis recover with medical treatment and do not have recurrences of acute disease, surgery is not routinely recommended. However, surgical management is necessary in 15% to 30% of patients, as diverticulitis can recur despite medical management. Elective surgical intervention should be considered after the second episode. Urgent surgical intervention is also sometimes necessary. Younger patients especially may require more aggressive management; in these patients surgery is sometimes recommended after the first attack, although this approach is still somewhat controversial.[20,22,23] Elective surgical management generally consists of a single-stage procedure to decrease morbidity and mortality. A laparoscopic approach has been used for sigmoid resection. This approach decreases hospitalization time and shortens recovery.[6]

COMPLICATIONS

Complications of diverticulitis include free perforation with fecal peritonitis, suppurative peritonitis secondary to ruptured abscess, abdominal or pelvic abscess, fistula, or obstruction. It is estimated that 20% to 30% of patients will have recurrent diverticulitis; patients who experience a second episode have more than a 50% chance of having a third episode.[2] The chance of recurrence after the first episode is 90% within 5 years.[6]

Patients between 40 and 50 years old are at increased risk for developing complications.[20,25] Medical management may not be successful, recurrences with complications are common, and aggressive treatment with early surgery when the patient is stabilized is sometimes recommended.[25] Immunosuppressed patients are at especially high risk for complications because they may not experience a normal inflammatory response and subsequently can develop spontaneous colon perforation and perforated diverticula.[10,23] Aggressive management of these patients includes emergency surgical intervention.[7]

INDICATIONS FOR REFERRAL/HOSPITALIZATION

The diagnosis of diverticulitis is, unfortunately, based on clinical findings that can be diagnostically nonspecific. The presentation, course of illness, and treatment plan can be challenging. Referral to a gastroenterologist is appropriate, if the diagnosis is unclear, attacks are recurrent, or if hospitalization is indicated. A surgical consultation is required for patients with suspected complications or who are readmitted for a second episode of diverticulitis.

PATIENT AND FAMILY EDUCATION

During the convalescent period, patients require a low-fiber diet (<15 g/day) and careful diet instruction. Whole grain breads and cereals, raw fruits and vegetables, nuts and seeds, and legumes should be avoided. Canned fruits and well-cooked vegetables are allowed in limited quantities. The diet can be liberalized as the patient's condition improves. Once stable and pain free, patients can reintroduce a high-fiber diet slowly, over several weeks, to avoid any abdominal distention or excess flatulence. Symptoms often guide the treatment plan. A fiber preparation may be necessary for patients who are unable to follow a diet reasonably high in fiber. Regardless of fiber supplementation, 27% of patients who have had surgical treatments will continue to experience symptoms.[6]

Patients should avoid laxatives and enemas because these substances increase colonic pressure. It is important that patients establish a regular bowel movement pattern of once or twice a day to once every 2 to 3 days. With a high-fiber diet the stools should be softer and thus easier to pass.

In addition, patients should be aware of the importance of reporting recurrent pain promptly, especially if the pain is associated with chills or fever. Urgent hospitalization may be necessary.

Diverticular Bleeding

DEFINITION/EPIDEMIOLOGY

Severe bleeding is a less common complication of diverticulosis. Hemorrhage from a colonic diverticulum generally begins without warning in an older individual with otherwise asymptomatic diverticulosis. Painless rectal bleeding is associated with diverticulosis in 15% to 40% of patients and is usually self-limited.[2,26] Massive bleeding occurs in approximately 5% of patients and may be sufficient to require transfusion.[17]

PATHOPHYSIOLOGY

Bleeding arises from the rupture of one of the branches of the vasa recta adjacent to a diverticulum. The most common site for massive bleeding is the right colon, particularly in older adults.[26] It is important to remember that diverticular bleeding is neither chronic nor occult. Iron deficiency anemia associated with occult blood in the stool can never be attributed to diverticulosis without an appropriate diagnostic evaluation.

CLINICAL PRESENTATION

Diverticular bleeding usually presents in an older patient with diverticulosis who has previously been asymptomatic or was not previously diagnosed. The patient may or may not experience abdominal cramping and passes a large volume of bright red to dark maroon blood with or without signs of hypovolemia. The patient may have one or two more of such movements and then no more, or the bleeding may continue for several days. Bleeding stops spontaneously in 80% of patients, with the rate of rebleeding after one episode between 20% and 25%.[27] There are no distinctive features by which to distinguish diverticular bleeding from other causes of lower gastrointestinal bleeding.

PHYSICAL EXAMINATION

The physical examination is generally normal, although the digital rectal examination can reveal anorectal lesions as the source of bleeding. If there is excessive blood loss, signs of hypovolemia with postural vital signs or shock may be present.

DIAGNOSTICS

A CBC will help determine not only the blood loss but also whether this bleeding has been ongoing. The initial assessment includes a rectal examination and a proctosigmoidoscopy, which may reveal bleeding from anorectal lesions, rectal cancer, and acute colitis. Upper gastrointestinal bleeding must be excluded by aspiration of gastric contents and in some instances esophagogastroduodenoscopy is indicated.[26] A barium enema should never be the initial test in patients with diverticular bleeding because angiography or colonoscopy is precluded until the contrast material is evacuated. With slow bleeding, colonoscopy is the best approach and a more recent study suggests that colonoscopy is an effective diagnostic adjunct even in aggressive bleeding.[26] Scintigraphic or angiographic localization is necessary with brisk bleeding. Mesenteric angiography can be used as a diagnostic tool for localizing the bleeding site and as a therapeutic intervention in which vasoconstrictive drugs or an artificial blood clot can be infused to control the hemorrhage.

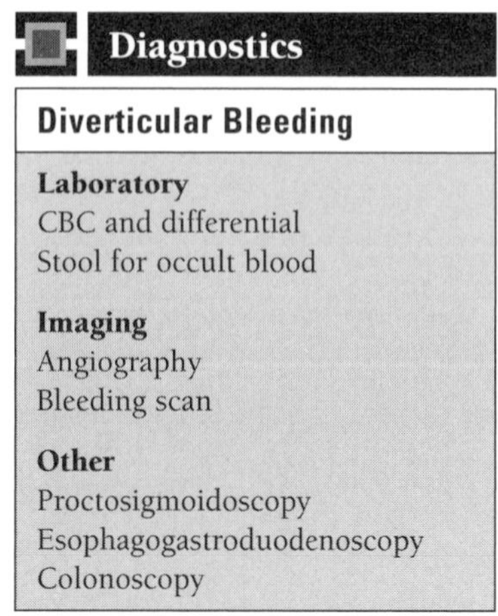

Diagnostics

Diverticular Bleeding

Laboratory
CBC and differential
Stool for occult blood

Imaging
Angiography
Bleeding scan

Other
Proctosigmoidoscopy
Esophagogastroduodenoscopy
Colonoscopy

DIFFERENTIAL DIAGNOSIS

Diverticular bleeding is a diagnosis of exclusion. Patients who present with a massive hemorrhage often have no prior history of diverticular complications. Bleeding is characteristically sudden and brisk and is usually self-limited. Any gastrointestinal lesion that has the potential for massive hemorrhage (e.g., a duodenal ulcer or Meckel's diverticulum) can present in a manner similar to diverticular bleeding and must be excluded. Gastric aspiration is a crucial part of the evaluation. Lower tract sources (vascular ectasias, inflammatory diseases, and anorectal lesions such as hemorrhoids, fissures, lacerations, polyps, ulcers, and neoplasms) must be considered.

MANAGEMENT

The prognosis for diverticular bleeding is generally favorable. Most bleeding stops spontaneously and does not recur. Therefore treatment of diverticular bleeding should begin with conservative medical management. Most patients can be observed without the need for urgent diagnostic or invasive therapeutic maneuvers. For those who do need intervention, the evaluation and treatment of diverticular bleeding are interrelated.

The primary interventions for diverticular bleeding are hemodynamic stabilization and resuscitation. Anal or rectal bleeding should first be excluded with a digital rectal examination and proctoscopy. Most cases of mild to moderate hemorrhage stop spontaneously with medical management that includes establishing IV access, placing a Foley catheter, and inserting a nasogastric tube to exclude an upper gastrointestinal source of bleeding. Laboratory tests should include electrolytes, CBC, coagulation studies, and blood type with cross-match.

Patients, especially older patients, who have massive, active bleeding require observation in an intensive care unit. As previously discussed, several diagnostic options are available and include radionucleotide scanning, angiography, and endoscopy. There are also several therapeutic options for the patient with persistent diverticular bleeding, including selective intraarterial infusion of vasopressin, angiographic embolization, or surgical resection.

Surgical intervention is required for massive and persistent bleeding that does not respond to medical treatment and interventional radiology. Surgery may also be recommended on an elective basis for patients with recurrent hemorrhages.

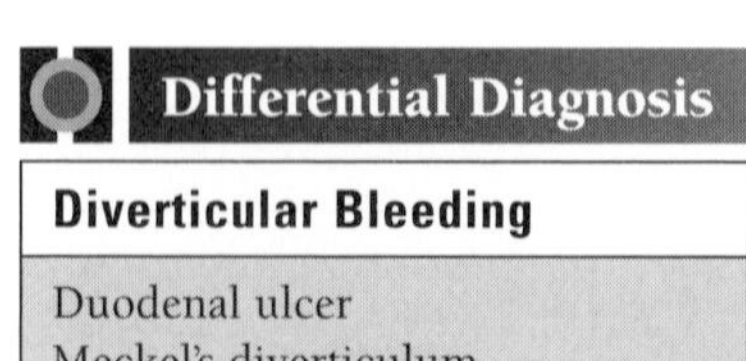

Differential Diagnosis

Diverticular Bleeding

Duodenal ulcer
Meckel's diverticulum
Vascular ectasia
Anorectal lesion
Inflammatory disease

COMPLICATIONS

The complications of diverticular hemorrhage are related to hypovolemia and circulatory collapse. Older patients tolerate the hemorrhage poorly because there is an ischemic risk to major organs with each bleeding episode.

INDICATIONS FOR REFERRAL/HOSPITALIZATION

Massive bleeding is an urgent situation and requires collaboration and referral to a gastroenterologist. Surgical intervention may also be necessary. In older patients with bleeding, transient hypovolemia can be a serious problem for major organs, and immediate hospitalization must be considered.

PATIENT AND FAMILY EDUCATION

Careful patient education is essential because there is a risk for recurrent bleeding after the first episode. It is important to advise patients to report symptoms in a timely fashion to avoid complications such as hypovolemia and circulatory collapse.

REFERENCES

1. Painter NS, Burkitt DP: Diverticular disease of the colon: a deficiency disease of western civilization, *Br Med J* 2(759):450-454, 1971.
2. Simmang CL, Shires GT: Diverticular disease of the colon. In Feldman M, Scharschmidt B, Sleisenger M, editors: *Sleisenger and Fordtran's gastrointestinal and liver disease pathophysiology/diagnosis/management*, ed 6, Philadelphia, 1997, WB Saunders.
3. Welch CE and others: An appraisal of the colon for diverticulitis of the sigmoid, *Ann Surg* 138:332, 1953.
4. Parks TG: Natural history of diverticular disease of the colon: a review of 521 cases, *Br Med J* 4(684):639-642, 1969.
5. Parks TG: Post-mortem studies on the colon with special reference to diverticular disease, *Proc R Soc Med* 61(9):932-934, 1968.
6. Ferzoco LB, Rapopoulos V, Silen W: Current concepts: Acute diverticulitis, *N Engl J Med* 338(21):1521-1526, 1998.
7. Farthmann EH, Ruckauer KD, Harng RU: Evidenced-based surgery: diverticulitis—a surgical disease? *Arch Surg* 385:143-151, 2000.
8. Burkitt MD, Painter MS: Dietary fiber and disease, *JAMA* 229(8): 1068-1074, 1974.
9. Gear JS and others: Symptomless diverticular disease and intake of dietary fibre, *Lancet* 1(8115):511-514, 1979.
10. Stemmermann GN, Yatani R: Diverticulosis and polyps of the large intestine: a necropsy study of Hawaii Japanese, *Cancer* 31(5):1260-1270, 1973.
11. Pemberton JH and others: Diverticulitis. In Yamata T et al, editors: *Textbook of gastroenterology*, ed 2, Philadelphia, 1995, JB Lippincott.
12. Hyland JM, Taylor I: Does a high fibre diet prevent the complications of diverticular disease? *Br J Surg* 67(2):77-79, 1980.
13. Taylor I, Duthie HL: Bran tablets and diverticular disease, *Br Med J* 1(6016):988-990, 1976.
14. Leahy AL et al: High fiber diet in symptomatic diverticular disease of the colon, *Ann R Coll Surg Engl* 67(3):173-174, 1985.
15. The ins and outs of diverticular disease, *Dig Health Nutr* 1:1, 1997.
16. Position of the American Dietetic Association: Health implications of dietary fiber: technical support paper, *J Am Diet Assoc* 88(2):217-222, 1988.
17. McGuire HH and others: Massive hemorrhage from diverticulosis of the colon: guidelines for therapy based on bleeding patterns observed in fifty cases, *Ann Surg* 175(6):847-855, 1972.
18. Marinella MA, Mustafa M: Acute diverticulitis in patients 40 years and younger, *Am J Emerg Med* 18(2):140-142, 2000.
19. McCarthy DW and others: Etiology of diverticular disease with classic illustrations, *J Natl Med Assoc* 88(6):389-390, 1996.
20. Ambrosetti P and others: Acute left colonic diverticulitis: a prospective analysis of 226 consecutive cases, *Surgery* 115(5):546-550, 1994.
21. Cho KC and others: Sigmoid diverticulitis: diagnostic role of CT: comparison with barium enema studies, *Radiology* 176(1):111-115, 1990.
22. Young-Fadok T, Pemberton JH: Treatment of acute diverticulitis. Retrieved June 11, 2002 from the World Wide Web: www.uptodate.
23. Ouriel K, Schwartz SI: Diverticular disease in the young patient, *Surg Gynecol Obstet* 156(1):1-5, 1983.
24. Zarling EJ and others: The effect of gastroenterology training on the efficiency and cost of care provided to patients with diverticulitis, *Gastroenterology* 112(6):1859-1862, 1997.
25. Gibert DN and others: *The Sanford guide to antimicrobial therapy*, ed 28, Hyde Park, Vt, 1997, Antimicrobial Inc.
26. Young-Fadok T, Pemberton JH: *Colonic diverticular bleeding*. Retrieved June 11, 2002 from the World Wide Web: www.uptodate.
27. Schoetz DJ: Uncomplicated diverticulitis: indications for surgery and surgical management, *Surg Clin North Am* 73(5):965-974, 1993.

CHAPTER 146

Gastroesophageal Reflux Disease

Nancy D. Bolton

DEFINITION/EPIDEMIOLOGY

Gastroesophageal reflux refers to the movement of gastric contents from the stomach to the esophagus. This occurs in virtually everyone several times a day without producing any symptoms or signs of damage. However, this normal physiologic process can be pathologic and can produce signs and symptoms of mucosal damage within the esophagus or in the pharynx, larynx, and respiratory tract. When this occurs or when there are chronic symptoms the individual is said to have gastroesophageal reflux disease (GERD).

GERD is one of the most prevalent clinical conditions affecting the gastrointestinal tract. If the prevalence of GERD is based on symptoms (primarily heartburn), the disease is very common in Western countries. Approximately 15% of adults use antacids more than once a week, with an estimated $3 billion dollars spent each year for these medications.[1] However, if the prevalence of reflux esophagitis is based on signs of esophageal injury, approximately 7% of symptomatic Americans have erosive esophagitis.[1] GERD is slightly more common in males than in females and is more common in Caucasians than in African-Americans.[1]

Reflux esophagitis is the most common form of GERD. The most common symptom is heartburn, which can range in severity from heartburn without esophageal mucosal damage to severe symptoms with esophageal mucosal damage in the form of erosions, ulcers, or a premalignant condition called Barrett's esophagus. The severity of symptoms is not always the best indicator of esophageal damage.

PATHOPHYSIOLOGY

There is not one single mechanism that explains all cases of GERD but there are four probable factors in the pathogenesis of reflux:

- Transient lower esophageal sphincter (LES) relaxation
- Low resting pressure of the sphincter
- Decreased ability of the esophagus to clear itself of reflux material[2]
- Delayed gastric emptying[3]

The extent of esophageal mucosal injury is determined by the length of time that the gastric contents are in contact with the esophageal mucosa. If the refluxate (hydrochloric acid, pepsin, bile, or pancreatic enzymes) are allowed sufficient time within the esophagus, the mucosal defenses are broken down. Symptomatic GERD results when the balance between the aggressive and defensive factors tilts in favor of the aggressive forces.[4]

The first factor, transient LES relaxation, has been shown to be the cause of most reflux events. LES relaxation allows the gastric contents to reflux back into the esophagus inappropriately, resulting in esophageal damage.

The second factor, low resting pressure of the sphincter, has been demonstrated in a minority of patients with reflux esophagitis. It remains unclear whether low LES pressure is a cause or consequence of esophagitis, because chronic inflammation may also reduce the ability of the sphincter to close. In addition, patients with chronic symptoms usually have the presence of a hiatal hernia. The combination of a hiatal hernia and reduced LES pressure appear to be co-factors that result in the greatest degree of reflux.[5] The presence of a hiatal hernia alone does not necessitate the presence of reflux esophagitis, because the majority of patients with hiatal hernias do not have any symptoms. In pregnancy, there is a 25% to 50% prevalence of reflux.[4] This reflux results from the relaxant effects that circulating estrogens and progesterones have on the LES.[1]

The next pathogenetic factor is the ability of the esophagus to clear itself of reflux material. Abnormalities in peristalsis increase the risk for esophagitis by failing to clear the refluxate, which increases contact time between mucosal acid and the esophagus. A decrease in esophageal peristalsis can be more pronounced in concomitant diseases such as diabetes mellitus or scleroderma, where the presence of neuromuscular dysfunction contributes to esophageal mucosal damage leading to esophagitis.

The last predisposing factor for the development of GERD is delayed gastric emptying, in which the gastric contents are allowed to backwash into the esophagus as a result of their increased time in the stomach. This condition is seen with diabetes, postviral infections, and most commonly a functional disorder.

Defense mechanisms include salivary secretion, which plays an important role in buffering reflux material in the esophagus, and the secretion of alkaline fluid by the esophageal glands.[2] Salivation is decreased during sleep, which contributes to prolonged acid clearance and increased symptoms during the night. Abnormalities of salivary secretion, such as sicca syndrome, can diminish salivary production and lead to esophagitis.

CLINICAL PRESENTATION

The most common symptom of GERD is heartburn, which is usually described as a burning discomfort experienced behind the breastbone.[4] (Other terms for heartburn include *indigestion, acid regurgitation, sour stomach,* and *bitter belching.*) The hot sensation usually begins inferiorly and radiates up the entire retrosternal area to the neck, occasionally to the back, and, rarely, into the arms. The sensation may become so intense that it is described as pain. Heartburn is usually relieved with antacids, baking soda, or milk, but this remedy is often short-lived. Heartburn is usually precipitated by food intake occurring within 1 hour of eating and particularly after the largest meal of the day.

Other foods that precipitate heartburn are foods high in fat or sugar, chocolate, coffee, and onions because they lower pressure in the LES (Box 146-1). Cigarette smoking and alcohol consumption may also lower pressure in the LES. Other foods that commonly cause heartburn are citrus products, tomato-based foods, and spicy foods. These foods do not affect LES pressure but instead are direct mucosal irritants. Other direct irritants include aspirin, nonsteroidal antiinflammatory drugs, potassium, or just pills themselves.

BOX 146-1

FACTORS AFFECTING HEARTBURN

LOW LES PRESSURE	DIRECT MUCOSAL IRRITANT	INCREASED INTRAABDOMINAL PRESSURE
Foods	Foods	Bending
Fat	Citrus based	Lifting
Chocolate	Tomato based	Straining
Onions	Coffee	Exercise
Coffee	Spicy food	
Sugars	Medications	
Medications	NSAIDs	
Calcium channel blockers	Acetylsalicylic acid	
Progesterone	Tetracycline	
Theophylline	Potassium chloride	
Alcohol	Tablets	
Cigarettes		

Patients may also complain of heartburn that increases after going to bed, especially after eating late in the evening. This usually occurs within 1 to 2 hours of bedtime. Several other maneuvers, including bending over, lifting, straining with a bowel movement, or exercising, may also precipitate heartburn because they increase intraabdominal pressure. Unfortunately, the frequency or severity of heartburn is not predictive of the degree of esophageal tissue damage seen at endoscopy. Some patients with erosions are asymptomatic, whereas other patients with frequent and even severe symptoms can have overall normal tissue.

Other symptoms of GERD include acid regurgitation, water brash, dysphagia, odynophagia, and chest pain. Acid regurgitation is the complaint of a bitter acidic fluid in the mouth that usually occurs at night or when bending over. This symptom should be differentiated from vomiting. Water brash is the appearance of salty-tasting fluid in the mouth because of stimulated saliva secretion. If delayed gastric emptying is the cause of GERD, abdominal fullness, nausea, and early satiety may be seen.[3]

Dysphagia and odynophagia are more predictive of severe disease and should be considered alarm symptoms. Dysphagia is an impairment of swallowing food into the stomach and is experienced immediately after swallowing. Patients may say that the food "sticks," "hangs up," or "stops." Odynophagia is pain on swallowing; this type of pain usually occurs under the sternum and has a sharp quality. Odynophagia is more commonly associated with infectious esophagitis or pill ulceration.

Chest pain can mimic angina, which is not surprising because of the shared neural pathways. Esophageal disorders are probably the most common cause of noncardiac chest pain.[4] Reflux is experienced by approximately 50% of patients with anginal-type chest pain but normal coronary arteries.[6] Symptoms that are more suggestive of esophageal problems include pain that continues for hours, interrupts sleep, or is non–exercise induced, retrosternal without lateral radiation, meal-related, or relieved with antacids.

Other nonesophageal or atypical symptoms of GERD include sore throat, earache, gingivitis, poor dentition, nocturnal cough, hoarseness, wheezing, bronchitis, asthma, and aspiration pneumonia. In children, GERD has been associated with sudden infant death syndrome and apnea.[1]

PHYSICAL EXAMINATION

A careful history is probably more important than the physical findings. Epigastric tenderness or heme-positive stools may be the result of esophageal erosions, ulcerations, or even severe inflammation. Weight loss may be a concern, particularly in patients who have dysphagia. Respiratory wheezes and cough may be seen if there is associated asthma. An association between dental erosions and GERD has been found; thus an oral examination may suggest GERD in a patient with extensive loss of enamel and exposed dentin.[7]

DIAGNOSTICS

A history of recurrent heartburn alone can be initially adequate to diagnose GERD in the absence of other warning signals of serious systemic disease such as weight loss, dysphagia, heme-positive stool, or anemia. Patients more than 50 years old with new onset of symptoms should not be initially placed on empiric therapy because of the increased incidence of gastric cancer with aging. As the severity of heartburn correlates poorly with the extent of tissue injury, this cannot be used to determine which patient requires an endoscopy. An upper gastrointestinal x-ray study is normal in 80% of patients with GERD, making endoscopy the "gold standard" for evaluation.[2]

Endoscopy is indicated for patients with any of the following:

- Age 50 years or older
- Unsuccessful empiric therapy
- Warning signs
- Long-standing symptoms requiring continuous therapy

Endoscopy with biopsy is required to search for intestinal metaplasia diagnostic of Barrett's esophagus, a premalignant condition requiring surveillance in the coming years. With dysphagia, an upper endoscopy is always indicated initially because dilation of a possible stricture can occur at the same time as the diagnostic procedure.

The standard diagnostic test for GERD is 24-hour pH monitoring, which detects the presence and amount of acid in the esophagus. However, this test is seldom used initially because it lacks the ability to demonstrate esophageal damage. It can confirm reflux in patients with persistent symptoms without evidence of esophagitis and with noncardiac chest pain or reflux associated pulmonary or upper airway symptoms. Esophageal manometry should be used to facilitate placement of pH probes and to guide antireflux surgery.[8]

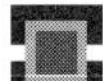

Diagnostics

Gastroesophageal Reflux Disease

Laboratory
CBC and differential*
H. pylori antibody
Stool for occult blood ×3

Other
Esophagoscopy with biopsies*

*If indicated.

DIFFERENTIAL DIAGNOSIS

The symptoms of GERD can be similar to those of cholelithiasis, peptic ulcer disease, gastritis, angina, and esophageal motility disturbances. These disorders can be distinguished from GERD through the use of ultrasound, upper gastrointestinal x-ray studies, endoscopy, esophageal manometry, ECG, or coronary angiography. GERD may be the most common cause of esophagitis, but there are other causes, including cytomegalovirus, herpes, or candida infections in patients who are immunocompromised. Medications such as tetracycline or potassium chloride, if dissolved in the esophagus, result in "pill esophagitis" (see Box 146-1). In unexplained cases of chest pain, cough, hoarseness or asthma, GERD should be considered.[8]

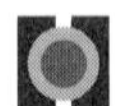

Differential Diagnosis

Gastroesophageal Reflux Disease

Cholelithiasis
Peptic ulcer disease
Gastritis
Angina
Esophageal motility disturbances
Esophagitis secondary infection
Tumor
Esophageal infection
Medication-induced "pill esophagitis"

MANAGEMENT

GERD progresses slowly and is rarely an acute or life-threatening condition. Therefore medical management is first-line treatment. The goals of GERD therapy include decreased symptoms and improved quality of life, prevention of complications, and cost-effective treatment.

The most effective treatment for uncomplicated GERD includes following lifestyle modifications and, if indicated, medical therapy. Lifestyle modifications are an essential component of patient education to reduce symptoms and prevent recurrence (Box 146-2). In addition, lifestyle modifications are cost-effective and promote a healthier lifestyle. Patients should be reminded that GERD is a chronic condition that will recur unless reflux is minimized with permanent lifestyle changes and hydrostatic measures.

Medications

Many heartburn sufferers do not seek medical care and choose antacids, over-the-counter acid suppressants, or do nothing about their symptoms. Antacids, in conjunction with lifestyle modifications, are an effective therapy for patients with minimal symptoms of heartburn (Figure 146-1). Antacids produce prompt but brief symptom relief by neutralizing acid in the stomach.[9] There have been no studies to evaluate the efficacy of therapy that combines lifestyle changes and antacids, but long-term trials suggest effectiveness in approximately 20% of patients.[10] The side effects of antacid therapy may include diarrhea produced by the magnesium-containing agents and constipation caused by the aluminum-containing agents. In the presence of significant renal disease, magnesium or aluminum products should not be used. Patients on salt-restricted diets should use low-sodium antacids such as magaldrate (Riopan).

BOX 146-2

LIFESTYLE CHANGES FOR THE MANAGEMENT OF GASTROESOPHAGEAL REFLUX DISEASE

- Smoking cessation
- Reduced alcohol consumption
- Reduced dietary fat
- Decreased meal size
- Weight reduction (if patient is overweight)
- Elevation of head of bed 6 inches
- Elimination of medications that are mucosal irritants or that lower esophageal pressure (see Box 146-1)
- Avoidance of chocolate, peppermint, coffee, tea, cola beverages, tomato juice, and citrus fruit juices
- Avoidance of supine position for 2 hours after meals
- Avoidance of tight-fitting clothes

Acid suppression is the mainstay of therapy for GERD. Proton pump inhibitors (PPIs) provide rapid symptomatic relief and healing of esophagitis in 6 to 8 weeks.[8] However H_2-histamine receptor antagonists (H_2RAs) in divided doses may also be used in patients with less severe GERD. These include cimetidine (Tagamet), ranitidine (Zantac), famotidine (Pepcid), and nizatidine (Axid). These products decrease the secretion of acid into the gastric lumen.[11] A review of the literature by the Practice Parameters Committee of the American College of Gastroenterology (ACG) found that twice-daily dosing of these agents in prescription strength gave symptomatic relief to only 60% of patients.[10] Unfortunately, symptom resolution has not correlated well with mucosal healing. These medications may be used as needed for intermittent heartburn. Only 48% of patients with esophagitis will heal on this regimen.[10] Higher and more frequent dosing (i.e., three times a day) is more effective for relieving symptoms and healing esophagitis. Caution should be observed with older patients or in the presence of preexisting renal or liver disease.

The Practice Parameters Committee of the ACG in 1999 therefore promoted the use of PPIs as first-line therapy for GERD.[8] This includes omeprazole (Prilosec), lansoprazole (Prevacid), pantoprazole (Protonix), rabeprazole (Aciphex), and most recently esomeprazole (Nexium). Nexium has increased bioavailability and is indicated as initial therapy or for patients on omeprazole who require twice-daily dosing.

PPIs are potent inhibitors of acid secretion and produce acid suppression superior to that of the H_2RAs, usually with only once-daily dosing.[9] Therefore they have a greater efficacy than the H_2RAs in relieving symptoms and in healing erosive esophagitis. Patients with moderate to severe esophagitis are usually treated for 8 weeks. PPIs are also superior in reducing

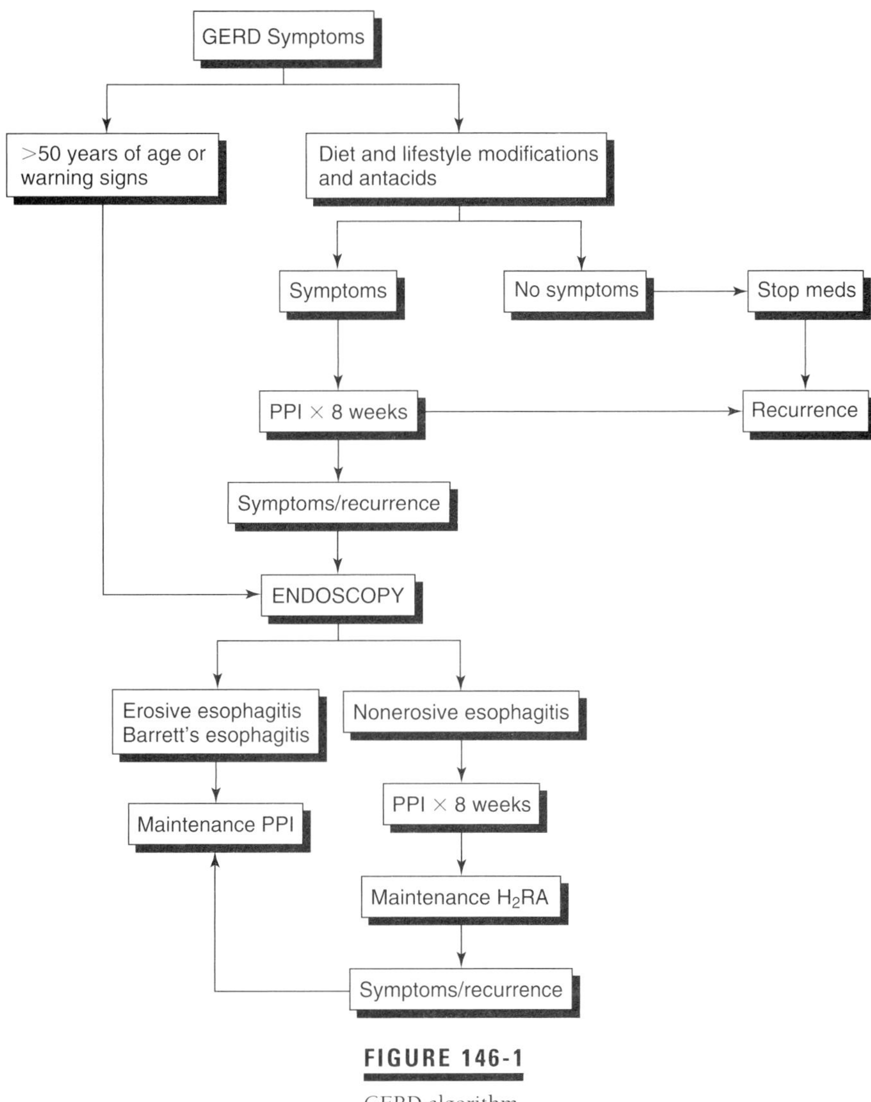

FIGURE 146-1

GERD algorithm.

the risk of relapse when continued for maintenance therapy.[1] The need for stricture dilation is reduced with the use of these agents.[11] The ACG guidelines consider chronic use of PPIs as an effective and appropriate form of maintenance therapy in many patients.[7]

The continued use of PPIs in GERD patients infected with *Helicobacter pylori* has shown a greater incidence of atrophic gastritis—a precursor in the carcinogenesis pathway.[12] For this reason, testing and treatment of *H. pylori* has been recommended but is controversial because it is not known if *H. pylori* treatment is protective or decreases the risk of gastric cancer. However, after eradication of *H. pylori*, GERD patients have had a rebound response. At the present time, it is unclear whether to treat GERD patients for *H. pylori*.

The ability of the esophagus to clear itself of reflux material is one of the pathogenetic factors of GERD. Metoclopramide (Reglan) has an efficacy similar to standard dose H_2RAs. Its mode of action includes increasing both gastric emptying and lowering esophageal sphincter pressure. Metoclopramide (Reglan) often produces side effects of the central nervous system, including drowsiness and extrapyramidal effects. In most cases there is little support for the use of this drug in combination with acid suppression.

Maintenance Therapies

With GERD, the goal of effective maintenance therapy is treatment that controls symptoms and prevents complications. There is a high rate of relapse, with 50% of symptoms recurring within 2 months and 82% recurring within 6 months without maintenance therapy.[6] If symptoms return after medical therapy is decreased or stopped, an esophagogastroduodenoscopy (EGD) should be performed. The ACG guidelines of 1999 consider chronic PPI therapy as effective and appropriate maintenance therapy.[7] If remission is maintained on maintenance therapy, it is thought that patients' quality of life will improve and that direct and indirect costs will be decreased.[6]

Patients with nonerosive GERD may be symptom free on full-dose H_2RAs as maintenance therapy. GERD refractory to medical therapy is very rare. The diagnosis should be confirmed before initiating chronic acid suppression therapy or antireflux surgery. Antireflux surgery performed by an experienced surgeon is a maintenance option for the patient with well-documented GERD.[8]

COMPLICATIONS

Complications of GERD include esophageal strictures, Barrett's esophagus, hemorrhage, and perforation. Strictures are bands of fibrous tissue in the distal esophagus and can impede the progress of food from the mouth to the stomach. These bands develop over months to years and are characterized by dysphagia and a possible reduction in heartburn because the stricture can act as a barrier to reflux. Initial treatment is with proton pump inhibitors to reduce inflammation. Dilation may be necessary if symptoms are persistent and may need to be repeated months to years later.

In Barrett's esophagus, the lower esophagus is lined with a simple columnar epithelium rather than with the normal stratified squamous epithelium.[1] This change results from chronic reflux—the columnar epithelium provides protection against acid. Although Barrett's esophagus is protective initially, it is a premalignant condition that can lead to the development of esophageal adenocarcinoma. Of the patients with esophagitis, 10% to 12% will develop Barrett's esophagus, with approximately 10% of these patients developing adenocarcinoma.[2] Barrett's esophagus occurs more often in Caucasian men at an average age of 55 years.[1] The presentation is commonly heartburn or dysphagia. Biopsies are required to confirm the diagnosis; if Barrett's esophagus is present, periodic upper endoscopies with biopsies are recommended to assess the development of dysplasia or malignancy.

Hemorrhage and perforation are rare complications of ulcerative esophagitis. However, chronic bleeding and iron deficiency anemia can develop and may be the only sign of GERD.

INDICATIONS FOR REFERRAL/HOSPITALIZATION

Although heartburn can be managed without a referral, it is important to identify patients who could profit from maximum long-term medical therapy or who have complications. Patients who initially received empiric treatment without success or whose symptoms recur when medications are stopped should have an upper endoscopy to determine if esophagitis is present. A gastroenterology referral is indicated if the patient is more than 50 years of age or has the warning signs of dysphagia (both solid and liquid), odynophagia, unexplained iron deficiency anemia, weight loss, fecal occult bleeding, obstructive symptoms (nausea, vomiting, and early satiety), or anorexia.

PATIENT AND FAMILY EDUCATION

Education is imperative for patients with GERD. If diet and lifestyle modifications are followed strictly, reflux symptoms may be kept to a minimum. There is no one particular diet for patients with reflux. Patients should avoid fatty foods, chocolate, peppermint, and excessive alcohol consumption. Food that may elicit symptoms for one person may not necessarily produce symptoms in another; therefore selective avoidance of foods that precipitate symptoms is necessary. Lifestyle modifications are numerous and have been outlined previously.

REFERENCES

1. Yamada T: *Textbook of gastroenterology,* ed 2, Philadelphia, 1995, JB Lippincott.
2. Gallup Organization National Survey: *Heartburn across America,* Princeton, NJ, 1998, Gallup Organization.
3. Christensen J: Gastroesophageal reflux disease: where do we stand? *Clin Focus*:11-17, 1995.
4. Champion MC: Prokinetic therapy in gastroesophageal reflux disease, *Can J Gastroenterol* 11(suppl B):55B-65B, 1997.
5. Sleisinger MH, Fortran JS: *Gastrointestinal disease,* ed 5, Philadelphia, 1993, WB Saunders.
6. Fennerty MB and others: The diagnosis and treatment of gastroesophageal reflux disease in a managed care environment, *Arch Intern Med* 156:447-484, 1996.
7. DeVault KR, Castell D: ACG treatments guideline: updated guidelines for the diagnosis and treatment of GERD, *Am J Gastroenterol* 94: 1434-1442, 1999.
8. Balazuda OV, Schneider FD: Evaluation and management of dyspepsia, *Am Fam Physician* 60:1773-1788, 1999
9. Devault KR, Castell D: Guidelines for the diagnosis and treatment of gastroesophageal reflux disease, *Arch Intern Med* 155:2165-2173, 1995.
10. Sachs G, Prinz C, Hersey SJ: *Acid related disorders: mystery to mechanism: mechanism to management,* Palm Beach, Fla, 1995, Sushu Publishing.
11. American College of Gastroenterology. Retrieved August 2002 from the World Wide Web: www.acg.gi.org.
12. Fennerty MB: *GERD as a chronic disease: why not use drugs for remission? Advances in gastroenterology, Virginia Gastroenterological Society meeting,* Williamsburg, Va, Sept 20-21, 1997.

CHAPTER 147

Gastrointestinal Hemorrhage

Joanne Marie Petrelli

DEFINITION/EPIDEMIOLOGY

Gastrointestinal (GI) bleeding is often reported to primary health care providers in both ambulatory and emergency settings. Patients often describe the symptoms as black tarry stools (melena), bright red stools (hematochezia), and even bright red vomitus (hematemesis). Some patients deny these symptoms, but fecal occult blood testing during regular health maintenance check-ups is positive.[1]

Gastrointestinal hemorrhage can occur anywhere in the GI tract from the mouth to the anus and can be overt or occult[2] (Table 147-1). Management of GI bleeding has remained constant over several decades, with only a few additions to the care plan. Hemodynamic stabilization of the patient, cessation of active bleeding, and prevention of recurrent bleeding have long remained the goals of medical management for this disorder, which results in approximately 100 cases per 100,000 per year.[3] Many of these patients require emergency treatment, hospitalization, and intensive care monitoring.

GI bleeding is subdivided into upper and lower GI bleeding according to its anatomic source. Patients with upper GI tract bleeding from a source proximal to the ligament of Treitz may be asymptomatic, have subtle signs of anemia and hypovolemia, or present dramatically with hematemesis, melena, or hematochezia.[4] Hemorrhage as a result of peptic ulcer disease, mucosal erosive disease, or esophageal varices constitutes 80% to 90% of upper GI bleeding.[4] These patients are more likely to be older, male (2:1), have co-morbid disease (cirrhosis, myocardial infarction) and be users of alcohol, tobacco, aspirin, anticoagulants, and/or nonsteroidal antiinflammatory drugs (NSAIDs).[5] Upper GI bleeding has been estimated to cause more than 350,000 hospitalizations per year and has a 10% mortality rate.[6]

Lower GI tract bleeding from a source distal to the ligament of Treitz can cause occult blood loss or massive hematochezia and shock. The most common cause of lower GI bleeding is diverticulosis, but other common sources include arteriovenous malformations, colorectal malignancy, inflammatory bowel disease, ischemic colitis, and hemorrhoids.[7]

TABLE 147-1 Bleeding Definitions

Type of Bleeding	Definition
Overt	Visible bright red or maroon colored blood in feces or emesis
Occult	No visible blood in feces or emesis. Patient may present with iron deficiency anemia (IDA) or have a positive fecal occult blood test (FOBT).
Obscure	IDA recurrent/persistent. FOBT positive. May or may not have visible bleeding. No bleeding source found at time of original endoscopy.
Obscure/Occult	IDA recurrent persistent. Positive FOBT. No visible blood in feces. No source identified.
Obscure/Overt	Blood visible in feces and emesis. Bleeding recurrent/persistent. No source found at original endoscopy.

Modified from Zuckerman GR, Prakash C, Askin MP, Lewis BS: American Gastroenterological Association practice guidelines, *Gastroenterology* 118(1): 210, 2000.

PATHOPHYSIOLOGY

The pathophysiology of GI bleeding can be associated with esophagitis, peptic ulcer disease, gastritis, *Helicobacter pylori*, esophageal or gastric varices, diverticulosis, gastric and colonic cancers, gastric and colonic polyps and angiodysplasia.[2-4] Peptic ulcers are defects in the mucosa of the duodenum or stomach that are caused by a breakdown in the normal mucosal defenses. Bleeding from peptic ulcers occurs when the ulcer erodes into a blood vessel.[2-4] Contributing factors include alcohol, NSAIDs, excess stomach acid production, and the presence of *H. pylori*.

Gastritis causes bleeding from diffuse superficial lesions in the gastric mucosa that are usually caused by local irritants or that occur in association with *H. pylori*. NSAIDs inhibit cyclooxygenase, decreasing the synthesis of protective prostaglandins, and may have direct effects on the gastric mucosa, causing both irritation and superficial lesions. Alcohol ingestion causes the production of leukotrienes by the gastric mucosa, which may be responsible for vascular stasis, engorgement, and increased vascular permeability, which leads to hemorrhage.[8,9] Gastritis can also be caused by major physiologic stressors, including burns, sepsis, trauma, and long-distance running, secondary to decreased splanchnic blood flow and the resultant decrease in mucus production, bicarbonate secretion, and prostaglandin synthesis, all leading to a breakdown in the normal mucosal defenses.[8]

H. pylori has received a formidable amount of public attention and research since it was first described in 1984. This gram-negative spiral bacterium has adaptive mechanisms to survive in the human stomach, including the conversion of urea, water, and acid to ammonia and bicarbonate; the use of adhesions and toxins; its motility; and the fact that it is microaerophilic. Its importance is that nearly 100% of cases of chronic, superficial gastritis, 90% to 95% of duodenal ulcers, and 80% of gastric ulcers are believed to be caused by *H. pylori*.[7,8] Treatment of this organism has been shown to cure ulcer disease, as well as decrease the incidence of ulcer recurrence and rebleeding.[10,11]

Esophageal varices, the second most common cause of upper GI bleeding, arise from obstruction of the portal venous system, leading to increased portal pressure, which over time results in the development of dilated venous collaterals.[12] The most common cause of portal hypertension in the United States is cirrhosis from alcoholic and chronic active hepatitis; however, worldwide the most common cause is parasitic liver disease (particularly schistosomiasis).[10-13] Approximately one third of all patients with cirrhosis will bleed from varices; overall mortality is 30%.[4,14]

Diverticulosis is present in 42% to 55% of the cases of acute lower GI bleeding.[3] Diverticula occur at the penetration site of nutrient vessels, with bleeding occurring as a consequence of arterial rupture into the diverticular sac.[8]

Angiodysplasia, small vascular tufts formed by capillaries, veins, and venules, representing an acquired arteriovenous malformation,[9] are the most common lesions found in the GI tract. A small percentage of these lesions are present at birth, but most angiodysplasias are detected in people older than 60 years.[15,16] Although massive bleeding is occasionally associated with these lesions, more often bleeding is slow, chronic, and occult.

CLINICAL PRESENTATION

Blood loss from the GI tract commonly manifests itself in one or more of several ways. Hematemesis is bloody vomitus that is either fresh and bright red or older and "coffee ground" in appearance. Melena is stool that is black, shiny, and foul smelling as a result blood degradation. Hematochezia is the passage of bright red to mahogany-colored blood from the rectum as pure blood, blood mixed with stool, blood clots, or bloody diarrhea. These manifestations are more overt or obvious, but occult blood loss is often more subtle. Occult blood loss can present as iron deficiency anemia (IDA) or as a positive routine fecal occult blood test using a chemical reagent.[16] The presentation can include symptoms associated with blood loss, such as presyncope, dyspnea, angina, postural hypotension, and shock with no overt bleeding source.

The history should include the amount, duration, and source of any bleeding, along with any associated symptoms including abdominal pain, chest pain, shortness of breath, diaphoresis, and weakness.[4] The patient should be questioned about prior episodes of bleeding and about other illnesses that may lead to bleeding such as cirrhosis, cancer, coagulopathies, or connective tissue disease. All significant past medical and surgical conditions should be elicited and documented, as well as any allergies and medication usage, including alendronate, potassium chloride, anticoagulants and over-the-counter preparations (especially aspirin and NSAIDs).[2] A careful history of alcohol, tobacco, and illicit drug use is also necessary.[2,4]

PHYSICAL EXAMINATION

The physical examination is brief and focused. The initial general appearance and a mental status evaluation of the patient should be noted. Vital signs should be obtained early and repeated frequently. The earliest sign of hypovolemia is tachycardia, with hypotension not occurring until volume loss approaches 40%.[17] The skin should be examined for color, temperature, turgor, moisture, and capillary refill. Cutaneous lesions on upper extremities, lips, and oral mucosa may reveal hereditary hemorrhagic telangiectasia or blue rubber bleb nevus syndrome. These can be related to a family history of GI bleeding.[2] Other cutaneous manifestations that should be noted on the physical examination include spider nevi, palmar erythema, scleral icterus, and parotid enlargement. The cardiovascular examination should focus on the heart rate and the character of the peripheral pulses. Postural change in blood pressure should be immediately noted. Orthostasis suggests a blood volume loss of 15% to 20%.[17] If the blood pressure falls more than 10 to 15 mm Hg and or the heart rate increases by more than 10 to 15 beats per minute when the patient stands from a supine position, consider immediate hospital admission. The abdomen should be auscultated and palpated to identify a mass, tenderness, guarding, or rigidity. A careful rectal examination can detect hemorrhoids, fissures, or rectal carcinoma. The stool should be examined for gross blood and melena, and tested for occult blood.[18] After the patient is stabilized, a thorough physical examination should be performed in search of non-GI sources of bleeding such as increased or irregular menstrual bleeding in the presence of IDA. The physical examination is an excellent time to have an IV catheter placed, perform initial laboratory studies, and begin IV electrolyte solutions if indicated.[19]

DIAGNOSTICS

The initial diagnostic step in the evaluation of GI bleeding should be insertion of a nasogastric (NG) tube, especially if the location of the bleeding is in question. Bright red blood from the NG tube indicates recent or active bleeding, although 16% of patients with actively bleeding lesions at endoscopy may not

Diagnostics

Gastrointestinal Bleeding

Laboratory	Imaging	Other
Stool for occult bleeding	Abdominal x-rays	Blood pressure tilts for orthostatic hypotension
CBC with differential	Bleeding scars or angiography*	ECG (if >40 years or if have cardiac history)
Platelets	Upright chest x-ray (for severe abdominal pain)	Endoscopy*
BUN	CT of abdomen and surgical consult (if all other tests remain negative and patient continues to have severe abdominal pain with intestinal bleeding)	Barium studies*
Creatinine		Air-contrast enema*
Serum glucose		Nuclear scintigraphy*†
Calcium		Selective mesenteric angiography*†
LFTs		Enteroscopy*
Serum electrolytes		Anoscopy†
Amylase level		Sigmoidoscopy†
PT/PTT		Colonoscopy†
ABGs		
Type and cross match		

*If indicated.
†For evaluation of lower GI bleeding.

demonstrate blood in the aspirate. The NG tube should be removed if there is no suggestion of active bleeding (no blood in stomach).[18,19] It is imperative that all heme-positive stools receive a full GI evaluation.

Laboratory evaluation of all patients with GI bleeding should include hemoglobin, hematocrit, and platelet count to assess baseline blood loss and platelet adequacy.[20] The patient's blood should be typed and cross-matched for 4 to 6 units of packed red blood cells, and laboratory studies for BUN, creatinine, glucose, calcium, LFTs, prothrombin time, and activated partial thromboplastin time should be done.[4] An increased BUN level with normal creatinine is suggestive of an upper GI source.[10] Arterial blood gases may be helpful in both assessing oxygenation and clarifying the acid-base status of the patient. An ECG should be obtained in all patients over 40 years old with chest or abdominal pain or a history of cardiac or pulmonary disease. Radiographic studies may include an acute abdominal series if there is suggestion of a perforated viscus or intestinal obstruction accompanying bleeding.

Further diagnostic studies such as endoscopy, barium studies, bleeding scans, or angiography should be performed at the discretion of the consulting gastroenterologist or surgeon.[18-21]

DIFFERENTIAL DIAGNOSIS

The sources of GI bleeding may be categorized as inflammatory, mechanical, vascular, neoplastic, systemic, or anomalous. Patients with an upper GI source of bleeding generally present with hematemesis and/or melena, a bloody NG aspirate, an elevated BUN-creatinine ratio (>36), and hyperactive bowel sounds. Patients with a lower GI source of bleeding generally present with hematochezia, a clear NG aspirate, a normal BUN-creatinine ratio, and normoactive bowel sounds.[20]

The presence or history of black or red hematemesis confirms an upper GI source after bleeding from the nose and oropharynx is excluded. Melena represents an upper GI source 85% to 95% of the time, and hematochezia from a briskly bleeding upper GI source accounts for 10% of cases.[4] Vomiting, coughing, wretching, or blunt abdominal trauma before bleeding suggests a Mallory-Weiss tear, the majority of which occur in the upper stomach. Painful upper GI bleeding is suggestive of peptic ulcer disease, gastritis, esophagitis, or duodenitis, with severe pain and peritoneal signs suggesting a perforated viscus. The bleeding of esophageal varices is suggested by a history of cirrhosis and painless bleeding.[4]

Lower GI sources of bleeding associated with abdominal pain include inflammatory bowel disease and aortoenteric fistula. Pain disproportionate to the physical findings is suggestive of ischemic bowel. Painless bleeding may be seen with diverticulosis, angiodysplasia, or hemorrhoids. Rectal pain may be associated with bleeding from anal fissures or hemorrhoids. Constipation may be a diagnostic clue for malignancy or hemorrhoids.

Inflammatory bowel disease or infectious diarrhea should not be overlooked in a patient presenting with bloody diarrhea. Enterohemorrhagic *Escherichia coli* (especially *E. coli* 0157:H7) are

Differential Diagnosis

Gastrointestinal Bleeding

UPPER GI BLEEDING (ORIGINATING ABOVE THE LIGAMENT OF TREITZ)

- Oral or pharyngeal lesions: swallowed blood from nose or oropharynx
- Swallowed hemoptysis
- Esophageal: varices, ulceration, esophagitis, Mallory-Weiss tear, carcinoma, trauma
- Gastric: peptic ulcer (including Cushing and Curling's ulcers), gastritis, angiodysplasia, gastric neoplasms, hiatal hernia, gastric diverticulum, pseudoxanthoma elasticum, Rendu-Osler-Weber syndrome
- Duodenal: peptic ulcer, duodenitis, angiodysplasia, aortoduodenal fistula, duodenal diverticulum, duodenal tumors, carcinoma of ampulla of Vater, parasites (e.g., hookworm), Crohn's disease
- Biliary: hematobilia (e.g., penetrating injury to liver, hepatobiliary malignancy, endoscopic papillotomy)

LOWER GI BLEEDING (ORIGINATING BELOW THE LIGAMENT OF TREITZ)

Small Intestine

- Ischemic bowel disease (mesenteric thrombosis, embolism, vasculitis, trauma)
- Small bowel neoplasm: leiomyomas, carcinoids
- Hereditary hemorrhagic telangiectasia (Rendu-Osler-Weber syndrome)
- Meckel's diverticulum and other small intestine diverticula
- Aortoenteric fistula
- Intestinal hemangiomas: blue rubber–bleb nevi, intestinal hemangiomas, cutaneous vascular nevi
- Hamartomatous polyps: Peutz-Jeghers syndrome (intestinal polyps, mucocutaneous pigmentation)
- Infections of small bowel: tuberculous enteritis, enteritis necroticans
- Volvulus
- Intussusception
- Lymphoma of small bowel, sarcoma, Kaposi's sarcoma
- Irradiation ileitis
- AV malformation of small intestine
- Inflammatory bowel disease
- Polyarteritis nodosa
- Other: pancreatoenteric fistulas, Schönlein-Henoch purpura, Ehlers-Danlos syndrome, systemic lupus erythematosus, amyloidosis, metastatic melanoma

Colon

- Carcinoma (particularly left colon)
- Diverticular disease
- Inflammatory bowel disease
- Ischemic colitis
- Colonic polyps
- Vascular abnormalities: angiodysplasia, vascular ectasia
- Radiation colitis
- Infectious colitis
- Uremic colitis
- Aortoenteric fistula
- Lymphoma of large bowel
- Hemorrhoids
- Anal fissure
- Trauma, foreign body
- Solitary rectal/cecal ulcers
- Long-distance running

From Ferri F: *Ferri's clinical advisor 2002*, St. Louis, 2002, Mosby.

responsible for up to 20,000 infections per year in the United States alone.[20] This is commonly associated with the ingestion of undercooked ground meat, contaminated water, or unpasteurized milk. This particular strain of *E. coli* has been linked to 250 deaths per year in the United States.[22]

MANAGEMENT

The most important concept in the management of acute GI bleeding is that resuscitation and stabilization must precede diagnostic and therapeutic interventions. The initial priorities are the establishment of an adequate airway, ensuring oxygenation and ventilation, followed by restoration of the circulatory status to normal (Figure 147-1).

Any patient thought to have significant bleeding should immediately have two large-bore IV lines or a central line placed. Fluid resuscitation should be vigorous and should consist of crystalloid infusions of either normal saline or lactated Ringer's solution at rates as rapid as the patient's cardiopulmonary system will allow in order to correct the volume deficit. Consideration for a central venous pressure line or a Swan-Ganz catheter should be given to patients with underlying cardiac, pulmonary, renal, or hepatic disease to prevent fluid overload.[4] A Foley catheter should be placed to assist with determining volume status with a minimum urine output of 30 to 50 ml/hr in the adult.

The blood product of choice initially is packed red blood cells for patients continuing to bleed, patients in shock, patients

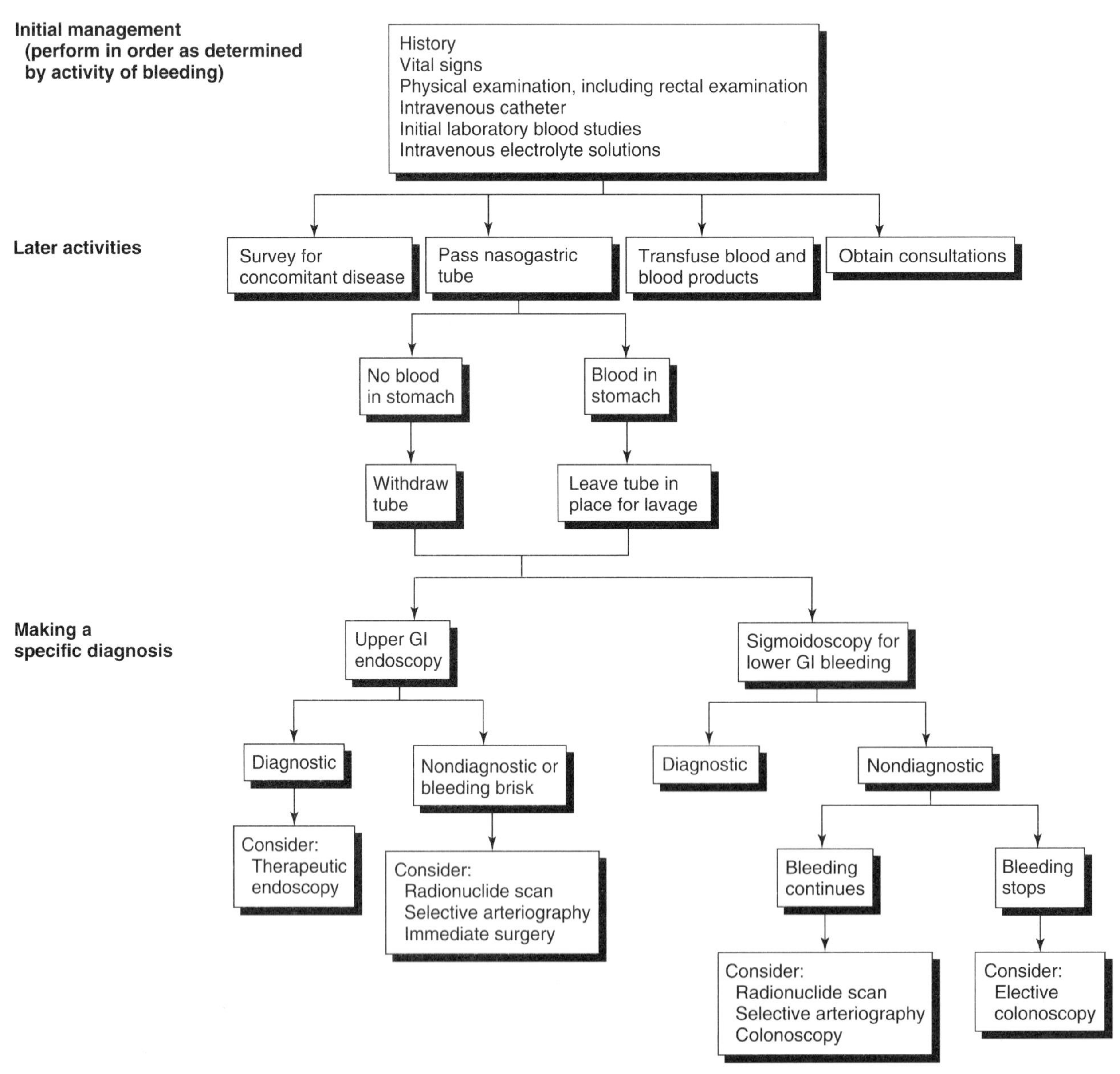

FIGURE 147-1

Management of gastrointestinal bleeding.(Modified from Stein JH, editor: *Internal medicine,* ed 5, St Louis, 1998, Mosby.)

with very low hematocrit values, or patients who have symptoms related to poor tissue oxygenation (e.g., angina).[18] For patients with massive blood loss, whole blood may be used. Close monitoring of coagulation parameters and serum calcium must accompany transfusion. Fresh frozen plasma may be used to correct coagulopathy and should be given at a rate of 1 units per every 5 to 6 units of blood transfused.[18]

The diagnostic test of choice in upper GI bleeding is endoscopy.[2,4,18] Endoscopy has the advantage of identifying patients with continued bleeding or high-risk lesions who will benefit from endoscopic therapy. High-risk endoscopic findings include arterial bleeding, adherent clot, visible vessels, and varices. Those at risk for rebleeding resulting in increased morbidity and mortality are patients over age 60 years, those with coagulopathies and other concurrent illnesses, and anyone hospitalized at the time of bleeding.[18]

The most common definitive therapy for esophageal varices is endoscopic sclerotherapy, which involves either intravariceal or paravariceal injection of a sclerosing agent. It has proved to be more effective than balloon tamponade or medical therapy. Balloon tamponade such as the Sengstaken-Blakemore tube have a success rate of 70% to 80% but may cause severe complications including aspiration, ulceration, and perforation if used improperly.[3]

Medical therapy with octreotide, a long-acting analogue of somatostatin, has become the vasoactive agent of choice for a patient experiencing acute GI bleeding. Octreotide decreases splanchnic and hepatic blood flow along with decreasing transhepatic and variceal pressures, thus reducing portal pressures. Acid suppression with H_2-blockers and proton pump inhibitors has no effect. Octreotide is given with a 100-μg IV bolus followed by a 50 μg/hr continuous infusion.[18]

Diagnostic modalities available for the evaluation of lower GI bleeding include anoscopy, sigmoidoscopy, colonoscopy, nuclear scintigraphy, selective mesenteric angiography (with vasopressin infusion or selective embolization), enteroscopy, and operative therapy.[14] The evaluation of the patient with lower GI bleeding depends on the rate (moderate, severe) and frequency (continuous, recurrent) of the bleeding.[18] If there is clinical suspicion of an upper GI source, the patient should undergo NG lavage. Vigorous fluid resuscitation should precede any diagnostic evaluation. As sigmoidoscopy in an unprepped patient may fail to produce the source of the bleeding, colonoscopy is now recommended for the evaluation of lower GI bleeding. If this fails to reveal a source of the bleeding, an endoscopy should be performed. Colonoscopy in this setting is the diagnostic procedure of choice because of its accuracy and therapeutic capability.[14,22] Barium studies are of little use in localizing acute lower GI bleeding and may actually yield misleading information.[3,23] Barium studies are usually reserved for high-risk patients who have contraindications to colonoscopy.

Radionuclide evaluation or a bleeding scan (red blood cell scan) is capable of detecting a hemorrhage as slow as 0.1 ml/min.[23] The tagged red blood cells circulate for 48 hours and gamma camera scanning is then used to detect the tagged cells in the bowel's lumen indicating lower GI bleeding. This test is positive 26% to 78% of the time.[3]

Enteroscopy, peroral or transnasal, is used for small bowel examination when both colonoscopy and endoscopy have not revealed a bleeding source. Causes of small bowel bleeding that can be detected by enteroscopy include large hiatal hernia sac erosions, peptic ulcer disease, and angioectasia.[24] Enteroscopy can also be used to evaluate suspected small bowel lesions, malabsorptive processes, and abnormal radiologic findings.

Indications for surgical management of lower GI bleeding include (1) transfusion of 4 or more units in 24 hours or greater than 10 units overall, and (2) significant rebleeding that occurs within 1 week of initial cessation and presence of co-morbid disease.[3] Emergency surgery can be lifesaving but associated with high morbidity and mortality if the location of the lesion is not identified before the surgical procedure. Surgical resection can be associated with rebleeding in up to 30% of the cases.[2]

Co-Management with Specialists

Asymptomatic patients in whom GI bleeding is suggested during routine screening or hemodynamically stable patients with minor bleeding may be appropriately evaluated on an outpatient basis with specialty referral for endoscopy and/or radiologic studies.[18]

LIFE SPAN CONSIDERATIONS

Upper GI bleeding has an overall mortality of 5% to 10%.[3] Mortality is significantly higher in older adults, primarily a result of co-morbid disease. Peptic ulcer bleeding accounts for 50% of the cases of upper GI bleeding. Variceal bleeding occurs in more than 40% of patients with chronic liver disease; 30% to 50% of patients die from a variceal bleeding episode.

The patient with lower GI bleeding tends to be older than the patient with upper GI bleeding and hence has more co-morbid illness. The incidence of lower GI bleeding is estimated to be approximately 20 to 27 per 100,000 cases per year. Acute lower GI bleeding is more common in men than women and escalates as age rises. This increase may be related to the increased incidence of diverticulosis, angiodysplasia, and neoplasms in older adults.[3]

COMPLICATIONS

Many of the complications of GI bleeding are associated with the diagnostic/therapeutic modalities used in its treatment. Serious complications of endoscopy, bleeding scans, and angiography include bowel ischemia and infarction.[8] Perforation of the gut can occur with upper or lower endoscopy. Extraintestinal complications of angiography include local hematoma formation, dye allergy, and the potential for renal failure.

INDICATIONS FOR REFERRAL/HOSPITALIZATION

All patients with acute upper GI bleeding require urgent consultation with a gastroenterologist.[4,23] Patients with hematochezia or signs of ongoing bleeding should also be immediately referred. A surgical consultation should be obtained for any patient who is hemodynamically unstable, has an abdominal aortic aneurysm or graft, or has a suspected perforation.[4,23]

Admission to the intensive care unit is recommended for all high-risk patients with hemodynamically unstable GI bleeding or rebleeding and for patients who have (1) red hematemesis or grossly bloody gastric aspirate, (2) an abdominal aortic aneurysm or a graft, (3) any bleeding with severe anemia, (4) a large drop in hematocrit, or (5) unstable co-morbid disease.[4,23]

Hospitalization is recommended for patients with melena who are hemodynamically unstable or who have had recent bleeding with significant but stable co-morbid disease.[4] A select group of patients may be discharged home after urgent endoscopy, provided they are hemodynamically stable, have no co-morbid disease, and have no high-risk endoscopic findings.[4]

PATIENT AND FAMILY EDUCATION

Patients should understand that NSAIDs, alcohol, tobacco, diet, and stress reduction can affect the disease. Substance abuse should be identified historically and patients actively encouraged to participate in alcohol/tobacco cessation programs. Stress management classes can be indicated for those patients whose life styles indicate that behavioral change in this area could be beneficial. General dietary guidelines should include (1) the need to avoid offending agents (i.e., generally spicy foods, alcohol, caffeine, chocolate), (2) the need to avoid late-night snacks in reflux disease, and (3) the fact that a low-fat, high-fiber diet low has shown benefit in diverticular disease and in the prevention of colon cancer. All patients should have thorough education and demonstrate an understanding of all medication use, interactions, and possible side effects.

HEALTH PROMOTION

Screening colonoscopy is recommended for all men and women of average risk to begin at age 50 years and for those with a strong family history of GI bleeding or colon cancer, screening should begin at age 40 years.[25]

REFERENCES

1. Spraycar M; *Steadman's medical dictionary* ed 26, Baltimore, Md, 1995, Williams and Wilkins.
2. Zuckerman GR and others: American gastroenterological association practice guidelines, *Gastroenterology* 118(1):201-221, 2000.
3. Fallah MA, Prakash C, Edmundowicz S: Acute gastrointestinal bleeding, *Med Clin North Am* 84(5):1183-1208, 2000.
4. McGuirk TD, Coyle WJ: Upper gastrointestinal tract bleeding, *Emerg Med Clin North Am* 14(3):523-545, 1996.
5. Chappell MS: Gastrointestinal bleeding associated with myocardial infarction, *Gastroenterol Clin* 29(2):423-444, 2000.
6. Eisen GM and others: An annotated algorithmic approach to upper gastrointestinal bleeding, *Gastrointest Endosc* 53(7):553-558, 2000.
7. Longstreth GF: Epidemiology of hospitalization for acute upper gastrointestinal hemorrhage: a population-based study, *Am J Gastroenterol* 90(2):206-210, 1995.
8. Longstreth GF: Epidemiology and outcome of patients hospitalized with acute lower gastrointestinal hemorrhage: a population-based study, *Am J Gastroenterol* 92(3):419-424, 1997.
9. Yardley JH, Hendrix TR: Gastritis, duodenitis, and associated ulcerative lesions. In Yamada T and others, editors: *Textbook of gastroenterology*, ed 3, Philadelphia, 1999, Lippincott.
10. Soll AH: Consensus conference. Medical treatment of peptic ulcer disease. Practice guidelines. Practice Parameters Committee of the American College of Gastroenterology, *JAMA* 275:622, 1996.
11. Hopkins RJ, Girardi LS, Turney EA: Relationship between helicobacter pylori eradication and reduced duodenal and gastric ulcer recurrence: a review, *Gastroenterology* 110:1244, 1996.
12. Jutabha R, Jensen DM: Management of severe upper gastrointestinal bleeding in the patient with liver disease, *Med Clin North Am* 80:1035, 1996.
13. Brewer TG: Treatment of acute gastroesophageal variceal hemorrhage, *Med Clin North Am* 77(5):993-1009, 1993.
14. Smith JL, Graham DY: Variceal hemorrhage. A critical evaluation of survival analysis, *Gastroenterology* 82:968, 1982.
15. Gunnlaugsson O: Angiodysplasia of the stomach and duodenum, *Gastrointest Endosc* 31:251, 1985.
16. Peterson WL, Laine L: Gastrointestinal bleeding. In *Gastrointestinal diseases*, ed 5, Philadelphia, 1993, WB Saunders.
17. Cook JD, Skikne BS: Iron deficiency: definition and diagnosis, *J Int Med* 226:349, 1989.
18. Pianka JD, Affronti J: Management principles of gastrointestinal bleeding, *Prim Care Clin Office Pract* 28(3): 557-575, 2001.
19. Ferri FF: Gastrointestinal bleeding. In *Ferri's clinical advisor*, St Louis, 2002, Mosby.
20. Bono MJ: Lower gastrointestinal bleeding, *Emerg Clin North Am* 14(3):547-556, 1996.
21. Oldfield EC, Wallace MR: The role of antibiotics in the treatment of infectious diarrhea, *Gastroenterol Clin North Am* 30(3):817-835, 2001.
22. Koutkia P and others: Enterohemorrhagic *Escherichia coli* 0157:H7: an emerging pathogen, *Am Fam Physician* 56(3):853-856, 1997.
23. Eisen GM and others: An annotated algorithmic approach to acute lower gastrointestinal bleeding, *Gastrointest Endosc* 53(7):859-863, 2001.
24. Eisen GM and others: Guidelines: enteroscopy, *Gastrointest Endosc* 53(7):871-873, 2001.
25. U.S. Preventive Screening Task Force: Screening for colorectal cancer. In *Guide to clinical preventive services*, ed 2, Baltimore, 1996, Williams and Wilkins.

CHAPTER 148

Hepatitis

Wendy L. Biddle

DEFINITION/EPIDEMIOLOGY

Hepatitis is a general term for inflammation in the liver. There are numerous causes of hepatitis, including viruses, alcohol, medications, autoimmune disease, and metabolic defects. Inflammation that continues for 6 months is considered chronic liver disease and can eventually result in cirrhosis, characterized by scarring and death of hepatocytes. There were more than 5.5 million cases of chronic liver disease and cirrhosis in 1998, for a rate of 2,030 cases per 100,000 population. Chronic liver disease accounts for $1.4 billion in direct health care costs per year.[1]

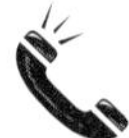

Physician consultation and referral is indicated for patients with newly diagnosed hepatitis

Viral Hepatitis

Viral hepatitis is attributed to five main groups of viruses that attack the liver: hepatitis virus A (HAV), B (HBV), C (HCV; previously known as non-A, non-B), D (HDV; previously known as delta and occurring only as co-infection with HBV), and E (HEV). The features of the viruses are described in Table 148-1. There is a sixth virus, G (HGV), which is new; it has been isolated, but little is known about it.[2] Other viruses can cause a secondary hepatitis that never becomes chronic. Acute viral hepatitis can range in severity from a clinically asymptomatic infection to fulminant liver failure and death. Chronic viral hepatitis is considered to be the presence of virus 6 months from initial exposure and can range in severity from mild disease with minimal inflammation to cirrhosis, liver failure, and/or hepatocellular carcinoma.

HAV is an RNA virus in the Picornaviridae family. In developed countries, hepatitis A accounts for up to one third of all cases of viral hepatitis. All strains of this virus belong to the same serotype; as a result, HAV immunoglobulin provides worldwide protection.[3] The virus can be inactivated by boiling for 1 minute or by exposure to formaldehyde, chlorine, or ultraviolet radiation. HAV occurs globally and is transmitted via the fecal-oral route, through person-to-person contact, and through the ingestion of contaminated food or water. Poor

TABLE 148-1 Features of Viral Hepatitis

	Hepatitis A	Hepatitis B	Hepatitis C	Hepatitis D	Hepatitis E
Incubation period	2-6 weeks	2-6 months	2-22 weeks	4-8 weeks	2-9 weeks
Onset	Usually acute	Usually insidious	Usually insidious	Usually acute	Usually acute
Symptoms					
Nausea and vomiting	Common	Common	Common	Common	Common
Fever	Common	Uncommon	Uncommon	Uncommon	Uncommon
Jaundice	50%	33%	25%	?	10%-20%
Arthralgias	Rare	Common	Rare	Rare	Rare
Diagnosis	IgM anti-HAV	HBsAg	Anti-HCV	IgM anti-HDV	Anti-HEV
Transmission					
Fecal-oral	Usual	Rare	No	?	Usual
Parenteral	Rare	Usual	Usual	Usual	No
Sexual	Yes	Yes	Yes	?	?
Perinatal	No	Yes	Yes	?	No
Sequelae					
Chronic carrier	No	5%-10%	Up to 75%	?Most	No
Chronic active hepatitis	No	Approximately 5%	75%	Up to 70%	No
Fulminant hepatitis	Approximately 0.1%	0.2%-1.0%	No	Up to 17%	2%-10%*
Recovery	>99%	85%-90%	—	?	90%-98%*
Epidemiology					
Epidemics	Foodborne or waterborne	Contaminated blood products	Intravenous drug abuse and contaminated blood products	Contaminated blood products	Foodborne or waterborne
Posttransfusion	Extremely rare	<5% of cases	85%-95% of cases	Possible	No
Prevention	ISG	HBIG vaccine	?ISG	Hepatitis B vaccine	?ISG from endemic areas

Modified from Stein JH and others: *Internal medicine,* ed 4, St Louis, 1994, Mosby.
ISG, Human immune globulin, *HBIG,* hepatitis B immune globulin.
*10%-20% fatalities in pregnant women.

sanitation, poor personal hygiene, and overcrowding increase the transmission rate.

HAV can be found in liver cells, bile, stool, and blood. Hepatitis A has an incubation period of 2 to 6 weeks, with patients being most infectious in the late incubation period. The virus can be found in the stool 2 to 3 weeks before and up to 1 week after the development of clinical jaundice. Despite the presence of HAV in the liver, viral shedding in feces, viremia, and infectivity rapidly decrease once jaundice appears.[4] Therefore most patients are contagious when they are asymptomatic and are no longer contagious by the time they become diagnosed with jaundice. An important exception involves neonates, who can be infectious for up to 6 months after clinical jaundice develops.[3] HAV infection never progresses to chronic hepatitis.

Hepatitis B is endemic worldwide, especially in Asia, where the carrier rate is estimated to be 1:4. It is less prevalent in the United States, but the Centers for Disease Control and Prevention (CDC) (www.cdc.gov/ncidad/diseases/hepatitis/index.htm) estimates there were 205,000 new infections and a total of 1.25 million cases of chronic hepatitis B in 1997.[5] Hepatitis B is endemic among Alaskan natives, with an estimated prevalence of 3% to 8%.[6]

HBV is a DNA virus that belongs to the Hepadnaviridae family. In Asia and Africa, HBV infection is seen mostly among newborns and young children and is spread via vertical transmission from mother to child. In North America and Europe, hepatitis B is more common among adolescents and young adults and is spread via sexual contact and percutaneous exposure. Each year, 10,000 hospital admissions and 250 to 300 deaths are attributed to HBV infection. More than 1 million people in the United States are chronic carriers, and almost 5000 people die from cirrhosis or hepatocellular carcinoma annually. The number of new cases of hepatitis B reported has declined each year since 1985. A safe and effective vaccine against HBV was introduced in 1982.[3]

Hepatitis B can present a clinical picture similar to that of the other subtypes, with a severity that can range from asymptomatic to fulminant and fatal liver failure; it can progress to chronic liver disease with cirrhosis and hepatocellular carcinoma.[4] HBV can be found in blood, tears, cerebrospinal fluid, breast milk, saliva, vaginal secretions, and seminal fluid. HBV is transmitted parenterally, via sexual contact, and perinatally. Heterosexual contact with a person infected with HBV is the most common mode of transmission, followed by IV drug use, homosexual activity and, last, vertical transmission from mother to child at the time of birth. Transmission from a blood transfusion is rare in the United States because of extensive screening processes. HBV is not transmitted via the fecal-oral route or by arthropod vectors. Compared with the general population, health care workers, especially surgeons, phlebotomists, and dialysis nurses, as well as spouses of infected persons, are at an increased risk for contracting HBV.

Hepatitis C, a primary reason for liver transplantation, has reached epidemic level in the United States, with an estimated 4 million people infected and anti-HCV seropositive (1% to 3% of the general population) and 2.7 million chronically viremic. Fortunately, new infections of HCV are uncommon; the primary cause of the approximately 38,000 new cases that occur per year is injection drug use.[7] Most infections occurred 10 to 30 years earlier. It is estimated that 20% to 40% of people with chronic hepatitis C will develop cirrhosis after 20 to 40 years. African Americans appear to have a slower disease progression with less cirrhosis than non–African Americans.[5,8]

HCV, first identified in 1989, is a single-strand RNA genome with a high rate of replication (10^{12} virions/day) and mutation. These characteristics lead to chronic infection, making it difficult to treat.[7] Currently six strains and multiple subtypes of the virus have been identified. Genotypes 2 and 3 respond better to treatment than does genotype 1, but 70% of people in the United States have genotype 1.

Once a person is infected, the body initiates humoral and cellular mechanisms. The Third National Health and Nutrition Examination Survey (NHANES III) found that approximately 75% of patients with HCV develop chronic infection. It is very rare to see fulminant hepatic failure with acute HCV. The 25% believed to have cleared the virus may have a strong cellular immune response to HCV. Ineffective cellular immune responses lead to inflammation and damage in the liver. Extrahepatic manifestations of HCV occur when humoral immune responses are continually stimulated. These can involve the skin, kidney, and nerves. Factors associated with rapid disease progression and cirrhosis include older age at time of infection, alcohol abuse, male gender, and co-infection with HIV.[7]

HCV is transmitted via transfusions, needle sticks, IV drug use, snorting cocaine, and tattoos. Sexual transmission is responsible for up to 20% of new cases, but the overall rate is believed to be low, less than 5%. Those with multiple partners have a 2 to 5 times higher risk of acquiring HCV through sexual contact. Long-term partners should be tested every 5 years. The rate of vertical transmission from mother to child during delivery is approximately 5%. Certain subgroups are believed to have an especially high rate: 20% of those on hemodialysis and even higher rates in prisoners.[7] People in certain occupations, such as emergency medical technicians, paramedics, rescue workers, and police and fire officers, may be at higher risk also. Co-infection of HCV and HIV is becoming more prevalent, creating unique challenges in management. There is no evidence that arthropod vectors transmit HCV.

HDV is a DNA virus that requires co-infection with HBV for replication. It can be transmitted with HVB or may superinfect an individual who is already infected with HBV. It is transmitted parenterally through IV drug use and rarely via sexual contact. Perinatal transmission is rare and can be prevented through HBV prophylaxis. When seen in the Mediterranean region, HDV is endemic with HBV. In nonendemic areas such as the United States, HDV is associated with percutaneous exposure and blood transfusions. HDV is not transmitted through the fecal-oral route or casual contact.

HEV is another RNA virus that has been identified as being responsible for some cases of non-A, non-B hepatitis. This virus has a short incubation period of 15 to 60 days and usually results in a self-limited disease. It is more common in children and young adults. Similar to HAV, HEV is enterically spread, most commonly via the ingestion of contaminated water. Areas endemic for HEV are Asia, Africa, and Central America. There have been no known cases in the United States, and international travelers are the only group at risk.[9] Infection during pregnancy can lead to liver failure, especially during the third trimester, with mortality rates as high as 30%.[3]

Alcoholic Hepatitis

Alcoholic hepatitis is a type of toxic liver injury associated with excessive alcoholic consumption on a chronic basis, usually 10 years or longer. It is estimated that 10% to 35% of heavy drinkers develop alcoholic hepatitis. There is some controversy on the levels of alcohol that constitute heavy drinking, but an average of two to three drinks a day for a man and one to two drinks a day for a woman is recognized as increasing the risk of liver disease.[10]

Toxic Hepatitis

Toxic hepatitis is also known as *drug-induced hepatitis* and is usually not dependent on preexisting liver disease. The full range of severity may be expressed in any setting in which drugs are taken. Drug-induced liver disease accounts for between 1:600 and 1:3500 hospital admissions and between 2% and 3% of all hospital admissions resulting from adverse drug reactions. Between 500 and 1000 therapeutic agents have been implicated in the etiology of a broad spectrum of hepatic diseases. Drugs account for approximately 15% to 30% of all fulminant hepatic failures.[11] A thorough drug history should include information about recent and past exposure to therapeutic agents. Details about the patient's occupation and work environment, as well as the use of herbal preparations and "traditional" medications, should be obtained.[11]

Cirrhosis

Cirrhosis is one of the leading causes of death in the United States, killing approximately 25,000 people per year (9.3 deaths per 100,000), and alcohol is responsible for close to 50% of cirrhosis-related deaths.[12] Studies suggest a genetic predisposition to alcoholic liver disease, and some ethnic groups are at higher risk, such as Native Americans. Heavy alcohol intake can affect nutritional status, producing primary and/or secondary malnutrition, which in turn can cause more liver damage.[13]

PATHOPHYSIOLOGY

Process of Inflammation and Development of Cirrhosis

The process of inflammation and development of scarring and cirrhosis is similar for all causes of hepatitis. The pathology of hepatitis involves inflammation and damage to the hepatocyte. Fibrosis and scarring with isolated hepatocyte injury and focal necrosis can develop. Mononuclear infiltration, which consists mostly of lymphocytes, invades the tissue, particularly around the portal triads. Cellular edema and death can occur. There may be a minor degree of periportal necrosis of hepatocytes around these triads, which gives the liver an appearance of piecemeal necrosis on microscopic examination. After the hepatocyte degenerates, its cytoplasm shrinks and condenses to form an acidophil body. The available space is then temporarily filled by monocytes. Although characteristic of acute viral hepatitis, these cytologic changes are not specific to this disease and can also be found with drug-induced injuries and other disease processes.[14]

The inflammatory and scarring processes can lead to "bridging" fibrosis between portal triads. This level of fibrosis and moderate inflammation is a sign that cirrhosis will develop if the damage continues. Increased numbers of liver cells begin to die; consequently, there may be more collapse and condensation of the liver stroma. This may occur over months in a severe acute injury but is more commonly seen in chronic infection, taking 10 or more years to develop.[14] Bridging necrosis and confluent necrosis can resolve, enabling complete regeneration and histologic recovery in acute hepatitis. Chronic hepatitis, however, can remain mild with little to no scarring ever developing. If scarring does develop it is unlikely to improve unless treatment is instituted. Over time, cirrhosis can lead to liver failure and/or hepatocellular carcinoma and death. Approximately 20% of people with cirrhosis from chronic hepatitis will develop a carcinoma.

Pathogenesis of Hepatitis

The exact pathogenesis of hepatitis A, C, D, and E is not clear. It seems that HBV involves immune complex–mediated tissue damage. Hepatitis B core antigen present on the hepatocyte cell membrane may act as a target for host antibody responses. Circulating immune complexes play an important role in explaining the extrahepatic diseases and serum sickness associated with HBV. These circulating complexes activate the complement system and can cause rash, fever, and angioedema when present as serum sickness or as other forms of immune complex disease such as glomerulonephritis and polyarteritis nodosa.[4]

Although the exact mechanism of alcohol damage to the liver is not known, there are several hypotheses. Ethanol is oxidized in the mitochondria, producing toxins that have harmful effects on lipid and carbohydrate metabolism. Acetylaldehyde is increased, causing hypoxia at the terminal veins in the liver, and oxygen-derived free radicals may cause damage of the liver cells. Proinflammatory cytokines are expressed, stimulating cells to produce collagen that leads to fibrosis.

Liver damage from hepatotoxins, such as chlorpromazine, rifampin, and estrogens, is variable depending on the drug, dose, and individual hypersensitivity. Damage can appear quickly or may take weeks to months after beginning the medication. Proposed mechanisms include alteration of the membranes, interference with the hepatic uptake process, and free radicals causing lipid peroxidation.[13]

CLINICAL PRESENTATION

Most people are not aware when they develop an acute hepatitis because the symptoms are similar to those of any other mild viral illness. Symptoms can include anorexia, fatigue, myalgias, nausea, fever, headaches, arthralgias, vomiting, and abdominal pain. Jaundice can occur, especially with HBV, but it is rare in other viral hepatitis illnesses.

Acute viral hepatitis occurs after an incubation period of varying lengths based on the specific virus. For HAV, the incubation period is 15 to 45 days with a mean of 4 weeks; for HBV and HDV, 30 to 180 days with a mean of 4 to 12 weeks; for HCV, 15 to 160 days with a mean of 7 weeks; and for HEV, 14 to 60 days with a mean of 5 to 6 weeks.[4] HDV infection can present as acute or chronic hepatitis and is dependent on HBV status; for HDV infection to occur, HBV must be present either chronically or simultaneously with HDV. These patients may have concomitant infection of both HBV and HDV acutely or a superimposed HDV infection with preexisting HBV. HBV and HDV are clinically indistinguishable from one another. The clinical suspicion for HDV infection should be high in patients who present with fulminant hepatic failure and a history of positive hepatitis B surface antigen (HBsAg); in such cases an anti-HDV test should be ordered. Unfortunately, acute HEV is difficult to diagnose because there are no commercially available tests. Suspicion of HEV should be increased in patients with clinical symptoms of hepatitis and a recent travel history to an underdeveloped country.[3]

People with alcoholic hepatitis commonly present with elevated liver function tests (LFTs) but can be asymptomatic. Often aspartate aminotransferase (AST [SGOT]) is higher than alanine aminotransferase (ALT [SGPT]), usually at a ratio of 2:1. Patients can have nonspecific symptoms such as nausea, vomiting, abdominal discomfort, or diarrhea. Those with advanced liver disease appear ill and malnourished and can be feverish.[10] There may be signs of cirrhosis such as jaundice, ascites, encephalopathy, and upper gastrointestinal bleeding.

The presentation of drug-induced liver disease can be a nonspecific febrile or viral-like illness. The diagnosis of chronic hepatitis can be challenging because patients often are not symptomatic until liver damage has progressed. Risk factors for the development of chronic hepatitis include a young age and immunosuppression.[3] Comparisons of the signs and symptoms of the hepatitis viruses are presented in Box 148-1.

BOX 148-1

SIGNS AND SYMPTOMS OF HEPATITIS

HAV
- May be asymptomatic
- Fever, jaundice, anorexia, nausea, malaise, myalgia
- Infectious 2 weeks before symptoms and 1 week after
- No carrier state or chronic illness

HBV
- May be asymptomatic
- Anorexia, nausea, myalgia, malaise, jaundice to fatal hepatitis
- Infectious 4 to 6 weeks before symptoms and for unpredictable time after symptoms
- Carrier state and chronic illness

HCV
- Few symptoms
- Anorexia, nausea, malaise, rarely jaundice, myalgia
- Infectious 4 to 6 weeks before symptoms and unpredictable after symptoms
- 75% progress to chronic hepatitis

HDV
- May be asymptomatic
- Anorexia, nausea, malaise, jaundice, myalgia
- Infectious 4 to 6 weeks before symptoms and unpredictable after symptoms
- Occurs only with HBV as co-infection or as superinfection in chronic HBV infection

HEV
- May be asymptomatic
- Fever, jaundice, anorexia, nausea, malaise, myalgia
- Infectious 2 weeks before symptoms and 1 week after symptoms
- No carrier or chronic state

From Dunn SA: *Primary care consultant*, St Louis, 1998, Mosby.

PHYSICAL EXAMINATION

A low-grade fever with acute hepatitis is far more common with HAV and HEV, although patients with HBV can develop a serum sickness–like syndrome that can include fever, arthralgias, and rash. Dark-colored urine and clay-colored stools may precede the onset of clinical jaundice by 1 to 5 days. With the onset of jaundice, these constitutional symptoms usually diminish.[3]

On examination, patients with jaundice often have both hepatomegaly and splenomegaly. The onset of jaundice or the icteric phase can be observed when the serum bilirubin is greater than 2.5 mg/dl and is most easily observed in the sclera or under the tongue. Symptomatic hepatitis is difficult to miss, but half of the patients with acute hepatitis do not develop jaundice. On the other end of the spectrum, a smaller portion of patients may develop fulminant hepatic failure.[3]

In alcoholic hepatitis, the physical findings may be consistent with cholestasis. Fever, jaundice, and leukocytosis may be present. Skin rashes are common and patients can have tender hepatomegaly, but splenomegaly is uncommon. Physical signs of alcoholic and nonalcoholic cirrhosis are similar, but it is believed that spider telangiectasia, especially on the trunk and upper extremities; parotid enlargement; gynecomastia; palmar erythema; and hepatomegaly are more common with alcoholic cirrhosis.[10]

The presence of extrahepatic manifestations can suggest toxic hepatitis. Fever, rash, and eosinophilia suggest drug hypersensitivity but are relatively nonspecific findings. Presenting signs may include pseudomononucleosis syndrome (phenytoin), systemic vasculitis (allopurinol and sulfonamides), and bone marrow suppression (nonsteroidal antiinflammatory drugs [NSAIDs]).[11]

DIAGNOSTICS

The first sign of hepatitis may be the elevation of the serum aminotransferases: AST/SGOT and ALT/SGPT. These enzymes increase proportionally during the prodromal phase of hepatitis and can reach 20 times normal. The total bilirubin can continue to increase as the aminotransferases decline and may reach 20 mg/dl. There are equal proportions of direct and indirect bilirubin in patients with hepatitis, and bilirubin will also be present in urine. The prothrombin time (PT) is usually normal in patients with acute hepatitis but may become prolonged in patients with severe hepatitis; thus PT can be used as a marker of prognosis. If the PT is greater than 3 times

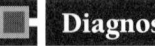

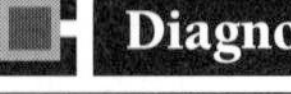
Diagnostics

Hepatitis

Laboratory
ALT, AST, alkaline phosphatase, bilirubin, globulin, protein, albumin, lactate dehydrogenase
CBC and differential, platelets
PT/INR
Hepatitis serologic tests
Genetic markers

Other
Abdominal ultrasound
Biopsy*

*If indicated.

normal (international normalized ratio [INR] >1.5), the patient should be evaluated for fulminant hepatic failure. The WBC count and hemoglobin/hematocrit are usually within normal limits. The platelet count is also normal but may be decreased in fulminant hepatic failure.[3]

Other laboratory tests that may be abnormal, indicating advancing liver damage, are platelet and albumin levels, which will be lower than normal. Anemia may be present. Lactate dehydrogenase and alkaline phosphatase levels are usually normal or mildly elevated. Alkaline phosphatase is not specific to the liver. An elevated alkaline phosphatase level can indicate a fatty liver or obstruction or disease in the bile ducts. If an elevated alkaline phosphatase level is documented, it is useful to determine how much of it is from the liver. Fractionation will show the percentages from the liver, bone, and intestines.

The elevation of aminotransferase levels does not seem to correlate with the histologic severity of the disease.[3] The only test that will provide information on the amount of inflammation and scarring in the liver is a biopsy. There are scoring mechanisms that can be used to provide a fairly standardized measure of the severity of liver disease.[15] Ultrasound and CT scan are both equally useful to document tumors, fatty tissue, and size of the liver. The ultrasound is more cost effective, providing screening information.

Hepatitis A should be suspected if hepatitis infection occurs after the ingestion of contaminated food or shellfish, after natural disasters, in institutionalized adults or children, in patients returning from travel to an endemic area, or in children or families of children in day care facilities. Diagnosis can be confirmed by the presence of immunoglobulin M (IgM) anti-HAV during the acute illness. Eventually, the IgM anti-HAV decreases over several months, and immunoglobulin G (IgG) anti-HAV rises and persists indefinitely.[3]

The diagnosis of acute HBV is dependent on the presence of HBsAg and IgM antibodies to hepatitis B core antigen (antibody) (IgM anti-HBc, or HBcAb), which appear approximately the same time as the symptoms. The antibody to HBsAg (HBs antibody, or anti-HBs) develops after infection (approximately 4 to 5 months after exposure) and serves as an indicator of immunity. Anti-HBs is also detectable in individuals who have received the hepatitis B vaccination series or who have passive immunity secondary to hepatitis B immune globulin (HBIG). Anti-HBc indicates prior exposure or infection and lasts for a prolonged period. The presence of IgM anti-HBc indicates recent infection with HBV, typically within the previous 4 to 6 months.

If hepatitis Be antigen (HBeAg) is detected, the virus is undergoing active viral replication and the patient is highly infectious. Antibodies to HBeAg (anti-HBe) develop in most people with HBV and indicate decreasing infectivity and replication of the virus (inactive phase).[3] Convalescence is suggested by normalization of elevated ALT; by loss of HBsAg, HBeAg, and HBV DNA; and by the development of anti-HBs. If this occurs within 6 months, the episode can be defined as acute hepatitis. Chronic infection occurs in approximately 2% to 5% of acutely infected individuals and is characterized by the persistence of HBsAg beyond 6 and the presence of HBeAg and HBV DNA for months to years.[14]

Clinically evident acute hepatitis C infection occurs less often than HAV or HBV, and often patients are asymptomatic or only mildly ill. The first level of testing is the antibody to hepatitis C (HCV Ab). If this is positive, the viral load should be tested by polymerase chain reaction (HCV RNA PCR). If the viral load is detectable, the patient is considered to have chronic hepatitis C; the serology is not available to distinguish acute from chronic HCV. There are at least six different strains of the virus known and the genotype can be tested as well. The genotype is useful to help determine potential response to treatment.[7]

HDV infection should be considered in patients with acute HBV infection who develop fulminant hepatic failure or in patients with chronic HBV who show evidence of deterioration. Anti-HDV can be detected to confirm the diagnosis of HDV infection. Patients co-infected with HDV have acute HBV and a positive anti-HDV test. Patients with chronic HBV and a positive anti-HDV test are superinfected. In patients who are superinfected, a high titer (>1:100) of anti-HDV indicates chronic hepatitis D.[3]

HEV infection should be considered in patients returning from travel to India, central and southeast Asia, and the Middle East. Unfortunately, there are no commercially available tests for HEV in the United States. If there is epidemiologic evidence of acute HEV infection and if other etiologies have been eliminated, serum should be sent to the CDC, and an expert in hepatitis should be consulted.[3]

In general, if acute viral hepatitis is suspected, the appropriate serologic tests should include IgM anti-HAV, IgM anti-HBc, HBsAg, and anti-HCV. In patients known to have fulminant hepatic failure or a known previous infection with HBV, an anti-HDV test is reasonable. HBsAg, HBcAb, HBsAb, and anti-HCV are the appropriate serologic tests for patients with chronic hepatitis.[3]

Typically, alcoholic hepatitis presents as a cholestasis type of liver disease, with abnormalities seen as elevations in bilirubin and alkaline phosphatase levels. The ratio of AST to ALT is often greater than 2.0, which is considered diagnostic of this disease. Anemia is present in more than 90% of patients with alcoholic hepatitis, and leukocytosis is seen in 41% of patients. In more severe disease, PT may be prolonged, and the albumin concentration is often low. These two proteins are measures of the capacity of the liver to synthesize proteins.

Laboratory testing in the diagnosis of suspected drug-induced liver disease is helpful in excluding other causes of liver disease. Liver biopsy is indicated when the diagnosis remains unclear. Diagnosis depends on the history of exposure; consistent clinical, laboratory, and liver biopsy findings in select cases; and the resolution of liver injury after the presumed toxin has been removed.[11]

Noninvasive markers for hepatic fibrosis have been developed and show promise as adjuncts to diagnosis and management of liver disease.[16] Currently a blood test is available that indicates whether fibrosis is present, absent, or indeterminate. It is hoped that this first-generation test will result in more specific and sensitive testing for liver disease.

DIFFERENTIAL DIAGNOSIS

It is always important that patients be evaluated for other causes of liver disease. For instance, chronically elevated LFTs may be a result of alcoholic liver disease, drug- or toxin-induced hepatitis, hepatic steatosis, cholestatic conditions, metabolic diseases, granulomatous hepatitis, pericholangitis associated with inflammatory bowel disease, or biliary or pancreatic disease. The most common cause of chronically elevated LFTs is fatty liver, affecting up to 20% of the general population. Fatty liver can progress to nonalcoholic steatohepatitis (NASH) and cirrhosis.

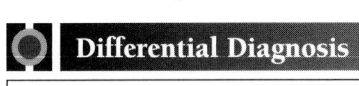

Hepatitis

- Alcoholic liver disease
- Autoimmune hepatitis
- Cholestatic conditions
- Granulomatous hepatitis (sarcoid)
- Hemochromatosis
- Hepatic steatosis
- Medication- or toxin-induced hepatitis
- Metabolic diseases
- Nonalcoholic steatohepatitis (NASH)
- Wilson's disease

The most common drugs known to cause hepatitis are acetaminophen, isoniazid, methotrexate, methyldopa, nitrofurantoin, rifampin, and the cholesterol-lowering statins. Regular monitoring of LFTs is necessary because LFT elevation indicates the presence of liver inflammation. Other viruses can also cause a secondary hepatitis, such as Epstein-Barr virus (EBV), cytomegalovirus (CMV), HIV, herpes simplex virus (HSV), varicella-zoster virus (VZV), adenovirus, and coxsackievirus.

Hemochromatosis, increased levels of iron, is the most common inherited disorder in the United States. Testing of iron saturation and ferritin is used for screening. If elevated levels of iron are found, the gene for hemochromatosis can be sought with a test. Autoimmune hepatitis, seen primarily in young women, can be screened with antinuclear antibodies (ANA) testing. Wilson's disease, an autosomal recessive condition that results in toxic copper accumulation in the liver and other organs, must also be considered. Low levels of serum ceruloplasmin, elevated levels of urinary copper, and Kayser-Fleischer rings in the eyes can establish a diagnosis of Wilson's disease.[3] Sarcoidosis can affect the liver and is seen primarily in African Americans. Obtaining an angiotensin-converting enzyme (ACE) level is used to screen for sarcoid.

MANAGEMENT

The management of acute HAV and HBV consists primarily of treating the acute symptoms and providing supportive care. The vast majority of patients do very well and experience no chronic sequelae. More than 99% of patients with HAV and up to 90% of patients with HBV recover without incident. Patients who recover from HAV infection do not develop chronic problems, whereas 6% to 10% of patients infected with HBV develop varying forms of chronic hepatitis.[3] If chronic hepatitis results from HBV infection, the HBsAg remains positive after the acute infection. In the acute, noncomplicated course the majority of patients do not require hospitalization, and only symptomatic care is needed. LFTs should be monitored every 2 weeks until normalization.

Before 1990 there was no effective treatment for chronic hepatitis. Interferon alfa-2b has since been approved for the treatment of chronic HBV and HCV, with varying success. With the onset of the antiviral age associated with the new anti-HIV drugs, many new chronic hepatitis drugs are currently under investigation.

Recommended treatment for chronic HBV infection in the active phase is subcutaneous injections of interferon alfa-2b 5 million U daily or 10 million U three times weekly for 16 weeks. A sustained response to interferon alfa-2b would be a disappearance of HBV DNA and normalization of ALT and AST that lasts at least 6 months after the completion of therapy. Sustained responses occur in approximately 25% to 40% of cases.[17,18] The side effect profile for interferon alfa-2b can be significant. Flu-like symptoms, fatigue, injection site reactions, and rash are the most common associated complaints.

Currently, the most promising treatment for chronic HCV is PEG-Intron A (interferon alfa-2b in a polyethylene glycol carrier, or peginterferon alfa-2b) and ribavirin. PEG-Intron A is a new formulation that is long acting and has better response rates. Ribavirin is an antiviral medication that improves response rates when combined with interferon. Dosing of the PEG-Intron A and ribavirin is done according to the patient's weight.[19] Recommended treatment time is 6 months for HCV genotypes 2 and 3 and 12 months for genotype 1. Side effects are similar to those for interferon but may be more intense. A sustained response is normalization of LFTs and undetectable viral load after treatment is stopped. Patients are followed periodically after treatment to watch for resurgence of the virus. Patients who relapse can be retreated.

The mainstay of therapy for alcoholic hepatitis is alcohol abstinence. Involvement of family, friends, and support groups may be helpful. Malnutrition is a strong contributor to the morbidity and mortality associated with alcoholic hepatitis, and therefore assessment by a dietitian, adequate diet therapy, and vitamin replacement for deficiencies are essential. Parenteral vitamin B is preferred over oral therapy for better absorption in alcoholic patients. Multivitamin preparations that include folic acid, thiamin, vitamins A and D, and essential minerals are also important. In the absence of hepatic encephalopathy, a high-protein diet is recommended. Corticosteroid therapy in the treatment of alcoholic liver disease is controversial. There are studies that show corticosteroids are beneficial for improvement in short-term survival in severe alcoholic hepatitis. However, if there is gastrointestinal bleeding, active infection, pancreatitis, or decompensated diabetes, corticosteroids are contraindicated. Transplants are considered in patients with proved long-term abstinence, but recidivism is a concern.[10]

The most important principle in the management of toxic liver disease is removal of the suspected drug or offending agent. Supportive care of acute hepatitis and liver failure is provided as necessary. In the case of severe, drug-induced liver failure, urgent liver transplantation can be lifesaving. Currently the only specific treatment available is the administration of *N*-acetylcysteine for acetaminophen overdose. In general, corticosteroids have no value in the treatment of drug-induced liver disease.[11]

LIFE SPAN CONSIDERATIONS

The liver is a remarkable organ that is capable of regeneration. The treatment of hepatitis has been shown to halt progression and improve liver histology. If hepatitis is treated and cirrhosis does not develop, patients can lead normal lives and their life span will be unaffected. If cirrhosis develops, the life span can be greatly reduced because cirrhosis is a leading cause of death.

Hepatitis is often insidious, and liver damage can be ongoing without the patient's knowledge. Often there are no signs or symptoms for many years. Lifestyle becomes an important factor, but it is not the sole issue in deteriorating liver disease. Some patients have very aggressive disease and treatment is difficult. Thus it is imperative that health care providers screen for risk factors and routinely monitor LFTs. Abnormal LFT results should never be ignored. The sooner identification and treatment can begin, the better is the prognosis.

COMPLICATIONS

The most significant complications of hepatitis are cirrhosis, liver failure, and cancer. HAV is an acute, self-limiting disease that does not develop into a chronic carrier state. The majority of patients who contract HBV recover without difficulty, although chronic hepatitis and fulminant hepatic failure can occur with HBV. The greatest risk with chronic HBV is the development of hepatocellular cancer. Fulminant hepatic failure does occur in a small percentage of patients (<1%) with acute HAV and HBV. Rapid elevation of PT (>3 times normal), hyperbilirubinemia, and hepatic encephalopathy indicate fulminant hepatic failure. Hospitalization with rapid organ transplantation is the only treatment option; without transplantation, the mortality rate is very high.

The majority of people (75%) infected with chronic HCV will do well, without complications. The most important factor in the progression of liver damage is alcohol intake. Those who drink regularly can increase their risk of developing cirrhosis to 50% in 5 years and their risk of cancer to 25%. Progression to cirrhosis can result in ascites, hepatic encephalopathy, peripheral edema, esophageal varices, and other complications of end-stage liver failure. Once cirrhosis is present, there is a risk for the development of hepatocellular carcinoma.

Alcoholic hepatitis has a significant risk of cirrhosis, liver failure, and/or cancer if the patient continues to drink alcohol. Physical and psychosocial problems as well as malnutrition are other complications are associated with alcoholism.

The prognosis of toxic liver disease is highly variable and depends on the clinical circumstances and the etiologic agent involved. The overall fatality rate is approximately 5%. There is a much poorer prognosis with some agents because they induce acute hepatic necrosis or cause progressive chronic liver disease and cirrhosis.[14]

INDICATIONS FOR REFERRAL/HOSPITALIZATION

Patients should be referred when abnormal LFT results are found (AST and/or ALT >40 or elevated alkaline phosphatase). Interpretation of testing, need for liver biopsy, and management require specialist input. Mild acute hepatitis can be managed with consultation, but follow-up with a gastroenterologist is necessary with HBV to determine the possibility of chronicity. Patients with chronic HCV should be referred after initial testing. Any patients with signs of decompensation should be emergently admitted to the hospital and gastroenterology consult should be obtained.

PATIENT AND FAMILY EDUCATION

All patients with hepatitis require careful education about the infection, prevention, transmission, treatment options, and complications. The benefit of rest, diet, avoidance of hepatotoxic substances, and medications should be emphasized.

Hepatitis A can be prevented. Contact with obviously contaminated food or water should be avoided, and infected individuals should not handle or prepare food. In addition, personal objects should not be shared, and hands should be washed thoroughly after patient contact. Health care workers should wear gloves when handling blood or body fluids. Travelers to underdeveloped countries should avoid eating uncooked shellfish, fruits, or vegetables or drinking water that could be contaminated.

Currently, the CDC recommends immune globulin for all travelers to developing countries where HAV is endemic. Hepatitis A immune globulin should be considered for travel that is going to be longer than 6 months. Prophylaxis against hepatitis A should be given as soon as possible after exposure (0.02 mg/kg IM), although it is of no benefit if not given within 2 weeks of exposure. Immunization with immune globulin lasts for 6 months. A hepatitis A vaccine is now currently available. The adult dose is 1.0 ml IM followed by a booster dose at 6 to 12 months. For children 2 to 18 years of age, 0.5 ml IM is given 1 month apart. The vaccine is protective for many years, but the total duration of immunity is unknown.[3]

The current plan to eliminate hepatitis B involves routine screening of pregnant women, prophylaxis of infants born to infected women, and routine infant immunization. The hepatitis B vaccine should also be offered to persons at occupational risk, adolescents, IV drug users, recipients of multiple blood products, sexually active individuals, household contacts of HBV carriers, hemodialysis patients, and international travelers. Two vaccines are currently available in the United States: Recombivax HB and Engerix-B. The vaccines are given in a series of three injections: the first two doses 1 month apart, and the third dose given 6 months after the second dose. There are two dosing options for infants: (1) at birth, 1 to 2 months of age, then 6 to 18 months of age; or (2) at 1 to 2 months of age, 4 months of age, then 6 to 18 months of age. If doses are inadvertently missed, the second and third doses should be given 3 to 5 months apart. Antibodies to HBV develop in approximately 90% to 95% of vaccinated individuals but may be as low as 50% to 70% among individuals who are immunocompromised. Checking a titer after the series is completed can determine immune status. Vaccines should be administered in the anterolateral thigh for infants and in the deltoid for adults and children. The vaccine is safe to administer during pregnancy and along with other childhood immunizations.[3]

To prevent transmission, therapy should be initiated immediately after exposure to HBV. It is recommended that infants born to HBsAg-positive women receive HBIG (0.5 ml) and the first dose of the hepatitis B vaccination series within 12 hours of birth, with two more doses of vaccine at 1 and 6 months of age. The recommendations for prophylaxis after sexual exposure to HBV include HBIG (0.06 ml/kg IM) within 14 days of exposure and simultaneous hepatitis B vaccination, with the second and third injections at 1 and 6 months, respectively. The HBIG and hepatitis B vaccines should always be given at different sites.[3]

HBV and HCV are transmitted by blood; therefore patients need to understand the importance of not sharing razor blades, toothbrushes, or nail clippers. Partners need to be tested because sexual transmission is possible. Barrier protection should be used, and partners should be told about the patient's hepatitis infection. Long-term monogamous partners can use their discretion if the partner is hepatitis negative, but all partners should be tested every few years to detect any seroconversion. Transmission from mother to baby during delivery is only about 5%, and it is not recommended to test children until age 16 years. Household contact has an extremely low risk. Patients with chronic hepatitis should clean up their blood spills with bleach and bag any bloodstained material before placing it in the trash.

All patients with liver disease should understand the significant risk of developing cirrhosis and cancer with alcohol ingestion. Patients should be counseled and resources provided to help drinking cessation. Referral to psychotherapy, substance abuse counselors, Alcoholics Anonymous, and support groups can be helpful. Family members and significant others need to be included in counseling and therapy.

Patients with chronic HBV and those with HCV with cirrhosis have a risk of developing hepatocellular carcinoma and need screening with ultrasound and alpha-fetoprotein tumor marker (AFP) every 6 months. Patients with chronic hepatitis should be vaccinated for both HAV and HBV as appropriate.

Treatment with interferon and PEG-Intron A and ribavirin can cause leukopenia and anemia. Patients must follow-up with scheduled appointments and blood tests. Patients must be taught how to administer the injections and need a full disclosure of the side effects of treatment, including depression.

HEALTH PROMOTION

Preventing hepatitis is possible with healthy lifestyles and avoidance of situations that increase risk. A healthy lifestyle includes alcohol and substance abuse avoidance, safe sexual practices, obtaining vaccinations, and regular checkups that include monitoring of LFTs.

Risk factors for hepatitis B and C include illicit IV drug use, intranasal cocaine use, tattoos, sexual contact with IV drug users and multiple sexual partners, blood transfusions before 1992, hemodialysis, occupational exposure to blood and needles, incarceration, and institutionalization.

Once hepatitis is diagnosed, complications and disease progression can be deterred by abstaining from alcohol and substance abuse, obtaining vaccinations, becoming knowledgeable about the disease, and maintaining regular follow-up with the health care provider.

REFERENCES

1. Sandler RS and others: The burden of selected digestive diseases in the United States, *Gastroenterology* 122:1500-1511, 2002.
2. Linnen J and others: Molecular cloning and disease association of hepatitis G virus: a transfusion-transmissible agent, *Science* 271:505-508, 1996.
3. Noskin GA: Prevention, diagnosis, and management of viral hepatitis: a guide for primary care physicians, *Arch Fam Med* 4:923-934, 1995.
4. Dienstag JL, Isselbacher KJ: Acute and chronic hepatitis. In Isselbacher KJ and others, editors: *Harrison's principles of internal medicine,* New York, 1994, McGraw-Hill.
5. Alter MJ and others: The prevalence of hepatitis C virus infection in the United States, 1988 through 1994, *N Engl J Med* 341:556-562, 1999.
6. McMahon BJ and others: Serologic and clinical outcomes of 1536 Alaska natives chronically infected with hepatitis B virus, *Ann Intern Med* 135:759-768, 2001.
7. Komanduri S, Cotler SJ: Hepatitis C: review, *Clin Perspect Gastroenterol* 4:91-99, 2002.
8. Wiley TE, Brown J, Chan J: Hepatitis C infection in African Americans: its natural history and histological progression, *Am J Gastroenterol* 97:700-706, 2002.
9. Zimmerman RK, Ruben FL, Ahwesh ER: Hepatitis B virus infection, hepatitis B vaccine, and hepatitis B immune globulin, *J Fam Pract* 45:295-315, 1997.
10. Walsh K, Alexander G: Alcoholic diver disease, *Postgrad Med J* 76: 280-286, 2000.
11. Zakim D, Boyer T: *Hepatology: a textbook of liver disease,* ed 3, Philadelphia, 1996, WB Saunders.
12. American Gastroenterological Association: *Hepatobiliary and pancreatic disorders in the burden of gastrointestinal diseases,* Bethesda, Md, 2001, The Association.
13. Tucker D: Normal and altered hepatobiliary and pancreatic exocrine function. In Bullock BA, Henze RL, editors: *Focus on pathophysiology,* Philadelphia, 2000, Lippincott Williams and Wilkins.
14. Ockner RK: Acute and chronic hepatitis. In Wyngaaden JB and others, editors: *Cecil textbook of medicine,* ed 19, Philadelphia, 1992, WB Saunders.
15. Albanis E, Friedman SL: Noninvasive markers of hepatic fibrosis, *Clin Perspect Gastroenterol* 5:182-187, 2002.
16. Davis GL: Hepatitis B: diagnosis and treatment, *South Med J* 90: 866-870, 1998.
17. Vail BA: Management of chronic viral hepatitis, *Am Fam Physician* 55:2749-2761, 1998.
18. Hoofnagle JH, Lau D: Chronic viral hepatitis: benefits of current therapies, *N Engl J Med* 334:1470-1471, 1996.
19. Manns MP and others: Peginterferon alfa-2b plus ribavirin compared with interferon alfa-2b plus ribavirin for initial treatment of chronic hepatitis C: a randomised trial, *Lancet* 358:958-965, 2001.

CHAPTER 149

Inflammatory Bowel Disease

Wendy L. Biddle

DEFINITION/EPIDEMIOLOGY

Inflammatory bowel disease (IBD) is a chronic inflammatory condition that affects approximately 2 million people in the United States.[1] There are two types of IBD: ulcerative colitis (UC) and Crohn's disease. Both involve the intestinal tract and typically have periods of remission and exacerbation. Although there are many similarities between UC and Crohn's disease, there are also some significant differences.

UC is a chronic inflammation of the lining of the colonic mucosa. Beginning in the rectum, the inflammation is diffuse and continuous and may involve the entire colon (pancolitis) or only part of the colon. Disease involving only the rectum (proctitis) or involving the rectosigmoid colon accounts for approximately 40% to 50% of the cases of UC. An additional 30% to 40% of patients have disease extending proximally to the splenic flexure (left-sided UC). Twenty percent of patients with UC have pancolitis.[2]

Crohn's disease is a chronic inflammation of all layers of the intestinal tract (transmural inflammation) and can involve any portion of the intestinal tract from the mouth to the anus. Approximately 30% to 40% of patients with Crohn's disease have disease only in the small intestine (ileitis or regional enteritis). The terminal ileum is almost always involved, and 40% to 45% of patients have disease in the small and large intestines (ileocolitis). Approximately 15% to 25% of patients have disease only in the colon (Crohn's colitis, not to be confused with UC). Crohn's disease occurs in the mouth, stomach, and duodenum in a very small percentage of patients.[3]

The transmural involvement in Crohn's disease is responsible for many of the complications that occur. Although the inflammation can be patchy (unlike UC, which is nearly always continuous), the involvement of all layers of the bowel wall creates many problems. Fibrosis occurs from the inflammation and can partially or completely obstruct the lumen of the intestinal wall. Weakening of the intestinal wall from inflammation results in sinus tracts or fistulas. Fistulas can develop from bowel to bowel (enteroenteric), bowel to skin (enterocutaneous), bowel to bladder (enterovesical), or bowel to vagina (enterovaginal).

The annual incidence of UC and the incidence of Crohn's disease are similar in both age of onset and worldwide distribution. The highest incidence of IBD is in North America, Europe, and Australia. The incidence in the developing countries is much less but has been increasing. The incidence in the United States is similar to that reported in Europe.[2,3] The range of reported incidence per 100,000 population in Europe is approximately 10.4 for UC and 5.6 for Crohn's disease. The prevalence in the United States is estimated to be 229 cases per 100,000 population for UC and 133 per 100,000 population for Crohn's disease.[4,5] IBD affects men and women equally, but approximately 20% more men have UC and 20% more women have Crohn's disease.[6] The peak age of onset is between 15 and 25 years, but IBD can appear at any age from infancy to older adulthood.

The cause of IBD is unknown. Research has suggested that UC and Crohn's disease are separate entities that may have different causes, although the mechanisms of inflammation and tissue damage may be similar. Although IBD has been considered an autoimmune process and can behave like an autoimmune disease, there is no strong evidence to suggest that this is the mechanism. It is thought that the intestines normally have a small amount of inflammation present to protect from infection. This normal state can be upset by a number of environmental triggers, resulting in IBD.[7]

In about 20% of persons with IBD, there seems to be a familial tendency in that these individuals have a first-degree relative with IBD.[1] In these families most have the same form of IBD, although both UC and Crohn's disease can occur in the same family. Persons of Jewish ethnicity originating in Europe have been shown to have a much higher risk of developing IBD.

During the past decade, cigarette smoking has been found to have different relationships to UC and Crohn's disease. A history of *current* smoking is a risk factor for Crohn's disease. Several studies have documented the association and an increased risk that is 2 to 5 times higher than that of nonsmokers. Smoking also appears to exacerbate Crohn's disease.[8] *Prior* smoking is a risk factor for the development of UC. More former smokers have UC than do in the general population. The onset of UC tends to occur a few years after quitting smoking.

PATHOPHYSIOLOGY

It is thought that inflammatory and immune cells are responsible for UC and Crohn's disease. A proposed mechanism of inflammation is an infection or other toxin that releases cell wall products that up-regulate macrophages and granulocytes. Macrophages and granulocytes activate circulating cells that migrate into the mucosa, releasing a variety of inflammatory factors such as cytokines, proteases, and oxygen-derived free radicals. These factors all promote inflammation, and the patient has no means of down-regulating the system to inhibit the inflammation. Either the tissue responds by resolving with scarring or other secondary immune reactions continue to create irreversible damage.[7] Many bacteria and other environmental factors have been suggested and studied, but no particular agent has been identified.

CLINICAL PRESENTATION

Both UC and Crohn's disease can have similar presentations and can be difficult to distinguish. Approximately 10% of patients do not have a definite diagnosis, and the disease is known as *indeterminate colitis*. People may complain of symptoms for varying lengths of time, and it is not unusual to have someone report abdominal pain intermittently for years before other symptoms develop. Abdominal pain may be the only presenting complaint. The symptoms of abdominal pain and diarrhea are present in most persons with either disease. The abdominal pain may be diffuse (generalized lower pain) or localized to the right or left lower quadrants. The pain is usually a cramping sensation and can be intermittent or constant.

Tenesmus, or spasms in the rectum, and fecal incontinence may be reported. Stools are often loose and/or watery and may have blood. Rectal bleeding is usually present with colitis, either UC or Crohn's colitis. Patients may report blood seen only on the toilet paper after wiping, blood present in the stool, or clots and large amounts of blood. With proctitis, rectal bleeding may be the only complaint, or constipation may be reported rather than diarrhea.

Other complaints may include fatigue, weight loss, anorexia, fever, chills, nausea, vomiting, joint pains, and mouth sores. Crohn's disease may present with only vague complaints of fatigue and abdominal cramping, but it can present with intestinal obstruction and symptoms of vomiting, bloating, and no stool, as well as with perianal disease of anal fissures, perirectal abscess, or fistula.[9] Pertinent history includes recent antibiotic use or travel, the health of other household members, family history of IBD, previous history of abdominal pain or diarrhea, and medication review.

PHYSICAL EXAMINATION

The patient can appear quite ill or seem to be in no distress. Fever and accompanying tachycardia can be present but often are not. All weight ranges can be seen, from underweight to obese. Conjunctival inflammation and/or oral aphthous ulcers may be present. Abdominal examination usually reveals a tender lower abdomen, which may be more prominent on one side or the other, although the abdomen can be diffusely tender. Hyperactive bowel sounds and palpation of loops of bowel may be noted, as well as a "mass" in the lower right quadrant. Rectal examination for occult blood may be positive, with frank blood and tenderness. Perianal lesions such as an abscess or purulent drainage from a fistulous tract may be present. Joints do not usually appear red or edematous. Skin lesions (e.g., erythema nodosum, pyoderma gangrenosum, or rashes) may also be noted.

DIAGNOSTICS

Blood Tests

A CBC is useful to determine the presence of anemia. The platelet count will often be elevated in the presence of active inflammation or infection. The erythrocyte sedimentation rate (ESR) can be elevated but is a nonspecific marker of inflammation. None of these tests are useful for diagnosis, although they have value in following a patient's progress. In addition, Crohn's disease may result in malabsorption, especially after a small bowel resection. Monitoring electrolytes, glucose, blood urea nitrogen (BUN), creatinine, and the vitamin B_{12} level is necessary to determine and treat deficiencies in Crohn's disease.

Genetic testing is now available as an adjunct to other diagnostics. Two markers, anti–*Saccharomyces cerevisiae* antibodies (ASCA) and perinuclear antineutrophil cytoplasmic antibodies (pANCA), have been developed for clinical use. From 60% to 80% of patients with UC and a subgroup of patients with UC-like CD are positive for pANCA. Sixty percent of patients with CD are positive for ASCA. A recent study examined the value of these markers for diagnosis in the group of patients with indeterminate colitis. The researchers were able to definitively diagnose 31 of 97 patients. Of those diagnosed, the sensitivity and specificity of pANCA and ASCA ranged from 66% to 78%.[10] Currently, the use of these markers is controversial, and further research is needed.

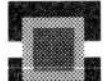
Diagnostics

Inflammatory Bowel Disease

Laboratory
CBC and differential
Platelet count
ESR
Electrolytes
Serum glucose
BUN, creatinine
Vitamin B-12
Genetic testing
- Anti–*Saccharomyces cerevisiae* antibodies (ASCA)
- Perinuclear antineutrophil cytoplasmic antibodies (pANCA)

Stool tests*
- *Giardia*
- *Campylobacter jejuni*
- *Clostridium difficile*
- *Yersinia enterocolitica*
- *Salmonella*
- *Shigella*

If immunocompromised
- Cytomegalovirus
- *Cryptosporidium*
- *Mycobacterium avium-intracellulare*

Imaging*
MRI
Endoscopy
Flexible sigmoidoscopy
Colonoscopy
Barium enema

Other
Biopsy

*If indicated.

Stool Tests

Initial presentation of diarrhea, as well as subsequent flares, should be evaluated for infection. Stool for ova and parasites should be obtained three times to eliminate the most common pathogens. Testing for *Clostridium difficile* is important during flares, especially if there has been recent antibiotic use. Special cultures for other organisms can be requested. Fecal leukocytes can be tested in the stool specimen and are present with inflammation.

Radiography

The barium enema is of limited use in diagnosing IBD and is most useful in detecting colonic distention, obstruction, fistulas, strictures, or tumors. It can detect an abnormal terminal ileum (useful in diagnosing Crohn's disease), but there are moderate false-positive and false-negative rates. A barium enema should not be used in patients with moderate to severe colitis because there is perforation risk when the colon is weakened from inflammation. MRI may be helpful in detecting fistulas and abscesses in patients with perianal Crohn's disease.

Endoscopy

Flexible sigmoidoscopy examines the lower 30 inches of the colon and is useful to determine the source of bright red rectal bleeding. It is more useful for UC than for Crohn's disease because UC almost always shows rectal inflammation; however, not all of the inflamed tissue may be visible if the disease extends beyond the splenic flexure. Flexible sigmoidoscopy can be done with or without cleansing the bowels first, although usually a cleansing preparation is used. An enema can be administered just before the procedure to remove stool in the lower portion of the colon.

Colonoscopy is useful in differentiating UC and Crohn's disease. Bowel cleansing is usually necessary for colonoscopy. Bowel preparations vary among institutions; many use a flavored osmotic salt solution that patients drink in large quantities the night before the colonoscopy.

Both UC and Crohn's disease may have distinguishing features endoscopically that, if found, may help differentiate one from the other. On endoscopy, UC inflammation will be continuous with disease in the rectum, up to the point that the inflammation stops. Crohn's disease can have "skip areas," sections of normal mucosa intermixed with inflamed mucosa. This skipping gives a cobblestone appearance to the mucosa. However, these distinguishing features may not be present, making the diagnosis difficult. Another useful endoscopic finding is an inflamed or abnormal terminal ileum that is almost exclusively present in Crohn's disease.

Mucosal biopsy samples, usually 3 to 4 mm, are especially helpful in diagnosis of IBD. Microscopically, acute and chronic inflammation can be seen. It may be difficult to distinguish UC from Crohn's disease, and in these patients the disease may be labeled "indeterminate colitis" until a clear diagnosis can be made. UC can have cryptitis and crypt abscesses, whereas Crohn's disease can show aphthous ulcers and granulomas.[2,3]

Virtual colonoscopy is being developed as an alternative to screening colonoscopy for colon cancer. This is done with a CT scan and requires the patient to be inflated with a large amount of air. The test is uncomfortable and costly and has a varying miss rate of polyps. It is not recommended as yet and has no role in diagnosing or managing IBD.

DIFFERENTIAL DIAGNOSIS

There are several diagnoses that should be excluded when a patient presents with the common symptoms of IBD: abdominal pain, rectal bleeding, and/or diarrhea.

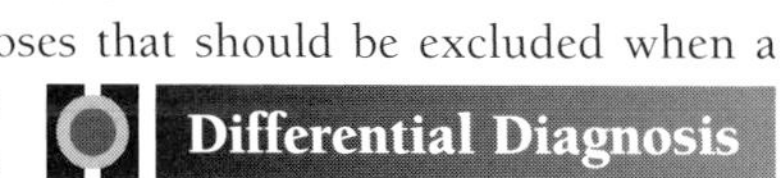

Inflammatory Bowel Disease

- Infectious causes
- Irritable bowel
- Pelvic inflammatory disease
- Appendicitis
- Ischemic colitis
- Radiation enteritis
- Lymphoma
- Systemic vasculitis
- Medications
- Bleeding from hemorrhoids, fissures, polyps

Rectal bleeding should never be ignored or assumed to be benign and should always be further evaluated. Bleeding may be from hemorrhoids, a fissure, or a colonic polyp. Abdominal pain in women may indicate endometriosis or pelvic inflammatory disease. Abdominal pain and diarrhea without bleeding may signify irritable bowel syndrome or appendicitis. Irritable bowel syndrome is a chronic, benign condition with no organic disease present.

Infectious causes of diarrhea need to be excluded. The most common pathogenic organisms to consider are *Giardia, Campylobacter jejuni, C. difficile* (especially with a history of recent antibiotic use), *Yersinia enterocolitica, Salmonella,* and *Shigella.* If a host is immunocompromised, infections with such organisms as cytomegalovirus, *Cryptosporidium,* and *Mycobacterium avium-intracellulare* should be excluded.[11]

Noninfectious causes include ischemic colitis (especially in patients over age 60 years), radiation enteritis or colitis (history of radiation to abdomen or pelvis; may be a late sequelae), lymphoma, and systemic vasculitis. Over-the-counter medications that can be a source of diarrhea include antacids with magnesium, mints with sorbitol, and laxatives. Medications that can produce an inflammatory colitis include antibiotics, chemotherapeutic agents, nonsteroidal antiinflammatory drugs (NSAIDs), and gold.[11]

MANAGEMENT

5-Aminosalicylic Acid

The primary medications for UC are the 5-aminosalicylic acid (ASA) products. Sulfasalazine has been used since the 1940s and has been proved to be safe and effective, even with long-term use. Sulfasalazine is a sulfapyridine and a 5-ASA product connected by a bond. The 5-ASA has been shown to be the active ingredient, and the sulfapyridine is responsible for most of the side effects. Several 5-ASA products have become available during the past 10 years (Table 149-1). Studies have shown that 4 g/day in divided doses is effective in establishing remission in colitis. 5-ASA suppositories are very effective for proctitis.

The 5-ASA products are also efficacious in treating UC and maintaining remission.[12] There is a rare occurrence of allergy to 5-ASA, and if this occurs, the drug should be stopped. Patients will present with a worsening of their colitis symptoms that will improve with discontinuation of the medication. 5-ASA medications are most useful for ulcerative colitis and disease in the colon. They have very limited use for small bowel disease, although occasionally a person with Crohn's disease of the small bowel will respond to 5-ASA. Some preparations of mesalamine (Pentasa, Asacol) may help inflammation that is present in the small bowel.

Corticosteroids

Oral and parenteral steroids are to be avoided if possible because of potential long-term side effects, including diabetes, osteoporosis, and cataracts. For disease that is not responding to 5-ASA or other medications, prednisone is usually started at doses of 40 to 60 mg PO q.d., although occasionally higher doses are used. Tapering to a lower dose is attempted within a few weeks. The tapering schedule depends greatly on the patient's response. A patient's symptoms may be improved within a few days to a week of beginning prednisone. If a response is not immediate, the higher dose may be continued until a response is noted or the patient is hospitalized. The goal is to use a minimal dose of prednisone for a minimal amount of time. Once remission is achieved, patients are tapered off of steroids

TABLE 149-1 Comparison of Medications for Ulcerative Colitis

Brand Name	Generic Name	How Supplied	Route	Daily Dose for Active Disease*	Daily Dose for Maintenance of Remission*	Common Side Effects
Azulfidine	Sulfasalazine	500-mg tablets	Oral	4 g (8 pills)	2 g (4 pills)	Headache, nausea, allergy to sulfa
Asacol	Mesalamine	400-mg delayed-release tablets	Oral	2.4 g (6 pills)	1.6 g (4 pills)	Dyspepsia, abdominal pain
Dipentum	Olsalazine	250-mg capsules	Oral	1 g (4 capsules)	1 g (4 capsules)	Diarrhea
Pentasa	Mesalamine	250-mg capsules	Oral	4 g (16 capsules)	1.5 g (6 capsules)	GI upset, headache
Rowasa	Mesalamine	4 g/60 ml	Rectal/retention enema	4 g (1 enema)	Every other night or less often	Hemorrhoids, rectal pain
Rowasa	Mesalamine	500-mg suppositories	Rectal	1 g (2 suppositories)	500 mg (1 suppository)	Rectal irritation

*Oral medications should be taken 2-4 times daily as indicated.

as soon as possible, although long, slow tapers may be necessary to prevent a flare. There is no proven use of steroids as maintenance therapy for Crohn's disease.

Rectal steroids in the form of a retention enema or foam are useful for colitis and can provide relief of urgency and spasm in the rectum, in addition to healing the inflamed mucosa. Rectal steroids are used for a few weeks, usually until there is an improvement of rectal symptoms. There is some absorption of the steroid systemically; thus long-term use (greater than a few months) is not routinely recommended.

Immunomodulators

There is a trend to use immunomodulators earlier in the course of disease than they have been used in the past. Azathioprine and 6-mercaptopurine (6-MP) may allow the patient to avoid steroids and are useful for steroid dependency. Some clinicians advocate using these medications as first-line treatment in CD.[13] These medications must be taken for 4 to 5 months before the full effect is seen. A CBC must be obtained periodically because of the risk of bone marrow suppression.[14] A CBC should be done weekly initially, then biweekly for 4 weeks, and then monthly. The development of leukopenia or thrombocytopenia warrants immediate discontinuation of the drug. Other adverse reactions, such as pancreatitis and hepatotoxicity, can also occur, requiring termination of treatment. Pancreatitis usually occurs within the first 2 months. An amylase level can be obtained after the first week of treatment and then 4 weeks later, but patients usually present with a clinical picture of pancreatitis, complaining of abdominal pain. Hepatotoxicity is rare, but monitoring liver function tests (LFTs) after the first month and then every 2 to 4 months is recommended. If an elevated liver enzyme level is found, the test should be repeated in 1 to 2 weeks. If the levels remain elevated or continue to rise, the drug should be discontinued and the patient referred to the gastroenterologist for further evaluation. Levels that are twice normal or higher are especially concerning and should prompt an immediate referral to a gastroenterologist.

Genetic testing can be used to monitor and optimize therapy with 6-MP. Thiopurine methyltransferase (TPMT) genotyping determines the patient's ability to produce the TPMT enzyme. The available testing can help identify those patients who would tolerate the drug and can also monitor drug metabolites to maximize the therapeutic effect.[13,15]

Parenteral methotrexate has been shown to be effective in CD, although there are less long-term data available than with 6-MP or azathioprine. Methotrexate has been shown to induce and maintain remission in CD. CBC values should be monitored periodically. Monitoring for hepatotoxicity with liver biopsies is controversial.[13]

Miscellaneous Medications

Metronidazole is effective in treating perianal disease and in healing fistulas associated with Crohn's disease. Other antibiotics such as ciprofloxacin are sometimes used, but sufficient data on efficacy are lacking. Research is ongoing on the use of antibiotics with IBD.

Biologics are the newest and most promising class of medications under development in the treatment of refractory CD. Infliximab, a tumor necrosis factor blocker, is indicated for refractory CD. It is administered intravenously at 2- to 3-month intervals. Serious adverse reactions include infection, infusion reactions, serum sickness–like reaction, and lupus-like syndrome. All patients must have a negative tuberculin test (PPD) before beginning therapy. Given alone or in combination with other immunomodulators, infliximab has induced remission in 25% to 35% and improvement in 45% to 54% of patients with refractory CD.[13] Studies are ongoing with infliximab and other patient populations. Other biologics and probiotics are under investigation, but probiotics are not recommended for IBD at this time.

Surgery

Approximately 20% of patients with UC and 66% of patients with Crohn's disease require surgery for refractory disease.[16] Patients with intractable disease are generally not responding to high doses of medications and may be systemically sick, with weight loss, anemia, nausea, and vomiting. Surgery is also indicated when dysplasia or cancer is found on biopsy. In UC a total colectomy is usually necessary. After surgery patients no longer have the colonic disease and can be taken off all IBD medications. Complications such as liver disease and ankylosing spondylitis may still be present, and treatment for these and other complications will need to be continued. Options for surgical treatment include an ileostomy and an ileal pouch–anal anastomosis (IPAA). With an IPAA the colon is removed except for some rectal tissue, the small intestine is anastomosed to the rectum, and an internal pouch is created to store stool. Patients have no external bag but will have several loose stools a day and can develop complications.

In Crohn's disease the average time from diagnosis to surgery is about 3 years. Surgery is indicated for medical therapy that failed, small bowel obstruction, fistulas, and abscesses. Up to 10% to 15% of patients are diagnosed with Crohn's disease by surgery. A small bowel or colonic resection is the most common surgical procedure, although colectomy may be necessary in some patients. Many patients do well after surgery, but recurrence can occur in up to 80% of patients within 6 months.[17] Approximately one third of patients who had a resection will require a second procedure, and a smaller number of patients will require additional surgical procedures.

LIFE SPAN CONSIDERATIONS

Studies have demonstrated an increased risk of colorectal cancer in patients with IBD, especially those with pancolitis. The risk in UC begins to increase after 10 years of disease and continually rises.[18] Surveillance with colonoscopy is recommended on a regular basis after 8 to 10 years of disease. Those patients with left-sided, limited colitis have a slight increase in risk but do not require as rigorous surveillance as do those with pancolitis.

Less is known about colorectal cancer in Crohn's disease. The risk in Crohn's disease also appears to be increased with disease duration.[19] It is thought that surveillance is necessary for Crohn's disease. Issues surrounding surveillance are controversial, and more extensive, long-term research is needed.

COMPLICATIONS

A number of extraintestinal manifestations can occur with IBD. These primarily involve the eyes, mouth, peripheral joints, skin, and blood vessels. Some are related to the inflammatory activity of the bowel. They become active when the bowel inflammation is active and resolve when the IBD is in remission. These manifestations include aphthous stomatitis, iritis, uveitis, episcleritis, arthritis, and skin lesions (pyoderma gangrenosum, erythema nodosum).

Peripheral arthritis occurs in 10% to 12% of patients with UC and in up to 22% of patients with Crohn's disease. Knees, ankles, and shoulders are most often affected. Between 1% and 26% of patients with UC and 3% to 16% of patients with Crohn's disease develop ankylosing spondylitis. Treatment of the underlying IBD is the best management approach for the arthritis, although symptomatic treatment can be used. Caution should be used in treating with NSAIDs because they can trigger a flare of IBD.[20]

Other complications include liver disease (sclerosing cholangitis), gallstones, malabsorption (Crohn's disease of the small bowel), and renal disease (stones, amyloidosis). Both men and women with IBD are at risk for osteoporosis, independent of steroid use. These complications are not associated with the inflammatory activity and need to be treated with standard management.

INDICATIONS FOR REFERRAL/HOSPITALIZATION

The diagnosis of IBD can be difficult and requires physician consultation. Referral for diagnostic and follow-up endoscopy procedures, as well as management, is the best approach. Once a patient is on a treatment regimen, primary care providers may be able to co-manage the IBD. Continual, close consultation with a gastroenterologist is necessary for optimal management and various treatment options.

Hospitalization is necessary at times for bowel rest, hydration, and parenteral medications. Patients who develop systemic symptoms such as weight loss, nausea, vomiting, severe abdominal pain, significant blood loss, or malnutrition should be evaluated and referred immediately.

PATIENT AND FAMILY EDUCATION

IBD has a significant impact on the quality of life for patients and their families. The stigma of a chronic bowel disease creates a unique set of problems. Patients may be afraid or unwilling to discuss their disease with loved ones, friends, and co-workers. Embarrassment about the symptoms and the need to be near a bathroom can prevent patients from participating in activities and outings. Fear of pain and diarrhea may keep them from eating, and they may become malnourished. Frequent visits and embarrassing, uncomfortable procedures may prevent them from seeking medical care when needed.

There is a great need for patient education for better disease management. Understanding the disease process, potential complications, medication side effects, and risks, such as cancer, is imperative. The need for regular health care visits and the importance of treatments and scheduled procedures should be emphasized. The patient should be educated about the need for a well-balanced diet and informed that there is no specific diet to follow for IBD. Written materials, videos, and educational meetings are available. The Crohn's and Colitis Foundation of America (CCFA) is a national patient organization that can provide information and support. There are also many local support groups that can provide a forum for learning, as well as support, for patients and their significant others.

When teaching patients with IBD, it is important to remember that they will be overwhelmed at first. Repetition is necessary to ensure that patients understand. Many visual aids are available that can be useful in helping patients understand the disease and the procedures and tests that are necessary. In addition, because patients can obtain a great deal of misinformation from the media and well-meaning friends, relatives, and others, correction of misinformation and misconceptions will help. Above all, establishing a trusting, comfortable relationship and listening carefully to patients are vital to the long-term management of IBD.

HEALTH PROMOTION

IBD is a disease of remission and exacerbation. The cause is unknown. Family history plays a limited role; only 20% of IBD patients have a family member with IBD. Cigarette smoking tends to exacerbate Crohn's disease but smoking cessation increases the risk of developing UC. Still, all patients should be encouraged to stop smoking because the risks of smoking far outweigh any benefit.

IBD is a chronic disease with no known cure. Patients should be encouraged to maintain a healthy lifestyle, which should include stress management. Compliance with the prescribed treatment regimen and regular follow-up are the two most important strategies a patient can implement to maximize health. Maintenance of remission can be achieved with medications, with the right dose. People with IBD are at higher risk for colon cancer and need regular colon cancer surveillance. Maintaining regular follow-up with their health care providers and contacting their provider with early signs of a flare will help to minimize problems. Patients need to understand their medication regimen, the importance of not self-adjusting doses, and what monitoring is necessary. Family members need to be a part of the health care team as well. Primary care providers can play a significant role in keeping the patient on task with their appointments, medications, and testing, ensuring the patient will obtain the highest level of wellness possible.

Patient Information

Crohn's and Colitis Foundation of America: http://www.ccfa.org, 1-800-932-2423

National Digestive Diseases Information Clearinghouse: http://www.niddc.nih.gov

REFERENCES

1. The American Society of Colon and Rectal Surgeons: Retrieved June 7, 2002, from the World Wide Web: http://www.fascrs.org.
2. Jewell DP: Ulcerative colitis. In Feldman M, Scharschmidt BF, Sleisenger MH, editors: *Sleisenger and Fordtran's gastrointestinal disease: pathophysiology/diagnosis/management,* ed 6, vol 2, Philadelphia, 1998, WB Saunders.
3. Kornbluth A, Sachar DB, Salomon P: Crohn's disease. In Feldman M, Scharschmidt BF, Sleisenger MH, editors: *Sleisenger and Fordtran's gastrointestinal disease: pathophysiology/diagnosis/management,* ed 6, vol 2, Philadelphia, 1998, WB Saunders.
4. Loftus EV and others: Ulcerative colitis in Olmsted County, Minnesota, 1940-1993: incidence, prevalence, and survival. *Gut* 46: 336-343, 2000.
5. Loftus EV and others: Crohn's disease in Olmsted county, Minnesota, 1940-1993: incidence, prevalence, and survival, *Gastroenterology* 114:1161-1168, 1998.
6. Lashner BA: Epidemiology of inflammatory bowel disease, *Gastroenterol Clin North Am* 24(3):467-474, 1995.
7. Sartor RB: Current concepts of the etiology and pathogenesis of ulcerative colitis and Crohn's disease, *Gastroenterol Clin North Am* 24(3):475-507, 1995.
8. Rhodes J, Thomas G: Nicotine treatment in ulcerative colitis: current status, *Drugs* 49(2):157-160, 1995.
9. Colonna T, Korelitz BI: Diagnosis and treatment of Crohn's disease, *Cortlandt Forum* August:169-177, 1995.
10. Joossens S and others: The value of serologic markers in indeterminate colitis: a prospective follow-up study, *Gastroenterology* 122(5): 1242-1247, 2002.
11. Young JL, Miner PB Jr: The differential diagnosis of inflammatory bowel disease, *Pract Gastroenterol* 19(2), 1995.
12. Sutherland LR, Roth DE, Beck PL: Alternatives to sulfasalazine: a meta-analysis of 5-ASA in the treatment of ulcerative colitis, *Inflamm Bowel Dis* 3(2):65-78, 1997.
13. Hanauer SB and others: The experts answer FAQs (frequently asked questions) in managing IBD, *Clinician* 20(1), 2002.
14. Griffin MG, Miner PB: Conventional therapy in inflammatory bowel disease, *Gastroenterol Clin North Am* 24(3):509-521, 1995.
15. Dubinsky MC and others: Pharmacogenomics and metabolite measurement for 6-mercaptopurine therapy in inflammatory bowel disease, *Gastroenterology* 115:822-829, 1998.
16. Platell C and others: Crohn's disease: a colon and rectal department experience, *Aust NZ J Surg* 65:570-575, 1995.
17. Hanauer SB: Refractory Crohn's disease. In Prantera C, Korelitz BI, editors: *Crohn's disease,* New York, 1996, Marcel Dekker.
18. Sugita A and others: Colorectal cancer in ulcerative colitis: influence of anatomical extent and age at onset on colitis-cancer interval, *Gut* 32:167-169, 1991.
19. Gillen CD and others: Crohn's disease and colorectal cancer, *Gut* 35:651-655, 1994.
20. Anderson M, Robinson M: Watching for—and managing—joint problems in inflammatory bowel disease, *J Musculoskel Med* November: 28-34, 1996.

CHAPTER 150

Irritable Bowel Syndrome

Elizabeth Friedlander

DEFINITION/EPIDEMIOLOGY

Irritable bowel syndrome (IBS) is a gastrointestinal (GI) condition that is classified as a "functional" GI disorder because there are no identifiable structural or biochemical etiologies by which to explain its development.[1] According to the 1997 American Gastroenterological Association medical position paper, IBS is defined as a combination of chronic or recurrent GI symptoms that are not explained by structural or biochemical abnormalities, are attributed to the intestines, and are associated with symptoms of pain and/or symptoms of bloating and distention.[2]

IBS has been defined using the Manning criteria (symptom-based criteria widely used in clinical research) and, more recently, the Rome II criteria.[3,4] Manning and others[5] identified six symptoms common in IBS: abdominal distention, relief of pain with defecation, sensation of incomplete evacuation, looser stools with the onset of pain, more frequent stools with the onset of pain, and the passage of mucus in the stools. The likelihood of the syndrome increases as the number of symptoms increase. The Rome II diagnostic criteria for IBS are listed in Box 150-1.[3]

IBS is known by a wide variety of names, including spastic colon, mucus colitis, nervous bowel, spastic colitis, and functional bowel. Although the term *functional bowel* is acceptable, the term *colitis* is misleading and should be avoided because inflammation is not part of the condition of IBS.[6]

Epidemiologic studies estimate that IBS affects 14% to 24% of females and 5% to 19% of males in the United States.[2,4] Symptoms typically have their onset in late adolescence to early adulthood; it is unusual to see an initial presentation of IBS in an individual older than 50 years.[7] The prevalence of IBS appears similar between whites and African Americans but is lower among Hispanics.[8] Studies indicate that IBS is also common in non-Western regions, including Japan, China, South America, and India.[9]

Although as many as 75% of persons with complaints of IBS do not seek health care for their symptoms, IBS still accounts for 12% of visits to primary care providers and 50% of gastroenterology referrals; this results in 2.4 to 3.5 million provider visits per year in the United States.[2,4,7,10] Persons with IBS miss 3 times as many work days as do healthy individuals, see health care providers more often for GI and non-GI complaints, and incur an estimated $8 billion in annual health care costs in the United States.[2,4,10]

To date, the approach to the diagnosis and management of IBS has been limited by an incomplete understanding of the pathogenesis, a lack of specific diagnostic criteria, and the absence of specific treatment recommendations.[4] The goals of clinical management are twofold: (1) to exclude the presence of underlying organic disease while considering the risk and expense of a diagnostic evaluation and (2) to provide support, education, and reassurance to maximize the well-being of those for whom IBS has become a chronic condition.

BOX 150-1

THE ROME II DIAGNOSTIC CRITERIA FOR IRRITABLE BOWEL SYNDROME

Abdominal discomfort or pain with two of three features:
- Relief with defecation
- Onset associated with change in frequency of stool
- Onset associated with change in appearance of stool

These symptoms must be present at least 12 weeks in the past 12 months (not necessarily consecutive weeks).

Modified from Thompson WG and others: Functional bowel habits and functional abdominal pain, *Gut* 45(suppl 2);1143-1147, 1999.

PATHOPHYSIOLOGY

Although the exact cause and pathogenesis of IBS remain unknown, recent research has improved understanding of the etiology of this disorder.[4] The signs and symptoms appear to be predominantly related to exaggerated normal intestinal motility patterns and/or sensory abnormalities in the colon, rectum, or small intestine.[2] Because none of these findings are present in all persons with IBS, it is possible that IBS encompasses a related group of disorders with different etiologies.[1]

Altered Motility

Although altered motility is often mentioned as a cause of IBS, much controversy remains regarding the exact electrical and contractile activity of the colon in IBS.[1] The types of motility patterns seen in the colon and small intestine of persons with IBS are similar to the contractions seen in healthy persons, and there is a lack of agreement on the motility patterns responsible for the diarrhea and constipation associated with IBS.[4] Normal bowel motility predominantly consists of segmenting contractions that function to inhibit the transit of bowel contents. Any increase in segmenting contractions results in constipation, whereas a decrease in contractions results in more frequent stools.[7]

More consistently demonstrated in IBS is an exaggeration of normal colonic motility in response to external and enteric stimuli such as psychologic stress, anxiety, anger, various drugs, and acute intestinal infection.[1,4]

Altered Visceral Sensation

Balloon distention studies of the sigmoid,[11] ileum, and colorectum demonstrate painful symptoms at significantly lower pressures and volumes in persons with IBS compared with healthy individuals.[1,4] This concept, known as *hyperalgesia,* suggests that altered visceral sensation plays a role in the pathogenesis of IBS.[4,11]

Research suggests that with IBS there is increased sensitivity to painful distention in the small bowel and colon, increased or unusual somatic referral of visceral pain, and increased sensitivity to normal intestinal functions. Several possible mechanisms of visceral afferent dysfunction have been suggested to explain the increased visceral sensitivity seen in IBS. These mechanisms include altered receptor sensitivity at the viscus, increased excitability of the dorsal horn neurons of the spinal cord, and altered central modulation of sensation.[1,4]

Role of Enteric Neurotransmitters

Some evidence suggests that abnormalities in extrinsic autonomic innervation of the viscera occurs with functional bowel disorders and that neuroimmune interactions may mediate stress-induced GI responses.[4,12,13] Recent research has focused on the role of enteric nervous system neurotransmitters, such as 5-hydroxytryptamine (5-HT [serotonin]), in controlling intestinal motility and visceral afferent (sensory) responses to normal stimuli (gas, sugars, bile acids, fatty acids) and noxious stimuli (allergens, infectious agents, balloon distention).[14] Ninety-five percent of the body's 5-HT is located in the gut, 3% is located in the brain, and 2% is located in platelets. 5-HT in the gut is manufactured and released from enterochromaffin cells located in the mucosa. Increases in intraluminal pressures result in the release of 5-HT. These neurotransmitters stimulate afferent fibers in the mucosa and initiate a peristaltic reflex, thereby enhancing GI motility and mediating visceral pain.[15] A preliminary study demonstrated increased plasma levels of postprandial 5-HT in women with IBS compared with healthy controls.[16] 5-HT may also play a role in mediating psychologic, stress-induced GI responses via the brain-gut axis.

Psychosocial Factors

Studies of the relationship between psychosocial factors and IBS suggest that although emotional responses to stress affect GI function and produce symptoms in all persons, these symptoms are produced to a greater extent in persons with IBS.[2,4] Although several studies report that persons with IBS have greater psychiatric diagnoses and more psychosocial difficulties than healthy individuals, persons with IBS who do not seek health care for their GI complaints are psychologically similar to healthy individuals.[1] In addition, patients with IBS seen in a primary care setting have fewer psychologic disturbances than those who request to be seen by a gastroenterologist.[4,17] Therefore psychosocial factors do not seem to *cause* IBS symptoms but rather influence how the illness is interpreted and expressed by the individual.[1,17]

Several studies have suggested an increased reporting of childhood physical and sexual abuse among persons with IBS.[1,4,18-20] Although the adverse effects of abuse on health status are independent of GI function, psychosocial trauma often leads to poor illness adjustment and is associated with increased pain reporting, increased provider visits, increased medication use, referral to specialists, and an overall poor clinical outcome.[2,4,19]

Permanent remission of IBS is experienced by 25% of patients; for the majority of patients IBS becomes a chronic illness.[7] As with any chronic illness, IBS has the potential to have an adverse impact on quality of life because it can lead to impairment of physical and psychosocial function, disability, work absenteeism, and increased provider visits.[2,4,21]

CLINICAL PRESENTATION

The symptoms of IBS usually begin in the late teens to 20s, are often gradual in onset, and are intermittent—lasting days, weeks, or months at a time.[1,7] After the exclusion of organic disease, the diagnosis is established according to the Rome II criteria (see Box 150-1), a set of symptom-based diagnostic criteria simplified from Rome I criteria.[2,3,22] Rome I criteria were derived from factor analysis that differentiated the symptoms of patients with IBS from healthy patients and patients with other GI disorders.[2-4,22]

The abdominal pain associated with IBS is usually described as a nonradiating, intermittent, crampy pain located in the lower abdomen (most commonly, the left lower quadrant). Although the location of the pain may vary, it often remains fairly constant for the individual.[7] The pain is typically worse 1 to 2 hours after meals; it is exacerbated by stress, relieved by a bowel movement, and does not interrupt sleep.[6] Establishment of the absence of nocturnal symptoms is critical to the diagnosis of IBS as a functional GI disorder.[7]

Diarrhea, constipation, or a pattern of alternating diarrhea and constipation may be reported with IBS. It is often necessary to clarify what is meant by these complaints. Mucus in the stool is commonly reported. Complaints of visible abdominal distention and bloating are also common.[6]

The likelihood of organic disease is indicated by an acute onset of GI symptoms or an onset of symptoms in patients older than 50 years. Nocturnal symptoms, bloody stools, weight loss, and fever are incompatible with a diagnosis of IBS and require immediate diagnostic evaluation and/or referral.[4,6,7] Although bleeding is not associated with IBS, it may occur secondary to an anal fissure or to hemorrhoids aggravated by the alteration in bowel habits associated with IBS.[7]

A complete health history should be elicited in the presence of an alteration in bowel habits. The history should include a thorough investigation of the presenting symptoms, any associated symptoms, and the presence of nocturnal symptoms. The patient should be questioned about previous diagnostic evaluations for similar symptoms. A past medical history and family history of GI problems, such as colon cancer and inflammatory bowel disease, should be obtained. The patient should be asked about the use of any prescription or over-the-counter medications that could cause diarrhea or constipation. A thorough review of diet, with particular emphasis on the presence of any food intolerances, should be discussed. The review of symptoms should focus on a consideration of the differential diagnoses for an alteration in bowel habits. A sensitive psychosocial history should be elicited to determine sources of stress, coping mechanisms, support systems, reactions to stress in the past, and the use of psychologic counseling services to cope with past stressors. A history of physical or sexual abuse as a child or an adult should also be explored.

PHYSICAL EXAMINATION

The physical examination should be performed to exclude organic disease and to reassure the patient.[4] With IBS, the physical examination is often unremarkable.[1] An abdominal, pelvic, and rectal examination should be performed. The presence of increased tympany to percussion; a palpable, tender, and cord-like sigmoid colon; and tenderness on rectal examination has been reported.[4,7]

DIAGNOSTICS

Several factors should be considered when planning a diagnostic strategy for the patient with an alteration in bowel habits. These factors include the duration and severity of symptoms, the demographic features, the presence of a family history of colon cancer, the nature and extent of psychosocial issues, and previous diagnostic evaluations for similar symptoms.[2,13] An initial approach should involve a limited diagnostic screen aimed at excluding organic disease.[4] Extensive testing is not required in the presence of positive symptom criteria without additional findings to suggest organic disease.[4,13] A diagnosis of IBS with adequate initial evaluation is rarely associated with a need for additional diagnostics in the future.[4] Repeated testing should be avoided because it often leads the patient to question the reliability of the initial diagnosis.[7]

Diagnostics

Irritable Bowel Syndrome

Laboratory
CBC and differential
ESR
TSH
Stool for occult blood/ova/parasites
Hydrogen breath test*
Serum glucose*
Serum electrolytes*
BUN*
Creatinine*

Imaging
Abdominal ultrasound*
Abdominal x-ray*
Barium enema*
KUB (flat plate and upright)*

Other
Flexible sigmoidoscopy or colonoscopy

*If indicated.

A limited screen for organic disease should include a CBC with differential, erythrocyte sedimentation rate (ESR), electrolytes, glucose, blood urea nitrogen (BUN), creatinine, thyroid-stimulating hormone (TSH), and a stool for occult blood and ova and parasites. Flexible sigmoidoscopy with or without a barium enema is indicated for most patients, and a colonoscopy should be performed for patients older than 50 years or patients with risk factors for colon cancer.[2,4,22] Examination of the proctosigmoid is generally unremarkable but often results in cramping and discomfort that may prevent complete advancement of the sigmoidoscope to the 60-cm level.[7] Additional diagnostic studies, such as a trial of a lactose-free diet or a hydrogen breath test to exclude lactase deficiency or an abdominal ultrasound to exclude gallstones, may be required depending on the constellation of symptoms. Complaints of excess gas and bloating should be evaluated with a plain x-ray examination of the abdomen.[4]

If the initial diagnostic screen is negative, treatment of symptoms should be initiated and reevaluated in 3 to 6 weeks. This diagnostic strategy allows for a more conservative and cost-effective evaluation. If the initial treatment fails, additional diagnostic studies or a referral to a gastroenterologist may be considered.[2,4] Patients older than 50 years with new or changed symptoms require a repeat evaluation.

DIFFERENTIAL DIAGNOSIS

A number of organic diseases have presentations similar to IBS, and it is essential that they be considered in the differential diagnosis. Colon cancer, inflammatory bowel disease, cholecystitis, causes and complications of chronic diarrhea or chronic constipation, intestinal parasites, lactase deficiency, malabsorption syndromes, thyroid disease, and psychiatric disorders, including anxiety, depression, somatization, panic disorder, and posttraumatic stress disorder, should be considered when evaluating the patient with a change in bowel habits.[1,2,6,7,19,23,24]

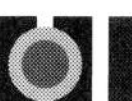

Differential Diagnosis

Irritable Bowel Syndrome

Colon cancer	Lactase deficiency
Inflammatory bowel disease	Malabsorption syndromes
Cholecystitis	Thyroid disease
Causes and complications of chronic diarrhea	Anxiety
Causes and complications of chronic constipation	Depression
Intestinal parasites	Somatization
	Panic disorder
	Posttraumatic stress disorder

MANAGEMENT

The treatment of IBS is purely symptomatic and includes dietary modifications, medications, behavioral therapy, education, and reassurance. To date, no one therapy has proved to be more effective than another. The most important factor in the successful management of IBS appears to be the establishment of a therapeutic relationship.[1,22] A nonjudgmental, attentive approach is essential to assist patients in shifting their focus from finding a cause for their symptoms to finding a way to cope with them.[4] Primary care providers must resist the urge to respond to chronic complaints with new or repeated diagnostic studies.[4,25]

Because both physiologic and psychosocial factors appear to play a role in the severity of symptoms and the expression of illness, both must be considered when developing a management plan.[4,22,26] Diagnosis and treatment of any underlying psychologic disorder, such as anxiety and depression, are essential.[7] Most patients (75%) with IBS have mild symptoms and can be managed in a primary care setting. They usually respond to education, reassurance, and dietary and lifestyle modifications.[4] A smaller number have moderate symptoms that are usually intermittent but can be disabling. They may have psychologic distress from their symptoms, but their symptoms correlate with gut physiology.[4] These patients often require gut-acting medications such as anticholinergic and antidiarrheal agents and, in some cases, psychologic counseling.[4] A very small number of patients have severe and refractory symptoms. They often report chronic, severe pain and psychosocial difficulties, and they require antidepressants, mental health referrals, and sometimes a pain management evaluation.[4] These patients require a team approach that includes comanagement with a gastroenterologist.

Dietary Modification

Food intolerance is a common cause of clinical symptoms in a number of patients with IBS. Gas, bloating, distention, and a change in bowel habits can be attributed to the intake of certain foods (Box 150-2). Dairy products and gas-forming foods are the most common offenders.[1,7] Other foods and beverages that may cause or aggravate symptoms include items artificially sweetened with fructose or sorbitol, as well as caffeine, alcohol, and fatty foods.[2,6]

BOX 150-2

COMMON GAS-FORMING FOODS

- Beans
- Beer
- Broccoli
- Brussels sprouts
- Cabbage
- Carbonated beverages
- Cauliflower
- Coffee
- Grapes
- Lentils and legumes
- Plums
- Raisins
- Raw onions
- Red wine

Although care should be taken to avoid unnecessary dietary restrictions, the initial recommendations should focus on eliminating foods suspected of causing or aggravating symptoms.[2] Use of a diary to record food intake and symptoms can help identify offending foods. Some patients may benefit from referral to a nutritionist.[8] Lactose intolerance should be excluded in all patients who initially present with symptoms of IBS.[1,27] Consideration should be given to hydrogen-breath testing or recommendation of a 3-week trial of a lactose-free diet.[1,27] Instructions should include a recommendation to avoid medications that could aggravate symptoms, such as laxatives and antacids with laxative effects.[6]

The role of fiber therapy in IBS remains controversial.[28] Fiber is likely to improve constipation-predominant IBS, but its role in relieving abdominal pain and diarrhea is less clear.[2] Clinical experience has demonstrated that many patients benefit from fiber after an initial period of bloating and abdominal discomfort. A trial of 20 to 30 g/day of fiber seems reasonable for the treatment of IBS.[1,6]

Synthetic fiber supplements are more soluble than natural fiber, cause less bloating, and may be better tolerated.[1] Slow introduction of the fiber load helps reduce gas and bloating. A number of commercial products are available as over-the-counter formulations. No one brand seems to have an advantage over another, although individual responses vary. Instruct patients to try a different brand if one seems ineffective or produces side effects. Supplementation may be accomplished by giving one tablet, rounded tablespoon, or packet of psyllium (Metamucil) or calcium polycarbophil (FiberCon) with food or 8 ounces of liquid q.d. to t.i.d. (according to response).[6] Another treatment option is methylcellulose (Citrucel) 1 scoop, q.d. to t.i.d.

Pharmacotherapy

Antispasmodics. Anticholinergics act to reduce sigmoid motility in response to a fatty meal.[4,29] Medications such as dicyclomine (Bentyl) 10 to 40 mg q.i.d. p.r.n. may be tried by patients who experience postprandial abdominal pain, gas, and bloating.[1] To achieve maximum effectiveness, the medication should be taken 30 to 60 minutes before meals.[4] Hyoscyamine sulfate, the active ingredient in Levsin and Donnatol, has several side effects, including urinary retention, tachycardia, and dry mouth.[6] Dicyclomine acts more selectively on the smooth muscle of the GI tract and may produce fewer side effects than the nonselective anticholinergics.[1] Although calcium channel blockers relax the smooth muscle of the GI tract, constipation is a reported side effect, and they have not been specifically approved for the treatment of IBS.[4]

Antidiarrheal Agents. Loperamide (Imodium) 2 to 4 mg q.i.d. p.r.n. decreases intestinal transit, enhances intestinal water absorption, and strengthens rectal sphincter tone, thereby improving the diarrhea, urgency, and fecal soiling of diarrhea-predominant IBS.[4] Patients may take a maximum of eight pills per day as needed to control symptoms. Polycarbophil (Fibercon) can be added to help increase stool bulk. Pepto-Bismal, Kaopectate, and bile acid sequestering agents, such as cholestyramine (Questran, Prevalite), should also be considered in the treatment of diarrhea-predominant IBS.[4] Alosetron, the 5-HT_3 receptor antagonist used for the treatment of diarrhea-predominant IBS in females,[3] was recently withdrawn from the market due to several cases of ischemic colitis.

Anticonstipation Agents. Synthetic fiber is helpful in treating constipation associated with IBS. In addition to fiber therapy, increasing fluids, and regular exercise, patients with constipation may benefit from stool softeners and osmotic laxatives such as lactulose and MiraLax (polyethylene glycol). Stimulant laxatives should be avoided whenever possible. Metoclopramide (Reglan), a promotility agent, has been used for years, has a minimum of side effects, and is considered safe in dosages of 5 to 10 mg q.i.d. However, patients should be referred to a gastroenterologist for a motility study to rule out a motility disorder before treating constipation with metoclopramide.

Tegaserod, a 5-HT_4 receptor antagonist manufactured by Novartis, is currently awaiting U.S. Food and Drug Administration (FDA) approval for the treatment of constipation-predominant IBS in females.[30]

Psychotropic Agents. Antidepressants, including tricyclic agents and selective serotonin reuptake inhibitors (SSRIs), are often used to treat IBS, particularly in patients with severe or refractory symptoms, impaired daily function, and associated depression or panic attacks.[4,23-25] The anticholinergic properties of the tricyclic antidepressants are believed to contribute to their effectiveness in treating the pain, gas, bloating, and frequent stools associated with IBS. Because of their tendency to cause constipation, tricyclic agents are probably best avoided in constipation-predominant IBS.

Because of their lower side effect profile, many providers are prescribing SSRIs instead of tricyclic agents, despite the fact that additional studies are still needed to assess their effects on patients with IBS.[4] A common side effect of SSRIs is diarrhea; therefore these drugs may prove most beneficial in treating constipation-predominant IBS. There is no clinical research to support the use of benzodiazepines in IBS; their use should be avoided because of their addictive potential.[1,4,7]

Alternative Therapies

Several alternative therapies have been studied in IBS, including cognitive-behavioral therapy, hypnosis, guided imagery, relaxation techniques, and stress management.[4,31,32] The data appear to support the value of alternative therapies in reducing anxiety and other psychologic symptoms and in decreasing GI symptoms.[4] Patients with underlying psychologic issues may benefit from a

BOX 150-3

EMERGENCY CRITERIA

Symptoms that are incompatible with IBS and require immediate diagnostic evaluation and/or referral:

- Nocturnal symptoms
- Bloody stools
- Fever
- Weight loss

BOX 150-4

INDICATIONS FOR REFERRAL

- Initial treatment failure
- Organic disease suspected
- Change in bowel habits in a patient older than 50 years
- Change in usual IBS symptom pattern

referral to a psychologist, mental health clinical nurse specialist, or psychiatric nurse practitioner. Patients with severe, refractory pain should be referred to a pain management program.[4]

Peppermint oil is a natural antispasmodic. With GI effects similar to calcium channel blockers, peppermint oil causes smooth muscle relaxation and can help with postprandial pain. Peppermint oil is also available in enteric-coated capsule form.

COMPLICATIONS

Serious complications from IBS are extremely rare. In some patients, the chronic nature of symptoms leads to a reduced quality of life and clinical depression. Chronic constipation may also result in hemorrhoids, anal fissures, fecal impaction, and, rarely, intestinal obstruction.

INDICATIONS FOR REFERRAL/HOSPITALIZATION

Nocturnal symptoms, bloody stools, fever, and weight loss are incompatible with a diagnosis of IBS and require immediate further diagnostic evaluation or referral (Box 150-3). Physician consultation and referral to a gastroenterologist are indicated if initial treatment of IBS fails, if organic disease is suspected or found, or if the patient who presents with a change in bowel habits is older than 50 years or has an established diagnosis of IBS and is reporting a change in the usual pattern of symptoms (Box 150-4). The gastroenterologist is also helpful in the comanagement of a patient with complex IBS.[2,6,7]

PATIENT AND FAMILY EDUCATION

Dietary and lifestyle modifications such as avoidance of food to which the patient is intolerant, increasing fluids and fiber, regular exercise, and alternative therapies should be discussed with patients.[7] Information regarding what constitutes "normal" bowel habits should be addressed. Bowel retraining can be accomplished by encouraging patients to sit on the toilet (without straining) for 15 to 20 minutes each morning after breakfast.[7] Medications for symptom control should be reviewed, and a discussion regarding laxative abuse included.[7]

Patients should be informed that the symptoms of IBS are very real. They should be taught that their symptoms arise from an increased sensitivity and reactivity of the gut to stimuli, resulting in pain and/or abnormal motility.[4] They should understand that IBS is a chronic condition that does not lead to cancer or colitis[7] and is characterized by periods of remission and exacerbation that often correlate with physical and psychologic stressors.[4] Reassurance has tremendous value in the treatment of IBS. Patients should be told that although there is no cure, there is help, and that the majority of patients learn to cope adequately with their symptoms and lead productive lives.[4]

HEALTH PROMOTION

The chronic nature of IBS symptoms may lead a patient with IBS to ignore a change in bowel habits resulting from an organic etiology. Patients need to be instructed that although IBS does not increase their risk for colorectal cancer, they should keep their screening current with recommended guidelines for colorectal screening in the general population, and they should immediately report a change in bowel habits that is atypical for their usual pattern of symptoms.

REFERENCES

1. Lynn RB, Friedman LS: Irritable bowel syndrome, *N Engl J Med* 329(26):1940-1943, 1993.
2. American Gastroenterological Association medical position paper: Irritable bowel syndrome, *Gastroenterology* 112(6):2118-2119, 1997.
3. Thompson WG and others: Functional bowel disorders and functional abdominal pain, *Gut* 45(suppl 2):1143-1147, 1999.
4. Drossman DA, Whitehead WE, Camilleri M: Irritable bowel syndrome: a technical review for practical guideline development, *Gastroenterology* 112(6):2120-2137, 1997.
5. Manning AP and others: Toward positive diagnosis of the irritable bowel, *Br Med J* 2:653-654, 1978.
6. Eastwood GL, Avundk C, editors: Irritable bowel syndrome. In *Manual of gastroenterology*, ed 2, Boston, 1994, Little, Brown.
7. Carlson E: Irritable bowel syndrome, *Nurse Pract* 23(1):83-93, 1998.
8. Zuckerman MJ and others: Health-care-seeking behaviors related to bowel complaints: Hispanics versus non-Hispanic whites, *Dig Dis Sci* 41(1):77-82, 1996.
9. Thompson WG: Functional bowel disorders and functional abdominal pain. In Drossman DA and others, editors: *Functional gastrointestinal disorders: diagnosis, pathophysiology and treatment*, McLean, Va, 1994, Degnon Associates.
10. Drossman DA and others: US householder survey of functional gastrointestinal disorders: prevalence, sociodemography, and health impact, *Dig Dis Sci* 38:1569-1580, 1993.
11. Munakata J and others: Repetitive sigmoid stimulation induces rectal hyperalgesia in patients with irritable bowel syndrome, *Gastroenterology* 112(1):55-63, 1997.
12. Heitkemper M and others: Increased urine catecholamines and cortisol in women with irritable bowel syndrome, *Am J Gastroenterol* 91(5):906-913, 1996.
13. Mayer EA, Raybould HE: The role of visceral afferent mechanisms in functional bowel disorders, *Gastroenterology* 99:1688-1704, 1990.
14. Bueno L and others: Mediators and pharmacology of visceral sensitivity; from basic to clinical investigations, *Gastroenterology* 112(4):1714-1743, 1997.
15. Goyal RK, Hirano I: The enteric nervous system, *N Engl J Med* 334:1106-1115, 1996.
16. Bearcroft CP, Perrett D, Farthing MJG: Postprandial 5-hydroxytryptamine in diarrhea predominant irritable bowel syndrome: a pilot study, *Gut* 42:42-46, 1998.

17. Dewsnap P and others: The prevalence of symptoms of irritable bowel syndrome among acute psychiatric inpatients with an affective diagnosis, *Psychosomatics* 37(4):385-389, 1996.
18. Drossman DA and others: Psychosocial aspects of the functional gastrointestinal disorders, *Gastroenterol Int* 8:47-90, 1995.
19. Irwin C and others: Comorbidity of post-traumatic stress disorder and irritable bowel syndrome, *J Clin Psychiatry* 57(12):576-578, 1996.
20. Drossman DA and others: Sexual and physical abuse in women with functional or organic gastrointestinal disorders, *Ann Intern Med* 113:828-833, 1990.
21. Whitehead WE, Burnett CK, Cook EW: Impact of irritable bowel syndrome on quality of life, *Dig Dis Sci* 41(11):2248-2253, 1996.
22. Dalton CS, Drossman DA: Diagnosis and treatment of irritable bowel syndrome, *Am Fam Physician* 55(3):875-885, 1997.
23. Masand PS and others: Irritable bowel syndrome and dysthymia: is there a relationship? *Psychosomatics* 38(1):63-69, 1997.
24. Zaubler TS, Katon W: Panic disorder and medical comorbidity: a review of the medical and psychiatric literature, *Bull Menninger Clin* 60(2 suppl A):A12-A38, 1996.
25. Bonis PA, Norton RA: The challenge of irritable bowel syndrome, *Am Fam Physician* 53(4):1229-1236, 1996.
26. Lembo T and others: Symptom duration in patients with irritable bowel syndrome, *Am J Gastroenterol* 91(5):898-905, 1996.
27. Tolliver BA and others: Does lactose maldigestion really play a role in the irritable bowel syndrome? *J Clin Gastroenterol* 23(1)15-17, 1996.
28. Bennett WG, Cerda JJ: Benefits of dietary fiber: myth or medicine? *Postgrad Med* 99(2):153-172, 1996.
29. Sullivan MA, Cohen S, Snape WJ: Colonic myoelectric activity in irritable bowel syndrome: effects of eating and anticholinergics, *N Engl J Med* 298:878-883, 1978.
30. Baker D: Tegaserod for the treatment of constipation-predominant irritable bowel syndrome, *Rev Gastroenterol Dis* 1(4):187-198, 2001.
31. VanDulmen AM, Fennis JF, Bleijenberg G: Cognitive-behavioral group therapy for irritable bowel syndrome: effects and long-term follow-up, *Psychosom Med* 58(5):508-514, 1996.
32. Houghton LA, Heyman DJ, Whorwell PJ: Symptomatology, quality of life and economic features of irritable bowel syndrome in hypnotherapy, *Ailment Pharmacol Ther* 10(1):91-95, 1996.

CHAPTER 151

Jaundice

Louise Meyer

DEFINITION/EPIDEMIOLOGY

Jaundice, or icterus, is a yellow or greenish discoloration of the skin, sclerae, and mucous membranes caused by bile pigments of conjugated or unconjugated bilirubin.[1] There are multiple causes of jaundice, requiring determination of the underlying disorder.

Jaundice can be divided into three categories. The first type involves unconjugated hyperbilirubinemia, which results when the indirect fraction of bilirubin exceeds 80% of the total bilirubin.[2] Hemolytic jaundice is an example of this type. The second type, obstructive jaundice, is produced by conjugated bilirubin. Conjugated bilirubinemia develops when the direct fraction of bilirubin ranges from 20% to 60% of the total bilirubin.[2] Hepatocellular jaundice is the third category and is caused by failure of the liver cells to conjugate bilirubin.[1]

The causes of jaundice are categorized according to (1) symptoms (acute or chronic), (2) evidence of bile duct dilation, and (3) jaundice of the conjugated or unconjugated varieties.[1] Jaundice is very common in newborns and occurs in 50% of term infants between the fourth and fourteenth day after birth.[3] In older children and young adults, common causes include viral hepatitis (accounts for 75% of jaundice in patients <30 years old), Gilbert's syndrome, drug-induced hepatitis, pregnancy, cirrhosis, and alcoholic hepatitis. In older patients, cirrhosis (accounts for 30% of jaundice in the 30- to 60-year-old age-group), pancreatic cancer, metastatic cancer to the liver, sepsis, common bile duct stone, and medication-induced hepatitis are the most common causes[2] (Box 151-1).

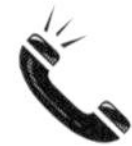

Physician consultation is indicated for patients with new-onset jaundice.

PATHOPHYSIOLOGY

The liver plays a major role in the metabolism of bile pigments. This process is divided into three distinct phases: (1) hepatic uptake, (2) conjugation, and (3) excretion.[1] A byproduct of hemolysis is bilirubin, which is produced through the breakdown of hemoglobin in RBCs.[4] There are two forms of bilirubin: indirect, or unconjugated, bilirubin (which is protein bound) and direct, or conjugated, bilirubin. The direct form circulates freely in the blood until it reaches the liver, where it is conjugated with glucuronide transferase and excreted into the bile.[1] An increase in unconjugated bilirubin is often associated with an increase in the destruction of RBCs. An increase in conjugated bilirubin is more likely seen with liver dysfunction or obstruction.[5] Disturbance in the passage of conjugated bilirubin from the liver to the intestine accounts for 60% of jaundice in patients older than 60 years.[2] With bile duct obstruction, bilirubin is conjugated by the hepatocytes but cannot flow into

BOX 151-1

CLASSIFICATION/CAUSES OF JAUNDICE

UNCONJUGATED HYPERBILIRUBINEMIA (PREDOMINANTLY INDIRECT-ACTING BILIRUBIN)

Increased bilirubin production
- Hemolytic anemias (thalassemias, sideroblastic anemias, some pernicious anemias), hematoma, infarction

Decreased hepatic uptake
- Posthepatitis, drug reactions, sepsis, prolonged fasting

Decreased bilirubin conjugation (decreased hepatic glucuronosyl transferase)
- Hereditary transferase deficiency (Gilbert's syndrome, Crigler-Najjar syndrome)
- Acquired transferase deficiency—drug inhibition (e.g., chloramphenicol), breast milk, hepatocellular disease
- Neonatal jaundice

CONJUGATED HYPERBILIRUBINEMIA (PREDOMINANTLY DIRECT-ACTING BILIRUBIN)

Impaired excretion—intrahepatic defects
- Familial defects (Dubin-Johnson syndrome, Rotor's syndrome), recurrent intrahepatic cholestasis, cholestatic jaundice of pregnancy
- Acquired disorders—viral or drug-induced hepatitis, cirrhosis, sepsis, postoperative complications, androgens, chlorpromazine, acetaminophen, sulfonamides, NSAIDs, aspirin), industrial poisons

Impaired excretion—extrahepatic defects
- Gallstones, biliary malformation, infection, biliary or pancreatic tumors, chronic pancreatitis, pancreatic pseudocyst

the duodenum.[1] Therefore bilirubin accumulates in the liver and enters the bloodstream, causing hyperbilirubinemia.

Extrahepatic obstructive jaundice develops if the common bile duct is occluded by gallstones or tumors, especially pancreatic carcinoma or strictures.[1,2] Because conjugated bilirubin is water soluble, it is excreted in the urine. This produces the characteristic orange urine with elevated conjugated bilirubin produced by inflammation.

Intrahepatic obstructive jaundice involves disturbances in hepatocyte function or obstruction of bile canaliculi. The uptake, conjugation, and excretion of bilirubin are affected, resulting in increased levels of conjugated and unconjugated bilirubin.[1]

Failure of liver cells to conjugate bilirubin causes hepatocellular damage, resulting in increased plasma concentrations of unconjugated bilirubin. In addition, bilirubin cannot pass from the liver to the intestine.[1] The etiologies of hepatitis include infections, medications, and genetic defects causing decreased enzyme production.

Hemolytic jaundice is caused by excessive hemolysis of RBCs. An increased amount of unconjugated bilirubin is formed through metabolism of the heme component of destroyed RBCs and exceeds the conjugation ability of the liver.[1] This causes the blood levels of unconjugated bilirubin to rise. Hemolysis can occur with blood transfusion reactions, after cardiopulmonary bypass, with sickle cell anemia, and with marrow or splenic destruction of RBCs. In sickle cell anemia, abnormal hemoglobin and a fragile cell membrane lead to hemolysis and an increase in the amount of free, unconjugated bilirubin.[1] Bone marrow development problems or defective erythropoiesis are conditions in which poorly manufactured erythrocytes are fragile and have a short life span. The result is an excess of unconjugated bilirubin that reaches the liver for conjugation.[1]

CLINICAL PRESENTATION

Jaundice is most commonly observed in the face, trunk, and sclera. Bilirubin is distributed uniformly in the sclera and is differentiated from the normal occurrence of the yellow subscleral fat that collects in the periphery.[1] In African Americans the mandibular frenum is a location to observe jaundice. Jaundice caused by carotene does not stain the sclera but rather is seen in the forehead, around the nasi, and in the palms and soles. The patient with jaundice may have pruritus, which often accompanies obstructive jaundice. The pruritus is caused by nerve injury in the skin by the bile pigments.[1] Cutaneous xanthomas may be seen in patients with jaundice from chronic cholestasis and suggest hypercholesterolemia. The presence of spider angiomas, palmar erythema, and ascites combined with malaise, anorexia, and right upper quadrant discomfort suggests chronic hepatocellular disease or cirrhosis. Colicky right upper quadrant pain, weight loss, and light-colored stools may be present in obstructive jaundice. Intermittent, colicky right upper quadrant pain before the onset of jaundice suggests choledocholithiasis.[2] Fever and chills may accompany biliary obstruction and virus- or drug-induced hepatitis. Occult blood in the stools suggests cancer as an etiology for jaundice.

Appropriate history includes determining whether the jaundice is acute or chronic as well as ascertaining associated symptoms. In acute jaundice, inquiry focuses on hepatitis risks, including recent travel; transfusions; tattoos; IV drug use; alcohol intake; medications (prescription, herbals, or over-the-counter); food, toxin, animal, or infected person exposures; unsafe sexual practices; and symptoms of biliary tract disease. Chronic jaundice may suggest viral hepatitis, biliary tract disease, pancreatitis, or chronic alcohol intake. Weight loss, anorexia, malaise, and other symptoms of cancer are noted. In addition, a list of medications taken by the patient and a complete family history, including cancer, Wilson's disease, hemochromatosis, and hereditary hemolytic anemias, provide vital information for an appropriate diagnosis.

PHYSICAL EXAMINATION

Acute jaundice requires a complete examination to determine the cause of the illness. Determination of vital signs, assessment of the cardiovascular system for congestive heart failure, and evaluation of the abdomen for ascites, organomegaly, guarding, and tenderness are essential.[5] Fever and right upper quadrant tenderness are most often associated with choledocholithiasis, cholangitis, or cholecystitis. An enlarged tender liver suggests acute hepatic inflammation or a rapidly growing hepatic tumor.[6] The presence of splenomegaly suggests portal hypertension from acute or active chronic hepatitis, as well as cirrhosis.[4,5]

Chronic jaundice mandates evaluation for chronic liver disease. Gynecomastia, testicular atrophy, and splenomegaly are strongly associated with cirrhosis. In addition, palmar erythema, facial telangiectasia, and Dupuytren's contractures are associated with cirrhosis from chronic ethanol ingestion.[7] Lymphadenopathy suggests malignancy and can be related to a pancreatic tumor obstructing the splenic vein or to a metastatic lymphoma. When malignancy is suspected, the investigation should concentrate on determining the location of the primary tumor as indicated by heme-positive stool, abdominal masses, breast masses, thyroid nodules, or supraclavicular lymphadenopathy. Physical findings associated with specific liver diseases include distended neck veins and hepatojugular reflux (right heart failure), xanthomas (primary biliary cirrhosis), and Kayser-Fleischer rings (Wilson's disease).[7]

DIAGNOSTICS

Liver function tests (LFTs), including albumin, aspartate aminotransferase (AST), and alanine aminotransferase (ALT); total and direct serum bilirubin; serum alkaline phosphatase; stool guaiac; and urine bilirubin, are obtained, in addition to a CBC with platelet count and a prothrombin time (PT). Elevated ALT and AST levels result from hepatocellular necrosis or inflammation.[5] An AST level that is more than twice the ALT level is typical with alcoholic liver injury. Elevated alkaline phosphatase levels suggest cholestasis, primary biliary cirrhosis, or infiltrative liver disease (e.g., tumor abscess, granulomas).[8] In obstructive liver disease the alkaline phosphatase may be greater than 3 times the normal level.[2]

A normal serum albumin suggests a more acute disease process than the chronic disease associated with low serum albumin.[9]

Unconjugated (indirect) hyperbilirubinemia suggests a hemolytic disorder, such as an autoimmune or microangiopathic hemolytic anemia. The most common cause of mild elevations of unconjugated bilirubin is Gilbert's syndrome, with physical stress, fever, fasting, or heavy alcohol ingestion as precipitants.[7]

Direct hyperbilirubinemia results from hepatocellular inflammation, cholestatic liver disease, or extrahepatic biliary obstruction. The presence of direct hyperbilirubinemia without liver enzyme abnormalities is uncommon but is seen in pregnancy or sepsis or after recent surgery.[7] Patients with elevated conjugated bilirubin should be evaluated for evidence of viral hepatitis, drug toxicity, or hepatic congestion. Serologic studies are used to diagnose hepatitis A, B, C, and D.[10] Common causes of toxic hepatitis include acetaminophen, allopurinol, androgenic steroids, aspirin and other salicylates, contraceptive steroids, chlorpromazine, erythromycin, glucocorticoids, mercaptopurine, methotrexate, plicamycin, nonsteroidal antiinflammatory drugs (NSAIDs), and sulfonamides.[11] Isolated conjugated direct hyperbilirubinemia is the primary symptom of two inherited disorders: Rotor syndrome and Dubin-Johnson syndrome.[7]

In patients with chronic liver disease lacking a defined cause, serum iron, transferrin saturation, and ferritin should be measured to screen for hemochromatosis. In hemochromatosis the serum ferritin is substantially elevated. Plasma iron may exceed 200 μg/dl, and transferrin saturation exceeds 70%.[2] In patients younger than 30 years with abnormal liver function test (LFT) results or in patients with hepatitis who test negative for viruses A, B, C, and D and neurologic dysfunction, measurements of serum ceruloplasmin and urine copper levels are recommended, to screen for Wilson's disease.[2]

Hepatobiliary imaging is recommended if the liver chemistry profile suggests cholestasis or extrahepatic obstruction. Ultrasound is greater than 90% specific and is close to 90% sensitive in detecting obstruction. A CT scan is indicated in cases where ultrasound is unsatisfactory.[2,7] However, ultrasonography is an effective means of detecting stones in the gallbladder and is somewhat more sensitive than a CT scan.[2] Endoscopic retrograde cholangiopancreatography (ERCP) or percutaneous transhepatic cholangiography (PTC) is indicated if extrahepatic obstruction is strongly suspected.[2] Percutaneous liver biopsy is the definitive study for determining the cause and extent of hepatocellular dysfunction or infiltrative liver disease, particularly if metastatic disease or a hepatic mass is suspected.[6]

DIFFERENTIAL DIAGNOSIS

The etiology of jaundice is multifactorial; consequently, the presence of coexisting disease is an important aspect of the evaluation. The finding of unconjugated hyperbilirubinemia can be related to increased bilirubin production (hemolytic anemia) or impaired bilirubin uptake and storage (hepatitis sequelae, posthepatitis, Gilbert's syndrome, drug reactions). Hereditary syndromes such as Crigler-Najjar and Gilbert's syndromes (resulting from impaired glucuronosyltransferase activity) and Dubin-Johnson and Rotor's syndromes (resulting from faulty excretion of bilirubin) are examples of causes of unconjugated bilirubin.[7] The presence of conjugated hyperbilirubinemia can be caused by hepatitis, cirrhosis, cholestasis, postoperative jaundice, spirochetal infections,

Diagnostics

Jaundice

Laboratory	**Imaging**
LFTs	Ultrasonography
CBC and differential, platelets	CT scan
PT	**Other**
Hepatitis profile*	ERCP*
Serum iron, transferrin saturation, ferritin	Liver biopsy
Serum ceruloplasmin	
Urine copper	
Urine bilirubin	

*If indicated.

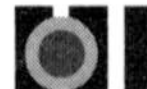

Differential Diagnosis

Jaundice

Hepatitis	Spirochete infection
Gilbert's syndrome	Infectious mononucleosis
Drug reaction	Sarcoidosis
Hemolytic anemia	Lymphoma
Hereditary syndromes	Toxins
Cirrhosis	Cholangitis
Cholestasis	Tumor
Postoperative jaundice	Choledochal cysts
Cholestatic jaundice of pregnancy	Choledocholithiasis
	Pancreatitis

infectious mononucleosis, sarcoidosis, lymphomas, and industrial toxins. Fever and chills suggest cholangitis. Etiologies of biliary obstructions include tumors, choledochal cysts, choledocholithiasis, pancreatitis, pancreatic neoplasms, and cholestatic jaundice of pregnancy. Jaundice during pregnancy is most commonly related to viral hepatitis.[5]

MANAGEMENT

The treatment of jaundice relates to the underlying disease process. Most patients with viral hepatitis can be treated symptomatically on an outpatient basis (see Chapter 148). When liver enzymes fail to return to normal levels within 6 months, liver biopsy is indicated.[2] Interferon alfa-2b may be useful in chronic hepatitis B and C after consultation with a gastroenterologist.[2] Cholangitis requires antibiotic therapy and surgical consultation. For patients with cholangitis, nonoperative biliary drainage can be performed via ERCP via transhepatically placed stents.[2] Surgical therapy is usually required for extrahepatic biliary obstruction. Gilbert's disease, Dubin-Johnson syndrome, and Rotor's syndrome beyond the neonatal period rarely require treatment to lower the bilirubin level. However, treatment for the primary disease process may require corticosteroids if the presentation of these diseases is complicated by hemolytic anemia.

The treatment for uncomplicated cirrhosis consists of voluntary restriction of activity if the patient has weakness and fatigue. The diet should be high in protein but low in sodium, and alcohol should be avoided. This regimen almost invariably results in improvement of hepatocellular function in patients with alcohol-induced cirrhosis.[7] Multivitamins and folic acid 1 mg/day may be given if the patient's diet is inadequate. Tranquilizers and sedatives should be avoided. When serum potassium falls below 3.5 mEq/L, the deficit of body potassium is approximately 300 to 500 mEq. This can be replaced over a few days with oral solutions of 10% potassium chloride, which provide 40 mEq of potassium/30 ml.[7] Protein can be restricted in stable cirrhotic patients to 45 g/day as long as there is a minimum of 400 g of carbohydrates ingested/day. Vegetable protein contains smaller amounts of ammonia, methionine, and aromatic acids and is better tolerated by these patients.[7] Lactulose is a nonabsorbable synthetic disaccharide that, when administered in dosages of 20 to 30 g t.i.d. to q.i.d., reduces blood ammonia and improves encephalopathy in the majority of patients. Patients with decompensated cirrhosis who are not responding to therapy should be considered for liver transplantation. Vitamin K 15 mg IV may improve prolongation of the PT.[7]

Pruritus, which is commonly associated with jaundice, may be disabling to some patients, resulting in depression. Early treatment with agents such as cholestyramine three times per day and antihistamines three or four times daily is highly recommended.[2] Fragrance-free soaps, less frequent bathing, and use of emollients may also help decrease the severity of pruritus.[4] Continued monitoring of LFTs, serologic tests, and hematologic studies of blood counts, platelets, and PTs as indicated are recommended for all patients with jaundice to detect complications.

COMPLICATIONS

The complications of jaundice are directly related to the underlying disease process. In cirrhosis, infection and gastrointestinal bleeding often precipitate decompensation. Potassium deficiency is common in cirrhosis and may contribute to hepatic encephalopathy.

Patients with hepatitis may experience one or two relapses during their recovery period. Complications of other underlying diseases associated with jaundice range from anemia to gastrointestinal infection, hepatocellular damage, encephalopathy, and postsurgical complications. The most serious complication of stenting is recurrent jaundice from stent occlusion and recurrent cholangitis.[12]

INDICATIONS FOR REFERRAL/HOSPITALIZATION

The management of patients with jaundice is often a complex process because of the myriad underlying disease processes, as well as the potential complications. The primary care physician is always consulted to determine the diagnosis and initial management plans. Consultation with a gastroenterologist, hepatologist, and/or surgeon is also often indicated.

Hospitalization of patients is indicated in cases of severe electrolyte imbalance or with evidence of severe hepatocellular failure, ascites, and prolonged PT unresponsive to treatment.[2]

PATIENT AND FAMILY EDUCATION

It is imperative that patients understand the underlying disease process and prevention regimens. Appropriate levels of activity and rest, the importance of medication adherence, and the need for avoidance of over-the-counter medications that interfere with hepatic function should be emphasized. Appropriate dietary instruction is essential for patients with hepatic disease, and referral to a dietitian for instruction of specific diets is desirable.

REFERENCES

1. McCance KL, Huether SE: *Pathophysiology: the biological basis for disease in adults and children,* ed 3, St Louis, 1998, Mosby.
2. Steiner GS, Lipsky MS: Jaundice. In Mengel MB, Schwiebert LP, editors: *Ambulatory medicine,* Norwalk, Conn, 1993, Appleton & Lange.
3. Seidel HM and others: *Mosby's guide to physical examination,* ed 4, St Louis, 1999, Mosby.
4. Horrell CJ: Jaundice. In Camo-Sorrell D, Hawkins RA, editors: *Clinical manual for the oncology advanced practice nurse,* Pittsburgh, Penn, 2000, Oncology Nursing Press, Inc.
5. Guss DA: Disorders of the liver, biliary tract, and pancreas. In Rosen P and others, editors: *Emergency medicine: concepts and clinical practice,* ed 4, St Louis, 1998, Mosby.
6. Wan-yea Lau FRS and others: A logical approach to hepatocellular carcinoma presenting with jaundice, *Ann Surg* 225(3):281-285, 1997.
7. Mezey E: Diseases of the liver. In Barker RL, Burton JR, Zieve PD, editors: *Principles of ambulatory medicine,* ed 4, Baltimore, 1995, Williams & Wilkins.
8. Driscoll CE and others: *The family practice desk reference,* ed 3, St Louis, 1995, Mosby.
9. Pratt DS: Approach to the patient with abnormal liver function tests. Retrieved June 14, 2002, from the World Wide Web: http://www.uptodate.
10. Gentilini P and others: Long course and prognostic factors of virus-induced cirrhosis of the liver, *Am J Gastroenterol* 92(1):66-72, 1997.
11. Clark JF, Queener SF, Karb VB: *Pharmacologic basis of nursing practice,* ed 5, St Louis, 1997, Mosby.
12. Oran NT, Oran I, Memis A: Management of patients with malignant obstructive jaundice, *Cancer Nursing* 23(2):128-133, 2000.

CHAPTER 152

Nausea and Vomiting

Sharon R. Smart

DEFINITION/EPIDEMIOLOGY

Nausea, vomiting, and diarrhea account for more than 2 million office visits and 220,000 hospitalizations each year.[1] The causes of nausea and vomiting are varied and present a challenge to health care providers. Not only do the symptoms need to be controlled to provide patient comfort and prevent complications, but the underlying cause must be diagnosed to provide proper treatment.

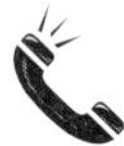

Physician consultation is indicated if nausea and vomiting are accompanied by pain, dehydration, acute abdomen, neurologic changes, or a metabolic imbalance.

PATHOPHYSIOLOGY

Vomiting is induced through stimulation of either the vomiting center (VC) or the chemoreceptor trigger zone (CTZ) of the central nervous system. Stimulation of the VC occurs through afferent vagal and sympathetic visceral pathways from delayed gastric emptying, distention, drugs, emotions, or ischemia.[2] Irritation of the CTZ can occur with metabolic disorders, rapid changes in motion, or medications.[2]

CLINICAL PRESENTATION

The presentation of nausea and vomiting varies from the gradual onset of symptoms noted with medication side effects, gastric retention, or early pregnancy to the acute episodes caused by viral gastroenteritis, food poisoning, increased intracranial pressure, or an acute abdominal emergency. Associated symptoms can include pain, headache, dizziness, tinnitus, diarrhea, fever, mental status changes, pregnancy, and anxiety. A thorough history should include the onset, duration, and severity of symptoms; associated symptoms; current medications; a history of medical problems (e.g., diabetes or irritable bowel syndrome); surgical history; and environmental exposures or therapies including radiation or chemotherapy. The relationship of nausea and vomiting to food, the force of vomiting (projectile vs. retching), and the quality of the emesis (bile, undigested food) should be assessed. A 24-hour dietary review, with bowel symptoms (diarrhea vs. constipation) and the time of the last void, should also be determined.

Acute episodes of nausea and vomiting may be associated with viral gastroenteritis, food poisoning, or medication overdose. Acute emergencies such as acute pancreatitis, appendicitis, bowel obstruction, peritonitis, or cholecystitis may be accompanied by fever or pain. These symptoms also occur in acute episodes of Crohn's disease, colitis, and diverticulitis. Chronic or recurrent nausea and vomiting may be psychogenic or the result of radiation or chemotherapy, gastric disorders, migraine headaches, diabetic gastroparesis, or a metabolic or endocrine abnormality.

PHYSICAL EXAMINATION

A thorough examination should include weight and temperature, as well as orthostatic vital signs to assess volume status. The skin should be assessed for turgor, color, moisture, or rashes; the head and neck should be assessed for evidence of dehydration, acute infection, lymphadenopathy, rigidity, or thyromegaly. A cardiovascular examination is necessary to determine the patient's response to the illness or other signs of infection; abdominal and rectal examinations are crucial to assess for distention, peristalsis, tenderness, rigidity, rebound, masses, fecal impaction, and bleeding. Mental status, gait, and cranial nerve function are also essential components of the evaluation, particularly if increased intracranial pressure is suspected.

DIAGNOSTICS

The presentation of nausea and vomiting, as well as the physical findings, will guide testing. Laboratory tests may include urine for specific gravity, erythrocyte sedimentation rate, serum glucose, electrolytes, ketones, BUN, creatinine, amylase, and LFTs, as well as drug levels if indicated. A serum human chorionic gonadotropin level should be obtained in women of childbearing age. Urinalysis with culture and sensitivity, CBC, thyroid-stimulating hormone, or further endocrine studies may be indicated in some cases.

Abdominal upright and plain x-ray films are necessary if an obstruction is suspected. An ultrasound, barium swallow, CT scan, or an endoscopic examination may be indicated for masses, dysphagia, or suspected gastrointestinal bleeding or ulceration. If a cerebral hemorrhage or mass is suspected, a head CT scan should be ordered after physician consultation. An ECG is indicated if myocardial infarction is considered to be the cause of the nausea and vomiting.

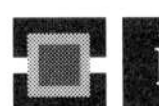

Diagnostics

Nausea and Vomiting

Laboratory
Urinalysis*
Serum electrolytes*
Serum glucose*
BUN*
Creatinine*
Serum ketones*
Amylase*
LFTs*
Drug levels*
Human chorionic gonadotropin*
CBC and differential*

Imaging
Abdominal x-ray studies*
Ultrasound*
Barium swallow*
Endoscopic examination*
Head CT scan*

Other
ECG*

*If indicated.

DIFFERENTIAL DIAGNOSIS

Nausea and vomiting may be caused by an acute or chronic process. Differentiation of the cause will assist in treatment of the underlying disease and in patient education efforts.

MANAGEMENT

Management of nausea and vomiting involves correction of the underlying cause, control of symptoms, and prevention of complications. The possibility of intestinal obstruction or acute abdomen should be eliminated before initiating other treatment options. Uncomplicated viral gastroenteritis (without metabolic imbalance or dehydration) can be managed with increased fluid intake and diet restrictions. A clear liquid diet should be followed for 24 hours, followed by 24 hours of the BRAT (banana, rice, applesauce, and toast) diet. This regimen will provide the bowels with sufficient rest. A bland diet is necessary the following week. Control of vomiting is important for patient comfort and prevention of complications. The use of antiemetics and/or IV hydration may be indicated. Antiemetic medication choices should be selected on the basis of the patient's past medical history and the suspected cause of the nausea and vomiting (Box 152-1). Adequate fluid intake must be maintained to prevent dehydration, especially if the illness is prolonged or severe. Intake should exceed output by at lease 500 ml in a 24-hour period. Assessment for hydration status should include postural vital signs along with the patient's ability to void every 2 to 3 hours. Oral hydration should be attempted in the office if the patient has postural hypotension and is able to tolerate fluid intake. If the patient is too nauseated or does not respond to oral fluid intake, IV hydration should be started. In general, 1 to 2 L of IV normal saline or lactated Ringer's solution over a few hours is well tolerated. Slower rates are recommended for older adults or patients who are debilitated. Physician consultation is recommended if postural hypotension is not corrected or if metabolic alkalosis or severe dehydration is present.

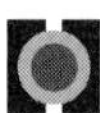

Differential Diagnosis

Nausea and Vomiting

Acute

Acute abdomen (appendicitis, ischemic bowel, peritonitis, abdominal aortic aneurysm, volvulus)
Acute labyrinthitis/Meniere's disease
Cholecystitis
Constipation
Increased intracranial pressure
Infection (viral, bacterial, or parasitic)
Intestinal obstruction
Medication (chemotherapy, toxic level of some medications, anesthesia, or side effect of medications)
Metabolic disturbances (diabetic ketoacidosis, adrenal crisis)
Migraine headache
Motion sickness
Myocardial infarction
Pain
Pregnancy
Uremia

Acute

Achalasia
Anorexia nervosa/bulimia
Cancer
Cirrhosis
Crohn's disease
Diabetic gastroparesis
Diverticular disease
Drug or alcohol use/withdrawal
Hepatitis
Irritable bowel syndrome
Pancreatitis
Peptic ulcer disease
Psychogenic

COMPLICATIONS

Complications of nausea and vomiting may be associated with the underlying condition. However, dehydration, hypokalemia, and metabolic acidosis are a concern. Although uncommon in alert patients, aspiration pneumonitis is a possibility in patients with decreased levels of consciousness. Continual vomiting may result in malnutrition and dental erosion. Forceful vomiting has been the cause of Mallory-Weiss syndrome and esophageal ruptures.

BOX 152-1

ANTIEMETIC MEDICATIONS

BISMUTH SUBSALICYLATE

For nausea with or without diarrhea: 30 ml PO q 30-60 min; maximum 8 doses in 24 hours; available over the counter

DIMENHYDRINATE

To prevent nausea and vomiting associated with motion sickness: 50-100 mg PO 30-60 minutes before travel; may be repeated q 4-6 hours p.r.n.; available over the counter

DRONABINOL

For nausea and vomiting: 5 mg/m2 PO 1-3 hours before chemotherapy; repeated q 2-4 hours p.r.n. to maximum 6 doses daily

METOCLOPRAMIDE HYDROCHLORIDE

For nausea related to diabetic gastroparesis: 10 mg PO 30 minutes before meals and at h.s. for 2-8 weeks, depending on response

For gastroesophageal reflux: 10-15 mg PO q.i.d. p.r.n. 30 minutes before meals and at h.s.; do not use for more than 12 weeks

For nausea and vomiting associated with chemotherapy: 1-2 mg/kg IV slowly over 1-2 minutes or infused over 15 minutes after diluting in 50 ml of D5W, D51/2NS, NS, Ringer's or lactated Ringer's solution; give first dose 30 minutes before chemotherapy, then q 2 hours p.r.n.; do not exceed 5 doses/day; may produce dystonic reaction when given IV; premedicate with diphenhydramine

PROCHLORPERAZINE

For severe nausea and vomiting: 5-10 mg PO t.i.d./q.i.d., 5-10 mg IM q 3-4 hours p.r.n. (maximum 40 mg/day), or 25 mg rectal suppository q 12 hours p.r.n.; may give 2.5-10 mg IV at a rate not to exceed 5 mg/min; IM injections should be given in the upper outer quadrant of the gluteal muscle; this drug should be used when only a few doses are required for treatment

PROMETHAZINE HYDROCHLORIDE

For nausea: 12.5-25 mg PO, IM, or rectally q 4-6 hours p.r.n.; use cautiously in ambulatory patients because of possible pronounced sedative effects.

TRIMETHOBENZAMIDE HYDROCHLORIDE

For mild to moderate nausea and vomiting: 250 mg PO t.i.d./q.i.d., 200 mg IM t.i.d./q.i.d., or 200 mg rectal suppository t.i.d./q.i.d.; IM injections should be given in the upper outer quadrant of the gluteal muscle; this drug is for short-term treatment

INDICATIONS FOR REFERRAL/HOSPITALIZATION

Nausea and vomiting accompanied by pain, dehydration, acute abdomen, neurologic changes, or a metabolic imbalance may require hospitalization, and the primary physician should be consulted. Hospitalization may also be indicated if the patient is unable to maintain hydration status at home. Referral to an appropriate specialist may be necessary if the nausea or vomiting is not controlled by supportive measures such as hydration, diet change, and antiemetics; if the patient's condition worsens or does not respond to treatment; or if a psychologic component is present.

Metabolic disturbances, pregnancy, altered medication, and drug or alcohol levels should be managed in consultation with the primary physician. Consultation is required for emergencies such as acute myocardial infarction or for patients with neurologic changes. Prolonged or recurring nausea or vomiting may indicate gastric paresis, irritable bowel, or pancreatitis and requires consultation with a gastroenterologist or appropriate specialist.

PATIENT AND FAMILY EDUCATION

Patients should be educated about adequate fluid intake, with special attention given to the types of fluid ingested. Oral rehydration solutions and broths are especially helpful in maintaining electrolyte balance. Dairy products and carbonated fluids should be avoided. A minimum of 96 to 120 ounces of fluid should be consumed each hour. An oral rehydration solution may be prepared by mixing 1 cup of orange juice, ¾ teaspoon salt, 1 teaspoon baking soda, 4 tablespoons of sugar, and 1 L of water.[3]

Because dehydration can occur easily and cause persistent vomiting, patients should be instructed to notify their primary care provider if any of the following occur:

- Vomiting persists despite antiemetic use
- Vomiting is accompanied by fever, severe abdominal pain, severe headache, neck pain, or lethargy
- Urine output becomes dark, or the patient does not void at least every 2 hours during the day
- Dizziness or light-headedness occurs with or without position change
- Patient is vomiting blood or fluid that has the appearance of coffee grounds

HEALTH PROMOTION

Patients should be instructed in the proper handling and storing of food products to prevent contamination and possible food poisoning. Patients traveling abroad should receive the necessary vaccinations and treatments appropriate for the country visited. Guidelines are available from the Centers for Disease Control and Prevention or through local travel clinics.

REFERENCES

1. Gavin N, Merrick N, Davidson B: Efficacy of glucose-based oral rehydration therapy, *Pediatrics* 98(1):45-51, 1996.
2. Hogan CM: Advances in the management of nausea and vomiting, *Nurs Clin North Am* 25(2):475-497, 1990.
3. Guerrant R, Bobak D: Bacterial and protozoal gastroenteritis, *N Engl J Med* 325(5):327-340, 1991.

CHAPTER 153

Oropharyngeal Dysphagia

Talli Craig McCormick

DEFINITION/EPIDEMIOLOGY

Oropharyngeal dysphagia is a swallowing disorder that involves dysfunction of one or more stages in the normal sequence of swallowing. This type of dysphagia differs from upper gastrointestinal disorders in that the dysfunction involves oral, pharyngeal, and laryngeal structures. The dysphagia may be mild or severe, resulting in malnutrition, dehydration, choking, aspiration, pneumonia, and even death. Estimates of incidence in the community vary, but in nursing homes, 60% of residents may have feeding difficulties.[1] Residents with aspiration are thought to have a 1-year mortality rate of 45%.[2]

PATHOPHYSIOLOGY

Dysphagia may be either oropharyngeal or esophageal. The etiology can be neurologic, neuromuscular, metabolic, pharmacologic, infectious, psychiatric, environmental, or structural. Identification of the causative agent or disease is paramount in the assessment and treatment of dysphagia. Structural causes are more common in esophageal dysphagia, and functional causes are more likely in oropharyngeal dysphagia (Box 153-1). Structural causes include trauma or surgery, tumor, webs, strictures or stenoses, diverticuli, infection, and, in some cases, cervical osteophytes or cricopharyngeal bars.[3]

To more fully understand dysphagia, it is essential to appreciate the anatomy and physiology of normal swallowing. Swallowing has three commonly described phases: oral, pharyngeal, and esophageal.[4] In addition to these three phases, there are preparatory phases to the act of eating. Most of us decide when we are hungry and what we would like to eat. We prepare it or go to a restaurant. We decide with whom we will eat. These decisions involve autonomy, fairly intact cognition, and neuromuscular function. Nursing home residents and homebound older adults may have significant limitations or restrictions in this preparatory phase.[5]

During the oral phase, a multitude of sensory information is gathered about the food and the involved structures. Quantity, shape, consistency, and moisture content are determined, along with the temperature, taste, and location of the food. The touch and pressure exerted on the oral structures, especially the tongue and hard and soft palates, are transmitted to the brainstem for further action and distribution. This continuous assessment by the sensory system allows for precise communication with the muscles of mastication.

Chewing (mastication) involves cranial nerves (CNs) V (trigeminal), VII (facial), IX (glossopharyngeal), and XII (hypoglossal), in addition to the muscles of the jaw, cheeks, tongue, and palate. The lips remain closed during chewing, while the tongue and teeth prepare the food into a bolus of the proper size and consistency. The soft palate descends to help hold the food within the mouth during chewing. The teeth close, the tongue

BOX 153-1

POTENTIAL CAUSES OF OROPHARYNGEAL DYSPHAGIA

IATROGENIC
Medication side effects (e.g., xerostomia, chemotherapy, neuroleptics)
Postsurgical muscular or neurogenic
Radiation
Corrosive (pill injury, intentional)

INFECTIOUS
Diphtheria
Botulism
Lyme disease
Syphilis
Mucositis (herpes, cytomegalovirus, *Candida*, etc.)

METABOLIC
Amyloidosis
Cushing's syndrome
Thyrotoxicosis
Wilson's disease

MYOPATHIC
Connective tissue disease
Myasthenia gravis
Myotonic dystrophy
Oculopharyngeal dystrophy
Polymyositis
Sarcoidosis
Paraneoplastic syndromes

NEUROLOGIC
Brain stem tumors
Head trauma
Stroke
Cerebral palsy
Guillain-Barré syndrome
Huntington's disease
Multiple sclerosis
Polio
Postpolio syndrome
Tardive dyskinesia
Amyotrophic lateral sclerosis
Parkinson's disease
Dementia

STRUCTURAL
Cricopharyngeal bar
Zenker's diverticulum
Cervical webs
Oropharyngeal tumors
Osteophytes and skeletal abnormalities
Congenital (cleft palate, diverticula, pouches)

PSYCHIATRIC
Grief
Depression
Globus

ENVIRONMENTAL
Poor positioning
Eating or being fed too quickly
Eating or being fed too large a bolus
Inappropriate consistency
Poor oral health or hygiene
Too distracted

Modified from Cook IJ, Kahrilal PJ: A technical review on management of oropharyngeal dysphagia, *Gastroenterology* 116(2):455-478, 1999; and Blackington E and others: Oropharyngeal dysphagia in the elderly, *Adv Nurse Pract* 7:45, 2001.

places the bolus in its central groove, and the bolus is then rapidly pushed, or transferred, through the pillars (fauces) into the pharynx.

At this point, the bolus passes a ring of sensory receptors at the base of the tongue, pillars, soft palate, and posterior pharyngeal wall. The transmission of a sensory impulse indicating the presence of a bolus is sent via CN IX (glossopharyngeal) to the swallowing center in the brainstem, which then initiates the involuntary phase of the swallow.[5-8]

Sensory input is also crucial to the pharyngeal stage. As the tongue pushes the bolus to the posterior pharynx, the soft palate flattens upward and backward (CN V), sealing off the nasopharynx. Simultaneously, the hyoid and larynx begin to move upward (CN X), tipping back the epiglottis. The pillars lower and the tongue presses against the posterior pharyngeal wall (CN IX) to block retrograde movement of the bolus into the oral cavity. Sensory fibers of CN X (vagus) transmit information to the swallowing center in the brainstem. The impulse returns via the motor component of the vagus nerve and initiates peristalsis of the pharyngeal constrictors to propel the bolus toward the esophagus, passing the valleculae and piriform sinuses. The soft palate descends, the larynx continues to rise, and the epiglottis descends. As the epiglottis descends to block the laryngeal opening, the upper esophageal sphincter (UES) or cricopharyngeal sphincter opens to allow the bolus to pass into the esophagus.[5-8]

As the food bolus enters the esophagus, these processes begin in reverse. Once in the esophagus, the UES closes and peristalsis and gravity propel the bolus toward the stomach. The lower esophageal sphincter (LES) opens and the bolus enters the stomach. Normal transit time varies depending on bolus consistency but is generally 2 to 4 seconds.[5-8]

CLINICAL PRESENTATION

Dysphagic patients can present with malnutrition, weight loss, dehydration, or pneumonia. Problems in the oral stage include poor bolus control, spillage either from the lips or into the pharynx, dry oral membranes, pocketing or oral residue, and difficulty with chewing. Pharyngeal dysphagia often results from weakness or poor coordination of the pharyngeal muscles. This can cause delayed swallow, failure of airway protection, nasal or oral regurgitation, or residue remaining in the pharynx after swallow, manifested as coughing, choking, or gurgling.

Xerostomia (dry mouth), either intrinsic or extrinsic, can be a contributing factor in dysphagia in 16% of older men and 25% of older women.[9] Globus, which is the sensation of a lump in the throat, can occur alone or coexist with esophageal dysphagia, particularly when accompanied by chest pain or heartburn.[10] Globus alone is merely a sensory experience; swallowing itself is unimpaired.

A detailed history is the most important step in differential diagnosis. Because dysphagia can be associated with neurologic disease, a thorough neuromuscular history is also important. Obtaining an accurate history can be complicated by reduced alertness as well as cognitive and speech impairments, which can also affect the patient's ability to participate in examination, diagnostics, and treatment strategies.

Onset, progression, location, duration, and food consistency aid in diagnosis. A short duration associated with weight loss can indicate malignancy.[3] Abrupt onset associated with neurologic impairment suggests a cerebrovascular accident. It is estimated that one third to one half of new stroke patients will have dysphagia, and in 10% to 15% of these, the dysphagia will persist beyond 1 month.[11] Swallowing thin liquids is often a problem after a stroke. Gradual progressive onset is more likely to be associated with Parkinson's disease, amyotrophic lateral sclerosis (ALS), sarcoidosis, myasthenia gravis, Alzheimer's dementia, or other chronic diseases.[3] Parkinson's disease is the most common movement disorder in older adults and leads to tongue rigidity and tremor, making bolus formation and transfer into the pharynx difficult. Difficulty swallowing only solids suggests a structural cause but not necessarily the location of the impairment. Ability to point to where the food "sticks" is useful for oropharyngeal obstructions and correlates well with radiographic studies. However, below the pharynx this information is less diagnostic.[12]

Eating or being fed too rapidly may result in either oral or nasal regurgitation and choking. Coughing up food after meals can indicate a pharyngeal diverticulum.[3] Frequent swallowing can indicate oral or pharyngeal residue. Patient positioning, degree of distraction, companions or assistants, utensils used, food consistency, and likes and dislikes can all provide information useful not only in differential diagnosis but also in deciding on treatment strategies.

A complete review of all medications is necessary because some medications can cause or contribute to swallowing dysfunction, whereas others, such as Fosamax (alendronate sodium), nonsteroidal antiinflammatory drugs (NSAIDs), and potassium, can cause direct damage to the esophageal mucosa (Box 153-2). Xerostomia, altered esophageal sphincter pressure, and reduced alertness are other medication side effects that can affect swallowing.[5]

PHYSICAL EXAMINATION

A thorough physical examination aids in the differential diagnosis, establishes the existence of deficits and impairments, and determines whether malnutrition or pneumonia is present.[3] A complete oral examination will reveal oral health and hygiene, including dentition, oral sensation, tongue strength, mobility, coordination, and specific CN function. Altered speech or voice, particularly nasal speech or a gurgling voice, should be noted. Nasal speech can indicate soft palate dysfunction, whereas a gurgling or wet voice is more indicative of weak pharyngeal constrictors. The presence or absence of the gag reflex is not predictive of swallowing dysfunction or risk of aspiration because the gag reflex may be absent in 20% to 40% of healthy adults.[13-15] Trial sips of water or spoonfuls of applesauce or pudding can reveal specific deficits. Observation and palpation of laryngeal elevation can detect delayed swallowing. The pharyngeal swallow should occur within approximately 1 second.

The complete neuromuscular examination includes CN function (particularly V, VII, IX, X, and XII) and assessment of muscle strength/weakness, muscle atrophy, or altered coordination. Involuntary movements, tremor, or gait disturbance should also be determined. A mental status assessment with particular emphasis on level of alertness and ability to concentrate and cooperate is important. Deformities of or past operations on the head, neck, or trunk may affect dysphagia or the ability to participate in diagnostic studies. Despite skillful and comprehensive physical examination, the risk for aspiration may not be fully appreciated without the use of radiographic study.[16]

BOX 153-2

MEDICATION-RELATED CONDITIONS THAT CAUSE OROPHARYNGEAL DYSPHAGIA

XEROSTOMIA
Antidepressants
Antispasmodics
Antihypertensives
Anticholinergics
Antihistamines
Bronchodilators
Sedatives

CENTRAL NERVOUS SYSTEM DEPRESSION
Anticonvulsants
Antianxiety agents (alprazolam, diazepam, chlordiazepoxide)
Antispasmodics (dantrolene, baclofen)
Antidepressants (trazodone, amitriptyline, desipramine)
Neuroleptics (haloperidol, chlorpromazine, thioridazine)
Sedatives

IMMUNOSUPPRESSION
Antibiotics
Cytotoxic agents

INCREASED SALIVATION
Anticholinesterase
Clonazepam
Clozapine

NEUROMUSCULAR JUNCTION BLOCKADE
Aminoglycoside antibiotics
Botulinum (Botox)

MYOPATHY
Corticosteroids
Lipid-lowering agents
Colchicine
L-Tryptophan

MUCOSAL INJURY
Fosamax
Tetracycline
NSAIDs
Potassium
Ferrous sulfate

LOWER ESOPHAGEAL SPHINCTER PRESSURE
Theophylline
Nitrates
Calcium channel blockers
Beta blockers
Hormone replacement therapy (HRT)
Anticholinergics

DIAGNOSTICS

Videofluoroscopy or modified barium swallow (MBS) is the most appropriate and commonly used imaging procedure. The primary purpose of the MBS is to determine if and to what degree aspiration occurs. Patients must be able to sit upright, hold still, and follow commands during the examination. Using contrast material, this radiographic study is designed to assess functional impairment of swallowing in four categories: delay in swallowing initiation, nasopharyngeal regurgitation, aspiration, and pharyngeal residue. Usually a variety of consistencies and bolus volumes are assessed during the MBS. This study not only aids in diagnosis but also helps determine the effectiveness of various positions, consistencies, or maneuvers used in treatment.

If a structural, rather than functional, cause is suspected, nasoendoscopy should be considered. Nasoendoscopy permits direct visualization of the oral cavity, nasopharynx, pharynx, and larynx. Lesion biopsy samples can be obtained during the procedure.

If muscle weakness or problems with sphincter relaxation are suspected, manometry can measure intraluminal pressures during the swallow. Manometry can be synchronized with videofluoroscopy (manofluorography) to distinguish more subtle findings.[17]

The fiberoptic endoscopic examination of swallowing, ultrasound, electromyography, and electroglottography are other diagnostic procedures that can be appropriate, although these tests are more limited. CT or MRI of the head and neck can aid in diagnosis but do not describe the actual swallow mechanism.

DIFFERENTIAL DIAGNOSIS

See the Differential Diagnosis box on p. 652.

MANAGEMENT

Structural causes of dysphagia such as tumors, strictures, webs, or diverticuli are usually treated with surgery or dilation. Chemotherapy and/or radiation may be used for tumors. No randomized controlled trials have been conducted, but a number of case series indicate that webs and strictures are amenable to dilation. Cricopharyngeal myotomy is the most common surgical treatment for oropharyngeal dysphagia of structural etiology, and consistent evidence of its beneficial effect is available.[18-25]

Studies exploring the use of myotomy for dysphagia of neurogenic origin are very different. Data are conflicting and are often methodologically weak and sometimes qualitative. Nonetheless, myotomy may offer benefit to 50% of patients with neurogenic dysphagia.[3] It is suggested that patients who benefit may be those with a higher preoperative hypopharyngeal intrabolus pressure related to resistance of flow across the UES.[26]

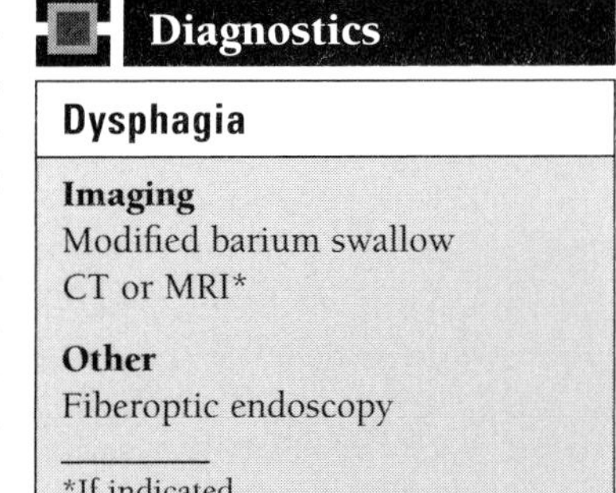
Diagnostics

Dysphagia

Imaging
Modified barium swallow
CT or MRI*

Other
Fiberoptic endoscopy

*If indicated.

Other structural radiographic abnormalities exist, but their impact on swallowing is unclear. Cervical osteophytes are a relatively common finding in older adults, but the incidence of actual dysphagia associated with them is less than 1%.[27] Cricopharyngeal bars are less common, and dysphagia is no more common in patients with bars than in patients without bars.[28] However, cricopharyngeal myotomy may relieve the dysphagia in patients who have no other abnormality of functional significance.[29]

Aspiration and Nonoral Feeding in Dysphagia of Functional Origin

Standard practice has been that patients who are found to have severe aspiration, which is not treatable with dietary or positional modifications, should receive nonoral feeding to prevent aspiration. It is clear that aspiration demonstrates severe swallowing dysfunction and that death is associated with aspiration pneumonia.[2,3] However, the relationship between aspiration and the risk of developing pneumonia is not as obvious. Smithard and others[30] found that dysphagic stroke patients were at significant risk for chest infections, malnutrition, and death, but aspiration did not predict this risk. Similarly, Johnson and others[31] discovered that 29 of 60 dysphagic stroke patients developed pneumonia within 1 year. However, this was not correlated with aspiration or pharyngeal pooling on videofluoroscopy. A recent study by Terpenning and others[32] suggests an increased risk of aspiration pneumonia in patients who have chronic obstructive pulmonary disease (COPD) or diabetes mellitus or who require assistance with feeding. Aspiration pneumonia was also more common in subjects with oral *P. gingivalis*, decayed teeth, and visible dental plaque.[32] Although Terpenning and others[32] hypothesized that poor healing associated with diabetes and poor pulmonary clearance could contribute to the development of pneumonia, they did not find an association with stroke. Langmore and others[33] propose that patients with compromised functional capacity may be fed too quickly or with too large a bolus. Croghan and others[2] found that the 15 of 22 dysphagic patients who received feeding tubes were at a significantly higher risk of pneumonia and death than were the 7 patients who did not receive them. In summary, it appears that aspiration probably contributes to the risk of pneumonia but may not be the only important contributor; nonoral feeding may not reduce this risk in all patients and, in some patients, may increase it.

The goal of differential diagnosis is identification of the disease process causing the dysphagia, if present. In Parkinson's disease, although there is little evidence that antiparkinsonian medications improve swallowing function in the long term, Bushmann and others[34] found short-term improvement in symptoms and videofluoroscopic findings. Thomas and Haigh[35] also offer case reports of a good response to antiparkinsonian medication. Improvement in dysphagia associated with thyrotoxicosis is more apparent; Branski and others[36] report resolution of dysphagia when patients become euthyroid.

Swallowing Strategies and Therapies

Head positioning, swallowing maneuvers, and dietary textural modifications seem to demonstrate the clearest evidence of benefit in the treatment of functional dysphagia.[3] Table 153-1 provides data on swallowing therapy techniques, indications, and rationale. Many therapeutic measures require autonomy and fairly intact cognitive function for memory and learning. For

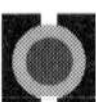

Differential Diagnosis

Dysphagia

Mechanical Problems
Acute inflammations
- Herpes simplex
- Tonsillitis, epiglottitis, pharyngitis, esophagitis
- Infectious and inflammatory bone and mucosal disorders

Chemical agents (aspirin, lozenges, gargles, alcohol)
Medications (see Box 153-2)
Skeletal anomalies
Muscle anomalies
Macroglossia
Pharyngoesophageal diverticulum
Carcinoma
Surgery
- Oral, palatal resections
- Glossectomy
- Supralaryngectomy; partial, total laryngectomy
- Tracheoesophageal puncture
- Chest surgery (coronary artery bypass graft)
- Endarterectomy
- Anterior cervical spine surgery

Irradiation
Cervical spine disease
Nasoenteric tubes
Tracheostoma tubes
Esophageal stenosis, webs, rings, stricture

Neurogenic Problems
Riley-Day syndrome
Acquired central nervous system disorders
- Stroke syndromes and vascular disorders
- Capsular infarct
- Pseudobulbar palsy
- Apraxias and agnosias
- Lacunar disease

Movement disorders
- Parkinson's disease
- Dystonias and dyskinesias
- Huntington's disease
- Palatal myoclonus

Poliomyelitis and other systemic infections
- Diphtheria
- Botulism
- Rabies
- Tetanus

Amyotrophic lateral sclerosis
Acquired peripheral nervous system disorders
Recurrent laryngeal neuropathies
Cranial nerve neuropathies
- Guillain-Barré syndrome
- Diabetes
- Leukemia
- Lymphoma
- Carcinoma
- Other neuropathies

Neurodevelopmental disorders
- Cerebral palsy
- Abnormal oral and pharyngeal reflexes
- Abnormal salivation
- Others

Myogenic Problems
Myasthenia gravis
Neuromuscular esophageal disorders
- Scleroderma
- Achalasia
- Diffuse spasm
- Others

Other Conditions
Dementias
Multiple sclerosis
Tuberculosis
Syphilis
Neoplasms
Degenerative disorders
Psychopathology
Feeding phobias
Atypical parent-child interactions
Sensory deficits

patients with certain strokes, Alzheimer's dementia, and some other neurologic diseases, this requirement may limit the usefulness of these techniques. Dietary modifications may be the best choice for many of these patients. Rasley and others[37] were able to prevent aspiration by altering head position in 25% of patients and to increase the volume of bolus tolerated without aspiration by 77% of patients. One randomized controlled trial studied the efficacy of alteration of diet consistency.[38] After 6 months of dietary modification (mechanical soft with thickened fluids), Groher[38] found an 80% reduction in episodes of pneumonia in dysphagic stroke patients compared with subjects consuming pureed foods and regular liquids.

COMPLICATIONS

Complications associated with dysphagia include impaired quality of life, coughing, choking, aspiration, malnutrition, dehydration, pneumonia, and death. Gastrostomy tube placement may be necessary and appropriate for some patients.

INDICATIONS FOR REFERRAL/HOSPITALIZATION

Dysphagic patients and/or their families should be offered dietary consultation. Other referrals will be dictated by the etiology of the dysphagia. A gastroenterologist should be consulted for a suspected gastroesophageal problem. Structural abnormalities may

TABLE 153-1 Swallowing Therapy Techniques, Indications, and Rationale

Technique	Execution (Rationale)	Indication
DIETARY MODIFICATION		
Thickened liquids	Reduced tendency to spill over tongue base	Disordered tongue function Preswallow spill/aspiration Impaired laryngeal closure
Thin liquids	Offers less resistance to flow	Weak pharyngeal contraction Reduced cricopharyngeal opening
MANEUVERS		
Supraglottic swallow	Breath hold, double swallow, forceful expiration (closes vocal folds before swallowing)	Aspiration: reduced/late vocal fold closures
Supersupraglottic swallow	Effortful breath hold (closes vocal folds before and during swallow) Increased anterior tilting of arytenoids	Aspiration (poor closure of laryngeal introitus)
Effortful swallow	Effortful tongue action (increases posterior motion tongue base)	Poor posterior tongue base motion
Mendelsohn maneuver	Prolong hyoid excursion guided by manual palpation (prolongs UES opening)	Poor pharyngeal clearance and laryngeal movement
POSTURAL ADJUSTMENTS		
Head tilt	Tilt posteriorly at swallow initiation (gravity clears oral cavity) Tilt laterally to unaffected side (directs bolus down stronger side)	Poor tongue control Unilateral pharyngeal weakness
Chin tuck	Chin down (widens valleculae, displaces tongue base and epiglottis posteriorly)	Aspiration, delayed pharyngeal response, reduced posterior tongue base motion
Head rotation	Rotate head to affected side (isolates damaged side from bolus path, reduces LES pressure) Rotate head to affected side with extrinsic pressure on thyroid cartilage (increases adduction)	Unilateral pharyngeal weakness Unilateral laryngeal dysfunction Unilateral pharyngeal dysfunction
Lying on side, elevation	Right or left lateral (bypass laryngeal introitus)	Aspiration, bilateral pharyngeal impairment or reduced laryngeal elevation
FACILITATORY TECHNIQUES		
Strengthening exercises	Various	Nonprogressive disease
Biofeedback	Augment volitional component	Poor pharyngeal clearance
Thermal stimulation	Cold, tactile stimulation to anterior faucial pillar	Delayed/absent swallow response
Gustatory stimulation	Sour bolus (facilitates swallow response)	Huntington's chorea, stroke

From Cook IJ, Kahrilas PJ: AGA technical review on management of oropharyngeal dysphagia, *Gastroenterology* 116(2):470, 1999.

require surgical intervention. Moderate to severe cases of oropharyngeal dysphagia require referral to a speech therapist, particularly if therapeutic swallowing techniques are needed. Referral to a neurologist is warranted for patients if the cause of the dysphagia is neurogenic. If oral health and hygiene are a concern, referral to a dentist for evaluation and treatment is indicated. Counseling or psychiatric consultation is necessary for patients experiencing grief or depression associated with the dysphagia.

Other co-morbid illnesses or conditions may affect dysphagia or contribute to the development of pneumonia. Pulmonary rehabilitation may be indicated for patients with concurrent lung disease. Suspected pneumonia should usually be evaluated at the hospital, especially if gastric fluid is thought to be the aspirate. Malnutrition or dehydration may require hospital admission.

PATIENT AND FAMILY EDUCATION

The most important aspects of education include patient feeding, positioning, maneuvers, and dietary textural modifications. Speech therapists can teach patients and families positioning and maneuvers to improve swallowing efficacy. The Silver Spoons Program,[39] which was designed to facilitate safe feeding, can also assist family members or institutional staff. Careful attention to bolus size, consistency, allowing plenty of time for meals, and proper patient positioning for meals improves safety.

Discussion concerning the risks and benefits of feeding tubes in specific disease entities is important for patients, families, and, often, staff. Although feeding tubes may not seem appropriate for patients with severe dementia,[40] cultural and religious preferences must be respected. Other concurrent illnesses may be important considerations. More research is needed, but for any given patient the decision to place a feeding tube must remain individualized and carefully considered.

HEALTH PROMOTION

Regular health screenings and recommendations regarding diet, exercise, and smoking cessation can prevent or delay the onset of disease, particularly in those with a strong family history of stroke. Once dysphagia is established, good oral hygiene, dental care, careful attention to positioning and swallowing techniques, and management of co-morbid illnesses, particularly respiratory and diabetes, can help to prevent pneumonia. Counseling can be beneficial for patients with a family history of hereditary neurologic or myopathic disorders associated with dysphagia. Support for families caring for dysphagic members may also help reduce caregiver stress.

Cook and Kahrilas provide an excellent recent review of oropharyngeal dysphagia.[3]

REFERENCES

1. Siebens H and others: Correlates and consequences of eating dependency in the institutionalized elderly, *J Am Geriatr Soc* 34:192-198, 1986.
2. Croghan JE and others: Pilot study of 12-month outcomes of nursing home patients with aspiration on videofluoroscopy, *Dysphagia* 9: 141-146, 1994.
3. Cook IJ, Kahrilas PJ: AGA technical review on management of oropharyngeal dysphagia, *Gastroenterology* 116(2):455-478, 1999.
4. Magendie F: *Precis elementaire de physiologie,* Paris, 1836.
5. Blackington E and others: Oropharyngeal dysphagia in the elderly, *Adv Nurse Pract* (7):42-49, 2001.
6. Kahrilas PJ: The anatomy and physiology of dysphagia. In Gelfand DW, Richter JE, editors: *Dysphagia: diagnosis and treatment,* New York, 1989, Igahu-Shoin.
7. Dodds W, Stewart E, Logemann J: Physiology and radiology of the normal oral and pharyngeal phases of swallowing, *Am J Radiol* 154: 953-963, 1990.
8. Perlman AL, Christensen J: Topography and functional anatomy of the swallowing structures. In Perlman AL, Schulze-Delrieu K, editors: *Deglutition and its disorders: anatomy physiology, clinical diagnosis and management,* San Diego, 1997, Singular Publishing Group, Inc.
9. Osterberg T, Landahl S, Hedergard M: Salivary flow, saliva, pH and buffering capacity in 70 year old men and women, *J Oral Rehabil* 11:157-170, 1984.
10. Moser G and others: High incidence of esophageal motor disorder in consecutive patients with globus sensation, *Gastroenterology* 101:1512-1521, 1991.
11. Gordon C, Hewer RL, Wade DT: Dysphagia in acute stroke, *Br Med J* 295:411, 1987.
12. Logemann JA: *Evaluation and treatment of swallowing disorders,* San Diego, 1983, College Hill.
13. Leder SB: Gag reflex and dysphagia, *Head Neck* 18:138-141, 1996.
14. Leder SB: Videofluoroscopic evaluation of aspiration with visual examination of the gag reflex and velar movement, *Dysphagia* 12:21-23, 1997.
15. Davies AE and others: Pharyngeal sensation and gag reflex in healthy subjects, *Lancet* 345:487-488, 1995.
16. Splaingard ML and others: Aspiration in rehabilitation patients: videofluoroscopy vs bedside clinical assessment, *Arch Phys Med Rehabil* 69:637-640, 1988.
17. Jacob P and others: Upper esophageal sphincter opening and modulation during swallowing, *Gastroenterology* 97:1469-1478, 1989.
18. Gagic NM: Cricopharyngeal myotomy, *Can J Surg* 26:47-49, 1983.
19. Duranceau A, Rheault MJ, Jamieson GG: Physiological response to cricopharyngeal myotomy and diverticulum suspension, *Surgery* 94:655-662, 1983.
20. Bonavina L, Nasir A, DeMeester T: Pharyngoesophageal dysfunctions: the role of cricopharyngeal myotomy, *Arch Surg* 120:541-549, 1985.
21. Lerut T, Van Raemdonck D, Guelinckx P: Pharyngo-oesophageal diverticulum (Zenker's): clinical therapeutic and morphological aspects, *Acta Gastrenterol Belg* 53:330-337, 1990.
22. Barthen W and others: Surgical therapy of Zenker's diverticulum: low risk and high efficiency, *Dysphagia* 5:13-19, 1990.
23. Lindgren S, Ekberg O: Cricopharyngeal myotomy in the treatment of dysphagia, *Clin Otolaryngol* 15:221-227, 1990.
24. Witterick IJ, Gullane PJ, Yeung E: Outcome analysis of Zenker's diverticulectomy and cricopharyngeal myotomy, *Head Neck* 17:382-388, 1995.
25. Shaw DW and others: Influence of surgery on deglutitive upper esophageal sphincter mechanics in Zenker's diverticulum, *Gut* 38: 806-811, 1996.
26. Ali GN and others: Predictors of outcome following cricopharyngeal disruption for pharyngeal dysphagia, *Dysphagia* 12:133-139, 1997.
27. Stuart D: Dysphagia due to cervical osteophytes, *Int Orthop* 13:95-99, 1989.
28. Curtis DJ, Cruess DF, Berg T: The cricopharyngeal muscle: a video-recording review, *Am J Radiol* 142:497-500, 1984.
29. Cruse JP and others: The pathology of cricopharyngeal dysphagia, *Histopathology* 3:223-232, 1979.
30. Smithard DG and others: Complications and outcome after acute stroke: does dysphagia matter? *Stroke* 27:1200-1204, 1996.
31. Johnson ER, McKenzie SW, Sievers A: Aspiration pneumonia in stroke, *Arch Phys Med Rehabil* 74:973-976, 1993.
32. Terpenning MS and others: Aspiration pneumonia: dental and oral risk factors in an older veteran population, *J Am Geriatr Soc* 49: 557-563, 2001.
33. Langmore SE and others: Predictors of aspiration pneumonia: how important is dysphagia? *Dysphagia* 13:69-81, 1998.
34. Bushmann M and others: Swallowing abnormalities and their response to treatment in Parkinson's disease, *Neurology* 39:1309-1314, 1989.
35. Thomas M, Haigh RA: Dysphagia, a reversible cause not to be forgotten, *Postgrad Med J* 71:94-95, 1995.
36. Branski D and others: Dysphagia as a primary manifestation of hyperthyroidism, *J Clin Gastroenterol* 6:437-440, 1984.
37. Rasley A and others: Prevention of barium aspiration during videofluoroscopic swallowing studies: value of change in posture, *Am J Roentgenol* 160:1005-1009, 1993.
38. Groher ME: Bolus management and aspiration pneumonia in patients with pseudobulbar dysphagia, *Dysphagia* 1:215-216, 1987.
39. Musson ND, Frye GD, Nash M: Silver Spoons: supervised volunteers provide feeding of patients, *Geriatr Nurs* 18:18-19, 1997.
40. Braun UK and others: Malnutrition in patients with severe dementia: is there a place for PEG tube feeding? *Ann Long-Term Care* 9(9):47-55, 2001.

CHAPTER 154

Pancreatitis

Terry Mahan Buttaro and JoAnn Trybulski

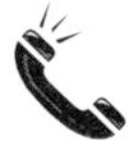

Physician consultation is indicated for patients with suspected pancreatitis.

Acute Pancreatitis

DEFINITION/EPIDEMIOLOGY

Acute pancreatitis, a severe inflammation of the pancreas, is characterized as edematous, hemorrhagic, or necrotizing, depending on the etiology, clinical presentation, and pathologic features. The clinical course and presentation range from mild, self-limiting abdominal pain to life-threatening, multisystemic complications with a high mortality rate. The diagnosis is often overlooked, but acute pancreatitis, which can occur at any age, is increasing, approximating 54 to 238 episodes per 1 million persons each year.[1] In the United States, alcohol abuse and biliary tract disease account for 65% to 80% of cases, although a number of factors have been implicated as precipitants[1] (Boxes 154-1 and 154-2). Biliary tract disease has also been associated with acute pancreatitis in pregnancy.[2]

PATHOPHYSIOLOGY

The exact mechanism of pancreatitis is not well understood. Disturbance to cystolic free ionized calcium, a substance in acinar cells, may initiate a series of intracellular events stimulating the conversion of trypsinogen to trypsin within the pancreatic acinar cell.[3] Once present, trypsin activates other proteolytic enzymes; chymotrypsin, elastase, lipase, and phospholipase, as well as the balance between the proteolytic and protease inhibitors, are disturbed. The resulting inflammation and necrosis

BOX 154-1

FACTORS ASSOCIATED WITH ACUTE PANCREATITIS

MOST FREQUENT CAUSES

Gallstones
Alcoholism
Idiopathic (may be related to diverse causes)

FREQUENT CAUSES

Toxins
- Ethyl alcohol
- Methyl alcohol
- Organophosphorous insecticides
- Scorpion venom

Medications
- ACE inhibitors
- Acetaminophen
- Aminosalicylates
- Asparaginase (Elspar)
- Azathioprine (Imuran)
- Chlorthalidone
- Cimetidine
- Corticosteroids
- ddI (2′,3′-dideoxyinosine: associated with concurrent pentamidine treatment)
- Erythromycin
- Estrogens (identified with type IV or V hyperlipidemia)
- Ethacrynic acid
- Furosemide (rare)
- Iatrogenic hypercalcemia
- IV lipids
- L-Asparaginase
- Methyldopa (rare)
- Metronidazole (rare)
- Nitrofurantoin
- Nonsteroidals
- Olsalazine 5-ASA (rare)
- Pentamidine (rare)
- Phenformin (rare)
- Ranitidine
- Sulindac
- Sulfonamides (rare)
- Tetracycline (rare)
- Thiazide diuretics
- Valproic acid

Blunt abdominal trauma
Crohn's disease of the duodenum
End-stage renal failure
Iatrogenic trauma: Cardiopulmonary bypass, endoscopic retrograde cholangiopancreatography, endoscopic sphincterotomy, manometry of the sphincter of Oddi, organ transplant, postoperative pancreatitis following abdominal or thoracic surgery
Hyperparathyroidism associated with hypercalcemia
Infection
- Parasitic: *Ascaris* worms, clonorchiasis
- Viral: Coxsackievirus, cytomegalovirus, mumps, and fulminant viral hepatitis
- Bacterial: *Campylobacter* jejuni, *Mycoplasma pneumoniae, Salmonella,* microlithiasis

Lipid abnormalities (hypertriglyceridemia)
Metabolic abnormalities: Hypercalcemia associated with excessive doses of vitamin D, parathyroid adenoma, familial hypocalciuric hypercalcemia, hypercalcemia associated with total parenteral nutrition
Pancreatic divisum
Pancreatic outflow obstruction: Afferent loop obstruction, annular pancreatitis
Penetrating peptic ulcer
Pregnancy
Surgery (endoscopic retrograde cholangiopancreatography)
Trauma
Tumor: Primary and metastatic

LESS FREQUENT CAUSES

Hereditary
Pancreatic cancer
Periampullary duodenal diverticulum
Refeeding after fasting
Rheumatologic disorders: Systemic lupus erythematosus, mixed connective tissue disorders, scleroderma
Thrombotic thrombocytopenic purpura
Vasculitis

BOX 154-2

FACTORS ASSOCIATED WITH ACUTE PANCREATITIS IN HIV-POSITIVE PATIENTS

INFECTION
Cytomegalovirus
Cryptococcus
Cryptosporidium
Mycobacterium avium and *Mycobacterium tuberculosis*
Toxoplasma gondii

MEDICATIONS
Didanosine
Pentamidine
Trimethoprim-sulfamethoxazole

may precipitate shock, hypocalcemia, coagulation disturbances, and pulmonary, renal, and cardiac dysfunction.

CLINICAL PRESENTATION

The sudden onset of constant, knifelike, increasingly severe epigastric or periumbilical pain is suggestive of acute pancreatitis. Although the pain can continue for several days and is usually excruciating, acute pancreatitis can be mild or even painless. The discomfort often radiates to the chest, left shoulder, left upper quadrant, lower abdomen, or flanks or in a bandlike fashion to the back. Nausea and vomiting invariably are present, and patients with pancreatitis appear ill and restless. Because the pain is aggravated in the supine position, afflicted patients may be sitting with their knees drawn up and the trunk flexed. Pertinent history includes pregnancy, human immunodeficiency virus (HIV) infection, recent alcohol ingestion, a heavy meal preceding the attack, previous history of blunt trauma, biliary colic or similar episodes, and a careful medication review.

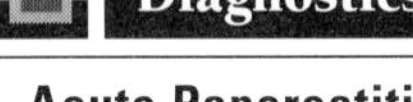

Diagnostics

Acute Pancreatitis

Laboratory
Chem 7 (electrolytes, BUN, creatinine)
Fasting lipid profile*
Serum and urinary trypsinogen-2
Trypsinogen activation peptide
C-reactive protein*
TSH*
Serum hCG in women of child-bearing age

Imaging
CT scan
Ultrasound
KUB
Chest x-ray
HIDA (hepato-iminodiacetic acid [lidofenin]) scan*

Other
ECG
ERCP*

*If indicated.

PHYSICAL EXAMINATION

Jaundice is rare, but scattered erythematous skin nodules, bibasilar rales, mild abdominal distention, low-grade fever, tachycardia, hypotension, or circulatory collapse may exist. A bluish hue in the periumbilical region (Cullen's sign) and ecchymotic discoloration in the flank area (Grey Turner's sign) suggest severe, necrotizing pancreatitis. Bowel sounds may be decreased or absent. Upper abdominal palpation may suggest the presence of a pancreatic pseudocyst. Epigastric tenderness is constant and profound, but guarding and rebound tenderness are variable.

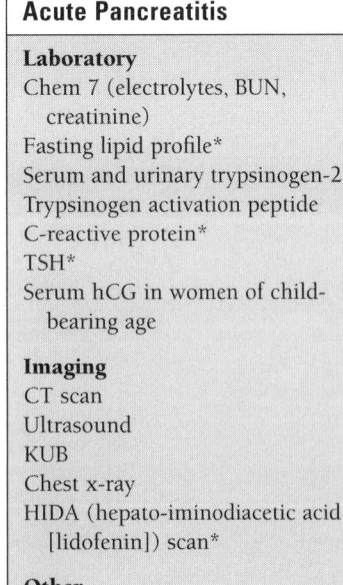

DIAGNOSTICS

An elevated serum amylase level is the standard diagnostic marker for pancreatitis. Rising 2 to 12 hours after the onset of symptoms, serum amylase may, however, remain normal and may not be acutely elevated in alcoholic or hypertriglyceridemia-associated pancreatitis. Serum amylase can be chronically elevated in other conditions, but in acute pancreatitis, the amylase levels usually return to normal within 2 to 3 days. The serum lipase level is more diagnostic in patients seen several days after the acute attack and is elevated in both alcoholic and nonalcoholic pancreatitis.[4] Serum and urinary trypsinogen-2 and trypsinogen activation peptide can be elevated in acute pancreatitis.[5] In the future, the urinary trypsinogen-2 test strip may offer rapid and reliable diagnosis for acute pancreatitis.[6]

Hemoconcentration, hyperglycemia, electrolyte abnormalities, and leukocytosis are commonly seen. Hypertriglyceridemia, hyperbilirubinemia, and transient hypocalcemia may also be present. Elevated liver enzyme levels combined with increased bilirubin and serum alanine aminotransferase indicate the probability of biliary pancreatitis, whereas an elevated C-reactive protein level indicates the possibility of pancreatic necrosis.[5]

An increase in serum calcium concentration combined with elevated alkaline phosphatase and decreased serum phosphatase levels may implicate hyperparathyroidism as a precipitant, whereas elevated triglyceride concentration combined with increased cholesterol concentration indicates hyperlipidemia. Hypoxemia is a worrisome sign that may indicate impending adult respiratory distress syndrome. Cardiac findings in acute pancreatitis include ST-segment and T wave abnormalities mimicking myocardial ischemia.

Abdominal radiographs are useful in the exclusion of pneumonia, a ruptured viscus, bowel obstruction, and gallstones. Chest x-ray studies are recommended and may show left lower lobe atelectasis or effusion. Although ultrasonography offers the most sensitive estimate of gallstone-induced pancreatitis, it may not be reliable because of abdominal distention.[5] Contrast-induced CT scanning is the most useful imaging technique, not only for diagnosis but also in calculating the size of a pancreatic phlegmon (accumulation of pancreatic fluid and possible necrosis), detecting a pseudocyst (collection of fluid around or within the pancreas), and recognizing pancreatic necrosis.

If the attack was not related to hyperparathyroidism, alcoholism, or familial tendency, it is essential that the underlying reason for the attack be determined. Endoscopic retrograde cholangiopancreatography (ERCP) may be advised for patients in whom no identifiable cause of acute pancreatitis is found after initial studies or if biliary obstruction is suspected.

DIFFERENTIAL DIAGNOSIS

Severe, sudden abdominal pain demands conscientious consideration. A ruptured viscus (particularly a perforated peptic ulcer), bowel obstruction, acute cholecystitis, biliary or renal colic, ascending cholangitis, leaking aortic aneurysm, myocardial infarction, pneumonia, vasculitic connective tissue disorders (e.g., lupus erythematosus or polyarteritis nodosa), diabetic ketoacidosis, and mesenteric infarction should all be considered when evaluating the patient with acute back or abdominal pain.

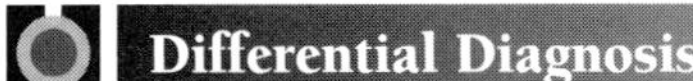

Acute Pancreatitis

Ruptured viscus
Bowel obstruction
Acute cholecystitis
Biliary/renal colic
Ascending cholangitis
Aortic aneurysm
Myocardial infarction
Pneumonia
Vasculitic connective tissue disorders
Diabetic ketoacidosis
Mesenteric infarction

MANAGEMENT

Recognition of underlying abdominal emergencies and the need for quick surgical intervention is essential. Hospitalization is usually indicated for analgesia and IV rehydration, as well as to monitor vital signs, volume status, and electrolytes. No oral medications, food, or fluids should be ingested, and precipitants of the attack, such as alcohol or medications, should be eliminated. Nasogastric suction can be suitable for patients with intractable vomiting or ileus, although routine nasogastric suction has not proved to be beneficial. Pain management includes the administration of meperidine hydrochloride if the patient is not allergic to this medication. Opiates, such as morphine sulfate, induce spasm of the sphincter of Oddi, exacerbating the pain, and should not be used. IV fentanyl can also be used for ongoing pain management to prevent complications associated with the long-term use of meperidine. Antibiotic therapy for acute pancreatitis is controversial but should be prescribed if secondary infection or necrotizing pancreatitis is present. Pain cessation, plus normalization of vital signs, radiographic studies, and laboratory values, indicates resolving pancreatitis. Liquids and the gradual addition of small amounts of food can be resumed once pain has subsided if serum amylase and lipase levels have also normalized. The recurrence of pain indicates the need to repeat serum amylase and lipase determinations and to again restrict oral intake.

Careful monitoring of fluid status, laboratory values, and cardiovascular, pulmonary, and renal status is indicated during the acute and convalescent phases of the attack. For patients with protracted attacks of pancreatitis, enteral feedings or total parenteral nutrition may be required. CT scanning is indicated for patients who do not respond to supportive measures. ERCP may be necessary for pancreatitis associated with gallstone pancreatitis, whereas surgical intervention may be necessary for necrotizing pancreatitis or infection.

COMPLICATIONS

Unfortunately, patients who have recovered from acute pancreatitis are at significant risk for recurrence. The development of continued pain, malabsorption, or new-onset diabetes mellitus signals the potential development of chronic pancreatitis and warrants immediate investigation. The majority of patients will recover with supportive therapy, although approximately 25% of patients will have complications.[7] These complications include hypocalcemia and other metabolic abnormalities, blindness (Purtscher's retinopathy), localized abscesses, phlegmons, pseudocysts, necrosis, hemorrhage, and multisystem organ failure.[7] The majority of deaths are caused by pulmonary failure or sepsis.

INDICATIONS FOR REFERRAL/HOSPITALIZATION

The treatment of acute pancreatitis is primarily supportive and requires physician consultation. Hospitalization for careful observation, frequent assessment of vital signs, laboratory analysis, IV therapy, normalization of electrolytes and glucose, and parenteral analgesia is indicated for all patients. Gastroenterology and surgical consultations are also recommended.

Hemodynamic monitoring, ERCP, or surgical intervention may be indicated for patients with cholangitis, worsening jaundice, a pseudocyst that is larger than 5 cm, pancreatic hemorrhage, abscess, or necrosis.[5] Although surgical debridement for pancreatic necrosis is indicated, the benefits of ERCP, surgery, antibiotics, and peritoneal lavage remain controversial.[5]

PATIENT AND FAMILY EDUCATION AND HEALTH PROMOTION

Patients should understand that severe abdominal pain with or without radiation, nausea, vomiting, or diaphoresis requires immediate evaluation. It is also important that patients understand the risk of repeated attacks of pancreatitis, the need to avoid possible precipitants, and the importance of adherence to prescribed therapy. Because the mortality rate from alcoholic pancreatitis is high, alcohol must be avoided. A low-fat diet, weight loss, exercise, and normalization of triglycerides should be the goal for patients with pancreatitis associated with hypertriglyceridemia. Medications that may have caused the pancreatitis should also be avoided.

Chronic Pancreatitis

DEFINITION/EPIDEMIOLOGY

Chronic pancreatitis, a chronic inflammation of the pancreas, is characterized by pain and histiologic changes in the gland. After the large reserve of pancreas secretory function is depleted by many years of gland destruction from inflammation, glandular changes may be accompanied by dysfunction, producing pancreatic insufficiency or diabetes. This is a progressive condition, in contrast to the inflammation of acute pancreatitis in which the gland can revert back to normal functioning (Table 154-1).

Alcohol is a major factor in both acute and chronic pancreatitis. Although the exact pathogenesis is not clearly understood, the initial pancreatic attack usually occurs after 10 years of heavy alcohol consumption.[8]

There can be other etiologies. Malnutrition or consumption of sorghum may play a role in the development of chronic pancreatitis in southern India, Indonesia, and central and south Africa.[8] In addition to severe malnutrition, uncommon etiologies include hereditary pancreatitis, hemochromatosis, trauma, sicca syndrome, radiation injury, gastric surgery, and tuberculosis. Biliary disease is rarely the primary cause of chronic pancreatitis.[4] Up to 25% of cases are truly idiopathic.[9] However, in patients older than 40 years, the finding of pancreatic dysfunction mandates an evaluation for pancreatic cancer.[9] Pancreatic dysfunction in adults aged 20 to 40 years should trigger an

TABLE 154-1 Comparison of Acute and Chronic Pancreatitis

Acute	Chronic
Neutrophil infiltration, diffuse involvement of large portion of pancreas	Monocyte infiltration, patchy focal fibrosis
Symptomatic	Long periods without symptoms, recurrent pain after meals
Abnormal amylase and lipase levels	Amylase and lipase levels may be normal
Gland may revert back to normal	Progressive changes are typical

From Freedman SD, Bishop MD: Etiology and pathogenesis of chronic pancreatitis. Retrieved March 2001 from the World Wide Web: http://www.uptodate.com.

investigation for cystic fibrosis because 85% of patients with cystic fibrosis have some pancreatic insufficiency.[9] Fifty percent of patients with chronic pancreatitis die within 25 years of diagnosis, with 15% to 20% of those deaths related to complications.[10] The remainder die of disease associated with chronic alcohol abuse.[10]

PATHOPHYSIOLOGY

Debate exists whether acute and chronic pancreatitis are two distinct disorders rather than stages of the same disease.[11] It is also postulated that the occurrence of pseudocysts or ductal strictures are risk factors for the progression of acute pancreatitis to chronic pancreatitis.

The exact pathogenesis of chronic pancreatitis is believed to be multifactorial (Box 154-3). Agreement exists on pathologic characteristics of the disease: irregular gland fibrosis, reduced number and size of acini and islets of Langerhans, and ductal obstruction by calcified protein precipitates. Based on pathologic features, three forms of chronic pancreatitis have been identified. The first form, alcoholic chronic pancreatitis, produces irregular dilation of pancreatic ducts with metaplasia or hyperplasia of the duct epithelium and fibrosis; this may be caused by the secretion of enzymatic proteins in a supersaturated state. These proteins may precipitate in ducts, producing intraductal calcifications, inflammation, and fibrosis. The second form is a consequence of main pancreatic duct obstruction by tumor, cyst, or trauma. This produces uniform ductal dilation and evenly distributed fibrosis, often without calcification or stones. Improvement in structure and function can be noted after the precipitating obstruction has been relieved. The final form, chronic inflammatory pancreatitis, produces fibrosis, atrophy of exocrine tissue, and mononuclear cell infiltration.

Primarily, two separate events have been postulated to initiate chronic pancreatitis: a decrease in the normal bicarbonate secretion and digestive enzyme conversion to an active form within the gland.[12] Mechanical obstruction produced by duct stones, tumors, or an alteration in duct function causes a decrease in bicarbonate production, as do genetic conditions that impair bicarbonate production. The activation of the digestive enzymes prematurely within the pancreas itself occurs with gland sphincter malfunction, ischemia, or antioxidant deficiency that produces free radical formation and cellular stress.[12]

BOX 154-3

ETIOLOGIES OF CHRONIC PANCREATITIS[12]

- Alcohol abuse
- Hereditary pancreatitis
- Ductal obstruction
- Tropical pancreatitis
- Autoimmune disease
- Cystic fibrosis
- Hyperparathyroidism
- Hereditary pancreatitis (mutation of trypsinogen gene)
- Idiopathic pancreatitis (associated with atherosclerotic disease)
- Nutritional deficiencies (of antioxidants, such as selenium or vitamin C or E)

From Freedman SD, Bishop MD: Etiology and pathogenesis of chronic pancreatitis. Retrieved March 2001 from the World Wide Web: http://www.uptodate.com.

CLINICAL PRESENTATION

Pain and pancreatic insufficiency characterize chronic pancreatitis. The pain of chronic pancreatitis may be absent or severe, recurrent or constant. Although often abdominal, the pain may be referred to the upper back, anterior chest, or flank. Usually the discomfort is not relieved by food or antacids and intensifies with alcohol or fatty food. Weight loss, diarrhea, and oily stools may be reported. Nausea, vomiting, or abdominal distention is less commonly seen. When the destruction of pancreatic function results in diabetes, the typical symptoms of polyuria, polydipsia, and polyphagia may be observed.

PHYSICAL EXAMINATION

Even in the presence of severe pain, physical examination may reveal few overt findings. Slight fever, weight loss, or abdominal tenderness may be present. Jaundice, signifying common bile duct obstruction, is less common. If pancreatic dysfunction results in severe malabsorption, signs of malnutrition will be evident. Painless chronic pancreatitis may present after years of silent gland destruction with steatorrhea (fatty stools) or diabetes. However, 90% of excretory function must be lost before signs and symptoms of malabsorption are evident.[9]

DIAGNOSTICS

Imaging studies and pancreatic function tests complement each other. Abdominal radiographs, endoscopic ultrasound (EUS), CT scan, MRI, and ERCP are diagnostic imaging studies that are useful in chronic pancreatitis. In one third of patients, abdominal radiographs (kidney-ureter-bladder [KUB]) may demonstrate pancreatic calcifications, thereby supporting the diagnosis.[8] However, abdominal ultrasound may expedite early diagnosis because pancreatic enlargement and calcifications can be seen earlier than on abdominal radiographs. Similar findings occur with pancreatic cancer. CT has been determined to have a test sensitivity of 90%.[9] Evidence of ductal dilation with focal enlargement, fluid collections, or calcifications on CT scanning or MRI indicates chronic pancreatitis. When there are no calcifications or evidence of pancreatic exocrine dysfunction (steatorrhea), ERCP demonstrates beading

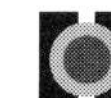

Diagnostics

Chronic Pancreatitis

Laboratory	Imaging
CBC and differential	CT scan
Serum amylase	KUB*, abdominal ultrasound*
Serum lipase	
Serum bilirubin	**Other**
Serum glucose	ERCP*
Serum alkaline phosphatase	Secretion stimulation test*
Stool for steatorrhea (fecal fat)	

*If indicated.

of the main pancreatic duct and ectatic side branches in chronic pancreatitis; the results of ERCP may be normal in early disease (symptoms <4 years).[13] With normal ERCP results and continued suspicion for chronic pancreatitis, pancreatic enzyme testing or EUS is the next step for evaluation. EUS requires a skilled endosonographer; stone formation on EUS is the most predictive feature of chronic pancreatitis.[14] Other EUS findings include visible side branches, cysts, lobularity, irregularity or dilation of main duct, hyperechoic foci, hyperechoic strands, and a main duct with hyperechoic margins.[14] The severity of chronic pancreatitis correlates with the number of EUS findings observed.

Laboratory data are useful to exclude other causes of abdominal pain and to determine whether pancreatic insufficiency exists. In contrast to acute pancreatitis, elevated serum amylase and lipase levels are not typically present. Although CBC and LFT (liver function tests) are typically normal, increased bilirubin and alkaline phosphatase levels can indicate compression of bile ducts and should prompt investigation for fibrosis, edema, or tumor. The presence of pancreatic insufficiency is indicated by elevated blood glucose if diabetes occurs, if stool exhibits fat with Sudan stain, or if there are elevated levels of fat in the 72-hour quantitative stool analysis. For the fat studies to be accurate, the patient must consume 100 g of fat/day.[10]

Tests to evaluate pancreatic function are also used in chronic pancreatitis and include the secretin stimulation and bentiromide tests. The secretin stimulation test is considered the "gold standard" and complements ERCP but is more invasive, involving measurement of the bicarbonate concentration of duodenum fluid after the administration of secretin.[13] The bentiromide test is less invasive. Bentiromide is absorbed from the gastrointestinal tract and excreted in the urine with the aid of the pancreatic enzyme chymotrypsin. Pancreatic insufficiency results in decreased levels of chymotrypsin; thus decreased levels (<50%) of the test substance are found in the urine, prompting further investigation. However, this test may not be sensitive enough to pick up mild pancreatic insufficiency. Liver disease, renal failure, and intestinal malabsorption can produce false-positive results. Additional tests of pancreatic function include measurement of chymotrypsin activity in the stool, trypsin-like serum immunoreactivity, and a modification of the Schilling test performed with and without the administration of pancreatic enzymes.

Differential Diagnosis

Chronic Pancreatitis

Pseudocysts	Pancreatic stones
Pancreatic cancer	Narcotics
Peptic ulcer disease	Pancreatic cancer
Cholelithiasis	Intestinal malabsorption
Biliary tract obstruction	Mesenteric vascular disease

DIFFERENTIAL DIAGNOSIS

A strong history of alcoholism suggests the diagnosis of chronic pancreatitis in the patient with abdominal pain. However, pseudocysts, pancreatic cancer, peptic ulcer disease, cholelithiasis, biliary tract obstruction, irritable bowel syndrome, and pancreatic stones should be excluded when considering the diagnosis of chronic pancreatitis.

In addition, because pancreatic cancer may present with signs and symptoms similar to those of chronic pancreatitis, patients may require ERCP or EUS for diagnosis. Pancreatic cancer should be suspected as a cause of chronic pancreatitis–like pain when a patient is older, has a negative history of alcohol use, has recent weight loss, has an extended duration of symptoms, and exhibits other constitutional signs and symptoms (e.g., fatigue, insomnia, anorexia). Consistent with the diagnosis of pancreatic cancer is a pancreatic duct stricture more than 10 mm long on ERCP.[13] Tumor markers (CEA, CA-19-9) may be normal or abnormal with pancreatic cancer.

Normal results on the D-xylose absorption test exclude the possibility of intestinal malabsorption. Angiography is used to exclude mesenteric vascular disease as the origin of chronic abdominal pain. Finally, the health care provider must recognize that chronic pancreatitis can occur in the setting of autoimmune diseases such as Sjögren's syndrome, systemic lupus erythematosus, and primary biliary cirrhosis and use appropriate testing to exclude associated conditions as warranted by the patient's history and presentation.

MANAGEMENT

The treatment of pancreatic dysfunction, pain control, and correction of symptomatic pancreatic structural abnormalities are the goals of chronic pancreatitis treatment. These management modalities require medical and possibly surgical intervention.

Pancreatic Dysfunction

The onset of diabetes mandates treatment according to established medical guidelines. Steatorrhea and diarrhea are produced by exocrine dysfunction; these are managed with a low-fat diet (<20 g/day), inhibition of gastric acid secretion with H_2 blockers, and pancreatic enzyme replacement. Enteric-coated pancreatic enzyme preparations include lipase, amylase, and protease. The dose should be cautiously titrated to relieve symptoms of steatorrhea: 4000 to 32,000 U of lipase with each meal and half this amount with snacks.[15] Pancreatic enzyme preparations are contraindicated in patients with allergy to pork and when flares of acute pancreatitis occur.[16] Dose changes are made prudently because bowel strictures, hyperuricosuria, and hyperuricemia can occur. Patients taking these enzyme preparations must maintain good hydration status. Additional nutritional support includes supplementation with fat-soluble vitamins and calcium.

Pain Control

The strong relationship between alcohol consumption and pancreatitis underscores the importance of alcohol abstinence to prevent further damage and reduce pain. The intense pain of chronic pancreatitis, coupled with inconsistent pain relief, is a risk factor for narcotic addiction. Nonnarcotic or nonsteroidal medications, coupled with careful assessment for surgical decompression of fluid accumulations or gland resection, may provide adequate pain management.[17] About 50% of patients who have nerve blocks for their chronic pancreatic pain report relief; the nerve block may need to be repeated in 2 to 6 months.[13] In addition, chronic pancreatitis pain management modalities should include pain clinics and relaxation techniques.

Dietary Interventions

Dietary interventions include fasting or small meals with decreased fat content. The administration of octreotide, a pancreatic secretion inhibitor, has yielded variant results for symptom relief.[18,19] With chronic pancreatitis, patients experience nutritional deficiencies as well as chronic pain. Antioxidants and dietary supplements containing medium-chain triglycerides are also under investigation to correct nutritional deficiencies and to relieve pain.[20]

Surgical Interventions

Pancreatic lithotripsy is used to treat duct stones, although it is not used commonly in the United States.[20] When a patient has pain nonresponsive to other treatments and dilated pancreatic ducts, a surgical procedure may relieve the obstruction causing pain. Pancreaticojejunostomy, or surgical decompression of dilated ducts, relieves pain in about 80% of individuals; however, pain often returns in 1 year.[20] Narrowing of the pancreatic ducts and sustained contraction of the duct sphincter muscles contribute to the chronic pain of chronic pancreatitis; duct stenting provides relief from these obstructive conditions.

The focal nature of chronic pancreatitis may allow partial resection of the gland in some patients, but this procedure has limitations because resection can compromise gland function. Autologous islet cell transplantation after entire gland resection is a topic under current exploration.[20]

Co-Management with Specialists

Consultation with a gastroenterologist is advised for diagnostic verification and collaborative management. Invasive studies may be indicated as the patient's condition changes or as complications ensue. Consideration for a pseudocyst drainage procedure, glandular resection, nerve block, or stenting procedure necessitates surgical consultation.

LIFE SPAN CONSIDERATIONS

Steatorrhea, diabetes, and pancreatic calcifications are complications commonly experienced by older adults with long-standing chronic pancreatitis. Also, idiopathic senile chronic pancreatitis may occur in adults older than 60 years. Two variants of senile chronic pancreatitis have been identified. In the first type, patients exhibit the typical symptoms of steatorrhea, weight loss, or diabetes; there is no pain. Primary inflammatory pancreatitis, the second and less common version, occurs primarily in women and presents with weight loss, steatorrhea, atypical or absent pain, fever, hypergammaglobulinemia, or chronic hepatitis.[21] For older adults, noninvasive testing with bentiromide is preferable to invasive techniques to determine pancreatic insufficiency.[21] Other causes of malabsorption in older adults should be considered. Celiac disease, small bowel contamination, and pancreatic cancer must be excluded.

COMPLICATIONS

Diabetes, exocrine insufficiency, malnutrition, and pain are complications associated with chronic pancreatitis. The development of extrahepatic biliary obstruction is signified by serum alkaline phosphatase levels that are twice the normal level for longer than 2 months.[9] Portal hypertension may occur as a result of thrombosis in the splenic or portal veins. Other complications include pseudocyst formation, pancreatic abscess, common bile duct obstruction, peptic ulcer, pseudoaneurysm of adjacent arteries, gastrointestinal bleeding, ascites from a leaking pseudocyst or damaged duct, and pancreatic cancer.

INDICATIONS FOR REFERRAL/HOSPITALIZATION

The primary care or collaborating physician is consulted for the initial diagnosis and management. Subsequent deterioration or complications in patient status warrant continued physician guidance.

Initial testing for stabile, uncomplicated patients can be accomplished in the outpatient setting. Hospitalization is required for the management of serious complications and for surgical drainage or resection procedures.

PATIENT AND FAMILY EDUCATION

It is vital that patients and families understand the recurrent, chronic character of the disease. Careful explanation of each individual's etiologic factors and the need for alcohol abstinence is necessary.

Patients with endocrine insufficiency should receive diabetic education because they are susceptible to macrovascular and microvascular complications. Patients with exocrine insufficiency must understand the origin of steatorrhea, the purpose and dosing of dietary supplements, components of a low-fat diet, and supplementation with fat-soluble vitamins and calcium. Guidelines for follow-up care, pain management, and symptoms requiring immediate attention are important to clarify and update.

Pancreatic Pseudocyst

DEFINITION/EPIDEMIOLOGY

Pancreatic pseudocysts contain blood, tissue, fluid, pancreatic digestive enzymes, and cellular debris accumulated in a cyst-like mass. The prefix *pseudo* is used because this localized collection of material does not have an epithelial lining, a hallmark for a true cyst.

Pseudocysts form as sequelae of acute pancreatitis or in association with chronic pancreatitis. Other, less common etiologies include gallbladder disease, surgery, and trauma.

Pseudocysts, occurring singularly or as multiple lesions, develop primarily in the body or tail of the pancreas but are found outside the pancreas.

PATHOPHYSIOLOGY

There are three explanations for the origin of pseudocysts, corresponding to clinically distinct conditions associated with pseudocyst formation. In acute pancreatitis, pseudocysts form when the inflamed gland produces fluid and exudate that fails to drain through ducts damaged by inflammation.[8] Chronic pancreatitis, characterized by duct enlargement, duct obstruction, and atrophy of duct epithelial lining, causes fluid to collect in a mass similar to a retention cyst.[8] A third etiology results from blunt or penetrating trauma damaging the pancreatic duct.

CLINICAL PRESENTATION

With acute pancreatitis, the persistence or recurrence of abdominal pain, nausea, vomiting, diarrhea, or weight loss prompts investigation for a pseudocyst. An increase in or recurrence of upper abdominal pain in a patient with a history of acute or chronic pancreatitis must be investigated for pseudocyst formation.[8] Other symptoms associated with pseudocyst formation include low-grade fever, jaundice, diaphragm inflammation, pleural effusion, and ascites. Pseudocysts are generally asymptomatic and cause symptoms through enlargement, producing duodenal or biliary obstruction, vascular occlusion, and fistula formation into adjacent viscera.[22] Gastrointestinal bleeding can result when a pseudoaneurysm forms from adjacent vessel necrosis and bleeds into a pancreatic duct.

DIAGNOSTICS

Diagnostics include pancreatic imaging by CT, MRI, or ultrasonography. With pleural effusion or ascites, the thoracentesis or paracentesis fluid has amylase levels above 1000 IU/L when there is a pseudocyst.[22] Biopsy samples of suspicious cystic lesions exclude premalignant growths or malignancies.[23] This is accomplished by CT-guided percutaneous needle biopsy. ERCP before surgery is indicated to determine ductal and pseudocyst anatomy; prophylactic antibiotics are given to decrease the risk of infection from pancreatic duct cannulation.[8]

Serologic analysis includes amylase, glucose, alkaline phosphatase, and bilirubin. Elevations of blood glucose and amylase are common. Increased serum alkaline phosphatase or bilirubin levels indicate compression of the common bile duct as it passes through the pancreas from extrahepatic biliary obstruction. With pancreatic pseudocyst, a CBC may show decreased hemoglobin and/or an elevated WBC count.

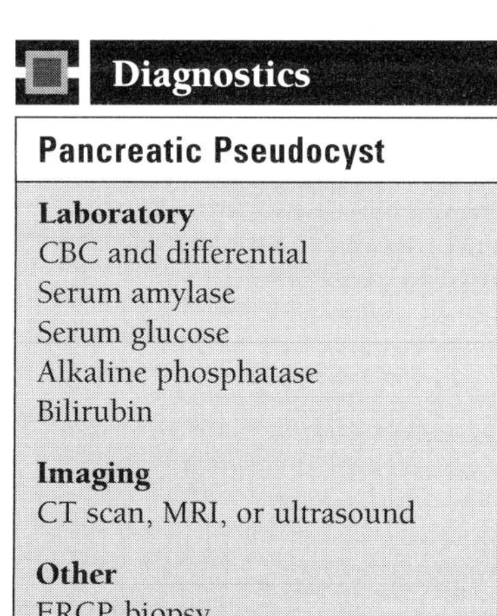

Diagnostics

Pancreatic Pseudocyst

Laboratory
CBC and differential
Serum amylase
Serum glucose
Alkaline phosphatase
Bilirubin

Imaging
CT scan, MRI, or ultrasound

Other
ERCP, biopsy

DIFFERENTIAL DIAGNOSIS

The presence of pancreatic fluid masses requires investigation. Pseudocysts can be confused with and should be distinguished from pancreatic abscesses, malignant cystadenomas, cystadenocarcinomas, retention cysts, congenital conditions, and desmoids. Concerns that a fluid collection is not a pseudocyst should be prompted when a patient has no prior history of acute pancreatitis, chronic pancreatitis, or pancreatic trauma; the absence of inflammatory changes on CT scan; and the presence of internal septae in the cyst.[22] EUS with fine needle aspiration is used to exclude malignancy in cystic lesions because pancreatic neoplasms may be cystic.

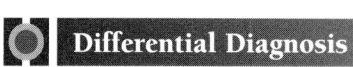

Differential Diagnosis

Pancreatic Pseudocyst

Pancreatic abscesses
Malignant cystadenomas
Cystadenocarcinomas
Retention cysts
Congenital conditions
Desmoids

MANAGEMENT

The decision process for pseudocyst management contains several steps. First, alternative diagnoses, particularly the risk that the cyst may represent a neoplasm, are excluded. Next, consideration of the presence of a complication of pseudocyst, a pseudoaneurysm, is entertained. This complication occurs in approximately 10% of patients with a pancreatic pseudocyst[22] (see Complications, below). In the past, prevailing clinical wisdom dictated that pseudocysts persisting for longer than 6 weeks required surgical decompression, based on the increased complication rate for these cysts.[22] However, two studies noted the resolution of pseudocysts after 6 weeks.[24,25] Currently there are several drainage options for pseudocysts, based on cystic location and patient symptoms. These options are multiple internal drainage procedures, percutaneous catheter drainage, or endoscopic approaches.

Co-Management with Specialists

Initial evaluation, laboratory tests, and imaging studies can be performed in the primary care setting. Complications, invasive diagnostics, and evaluation for surgery require collaboration with specialists in radiology, surgery, and gastroenterology.

COMPLICATIONS

Occasionally confused with pancreatic abscesses, infected pseudocysts cause severe pain, a fever with a high temperature, chills, and leukocytosis. However, on ultrasound or CT scan, infection is viewed as a diffuse area of necrosis, whereas an abscess is seen as a well-defined area of purulence.[8] Furthermore, pseudocysts may erode and perforate structures, resulting in rupture into the peritoneal cavity or gastrointestinal tract. Stomach perforation can present with few symptoms and require no treatment; peritoneal perforation necessitates surgical intervention and can be fatal. Colon perforation presents with abdominal pain and self-limited bloody diarrhea. Pseudocysts can also erode blood vessels, creating a pseudoaneurysm and producing hemorrhage and shock.[8] Three clinical findings are associated with pseudoaneurysm formation: gastrointestinal bleeding, sudden pseudocyst enlargement, and an unexplained decrease in hematocrit.[22] Elevated serum amylase levels and ascitic fluid containing amylase and protein suggest a leaking pseudocyst.[9]

INDICATIONS FOR REFERRAL/HOSPITALIZATION

If a pseudocyst or another complication is suspected, the collaborating physician is consulted during the initial visit. Long-term management requires careful and continued collaboration with the primary care physician.

PATIENT AND FAMILY EDUCATION

Patients at risk for pseudocyst formation should be educated about the symptoms of a pseudocyst and the necessity to contact their primary care provider for increased or persistent pain. Patients with known pseudocysts should receive instruction concerning the etiology of their condition, explanation of complications and their symptoms, and indications to seek medical attention.

REFERENCES

1. Gupta PK, Al-Kawas FH: Acute pancreatitis, *Am Fam Physician* 52(2):435-443, 1995.
2. Ramin KD and others: Acute pancreatitis in pregnancy, *Am J Obstet Gynecol* 173(1):187-191, 1995.
3. Cappel MS, Marks M: Acute pancreatitis in HIV seropositive patients: a case control study of 44 patients, *Am J Med* 98(3):243-248, 1995.
4. Sterby B and others: What is the best biochemical test to diagnose acute pancreatitis? a prospective study, *Mayo Clin Proc* 71(1138), 1996.
5. Tenner S and others: Urinary trypsinogen activation peptide (TAP) predicts severity in patients with acute pancreatitis, *Int J Pancreatol* 21(105), 1997.
6. Ballie J: Treatment of acute biliary pancreatitis (editorial), *N Engl J Med* 336:286-287, 1997.
7. Steinberg W, Tenner S: Acute pancreatitis, *N Engl J Med* 330(17): 1198-1210, 1994.
8. Grendell JH, Cello JP: Chronic pancreatitis. In Sleisenger MS, Fordtran JS, editors: *Gastrointestinal disease: pathology, diagnosis, management,* ed 5, Philadelphia, 1993, WB Saunders.
9. Greenberger NJ: Chronic pancreatitis. In Noble J, editor: *Textbook of primary care medicine,* St Louis, 1996, Mosby.
10. Steer ML, Waxman I, Freedman S: Chronic pancreatitis, *N Engl J Med* 332:1482-1489, 1995.
11. Ammann RW, Heitz PU, Kloppel G: Course of alcoholic chronic pancreatitis: a prospective clinicomorphological long-term study, *Gastroenterology* 111:224-231, 1996.
12. Freedman SD, Bishop MD: Etiology and pathogenesis of chronic pancreatitis. Retrieved March 2001 from the World Wide Web: http://www.uptodate.com.
13. Freedman SD: Clinical manifestations and diagnosis of chronic pancreatitis. Retrieved March 2001 from the World Wide Web: http://www.uptodate.com.
14. Wallace MB and others: The reliability of EUS for the diagnosis of chronic pancreatitis: interobserver agreement among experienced endosonographers, *Gastrointest Endosc* 53(3):294-299, 2001.
15. *Physicians' desk reference,* ed 50, Montvale, NJ, 1996, Medical Economics.
16. *Nursing 96: drug handbook,* Springhouse, Pa, 1996, Springhouse Press.
17. Barnes SA and others: Pancreaticoduodenectomy for benign disease, *Am J Surg* 171:131-135, 1996.
18. Freiss H and others: Randomized controlled multicenter study of prevention of complications by octreotide in patients undergoing surgery for chronic pancreatitis, *Br Surg J* 82:1270-1273, 1995.
19. Malfertheiner P and others: Treatment of pain in chronic pancreatitis by inhibition of pancreatic secretion with octreotide, *Gut* 36:450-454, 1995.
20. Freedman SD: Patient Information: Chronic pancreatitis. Retrieved January 2001 from the World Wide Web: http://www.uptodate.com.
21. Gullo L, Sipahi HM, Pezzilli R: Pancreatitis in the elderly, *J Clin Gastroenterol* 19:64-68, 1994.
22. Howell DA, Shah RJ, Parsons WG: Diagnosis and management of pseudocysts of the pancreas. Retrieved April 2001 from the World Wide Web: http://www.uptodate.com.
23. Rosenfeld AT: The evaluation of pancreatic cysts, *J Clin Gastroenterol* 20:94-95, 1995.
24. Yeo CJ and others: The natural history of pancreatic pseudocysts documented by computed tomography, *Surg Gynecol Obstet* 170:41, 1990.
25. Howell DA and others: Pancreatic ductal anatomy in patients undergoing endoscopic pseudocyst drainage: implications of follow-up data (abstract), *Gastrointest Endosc* 43:467, 1996.

CHAPTER 155

Tumors of the Gastrointestinal Tract

Louise Meyer

Tumors of the gastrointestinal tract may be benign or malignant. It is essential that malignant tumors be identified as early as possible and treated appropriately. This chapter focuses on the common malignancies of the esophagus, stomach, small intestine, and colon; common benign tumors of the gastrointestinal tract are also mentioned.

Tumors of the Esophagus

DEFINITION/EPIDEMIOLOGY

Esophageal carcinoma most commonly occurs during the sixth decade of life and is one of the most lethal of all cancers, with a 5-year survival rate of 12%.[1-3] In the past, most esophageal malignancies were squamous cell carcinomas. However, there has been a significant increase in the incidence of adenocarcinoma that arises from the columnar cells found in Barrett's esophagus.[4-6] The worldwide incidence of squamous cell carcinoma of the esophagus ranges from 2.5 to 5 per 100,000 population for men and 1.5 to 2.5 per 100,000 population for women.[1] Endemic areas include regions of northern China, South Africa, the Normandy and Brittany provinces of France, northern Iran, India, and areas of Asia.[1,4]

Risk factors for the development of esophageal cancer include chronic smoking, primary squamous cell carcinoma of the head and neck, alcohol consumption, thermal injury from the ingestion of hot liquids, and exposure to aflatoxin, asbestos fibers, and nitrosamines.[4,7] Nutritional deficiencies of riboflavin, niacin, zinc, protein, and vitamins A, E, and C have also been implicated.[3,4,7,8] The major risk factors for squamous cell esophageal carcinoma are chronic smoking and alcohol consumption, as well as celiac sprue, Plummer-Vinson syndrome, and tylosis.[4,6,8,9] The single most important risk factor for the development of adenocarcinoma of the esophagus is esophageal reflux leading to the premalignant condition of Barrett's esophagus.[6-8,10]

PATHOPHYSIOLOGY

Squamous cell carcinomas of the esophagus involve the middle third of the esophagus in 50% of cases and can be polypoid, ulcerative, or infiltrative.[4] Polypoid tumors are the most common and may project into the lumen, causing obstruction. Ulcerating tumors may penetrate into the mediastinum, causing hemorrhage rather than obstruction. Infiltrative tumors may have circumferential involvement, causing thickening and stenosis of the esophageal wall.[4] Esophageal adenocarcinomas arise in Barrett's esophagus—a metaplasia of the distal esophagus in which the gastric mucosa and intestinal epithelium occur in association with long-term gastroesophageal reflux. Its extensive lymphatic system allows cancers of the esophagus to spread locally and into adjacent mediastinal structures regardless of tumor type.[3]

CLINICAL PRESENTATION

Dysphagia is the classic presenting symptom of esophageal carcinoma. This symptom indicates that the esophageal lumen has been reduced by at least half of its normal diameter.[7] Other symptoms include anorexia, weight loss, and odynophagia with radiation to the back. Hoarseness results from tumor involvement of the recurrent laryngeal nerve, and a tracheoesophageal fistula may produce a chronic cough.[4,7] The clinical features of esophageal adenocarcinoma are similar to those of squamous cell carcinoma but may also produce early satiety, nausea, vomiting, and bloating because of tumor encroachment into the stomach.

PHYSICAL EXAMINATION

Fixed supraclavicular, cervical lymphadenopathy, and axillary lymph node metastasis are signs of advanced disease. Both hepatomegaly secondary to metastatic disease and superior vena cava syndrome indicate a poor prognosis.[3,7]

DIAGNOSTICS

New-onset dysphagia should prompt an evaluation for an esophageal tumor. Diagnostic evaluation of the patient with a suspected esophageal carcinoma is a two-step procedure that begins with a barium esophagram and is followed by an upper gastrointestinal endoscopy with biopsy and cytologic tests.[2,3,7,8] The barium esophagram and endoscopy are used in evaluating the primary tumor. Endoscopic ultrasound will help determine the extent of disease locally.[8] A clinical examination, biochemical assay, chest x-ray examination, CT scan, radionuclide bone scan, ultrasonography, and biopsy of suspicious lesions may be useful in the metastatic evaluation.[2,3,7,8]

DIFFERENTIAL DIAGNOSIS

In the adult patient with new onset of progressive, solid dysphagia, the differential diagnosis includes esophageal squamous cell carcinoma, esophageal adenocarcinoma, adenocarcinoma of the gastric cardia, benign peptic stricture, corrosive stricture, and esophageal motor disorders such as achalasia or scleroderma. Symptoms of dysphagia, especially in a patient older than 45 years, mandate a complete evaluation to exclude esophageal carcinoma.

MANAGEMENT

Gastroenterologic, oncologic, and surgical consultations are critical for the evaluation of esophageal tumors. A total thoracic esophagectomy with gastric pull-up or colon interposition is usually required for surgical intervention of esophageal carcinoma.[2] Although still somewhat controversial, concurrent radiation and chemotherapy before surgery may provide the best potential

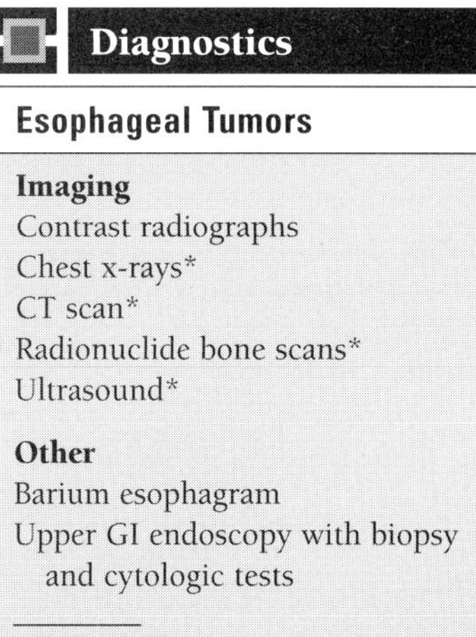
Diagnostics

Esophageal Tumors

Imaging
Contrast radiographs
Chest x-rays*
CT scan*
Radionuclide bone scans*
Ultrasound*

Other
Barium esophagram
Upper GI endoscopy with biopsy and cytologic tests

*If indicated.

for cure in locally advanced disease.[3,8] However, palliation for dysphagia may be the only realistic goal because most patients have incurable disease at the time of diagnosis. Palliation can be accomplished by peroral stenting through the stenosis and transendoscopic ablation of obstructing tumors by laser photocoagulation. For advanced disease, esophagectomy provides superb palliation.[6] Radiation therapy may provide palliation for patients who are not candidates for surgery.[6] Postoperative elevation of serum carcinoembryonic antigen (CEA) levels may be the first objective sign of recurrent disease and should prompt additional therapy such as surgery or chemotherapy.[9,11]

Differential Diagnosis

Esophageal Tumors

- Benign esophageal leiomyomata
- Esophageal carcinoma
- Esophageal adenocarcinoma
- Adenocarcinoma of the gastric cardia
- Benign peptic stricture
- Corrosive stricture
- Esophageal motor disorders

COMPLICATIONS

Because of the distensibility of the esophagus, esophageal carcinoma tends to be silent until late in its course. Complications are usually related to mediastinal extension or esophageal narrowing and may include obstruction, hemorrhage, perforation, and fistula formation. Because the esophagus lacks a true serosa, cancer is often not contained at the time of diagnosis. The lungs and liver are the most common sites of hematogenous metastasis. Complications of esophageal resection include torsion or gangrene of the gastric, colonic, or jejunal "pull-up"; anastomotic leak; anastomotic stricture; subphrenic abscess; hemorrhage; wound infection and dehiscence; sepsis; dumping syndrome; and reflux esophagitis.

PATIENT AND FAMILY EDUCATION

Dietary instructions should be consistent with the degree of dysphagia that is experienced. Patients who have responded to therapy but continue to use alcohol and tobacco products during treatment demonstrate a poor response to treatment and an increased rate of local recurrence.[9] Therefore patients should be encouraged to discontinue the use of these products and should be provided with therapeutic interventions for alcohol and tobacco cessation.[6,10]

HEALTH PROMOTION

Primary prevention of esophageal cancer includes avoidance of all tobacco products and of heavy alcohol consumption. It is also important to consume a diet that is rich in fruits and vegetables and to maintain a normal weight. With obesity, there can be increased acid reflux, thus multiplying the risk for adenocarcinoma of the lower esophagus and stomach.[6,10]

Tumors of the Stomach

DEFINITION/EPIDEMIOLOGY

During the past 50 years there has been a dramatic decline in the incidence of gastric cancer in the United States.[4] This decrease has been attributed to improved refrigeration and the reduced consumption of preserved foods.[4] The incidence of gastric carcinoma is high in Japan and Chile, where rates are 7 to 8 times higher than those in the United States.[4] In the United States, gastric carcinoma occurs more often in African-Americans, Hispanics, and Native Americans.[9] Common benign tumors of the stomach include leiomyomas and epithelial polyps.

Risk factors for gastric adenocarcinoma include *Helicobacter pylori* gastritis, chronic atrophic gastritis, pernicious anemia, and gastric polyps.[4,9] Dietary risk factors include a decreased consumption of fruits and vegetables and an increased intake of salt, nitrates and nitrites, and smoked and poorly preserved foods.[4,9] Genetic factors linked to gastric carcinoma include hereditary nonpolyposis colorectal cancer, familial polyposis, and first-degree relatives of patients with gastric cancer. A partial gastrectomy for peptic ulcer disease is also associated with an increased risk of gastric carcinoma.

PATHOPHYSIOLOGY

Gastric cancer is divided into intestinal and diffuse types. The intestinal type of gastric adenocarcinoma has distinct, large glands lined by columnar cells with a well-defined brush border; this type tends to occur in the distal stomach and may be polypoid or ulcerated.[12] The diffuse type of gastric cancer extends widely without distinct margins and infiltrates and thickens the stomach wall without forming a mass. Gastric carcinomas spread via direct extension, lymphatic spread, hematogeneous metastasis, and peritoneal seeding.

CLINICAL PRESENTATION

Weight loss, abdominal pain, anorexia, and vomiting are the most common symptoms of advanced gastric carcinoma.[4,9,13] The abdominal pain begins as insidious upper abdominal discomfort that ranges in intensity from a vague sense of postprandial fullness to a severe, steady pain.[14] Other symptoms include a change in bowel habits, dysphagia, melena, anemic symptoms, and hemorrhage.[9,15]

PHYSICAL EXAMINATION

Patients with advanced gastric cancer may present with cachexia, small bowel obstruction, epigastric mass, ascites, hepatomegaly, or lower extremity edema. Metastases may also manifest as an enlarged left supraclavicular lymph node (Virchow's node) or an enlarged left anterior axillary lymph node, enlarged periumbilical lymph nodes (Sister Mary Joseph's node), an enlarged ovary (Krukenberg's tumor), or a mass on Blumer's shelf on rectal examination.

DIAGNOSTICS

An upper gastrointestinal endoscopy is the imaging modality of choice for stomach tumors because it allows direct visualization and biopsy of the tumor.[16] A minimum of four biopsies of the lesion should be made; diagnostic

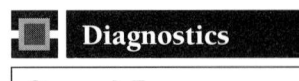

Diagnostics

Stomach Tumors

Laboratory
- LFTs
- CBC and differential
- Stool for occult blood

Imaging
- Contrast radiographs
- CT scan of abdomen

Other
- Endoscopy and biopsy

accuracy approaches 100% with 10 biopsies.[16] After diagnosis, staging is performed to determine the presence of local spread or distant metastasis. The metastatic evaluation includes liver biochemical assays, abdominal CT scanning, and biopsy of suspected nodes.[9] Blood studies may reveal hypochromic, microcytic anemia secondary to iron deficiency. The stool is often positive for occult blood.

DIFFERENTIAL DIAGNOSIS

The differential diagnosis for tumors of the stomach includes gastric lymphoma, leiomyosarcoma, and gastric metastasis from the lung, breast, and melanoma. Kaposi's sarcoma of the stomach, which may be present in patients with AIDS, and hypertrophic gastropathy (Menetrier's disease) are also included in the differential diagnosis.

MANAGEMENT

Gastroenterologic, surgical, and oncologic consultations are essential for a patient with gastric cancer. Complete resection of the gastric carcinoma and adjacent lymph nodes offers the only chance for cure. A palliative resection should be considered for patients with advanced lesions who present with obstruction or bleeding. Obstruction and dysphagia from large carcinomas of the gastric cardia can be managed by laser coagulation, which results in recanalization of the lumen and the relief of obstructive symptoms.[17]

Because gastric cancers are radioresistant, adequate control of the tumor requires doses of radiation that exceed the tolerance of the surrounding structures.[12] Therefore moderate doses of radiation are used only for symptom palliation. Adjuvant chemotherapy in gastric cancer appears to offer no advantage for survival after a curative resection.[9,14]

COMPLICATIONS

Gastric carcinomas are detected at an advanced stage, and the prognosis of this neoplasm remains poor. Ovarian metastases occur in approximately 10% of gastric cancers and may be associated with ovarian dysfunction such as virilization.[12] Intraperitoneal dissemination of the tumor may occur with involvement of the omentum, peritoneum, and serosa of the intestine.

PATIENT AND FAMILY EDUCATION

Although gastric tumors and small colon tumors may be associated with aging, cancer can affect younger patients. Weight loss, anorexia, difficulty swallowing, abdominal pain, a change in bowel habits, and blood in the stool are all signs of gastrointestinal cancers. Patients should be reminded to notify their primary care provider if any of these symptoms occur. In addition, patients should routinely be asked about a family history of gastrointestinal or other cancers.

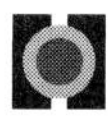

Differential Diagnosis

Stomach Tumors	
Gastric lymphoma	Kaposi's sarcoma of the stomach
Leiomyosarcoma	Hypertrophic gastropathy
Gastric metastasis	

HEALTH PROMOTION

A well-balanced diet rich in fruits and vegetables is very important for overall good health. Such a diet will provide sufficient vitamins and antioxidants to maintain health. Consumption of smoked and highly salted, nitrated food should be avoided or severely limited. Only food that is refrigerated and kept under safe conditions should be consumed. Avoidance of all tobacco products is strongly recommended.[10,18]

Because infectious agents have been associated with gastric cancer, it is important that good hygiene is practiced. Diagnosis of *H. pylori* infection and subsequent treatment also contribute to a reduction in the incidence of gastric cancer.[18]

Exposure to glycol ethers, hydraulic fluids, and leaded gasoline should also be limited. Education of the public along with increasing protection and surveillance in the workplace will limit or eliminate exposure to these products.[18]

Tumors of the Small Intestine

DEFINITION/EPIDEMIOLOGY

Adenocarcinomas of the small intestine account for up to half of all malignancies of the small bowel.[3,16] After resection of small bowel adenocarcinomas, there is a 5-year survival rate of 20%.[19] The peak incidence of symptomatic tumors is in the sixth decade of life.[19] The highest rate of small bowel adenocarcinoma occurs in African-American men.[19] Other malignant neoplasms of the small intestine include carcinoid tumors, lymphomas, and leiomyosarcomas.[4] All carcinoid tumors should be considered malignant. Metastasis occurs in up to 90% of patients with carcinoid tumors larger than 2 cm.[19] More than 95% of all gastrointestinal carcinoids occur in the appendix, rectum, and small intestine.[20]

The three most common benign tumors of the small intestine are adenomas, leiomyomas, and lipomas.[4,19] Multiple adenomas may occur in the small intestine in Peutz-Jeghers syndrome and are considered benign; however, in 2% to 3% of these patients, adenocarcinoma develops.[4]

Risk factors for adenocarcinoma of the small bowel include Crohn's disease, sprue, ileostomy stomas, pouches and conduits, familial adenomatous polyposis, and Peutz-Jeghers syndrome.[9,20] Patients with Crohn's disease have a 100-fold increased risk of the development of carcinoma of the small bowel and adenocarcinoma develops 10 years earlier than expected for this malignancy.[4]

PATHOPHYSIOLOGY

Adenocarcinomas of the small intestine may be polypoid, ulcerative, or annular and stenosing. Adenocarcinomas of the small intestine infiltrate through the bowel wall and invade adjacent organs. Venous invasion of the lymph nodes occurs via either metastasis or direct extension of the tumor.

Carcinoid tumors are well-differentiated endocrine tumors that arise from the enterochromaffin cells at the base of Lieberkühn's crypts. These cells give the tumor its most clinically distinctive feature—its ability to secrete tumor products that induce the carcinoid syndrome.[4,19,20] Serotonin is believed to be the humoral mediator responsible for the diarrhea that occurs with carcinoid syndrome.[4] Serotonin is deaminated by monoamine oxidase to 5-hydroxyindoleacetic acid (5-HIAA), which is excreted in the urine.[4] The right side of the heart is exposed to the effects of tumor products that have been released into the vena cava from hepatic metastases. Endocardial fibrosis may occur as a result, forming plaques on the tricuspid and pulmonic valves, the endocardium of the right-sided cardiac chambers, the vena cava, the coronary sinus, and the pulmonary artery.[4]

CLINICAL PRESENTATION

With both benign and malignant small bowel tumors, abdominal pain is the most common symptom. Other symptoms include nausea, vomiting, cramping abdominal pain, abdominal distention aggravated by eating, and weight loss. Unless patients manifest the carcinoid syndrome—characterized by flushing, diarrhea, wheezing, and sweating—no specific signs or symptoms suggest the diagnosis.[16]

PHYSICAL EXAMINATION

A palpable abdominal mass may be present in up to 40% of patients with a small bowel malignancy.[20] Duodenal adenocarcinomas that involve Vater's ampulla may cause obstructive jaundice or pancreatitis.[4,19] Hepatomegaly, ascites, and jaundice indicate advanced metastatic disease. Pulmonic stenosis may cause a systolic murmur in patients with carcinoid syndrome.[4]

DIAGNOSTICS

In the evaluation of small bowel tumors, the stool should be tested for occult blood. However, the diagnostic modality of choice is a small bowel follow-through (SBFT), an extension of the conventional barium meal in which the barium is ingested orally.[20] Enteroclysis, synonymous with a small bowel enema, may be performed by infusing approximately 1 L of barium until bowel distention occurs and the barium reaches the terminal ileum.[20] Enteroclysis is superior to SBFT in the diagnosis of small bowel disease, except for lesions of the terminal ileum.

Additional studies after barium radiology may be indicated and include endoscopy, CT scanning, arteriography, serotonin and metabolite levels, and scintigraphy.[20] Endoscopy is indicated for duodenal lesions that are accessible with gastroduodenoscopy and for terminal ileal lesions accessible with colonoscopy. A CT scan is indicated to determine metastasis, including hepatic involvement, by possible malignant tumors. Arteriography is indicated in cases of obscure gastrointestinal bleeding. Serotonin and metabolites (5-HIAA), as well as scintigraphy, may be necessary for suspected carcinoid tumors.[20] A laparotomy may be necessary when the diagnostic modalities are insufficient.

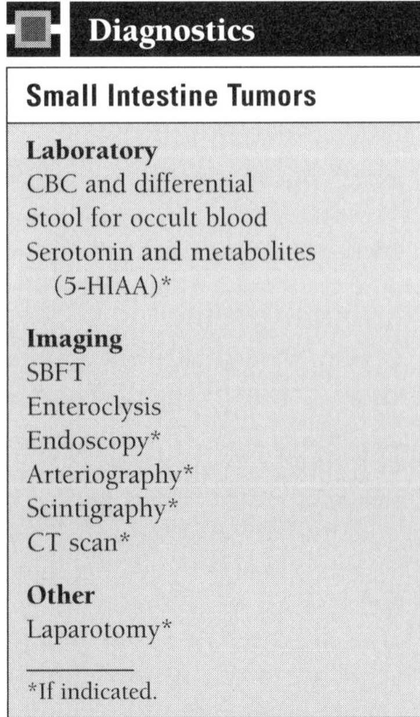

Diagnostics

Small Intestine Tumors

Laboratory
CBC and differential
Stool for occult blood
Serotonin and metabolites (5-HIAA)*

Imaging
SBFT
Enteroclysis
Endoscopy*
Arteriography*
Scintigraphy*
CT scan*

Other
Laparotomy*

*If indicated.

DIFFERENTIAL DIAGNOSIS

Small bowel tumors may be considered one of the less common causes of intestinal obstruction, occult gastrointestinal blood loss, weight loss, and unexplained abdominal pain. The diagnosis of a small bowel tumor often is not made before laparotomy. Therefore the differential diagnosis includes adhesions, hernias, intussusception, volvulus, intraabdominal abscesses and hematomas, endometriosis, pelvic inflammatory disease, Crohn's disease, ischemia, hematoma associated with oral anticoagulant therapy, radiation enteritis, amyloidosis, ingested foreign bodies, gallstones, bezoars, and worms.

MANAGEMENT

Gastroenterologic, oncologic, and surgical consultations are essential to provide optimal care for patients with small bowel tumors. These cancers are managed surgically, which offers the only hope for cure. Because adenocarcinomas metastasize early to regional lymph nodes, a wide resection is undertaken.[20] If the lesions cannot be resected for cure, a palliative resection of the main lesion is recommended. Chemotherapy and radiation therapy yield minimal benefit.[20] The 5-year survival rate for adenocarcinoma of the small bowel is not greater than 20%, even after curative resection.[20]

Because carcinoid tumors greater than 1 cm in diameter are capable of metastasizing, a wide resection should be undertaken. Nonresectable intestinal and hepatic metastatic carcinoids should have aggressive debulking to alleviate symptoms of the carcinoid syndrome and possibly prolong survival.[20] Carcinoid syndrome may be treated with injections of octreotide (a synthetic somatostatin analog that is a serotonin antagonist) to provide symptomatic relief until surgical management of the carcinoid tumor can be performed.[16,20,21] Hepatic artery embolization with combination chemotherapy and interferon-γ may control symptoms of carcinoid syndrome.[21]

INDICATIONS FOR REFERRAL/HOSPITALIZATION

Large lesions of the small intestine may produce partial or intermittent obstruction, bleeding, intussusception, and volvulus. Carcinoid tumors spread locally to regional lymph nodes,

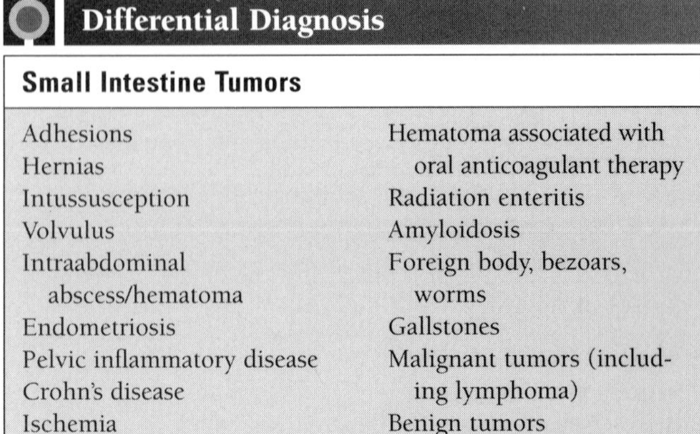

Differential Diagnosis

Small Intestine Tumors

Adhesions	Hematoma associated with oral anticoagulant therapy
Hernias	Radiation enteritis
Intussusception	Amyloidosis
Volvulus	Foreign body, bezoars, worms
Intraabdominal abscess/hematoma	Gallstones
Endometriosis	Malignant tumors (including lymphoma)
Pelvic inflammatory disease	Benign tumors
Crohn's disease	
Ischemia	

the liver, other intraabdominal organs, and the lung. Small carcinoid tumors normally do not invade or obstruct the bowel lumen but can penetrate the muscle layer and lead to adhesions, bowel kinking, angulation, and obstruction. Massive fibrosis of the mesenteries, omentum, and peritoneum may result from the leakage of serotonin and other vasoactive substances. High serum levels of 5-HIAA may cause endocardial fibrotic plaques that stiffen and fix the tricuspid and pulmonic valves, which may lead to right-sided heart failure.[4]

PATIENT AND FAMILY EDUCATION

Patient and Family education for tumors of the small intestine is the same as for tumors of the stomach (see p. 665).

HEALTH PROMOTION

Please see the Health Promotion section for tumors of the colon (see p. 668).

Tumors of the Colon

DEFINITION/EPIDEMIOLOGY

Colorectal cancer is the third most common cancer in the United States and is the second leading cause of cancer deaths.[9,22] Adenocarcinomas account for more than 95% of all malignant tumors of the large bowel.[9] Risk factors for the development of colorectal cancer include prior colorectal cancer, ulcerative colitis, hereditary and genetic factors, familial polyposis syndromes, history of breast or female genital cancer, and a high-fat, low-bulk diet. Benign tumors of the colon include polyps and polyposis syndromes.

PATHOPHYSIOLOGY

Colorectal adenocarcinomas may be polypoid, ulcerating, or infiltrative. Adenocarcinomas of the colon form well-differentiated glands and secrete large amounts of mucin.[22] Signet-ring cells, in which a large vacuole of mucin displaces the nucleus to one side, may be present in some tumors.[4,21,22] Colorectal carcinoma can spread intraluminally or via direct extension, hematogenous spread, lymphatic dissemination, or transperitoneal seeding.

Genetic alterations in malignancy include deletions, amplifications, and single-nucleotide mutations. *ras* point mutations are observed in almost half of all colon cancers and in approximately one third of patients with familial adenomatous polyposis. The *ras* genes encode for proteins located on the inner surface of the plasma membrane, bind guanine nucleotides, and are involved in signal transduction from the cell membrane to the nucleus.[21] Mutations located at critical positions in the gene alter the *ras* protein so that signal transduction is unregulated, which leads to additional cell growth. A mutation at just one of three codons—12, 13, and 61—of the *K-ras2* gene is the mechanism via which the *ras* oncogene is activated in many colorectal neoplasms.[23]

The gene most responsible for malignant conversion of benign colonic neoplasms appears to be *p53*. The tumor suppressor *p53* gene prevents nuclear replication after injuries that are likely to damage the DNA. In the presence of damaged DNA, the level of *p53* protein rises in the cell, and progression into the cell cycle is prevented.[21] The cell then repairs the damage, or programmed cell death ensues. Inactivation of the *p53* gene permits mutated DNA to be replicated and removes the restraint on abnormal cell behavior. Mutations of the *p53* gene are probably some of the most common and most powerful tumor-causing genetic lesions.

Other genetic abnormalities in malignant colonic tumors include the high expression of the c-*myc* oncogene, deletion of the *DCC* ("deleted in colon cancer") gene, and mutation of the *MCC* ("mutated in colon cancer") gene.[4,23] The loss of heterozygosity, which refers to the deletion of one chromosomal allele, has been observed in colon carcinoma on the genes of chromosomes 17 and 18.[23] The *MCC* gene has shown mutations in colon cancer and is located on chromosome 5 in the same region as the familial adenomatous polyposis gene.[4]

CLINICAL PRESENTATION

The symptoms of colon carcinoma depend on the location of the tumor. Cancers of the proximal colon usually attain a larger size before becoming symptomatic compared with cancers of the left colon and rectum. Fatigue, shortness of breath, angina due to hypochromic, microcytic anemia, and a melanotic, liquidy stool may be the principal means of presentation of right-sided colonic masses. Abdominal discomfort may be present as the tumor increases in size. Obstruction is uncommon because of the large diameters of the cecum and ascending colon. The left colon has a smaller lumen than the proximal colon, and therefore obstructive symptoms may occur. Left-sided symptoms include cramps, gas pain, and a decrease in the caliber of the stool. Carcinomas of the descending and sigmoid colon are often circumferential and may also cause obstruction.

Patients with colon carcinoma may experience colicky abdominal pain, especially after meals, as well as a change in bowel habits. Constipation may alternate with an increased frequency of defecation. Hematochezia may be present with distal rather than proximal lesions, and bright red blood passed via the rectum may be seen with cancers that involve the left colon and rectum. Approximately one half of patients with colon cancer experience anorexia and weight loss.

PHYSICAL EXAMINATION

Patients may present with a palpable abdominal mass and signs of distention or intestinal obstruction. Supraclavicular nodes may be positive with left-sided cancer, and the liver may be enlarged because of metastasis.[4,21]

DIAGNOSTICS

Visual inspection and digital examination of the anus and distal rectum are important in the evaluation of colorectal tumors to permit palpation of a possible tumor and to obtain stool to test for occult blood. A CBC should also be obtained. The air-contrast barium enema is used initially to detect polyps and cancers of the colon.[16,23] However, the sensitivity of the barium enema is directly related to the diligence of the radiologist. If the air-contrast barium enema is negative, a colonoscopy must be performed.[23] A colonoscopy, as well as flexible sigmoidoscopy, allows for direct visualization and biopsy of the colon.[16] Virtual colonoscopy, which is a high resolution CT scan, is a promising new screening tool that is in trial.[24] However, there are continued concerns that virtual colonoscopy may not detect small tumors. The CEA is not a useful screening test but is a valuable marker for recurring cancer.[2] The metastatic evaluation includes a CT scan, a chest x-ray study, and liver function tests (LFTs).[3,16]

DIFFERENTIAL DIAGNOSIS

The differential diagnosis of colon carcinoma includes benign tumors, diverticulitis, ulcerative colitis, Crohn's disease, tuberculosis, amebiasis, fungal masses, schistosomiasis, viral lesions such as cytomegalovirus, feces, lymphoid polyps and lymphoma, carcinoid tumors, metastatic lesions, and Kaposi's sarcoma. Obstructing lesions may include strictures from inflammation, radiation and ischemic colitis, and volvulus. In addition, extrinsic compression may occur from endometriosis and pancreatitis.

MANAGEMENT

Gastroenterologic, oncologic, and surgical consultations are necessary to provide optimal care for patients with colorectal tumors. The primary treatment of colorectal cancer is surgical intervention with wide resection (hemicolectomy) and removal of regional lymph nodes.[23] Adjuvant chemotherapy for colon cancer has been used in an attempt to reduce the recurrence rate of metastatic disease.[23] It has been shown to decrease the recurrence rate by 30% and to decrease distant metastasis by 50% in stage II and III disease.[25]

The use of radiation therapy as an adjunctive treatment is not beneficial for colon cancers outside of the rectum.[23] The CEA sample should be drawn before removal of a primary tumor because not all cancers produce this glycoprotein. If the preoperative value is not elevated, the test is not informative in the postoperative period. If the CEA is elevated before surgery, the CEA should be repeated 1 month after surgery for tumor recurrence (if the physician and patient are willing to undertake repeat surgery).[23] Detection of recurrence by serial CEA has been shown to occur between 1 and 18 months, with a median of 3 months.[26]

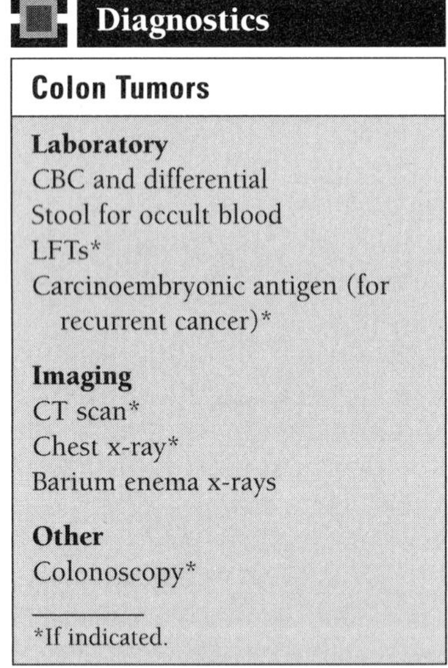

Diagnostics

Colon Tumors

Laboratory
CBC and differential
Stool for occult blood
LFTs*
Carcinoembryonic antigen (for recurrent cancer)*

Imaging
CT scan*
Chest x-ray*
Barium enema x-rays

Other
Colonoscopy*

*If indicated.

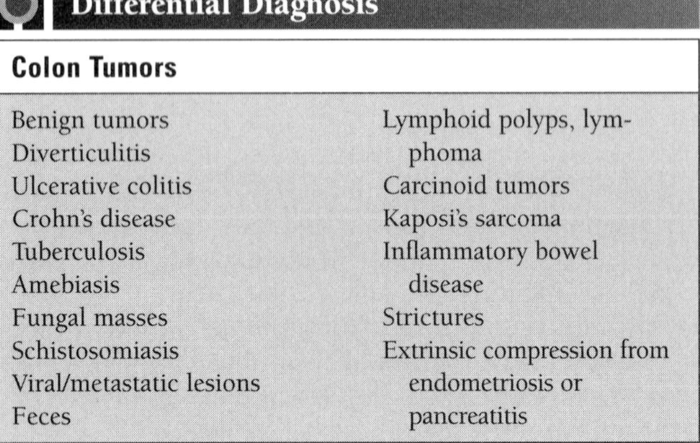

Differential Diagnosis

Colon Tumors

Benign tumors
Diverticulitis
Ulcerative colitis
Crohn's disease
Tuberculosis
Amebiasis
Fungal masses
Schistosomiasis
Viral/metastatic lesions
Feces
Lymphoid polyps, lymphoma
Carcinoid tumors
Kaposi's sarcoma
Inflammatory bowel disease
Strictures
Extrinsic compression from endometriosis or pancreatitis

COMPLICATIONS

Colorectal cancer may cause large bowel obstruction or perforation in cancers that reach an advanced stage.[4] Rate of recurrence within the abdominal cavity, including liver metastasis, is high.[26] Distant metastases, which are thought to be disseminated via hematogenous spread, may occur to the lungs, adrenal glands, bones, and brain.[26] Weight loss, fatigue, rectal bleeding, abdominal and pelvic pain, coughing, a change in bowel habits, and bone pain may signal recurrent disease.

PATIENT AND FAMILY EDUCATION

Because 10% of tumors are palpated rectally, annual digital rectal examinations should be started at 40 years of age.[2] Annual testing for fecal occult blood should also start at age 40. Also recommended is a sigmoidoscopy at age 45 or 8 years younger than the youngest family member afflicted with colon cancer, and then every 3 years thereafter. In patients with familial polyposis of the colon, colorectal cancer is inevitable 10 to 15 years after the onset of polyposis, and elective complete colectomy is required. Other family members must be screened for the dominant inheritance pattern.[9] The American Cancer Society recommends that routine screening for colon cancer begin at 50 years of age with annual fecal occult blood testing, a sigmoidoscopy every 5 years, and a colonoscopy every 10 years.[27] If polyps are present, a repeat flexible sigmoidoscopy is indicated in 3 years.

Individuals at high risk for the development of colon carcinoma, such as those with familial polyposis syndrome, prior adenomatous colonic polyps or cancer, or long-standing ulcerative colitis involving the entire colon, should be screened periodically with examination of the entire colon.[9]

Healthy diets with increased fiber and decreased fat intake may help prevent colon cancer, and therefore these diets should be explained routinely.

To detect the postoperative recurrence of colorectal carcinoma, patients should be evaluated every 3 months for 2 years with history, CEA, and physical examination and then every 6 months for 2 more years.[2] A screening colonoscopy should also be performed 1 year after surgery and, if normal, then every 3 years.[2]

HEALTH PROMOTION

Promotion of a healthy lifestyle is essential in the prevention of colorectal cancer. Patients should be encouraged to exercise on a regular basis: it is recommended that they exercise for 30 minutes at least 3 times weekly. More vigorous exercise may provide more benefit. A diet that provides five servings of fruits and vegetables and is low in red meat will help minimize the risk of colorectal cancer. It is important to limit the fat intake to 25% to 30% of the total caloric intake and to increase the amount of fiber to 20 to 30 g/day. These recommendations will help maintain a normal body weight. Avoidance of tobacco products and heavy alcohol consumption is also important.[10]

REFERENCES

1. Kirby TJ, Rice TW: The epidemiology of esophageal carcinoma: the changing face of a disease, *Chest Surg Clin North Am* 4(2):217-225, 1994.
2. Blackbourne LH: Thoracic surgery: esophageal carcinoma. In Blackbourne LH, editor: *Surgical recall*, Baltimore, 1994, Williams & Wilkins.
3. Fox JR, Kuwada S: Today's approach to esophageal cancer. What is the role of the primary care physician? *Postgrad Med* 107(5):109-114, 2000.
4. Rubin E, Farber JL: The gastrointestinal tract. In Rubin E, Farber JL, editors: *Pathology*, ed 2, Philadelphia, 1994, JB Lippincott.
5. Blot WJ, Devesa SS, Fraumeni JF: Continuing climb in rates of esophageal adenocarcinoma: an update, *JAMA* 270(11):1320, 1993.
6. Brooks-Brunn J: Esophageal cancer: an overview, *Med Surg Nurs* 9(5):248-254, 2000.
7. Reid BJ, Thomas CR: Esophageal neoplasms. In Yamada T, editor: *Textbook of gastroenterology*, ed 2, Philadelphia, 1995, JB Lippincott.
8. Quinn KL, Reedy A: Esophageal cancer: therapeutic approaches and nursing care, *Semin Oncol Nurs* 15(1):17-25, 1999.
9. Barron T and others: Gastrointestinal disease. In Andreoli TE and others, editors: *Cecil's essentials of medicine*, ed 4, Philadelphia, 1997, WB Saunders.
10. Byers T and others: American Cancer Society guidelines on nutrition and physical activity for cancer prevention: reducing the risk of cancer with healthy food choices and physical activity, *Cancer* 52(2): 92-119, 2002.
11. Clark GWB and others: Carcinoembryonic antigen measurements in the management of esophageal cancer: an indicator of subclinical recurrence, *Am J Surg* 170(6):597-600, 1995.
12. Davis GR: Neoplasms of the stomach. In Sleisenger MH, Fordtran J, editors: *Gastrointestinal disease*, ed 5, Philadelphia, 1993, WB Saunders.
13. Orringer MB: Complications of esophageal surgery. In Zuidema GD, editor: *Shackelford's surgery of the alimentary tract*, ed 4, Philadelphia, 1996, WB Saunders.
14. Hermans J and others: Adjuvant therapy after curative resection for gastric cancer: meta-analysis of randomized trials, *J Clin Oncol* 11(8):1441-1447, 1993.
15. Albert C: Clinical aspects of gastric cancer. In Rustgi AK, editor: *Gastrointestinal cancers: biology, diagnosis, and therapy*, Philadelphia, 1995, Lippincott-Raven.
16. Karp SJ, Morris J, Soybel D: Esophagus. In Marino BS, editor: *Blueprints in surgery*, Malden, MA, 1988, Blackwell Science.
17. Fuchs CS, Mayer RJ: Gastric carcinoma, *N Engl J Med* 333(1):32-41, 1995.
18. Christian TK, Stadlander H, Waterbor JW: Molecular epidemiology, pathogenesis and prevention of gastric cancer, *Carcinogenesis* 20(12):2195-2207, 1999.
19. Greager JA and others: Neoplasms of the small intestine. In Zuidema GD, editor: *Shackelford's surgery of the alimentary tract*, ed 4, Philadelphia, 1996, WB Saunders.
20. Lance PL: Tumors and other neoplastic diseases of the small bowel. In Yamada T, editor: *Textbook of gastroenterology*, ed 2, Philadelphia, 1995, JB Lippincott.
21. Marshall JB, Bodnarchuk G: Carcinoid tumors of the gut: our experience over three decades and review of the literature, *J Clin Gastroenterol* 16(2):123-129, 1993.
22. Bresalier RS, Kim YS: Malignant neoplasms of the large intestine. In Sleisenger MH, Fordtran JS, editors: *Gastrointestinal disease: pathophysiology, diagnosis, management*, ed 5, Philadelphia, 1993, WB Saunders.
23. Boland CR: Malignant tumors of the colon. In Yamada T, editor: *Textbook of gastroenterology*, ed 2, Philadelphia, 1995, JB Lippincott.
24. Kuwada S: Colorectal cancer 2000, *Postgrad Med* 107(5):96-107, 2000.
25. Stefanik DC, Muscari E: Colon cancer, *Am J Nurs*, April (Suppl):36-40, 2000.
26. Averbach AM, Sugarbaker PH: Use of tumor markers and radiologic tests in follow-up. In Cohen AM, Winawer SJ, editors: *Cancer of the colon, rectum, and anus*, New York, 1995, McGraw-Hill.
27. Ransohoff DF, Sandler RS: Screening for colorectal cancer, *N Engl J Med* 346(1):40-44, 2002.

CHAPTER 156

Ulcer Disease

Donna M. Glynn and Nancy D. Bolton

Duodenal Ulcers

DEFINITION/EPIDEMIOLOGY

Ulcer disease is a pathologic, destructive, chronic disorder characterized by ulceration of the gastric and duodenal mucosa. The incidence of duodenal ulcers continues to rise. This increase is related to uncontrolled risk factors, increasing use of nonsteroidal therapy, and *Helicobacter pylori* infections. Duodenal ulcers have had a serious impact on the economics of health care and society because of recurrence, increased office visits, medication costs, diagnostic costs, and patient quality of life. Therefore it is essential to obtain a thorough health history, identify potential risk factors, and provide cost-effective diagnosis and treatment of duodenal ulcers, as well as to prevent recurrence of this common disorder.

Duodenal ulcer disease may be defined as an imbalance both in the amount of acid-pepsin production delivered from the stomach to the duodenum and in the ability of the duodenal lining to protect itself. Duodenal ulcers may also occur from an infection caused by *H. pylori*, the most common bacterial infection found in adults.[1]

Risk factors for ulcer disease include stress, cigarette smoking, chronic obstructive pulmonary disease, alcohol, and alcoholic cirrhosis.[2] Certain drug preparations have also been shown to increase the incidence of duodenal ulcers. Chronic use of aspirin and nonsteroidal antiinflammatory drugs (NSAIDs) has been shown to produce mucosal damage, and these drugs are readily available over-the-counter.

Certain conditions and genetic factors have also been identified as risk factors for the development of duodenal ulcer disease. Zöllinger-Ellison syndrome, a condition that causes increased acid production, results in ulcer disease. Genetic risk factors include first-degree relatives with duodenal ulcer disease, blood group O, elevated levels of pepsinogen I, the presence of HLA-B5 antigen, and decreased RBC acetylcholinesterase.[3]

Duodenal ulcer disease affects approximately 5 million people in the United States annually, and 16 million individuals will have the disease at some point during their lifetime.[4] Duodenal ulcers continue to be more common than gastric ulcers. The peak incidence for duodenal ulcer occurrence is in the fifth decade for men and the sixth decade for women, with an estimated recurrence rate of 75% to 80% within 1 year of diagnosis if maintenance therapy is not administered.[2] Current statistics regarding *H. pylori* infections report that 10% of whites younger than age 35 are infected, with percentages rising to 80% by age 75.[5] More than 90% of duodenal ulcers are caused by *H. pylori*, and the prevalence is believed to be significantly higher because of inadequate screening and the high number of individuals who do not seek medical care or who self-treat with over-the-counter preparations.[6]

PATHOPHYSIOLOGY

The function of the gastrointestinal tract is digestion of food and absorption of nutrients. This process is achieved by high concentrations of acid and pepsin that are secreted from the parietal cells of the stomach. The surface of the mucosa secretes an alkaline mucus that protects the mucosa from self-digestion. However, when this system is interrupted, the protective tissue is damaged and erosion or ulcer formation occurs. Duodenal ulcers are primarily located in the duodenal bulb or within 3 cm of the pyloric duodenal junction and are usually less than 1 cm in diameter. Reducing the production of acid and pepsin is key to the promotion of healing and prevention of recurrence.

H. pylori, a spiral-shaped flagellated organism, was first discovered in 1983 and is strongly associated with duodenal ulcer disease. The infection is acquired via the orofecal route. Once ingested, *H. pylori* attaches to the gastric mucosa and produces local tissue injury, resulting in the release of cytotoxins and proteases.[5]

CLINICAL PRESENTATION

The most common presenting chief complaint is epigastric pain. This discomfort is often described as a sharp, burning, aching, gnawing pain occurring $1\frac{1}{2}$ to 3 hours after meals or in the middle of the night. The patient will report that the pain is usually relieved with the ingestion of food or antacids; however, the symptoms are recurrent, with episodes that from several days to months. Changes in the intensity, duration, or location of the pain may indicate penetration or perforation of an ulcer. Symptoms of nausea and vomiting are rare. Ironically, weight gain is not uncommon because the ingestion of food alleviates the pain.

PHYSICAL EXAMINATION

Inspection, auscultation, and percussion will generally yield negative findings. In rare presentations, auscultation may reveal a succussion splash 4 hours or longer after meals, which would indicate a duodenal or pyloric channel ulcer, causing gastric outlet obstruction. Palpation may produce epigastric tenderness midline between the umbilicus and the xiphoid process. If a perforation has occurred, the patient will have a rigid abdomen and generalized rebound tenderness. Rectal examination should be included with testing for melena.

DIAGNOSTICS AND DIFFERENTIAL DIAGNOSIS

A CBC will exclude the presence of anemia. Serum culture for *H. pylori* is also indicated initially. Differential diagnosis for duodenal ulcer disease is based on the symptoms reported and the location of the pain. Cholecystitis presents as right upper quadrant abdominal discomfort. Vague abdominal pain with reports of diarrhea or constipation may be associated with diverticulosis, irritable bowel syndrome, or nonulcer dyspepsia. Gastroesophageal reflux disease (GERD), pancreatitis, and malignancy should also be considered.

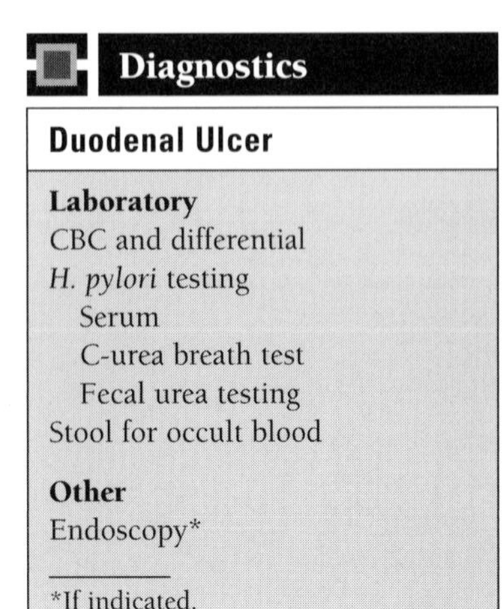
Diagnostics

Duodenal Ulcer

Laboratory
CBC and differential
H. pylori testing
Serum
C-urea breath test
Fecal urea testing
Stool for occult blood

Other
Endoscopy*

*If indicated.

Zöllinger-Ellison syndrome is a condition of excessive acid production. This should be considered if the individual does not respond to the traditional diet, smoking cessation, and pharmacologic therapy.

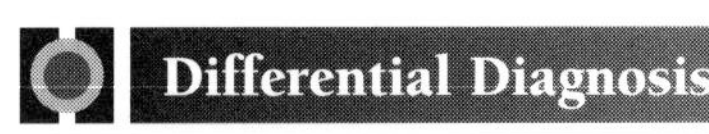

Duodenal Ulcer

Cholecystitis
Diverticulosis
Irritable bowel syndrome
Nonulcer dyspepsia
GERD
Pancreatitis
Malignancy
Zöllinger-Ellison syndrome

MANAGEMENT

First-line treatment of duodenal ulcer disease is a 2-week trial of antiulcer therapy. If NSAID use is documented, the medications should be discontinued. If objective findings include anemia, gastrointestinal bleeding, rigid abdomen, weight loss, or new-onset dyspepsia in an individual older than 50 years, an immediate physician consultation is indicated. If symptoms persist after the 2-week course of therapy, referral to a gastroenterologist for endoscopy is appropriate. Recent studies support endoscopy over barium-contrast radiography as having higher rates of detecting pathology through direct observation and biopsy.[3] The presence of *H. pylori* may be determined during the endoscopy or by noninvasive techniques of serology or carbon isotope–urea breath test.[7]

The most widely accepted antiulcer therapy is the use of H_2-receptor antagonists. These preparations inhibit gastric acid secretion by blocking the H_2-receptors of the parietal cells. H_2-receptor antagonists are associated with a 75% to 90% healing rate over a 4- to 6-week period, which is then followed by maintenance dosing at bedtime for 1 year. Cimetidine was the first product developed and continues to be the most cost effective. However, awareness of potential drug interactions caused by the inhibition of cytochrome P-450 pathway is an important consideration. Other H_2-receptor antagonists include ranitidine, famotidine, and nizatidine.

The recent approval by the U.S. Food and Drug Administration (FDA) of over-the-counter H_2-receptor antagonists for acid control presents new challenges for primary care providers. Again, an in-depth history that includes over-the-counter medication use is extremely important when contemplating treatment options.

Proton pump inhibitors omeprazole and lansoprazole are the most potent and most expensive treatment option for duodenal ulcer therapy. These preparations block the production of acid secretion. Daily dosing eliminates acid production and has been proved to be highly effective in the treatment of duodenal ulcers, although long-term studies regarding prolonged effects of acid production elimination are pending.

Prostaglandin therapy protects the gastric/duodenal mucosa and should be considered for individuals unable to discontinue NSAID use. Misoprostol is the only available agent at the present time. To effectively inhibit acid production and prevent duodenal damage, the therapeutic dose has been shown to produce transient side effects of cramping and diarrhea, which can be eliminated with a lower initial dose.[8]

Treatment options for *H. pylori* eradication continue to be closely evaluated. A combination of bismuth and metronidazole, with either amoxicillin or tetracycline, has been the most widely studied and produces a greater than 90% cure rate with 2 weeks of therapy.[9] However, shorter courses of therapy are being prescribed; other antibiotics such as clarithromycin (Biaxin) can be substituted for amoxicillin or tetracycline. Proton pump inhibitor therapy has documented improved efficacy over the H_2-receptor antagonist blockers, but cost and adherence must be considered before initiating therapy (Box 156-1).

COMPLICATIONS

Perforation of duodenal ulcer is a life-threatening complication of chronic ulcer disease. This is most common in older patients and requires emergency care. Other complications include hemorrhage, gastric ulcer obstruction, and ulcers refractory to treatment.

INDICATIONS FOR REFERRAL/HOSPITALIZATION

Gastroenterology referral is indicated for endoscopy if bleeding is suspected or for examination of the duodenum and associated structures. Surgical referral is indicated for emergency intervention and in cases of prolonged refractory ulcer disease.

PATIENT AND FAMILY EDUCATION

Patient education involves the identification and modification of risk factors, specifically cigarette smoking. Once a diagnosis of ulcer disease has been established, education should also include the signs and symptoms of hemorrhage, perforation, gastrointestinal bleeding, and anemia. In addition, the consequences of medication nonadherence related to the treatment of duodenal ulcer disease and *H. pylori* infection should be carefully reviewed.

Gastric Ulcers

PATHOPHYSIOLOGY

As stated, *H. pylori* is a spiral-shaped bacterium that was discovered in 1983.[10] The organisms live within or beneath the gastric mucous layer. *H. pylori* is not an invasive bacterium but causes damage by making the mucosa vulnerable to peptic acid damage. The process of emitting enzymes and toxins that can alter the gastric epithelium disrupts the mucous layer. Gastritis results from *H. pylori* colonization, but many patients are asymptomatic and the gastritis does not progress. In other patients the gastritis will progress to peptic ulcer disease (PUD), and in 2% to 4% of patients, gastric cancer will develop.[11] Why *H. pylori* infection is a benign condition in some and a causative agent for PUD or cancer in others is not clearly understood. However, *H. pylori* has been identified in 65% to 75% of patients with non-NSAID use and gastric ulcers.[12]

NSAID/aminosalicylic acid (ASA) use is a major causative factor in the development of gastric ulcers. Approximately 15% to 25% of patients taking NSAIDs will develop gastric ulcers, with 50% of these patients having *H. pylori* as a coexisting factor.[13] Patients taking NSAIDs have a threefold greater risk of developing a serious gastrointestinal event, and those older than 60 years have a fivefold increased risk.[14] Others at increased risk include those patients with a previous ulcer history, patients in

BOX 156-1

***HELICOBACTER PYLORI* TREATMENT OPTIONS**

1. Bismuth, 2 tablets q.i.d.
   Metronidazole, 250 mg t.i.d./q.i.d.
   Tetracycline, 500 mg q.i.d.
   Omeprazole, 20 mg b.i.d.
   Duration: 1 week
   Cost: $
   Efficacy 94%-98%
2. Bismuth, 2 tablets q.i.d.
   Metronidazole, 250 mg t.i.d./q.i.d.
   Tetracycline, 500 mg q.i.d.
   H_2-receptor antagonist therapy as directed for 1 month
   Duration: 2 weeks
   Cost: $
   Efficacy >90%
3. Bismuth, 2 tablets q.i.d.
   Tetracycline, 500 mg q.i.d.
   Clarithromycin, 500 mg t.i.d.
   H_2-receptor antagonist h.s.
   Duration: 2 weeks
   Cost: $$$
   Efficacy >90%
4. Bismuth, 2 tablets q.i.d.*
   Tetracycline, 500 mg q.i.d.
   Metronidazole, 500 mg t.i.d.
   Omeprazole, 20 mg b.i.d.
   Duration: 1 week
   Cost: $
   Efficacy >90%
5. Bismuth, 2 tablets q.i.d.
   Clarithromycin, 500 mg t.i.d.
   Tetracycline, 500 mg q.i.d.
   Duration: 1-2 weeks
   Cost: $ 1 week
   $$ 2 weeks
   Efficacy >90%
6. Ranitidine bismuth citrate, 400 mg b.i.d. for 1 month
   Clarithromycin, 500 mg t.i.d. for 2 weeks
   Duration: As above
   Cost: $$
   Efficacy 82%

Modified from NIH Consensus Development Panel on *Heliobacter pylori* in Peptic Ulcer Disease: NIH consensus conference: *Helicobacter pylori* in peptic ulcer disease, *JAMA* 272, 1994.
Cost: $, $100; $$, $100-$200; $$$ >$200.
*Requires 3 days of pretreatment with omeprazole before antibiotic therapy.

poor general health, and patients using steroids or anticoagulants.[15] In addition, the longer a person remains on NSAIDs, the greater is the cumulative risk.

Endoscopic studies show that gastric erosions will develop in virtually everyone who ingests therapeutic doses of ASA on a regular basis. NSAID/ASA use inhibits the synthesis of prostaglandin, which plays an important role in mucosal defense. These products also reduce mucus secretion, which is protective, thus allowing acid to damage the lining of the stomach. The selective inhibitors of cyclooxygenase-2 (COX-2) (e.g., celecoxib and rofecoxib) seem to reduce but not eliminate the incidence of gastric ulcers in NSAID users.[16]

Malignancy is the last major cause of gastric ulcers. Duodenal ulcers are rarely malignant. Gastric ulcers are most commonly not seen in areas other than the antrum. Ten percent of all gastric ulcers are idiopathic, but this group may include undiscovered NSAID users.[12,17]

Other etiologic risk factors for PUD include caffeine/coffee ingestion, alcohol use, smoking, and family history. Caffeine stimulates acid and pepsin secretion. Coffee (both regular and decaffeinated) stimulates these enzymes more than does caffeine alone; this suggests that there is something in coffee besides caffeine that increases acid secretion.

Alcohol damages the mucosa of the stomach. It is dose dependent and is associated with upper gastrointestinal bleeding in about one third of patients.[18]

Smokers have up to a fivefold risk over nonsmokers for the development of ulcers.[11] They are also more likely to develop complications, to have less spontaneous healing, and to have slower healing rates with medications.

There is a twofold to threefold increased risk of developing a gastric ulcer if a first-degree relative has had a gastric ulcer.[18] The site of formation is also fairly consistent in family members. If a family member has a gastric ulcer, there is an increased risk of the development of a gastric ulcer rather than of a duodenal ulcer.

CLINICAL PRESENTATION

Most patients with PUD have variable abdominal pain. Unfortunately, abdominal pain can be associated with other conditions, such as GERD, pancreatitis, or cholecystitis. A patient with a duodenal ulcer typically has epigastric pain that is most apparent a few hours after eating or at night. One third of the patients with gastric ulcers and two thirds of the patients with duodenal ulcers describe the presence of pain that awakens them from sleep, usually between 12 and 3 AM. This gnawing, burning pain is usually relieved with antacids or food.

Gastric ulcer pain is similar, but the pain may be increased by food and may also be located in the upper left quadrant, as well as radiating to the back. Bloating, belching, nausea, vomiting, and weight loss may be present.[19] Pain persists for an average of 6 to 8 months before the patient seeks medical attention.[18] NSAID-induced ulcers are often painless, with the most common presentation being melena or iron deficiency anemia.

Patients with gastroduodenitis can have symptoms that cannot be distinguished from ulcer disease. The etiology of PUD/gastritis abdominal pain is not clearly understood. About 30% of patients have nonhealed ulcers and are symptom free or have healed ulcers but continue to have symptoms.[12]

PHYSICAL EXAMINATION

There may be no abnormal findings, but epigastric or left upper quadrant tenderness is most commonly found on examination. Weight loss may also be observed. Rectal examination may reveal a heme-positive stool. An acute abdomen with heme-positive stool is a more obvious sign of gastrointestinal bleeding.

DIAGNOSTICS

A CBC is indicated for the determination of anemia. If NSAID use is not part of the patient's history, or if the patient has "alarm" markers, such as anemia, gastrointestinal bleeding, anorexia, early satiety, or weight loss, a diagnostic evaluation should be performed.[13] Immediate investigation is also indicated for patients older than 50 years with new-onset dyspepsia to exclude gastric neoplasia. Upper endoscopy is superior to barium contrast radiography in detection rates and for diagnosis.

A positive serology for *H. pylori* represents exposure to the bacterium but not necessarily its presence in the stomach. A carbon-labeled breath test is now FDA approved, is noninvasive, and has a high rate of sensitivity. This can confirm the presence of *H. pylori* if endoscopy is not indicated. If endoscopy is indicated, a biopsy sample is taken and placed in a rapid urease test to determine the organism's presence. This can be performed without the expense of sending the biopsy sample to the pathologist.

If a gastric ulcer is present on endoscopy, the margins should be included in a biopsy to exclude malignancy. Several studies indicate that a single endoscopic examination with careful inspection and expert pathologic interpretation of adequate multiple biopsy specimens will yield greater than 98% sensitivity for cancer.[13,20] A follow-up endoscopy should be performed to confirm healing.

DIFFERENTIAL DIAGNOSIS

Malignancy is a potential consideration, particularly with gastric ulcers. In addition, gastrointestinal reflux, cholecystitis, pancreatitis, and diverticulitis should be considered.

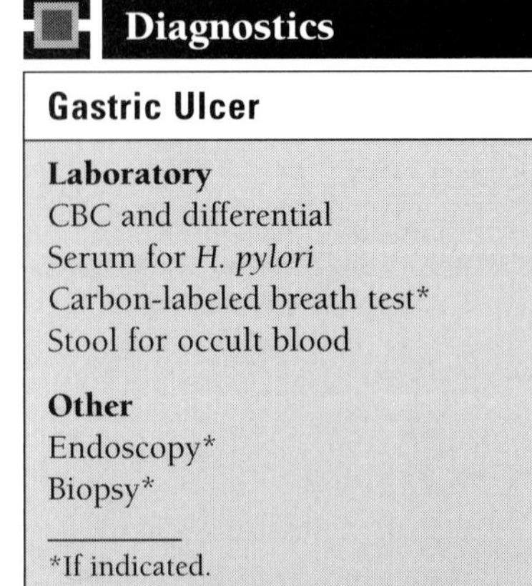
Diagnostics

Gastric Ulcer

Laboratory
CBC and differential
Serum for *H. pylori*
Carbon-labeled breath test*
Stool for occult blood

Other
Endoscopy*
Biopsy*

*If indicated.

MANAGEMENT

The goals of treatment for PUD include relief of symptoms, avoidance of complications, and prevention of recurrence.

If *H. pylori* is identified in an ulcer patient, antibiotic therapy is in-

Differential Diagnosis

Gastric Ulcer

Malignancy	Pancreatitis
Gastrointestinal reflux	Diverticulitis
Cholecystitis	

dicated, as well as antisecretory therapy. There is no particular "ulcer diet," but decreasing caffeine/coffee ingestion, alcohol use, and smoking will aid healing. Most studies have shown that proton pump inhibitors have superior healing rates compared with H_2-receptor antagonists. Once-daily use of proton pump inhibitors shows healing rates of 60% to 74% after 4 weeks and 85% to 96% at 8 weeks.[17] More potent acid inhibition results in better ulcer healing.[21] Therefore gastric ulcer therapy takes longer than duodenal ulcer therapy. Increased doses of proton pump inhibitors are sometimes needed for large, slow-healing, or complicated ulcers. NSAIDs should be discontinued if possible, with acetaminophen substituted. COX-2 inhibitors should be used cautiously.

Ulcer recurrence rates are decreased to 4% versus 59% if *H. pylori* is eradicated[22] (see Management under Duodenal Ulcers [p. 670] for recommended treatment). Maintenance therapy is not indicated if *H. pylori* is eradicated or NSAID use is discontinued in a patient who does not have complications. If patients need to restart NSAIDs, misoprostol 800 μg/day may reduce the risk of ulcer complications.[23-25] The use of proton pump inhibitors while continuing NSAIDs may prevent ulcer recurrence.[25,26] Patients who have no known etiology for their gastric ulcer, especially those with complications, should be considered for maintenance therapy with full-dose H_2-receptor antagonists or long-term proton pump inhibitors.

COMPLICATIONS

Hemorrhage is the most common complication and occurs in about 15% of patients with ulcers.[12] It is more common in patients older than 50 years. This may be due to increased NSAID use in this age-group, particularly in women. From 10% to 20% of these patients bleed from an ulcer without any prior symptoms.[12] Eradication of *H. pylori* usually prevents duodenal ulcers and non–NSAID-induced gastric ulcers from recurring, and this may prevent recurrent hemorrhage.[27]

Perforation occurs in about 7% of patients with PUD.[12] This complication is increased with the use of NSAIDs. Gastric outlet obstruction or pyloric stenosis can lead to gastric retention.[18,28] This can be caused by inflammation, edema, or scarring secondary to chronic recurrent ulcers.

INDICATIONS FOR REFERRAL/HOSPITALIZATION

Hospitalization and gastroenterology referral are indicated for evaluation of bleeding ulcers. Consultation with a gastroenterologist is also warranted for suspected malignancy or if symptoms continue after treatment.

PATIENT AND FAMILY EDUCATION/HEALTH PROMOTION

It is important that patients and families understand the physiology of the disease, potential complications, and the importance of therapy. Careful explanation of the need to stop smoking; to avoid alcohol, ASA, and NSAIDs; and the side effects of medications is also necessary.

REFERENCES

1. Digestive Health Initiative: International update conference on Helicobacter pylori, *Digestive Disease Week,* May 1997.
2. Keithley JK: Histamine H_2-receptor antagonists, *Nurs Clin North Am* 26(2):361-373, 1991.
3. Soll AH: Consensus conference: medical treatment of peptic ulcer disease: practice guidelines, *JAMA* 275(8):622-629, 1996.
4. Saltiel E: Peptic acid disorders: developing a disease management program, *J Managed Care Pharmacol* 2(5):569-575, 1996.
5. Damianos AJ, McGarrity TJ: Treatment strategies for Helicobacter pylori infection, *Am J Gasteroenterol* 55(8):2765-2786, 1997.
6. Marshall BJ: Helicobacter pylori, *Am J Gastroenterol* 89(8):116-128, 1994.
7. Culter AF and others: Accuracy of invasive and noninvasive tests to diagnose Helicobacter pylori infection, *Gastroenterology* 109:136-141, 1995.
8. Graham DY and others: Duodenal and gastric ulcer prevention with misoprostol in arthritis patients taking NSAIDs, *Ann Intern Med* 119:257-262, 1993.
9. Chiba N and others: Meta-analysis of the efficacy of antibiotic therapy in eradicating H. pylori, *Am J Gastroenterol* 87:1716-1727, 1992.
10. Peura DA: *Helicobacter pylori: 1997 and beyond: advances in gastroenterology,* Williamsburg, Va, September 20-21, 1997, American College of Gastroenterology, Virginia Gastroenterological Society.
11. Kimmey MB: Gastritis and peptic ulcer disease. In Rakel RE, editor: *Conn's current therapy,* Philadelphia, 1998, WB Saunders.
12. Yamada T: *Textbook of gastroenterology,* ed 2, Philadelphia, 1995, JB Lippincott.
13. Soll AH, for the Practice Parameters Committee of the American College of Gastroenterology: Medical treatment of peptic ulcer disease: practice guidelines, *JAMA* 275:622-629, 1996.
14. Lanza FL: ACG Treatment Guideline: treatment and prevention of NSAID induced ulcers, *Am J Gastroenterol* 93:2037-2046, 1998.
15. Griggin MR, Scheiman JM: Prospects for changing the burden of NSAID toxicity, *Am J Med* 110:33S-37S, 2001.
16. Bazzoli F, De-Luca L, Graham DY: Helicobacter pylori infection and the use of NSAIDs, *Best Pract Res Clin Gastroenterol* 15:775-785, 2001.
17. Sachs G, Prinz C, Hersey SJ: *Acid related disorders: mystery to mechanism: mechanism to management,* Palm Beach, Fla, 1995, Sushu Publishing.
18. Molinoff PB: Pathophysiology and clinical aspects of peptic ulcer disease. In *Peptic ulcer disease: mechanisms and management,* Rutherford, NJ, 1990, Healthpress Publishing.
19. Sontag SJ: Guilty as charged: bugs and drugs in gastric ulcer, *Am J Gastroenterol* 92(8):1255-1261, 1997.
20. Sleisinger MH, Fordtran JS: *Gastrointestinal disease,* ed 6, Philadelphia, 1993, WB Saunders.
21. Hunt RH: Eradication of H. pylori infections, *Am J Med* 100(5A): 42S-50S, 1996.
22. Hopkins RJ, Girardi LS, Turney EA: Relationship between *H. pylori* eradication and reduced duodenal and gastric ulcer recurrency: a review, *Gastroenterology* 110(4):1244-1252, 1998.
23. Mohamed AH, Salena BJ, Hunt RH: NSAID-induced gastroduodenal ulcers: exploring the silent dilemma, *J Gastroenterol* 29(suppl 7): 34-38, 1994.
24. Zfass AM, McHenry L Jr, Sanyal AJ: Nonsteroidal antiinflammatory drug–induced gastroduodenal lesions: prophylaxis and treatment, *Gastroenterology* 1(2):165-169, 1993.
25. Rostom A: The prevention of chronic NSAID induced upper GI toxicity: a Cochrane collaboration metaanalysis of randomized controlled trials, *J Rheumatol* 27:2203-2214, 2000.
26. Bianchi, PG: Efficacy of pantoprazole in prevention of peptic ulcers induced by NSAID: a prospective, placebo controlled, double blind, parallel group study, *Dig Liver Dis* 32:207-208, 2000.
27. Bjorkman DJ, Ziebert J: Non-steroidal anti-inflammatory drug, nonmalignant gastric ulcers, *Gastrointest Endosc Clin North Am* 6(3): 527-544, 1996.
28. Mohamed AH, Hunt RH: The rationale of acid suppression in the treatment of acid-related disease, *Aliment Pharmacol Ther* 8(suppl): 3-10, 1994.

PART 13

Evaluation and Management of Genitourinary Disorders

PATRICIA POLGAR BAILEY, Section Editor

CHAPTER 157

Erectile Dysfunction

Laura Stempkowski

DEFINITION/EPIDEMIOLOGY

Erectile dysfunction (ED) is the consistent inability to achieve and maintain a firm erection for satisfactory sexual activity.[1] Since the National Institutes of Health Consensus Conference in 1988, the term *erectile dysfunction* has replaced the term *impotence*.[2] ED is now recognized as a medical problem with potential psychologic consequences that may interfere with a man's self-esteem and interpersonal relationships.

In the United States, approximately 10 to 20 million men have ED.[3] The majority of these men are older than 65 years. The Massachusetts Male Aging Study conducted between 1987 and 1989 found an overall rate of ED of 52%.[1] The overall probability of ED was 39% at age 40 and 67% at age 70.[1] Men with ED are often embarrassed to discuss their problem openly with health care providers; consequently, most men seek treatment only after being referred by a family physician. Embarrassment and lack of adequate information are the two most commonly cited reasons for failing to seek treatment.[1] The advent of new pharmacologic agents for treating ED and their associated publicity have increased the awareness of the scope of this problem and resulted in an increased number of men seeking treatment.

PATHOPHYSIOLOGY

Erectile function is a neurovascular event that is initiated by cognitive or tactile stimulation that is processed in the brain. Chemical mediators cause the essential relaxation of tissue and perfusion of the corpora cavernosum and corpus spongiosum. Nitric oxide (NO) and cyclic guanosine monophosphate (cGMP) are the primary noncholinergic and cholinergic mediators responsible for the neurogenic aspect of erection. Engorgement of the corpora and corpus spongiosum in turn compresses the veins to prevent the venous outflow of blood. This is how the erection is maintained and accounts for the vascular component of erection.[4] Any factor that interferes with this process may lead to ED.

The etiology of ED may be clearly identified (e.g., radical prostatectomy) or may be multifactorial, requiring comprehensive assessment. Although in the past ED was believed to be psychogenic, it has been shown that more than 70% of cases have a physiologic origin.[4] Alterations in vascular supply, hormonal changes, neurologic dysfunction, or medications and associated systemic disease may contribute to ED.

Psychogenic

Psychologic factors that may be of etiologic significance include performance anxiety, guilt, and strict religious constraints. Life events, such as a business failure, loss of health, or deterioration in the partner relationship, may also contribute to ED because of their impact on mood, anxiety, self-esteem, and depression. Developmental vulnerabilities, such as a history of child abuse, may have a profound effect on sexual function.[5] When combined with physiologic problems, psychologic issues can result in significant erectile difficulties.

Hormonal

Testosterone deficiency may be caused by hypothalamic or pituitary tumors or by treatment aimed at suppressing testosterone, such as hormonal therapy in the treatment of prostate cancer. Although the primary effect of testosterone deficiency is decreased libido, ED may result as well. Other conditions that may precipitate decreased libido or ED because of their hormonal effects include hyperprolactinemia, hyperthyroidism, hypothyroidism, Cushing's syndrome, and Addison's disease.[5]

Vasculogenic-Neurogenic

Vasculogenic-neurologic disorders that cause ED may be related to the stage of erection—a failure to initiate erection, a failure to achieve erection, or a failure to sustain erection. Potential cause of vasculogenic-neurogenic ED and the major associated conditions are listed in Box 157-1.

Pharmacologic Risk Factors

The major classes of drugs that affect erectile function include antihypertensives, antidepressants, and major tranquilizers. ED may result from pharmacologic effects on central nervous system, vascular system, hormone levels, and libido (Box 157-2).

Surgical Risk Factors

ED may occur after major surgery that potentially alters either the innervation or blood flow to the penis. These procedures may also affect a man's body image and self-perception of masculinity. Examples of such procedures are the radical prostatectomy, radical cystectomy, and abdominal-perineal resection. Nerve-sparing techniques minimize this risk and may result in the preservation of erectile function.

Other

Pelvic radiation therapy (e.g., to treat prostate cancer) may damage nerves and blood vessels, potentially resulting in ED.

BOX 157-1

CAUSES OF ERECTILE DYSFUNCTION

NEUROGENIC
- Multiple sclerosis
- Peripheral neuropathy
- Radical prostatectomy
- Spinal cord injury
- Stroke

VASCULAR
- Cardiovascular or peripheral vascular disease
- Congestive heart failure
- Cigarette smoking
- Diabetes mellitus
- Trauma to perineum or pelvis

HORMONAL
- Decreased testosterone, LH, or increased prolactin

PSYCHOGENIC
- Anxiety
- Depression
- Stress

MEDICATIONS
- See Box 157-2

Data from Albaugh J, Lewis J: Insight into the management of erectile dysfunction: part I, *Urol Nurs* 19(4):242, 1999.

CLINICAL PRESENTATION

Men may be reluctant to discuss such a sensitive and personal subject. Care must be taken to reassure them that ED affects many men and that there is effective treatment available.[6] It is important for health care providers to include sexual assessment as a component of routine health care surveillance and to become comfortable in eliciting the information that will help identify ED, give insight into its etiology, and guide further intervention.

The patient history should include questions that address the onset of ED (gradual or abrupt); whether there is difficulty achieving or maintaining an erection, or both; and the presence and quality of nocturnal erections. In addition, the onset of ED, particularly if associated with a specific event (e.g., stress), should be determined. A urologic questionnaire may be helpful in obtaining information of such a personal nature. The clinical history should include current health problems, a review of systems, and current medications, including nonprescription drugs and herbal formulations.

PHYSICAL EXAMINATION

The physical examination is focused on detecting signs of endocrine, vascular, or neurologic deficit and penile abnormality. Testicular atrophy, gynecomastia, or signs of hypothyroidism or hyperthyroidism may indicate hormonal abnormalities. Vascular assessment includes checking pulses in the lower extremities and observing for vascular skin changes in the lower extremities (e.g., hair loss). Neurologic assessment is focused on testing for genital reflexes (bulbocavernosus, cremasteric, scrotal, sphincter tone) and light touch discrimination.[5] During the genital examination, it is important to palpate for penile plaques, which may indicate Peyronie's disease. The presence of plaques in the tunica albuginea limits penile distensibility, causing a bend in the penis with erection. This may interfere with sexual activity by making penetration difficult.[7]

BOX 157-2

DRUGS THAT AFFECT ERECTILE DYSFUNCTION

ANTIHYPERTENSIVES

Beta blockers: propranolol, atenolol
Diuretics: hydrochlorothiazide, amiloride, chlorthalidone, spironolactone
ACE inhibitors: enalapril, lisinopril
Centrally acting agents: clonidine, methyldopa
Peripherally acting agents: guanethidine
Miscellaneous: labetalol, reserpine

ANTIDEPRESSANTS

Tricyclic: amoxapine, imipramine, clomipramine
Miscellaneous: bupropion, tranylcypromine, venlafaxine

OTHER DRUGS

Antipsychotics: chlorpromazine, fluphenazine, lithium, thioridazine, sulpiride
Antianxiety: chlordiazepoxide
Antiarrhythmics: digoxin, phenytoin
Anticonvulsants: acetazolamide, carbamazepine, phenytoin, phenobarbital, primidone
Anticholinergics: atropine, dicyclomine, ipratropium, scopolamine
Histamine H_2 agonists: cimetidine, ranitidine, famotidine
Miscellaneous medications: clofibrate, dichlorphenamide, fenfluramine, ketoconazole, methadone, methazolamide, norethindrone, thiabendazole
Illicit and abused drugs: alcohol, amphetamines, cocaine, marijuana, tobacco

Data from Albaugh J, Lewis J: Insight into the management of erectile dysfunction: part I, *Urol Nurs* 19(4):242, 1999.

DIAGNOSTICS

Initially, nocturnal penile tumescence is evaluated to determine whether erectile dysfunction is attributed to a psychogenic or an organic condition.[8] The Snap-Gauge (Dacomed Corp., Minneapolis, MN), a Velcro band with three colored films arranged parallel to each other, is fitted around the penis. Each films ruptures to correspond with the intracavernosal pressures found in erection. Response is gauged by the number of films broken, with 0 to 1 indicating absent rigidity and 2 to 3 indicating rigid erections. Studies have shown the Snap-Gauge results to be inaccurate up to one third of the time.[8]

The Rigi-Scan (Dacomed Corp.) is a more sophisticated device that provides continuous tumescence monitoring and can distinguish functional from inadequate erections in the majority of cases.[8]

Studies to evaluate penile vasculature include the intracavernosal injection of a vasoactive drug (e.g., alprostadil) or color duplex Doppler ultrasound (CDDU). CDDU evaluates anatomic abnormalities as well as measuring both penile inflow and outflow.[9]

In the absence of a reliable test, the clinician must rely on the patient's history, physical examination, and laboratory testing—thyroid stimulating hormone (TSH), luteinizing hormone (LH), serum electrolytes, serum glucose, BUN, creatinine, serum testosterone, prolactin, and cholesterol—to determine the etiology of ED.

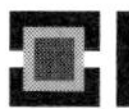

Diagnostics

Erectile Dysfunction

Laboratory
CBC and differential
Serum glucose and/or HbA_{1C}
Serum electrolytes
BUN and creatinine
Cholesterol
TSH
Prolactin
Serum testosterone
Luteinizing hormone

Other
As indicated (see Diagnostics, above)

DIFFERENTIAL DIAGNOSIS

See Differential Diagnosis box for Erectile Dysfunction.

Differential Diagnosis

Erectile Dysfunction

Decreased libido
Anorgasmia
Ejaculatory dysfunction

Data from Ellsworth P, Rous S: *Primary care essentials: urology,* Maldern, Mass, 2001, Blackwell Science, Inc, p 134.

MANAGEMENT

Treatment options for ED are dependent on the etiology and patient/partner preference. The range of options includes psychotherapy, medication, sexual counseling, and surgery. Patients usually choose the least invasive treatment at first and progress to more invasive treatments until an acceptable method is found.[3]

Psychotherapy is the preferred treatment for psychogenic ED. Sexual counseling can enhance communication, ease some of the stress associated with ED, and dispel myths. In mixed psychogenic and organic ED, psychotherapy may relieve anxieties and increase the success of medical or surgical intervention.

For men whose only difficulty is maintaining an erection, a constriction band (e.g., ACTIS venous flow controller; Vivus Pharmaceuticals, Mountainview, Calif.), applied at the base of the penis after erection, may be all that is needed.[10]

Vacuum devices are associated with an 80% to 90% success rate and are among the least invasive and least expensive of the current treatment options. They produce an erection by creating a vacuum around the penis that triggers passive blood flow into the corpora cavernosa. Erection is then maintained by a constriction band applied at the base of the penis.

Sildenafil (Viagra) is an oral medication that facilitates erection by enhancing the effects of nitric oxide and blocking the degradation of cGMP. Sildenafil must be taken 30 minutes to 1 hour before sexual activity and must be combined with stimulation to be successful. Evidence has shown sildenafil to be effective in a wide range of patients with ED.[11] It is not the preferred option for men with neurogenic ED and is absolutely contraindicated in patients who are taking nitrates.

Alprostadil (prostaglandin E_1) is indicated for the treatment of ED related to vasculogenic, neurogenic, psychogenic, or mixed etiologies. Alprostadil is available as a urethral suppository (MUSE) or as a solution for intracavernosal injection (Caverject/Edex).[10] The dose is highly individualized and requires the patient to have a test dose in the clinical setting. For this reason, patients wishing to pursue this option are usually referred to a urologist.

Only 5% to 10% of ED is caused by hormone imbalance, such as low levels of testosterone or high levels of prolactin.[10] Testosterone replacement therapy is available by injection or transdermal patch with the goal to keep the serum testosterone level with normal limits.

Surgical management includes vascular surgery or implantation of a penile prosthesis. The goal of vascular surgery is to increase arterial inflow to the corpora cavernosa and to increase venous outflow resistance. Candidates are selected only after careful vascular examination, measurement of intracavernous pressures, and observation of the patient's response to certain pharmacologic agents. Younger men with discrete lesions, usually sustained from pelvic or perineal trauma, seem to be the best candidates for vascular surgery.

Penile prostheses may be malleable, mechanical, or inflatable devices and provide girth and rigidity; they do not provide increased length. The decision to proceed with implant therapy often comes after treatment with the less invasive options has failed. Complications of penile implants are infection, erosion, and component failure. Because of improvements in design and more durable materials, the complication rated has significantly decreased over the past few years and patient/partner satisfaction has been shown to be 80% to 90%.[10]

Current research may lead to the development of new oral agents for ED and offer insight into combination therapy that may lead to successful therapy when single-agent treatment has failed.

COMPLICATIONS

Unfulfilled or even destroyed relationships, lack of self-esteem, and depression are common complications of ED. Unsatisfactory results or treatment failure are ongoing concerns.

INDICATIONS FOR REFERRAL/HOSPITALIZATION

For medical and surgical management, the patient with ED is referred to a urologist with a subspecialty in sexual dysfunction. Patients with hormonal abnormalities should be referred to an endocrinologist or urologist. Referral for sexual counseling or psychotherapy should be considered when appropriate.

PATIENT AND FAMILY EDUCATION

Patient education is key to the success of treatment for ED. The primary care provider must take the necessary time to counsel patients regarding the available options appropriate to their individual needs. It is important to remember that ED is a couple's problem and to include the partner whenever possible. The patient and partner should have realistic expectations of treatment and understand their role in its success.

Whether the patient is using a vacuum device, taking an oral medication, urethral suppository, or penile injection therapy, it is important that they are instructed in its use. If the patient has elected injection therapy, it is essential that the patient and partner feel comfortable with the injection process and are able to demonstrate accurate administration. Instructions should be provided in writing along with telephone numbers to call should they have further questions or problems. Follow-up is important to determine if further intervention is needed.

REFERENCES

1. Mulhall JP, Goldstein I: Epidemiology of erectile dysfunction. In Mulcahy JJ, editor: *Diagnosis and management of male sexual dysfunction*, New York, 1997, Igaku-Shoin.
2. NIH Consensus Conference: Impotence, NIH Consensus Development Panel on Impotence, *JAMA* 270(1):83-90, 1993.
3. Lue TF: Physiology of penile erection and pathophysiology of erectile dysfunction and priapism. In Walsh PC and others, editors: *Campbell's urology*, ed 7, vol 2, Philadelphia, 1998, WB Saunders.
4. Albaugh J, Lewis J: Insights into the management of erectile dysfunction: part I, *Urol Nurs* 19(4):241-245, 1999.
5. Maurice WL: *Sexual medicine in primary care*, St Louis, 1999, Mosby.
6. Lue TF: Male sexual dysfunction. In Tanagho EA, McAnin JW, editors: *Smith's general urology*, ed 14, Norwalk, Conn, 1995, Appleton & Lange.
7. Carson CC: Peyronie's disease: etiology, diagnosis, and treatment. In Mulcahy JJ, editor: *Diagnosis and management of male sexual dysfunction*, New York, 1997, Igaku-Shoin.
8. Daitch JA, Lakin MM, Montague DK: Nocturnal penile tumescence monitoring. In Mulcahy JJ, editor: *Diagnosis and management of male sexual dysfunction*, New York, 1997, Igaku-Shoin.
9. Brodereick GA: Noninvasive arterial evaluation of the patient complaining of erectile dysfunction with color duplex Doppler ultrasound. In Mulcahy JJ, editor: *Diagnosis and management of male sexual dysfunction*. New York, 1997, Igaku-Shoin.
10. Albaugh J, Lewis J: Insights into the management of erectile dysfunction: part II, *Urol Nurs* 20(1), 2000.
11. Padma-Nathan H, Steers WD, Wicker PA: Efficacy and safety of oral sildenafil in the treatment of erectile dysfunction: a double-blind, placebo-controlled study of 329 patients, *Int J Clin Pract* 52(6):375-380, 1998.

CHAPTER 158

Hypokalemia and Hyperkalemia

Carol A. Whelan

DEFINITION/EPIDEMIOLOGY

The amount of potassium present in the average human body is approximately 50 mEq/kg. Of this, 90% is found in intracellular fluid, 8% in skin and bones, and 2% in extracellular fluid.[1-5] The maintenance of this relatively small amount of extracellular potassium is critical; small changes can cause serious clinical consequences.

The definitions of *hypokalemia* and *hyperkalemia* are stated in terms of extracellular (or serum) potassium. Normal values for serum potassium are dependent on individual laboratories, but the usual range for normal values is approximately 3.5 to 5 mEq/L. Potassium imbalances can be defined as acute or chronic and can be further defined by the degree of severity.

Chronic hypokalemia and hyperkalemia develop in a minimum of weeks to months, and acute hypokalemia and hyperkalemia occur over hours to days. Mild hypokalemia occurs at serum levels of 3.5 to 4 mEq/L; moderate hypokalemia, 3 to 3.5 mEq/L; and severe hypokalemia, below 3 mEq/L. *Mild to moderate hyperkalemia* is defined as a serum level of 5.5 to 6.9 mEq/L, and *severe hyperkalemia* is defined as a serum level of 7 mEq/L or greater.

Levels of potassium in the intracellular and extracellular fluids do not always correlate, as seen in diabetic ketoacidosis. Severe depletion of intracellular potassium (termed *potassium deficiency*) as a result of osmotic diuresis (which leads to increased renal loss of potassium), despite normal or even elevated extracellular (serum) levels of potassium, is caused by insulin deficiency.[6] Once exogenous insulin is administered, clinical hypokalemia may develop rapidly.[6]

In the vast majority of cases, hypokalemia is drug induced; approximately 30% of all patients who are treated with non–potassium-sparing diuretics develop low serum potassium levels.[5] Most cases of chronic hyperkalemia are caused by renal failure.

Physician consultation is indicated for serum potassium levels lower than 3 mEq/L or higher than 6 mEq/L.

PATHOPHYSIOLOGY

Potassium balance is affected by intake, excretion, and internal potassium regulation.[1-3] The minimum daily requirement for potassium intake in the normal adult is approximately 40 to 50 mEq.[1-3] Excretion occurs primarily in the kidneys and gastrointestinal tract, with a small amount excreted in perspiration. Internal potassium regulation is dependent on acid-base balance, plasma insulin levels, plasma catecholamine levels, and aldosterone activity.[3]

Because the kidneys are normally able to conserve potassium quite efficiently, hypokalemia is rarely due to inadequate intake. The main causes of hypokalemia are increased renal loss from exogenous drug administration, primary or secondary hyperaldosteronism, and internal shifting of potassium from the extracellular to the intracellular space, which can occur with insulin administration or catecholamine excess (Box 158-1). Although vomiting may cause hypokalemia, it is not because of a loss of potassium from the gastrointestinal tract but rather because of secondary hyperaldosteronism related to volume depletion[7] or, more rarely, metabolic alkalosis from loss of gastric secretions.[5]

The ability of the kidneys to maintain potassium homeostasis is preserved until the glomerular filtration rate (GFR) falls below 10 ml/min.[7] Therefore chronic hyperkalemia in patients with GFRs exceeding 20 ml/min is most likely caused by either a defect in mineralocorticoid activity or a lesion within the cortical collecting system.[2] Causes of hyperkalemia are listed in Box 158-2.

CLINICAL PRESENTATION

The prevention of clinically significant hypokalemia and hyperkalemia is essential. In the absence of early detection and treatment, hypokalemia can cause serious complications and even death. The major symptoms are associated with skeletal muscle.[2,4] Hypokalemia causes hyperpolarization, which decreases impulse conduction and muscular contraction.[2] Flaccid

BOX 158-1

CAUSES OF HYPOKALEMIA

Non–potassium-sparing diuretics
Antibiotics
Alcoholism
Osmotic diuresis
Primary hyperaldosteronism
Secondary hyperaldosteronism
Glucocorticoid-induced hypertension
Malignant hypertension
Renovascular hypertension
Renin-secreting tumor
Liddle's syndrome
11-Beta-hydroxysteroid dehydrogenase deficiency
Excess licorice ingestion
Congenital adrenal hyperplasia
Type I RTA
Type II RTA
Bartter's syndrome
Gitelmans' syndrome
Hypomagnesemia
Exogenous insulin administration
Catecholamine excess
Familial periodic hypokalemic paralysis
Thyrotoxic hypokalemic paralysis
Leukemia
Beta-adrenergic agonists
Trauma

paralysis, beginning in the extremities and moving centrally, can eventually lead to respiratory paralysis. Possible cardiac complications include ventricular arrhythmias. Typical ECG findings include ST-segment depression, flattening and inversion of the T wave, and the appearance of a prominent U wave.[2,4] The appearance and severity of these ECG abnormalities do not correspond to the degree of hypokalemia and should not be used as a substitute for monitoring of serum levels.[4]

Clinical manifestations of hyperkalemia are chiefly cardiac, although neuromuscular complications can also occur.[2] ECG changes associated with hyperkalemia include peaked T waves (often the first ECG finding), ST-segment depression, widening of the QRS and PR intervals, and loss of the P wave.[2] A late ECG sign is the appearance of a sine-wave pattern,[2,4] which is usually indicative of impending ventricular fibrillation and asystole.[2]

Although cardiac manifestations are obviously the most dangerous sequelae of hyperkalemia, neuromuscular complications, including paresthesias and fasciculations in the extremities, may be seen. Peripheral paralysis can occur, but paralysis of the respiratory muscles is rare.[2]

PHYSICAL EXAMINATION

A thorough history is the most important part of the physical examination. Any history of diuretic use, laxative use, vomiting, diarrhea, abnormal urine output, diabetes mellitus, or hypertension, as well as a thorough diet and medication history, should be elicited. The physical examination should include a full assessment of vital signs (including orthostatic blood pressures), assessment of volume status,[5] and examination of the neuromuscular system, including assessment of muscular strength and reflexes.

BOX 158-2

CAUSES OF HYPERKALEMIA

- Pseudohyperkalemia
  - Traumatic venipuncture
  - Severe leukocytosis
- True hyperkalemia
  - Renal failure
  - Angiotensin-converting enzyme inhibitors
  - Potassium-sparing diuretics
  - NSAIDs
  - Bactrim
  - Heparin
  - Beta blockers
  - Hypoaldosteronism
  - Type IV RTA
  - Adrenal insufficiency (Addison's disease)
  - Sickle cell anemia
  - Systemic lupus erythematosus
  - Insulin deficiency
  - Acidosis
  - Familial hyperkalemic periodic paralysis
  - Rhabdomyolysis
  - Tumor lysis syndrome

DIAGNOSTICS

Diagnostics should assess the degree of the potassium imbalance, as well as the cause. Serum electrolytes, BUN, serum creatinine, and serum glucose, as well as a 12-lead ECG and urinary electrolytes, should be obtained.

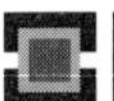

Diagnostics

Hypokalemia

Laboratory
Serum electrolytes
BUN
Creatinine
Serum glucose
Serum magnesium
Plasma osmolality*
Urinary potassium—random
24-hour urine collection for potassium*
Urine osmolity*
Early-morning urinary pH*
Plasma renin activity*
Plasma aldosteronism*

Other
ECG*
ABGs

*If indicated.

Hypokalemia

Patients whose hypokalemia is not iatrogenic (i.e., drug induced) or the result of vomiting, diarrhea, alcoholism, or excess licorice ingestion should be evaluated to determine the underlying cause of the hypokalemia. To effectively organize the diagnostic evaluation, hypokalemic patients may be subdivided into three groups: those with increased renal potassium excretion (>20 mEq/L) and hypertension, those with increased renal potassium excretion but without hypertension, and those with normal or decreased renal potassium excretion.

If the patient is hypertensive, plasma renin activity (PRA) and plasma aldosterone levels should be measured but only *after* the hypokalemia has been corrected. Primary hyperaldosteronism is suggested if the PRA is suppressed and the plasma aldosterone levels are elevated. Secondary hyperaldosteronism will result in both a high PRA and a high plasma aldosterone level. Liddle's syndrome will also cause hypokalemia and hypertension, but both PRA and plasma aldosterone levels will be suppressed.[3]

When patients with hypokalemia are normotensive, measurement of serum bicarbonate helps further define the differential diagnosis.[5] Low serum bicarbonate levels are consistent with diabetic ketoacidosis, metabolic acidosis, or renal tubular acidosis (RTA).[5] Hypokalemia associated with hyperchloremic metabolic acidosis is suggestive of type I RTA; a morning urinary pH should be checked. Levels higher than 6 are consistent with type I RTA.[3]

High serum bicarbonate levels in normotensive patients are consistent with Bartter's syndrome.[5] Bartter's syndrome will also result in high PRA and plasma aldosterone levels, but this is quite rare and is usually seen only in children or young adults. In addition to the abnormal laboratory findings, patients with Bartter's syndrome typically are of short stature, have muscle weakness, and are normotensive.[3]

Hypokalemia and normal serum bicarbonate levels in normotensive patients may also be caused by magnesium deficiency.[3] Alcoholic patients, chemotherapy patients, and patients with malabsorption syndrome are at risk for developing magnesium deficiency.[3]

Occasionally hypokalemia is not due to increased renal loss; these patients will have low urinary potassium (<20 mEq/L).[5]

The differential diagnosis is fairly limited and generally involves some sort of gastrointestinal loss, through laxative abuse, villous adenoma, or severe diarrhea.[5] Patients previously treated with non–potassium-sparing diuretics who are potassium depleted will also have low urinary potassium.[5] Catecholamine excess, whether endogenous (as seen in acute myocardial infarction) or exogenous (as in beta-adrenergic agonist administration), may also cause transient hypokalemia because of an increased cellular uptake of potassium.[5]

If after thorough investigation of the patient's history and medication profile, in addition to completion of the appropriate evaluation, the etiology of the hypokalemia is still unknown, referral to an endocrinologist is appropriate.

Hyperkalemia

In cases of hyperkalemia, renal status should be determined. Individuals with chronic renal failure (CRF) who previously had normal potassium levels should have a 24-hour urine collection to assess for creatinine clearance and be questioned thoroughly regarding any diet changes, infection, trauma, or the use of nonsteroidal antiinflammatory drugs (NSAIDs) and other medications. Numerous cases of trimethoprim-sulfamethoxazole–induced hyperkalemia have been reported. Patients with preexisting renal impairment or disturbances in potassium excretion or with human immunodeficiency virus (HIV) infection and those treated with angiotensin-converting enzyme (ACE) inhibitors appear to be most at risk.[8]

Persons without renal failure and hyperkalemia should be assessed for adrenocortical insufficiency (Addison's disease), which almost always results in hyponatremia, hypertension, hypovolemia, and renal insufficiency.[3] A cosyntropin stimulation test should be performed if Addison's disease is suspected.

Hyperkalemia may also result from hypoaldosteronism and is twice as common in patients with diabetes mellitus.[3] PRA and plasma aldosterone levels are diagnostic. Secondary hypoaldosteronism can result from the prolonged use of heparin, but in general the hyperkalemia is mild.[3] ACE inhibitors also decrease aldosterone levels and can cause hyperkalemia. Tubular unresponsiveness to aldosterone may also cause hyperkalemia and may be seen in sickle cell disease, systemic lupus erythematosus, and amyloidosis.[3]

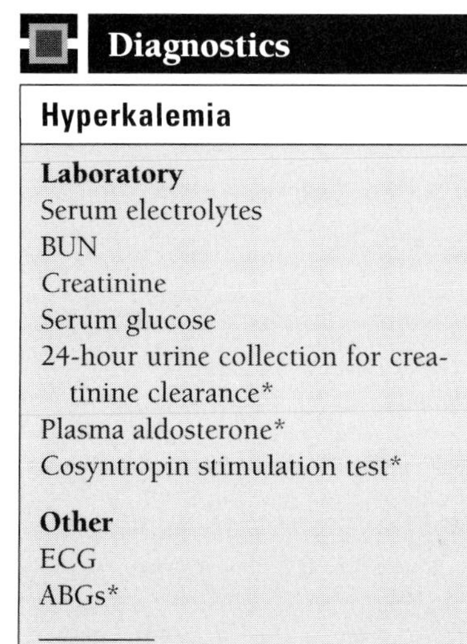
Diagnostics

Hyperkalemia

Laboratory
Serum electrolytes
BUN
Creatinine
Serum glucose
24-hour urine collection for creatinine clearance*
Plasma aldosterone*
Cosyntropin stimulation test*

Other
ECG
ABGs*

*If indicated.

DIFFERENTIAL DIAGNOSIS

Hypokalemia and hyperkalemia are caused by a variety of disorders. Hypokalemia is usually related to one or more of the following: inadequate potassium intake (rare), extracellular-to-intracellular potassium shift, or renal and extrarenal potassium losses. Hyperkalemia is related to inadequate potassium excretion, excessive potassium intake, or an intracellular shift of potassium from tissue to serum.

Differential Diagnosis

Hypokalemia and Hyperkalemia

Hypokalemia
Inadequate dietary intake
Extracellular-to-intracellular potassium shift
Renal and extrarenal potassium loss

Hyperkalemia
Inadequate potassium excretion
Excessive potassium intake
Intracellular shift of potassium to serum

MANAGEMENT

The management of hypokalemia and hyperkalemia should begin with identification of the underlying cause, and except for patients who are surreptitiously inducing vomiting or using large amounts of diuretics or laxatives, the cause of the potassium imbalance is usually readily apparent.[3] Most cases are a result of either diuretic use or renal failure. Hyperkalemia can also be a pseudohyperkalemia, which may be caused by traumatic venipuncture or, rarely, leukocytosis in the setting of leukemia.[3]

All at-risk patients should be frequently screened using laboratory analysis. When diuretics are being prescribed, the patient's serum potassium concentration should be checked before initiation of treatment and then 1 and 4 weeks after the initiation of therapy.[5]

In persons with chronic hyperkalemia, any use of ACE inhibitors, NSAIDs, potassium-sparing diuretics, or salt substitutes (those containing potassium chloride) should be reassessed and most likely discontinued.[3]

Acute Hypokalemia

The treatment of acute hypokalemia involves the administration of oral or IV potassium supplements. If life-threatening arrhythmias or neuromuscular symptoms are present, IV potassium supplementation should be initiated.[3] IV potassium concentration should not exceed 40 mEq/L. IV potassium is usually infused at a rate of less than 10 mEq/hr.[9] Cardiac monitoring and frequent serum potassium assessment (every 3 to 6 hours) are essential. Once all cardiac arrhythmias and neuromuscular symptoms are absent, the patient may be switched to oral replacement. The normal dosage for oral potassium is 20 to 40 mEq b.i.d. to q.i.d.[3]

Chronic Hypokalemia

The primary goal of treatment of chronic hypokalemia is identification of the underlying cause. In cases of drug-induced hypokalemia, the medication should be changed, if possible. If the clinical status prohibits this, then treatment is dependent on the degree of hypokalemia. Some controversy exists as to whether patients with mild hypokalemia (3.5 to 4 mEq/L) should be aggressively treated[3,5]; however, these patients can certainly benefit from dietary teaching. In patients with potassium levels lower than 3.5 mEq/L, oral supplementation should be given, with normal dosages ranging between 20 and

80 mEq/day. Patients with hyperaldosteronism should be referred to an endocrinologist and may be successfully managed with spironolactone; however, if an aldosterone-secreting tumor is identified, surgical removal may be preferred.

Acute Hyperkalemia

Treatment of acute hyperkalemia with life-threatening symptoms (generally seen at potassium levels of ≥7 mEq/L) is accomplished by the administration of IV calcium.[2-4] The usual recommended dose is 10 ml of a 10% calcium solution such as calcium chloride. The ECG should be monitored while the calcium is administered. Calcium should be administered only when ECG changes such as a widening QRS have occurred.[3,4] Calcium does not correct the underlying hyperkalemia; it only counters the adverse neuromuscular effects of hyperkalemia.[4] Calcium infusion should always be followed with specific therapy aimed at lowering the plasma potassium level (i.e., insulin and glucose infusion).

The treatment of acute hyperkalemia that has not yet resulted in life-threatening sequelae is most quickly accomplished by the administration of IV glucose and insulin.[3,4] This results in a shift of extracellular potassium into the cell.[4] Care should be taken in diabetic patients with hyperkalemia, because glucose infusion that is not accompanied by a matching infusion of insulin can actually result in increased hyperkalemia because of extracellular hyperosmolarity.[2]

When the patient is able to safely take medication orally and life-threatening sequelae have not developed, treatment with Kayexalate in sorbitol solution may be used. This may be the treatment of choice in outpatients who are stable but have potassium levels in the 5.5 to 6.9 mEq/L range. In patients unable to tolerate oral administration, Kayexalate may be given rectally.[3]

Sodium bicarbonate is occasionally used in the treatment of hyperkalemia, both to treat the acidosis that may accompany hyperkalemia and to correct the hyperkalemia itself by causing a pH-dependent shift of potassium from the extracellular to the intracellular space.[4] Sodium bicarbonate should be used with caution, and care should be taken not to cause sodium overload or metabolic alkalosis.[3]

Chronic Hyperkalemia

The most common cause of chronic hyperkalemia is renal failure; therefore the most common management of chronic hyperkalemia is dialysis. It is quite rare for intake alone to account for hyperkalemia because renal excretion increases with increased intake in patients with normal renal function. Diet modification is essential, however, in patients with renal failure and chronic hyperkalemia. Referral to a dietitian can be quite helpful.

The treatment of chronic hyperkalemia caused by hypoaldosteronism may be accomplished with oral Kayexalate or furosemide, but the preferred treatment is the administration of fludrocortisone acetate (Florinef).[3] If Addison's disease is diagnosed, treatment with replacement hydrocortisone should correct the hyperkalemia.

COMPLICATIONS

Potassium abnormalities are potentially life threatening. Cardiac conduction defects, arrhythmias, ileus, paralysis, muscle weakness, increased blood pressure, and renal injury are consequences of hypokalemia. Hyperkalemia also causes cardiac arrhythmias, as well as heart block, ventricular fibrillation, muscle weakness, and paralysis.

INDICATIONS FOR REFERRAL/HOSPITALIZATION

Any patient found to have an underlying metabolic disorder as a cause of hypokalemia or hyperkalemia and patients in whom the etiology of the hypokalemia or hyperkalemia is unknown should be referred to an endocrinologist. Patients with hyperkalemia and renal disease should always be referred to a renal specialist. All patients with life-threatening symptoms of hypokalemia or hyperkalemia should be evaluated for possible hospitalization. Also, patients with hyperkalemia and acute renal failure should be urgently hospitalized.

PATIENT AND FAMILY EDUCATION

Patient education for hypokalemia or hyperkalemia should center on diet education and awareness of the importance of continued chronic supplementation therapy and laboratory monitoring. Education regarding potential drug effects on hypokalemia or hyperkalemia is also important. Chronic laxative use should be avoided because this has been associated with potassium loss. Patients with chronic hypokalemia should avoid large amounts of licorice because licorice has also been associated with hypokalemia. Patients taking potassium supplements should be advised not to crush the potassium tablets and to swallow the tablet with a large glass of fluid. If untoward effects of potassium occur, the patient should be advised to call or see a primary care provider.

HEALTH PROMOTION

Because hyperkalemia is usually secondary to renal failure and hypokalemia is usually the result of diuretic use, health promotion should focus on the prevention of renal failure and hypertension. When prevention is no longer possible, patient education regarding the need for monitoring and prevention of complications is paramount.

REFERENCES

1. Brenner BM: *The kidney,* ed 5, Philadelphia, 1996, WB Saunders.
2. Levine DZ: *Caring for the renal patient,* ed 3, Philadelphia, 1997, WB Saunders.
3. Mandal AK: Hematuria and hypokalemia, *Med Clin North Am* 81(3):641-652, 1997.
4. Braunwauld E and others: *Harrison's principles of internal medicine,* ed 15, New York, 2001, McGraw-Hill.
5. Barker RL, Burton JR, Zieve PD: *Principles of ambulatory medicine,* ed 4, Baltimore, 1995, Williams & Wilkins.
6. Whelan CA: Chronic renal failure: nondialysis care, *Am J Nurse Pract* 2(7):21-31, 1998.
7. Greenberg A: *Primer on kidney diseases,* ed 2, New York, 1994, Academic Press.
8. Perazella MA: Trimethoprim-induced hyperkalaemia: clinical data, mechanism, prevention and management, *Drug Safety* 22(3):227-236, 2000.
9. Kruse JA, Carlson RW: Rapid correction of hypokalemia using concentrated intravenous potassium chloride infusion, *Arch Intern Med* 150(3):613-617, 1990.

CHAPTER 159

Incontinence

Updated by Joanne Sandberg-Cook

DEFINITION/EPIDEMIOLOGY

Urinary incontinence is the transient or persistent loss of urine; it affects approximately 17 million Americans.[1] There are four main types of persistent incontinence: urge incontinence, overflow incontinence, mixed incontinence, and functional incontinence. Transient incontinence, which is usually abrupt in onset and is often reversible, has many causes (Boxes 159-1 and 159-2).

Incontinence is experienced by 15% to 35% of noninstitutionalized adults older than 60 years.[1] The incidence of this disorder ranges from 4% in young community dwellers to 50% in older nursing home residents.[2] Urinary incontinence is considered to be one of the major causes of institutionalization of older adults. The annual cost of managing this disorder is more than $10 billion.[3]

BOX 159-1

PERSISTENT INCONTINENCE

Stress incontinence A loss of urine with activities that result in increased intraabdominal pressure.

Urge incontinence An involuntary loss of urine preceded by a strong, unexpected urge to void.

Overflow incontinence An involuntary loss of urine associated with a distended bladder.

Mixed incontinence A combination of urge and stress incontinence that is more common in older women.[1]

BOX 159-2

CAUSES OF TRANSIENT INCONTINENCE

FUNCTIONAL INCONTINENCE
- Chronic illness
- Confusion
- Psychologic disorder
- Restricted mobility

INCREASED URINARY PRODUCTION
- Congestive heart failure
- Excessive fluid intake
- Hypercalcemia
- Hyperglycemia
- Venous insufficiency with edema

LOWER URINARY TRACT CONDITIONS
- Atrophic vaginitis
- Pregnancy
- Prostatectomy
- Stool impaction
- Urethritis
- Urinary tract infection

MEDICATIONS
- Alpha-adrenergic blockers
- Anticholinergics
- Caffeine
- Calcium channel blockers
- Diuretics
- Psychotropics

Adult urinary incontinence should not be considered normal at any age and is not an expected outcome of aging. However, impaired mobility, weakened pelvic floor muscles, benign prostatic hypertrophy, increased incidence of urinary tract infections, and conditions related to aging may increase the incidence of incontinence.[4]

PATHOPHYSIOLOGY

Urinary incontinence is usually the symptom of an underlying bladder or sphincter problem that can be treated. There are several major causes of dysfunction.

Overactive Bladder

Overactive bladder (OAB) is the most common cause of incontinence in older adults.[5] It results in involuntary bladder contraction, which leads to *urge incontinence*. It is associated with increased spontaneous activity of the detrusor smooth muscle and specific cellular changes.[3]

Urethral Obstruction

Urethral obstruction results in overflow incontinence and occurs when the bladder is unable to empty normally despite normal filling. In men, it is often the result of outflow obstruction caused by benign prostatic hyperplasia. The bladder becomes overdistended, resulting in increased intravesicular pressure that leads to *overflow incontinence* (see Chapter 161).

Stress Incontinence

Stress incontinence is more common in women than in men. In women stress incontinence results from the loss of muscle tone and the descent of the bladder after childbirth. In men it may be the result of rapid weight gain or a radical prostatectomy.

Functional Incontinence

Functional incontinence is related to factors other than pathology of the urinary tract. This can include impaired mobility, confusion, fecal impaction, chronic illness and weakness, and psychologic disorders.

CLINICAL PRESENTATION

The presentation of incontinence can differ and is somewhat dependent on etiology. A careful history and physical examination should exclude the causes of transient incontinence that can be easily treated. Each type of persistent incontinence may have a different presentation; a careful history indicates the type of incontinence being experienced.

The patient history should include a review of medications; a focused medical, neurologic, and genitourinary history; and a detailed review of the symptoms related to urinary incontinence.[1] The frequency, timing, amount, duration, characteristics, and precipitants of the incontinence should be recorded in a voiding diary for several days. Alterations in bowel and bladder habits, the number of pads or briefs used, and the response to previous treatments should be noted.

PHYSICAL EXAMINATION

The examination should include an evaluation for the presence of edema, neurologic conditions, and assessment of functional ability. Abdominal, pelvic, rectal, and genital examinations are also important. A mental status evaluation and an assessment of mobility and social factors should be performed in older adults.

The environmental, physical, and mental assessments may indicate functional incontinence. However, other types of incontinence must be considered before making a diagnosis of functional incontinence.

Stress incontinence is characterized by the loss of small amounts of urine during coughing, lifting, or any activity that increases intraabdominal pressure. Observing for urine loss when the patient has a full bladder and is asked to cough may help to establish this diagnosis. The medical history may be significant for previous bladder or vaginal surgery; in men a history of radical prostatectomy may be reported. Weakened pelvic floor musculature may be evident on physical examination.

Urge incontinence is characterized by the loss of urine after a sense of urgency to void and the inability to hold urine long enough to reach to the bathroom. Neurologic problems such as a cerebrovascular accident, Parkinson's disease, multiple sclerosis, spinal cord lesions, upper motor neuron lesions, and urinary tract infections must be excluded.

Urinary frequency and a sensation of incomplete emptying characterize overflow incontinence. There is a loss of urine when the bladder is overdistended. The distended bladder may be palpable on physical examination. The medical history may include peripheral neuropathy from diabetes, pelvic surgery, or disk compression.

Mixed incontinence should be considered in the presence of symptoms related to urine storage and bladder emptying. Mixed incontinence can be difficult to diagnose and treat.

DIAGNOSTICS

Urinalysis and urine cultures are important to exclude a urinary tract infection when incontinence is present. Urine cultures may be reserved for patients with symptoms (fever, urgency, frequency, or dysuria) or a positive urinalysis or urine dipstick result. A BUN and creatinine level should be obtained if compromised renal function is suspected, especially with overflow incontinence. If polyuria is suspected, serum glucose and calcium tests are recommended.

Postvoid residual (PVR) urine is helpful to exclude difficulty in bladder emptying—a condition that is noted in overflow incontinence. Pelvic ultrasound or catheterization can evaluate a PVR. Generally, a PVR of less than 50 to 100 ml is considered normal; residuals greater than 100 ml suggest inadequate emptying.[1]

Further testing is usually not necessary for the basic evaluation of urinary incontinence unless the onset is sudden, associated with severe symptoms, or accompanied by suprapubic pain or unless there are risk factors for bladder cancer (e.g., smoking). A urine cytologic test should be considered in patients with risk factors or symptoms that suggest bladder cancer.[6]

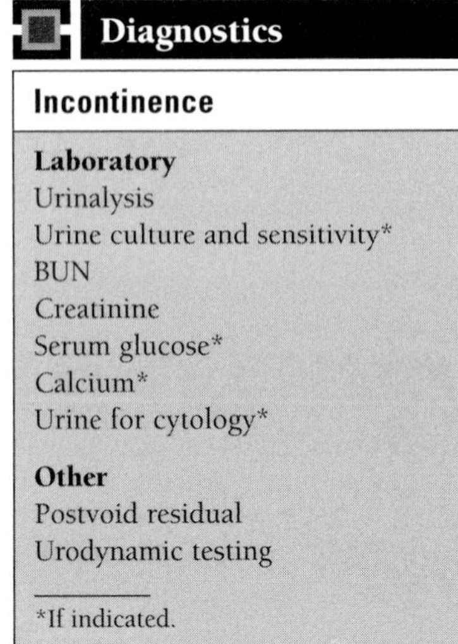
Diagnostics

Incontinence

Laboratory
Urinalysis
Urine culture and sensitivity*
BUN
Creatinine
Serum glucose*
Calcium*
Urine for cytology*

Other
Postvoid residual
Urodynamic testing

*If indicated.

In older adults it is important to consider causes outside the urinary tract. In the younger population, incontinence is usually associated with deficits in the urinary tract. The patient should be referred to a urologist if further diagnostic testing (e.g., simple cystometry and urodynamics, including complex cystometry and uroflowmetry) is necessary.[6] Further testing is warranted when the diagnosis is uncertain and the primary care provider is unable to develop an effective management plan based on the available data, when hematuria without infection is present, when a surgical intervention is being considered, or when therapy has failed.

DIFFERENTIAL DIAGNOSIS

The type of incontinence, either transient or persistent, is based on the history, physical, and diagnostic data. Once the cause of the incontinence has been identified, a management plan can be initiated.

MANAGEMENT

The treatment of incontinence varies according to the cause. Medical conditions that may be exacerbating the incontinence should be treated, and medications that contribute to the incontinence should be decreased or discontinued if possible. Behavioral and pharmacologic therapies are the main treatments of urinary incontinence. Surgery is indicated in some individuals.

Stress Incontinence

Pelvic muscle exercises (PMEs), or Kegel's exercises, are effective in strengthening the voluntary periurethral and perivaginal muscles. PMEs are performed by tightening the perivaginal muscles and anal sphincter as if controlling defecation and urination. Tightening of the abdominal or thigh muscles should be avoided. Contractions should be held for 10 seconds followed by a period of relaxation. It is recommended that the exercises be performed 30 to 80 times daily for at least 8 weeks. Patients should be advised to begin the exercises gradually. They may need support from their primary care provider to maintain the motivation to continue these exercises, which may need to be continued indefinitely.

In premenopausal patients with stress incontinence, PMEs may be augmented with vaginal weights for the purpose of strengthening the pelvic muscles.[1] Vaginal weights range from 20 to 100 g. Patients are instructed to insert a weight intravaginally, which should then be retained during ambulation by contracting the pelvic muscles. This exercise should be performed

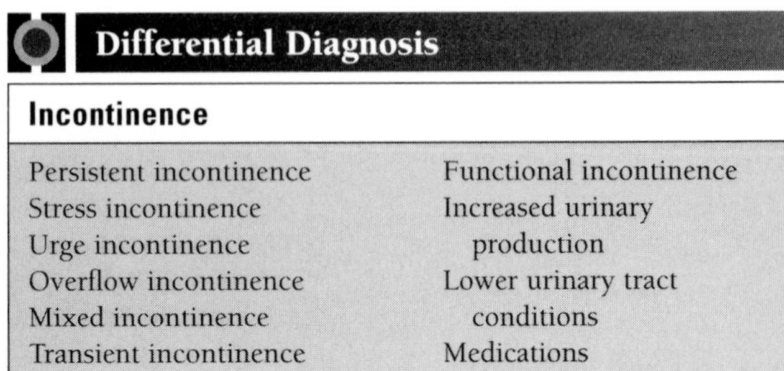
Differential Diagnosis

Incontinence

Persistent incontinence	Functional incontinence
Stress incontinence	Increased urinary production
Urge incontinence	Lower urinary tract conditions
Overflow incontinence	Medications
Mixed incontinence	
Transient incontinence	

for 15 minutes twice daily. The weights are increased gradually to strengthen the pelvic muscles. Pessary placement may be helpful.

Alpha-adrenergic agonists such as pseudoephedrine (Sudafed), which increase the pressure exerted by the muscles of the bladder neck, can be tried for stress incontinence. Although not curative, these drugs may provide some improvement in symptoms.[1] Oral or vaginal estrogen can be used in women with postmenopausal stress incontinence. Conjugated estrogens may be administered orally (0.3 to 1.25 mg/day), or estrogen cream may be administered vaginally (2 g/day; one applicator daily for 2 weeks and then twice weekly). Progesterone 2.5 to 10 mg/day PO continuously or intermittently should be administered to women with an intact uterus to prevent endometrial hyperplasia.[1]

Imipramine 10 to 50 mg q.d. or other tricyclic antidepressants may also be recommended, especially in younger patients, if other therapies are ineffective.

Surgery should be considered if treatment regimens are ineffective or if patients are not able to adhere to other treatment plans. Stress incontinence is the most common type of incontinence treated with surgery. Surgery is performed to lift and support the connection between the bladder and the urethra. Choices include retropubic suspension, needle endoscopic suspension, urethral, sling, urethral bulking, and an artificial sphincter. Injections of collagen into the bladder neck may also be helpful. Referral to an urologist is recommended if surgery is being considered.

Urge Incontinence

Behavioral methods of treating urge incontinence include bladder training and timed voiding. These techniques have been shown to improve the condition. Bladder training requires the patient to postpone voiding, resist the sense of urgency, and void on a predetermined schedule. Intervals of 2 to 3 hours are the initial goal set for voiding. Gradually the interval is increased as tolerated. The bladder should be emptied at the scheduled intervals, and voiding should be delayed if the urge occurs between the scheduled times. Training should continue for several months. During this time patients benefit from the support and encouragement of their primary care provider.

Scheduled voiding by the caregiver may be effective when a patient cannot use the toilet independently. Assistance with toileting should be provided every 2 to 4 hours during the day and night to minimize incontinence. Habit training is another method by which to decrease incontinence in dependent patients. In this strategy a toileting schedule is developed according to the patient's past voiding habits. Based on a record of incontinence, a schedule can be developed to decrease episodes of incontinence. PMEs, biofeedback, and pelvic muscle stimulation may also be effective in improving the symptoms of urge incontinence.

Medications may be helpful in the treatment of urge incontinence.[5] Antimuscarinic agents decrease involuntary bladder contraction. Newer drugs include tolterodine tartrate (Detrol; 1 to 2 mg b.i.d. and Detrol LA 4 mg q.d.) and oxybutynin chloride (Ditropan XL) 5 mg q.d. These agents can be used safely for both younger and older patients with overactive bladder and urge incontinence.[7] However, oxybutynin has more anticholinergic side effects. Anticholinergics are often poorly tolerated in older adults because of side effects of confusion, constipation, dizziness, blurred vision, and tachycardia. Medication dosages in older adults should be started at a low dose and increased gradually.

Hyoscyamine sulfate (Levsin, Levbid) may be used as an alternative medication in the treatment of urge incontinence. Because there are limited studies related to its effectiveness, it is not recommended as a first-line agent.[1] It functions as both an anticholinergic and a smooth muscle relaxant. Anticholinergic side effects make this a poor choice for older patients.

Tricyclic agents may be helpful for certain patients with urge incontinence. In general, low doses of these drugs should be used in older adults because of the potential for adverse effects. Cardiac and anticholinergic side effects are common. Orthostatic hypotension with an increased risk of falls is common in older adults who take these medications.

Overflow Incontinence

With overflow incontinence, surgery is often indicated to relieve urethral obstruction due to either benign prostatic hypertrophy (BPH) or nonreducible prolapse. Occasionally a pessary is helpful for prolapses that may cause partial urethral obstruction. Both finasteride (Proscar; 5 mg q.d. and tamsulosin hydrochloride (Flomax; 0.4 to 0.8 mg q.d.) have been used with some success in the treatment of BPH. These drugs are contraindicated in women and should be avoided in the presence of known bladder outlet obstruction. Clean intermittent catheterization (CIC) is recommended for patients who have urethral obstruction and are not good surgical candidates.

Mixed Incontinence

After careful diagnostic evaluation that identifies the primary cause of the incontinence, mixed incontinence is treated using one or a combination of previously described methods of treatment.

Functional Incontinence

Functional incontinence can be resolved through treatment of the underlying cause and through the use of behavioral techniques.

LIFE SPAN CONSIDERATIONS

Incontinence can occur at any age but is more common in older adults. Changes in the urinary tract that occur with aging contribute to the development of incontinence. Bladder capacity, contractility, and the ability to postpone voiding are thought to decline with age. Prostate size increases, involuntary bladder contractions increase, and the PVR may increase to 50 to 100 ml.[3] These changes—as well as the increased presence of chronic health problems and the use of medications that may have an effect on the urinary tract—explain why incontinence is so common in the older population.

COMPLICATIONS

Incontinence can lead to skin breakdown, infections, and problems with self-esteem, anxiety, depression, and social isolation.[8] Patients who have overflow incontinence are at increased risk for developing renal problems because of urinary retention. There also is an increased incidence of institutionalization in older

adults who are incontinent. Patients often limit fluids in an effort to control symptoms, thereby putting themselves at risk for dehydration.

INDICATIONS FOR REFERRAL/HOSPITALIZATION

Consultation with a physician is important when there is difficulty in determining the type of incontinence, when mixed incontinence is suspected, and when traditional treatment regimens provide inadequate relief of symptoms.

An urology referral is indicated when the following conditions are present with incontinence: abnormal PVR, a prostate examination that suggests prostate cancer, a neurologic condition, symptomatic pelvic prolapse, recurrent symptomatic urinary tract infection, a history of radical pelvic or incontinence surgery, or persistent symptoms of difficult bladder emptying.[1] Further testing is warranted when the diagnosis is uncertain, when hematuria without infection is present, when surgical intervention is being considered, or when therapy has failed.

Incontinence that does not respond adequately to initial treatment may be managed more effectively in collaboration with a provider who specializes in the care of patients with incontinence. This can include continence nurses, physical and occupational therapists. Biofeedback is sometimes used to augment PMEs in patients with stress or urge incontinence. Biofeedback can be used to increase awareness of pelvic muscle function and to change responses in an attempt to improve urination. Stimulation of the pelvic floor muscles may also be effective in treating stress, urge, and mixed incontinence and must be performed by a professional skilled in the procedure.

PATIENT AND FAMILY EDUCATION

The effectiveness of behavioral strategies in the treatment of incontinence is dependent on the education of patients, families, and caregivers. Plans for behavioral interventions should be realistic and should meet the needs of the patient and caregivers. Follow-up visits for reinforcement, support, and opportunities for the modification of plans should be performed on a regular basis until the incontinence is controlled.

REFERENCES

1. Urinary Incontinence in Adults Guideline Panel, Urinary Incontinence in Adults: *Acute and chronic management: clinical practice guideline*, Washington, DC, March 1996, US Department of Health and Human Services, publication No. 96-0682.
2. Newman DK, Burns PA: Significance and impact of urinary incontinence, *Nurse Pract Forum* 5(3):130-133, 1994.
3. Resnick NM: Urinary incontinence, *Lancet* 346:255-260, 1995.
4. Brundage DJ, Linton AD: Age-related changes in the genitourinary system. In Matteson MA, McConnell ES, Linton AD, editors: *Gerontological nursing*, Philadelphia, 1997, WB Saunders.
5. Newman DK, Giovannini D: The overactive bladder: a nursing perspective, *Am J Nurs* 102(6):36-44, 2002.
6. Penn C and others: Assessment of urinary incontinence, *J Gerontol Nurs* 22(1):8-19, 1996.
7. Zinner NR, Mattiasson A, Stanton SL: Efficacy, safety, and tolerability of extended-release once daily tolterodine treatment for the overactive bladder in older vs younger patients, *J Am Geriatr Soc* 50(5):799-807, 2002.
8. Gallo ML, Fallon PJ, Staskin DR: Urinary incontinence: steps to evaluation, diagnosis, and treatment, *Nurse Pract* 22(2):21-44, 1997.

CHAPTER 160

Infectious Processes: Urinary Tract Infections and Sexually Transmitted Diseases

Marilyn Bleiler Green and Patricia Polgar Bailey

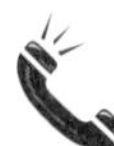

Physician consultation is recommended for newly diagnosed syphilis.
Physician/obstetric consultation is indicated for pregnant women with suspected pyelonephritis.

Urinary Tract Infections

DEFINITION/EPIDEMIOLOGY

Urinary tract infection (UTI) is a broad term used to describe bacterial infection or inflammation of the bladder (cystitis), urethra (urethritis), or renal pelvis/kidneys (pyelonephritis) and microbial colonization of the urine. All of these structures, as well as adjacent structures such as the epididymis and prostate, are at risk of acquiring infection from the common urinary stream. A lower UTI is an infection or inflammation of the bladder or urethra. Upper or ascending UTIs include infections of the ureters and kidneys. Simple or uncomplicated UTIs are infections experienced by women with no significant history of UTIs and characterized by recent onset of mild to moderate symptoms. All other UTIs are considered complicated or nonsimple. In addition, UTIs can be due to acute or chronic infections.

Infection of the urinary tract is a common problem, second in frequency only to respiratory infections. Direct medical costs associated with UTI are estimated at $1.6 billion annually in the United States and are responsible for over 8 million office visits yearly. Half of all women will be affected by a UTI at least once during their lifetime.[1]

UTIs are a particular problem in certain patient groups. Young sexually active women are disproportionately affected. The incidence of cystitis among premenopausal sexually active women is 0.5 to 0.7 infections per person-year (7 to 8 million cases yearly) and an estimated 40% of women will experience cystitis at some point in life. Of those about 20% will develop recurrent infections, mostly as a result of reinfection (rather than relapse). UTIs remain a significant problem in older women, both in terms of asymptomatic bacteriuria and symptomatic infections.[3,4] UTIs are unusual in men less than 50 years old with normal urologic structures. During the mid-1950s and 1960s, the incidence of UTIs increased, largely as a result of prostate hypertrophy and obstruction of the urinary tract. Additional common reasons for UTIs in men include instrumentation, anatomic and functional abnormalities, suppressed host defense mechanisms, and anal intercourse. After age 65 years, the incidence of UTIs in men begins to equal that in women because of benign prostatic hypertrophy.[4]

PATHOPHYSIOLOGY

Most UTIs in women are secondary to ascending infection from the periurethral or perianal area. Cystitis in women is more common than in men because of the proximity of the urethral opening and vagina to the perianal area. Bacteria reach the bladder through the urethra and may ascend to the kidneys through the ureters. Colonization of the vaginal introitus plays an important role in recurrent infections.

A relatively narrow spectrum of microorganisms causes the majority of UTIs; the most prominent pathogens include *Escherichia coli* (approximately 28% of cases), gram-negative organisms including *Klebsiella, Proteus, Enterobacter,* and *Serratia* spp. (approximately 40%) and gram-positive cocci such as *Enterococcus* and *Staphylococcus* spp. (approximately 20%). Approximately 95% of simple lower UTIs are caused by autoinoculation with Enterobacteriaceae from the bowel. *E. coli* is the causative bacterium in approximately 90% of cases of uncomplicated, acute cystitis (i.e., healthy females with anatomically normal urinary tract) and 30% of nosocomial infections in men and women. *Staphylococcus saprophyticus* is also common in young women in ambulatory settings and can account for as much as 10% of UTIs, especially during the summer months.[5]

Complicated UTIs may be due to a number of infectious agents other than *E. coli*. Common aerobes include *Klebsiella pneumoniae, Proteus mirabilis, Pseudomonas aeruginosa,* and *Enterococcus* species. *Enterococcus* organisms are particularly common in nosocomial UTIs of either sex.[5] Most UTIs in women are not due to complicating conditions or serious problems. Sexual intercourse and diaphragm use have been the two behaviors most consistently associated with UTIs in many studies, but not in all. In addition, in some studies voiding within 10 to 15 minutes of coitus has been found to be protective when compared with control subjects. Prior infection and exposure to vaginal spermicide are also risk factors.[3,6] Single studies have found an association between UTIs and certain behavioral factors, including purposely resisting the urge to void, decreased fluid intake and wearing synthetic underwear. However, these associations have not held up in multiple studies. Factors not associated with UTIs include direction of wiping the perineum after defecation, tampon use, bubble baths, douching, tight clothing, and intake of carbonated beverage, coffee, or tea.[7]

Because UTIs are uncommon in men less than 50 years old, they are considered "complicated" infections in men.[3] The incidence is higher in newborns, infants, and older men, all of whom are more likely to have anatomic abnormalities of the urinary tract. Some data suggest that lack of circumcision may contribute to the increased incidence of UTI among young men; however, this was not confirmed in subsequent studies in which the majority of men with acute cystitis had been circumcised.[8] Homosexuality has been identified as a risk factor for UTI in men and heterosexual anal coitus may also increase the risk of UTI in young, healthy men. Prostatic hypertrophy significantly increases the risk of UTI in older adults.[9] Risk factors for UTIs in women and men are listed in Box 160-1.

BOX 160-1

RISK FACTORS FOR URINARY TRACT INFECTIONS

WOMEN

Inherent anatomic risk (4-cm female urethra vs. 20-cm male urethra)
Fecal contamination
History of recent UTI
Decreased fluid intake
Irregular bladder emptying
Vaginal pH >4.5
Sexual intercourse
Failure to void within 10 to 15 minutes of coitus
Diaphragm/spermicide use
Symptomatic partner
Pregnancy
Menopause
Hyperuremia
Neurogenic bladder
Kidney disease
Urologic abnormalities
Instrumentation
Immunosuppression

MEN

Urologic abnormalities
Neurogenic bladder
Instrumentation
Benign prostatic hypertrophy
Anal intercourse
Immunosuppression

CLINICAL PRESENTATION

UTIs can be subdivided into several distinct types of infection: acute uncomplicated UTIs, recurrent UTIs, complicated UTIs, urethritis, pyelonephritis, and asymptomatic bacteriuria, with different characteristics associated with each of these syndromes.

Acute uncomplicated UTIs are characterized by signs and symptoms of bladder irritation: increased frequency, urgency, dysuria, and occasionally hematuria. The term *uncomplicated infection* implies that this is a relatively uncommon occurrence in the affected individual who is also otherwise healthy, that there are a small number of responsible pathogens that are susceptible to first-line narrow-spectrum antimicrobial agents, and that there are no underlying urologic or gynecologic abnormalities. A more acute presentation, including high fever, chills, flank pain, costovertebral angle (CVA) tenderness, nausea, and vomiting, is suggestive of pyelonephritis or urosepsis.

An estimated 40% of women will have a UTI at some point in life and approximately 20% will have recurrent infections. There are two basic patterns of recurrence: relapse and reinfection. Relapse refers to infection caused by bacterial persistence—infection by the previously treated pathogen, which was not completely eradicated by the course of antimicrobial therapy. Reinfection refers to recurrence of infection by introduction of a new bacterial strain. In the majority of women, recurrent UTIs are due to reinfection rather than relapse.

Groups often bothered by recurrent infections include sexually active women who report a temporal relationship of urinary symptoms to intercourse, those with compromised host defenses because of underlying systemic illness or immunosuppressive therapy, those with a history of upper UTIs, and pregnant women. Infections caused by relapse are usually caused by certain pathogens including *Klebsiella, Pseudomonas, Proteus,* and *Enterococcus* organisms.

Complicated UTIs are those that occur in patients with underlying urologic or gynecologic abnormalities or that are caused by pathogens that have developed antimicrobial resistance. UTIs are also considered complicated when co-morbidity or other factors increase the risk of persistence, recurrence, or treatment failure. Common causes of complicated infections include functional or anatomic abnormalities of the urinary tract (e.g., a history of polycystic renal disease, nephrolithiasis, neurogenic bladder), underlying disease (e.g., diabetes mellitus, acquired immunodeficiency syndrome [AIDS], or any other immuncompromising illness), use of immune-modifying drugs, pregnancy, the presence of an indwelling catheter, recent instrumentation (e.g., catheterization or cystoscopy), and older age.[10] However, these complicating factors are not always immediately apparent and do not necessarily predict the initial presentation, which can range from a mild cystitis to an acutely toxic presentation. Differentiating between types of UTI and underlying causes is important in determining effective treatment regimens. UTIs in men are uncommon and often represent underlying abnormalities; therefore they are considered at least partially complicated.

Pyelonephritis refers to bacterial infection of the upper urinary tract, which includes the kidneys and the ureters, and usually results from ascending infection. A sustained bladder infection and the presence of reflux increase the risk of ascending infection. High fever, chills, flank pain, CVA tenderness, nausea, and vomiting in the presence of urinary symptoms are suggestive of pyelonephritis. However, kidney infection may also present with only bladder irritation and the absence of any of the classic signs or symptoms. The presence of white blood cell (WBC) casts on microscopy is considered pathognomonic for pyelonephritis. *E. coli* accounts for more than 80% of acute uncomplicated cases of pyelonephritis.[3] Pyelonephritis in male patients suggests an underlying urologic structural abnormality. Renal calculi and embolic infarction can also cause flank pain and hematuria, mimicking pyelonephritis. However, unlike the case with UTIs, urine cultures are sterile and no bacteria are seen on Gram's stain.

Urethritis is characterized by an inflammation (mechanical, chemical, or bacterial) of the urethra alone. Infection of the urogenital tract by sexually transmitted diseases, especially chlamydia, has reached epidemic proportions. Prevalence is highest among sexually active adolescents and young adults. Urethritis is generally classified as gonococcal or nongonococcal in etiology. Nongonococcal urethritis (NGU) is most common, with *Chlamydia* being the most frequent causative organism. Other urethral pathogens include *Ureaplasma urealyticum, Mycoplasma hominis,* and, in women, *Trichomonas vaginalis* and *Gardnerella vaginalis.* Symptoms are usually mild and gradual in onset. Women may experience vaginal discharge or bleeding from concomitant cervicitis and lower abdominal pain. Signs and symptoms of urethritis may include dysuria and irritative symptoms, frequency, urethral discharge, and pruritus at the distal end of the penis. Urinalysis often demonstrates pyuria and, less commonly, hematuria. Urine cultures generally show a colony count $<$100/ml. A low colony count in the presence of the aforementioned symptoms is suggestive of urethritis. Approximately 1% to 2% of women have urethritis and in postmenopausal women, urethritis and atrophic vaginitis are common causes of lower urinary tract symptoms.[11]

Asymptomatic bacteriuria refers to a colony count $\geq$100,000/ml in the absence of symptoms. Asymptomatic bacteriuria is more common in women, increases in both sexes with advancing age, and is found in as many as 40% of older men and women, especially those living in nursing homes. In addition to advancing age and nursing homes, asymptomatic bacteriuria is also associated with a history of indwelling catheterization, instrumentation, urinary incontinence, multiple medical illnesses, and impaired functional and mental status. It is several-fold more common in women with diabetes mellitus.[12] Screening for asymptomatic bacteriuria is recommended only for pregnant women and before urologic surgery. Treatment of asymptomatic bacteriuria before urologic surgery decreases the risk of postsurgical complications. Treatment of pregnant women with asymptomatic bacteriuria, particularly during the first trimester, reduces the risk of acute pyelonephritis and the risks of prematurity and low birth weight in their infants.[13]

PHYSICAL EXAMINATION

Important history to elicit from the woman with a complaint of UTI symptoms should include an assessment of urine frequency, nocturia, dysuria or burning on urination, pruritus, fever or chills, hematuria, vaginal or pelvic signs and symptoms, last menstrual period, and any prior history of UTIs or cervicitis/pelvic inflammatory disease (PID). Patients should be queried about medical history, specifically history of immunocompromising disease, use of immune-modifying drugs, and recent instrumentation. It is worth noting that most women know when they have a UTI; women with a previous history of UTI correctly diagnosis (as confirmed by urine culture) themselves as having a UTI more than 90% of the time.[4]

Vaginal symptoms, external irritation on urination, and the presence of dyspareunia are helpful in sorting out vaginal etiologies from those referable to the urinary tract. Male patients should be assessed for urethral discharge, penile lesions, a history of UTIs or sexually transmitted diseases, and previous prior treatment, if any. It is important to ask all patients about sexual history and risk factors for gonorrhea or chlamydia, including new or symptomatic sexual partners.

The physical examination should include assessment of vital signs, signs and symptoms of acute illness, and dehydration. An examination of the female patient should include a pelvic examination if there is any indication that infection is not solely associated with the urinary tract. The vulva, vagina, cervix, periurethral area, and perianal area should be assessed for discharge, excoriations, tenderness, and ulcerations. In male patients the penis should be checked for discharge, lesions, ulcerations, and swelling. The prostate should be checked for tenderness, swelling, masses, or nodules.

The pace, extensiveness, and order of the evaluation is largely dictated by the clinical presentation. The diagnosis of UTI is suggested by the history and physical examination and confirmed by examination of the urine.

DIAGNOSTICS

The urinalysis is the most important initial study. A urine dipstick is a reasonable rapid diagnostic aid. A clean-voided specimen minimizes contamination from vaginal and labial sources. Leukocyte esterase reflects the presence of WBCs in the urine. However, not all UTIs are associated with WBCs in the urine. The nitrite test reflects the presence of urinary nitrite, which is reduced from urinary nitrate by certain bacteria, although not all bacteria reduce nitrate to nitrite. If both the nitrate test and the leukocyte esterase test are positive, then a UTI is present more than 90% of the time. In addition to the information obtained from the dipstick, urine can be examined microscopically, which allows for easier detection of red blood cells, WBCs, bacteria, and WBC casts. Correlation with subsequent culture is approximately 90%. Uncentrifuged urine can be examined under a coverslip with an oil immersion lens. A WBC count $>7/mm^3$ on low power is abnormal, although not specific for infection. A WBC count $\leq 7/mm^3$ suggests that infection is not present. A count of greater than 2 to 5 WBCs per high-powered field of spun urine is suggestive of a UTI. Sheets of numerous crystal suggest calculi and the presence of WBC casts (a renal cylindric plug of tightly packed leukocytes) are considered proof positive of kidney involvement (either stones or infection). Abnormalities for pH, protein, and blood are nonspecific with respect to UTIs. In the presence of symptoms but a negative dipstick, direct demonstration by microscopy or culture should be done before excluding the possibility of infection.

Urine culture is the "gold standard" and should be obtained in all patients who are febrile, seriously ill, have a history of frequent UTIs, have recently been hospitalized, or for whom empiric treatment has failed. Infections in pregnant women should always be cultured.[14] In addition, cultures should be obtained in young men because infections are unusual and suggestive of underlying problems. If prostatitis is suspected in men, segmental urine and expressed prostatic secretions should be obtained, viewed microscopically, and cultured. There are differing views regarding the need for urine cultures in otherwise healthy women with mild to moderate symptoms. A 100,000/ml colony count is no longer considered a useful parameter for symptomatic women; this traditional criterion for infection provides for high specificity but poor sensitivity (as low as 50% in young women). A colony count as low as 10,000/ml can cause symptomatic infections in some people and most experts agree that UTIs can even occur with bacterial counts as low as 100/ml. Some of these individuals, if untreated, may tend to return with even more severe infections at even higher colony counts.[3,9]

Diagnostics

Urinary Tract Infections

Laboratory
- Urinalysis (clean-voided specimen)
- Urine culture and sensitivity*
- Sexually transmitted disease cultures*
- Segmented urine and expressed prostatic secretions in men*

Imaging
- Renal ultrasound*
- IV pyelography*
- CT scan/MRI*
- Radiography of kidney*

Other
- Cystoscopy*
- Voiding cystourethrogram*

*If indicated.

The bacterial species identified by the culture is as important as the colony count. The presence of multiple species suggests contamination of the specimen, except in the case of catheterization or other special circumstances. Small numbers of certain pathogens, including *Klebsiella* organisms and *E. coli,* should be regarded as suspicious. Large numbers of skin flora, such as *Staphylococcus epidermidis,* dipthroids, and beta-hemolytic streptococci, can usually be ignored. Anaerobic bacteria do not usually cause UTIs; their presence suggests communication with the bowel. The presence of *Candida* organisms usually suggests vaginal contamination.

Sterile pyuria is defined as a negative urine culture despite a positive urinalysis (e.g., positive leukocyte esterase). This condition requires further investigation, as the absence of pathogens on culture does not imply the absence of infection. Some infectious organisms, such as NGU, do not grow on standard laboratory media. Cultures specific for these organisms, such as antigen and DNA detection techniques, should be considered if the history and physical examination suggest a chlamydial or nongonococcal cause. However, many patients with urethral syndrome do not have a demonstrable infectious agent even when special culture media are used. Gram-negative intracellular diplococci on Gram's stain is diagnostic for gonococcal urethritis. Renal tuberculosis, systemic illness, vaginal contamination, and kidney stones can also cause leukocytosis in the absence of a positive culture.[15]

"Test of cure" urine cultures should be obtained in men and whenever there is suspicion that an infection may not have been eradicated. Routine "test of cure" cultures are generally not indicated unless a persistent (as opposed to a recurrent) UTI is suspected. The recurrence of a UTI within 2 weeks is suggestive of a persistent UTI. One posttreatment urinalysis may be helpful to exclude hematuria, as persistent hematuria requires further diagnostic evaluation to exclude renal calculi and tumors.[7]

Persistent UTIs require more extensive urologic evaluation. Renal ultrasonography is a quick, noninvasive way to evaluate renal function; it can detect kidney size, scarring, calculus, renal tumors, and hydronephrosis. Indications for evaluating patients with UTIs with ultrasound include frequent recurrent UTIs in female patients or failure to eradicate infection despite appropriate therapy; acute pyelonephritis in male patients; recurrent pyelonephritis in female patients; or acute infection with systemic symptoms, palpable bladder or renal mass, and signs and symptoms suggestive of renal calculi or *Proteus* infection (e.g., pH >7, posttreatment pyuria).[7,16]

Intravenous pyelogram (IVP) scanning and CT scanning may be useful if the ultrasound examination is noninformative or nonspecific. Both can provide additional detail to help guide treatment. CT scans are better than either ultrasound or IVP for imaging certain conditions, including lymphadenopathy and renal abscesses and masses. MRI provides even sharper imaging but at considerably greater expense. Radioisotope scans of the kidney may be required to further define anatomic abnormalities.[5] Cystoscopy involves a visual examination of the interior of the bladder by means of a cystoscope and is used to exclude bladder disease. A voiding cystourethrogram is the study of choice for demonstrating and determining the degree of vesicourethral reflux (i.e., the retrograde flow from the bladder to the ureters). Retrograde flow is associated with, but not necessarily the cause of, infection.

DIFFERENTIAL DIAGNOSIS

The differential diagnosis of an acute uncomplicated UTI includes urethritis, vaginal infections (e.g., *Gardnerella, Candida albicans* or *Trichomonas* organisms), sexually transmitted diseases that may lead to cervicitis or PID (e.g., *Chlamydia trachomatis, Neisseria gonorrhoeae*), and other sexually transmitted disease (e.g., herpes simplex virus) that may mimic symptoms of UTI but are considered distinct from UTIs.[11] The diagnosis is usually made on the basis of the history, presenting signs and symptoms, and findings on urinalysis and other laboratory work. In the case of a negative urine dipstick in the presence of urinary symptoms, microscopic evaluation or culture should be performed before it is determined that a UTI is not present. A pelvic examination should be considered in a female patient if the history is suggestive of vulvovaginitis from candidiasis, trichomoniasis, or another infection such as herpes simplex. Chlamydial and gonorrheal cultures should be obtained in a sexually active female patient to exclude urethritis. The combination of cervical discharge, cervical motion tenderness, and adnexal tenderness suggests cervicitis or PID. Atrophic vaginitis should be considered in a postmenopausal woman not using topical estrogen therapy. A woman who presents with one or more symptoms of UTI has a probability of infection of at least 50%. Specific combinations of symptoms (e.g., dysuria and frequency without vaginal discharge) substantially increase the likelihood of UTI. In contrast, the history and physical examination are less reliable in accurately excluding UTI in women who present with urinary symptoms. A urine culture and pelvic examination should be considered in women who present with symptoms of UTI but whose history and physical are essentially negative.[10]

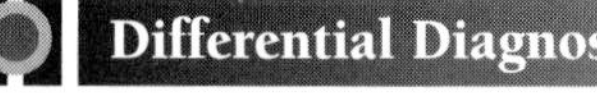

Urinary Tract Infections

Acute Infections
Urethritis
Vaginitis
Cervicitis
Pelvic inflammatory disease
Herpes simplex
Acute urethral syndrome
Interstitial cystitis

Chronic Infections
Structural abnormalities
Neurologic dysfunction
Renal calculi/masses
Intrarenal/perirenal abscess
Bladder tuberculosis
Prostate enlargement

Clinical syndromes in women that mimic UTIs include acute urethral syndrome (also referred to as symptomatic abacteriuria) and interstitial cystitis. Clinical presentation is characterized by bladder irritation, frequency, urgency, and dysuria. The urinalysis is often unimpressive, with few leukocytes and no bacteria. Urine cultures show no significant colony counts, and urethral cultures are often negative. Studies have shown that some women have bacterial infection with very low colony counts; these women respond to the standard therapy for an uncomplicated UTI. Approximately 30% of these women have no pyuria and no detectable infection. A subset of these women may have interstitial cystitis, which some postulate to be an advanced stage of infection of the lower urinary tract resulting either from conventional pathogens or organisms established earlier in the urethra and tissues below the bladder as a result of repeated and prolonged administration of antibiotics. No treatment has been found to be effective once the histologic changes have become established.[17] Symptoms include suprapubic discomfort, especially with a full bladder, and symptoms are often relieved with voiding. Urinalysis is often normal, but hematuria may be present. Urine cultures are sterile. The etiology of symptoms is difficult to diagnose; if hematuria is present and persists, other causes of hematuria, such as bladder cancer, should be excluded. No definitive therapy for interstitial cystitis has been developed. It is hoped that improved diagnosis and management at initial stages of infection or inflammation will decrease the prevalence of this chronic condition. Tricyclics may provide some symptomatic relief for women with interstitial cystitis.[17]

The differential diagnosis for recurrent UTIs includes structural abnormalities (such as obstructive uropathy, congenital anomalies, urinary tract fistulas), neurologic dysfunction, renal calculi and renal masses, intrarenal and perirenal abscesses, bladder tuberculosis, and prostate enlargement in men. Patients with recurrent UTIs or infections that do not respond to standard antimicrobial therapy should be referred to the urologist to exclude underlying causes.[16]

MANAGEMENT

A wide range of antibiotic agents are effective in treating UTIs; nonetheless, drug selection must be made carefully. Common and avoidable reasons for treatment failure include inappropriate antibiotic selection, adverse reactions, subtherapeutic dosing, and inadequate treatment duration. The choice of antibiotic should be determined by the criteria listed in Box 160-2. Classes of antibiotics used to treat routine UTIs include trimethoprim/sulfamethoxazole (TMP-SMX), ampicillin, cephalosporins, fluoroquinolones, and nitrofurantoin. Based on the criteria listed in Box 160-2, however, certain antibiotics may not be appropriate in all situations.

TMP-SMX is bacteriolytic and relatively inexpensive and therefore considered the drug of choice for the treatment of community-acquired acute uncomplicated cystitis. Reported bacterial eradication and cure rates are higher than 85% to 90%.

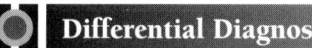

BOX 160-2

CRITERIA FOR ANTIBIOTIC SELECTION

Type of UTI (acute uncomplicated, complicated, recurrent)
Microorganism susceptibility (culture and sensitivity [C&S])
Likelihood of bacterial resistance
Adequate antimicrobial concentration achieved in urine
Toxicity
Side effects
Renal function
Concomitant conditions

Most of the side effects and allergic reactions to this drug combination are due to the sulfur component. Trimethoprim alone provides antimicrobial coverage that is comparable to that of the combination and therefore can also be used alone.[18] Acute uncomplicated UTIs should usually be treated with an antibiotic for 3 days; 3-day regimens have been shown to give the same cure rate as traditional 7- to 10-day courses. Single-dose treatment of an uncomplicated UTI is less effective than a 3-day course.[9]

There is, however, an increasing prevalence of antimicrobial resistance among women with community-acquired infections, increasing from 9% in 1992 to more than 18% in 1996. Studies suggest that the prevalence of TMP-SMX may be as high as 29%. Therefore TMP-SMX is not recommended as the empiric drug for UTI treatment in areas where 10% to 20% of strains demonstrate resistance.[19]

Additional first-line antimicrobial agents (both effective and inexpensive) include ampicillin, amoxicillin, and amoxicillin clavulanate. However, TMP-SMX-resistant organisms are often resistant to multiple drugs including ampicillin, amoxicillin, and first-generation cephalosporins. In fact, *E. coli* resistance to these drugs exceeds 30% in most locations. Resistance to amoxicillin clavulanate is only slightly lower than resistance to amoxicillin alone and is often independent of beta-lactamase activity.[18-20]

Fluoroquinolones (e.g., ciprofloxacin, ofloxacin, norfloxacin, levofloxacin) are an appropriate alternative to TMP-SMX. They provide good coverage and tend to be well tolerated; however, they are generally significantly more expensive than other commonly used drugs. At present, the *E. coli* that cause community-acquired infections are still susceptible to fluoroquinolones, although there are reports of increased fluoroquinolone resistance. More widespread use of these drugs will likely result in increasing antimicrobial resistance, which is the basis for reserving this class of drugs for treatment of complicated infections. Fluoroquinolones are also generally effective against Enterobacteriaceae, as well as staphylococci, *P. aeruginosa, Mycoplasma, Chlamydia,* and some streptococci.

Additional treatment options include the cephalosporins and nitrofurantoin. Cephalosporins (e.g., cefuroxime) are also effective in treating typical pathogens but tend to be relatively expensive. Their side effect profile is similar to that of the aminopenicillins.[9] Nitrofurantoin (50 to 100 mg every 12 hours) is a synthetic antibacterial agent and is indicated for the treatment of acute uncomplicated UTIs caused by susceptible strains of *E. coli* or *S. saprophyticus,* as well as several other gram-positive aerobes such as *S. epidermidis* and *Staphylococcus aureus*. It is also effective for prophylaxis of recurrent UTI. Side effects of nitrofurantoin are relatively rare but significant, including pulmonary complications and hepatitis. Although nitrofurantoin is pregnancy category B during the first trimester, it is category X at term because of the increased risk of CPD6 anemia. Table 160-1 includes a list of antibiotics effective in treating UTI.

Suboptimal candidates for short-course therapy include those with diabetes mellitus, a history of relapses or more than three UTIs during the past year, and those who are immunocompromised. Such patients require more conventional antimicrobial therapy of 10 to 14 days for what are considered complicated UTIs. In addition, men should be treated with a 7- to 10-day course of therapy because all UTIs in men are considered complicated.

Given the global problem of increasing antimicrobial resistance, the use of broad-spectrum antibiotics for uncomplicated UTIs should be avoided if possible. The value of broad-spectrum antibiotics such as the fluoroquinolones should be reserved for the treatment of infections caused by resistant gram-negative pathogens, where their use has been shown to decrease hospitalization time and the need for IV therapy.[8]

Phenazopyridine (Pyridium), a urinary tract analgesic, is sometimes used in patients with dysuria. It is often prescribed alone or concurrently with an antimicrobial agent. A dose of 200 mg t.i.d. for 48 to 72 hours may relieve dysuria in true UTIs; however, the use of phenazopyridine and an antibiotic has not demonstrated more effective or rapid relief of symptoms than the use of an antibiotic alone. Phenazopyridine is a dye (urine will turn orange in color and can stain fabric) and can accumulate in older adults or in anyone with impaired renal function, precipitating renal failure. It should be avoided in persons with hepatitis and hemolytic anemia and is contraindicated in all those with glucose-6-phosphate dehydrogenase deficiency.

The effectiveness of specific nonpharmacologic therapies, especially cranberry juice, is still unclear, although the general consensus in the lay public is that cranberry juice is helpful in treating and preventing UTIs. Recent studies suggest that cranberry juice may have some beneficial effect in the management and prevention of UTIs and have a variable effect in their treatment. The assumption has been that cranberry juice's acidification of urine is responsible for its antibacterial effect; however, increased urine acidification does not appear to play a role. Rather, the inhibition of bacterial adherence to uroepithelial cells seems to explain the beneficial effect of cranberry juice supplementation. In

TABLE 160-1 Antibiotic Treatment for Urinary Tract Infections

Antibiotic	Drug Category	Dose
Trimethoprim-sulfamethoxazole	C *	160/800 mg b.i.d.
Trimethoprim	C*	100 mg b.i.d.
Ampicillin	B	250 mg-500 mg (t.i.d., q.i.d.)
Amoxicillin	B	250 mg-500 mg (t.i.d., q.i.d.)
Amoxicillin-clavulanate	B	250 mg-500 mg (t.i.d., q.i.d.)
Erythromycin	B	250 mg-500 mg q.i.d.
Cefuroxime	B	125-250 mg b.i.d.
Cephalexin	B	250 mg b.i.d.
Nitrofurantoin	B (1st trimester) X (at term)	50-100 mg b.i.d.
Ciprofloxacin	C	250 mg-500 mg, b.i.d., q.i.d.
Levofloxacin	C	250 mg q day
Norfloxacin	C	400 mg b.i.d.
Ofloxacin	C	300 mg b.i.d.

*Should not be prescribed for pregnant women in the third trimester.

addition, at least two studies have shown that drinking cranberry juice daily reduces the recurrence rate of UTIs compared to *Lactobacillus* sp. and placebo ingestion.[21-24]

Recurrent UTIs should be treated as outlined in the preceding paragraphs and documented by at least one urine culture. If there are frequent recurrences, such as three or more in a year, the urinary tract should be evaluated for abnormalities; patients with structural problems should be referred to the appropriate specialist, usually a urologist or gynecologist. Three or more infections per year in the absence of urologic abnormalities is an indication for antibiotic prophylaxis. Recurrent cystitis can be managed by one of several strategies: continuous prophylaxis, postcoital prophylaxis, or therapy initiated by the patient. Of the prophylactic regimens that have been used, continuous low-dose prophylaxis is the most well established. This type of regimen consists of daily or three times a week subtherapeutic doses of an antibiotic known to be effective in the treatment of UTI. In addition, these antibiotics can also be taken after intercourse, or they can be initiated by the patient on experiencing symptoms. Patient-initiated therapy may be prescribed in the form of multiple 3-day courses of antibiotics to be started at the onset of UTI symptoms; such treatment has been found to be both cost-effective and safe with respect to drug toxicity.[6] The most commonly used agents for continuous prophylaxis include TMP-SMX 40 to 200 mg (half a single-strength tablet), trimethoprim 40 to 80 mg, nitrofurantoin 50 to 100 mg, norfloxacin 200 mg, or cephalexin 250 mg. Postmenopausal women who experience recurrent UTIs may find symptomatic relief with topical estrogen cream. Studies on oral estrogen therapy and its effect on recurrent UTI symptoms are nonconclusive.[7]

Complicated UTIs are those that occur in patients with urologic abnormalities or other co-morbidity that increase the risk of infections caused by pathogens resistant to antibiotics. These complications may not be completely obvious and do not necessarily predict the severity of infection on presentation. The clinical spectrum ranges from a mild cystitis to an acute pyelonephritis with systemic complications, but can also include long periods of asymptomatic bacteriuria. Treatment of complicated UTIs should be extended for at least 7 days and must be based on urine culture and susceptibility testing. SMF-TMX is a reasonable empiric first choice while results of the culture and sensitivity are pending. A posttreatment test of cure is not necessary as long as symptoms have completely resolved. If culture-directed therapy fails, a repeat urine culture and further evaluation are indicated.[9]

Diabetes mellitus is one of the most common primary care problems associated with a significant increased risk of developing complications of UTI and/or unusual forms of infections. Individuals with diabetes are also more likely to develop rare complications, such as emphysematous cystitis and pyelonephritis, abscess formation, and renal papillary necrosis than those who do not have diabetes mellitus. In addition, the prevalence of urinary tract anatomic or physiologic abnormalities seems to be greater among those with diabetes. The most common pathogen is *E. coli,* but unusual pathogens and fungal infections, particularly *Candida* species, are more common among persons with diabetes. For these reasons, the initial choice of empiric antibiotic should be based on the Gram's stain of the urine and by results of recent urine cultures if available. Fungal infection should also be considered if it has occurred before or if there is a history of recent instrumentation or broad-spectrum antibiotic use. The majority of pathogens in this population are still sensitive to the fluoroquinolones, and reasonable empiric first choices include ciprofloxacin, levofloxacin, and gatifloxacin. Additional options include imipenem, ticarcillin-clavulanate, and piperacillin-tazobactam. Therapy should be continued for 7 days or possibly longer depending on individual circumstances.[25]

Asymptomatic bacteriuria should be treated in pregnancy and before urologic surgery. Antimicrobial therapy should be based on urine culture and antibiotic susceptibility. Most infections respond to 3-day courses of amoxicillin, TMP-SMX (contraindicated in third trimester of pregnancy), an oral cephalosporin, or nitrofurantoin (contraindicated at term). In most other adults, asymptomatic bacteriuria does not cause symptomatic infection, renal failure, urosepsis, or increased mortality; therefore routine screening and treatment in other adult groups are not recommended.[3]

Treatment of urethritis depends on suspicion, if not confirmation, of the causative agent. Diagnosis of urethritis is confirmed by culture, but treatment is often empiric, based on the history, symptoms, and a urine culture significant for sterile pyuria. The most common cause of urethritis is *C. trachomatis,* which responds to both doxycycline 100 mg PO b.i.d. for 7 days, azithromycin 1 g in a single dose, and ofloxacin 400 mg PO every 12 hours for 5 days. These drugs are usually also effective against *Ureaplasma* organisms. Pregnant women, for whom these drugs are contraindicated, can be treated with erythromycin base 500 mg PO q.i.d. for 7 days (erythromycin estolate is contraindicated in pregnancy). Less common causes of urethritis include *N. gonorrhoeae,* which requires a dose of ceftriaxone (Rocephin) 250 mg IM. Treatment of *N. gonorrhoeae* should include simultaneous treatment of NGU with both ceftriaxone and doxycycline or ofloxacin as a single agent. Infection with *Trichomonas* organisms, if identified, should be treated with metronidazole 250 mg PO t.i.d. for 1 week.

Treatment of pyelonephritis depends on the acuity and severity of symptoms, presence of complicating risk factors, susceptibility of the pathogen to oral antimicrobial agents, and presence of the patient's social supports. Antimicrobial therapy is based on Gram's stain and antibiotic susceptibility. Patients who are otherwise healthy can be treated on an outpatient basis with 10 to 14 days of oral antibiotics, provided that the patient is reliable, can take oral antibiotics, and has a phone and means of transportation should signs and symptoms worsen. Older adults and those with acute, severe symptoms and possibly urosepsis are candidates for hospitalization and often require parenteral therapy. A history of diabetes mellitus, sickle cell anemia, nephrolithiasis, or excessive analgesic use increases the risk of renal papillary necrosis and subsequent obstruction and can be considered an indication for hospitalization.

Co-Management with Specialists

Patients with frequent recurrent or relapsing UTIs should be referred for further evaluation, especially if underlying urologic or gynecologic abnormalities have not been excluded. Those with underlying functional, metabolic, or structural urologic abnormalities, which increase the risk of UTIs, should be managed in conjunction with a specialist. Patients with co-morbidity that does not affect the risk of UTIs but that increases the severity of infection once contracted may benefit from collaboration with a specialist.

LIFE SPAN CONSIDERATIONS

Asymptomatic UTIs are more prevalent in pregnant women; screening for and treatment of infection are indicated in these women to decrease the risk of acute pyelonephritis and premature delivery and low birth weight. Refer to Table 160-1 for a list of treatment options during pregnancy.

UTIs are the most common cause of bacterial infection in older adults but are often not accompanied by the classic signs and symptoms. Symptoms are often subtle and may include a vague change in mental status, decreased appetite, lethargy, and increased falls (sustained during efforts to get to the bathroom). UTIs are also the most common cause of sepsis, the second most common cause of bacteremia in the geriatric population and an important cause of morbidity and mortality in nursing facilities.[26]

COMPLICATIONS

The most common complication of UTI is pyelonephritis, a bacterial infection of the kidney resulting from ascending untreated or inadequately treated lower UTI. Urosepsis is a potentially life-threatening systemic complication of UTI that requires high-dose parental antimicrobial therapy.

INDICATIONS FOR REFERRAL/HOSPITALIZATION

Any patient who appears acutely ill or with signs and symptoms of obstruction or urosepsis requires immediate hospitalization. Specific signs and symptoms requiring consideration for hospitalization or referral include rigors, high fever, flank pain, nausea, and vomiting.

PATIENT AND FAMILY EDUCATION

There are nonpharmacologic measures that have been demonstrated to prevent episodic or recurrent UTIs. Sexual intercourse and not voiding within 10 to 15 minutes after coitus are the two factors most consistently associated with UTIs. In discussing the association between these two factors and UTIs with a patient, it is important to distinguish between UTIs and sexually transmitted diseases. Explanations and suggestions must be offered in a way that is nonjudgmental and does not imply guilt. There is no basis for suggesting changes in a patient's sex life; however, recommending that a woman void within 10 to 15 minutes after coitus may decrease the frequency of UTIs. Drinking plenty of fluids (64 to 80 oz), urinating frequently, wiping from front to back, and avoiding feminine hygiene products (for the genital area) that contain deodorants may also be helpful in preventing urinary tract infections.[27,28] Women who have had previous UTIs should be encouraged to seek treatment as soon as symptoms are recognized.

Women who use a diaphragm/spermicide may wish to consider an alternative form of birth control to avoid UTIs. This discussion must include the risks and benefits of other contraceptive options. Given the other options, some women may prefer to continue diaphragm use and use antibiotic prophylaxis as a way to minimize recurrent infections.

Women who suffer from recurrent UTIs should be educated about the possible benefits of antimicrobial suppression or postcoital prophylaxis, depending on the situation. Intravaginal estrogen cream may be helpful for postmenopausal women who suffer from recurrent UTIs. Daily ingestion of cranberries, whether in juice, concentrate, cocktail formulation, or capsule supplementation, may have a beneficial role in prevention of UTIs, especially in women experiencing recurrent infections.

Other behavioral changes commonly recommended, such as avoiding tight or synthetic underwear, vaginal douching, and tampon use, have not been substantiated. Providers should refrain from suggesting lifestyle changes that may be more of a reflection of their biases than of clinical research.

Additional patient information can be obtained from the following sources:

National Kidney and Urologic Diseases
Information Clearinghouse
3 Information Way
Bethesda, MD 20892-3580
(301) 654-4415
http://www.niddk.nih.gov

American Foundation for Urologic Disease
Answers to Your Questions about Urinary Tract Infections
(800) 242-2383
http://www.afud.org

National Kidney Foundation
(800) 622-9010
Cleveland Clinic
http://www.ccf.org/education/pated

Sexually Transmitted Diseases

DEFINITION/EPIDEMIOLOGY

The term *sexually transmitted disease* (STD) encompasses more than 25 infectious organisms that are transmitted through sexual activity and the dozens of clinical syndromes associated with these organisms. Since 1980 eight new sexually transmitted pathogens have been identified in the United States.[29,30] Excluding the human immunodeficiency virus (HIV), the most common STDs in the United States are *Chlamydia,* gonorrhea, genital herpes, human papillomavirus, trichomoniasis, and bacterial vaginosis.[31]

The health consequences of STDs vary. Left untreated, bacterial STDs can produce painful anogenital symptoms such as urethritis or cervicitis, as well as more serious complications such as PID or life-threatening tertiary syphilis.[32]

STDs are almost always transmitted from person to person by sexual intercourse. STDs are spread most efficiently by anal or vaginal intercourse and less effectively by oral intercourse. Pregnant women infected with an STD may infect infants in utero, during birth, or through breastfeeding.[29] Women are more vulnerable to STDs because they are more biologically susceptible to certain STDs than men and are more likely to have asymptomatic infection.

The management of STDs is often confounded by the inclusiveness of the term itself. A number of different organisms may be associated with different syndromes; for example, genital ulcers can result from herpes, chancroid, syphilis, or other infections.

Over the past decade the epidemiology of STDs has changed dramatically. As a group STDs are considered to be at epidemic proportions.[29] Five of the top 10 reportable diseases in the United States are STDs (chlamydial infection, gonorrhea, AIDS, primary and secondary syphilis, and hepatitis B virus infection).[33] There are approximately 15 million new cases of STDs annually in the United States.[31] Rates of many STDs, particularly viral STDs (genital herpes, HIV, and human papillomavirus), are higher now than they were three decades ago. Syphilis continues to remain a problem in the United States, with rates reaching epidemic proportions in the mid-1980s and early 1990s.[34] Rates have recently begun to decrease, with most increases now noted in populations such as crack cocaine users and their sexual partners.[29] In the United States the reported rate of syphilis is at the lowest level since reporting began in 1941.[31]

STDs affect persons of all racial, cultural, and socioeconomic groups, but with wide discrepancies among these groups. The rate of gonorrhea in African-American adolescents is more than 30 times the rate in Caucasian adolescents and 11 times higher than rates among Hispanics.[31,35] The rate of primary and secondary syphilis in African-Americans is nearly 30 times that in Caucasians.[31] Although the rates of primary and secondary syphilis have declined between 1997 and 1999, they continue to remain considerably higher for African-American and Hispanics than for Caucasians. Despite this recent decline there still exists a disparity between these groups, with syphilis being one of the most glaring examples of the existing gaps in minority health status.[31] Congenital syphilis has decreased nationally in recent years.

Adolescents and young adults are at the greatest risk of acquiring an STD. Approximately 3 million teenagers acquire an STD each year. The incidence of gonorrhea and chlamydia is highest in 15- to 19-year-olds. Young men and women under age 25 account for two thirds of all cases of chlamydia and gonorrhea in the United States. Sexual behavior that includes multiple partners, inconsistent use of condoms, and endocervical ectopy in female patients contribute to the higher risk in this age-group.[29,31,32,36]

CLINICAL PRESENTATION

A significant number of persons with STDs have no apparent signs or symptoms.[37] More than one site may be infected simultaneously (e.g., cervix plus urethra), and symptoms may overlap and involve more than one pathogen. Diseases are tentatively classified into syndromes to narrow the field of possible pathogens.[30,37,38]

Because STDs do not always present with distinct clinical features, determining which patients are at risk necessitates a thorough sexual history. Practitioners are advised to adopt a standardized approach to anyone at risk for an STD. Eliciting a history for an STD needs to be routine, standardized, and guided by the individual's age. An effective sexual history is critical for diagnosis and for counseling individuals with regard to risk-reduction behaviors. Sexual orientation and sexual behavior can be sensitive topics. Questions are best phrased in an open-ended, nonjudgmental, and nontechnical format and must address pertinent data (Box 160-3). Consideration of age-related developmental characteristics, particularly those associated with adolescence, is critical. Female adolescents may protect themselves against pregnancy with oral contraceptives yet forego condoms.[37,39,40]

All adolescents in the United States can be provided with confidential diagnosis and treatment of STDs without parental consent or knowledge.[38] In many states adolescents can be provided with HIV counseling and testing without parental consent or knowledge.[41]

PHYSICAL EXAMINATION

The physical examination for an STD incorporates the same principles as the history. It is routine, standardized, and sensitive to the patient's age, individual needs, and cultural heritage. Consistently examining all areas reduces the chance of a missed diagnosis. Minimum physical examination procedures for women and men are listed in Box 160-4.

Every effort should be made to allay anxiety. All steps of the examination should be explained before beginning. Female patients normally void before the examination. However, when collecting specimens it is important to follow manufacturer's recommendations to ensure proper specimen collection technique. Female patients may or may not void before examination

BOX 160-3

SEXUAL HISTORY

Condoms—consistency of use, and for what sexual practices
Previous STDs
Medication allergies
Most recent sexual encounter and number of partners in past 2 months and past year
High-risk behaviors, including use of drugs and alcohol (or use of by partners), including which drugs, how often, and what route
Does patient have sex with men, women, or both?
Do partners have sex with men, women, or both?
Travel and location
Dysuria, frequency, hematuria
Adenopathy
Fatigue, weight loss, night sweats, unexplained diarrhea, fever

ADDITIONAL HISTORY FOR WOMEN

Vaginal discharge, bleeding, color
Skin rash, lesions, sores; location
Pruritus (vulvar, anal, oral, other)
Pain (abdominal, vaginal, vulvar, anal, headache, joints)
Rectal discharge, pain, blood
Birth control methods, consistency of use
Last menstrual period, description, changes

ADDITIONAL HISTORY FOR MEN

Penile discharge
Lesions (penis, scrotum, oral cavity, other)
Skin rash
Pruritus (urethra, anus, skin)
Pain (testes, joints, headache, anal)
Adenopathy
Rectal discharge, bleeding, constipation

depending on the diagnostic test used. Urine ligase chain reaction (LCR) specimens for chlamydia and gonorrhea from women and men should be first-voided specimens. Male patients should be instructed not to void before the examination.

DIAGNOSTICS

After completing the routine screening history and examination, it may be possible to classify the patient in one of several clinical syndromes. This narrows the field of possible pathogens that cause the syndrome and guides treatment. If the patient is asymptomatic, therapy is determined by the laboratory results. Partners of persons with identified STDs are evaluated and treated on the basis of their last sexual encounter and the particular STD in question. Early, specific diagnosis and treatment of symptomatic and asymptomatic persons will prevent further transmission of disease to their partners. However, appropriate diagnosis of an STD often requires multiple specific diagnostic tests because of the variety of STDs. "Syndromic diagnosis," which uses the patient's history, results of physical examination, and laboratory test results can be used for the diagnosis of clinical syndromes.[29] Table 160-2 outlines the STDs and their associated pathogens and syndromes, appropriate diagnostics, and differential diagnoses.

BOX 160-4

MINIMUM PHYSICAL EXAMINATION FOR SEXUALLY TRANSMITTED DISEASES

WOMEN

Examination of the mouth
Examination of the lymph nodes
Examination of the skin on the thorax, abdomen, limbs, palms, soles
Examination of the anogenital area
Pelvic examination, including speculum examination and bimanual examination
Assessment for cervical motion tenderness
Palpation for inguinal and femoral adenopathy

MEN

Examination of the mouth
Examination of the lymph nodes
Examination of the skin of the thorax, abdomen, limbs, palms, soles
Examination of the external genitalia and anus

MANAGEMENT

The major curable syndromes in adults include urethritis in men; vaginal discharge, cervicitis, and PID in women; and genital ulcers in both men and women. In the United States it is common to initiate syndromic treatments effective against all common bacteria causing these syndromes while laboratory results are pending. Co-infection with more than one organism is common. Treatment is usually reserved for symptomatic individuals. It is not useful for mild or asymptomatic infection. In addition, the predictive value of any test will vary depending on the prevalence of the disease in the population.[9]

Antimicrobial therapy is available for all bacterial STDs, as well as those caused by protozoa and ectoparasites. Drugs for viral STDs are largely limited to symptom alleviation because they cannot eradicate the organism. The standards published by the Centers for Disease Control and Prevention (CDC)[41] in 2002 use the regimens listed in Box 160-5.

For most STDs the partners of patients should be examined. According to the standards published by the CDC,[41] when exposure to a treatable STD is considered likely, appropriate antimicrobial agents should be administered, even though clinical signs of infection are not evident and laboratory tests are not yet available. Evidence exists suggesting benefit for the regimens recommended by the CDC for specific STDs.[41,42] In many states the local state or health department can assist in partner notification for selected STDs (e.g., HIV infection, syphilis, gonorrhea, hepatitis B, and chlamydia).

TABLE 160-2 Treatment Profile for Sexually Transmitted Diseases

Pathogen	Clinical Presentation	Diagnosis	Consultation/ Co-Management	Complications	Other
CHLAMYDIA					
Chlamydia trachomatis *Differential diagnosis:* Pelvic inflammatory disease (PID); gonorrhea	Often asymptomatic *Female:* Endocervical mucus (yellow or green), cervical ectopy, or edema *Male:* dysuria, mucoid purulent discharge, itching	Ligase chain reaction (LCR) swab Polmerase chain reactor (PCR) swab DNA probe Direct fluorescence antibody (DFA) Enzyme immunoassay (EIA), enzyme-linked immunosorbent assay (ELISA) Urine LCR Leukocyte esterase test (LET)	Treatment failure HIV-positive patients	PID Perihepatitis Reiter's syndrome Chronic conjunctivitis Chronic pelvic pain Infant infection Epididymitis	Collect specimen for chlamydia. Treat presumptively with PID, nongonococcal urethritis (NGU), gonococcal infection, epididymitis in men <35 years old. Syphilis serology. Offer HIV counseling and testing.

continued

TABLE 160-2 Treatment Profile for Sexually Transmitted Diseases—cont'd

Pathogen	Clinical Presentation	Diagnosis	Consultation/ Co-Management	Complications	Other
GONORRHEA					
Neisseria gonorrhoeae *Differential diagnosis:* NGU; PID	Purulent urethral discharge Dysuria Pruritus Anorectal burning Skin lesions *Female:* Frequently asymptomatic; dysuria; leukorrhea; abnormal uterine bleeding; cervical motion tenderness (CMT); vaginal discharge; pharyngeal edema/erythema	Gram's stain Direct culture LCR PCR swab Gen Probe EIA LET (requires confirmation)	Treatment failure Complications	Prostatitis Epididymitis Cystitis PID Disseminated gonorrhea Gonococcal conjunctivitis	Treat presumptively for chlamydia. Specimen testing for gonorrhea should occur before other testing. Partners are evaluated and treated. Syphilis serology. Offer HIV counseling and testing.
NONGONOCOCCAL URETHRITIS					
C. trachomatis (23%-55% of cases) *Ureaplasma urealyticum* (20%-40% of cases) *Trichomonas vaginalis* (25% of cases) Herpes simplex virus *Differential diagnosis:* Gonorrhea	Dysuria Mucoid or purulent discharge Pruritus Hematuria Frequency Urgency Endocervical exudate, friability	Gram's stain Wet mount Tests for gonorrhea and chlamydia	Treatment failure Complications	Epididymitis Penile edema Reiter's syndrome Tenosynovitis	If microscopic tests are not available, treat for both gonorrhea and chlamydia.
PRIMARY SYPHILIS					
Treponema pallidum *Differential diagnosis:* Genital herpes; chancroid; lymphogranuloma venereum; balantitis, excoriation of nonulcerative lesions; squamous cell carcinoma	Painless chancre at site of inoculation Discrete, enlarged, painless regional lymph nodes Incubation (10-90 days: average 21 days)	Darkfield microscopy Nontreponemal serology (RPR, VDRL) Confirm with treponemal serology (MHA-TP, FTA-ABS) Sequential serologic testing; use same testing method and laboratory	Positive diagnosis of disease All HIV-positive patients	Secondary syphilis Meningitis Cardiovascular or neurologic disease Facilitates HIV transmission Left untreated, can cause perinatal death or congenital syphilis in infants	Systemic disease: average incubation is 3 weeks. Chancre is unnoticed in 15%-39% of cases. Nontreponemal serology and clinical follow-up at 6 and 12 months. Note fourfold drop in titer; evaluate for HIV infection. Treatment failure: retreat/consultation with specialist is indicated; patients may need lumbar puncture.
SECONDARY SYPHILIS					
T. pallidum *Differential diagnosis:* All undiagnosed mucocutaneous skin eruptions (e.g., drug eruption, pityriasis rosea, scabies)	Ulcerations: symmetric papillosquamous eruption on palms, soles, mucous membranes, trunk Appears 2-8 weeks after appearance of chancre Generalized adenopathy Malaise, arthralgias Oral mucous patches Condylomata lata Hepatosplenomegaly Symptoms of UTI	As with primary syphilis	As with primary syphilis	As above	Increased incidence associated with crack cocaine use and illicit drug use. At 6 and 12 months follow-up, assess for fourfold drop in titer. A fourfold increase in titer at any time may represent treatment failure or reinfection.

TABLE 160-2 Treatment Profile for Sexually Transmitted Diseases—cont'd

Pathogen	Clinical Presentation	Diagnosis	Consultation/ Co-Management	Complications	Other
LATENT SYPHILIS (EARLY LATENT, LATE LATENT)					
T. pallidum	Positive serology without evidence of clinical disease Evaluate for aortitis, neurosyphilis iritis	Reactive VDRL or RPR Reactive FTA-ABS or MHA-TP	All cases managed with specialist	Progression of disease	Latent syphilis is diagnosed as probable on the basis of documented seroconversion or on a fourfold increase in titer of nontreponemal test. History of symptoms or exposure to partner during previous 12 months.
CHANCROID					
Haemophilus ducreyi *Differential diagnosis:* Genital herpes; primary syphilis; lymphogranuloma venereum; infected or traumatic lesions	One or more painful genital ulcers with tender inguinal adenopathy May have supportive inguinal adenopathy and undermined ulcer borders	Isolation of *H. ducreyi* Most cases diagnosed on clinical grounds Painful ulcers 4-7 days after exposure Usually coronal sulcus in men Prepuce in women	Treatment failure	Successful treatment cures infection In extensive cases, scarring can result despite successful therapy	Patients reexamined at 3-7 days. Larger ulcers heal more slowly. No evidence of *T. pallidum* on darkfield examination or by serology. Culture negative for HSV. Partner contact: examine and treat within 10 days. Syphilis serology. HIV counseling.
GENITAL HERPES (PRIMARY, RECURRENT)					
Herpes simplex virus 2 (HSV-2) and sometimes HSV-1 *Differential diagnosis:* Primary syphilis; chancroid; fixed drug eruption; folliculitis	*Primary:* Vesicular lesions on erythematous base *Male:* Penis shaft, glans, urethra, rectum *Female:* Vulva, vagina, anus, cervix Lesions painful, with malaise, fever, painful adenopathy Lesions ulcerative to superficial ulcers *Recurrent:* Clinical prodrome—pain, itching, burning, tingling Constitutional symptoms rare Vesicles Superficial ulcers	History and physical with confirmation by viral culture Moist swab of unroofed or weeping vesicle from base of ulcer Tzanck smear of scrapings from lesion looking for multinucleated giant cells Testing for HSV should be routine in all atypical and all undiagnosed genital ulcers	Secondary infection Ocular infection Persistent constitutional symptoms Urinary retention Primary or recurrent infection during pregnancy HIV-positive patients	Secondary infection Ocular infection Neonatal infection Premature delivery Spontaneous abortion Intrauterine growth retardation Fetal infection	Treatment is symptomatic. Infection may recur. May be transmitted to sex partners even when no lesions are present. Support groups are available. Many educational resources are available.

BOX 160-5

TREATMENT OF SEXUALLY TRANSMITTED DISEASES

TREATMENT OF DISEASES CHARACTERIZED BY URETHRITIS OR CERVICITIS

UNCOMPLICATED GONOCOCCAL INFECTIONS

Recommended regimens

A single dose of:
Cefixime, 400 mg PO, *or*
Ceftriaxone, 125 mg IM, *or*
Ciprofloxacin, 500 mg PO, *or*
Ofloxacin 400 mg PO *or*
Levofloxacin 250 mg PO

Plus

A regimen effective against co-infection with *Chlamydia trachomatis,* such as:
Azithromycin, 1 g PO in a single dose, *or*
Doxycycline, 100 mg b.i.d. for 7 days

CHLAMYDIA

Recommended regimens

Azithromycin, 1 g PO in a single dose, *or*
Doxycycline, 100 mg PO b.i.d. for 7 days

Alternative regimens

Erythromycin base, 500 mg PO q.i.d. for 7 days, *or*
Erythromycin ethylsuccinate, 800 mg PO q.i.d. for 7 days, *or*
Ofloxacin, 300 mg PO b.i.d. for 7 days *or*
Levofloxacin 500 mg PO once a day for 7 days

NONGONOCOCCAL URETHRITIS

Recommended regimens

Azithromycin, 1 g PO in a single dose, *or*
Doxycycline, 100 mg PO b.i.d. for 7 days

Alternative regimens

Erythromycin base, 500 mg PO q.i.d. for 7 days, *or*
Erythromycin ethylsuccinate, 800 mg PO q.i.d. for 7 days, *or*
Ofloxacin, 300 mg PO b.i.d. for 7 days *or*
Levofloxacin 500 mg PO for 7 days

TREATMENT OF DISEASES CHARACTERIZED BY GENITAL ULCERS

Genital Herpes: First Clinical Episode

Recommended regimens

Acyclovir, 400 mg PO t.i.d. for 7-10 days, *or*
Acyclovir, 200 mg PO five times daily for 7-10 days *or*
Famciclovir, 250 mg PO t.i.d. for 7-10 days, *or*
Valacyclovir, 1 g PO b.i.d. for 7-10 days

Genital Herpes: Recurrent Episodes

Recommended regimens

Acyclovir, 400 mg PO t.i.d. for 5 days, *or*
Acyclovir, 200 mg PO five times daily for 5 days, *or*
Acyclovir, 800 mg PO b.i.d. for 5 days, *or*
Famciclovir, 125 mg PO for 5 days, *or*
Valacyclovir, 500 mg PO b.i.d. for 3-5 days *or*
Valacyclovir 1.0 g PO daily for 5 days

Primary, Secondary, or Latent Syphilis of Less Than 1 Year's Duration

Recommended regimens

Benzathine penicillin G, 2.4 million U IM in a single dose
If allergic to penicillin:
Doxycycline, 100 mg b.i.d. for 14 days *or*
Tetracycline, 500 mg PO q.i.d. for 14 days

Early Latent Syphilis

Recommended regimens

Benzathine penicillin G 2.4 million U IM in a single dose

Late Latent Syphilis of More Than 1 Year's Duration or Unknown Duration

Recommended regimens

Benzathine penicillin G, 7.2 million U total, administered as 3 doses of 2.4 million U IM each, at 1-week intervals

Chancroid

Recommended regimens

Azithromycin, 1 g PO in a single dose, *or*
Ceftriaxone, 250 mg IM in a single dose, *or*
Ciprofloxacin, 500 mg PO b.i.d. for 3 days, *or*
Erythromycin base, 500 mg PO t.i.d. for 7 days

From Centers for Disease Control and Prevention: Sexually transmitted diseases treatment guidelines—2002, *MMWR* 51(RR06):1-80, 2002. Consult these guidelines for more detailed recommendations, including guidelines for treatment of pregnant patients, HIV-infected patients, allergic patients, and other specific groups.

Co-Management with Specialists

All pregnant and HIV-positive patients should be co-managed with a specialist or collaborating physician. All treatment failures necessitate management with a specialist. Consultation or co-management with a specialist is necessary for all cases of syphilis (see Table 160-2).

LIFE SPAN CONSIDERATIONS

Adolescents or young adults under 20 years of age are at the highest risk for acquiring an STD. They are more likely than other groups to have unprotected sex and multiple sex partners, and young women may also choose partners older than themselves. In addition young women are biologically more susceptible to chlamydia, gonorrhea, and HIV. Among adolescents, gonorrhea increased 13% between 1997 and 1999, with young African-American women and men at extremely high risk.[31] Screening of asymptomatic high-risk patients with sensitivity to age-related developmental and cultural characteristics is required. STD prevention should be initiated before sexual activity begins, with education about healthy, safe sexual practices and continual reinforcement throughout the life span. Additional life span considerations relate to the development of PID in women, with possible consequences of infertility, ectopic pregnancies, and chronic pelvic pain.

Prevention of viral STDs requires the adoption of lifelong healthy sexual behaviors to help avoid acquisition and spread of infection. The prevalence of herpes increases with age because the disease, once acquired, stays within the body. The rate of new infections of herpes and human papillomavirus are typically highest in the late teens and early twenties.[31] Factors related to the spread and acquisition of STDs often include other high-risk behaviors, such as multiple partners, use of illicit drugs, and unsafe sexual practices, such as not using condoms. Prevention of reinfection often necessitates other lifestyle behavior changes that address these specific risk factors.[29,32]

Diseases Characterized by Cervicitis and Urethritis

Urethritis, or inflammation of the urethra, is caused by an infection characterized by the discharge of mucoid or purulent material and by burning during urination. Urethritis is the most common STD syndrome in men. Asymptomatic infections are common.[38] Urethritis is classified as gonococcal if caused by *N. gonorrhoeae* (gonorrhea) or NGU if *N. gonorrhoeae* is not detected. The frequency of gonococcal urethritis and NGU varies by population studies.[29,31,41]

GONORRHEA

Gonorrhea is a reportable disease caused by the gram-negative diplococcus *N. gonorrhoeae*. It primarily involves mucocutaneous surfaces of the genitourinary tract, pharynx, conjunctiva, and anus. In men it is often characterized by a purulent urethral discharge, whereas in up to 80% of women it is asymptomatic. The causative agent, *N. gonorrhoeae,* was discovered in 1879 by Albert Neisser.[31,38,41,43-45] Left untreated, it can result in a range of complications from acute salpingitis in female patients, to perihepatitis (Fitz-Hugh–Curtis syndrome), to disseminated gonococcal infections, to ophthalmia neonatorum in newborns. Infections caused by gonorrhea are a major cause of PID, ectopic pregnancy, and chronic pelvic pain in the United States.[29]

An estimated 650,000 cases of gonorrhea occur each year in the United States.[31] Populations at risk for gonorrhea include young, sexually active individuals (such as teenagers), nonwhite urban poor, and other individuals who engage in high-risk behaviors such as use of illegal drugs or prostitution. Recently, researchers have seen indications that gonorrhea may be on the increase among gay and bisexual men. Gonorrhea rates are highest in females between the ages of 15 and 19 years and males between the ages of 20 and 24 years. Overall gonorrhea rates have increased in both males and females between 1997 and 1999.[31] Geographic variation is substantial, with the highest rates of infection occurring in poor, minority communities in large cities and in rural southeastern states.[31,32]

Carriers with no symptoms or those who have ignored symptoms usually spread gonorrhea.[43] Up to 50% of persons with gonorrhea have a coexistent chlamydia infection.[29,31,32]

Pathophysiology

N. gonorrhoeae is a human pathogen that infects mucus-secreting columnar and transitional epithelium. The portal of entry can be the genitourinary tract, eyes, oropharynx, anorectum, or skin. Transmission by vaginal or anal intercourse is more efficient than orogenital transmission. Autoinoculation of the organism to the eyes is possible. Neonates can acquire the infection during passage through the birth canal. The incubation period is 1 to 14 days after exposure, with a peak of 2 to 5 days in male patients. Longer intervals between exposure and the onset of symptoms are common. Some men never develop symptoms. In women the infection typically becomes evident 2 to 7 days after exposure. The infection generally begins in the anterior urethra, accessory urethral glands, Bartholin's or Skene's glands, and the cervix. If untreated, gonorrhea spreads from its initial sites upward into the genital tract, prostate, and epididymis in men and into the fallopian tubes in women. Pharyngitis may develop after orogenital contact. The organism may also invade the bloodstream, leading to bacteremic involvement of other tissues, including joint spaces, heart valves, meninges, and other tissues. Menstruation increases the risk of intraluminal ascent from the cervix and predisposes the patient to gonococcal bacteremia.[38,46]

Clinical Presentation

Although customarily categorized as gonococcal urethritis or NGU, one fourth of male patients with gonococcal urethritis may also have simultaneous infection with *Chlamydia* organisms.[30] Signs and symptoms of infection with *N. gonorrhoeae* include urethritis, with purulent urethral discharge (drip) in 75% of men, as well as dysuria and pruritus. Urethral discharge can range from clear to purulent and copious. Discharge with gonococcal urethritis is most often purulent, whereas that with NGU tends to be clear or mucoid. It is impossible to distinguish between the two on clinical grounds alone. Less commonly seen is hematuria, frequency, or urgency. Asymptomatic infections can occur but are less typical with gonococcal infections than with NGU. Pharyngeal infection usually occurs in association with anogenital gonorrhea. The majority of pharyngeal infections are asymptomatic. Infection may be transmitted to genital sites through oral sex or progress to disseminated gonococcal infection. Anorectal infection may present with anorectal burning, mucopurulent discharge, and painful bowel movements.[32,44,47] Fewer than 5% of men have no symptoms.[29]

In female patients gonorrheal infection is often asymptomatic in the early stage of disease (up to 80% of cases) and may not present until the disease is more advanced. Initial symptoms in women (2 to 7 days after exposure) include dysuria, leukorrhea, lower abdominal discomfort, abnormal uterine bleeding, and dysuria. Later signs may include adnexal tenderness, cervical motion tenderness, purulent vaginal discharge, elevated temperature, right upper quadrant pain, joint pain or swelling, skin lesions, nausea, and vomiting. Signs of disseminated disease occur most often when gonorrhea is acquired during menses or pregnancy and include tenosynovitis, skin lesions, fever, and polyarthralgias.[47-49] Pharyngitis can occur with orogenital contact, and anorectal signs may be present with rectal involvement.

Transmission risk from an infected man to a woman is 70% after one exposure. Transmission from an infected woman to a man is as low as 20% with one exposure but rises to 60% to 90% with four exposures.[47]

Diagnostics

Laboratory diagnosis of gonorrhea is dependent on the setting and on the availability of diagnostic laboratory facilities. Microscopic examination of gram-stained urethral or cervical specimens can detect infection with *N. gonorrhoeae*. The sensitivity of Gram's stain is higher in symptomatic men (90% to 95%) than in asymptomatic men (70%). Gram's stain is less sensitive for cervical infections in women (30% to 65%) and is not useful in diagnosing pharyngeal and rectal infections.[50]

The most sensitive and specific test for detecting gonococcal infection is direct culture from sites of exposure (urethra, endocervix, throat, rectum). However, other methods are becoming increasingly popular because of the difficulty of handling and storing the culture medium. In women, endocervical canal culture sensitivity is 86% to 96%. Urethral sensitivity is 94% to 98% in symptomatic men and 84% in asymptomatic men.[32,50,51] Male patients should refrain from voiding for at least 2 hours before testing. Female patients should void unless urethral samples are anticipated.[50,51]

In clinical settings where handling and storage of culture medium are difficult, nonculture methods of testing are popular. The most widely used methods include DNA probes and enzyme immunoassays (EIAs). EIAs are generally less accurate in low-risk populations.[32] The accuracy in a primary care population may not be as high and may result in false-positive findings in low-risk, asymptomatic individuals. The same swab can also be used to test for chlamydia. Because chlamydia and gonorrhea cause similar symptoms and often occur simultaneously (50%), diagnostic and screening tests for the two infections are usually performed together. In women who have had a hysterectomy, urethral specimens should be obtained.[51] DNA probes may only be used to test the cervix and urethra. They do not provide information on antibiotic susceptibility, are not used for tests of cure, and are not used for medicolegal purposes.[32,50]

Nucleic acid amplification tests, such as the polymerase chain reaction (PCR) and LCR, are increasingly being used for the diagnosis of many STD infections, including gonorrhea. As with chlamydia all urine LCR samples should be first-void or first-pass urine specimens (refer to the manufacturer's directions).

CHLAMYDIA

Chlamydia is an STD caused by an intracellular, parasitic organism, *C. trachomatis*. Currently there are at least 15 recognized serotypes of *C. trachomatis*. Clinical syndromes associated with certain *C. trachomatis* serotypes include NGU, mucopurulent cervicitis, PID, lymphogranuloma venereum, acute urethral syndrome in female patients, ocular infections, proctocolitis, epididymitis, and Reiter's syndrome in adults. *C. trachomatis* may be acquired by infants through an infected birth canal, causing pneumonia and conjunctivitis in newborns.[48,52]

Chlamydia is the most prevalent bacterial STD in the United States. Each year, an estimated 3 million new cases of genital infection caused by *C. trachomatis* occur in the United States at a cost of $2.4 billion.[29,31,50] Chlamydial infection is especially prevalent among adolescents. In the last two decades, genital chlamydial infection has been identified as a major public health problem because of its association with several disease syndromes, including NGU, mucopurulent cervicitis, and PID.[45,52]

In female patients these infections often result in serious reproductive tract complications. A number of factors limit documentation of the incidence and prevalence of genital chlamydial infection, including large numbers of asymptomatic persons in whom infection can be detected only through screening.[31,52,53]

Pathophysiology

C. trachomatis can be serologically divided into types A, B, and C, which are associated with trachoma; types L1, L2, and L3, which are associated with lymphogranuloma venereum; and types D through K, which are associated with genital infections and their complications.[46] The organism infects the genital tract of women most commonly at the transition zone of the endocervix.[48] Chlamydia should be suspected in female patients with probable cervicitis on the basis of mucopurulent discharge from the cervical os, easily induced bleeding, and edema in the area of ectopy.[10] In male patients symptoms often resemble those of gonorrhea. Up to 85% of women and 25% of men with chlamydia are asymptomatic (see Table 160-1).[29]

Diagnostics

Chlamydia organisms, which are obligate and intracellular, are found within urethral, cervical, and rectal epithelial cells, but not in exudate or pus. Because a specimen containing purulent discharge is inadequate for identification of the organism, the cervical os must be cleaned to remove debris and secretions. The DNA probe can be used to test for both chlamydia and gonorrhea. In the future, nucleic acid amplification tests, such as PCR and LCR, are likely to be considered the standard for diagnosis of STDs, including chlamydia. Regardless of the method used, it is important to closely follow the manufacturer's instructions for specimen collection and transport.[31,50,52]

The sensitivity of the LCR and PCR techniques has led to increased ease in specimen collection, such as simple urine and vaginal swabs rather than the more invasive sampling techniques. Screening methods using a patient-obtained vaginal swab, tampons, and sanitary napkins of self-collected samples has also been studied.[31,54,55]

Diseases Characterized by Genital Ulcers

In the United States most young, sexually active patients who have genital ulcers have either genital herpes, syphilis, or chancroid. More than one of these diseases can be present in a patient who has genital ulcers. Each has been associated with an increased risk of HIV infection.[41]

SYPHILIS

Syphilis is a complex systemic STD caused by *Treponema pallidum*. Syphilis has been classified by the CDC into several stages, depending on the length of infection (Box 160-6).[56] Patients may present with signs and symptoms of primary infection (ulcer or chancre at the infection site; see Color Plate 6), secondary infection (rash, mucocutaneous lesions, and adenopathy), or tertiary infection (cardiac, neurologic, ophthalmic, auditory, or gummatous lesions).[41]

The reemergence of syphilis between 1987 and 1990 was most notable among populations that included illicit drug users, particularly crack cocaine users and their sex partners.[29,57] At

BOX 160-6

STAGES OF SYPHILIS

Primary syphilis	Latent syphilis, unknown duration
Secondary syphilis	Neurosyphilis
Latent syphilis	Late syphilis
Early latent syphilis	Syphilitic stillbirth
Late latent syphilis	

present the reported rate of syphilis is at the lowest level since reporting began in 1941. The number of cases of primary and secondary syphilis declined by more than 22% form 1997 to 1999.[31]

Pathophysiology

Syphilis is usually spread through contact with infectious lesions that can enter the host during sexual activity through sites where the epithelium has been disrupted from minor trauma. Sexual contact with a partner who has early syphilis is associated with the highest risk of developing the disease. The mean time from exposure to the development of active infection (chancre formation) is 21 days (range 7 to 60 days). At this time the individual becomes actively infectious.[58]

Chancres typically develop at the site of inoculation. Since syphilitic lesions are painless, in contrast to lesions associated with chancroid, some patients may not be aware of them. Secondary syphilis, the hematogenous dissemination of *T. pallidum,* causes more widespread findings, including macules and papules on the trunk, neck, palms, and soles. Condylomata lata, which are raised, flat, broad, grayish papular lesions, may occur in moist areas such as the anus, scrotum, and vulva. Mucous patches (small, asymptomatic, shallow ulcerations) may occur in the oral or genital mucosa or at the angles of the mouth.[44,58,59]

The signs of primary and secondary syphilis may resolve spontaneously even without treatment. The patient then enters the latent stage of the disease, in which there are generally no clinical signs or symptoms of infection and diagnosis is made on the basis of serology. A pregnant woman with latent disease can infect her fetus.[58]

Tertiary syphilis is manifested after a variable period of latency in approximately one third of patients who fail to receive treatment. Late-stage syphilis may occur 10 to 20 years after initial infection. It may present as gummatous disease (rubbery lumps or lesions found in subcutaneous tissue), cardiovascular disease, or neurosyphilis in one third of untreated patients. Neurosyphilis can occur in all stages of syphilis. The diagnosis of neurosyphilis is based on clinical findings and examination of the serum and cerebrospinal fluid.[58]

Diagnostics

Darkfield examinations and direct fluorescent antibody tests of lesion exudate or tissue are the definitive methods for diagnosing early syphilis. Serologic testing using nontreponemal tests (e.g., Venereal Disease Research Laboratory [VDRL] and rapid plasma reagin) and treponemal tests (e.g., fluorescent treponemal antibody absorbed and microhemagglutination assay for antibody to *T. pallidum*) is done for presumptive diagnosis. The use of one test alone is not sufficient. The nontreponemal test, the initial screening test, correlates with disease activity and is reported quantitatively. The treponemal test is used to confirm the diagnosis,[37] as false-positive nontreponemal test results are associated with hepatitis, viral pneumonia, pregnancy, infectious mononucleosis, and other viral infections. Chronic false-positive findings are associated with connective tissue diseases such as systemic lupus erythematosus.[58] Patients treated for early syphilis whose nontreponemal test either shows an increase or fails to show a fourfold decline in *T. pallidum* within 6 months should be retreated. Further evaluation may also be indicated.

GENITAL HERPES

Herpes simplex virus (HSV) infection is a condition characterized by primary infection of genital or anal area with visible, painful, genital, or anal lesions or grouped vesicles at the site of inoculation and regional lymphadenopathy. Recurrent HSV infections is characterized by a normal course of recurring outbreaks of vesicles at the same site.[24] Both HSV-1 and HSV-2 can infect the genitalia. HSV-2 causes the majority of cases of genital herpes infections. It is estimated that 16% (approximately 1 in 5) of the U.S. adult population is HSV-2 seropositive.[32,60] In 1999 the estimated prevalence was 19% among the general population between 14 and 49 years old. As many as 1 million people in the United States become infected each year.[31]

Spread of genital herpes is by direct contact, with transmission by infected secretions. Transmissibility is higher with active lesions, but asymptomatic shedding of virus with transmission is also probable. Asymptomatic shedding occurs more often during the first 3 months after primary infection.[40] Most neonatal HSV-2 infections occur during delivery in women who have acquired HSV-2 during pregnancy. Neonatal HSV infections range from mild and localized infection to fatal and disseminated disease. One fourth of HSV-infected neonates develop disseminated disease, and one third have encephalitis. Even with treatment, the mortality rate is 57% among infants with disseminated disease and 15% among those with encephalitis.[32,34,60]

Pathophysiology

After an inoculation onto a mucosal surface, the virus undergoes primary replication resulting in the production of the characteristic lesion (a thin-walled vesicle on an erythematous base). With primary infection the HSV travels along sensory nerves and establishes latency within sensory nerve fibers for life. Reactivation occurs via spread down peripheral sensory nerve pathways, with further replication occurring at cutaneous sites corresponding to distributions of the sensory nerves. Reactivation can be symptomatic or asymptomatic. The sexual contacts of individuals with either symptomatic or asymptomatic disease are at risk of becoming infected.[34,43,60]

Diagnostics

Diagnosis of HSV is often a clinical decision based on the patient's history and the morphology of the lesions. The diagnosis is confirmed with a Tzanck test on tissue taken from the base of a lesion or unroofed vesicle.[44,60] Unfortunately healing lesions affect the sensitivity of virologic testing. Recently several serologic tests have been developed based on antibody to

HSV glycoproteins G1 and G2, which have antigenic specificities to HSV-1 and HSV-2.[61-63] The CDC recommends that any serologic testing for herpes simplex should use type-specific assays.[64] A new product to detect HSV-2 is the POCkit HSV-2, which allows for point-of-care testing. This test is sensitive for established HSV-2 infections only. It has no value in the diagnosis of a primary HSV-2 infection.[31,61] A number of other products are now available for serologic testing. With the newer tests, however, it may take a number of weeks for the antibody to develop, so the test will not be positive at the time of a primary outbreak.

CHANCROID

Chancroid is an STD characterized by painful genital ulceration and inflammatory inguinal adenopathy. The disease is characterized by infection with *Haemophilus ducreyi*.[56]

From 1987 to 1995, cases of chancroid in the United States have steadily declined, with approximately 3500 cases reported in 1991 and 606 cases reported in 1995.[35] In 1999 only 143 cases were reported.[11] Cases are not consistently reported from state to state.

Pathophysiology

Chancroid is a genital ulcer disease characterized by one or a few painful ulcers that develop after an incubation of 4 to 7 days. The most distinguishing feature is deep, raw, painful ulcerations. Painful inguinal adenopathy, often unilateral, develops in 50% of patients 1 to 2 weeks after the primary lesion. Buboes occur and may drain spontaneously.[44]

Diagnostics

Diagnosis is often clinical. Confirmation is based on isolation of *H. ducreyi* from a clinical specimen.[44]

OTHER ULCERATIVE DISEASES

Lymphogranuloma venereum and granuloma inguinale are two other causes of genital ulcers. The incidence of these genital ulcers is rare in the United States, with no cases of granuloma inguinale reported in 1995 and 186 cases of lymphogranuloma venereum reported in 1995.[29,35] Suspicion of either of these conditions requires consultation and often referral to a practitioner skilled in the diagnosis of STDs.[65]

Patient Education

Patient education efforts need to focus on preventing the establishment of high-risk behaviors before sexual activity is initiated. The general public is largely unaware of the health consequences of STDs because many infections are asymptomatic; major health consequences, such as infertility and chronic disease, occur years after initial infections; and the stigma associated with STDs often inhibits frank and open discussion about STDs and their consequences. Population-specific educational efforts and screening for specific STDs must be established to help curb this hidden epidemic.[29]

Many resources for patient education are available. A great deal of information is available on the Internet for both the primary care provider and the patient. The CDC, Division of STD Prevention, has not only the current treatment guidelines, but also STD fact sheets and valuable links to other sites, including the American Social Health Association. The Web site address is www.cdc.gov/nchstp/dstd/dstdp.html.

REFERENCES

1. Foxman B and others: Urinary tract infection: self-reported incidence and associated costs, *Ann Epidemiol* 10:509-515, 2000.
2. Reference deleted in galleys.
3. NCHS, CDC, DHHS: Ambulatory care visits to physician offices, hospital outpatient departments, and emergency departments: United States, 1997. Vital and Health Statistics Series 13(143), 1999.
4. Hooten TM and others: A prospective study of risk factors for symptomatic urinary tract infections in young women, *N Engl J Med* 335:468-474, 1996.
5. Stamm WE: Towards control of urinary tract infections, *Lancet Infectious Diseases* 2(2): 120-122, 2002.
6. National Nosocomial Infections Surveillance (NNIS) Systems report, Data summary from October 1986-April 1998. A report from the NNIS System, CDC, Atlanta GA, 1998.
7. Stapleton A: Prevention of recurrent urinary tract infections in women, *Lancet* 353:7-8, 1999.
8. Leiner S: Recurrent urinary tract infections in otherwise healthy women: rational strategies for work-up and management, *Nurse Pract* 20(2):48-56, 1995.
9. Krieger JN and others: Urinary tract infections in healthy university men, *J Urol* 149:1046-1048, 1993.
10. Campbell J and others: "Telephone treatment" of uncomplicated acute cystitis, *Cleve Clin J Med* 66(8):495-501, 1999.
11. Bent S and others: Does this woman have an acute uncomplicated urinary tract infection? *JAMA* 287(20):2701-2710, 2002.
12. Raz R and others: Recurrent urinary tract infection in post-menopausal women, *Clin Infect Dis* 30:152-156, 2000.
13. Ronald A, Ludwig E: Urinary tract infections in adults with diabetes, *Int J Antimicrob Agents* 17:287-292, 2001.
14. Delzell JE, Lefevre ML: Urinary tract infection during pregnancy, *Am Fam Physician* 62:713-720,2000.
15. Stapleton A, Stamm WE: Prevention of urinary tract infection, *Infect Dis Clin North Am* 11(3):719-733, 1997.
16. Hassay K: Effective management of urinary discomfort, *Nurse Pract* 20(2):36-44, 1995.
17. Gantz NM, Noskin GA: Complicated UTI: targeting the pathogens, *Patient Care* 31(7):212-223, 1997.
18. Maskell R: Broadening the concept of urinary tract infection, *Br J Urol* 76:5, 1995 (letter).
19. Kunin CM: Urinary tract infections: detection, prevention and management, ed 5, Baltimore, 1997, Williams & Wilkins.
20. Raz R and others: Empiric use of trimethoprim-sulfamethoxazole (TMP-SMX) in the treatment of women with uncomplicated urinary tract infections, in a geographical area with a high prevalence of TMP-SMX resistant uropathogens, *Clin Infect Dis* 32:1165-1169, 2002.
21. Gupta K and others: Antimicrobial resistance among uropathogens that cause community-acquired urinary tract infections in women: a nationwide analysis, *Clin Infect Dis* 33:89-94, 2001.
22. Lowe FC and Fagelman E: Cranberry juice and urinary tract infections: What is the evidence? Urology 57:407-413, 2001.
23. Triezenberg DJ: Can regular intake of either cranberry juice or a drink containing *Lactobacillus* bacteria prevent urinary tract infection (UTI) recurrence in women after an initial episode, *J Fam Pract* 50(10):841, 2001.
24. Kontiokari T and others: Randomized trial of cranberry-lingonberry juice and lactobacillus GG drink for the prevention of urinary tract infections in women, *BMJ* 322:1571, 2001.
25. Stapleton A: Urinary tract infections in patients with diabetes, *Am J Med* 133(1A):80S-84S, 2002.
26. Yoshikawa TT and others: Management of complicated urinary tract infection in older patients, *J Am Geriatr Soc* 44:1235-1241, 1996.

27. Anonymous: JAMA patient page: urinary tract infections, *JAMA* 283(12):1646, 2000.
28. Anonymous: Patient information: urinary tract infections, *Cleve Clin J Med* 66(8): 502, 1999.
29. Institute of Medicine, Committee on Prevention and Control of Sexually Transmitted Diseases: *The hidden epidemic: confronting sexually transmitted diseases,* Washington DC, 1997, National Academy Press.
30. Celum CL and others: *The management of sexually transmitted diseases,* ed 2, Seattle, 1994, Health Sciences Center for Educational Resources.
31. Center for Disease Control and Prevention: *Tracking the hidden epidemics: trends in STDs in the United States,* Bethesda, 2000, CDC.
32. US Preventive Services Task Force: *Guide to clinical preventive services,* ed 2, Baltimore, 1996, Williams & Wilkins.
33. Centers for Disease Control and Prevention: Summary of notifiable diseases, United States, MMWR 43:3-12, 1996.
34. Hook EW: Biomedical issues in syphilis control, *Sex Transm Dis* 23: 5-8, 1996.
35. Centers for Disease Control and Prevention, Division of STD Prevention: *Sexually transmitted disease surveillance,* 1995, Atlanta, 1996, US Department of Health and Human Services, Public Health Service, Centers for Disease Control and Prevention.
36. Gunn RA, Veinbergs E, Freidman LS: Adolescent health care providers: establishing a dialogue and assessing sexually transmitted disease prevention practices, *Sex Transm Dis* 24:90-93, 1997.
37. Borgatta L and others: A contemporary approach to curbing STDs, *Patient Care* 30(20):30-42, 1996.
38. Centers for Disease Control and Prevention: 1993 Guidelines for treatment of sexually transmitted diseases, *MMWR* 42(RR-14):1-102, 1993.
39. History taking. In STD/HIV Prevention Training Center of New England: Home study module, 3-day intensive course, 1997.
40. Hook EW, Sondheimer S, Zenilman J: Today's treatment for STDs, *Patient Care* 29(3):40-56, 1995.
41. Centers for Disease Control and Prevention: 2002 Guidelines for treatment of sexually transmitted diseases, *MMWR* 51(RR06):1-80, 2002.
42. Barton S and others, editors: *Clinical evidence 5,* London, 2001, British Medical Journal Publishing Group.
43. Holmes KK, Morse SA: Gonococcal infections. In Fauci A and others, editors: *Harrison's principles of internal medicine,* New York, 1998, McGraw-Hill.
44. Fitzpatrick TB and others: *Color atlas and synopsis of clinical dermatology,* ed 3, New York, 1997, McGraw-Hill.
45. Fiumara NJ: *Pictorial guide to sexually transmitted diseases,* New York, 1989, Reed Publishing.
46. Mehring PC: Sexually transmitted diseases. In Porth CM, editor: *Pathophysiology: concepts of altered health states,* ed 4, Philadelphia, 1994, JB Lippincott.
47. Rice P: Gonococcal and chlamydial infection 1996. In STD/HIV Prevention Training Center of New England: Home study module, 3-day intensive course, 1997.
48. Uphold CR, Graham MV: *Clinical guidelines in family practice,* ed 2, Gainesville, Fla, 1994, Barmarrae Books.
49. Hawkins JW, Roberto-Nichols DM, Stanley-Haney JL: *Protocols for nurse practitioners in gynecologic settings,* ed 5, New York, 1995, The Tiresias Press.
50. Sexually transmitted diseases and HIV infection. In US Department of Health and Human Services: *The clinician's handbook of preventive services,* Alexandria, Va, 1994, International Medical Publishing.
51. Sexually transmitted diseases and HIV infection. In US Department of Health and Human Services: *The clinicians' handbook of preventive services: put prevention into practice,* Alexandria, Va, 1994, International Medical Publishing.
52. Peeling RW: Chlamydia as pathogens: new species and new issues, emerging infections, *CDC* 2(4):307-319, 1996.
53. Centers for Disease Control and Prevention: Chlamydia trachomatis genital infections: United States, 1995, *MMWR* 46(9):193-198, 1997.
54. Hook EW and others: Screening for chlamydia with patient obtained vaginal swabs, *J Clin Microbiol* 33:2133-2135, 1997.
55. Cohen M: STDs: forgotten but not gone, 40th Interscience Conference on Antimicrobial Agents and Chemotherapy, Day 1, September 17, 2000.
56. Centers for Disease Control and Prevention: Case definitions for infectious conditions under public health surveillance, *MMWR* 46(RR-10): 34-37, 1997.
57. Hook EW, Marra CM: Acquired syphilis in adults, *N Engl J Med* 326(16):1060-1066, 1992.
58. Larson S, Steiner B, Rudolph A: Laboratory diagnosis and interpretation of tests for syphilis, *Clin Microbiol Rev* 8(1):1-19, 1995.
59. Felenstein D: Syphilis 1996. In STD/HIV Prevention Training Center of New England: Home study module, 3-day intensive course, 1997.
60. Dorsky D: Herpes simplex virus infections. In STD/HIV Prevention Training Center of New England: Home study module 3-day intensive course, 1997.
61. Ashley RL, Wald A, Eagleton M: Premarket evaluation of the POCkitTM HSV-2 type specific serologic test in culture documented cases of genital herpes simplex virus type 2, *Sex Transm Dis* 27(5): 266-269, 2000.
62. Whittington WL, Celum CL, Cent A, Ashley RL: Use of glycoprotein G-based type-specific assay to detect antibodies to herpes simplex virus type 2 among persons attending sexually transmitted disease clinics, *Sex Transm Dis* 28(2):99-104, 2001.
63. Cowan FM: Testing for type specific antibody to herpes simplex virus-implications for clinical practice, *J Antimicrob Chemother* 45(Suppl T-3): 9-13, 2000.
64. Division of STD Prevention. Prevention of genital HPV infection and sequelae: *Report of an external consultants meeting.* Department of health and human services, Atlanta, 1999, CDC.
65. Schmid P: Approach to the patient with genital ulcer disease, *Med Clin North Am* 74(6):1559-1572, 1990.

CHAPTER 161

Obstructive Uropathy

Joanne Sandberg-Cook

DEFINITION/EPIDEMIOLOGY

Obstructive uropathy refers to the structural or functional changes in the urinary tract that impair the flow of urine. The degree, duration, and location of the obstruction determine the extent of functional and pathologic changes in the kidney.

Obstructive uropathy is relatively common and occurs at all ages. The incidence depends directly on the causative lesion; in 1992 obstructive uropathy was the fourth leading diagnosis at discharge from hospital among men with renal or urologic disorders.[1] Obstructive uropathy accounted for 1.9% of new cases of end-stage renal disease in the United States in 1992.[1] Men are affected 3 times as often as women, with the peak incidence occurring between the ages of 75 and 79.[1]

BOX 161-1

COMMON CAUSES OF OBSTRUCTIVE UROPATHY

INTRINSIC CAUSES	EXTRINSIC CAUSES
Intraluminal	Abdominal
Stones	Ileum, left colon, duodenum
Papilla	Aneurysms
Clots	Pelvic
Fungal balls	Prostatic hypertrophy
Structural	Cysts, tumors of uterus, ovaries
Stricture	Endometriosis
Tumors, polyps	Pregnancy
Infection: granuloma	Phimosis, meatal stenosis
Anatomic defects	Retroperitoneal
Valve or sphincter abnormalities	Fibrosis
Functional	Tumor, lymphoma
Ureterovesical reflux	
Adynamic ureters	
Neurogenic bladder	

PATHOPHYSIOLOGY

Obstruction to urine flow can result from intrinsic or extrinsic mechanical blockage, as well as from functional defects not associated with a fixed occlusion. Lesions causing mechanical obstruction can occur at any level of the tract from the renal calyces to the external meatus. When the lesion is above the level of the bladder, unilateral dilation of the ureter and kidney (hydronephrosis) can occur; when the lesion is below the level of the bladder, bilateral involvement of the kidneys is the rule. Common forms of mechanical obstructions are listed in Box 161-1. In adults urinary tract obstruction is generally the result of acquired defects, whereas it is usually the result of congenital defects in children.[2] Obstruction to urine flow causes increased pressure and urine volume proximal to the obstruction. Significant or prolonged increases in pressure can cause significant damage to renal tissue, resulting in renal insufficiency and/or failure.

Functional impairment of urine flow can result from disorders that involve both the ureter and bladder. Common lesions include neurogenic bladder with adynamic ureter and vesicoureteral reflux.[2] Neurogenic bladder can be caused by upper neuron damage, which may produce involuntary micturition, or by lower spinal tract injury causing an atonic bladder. In both cases a significant urinary residual may occur, resulting in reflux of urine into the ureters and increased pressure in the upper urinary tract. This increased pressure, with its resultant decreased renal blood flow and ischemia, can result in significant injury and even death of renal tissue.

CLINICAL PRESENTATION

Pain is the most common presenting symptom. Flank pain occurring in a crescendo/decrescendo pattern radiating to the lower abdomen, testes, or labia is not uncommon in acute obstruction. Chronic or slowly developing obstructive lesions may be asymptomatic. Flank pain that occurs only with urination is pathognomonic of vesicoureteral reflux.[2] Polyuria and nocturia can be seen in chronic partial obstruction. Total complete bilateral obstruction results in total anuria. Hesitancy and straining to initiate a urinary stream, postvoid dribbling, frequency, and overflow incontinence are common complaints of patients with obstruction at or below the bladder level. Noting the pattern of urinary output, particularly whether the pattern has changed abruptly, has gradually declined, or fluctuates, is important. Recurrent urinary tract infections can also be seen with chronic partial obstructions. A past medical history of renal calculi is relevant. A medication history or a history of illicit drug use should also be elicited.

PHYSICAL EXAMINATION

A general physical examination should be performed on all patients. Blood pressure measurement is critical because both acute and chronic hydronephrosis can be accompanied by severe hypertension. A fever may indicate infection. Palpation and percussion of the abdomen often reveal bladder distention. An enlarged, tender kidney may be noted, especially in thin patients. This will manifest as a flank mass or increased abdominal girth. In men a rectal examination will determine the size of the prostate gland and the presence of nodules. The penis should be inspected for evidence of meatal stricture or phimosis. In women a pelvic examination, including careful inspection of the external genitalia, will reveal vaginal, uterine, or rectal lesions that might cause urinary tract obstruction. Signs of azotemia, including pallor, skin changes, volume expansion, or depletion can be seen.

DIAGNOSTICS

In the office setting, ascertaining postvoid residual urine will provide information about the residual volume. Catheterization will provide a sterile urine specimen for analysis. Routine blood studies are often nonspecific, but a CBC (looking for anemia) and electrolytes, BUN, and creatinine (to determine renal function) may be helpful. Urinalysis is necessary for all patients in whom an obstructive uropathy is suspected. Gross

Diagnostics

Obstructive Uropathy

Initial
Postvoid residual
Urine dip for leukocytes, nitrites, blood

Laboratory
CBC and differential
Serum electrolytes
BUN
Creatinine
Serum glucose
Urinalysis
Urine cultures*
Blood cultures*

Imaging
KUB
IV pyelogram
Ultrasound
CT scan

Other
Antegrade/retrograde pyelography
Whitaker's test
Cystoscopy
Urodynamics

*If indicated.

hematuria can be seen in acute obstruction, especially when the obstruction is caused by calculi or a bladder tumor. Uric acid crystals in the urine sediment raise the suspicion of uric acid nephropathy or calculi. A urine culture will exclude infection. A blood glucose or hemoglobin A_{1c} level can help exclude diabetes. The need for further studies depends on the symptom complex and results of the previously mentioned studies.

In patients with flank pain, renal calculus must be excluded. This can be done with plain (kidney-ureter-gladder [KUB]) films of the abdomen. If calculus is found, an IV pyelogram will help determine the degree of obstruction. If renal function is impaired, diagnostic ultrasound evaluation is the preferred procedure for visualization of the renal pelvis and for the diagnosis of hydronephrosis.[1] Urodynamics may be helpful in diagnosing lower tract obstruction. CT scanning can be helpful in uncertain diagnostic circumstances but can be costly and is not always available. Other procedures useful in determining the site of obstruction include antegrade or retrograde pyelography. Pressure flow studies (Whitaker's test) may be required to diagnose upper tract obstruction or in those cases in which a partial obstruction of uncertain clinical significance is discovered.[3] Finally, cystoscopy provides direct visualization of the bladder, urethra, prostate, and ureteral openings.

DIFFERENTIAL DIAGNOSIS

A history of difficulty in voiding, recurrent infection, pain, or changes in urinary volume are common. Causes of obstruction can be congenital, acquired intrinsic defects, or acquired extrinsic defects. Obstruction can occur at any level of the urinary tract but is most common at the level of the ureter, the bladder outlet, and the urethra. Some of the more common causes of obstructive uropathy are listed in Box 161-1.

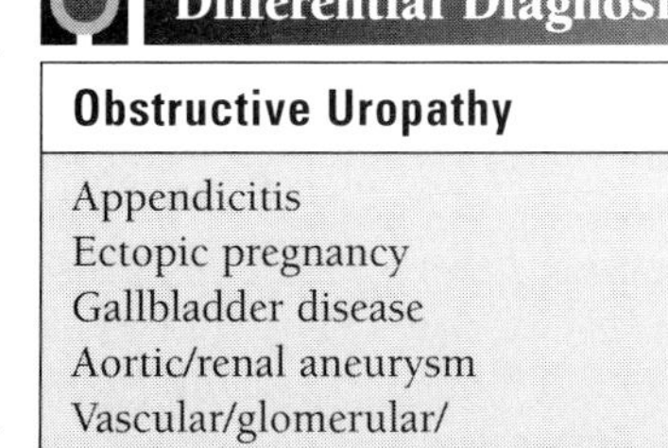

Differential Diagnosis

Obstructive Uropathy

Appendicitis
Ectopic pregnancy
Gallbladder disease
Aortic/renal aneurysm
Vascular/glomerular/tubulointerstitial disease

In patients with flank pain, abnormalities of adjacent structures and referred pain should be considered. This can include appendicitis, ectopic pregnancy, gallbladder disease, aortic aneurysm, and renal aneurysm. In patients with renal insufficiency, other causes of renal failure must be considered, including vascular, glomerular, and tubulointerstitial diseases.[3]

MANAGEMENT

Treatment to relieve partial obstruction is indicated when the patient has (1) repeated infections, (2) significant symptoms, (3) urinary retention, and (4) impairment of renal function. Urinary tract obstruction complicated by infection should be relieved as soon as possible to prevent the development of sepsis, preserve renal function, normalize blood pressure, correct imbalances in fluid and electrolytes, and treat pain.

The acute treatment of lower tract obstruction is catheterization. Obstruction caused by prostatic hypertrophy is not always progressive, and the patient need not be treated unless there is retention, recurrent infection, or symptoms not acceptable to the patient. These might include frequency, nocturia, difficulty initiating a urinary stream, dribbling, or overflow incontinence. Chronic urinary retention due to prostatic hypertrophy may respond to alpha$_1$-blockers such as terazosin (Hytrin), tamsulosin hydrochloride (Flomax), or doxazosin mesylate (Cardura). Finasteride (Proscar) can be effective for relieving symptoms of benign prostatic hypertrophy (BPH) by reducing the size of the prostate, thereby increasing the urinary flow (see Chapter 163).

The decision to undertake surgical or instrumental procedures for the relief of obstruction depends on the location of the obstruction, the presence of infection, and the patient's renal function. Relief of a complete obstruction should occur as soon as possible after diagnosis. Infection raises the risk of sepsis; therefore infection should be treated before surgical procedures whenever it is possible to wait. If the patient is in renal failure, dialysis may be necessary before instrumentation. In patients with calculi, it may be possible to wait while providing pain relief, fluids, and ongoing evaluation of renal function (see Chapter 165).

LIFE SPAN CONSIDERATIONS

Obstructive uropathy occurs at all ages. New ultrasound techniques have made it possible to diagnose obstruction in the fetus during pregnancy. In the young and middle-aged, acute obstruction is most likely caused by calculi. In women, pelvic cancer is an important cause. In the older man, the most common association is with BPH or cancer.

COMPLICATIONS

Complications of untreated urinary tract obstruction include azotemia, life-threatening sepsis, nocturia, fluctuating urine volume, and obstructive nephropathy that can lead to chronic renal insufficiency or renal failure. The development of renal failure secondary to obstruction is related to the development of interstitial fibrosis. Recent studies have suggested that the administration of ACE inhibitors may slow the development of interstitial fibrosis.[4]

Complications of surgical procedures include infection, sepsis, bleeding, difficulty voiding, and pain. A profound and prolonged diuresis known as postobstructive diuresis can follow the relief of obstruction. This diuresis is characterized by marked losses of water and sodium as well as an inability to acidify the urine.[4] The exact mechanisms that account for this are unknown. Careful replacement of fluids while monitoring weight, plasma, and urine electrolytes is necessary.[1]

INDICATIONS FOR REFERRAL/HOSPITALIZATION

Renal calculi greater than 7 mm usually do not pass spontaneously and should be treated surgically. These patients should be referred to an urologist or a lithotripsy center. Patients with anuria and acute renal failure should be referred to a nephrologist for management. Hospitalization and/or dialysis may be indicated. Patients with chronic or intermittent urinary retention may benefit from consultation with technicians or urologic nurses who can teach self-catheterization.

PATIENT AND FAMILY EDUCATION

Patients with urinary tract obstruction are often uncomfortable and often frightened. Every effort should be made to alleviate their discomfort and to provide information and reassurance. All patients with obstruction should be taught the signs and symptoms of infection, including how to take their own temperature. Patients whose obstruction is caused by calculi need to understand that the likelihood of recurrence is high. Adequate daily fluid intake may help prevent recurrence. Dietary modification, depending on the type of stone, may be indicated.[5] Patients with prostatic hypertrophy taking alpha-blockers need to be advised of the potential for postural hypotension and confusion, especially in older adults. All patients need to know how to access the health care system in an emergency situation whether at home or while traveling.

REFERENCES

1. Klahr S: Obstructive uropathy. In Stein J and others, editors: *Internal medicine,* ed 5, St Louis, 1998, Mosby.
2. Seifter J, Brenner B: Urinary tract obstruction. In Isselbacher KJ and others, editors: *Harrison's principles on internal medicine,* ed 13, New York, 1994, McGraw-Hill.
3. Garrick R: Obstructive nephropathy. In Hurst JW, editor: *Medicine for the practicing physician,* ed 4, Stamford, Conn, 1996, Appleton & Lange.
4. Klahir S: Obstructive nephropathy, *Intern Med* 39(5):355-361, 2000.
5. Gray M: *Genitourinary disorders,* St Louis, 1992, Mosby.

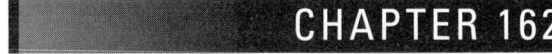

CHAPTER 162

Pregnancy in Renal Disease

Patricia Polgar Bailey and Terry Mahan Buttaro

DEFINITION/EPIDEMIOLOGY

Advances in the management of pregnancy in women with renal disease during the past two decades have resulted in remarkably improved maternal and neonatal outcomes. The effect of renal dysfunction on pregnancy depends on several factors, including the degree of maternal renal impairment at the time of conception, the presence of hypertension at the time of conception and during pregnancy, the type of underlying renal disease, and maternal co-morbidity.[1] Fetal survival rates in women with mild renal insufficiency are approximately 95%. In women with more serious renal disease, fetal survival rates are as low as 50% to 75%, with a high proportion of premature deliveries and low-birth-weight infants. Pregnancy in women with end-stage renal disease (ESRD) occurs rarely; only approximately 1% of women of childbearing age on dialysis become pregnant. The overall success rate of pregnancies in women with ESRD averages 50%.[2]

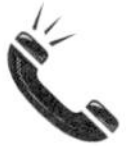

Physician consultation is indicated for the pregnant woman with underlying renal disease, deteriorating renal function, and suspected pyelonephritis.

PATHOPHYSIOLOGY

During a normal pregnancy, renal function changes significantly. Maternal extracellular fluid, especially plasma volume, increases (by 30% to 50%) to provide adequate blood supply to the fetoplacental unit. Renal plasma flow increases by 80%, and the glomerular filtration rate (GFR) increases by 50% from the end of the first trimester.[3] As a result of these changes, serum creatinine falls to approximately 0.7 mg/dl and BUN falls to 9 mg/dl. Blood pressure also drops during pregnancy to an average of 105/60 mm Hg. Hyperfusion causes an increase in kidney size of 1 to 1.5 cm. High plasma levels of progesterone contribute to dilation of the ureters and renal calices, which is referred to as *hydronephrosis of pregnancy.* There is an increased chance of the development of bacteriuria because of the sluggish urine flow through the dilated renal tubules. These changes remain throughout pregnancy and return to baseline values at the end of the pregnancy. Identifying renal disease in pregnancy must take into consideration the normal physiologic changes during pregnancy because what might be considered normal blood pressure and renal function values in many adults are clearly elevated values in pregnant women.[2]

The effect of pregnancy on the course of chronic renal disease has not been clearly established. In women with primary glomerulonephritis and mild renal insufficiency (serum creatinine <1.4 mg/dl) at the time of conception, pregnancy may induce an increase in serum creatinine and increasing hypertension. However, renal function generally returns to baseline postpartum. Fetal loss (not considering therapeutic abortions), according to several recent large studies, is approximately 21%, with a preterm delivery rate of 19% in this population. In women with more advanced renal disease, pregnancy may induce an acceleration in renal failure, as well as a worsening fetal outcome.[2,3]

It is generally accepted that the fetal prognosis is not determined by the type of glomerular disease; rather it is determined by the presence or absence of risk factors associated with the nephropathy, including the level of proteinuria, hypertension, and the degree of renal function impairment at the time of conception. In women with primary nonglomerular kidney disease, maternal and fetal morbidity correlates most significantly with the level of renal functioning at the time of conception. In certain diseases such as autosomal dominant polycystic kidney disease (ADPKD), pregnancy outcomes are generally uncompromised because the majority of women with ADPKD of childbearing age have normal renal function. In contrast, fetal and maternal outcomes are at greater risk in women with diabetes who have overt nephropathy and impaired renal function.[3]

In women with renal impairment due to systemic disease, pregnancy can be quite problematic, with poor maternal and fetal outcomes. Disease activity may exacerbate during the pregnancy; in addition, the sequelae associated with the multisystem disease may add to those risk factors specific to the renal disease.[3]

CLINICAL PRESENTATION AND PHYSICAL EXAMINATION

Irregular menses are common among women with renal disease; because renal impairment progresses to ESRD, increasing numbers of women do not ovulate and are amenorrheic. However, during the past decade there have been significant advances in medical therapies for women with renal disease. The use of recombinant human erythropoietin therapy—a therapy that in addition to its effects on hypothalamic function may also improve sexual interest and function—has been introduced. In addition, increasing percentages of women with advanced renal disease are menstruating compared with earlier reports: approximately 40% compared with 10% a decade ago. A significant percentage of those women who are sexually active report not using any method of birth control, perhaps because of their misperception regarding infertility.[4]

Women with renal impairment may assume that missed menses are due to the menstrual irregularity associated with their disease. Increasingly, women with renal disease are able to conceive; thus all sexually active women of childbearing age with renal impairment who present with missed menses should have a serum human chorionic gonadotropin (hCG) sample drawn to exclude pregnancy. However, serum hCG can be elevated in women with severe renal disease (and increased serum creatinine), so ultrasound may be necessary to determine viable pregnancy.[5] Menstrual irregularities and amenorrhea occur most often in women with higher serum creatinine levels. After renal transplantation, menstrual irregularities may improve. Providers should maintain a high index of suspicion that amenorrhea may be due to pregnancy in women with milder renal insufficiency and in those with renal transplants. The physical examination should include the standard prenatal evaluation and renal function tests.

In some women renal disease first manifests itself during pregnancy. A presentation that includes proteinurea, hypertension, or an elevated serum creatinine level is suspicious for renal disease. Such a constellation of signs also mimics preeclampsia, especially when it occurs during the latter half of pregnancy, and accurate diagnosis depends on further evaluation.

DIAGNOSTICS AND DIFFERENTIAL DIAGNOSIS

Urinalysis and renal function should be monitored regularly. Because anemia is associated with both pregnancy and renal disease, the hemoglobin and hematocrit should be checked at regular intervals to determine the need for erythropoietin. Pregnancy in women with lupus nephritis requires screening for lupus anticoagulant activity.[5]

MANAGEMENT

Multidisciplinary management of pregnancy in women with renal disease, preferably in a tertiary care facility, with close coordination among a specialist in high-risk obstetric care, an attendant neonatal intensive care unit, and a nephrologist, is essential. Referrals should be made at the beginning of gestation, and close multidisciplinary care should continue throughout the pregnancy.[2]

Maternal renal function and blood pressure control are the two most important determinant factors of fetal outcome. There is general agreement that high blood pressure in pregnant women with renal disease should be treated more aggressively than in patients with isolated essential hypertension. What constitutes optimal blood pressure control in these women is still being debated; however, research suggests that the diastolic blood pressure maintained between 80 and 90 mm Hg may be a useful criterion.[3] In general, the blood pressure goal should be less than 120/80 mm Hg to preserve renal function.

Monthly monitoring of renal status for asymptomatic bacteriuria, proteinuria, and preeclampsia are also important components of management.[5] Progress in obstetric and neonatal care has increased the probability that women with impaired renal function will be able to give birth to living infants, albeit often premature infants of low birth weight, without a prohibitive risk of worsening the mother's renal function. Crucial to the best possible maternal and fetal outcome is closely coordinated care between the obstetrician and the nephrologist, and optimal blood pressure control.[6]

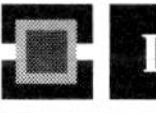

Diagnostics

Pregnancy in Renal Disease

Laboratory
Hemoglobin and hematocrit
Serum hCG
Urinalysis*
24-Hour urine for proteinuria*
BUN, creatinine*

Imaging
Ultrasound as determined by obstetrician

*As determined by nephrologist.

COMPLICATIONS

The two most significant complications of pregnancy in women with chronic renal disease are an acceleration of maternal renal disease and poor fetal outcome. Maternal morbidity is due primarily to the increased risk of preeclampsia, hypertension, or both. Fetal morbidity is principally related to the increased risk of preterm delivery and intrauterine growth retardation (IUGR).[2]

The effect of pregnancy in women with renal disease depends on several factors, including whether renal impairment is the primary disease or is associated with a systemic process and on the level of renal function at the time of conception.[3] Pregnancy in women with renal insufficiency but with preserved renal function and normal blood pressure at the time of conception generally does not result in a worsening of the maternal renal condition.[4] However, IUGR is seen even with mild renal disease (serum creatinine <1.4 mg/dl).[2] In contrast, if renal function is significantly impaired and/or there is coexisting hypertension at the time of conception, the probability of poor maternal and fetal outcome is significantly increased. An accelerated deterioration of maternal renal function during pregnancy has been reported in one third or more of women with significantly compromised renal function. In addition, the fetal loss rate is as high as 16% to 33% (not including first-trimester abortions), and a high proportion of premature deliveries and low-birth-weight infants has been reported in this population.[6] Pregnancy in women with ESRD on maintenance dialysis is rare. Fertility is decreased in these women as a result of uremia-associated hypothalamopituitary dysfunction, which results in ovarian dysfunction and anovulatory cycles.[2] The diagnosis of pregnancy can be difficult and is generally made late. The perinatal course is generally complicated, with a poor fetal outcome. In addition, the high risk of an unsuccessful outcome can precipitate an emotional crisis in women who are already experiencing significant stress in association with their chronic illness. However, with improved dialysis efficacy and as the general condition of patients on dialysis improves, fertility has been augmented and there is reason to have a more optimistic view about the course of pregnancy. Appropriate contraception is necessary for all women with renal dysfunction who are of childbearing age to prevent unplanned or unwanted pregnancies.[2,3]

INDICATIONS FOR REFERRAL/HOSPITALIZATION

Pregnant women with underlying renal disease or women who develop renal dysfunction during pregnancy require careful management by specialists. All pregnant women with underlying renal disease or deteriorating renal function should be referred to a nephrologist and a specialist in high-risk obstetric care. Because the risk of fetal mortality is significantly higher for these women, hospitalization in a tertiary care facility is advised for delivery or for any other problems associated with the pregnancy.

PATIENT AND FAMILY EDUCATION

Women with preexisting renal disease who are considering pregnancy should have preconception counseling about their prospects for a successful pregnancy and the effect of pregnancy on their underlying disease. Pregnancy in all women with renal disease should, insofar as possible, be planned so that conception takes place at a time when risks are minimal. Patients with primary renal disease and normal or near-normal renal function have few contraindications to pregnancy. The best time for patients with systemic renal disease, such as systemic lupus erythematosus, to conceive is after stable remission of the disease process for at least 1 year. Diabetic women with nephropathy should achieve optimal glycemic control before conceiving. Women with diabetes and hypertension are at particularly high risk for poor pregnancy outcomes. These higher risks should be discussed when counseling women who are considering childbearing. In addition, women should be counseled about the importance of optimal blood pressure control and close follow-up from the time of conception and throughout the pregnancy.[1,3]

REFERENCES

1. Holley JL and others: Pregnancy outcomes in a prospective matched control study of pregnancy and renal disease, *Clin Nephrol* 45(2):77-82, 1996.
2. Clark EC, Sterns RH: Chronic renal disease. In Leppert PC, Howard R, editors: *Primary care for women,* Philadelphia, 1997, Lippincott-Raven.
3. Jungers P, Chauveau D: Pregnancy in renal disease, *Kidney Int* 52(4):871-875, 1997.
4. Holley JL and others: Gynecologic and reproductive issues in women on dialysis, *Am J Kidney Dis* 29(5):685-690, 1997.
5. Rose BD and other: *Pregnancy in women with underlying renal disease.* Retrieved September 6, 2002, from the World Wide Web: www.uptodate online.com.
6. Jungers P and others: Pregnancy in women with impaired renal function, *Clin Nephrol* 47(5):281-288, 1997.

CHAPTER 163

Prostate Disorders

Carol A. Whelan

Benign Prostatic Hyperplasia

DEFINITION/EPIDEMIOLOGY

Benign prostatic hyperplasia (BPH) is a noncancerous enlargement of the prostate gland. BPH is an almost ubiquitous phenomenon, occurring in up to 90% of all men by the eighth decade of life.[1]

PATHOPHYSIOLOGY

The prostate gland undergoes its first growth spurt during puberty and attains an average size of 20 g by age 20. The gland then undergoes a second growth spurt during the fifth decade of life. This growth is characterized by localized proliferation in the periureteral region, leading to glandular compression, which may cause ureteral compression.[1]

The development of the prostate gland is dependent on androgen secretion, and both the presence of testes and advancing age are necessary for the development of BPH.[1] Dihydrotestosterone (DHT) is the main mediator of the growth and secretory function of the prostate and is the active metabolite that results from testosterone conversion.[2] BPH seems to be related to a complex interaction between androgen and estrogen secretion; abnormal serum elevations of androgen and estrogen stimulate prostatic growth. Other factors that contribute to prostatic enlargement appear to be related to the elaboration of certain growth factors, the formation and maintenance of DHT levels, and the functioning of androgen receptors.[2]

CLINICAL PRESENTATION

Symptoms of BPH are either obstructive or irritative in character. Obstructive symptoms include urinary hesitancy, decreased caliber and force of the stream, and postvoid dribbling. These symptoms are related to bladder outlet obstruction. Irritative symptoms include frequency, urgency, and nocturia and occur as a result of decreased functional bladder capacity and instability, or infection. Occasionally, hematuria accompanies BPH. Episodic symptoms may be present over many years with a very gradual increase in the intensity of symptoms over time.

A thorough history is important. Current over-the-counter and prescription medication use should be explored to determine the presence of anticholinergics, which can impair bladder contractility, or sympathomimetics, which increase outflow resistance. Diuretics, which can cause an increased output of urine, may lead to urinary retention, especially in the presence of partially decompensated detrusor muscle.

BPH symptoms may be quantified using a symptom index developed by the American Urologic Association (Table 163-1)[3] to aid in classifying symptom severity and in developing a treatment plan. Symptoms are rated according to frequency of occurrence. A score of 0 to 7 indicates mild symptoms; 8 to 19, moderate symptoms; and 20 to 35, severe symptoms.

PHYSICAL EXAMINATION

A digital rectal examination (DRE) and a focused neurologic examination assessing sacral nerve roots are recommended to evaluate for rectal or prostate malignancy, to determine neurologic

TABLE 163-1 American Urologic Association Symptom Index for BPH

Questions to Be Answered	Not at All	Less than One Time in Five	Less than Half the Time	About Half the Time	More than Half the Time	Almost Always
Over the past month, how often have you had a sensation of not emptying your bladder completely after you finish urinating?	0	1	2	3	4	5
Over the past month, how often have you had to urinate again less than 2 hours after you finished urinating?	0	1	2	3	4	5
Over the past month, how often have you found you stopped and started again several times when you urinated?	0	1	2	3	4	5
Over the past month, how often have you found it difficult to postpone urination?	0	1	2	3	4	5
Over the past month, how often have you had a weak urinary stream?	0	1	2	3	4	5
Over the past month, how often have you had to push or strain to begin urination?	0	1	2	3	4	5
Over the past month, how many times did you most typically get up to urinate from the time you went to bed at night until the time you got up in the morning?	0 (None)	1 (1 time)	2 (2 times)	3 (3 times)	4 (4 times)	5 (5 times)

From Barry MJ and others: The American Urologic Association symptom index for benign prostatic hyperplasia, *J Urol* 148(5):1549-1557, 1992.

problems that may result in bladder symptoms, and to evaluate anal sphincter tone. A lower abdominal examination is necessary to ascertain bladder distention from urinary retention. Prostatic nodules or induration should be noted on rectal examination because these findings suggest prostate cancer. The normal prostate is heart shaped and measures approximately 4 × 3 × 2 cm. With BPH there may be uniform or focal enlargement of the prostate. The size of the prostate does not always correlate with symptom severity, however, and should not direct therapy. The median sulcus is often obliterated in BPH, and it is often difficult to palpate over the base of the prostate because of the gland's enlarged size in advanced stages. With BPH the gland is nontender and should be rubbery and smooth in consistency.

DIAGNOSTICS

A urinalysis should be performed to exclude a urinary tract infection or the presence of hematuria. Determination of the creatinine level is necessary to assess renal function. Elevation of the creatinine level is an indication for urologic evaluation of the upper urinary tract.[4] Measurement of serum prostate-specific antigen (PSA) is considered an optional test in the assessment of patients with BPH unless physical findings on DRE are suspicious of prostate cancer.[4] The PSA test is a less specific indicator of prostate cancer in men who have BPH, but men should be advised that they have a 10% to 15% risk of having coexistent prostate cancer and that the PSA test is available for screening.[5] Assessment of free PSA may help increase specificity for prostate cancer.

DIFFERENTIAL DIAGNOSIS

Symptoms of bladder outlet obstruction mandate evaluation for bladder calculi, urethral stricture, cancer of the prostrate, and bladder neck contracture. Bladder cancer should be a consideration in a male patient with unexplained hematuria. Urinary tract infection must be excluded if there are complaints of irritative voiding symptoms. If abnormalities are found on neurologic examination and problems with urinary retention are present, neurologic disease must be considered.[6] Prostate cancer should be considered when an asymmetric enlargement, nodule, or induration is palpated on rectal examination.

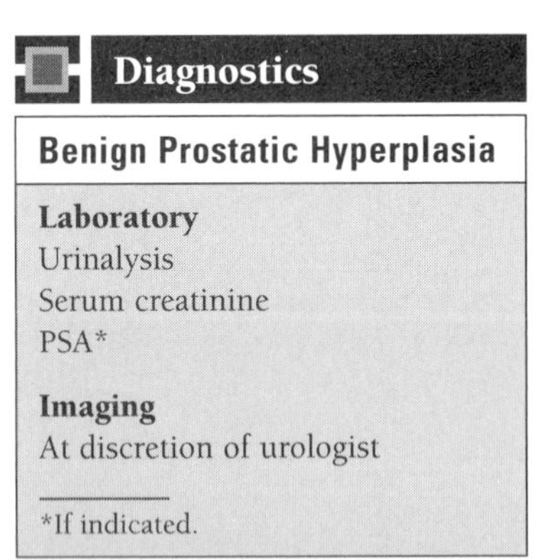
Diagnostics

Benign Prostatic Hyperplasia

Laboratory
Urinalysis
Serum creatinine
PSA*

Imaging
At discretion of urologist

*If indicated.

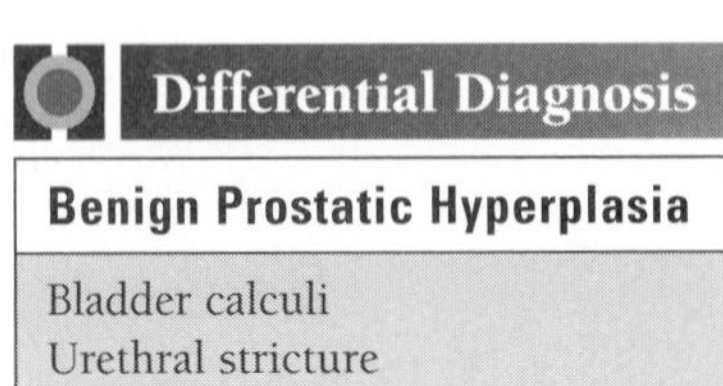
Differential Diagnosis

Benign Prostatic Hyperplasia

Bladder calculi
Urethral stricture
Bladder neck contracture
Cancer
Urinary tract infection
Neurologic disorder

MANAGEMENT

The management goal for treatment of BPH is relief of symptoms. Treatment options include watchful waiting, finasteride therapy, alpha$_1$-adrenergic antagonist therapy, balloon dilation, or surgery.[4] The benefits and risks associated with each treatment should be carefully explained to the patient. It is important to advise the patient that if a choice of watchful waiting is made, consideration of other treatment approaches is possible at any time if symptoms increase.

Alpha$_1$-adrenergic antagonists lower bladder neck and ureteral resistance. Finasteride (a 5-alpha-reductase enzyme inhibitor) shrinks prostatic glandular hyperplasia by decreasing tissue DHT levels.[1] Evidence for benefit exists for the use of both finasteride and alpha$_1$-adrenergic antagonist therapy[1,7,8]; however, in men with BPH of less than 40 g, alpha$_1$-adrenergic therapy appears to be superior to therapy with finasteride.[7] Recent studies suggest that finasteride may be superior in patients with prostatic enlargement greater than 40 g and in patients with hematuria from BPH.[1,9]

Limited evidence exists for benefit regarding the use of saw palmetto extract in the treatment of mild BPH.[10,11] Therapy with saw palmetto extract appears to be safe with little or no adverse effects.[10,11]

Balloon dilation reduces symptoms in the short term, but the long-term follow-up of the procedure has not been adequately studied. Transurethral resection of the prostate (TURP), transurethral incision of the prostate (TUIP), and open prostatectomy are surgical procedures that are effective for severe BPH.

COMPLICATIONS

Urinary tract infection and urinary retention are common sequelae of BPH. In addition, urinary retention can result in renal problems if not detected early.

INDICATIONS FOR REFERRAL/HOSPITALIZATION

Referral to a urologist is necessary for surgical intervention. Indications for surgery include urinary retention; intractable symptoms related to obstruction; recurrent or persistent urinary tract infection; recurrent prostatic bleeding; significant postvoid residual; changes in the kidneys, ureters, or bladder caused by prostatic obstruction; an abnormally low urinary flow rate; or bladder calculi. IV urography, filling cystometry, uroflowmetry, urethrocystoscopy, pressure-flow studies, and postvoid residuals may be helpful in individual situations, and their need can best be determined by a urologist. They are not recommended as standard tests for the evaluation of BPH.[4]

Acute urinary retention with a distended bladder confirmed by palpation or catheterization increases the risk of infection and renal complications, and hospitalization may be indicated.

PATIENT AND FAMILY EDUCATION

Patients should understand the advantages and risks of each treatment option so that informed decisions can be made. The patient should be advised of the importance of monitoring symptom progression and to report any abrupt change in symptom pattern, which may indicate a complication or another pathologic process.

Prostatitis

DEFINITION/EPIDEMIOLOGY

Prostatitis, or inflammation of the prostate gland, is a common problem in the adult male population. There are four basic types of prostatitis: acute bacterial, chronic bacterial, nonbacterial, and prostatodynia. Accurate diagnostic differentiation of these is a prerequisite for effective management.

The prostate gland, through which the urethra passes, is an organ that is located adjacent to and at the inferior aspect of the bladder. Bacterial prostatitis (both acute and chronic) is caused by bacterial inflammation. However, nonbacterial prostatitis, for which there is no identifiable etiology, is the most common cause of prostatic inflammation. Prostatodynia is characterized by symptoms of prostatic inflammation but without signs of inflammation on physical examination. It has been estimated that 25% of male primary care visits with genitourinary complaints are related to prostatitis.[12]

PATHOPHYSIOLOGY

The organisms responsible for acute and chronic prostatitis are usually gram-negative organisms and include *Escherichia coli, Klebsiella, Pseudomonas, Proteus,* and *Enterobacter* species, with *E. coli* being the most common.[13] Other enterococci that are normally found in feces can also cause prostatitis. A zinc-containing antibacterial factor present in normal prostatic fluid aids in resisting infection. Abnormally low levels of this factor have been associated with bacterial prostatitis.[2]

Acute bacterial prostatitis results from the ascent of organized, colonized bacteria from the lower urethra to the prostate. The urethral bacteria may be a result of infection or normal fecal flora. Increases in intraurethral pressure as a result of intercourse can result in bacterial deposition into the prostate. Difficulty in bacterial eradication increases the risk of chronic infection. Urologic instrumentation is another common cause of acute bacterial prostatitis.

The cause of nonbacterial prostatitis is less clear. *Ureaplasma urealyticum, Chlamydia, Gardnerella,* and *Mycoplasma* organisms have occasionally been found on urine and prostatic secretion cultures and are considered potential causative agents. However, their actual significance is unknown. Nonbacterial prostatitis may have a noninfectious inflammatory etiology that is possibly related to autoimmune dysfunction.[6]

The cause of prostatodynia is also unknown. There is some evidence that it may be related to a neurologic disorder that results in voiding dysfunction and in dysfunction of the pelvic floor musculature.[6,14]

CLINICAL PRESENTATION

Fever, chills, malaise, myalgias, and arthralgias are common with acute bacterial prostatitis. Genitourinary symptoms include hesitancy, frequency, urgency, nocturia, dysuria, and a sensation of incomplete bladder emptying. Accompanying complaints may be low back pain, perineal pain, or suprapubic pain. PSA levels are often markedly elevated and should not be checked in prostatitis because they are not reliable indicators of either infection or cure.

The presentation of chronic prostatitis tends to be more varied than acute prostatitis and may include a history of recurrent urinary tract infection (usually with the same organism) and complaints of urinary frequency, urgency, and burning on urination. Perineal, inguinal, or suprapubic pain may be present.[15]

Nonbacterial prostatitis is characterized by prostatic pain or vague discomfort of the suprapubic, scrotal, inguinal, lower back, or perineal areas. Pain on ejaculation may also occur. Urinary symptoms such as hesitancy, a decrease in the urinary stream, frequency, urgency, and burning on urination may also be present.

Symptoms suggestive of prostatodynia include pain and discomfort in the pelvic area and problems related to urinary flow. Urinary symptoms may include hesitancy, an interrupted flow, postvoid dribbling, and decreased flow. Frequency, urgency, and nocturia may be present. Penile and urethral pain, as well as discomfort in the lower back, suprapubic area, testicles, groin, and perineum, is often reported. There usually is no history of urinary tract infection, but there may be a lifetime history of voiding difficulties.

PHYSICAL EXAMINATION

An abdominal examination and a rectal examination are important components of the physical examination for symptoms related to the prostate. The abdominal examination should exclude bladder distention, and the prostate gland should be examined for size, consistency, and the presence of tenderness. Normally, the prostate is heart shaped and measures approximately 4 × 3 × 2 cm.

In acute bacterial prostatitis the prostate is typically enlarged, with tenderness and induration. The prostate examination should be performed gently, and excessive manipulation of the prostate should be avoided to avoid inducing bacteremia. Urinary retention and fever may be present.

The prostate examination in chronic bacterial prostatitis may be nonspecific or may reveal a tender or boggy prostate. In nonbacterial prostatitis the prostate examination is usually normal, but occasionally a soft, boggy prostate with tenderness may be present. Physical examination in prostatodynia is unremarkable with the exception that increased anal sphincter tone and paraprostatic tenderness may be present.

DIAGNOSTICS

The history and physical examination are often adequate to diagnose prostatitis. Examination of expressed prostatic secretions (EPS) may be helpful to both diagnose and determine the type of prostatitis, but it should not be done if acute prostatitis is suspected. Segmented urine specimens representing the urethral (voided bladder [VB] 1), bladder (VB2), EPS, and postprostatic massage (VB3) contents are obtained and viewed for the presence of WBCs. More than 10 WBCs per high-power field on the EPS or spun VB3 is suggestive of bacterial prostatitis. Cultures of the EPS and VB3 specimens should show significant growth of colonies (>5000/ml) with bacterial prostatitis.

The segmented urine specimens are collected after foreskin retraction and cleaning of the glans penis. The first 10-ml specimen is labeled VB1. A midstream urine specimen is labeled VB2. The practitioner should then ask the patient to bend over while the patient is retracting the foreskin and holding a specimen container in front of the meatus. The practitioner should press on the lateral lobe of the prostate and slide the examining

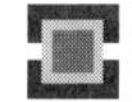 **Diagnostics**

Prostatitis

Laboratory
Segmented urine specimens for culture and sensitivity
CBC and differential
BUN
Creatinine

Imaging
At discretion of urologist

finger toward the midline 6 or 7 times on each side of the prostate. Milking the secretions by applying gentle pressure on the bulbous urethra may be necessary to obtain the prostatic secretion (EPS). The VB3 specimen is the 5 to 10 ml of urine passed immediately after prostatic massage. Because bacterial prostatitis is almost always caused by gram-negative organisms, many clinicians choose to initially treat suspected prostatitis empirically based on history and physical examination.

If acute bacterial prostatitis is suspected, prostatic massage should be avoided to minimize a risk of bacteremia. In acute bacterial prostatitis the urinalysis results may reveal pyuria, bacteriuria, and varying degrees of hematuria, with urine culture necessary for organism identification. A CBC is significant for increased numbers of leukocytes with a left shift.

In chronic bacterial prostatitis the urinalysis is normal unless there is a coexistent cystitis. However, both the EPS and VB3 specimens show increased numbers of leukocytes. Culture of the organisms in the VB3 specimen is necessary for diagnosis.

Urine cultures are negative with nonbacterial prostatitis, but increased numbers of leukocytes are seen in the EPS specimen. In prostatodynia the urine and EPS specimens are normal. Urodynamic testing may show signs of dysfunctional voiding.

DIFFERENTIAL DIAGNOSIS

The diagnosis of acute prostatitis is usually made on the basis of the clinical presentation and the markedly tender prostate on physical examination. It can be distinguished from acute pyelonephritis, acute epididymitis, and acute diverticulosis by a careful history, physical examination, and urinalysis. Prostatic enlargement from BPH or prostate cancer causing urinary retention can usually be distinguished from acute bacterial prostatitis on rectal examination.

Chronic bacterial prostatitis can be differentiated from chronic urethritis and cystitis with segmented urine cultures. Other common causes of urinary outflow problems, such as BPH, urethral stricture, and prostate cancer, need to be considered. Bladder carcinoma, sphincter dyssynergia, and neurogenic bladder also can cause lower urinary tract irritative symptoms.[16] Rectal examination should help to exclude anal disease, such as tumors, which may present similarly to chronic prostatitis.

The primary condition to be considered in the differential diagnosis of nonbacterial prostatitis is chronic bacterial prostatitis. The absence of positive cultures and a negative history of urinary tract infection support the diagnosis of nonbacterial prostatitis. A urinary cytologic examination and cystoscopy are indicated in the older man with irritative voiding symptoms and negative cultures, to exclude bladder cancer.[6] Interstitial cystitis and carcinoma in situ of the bladder may present with similar symptoms in the younger man.

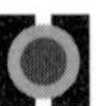

Differential Diagnosis

Prostatitis

Acute/chronic bacterial prostatitis	Benign prostatic hyperplasia
Acute pyelonephritis	Urethral stricture
Acute epididymitis	Sphincter dyssynergy
Acute diverticulitis	Neurogenic bladder
Prostatic cancer or bladder cancer	Interstitial cystitis
	Obstructive calculus

MANAGEMENT

Many patients with acute prostatitis are severely ill and require broad-spectrum antibiotic therapy. Depending on the severity of the illness, hospitalization and IV antibiotic therapy may be indicated. Evidence exists for benefit of the use of fluoroquinolones.[17] A patient who is afebrile for 24 to 48 hours should be switched from IV to oral therapy.

Those who are less acutely ill may be treated on an outpatient basis with oral antibiotics. Trimethoprim-sulfamethoxazole and fluoroquinolones are effective in treating the illness,[18] but penicillins and cephalosporins do not penetrate the prostatic epithelium. The length of appropriate treatment ranges from 2 to 6 weeks. In general, acute bacterial prostatitis requires antibiotic therapy for a minimum of 3 weeks to prevent the development of chronic bacterial prostatitis.[13,16,19] Follow-up segmented urine cultures, including prostatic secretions, are necessary after treatment is completed. Local measures may be helpful in reducing discomfort. Sitz baths, 3 times per day, may reduce perineal pain. Analgesics, antipyretics, stool softeners, and bed rest may also be beneficial.

The treatment of chronic bacterial prostatitis is more complex because of the difficulty in attaining therapeutic intraprostatic antibiotic levels in a noninflamed prostate. The antibiotics that have demonstrated the highest effectiveness include trimethoprim-sulfamethoxazole, the fluoroquinolones, and erythromycin. Trimethoprim-sulfamethoxazole for 4 to 16 weeks generally provides effective treatment.[19] Fluoroquinolones have good prostatic penetration and are effective against most of the causative organisms. Treatment length is often 3 weeks to 4 months.[19] It is recommended that a segmented urine culture be conducted on all men being treated with antibiotics 4 weeks into treatment. If the urine is not sterile at that time, treatment should be changed.[14]

Curing chronic bacterial prostatitis may be difficult. A cure is demonstrated by negative segmented urine cultures 6 months after completion of therapy.[20] However, the WBC count may remain elevated long after a cure. If a relapse occurs, a longer course of antibiotic therapy is necessary.

If a cure is not achieved, a low dose of antibiotics may be prescribed to prevent symptomatic infection. Commonly used medications include trimethoprim/sulfamethoxazole DS (160 mg/800 mg, 1 tablet/day or q.o.d.) or nitrofurantoin (50 to 100 mg/day).

Supportive measures such as warm water baths may be helpful in the treatment of chronic bacterial prostatitis. Beverages that produce rapid bladder expansion, such as coffee, tea, and alcohol, should be avoided. The use of medications that impair bladder function (e.g., anticholinergics, sedatives, antidepressants) should be assessed.

The treatment of nonbacterial prostatitis is controversial because of the inability to isolate a causative organism. If *Ureaplasma* or *Chlamydia* organisms are suspected, doxycycline, erythromycin, or a fluoroquinolone should be prescribed for 2 to 4 weeks.[13] If there is no response to treatment, antibiotic therapy should be discontinued and the emphasis shifted to symptomatic relief.

Supportive measures as described previously may be helpful, including warm tub baths and the use of nonsteroidal antiinflammatory drugs (NSAIDs). Normal sexual activity is not contraindicated. If patients complain of irritative voiding problems, a trial of anticholinergic medications, such as oxybutynin chloride, may be effective. If spicy foods, alcohol, or caffeine aggravate symptoms, they should be avoided.

The treatment of prostatodynia includes the use of alpha-blocking agents that relax the muscles of the bladder neck. To minimize the risk of hypotension, therapy should be initiated with a low dose.

The use of biofeedback, referral to a mental health professional for stress and emotional problems, and the use of sitz baths and NSAIDs may also be helpful in prostatodynia.

LIFE SPAN CONSIDERATIONS

The risk of sexually transmitted diseases, which can be difficult to identify by culture and may need to be treated empirically, should be assessed. In the older man, the possibility of coexistent BPH or prostate cancer, which can potentiate the signs and symptoms of prostatitis, should be considered.

COMPLICATIONS

A prostatic abscess rarely occurs as a complication of acute bacterial prostatitis except in immunocompromised patients. The symptoms are similar to those of acute bacterial prostatitis, but on rectal examination there is a fluctuance of the affected lobe. Diagnosis can be confirmed with transrectal ultrasound (TRUS). The treatment usually includes surgical drainage and antibiotics. Other complications of acute bacterial prostatitis may include pyelonephritis, epididymitis, seminal vesiculitis, and bacteremia.

INDICATIONS FOR REFERRAL/HOSPITALIZATION

Because of the severity of the illness associated with acute bacterial prostatitis and the potential chronicity of bacterial and nonbacterial prostatitis and prostatodynia, co-management with a urologist is often indicated. Urologic referral is indicated for severe cases of acute bacterial prostatitis, when comorbidity increases the risk of sequelae or signs of urinary retention are present. Refractory chronic prostatitis in the presence of prostatic stones also requires urologic referral. If symptoms do not resolve after the treatment of nonbacterial prostatitis or prostatodynia, a urologic referral is necessary to exclude cystitis[21] or bladder cancer and to confirm the diagnosis of nonbacterial prostatitis or prostatodynia.

Hospitalization is indicated for acute illness. If prostate enlargement results in urinary retention, urinary catheterization is contraindicated and a percutaneous suprapubic tube is necessary until the prostatic enlargement subsides.

PATIENT AND FAMILY EDUCATION

Education regarding the cause of patients' symptoms and treatment is necessary. The long duration of antibiotic treatment in several of these conditions requires that patients understand the necessity of maintaining an adequate therapeutic level for the duration of therapy. The importance of follow-up should be stressed, as well as the importance of using condoms to prevent the reintroduction of bacteria into the urethra with sexual intercourse. Anal intercourse should be avoided with acute bacterial prostatitis.

Prostate Cancer

DEFINITION/EPIDEMIOLOGY

Cancer of the prostate is the most common malignancy in men in the United States and the second leading cause of cancer death in men over the age of 55.[1] In the United States in 1998 there were 184,500 new cases diagnosed and 39,200 known deaths from prostate cancer.[22] Risk factors include advancing age and a positive family history of prostate cancer. As a result of effective screening and the aging of the U.S. population, the number of prostate cancer cases diagnosed has increased.[23]

Eighty percent of cases are diagnosed in men over age 65, with incidence rates being 66% higher in African-American men than in white men.[24,25] The mortality rate of African-American men is estimated to be twice that of white men.[24] The 5-year survival rate for prostate cancer is greater than 80% when it is detected at an early stage.[26]

PATHOPHYSIOLOGY

The most common type of prostate cancer is adenocarcinoma. It develops in the acinar glands located in the posterior peripheral zone of the prostate. Histologic grading is an important predictor of prognosis. The Gleason system incorporates clinical and physiologic parameters for grading of the malignancy[27] (Table 163-2).

Tumors can arise in one or both lobes of the prostate and can spread within the prostate, through the prostatic capsule, and

TABLE 163-2 Gleason Grading Scale

Stage	Description
A1	Clinically undetectable, lesion is confined to one lobe of prostate; well-differentiated local adenocarcinoma found on pathologic examination
A2	Clinically undetectable, diffuse or multifocal distribution of well-differentiated tumor found on pathologic examination
B1	May be palpable on rectal examination; limited to one lobe of prostate; confined within prostate capsule; nodule less than 1.5 cm; metastasis to lymph nodes in 10% to 20% of patients
B2	Involves both lobes of prostate; metastasis to lymph nodes in 15% to 40%; nodules greater than 1.5 cm
C	Local extension outside of prostate capsule into vesicles or surrounding tissue; lymph node metastasis in 40% to 80%; no metastasis to other sites
D1	Metastatic involvement of pelvic lymph nodes; lesions may extend into bladder, rectum or pelvis
D2	Distant metastases

From Vetrosky DT, Gerdom L, White GL Jr: Prostate cancer: pathology, diagnosis, and management, *Clin Rev* 7(5):79-100, 1997.

through the seminal vesicles or the base of the bladder, with metastasis occurring via the lymphatic and circulatory systems.[26]

CLINICAL PRESENTATION

Presenting symptoms of prostate cancer may include urinary hesitancy, urgency, nocturia, and frequency, although in early stages of the disease the patient is usually asymptomatic. Symptoms tend to increase in intensity over a 1- to 2-month period, which is different from the slow, gradual progression in symptoms that occurs in BPH. In more advanced disease, presenting symptoms may include back pain, impotence, and other bone pain that suggests metastasis. Other symptoms of metastasis include weight loss, constipation, malaise, hematuria, and rectal pain or symptoms related to nerve root compression, such as paresthesias or extremity weakness.

PHYSICAL EXAMINATION

A firm nodule on rectal examination, induration, or a stony, asymmetric prostate is suspicious for prostate cancer. In the early disease stage, the prostate examination will generally be normal. Routine DRE is recommended for men over the age of 50. The American Cancer Society recommends that African-American men older than age 45 and men over the age of 40 with a family history of prostate cancer be screened annually for prostate cancer with a DRE.[23]

DIAGNOSTICS AND DIFFERENTIAL DIAGNOSIS

Measurement of the PSA combined with DRE is considered the most sensitive and specific screening method for prostate cancer. The PSA is a protease enzyme secreted by the prostate gland, and levels may be elevated in benign and malignant conditions of the prostate. A PSA level below 5 μg/L is considered normal. Values between 5 and 10 μg/L may be seen in early prostate cancer and other benign conditions, and values over 10 μg/L suggest prostate cancer. Values above 80 μg/L may indicate advanced or metastatic disease. The PSA test has a 96% sensitivity and 95% specificity for the detection of early prostate cancer.[23] The use of the free PSA test may increase specificity for prostate cancer.

An alternative method of considering normal ranges for the PSA test is according to age:

AGE (yr)	*NORMAL RANGE (μg/L)*
40-49	0-2.5
50-59	0-3.5
60-69	0-4.5
70-79	0-6.5

Studies suggest that different age-specific reference ranges should be considered for African-American men because many cases in this population would be missed using the traditional reference ranges. For the test to have 95% sensitivity in African-American men, the following reference ranges are suggested:[28]

AGE (yr)	*NORMAL RANGE (μg/L)*	*SPECIFICITY (%)*
40-49	0-2.0	93
50-59	0-4.0	88
60-69	0-4.5	81
70-79	0-5.5	78

The American Cancer Society and the American Urologic Association recommend measurement of the PSA in all men over 50 years of age except for those with a family history of prostate cancer or African-American men. In these groups, PSA testing is recommended beginning at age 40.

If the PSA test or DRE is abnormal, TRUS of the prostate with a TRUS-guided biopsy is recommended. The TRUS allows for guided biopsy of suspicious hypoechoic areas.

In cases with a positive biopsy of the prostate and a PSA above 10 μg/L, a radionuclide bone scan may be necessary to determine the presence of bone metastases. A CT scan or MRI of the abdomen and pelvis is important to assess the regional lymph nodes. A chest x-ray study can exclude metastasis to the lungs. An elevated alkaline phosphatase level suggests bone metastasis, and an elevated acid phosphatase level is correlated with extension outside the prostatic capsule.[23] The differential diagnosis includes BPH and prostatitis when there is an abnormal DRE and PSA test.

Diagnostics

Prostate Cancer

Laboratory	**Other**
PSA	Needle biopsy
CBC and differential*	

*If indicated.

MANAGEMENT

Treatment decisions are based on the stage at diagnosis, prognostic features of the tumor, and the patient's age, medical condition, and treatment preference. Decisions regarding therapy are complex and controversial. The current therapy with disease classified as stage A or B is radical prostatectomy or radiation therapy. Long-term survival rates are 80% to 90% with either treatment.[29] Cryotherapy is being used more commonly in localized prostate cancer.

Hormonal therapy has been used for symptomatic patients with advanced disease, but evidence of benefit is unclear as to whether androgen suppression improves long-term outcome.[30] Hormone treatments include oral estrogens, orchiectomy, luteinizing hormone–releasing hormone (LHRH) agonists, antiandrogens, and progestational agents. LHRH agonists act by initially stimulating pituitary gonadotropin production and later inhibiting it.

Pain management is often an important treatment issue in more advanced disease. Palliative treatment with radiation and medication may be helpful to relieve the pain.

LIFE SPAN CONSIDERATIONS

PSA screening is not recommended for men over the age of 70 because of the typically slow progression of the disease and because men over the age of 70 are generally less likely candidates for radical prostatectomy. Early hormonal treatment for asymptomatic

Differential Diagnosis

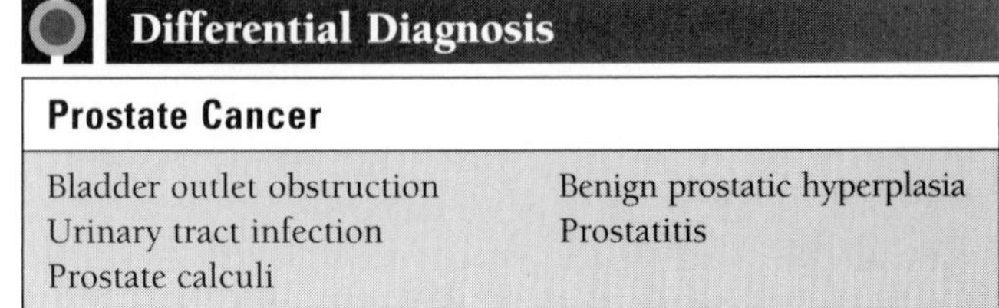

Prostate Cancer

Bladder outlet obstruction	Benign prostatic hyperplasia
Urinary tract infection	Prostatitis
Prostate calculi	

disease is still controversial. For the same reasons, treatment for asymptomatic older men with localized disease is often deferred. Although PSA screening is still somewhat controversial, clinicians should remember that prostate cancer is the second leading cause of cancer death in men in the United States.[22]

COMPLICATIONS

The major complication of prostate cancer is metastatic disease. Risks of surgery include hemorrhage or injury to the obturator nerve, ureter, or rectum. The long-term complications of surgery include incontinence and impotence.[23] Problems associated with radiation therapy include urinary problems, intestinal sequelae, impotence, and transient edema. Intestinal problems include diarrhea, fecal incontinence, rectal bleeding, intestinal obstruction, rectal strictures, mucus discharge, and tenesmus. Potential urologic problems include cystitis, hematuria, frequency, dysuria, and urethral stricture. The main complications of cryotherapy include urethral stricture, irritative symptoms, urinary incontinence, impotence, rectourethral fistula, bladder neck contracture, and urinary retention.

INDICATIONS FOR REFERRAL/HOSPITALIZATION

A referral should be made to a urologist when a suspicious finding is found on DRE or the PS is elevated. After treatment, the primary care provider can offer follow-up care that includes monitoring of the PSA levels. After radical prostatectomy, the PSA levels fall to less than 0.2 μg/L. PSA levels also fall after radiation therapy and continue to decrease for 12 months after completion of therapy. PSA levels should be tested at 6 and 12 months after treatment and annually thereafter. An increase in PSA should be evaluated with a TRUS and biopsy. Hospitalization may also be necessary in the case of advanced metastatic disease.

PATIENT AND FAMILY EDUCATION

Education includes the importance of screening for prostate cancer, the strengths and limitations of PSA screening, and the implications of an abnormal prostate examination or PSA test.

HEALTH PROMOTION

Patient education is an important aspect of maintaining good prostate health. It is fortunate that there are many new resources available. Web-based information varies in accuracy and content, but there are many reliable sites, such as http://web.health.aol.thriveonline.oxygen.com/medical/prostate.index.html. Simply making patients aware of the symptoms of prostate disorders via waiting room literature may help increase the willingness of patients to discuss prostate symptoms. To help prevent prostate cancer, limited evidence for benefit exists for diets high in lycopene (found in tomatoes) and low in fat.[31,32]

REFERENCES

1. Braunwald E. and others: *Harrison's Principles of Internal Medicine*, ed 15, New York, 2001, McGraw Hill.
2. Kelley WN, editor: *Essentials of internal medicine*, Philadelphia, 1994, JB Lippincott.
3. Barry MJ and others: The American Urologic Association symptom index for benign prostatic hyperplasia, *J Urol* 148(5):1549-1557, 1992.
4. Benign Prostatic Hyperplasia Guideline Panel: *Benign prostatic hyperplasia: diagnosis and treatment*, Washington, DC, February 1994, US Department of Health and Human Services, publication No. 94-0582.
5. Goodson JD, Barry MJ: Management of benign prostatic hyperplasia. In Goroll AH, May LA, Mulley AG Jr, editors: *Primary care medicine: office evaluation and management of the adult patient*, ed 3, Philadelphia, 1995, JB Lippincott.
6. Presti JC Jr, Stoller ML, Carroll PR: Urology. In Tierney LM Jr, McPhee SJ, Papadakis MA, editors: *Current medical diagnosis and treatment*, ed 34, Norwalk, Conn, 1995, Appleton & Lange.
7. Lepor H and others: The efficacy of terazosin, finasteride, or both in benign prostatic hyperplasia, *N Engl J Med* 335:533-539, 1996.
8. Hudson BP and others: Efficacy of finasteride is maintained in patients with benign prostatic hyperplasia treated for years. The North American Finasteride Study Group, *Urology* 53:690-695, 1999.
9. Wilde MI, Goa KL: Finasteride: an update of its use in the management of symptomatic benign prostatic hyperplasia, *Drugs* 57:557-581, 1999.
10. Marks LS and others: Effects of saw palmetto herbal blend in men with symptomatic benign prostatic hyperplasia, *J Urol* 163:1451-1456, 2000.
11. Gerber GS: Saw palmetto for the treatment of men with lower urinary tract symptoms, *J Urol* 163:1408-1412, 2000.
12. Meares EM Jr: Prostatitis, *Med Clin North Am* 75(2):405-424, 1991.
13. Criste G, Gray D, Gallo B: Prostatitis: a review of diagnosis and management, *Nurse Pract* 19(7):32-38, 1994.
14. Denman SJ, Murphy PA: Genitourinary infections. In Barker LR, Burton JR, Zieve PD, editors: *Principles of ambulatory medicine*, ed 4, Baltimore, 1995, Williams & Wilkins.
15. Krieger JN and others: Chronic pelvic pains represent the most prominent urogenital symptoms of chronic prostatitis, *Urology* 48(5):715-722, 1996.
16. Goodson JD: Management of acute and chronic prostatitis. In Goroll AH, May LA, Mulley AG Jr, editors: *Primary care medicine: office evaluation and management of the adult patient*, ed 3, Philadelphia, 1995, JB Lippincott.
17. Chow RD: Prostatitis. Work-up and treatment of men with telltale symptoms, *Geriatrics* 56:32-36 April 2001.
18. Berg D: *Handbook of primary care medicine*, Philadelphia, 1993, JB Lippincott.
19. Donovan DA, Nicholas PK: Prostatitis: diagnosis and treatment in primary care, *Nurse Pract* 22(4):144-156, 1997.
20. Berger PE, Hanno PM: A spectrum of prostatitis syndromes, *Patient Care*, pp 95-111, May 15, 1990.
21. Miller JL and others: Prostatodynia and interstitial cystitis: one and the same? *Urology* 45(4):587-590, 1995.
22. Lee JJ: Design considerations for efficient prostate cancer chemoprevention trials, *Urology* 58(suppl 1):205-212, 2001.
23. Pinto HA: Prostate cancer. In Fishman MC and others, editors: *Medicine*, Philadelphia, 1996, Lippincott-Raven.
24. American Cancer Society: *Cancer facts and figures—1997 and addendum*, Atlanta, 1997, The Society.
25. Nicoll LH, Carroll P: The prostate, *Lippincott Health Promotion Lett* 2(1):1-8, 1997.
26. Vetrosky DT, Gerdom L, White GL Jr: Prostate cancer: pathology, diagnosis, and management, *Clin Rev* 7(5):79-100, 1997.
27. Gleason DF, Melligor GT: Prediction of prognosis of prostatic adenocarcinoma by combined histologic grading and clinical staging, *J Urol* 111:58-64, 1974.
28. Tewari A and others: Prostate neoplasms. In Lonergan ET, editor: *Geriatrics: a Lange clinical manual*, Norwalk, Conn, 1996, Appleton & Lange.
29. Berger RE, Hanno PM: The fine points of prostatitis care, *Patient Care*, pp 91-107, Sept 15, 1992.
30. Theyer G, Hamilton G: Current status of intermittent androgen suppression in the treatment of prostate cancer, *Urology* 52:353-359, 1998.
31. Arab L, Steck S: Lycopene and cardiovascular disease, *Am J Clin Nutr* 72:1691S-1695S, 2000.
32. Moyad MA: Fat reduction to prevent prostate cancer: waiting for more evidence? *Curr Opin Urol* 11:457-461, 2001.

CHAPTER 164

Proteinuria and Hematuria

Carol A. Whelan

Proteinuria and hematuria are relatively common findings on routine urinalysis. However, these findings can also be signs of serious disease or neoplasm, and therefore a careful, systematic evaluation is essential.[1-5]

Proteinuria

DEFINITION/EPIDEMIOLOGY

Approximately 15 kg of protein are filtered through the adult kidney each day, with normally less than 150 mg excreted.[1,3,4] Although proteinuria is generally defined as an excretion rate >150 mg/day, the term *microalbuminuria* is often used to describe proteinuria that occurs at rates of 30 to 300 mg/day; the term *macroalbuminuria* is occasionally used to describe rates of >300 mg/day. Common causes of proteinuria are listed in Box 164-1.

Although isolated proteinuria is not necessarily associated with excess morbidity and mortality, it is often a sign of serious systemic disease. End-stage renal disease has a yearly mortality rate of 20%, and nephrotic syndrome carries a high risk of morbidity and mortality.

PATHOPHYSIOLOGY

Normal urine proteins are composed of approximately 40% to 50% Tamm-Horsfall proteins, 30% to 40% albumin, and 20% to 30% various plasma proteins.[3,4] Protein excretion is affected by three factors: (1) prevention of excretion by the glomerular capillary wall, (2) resorption and catabolism by the proximal tubule cells, and (3) production of low-molecular-weight proteins.[3,4] Therefore proteinuria is classified as either glomerular, tubular, or overflow in origin.[1,3] Proteinuria may be further defined as transient or persistent.[1] Transient proteinuria is caused by hemodynamic changes and is generally benign, whereas persistent proteinuria (defined as three or more positive specimens) indicates a pathologic process that requires investigation to identify the cause.[1]

BOX 164-1

COMMON CAUSES OF PROTEINURIA

DRUG-INDUCED
- Lithium
- Cyclosporin
- Cisplatin
- NSAIDs

HEREDITARY
- Polycystic kidney disease
- Medullary kidney disease

IMMUNE
- Drug allergies
- Collagen/vascular disorders
- Immunoglobulin A nephropathy
- Sarcoidosis

INFECTION
- Bacterial, fungal, or parasitic infection
- Tuberculosis

METABOLIC
- Hyperuricemia
- Hypercalcemia
- Amyloid

VASCULAR
- Diabetes mellitus
- Hypertension
- Sickle cell disease
- Radiation nephritis

INCREASED PRODUCTION
- Multiple myeloma

CLINICAL PRESENTATION

The clinical presentation of the patient with proteinuria can vary from healthy young adults with functional proteinuria related to prolonged exercise to seriously ill diabetic patients with nephrotic syndrome. Therefore all individuals should be screened for proteinuria by routine dipstick testing. Especially important is the routine screening of pregnant women. Proteinuria before 24 weeks' gestation indicates a likely glomerulonephritis, whereas proteinuria after 24 weeks' gestation is usually a sign of preeclampsia.[5]

Persistent proteinuria in patients with diabetes is usually a result of diabetic nephropathy. However, uncontrolled diabetes mellitus may cause transient proteinuria, most likely as a result of hyperfiltration and decreased tubular reabsorption.[6]

PHYSICAL EXAMINATION

With proteinuria, a complete and thorough history is essential. Specific areas of focus should include recent acute or chronic illness, surgery, diagnostic procedures (especially those requiring contrast media), urinary frequency or symptoms suggesting infection, risk factors for human immunodeficiency virus (HIV) infection, medications taken (including over-the-counter medications), a family history of renal disease or diabetes, and recent physical activity (especially exercise or cold-weather activities). The physical examination should be comprehensive and thorough; in the case of coexistent diabetes, the severity of the diabetes should be assessed to determine if it correlates with the severity of proteinuria. Diabetic retinopathy is often present in patients with diabetic renal disease.[1]

DIAGNOSTICS AND DIFFERENTIAL DIAGNOSIS

Proteinuria is usually detected on routine dipstick testing, and any value of 1 or greater on two or more occasions should be investigated. Limitations of dipstick testing include false-negative results resulting from dilution, the inability of dipstick testing to detect microalbuminuria, false-positive results caused by certain medications, and the limitation of dipstick reagents to detect light-chain proteins.[1]

Once proteinuria has been identified, the urine should be tested for Bence Jones proteins (the presence of which suggests multiple myeloma).[1] In addition, a full blood chemistry panel with fasting blood sugar, a lipid profile, urine culture and sensitivity, and CBC with differential are indicated. A diagnostic flowchart for the evaluation of proteinuria is provided in Figure 164-1.

Once proteinuria has been identified, it is important to determine if it is persistent or transient.[1] Transient proteinuria in an otherwise healthy patient that is secondary to an identifiable cause (e.g., exercise, fever, congestive heart failure) may

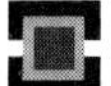 Diagnostics

Proteinuria

Laboratory
Urine dipstick
Urine for Bence-Jones proteins
CBC and differential
Serum electrolytes
Serum glucose
BUN
Creatinine
Serum albumin
Calcium phosphorus
Lipid profile
Urinalysis
Urine culture and sensitivity*
24-hour urine for volume, protein, and creatinine clearance*
Three early morning urines for protein*
Serum protein electrophoresis*
Urine protein electrophoresis*
Consider the following: ESR, ANA, lupus preparation (if collagen disease is suspected)
Antistreptolysin-O (ASO) titer, complement (C3, C4) (if glomerulonephritis is suspected)
Hepatitis B surface antigen (if hepatitis vaculitis is suspected)

Imaging
Renal ultrasound
IV pyelogram*

Other
Renal biopsy*

*If indicated.

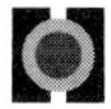 Differential Diagnosis

Proteinuria

Transient proteinuria
Persistent proteinuria
Orthostatic proteinuria/nonorthostatic proteinuria
Glomerulonephritis
Diabetic nephropathy
Nephrotic syndrome
Vasculitis
Medications

be classified as functional proteinuria and does not require further diagnostic testing or evaluation.[1,3]

Persistent proteinuria that cannot be classified as functional proteinuria requires further investigation. Investigation should begin with a 24-hour measurement of urine protein and creatinine clearance to determine the urinary protein excretion and the protein-creatinine ratio.[4] If the excretion rate is >3.5 g/day, the patient by definition has nephrotic syndrome,[4] which is usually accompanied by hypoalbuminemia, hyperlipidemia, and edema; nephrotic syndrome mandates a nephrologist's evaluation. It is important to remember that diabetes is the leading cause of nephrotic syndrome and accounts for 75% of all cases.[1]

If the 24-hour urinary protein excretion rate is >3.5 g/day, patients should be classified as having normal or abnormal renal function. Proteinuria in the presence of normal renal function is defined as "isolated" proteinuria; in these patients the next step is to determine if the proteinuria is orthostatic or nonorthostatic.[1] Urinary protein excretion can increase after prolonged standing, and therefore three early-morning voids should be checked for protein. If all the results are negative, a diagnosis of orthostatic proteinuria can be made, and no further diagnostic tests are necessary.[1] However, referral to a renal specialist is also appropriate because this is a poorly understood, although generally benign and self-limited, condition.[1,3]

Patients with nonorthostatic proteinuria and normal renal function and without an elevation in Bence Jones proteins should be referred to a renal specialist. A renal biopsy may be needed to determine the cause of the proteinuria. The presence of Bence Jones proteins warrants a serum protein electrophoresis, and a referral for further evaluation to exclude multiple myeloma is necessary.

Other diagnostic tests are dependent on presentation and differential. Collagen disease, glomerulonephritis, hepatitis-induced vasculitis, urate-related renal disease, diabetes, and other systemic disease or structural abnormalities should be considered in the evaluation of proteinuria.[5]

MANAGEMENT

Management of proteinuria is obviously dependent on the underlying cause, but some general principles apply. A careful medication review should be performed, and any medications implicated in proteinuria should be discontinued. Angiotensin-converting enzyme agents have been found to reduce proteinuria, most likely by decreasing interglomerular pressure, and thus may be indicated.[1] Diabetes and hyperlipidemia, if present, should be aggressively managed; blood pressure control is also important. Patients with chronic renal failure should be managed aggressively to help prevent or delay the onset of end-stage renal disease (see Chapter 165). Sodium- and protein-restricted diets may be indicated for some patients.

COMPLICATIONS

Nephrotic syndrome with associated edema, hypoalbuminemia, and extrarenal complications is a potential consequence of proteinuria. Immobilization, hyperlipidemia, hypercoagulability, and electrolyte disturbances are additional risks.

INDICATIONS FOR REFERRAL/HOSPITALIZATION

All patients with renal disease or abnormal renal function should be referred to a renal specialist for consultation and management guidance. Referrals for patients with isolated orthostatic proteinuria should be based on a thorough risk assessment and evaluation of their general health, life span considerations, and concerns for aggressive management.

Any patients presenting with nephrotic syndrome, acute renal failure, renal failure of unknown origin, or unstable vital signs should be urgently referred for hospitalization. New-onset proteinuria in pregnant women should be considered a medical emergency, and urgent referral to exclude eclampsia is indicated.

PATIENT AND FAMILY EDUCATION

Patient education depends on the cause of proteinuria, but diet education, diabetic teaching for patients with diabetes, and education concerning blood pressure management are usually necessary. Especially important is that the patient and family

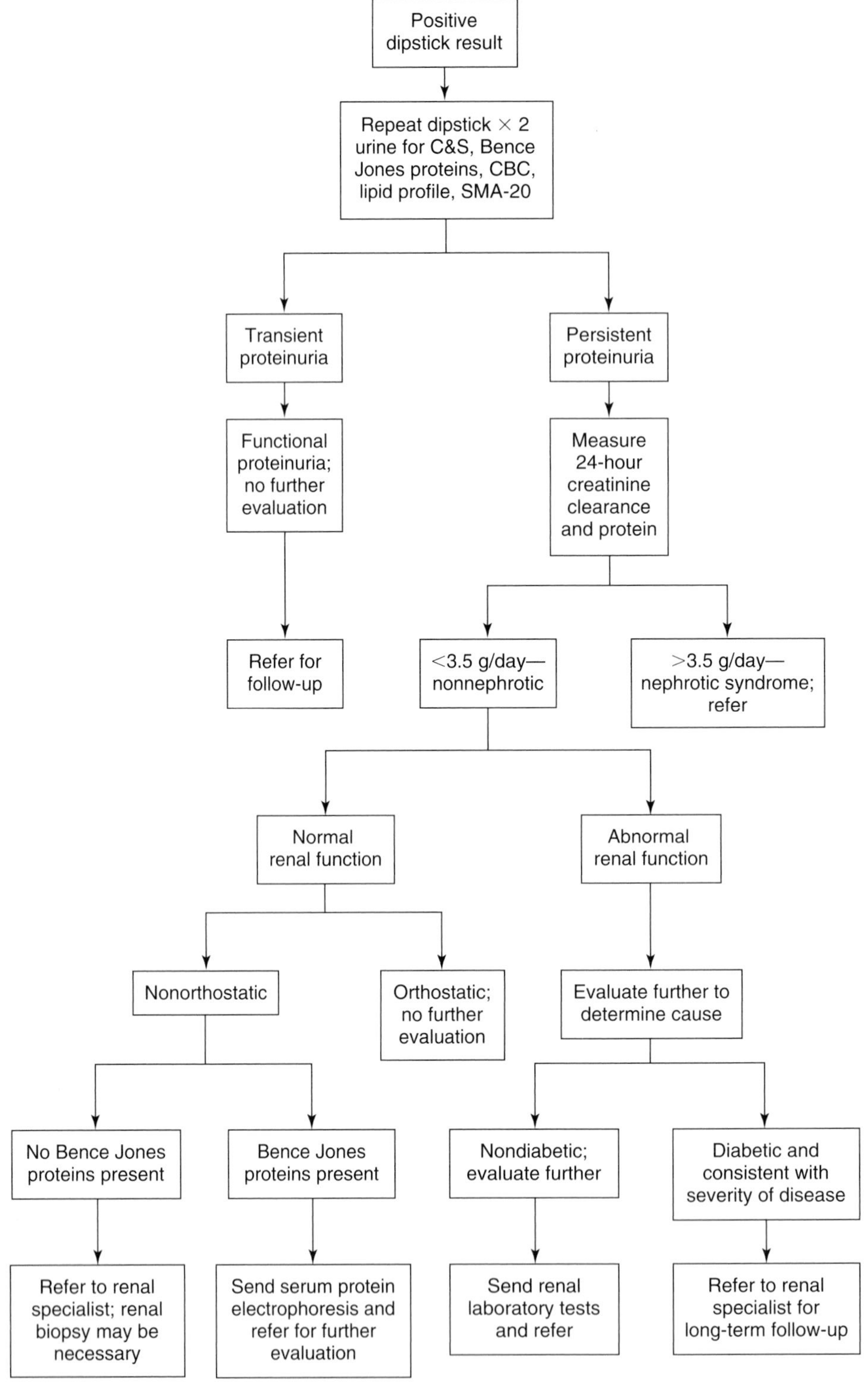

FIGURE 164-1

Evaluation of proteinuria. *C&S*, Culture and sensitivity; *SMA-20*, sequential multiple analysis of 20 chemical constituents.

understand the importance of diagnostic testing and the need for regular follow-up care.

Hematuria

DEFINITION/EPIDEMIOLOGY

Hematuria is generally defined as three or more red blood cells (RBCs) per high-powered field (HPF).[2,3] Transient hematuria is defined as hematuria that occurs on one occasion, whereas persistent hematuria is defined as hematuria that occurs on two or more consecutive occasions.[1] Exercise-induced hematuria in healthy young adults has no known morbidity or mortality, but both transient and persistent hematuria can be signs of serious disease. Common causes of hematuria are listed in Box 164-2.

The rates for hematuria in the general population vary with gender and age. One study of 1000 men ages 18 to 33 years had documented rates of transient hematuria of 38.7%, with virtually all patients found to have no serious disease.[3] Other studies have documented rates of transient hematuria up to 13% in postmenopausal women, with again relatively no serious pathologic conditions identified.[1] However, in men over 50 years old, even transient hematuria is often an indication of more serious disease, with up to 2.4% of this population having urinary tract malignancy.[1] Gross hematuria in older men denotes a significant risk of malignancy, with documented rates as high as 20%.[3]

PATHOPHYSIOLOGY

Normal urinary excretion of RBCs is 2 million/day, which results in 2 to 3 RBCs/HPF.[5] Isolated hematuria (hematuria unaccompanied by any other abnormal urine components) can result from bleeding anywhere from the renal pelvis to the urethra but is rarely caused by systemic disease.[5] Hematuria related to renal disease enters the tubular field along the nephron and produces RBC casts that are indicative of the renal origin.[2,4,5] Bacterial infections are a common cause of hematuria, and the presence of bacteria on urinalysis is suggestive of an infectious cause. Acute cystitis or urethritis can cause gross hematuria and is more common in women than in men.[2,7] The presence of proteinuria and hematuria is suggestive of glomerular or interstitial nephritis.[4]

BOX 164-2

COMMON CAUSES OF HEMATURIA

GLOMERULAR
- Glomerulonephritis
- Lupus nephritis
- Interstitial nephritis
- Pyelonephritis
- Vasculitis
- Alport's syndrome

NONGLOMERULAR
- Infection
- Neoplasm of the bladder, ureter, prostate, or kidney
- Renal or bladder calculi
- Polycystic kidney disease
- Sickle cell (disease or trait)
- Trauma
- Increased bleeding time
- Hemorrhagic cystitis
- Schistosomiasis

MISCELLANEOUS
- Drug-induced
- Exercise
- Endometriosis

PSEUDOHEMATURIA
- Menstrual contamination
- Hemoglobinuria
- Myoglobinuria
- Porphyrins
- Red food dyes
- Dilantin
- Quinine
- Phenothiazines
- Rifampin

CLINICAL PRESENTATION

Hematuria is often accompanied by clinically significant symptoms or by abnormalities in the urinalysis that can aid in identifying the source of bleeding. The patient's age, gender, and level of physical activity should always be considered (long-distance runners have been documented to have rates of hematuria as high as 18%).[5] Hematuria associated with pyuria suggests an infectious process, whereas colicky flank pain suggests pain originating from a ureter.[5] A prostatic or urethral source is likely when bleeding occurs only at the beginning or end of micturition.[4,8] The presence of hemoptysis, acute renal failure, and hematuria is highly suggestive of Goodpasture's syndrome.[2] Glomerulonephritis is signified by hematuria accompanied by edema, hypertension, and a sore throat or skin infection.[3,7]

PHYSICAL EXAMINATION

A thorough patient history should be obtained and should include urinary patterns, urine color, timing of hematuria (beginning, end, or throughout micturition, as well as transient or persistent), flank pain, history of renal calculi, urinary tract infections (UTIs), hemoptysis or bloody nasal secretions, recent acute or chronic illness, medications (including over-the-counter and illicit drugs), history of sexually transmitted disease, risk for HIV infection, or a history of travel to areas with endemic schistosomiasis (the leading cause of hematuria worldwide).[2] A complete family history specifically related to renal disease, sickle cell disease or traits, and congenital deafness (indicating Alport's syndrome) is also necessary. A comprehensive physical examination, including a pelvic examination in women and a prostate examination in men, is warranted.

DIAGNOSTICS AND DIFFERENTIAL DIAGNOSIS

The most important diagnostic element for hematuria is the urinalysis (Figure 164-2).[2] A urinalysis with RBC casts indicates hematuria originating from the renal parenchyma.[2] Further evidence of a renal source is the presence of large amounts of proteinuria (>1 g/24 hr), dysmorphic RBCs, cola-colored urine, or renal insufficiency.[2-5] One major limitation of dipstick testing is that it detects the presence of heme, not RBCs, in the urine. If the dipstick is positive for heme but no increased numbers of RBCs are seen by microscopic examination, the urine should be tested for myoglobinuria and hemoglobinuria.[8]

In addition, an attempt to localize the source of the hematuria can be made by the three glass test or segmented urine specimens (see Chapter 163). Hematuria in voided bladder 1 (VB1) indicates anterior urethral lesions or urethritis as the source; hematuria only in VB3 may be produced by lesions in the posterior urethra, bladder neck, or trigone. Hematuria in

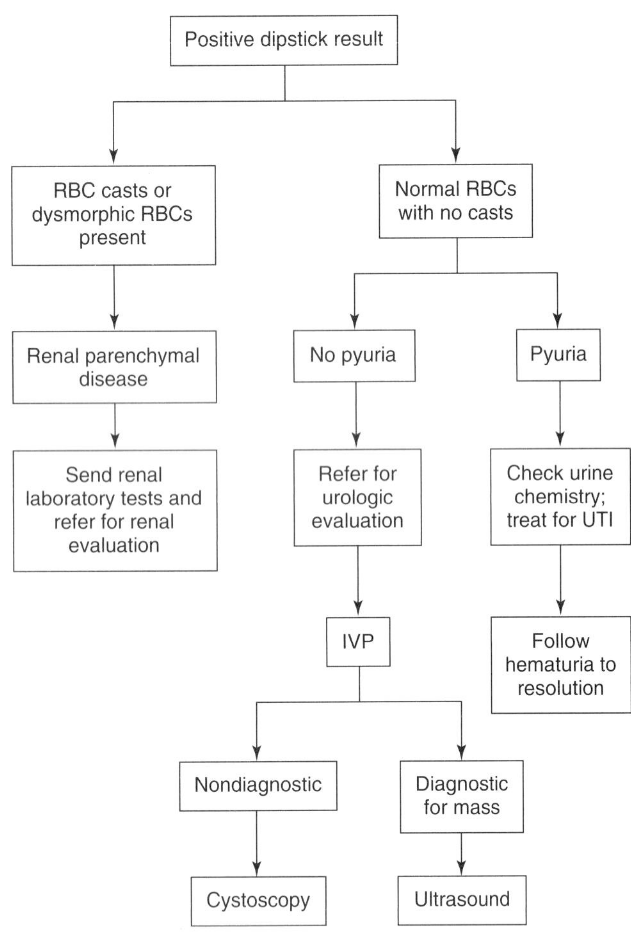

FIGURE 164-2

Evaluation of hematuria.

Diagnostics

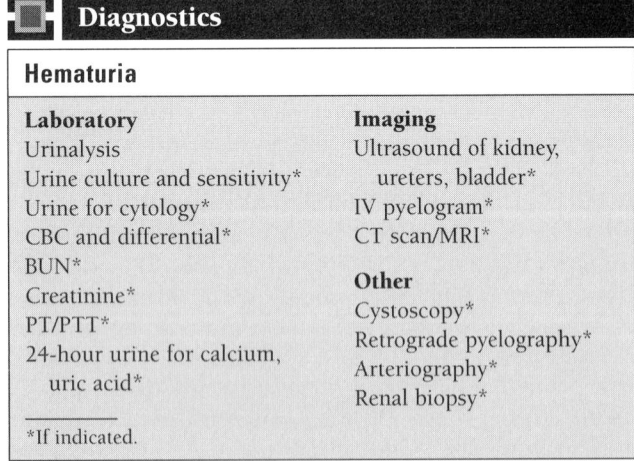

Hematuria	
Laboratory	**Imaging**
Urinalysis	Ultrasound of kidney, ureters, bladder*
Urine culture and sensitivity*	IV pyelogram*
Urine for cytology*	CT scan/MRI*
CBC and differential*	
BUN*	**Other**
Creatinine*	Cystoscopy*
PT/PTT*	Retrograde pyelography*
24-hour urine for calcium, uric acid*	Arteriography*
	Renal biopsy*

*If indicated.

all three specimens (VB1, VB2, VB3) is consistent with an etiology at or above the bladder.

A referral to a urologist is indicated when a renal origin is suggested. Antinuclear antibodies, immunoglobulins, cryoglobulins, cytoplasmic-antinuclear cytoplasmic antibodies, antiglomerular basement membrane antibodies, serum electrolytes, serum glucose, BUN, creatinine, antistreptolysin O titer, serum protein electrophoresis, and Venereal Disease and Research Laboratory (VDRL) tests[2,6] are indicated.

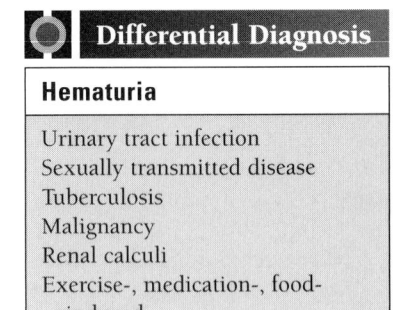

Differential Diagnosis

Hematuria
Urinary tract infection
Sexually transmitted disease
Tuberculosis
Malignancy
Renal calculi
Exercise-, medication-, food-induced
Glomerular disease
Bladder outlet obstruction

When hematuria originates from the lower urinary tract, intact and uniform RBCs should be present.[2,3,8] The presence of intact RBCs, white blood cells (WBCs), and bacteria suggest hematuria resulting from a UTI. The decision to obtain a urine culture and sensitivity should be guided by the patient's age and gender and the presence of resistant organisms in the local population. After treatment has been completed, a repeat urinalysis is necessary to ensure that the hematuria has resolved. Failure to follow hematuria to resolution may result in failure to diagnose a serious condition (that in fact may have contributed to the development of the original UTI). If symptoms are suggestive of a UTI despite a negative urine culture, a diagnosis of chlamydia or tuberculosis should be investigated.[4,5]

If the hematuria resolves after treatment of the UTI, no further diagnostic testing is indicated, although the presence of repeat UTIs in low-risk populations such as young men should always be fully investigated. If hematuria fails to resolve despite resolution of the UTI, referral for a urologic evaluation is required.[2]

In the absence of RBC casts or bacteria and WBCs, a urologic evaluation should be performed, usually with IV pyelography (IVP).[2,3,5,6] If the IVP is diagnostic for a mass, an ultrasound or CT scan to determine if the mass is cystic or solid is suggested. A cystic mass may be aspirated, but a solid mass should either be further evaluated by arteriography or referred to a urologic surgeon for excision and pathologic testing. If the IVP is nondiagnostic, the next step in the evaluation is cystoscopy, which includes inspection, biopsy, and culture of the bladder tissue. Cystoscopy is highly diagnostic for uroepithelial neoplasms. If the cystoscopy is nondiagnostic, the urologist may request a retrograde pyelography, arteriography, or renal biopsy (see Figure 164-2).

MANAGEMENT

Management of hematuria consists mainly of identification, diagnosis, and referral. Further management considerations are based on the underlying pathologic condition and not on the presence of the hematuria itself.

COMPLICATIONS

Complications of hematuria are dependent on the underlying pathologic condition. Urinary obstruction, renal failure, anemia, infections, and hydronephrosis are potential complications.

INDICATIONS FOR REFERRAL/HOSPITALIZATION

Isolated, transient hematuria or hematuria related to a UTI does not require a urology consultation. Referral to a renal or urology specialist is indicated to evaluate other causes of hematuria. Patients with large amounts of frank hematuria, severe flank pain suggestive of renal calculi, unstable vital signs, signs of urologic obstruction, or acute renal failure should be referred for urgent evaluation and possible hospitalization.

PATIENT AND FAMILY EDUCATION

Patient education is largely dependent on the cause of the hematuria; specific advice and educational material specific to the underlying pathologic process are appropriate. One of the major goals of education in asymptomatic hematuria is to reinforce the importance of the diagnostic evaluation. Other guidance should focus on the explanation of tests, medications, untoward effects, and the need for careful follow-up evaluation when indicated.

REFERENCES

1. Hassan A: Proteinuria, *Post Grad Med* 101(4):173-180, 1997.
2. McCarthy JJ: Outpatient evaluation of hematuria, *Post Grad Med* 101(2):125-131, 1997.
3. Ahmed Z, Lee J: Asymptomatic urinary abnormalities: hematuria and proteinuria, *Med Clin North Am* 81(3):641-652, 1997.
4. Isselbacher KJ and others: *Harrison's principles of internal medicine*, ed 13, New York, 1994, McGraw-Hill.
5. Barker RL, Burton JR, Zieve PD: *Principles of ambulatory medicine*, ed 4, Baltimore, 1995, Williams & Wilkins.
6. Mandal AK, Jennette JC: *Diagnosis and management of renal disease and hypertension*, Philadelphia, 1988, Lea & Febiger.
7. Gambrell RC, Blount BW: Exercise induced hematuria, *Am Fam Physician* 53(3):905-912, 1996.
8. Levine DZ: *Caring for the renal patient*, ed 3, London, 1997, WB Saunders.

CHAPTER 165

Renal Failure

Carol A. Whelan

DEFINITION/EPIDEMIOLOGY

Renal failure is a complex and challenging health issue that demands the involvement of both specialists and primary care providers. Defined as a glomerular filtration rate (GFR) of less than 50% of normal, renal failure consists of two distinct types: chronic renal failure and acute renal failure.[1,2]

Chronic renal failure (CRF) is defined as a reduction in GFR that has been present for at least 2 to 3 months.[1-3] However, CRF should not be viewed in simple mathematic terms but rather as an ongoing process of renal injury that causes compensatory hyperfiltration in less-affected glomeruli, which eventually leads to the destruction of those glomeruli as well.[1] This ongoing destruction results in a steady and predictable decline in renal function, which eventually affects every organ system in the body.[1,2]

Acute renal failure (ARF) is defined as an increase in serum creatinine of 0.5 mg/dl or more within 24 hours or as a loss of renal function that has occurred over a period of hours or days. ARF can be classified either by the physiologic cause (prerenal, intrarenal, or postrenal) or by the amount of urine produced (anuric, oliguric, or nonoliguric).[4]

Mild renal failure is usually defined as a GFR of approximately 35% to 50% of normal, whereas moderate renal failure is defined as a GFR of approximately 20% to 35% of normal.[1] Severe renal failure occurs at a GFR of 10% to 20% of normal, with rates below 10% being classified as end-stage renal disease (ESRD).[1] Patients with GFRs of 51% to 79% of normal may be classified as having chronic renal insufficiency (CRI). It is important to identify all patients with impaired renal function to prevent or slow the onset of CRF.

Although exact statistics regarding the prevalence of mild to moderate renal failure are not available, the epidemiology of ESRD has been widely documented by the U.S. Renal Data System (USRDS), which collects statistics on all Medicare patients on dialysis. Since 1974 the United States has extended Medicare coverage to virtually all patients on dialysis in the United States; therefore these data are highly representative of the current dialysis population in the United States. According to the USRDS, almost 80,000 patients began treatment for ESRD in 1997, twice the number of patients in 1988. By January of 1998 almost 300,000 patients were receiving treatment for ESRD.[5] The two leading causes of ESRD are hypertension (28.5%) and diabetes mellitus (33.1%).[3] Other causes of ESRD include glomerulonephritis (14.9%), interstitial nephritis (3.7%), cystic kidney disease (3.6%), and collagen vascular disease (2.3%).[3] Diabetic ESRD continues to increase at the rate of 11% per year.[6] Statistically, non-Caucasians are four times more likely to require dialysis, and although African-Americans make up 13% of the U.S. population, they represent 32% of patients with ESRD.[7] The current cost of treating ESRD is close to $10 billion, and this figure is expected to continue to rise.[6,7]

ARF is primarily an iatrogenic disease of hospitalized patients. It is estimated that up to 5% of all hospitalized patients will develop some degree of ARF.[4]

Immediate emergency department referral/physician consultation is indicated for patients with acute renal failure.

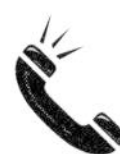

Nephrology consultation is indicated for patients with chronic renal failure.

PATHOPHYSIOLOGY

The basic pathophysiology of CRF is that of renal injury and loss of functioning nephrons (the mechanism of which depends on the underlying cause). This results in hyperfiltration in the surviving glomeruli (in an attempt by the body to increase GFR), which then causes ongoing glomerular stress and renal injury, resulting in glomerular destruction.[1,3] The result is a decrease in GFR and a continuance of the hyperperfusion-destruction syndrome. If this process is allowed to progress, uremic syndrome (a constellation of symptoms that occurs in severe renal failure) occurs.

The pathophysiology of ARF is dependent on the site of occurrence. Prerenal ARF, the most common type of ARF, is caused by renal hypoperfusion and does not result in structural kidney damage.[4] Intrarenal ARF, the result of damage to the renal parenchyma, may be a result of prolonged prerenal ARF (which leads to acute tubular necrosis), toxins, interstitial nephritis, or acute glomerulonephritis.[4] Postrenal (obstructive) ARF results from physical obstruction of urine outflow and may be caused by neoplasm, prostatic enlargement, bladder dysfunction, or nephrolithiasis.[4,8]

CLINICAL PRESENTATION

The clinical presentation of CRF is often subtle, and symptoms are uncommon with a GFR above 35%. Therefore suspicion for mild renal disease should be based on recognition of the primary pathologic mechanism responsible for renal injury, particularly in patients with diabetes mellitus and hypertension.

Once the GFR falls below 35%, a variety of metabolic, psychiatric, hematologic, cardiovascular, and acid-base regulatory problems occur. Clinical presentation at this point is dependent on the particular complication, as well as on the underlying cause of the renal failure (Box 165-1).[1-3,8,9]

The usual clinical presentation of ARF is that of prerenal ARF in a hospitalized patient who has undergone surgery, been exposed to radiocontrast dye, received aminoglycoside antibiotics, or developed sepsis.[4] Most of these patients have identifiable risk factors, such as CRI, CRF, advanced age, liver disease, diabetes, or vascular disease.[4] Therefore it is essential to identify those at high risk *before* ARF develops. It is equally important to begin early screening for all of the complications of renal disease in order to prevent morbidity and to establish a credible baseline for the individual patient.

PHYSICAL EXAMINATION

The physical examination should include both a focused examination that serves to identify pathologic processes caused by the primary disease entity (e.g., diabetes mellitus or hypertension) and a broader examination that attempts to identify the effects of progressive renal failure. Areas of importance include assessment of vital signs (including measurement of bilateral and orthostatic blood pressure); funduscopic evaluation for signs of arteriovenous nicking, diabetic retinopathy, and papilledema; assessment of volume status by determination of jugular vein distention; auscultation of lung sounds; assessment for the presence of edema or ascites; and assessment of heart sounds to screen for volume overload and pericarditis. A full abdominal examination should include auscultation for renal artery bruits; examination of the skin for ecchymosis, rashes (especially those suggesting collagen-vascular disorders), or uremic frost; percussion of the bladder (to exclude distention); rectal examination; and evaluation of the prostate (to exclude obstruction) in male patients.[8] Formal and informal mental status examinations should be included to screen for depression and other psychiatric complications.

BOX 165-1

MAJOR COMPLICATIONS OF CHRONIC RENAL FAILURE

CARDIOVASCULAR COMPLICATIONS
- Atherosclerosis
- Congestive heart failure (CHF)
- Hypertension
- Pulmonary edema
- Pericarditis

METABOLIC COMPLICATIONS
- Hyperkalemia
- Metabolic acidosis
- Alterations in vitamin D, calcium, and phosphorus metabolism and absorption
- Hyperparathyroidism
- Renal osteodystrophies
- Hyperlipidemia
- Nausea, vomiting
- Anorexia

PSYCHOSOCIAL COMPLICATIONS
- Depression
- Insomnia
- Suicide
- Sexual dysfunction
- Impoverishment
- Unemployment

HEMATOLOGIC COMPLICATIONS
- Anemia
- Leukopenia
- Erythropoietin (EPO) deficiency

DIAGNOSTICS

A full chemistry panel should be obtained, including electrolytes, fasting blood sugar, magnesium, phosphorus, ionized calcium, total protein and serum albumin, liver enzymes, lipid profile, CBC, and intact parathyroid hormone (PTH). Further studies include renal biopsy and nuclear imaging. However, the risks associated with arteriography compel consultation with a nephrologist before subjecting the patient to potential complications.

Although imaging studies are not particularly useful in diagnosing the extent of renal disease, renal ultrasound is recommended to determine the presence of cysts or obstruction, as well as to document the size of the kidneys.[8,9] This is necessary, as CRF characteristically results in smaller than average kidneys, whereas ARF is characterized by normal or even enlarged kidneys. Asymmetry may be a result of unilateral renal artery stenosis.[9]

Diagnostics

Renal Failure

Laboratory
- Urinalysis and urine osmolality
- 24-hour urine collection for volume, protein, creatinine clearance
- CBC and differential
- Serum electrolytes
- Serum glucose
- BUN
- Creatinine
- Calcium/ionized calcium
- Albumin
- Total protein
- Phosphorus
- Magnesium
- Uric acid
- PTH
- Serum complement levels (C3 and C4)*
- Antinuclear antibodies*
- Rheumatoid factor*
- Cryoglobulins*
- Antistreptococcal antibodies*
- Antineutrophil cytoplasmic antibodies (ANCAs)*
- Hepatitis B*
- HIV*

Imaging
- Ultrasound
- CT or MRI

Other
- Renal biopsy
- ECG

*If indicated.

DIFFERENTIAL DIAGNOSIS

The main issue in the diagnosis of CRF is exclusion of ARF. ARF is a potentially reversible, life-threatening condition, and all patients with ARF should be hospitalized and managed by specialists. The most common type of ARF seen in primary care is prerenal ARF (caused by renal hypoperfusion) related to volume depletion, hypotension, aminoglycoside antibiotic use, and radiocontrast dye exposure.[4] Often these patients have preexisting risk factors, such as CRI, CRF, advanced age, liver disease, diabetes, or vascular disease.[4] In addition, some patients with CRF will have a small degree of reversible prerenal ARF caused by hypovolemia or alterations in renal hemodynamics that result in renal hypoperfusion (e.g., from nonsteroidal antiinflammatory drugs or angiotensin-converting enzyme [ACE] inhibitors).

Urinalysis is highly diagnostic in differentiating between ARF and CRF. Prerenal ARF is usually accompanied by urine osmolality of >500, specific gravity of >1.020, and hyaline casts. Intrarenal ARF results in a urine osmolality of ~300, a specific gravity of ~1.010, tubular casts, tubular cells, and a very distinctive brownish, muddy appearance that is due to brown granular casts.[4,8]

Occasionally outpatients will present with postrenal obstructive ARF. A distended bladder, flank pain, and prostatic enlargement are potential causes. Ultrasound imaging virtually always detects obstruction.[8]

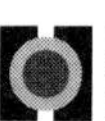

Differential Diagnosis

Renal Failure

- Acute renal failure
  - Prerenal failure
  - Intrarenal failure
  - Postrenal failure
- Chronic renal failure

If, after a thorough history and physical examination, ARF is still considered a potential diagnosis, the patient should be urgently referred to a renal specialist. Renal ultrasound evaluation and/or biopsy may be necessary for a definitive diagnosis.

Vigilance is necessary to determine any underlying correctable pathologic process that may be causing renal failure. Renal vascular hypertension should always be considered when renal function deteriorates rapidly with the initiation of ACE inhibitors or when abdominal bruits are heard on auscultation.

MANAGEMENT AND COMPLICATIONS

Mild to Moderate Chronic Renal Failure

In January 2000, the National Kidney Foundation (NKF) launched the Kidney Disease Outcomes Quality Initiative, whose purpose is to develop and publish evidence based clinical practice guidelines. These guidelines are available on the NKF's website at http://www.kidney.org.

Although mild to moderate CRF produces relatively few symptoms, interventions to decrease morbidity and mortality, as well as interventions to slow or even halt the progression of renal failure, are most effective at this stage. Therefore the first goal of treatment is the identification of patients with mild to moderate CRF via screening tools such as urinary dipstick testing for protein, the measurement of urinary albumin excretion (rates greater than 30 mg/24 hr are considered abnormal and have been shown to be a precursor for diabetic nephropathy), and the measurement of urinary creatinine clearance via timed urine collection (preferably a 24-hour collection).[10]

Progression of CRF should be monitored via 24-hour urine measurements of creatinine clearance, as the practitioner should not rely solely on estimates of renal function based on serum creatinine. The urine should also be regularly examined by dipstick and microscopic analysis, with measurement of specific gravity, proteinuria, hematuria, pyuria, and sediment. When a 24-hour urine sample is being collected for creatinine clearance, measurement should also be made of microalbumin unless frank proteinuria is present.

If the patient is diabetic, glycosylated hemoglobin should be monitored. Once the hematocrit falls below 32%, erythropoietin (EPO) levels should also be obtained. The clinical decision as to how often the previously mentioned laboratory values should be monitored depends on the severity of the renal disease and the presence of abnormalities in laboratory values.

Cardiovascular Management and Complications. Cardiovascular complications are the leading cause of death among patients with ESRD, accounting for more than 50% of deaths in the first year of dialysis.[5] The current annual mortality rate for U.S. patients with ESRD is more than 20% per year.[5] Therefore prevention of cardiovascular complications is of the utmost priority. Unfortunately, 70% of patients who begin dialysis treatment already have left ventricular hypertrophy and 40% have congestive heart failure (CHF).[5,11]

Once CRF has been identified, management of hypertension (if present) is extremely important. *Evidence exits for benefit* of adequate blood pressure control.[5] Ideally, the patient's blood pressure should be reduced to 130/80. *Evidence exists for benefit* of the use of ACE inhibitors in patients with diabetic nephropathy, and benefit for patients with nondiabetic renal disease and proteinuria.[12-15] ACE inhibitors must be used cautiously in patients at risk for hyperkalemia and should not be used in patients with renal artery stenosis unless prescribed by a renal specialist, in which case close monitoring of renal function is absolutely essential.[9,10] It is necessary to repeat a serum potassium, BUN, and serum creatinine measurement 1 week after initiation of ACE inhibitor therapy. In addition, careful blood pressure monitoring is important, both to ensure achievement of control of hypertension (with a maximum blood pressure of 135/85) and to guard against hypotensive responses to ACE inhibitor therapy.

Hyperlipidemia is both a complication of CRF and a potential factor in the progression of the disease.[16] *Evidence exists for benefit* of lowering low-density lipoprotein (LDL) cholesterol in patients with coronary artery disease (CAD).[17] A wide variety of agents are available for the treatment of lipid disorders, although most have dosing limitations dependent on the degree of CRF present. When appropriate lipid goals are being determined, any patient with diabetes and CRF should be viewed as having CAD; therefore secondary prevention goals (i.e., LDLs <100 mg/dl) should be sought.

Dietary Management and Metabolic Complications. An essential component of management is diet modification (Table 165-1). Dietary referral is beneficial for optimal care. This is especially true in patients with underlying diabetes and in patients who are under or over ideal body weight, as the dietary recommendations must be modified for these patients. American Dietetic Association (ADA) guidelines for renal failure diets are available in the *Manual of Clinical Dietetics*, published by the ADA.

Although protein restriction is widely recommended, the issue of how much to restrict protein remains controversial. Although a protein restriction of approximately 0.6 to 0.8 g/kg/day is widely recommended, it is important to monitor nutritional status via measurement of serum albumin and total protein.[2,8,18] A statistical correlation has been established between patients who present for initiation of dialysis with low serum albumin and total protein levels, and increased mortality.[7] Although this relationship has been established only as a temporal and not a causal relationship, maintaining serum albumin and protein levels within normal limits would appear to be prudent management.[18]

Evidence exists for benefit of tight glycemic control in halting or slowing the progression of diabetic renal disease.[2,6,8,9,19] Glycosylated hemoglobin levels within 10% of normal have been shown to be highly protective and associated with a lack of target organ damage.[9,10,19]

Although hyperkalemia is not usually a major issue in mild to moderate renal failure, monitoring of serum potassium (especially in patients taking ACE inhibitors) is mandatory. Patients receiving ACE inhibitor therapy may require decreased dosages to maintain serum potassium within normal limits. Some patients may not tolerate ACE inhibitor-induced hyperkalemia, and the medication will have to be discontinued. Most patients should be instructed to avoid potassium-containing salt substitutes, particularly as many hypertensive patients will have been told to restrict salt and may use salt substitutes without realizing that these substitutes contain almost pure potassium. Dietary potassium can also be restricted to less than 60 mEq/day. If necessary, sodium polystyrene (Kayexalate) should be prescribed to maintain serum potassium levels below 6 mEq/L.

Control of serum phosphorus and calcium is crucial in preventing metabolic complications, and many patients with CRF ultimately develop secondary hyperparathyroidism and renal osteodystrophy, even though these are often preventable entities. In addition, *evidence for benefit exists* that diets low in phosphorus (0.8 to 1 g/day) can delay the progression of renal failure, likely as a result of the prevention of deposition of phosphate and calcium in the interstitium of the kidney.[18]

In addition to limiting intake of phosphorus, supplemental calcium is required. Calcium taken with meals helps to decrease absorption of phosphorus, and calcium taken between meals helps to raise serum calcium levels.[8] A normal starting dose of calcium is usually 600 mg PO b.i.d. with meals and can be adjusted on the basis of ionized calcium values, intact PTH, and serum phosphorus. Patients with CRF should receive 800 IU of vitamin D per day, and serum levels should be monitored. Use of aluminum or magnesium antacids should be avoided, as these can cause aluminum or magnesium toxicity.

Because of alterations in metabolism and renal function, many drugs must be avoided or adjusted on the basis of renal function. When any drug is being prescribed for a patient with CRF, manufacturer's recommendations regarding use in CRF should be determined and creatinine clearance should be estimated:

$$\text{Creatinine clearance} = (140 - \text{Age}) \times \text{Weight [kg]}/72 \times \text{Serum creatinine (mg/dl)} \times (0.85 \text{ if the patient is female})$$

A partial listing of drugs requiring dosing adjustments is presented in Box 165-2. For female patients the value obtained in this equation should be multiplied by 0.85 to accurately estimate creatinine clearance.

TABLE 165-1 Dietary Recommendations for Adult Patients with Chronic Renal Failure Who Are Not on Dialysis

	Recommendation
Protein	0.6-0.8 g/kg/day
Calories	35 kcal/kg/day
Phosphorus	8-12 mg/kg/day
Calcium	1200-1600 mg/day
Sodium	1-3 g/day
Potassium	Not restricted unless serum potassium level is elevated or urine output <1 L/day

Data from The American Dietetic Association: *Manual of clinical dietetics,* ed 5, Chicago, 1996, The Association.

BOX 165-2

DRUGS REQUIRING DOSAGE ADJUSTMENT IN CHRONIC RENAL FAILURE*

Antibiotics	Antihypertensives
NSAIDs	Antifungals
Digoxin	Antivirals
Phenobarbital	Librium
Narcotics	Lithium carbonate
Antiarrhythmics	

*Always consult the manufacturer's instructions when prescribing any drugs for patients with CRF.

Hematologic Management and Complications. EPO production is usually normal, with GRF rates above 20%. However, the CBC should be monitored, and if the hematocrit level falls below 32% (the level at which EPO production is stimulated), serum EPO levels should be monitored to determine if this is the cause of the anemia. If serum EPO is low despite the presence of anemia, exogenous EPO should be given. To avoid transfusion-related hepatitis B, immunization should be given to those patients who are antibody negative.

Psychosocial Management and Complications. Although the medical management of CRF may seem overwhelming to even veteran primary care providers, it is often devastating to the victim of CRF. Therefore it is essential for adequate social and psychiatric support to be provided. Referral to a social worker is often advantageous to help provide adequate social support and assist the patient in applying for financial assistance and entitlement programs. Even with Medicare coverage, the cost of medical care can be devastating, and many patients with CRF are unable to continue working because of medical complications.

Severe Renal Failure

When GRF falls below 20%, the progression to ESRD is virtually inevitable. Therefore as prevention of progression is improbable, prevention of complications becomes paramount. Although continued control of hypertension, hyperglycemia, hyperlipidemia, serum potassium, phosphorus, magnesium, and calcium is important, the goals become more difficult as the GRF approaches 10%. Consultation with a renal specialist aids in management.

Cardiovascular Management and Complications. Despite careful management, complications and management issues may develop. The onset of CHF and pulmonary edema may indicate the need for dialysis. Hypertension may escalate, and increasingly higher doses of both diuretics and antihypertensive medications may be needed. However, at this point ACE inhibitors may not be tolerated, and if hyperkalemia is present, these drugs should probably be discontinued.

Dietary Management and Metabolic Complications. The National Kidney Foundations Disease Based Outcomes Quality Initiative (DOQI) lists guidelines for advanced CRF patients treated without dialysis. The guidelines state that evidence *suggests* that low-protein diets "may retard the progression of renal failure or delay the need for dialysis therapy."[20] The guidelines call for approximately 0.60 g protein/kg/day. The guidelines acknowledge that confusion remains within the nephrology community as to the role of protein restriction, partly because of the previously mentioned correlation with lower serum albumin levels and higher mortality rates. The guidelines further suggest that maintenance of adequate caloric intake (35 kcal/kg/day) may help maintain nutritional status.

The maintenance of calcium and phosphorus values within as normal a range as possible is also important. Nausea and vomiting may become problematic, and the use of high-calorie supplements may be necessary. Although restriction of salt and potassium may not have been previously necessary, these elements now must be restricted. Intact PTH levels should be monitored, and levels two to three times normal can be expected, but levels above this range indicate the need for endocrinology referral.

Hematologic Management and Complications. Anemia will become apparent, and endogenous EPO production will likely be inadequate. If EPO therapy is required, the DOQI states that *evidence exists for benefit* of a target hematocrit of 33% to 36%. EPO is available in vials of 10,000 units/ml. Given subcutaneously, the dosage should be calculated on the basis of the patient's weight (50 units/kg/week). Monthly hematocrit measurements are necessary during therapy so that the dosage can be appropriately increased if necessary. Measurements of serum iron and ferritin levels are recommended before initiating EPO therapy and periodically to indicate whether iron therapy should be initiated.

Psychosocial Management and Complications. One of the major tasks to be accomplished during this phase is planning for dialysis. This may be quite traumatic for the patient but is crucial for the prevention of major complications. A referral to a nephrologist is now indicated if one has not already been made. The type of dialysis should be determined, and the appropriate type of access established (arteriovenous fistulas take up to 3 months to heal and therefore should be placed well in advance). If continuous ambulatory peritoneal dialysis (CAPD) is elected, training is required and should be started as early as possible. Patients should visit the dialysis unit that will be managing their care to familiarize themselves with both the routine and the staff.

Depression and suicide are major considerations, and every effort should be made to provide psychosocial support. Selective serotonin reuptake inhibitor antidepressants can be used, and the dosage does not have to be adjusted for CRF. If transplantation is a possibility, discussions regarding this issue can begin.

End-Stage Renal Disease

Cardiovascular Management and Complications. Hypertension and hyperlipidemia should continue to be aggressively managed. Whereas the renal specialist may be concerned with fluid and electrolyte balance, the primary care provider should consider the potential for cardiovascular complications, as these are leading causes of death in patients with ESRD.[2] Hypertension should be aggressively managed.

Pulmonary edema and CHF are major concerns in ESRD, and if the patient is unstable, hospitalization and urgent dialysis may be necessary. All episodes of CHF and pulmonary edema should be reported to the renal specialist, as adjustments can be made in the dialysate fluid to compensate for fluid overload.

Dietary Management and Metabolic Complications. Dietary management should be aimed at control of electrolytes (including calcium, phosphorus, and potassium), prevention of malnutrition, and maintenance of acceptable fluid volume status.[16] Daily dietary requirements for patients with ESRD are dependent on the type of dialysis chosen (CAPD vs. hemodialysis). Current ADA guidelines for patients on CAPD or hemodialysis are outlined in Table 165-2. All patients with ESRD should be referred to a dietitian for optimization of nutritional status.

Hematologic Management and Complications. EPO replacement therapy will be necessary. EPO given subcutaneously is more effectively absorbed than EPO given intravenously (or into extracorporeal blood during hemodialysis).

Psychosocial Management and Complications. The stress of dealing with severe chronic illness can be psychologically devastating. Patients with ESRD are known to suffer from high rates of depression, insomnia, and anxiety (especially patients on hemodialysis).[8] Often ignored, sexual dysfunction occurs at high rates in both male and female patients with ESRD.[8] The treatment of these and other psychiatric complications should begin before the onset of ESRD.

INDICATIONS FOR REFERRAL/HOSPITALIZATION

All patients with CRF should be referred as early as possible to a renal specialist for consultation. If access to a dietitian is available, referral should be made as soon as CRF is identified.

Hospitalization should be considered for any acute, life-threatening disorder, and potential problems are innumerable. More common causes include acute fluid and electrolyte disorders, acute hypertensive emergency, pulmonary edema, acute CHF, pericarditis, and metabolic acidosis.

PATIENT AND FAMILY EDUCATION

Patient education in renal failure is highly complex. CRF and ESRD require carefully coordinated care. Enrollment in diabetic classes when appropriate, renal diet cooking classes, and support groups can be of tremendous benefit. By gradually introducing different educational materials and enabling the patient to help control the course of the disease, the primary care provider can help restore a sense of independence and confidence in the patient.

TABLE 165-2 Dietary Recommendations for Adults with End-Stage Renal Disease (Based on Dialysis Method)

	Recommendation for Hemodialysis	Recommendation for Peritoneal Dialysis
Protein	1.1-1.4 g/kg/day	1.2-1.5 g/kg/day
Calories	30-35 kcal/kg/day	25-35 kcal/kg/day
Phosphorus	<17 mg/kg/day	<17 mg/kg/day
Calcium	1.0-1.8 g/day	1.0-1.8 g/day
Fluid	Daily urine output +500-750 ml/day	2-3 L/day based on weight and blood pressure
Sodium	2-3 g/day	3-4 g/day based on weight
Potassium	40 mg/kg	Unrestricted unless elevated

Data from The American Dietetic Association: *Manual of clinical dietetics,* ed 5, Chicago, 1996, The Association.

REFERENCES

1. Isselbacher KJ and others: *Harrison's principles of internal medicine,* ed 13, New York, 1994, McGraw-Hill.
2. Malhotra D, Tzamaloukas AH: Non-dialysis management of chronic renal failure, *Med Clin North Am* 81:749-766, 1997.
3. Barker RL, Burton JR, Zieve PD: *Principles of ambulatory medicine,* ed 4, Baltimore, 1995, Williams & Wilkins.
4. Mindell JA, Chertow GM: A practical approach to acute renal failure, *Med Clin North Am* 81:731-748, 1997.
5. Eknoyan G and others: The national epidemic of chronic kidney disease, *Postgrad Med* 110(3):23-29, 2001.
6. Owen WF: *Primary care of patients with chronic renal failure,* Unpublished manuscript, 1997.
7. Hood VL, Gennari FJ: End stage renal disease: measures to prevent or slow its progression, *Postgrad Med* 100:163-176, 1996.
8. Levine DZ: *Caring for the renal patient,* ed 3, Philadelphia, 1997, WB Saunders.
9. Avram MM, Klahr S: *Renal disease progression and management,* Philadelphia, 1996, WB Saunders.
10. Bennett PH and others: Screening and management of microalbuminuria in patients with diabetes mellitus: recommendations to the Scientific Advisory Board of the National Kidney Foundation from an ad hoc committee of the Council on Diabetes Mellitus of the National Kidney Foundation, *Am J Kidney Dis* 25:107-112, 1995.
11. London GM: Left ventricular alterations and end-stage renal disease, *Nephrol Dial Transplant* 17(1 suppl): S29-S36, 2002.
12. Parving HH: Benefits and costs of antihypertensive treatment in incipient and overt diabetic nephropathy, *J Hypertension* 16(1 suppl): S99-S101, 1998.
13. Bernadet-Monrozies P and others: The effect of angiotensin-converting enzyme inhibitors on the progression of chronic renal failure, *Presse Med* 31(36): 1714-1720, 2002.
14. Porush JG: Hypertension and chronic renal failure: the use of ACE inhibitors, *Am J Kidney Dis* 31(1): 177-184, 1998.
15. Mogensen CE: Preventing end-stage renal disease, *Diabetic Medicine Supplement* 15(4): S51-S56, 1998.
16. Degroot PJ, Kenler SR, Dwyer JT: Optimizing dialysis: past, present and future, *Nutr Today* 32:30-36, 1997.
17. Stein EA: Managing dyslipidemia in the high risk patient, *Am J Cardiol* 89(5A), 50C-57C, 2002.
18. The American Dietetic Association: *Manual of clinical dietetics,* ed 5, Chicago, 1996, The Association.
19. The Diabetes Control and Complications Trial Research Group: The effect of intensive treatment of diabetes on the development and progression of long-term complications in insulin-dependent diabetes mellitus, *N Engl J Med* 329:977-986, 1993.
20. National Kidney Foundation Clinical Guidelines; published 2000 on http://www.nkf.org.

CHAPTER 166

Testicular Disorders

Updated by Patricia Polgar Bailey

DEFINITION/EPIDEMIOLOGY

Scrotal pain may be a symptom of an underlying pathologic condition of the scrotum or testis. The pain may be described as sharp, dull, aching, uncomfortable, or tender; and it is characterized as mild, moderate, or severe. The pain may be sudden in onset, remitting, or progressively escalating in severity. Scrotal pain may be the chief complaint or a serendipitous finding during the history and physical examination. It is necessary to determine the cause of the pain to evaluate the need for emergent referral or intervention and to exclude potentially life-threatening conditions.

Scrotal masses may be nodules or cystic changes on the skin of the scrotum; may involve intrascrotal contents such as the testis, epididymis, spermatic cord, or tunica vaginalis; or may be the result of abdominal structures herniated into the scrotal sac. Palpation may reveal single or multiple nodules of varying sizes with consistencies that range from soft to firm. The mass may be freely moveable or fixed and may range from nontender to extremely painful to touch or manipulation. Masses are found during testicular self-examination (TSE) or are discovered during examination and palpation of the scrotum by a health care provider. The mass may go undetected if it is small, if enlargement is gradual, and/or if discomfort is minimal or absent.

Scrotal swelling, or edema, may involve only one scrotum (left or right hemiscrotal edema) or both scrota (bilateral scrotal edema) and may indicate the presence of an underlying pathologic condition. Edema caused by a hydrocele may be benign, whereas swelling related to testicular torsion or a malignant tumor of the testis may be potentially life threatening. The clinical presentation of testicular cysts and dysplasias is enlarged testes, and both are clinically interpreted as neoplasms until otherwise evaluated.[1] Testicular tumors are usually malignant and account for approximately 1% of all malignancies in men.

The epidemiology of scrotal pain, masses, and swelling is dependent on the etiology of the disorders that manifest these symptoms. Specific disorders may occur more often in certain age-groups. The causes of scrotal pain, masses/tumors, or swelling discussed in this chapter are limited to those most commonly encountered in primary care: varicocele, epididymitis, epididymo-orchitis, spermatocele, hydrocele, torsion of the spermatic cord, trauma, scrotal hernia, and testicular tumors.

Immediate emergency department referral/ physician consultation is indicated for patients with sudden-onset unilateral scrotal pain or testicular torsion.

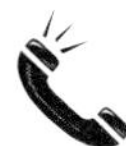

Physician consultation is indicated for epididymitis or right varicocele.

PATHOPHYSIOLOGY

A varicocele is caused by incompetent valves within the veins arising from the pampiniform plexus. This condition allows the reflux of blood from the spermatic vein, which results in dilated, tortuous varicose veins in the spermatic cord.[2] The incidence of varicocele is approximately 10% in young men and most often affects the left side.[3]

Epididymitis is an acute or chronic inflammation of the epididymis. The etiology may be bacterial, viral, parasitic, chemically induced, or related to trauma,[4] and it is further categorized as a nonspecific or specific infection or traumatic injury.[4] Nonspecific infections are caused by gram-negative rods, gram-positive cocci, or anaerobic bacteria associated with a group of diseases with similar symptoms.[5] Inflammation of the epididymis is occasionally caused by trauma or urinary reflux from the urethra through the vas deferens.[5] In men less than 35 years old, the cause is often related to sexual transmission of *Neisseria gonorrhoeae, Chlamydia trachomatis,* or *Escherichia coli.*[2] In men over 35 years old, epididymitis is most often associated with gram-negative rods or urologic procedures such as transurethral resection of the prostate or urethral catheterization. Epididymal inflammation may result as an asymptomatic complication of secondary syphilis, whereas tubercular epididymitis results from involvement of the prostate. Epididymitis can also occur in conjunction with inflammation of the testis (epididymo-orchitis) as a result of reflux of urine from straining, although the exact cause is unclear.[2]

Orchitis is a systemic, blood-borne infection that results in inflammation of the testis. It may coexist with epididymitis, be a consequence of viral infections such as mumps, or be a complication of syphilis, mycobacterial infections, or fungal infections.[2] Epididymo-orchitis is a complication in 20% to 35% of adolescent boys and young men with mumps[5] and can occur as a complication of many infectious diseases.[2,5]

A spermatocele is a sperm-filled cyst that arises from the tubules that connect the rete testis to the head of the epididymis. The etiology of this condition is unclear. Spermatoceles are usually small but can enlarge to several centimeters.[3]

A hydrocele is an accumulation of fluid within the tunica vaginalis as seen in adults; it may also result from a patent processus vaginalis at birth. In the adult, a hydrocele is often the result of trauma, a hernia, a testicular tumor, or as a complication of epididymitis.

Torsion of the spermatic cord is most often seen in the left testis. The left spermatic cord is longer and becomes twisted twice as often as that on the right side. Trauma may be the precipitating factor in young males. The torsion can be intermittent or complete and at times may resolve spontaneously. This condition results in congestion of venous blood flow and concomitant edema of the testis. If not resolved spontaneously or surgically, torsion can result in complete venous obstruction and necrosis of the testicular tissues.[6]

Trauma to the scrotum can be caused from burns or blunt force, or it may be penetrating and involve the testicle. Although only 2% to 3% of male patients presenting for medical care have genitourinary trauma injury, most of these injuries involve the scrotum and/or testis. A scrotal hernia results when a segment of the bowel slips through the internal inguinal ring, where it may remain in the inguinal canal or pass into the scrotal sac.[2] The hernia may spontaneously reduce by digital manipulation or when the patient lies supine, or it may become strangulated and require surgical reduction.

The origin of testicular tumors can be divided into three primary categories: germ cell origin, gonadal sex cord/stromal origin, and miscellaneous origin. On the basis of the histologic and genetic origin of the tumor, neoplasms of germ cell origin may be further divided into seminomas, nonseminomas, and non–germ-cell tumors.[7]

Testicular malignancies are relatively uncommon in the general population, occurring in only two to three men per 100,000 each year.[8] The most common age of occurrence is between 25 and 35 years,[8] although these tumors have also been reported in infants and in older men.[9] Testicular tumors appear to occur more often in white than in nonwhite populations, with a 35 times greater incidence in men who have a history of cryptorchism.[10] Seminomas are the most common type of testicular tumor and account for 90% to 95% of all primary malignancies.[8,9] Testicular nonseminomas are often associated with the presence of serum tumor marker products, particularly alpha-fetoprotein (AFP) and human chorionic gonadotropin (hCG). These markers are sensitive to changes in body tumors and can be used for diagnosis, prognosis, and monitoring of treatment response.

Although the exact cause of testicular tumors is unknown, tumors have been associated with scrotal trauma, atrophy, cryptorchism, and exogenous estrogen exposure.[7] Approximately 50% of patients diagnosed with a malignant testicular tumor have a history of cryptorchism, and 10% to 15% of patients have a history of scrotal trauma.[10,11] Studies also support an increased risk of tumor development in the sons of women exposed to diethylstilbestrol, estrogen, or estrogen-progestin combinations in the first 2 months of pregnancy.[7] In 10% of the cases studied, the development of testicular cancer has been linked with metastatic disease elsewhere in the body.[10] Studies also suggest a link between the development of testicular cancer and exposure to toxic chemicals or viruses.[7,9]

The development of testicular tumor cells is believed to occur during embryonic germ cell development within the testes. During normal male embryonic development, germ cells become spermatocytes. Tumor cells develop when embryonic germ cells undergo an abnormal pattern of differentiation. Germ cell tumors represent approximately 90% to 95% of all testicular tumors; nongerminal cell tumors such as Leydig's and Sertoli's cell tumors represent fewer than 5% of all testicular tumors.[7] Leydig's cell tumors are the most common and occur in both children and young adults. Metastasis from testicular tumors occurs primarily via the lymphatic system to other parts of the body.[8]

CLINICAL PRESENTATION

With testicular disorders, the history and presenting symptoms often suggest the underlying pathologic condition. Because some disorders may not cause significant discomfort, however, all male patients should be queried about changes in testicular size or the presence of nodules, pain, or penile discharge. The following disorders may be identified by the presenting complaint:

Varicocele—There are usually no visible outward signs other than a blue color through light-colored scrotal skin. The patient may complain of a dull pain or ache in the affected hemiscrotum or may be asymptomatic.[2]

Epididymitis—The patient presents with history of sudden onset of severe pain that is partially relieved by elevating the scrotum (Prehn's sign). Accumulation of scrotal edema is rapid and accompanied by fever.[2]

Orchitis—The patient presents with a history of sudden onset of acute or moderate pain, testicular swelling, and fever; the patient may have concomitant hydrocele.[2]

Spermatocele—A spermatocele is most often found on examination and usually is not painful. Enlarged and movable, a spermatocele may feel like a third testis or be mistaken for a hydrocele.[2]

Hydrocele—The patient may report a gradual enlargement that has become bothersome as a result of bulk in the scrotum.[2] There is marked edema, which may be uncomfortable to the patient because of the added weight. Hydroceles are usually painless and may be present for long periods, partially resolve, and recur before the patient seeks medical attention. A hydrocele may occur secondary to a tumor when excess serous fluid accumulates in the scrotal sac. A large scrotal mass that develops after minimal trauma to the testicles may suggest rupture of a testicular neoplasm.

Torsion of the spermatic cord—This condition is sudden in onset, extremely painful, and may awaken the patient from sleep or be trauma induced. In addition to testicular pain, the patient may experience abdominal pain, nausea, and vomiting with no fever.[2]

Trauma—There may be a history of blunt and/or penetrating injury to the scrotum that may involve the scrotal contents. Bruising, bleeding, and/or edema may be visible. Depending on the type and extent of the injury, the patient may be in excruciating pain or have little pain other than extreme tenderness to manipulation. If the trauma results in injury and inflammation of the epididymis, fever may also be present.

Scrotal hernia—Scrotal swelling and pain on straining are common complaints.[2] The edema is increased after standing in an erect position but decreases when the patient is in a recumbent position.

Testicular tumors—The patient generally seeks medical care for evaluation of an abnormal mass found during self-examination. Approximately 10% of patients complain of pain/discomfort in the testicles. Rarely, infertility is the presenting complaint.[4] The most common symptom or finding associated with a testicular tumor is the presence of a palpable mass that is often accompanied by edema or a sensation of fullness or heaviness in the scrotum. Patients may complain of scrotal pain; on rare occasions, an abdominal mass may be palpable. Other complaints such as back or abdominal pain, nausea, anorexia, or bowel and bladder symptoms may occur with retroperitoneal lymph node involvement.[4,5] Systemic endocrine effects may cause gynecomastia; as a result, associated lymph nodes may be enlarged and tender.

PHYSICAL EXAMINATION

Examination begins with inspection of the scrotum. Scrotal size can change with temperature variations because of the cremaster muscle mechanism. Asymmetry is expected because the left hemiscrotum is normally lower than the right. The skin of each hemiscrotum should be inspected carefully, spreading the rugae between the fingers. Care should be taken to inspect both the anterior and posterior surfaces to detect any lesions. It is common to find multiple sebaceous cysts on the scrotal skin that are small, firm, nontender, and white to yellowish in color.[2]

Each hemiscrotum should be palpated with the thumb and first two fingers of both hands. The scrotal contents should be easily movable in a sliding fashion. The testes should be oval in shape, smooth, equal, and firm but rubbery. The normal epididymis is softer than the testis, nontender, and smooth. To palpate the spermatic cord, the practitioner should slide the fingers and thumb up from the epididymis. The cord should feel smooth and nontender. Documentation should include any tenderness or pain, discoloration, edema, or abnormal findings, such as are found in the following conditions:

Varicocele—The patient presents with bluish color that shows through the scrotal skin; when the patient stands, palpation of the soft mass reveals a "bag of worms" on the proximal spermatic cord.[2] Right varicoceles may indicate venous obstruction or renal cancer. Varicoceles decrease when the patient is in the supine position.

Epididymitis—The scrotum is red, enlarged, and extremely tender. The epididymis may be enlarged and difficult to distinguish from the testis. The scrotal skin over the affected area may be edematous and thickened. Tubercular epididymitis manifests as a characteristic beading of the vas deferens. A history of prostatitis may be a precursor to the development of epididymitis.

Orchitis—As with epididymitis, testicular edema may be so pronounced that it is difficult to distinguish the testes from the epididymis. Palpation may reveal swollen, very tense testes that are painful, and the patient may be febrile.

Spermatocele—The spermatocele is palpated as a small, nontender, freely movable mass above and behind the testis. The mass may arise from the vasa efferentia (tubules that connect the rete testis to the epididymis), the epididymis, or cystic structures on the upper pole of the testis.[2] Transillumination of the mass in a darkened room may help visualize the mass.

Hydrocele—Palpation reveals a nontender mass, unless there is an underlying inflammatory process such as an epididymal infection.

Torsion of the spermatic cord—The scrotum may be edematous and erythematous, and the affected scrotum may be higher as because of shortening that occurs as a result of rotation. Torsion usually occurs in the left hemiscrotum. The spermatic cord is swollen and extremely tender, and the epididymis may be felt anteriorly. The cremaster response is absent on the affected side.[2]

Trauma—Bruising, bleeding, and edema may be present. Inspection should include careful comparison of coloration to determine the extent of bruising and/or expanding hematoma. A ruptured testis should be suspected if there is evidence of increasing hematoma, edema, and pain. Palpation should include external skin and scrotal contents. Documentation includes the time/date of injury, type of trauma, and any change in signs/symptoms since the time of injury.

Scrotal hernia—Inspection reveals an enlarged hemiscrotum that may spontaneously reduce when supine. Palpation reveals an enlarged mass in the scrotum that may spontaneously reduce when the patient is reclining. The practitioner will not be able to move the fingers above the mass, which should be soft and mushy but painless unless incarcerated and ischemic. Scrotal hernias do not transilluminate. Auscultation of bowel sounds over the mass is significant for the diagnosis of bowel in the scrotal sac.

Testicular tumor—Inquiry should focus on previous trauma to the scrotum or perineal area and the history or presence of cryptorchism, pain, swelling, or sensations in the scrotum. The physical examination should include inspection and palpation of the abdomen, perineal area, scrotal sac, testes, and surrounding lymph nodes. Palpation should be performed using both hands to assist in differentiating between a mass located on the body of the testicle and a mass located on or within the epididymis. The location, size, mobility, and degree of tenderness of normal structures, as well as any abnormal findings, should be noted.

Any solid, firm mass within the body of the testicle should be considered a tumor unless proven otherwise. A painless mass in one or both hemiscrotums with or without a hydrocele suggests malignancy.[8] Supraclavicular, scalene, and inguinal nodes are often enlarged.[8] Back pain may be present if masses are located in the retroperitoneal area. Scrotal transillumination performed in a darkened room may be used to visualize abnormalities and detect solid vs. fluid-filled masses.[9]

DIAGNOSTICS

Many testicular disorders are readily recognized at the time of presentation and do not require further evaluation. In general, clinical presentation and physical examination guide the choice of appropriate diagnostics:

Varicocele—Semen analysis may reveal oligospermia or azoospermia but can be normal.

Epididymitis—Doppler ultrasound may show increased sound waves caused by hyperemia.[4] Laboratory tests reveal white blood cells and bacteriuria.[2]

Orchitis—Doppler ultrasound may show increased sound waves caused by hyperemia.[4]

Spermatocele—A mass is located at the proximal aspect of the spermatic cord. Transillumination of the mass is expected.

Hydrocele—A hydrocele will transilluminate in a darkened room. (A cystic mass transilluminates; a tumor does not.)

Torsion of the spermatic cord—Doppler ultrasound may show diminished sound waves caused by ischemia.[4]

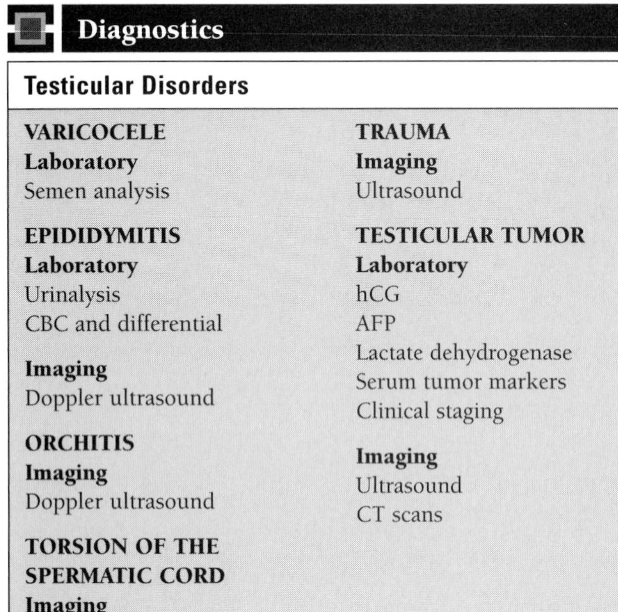

Diagnostics

Testicular Disorders

VARICOCELE
Laboratory
Semen analysis

EPIDIDYMITIS
Laboratory
Urinalysis
CBC and differential

Imaging
Doppler ultrasound

ORCHITIS
Imaging
Doppler ultrasound

TORSION OF THE SPERMATIC CORD
Imaging
Doppler ultrasound

TRAUMA
Imaging
Ultrasound

TESTICULAR TUMOR
Laboratory
hCG
AFP
Lactate dehydrogenase
Serum tumor markers
Clinical staging

Imaging
Ultrasound
CT scans

Trauma—The patient presents with visible bruising. Ultrasonography may be used to determine if the testis is intact.

Scrotal hernia—A scrotal hernia does not transilluminate.

Testicular tumor—The diagnosis of testicular cancer is generally confirmed through direct surgical exploration of the testes. Serum tumor markers, hCG, AFP, and lactic acid dehydrogenase may be used to support the history and physical examination findings. Tumor markers elevate when disease is present and return to normal during recovery.[11] A negative marker does not necessarily exclude disease, but an elevated marker is considered clinically significant.[9] High levels of hCG are seen in both seminomatous and nonseminomatous tumors, whereas AFP levels are elevated only in seminomas.[7] Ultrasonography is useful in detecting nonpalpable testicular masses and in confirming the size and location of palpable tumors. Differentiation of intratesticular masses from extratesticular masses may also be accomplished using ultrasound.[12] Abdominopelvic CT or other x-ray studies may be necessary to determine the extent and location of metastasis.

To assist practitioners in assessing the extent of testicular disease, various clinical staging systems have been developed and are based on surgical findings and histologic examination of retroperitoneal lymph nodes: stage I, tumor confined to testis; stage II, tumor spread to regional lymph nodes; stage III, tumor spread beyond retroperitoneal nodes.[7] Numerous other staging systems have been developed and are useful for describing and standardizing the clinical stages of testicular tumors.

DIFFERENTIAL DIAGNOSIS

The differential diagnosis for any testicular disorder should first exclude the possibility of a testicular tumor. It is often difficult to differentiate between epididymitis and orchitis because the symptoms are similar. A varicocele is more discernible than other scrotal masses because palpation of this mass classically resembles a bag of worms. However, many of the other conditions may have hydrocele development as a symptom.

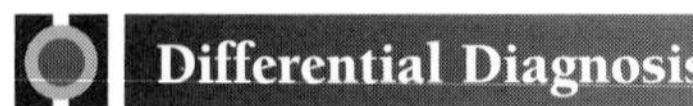
Differential Diagnosis

Testicular Disorders
Tumor
Cysts
Testicular torsion
Epididymitis
Orchitis
Hydrocele
Varicocele
Hernia
Hematoma
Spermatocele

The differential diagnosis for testicular tumors includes cysts, testicular torsion, epididymitis, or epididymal orchitis. A hydrocele, hernia, hematoma, or spermatocele may also mimic a testicular tumor.[11] The presence of a testicular mass is suggestive of a tumor and indicates the need for immediate referral.

Various diagnostics such as urine culture, urinalysis, Doppler ultrasound, and nuclear scan may be indicated to determine the cause of pain, mass, or edema. The history is probably equal to the physical examination in making a definitive diagnosis of the condition on the basis of signs, symptoms, precipitating factors, and length of time these have been present (or if they have changed over time).

MANAGEMENT

Management of testicular disorders depends on the specific type of disorder:

Varicocele—Treatment is ligation of the spermatic vein by a surgeon. However, recent review of the literature found insufficient evidence that ligation of the varicocele improves pregnancy rate in couples with unexplained fertility, whereas several studies in this review demonstrated improvement in semen quality after varicocele treatment.[13]

Epididymitis/orchitis—Antiinfective therapy is recommended, and guidance by sensitivity reports is suggested. In severe cases it may be necessary to use parenteral antibiotics.[4] With tubercular epididymitis, an epididymectomy may be performed to eradicate the condition.[4] Antipyretics should be used to reduce discomfort and fever, and an antiinflammatory agent should be prescribed. An antiemetic can also be prescribed for nausea and vomiting.

Spermatocele—No treatment is required unless the patient complains of discomfort or concern because of the increasing size of the mass. Treatment, if warranted, is excision of the mass.

Hydrocele—Active treatment is not warranted unless complications are present. If indicated, the hydrocele should be drained surgically and the hydrocele sac reanastomosed. Unfortunately, hydroceles may recur.[3] Some recent investigations for treatment have included sclerosing hydroceles to reduce recurrence rates.[14]

Torsion of the spermatic cord—Treatment is immediate surgical exploration and intervention to prevent ischemia and restore blood flow.

Trauma—If all scrotal contents are intact, trauma injuries can be treated symptomatically with ice and elevation. However, if there is concern that the testicle has been ruptured or penetrated, or if other contents are not palpated as intact, immediate surgical exploration and intervention should be sought.

Scrotal hernia—If the herniated bowel is reducible, surgical referral for possible future repair is indicated. However, the presence of pain may indicate incarceration of the bowel, in which case immediate emergency department referral/surgical consultation is indicated.

Testicular tumor—Prompt evaluation is essential. Surgical exploration and intervention are indicated if a mass in or adjacent to the testis cannot be satisfactorily evaluated with physical examination, transillumination, and ultrasonography. Primary treatment for seminomas involves radical orchiectomy followed by irradiation of the retroperitoneal lymph for low-stage seminomas and chemotherapy for more advanced stage seminomas. Nonseminomas are also treated with radical orchiectomy followed by retroperitoneal lymphadenectomy. Chemotherapy may be used for more advanced stage nonseminomas.[7] Follow-up visits should include a thorough physical examination, a chest x-ray study, and measurement of serum tumor markers monthly for the first year, every 2 months for the second year, and every 3 to 6 months for up to 5 years.

After a malignancy has been confirmed, the patient with testicular cancer may be placed on chemotherapy. In addition, the use of nonsteroidal antiinflammatory drugs and other analgesic agents may be necessary to relieve pain and inflammation.

LIFE SPAN CONSIDERATIONS

Four issues should be considered in the assessment and treatment of conditions involving the scrotum or testes: threat to life, immediate pain or discomfort, potential for infertility and/or impotence, and quality of life. Treatment success may depend on the overall health of the patient, available treatment options, and age-related issues affecting treatment decisions. Although the age of the patient may influence concerns regarding fertility, the potential loss of potency should not be disregarded in men of advanced age.

Surgical intervention for testicular tumors may result in body image disturbances and altered sexuality in adolescence and later life. After an orchiectomy, counseling may be indicated to assist in coping with loss related to alterations in the genitals and reproductive system. Education related to chemotherapy and surgical intervention is important to promote understanding and acceptance of the disorder and treatment.

COMPLICATIONS

Varicoceles can cause infertility because sperm concentration and motility are decreased in 65% to 75% of patients. The condition can be reversed if the varicocele is surgically corrected.[3] Infertility is also the most serious complication of epididymitis, orchitis, and spermatocele. In orchitis, testicular atrophy may develop in 50% of patients; on palpation, the testes are small and soft.[4] If a hydrocele is large, bowel herniation is likely and should be considered. Testicular tumors and epididymitis should be excluded. Unless complications such as diminished blood supply to the testis or hemorrhage resulting from trauma are present, active therapy for hydrocele is not required.[3]

Torsion of the spermatic cord is a medical emergency and should be surgically explored and relieved as quickly as possible to prevent the development of gangrene. A delay in treatment could result in testicular infarction and loss of the affected testicle. In scrotal trauma, the most pressing concern is whether the testis has been ruptured or the blood supply compromised from trauma-induced torsion of the spermatic cord. A referral to a urologist is required to verify that the testis and other scrotal contents are intact, with the injury treated symptomatically. Scrotal hernia with pain may indicate incarceration of the bowel and danger of ischemia, necrosis, and subsequent gangrene.

Testicular tumors are the most common malignancy and the third leading cause of death in young men.[10] Unlike other cancers, testicular cancer is potentially curable, even in an advanced stage. Improvements in diagnostic techniques and treatments over the past 25 years have resulted in an increased survival rate of approximately 90%.[11] The occurrence of testicular cancer in men over age 60 years is uncommon.[11] Prognosis with treatment may depend on the presence of other age-related or chronic health conditions at the time of treatment.

INDICATIONS FOR REFERRAL/HOSPITALIZATION

Patients suspected of having a testicular mass, torsion of the spermatic cord, or an incarcerated scrotal hernia require immediate referral. Epididymitis and minor scrotal trauma can be managed by the primary care provider unless complications are present or the testis is involved in a traumatic injury. A spermatocele should be referred for possible excision, as should the hydrocele that is expanding, causing pain, or may be caused by a scrotal tumor.

Hospitalization should be considered if the pain is unremitting, if a testicular mass is suspected, or if edema from testicular involvement cannot be excluded. Decisions regarding treatment alternatives may require in-depth discussion and consideration.

PATIENT AND FAMILY EDUCATION

Diagnosis, treatment options, potential outcomes, and the need for follow-up care should be carefully explained to patients. All patients should be encouraged to discuss their concerns or fears regarding the diagnosis and treatment or treatment options. These concerns and fears should be addressed truthfully regarding potential complications and the severity of the condition.

Patients with testicular masses require ongoing education and support from the time of diagnosis through all phases of treatment. Whenever possible, the spouse and/or significant other should be educated about the disease process, prognosis, treatment, and effects of treatment on relationships and sexuality. The patient and family should be encouraged to verbalize feelings and to support each other throughout the process.

HEALTH PROMOTION

Male patients, from adolescents to older adults, should be instructed on the correct method of TSE, asked to do a return demonstration, and encouraged to teach other males in their family the method and importance of the examination. The TSE should be performed monthly; patients should see their primary care provider if any abnormalities are detected.

REFERENCES

1. Peterson RO: Testicular neoplasms. In Caputo GM, Wight A, editors: *Urologic pathology,* ed 2, Philadelphia, 1992, JB Lippincott.
2. Jarvis C: Male genitalia. In Jarvis C, editor: *Physical examination and health assessment,* ed 2, Philadelphia, 1996, WB Saunders.
3. McAninch JW: Disorders of the testis, scrotum, and spermatic cord. In Tanagho EA, McAninch JW, editors: *Smith's general urology,* ed 14, Norwalk, Conn, 1995, Appleton & Lange.
4. Gray M: Scrotal inflammation. In Gray M, editor: *Genitourinary disorders,* St Louis, 1992, Mosby.
5. Meares EM: Nonspecific infections of the genitourinary tract. In Tanagho EA, McAninch JW, editors: *Smith's general urology,* ed 14, Norwalk, Conn, 1995, Appleton & Lange.
6. Sugar EC, Hoyler-Grant C: Disorders of the external genitalia in children. In Karlowizc KA, editor: *Urologic nursing: principles and practice,* Philadelphia, 1995, WB Saunders.
7. Klimaszewski AD, Karlowicz KA: Cancer of the male genitalia. In Karlowicz KA, editor: *Urologic nursing: principles and practice,* Philadelphia, 1995, WB Saunders.
8. Gray MR: Testicular tumors. In Gray M, editor: *Genitourinary disorders,* St Louis, 1992, Mosby.
9. Rowland RG, Fosta RS, Donohue J: Scrotum and testis. In Gillenwater JY and others, editors: *Adult and pediatric urology,* ed 3, St Louis, 1996, Mosby.
10. Spirnack JP: Adult scrotal mass. In Resnick MI, Caldamone AA, Spirnack JP, editors: *Decision making in urology,* ed 2, Philadelphia, 1991, BC Decker.
11. Richie JP: Detection and treatment of testicular cancer, *CA Cancer J Clin* 43(3):151-175, 1993.
12. Comiter CV and others: Nonpalpable intratesticular masses detected sonographically, *J Urol* 154:1367-1369, 1995.
13. Evers JLH, Collins JA, Vandekerckhove P: Surgery or embolisation for varicocele in subfertile men, *The Cochrane Database* of Systematic Reviews Issue 3, 2002, Retrieved September 2, 2002 from the World Wide Web: http://gateway2.ovid.com/oviedweb.cgi.
14. Yilmaz U and others: Does pleurodesis for pleural effusions give bright ideas about agents for hydrocele sclerotherapy? *Int Urol Nephrol* 32(1):89-92, 2000.

CHAPTER 167

Tumors of the Genitourinary Tract (Kidneys, Ureters, Bladder)

Laura Stempkowski

DEFINITION/EPIDEMIOLOGY

Tumors of the urinary tract may be benign or malignant. Benign renal tumors include adenomas, oncocytomas, and angiomyolipomas and are often incidentally found on imaging studies. Adenomas are small tumors of the renal cortex and are most often asymptomatic. Oncocytomas are adenomas of the renal collecting tubule and represent 1% to 14% of renal tumors. Although considered benign, on rare occasions they have demonstrated malignant potential. Angiomyolipomas, as the name implies, contain vascular tissue, smooth-muscle cells, and fatty elements. Because of the potential for hemorrhage, patients may become symptomatic presenting with pain, hematuria, or hypertension.[1]

Renal cell carcinoma (RCC) is the most prevalent malignant renal tumor in adults and constitutes more than 90% of all adult renal cancers. Wilms' tumor is a childhood renal tumor affecting approximately 1 in 10,000 children under the age of 15 years.[2]

Cancer of the bladder is the second most common cancer of the genitourinary tract.[3] The male-female ratio is 3:1, and the average age at diagnosis is 65 years.[4] As the population ages, the incidence of bladder cancer is increasing, but the incidence of advanced bladder cancer and the mortality rate are decreasing.[4] The etiology is unknown, but known risk factors include cigarette smoking and occupational exposures to chemicals, dyes, rubber, petroleum, leather, and printing chemicals. Chronic infection has been associated with bladder cancer, secondary to neurogenic bladder, stones, or long-term indwelling catheter use.[5]

PATHOPHYSIOLOGY

Renal Cell Carcinoma

In all, 85% of renal tumors are parenchymal tumors; the remainder have a uroepithelial origin or arise from supporting structures. RCC is an adenocarcinoma of the kidney that most often originates from the proximal tubule.[6] Evidence of metastasis is present in one third of patients at the time of diagnosis. The most common site of metastasis is the lungs.[6] Renal cell carcinomas are often associated with paraneoplastic syndromes, which may produce the initial symptoms (e.g., fever, anemia, cachexia, hypercalcemia, erythrocytosis, hypertension, hepatic dysfunction).[6]

RCC occurs with equal frequency in either kidney and may occur in the upper, mid, or lower poles. Tumor size at presentation varies from 1 to 10 cm or larger, and tumor size has been inversely correlated with survival.[1] Prognosis and treatment recommendations are based on the stage of disease. Two systems are commonly used to define the extent of disease: the Robson staging system and the TNM (tumor-nodes-metastasis) classification for kidney cancer.[6]

Wilms' Tumor

Wilms' tumor is unilateral in 95% of cases and is associated with several congenital anomalies, including cryptorchidism, ureteral duplication, and hypospadias.[6] Acquired von Willebrand disease has been associated with Wilms' tumor and should be considered in children with coagulation abnormalities or bleeding symptoms.[2]

Wilms' tumor may be familial or sporadic in occurrence and is associated with chromosomal abnormalities. The familial type is thought to be inherited by autosomal dominant transmission.[3]

Wilms' tumors are usually large and multi-lobulated with focal areas of hemorrhage and necrosis. Metastasis (e.g., lungs, liver) is present in 10% to 15% of cases at the time of diagnosis.[3] Staging of Wilms' tumor is based on the National Wilms' Tumor Society staging system and consists of five stages: from stage I (tumor limited to kidney and completely excisable) to stage IV (hematogenous metastasis to lung, liver, bone, and brain) and stage V (bilateral renal involvement).[3]

Bladder Cancer

Bladder cancer develops within the urothelium, the lining of the urinary tract. The urothelium is composed of three to seven layers of transitional cells that cover the muscular layers of the bladder wall. Proliferative changes of the transitional cells may result in cancer, which may remain superficial or progress to invasive or metastatic disease.

Transitional cell carcinoma (TCC) accounts for approximately 90% of all bladder cancers and may appear as papillary lesions or, less commonly, as sessile or ulcerated lesions.[3] A papilloma or papillary tumor is a less aggressive transitional cell tumor. Nontransitional cell carcinomas include adenocarcinomas, squamous cell carcinomas, undifferentiated carcinomas, and mixed carcinomas. Squamous cell carcinomas account for 2% to 5% of bladder cancers and are more resistant to treatment.[7]

Carcinomas of the bladder are graded and staged in an effort to define the aggressiveness and extent of disease. Staging defines the depth of invasion within the bladder and progression of disease—stage 0 (mucosal changes) to stage D (lymph node involvement). The depth of invasion into muscle layers and perivesical fat increases the risk of metastasis.[4]

Grading refers to the degree of cellular differentiation from normal urothelium. Transitional cell carcinomas are graded on a numerical scale from 1 to 4, with the higher grade tumors being more invasive and aggressive in behavior.

It is important to remember that transitional cell carcinoma can progress to, or present as, upper tract lesions. At least 90% of malignancies arising within the renal pelvis and ureter are TCCs. TCC of the upper tract is seen in nearly 5% of patients who have had bladder cancer.[8]

CLINICAL PRESENTATION

The average age at diagnosis of RCC is 55 to 60 years, with a male-female ratio of 2:1.3. The classic triad of flank pain, hematuria, and renal mass occurs in less than 10% of patients and, consequently, RCC is often not diagnosed until metastasis has occurred. A significant number of RCCs are found incidentally on imaging for other clinical problems.

Wilms' tumor affects children, with a mean age at diagnosis of 3.5 to 4 years.[2] In Wilms' tumor, the prevalent feature is an abdominal mass. Abdominal pain occurs in 30% to 40% of these patients, which may suggest an acute abdomen.

More than 70% of bladder cancer patients present with intermittent painless gross hematuria that is often described as continuing throughout urination. Irritative voiding symptoms (e.g., urgency, frequency, dysuria) may or may not be present.[5] The presence of microhematuria also may herald a urothelial malignancy and requires further investigation.

PHYSICAL EXAMINATION

Approximately 80% of children will have a large, smooth, firm, flank mass that often extends across the midline.

DIAGNOSTICS

See the Diagnostics box below.

DIFFERENTIAL DIAGNOSIS

See the Differential Diagnosis box on p. 734.

MANAGEMENT

Renal Cell Carcinoma

The prognosis for RCC is poor unless it is diagnosed and treated before metastasis occurs. Surgical intervention for localized disease offers the only potential for cure.[9] Surgical options include a radical nephrectomy, which may be done as either a laparoscopic or open procedure. A nephron-sparing partial nephrectomy may be an option in select situations.[10]

Preoperative renal artery embolization may be used to minimize blood loss, or pain or hematuria in the event of a nonre-

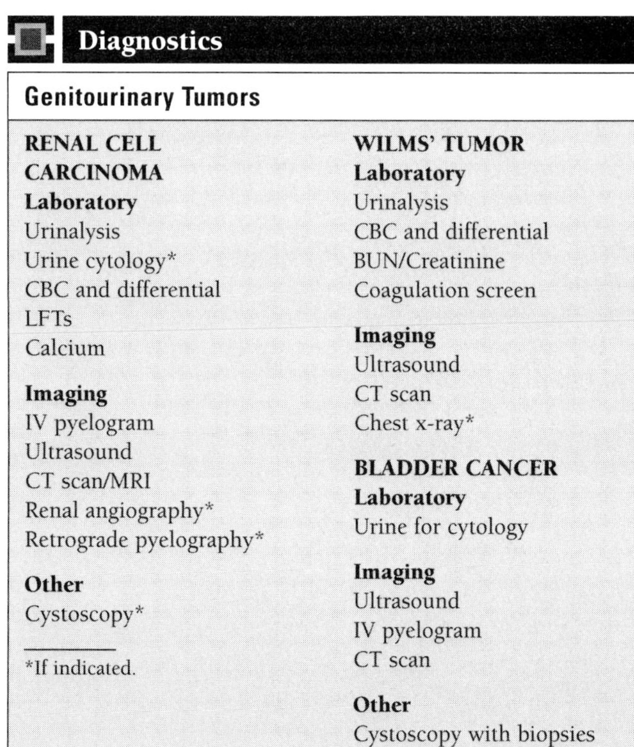

Diagnostics

Genitourinary Tumors

RENAL CELL CARCINOMA
Laboratory
Urinalysis
Urine cytology*
CBC and differential
LFTs
Calcium

Imaging
IV pyelogram
Ultrasound
CT scan/MRI
Renal angiography*
Retrograde pyelography*

Other
Cystoscopy*

WILMS' TUMOR
Laboratory
Urinalysis
CBC and differential
BUN/Creatinine
Coagulation screen

Imaging
Ultrasound
CT scan
Chest x-ray*

BLADDER CANCER
Laboratory
Urine for cytology

Imaging
Ultrasound
IV pyelogram
CT scan

Other
Cystoscopy with biopsies

*If indicated.

Differential Diagnosis

Genitourinary Tumors

Renal Cell Carcinoma
Simple cyst
Angiomyolipoma
Renal abscess
Arteriovenous malformations
Renal lymphoma
Transitional cell carcinoma of renal pelvis
Adrenal cancer
Oncocytoma

Wilms' Tumor
Neuroblastoma
Hydronephrosis
Mesoblastic nephroma
Fecal mass
Renal tumor, non-Wilms' tumor

Bladder Cancer
Urinary tract infection
Interstitial cystitis
Hemorrhagic cystitis
Fibrous polyp
Endometriosis
Hematoma
Bladder calculi

sectable tumor.[9] For patients with disseminated disease, radiation therapy is used for palliation of metastatic lesions (e.g., to the brain, bone, or lungs). RCC has shown limited response to biologic response modifiers (e.g., interferons, interleukin). Interleukin-2 has been the most effective of these for treating metastatic RCC. Clinical trials investigating vaccine therapy are promising and ongoing.[11]

Wilms' Tumor

For the child with Wilms' tumor, multimodality therapy has been successful, with cure rates currently approaching 90%.[2]

Bladder Cancer

Transurethral resection of the bladder tumor is usually the initial treatment for superficial bladder cancer. In cases of less aggressive cancer, follow-up surveillance may include interval urine cytologies and repeat cystoscopy with transurethral resection as necessary. Adjuvant intravesical therapy (e.g., bacillus Calmette-Guérin, mitomycin C, thiotepa, doxorubicin) may be used for tumors with unfavorable prognostic features (e.g., frequent recurrence, multifocal tumors, carcinoma in situ).[9] For muscle-invasive bladder tumors, a radical cystectomy with urinary diversion remains the standard therapy. Options for urinary diversion include ileal conduit, continent diversion, and orthotopic neobladder. Bladder conservation therapy, with combined-modality therapy with radiation and chemotherapy, may be an option for some patients.[12]

COMPLICATIONS

See Box 167-1.

INDICATIONS FOR REFERRAL/HOSPITALIZATION

A history and clinical presentation suspicious for genitourinary tumors mandate specialist referral and consultation. Hospitalization may be indicated for cases of acute illness or advanced disease.

PATIENT AND FAMILY EDUCATION

Patient education regarding tumors of the genitourinary tract should include information regarding prevention, the disease process, diagnostic and staging procedures, treatment options, prognosis, and symptom management. The importance of lifelong surveillance and follow-up care must be emphasized.

BOX 167-1

COMPLICATIONS OF COMMON GENITOURINARY TUMORS

RENAL CELL CARCINOMA
Complications of metastasis
Anemia
Pain
Hypercalcemia
Erythrocytosis
Hypertension
Hepatic dysfunction

WILMS' TUMOR
Treatment-related morbidity
Metastasis-related morbidity
Complications of associated congenital anomalies

BLADDER CANCER
Bladder perforation
Hematuria
Clot retention
Metastasis
Treatment-related morbidity
Obstruction

REFERENCES

1. Langdon DR, Liang BA, Harris RD: Imaging of renal tumors. In Ernstoff MS, Heaney JA, Peschel RE, editors: *Urologic cancer,* Cambridge, 1997, Blackwell Science.
2. Williams JA, Greenwald CA, Rao BN: Wilms' tumor. In Vogelzang NJ and others, editors: *Genitourinary oncology,* ed 2, Philadelphia, 2000, Lippincott Williams & Wilkins.
3. Carroll PR: Urothelial carcinoma: cancers of the bladder, ureter, and renal pelvis. In Tanagho EA, McAninch JW, editors: *Smith's general urology,* ed 14, Norwalk, 1995, Appleton & Lange.
4. Hudson MA, Catalona WJ: Urothelial tumors of the bladder, upper tracts, and prostate. In Gillenwater JY and others, editors: *Adult and pediatric urology,* ed 3, vol 1, St Louis, 1996, Mosby.
5. Hawkins CA: Diagnosis of and screening for urothelial cancer. In Ernstoff MS, Heaney JA, Peschel RE, editors: *Urologic cancer,* Cambridge, 1997, Blackwell Science.
6. McDougal WS, Garnick MB: Clinical signs and symptoms of renal cell carcinoma. In Vogelzang NJ and others, editors: *Genitourinary oncology,* ed 2, Philadelphia, 2000, Lippincott Williams & Wilkins.
7. Flynn SD, Kacinski B, Peschel RE: Pathology and staging of urothelial cancer. In Ernstoff MS, Heaney JA, Peschel RE, editors: *Urologic cancer,* Cambridge, 1997, Blackwell Science.
8. Heney NM: Management of tumors in the renal pelvis and ureter. In Ernstoff MS, Heaney JA, Peschel RE, editors: *Urologic cancer,* Cambridge, 1997, Blackwell Science.
9. Dreicer R, Williams RD: Renal parenchymal neoplasms. In Tanagho EA, McAninch JW, editors: *Smith's general urology,* ed 14, Norwalk, 1995, Appleton & Lange.
10. Franklin JR, de Kernion JB: Surgical approaches to renal cell carcinoma. In Ernstoff MS, Heaney JA, Peschel RE, editors: *Urologic cancer,* Cambridge, 1997, Blackwell Science.
11. Gorsch SM, Ernstoff MS: Biologic therapy of renal cell carcinoma. In Ernstoff MS, Heaney JA, Peschel RE, editors: *Urologic cancer,* Cambridge, 1997, Blackwell Science.
12. Heaney JA: Future directions in urothelial cancer. In Ernstoff MS, Heaney JA, Peschel RE, editors: *Urologic cancer,* Cambridge, 1997, Blackwell Science.

CHAPTER 168

Urinary Calculi

Carol A. Whelan

DEFINITION/EPIDEMIOLOGY

Urinary calculi, or stone disease, is the third most common disorder of the urinary tract, with a prevalence rate of up to 10% in industrialized nations.[1,2] The incidence of stone formation may be related to geography, climate, season, age, gender, and heredity.[3] The majority of stones are found within the kidney, but stone formation may also occur in the ureter and bladder and urinary diversion structures (e.g., ileal conduit, orthotopic bladder). Although many questions about stone formation remain unanswered, understanding of the etiologies has improved in recent years. As a result, greater emphasis is directed at the prevention of stone formation.

In the United States, the incidence of urinary calculi is highest in the Southeast but is also prevalent in the Northwest and Southwest. Symptoms of stone complications tend to occur more often during the summer season. The peak age of onset is 20 to 30 years, with the incidence tapering after age 50 years. There is a male-to-female predominance of 3 to 4:1.[2] Excessive ingestion of substances that produce stones, such as purines (e.g., seafood, organ meats), oxalates (e.g., colas, chocolate), calcium (e.g., dairy products), and phosphate increase the incidence of stone formation. In the United States, stone disease in children is usually related to metabolic alterations or a tendency to develop stones after urinary diversion. The genetic predisposition to stones is controversial, except for stones resulting from enzyme deficiencies (e.g., cystinuria and xanthinuria). Other predisposing factors include occupation (e.g., sedentary activity, risks of dehydration), a family history of urinary stone formation, and medications (e.g., acetazolamide, antacids, ascorbic acid in dosages of 2 g or more daily, hydrochlorothiazide, and indinavir [Crixivan]).

PATHOPHYSIOLOGY

The formation of urinary calculi is a multifaceted process. The natural sequence of urine changes leading to stone development include urine saturation, urine supersaturation, formation of crystalline materials, crystal nucleation, aggregation, retention of crystals by the urothelium, and continued growth of the stone on retained crystals.[4] The entire process is influenced by multiple chemical, physical, physical-chemical, biochemical, and physiologic events. The components of urinary stones include calcium oxalate, calcium phosphate, bacteria, purines, or cystine; the majority of stones are mixtures of two or more components.

The various types of stones include calcium, uric acid, ammoniomagnesium phosphate (struvite), cystine, and xanthine.[2] Calcium stones are the most common type and account for approximately 70% of all stones formed.[2] Approximately 26% of these stones are composed of pure calcium oxalate; 7% are pure calcium phosphate, and the remainder are a combination of calcium oxalate and calcium phosphate, a few of which may contain a uric acid core.[2] Calcium stones are radiopaque, tend to be limited to 1 cm in size, and differ in etiology. Urine levels of oxalate, normally a metabolic byproduct, may increase as a result of the ingestion of foods high in oxalate such as rhubarb, nuts, cocoa, tea, beans, lime peel, and green leafy vegetables; this condition is termed *hyperoxaluria*. Hyperoxaluria may also develop with certain malabsorptive small bowel disorders, including Crohn's disease, jejunoileal bypass, celiac sprue, chronic pancreatitis, and biliary obstruction. The ingestion of ethylene glycol, a major component of antifreeze, can also result in hyperoxaluria. Primary hyperoxaluria, an enzyme deficiency, is one of the most severe of the diseases causing stone formation.[2] Urine saturation with uric acid, known as hyperuricosuria, may result in urate crystals that serve as a nidus for calcium oxalate nucleation. Hypocitraturia, which forms a highly soluble complex with calcium, is an important inhibitor of stone formation.

Conditions that cause reduced citrate excretion include distal renal tubular acidosis (RTA), diarrheal disorders, infection, exercise starvation, and androgen and magnesium deficiency. RTA results in metabolic acidosis, defective urinary acidification, hypokalemia, and reduced urinary citrate concentrations. Metabolic acidosis increases bone resorption, resulting in increased calcium and phosphate concentration. Favorable conditions for calcium phosphate stone formation are high urine pH, reduced citrate excretion, and increased urinary concentration of calcium and phosphate. Stone formation is also encouraged by anatomic abnormalities that reduce urine flow or cause stasis, including horseshoe kidney, genitourinary diverticula, obstructive disorders, and medullary sponge kidney.

Uric acid stones account for 5% to 10% of all stones and are more prevalent in men. Uric acid is an end-product of purine metabolism; increased uricosuria is often due to dehydration and excessive purine intake. Other risk factors include a consistently low urine pH, gout, myeloproliferative disorders, cytotoxic drugs, and conditions that predispose a patient to concentrated urine. Uric acid stones are radiolucent and appear as filling defects on the x-ray study.[2] Prevention involves reducing dietary purines, administering allopurinol to reduce uric acid excretion, and maintaining a urine volume greater than 2 L/day and a urinary pH greater than 6.0.[1] Alkalization of urine may help to prevent and dissolve stones.

Struvite stones, composed of magnesium, ammonium, and phosphate (MAP), are also referred to as *infection stones*. Struvite stones account for approximately 10% to 15% of all stones, are more prevalent in women, and are often present as renal staghorn calculi. Struvite stones grow rapidly and recur frequently. Urease, a bacterial enzyme, precipitates urea splitting and results in high ammonium concentration and alkaline urine (pH range of 6.8 to 8.3). This elevated pH causes the MAP crystals to precipitate, creating the struvite stone. Struvite does not form in the absence of infection; the urinary infection is usually from *Proteus* organisms.

Cystinuria is a genetic abnormality in which there is an excessive urinary excretion of the amino acids cystine, ornithine, lysine, and arginine. The low solubility of cystine results in stone formation, accounting for 1% to 2% of all stones. Cystine stones are radiopaque and tend to be round. The peak incidence of cystine stones is in the second and third decade of life.

Cystinuria should be suspected with stone formation in children.

Xanthinuria is caused by a congenital deficiency of the enzyme xanthine oxidase, which results in stone formation and increased excretion of xanthine. These stones are radiolucent and are often mistaken for uric acid stones.

CLINICAL PRESENTATION

Patients with renal colic often present with severe flank pain that may migrate anteriorly and into the groin as the stone moves from the kidney toward the bladder. Renal or ureteral colic is a result of the stone obstruction of the urinary tract. This obstruction is usually in one or more of five locations: (1) the calyx; (2) the ureteropelvic junction; (3) at or near the pelvic brim, where the ureter begins to arch over the iliac vessels; (4) the posterior pelvis, where the ureter is crossed anteriorly by the pelvic blood vessels and the broad ligament; and (5) the ureterovesical junction, which is the most constricted area.[4] Renal or ureteral colic is often associated with nausea and vomiting, gross hematuria, and dysuria. Fever may be present if infection occurs with the stone. Patients are often extremely restless as they attempt to find a comfortable position. Less often there may be persistent microhematuria or intermittent dull pain that extends over weeks or months.

PHYSICAL EXAMINATION

A careful medical history should be obtained and should include stone history, medical problems, medications, family history, occupation, diet, and fluid intake. The physical examination includes assessment of systemic symptoms; meticulous abdominal examination to exclude other sources of pain is essential. Typical examination findings include fever, tachycardia, diaphoresis, and costovertebral angle tenderness.

DIAGNOSTICS

Proper evaluation can identify the underlying cause of stone formation in up to 97% of patients.[5] Furthermore, up to 50% of all first-time stone formers will have a recurrence.[5] The cornerstone of diagnostics is a detailed history and physical, after which the appropriate laboratory work can be ordered.

Urinalysis is necessary to determine pH and to identify the presence of bacteria, crystals, and red blood cells. Urine should be strained for stone analysis. CBC, a complete metabolic panel (SMA-20), and an intact parathyroid hormone (PTH) level should be obtained. If the cause is still unknown, a 24-hour urine on the patient's usual diet should be obtained and measured for calcium, oxalate, citrate, magnesium, sodium and sulfate.

Urine pH above 6.5 suggests infection, and a follow-up culture is necessary.[5] Urine pH below 5.4 associated with metabolic acidosis is almost always RTA, whereas the presence of benzene crystals is diagnostic of cystinuria.[5] Elevated intact PTH levels and hypercalcemia are the result of either hyperparathyroidism (either primary or secondary) or sarcoidosis.[5]

Either an abdominal x-ray study (KUB) or an ultrasound will aid in diagnosis. An IV pyelogram may also be considered. An IVP is contraindicated in patients with sensitivity to radiologic dye.

Diagnostics

Urinary Calculi

Laboratory	Imaging
Urinalysis	Ultrasound
CBC and differential	IV pyelogram and IM pyelogram with tomography*
Complete metabolic panel	CT scan*
PTH	Retrograde pyelography*
24-hour urine (for calcium oxalate, citrate, magnesium, sodium, and sulfate)*	**Other**
Urine culture*	Urine strain for stone analysis

*If indicated.

DIFFERENTIAL DIAGNOSIS

See the Differential Diagnosis box below.

MANAGEMENT

Nonpharmacologic means of treatment should be used initially for all patients regardless of stone type. All patients with recurrent stones should have stone analysis to plan appropriate treatment. Urinary calculi 5 mm or less in diameter are usually passed spontaneously, sometimes only after aggressive hydration. Larger stones were considered a major problem before the 1980s, when extensive surgical procedures were often needed. The morbidity associated with stone disease has been greatly reduced with the advent of extracorporeal techniques for stone treatment and with the refinement of endoscopic surgery. The three major endourologic procedures include extracorporeal shock-wave lithotripsy (ESWL), percutaneous nephrolithotomy (PCNL), and ureteroscopy. ESWL is the least invasive treatment and the treatment of choice for 80% to 85% of stones.[6] It is indicated for stones that cannot be passed spontaneously, can be visualized on x-ray film, are located in the proximal ureter or kidney, and are less than 2.5 to 3.0 cm. PCNL is the treatment of choice for renal and proximal ureteral stones larger than 2.0 to 3.0 cm. Ureteroscopy, an emergency procedure, may be performed to relieve obstruction, to allow basket extraction of stones, or to allow lithotripsy of stones in the distal ureter.

Calcium stones are the most complex of all stones in their causes and treatments. The accepted theory of etiology is an

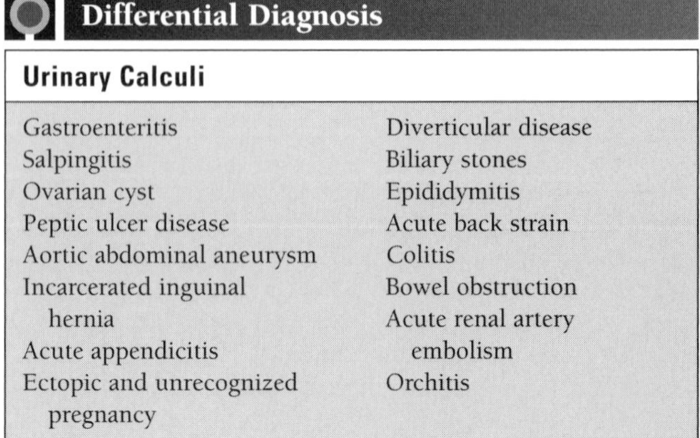

Differential Diagnosis

Urinary Calculi

Gastroenteritis	Diverticular disease
Salpingitis	Biliary stones
Ovarian cyst	Epididymitis
Peptic ulcer disease	Acute back strain
Aortic abdominal aneurysm	Colitis
Incarcerated inguinal hernia	Bowel obstruction
Acute appendicitis	Acute renal artery embolism
Ectopic and unrecognized pregnancy	Orchitis

imbalance between urinary excretion of insoluble salts and water, which results in an environment of supersaturation.[6] Therefore treatment is aimed at raising urine flow rate and reducing excretions of stone-forming salts. Stone formation associated with idiopathic hypercalciuria can be decreased with a twice-daily dose of thiazides and a low-calcium, low-protein, low-sodium diet. Evidence for benefit exists for the use of thiazides and the prevention of renal stones.[7] Calcium stones associated with hyperparathyroidism are best prevented through surgical removal of parathyroid adenoma or parathyroid tissue. Administration of oral citrate or alkali replacement decreases the chances for stone formation.

The main cause of hyperoxaluria seems to be related to diet and is most easily regulated by omitting foods high in oxalate, such as colas, chocolate, and peanuts. Management of hyperoxaluria related to malabsorption syndromes is multifaceted and may include improvement of bowel function, reduced fat and oxalate intake, and the administration of calcium and cholestyramine.

Hyperuricosuria, which is associated with calcium oxalate stones, is most simply managed by reducing the intake of foods that cause elevated uric acid excretion. Persistent stone formation may be treated with allopurinol, which lowers uric acid, but limited evidence exists for its benefit.[7]

Uric acid stones are managed most practically by maintaining a urine output greater than 2 L/day and alkalinizing the urine.[8] Maintaining a urinary pH above 6.0 increases the solubility of urate ions, thereby decreasing stone formation. Avoidance of excessive purine intake may be beneficial. Commonly used alkalinizing agents are sodium bicarbonate and potassium citrate,[8] but very limited evidence exists for their benefit.[7] Allopurinol, which inhibits the formation of uric acid, is commonly used when there is a lack of response to diet control and alkalinizing agents, but again, only limited evidence exists for its benefit.[7]

Management of ammoniomagnesium phosphate (struvite) stones may require medical and/or surgical interventions. Antimicrobial therapy to sterilize the urine—thereby slowing the growth of stones or preventing the formation of new stones—is not a definitive therapy but provides valuable adjuvant therapy. Urease inhibitors may be used to prevent struvite formation or to slow the growth of existing calculi.[9] The most commonly used urease inhibitor is acetohydroxamic acid. Hydroxyurea, once thought to be a potent inhibitor, is no longer considered effective and also has demonstrated high toxicity rates. Irrigation with chemical solutions to dissolve the stone or stone fragments, called *chemolysis,* is no longer considered effective because of the risks of treatment and the length of time necessary for stone dissolution.[9] Surgical options include nephrolithotomy, ESWL, and PCNL. The American Urologic Association Nephrolithiasis Guidelines Panel recently recommended that PCNL or a combination of PCNL and ESWL be the first-line treatment for struvite calculi.[9] ESWL is considered appropriate for small (2.0 cm) struvite calculi, and nephrolithotomy is an acceptable option for complex struvite calculi.

Prevention of cystine stones includes reduced intake of protein-rich foods and high intake of fluids (3 L/day). Alkalinization of urine may be of limited value given its tendency to precipitate the formation of calcium stones. D-Penicillamine or tiopronin (Thiola) may be prescribed to reduce stone formation. Among the more common side effects of long-term D-penicillamine therapy is B_{12} deficiency. Thiola has fewer side effects but still poses some risk for hematologic changes, fever, proteinuria, and rash. Prevention of xanthine stones includes high fluid intake and urinary alkalization.

COMPLICATIONS

Renal calculi are associated with an increased risk of urinary tract infection with the potential for progression to sepsis. Hydronephrosis, which is associated with partial or complete obstruction of the renal pelvis or ureter, is another possible complication. Additional potential sequelae include renal tissue damage and renal failure as a result of obstruction or stone movement and nephrocalcinosis as a result of deposition of calcium phosphate in the renal parenchyma.[3]

INDICATIONS FOR REFERRAL/HOSPITALIZATION

Management of kidney or urinary tract stones often requires both medical and surgical intervention. Specific treatment depends on a number of factors including stone type and location. The presence of infection or obstruction is an indication for urologic referral. Patients with persistent pain, gross hematuria, fever, or chills should be referred. Severe obstruction, infection, pain, and serious bleeding may require hospitalization.

PATIENT AND FAMILY EDUCATION

Patients suspected of having stones should be instructed to increase fluid intake, strain all urine, and use analgesics as necessary. An emphasis on healthy lifestyle habits such as regular exercise, generous fluid intake (2 to 4 L/day), and a balanced diet high in fiber is preliminary to stone prevention. Specific patient education is based on individual risk factors, the type of stone produced by the patient, a prescribed medical regimen, and co-morbidities.

REFERENCES

1. Stoller ML, Bolton DM: Urinary stone disease. In Tanagho EA, McAninch JW, editors: *Smith's general urology*, ed 14, Norwalk, Conn, 1995, Appleton & Lange.
2. Monk RD: Clinical approach to adults, *Semin Nephrol* 16(5):375-388, 1996.
3. Bruton DS and others: Urinary calculi. In Karlowicz KA, editor: *Urologic nursing: principles and practice*, Philadelphia, 1995, WB Saunders.
4. Menon M, Parulkar BG, Drach G: Urinary lithiasis: etiology, diagnosis and medical management. In Walsh PC and others, editors: *Campbell's urology*, ed 7, vol 2, Philadelphia, 1998, WB Saunders.
5. Rivers K, Shetty S, Menon M: When and how to evaluate a patient with nephrolithiasis, *Urol Clin North Am* 27(2):203-213, 2000.
6. Lingerman JE: Lithotripsy and surgery, *Semin Nephrol* 16(5):487-498, 1996.
7. Pearle MS, Roehrborn CG, Pak CY: Meta-analysis of randomized trials for the prevention of calcium oxalate nephrolithiasis, *J Endourol* 13(9):679-685, 1999.
8. Parks JH, Coe FL: Pathogenesis and treatment of calcium stones, *Semin Nephrol* 16(5):398-411, 1996.
9. Asplin JR: Uric acid stones, *Semin Nephrol* 16(5):412-425, 1996.

PART 14

Evaluation and Management of Gynecologic Disorders

PATRICIA POLGAR BAILEY, Section Editor

CHAPTER 169

Amenorrhea

Marie Elena Botte

DEFINITION/EPIDEMIOLOGY

Amenorrhea is the absence of menstrual bleeding. Primary amenorrhea has been defined as the absence of both spontaneous uterine bleeding and secondary sexual characteristics (delayed puberty) at age 14, by 2 years after sexual maturation,[1] or the absence of menarche at age 16 regardless of the presence of secondary sexual characteristics.[2,3] Secondary amenorrhea refers to the absence of menstrual bleeding by 18 months after menarche,[1] for 12 months, or three cycle lengths, in a woman with prior oligomenorrhea,[3] and the cessation of menstrual bleeding for 6 months in a woman with prior regular menses. Although the average age for menarche in the United States is 12.7 years[4] (12.8 years for white adolescents and slightly earlier, 12.6 years, for their black counterparts), there is a range of 9 to 16 years, and factors besides race such as nutritional status, body fat, and maternal age at menarche are also contributory.[1]

Primary amenorrhea has an estimated prevalence of between 0.1% and 0.3%.[3] Secondary amenorrhea is much more common, affecting between 1% and 3% of women of reproductive age in the general population.[5] Higher prevalence has been noted in specific subgroups of women, such as college students, U.S. ballet dancers (there is a much lower prevalence in dancers from the Netherlands), and endurance athletes, particularly runners.[6,7] Studies have found the relative risk of amenorrhea to be highest in younger women[8] who are more educated and older at menarche than control subjects, as well as in users of oral contraceptives.[8]

Amenorrhea is one of the cardinal features of anorexia nervosa, and one study found a subgroup of amenorrheic runners who scored in the extreme range on measures of both depression and eating disorders.[7] Women with systemic lupus erythematosus receiving pulse cyclophosphamide therapy are at increased risk of sustained amenorrhea, and women diagnosed with type 1 (insulin-dependent) diabetes mellitus before menarche have an increased probability of delayed menarche and menstrual disturbances, including amenorrhea.[9] Approximately 2.5 % of healthy adolescents will experience pubertal delay.[2]

PATHOPHYSIOLOGY

Aside from physiologic amenorrhea resulting from constitutional delay, pregnancy, lactation, or menopause, the pathophysiologic mechanisms for amenorrhea generally involve disorders of the sex chromosomes, hypothalamic-pituitary-ovarian axis, and related hormone production; the responsiveness of the uterine endometrium to various hormones; and the patency of the outflow tract. Because normal ovarian development is dependent on the presence of at least two X chromosomes, abnormalities involving X and Y chromosomes can result in gonadal failure, agonadism, gonadal dysgenesis, and androgen resistance (testicular feminization). Problems with hypothalamic synthesis or release of gonadotropin-releasing hormone (GnRH) can result in hypogonadotropic hypogonadism. Müllerian agenesis, obstruction of the vaginal outflow tract (such as with an imperforate hymen), cervical stenosis, or transverse vaginal septa are structural etiologies for primary amenorrhea. Transient amenorrhea can also result from administration of leuprolide (Lupron) in the treatment of fibroids or endometriosis. Physiologic lesions such as tumors or adenomas, systemic illness, or total-body and nodal irradiation may also contribute to the problem.[10-13]

Disorders of the hypothalamic-pituitary-ovarian axis can cause primary, as well as secondary, amenorrhea. Hypothalamic causes for dysfunction of this axis that can result in pubertal delay or insufficiency commonly include stress, starvation, chronic illness, depression, intensive athletic training, weight loss, and eating disorders; up to 25% of female athletes experience exercise-induced amenorrhea.[14] The Female Athlete Triad involves the combination of amenorrhea, osteoporosis, and disordered eating, and in female college athletes disordered eating is estimated to be between 15% and 62%.[15] The majority of young women with amenorrhea are estrogen deficient; a minority have normal estrogen levels that are unopposed by progesterone secondary to anovulation.[5]

Amenorrhea resulting from weight loss has been linked to a deranged process of prolactin secretion as a result of both neuroendocrine alterations and low plasma levels of gonadal steroids, as well as changes in the growth hormone-releasing hormone-induced growth hormone response.[16] One study found that among anorectic and bulimic women, those with amenorrhea had a mean percent of ideal body weight, as defined by Metropolitan Life Insurance Company criteria, of 74% ± 1%, compared with 102% ± 19% for those who were menstruating.[17] Another study found no statistically significant association between amenorrhea and body mass index but did note an association between amenorrhea and fasting or purging behaviors in normal and above-weight teenagers that was most evident in the heaviest subjects.[18] The physiologic mechanism resulting in amenorrhea and hypothalamic dysfunction associated with anorexia nervosa has yet to be fully elucidated, but it is believed that neurotransmitter abnormalities (central dopaminergic and opioid activity) may modulate the response of luteinizing hormone (LH) to GnRH.[19] Amenorrhea can also be seen in obese patients; reduction of body fat can bring about return of regular menstrual flow.

Persistent amenorrhea has been correlated with a longer duration of eating disorders and the presence of a concomitant anxiety disorder.[17] There has also been support for an association between stressful life events and the onset of hypogonadotropic-type secondary amenorrhea.[20] There may also be a causal role for increased melatonin secretion in hypogonadotropic hypogonadism.[21]

Prolactinemia associated with amenorrhea following normal puberty may be caused by breastfeeding, microadenomas or macroadenomas of the pituitary, renal failure, or the use of medications (e.g., psychoactive drugs such as haloperidol, amitriptyline, benzodiazepines, cocaine). Studies have suggested that (1) suppression of normal ovarian cyclic activity in women with pituitary microadenomas may be mediated by hyperprolactinemia, which blocks the action of gonadotropin at the ovarian level, and (2) that anovulation associated with hyperprolactinemic amenorrhea is primarily caused by both impaired gonadotropin pulsatility and derangement of the estrogen-positive feedback effect on LH in the face of a continued ovarian response to gonadotropin.[22,23]

Certain drugs, such as chemotherapeutic agents, may affect menstruation. Autoimmune disorders, such as Addison's disease, hypothyroidism, and toxic thyroiditis, have also been associated with amenorrhea, perhaps as a result of connections between genes controlling reproductive function and genes associated with autoimmune conditions on a segment of the major histocompatibility complex.[24] In thalassemic patients with secondary amenorrhea, severe and progressive damage to the hypothalamic-pituitary axis has been demonstrated by gonadotropin pulse abnormalities, marked reduction in GnRH-stimulated gonadotropin levels, and even apulsatility.[25]

CLINICAL PRESENTATION

Relevant history in the evaluation of amenorrhea includes a thorough menstrual history (age at menarche, frequency, duration, flow, last menstrual period, history of missed menses). A complete sexual history (number of partners; date of last intercourse; method of birth control and percentage of use; number of pregnancies, abortions, miscarriages, or ectopic pregnancies; and surgical history), as well as the age at menarche and menopause for family members and any family history of infertility, is also necessary.

Probable signs of past ovulatory cycles include breast tenderness, cyclic abdominal pain or bloating, and changes in the cervical mucus. The past medical history should be examined specifically for autoimmune disorders, childhood onset of type 1 diabetes mellitus, previous irradiation or chemotherapy, frequent fractures or osteoporosis, and thyroid or adrenal dysfunction. A complete medication history regarding prescribed, over-the-counter, and illicit drug use should be obtained. Nutritional and exercise factors, including disordered eating behavior, recent weight loss or gain, and athletic training are evaluated, along with endocrinologic markers of growth and development (growth charts and the presence or absence of secondary sexual characteristics, specifically breast development and pubic hair).

A review of systems may reveal indications of systemic illness such as thyroid dysfunction, headaches, or visual disturbances (possibly indicating a cranial mass in the area of the pituitary or hypothalamus), galactorrhea, or signs of hyperandrogenism (hirsutism, truncal obesity, deepening of the voice) or hypoestrogenism (hot flashes, vaginal dryness, headaches, depression, dyspareunia, decreasing breast size). A social history may indicate substance abuse or stressful life events (e.g., going away to college, entering religious life or the armed forces, sudden changes in the environment, death or divorce in the family), which have been linked with amenorrhea.[10,12]

PHYSICAL EXAMINATION

In addition to an evaluation of general growth and development (congenital short stature together with neck webbing and a pigeon chest suggests Turner's syndrome), the physical examination may reveal signs of androgen excess (hirsutism, acne, male pattern hair loss, truncal obesity, clitoromegaly >1 cm), androgen insensitivity (complete absence of axillary and pubic hair), hyperprolactinemia (galactorrhea on breast examination), decreased estrogen status (pale, dry vaginal mucosa; scant cervical mucus), or eating disorders (cachexia, hypothermia, lanugo hair, decreased blood pressure, bradycardia, dry skin, tooth decay, chipmunk cheeks, Chvostek's sign). Visual acuity and a funduscopic examination are important, because vision changes or retinal abnormalities may reflect an intracranial mass. The thyroid is palpated for masses or nodules. A pelvic examination assesses estrogen status via vaginal epithelium and cervical mucus, may identify an imperforate hymen, and also provides a gross evaluation of the cervix, uterus, and ovaries. Presumptive signs of pregnancy include breast tenderness, a bluish-colored cervix (Chadwick's sign), fatigue, nausea, vomiting, and urinary frequency. Probable signs of pregnancy are an enlarged uterus, a positive pregnancy test, and softening of the lower uterine segment (Goodell's and Hegar's signs). Enlarged ovaries are palpable in 60% of women with polycystic ovary disease[12] and in combination with acne, obesity and acanthosis nigricans suggest this diagnosis. Abdominal striae on nulliparous women may be indicative of hypercortisolism[3] and skin tags, fissures, and fecal occult blood may indicate inflammatory bowel disease.[1]

DIAGNOSTICS

The possibility of pregnancy or lactation-induced amenorrhea must be excluded in all women before any other diagnostic evaluation is initiated. Next, follicle-stimulating hormone (FSH), LH, thyroid-stimulating hormone (TSH), and prolactin levels should be checked for anovulation, hypothyroidism, or hyperprolactinemia, respectively, or possibly for an early presentation of acromegaly, which produces excess prolactin, as well as growth hormone. The best time to obtain a prolactin level is early in the morning after a 12-hour fast. There should be no stimulation of the breasts before the serum level is drawn. If prolactin levels are elevated, a CT scan of the sella turcica to identify microadenomas and macroadenomas is necessary. If these tests are normal, a progesterone challenge test, which classically consists of 10 mg of medroxyprogesterone administered daily for 5 to 7 days, can further evaluate estrogen status. Any vaginal bleeding within 2 to 7 days after the cessation of progesterone signals a positive progesterone challenge, indicating both adequate estrogen stores and patency of the outflow tract. A negative progesterone challenge (i.e., no bleeding 2 to 7 days after cessation of progesterone) indicates either inadequate estrogen stores or an obstruction of the outflow tract. To further differentiate hypoestrogenism from obstruction, the test can be repeated after daily administration of 2.5 mg of estrogen for 21 days, followed by 10 mg of progesterone for the next 5 days. If there is still no withdrawal bleeding, investigation into structural or outflow reasons for the amenorrhea should ensue.

If amenorrhea is secondary to anovulation, potential causes include Cushing's syndrome, adrenal or ovarian tumors, premature ovarian failure, or, more commonly, polycystic ovary syndrome. An FSH level elevated beyond 20 IU/L after repeated measurements is indicative of ovarian failure. An elevated LH/FSH ratio (>2) is suggestive of polycystic ovary syndrome; an FSH >40 indicates menopausal status.

To differentiate between pituitary and hypothalamic amenorrhea, a luteinizing hormone-releasing hormone test is generally performed in conjunction with imaging of the sellar region by CT or MRI. Recent research indicates that long-term administration of pulsatile GnRH can differentiate hypothalamic amenorrhea by an ovulatory response within two treatment cycles and confirms the diagnosis in an area where diagnosis has generally been made by exclusion.[26] In the absence of an ovulatory response, a pituitary cause for the amenorrhea should be suspected.

MRI has been shown to be an effective and accurate tool for evaluating the cause of primary amenorrhea and planning for surgery, particularly when this involves congenital disorders of sexual differentiation and localization of the gonads.[27] MRI of the sellar region is also important in the assessment of pituitary adenomas and is more effective than CT in detecting empty sella syndrome.[26] A hysterosalpingogram or sonohystogram can be used to outline the uterine cavity if a bicornuate uterus or double cervix is suspected.

Other diagnostic tests that may be useful in particular situations include the clomiphene challenge test, which may provide information necessary to make an early diagnosis of waning ovarian function in hypergonadotropic amenorrhea.[28] Increased serum dehydroepiandrosterone (DHEA) (>700 mg/dl) indicates an adrenal origin for androgens in women with hirsutism, and elevated plasma testosterone levels (>90 ng/dl) suggests tumors of adrenal and ovarian origin or congenital adrenal hyperplasia[1]; levels above 200 ng/dl are found in the rare Sertoli-Leydig cell tumors.[29] The level of sex hormone-binding globulin, which binds potent androgens such as testosterone and therefore controls the level of active androgens in circulation, may also provide useful clinical information.

Chemistry profiles (including serum electrolytes, serum glucose, BUN, and creatinine), urinary free cortisol, thyroid antibodies, an erythrocyte sedimentation rate, and a glucose tolerance test can help differentiate possible causes of autoimmune-related amenorrhea, such as Addison's disease, diabetes mellitus, thyroiditis, and hypoparathyroidism. This is especially important, considering that 20% to 40% of cases of premature ovarian failure are associated with autoimmune disease.[3] The diagnosis of premature ovarian failure in a young woman (generally under age 25 or 30 years) warrants karyotyping to exclude the presence of a Y chromosome.

DIFFERENTIAL DIAGNOSIS

Primary Amenorrhea

Physiologic primary amenorrhea may be attributable to constitutional delay, although 97% to 99% of young women experience menarche by age 16 years[12,30] and 95% by 14.5 years.[4] Failure of the gonads to develop normally accounts for half of all cases of primary amenorrhea.[31] Other possible causes include Turner's syndrome (45, X), mosaicism, abnormal X chromosomes, the presence of an intact or fragmented Y chromosome, pure gonadal dysgenesis (may present with hyperandrogenism), and the rare 17-alpha hydroxylase deficiency, which presents with hypernatremia, hypokalemia, and hypocortisolism.[31]

Additional causes of primary amenorrhea include structural abnormalities (imperforate hymen, transverse septum, congenital absence of the uterus or vagina), premature ovarian failure (may be idiopathic or secondary to radiation or chemotherapeutics), malnutrition, systemic illness, tumors (ovarian, hypothalamic, parasellar, or adrenal), and any of the disturbances in the hypothalamic-pituitary-ovarian axis that also cause secondary amenorrhea. In one retrospective study the most common causes of primary amenorrhea were hypergonadotropic amenorrhea secondary to ovarian failure and congenital absence of the uterus and vagina.[32]

Rare causes of primary amenorrhea include gonadal dysgenesis caused by chromosomal translocation, mutations in the beta subunit of FSH, vaginal inversion and uterine acollis, multiple endocrine neoplasia, progesterone-producing adrenal adenoma, increased melatonin secretion from a cystic pineal lesion, and childhood trauma.

Secondary Amenorrhea

Pregnancy is the most common cause of secondary amenorrhea; lactation and early menopause are other physiologic possibilities. Transient amenorrhea may occur in the first 2 postmenarchal years, after discontinuation of oral contraceptives, and in the majority of women who receive medroxyprogesterone (Depo-Provera) for contraception.[12,33] Aside from these causes, secondary amenorrhea is most often linked to disor-

Diagnostics

Amenorrhea

Laboratory	
Serum HCG	BUN
Thyroid profile	Creatinine
Thyroid antibodies*	ESR
LH	Urinary free cortisol*
FSH	**Imaging**
Prolactin	CT or MRI*
DHEA	**Other**
Serum electrolytes	Clomiphene challenge test
Serum glucose	

*If indicated.

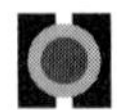

Differential Diagnosis

Amenorrhea

Primary Amenorrhea	Secondary Amenorrhea
Structural abnormalities	Pregnancy
Premature ovarian failure	Lactation
Malnutrition	Menopause
Systemic illness	Medications (oral contraceptives, reserpine, metoclopramide, Depo-Provera)
Tumors: ovarian, hypothalamic parasellar, or adrenal	Disorder of hypothalamic-pituitary-ovarian axis
Disturbance of hypothalamic-pituitary-ovarian axis	Premature ovarian failure
Gonadal dysgenesis (chromosomal translocation)	Chronic anovulatory disorder (polycystic ovary disease, obesity-related disorder, idiopathic disorder)
Vaginal inversion	Sheehan's syndrome
Uterine acollis	Hypogonadotropic hypogonadism
Multiple endocrine neoplasia	Thyroid disease
Trauma	Tuberculosis
Cystic pineal lesion	Late-onset 21-hydroxylase deficiency
Turner's syndrome	Pituitary tumor
17-alpha hydroxylase deficiency	Hyperprolactinemia

dered functioning somewhere along the hypothalamic-pituitary-ovarian axis.

Other causes of secondary amenorrhea include premature ovarian failure and chronic anovulatory disorder (polycystic ovary disease, obesity-related disorder, idiopathic disorder). Less common conditions include pituitary tumors, hyperprolactinemia, Sheehan's syndrome (postpartum pituitary necrosis), hypogonadotropic hypogonadism, thyroid disease, tuberculosis, and late-onset 21-hydroxylase deficiency. For the majority of women a clinical history, physical examination, and laboratory determination of TSH, LH, FSH, and prolactin levels are sufficient for diagnosis.

Categorization of amenorrhea by etiology (hyperprolactinemic, hyperandrogenic, hypergonadotropic, and hypogonadotropic) provides a helpful framework for consideration of the differential diagnosis, evaluation, and management.

Hyperprolactinemic amenorrhea can be caused by drugs (including reserpine, phenothiazines, oral contraceptives, metoclopramide, and alpha-methyldopa), prolactin-secreting tumors of the pituitary, or systemic illnesses such as acromegaly or hypothyroidism. Physiologic causes for increased prolactin levels include lactation and nipple stimulation. For this reason, prolactin levels are most helpful when drawn before a clinical breast examination.

Hyperandrogenic amenorrhea is seen most commonly in women with polycystic ovary disease (also called hyperandrogenic chronic anovulation or Stein-Leventhal syndrome) but may also be caused by obesity, Cushing's syndrome, hyperprolactinemia, thyroid disease, adrenal disease (hyperplasia, adenoma, carcinoma), androgen-secreting ovarian tumors, or drug abuse.[3,11]

Hypergonadotropic amenorrhea affects about 1% of women under the age of 40 years. The differential diagnosis for ovarian failure includes chromosomal (mosaicism and gonadal dysgenesis), autoimmune (Hashimoto's thyroiditis, Addison's disease, diabetes mellitus, hypoparathyroidism), metabolic (ovarian enzymatic defects), familial, infectious (mumps), idiopathic, or iatrogenic (irradiation, chemotherapy) causes, as well as resistant ovary syndrome.[34]

Hypogonadotropic amenorrhea can be a result of emotional or physical stress (including athletic training), depression, nutritional deficiency, weight loss, eating disorders, thyroid or adrenal dysfunction, isolated gonadotropin deficiency (Kallmann's syndrome), or hypothalamic or pituitary lesions (craniopharyngiomas, germinomas, pituitary adenomas, endodermal sinus tumors, pituitary apoplexy, empty sella syndrome, postpartum ischemia, necrosis of the pituitary gland).[3,34] Head injuries (especially head-on automobile collisions resulting in whiplash) and external irradiation can damage the hypothalamus[35]; infections (tuberculosis, HIV) can disrupt pituitary function.[36]

In addition to disorders of the hypothalamic-pituitary-ovarian axis, secondary amenorrhea can be due to uterine pathology, including endometrial hyperplasia, postpartum uterine adhesions, or iatrogenic Asherman's syndrome. Rare causes of secondary amenorrhea include hydrocephalus, Pendred's syndrome, onchocerciasis, and neurosarcoidosis.

MANAGEMENT

Amenorrhea caused by systemic illness or endocrinopathy, treatment of the underlying cause, such as diabetes mellitus or hypothyroidism, generally resolves as a result of renewed ovarian function.[1] Spontaneous recovery of menses after prolonged irradiation-induced ovarian failure after treatment of Hodgkin's disease, as well as in cases of chemotherapy-induced ovarian failure, does also occur.[13,36] Gonadal function should be reassessed periodically in these women, and oral contraceptives are a good choice for hormone replacement in women not desiring pregnancy.[36]

Menses return between 6 and 14 months after a last injection of Depo-Provera and within 6 months after stopping oral contraceptives in postoral contraceptive amenorrhea. Eventual return of menstruation has been shown, after a variable interval, for less than half of women with medically refractory menorrhagia after endometrial ablation and uterine resection.[37] In perimenopausal women amenorrheic intervals are common and do not require any treatment aside from adequate contraception when pregnancy is not desired (in these women unplanned pregnancy is a potential event unless FSH levels have been consistently elevated (>30 mIU/ml) and the amenorrhea has been present for more than 1 year).[38]

Several studies have demonstrated the effectiveness of lifestyle modifications, including diet and exercise, for the recovery of regular menses.[39] One study found that menses returned at approximately 90% of standard body weight and that 86% of women who attained this weight gain experienced menstrual return within 6 months.[39] However, whereas women with anorexia/eating disorders and endurance athletes have benefited from increased caloric intake and decreased exercise,[11] some overweight and hirsute women with hyperandrogenism may recover normal menses with control of excess body weight via caloric restriction.[3] Adequate calcium intake or supplementation and weight-bearing exercise should be encouraged in women who are amenorrheic for any reason to help maintain bone density.

Supplemental estrogen and progesterone (such as with oral contraceptives) have been recommended for the prevention of further bone loss and subsequent fracture development in women with decreased estrogen levels,[40] although normalizing body weight is the single most important factor in regaining bone density.[41] Irreversible bone loss can occur after 3 years of amenorrhea, although scant direct evidence supports the use of hormone replacement therapy in amenorrhic women.[15] Administration of estrogen and progesterone is also necessary after hysteroscopic adhesiolysis to reestablish a functional endometrium in women with Asherman's syndrome.[5] No treatment is required if women maintain normal estradiol and prolactin levels in postoral contraceptive amenorrhea.[42] Amenorrhea caused by onchocerciasis has been reversed with Mectizan.[43]

Bromocriptine has been widely studied with demonstrated effectiveness for promoting menstrual bleeding and ovulation and is the drug of choice for hyperprolactinemic amenorrhea and the syndrome of galactorrhea-amenorrhea.[42,44] In case of relapse, this treatment should be resumed and continued. Cabergoline has been shown in one multicenter, randomized, double-blind study to be more effective and better tolerated than bromocriptine, with fewer gastrointestinal symptoms.[45] Subcutaneous pulsatile GnRH therapy combined with human chorionic gonadotropin has also been proposed as a method of ovulation induction if these women should desire pregnancy.[23]

Naltrexone hydrochloride, an oral antiopioid, has been studied as an agent in the management of amenorrhea resulting from hypogonadotropic syndromes.[46] Use of oral contraceptives by these women has been shown to improve lumbar spine and total body bone mineral.[47] Interestingly, naltrexone was less effective than a placebo in eliciting menstrual bleeding in functional hypothalamic amenorrhea in one study that stressed the importance of psychosomatic effects in the treatment of this disorder.[46]

Restoration of hypothalamic-pituitary-ovarian function is necessary for resumption of menses in women with weight loss-related amenorrhea.[39] Intramuscular GnRH administration on alternate days has been used to increase FSH levels, reinstate LH pulsatility, and, in conjunction with clomiphene therapy, induce ovulation in women with weight loss-associated amenorrhea.[48]

Women with eating disorders, such as anorexia nervosa, are best managed in collaboration with psychiatric or other specialized eating disorder services. Evidence of anatomic or endocrinologic abnormalities mandates co-management with the appropriate specialist.

LIFE SPAN CONSIDERATIONS

The prognosis regarding present or future fertility is a major concern of many women with amenorrhea and will guide the treatment plan in most instances. For women with hypothalamic amenorrhea resulting from stress, weight loss, or exercise, reassurance regarding the reversible nature of the problem on requisite lifestyle modification may be all that is necessary. For other women, such as those with premature ovarian failure or structural or chromosomal abnormalities incompatible with achieving a natural pregnancy, alternatives such as adoption, egg donation, or surrogacy may need to be considered.

COMPLICATIONS

Untreated amenorrhea is associated with significant long-term morbidity, especially when it occurs in younger women.[5] Loss of body weight is adversely related to pituitary-ovarian function, and in 20% to 30% of women with weight loss-related amenorrhea no restoration of function is attained despite recovery of body weight.[48]

Hypoestrogenemic amenorrhea has been associated with an increased risk of osteoporosis and fractures.[15,49] One study found that the bone density of women with primary amenorrhea was significantly lower than the bone density of women with secondary amenorrhea and that 21 out of 27 patients studied had osteopenia, a higher rate than that reported for postmenopausal women.[40]Another study of women with amenorrhea found hypoestrogenism and lower spine, wrist, and metatarsal bone mineral density, which remained below control levels despite a return of menses in some subjects.[49] Although some improvements in bone mineral density have been observed with appropriate treatment for amenorrhea, this recovery in bone mass has not been substantial,[50] again emphasizing the importance of early diagnosis and treatment.

The hypoestrogenemic state has also been associated with unfavorable lipid profiles and a significantly increased risk of cardiovascular events. Anovulatory amenorrhea puts women at increased risk for endometrial hyperplasia and endometrial carcinoma. Women with polycystic ovary syndrome have a threefold increased risk for developing hypertension and a sixfold increased risk for developing type 2 (non–insulin dependent) diabetes mellitus; a sevenfold increased risk for coronary heart disease is seen in women with chronic hyperandrogenic anovulation.[3]

INDICATIONS FOR REFERRAL/HOSPITALIZATION

Suspected or confirmed genetic abnormalities that result in primary or secondary amenorrhea warrant referral to a specialist for more thorough evaluation. Young women with either Y-chromosome fragments or an entire Y chromosome will need to have their gonads removed after pubertal development is complete, because of the increased risk of malignant gonadoblastoma.[31] Referral to an infertility specialist is particularly indicated for women with ovarian reserve factors, anovulatory cycles, hyperprolactinemia, and genetic or structural factors.

Hospitalization may be necessary for women with anorexia nervosa who have lost more than 30% of their desired body weight and fail to gain weight, as well as for those with suicidal ideation.[33] Inpatient surgical care may be indicated for women with tumors or adenomas associated with amenorrhea.

PATIENT AND FAMILY EDUCATION/HEALTH PROMOTION

Women will have varying educational needs depending on the cause of their amenorrhea, but all women should receive basic nutritional counseling with an emphasis on obtaining sufficient calcium via either food sources or supplementation. Women should also be reminded that pregnancy can occur in the presence of amenorrhea; sexually active women not desiring pregnancy, especially adolescents, should receive appropriate contraceptive counseling. Women with genetic or congenital abnormalities may wonder about their ability to become pregnant and need to be appraised of their reproductive potential. The necessity for gonadectomy to prevent future malignancies should be discussed with women who have Y-chromosome fragments or Y chromosomes.

The reversible nature of most cases of hypothalamic amenorrhea resulting from stress, weight changes, or exercise, as well as the temporary (6 months or less) duration of postoral contraceptive amenorrhea can be stressed to women for whom these factors are relevant. When counseling athletes, it is important to remind them that amenorrhea can be an indication of overtraining, as well as possibly contribute to poorer future performance deficits, especially in light of the long-term health consequences, such as fractures and osteoporosis.[51] As with hypoestrogenemic women, women with androgen excess are at increased risk of lipid abnormalities and coronary artery disease.[34] Counseling may be required in an effort to reduce other contributing risk factors, such as obesity.

REFERENCES

1. Pletcher J, Slap G: Menstrual disorders: amenorrhea, *Pediatr Clin North Am* 46(3):505-518, 1999.
2. Rosen D, Foster C: Delayed puberty, *Pediatr Rev* 22(9): 2001.
3. Kiningham RB, Apgar BS, Schwenk TL: Evaluation of amenorrhea, *Am Fam Physician* 53(4):1185-1194, 1996.
4. Mitan L, Slap G: Adolescent menstrual disorders, *Med Clin North Am* 84(4):851-868, 2000.

5. Schachter M, Shoham Z: Amenorrhea during the reproductive years: is it safe? *Fertil Steril* 62(1):1-16, 1994.
6. Fogelholm M and others: Amenorrhea in ballet dancers in the Netherlands, *Med Sci Sports Exerc* 28(5):545-550, 1996.
7. Klock SC, DeSouza MJ: Eating disorder characteristics and psychiatric symptomology of eumenorrheic and amenorrheic runners, *Int J Eating Dis* 17(2):161-166, 1995.
8. Skierska E, Lesczynska-Bystrzanowska J, Gajewski AK: Risk analysis of menstrual disorders in young women from urban population (Polish), *Przegl Epidemiol* 50(4):467-474, 1996.
9. Yeshaya A and others: Menstrual characteristics and women suffering from insulin-dependent diabetes mellitus, *Int J Fertil Menopausal Stud* 40(5):269-273, 1995.
10. Tolis G, Diamante E: Distress amenorrhea, *Ann NY Acad Sci* 771: 660-664, 1995.
11. Epp SL: The diagnosis and treatment of athletic amenorrhea, *Physician Assist* 4(3):129-144, 1997.
12. Chikotas N: Secondary amenorrhea, *J Am Acad Nurse Pract* 7(9): 453-460, 1995.
13. Halyard MY and others: Prolonged amenorrhea associated with total nodal irradiation for Hodgkin's disease, *JAMA* 88(6):391-393, 1996.
14. Warren M, Freid J: Hypothalamic amenorrhea, *Endocrin Metabol Clin* 30(3):611-629, 2001.
15. Hobart J, Smucker D: The female athlete triad, *Am Fam Physician* 61(11):3357-3364, 2000.
16. Genazzani AD and others: Growth hormone (GH)-releasing hormone-induced GH response in hypothalamic amenorrhea: evidence of altered central neuromodulation, *Fertil Steril* 65(5):935-938, 1996.
17. Copeland PM, Sacks NR, Herzog DB: Longitudinal follow-up of amenorrhea in eating disorders, *Psychosomatic Med* 57(2):121-126, 1995.
18. Selzer R and others: The association between secondary amenorrhea and common eating disordered weight control practices in an adolescent population, *J Adolescent Health* 19(1):56-61, 1996.
19. Golden NH, Shenker IR: Amenorrhea in anorexia nervosa. Neuroendocrine control of hypothalamic dysfunction, *Int J Eating Dis* 16(1):53-60, 1994.
20. Fioroni L and others: Life events impact in patients with secondary amenorrhoea, *J Psychosomatic Res* 38(6):617-622, 1994.
21. Walker AB and others: Hypogonadotrophic hypogonadism and primary amenorrhea associated with increased melatonin secretion from a cystic pineal lesion, *Clin Endocrinol* 45(3):353-356, 1996.
22. Luboshitzky R and others: Nocturnal melatonin and leuteinizing hormone rhythms in women with hyperprolactinemic amenorrhea, *J Pineal Res* 20(2):72-78, 1996.
23. Matsuzaki T and others: Mechanism of anovulation in hyperprolactinemic amenorrhea determined by pulsatile gonadotropin-releasing hormone injection combined with human chorionic gonadotropin, *Fertil Steril* 62(6):1143-1149, 1994.
24. Jin K and others: Reproductive failure and the major histocompatibility complex, *Am J Hum Genet* 56(6):1456-1467, 1995.
25. Chatterjee R and others: Prospective study of the hypothalamic-pituitary axis in thalassaemic patients who developed secondary amenorrhea, *Clin Endocrinol* 39(3):287-296, 1993.
26. Grana M and others: Long-term administration of pulsatile gonadotropin-releasing hormone for exploration of pituitary functionality in amenorrheic patients, *Gynecol Endocrinol* 11(2):91-99, 1997.
27. Reinhold C and others: Primary amenorrhea: evaluation with MR imaging, *Radiology* 203(2):383-390, 1997.
28. Lin J, Yu C: Hypergonadotropic secondary amenorrhea: clinical analysis of 126 cases, *Am J Obstet Gynecol* 31(5):278-282, 1996.
29. Tsai CC, Collins SH, Swanger SJ: Ovarian Sertoli-Leydig cell tumor in an amenorrheic hirsute patient, *Chang Keng i Hsueh-Chang Gung Med J* 19(2):191-195, 1996.
30. Aloi JA: Evaluation of amenorrhea, *Compr Ther* 21(10):575-578, 1995.
31. Mishell DD and others: *Comprehensive gynecology*, St Louis, 1997, Mosby-Year Book, Inc.
32. Seshadri L and others: Endocrine profile of women with amenorrhea and oligomenorrhea, *Int J Gynaecol Obstet* 45(3):247-252, 1994.
33. McGee C: Secondary amenorrhea leading to osteoporosis: incidence and prevention, *Nurse Pract* 22(5):38-45, 48, 51-52, 57-58, 63-64, 1997.
34. Warren MP: Clinical review 77: evaluation of secondary amenorrhea, *J Clin Endocrinol Metab* 81(2):437-442, 1996.
35. Yen SSC: Female hypogonadotropic hypogonadism, *Endocrinol Metab Clin North Am* 22(1):29-57, 1993.
36. Nasir J and others: Spontaneous recovery of chemotherapy-induced primary ovarian failure, *Clin Endocrinol* 46(2):217-219, 1997.
37. Seeras RC, Gilliland GB: Resumption of menstruation after amenorrhea in women treated by endometrial ablation and myometrial resection, *J Am Assoc Gynecol Laparosc* 4(3):305-309, 1997.
38. Society TNAM: Clinical challenges of perimenopause: consensus opinion of the North American Menopause Society, *Menopause* 7(1): 5-13, 2000.
39. Golden NH and others: Resumption of menses in anorexia nervosa, *Arch Pediatr Adolesc Med* 151(1):16-21, 1997.
40. Ulrich U and others: Osteopenia in primary and secondary amenorrhea, *Horm Metab Res* 27(9):423-435, 1995.
41. Kaplan Seidenfeld M, Rickert V: Impact of anorexia, bulemia, and obesity on the gynecologic health of adolescents, *Am Fam Physician* 64(3):445-450, 2001.
42. Karaman AS, Uran B, Erler A: Serum prolactin levels in postpill amenorrheic patients, *Int J Gynaecol Obstet* 43(2):177-180, 1993.
43. Anosike JC, Abanobi OC: Reversal of amenorrhoea after Mectizan treatment, *Trop Geographical Med* 47(5):222-224, 1995.
44. Tartagni M and others: Long-term follow-up of women with amenorrhea-galactorrhea treated with bromocriptine, *Clin Exp Obstet Gynecol* 22(4):301-306, 1995.
45. Pascal-Vigneron V and others: Hyperprolactinemic amenorrhea: treatment with cabergoline versus bromocriptine. Results of a national multicenter randomized double-blind study, *Presse Med* 24(16): 753-757, 1995.
46. Manieri C and others: Naltrexone must not be considered a real therapy in functional hypothalamic amenorrhea. The results of a double blind controlled study, *Panminerva Med* 35(4):214-217, 1993.
47. Hergenroeder AC and others: Bone mineral changes in young women with hypothalamic amenorrhea treated with oral contraceptives, medroxyprogesterone, or placebo over 12 months, *Am J Obstet Gynecol* 176(5):1017-1025, 1997.
48. Kotsuji F and others: Alternate-day GnRH therapy for ovarian hypofunction induced by weight loss: treatment of six patients who remained amenorrhoeic after weight gain, Clin Endocrinol 39(6): 641-648, 1993.
49. Jonnavithula S and others: Bone density is compromised in amenorrheic women despite return of menses: a 2-year study, *Obstet Gynecol* 81(5 (part 1)):669-674, 1993.
50. Gulekli B, Davies MC, Jacobs HS: Effect of treatment on established osteoporosis in young women with amenorrhea, *Clin Endocrinol* 41(3):275-281, 1994.
51. Dueck CA and others: Treatment of athletic amenorrhea with a diet and training intervention program, *Int J Sport Nutr* 6(1):24-40, 1996.

CHAPTER 170

Bartholin's Gland Cysts and Abscesses

Marie Elena Botte

DEFINITION/EPIDEMIOLOGY

The Bartholin's glands, also known as the greater vestibular or vulvovaginal glands,[1] were first discovered by the French anatomist Joseph Guichard du Verney in the late seventeenth century[2]; their physiology was described by the Danish anatomist Gaspard Bartholin in 1677.[3] These paired glands, homologous to the male bulbourethral glands in structure, placement, and function,[1] have ducts about 1 inch long that open into the vestibule just distal to the hymenal ring[4] at the 5-o'clock and 7-o'clock position. The glands continually secrete mucus, which lubricates the vulva. Bartholin's gland cysts are generally noninfectious enlargements of the gland related to ductal obstruction,[5] which can occur as a result of inflammation, mucus, or congenitally narrowed ducts.[6] Bartholin's gland abscesses, also called bartholinitis or Bartholin's adenitis[1] are the result of acute infection followed by obstruction.[7]

Bartholin's gland cysts occur most often during women's reproductive years[3,8]; one study found that 83% of patients were between 20 and 50 years.[3] Clinicians are likely to encounter cysts of this gland in approximately 2% to 3% of new gynecologic patients and once per 46 pelvic examinations.[9]

PATHOPHYSIOLOGY

Cysts of the Bartholin's gland are related to obstruction of the duct orifice.[5,8] They are most commonly the result of trauma, parturition, or episiotomy[10] and can be the result of inflammatory scarring, epithelial metaplasia, or inspissated secretions that accumulate.[8] In the presence of an infectious process, inflammation of the gland's acinus may lead to abscess.[6,7] Most cases are self-limited but can be severely discomforting.[1]

Any opportunistic genital or genitourinary organism can be the cause of an acute inflammation. Studies have demonstrated the presence of *Chlamydia* trachomatis,[11] *Haemophilus influenzae*[11] (both the more virulent type b and a nontypable beta-lactamase positive strain),[12] and *Neisseria sicca*.[13] Bacteroides species have been detected in cultures from abscess formations in HIV antibody-positive women; capnophilic bacteria,[14] *Streptococcus* pneumoniae,[14] pure gram-negative cultures (*Escherichia coli* and *Proteus*), *Neisseria gonorrhoeae*, and polymicrobial flora including gram-negative and gram-positive anaerobes. Aerobic and facultative organisms[7] have also been implicated in abscess formation. One study emphasizing the polymicrobial nature of Bartholin's gland abscess found an average of 2.6 isolates per specimen,[15] 1.7 anaerobic (mostly *Bacteroides* species with some peptostreptococcus), and 0.9 aerobic and facultatives (*E. coli* and *N. gonorrhoeae*).

CLINICAL PRESENTATION

Bartholin's gland cysts are often asymptomatic,[9] generally unilateral,[1] and range in size from 1 to 3 cm[16]; they can be chronic or recurrent. Associated pain is generally a signal of an infectious process and development of an abscess, which can often grow large and rapidly over 2 to 4 days.[16] Women may present with pain, especially while walking or standing, swelling, dyspareunia, or tenderness. Specific inquiry into recent history of infectious process may yield clues to etiology. A recent vaginal delivery or history of localized trauma can be explored.

PHYSICAL EXAMINATION

Physical examination includes vital signs, visualization of the affected area, and assessment of accompanying inguinal node involvement. Patients usually exhibit a unilateral, erythematous, edematous mass located lateral to the vestibule that ranges from tender to extremely painful. The size may vary and discharge is usually present. A speculum or bimanual examination may be too painful until the cyst or abscess has been treated.

DIAGNOSTICS

Culturing of cystic contents and the cervix for sexually transmitted infections has been recommended[17] to ensure adequate treatment of women and their sexual contacts. A CBC can identify leukocytosis.

DIFFERENTIAL DIAGNOSIS

Cysts or abscesses of the Bartholin's gland compose the majority of cysts in the vulvar region[9] and are the most common diseases of the gland.[10] While solid benign tumors,[18,19] adenocarcinoma,[20] neuroendocrine carcinomas,[21] adenoid cystic carcinoma,[22,23] mixed tumors, leiomyomas, adenofibromas, mucinous cystadenomas, papillary tumors, mucocele-like changes, endometriosis, and malakoplakia all can originate in the Bartholin's gland,[9] these presentations are rare. Carcinoma of the Bartholin's gland, which can be primary,[24] accounts for less than 1% of all female genital neoplasms.[25] Tuberculosis of the Bartholin's gland is also very rare (vulval and vaginal infections compose less than 2% of genital tuberculosis) but should be considered a Bartholin's gland if swelling does not resolve after excision.[26]

MANAGEMENT

Antibiotics

When initiated early, empiric antibiotic treatment can potentially prevent full-blown abscess formation and should focus on both aerobic and anaerobic organisms as potential sources of infection.[1] Treatment is generally initiated with broad-spectrum antibiotics to decrease the chance of abscess formation or the need for surgical intervention. Erythromycin 250 mg q.i.d. for 10 days is a usual first-line therapy, followed by doxycycline 100 mg b.i.d. for 10 days (not for pregnant women) or cephalexin 250 mg q.i.d. for 10 days for those who are

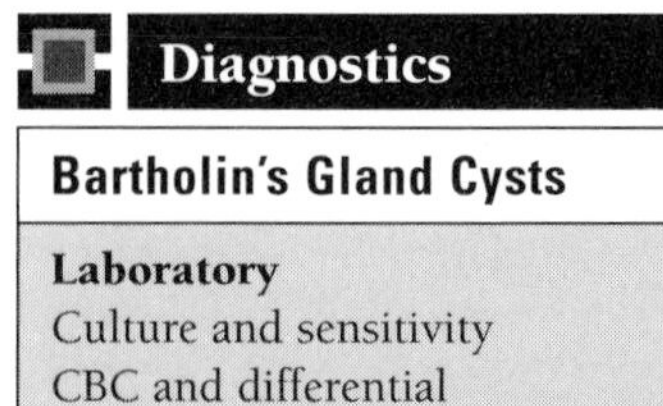

Diagnostics

Bartholin's Gland Cysts

Laboratory
Culture and sensitivity
CBC and differential

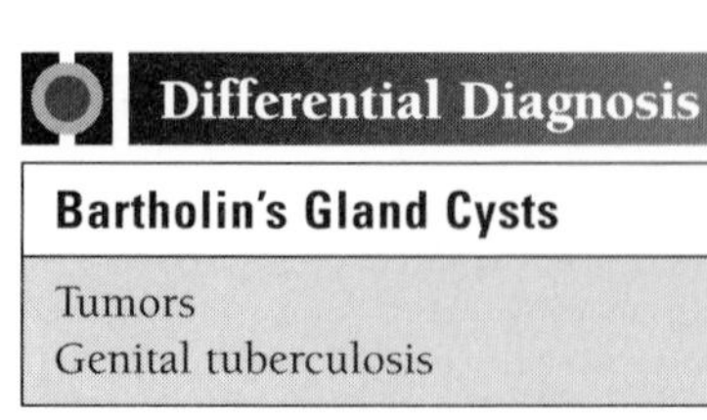

Differential Diagnosis

Bartholin's Gland Cysts

Tumors
Genital tuberculosis

allergic to or cannot tolerate erythromycin. Follow-up evaluation after antibiotic therapy is recommended at 7 to 10 days.

Surgical Treatments

A variety of surgical options to treat Bartholin's gland cysts and abscesses have been cited in the literature and range from simple incision and drain and drainage techniques (with and without the insertion of a catheter) to visualization and expression of cyst contents using ultrasound imaging,[27] and the application of silver nitrate or CO_2 lasers. Adequate pain control is an important issue for all women who have surgical intervention for Bartholin's cysts and abscesses. Because sufficient local anesthetic is often difficult to obtain for cyst drainage, the pudendal block, which anesthetizes the lower vagina and posterior vulva, has been recommended as an adjunct for regional anesthesia.[28]

Incision and Drainage

Incision and drainage followed by packing with gauze is a commonly used management strategy for Bartholin's cysts and abscesses and was once the mainstay of treatment.[4] The procedure requires a minimum of surgical skill but is not without disadvantages. Although the procedure is effective for temporary relief of symptoms, the recurrence rate is high.[4] Weekly follow-up monitoring is recommended after placement of a drain.

Excision of the Bartholin's Gland

Removal of the entire gland, once standard procedure,[5] is now recommended only when there is suspicion of malignancy[3] or for recurrent abscess.[16] Current surgical practices emphasize preservation of the gland's function.

Marsupialization and Window Operation

Both of these treatments seek to create and maintain a patent fistula for drainage of the cyst or abscess. The techniques differ significantly only in that the cyst is excised in the marsupialization procedure versus the "window" cut unto the cyst or abscess in the latter. In both marsupialization and window techniques pudendal or local anesthesia is used and the edges of the opened cyst cavity are sutured to the adjacent labial skin to make a permanent opening. The gland remains functional after both procedures,[4,8] and the size of the fistulas created gradually decreases over time. Recurrence rates for marsupialization are between 2% and 24%.[4] Recommended follow-up care after marsupialization is 4 to 6 weeks.

Catheter/Drain Placement

The goal of catheter or drain placement is the creation of a fistula through which the gland can continue to drain. The drain can be placed after a simple stab wound or a marsupialization procedure and generally is left in place for 6 to 8 weeks to ensure fistula patency.[4,10] Recurrence rate is about 24%.[10]

Carbon Dioxide Laser Therapy

With the patient under local anesthesia, the carbon dioxide (CO_2) laser is used first to create a defect from the vulvar skin to the cystic cavity as near as possible to the original duct tract. Mucus is released from the cyst on entering the cavity and the gland is gently massaged to express the remaining free mucus. The neostoma that is created allows for continued drainage after the procedure without the presence of sutures or mechanical devices such as catheters or drains and allows an epithelial-lined tract to form. Glandular function is maintained, sexual function is not impaired after a 2-week healing period, and the size of the created defect is substantially reduced with complete healing (from approximately 1.5 to 0.2 cm).[5]

In a second type of procedure that occurs with the patient under general anesthesia, the CO_2 laser is used to vaporize the internal capsule of the cystic formation after a simple incision.[3,29] Both procedures take about 10 minutes or less,[5,29] and healing generally occurs without scarring. A disadvantage of these approaches is that the laser equipment is expensive to install and maintain.

Silver Nitrate

Insertion of silver nitrate ($AgNO_3$) into a scalpel-formed incision has been shown in several studies to be a simple and inexpensive option for treatment,[30,31] as effective as traditional excision techniques and with fewer complications.[30,32] However, chemical burning of the vulva has been observed.[30]

LIFE SPAN CONSIDERATIONS

Bartholin's gland cysts and abscesses are most common in women of reproductive age, yet, when adequately treated, women maintain function without reproductive or other sequelae such as dyspareunia.

COMPLICATIONS

Incision and drainage are often followed by cyst recurrence[29] and gland excision may be accompanied by hemorrhage, hematoma formation, trauma to surrounding tissues, scarring, a long healing process, and subsequent dyspareunia from loss of vaginal lubrication.[4,29,30] Toxic shock syndrome, a very rare complication, has been noted in the literature,[33] both before and after a corrective surgical procedures.[7] True necrotizing fasciitis[34] has been noted in one case after an abscess that drained spontaneously.

INDICATIONS FOR REFERRAL/HOSPITALIZATION

Primary care providers not comfortable managing Bartholin's cysts and abscesses are encouraged to refer these cases to more experienced surgeons for appropriate therapy. Bartholin's gland cysts or abscesses are generally managed successfully on an outpatient basis, but systemic infection or other complications remain valid indications for hospitalization.

Women who have been treated by surgeons for Bartholin's gland cysts or abscesses should have continued follow-up care with their primary care providers. Providers can also check for possible sequelae to treatment including dyspareunia in the course of routine gynecologic or other primary care provision.

PATIENT AND FAMILY EDUCATION

Explaining to patients the basic physiology of the Bartholin's gland and the pathophysiology involved in cyst or abscess may help to demystify the occurrence of the condition and the treatment experience. Women may also benefit from an explanation of what to do and expect after a various treatment strategy is used. After CO_2 therapy, for example, patients are instructed to refrain from sexual intercourse for 2 weeks; potential postoperative discomfort is managed with salt water soaks.[5] Women should be counseled to expect drainage of mucus for 2 to 3 days after certain procedures while the cyst or abscess resolves. Proper hygiene, sitz baths or soaks, and condom use are also helpful in the treatment and prevention of future Bartholin's gland cysts and abscesses.

REFERENCES

1. Cunha B: Bartholin's gland abscess, *Emerg Med* 26(5):85-86, 1994.
2. Bouchet A: Gaspard II Bartholin et la glande vulvovaginale, *Ann Chirurgie* 125(5):483-488, 2000.
3. Heah J: Methods of treatment for cysts and abscesses of Bartholin's gland, *Br J Obstet Gynaecol* 95:321-322, 1998.
4. Downs MC, Randall HW: The ambulatory surgical management of Bartholin duct cysts, *J Emerg Med* 7(6):623-626, 1989.
5. Davis GD: Management of Bartholin duct cysts with the carbon dioxide laser, *Obstet Gynecol* 65(2):279-280, 1985.
6. Quint E, Smith Y: Adolescent gynecology, part 1- common disorders, *Pediatr Clin North Am* 46(3):593-606, 1999.
7. Lopez-Zeno JA, Ross E, O'Grady JP: Septic shock complicating drainage of a Bartholin gland abscess, *Obstet Gynecol* 76(5):915-916, 1990.
8. Cho JY, Myoung OA, Cha KS: Window operation: an alternate treatment method for Bartholin gland cysts and abscesses, *Obstet Gynecol* 76(5) (part 1):886-888, 1990.
9. Enghardt MH, Valente PT, Day DH: Papilloma of Bartholin's gland duct cyst: first report of a case, *Int J Gynecol Pathol* 12(1):86-92, 1993.
10. Yavetz H and others: Fistulization: an effective treatment for Bartholin's abscesses and cysts, *Acta Obstet Gynecol Scand* 66:63-64, 1987.
11. Hoosen AA and others: Sexually transmitted diseases including HIV infection in women with Bartholin's gland abscesses, *Genitourinary Med* 71(3):155-157, 1995.
12. van Bosterhaut B and others: *Haemophilus influenzae* bartholinitis, *Eur J Clin Microbiol Infect Dis* 9(6):442, 1990.
13. Berger SA and others: Bartholin's gland abscess caused by *Neisseria sicca*, *J Clin Microbiol* 26(6):1589, 1988.
14. Quentin R and others: Frequent isolation of capnophilic bacteria in aspirate from Bartholin's gland abscesses and cysts, *Eur J Clin Microbiol Infect Dis* 9(2):138-141, 1990.
15. Brook I: Aerobic and anaerobic microbiology of Bartholin's abscess, *Surg Gynecol Obstet* 169(1):32-34, 1989.
16. Schroeder B: Vulvar disorders in adolescents, *Obstet Gynecol Clin* 27(1):35-48, 2000.
17. Bleker OP, Smalbraak DJ, Schutte MF: Bartholin's abscess: the role of *Chlamydia trachomatis*, *Genitourinary Med* 66(1):24-25, 1990.
18. Foushee JHS, Reeves WJ, McCool JA: Benign masses of Bartholin's gland, *Obstet Gynecol* 31(5):695-701, 1968.
19. Mandsager NT, Young TW: Pain during sexual response due to bilateral Bartholin's gland adenomas. A case report, *J Reprod Med* 37(12):983-985, 1992.
20. Hastrup N, Andersen ES: Adenocarcinoma of Bartholin's gland associated with extramammary Paget's disease of the vulva, *Acta Obstet Gynecol Scand* 67(4):375-377, 1988.
21. Jones MA and others: Small cell neuroendocrine carcinoma of Bartholin's gland, *Am J Clin Pathol* 94(4):439-442, 1990.
22. Kiechle-Schwartz M and others: Cytogenic analysis of an adenoid cystic carcinoma of the Bartholin's gland. A rare, semimalignant tumor of the female genitourinary tract, *Cancer Genet Cytogenet* 61(1): 26-30, 1992.
23. Amichetti M, Aldovini D: Primary adenoid cystic carcinoma of the Bartholin's gland: a clinical, histological and immunocytochemical study of a case, *Eur J Surg Oncol* 14(4):335-339, 1988.
24. Obermair A: Primary Bartholin gland carcinoma: a report of seven cases, *Aust N Z J Obstet Gynaecol* 41(1):78-81, 2001.
25. Copeland LJ and others: Bartholin gland carcinoma, *Obstet Gynecol* 67(6):794-801, 1986.
26. Dhall K, Das SS, Dey P: Tuberculosis of Bartholin's gland, *Int J Gynecol Obstet* 48:223-224, 1995.
27. Eppel W: Ultrasound imaging of Bartholin cysts, *Gynecol Obstet Invest* 49(3):179-82, 2000.
28. Anderson GV Jr: The forgotten block, *J Emerg Med* 8(4):505-506, 1990.
29. Lashgari M, Keene M: Excision of Bartholin duct cysts using the CO_2 laser, *Obstet Gynecol* 67(5):735-736, 1986.
30. Mungan T and others: Treatment of Bartholin's cyst and abscess: excision versus silver nitrate, *Eur J Obstet Gynecol Reprod Biol* 63(1):61-63, 1995.
31. Ergeneli M: Silver nitrate for Bartholin gland cysts letter, *Eur J Obstet Gynecol Reprod Biol* 82(2):231-232, 1999.
32. Bulatovic S: Therapy of inflammatory changes in Bartholin's glands (Serbo-Croatian), *Medicinski Pregled* 53(5-6):289-292, 2000.
33. Shearin RS, Boehlke J, Karanth S: Toxic shock-like syndrome associated with Bartholin's gland abscess: case report, *Am J Obstet Gynecol* 160(5 pt 1):1073-1074, 1989.
34. Frohlich EP, Schein M: Necrotizing fasciitis arising from Bartholin's abscess. Case report and review of the literature, *Isr J Med Sci* 25(11):644-647, 1989.

CHAPTER 171

Breast Disorders

Cynthia J. Gantt

It is estimated that at least 50% of all women will experience some sort of breast symptoms in their lifetime.

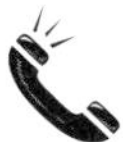

Surgical referral is indicated for patients with persistent symptoms of mastitis (despite antibiotic therapy), unilateral spontaneous nipple, or a dominant mass.

Breast Pain and Infections

DEFINITION/EPIDEMIOLOGY

Breast pain is often referred to as mastalgia or mastodynia. Mastalgia is the most common breast problem encountered in primary care. The incidence of mastalgia is estimated to be as high as 70%.[1] Premenstrual, cyclic breast pain is the most common type of mastalgia.[2] Noncyclic mastalgia is most common in women 40 to 50 years old. Mastalgia may be associated with fibrocystic breast changes and usually resolves spontaneously without treatment. Breast infections are generically known as mastitis. Mastitis is overwhelmingly associated with lactation but must always be differentiated from inflammatory breast cancer.

PATHOPHYSIOLOGY

Although the breasts are hormonally influenced, little is known about the mechanisms of action and interaction of hormones and their effect on breast tissue.[2] Reports of response to bromocriptine, a prolactin inhibitor and dopamine agonist in alleviating mastalgia seems to implicate prolactin, even in women with normal laboratory levels. Furthermore, women during the menarche and perimenopause have a high incidence of breast problems. A decreased ratio of progesterone to estrogen, which is seen in physiologic anovulatory cycles during these periods, has also been suggested, but not proven.[2] Fluid retention has not been shown to correlate with mastalgia.[3] Breast pain is not related to breast size, weight, or fluid retention. Mastalgia is sometimes associated with a solitary cyst or diffuse fibrocystic changes, yet no specific histologic findings differentiate women who do from women who do not experience breast pain.[2,4,5]

In lactational, or puerperal mastitis, organisms enter the breast ductal system from the infant through the nipple and cause infection in a segment of the breast where milk drainage is poor. Breast milk provides a good culture medium for these microorganisms. Puerperal mastitis is most commonly caused by *Staphylococcus aureus;* however, other organisms also have been implicated in puerperal mastitis. Nonlactational mastitis is rare and can have several origins, including squamous metaplasia of the lactational ducts, periareolar abscesses, or cellulitis.[6]

Histologic findings associated with fibrocystic breast changes include macrocysts, microcysts, proliferation of epithelial tissue, duct hyperplasia, and connective tissue fibrosis.[7]

CLINICAL PRESENTATION

Cyclic mastalgia is usually bilateral and poorly localized. Women will describe a heaviness or soreness that may radiate to the axilla and arms. In contrast, noncyclic mastalgia is often unilateral, localized, and described as a sharp, burning pain. Mastalgia is the sole presenting symptom of breast cancer approximately 7% of the time.[1]

Lactational mastitis is usually unilateral and most commonly develops during the second to fourth week after delivery, but may occur any time during lactation.[6] Women with lactational mastitis often present with breast engorgement and tenderness, fever, chills, anorexia, headache, and malaise. Erythema is usually confined to the area of a single breast lobule. A discrete mass is suggestive of abscess formation. The axillary lymph nodes may be tender and enlarged. Nonlactational mastitis is a rare condition most often seen in women who are immunocompromised (e.g., women with diabetes), those with autoimmune disorders, and people who have undergone radiation treatment.[5] Nonlactational mastitis may also be accompanied by nipple discharge (see Nipple Discharge and Galactorrhea p. 752).

Pain and erythema involving the entire breast, accompanied by increased breast firmness and size is suggestive of inflammatory breast carcinoma and requires immediate referral. Some patients with inflammatory carcinoma present with a red, swollen breast with thickened, edematous skin (peau d'orange), with or without a palpable mass.

Several well-established risk factors are associated with the development of breast cancer, primarily age and female sex. Family history is highly significant in a first-degree relative (mother, sister, daughter), especially if the cancer was diagnosed before menopause. Women with premenopausal first-degree relatives with breast cancer have a threefold to fourfold increased risk of developing breast cancer. Early menarche and late menopause may also increase the risk of breast cancer by increasing lifetime exposure to hormones. Similarly, women who gave birth to their first child after age 30 years or who never became pregnant are also at increased risk. Apparently, this is due to an increase in female reproductive hormones accelerating cell division in breast tissue, which in turn augments the risk of mutations. A history of atypical hyperplasia on biopsy (see Breast Masses, p. 754) or a history of benign breast disease requiring at least two breast biopsies. Other risk factors identified for developing breast cancer include those with high social economic status, white race, and history of exposure to ionizing radiation. It is important to note that most women with breast cancer do not have any identifiable risk factors.[8]

A thorough history and breast cancer risk assessment should be obtained from every woman who presents with a breast complaint. Current symptoms such as nipple discharge, breast mass, change in mass with the menstrual cycle, mass in axilla, skin dimpling, ulceration, inflammation and noncyclic pain; current medications, including hormone therapy; history of previous breast cancer or other breast problems; history of breast implants or breast reduction; age at menarche and menopause; history of trauma; history of other types of cancer; and in premenopausal women, pregnancy and lactation history. Breast cancer screening history should include the date and results of the last clinical breast examination (CBE) and mammography.[5]

Only an estimated 7% of breast cancers are hereditary. A woman with a BRCA-1 mutation is estimated to have a 56% to 87% lifetime risk of developing breast cancer. Half of women with the BRCA-1 mutation are diagnosed with breast cancer by age 41. The majority of hereditary ovarian cancers are thought to be due to mutations in BRCA-1.[9] A recent study has found that the risk of breast cancer is significantly lower for those with the BRCA-2 mutation. An increased risk of breast cancer was 15% by age 50 years and 35% at age 70 years, compared with 2% and 8% at these ages in noncarriers. BRCA-2 mutations also increase the risk of male breast cancer.[10]

PHYSICAL EXAMINATION

A thorough breast examination must be performed on every woman who presents with a breast problem. Breast examination must be methodical and carefully executed to include all breast tissue. The breasts should be inspected for differences in size, skin changes, retraction or dimpling of the skin or nipple, prominent venous patterns, pain, lesions, and signs of inflammation. The axillary and supraclavicular and infraclavicular areas should be palpated in the sitting position. Examination of the breasts should be performed in both the sitting and supine positions, with the woman's hands behind her head. The flat surface of the fingertips should be used to palpate all of the breast tissue against the chest wall. In women with a history of nipple discharge, the nipple-areolar complex is compressed very gently in the horizontal and vertical directions. If this technique does not elicit discharge, firm, equal pressure should be applied from the periphery toward the nipple. To distinguish multiple from single discharges, pressure must be distributed evenly so that the duct system is milked for each number on the clock. Skin changes that may signify carcinoma include erythema, retraction, or dimpling, as well as nipple excoriation or crustiness.

DIAGNOSTICS

Noncyclic breast pain is initially investigated with a bilateral mammogram in postmenopausal women. An ultrasound is usually performed for young women with persistent, noncyclic mastalgia. Mammography is not indicated in lactating women with an initial presentation of mastitis but should be considered in any woman with a breast infection that does not respond to appropriate antibiotic therapy within 3 to 7 days. Ultrasound may detect abscess formation in a lactating woman with suspected mastitis but is not required.

Diagnosis of inflammatory breast cancer cannot be made with radiographic examination alone; pathologic examination is required for confirmation. A skin biopsy reveals dermal lymphatics congested with cancer cells.

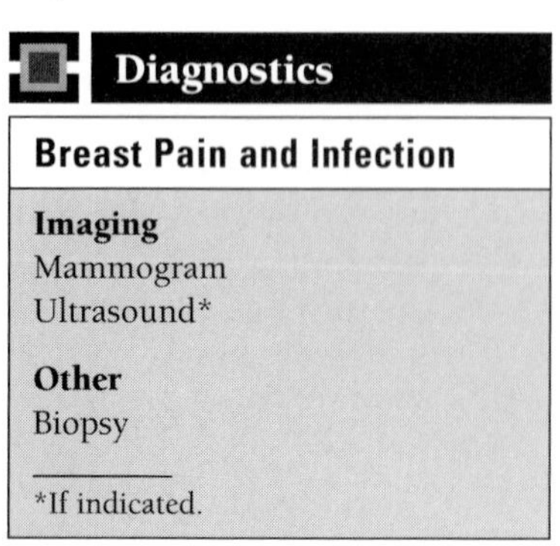

Diagnostics

Breast Pain and Infection

Imaging
Mammogram
Ultrasound*

Other
Biopsy

*If indicated.

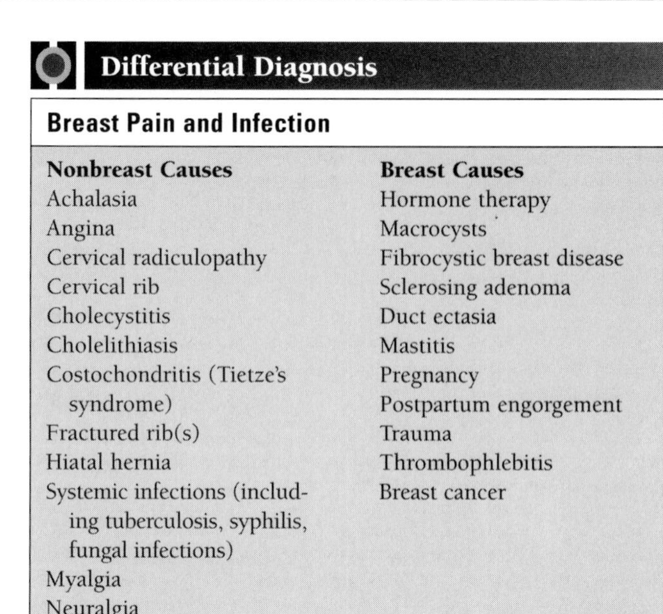

Differential Diagnosis

Breast Pain and Infection

Nonbreast Causes	Breast Causes
Achalasia	Hormone therapy
Angina	Macrocysts
Cervical radiculopathy	Fibrocystic breast disease
Cervical rib	Sclerosing adenoma
Cholecystitis	Duct ectasia
Cholelithiasis	Mastitis
Costochondritis (Tietze's syndrome)	Pregnancy
Fractured rib(s)	Postpartum engorgement
Hiatal hernia	Trauma
Systemic infections (including tuberculosis, syphilis, fungal infections)	Thrombophlebitis
Myalgia	Breast cancer
Neuralgia	
Peptic ulcer disease	
Pleurisy	
Trauma (nonbreast)	

DIFFERENTIAL DIAGNOSIS

The differential diagnosis of breast pain includes a normal physiologic event, a hematoma or fat necrosis often related to past trauma, a ruptured cyst, a nonruptured cyst under tension, infection, a tumor, and an idiopathic condition. Chest wall or nonbreast pain accounts for about 7% of women presenting with complaints of mastalgia. Tietze's syndrome or costochondritis is an inflammation of the costochondral junction that can occur spontaneously or after radiation therapy.[2] The pain can be reproduced with pressure over the costal cartilage rather than the more generalized pattern of mastalgia. Movement may also precipitate chest wall pain, and there is no relationship to the menstrual cycle.[1]

In lactating women, the differential diagnoses for mastitis include breast engorgement, which is usually bilateral unless only one breast is being used for feedings, and the rare inflammatory carcinoma. In nonlactating women, acute mastitis must be differentiated from inflammatory breast cancer, which represents only 0.5% of all breast cancers.[4] In inflammatory breast cancer the erythema and induration are usually more diffuse and skin changes are more common. The principle indication of cancer, however, is the failure to respond to appropriate antibiotic therapy. Other differential diagnoses include mammary duct ectasia (also known as plasma cell mastitis and nonlactational chronic breast abscess), unrecognized gross cystic disease, other extrinsic infections, numerous skin diseases, and other thoracic diseases such as metastatic lung cancer and lung granulomas.[2]

MANAGEMENT

After a thorough history, evaluation, and risk assessment, reassurance will be all that is needed for 85% of women with cyclic mastalgia. For the 15% of the women not helped with reassurance alone, use of a pain chart for at least 2 cycles may be helpful in elucidating any patterns of mastalgia. Patients can also be reassured that breast pain has a high spontaneous remission rate (60% to 80%).[6] Relief of symptoms may come for these women after some hormonal event such as pregnancy, menopause, or the use of oral contraceptives.[2] Management of cyclic mastalgia should also include reevaluation of the breast pain at a different time during the menstrual cycle, preferably soon after the menses.

Evidence Exists for Benefit

Proven benefits for the treatment of cyclic mastalgia are few. Because of the extreme variability in mastalgia, only treatments that have been tested in randomized, controlled trials (RCT) can be confidently considered. Danazol (Danocrine) an antigonadotropin, is the only drug labeled by the U.S. Food and Drug Administration for the treatment of mastalgia. RCTs have demonstrated a response rate of 50% to 75% in women with cyclic breast pain who received danazol 100 to 400 mg/day PO in two divided doses. Approximately 75% of women with noncyclic pain responded to the drug.[3] The severe side effect profile and teratogenic potential of danazol support referral or collaboration before initiation of treatment.

For lactational mastitis, empirical treatment with dicloxacillin 500 mg every 6 hours for 7 to 10 days or clindamycin 300 mg every 6 hours for penicillin-allergic patients is appropriate. The woman should be encouraged to continue nursing during therapy, as adequate drainage of the infected area is important.[11] Improved drainage and emptying of the breast may be accomplished by altering positioning while breastfeeding. Breast emptying by manual expression or hand pump, breast massage, and hot showers may also improve drainage, thereby decreasing discomfort. Cool compresses after breastfeeding may decrease inflammation. Women should be discouraged from weaning at this time, as the resulting breast engorgement can increase the severity of the mastitis. Reevaluation should be performed 3 days after initiation of treatment if significant improvement has not been seen during that interval.[6]

In the older, nonlactating woman with suspected mastitis, outpatient antibiotic therapy with clindamycin 300 mg every 6 hours, or amoxicillin/clavulanate (Augmentin) 500 mg every 12 hours, or cephalexin 500 mg every 6 hours each for 7 days should be prescribed.[11] The increased risk of inflammatory carcinoma in this population mandates close follow-up monitoring. Failure to fully respond to antibiotics requires immediate referral. Overall prognosis and survival from inflammatory breast cancer are directly affected by timely diagnosis and treatment. Therefore prompt referral for a definitive tissue diagnosis is required.

Limited Evidence Exists for Benefit

Supportive bras can be helpful. Some women report some temporary relief with nonsteroidal antiinflammatory drugs (NSAIDs) and acetaminophen.[4] Pharmacologic treatment options without significant adverse reactions include oral contraceptives (which, if thought to be a contributing factor to cyclic mastalgia may be discontinued or changed to an alternative agent with a lower estrogen and higher progesterone content).

In both lactational and nonlactational mastitis, acetaminophen or NSAIDs and moist heat may be beneficial.

Evidence of Benefit Unclear

Caffeine avoidance has been a popular treatment measure in women with breast pain. Two RCTs and one case-control study failed to demonstrate a therapeutic benefit for caffeine restriction. Vitamin E supplementation has also been advocated as a treatment for breast pain. However, two double-blind, placebo-controlled, randomized clinical trials demonstrated no benefit to this approach.[3] Diuretics, salt restriction, pyridoxine, decreased dietary intake of fat, high fiber and soy isoflavone, and smoking cessation, although often recommended, have not been proven to be effective.[10]

LIFE SPAN CONSIDERATIONS

Benign breast symptoms generally occur in women during the menstruating years, with a mean age of 39 years and a range of 16 to 67 years.[2] Because the incidence of carcinoma increases with age, any breast complaint in a postmenopausal woman is worrisome. Lactational mastitis is by far the most common type of mastitis and often exacerbates the fatigue, discomfort, and stress normally associated with the postnatal period.

COMPLICATIONS

Mastalgia may be associated with a benign macrocyst (see Breast Masses, p. 754). Mastitis may either present with or progress to include abscess formation. An abscess occurs in approximately 10% of puerperal mastitis cases. Abscess formation is also a risk in nonlactational mastitis and requires referral. If the patient's symptoms do not respond to appropriate antibiotic therapy within a few days, the possibility of a breast abscess or inflammatory breast cancer must be considered.[4,6]

INDICATIONS FOR REFERRAL/HOSPITALIZATION

Treatment of cyclic mastalgia with antigonadotropic agents should be managed by, or in consultation with, a specialist because of the severity of the side effect profile and the teratogenicity of this class of drugs.

Surgical intervention for incision and drainage is also needed when a fluctuant mass, suspicious for an underlying abscess, accompanies mastitis. Intravenous antibiotics may be required to treat acute mastitis unresponsive to oral agents. In-home IV therapy or hospitalization is required for administration of appropriate antibiotics. Surgical referral is also indicated when inflammatory breast cancer is suspected. The diagnosis is made after an incisional skin biopsy.

Because the only currently available putative form of primary prevention is bilateral prophylactic mastectomy, a family history that includes a first-degree relative who was diagnosed when premenopausal and/or diagnosed with bilateral disease or two or more family members who have been affected with breast cancer suggests possible familial clustering. In such cases referral for possible genetic counseling and gene mapping should be discussed.

PATIENT EDUCATION

Many women present with mild forms of mastalgia, fearful that they have cancer. Premenopausal women who experience breast pain should receive a thorough CBE and education and should be reassured that pain is rarely a presenting symptom of breast cancer. Lactating women should also be reassured that mastitis is a common complication of lactation, the nutrition of the breast milk is unaffected by the infection, and that a history of mastitis is not associated with an increased risk of breast cancer.

Although women themselves first detect 70% to 90% of masses, there is much debate over whether routine BSE screening reduces the risk of mortality from breast cancer. Yet for women who have presented with a breast complaint, encouraging self-monitoring is often an important part of follow-up care. Menstruating women should be advised to perform BSE during the week after menses.[4]

Nipple Discharge and Galactorrhea

DEFINITION/EPIDEMIOLOGY

Nipple discharge most often involves a benign process. Nipple discharge has been reported in 10% to 15% of women with benign breast disease, and is found in 2.5% to 3% of women with breast cancer. Nipple discharge encompasses all breast secretions, both spontaneous and those requiring manual expression. Galactorrhea includes spontaneous, nonpuerperal and nonlactational nipple discharge that is either grossly milky or composed of fat droplets identified microscopically. Galactorrhea is usually caused by stimulation of the breast by elevated prolactin secretions from the pituitary. Galactorrhea is not a symptom of breast cancer.[4] All patients with spontaneous or unilateral nipple discharge, regardless of the characteristics of the discharge, should be referred for surgical evaluation.

Bilateral nipple discharges usually have physiologic causes, such as hyperprolactinemia associated with infertility that may lead to galactorrhea, but can occur in bilateral breast disease such as mammary duct ectasia. Mammary duct ectasia is a benign condition occurring in postmenopausal women, characterized by dilation of the ducts, nipple secretions (may be spontaneous or nonspontaneous) and periductal inflammation.[5] Nipple secretions associated with mammary duct ectasia are multicolored, sticky, and heme-negative.[4]

Pathologic nipple discharges occur spontaneously, are unilateral, come from a single duct opening on the nipple, and are serous or bloody. This type of discharge is most commonly associated with a benign intraductal papilloma. An intraductal papilloma is a neoplastic growth within a major breast duct.[2,4]

Galactorrhea may be physiologic, idiopathic, a side effect of certain medications, or related to neoplasms or central nervous system (CNS) disorders, but its incidence is most commonly associated with several drugs and secondly with pituitary or CNS lesions. Hormonal agents, primarily oral contraceptives, are the most common pharmacologic cause of nipple discharge. Galactorrhea is often associated with pregnancy and can persist for 1 to 2 years postpartum, but it may also coexist with anovulatory syndromes.

PATHOPHYSIOLOGY

Most nipple discharge is physiologic in nature and is not symptomatic of any pathologic condition. The breast of a nonlactating woman secretes fluid into the ductal system of the breast. Usually this fluid is absorbed into the blood and lymphatic systems.[4] Stimulation of estrogen, progesterone, and prolactin, as well as the presence of growth hormones, insulin, and adrenal hormones, may initiate nipple discharge. When the physiologic fluid is secreted through the nipple, it is generally bilateral, serous, arising from multiple ducts, and not spontaneous.

The most common cause of pathologic nipple discharge is intraductal papilloma, followed by duct ectasia. The presence of an associated palpable mass increases the likelihood of cancer.[3] The most common causes of occult blood in nipple discharge are, in order of frequency, intraductal papilloma, mammary duct ectasia, fibrocystic changes, and carcinoma.[2]

Prolactin is a stress hormone known to transform mammary epithelial cells from a presecretory to a secretory state. Because lactogenesis can occur in breast tissue that is metabolically stimulated by various hormones such as estrogen, progesterone, corticosteroids, insulin, growth, and thyroid hormones, disruptions of any of these underlying systems can result in galactorrhea.[12]

CLINICAL PRESENTATION

The first step in evaluating nipple discharge is to determine whether it is physiologic or pathologic. Nipple discharges are considered pathologic if they are spontaneous, bloody, or associated with a mass. Pathologic discharges are usually unilateral and involve a single duct. Physiologic nipple discharges are characterized by discharge only with compression and by multiple duct involvement. These discharges are often bilateral. With either pathologic or physiologic discharges, the fluid may be clear, yellow, white, or dark green.[3] The duration of the discharge should also be determined. Any personal or family history of breast cancer must also be elicited.

A complete medication and past medical history, including endocrine and reproductive histories, should be obtained to exclude lactational discharge. Although it is not common, lactational secretions may persist for years after weaning if the breasts continue to be manually stimulated.

Mammary duct ectasia often presents with dark green, brown or blackish multiple duct discharge. It is seen in the perimenopausal period. Pituitary prolactinomas are associated with elevated prolactin levels. Clinical signs and symptoms in addition to galactorrhea include headache, amenorrhea, defects in peripheral vision, hirsutism, acne, and hypogonadism presenting as decreased libido, decreased fertility, or decreased bone density.[12,13]

PHYSICAL EXAMINATION

A thorough breast examination as previously described should be performed to assess for an underlying breast mass and should include gentle compression of the nipple-areolar complex between the thumb and index finger. Milking the ducts with equal pressure from various directions is required to determine the origin of the discharge from either a single duct or multiple ducts.

In the presence of galactorrhea, funduscopic examination to exclude papilledema, as well as evaluation of visual acuity, visual fields by confrontation, and extraocular movements, are indicated to detect a bitemporal field defect and asymmetry of field loss, which are common in parapituitary lesions. Neurologic and thyroid examinations should also be performed.

DIAGNOSTICS

Nipple discharge should be tested for occult blood. Cytology is not recommended because the absence of malignant cells does not exclude malignancy or distinguish intraductal from invasive cancer. A diagnostic mammogram should be obtained in the evaluation of unilateral, spontaneous, clear, serous, or bloody discharge to discern nonpalpable masses or calcifications. Any mammographic abnormality should correspond to the quadrant of the breast from which the discharge originates to be considered relevant to the cause of the discharge. Most of these mammograms are normal and should not deter surgical referral.[5]

Diagnostics

Nipple Discharge and Galactorrhea

Laboratory
Microscopy
Prolactin level, TSH (or thyroid profile)
Serum HCG

Imaging
Mammograms
Ductogram*
MRI for hyperprolactinemia

*If indicated.

Pregnancy should be excluded by obtaining a human chorionic gonadotropin level in all premenopausal women experiencing amenorrhea and galactorrhea. Serum prolactin is the single most important test that can establish a lesion of pituitary or CNS origin. The serum prolactin level may be artificially elevated if performed after breast stimulation, including clinical examination and is more accurate when obtained in the fasting state. If serum prolactin is only marginally elevated, repeat or serial testing should be performed to document accurate results. The majority of women with hyperprolactinemia have microadenomas of the pituitary. Serum prolactin may be normal or only slightly elevated when galactorrhea is drug related. Thyroid profiles should also be obtained, as primary hypothyroidism can cause elevation of serum prolactin and galactorrhea.

MRI of the brain is indicated for the patient with symptoms suggestive of an intracranial mass, galactorrhea with amenorrhea, or an elevated prolactin level (>20 ng/ml). An MRI may be obtained when galactorrhea is associated with amenorrhea or oligomenorrhea even with a normal prolactin level, as the risk of pituitary adenoma is still significant.[12]

DIFFERENTIAL DIAGNOSIS

Duct ectasia, nonpuerperal mastitis, intraductal papilloma, and breast cancer must be considered in the presence of a nonmilky nipple discharge. Pseudonipple discharges can be caused by inverted nipples, eczema, or infection (see Breast Abnormalities, p. 756).

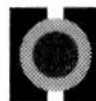
Differential Diagnosis

Nipple Discharge and Galactorrhea

Duct ectasia
Nonpuerperal mastitis
Intraductal papilloma
Breast cancer

Chemical Agents
Amphetamines
Anesthetics
Arginine
Atypical antipsychotics (clozapine, loxapine, risperidone)
Benzamides (metoclopramide, sulpiride)
Benzodiazepines
Butyrophenones (haloperidol)
Cimetidine
Danazol
Dronabinol
Estrogen
Flunarizine
Isoniazid
Methyldopa
MAO inhibitors
Opiates
Oral contraceptives
Phenothiazines
Progestins
Rauwolfia alkyloids
Reserpine
Selective serotonin reuptake inhibitors (SSRIs)
Thioxanthenes
Thyrotropin-releasing hormone
Tricyclic antidepressants
Verapamil

Idiopathic Causes
Conditions related to abnormal dopamine secretion

Medical (Nonmalignant) Conditions
Addison's disease
Ahumada-del Castillo syndrome*
Chiari-Frommel syndrome*
Chronic renal failure
Chest wall lesions
CNS lesions (involving hypothalamus or pituitary)
Cushing's disease
Endocrine anovulatory syndromes
Forbes-Albright syndrome
Hand-Schüller-Christian disease
Head trauma
Liver failure
Multiple sclerosis
Polycystic ovaries
Postencephalitis
Primary hypothyroidism
Renal failure
Sarcoidosis
Thoracic herpes zoster

Medical (Malignant) Conditions
Adrenal carcinoma
Breast carcinoma (rare)
Bronchogenic carcinoma
Chest wall lesions
CNS lesions (involving hypothalamus or pituitary)
Ovarian cystic teratoma
Renal adenocarcinoma

Physiologic Conditions
Cyclic menstrual hormone variations
Pregnancy (after first trimester)
Postlactation (few months to 5 years)
Nipple stimulation
Stress

Surgical Procedures†
Implantation of breast prostheses
Postthoracotomy
Reduction mammoplasty

Pseudodischarges
Atopic dermatitis
Herpes simplex
Infected Montgomery's glands
Inverted nipples
Lactiferous sinuses
Molluscum contagiosum
Nipple trauma
Paget's disease
Sebaceous cysts of the nipple

*May be associated with pituitary tumors.
†Procedures that may result in irritation to the afferent arc.

The differential diagnosis of galactorrhea includes pituitary adenomas, neurologic disorders, hypothyroidism, numerous medications, breast stimulation, chest wall irritation (e.g., clothing, breast implants, and postreduction), and physiologic causes.[13]

MANAGEMENT

Treatment of underlying infection, as previously described, is required if nipple discharge is related to acute mastitis. When a chemical origin for galactorrhea is suspected, discontinuation or substitution with a comparable pharmacologic agent may be attempted when possible. Restoration to the euthyroid state is indicated if hypothyroidism is present. Minimal intervention is required for galactorrhea of idiopathic, drug-related, or physiologic in origin.

Mammary duct ectasia is self-limited and not related to neoplasms. Treatment is not necessary unless the patient insists, and then the only effective treatment is surgical removal of all the involved ducts. Because intraductal papillomas usually present with a spontaneous bloody discharge, excision is required to exclude carcinoma.[4]

Co-Management with Specialists

In the past, bromocriptine was routinely used to treat galactorrhea, including the treatment of pituitary microadenomas. Recently, however, increased concern has been raised related to the use of bromocriptine. Increased rates of hypertensive crises and stroke have been documented when used in postpartum women who used the drug.[4] Therefore this medication, if used at all, should be used in consultation with a specialist.

Controversy also exists regarding the frequency of follow-up care for pituitary microadenomas. Repeat MRI examinations are often recommended until the growth of the lesion is established, and these should be performed in conjunction with the consulting specialist.

LIFE SPAN CONSIDERATIONS

Most women are concerned about getting breast cancer, and nipple discharge usually heightens concerns about possible malignancy. Although nipple discharge is not commonly associated with cancer, careful attention must be taken to ensure that a complete workup is conducted. Galactorrhea is more common in premenopausal women, and duct ectasia is seen more often in perimenopausal and postmenopausal women.

INDICATIONS FOR REFERRAL/HOSPITALIZATION

All patients with spontaneous or unilateral nipple discharge, regardless of color, should be referred for surgical evaluation. Intraductal papillomas require surgical biopsy and excision.[3] Galactorrhea accompanied by decreased visual fields, deterioration in visual acuity, papilledema, progressive headache, and nausea or vomiting should be promptly discussed and referred to a neurologist, endocrinologist, or neuroendocrinologist. When idiopathic galactorrhea is suspected, referral to a specialist for confirmation of the diagnosis is also indicated.

PATIENT AND FAMILY EDUCATION

Patients should be reassured that most causes of breast discharge are nonmalignant. In the presence of a normal prolactin level and menses, women with galactorrhea should be informed of its normal physiologic association with nipple and breast stimulation. Patients with pituitary adenoma should be reassured of the generally favorable response to treatment. Accurate and clear information, support, and close follow-up monitoring will help minimize the anxiety that often accompanies the presence of breast discharge.

Breast Masses

DEFINITION/EPIDEMIOLOGY

Although a breast mass is the most common presentation of breast cancer, 90% of breast masses are caused by benign lesions such as cysts, fibroadenomas, and fibrocystic changes.[6] Nonetheless, every woman, regardless of age presenting with a breast mass, should be evaluated and monitored to exclude or establish a diagnosis of cancer. The average lifetime risk of breast cancer is 12% or approximately 1 in 8 women. The decision to evaluate a palpable breast mass should not depend on the presence or absence of risk factors. More than 75% of women with newly diagnosed breast cancer have no identifiable risk factors.[7]

Benign gross cysts are the most common type of dominant lump and are characterized as a distinct entity consisting of a palpable, fluid-filled sac within the breast tissue. Although gross cysts may be found in younger women, they are most commonly found in women between 35 and 50 years old. Cysts are rare in postmenopausal women not on HRT and should be viewed as breast cancer until proven otherwise. Fibroadenomas are the most common benign solid lesion of the female breast. Characteristically, fibroadenomas are painless, well-circumscribed, freely movable masses with a rounded, lobulated, or discoid configuration. They usually have a rubbery feeling, but may appear hard, especially if calcified. Fibroadenomas occur most often in women in their twenties and thirties but may occur anytime after puberty, and even during menopause. They are hormonally responsive and may increase in size during the end of the menstrual cycle.

It is impossible to distinguish between fibroadenomas and cysts on CBE alone; therefore imaging (ultrasound and/or mammography) and tissue sampling (e.g., fine needle aspiration [FNA]) are required for diagnosis. This combination of diagnostic measures is referred to as the "triple test." Fibrocystic changes include a compilation of nondiscrete breast masses that are often accompanied by breast pain. Fibrocystic changes tend to occur most commonly in women in their twenties and thirties. Tissue diagnosis and imaging are required less often in these women.[2]

PATHOPHYSIOLOGY

Breast cysts are fluid-filled, and are thought to arise from dilation or obstruction of collecting ducts. Rarely, a cyst with an irregular wall may signify intracystic carcinoma or a carcinoma adjacent to the cyst.[6] Debate continues about any increased risk of developing breast cancer in women with a history of breast cysts. Evidence exists associating some forms of atypical hyperplasia found on breast biopsy with an increased risk of later breast cancer development.[4] Therefore women with a history of cystic breasts who present with a dominant mass should not be ignored or labeled as having "just another cyst."

Fibroadenomas occur when periductal stromal connective tissue proliferates within the lobules of the breast. Estrogen receptors are present in fibroadenomatous tissue. Exogenous estrogen, progesterone, pregnancy, and lactation can stimulate the growth of fibroadenomas.[2] The relationship between fibroadenomas and breast cancer is complicated. Histologically, when a mass is composed of microscopic elements beyond the basic glandular tissue that make up simple fibroadenomas, the lesion is labeled as a complex fibroadenoma. Simple fibroadenomas do not appear to increase the risk of developing breast cancer. One third of fibroadenomas are thought to be complex and, in the presence of a family history of breast cancer, seem to increase the risk of future breast cancer development.[4]

CLINICAL PRESENTATION

A discrete, palpable mass is three-dimensional, different from surrounding tissues, and usually asymmetric compared with normal glandular tissue that is generally mirrored in the contralateral breast. Clinical signs that suggest (but are not diagnostic) of a benign condition include a mass that is soft or rubbery and mobile. Features suggestive of malignancy include a mass that feels firm or hard, has an irregular shape, is solitary, and feels different from surrounding breast tissue. Occasionally breast cancers are fixed and associated with other signs such as skin retraction, dimpling, erythema, nipple discharge, nipple retraction, and skin changes including erythema.[4-6]

Cysts are dominant, discrete masses that are fluid-filled and round, and usually change cyclically on a monthly basis, with enlargement and pain occurring before menses. Pain associated with breast cysts often occurs in the upper, outer quadrants and radiates to the axilla. Cysts are most commonly found in women between 35 and 50 years old.[2] Fibroadenomas are solid, encapsulated, and usually nontender masses. They are most commonly found in the upper outer quadrant and tend to be unilateral, although they can exist anywhere in either breast, and there can be more than one present at a time. While they can enlarge cyclically before menses, they tend to be uniform in size over time or increase in size at a gradual rate. They are most commonly found in women in their twenties, although they can be present anytime from puberty through menopause.[4]

Fibrocystic changes present as prominent, rubbery, thickened, symmetric plaques of glandular breast tissue that lacks discreteness and blend into the surrounding breast tissue. Pain is the most common complaint and can be cyclical. The pain is often bilateral, poorly localized, and extends to the shoulder, axilla, or arm.[2]

PHYSICAL EXAMINATION

Key historical features in the evaluation of a breast lump are the length of time the mass has been present, presence of pain, change in size or texture over time, relationship to menstrual cycle, and nipple discharge. Risk factors for breast cancer (see Breast Pain and Infections p. 749) should be assessed. Also important is pathologic information on any previous breast cyst aspirations, including a personal history of atypical hyperplasia, which can increase the risk of breast cancer three to five times and double that in women with a strong family history.[2]

CBE of a woman with a complaint of a dominant breast mass should include assessing for a symmetric finding in both breasts, the consistency or texture of any mass, mobility, size, and shape.[5] Nipple discharge should also be assessed if reported (see Breast Pain and Infections, p. 749).

DIAGNOSTICS

CBE is a method of detection, not an independent diagnostic test. Diagnostic mammography usually is the initial test for a palpable mass in women over 35 to 40 years. A negative mammogram should not deter follow-up evaluation, as 15% to 18% of mammograms appear negative in the presence of a palpable cancer. Mammography is usually performed, as hematoma formation secondary to biopsy procedures may obscure radiographic findings. For younger women the dense glandular tissue lowers the sensitivity of mammograms, and ultrasound directed at the area of concern is the preferred imaging study.[2] In diagnosing any dominant mass, FNA is usually performed to determine if the mass is cystic or solid. If the lesion is cystic, the fluid is aspirated, and the cyst is collapsed. If no fluid is obtained, or an underlying mass is palpated after aspiration, it is assumed that it is a solid lesion requiring open biopsy.[2] FNA also has the potential benefit of decreasing the size of the cyst and relieving any accompanying pain. Cysts require surgical biopsy only if the aspirated fluid is bloody, the palpable abnormality does not resolve completely after the aspiration of fluid, or the same cyst recurs multiple times in a short time period.[4]

DIFFERENTIAL DIAGNOSIS

The differential diagnosis of a dominant breast mass includes invasive breast cancer, macrocyst (clinically evident cyst), and fibroadenoma. In addition, prominent areas of fibrocystic change, fat necrosis as a result of surgical or extraneous trauma, and a galactocele (a milk cyst in a lactating woman) may present as a breast mass.[3,4]

MANAGEMENT

Management of the patient with a breast mass varies according to age, clinical history, and clinical findings. Detection of a breast mass usually creates significant anxiety in a woman and her family and requires sensitive communication.[5] If a cyst is detected, aspiration is often offered and requested by women for both diagnosis and relief of pain.

Cysts require cytology of aspirate fluid and surgical biopsy only if the aspirated fluid is bloody, the palpable abnormality does not resolve completely after the aspiration of fluid, or the cyst recurs. This approach has been supported by large studies of benign-appearing cyst fluid aspirates. No cancers were

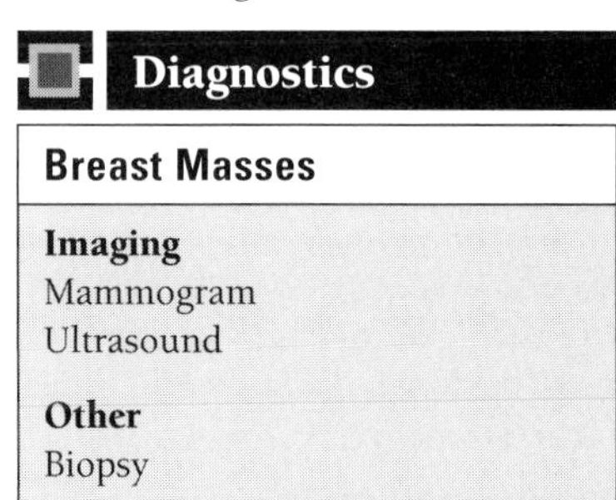

Diagnostics

Breast Masses

Imaging
Mammogram
Ultrasound

Other
Biopsy

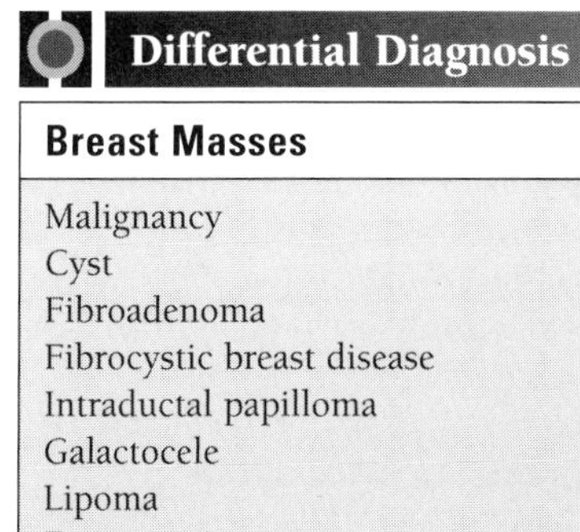

Differential Diagnosis

Breast Masses

Malignancy
Cyst
Fibroadenoma
Fibrocystic breast disease
Intraductal papilloma
Galactocele
Lipoma
Fat necrosis

ultimately identified in 6782 aspirates of low-probability samples. Patients with a solitary breast cyst must be reexamined 4 to 6 weeks after cyst aspiration to determine if the cyst has recurred.[3]

Noncystic masses in premenopausal women that are different from the surrounding breast tissue require histologic sampling by FNA, core cutting, or needle or excisional biopsy. Observation for one or two menstrual cycles is appropriate only for vague asymmetry or nodularity when it is unclear that a dominant breast mass is present.[3]

Evidence Exists for Benefit

The accuracy for FNA alone are high. One review of 4943 FNAs reported 87% sensitivity for carcinoma. In another review of 3545 such procedures a 9.6% false-negative rate was reported. When the triple test approach—CBE, imaging (ultrasound or mammography) and FNA—indicates benign breast disease, one review found that the likelihood of cancer was only 0.6%.[3]

Routine practice has been to excise fibroadenomas. However, there is increasing support for observation in women younger than 35 to 40 years when the lesion can be diagnosed by nonsurgical procedures: CBE, ultrasonography, and FNA.[4,7,12]

LIFE SPAN CONSIDERATIONS

In approximately 78% of women, breast cancer is diagnosed over age 50 years. Approximately 22% percent of breast cancers are diagnosed in women under 50 years of age. An estimated 7% of invasive breast cancers are diagnosed in women younger than 40 years.[7] Because the risk of breast carcinoma increases with age, any dominant mass or asymmetric thickening in postmenopausal woman should raise the index of suspicion for malignancy. Therefore abnormalities detected on physical examination in women over 40 years old should be regarded as possible cancers until they are documented to be benign.[4]

Physical examination and mammography of the breasts of young premenopausal women can be challenging because of breast lumpiness from the increased glandular-to-fat ratio when compared to the more homogenous breasts of postmenopausal women.[6]

Cystic findings become less common after menopause, although cysts, pain, and discharge can be found in women taking HRT.[5] Fibrocystic symptoms may remain stable or worsen until menopause. Up to 20% of women may experience spontaneous resolution.[7] Approximately 1 in 3000 pregnant women will develop invasive breast cancer.[7] Any breast mass discovered during pregnancy or lactation must be thoroughly evaluated as suggested for all premenopausal women.

INDICATIONS FOR REFERRAL/HOSPITALIZATION

A palpable solid mass in all women, regardless of age, requires both consultation by a specialist and referral for surgical evaluation. Women should be referred for mammography/ultrasound and FNA so that "triple testing" including CBE is provided. The triple test helps make a decision about whether further studies (e.g., open surgical biopsy) are needed in the workup to avoid delays in the diagnosis and treatment of breast cancer.[5] Even when fibrocystic changes are suspected, surgical evaluation of a persistent, palpable dominant mass or lump is required. Tissue diagnosis alone will provide a definitive diagnosis and determine the presence of atypical hyperplasia.

Women with a strong family history of breast cancer may be candidates for genetic testing for BRCA mutations. Increased surveillance and prophylactic mastectomies are the current approaches for women with these genetic mutations. This raises many psychosocial and ethical issues.

PATIENT AND FAMILY EDUCATION

Most women are worried about developing breast cancer. Women need reassurance regarding the benign nature of breast lesions that wax and wane with hormonal variation, as well as the rationale behind conservative vs. surgical management. Education must also focus on the need for prudent breast evaluation of all breast symptoms and/or lesions regardless of the improbability of malignancy.

Breast Abnormalities

DEFINITION/EPIDEMIOLOGY

Paget's disease of the nipple (PDN) is a superficial manifestation of an underlying breast carcinoma most often of ductal origin. PDN is believed to represent 1% to 3% of all breast cancers. PDN is rare in men but, unfortunately, it is associated with a poorer prognosis in men.[14]

Gynecomastia is an enlargement of the male breast caused by the proliferation of glandular tissue and should prompt investigation for a cause. Benign gynecomastia is an almost universal finding among boys in middle to late puberty.[15]

PATHOPHYSIOLOGY

Controversy exists regarding the origin of the malignant cells seen in PDN. They may represent malignant breast ductal epithelial cells, which then migrate into the epidermis of the nipple.[14]

Gynecomastia in the older male is associated with an altered ratio of estrogen to androgens in a number of conditions, including aging, malnutrition, testicular pathology, hypogonadism, cirrhosis, and thyrotoxicosis. Hormonal secretions from neoplasms in the testis or adrenal glands may cause gynecomastia. Other tumors may secrete ectopic hormones such as those from bronchogenic carcinoma or hepatoma.[2] Drugs most commonly implicated in causing gynecomastia include digoxin, cimetidine, ketoconazole, flutamide, estrogen, and related drugs and anabolic steroids.[15] Pubertal gynecomastia may be related to an estradiol-testosterone imbalance.[2]

CLINICAL PRESENTATION

Clinically, PDN appears as a unilateral, well-demarcated, erythematous, scaly plaque first appearing on the nipple and subsequently spreading to the areola. The surrounding skin is usually spared. Serous or sanguinous discharge, pain, crusting, pruritus, burning, epithelial thickening, erythema, ulceration, nipple retraction, and an underlying breast mass (in up to 60% of patients) may be seen. A small vesicular lesion on the nipple, persistent soreness, pain, or pruritus of the nipple-areolar complex in the absence of other clinical symptoms should be evaluated thoroughly because these may be early manifestations of PDN.[14]

Males with gynecomastia present with asymmetric or symmetric breast enlargement. Gynecomastia is a common clinical condition, with peak prevalence in the forties to seventies, and ranges from 30% to 55% in adult men. In benign gynecomastia of adolescence, the breast tissue is usually asymmetric and often tender.[15]

PHYSICAL EXAMINATION

A thorough breast examination as described previously must be conducted. Paget's disease of the breast may present solely with scaling of the nipple, but it may also be accompanied by erythematous and excoriated, retracted nipples. The erosion of the areolar tissue may produce copious clear or viscous yellow exudate. As the disease steadily progresses, the excoriated surface of the nipple may result in a bloody discharge and associated adenopathy.

A detailed history, including medication and alcohol use, is essential in assessing gynecomastia. The breast area is palpated while the patient lies supine. The presence of a rubbery mass below the areola usually indicates the presence of mammary tissue, not just fatty tissue. Any dominant firm, fixed, unilateral mass should raise suspicion for breast carcinoma.[15]

DIAGNOSTICS

If Paget's disease is suspected, punch biopsy of the nipple either may be performed as an office procedure or referred to a surgeon. As with all breast abnormalities, mammography is indicated, but should not delay referral to a specialist.

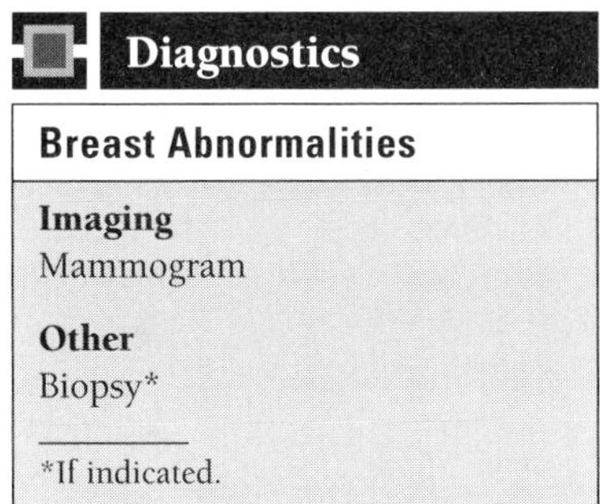
Diagnostics

Breast Abnormalities

Imaging
Mammogram

Other
Biopsy*

*If indicated.

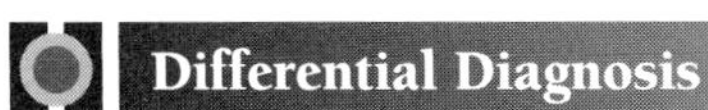
Differential Diagnosis

Breast Abnormalities

Paget's disease
Eczema
Psoriasis
Contact dermatitis
Lichen sclerosis
Nevoid hyperkeratosis of areola
Malignant melanoma
Bowen's disease
Carcinoma
Intraductal papilloma
Herpes
Tinea versicolor

In evaluating gynecomastia, history, physical examination, and laboratory studies to determine signs of thyroid excess, liver disease, lung cancer, and hypogonadism are indicated. This evaluation usually indicates the possible cause of gynecomastia. If no cause is found, further evaluation may involve testing for serum human chorionic gonadotropin, testosterone, estradiol, and luteinizing hormone to exclude other causes of hormonal disruption.[15]

DIFFERENTIAL DIAGNOSIS

Paget's disease should be suspected until proven otherwise. This is true even in a lesion that has healed spontaneously because patients have been identified with healed nipple lesions that were subsequently diagnosed as PDN. PDN is most commonly misdiagnosed as eczema. (Table 171-1). Eczema involving the nipple (vs. the areola) is rare and, when present, is usually bilateral. The differential diagnosis of PDN includes psoriasis, contact dermatitis, tinea, basal cell carcinoma, Bowen's disease, and benign intraductal papilloma of the nipple. Direct spread of invasive carcinoma from the underlying breast may be considered after Paget's disease is excluded.[14]

TABLE 171-1 Eczema vs. Paget's Disease of the Nipple

Eczema	Paget's Disease of the Nipple
Usually bilateral	Unilateral
Intermittent history with rapid progression	Continuous history with slow progression
Moist initially	Moist or dry
Indistinct border	Irregular but distinct border
Areola involved, nipple may be spared	Nipple always involved and disappears in advanced cases
Itching common	Itching common

Male breast cancer, although uncommon (fewer than 1% of male cancers), must be excluded in men 40 years and older presenting with unilateral breast mass. The risk of breast cancer in patients with Klinefelter's syndrome with gynecomastia is increased approximately 20-fold.[15] True gynecomastia needs to be differentiated from pseudogynecomastia, the enlargement in the area of the breasts caused by excess fatty tissue, which is due to obesity, not iatrogenic factors.

MANAGEMENT

Paget's disease is treated with mastectomy or breast conservation surgery and may be followed with radiation treatments.[14] In the case of possible drug effect and gynecomastia, the suspected agent should be stopped to assess for resolution. If there is suspicion that the gynecomastia is related to a medication, the suspected agent should be discontinued and the breast reassessed for resolution of the gynecomastia.

INDICATIONS FOR REFERRAL/HOSPITALIZATION

Because histologic diagnosis of Paget's disease is required, surgical referral for skin biopsy or excisional biopsy of the underlying mass is indicated. Biopsy-proven Paget's disease should be viewed as an invasive breast cancer and must be referred to an oncologist for management.[14]

Patients presenting with gynecomastia should be referred when breast cancer is suspected or when concern exists for other serious disease processes (e.g., alcoholism, liver disease).

PATIENT AND FAMILY EDUCATION

Patients undergoing evaluation for Paget's disease require the same accurate information, support, and well-coordinated care that all patients anticipating a possible diagnosis of cancer deserve.

Men should be advised that gynecomastia associated with chemical agents should resolve when the agents are stopped. Men may need reassurance because of the altered body image issues that may accompany gynecomastia. Gynecomastia of adolescence typically resolves spontaneously within 2 years.[2]

REFERENCES

1. Padden DL: Mastalgia: evaluation and management, *Nurse Pract Forum* 11(4):213-218, 2000.
2. Johnson C: Benign breast disease, *Nurse Pract Forum* 10(3):137-144, 1999.
3. Morrow M: The evaluation of common breast problems, *Am Fam Physician* 61(8):2371-2378, 2000.
4. McCool WF and others: Breast health care: a review, *J Nurse Midwifery* 43(6):406-430, 1998.
5. Clinical Breast Protocols Workgroup, California Department of Health Services: *Breast diagnostic algorithms for primary care clinicians*, Davis, Calif, 2000, UC Davis.
6. Apantaku LM: Breast cancer diagnosis and screening, *Am Fam Physician* 62(3):929-934, 2000.
7. Pruthi P: Detection and evaluation of a palpable breast mass, *Mayo Clin Proc* 76(6):641-648, 2001.
8. Shepherd JE, Muto, MG: Testing for genetic susceptibility to ovarian and breast cancer, *Patient Care* 34(11):131-153, 2000.
9. Eyfjord JE: Risk of breast cancer among BRCA2 mutation carriers lower than previously estimated, *Evidence-based Oncol* 1(1):6-9, 2000.
10. Horner NK, Lampe JW: Potential mechanisms of diet therapy for fibrocystic conditions show inadequate evidence of effectiveness, *J Am Diet Assoc* 100(11):1368-1380, 2000.
11. Gilbert DN and others: *The Sanford guide to antimicrobial therapy*, Vienna, Va, 2001, Antimicrobial Therapy.
12. Whitman-Elia GF, Windham NQ: Galactorrhea may be clue to serious problem, *Postgrad Med* 107(7):165-171, 2000.
13. Pena KS, Rosenfeld, JA: Evaluation and treatment of galactorrhea, *Am Fam Physician* 63(9):1763-1770, 2001.
14. Whitaker-Worth DL and others: Dermatologic diseases of the breast and nipple, *J Am Acad Dermatol* 43(5 Pt 1):733-751, 2000.
15. Bakshi S, Miller DK: Assessment of the aging man, *Med Clin North Am* 83(5):1131-1149, 1999.

CHAPTER 172

Chronic Pelvic Pain

Cynthia M. Williams

DEFINITION/EPIDEMIOLOGY

Chronic pelvic pain (CPP) is a continuous or episodic, noncyclic pain that persists for more than 6 months and is severe enough to alter a woman's lifestyle and behavior.[1,2] The pain is considered chronic under several conditions: (1) it is refractory to medical management, (2) there is impairment of physical functioning (including sexual), (3) signs of depression are present, and (4) the pain becomes the highest priority for both the patient and her family.[3]

In some studies, prevalence rates for CPP from 14% to 39% have been reported, with an estimated 9.2 million women experiencing CPP in the United States at an annual direct cost of $880 million.[4,5] Women have a 5% risk of developing CPP at some point during their lifetime. This risk increases to approximately 20% if there is a history of pelvic inflammatory disease (PID).[1] It has been estimated that approximately 10% of all referrals to gynecologists are for CPP, with an estimated 10% to 35% of laparoscopies performed in the United States for the diagnosis of CPP. Approximately 80,000 hysterectomies are performed annually for CPP without any documented long-term efficacy.[6] The typical woman with CPP is in her late 20s to early 30s, with first intercourse at an early age, multiple sexual partners, previous pregnancies, and multiple major and minor surgical procedures.[6] She has a higher lifetime incidence of major sexual abuse and more global histories of physical and sexual abuse from childhood.[7]

PATHOPHYSIOLOGY

CPP is a poorly understood entity. It does not follow the classic pain theory patterns of centrally mediated pain. Possible explanations include undetected irritable bowel syndrome, pelvic venous congestions with reduced blood flow, and altered spinal cord and brain processing of stimuli.[8] Because the pathogenesis is so complex and uncertain, a biopsychosocial model for pain expression is followed in which the physical, emotional, and psychologic aspects of the pain overlap to produce and modulate the syndrome.[1]

CLINICAL PRESENTATION

The evaluation of CPP can take many office visits and become a highly frustrating experience for both patient and provider. A complete and thorough history and physical examination is crucial in developing a rational approach to women with CPP. It is important that the patient understand early on that visits are not only for evaluation and treatment but also for the formation of a continued therapeutic relationship between patient and provider.[2,9]

The history should include a description of the nature, intensity, distribution, radiation, location, and daily pattern of the pain. Associated events, including complaints of fever, sweats, fatigue, anorexia, nausea, vomiting, and constipation, should be elicited. The relationship of the pain to posture, meals, bowel movements, voiding, menstruation, intercourse, medications, as well as any factors that aggravate or alleviate the pain, should be determined. Past surgeries, pelvic infections, and a history of infertility are important diagnostic clues to the origin of the pain.[10]

The role that the pain has taken in an individual's life, including its impact on relationships and work, should be discussed. A history of both physical and sexual abuse and any coexisting neuropsychiatric history should be explored.[3]

PHYSICAL EXAMINATION

The physical examination should be thorough, complete, and guided by the history. The initial part of the examination should begin with observation of the patient's general demeanor during the interview. Particular attention should be given to the abdominal, pelvic, and neuromuscular examination because CPP has numerous and diverse etiologies (see the Differential Diagnosis box).

The abdomen should be examined to elicit a point or area of tenderness. It is important that the patient be allowed to indicate the location of the pain and the depth of palpation necessary to elicit the discomfort. If pain is experienced during palpation of the abdomen, a trigger point, hernia, endometriosis, or hematoma is likely. Costovertebral angle tenderness should also be elicited if there is tenderness with suprapubic palpation. The groin should be evaluated for inflamed lymph nodes and hernias.

The back should be examined for lordosis, scoliosis, and any tenderness over the paraspinal musculature, sacroiliac joints, or spine prominence. Range of motion should be evaluated. By having the patient lie in the lateral decubitus position, passive thigh extension can be accomplished and may reveal psoas muscle tenderness.

The pelvic examination should be performed in a gentle, stepwise manner. Attention should be given to any evidence of a vulvar pathologic condition. Pelvic relaxation should be evaluated by having the patient bear down while the practitioner separates the labia and observes for a significant cystocele, rectocele, enterocele, or cervical or uterine prolapse.

A single-digit transvaginal examination (monomanual) is necessary to elicit any tenderness in the adnexa, cervix, or posterior vagina; along the vaginal side walls; or near the base of the bladder or urethra. Special attention during palpation of the levator ani muscles, piriformis muscles, and the coccyx is important, because all have been implicated as a cause of chronic pelvic pain and discomfort.

A careful speculum examination is performed to visualize the cervix and vagina and to inspect for neoplasms, prolapse, or infections. This examination may reveal vaginismus, with involuntary spasms of the vaginal musculature that make insertion of the speculum difficult.

The bimanual examination and rectovaginal examination complete the genitourinary evaluation. Particular attention should be given to areas of tenderness. Cervical motion tenderness has been associated with endometriosis, pelvic adhesive disease, inflammatory bowel disease, and ureteral colic. A fixed retroverted uterus or an enlarged boggy uterus, the hallmark of adenomyosis, may be noted. Uterine fibroids do not classically cause pain unless they are degenerating or infarcting, but their enlargement may cause a feeling of heaviness and pressure on nerve endings in the lower abdomen and pelvis. Finally, the rectovaginal examination may reveal nodularity in the cul-de-sac that is associated with endometriosis. The examination may also help identify any rectal masses, and the piriformis muscle can be evaluated for spasms and tenderness.

DIAGNOSTICS

Laboratory studies should be based on the history and physical findings. The usual evaluation for CPP should include vaginal cultures, urinalysis, a urine culture, and CBC. In the absence of physical findings, IV pyelograms, barium enemas, small bowel studies, CT, and transvaginal ultrasounds are rarely, if ever, indicated.[3] A pelvic ultrasound may be beneficial if the bimanual examination was difficult or unsatisfactory; in some cases the vaginal ultrasound may be used as a diagnostic tool in place of laparoscopy for unclear presentations of CPP.[1,11]

Laparoscopy is generally indicated, especially if the pelvic examination is abnormal. Commonly found abnormalities include endometriosis, adhesions, and chronic PID. Thus this modality is appropriate in the diagnosis and treatment of CPP.[9,12]

Another technique that is diagnostic for CPP is trigger point injection.[13] This technique is also therapeutic for patients whose pain is caused by abdominal wall trigger points. The trigger point can be injected with 1% lidocaine (Xylocaine) or 0.25% bupivacaine with a 25-gauge, 1.5-inch needle.[3] By eliminating the abdominal trigger point, the pelvic examination can be repeated to identify any pelvic pathologic condition. Other locally tender points such as the vaginal cuff have been successfully injected for pain management.

DIFFERENTIAL DIAGNOSIS

The differential diagnosis is extensive for CPP. From a primary care perspective, a good history and physical examination aid in the differential diagnosis. The most common cause of CPP is probably gastrointestinal.[5,14] Irritable bowel syndrome (IBS) is believed to account for 50% of all cases of CPP.[10] IBS is a chronic functional bowel disorder that is often accompanied by gynecologic complaints and labeled as CPP. IBS consists of a constellation of symptoms, including abdominal pain or discomfort that

Diagnostics

Chronic Pelvic Pain

Laboratory
Vaginal cultures*
CBC and differential
Serum human chorionic gonadotropin
ESR
Urinalysis*
Culture and sensitivity*

Imaging
Pelvic ultrasound
Transvaginal ultrasound*
Kidney ultrasound
Ureter ultrasound
Kidney and upper bladder*
Barium enema*
MRI or CT scan

Other
Laparoscopy*
Trigger point injection*

*If indicated.

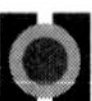

Differential Diagnosis

Chronic Pelvic Pain

Musculoskeletal	Gynecologic
Myofascial	Dysmenorrhea
Coccygodynia	Pain with ovulation
Low back pain	Chronic pelvic inflammatory disease
Scoliosis and other postural problems	Adhesions
Spasm of the pelvic floor	Endometriosis
Gastrointestinal	**Other**
Irritable bowel syndrome	Nerve entrapment of lower abdominal wall
Constipation	
Diverticulosis/diverticulitis	
Urologic	
Cystitis	
Urethral syndrome	
Bladder spasms	
Chronic pyelonephritis	
Stones	

is relieved with defecation; it is usually associated with alternating constipation and diarrhea. The pain of IBS is usually worse around the time of menstruation and may be associated with dyspareunia.

CPP and IBS share many of the same psychosocial factors, including a high prevalence of depression, somatization, and a history of physical or sexual abuse.[14] A diagnosis of IBS should be included in any differential diagnosis of CPP. As with any other gastrointestinal complaint, more serious disease entities need to be excluded, including inflammatory bowel disease, diverticulitis, and malignancy.

Urinary tract problems may present as CPP. Because the gynecologic and urinary systems share embryologic origins, differentiating the source of pain can be difficult. A pathologic condition of the urinary tract can present with a constellation of symptoms, including pelvic pain, dysuria, urgency, hesitancy, dyspareunia, postcoital voiding difficulties, and incontinence. Urethral syndrome, chronic urethritis, interstitial cystitis, and bladder spasms should be considered in the differential diagnosis.[15]

Musculoskeletal diseases are also associated with CPP. These conditions can range from postural problems, herniated disk disease, chronic pelvic tilt, degenerative joint disease, or myofascial trigger points. Levator ani muscle spasms and piriformis muscle spasms are two conditions that are easy to evaluate on physical examination and may be a source of pain and discomfort.

Levator ani muscle spasms are perhaps one of the most overlooked causes of CPP.[3] They usually present as sacral pain. The pain is caused by contraction and spasm of the levator ani muscles. Palpation of this muscle group reveals tenderness and increasing pain with voluntary contraction. Teaching the patient to relax these muscles and the vaginal muscles will help alleviate the discomfort.

Piriformis syndrome or spasms of the piriformis muscle during external rotation of the leg can be reproduced by contraction of the externally rotated leg against resistance. Because the piriformis muscle can be palpated transvaginally, tenderness along the muscle should be evaluated during bimanual examination. Physical therapy is usually indicated in helping to relieve the spasms.

A gynecologic source of pain should always be considered. Although a pathologic condition is more likely with acute pain, certain entities are more commonly seen with CPP.

Endometriosis is a chronic condition often seen during laparoscopy for CPP.[3] Endometriosis is caused by the development of implants outside the endometrium. Because these implants can be found anywhere and are responsive to the cyclic hormonal cycle, the point source of the pain can be elusive. On physical examination, either tenderness in the cul-de-sac or along the uterosacral ligaments (early finding) or nodularity in the same locations (late finding) may be noted. The diagnosis should be confirmed by laparoscopy.

Adhesions are scar tissue that can form between any two abdominal organs, usually after surgery or intraabdominal infections such as PID. The pain occurs because of the stretching of usually mobile structures that are now scarred. Patients usually complain of a substantial positional component to the pain. The diagnosis can be confirmed by laparoscopy.

Other gynecologic origins of CPP to consider are pain with ovulation, dysmenorrhea, functional ovarian cysts, ovarian torsion, chronic PID, pelvic congestion of the reproductive organ venous system, adenomyosis, and leiomyomata.

Finally, a psychiatric component such as clinical depression or somatization disorder should be considered if no other pathologic entity or explanation can be found for the pain. A screening for depression and a referral to a psychiatrist can assist in this area.

MANAGEMENT

Information for sound evidence-based practice is not widely available.[8] There appears to be support for the use of ultrasound scanning as an aid to counseling and reassurance, the use of a multidisciplinary approach to assessment and treatment with the aim of improving function and the use of progesterone (medroxyprogesterone acetate) for ovarian cycle suppression. Adhesiolysis and the use of sertraline were not shown to be of benefit.

In general, positive reinforcement and general psychologic support are important in the early diagnostic phase of CPP. Women suffer for years, and many are told the problem is psychosomatic. Consideration of depression and sleep disorders is important, because treatment of these conditions enhances management of the chronic pain syndrome. If a cause for the pain is identified, appropriate management should be undertaken with the assistance of the appropriate physician specialist.

During the diagnostic evaluation, the pain component should be treated effectively and promptly. Nonsteroidal anti-inflammatory drugs can be prescribed to address the discomfort and pain. These medications should be given on a routine schedule, not on an as-needed basis.

Regular office visits are quite important. These visits enable discussion of the progress of the diagnostic process and assessment of therapy, and they provide reassurance and support during the evaluation period.[9,10]

LIFE SPAN CONSIDERATIONS

CPP usually occurs during a woman's late 20s and early 30s but can present itself in the adolescent years.[16] This can be a stressful period in a woman's life—she may be married, considering pregnancy, raising children, and/or involved in a career. CPP can profoundly impact a woman's personal and professional life. An open mind and the pursuit of appropriate diagnostics, as well as support for the patient's fears, anxieties, and stresses, can have a profound impact on the understanding of CPP and ultimate pain control.[15]

COMPLICATIONS

Numerous pathologies have been identified with CPP, and therefore the potential for complications is incalculable. For many women the frustration associated with the diagnosis and treatment of this disorder can be arduous. In addition, there is often a psychogenic component to the disorder that is not easily addressed.

INDICATIONS FOR REFERRAL/HOSPITALIZATION

The etiology of CPP is often complex and multifaceted, and treatment may involve several specialists. A coordinated multidisciplinary approach has been advocated.[9,10] Consultation with a physician is appropriate to ensure coordination of care with appropriate referrals to specialists as needed.[17]

PATIENT AND FAMILY EDUCATION

Reassurance that the causes of CPP, although real and concerning, tend to be less urgent than those causing acute pelvic pain can be helpful. In addition, it is important that the patient understand that additional diagnostic testing may not be indicated. Education should include information about the possible sources of pain and an explanation that the alleviation of pain may be best achieved by a combination of therapies, including medical, psychologic, and behavioral treatments.

HEALTH PROMOTION

Helping a woman to understand her body and the sources of possible pain can assist her in coping. As always, a healthy diet, regular exercise, moderation of alcohol intake, and relaxation techniques can go a long way in improving a woman's management of the stress and anxiety associated with CPP.

REFERENCES

1. Ryder RM: Chronic pelvic pain, *Am Fam Physician* 54(7):2225-2232, 1996.
2. Rosenfeld JA: Chronic pelvic pain: an integrated approach, *Am Fam Physician* 54(7):2187-2193, 1996.
3. Steege JF: Office assessment of chronic pelvic pain, *Clin Obstet Gynecol* 40(3):554-563, 1997.
4. Jamieson DJ, Steege JF: The prevalence of dysmenorrhea, dyspareunia, pelvic pain, and irritable bowel syndrome in primary care practices, *Obstet Gynecol* 87(1):55-58, 1996.
5. Mathias SD and others: Chronic pelvic pain: prevalence, health-related quality of life, and economic correlates, *Obstet Gynecol* 87(3):321-327, 1996.
6. Reiter RC: A profile of women with chronic pelvic pain, *Clin Obstet Gynecol* 33(1):130-136, 1990.
7. Walling MK and others: Abuse history and chronic pain in women. I. Prevalence of sexual abuse and physical abuse, *Obstet Gynecol* 84(2):193-199, 1994.
8. Stones RW, Mountfield J: Interventions for treating chronic pelvic pain in women, *Cochrane Database Syst Rev* (4):CD000387, 2000.
9. Price JR, Blake R: Chronic pelvic pain: the assessment as therapy, *J Psychosom Res* 46(1):7-14, 1999.
10. Smith RP: *Chronic pelvic pain, ACOG Technical Bulletin,* no 223, Washington, DC, 1996, American College of Obstetrics and Gynecology.
11. Nolan TE, Elkins TE: Chronic pelvic pain: differentiating anatomic from functional causes, *Postgrad Med* 94(8):125-138, 1993.
12. Roseff SJ, Murphy AA: Laparoscopy in the diagnosis and therapy of chronic pelvic pain, *Clin Obstet Gynecol* 33(1):137-144, 1990.
13. Slocumb JC: Chronic somatic, myofascial, and neurogenic abdominal pelvic pain, *Clin Obstet Gynecol* 33(1):145-153, 1990.
14. Longstreth GF: Irritable bowel syndrome and chronic pelvic pain, *Obstet Gynecol Surv* 49(7):505-507, 1994.
15. Lipscomb GH, Ling FW: Chronic pelvic pain, *Med Clin North Am* 79(6):1411-1425, 1995.
16. Hewitt GD, Brown RT: Acute and chronic pelvic pain in female adolescents, *Med Clin North Am* 84(4):1009-1025, 2000.
17. Parker P, Rosenfeld JA: Dyspareunia and pelvic pain. In Rosenfeld JA, editor: *Women's health in primary care,* Baltimore, 1997, Williams & Wilkins.

CHAPTER 173

Dysmenorrhea

Jackie S. Fantes; updated by Terry Mahan Buttaro

DEFINITION/EPIDEMIOLOGY

The term *dysmenorrhea,* from the Greek language, meaning "difficult monthly flow" refers to painful menstruation. Dysmenorrhea is classified as either primary or secondary. Primary dysmenorrhea usually occurs within 6 to 12 months after menarche begins and has no organic cause. Secondary dysmenorrhea usually presents later in life and generally has an organic cause such as endometriosis, uterine fibroids, adenomyosis, or an intrauterine contraceptive device (IUD).[1,2]

Dysmenorrhea is one of the most commonly encountered gynecologic disorders and at one time was considered psychologic.[1] Statistics estimate that 60% to 93% of adolescents and 30% to 50% of childbearing women in the United States suffer from dysmenorrhea.[1-3] Approximately 10% to 15% of these women experience discomfort that inhibits normal daily activity for 1 to 3 days each month.[1,2] The peak age incidence of dysmenorrhea is during the late teenage years and early twenties.[3]

PATHOPHYSIOLOGY

Primary dysmenorrhea has been attributed to uterine contractions or ischemia, psychologic influences, and cervical factors.[4] Contractions in the menstruating uterus have been attributed to the production of prostaglandins (PG), specifically $PGF_{2\alpha}$ and PGE_2.[4] The prostaglandins also cause the nausea and diarrhea associated with dysmenorrhea.[1] Current evidence shows that the menstrual fluid of women with primary dysmenorrhea has higher than normal levels of these prostaglandins.[4] Normal menstruation produces contractions of 50 to 80 mm Hg, lasting 15 to 30 seconds, that help to expel the menstrual fluids. The resting uterine pressures are normally 5 to 15 mm Hg. However, in women with primary dysmenorrhea, contractions may exceed 400 mm Hg and last longer than 90 seconds, with resting pressures as high as 80 to 100 mm Hg.[3] This prostaglandin hypothesis can also explain the extragenital symptoms of primary dysmenorrhea. It has been shown that IV injection of prostaglandins causes nausea, vomiting, diarrhea, headache, and syncope, which are symptoms often seen in severe primary dysmenorrhea.[5]

There is no convincing evidence that mechanical cervical obstruction or severe uterine flexion causing obstructed uterine flow is present in patients with primary dysmenorrhea.[6] Psychologic considerations have not been convincingly demonstrated to be the initial cause of primary dysmenorrhea but should be considered in patients who do not respond to medical therapy.[2]

Secondary dysmenorrhea is caused by a pathologic process that affects the uterus, fallopian tubes, ovaries, or pelvic peritoneum. These processes can cause pain by altering pressures in or around pelvic structures, changing or restricting blood flow, or irritating the pelvic peritoneum. They can occur with the normal physiology of menstruation or act completely independently, with symptoms presenting during specific points in the menstrual cycle.[3]

CLINICAL PRESENTATION

The diagnosis of primary dysmenorrhea is based on clinical features. The initial onset of symptoms is usually within 6 to 12 months of menarche, with 90% of women with primary dysmenorrhea experiencing symptoms within 2 years of menarche. Women will complain of recurrent sharp, cramplike lower abdominal pain that is usually over the suprapubic area. The pain will often radiate to the back, sacrum, or inner thighs. The pain usually begins a few hours before or just after the onset of menstruation and lasts the first 1 to 3 days of menstruation; it can be associated with nausea, vomiting, diarrhea, low back pain, or headache.[1,2,4]

The signs and symptoms of secondary dysmenorrhea are determined by the underlying pathologic process. Some clues that may distinguish primary dysmenorrhea from secondary dysmenorrhea include the age of onset. Secondary dysmenorrhea usually occurs in older women, 30 or 40 years of age. The pain is often not limited to the menses and is less related to the first day of flow. There may be an array of associated symptoms, which include dyspareunia, infertility, and abnormal bleeding.[4] The history should include age at menarche, menstrual history, last menstrual period, location and severity of discomfort, associated symptoms (headache, dizziness, nausea, vomiting, diarrhea, dyschezia), amount of school/work missed, medications, method of birth control, and the adequacy of its use.[1] Abdominal and pelvic pain not related to the menstrual cycle should also be explored.

PHYSICAL EXAMINATION

Physical examination findings are normal in primary dysmenorrhea. The diagnosis is based on a careful history.[4]

The physical examination for secondary dysmenorrhea must include a thorough abdominal, pelvic, and rectovaginal examination. Clues to diagnosis may be asymmetric enlargement of the uterus or adnexa (indicates myomas or other tumors), symmetric enlargement (indicates adenomyosis), the presence of painful nodules in the posterior cul-de-sac together with restricted motion of the uterus (indicates endometriosis), cervical stenosis (suggesting retrograde menstruation), or restricted motion of the uterus together with thickened adnexal structures (indicates pelvic scarring or adhesions).[3]

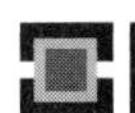
Diagnostics

Secondary Dysmenorrhea

Laboratory
CBC and differential
Erythrocyte sedimentation rate
Urinalysis*
Gonococcal, *Chlamydia* cultures
Pap test

Imaging
Pelvic ultrasound (transvaginal, vaginal)*

Other
Laparoscopy*
Hysterosalpingogram*
Hysteroscopy*
D&C*

*If indicated.

DIAGNOSTICS

No diagnostic studies are needed for the diagnosis of primary dysmenorrhea. However, if the diagnosis of primary versus secondary dysmenorrhea is not clear, certain diagnostic tests may be helpful. Laboratory evaluation may include a CBC, erythrocyte sedimentation rate, and genital cultures for pathogens. Radiologic evaluation may include pelvic ultrasound or a hysterosalpingogram. If the final diagnosis is still unconfirmed, the patient may require a laparoscopy, hysteroscopy, or dilation and curettage.[2]

DIFFERENTIAL DIAGNOSIS

Although the diagnosis of primary dysmenorrhea is made by a careful history/clinical presentation, the etiology of secondary dysmenorrhea can be difficult, and it is important to be aware of the causes. These causes can be broadly classified as intrauterine or extrauterine. Intrauterine causes include myomas, adenomyosis, polyps, an IUD, infection, cervical stenosis, and cervical lesions. Extrauterine causes include endometriosis, tumors (myomas or malignant), inflammation, adhesions, psychogenic causes, pelvic congestion syndrome, or nongynecologic causes, which include urologic, gastrointestinal, musculoskeletal, and psychiatric etiologies.[3]

MANAGEMENT

The mainstay of treatment for primary dysmenorrhea includes nonsteroidal antiinflammatory drugs (NSAIDs), which are antiprostaglandins, and oral contraceptives. Although more studies need to address the efficacy of oral contraceptives in the management of dysmenorrhea, it is theorized that oral contraceptives reduce menstrual flow and inhibit ovulation, thus reducing the pain of primary dysmenorrhea.[4,5] Many studies have shown NSAIDs, including the cyclooxygenase (COX)-2 inhibitors, beneficial in the treatment of dysmenorrhea, although no studies have clearly determined which NSAIDs are the most efficacious.[1] Typical examples of NSAIDs that are approved by the U.S. Food and Drug Administration for treating primary dysmenorrhea are listed in Box 173-1. If the discomfort of primary dysmenorrhea is not controlled with NSAIDs and oral contraceptives, further diagnostic evaluation is indicated to exclude pelvic pathology.

Other approaches used in the management of dysmenorrhea include calcium channel blockers (such as nifedipine or diltiazem), tocolytic agents (such as albuterol [salbutamol]), progestogens, transcutaneous electrical nerve stimulation (TENS), acupuncture, herbal remedies, exercise, low-fat vegetarian diet, castor oil packs to the abdomen, vitamin E (500 IU for 2 days before and 3 days after the onset of menses), fish oil supplement, psychotherapy, and hypnosis. TENS units, vitamin E, and exercise have proven beneficial in some studies, but more and larger studies are necessary to determine the effectiveness of other treatments.[1,5] Presacral neurectomy and uterosacral ligament division were used in the past to treat dysmenorrhea but are rarely performed today.[2,4,7]

These treatments for primary dysmenorrhea may also assist in the treatment of secondary dysmenorrhea. However, ultimately the only successful management of secondary dysmenorrhea is to treat the underlying disease.[3]

COMPLICATIONS

Dysmenorrhea may be a difficult and frustrating condition to treat in some patients. If patients diagnosed with primary dysmenorrhea do not respond to conventional treatment, the diagnosis may need to be reassessed.[4]

INDICATIONS FOR REFERRAL/HOSPITALIZATION

Patients with recalcitrant primary dysmenorrhea and no apparent secondary causes found by physical examination, laboratory studies, and radiologic studies need to be referred for gynecologic evaluation for possible surgical diagnostic evaluation/treatment. Referral is also necessary if a secondary cause is found and requires surgical intervention.[4] In difficult cases psychologic factors must be considered, and psychiatric referral may be warranted.[2]

PATIENT AND FAMILY EDUCATION

Patients with dysmenorrhea must be educated about their disease and specifically about why certain treatments are being implemented. Women on NSAID therapy should understand the potential gastrointestinal adverse effects associated with NSAIDs. One study has shown that risk factors for dysmenorrhea include early age at menarche, long menstrual periods, smoking, alcohol intake, and weight greater than the 90th percentile. Therefore patient education concerning a healthy lifestyle needs to be included.[7]

Differential Diagnosis

Dysmenorrhea

Intrauterine Causes
Myomas
Adenomyosis
Polyps
Intrauterine contraceptive device
Infection
Cervical stenosis
Cervical lesions

Extrauterine Causes
Ectopic pregnancy
Endometriosis
Tumors
Fibroids
Inflammation
Adhesions
Imperforate hymen

Psychogenic Causes
Pelvic congestion syndrome

Nongynecologic Causes
Urologic etiologies
Gastrointestinal etiologies
Musculoskeletal etiologies
Psychiatric etiologies

BOX 173-1

EXAMPLES OF NSAIDS FOR TREATING DYSMENORRHEA

- Ibuprofen, 400-800 mg PO q 6 hours × 3 days
- Naproxen, 500 mg as initial dose, then 250 mg q 6-8 hours × 3 days
- Naproxen sodium, 550 mg as initial dose, then 275 mg q 6-8 hours × 3 days
- Mefenamic acid, 500 mg as initial dose, then 250 mg q 4-6 hours × 3 days
- Meclofenamate, 100 mg as initial dose, then 50-100 mg q 6 hours (not to exceed 400 mg/day) × 3 days
- Valdecoxib 10-20 mg q.d. or b.i.d. × 3 days
- Rofecoxib 50 mg q.d. for 3 to 5 days

REFERENCES

1. Barbieri RL: Primary dysmenorrhea in adults. Retrieved Spetember 9, 2002 from the World Wide Web: www.uptodateonline.
2. Smith RP: Cyclic pelvic pain and dysmenorrhea, *Obstet Gynecol Clin North Am* 20(4):753-764, 1993.
3. Maxson WS, Rosenwaks Z: Dysmenorrhea and premenstrual syndrome. In Copeland LJ, editor: *Textbook of gynecology,* Philadelphia, 1993, WB Saunders.
4. *Dysmenorrhea,* ACOG Tech Bull 68, 1983.
5. Proctor M, Farquhar C: Dysmenorrhea. In Barton S, editor: *Clinical evidence,* London, 2001, BMJ Publishing Group.
6. Eden JA: Dysmenorrhea and premenstrual syndrome. In Hacker NF, Moore JG, editors: *Essentials of obstetrics and gynecology,* ed 2, Philadelphia, 1992, WB Saunders.
7. Kennedy S: Primary dysmenorrhea, *Lancet* 349(9095):1116, 1997.

CHAPTER 174

Dyspareunia

Marie Elena Botte

DEFINITION/EPIDEMIOLOGY

Dyspareunia is defined as recurrent or persistent genital pain associated with sexual intercourse.[1] Although the condition is not unique to women, and men can have dyspareunia from a variety of causes such as dermatologic infections or structural abnormalities,[2] it is much more commonly encountered in women and is therefore almost exclusively described as a women's health issue. Dyspareunia can develop secondary to other vulvar problems such as vulvar vestibulitis, vaginismus, or vulvodynia. *Vulvar vestibulitis* refers to severe pain on vestibular contact or with attempted vaginal entry, tenderness to pressure within the vestibule, and vulvar erythema.[3] *Vaginismus* is involuntary spasm of the muscles surrounding the outer third of the vagina brought on by real, imagined, or anticipated attempts at vaginal penetration.[4] *Vulvodynia* refers to chronic vulvar discomfort that may involve complaints of rawness, burning, stinging or irritation, and is not necessarily related to sexual activity.

Dyspareunia is a common gynecologic complaint, with an estimated prevalence of between 46%[5,6] and 60%.[7] Factors influencing dyspareunia include spontaneous and postabortive pelvic inflammatory disease[8] and psychosocial factors such as rigid religious upbringing, low physical and emotional satisfaction, decreased general happiness, or previous painful sexual experience. Dyspareunia has not been consistently associated with factors such as age, parity, marital status, race, income, education, psychopathology, or prior sexual abuse.[5]

PATHOPHYSIOLOGY

Dyspareunia is often due to inadequate vaginal lubrication. This can often be attributable either to insufficient stimulation or arousal during sexual activity or can be related to decreased estrogen, a condition noted in postmenopausal women and breast cancer survivors.[9] Superficial dyspareunia has been associated with trauma or inflammation,[10] vaginal and hymenal abnormalities, postobstetric or postoperative vulvar outlet stenosis, factitious urticaria,[11] urinary tract infections,[12] occlusion of the Bartholin gland duct,[13] stenosing lichen planus, Bowen's disease, and focal vestibulitis. Aortoiliac or atherosclerotic disease can diminish pelvic blood flow and lead to vaginal wall and clitoral smooth muscle fibrosis.[1]

Tiny *mucosal tears* have been implicated in focal vulvitis[14] and *perivascular inflammation* has been proposed as a mechanism causing dyspareunia in women with Sjögren's syndrome.[10] Dyspareunia after a normal pelvic examination has been linked with *overexertion of the levator ani muscles* and subsequent myalgia after the initiation of Kegel exercises.[15] When the levator ani muscles are hypertonic, vaginismus can result.[1] Various infectious processes, structural abnormalities, nonalcoholic liver disease (by decreasing vaginal lubrication), glomus tumors, ciguatera (human semen carries the irritating toxin), horseback riding, fibroids, interstitial cystitis, urethral disorders, and vulvodynia have also been noted in the literature.[12] Pelvic floor surgery can either ameliorate preexisting dyspareunia or cause it.[15] Episiotomies have been tied to significant increases in dyspareunia, particularly those involving the mediolateral technique[16] and glycerol-impregnated chromic catgut.[14,17] Obstetric instrumentation and perineal trauma contribute to postpartum dyspareunia.[18]

One study found a group of women with progressively worsening dyspareunia who had been treated unsuccessfully for nonspecific vulvitis and vaginitis whose external genitalia appeared normal to close visual inspection but under magnification revealed *erythema around the Bartholin duct openings.*[19] In another study, each of 21 women treated surgically for dyspareunia and vulvodynia, Barbero and colleagues[20] found stricture of the vaginal introitus secondary to *membranous hypertrophy* of the posterior fourchette. In addition to histologic findings of *chronic nonspecific inflammation* in many of the women and two with changes suggestive of human papillomavirus infection, 80% of these women had erythema and tenderness of the vestibule. Hormonal and sexual history factors (oral contraception use before age 17 years and first intercourse before age 15 years) have been proposed as causes for vulvar vestibulitis syndrome.[21]

CLINICAL PRESENTATION

Health care providers need to take an active role in inquiring specifically about discomfort during or after sexual intercourse and not simply assume that women will raise the issue if it is a problem. Women often will not voice this concern even if it is the main reason for their visit.[14,22] Research has shown that although some women will discuss dyspareunia with their partner, far fewer consult a health care provider for the problem. Of women who seek medical help, only 15% receive a specific diagnosis or effective treatment.

A thorough symptom analysis will guide the physical examination and should specifically include questioning about the onset of the discomfort and its relationship to particular partners, positions, times in the menstrual cycle, contraceptive devices, and substances (such as latex condoms, spermicides or lubricants), and products such as douches, soaps, tampons, or detergents. Women may report pain with tampon use or pelvic examinations. Important information to gather includes number of pregnancies and type of delivery, surgical history, history of rape or sexual abuse, and menopausal signs and symptoms. Knowing whether the pain is on entry, postcoital, generalizable to the entire vulva, felt only with deep thrusting, or localized to a particular anatomic structure or area is helpful in determining the etiology of the discomfort.

PHYSICAL EXAMINATION

A thorough pelvic examination is necessary for all complaints of dyspareunia. The experience can be educational for the woman and more informative for the clinician if the patient sits somewhat upright and holds a small hand mirror; this allows the woman, who then can see what is happening, to feel more in control.[23] It is important to correlate the discomfort elicited during the pelvic examination with specific physical findings whenever possible. In addition, clarification should be sought regarding pain elicited to determine if it is similar to what the woman has been experiencing during intercourse, as many women find pelvic examinations generally uncomfortable.

The external genitalia should be examined for erythema, pigment changes, lesions (including herpes and condyloma), and indications of trauma or abuse. Touching the vestibule and the hymen with a moistened cotton swab may elicit the pain of vulvar vestibulitis, a condition in which there is exquisite tenderness to pressure at specific sites[3] and is often accompanied by erythema.

A finger inserted gently into the introitus and gradually pressed in a posterior direction may elicit the spasms of vaginismus; conscious control of the pelvic floor musculature can be evaluated by asking the woman to squeeze and relax the muscles around the examiner's finger. The Bartholin glands, which are normally not palpable, may be tender and enlarged. A narrow, well-lubricated speculum should be used to evaluate the vagina. A bimanual examination can assess for uterine and ovarian size, fibroids, ovarian cysts, other pelvic masses, as well as cervical motion tenderness (seen with pelvic inflammatory disease) and the position of the uterus. Hemorrhoids or prolapse of the uterus, bladder, or rectum may be evident. A rectal or rectovaginal examination is generally not necessary.

DIAGNOSTICS

Wet mounts, potassium hydroxide prep and cultures of vaginal discharge as well as endocervical Pap smear, *Chlamydia trachomatis*, and *Neisseria gonorrhoeae* cultures will help to rule out infection as a cause for either superficial or deep dyspareunia.[14] A CBC and erythrocyte sedimentation rate can help to identify inflammation and infection; a urinalysis evaluates for urinary tract infection, and a human chorionic gonadotropin can exclude ectopic pregnancy.

DIFFERENTIAL DIAGNOSIS

Potential causes for dyspareunia include both psychologic and pathophysiologic etiologies. Most cases are probably a combination of both. A problem that is initially physical often has a continued and escalating psychologic impact. Potential causes for dyspareunia are listed in the Differential Diagnoses box and are arranged according to the phase of intercourse during which the symptom is experienced.

MANAGEMENT/HEALTH PROMOTION

Women with dyspareunia resulting from insufficient lubrication may benefit significantly from education regarding the physiology of female arousal and the importance of allowing

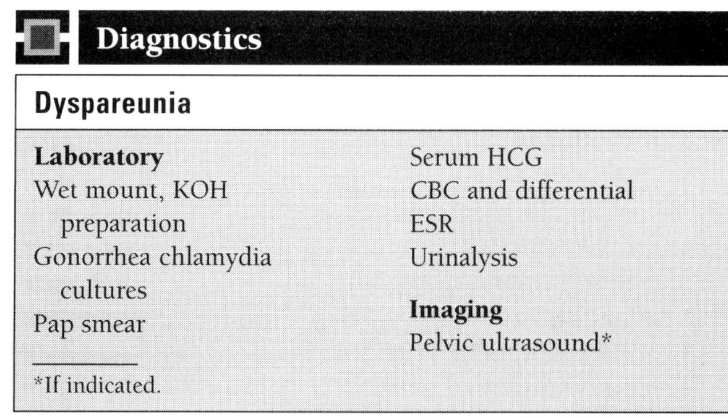

Diagnostics

Dyspareunia

Laboratory	
Wet mount, KOH preparation	Serum HCG
Gonorrhea chlamydia cultures	CBC and differential
Pap smear	ESR
	Urinalysis
	Imaging
	Pelvic ultrasound*

*If indicated.

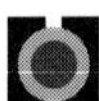

Differential Diagnosis

Dyspareunia

Surface (Occurs with Penetration)
Insufficient arousal
Hypoestrogenic mucosal
Vaginitis
Vaginismus
Hymenal abnormalities
Dermatopathology
Postherpetic neuralgia

Focal
Vulvar vestibulitis
Bartholin's gland cyst or abscess
Episiotomy scar
Residual sutures
Introital tear
Herpetic lesions
Urethral problems

Deep (Occurs with Penile Thrusting)
Pelvic inflammatory disease
Fibroids
Endometriosis
Hemorrhoids
Inflammatory bowel disease
Retroverted uterus
Uterine prolapse
Pelvic adhesions or masses

Postcoital
Urinary tract infection
Vulvodynia

Irritants
Contraceptive devices
Spermicides
Douches
Feminine hygiene products
Soaps

Psychosocial Factors
Anxiety
Prior painful sexual experience
Rigid upbringing

adequate time before vaginal penetration for the vascular engorgement of genital tissues that results in glandular secretions. If the problem is estrogen-insufficient vaginal dryness, national guidelines[24-27] suggest topical estrogen cream or hormone replacement therapy (HRT) as the most effective way to build up the vascularity of the vaginal epithelium and thereby induce physiologic lubrication. Alternative vaginal lubrication (water-based products such as glycerin [Astroglide]) for those women using condoms or diaphragms) is suggested for those women for whom supplemental estrogen is contraindicated. Alternative sexual positioning (female astride to control penetration) or position changes can alleviate the pain of dyspareunia for some women, as can nonsteroidal agents, topical application of lidocaine, or a warm bath before sex.[28]

Dyspareunia secondary to endometriosis has been treated successfully during therapy and for 6 months afterward with both nafarelin acetate and danazol.[29] Treatment of vaginismus-related dyspareunia focuses on helping the woman to regain voluntary control of the muscles of the pelvic floor.[4] Vulvar vestibulitis has been treated successfully with topical estrogen cream applied twice a day for 4 to 8 weeks and intralesional injections of interferon.[30] Treatments for vulvodynia include a low-oxalate diet and calcium citrate supplementation to neutralize urinary oxalates and tricyclic agents.[30,31] Behavioral approaches are most often used and often involve pelvic floor contraction/relaxation exercises as well as using fingers or dilators to progressively desensitize the woman to vaginal penetration. Surgical intervention is rarely required and may be detrimental[4] to the resolution of the vaginismus. Behavioral treatment is also first-line therapy for vulvar vestibulitis syndrome, as research documents no statistical difference in effect between this option and corrective surgery.[32]

LIFE SPAN CONSIDERATIONS

Dyspareunia effects sexually active women of all ages but may become increasingly evident at times of major transition in a woman's life, including onset of sexual activity, childbirth, and menopause.

COMPLICATIONS

Dyspareunia is known to have a detrimental effect on relationships and can continue unacknowledged and unaided for years in the absence of clinician inquiry and therapeutic involvement. Although the morbidity associated with dyspareunia varies widely with its attendant cause, the impact on a woman's quality of life can be profound and should not be underestimated.

INDICATIONS FOR REFERRAL/HOSPITALIZATION

Women with dyspareunia related to severe psychologic distress or anxiety may be best managed in collaboration with psychiatric or other counseling services. For severe vulvar vestibulitis unresponsive to conservative behavioral-based therapies, perineoplasty or posterior vestibulectomy can be performed as a last resort[3,33] and involves a crescent-shaped posterior vestibular excision followed by vaginal advancement.[33] Surgery is less successful if there is concomitant vaginismus (unless the vaginismus is treated first),[3] in dyspareunia since first intercourse, and in women with associated persistent vulvar pain.[34]

One treatment guideline suggests that hysterectomy may be indicated for women with documented pelvic adhesions unresponsive to lysis or for women over 30 years with more than 6 months of moderate to severe idiopathic dyspareunia unresponsive to nonsteroidal drugs and/or HRT who do not desire further children, but only after other potential causes have been excluded by laparoscopy/laparotomy, colonoscopy/barium enema, cystoscopy/IV pyelography and psychologic evaluation.[35] For some women in whom dyspareunia is related to prior hysterectomy, surgical excision of the vaginal apex has been a successful surgical procedure.[36]

PATIENT AND FAMILY EDUCATION

Education is central in the management of dyspareunia, particularly when the cause of discomfort is attributable to insufficient sexual arousal time and lubrication, spasms of vaginismus, control of concomitant infections, or the use of irritating or allergenic products. Taking the time to educate individuals about their bodies and the particular strategies necessary to attain or resume sexual activity without discomfort is an important aspect of comprehensive, holistic primary care.

REFERENCES

1. Berman J, Goldstein I: Female sexual dysfunction, *Urol Clin North Am* 28(2):405-416, 2001.
2. Shechet J, Tanenbaum B, Freid SM: Male dyspareunia in the uncircumcised patient, *Am Fam Physician* 60(1):54-56, 1999.
3. Abramov L, Wolman I, David MP: Vaginismus: an important factor in the evaluation and management of vulvar vestibulitis syndrome, *Gynecol Obstet Invest* 38(3):194-197, 1994.
4. Biswas A, Ratnam SS: Vaginismus and outcome of treatment, *Ann Acad Med Singapore* 24(5):755-758, 1995.

5. Heim LJ: Evaluation and differential diagnosis of dyspareunia, *Am Fam Physician* 63(8):1535-1544, 2001.
6. Jamieson DJ, Steege JF: The prevalence of dysmenorrhea, dyspareunia, pelvic pain, and irritable bowel syndrome in primary care practices, *Obstet Gynecol* 87(1):55-58, 1996.
7. Glatt AE, Zinner SH, McCormack WM: The prevalence of dyspareunia, *Obstet Gynecol* 75(3, part 1):433-436, 1990.
8. Heisterberg L: Factors influencing spontaneous abortion, dyspareunia, dysmenorrhea, and pelvic pain, *Obstet Gynecol* 81(4):594-597, 1993.
9. Loprinzi CL and others: Phase III randomized double blind study to evaluate the efficacy of a polycarbil-based vaginal moisturizer in women with breast cancer, *J Clin Oncol* 15(3):969-973, 1997.
10. Skopouli FN and others: Obstetric and gynaecologic profile in patients with primary Sjogren's syndrome, *Ann Rheum Dis* 53(9):569-573, 1994.
11. Lambris A, Greaves MW: Dyspareunia and vulvodynia are probably common manifestations of factitious urticaria, *Br J Dermatol* 136(1):140-141, 1997.
12. Jones KD, Lehr ST, Hewell CW: Dyspareunia: three case reports, *J Obstet Gynecol Neonat Nurs* 26(1):19-23, 1997.
13. Sarrel PM and others: Pain during sex response due to occlusion of the Bartholin gland duct, *Obstet Gynecol* 62(2):261-264, 1983.
14. Sarazin SK, Seymour SF: Causes and treatment options for women with dyspareunia, *Nurse Pract* 16(10):30, 35-38, 41, 1991.
15. DeLancey JOL, Sampselle CM, Punch MR: Kegel dyspareunia: levator ani myalgia caused by overexertion, *Obstet Gynecol* 82(4):658-659, 1993.
16. Bex PJ, Hofmeyer GJ: Perineal management during childbirth and subsequent dyspareunia, *Clin Exp Obstet Gynecol* 14(2):97-100, 1987.
17. Grant A: Dyspareunia associated with the use of glycerol-impregnated catgut to repair perineal trauma. Report of a 3-year follow up study, *Br J Obstet Gynaecol* 96(6):741-743, 1989.
18. Signorello L: Postpartum sexual functioning and its relationship to perineal trauma: a retrospective cohort study of primiparous women, *Am J Obstet Gynecol* 184(5):881-890, 2001.
19. Lopez-Zeno JA, Ross E, O'Grady JP: Septic shock complicating drainage of a Bartholin gland abscess, *Obstet Gynecol* 76(5):915-916, 1990.
20. Barbero M and others: Membranous hypertrophy of the posterior fourchette as a cause of dyspareunia and vulvodynia, *J Reprod Med* 39(12):949-952, 1994.
21. Bazin S and others: Vulvar vestibulitis syndrome: an exploratory case-control study, *Obstet Gynecol* 83(1):47-50, 1994.
22. Jarvis GJ: Dyspareunia, *BMJ* 288:1555-1556, 1987.
23. Steege JF, Ling FW: Dyspareunia: a special type of chronic pelvic pain, *Obstet Gynecol Clin North Am* 20(4):779-793, 1993.
24. Clinical challenges of perimenopause: consensus opinion of the North American Menopause Society, *Menopause* 7(1):5-13, 2000.
25. A decision tree for the use of estrogen replacement therapy or hormone replacement therapy in postmenopausal women: consensus of the North American Menopause Society, *Menopause* 7(2):76-86, 2000.
26. United States Preventive Services Task Force: *Postmenopausal hormone prophylaxis*, Baltimore, Md, 1996, Williams & Wilkins.
27. AACE medical guidelines for clinical practice for management of menopause, *Endocr Pract* 5(6):355-366, 1999.
28. Phillips N: Female sexual dysfunction: evaluation and treatment, *Am Fam Physician* 62(1):127-136, 2000.
29. Adamson GD, Kwei L, Edgren RA: Pain of endometriosis: effects of nafarelin and danazol therapy, *Int J Fertil Menopausal Stud* 39(4): 215-217, 1994.
30. Metts J: Vulvodynia and vulvar vestibulitis: challenges in diagnosis and management, *Am Fam Physician* 59(6):1547-1556, 1999.
31. Quint E, Smith Y: Adolescent gynecology, part 1: common disorders, *Pediatr Clin North Am* 46(3):593-606, 1999.
32. Weijmar Schultz WC and others: Behavioral approach with or without surgical intervention to the vulvar vestibulitis syndrome: a prospective randomized and non-randomized study, *J Psychosom Obstet Gynaecol* 17(3):143-148, 1996.
33. Berville S, Moyal-Barracco M, Paniel BJ: Treatment of vulvar vestibulitis by posterior vestibulectomy. Twelve case reports, *J Gynecol Obstet Biol Reprod (Paris)* 26(1):71-75, 1997.
34. Bornstein J and others: Predicting the outcome of surgical treatment of vulvar vestibulitis, *Obstet Gynecol* 89(5 pt 1):695-698, 1997.
35. *Hysterectomy*, Lexington, Mass, 1997 (revised 1999), Optimed Clinical Development Group.
36. Sharp H: The role of vaginal apex excision in the management of persistent posthysterectomy dyspareunia, *Am J Obstet Gynecol* 183(6): 1385-1388, 2000.

CHAPTER 175

Ectopic Pregnancy

Marie Elena Botte

DEFINITION/EPIDEMIOLOGY

Ectopic pregnancy occurs when a fertilized ovum implants anywhere outside of the uterus. Occurring in 1 out of 100 pregnancies,[1] ectopic pregnancy is the second leading cause of maternal mortality[2] and the leading cause of pregnancy-related death in the first trimester.[3] The rate of ectopic pregnancy in the United States has risen dramatically in the past three decades[4]; prevalence has risen sixfold since 1970, perhaps because of an attendant increase in sexually transmitted diseases, increased frequency of sterilization procedures, and delayed childbearing.[5] The rate of ectopic pregnancy has been found to increase dramatically after the age of 30, especially beyond the age of 35.[6] The mortality rate related to ectopic pregnancy for African Americans is twice that of white women; among adolescents of minority race the rate is 5 times that of their white counterparts, a difference not entirely explained by the difference in prevalence between these groups.[7]

Immediate emergency department referral/physician consultation is indicated for female patients with a positive test for serum human chorionic gonadotropin (hCG) and abdominal pain and bleeding.

PATHOPHYSIOLOGY

Proposed pathophysiologic explanations for ectopic pregnancy include abnormal embryogenesis[8,9] (with serious chromosomal aberration in one third of cases),[10] ascending *Chlamydia trachomatis* infection that scars the fallopian tubes,[11] and luteal phase defects.[12] History of or current pelvic inflammatory disease (PID) and in utero diethylstilbestrol (DES) exposure may also result in ectopic gestation. Cases have been reported that involve clear cell hyperplasia of the fallopian tube[13] and development in a cesarean section scar.[14] Although implantation can occur anywhere on the cervix, in the abdomen, or on the ovary, 95% of ectopic pregnancies implant in the fallopian tube.[2]

Cervical pregnancy, which accounts for less than 1.0% of all ectopic pregnancies, has been associated with cervicouterine instrumentation[8]; ovarian pregnancy has been associated with ovulation induction and intrauterine insemination.[15] Persistent ectopic pregnancy involves residual trophoblastic activity and a beta-hCG level that rises or plateaus, whereas chronic ectopic pregnancy contains no active trophoblastic tissue and results in an hCG level that is low or absent.[16] One retrospective study found that chronic ectopic pregnancy accounts for as much as 20.3% of all ectopic pregnancies.[17]

CLINICAL PRESENTATION

Risk factors for ectopic pregnancy should be elicited for any woman when pregnancy is suspected, although identifiable factors may be absent in many women with ectopic pregnancies.[18] There is strong evidence for the following risk factors, which interfere with fallopian tube function, and include past or current history of the following: sexually transmitted infections and PID,[19,20] including recurrent chlamydial infection[21]; pregnancy occurring while on oral contraceptives (because of the mechanism of action of the birth control pill on the ciliary movement of the fallopian tube); previous history of ectopic pregnancy[18,22]; history of infertility[18]; in utero DES exposure[22]; documented tubal pathology[22]; prior appendectomy or pelvic operation[18]; cesarean section[23]; prior tubal sterilization or operation[18,22,24-26]; history of in vitro fertilization[2]; and congenital malformation of the fallopian tubes.[2] Cigarette smoking,[2,27] vaginal douching,[28,29] multiple sexual partners, and early age at first intercourse have weaker evidence for association. Although intrauterine contraceptive devices (IUDs) per se do not increase the risk for ectopic pregnancy, pregnancies that do occur with these devices in place are more likely to be ectopic.[30] Previous induced abortion has not been associated with subsequent ectopic pregnancy.[31,32]

Symptoms of nonruptured ectopic pregnancy can be vague and subacute. The most common symptom of ectopic pregnancy is abdominal pain, which may present in isolation or in combination with vaginal bleeding or spotting, dizziness, and shoulder pain[33] (which suggests blood irritating the diaphragm); symptoms generally appear between 6 and 12 weeks' gestation. Amenorrhea for 1 to 2 months and the usual early signs of pregnancy (nausea, fatigue, breast heaviness) are often part of the initial presentation. Women can also present with generalized or unilateral pelvic or abdominal pain described as sharp, cramping, continuous, or intermittent. Less common presenting symptoms include acute urinary retention[34] and abnormal dark, scant vaginal bleeding. Painless vaginal bleeding is the most common presentation for cervical pregnancy.[35] Pain that radiates to the shoulder is more common in a ruptured ectopic pregnancy. Acute syncopal episodes and hypotension are possible secondary to rupture-induced peritoneal hemorrhage. Chronic ectopic pregnancy generally presents as a pelvic mass, with minimal symptoms such as intermittent pain, and a low or absent hCG titer.[17,36]

PHYSICAL EXAMINATION

Any suspicion of ectopic pregnancy requires a thorough physical examination, although the history and physical examination, with a combined sensitivity of 50%, can neither exclude nor establish the presence of an ectopic pregnancy. Postural vital signs and temperature are essential to indicate the presence of hypotension or infection. Speculum examination may reveal a bulging cul-de-sac (indicative of hemoperitoneum in rupture), a bluish coloration of the cervix (a normal finding in any pregnancy), and evidence of vaginal bleeding. Uterine enlargement occurs in roughly one fourth of women with ectopic pregnancy, but its size may be less than expected according to dates (generally smaller than 8 weeks' size). Approximately 75% of women with ectopic pregnancies have abdominal tenderness,[2] but the abdominal examination may be normal if the ectopic pregnancy has not ruptured; cervical motion tenderness may also be present. An adnexal mass and peritoneal signs, although uncommon, are highly predictive of ectopic gestation. The pelvic examination may also reveal signs that suggest a cause other than ectopic pregnancy as the source of the bleeding, such as hemorrhoids, urethral irritation, cervical lesions, or condyloma. Although tissue at the os is a sign of spontaneous abortion and an open os and heavy vaginal bleeding are predictive of an abnormal intrauterine pregnancy, absence of these signs does not differentiate ectopic from intrauterine gestation.[37]

DIAGNOSTICS

Pregnancy tests have become increasingly sensitive in recent years and are the first step in the diagnosis of any suspected ectopic pregnancy. The slope of a rising hCG titer has been found to be a useful determinant of early ectopic pregnancy below the ultrasonographic discriminatory zone.[38,39] In normal pregnancy, this titer doubles every 1.4 to 3.5 days,[5] with a minimum of 66% increase suggesting viable pregnancy in clinical practice; a titer that plateaus or falls suggests either ectopic pregnancy or miscarriage, although some ectopic pregnancies (and nonviable intrauterine pregnancies) do present with abnormally rising hCG levels. Because nearly all ectopic pregnancies have hCG titers <50,000 mIU/ml, a single value above this level can help to rule out ectopic pregnancy.

Initial diagnostic tests also include a CBC, because women with ectopic gestation are often anemic, as well as a blood type and Rh determination. Serum progesterone is a useful marker of viable pregancy[1,5]; levels >25 ng/ml are highly predictive of successful intrauterine pregnancy and correlate with low risk of ectopic pregnancy,[40] and levels <5 ng/ml identify nonviable pregnancies with nearly 100% sensitivity. Other potential markers for ectopic pregnancy include leukemia inhibitory factor (involved in the implantation process) and smooth muscle heavy-chain myosin (implicated in smooth muscle destruction), but at the present neither of these indices is sufficiently discriminatory to be useful in clinical practice.[41,42]

Ultrasonography is particularly useful for demonstrating viable intrauterine pregnancy; spontaneous heterotopic pregnancy (coexistent uterine and ectopic gestation) is so rare that detection of intrauterine pregnancy on ultrasound essentially rules out ectopic gestation.[5,43] Transvaginal ultrasound can detect ectopic pregnancy in one third of women with beta-hCG levels <1000 mIU/ml,[44] and 3 weeks after missed menses, virtually all viable intrauterine pregnancies, half of nonviable intrauterine and viable ectopic pregnancies, and one fourth of nonviable ectopic pregnancies can be detected with this method.[45] At low hCG levels, ultrasound is often nondiagnostic, but when hCG levels are >1800 mIU/ml, sonography is helpful in establishing the location and viability of the pregnancy.

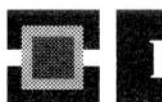

Diagnostics

Ectopic Pregnancy

Laboratory
Serum HCG (beta-hCG)
CBC and differential
Type and crossmatch*
Rh titers*

Imaging
Pelvic ultrasound
Pelvic CT or MRI*

*If indicated.

Many clinicians therefore advocate the combined use of transvaginal sonography and beta-hCG levels, citing an ability to detect earlier and smaller ectopic pregnancies without the attendant risks of a surgical procedure.[1,5,38,46] At hCG levels of 1500 to 1800 mIU/ml, a gestational sac should be visible[30]; at >5000 mIU/ml, a yolk sac.[47] When ultrasound findings are indeterminate, diagnostic laparoscopy is considered by many to be the "gold standard" for the diagnosis of ectopic pregnancy.[46] However, the advent of new strategies, particularly very sensitive pregnancy tests and ultrasonography, contribute to "near perfect" noninvasive diagnostic acumen[2,22] and permit medical management of the condition in carefully selected instances.

DIFFERENTIAL DIAGNOSIS

Ectopic pregnancy must be considered a likely possibility in any woman of childbearing age with abdominal pain (and/or bleeding) until proved otherwise.[48] Other possible differentials include appendicitis, salpingitis, cholecystitis, PID, intrauterine pregnancy with inaccurate dates, corpus luteum cyst, gestational trophoblastic neoplasm, incomplete or missed spontaneous abortion, endometriosis, pelvic mass, ureteral calculi, and adnexal torsion. A twisted cystic teratoma[49] or a ruptured malignant ovarian tumor[50] may present similarly to a ruptured ectopic pregnancy.

MANAGEMENT

Spontaneous resolution is not an uncommon phenomenon, and it occurs in up to 88% of cases that are less vascular and less advanced (1 to 3.5 cm) and in which declining hCG levels are initially low (<200 mIU/ml).[5] During the course of resolution, associated beta-hCG levels become undetectable in 3 to 45 days (mean, 15.8 days).

Methotrexate therapy, with and without leucovorin rescue or accompanying mifepristone, has been widely used as a nonsurgical intervention for nonruptured ectopic pregnancies of <3.5 cm^2.[51,52] A folic acid antagonist that inhibits purine and pyrimidine synthesis, methotrexate interferes with DNA synthesis and cellular multiplication. Rapidly growing tissues such as fetal and trophoblastic cells are most susceptible. Various dosage strategies have been explored, with decreased occurrence and severity of side effects observed in single, low-dose intramuscular injections.[2] Methotrexate has also been used successfully to decrease the incidence of persistent ectopic pregnancy after salpingostomy,[53] in cervical pregnancy,[54] and in women eligible for expectant management.[55] Appropriate candidates for methotrexate therapy should be hemodynamically stable, have no active renal or hepatic disease, and have no evidence of thrombocytopenia or leukopenia. Initial hCG levels in this population should be low, the gestational sac should be small (<3.5 cm), and there should be no discernible fetal cardiac activity on ultrasound. Methotrexate therapy has a 94% success rate as long as the woman fits the appropriate criteria. Methotrexate 50 mg/m^2 is given IM, followed by a repeat hCG and symptom assessment on day 4 and another hCG on day

Differential Diagnosis

Ectopic Pregnancy

Appendicitis	Incomplete abortion
Salpingitis	Endometriosis
Cholecystitis	Pelvic mass
Pelvic inflammatory disease	Ureteral calculi
Intrauterine pregnancy	Adnexal torsion
Corpus luteum cyst	Cystic teratoma
Gestational trophoblastic neoplasm	Ruptured malignant ovarian tumor

7. For women whose hCG titers do not decline significantly by 15%, a second injection of methotrexate is indicated. If a woman's hCG titer declines by the seventh day, she should be followed weekly until it is undetectable. Side effects of treatment with methotrexate include diarrhea, nausea, perioral irritation, and transient transaminase elevations.

Surgical laparoscopy or laparotomy remains the only treatment choice for ruptured ectopic pregnancy.[2] Although laparoscopy is the standard treatment for all ectopic pregnancies,[56] attendant risks include perioperative and postoperative complications (24% in one study),[57] including uncontrollable hemorrhage, adhesion formation,[2] subcutaneous emphysema and pneumothorax,[58] and reduced subsequent fertility.[2]

LIFE SPAN CONSIDERATIONS

All sexually active women of reproductive age are theoretically at risk for ectopic pregnancy, especially those with one or more of the risk factors mentioned earlier. Women in their 20s are more likely to have ectopic gestation, but adolescents and perimenopausal women are also at risk.[20] Women, including those for whom infertility is an issue, may require the support of the clinician in expressing and grieving the loss of the pregnancy and the baby who was expected.[59]

COMPLICATIONS

Ruptured ectopic pregnancy can result in acute, massive bleeding and poses an immediate threat to life.[2] Rupture is more likely at higher presenting levels of hCG and multiple ovulation/ovulation induction.[60] Misdiagnosis, which is as high as 12% of cases, can result in sudden death secondary to internal hemorrhage and infection. Nonfatal sequelae of delayed diagnosis include infection and an increased rate of salpingectomy, potentially affecting future fertility.[61] Missed or delayed diagnoses and subsequent ruptures occur more often in women previously treated with therapeutic abortions when ectopic pregnancies were not suspected. In addition, the risk of a missed or delayed diagnosis is higher in women considered to be less at risk for an ectopic pregnancy, including those with no history of ectopic pregnancy and those with at least one child.[33,62,63]

Methotrexate administration has been associated with cases of alopecia[64] and life-threatening neutropenia[65]; high doses can cause bone marrow depression, hepatotoxicity, stomatitis, pulmonary fibrosis, and photosensitivity.[2] The risk of persistent ectopic pregnancy ranges from 3% to 20% after conservative surgical therapy and 9.8% for treatment with methotrexate.[66] Research has shown a significantly reduced fertility rate postoperatively for some women after ectopic pregnancy[67] and a relationship between advancing age, prior ectopic pregnancy, and declining future pregnancy rates.[68]

INDICATIONS FOR REFERRAL/HOSPITALIZATION

All women with suspected ectopic pregnancy should be referred immediately to an attending physician or a gynecologist for evaluation because the consequences for missed or delayed diagnosis can be dire. Ruptured ectopic pregnancy is a surgical emergency and requires immediate admission and attention. Suggestive hCG levels (<1000 mIU/ml) and an indeterminate vaginal ultrasound necessitate further evaluation, preferably as an inpatient.[69] Although transient abdominal pain is common in the second week after methotrexate administration and generally resolves within 24 hours,[51] severe pain is an indication for hospital-based observation because it may indicate tubal rupture.

PATIENT AND FAMILY EDUCATION

All women should be appraised of their subsequent risk of reduced fertility and recurrent ectopic pregnancy. Condom use should be encouraged to reduce the likelihood of infection and PID because declining rates of chlamydial infection have been associated with declining rates of ectopic pregnancy.[70] Women on birth control pills should be reminded to take them as directed. Women at risk for ectopic pregnancy should alert their provider when they become pregnant. Women who have received methotrexate therapy for nonruptured ectopic pregnancy need to refrain from sexual activity and consuming alcohol or vitamins containing folic acid until after the resolution of the ectopic pregnancy. These women should also be alerted to the possibility that they may experience increased abdominal pain 5 to 10 days after therapy. Further clinical evaluation would be necessary at this point because severe pain may indicate tubal abortion and rupture.

REFERENCES

1. Eisenger S: Early pregnancy bleeding: a rational approach, *Clin Fam Pract* 3:225-249, 2001.
2. Maiolatesi CR, Peddicord K: Methotrexate for nonsurgical treatment of ectopic pregnancy: nursing implications, *J Obstet Gynecol Neonatal Nurs* 25:205-208, 1996.
3. Ectopic pregnancy—United States, 1990—1992, *MMWR Morb Mortal Wkly Rep* 44:46-48, 1995.
4. Morgan A: Adnexal mass evaluation in the emergency department, *Emerg Med Clin North Am* 19:799-813, 2001.
5. Carr R, Evans P: Ectopic pregnancy, *Prim Care Clin Office Pract* 27:169-183, 2000.
6. Coste J and others: Incidence of ectopic pregnancy: first results of a population-based register in France, *Hum Reprod* 9:742-745, 1994.
7. Bernstein J: Ectopic pregnancy: a nursing approach to excess risk among minority women, *J Obstet Gynecol Neonatal Nurs* 24:803-810, 1995.
8. Ushakov FB and others: Cervical pregnancy: past and future, *Obstet Gynecol Surv* 52:45-59, 1997.
9. Toikkanen S, Joensuu H, Erkkola R: DNA anuploidy in ectopic pregnancy and spontaneous abortions, *Eur J Obstet Gynecol Reprod Biol* 51:9-13, 1993.
10. Karikoski R, Aine R, Heinonen PK: Abnormal embryogenesis in the etiology of ectopic pregnancy, *Gynecol Obstet Invest* 36:158-162, 1993.
11. Lan J and others: Chlamydia trachomatis and ectopic pregnancy: retrospective analysis of salpingectomy specimens, endometrial biopsies, and cervical smears, *J Clin Pathol* 48:815-819, 1995.
12. Guillaume AJ and others: Leuteal phase defects and ectopic pregnancy, *Fertil Steril* 63:30-33, 1995.
13. Tziorttziotis DV and others: Clear cell hyperplasia of the fallopian tube epithelium associated with ectopic pregnancy: report of a case, *Int J Gynecol Pathol* 16:79-80, 1997.
14. Godin PA, Bassil S, Donnez J: An ectopic pregnancy developing in a previous cesarean section scar, *Fertil Steril* 67:398-400, 1997.
15. Bontis J and others: Intrafollicular ovarian pregnancy after ovulation induction/intrauterine insemination: pathophysiological aspects and diagnostic problems, *Hum Reprod* 12:376-378, 1997.
16. Dunn RC, Taskin O: Chronic ectopic pregnancy after clinically successful methotrexate treatment of ectopic pregnancy, *Int J Gynaecol Obstet* 51:247-249, 1995.
17. Turan C and others: Transvaginal sonographic findings of chronic ectopic pregnancy, *Eur J Obstet Gynecol Reprod Biol* 7:115-119, 1996.

18. Garrett AM, Vukov LF: Risk factors for ectopic pregnancy in a rural population, *Fam Med* 28:111-113, 1996.
19. Coste J and others: Sexually transmitted diseases as a major cause of ectopic pregnancy: results from a large case-control study in France, *Fertil Steril* 62:289-295, 1994.
20. Ramirez NC, Lawrence WD, Ginsburg KA: Ectopic pregnancy: a recent five-year study and review of the last 50 years' literature, *J Reprod Med* 41:733-740, 1996.
21. Hillis SD and others: Recurrent chlamydial infections increase the risks of hospitalization for ectopic pregnancy and pelvic inflammatory disease, *Am J Obstet Gynecol* 176:103-107, 1997.
22. Ankum WM and others: Risk factors for ectopic pregnancy: a meta-analysis, *Fertil Steril* 65:1093-1099, 1996.
23. Hemminki E, Merilainen J: Long-term effects of cesarean sections: ectopic pregnancies and placental problems, *Am J Obstet Gynecol* 174:1569-1574, 1996.
24. Peterson HB and others: The risk of ectopic pregnancy after tubal sterilization. U.S. Collaborative Review and Sterilization Working Group, *N Engl J Med* 336:762-767, 1997.
25. Mol BW and others: Contraception and the risk of pregnancy: a meta-analysis, *Contraception* 52:337-341, 1995.
26. Napolitano PG, Vu K, Rosa C: Pregnancy after failed tubal sterilization, *J Reprod Med* 41:609-613, 1996.
27. Saraiya M and others: Cigarette smoking as a risk factor for ectopic pregnancy, *Am J Obstet Gynecol* 178:493-498, 1999.
28. Kendrick JS and others: Vaginal douching and the risk of ectopic pregnancy among black women, *Am J Obstet Gynecol* 176:991-997, 1997.
29. Zhang J, Thomas AG, Leybovich E: Vaginal douching and adverse health affects: a meta-analysis, *Am J Public Health* 87:1207-1211, 1997.
30. Tenore J: Ectopic pregnancy, *Am Fam Phys* 61:1080-1088, 2000.
31. Skjeldestad FE, Atrash HK: Evaluation of induced abortion as a risk factor for ectopic pregnancy: a case-control study, *Acta Obstet Gynecol Scand* 76:151-158, 1997.
32. Altrash HK and others: The relation between induced abortion and pregnancy, *Obstet Gynecol* 89:512-518, 1997.
33. Diamond MP and others: Failure of standard criteria to diagnose nonemergency ectopic pregnancies in a noninfertility patient population, *J Am Assoc Gynecol Laparosc* 1:131-134, 1994.
34. David P, Gianotti A, Garmel G: Acute urinary retention due to ectopic pregnancy, *Am J Emerg Med* 17:44-45, 1999.
35. Acosta DA: Cervical pregnancy: a forgotten entity in family practice: *J Am Board Fam Pract* 10:290-295, 1997.
36. Abramov Y and others: Doppler findings in chronic ectopic pregnancy: a case report, *Ultrasound Obstet Gynecol* 9:344-346, 1997.
37. Dart R, Kaplan B, Varalkis K: Predictive value of history and physical examination in patients with suspected ectopic pregnancy, *Ann Emerg Med* 33:283-290, 1999.
38. Dart R, Mitterando J, Dart L: Rate of change of serial beta-human chorionic gonadotropin values as a predictor of ectopic pregnancy in patients with indeterminate transvaginal ultrasound findings, *Ann Emerg Med* 34:703-710, 1999.
39. Gronlund B, Marushak A: Serial human chorionic gonadotrophin determination in the diagnosis of ectopic pregnancy, *Austral N Z J Obstet Gynaecol* 33:312-314, 1993.
40. Buckley R and others: Serum progesterone testing to predict ectopic pregnancy in symptomatic first-trimester patients, *Ann Emerg Med* 36:95-100, 2000.
41. Birkhahn R and others: Serum levels of smooth muscle heavy-chain myosin in patients with ectopic pregnancy, *Ann Emerg Med* 36: 101-107, 2000.
42. Wegner N, Mershon J: Evaluation of leukemia inhibitory factor as a marker of ectopic pregnancy, *Am J Obstet Gynecol* 184:1074-1075, 2001.
43. Durston W and others: Ultrasound availability in the evaluation of ectopic pregnancy in the ED: comparison of quality and cost-effectiveness with different approaches, *Am J Emerg Med* 18:408-417, 2000.
44. Dart RG, Kaplan B, Cox C: Transvaginal ultrasound in patients with low beta-human chorionic gonadotropin values: how often is the study diagnostic? *Ann Emerg Med* 30:135-140, 1997.
45. Popp LW, Colditz A, Gaetje R: Diagnosis of intrauterine and ectopic pregnancy at 5-7 postmenstrual weeks, *Int J Gynaecol Obstet* 44:33-38, 1994.
46. Atri M and others: Role of endovaginal sonography in the diagnosis and management of ectopic pregnancy, *Radiographics* 16:755-774, 1996.
47. Scroggins K, Smucker W, Krishen A: Spontaneous pregnancy loss, *Prim Care Clin Office Pract* 27:153-167, 2000.
48. Gaeta TJ, Raderos M, Izquierdo I: Atypical ectopic pregnancy, *Am J Emerg Med* 11:233-234, 1993.
49. Pothula V, Matseoane S, Godfrey H: Gonadotropin-producing benign cystic teratoma simulating a ruptured ectopic pregnancy, *J Natl Med Assoc* 86:221-222, 1994.
50. Riley GM, Babcock C, Jain K: Ruptured malignant ovarian tumor mimicking ruptured ectopic pregnancy, *J Ultrasound Med* 15:871-873, 1996.
51. Gazvani M, Emery S: Mifepristone and methotrexate: the combination for medical treatment of ectopic pregnancy, *Am J Obstet Gynecol* 180:1599-1600, 1999.
52. Barnhart K, Esposito M, Coutifaris C: An update on the medical treatment of ectopic pregnancy, *Obstet Gynecol Clin* 27:653-657, 2000.
53. Graczykowski JW, Mishell DR: Methotrexate prophylaxis for persistent ectopic pregnancy after conservative treatment by salpingostomy, *Obstet Gynecol* 89:118-121, 1997.
54. Kung F: Efficacy of methotrexate treatment in viable and nonviable cervical pregnancies, *Am J Obstet Gynecol* 181:1438-1444, 1999.
55. Korhonnen J, Stenman U-H, Ylostalo P: Low-dose oral methotrexate with expectant management of ectopic pregnancy, *Obstet Gynecol* 88:775-778, 1996.
56. Buster JE, Carson SA: Ectopic pregnancy: new advances in diagnosis and treatment, *Curr Opin Obstet Gynecol* 7:168-176, 1995.
57. Clasen K and others: Ectopic pregnancy: let's cut: strict laparoscopic approach to 194 consecutive cases and review of literature on alternatives, *Hum Reprod* 12:596-601, 1997.
58. Perko G, Fernandes A: Subcutaneous emphysema and pneumothorax during laparoscopy for ectopic pregnancy removal, *Acta Anaesthesiol Scand* 41:792-794, 1997.
59. Wheeler SR: Psychosocial needs of women during miscarriage or ectopic pregnancy, *AORN J* 60:221-227, 1994.
60. Job-Spira N and others: Ruptured tubal ectopic pregnancy: risk factors and reproductive outcome. Results of a population-based study in France, *Am J Obstet Gynecol* 180:938-944, 1999.
61. Robson SJ, O'Shea RT: Undiagnosed ectopic pregnancy: a retrospective analysis of 31 "missed" ectopic pregnancies at a teaching hospital, *Austral N Z J Obstet Gynaecol* 36:182-185, 1996.
62. Li L, Smialek JE: Sudden death due to rupture of ectopic pregnancy concurrent with therapeutic abortion, *Arch Pathol Lab Med* 117: 698-700, 1993.
63. Saxon D and others: A study of ruptured tubal ectopic pregnancy, *Obstet Gynecol* 90:46-49, 1997.
64. Trout S, Kemmann E: Reversible alopecia after single-dose methotrexate treatment in a patient with ectopic pregnancy, *Fertil Steril* 64: 866-867, 1995.
65. Isaacs JDJ, McGehee RP, Cowan BD: Life-threatening neutropenia following methotrexate treatment of ectopic pregnancy: a report of two cases, *Obstet Gynecol* 88:694-696, 1996.
66. Yao M, Tulandi T: Current status of surgical and nonsurgical management of ectopic pregnancy, *Fertil Steril* 67:421-433, 1997.
67. Korell M, Albrich W, Hepp H: Fertility after organ preserving surgery of ectopic pregnancy: results of a multicenter study, *Fertil Steril* 68:220-223, 1997.
68. al-Nuaim L and others: Reproductive potential after an ectopic pregnancy, *Fertil Steril* 64:942-946, 1995.
69. Kaplan BC and others: Ectopic pregnancy: prospective study with improved diagnostic accuracy, *Ann Emerg Med* 28:10-17, 1996.
70. Egger M and others: Screening for chlamydial infections and the risk of ectopic pregnancy in a county in Sweden: ecological analysis, *BMJ* 1:22-23, 1999.

CHAPTER 176

Fertility Control

Elizabeth Renee Thomas; updated by Patricia Polgar Bailey and Terry Mahan Buttaro

DEFINITION/EPIDEMIOLOGY

In the United States, 95% of sexually active women have used contraception at some time in their lives. Many of these women have tried more than one method of contraception. In 1995, 64% of women ages 15 to 44 years were using some type of contraception, an increase from 60% in 1988 and 56% in 1982. Of the 36% of women in this age-group not practicing contraception, approximately 5% were sterile because of hysterectomy or some other noncontraceptive reason; another 9% were pregnant, postpartum, or trying to become pregnant; and 11% had never had intercourse.[1] Thus of the women who might have had reason to practice some method of fertility control, 85% were doing so.

In 1995, the most commonly used contraceptive methods were female sterilization (10.7 million women) and oral contraceptive pills (10.4 million women). The next most widely used forms of fertility control were the male condom and male sterilization. Fewer than 1 million women reported using hormonal implants, intrauterine devices (IUDs), diaphragms, foam, natural family planning, or "other" methods. Fewer than half the women who reported using the diaphragm and IUD in 1982 were using it in 1995.[1]

Many of the women currently using some method of fertility control express concern over the potential side effects and health risks associated with contraceptive use.[2] Because almost half the pregnancies in this country are unintended, it is essential that primary care providers educate and counsel women and their partners on the variety of feasible options. It is imperative that the woman (and her partner if desired) be involved in the plan of care rather than be merely a recipient of the provider's expertise and advice. Discussion should include information about the risks and benefits of contraceptive options, their potential side effects, their rate of efficacy, and effects on future fertility.

HORMONAL CONTRACEPTION

Oral Contraceptives

The oral contraceptive pill (OCP) is a highly effective means of preventing pregnancy and has played an important role in contraception since its approval by the U.S. Food and Drug Administration (FDA) in 1960. The terms *birth control pill, combined oral contraceptive,* and *oral contraceptive* generally refer to pills containing both estrogen and progestin. In this chapter, these terms are not used to refer to progestin-only pills, also known as *minipills.* OCPs prevent pregnancy by suppressing ovulation. They also thicken the cervical mucus to hamper the ability of the sperm to reach the egg, accelerate ovum transport through the fallopian tube, and alter the endometrium in a way that makes it unreceptive to the implantation of a fertilized egg. Thus should ovulation take place, the risk of pregnancy remains minimal.

Only two estrogenic compounds are used currently in the United States: (1) ethynyl estradiol, which is pharmacologically active, and (2) mestranol, which must be converted by the liver into ethinyl estradiol before it is pharmacologically active.[3] The dose of estrogen used in combination OCPs has decreased dramatically since they first became available; in the United States combination OCPs currently contain 20 to 50 μg of estrogen, with those most widely prescribed containing 30 to 35 μg. The lower dose formulations have the same rate of efficacy but fewer adverse effects.[2] OCPs also contain one of several progestins, including norethindrone, levonorgestrel, norgestrel, norethindrone acetate, ethynodiol diacetate, norgestimate, and desogestrel. The latter two progestins, norgestimate and desogestrel, are less androgenic progestins; the OCP formulations that use them are referred to as third-generation contraceptives.

Several different types of OCPs are available and vary according to the dose of hormones and the formulations within each cycle pack. Monophasic OCPs have a constant dose of estrogen and progestin in each of the 21 active tables of each cycle pack. Phasic OCPs have altering doses of progestin and, in some cases, estrogen throughout the cycle. The aim of manufacturers in lowering the total monthly exogenous hormone dose while trying to simulate a woman's normal menstrual cycle is to reduce the metabolic side effects associated with OCP use.

With perfect use, OCPs are 99.5% to 99.9% effective in preventing pregnancy. However, with typical use in the United States, the rate of efficacy drops to 97%.[3] (All efficacy rates are based on a 1-year time frame.) An important reason for the decreased efficacy of OCPs is the high rate of women who discontinue taking the pill. Adherence failure is multifactorial. For some women, spotting or other side effects contribute to pill failure; for others, there is a misunderstanding about the importance of taking the pill on a regular basis.[4] After 1 year of use, usually only 50% to 70% of women are still taking OCPs.[3] Because of these high rates of discontinuation, it has been recommended that all women who are prescribed OCPs be provided with an additional method of birth control.

The regimen of OCPs should be initiated on either the first day of menses or on the first Sunday after menses begin. Women should be encouraged to take OCPs at the same time every day and to associate pill taking with a certain daily habit or ritual if that helps to facilitate compliance. Daily compliance is essential to ensuring efficacy. Women who miss one or two tablets should take two tablets for each of the missed days. Women who miss more than 2 days should continue taking the pills as prescribed but use an additional form of birth control for the remainder of the cycle. Women who often miss doses of OCPs should be encouraged to consider a form of fertility control that does not depend on daily compliance.[2]

The side effects of OCPs are a major reason for noncompliance and discontinuation. Just over half of all OCP users are satisfied with the method. Of the dissatisfied users, 94% mention side effects that include nausea, headaches, weight gain, depression, and menstrual problems.[5] Nausea and breast tenderness resulting from the estrogen component of OCPs are common side effects. OCPs cause an increase in blood pressure, which should be monitored once or twice a year in all women and more often in women with a history of hypertension. Menstrual changes, including intermenstrual (breakthrough) spotting or bleeding, occur in 25% of women during the first 3 months of OCP use and decrease significantly during subsequent use. Women with persistent intermenstrual bleeding after 3 months of OCP use should be evaluated for possible causes of bleeding unrelated to OCP use, including infection or neoplasia.[2] Amenorrhea may also occur, especially in women who have been using OCPs for a prolonged period. A decreased libido—a decreased interest in sex or a decreased ability to have an orgasm—is another possible side effect of OCPs. Other possible side effects include fluid retention, leukorrhea, and pruritus. Headaches are an additional side effect reported by OCP users. Tension headaches are not considered to be related to OCP use and should be evaluated and managed accordingly. Migraine headaches are known to both improve and worsen while taking OCPs. Women who experience "classic migraines" and women who experience increased frequency or intensity of migraines while taking OCPs should be advised to use some other form of fertility control.

Substantial contraceptive and noncontraceptive benefits are associated with OCPs. Menstrual improvements associated with OCPs include more regular and predictable menses, a 25% reduction in anemia resulting from menorrhagia, less dysmenorrhea, fewer days for menses, a reduced flow, and the restoration of regular menses in anovulatory women. There is a 50% decrease in functional ovarian cysts among OCP users, with a 75% reduction in functional cyst-related hospital admissions. Additional gynecologic benefits include a decrease in the incidence of gynecologic cancers, including epithelial ovarian cancer (50% reduction) and endometrial adenocarcinoma (50% reduction), and the prevention and treatment of endometriosis (30% reduction). Certain conditions occur less often in women taking OCPs; there is a 50% combined reduction in breast fibroadenoma and fibrocystic changes, a 50% reduction in pelvic inflammatory disease (with the exception of infections caused by *Chlamydia trachomatis)*, and a 90% reduction in ectopic pregnancies. Additional benefits may include maintenance of or increased bone mineral density, a decreased risk of atherosclerosis and severe rheumatoid arthritis, acne improvement, and enhanced sexual enjoyment.[2,3,6]

There are significant health risks with and disadvantages to the use of OCPs, including a lack of protection against HIV infection—a greater threat to the health of many sexually active individuals than an unplanned pregnancy. To protect against HIV infection, barrier methods (e.g., condoms) must be used in conjunction with OCPs. Other possible untoward side effects resulting from the estrogen component in pills includes increased breast size (ductal and fatty tissue), stimulation of breast neoplasia, cervical erosion or ectopia, thromboembolic complications, pulmonary emboli, cerebrovascular accidents, hepatocellular adenomas and cancer, the growth of leiomyomata, telangiectasia, and a rise in the cholesterol concentration in gallbladder bile.[3]

The risk of cardiovascular disease (CVD) associated with OCP use has been a concern since the first cases were reported among pill users. Several large World Health Organization studies have demonstrated that the added risk of an adverse cardiovascular outcome is very small among low-dose pill users who were at low risk for CVD before taking the pill. Data from these studies suggest that, in women using OCPs containing the second-generation progestins levonorgestrel and norethisterone, there is an excess risk of 4 to 10 cases of venous thromboembolism per 100,000 women; this results in one to two extra deaths per million women per year. The risk seems to double if pills containing the third-generation progestins desogestrel and gestodene are used. Despite the scare in 1995 regarding these newer progestins, the risk attributable to them is still relatively small given the excess mortality of only 1 to 2 per million per year. This increased risk of thromboembolism is still less than the risk associated with high-dose estrogen OCPs. There is also tentative evidence that these less androgenic progestins do not carry the increased risk of myocardial infarction (MI) seen with levonorgestrel, a second-generation progestin.[6-8]

Studies on stroke and OCPs have demonstrated no increase in risk or an increased risk of only 0.5 per 100,000 woman-years for low-dose pill users less than 35 years of age who have no cardiovascular risk factors. In addition, the type of progestin does not seem to influence the risk. Thus in the absence of risk factors, low-dose pills may carry no excess risk of stroke. For women using high-dose pills, the excess risk for cerebrovascular accidents is 8 per 100,000; in low-dose pill users older than 35 years, the risk is 2 per 100,000. Evidence suggests that the use of OCPs raises the risk of acute MI by less than 1 per 100,000 woman years, which translates into fewer than three additional cases per year. The risk may be greater in older women who smoke. Appropriate screening, particularly of blood pressure, before initiating and during OCP use will likely reduce this risk.[7]

The potential impact of OCP use on breast cancer is a concern for a great number of women interested in this form of fertility control. Epidemiologic data suggest that current OCP users have an increased relative risk of breast cancer of 1.24; this risk seems confined largely to tumors localized to the breast. Women who begin taking OCPs before age 20 years have a somewhat higher risk than those who start later. For women who use the pill when older, for example up to the age of 40 years, the estimated cumulative incidence is 199 per 10,000 women at age 50 years (an excess of 19 cases per 10,000) and 394 per 10,000 women at age 60 (an excess of 14 cases per 10,000). The patterns of breast cancer risk seem similar for both progestin-only and combined OCPs, with no difference between oral and injectable preparations.[7]

Both the estrogen and progestin components of OCPs may potentially increase breast tenderness, headaches, hypertension, and the risk for MI. The androgenic effects of the progestin in OCPs may be associated with increased appetite and weight gain, depression, fatigue and tiredness, decreased libido and sexual pleasure, acne and oily skin, increased breast size (alveolar tissue), an increase in low-density lipoprotein cholesterol, a decrease in high-density lipoprotein (HDL) cholesterol, glucose intolerance, and decreased carbohydrate tolerance.[3]

OCPs should not be prescribed for women with the following conditions: a history of thrombophlebitis or thromboembolic disorder, cerebrovascular accident, coronary artery or ischemic heart disease, breast cancer or suspected breast cancer, suspected estrogen-dependent neoplasia, pregnancy or suspected pregnancy, concomitant hepatic adenoma or liver cancer, and markedly impaired liver function. Caution should be used in prescribing OCPs to women older than 35 years old who smoke more than 15 cigarettes per day, women who develop migraines after the initiation of OCPs, or women with blood pressure greater than 140/90 mm Hg, diabetes mellitus, obesity with a body mass index >30 kg/m^2, immobilization pending within the next 4 weeks, undiagnosed vaginal or uterine bleeding, sickle cell disease or sickle cell–hemoglobin C disease, lactation, gestational diabetes, active gallbladder disease, congenital hyperbilirubinemia, a history of cardiac or renal disease, or a family history of hyperlipidemia or death of a parent or sibling from MI before age 50 years. In addition, caution should be used when considering OCPs for women before the third postpartum week or for those older than age 50 years.[3,7]

The warning signs to teach OCP users can be summarized with the acronym *ACHES*, which refers to *A*bdominal pain (severe); *C*hest pain (severe), cough, or shortness of breath; *H*eadaches (severe), dizziness, weakness, or numbness; *E*ye problems (vision loss or blurring) or speech problems; and *S*evere leg pain (calf or thigh). Women who experience any of these signs or symptoms or who develop depression, jaundice, or a breast lump should discontinue taking the pill and consult their provider. OCP users who smoke should be encouraged to quit smoking; if quitting is not possible, they should consider discontinuing the use of OCPs after age 35 years and definitely by age 40 years.[3]

Progestin-Only Pills (Minipills). Progestin-only pills were introduced approximately 10 years after OCPs appeared on the market. A number of preparations that use a variety of different progestins are now available. Progestin-only pills prevent pregnancy by inhibiting ovulation, thickening and decreasing the amount of cervical mucus (which inhibits sperm penetration), contributing to the development of a thin and atrophic endometrium, and promoting premature luteolysis. Progestin-only pills are taken on a daily basis, with no pill-free days. Progestin-only pills are most effective if ovulation is inhibited and are generally considered less effective than OCPs. Failure rates vary from 1.1% to 13.2% during the first year of use. Minipills do not adversely affect lactation; they also represent an effective form of contraception for lactating women, because in these women the efficacy rate is close to 100%. Progestin-only pills are also useful for women who wish to use an OCP but have contraindications to combined pills. Disadvantages include the potential for progestogenic side effects, including menstrual cycle disturbances, weight gain, breast tenderness, an increase in functional ovarian cysts, ectopic pregnancy, interactions with anticonvulsants, and bone density decrease.[3]

Spironolactone Analogues. Drospirenone (3 mg), a new progesterone, has been combined with ethinyl estradiol (30 μg) as the components of a new monophasic oral contraceptive (Yasmin). Hyperkalemia is a potential adverse effect related to the potassium-sparing effects of drospirenone. Pregnancy should be excluded before this oral contraceptive is started.

Injectable Contraception

One injectable form of contraception available in the United States is medroxyprogesterone acetate (MPA) (Depo-Provera). MPA prevents pregnancy by inhibiting ovulation and is used by more than 14 million women worldwide.[6] A 150-mg injection of MPA suppresses ovulation for 14 weeks. With a prescribed dose given every 3 months, contraceptive efficacy is 99.7%. The recommended time to initiate MPA is within 5 days of the onset of menses, partly to ensure that the woman is not pregnant but also because administration at this time prevents ovulation during the first month of use. MPA injections should be administered every 12 weeks, which provides a 2-week "grace" period given the 14-week duration of action. The possibility of pregnancy should be first excluded for any woman who is more than 2 weeks late for her MPA injection.[2]

Medroxyprogesterone acetate/estradiol cypionate suspension (Lunelle [MPA/E_2C]) is the first monthly injectable contraceptive to be prescribed in the United States. Administered into the deltoid, gluteus maximus, or anterior thigh, a 0.5 ml IM injection is given within 5 days of the onset of the menstrual period and every 28 to 30 days thereafter. Amenorrhea, common in MPA, is not associated with MPA/E_2C. There seems to be a high level of satisfaction with MPA/E_2C, and studies have shown it to be highly effective (in a 12-month study no pregnancies occurred).[4] Unfortunately, manufacturing problems have affected the availability of Lunelle. It is expected, however, that it will be available in the future.

Menstrual changes occur in almost all women who use MPA and are the most the most common cause for dissatisfaction and discontinued use of this form of fertility control. Irregular bleeding usually resolves within the first month of use. Amenorrhea is the most common menstrual change with persistent use of MPA. Women for whom menstrual irregularities are disconcerting should be counseled regarding alternative contraceptive choices. Other side effects of MPA include headache, abdominal or breast bloating, fatigue, depression, decreased libido, and a 1- to 3-lb weight gain.[2] MPA is a reversible form of contraception, but a return to fertility is often delayed after discontinuation of MPA. Within 10 months of the last injection, 50% of women who discontinue MPA to become pregnant are able to conceive, but in others fertility may not be restored for as long as 18 months.[2]

MPA is associated with certain noncontraceptive benefits, such as a reduction in or elimination of premenstrual symptoms, a reduced risk of pelvic inflammatory disease (PID), a decreased risk of endometrial cancer, hematologic improvement in women with sickle cell disease, and reduced seizures in women with seizure disorders. MPA-induced amenorrhea may make MPA a good contraceptive choice for women with menorrhagia, dysmenorrhea, and iron deficiency anemia, as well as for women with mental deficits who have menstrual hygiene problems.

Both MPA and MPA/E_2C are associated with certain health risks. As is the case with OCPs, MPA and MPA/E_2C provide no protection from many sexually transmitted diseases (STDs), including HIV. Presently no data suggest that either of these products is associated with an increased risk of breast, endometrial, ovarian, and cervical carcinoma. HDL cholesterol levels tend to fall in women using MPA.[3] Decreased bone density has been noted among some MPA users, but this was reversed with discontinuation of MPA.[6]

Women should be counseled to use an additional form of contraception for the first 2 weeks after the first MPA or MPA/E_2C injection. Women who are at risk for STDs should use a barrier method of contraception, preferably condoms. Women who become concerned about their menstrual irregularities on

MPA or who develop signs or symptoms of infection should consult their primary care provider. Women need to be informed about the likely delay in fertility after discontinuation of MPA. MPA is not the best choice for women who wish to become pregnant within the next 1 to 2 years; these women should be counseled regarding alternative contraceptive options. MPA/E_2C has not seemed to delay fertility.

Contraceptive Implants

The contraceptive implant levonorgestrel (Norplant), which consists of six 34 × 2.4 progestin-coated Silastic implants filled with 36 mg of crystalline levonorgestrel is no longer being manufactured.[9] In late 2000, the manufacturer announced that any implant distributed after October 1999 may not be effective and suggested that women with Norplant implants use backup contraception or have the implants removed.[9]

The progestin released from contraceptive implants resulted in circulating levels sufficient to prevent pregnancy. The released progestin also thickened and decreased the amount of cervical mucus, inhibiting the penetration of sperm, making the endometrium thin and inactive. The efficacy rate of levonorgestrel implants was approximately 99.2% to 99.7% per 100 women per 5 years of use. Pregnancy rates gradually increased over time, with annual pregnancy rates of 2% during the sixth year of use. For this reason, Norplant was recommended for only 5 years of use. Menstrual changes were the most common side effect associated with contraceptive implants and tended to be the most problematic during the first year of use. In contrast to MPA, amenorrhea occurred in a minority (5% to 10%) of implant users. Headache was another common side effect and one of the most common reasons for implant removal.

For women who still have a contraceptive implant, the risk of pregnancy should be reiterated and a pregnancy test obtained if amenorrhea develops. Fertility return is rapid once Norplant has been removed as progestin levels fall to undetectable levels within 1 week. The insertion and removal of implants are minor office procedures performed by a practitioner specifically trained in the procedure.

BARRIER METHODS

Barrier methods of fertility control are so named because they act as mechanical barriers and prevent pregnancy by blocking the passage of sperm through their surfaces. In addition, they prevent or reduce contact with genital lesions, discharges, or secretions.

Condoms

Most condoms made in the United States are manufactured from latex; approximately 5% are made from animal skin (usually lamb intestine). Although both types of condoms interfere with the passage of sperm, only latex condoms protect against STDs, HIV, and viral infections (hepatitis B and herpes simplex). Failure rates with condoms are as low as 3% with perfect use and as high as 12% with typical use (based on 1 year of use).[2,3] A polyurethane female condom (Reality) is now available and has the benefit of affording women direct control of contraception and disease prevention. However, failure rates for the female condom are significantly higher (5% with perfect use, 21% with typical use) than for male condoms. Among women using some form of fertility control during the last decade, male condom use has increased from 15% in 1988 to 20% in 1995. Condoms are the only immediately reversible method of contraception for men. Patient education regarding condom use should include information about how to put on and remove a condom, the need to leave a receptacle at the tip of the condom to avoid breakage, what to do in case of condom slippage or damage, and the importance of avoiding oil-based products (e.g., petroleum jelly, cold cream) when extra lubrication is needed.

Diaphragms and Cervical Caps

Diaphragms and cervical caps are female barrier methods of contraception. Both must be individually fitted to be effective; even with correct use, failure rates are as high as 5% to 9% for nulliparous users and 5% to 26% for parous users during the first year of use. Diaphragm use has steadily decreased during the last 15 years. In 1982, 8.1% of contraceptive users ages 15 to 44 years used a diaphragm; this number dropped to 2.0% in 1988 and 0.8% in 1995.[4] Both the diaphragm and the cervical cap are used with spermicidal cream or jelly. The diaphragm is a dome-shaped rubber cap that comes in a variety of sizes. It fits into the vagina, covering the cervix and the anterior vagina from the pubic symphysis to the posterior fornix. The diaphragm should remain in place for at least 6 hours after intercourse, but no more than 24 hours (to minimize the risk of toxic shock syndrome). Once in position, the diaphragm provides effective contraception for 6 hours, after which fresh spermicide must be applied if additional contraceptive protection is desired. A weight gain of more than 25% requires a refitting. The cervical cap is a deep, soft rubber cup that covers the surface and fits snugly around the base of the cervix. The cap provides continuous contraceptive protection over 24 hours regardless of how often intercourse occurs. Additional spermicide or jelly is not needed for repeated intercourse.

Advantages of the female barrier methods include a lack of dependence on partners for contraception and none of the side effects of systemic hormones. With the exception of the female condom, all female vaginal barrier methods are used in conjunction with spermicides. Some protection against HIV is afforded if the spermicide contains nonoxynol-9. On the other hand, research has demonstrated that vaginal irritation caused by nonoxynol 9 may *increase* HIV susceptibility. Reduction in the risk of other STDs, including gonorrhea and chlamydia, varies from 10% to 50% depending on the study. Risks associated with the use of diaphragms and cervical caps include latex allergy, toxic shock syndrome, and recurrent urinary tract infections.[2,3]

Spermicides

A variety of over-the-counter spermicidal products are available in the United States and include foams, creams, gels, suppositories, and films. The active ingredient in all spermicides available in the United States is nonoxynol-9 or a similar agent that destroys the membrane of the sperm cell. Spermicides can be used alone but, as noted earlier in this chapter, are also essential for the effective functioning of diaphragms and cervical caps. Effectiveness varies with the type of usage and compliance; failure rates vary from 20% with typical use to 10% with educated, motivated couples.[2]

One major advantage of spermicides is that they are available over the counter. Many women also appreciate that there is no partner involvement with this method. Spermicides provide some protection against gonorrhea and chlamydia. Side effects include allergic reactions to the active ingredient or to the particular spermicide base or vehicle, which generally manifests itself as vulvar pruritus or a rash. Women who are prone to yeast infections may notice an increased frequency of this problem when spermicides are used. Although women do not need to consult a health care provider to use spermicides, it is nonetheless important for this option to be discussed in any family planning session.

Intrauterine Devices

Intrauterine contraceptive devices currently available in the United States include (1) the Copper T380A, a T-shaped, polyethylene device with a stem and cross arms partly covered by copper wire and tubing; (2) the progesterone-releasing IUD (Progestasert), a plastic, T-shaped device that releases 65 μg of progesterone per day for at least 1 year; and (3) the levonorgestrel-containing IUD (Mirena), a recently approved slow-releasing pump device.[2,4] Copper IUDs prevent fertilization primarily by creating a spermicidal environment. The IUD causes the endometrium to initiate a foreign body reaction, which results in sterile inflammation and inhibits sperm from reaching the fallopian tube. As the inflammatory response is heightened, local prostaglandin response is increased, and endometrial enzyme production is inhibited. Progesterone-releasing IUDs thicken the cervical mucus, reduce sperm penetration, and inhibit sperm survival and implantation. The Copper T380A, with a failure rate of only 0.5% to 0.8% during the first year of use, is more effective in preventing pregnancy than Progestasert, which has a failure rate of approximately 3% during the first year of use. IUD use has declined from 7.1% in 1982 to 0.8% in 1995.[1]

The IUDs currently in use are associated with far fewer complications than the early copper-containing IUDs (including the Dalkon Shield) of the 1980s. Possible disadvantages to and complications of IUD use include an increased risk of PID, with the greatest risk occurring at the time of insertion. Some experts believe that this insertion-related infection may be prevented by administering 200 mg doxycycline to the woman 1 hour before insertion. Women who develop asymptomatic gonorrhea or chlamydia infections may be treated with the IUD in place. Removal of the IUD is recommended if the infection does not respond to therapy or if actual PID develops as a result of the infection. It is unclear whether IUDs increase the rate of transmission of HIV. IUDs may increase uterine lining bleeding, making transmission of the virus easier, but this has not been demonstrated by research. Other potential side effects include increased dysmenorrhea, bleeding, or spotting; 10% of IUDs are removed for these reasons.

Of the pregnancies that do occur with IUDs in place, 50% result in spontaneous abortion. In contrast to the older-generation IUDs, the Copper T380A decreases rather than increases the overall risk of ectopic pregnancy by 90% as compared with the risk for noncontraceptive users. On the other hand, the progesterone-releasing IUD has an ectopic pregnancy rate that is 50% to 80% *higher* than that for women not using contraception. Reduction of ectopic pregnancies is greatest with contraceptive methods that inhibit ovulation. When an IUD user does become pregnant, there is an increased ratio of ectopic to intrauterine gestations.[2]

IUDs should not be prescribed for women with a history of ectopic pregnancy, nulliparous women, or women with active, recent, or recurrent pelvic infections, including postpartum endometriosis or infection after an abortion or known or suspected pregnancy. Caution should be exercised if an IUD is being considered for a woman with risk factors for PID or STDs; undiagnosed irregular, heavy, or abnormal vaginal bleeding; a cervical or uterine malignancy; or an unresolved Papanicolaou's (Pap) test. Additional precautions include a history of previous problems with IUDs (e.g., pregnancies, expulsion, perforation, pain, or heavy bleeding), a past history of vasovagal reactivity or fainting, valvular heart disease (e.g., aortic stenosis), uterine anatomic abnormalities, and a history of anemia.

For most nulliparous women there are better contraceptive options than an IUD; nulliparous women tend to tolerate IUDs less well than women who have carried at least one pregnancy to term. There may also be a slightly increased risk of infertility in women with a history of IUD use.[3] Patient education should include information about checking for the IUD string as well as the signs and symptoms of possible complications, including pain, bleeding, odorous discharge, fever, or missed menses.[2]

Vaginal Ring

Etonogestrel/ethinyl vaginal ring (Nuva Ring) is a vaginal contraceptive ring that delivers 15 μg ethinyl estradiol and 120 μg of etonogestrel each day. Inserted into the vagina by the patient, the ring is removed after 3 weeks for 1 ring-free week. Menses commences in 2 to 3 days. To prevent pregnancy, a new ring must be inserted after the ring-free week (7 days). In a study of 1145 women monitored through 12,109 cycles, six pregnancies occurred.[9] The vaginal ring provides contraception using lower hormonal doses than other contraceptive methods, is readily reversible, and is easy for patients to use. Headache, nausea, and vaginal discomfort have been reported in 15% of patients.[9]

CONTRACEPTIVE PATCH

Norelgestromin/ethinyl estradiol transdermal system (Ortho Evra) is the first contraceptive patch available in the United States. The patch delivers 20 μg of ethinyl estradiol and 150 μg of norelgestromin daily and is 99% effective. Each cycle consists of a contraceptive patch applied to the abdomen, buttock, upper outer arm, or torso once a week for 3 weeks. After the third week the patch is removed for a contraceptive-free week during which menstrual bleeding occurs.

The contraceptive patch may be less effective in women weighing more than 198 pounds, but reported advantages include ease of use, improved adherence, reversibility, and steady-state hormonal levels. Side effects include breast discomfort, headache, nausea, dysmenorrhea, and skin irritation at the patch site.

POSTCOITAL CONTRACEPTION

Postcoital contraception, also referred to as emergency contraception or the "morning-after pill," is intended for women who have experienced a single episode of unprotected intercourse within a given menstrual cycle. Postcoital contraception can also be used in cases of sexual assault.[2,6,7] Several contraceptive regimens have been used for this purpose (Table 176-1). Preven and Plan B, emergency contraceptive kits, are also available. All of these methods prevent implantation, but to be effective, they must be taken within the first 72 hours after unprotected intercourse. The side effects of all emergency contraceptive regimens include nausea and vomiting, breast tenderness, dizziness, menorrhagia, and abdominal pain. The combination method (ethynyl estradiol and norgestrel [Ovral]) uses a relatively lower steroid dose than others, thus mitigating the side effects but retaining a demonstrated efficacy rate of 98%. Women should be educated about the availability of postcoital contraception to prevent unplanned or unwanted pregnancies in the event that an "emergency" occurs.

SURGICAL STERILIZATION

Methods of surgical sterilization include tubal sterilization and vasectomy. Sterilization is the most commonly reported method of fertility control; in the United States in 1995, it was the method used by 38.6% contraceptive users ages 15 to 44 years.[1] Advantages of both male and female sterilization include its permanence, high rate of efficacy (0.4% failure rate for women and 0.15% for men), cost-effectiveness, lack of significant long-term side effects, and lack of need for partner compliance. Permanence is also a disadvantage of sterilization because reversibility is difficult and expensive. In addition, sterilization provides no protection against STDs, including HIV.[3]

NATURAL FAMILY PLANNING

Natural family planning (NFP) includes any method of family planning that is based on observations of the signs of fertility rather than on interference with physiologic function. It is important for primary care providers to suggest NFP to their patients, because it may be an attractive option for many women who might otherwise be unaware of its benefits. The two major forms of NFP practiced in the United States are the ovulation method and the symptothermal method.

The Ovulation Method

The ovulation method is based on a single fertility sign: the changes in the mucus secreted by a woman's cervix. Hormonal changes cause the cervical mucus to vary in appearance and consistency throughout the menstrual cycle, forming a recognizable pattern that corresponds to her fertility. During menstruation, estrogen and progesterone levels are at their lowest. This low hormonal level allows the pituitary gland to release follicle-stimulating hormone, thus initiating the growth of several ova. The follicles release estrogen as they develop. Estrogen causes the endometrium to thicken in anticipation of the possibility of pregnancy, and it also influences the characteristics of the cervical mucus. When the level of estrogen is low, a woman will experience vulvar dryness; an opaque, sticky mucus appears as estrogen increases. Fertile mucus forms channels within itself to allow for the passage of sperm. By contrast, the opaque sticky mucus seen before and after ovulation has a closely woven microstructure that hinders the passage of sperm and forms a plug in the cervical os. In absence of fertile cervical mucus, sperm can live in the vaginal tract for only 30 minutes to 24 hours. In the presence of cervical mucus, sperm remain viable for up to 5 or 6 days.[10]

With the ovulation method, the average cycle is divided into four phases: (1) menstruation, (2) the postmenstrual infertile days, (3) the fertile period, and (4) the 2-week infertile period of postovulation. Any day of bleeding is considered a fertile period because bleeding may mask the presence of mucus, but most women do not secrete cervical mucus until several days after menstruation has ended. As long as cervical mucus is not present, intercourse can occur every other evening in the postmenstrual period. Intercourse is confined to the evening because the absence of cervical mucus must be ensured if pregnancy is to be avoided. The absence of mucus in the morning might be a postural rather than a true absence. Intercourse is further restricted to every other evening because semen can take 24 hours to leave the vaginal area and can mask the presence of mucus. Cervical mucus can be checked and examined by wiping a toilet tissue across the vaginal opening either before or after urination. Cervical mucus, if present, remains on top of the tissue without being absorbed; its character should be examined for elasticity and translucence. At the first sign of mucus the couple should abstain from sexual intercourse and genital-to-genital contact of any type. The period of abstinence extends until the evening of the fourth day after the appearance of clear, stretchy, lubricating mucus (peak mucus), at which time intercourse is not restricted again until menstruation. Ovulation typically occurs within 1 day before, during, or after the appearance of peak mucus.[3]

The Symptothermal Method

The second method of family planning, the symptothermal method (STM), is similar to the ovulation method but uses two other fertility signs besides cervical mucus: basal body temperature and the position, shape, and consistency of the cervix.

TABLE 176-1 Postcoital Contraceptive Regimens

Drug	Trade Name	Dosage
Ethinyl estradiol	*	2.5 mg PO b.i.d. for 5 days
Norgestrel and ethinyl estradiol	Ovral	2 doses PO 12 hours apart
	Lo/Ovral, Nordette, Levlen, Triphasil Tri-Levlen (yellow pills only)	4 doses PO 12 hours apart
Ethinyl estradiol plus levonorgestrel†	Preven	2 tablets within 72 hours of unprotected intercourse; 2 or more tablets 12 hours later

*Not available in the United States as a single preparation.
†Considered to be 75% effective.

STM is the most widely used method of NFP in the United States. Advocates of this method place particular emphasis on the cooperation of man and woman in fertility regulation.

With STM, the menstrual cycle is separated into three phases. The relatively infertile phase lasts from the beginning of menstruation to the onset of any mucus. The fertile phase lasts from the first sign of mucus until the beginning of the third phase. The third phase, known as the postovulatory infertility phase (also known as the absolute infertility phase), begins on the fourth day of a temperature elevation and the fifth day of the drying of the cervical mucus.[10] A basal thermometer (useful for measuring subtle variations in body temperature between 35.5° and 37.7° C [96° and 100° F]) is used to record morning body temperatures. Typically, a biphasic curve is observed over the course of the menstrual cycle, with low temperatures recorded before ovulation and slightly higher temperatures recorded after ovulation. A typical postovulatory elevation ranges between 0.4° F and 1.0° F above the average of the last 6 ovulatory days.[11] The temperature rise is caused by the presence of progesterone, which is released by the empty follicle after ovulation. At least 3 days of elevated temperatures must be recorded before the postovulatory infertile phase begins on the evening of that third day. Basal body temperature does not give any advance warning of ovulation but indicates when ovulation has passed.

Palpation of the cervix is performed as an adjunct to the other signs of fertility. During the infertile period the cervix is firm and low in the vagina, and the cervical os is closed. As ovulation approaches, the cervix softens and elevates until it is almost out of reach, and the cervical os opens. Some women find this to be a helpful sign; others do not. In some cycles these signs provide information as to when the woman is capable of conceiving. Couples who wish to avoid pregnancy should wait to have intercourse until all signs indicate that the fertile time has passed.

Conscientious application of the principles of NFP is an effective method of family planning, with failure rates of 3% for the ovulation method, 2% for the symptothermal method, and 1% when intercourse is confined to the postovulation period.[3] Undoubtedly, abstinence is a major stumbling block for many couples when first considering NFP. Nevertheless, couples who choose NFP grow to appreciate abstinence as a significant avenue for personal growth in their relationship by fostering emotional intimacy and encouraging balance within the sexual relationship.

REFERENCES

1. Piccinino LJ, Moser WD: Trends in contraceptive use in the United States: 1982-1995, *Fam Plan Perspect* 30(1):4-10, 1998.
2. Kaunitz AM and others: Contraception: a clinical review for the internist, *Med Clin North Am* 7(6):1377-1409, 1995.
3. Hatcher RA and others, editors: *Contraceptive technology*, ed 16, New York, 1994, Irvington Publishers.
4. Moore A: Adherence issues with contraceptive regimens: old problems, added options, *Women's Health Care* 1(4):9-14, 2002.
5. Rosenfeld A and others: Women's satisfaction with birth control, *J Fam Pract* 36(2):169-173, 1993.
6. Kubba AA: Contraception: a review, *Int J Clin Pract* 52(2):102-105, 1998.
7. Mazza D: Recent advances in contraception, *Aust Fam Physician* 27(5):347-352, 1998.
8. Chasan-Taber L, Stampfer MJ: Epidemiology of oral contraceptives and cardiovascular disease, *Ann Intern Med* 128(6):467-477, 1998.
9. Martin KA, Barbieri RL: Overview of contraception. Retrieved September 19, 2002 from the World Wide Web: www.uptodate.com.
10. Hamilton K: The symptothermal method of natural family planning, *Physician Assist* 8(11), 1984.
11. Geerling JH: Natural family planning, *Am Fam Physician* 52(6): 1749-1760, 1995.

CHAPTER 177

Genital Tract Cancers

Denise T. Bynum

DEFINITION/EPIDEMIOLOGY

Gynecologic malignancies include vulvar, vaginal, cervical, endometrial, ovarian, and fallopian tube cancers; endometrial, ovarian, and cervical cancers are the most commonly diagnosed. Cervical and endometrial cancers have a high cure rate because of several factors, including (1) premalignant changes that lead to early diagnosis (especially with cervical cancer) and (2) metastatic spread that is local and regional in the early stages (in cervical and endometrial cancer). In addition, these cancers are sensitive to radiation (cervical and endometrial cancer) and chemotherapy (choriocarcinoma and, sometimes, ovarian cancer). The terminology for cervical dysplasia and carcinoma in situ has changed to *cervical intraepithelial neoplasia* (CIN). Similarly, the terminology for preinvasive vulvar and vaginal lesions has changed to *vulvar intraepithelial neoplasia* (VIN) and *vaginal intraepithelial neoplasia* (VAIN), respectively.[1]

All suspicious lesions in the genital tract require referral to a gynecologist for biopsy. Surgical management is usually the initial treatment and is often curative, particularly in the early stages.[1] If cancer is confirmed, a gynecologic oncologist should be consulted. The gynecologic oncologist has extensive surgical experience and expertise in radiation and medical oncology.

Vulvar Cancer

DEFINITION/EPIDEMIOLOGY

The National Cancer Institute (NCI) estimates 3600 new cases with 800 deaths attributed to vulvar cancer occurred in 2001.[2] Vulvar cancer accounts for 4% of all female genital tract cancers and 0.6% of all cancers in women.[3] Lymph node status is the most significant prognostic factor. The 5-year survival rate is 90% for women without nodal involvement and decreases to 30% to 55% for women with positive nodes.[3]

PATHOPHYSIOLOGY

Risk factors for vulvar cancers include cigarette smoking, human papillomavirus (HPV) infection, HIV infection or other conditions that cause immunosuppression, low socioeconomic status, VIN, chronic vulvar inflammation, other genital tract cancers, genital herpes infections, lichen sclerosis, chronic granulomatous disease, and syphilis. Patients with a family history of melanoma or atypical moles have an increased risk of melanoma. There are several types of vulvar cancers. Squamous cell carcinomas account for the majority of invasive cancers. Verrucous carcinoma is a subtype of invasive squamous cell that causes cauliflower-like growths similar to genital warts.[3] Paget's disease is a lesion of unknown cause that arises from the apocrine-bearing part of the vulvar skin. Paget's disease presents with pruritus, soreness, erythematous skin, and hyperkeratotic plaques and may be confused with candidiasis. Bartholin's gland carcinoma is a carcinoma of the mucin-secreting glands on either side of the lower vagina. The tumor may present as a unilateral deep mass and is often diagnosed as a cyst or an abscess. Bartholin's gland carcinoma accounts for 2% of vulvar malignancies and occurs in a younger age-group than vulvar squamous carcinoma.[1] Adenocarcinoma cells are found within the epidermis and skin appendages.

CLINICAL PRESENTATION

Most patients have a history of vulvar irritation, burning and/or pain, pruritus, local discomfort, excoriation, fissuring, painful irritation, bleeding and discharge, and/or a painful vulvar lump. The lesion may be white, raised, hyperkeratotic, or pigmented. Invasive cancers may present with a foul discharge. Many tumors are detected late and may present with rectal bleeding, urethral obstruction, and/or large involved inguinal lymph nodes.

PHYSICAL EXAMINATION

Early diagnosis in vulvar cancer is important. The initial lesion may appear as a small raised area or as an ulceration that will not heal, or it may be associated with a secondary infection. The cancer spreads along the labia. Regional lymph nodes require examination because the cancer will metastasize freely as a result of the many lymph channels in that area. The presence of palpable lymph nodes usually represents malignant spread.

DIAGNOSTICS AND DIFFERENTIAL DIAGNOSIS

Vulvar carcinoma can be mistaken for other conditions, including eczema or dermatitis, ulcerative lesions such as syphilis, or granuloma inguinale. The definitive diagnosis requires a biopsy. Metastatic disease may increase serum calcium levels. Crohn's disease can present as an ulcerative area on the vulva, and a lesion, on rare occasion, could be a metastasis from a distant site.

MANAGEMENT AND INDICATIONS FOR REFERRAL/HOSPITALIZATION

All patients with a suspicious lesion of the vulva require referral for biopsy. Treatment is primarily wide surgical excision, vulvectomy, or pelvic exenteration. Treatments for preinvasive lesions include local chemotherapy or laser therapy. Cystoscopy and sigmoidoscopy are often indicated to exclude invasive disease. During the past 20 years, treatment has changed from radical vulvectomy with inguinal and deep pelvic lymphadenectomy to a much less extensive vulvectomy and selective groin resection. Pelvic lymphadenectomy is rarely done.[4]

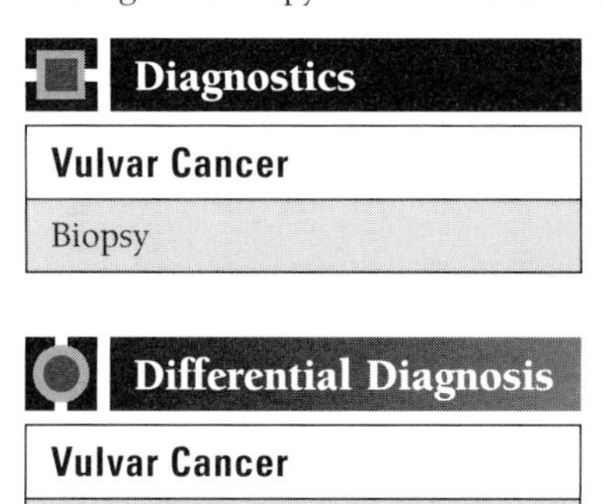

Diagnostics

Vulvar Cancer
Biopsy

Differential Diagnosis

Vulvar Cancer
Carcinoma Dermatitis Syphilis Granuloma inguinale Eczema Crohn's disease

LIFE SPAN CONSIDERATIONS

Invasive vulvar cancer occurs most often between the ages of 65 and

70, with noninvasive vulvar cancer occurring most often in women aged 20 years or younger. Seventy-five percent of vulvar cancers occur in women older than 50.[2] The preinvasive lesions can occur at any age but are more common in younger patients and are associated with HPV infection.

COMPLICATIONS

Complications after genital tract cancer depend on the stage of the cancer and method of treatment. Usual complications include those associated with radiation, chemotherapy, or surgery. Metastasis can occur if the cancer is invasive. (For further information, see Chapter 258.)

PATIENT AND FAMILY EDUCATION

All patients should understand the necessity of screening to ensure early detection of vulvar and vaginal cancer. Screening methods include an annual pelvic examination and Papanicolaou (Pap) test, monthly genital self-examination, and prompt reporting of unusual symptoms.[5] The American Cancer Society recommends that all sexually active or women who have reached 18 years of age have an annual Pap smear and pelvic examination. After 3 normal examinations in a row, women aged 18 to 40 years can have an annual Pap/pelvic examination every 1 to 3 years at the judgment of their health care provider. After 40 years of age, annual examinations are recommended.[3]

Vaginal Cancer

DEFINITION/EPIDEMIOLOGY

Vaginal cancer is an uncommon genital tract tumor that accounts for 3% of genital tract cancers.[3] More than 1 million women have been exposed to diethylstilbestrol (DES), which was commonly used between 1940 and 1971 for the prevention of spontaneous abortions.[3] The incidence of vaginal cancer in exposed daughters is estimated at 1:1000.[3] The prognosis for vaginal cancer depends on the stage and involvement of lymph nodes. The 5-year survival rate is 96% for stage 0, 73% for stage I disease, 58% for stage II disease, 36% for stage III/IV disease, and 14% for melanoma.[3]

PATHOPHYSIOLOGY

Squamous cell carcinomas account for 85% of tumors, with the remaining 15% consisting of adenocarcinomas, sarcomas, leiomyosarcomas, and melanomas.[1] Squamous cell carcinomas arise from surface epithelial cells, adenocarcinomas arise from glandular cells, sarcomas arise from connective tissue, and melanomas arise from melanocytes. Non–clear cell adenocarcinoma is very rare, occurs predominantly in postmenopausal women, and has a worse prognosis than squamous cell carcinoma.[5] Clear cell adenocarcinoma is usually associated with DES exposure in utero. VAIN occurs in the upper third of the vagina and presents with an abnormal Pap test. Primary vaginal tumors are rare. If the tumor is primary, it is usually a squamous cell carcinoma. However, these are usually extensions from endometrial, ovarian, vulvar, renal, or colorectal cancers. Primary adenocarcinoma of the vagina is rare and most often related to DES exposure. These cancers were diagnosed more often in the 1970s and 1980s.[1] Box 177-1 presents risk factors for vaginal cancer.

BOX 177-1

RISK FACTORS FOR VAGINAL CANCER

- HPV infection
- Sexually transmitted diseases (genital herpes simplex)
- Prior irradiation of pelvis
- Smoking
- Immunosuppressive therapy
- Chemotherapy for other malignancy
- Prolonged use of pessary
- Previous malignancy of uterus, cervix, or vulva
- DES exposure in utero
- Age
- Vaginal adenosis or irritation

CLINICAL PRESENTATION

Twenty percent of vaginal carcinomas are asymptomatic and found on a routine pelvic examination. The most common symptom is abnormal bleeding; however, the patient may also complain of vaginal, back, leg, or pelvic pain; dyspareunia; dysuria; constipation; or vaginal discharge and/or mass. A patient with an advanced tumor usually complains of continuous pain or urinary and/or bowel problems. The most common site for a primary tumor is the upper third of the vagina.

PHYSICAL EXAMINATION

The tumor can develop anywhere but is most often found on the lower anterior and lateral vaginal wall. Late-stage signs, such as leg edema or lymph node involvement, are found with adenocarcinoma in more than 95% of cases.[1]

DIAGNOSTICS AND DIFFERENTIAL DIAGNOSIS

The patient should be referred for colposcopy (the study of the transformation zone using a microscope with low magnification) and to exclude primary disease elsewhere. The Pap test has a low sensitivity for detecting clear cell carcinoma; thus DES-exposed women without symptoms should be seen by a gynecologist for inspection of the vagina and cervix, biopsy, and colposcopy. The differential diagnosis includes VAIN, a metastatic lesion, and, if the woman is of childbearing age, trophoblastic disease.

MANAGEMENT AND INDICATIONS FOR REFERRAL/HOSPITALIZATION

Patients with suspicious lesions require colposcopy and biopsy. Wide excision with the patient under anesthesia, as well as cystoscopy and sigmoidoscopy, may be necessary to ensure that the cancer is not invasive. The treatment depends on the type and stage of the disease and may include radiation or pelvic exenteration. Vaporization with a carbon

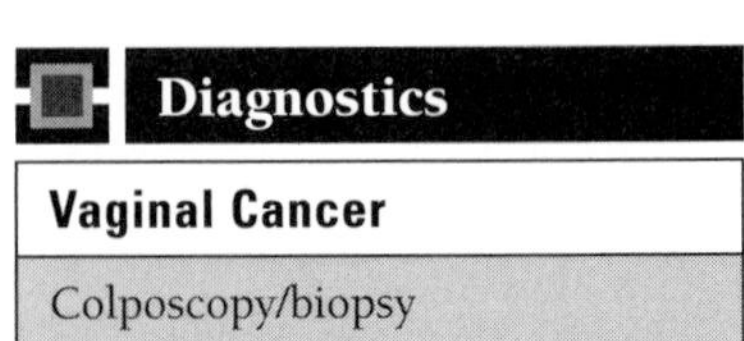
Diagnostics

Vaginal Cancer
Colposcopy/biopsy

Differential Diagnosis

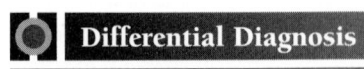

Vaginal Cancer
Vaginal intraepithelial neoplasia Metastatic lesion Trophoblastic disease

dioxide laser or intravaginal application of 5-fluorouracil (5-FU) may be used for premalignant lesions. Chemotherapy has not been proved effective for vaginal cancer.[2]

LIFE SPAN CONSIDERATIONS

Age is a risk factor for squamous cell cancer of the vagina. Most patients with this type of cancer are between 50 and 70 years of age.[3] In contrast; clear cell adenocarcinoma has a patient age range of 7 to 29 years, with the average age at diagnosis of 19. The peak incidence is between 14 and 20 years and is associated with DES exposure in utero. With most of the women exposed to DES now between the ages of 30 and 60, the number of new cases of this type of cancer has decreased.[3]

COMPLICATIONS

Complications after genital tract cancer depend on the stage of the cancer and method of treatment and include those associated with radiation, chemotherapy, or surgery. (For further information, see Chapter 258.)

PATIENT AND FAMILY EDUCATION

After vaginal cancer, follow-up will include a pelvic examination and Pap test every 3 months for 2 years and then every 6 months for 3 years, with a chest x-ray study annually. Patients with vaginal cancer require a careful explanation that they are more likely to develop a malignancy in the cervix or vulva. Even after a hysterectomy, a Pap test should be done at least every 1 to 2 years. DES-exposed women should be vigilantly followed with yearly Pap tests. Female patients exposed to DES in utero who have symptoms should be examined despite their age, and beginning at age 14 (or menarche) these patients should have examinations twice a year or more often if epithelial changes are present.

Cervical Cancer

DEFINITION/EPIDEMIOLOGY

The NCI estimates that 12,900 new cases of cervical cancer occurred in 2001, with 4400 deaths annually.[2] For all women in the United States, the incidence is 8:100,000. A Pap test is a widely used cancer screen. This cancer is the easiest to cure if found early. The incidence of invasive cancer of the cervix has decreased, but that of CIN has increased.

The mortality rate has decreased in African-American women but is still twice that of white women (6.7% compared with 2.5%). The mortality rate has decreased with the use of Pap tests and colposcopy. Cervical cancer has a 5-year survival rate of 100% for preinvasive cancer, 92% for localized cancer, and 70% for all stages.[3]

PATHOPHYSIOLOGY

Squamous cell carcinomas account for 85% to 90% of cervical cancers.[1] Adenocarcinoma can also occur in the cervix. This cancer arises from precursor lesions that begin with atypical cervical cells and gradually progress to CIN and eventually to invasive cancer of the cervix. These precursor lesions can regress or progress into malignancy.[1] As mentioned earlier, the terminology for noninvasive cervical squamous epithelial lesions has changed from carcinoma in situ and dysplasia to CIN. The CIN system grades the lesion according to the involvement of the epithelial thickness:

- **CIN grade I (mild dysplasia):** Lesion well differentiated; involves initial third of the epithelial layer
- **CIN grade II (moderate dysplasia):** Less differentiated; involves one to two thirds of the epithelial layer
- **CIN grade III (severe dysplasia):** Undifferentiated two thirds, full-thickness (carcinoma in situ) involvement

Cervical cancer has a long latency during the preinvasive period. The immature transformation zone of the cervix is particularly sensitive to viral infections. This may explain why those who are sexually active early have an increased incidence of cervical cancer.[1] Box 177-2 presents risk factors for cervical cancer.

CLINICAL PRESENTATION

Early symptoms include abnormal uterine bleeding (postmenopausal, postcoital, after douching, or intermenstrual) or foul vaginal discharge. Bleeding usually begins as light and serosanguineous and becomes heavier and more persistent as the tumor enlarges. Late symptoms include pain, leg edema, and urinary and rectal symptoms.

PHYSICAL EXAMINATION

A vaginal examination may reveal an enlarged cervix; friable tumor on the cervix, or ulcerative lesion that bleeds easily on contact. A Pap test will detect precancerous and cancerous lesions on the cervix or within the endocervix even if the cervix appears normal. The Pap test should include a scraping from the cervical os and a brushing from the endocervical canal. The specimen should be sent for interpretation by an experienced cytopathologist. The patient should be assessed for anemia if she has persistent heavy bleeding. A lesion on the cervix requires biopsy even if the Pap test is negative.

DIAGNOSTICS AND DIFFERENTIAL DIAGNOSIS

Epithelial cell abnormalities require diligent follow-up. If an infection is likely, the infection should be treated, and the test repeated in 3 months. If an infection is unlikely, the test should be repeated in 3 months. If atypical cells continue at that point, the patient should be referred for colposcopy, endocervical curettage, or cone biopsy to locate the lesion. Atypical cells are always significant and require intervention. High-grade changes on the

BOX 177-2

RISK FACTORS FOR CERVICAL CANCER

- Early sexual activity (younger than ages 16-18 years)
- Multiple sexual partners (four or more)
- Young age at first pregnancy
- Short intervals between pregnancies
- Sexually transmitted diseases (including human papillomavirus and herpes simplex)
- Low socioeconomic status
- Cigarette smoking
- Oral contraceptive use
- HIV infection
- Immunosuppression
- Increased parity
- Poor personal hygiene
- Uncircumcised partner
- Promiscuous male partners
- DES exposure
- Age

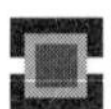

Diagnostics

Cervical Cancer
Pap test
Biopsy/colposcopy

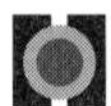

Differential Diagnosis

Cervical Cancer
Cervicitis
Infection
Cervical polyp
Endometrial cancer/metastatic carcinoma

Pap smear require immediate referral for colposcopy. The differential diagnosis includes severe cervicitis, a cervical polyp, carcinoma of the endometrium with cervical extension, and metastatic carcinoma.

MANAGEMENT AND INDICATIONS FOR REFERRAL/ HOSPITALIZATION

The patient should be referred for radiation, electrocautery, cryotherapy, conization, or hysterectomy. The treatment choices are based on the size, location, and histology of the lesion and the patient's age, parity, and reliability for follow-up.

LIFE SPAN CONSIDERATIONS

The NCI reports that women 65 years old and older account for 24% of all cases and 41% of deaths.[2] Lower screening rates are viewed as the cause. Some sources recommend that screening can cease after age 65 if there is a history of regularly obtained negative smears and the patient has no high-risk characteristics. There is debate about this because of the number of malignancies seen in older adults. Pap tests should be performed annually if not performed regularly before age 65 years or if the smear has been abnormal. The incidence of carcinoma in situ peaks between the ages of 20 and 30 years. After age 25 years, the cases of invasive cervical cancer increase with age, along with the chance of dying from the disease.[2]

COMPLICATIONS

Complications after genital tract cancer depend on the stage of the cancer and method of treatment and include those associated with radiation, chemotherapy, or surgery. (For further information, see Chapter 258.)

PATIENT AND FAMILY EDUCATION

Women who are sexually active or have reached age 18 years should have an annual Pap test and a pelvic examination (according to the American Cancer Society and the American College of Obstetricians and Gynecologists). After three or more consecutive satisfactory annual examinations, the test may be done less often at the primary care provider's discretion.[1]

Endometrial Cancer

DEFINITION/EPIDEMIOLOGY

Endometrial cancer is the most common female genital tract cancer and the fourth most common malignancy in women.[1] The NCI estimated that 38,300 new cases occurred with 6600 deaths for 2001.[2] Providers need to be aware of risk factors, diagnostic tests, pertinent history, and symptoms. The American Cancer Society notes the 5-year survival rate for all cases to be 84%.[2] The survival rate for white women exceeds that for African-American women by 15% at each stage.[2]

PATHOPHYSIOLOGY

Excess estrogen is the biggest risk factor for endometrial cancer. Most women who develop endometrial cancer have a history of exposure to abnormal estrogen levels. The risk of taking estrogen is neutralized with the addition of progestin. The risk is increased among first-degree relatives of patients with endometrial cancer and is associated with breast and colon cancer. Unopposed estrogen causes the endometrium to become thicker and more vascular (hyperplasia). Endometrial hyperplasia is divided into three groups: simple, complex, and atypical. Endometrial carcinoma develops in 20% to 30% of women with untreated atypical hyperplasia.[1] Without progesterone, the structural support needed to sustain vascularity is not present and spontaneous superficial random hemorrhages occur.[6] Box 177-3 presents risk and protective factors associated with endometrial cancer.

CLINICAL PRESENTATION AND PHYSICAL EXAMINATION

The symptoms of endometrial cancer often present when cure is still possible. Patients may present with painless, postmenopausal bleeding, discharge, painful or difficult urination, dyspareunia, or pelvic pain. Later signs of uterine cancer include cramping, pelvic discomfort, postcoital bleeding, lower abdominal pressure, and enlarged lymph nodes. A detailed history of menstruation, dyspareunia, pelvic pain, fever, trauma, and intrauterine contraceptive device (IUD) use should be elicited, and risk factors for endometrial cancer reviewed. The physical examination includes a bimanual pelvic examination, Pap test, and assessment for abdominal masses, signs of bleeding disorders, and thyroid abnormalities.

BOX 177-3

ENDOMETRIAL CANCER: RISK AND PROTECTIVE FACTORS

RISK FACTORS
- Obesity
- Menstruation span
  - Early menarche
  - Late menopause
  - No children
- Age (greater than 50)
- Polycystic ovary syndrome (Stein-Leventhal syndrome)
- Ovulation failure/infertility
- Estrogen-secreting tumors
- Other endocrine disorders
- Hypertension
- Diabetes mellitus
- Immunodeficiency
- Endometrial hyperplasia
- Diet high in animal fat
- Ovarian cancer
- Breast cancer
- Caucasian race
- Estrogen replacement therapy without progesterone (long term, high doses)
- Tamoxifen therapy
- Sequential oral contraception
- Hormonal therapy
- Previous radiation therapy (pelvic)
- DES exposure
- History of inherited form of colorectal cancer

PROTECTIVE FACTORS
- Combined oral contraception
- High parity

DIAGNOSTICS

The Pap test is not usually effective in detecting endometrial cancer. If endometrial cancer is suspected or if the patient is at high risk for its development, referral for a pelvic examination, transvaginal ultrasound, endometrial biopsy, hysteroscopy, and/or dilation and curettage (D&C) is necessary. Endometrial aspiration is a more direct sampling of the uterine cavity and is less painful than a D&C. If endometrial cancer is suspected, the following tests are required: serum human chorionic gonadotropin (hCG) (if the patient is of reproductive age), CBC, BUN, creatinine, platelet count, cultures to exclude infection, saline and potassium hydroxide (KOH) preparations of vaginal secretions, clotting studies, and hormone levels to detect menopausal status.[2,7]

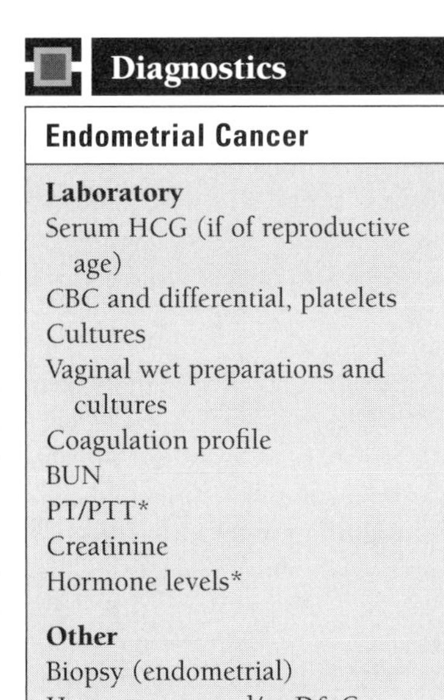

Diagnostics

Endometrial Cancer

Laboratory
Serum HCG (if of reproductive age)
CBC and differential, platelets
Cultures
Vaginal wet preparations and cultures
Coagulation profile
BUN
PT/PTT*
Creatinine
Hormone levels*

Other
Biopsy (endometrial)
Hysteroscopy and/or D&C
Transvaginal ultrasound

*If indicated.

DIFFERENTIAL DIAGNOSIS

Benign causes of bleeding include atrophic vaginitis, cervicitis, cervical polyps, ovarian cysts, inflammation, infection, endometriosis, uterine fibroids, uterine prolapse, polyps, erosions, PID, trauma (foreign body, sexual abuse, tampon), and complications of pregnancy (retained products of conception). In addition, systemic diseases (bleeding, thyroid, liver, renal disorders) and medications (oral contraceptives, steroids, anticoagulants, neuroleptics, major tranquilizers) can cause bleeding.

MANAGEMENT AND INDICATIONS FOR REFERRAL/HOSPITALIZATION

An endometrial biopsy is essential for any patient with postmenopausal bleeding. Women at risk because of hormonal therapy require an annual endometrial sampling and other diagnostic interventions. Surgery is the treatment of choice for endometrial cancer except in late-stage disease. Treatment also includes radiation, hormonal therapy, and chemotherapy and depends on the type and stage of cancer as well as the patient's overall medical condition.

Differential Diagnosis

Endometrial Cancer	
Atrophic vaginitis	Uterine fibroids
Cervicitis	Uterine prolapse
Cervical polyp	Uterine polyp
Ovarian cyst	Pelvic inflammatory disease
Inflammation	Trauma
Infection	Medications
Endometriosis	Pregnancy
Systemic disease	

LIFE SPAN CONSIDERATIONS

The average age for the diagnosis of endometrial cancer is 60, with 95% of patients 40 years old or older.[3] The incidence increases with advancing age. When endometrial cancer occurs before the age of 40 years, it is usually associated with chronic obesity and/or anovulation.[7]

COMPLICATIONS

Complications after genital tract cancer depend on the stage of the cancer and method of treatment and include those associated with radiation, chemotherapy, or surgery. (For further information, see Chapter 258.)

PATIENT AND FAMILY EDUCATION

Patients should understand that the use of estrogen plus progesterone for postmenopausal hormone replacement therapy does not increase the risk of endometrial cancer. It is also necessary that women understand the importance of evaluation for unusual bleeding.

Ovarian Cancer

DEFINITION/EPIDEMIOLOGY

Ovarian cancer has a high fatality rate and is the fifth leading cause of death from cancer in women.[2] The NCI estimated that 23,400 new cases with 13,900 deaths occurred in 2001.[2] The National Ovarian Cancer Coalition (NOCC) notes that ovarian cancer accounts for 4% of all cancers among women. The death rates have not changed significantly in the past 50 years, with only 25% of ovarian cancers found early.[8] The 5-year survival rate is 90% for stage I, 70% for stage II, and 15% to 20% for stage III or IV.[8]

PATHOPHYSIOLOGY

Tumors primarily arise from the epithelial cells; however, they can also arise from the germinal or stromal cells of the ovary. Increased age and family history are risk factors, with family history being the best predictor of risk. One second-degree relative with ovarian cancer increases the lifetime risk to 2.9%; one first-degree relative with ovarian cancer increases the lifetime risk to 4% to 5%; and two or more affected first-degree relatives increases the risk to 30% to 50%.[6] The *BRCA1* gene, identified in 1994, has been linked to breast and ovarian cancer.[9] However, these hereditary syndromes occur in very few cases of ovarian cancer. Box 177-4 presents risk and protective factors associated with ovarian cancer.

CLINICAL PRESENTATION

If the patient presents with signs and symptoms, metastasis has occurred in 75% of the cases.[1] Only 25% of ovarian carcinomas are diagnosed at a time when they are curable.[1,3] There are no early warning symptoms. Early-stage disease is usually diagnosed from an asymptomatic mass noted on a routine pelvic examination. The usual presenting symptoms are the result of

BOX 177-4

EPITHELIAL OVARIAN CANCER: RISK AND PROTECTIVE FACTORS

RISK FACTORS
- Advancing age
- Northern European or North American descent
- Nulliparity*
- Personal history of breast,* endometrial, or colon cancer
- Family history of ovarian cancer
- Infertility*
- Fertility drugs
- Dietary fat consumption*
- Milk product consumption
- Coffee consumption
- Perineal talc usage*
- Menstrual history (more periods* = increased risk)

PROTECTIVE FACTORS
- Pregnancy
- Tubal ligation or hysterectomy
- Oral contraceptives

Data from Griffiths CT and others: *Gynecologic oncology,* London, 1997, Mosby-Wolfe.
*Each of these risk factors increases the lifetime risk by 2%.

advanced disease and include abdominal pain, distention, bloating, nausea, pelvic discomfort, pressure or pain, weight loss, urinary frequency, leg pain, bleeding between periods or after menopause, and shortness of breath.

PHYSICAL EXAMINATION

A pelvic examination for an adnexal mass should be done but is not sensitive for detecting ovarian cancer. The assessment should include all possible conditions in the differential diagnosis.

DIAGNOSTICS

CA-125 is an antigenic determinant on a serum glycoprotein that is elevated in most women with epithelial ovarian cancer. CA-125 is also elevated in late-stage endometrial cancers and in about 60% of pancreatic cancers. A value above 35 units/ml is abnormal but nonspecific. Elevations may be the result of cervical, endometrial, or fallopian tube carcinoma or pregnancy; benign ovarian cysts; PID; endometriosis; or uterine leiomyoma.[1,6] Elevated CA-125 levels may require transabdominal or transvaginal ultrasound evaluation. Invasive diagnostic evaluation, often including laparotomy, may be necessary.

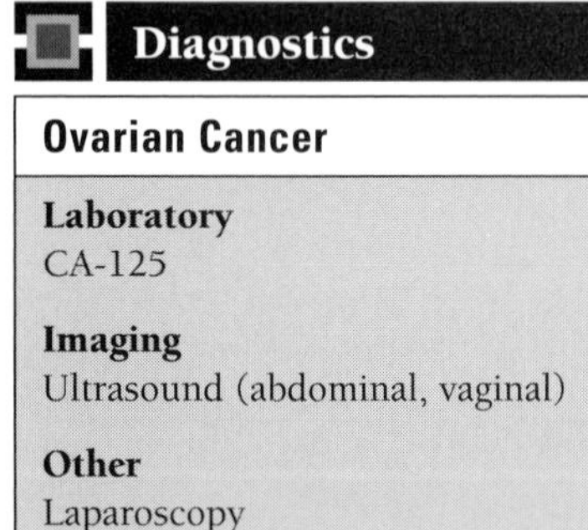
Diagnostics

Ovarian Cancer

Laboratory
CA-125

Imaging
Ultrasound (abdominal, vaginal)

Other
Laparoscopy
Biopsy

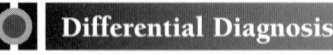

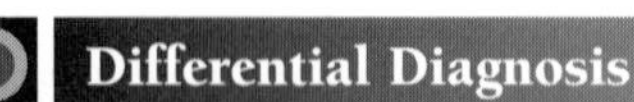
Differential Diagnosis

Ovarian Cancer

- Sigmoid diverticulitis
- Pregnancy
- Distended bladder
- Distended cecum
- Stool in sigmoid colon
- Pelvic kidney
- Fallopian tube, uterine, or gastrointestinal tumor

DIFFERENTIAL DIAGNOSIS

Other conditions can present as a pelvic mass. These include sigmoid diverticulitis, pregnancy, a distended bladder, a low-lying distended cecum, stool in the sigmoid colon, a pelvic kidney, and a fallopian tube, uterine, or gastrointestinal tumor.[1] Carcinoma of the fallopian tube is so rare (0.3% of gynecologic cancers) that it is considered an appendage of ovarian cancer.[1] It should be suspected with atypical presentations (i.e., women with abnormal vaginal bleeding that does not respond to hormone therapy after a D&C).[10]

MANAGEMENT AND INDICATIONS FOR REFERRAL/HOSPITALIZATION

All patients with suspected ovarian carcinoma are referred for surgery, radiation, and/or chemotherapy. Older female patients with gastrointestinal symptoms need an evaluation for ovarian cancer if a gastrointestinal etiology for the symptoms is not isolated.

LIFE SPAN CONSIDERATIONS

Advancing age correlates with increased incidence of the disease and its virulence. The survival rate for women older than 65 years is half that for younger women.[1]

COMPLICATIONS

Complications after genital tract cancer depend on the stage of the cancer and method of treatment and include those associated with radiation, chemotherapy, or surgery. (For further information, see Chapter 258.)

PATIENT AND FAMILY EDUCATION

Patients with a familial history of the rare hereditary form of ovarian cancer should be referred to a gynecology specialist to determine appropriate screening and follow-up. Patients with a family history of sporadic ovarian cancer may benefit from screening and should be referred for consultation. Routine screening of the population is not necessary.

REFERENCES

1. Griffiths CT and others: *Gynecologic oncology,* London, 1997, Mosby-Wolfe.
2. National Cancer Institute website. Retrieved August 12, 2002, from the World Wide Web: http://www.nci.nih.gov.
3. American Cancer Society website. Retrieved August 12, 2002, from the World Wide Web: http://www.cancer.org.
4. Echt ML and others: Detection of sentinel lymph nodes with lymphazuria in cervical, uterine and vulvar malignancies, *South Med J* 92:204-208, 1999.
5. Bynum DT: Vaginal carcinoma: a rare but treatable cancer, *J Soc Gynecol Nurse Oncol* 6:24-36, 1996.
6. Driscoll CE and others: *The family practice desk reference,* ed 3, St Louis, 1996, Mosby.
7. Elliott JL and others: Endometrial adenocarcinoma and polycystic ovary syndrome: risk factors, management, and prognosis, *South Med J* 94:529-531, 2001.
8. National Ovarian Cancer Coalition website. Retrieved August 12, 2002, from the World Wide Web: http://www.ovarian.org.
9. Olopade OI: Genetics in clinical cancer care: the future is now, *N Engl J Med* 335:1455-1456, 1996.
10. Raychaudhuri K, Hirsh PJ: Atypical presentation of primary fallopian tube carcinoma, *J Obstet Gynaecol* 17(4):403-406, 1997.

CHAPTER 178

Infertility

Marie Elena Botte

DEFINITION/EPIDEMIOLOGY

Infertility is defined as a couple's inability to conceive after 1 year of unprotected intercourse[1-3] or to carry a pregnancy to live birth.[4] Infertility affects one couple in six and prevalence increases dramatically with maternal age.[1] In this chapter, infertility is contrasted with *sterility,* which is a term that applies to those members of a population for whom there is no possibility of attaining a natural pregnancy.[5] Although as many as 12% to 28%[6] of couples experience transient or persistent infertility at some point in their lives and 1 in 10 couples seek medical help for the problem of subfertility,[7] 10% to 50% of involuntarily childless people never seek professional help.[6] The recent increase in the numbers of individuals who present to health care professionals for help with infertility is most likely attributable to a combination of factors, including an increasing number of women delaying the birth of their first child and widespread media attention regarding new reproductive technologies and possibilities. An estimated 15% of all couples will experience infertility, and half of these couples will remain unable to have a biologic child of their own.[3]

PATHOPHYSIOLOGY

Physiologic dysfunction in men accounts for approximately 20% to 50% of all cases of infertility[2,6]; ovulation dysfunction in women contributes to 25% of infertility cases; and tubal factors (20%), endometriosis (5%) and unexplained causes (between 10% and 25%) are other factors. Multiple factors contribute to infertility in 40% of couples,[2] and combined male and female factors occur in about 30%.[6] In 10% to 25% of cases, no specific factor can be identified.[3,6,8] The odds of delivering a healthy infant drop 3.5% per year after age 30 years. For women younger than 25, the rate of impaired fertility is 11.7%; this rate rises to 42.1% for women older than 35 years.

Male-factor infertility can generally be attributable to chromosomal or structural defects or to endocrine abnormalities of the hypothalamic-pituitary-testicular axis. Contributing hypothalamic-pituitary disorders include congenital gonadotropin-releasing hormone (GnRH) deficiency (Kalman's syndrome), hemochromatosis, pituitary and hypothalamic tumors, infiltrative disorders (tuberculosis, sarcoidosis), hormonal disturbance (androgen, cortisol, and estrogen excess, hyperprolactinemia), or systemic disorders such as chronic illness, obesity, and nutritional deficiencies.[9] Structural causes include cryptorchism, aplasia or obstruction in the male genital tract, varicoceles (generally only a problem when accompanied by other factors such as abnormal semen analysis), congenital bilateral absence of the vas deferens (which can indicate partial expression of a gene mutation for cystic fibrosis), impotence, or ejaculatory dysfunction. Factors influencing spermatogenesis or motility include inflammation or infection (postpubertal mumps, gonorrhea, *Chlamydia*) direct injury/trauma (including postoperative), radiation, chemotherapy, heat, medications, toxic exposures, and abuse of substances, including alcohol, cocaine, steroids, and marijuana.

Exposure, possibly in an occupational setting, to solvents, pesticides, heavy metals, pharmaceuticals, anesthetic gases, ionizing radiation, heat, and lead[10,11] are established reproductive hazards for both men and women. Occupational exposures in male workers can affect the male reproductive system, leading to sperm abnormalities, hyperestrogenism, impotence, infertility, or increased spontaneous abortions in the partners of exposed workers.[12] In women, cigarette smoking, shift work, and occupational exposure to chemotherapeutic drugs have also been associated with an increased subsequent risk of infertility.[13] Primary care practitioners can consult websites of the National Institute for Occupational Safety and Health (NIOSH) (http://www.cdc.gov/niosh/homepage/html) and the Occupational Safety and Health Administration (OSHA) (www.OSHA.gov) for further information on reproductive hazards and their management.

Tubal infertility has been associated with lower family income.[14] Ovulatory dysfunctions range from congenital absence of the ovaries and premature ovarian failure to various disruptions in the hypothalamic-pituitary-ovarian axis and other metabolic/endocrine conditions such as hypothyroidism and hyperthyroidism. Uterine and fallopian pathology includes current or past PID resulting in salpingitis, endometriosis, iatrogenic Asherman's syndrome after overly vigorous curettage, fibroids, bicornuate uterus, and postinfectious or operative tubal scarring and adhesions. Preembryonic developmental problems and implantation problems have been postulated as possible etiologies for idiopathic infertility.[15]

Pathophysiology involved in infertility includes interference with circadian rhythms and the temporal pattern of endocrine functions in shift work.[16] In addition, endogenous opioid-mediated inhibition of the hypothalamic GnRH pulse generator[17] has been implicated in hypothalamic ovarian failure. The link between infertility and various autoimmune disorders may be related to the fact that the segment of the major histocompatibility complex (MHC) that contains genes that affect reproduction also contains genes associated with various autoimmune disorders.[18] The connection with diabetes mellitus has been linked at least in part to a functional deficit of hypothalamic noradrenergic neurons[19] and in cystic fibrosis to congenital bilateral absence of the vas deferens.[20]

CLINICAL PRESENTATION

Ideally, both members of the couple are present for the initial interview; this is invaluable not only for the comprehensiveness of the medical history but also for providing insight into the couple's communication and decision-making style, emotional status, ability to support each other, coping strategies, and current level of functioning.[21] Subsequent interviews with either partner alone may reveal information (e.g., previous pregnancies, abortions, or infections) that the individual is not comfortable disclosing otherwise. Essential components of relevant history to elicit include duration of the couple's infertility, previous pregnancy or siring of children, and the woman's age because these factors have been consistently demonstrated to affect the prognosis.

Other relevant historical information includes a thorough obstetric and gynecologic history (contraceptive use, prior pregnancy, therapeutic abortion, miscarriage, infection, pathology, or procedures). Particular attention is given to the menstrual history for cues related to ovulatory cycles, including mid-cycle discomfort, regular menses, premenstrual symptomatology, and periods that occur every 27 to 30 days.[1] The past medical history focuses on infections, surgeries, medications, and systemic and autoimmune disorders. Family history is assessed for relatives with infertility or early menopause, autoimmune disorders such as lupus and maternal diethylstilbestrol (DES) exposure. A review of systems may reveal weight changes, signs of estrogen deficiency or excess, signs of thyroid imbalance, hyperandrogenism or virilism, hyposmia (which may be related to Kallman's syndrome),or of galactorrhea, headaches, or visual disturbances (which are possibly suggestive of pituitary pathology).

Social history should include patterns of smoking, alcohol or other substance use such as caffeine, exercise patterns, level of stress and coping strategies, potential eating disorders, and frequency of intercourse. Occupational history may reveal a host of potential reproductive threats, including the prolonged waiting time to pregnancy observed in female shift workers.[16] Laboratory workers, health care workers (including anesthetists, dental assistants, and hospital personnel), farmers, painters, and construction workers may be exposed to reproductive toxins such as lead, nitrous oxide and solvents; domestic exposures include recent home renovation, contaminated air or ground water, and domestic pesticide use.[11] Various population-based studies have failed to find a correlation between consanguinity (uncle-niece, first cousins, and first-degree cousins once removed) and primary sterility.[22] Infertility has also been shown not to be related to prior cervical laser surgery.[23]

PHYSICAL EXAMINATION

Examination of the male partner includes inspection of the genitals for abnormalities, including phimosis, varicocele (the most commonly identified genital abnormality in subfertile men), and hypospadias. The bilateral presence of the vas deferens is established, and the testes are palpated for maldescent, consistency, and size. Decreased testicular size is related to impaired spermatogenesis; the length of the testes (measured in a warm room, after the patient has been standing for several minutes) should be more than 4 cm and the volume more than 20 ml by orchidometry.[24]

Physical examination of the female partner includes palpation of the thyroid, a breast examination to check for galactorrhea, and evaluation of signs of hypoestrogenic status (dry, pale vaginal mucosa), androgen excess (hirsutism, male pattern hair loss, acne, obesity), or virilization (changes in body fat distribution, a lowering of the voice, or clitoromegaly). A pelvic examination also provides a gross indication of the state of the reproductive organs and may detect enlarged ovaries or other masses such as uterine fibroids. Changes in visual acuity or visual fields may be indicative of a cranial (pituitary) mass.

DIAGNOSTICS

Considerable debate surrounds the selection and interpretation of diagnostic studies in the context of a basic fertility workup[5,25] because of the difficulty in establishing cutoff points for "abnormal" in investigations such as semen analysis and the demonstrated inability of many analyses to differentiate between fertile and infertile individuals.[26,27] Complicating the issue is the likelihood that many couples present with a constellation of factors, such as varicoceles and low-normal sperm count; although each may be relatively insignificant in isolation, they combine synergistically to produce clinical infertility.

According to published World Health Organization (WHO) guidelines,[5] semen analysis should be performed early on in the evaluation, after 36 to 48 hours of abstinence. National Guidelines from England[28] and the U.S. Institute for Clinical Systems Improvement[29] suggest a repeat semen analysis after 4 months if the first test was normal and there has been no intervening pregnancy. If semen analysis indicates oligospermia, a follicle-stimulating hormone (FSH) and testosterone level should be obtained before referral to a male infertility specialist; if the serum testosterone level is low or the patient has other symptoms of hypogonadism (decreased libido and/or potency), a prolactin level should also be obtained. Testicular volume assessment with an orchidometer combined with basal serum FSH level can also be used to estimate future fertility in individuals who are long-term survivors of malignancy in childhood or adolescence.[30] The postcoital test (PCT) has received mixed reviews in the literature and is generally not recommended.[28,29] It can be useful to confirm that intercourse has taken place, but it has poor sensitivity, specificity, positive predictive value, and negative predictive value.[1]

Although the only definitive proof of ovulation in a particular cycle remains a subsequent pregnancy, ovulatory assessment has traditionally been done with basal body temperature charting.[31] A biphasic curve demonstrating a consistently raised temperature in the later half of the cycle is one of the simplest, most inexpensive, and practical ways to assess ovulatory function.[32] Plasma mid-luteal progesterone concentration[5] (a level >3 ng/ml is confirmatory but cannot assess the quality of the luteal

Diagnostics

Infertility

MEN
Laboratory
Semen analysis
FSH
Testosterone level*
Prolactin level*
Hepatitis screen
HIV

Other
Testicular volume assessment

WOMEN
Laboratory
Rubella titer*
Pap smear
Chlamydia culture or serum antibody
Gonococcal culture
FSH
LH
TSH
RPR*
CBC and differential
PPD
Antiphospholid antibody*
ANA*
Clomiphene stimulation test
DHEA
ESR*
Hepatitis screen
HIV
Rubella titer

Other
Hysterosalpingography

*If indicated.

phase[1]), and home kits for measuring the luteinizing hormone (LH) surge in urine[2] can be useful to help confirm ovulation. All female patients merit a rubella titer (if indicated), cervical cytology (Pap), and *Chlamydia* culture[2] or serum antibody[1] (found in 73% of patients with distal tubal occlusion and in no patients with normal fallopian tubes in one study of women undergoing an infertility evaluation[1]). Evaluation of tubal patency is most commonly done by hysterosalpingography (HSG) and can even be therapeutic in that women have been known to conceive soon after this procedure.[2] For women more than 35 years of age, a day-3 FSH level and an estradiol level are indicated to assess ovarian reserve (elevated day-3 FSH levels indicate a poorer outcome with assisted reproductive technologies).

Additional laboratory assessment is indicated by the patient's history and physical examination and is *not* warranted for all women concerned about their fertility, especially those with regular menstrual cycles. These tests include prolactin and thyroid assays,[28] testosterone, and dehydroepiandrosterone (DHEA) and 17-hydroxyprogesterone tests where indicated and clomiphene challenge to evaluate ovarian reserve. An anticardiolipin antibody, antiphospholipid antibody, and antinuclear antibody (ANA) can be performed to exclude lupus.

DIFFERENTIAL DIAGNOSIS

A wide range of conditions can contribute to infertility, including genetic, structural, and endocrine disorders; acquired infections; treatment of other conditions with radiation or chemotherapy; body mass index; personal behaviors like alcohol consumption and maternal cigarette smoking; medications; sexual dysfunction; antisperm antibodies; previous genital or pelvic surgery; and exposure to reproductive toxins. Congenital causes include gonadal dysgenesis, chromosomal mosaicism, congenital bilateral absence of the vas deferens or the uterus, Kleinfelter's syndrome (small hard testes, gynecomastia), Turner's syndrome (short stature, pigeon chest, webbed neck), deletions in the Y chromosome genes, and isolated corticotropin (ACTH) deficiency,[33] which is rare but treatable. Male factors contributing to infertility are generally determined by semen analysis.

Ovulatory dysfunction can be attributable to hyperprolactinemia, hypogonadotropic hypogonadism (these women have decreased serum estradiol levels and no withdrawal bleeding after a progesterone challenge), hypergonadotropic hypogonadism (elevated FSH levels indicating premature ovarian failure and possible presence of Y chromosome in young women), and normogonadotropic anovulatory conditions including polycystic ovary syndrome (a hyperandrogenic condition often presenting with acne, weight gain, hirsutism, or acanthosis nigrans when hyperinsulinemia is also contributing), luteal phase defects, and multifollicular ovaries.

Differential Diagnosis

Infertility

Genetic disorder	Alcohol
Structural disorder	Smoking
Endocrine disorder	Antisperm antibody
Co-morbid illness	Sexual dysfunction
Infection	Chemical exposure
Body mass index	Radiation
Medications (including chemotherapy)	

MANAGEMENT

Although the provision of infertility services is beyond the scope of practice of most primary care providers, they nevertheless perform an important initial exploration of historical, physical examination, and selected diagnostic factors that can facilitate expedient and timely referral to appropriate specialists when indicated. Primary care providers can also intervene early in terms of improving modifiable lifestyle risk factors, improving coping mechanisms, providing basic preconceptual education and care, and improving overall health for all patients who are attempting conception.

According to the American Society of Reproductive Medicine, an infertility evaluation is warranted after 1 year of coital exposure for couples in which the woman is younger than 35 years and after 6 months when she is older than 35 years.[34] Individuals warranting an expedited workup/referral to a specialist include women without periods, with irregular periods, or with bleeding between periods, as well as those who have pain with intercourse and a history of abdominal surgery, ruptured appendix, or upper genital tract infection.[1] Men for whom similar expedited workup and referral to reproductive specialist is appropriate include those with difficulty sustaining an erection or who are unable to ejaculate during intercourse and those with a history of testicular injury, infection, or maldescension.[1]

Of all couples diagnosed as infertile, 15% to 60% will experience pregnancy without treatment of any kind within 1 year[2,5] and 25% to 80% will be successful within 2 years.[5] Prognosis in these instances is more encouraging if the duration of infertility has been less than 3 years, if the woman is younger than 32 years, and if the couple has previously conceived a child[35]; prognosis is worse for situations involving endometriosis, male-factor infertility, and tubal pathologies[5] or multiple factors.[35]

It is essential from the outset to reinforce with any couple seeking treatment that appropriately directed therapy, excluding advanced reproductive technologies, is *unsuccessful* up to 50% of the time.[2,5] More elaborate assisted reproductive technologies (ARTs) such as in vitro fertilization (IVF) and the newer intracytoplasmic sperm injection (ICSI) along with donor gametes and surrogacy may provide hope for pregnancy otherwise unattainable through more conventional means. However, these approaches can be expensive and risky, and they often raise moral and ethical dilemmas regarding their use.[36]

Any treatment plan should follow a full discussion regarding all possible treatment options, including adoption, childfree living without intervention of any kind, and the possibility of stopping at any time in the treatment process. Discussion must address attendant benefits, risks, time required for participation, and costs, along with reasonable estimations of probability for achieving pregnancy based on relevant infertility factors[37] both with and without treatment. Ongoing counseling for the couple should be offered and encouraged. Counseling may help the couple to discontinue treatment when appropriate, to support the solicitation of second opinions, to participate in support groups, to establish a (necessarily arbitrarily determined) time limit for treatment, and to take time *off* from treatment to give them a sense of control and balance in their lives. Patients are referred to a specialist for evaluation and management of ARTs.

LIFE SPAN CONSIDERATIONS

Normalizing weight, improving nutritional status, folate supplementation, reducing stress, and eliminating potential detrimental factors such as cigarette smoking, caffeine and alcohol intake, illicit drug use, and exposure to potential reproductive toxins are general health-promoting interventions for the couple. These interventions, which may raise a couple's chances of attaining pregnancy, might also improve their psychologic health.[38]

PHARMACOLOGIC THERAPY

When infertility is due to hypothalamic-pituitary insufficiency in the male partner (as is the case in 1% to 2% of male-factor infertility), these men often respond well to gonadotropin or GnRH therapy.[9] Induction of ovulation according to a variety of protocols involving gonadotropins has been used for hypogonadotropic hypogonadism in women.[39,40] Chronic *opiate agonist* administration (naltrexone) can normalize ovarian function[17,41] for women with hypothalamic ovarian failure. Another approach, which requires referral to a specialist, entails pulsatile administration of GnRH,[41] specifically at frequencies of 90 or 120 minutes, which more reliably induce follicular development, ovulation, and normal luteal function.[42] *Bromocriptine* or other, newer dopamine agonists such as cabergoline are indicated in the treatment of hyperprolactinemia.

Antiestrogens such as *clomiphene citrate* or *tamoxifen* are used for the induction of ovulation in women with polycystic ovary syndrome.[5] *Estrogen replacement* for women with hypergonadotropic hypogonadism is important to prevent osteoporosis; ovulation-inducing therapies are neither useful nor indicated for these women. For women with chemotherapy-induced ovarian failure, ovarian function should be reassessed periodically[43] because spontaneous recovery has been noted. Clomiphene citrate, human menopausal gonadotropin, and various ART procedures are often used empirically for unexplained infertility.

ARTs include such technologies as Gamete intrafallopian transfer (GIFT), IVF, direct intraperitoneal injection of sperm, and intrafollicular injection of sperm. The induction of superovulation is often followed by artificial insemination of some kind; success is highly influenced by the woman's age, with cycle fecundity dropping from an average of 0.23 to 0.05 after age 40 years.[44]

Women or men being managed by specialists for infertility still require basic primary care services. This enables the primary care provider to assess and intervene on behalf of the couple's functional, emotional, and psychospiritual responses to continuing therapy. Somatization is a common manifestation of the psychologic stress of infertility,[6] as are sexual problems, depressive reactions, emotional instability, relationship difficulties, reduced self-confidence/esteem, and feelings of anger, guilt, grief, isolation, and anxiety.

COMPLICATIONS

Women with polycystic ovary syndrome do not generally respond as well to ovulation induction as do women with other ovulatory disorders and have an increased risk of ovarian hyperstimulation when they do respond.[5] Other infertility treatment–related complications include a controversial association between fertility drugs and ovarian cancer[5] and the protracted psychic anguish that can accompany successive failed treatment cycles. The risks of multiple gestation associated with ARTs have been well documented in the literature, but even resultant singleton pregnancies represent obstetric risks, given an increased incidence of pregnancy-induced hypertension, placenta previa, elective cesarean, preterm labor, and a lower mean birth weight than controls.[45]

INDICATIONS FOR REFERRAL/HOSPITALIZATION

Referral to a reproductive urologist is indicated for male factors identified on semen analysis.[2] Referral to a reproductive endocrinologist or fertility specialist is indicated for an abnormal PCT, for a basic infertility workup that does not disclose the source of the problem, or for any of the various ART procedures should they be a couple's only hope for conception. Couples interested in exploring complementary therapeutic options may find some success with acupuncture.[46]

Pathologic conditions, including adhesiolysis and various testicular, uterine, or tubal pathologies, may require surgical repair. In addition, complications from therapy (moderate to severe ovarian hyperstimulation syndrome) may require hospitalization.

PATIENT AND FAMILY EDUCATION

Infertility and its often unsuccessful medical treatment present a conglomerate of stresses and losses with which the couple must contend,[21] including the loss of biologic children and the experiences of pregnancy and breastfeeding. Individuals endure the stresses of complicated, expensive, and invasive treatment interventions, which can be experienced as humiliating or embarrassing. Adjusting to infertile status is easier for individuals with positive self-esteem, an internal locus of control, and higher socioeconomic status, whereas increased anxiety and distress have been associated with advancing age, undifferentiated sex-role identity, and low self-esteem.[47] Several studies have supported the contention that motherhood, identity development, personal happiness, and well-being are involved in many women's desires for having children[48]; this desire for children often remains strong after many years of infertility.[48]

Motives for medical consultation by infertile couples, in addition to the desire to have a child, include education and understanding regarding the cause of the infertility.[49] Primary care providers should be aware of recent research indicating a disparity between medical diagnosis and what is perceived as the diagnosis by 38% of infertile individuals[50] along with a tendency for patients to blame themselves for the infertility. Basic education for infertile persons includes advising intercourse about twice a week[2] and avoiding lubricants that may be spermicidal such as K-Y Jelly, petroleum jelly, and Surgilube. In contrast, raw egg white and vegetable oil do not seem to affect sperm motility.[24] Education should also encourage cessation of alcohol or illicit drug use, smoking cessation,[51,52] proper nutrition, and normalization of body mass index (especially for women), as well as strategies for stress reduction. Primary care providers can also provide an initial infertility work-up that focuses on explaining the various diagnostic procedures as well as addressing couples' concerns and questions as they arise. The American Society of Reproductive Medicine (ASRM) website (www.asrm.org) is a good source of patient information.

It is particularly important to provide couples with an accurate estimation of the success rates that are expected by various procedures and the concordant risks, discomforts, and expenses entailed.[53] Unfortunately, there have been fewer randomized clinical trials in the area of infertility management than in other branches of medical science, and many studies have small sample sizes, inappropriate design, and pseudorandomization.[54] Although the incidence and medical problems associated with ART-associated multiple gestations have been widely emphasized in the medical literature, one study found that 67% to 90% of infertile couples expressed a desire for twins, and fear about multiple gestations was rejected by the majority of these couples.[55] This clearly indicates a need for additional education about the risks associated with ARTs.

For couples who are able to conceive with treatment, providers of primary care can stress the normalcy of the pregnancy and help the couple through the normative developmental processes of pregnancy and parenthood.

Many clinicians emphasize the importance of helping couples to determine their own end point and timeline for intervention attempts[37] because there always seems to be some promising or potential development around the corner.[31] Some research has indicated increased social support and greater contentment over time for infertile couples,[4] but continuing interventional attempts can also have a detrimental effect on the well-being of individuals and the couple,[56,57] with one study finding a greater psychologic than physiologic burden sustained when undergoing infertility treatment with IVF.[58]

Because the length of time that a woman has been infertile is related to her future fecundability[59] and because fertility decreases exponentially with increasing age,[34] many infertile individuals find themselves confronted with the necessity of redefining their expectations and goals related to establishing a family. Clinicians play an important role in facilitating the grieving process for the many losses sustained throughout the experience of diagnosis and treatment. This process is important because it constitutes the experiential prerequisite to acceptance and is essential for the couple to move on with their lives. Clinician support can enforce an "unsuccessful" couple's eventual realization that they have been thorough and have tried sufficient therapeutic intervention and that cessation of such interventions is reasonable and advisable. Couples can then be supported in their efforts to plan their lives in ways that may include consideration of adoption or child-free living as valid alternatives to biologic parenthood.

REFERENCES

1. Penzias AS: Infertility: contemporary office-based evaluation and treatment, *Obstet Gynecol Clin North Am* 27:473-486, 2000.
2. Morell V: Basic infertility assessment, *Prim Care* 24:195-204, 1997.
3. Templeton A: Infertility: epidemiology, aetiology and effective management, *Health Bull (Edinb)* 53:294-298, 1995.
4. Hirsch AM, Hirsch SM: The long-term psychosocial effects of infertility, *J Obstet Gynecol Neonatal Nurs* 24:517-522, 1995.
5. Eshre CW: Infertility revisited: the state of the art today and tomorrow. The ESHRE Capri Workshop. European Society for Human Reproduction and Embryology, *Hum Reprod* 11:1779-1807, 1996.
6. Himmel W and others: Management of involuntary childlessness, *Br J Gen Pract* 47:111-118, 1997.
7. de kreser D, Baker H: Infertility in men: recent advances and continuing controversies, *J Clin Endocrinol Metab* 84:3443-3450, 1999.
8. Organization WH: Towards more objectivity in diagnosis and management of male fertility, *Int J Androl* 7(suppl):1-53, 1997.
9. Khorram O and others: Reproductive technologies for male infertility, *J Clin Endocrinol Metab* 86:2373-2379, 2001.
10. Frazier L: Workplace reproductive problems, *Prim Care* 27:1039-1056, 2000.
11. Solomon GM: Reproductive toxins: a growing concern at work in the community, *J Occup Environ Med* 39:105-107, 1996.
12. Baranski B: Effects of the workplace on fertility and other related reproductive outcomes, *Environ Health Perspect* 101(suppl 2):81-90, 1993.
13. Valanis B and others: Occupational exposure to antineoplastic agents and self-reported infertility among nurses and pharmacists, *J Occup Environ Med* 39:574-580, 1997.
14. Collins JA, Burrows EA, Willan AR: Occupation and the clinical characteristics of infertile couples, *Can J Public Health* 85:28-32, 1994.
15. Martin JS and others: The pregnancy rates of cohorts of idiopathic infertility couples gives insights into the underlying mechanism of infertility, *Fertil Steril* 64:98-102, 1995.
16. Bisanti L and others: Shift work and subfertility: a European multicenter study. European Study Group on Infertility and Subfertility, *J Occup Environ Med* 38:352-358, 1996.
17. Wildt L and others: Treatment with naltrexone in hypothalamic ovarian failure: induction of ovulation and pregnancy, *Hum Reprod* 8: 350-358, 1993.
18. Jin K and others: Reproductive failure and the major histocompatibility complex, *Am J Hum Genet* 56:1456-1467, 1995.
19. Bitar MS: The role of catecholamines in the etiology of infertility in diabetes mellitus, *Life Sci* 61:65-73, 1997.
20. Lissens W and others: Cystic fibrosis and infertility caused by congenital absence of the vas deferens and related clinical entities, *Hum Reprod* 11(suppl 4):55-78, 1996.
21. Boxer AS: Images of infertility, *Nurse Pract Forum* 7:60-63, 1996.
22. Edmond M, De Braekeleer M: Inbreeding effects on fertility and sterility: a case-control study in Saguenay-Lac-Saint-Jean (Quebec, Canada) based on a population registry 1838-1971, *Ann Hum Biol* 20:545-555, 1993.
23. Spitzer M and others: The fertility of women after cervical laser surgery, *Obstet Gynecol* 86(4 Pt 1):504-508, 1995.
24. Spitz A, Kim ED, Lipshultz LI: Contemporary approach to the male infertility evaluation, *Obstet Gynecol Clin North Am* 27:487-516, 2000.
25. Puttermans P, Ombelet W, Brosens I: Reflections on the way to conduct an investigation of subfertility, *Hum Reprod* 10(suppl 1):80-89, 1995.
26. Guzick DS and others: Infertility evaluation in fertile women: a model for assessing the efficacy of infertility testing, *Hum Reprod* 9: 2306-2310, 1994.
27. Guzick DS: Do infertility tests discriminate between fertile and infertile populations? *Hum Reprod* 10:2008-2009, 1995.
28. Royal College of Obstetricians and Gynaecologists: *The initial investigation and management of the infertile couple,* London, 1998, The College.
29. Institute for Clinical Systems Improvement: *Diagnosis and management of infertility,* Bloomington, MN, 2000 (updated 4/2001), The Institute.
30. Muller HL and others: Gonadal function of young adults after therapy of malignancies during childhood or adolescence, *Eur J Pediatr* 155:763-769, 1996.

31. Mastroianni LJ: Forty years of infertility management: exponential progress and a demanding future, *Nurse Practitioner Forum:* 7:87-91, 1996.
32. Ayres-de-Compos D and others: Inter-observer agreement in analysis of basal body temperature graphs from infertile women, *Hum Reprod* 10:2010-2016, 1995.
33. Atkin SL, Masson EA, White MC: Isolated adrenocorticotropin deficiency presenting as primary infertility, *J Endocrinol Invest* 18:456-459, 1995.
34. Stansberry J: The infertile couple: an overview of pathophysiology and diagnostic evaluation for the primary care provider, *Nurse Pract Forum* 7:76-86, 1996.
35. Moran C and others: Prognosis for fertility analyzing different variables in men and women, *Arch Androl* 36:197-204, 1996.
36. Baird PA: Ethical issues of fertility and reproduction, *Annu Rev Med* 47:107-116, 1996.
37. Paulson RJ, Sauer MV: Counseling the infertile couple: when enough is enough, *Obstet Gynecol* 78(3 pt 1):462-464, 1991.
38. Galletly C and others: A group program for obese, infertile women: weight loss and improved psychological health, *J Psychosom Obstet Gynaecol* 17:125-128, 1996.
39. Balen AH and others: Cumulative conception and live birth rates after the treatment of anovulatory infertility: safety and efficacy of ovulation induction in 200 patients, *Hum Reprod* 9:1563-1570, 1994.
40. Fox R, Ekeroma A, Wardle P: Ovarian response to purified FSH in infertile women with long-standing hypogonadotropic hypogonadism, *Aust N Z J Obstet Gynecol* 37:92-94, 1997.
41. Leyendecker G, Waibel-Treber S, Wildt L: Pulsatile administration of gonadotropin-releasing hormone and oral administration of naltrexone in hypothalamic amenorrhea, *Hum Reprod* 8(Suppl 2):184-188, 1993.
42. Letterie GS and others: Ovulation induction using S.C. pulsatile gonadotropin-releasing hormone: effectiveness of different pulse frequencies, *Hum Reprod* 11:19-22, 1996.
43. Nasir J and others: Spontaneous recovery of chemotherapy-induced primary ovarian failure, *Clin Endocrinol* 46:217-219, 1997.
44. Lobo RA: Unexplained infertility, *J Reprod Med* 38:241-249, 1993.
45. Tanbo T and others: Obstetric outcome in singleton pregnancies after assisted reproduction, *Obstet Gynecol* 86:188-192, 1995.
46. Mo X and others: Clinical studies in the mechanism for acupuncture stimulation of ovulation, *J Tradit Chin Med* 13:115-119, 1993.
47. Koropatnick S, Daniluk J, Pattinson HA: Infertility: a non-event transition, *Fertil Steril* 59:163-171, 1993.
48. van Balen F, Trimbos-Kemper TC: Involuntarily childless couples: their desire to have children and their motives, *J Psychosom Obstet Gynaecol* 16:137-144, 1995.
49. van Balen F, Verdurmen J, Ketting E: Choices and motivations of infertile couples, *Patient Educ Couns* 31:19-27, 1997.
50. van Balen F, Trimbos-Kemper T, Verdurmen J: Perception of diagnosis and openness of patients about infertility, *Patient Educ Couns* 28: 247-252, 1996.
51. Hughes EG, Brennan BG: Does cigarette smoking impair natural or assisted fecundity? *Fertil Steril* 66:679-689, 1996.
52. Bolumar F, Olsen J, Boldsen J: Smoking reduces fecundity: a European multicenter study on infertility and subfecundity. The European Study Group on Infertility and Subfecundity, *Am J Epidemiology* 143: 578-587, 1996.
53. Stovall DW, Guzick DS: Current management of unexplained infertility, *Curr Opin Obstet Gynecol* 5:228-233, 1993.
54. Vandekerckhove P and others: Infertility treatment: from cookery to science. The epidemiology of randomised controlled trials, *Br J Obstet Gynaecol* 100:1005-1036, 1993.
55. Gleicher N and others: The desire for multiple births in couples with infertility problems contraindicates present practice patterns, *Hum Reprod* 10:1079-1084, 1995.
56. Van Balen F, Trimbos-Kemper TC: Factors influencing the well-being of long-term infertile couples, *J Psychosom Obstet Gynaecol* 15:157-164, 1994.
57. Berg BJ, Wilson JF: Patterns of psychological distress in infertile couples, *J Psychosom Obstet Gynaecol* 16:65-78, 1995.
58. van Balen F, Naaktgeboren N, Trimbos-Kemper TC: In vitro fertilization: the expense of treatment, pregnancy, and delivery, *Hum Reprod* 11:95-98, 1996.
59. Jansen RP: Relative infertility: modeling clinical paradoxes, *Fertil Steril* 59:1041-1045, 1993.

CHAPTER 179

Menopause

Mary J. Attardo

DEFINITION/EPIDEMIOLOGY

Menopause is defined as ovarian failure with associated reduction of estrogen production; it is confirmed by a period of 1 year without menses and a follicle-stimulating hormone (FSH) level of greater than 40 mIU/ml.[1] Menopause can be abruptly induced surgically with bilateral oophorectomy. Hysterectomy without oophorectomy results in cessation of menses but not necessarily ovarian failure. Menopause in this case must be measured by FSH levels and associated symptoms.[2]

In 1981 the World Health Organization defined three stages of menopausal status[3]:

Stage I—Premenopause: the reproductive years before menopause

Stage II—Perimenopause: the time period immediately before menopause, when clinical, biologic, and endocrinologic symptoms and signs indicate approaching menopause, until menopause is confirmed

Stage III—Postmenopause: the time from the date considered to be menopause, as determined by 12 months of amenorrhea, throughout the rest of life

The average age of menopause in the United States is 51 years.[1] Based on an average life expectancy of 75 to 83 years, most women will live one third of their life in a postmenopausal state. Heart disease incidence in women increases dramatically after menopause and causes more deaths than breast, uterine, and ovarian cancers combined.[4] Osteoporosis, a condition of metabolic bone mass reduction resulting in increased risk of bone fracture, accelerates in progression at the time of menopause and throughout the postmenopausal years.[5,6] Hot flashes, sleep disturbances, dermal and urogenital changes, menstrual irregularities, dyspareunia, poor concentration, memory difficulties, and mood alterations are often reported in the perimenopausal and postmenopausal stages, provoking women to seek care.

PATHOPHYSIOLOGY

Estrogen deficiency affects many physiologic functions as a result of the vast distribution of estrogen receptors throughout the body. Diminished ovarian function and reduction of ovarian follicle production result in diminished secretion and circulation of estradiol, the principal endogenous form of estrogen in premenopausal women. Ovarian production of progesterone is reduced as well.[7] Estrone, which is produced in adipose tissue from adrenal androstenedione, thus becomes the main source of estrogen after menopause.[8]

Menstrual irregularity is one of the first symptoms that women experience in perimenopause. Some cycles are shortened in association with a shorter follicular phase of 6 to 10 days, which may be followed by a normal duration of the luteal phase. Some cycles become anovulatory and can last 40 to 60 days. It is possible that a woman will fluctuate from the perimenopausal stage back to the premenopause state for some months as menstrual patterns vary from irregular to regular. Menstrual bleeding also changes in perimenopause. Oligomenorrhea (abnormal menstrual periods of more than 30 and even up to 90 days between periods) and hypomenorrhea (regular menses but decreased amount of bleeding) are quite common. Menorrhagia (heavier and/or longer bleeding during a normal menstrual period) and metrorrhagia (bleeding between periods) are less common but can be troubling.[3] As the number of ovarian follicles decrease, the FSH level elevates in an effort to promote increased ovarian function. FSH usually will remain elevated through perimenopause, although levels can be normal despite the presence of menopausal symptoms. Luteinizing hormone may or may not increase during this stage, although it is less reliable as a menopause marker.[3]

Hot flashes and flushes are common during perimenopause and may continue in the menopausal years. It is theorized that estrogen deficiency causes an increase in norepinephrine, thereby stimulating the thermoregulatory center of the hypothalamus.[7] The resultant hot flash or flush presents suddenly as a sensation of intense heat, lasting from 30 seconds to 5 minutes. Associated symptoms include palpitations, nausea, headache, and dizziness. These symptoms can occur during sleep, causing night sweats and sleep disruption.[1] When a pattern of interrupted sleep develops, irritability, fatigue, and a compromised sense of well-being may be experienced.[9]

Genitourinary changes also occur as a result of estrogen deficiency. The vagina contains the highest concentration of estrogen receptors in the female body. During menopause, vaginal mucosa thins, loses rugae, and becomes friable. The vaginal shape becomes narrow and shorter, causing dyspareunia and loss of support for pelvic structures. Vaginal pH increases to 6.5 to 7.5, creating an environment with less resistance to pyogenic organisms. Atrophy occurs at the vulva, labia majora and minora, urethra, trigone of the bladder, and pubococcygeal muscle, often resulting in vulvar pruritis, cystitis, urinary tract infections, and stress incontinence.[7] Prolapses of the uterus, bladder, and rectum occur as a result of lost tone over time. Reduced vaginal secretions produced with sexual arousal can lead to dyspareunia and diminished sexual interest.[10]

Estrogen deficiency also affects the skin and bones. An overall reduction in collagen occurs, resulting in some loss of skin tone. Skin thickness is reduced, and dryness increases. Bone mass loss begins around age 35 years but significantly escalates at the time of menopause. Trabecular bone found at the hip and spine is the most common site of loss associated with estrogen deficiency. A woman may be asymptomatic for many years after menopause before a fracture occurs or an x-ray film reveals extensive bone loss. However, spinal deformity may be observed in the form of height loss and a dowager's hump.

The link between the presence of estrogen and a low incidence of atherosclerosis is not completely understood; however, research suggests that estrogen provides protection from elevations of low-density lipoprotein (LDL) cholesterol, as well as maintenance of higher levels of high-density lipoprotein (HDL) cholesterol.[11] Estrogen may also prevent coronary disease in other ways by reducing the plaque deposition on blood vessel linings and possibly by promoting dilation of the coronary arteries, thereby improving coronary blood flow.[1]

Once the endogenous estrogen supply diminishes, a rise in total cholesterol and LDL, as well as a fall in HDL, commonly occurs. This is not entirely responsible for the increased incidence of coronary heart disease in postmenopausal women, but when it is considered in conjunction with smoking, hypertension, a high-fat diet, obesity, inactivity, or diabetes, coronary artery disease becomes more probable.

CLINICAL PRESENTATION

Women experiencing dysmenorrhea, menorrhagia, hot flashes, or sleep disturbances may seek assistance in managing these discomforts. However, many women during perimenopause do not seek health care, despite symptoms. It is important to ask the woman about menopause status, symptoms she is experiencing, and how she manages them. It is also important to clarify normal vs. abnormal symptoms. Obtaining a thorough health history, family history, medication history (including use of all home remedies and over-the-counter medications), gynecologic history, and sexual history is important to identify risk factors for future disease.

Depression has long been associated with menopause. Several studies support the idea that this may be less related to estrogen deficiency and more related to multiple psychosocial stressors commonly occurring at midlife. Inquiries should be made into the patient's perception of her well-being at this time of social stress and physical change.

Consideration should be made for cultural differences in the meaning of menopause. In cultures that view the primary value of women as being in roles of childbearing and child rearing, menopause can signify an end to a woman's sense of value.[12] In many cultures women care for other family members before they care for themselves. For this reason, women may not seek care for perimenopausal symptoms, losing an opportunity to address health risks.

PHYSICAL EXAMINATION

A complete physical examination is indicated, including height and weight for baseline measures, and inspection of posture for skeletal abnormalities. Thyroid palpation for nodules and cardiac auscultation for heart sounds may uncover asymptomatic abnormalities. A breast examination, pelvic examination, and Papanicolaou's (Pap) test are necessary to evaluate for early signs of gynecologic problems. Abdominal and rectal examinations are important for disease screening. Peripheral vascular palpation and inspection can reveal circulatory deficits, and skin inspection will detect evidence of inflammation or excess sun exposure.

DIAGNOSTICS

In addition to FSH and luteinizing hormone to confirm menopause, diagnostic testing should include a CBC to assess for anemia, which may result from prolonged menorrhagia. A complete chemistry profile, including serum electrolytes, serum glucose, BUN, creatinine, fasting blood sugar, fasting cholesterol (including HDL-LDL ratio and triglycerides), and liver enzymes (including lactate dehydrogenase and alkaline phosphatase), should be obtained, particularly if hormone replacement therapy (HRT) may be considered. A thyroid-stimulating hormone level to exclude hypothyroidism as a cause of menstrual irregularity or other symptoms and urinalysis to detect microscopic hematuria or proteinuria are necessary.[10] Additional screening tests such as mammograms should be ordered in accordance with current recommendations.

For women at risk for osteoporosis, a baseline bone density measurement using dual energy x-ray absorptiometry is necessary to predict the extent of intervention needed to prevent osteoporosis.[5] An ECG may be necessary to exclude cardiac abnormality for women who are experiencing palpitations. If menopause is questionable, an FSH level is recommended if there are symptoms. Pregnancy can be a possibility; therefore pregnancy testing is recommended.[10]

DIFFERENTIAL DIAGNOSIS

Although many somatic changes reported by women in midlife can be attributed to estrogen deficiency, other processes should be considered. Amenorrhea may be related to pregnancy, a thyroid disorder, obstruction of the uterine outflow tract, or polycystic ovaries, whereas the night sweats experienced in menopause may be related to an infectious process. Palpitations may be cardiogenic in origin or related to medications, infection, smoking, caffeine, alcohol, anxiety, anemia, or thyrotoxicosis. Mood disturbances may indicate depression or anxiety and should not be simply attributed to menopause.

MANAGEMENT

The primary care provider should initiate a discussion with the patient to investigate her feelings about menopause, to encourage verbalization of anxieties or concerns, and to dispel any myths or misunderstandings. Choosing the approach for managing midlife symptoms or preventing future disease is a collaborative decision between the primary care provider and the patient. HRT has been commonly prescribed. However, uncertainty remains regarding safety and side effects. Many alternative therapies can be used to

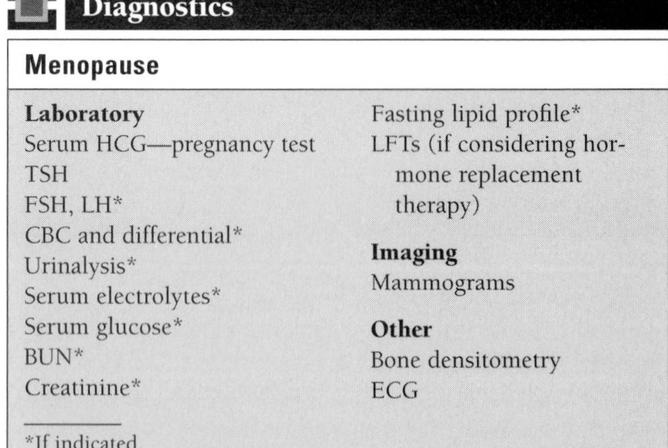

Diagnostics

Menopause

Laboratory	Fasting lipid profile*
Serum HCG—pregnancy test	LFTs (if considering hormone replacement therapy)
TSH	
FSH, LH*	**Imaging**
CBC and differential*	Mammograms
Urinalysis*	
Serum electrolytes*	**Other**
Serum glucose*	Bone densitometry
BUN*	ECG
Creatinine*	

*If indicated.

Differential Diagnosis

Menopause

Amenorrhea	Uterine outflow obstruction
Menstrual irregularity	Hypothalamic dysfunction
Pregnancy	Polycystic kidney disease
Thyroid disorder	Cancer

alleviate individual symptoms. Often a combination of these approaches may be necessary.

Evidence Exists for Benefit

Perimenopausal Oral Contraceptives. For women experiencing perimenopausal menstrual irregularity, use of low-dose oral contraceptives can have multiple benefits. Oral contraceptives help regulate bleeding to a more predictable pattern and reduce heavy bleeding, manage perimenopausal symptoms, and minimize the risk of pregnancy. Research has shown a decreased risk of endometrial and ovarian cancer, benign breast disease, ovarian cysts, and leiomyoma development with the use of oral contraceptives. Before a woman begins taking oral contraceptives during perimenopause, an FSH level should be measured on the third day of the menstrual cycle to assess ovarian function. Pregnancy should be excluded, as it is still a possibility with FSH levels between 20 and 30 mIU/ml. Dosages as low as 0.20 mg of estrogen in oral contraceptives are satisfactory for perimenopause.[12] Oral contraceptives are not recommended for perimenopausal women who have a history of smoking, thromboembolism, hypertension, coronary artery disease, or diabetes, or for those who are obese.[8] Warning signs of complications with oral contraceptives must be reviewed with women despite the lower estrogen dose. Transition to HRT can be discussed when menopause is confirmed. Menopause may be difficult to assess, as withdrawal bleeding will be induced by oral contraceptives. Annual FSH levels measured on the sixth or seventh day of nonhormone use are necessary to determine menopause. Transition to HRT is safe if the FSH level is >40 mIU/ml.[8,13]

Hormone Replacement Therapy. Many preparations and combinations of HRT have been used by perimenopausal and postmenopausal women to relieve discomforts associated with estrogen deficiency. HRT is still appropriate for the short-term management (less than 5 years) of vasomotor symptoms and genitourinary changes associated with menopause. Individual needs, concerns, and risk factors should be considered when choosing a preparation (Table 179-1).

Oral Estrogen and Progestins. Oral estrogen, used for noncontraceptive purposes, is a natural steroidal compound derived from animal sources or created synthetically to mimic estrogen. It differs from estrogen found in oral contraceptives, which is synthetic and nonsteroidal.[8] In premenopausal women endogenous estrogen exists in the potent form of estradiol. At menopause and after menopause, estrone, which is produced in adipose tissue, becomes the most available estrogen. Estriol, which results from the metabolism of estrone, is a weak form of postmenopausal endogenous estrogen.[8] Exogenous oral estrogen preparations are available in similar forms, but once it is absorbed by the intestinal wall, this estrogen is

TABLE 179-1 Hormone Replacement Therapy Regimens

Type of Administration	Hot Flash Management	Treatment of Vaginal Dryness	Prevention of Osteoporosis	Favorable Lipid Effect	Advantages	Disadvantages
Transdermal estradiol (may be considered with smokers, migraines, high triglycerides, hepatic disease, GI problems, or history of thrombophlebitis)	+	+	+	Minimal	Fewer hepatic effects; less accumulation of estrogen in body; no triglyceride rise; fewer headaches	Need progestin delivery for women with uterus; local skin irritation/reaction
Vaginal cream	−	+	−	−	Fewer systemic effects; fewer somatic side effects	Possible endometrial hyperplasia
Vaginal ring	−	+	−	−	Can deliver progestins in same system	Limited data
Continuous estrogen and progestin	+	+	+	+	Easy to follow—no long-term withdrawal bleeding; lower dose of progestin; therefore fewer side effects; possibly less trigger of migraines	Erratic vaginal bleeding for first few months Possible increased risk for breast cancer and cardiovascular disease when used longer than 5 years
Continuous estrogen, cyclic progestin	+	+	+	+	Abnormal bleeding easier to assess; able to adjust timing of progestin to change pattern of bleeding	Higher dose of progestin—more systemic side effects; monthly cyclic withdrawal bleeding
Sequential estrogen and progestin	+	+	+	+	Used for many years in the United States	Monthly cyclic withdrawal bleeding; higher dose of progestin; increased chance of error

+, Therapeutic effect on signs and symptoms; −, no effects on signs and symptoms.

transported to the portal circulation and undergoes a first-pass effect in the liver, where it is converted to estrone sulfate and metabolized.[14]

Commonly used oral estrogens are conjugated equine estrogen (Premarin) 0.625 mg, estropipate (Ogen) 0.625 mg, esterified estrogen (Estratab) 0.625 mg, micronized estradiol (Estrace) 1 mg, ethinyl estradiol (FemHRT) 5 μg, and 17β-estradiol (Activella and Ortho-prefest) 1 mg.[15] These are standard dosages based on results from research studies proving maintenance of bone mass.[8] Unopposed estrogen is taken continuously or in a cyclic manner of 3 weeks of daily use with 1 week of omission per month. Estrogen should be taken at the same time each day and is less likely to cause nausea if taken with food or taken at night. Benefits include management of hot flashes, bone mass protection, and prevention of urogenital symptoms. Unopposed estrogen alone is most effective in the elevation of HDL levels, with reduction of LDL and total cholesterol levels, although an increase in triglycerides may occur. It may also play a role in prevention of memory loss with dementia.[16] Side effects can include nausea, gastrointestinal upset, and temporary breast tenderness in the weeks after initiating use. It also can cause exacerbation of fibroids and endometriosis. Oral estrogens may exacerbate cholelithiasis. Endometrial hyperplasia, which may lead to endometrial cancer, can occur in women who have not had a hysterectomy as a result of the endometrial proliferative effects of unopposed estrogen. This is prevented by adding a progestin in a sufficient dosage and frequency. For this reason, estrogen without opposing progestin should be used only in women who have had a hysterectomy.[17] Research studies have found that estrogen may change the distribution of fat to a more female pattern involving the hips and thighs, but estrogen has not been associated with overall weight gain.[8] Alteration in corneal curvature has been reported with estrogen use and may affect the fit of contact lenses.[8] Although hypertension has been associated with oral contraceptives and with higher dosages of estrogen, it is not considered to be a side effect of HRT.[14]

Commonly used formulations of progestins are medroxyprogesterone acetate (Provera) 2.5 mg or 5 mg, norgestimate (Ortho-prefest) 0.09 mg, and norethindrone acetate (Activella and FemHRT) 0.5 mg or 1 mg.[15] Unfortunately, progestins may cause breast tenderness, abdominal and pelvic cramping, bloating, irritability, anxiety, weight gain, and mood alterations. These symptoms tend to be more severe with higher dosages of progestin; therefore lower dosages are better tolerated. Progestins may limit the lipid benefits achieved with estrogen.

HRT preparations of combined estrogen/progestin are given cyclic or continuously. Cyclic HRT results in predictable withdrawal vaginal bleeding for as long as HRT is used. Continuous HRT produces unpredictable vaginal bleeding in the first several months of use, but all bleeding usually disappears by 1 year of consistent use. Bleeding and spotting associated with HRT can be distressing, especially when it is unpredictable, and is the most common reason for discontinuation of HRT. Women need to understand that this may be expected and will be unpredictable temporarily. Heavy bleeding or prolonged intermittent bleeding after initiation of therapy, or random vaginal bleeding after 6 to 12 months on continuous HRT, warrants evaluation.[8] Transvaginal ultrasound examination to measure endometrial thickness may be indicated. Endometrial biopsy is often necessary to exclude carcinoma.[16]

Transdermal Estradiol. Transdermal estradiol is estrogen provided by a patch placed on the skin. With this delivery system, the first-pass hepatic effect is avoided, resulting in fewer hepatic effects and gastrointestinal symptoms. Transdermal estradiol delivery is constant and is absorbed into the systemic circulation. Lower dosages are used for this reason. Modest improvements have been noted in HDL, LDL, and total cholesterol levels, but no elevations in triglyceride levels occur with transdermal estrogen. Research studies support the benefits of preventing osteoporosis, genitourinary changes, and vasomotor symptoms as being comparable to those seen with oral estrogen.[14] Studies show less estrogen accumulation after cessation of patch use than with oral estrogen. The patch is favorable for women who have hepatic concerns, reduced gastrointestinal absorption, nausea with oral estrogen, or poor symptom control with oral estrogen.[8]

For women with an intact uterus who use transdermal estrogen, an oral progestin can be prescribed for 10 to 12 consecutive days per month. Combi-patch (estradiol/norethindrone acetate) provides both estrogen and progestin in an easy-to-use transdermal patch that is changed twice a week.

Patches are available in estrogen dosages of 0.05 to 0.25 mg/day. Estraderm patches are changed every 3 days and Climara patches are changed weekly. Patches can be applied to intact skin on the abdomen, lower back, buttock, lateral thorax, or upper arm, but never to the breast. Rotating sites with each application prevents damage to the skin. Mild erythema or pruritus is a common side effect. Severe skin reactions can occur, often resulting in discontinuation of use.[8]

Vaginal Estrogen. For treatment of urogenital symptoms only, the application of vaginal cream directly to the vagina is favorable because of its limited systemic absorption and associated side effects. Available preparations are conjugated equine estrogen (Premarin) 0.625 mg/g, estradiol-17β, 0.1 mg/g (Estrace 0.01% vaginal cream), and estropipate (Ogen) 1.5 mg/g. Depending on the preparation, 0.5 to 4 g is applied daily for 4 weeks. The dosage can then be given cyclically—3 weeks on, 1 week off—or reduced to one or two times per week. Routine tapering of the medication is recommended at 3-month intervals. The effect that topical estrogen has on the endometrium is unclear. With projected long-term use of vaginal estrogen, the use of a progestin is currently advised.[8] Although they are still being studied, vaginal rings have been introduced as a source of vaginal estrogen to be used for up to 3 months at a time, but they must be removed for intercourse. A progestin can be used via this delivery system, which may prove to be advantageous.[8]

Raloxifene. Raloxifene, a selective estrogen receptor modulator, is approved for prevention and treatment of osteoporosis. Although it is not approved for treating menopause, it is an option for preventing bone loss when HRT is contraindicated. Because raloxifene may exacerbate hot flashes, it should not be used in women experiencing these symptoms during menopause. Lipid benefits have been proven in research studies that are similar to those of HRT.[18]

Nonpharmacologic Interventions. Habit modifications can be made to alleviate the symptoms of menopause without medication. Limiting caffeine intake can reduce the severity of hot flashes and may relieve some sleep disturbances. Daily exercise can help with improving quality of sleep as well. For vaginal dryness, several water-based lubricants are available to prevent dyspareunia.

Limited Evidence Exists for Benefit

For those who choose not to take HRT, several alternative herbal therapies are available for management of menopausal symptoms, as well as for prevention of complications of estrogen deficiency. However, scientific data about the effectiveness, safety, and long-term effects are lacking, as herbal medications are not regulated by the FDA. Ginseng, in the form of tea, capsules, and powder, has been used to reduce hot flashes and improve concentration, possibly as a result of its estrogen derivative content. This herb should be used cautiously, as high doses can cause hypertension.[12,19] Dong Quai, another Asian root, has been promoted as an agent to reduce hot flashes, insomnia, and irritability. It is not recommended for women who take anticoagulants or have heavy menstruation and fibroids. It has been found to cause breast tenderness.[8] Vitamin E and evening primrose may be helpful to reduce hot flashes.[19] Low doses of black cohosh may also be beneficial.[20] Homeopathy, using a self-healing approach, considers a variety of symptoms and offers several treatment modalities. Acupuncture has also been suggested as a means to manage symptoms.[8] If alternative therapies are chosen, it is important to convey support and regularly inquire about the outcome.

Evidence of Benefit Unclear

Recently, many studies have focused on the use of phytoestrogens for symptom relief and disease prevention, including osteoporosis and estrogen deficiency-related symptoms. Structurally, phytoestrogens resemble 17β-estradiol, thereby having affinity to beta-estrogen receptors. Phytoestrogens may alter circulating endogenous estrogen levels, although this has yet to be proven in studies. Isoflavones are the most common type of phytoestrogen and are primarily found in soy. There appear to be health benefits with increasing dietary intake of isoflavones.[21] A minimum of 6.25 g of soy protein four times a day is necessary for beneficial results.[22] Studies are ongoing with endpoints on several disease processes that may elicit more data regarding indications for soy and other plant-derived estrogens. However, patients should understand that there might be an increased risk of breast cancer and other diseases with the phytoestrogens.

LIFE SPAN CONSIDERATIONS

Lifestyle modifications at midlife are important for promoting health and well-being. Use of alcohol, tobacco, or recreational drugs should be evaluated. Healthy dietary habits and exercise should be encouraged for prevention of osteoporosis, heart disease, and obesity. Health beliefs and wellness practices should be discussed to identify misuse of alternative treatments. With the risk of pregnancy eliminated by menopause, birth control is no longer a concern; however, for women in nonmonogamous relationships, the use of condoms is still important and should be encouraged. The risk of STDs and HIV with unprotected sex is a continuous lifelong potential, regardless of age or menopausal status.

COMPLICATIONS

The relationship of estrogen to the development of breast cancer is still not clear. Estrogen is known to be a promoter for estrogen-dependent tumors; thus it is contraindicated for use in women who have or have had breast cancer. The Nurses Health Study has shown a slight increased risk of breast cancer in women who use HRT for more than 5 years. Although results of other studies focusing on long-term use of HRT have been variable, the Women's Health Initiative results suggest that long-term estrogen/progestin combination therapy could result in increased breast cancer and cardiovascular disease.[8,23] HRT is still indicated short term for vasomotor and urogenital symptoms associated with menopause, but they should not be used for more than 5 years. HRT is no longer the drug regimen of choice to prevent osteoporosis. Ongoing studies may yield more definitive results to assist in helping to understand this risk. It has been postulated that the effect of HRT use is similar to the increased risk for breast cancer associated with a late menopause onset. After discontinuation of HRT, any increased risk of breast cancer essentially disappears. HRT does not increase recurrence rate or mortality rate from breast cancer. In fact, HRT users are more likely to be diagnosed with localized vs. advanced disease. Individual risk must be considered when evaluating candidacy for HRT.[15,16] Consideration of other medications for bone loss (e.g., bisphosphonates, calcium, vitamin D) and vasomotor symptoms (venlafaxine) should be explored with the patient.

Absolute contraindications to use of HRT include a history of or the presence of breast cancer, a history of advanced endometrial cancer, undiagnosed vaginal bleeding, a recent myocardial infarction or cerebrovascular accident, acute liver disease, a history of thromboembolic disease, and pregnancy.[16,24] Recent reevaluation of prior studies reveals what may be an increased risk of cardiac events in the first year of use by women with preexisting coronary artery disease. That risk reduces significantly after the first year of use of HRT. This suggests that there may be an early thrombogenic effect followed by a later antiatherogenic effect by HRT,[16] and studies are ongoing to study this effect. Deep vein thrombosis (DVT) and pulmonary emboli occur at a slight increased frequency shortly after initiating HRT, especially in smokers. Efforts should be made to caution patients who smoke or have prolonged immobility because of injury or lengthy air travel to prevent DVT. This increased risk of DVT dissipates within the first year after initiating HRT. Precautions for HRT use include pancreatitis, migraine headaches, gallbladder disease, elevated liver enzymes, smoking, excessive alcohol intake, use with psychotropic drugs, uterine fibroids, endometriosis, diabetes, and a significant family history of breast cancer. Research supports no increased risk with use of estrogen in stage I, grade I endometrial cancer. Postmenopausal bleeding must be evaluated and carcinoma excluded before a woman may begin HRT.[8]

INDICATIONS FOR REFERRAL/HOSPITALIZATION

Women who have little or no relief of symptoms may need evaluation by a gynecologist or endocrinologist. Patients with clinical depression should be referred for psychiatric evaluation and treatment to minimize risk of chronic depression or self-harm. Collaboration with an oncologist is recommended for women with a history of breast cancer or advanced endometrial cancer.

PATIENT AND FAMILY EDUCATION

Menopause teaching is most beneficial if it is started before perimenopausal symptoms begin.

Teaching points should include:

- Cotton clothing worn in layers can give more comfort while hot flashes occur.
- Sleep may be improved by keeping consistent rising and retiring times, exercising early in the day, and planning quiet, relaxing activities for the evening. Sedatives should be avoided.
- Vaginal dryness can be less problematic if intercourse occurs regularly and more time is allowed for foreplay. Water-based lubricants can be helpful.
- It is common, not unusual, for women to feel overwhelmed with the psychosocial and physical changes of midlife. Reinforcement that these symptoms are normal is necessary.
- Kegel exercises should be done daily to maintain tone and support of the bladder and vagina.
- Recommended calcium intake during perimenopause is 1000 mg/day. After menopause 1500 mg/day is recommended.
- Detailed explanation of the risks and benefits of HRT and a review of expected symptoms vs. abnormal symptoms are needed.
- Pregnancy prevention is important until menopause is confirmed.
- Menopause does not mean that youth, attractiveness, sexuality, and purpose are lost.
- Recommended web sites for reliable information: www.ama-assn.org:80; www.fore.org; www.drweil.com (herbal and vitamin information); www.mayo.ivi.com; and www.eatright.com (diet and exercise information).
- Another source of information is the American Menopause Foundation, Empire State Building, Suite 2822, 350 Fifth Avenue, New York, NY 10118; (212) 714-2398.

HEALTH PROMOTION

A sense of investing in future health to preserve the quality of life should be conveyed. Smoking cessation, limited intake of caffeine and alcohol, and regular exercise can reduce triggers of hot flashes and sleep disturbances. Maintenance of normal blood pressure, a low-cholesterol diet, and regular aerobic exercise will help to prevent cardiac disease. Adequate calcium intake, regular exercise, smoking cessation, and limited intake of caffeine and alcohol will help to prevent osteoporosis. Annual mammograms and Pap tests are needed.

REFERENCES

1. Milonig V: Menopause: health promotion opportunities, *AAOHN J* 44(12):585-594, 1996.
2. Youngkin E, Davis M: *Women's health: a primary care clinical guide,* Norwalk, 1994, Appleton & Lange.
3. Li S and others: Perspectives on menopause, *Clin Nurse Spec* 9(3): 145-148, 1995.
4. American Heart Association: *Heart and stroke facts: 1995 statistical supplement,* Dallas, 1995, The Association.
5. National Osteoporosis Foundation: *Osteoporos Rep* 13(1), 1997.
6. Drugay M: Breaking the silence, *J Gerontol Nurs* 23(6):36-43, 1997.
7. McKeon V: Hormone replacement therapy: evaluating the risks and benefits, *JOGNN* 23(8):647-656, 1994.
8. Lichtman R: Perimenopausal and postmenopausal HRT, part 2, *J Nurse Midwifery* 41(1):3-23, 1996.
9. Clark AJ and others: Sleep disturbances in midlife women, *J Adv Nurs* 22(3):562-568, 1995.
10. Hawkins J, Roberto-Nichols D: *Protocols for the nurse practitioner in gynecologic settings,* ed 5, New York, 1995, Tiresias Press.
11. King K, Kerr J: Evolution of hormone replacement therapy as a treatment and prophylaxis for coronary artery disease, *J Adv Nurs* 23(5):984-991, 1996.
12. Jones J: Embodied meaning: menopause and the change of life, *Soc Work Health Care* 19(3/4):43-65, 1994.
13. Bachman G: The change before the change, *Postgrad Med* 95(4): 113-121, 1994.
14. National Osteoporosis Foundation: *Osteoporos Clin Updates* 1(6), 1997.
15. Mattox, JH, Schulman LP: Combined oral hormone replacement therapy formulation, *Am J Obstet Gynecol* 185(2 Suppl):S38-46, 2001.
16. Burkman RT, Collin JA, Greene RA: Current perspectives on benefits and risks of hormone replacement therapy, *Am J Obstet Gynecol* 185 (2 Suppl):S13-23, 2001.
17. The Writing Group for the PEPI Trial Effects of Estrogen or Estrogen/Progestin Regimens on Heart Disease Risk Factors in Postmenopausal Women: The Postmenopausal Estrogen/Progestin Interventions (PEPI) trial, *JAMA* 273:199-208, 1995.
18. Gafs M, Taylor M: Alternatives for women through menopause, *Am J Obstet Gynecol* 185:S47-56, 2001.
19. Wasaha S, Angelopoulos F: What every woman should know, *Am J Nurs* 96(1):25-32, 1996.
20. Peters S: Menopause: a new era, *Adv Nurse Pract* 6(7):61-64, 1998.
21. Tham DM, Gardner CD, Haskell WL: Potential health benefits of dietary phytoestrogen: a review of clinical, epidemiological and mechanistic evidence, *J Clin Endocrinol Metab* 83(7):2223-2235, 1998.
22. Henkel J: Soy. Health claim for soy protein, questions about other components, *FDA Consumer* 34(3):13-15, 18-20, 2000.
23. Writing Group for the Women's Health Initiative Investigators: Risks and benefits of estrogen plus progestin in healthy postmenopausal women: principal results from the Women's Health Initiative randomized controlled trial, *JAMA* 288:321-333, 2002.
24. Scura K, Whipple B: How to provide better care for the postmenopausal woman, *Am J Nurs* 97(4):36-43, 1997.

CHAPTER 180

Pap Smear Abnormalities

Updated by Joanne Sandberg-Cook

DEFINITION/EPIDEMIOLOGY

The Papanicolaou (Pap) test is a screening test that uses cytologic examination of exfoliated cells to detect cervical cancer and precursor lesions. Use of the Pap smear has resulted in a significant decrease in deaths from cervical cancer by identifying localized and precursor lesions, which can then be treated. The 5-year survival rate for localized cervical cancer is approximately 90%, whereas it is only 14% for women with advanced disease (stage IV).[1] The Pap smear is not sufficient for evaluating grossly abnormal lesions of the cervix; these lesions must undergo a biopsy for a definitive diagnosis to be made.

The Bethesda System, which was revised in 2001 (Box 180-1), is widely used to report Pap smear results.[2] This classification system attempts to use clear and concise terminology to assist in the management of women with abnormal Pap smears. It includes a statement of specimen adequacy, general categorization, and interpretation/results.

Cervical cancer is the most common cancer in women worldwide. Recent estimates indicate that 14,500 new cases of and 4800 deaths due to cervical cancer will occur yearly.[3] The median age of cervical cancer diagnosis is 54 years, although the range extends from the adolescent years into the 90s.[4] Each year approximately 600,000 women are diagnosed with premalignant changes that are referred to as *squamous intraepithelial lesions* (SILs). An estimated 3% to 10% of all women undergoing Pap smears are given the diagnosis of ASC-US (atypical squamous cells of undetermined significance).[5]

Risk factors for cervical cancer include infection with certain types of human papillomavirus (HPV), a history of multiple sex partners, early age of first intercourse (<18 years), exposure to cigarette smoke, HIV infection, low socioeconomic status, and poor nutrition.[6,7] Exposure to diethylstilbestrol (DES)—a hormonal therapy that was used from the 1940s until the early 1970s to prevent spontaneous abortion and preterm labor—in utero increases the risk for cervical adenocarcinoma. Women exposed to DES in utero should have Pap smears, including vaginal smears, every 6 months and should be monitored in conjunction with a gynecologist for periodic colposcopy.

PATHOPHYSIOLOGY

The uterine cervix is composed of two distinct epithelial cell types: squamous and columnar. The squamous cells line the distal ectocervix and vagina. Columnar cells line the endocervical canal and the proximal ectocervix. The approximately circular line on the ectocervix where the two cell types meet is called the *squamocolumnar junction*. At puberty, hormonal changes initiate the transformation of the distal columnar epithelia into squamous cells; this process is referred to as *squamous metaplasia*. The transformation zone is the area in which

BOX 180-1

THE 2001 BETHESDA SYSTEM (ABRIDGED)

ADEQUACY OF SPECIMEN

Satisfactory for evaluation (note presence/absence of endocervical/transformation zone component)

Unsatisfactory for evaluation (specify reason)

GENERAL CATEGORIZATION

Negative for intraepithelial lesion or malignancy

Epithelial cell abnormality

Other

INTERPRETATION/RESULT

Negative for Intraepithelial Lesion or Malignancy

Includes findings of the following:

- Trichomonas, bacterial, viral, and fungal organisms
- Nonneoplastic changes, including reactive cellular changes associated with inflammation, radiation, and IUD; glandular cells (posthysterectomy); and atrophy

Epithelial Cell Abnormalities

Squamous cell

- Atypical squamous cells of undetermined significance (ASC-US) cannot exclude high-grade squamous intraepithelial lesion (ASC-H)
- Low-grade squamous intraepithelial lesion (LSILs) encompassing human papillomavirus (HPV), mild dysplasia, cervical intraepithelial neoplasia (CIN) 1
- High-grade squamous intraepithelial lesions (HSILs) encompassing moderate and severe dysplasia, carcinoma in situ, CIN 2 and CIN 3
- Squamous cell carcinoma

Glandular cell

- Atypical glandular cells (AGC)
  - Endocervical
  - Endometrial
  - Not otherwise specified
- Atypical glandular cells, favor neoplastic
  - Endocervical
  - Not otherwise specified
- Endocervical adenocarcinoma in situ (AIS)
- Adenocarcinoma
  - Endocervical
  - Endometrial
  - Extrauterine
  - Not otherwise specified

Other (list not comprehensive)

Endometrial cells in a woman >40 years of age

Modified from Solomon D and others: The 2001 Bethesda System: terminology for reporting results of cervical cytology, *JAMA* 287:2114-2119, 2002.

squamous metaplasia occurs and is the site of most squamous cell abnormalities.

There is clear evidence that sexually transmitted carcinogens are associated with the development of cervical cancer and SILs. The viral DNA of HPV has been found to be integrated into the cellular genomes of approximately 95% of invasive cervical cancers, although direct causation has yet to be demonstrated.[4] Certain viral types of HPV are considered to be high risk for causing invasive disease, particularly types 16, 18, 45, and 46; types 31, 33, 35, 51, and 52 have been identified in approximately 15% of cancerous lesions.[8] Additional sexually transmitted factors may have a co-causative role.

SILs may persist, spontaneously regress, or advance to invasive disease. Concurrent HIV infection is associated with a more aggressive disease course.

MANAGEMENT

The management of abnormal Pap smears can be approached using the following guidelines. Treatment decisions must take the patient's individual risk factors and ability to follow-up into consideration. Routine follow-up implies repeat Pap smears appropriate to the patient's history and findings. For women with no history of abnormal results, a low-risk profile, and at least three prior negative smears, routine follow-up is every 2 to 3 years.[9] Women with an increased risk should have yearly Pap smears. Women with previous epithelial abnormalities should have a yearly screening after initial treatment and surveillance. Patients with HIV infection should have Pap smears every 6 months for the first year and then annually if all previous smears have been normal.[7] HIV-positive patients with a history of HPV infection, previous Pap smears with epithelial cell abnormalities, or symptomatic HIV disease should have Pap smears every 6 months.[7] Women ages 65 or older with no history of abnormal results and three prior negative smears can discontinue testing, provided they do not have continued risk factors for developing cervical cancer (e.g., multiple sex partners, HIV infection). Follow-up guidelines are presented in Box 180-2.

BOX 180-2

FOLLOW-UP GUIDELINES FOR A PAP SMEAR

MANAGEMENT OF ATYPICAL SQUAMOUS CELLS OF UNDETERMINED SIGNIFICANCE (ASC-US)

Negative results: Repeat screening at 12 months

ASC-US: Repeat screening in 6 months

Two consecutive negative results: Routine screening in 12 months

ASC-US on two repeat tests: Refer for colposcopy or DNA testing for high risk types of human papillomavirus (HPV)

MANAGEMENT OF ASC-H

Low-grade squamous intraepithelial lesions (LSILs), high-grade squamous intraepithelial lesions (HSILs), and atypical glandular cells: Refer for colposcopy

Modified from ASCCP 2001 consensus guidelines for the management of women with cervical cytological abnormalities, *JAMA* 287:2120-2129, 2002.

INDICATIONS FOR REFERRAL/HOSPITALIZATION

Patients with low-grade squamous intraepithelial lesions (LSILs), high-grade epithelial lesions (HSILs), carcinoma in situ, or squamous cell carcinoma should be referred to a gynecologist for colposcopy, endocervical curettage, or intrauterine biopsy.

PATIENT AND FAMILY EDUCATION

Patients who receive an abnormal Pap smear result deserve accurate and complete information regarding their diagnosis and expected course of evaluation and treatment. The Pap smear is often referred to as the "test for cervical cancer"; therefore anticipatory guidance at the time of the Pap smear regarding possible results other than cancer can greatly facilitate patient comprehension when the result is abnormal. Information needs to be given to allay a woman's fear of cancer, and primary care providers need to provide assistance in dealing with the feelings of uncertainty that such a result can cause. Providing patients with information regarding the optimal timing of and preparation for a Pap smear can help minimize the number of additional studies needed and therefore lessen patient anxiety. These strategies include collection of the Pap smear at midcycle (if the patient still menstruates), avoidance of intercourse for 24 hours before the test, and avoidance of intravaginal preparations for 48 hours before the test.

Education must include information recommending decreased exposure to cigarette smoke, the use of barrier contraception with spermicide to decrease the chance of exposure to HPV, and immune system enhancement. The immune system benefits from adequate sleep; balanced nutrition, including adequate intake of carotene, vitamins C and E, and folate; limited exposure to alcohol and drugs; and stress reduction. Providing patients with this information can help them to cope with the abnormal Pap smear result well after they are initially notified.

REFERENCES

1. US Preventive Services Task Force: Screening for cervical cancer. In *Guide to clinical preventive services*, ed 2, Washington, DC, 1996, US Department of Health and Human Services.
2. Solomon D and others: The 2001 Bethesda System: terminology for reporting results of cervical cytology, *JAMA* 287:2114-2119, 2002
3. Parker SL and others: Cancer statistics, *CA Cancer J Clin* 47:5-27, 1997.
4. Cox JT and others: Human papillomavirus testing by hybrid capture appears to be useful in triaging women with a cytologic diagnosis of atypical squamous cells of undetermined significance, *Am J Obstet Gynecol* 172:946-954, 1995.
5. Wertheim I, Soto-Wright VJ, Goodman HM: Gynecologic cancers. In Carlson KJ, Eisenstadt SA, editors: *Primary care of women*, St Louis, 1995, Mosby.
6. Schafer A and others: The increased frequency of cervical dysplasia-neoplasia in women with the human immunodeficiency virus is related to the degree of immunosuppression, *Am J Obstet Gynecol* 164:593-599, 1991.
7. El-Sadr W and others: *Evaluation and management of early HIV infection: clinical practice guideline*, no 7, Rockville, MD, 1994, Agency for Health Care Policy and Research, publication No. 94-0572.
8. The Task Force on HPV and Other STDs of the American College Health Association: *Genital human papillomavirus disease*, Baltimore, 1997, The Association.
9. Wright TC and others. ASCCP 2001 consensus guidelines for the management of women with cervical cytological abnormalities, *JAMA* 287:2120-2129, 2002.

CHAPTER 181

Pelvic Inflammatory Disease

Updated by Joanne Sandberg-Cook

DEFINITION/EPIDEMIOLOGY

Pelvic inflammatory disease (PID) refers to a spectrum of inflammatory disorders of the upper genital tract in women. It can include any combination of endometritis, salpingitis, tubo-ovarian abscess (TOA), and pelvic peritonitis.

Although PID is not a reportable disease, it is estimated that there are approximately 1 million cases of PID annually in the United States.[1] Hospitalizations for PID have continued to decline since the early 1980s, but the number of initial office visits for the evaluation and treatment of PID has remained relatively constant.[2] Risk factors for PID include age younger than 25, multiple sexual partners, no current use of contraception, and living in an area with a high prevalence of sexually transmitted diseases (STDs). There is a strong correlation between the incidence of STDs and PID in any given population. Other risk factors for PID include penetration of the cervical mucus barrier during medical procedures, including the insertion of an intrauterine contraceptive device (IUD), and vaginal douching. A woman's risk for PID is decreased if she uses barrier contraception, takes oral contraceptives, or has had a tubal sterilization.

The risk of PID in young women is significant; 75% of all cases of PID occur in women under the age of 25.[1] Contact with multiple sexual partners and inconsistent use of contraception can account for the increased incidence of STDs in women younger than 25, although it does not fully account for the increased incidence of PID. Younger women with chlamydial infections of the cervix have a higher incidence of upper genital tract infection than do older women.[1]

Previous diagnosis of PID is a risk factor for subsequent episodes, with approximately 15% to 25% of all women with PID experiencing more than one episode.[1] These subsequent infections are generally new, primary attacks of PID, not flares of latent or chronic infection.[1] Reinfection is often related to contact with untreated sexual partners.

PATHOPHYSIOLOGY

PID is usually a polymicrobial infection, caused by organisms that ascend from the vagina and cervix along the mucosa of the endometrium to infect the mucosa of the fallopian tubes. The most common organisms implicated in PID include *Neisseria gonorrhoeae* and *Chlamydia trachomatis;* however, microorganisms that can be part of the normal vaginal flora (e.g., anaerobes, *Gardnerella vaginalis, Haemophilus influenzae,* enteric gram-negative rods, and *Streptococcus agalactiae*) can also cause PID.[3] *Mycoplasma hominis* and *Ureaplasma urealyticum* are also possible etiologic agents.[3] The mildest form of salpingitis involves tubal hyperemia, edema of the tubal wall, and exudate on the tubal surface and fimbriated ends.[4] If salpingitis is left untreated, further inflammatory changes of the pelvic organs occur, including tubal adhesions, pyosalpinx, or TOA.

The Fitz-Hugh–Curtis syndrome (FHCS) involves perihepatic inflammation that is due to the transperitoneal, lymphatic, or vascular spread of *N. gonorrhoeae* or *C. trachomatis.* There is inflammation of the liver capsule without parenchymal involvement.[4] FHCS develops in 5% to 10% of women with PID.[1] Chronic FHCS is characterized by adhesions between the anterior liver surface and the parietal peritoneum beneath the diaphragm. The treatment is the same as for PID.

The increased incidence of PID in young women may be explained by a larger cervical squamocolumnar junction, allowing for easier colonization with *N. gonorrhoeae* or *C. trachomatis,* and by a decreased antibody response.[1] However, PID is uncommon in pregnancy because of the physiologic changes in the uterus. The uterotubal junction is closed as early as the seventh week of gestation, and the chorioamnion covers the endocervix around the twelfth to fifteenth week. An ascending infection before the twelfth week often leads to endometritis and spontaneous abortion. After the twelfth week, it results primarily in chorioamnionitis.

Very rarely, PID can result from secondary extension of infection of adjacent organs, as in appendicitis or diverticulitis. It may also result from hematogenous dissemination of tuberculosis or as a rare complication of a tropical disease such as schistosomiasis. The following discussion refers only to ascending infections resulting in PID.

CLINICAL PRESENTATION

The clinical presentation of PID varies widely. Although some women are truly asymptomatic, others remain undiagnosed because of their mild or nonspecific signs and symptoms. These can include abnormal vaginal bleeding, dyspareunia, and vaginal discharge. Lower abdominal and pelvic pain of less than 2 weeks' duration is the most common presenting symptoms. It is usually described as dull and constant and is worsened by movement and sexual intercourse. The onset of symptoms occurs most commonly in the first half of the menstrual cycle. Complaints of fever or abnormal vaginal discharge may also be present.

Women with FHCS present with right upper quadrant pain, pleuritic pain, and tenderness with liver palpation. These symptoms are often mistaken for cholecystitis or pneumonia.

PHYSICAL EXAMINATION

According to the Centers for Disease Control and Prevention (CDC), the following three clinical criteria for PID must be met before antibiotic therapy can be initiated: (1) lower abdominal tenderness, (2) adnexal tenderness, and (3) cervical motion tenderness. In addition, no other cause for the illness should be evident (e.g., diverticulitis, ectopic pregnancy, or appendicitis).

DIAGNOSTICS

The diagnosis of PID is imprecise; the clinical diagnosis of symptomatic PID has a positive predictive value for salpingitis of 65% to 90% of what is predicted with laparoscopy.[3] A pregnancy test should be obtained immediately to assess for the possibility of ectopic pregnancy, although a negative result is not conclusive. Pelvic ultrasound evaluation is indicated when TOA is suspected. Additional studies to consider include syphilis (rapid plasma reagin [RPR]) and HIV serologies.

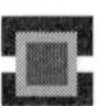

Diagnostics

Pelvic Inflammatory Disease

Laboratory
Serum hCG
CBC and differential
ESR
Laboratory confirmation of cervical infection with *Neisseria gonorrhoeae* or *Chlamydia trachomatis*
RPR (to exclude concurrent syphilis infection)
HIV serology*

Imaging
Pelvic ultrasound

Other
Laparoscopy

*If indicated.

An accurate diagnosis of PID is difficult, given the wide variation in symptoms on presentation. However, the potential damage to the reproductive health of women with even mild or atypical PID is well documented.[3] Diagnosis and management of other causes of lower abdominal pain are unlikely to be affected by the initiation of empiric therapy for PID.

DIFFERENTIAL DIAGNOSIS

The most important conditions in the differential diagnosis for PID are ectopic pregnancy, acute appendicitis, ovarian torsion, and ovarian cyst. Other conditions to consider include endometriosis, corpus luteum bleeding, pelvic adhesions, benign ovarian tumor, irritable bowel syndrome, diverticulitis, pyelonephritis, and cystitis.

MANAGEMENT

Treatment regimens for PID must provide empiric, broad-spectrum antimicrobial coverage, including anaerobic coverage. No single antibiotic agent is adequate; thus combination therapy is necessary. In choosing a therapy, the provider should consider availability, cost, patient acceptance, and antimicrobial susceptibility. The CDC provides periodic treatment recommendations for PID and other STDs.

Oral and parenteral therapy for PID is outlined in Box 181-1.[3] Patients receiving oral therapy should be reevaluated within 72 hours. Clinical improvement is indicated by defervescence, reduction in direct or rebound abdominal tenderness, and reduction in uterine, adnexal, and cervical motion tenderness. If significant clinical improvement is not seen within 72 hours after initiating therapy, the patient should be reevaluated to confirm the diagnosis and receive parenteral therapy and/or surgical intervention. Patients should be tested for cure of infection with *C. trachomatis* and *N. gonorrhoeae* 4 to 6 weeks after the completion of therapy.

Patients receiving parenteral therapy should show substantial improvement within 72 hours after therapy is initiated. Those who do not receive parenteral therapy usually require further diagnostic evaluation and/or surgical intervention.

Treatment of sexual partners of women with PID is imperative because of the risk for re-infection of the patient and the high incidence of urethral gonococcal or chlamydial infections in the male sexual partner. Sexual partners who had sexual contact with the patient during the 60 days preceding the onset of symptoms should be treated empirically with regimens effective against *C. trachomatis* and *N. gonorrhoeae*, regardless of the apparent etiology of PID or pathogens isolated from the patient.[3] Sexual abstinence should be recommended until both partners have completed treatment.

Differential Diagnosis

Pelvic Inflammatory Disease

Ectopic pregnancy	Pelvic adhesion
Acute appendicitis	Benign ovarian tumor
Ovarian torsion	Irritable bowel syndrome
Ovarian cyst	Diverticulitis
Endometriosis	Pyelonephritis
Corpus luteum bleeding	Cystitis

COMPLICATIONS

Sequelae of PID include a significantly increased risk of tubal factor infertility, ectopic pregnancy, and chronic pelvic pain. There are a small number of deaths annually that are the result of a ruptured TOA. Furthermore, the duration, severity, and number of episodes of PID are proportional to the prevalence of long-term sequelae.

INDICATIONS FOR REFERRAL/HOSPITALIZATION

Referral for hospitalization of the patient with PID is indicated if:

- Surgical emergencies, such as appendicitis or ectopic pregnancy, cannot be excluded.
- The patient is pregnant.
- The patient has failed to respond clinically to outpatient therapy.
- The patient is unable to follow or tolerate an outpatient regimen.
- The patient has severe illness, nausea and vomiting, or a high fever.
- The patient has a TOA.
- The patient is immunodeficient (i.e., HIV-positive with a low CD4 count or is receiving immunosuppressive therapy).

In early observational studies, HIV-infected women with PID were more likely to require surgical intervention.[3] A subsequent and more comprehensive study showed that despite a more severe clinical presentation, HIV-infected women with PID responded equally well to standard parenteral therapies.[3]

Gynecologic or surgical consultation is indicated when the diagnosis is unclear. Unilateral pelvic pain or a mass is a strong indication for laparoscopy.

PATIENT AND FAMILY EDUCATION

Patient education is an extremely important component in the treatment of the woman with PID. It must include clear information regarding the diagnosis, including transmission and sequelae. The need for completion of therapy regardless of symptoms, timely follow-up, and partner treatment cannot be overemphasized. It is also helpful to encourage the patient in appropriate medical care–seeking behavior, including seeking care immediately when symptoms recur. The behaviors that increase the risk of PID also increase the risk for HIV infection. Referral for HIV testing and counseling is recommended. Finally, information regarding prevention of future infections must be reviewed and repeated at all follow-up visits.

BOX 181-1

ORAL AND PARENTERAL THERAPY FOR PELVIC INFLAMMATORY DISEASE

PARENTERAL REGIMEN A

Cefotetan 2 g IV every 12 hours
OR
Cefoxitin 2 g IV every 6 hours
PLUS
Doxycycline 100 mg orally or IV every 12 hours

NOTE: Because of pain associated with infusion, doxycycline should be administered orally when possible, even when the patient is hospitalized. Both oral and IV administration of doxycycline provide similar bioavailability.

Parenteral therapy may be discontinued 24 hours after a patient improves clinically, and oral therapy with doxycycline (100 mg b.i.d.) should continue to complete 14 days of therapy. When tubo-ovarian abscess is present, many health care providers use clindamycin or metronidazole with doxycycline for continued therapy rather than doxycycline alone because it provides more effective anaerobic coverage.

PARENTERAL REGIMEN B

Clindamycin 900 mg IV every 8 hours
PLUS
Gentamicin loading dose IV or IM (2 mg/kg of body weight) followed by a maintenance dose (1.5 mg/kg) every 8 hours. Single daily dosing may be substituted.

NOTE: Parental therapy can be discontinued 24 hours after a patient improves clinically; continuing oral therapy should consist of doxycycline 100 mg PO b.i.d. or clindamycin 450 mg PO q.i.d. to complete a total of 14 days of therapy. When tubo-ovarian abscess is present, clindamycin may be preferable to doxycycline because clindamycin provides more anaerobic coverage.

ALTERNATIVE PARENTAL REGIMENS

Ofloxacin 400 mg IV every 12 hours
OR
Levofloxacin 500 mg IV q.d.
WITH OR WITHOUT
Metronidazole 500 mg IV every 8 hours
OR
Ampicillin-sulbactam 3 g IV every 6 hours
PLUS
Doxycycline 100 mg orally or IV every 12 hours.

NOTE: Preliminary data suggest that levofloxacin is as effective as ofloxacin and may be substituted; its single daily dosing makes it advantageous from a compliance perspective. Ampicillin-sulbactam plus doxycycline has good coverage against *C. trachomatis, N. gonorrhoeae,* and anaerobes and is effective for patients who have tubo-ovarian abscess.

ORAL TREATMENT

Regimen A

Ofloxacin 400 mg orally b.i.d. for 14 days
OR
Levofloxacin 500 mg orally q.d. for 14 days
WITH or WITHOUT
Metronidazole 500 mg orally b.i.d. for 14 days

Regimen B

Ceftriaxone 250 mg IM in a single dose
OR
Cefoxitin 2 g IM in a single dose and probenecid 1 g orally administered concurrently in a single dose
OR
Other parenteral third-generation cephalosporin (e.g., ceftizoxime or cefotaxime)
PLUS
Doxycycline 100 mg orally b.i.d. for 14 days
PLUS
Metronidazole 500 mg orally b.i.d. for 14 days

NOTE: The optimal choice of a cephalosporin for Regimen B is unclear; although cefoxitin has better anaerobic coverage, ceftriaxone has better coverage against *N. gonorrheae.* Clinical trials have demonstrated that a single dose of cefoxitin is effective in obtaining short-term clinical response in women who have PID; however, the theoretical limitations in its coverage of anaerobes may require the addition of metronidazole to the treatment regimen. The metronidazole also will effectively treat bacterial vaginosis, which is often associated with PID.

ALTERNATIVE ORAL REGIMENS

There are data to suggest that amoxicillin-clavulanic acid plus doxycycline is effective in obtaining short-term clinical response; however, gastrointestinal symptoms might limit compliance with this regimen. Azithromycin has been evaluated in the treatment of upper reproductive tract infections; however, data are insufficient to recommend this agent as a component of any of the oral treatment regimens for PID.

From the Centers for Disease Control and Prevention: Sexually transmitted diseases treatment guidelines—2002, *MMWR* 51(RR06):1-80, 2002.

REFERENCES

1. Mishell DR and others: *Comprehensive gynecology,* ed 3, St Louis, 1997, Mosby.
2. Centers for Disease Control and Prevention, Division of STD Prevention: *Sexually transmitted disease surveillance, 1994,* Atlanta, Sept 1995, US Department of Health and Human Services, Public Health Service.
3. Centers for Disease Control and Prevention: Sexually transmitted diseases treatment guidelines 2002, *MMWR* 51(RR-6):1-78, 2002.
4. Soper DE: Pelvic inflammatory disease. In Rock JA and others, editors: *Advances in obstetrics and gynecology,* vol 1, St Louis, 1994, Mosby.

CHAPTER 182

Periconception Care

Debra Hobbins

DEFINITION/EPIDEMIOLOGY

Periconception care has been proposed as an innovative and preventive strategy of identifying and modifying risks or behaviors through appropriate education, management, or referral to reduce reproductive risks before conception, improve the mother's long-term health, and decrease rates of infant morbidity and mortality.[1,2] It is estimated that 40% to 60% of all births are unintended at conception, with 95% of pregnancies in teenagers unplanned. These numbers emphasize the need to incorporate preconception health practices into health education and counseling of all women of reproductive age and in whatever settings they may present.[3-7] The critical phase of organogenesis occurs during days 17 to 56 after conception—before most women know they are pregnant.[8] Optimal prenatal care is initiated through periconception care.

Traditionally, women's health care has been segmented, with childbearing separated from the overall health promotion and management of chronic health issues. Pregnancy has been viewed as a discrete event, with little relationship to a woman's health before or after. Periconception care recognizes the links between childbearing and women's health across the life span.[9]

PARTNER INVOLVEMENT

Partner involvement in preconception counseling contributes to the emotional well-being of the couple; it is important for family, genetic, and psychosocial histories; and it provides an opportunity to educate the woman and her partner equally about the potential influences of their lifestyle and health status on a future pregnancy.[10,11] Smoking and alcohol use by the father are implicated in low birth weight and subfertility. Advanced paternal age is associated with new, single-gene mutations such as neurofibromatosis. Paternal chemical or substance exposures may contribute to adverse reproductive outcomes and affect the maternal environment, contributing to subfertility and spontaneous abortion.[12] Partner promiscuity, IV drug use, or bisexuality puts the woman and fetus at risk for all sexually transmitted diseases.[1,13,14]

HEALTH ASSESSMENT: HISTORY

Advanced maternal age is becoming more common. Women older than 35 years are at increased risk of the following:[15]

- Subfertility due to medical illness
- Premature menopause
- Anovulation and endometriosis
- Chromosome abnormalities
- Chronic illness
- Pregnancy complications such as gestational diabetes, hypertension, and placental abnormalities
- Cesarean section
- Fetal death

Teen-aged mothers have an increased risk of low-birth-weight infants, preterm infants, and infants who die before 1 year of age.[16]

All individuals are estimated to carry five to seven lethal recessive genes.[17] Preconception education regarding genetic conditions provides the couple with information for understanding the opportunities for antenatal diagnosis, its limitations, and the risks involved. The couple can use this information to consider their reproductive options and to make knowledge-based decisions about the reproductive risks they are willing to take or whether they should avoid a pregnancy.[1,18] Questioning all couples about personal or family histories of birth defects, mental retardation, consanguinuity, and genetic diseases is critical.[5,18] Ethnic background is emerging as an indication for genetic screening[1,10,16] (Box 182-1).

Housing, home environment, family and social support, and safety need to be addressed. It is estimated that 17% to 37% of pregnant women experience domestic abuse; this abuse is more common than gestational diabetes, hypertension, and birth defects.[19] Victims of domestic abuse are at increased risk for placental separation; perinatal hemorrhage; rupture of the uterus, liver, or spleen; and preterm birth.[10] Screening for domestic violence must be incorporated into a routine history (see Chapter 21).[20] Cultural and extended family issues surrounding childbearing deserve exploration and may alert the primary care provider to potential marital problems, parenting issues, beliefs of grandparents, and influences that may affect the woman's psychosocial status.

Fetal alcohol syndrome is more prevalent than both Down's syndrome and spina bifida and is the leading cause of mental retardation. Because alcohol is a known teratogen and no amount has been proved safe, many primary care providers advocate alcohol abstinence during attempts for conception and during pregnancy.[10,16] Alcohol use is associated with stillbirth, low birth weight, and spontaneous abortion. Smoking, the leading preventable cause of low birth weight, increases the risk of spontaneous abortion, preterm labor, upper respiratory infections in infants, and deaths from sudden infant death syndrome (SIDS). Limiting caffeine to 300 mg/day (the amount in 2 cups of coffee, 15 cups of cocoa, or two 32-ounce cola drinks) is recommended.[10]

Recreational and IV drug use carries an overall increased risk of nutritional deficiencies. Marijuana use may contribute to low birth weight, preterm birth, and congenital malformations.[1,7] Cocaine or crack use can lead to placental abruption, preterm birth, intrauterine growth restriction, congenital malformations, and dysfunction of the central nervous system in newborns; heroin or methadone use can cause neonatal withdrawal syndrome.[1,7,11,21] In addition, IV drug use increases the risks for infection with HIV, hepatitis viruses B and C, and skin abscesses.[11,16]

Employment and financial concerns need to be discussed at preconception. Long work hours, work-related stress, strenuous physical work, and prolonged standing contribute to preterm births.[22] Ascertaining the nature of employment provides clues about exposure to environmental toxins and work hazards. Pregnancy and childbirth are often the first major medical expenses that parents incur, and these costs are often underestimated. It is critical that the primary care provider

BOX 182-1

PERICONCEPTION HEALTH ASSESSMENT: HISTORY

DEMOGRAPHICS

Age <15 or >35 years

FAMILY HISTORY

Birth defects
Mental retardation
Hemoglobinopathies
Cystic fibrosis
Tay-Sachs disease
Duchenne's muscular dystrophy
Fragile X syndrome
Hemophilia
Phenylketonuria
Sickle cell disease
Consanguinity

ETHNIC BACKGROUND: CARRIER TESTING

Sickle cell anemia: African, African-American, Middle Eastern, Indo-Pakistani, Latino, Mediterranean
Tay-Sachs disease: Ashkenazi Jew, French Canadian, Cajun
Cystic fibrosis: Caucasian
Alpha-thalassemia: African, Southeast Asian, Filipino
Beta-thalassemia: African, Mediterranean, Southeast Asian, Indo-Pakistani, Asian, African-American

SOCIAL HISTORY

Housing
Home environment/safety
Family/social support
Cultural beliefs/issues
Alcohol/tobacco
Recreational/IV drugs
Caffeine
Life stresses
Financial concerns
Employment

NUTRITION HISTORY

Weight for height
Diet and supplements
Anorexia/bulimia/pica
Exercise
Folic acid
Vitamin D

MEDICAL HISTORY

Diabetes
Seizure disorder
Asthma
Recurrent urinary tract infections/renal disease
Anemia
Tuberculosis
Thyroid disease
Systemic lupus erythematosus/autoimmune disease
Chronic hypertension
Thromboembolic disease
Heart disease
Pulmonary hypertension
Marfan's syndrome
Surgery/trauma/cancer

INFECTIOUS DISEASE HISTORY

Immunization status
Rubella/proven immunity
Varicella-zoster
Tuberculosis
Human parvovirus B19 (fifth disease)
Cytomegalovirus
Toxoplasmosis/outdoor cat
Hepatitis C (particularly IV drug users)

Sexually Transmitted Infections

Human papillomavirus
Chlamydia
Gonorrhea
Syphilis
Herpes simplex virus
Hepatitis B
HIV/AIDS

ENVIRONMENTAL EXPOSURES

Hyperthermia
Home: Oven cleaners, paint, bleach, wood finishing items
Work: Pesticides, cytotoxics, heavy metals, gases, solvents, radiation, vibrating machines

REPRODUCTIVE HISTORY

Menstrual dysfunction
Contraceptive method
Uterine malformations
Cervical abnormality
Diethylstilbestrol (DES) exposure
Pelvic infections
Subfertility
Prior fetal losses
NICU/neonatal death
Birth-related complications
Cesarean section
Gestational diabetes
Preeclampsia
Previous child with birth defect
Birth of child <5.5 or >9 pounds
Preterm birth

MEDICATION HISTORY

Prescription Teratogens

Gold
Lithium
Isotretinoin (Accutane)
Etretinate (Tegison)
Phenytoin
Divalproex sodium (Depakote)
Carbamazepine
Trimethadione
Phenobarbital
Primidone
Warfarin (Coumadin)
Cytotoxics
Androgenic steroids
Angiotensin-converting enzyme (ACE) inhibitors

Over-the-Counter Teratogens

Vitamin A >10,000 IU/day
Aspirin
Ibuprofen

initiate dialogue regarding childbearing costs and the need to investigate insurance coverage and family leave policies.[1,10,11] The provider should also determine underweight or overweight status, eating disorders, pica, and vegetarian eating habits. Neural tube defects occur in the first 17 to 30 days after conception.[23] Obesity at conception is linked to an increased risk of neural tube defects, independent of folic acid intake; women who are underweight at conception are at an increased risk for a preterm birth.[5,24,25] All women capable of becoming pregnant should consume 0.4 mg/day of folic acid to reduce the risk of neural tube defects and orofacial clefts in offspring.[26-28] It has been suggested that women who are

BOX 182-2

PERICONCEPTION HEALTH ASSESSMENT: PHYSICAL EXAMINATION AND LABORATORY TESTS

PHYSICAL EXAMINATION

In All Patients

Height
Weight
Blood pressure
Pulse
Thyroid examination
Cardiac examination
Respiratory examination
Breast examination
Pelvic examination
Pelvimetry

As Indicated

Ophthalmoscopic
Neurologic
Lower extremities

LABORATORY TESTS

In All Patients

Blood type, Rh factor
Antibody titer (direct Coombs' test)
Hemoglobin/hematocrit
Rubella titer
Syphilis
Dipstick or urinalysis
Culture and sensitivity (asymptomatic bacteriuria)
Papanicolaou's (Pap) test
Chlamydia
Gonorrhea
Wet mount of vaginal discharge (bacterial vaginosis)
Hepatitis B surface antigen
HIV

As Indicated

Tuberculosis (PPD)
Genetic testing
Hemoglobin electrophoresis
Drug screen
Toxoplasma titer
Cytomegalovirus titer
Varicella-zoster titer
Herpes simplex
Toxicology screen
Lead level
Drug screen
Thyroid function studies
HbA_{1C}
Hepatitis C Ab

young, unmarried, and obese; who smoke and eat few fruits and vegetables; or who have a low level of education be targeted for this intervention.[23] Folic acid is now added to all enriched cereal grain products.[29] Folic acid supplements provide greater elevation in serum folate levels than dietary food intake.[30] Supplements of elemental iron, 30 to 60 mg/day, are appropriate for women with anemia.[31] Prenatal vitamins are often prescribed at periconception because of the difficulty of determining a patient's nutritional status, but their routine use is not recommended.[32,33] However, recent research suggests that periconception ingestion of folic acid–containing multivitamin supplements reduces the occurrence of the first neural tube defect, urinary tract and cardiovascular congenital abnormalities, and congenital limb deficiencies more than does folic acid alone.[34] Exercise is to be encouraged as a part of wellness care.

In a woman with significant medical problems, the potential risk to the woman and her fetus is assessed (see Box 182-1). This is especially necessary if the woman's life expectancy could be markedly reduced by pregnancy or if the fetus could have a high likelihood of complications. Maternal conditions that pose risk include hypertension, Marfan syndrome, cardiomyopathy, renal insufficiency, and coarctation of the aorta.[10] Diabetic teratogenesis is related to first-trimester hyperglycemia.[35] Women with diabetes need to be educated about the importance of developing and continuing good general health practices and optimal glycemic control before conception and throughout pregnancy. Glycosylated hemoglobin is an excellent marker of glycemic control for the prior 6 weeks. Because only one third of women with diabetes seek preconception care, contraceptive management and preconception counseling should occur at each visit.[36-38] Other chronic illnesses need to be under control before conception[10,11,14] (see Box 182-1). Exposure or immunity to infectious diseases, including sexually transmitted diseases, needs to be investigated; strategies to treat these diseases and/or to minimize the risks should be discussed with the couple[3,10,11,39] (Box 182-2; see also Box 182-1). Preconception toxic exposures may result in infertility, spontaneous abortions, or congenital malformations in offspring. The toxic, mutagenic, teratogenic, and carcinogenic effects may not become apparent until childhood or adulthood in the form of behavioral disorders and neoplasms.[40]

Hyperthermia and temperatures of greater than 38.9° C (102° F), during the first weeks of pregnancy have been associated with neural tube defects.[14] Factors that have contributed to previous poor pregnancy outcomes or that could affect future pregnancies and may be amenable to intervention are identified before conception[41] (see Box 182-1). A list of both prescription and over-the-counter drugs, including homeopathic remedies, should be obtained from the couple. Couples must be informed about medications with teratogenic potential (see Box 182-1) to enable them to plan carefully for pregnancy. The woman may be able to modify, substitute, or eliminate these drugs before conception.[39]

Periconception care seeks to improve health outcomes for the mother and her infant by identifying risks, providing education to facilitate knowledge-based decision making, and instituting appropriate interventions (Box 182-3). Periconception care emphasizes good health care for all women. The current expectation is that in each "routine visit" with a primary care provider, periconception care is provided in some form to every woman capable of conceiving and documented in the medical record.[42,43] A comprehensive approach also includes community-based initiatives.[44] Most infants are born healthy, but fetal, neonatal, and maternal complications can occur under the best of circumstances. Periconception care does not guarantee a good pregnancy outcome, but it does assist families in maximizing resources and minimizing risk.

BOX 182-3

PERICONCEPTION COUNSELING INTERVENTIONS

EDUCATION

Menstrual cycle and calendar
Fertile period/sexuality
Plans for childbearing
Family planning methods
Discontinuing method
Intercourse frequency/timing
Subfertility evaluation if no conception after 12 months (or 6 months if >37 years)
Control of chronic illness
Risk factors for sexually transmitted diseases, pelvic inflammatory disease
Lifestyle/employment risks
Substance abuse risks
Environmental exposures
Healthy diet
Health insurance, benefits, family leave policies
Partner/family/social support
Hyperthermia risks

LIFESTYLE CHANGES

Smoking cessation
Elimination of alcohol, illicit drugs
Limiting of caffeine to 300 mg/day
Limiting of over-the-counter medications
Folic acid 0.4 mg/day (supplement)
Prenatal vitamins and vitamin D as indicated
Calcium supplement 1200 mg/day
Iron 30-60 mg/day
Regular exercise 15-30 minutes, interspersed with rest, water
Avoidance of hot tub/sauna
Treatment of fever

IMMUNIZATION INFORMATION

MMR, varicella, polio: Contraindicated in pregnancy; contraception should be avoided for 3 months after immunization
Td: Not contraindicated; booster q 10 years
Hepatitis B: If indicated

POSSIBLE REFERRAL

Genetic counseling
Nutrition counseling to attain appropriate weight or if an eating disorder is present
WIC
Cooperative extension services
Management of chronic illness
Substance abuse counseling
Substitution/elimination of teratogenic medications
Specialists as indicated
Dentist
Laboratory studies
Domestic violence assistance or counseling
Financial/medical assistance

REFERENCES

1. Cefalo RC, Bowes WA, Moos MK: Preconception care: a means of prevention, *Baillieres Clin Obstet Gynaecol* 9:403-416, 1995.
2. Schrander-Stumpel C: Preconception care: challenge of the new millennium? *Am J Med Genet* 89;58-61, 1999.
3. State-specific pregnancy and birth rates among teenagers—United States, 1991—1992, *MMWR Morb Mortal Wkly Rep* 44:676-684, 1995.
4. Institute of Medicine: *The well-being of children and families*, Washington, DC, 1995, National Academy Press.
5. American Academy of Pediatrics and The American College of Obstetricians and Gynecologists: *Guidelines for perinatal care*, ed 4, Elk Grove Village, IL, 1997, The Academy.
6. Adams MM and others: Pregnancy planning and pre-conception counseling: the PRAMS Working Group, *Obstet Gynecol* 82:955-959, 1993.
7. Morrow CE: Preventive care in pregnancy, *Prim Care* 22:775-784, 1995.
8. Leavitt C: Preconception health promotion, *Prim Care* 20:537-549, 1993.
9. Walker LO, Tinkle MB: Toward an integrative science of women's health, *J Obstet Gynecol Neonatal Nurs* 25:379-382, 1996.
10. Cheng D: Preconception health care for the primary care practitioner, *Md Med J* 45:297-304, 1996.
11. Swan LL, Apgar B: Preconceptual obstetric risk assessment and health promotion, *Am Fam Physician* 51:1875-1885, 1995.
12. Frazier LM, Jones TL: Managing patients with concerns about workplace reproductive hazards, *J Am Med Womens Assoc* 55:80-83, 105, 2000.
13. Summers L, Price RA: Preconception care: an opportunity to maximize health in pregnancy, *J Nurse Midwifery* 38:188-198, 1993.
14. Olsen ME: Preconception evaluation and intervention, *South Med J* 87:639-645, 1994.
15. van Montfrans JM and others: Are elevated concentrations in the preconceptional period a risk factor for Down's syndrome pregnancies? *Hum Reprod* 16:1270-1273, 2001.
16. Leuzzi RA, Scoles KS: Preconception counseling for the primary care physician, *Med Clin North Am* 80:337-369, 1996.
17. Vogel F, Jotulsky AG: *Human genetics*, ed 3, New York, 1995, Springer.
18. Eng CM and others: Prenatal genetic carrier testing using triple disease screening, *JAMA* 278:1268-1272, 1997.
19. McFarlane J and others: Assessing for abuse during pregnancy, *JAMA* 267:3176-3178, 1992.
20. American Medical Association, Council on Scientific Affairs: Violence against women: relevance for medical practitioners, *JAMA* 267: 3184-3189, 1992.
21. American College of Obstetricians and Gynecologists: *Exercise during pregnancy and the postpartum period;* technical bulletin No. 189, Washington, DC, 1994, The College.
22. Luke B and others: The association between occupational factors and preterm birth: a United States Nurses Study, *Am J Obstet Gynecol* 173:849-862, 1995.
23. Centers for Disease Control and Prevention: Knowledge and use of folic acid among women of reproductive age—Michigan, 1998, *MMWR Morb Mortal Wkly Rep* 50(10): 185-9, 2001.
24. Werler MM and others: Prepregnant weight in relation to risk of neural tube defects, *JAMA* 275:1089-1092, 1996.
25. Siega-Riz AM, Adair LS, Hobel CJ: Maternal underweight status and inadequate rate of weight gain during the third trimester of pregnancy increases the risk of preterm delivery, *J Nutr* 126:146-153, 1996.
26. U.S. Preventive Services Task Force: *Guide to clinical preventive services: report of the U.S. Preventive Services Task Force*, ed 2, Baltimore, 1996, Williams & Wilkins.
27. Hurren C and others: Folic acid and prevention of neural-tube defects, *Lancet* 350:664, 1997.
28. Shaw GM and others: Risks of orofacial clefts in children born to women using multivitamin-containing folic acid periconceptionally, *Lancet* 346:393-396, 1995.
29. Centers for Disease Control and Prevention: Knowledge and use of folic acid by women of childbearing age: United States 1997, *MMWR Morbid Mortal Wkly Rep* 46:721-723, 1997.
30. Elkin AC, Higham J: Folic acid supplements are more effective than increasing dietary folate intake in elevating serum folate levels, *Br J Obstet Gynecol* 107(2):285-9, 2000.

31. Freightner JW: *Routine iron supplementation during pregnancy: the Canadian guide to clinical preventive health care,* Ottawa, 1994, Publications Canada, The Canadian Task Force on the Periodic Health Examination.
32. Kolasa KM, Weismiller DG: Nutrition during pregnancy, *Am Fam Physician* 56:205-212, 1995.
33. Yu SM and others: Preconceptional and prenatal multivitamin mineral supplement use in the 1988 National Maternal and Infant Health Study, *Am J Public Health* 86:240-242, 1996.
34. Czeizel AE: Primary prevention of neural-tube defects and some other major congenital abnormalities: recommendations for the appropriate use of folic acid during pregnancy, *Paediatr Drugs* 2:437-439, 2000.
35. Rodgers BD, Rodgers DE: Efficacy of preconception care of diabetic women in a community setting, *J Reprod Med* 41:422-426, 1996.
36. Janz NK and others: Diabetes and pregnancy, *Diabetes Care* 18: 157-165, 1995.
37. American Diabetes Association: Preconception care of women with diabetes, *Diabetes Care* 20(suppl 11):840-843, 1997.
38. Holing EV: Preconception care of women with diabetes: the unrevealed obstacles, *J Matern Fetal Med* 9:10-13, 2000.
39. Centers for Disease Control and Prevention: US Public Health Service recommendation for human immunodeficiency virus counseling and voluntary testing for pregnant women, *MMWR Morbid Mortal Wkly Rep* 44:RR-7, 1995.
40. Berkowitz GS, Marcus M: Occupational exposures and reproduction. In Lee RV, editor: *Current obstetric medicine,* St Louis, 1993, Mosby.
41. Cefalo KC, Moos MK: *Preconceptional health care: a practical guide,* ed 2, St Louis, 1995, Mosby.
42. Morrison EH: Preconception care, *Prim Care* 27:1-12, 2000.
43. Bernstein PS, Sanghvi T, Merkatz IR: Improving preconception care, *J Reprod Med* 45:546-552, 2000.
44. Stanford JB, Hobbins D: Obstetric risk assessment, section A: preconception risk assessment. In Ratcliffe SD and others, editors: *Family practice obstetrics,* ed 2, Philadelphia, 2001, Hanley & Belfus.

CHAPTER 183

Sexual Dysfunction

Cynthia M. Williams

DEFINITION/EPIDEMIOLOGY

Human sexual expression is complex and changes throughout the life cycle. It is strongly influenced by culturally defined roles, religious beliefs, and the physical and emotional health of the individual.[1] Sexual dysfunction has no singular explanation; it is influenced by both internal and external forces. However, a useful definition for sexual dysfunction is any sexual behavior or problem that makes sexual expression difficult or constantly dissatisfying to the individual or partner.[2]

A recent consensus development conference on female sexual dysfunction (FSD) further classified the sexual dysfunction into four major categories (1) sexual desire disorders that include hypoactive sexual desire and sexual aversion, (2) sexual arousal disorder, (3) orgasmic disorder, and (4) sexual pain disorders, including dysparunia, vaginismus, and noncoital sexual pain.[3]

Sexual problems probably exist in one form or another throughout a woman's life. For many reasons, including their own attitudes and beliefs, personal comfort, experience, and knowledge, health professionals are reluctant to make inquiries into the sexual health of their patients.[4,5] The epidemiologic studies of FSD are few and flawed. In a recent analysis of the National Health and Social Life Survey the prevalence of sexual dysfunction was found to be 43% for women younger than 60 years.[6] Poor physical and emotional health and negative sexual experiences and overall well-being greatly influenced FSD.[6] FSD is associated with many of the same disease processes that are associated with male erectile dysfunction, including aging, hypertension, atherosclerotic disease, cigarette smoking, and pelvic operations.[3] The most commonly encountered sexual concerns range from painful intercourse, misinformation, psychosexual dysfunction, failure to achieve orgasm, extramarital sex, and organic sexual dysfunction to sexual abuse to sexual preference concerns.[7]

PATHOPHYSIOLOGY

Insight into sexual problems and dysfunction depends on an understanding of the human sexual response cycle.[8] The *sexual response cycle* includes the desire, arousal (vascular), orgasm (muscular), and resolution (in men) phases. Desire is the factor that initiates the overall sexual response cycle. Others have stressed the need for a different model to explain the sexual response cycle in women.[9] The classic sexual response model first defined by Masters and Johnson may not fully explain the underpinnings of a woman's sexual health to include a lower biologic urge to be sexual for release of sexual tension; the motivation, or "drive," to be sexual may be tied to nonsexual gains or rewards; sexual arousal is a subjective mental excitement; and, finally, orgasmic release of sexual tension may or may not occur in every sexual encounter. An understanding of sexual dysfunction should recognize that any of the above may overlap in a positive or negative manner and affect further sexual encounters.

Several etiologies should be considered in the evaluation of FSD. Vasculogenic impotence in men may be analogous to clitoral and vaginal vascular insufficiency in women. Spinal cord injury or any diseases of the central or peripheral nervous system can result in neurogenic FSD, especially as it concerns lubrication and orgasm. Any dysfunction of the hypothalamic-pituitary axis from either surgical or medical castration, natural menopause, premature ovarian failure, or chronic birth control use can result in hormonally based FSD. Finally, psychogenic origins, whether in the presence or absence of organic disease, can lead to FSD. This also includes medications used to treat depression, especially the selective serotonin reuptake inhibitors (SSRIs).[10,11]

CLINICAL PRESENTATION

The sexual history is an important component of care, but neither patients nor primary care providers should be forced to discuss sexuality.[4,5] Providers need to be comfortable with their own sexuality and willing to discuss the subject. An open, understanding, nonjudgmental attitude and a willingness to explore sexual health will allow the patient to discuss sexuality concerns.

A brief sexual history should include the gynecologic history, sexual activity, number of partners, homosexual/heterosexual relationships, difficult or abusive sexual experiences, and satisfaction with sexual experiences. Problems with desire, arousal, lubrication, orgasm, pain, bleeding, or lesions; sexually transmitted disease (STD) exposure; and the need for contraception should also be reviewed. In addition, exploration of recent life events (e.g., divorce, separation, or recent losses) and cultural attitudes toward sexual activity should be considered. Because medications can affect all phases of the sexual cycle, a drug review is imperative.

When a sexual problem is elicited, the history should include a detailed description of symptoms, as well as the onset, course, patient's perception of the disorder, past medical history, and past treatments and outcomes. It is also important to determine the patient's expectations and goals for treatment.

PHYSICAL EXAMINATION

A complete physical examination is indicated, with particular attention to the genitourinary, vascular, and neurologic systems. The examination should determine the presence of galactorrhea and nipple erection; vulvar lesions, anomalies, or tenderness; labial thickness or thickening; and any notable rectocele or cystocele. The clitoris, hymen, vagina, and cervix should be examined for signs of infection, injury, atrophy, adhesions, or discharge. Gentle squeezing will allow evaluation of the bulbocavernosus reflex, which demonstrates integrity of the S2 to S4 sacral nerves, part of the neurologic foundation of the sexual response cycle. A bimanual examination is necessary to palpate the vagina, cervix, uterus, and adnexa. Vaginal muscle tone can be evaluated by having the patient squeeze the examiner's fingers and may indicate vaginismus.

DIAGNOSTICS

Specific laboratory tests are indicated for physiologic phase disorders, although no one battery of tests is recommended.[4,5] Diagnostic studies are guided by the history and physical examination and may include cultures, a thyroid panel, CBC, hormonal studies, serum corticosteroids, fasting blood sugar (FBS), and renal and liver function studies. Screening for depression may also be indicated.

DIFFERENTIAL DIAGNOSIS

Psychosocial difficulties; depression; posttraumatic stress disorder (PTSD); hormonal imbalance; thyroid, adrenal, liver, and kidney disorders; diabetes; infection; injury; substance abuse; arterial insufficiency; and neurologic disease or injury should be considered in the differential diagnosis. In addition, many common diseases and medications can affect sexual functioning (Table 183-1).[4]

MANAGEMENT

The management of FSD can be frustrating for both the woman and her clinician. Recently the Food and Drug Administration (FDA) approved a vacuum therapy device to enhance clitoral engorgement.[12] The Clitoral Therapy Device (EROS-CTD) was effective, especially in postmenopausal women, in increasing genital sensation and lubrication, achieving orgasm, and improving overall sexual satisfaction. More research is needed to evaluate long-term and prophylactic use of this device.

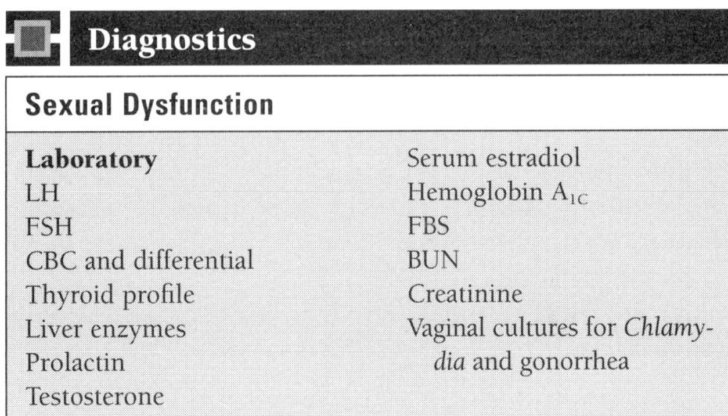

Diagnostics

Sexual Dysfunction

Laboratory	Serum estradiol
LH	Hemoglobin A_{1C}
FSH	FBS
CBC and differential	BUN
Thyroid profile	Creatinine
Liver enzymes	Vaginal cultures for *Chlamydia* and gonorrhea
Prolactin	
Testosterone	

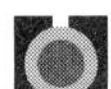

Differential Diagnosis

Sexual Dysfunction

Diseases and Other Factors That Affect Sexual Function
- Diabetes
- Thyroid disease
- Coronary artery disease
- Congestive heart failure
- Vascular disease
- Dementia
- Chronic obstructive pulmonary disease

Psychologic Factors That Decrease Libido
- Depression
- Anxiety
- Posttraumatic stress disorder
- Fatigue

Conditions That Cause Painful or Uncomfortable Intercourse
- Inadequate vaginal lubrication
- Introital dyspareunia
- Scarring
- Thick or intact hymen
- Vaginismus
- Clitoral hyperstimulation
- Endometriosis
- Ovarian cysts
- Arthritis
- Psychogenic pain from previous trauma

TABLE 183-1 Common Medications Causing Sexual Dysfunction

Class of Drugs	Example
Antihypertensives	Thiazide diuretics, clonidine, methyldopa, captopril, beta blockers
Antidepressants	Amitriptyline, imipramine, trazodone, monoamine oxidase inhibitors, selective serotonin reuptake inhibitors
Hormonal agents	Estrogen, progesterone
Anticholinergics	Atropine, hydroxyzine
H_2-receptor antagonists	Cimetidine
Antipsychotics	Chlorpromazine, thiothixene, haloperidol
Sedatives	Alcohol, barbiturates
Anxiolytics	Valium

Not all complaints of FSD are psychologic, but the clinical and basic science of the study of FSD is in its infancy. There are currently no FDA-approved medication therapies, but many medications used for the treatment of male erectile dysfunction are being used in clinical protocols with women.[10]

Estrogen replacement therapy can improve clitoral sensitivity, increase libido, and decrease painful intercourse. In addition, local or topical estrogens (estrogen vaginal cream and the vaginal estradiol ring) can relieve symptoms of vaginal dryness, burning, and urinary frequency and urgency.

Methyl testosterone has been used in postmenopausal women for symptoms ranging from lack of desire to lack of vaginal lubrication. Potential benefits of therapy included increases in clitoral sensitivity, vaginal lubrication, libido, and arousal. The potential side effects of weight gain, clitoral enlargement, increased facial hair, and hypercholesterolemia may outweigh the benefits.

Sildenafil (Viagra), a selective type V phosphodiesterase inhibitor, appears to improve both subjective and physiologic parameters in a small study of women who were administered Sildenafil.[13] Sildenafil also appears to benefit women with SSRI-precipitated sexual dysfunction.[14]

Phentolamine (Vasomax), an alpha-adrenergic blocker that causes vascular smooth muscle relaxation has been studied in men. A small pilot study in menopausal women with sexual arousal disorder noted an improvement in lubrication and pleasurable sensations in the vagina.[15]

COMPLICATIONS

Many sexual concerns involve pregnancy issues. Methods of contraception may influence a woman's sexual response and cause problems or dysfunction. Hormonal contraception may affect desire, libido, or performance, although many women discover enhanced sexuality, knowing pregnancy is unlikely. For women desiring pregnancy, the stress and timing of intercourse may interfere adversely with both pleasure and communication.

INDICATIONS FOR REFERRAL/HOSPITALIZATION

Many sexual concerns and dysfunctions can be treated with good anticipatory guidance and education about sexuality and sexual health. With other patients, the underlying medical condition is treated. For those who may require extensive general or sex therapy, referral to a reputable certified sex therapist is warranted. In addition, if available evaluation in a women's sexual health clinic may allow for a better elucidation of the problem, validate the individual, and lead to a more comprehensive treatment approach.[10]

PATIENT AND FAMILY EDUCATION/HEALTH PROMOTION

The opportunity to explore sexual concerns through an open dialogue is the most therapeutic approach. Education should be directed toward understanding normal sexual response and the stages associated with the sexual response cycle. The importance of diet, exercise, and adequate sleep cannot be overstated because stress and fatigue are significant co-factors that affect sexual desire. Promoting cholesterol reduction, tobacco cessation, and blood pressure and glycemic control may go a long way in the prevention of potential vasculogenic causes of FSD.

The following resources can assist patients with sexual dysfunction:

- Barbach L: *For yourself: fulfillment of female sexuality,* New York, 2000, Signet.
- Berman JL: *For women only: a revolutionary guide to overcoming sexual dysfunction and reclaiming your sex life,* New York, 2001, Henry Holt & Co.
- Butler R: *Love and sex after sixty,* New York, 1993, Ballantine.
- Kaplan HS: *The illustrated manual of sex therapy,* New York, 1988, Brunner/Mazel.
- Zilbergeld B: *The new male sexuality,* New York, 1999, Doubleday.
- American Association of Sex Educators, Counselors and Therapists (AASECT) website: http//:www.aasect.org.
- American Psychological Association website http//:www.apa.org.
- Kinsey Institute for Research in Sex, Gender, and Reproduction website http//:www.indiana.edu/~kinsey.

REFERENCES

1. Bullard DG, Caplan H: Sexual problems. In Feldman MD, Christensen JF, editors: *Behavioral medicine in primary care,* Stamford, Conn, 1997, Appleton & Lange.
2. Klingman EW: Office evaluation of sexual function and complaints, *Clin Geriatr Med* 7:15-39, 1991.
3. Basson R and others: Report of the international consensus development conference on female sexual dysfunction: definitions and classifications, *J Urol* 163:888-893, 2000.
4. Phillips NA: Female sexual dysfunction: evaluation and treatment, *Am Fam Physician* 62;127-136, 141-142, 2000.
5. MacLaren A: Primary care for women: comprehensive sexual health assessment, *J Nurse Midwifery* 40:104-119, 1995.
6. Laumann EO, Paik A, Rosen RC: Sexual dysfunction in the United States: prevalence and predictors, *JAMA* 281:537-544, 1999.
7. Driscoll CE: Assisting patients with sexual problems. In Taylor RB, editor: *Family medicine,* New York, 1994, Springer-Verlag.
8. Berman JR, Goldstein I: Female sexual dysfunction, *Urol Clin North Am* 28:405-415, 2001.
9. Basson R: The female sexual response: a different model, *J Sex Marital Ther* 26:51-65, 2000.
10. Berman JR, Berman L, Goldstein I: Female sexual dysfunction: incidence, pathophysiology, evaluation and treatment options, *Urology* 54:385-391, 1999.

11. Gitlin MJ: Psychotropic medications and their effects on sexual function: diagnosis, biology, and treatment approaches, *J Clin Psychiatr* 55:406-413, 1994.
12. Billups KL and others: A new non-pharmacological vacuum therapy for female sexual dysfunction, *J Sex Marital Ther* 27: 435-441, 2001.
13. Berman JR and others: Effect of sildenafil on subjective and physiologic parameters of the female sexual response in women with sexual arousal disorder, *J Sex Marital Ther* 27:411-420, 2001.
14. Rosen RC, Lane RM, Menza M: Effects of SSRI on sexual dysfunction: a critical review, *J Clin Psychopharmacol* 19:67-85, 1999.
15. Rosen R and others: Oral phentolamine and female sexual arousal disorder: a pilot study, *J Sex Marital Ther* 25:137-144, 1999.

CHAPTER 184

Unplanned Pregnancy

Leslie J. Collins; Updated by Patricia Polgar Bailey

A positive pregnancy test can generate a variety of responses. For some patients, the news brings joy and excitement; for others, the news can be a crisis of varying proportion. Although many personal and socioeconomic factors may affect a woman's individual reaction, one common denominator is ensured—the woman's life is changed.

Although the use of contraceptives is widespread, one study found that only 51% to 63% of adults discuss contraception with a health care provider.[1] Moreover, a majority of pregnancies in the United States are unplanned.[2]

The primary care provider is often the patient's first confidante in the first few minutes surrounding the news of an unplanned pregnancy and is in a unique position to assist her in meeting her total health and wellness needs. For women for whom the pregnancy represents a crisis, several types of reactions can occur.

An unplanned pregnancy is a situation in which the response of the primary care provider is critical to establishing and maintaining an environment that feels safe and supportive to the patient. The initial role of the provider is to listen; both verbal and nonverbal communications provide information that is useful in developing the care plan. The patient needs to be allowed time to express her feelings.

After the patient has expressed herself, the primary care provider can assist with prioritizing the patient's concerns and needs by focusing on one issue at a time. By exhibiting a willingness to listen and help, the provider helps to build the patient's confidence. An exploration of the patient's feelings about pregnancy, the child, abortion, and abortion alternatives provides an opportunity to further process the situation. It is also helpful for the provider to know if the patient has previously experienced an unplanned pregnancy or if she knows anyone who has dealt with an unplanned pregnancy and the decision to either have an abortion, raise the child, or surrender the child for adoption. A critical piece of information concerns the woman's support system and the role of the child's father in the woman's life and in the decisions about this pregnancy. Although patients seek a rapid solution to the crisis of an unplanned pregnancy, the provider should encourage the patient to take the time necessary to make an informed decision regarding this life-changing situation, because even a decision to end the pregnancy can have long-term effects.

In many cases, the pregnancy is not the only issue that concerns the patient. In fact, the patient's reaction to the pregnancy may be concealing her real concerns—finances, domestic violence, sexual abuse, or other issues. Assessing these concerns is essential in the decision-making process.

Patients may need time to process their emotions and discuss the pregnancy with the significant people in their lives. A scheduled follow-up visit provides an opportunity to further discuss with the patient her reactions and their effect on decision making, as well as to provide information and available support services. These initial meetings play an important role in how patients react to their pregnancy and assist with the decision-making process.

Patients feel especially vulnerable and pressured to find a quick and easy solution. Many report feeling as if they are racing against the clock, and they look to the significant people in their life for support and advice. Support may be lacking, or advice from these sources may differ from what the patient desires.

The primary care provider should inform the patient of the full range of available options. For someone experiencing an unplanned or a crisis pregnancy, abortion is often viewed as the only solution. However, other viable options do exist and may effectively counter the automatic assumption that an abortion is the only and/or best solution. Referrals to crisis pregnancy centers can provide patients with the expertise of trained staff and can broaden options. If the patient does not want to go to a crisis pregnancy center or if one is not accessible to her, a referral to a professional counselor is appropriate. The more informed the patient, the less likely it is that the patient will regret the eventual decision. Regardless of the decision, continued and unconditional acceptance of and compassion toward the patient will contribute to her overall wellness at this critical time.

Counseling a patient who is experiencing a crisis pregnancy can be very challenging. The following framework, which contains lists of questions for the primary care provider to ask the patient, may help to make this interaction fruitful for both patient and provider:

Focus on the patient. There is often a great deal of conversation about and concern for the infant. However, it is the woman who is experiencing the crisis, and it is she who ultimately makes the most adjustments.

Inquire about the patient's feelings.

- What does the pregnancy mean to you?
- Who knows that you are pregnant?
- What is your relationship with the father of the baby? How involved is he in the decision making? How supportive will he be with your decision?
- Who is your support system?
- Are you considering an abortion?
- Would you consider alternatives to abortion?

Make abortion real. If a patient is considering an abortion, it is important that she have as much accurate information as possible about the procedures involved, the risks, and the possible complications:

- Have you ever been pregnant before?
- Have you ever had an abortion?
- What does abortion mean to you?
- Do you know how abortions are performed?
- Do you know the physical risks that can result from abortion?
- Do you know anyone who has had an abortion?
- What were your opinions about abortion before you learned you were pregnant?

Make the infant real. To make an informed decision, the patient needs to learn about the development of the fetus. The primary care provider should be prepared to discuss the different stages of fetal development:

- Do you know the present physical development of your baby?

Focus on the woman and her future. The primary care provider should do the following:

- Ask the patient if she ever plans to have children.
- Ask the patient how she would feel if this were to be her only pregnancy.
- Remind the patient that she has time to make her decision.
- Discuss the hormones of pregnancy and how they affect the decision-making process, especially during the first few months.

Use caution when mentioning adoption as an option, because the word "adoption" can generate negative or even painful feelings. When counseling patients, it is helpful to listen for any hints as a guide to the patient's feelings about this topic. Both the primary care provider and the patient need to remember that adoption is an option. It is not a quick decision but rather a process to work through.

For patients who are committed to continuing the pregnancy, a care plan needs to be developed and should cover the following topics:

- Referral to an obstetrician for prenatal care
- Prenatal vitamins for the patient to take while awaiting her first prenatal visit
- Information on diet and healthy lifestyle
- Financial resources
- Type of aid available to the patient, if needed, before and after birth
- Plans with regard to work or school
- Type of housing arrangements available during the pregnancy and after delivery
- The patient's relationship with the father of the baby
- Marriage
- Single-parenting issues
- Adoption (even if the patient plans to keep her infant, she needs to consider the issues involved in adoption and the impact of adoption on herself and the infant)
- Child support
- Day care
- Support from family and friends

For the patient who has decided to have an abortion, the complexities involved should be realistically reviewed. For example, a woman who is being pressured by the father of the child to have an abortion runs the same risk of being abandoned after the abortion as if she keeps the child. The woman who has repeated abortions needs to consider the possibility of future gynecologic, obstetric, and psychologic complications. It is not uncommon for women who have had an abortion to experience a subsequent miscarriage, ectopic pregnancy, placenta previa, abruptio placentae, or premature birth. Psychologic problems can include guilt, remorse, anger, eating disorders, addictions, and spiritual alienation. These manifestations are categorized under a condition called *postabortion stress syndrome* and may be similar to those of posttraumatic stress disorder (see Chapter 265).

The primary care provider should provide factual information and be understanding as the patient makes plans and considers her options. The provider should avoid exerting pressure or being judgmental. The decision must be made by the patient; preparation is directed toward making the decision one that the patient can live with in the future.

If the patient plans to place the infant for adoption, assistance should be provided to establish future life goals. Professional counseling and support services are critical to prepare for the legal termination of parental rights and to assist the woman with some of the psychologic aspects of releasing her infant. The patient should be encouraged not to view adoption as an indication of lack of love for her infant or as an indication that she is any less of a mother than a woman who keeps her infant. In addition, the decision for adoption can be viewed as providing both the patient and the infant with opportunities not otherwise present.

Attempts should be made to thoroughly explore the possibilities of keeping the infant. Failure to go through this thinking and feeling process may contribute to future regrets concerning this decision.

REFERENCES

1. Delbanco S and others: Public knowledge and perceptions about unplanned pregnancy and contraception in three countries, *Fam Plann Perspect* 29:70-75, 1997.
2. Rosenfeld JA, Everett KD: Factors related to planned and unplanned pregnancy, *J Fam Pract* 43:161-166, 1996.

CHAPTER 185

Vulvar and Vaginal Disorders

Elizabeth C. Sensenig and Patricia Polgar Bailey

Nonneoplastic Epithelial Disorders

DEFINITION/EPIDEMIOLOGY

Benign vulvar disorders account for significant patient concern. Signs and symptoms include pruritus, pain, burning, and irritation. Pruritus is often the chief patient complaint.

Vulvar pruritus is a common vulvar symptom that may be unrelated to vaginitis, sexually transmitted infections (STIs), Bartholin's duct cysts, or neoplasms. Proper treatment of vulvar pruritus depends on an accurate diagnosis. Women with vulvar pruritus often receive multiple treatments in the absence of a correct diagnosis; women are commonly prescribed therapy over the phone without ever having been examined, even if symptoms have been recurrent.[1]

In examining women with vulvar pruritus, it is advisable to ask about and inspect other areas of the body; many conditions affecting other organ systems can have vulvar manifestations, including tuberculosis, Crohn's disease, and endometriosis. For example, vulvar psoriasis may have an unusual presentation, but more typical psoriatic lesions are often seen simultaneously elsewhere on the body and may provide a diagnostic clue.

The visual inspection is essential in identifying vulvar changes. A handheld microscope, or in some cases a colposcope, may allow for more detailed inspection. Washing the vulvar area with 3% to 5% acetic acid will highlight lesions, especially those related to human papillomavirus (HPV) and neoplastic changes. Vaginitis, cervicitis, and other STIs should be excluded. Some of the other common vulvar conditions causing pruritus are presented in this chapter.

Nonneoplastic epithelial disorders were formerly referred to as vulvar dystrophies. They were renamed under a classification scheme adopted in 1987 by the International Society for the Study of Vulvar Disease to include the following:

- Lichen sclerosus
- Squamous hyperplasia
- Other dermatoses

Lichen Sclerosus

PATHOPHYSIOLOGY

Lichen sclerosus (LS) (formerly lichen sclerosus et atrophicus) is no longer thought to be an atrophic disease, but the etiology of this chronic condition remains unknown. Some theories suggest that LS may be triggered by an infectious process, excessive friction, an autoimmune process, abnormal hormonal levels (especially testosterone), or genetic predisposition.[2,3]

Although primarily seen in perimenopausal and postmenopausal white women, LS does occur in females of all ages, including young girls. It does affect males but at rates much lower than in females. LS is primarily found in the anogenital region, but it can be seen elsewhere on the body, such as the neck and shoulders.

CLINICAL PRESENTATION AND PHYSICAL EXAMINATION

Although it is sometimes asymptomatic, LS often results in severe vulvar pruritus or dyspareunia. Affected areas include the labia minora, vulvar vestibule, perineum, and clitoris; the vagina is usually spared. Early LS can be particularly difficult to diagnose. On examination white papules can be seen, and the epithelium may appear normal or thin, resembling parchment paper. There is also typically decreased tissue elasticity, and edema may be present, depending on the disease stage. Fissures and secondary infections may develop, especially with sexual activity or scratching, which may make diagnosis especially difficult.[4] With disease progression, papules develop into large, hypopigmented, symmetric plaques, often hourglass or keyhole shaped, on the labia minora and vulva, which can resemble hyperplasia. If these are not treated, there is eventual loss of vulvar architecture such that the labia minora are no longer seen and introital stenosis may develop, resulting in dyspareunia.[4,5]

DIAGNOSTICS AND DIFFERENTIAL DIAGNOSIS

The differential diagnosis for LS includes lichen planus, which is more likely to involve erosive lesions in the vagina, or vitiligo, which is similar to white plaques, but with no epithelial thinning.[4] The diagnosis is made by examination, and although vulvar biopsy may not be needed in clear-cut cases, it is important to exclude atypia or mixed diagnoses.[6] In addition, thyroid studies are recommended because approximately one third of women with LS are hypothyroid, although this relationship is unclear.[5]

MANAGEMENT

The current treatment of choice is clobetasol propionate 0.05%, which has been shown to improve histologic changes, as well as control symptoms after twice-daily application for 3 months, with the dose gradually tapered.[7-10] Contact dermatitis is a rare but reported side effect of this medication. Subsequent LS recurrences are managed by reinstating the clobetasol therapy.[10] Long-term sequelae of potent topical corticosteroids (atrophy, and thinning of skin and subcutaneous tissues) have not been clinically significant in this disorder.[10] Hydroxyzine 25 to 50 mg h.s. may also help relieve pruritus associated with LS.

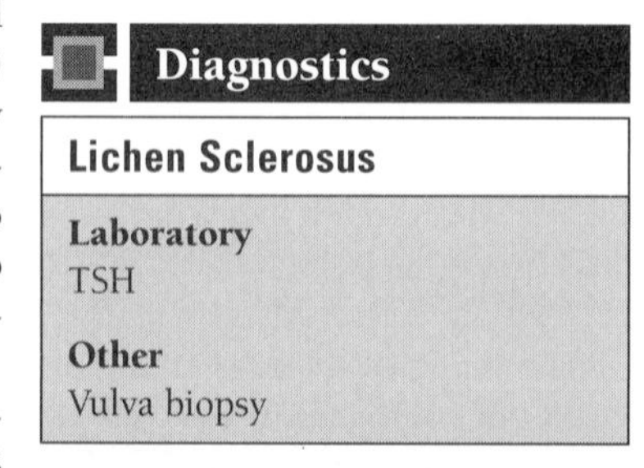
Diagnostics

Lichen Sclerosus

Laboratory
TSH

Other
Vulva biopsy

Until recently, standard treatment for LS was testosterone propionate, 2% in petroleum applied to the vulva or affected area two to three times per day for 2 to 6 months, followed by a taper to less frequent applications for maintenance therapy.[5] Increased serum androgens are seen in adults after 4 weeks of using testosterone, and many develop symptoms of clitoromegaly, acne, hair loss, voice changes, and increased libido, requiring cessation of medication.[11,12] Despite these known side effects, this regimen is still commonly prescribed.

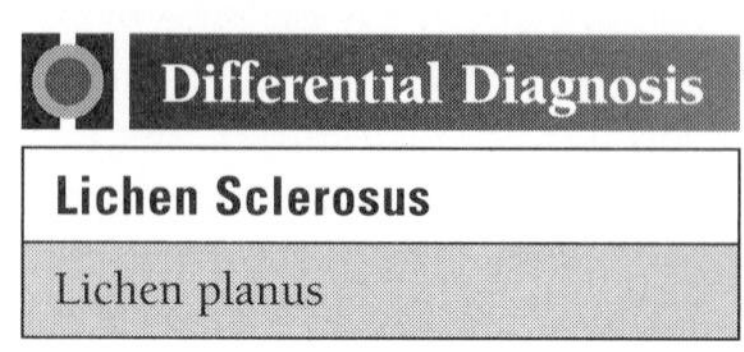
Differential Diagnosis

Lichen Sclerosus

Lichen planus

COMPLICATIONS AND INDICATIONS FOR REFERRAL/HOSPITALIZATION

There have been controversial reports that LS results in an increased risk of squamous cell carcinoma, but this has not been supported by research. If there is any question of hyperplasia or a mixed diagnosis, a gynecologic referral for a biopsy to exclude atypia is indicated, especially in older women. LS is often seen in combination with hyperplasia and requires closer follow-up monitoring.[5] Prophylactic surgery, previously recommended to prevent conversion to cancer, is no longer considered appropriate management.[2,3,13] The role of surgery is quite defined in LS and should be limited to repair of introital stenosis or confirmed malignant disease.[11,13] Although surgery is sometimes advocated for management of recalcitrant symptoms, it should be remembered that women are still at risk for LS recurrence even after vulvectomy.

PATIENT AND FAMILY EDUCATION

The likelihood of recurrence of LS should be discussed; however, connections between childhood LS and future outbreaks or increased risk of neoplastic changes are unclear.[3] Adherence to treatment regimens and follow-up visits should be encouraged. The affected area should be kept as clean and dry as possible, and application of a thin layer of petroleum jelly to the affected area to limit moisture loss may be helpful. The patient should be taught vulvar self-examination and to report early symptoms so that recurrences may be controlled with the lowest-potency medication possible.

Squamous Cell Hyperplasia

PATHOPHYSIOLOGY

Generally, squamous cell hyperplasia is the result of repetitive surface trauma form irritants that cause scratching or rubbing, the notorious itch-scratch cycle. Squamous cell hyperplasia is characterized histologically by epithelial thickening and hyperkeratosis, lengthening and thickening of the rete pegs, and an inflammatory reaction in the dermis. It presents, as do most of the nonneoplastic epithelial disorders, as pruritus, which may be secondary to degeneration and inflammation of terminal nerve fibers. The diagnosis is one of exclusion, and because the condition is often thought to be the equivalent to lichen simplex chronicus, there is some diagnostic confusion.[14]

CLINICAL PRESENTATION AND PHYSICAL EXAMINATION

The affected woman may complain of pain, limitation of movement because of strictures, and dyspareunia. Squamous cell hyperplasia has a varied gross appearance, as it may be affected by moisture, scratching, and/or medications. The skin may look red or white depending on the amount of hyperkeratosis.

It may affect the labia majora, intralabial sulci, outer aspect of the labia minora, and clitoris. The skin may exhibit thickening, fissures, or excoriations. Lesions may be localized or poorly defined.

DIAGNOSTICS AND DIFFERENTIAL DIAGNOSIS

It can be difficult to differentiate among the nonneoplastic epithelial disorders. A biopsy should be performed for histologic diagnosis; a punch biopsy, using adequate local analgesia, is generally the easiest type. Suturing of the biopsy site is rarely needed, as adequate hemostasis can be achieved with silver nitrate. The most important areas from which biopsy specimens should be taken are those of fissuring, ulceration, induration, or thick plaques. An additional reason for performing a biopsy is to exclude atypia, as both LS and squamous cell hyperplasia have a risk of carcinogenic transformation of 1% to 5%.[3]

MANAGEMENT

Treatment, as with LS, is aimed at relieving the itch-scratch cycle. General attention to proper hygiene is important. If the skin is moist or macerated, 5% Burow's solution applied three to four times daily for 30 to 60 minutes is beneficial.[14] Systemic antihistamines or tricyclic antidepressants, especially taken at bedtime, may help. As in LS the treatment of choice is application of a potent corticosteroid cream. Clobetasol propionate 0.05% and betamethasone have both been studied.[2] Unlike in LS, close monitoring for signs of long-term, adverse sequelae is essential.[14] For refractory lesions, intralesional injections of triamcinolone acetonide may be used.[14] Surgical treatment should be avoided if possible, because the recurrence rate can be 40% to 50%.[14]

Complications, considerations for referral, and patient education are the same as for LS.

Contact or Allergic Dermatitis

The description of symptom onset can distinguish contact dermatitis from allergic dermatitis.[9] Contact dermatitis occurs when there is an immediate irritation of the area after exposure to an offending substance. Allergic responses, however, develop several days after exposure. The diagnosis of these conditions is made by history and physical examination findings that include erythema or edema. Both of these conditions are relieved when the triggering substance is identified and eliminated. The list of possible irritants is extensive. Women should be asked about treatments to the vulva (either prescribed or over-the-counter medications), as well as use of feminine hygiene products such as douches, sprays, and deodorants; tampons/pads; condoms; spermicides; lubricants; laundry detergents; soaps; and shampoos. Burow's compresses, sitz baths, or emollients may improve symptoms. Allergic dermatitis usually takes a long time to resolve after exposure is terminated; resolution may be facilitated by a short course of topical steroids.

Eczema

Similar to eczema elsewhere on the body, vulvar eczema is typically a result of persistent scratching or aggravation of an area after an allergic trigger and can be an acute or chronic condition. The typical presentation includes severe pruritus lasting several weeks or more. A red rash or erythema without distinct borders is usually observed on examination and, if left untreated, can progress to the thickened scaly plaques seen in squamous cell hyperplasia.[5] The diagnosis is made by the symptom history, vulvar examination, and presence of eczema on other parts of the body; biopsies are not beneficial. Psoriasis and seborrhea are often confused with eczema, and any diagnosis will be hampered if there has been scratching of the area. The practitioner should be alert to the possibility of secondary infection with continued dermal irritation.[5]

Treatment of pruritus includes cold compresses, Burow's solution, and antihistamines. In addition, acute exacerbation of symptoms can be treated with an oral prednisone taper, which can be followed by topical betamethasone 0.1%, b.i.d. to t.i.d. for 2 weeks, and then tapered. Less potent topical steroids, such as triamcinolone cream 0.1%, may also provide relief. Triamcinolone acetonide injections can be used for recalcitrant eczema. Secondary infections must also be treated. Any known triggers should be avoided. The use of mild soaps and a moisturizer to improve skin hydration may be helpful.

Psoriasis

Often seen on the knees or elbows, psoriasis is an inherited chronic condition that presents as a pruritic, red and scaly, or thick white fissured plaque with clear-cut borders. It is often exacerbated by stress and occurs simultaneously in various parts of the body. In addition, new psoriatic lesions may develop at an injury site (referred to as Koebner's phenomenon). Biopsies are rarely useful for diagnosis, but candidiasis, eczema, seborrhea, and Paget's disease should be excluded.[5]

Treatment for psoriasis is aimed at symptom relief. Calcipotriene ointment (Dovonex), a topical vitamin D_3 preparation, is effective without the risk of skin atrophy.[14] Low-potency corticosteroid creams can be used but are seldom effective by themselves. Ultraviolet treatments are used to treat psoriasis; efficacy for vulvar lesions may be limited. Tar preparations are irritating to the vulvar skin and should be avoided.[14] Referral should be made to a gynecologist or dermatologist for recalcitrant symptoms when steroid injections, methotrexate, retinoids, or cyclosporine therapy may be helpful.[15] Patient education should include stress management, which may reduce recurrence.

Lichen Planus

Lichen planus can be an acute or chronic dermatosis affecting the skin, mucous membranes, or both. The cause is uncertain, but evidence suggests that it is immunologically mediated.[16] In the genital area, the appearance ranges from delicate, white reticulated papules to an erosive, desquamating process. Large denuded areas may lead to profuse leukorrhea or can become adherent, causing stenosis of the vaginal introitus. Diagnosis is confirmed by biopsy.

Initial treatment consists of topical high-potency corticosteroid ointments or intralesional corticosteroid injections for symptomatic relief. Short courses of systemic corticosteroids may be needed for severe symptoms or flares of disease.[17,18]

In addition there are other nonneoplastic epithelial disorders. The "dark lesions" of lentigo melanosis (a frecklelike concentration of melanocytes), nevi, carcinoma, and melanoma result form stimulation of the number or function of the melanocytes. Paget's disease, a red, scaly localized eczematous lesion, is characterized by nests of clear cells at the tips of the rete pegs and hyperkeratosis. Early in the disease the gross appearance is characterized as "velvety" and then later as "mottled." Paget's disease has a 20% to 30% risk of transformation to cancer.[14]

Vulvar Pain

In 1983 the International Society for the Study of Vulvar Disease recommended that the term *vulvodynia* be used to describe burning vulvar pain.[20] Although burning vulvar symptoms can be attributed to conditions such as vaginitis, HPV, or dermatoses such as those described in this chapter, the term is generally reserved for conditions such as vulvar vestibulitis syndrome and dysesthetic (essential) vulvodynia, which have no known cause. It is hoped that increased understanding of these conditions will be accompanied by more precise nomenclature.

Vulvar Vestibulitis Syndrome

DEFINITION/EPIDEMIOLOGY

Vulvar vestibulitis syndrome (VVS) is a chronic inflammatory condition of the vulvar vestibule that is characterized by burning pain on touch, which can persist for several days after the touch is removed. In 1987 Friedrich defined the condition and included three criteria for diagnosis: (1) severe pain on vestibular touch or attempted vaginal entry, (2) tenderness to pressure localized within the vulvar vestibule, and (3) physical findings confined to the vestibular erythema of various degrees.[21] Although VVS is now better understood, the etiology and most appropriate treatment of this condition remain unknown.

Vulvar vestibulitis is found almost exclusively in women of reproductive age who are or have been sexually active. The true prevalence is unknown. The majority of affected women are white (97%) and nulliparous (75%).[22] Primary (no identifiable initial trigger or time of onset) and secondary (such as post-HPV or vaginitis treatment or postpartum) categories of VVS have been suggested.

PATHOPHYSIOLOGY

For reasons that are unclear but that may suggest a genetic etiology or selection bias, VVS is predominantly seen in white women, many of whom report having a relative who experienced similar symptoms or at least difficulty with tampon insertion.[23,24]

Etiologies of VVS, including HPV and a *Candida*-triggered autoimmune response, have been suggested but not supported in the literature. In fact, treatments for HPV, such as topical acid or laser therapy, can lead to secondary VVS. A causal association between VVS and *Candida* organisms has not been established, but as more women treat themselves repeatedly with over-the-counter vaginal antifungicides, sensitivity to ingredients in these preparations may develop, increasing women's risk of developing VVS. Other theories include an association between VVS and interstitial cystitis, both of which are inflammatory conditions of tissues that share embryologic origins. Many of these women have overlapping urinary and vulvar symptoms.[25,26] VVS may also be associated with a sympathetically maintained pain feedback loop that is perpetuated by an underlying pelvic floor muscle instability or hypertonicity that is initially triggered by a superficial tissue insult.[27,28] The association between VVS and oral contraceptives remains controversial. It has been suggested that oral contraceptives downregulate receptors enough to cause epithelial thinning, but research has not demonstrated a clear association between oral contraceptives and the incidence of VVS. Although reports include exacerbation of symptoms related to the menstrual cycle or pregnancy, no mechanism has been identified.[23] In addition, various hormonal creams have been shown to be generally ineffective in treating VVS.[15]

Given the lack of obvious clinical findings, VVS was long thought to be a result of sexual dysfunction, childhood trauma, or some other psychologic disorder, theories now recognized as fallacious. A chronic pain syndrome that heavily impacts sexual relationships and daily activities is apt to be, not surprisingly, accompanied by anxiety or depression. These issues should be addressed, but to assume a causal link with VVS is inappropriate.

CLINICAL PRESENTATION

A thorough history is essential to managing VVS. Presentation commonly includes complaints of severe, burning vulvar pain during introital penetration with sexual intercourse or tampon use, during bicycle or horseback riding, or when wearing tight or bulky clothing. Pain may last a few minutes or as long as a few days after the trigger has been removed. Symptoms have often been present for months or years, resulting in a long history of frequent consultations. The history should include information about the initial onset of symptoms (if an initial onset can be identified), along with symptom characteristics, duration, and frequency. The impact of symptoms on sexual function should be determined, including how often intercourse is attempted and how often it is stopped because of pain. Assessment should also be made as to the impact of symptoms on daily activities and how often thoughts are distracted by symptoms during the course of a day. The presence of back pain, muscle soreness, and bowel and urinary patterns may be helpful in identifying related disorders. Previous ineffective treatment should be documented. Prior management has often included repeated treatment for yeast or bacterial infections; determining whether treatment was empiric or culture based is essential. A review of previous medical records can be helpful. Women should also be asked if they have developed any techniques of their own to ease discomfort.

PHYSICAL EXAMINATION AND DIAGNOSTICS

Generally, visual examination of the vulva and introitus is unremarkable, although erythema near the vestibular glands may be present. The most revealing test is the use of a water- or saline-moistened cotton-tipped applicator to test for sensitivity to touch. This is done by simply touching with the applicator in multiple locations around the labia minora, vestibule, clitoris, and urethra to determine any areas of tenderness, to elicit burning, and to rate the degree of discomfort. With VVS, tenderness or burning is usually triggered near Bartholin's glands, the posterior fourchette, and to either side of the urethral opening. Use of the smallest speculum possible and a gentle, unhurried examination with extra lubrication will be better tolerated. Colposcopic evaluation of the involved areas, although advocated by some, is generally not appropriate unless physical findings suggest HPV or vulvar intraepithelial neoplasia. Vulvar biopsies typically show inflammation and should be performed only if a pathologic condition is suggested by the physical examination.[29]

DIFFERENTIAL DIAGNOSIS

STIs should be excluded and cultures performed for beta-streptococcus and *Candida* and *Ureaplasma* organisms.[30,31] The diagnosis of VVS is made on the basis of the history, positive physical examination findings, and negative cultures.[32]

MANAGEMENT

Although spontaneous resolution of symptoms is possible, treating VVS is often a matter of trial and error and requires a solid provider-patient relationship.[33] Although many treatments are aimed at what is thought to be the underlying problem, the fact that the primary symptom is pain cannot be forgotten. Reassurance that this condition is real and that the concerns are legitimate is important. Women should be informed that partial symptom relief is likely, but that it will take time for adequate treatment trials. Realistic goals and time frames should be established, and extra time planned for appointments.[34] Each woman should be involved as much as possible and should keep a daily symptom log, noting any possible pain triggers and rating the severity and duration of symptoms. Decisions to seek alternative forms of treatment, such as acupuncture, should be supported and incorporated into the overall management plan.

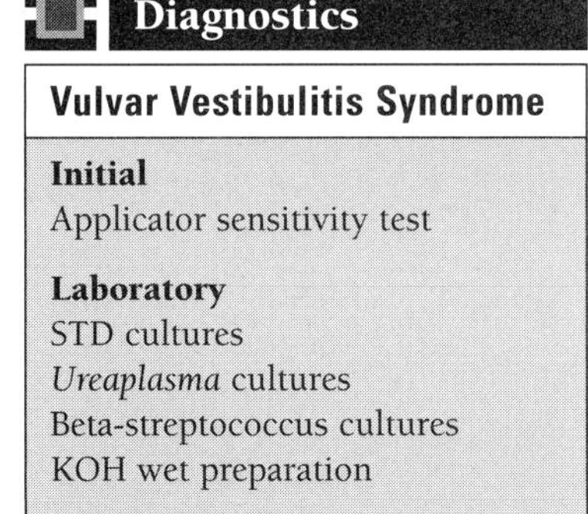

Diagnostics

Vulvar Vestibulitis Syndrome

Initial
Applicator sensitivity test

Laboratory
STD cultures
Ureaplasma cultures
Beta-streptococcus cultures
KOH wet preparation

Other
Biopsies
Colposcopy*

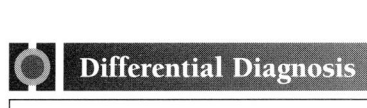

*If indicated.

Treatment of VVS is dictated by the woman's history. If recurrent candidiasis is suspected, a trial of fluconazole 150 mg weekly for 2 months, then biweekly for another 2 months, followed by one dose monthly. Liver function tests generally do not need to be performed, but careful evaluation for possible drug interactions (e.g., oral hypoglycemics, anticoagulants) is required.[22] Topical antifungal creams such as terconazole, miconazole, and clotrimazole may further irritate the vestibule.

Differential Diagnosis

Vulvar Vestibulitis Syndrome

Sexually transmitted diseases
Infection with *Candida* or *Ureaplasma* organisms
Infection with beta-streptococcus

Other oral treatments aimed at interfering with the pain feedback loop include antihistamines (e.g., hydroxyzine 25 mg h.s.) or antidepressant medications. Low-dose antidepressants have long been used to manage pain, and it should be carefully explained that this is the indication for which the antidepressant is being prescribed. Suggested antidepressant regimens include amitriptyline or nortriptyline 10 mg h.s., with a gradual increase every 2 to 4 weeks (while monitoring for side effects) to a total dose of 75 to 100 mg h.s.[35] Often patients will notice improvement with a dosage of 50 mg every day or less.

Another noninvasive approach involves education about calcium oxalate restriction and calcium citrate supplementation. Many common foods, such as peanut butter, are high in calcium oxalates, and although restricting intake may be difficult, some have found it helpful. Symptom reduction has been achieved with calcium citrate and a low-oxalate diet.[36] Additional information on low-oxalate diets can be obtained from national VVS groups.

COMPLICATIONS

Patients with vulvar pain may be reticent to discuss physical and sexual concerns and reluctant to have pelvic examinations. The disorder may be embarrassing and frustrating and may prohibit some patients from enjoying life or an intimate sexual relationship. These patients require considerable support and understanding and often will benefit from psychologic counseling.

INDICATIONS FOR REFERRAL/HOSPITALIZATION

Consultation with a physical therapist is helpful to evaluate for pelvic asymmetry and pelvic floor musculature, which typically shows instability and increased resting tone in patients with VVS.[27,28] Trigger point physical therapy for myofascial release may be therapeutic, especially for patients complaining of back pain or persistent muscle soreness.[36,37] Continued pelvic floor muscle dysfunction may perpetuate the sympathetically maintained pain feedback loop. Twice-daily biofeedback exercises may help reestablish muscle stability over the course of many months and provide significant, if not complete, symptom relief.[27]

If the response to any of the aforementioned interventions has been inadequate, referral should be made to a gynecologist knowledgeable about different treatment options, such as interferon injections, laser surgery, and vestibulectomy.[38] Interferon therapy involves vestibular injections three times a week for 4 weeks. Mixed results have been realized with both interferon therapy and laser surgery.[39,40] Vestibulectomy remains the final option and has a success rate of 50% to 60% (complete symptom relief), which is thought to improve with the use of newer surgical methods and appropriate screening of patients.[41] Counseling and preoperative or postoperative treatment of vaginismus using dilators have been shown to improve surgical outcomes.[41,42]

PATIENT AND FAMILY EDUCATION

The impact of VVS on intimate relationships is significant, and the woman's partner should be included in discussions when possible and appropriate. Counseling referrals should be offered with the understanding that the primary care provider does not believe symptoms are psychogenic in nature, but rather that there are real emotional challenges to living with a chronic pain syndrome; the provider should also acknowledge that hope often gives way to disappointment before symptom relief is experienced. Local peer support groups can be found in some areas, and women can contact national groups for more information (Box 185-1).

When treatment options are being discussed, women should first be counseled to avoid vulvar irritants and implement the self-care measures described in Box 185-1. Many topical treatment options have been tried, including estrogen and progesterone creams and topical anesthetics such as lidocaine 2% jelly. Although some women may respond to these therapies, others will experience an exacerbation of symptoms with any topical medication.[33]

Dysesthetic (Essential) Vulvodynia

Dysesthetic vulvodynia (DV) is characterized by spontaneous and constant vulvar pain without the focal tenderness typically seen in VVS. In DV, pain is not confined to coital attempts or other known triggers. Complaints of concomitant urethral, rectal, or back pain are more common than with VVS.[35] This condition may represent a neuropathic process such as a reflex sympathetic dystrophy or pudendal neuralgia.[43] Other than more widespread symptom distribution, physical findings on examination are similarly unremarkable, as with VVS.

The goal of treatment in DV is pain management. If initial attempts at treating symptoms are not successful, consultation with a pain management specialist may be helpful. As with VVS, attention should be given to pain and the emotional impact chronic pain can have on a person's life. Counseling referrals should be offered. Topical or oral estrogen may be useful in some cases, but women with DV are more likely than those with VVS to respond well to antidepressant therapy.[35] Dosages are the same as those used for VVS. If antidepressants are unsuccessful, anticonvulsants such as phenytoin or carbamazepine may be helpful, but their use requires strict monitoring of blood levels. A 50% success rate with nerve blocks of three to six injections has been demonstrated. Surgery is a final option and is thought to be more effective for DV than laser surgery or alcohol injections.[35] Alternative forms of chronic pain management, such as guided imagery or acupuncture, may be useful as well, but outcome data are not yet available.

Genital Human Papillomavirus

DEFINITION/EPIDEMIOLOGY

Genital HPV is a group of at least 20 HPV types that have an affinity for the anogenital region. Clinical genital HPV infections are well known as genital warts, or condylomata acuminata, which are benign tumors often caused by HPV types 6 and 11, which have a low risk for oncogenicity. Infections with HPV types 16 and 18, with a high risk for oncogenicity, have been associated with high-grade intraepithelial neoplasia and genital cancers, particularly cervical cancer.

Genital HPV is the most common viral STI. The exact prevalence and incidence of HPV infection are unknown. However, it has been estimated that at any given time approximately 1% of sexually active women have external genital warts and that 20% to 50% have subclinical or latent genital HPV infection.[40] Approximately 50% to 80% of men who have sexual intercourse with women with HPV will develop HPV infection.[41]

BOX 185-1

PATIENT EDUCATION AND RESOURCES

1. Wear loose, soft clothing as much as possible, such as skirts without underwear while at home. Avoid spandex and stockings or try thigh-high or shorter stockings.
2. Wear all-white, all-cotton underwear always (not just cotton crotch panel).
3. Use only white, unscented toilet paper.
4. Use mild laundry detergent and rinse underwear a second time in hot water.
5. When bathing, use mild soap and carefully rinse vulvar area with plain water, and make sure all other soaps and shampoos are completely rinsed from area.
6. Avoid deodorant tampons and pads; instead of panty liners on light days, wear old underwear that can get stained. Another option is reusable cotton menstrual pads, available from Glad Rags, PO Box 12648, Portland, OR 97212; (800) 799-4523.
7. Avoid douches and deodorant sprays or powders in the groin area.
8. Use pure vegetable oil or mineral oil for lubrication with sex, and avoid other commercial lubricants and spermicides.
9. Maintain as much nonpenetrating sexual activity as possible.
10. Rinse vulva after voiding with plain water spray bottle.
11. Keep detailed symptom diary that includes at least the following: characteristics of symptoms, their severity and duration, and triggering event if identified.
12. Contact national resources for local support groups and additional information and newsletters:

Vulvar Pain Foundation
PO Drawer 177
Graham, NC 27253
(910) 226-0704
Website: www.vulvarpainfoundation.org

National Vulvodynia Association
PO Box 19288
Sarasota, FL 34276-2288
(941) 927-8503; fax: (941) 927-8602
Website: www.nva.org

PATHOPHYSIOLOGY

The pathophysiology of genital HPV infection is not clearly understood.[42] It seems, however, that HPV enters the genital epithelium through an area of microtrauma. Patients exposed to genital HPV may develop clinical, subclinical, or latent infections. Clinical infection results from productive infection in which the cells have altered differentiation and/or transit time and the development of warts. In subclinical infection, HPV viral proteins and infectious particles are present, but there is no overtly visible change in the skin. In latent infection, HPV DNA is in the cell, but the complete viral particles are not assembled. The vast majority of latent HPV infections are transient and self-limiting.[43]

As indicated previously, genital HPV is considered an STI. It is most often spread by genital skin-to-genital skin contact. Although the incidence is infrequent, nonsexual routes of transmission, including autoinoculation and vertical and perinatal transmission, are also possible. Infection with HPV may be followed by a latency period ranging from 2 weeks to several years. The long latency or incubation period makes it challenging to determine the origin of the virus and its mode of transmission. The degree to which transmission is possible in latent and subclinical infection is not known; however, it has been proposed that individuals with HPV are less infectious when they are free of visible warts.[44] Although much remains unknown about the specifics of infectivity, condom use is encouraged. Female condoms may be more helpful than male condoms during heterosexual intercourse because, when used properly, they substantially decrease the area of potentially exposed genital skin.[45]

CLINICAL PRESENTATION

Genital Warts

Genital warts, also known as condylomata acuminata, are benign tumors that often have a pointed, irregular fissured appearance. Their appearance ranges from single, small, painless, smooth, flat, skin-colored warts to fleshy papules that may become confluent cauliflower-like growths (see Color Plate 7). Although they are often asymptomatic, genital warts can be associated with pruritus, burning, pain, and bleeding. They usually regress spontaneously but may last anywhere from a month to several years.

Genital warts in women occur most often on the vulva, but they may also be seen on the introitus, vagina, perineum, perianal area, urethra, and cervix. In men genital warts often occur on the distal third of the penis and on the urethral meatus, urethra, scrotum, and perianal area. Some men with urethral lesions have hematuria. Rarely, condylomata acuminata can be found on the oral mucosa, larynx, trachea, rectum, or bladder.

Intraepithelial Neoplasia

HPV infection can lead to intraepithelial lesions, which are dysplastic changes of the anogenital epithelium. HPV is most often associated with the development of intraepithelial lesions of the cervix, referred to as cervical intraepithelial neoplasia; however, it is also associated with intraepithelial lesions of the vulva, vagina, anus, and penis. The vast majority of HPV infections will not become malignant even if left untreated.[46]

DIAGNOSTICS

The diagnosis of genital warts is usually made during visual inspection on the basis of the typical clinical appearance. A biopsy and histologic examination should be performed when patients have frequent recurrences or resistant, large, or pigmented warts. The threshold for biopsy should be lowered in patients who are immunosuppressed, because these patients are at greater risk of developing squamous cell carcinoma. Because of the risk of developing anal cancer associated with the presence of intraanal warts, anoscopy may be considered for patients who have genital warts and a history of anal-receptive intercourse. All women with genital warts should have a Pap test performed to screen for cervical HPV infection. Screening for syphilis (rapid plasma reagin), other STIs, and HIV should be offered, as infection with genital warts may be a marker of unsafe sexual practices.

The application of 5% acetic acid causes most tissue infected with HPV to whiten. This is called acetowhitening. False-positive acetowhitening may occur with many inflammatory conditions, including candidiasis, genital irritation, and skin previously treated for warts.

Magnification (often with a colposcope) and directed cytologic and histologic examination of acetowhite areas allow practitioners to diagnose subclinical HPV infection. Cytologic evidence of HPV infection is determined by the presence of koilocytosis; histologic evidence of HPV infection is characterized by hyperkeratosis, parakeratosis, and koilocytosis.

Latent genital HPV infection can be diagnosed by way of molecular testing and typing of genital HPV DNA. The utility of HPV DNA testing and typing in clinical practice is currently under debate and not yet routinely recommended.[47]

DIFFERENTIAL DIAGNOSIS

See the Differential Diagnosis box on p. 818.

MANAGEMENT

There is no cure for genital HPV infection. Current treatment for clinical HPV infection is aimed at removal of genital warts. Although wart-free periods are often achieved, recurrences are common with all therapies. The topical treatments considered first-line agents for most genital wart infections are discussed in Box 185-2. If a patient has extensive, large, vaginal, urethral, cervical, or rectal warts, or if treatment with the agents in Box 185-2 is ineffective, then another method of treatment should be tried and the patient referred to a facility experienced with

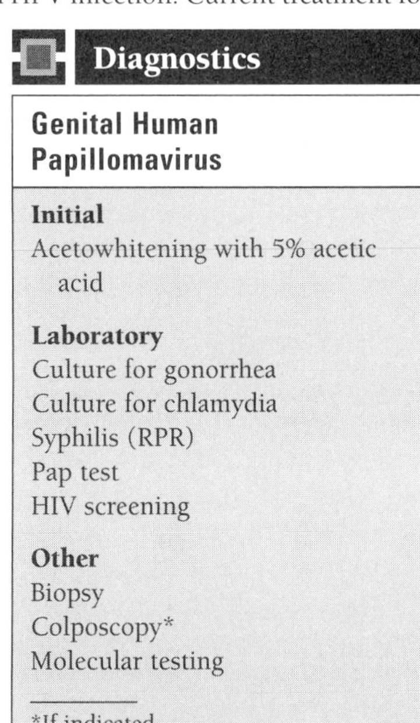

Diagnostics

Genital Human Papillomavirus

Initial
Acetowhitening with 5% acetic acid

Laboratory
Culture for gonorrhea
Culture for chlamydia
Syphilis (RPR)
Pap test
HIV screening

Other
Biopsy
Colposcopy*
Molecular testing

*If indicated.

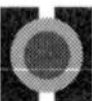

Differential Diagnosis

Genital Human Papillomavirus

Condylomata lata	Sebaceous cysts
Molluscum contagiosum	Benign pearly penile papules
Herpes simplex virus	Lichen planus
Nevi	Psoriasis
Skin tags	Bowenoid papulosis*
Folliculitis	Intraepithelia neoplasm*
Vestibular papillae	Malignant melanoma*
Seborrheic keratosis	

*Bowenoid papulosis, malignant melanoma, and giant condyloma (Buschke-Lowenstein tumor) are neoplasms that, if suspected, require biopsy.[48]

modalities such as the loop electroexcisional procedure, carbon dioxide laser, electrodesiccation, electrocauterization, surgical excision, intralesional interferon-alpha or topical 5-fluorouracil cream.

LIFE SPAN CONSIDERATIONS

Genital warts tend to grow faster and larger during pregnancy; however, elective cesarean delivery is not recommended for women with genital HPV unless warts present mechanical obstruction. Vertical or perinatal transmission occurs infrequently. There is an association between genital warts in the mother and the development of juvenile laryngeal papillomatosis and/or external anogenital, nasooral, respiratory, and conjunctival warts in the child. In addition to vertical transmission from infected mothers, possible modes of HPV transmission in children include autoinoculation, casual social contact, and sexual abuse.

COMPLICATIONS

The development of cervical cancer remains the largest threat of all HPV-associated neoplasia. (See Chapter 180 for further discussion.)

INDICATIONS FOR REFERRAL/HOSPITALIZATION

A biopsy should be performed on any lesions that appear atypical, pigmented, or persistent, to exclude malignancy. Pathologists interpreting biopsies need to be informed of previous treatment of affected areas, as podophyllum and 5-fluorouracil can cause atypical-appearing cells that could be falsely diagnosed as advanced intraepithelial neoplasia or cancer.

PATIENT AND FAMILY EDUCATION

Diagnosis and treatment of HPV can be traumatic, negatively affecting relationships, employment, self-concept, self-esteem, sexuality, and mental health. Because of the potential psychosocial and psychosexual sequelae of HPV infection, the personal impact of the disease on the lives of patients should be assessed.

Information related to the nature of the virus and its incurability, potential recurrences, modes of transmission, and treatment, as well as the benefits of follow-up care, should be presented to patients verbally and in written format. Sexual practices and safer sex should be discussed in an open and nonjudgmental manner. Anticipatory guidance or role playing with patients to help them disclose their HPV status to future or current partners may also be helpful. Encouraging patients and their partners to perform genital self-examination is suggested as well.

BOX 185-2

COMMON TOPICAL TREATMENTS FOR GENITAL WARTS

Cryotherapy with liquid nitrogen or probe—Applied weekly or biweekly to wart and 1-mm area of surrounding skin until warts are cleared. Some pain may be experienced during and after therapy.

Podofilox 0.5% (Condylox)—Approved for self-treatment of external genital warts; applied to warts twice a day for 3 days, followed by a 4-day period of no treatment. This cycle can be repeated 4 times if necessary. Primary care provider applies first treatment to teach technique. There is mild to no discomfort with treatment. It is contraindicated in pregnancy.

Podophyllum 10%-20%—In a compound or tincture of benzoin. Applied to warts and washed off in 1-4 hours. It can be repeated once a week for a maximum of 6 weeks. Discomfort may be mild. It is contraindicated in pregnancy and is not to be used on the cervix, vagina, or urethra. Systemic reactions have occurred with extensive use.

Trichloracetic acid (TCA) 80%-90%—Applied to warts (normal tissue should be carefully avoided) and powdered with talc or baking soda to remove excess acid. Treatment can be weekly or biweekly and is limited to 6 applications. Sharp pain is common and may be decreased by applying lidocaine jelly or spray to skin around the wart.

Imiquimod 5% (Aldara)—Self-applied cream for treatment of external and perianal genital warts. Applied to affected area, rubbed in completely, 3 times a week for a maximum of 16 weeks. Patient should avoid intercourse on nights cream is applied and wash off cream 6-10 hours after application. The cream can weaken condoms and diaphragms. Side effects of erythema, flaking, and edema may occur.

HEALTH PROMOTION

Health-promoting practices, such as limiting alcohol consumption, eating a well-balanced diet, quitting smoking, getting regular sleep and exercise, and reducing stress help to decrease the progression and recurrence of HPV infections.

The American Social Health Association* has a quarterly newsletter, *HPV News*, designed to address the concerns of people with genital HPV infection.

Vaginitis and Vaginosis

DEFINITION/EPIDEMIOLOGY

Vaginitis and vaginosis are disorders of the vagina that are characterized by vaginal discharge, odor, or vulvovaginal irritation. Vaginitis involves inflammation, whereas vaginosis does

*American Social Health Association, PO Box 13827, Research Triangle Park, NC 27709; (919) 361-8400; http://www.ashastd.org.

not. Both have historically been grouped under the term *vaginitis*. They result from an imbalance in the vaginal ecosystem, which may be caused by bacterial, fungal, protozoan, or viral infection; hypoestrogenic states; foreign bodies; contact dermatitis; or allergy. Recurrent vaginitis is defined as four or more episodes within a year.

Affecting women of all ages, vaginitis is the most common gynecologic problem encountered by primary care providers. Bacterial vaginosis is the most common cause of vaginitis, with an incidence of 15% to 65%, depending on the location of practice.[48] Of note is the fact that approximately 50% of the women meeting the diagnostic criteria for bacterial vaginosis are asymptomatic.[46] The second most common cause of vaginitis is vulvovaginal candidiasis, with an estimated 1.3 million cases annually in the United States.[44] An estimated 75% of all women will experience at least one episode of vulvovaginal candidiasis in their lifetime, and 40% to 45% will experience more than one episode.[46] The third most common cause of vaginitis is trichomoniasis, which is also commonly asymptomatic.

Bacterial Vaginosis

PATHOPHYSIOLOGY

Bacterial vaginosis (BV) is characterized by the replacement of the normal, hydrogen peroxide-producing *Lactobacillus* organisms in the vagina with high concentrations of anaerobic bacteria, *Gardnerella vaginalis*, and *Mycoplasma hominis*.[46] In the presence of BV infection, protective hydrogen peroxide-producing lactobacilli are significantly reduced. These changes are accompanied by an elevated pH, which facilitates the growth of the pathogenic organisms and their adherence to vaginal epithelia, seen as "clue" cells on a saline wet mount. The anaerobes facilitate the release of amines, which produce the characteristic "fishy" odor, especially on alkalization of the vaginal discharge.

The cause of microbial alterations in BV is not fully understood. It is associated with sexual activity, as women who have never been sexually active rarely get BV, and women with multiple male sexual partners are at higher risk. See Box 185-3 for other suspected risk factors for BV. However, it cannot be strictly classified as an STI. The principal argument against sexual transmission of BV is the reported lack of benefit from treating male partners.[45]

BOX 185-3

SUSPECTED RISK FACTORS FOR BACTERIAL VAGINOSIS

- New sexual partner in the past month
- Multiple sexual partners
- Presence of an STD
- Oral receptive sex
- Lesbian sexual relationship
- Early first coitus
- Douching
- IUD use
- Black race
- Cigarette smoking

BV, Bacterial vaginosis; *STD*, sexually transmitted disease; *IUD*, intrauterine device.

CLINICAL PRESENTATION

Symptoms of BV most often include an increased quantity of malodorous vaginal discharge, most noticeable after intercourse and during menses, because of the alkaline nature of semen and blood. Some patients experience mild to moderate vulvovaginal irritation.

On examination the vaginal discharge is often thin, homogeneous, and adherent to the vaginal walls and cervix. The fishy amine odor may be present, and rarely there is vaginal inflammation.

PHYSICAL EXAMINATION

The physical examination begins with visual inspection of the pubic area and vulva, and vaginal examination. Assessment of the skin turgor and elasticity, the presence of normal or sparse pubic hair, and whether the labia are full, atrophic, or dry are important. Any vulvovaginal erythema, lesions, discharge, or prolapse should be noted. A speculum examination is necessary to determine the color, consistency, viscosity, and odor of any vaginal or cervical discharge. In addition, the pH of any vaginal fluid should be tested. Erythema, lesions, erosion, or friability of the cervical surface or vaginal walls can be helpful in determining the diagnosis. A bimanual examination is done to assess for cervical motion tenderness and for uterine or adnexal masses or pain.

DIAGNOSTICS

The diagnosis of BV can be made by clinical or Gram's stain criteria. Clinical criteria require the presence of three of the following[46]:

1. Homogeneous, white, noninflammatory discharge that adheres to the vaginal walls
2. The presence of clue cells on microscopic examination
3. pH of vaginal fluid >4.5
4. Vaginal discharge with a fishy odor before or after the addition of 10% potassium hydroxide (KOH) (positive whiff test)
5. Gram's stain may be used for diagnosis to determine the relative concentration of the bacterial morphotypes characteristic of BV, which will be increased 100-fold to 1000-fold. Culture is not recommended because it is not specific.

DIFFERENTIAL DIAGNOSIS

See the Differential Diagnosis box on p. 823.

MANAGEMENT

Treatment options for BV are outlined in Box 185-4. The most common side effect of oral metronidazole is gastrointestinal upset. Patients taking metronidazole should be advised to avoid the use of alcohol during treatment

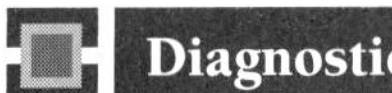

Diagnostics

Bacterial Vaginosis

Initial
pH >4.5

Laboratory
Wet mount with normal saline or 10% KOH
KOH whiff test
Gram's stain

and for 24 hours thereafter to avoid a disulfiram-like reaction (severe nausea and vomiting). Oral clindamycin has been shown to be as effective as oral metronidazole, but it is more expensive and may cause diarrhea.[46] Single-dose metronidazole therapy has a lower efficacy than 7-day metronidazole therapy or than the topical therapies.[46] Flagyl ER, 750 mg once daily has been approved by the U.S. Food and Drug Administration (FDA) for treatment of BV, although data regarding clinical equivalency have not been published. Routine treatment of sexual partners is not recommended.

Treatment of BV in pregnancy is of particular importance because of its association with preterm and low-birth-weight deliveries. Treatment should use one of the oral therapies outlined in Box 185-4 to penetrate the chorion, amnion, and decidua.[47] Intravaginal clindamycin is not recommended in pregnancy because of an increased risk of preterm delivery.[46] Although metronidazole was previously contraindicated in the first trimester, a recent meta-analysis disputes this claim.[48] The lower recommended doses further limit fetal exposure. Treatment in pregnancy should be followed by a test of cure 1 month after completion of therapy and by retreatment if necessary. Screening of the asymptomatic pregnant woman for BV remains controversial, although most agree that women at high risk for preterm delivery should be screened and treated in the early second trimester.[46,48] A large, randomized clinical trial is underway to clarify the benefits of therapy for BV in pregnancy.[46]

BV recurs within a month in about 30% of women.[49] Persistence of pathogens, an unidentified host factor, failure of lactobacilli to recolonize the vagina, and reinfection from a male partner are possible explanations. Consider performing a routine "test of cure" (vaginal pH, whiff test, and a saline wet mount) 2 to 3 weeks after therapy to ensure that infection is resolved and to confirm regrowth of lactobacilli. For recurrent BV infections, defined as three or more episodes yearly, alternate first line agents; suggest prophylactic use of intravaginal metronidazole, twice a week for 3 to 6 months.[50]

BOX 185-4

TREATMENT OF BACTERIAL VAGINOSIS

STANDARD TREATMENT

Metronidazole, 500 mg PO b.i.d. for 7 days

Or

Clindamycin cream 2%, 1 full applicator (5 g) intravaginally h.s. for 7 days

Or

Metronidazole gel 0.75%, 1 full applicator (5 g) intravaginally q day or b.i.d. for 5 days

ALTERNATIVE REGIMENS

Metronidazole, 2 g PO in a single dose

Or

Clindamycin, 300 mg PO b.i.d. for 7 days

Or

Clindamycin ovules, 100 g intravaginally q.h.s. for 3 days

TREATMENT IN PREGNANCY*

Metronidazole, 250 mg PO t.i.d. for 7 days

Or

Clindamycin, 300 mg PO b.i.d. for 7 days

Modified from Centers for Disease Control and Prevention: Sexually transmitted diseases treatment guidelines, *MMWR* 51(RR-6), 43-44, 2002.
*See text for discussion.

COMPLICATIONS

Once considered benign, BV is now associated with many serious gynecologic and obstetric complication (Box 185-5). Perhaps of greatest concern is the possible link between BV and infection with human immunodeficiency virus (HIV), as supported by several recent studies.[51-55] The shift in vaginal pH from acidity to alkalinity associated with the presence of semen may favor male-to-female transmission of HIV, and HIV infection is consistently associated with reduced levels of vaginal lactobacilli.[56]

The bacterial flora of BV have been implicated in pelvic inflammatory disease (PID) and have also been associated with endometritis, PID, and vaginal cuff cellulitis after invasive procedures. Evidence supports the screening and treatment of BV before therapeutic abortion,[46] and hysterectomy and should be considered for patients at high risk for preterm labor.

INDICATIONS FOR REFERRAL/HOSPITALIZATION AND PATIENT AND FAMILY EDUCATION

See Indications for Referral/Hospitalization and Patient and Family Education, p. 824.

Vulvovaginal Candidiasis

PATHOPHYSIOLOGY

Vulvovaginal candidiasis (VVC) is caused by growth of the fungus *Candida* in the vagina. Most infections involve *C. albicans*, although up to 17% may be caused by non-*albicans* species.[57]

BOX 185-5

COMPLICATIONS ASSOCIATED WITH BACTERIAL VAGINOSIS

GYNECOLOGIC

- Increased risk of HIV
- Recurrent cystitis
- PID, including postabortion and subclinical PID
- Cervicitis
- Abnormal Pap smears
- Postsurgical gynecologic infections

OBSTETRIC

- Early spontaneous abortion
- Preterm labor
- Premature rupture of membranes
- Chorioamnionitis
- Postpartum endometritis

BV, bacterial vaginosis; *PID*, pelvic inflammatory disease.

The most common non-*albicans* species involved in VVC are *Torulopsis glabrata* and *Candida tropicalis*, which may present atypically and be more resistant to standard therapies. Women with HIV infection or recurrent VVC are twice as likely to have non-*albicans* VVC.[57] In all, 10% to 20% of asymptomatic women with a healthy vaginal ecosystem harbor *Candida* organisms.[49] Several factors may trigger the change from colonization to proliferation, which results in the development of symptomatic VVC. These include changes in the vaginal ecosystem and possible phenotypic changes in the *Candida* organism. Symptomatic VVC involves candidal tissue invasion, causing inflammation, mucosal swelling, erythema, and exfoliation of epithelia. Factors that cause an increased susceptibility to VVC include antibiotic therapy, pregnancy, diabetes, use of oral contraceptives (especially high-dose formulations), immunosuppression, and occlusive, synthetic clothing.

Recurrent VVC is defined as four or more documented episodes of VVC in 1 year. The pathophysiology of recurrent or chronic VVC remains controversial. It affects less than 5% of women annually, and the majority have no predisposing condition, such as diabetes or immunosuppression. Earlier theories on the cause of recurrent VVC have included reinfection from an intestinal reservoir, sexual transmission, and the "vaginal relapse theory," which proposes that incomplete eradication of *Candida* occurs after treatment and that the small numbers of *Candida* organisms present then multiply and result in recurrence. More recent theories propose deficiencies in the normal protective vaginal flora, a deficiency in antigen-specific, cell-mediated immunity to *Candida*, and a possible local hypersensitivity to *Candida*, predisposing the patient to recurrences.

CLINICAL PRESENTATION

Typical symptoms of VVC include pruritus and vaginal discharge. Other symptoms may include vulvar burning, dyspareunia, vulvar dysuria, and vaginal irritation. It is important to assess for recent use of over-the-counter preparations.

PHYSICAL EXAMINATION

On physical examination the vulva and vagina may be hyperemic and edematous. Vulvar excoriation may be present. The vaginal discharge is usually whitish, curdlike, and adherent to the vaginal walls. Variations in the vaginal discharge are possible, although care must be taken to exclude concurrent infections.

DIAGNOSTICS

The diagnosis of VVC can be made on demonstration of pseudohyphae or yeast on a 10% KOH wet mount or Gram's stain, or by culture. Use of KOH in microscopy improves visualization by disrupting cellular material, which may obscure the yeast forms. The vaginal pH in VVC is normal (4 to 4.5). Identification of yeast in the absence of symptoms is not an indication for treatment.

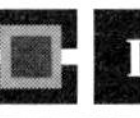

Diagnostics

Vulvovaginal Candidiasis

Initial
pH <4.5

Laboratory
Wet mount with normal saline or 10% KOH
Gram's stain
Culture

DIFFERENTIAL DIAGNOSIS

See the Differential Diagnosis box on p. 823.

MANAGEMENT

Treatment options for VVC are outlined in Box 185-6. The single-dose topical therapies should be reserved for mild VCC because of their slightly lower effectiveness. Multiday regimens are more appropriate for moderate to severe VVC, and the use

BOX 185-6

RECOMMENDED REGIMENS FOR TREATMENT OF VULVOVAGINAL CANDIDIASIS

INTRAVAGINAL AGENTS

Butoconazole: 2% cream 5 g intravaginally for 3 days*
or
Butoconazole: 2% cream 5 g (Butaconazole sustained release), single intravaginal application
or
Clotrimazole: 1% cream 5 g intravaginally for 7-14 days*
or
Clotrimazole, 100 mg vaginal tablet for 7 days
or
Clotrimazole: 100 mg vaginal tablet, two tablets for 3 days
or
Clotrimazole: 500 mg vaginal tablet, one tablet in a single application
or
Miconazole: 2% cream 5 g intravaginally for 7 days*
or
Miconazole: 100 mg vaginal suppository, one suppository for 7 days*
or
Miconazole: 200 mg vaginal suppository, one suppository for 3 days*
or
Nystatin: 100,000-unit vaginal tablet, one tablet for 14 days
or
Tioconazole: 6.5% ointment 5 g intravaginally in a single application*
or
Terconazole: 0.4% cream 5 g intravaginally for 7 days
or
Terconazole: 0.8% cream 5 g intravaginally for 3 days
or
Terconazole: 80 mg vaginal suppository, one suppository for 3 days

ORAL AGENT

Fluconazole: 150 mg oral tablet, one tablet in a single dose

Modified from Centers for Disease Control and Prevention: Sexually transmitted diseases treatment guidelines, *MMWR* 51(RR-6), 43-44, 2002.
*Over-the-counter (OTC) preparations
NOTE: The creams and suppositories in this regimen are oil-based and may weaken latex condoms and diaphragms.

of a cream is preferred in the presence of vulvar symptoms. Use of terconazole is more effective in non-*albicans* VVC. The choice of an oral vs. topical therapy can be based on patient preference. However, increased cost and a small risk of liver toxicity cause some health care providers to reserve oral fluconazole for recurrent or recalcitrant VVC. Treatment of VVC in pregnancy should use one of the topical azoles, preferably for 7 days.[46] Treatment of sexual partners is not indicated except in cases of symptomatic balanitis or penile dermatitis.

In recurrent VVC it is necessary to assess for predisposing conditions and to confirm the diagnosis by culture. Evaluation should include a fasting blood sugar in nonpregnant patients or a glucose tolerance test if the patient is pregnant. Routine HIV testing is not indicated in patients without identifiable risk factors.[46]

An optimal treatment strategy for recurrent VVC has not been identified. A reduction in recurrences has been shown with an initial intensive regimen of topical therapy for 10 to 14 days, followed by oral ketoconazole, 100 mg every day for ≤6 months.[46] Current studies are evaluating the use of weekly clotrimazole, itraconazole, and fluconazole in recurrent VVC.[46] Patients taking oral antifungal agents should have their liver function tests monitored regularly.

COMPLICATIONS

Complications are uncommon. Superficial lesions and lacerations may occur in the vagina and vulva. Severely immunosuppressed patients may develop systemic infection. Patients with type 2 (non-insulin-dependent) diabetes who are taking oral hypoglycemic medications and are being treated with fluconazole may develop severe hypoglycemia. Interactions of fluconazole with other drugs, particularly warfarin, are potentially serious.

INDICATIONS FOR REFERRAL/HOSPITALIZATION AND PATIENT AND FAMILY EDUCATION

See Indications for Referral/Hospitalization and Patient and Family Education, p. 824.

Trichomoniasis

PATHOPHYSIOLOGY

Trichomoniasis results from vaginal infection with the flagellated protozoan *Trichomonas vaginalis,* which is predominantly sexually transmitted. Transmission through contact with fomites may occur rarely.

CLINICAL PRESENTATION AND PHYSICAL EXAMINATION

Symptoms of trichomoniasis include vulvovaginal irritation, increased vaginal discharge, and occasional dysuria. On examination the discharge can be yellow-green, copious, and frothy. Vaginal inflammation is present, and punctate hemorrhages on the cervix are occasionally seen, producing the so-called strawberry cervix.

DIAGNOSTICS

In trichomoniasis the vaginal pH is greater than 4.5. Motile, flagellated trichomonads, and leukocytes are seen on a saline wet mount. Diagnosis by wet mount has approximately 30% to 70% sensitivity.[47] Diagnosis by culture is more sensitive and should be considered if there is suspicion of trichomoniasis, but the wet mount is negative. Polymerase chain reaction testing is also available, although it is not commonly used at this time. The diagnosis can also be made incidentally if the organisms are found on a Pap test.

DIFFERENTIAL DIAGNOSIS

See the Differential Diagnosis box on p. 823.

MANAGEMENT

Treatment options for trichomoniasis are outlined in Box 185-7. Concurrent treatment of sexual partners is necessary, and the patient and her partner(s) should refrain from sexual activity until all have completed treatment and are symptom free. Patients and their partners must be instructed to avoid alcohol during treatment with metronidazole and for 24 hours after its completion to avoid a disulfiram-type reaction (severe nausea and vomiting). The FDA has approved metronidazole (Flagyl) 375 mg b.i.d. for 7 days for treatment of trichomoniasis on the basis of its pharmacokinetic equivalency with metronidazole 250 mg t.i.d. for 7 days. No clinical data are available to demonstrate clinical efficacy.

Patients with culture-documented trichomoniasis who do not respond to treatment as outlined in Box 185-7 and in whom reinfection has been excluded should be managed with expert consultation, including metronidazole susceptibility testing, which is available through the Centers for Disease Control and Prevention.[46]

Diagnostics

Trichomoniasis

Initial
pH ≥5

Laboratory
Wet mount with normal saline or 10% KOH
Culture
Pap test
Direct immunofluorescent antibody staining*

*If indicated.

BOX 185-7

TREATMENT OF TRICHOMONIASIS

RECOMMENDED REGIMEN
Metronidazole, 2 g PO in a single dose

ALTERNATIVE REGIMEN
Metronidazole, 500 mg PO b.i.d. for 7 days

IN THE EVENT OF TREATMENT FAILURE
The patient and her partner(s) should be retreated with metronidazole, 500 mg PO b.i.d. for 7 days

IF TREATMENT IS AGAIN UNSUCCESSFUL
Retreat patient with metronidazole, 2 g PO q.d. for 3-5 days

Modified from Centers for Disease Control and Prevention: 1998 Guidelines for treatment of sexually transmitted diseases, *MMWR* 47(RR-1): 70-79, 1998.

COMPLICATIONS

Trichomoniasis in pregnancy has been associated with such adverse outcomes as premature rupture of membranes, preterm delivery, and low birth weight. Its treatment in pregnancy has been controversial because of concerns regarding the safety of metronidazole in pregnancy. As discussed earlier under Bacterial Vaginosis, this stance has been increasingly challenged. More conservative sources recommend waiting until the second trimester to treat with metronidazole, 2 g PO in a single dose, whereas some newer data suggest that waiting is not necessary.[57] If waiting until the second trimester to treat is preferred, clotrimazole can be used intravaginally for symptomatic relief. A test of cure should follow treatment of trichomoniasis in pregnancy.

INDICATIONS FOR REFERRAL/HOSPITALIZATION AND PATIENT AND FAMILY EDUCATION

See Indications for Referral/Hospitalization and Patient and Family Education, p. 824.

Atrophic Vaginitis

PATHOPHYSIOLOGY

Atrophic vaginitis is caused by reduced endogenous estrogen levels. This is most commonly found in the postmenopausal patient, although lactation, antagonistic medications, and ovarian failure resulting from disease processes also induce hypoestrogenic states. The lower estrogen level causes the vaginal epithelium to become thin and fragile, with a decreased glycogen content. There is an increased pH as a result of decreased lactic acid production, leading to an environment prone to an overgrowth of pathogenic organisms and to a lowered concentration of lactobacilli. Despite these changes, most women with vaginal atrophy are not symptomatic.

CLINICAL PRESENTATION AND PHYSICAL EXAMINATION

Women with atrophic vaginitis present with vaginal soreness, vulvovaginal dryness, occasional vaginal discharge or spotting, and dyspareunia. The vulvar skin is thin, with decreased subcutaneous tissue and variable pubic hair loss. The vaginal walls are pale with decreased or absent rugae, with occasional petechiae. Vaginal discharge can be thick, watery, or blood tinged.

DIAGNOSTICS

The vaginal pH in atrophic vaginitis is usually 5.5 to 7. The saline wet mount reveals increased leukocytes and small, round epithelia. If unexplained vaginal bleeding is present, endometrial biopsy is necessary. Similarly, if vulvar pruritus is present, a biopsy is indicated to exclude vulvar dystrophy or carcinoma. Cultures to exclude concurrent infections are done as indicated.

DIFFERENTIAL DIAGNOSIS

Although the majority of patients with vaginitis have one of the conditions outlined in the preceding material, there are other important, although less common, conditions to be considered in the differential diagnosis.

Cytolytic Vaginosis

Cytolytic vaginosis (CV) is an important condition to consider in the differential diagnosis for recurrent VVC. It is caused by an overgrowth of *Lactobacillus* organisms in the vagina, which causes a decreased pH. This increased acidity is believed to be responsible for the irritative symptoms. Patients present with vulvovaginal pruritus, dyspareunia, clumpy white discharge, and vulvar dysuria. There tends to be an increase in symptoms during the luteal phase of the menstrual cycle. Most patients have tried numerous antifungal therapies to treat their symptoms, with only limited relief.

The diagnosis of CV is primarily by saline wet mount. There is an absence of trichomonads, "clue cells," and *Candida* organisms. There is an increase in lactobacilli, which may adhere to the epithelial cells, producing a "false clue cell." There may be bare or "naked" nuclei, the products of cytolysis. The pH is generally 3.5 to 4.5.

Treatment of CV involves raising the vaginal pH. The patient should be encouraged to discontinue all antifungal treatments. The use of tampons should be discontinued, thus allowing the alkaline menstrual blood to bathe the vaginal walls.[53] Baking soda sitz baths can decrease the irritative vulvar symptoms by neutralizing the acidic secretions. The patient can add 2 to 4 tablespoons of baking soda to 1 to 2 inches of warm bathwater for the sitz bath. Finally, if these conservative measures do not provide relief, the patient can use baking soda douches once or twice a week as needed.[58] These can be prepared using 1 to 2 teaspoons of baking soda in a pint of warm water.

Viral Infections

Viral infections such as herpes simplex virus (HSV) and HPV can also cause vaginal complaints. HSV can affect the cervix, causing profuse vaginal discharge, along with pain and ulceration. HPV can produce exophytic vaginal lesions, and larger condylomas can produce vaginal discharge, postcoital bleeding, and pruritus. The diagnosis and treatment of these viruses are outlined elsewhere in this text.

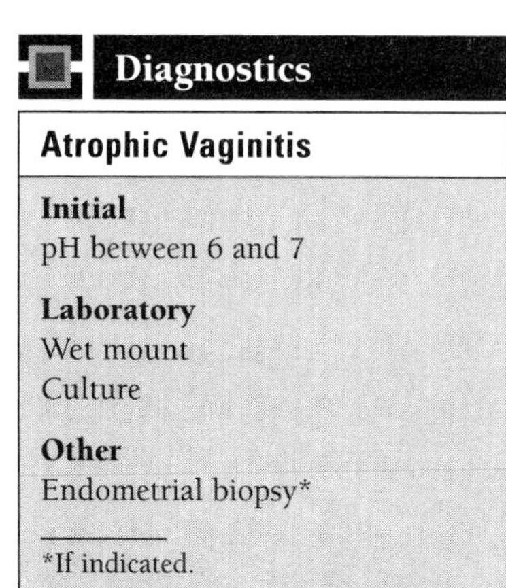

Diagnostics

Atrophic Vaginitis

Initial
pH between 6 and 7

Laboratory
Wet mount
Culture

Other
Endometrial biopsy*

*If indicated.

Differential Diagnosis

Vaginitis and Vaginosis

Bacterial vaginosis	Viral infections
Trichomoniasis	Foreign bodies
Candidiasis	Cervicitis
Gonorrhea	Hypersensitivity
Chlamydia	Physiologic discharge
Cytolytic vaginosis	

Foreign Body

Vaginal foreign bodies can cause inflammatory reactions leading to malodorous discharge, risk of ulceration, and fissures secondary to pressure necrosis. The symptoms generally resolve with the removal of the foreign body.

Cervicitis

Mucopurulent cervicitis is another cause of vaginal discharge that may also cause irritative vaginal symptoms. Cultures for gonorrhea and chlamydia should be performed.

Hypersensitivity

Allergy and contact dermatitis are possible causes of vaginitis symptoms. A thorough history can help identify any offending agents, especially spermicides, latex, bubble baths, "feminine hygiene" products, and soaps. Latex sensitivity should be suspected if the patient's symptoms are reproduced with a gynecologic examination using latex gloves. The elimination of the offending agent, short-term use of a mild corticosteroid cream, cool compresses, and use of a bland emollient such as mineral oil should provide relief of the symptoms. Avoidance of latex can be challenging. Use of nonlatex condoms or the "female condom" should be recommended, although nonlatex male condoms are less protective for HIV. The patient's chart should be labeled in cases of latex sensitivity to avoid future use of latex gloves or other products during examinations. Referral is indicated if symptoms do not resolve within 1 to 2 weeks and other etiologies cannot be identified.

Physiologic Discharge

Finally, the patient presenting with increased vaginal discharge in the absence of malodor or irritative symptoms may simply need education regarding physiologic discharge and the cyclic variations that are possible.

MANAGEMENT

Treatment of atrophic vaginitis involves estrogen therapy, which causes maturation of the epithelium, reversing the changes that resulted in the vaginitis. Regimens may include standard postmenopausal oral estrogen or estrogen with progestin therapy if this is not contraindicated and if other therapeutic benefits are desired. Otherwise, treatment usually involves topical estrogen cream, tablets, or vaginal rings. Recommended regimens include estradiol cream 0.1%, 2 to 4 g intravaginally every day for 1 to 2 weeks, then 1 to 2 g intravaginally every day for 1 to 2 weeks, then 1 g intravaginally one to three times per week for maintenance; *or* conjugated estrogen cream, 2 to 4 g intravaginally every day for 1 to 2 weeks, then 2 to 4 g intravaginally every other day for 1 to 2 weeks. The conjugated estrogen cream is then tapered and discontinued. A pill form of estradiol is also available and is used intravaginally every day for 1 to 2 weeks, then twice weekly for 2 to 4 weeks then tapered and discontinued. A vaginal estrogen ring is available that is placed in the vagina and remains in place for 90 days.

An effort to taper and discontinue any regimen should be attempted after 3 months, as continued therapy may not be necessary. If treatment continues for more than 3 months, the addition of periodic progestin therapy is indicated in the patient with an intact uterus (e.g., medroxyprogesterone acetate, 10 mg PO every day for the first 7 days of each month). Patients with atrophic vaginitis in whom estrogen is contraindicated may benefit from the use of lubricants or acidifying agents, although success has been limited.

INDICATIONS FOR REFERRAL/HOSPITALIZATION

Consultation with a gynecologist is indicated in cases of treatment failure as previously indicated. Postmenopausal women with unexplained vaginal bleeding or vulvar pruritus require referral for appropriate biopsy. Gynecologic consultation is also indicated in cases with an unusual presentation or in which the etiology is unknown or unclear.

PATIENT AND FAMILY EDUCATION

Thorough patient education is necessary regarding diagnosis, transmission, treatment, prevention, need for treatment of sexual partners, need for test of cure, and the sequelae of remaining untreated. Anticipatory guidance regarding medication side effects is essential. Furthermore, patients need counseling regarding the time by which relief can be expected and the indications for reevaluation. HIV testing and counseling should be considered in patients whose sexual activities have put them at higher risk.

REFERENCES

1. Nunns D, Mandel D: The chronically symptomatic vulva: prevalence in primary health care, *Genitourin Med* 72:343-344, 1996.
2. Meffert L, Davis B, Grimwood R: Lichen sclerosus, *J Am Acad Dermatol* 32(3):393-416, 1995.
3. Thomas R and others: Anogenital lichen sclerosus in women, *J R Soc Med* 89:694-698, 1995.
4. Leibowitch M: Lichen sclerosus, *Semin Dermatol* 15(1):42-46, 1996.
5. Wilkinson E, Stone K: *Atlas of vulvar disease*, Baltimore, 1995, Williams & Wilkins.
6. O'Keefe R and others: Audit of 114 non-neoplastic vulvar biopsies, *Br J Obstet Gynaecol* 102:780-786, 1995.
7. Bracco G et al: Clinical and histologic effects of topical treatments of vulvar lichen sclerosus: a critical evaluation, *J Reprod Med* 38(1): 37-40, 1993.
8. Bornstein J and others: Clobetasol dipropionate 0.05% versus testosterone propionate 2% topical application for severe lichen sclerosus, *Am J Obstet Gynecol* 178:80-84, 1998.
9. Lorenz B and others: Lichen sclerosus: therapy with clobetasol propionate, *J Reprod Med* 43(9): 790-794, 1998.
10. Sinha P and others: Lichen sclerosus of the vulva: long-term steroid maintenance therapy, *J Reprod Med* 44(7):621-624, 1999.
11. Zellis S, Pincus S: Treatment of vulvar dermatoses, *Semin Dermatol* 15(1):71-76, 1996.
12. Joura E and others: Short-term effects of topical testosterone in vulvar lichen sclerosus, *Obstet Gynecol* 89(2):297-299, 1997.
13. Abramov Y and others: Surgical treatment of vulvar lichen sclerosus: a review, *Obstet Gynecol Surv* 51(3):193-199, 1996.
14. Larrabee R, Kylander J: Benign vulvar disorders: identifying features, practical management of nonneoplastic conditions and tumors, *Postgrad Med* 109(5):151-164, 2001.
15. Kaufman RH, Faro S: *Benign diseases of the vulva and vagina*, ed 4, St Louis, 1994, Mosby.
16. Fitzpatrick TB and others: Disorders of cell kinetics and differentiation. In *Color atlas and synopsis of clinical dermatology: common and serious disease*, ed 5, New York, 1997, McGraw Hill.

17. Hopkins MP, Snyder MK: Benign disorders of vulva and vagina. In Curtis MG, Hopkins MP, editors: *Glass's office gynecology,* ed 5, Baltimore, 1999, Williams & Wilkins.
18. Lewis FM: Vulvar lichen planus, *Br J Dermatol* 138(4):569-575, 1998.
19. Reference deleted in galleys.
20. Lynch P: Vulvodynia: a syndrome of unexplained vulvar pain, psychologic disability and sexual dysfunction: the 1985 ISSVD presidential address, *J Reprod Med* 31(9):773-780, 1986.
21. Friedrich EG: Vulvar vestibulitis syndrome, *J Reprod Med* 32:110-114, 1987.
22. Davis G, Hutchison C: Clinical management of vulvodynia, *Clin Obstet Gynecol* 42(2):221-233, 1999.
23. Goestch M: Vulvar vestibulitis: prevalence and historic features in a general gynecologic population, *Am J Obstet Gynecol* 164(6):1609-1616, 1991.
24. Furlonge C and others: Vulvar vestibulitis syndrome: a clinico-pathological study, *Br J Obstet Gynaecol* 98:703-706, 1991.
25. Fitzpatrick C and others: Vulvar vestibulitis and interstitial cystitis: a disorder of urogenital sinus-derived epithelium? *Obstet Gynecol* 81(5):860-861, 1993.
26. Foster D, Robinson J, Davis K: Urethral pressure variation in women with vulvar vestibulitis syndrome, *Am J Obstet Gynecol* 169(1):107-112, 1993.
27. Glazer H and others: Treatment of vulvar vestibulitis syndrome with electromyographic biofeedback of pelvic floor musculature, *J Reprod Med* 40(4):284-290, 1995.
28. White G, Jantos M, Glazer H: Establishing the diagnosis of vulvar vestibulitis, *J Reprod Med* 42(3):157-160, 1997.
29. Mann M and others: Vulvar vestibulitis: significant clinical variables and treatment outcomes, *Obstet Gynecol* 79(1):122-125, 1992.
30. Bazin S and others: Vulvar vestibulitis syndrome: an exploratory case-control study, *Obstet Gynecol* 83(1):47-50, 1994.
31. Sjöberg I, Lundqvist E: Vulvar vestibulitis in the north of Sweden: an epidemiologic case-control study, *J Reprod Med* 42(3):166-168, 1997.
32. Friedrich E: Vulvar vestibulitis syndrome, *J Reprod Med* 32(2): 110-114, 1987.
33. Foster D and others: Long-term outcome of perineoplasty for vulvar vestibulitis, *J Women Health* 4(6):669-675, 1995.
34. Julian T: Essential "dysesthetic" vulvodynia: (1) diagnosis and evaluation; (2) a rational approach for management, *Adv Colposcopy* 1-8, 1994.
35. McKay M: Dysesthetic ("essential") vulvodynia: treatment with amitriptyline, *J Reprod Med* 38(1):9-13, 1993.
36. Edwards L: Vulvodynia: an addendum by Libby Edwards, MD, *Fitzpatrick's J Clin Dermatol* 3(5):10-12, 1995.
37. Solomons C, Melmed M, Heitler S: Calcium citrate for vulvar vestibulitis: a case report, *J Reprod Med* 36(12):879-882, 1991.
38. Pomerantz E: Vulvodynia: etiology and treatment strategies, *J ObGyn Patient* 18(3):10-12, 1994.
39. Spadt S: Suffering in silence: managing vulvar pain patients, *Contemp Nurse Pract* 32-38, 1995.
40. Marinoff S and others: Intralesional alpha interferon: cost-effective therapy for vulvar vestibulitis syndrome, *J Reprod Med* 38(1):19-24, 1993.
41. Reid R and others: Flashlamp-excited dye laser therapy of idiopathic vulvodynia is safe and efficacious, *Am J Obstet Gynecol* 172(6):1684-1701, 1995.
42. Abramov L, Wolman I, David M: Vaginismus: an important factor in the evaluation and management of vulvar vestibulitis syndrome, *Gynecol Obstet Invest* 38:194-197, 1994.
43. Schover L, Youngs D, Cannata R: Psychosexual aspects of the evaluation and management of vulvar vestibulitis, *Am J Obstet Gynecol* 167(3):630-636, 1992.
44. Jones K, Lehr S: Vulvodynia: diagnostic techniques and treatment modalities, *Nurse Pract* 19(4):34-46, 1994.
45. Wakamatsu MM: Vaginitis. In Carlson KJ, Eisenstat SA, editors: *Primary care of women,* St Louis, 1995, Mosby.
46. Colli E and others: Treatment of male partners and reoccurrence of bacterial vaginosis: a randomized trial, *Genitourin Med* 73:267-270, 1997.
47. Centers for Disease Control and Prevention: 1998 Guidelines for treatment of sexually transmitted diseases, *MMWR* 47(RR-1):70-79, 1998.
48. Mead PB and others: Screening for lower genital tract pathogens in the OB patient, *Contemp Ob/Gyn* 42(5):126-145, 1997.
49. Burtin P and others: Safety of metronidazole in pregnancy: a meta-analysis, *Am J Obstet Gynecol* 172:525-529, 1995.
50. Hay P: Recurrent bacterial vaginosis, *Curr Infect Dis Rep* 2:506-512, 2000.
51. Sobel JD, Leaman D: Suppressive maintenance therapy of recurrent bacterial vaginosis utilizing 0.75% metronidazole gel, *Int J Gynaecol Obstet* 67(suppl):41, 1999.
52. Taha TE et al: Bacterial vaginosis and disturbances of vaginal flora: association with increased acquisition of HIV, *AIDS* 12:1699-1706, 1998.
53. Royce RA and others: Bacterial vaginosis associated with HIV infection in pregnant women from North Carolina, *J Acquir Immune Defic Syndr Hum Retrovirol* 20:382-386, 1999.
54. Taha TE et al: HIV infection and disturbances of vaginal flora during pregnancy, *J Acquir Immune Defic Syndr Hum Retrovirol* 20:52-59, 1999.
55. Martin HL and others: Vaginal lactobacilli, microbial flora and risk of human immunodeficiency virus type 1 and sexually transmitted disease acquisition, *J Infect Dis* 180:1863-1868, 1999.
56. Tevi-Benissan C and others: In vivo semen-associated pH neutralization of cervicovaginal secretions, *Clin Diagn Lab Immunol* 4:367-374, 1997.
57. Spinillo A and others: Prevalence of and risk factors for fungal vaginitis caused by non- albicans species, *Am J Obstet Gynecol* 176:138-141, 1997.
58. Secor RMC: Cytolytic vaginosis: a common cause of cyclic vulvovaginitis, *Nurse Pract Forum* 3(3):145-148, 1992.

PART 15

Evaluation and Management of Musculoskeletal and Arthritic Disorders

JOANNE SANDBERG-COOK, Section Editor

CHAPTER 186

Ankle and Foot Pain

Marie-Eileen Onieal

The foot contains 26 bones. Twelve of these bones are components of the medial and lateral longitudinal arches. In conjunction with the ankle, the foot plays a major role in supporting the body and providing locomotion. These functions can cause painful conditions of the foot that develop in the heel, arch, or forefoot. Improper or ill-fitting footwear is often the culprit.

In the United States, foot and ankle problems are the reason for more than 5.3 million visits every year to health care providers. Approximately 1.6 million visits are for ankle sprains and 950,000 visits are for ankle fractures.[1] Sports injuries are often the cause, but even activities of daily living stress the foot and ankle. Walking alone puts up to 1.5 times body weight on the foot. The average person logs roughly 1000 miles yearly. During 1 hour of strenuous exercise, feet cushion up to 1 million pounds of pressure.

The specific functions of the ankle and foot predispose them to injuries and disorders that can result in chronic problems if not identified quickly and managed properly.

Ankle Sprains

DEFINITION AND EPIDEMIOLOGY

The uniaxial ankle joint, or ankle joint, is the most primitive joint in the body and is crucial to walking, running, and the performance of all sports. The limited motion of the ankle gives it stability. The ankle joint consists of three major bones: the tibia, fibula, and talus. The tibia and fibula form the ankle mortise, and the talus fits into this mortise. The talus, which has no muscle or tendon attachment, gives the ankle its hinge motion. The talus also bears the entire weight of the extremity during walking. The deltoid, anterior talofibular, calcaneal fibular, and the posterior talofibular ligaments hold the ankle bones in the mortise.

Ankle sprains occur in all ages and are the most common problem encountered by primary care providers. A sprain is a ligamentous injury caused by an abnormal motion, a sudden change in direction, or a misstep on an uneven surface. Even a minor ankle sprain can jeopardize joint stability. The severity of the physical findings determines the sprain category (Table 186-1). The categories define the management of the injury, but the category parameters are indistinct. Previous ankle sprains can increase the potential for injury recurrence. Early diagnosis, treatment, and rehabilitation decrease the recurrence of a sprain in a previously injured ankle.

PATHOPHYSIOLOGY

Two types of injuries cause an ankle sprain. The most common is the inversion injury, in which the foot plantar flexes and internally rotates as the ankle inverts. The "roll" of the ankle injures the lateral ligaments and can also cause a lateral avulsion fracture. The less common eversion injury occurs when the ankle sustains an external rotation mechanism. Eversion stress injures the medial structures of the ankle, damaging the deltoid ligament or the syndesmosis.

CLINICAL PRESENTATION

The most common presentation of an ankle sprain is a swollen and painful joint. Ecchymosis and decreased range of motion are generally present. In many instances, weight bearing causes pain; some patients are unable to bear any weight on the affected joint.

When obtaining the history, it is important to determine if the patient heard any audible sounds at the time of injury. An audible "snap" or "pop" indicates the potential for a more serious injury. Immediate swelling or ecchymosis raises the suspicion of a fracture or the amount of joint involvement. Patients also commonly report a sensation of light-headedness, nausea, or diaphoresis immediately after the injury.[2]

PHYSICAL EXAMINATION

With a sprain, the ankle joint is often swollen and ecchymotic, and the edema can create an illusion of deformity. Limited active and passive motion and point tenderness at the site of injury are common. Joint laxity is present in more severe sprains. Muscle spasm often prevents accurate testing of strength and stability. If the injury is not acute, swelling and ecchymosis at the lateral aspect of the foot and the toes are common. With severe ankle sprains, tenderness may extend up the extremity. The entire lower limb should always be palpated.

DIAGNOSTICS

Although guidelines for radiographs are controversial, plain radiographs are necessary for severe injuries. An x-ray study of the lower leg should also be performed if there is tenderness at the fibular head. With less severe injuries, radiographs are used to exclude an avulsion injury. More extensive radiologic examinations such as stress films, CT scans, and MRIs are considered in consultation with an orthopedic surgeon.

DIFFERENTIAL DIAGNOSIS

Ankle injuries range from simple strains to severe injury. The possibility of associated fibula fracture, stress fracture, avulsion fracture, or dislocation should be considered. Bursitis and tendinitis should be included in the differential diagnosis.

MANAGEMENT

The severity of the sprain dictates the management (see Table 186-1). TED (thromboembolic disease) hose provide support to the entire lower limb, aid circulation, and are less bulky. All sprains require rehabilitation to restore the ankle to a

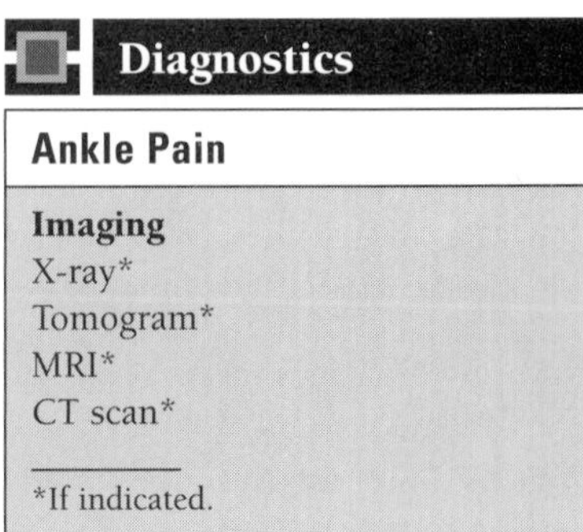

Diagnostics

Ankle Pain

Imaging
X-ray*
Tomogram*
MRI*
CT scan*

*If indicated.

TABLE 186-1 Classification and Treatment of Ankle Sprains

First Degree	Second Degree	Third Degree
PATHOLOGY		
Stretching/minor tearing of ligament fibers	Partial tearing of ligament fibers	Complete tearing of ligament fibers
FINDINGS		
Minimal pain	Mild to moderate pain	Severe pain
Mild swelling	Moderate swelling	Significant swelling*
Mild ecchymosis	Moderate ecchymosis	Severe ecchymosis*
Full range of motion (ROM)	Painful, slightly limited motion	Loss of function
Mild point tenderness	Point tenderness over joint	Severe pain (difficult examination)
Stable joint	Mild joint laxity with stress	Abnormal joint movement
Ability to bear weight	Painful to bear weight (may be unable to do so)	Inability to bear weight
TREATMENT		
RICE; active ROM exercises	RICE; active ROM exercises as tolerated	Referral to orthopedic surgeon (may require surgery)
Non–weight-bearing activity (swimming, stationary bike)	Partial weight bearing (crutches/cane) as tolerated	Cast for 4-6 weeks
		No weight bearing
Return to sports in 2-3 weeks	Gradual progression to full weight bearing	Gradual progression to full weight bearing
	Return to sports in 4-8 weeks with ankle support (Aircast or taping)	Rehabilitation before returning to sports with ankle support (Aircast or taping)
SEQUELAE		
Tends to recur in first month if not fully rehabilitated	Recurrent sprains, joint instability, traumatic arthritis	Persistent instability (nonsurgical treatment), traumatic arthritis

Created by Marie-Eileen Onieal, PhD (c), MMHS, RNC, PNP, FAANP.
*Occurs rapidly, usually within the first 30 minutes.

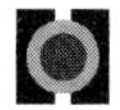

Differential Diagnosis

Ankle Pain

Trauma/fracture	Dislocation/subluxation
Strain	Tendinitis
Sprain (first, second, or third degree)	Achilles tendonitis
Bursitis	Achilles bursitis

stable and pain-free state. It is important that patients understand that the treatment and recovery process will take weeks. Rehabilitation should begin as soon as possible after the injury and should include range-of-motion and strengthening exercises.[3] Even a severely edematous ankle can be mobilized with the simple exercise of "writing the alphabet" with the affected foot. A program of active and passive resistive exercises progresses as range of motion and strength improves. Patients can return to sports when they are pain free and are able to balance on the injured leg. The patient with a second- or third-degree sprain should wear an external ankle support such as the Aircast stirrup for the remainder of the season.[3]

COMPLICATIONS

Most ankle sprains tend to recur within the first month if the ankle has not been fully rehabilitated. Second- and third-degree sprains carry with them an increased risk of joint instability and traumatic arthritis. A weak ankle joint is at risk for fracture when stressed.

INDICATIONS FOR REFERRAL/HOSPITALIZATION

Fractures, dislocations/subluxations, and grade 3 sprains require an orthopedic referral. Physical therapy may also be indicated to promote rehabilitation and a safe return to sports or work-related activities.

PATIENT AND FAMILY EDUCATION

Patients need to understand the importance of RICE (rest, ice, compression, and elevation), as well as the necessity of preventing weight bearing on the injured ankle. Patients and family members should also be instructed in medication dosages and side effects, proper Ace bandages wrapping technique, cast care, and crutch usage. The recuperative process and the risk of recurrence also require explanation.

Achilles Tendinitis

DEFINITION/EPIDEMIOLOGY

The Achilles tendon is posterior to the ankle joint and is responsible for flexion and extension of the ankle. It attaches the gastrocnemius and the soleus of the calf to the calcaneus, and it is palpated from the distal pole of the calf to the calcaneus.[4] The two most common injuries of the Achilles tendon are tendinitis and rupture.

Achilles tendinitis is a painful inflammation with or without swelling around the Achilles tendon. Unlike other tendons, the Achilles tendon does not have a synovial sheath but instead has a paratenon, which has a similar function. Except for severe cases, true Achilles tendinitis primarily affects the paratenon.[5] A nodule of mucoid degeneration forms in the body of the tendon in severe or chronic Achilles tendinitis.[6]

PATHOPHYSIOLOGY

Improper training, running up hills, or wearing shoes with soles that are too rigid often causes Achilles tendinitis. Shoes or boots with a high back can also irritate the tendon, causing inflammation. Wearing shoes with heels that maintain plantar flexion for long periods causes the tendon to shorten. Changing to flat or running shoes then increases stress on the tendon. Occasionally, Achilles tendinitis is caused by an anatomic abnormality such as excessive foot pronation or tight hamstrings or gastrocnemius muscles.[6]

CLINICAL PRESENTATION

Patients with Achilles tendinitis may have intermittent symptoms and may describe a pain that subsides during exercise but increases in severity while at rest. Morning stiffness or severe pain when climbing stairs is also common. Most patients have an abnormal gait. Some limp and some walk on their toes to avoid the heel-strike phase of walking.

PHYSICAL EXAMINATION

Localized swelling may be present around the tendon. A palpable nodule and crepitus may be present in severe or chronic cases.[7]

DIAGNOSTICS

Radiologic or laboratory tests are usually unnecessary, but the appropriate diagnostic tests should be guided by the history. MRI may be useful in diagnosing a ruptured tendon.

DIFFERENTIAL DIAGNOSIS

Heel pain may have varied causes. Sprains, infection, fracture, plantar fasciitis, and partial tendon rupture should be considered in the differential diagnosis of Achilles tendinitis.

MANAGEMENT

Treatment of the acute phase of Achilles tendinitis begins with the cessation of all sports activities and exercise. Tendon rest is imperative to avoid further injury. In severe tendinitis, crutches and partial weight bearing are indicated. Nonsteroidal antiinflammatory drugs (NSAIDs) and an ice massage for 20 minutes three to four times a day help to decrease inflammation and pain. A simple shoe insert that raises the heel approximately 2 cm also helps to ease strain on the tendon. In more severe or chronic cases, ultrasound is an adjunct therapy. Regular follow-up visits to assess progress and to discourage the patient from returning to activity prematurely are necessary. Resolution of acute tendinitis can take 8 weeks or longer. A program of stretching and strengthening begins when pain and swelling have subsided. To prevent recurrence or rupture, it is essential that patients do stretching exercises before engaging in any exercise.

COMPLICATIONS

Achilles tendon rupture is the most common complication of Achilles tendinitis. Shortening of the tendon, chronic tendinitis, and injuries as a result of the commonly associated abnormal gait also may result from acute tendinitis.

INDICATIONS FOR REFERRAL/HOSPITALIZATION

Patients with severe tendinitis or suspected tendon rupture require immediate referral to the orthopedic surgeon. In addition, patients who fail conservative therapy or who have significant tightness in the hamstrings or gastrocnemius require referral.

PATIENT AND FAMILY EDUCATION

Achilles tendinitis can be a frustrating, slowly resolving, and recurrent problem. Patients with this condition need support during rehabilitation and need to be educated about proper retraining and stretching programs. During the rehabilitative phase, alternative activities such as swimming or cycling can be pursued as long as participation does not cause pain.

Achilles Tendon Rupture

DEFINITION AND EPIDEMIOLOGY

Achilles tendon rupture is a sudden event that results from a forced stretch on an already degenerating tendon; it is a soft tissue emergency. Although Achilles tendon ruptures are not common, there is an increased risk for this injury in poorly conditioned athletes more than 30 years old. In all, 80% of those injured are men; moreover, because most right-handed people begin their gait with their left foot, there is a higher incidence of left tendon ruptures.[8]

PATHOPHYSIOLOGY

Despite being the thickest and strongest tendon in the body, the Achilles tendon is the one most commonly ruptured, possibly as a result of underlying tendon degeneration or weakness that predisposes the tendon to rupture. In persons over age 30 years, there is a decreased blood supply to the area where the tendon most often ruptures. Often the offending event is a jump, a sudden change in direction, or simply a push off in stride. The pop of a tendon rupture is audible to others nearby.

CLINICAL PRESENTATION

The classic comment by patients with an Achilles tendon rupture is, "I thought I was shot in the calf." There is sudden weakness in the ankle. It is impossible to rise up on the toes and most people will limp; pain, however, is not common.

PHYSICAL EXAMINATION

There is a visible and palpable "gap" overlying the tendon where the rupture occurred, usually about $1\frac{1}{2}$ inches above the calcaneal prominence. The definitive evaluation is the Thompson test, which is performed with the patient kneeling on a chair or prone with the knee in flexed position. The tendon is intact if the foot plantar flexes when the calf is squeezed (negative Thompson). If there is no movement, the tendon is ruptured (positive Thompson). The Thompson test can be negative if the tear is partial.

DIAGNOSTICS

Radiologic examinations are not helpful because tendons are not radiopaque. MRI will demonstrate the rupture and can be used if indicated.

DIFFERENTIAL DIAGNOSIS

The classic presentation and physical findings that characterize a ruptured Achilles tendon simplify the diagnosis. However, the diagnosis may be more complex with a partial tear. Achilles tendinitis or Achilles bursitis is not usually associated with a sudden onset.

MANAGEMENT

There are two accepted treatments for the ruptured Achilles tendon. The conservative, nonsurgical approach requires a long-leg cast with the foot in a plantar-flexed position. The cast stays on for approximately 6 weeks, allowing the tendon to heal by scar formation. Wearing a heel lift for 2 months helps to prevent undue stress on the new scar after casting. Unfortunately, this method has multiple disadvantages. The tendon heals longer in length, which weakens the calf muscle and the push-off power. Calf muscles also atrophy in a cast (usually about 20%), which adds to the decreased strength and size. In addition, 20% of the tendons allowed to heal in this manner rupture again once activities resume.[9] Patients with chronic pain who are not surgical candidates may benefit from an ankle-foot orthosis.

The second method of treatment for a ruptured Achilles tendon is surgical repair. The patient is in a long-leg cast for 6 weeks after surgery; then the patient wears a short-leg, walking cast for an additional 4 weeks.[10] As in the nonoperative method, a heel lift is used to prevent undue stress on the tendon. The surgical method is superior to the nonoperative method because it restores 95% of the normal power of the calf muscle.[9]

COMPLICATIONS

Weakened or atrophied muscles are a common complication of tendon ruptures. Close attention to rehabilitation and muscle strengthening after the injury helps reduce the magnitude of these complications.

INDICATIONS FOR REFERRAL/HOSPITALIZATION

An Achilles tendon rupture is a soft tissue emergency. Immediate referral to an orthopedic surgeon is required.

PATIENT AND FAMILY EDUCATION

The most important education regarding Achilles tendon rupture is preventive. Patients who are beginning to exercise should be instructed to follow a simple, gentle stretching program before exercising. For example, patients can stand on a slanted board or on the edge of a step and let their heels drop below the level of the step. This stretched position is held for 10 to 15 seconds, and the exercise is repeated for 10 to 15 minutes. If patients cannot feel a pull on the Achilles tendon, the stretch is not being done properly. Bouncing is counterproductive.

Osteochondritis Dissecans

DEFINITION AND EPIDEMIOLOGY

With osteochondritis dissecans, a small fragment of bone underlying the articular cartilage becomes avascular and necrotic. In some cases, this necrotic area dislodges from the surface. Repeated stress on the joint causes a separation of the articular surface of the joint. Osteochondritis dissecans is seen more in adolescents and young adults and usually in males. It is common in athletes who participate in activities in which the stress on the ankle is greater (ballet dancers, runners, basketball players). This condition also occurs at the knee and elbow.

PATHOPHYSIOLOGY

The etiology of this condition is unknown. Several theories have suggested various causes—trauma, nonunion of a fracture line, and ischemic necrosis have been implicated. Additionally noted are a familial tendency, certain skeletal abnormalities, or endocrine abnormalities.[11]

CLINICAL PRESENTATION

The usual presentation of osteochondritis dissecans is chronic pain and swelling that develops gradually over months. Activity increases the swelling and the pain, which intensifies as the ankle stiffens. Rest relieves the symptoms. Occasionally, the athlete will recall a trauma.

PHYSICAL EXAMINATION

Range of motion is usually normal, and the joint is stable. Because the damaged area is within the joint, it is often difficult to palpate an area of tenderness.

DIAGNOSTICS

Radiologic examination alone provides the definitive diagnosis. Plain x-ray films of the ankle occasionally reveal a loose bone fragment or an area of sclerotic bone. Tomograms or MRIs help to better define the lesion and the staging of the injury.

DIFFERENTIAL DIAGNOSIS

As in any joint, trauma or fracture should be considered. Tendinitis and recurrent sprain should also be considered.

MANAGEMENT

Osteochondritis dissecans warrants close observation by an orthopedic surgeon. Because the injured area has decreased or no capacity to heal itself, surgery is often necessary. In the younger child with a shorter duration of pain, immobilization in a cast for 4 to 6 weeks may resolve the problem. Older patients, patients with a longer duration of injury, or patients with a loose bone fragment require surgery.

COMPLICATIONS

Degenerative arthritis, decreased range of motion, and chronic pain are all potential sequelae of this condition.

INDICATIONS FOR REFERRAL/HOSPITALIZATION

Osteochondritis dissecans is a potentially serious condition. Orthopedic consultation is recommended to prevent complications.

PATIENT AND FAMILY EDUCATION

The exact cause of osteochondritis dissecans is unknown. Therefore it is important that patients and families understand that any joint pain that occurs during exercise or interferes with normal activities of daily living requires medical assessment. Careful explanation of the potential sequelae of this condition, including degenerative arthritis, decreased range of motion, and chronic pain, is also necessary.

Plantar Fasciitis

DEFINITION AND EPIDEMIOLOGY

Plantar fasciitis is a painful disorder that involves the plantar aspect of the heel. It can be acute or chronic and is characterized by pain in the bottom of the foot—along the arch and the heel bone. A dense fibrous tissue, the plantar fascia, extends from the calcaneal tuberosity to the metatarsal heads. The fascia can become irritated from overuse, trauma, or the wearing of shoes with poor arch support. People with flat or cavus feet are especially vulnerable to this condition.

PATHOPHYSIOLOGY

The plantar fascia supports the arch and the sole of the foot. High impact or stress, such as running and jumping, increases the pressure exerted on the fascia by spreading the toes or flattening the arch; this tears the fascia. Four common causes of fascia tears or inflammation are a sudden turn that causes increased pressure on the sole of the foot, shoes without adequate support, shoes with stiff soles, and feet that pronate excessively. Patients not uncommonly have heel spurs. The pain is gradual in onset and increases as the inflammation worsens or as the tear extends.

CLINICAL PRESENTATION

Patients with plantar fasciitis complain of pain with weight bearing the first thing in the morning or after periods of rest. High-impact activities, running, and rising up on toes aggravate the pain or make it unbearable. Occasionally patients limp or avoid planting the heel when walking.

PHYSICAL EXAMINATION

With plantar fasciitis, there is point tenderness at the insertion of the fascia to the calcaneus. There may be fullness along the arch. There may be pain along the body of the fascia, at the medial and lateral aspects of the heel, or at the metatarsal heads.

DIAGNOSTICS

X-ray studies are indicated to rule out any bony abnormality or underlying other cause such as a foreign body. Radiographs often reveal a bone spur that points forward from the heel.

DIFFERENTIAL DIAGNOSIS

A history of early morning heel discomfort that resolves after several minutes but returns later in the day is usually clinically diagnostic of plantar fasciitis. However, other causes of heel pain, including calcaneal fracture, retrocalcaneal or infracalcaneal bursitis, gout, infection of the calcaneal fat pad, arthritis, Reiter's syndrome, plantar warts, and tarsal tunnel syndrome, should be considered.

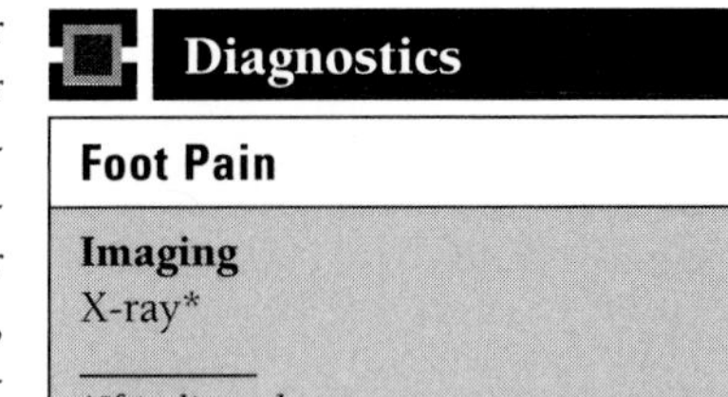

Diagnostics

Foot Pain

Imaging
X-ray*

*If indicated.

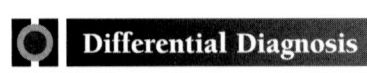

Differential Diagnosis

Foot Pain

Heel
Plantar fasciitis
Calcaneal fracture
Retrocalcaneal or infracalcaneal bursitis
Gout
Infection
Reiter's syndrome
Tarsal tunnel syndrome

Forefoot Pain
Morton's neuroma
Fracture
Infection
Ganglion
Ledderhose syndrome
Flat feet
Corn
Bunion
Peripheral neuritis

MANAGEMENT

A conservative approach to managing this condition begins with complete rest from high-impact activities. All shoes should have good arch support, which can be achieved with commercially available arch supports. Some patients do well with a heel cup or heel pad that raises the heel approximately $\frac{1}{4}$ inch. NSAIDs and ice massage help to reduce inflammation and pain. A key component of treatment is a program of exercises that stretch the heel cord and plantar fascia.

COMPLICATIONS

Usually there are no complications associated with plantar fasciitis. However, an alteration in gait can cause other musculoskeletal problems such as hip or back pain. Plantar fasciitis can be a lingering problem that frustrates both the patient and provider.

INDICATIONS FOR REFERRAL/HOSPITALIZATION

Any patient who fails to respond to conservative therapies should be referred to an orthopedic surgeon or a podiatrist. Ultrasound treatment by a physical therapist helps in severe cases; some patients benefit from custom-made orthotics, whereas others require cortisone injections. In rare cases, the fascia is surgically released.

PATIENT AND FAMILY EDUCATION

See Patient and Family Education under Morton's Neuroma, p. 833.

Morton's Neuroma

DEFINITION AND EPIDEMIOLOGY

A neuroma is a nerve tumor that can result from external pressure on a nerve. Morton's neuroma is a result of perineural fibrosis of the plantar nerve at the point where the medial and lateral branches of the plantar nerve converge. This condition is seen primarily in females, with the most common cause being tight or high-heeled shoes.[12] This condition can also develop in people with claw toes and bunions.

PATHOPHYSIOLOGY

Compression of the interdigital plantar nerves causes repeated trauma, which in turn causes fibrosis of the nerve. Tight, pointed-toe shoes aggravate the irritation once the neuroma has formed.

CLINICAL PRESENTATION

Patients with Morton's neuroma complain of severe pain and burning in the region of the third web space. Going barefoot and foot massages relieve the discomfort. Elevation of the foot aggravates the condition.

PHYSICAL EXAMINATION

With Morton's neuroma, there is point tenderness and often edema over the third web space—between the third and fourth metatarsals. Compressing the metatarsals toward the midline of the foot reproduces the pain. Occasionally, there is paresthesia at the reciprocal surfaces of the toes. The examination is otherwise unremarkable.

DIAGNOSTICS

Radiographs are indicated in the absence of a clear-cut history. X-ray studies occasionally reveal a narrowing of the space between the metatarsals, which creates the underlying cause.[12]

DIFFERENTIAL DIAGNOSIS

The plantar surface of the foot should be smooth and nontender. Calluses and plantar warts on the ball of the foot may be tender as well as rough and nodular. Ganglions are cystlike in appearance, whereas infectious processes will classically have edema, erythema, warmth, and tenderness. Ledderhose syndrome is characterized by a painless, thickened palmar fascia and is often associated with Dupuytren's contracture (see Chapter 192) and Peyronie's disease. The presence of edema and tenderness between the third and fourth metatarsal heads strongly suggests Morton's neuroma; however, stress fractures should be considered in the differential diagnosis.

MANAGEMENT

Conservative treatment can resolve this condition. Wider toed shoes, separation of the toes with a small pad, and NSAIDs all help to reduce the inflammation. In persistent cases, injection with steroids is often effective.

COMPLICATIONS

Removal of the neuroma causes the toes to become permanently numb.

INDICATIONS FOR REFERRAL/HOSPITALIZATION

If conservative treatment and/or steroid injections are not effective, a referral for excision of the neuroma is advised.

PATIENT AND FAMILY EDUCATION

Patients should be encouraged to wear properly fitting shoes that have adequate toe room, good arch support, and a low or flat heel. Shoes should be bought at the end of the day, when feet are bigger and should be replaced when support wears out. Shoes should be fitted to ensure proper size. Metatarsal arch pads, if used correctly, may ease the discomfort associated with Morton's neuroma and metatarsalgia.

Other Common Foot Problems

Bunions, bunionettes, corns, calluses, hammertoes, hallux rigidus, hallux valgus, plantar warts, and ingrown toenails are discussed in Table 186-2; their differential diagnoses and management are also discussed.

TABLE 186-2 Other Common Foot Problems

Problem	Presentation	Examination and Diagnostics*	Differential Diagnosis* and Management
BUNION An inflammatory deformity of the first metatarsophalangeal (MTP) joint related to flat feet or laxity of the first toe and first metatarsal bone	Intense pain over the first MTP joint	Edema, deformity, and tenderness of the first metatarsal head; joint crepitus may be palpated *Diagnostics:* If gout is suspected, uric acid levels and joint aspiration are considered; x-ray studies are not diagnostic	*Differential diagnosis:* Gout *Management:* Warm packs or soaks, NSAIDs, and well-fitted shoes with adequate toe space Podiatry referral indicated for custom-made protective shield or foot mold Orthopedic/podiatry referral necessary for surgical correction if conservative management does not control pain
BUNIONETTE Pressure over the bony prominence on the fifth metatarsal head that results in bursa or ulceration	Painful, edematous lesion on the MTP joint of the fifth toe	Edema and erythema over the lateral aspect of the MTP of the fifth toe; may be accompanied by a cyst-like, fluid-filled lesion	*Management:* Properly fitting shoes with adequate toe room, bunion padding Hard lesions can be filed down

*Because of the classic presentation of these disorders, diagnostic testing and differential diagnoses are noted only when indicated.

continued

TABLE 186-2 Other Common Foot Problems—cont'd

Problem	Presentation	Examination and Diagnostics*	Differential Diagnosis* and Management
CORN *Hard corn (heloma durum):* Hyperkeratotic lesions caused by pressure or friction; usually found on the toes or other bony prominence *Soft corn (heloma molle):* Macerated, interdigital, and painful; caused by pressure	Painful lesion between toes or on dorsal surface of toes	Erythematous, painful lesion; hammertoes may also be present	*Management:* Avoidance of tight-fitting shoes, use of corn pads to relieve pressure, routine paring of corns with file or scalpel Powder and lambswool or soft cotton between toes to prevent excessive moisture Referral to orthotics for customized orthotic device Surgical repair for accompanying hammertoe or arthroplasty p.r.n. Patients with diabetes or peripheral vascular disease (PVD) require vigilant care to prevent corns/calluses and ulceration or infection
CALLUS Hypertrophied area of skin on sole of foot related to excessive supination, pronation, or other abnormality	Usually asymptomatic	Dried, hypertrophied epidermal layer; may surround or protect a plantar wart or foreign body	*Management:* Daily skin cream or lanolin, use of pumice stone by patient Painful calluses can be debrided with a scalpel to relieve pressure Orthotic device as indicated For patients with diabetes or PVD, see Corn
HALLUX FLEXUS (HAMMERTOE OR CLAW TOE) Proximal joint of second toe is dorsiflexed while middle joint is plantar flexed	Painful corn is most common complaint	Dorsal flexion of first phalanx of second toe (either foot), with plantar flexion in second phalanx; may be accompanied by painful callus on metatarsal head and/or at nail end, as well as painful corn on dorsal surface proximal interphalangeal joint	*Management:* See Corn Referral to podiatrist or orthopedic surgeon for surgical repair
HALLUX RIGIDUS Inflexible great toe, usually a result of arthritic changes	Pain with ambulation, climbing stairs	Immobile, fixated first MTP joint; may be slightly edematous with accompanying irregularity of joint edges related to osteophyte formation; diminished active/passive range of motion caused by immobility and pain *Diagnostics:* X-ray (anteroposterior, lateral views)	*Management:* NSAIDs for pain Podiatry or orthopedic referral for surgical repair
HALLUX VALGUS/HALLUS VARUS *Hallux valgus:* Great toe is laterally displaced toward other toes *Hallux varus:* Great toe is medially displaced away from other toes	Painful bunion of first MTP joint	*Hallux valgus:* Great toe laterally displaced with possible accompanying bunion, hammertoe; second toe may extend over great toe *Hallux varus:* Great toe is medially displaced	*Management:* Bunion care as described under Bunion Surgical or podiatry referral as indicated

*Because of the classic presentation of these disorders, diagnostic testing and differential diagnoses are noted only when indicated.

TABLE 186-2 Other Common Foot Problems—cont'd

Problem	Presentation	Examination and Diagnostics*	Differential Diagnosis* and Management
PLANTAR WARTS Viral infection causes warty growth on plantar surface	May be asymptomatic or may be complaints of pruritic, painful lesion on sole of foot; pain increases with weight-bearing activities	Callus may obscure wart, which commonly is 1 mm to 1 cm in size Paring of callus reveals rough lesion with numerous small, black spots in center of lesion	*Differential diagnosis:* Porokeratotic lesion, foreign body *Management:* Warts may resolve spontaneously For patients without diabetes or PVD: daily debridement with pumice stone, application of salicylic acid solution nightly to affected area, and gentle debridement of lesion each morning with an emery board may be sufficient Patients should be reminded that lesions can spread; therefore debrided tissue must be carefully discarded Referral to podiatry is indicated if conservative measures fail
ONYCHOCRYPTOSIS (INGROWN TOENAIL) Usually related to poor nail trimming or tight-fitting shoes	Pain and edema of great toe	Tender, edematous, erythematous area at corner of distal nailbed; lateral nailbed is usually involved and obscured by hypertrophied tissue Purulent discharge may be evident Careful examination for lymphangitis and range of motion is necessary	*Management:* For minimal ingrown toenail, wedge removal of nail edge will relieve discomfort If infection is present, patient is immunocompromised, or nail is severely ingrown, podiatry or surgical consult is warranted for nail excision and possible matricectomy Infection should be treated with appropriate antibiotic and patient instructed to soak foot in warm water several times daily, elevate foot, apply bandage, and wear open-toed shoes or soft slippers Further instruction regarding nail care is also necessary

*Because of the classic presentation of these disorders, diagnostic testing and differential diagnoses are noted only when indicated.

REFERENCES

1. American Academy of Orthopaedic Surgeons: *Fact sheet: the foot and ankle,* Retrieved July 2001 from the World Wide Web: http://orthoinfo.aaos.org.
2. Mercier LR: The ankle and foot. In *Practical orthopedics,* Chicago, 1980, Year Book.
3. American Academy of Orthopaedic Surgeons: The foot. In: *Athletic training and sports medicine,* ed 2, Park Ridge, Ill, 1991, The Academy.
4. American Academy of Orthopaedic Surgeons: Physiology of tissue repair. In *Athletic training and sports medicine,* ed 2, Park Ridge, Ill, 1991, The Academy.
5. Southmayd W, Hoffman M: The foot. In *Sports health: the complete book of athletic injuries,* New York, 1989, Quickfox.
6. Harwood-Nuss A and others: *The clinical practice of emergency medicine,* Philadelphia, 1991, JB Lippincott.
7. American Academy of Orthopaedic Surgeons: The ankle. In: *Athletic training and sports medicine,* ed 2, Park Ridge, Ill, 1991, The Academy.
8. Onieal ME: Ankle sprains (question and answer), *J Am Acad Nurse Pract* 5(5):226-227, 1993.
9. Hoppenfeld S: Physical examination of the foot and ankle. In: *Physical examination of the spine and extremities,* New York, 1976, Appleton-Century-Crofts.
10. Brody DM: Running injuries, *Clin Sympos* 32(4):1-36, 1980.
11. Graham J: Injuries to the knee and leg. In McLatchie BR, editor: *Essentials of sports medicine,* New York, 1993, Churchill Livingstone.
12. Southmayd W, Hoffman M: The ankle. In *Sports health: the complete book of athletic injuries,* New York, 1989, Quickfox.

CHAPTER 187

Bone Tumors

Sharon G. Childs

DEFINITION/EPIDEMIOLOGY

The incidence of skeletal neoplasms is increasing every year. Metastatic bone disease is significant and occurs in more than half of diagnosed cancers. The best patient outcomes occur with accurate diagnosis, staging, medical/surgical treatment, pharmacotherapy, psychosocial counseling, and adjuvant therapies for the management and treatment of pain.

Bone tumors may be benign or malignant. Common primary tumors include breast, kidney, lung, multiple myeloma, prostate, and thyroid. Batson's vertebral vein plexus may facilitate the spread of malignant cells from the breast, kidney, lung, prostate, and thyroid.[1] Bone metastases disseminate to pelvis, proximal long bones, ribs, skull, and spine.

Current data from the Surveillance, Epidemiology, and End Results program of the National Cancer Institute indicate that multiple myeloma is the most commonly occurring primary musculoskeletal malignancy, followed by soft tissue tumors, and then bone/joint tumors. The incidence of primary sarcoma is low (approximately 10,000/year).[2] Among bone cancers, osteosarcoma, chondrosarcoma, and Ewing's sarcoma account for 83% of all bone tumors. There is a higher incidence of bone cancer in males, with equal distribution in African-American and white males.

Primary bone tumors are uncommon, are usually malignant, and are seen in the 20- to 40-year age range. Metastatic bone lesions exceed primary tumors in later life. Metastases originate from bladder, breast, cervical, lung, kidney, lymphoma, prostate, and thyroid primary sites.[3,4]

PATHOPHYSIOLOGY

The pathogenesis of bone tumors is determined by the specific cytologic features and histomorphologic makeup of the cancer cell. Classifications of neoplastic cells arise from chondrogenic (cartilage), osteogenic (bone), and fibrogenic (fibrous tissue) cells. Osteosarcomas are the most common type of osseous tumor.[5] Research concerning the molecular basis of tumor suppressor genes and their effects on abnormal proliferation and malignant conversion of cells has led to more defined pathogenesis of cancer.[6] Increased expression of oncogenes precipitated by the mutation in DNA sequences leads to the development of the cancer cell. Mutation, environmental exposure (chemicals, carcinogens, viruses), ionizing radiation, genetic predisposition, and immunodeficiency all precipitate the development of neoplasms.[2,5]

CLINICAL PRESENTATION

The most common presenting symptom is pain. The expression of pain may vary from mild to moderate to unrelenting/intense. Lytic (metastatic) lesions may be monostotic (localized) or polyostotic (diffuse, involving many bones). Bone metastasis is also referred to as blastic or mixed depending on x-ray appearance.[6] The patient may complain of local swelling or limitation in movement of the affected limb/joint. In patients with bone tumor arising from Ewing's sarcoma, the effects of tumor necrosis factor (TNF) precipitate a pyogenic (febrile) response.[7] Symptom experience and distress are related to a wide range of patient descriptors. The paraneoplastic syndromes are related to aberrant hormonal and metabolic effects of tumor products and immune complexes stimulated by tumor growth.[7] A myriad of signs and symptoms such as anorexia, fever, malaise, or weight loss may be exhibited. Toxic metabolic effects such as hypercalcemia or hyponatremia may be life threatening. Coagulopathy, thrombophlebitis, and hypoglycemia may also be present. Patients may initially present with signs of hypercalcemia (tetany, seizure, weakness, arrhythmia, decreased deep tendon reflexes), and hyperuricemia. Patients may also exhibit signs and symptoms of spinal cord nerve root compression, pathologic fracture, and questionable hematopoiesis (anemia, leukocytosis/leukopenia).[7]

PHYSICAL EXAMINATION

After obtaining complete family, social, and occupational histories, the patient is examined with attention focused on the affected bone lesion. Local/surrounding tissues should be palpated for swelling, mass, and pain. Regional lymph nodes should be palpated for consistency and quality. Assessment of vital signs and surveillance of paraneoplastic signs and symptoms should be performed.

DIAGNOSTICS

Depending on the suspected cancer, diagnostic studies may include serum immunoelectrophoresis (to detect multiple myeloma), a CBC with differential, erythrocyte sedimentation rate, prostate-specific antigen (PSA), urinalysis (to detect renal/bladder cancer), alkaline phosphatase, serum calcium, uric acid, chest x-ray study, focused radiographic study of the

Diagnostics

Bone Tumors

Laboratory	Imaging
Serum and urine protein immunoelectrophoresis	X-ray—2 plane
CBC and differential	Chest x-ray
ESR	Bone scan
PSA*	CT scan/MRI
Urinalysis	Arthrography
Alkaline phosphatase	Angiography
Calcium	Skeletal survey
Uric acid	**Other**
5-HIAA	Bone biopsy
CEA	
CA-125	
$Alpha_1$-fetoprotein	
Phosphorus	
LFTs	

*If indicated.

affected area (Box 187-1), bone biopsy (for histopathology and staging), and bone scintigraphy (scan) to ascertain skeletal involvement and activity of the lesion. Serologic tumor markers, which quantify tumor products or substances, such as PSA, 5-hydroxyindoleacetic acid, carcinoembryonic antigen (CEA), CA-125, and alpha$_1$-fetoprotein should be obtained.[1] Other invasive diagnostic imaging studies include CT (to determine the anatomic extent of destruction of cortical vs. cancellous bone, compartment changes, and neurovascular impingement), MRI (defines tumor, soft tissue extension, and marrow involvement),[6] arthrography (determines joint involvement, cartilaginous tumors of intraarticular vs. extraarticular origin), and angiography (performed perioperatively to determine vascular status before limb salvage surgery).

DIFFERENTIAL DIAGNOSIS

The differential diagnoses include arthritis, both monoarticular and polyarticular; avascular necrosis and bone infarcts; cellulitis; deep vein thrombosis; ganglion and epidermoid cysts; heterotopic ossification; leukemia; neurogenic arthropathy (Charcot's joint); osteomyelitis; Paget's disease; pigmented villonodular synovitis and stress fracture.

BOX 187-1

RADIOGRAPHIC FINDINGS ASSOCIATED WITH BONE TUMORS

BENIGN, SLOW-GROWING TUMORS

Minimal to no soft tissue involvement
Cortical margin well defined
Distinct demarcation to boundary of lesion
Sclerotic margins
Solid and continuous reaction about periosteum

MALIGNANT LESIONS

Cortical destruction and erosion
Absence of sclerotic boundaries
Accompanying soft tissue mass
Irregular periosteal involvement
Codman's triangle (periosteal elevation, extension of calcification into soft tissue, "onion peeling," moth-eaten, sunburst pattern)
Indistinct boundaries to tumor mass involving bone and soft tissue
Poor margination, periosteal irregularity

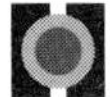

Differential Diagnosis

Bone Tumors

Arthritis (monoarticular and polyarticular)	Heterotopic ossification
Avascular necrosis and bone infarcts	Leukemia
Bursitis	Neurogenic arthropathy (Charcot's joint)
Cellulitis	Osteomyelitis
Deep vein thrombosis	Paget's disease
Ganglion and epidermoid cysts	Pigmented villonodular synovitis
	Stress fracture

MANAGEMENT

Treatment of bone tumors depends on the stage of the disease, cell morphology (primary or secondary site), and type of cancer. Surgical excision with subsequent external beam radiation is usually performed. Amputation, debulking procedures, grafting, open reduction internal fixation with a prosthesis, and limb salvage/sparing procedures may be performed. *Strong evidence exists* for the treatment of malignant bone tumor by incorporating preoperative neoadjuvant chemotherapy for 8 to 12 weeks and maintenance chemotherapy for 6 to 12 months.[1] Hormones, vaccines, growth factors, cytokines, monoclonal antibodies, and gene receptor-focused therapy may also be included in the patient's treatment.[3,8] Radiopharmaceuticals are used to destroy cancer cells, as an aid for pain relief, and as an alternative modality to wide field radiation.[7] These drugs include iodine-labeled diphosphonate, phosphorus-32, samarium 153-lixidronam, and strontium-89.[7,8]

Pain medication is prescribed and administered as a regimen and never by p.r.n. dosing. Opiates are the drug of choice for bone and musculoskeletal pain, in combination with nonsteroidal antiinflammatory drugs. Other adjuvant drugs, such as antidepressants and anticonvulsant drugs, may be helpful in managing pain. Specific drug and dosage scheduling is patient specific. Dosages are titrated according to patient need and response.

Nonpharmacologic modalities, such as acupuncture, biofeedback, distraction, guided imagery, hypnosis, and transcutaneous electrical nerve stimulation, are also used.[7,8]

LIFE SPAN CONSIDERATIONS

Growth and development issues across the life span are affected by bone tumors. Physical demands associated with cancer affect actual physical growth in children and adolescents. Socialization and peer relationships may be altered. Sexually active patients of childbearing age who are receiving teratogenic drugs are placed on reliable birth control. Sperm banking should be discussed.[3] Career/vocation, health insurance, fatigue/stamina, and increased dependency concerns for middle-aged and older adults, and psychosocial issues across the life span need to be addressed.

COMPLICATIONS

Associated complications related to the presence of malignant bone tumor include bleeding diathesis, bone marrow suppression, infection, and toxicities secondary to chemotherapy and radiation.[3,6,7,9] Late effects in childhood and adolescent survivors may include auditory, cardiac, pulmonary, renal, development of secondary malignancies, fertility and psychosocial outcomes as mentioned previously.[9]

INDICATIONS FOR REFERRAL/HOSPITALIZATION

Patients with primary cancers are referred to an oncologist for definitive tumor staging, diagnosis, and treatment. Patients with metastasis or recurring bone tumor also require referral. Other specialists involved in treatment include advanced practice oncologic nurses, general surgeons, neurosurgeons, orthopedic surgeons, physical/occupational therapists, psychiatric/mental health practitioners, and pharmacists.

Patients with progressive dyspnea, cardiopulmonary involvement, and those with neurologic, spinal cord, cauda equina syndrome, gastrointestinal or genitourinary hemorrhage, or acute renal failure require hospitalization.

PATIENT AND FAMILY EDUCATION

Bone cancer involves acute and chronic treatment and creates many lifestyle changes. Patients and family need education regarding disease process, treatment regimen, medications, complications, and prognosis. Nutritional consultation can help with meeting nutritional requirements even when appetite is affected by disease or treatment. Restrictions regarding activity and weight bearing, transfers (with assistive devices), and general exercise regimen are addressed with patients and family.

REFERENCES

1. Frassica F, Frassica D, McCarthy E: *Orthopaedic pathology,* In Miller M, Brinker M, editors: *Review of orthopaedics,* ed 3, Philadelphia, 2000, WB Saunders.
2. Praemer A, Furner S, Rice D: *Musculoskeletal conditions in the United States,* Rosemont, Ill, 1999, American Academy of Orthopaedic Surgeons.
3. Haynes K: *Tumors of the musculoskeletal system.* In Schoen D, editor: *Core curriculum for orthopaedic nursing,* ed 4, Pitman, NJ, 2001, NAON.
4. Arce D, Sasa P, Abul-Khoudoud H: Recognizing spinal cord emergencies, *Am Fam Physician* 64(4):631-638, 2001.
5. Hawkins R: Mastering the intricate maze of metastasis, *Oncol Nurs Forum* 28(6):959-965, 2001.
6. Bertoni F, Bacchini P: Classification of bone tumors, *Eur J Radiol* 1(suppl):S74-76, 1998.
7. Maxwell T, Givant E, Kowalski M: Exploring the management of bone metastasis according to the Roy adaptation model, *Oncol Nurs Forum* 28(7):1173-1181, 2001.
8. Struthers C, Mayer D, Fisher G: Nursing management of the patient with bone metastasis, *Semin Oncol Nurs* 14(3):199-209, 1998.
9. Mosher R, Mcarthy B: Late effects in survivors of bone tumors, *J Pediatr Oncol Nurs* 15(2):72-89, 1998.

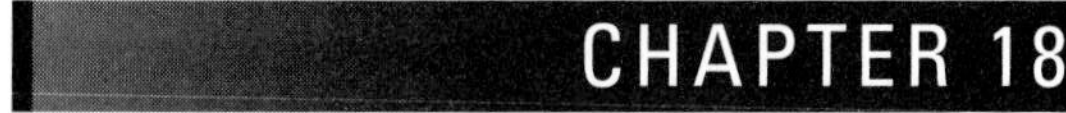

Bursitis

Scott W. Shiffer

Bursitis is a pathologic, inflammatory disorder of the bursae caused by varied acute or insidious processes. In response to overuse, autoimmune diseases, crystal deposits, infection, hemorrhage, or even without an obvious cause, bursitis can result in mild pain or a disabling condition.[1,2] There are numerous bursae throughout the body, but only a few ever become inflamed or problematic. The most commonly affected bursae are located at the shoulder, hip, knee, elbow, and heel.

Shoulder Bursitis

DEFINITION/EPIDEMIOLOGY

The four major bursae around the shoulder include the subacromial (subdeltoid), subcoracoid, subscapularis, and scapular bursae. The subacromial-subdeltoid bursa is located between the deltoid muscle and rotator cuff and extends under the acromion and coracoacromial arch. Subacromial bursitis is the most common type of bursitis and is commonly seen in older adults and in athletes less than 25 years of age.[1,3] This condition is generally caused by mechanical irritation resulting from overhead activities, and it leads to rotator cuff tendinitis. If left untreated, the condition progresses into an irreversible impingement condition.[3]

CLINICAL PRESENTATION AND PHYSICAL EXAMINATION

Anterior or lateral shoulder pain with acute or insidious onset is the most common presenting complaint of shoulder bursitis. The pain is exacerbated by overhead activities, and there may be a deep aching that interrupts sleep at night.[4,5] Increased pain with active abduction and internal rotation of the arm, plus tenderness below the acromion, is demonstrated. Weakness can often be established with internal rotation. A complete neuromuscular examination with careful palpation and passive and active range of motion should be performed. The Neer's and Hawkins' impingement signs are diagnostic and indicate inflammation of the subacromial bursa and rotator cuff (Box 188-1).[3,4]

DIAGNOSTICS AND DIFFERENTIAL DIAGNOSIS

Plain radiographs are often normal in the early stages of shoulder bursitis.[1,3,6] X-ray studies may demonstrate a hooked acromion, calcification of the supraspinatus tendon, osteopenia of the humerus greater tuberosity, and a distance of less than 5 mm between the acromion and humerus.[4] MRI is useful in the latter stages of the disease.[1] If the condition is related to an autoimmune or inflammatory process, serologic tests may reveal an elevated erythrocyte sedimentation rate, a positive rheumatoid factor, or antinuclear antibodies. If a septic cause is suspected, a Gram's stain and culture of the bursa fluid should be

Differential Diagnosis

Shoulder Bursitis

Fracture or dislocation
Trauma
Arthritis (osteoarthritis or rheumatoid arthritis)
Adhesive capsulitis
Rotator cuff tendonitis or tear
Strain
Referred pain
Subacromial spur
Neoplasm

obtained. If an aseptic condition is the cause of the bursitis, crystals may be observed in the bursa aspirate (Box 188-2).[4] The differential diagnosis includes tubercular effusion, infection, arthritis, hemarthrosis, and gout or pseudogout.

The impingement injection test is one method of differentiating between impingement and other shoulder disorders.[3,7] With this test, 10 ml of 1% lidocaine (Xylocaine) is injected into the subacromial space; after 5 to 10 minutes, the tests for impingement are repeated. If the pain is

BOX 188-1

NEER'S AND HAWKINS' IMPINGEMENT SIGNS

NEER'S IMPINGEMENT SIGN

Raise and pull on straightened arm forcibly from the side to full abduction above the head.

A positive test will cause pain.

HAWKINS' IMPINGEMENT SIGN

Flex the elbow to 90 degrees and raise the upper arm to 90 degrees abduction (parallel to the floor). Then rotate the arm internally across the front of the body causing compression of the rotator cuff and subacromial bursa between the head of the humerus and coracoacromial ligament.

A positive test will cause pain.

Data from Neer CS: Impingement lesions, *Gen Orthop* 173:70-77, 1983; and Hawkins RJ, Kennedy JC: Impingement Syndrome in athletes, *Am J Sports Med* 8:151-157, 1980.

BOX 188-2

GUIDELINES FOR BURSA ASPIRATION AND INJECTION

PURPOSE

The purpose of bursae aspiration and injection is to evaluate the bursae fluid to determine the etiology of the inflammation and to drain abnormal fluid accumulation to relieve pain. Local anesthetics such as lidocaine or corticosteroids may be introduced into the bursae for symptomatic management of inflammation. Subacromial, trochanteric, anserine, and prepatellar bursitis are conditions that improve with local corticosteroids injection.

CONTRAINDICATIONS

Contraindications to aspiration and injection include, but are not limited to, cellulitis at the injection site, primary coagulopathy or uncontrolled anticoagulant therapy, septic effusion of a bursa or periarticular structure, more than three previous injections at the same site in the previous 12 months or lack of improvement after two prior injections, suspected bacteremia from another site, unstable joints (for corticosteroids injection), tumors, fractures, joint prosthesis, or inaccessible joints.

PATIENT EDUCATION AND CONSENT

Patient education and consent are necessary before the procedure. The risks and benefits of bursae aspiration should be explained. Adverse effects of introducing a needle into the bursae include infection, bleeding, and pain. Potential complications of corticosteroid therapy include postinjection flare (increased pain for 1 or 2 days), arthropathy, tendon rupture, facial flushing, skin atrophy and depigmentation, transient paresis, hypersensitivity reaction, pericapsular calcification, and acceleration of cartilage attrition.

TECHNIQUE

Aseptic technique for bursae aspiration and injection begins by prepping the site for aspiration or injection with povidone-iodine and draping accordingly. The appropriate needle for the procedure is selected: an 18- or 20-gauge needle for aspiration, and a 22- or 25-gauge $1\frac{1}{2}$ inch needle for injection. A 5- or 10-ml Luer-Lok syringe is recommended. Figures 188-1 to 188-7 demonstrate techniques for aspirating and injecting bursae.

A variety of corticosteroid preparations are available in different potencies. The three common corticosteroid local injection therapies used to treat bursae are hydrocortisone acetate (25 or 50 mg/ml), which is short acting (use 8-40 mg); Triamcinolone acetonide (40 mg/ml), an intermediate-acting preparation (use 4-10 mg); and long-acting dexamethasone sodium acetate (8 mg/ml) (use 1.5-3 mg).

Lidocaine is combined with the steroid of choice to disperse the steroid in the injection site. A history of lidocaine allergy must first be obtained. Lidocaine (5 ml) is combined with the steroid for subacromial, trochanteric, or calcaneal bursae. For smaller bursae, such as the olecranon and prepatellar, up to 3 ml of lidocaine combined with the chosen steroid is recommended.

FOLLOW-UP

Procedure after-care includes applying a bandage over the aspiration/injection site and reminding the patient that the procedure is provided in addition to other conservative measures and is not a cure in itself. Oral NSAIDs are continued. Symptoms of infection should be reported immediately.

Data from Pfeninger JL: Joint and soft tissue aspiration and injection. In Pfeninger JL, Fowler GC, editors: *Procedures for primary care physicians*, St Louis, 1994, Mosby.

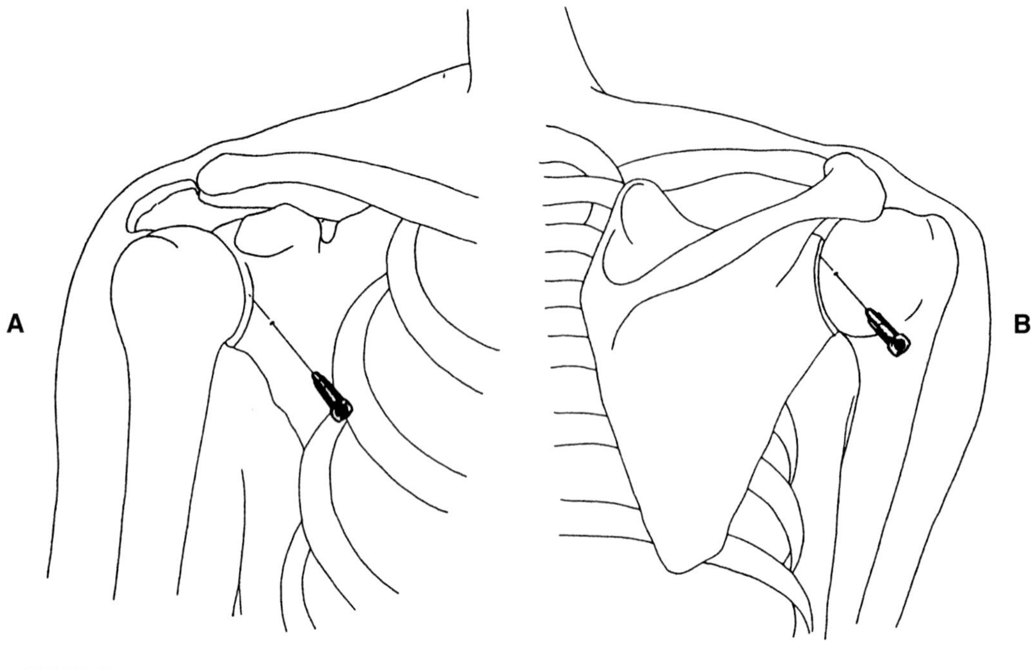

FIGURE 188-1

Arthrocentesis of the shoulder. **A**, Anterior approach. **B**, Posterior approach. (From Noble JP: *Textbook of primary care medicine,* ed 2, St Louis, 1996, Mosby.)

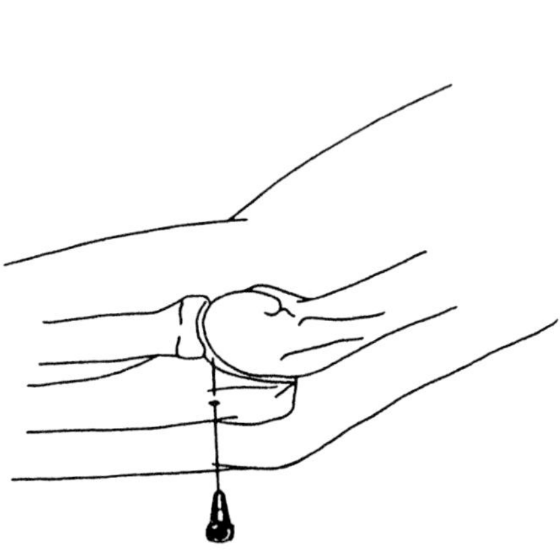

FIGURE 188-2

Arthrocentesis of the elbow. (From Noble JP: *Textbook of primary care medicine,* ed 2, St Louis, 1996, Mosby.)

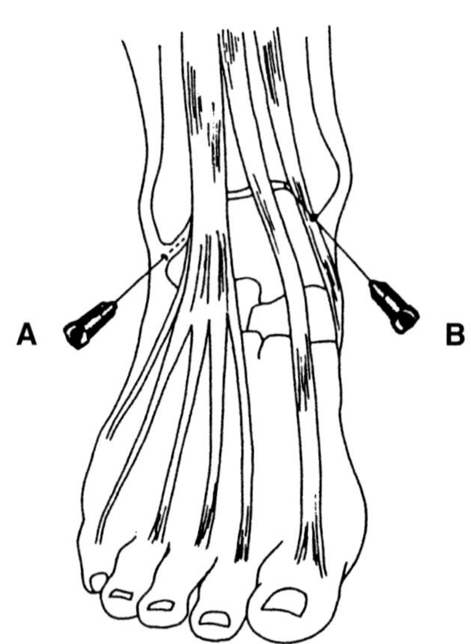

FIGURE 188-3

Arthrocentesis of the ankle. **A**, Medial approach. **B**, Lateral approach. (From Noble JP: *Textbook of primary care medicine,* ed 2, St Louis, 1996, Mosby.)

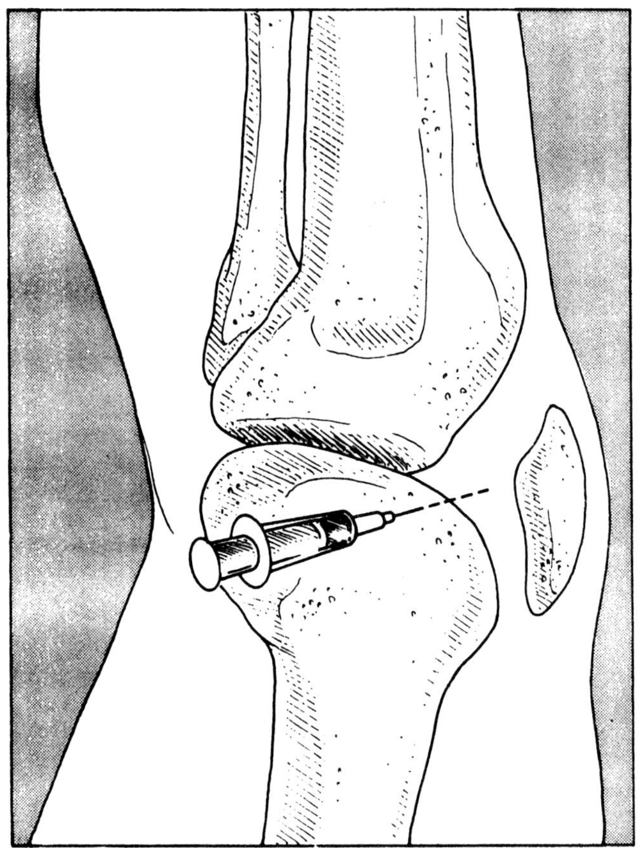

FIGURE 188-4

Arthrocentesis of the knee. (From Noble JP: *Textbook of primary care medicine,* ed 2, St Louis, 1996, Mosby.)

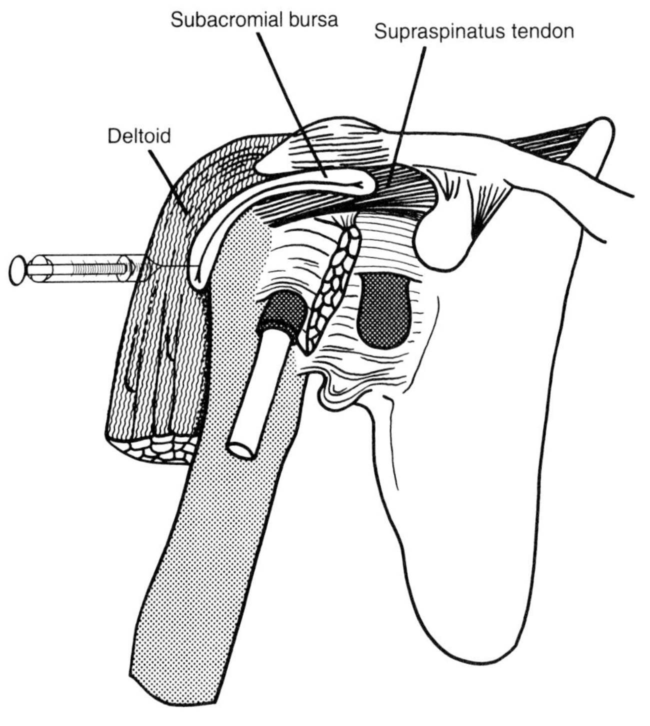

FIGURE 188-5

Injection of the subacromial bursa. (From Noble JP: *Textbook of primary care medicine,* ed 2, St Louis, 1996, Mosby.)

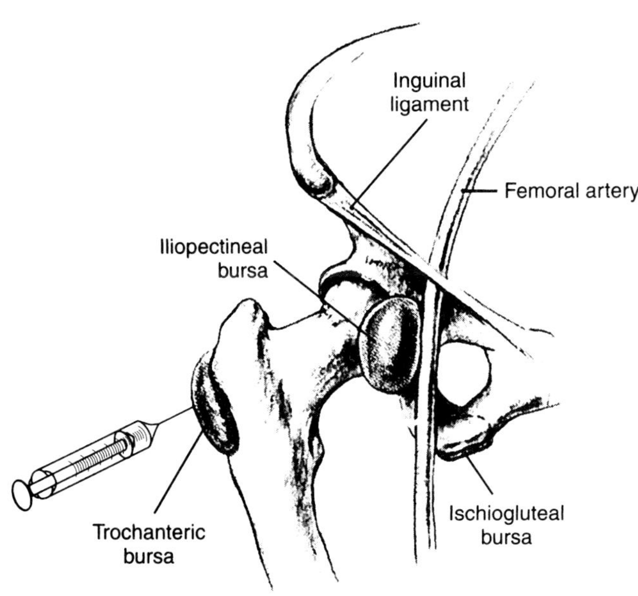

FIGURE 188-6

Injection of the trochanteric bursa. (From Noble JP: *Textbook of primary care medicine,* ed 2, St Louis, 1996, Mosby.)

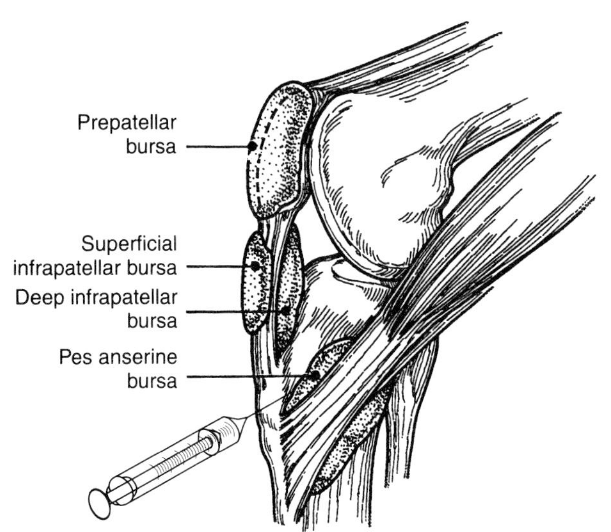

FIGURE 188-7

Injection of the anserine bursa. (From Noble JP: *Textbook of primary care medicine,* ed 2, St Louis, 1996, Mosby.)

reduced 50%, the shoulder pain is secondary to subacromial bursitis and tendinitis.[3,5]

MANAGEMENT

Except for autoimmune and septic shoulder conditions, treatment is directed at rehabilitating the rotator cuff. More than 90% of patients with subacromial bursitis respond to periodic gentle range-of-motion joint activities, avoidance of activities that exacerbate the pain, thermal modalities, either heat or ice, and nonsteroidal antiinflammatory drugs (NSAIDs). Additional pain relief may be provided by scheduled doses of acetaminophen. Stronger analgesics are occasionally necessary, especially at night.[3,4] Immobilization, which may worsen the condition by causing adhesions, should be avoided.[3] Severe cases of shoulder bursitis may be managed with corticosteroid injections, which are limited to three injections in a 12-month period no fewer than 30 days apart.[4,8] Physical therapy for appropriate exercises, ultrasound, and electrical stimulation are also appropriate methods of treatment. A demonstrated rotator cuff tear or subacromial fibrosis warrants an orthopedic referral.[3,9]

Elbow (Olecranon) Bursitis

Located on the posterior, extensor aspect of the elbow, olecranon bursitis is the most common type of elbow bursitis. The bursa is swollen and tender but no elbow motion is lost. There are four classifications of olecranon bursitis: chronic, acute, septic, and aseptic. Most cases result from trauma; chronic olecranon bursitis is related to repetitive trauma that results in thickening of the bursa wall. One third of all cases of olecranon bursitis are septic.[10] Other common etiologies include trauma, rheumatoid arthritis, gout, and pseudogout. For a more thorough discussion of elbow bursitis, see Chapter 189.

Differential Diagnosis

Elbow (Olecranon) Bursitis	
Septic bursitis	Effusion
Gout	Fracture
Arthritis (osteoarthritis or rheumatoid arthritis)	Epicondylitis
	Sprain
Tendinitis	Trauma

Hip Bursitis

DEFINITION/EPIDEMIOLOGY

Hip bursitis is a common disorder that results from acute or recurrent trauma, musculotendinous overuse, degenerative changes, biomechanical abnormalities, or systemic disease. The trochanteric, iliopsoas, and ischiogluteal groups are the major structures of bursae around the hip. Trochanteric bursitis is a very common disorder affecting women somewhat more often than men (Table 188-1). Conditions that can contribute to trochanteric bursitis include osteoarthritis (OA) of the spine, leg length discrepancy, and scoliosis.

CLINICAL PRESENTATION

Hip bursitis is characterized by pain over the affected bursa. The pain may be sudden or gradual in onset and results from overuse or trauma. Depending on which bursa is inflamed, the pain can have a pseudoradicular quality with radiation down the lateral thigh, knee, or anteriorly to the groin. Pain is often worse at night. Passive joint mobility is usually not affected, although guarding may limit active mobility.

MANAGEMENT

Hip bursitis is managed with NSAIDs, rest, heat, and ice application. A steroid injection may be helpful if more conservative

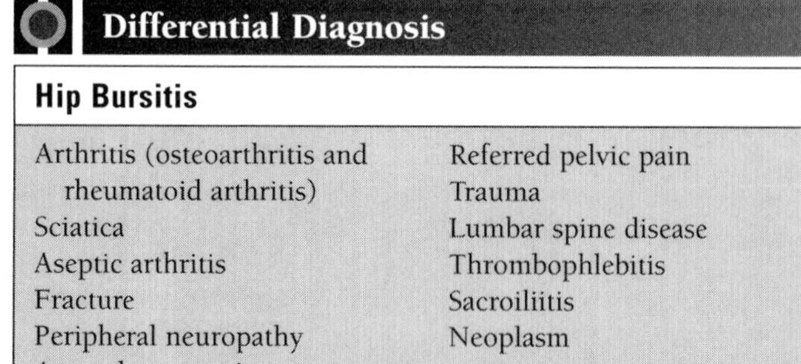

Differential Diagnosis

Hip Bursitis	
Arthritis (osteoarthritis and rheumatoid arthritis)	Referred pelvic pain
	Trauma
Sciatica	Lumbar spine disease
Aseptic arthritis	Thrombophlebitis
Fracture	Sacroiliitis
Peripheral neuropathy	Neoplasm
Avascular necrosis	

TABLE 188-1 Hip Bursitis

	Hip Bursae		
	Trochanteric	Ischiogluteal	Iliopsoas
Location of pain	Lateral hip to lateral thigh and buttock	Ischial tuberosity into posterior thigh; worse with sitting	Groin, with radiation to anterior hip
Examination	Pain worse with hip rotation; may be soft tissue swelling	Tenderness over the ischial tuberosity	Pain worse with resisted hip flexion and hyperextension
Diagnostics	X-rays are usually normal and noncontributory for hip bursitis; a bone scan may be helpful only in refractory conditions		
Differential diagnosis*	Fracture of the greater trochanter	Fracture	Hip arthritis

Data from Steinberg GG: Hip, pelvis, and proximal thigh. In Steinberg GG, Akins CM, Baron DT, editors: *Ramamurti's orthopedics in primary care,* ed 2, Baltimore, 1992, Williams & Wilkins.
*Consider herniated disk, avascular necrosis, or systemic disease.

treatment is unsuccessful. Physical therapy with ultrasound treatments will maximize the rehabilitation regimen.

Knee Bursitis

DEFINITION/EPIDEMIOLOGY

There are numerous bursae around the knee. Anserine bursitis is commonly seen in middle-aged to older women with big legs. Pain is characteristically located over the medial aspect of the knee about 2 inches below the knee margin. The prepatellar bursa is located between the skin and the patella and is one of the most common sites of pyogenic bursitis. Prepatellar bursitis is sometimes referred to as "housemaid's knee" and commonly affects occupations that require excessive kneeling, such as carpentry or carpet laying.[2,11]

CLINICAL PRESENTATION AND PHYSICAL EXAMINATION

Except in infectious cases, severe pain is unusual in prepatellar bursitis.[12] There is, however, tenderness over the anterior knee that is accompanied by localized edema over the lower half of the patella and upper body of the patella ligament (prepatellar bursitis) or on both sides of the patella ligament (infrapatellar bursitis). Often there is bursa thickening that feels rough, like nodules or bone chips.[2] Although the inflamed bursa causes swelling, the edema is different from that noted when there is fluid in the knee joint. Because knee effusion is absent, a ballottement test for a floating patella will be negative (Figure 188-8). A pyogenic prepatellar bursitis may appear cellulitic. Anserine bursitis is exquisitely tender to palpation and often associated with OA of the knee, especially if the patient had a valgus (knock-knee) deformity.

The differential diagnosis includes tubercular effusion, infection, arthritis, hemarthrosis, and gout or pseudogout.

MANAGEMENT

Acute and chronic knee bursitis is best managed initially with conservative treatment including rest, physical therapy, and NSAIDs. Acute bursitis may also respond to ice application and aspiration of the affected site and injection of steroids. Septic prepatellar bursitis, commonly caused by staphylococci, often responds well to immobilization, one of two daily aspirations, and appropriate antibiotic coverage.[11,12]

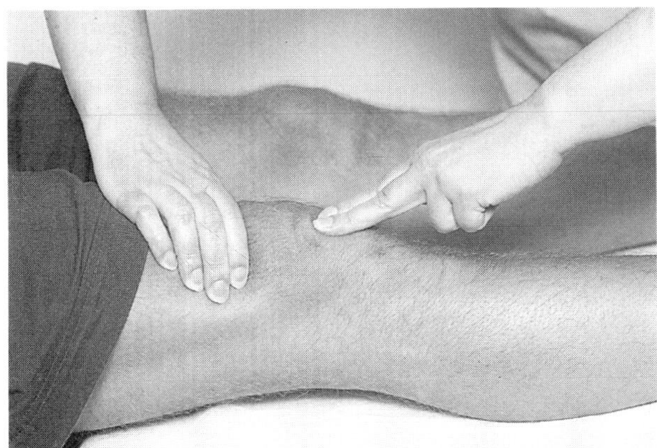

FIGURE 188-8

Ballottement of the knee. (From Barkauskas VH: *Health and physical assessment*, ed 2, St Louis, 1998, Mosby.)

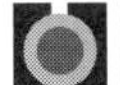

Differential Diagnosis

Knee (Prepatellar) Bursitis	
Effusion	Osteochondritis dissecans
Arthritis (osteoarthritis or rheumatoid arthritis)	Referred pain
Fracture	Overuse syndrome
Gout	Chondromalacia
Sprain	Patellofemoral joint instability
Ligament or meniscus injury	Trauma
Retropatellar bursitis	Septic bursitis
Pes anserinus bursitis	

Heel (Calcaneal) Bursitis

DEFINITION/EPIDEMIOLOGY

There are two clinically significant bursae in the posterior heel. The retrocalcaneal bursa lies between the calcaneus and the Achilles' tendon and is usually associated with systemic inflammatory diseases such as the spondyloarthropathies, rheumatoid arthritis, and gout.[13] The posterior calcaneal bursa is located between the Achilles' tendon and the skin. Calcaneal bursitis is the result of local mechanical irritation to the posterior heel and affects ice skaters (primarily female) and long-distance runners.[12]

CLINICAL PRESENTATION AND PHYSICAL EXAMINATION

The usual presentation of calcaneal bursitis includes a history of poor-fitting shoes. This causes the heel to rub on the back of the shoe and results in heel pain.[14] Physical findings include a palpable, swollen bursa that is tender at the Achilles' tendon insertion site at the posterior heel. There may also be erythema of the affected area.

DIAGNOSTICS AND DIFFERENTIAL DIAGNOSIS

Reiter's syndrome, fracture, os trigonum syndrome, loose bodies, or calcaneal apophysitis are possible causes of calcaneal pain. In addition

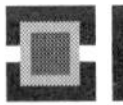

Diagnostics

Bursitis

Laboratory
CBC and differential*
ESR*
Rheumatoid factor*
Uric acid*
ANA*
Culture and sensitivity (of bursa fluid)*
Gram's stain (of bursa fluid)*
Analysis of bursa aspirate for crystals*

Imaging
X-ray
Ultrasound
MRI

Others
Joint aspiration

*If indicated.

tubercular effusions, infection, inflammatory arthritis, hemarthrosis, and gout or pseudogout should be considered. Achilles tendinitis and osteomyelitis can both cause heel pain.

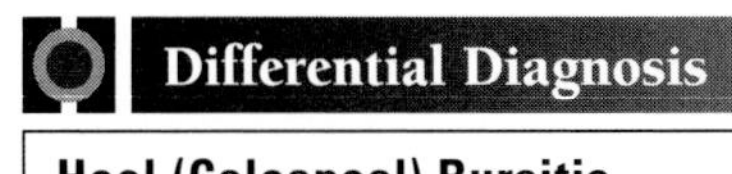

Heel (Calcaneal) Bursitis

Trauma/fracture
Achilles tendonitis
Plantar fasciitis

MANAGEMENT

Conservative management of calcaneal bursitis requires rest, NSAIDs, and the avoidance of poorly fitting shoes. Application of heat and cold may alleviate some pain. Physical therapy for Achilles' tendon stretching and ankle flexion/extension exercises may also be helpful. In some cases, a corticosteroid injection to the affected bursa is beneficial.[8] However, caution is advised to avoid injecting and subsequently weakening the Achilles' tendon.[12] An ultrasound-guided steroid injection may be beneficial if a nonguided ultrasound injection is not successful.[15]

LIFE SPAN CONSIDERATIONS

With aging, tendons become less elastic making them more susceptible to injury. Also with aging or disuse atrophy, the muscles become weaker, exhibit less bulk and endurance, and are less able to absorb mechanical forces. There may be a genetic predisposition to these syndromes related to inherited variations in anatomy resulting in altered biomechanics. There is no impact on longevity.

COMPLICATIONS

The pain of bursitis can be particularly disabling for many patients. Some patients with shoulder or elbow bursitis stop using the affected extremity, resulting in increased disability; others do not bear weight on the affected extremity to avoid pain. Unfortunately, recurrent episodes of acute bursitis can develop into chronic bursitis. The adjacent tissue may be compromised in cases of severe bursal swelling, and it may be difficult to determine the true etiology of the patient's discomfort. Infection of the bursa and/or surrounding tissue is not uncommon. Oral antibiotic therapy may be sufficient for some patients with septic bursitis, but many patients require IV antibiotic therapy, hospitalization, and daily aspiration of the bursa fluid.

INDICATIONS FOR REFERRAL/HOSPITALIZATION

Patients with suspected septic bursitis should be referred to a physician or orthopedic specialist expediently. Aspiration of the infected bursa for fluid analysis and antibiotic therapy are indicated. Hospitalization may be required for some patients, particularly those who have diabetes or are immunosuppressed.

A referral to an orthopedist or a rheumatologist is appropriate for patients who do not respond to conservative measures within a reasonable period of time. Physical therapy often expedites recovery, minimizes pain, and prevents joint immobility.

PATIENT AND FAMILY EDUCATION

Because bursitis is related to repetitive activities, such as the kneeling associated with prepatellar bursitis, recurrence is possible. Patients should understand this and try to avoid activities that may exacerbate the disorder. Knee pads should be used by patients with prepatellar bursitis. Rest is indicated during the acute process, but gentle stretching and range-of-motion exercises should begin as soon as possible and continue indefinitely to prevent stiffness and maintain mobility. Ice or heat plus NSAIDs help decrease joint inflammation. A joint that becomes erythematous, tender, and swollen with associated fever requires assessment by a primary care provider. If corticosteroid injections are necessary, the risks and benefits should be discussed before injection.

REFERENCES

1. Reveille JD: Soft tissue rheumatism: diagnosis and treatment, *Am J Med* 102(1A):23S-29S, 1997.
2. Mercier LR, editor: The knee. In *Practical orthopedics*, ed 4, St Louis, 1995, Mosby.
3. Hunter DM: Shoulder pain. In Tintinalli JE, Ruiz E, Krome RL, editors: *Emergency medicine*, New York, 1996, McGraw-Hill.
4. Salzman KL, Lillegard WA, Butcher JD: Upper extremity bursitis, *Am Fam Physician* 56(7):1797-1806, 1997.
5. Belzer JP, Durkin RC: Common disorders of the shoulder, *Prim Care* 23(2):365-388, 1996.
6. Bureau NJ, Dussault RG, Keats TE: Imaging of bursae around the shoulder joint, *Skeletal Radiol* 25(6):513-517, 1996.
7. Pfeninger JL: Joint and soft tissue aspiration and injection. In Pfeninger JL, Fowler GC, editors: *Procedures for primary care physicians*, St Louis, 1994, Mosby.
8. Larson HM, O'Connor FG, Nirschl RP: Shoulder pain: the role of diagnostic injections, *Am Fam Physician* 53(5):1637-1647, 1995.
9. Green A: Arthroscopic treatment of impingement syndrome, *Orthop Clin North Am* 26(4):631-641, 1996.
10. Stell IM: Septic and non-septic olecranon bursitis in the accident and emergency department: an approach to management, *J Accid Emerg Med* 13(5):351-353, 1996.
11. Crenshaw AH Jr: Tendinitis and bursitis. In Canale ST: *Campbell's operative orthopedics*, ed 9, St Louis, 1998, Mosby.
12. Butcher JD, Salzman KL, Lillegard WA: Lower extremity bursitis, *Am Fam Physician* 53(7):2317-2324, 1996.
13. Liu NYN, Canoso JJ: Periarticular rheumatic disorders. In Noble J, editor: *Textbook of primary care medicine*, ed 3, St Louis, 2001 Mosby.
14. Quirk R: Common foot and ankle injuries in dance, *Orthop Clin North Am* 25(1):123-133, 1994.
15. Cunnane G and others: Diagnosis and treatment of heel pain in chronic inflammatory arthritis using ultrasound, *Semin Arthritis Rheum* 25(6):383-389, 1996.

CHAPTER 189

Elbow Pain

Denise A. Vanacore

DEFINITION/EPIDEMIOLOGY

A hinged joint that allows flexion and rotation of the forearm, the elbow provides a wide, stable arc of motion for the hand.[1] Microtears of the muscles, ligaments, and tendons from inflammation and trauma are common causes of acute and chronic elbow pain.

Most elbow injuries result from overuse during high force and/or repetitive motion activities. Two groups of people seem to be at increased risk for elbow disorders. The first is high-performance athletes, especially in racket and throwing sports such as baseball, tennis, and basketball. The second group includes those with jobs that require forceful or repetitive wrist and elbow rotation, lifting, gripping, or torquing motions. High-risk occupations include factory workers, laborers, carpenters, and grocery checkers. The prevalence of occupational epicondylitis is as high as 5%.[2] In the general population, injuries may occur from pursuing recreational hobbies; improper preparation, lack of strength or conditioning, or overzealousness can all contribute to elbow pain.

PATHOPHYSIOLOGY

The elbow is formed by the articulations of the humerus, radius, and ulna. The humeroulnar articulation is a hinge joint and allows elbow flexion and extension. The humeroradial and radioulnar articulations are partially ligamental; their flexibility allows rotation of the radius and pronation/supination of the forearm.

Full range of motion of the elbow is 140 degrees of flexion, zero degrees of extension, and 90 degrees each of pronation and supination.[3] Functional range of motion for normal activities of daily living is 30 to 130 degrees of flexion, with the greatest strength and greatest stress on the elbow at 70 degrees.[4] In athletes, full range of motion may be required, especially for arm weight-bearing sports.[4]

Stability of the elbow is accomplished through bones, ligaments, and muscles. The humeroulnar joint is the main stabilizer for flexion/extension of the elbow. Rotational stability is divided into valgus and varus stabilizers. A valgus stress is a force on the medial elbow from throwing or axial compression. Primary valgus stabilizers are the medial (ulnar) collateral ligaments and their supporting muscles. A varus stress is a force on the lateral elbow. The lateral (radial) collateral ligaments stabilize for varus stress.

Elbow injuries may be classified as acute or chronic. Acute injuries result from a single high force, such as a fall or direct blow, that is greater in strength than the tendon, ligament, or bone affected.[1,4] However, the vast majority of injuries are chronic. Chronic injuries occur from repetitive, submaximal forces that overload the elbow's ability to adequately heal, causing recurrent pain.

CLINICAL PRESENTATION

Elbow pain may be traced to a specific activity or chain of events, or present insidiously, with no identifiable trigger. Once an injury has occurred, everyday activities such as picking up groceries, or reaching or pulling, can cause pain. A thorough history, including occupational and recreational activities, as well as any prior elbow injury, is essential. A history of other joint pain or swelling is also needed to exclude rheumatoid arthritis, psoriasis, or other systemic diseases.

PHYSICAL EXAMINATION

Physical examination is performed on both elbows to assess for alteration in carrying angle, posture, strength, and range of motion. Bony and soft tissue landmarks should be assessed for asymmetry, misalignment, erythema, and tenderness. Bony landmarks for examination are the medial and lateral epicondyles of the humerus and the olecranon process of the ulna. When the elbow is flexed at 90 degrees, the olecranon and the medial and lateral epicondyles form an isosceles triangle. When the elbow is fully extended, these points lie in a straight line. Any deviation from this suggests a pathologic condition.[3]

Posteriorly the olecranon bursa overlies the olecranon process. Medially ligaments run from the epicondyle to the trochlear notch of the ulna. The ulnar nerve sits in a groove between the medial epicondyle and the olecranon process.[3] Muscles for wrist flexion and pronation originate via tendons from the medial epicondyle, then spread out along the palmar surface of the forearm. The supracondylar and epitrochlear lymph nodes lie along the medial surface of the humerus. Laterally the radial head is about 1 inch distal to the lateral epicondyle. The lateral ligaments run between these points. Wrist extensor and supinator muscles originate via the lateral epicondyle, then spread down the dorsal forearm. Physical examination should include the wrist and shoulder, as they may cause referred pain to the elbow.

DIAGNOSTICS

Testing is based on the mechanism of injury and/or duration of symptoms. X-rays studies of the elbow are the most common tests ordered. Standard x-ray studies include an anteroposterior film with the elbow fully extended and supinated and a lateral view with the elbow flexed at 90 degrees and the forearm supinated. Oblique views may be needed to better study the radial head and shaft, the humeral condyles, and the coronoid process of the ulna.[5] Laboratory testing is based on the clinical history. A CBC, erythrocyte sedimentation rate, rheumatoid

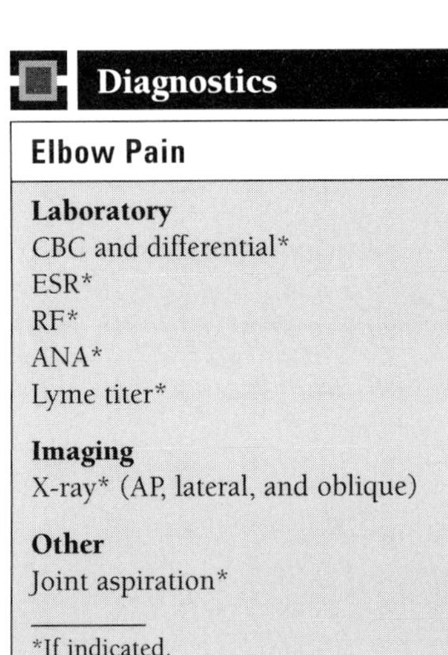
Diagnostics

Elbow Pain

Laboratory
CBC and differential*
ESR*
RF*
ANA*
Lyme titer*

Imaging
X-ray* (AP, lateral, and oblique)

Other
Joint aspiration*

*If indicated.

factor, antinuclear antibody test, Lyme titer, or elbow joint aspiration may be indicated to exclude infection or systemic disease. Joint aspirate should be evaluated with a culture, Gram's stain, and crystals. Based on an examination with neurologic findings, electromyographic and nerve conduction studies may be indicated.

DIFFERENTIAL DIAGNOSIS

The most common causes of elbow pain are sprains, fractures, bursitis, epicondylitis (lateral or medial), and ulnar neuritis (Table 189-1). Elbow pain is usually due to local injury but may result from a referred, external condition. Based on the history, the differential diagnosis for referred pain should include cervical disk or nerve root problems, thoracic outlet or brachial plexus disease, radicular pain from the shoulder, neck or wrist overuse injuries, diabetes, cardiovascular disease, and peripheral nerve entrapment syndromes.[4,5] Systemic diseases that may cause elbow pain, such as rheumatoid arthritis, osteoarthritis, psoriatic arthritis, and Lyme disease, should also be considered. Gout can cause either a true joint arthritis or an olecranon bursitis.

MANAGEMENT

Ideally, treatment begins before injury occurs. Injury prevention strategies include flexibility, strength, and endurance training; warm-up and cool-down stretching exercises; and avoidance of fatigue through limiting total activity time. Proper equipment, body mechanics, and ergonomics are also important to prevent injuries from occurring.

Once injury occurs, general goals of treatment are pain management, healing of microtears, and prevention of reinjury. RICE therapy (rest, ice, compression, and elevation) should be initiated

Differential Diagnosis

Elbow Pain

- Arthritis (rheumatic or osteoarthritis)
- Brachial plexus disease
- Bursitis
- Cardiovascular disease
- Cervical disk disease
- Cubital tunnel syndrome
- Diabetes
- Digital biceps tendon rupture
- Dislocation
- Epicondylitis lateral (tennis elbow)
- Epicondylitis medial (golfer's elbow)
- Fracture
- Gout
- Impingement
- Lyme disease
- Osteochondrosis
- Osteophytes
- Overuse injuries
- Peripheral nerve entrapment
- Pseudogout
- Psoriatic arthritis
- Radicular pain
- Septic joint
- Sprain
- Tendinitis
- Thoracic outlet syndrome
- Triceps rupture
- Ulnar neuritis

TABLE 189-1 Common Elbow Ailments*

Ailment	Presentation	Examination	Differential Diagnosis/Management
EPICONDYLITIS			
Inflammatory condition characterized by pain at tendon origin of muscle groups at medial (golfer's elbow) or lateral (tennis elbow) aspects of elbow; usually self-limiting, but may take several months for full recovery	Gradual or acute onset of pain along affected epicondyle, with or without radiation; history may include heavy lifting, hammering, screwing, or gripping	Local tenderness over or just distal to affected epicondyle; possible tenderness of flexor and extensor muscles; range of motion (ROM) and distal neurovascular examination within normal limits *Lateral epicondylitis:* Pain at or around lateral epicondyle is reproduced by resistive wrist extension (examiner applies pressure to force wrist into flexion while patient extends wrist) *Medial epicondylitis:* Pain is exacerbated by resistive wrist flexion	*Differential diagnosis:* Carpal tunnel syndrome, cervical radiculopathy, rotator cuff tendinitis, lateral or medial collateral ligament sprains, osteoarthritis, or avulsion fracture *Management:* Conservative treatment: NSAIDs, tennis elbow splint, "palms-up" lifting, toning exercises of wrist extensors; steroid injection may be helpful if above treatment is unsuccessful; orthopedic referral for surgical evaluation if treatment fails
SPRAINS			
Tearing or stretching of lateral or medial collateral ligaments from varus or valgus stretch	Pain occurs after throwing, overhead, or weight-bearing activity (medial) or fall onto extended elbow (lateral)	Tenderness of overlying affected ligaments; medial tenderness is maximal 2 cm distal to epicondyle, with pain and/or instability with valgus stretch at 30 degrees of elbow flexion; lateral tenderness is vague, reproduced only with arm extended and supinated	*Differential diagnosis:* Epicondylitis, radial/ulnar nerve irritation, avulsion fracture, or ligament tear *Management:* RICE; may use sling/splint for 48 hours if significant pain/edema

*Created by Terry Mahan Buttaro, MS, APRN, BC, ANP, GNP, CEN, CCRN.

TABLE 189-1 Common Elbow Ailments*—cont'd

Ailment	Presentation	Examination	Differential Diagnosis/Management
RADIAL HEAD FRACTURES			
Usually caused by fall onto outstretched hand; commonly involves superior portion of radial bone	Affected arm is usually cradled at 90 degrees; pain decreases 30 minutes after injury, then recurs several hours later because of bleeding in joint	Local or diffuse edema; tenderness over radial head; ROM limited, rotation quite painful; grasp strength diminished; intact radial pulse and normal neurologic examination of hand and wrist	*Differential diagnosis:* Acute lateral epicondylitis, capsular tears, cartilage injury, subluxation/dislocation of radial head, fracture of olecranon or humerus *Management:* Ice, immobilization with posterior splint or sling with elbow flexed at 90 degrees; displaced or complicated fractures often require surgical repair
ULNAR NEURITIS			
(Cubital Tunnel Syndrome) Compression of ulnar nerve causing numbness or tingling in nerve's distribution	May be complication of rheumatoid arthritis, ganglion, elbow fracture, repeated irritation, or medial ligament sprain; pain usually localized to medial elbow; may radiate down forearm or cause clumsiness of hand; numbness and tingling may replace pain in severe cases	Tenderness over ulnar groove; sensory loss of fifth digit; diminished motor strength of fourth and fifth digits; positive Tinel's sign (tingling sensation down forearm and hand in ulnar distribution when tapping over ulnar groove); in severe cases may be forearm motor weakness and muscle atrophy; diagnostics: electromyographic studies	*Differential diagnosis:* Medial epicondylitis, cervical disk disease, thoracic outlet syndrome *Management:* Rest of affected hand; elbow pads; wrist/elbow splint/support in neutral position; ice, NSAIDs, physical therapy; conservative treatment is rarely effective; referral to orthopedics or neurology is appropriate
OLECRANON BURSITIS			
Swelling of bursal sac underlying olecranon process; may be acute, chronic, septic, or aseptic and associated with history of trauma, rheumatoid arthritis, or gout	After acute injury, development of painful, edematous elbow; in chronic inflammation, soft, edematous nontender elbow; ROM often intact	Edema, possible tenderness over posterior elbow; full ROM and normal neurologic examination; in chronic bursitis, rough nodular consistency may be noted; if secondary infection, fever, warmth, erythema, and tenderness will be present	*Differential diagnosis:* Consider tendonitis; synovitis if edema is diffuse with limited elbow extension; infection; fracture with history of trauma; gout if extremely tender and erythematous; osteophytes; osteochondrosis *Management:* X-rays if indicated; aspiration of bursal fluid for diagnosis; hospitalization of patients with septic bursitis for aspiration, IV antibiotics p.r.n.; otherwise, RICE, NSAIDs, antibiotics if indicated; steroid injection p.r.n.; orthopedic referral if no response to treatment in 1 week

*Created by Terry Mahan Buttaro, MS, RN, CS, CEN, CCRN, ANP, GNP.

to protect the elbow from further injury. NSAIDs can be used to reduce pain and tissue inflammation. Physical therapy with ultrasound or electrical stimulation can be used acutely, followed by rehabilitation exercises and a gradual return to activity. Changes in technique, equipment, and ergonomics should also be implemented to prevent injury recurrence.

COMPLICATIONS

Recurrent epicondylitis or tendonitis may cause cumulative weakening of those tissues, resulting in impairment of grip function, lifting ability, or nerve entrapment of the arm.[5,6] Limitation of elbow range of motion, arthritis, and chronic elbow pain may be caused from improper diagnosis or treatment of the underlying elbow disorder.

INDICATIONS FOR REFERRAL/HOSPITALIZATION

Acute trauma resulting in fracture, dislocation, vascular, or neurologic clinical findings should be referred to an orthopedist. Recurrent injury, failure to improve with basic management, chronic pain with activity, or complaints of arm weakness should also be referred. A septic elbow joint may require intravenous antibiotics.

PATIENT AND FAMILY EDUCATION

Injury prevention and early recovery are assisted by teaching about proper stretching and conditioning exercises, the need for rest at early symptoms of pain, use of ergonomic redesign (in rackets, workplace, power tools), and proper body mechanics for sports and repetitive motion activities. Individuals with recurrent injury or any change in elbow function or mobility should be advised to seek prompt medical attention to minimize complications.

REFERENCES

1. Caldwell GL, Safran MR: Elbow problems in the athlete, *Orthop Clin North Am* 26(3):465-485, 1995.
2. Hales TR, Bernard BP: Epidemiology of work-related musculoskeletal disorders, *Orthop Clin North Am* 27(4):679-710, 1996.
3. Hoppinfield S: *Physical examination of the spine and extremities*, Norwalk, Conn, 1976, Appleton-Century-Crofts.
4. Safran MR: Elbow injuries in athletes: a review, *Clin Orthop* 310: 257-277, 1995.
5. Mercier LR: *Practical orthopedics*, ed 4, St Louis, 1995, Mosby.
6. Anderson BC: *Office orthopedics for primary care: diagnosis and treatment*, Philadelphia, 1995, WB Saunders.

CHAPTER 190

Fibromyalgia

Susan R. Tussey

DEFINITION/EPIDEMIOLOGY

Fibromyalgia syndrome (FS) is a controversial rheumatologic disorder characterized by symptoms of fatigue, nonrestorative sleep, generalized muscle aches, depression, migraines, and gastrointestinal complaints. FS gained acceptance as a disorder in 1990 after the American College of Rheumatology developed diagnosis criteria for diagnosis, although many people with FS vary with their symptoms.

Fibromyalgia is characterized by chronic, widespread musculoskeletal aches or stiffness and soft tissue tender points greater than 3 months' in duration and without an identifiable source (Box 190-1 and Figure 190-1). Usually accompanied by profound fatigue and sleep disturbance, fibromyalgia may occur in the presence of other rheumatologic disorders such as chronic fatigue syndrome, myofascial pain syndrome, and rheumatoid arthritis.[1]

FS is eight to nine times more prevalent in women than men in all age-groups, with onset generally at age 40 to 50 years, but may occur across the life span. Approximately 2% of the total population is affected, and the incidence is 8% in women 60 to 69 years old.[2] FS affects 3 to 6 million Americans, and accounts for 2% of all primary care visits, 10% of all internal medicine referrals, and up to 20% of rheumatology referrals.[1,2] Symptoms start gradually in adulthood or rarely, in childhood, and wax and wane in intensity; remissions are rare.[1]

PATHOPHYSIOLOGY

Although the cause of FS is unclear, new research has implicated central nervous system dysfunction instead of primary muscle pathology as once thought. Neuroendocrine disturbances at the level of the hypothalamus and/or pituitary involving growth hormone (GH), insulin-like factor (IGF) and possible prolactin are decreased in FS patients.[3] Hormones are released during the stages of sleep, specifically GH in stage 3 and stage 4 of non-REM sleep. In sleep studies patients with FS have disturbances in non-REM sleep and infrequent progression to stage 3 and stage 4 sleep, resulting in morning fatigue. One third of FS patients have low IGF, an indication of low GH secretion, which suggests that symptoms of FS may be caused by disturbing non–REM sleep. Treatment with GH increased IGF levels and improved pain and sleep, and reduced overall symptoms; however the cost is prohibitive.[3,4]

Other neuroendocrine abnormalities include elevation of cerebral spinal fluid substance P levels and decreased cortisol production. FS patients have three times the levels of substance P, which is significant, as this neurotransmitter plays a role in enhanced pain perception. This may be the reason for the heightened pain perception experienced by fibromyalgia patients. Alteration in the hypopituitary-adrenal axis with low production of cortisol, perhaps secondary to the stress response, contrasts with depression where high production of cortisol is found. These

BOX 190-1

AMERICAN COLLEGE OF RHEUMATOLOGY 1990 CRITERIA FOR THE CLASSIFICATION OF FIBROMYALGIA*

- History of widespread pain.
  Pain is considered widespread when all of the following are present: pain on the left side of the body, pain on the right side of the body, pain above the waist, and pain below the waist. In addition, axial skeletal pain (cervical spine or anterior chest or thoracic spine or low back) must be present. In the definition, shoulder and buttock pain is considered as pain for each involved side. "Low back" pain is considered lower segment pain.
- Pain in 11 of 18 tender point sites on digital palpation. Digital palpation should be performed with an approximate force of 4 kg. For a tender point to be considered "positive," the subject must state that the palpation was painful. "Tender" is not to be considered "painful." Pain, on digital palpation, must be present in at least 11 of the following 18 tender point sites:
  Occiput: bilateral, at the suboccipital muscle insertions
  Low cervical: bilateral, at the anterior aspects of the intertransverse spaces at C5-C7
  Trapezius: bilateral, at the midpoint of the upper border
  Supraspinatus: bilateral, at origins, above the scapula spine near the medial border
  Second rib: bilateral, at the second costochondral junctions, just lateral to the junctions on upper surfaces
  Lateral epicondyle: bilateral, 2 cm distal to the epicondyles
  Gluteal: bilateral, in upper outer quadrants of buttocks in anterior folds of muscle
  Greater trochanter: bilateral, posterior to the trochanteric prominence
  Knee: bilateral, at the medial fat pad proximal to the joint line.

From Wolfe FW and others: *Arthritis Rheum* 33:160, 1990.
*For classification purposes, patients are said to have fibromyalgia if both criteria are satisfied. Widespread pain must have been present for at least 3 months. The presence of a second clinical disorder does not exclude the diagnosis of fibromyalgia.

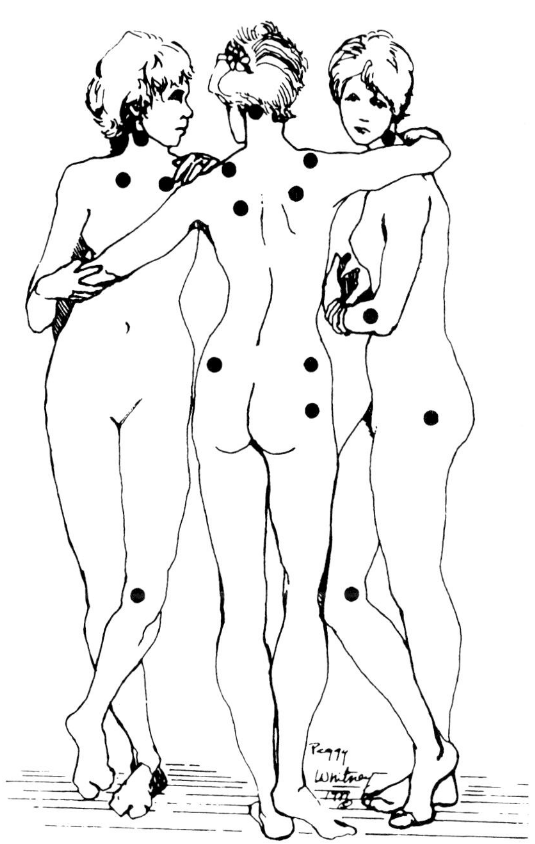

FIGURE 190-1

Tender point locations for the 1990 classification criteria for fibromyalgia. (From Wolfe FW and others: The American College of Rheumatology 1990 criteria for the classification of fibromyalgia: report of the multicenter criteria committee, *Arthritis Rheum* 33(2):160-172, 1990.)

results suggest that the etiology of FS may be a product of disturbances in the autonomic and endocrine stress response systems.[4]

Other theories include trauma as the onset of fibromyalgia and myofascial pain, low central levels of serotonin synthesis, and myriad complex psychosocial factors in several disorders of the FS spectrum. More controlled studies are needed, which is difficult given the multifactorial presentations of each patient.

CLINICAL PRESENTATION

Persistent widespread pain is the hallmark of the syndrome, along with chronic fatigue. A variety of other somatic complaints include poor sleep, cognitive difficulties, auditory/vestibular/ocular complaints, chronic rhinitis/"allergies," migraines, palpitations, irritable bowel syndrome, subjective sense of joint swelling, and mood disorders.[5]

PHYSICAL EXAMINATION

With fibromyalgia, muscle strength is typically normal, and there is no evidence of synovitis or soft tissue inflammation. Making the diagnosis depends on findings from the history and physical examination, and FS should be considered with any musculoskeletal pain not explained with a clearly defined anatomic lesion .

The American College of Rheumatology developed criteria characteristic of FS symptoms (see Box 190-1). Pressure point evaluation of sites using 4 kg of pressure, with the report of pain, not tenderness, at 11 of the 18 sites; widespread pain on the left and right side; and pain above and below the waist. (A pressure of 4 kg is achieved by digital palpation of the thumb with enough pressure to blanch the thumbnail.) Shoulder and buttock pain qualifies for the definition of pain of each side, and low back pain must be present. Pain of the cervical spine, anterior chest, and thoracic spine (axial skeletal pain) also is required for diagnosis.[6] However, these criteria were not meant to be rigid, and some patients will not exhibit all 11 pressure points and still have the diagnosis of FS.

DIAGNOSTICS

An in-depth history and physical examination reduce the need for extensive and expensive objective tests. Typically laboratory values and electromyography findings are normal, CBC, erythrocyte sedimentation rate, rheumatoid factor, antinuclear antibodies, and thyroid-hormone are of value in excluding underlying autoimmune disorders such as rheumatoid arthritis and polymyalgia rheumatica. Sleep studies may be warranted for some patients. Radiographs are of limited value.[3,4]

DIFFERENTIAL DIAGNOSIS

Symptoms of fibromyalgia often overlap with those of myofascial pain syndrome, chronic fatigue syndrome, hypothyroidism, bursitis/tendinitis, depression, and anxiety. Connective tissue diseases that should be included in the differential diagnosis include rheumatoid arthritis, systemic lupus erythematosus, polymyalgia rheumatica, giant cell arteritis, and polymyositis. Certain medications can also cause increased pain sensitivity.

MANAGEMENT

Treatment of FS does not fit a specific algorithm or paradigm and is as much of an art as a science. The goal of therapy should be patient empowerment to control pain, enhance sleep, and maintain mobility. Education allows the patient opportunities to individualize treatment and reduce symptoms, and may incorporate pharmacologic, cognitive, exercise, and alternative therapies.[7]

Diagnostics

Fibromyalgia

Serum electrolytes*	ESR
BUN*	Rheumatoid factor
Creatinine*	TSH*
Serum glucose*	Antinuclear antibody*
CBC and differential	

*If indicated.

Pharmacology

Low doses of tricyclic drugs have been studied, most particularly amitriptyline 10 mg taken 2 to 3 hours before bedtime, allowing peak sedative effect and reducing sedation on awakening. One study noted synergistic effects with amitriptyline and cyclobenzaprine started slowly and increased 10 mg every 1 to 2 weeks (maximum doses of 70 to 80 mg amitriptyline and 40 mg of cyclobenzaprine). Also studied were selective serotonin reuptake inhibitors such as fluoxetine 20 mg (Prozac) and amitriptyline, but results are conflicting. Sertraline and venlafaxine also may be of some benefit, indicating medications that augment central adrenergic tone may be more effective than drugs that work by serotonergic mechanisms (Table 190-1).

Other medications that have proved helpful for pain include gabapentin (Neurontin) and trazodone (Desyrel) and for sleep zolpidem (Ambien). Nonsteroidal antiinflammatory agents and acetaminophen are commonly prescribed and, although they have not been proven to be effective as once thought, can play a role in pain management.[4,7]

Cognitive Behavioral Therapy

Because FS is complex, cognitive behavioral therapy uses different approaches to integrate coping skills, relaxation training, activity pacing, visual imagery techniques, and goal setting to allow the patient control to improve function and pain. The Arthritis Foundation and other web sites can help direct patients to self-help books and classes.[4,5,7]

Exercise

Aerobic exercise can improve pain as well as have an antidepressant effect.[8] Usually patients with fibromyalgia have not been active physically and experience increased pain when they begin an aerobic exercise program. Gentle stretching is a must before engaging in a low-impact activity such as biking,

Differential Diagnosis

Fibromyalgia

Medication-induced condition	Metabolic disorder
Chronic fatigue syndrome	Tendinitis/bursitis
Polymyalgia rheumatica	Myofascial pain syndrome
Depression/anxiety	Hypothyroidism
Connective tissue disorders	

TABLE 190-1 Pharmacologic Therapy for Fibromyalgia

Medication	Proposed Action
Amitriptyline 10-20 mg q h.s., gradually increasing to 70 mg	Restoration of sleep
Cyclobenzaprine 10 mg t.i.d. p.r.n. or in combination with amitriptyline	Pain relief
Selective serotonin reuptake inhibitor—20 mg fluoxetine (Prozac) alone or in combination with amitriptyline	
Venlafaxine 75 mg PO b.i.d.-t.i.d.	Augment central adrenergic to decrease pain
Gabapentin 300 mg t.i.d.	Pain relief
Trazodone 50 mg PO q.h.s.	Pain relief
Zolpidem tartrate (Ambien) 5-10 mg PO q.h.s.	Improve sleep
Lidocaine 1% 2-3 ml equal parts IM in tender point areas	Pain relief for recalcitrant tender point pain

swimming, and walking. Massage aids in relaxation and produces physiologic benefits. Encouragement to continue the exercise program is needed to combat the continued muscle wasting often associated with fibromyalgia, as well as to alleviate patients' perception that pain is inevitable. Consider a one-on-one therapist or exercise partner for any program to improve success.[4,5]

Alternative Therapies

Acupuncture, chiropractic manipulation, and trigger point injections have been studied, and are reported to be effective adjuncts to a treatment regimen. The injection of tender points with lidocaine (Xylocaine) or bupivacaine (Marcaine) has been attempted for symptoms not controlled with other medications with some success.[9]

Chronic Opioid Analgesic Therapy

Reserved for those with severe pain and significant functional impairment, controlled clinical trials show chronic opioid analgesic therapy to be effective in non–cancer-related pain. Oxycodone (Roxicodone) or morphine sulfate (Duramorph) have been used for intermittent pain, but patients need to be aware of the high dependence possibility and be monitored closely.[4,5]

Multidisciplinary Approach

These group therapy programs are based on cognitive behavioral therapy approaches for living day to day effectively and increasing endurance and strength. An evidenced-based clinical review evaluated seven trials and found insufficient evidence that these programs are effective by themselves and worked better as an adjunct to a primary provider. The studies were of low quality and variables tested were so varied it was difficult to standardize the trials for comparison. More research is needed to establish the effects of a multidisciplinary approach as a treatment for FS.[10,11]

COMPLICATIONS

Disability is one of the most serious complications of this painful syndrome and very often difficult to document or receive compensation. Other complications include depression, insomnia, muscle atrophy, misdiagnosis, and drug-seeking behavior.

INDICATIONS FOR REFERRAL/HOSPITALIZATION

FS patients can be managed in primary care; however management requires individualized plans of care and willingness for creativity in treatment plans, perhaps including alternative treatments. Pain management clinics for pain control and transcutaneous electrical nerve stimulation units have been effective for chronic pain. Psychologists, physiologists, physical therapists, and chiropractors may aid in symptom control.

Hospital admissions generally are associated with conditions that are coexistent with fibromyalgia, such as gastrointestinal and depressive manifestations.

PATIENT AND FAMILY EDUCATION

Education is imperative for improved patient understanding of fibromyalgia and the development of individual strategies to cope with the pain, fatigue, and chronic nature of the syndrome. The importance of regular exercise and adequate rest should be emphasized. Family members are affected and should be involved in education to understand this complex, disabling disorder to maximize support for these patients. Support groups can be invaluable. Information abounds on the Internet, and careful evaluation is needed to evaluate the material. Available resources include the following:

The Arthritis Foundation
1330 West Peachtree Street
Atlanta, GA 30309
(404) 872-7100
http://www.arthritis.org

National Institute of Arthritis and Musculoskeletal and Skin Diseases (NIAMS)
National Institute of Health
http://www.niams.nih.gov

The Fibromyalgia Network Newsletter
PO Box 31750
Tucson, AZ 85751
(800) 853-2929
http://www.fmnetnews.com

Oregon Fibromyalgia Foundation
1221 SW Yamhill, Suite 303
Portland, OR 97205
http://www.myalgia.com

American Association of Medial Acupuncture
5820 Wilshire Blvd., Ste. 500
Los Angeles, CA 90036
http://www.medicalacupuncture.org

HEALTH PROMOTION

Modifiable risk factors include exercise for pain control and maintaining flexibility, support systems for improving mental health, and self-esteem. FS is a multifactorial syndrome that requires empowering patients with the tools needed for improving activities of daily living.

REFERENCES

1. Wolfe F: The fibromyalgia problem (editorial), *J Rheumatol* 24(7): 1247-1249, 1997.
2. Wolfe F and others: The prevalence and characteristic of fibromyalgia in the general population, *Arthritis Rheum* 38:19-28, 1995.
3. Landis C and others: Decreased nocturnal levels of prolactin and growth hormone in women with fibromyalgia, *J Clin Endocrinol Metab* 86:1672, 1978.
4. Millea P: Treating fibromyalgia, *Am Fam Physician* 62(7):1572-82, 1987.
5. Winfield J: Pain management in the rheumatic diseases, *Rheum Dis Clin North Am* 25:55-79, 1999.
6. Wolfe F and others: The American College of Rheumatology 1990 criteria for the classification of fibromyalgia: report of the multicenter criteria committee, *Arthritis Rheum* 33(2):160-172, 1990.
7. Ruddy: *Kelley's textbook of rheumatology*, ed 6, Philadelphia, 2001, WB Saunders.
8. Karper WB and others: Exercise program effects on women with fibromyalgia syndrome, *Clin Nur Spec* 15(2):67-75, 2001.
9. Berman B: The evidence for acupuncture as a treatment for rheumatologic conditions, *Rheum Dis Clin North Am* 26(1):103-115, 2000.
10. Bennett R: Multidisciplinary group programs to treat fibromyalgia patients, *Rheum Dis Clin North Am* 22(2):351-367, 1996.
11. Shae W and others: Evidence based clinical practice, *Evidence-based Healthcare* 4(4): 2000.

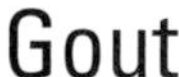 CHAPTER 191

Gout

Denise T. Bynum

DEFINITION/EPIDEMIOLOGY

Gout is a hereditary metabolic disease caused by hyperuricemia that affects 13.6 per 1000 men and 6.4 per 1000 women in the United States.[1] Prevalence has increased over the last few decades in the United States and other countries with a high standard of living.

Joint, bone, and subcutaneous inflammation resulting from monosodium urate crystal deposition in the joints marks this common form of acute monarticular arthritis. Gout is rare in childhood, affecting men mostly in the third and fourth decade, with a peak incidence in the fifth decade. It is unusual in women until after menopause (ages 50 to 70 years) unless a woman has renal insufficiency or uses diuretics.[1] The low incidence in women is likely due to estrogen's effect on the renal tubules, where it expedites the renal excretion of uric acid.[1]

PATHOPHYSIOLOGY

Gout is related to a genetic defect in the production or excretion of uric acid, a crystalline acid that is an end-product of purine metabolism. Gout is due to either increased production of uric acid (metabolic origin) or decreased excretion of uric acid (renal origin). Uric acid cannot be metabolized; therefore it must be excreted. Excess uric acid crystallizes, infiltrates the joints, deposits in synovial cells in joint lining, and causes an inflammatory response. The risk for developing primary gout is directly proportional to the severity and duration of hyperuricemia. The majority of patients with primary gout have an inherited faulty uric acid metabolism. Acute gout progresses to chronic gouty arthritis in a small majority of patients. The intercritical period is the asymptomatic period between attacks, which may last for several months or years.

As the disease progresses, the asymptomatic intervals become shorter and more joints become involved. In chronic gout there is inflammation owing to the urate crystal deposits called tophi. These chalky deposits of sodium urate are surrounded by giant cell inflammatory reactions and can develop at sites of irritation, such as the Achilles tendon, joints of the hand, pinna of the ear, synovium, subchondral bone, infrapatellar tendon, olecranon bursa, and the subcutaneous tissue on the extensor surface of the forearms. Tophi have also been found in the aortic walls, heart valves, nasal and ear cartilage, eyelids, cornea, and sclera. Tophi do not develop if there is adequate treatment.[2]

Secondary hyperuricemia is caused by a variety of diseases where there is an increase in cell turnover. These conditions include leukemia, multiple myeloma, myeloproliferative disease, lymphoproliferative disease, hemolytic or pernicious anemia, glycogen storage disease, psoriasis, renal insufficiency, and sarcoidosis. Certain drugs can alter renal tubular function and contribute to a decrease in uric acid excretion. These include cyclosporine, salicylate, lead acetate, diuretics (thiazides and furosemide), pyrazinamide, ethambutol, nicotinic acid, and alcohol.

CLINICAL PRESENTATION

The acute phase of gout usually presents in one joint, and in 50% to 75% of patients, it is the metatarsophalangeal joint of the great toe that is edematous, red, warm, and extremely painful (also called podagra).[3] Other common sites include the tarsal joint (instep of the foot), ankle, knee, and less commonly in the fingers, wrist, or elbow. The first attack often begins suddenly at night as a result of water being absorbed from the joint spaces, leaving an increased saturation of monosodium urate. The painful attack peaks within 12 to 24 hours, and subsides spontaneously in 3 to 10 days.[2] The second attack may not occur for years. Attacks are usually recurrent, lasting longer and occurring more often with each recurrence. Precipitating causes include intake of certain medications or alcohol, recent changes in diet, trauma, surgical stress, illness, or exposure to lead. The number, duration, and characteristics of previous attacks, as well as adherence to treatment, should be determined. Gout is sometimes associated with hypertension, hyperlipidemia, renal disease, obesity, alcohol use, starvation, lead intoxication, surgery, trauma, diabetes, hypothyroidism, hyperparathyroidism or hypoparathyroidism, Paget's disease, psoriasis, or Down syndrome. Gout may be a risk factor for coronary artery disease. Gout should be suspected in patients with vague musculoskeletal aches that respond promptly to nonsteroidal anti-inflammatory drugs (NSAIDs). The presence of these conditions and a family history of gout should be determined during the history and physical examination.

PHYSICAL EXAMINATION

The patient with gout can present with chills and fevers, with joints that are warm, tender, and erythematous. The joints occasionally have deformities. Tophi, irregular subcutaneous nodules that may have a creamy white discharge composed of urate crystals, may become visible 10 to 12 years after the initial attacks (range 3 to 42 years).[3] Tophi appear as irregular subcutaneous nodules and may have a creamy white discharge composed of urate crystals (Color Plate 39). Tophi may resemble the nodules of rheumatoid arthritis. Over time, symptoms such as morning aching and stiffness, synovial tissue thickening, and joint deformity occur. Ocular manifestations include episcleritis, uveitis, and uric acid crystals in the cornea.

DIAGNOSTICS

Serum uric acid levels >7 mg/dl support the diagnosis of gout but are not specific, as a few patients with gout will be normouricemic. Attacks seem to be related to sudden changes in serum uric acid levels. Some patients with hyperuricemia may never experience an attack. In asymptomatic hyperuricemia the serum uric acid level is >7 mg/dl (normal for men is 5 ± 1 mg/dl; normal for women is 4 ± 1 mg/dl). Serum uric acid levels can be used to assess the risk for urate stones and the need for aggressive therapy. During the attack, the erythrocyte sedimentation rate and white blood cell count may be elevated, especially if large or numerous joints are involved. A rheumatoid factor titer is additionally indicated to exclude rheumatoid arthritis. Because of the possibility of renal and cardiovascular effects, a CBC,

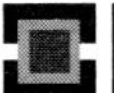

Diagnostics

Gout
Laboratory
CBC and differential
ESR
Serum uric acid
BUN, creatinine
Urinalysis
Rheumatoid factor*
24-hour urine collection for uric acid (without dietary restrictions)
Serum creatinine
BUN
Imaging
X-ray*
Other
Joint aspirate

*If indicated.

urinalysis, serum creatinine and BUN should be included.[3]

If a single joint is involved, aspirate from the acutely inflamed joint should be obtained and a wet mount prepared for examination under a compensated polarizing microscope. A 24-hour urine collection to measure uric acid excretion should be considered. Uric acid excretion is normally between 600 and 900 mg on a regular diet (>900 mg suggests overproduction of urate). X-ray studies may be indicated to exclude other conditions but are helpful in differentiating gout from other diseases only in advanced cases. Drugs that induce hyperuricemia, such as low-dose aspirin or probenecid, may alter laboratory results.

DIFFERENTIAL DIAGNOSIS

If there is no response to gout treatment within 48 hours, an infection or another disease must be considered. Pseudogout is another crystal deposition disease that is caused by the presence of calcium pyrophosphate dihydrate (CPPD) in the joints. Pseudogout has an asymptomatic phase and causes acute and chronic arthritis similar to that seen with gout, but tophi rarely occur. Pseudogout tends to occur in older patients. Unlike with gout, with pseudogout there is no way to remove the CPPD crystals from the joints, nor is there a medication available to prevent CPPD crystal formation. The treatment for pseudogout includes NSAIDs, colchicine, aspiration, and intraarticular corticosteroids.

Other conditions to consider include cellulitis, septic arthritis, amyloidosis, or bursitis related to a bunion; joint infection; Reiter's syndrome; ankylosing spondylitis; psoriatic arthritis; arthritis of inflammatory bowel disease; and arthritis of sarcoidosis. Infection or diabetic foot ulcer should be considered in the differential diagnosis if the skin over a joint is red and peeling.

MANAGEMENT

Asymptomatic hyperuricemia (>13 mg/dl in men and >10 mg/dl in women) is generally not treated but monitored closely and the cause investigated. For the acute phase of gout, prompt institution of antiinflammatory therapy will relieve acute symptoms. Antiinflammatory therapy should be given for 3 to 6 months or until all visible urate deposits have disappeared to reduce the risk of an acute attack of gout.

In chronic gout (more than three attacks per year) or in patients who are difficult to treat because of allergies or toxicity, therapy should include a urate-lowering agent, such as allopurinol or probenecid.[4] Urate-lowering agents should be initiated at least 1 month after an acute attack, as these drugs

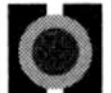

Differential Diagnosis

Gout	
Gonococcal arthritis	Arthritis of sarcoid
Osteoarthritis	Septic arthritis
Rheumatoid arthritis	Bursitis
Infectious arthritis	Reiter's syndrome
Rheumatic fever	Psoriatic arthritis
Pseudogout	Arthritis of inflammatory bowel
Lyme disease (in selected geographic areas)	Amyloidosis
Cellulitis	Ankylosing spondylitis
Joint infection	

can trigger acute gout. Joint immobilization, decreased weight bearing, cold applications, and protection from trauma may also be helpful. Patients with acute gout should be reassessed or contacted in 24 hours. The patient should be assessed and treated for the diseases that are associated with gout, such as hypertension, hyperlipidemia, and heart disease. Annual physical examinations that include uric acid levels are necessary for chronic gout. Table 191-1 lists the medications for use in acute and chronic gout.[2,5-7] A drug reference should be consulted for complete prescribing information.

COMPLICATIONS

Complications include renal infection, nephropathy, and nephrolithiasis. Deposits of uric acid crystals collect in the kidneys causing renal uratelithiasis in 10% to 25% of patients with primary gout.[3] The incidence of this renal uratelithiasis is two times higher in secondary gout than primary gout and can contribute to chronic renal disease.[2] Acute gouty nephropathy is caused by massive cell turnover with precipitation of uric acid in collecting ducts and ureters causing blockage of urine and acute renal failure. Chronic urate nephropathy is caused by microtophi that leads to a giant cellular inflammatory response resulting in proteinuria and the inability to concentrate urine. Hypersensitivity to allopurinol occurs primarily with concurrent renal insufficiency; it is uncommon, but can be fatal. Tophi can cause pain, impaired skin integrity, soft tissue deformities, joint destruction, and nerve compression syndromes (e.g., carpel tunnel syndrome).

INDICATIONS FOR REFERRAL/HOSPITALIZATION

Corticosteroid injections into the affected joints may require referral, depending on the primary care provider's experience, state practice acts, and the agreement with the collaborating physician. Contraindications for drug therapy or signs of side effects require consultation for management. Hospitalization is rarely necessary unless the pain cannot be managed on an outpatient basis or complications resulting from the disease (such as joint infection) or drug therapy occur.

PATIENT AND FAMILY EDUCATION

Gradual weight loss is helpful and should be encouraged if the patient is obese. Fasting or very-low-calorie diets can precipitate an attack. Patients should also reduce alcohol consumption

TABLE 191-1 Gout Pharmacotherapy

Class	Generic Name	Brand Name	Action	Dose/ Frequency/ Directions	Contraindications	Adverse Reactions	Precautions
NSAID	Indomethacin	Indocin	Inhibits prostaglandin synthesis; analgesic; antiinflammatory; antipyretic	50 mg q 8 hr until pain is tolerable, then discontinue; give with food or milk; take whole (do not crush or chew)	Aspirin allergy, asthma, severe hepatic or renal disease, ulcer disease	GI ulcers, bleeding, or perforation; headache; nausea; dizziness; cholestatic hepatitis; nephrotoxicity; blood dyscrasias	GI disorders, impaired renal or hepatic function, cardiac disorders, hypertension, edema, sepsis, depression, Parkinsonism, bleeding disorders, pregnancy, lactation, children, older adults
	Naproxen	Naprosyn	See Indomethacin	750 mg initially, followed by 500 mg q 12 hr; give with food or milk; take whole (do not crush or chew)	Aspirin allergy, third-trimester pregnancy, asthma, severe renal or hepatic disorder, ulcer disease	GI bleeding, peptic ulcer, abdominal pain, constipation, heartburn, dizziness, cholestatic hepatitis, nephrotoxicity, blood dyscrasias	Active peptic ulcer, history of upper GI disease, impaired renal or hepatic function, elders, pregnancy, lactation, children <2 years, bleeding or cardiac disorders
Antigout	Colchicine		Inhibits formation of leukocytes; decreases phagocytosis and inflammation in joints Lowers deposit of uric acid	0.5 mg q 1 hr until total dose of 7.2 mg or 16 doses, symptoms abate, or GI symptoms; give on empty stomach	Allergy; serious GI, renal, hepatic, or cardiac disorder; blood dyscrasia	Diarrhea, abdominal cramping, anorexia, nausea or vomiting, malaise, blood dyscrasias (drug of choice in past/not used as frequently now because of side effects) Prolonged use may decrease vitamin B_{12} absorption	Severe renal disorders, blood dyscrasias, hepatitis, elders, pregnancy, lactation, children
Xanthine oxidase inhibitor	Allopurinol	Zyloprim	Inhibits breakdown of purine reducing uric acid synthesis; goal is to keep uric acid <6.5 mg/dl	100 mg for 1 week, then increase by 100 mg/day at weekly intervals with 300 mg/dose and 800 mg/day maximum	Asymptomatic hyperuricemia, hypersensitivity	GI upset, abdominal pain, nausea, vomiting, anorexia, blood dyscrasias, cholestatic jaundice, acute gout, fever, headache, renal failure, allopurinal hypersensitivity reaction consisting of fever, rash, decreased renal function, liver damage, or leukocytosis; stop drug at earliest sign of bone marrow suppression or Stevens-Johnson syndrome	Pregnancy, lactation, children; reduce dose for patients with renal or hepatic insufficiency; no benefit in acute gout and may precipitate an attack during early stages of therapy; potential toxicity enhanced in elders or patients taking diuretics or PCN

Uricosuric	Sulfinpyrazone	Anturane	Inhibits tubular reabsorption of urates; increases excretion of uric acids	100-200 mg b.i.d. × 1 wk, then 200-400 mg b.i.d.; do not exceed 800 mg/day	Hypersensitivity to pyrazolone derivatives, severe hepatic or renal disease, creatinine clearance <50 mg/min, active peptic ulcer disease (PUD), GI inflammation, renal calculi	Gastric irritation; nausea, vomiting, anorexia, hepatic necrosis, agranulocytosis, convulsions, apnea, coma	Pregnancy, lactation
	Probenecid	Benemid	Promotes renal excretion of uric acid; inhibits renal tubular reabsorption of urates; preferred in interval gout with no risk of stones and adequate renal function	250 mg b.i.d. × 1 week, then increase to 500 mg b.i.d.	Hypersensitivity, severe hepatic disease, blood dyscrasias, severe renal disease, CrCl <50 mg/min, history of uric acid calculus	Rash, GI upset, headache, dizziness, nephrotic syndrome, hepatic necrosis, urinary frequency, sore gums, uric acid kidney stones, hematuria, renal colic, fever, hemolytic anemia, acidosis, hypokalemia, hyperchloremia, apnea, constipation	Pregnancy, severe respiratory disease, lactation, cardiac edema, children <2 years
Uricosuric combination	Probenecid, 500 mg, plus colchicine, 0.5 mg		See individual drugs above	1 tablet daily for 1 week, then 1 tablet b.i.d.	See individual drugs above	See individual drugs above	See individual drugs above
Corticosteroid	Prednisolone	Prednisone, Medrol	Decreases inflammation by suppressing migration of polymorphonuclear leukocytes	20-60 mg for 3-4 days, then taper off	Psychosis, hypersensitivity, idiopathic thrombocytopenia, acute glomerulonephritis, fungal infections, children <2 years, AIDS, tuberculosis (TB)	Depression mood changes, circulatory collapse, thrombophlebitis, embolism, nausea, increased appetite, diarrhea, GI ulceration, pancreatitis, thrombocytopenia	Pregnancy diabetes, glaucoma, osteoporosis, seizures, ulcerative colitis, congestive heart failure (CHF), renal disease, esophagitis, PUD
Pituitary hormone	Corticotropin	ACTH	Stimulates release of several hormones and more effective than prednisone alone; one of the safest agents for renal insufficiency, GI disease, or CHF	40 IU IM q 12 hr; give no more than 3 days	Scleroderma, CHF, PUD, hypertension	Convulsions, peptic ulcer perforation, impaired wound healing, nausea, vomiting, water retention	Pregnancy, TB, hepatic disorder, hypothyroidism, psychiatric disorder

and avoid salicylates and diuretics. Only small amounts of circulating purine are from dietary sources; therefore a diet low in purine is usually not recommended. However, several sources recommend avoiding foods that are extremely high in purine, such as sardines, anchovies, salmon, herring, caviar, organ meats, bacon, turkey, shellfish, red meat, meat broths, smoked or pickled meat, yeast, legumes, beer, and wine. All alcohol should be avoided, as it can interfere with the elimination of uric acid. Servings should be limited to one a day for foods that are moderately high in purine content, such as dry cereals, asparagus, cauliflower, and mushrooms. Information on the risks and benefits of a prophylactic medication program and the need to increase fluid intake to 2 to 3 L/day should be carefully explained. The patient should be referred to the Arthritis Foundation and instructed to keep an extra supply of medication for use in acute attacks.[8,9]

REFERENCES

1. Klippel JH: *Primer on the rheumatic diseases,* ed 12, Atlanta, 2001, The Arthritis Foundation.
2. Smelzer SC, Bare BG: *Brunner & Suddarth's textbook of medical surgical nursing,* ed 9, Philadelphia, 2000, Lippincott.
3. Pittman JR, Bross MH: Diagnosis and management of gout, *Am Fam Physician* 59(7):1799-1806, 1999.
4. Canoso JJ, Kalish RA: Gout: effective drug therapy for acute attacks and for the long term, *Consultant* 36(8):1752-1755, 1996.
5. Murphy J, editor: *Nurse practitioner's prescribing reference,* London, 2001, Prescribing Reference.
6. Skidmore-Roth L: *Mosby's drug guide for nurses,* ed 3, St Louis, 2001, Mosby.
7. Christ P: Gout: a complex disorder, *Ostomy Q* 37(3):20-21, 2000.
8. Mayo Foundation for Medical Education and Research: Retrieve February 28, 2002, from the World Wide Web: http://www.mayoclinic.com.
9. American College of Rhematology: Retrieved 2000 from the World Wide Web: http://www.rheumatology.org/patients/factsheet/gout/html.

CHAPTER 192

Hand and Wrist Pain

Karin C. Dieselman

DEFINITION/EPIDEMIOLOGY

Fractures, strains, and sprains of the hands and fingers are injuries commonly seen in primary care (see Chapter 204). Hand disorders may result from either recreational or work-related activities. Job specialization, repetitious tasks, and workplace demographics have contributed to an increased incidence of cumulative hand and wrist injuries. In 1992, 60% of new work-related disorders were associated with repetitive movement.[1,2] These injuries, which are also known as cumulative trauma disorders (CTDs), account for 56% of occupational injuries and are defined as muscle, tendon, osseous, or neurologic conditions produced or exacerbated by repetitive movements.[3] Many factors, including obesity and various medical conditions, contribute to the development of these conditions.

Immediate orthopedic referral is indicated if the finger cannot be passively extended (trigger finger).

PATHOPHYSIOLOGY

Injuries from CTDs include sprains and strains, but CTDs usually result from microtraumas that over time affect the tendons, tendon sheaths, and connective tissues. The exact pathologic mechanism is not clearly understood.[1,4] In the past, it was thought that overuse syndromes represented an inflammatory process, but more recent studies have shown no identifiable inflammation or tissue damage.[1,5]

CLINICAL PRESENTATION

Localized pain, numbness, tingling, weakness, or immobility are the common reasons that patients with hand or wrist disorders seek care.[6] The symptoms may be intermittent or constant and often affect quality of life. The diagnosis of any hand or wrist disorder is facilitated by a comprehensive medical, recreational, and occupational history. The precise anatomic location of the problem, as well as onset, quality, intensity, radiation, evolution, and exacerbating and relieving factors, should be documented. It is usually helpful to have the patient draw a hand diagram and document the areas of numbness, tingling, pain, and sensory loss. The history should include work environment, job tasks, dominant hand, history of injury, co-morbid illnesses, recreational activities, hobbies, allergies, and current medication use. If the patient is a woman of childbearing age, the date of the last menstrual period should be noted.

Trigger finger, or stenosing tenosynovitis, is a disorder of the flexor tendons of the fingers or thumb. This condition, which may be more prevalent in patients with diabetes, occurs when a nodule or thickening in the tendon catches on the edge of the tendon sheath as the tendon attempts to glide during movement.

This thickening narrows the fibrous/osseous canal, which impedes tendon movement. The pulley action is impaired, causing a painful locking or triggering of the affected digit or thumb during extension. Although any digit may be affected, the middle or ring finger is most commonly involved.

Chronic stenosing tenosynovitis of the wrist, or de Quervain's disease, is typically encountered in occupations that require repetitive wrist and thumb movements. Initially the patient may describe a catching sensation as thumb extension is attempted after flexion. As the condition progresses, the thumb may become locked in flexion.

Dupuytren's contracture, or palmar fibrosis, may be a hereditary process that initially develops as a painless nodule on the palmar fascia at the base of a digit. An inflammatory fibrosis subsequently expands into a bandlike cord under puckered skin and causes a flexion contracture. Although any finger (and both hands) may be affected, the resultant contracture most often affects the ring finger. The little finger may also be involved.

Carpal tunnel syndrome (CTS) is one of many nerve entrapment neuropathies and results from compression of the median nerve in the carpal tunnel of the wrist. An opening under the carpal ligament on the palmar side of the carpal bones, the carpal tunnel is the passageway for the nine digital flexor tendons, blood vessels, and the median nerve of the hand. Pregnancy, menopause, arthritis, diabetes, hypertension, hypothyroidism, trauma, and a history of occupational or sports-related activities are some of the conditions that affect these structures and result in nerve entrapment. The tendons swell with overuse, which decreases the cross-sectional area in the tunnel. Synovial fluid increases to decrease friction, but the resultant pressure in the small tunnel causes pressure on the median nerve. Conduction is impeded, muscle strength is decreased because of the disturbance in motor fibers, and pain and paresthesia occur because of the disturbance in the sensory fibers.

Intermittent wrist pain with numbness and tingling that radiates from the palm to the thumb, index finger, middle finger, and/or ring finger often are common presenting complaints of CTS. Additionally, the patient may awaken during the night with numbness, may complain of pain and tightness at the wrist and forearm that increases with activity, and may describe an inability to hold objects or a tendency to drop things. If the compression continues, the motor component of the median nerve is affected, and the ability to grasp with the thumb and index finger may be lost.

Cubital tunnel syndrome is a nerve entrapment neuropathy that results from ulnar nerve compression below the notch of the elbow. Pain that radiates from the elbow to the ring or little finger, numbness, and tingling are characteristics of this syndrome. A diminished grasp indicates motor dysfunction (see Chapter 189).

Trapeziometacarpal arthritis is a common site of arthritis in women. Common complaints include pain at the base of the thumb and weakness and pain with pinching. Table 192-1 presents other common hand problems.

PHYSICAL EXAMINATION

Muscle wasting, arm shortening, edema, point tenderness, deformity, pulses, and skin color and temperature should be noted when examining patients with hand or wrist pain. Passive and active range of motion, muscle strength, and sensory and motor testing are also necessary. Additional specific tests may be indicated.

TABLE 192-1 Other Common Hand Problems

Disorder	Clinical Presentation	Physical Examination/ Diagnostics	Management/Referral
GANGLION Benign cystic tumor of the hand or wrist; also found on foot or ankle	May be sudden or gradual onset of pain, or may be totally asymptomatic	Round, broad-based, translucent cyst on digit or wrist; may be obscured with movement Diagnostics are usually unnecessary, but ultrasound may be valuable for some patients[7]	*Referral:* If symptomatic, referral to physician for aspiration or cortisone injection, orthopedic referral for surgical excision
RAYNAUD'S DISEASE See Chapter 240 Intermittent vasoconstriction of digital arteries that causes blanching, numbness, and pain on fingertips or toes; commonly occurs in women Raynaud's phenomenon has similar presentation but is secondarily related to *Helicobacter pylori;* estrogen replacement therapy; hematologic dyscrasias; vasospastic, arterial, or connective tissue disorder; neurovascular or hematologic syndrome; medication; or repetitive trauma[8,9]	Intermittent digital pain often exacerbated by cold, stress	Blanched white fingertips (or toes) lasting several minutes to an hour, followed by severe pain and digital hyperemia, may be present Complete physical examination and vital signs are necessary to determine presence of bruits, peripheral pulses, telangiectasias under nailbeds, digital tip ulceration, and gangrene If secondary disease is not suspected, CBC, ESR, LFTs, ANA, chemistry profile, and serum protein electrophoresis may be indicated; EMG studies if carpal tunnel is suspected	*Management:* Smoking cessation; avoidance of medications that may induce vasospasm; keeping fingers/toes warm, covered; avoidance of precipitants; acupuncture[10] *Referral:* If secondary Raynaud's syndrome is suspected, physician referral for appropriate testing is necessary; diagnostics may include chest x-ray, angiography Referral to a hand specialist may also be warranted in severe cases for adventitial stripping[11]

Trigger Finger

The proximal interphalangeal joint (PIP) of the affected finger or thumb is flexed at 90 degrees. The digit can usually be extended, but there may be considerable pain with extension. With trigger thumb, resisted thumb extension can exacerbate the pain over the affected tendons. The nodule may be palpable.

Tenosynovitis

On inspection, there may be a palpable nodule at the base of the thumb. Edema and tenderness may be present over the radial stylus. A positive Finklestein's test is confirmed if pain over the radial stylus is reproduced when the patient folds the thumb across the palm, flexes the fingers over the thumb, and then the clinician deviates the hand in the direction of the ulna. Grip and pinch strength should also be assessed.

Palmar Fibrosis

Contracture may be evident on one or both hands, as well as on the feet, and may interfere with function. Painless edema along the nodule is also present.

Carpal Tunnel Syndrome

Atrophy of the thenar eminence may be evident, but generally edema is not present. Tenderness, motor strength (including grip and pinch), and sensory deficits must be determined. Phalen's maneuver and Tinel's sign may reproduce symptoms (Figures 192-1 and 192-2).

Trapeziometacarpal Arthritis

Pain is elicited by adducting the first metacarpal and hyperextending the first metacarpal phalange. The grind test will also elicit pain.

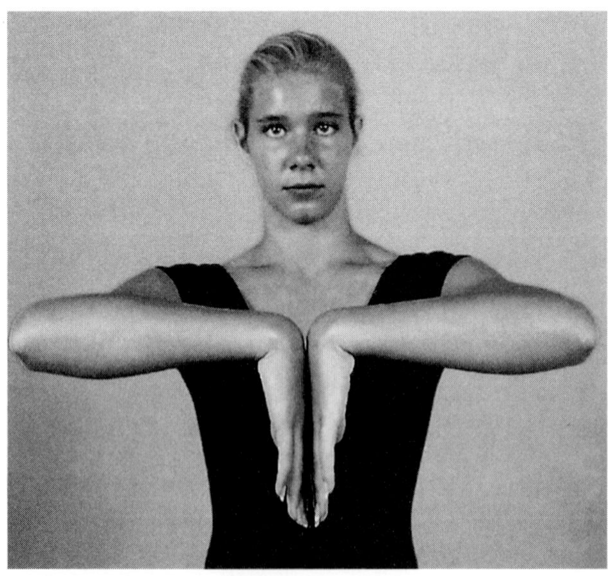

FIGURE 192-1

Phalen's maneuver for carpal tunnel syndrome. (From Barkauskas VH: *Health and physical assessment,* ed 2, St Louis, 1998, Mosby.)

DIAGNOSTICS AND DIFFERENTIAL DIAGNOSIS

An x-ray study may be indicated if bony abnormalities are suspected. Laboratory studies are rarely necessary. However, serum glucose, thyroid-stimulating hormone (TSH), erythrocyte sedimentation rate (ESR), antinuclear antibodies (ANA), and rheumatoid factor may be indicated. An electromyogram (EMG) may be ordered by a specialist.

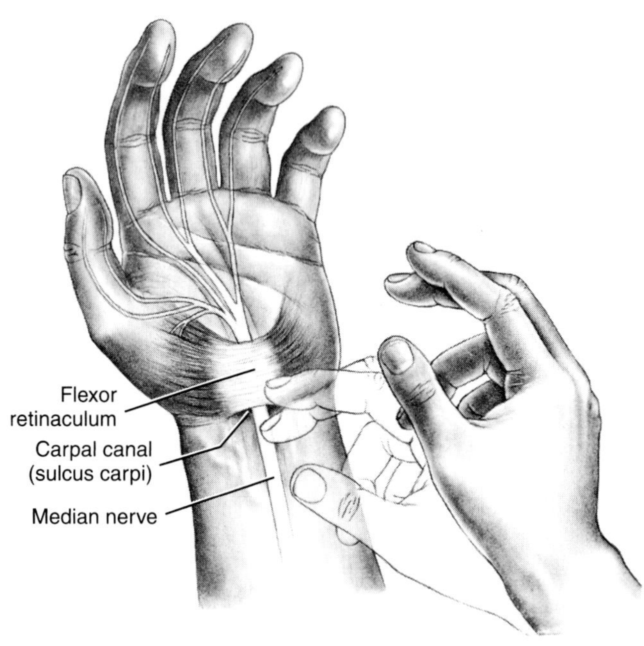

FIGURE 192-2

Eliciting Tinel's sign. (From Barkauskas VH: *Health and physical assessment,* ed 2, St Louis, 1998, Mosby.)

Diagnostics

Hand and Wrist Pain

Laboratory	Imaging
Serum glucose*	X-ray*
TSH*	Ultrasound*
ESR*	**Other**
ANA*	EMG
Rheumatoid factor*	

*If indicated.

Differential Diagnosis

Hand and Wrist Pain

Fracture	Dupuytren's contracture
Sprain	Carpal tunnel syndrome
Strain	Cubital tunnel syndrome
Ganglion	Trapeziometacarpal arthritis
Stenosing tenosynovitis	Rheumatoid arthritis
de Quervain's disease	Osteoarthritis

Trigger Finger
Diagnostic tests are not indicated unless associated conditions are suspected. The differential diagnosis should include joint arthrosis, rheumatoid arthritis, flexor tendon rupture, tendon sheath cysts, or Dupuytren's contracture. Associated conditions include diabetes, rheumatoid arthritis, and vibration exposure.

Tenosynovitis
X-ray studies are indicated to exclude fracture or arthritis. CBC, ESR, ANA, and rheumatoid factor may also be indicated if rheumatoid arthritis is suspected. The differential diagnosis includes stenosing tenosynovitis of the thumb, fracture, or arthritis.

Palmar Fibrosis
Dupuytren's contracture has a classic appearance. The diagnosis is based on a history of painless swelling plus inspection and palpation of the nodule. Diagnostic tests and a differential diagnosis are usually unnecessary.

Carpal Tunnel Syndrome
An x-ray study of the wrist is recommended to exclude bony abnormalities; cervical films are used to exclude cervical radiculopathy. Electrodiagnostic studies, such as EMG and nerve conduction studies, may be necessary for both carpal tunnel and cubital tunnel syndrome if symptoms do not respond to conservative treatment. Laboratory studies are rarely indicated, but serum glucose, CBC, ESR, ANA, rheumatoid factor, and TSH may be required for certain patients. The differential diagnosis includes cervical radiculopathy, basal joint arthritis of the thumb, thoracic outlet syndrome, and polyneuropathy.

Trapeziometacarpal Arthritis
X-ray studies are indicated to exclude fracture. The differential diagnosis should also include infection, radial bursitis, tenosynovitis, and sprain.

MANAGEMENT AND INDICATIONS FOR REFERRAL/HOSPITALIZATION
The potential personal and economic ramifications of CTDs are significant. Treatment should be expedient and multidisciplinary to avoid prolonged disability. Reduction of risk factors, prevention of further injury, management of pain, restoration of function, and strengthening of muscle should be the primary goals of treatment[1,5,6] (Box 192-1).

BOX 192-1

TREATMENT OF CARPAL TUNNEL DISEASE

- Rest or reduce activity
- Ice or cold packs to affected area
- Nonsteroidal antiinflammatory drugs (if no contraindications)
- Splinting at night
- Physical or occupational therapy
- Orthopedic or neurosurgical referral, if persistent symptoms

Trigger Finger
Immediate orthopedic referral is indicated if the finger cannot be passively extended. Treatment of an associated condition, rest, NSAIDs, and splinting of the PIP of the affected finger is an appropriate intervention. A thumb spica splint should be applied to affected thumbs. If there is no improvement after 2 weeks, an orthopedic evaluation is indicated for possible corticosteroid injection or surgical release of the tendon.

Tenosynovitis
Ice, NSAIDs, and continuous immobilization in a padded gutter splint are initially indicated; cortisone injection of the nodule may offer the greatest relief. An orthopedic referral is necessary if there is no improvement after 2 weeks.

Palmar Fibrosis
If contractures are interfering with function, a referral to a hand specialist for surgical excision of the fascia may be warranted. Passive extension, NSAIDs, and cortisone injections have had less than impressive results and are not recommended.

Carpal Tunnel Syndrome
Treatment consists of neutral wrist splints, NSAIDs, ice, and work/home modification. If there is no improvement in 3 weeks, a referral to a hand specialist is indicated for steroid injection or surgical evaluation.

Trapeziometacarpal Arthritis
The use of splinting and NSAIDs for 3 weeks is appropriate initially. If relief is not achieved, a referral to an orthopedist for steroid injection is warranted.

COMPLICATIONS
Contractures and pain are significant complications of hand and wrist disorders. In addition, nerve compression can jeopardize the sensory function, motor function, and reflexes of the affected hand. These problems affect quality of life, work, and recreational activities. Although surgery is indicated for hand disorders that are not responsive to conservative therapies, there is an inherent risk in any surgical procedure. Continued symptoms, reflex sympathetic dystrophy, nerve damage, and disfigurement are additional hazards associated with any surgical procedure of the hand or wrist.

PATIENT AND FAMILY EDUCATION
Patients should understand the importance of hourly 10-minute rest periods during activities that require repetitive hand movements. Splints that keep the wrist straight or slightly extended should be worn at night and, if necessary, during the day. Careful explanation of splint use is important because patients often remove the splint during activity, which results in further inflammation and a prolonged recovery period. Wrist splints can also be worn while sleeping to relieve discomfort during the night.

The use of cold packs and NSAID therapy should also be explained. Hand weakness, symptoms that increase in severity, or symptoms not relieved by conservative therapies should be reported to the primary care provider.

HEALTH PROMOTION

Avoiding overexertion of the hand and wrist can prevent many cases of injury. Warming up and stretching these muscles before activity may help to decrease the risk of injury.[12] The use of proper body mechanics may also reduce the risk of injury. It may be necessary to arrange the work environment to allow for more comfort and less strain on the body.[13] Taking frequent rest breaks during repetitive activities and doing strengthening exercises may help as well.

REFERENCES

1. Mooney V: Overuse syndromes of the upper extremity: rational and effective treatment, *J Musculoskel Med* 15(8):11-18, 1998.
2. Siverstein BA and others: Work-related musculoskeletal disorders: comparison of data sources for surveillance, *Am J Ind Med* 31(5): 600-608, 1997.
3. Melhorn JM: Cumulative trauma disorders and repetitive strain injuries: the future, *Clin Orthop* (351):107-126, 1998.
4. Higgs PE, Young VI: Cumulative trauma disorders, *Clin Plast Surg* 23:30, 421-433, 1996.
5. Downs DG: Nonspecific work-related upper extremity disorders, *Am Fam Physician* 55(4):1296-1302, 1997.
6. Sheon RP: Repetitive strain injury. Part 2. Diagnostic and treatment tips on six common problems: The Goff Group, *Postgrad Med* 102(4):72-78, 1997.
7. Hoglund M, Tordai P, Muren C: Diagnosis of ganglions in the wrist and hand, *Acta Radiol* 35(1):35-39, 1999.
8. Appiah R and others: Treatment of primary Raynaud's syndrome with traditional Chinese acupuncture, *J Intern Med* 241(2):119-124, 1997.
9. Gasbarrini A and others: *Helicobacter pylori* eradication ameliorates primary Raynaud's phenomenon, *Dig Dis Sci* 43(8):1641-1645, 1998.
10. Fraendel I and others: The association of estrogen replacement therapy and the Raynaud phenomenon in postmenopausal women, *Ann Intern Med* 129(3):208-211, 1998.
11. Yee Am, Hotchkiss RN, Paget SA: Adventitial stripping: a digit saving procedure in refractory Raynaud's phenomenon, *J Rheumatol* 25(2):269-276, 1998.
12. Farnsworth EM: Diagnosis and management of repetitive strain injury, *Adv Nurse Pract* 9(8):32-38, 2001.
13. LoBuano C: Identifying entrapment and compression neuropathies, *Patient Care Nurse Pract* 2(12):28-36, 1999.

CHAPTER 193

Hip Pain

Diana G. French

DEFINITION/EPIDEMIOLOGY

Hip pain is a common complaint in primary care and a major source of discomfort and pain and of functional limitation, especially among older adults. Considering that hip pain is a symptom of an underlying pathologic process and not a disease, numerous underlying causes of hip pain may be described. An accurate diagnosis and the appropriate management of hip pain are important in reducing the burden for both the patient and the family.

The patient who presents with a chief complaint of hip pain may be a diagnostic challenge for the primary care provider. The anatomy of the hip encompasses a large area, and the patient may not be able to localize the area of pain. Hip pain may be broadly defined as any sensation of pain immediately surrounding or within the pelvic girdle. It may also be accompanied by limitation of range of motion secondary to the pain, and there may be an increase in pain with activity or weight bearing.

Because hip pain is a symptom and not a specific disease entity, there is no epidemiologic pattern that describes the prevalence and incidence. Major causes of hip pain differ across age-groups and may be categorized as traumatic or nontraumatic (Table 193-1). In adults and older adults, major causes of nontraumatic hip pain include osteoarthritis (OA) and bursitis. An important cause of hip pain in the adolescent is slipped capital femoral epiphysis (SCFE), which may or may not be associated with trauma. Although the underlying cause is unclear, SCFE is most likely to be seen during the growth spurt between the ages of 10 and 15 years. The typical patient is an obese male adolescent.[1] Hip pain secondary to trauma includes strains and sprains of ligamentous structures, contusions, fractures, and dislocations.

TABLE 193-1 Causes of Hip Pain and Age-Groups Commonly Affected

Age-Group	Traumatic Cause*	Nontraumatic Cause
Adolescents and young adults	SCFE† Stress fracture Sprains, strains	SCFE Arthritis—rheumatoid, degenerative
Adults	Stress fracture Sprains, strains	Bursitis Neuropathy Fasciitis
Older adults	Hip fracture Dislocation	Osteoarthritis Bursitis Neuropathy Fasciitis Spinal stenosis

*Avascular necrosis should *always* be ruled out for hip pain caused by trauma.
†Slipped capital femoral epiphysis (SCFE) may occur with or without trauma.

In the adult population a major cause of hip pain is OA.[2] Approximately 43 million Americans are currently affected by arthritis. Because of the aging of the U.S. population, it is estimated that by 2020 arthritis may affect more than 60 million people.[3] This represents a tremendous impact on functional capabilities, quality of life, and economic burden.

Another common condition among adults that produces a painful hip is bursitis. Bursitis may be related to overuse syndromes, injury, or degeneration of muscles and tendons that support the hip.[2]

Infection of the hip joint is rare in adults, although this should be considered in patients with a prosthetic hip and new-onset hip pain. Patients in whom septic arthritis of the hip develops are typically immunocompromised—taking corticosteroids or chemotherapeutic agents. IV drug users are also at increased risk for joint infection.[2]

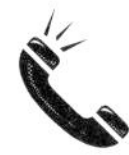

Orthopedic consultation is indicated for patients with suspected hip dislocation, fracture, or sepsis.

PATHOPHYSIOLOGY

Understanding the mechanisms of hip pain requires a review of the anatomy of the hip joint and structures of the pelvic girdle. The hip, like the shoulder, is a ball and socket and is classified as a diarthroidal or synovial joint. A fibrous capsule of ligaments and cartilage covers the points at which the bones articulate. A membrane that secretes synovial fluid provides lubrication for motion. Spaces between the tendons, ligaments, and bones, called *bursae,* permit ease of motion and reduce friction.[4]

The ball and socket of the hip joint itself is made up of the head of the proximal femur and the acetabulum, which is formed by the ischium, pubis, and ilium. Strong ligaments form the capsule that covers the entire hip joint. Completely lining the capsule and extending down the neck of the femur is the synovial membrane.

The primary functions of the hip are weight bearing and locomotion. The muscles of the hip are essential in maintaining upright stability and gait. The muscles of the hip may be classified into five functional groups according to their action: the abductors, flexors, adductors, extensors, and rotators. Musculotendinous pain of the hip may contribute to distortions of gait, which may produce a limp.[2]

The underlying cause of the pain determines the actual mechanisms of the pathophysiology. Arthralgia secondary to degenerative joint disease results from the breakdown and loss of cartilage at the points of stress and motion in the joint. A loss of joint space with the destruction of protective structures contributes to the pain and deformity associated with OA. Bursitis, a common cause of hip pain, is caused by inflammation of the bursae of the joint capsule. Inflammation may be the result of prior trauma or an extension of an inflammatory process.[2]

CLINICAL PRESENTATION

For the patient who presents with a chief complaint of hip pain, a careful history must be obtained with particular attention given to the history of the present illness. Any history of joint replacement and recent or old trauma to the hip and lower back should be obtained. Pertinent questions related to location, onset, duration, severity, setting, associated manifestations, and aggravating/alleviating factors will be useful in narrowing the diagnosis.

For most patients with hip pain, the pain is increased with activity. Pain at rest may indicate inflammatory, infectious, or neoplastic disease. With degenerative joint disease (OA), the pain will become progressively more severe and can occur in the groin, buttock, anterior or lateral thigh, or knee. Often the patient may not be able to localize the exact location of the pain as synovitis, muscle spasm, and capsular contracture progress. The pain will often be accompanied by stiffness on first arising in the morning and after long periods of inactivity. The duration of stiffness with OA is usually short, lasting only 5 to 30 minutes. Walking or prolonged standing will tend to aggravate the pain, and rest relieves it. When OA is the cause, pain may also occur in other joints of the body, especially the knees and the joints of the hands.[5]

Bursitis, another common cause of hip pain in adults, presents with point tenderness and focal pain over the bursa. Any of the three major bursae surrounding the hip may be affected. Patients with trochanteric bursitis will complain of pain in the lateral hip posterior to the greater trochanter with frequent radiation down the lateral thigh to the knee.[2,6] Ischiogluteal bursitis presents as pain over the ischial tuberosity with radiation to the posterior thigh. Pain in the groin with radiation to the anterior thigh may indicate iliopsoas bursitis. Pain will be aggravated with walking.

The patient with septic or infectious arthritis of the hip may present after an incident of trauma or after surgery. A contiguous site of bacterial infection may also create a route for bacterial invasion of the joint. High fever, excruciating pain, and limited range of motion may be present. In the adolescent and young adult, *Neisseria gonorrheae* is the most common causative organism. In adults of all ages, *Staphylococcus aureus* is the usual source of infection, although other pathogens may be implicated.[7]

Avascular necrosis, often associated with trauma, alcohol abuse, corticosteroids, rheumatoid arthritis, or systemic lupus erythematosus, is often bilateral. The patient will report a gradual onset of dull aching or throbbing pain in the groin, lateral hip, or buttock.[8]

An insidious onset of moderate to severe hip, thigh, or knee pain associated with a limp or an acute onset of hip pain after injury, especially in an adolescent, should raise the suspicion of SCFE. SCFE is also associated with obesity; more than half of affected adolescents exceed the 95th percentile for weight and age. Delayed sexual maturity may also be evident.[2,9]

PHYSICAL EXAMINATION

Two tests of hip function during physical examination are essential: gait and range of motion. The gait may be affected by a limp (antalgic gait) that is characterized by an exaggerated swaying motion of the upper body toward the painful hip while walking. Motion restriction of abduction and internal rotation are usually more pronounced than restriction of adduction and external rotation. Pain, muscle spasm, and guarding are noted with passive and active full range of motion. Inspection may reveal a flexion-contracture of the hip and atrophy of the musculature of the buttocks. Crepitus of the joint may be evident on palpation.[2,10]

Pain on palpation that is well localized (point tenderness) and accompanied by redness, warmth, and swelling may indicate bursitis. Hip flexion and internal rotation will exacerbate the pain.[4] In the older patient, fracture may be suspected if there is a history of a fall or rotational injury to the hip. The patient will complain of hip, groin, or thigh pain and will be unable to bear weight or move the leg. The affected extremity will usually be shortened and externally rotated. In the adolescent patient with SCFE, significant muscle spasm and restricted internal rotation will be evident.[2,8]

DIAGNOSTICS

The diagnosis of hip pain is often made on the basis of clinical examination of the patient. However, diagnostic testing is warranted if there has been trauma or to exclude more serious causes of hip pain, such as avascular necrosis of the femur. X-ray studies should include an anteroposterior (AP) view of the pelvis, frog-leg and AP views of the hip, and two views of the lumbosacral spine.[9,11] Weight-bearing films are important to assess the extent of joint degeneration and joint space narrowing. If avascular necrosis is suspected, MRI is the diagnostic test of choice. MRI is not as sensitive in identifying cartilaginous changes of the joint.[12] If rheumatic causes are suspected, a CBC, erythrocyte sedimentation rate (ESR), and rheumatic factor analysis should be obtained. With radiographic evidence of effusion, joint aspiration, performed under fluoroscopic guidance, is indicated. Aspirate is sent for culture and sensitivity, a cell count with differential, and identification of crystalline deposits.[8]

DIFFERENTIAL DIAGNOSIS

Although the most common cause of hip pain in the adult is OA, other diagnostic possibilities should be considered if there is no relief of symptoms with standard treatment. Fractures, dislocations, inflammatory conditions, rheumatoid arthritis, infections, and avascular necrosis are other important causes of hip pain.[8]

Minimal force applied to the hip joint may produce a fracture, especially in the older woman with osteoporosis. Traumatic dislocations are more often seen in young patients who engage in activities with a risk for violent injury. Joint infection or avascular necrosis should be excluded for any patient who has a history of trauma to the hip or risk factors such as alcohol abuse, a suppressed immune system, corticosteroid use, or IV drug use.[2,8]

Diagnostics

Hip Pain

Laboratory
CBC and differential
ESR
Rheumatoid factor*

Imaging
X-ray
MRI*

Other
Joint aspiration for culture and sensitivity, crystalline deposits, and cell count*

*If indicated.

Extraarticular causes of hip pain include bone diseases, such as osteoporosis, malignancy, Paget's disease, and osteomyelitis; neuropathic pain of diabetes, alcoholism, and vitamin B_{12} deficiency; and vascular diseases, such as atherosclerosis, diabetes, and vasculitis. In patients who are runners or who participate in sports, a femoral stress fracture should also be considered.[6]

MANAGEMENT

Hip pain is a symptom of an underlying pathophysiologic process. Although hip pain has the potential to produce functional limitations and to impair quality of life, the management should be directed toward identifying and treating the underlying cause of the pain. Evidence-based practice in treating the adult patient with hip pain is focused on the various causes of the hip pain such as OA (see Chapter 199). Pain management is a major issue for patients with OA involving the hip. Although most randomized controlled trials have focused on OA of the knee, some have demonstrated that evidence exists for benefit with the use of nonsteroidal antiinflammatory drugs (NSAIDs) and acetaminophen analgesics in relief of hip pain. Both classes of analgesics have been shown to provide reduction in pain secondary to OA. There is no clear evidence that either class of analgesic is superior in reducing OA pain. Capsaicin, an over-the-counter topical analgesic, has also been shown to provide short-term pain relief and has fewer side effects than oral agents.[13] The adverse effect most commonly reported for topical agents is local skin irritation. For pain related to bursitis, tendonitis, or traumatic injury, NSAIDs will likely be more effective in controlling the pain and promoting mobility.

Nonpharmacologic measures are aimed at restoring and maintaining function of the joint and as an adjunct to pharmacologic therapy. Recommendations for complete rest or inactivity of the joint should be given only after careful weighing of the risk versus benefit. Muscular atrophy and weakness may result and contribute to the primary problem. Evidence for benefit does exist for exercise and education in reducing pain, with exercise demonstrating the strongest evidence for benefit.[13] Exercise also improves functional status and provides a sense of well-being. Range of motion and low-stress, low-impact exercises should be prescribed. An aquatic exercise program, as recommended by The Arthritis Foundation, promotes mobility while relieving mechanical weight bearing on the joint. Use of heat before and ice after exercise may also alleviate pain.[2,14]

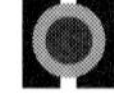

Differential Diagnosis

Hip Pain

Rheumatoid arthritis	Septic sacroiliitis
Osteoarthritis	Osteomyelitis
Septic arthritis	Cellulitis
Joint infection	Gout
Malignancy	Pseudogout
Sprain	Sickle cell disease
Strain	Avascular necrosis
Stress fracture	Osteoporosis
Traumatic dislocation	Paget's disease
Bursitis/tendonitis	Neuropathy
Fasciitis	Vascular disease

COMPLICATIONS

Complications of hip pain are dependent on the cause. Osteoporosis of the hip may result in a spontaneous fracture with or without trauma. Degenerative joint disease and the various inflammatory and traumatic conditions that are accompanied by loss of function and mobility may result in falls with injury and numerous cardiovascular effects of deconditioning. Older patients in particular should be monitored for gastrointestinal irritation if taking NSAIDs. An adolescent with SCFE has a guarded long-term prognosis for repeat injury and complications. A serious complication, avascular necrosis of the femur, may occur in approximately 30% of patients with SCFE. Premature development of degenerative arthritis may occur with or without avascular necrosis.[1]

INDICATIONS FOR REFERRAL/HOSPITALIZATION

Hip pain requires an ongoing assessment of the patient's functional capabilities and relief of painful symptoms. A multidisciplinary approach involving a physical therapist or an occupational therapist is indicated. Physical therapy improves joint mobility and prevents the complications of joint disuse. Occupational therapists may assist patients with limitations of function in adapting activities of daily living for optimal independence. Referral to an orthopedic surgeon is indicated for patients suspected of having joint infection or avascular necrosis or for those with progressive loss of function or refractive chronic pain. Urgent referral is required for patients with hip fracture and dislocation.[8]

PATIENT AND FAMILY EDUCATION/HEALTH PROMOTION

Chronic joint pain can be mentally and physically wearing on the patient. A multidisciplinary approach to care with the patient as an active participant in the decision-making process may prove more satisfactory for the patient and provider over the long term. The patient is entitled to an explanation regarding the source of the pain and whether it is likely to be temporary or chronic in nature. Facilitating patient understanding of anticipated outcomes and prognosis is extremely beneficial in strengthening the patient-provider relationship.

Health-promoting activities should be directed toward maintaining and preserving function of the joint. The management of a painful hip may include range of motion and muscle strengthening exercises as recommended by the physical therapist. Maintenance of optimal weight should be encouraged because the excess weight of obesity places tremendous stresses on the hip. The patient taking NSAIDs should take medications with food and be knowledgeable of the signs and symptoms of gastrointestinal irritation. Because the risk of falls may be increased with hip pain, especially among older adults, an assessment of the home environment for potential risk is warranted.

REFERENCES

1. Eilert RE: Orthopedics. In Hay WW and others, editors: *Current pediatric diagnosis and treatment,* New York, 2001, McGraw-Hill.
2. Steinberg GG: Pelvis, hip, and proximal thigh. In Steinberg GG, Akins AM, Baran DT, editors: *Orthopaedics in primary care,* Baltimore, 1999, Williams & Wilkins.
3. Centers for Disease Control and Prevention: Facts about arthritis, 1997, MMWR Fact Sheet. Retrieved August 12, 2002, from the World Wide Web: http://www.cdc.gov/od/oc/media/fact/arthriti.htm.
4. Seidel HM: *Mosby's guide to physical examination,* ed 4, St Louis, 1999, Mosby.
5. Brandt K: Osteoarthritis. In Braunwald E and others, editors, *Harrison's principles of internal medicine,* ed 15, New York, 2001, McGraw-Hill.
6. Jones DL, Erhard RE: Diagnosis of trochanteric bursitis versus femoral neck stress fracture, *Phys Ther* 77:58-67, 1997
7. Thaler SJ, Maguire JH: Infectious arthritis. In Braunwald E and others, editors, *Harrisons' principles of internal medicine,* ed 15, New York, 2001, McGraw-Hill.
8. Berry DJ, Bono JV, Mason JB: Hip and thigh. In Greene WB editor: *Essentials of musculoskeletal care,* Rosemont, Ill, 2001, American Academy of Orthopaedic Surgeons.
9. Koop S, Quanbeck D: Three common causes of childhood hip pain, *Pediatr Clin North Am* 43:1053-1066, 1996.
10. Willms JL, Schneiderman H, Algranati PS: *Physical diagnosis,* Baltimore, 1994, Williams & Wilkins.
11. Mansour ES, Steingard MA: Anterior hip pain in the adult: an algorithmic approach to diagnosis, *J Am Osteopath Assoc* 97:32-38, 1997.
12. Edwards DJ, Lomas D, Villar RN: Diagnosis of the painful hip by magnetic resonance imaging and arthroscopy, *J Bone Joint Surg Br* 77: 374-376, 1995.
13. Dieppe P and others: Osteoarthritis. In Barton S, editor, *Clinical evidence,* London, 2001, BMJ Publishing.
14. Kraus V: Pathogenesis and treatment of osteoarthritis, *Med Clin North Am* 81:85-112, 1997.

CHAPTER 194

Infectious Arthritis

Thomas H. Taylor

DEFINITION/EPIDEMIOLOGY

Any inflammation of the joint space is called arthritis. Infectious arthritis is one type of arthritis and is always associated with inflammation, whereas arthralgia is pain in and around the joint. Redness, warmth, swelling, and joint effusion always merit consideration of infectious arthritis, even if another cause of arthritis, such as osteoarthritis or rheumatoid arthritis, precedes the acute worsening of symptoms. Infectious arthritis may occur throughout life but its peak incidence is in childhood and old age.[1] Many different organisms may cause infectious arthritis. Although the presentation of bacterial or viral arthritis is often acute, Lyme disease, mycobacterial, fungal, filarial, and some forms of bacterial arthritis (gonococcal, meningococcal) are often more chronic.

PATHOPHYSIOLOGY

Synovial tissue is vascular and is susceptible to hematogenous seeding by bacteria. Bacterial toxins induce leukocytes and chondrocytes to produce proteases, which are destructive to cartilage.[2] It is no accident that *Staphylococcus aureus* is the most common cause of infectious arthritis. This organism has receptors for the glycoproteins found in joints and has frequent access to hematogenous seeding from minor wounds and abrasions.[3] Streptococci are also normal skin flora, second only to *S. aureus* as etiologic agents of infectious arthritis. *Neisseria gonorrhoeae* is the major cause of infectious arthritis in sexually active adults under 30 years old. This is not unexpected given the ease with which *N. gonorrhoeae* invades the bloodstream during menses or parturition and after acute urethritis. Gram-negative bacilli cause approximately 10% of cases, often in older adults and neonates, and are associated with a better outcome than gram-positive infections.[4] Anaerobes are an uncommon but previously unrecognized cause of infectious arthritis, and are associated with human bites, intraabdominal abscess, and adjacent decubitus ulcer.

CLINICAL PRESENTATION

Septic arthritis presents as abrupt onset of a painful, swollen, and erythematous joint that is warm to the touch. Discomfort in the resting position, without any motion, is a distinguishing feature of infectious arthritis. Most other forms of arthritis are relieved when motion is stopped.[5] Fever is usually present, but may be low grade or absent. Rigors are present in approximately 25% of patients and signify bacteremia. Although any joint may be involved, the knee is most commonly affected, followed by the other weight-bearing joints.[6] Patients who are bedridden and push themselves around on their elbows often sublux the sternoclavicular joint. There is a high incidence of infectious arthritis at the collar bone in these patients. Infectious arthritis is more likely to occur in a joint previously afflicted with some other form of arthritis. A monarticular presentation (90%) is the rule; this condition should be suspected when the flare-up of one joint is superimposed on an underlying polyarticular arthritis (e.g., rheumatoid arthritis). Polyarticular infectious arthritis is sometimes seen with streptococcal or staphylococcal infections, but involves only two or three joints (pauciarticular). Fever and arthritis are less impressive in gonococcal arthritis, which is distinguished by a migrating polyarticular presentation.

PHYSICAL EXAMINATION

The affected joint is erythematous, warm to the touch, and swollen. Synovial effusion is evident and may be detected in the knee as a bulge sign (the medial side of the knee is milked upward to displace fluid, and the medial space is observed for a bulge, which signifies fluid return) or patellar ballottement (floating patella sign). Decreased range of motion and muscle spasm are prominent. The proximal lymph node may be enlarged and tender. An original source of infection, such as a boil, foot ulcer, gonococcal urethritis, pneumonia, or endocarditis, should be searched for. Distinct clinical presentations are seen in special situations, which are discussed next.

Gonococcal Arthritis

N. gonorrhoeae is the most common pathogen in sexually active young adults with infectious arthritis. There appear to be two clinical presentations. Group I is distinguished by tenosynovitis and dermatitis. Skin lesions are present in countable numbers and multiple stages; these lesions are most often maculopapular but are sometimes necrotic, pustular, or vesicular. A migratory polyarthralgia is more predominant than true polyarthritis, and inflammation extends up the tendon sheaths. Synovial fluid cell counts are lower than those commonly seen in bacterial arthritis, and the synovial fluid culture is often negative. The blood culture may be positive, but only 20% of patients have genitourinary symptoms of gonorrhea.

Group II may occur after a migratory polyarthritis, tenosynovitis, or dermatitis, but now the arthritis has settled in one or two joints. The synovial fluid is more purulent, and the culture is more likely to be positive. Blood cultures have become negative. Cultures of the cervix, urethra, and rectum are positive in 90% of patients if obtained early on selective media (e.g., Thayer-Martin). Synovial fluid cultures should be plated directly onto chocolate agar. DNA amplification tests may be used to detect *N. gonorrhoeae* in synovial fluid.[7]

Whether these groups represent sequential stages of disease or distinct presentations in different hosts is still debated.[8] Often one or the other condition is present, but the cultures are negative. In this situation, a response to ceftriaxone, 1 g/day IV over 48 hours, may be considered diagnostic.

Prosthetic Joint Infection

Millions of people have prosthetic joints, and 1% to 5% of these will become infected depending on the predisposing factors. In approximately half of the cases, the infection is locally introduced at the time of surgery but may not become apparent until months to years later. Coagulase-negative staphylococci are common in this clinical setting and produce an indolent course. Hematogenous seeding at the bone-cement interface with *S. aureus* or group A streptococci may present more acutely and with sepsis or toxic shock, which is characteristic of these more virulent organisms. Infections in older patients with underlying disease may include gram-negative bacilli (20%) and anaerobes (7%).[9]

Infection in a prosthetic joint is difficult to diagnose, but 95% of the patients have joint pain. Less than 50% of patients have fever, swelling, or sinus drainage. An infectious prosthetic joint must be differentiated from a noninfectious inflammation, such as a reaction to cement or metal or a mechanical problem (e.g., loosening, dislocation, hemarthrosis, and malposition). Mechanical problems are painful during motion, weight bearing, and pivoting but are comfortable while at rest. Constant joint pain suggests an infection. Plain radiographs are abnormal in 50% of patients, with lucencies greater than 2 mm along the bone-cement interface, migration of the prosthesis, and periosteal reactions. A technetium bone scan should become negative 8 months after surgery; the negative bone scan provides strong evidence against an infectious prosthetic joint. However, positive bone scans or indium leukocyte scans are nonspecific and may be positive because of noninfectious or mechanical problems.[10] Thus the diagnosis of a prosthetic joint infection relies on aggressive attempts to isolate an organism by aspiration of joint fluid or arthrotomy tissue.

Lyme Disease

Only 50% of patients with Lyme disease recall a tick bite, but in the setting of known tick exposure, 80% of patients with stage I Lyme disease suffer arthralgias or migratory arthritis. During stage I the characteristic rash (erythema chronicum migrans) appears with an expanding red border, central clearing, and secondary smaller lesions. Fever, headache, myalgias, and lymphadenopathy are more noticeable than the skin lesions, which are painless. Stage II disease includes multiple systemic features: cardiac problems (heart block) in 10% of patients, neurologic problems (Bell's palsy, meningitis, cranial neuritis, encephalitis, radiculitis with neuropathy) in 15%, and arthritis in 60%. More prolonged attacks of true arthritis develop in a few joints. Persistent stage III arthritis (10% of patients) evolves over 1 year and settles in one or two large joints.

In Lyme disease the causative spirochete, *Borrelia burgdorferi,* is difficult to culture from synovial fluid, but sensitive methods of antigen detection or polymerase chain reaction (PCR) reveal its presence. Having a high index of suspicion in the right clinical setting makes the diagnosis. In the wrong clinical setting (without prior probability), serologic tests for Lyme disease are misleading because of the high false-positive rate; therefore such tests should not be ordered indiscriminantly.[11] All patients with true arthritis, stage II or III Lyme disease, should be positive on the Lyme enzyme-linked immunosorbent assay and confirmed by Western blot. The outcome is better if diagnosis and treatment are rendered early in this form of infectious arthritis. Medical therapy fails in approximately 50% of patients with stage III Lyme arthritis; progressive joint destruction may then merit synovectomy or total joint arthroplasty.[12]

Intravenous Drug Use

Infectious arthritis in unusual locations (e.g., sacroiliac joint, sternoclavicular joint, symphysis pubis) should raise suspicion of IV drug use. The presence of *Pseudomonas aeruginosa, Serratia marcescens,* and *Candida* species should lead to open-ended and nonjudgmental queries regarding recreational drug use.[13] However, most of the infections in these joints are due to *S. aureus* with or without IV drug use. Hips and shoulders are other common sites in heroin addicts; disseminated gonococcal disease and syphilis should also be considered. The response to antibiotic therapy alone is good (90%), and few patients require surgical drainage despite usually aggressive organisms (e.g., *P. aeruginosa* and *S. aureus*).

Septic Sacroiliitis

Septic sacroiliitis confuses many primary care providers. Although 75% of patients present with acute fever and continuous low back pain that is exacerbated by motion and weight bearing, the symptoms are generally diffuse and bilateral. The physical examination alone is inadequate in distinguishing sacroiliitis from muscle pain, disk disease, femoral nerve entrapment in the buttocks, bursitis, or intraabdominal process. Plain radiographs are not helpful in early diagnosis. Focal pain that occurs when shear forces are applied to the sacroiliac joint may indicate septic sacroiliitis, in which case the patient should be referred immediately for a CT scan or MRI. An MRI is uniquely suited to this difficult diagnosis because it alone has the potential to define fluid in the sacroiliac joint, adjacent bone marrow inflammation, and soft tissue abscesses that may extend into the abdominal cavity and the psoas, iliac, and pyriform muscles. These collections need pigtail catheter drainage or surgical debridement.[14]

DIAGNOSTICS

Peripheral blood leukocytosis is present in only 50% of patients with infectious arthritis, is rarely greater than 14,000/mm^3, and correlates only with acute presentation and fever. Erythrocyte sedimentation rate is often elevated but is also nonspecific. Peripheral blood cultures are positive in 40% of cases and are the only sources of microorganism in 10% of cases.[15] Younger patients suspected of having gonococcal arthritis should have pharyngeal, rectal, and cervical or urethral cultures on specialized gonococcal media. The most important examination for the diagnosis of infectious arthritis is synovial fluid, not only for culture but also for cellular and chemical analysis. Aspiration of inflamed joints provides three important pieces of information: diagnosis of crystal induced arthritis, degree of inflammation (cell count), and specimen for culture. Any joint suspected of infection should be aspirated without delay, because the outcome of infectious arthritis is dependent on early diagnosis and treatment. Sterile

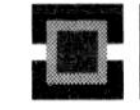
Diagnostics

Infectious Arthritis

Laboratory
CBC and differential
Erythrocyte sedimentation rate
Blood cultures
Rectal, cervical, urethral, or pharyngeal cultures*
Lyme ELISA/Western blot test*

Imaging
X-ray
CT scan/MRI*

Other
Joint aspirate of synovial fluid for crystals, culture, cell count, protein, glucose, and Gram's stain

*If indicated.

technique should be used, and the provider should avoid entering the joint through an area of skin that may be infected. It is important to send blood and synovial fluid cultures for analysis before starting antibiotics.

Synovial fluid analysis consists of evaluation for crystals, cell count and differential, protein, glucose, Gram's stain, and cultures (aerobic and anaerobic). With chronic synovitis, fungal and mycobacterial cultures are also sent for analysis, and special stains for acid fast bacteria and fungi are performed. Synovial fluid leukocyte counts will be very high (Table 194-1); cell counts in the 100,000/mm^3 range are considered infectious until proven otherwise.[5,6] Gout, Reiter's syndrome, and rheumatoid arthritis may cause similarly high cell counts, whereas early infectious arthritis or established gonococcal arthritis may cause relatively low cell counts. The predominance of polymorphonuclear leukocytes in synovial fluid is a clue, but is specific only if it exceeds 85%. Synovial fluid glucose less than 40 mg/dl or less than 50% of a simultaneous blood glucose is supportive evidence for bacterial arthritis and is found in 50% of cases. Intracellular crystals and the profusion of polymorphonuclear cells suggest gout, but free-floating crystals are sometimes seen in infectious arthritis.[16] Synovial fluid protein is markedly elevated in both infectious arthritis and other forms of inflammatory arthritis. Synovial fluid PCR may be used to diagnose gonococcal arthritis and Lyme arthritis.

Radiographs take 2 weeks to demonstrate joint space narrowing and marginal erosions—too late to salvage a functional joint. However, the underlying arthritis or osteomyelitis is identifiable early. Gas formation in or around a joint is an important clue to anaerobic organisms or *Escherichia coli*.[17] Such a finding requires early surgical intervention and the removal of any prosthetic material. A three-phase technetium bone scan is helpful in differentiating cellulitis, infectious arthritis, and osteomyelitis.[18] However, arthrocentesis is better. Thus a bone scan, gallium scan, and indium leukocyte scan are of little practical value. A CT scan or MRI is advantageous in difficult diagnostic situations (e.g., sternoclavicular or sacroiliac joints) and as a guide to joint aspiration and anatomic definition of an infected hip.[19]

DIFFERENTIAL DIAGNOSIS

Inflammatory arthritis is marked by a leukocyte count of more than 2000/mm^3. Other types of inflammatory arthritis are distinguished from infectious arthritis by culture and Gram's stains; however, gout, Reiter's syndrome, and rheumatoid arthritis may accrue cell counts in the infectious arthritis range (cell count near 100,000/mm^3). In such situations, antibiotics should be initiated until cultures are finalized. Cellulitis, bursitis, acute osteomyelitis, and angioedema should be distinguished by their greater range of motion and less-than-circumferential swelling. Polyarticular infectious arthritis is sometimes seen with staphylococci and streptococci, but also suggests metastatic foci resulting from subacute bacterial endocarditis.[20] Polyarticular noninfectious arthritis is seen with rheumatic fever or poststreptococcal reactive arthritis. In either case, the joint is not the focus of the streptococcal infection. The arthritis of rheumatic fever is migratory and resolves spontaneously in 1 month. Another form of acute reactive arthritis, Reiter's syndrome, is accompanied by urethritis, conjunctivitis, and enthesopathy (i.e., inflamed tendon insertions).

MANAGEMENT

Early initiation of antimicrobial therapy and drainage are the hallmarks of treatment for infectious arthritis. If this condition remains undiagnosed or untreated longer than 5 to 7 days, the prognosis for a functional joint is poor. The appropriate antibiotic is chosen on the basis of the Gram's stain and culture

Differential Diagnosis

Rheumatic Disorders

Bursitis	Angioedema
Gout	Rheumatic fever
Pseudogout	Osteoarthritis
Rheumatoid arthritis	Osteomyelitis
Reiter's syndrome	Cellulitis

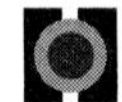

Differential Diagnosis

Infectious Arthritis

Staphylococcus aureus and *Streptococcus* sp	Prosthetic joint (coagulase-negative staph [CANS])
Gram-negative (IV drug use, neonatal, older adults)	Lyme disease
Gonococcal arthritis	Septic sacroiliitis
	Viral
	Mycobacteria or fungal

TABLE 194-1 Synovial Fluid Analysis

Characteristic	Normal	Noninflammatory (Osteoarthritis)	Inflammatory (Rheumatoid)	Septic (Infection)
Volume	<3.5 ml	>3.5 ml	Large	Large
Clarity	Clear	Transparent	Translucent	Opaque
WBC/mm^3	<200	200-2000	2000-75,000	50,000-100,000
PMN leukocytes	<25%	<25%	>50%	>75%
Culture	Negative	Negative	Negative	Positive
Glucose	Equal to blood	Equal to blood	>50% blood glucose	<50% blood glucose
Protein	1.7 g/dl	<3.0 g/dl	>3.0 g/dl	>3.0 g/dl

PMN, Polymorphonuclear.

(Table 194-2). Older children and adults do well with nafcillin or oxacillin, especially if the Gram's stain suggests *S. aureus*. To cover gonococcal arthritis, sexually active young adults should receive ceftriaxone, 1 g IV daily for 7 to 10 days.[21] Pending culture results, infectious arthritis in a prosthetic joint after recent surgery may require empiric vancomycin to cover coagulase-negative staphylococci or methicillin-resistant *S. aureus*. Aminoglycosides are sometimes added for synergism in patients who are infected with *S. aureus* or IV drug users where *P. aeruginosa* is suspected, but aminoglycosides do not work well in abscesses or joints in which the pH is low.[22] Cefazolin is a good alternative for treating *S. aureus* in individuals who are allergic to penicillin.

Duration of therapy is 2 weeks for *Haemophilus influenzae* and streptococci and 3 weeks for staphylococci or gram-negative bacilli. Shorter courses and oral regimens are often effective in children. Gonococcal arthritis responds quickly and may be treated entirely on an outpatient basis with 2 to 3 days of IV ceftriaxone followed by early conversion to oral cefixime 400 mg b.i.d. or ciprofloxacin 500 mg b.i.d. to complete a 7- to 10-day course. Patients with underlying rheumatoid arthritis and virulent organisms should be treated for 4 weeks.[23] New fluoroquinolones with improved gram-positive coverage are becoming available. These include gatifloxacin, moxifloxacin, levofloxacin, and trovafloxacin. These oral agents may have a possible use in infectious arthritis of adults but are not approved for use in children.[24] Antibiotics have ready access to inflamed joints and should not be given by intraarticular injection or added to solutions for irrigating joints. Antibiotics injected directly into joints may initiate chemical synovitis and prolong postinfectious arthritis.[3]

An infected joint is similar to an abscess that needs daily drainage until the inflammation has resolved. Proteolytic enzymes, which destroy cartilage, are produced by activated leukocytes. Therefore it is important that purulent material and bacterial toxins be removed to preserve cartilage. This is accomplished equally well with either daily arthrocentesis or arthroscopic lavage with placement of drains. Daily arthrocentesis is less expensive and is not complicated by instrumentation morbidity; it also offers the possibility of serial culture and cell counts of synovial fluid to gauge response to therapy. Arthroscopic lavage with debridement and placement of drains or open arthrotomy is appropriate if there is persistence of recurrent effusion and elevation of cell counts after 5 days of daily arthrocentesis. Hips should be surgically drained at the outset because of their anatomic complexity.[25]

An infected prosthetic joint requires drainage, debridement, and removal of all prosthetic components and cement. Even with sensitive organisms, retention of the prosthesis and antibiotic therapy with limited surgical debridement is successful in only about 20% of cases. If revision arthroplasty is attempted at the primary surgery, the success rate is less than 70%. The best approach is a two-step procedure, with removal of prosthesis and cement and 6 weeks of antibiotics followed by revision arthroplasty. Antibiotic-impregnated beads may be used to manage the dead space pending reimplantation with an antibiotic-impregnated cement. Six weeks of IV antibiotics are crucial to achieve the 90% success rate.[26]

TABLE 194-2 Therapy for Bacterial Arthritis

Infectious Organisms	Therapy
SEEN ON GRAM'S STAIN	
Gram-positive cocci	
S. aureus, S. epidermidis, streptococci	Nafcillin or oxacillin
If MRSA or MRSE are likely	Vancomycin
Gram-negative cocci	
N. gonorrhoeae	Ceftriaxone
Gram-negative bacilli	
Enterobacteriaceae, *H. influenzae*	Piperacillin and aminoglycoside *or* Third-generation cephalosporin
NEGATIVE GRAM STAIN (PENDING CULTURE AND SENSITIVITIES)	
Older than 5 years	
S. aureus, group A streptococcus	Nafcillin or oxacillin
If MRSA or MRSE likely	Vancomycin
Compromised hosts, older adults	
S. aureus, streptococcal species, gram-negative bacilli	Third-generation cephalosporin *or* Piperacillin/tazobactam
If MRSA or MRSE likely	Add vancomycin
IV drug use	
S. aureus, Pseudomonas, Serratia	Ceftazidime *or* Piperacillin/tazobactam
Sexually active young adult with dermatitis-arthritis syndrome	
N. gonorrhoeae, N. meningitidis	Ceftriaxone

Cefazolin or vancomycin may be substituted for nafcillin in patients who are allergic to penicillin. *MRSA,* Methacillin-resistant *S. aureus; MRSE,* methacillin-resistant *S. epidermidis.*

LIFE SPAN CONSIDERATIONS

Mortality is low when infectious arthritis is diagnosed and treated appropriately. The associated infection carries a significant mortality in older patients or immunocompromised hosts. Toxic shock or a continuing infectious syndrome despite a sterile blood culture is attributable to toxin production by small residual foci of staphylococci or streptococci around dead cartilage or prosthetic joints. There should be no delay in prosthetic joint removal and surgical debridement in the setting of toxic shock or sepsis syndrome, because death may result. Surgery should not be delayed because the problem is typically an abscess, which is unlikely to respond to a continued course of antibiotics.

COMPLICATIONS

Progressive loss of joint function develops in 25% to 50% of patients.[3] A relapse of infectious arthritis may occur if the selection or duration of the antibiotic therapy is inappropriate. Recurrent aseptic joint effusion is common and is referred to as postinfectious synovitis. Minor trauma may exacerbate such synovitis. More immediate complications include an associated abscess or bursa infection, which must be drained, and associated osteomyelitis. Ankylosis or fibrous fusion, ligamentous instability, and joint contracture are consequences of delayed diagnosis. A total joint arthroplasty can provide for mobility in such joints but cannot reverse ligamentous instability or joint contracture. Secondary osteoarthritis is a delayed complication that does respond to total joint arthroplasty. The factors that determine outcome are listed in Box 194-1.[27,28]

INDICATIONS FOR REFERRAL/HOSPITALIZATION

All patients with infectious arthritis should be hospitalized initially, because they need to adhere to strict non–weight-bearing activities to preserve cartilage, for daily aspiration, or for initial surgical drainage. For patients who have been prescribed bed rest, early mobilization with a passive mobilization device helps prevent adhesions. Infectious disease and orthopedic consultation is facilitated when the patient is hospitalized. A physical therapist should be involved, because early mobilization to prevent contracture and eventual weight bearing are important. Cartilage has no blood supply and is dependent on compression through early mobilization for nutritional requirements and integrity of structure. When the effusion has subsided, early discharge with a home IV therapy or oral antibiotics is feasible.

Gonococcal arthritis may, in some cases, be managed with outpatient therapy. However, gonococcal arthritis may be confused with Reiter's syndrome—a triad of urethritis, conjunctivitis, and arthritis. If cultures are negative, a rapid response to IV ceftriaxone is diagnostic of gonococcal arthritis. Therefore close observation in a hospital could be essential.[29]

PATIENT AND FAMILY EDUCATION

Patients should be instructed to be sure that any necessary dental work is done, teeth extractions completed, prostate obstruction relieved, and wounds or ulcers healed before undergoing a total joint arthroplasty. These procedures remove potential sources of bacteremia. Antibiotic prophylaxis before surgery for total joint arthroplasty is advised to prevent postsurgical infectious arthritis, but prophylaxis before dental work is not advised unless otherwise indicated by the patient's status.[30] Patients with rheumatoid arthritis should be aware that superimposed infectious arthritis is possible. They should disclose any monarticular flare to their physician for early diagnostic arthrocentesis. Cellulitis, wounds, and ulcers should receive prompt medical attention to prevent bacteremia. Patients recovering from infectious arthritis must be instructed in home physical therapy to prevent contracture and to advance weight bearing after inflammation has subsided. The potential side effects of antibiotics need to be explained, antibiotic associated diarrhea should be anticipated, and patients with indwelling central lines must be instructed in line care and signs of line infection.

BOX 194-1

FACTORS AFFECTING OUTCOME IN INFECTIOUS ARTHRITIS

- Delay in diagnosis and treatment beyond 7 days
- Persistently positive culture and effusion after 5 days of treatment
- Prior arthritis, especially rheumatoid arthritis
- Compromised host and older patients
- Virulence of organism: *S. aureus* vs. coagulase-negative staphylococcus
- Specific joint involved: hips worse than knees
- IV drug use: good prognosis with aggressive organisms
- Appropriate antibiotics
- Effective drainage and debridement
- Physical therapy: initially non–weight bearing, early mobilization, splint contractures

REFERENCES

1. Gillespie WJ: Epidemiology in bone and joint infection, *Infect Dis Clin North Am* 4(3):361-76, 1990.
2. Goldenberg AL: Pathophysiology: nongonococcal bacterial arthritis. In Espinoza L, editor: *Infections in the rheumatic diseases: a comprehensive review of microbial relations to rheumatic disorders,* Orlando, Fla, 1988, Grune & Stratton.
3. Goldenberg DL: Septic arthritis, *Lancet* 351:197-202, 1998.
4. Blackburn WD Jr: Gram-negative septic arthritis. In Espinoza L, editor: *Infections in the rheumatic diseases: a comprehensive review of microbial relations to rheumatic disorders,* Orlando, Fla, 1988, Grune & Stratton.
5. Bourne Collo MC and others: Evaluating arthritic complaints, *Nurse Pract* 16(2):9-20, 1991.
6. Goldenberg DL: The evaluation of patients with nongonococcal bacterial arthritis. In Espinoza L, editor: *Infections in the rheumatic diseases: a comprehensive review of microbial relations to rheumatic disorders,* Orlando, Fla, 1988, Grune & Stratton.
7. Liebling MR and others: Identification of *Neisseria gonorrhoeae* in synovial fluid using polymerase chain reaction, *Arthritis Rheum* 37:702-709, 1994.
8. Goldenberg DL: Gonococcal arthritis. In Espinoza L, editor: *Infections in the rheumatic diseases: a comprehensive review of microbial relations to rheumatic disorders,* Orlando, Fla, 1988, Grune & Stratton.
9. Gillespie WJ: Infection in total joint replacement, *Infect Dis Clin North Am* 4:465-484, 1990.
10. Brause BD: Infections with prostheses in bones and joints. In Nundell GL, Bennett JE, Dolin J, editors: *Principles and practice of infectious diseases,* ed 4, New York, 1995, Churchill Livingstone.
11. Steere AC and others: The overdiagnosis of Lyme disease, *JAMA* 269:1812-1816, 1993.
12. Steere AC: Musculoskeletal manifestations of Lyme disease, *Am J Med* 98(4A):44S-51S, 1995.
13. Brancos MA and others: Septic arthritis in heroin addicts, *Semin Arthritis Rheum* 21:81-87, 1991.
14. Zimmerman B, Mikolich DJ, Lally EV: Septic sacroiliitis, *Semin Arthritis Rheum* 26:592-604, 1996.
15. Smith JW: Infectious arthritis, *Infect Dis Clin North Am* 4(3):523-537, 1990.
16. Baer PP and others: Coexistent septic and crystal arthritis: report of four cases and literature review, *J Rheumatol* 13:604-607, 1986.
17. Ranjan R, Matei D, Kaufman L: Emphysematous septic arthritis: case report and review of the literature, *J Rheumatol* 22:1776-1778, 1995.
18. Sutter CW, Shelton DK: Three-phase bone scan in osteomyelitis and other musculoskeletal disorders, *Am Fam Physician* 54:1639-1647, 1996.
19. Greenspan A, Tehranzadeh J: Imaging of infectious arthritis, *Radiol Clin North Am* 39(2):267-276, 2001.
20. Dubost JJ and others: Polyarticular septic arthritis, *Medicine* 72:296-310, 1993.
21. Wise CM and others: Gonococcal arthritis in an era of increasing penicillin resistance: presentations and outcomes in 41 recent cases (1985-1991), *Arch Intern Med* 154:2690-2695, 1994.

22. Hamed KA, Tami Y, Proloer CG: Pharmacokinetic optimization of the treatment of septic arthritis, *Clin Pharmacokinet* 31:156-163, 1996.
23. Nolla JM and others: Pyarthrosis in patients with rheumatoid arthritis: a detailed analysis of 10 cases and literature review, *Semin Arthritis Rheum* 30(2):121-126, 2000.
24. Wuldvogel FN: Use of quinolones for the treatment of osteomyelitis and septic arthritis, *Rev Infect Dis* 11(suppl 5):S1259-S1263, 1989.
25. Redfield D, Hayes T: Orthopedic infections, *Crit Care Nurs Q* 21(2):24-35, 1998.
26. Harris JM III: Orthopedic aspects of septic arthritis. In Espinoza L, editor: *Infections in the rheumatic diseases: a comprehensive review of microbial relations to rheumatic disorders,* Orlando, Fla, 1988, Grune & Stratton.
27. Esterhal JL, Gello I: Adult septic arthritis, *Orthop Clin North Am* 22:503-514, 1991.
28. Kaandorp CJE and others: The outcome of bacterial arthritis, prospective, community-based study, *Arthritis Rheum* 40:884-892, 1997.
29. Keat H: Sexually transmitted arthritis syndromes, *Med Clin North Am* 74:1617-1631, 1990.
30. Wahl MJ: Myths of dental-induced prosthetic joint infections, *Clin Infect Dis* 20:1420-1425, 1995.

CHAPTER 195

Knee Pain

Marie-Eileen Onieal

DEFINITION/EPIDEMIOLOGY

About 10.8 million visits are made to health care provider offices because of a knee problem. It is the most often treated anatomic site by orthopedic surgeons.[1] The multiple structures within the knee make it vulnerable to various types of injuries and degenerative change. Many injuries can be treated conservatively; others require surgery. There also are many extraarticular structures that can become inflamed or injured, causing knee pain.

Musculoskeletal injuries are usually sports specific rather than gender specific; however, anatomic differences can contribute to susceptibility to injury. Injuries to the anterior cruciate ligament (ACL), for example, often occur in soccer, basketball, and volleyball participants. Data collected since 1995 demonstrate that men and women who participate in the same sport have different ACL injury patterns. The incidence of ACL injuries among women basketball players is twice that for men, and female soccer players are 4 times more likely to experience an ACL tear than their male counterparts. Both women and men incur ACL injuries in noncontact situations. Nearly 60% of ACL injuries in female basketball players occur when landing from a jump.[1]

Knee Pain

The knee is a modified hinge joint that has some rotational mobility when flexed. The knee joint contains three bones, three articulations, five major tendons, four major ligaments, and two menisci. The lateral and medial articulations are between the femoral and tibial condyles. The intermediate articulation is between the patella and the femur. A relatively weak joint, the knee gains its strength from the strong ligaments that attach the femur to the tibia. There are five intrinsic ligaments that assist in strengthening the articular capsule. The cruciate ligaments connect the femur and tibia within the articular capsule, crossing each other in the form of an X.

As a major weight-bearing joint, the knee is susceptible to many injuries. Torsion is limited in the joint, and any motion that extends beyond the defined range results in a ligamentous injury. Because the knee depends on the integrity of the ligaments to provide its stability, a knee injury can be a calamitous event.

Collateral Ligament Sprains

There are two collateral ligaments: the medial collateral ligament (MCL) and the lateral collateral ligament (LCL). The MCL attaches to the medial condyle of the femur and the tibia. The LCL attaches to the lateral femoral condyle and extends to the lateral tibial plateau. The MCL and the LCL are injured when the valgus (MCL) or varus (LCL) stress to the joint extends beyond the normal range of motion. MCL injuries are more common and often include an injury to the medial meniscus. Football players and skiers are more prone to ligamentous injuries, but they can occur just as easily on the dance floor or in the bathroom.

PATHOPHYSIOLOGY

A wrenching motion of the knee while the foot stays firmly planted causes injury to the MCL. In these injuries the knee is in flexion and in a slight internal rotation. LCL injuries occur when the varus stress applied to the knee causes a "bend" toward the outside.[2] The injuries are graded as first-, second-, or third-degree sprains (Table 195-1).

CLINICAL PRESENTATION

The knee is painful and often swollen and may or may not be ecchymotic over the body of the ligament. Some patients report a feeling that the knee "bent the wrong way" and that the knee became edematous within 20 to 30 minutes. More rapid swelling is an ominous sign.[2]

PHYSICAL EXAMINATION

An examination that occurs immediately after the injury is easier and helps to ascertain the severity of the injury. The examination of the knee is more difficult once the joint swells. Both knees should be observed for edema, deformity, muscle atrophy, and patella placement. Fluctuance should be determined with patient first standing and then supine. Tenderness and bony landmarks should be ascertained as well. In the suspected collateral ligament sprain, there is tenderness along the body of the ligament, and point tenderness at the attachment site is commonly present. In the MCL injury, there may be tenderness at the medial joint line because the MCL attaches to the medial meniscus. Pain at the lateral joint line is equivalent to a joint injury.

Varus or valgus stress on the knee joint determines joint laxity (Figure 195-1). Active range of motion in extension and flexion should be assessed. If active range of motion is not possible, passive extension and flexion should be determined. The unaffected knee should always be examined first to establish the baseline and to allay any anxiety about the evaluation.

TABLE 195-1 Collateral Ligament Sprains

First Degree	Second Degree	Third Degree
PATHOLOGY		
Ligament fibers attached	Partial avulsion of fibers from femoral condyle	Complete rupture of ligament (often associated with ACL/PCL tears or tibial plateau fractures)
FINDINGS		
Tenderness along body of ligament	Pain at joint line of ligament insertion	Significant pain at ligament insertion and joint line
Minimal to no swelling	Swelling with tenderness localized to attachment point	Significant swelling with ecchymosis
No joint widening with ligament stress	Slight to moderate increase in joint widening with stress	Increased joint widening with minimal stress

DIAGNOSTICS

Plain radiographs exclude fractures and dislocations. More extensive radiologic examinations, such as stress films, CT scans, and MRIs, should be considered in consultation with an orthopedist. It is important to note that in the acutely swollen joint, MRIs are often inconclusive.

DIFFERENTIAL DIAGNOSIS

As with any joint injury, a fracture or dislocation must be considered. In the knee, consider an ACL or a posterior cruciate ligament (PCL) injury as well.

MANAGEMENT

Isolated first- and second-degree sprains can be managed with RICE (*r*est, *i*ce, *c*ompression [or immobilization], and *e*levation). If the knee is unstable, an external knee immobilizer is worn at all times. The patient should avoid weight bearing on a swollen or acutely painful knee. Simple straight leg raises and quadriceps-tightening exercises, as well as adductor-strengthening exercises, can be done, even in the immobilizer. Once the swelling and pain subside, a more progressive rehabilitation program should begin.

COMPLICATIONS

Without accurate diagnosis and treatment, the injury can extend, jeopardizing the joint's stability and other structures. The incompletely rehabilitated knee will be weak and potentially unstable. Traumatic arthritis can be a sequel in any joint injury.

INDICATIONS FOR REFERRAL/HOSPITALIZATION

All severe sprains and fractures should be referred to an orthopedist. Referral to a physical therapist should be considered, to assist in complete rehabilitation.

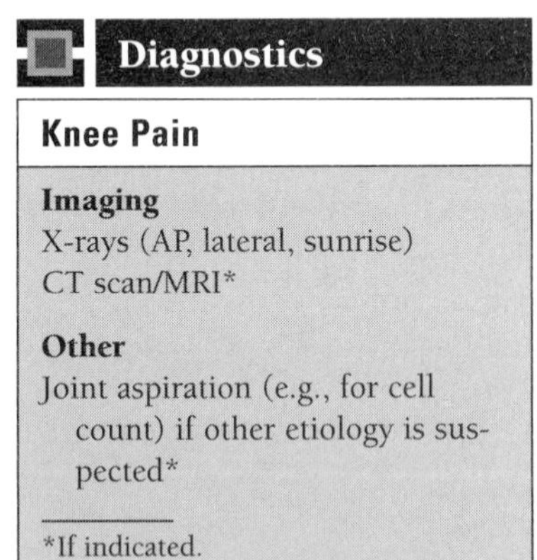

Diagnostics

Knee Pain

Imaging
X-rays (AP, lateral, sunrise)
CT scan/MRI*

Other
Joint aspiration (e.g., for cell count) if other etiology is suspected*

*If indicated.

PATIENT AND FAMILY EDUCATION

Explanation of the importance of adherence to the rehabilitative process is imperative. In some instances a knee support for sports is necessary. Pain and swelling are

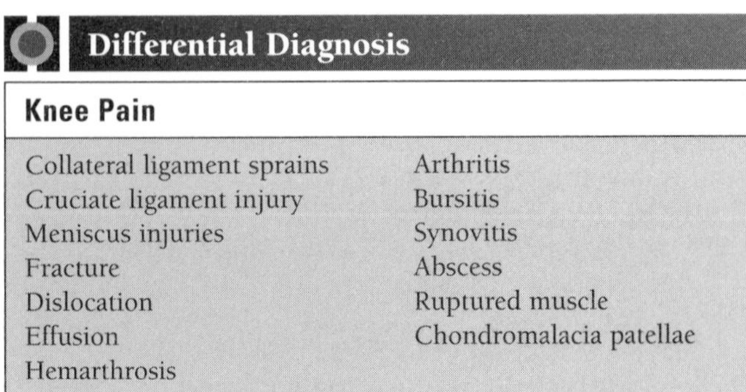

Differential Diagnosis

Knee Pain

Collateral ligament sprains	Arthritis
Cruciate ligament injury	Bursitis
Meniscus injuries	Synovitis
Fracture	Abscess
Dislocation	Ruptured muscle
Effusion	Chondromalacia patellae
Hemarthrosis	

indicators that the knee is being overstressed or has been reinjured.

Cruciate Ligament Injuries

There are two cruciate ligaments: the ACL and the PCL. The ACL attaches to the anterior part of the intercondylar area of the tibia, posterior to the medial meniscus, and rises superiorly, posteriorly, and laterally to attach to the posterior section of the medial side of the lateral condyle of the femur. The ACL restrains the anterior-to-posterior alignment of the knee, keeping the proper relationship of the femur to the tibia. It is loose with the knee in flexion and tight when the knee is fully extended. It is the weaker of the two cruciate ligaments.

The PCL originates at the posterior part of the intercondylar area of the tibia. It crosses superiorly and anteriorly on the medial side of the ACL and attaches to the anterior part of the lateral surface of the medial femoral condyle. The PCL is tight with the knee in flexion.

A cruciate ligament injury can be a sprain, a partial tear, or a complete disruption of the ligament. Physical examination and radiologic tests as indicated are used to determine the degree of the injury. The ACL is the most commonly involved structure in severe knee injuries. In 70% of patients presenting with acute, traumatic hemarthrosis, it is the injured structure.[3] The PCL is less often injured.[2]

PATHOPHYSIOLOGY

The PCL is the stronger ligament and is usually injured through trauma to the anterior surface of the proximal tibia (as in hitting the dashboard).[3] The ACL injury often occurs in combination with ruptures of the MCL and the medial meniscus (O'Donaghue's triad). Once the ligament is torn, the knee is unstable. Swelling occurs rapidly in an ACL or a PCL injury because of bleeding from the ligament tear.[4]

CLINICAL PRESENTATION

The patient often recalls hearing a "pop" or feeling the knee "snap" and has an instantaneous sensation of something being "terribly wrong." Pain from the injury prevents a return to the activity. Patients report a "distrust" of the knee during activities and that the knee "gives out," especially during exertion.

PHYSICAL EXAMINATION

The knee is swollen, and the patient is unable to fully flex or extend the knee. Four standard tests ascertain the integrity of the ligaments. Hamstring spasms and the posterior horn of the meniscus can stabilize the knee, falsely indicating a stable

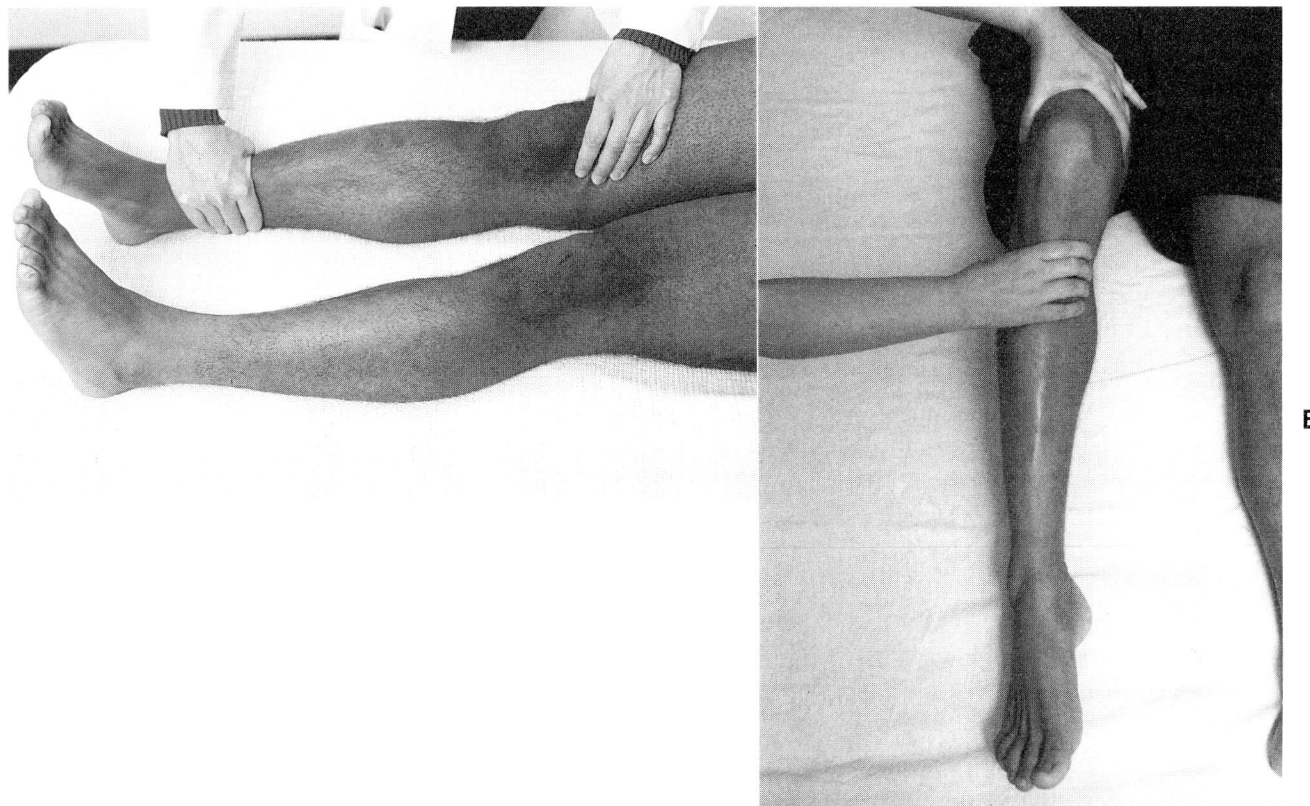

FIGURE 195-1

Varus and valgus stress test of the knee. **A**, Knee extended. **B**, Knee flexed. (From Seidel HM and others: *Mosby's guide to physical examination*, ed 4, St Louis, 1999, Mosby.)

joint; thus it is important for the patient to relax. The normal knee should be examined first to allay anxiety and to establish a baseline because most people have some degree of laxity in the ligaments.

Lachman's test is used to assess the ACL. The knee should be flexed to about 15 to 30 degrees. One hand is placed just below the knee joint on the posterior aspect of the tibia/fibula. The other hand is placed on the anterior aspect of the femur just above the joint. The examiner lifts up the lower leg while pushing down on the upper leg. If the ACL is intact, the examiner should feel a "knock" or a firm "stop" as the ACL prevents the tibia from sliding forward. In the absence of a firm end point, a ligament tear should be suspected.

The anterior drawer test also is used to assess the ACL (Figure 195-2). The knee should be flexed to about 90 degrees, and the foot should be kept flat on the examination surface. The examiner sits on the patient's foot and firmly grasps the lower leg, placing the fingers below the popliteal space and the thumbs on the tibial tuberosity. The examiner pulls gently but firmly on the tibia, attempting to slide the tibia forward. A "soft" or absent end point indicates a tear.[3]

The posterior drawer test also is used to assess the PCL (see Figure 195-2). The patient should be positioned the same as in the anterior drawer test. The examiner pushes posteriorly on the tibia. A torn PCL allows the tibia to slide backward.[5]

The pivot shift test also is used to assess the ACL. It is a more difficult test to master. The examiner grabs the lower leg, flexes the knee, and pushes down on the tibia while flexing and extending the knee. If the ACL is torn, the bones shift erratically with this maneuver.

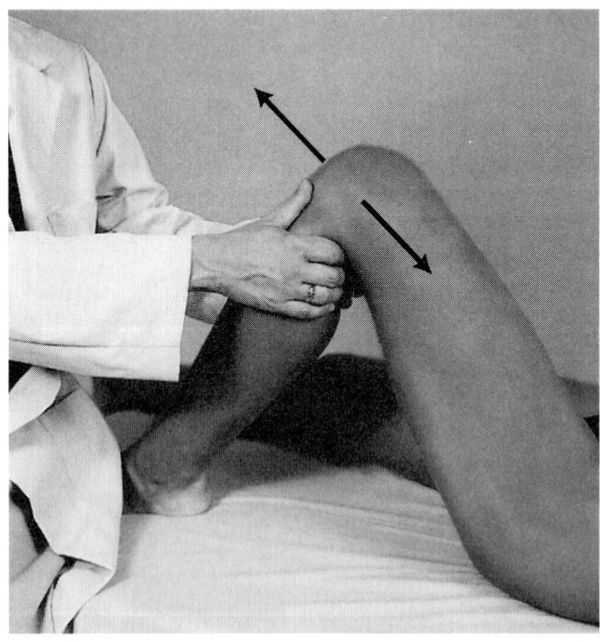

FIGURE 195-2

Drawer test for anterior and posterior stability of the knee. (From Barkauskas VH and others: *Health and physical assessment,* ed 2, St Louis, 1998, Mosby.)

DIAGNOSTICS

X-ray studies of the knee are indicated. Plain films demonstrate effusions, loose bodies, and avulsion fractures. Segund's fracture, an avulsion of the lateral aspect of the tibial plateau, is pathognomonic of an ACL tear. MRI provides a definitive evaluation of the ligaments.

DIFFERENTIAL DIAGNOSIS

As with any knee injury, damage to other intraarticular structures must be considered. Fracture-dislocations are included in the differential diagnosis.

MANAGEMENT

The degree of the tear with or without instability guides the treatment plan. Partial tears and tears without a concurrent fracture or meniscus tear can often be managed conservatively.[6] An acutely injured knee requires immobilization to decrease swelling and pain. Weight bearing on the affected knee should be avoided. The quadriceps muscle begins to atrophy quickly with inactivity; therefore strengthening exercises should begin as tolerated, starting with the simple straight leg raise. The quadriceps muscles are adjunct stabilizers to the ACL, and rehabilitation should stress regaining full range of motion and strength.[2]

COMPLICATIONS

The patient with an unstable knee is in jeopardy of fracture, aggravation of the initial injury, or falls as a result of the instability, resulting in other injuries. A knee that has sustained severe trauma is susceptible to the development of arthritis.

INDICATIONS FOR REFERRAL/HOSPITALIZATION

All persons who have sustained an injury to the cruciate ligaments require an evaluation by an orthopedic surgeon. The timing of surgical repair is controversial, and many patients function normally without surgery.

PATIENT AND FAMILY EDUCATION

It is important that the patient understand that despite reconstruction and rehabilitation, the knee is never perfectly normal. The knee can be functional but in some cases will require the use of a custom-made brace.[4]

Meniscus Injuries

The menisci are crescent-shaped fibrocartilaginous structures on the articular surface of the tibia. They act as shock absorbers for the knee and help to control normal knee motion. Meniscus tears are the third most common of all knee injuries. The medial meniscus is injured or torn more often than the lateral meniscus because of its structure, mobility, and attachment.

PATHOPHYSIOLOGY

The menisci maintain the space between the bones in the knee joint. They are injured when the knee is twisted while in the flexed position. The femur compresses against the tibia and grinds against the meniscus. This grinding motion tears the meniscus as the force exceeds the strength of the fibrocartilage. Once torn, the menisci cannot heal. Menisci tear as a direct result of injury or indirectly as a result of the normal wear and tear on the knee.

CLINICAL PRESENTATION

In an acute injury, joint effusion is always present. There is tenderness along the joint line, and often the person has a sense of instability. Those with a degenerative tear will complain of joint line discomfort and a sense of locking or giving way, especially on descending stairs or walking on uneven surfaces.

PHYSICAL EXAMINATION

Along with effusion in the acute state, quadriceps atrophy is often evident. The joint is stable, but palpating the joint line produces tenderness. McMurray's test helps to ascertain a tear in the cartilage (Figure 195-3). To perform McMurray's test, the examiner has the patient lie supine with the legs straight. The examiner firmly grasps the heel with one hand and places the other hand on the knee joint, with the fingers on the medial side and the thumb at the lateral side. The examiner flexes the knee while rotating the tibia internally and externally on the femur. This maneuver will loosen the joint. Then, while flexing and externally rotating the leg, the examiner applies valgus stress to the lateral side of the knee. The examiner holds the valgus stress on the joint while extending the leg and palpating the medial joint line. If a "click" or "pop" is heard or felt, the medial meniscus is torn.

McMurray's test can also be performed with the patient in a sitting position and the knee flexed to 90 degrees (see Figure 195-3). The patient should internally rotate the affected leg while the practitioner slowly extends the leg. While performing the maneuver, the practitioner should apply resistance to the knee medially to test the medial meniscus. The practitioner should repeat the maneuver, applying resistance to the knee laterally to test the lateral meniscus. The test is positive if the knee cannot be extended.

In addition to McMurray's test, a simpler test is Apley's compression test (Figure 195-4). This test should be done with the patient prone and the affected leg flexed to 90 degrees. The examiner places his or her knee on the patient's posterior thigh to stabilize it, grabs the foot firmly, leans on the heel to squeeze the menisci between the femur and the tibia, and rotates the tibia. If pain is elicited, there is a tear in the meniscus. The patient should be asked to describe the location of the pain to distinguish a medial meniscus tear from a lateral meniscus tear.

DIAGNOSTICS

The definitive diagnostic test is MRI. Plain films should be obtained to exclude any bony abnormalities.

DIFFERENTIAL DIAGNOSIS

Many times there is a sense of joint instability in addition to joint line tenderness; thus the potential for fracture or other structural injury must be considered.

MANAGEMENT

With a minor tear in the meniscus, the treatment is usually conservative. RICE and the use of crutches help quiet the acute phase. Rehabilitation to improve the strength of the quadriceps

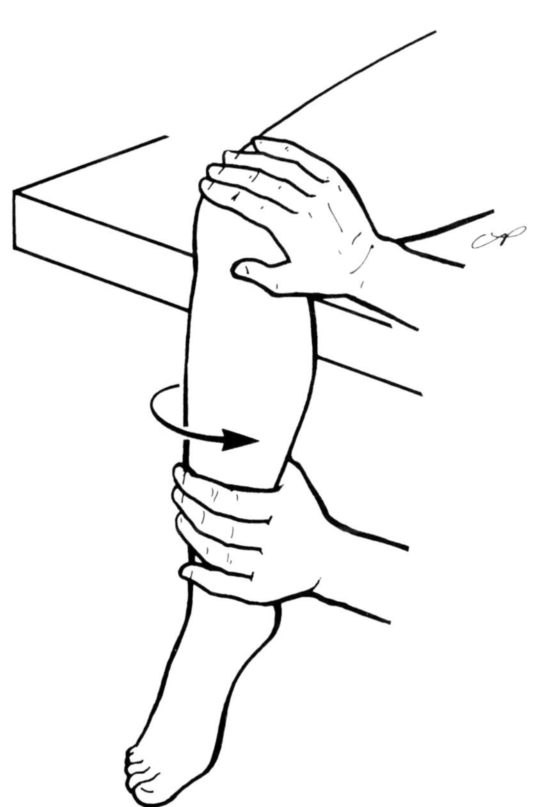

FIGURE 195-3

McMurray's test of the knee. (From Barkauskas VH and others: *Health and physical assessment,* ed 2, St Louis, 1998, Mosby.)

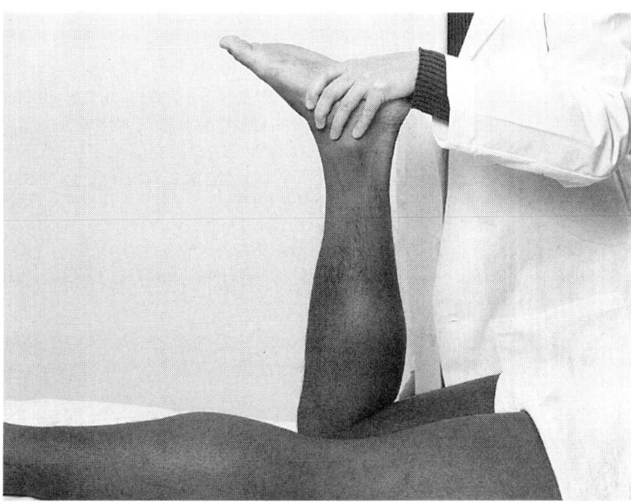

FIGURE 195-4

Apley's assessment of the knee. (From Seidel HM and others: *Mosby's guide to physical examination,* ed 4, St Louis, 1999, Mosby.)

muscle is imperative. Straight leg raises with the knee in extension, but not locked, can be started immediately and weight bearing gradually increased. Non–weight-bearing activities such as swimming and riding a stationary bicycle are excellent for increasing range of motion and strength.

COMPLICATIONS

Articular damage from the meniscus tear may result in arthritis (see Chapter 199). Because the menisci are stabilizers for the knee, loss of their integrity can lead to more extensive injuries.

INDICATIONS FOR REFERRAL/HOSPITALIZATION

Orthopedic referral is necessary for patients with persistent locking or swelling in the knee. An orthopedic surgeon or sports medicine specialist should be consulted when persistent effusions do not resolve or respond to conservative measures.

PATIENT AND FAMILY EDUCATION

Maintaining quadriceps strength is essential to minimize the disabilities associated with this injury. Although the knee may not be 100% normal, participation in sports with proper warm-up and equipment can be enjoyed. Achiness and swelling after a particularly strenuous workout or game can be normal. Ice and NSAIDs can help control the symptoms. A patient with persistent swelling, pain, or episodes of instability should be reevaluated.

Inflammatory and Degenerative Disorders

As people age or become deconditioned as a result of chronic injury or disease, knee pain can be caused by a variety of inflammatory, extraarticular conditions as well as age-related degeneration. Anserine bursitis is commonly seen in middle-aged women with osteoarthritis of the knee and a valgus deformity. This disorder produces pain and tenderness over the medial aspect of the knee about 2 inches below the joint line. Obvious swelling is not uncommon. Anserine bursitis is treated conservatively with ice and nonsteroidal antiinflammatory drugs (NSAIDs), but steroid injections may be necessary to alleviate pain in particularly severe cases.

Prepatellar bursitis ("housemaid's knee") manifests as a swelling superficial to the patella. This condition results from trauma such as occurs with frequent kneeling and is seen commonly in workers who work on their knees, such as floor or carpet layers. Pain is mild unless direct pressure is applied over the bursa, and there is no pain with weight bearing or range of motion of the knee. The condition is treated with rest, ice, and NSAIDs and is prevented by protecting the knee from repeated trauma.

Popliteal cysts ("Baker's cysts") are commonly seen in conjunction with rheumatoid arthritis, osteoarthritis, or internal derangements of the knee. Initially a cystic swelling in the popliteal space may be the only finding. As the cyst increases in size, the possibility of rupture increases. A ruptured cyst will drain into the calf, causing pain, erythema, and swelling, mimicking phlebitis. An ultrasound examination will provide a definitive diagnosis of this condition.

Osteoarthritis is probably the most common cause of knee pain in the older population (see Chapter 199). Pain, stiffness, and decreased function are all cardinal signs. Pain is generally insidious in onset and characterized as mild to moderate. Resting the knee usually alleviates the pain. Osteoarthritis is progressive, and the cartilage damage is permanent. However, conservative treatment including muscle strengthening, weight loss, analgesics, and NSAIDs is often effective. Injections of steroids or hyaluronan may provide temporary relief. Severe disease, manifested by resting or night pain and increasing difficulty with ambulation, may require joint replacement surgery.

REFERENCES

1. American Academy of Orthopaedic Surgeons: Your orthopedic connection. Retrieved August 12, 2002, from the World Wide Web: http://www.ortheoinfo.aaos.org.
2. Schenck R, editor: *Athletic training and sports medicine,* ed 2, Park Ridge, Ill, 1991, American Academy of Orthopedic Surgeons.
3. Harwood-Nuss A and others: Knee injuries. In *The clinical practice of emergency medicine,* Philadelphia, 1991, JB Lippincott.
4. Levin S: ACL reconstruction: the best treatment option? *Physician Sportsmed* 20:141-161, 1992.
5. Gates SJ, Mooar PA: The thigh, knee and patella. In: *Orthopaedics and sports medicine for nurses,* Baltimore, 1989, Williams & Wilkins.
6. Klippel JH: *Primer on the rheumatic diseases,* ed 12, Atlanta, 2001, The Arthritis Foundation.

CHAPTER 196

Low Back Pain

Michele DuBois Finnell and Virginia McNally Minichiello

DEFINITION/EPIDEMIOLOGY

Low back pain (LBP) is one of the most common complaints of patients seen in ambulatory care settings. It is estimated that in the adult population, 50% to 70% of persons will experience musculoligamentous or musculoskeletal back pain at some point in their adult life.[1] The risk is increased when the individual is involved in an occupation that requires either prolonged sitting or excessive, repetitive lifting, bending, twisting, or reaching. The most common causes of LBP are ligamentous/muscular injury, degeneration of the spine (osteoarthritis or spondylolysis), and disk herniation. Older individuals may develop *spinal stenosis,* which is a narrowing of the spinal canal often caused by bone spurs or *spondylolisthesis* (slipping of one vertebra over another).

LBP is commonly associated with overuse or an incompetence of the soft tissue structures. Acute low back pain (ALBP) is pain that persists for less than 3 weeks, and chronic low back pain (CLBP) is defined as that lasting longer than 7 weeks.[1]

LBP is a problem of great magnitude, second only to headache as the most common complaint of pain. Chronic impairment of the back and spine is the most common cause of physical disability in adults younger than 45 years in the United States.[2] At any given time, 31 million Americans will be experiencing some sort of LBP. It is one of the most common causes of disability and lost work time. Although men reportedly have a higher incidence of back pain over their lifetime, women now represent more than 60% of the workforce, and their incidence of back pain will eventually equal that of the men. In addition, a woman's likelihood of experiencing LBP is increased after two or more pregnancies.[3] Back pain in nurses younger than 45 years represents the number one cause of disability in this professional group.[4]

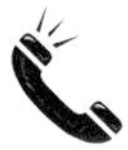

Physician consultation is indicated if back pain is associated with a neurologic deficit, decreased or absent pulses, or bowel or bladder dysfunction.

PATHOPHYSIOLOGY

Structurally, the posterior longitudinal ligaments and opposing anterior longitudinal ligaments provide spinal support at the surface of the vertebral column in addition to the supraspinous and interspinous ligaments.[5] In fact, the integrity of the spinous processes is maintained by the interlocking of the facet joints in the vertebral column. The spinal column houses the spinal nerves and is cushioned by the intravertebral disks.

Discerning the source of the back pain may be a challenge to the primary care provider because the source is often masked by the reaction of the varied tissues. Degenerative changes in the disk are responsible for most of the pathophysiology of LBP. The impact of stress at the lumbosacral area varies with positioning. The exact amount of pressure being delivered to the area with varied loads shows the vulnerability of this area. The difference in pressure in L3 and L4 disks varies with positioning. There is an increase in pressure of more than 43% between sitting upright or standing compared with being in the supine position.

With repetitive stress, disruption of the muscle fibers or attachments of the ligaments may occur. Injuries such as these will result in bleeding or spasm, causing tenderness and swelling of the affected areas.

As the disk weakens, it may bulge, causing irritation of a nerve root, generally at or below the level of herniation. This results in radicular (sciatic) pain, described as a burning, sharp, intense, or stabbing pain evolving from either the lumbar or sacral area. Radicular pain is worsened by activities that increase intraabdominal pressure, such as coughing, sneezing, or straining at stool. Pain radiating down one or both legs is suggestive of nerve root irritation and is highly sensitive for disk herniation. It can also be suggestive of spinal stenosis with radiation to the buttocks. The pain may be due to either the direct compression of the dural sac or the nerve root exiting from the involved area. Stenosis will impede flow of cerebrospinal fluid; standing does not provide relief but sitting or bending forward will because the spinal canal size is increased with this maneuver. Incidental findings of stenosis on x-ray studies or CT scans must be correlated with clinical findings because older patients may have claudication due to both peripheral vascular disease and spinal stenosis. Surgery may be indicated after conservative measures fail and disabling pain escalates.[6]

Neurogenic claudication may be present and described as numbness and weakness with activity. This must be differentiated from vascular claudication, which is associated with decreases in peripheral pulses. If bowel or bladder incontinence is reported, immediate evaluation is essential to exclude cauda equina syndrome, suggesting involvement of the S2-4 nerve roots.

CLINICAL PRESENTATION

A complete medical history, including the chief complaint, history of the present illness, past medical history, family history, occupational and social history, and a review of systems, is essential if an injury has precipitated the LBP. It is important to understand the mechanism of injury, which can be achieved with a complete symptom analysis (Box 196-1).

The symptom analysis (e.g., fever, bowel or bladder dysfunction, saddle anesthesia, persistent pain unresponsive to bed rest), when used properly, will provide a wealth of knowledge about the patient's condition. A history of recent trauma, cancer, recent lumbar puncture, concurrent infection, or chronic use of high-dose corticosteroids will help establish an accurate diagnosis.

PHYSICAL EXAMINATION

It is important to evaluate the patient during activity and in several positions. Gait should be observed as the patient walks into the examination room. The examiner should watch for an antalgic gait, foot drop, a widened base of support, or joint instability, as well as posture.

Symmetry of musculature, obvious curvature, and loss of lordosis are assessed with the patient in standing position. Curvature of the spine does not usually cause back pain, and loss of lordosis is often caused by muscle spasm. The spinous processes, sacroiliac joint (SIJ), sciatic notch, and paraspinal musculature should be palpated to assess for focal tenderness and spasm.

Range of motion and flexibility, including the ability to perform lateral bends, back extension, and toe touches, are examined. Partial assessment of lower extremity strength can be accomplished by asking the patient to walk on his or her heels (anterior tibialis, L4) and toes (gastrocnemius, S1) in addition to tandem walking for hip girdle stability.

Motor strength is assessed by testing hip flexor strength (T12 to L3), quadriceps strength (L2-4), and hamstring strength (L5 to S1), as well as hip abductor (L5) and adductor (L2-4) muscle groups. Comparison of strength from one side to the other is very important; the two sides should be equal. Sensation to light touch and pinprick and deep tendon reflexes (DTRs) should also be assessed[7] (Figure 196-1). DTRs are almost always symmetric; however, asymmetric reflexes may be normal for that patient based on a history of previous trauma. It is also very helpful to use augmentation (distraction) techniques when testing reflexes to truly assess their presence or absence. Documentation of DTRs with augmentation is essential.[8]

Before examining the patient in a supine position, the examiner should perform a straight leg raise (SLR) with the patient in the sitting position. If the sciatic nerve is irritated, the SLR test will be positive in both the sitting and lying positions (Figure 196-2). The SLR test by itself does not indicate significant nerve root tension/irritation. Pain below the knee at less than 70 degrees of SLR that is aggravated by ankle dorsiflexion or extension and rotation of the limb is suggestive of L5, S1 nerve root tension related to disk herniation. Crossover pain is a stronger indicator of nerve root compression than SLR pain on the affected side. Ninety percent of radiculopathy due to lumbosacral disk herniation involves nerve roots L4, L5, or S1 at the L4, L5, or S1 disk level.[1,9]

With the patient in the supine position, the lower extremity should be inspected for passive range of motion. If range of motion is painful without stretching the sciatic nerve, osteoarthritis should be considered in the differential diagnosis. A positive SLR test in both the sitting and lying positions suggests nerve root tension/irritation, which may be caused by a herniated disk. If bladder or bowel dysfunction is present, examination of rectal sphincter tone should also be done to exclude cauda equina syndrome (S2, S3, or S4 injury).

BOX 196-1

SYMPTOM ANALYSIS

ONSET
When did the back pain start? What precipitated the pain? Was there an injury? Sudden onset or chronic? Prior history? What treatment has been tried in the past? Does it help? Is it better now, or when it started?

QUALITY
What is the pain like? Describe it.

QUANTITY/SEVERITY
Rate the pain on a 0-10 scale now and when it first started.

CONSISTENCY
When does the pain occur? Does it awaken you from sleep? Does it get better with rest?

LOCATION
Point to where the pain is. Does it move? Does it get better with sitting? With standing?

TIMING
Is the pain constant? Cyclic? Intermittent? How long does each episode of back pain last?

AGGRAVATING/ALLEVIATING SYMPTOMS
What makes the pain worse? What makes it better?

ASSOCIATED SYMPTOMS
Any bowel or bladder problems? Any numbness or tingling in extremities?

PRESENT STATUS
Current symptoms? Currently working? What type of work? What other activities are you involved with in your personal life (e.g., taking care of children, elders, house work, weight lifting)?

DIAGNOSTICS

With a complete symptom analysis and the physical examination, a diagnosis can usually be made without further diagnostic tests. Routine radiographs of the lumbosacral spine are neither cost-effective nor useful in decision making in patients aged 20 to 50 years. Finding normal disk spaces does not exclude a herniated disk, and encountering a narrowed disk space cannot distinguish between disk rupture and asymmetric degeneration. Osteophytes extending from the vertebral bodies indicate little more than long-existing disk degeneration and attempts of the body to heal itself.

However, certain situations do require x-ray studies to aid in the differential diagnosis (Box 196-2).

MRI may be indicated to pinpoint the source of the radiculopathy or if back pain without radiculopathy continues for longer than 6 weeks without improvement despite physical therapy or use of nonsteroidal antiinflammatory drugs (NSAIDs). However, many individuals without back pain have disk bulges or protrusions that may be discovered coincidentally on MRI.[10] Therefore without the accompanying findings of radiculopathy or abnormalities on physical examination, the MRI findings may prove to be nondiagnostic and expensive.

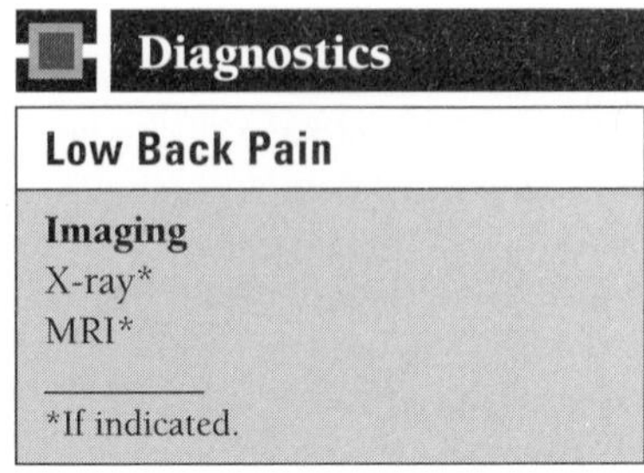
Diagnostics

Low Back Pain

Imaging
X-ray*
MRI*

*If indicated.

DIFFERENTIAL DIAGNOSIS

Because back pain is one of the more common primary care complaints, it is important to exclude the possibility of other sources of LBP, particularly osteoporotic

Nerve root	L4	L5	S1
Pain	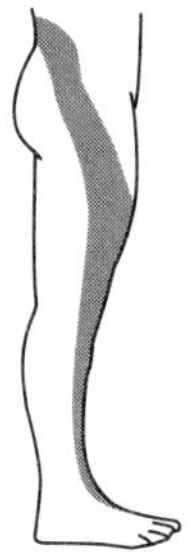	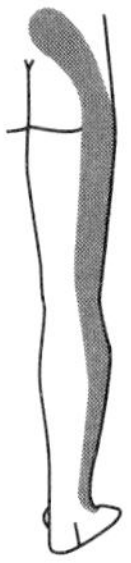	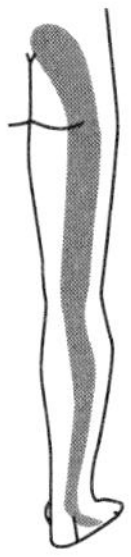
Numbness	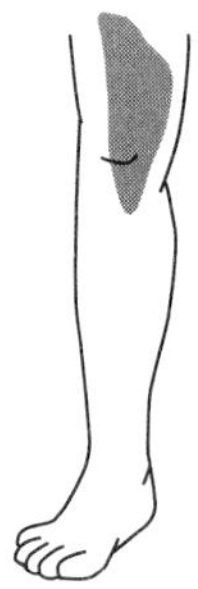	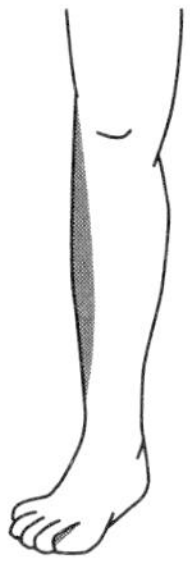	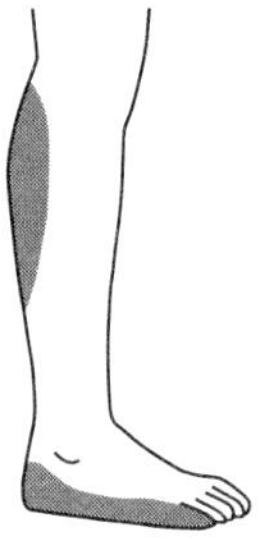
Motor weakness	Extension of quadriceps	Dorsiflexion of great toe and foot	Plantar flexion of great toe and foot
Screening examination	Squat and rise	Heel walking	Walking on toes
Reflexes	Knee jerk diminished	None reliable	Ankle jerk diminished

FIGURE 196-1

Reflex testing. (From Nordin M, Andersson GBJ, Pope MH: *Musculoskeletal disorders in the workplace: principles and practice,* St Louis, 1997, Mosby.)

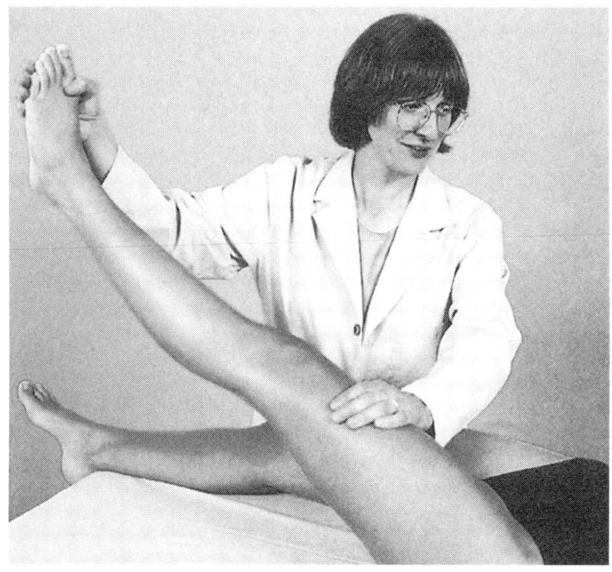

FIGURE 196-2

Straight leg-raising test (supine position). (From Barkauskas VH and others: *Health and physical assessment,* ed 2, St Louis, 1998, Mosby.)

BOX 196-2

INDICATIONS FOR IMAGING STUDIES

MAJOR TRAUMA

Suspicion of malignancy: Over age 50, focal persistent bone pain unrelieved by rest, or a history of malignancy

Suspected compression fracture: Prolonged steroid use, postmenopausal woman, or severe trauma

Suspected ankylosing spondylitis: Young male patient, limited spinal range of motion, SIJ pain

Worsening chronic osteomyelitis: Low-grade fever, high sedimentation rate, focal tenderness, especially after a spinal tap

MAJOR NEUROLOGIC DEFICIT

Localized back pain to the higher lumbar and thoracic regions—compression fractures and metastatic tumors are common in these areas compression fracture, infection, trauma, inflammatory disease, myositis, fibromyalgia, neoplasm, malignancy, spinal stenosis, and acute abdominal aneurysm in patients older than 50 years.

The majority of patients with back pain have musculoligamentous injury or degenerative changes resulting in pain. Other sources of LBP include referred pain from other systems (e.g., the genitourinary system or reproductive organs). Metabolic diseases, such as diabetes, may cause peripheral neuropathies that result in leg pain, and of course, psychologic stressors cannot be overlooked.

MANAGEMENT

In the acute stage of back pain, the initial treatment should attempt to decrease the inflammatory response to the injury, trauma, and stress in the area. Analgesia and control of inflammation will provide comfort (see Table 199-1). Regularly scheduled acetaminophen (Tylenol) is appropriate and beneficial for many patients. Many patients self-treat, having access to NSAIDs over the counter. They may wait to see their primary care provider until they no longer can attain relief from pain or they are frustrated with limitations to their mobility. The benefit of the nonsteroidal medications is that they do provide some analgesia along with their antiinflammatory effects. If relief is not adequate with NSAIDs or the patient is unable to tolerate them, the newer cyclooxygenase-2 (COX-2) inhibitors as well as muscle relaxants may be added. The addition of a muscle relaxant precludes operating machinery and driving; therefore the patient may be restricted in work assignments. Patients need to be advised that analgesia is only for the short term; the key to improvement is mobilization and activity.

Conservative treatment, including antiinflammatory agents and possibly muscle relaxants and analgesics, is the hallmark of management for musculoskeletal LBP. With the initial onset of ALBP, bed rest is indicated, but only for 2 to 3 days, and is followed by a return to normal activities of daily living. The use of intermittent heat and/or ice, massage, an aerobic exercise program, abdominal strengthening exercises, and, in some cases, reconditioning exercises with physical therapy are all essential to successful recovery. A walking program can be initiated very early in the rehabilitation for generalized conditioning and toning. Exercise has been shown to be an effective adjunct to analgesia and is necessary to facilitate recovery.[11] It is very helpful to address the patient's fears of reinjury or further exacerbation. Newer modalities for treating back pain, such as acupuncture, may be an appropriate complementary treatment in some patients and requires exploration with the provider to determine appropriate timing and to evaluate response to the therapy.[4]

Differential Diagnosis

Low Back Pain

Osteoporotic compression fracture	Neoplasm
Infection	Malignancy
Trauma	Acute abdominal aneurysm
Inflammatory disease	Referred pain
Myositis	Peripheral neuropathy
Fibromyalgia	Spinal stenosis

LIFE SPAN CONSIDERATIONS

In the developing spine, contortions associated with spinal malformations present when the child assumes the erect position and begins weight bearing. Numerous structural deficits will be readily visible, and assessment of the patient from early childhood into adolescence requires good assessment of the musculoskeletal system. Early identification of structural deficits may well permit correction.

In the young adult, changes in spinal structures may indicate spondylolisthesis (slipping forward of a vertebra over the adjoining vertebrae). Spinal changes such as spondylolisthesis, caused by excessive extension and flexion as occurs in gymnasts and some other athletes, present challenges to the examiner in determining the source of the pain and the long-term possibility of improvement. Congenital spinal stenosis may be seen, as occurs in achondroplastic dwarfs.[6]

Degenerative changes of the spine occur with the aging process but may not be wholly responsible for back pain. Older individuals may develop degenerative disease that will present with lumbago (LBP), leg pain (sciatica), or both. Spinal stenosis (acquired) in the older adult is not uncommon and may affect mobility and lifestyle. The pain associated with spinal stenosis is often claudicating and may be alleviated by stooping forward into an abnormal posture (much like when pushing a grocery cart).[12]

Mechanical/structural changes in the individual may also be responsible for back pain. These involve weight changes, pregnancy, sudden growth spurts in the child or adolescent, and osteoporotic deformities in the aging adult.

COMPLICATIONS

The management of mechanical LBP is uncomplicated and can be accomplished by the primary care provider. If a patient has asymmetric reflexes but no other symptoms of a herniated disk other than back pain, no referral is necessary unless symptoms persist for longer than 6 weeks. However, if neurologic symptoms occur or seem to be progressing (e.g., a new onset of sciatica, which may cause a loss of reflexes, muscle weakness, or atrophy) (see Figure 196-1), then treatment options are altered. At that time, further diagnostic testing and referral to an orthopedist or a neurologist are appropriate.

INDICATIONS FOR REFERRAL/HOSPITALIZATION

In general, mechanical LBP is not an indication for hospitalization. However, cauda equina syndrome or incapacitating back pain that prohibits management at home requires emergent evaluation and possible hospitalization. The onset of neurologic symptoms requires an urgent evaluation but not necessarily admission.

If a patient has a motor or sensory loss, as well as asymmetric reflexes, then referral to a neurologist or an orthopedist is appropriate. Surgery is considered when there is a neurologic deficit or when chronic LBP does not resolve and there is a clear pathologic finding that correlates directly with the clinical examination. If surgery is the recommended treatment option, the surgeon will also make physical therapy recommendations. Physical therapy referral will assist the patient in learning proper body mechanics and physical reconditioning.

A second referral to the specialist should be considered if symptoms return or persist. In many major medical centers, specialized, multidisciplinary spine centers are available to evaluate and treat patients with chronic back pain.

PATIENT AND FAMILY EDUCATION

Patients should be informed that 85% of those with LBP will recover in 3 to 5 days and will be completely back to normal within 6 to 8 weeks. Problems with bowel or bladder control, leg weakness or persistent leg pain below the knee, symptoms of a urinary tract infection, or an inability to stand on toes should be reported immediately.

Enhanced patient understanding plays a crucial role in reducing and improving back pain and reducing emergency department use. Patients are encouraged to take control of their pain by using the treatment modalities outlined for them, following their medication regimen, and reporting changes in symptoms.

Aerobic activity and physical reconditioning are recommended to all individuals with LBP without radicular symptoms because inactivity and immobilization have not been shown to improve outcomes. Continuation of usual activity maintains conditioning and reduces lost work time. Proper body mechanics for work and home cannot be ignored. Physical therapists will help teach proper body mechanics and provide physical reconditioning exercises. Patients should be encouraged to maintain stretching exercises, abdominal strengthening, and physical activity to reduce the recurrence rate of LBP.[2]

REFERENCES

1. Schnare S: Evaluating and managing low back pain, *Contemp Nurse Pract* 10:10-15, 1995.
2. Schoen DC: *Adult orthopaedic nursing,* Philadelphia, 2000, JB Lippincott.
3. Finnell M: *Primary care seminar,* Beth Israel Hospital, lecture on back pain in the primary care setting, Nov 22, 1994, Boston.
4. Smith-Fassler ME, Lopez-Bushnell K. Acupuncture as complementary therapy for back pain, *Holist Nurs Pract* 15:35-44, 2000.
5. Sulco TP: Musculoskeletal dysfunction and treatment. In *Orthopedic care of geriatric patients,* St Louis, 1985, Mosby.
6. Esses SI: *Textbook of spinal disorders,* Philadelphia, 1995, JB Lippincott.
7. Nordin M, Andersson GBJ, Pope MH: *Musculoskeletal disorders in the workplace: principles and practice,* St Louis, 1997, Mosby.
8. Barkauskas VH and others: *Health and physical assessment,* ed 2, St Louis, 1998, Mosby.
9. McCance KL, Heuther SE: *Pathophysiology: the biologic basis of disease in adults and children,* ed 3, St Louis, 1998, Mosby.
10. Jensen MC and others: Magnetic imaging of the lumbar spine in people without back pain, *N Engl J Med* 331:69-73, 1994.
11. McLain K and others: Effectiveness of exercise versus normal activity on acute low back pain: an integrative synthesis and meta-analysis, *Online Journal of Knowledge Synthesis for Nursing* 6(7), 2001. http://www.stti.iupui.edu/library/ojksn/ (accessed 10/19/01).
12. Braddom R: Conservative approach to uncomplicated back pain. In Young MA, Lavin RA, editors: *Physical medicine and rehabilitation in state of the art reviews,* Philadelphia, 1995, Hanley & Belfus, Inc.

CHAPTER 197

Myofascial Pain Syndrome

Sharon G. Childs

DEFINITION/EPIDEMIOLOGY

Fibrositis, muscular rheumatism, lumbago, interstitial myofascitis, and *fibromyositis* are a few of the terms included in the nomenclature used to describe a painful muscular disorder called myofascial pain syndrome (MPS).[1,2] This intriguing and often misdiagnosed condition presents challenges for diagnosis and treatment. Although it is not a deforming disease, patients express varying levels of disability (physical and emotional) as a result of dealing with chronic pain from what they suspect is an essentially unknown etiology. In the past, health care providers may have inadvertently engendered paternalistic behaviors that created nonmilieu and learned helplessness in patients affected with MPS.[3]

MPS is a muscle disorder characterized by localized nonarticular musculoskeletal pain, sleep disorder related to pain, and regional musculoskeletal pain originating from trigger points (TPs).[1,4] TPs are nonpathologic masses in fascia or skeletal muscle that may be palpated by applying moderate to firm pressure. TPs cause local autonomic dysfunction (e.g., coroyza, diaphoresis, hyperemia after TP palpation, local vasoconstriction, lacrimation, piloerection, and proprioceptive disturbances).[1,3,4]

MPS occurs equally among the two sexes. It is not associated with any particular age-group. The myofascial pain and TPs can be precipitated by traumatic injury, viral illness, or repetitive strain trauma to the affected musculoskeletal tissues. There are no data to support a connection of family history, race, or socioeconomic factors with MPS. Precipitating factors are listed in Box 197-1.

PATHOPHYSIOLOGY

There is no definitive neurochemical or neurophysical rationale to explain MPS. However, the two most suspected pathogeneses

BOX 197-1

PRECIPITATING FACTORS ASSOCIATED WITH MYOFASCIAL PAIN SYNDROME

- Chronic infections
- Metabolic and endocrine pathology (hyperglycemia, hyperuricemia, hypothyroid)
- Mechanical stressors (physical biomechanical dysfunction, poor posture, poor ergonomics, repetitive strain injury)
- Neurologic pathology (entrapment neuropathies, peripheral neuropathy, radiculopathy)
- Nutritional deficiencies
- Rheumatologic pathology (rheumatoid arthritis, systemic lupus erythematosus, osteoarthritis, polymyalgia rheumatica)
- Psychosocial factors (persistent anxiety, depression, secondary gain issues)

of MPS are: dysfunction in Ca^{++} pump mechanism and the effects of substance P (a neurotransmitter stored within afferent nociceptive fibers). The most widely accepted hypotheses are (1) the occurrence of microtrauma with subsequent overload in skeletal muscle, which leads to repetitive ionic exchange of calcium, precipitating sarcomere shortening, and continuous muscle contraction and (2) peripheral hyperactivity of the peptidergic nervous system secondary to the immunoreactivity of substance P.[5] Increased local metabolic demand using energy stores of oxygen and adenosine triphosphate (ATP) results in an ischemic process within muscle. Inflammatory mediators irritate chemoreceptors, causing pain, as well as a cycle of cellular irritability.[1]

Pain is modulated and stimulated by algogenic substances around nociceptors. With continuous stimulation of nociceptors and other receptors about TPs, a state of hyperalgesia and referred pain compounds cellular dysfunction.

CLINICAL PRESENTATION

MPS is a common problem that is seen in the outpatient setting. Thorough occupational, physical, and psychosocial histories should be obtained, including the mechanism of injury related to the patient's complaints. TPs associated with pain in muscle affect ligaments, subcutaneous tissue, and tendon insertions according to the pattern of referred pain. These symptoms are pathognomonic for MPS. Patients may complain of deep aching or burning pain. Pain does not generally travel along dermatomal or myotomal pathways. Although referred pain may be precipitated by nerve entrapment–like pain, myofascial pain is not radicular in origin. Other complaints include muscle fatigue, stiffness, spasm, and poor, nonrestful sleep.

PHYSICAL EXAMINATION

Affected musculoskeletal tissues should be inspected and palpated for erythema, warmth, lesions, spasms, and edema. TPs are palpated as taut fibrous bands or "knots" in the subcutaneous tissue. A pressure threshold algometer can be used to quantify TP sensitivity, monitor resolution of TP pain, and diagnose MPS.[1,2]

DIAGNOSTICS

Laboratory studies for serum chemistries, serum glucose, BUN, creatinine, CBC, erythrocyte sedimentation rate (ESR), myoglobin level, serum vitamin levels, and thyroid panel are recommended. Plain radiographs, thermography, electromyography (EMG), and nerve conduction studies (NCS) may be warranted. Structural defects (leg length discrepancy, spine dysfunction such as scoliosis or hip dysplagia), poor posture, systemic medical illness (e.g., diabetes mellitus, hypothyroidism), nutritional deficiencies, and behavioral components may be associated with recalcitrant pain situations that affect musculoskeletal tissues.

DIFFERENTIAL DIAGNOSIS

Fibromyalgia and MPS have similar presentations. However, MPS is characterized by pain that is regionally referred by palpation of TPs. Fibromyalgia is distinguished by multiple paired tender points above and below the waist. Other conditions that should be included in the differential diagnosis include arthritis, bacterial/viral/spirochetal infections, bursitis/tendonitis, chronic fatigue syndrome, collagen disorders, metabolic myopathy, muscle strain, polymyalgia rheumatica, sciatica, and electrolyte, nutritional, and metabolic imbalances.

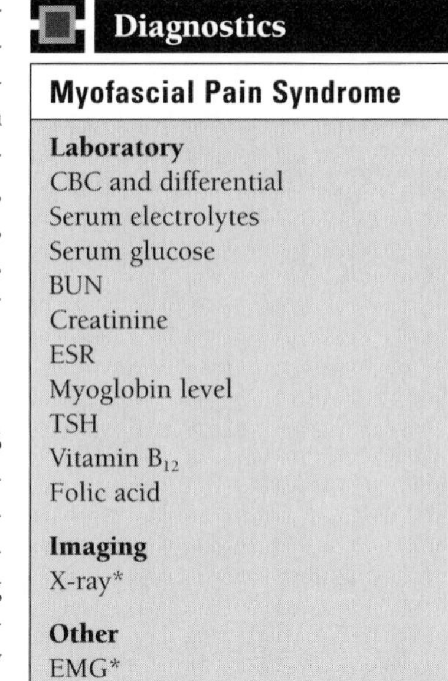

Diagnostics

Myofascial Pain Syndrome

Laboratory
CBC and differential
Serum electrolytes
Serum glucose
BUN
Creatinine
ESR
Myoglobin level
TSH
Vitamin B_{12}
Folic acid

Imaging
X-ray*

Other
EMG*
NCS*

*If indicated.

MANAGEMENT

The treatment of MPS is focused on individualized and etiology-specific modalities. Psychosocial issues dealing with chronic pain, malingering for secondary gain, and underlying behavioral issues that influence the patient's behavior should be addressed early in the treatment regimen. Psychosocial counseling may be indicated.

Management includes "spray and stretch," which incorporates spraying the skin with a vapor coolant such as Fluori-Methane while at the same time stretching affected muscle tissue. Ice compresses also provide adequate cooling. This maneuver releases taut bands as the tissue stretching decreases muscle tension and releases TPs. Evidence exists for the benefit of physical therapy treatment such as thermal (cool/warm) modalities and flexibility and strengthening exercises.[6-8]

Other therapeutic treatments that have proven beneficial for MPSs include TP injection with local anesthetics (1% to 2%

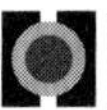

Differential Diagnosis

Myofascial Pain Syndrome

Acute cervical strain	Metabolic imbalance
Angina	Metabolic myopathies
Appendicitis	Muscle strain
Atypical facial neuralgia	Nutritional (vitamin) deficiency
Arthritis	Occipital neuralgia
Back pain (radicular)	Osteomalacia
Bacterial infection	Otitis
Bursitis/tendonitis	Pelvic pain
Cephalgia	Polymyalgia rheumatica
Chronic fatigue syndrome	Psychogenic rheumatism
Collagen disorders	Sciatica
Dermatomyositis	Subdeltoid bursitis
Early collagen disease	Thoracic outlet syndrome
Electrolyte imbalance	Trochanteric bursitis
Epicondylitis	Viral syndromes
Hypothyroidism	
Heel spur	
Infectious process (bacterial, viral, spirochete)	

lidocaine, 0.25% mepivacaine, and 0.0625% bupivacaine) and a dry needling technique in which a sterile needle is used to stimulate a TP to interrupt spontaneous electrical activity (and thus terminate taut muscle bands).[8,9] Multiple injections may be necessary. Injectable corticosteroid preparations are contraindicated because of possible side effects, which can include muscle weakness, tendon rupture, dermal depigmentation, and atrophy of adipose tissue. Unless local inflammation of structures is suspected, corticosteroids are not injected in TPs.

Pharmacotherapy is included in the treatment regimen. Nonsteroidal antiinflammatory drugs (NSAIDs) may relieve posttherapy tissue and muscle soreness (see Table 199-1). With acute muscle spasm, muscle relaxants such as carisoprodol (350 mg t.i.d.), cyclobenzaprine (10 mg every 12 hours), or metaxalone (400 to 800 mg t.i.d.) may be prescribed. Tricyclic antidepressants and antiseizure drugs may also be helpful in treating patients with underlying psychopathology and/or neuropathic pain and to improve sleep. The choice of drug, dosing, and duration of treatment are patient specific and titrated to patient response. Acute pain is treated with tramadol (50 to 100 mg every 4 to 6 hours p.r.n.), hydrocodone, or acetaminophen in combination with other drugs.

Other adjunctive therapies include acupuncture, biofeedback, deep muscle massage and myofascial release, transcutaneous electrical nerve stimulation (TENS), and ultrasound. One or several modalities may be used.

COMPLICATIONS

There are no complications. Misdiagnosis can lead to chronic pain with emotional and affective determinants that often accompany chronic illness and pain. In severe pain, a disuse condition can occur; this includes atrophied muscle tissue, general deconditioning, and, in cases of psychogenic overlay, flexed posturing of the spine called camptocormia.

INDICATIONS FOR REFERRAL/HOSPITALIZATION

Patients who fail to respond to treatment require referral to physicians/specialists, including but are not limited to physiatrists for EMG, NCS (studies do not show abnormalities related to MPS), or invasive injections; psychiatric health care practitioners; social workers; nutritionists; neurologists; anesthesiologists; and orthopedists. Hospitalization may be necessary for invasive injections or procedures.

PATIENT AND FAMILY EDUCATION

Body ergonomics, proper lifting, and the use of equipment are important to prevent reinjury. Patients require education regarding issues of repetitive lifting, end-range muscle straining, ergonomics, and inappropriate body maneuvers for activities of daily living, work, and recreation.

REFERENCES

1. Auleciems L: Myofascial pain syndrome: a multidisciplinary approach, *Nurse Pract* 20:18-31, 1995.
2. Harden R and others: Signs and symptoms of the myofascial pain syndrome: a national survey of pain management providers, *Clin J Pain* 16:64-72, 2000.
3. Arnoff G: Myofascial pain syndrome and fibromyalgia: a critical assessment and alternate view, *Clin J Pain* 14:74-85, 1998.
4. Travell J, Simons D: *Myofascial pain and dysfunction: the trigger point manual,* vols 1 and 2, Baltimore, 1999, Williams & Wilkins.
5. DeStafano R and others: Image analysis quantification of substance P immunoreactivity in the trapezius muscle of patients with fibromyalgia and myofascial pain syndrome, *J Rheum* 27:2906-2910, 2000.
6. Esenyel M, Caglar N, Aldemir T: Treatment of myofascial pain, *Am J Phys Med Rehab* 79:48-52, 2000.
7. Hanten W and others: Effectiveness of a home program of ischemic pressure followed by sustained stretch for treatment of myofascial trigger points, *Phys Ther* 80:997-1003, 2000.
8. Cummings T, White A: Needling therapies in the management of myofascial trigger point pain: a systematic review, *Arch Phys Med Rehab* 82:986-992, 2001.
9. Iwami H and others: Water-diluted local anesthetic for trigger point injection in chronic myofascial pain syndrome: evaluation of types of local anesthetics and concentration of water, *Reg Anesth Pain Med* 26:333-336, 2001.

CHAPTER 198

Neck Pain

Rita Beckman-Williams and Robert J. Riggen

DEFINITION/EPIDEMIOLOGY

Neck pain is one of the most common patient complaints in primary care. Disorders of the musculoskeletal structures of the neck are responsible for most painful neck conditions, including neck strain, torticollis ("wry neck"), degenerative cervical spine disease, and cervical disk disease.[1] Thoracic pathology, particularly coronary artery disease and esophageal disease, may cause referred neck pain. Neck pain is considered chronic if it lasts longer than 3 months. Factors that may predispose to chronic pain are prolonged postural malalignment, repeated strain, facet subluxation, disk herniation, facet joint disease, and physical factors such as repetitive neck movement, cold exposure, and vibrations.[2,3] Pending litigation and disability claims may also contribute to the chronicity of symptoms. With cervical fracture and cord damage, the clinical course may be characterized by long-term morbidity, paraplegia, or, rarely, death.

Immediate emergency department referral/physician consultation is indicated for patients with a suspected cervical fracture, new-onset neurologic findings, or signs of meningeal irritation.

PATHOPHYSIOLOGY

The neck muscles surround the trachea and esophagus anteriorly and the seven cervical vertebrae posteriorly. The sternocleidomastoid and trapezius muscles form a triangle laterally, thereby supporting the head and allowing movement. The facet joints extend laterally from the spinous processes of the vertebrae and allow rotational movement. Forceful extension and flexion of the neck result in microtears of the muscles and ligaments with secondary hemorrhage, edema, and inflammation.[4]

Both the changes of aging and arthritis may contribute to neck pain. The cervical disks normally begin to show signs of degeneration in the fourth decade of life. Osteoarthritis causes breakdown of the articular cartilage of the facet joints as well as microfractures and subsequent cyst and bony spur formation, leading to joint space narrowing. The inflammatory response and granulation tissue associated with rheumatoid arthritis erode both bones and ligaments. All of these conditions may cause impingement on the nerve roots as they emerge from the spinal cord through the neuroforamina with resulting radicular pain. Cervical disk injury often causes radicular pain as well and is often associated with trauma, although it may occur with no history of trauma. Headache and pain referred to the arm and shoulder may be associated with neck pain, as may nondermatomal parasthesias, dizziness, and blurred vision, possibly because of damage to the cervical sympathetic plexus.

CLINICAL PRESENTATION

Sharp neck pain, at times radiating to the head, shoulder, arm, or hand, occurs within hours to days after an acute injury sustained during a motor vehicle accident, sports activity, or acute disk injury. After a motor vehicle accident, pain may be accompanied by mild amnesia and transient mental dullness. Sudden movement of the head during a sports injury or accident may be the causative factor for a strain or hematoma and aggravate an existing injury. Sharp, typically burning or achy pain, with or without radiation to shoulder, arm, and hand, occurs with chronic pain. After prolonged pain the patient may complain of dizziness, occipital headache that may radiate temporally, blurred vision, specific point tenderness, or spasm; the patient may be grimacing, with shrugged shoulders, hand on chin, and the head held in lateral flexion.[5]

Point tenderness of a muscle indicates strain, tear, or hematoma of the muscle palpated or of a deeper muscle. Ropy nodules on muscles and ligaments may be a result of chronic strain and microtears. Cold drafts and tension have also been known to adversely affect muscles. Neck pain is aggravated by prolonged sitting with the neck flexed anteriorly or laterally as when typing or using the telephone, sleeping with the head hyperextended, lifting weights, sneezing, and coughing. A complete history that includes the mechanism of injury, usual posture, sports played, current weight-lifting practices at home and at work, use of seat belts, presence of osteoporosis, rheumatoid arthritis, or osteoarthritis and a review of symptoms and past medical history ensure appropriate diagnostic studies, education, referral, and plan of care. Neurologic history should include the presence and distribution of pain, functional limitations, weakness, parasthesias, numbness, and bladder or bowel dysfunction. The presence of fever, unexplained weight loss, previous malignancy, prolonged use of steroids, IV drug use, immunosuppression, and psychologic problems should also be noted.

PHYSICAL EXAMINATION

Inspection of the neck begins when the patient is introduced (Table 198-1). The patient should be assessed for the presence of a grimace when shaking hands, during removal of garments, and during demonstration of range of motion. Palpation may reveal tenderness, swelling, abnormal masses, and facet alignment. The examiner begins at C2 and palpates each of two lateral facet joints for each spinous process. Cervical lymph node examination may be done while palpating the trapezius.

The neck is inspected for neutral alignment of the head and visual enlargement of the lymph nodes and thyroid gland. The parotid gland, palpable only with disease, is found at the posterior angle of the mandible. After range of motion is assessed, the strength of the intrinsic muscles of the neck is tested by requesting that the patient repeat each motion while the examiner provides resistance with one hand on the patient's head and the other hand on the patient's sternum for forward flexion and on the patient's shoulder for all other motions.

Several special maneuvers assist with assessing the integrity of the spine and locating the point of injury (Box 198-1). Axial compression and the Valsalva maneuver assess for increased

TABLE 198-1 Physical Examination of the Cervical Spine

Physical Examination	Possible Diagnosis
INSPECTION	
Note rash, papules, prominent superior vertebrae, scars, swelling, hematomas, symmetry	Asymmetry, prominent vertebrae, or swelling due to fracture, subluxation; scars due to surgery, old trauma; ecchymosis after trauma
Lordotic cervical spine should be aligned and rest over relaxed shoulders; should be smooth range of motion and movement when disrobing	Inability to rotate; fracture of odontoid process
Normal range of motion: Forward flexion: 45 degrees—chin to chest Extension: 55 degrees—eyes parallel to ceiling Lateral band: 45 degrees—ears toward shoulder Rotation: 70 degrees—chin almost touching shoulder	Rotated head: may be spasm, torticollis or, rarely, subluxation of atlantoaxial joint; limited range due to whiplash pain after motor vehicle accident, fused vertebrae, lymph node enlargement, fracture, and referred pain
POSTERIOR PALPATION	
(Supine patient relaxes muscles) C2 through large T1 should be aligned; should be pain free; should be immobile spine	Spinous process pain due to disk herniation or fracture, lateral mobility of spinous process, and crepitus due to fracture
Lateral facet joint tenderness or swelling	Subluxation
Occipital nerves and nuchal ligament from base of skull to C7; head forward flexed	Ruptured ligament if tenderness; presence of nodules may indicate trigger points
Trapezius (large muscle) should be bilaterally equal from T12 and laterally to acromion (palpate with hand; turn head away from tested side)	Hard muscle due to spasm; tenderness due to muscle strain; point tenderness due to fibromyalgia; presence of nodules may indicate trigger points
Splenius cervicis (small muscle), located superiorly in triangular space between trapezius and sternocleidomastoid	Spasm; presence of nodules may indicate trigger points
Levator scapulae, scalene posterior, and scalene medial inferior to splenius cervicis (difficult to palpate)	Strain or spasm, point tenderness fibromyalgia; presence of nodules may indicate trigger points
ANTERIOR PALPATION	
Examination aids in identifying location of posterior landmarks	May be thyroid, lymph node, and parotid enlargement
Superior midline hyoid bone corresponds to C3 posteriorly; smooth thyroid cartilage corresponds to C4-5	
Sternocleidomastoid reaches from sternoclavicular joint to mastoid process	Injury after motor vehicle accident, swelling may indicate hematoma and produce torticollis
AUSCULTATION	
Spinous processes for crepitus	Cervical spondylosis, rheumatoid arthritis

cervical pressure and may cause radiating pain from different origins. Lifting the head at the chin and occiput may decrease the pain of contracted muscles. Adson's test evaluates the integrity of the subclavian artery and C5 to T1 nerves. Radicular symptoms may become apparent while performing Adson's test, indicating compression of C5 to T1 nerves traveling through the brachial plexus, and aids in the diagnosis of thoracic outlet syndrome. Carpal tunnel syndrome or another distal problem may contribute to arm pain or radiation; therefore, the shoulder, elbow, and hand should also be examined.[4]

Absent or diminished sensation, reflex, and strength may occur with disk injury. The sensory, motor, and reflex testing of these nerves aids in evaluating the integrity of the spine (Table 198-2). Evaluation of the cranial nerves, as well as the upper and lower extremities, is indicated. The presence of hyperreflexia in the lower extremities, muscle spasticity, or a gait disturbance suggests upper motor neuron dysfunction, possibly caused by cervical myelopathy from cord compression by a tumor or bony spur.

BOX 198-1

SPECIAL MANEUVERS—CERVICAL SPINE

Compression test—Press down on top of head to increase cervical pressure. Note pain in dermatone to determine location of cervical injury.

Valsalva's test—Increases cervical pressure. Pain caused by disk herniation or mass. Note location of neck pain and dermatone pain.

Swallow test—Pain due to anterior spine mass or infection.

Adson's test—Evaluates integrity of subclavian artery and C5 to T1 nerves. Abduct and externally rotate shoulder while rotating head toward arm tested. Radicular symptoms indicate that origin of pain is at subclavian artery where C5-T1 nerves travel. Diminished pulse indicates compression of radial artery.

DIAGNOSTICS

The primary care provider will generally see a trauma patient for a follow-up visit after initial emergency care. However, if the initial assessment in the provider's office indicates objective neurologic deficit, spinal tenderness to palpation, head injury, or prolonged confusion, a series of x-ray studies is warranted with patient's neck properly immobilized.[5]

Several x-ray projections show different views of the spine and are used to determine the area of the spine that is injured. The anteroposterior view details spinal alignment, uniformity of the disk spaces and vertebrae, and facet dislocation. The open-mouth odontoid view reveals C1 and C2. The cross-table lateral view allows for inspection of the C1 to T1 spine malalignment or fracture and narrowing of the disk space. Widening of the disk space may indicate a posterior ligament tear. The right and left oblique views provide inspection of the neuroforamina and facets.[4] If plain x-rays suggest fracture, or if clinical suspicion for fracture or instability is high and plain films are non-diagnostic, additional studies including flexion-extension views, CT or MRI are indicated.

One half of patients with new-onset, acute cervical pain present without a history of trauma. In an alert patient with normal physical examination findings and absence of neck tenderness and neurologic deficits, diagnostic studies are unnecessary. However, patients with neck pain greater than 1 month's duration, arm pain, weakness, absent or diminished reflexes, or a history of spondylosis will benefit from MRI to exclude nerve damage, even in the absence of findings on plain x-rays.[6,7] It has been shown that 76% of these patients have had diagnostic abnormalities, although not all are clinically relevant. Electrophysiologic studies may be needed to assess patients with suspected radiculopathy (nerve root irritation) or myelopathy (spinal cord compromise).

TABLE 198-2 Neurologic Testing of Cervical Spine

Neurologic Level	Motor	Reflex
C5	Biceps Deltoid	Biceps
C6	Biceps Wrist extensors	Radial
C7	Triceps Wrist flexors Finger extensors	Triceps
C8	Finger flexors interossei muscles (abduct, adduct fingers)	None
T1	Interossei muscles	None

Diagnostics

Neck Pain

Imaging	**Other**
X-ray*	Electromyelogram*
CT scan or MRI*	

*If indicated.

DIFFERENTIAL DIAGNOSIS

Acute neck pain may become a chronic problem. Evaluation for fracture or subluxation after trauma may reveal degenerative changes, particularly in older adults. Infection of the bones due to septic arthritis, syphilis, or tuberculosis is an uncommon cause of cervical pain. Infection of the meninges will likely be accompanied by headache, fever, and cognitive deficits. A review of systems, past medical history, and physical examination may indicate that pain is referred.

MANAGEMENT

The goals of management are pain modification, maintaining or restoring strength and flexibility, and assistance with return-to-work issues. Immediate care of simple neck strain or chronic, aggravated disk herniation includes ice treatment for 15 minutes every 2 hours while awake, strategies for relaxation, and gentle range-of-motion exercises performed while showering or after medication. Simple activities of daily living are allowed; however, lifting, pulling, pushing, and lying on a couch are prohibited. Use of a cervical pillow, preferably water based, that aligns the spine in a lordotic position decreases pain and improves the quality of sleep.[8] Two or 3 days after injury, cervical resistance exercises and back strengthening exercises should begin. Nonsteroidal antiinflammatory drugs (NSAIDs), as well as low-dose muscle relaxants, will decrease pain and improve function. Narcotic pain medications may be necessary initially in some cases, but their use should be time limited. Trauma patients must be observed for deteriorating neurologic status; therefore muscle relaxants are contraindicated. Although soft collars are often used, their effectiveness in reducing persistent pain or the length of rehabilitation has not been proved.[9]

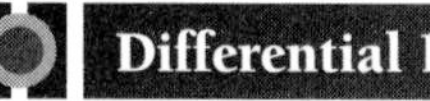

Neck Pain

Acute Neck Pain
- Dislocation/fracture/subluxation
- Disk herniation
- Arthritis (acute flair)
- Hematoma/myositis
- Infection
- Wry neck
- Myalgia
- Polio
- Subarachnoid hemorrhage
- Tetanus
- Referred pain from:
  - Aortic aneurysm
  - Heart/lung
  - Gallbladder
  - Brain/spinal cord (meningitis)

Chronic Neck Pain
- Osteoporosis/osteomalacia
- Osteitis of syphilis and osteophytes
- Paget's disease
- Tumor
- Tuberculosis
- Disk herniation
- Ankylosing spondylosis
- Osteoarthritis
- Chronic muscle sprain
- Fibromyalgia
- Trauma
- Headache
- Myofascial pain syndrome
- Referred pain from:
  - Aortic aneurysm
  - Cancer of esophagus
  - Carpal tunnel syndrome
  - Glenohumeral ganglion
  - Infection of mandible teeth/temporomandibular joint pain
- Lymph enlargement
- Spinal cord tumor

Co-Management with Specialists

Patients with a history of disk herniation should be wary of returning to work or beginning employment that requires heavy lifting or sitting in a position where posture is other than neutral until a work capacity evaluation is performed by a physical therapist and activity parameters are established. The work capacity evaluation will benefit the employee and employer by establishing realistic goals for return to work. If there is no improvement of pain within 3 days of an acute injury or if a patient complains of recurring pain, referral to a physical therapist for soft tissue mobilization, traction, muscle energy techniques, ultrasound treatment, electrical stimulation, and review of cervical as well as back exercises is indicated. Traction, provided by the physical therapist, is useful for chronic degenerative disease. Patients requiring a change in occupation will benefit from occupational therapy referral. Chiropractic manipulation may also be efficacious in the reduction of pain. If subjective pain symptoms and improved neurologic status do not occur after several physical therapy sessions, referral to a neurologist is indicated for patients with a herniated disk. The patient with facet subluxation will benefit from a minimum of six physical therapy visits. Symptom relief may require as many as 10 visits for patients with arthritis. Psychologic consultation may be helpful if depression, anxiety, or adjustment disorder complicates recovery.[10]

COMPLICATIONS

Simple muscle strain is usually self-limiting. Extension-flexion ("whiplash") injuries may result in continued pain, sometimes for years, possibly because of accelerated disk degeneration, facet disease, or other poorly understood mechanisms. Headache may develop as a result of tight, short muscles at the atlantoaxial junction. Altered proprioception and/or dizziness accompanies chronic neck pain. Exacerbation of injuries occurs with chronic poor posture, continued poor sleep habits, ergonomically unfit work sites, repeated trauma, or accelerated cervical deterioration. New-onset psychologic disturbances have been documented in more than 50% of patients with chronic neck pain.[10]

INDICATIONS FOR REFERRAL/HOSPITALIZATION

Supportive care in an emergency department and orthopedic or neurosurgical consultation are mandatory for all patients with a cervical fracture. Stabilization, traction, and immobilization are essential to decrease the potential for further injury.[5] C1 vertebral fracture is a life-threatening emergency. Immediate immobilization, stabilization, and transfer to an emergency department are indicated. Shallow dive injuries may cause C5 fractures resulting in quadriplegia and possibly death. Although rare, C7 fracture and ipsilateral pupil dilation may occur with rear-end whiplash. Trauma patients with neurologic deficits require immediate neurologic consultation. Chronic pain syndrome, characterized by prolonged disability or prescription drug use, may require referral to a chronic pain clinic. A small percentage of patients with neurologic symptoms may benefit from surgery. Consultation with a physiatrist is indicated for persistent point tenderness to evaluate the need for trigger point injections with lidocaine and/or steroids.

PATIENT AND FAMILY EDUCATION

Maintaining the neck in a neutral posture, demonstrating proper body mechanics, and performing daily back and neck exercises are important practices for patients with a history of neck pain and are essential for patients with a herniated disk. The use of a mirror enables the patient to correct his or her posture with visual feedback. The cervical spine is in correct position when the neck is in alignment with the thoracic spine rather than jutting forward. The shoulders should be relaxed, with the chest held forward and the mandible relaxed. If the patient can visualize a string on the top of the scalp, gently pulling the head superiorly, pressure may be alleviated.

New onset of arm or shoulder paresthesias or severe headache after an injury should be viewed as a warning to return for follow-up. Family members should be given a list of warning signs for decreased level of consciousness and instructed to seek emergency department care without hesitation. A medication education sheet and exercise sheet provide needed sources for reference. Finally, reassurance that discomfort is a normal part of recovery is helpful to patients and families.

HEALTH PROMOTION

Counseling concerning the avoidance of alcohol while swimming and diving, the use of properly adjusted seat belts and headrests, and the use of helmets while riding bicycles or motorcycles are important strategies for the prevention of neck injuries. Proper workplace ergonomics, sleeping posture, and reaching and lifting techniques also minimize stress on cervical structures.

REFERENCES

1. Squires B, Gargan MF, Bannister GC: Soft-tissue injuries of the cervical spine: 15-year follow-up, *J Bone Joint Surg Br* 78:955-957, 1996.
2. Lord SM and others: Chronic cervical zygapophysial joint pain after whiplash: a placebo-controlled prevalence study, *Spine* 21:1737-1745, 1996.
3. Marchiori DM, Henderson CN: A cross-sectional study correlating cervical radiographic degenerative findings to pain and disability, *Spine* 21:2747-2751, 1996.
4. Monahan JJ: Cervical spine. In Steinberg GG, Akins CM, Baran DT, editors: *Ramamurti's orthopaedics in primary care*, Baltimore, 1992, Williams & Wilkins.
5. Hussey RW: Spinal cord injuries. In May HL and others, editors: *Emergency medicine*, Boston 1992, Little, Brown.
6. Haldeman S: Diagnostic tests for the evaluation of back and neck pain, *Neurol Clin* 14:103-117, 1996.
7. Mirza SK, White AA III, Panjabi MM: The lower cervical spine: evaluating instability in cervical spine injuries, part 2, J *Musculoskel Med* 13:12-24, 1996.
8. Lavin RA, Pappagallo M, Kuhlemieer KV: Cervical pain: a comparison of three pillows, *Arch Phys Med Rehabil* 78:193-198, 1997.
9. Gennis P and others: The effect of soft cervical collars on persistent neck pain in patients with whiplash injury, *Acad Emerg Med* 3:568-573, 1996.
10. Radanov BP and others: Course of psychological variables in whiplash injury—a 2-year follow-up with age, gender and education pair-matched patients, *Pain* 64:429-434, 1996.

CHAPTER 199

Osteoarthritis

Ann S. Bruner-Welch

DEFINITION/EPIDEMIOLOGY

Osteoarthritis (OA) is a progressive degenerative joint process. It involves degeneration of the articular (hyaline) cartilage layer on the ends of bones at the joints.[1-3] OA presents as a mono or polyarticular phenomenon and is often asymmetric. Occasionally it can present as a more generalized disease.[4]

OA is the most common type of arthritis, and it usually begins asymptomatically in the second or third decade of life. By the fourth decade of life, most people have some degree of pathologic change on articular weight-bearing surfaces.[3-5] Symptoms typically begin to appear in the fourth through sixth decades of life. Some degree of symptomatic arthritis is extremely common by the seventh decade.[3-5] Men and women are equally affected.[3] Risk factors include obesity, prior trauma, genetics, repetitive activities, and metabolic, neurologic, or hematologic conditions.[2,4,5]

The carpal metacarpal (CMC) joints of the thumbs, distal interphalangeal (DIP) joints of the fingers, first metatarsophalangeal (MTP) joints of the feet, cervical and lumbar spine, and weight-bearing joints such as the hips and knees are most commonly affected.[1-3,5] It can also affect previously injured joints.[1,2,4,5] Pain, stiffness, and limited range of motion are the most common reasons for seeking medical care. The degenerative effects of OA result in physical disability and can have a profound impact on the quality of life.[5]

PATHOPHYSIOLOGY

Initially, the cartilage softens and becomes overhydrated and boggy, with decreased quantity and size of proteoglycans within the matrix.[3-5] Collagen also loses its stiffness with fewer cells and loss of crosslinks as degradation continues.[4,5] The surface layers fibrillate and the cartilage loses its thickness, develops surface crevices, and then loses integrity. Loose cartilaginous fragments (known as *loose bodies*) can flake off, blocking range of motion and contributing to pain and disability.[2,3,5]

Chondrocytes proliferate with increased metabolic activity as the subchondral bone scleroses under the damaged areas. It thickens, stiffens, and then produces cysts, microfractures, and osteophytes at the joint margins.[1-5] These later findings are often seen on radiographs. The associated increased metabolic activity can be picked up on a bone scan.

The cartilage surface is completely aneural, making the pathogenesis of pain from OA is speculative. It is thought to be secondary to increased venous pressure within the bony capillaries and irritation of surrounding supportive tissue.[2,3] As a result of the joint degradation, the joint capsule may also tighten, resulting in the development of a reactive synovitis and pain. This synovitis is usually sparse in cellular infiltrate and fibrotic in nature. However, it causes an effusion that can stretch and further destabilize the joint capsule.[6]

CLINICAL PRESENTATION AND PHYSICAL EXAMINATION

Insidious, progressive pain or stiffness of one or more joints may be the initial presenting complaint. Symptoms are most prevalent on arising and after a prolonged activity and relieved by rest.[1,3-5] Weight-bearing activities, such as going up or down stairs, getting up from a sitting position, walking, prolonged standing, or a change in activity level, can be particularly troublesome.[3-6] The patient may also complain of crepitus (grinding), swelling, and gradual loss of motion as the disease progresses.[2-4]

When OA involves the cervical or lumbar spine, neuropathy and radiculopathy may develop as nerves are compressed.[2,3] OA involving the hip presents with groin or buttock pain that can radiate to the knee.[2,3] The pain can cause the patient to "favor" the hip, which in turn can contribute to specific muscle weakness. The resultant gait is known as a Trendelenburg gait. OA of the knee involves the medial joint compartment 70% of the time, leading to a varus deformity of the extremity.[2,3] It can then progress to include the lateral joint compartment and patellofemoral articulations as well. Pain on palpation of the medial and lateral joint lines and joint effusions are often seen. Quadriceps muscle atrophy is common on the affected side.

OA of the hands presents as Heberden's nodes (deformity of the DIP joints) and Bouchard's nodes (deformity of the proximal interphalangeal [PIP] joints). A compression test, as well as pain with palpation of the joint, can detect OA of the CMC joint. Contracture, deformity, and even joint fusion are common as the disease progresses.[2] Fortunately, OA of the hands is seldom completely disabling.

DIAGNOSTICS

In the early stages of OA, radiographic findings may not be evident.[2,3,7] As the disease progresses and joint space is lost, radiographic changes become more prominent.[2-4] A bone scan may show increased metabolic activity within an arthritic joint.

OA is a nonsystemic disease. There are no serologic markers for OA, but serologic tests are commonly performed to rule out other disorders. See the Diagnostics box for optional testing.

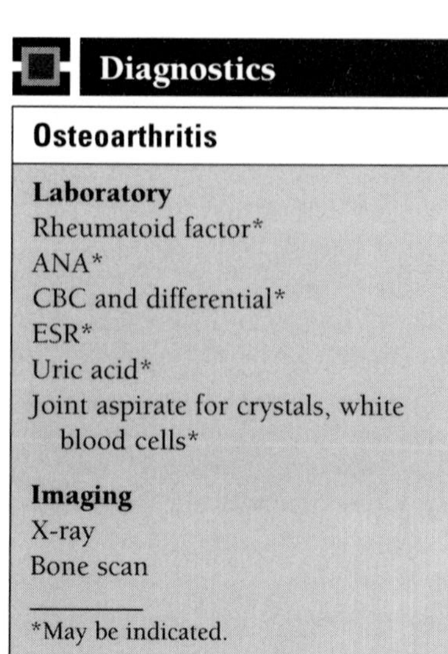

Diagnostics

Osteoarthritis

Laboratory
Rheumatoid factor*
ANA*
CBC and differential*
ESR*
Uric acid*
Joint aspirate for crystals, white blood cells*

Imaging
X-ray
Bone scan

*May be indicated.

DIFFERENTIAL DIAGNOSIS

The Differential Diagnosis box denotes other diseases that should also be considered and excluded when appropriate. Other arthritic conditions such as rheumatoid arthritis, gout, and pseudogout are commonly seen with OA.

MANAGEMENT

Strong Evidence for Good Benefit

Acetaminophen. Acetaminophen has long been the mainstay of initial

Differential Diagnosis

Osteoarthritis	
Lupus erythematosus	Arthritis
Lyme disease	Bursitis
Malignancy	Tendinitis
Fracture/dislocation	Gout
Neuropathy	Paget's disease
Osteomyelitis	Fibromyalgia
Osteonecrosis	Soft tissue disease
Avascular necrosis	

treatment for early OA. The analgesic properties can reduce discomfort without the additional risks of antiinflammatory medications.[2-4,7-10] One gram 4 times daily has been suggested.[3] The maximum daily dose is 4 g (1000 mg PO every 6 hours) for adults. Hepatotoxicity is a concern, particularly if acetaminophen is used in conjunction with alcohol. The maximum daily dose of acetaminophen in patients receiving warfarin therapy should not exceed 2500 mg PO.

Tramadol Hydrochloride (Ultram). Ultram is another nonopioid pain reliever that is indicated for moderate to moderately severe pain; Ultram is not a nonsteroidal antiinflammatory drug (NSAID). The packaging insert should be followed for dosing and precautions.[11] It is also available as a combination drug with acetaminophen. The combination is synergistic and can be given in addition to NSAIDs.

NSAIDs. NSAIDs have long been part of the treatment regimen for OA. NSAIDs are believed to be most beneficial for their analgesic rather than their antiinflammatory properties. The concern with NSAID therapy is the associated risk of gastrointestinal bleeding, especially in older adults.[2-6,8-10]

The COX-2 selective inhibitors were designed to reduce joint pain and inflammation with fewer adverse effects on the stomach or platelets.[12-20] The newer COX-2 specific antiinflammatory drugs have a gastrointestinal bleed rate equal to that of placebo in clinically controlled trials.[12,13] The safety and efficacy have been demonstrated in a number of double-blind, placebo-controlled studies; this includes use in cardiovascular and renally impaired patients.[12-20] Fluid retention is a potential side effect. In debilitated or older patients, kidney and liver function and blood pressure changes should be monitored closely.[13]

Despite the demonstrated safety and efficacy of COX inhibitors, many health insurance companies require traditional NSAIDs as first-line therapy and reserve the use of COX-2 specific medications for a select group of high-risk patients, including patients taking anticoagulant drugs, those with a history of gastrointestinal bleeding or peptic ulcer disease, or those receiving chronic steroid therapy.

Because there is some concern that patients on COX-2 inhibitors may have a higher incidence of vascular events, patients at risk of stroke or myocardial infarction should continue to receive prophylactic aspirin. Meloxicam (Mobic) is a preferential inhibitor of COX-2, but it is not a true COX-2 inhibitor according to the criteria of the Food and Drug Administration (FDA). Nonetheless, it seems to be well tolerated, with few side effects or drug-drug interactions.[20]

Of the traditional antiinflammatory drugs, choline salicylate/magnesium salicylate (Trilsate), etodolac (Lodine), salsalate (Disalcid), diclofenac/misoprostol (Arthrotec), and nabumetone (Relafen) are touted as having better gastrointestinal tolerance. They might be considered if the COX-2 drugs are not tolerated or available, particularly if a patient is going to be on long-term therapy. See Table 199-1 for NSAID dosing.

Good Evidence for Potential Benefit

Glucosamine with or without Chondroitin. Several studies now support the use of glucosamine for OA of the knees. The recommended dosage is 500 mg of glucosamine sulfate t.i.d. If patients fail to feel a benefit from this regimen, they may consider adding chondroitin with some improvement in symptoms. There are few side effects or known drug-drug interactions. Because it is a dietary supplement and is not regulated by the FDA, the potency and quality may not be consistent between different brands. If one brand is not helpful, the patient may try another with good results.[22-24]

Hyaluronans. Intraarticular injections of exogenous hyaluran can also help reduce the pain of OA of the knees.[25,26] It seems to be most effective in mild to moderate OA and acts as a lubricant as it improves viscosity within the joint. It has been compared favorably with naproxen (Naprosyn) in efficacy in double-blinded, placebo-controlled studies with fewer adverse reactions.[26] It is injected once a week for 3 to 5 weeks depending on the preparation, and it may provide benefit for 6 months or longer.[25,26]

Intraarticular Corticosteroid Injections. Intraarticular corticosteroid injections can also provide significant pain relief for mild to severe disease.[3,4] The duration of benefit varies widely. Even in severe disease, injections are not recommended more often than every 3 to 4 months. Caution should be used with patients who are on oral prednisone preparations or who have diabetes. All patients should be warned about transient increased pain, warmth, and/or redness of the joint after an injection. If these symptoms persist, the patient should seek follow-up.

Kenalog (triamcinolone acetonide) and Depo-Medrol (methylprednisolone acetate) are the preferred corticosteroid preparations because they remain in solution within the joint and do not leave behind crystalline particulate debris. Diabetic patients should be warned to expect a transient elevation in blood glucose levels for about 3 to 4 days.

Limited Evidence Exists for Benefit

Acupuncture. A growing body of evidence suggests that acupuncture may be beneficial as adjunctive treatment for OA as well as a number of other ailments.[27]

Other Medications Helpful for Chronic Pain. Other medications, such as gabapentin (Neurontin), selective serotonin reuptake inhibitors (SSRIs), and tricyclic antidepressants (TCAs), have also been used successfully in the management of chronic pain associated with OA.[28]

TABLE 199-1 Nonsteroidal Antiinflammatory Cost Analysis and Dosing Chart

Class	Medication	OA Dosing	
Cox 2 Inhibitor	Celebrex (celecoxib)	100 mg q.d.-b.i.d. $2.00/pill $2.00-$4.00/day	200 mg q.d. $2.00/pill $2.00/day
	Vioxx (rofecoxib)	12.5 mg q.d.-b.i.d. $2.00/pill $2.00-$4.00/day	25 mg q.d. $2.00/pill $2.00/day
	Bextra (valdecoxib)	10 mg q.d. $3.60/pill $3.60/day	
Indoleacetic Acid and Related Compounds	Clinoril (sulindac)	150 mg b.i.d. $1.25/pill $2.50/day	200 mg b.i.d. $1.40/pill $2.80/day
	Indocin (indomethacin)	25 mg b.i.d.-t.i.d. $0.66/pill $1.22-$1.88/day	50 mg b.i.d.-t.i.d. $1.05/pill $2.10-$3.15/day
	Indocin SR (indomethacin)	75 mg q.d. $1.70/pill $1.70/day	
	Lodine (etodolac)	300 mg b.i.d. $1.55/pill $3.10/day	500 mg b.i.d. $1.55/pill $3.10/day
	Lodine XL (etodolac)	400-1000 mg q.d.	
Naphthylalkanone	Relafen (nabumetone)	500 mg b.i.d. $1.20/pill $2.40/day	750 mg b.i.d. $1.40/pill $2.80/day
NSAID/GI Mucosal Protective Combo.	Arthrotec (diclofenac/misoprostol)	50 mg q.d. $1.40/pill $1.40/day	75 mg q.d. $1.40/pill $1.40/day
Oxicams	Feldene (piroxicam)	10 mg b.i.d. $1.75/pill $3.50/day	20 mg q.d. $2.87/pill $2.87/day
	Mobic (meloxicam)	7.5 mg q.d.-b.i.d. $1.90/pill $1.90-$3.80/day	
Phenylacetic Acids	Cataflam (diclofenac potassium)	50 mg b.i.d.-t.i.d. $1.85/pill $3.70-$5.55/day	
	Voltaren (diclofenac sodium)	50 mg b.i.d.-t.i.d. $1.21/pill $2.40-$3.60/day	75 mg b.i.d. $1.45/pill $2.90/day
	Voltaren XR (diclofenac)	100 mg q.d.	

Data from Searle: Quick Reference to selected branded prescription nonsteroidal agents, 2000; and Epocrates palm reference, www.ePocrates.com October 2001.

Evidence and Benefits Unclear

MSM (methyl sulfonyl methane) and SAM-e (S-adenosyl methionine) are other dietary supplements that a number of patients with OA are trying to help control the pain of moderate to severe disease.[28] Therapeutic magnets are touted to help reduce the chronic pain of OA. Although there is no current scientific evidence to support their efficacy, they seem to cause no further harm other than to the pocketbook. There is anecdotal evidence that some patients may benefit.

Nonpharmacologic Measures

Exercise has a number of potential benefits for OA management. Aerobic exercise can help with cardiovascular conditioning as well as weight reduction (if indicated). Physical and/or occupational therapy can improve muscle strength and

TABLE 199-1 Nonsteroidal Antiinflammatory Cost Analysis and Dosing Chart—cont'd

Class	Medication	OA Dosing		
Propionic Acids	Anaprox (naproxen sodium)	275 mg t.i.d.-q.i.d. $0.85/pill $2.55-$3.40/day		
	Anaprox DS (naproxen sodium)	550 mg q.d.-b.i.d. $1.33/pill $1.33-$2.66/day		
	Ansaid (fluriprofen)	50 mg b.i.d.-t.i.d. $1.22/pill $2.44-$3.66/day	100 mg b.i.d.-t.i.d. $1.75/pill $3.50-$4.25/day	
	Daypro (oxaprozin)	2-600 mg q.d. $1.42/pill $1.42/day		
	Motrin (ibuprofen)	400 mg t.i.d.-q.i.d. $0.30/pill $0.90-$1.20/day	600 mg t.i.d.-q.i.d.	800 mg t.i.d.-q.i.d.
	Naprelan (Naproxen sodium)	2-375 mg q.d. $1.33/pill $2.66/day	2-500 mg q.d. $1.66/pill $3.22/day	
	Naprosyn (naproxen)	250 mg b.i.d. $0.84/pill $1.68/day	500 mg b.i.d. $1.20/pill $2.40/day	
	Orudis (ketoprofen)	75 mg t.i.d. $1.27/pill $3.81/day		
	Oruvail (ketoprofen)	100-200 q.d.		
	Toradol (ketorolac)	10 mg q.i.d. $1.00/pill $4.00/day		
Pyrroleacetic Acids	Tolectin (tolmetin)	200 mg 1-3 t.i.d. $0.74/pill $2.25-$6.66/day	600 mg t.i.d. $1.58/pill $4.74/day	
Salicylic Acids	Disalcid (salsalate)	500 mg 2 t.i.d. $0.62/pill $2.48/day	750 mg q.i.d. $0.79/pill $3.16/day	
	Dolobid (diflunisal)	250 mg b.i.d. $1.14/pill $2.28/day	500 mg b.i.d. $1.42/pill $2.83/day	
	Trilsate (choline magnesium trisalicylate)	500 mg 3 b.i.d. $0.97/pill $3.60/day	750 mg t.i.d. $1.50/pill $2.91	

functional capacity. Stretching programs can help re-balance joints and reduce contractures that lead to excess joint wear. Supportive, well-cushioned shoe wear with lifts or wedges can help adjust for angular deformities. Assistive devices such as canes or walkers can help reduce the load of lower extremity joints.[1-10] Heat and/or ice may also provide symptomatic relief and improve exercise tolerance.

LIFE SPAN CONSIDERATIONS

OA is not a terminal disease, but it can cause significant disability. The primary goal of management, both conservative and surgical, is to improve the quality of life. See Management for specific recommendations.

COMPLICATIONS

Pain and immobility that affect the patient's functional capacity and quality of life are the main complications associated with OA.

Other complications are directly related to the treatment of the disease, including medication side effects, infection or microfractures of damaged joints, or failure involving prosthetic components.

INDICATIONS FOR REFERRAL/HOSPITALIZATION

When conservative measures fail, the patient's quality of life can be significantly diminished. Frequent or constant disabling pain, especially pain at rest, and functionally limiting symptoms are the most important criteria for orthopedic consultation.[1-10]

There are a number of pain-relieving procedures that can be done in a specialty office, including conservative measures such as repeat intraarticular corticosteroid injections or bracing. Arthroscopic surgical procedures can include joint lavage, partial medial or lateral meniscectomy or chondroplasty as indicated, lateral patellar retinacular release, fracture drilling of full-thickness defects, or chondral grafts. Larger or open surgical procedures could include osteotomy and partial or total joint arthroplasty.[7]

Once a patient has undergone total joint replacement, long-term management may include prophylactic antibiotics for dental work or endoscopy. This remains controversial and should be based on local protocols. Annual x-rays to evaluate the position and fixation of prosthetic components may also be recommended.[29]

Researchers continue to develop new technologies to manage this disease. Newer medications, different prosthetic joint components, osteochondral replacement procedures, and gene therapy for rare hereditary forms of OA are some of the newer treatment modalities being evaluated.[8]

PATIENT AND FAMILY EDUCATION

The treatment of OA is comprehensive and should begin with a clear explanation of the disease process and likely progression of the disease. Instruction on joint protection or lifestyle modification to protect the painful joint should include job or lifestyle modifications. The use of assistive devices, such as a cane, crutches, or a walker, can be helpful. Patients are encouraged to be realistic about their limitations to avoid exacerbations of symptoms.[1-10]

There are a number of good websites on the Internet that can help further educate the patient on the disease process as well as newer treatment options.

HEALTH PROMOTION

Obesity and repetitive stress/trauma are specific modifiable risk factors for the development of OA; reduction in one or both may substantially reduce symptoms and disease progression.[2,3] Maintaining an active lifestyle can significantly improve the quality of life for these individuals.

REFERENCES

1. Snider RK: *Essentials of musculoskeletal care,* Park Ridge, Ill, 1997, American Academy of Orthopedic Surgeons.
2. Cecil RL, Goldman L, Bennett JC: *Cecil's textbook of medicine,* ed 21, Philadelphia, 2000, WB Saunders.
3. Beers M and others: *The Merck manual of diagnosis and therapy,* ed 17, Rahway, NJ, 1999, Merck & Co.
4. Loeser RF: Aging and the etiopathogenesis and treatment of osteoarthritis, *Rheum Dis Clin North Am* 26:547-567, 2000.
5. Fife RS: Osteoarthritis and related diseases, *Best Practice of Medicine,* 2002. Retrieved August 12, 2002, from the World Wide Web: http://www.merck.praxis.md/bpm/bpm.asp?page=CPM02RH401§ion=report&ss=2&hilight=Fife.
6. Bluestone R: Assessing the patient with OA: a regional approach, *J Musculoskel Med* (suppl):7, 1996.
7. Felson DT: The course of osteoarthritis and factors that affect it, *Rheum Dis Clin North Am* 19:607-615, 1993.
8. Ramont IL: *Clinical guidelines on hip pain,* American Academy of Orthopedic Surgeons/American Association of Neurologic Surgeons/American College of Rheumatology/American College of Physical Medicine and Rehabilitation; 1999 National Guidelines Clearinghouse. Retrieved August 12, 2002, from the World Wide Web: http://www.guideline.gov.
9. *Clinical guidelines to knee pain,* American Academy of Orthopedic Surgeons/American Association of Neurologic Surgeons/American College of Rheumatology/American College of Physical Medicine and Rehabilitation; 1999 National Guidelines Clearinghouse. Retrieved August 12, 2002, from the World Wide Web: http://www.guideline.gov.
10. *Clinical guidelines on wrist pain,* American Academy of Orthopedic Surgeons/American Association of Neurologic Surgeons/American College of Rheumatology/American College of Physical Medicine and Rehabilitation; 1999 National Guidelines Clearinghouse. Retrieved August 12, 2002, from the World Wide Web: http://www.guideline.gov.
11. Ortho-McNeil Pharmaceutical, Inc: *Information for you about Ultram,* Raitan, NJ, December 1999, Ortho-McNeil Pharmaceutical, Inc.
12. Silverstein FE and others: Gastrointestinal toxicity with celecoxib vs nonsteroidal anti-inflammatory drugs for osteoarthritis and rheumatoid arthritis: the CLASS study: a randomized controlled trial. Celecoxib Long-term Arthritis Safety Study, *JAMA* 284:1247-1255, 2000.
13. Bombardeoer C and others: Comparison of upper gastrointestinal toxicity of rofecoxib and naproxen in patients with rheumatoid arthritis: VIGOR Study Group, *N Engl J Med* 343:1520-1528, 2000.
14. Lipsky and others: Analysis of the effect of Cox-2 specific inhibitors and recommendations for their use in clinical practice, *J Rheumatol* 27:6, 2000.
15. Rossat J and others: Renal effects of selective cyclooxygenase-2 inhibition in normotensive salt-depleted subjects, *Clin Pharmacol Ther* 7:76-84, 1999.
16. Whelton A and others: Cyclooxygenase-2-specific inhibitors and cardiorenal function: a randomized, controlled trial of celecoxib and rofecoxib in older hypertensive osteoarthritis patients, *Am J Ther* 8: 85-95, 2001.
17. Goldstein JL, Moskowitz R: *Cox-2 inhibitors in arthritis management: data driven clinical decisions,* audioconference, October 2000. Sponsored by the University of Texas Southwestern Medical Center at Dallas, and supported by an unrestricted educational grant from Pharmacia and Pfizer, Inc.
18. Moskowitz R and others: *The use of Cox-2 specific inhibitors in patients with renal and/or cardiovascular risk factors,* audioconference, August 1, 2001. Sponsored by the University of Texas Southwestern Medical Center at Dallas, and supported by an unrestricted educational grant from Pharmacia and Pfizer, Inc.
19. Simon LS, Gitlin N: Challenges in the management of osteoarthritis: a case-based discussion, interactive program, August 2, 2001. Presented by the Foundation of Better Health Care in Santa Rosa, Calif, for and with local physicians and health care provider participation.
20. Hawkey C and others: Gastrointestinal tolerability of meloxicam compared to diclofenac in osteoarthritis patients, *Br J Rheumatol* 37:937-945, 1998.
21. Blue Cross of California, Health Net, and Health Plan of the Redwoods: *Prior authorization for selective Cox-2 NSAIDs,* April 2000, Blue Cross.
22. Reginster JY and others: Long term effects of glucosamine sulfate on osteoarthritis progression: a randomized, placebo controlled clinical trial, *Lancet* 357:251-256, 2001.
23. McAlindon T: Glucosamine for osteoarthritis: dawn of a new era? *Lancet* 357:247-248, 2001.
24. McAlindon TE and others: Glucosamine and chondroitin for treatment of osteoarthritis: a systematic quality assessment and meta-analysis, *JAMA* 283:1469-1475, 2000.
25. Scali JJ: Intra-articular hyaluronic acid in the treatment of osteoarthritis of the knee: a long term study, *Eur J Rheumatol Inflamm* 15(1): 1995.

26. Oster DM and others: *The evolving treatment of osteoarthritis of the knee: a new perspective on hyaluronans*, a CME Satellite Symposium, February 28, 2001.
27. Acupuncture Office of Medical Applications of Research (NIH)/ National Center for Complimentary and Alternative Medicine, 1997, National Guidelines Clearinghouse. Retrieved August 12, 2002, from the World Wide Web: http://www.guideline.gov.
28. Schneider MS: *Pain perception and management*, Cortext educational seminar, August 6, 2001. Cortext Educational Seminars, a division of Medical Education Collaborative, CorText/Mind Matters Educational Seminars (888) 671-9335; website: http://www.cortext.com.
29. Total hip replacement, Office of Medical Applications of Research (NIH)/National Institute of Arthritis and Musculoskeletal and Skin Diseases, September 1994 (reviewed 1998), National Guidelines Clearinghouse. Retrieved August 12, 2002, from the World Wide Web: http://www.guideline.gov.

CHAPTER 200

Osteomyelitis

Thomas H. Taylor

DEFINITION/EPIDEMIOLOGY

Infection of bone has been classically divided into three groups: (1) hematogenous osteomyelitis, seeded from bacteremia; (2) osteomyelitis associated with a contiguous focus, such as a puncture wound, foreign body, or adjoining soft tissue infection; and (3) osteomyelitis associated with peripheral vascular disease, such as diabetic foot infections or other vascular insufficiency.[1] Osteomyelitis may be further divided into acute and chronic varieties. *Acute* disease is defined by the sudden onset of inflammation, warmth, redness, and edema. Hematogenous osteomyelitis in the young is most likely to present acutely, usually with one organism seeding the medullary cavity, and a good prognosis can be predicted. Children between 1 and 15 years of age and adults older than 50 are predisposed to hematogenous osteomyelitis. There is an increasing incidence of acute osteomyelitis throughout childhood and into adolescence.[2] Osteomyelitis with vascular insufficiency in older adults is more likely to present as *chronic* or indolent infection. An external focus erodes the superficial periosteum. The flora are usually mixed, and the prognosis varies greatly with factors such as the extent of bone involvement, sequestra, organisms, and host conditions. Acute osteomyelitis not diagnosed or treated well will advance to chronic osteomyelitis, resulting in a poorer prognosis and complications in approximately 5% of patients.

More recent classification by Cierny and others[3] takes into consideration the extent of anatomic involvement and systemic or local factors, providing a guide to determining the prognosis, the extent of surgical intervention, and antibiotic treatment. Various anatomic stages require further surgical resection, revascularization, muscle flaps, skin grafts, management of dead space, and bone grafts, as outlined in Table 200-1. Physiologic class is defined by A, B, or C hosts.[4] A favorable prognosis accompanies A hosts with normal vasculature and metabolic factors and a normal immune system. B hosts carry a worse prognosis by virtue of local or systemic compromise. Systemic factors, such as diabetes, smoking, malnutrition, hypoxia, immunosuppression, and immunodeficiency, must be addressed. Local factors, such as lymphadema, venous stasis, arterial insufficiency, and sensory deficits, must be managed (Box 200-1). Revascularization, in terms of vascular grafts or muscle flaps, is crucial. The Cierny-Mader staging system is important to medical and surgical management but also guides prognosis and education.

PATHOPHYSIOLOGY

Metaphyseal bone, just beneath the epiphysis, or growth plate, is where growing beds of terminal arterioles are prone to deposition of bacteria. Thus the ends of long bones are the most common location of hematogenous osteomyelitis in young patients. In children the infection spreads laterally, beneath the epiphysis, through the thin cortex, and under loosely applied

TABLE 200-1 Anatomic Classification of Adult Long Bone Osteomyelitis (Cierny-Mader System)

Stage	Description	Etiologies	Treatment
I. *Medullary*	Necrosis limited to medullary contents and endosteal surfaces	Hematogenous infection	**Pediatric**—Antibiotics; host alteration (e.g., nutritional support) **Adult**—Unroofing; intramedullary reaming
II. *Superficial*	Bone necrosis limited to exposed surface	Contiguous soft tissue infection	**Pediatric**—Antibiotics; host alteration **Adult**—Superficial debridement; local or microvascular flap coverage; possible ablation
III. *Localized*	Full-thickness cortical sequestration; infection is well marginated, and bone is stable before and after debridement	Trauma; evolution of stage I or II; iatrogenic	Antibiotics; host alteration; debridement; dead-space management; temporary stabilization; bone graft optional
IV. *Diffuse*	Circumferential and/or permeative infection; bone is unstable before or after debridement	Trauma; evolution of stage I or II; iatrogenic	Antibiotics; host alteration; debridement; dead-space management; stabilization (internal or external fixation); possible ablation

Modified from Mader JT, Calhoun J: Long-bone osteomyelitis, diagnoses, and management, *Hosp Pract* 29(10):71-76, 1994.

BOX 200-1

PHYSIOLOGIC CLASSIFICATION OF HOSTS WITH OSTEOMYELITIS (CIERNY-MADER SYSTEM)

A—Normal hosts with osteomyelitis

B_S—Systemic compromise
- Diabetes mellitus
- Extremes of age
- Hypoxia (chronic)
- Immunosuppression
- Immune deficiency
- Malignancy
- Malnutrition
- Renal failure
- Hepatic failure

B_L—Local compromise
- Arteritis
- Extensive scarring
- Sensory loss
- Lymphedema
- Major-vessel compromise
- Small-vessel disease
- Venous stasis
- Tissue irradiation
- Tobacco abuse

C—Fragile host: treatment worse than osteomyelitis

periosteum, giving rise to the characteristic *involucrum,* or subperiosteal abscess. *Brodie's abscess* is a central cortical abscess with a surrounding rim of reactive bone that is more common in adolescents and adults. As the epiphysis closes and capillary loops mature, more central metaphyseal and diaphyseal locations become common. Now the periosteum is firmly adherent to less vulnerable thick cortex, and infection is contained within metaphyseal bone, forming *sequestrum,* or central nidus of dead bone.[5]

Infecting organisms also differ according to the age of the patient, contiguous or hematogenous focus, and host condition. A single focus and a single organism are the norm for hematogenous osteomyelitis. Infants most often harbor *Staphylococcus aureus,* group A and B streptococci, and gram-negative enteric organisms. Children over the age of 1 have most often been infected with *Staphylococcus aureus* and *Streptococcus pyogenes.* With the advent of Hib conjugate vaccine, *Haemophilus influenzae* is now uncommon in children over the age of 1 year. *S. aureus* is dominant in both hematogenous and contiguous focus osteomyelitis, but vascular insufficiency with chronic ulcer causes mixed infection with *S. aureus,* streptococci, anaerobes, and gram-negative bacilli.[6]

CLINICAL PRESENTATION

Acute hematogenous osteomyelitis in children or young adults is associated with fever, leukocytosis, local edema, erythema, and tenderness. A soft tissue abscess and sinus tract, sometimes exiting many centimeters from the infected bone, may cause practitioners not to consider deeper infection of bone. The fever may be quite indolent and mild, or high and spiking. On the other hand, chronic osteomyelitis is seldom associated with fever or leukocytosis. Adjacent ulcer and soft tissue cellulitis may mask bone tenderness. In such a situation, the diagnosis of chronic osteomyelitis is difficult. Subacute presentation of osteomyelitis may challenge primary care providers caring for patients with fever of unknown origin.

PHYSICAL EXAMINATION

Physical findings are indistinguishable from the clinical presentation. Deep palpation may be necessary to elicit bone tenderness. Ulcers with visible bone or sinus tracks that probe to bone are diagnostic of osteomyelitis.[7] Special situations and clinical syndromes are important to recognize and are briefly discussed.

Vertebral Osteomyelitis

Low back pain is a common problem for which a precise source may not be discovered in 80% of patients. Primary care providers should be content with ambiguity, but warning signs merit further investigation[8] (Box 200-2). Osteomyelitis may be recognized by a radiologic process that involves both sides of the disk and adjacent vertebrae symmetrically. Malignancy does not cross the disk to involve adjacent vertebrae.[9] Early recognition is important because posterior extension causes epidural abscess and cord compression. Collapsed vertebrae may also threaten the spinal cord. The course may be complicated by paravertebral, retropharyngeal, mediastinal, and subphrenic abscesses, which must be drained.[10]

Pyogenic vertebral osteomyelitis is common in adults and is usually hematogenous and insidious in onset. Pain evolves gradually over weeks to months. Fever and leukocytosis are absent in 50% of cases. Although *S. aureus* is the predominant organism, a

BOX 200-2

LOW BACK PAIN: WARNING SIGNS SUGGESTING MALIGNANCY OR OSTEOMYELITIS

- Previous cancer
- Weight loss
- Elevated erythrocyte sedimentation rate (ESR)
- Fever, other constitutional symptoms
- Localized tenderness over vertebral body
- Lack of positional relief
- Lack of improvement over time
- Distant foci of infection (endocarditis)
- Indwelling IV catheters
- IV drug abuse
- Neurologic signs (weakness, sensory loss, asymmetric reflexes, loss of bowel or bladder function)

unique feature of vertebral osteomyelitis is a relatively high rate (30%) of gram-negative infection with a urinary focus in older patients.[11] Young patients with *Pseudomonas aeruginosa* may attribute their vertebral osteomyelitis to IV drug use. Unusual pathogens, such as *Candida* species, other fungi, mycobacteria, and gram-negative organisms, emphasize the need to make an etiologic diagnosis if treatment is to be successful.

Diabetic Foot

A diabetic foot ulcer is the best example of contiguous focus osteomyelitis and vascular insufficiency. Although the pulses may be palpable and arterial Doppler studies show good waveforms, 60% of these lesions are associated with relatively high-grade large-vessel obstruction on arteriography.[12] Thus, recognition of arterial insufficiency and revascularization are important. In the age of diagnostic-related categories for reimbursement and short hospital stays, the role of amputation in diabetes has, unfortunately, increased. Primary care providers must promote prevention, early recognition, and adequate care of diabetic foot ulcers.[13]

Recognition of osteomyelitis in a diabetic foot may be difficult. Ingrown toenails, stubborn cellulitis, neuropathic ulcer, and simple edema can be associated signs. Concurrent peripheral neuropathy will mask focal tenderness. Fever, leukocytosis, increasing hyperglycemia, and systemic toxicity may all be absent. Because of reactive bone formation in neuropathic feet (Charcot's joint), both plain films and bone scans are problematic.[14] Biopsy of bone is the definitive diagnostic study and supplies good microbiology to direct antibiotic treatment.[15] However, poor healing at the biopsy site may lead to further compromise of the foot. Thus empiric therapy is often undertaken unless debridement is indicated by anatomic criteria. Failure of therapy in later stages is greater than 50%. In those cases, suppression with oral antibiotics or amputation may be a reasonable alternative.[16]

Pseudomonas Infection

Pseudomonas osteomyelitis of the foot in children is a unique form of infection following a puncture wound such as a nail through the shoe. Sneakers provide a wet, fertile environment for *Pseudomonas aeruginosa*. The resultant acute osteochondritis presents within days, before osteomyelitis has really established itself. Thus a few days of an IV antipseudomonal antibiotic followed by oral antibiotics is effective.[17] *Pseudomonas* and *Serratia* are associated with IV drug abuse and may involve unusual sites, such as sacroiliac, sternoclavicular, pubic joints, and contiguous bone.

Salmonella Infection

Patients with sickle cell disease are susceptible to osteomyelitis because an expanded bone marrow with marginal sinusoidal blood flow causes ischemic foci for bacteria to seed. Bowel ischemia, due to intravascular sickling, encourages enteric flora to enter the circulation. *S. aureus* is most common, but enteric gram-negative organisms, especially *Salmonella* organisms, are often encountered.[18]

DIAGNOSTICS

Given the spectrum of disease and varied microbiology of osteomyelitis, cultures of bone and blood are essential to diagnosis and management. Cultures from sinus tracts or ulcers are not indicative of organisms in underlying bone.[19,20] Blood cultures are positive in 40% of cases of acute osteomyelitis but are rarely positive in chronic osteomyelitis. In adults with contiguous focus chronic osteomyelitis, culture specimens can be obtained with surgical debridement from bone and soft tissue. Leukocyte counts and erythrocyte sedimentation rates (ESRs) are elevated in acute disease and should be monitored for improvement. Visible bone or sinus tracts that probe to bone are diagnostic of chronic osteomyelitis.[7] Radiographic plain films usually begin to demonstrate destructive processes within 2 weeks of onset in acute osteomyelitis. They are helpful in determining extent and activity in chronic osteomyelitis but may be difficult to interpret in the diabetic foot, where neuropathic osteoarthritis is common. Plain films are sufficient follow-up for well-treated disease. The primary care provider should complete all the above-mentioned studies.

In cases where conventional radiography is ambiguous (i.e., at less than 2 weeks in acute osteomyelitis or with confounding bone disease in chronic osteomyelitis), radiographs may be followed by a technetium bone scan. Bone scans have high sensitivity (90%) but low specificity (70%) because of their inability to distinguish fracture, osteoarthritis, tumor, gouty tophi, and neuropathic bone formation from infection. Gallium scans or indium leukocyte scans provide greater specificity: gallium binds to transferrin and other proteins associated with inflammation

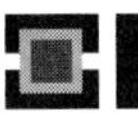
Diagnostics

Osteomyelitis

Laboratory
CBC and differential
Blood cultures
ESR

Imaging
X-ray
Bone scan*
Gallium or indium scan*
CT scan/MRI*

Other
Open bone biopsy or needle aspiration of bone with culture and sensitivity*

*If indicated.

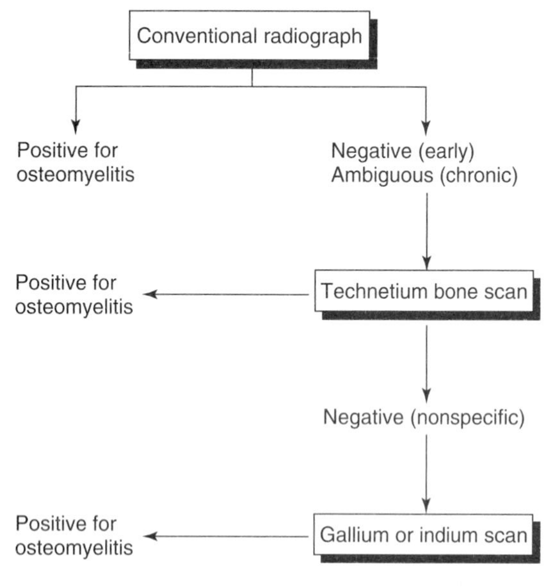

FIGURE 200-1

Imaging studies in osteomyelitis.

or infection, indium-labeled leukocytes are uniquely focused in sites of infection. The disadvantages of gallium scans are poor imaging detail and the need to wait 48 to 72 hours after injection before imaging. The disadvantages of indium scans are the expense of white blood cell labeling and the need to draw 40 ml of blood from the patient for in vitro labeling.[9,21]

Radionucleotide scans (technetium, gallium, indium) do not show anatomic detail. If surgery is contemplated in an adult with chronic or acute osteomyelitis, then CT or MRI will best define sequestra, the anatomic stage, and associated abscess. Both allow for guided needle aspiration of bone. A CT scan is the modality of choice to define bone sequestra, cortical erosion, and anatomical stage, but MRI may be preferred in cases of vertebral osteomyelitis or diabetic foot because of its better soft tissue resolution. Both imaging modalities are disturbed by metallic joint prostheses or internal fixation hardware.[9,21] Traumatic changes and neoplasm may not be distinguishable from osteomyelitis (Figure 200-1).

DIFFERENTIAL DIAGNOSIS

Osteomyelitis at the metaphysis of long bones approximates the joint and must be distinguished from septic arthritis. Examination for joint effusion and arthrocentesis will diagnose a septic joint, and radiologically the bone will be normal. Gout may cause cystic erosion in bone associated with a draining tophus. Although cultures are often positive for skin flora, the drainage is laden with crystals rather than neutrophils. Tophaceous gout is antibacterial and unlikely to be infected. Bone infarcts in hemoglobinopathy are multiple and recurrent, unlike the case with unifocal osteomyelitis. Posttraumatic periosteal reaction may mimic early osteomyelitis radiologically or may serve as a site for osteomyelitis secondary to recent trauma. Nonspecific periosteal or cortical change due to adjacent bursitis, abscess, or ulcer is difficult to distinguish from contiguous focus osteomyelitis. Tumor may or may not have distinguishing features on plain films. Old, inactive osteomyelitis may be indistinguishable from active infection radiologically. Finally, a focus of osteomyelitis secondary to subacute bacterial endocarditis must be considered if blood cultures are positive and a new cardiac murmur is appreciated.

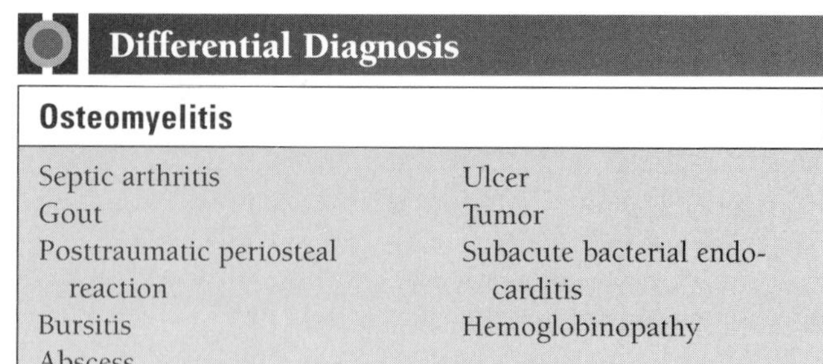

Differential Diagnosis

Osteomyelitis

Septic arthritis	Ulcer
Gout	Tumor
Posttraumatic periosteal reaction	Subacute bacterial endocarditis
Bursitis	Hemoglobinopathy
Abscess	

MANAGEMENT

Anatomic considerations define surgical management. Antibiotics alone often manage acute hematogenous medullary infection in children. Later stages with involucrum will need to be surgically unroofed. All more destructive stages require surgical intervention as defined in Figure 200-1, as well as prolonged antibiotic therapy based on the sensitivity of organisms obtained by culture of bone at surgery. In stage IV disease, extensive removal of infected bone may require orthopedic rod internal fixation, external fixation, bone graft, and dead space management with antibiotic-impregnated beads and two-phase joint replacement. Plastic surgery may be required to bring skin grafts or tissue flaps over bone to fill defects and revascularize. Vascular surgery may be required to revascularize with bypass grafts or to reroute major vessels away from infected areas.

For the most part, osteomyelitis is treated with 4 to 6 weeks of IV antibiotic therapy and will require placement of a central line.[22] Innovative home infusion pumps allow for early discharge but require a visiting nurse or patient education to administer.[23,24] Occasionally, sensitive organisms will respond to oral antibiotics, but serum bactericidal levels of antibiotics in blood should be determined before discharge.[25] Children with acute osteomyelitis may be successfully treated with oral antibiotics, after 5 to 10 days of parenteral antibiotic.[26] The doses of oral penicillins and cephalosporins are higher than doses used for common infection. Adults may not tolerate these doses, and only fluoroquinalones and clindamycin for sensitive pathogens have proven efficacy for oral regimens in adults.[27]

As opposed to vertebral osteomyelitis, in which hematogenous focus yields a single organism, diabetic contiguous focus osteomyelitis yields mixed flora. Counterintuitively, the organisms and antibiotic coverage are easier to predict. Coagulase-positive and -negative staphylococci, streptococci, anaerobes, and gram-negative bacilli are predictably present in necrotic tissue. An accompanying cellulitis is usually due to streptococci or staphylococci and may be treated with nafcillin or cefazolin alone. However, to treat the ulcer or underlying osteomyelitis, coverage of all organisms is necessary (i.e., monotherapy with cefotetin, ampicillin/sulbactam, ticarcillin/clavulanate, piperacillin/tazobactam, or imipenem/cilastatin). Oral therapy with ciprofloxacin/clindamycin combination therapy, new oral fluoroquinolones (gatifloxacin, moxifloxacin, trovafloxacin), or amoxicillin/

TABLE 200-2 Empiric Therapy of Osteomyelitis in Adults

Classification	Organism	Antibiotic
Acute hematogenous osteomyelitis	*Staphylococcus aureus,* streptococci	Nafcillin, cefazolin
Contiguous focus vascular insufficiency, diabetic foot, neuropathic ulcer	*S. aureus,* steptococci, gram-negative bacilli, anaerobes	Cefotetin, ampicillin/sulbactam, ticarcillin/clavulanate, piperacillin/tazobactam, imipenem/cilastatin

Additional considerations in special hosts:
IV drug abuse: *S. aureus, Pseudomonas, Serratia, Enterobacter* organisms
Hemoglobinopathies: *Salmonella* organisms
Immunosuppression: *Enterobacter,* mycobacteria, fungi

clavulanate may be used in some infections.[28] Diabetics who have been soaking their ulcer in tap water, which is not advised, may have acquired *Pseudomonas* organisms. This will necessitate the addition of an antipseudomonal antibiotic, such as piperacillin, ceftazidime, or ciprofloxacin[29] (Table 200-2). Aminoglycosides have poor penetration into bone and do not work well in abscesses, where pH is low.

The primary care provider must follow the patient for allergic reaction and toxicity of antibiotics, diarrhea due to *Clostridium difficile,* thrombosis and infection of central lines, and response to therapy. Central lines should be removed soon after completion of antibiotics so as not to provide a focus for further infection. Primary care should address nutrition, control of diabetes, reduction of immunosuppressive drugs, rehabilitation for alcohol and substance abuse, smoking cessation in vascular insufficiency, treatment of ulcers, and monitoring patients who are at high risk for the development of foot infection. Regular visits to a podiatrist may provide nail care, attention to footwear, wound care, and prophylactic surgery.[30]

LIFE SPAN CONSIDERATIONS

Osteomyelitis is usually not a lethal infection, but associated sepsis may be life threatening. Amputation is a special problem that may require physical therapy, prosthetics, and psychiatric counseling. Chronic use of a suppressive antibiotic is an option if surgery is too life threatening or amputation is being contemplated with understandable reluctance. The patient's quality of life is certainly altered by amputation. However, primary care providers may need to provide information regarding below-the-knee amputation and a prosthesis, which may be more functional than a chronically draining site of osteomyelitis in a foot with marginal blood flow.

COMPLICATIONS

Failure of aggressive therapy and relapse are common in patients with diabetes or vascular insufficiency or in compromised hosts. *S. aureus* is noted for associated cellulitis, sepsis, and metastatic foci of infection. Fracture through advanced anatomic disease should be preventable by orthopedic evaluation. Sinus tracts, abscesses, and hematomas need to be diagnosed and drained. Infection may threaten adjacent vessels, tendons, and nerves. Chronic osteomyelitis can cause squamous cell carcinoma at the site of chronic drainage. Amyloidosis has been caused by the systemic response to chronic osteomyelitis.

INDICATIONS FOR REFERRAL/HOSPITALIZATION

Patients with acute osteomyelitis are sick, often septic, and require IV antibiotics and evaluation by specialists, which often includes an infectious disease specialist and orthopedic surgeon. There is no question about the need for initial hospitalization, although prolonged antibiotic therapy may be continued at home. Curative therapy for chronic osteomyelitis involves elective admission with surgical debridement, culture of bone, and consultation as defined by individual needs. Same-day surgery programs sometimes accomplish this without hospitalization. Suppressive antibiotic therapy for chronic osteomyelitis may be administered on an outpatient basis.

PATIENT AND FAMILY EDUCATION

In addition to receiving an explanation of the various diagnostic and therapeutic options, patients should understand that "cure" is an elusive concept. Acute osteomyelitis may relapse years after treatment, and chronic osteomyelitis may smolder indefinitely in a subacute fashion with intermittent drainage. Patients with extensive bony defects must take precautions against fracture. Patients need to be educated regarding prolonged therapy, central venous lines, relapses, antibiotic complications, amputation, and suppression. Preventive measures include teaching daily foot inspection to patients with diabetes, arthritis, vascular insufficiency, or neuropathy, because these patients are particularly prone to infections in the feet. Diabetic and neuropathic ulcers require prompt medical attention. Insensate feet must be protected from heat, cold, and trauma. Control of diabetes, management of edema, good nutrition, and smoking cessation are all important.

REFERENCES

1. Lew DP, Waldvogel FA: Osteomyelitis, *N Engl J Med* 336:999-1007, 1997.
2. Gillespie WJ: Epidemiology in bone and joint infection, *Infect Dis Clin North Am* 4:361-376, 1990.
3. Cierny C, Mader JT, Pemnick H: A clinical staging system of adult osteomyelitis, *Contemp Orthop* 10:17-37, 1985.
4. Mader JT, Shirtliff M, Calhoun JH: Staging and staging application in osteomyelitis, *Clin Infect Dis* 25:1303-1309, 1997.
5. Mader JT, Calhoun J: *Osteomyelitis, principles and practice of infectious disease,* ed 4, New York, 1995, Churchill Livingstone.
6. O'Hanley P, Swartz MN: Osteomyelitis, *Sci Am Med,* 1995.
7. Grayson ML and others: Probing to bone in infected pedal ulcers: a clinical sign of underlying osteomyelitis in diabetic patients, *JAMA* 273:721-723, 1995.

8. Mazanec D: Low back pain: living with ambiguity, *Cleve Clin J Med* 64:407-410, 1997.
9. Haas DW, McAndrew MP: Bacterial osteomyelitis in adults: evolving considerations in diagnosis and treatment, *Am J Med* 101:550-561, 1996.
10. Stravebaugh LJ: Vertebral osteomyelitis, *Postgrad Med* 97:147-154, 1995.
11. Sapico Fl, Montgomerie JZ: Vertebral osteomyelitis, *Infect Dis Clin North Am* 4:539-550, 1990.
12. Caputo GM and others: Assessment and management of foot disease in patients with diabetes, *N Engl J Med* 331:854-860, 1994.
13. Culleton JL: Preventing diabetic foot complications, *Postgrad Med* 106:74-83,1999.
14. Longmaid HE, Kruskal JB: Imaging infections in diabetes patients, *Infect Dis Clin North Am* 9:163-182, 1995.
15. Khatri G et al: Effect of bone biopsy in guiding antimicrobial therapy of osteomyelitis complicating open wounds, *Am J Med Sci* 321: 367-371, 2001.
16. Karchmer AW, Gibbons GW: Foot infections in diabetes: evaluation and management, *Curr Clin Top Infect Dis* 14:1-22, 1994.
17. Jacobs RF, McCarthy RE, Elser JM: Pseudomonas osteochondritis complicating puncture wounds of the foot in children, *J Infect Dis* 160:657-661, 1989.
18. Anand AJ, Glatt AE: Salmonella osteomyelitis and arthritis in sickle cell disease, *Semin Arthritis Rheum* 24:211-221, 1994.
19. Mackowiak PA, Jones SR, Smith JW: Diagnostic value of sinus-tract cultures in chronic osteomyelitis, *JAMA* 239:2772-2775, 1978.
20. Perry CR, Pearson RL, Miller GH: Accuracy of cultures of material from swabbing of the superficial aspect of the wound and needle biopsy in the preoperative assessment of osteomyelitis, *J Bone Joint Surg* 73:745-749, 1991.
21. Tehranzadeh J and others: Imaging of osteomyelitis in the mature skeleton, *Radiol Clin North Am* 39:223-250, 2001.
22. Lientry LO: Antibiotic therapy for osteomyelitis, *Infect Dis Clin North Am* 4:485-499, 1990.
23. Tice AD: Outpatient parenteral antimicrobial therapy for osteomyelitis, *Infect Dis Clin North Am* 12:903-919, 1998.
24. Williams DN and others: Practice guidelines for community-based parenteral anti-infective therapy, *Clin Infect Dis* 25:787-801, 1997.
25. Weinstein MP and others: Multicenter collaborative evaluation of a standard serum bactericidal test as a predictor of therapeutic efficacy in acute and chronic osteomyelitis, *Am J Med* 83:218-222, 1987.
26. Nelson JD: A critical review of the role of oral antibiotics in the management of hematogenous osteomyelitis. In: Remington RS, Swartz MN, editors. *Clinical topics in infectious disease,* Vol 4, New York, 1996, McGraw-Hill.
27. Greenberg RN and others: Ciprofloxacin, lomefloxacin, levofloxacin as treatment for chronic osteomyelitis, *Antimicrob Agents Chemother* 44:164-166, 2000.
28. Rissing JP: Antimicrobial therapy for chronic osteomyelitis in adults: role of the quinolones, *Clin Infect Dis* 25:1327-1333, 1997.
29. Grayson ML: Diabetic foot infections: antimicrobial therapy, *Infect Dis Clin North Am* 9:143-161, 1995.
30. Muha J: Local wound care in diabetic foot complications, *Postgrad Med* 106:97-102, 1999.

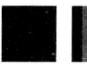

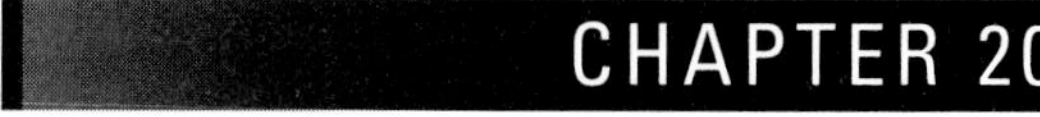

Osteoporosis

Alan Ona Malabanan

DEFINITION/EPIDEMIOLOGY

Osteoporosis is characterized by increased bone fragility and increased susceptibility to fracture. This increased bone fragility results from decreases in bone mass and deterioration of bone microarchitecture that occur as the result of estrogen deficiency and aging. Osteoporosis is the most common metabolic bone disease, with more than 28 million Americans either having the condition or at risk for it. It is the leading cause of fractures, accounting for approximately 1.5 million fractures yearly.[1] Osteoporotic fractures are more common than heart attack, stroke, or cancer.[2,3]

Osteoporosis is also defined, by the World Health Organization, as a bone mineral density (BMD) ≤2.5 SDs below the young normal mean (i.e., T score ≤–2.5).[4] In the absence of osteoporotic fracture, this densitometric definition is the most clinically relevant but should not be used as the sole criterion for treatment decision. Much like elevated cholesterol is one risk factor for heart attack, osteoporosis is but one risk factor for osteoporotic fracture. There is no definitive BMD threshold at which osteoporotic fractures occur—only an increasing likelihood of fracture with decreasing BMD. Other risk factors, such as increasing age, family history of hip fracture, current cigarette smoking, or prior fracture, have an impact on this fracture likelihood independent of the BMD.[5]

PATHOPHYSIOLOGY

Bone serves as a large calcium reservoir, in addition to providing a supportive and protective framework for the body. Calcium is necessary for proper neural, musculoskeletal, and cardiac function. Normal bone remodeling allows both access to the calcium reservoir and replacement and repair of old and damaged bone. Bone remodeling has two main phases: bone resorption and bone formation.

Bone *resorption,* which releases calcium into the circulation, is the removal of damaged or old bone by osteoclasts, cells derived from macrophages and monocytes. This process is rapid and occurs in a matter of days to weeks. Osteoblasts, in response to parathyroid hormone and other cytokines, secrete RANK ligand (receptor for activation of nuclear factor kappa beta) and mCSF (monocyte-colony stimulating factor), which cause monocytes/macrophages to differentiate into osteoclasts and proliferate. Osteoclasts produce powerful degradative enzymes, such as cathepsin K, to break down bone, releasing calcium, phosphorus, and type I collagen crosslinked products into the circulation.[6]

Bone formation occurs when osteoblasts lay down osteoid, an organic matrix composed of type I collagen and other proteins. Bone formation, occurring over months, is a slow process. It is estimated that the skeleton is completely replaced over approximately 4 years. Osteoblasts are also responsible for mineralizing the bone, depositing calcium and phosphorus into the osteoid.

This process is dependent on the presence of adequate amounts of calcium and phosphorus and alkaline phosphatase activity. Poor bone mineralization leads to *osteomalacia,* a painful softening of the bone.

Normally, bone resorption and bone formation proceed at equal rates. In osteoporosis, however, the rate of bone resorption exceeds that of bone formation producing a net loss of bone. This uncoupling of bone resorption and bone formation is a consequence of estrogen deficiency and is most pronounced in the first 5 to 10 years after menopause.

Glucocorticoid use is the most common cause of secondary osteoporosis. It causes osteoblast death, decreases levels of estrogen and testosterone, increases the metabolism of vitamin D, and decreases the intestinal absorption of calcium.[7] This increased bone resorption/decreased bone formation leads to a very rapid loss of bone, the majority of which occurs in the first 6 months of glucocorticoid use. Other drugs, such as chronic opiates, anticonvulsants, heparin, excessive thyroid hormone, leuprolide, cancer chemotherapeutics, and cigarettes, lead to similar changes in bone metabolism.[8]

Risk Factors

Risk factors, both nonmodifiable and modifiable, increase the risk of bone loss or osteoporotic fracture (Box 201-1). These risk factors should be considered when deciding on osteoporosis screening or therapy. Nonmodifiable risk factors for osteoporosis include increasing age, personal history of fracture as an adult, white or Asian race, female gender, and history of fracture in a first-degree relative. Potentially modifiable risk factors for osteoporosis include estrogen deficiency, associated with menopause at younger than age 45 or bilateral ovariectomy and premenopausal amenorrhea, cigarette smoking, low calcium intake, low body weight (<127 lb), excessive alcohol intake, inadequate physical activity, visual impairment, poor health/frailty, or falls.[1] Minor risk factors for hip fracture in older women include tall height at age 26, fair to poor self-related health, previous hyperthyroidism, use of long-acting benzodiazepines, excessive caffeine intake, not walking for exercise, weight loss since age 25, on feet for less than 4 hours per day, inability to rise from a chair without using arms, poor depth perception, poor contrast sensitivity, and tachycardia at rest.[5,9]

BOX 201-1

RISK FACTORS FOR BONE LOSS OR OSTEOPOROTIC FRACTURE

NONMODIFIABLE

Advanced age
Female gender
White or Asian race
Personal history of fracture
History of fracture in a first-degree relative
Dementia

MODIFIABLE

Hypogonadism
Current cigarette smoking
Excessive alcohol or caffeine use
Low calcium intake
Low body weight (<127 lb)
Inadequate physical activity
Visual impairment
Glucocorticoid or anticonvulsant use
Thyrotoxicosis
Recurrent falls
Poor health or frailty

CLINICAL PRESENTATION

Unless an osteoporotic fracture is present, osteoporosis is *clinically silent.* Low BMD, in the absence of osteoporotic fracture, *does not* cause pain. If pain is present, the presence of fracture should be confirmed or a secondary cause of the low BMD, such as osteomalacia, ruled out.

The sine qua non of osteoporosis is an osteoporotic fracture, a fracture occurring with no or minimal trauma. The presence of a typical osteoporotic fracture in a postmenopausal woman is usually sufficient to diagnose osteoporosis. The typical sites of fractures include the vertebra, the distal wrist, the proximal femur, and the ribs. Unfortunately, even in the presence of a typical osteoporotic fracture, the diagnosis of osteoporosis is often missed and treatment is never initiated.[10-12] Osteoporosis occurring in men, premenopausal women, or perimenopausal women should lead to a consideration of secondary causes of osteoporosis.[8,13]

PHYSICAL EXAMINATION

Severe or established osteoporosis, that is, osteoporosis with fractures, is readily identifiable. The "dowager's hump" is a thoracic spine kyphotic deformity that occurs with multiple vertebral compression fractures. Vertebral compression fractures may also lead to scoliosis and height loss. A height loss of >5 cm (2 inches) or >4 cm (1.6 inches) over 10 years has been associated with low bone density and an increased incidence of vertebral compression fractures.[14-16]

The physical examination in osteoporosis should be directed toward finding signs of secondary osteoporosis. The presence of band keratopathy may suggest a diagnosis of primary hyperparathyroidism. Exophthalmos or lid lag, goiter, tremor, warm moist skin, weight loss, or pretibial myxedema may indicate a diagnosis of hyperthyroidism. The presence of dorsal fat, facial plethora, supraclavicular fat, hypertension, centripetal obesity, proximal muscle weakness, edema, or violaceous abdominal striae may suggest a diagnosis of Cushing's syndrome. Gynecomastia, or decreased facial or axillary hair, and testicular atrophy may suggest hypogonadism. The presence of blue sclera may suggest a diagnosis of osteogenesis imperfecta.

Fall risk should be assessed in each patient presenting with osteoporosis. Lower extremity strength, balance, gait, and postural reflexes should be carefully assessed. Poor visual acuity, weak grip strength, difficulty arising from a chair, the presence of a Romberg sign, excessive body sway, and an unsteady gait may all be signs of increased fall risk that may benefit from physical therapy evaluation or evaluation in a specialty fall clinic.

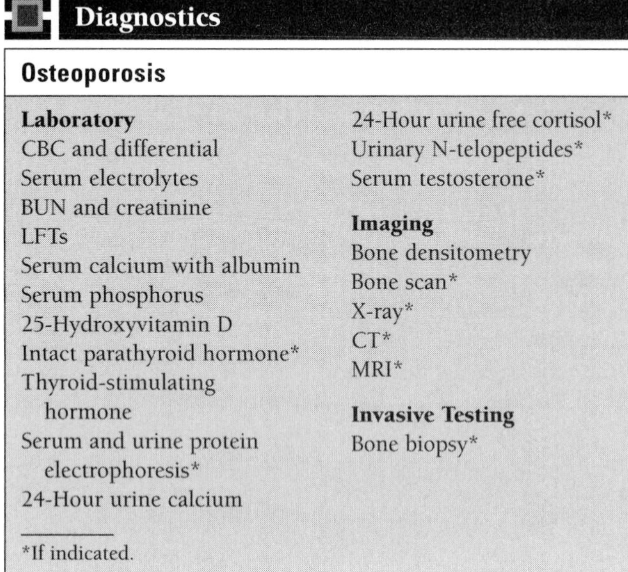

Diagnostics

Osteoporosis

Laboratory
CBC and differential
Serum electrolytes
BUN and creatinine
LFTs
Serum calcium with albumin
Serum phosphorus
25-Hydroxyvitamin D
Intact parathyroid hormone*
Thyroid-stimulating hormone
Serum and urine protein electrophoresis*
24-Hour urine calcium
24-Hour urine free cortisol*
Urinary N-telopeptides*
Serum testosterone*

Imaging
Bone densitometry
Bone scan*
X-ray*
CT*
MRI*

Invasive Testing
Bone biopsy*

*If indicated.

DIAGNOSTICS

Routine chemistry profiles (serum electrolytes, fasting serum calcium and phosphorus, serum glucose, BUN, and creatinine) are usually normal in idiopathic osteoporosis. However, screening laboratory tests may be indicated to exclude underlying pathologic processes suggested by physical examination or presenting symptoms. Low vitamin D levels and vitamin D deficiency are a coexisting condition in many patients with osteoporosis,[17] as well as in general medical inpatients.[18] A 25-hydroxyvitamin D (*not* 1,25-dihydroxyvitamin D) assessment should be part of the initial evaluation of osteoporosis. The normal range for 25-hydroxyvitamin D in New England is 9 to 52 ng/ml; however, a normal 25-hydroxyvitamin D may still be consistent with vitamin D insufficiency.[19] Choosing a value in the middle of the normal range to indicate adequacy (i.e., approximately 30 ng/ml) may be a reasonable rule of thumb. A safe and effective method of repleting vitamin D stores in those with normocalcemia and normal renal function is to give 50,000 units of vitamin D weekly for 8 weeks.[19]

Biochemical markers are urine and blood tests that measure breakdown products of bone and collagen. A *biochemical marker* is an indirect measurement of bone turnover (i.e., bone resorption and formation). Bone resorption markers (N-telopeptides and C-telopeptides) evaluate osteoclast activity, and bone formation markers (bone-specific alkaline phosphatase, osteocalcin, procollagen I extension peptides) evaluate osteoblast activity. High levels imply increased bone turnover. At this time the role of bone markers in primary care is unclear, although specialists may use them. Bone resorption markers help identify response to antiresorptive drug treatment. Six-month intervals are the usual frequency for testing bone markers.

Plain radiographs are useful primarily in confirming the presence of fracture. They are very insensitive to decreases in bone mass. In the absence of fracture, the "gold standard" for diagnosing osteoporosis is bone densitometry, by dual energy x-ray absorptiometry, of the hip and posteroanterior lumbar spine. Indications for bone densitometry are listed in Box 201-2. Bone density assessment of other sites such as the finger, wrist, and ankle and the use of other technologies, such as ultrasound, are useful in diagnosing osteoporosis and predicting fracture risk (particularly in woman over 65 years of age) but may not be as useful in ruling out osteoporosis.[20,21]

Bone density provides three pertinent numbers. The first is the actual area density in grams per centimeters squared. This density is then compared with the manufacturer database for young normal adults and age-matched adults. This comparison results in a T score and a Z score, respectively. The T score is used in diagnosing osteopenia (T score, <-1.0 and >-2.5) and osteoporosis (≤ -2.5). The Z score is ignored, unless it is <-2.0.

Only bone density of the posteroanterior lumbar spine and hip is recommended for monitoring osteoporosis treatment efficacy, and it is generally performed at 1- to 2-year intervals, depending on the precision of the scan. In general, a 5% density change is considered significant and not caused by measurement statistical variation.[22] Some disease states such as chronic glucocorticoid therapy or paraplegia may lead to more rapid bone density changes. In these cases, assessing bone density every 6 months to 1 year may be indicated.

BOX 201-2

INDICATIONS FOR BONE DENSITOMETRY

WOMEN
Age $\geq$65 yr
Postmenopausal age <65 yr with risk factors
Postmenopausal with a fracture
Considering osteoporosis therapy
Receiving long-term hormone-replacement therapy (HRT)

MEN
Age $\geq$70 yr
Low trauma fractures
Hypogonadism
Prevalent vertebral deformities
Radiographic osteopenia

BOTH
Hyperparathyroidism
Chronic glucocorticoid therapy

Data from National Osteoporosis Foundation: *Physician's guide to prevention and treatment of osteoporosis*, Belle Mead, NJ, 1999, Exerpta Medica, Inc; Orwoll ES: Osteoporosis in men, *Endocrinol Metab Clin North Am* 272:349-367, 1998; and Bennell K and others: The role of physiotherapy in the prevention and treatment of osteoporosis, *Manage Ther* 54:198-213, 2000.

DIFFERENTIAL DIAGNOSIS

Osteoporosis is classified as either primary or secondary. Primary osteoporosis includes bone loss arising from menopausal estrogen deficiency or aging. Secondary osteoporosis results from an acquired or inherited disease that interferes with bone remodeling or increases bone turnover.

Postmenopausal osteoporosis should be distinguished from secondary causes of osteoporosis (Box 201-3). A secondary cause of osteoporosis may indicate potentially reversible osteoporosis.

Differential Diagnosis

Osteoporosis

Aging	Eating disorders/ malnutrition
Estrogen or testosterone deficiency	Malignancy, including metastatic diseases, multiple myeloma, lymphoma, leukemia
Diabetes mellitus	Medications
Cushing's syndrome	Osteopetrosis
Hyperthyroidism	Paget's disease
Hyperparathyroidism	Rheumatoid arthritis
Hyperprolactinemia	Osteogenesis imperfecta
Acromegaly	Marfan's syndrome
Hypercalcinuria	Turner's syndrome
Chronic renal disease	Klinefelter's syndrome
Renal transplantation	
Liver disease	
Malabsorption	

Suspicion of secondary causes of osteoporosis should be high in premenopausal and perimenopausal women, men, those with bone density Z scores <-2, and those with bone pain in the absence of fracture.

The presence of a fragility fracture in the absence of low bone density should raise the concern of localized bone destruction, as with metastatic disease or plasmacytoma. Thoracic spine fractures caused by metastasis are more likely when they involve vertebrae above T7.[23] There also are less common metabolic bone diseases such as Paget's disease and osteopetrosis that may lead to pathologic fractures, despite normal or even high bone density. Further testing, which can include CT scanning, MRI, nuclear medicine bone scanning, or even bone biopsy, may be indicated.

MANAGEMENT

Much of the bone loss of osteoporosis is *irreversible* and prevention should be the major focus of primary care providers. Ideally, efforts at preventing osteoporosis should begin before puberty and should consist of adequate calcium and vitamin D intake, adequate weight-bearing exercise, and avoidance of cigarette smoking and excessive alcohol. These preventive efforts are also recommended in adults and in those in whom osteoporosis has already developed.

The National Academy of Science recommends between 1000 and 1300 mg of elemental calcium (between 3 and 5 cups of milk daily) and between 200 and 600 units of vitamin D daily for adults (Table 201-1).[24] Those who are unable to tolerate dairy may have to use calcium supplements, such as calcium carbonate and calcium citrate. A recent study[25] found that several preparations of calcium carbonate, both oyster shell– and non–oyster shell–based preparations, have trace amounts of lead, of which the long-term implications are unclear.[26] Some recommend taking two multivitamins daily (approximately 800 IU of vitamin D/day) to provide adequate vitamin D. This practice may lead to excessive vitamin A intake, which has been associated in retrospective studies with osteoporosis and hip fracture.[27,28] A combination of confirmed lead-free calcium/vitamin D preparation and one multivitamin daily is probably the best therapeutic alternative.

BOX 201-3

SECONDARY CAUSES OF LOW BONE MASS

ENDOCRINE CAUSES
Hypogonadism
Cushing's syndrome
Hyperparathyroidism
Hyperthyroidism
Hyperprolactinemia
Diabetes mellitus type 1
Acromegaly

GASTROINTESTINAL CAUSES
Gastrectomy
Celiac disease
Malabsorption
Inflammatory bowel diseases
Primary biliary cirrhosis
Hemochromatosis
Anorexia nervosa

NEUROLOGIC CAUSES
Multiple sclerosis
Parkinson's disease
Spinal cord injury

OSTEOMALACIAS
Vitamin D deficiency
Chronic renal failure
Hypophosphatasia
Fanconi's syndrome
Oncogenic osteomalacia
X-linked hypophosphatemic rickets

MALIGNANCY (MARROW ASSOCIATED)
Multiple myeloma
Leukemias and lymphomas
Systemic mastocytosis
Tumoral hypercalcemia

CONNECTIVE TISSUE DISEASES
Rheumatoid arthritis
Ankylosing spondylitis
Osteogenesis imperfecta
Ehlers Danlos syndrome
Sarcoidosis
Homocystinuria

DRUGS
Glucocorticoids
Heparin
Cyclosporin A
Anticonvulsants
GnRH analogues
Lithium
Methotrexate
Cigarette smoking
Excessive alcohol
Excessive thyroxine
Chronic opiates
Tamoxifen premenopausal use

Data from National Osteoporosis Foundation: *Physician's guide to prevention and treatment of osteoporosis,* Belle Mead, NJ: Exerpta Medica, Inc.; Harper KD and Weber TJ: Secondary osteoporosis: diagnostic considerations, *Endocrinol Metab Clin North Am* 272:349-367, 1998.

The major source of vitamin D is sunlight exposure, with cutaneous synthesis of vitamin D from exposure to ultraviolet-B radiation. Sunlight exposure (without sun block) to hands, arms, and face for 10 to 15 minutes 2 or 3 times a week is recommended by many experts, although the adequacy of this regimen is dependent on season, latitude, and skin pigmentation.[29] Those at risk for skin cancer may also wish to forgo this source of vitamin D. Studies of calcium and vitamin D intake have shown a modest increase in bone density, with a significant decrease in fracture in both older men and women.[30,31]

Bone is a dynamic tissue that adapts to loading (i.e., weight-bearing exercise) with hypertrophy and increased strength. Exercise is an important part of any osteoporosis therapy and was recently reviewed.[32,33] Unloading of the skeleton, as occurs with bed rest, space flight, and spinal cord injury, results in dramatic decrements in bone mass.[34,35] Conversely, weight-bearing exercise and weight training may increase bone density and their effects are dependent on estrogen status. Exercise alone has not

TABLE 201-1 Recommended Calcium and Vitamin D Daily Intake

Age (yr)	Calcium (mg/day)	Vitamin D (IU/day)
1-3	500	200
4-8	800	200
9-13	1300	200
14-18	1300	200
19-30	1000	200
31-50	1000	200
51-70	1200	400*
>70	1200	600*

Data from Institute of Medicine: *Dietary reference intakes: calcium, phosphorus, magnesium, vitamin D and fluoride,* Washington, DC, 1997, National Academy Press.
*Evidence exists to recommend a vitamin D daily dosage of 400 to 900 IU/day for these age-groups.

BOX 201-4

FDA-APPROVED THERAPIES FOR OSTEOPOROSIS*

PREVENTION	TREATMENT
Estrogen with or without progesterone	Raloxifene
Raloxifene	Alendronate
Alendronate	Risedronate
Risedronate	Calcitonin

*At the time of this writing.

been shown to prevent menopausal bone loss, and there is no evidence showing a decrease in fracture risk with exercise alone. There are some exercise regimens such as Tai Chi, lower limb strengthening, and balance training that may decrease risk of fall.[36,37] Exercises to be avoided include high-impact loading, abrupt or explosive movements, resistive trunk flexion, twisting movements, and dynamic abdominal exercises.[32] Referral to a physical therapy for guided exercise may be helpful.

Hip protector pads have been proved to prevent hip fractures. They are indicated for patients with high risk for fall, those with decreased fat and muscle stores, and those with previous fractures. A study by Cameron and others[38] showed that the use of hip protectors decreased the number of hip fractures from 46.0 to 21.3 fractures per 1000 person-years.

In those with osteoporosis, preventive measures of calcium, vitamin D, and exercise alone are not sufficient to prevent osteoporotic fracture. For those with densitometric osteoporosis (T score <-2.5), densitometric osteopenia (T-score <-1.0 and >-2.5) with multiple risk factors and particularly those already with osteoporotic fracture, pharmacologic therapy is imperative. The National Osteoporosis Foundation issued guidelines in 1998, which apply to Caucasian post-menopausal women, suggesting treatment for those with T-scores <-2 regardless of presence of risk factors, and those with T-scores <-1.5 in the presence of risk factors.[1] FDA-approved therapies at the time of this writing are listed in Box 201-4.

The only class of FDA-approved agent at this time that has been proved to prevent both vertebral and nonvertebral fractures in prospective studies is the bisphosphonate. Bisphosphonates, which are synthetic analogues of pyrophosphate, reduce bone resorption and bone loss by binding to bone and poisoning active osteoclasts. There are two bisphosphonates currently FDA approved for the prevention and treatment of postmenopausal osteoporosis and glucocorticoid-induced osteoporosis: alendronate and risedronate. Only alendronate is approved for male osteoporosis, although both bisphosphonates are approved for treatment of males with glucocorticoid-induced osteoporosis. Studies with these agents have shown yearly bone density increases of 2% to 3% at the lumbar spine, which is the skeletal site most responsive to these agents.[39-42] Contraindications include disorders of esophageal motility or active gastroesophageal bleeding, hypocalcemia, and renal disease. The recommended dosage of alendronate for the prevention is 5 mg/day (or 35 mg per week). For the treatment of osteoporosis, the dosage is 10 mg/day or 70 mg per week. With risedronate, the prevention and treatment dosages are the same: 5 mg/day or 35 mg once a week. Bisphosphonates should be taken on an empty stomach, with 6 to 8 ounces of water, 30 minutes before eating, taking other medications or lying down. To decrease gastrointestinal effects, it is important that patients be given explicit instructions on proper administration; esophagitis can be problematic. The weekly dose of a bisphosphonate may be better tolerated than the daily dose,[43] and there is some evidence of decreased gastrointestinal toxicity with daily 5 mg risedronate compared with 10 mg alendronate.[44] At higher daily doses, 30 mg risedronate and 40 mg alendronate, the effects on the gastric and duodenal mucosa were similar for the two bisphosphonates, and much less than for aspirin 650 mg q.i.d.[45]

Raloxifene is FDA approved for postmenopausal osteoporosis prevention and treatment at a dosage of 60 mg/day. Raloxifene is a selective estrogen receptor modulator (SERM), which acts as an estrogen receptor agonist on the skeleton but as an antagonist on breast and uterine tissue. Raloxifene has been shown to produce roughly a 1.5% to 3% increase in spine and femoral neck density after 3 years, with a 30% reduction in new vertebral fractures.[46] No reduction in nonvertebral fractures has been shown yet. There is an increased risk of venous thromboembolic disease, hot flashes, and leg cramps with raloxifene. Notably, there also is an 84% reduction in the risk of estrogen receptor–positive invasive breast cancers over 4 years,[47] and there are ongoing studies to see if this risk reduction is present in women with a high risk for breast cancer.

Hormone replacement is currently FDA approved only for the prevention of osteoporosis, not for its treatment. Estrogen inhibits bone resorption, decreases bone remodeling, and enhances absorption of calcium. Although there are substantial data showing BMD increases with estrogen use,[48,49] there are insufficient prospective data showing a decreased fracture risk with estrogen use. Those women with an intact uterus will require a regimen with progesterone, either daily or cycled (0.625 mg of conjugated equine estrogen daily with 2.5 mg of medroxyprogesterone acetate daily or 5 mg of medroxyprogesterone acetate for 10 to 15 days of a 30-day cycle).

Contraindications to the use of estrogen include undiagnosed vaginal bleeding, pregnancy, active thrombosis or thrombophlebitis, active liver disease, endometrial adenocarcinoma, breast cancer, and other estrogen-dependent tumors. Caution should be taken with a medical diagnosis of endometriosis, uterine leiomyoma, gallbladder disease, migraine headaches, a family history of breast cancer, or a history of thrombophlebitis. Once estrogen therapy is stopped, bone loss resumes at the same rate as in untreated women.[50,51] With long-term use of estrogen, those at risk for breast cancer and those with a history of uncomfortable side effects should be monitored closely. Most endocrinologists believe that any increase in bone mass is beneficial in preventing further bone loss, regardless of age. Therefore the older woman not previously treated with hormone replacement may benefit from the initiation of hormones to prevent further bone fractures.[52] Concerns about the increased risk of breast cancer and cardiovascular disease associated with long-term (more than 5 years) hormone replacement therapy (estrogen plus progesterone) should be discussed with the patient if hormone replacement therapy is considered.

Subcutaneous parathyroid hormone (PTH) is an anabolic bone agent. Anabolic agents stimulate bone formation and increase bone-remodeling rates. Intermittent PTH administration shows an anabolic effect increasing bone mass, whereas continuous PTH administration leads to bone loss as in primary hyperparathyroidism. A PTH analogue (PTH 1-34), administered subcutaneously, has been shown to increase bone density at the hip and spine in women,[53] men,[54] and postmenopausal women on glucocorticoid therapy.[55] An international multicenter study showed that 20 μg of PTH daily administered to postmenopausal women with established osteoporosis increased spine density by approximately 8% and approximately 2% at the femoral neck at the end of 1 year. It was shown to decrease vertebral fractures by approximately 65% and nonvertebral fractures by 35%.[53] Adverse effects included nausea, headache, and temporary hypercalcemia. It is expected to be approved by the FDA for use in osteoporosis in the spring of 2003.

Etidronate, a first-generation bisphosphonate, is also used for osteoporosis, although it does not have FDA approval for this indication. It increases bone density and decreases the risk of vertebral fractures in postmenopausal women.[56,57] It also has been shown to decrease bone loss in individuals treated with corticosteroids.[58] The recommended daily dose is 5 to 10 mg/kg for 2 weeks (usually 400 mg q.h.s.), followed by 11 to 13 weeks of 1000 to 1500 mg calcium supplementation.

IV pamidronate has also been used for osteoporosis because of its effects on increasing bone density. It has been shown to be useful in children with osteogenesis imperfecta in uncontrolled studies, decreasing the risk of fracture and improving the quality of life.[59] It has been studied in heart transplant recipients[60] and in men with prostate cancer.[61] It is FDA approved for the treatment of bone disease associated with multiple myeloma[62] and breast cancer.[63] Regimens for breast cancer and myeloma generally involve doses of 90 mg IV administered over 2 to 4 hours monthly. It should not be used in patients with hypocalcemia, uncorrected vitamin D insufficiency, renal failure, or allergy to bisphosphonates. It should be used with caution in those with mild renal insufficiency. It has been associated with myalgias, fevers, leukopenia, and bone pain after the first dose ("Aredia flu") in younger patients.

Calcitonin is a peptide hormone that appears to slow bone loss and temporarily increase vertebral bone mass by decreasing osteoclastic activity. The drug's effect on bone is more pronounced with trabecular bone. The nasal spray produces a 3% increase in vertebral bone only[64] and is not as effective as estrogen and alendronate in forming new bone. Drug delivery is via injection or nasal spray, with the recommended dosage being 50 to 100 units/day 3 times per week for the injection and 200 units/day, alternating nostrils, for the nasal spray. It is FDA approved for use in postmenopausal women (>5 years postmenopause) with osteoporosis. The supplementation of calcium and vitamin D enhances therapy. Most osteoporosis experts do not advise the use of calcitonin therapy alone in treating established osteoporosis.

Calcitriol therapy has been shown to decrease vertebral fractures after 3 years from (31.5 per 1000 person-years to 9.9 per 1000 person-years) in postmenopausal women,[65] but adverse effects such as hypercalciuria and hypercalcemia limit its use. Testosterone therapy in hypogonadal older men is useful in increasing bone density.[66] Its efficacy in preventing fractures is not yet established.

Combinations of therapies (e.g., bisphosphonates and estrogen, PTH and estrogen, and PTH and bisphosphonates) may have additive effects on bone density increases.[67-69] It is not clear whether these bone density increases are associated with decreased fracture risk.

Sodium fluoride is an anabolic agent that causes marked increases in bone formation. However, excessive fluoride use may lead to increased fracture risk, despite bone density increases (fluorosis). Data regarding its efficacy in preventing fracture with slow-release preparations are conflicting,[70] and its use is not recommended.

Co-Management with Specialists

Co-management is dependent on the particular needs of each patient. Fracture management and pain control are the primary reasons for referral. Referrals may also be made to the following specialists:

- *Endocrinologists* or *rheumatologists* specializing in metabolic bone disease for persistent fractures, patients with secondary osteoporosis, premenopausal women or children with osteoporosis, or those with osteoporosis intolerant of FDA-approved therapies
- *Pain specialist* to manage escalating chronic pain associated with debilitating bone and muscle changes associated with fractures
- *Physical therapist* for management of exercise for osteoporosis, spinal and posture strengthening, pain management, and fall/fracture prevention
- *Nutritionist* for balanced diet guidelines regarding calcium and vitamin D intake appropriate for the individual's age and activity level
- *Orthopedic surgeon* for surgical correction of bone fractures

LIFE SPAN CONSIDERATIONS

Osteoporotic fractures, especially those of the hip, are associated with increased morbidity and increased mortality. In the first year after hip fracture, one third are discharged to nursing homes, 50% are unable to walk without assistance, and 24% die.[71-73] Mortality rates in men with hip fracture are higher because of co-morbid conditions.[13] In women with vertebral fractures, those with one or more fractures had a 1.23-fold greater age-adjusted mortality rate, with mortality increasing with greater numbers of vertebral fractures.[74]

TABLE 201-2 Physical Therapy: Spinal Support

Area	Support
Thoracolumbar area	Body jacket clamshell brace Jewett three-point brace Boston brace
Lumbosacral area	Lumbosacral corset

COMPLICATIONS

Eighty-four percent of those with clinically diagnosed vertebral compression fractures complain of pain. The acute pain of vertebral fracture usually lasts between 2 weeks and 3 months. Chronic back pain from spinal changes, microfractures, and muscle spasms can develop. Patients may develop reduced exercise tolerance and pulmonary reserve. Abdominal protuberance due to loss of height at the lumbar spine may result leading to early satiety and resultant weight loss. There is loss of self-esteem and a distortion of body image.[75]

Altered activity or inability to participate in activities of daily living because of pain may persist for a much longer period. In these cases, bed rest and decreased activity for a few days are warranted. The individual should be instructed in proper positioning—either lying supine or side lying with pillows positioned under the knees or between the knees. Medications for pain, such as muscle relaxants for spasms, nonsteroidals (cyclooxygenase-1 [COX-1] and COX-2 inhibitors), and acetaminophen for pain and inflammation, should be prescribed as needed. Narcotics should be used sparingly because of the potential for addiction and associated fall risk. Moist heat or ice may help with pain relief. Moist heat is generally recommended for muscle spasms, and ice is recommended for bone inflammation and/or pain. The individual in acute pain may need to use a cane or walker to ambulate safely. Short-term use of a spinal support may be beneficial (Table 201-2). Also available is a posture training support (PTS) designed to pull the shoulders back with weights as the muscles become stronger.

Chronic pain management may be enhanced with physical therapy. Modalities include transcutaneous electrical nerve stimulation (TENS), electrical muscle stimulation, ultrasound with healed fractures, iontophoresis, and heat or ice. Manual therapy, including joint mobilization, muscle energy techniques, myofascial release, and strain/counterstrain on trigger points in muscle, is beneficial in mobilizing soft tissue and improving muscle imbalance of the spine.

Vertebroplasty and kyphoplasty are new minimally invasive techniques in which polymethylmethacrylate (PMMA) cement is injected into the fractured vertebrae, thereby stabilizing it. The two techniques differ in that vertebroplasty uses a high-pressure injection system and kyphoplasty uses a balloon to expand the collapsed vertebrae and produce a space for the PMMA. Vertebroplasty has a reported rate of success in pain relief of 70% to 90%, and kyphoplasty, 90%. Kyphoplasty has the added benefit of significantly increasing vertebral height. Complication rates are low and include radiculopathy and cord compression. Cement leakage is common, however, particularly in vertebroplasty.[76] This appears an effective therapy for pain relief of vertebral fractures, although the biomechanical effects on the adjacent nonfractured vertebra are not yet clear.

BOX 201-5

FALL PREVENTION MEASURES

- Regular eye examinations and correction for inadequacies
- Hearing evaluation for sound detection
- Use of assistive devices cane or walker as needed
- Use of rubber-soled/flat-soled fully enclosed shoes
- Use of handrails and steady pieces of furniture
- Use of grab bars, tub seats, and elevated toilets in the bathroom
- Walkways clear of objects and throw rugs
- Use of proper lighting in hallways and stairways

INDICATIONS FOR REFERRAL/HOSPITALIZATION

The treatment for fractures is primarily supportive and requires physician consultation. Hospitalization for severe pain or setting of fractures (e.g., hip fractures) requires consultation with a specialist. Monitoring for potential complications after hip fractures or for parenteral analgesia is indicated.

PATIENT AND FAMILY EDUCATION

Patient education is essential for the prevention and treatment of fractures. Education encompasses nutrition, psychosocial issues, risk factor modification, proper body mechanics and positioning, safety, and fall prevention. Most accidents occur in the home and are related to poor vision, decreased hearing, slowed reflexes, impaired mental status, limited spinal flexibility, decreased lower extremity strength, and unsteady gait. These factors, coupled with decreased muscle and fat mass to cushion the fall, place the individual at jeopardy for injury.[77] Education of individuals prepares them to take an active role in their care (Box 201-5). Family members should be informed of their risk of osteoporosis and encouraged to take preventive measures.

Resources available include the following:

- Information for both the patient and the primary care provider is available from the National Osteoporosis Foundation, 1150 17th Street NW, Suite 500, Washington, DC 20036 http://www.nof.org.
- *Boning up: a guide to osteoporosis prevention* has illustrations of good posture and helpful hints. It is available from the National Osteoporosis Foundation.
- *Living it safe,* an informational guide for patients on fall prevention, is available from the American Academy of Orthopedic Surgeons, PO Box 1998, Des Plaines, IL 10017.

REFERENCES

1. National Osteoporosis Foundation: *Physician's guide to prevention and treatment of osteoporosis,* Belle Mead, NJ, 1999, Exerpta Medica, Inc.
2. American Heart Association: *2002 Heart and stroke statistical update,* Dallas, 2001, The Association.
3. American Cancer Society: *Cancer facts & figures 2002,* Atlanta, 2002, The Society.

4. Kanis JA and others: The diagnosis of osteoporosis, *J Bone Miner Res* 9:1137-1141, 1994.
5. Cummings SR and others: Risk factors for hip fracture in white women. The study of osteoporotic fractures research group, *N Engl J Med* 332:767-773, 1995.
6. Teitelbaum SL: Bone resorption by osteoclasts, *Science* 289:1504-1508, 2000.
7. Lane NA and others: The science and therapy of glucocorticoid-induced bone loss, *Endocrinol Metab Clin North Am* 27:465-483, 1998.
8. Harper KD, Weber TJ: Secondary osteoporosis: diagnostic considerations, *Endocrinol Metab Clin North Am* 27:349-367, 1998.
9. Garnero P and others: Markers of bone resorption predict hip fracture in elderly women: the EPIDOS Prospective Study, *J Bone Miner Res* 11:1531-1538, 1996.
10. Hajcsar EE and others: Investigation and treatment of osteoporosis in patients with fragility fractures, *CMAJ* 163:819-822, 2000.
11. Freedman KB and others: Treatment of osteoporosis: are physicians missing an opportunity? *J Bone Joint Surg* 82A:1063-1070, 2000.
12. Mallmin H and others: Fracture of the distal forearm as a forecaster of subsequent hip fracture: a population-based cohort study with 24 years of follow-up, *Calcif Tissue Int* 52:269-272, 1993.
13. Orwoll ES: Osteoporosis in men, *Endocrinol Metab Clin North Am* 27:349-367, 1998.
14. Pluijm SM and others: Consequences of vertebral deformities in older men and women, *J Bone Miner Res* 15:1564-1572, 2000.
15. Lunt M and others: Bone density variation and its effects on risk of vertebral deformity in men and women studied in thirteen European centers: the EVOS study, *J Bone Miner Res* 12:1883-1894, 1997.
16. Sanila M and others: Height loss rate as a marker of osteoporosis in postmenopausal women with rheumatoid arthritis, *Clin Rheumatol* 13:256-260, 1994.
17. Leboff MS and others: Occult vitamin D deficiency in postmenopausal US women with acute hip fracture, *JAMA* 281:1505-1511, 1999.
18. Thomas MK and others: Hypovitaminosis D in medical inpatients, *N Engl J Med* 338:777-783, 1998.
19. Malabanan A and others: Redefining vitamin D insufficiency, *Lancet* 351:805-806, 1998.
20. Siris ES and others: Identification and fracture outcomes of undiagnosed low bone mineral density in postmenopausal women: results from the National Osteoporosis Risk Assessment, *JAMA* 286:2815-2822, 2001.
21. Malabanan AO and others: The utility of portable dual energy x-ray absorptiometry of the wrist in patients referred to a bone health clinic, a pilot study, *J Clin Densitom* 1:245-250, 1998.
22. Health Care Financing Administration: Medicare coverage of and payment for bone mass measurements, *Fed Reg* 63:34320-34328, 1998.
23. Biyani and others: Thoracic spine fractures in patients older than 50 years, *Clin Orthop* 328:190-193, 1996.
24. Institute of Medicine: *Dietary reference intakes: calcium phosphorus, magnesium, vitamin D and fluoride,* Washington, DC, 1997, National Academy Press.
25. Ross EA and others: Lead content of calcium supplements, *JAMA* 284:1425-1429, 2000.
26. Heaney R: Lead in calcium supplements: cause for alarm or celebration? *JAMA* 284:1432-1433, 2000.
27. Melhus H and others: Excessive dietary intake of vitamin A is associated with reduced bone mineral density and increased risk for hip fracture, *Ann Intern Med* 129:770-778, 1998.
28. Feskanich D and others: Vitamin A intake and hip fractures among postmenopausal women, *JAMA* 287:47-54, 2002.
29. Holick MF: Vitamin D: photobiology, metabolism, mechanism of actions, and clinical applications. In Favus MJ, editor: *Primer on the metabolic bone diseases and disorders of mineral metabolism,* Philadelphia, 1999, Lippincott Williams & Wilkins.
30. Chapuy MC and others: Vitamin D_3 and calcium to prevent hip fractures in elderly women, *N Engl J Med* 327:1637-1642, 1992.
31. Dawson-Hughes B and others: Effect of calcium and vitamin D supplementation on bone density in men and women 65 years of age or older, *N Engl J Med* 337:670-676, 1997.
32. Bennell K and others: The role of physiotherapy in the prevention and treatment of osteoporosis, *Manage Ther* 5:198-213, 2000.
33. Marcus R: Role of exercise in preventing and treating osteoporosis, *Rheum Dis Clin North Am* 27:131-141, 2001.
34. Arnaud SB and others: Effects of 1-week head-down tilt bed rest on bone formation and the calcium endocrine system, *Aviat Space Environ Med* 63:14-20, 1992.
35. Biering-SF and others: Longitudinal study of bone mineral content in the lumbar spine, the forearm and the lower extremities after spinal cord injury, *Eur J Clin Invest* 20:330-335, 1990.
36. Wolf SL and others: Reducing frailty and falls in older persons: an investigation of Tai Chi and computerized balance training, *J Am Geriatr Soc* 44:489-497, 1996.
37. Campbell AJ and others: Falls prevention over 2 years: a randomized controlled trial in women 80 years and older, *Age Ageing* 28:513-518, 1999.
38. Cameron ID and others: Prevention of hip fracture with use of a hip protector, *N Engl J Med* 344:855-857, 2001.
39. Liberman UA and others: Effect of oral alendronate on bone mineral density and the incidence of fractures in postmenopausal osteoporosis: the Alendronate Phase III Osteoporosis Treatment Study Group, *N Engl J Med* 333:1437-1443, 1995.
40. Black DM and others: Randomised trial of effect of alendronate on risk of fracture in women with existing vertebral fractures, *Lancet* 348:1535-1541, 1996.
41. Orwoll E and others: Alendronate for the treatment of osteoporosis in men, *N Engl J Med* 343:604-610, 2000.
42. Harris ST and others: Effects of risedronate treatment on vertebral and nonvertebral fractures in women with postmenopausal osteoporosis: a randomized controlled trial, *JAMA* 282:1344-1352, 1999.
43. Schnitzer T and others: Therapeutic equivalence of alendronate 70 mg once-weekly and alendronate 10 mg daily in the treatment of osteoporosis. Alendronate Once-Weekly Study Group, *Aging* 12:1-12, 2000.
44. Lanza FL and others: Endoscopic comparison of esophageal and gastroduodenal effects of risedronate and alendronate in postmenopausal women, *Gastroenterology* 119:866-869, 2000.
45. Lanza F and others: An endoscopic comparison of the effects of alendronate and risedronate on upper gastrointestinal mucosae, *Am J Gastroenterol* 95:3112-3117, 2000.
46. Ettinger B and others: Reduction of vertebral fracture risk in postmenopausal women with osteoporosis treated with raloxifene: results from a 3-year randomized clinical trial. Multiple outcomes of raloxifene evaluation (MORE) investigators, *JAMA* 282:637-645, 1999.
47. Cauley JA and others: Continued breast cancer risk reduction in postmenopausal women treated with raloxifene: 4-year results from the MORE trial. Multiple outcomes of raloxifene evaluation, *Breast Cancer Res Treat* 65:125-134, 2001.
48. PEPI Investigators: Effects of hormone therapy on bone mineral density: results from the Postmenopausal Estrogen/Progestin Interventions PEPI Trial, *JAMA* 276:1389-1396, 1996.
49. Villareal DT and others: Bone mineral density response to estrogen replacement in frail elderly women: a randomized controlled trial, *JAMA* 286:815-820, 2001.
50. Felson DT and others: The effect of postmenopausal estrogen therapy on bone density in elderly women, *N Engl J Med* 329:1141-1146, 1993.
51. Belchetz PE: Hormonal treatment of postmenopausal women, *N Engl J Med* 330:1062-1071, 1994.
52. Grey AB, Cundy TF, Reid IR: Continuous combined oestrogen/progestin therapy is well tolerated and increases bone density at the hip and spine in post-menopausal osteoporosis, *Clin Endocrinol* 40:671-677, 1994.
53. Neer RM and others: Effect of parathyroid hormone (1-34) on fractures and bone mineral density in postmenopausal women with osteoporosis, *N Engl J Med* 344:1434-1441, 2001.
54. Bilezikian JP, Kurland ES: Therapy of male osteoporosis with parathyroid hormone, *Calcif Tissue Int* 69:248-251, 2001.
55. Lane NE and others: Bone mass continues to increase at the hip after parathyroid hormone treatment is discontinued in glucocorticoid-induced osteoporosis: results of a randomized controlled clinical trial, *J Bone Miner Res* 15:944-951, 2000.

56. Storm T and others: Effect of intermittent cyclical etidronate therapy on bone mass and fracture rate in women with post menopausal osteoporosis, *N Engl J Med* 322:1265-1271, 1990.
57. Watts NB and others: Intermittent cyclical etidronate treatment of postmenopausal osteoporosis, *N Engl J Med* 323:73-79, 1990.
58. Adachi JD and others: Intermittent etidronate therapy to prevent corticosteroid-induced osteoporosis, *N Engl J Med* 337:382-387, 1997.
59. Glorieux FH and others: Cyclic administration of pamidronate in children with severe osteogenesis imperfecta, *N Engl J Med* 339:986-987, 1998.
60. Shane ES and others: Prevention of bone loss after heart transplantation with antiresorptive therapy: a pilot study, *J Heart Lung Transplant* 17:1089-1096, 1998.
61. Smith MR and others: Pamidronate to prevent bone loss during androgen-deprivation therapy for prostate cancer, *N Engl J Med* 345:948-955, 2001.
62. Berenson JR and others: Efficacy of pamidronate in reducing skeletal events in patients with advanced multiple myeloma, *N Engl J Med* 334:488-493, 1996.
63. Hortobagyi GN and others: Efficacy of pamidronate in reducing skeletal complications in patients with breast cancer and lytic bone metastases, *N Engl J Med* 335:1785-1792, 1996.
64. Overgaard K and others: Effect of salcatonin given intranasally on bone mass and fracture rates in established osteoporosis: a dose-response study, *Br Med J* 305:556-561, 1992.
65. Tilyard MW and others: Treatment of postmenopausal osteoporosis with calcitriol or calcium, *N Engl J Med* 326:357-362, 1992.
66. Snyder PJ and others: Effect of testosterone treatment on bone mineral density in men over 65 years of age, *J Clin Endocrinol Metab*, 84: 1966-1972, 1999.
67. Wimalawansa SJ: Prevention and treatment of osteoporosis: efficacy of combination of hormone replacement therapy with other antiresorptive agents, *J Clin Densitom* 3:187-201, 2000.
68. Lindsay R and others: Randomised controlled study of effect of parathyroid hormone on vertebral-bone mass and fracture incidence among postmenopausal women on oestrogen with osteoporosis, *Lancet* 350:550-555, 1997.
69. Rittmaster RS and others: Enhancement of bone mass in osteoporotic women with parathyroid hormone followed by alendronate, *J Clin Endocrinol Metab* 85:2129-2134, 2000.
70. Haguenauer D and others: Fluoride for treating postmenopausal osteoporosis, *Cochrane Database Syst Rev* CD002825, 2000.
71. Kannus P and others: Epidemiology of hip fractures, *Bone* 18(1 suppl):57S-63S, 1996.
72. Riggs BL, Melton LJ: The worldwide problem of osteoporosis: insights afforded by epidemiology, *Bone* 17(5 suppl):505S-511S, 1995.
73. Ray NF and others: Medical expenditures for the treatment of osteoporotic fractures in the United States in 1995: report from the National Osteoporosis Foundation, *J Bone Miner Res* 12:24-35, 1997.
74. Kado DM and others: Vertebral fractures and mortality in older women: a prospective study, *Arch Intern Med* 159:1215-1220, 1999.
75. Silverman SL: The clinical consequences of vertebral compression fracture, *Bone* 13:S27-S31, 1992.
76. Garfin SR and others: New technologies in spine: kyphoplasty and vertebroplasty for the treatment of painful osteoporotic compression fractures, *Spine* 26:1511-1515, 2001.
77. Swezey RL: Site-specific isometric exercises can be done safely at home: preventing osteoporotic fractures: the role of exercise, posture, and safety, *J Musculoskel Med* 14:9-23, 1997.

CHAPTER 202

Paget's Disease of the Bone

Julie P. Fago

DEFINITION/EPIDEMIOLOGY

Paget's disease is the second most common metabolic bone disease in older adults. Traditionally, medical and surgical specialists have managed the various manifestations of the disease, but now with more effective treatments available, the primary care team can provide complete management in most cases.

Paget's disease is uncommon before the age of 40 years; however, by the age of 80 years, 1 out of 10 persons are affected by the disease. Between 18% and 25% of the population have at least one family member with Paget's disease, leading to speculation of a genetic (or environmental) component. Paget's disease is common in England, Western Europe, New Zealand, Australia, and the United States; it is uncommon in Asia, Africa, India, and Scandinavia.

PATHOPHYSIOLOGY

Paget's disease is characterized by a localized increase in bone turnover and blood flow. It can affect one or more sites (monostotic vs. polyostotic). Once the disease is fully established, previously unaffected bones are usually spared. For reasons that are still not well understood, osteoclasts in the affected area are increased in number, size, and activity and cause breakdown of focal areas of bone at great speed. The osteoblasts, which are unaffected by the disease process, try to keep up with the bone degradation by laying down new osteoid as fast as they can. However, the newly formed bone is disorganized and lacks the architectural integrity of normal bone. This results in mechanically weak, highly vascular bone that is prone to deformity and fractures, especially if weight-bearing parts of the skeleton are affected.[1]

CLINICAL PRESENTATION

Although Paget's disease is usually asymptomatic, bone pain is the most common presenting symptom. The pain can be misinterpreted as part of the "aging process" or as part of another disease process. In one study, one third of patients presenting with bone pain were misdiagnosed as having osteoarthritis.[2] Failure to diagnose and initiate early treatment can result in irreversible consequences and significant morbidity.

The degree and character of the bone pain vary with the location and activity of Paget's disease. The most commonly involved sites are the pelvis, femur, tibia, spine, and skull. The hands and feet are only rarely involved. Generally, the affected bone is moderately painful both at rest and during motion. Most patients describe the pain as a deep ache (like a toothache) that can become severe and sharp with weight bearing and when the area is warmed. Hot baths and even warm bedclothes can intensify the pain.[3]

PHYSICAL EXAMINATION

On examination, the affected area is often tender to the touch and may be warm as a result of increased new blood vessel growth within the bone itself. The pagetic bone can be noticeably enlarged. Affected bones may be deformed in a bow shape either from the effects of gravity or from the tension of the attached musculature on the architecturally incompetent pagetic bone. When bones in the lower extremity become deformed, the patient will have an abnormal gait and, often, arthritic changes within the surrounding joints as a result of the mechanical stress.[4] When the skull is involved, the head size may increase, and frontal bossing may be evident.

Nerve entrapments can occur as a result of bony overgrowth, resulting in a variety of neuropathies, including cranial nerve palsies. Hearing loss may occur as a result of sensory neuropathy and/or conduction impairment resulting from pagetic involvement of the ossicles of the inner ear. When the spine is involved, bony overgrowth can result in spinal stenosis with attendant radiculopathies and/or motor impairments.[5]

DIAGNOSTICS

Diagnosis is confirmed by checking the serum alkaline phosphatase (SAP) and/or urinary N-telopeptide (NTx) level, both of which will be quite elevated in active disease. Their levels correlate with the extent and activity of the disease. Radiographic studies of the affected area(s) usually show a classic mixed sclerotic/lytic ("cotton-wool") pattern, cortical thickening, and bony enlargement. Bone scans show increased uptake in affected areas, but this pattern can be difficult to differentiate from other processes such as cancer and arthritis.

DIFFERENTIAL DIAGNOSIS

The symptoms and signs of Paget's disease must be distinguished from several other conditions. When the joints are involved, the differential diagnosis includes osteoarthritis, gout, and pseudogout. Ironically, these three diagnoses can coexist with Paget's disease, can be a complication of Paget's disease, or can mimic the symptoms of Paget's disease when the latter affects the bone adjacent to a joint.

Bone pain that occurs with an elevated SAP level and positive bone scan must be distinguished from malignancy, most commonly a metastasis from a distant site. In early, active Paget's disease the initial wave of osteoclastic resorption can appear as lytic lesions on plain radiographs and thus may mimic such malignancies as multiple myeloma. However, in the great majority of cases, the radiograph will show changes pathognomonic of Paget's disease.

Diagnostics

Paget's Disease

Laboratory
Serum alkaline phosphatase
Urinary N-telopeptide

Imaging
Plain x-ray studies of affected areas
Bone scan
MRI (if neurologic symptoms)

Differential Diagnosis

Paget's Disease

Osteoarthritis	Pseudogout
Gout	Malignancy

MANAGEMENT

The goals of treatment are to suppress osteoclastic activity, allowing the osteoblasts to catch up and lay down architecturally normal bone, which in turn reduces symptoms and prevents disease progression. All patients with bone pain or neurologic impingements, or who are at risk for complications based on the site of disease (femoral head, tibia, skull) should receive therapy (Box 202-1). Although some controversy remains about whether to treat patients solely on the basis of an elevated SAP level, most agree that values three to four times the normal range merit treatment. Bone pain usually responds within 2 to 3 weeks of active drug treatment. (See Table 202-1 for pharmacologic treatment of Paget's disease.) Neuropathies, if detected early, may also respond, but arthropathy will not, because it represents fixed-joint degradation. Efficacy of treatment is determined by the amount and duration of the reduction in SAP or NTx.

Bisphosphonates

Bisphosphonates are the most effective long-term treatment. Although initially they may cause a transient increase in pain, symptoms generally abate within weeks. Etidronate (Didronel), the first bisphosphonate approved for use in Paget's disease, produces moderate improvement in both symptoms and biochemical markers but because it may cause osteomalacia and increase the risk of fracture, it is no longer commonly used.[6]

Alendronate (Fosamax) and risedronate (Actonel) are the bisphosphonates of choice for treating Paget's disease in the United States. Clear evidence from randomized controlled trials have shown that compared to etidronate, both achieve quicker normalization of biochemical markers and pain reduction, have prolonged posttreatment effects, and reduced relapse rates.[7,8] The main side effects are stomach upset and, rarely, in the case of alendronate, esophageal ulceration.

Pamidronate (Aredia) is another potent treatment option, although it is available only in an IV form. Studies have shown that one 3-day treatment course (180 mg total) will induce a clinical and biochemical remission lasting an average of 14 months in the majority of patients.[9] In those with mild disease, one 60-mg infusion may be all that is needed. More severe disease may require titration of up to 480 mg given over several weeks. Because of its rapid onset of action, pamidronate is the drug of choice for patients with impending fracture, neurologic impingements, or severe refractory disease.[3] The side effects are

BOX 202-1

INDICATIONS FOR DRUG THERAPY IN PAGET'S DISEASE

- Bone or joint pain
- Pagetic lesions in weight-bearing sites
- Involvement of the skull
- Nerve entrapments
- Preparation for elective joint replacement
- Serum alkaline phosphatase levels >3 to 4 times normal

TABLE 202-1 Pharmacologic Treatment for Paget's Disease

Drug	Dose	Side Effects
BIPHOSPHONATES		
Alendronate	40 mg PO qd for 6 months	Nausea, esophageal ulcers
Risedronate	30 mg PO qd for 2 months	Nausea
Etidronate	400 mg PO qd for 6 months*	Nausea, osteomalacia
Pamidronate	30-60 mg IV qd for 3 days or 60 mg IV once for mild disease (maximum 480 mg)	Mild fever, hypocalcemia, flulike symptoms, transient leukopenia
CALCITONIN		
Salmon	50-100 IU SQ qd for 3-6 months, then three times per week†	Flushing, nausea, loss of efficacy
Human	0.5-1 mg SQ as above	Flushing, nausea, loss of efficacy
Nasal	200-400 IU qd as above	Nasal irritation, loss of efficacy
Plicamycin	15-25 μg/kg IV qd for 10 days	Bone marrow, kidney, liver toxicity

*Etidronate should be given cyclically with at least 6 month of no treatment between courses.
†Patients with mild disease may need <1 year of treatment; those with moderate to severe disease may need to be treated indefinitely.

generally minor, but a transient hypocalcemia, leukopenia, and flulike symptoms can be seen.

Calcitonin

Calcitonin, although not as potent or long-lasting as the bisphosphonates, remains an effective, well-tolerated treatment option.[3] Pain generally remits after 2 to 3 weeks, and as treatment continues, lytic lesions fill in with new normal bone, vascularity decreases, and neurologic deficits (if any) improve remarkably.[10] However, the effect of calcitonin wears off with time because of the development of antibodies (in the case of salmon or porcine calcitonin) and/or downregulation of calcitonin receptors.[11] The effective dose of salmon calcitonin is 50 to 100 IU SC every day for 1 month followed by injections three times a week for 3 to 6 months as dictated by clinical symptoms and biochemical markers. Nasal salmon calcitonin (200 IU) and human calcitonin (0.5 mg SC) can be used in a similar schedule. The main side effects of injectable calcitonin are transient flushing and nausea. Vomiting, diarrhea, and abdominal pain can also occur. Nasal calcitonin is generally better tolerated but can cause nasal irritation.

Plicamycin

Although not labeled for the treatment of Paget's disease, plicamycin (formerly called mithramycin) has been used for severe Paget's disease, particularly in cases with extensive basilar skull involvement. An IV infusion of 15 to 25 μg/kg body weight over 10 days can induce a rapid fall in SAP and improvement in symptoms. However, because of its significant side effects, including bone marrow suppression and liver and kidney toxicity, IV pamidronate has become the preferred agent for cases needing urgent intervention.[3]

Adjuvant Therapy

Nonsteroidal antiinflammatory drugs or cylcooxygenase-2 inhibitors can be useful adjuncts for patients with joint or bone pain. When pain is severe, opioids may need to be used until the Paget's disease is controlled. Assistive devices, including shoe lifts, walkers, and canes for equalizing leg length discrepancies, as well as physical therapy for joint symptoms, are often quite helpful. Calcium and/or vitamin D supplements should be considered for those with low dietary intake to ensure adequate bone mineralization.

Ongoing Monitoring

Patients with Paget's disease need to be evaluated periodically. Those with asymptomatic disease in areas of the skeleton where there is little or no risk (e.g., the iliac crest) can be monitored less closely. Conversely, those with active disease in weight-bearing bones or the skull require aggressive follow-up care. Disease activity is monitored by using biochemical markers (SAP or NTx), which are usually measured at 3- to 6-month intervals in active disease or yearly in inactive disease. In addition, pain, joint symptoms, neurologic function, and medication side effects need to be assessed at every visit.

LIFE SPAN CONSIDERATIONS

Although untreated Paget's disease can cause pain and deformity, the life span is unaffected unless the patient develops osteosarcoma or severe flattening of the base of the skull with spinal cord compression.

COMPLICATIONS

Bone pain typical of Paget's disease must be distinguished from other long-term consequences of untreated Paget's disease, including neural compromise, fractures, joint deterioration, and sarcomatous transformation. Nerve compression is most common when the spine or skull is involved. Enlarging bone in the vertebrae can compress spinal nerve roots or even the spinal cord itself, resulting in neuropathic pain and/or myelopathies. Cranial nerves, which exit the skull through tiny foramina, can also be compressed, resulting in facial pain, paralysis, or deafness. Involvement of the base of the skull can result in hydrocephalus (often presenting as dementia) or brainstem compression.

Pagetic fractures present with sudden, severe knifelike pain. They may be traumatic, or if the pagetic bone is weakened by extensive lytic disease, can occur spontaneously. Until Paget's disease is controlled, healing is difficult and slow. Pagetic arthropathy occurs when bone adjacent to joint surfaces (e.g., the femoral head or the acetabulum) is affected, resulting in abnormal joint architecture and subsequent degenerative arthritis.

The most dreaded consequence of long-term Paget's disease is osteosarcoma. This is heralded by a sudden increase in pain intensity at a pagetic site. Although it is rare, osteosarcoma has an extremely poor prognosis. The majority of patients die within 1 to 3 years.

INDICATIONS FOR REFERRAL/HOSPITALIZATION

Medical management of straightforward cases can be easily handled by the primary care provider. However physical therapists are invaluable members of the management team because of their expertise in maximizing physical function and knowledge of assistive devices. Referral to a rheumatologist is indicated if the patient's disease is unresponsive to usual treatment. Orthopedic referral is indicated when an associated arthropathy or spinal stenosis causes unremitting pain or loss of function.

Severe neurologic complications such as hydrocephalus requires aggressive inpatient antipagetic therapy combined with neurosurgical intervention. Other causes of hospitalization include fracture, elective joint replacement, or spinal decompression.

PATIENT AND FAMILY EDUCATION

Patients and their families must understand the disease process and medical management to manage Paget's disease optimally. First, they need to be informed about how to take their medications and what side effects could occur. Second, patients need to promptly report any worsening of their symptoms, which could herald disease progression, fracture, or sarcomatous transformation. Those with skull involvement need to understand what neuropathic symptoms to look for and the importance of prompt reporting. For example, progressive hearing loss should not be blamed on age.

In addition, family members should inform their own primary care team of their family history of Paget's disease and should be cautioned to report bone pain or symptoms of nerve compression.

HEALTH PROMOTION

Patients should be encouraged to remain as physically active as possible. If the tibia or proximal femur is affected, heavy weight-bearing exercise should be avoided until the disease is in remission. Swimming, bicycling, and Tai Chi are excellent alternatives for patients with painful arthropathy. Adequate dietary (or supplemental) calcium and vitamin D are important to help maintain bone density.

REFERENCES

1. Sirus ES: Extensive personal experience: Paget's disease of the bone, *J Clin Epidemiol Metab* 80(2):335-339, 1995.
2. Hamdy RC, Moore S, LeRoy J: Clinical presentation of Paget's disease of the bone in older patients, *South Med J* 86(10):1097-1100, 1993.
3. Sirus ES: Paget's disease of the bone, In Favus MJ, editor: *Primer on the metabolic bone diseases and disorders of mineral metabolism*, ed 4, Philadelphia, 2000, Lippincott-Raven.
4. Altman RD: Arthritis in Paget's disease of the bone, *J Bone Metab Res* 14(Suppl 2):85-87, 1999.
5. Poncelet A: The neurologic complications of Paget's disease, *J Bone Metab Res* 14(Suppl 2):88-91, 1999.
6. Drake WM and others: Consensus statement on the modern therapy of Paget's disease of the bone from a Western Osteoporosis Alliance Symposium, *Clin Ther* 23 (4):620-626, 2001.
7. Sirus ES and others: Comparative study of alendronate versus etidronate for the treatment of Paget's disease of the bone, *J Clin Endocrinol Metab* 81:961-967, 1996.
8. Miller PD and others: A randomized, double-blind comparison of risidronate and etidronate in the treatment of Paget's disease of the bone, *Am J Med* 106(5):513-520, 1999.
9. Grauer A and others: Long-term efficacy of IV pamidronate in Paget's disease of the bone, *Semin Arthritis Rheum* 23(4):283-284, 1994.
10. Wallach S: Calcitonin: history and prospects—a personal view, *Semin Arthritis Rheum* 23(4):256-260, 1994.
11. Singer FR, Fredericks RS, Minkin C: Salmon calcitonin therapy for Paget's disease of the bone: the problem of acquired clinical resistance, *Arthritis Rheum* 23:1148-1154, 1980.

CHAPTER 203

Shoulder Pain

Kathy J. Fabiszewski

DEFINITION/EPIDEMIOLOGY

Shoulder pain and dysfunction are among the most common musculoskeletal complaints encountered in primary and emergency care, representing the sixth and ninth most common reasons given for consulting the primary care provider and internist, respectively, and they are second only to knee pain as a source of impairment in sports and recreational activities.[1,2] Trauma or disease may cause shoulder pain. Injury, coupled with pain, predisposes the individual to functional impairment or disability. The prevalence of shoulder pain ranges from 8% to 20% in the those 30 years and older; it is most prevalent in middle and older age.[1]

Immediate emergency department referral or orthopedic consultation are indicated for patients with suspected shoulder dislocation. Physician consultation is indicated for patients with acromioclavicular separation and rotator cuff tears.

PATHOPHYSIOLOGY

The shoulder comprises four separate joints or articulations that are composed of only three bones: the scapula, clavicle, and humerus. The shoulder or glenohumeral joint (the articulation of the humerus and the glenoid fossa of the scapula) is a closely fitted, complex ball-and-socket joint that is capable of a wide, almost global, range of motion. Adjacent to the glenohumeral joint are the acromioclavicular joint (the articulation between the acromion process and the clavicle) and the sternoclavicular joint (the articulation between the manubrium of the sternum and the clavicle), which form the shoulder girdle. At the scapulothoracic joint, the scapula is suspended from the posterior thoracic wall by muscular attachments to the ribs and spine.[3] Normal shoulder motion is dependent on the smooth, integrated movement of these articulations.

The primary movers of the glenohumeral joint are the pectoralis major and minor (adducts the shoulder), deltoid (abducts the shoulder), teres major, and latissimus dorsi.[3] The trapezius muscles elevate and rotate the scapula. The shoulder joints are stabilized by the soft tissues of the shoulder girdle, including the joint capsule, glenoid labrum, muscles of the rotator cuff, long head of the biceps, and scapular stabilizers.[3] The shoulder socket (glenoid) is shallow and subsequently has little inherent bony stability. This anatomic arrangement provides for greater mobility but is accomplished by compromising some stability, making the shoulder one of the most commonly dislocated joints in the body.

The rotator cuff consists of the musculotendinous attachments of the supraspinatus, infraspinatus, and teres minor muscles that come together and attach on the greater and lesser tuberosities.[4] The primary functions of the rotator cuff are rotation of the humeral head and dynamic stabilization of the glenohumeral joint.[4]

The greater tuberosity of the humerus, tendons of the rotator cuff muscles that elevate the arm, and the subacromial bursa move back and forth through a tight archway of bone and ligament known as the coracoacromial arch. When the arm is raised, the archway becomes smaller, impinging these structures and making them prone to inflammation and degeneration.

CLINICAL PRESENTATION

The patient with a shoulder problem typically complains of shoulder pain, which is aggravated by movement and is often accompanied by limitation of movement. There may or may not be a history of trauma or overuse. Surprisingly, many individuals will fail to recollect trauma unless specifically asked. Patients often report difficulty with activities of daily living such as bathing, combing their hair, or dressing, as well as driving, carrying groceries, or exercising. Other symptoms may include stiffness, crepitation, and aching discomfort related to vigorous or sustained use.

Inquiring about hand dominance, employment (lifting, chronic stress on joints, safety precautions, etc), exercise and recreational activities (extent, type, and frequency), and self-care capacity facilitates identification of contributing factors, potential etiologies, and the functional impact of the symptomatology. Identifying any history of recent or remote trauma is vital. Determining previous diagnostic studies, hospitalizations/surgeries, or therapies guides diagnostic evaluation.

It is also critical to ascertain the exact location and distribution of the pain. It is unusual for pain originating in the shoulder, for example, to radiate below the elbow.[3] Pain involving other joints is suggestive of a generalized arthritic process. Characterization of the type, intensity, timing, and duration of pain, as well as identification of ameliorating and exacerbating factors, is also essential. The American Shoulder and Elbow Surgeons Standardized Form for Assessment of the Shoulder (Figure 203-1) incorporates a synopsis of both patient self-evaluation data and physical examination parameters and is useful in organizing a primary care approach to shoulder pain.

PHYSICAL EXAMINATION

Physical examination begins with visual inspection of the shoulder. Anterior and posterior examination for surgical scars, displacement of bony prominences, warmth, swelling, changes in skin color or texture, muscular atrophy, and winging of the scapula is necessary. Asymmetry with the uninvolved shoulder should be noted. Classically, there is focal tenderness. Before any shoulder movement is initiated, the examiner should palpate for tenderness in the sternoclavicular joint, the acromioclavicular joint, and the shoulder itself. Both shoulders can be palpated simultaneously to compare the affected side with the unaffected side.[3] Palpating bony landmarks is especially valuable in excluding a joint disorder; palpating the muscular structures is useful in excluding spasm. A simple shoulder examination checklist is provided in Box 203-1.

Active motion should be performed first to determine the integrity of the rotator cuff and to ascertain the location of the

SHOULDER ASSESSMENT FORM
AMERICAN SHOULDER AND ELBOW SURGEONS

Examiner:

Name:	Date:
Age: Hand dominance: R L Ambi	Gender: M F
Diagnosis:	Initial Assess? Y N
Procedure/Data:	Follow-up: M; Y;

PATIENT SELF-EVALUATION

Are you having pain in your shoulder? (circle the correct answer)	Yes	No

Mark where your pain is

FRONT BACK

Do you have pain in your shoulder at night?	Yes	No
Do you take pain medication (aspirin, Advil, Tylenol, etc.)?	Yes	No
Do you take narcotic pain medication (codeine or stronger)?	Yes	No
How many pills do you take each day (average)?		pills

How bad is your pain today (mark line)?

0 ——————————— 10

No pain at all — Pain as bad as it can be

Does your shoulder feel unstable (as if it is going to dislocate)?	Yes	No

How unstable is your shoulder (mark line)?

0 ——————————— 10

Very stable — Very unstable

Circle the number in the box that indicates your ability to do the following activities:
0 = unable to do; 1 = very difficult to do; 2 = somewhat difficult; 3 = not difficult

ACTIVITY		RIGHT ARM	LEFT ARM
1. Put on a coat		0 1 2 3	0 1 2 3
2. Sleep on your painful or affected side		0 1 2 3	0 1 2 3
3. Wash back/do up bra in back		0 1 2 3	0 1 2 3
4. Manage toileting		0 1 2 3	0 1 2 3
5. Comb hair		0 1 2 3	0 1 2 3
6. Reach a high shelf		0 1 2 3	0 1 2 3
7. Lift 10 lb above the shoulder		0 1 2 3	0 1 2 3
8. Throw a ball overhand		0 1 2 3	0 1 2 3
9. Do usual work. List:		0 1 2 3	0 1 2 3
10. Do usual sport. List:		0 1 2 3	0 1 2 3

FIGURE 203-1

The American Shoulder and Elbow Surgeon's Standardized Form for Assessment of the Shoulder.(Reprinted with permission from the American Shoulder and Elbow Surgeons.)

PHYSICIAN ASSESSMENT				
RANGE OF MOTION	Right		Left	
Total shoulder motion goniometer preferred	Active	Passive	Active	Passive
Forward elevation (maximum arm-trunk angle)				
External rotation (arm comfortably at the side)				
External rotation (arm at 90 degrees of abduction)				
Internal rotation (highest posterior anatomy reached with the thumb)				
Cross-body adduction (antecubital fossa to the opposite acromion)				

SIGNS	0 = none; 1 = mild; 2 = moderate; 3 = severe		
SIGN		Right	Left
Supraspinatus/greater tuberosity tenderness		0 1 2 3	0 1 2 3
Anteroclavicular joint tenderness		0 1 2 3	0 1 2 3
Biceps tendon tenderness (or rupture)		0 1 2 3	0 1 2 3
Other tenderness—List:		0 1 2 3	0 1 2 3
Impingement I (passive forward elevation in slight internal rotation)		Y N	Y N
Impingement II (passive internal rotation with 90 degrees of flexion)		Y N	Y N
Impingement III (90 degrees of active abduction—classic painful arc)		Y N	Y N
Subacromial crepitus		Y N	Y N
Scars—location		Y N	Y N
Atrophy—location		Y N	Y N
Deformity—describe		Y N	Y N

STRENGTH (record MRC grade)

0 = no contraction; 1 = flicker; 2 = movement with gravity eliminated; 3 = movement against gravity; 4 = movement against some resistance; 5 = normal power

	Right	Left
Testing affected by pain?	Y N	Y N
Forward elevation	0 1 2 3 4 5	0 1 2 3 4 5
Abduction	0 1 2 3 4 5	0 1 2 3 4 5
External rotation (arm comfortably at the side)	0 1 2 3 4 5	0 1 2 3 4 5
Internal rotation (arm comfortably at the side)	0 1 2 3 4 5	0 1 2 3 4 5

INSTABILITY

0 = none; 1 = mild (0–1 cm translation); 2 = moderate (1–2 cm translation or translates to glenoid rim); 3 = severe (>2 cm translation or over rim of glenoid)

	Right	Left
Anterior translation	0 1 2 3	0 1 2 3
Posterior translation	0 1 2 3	0 1 2 3
Inferior translation (sulcus sign)	0 1 2 3	0 1 2 3
Anterior apprehension	0 1 2 3	0 1 2 3
Reduces symptoms?	Y N	Y N
Voluntary instability?	Y N	Y N
Relocation test positive?	Y N	Y N
Generalized ligamentous laxity?	Y N	Y N
Other physical findings:		

FIGURE 203-1, cont'd

For legend, see previous page.

BOX 203-1

SHOULDER EXAMINATION

INSPECTION

1. Visual inspection comparing affected shoulder with the uninvolved shoulder
2. Range of motion of the cervical spine
3. Active range of motion of the shoulder
   - Wall push (look for winging)
   - Forward elevation/flexion
   - Extension
   - External rotation
   - Internal rotation
   - Abduction
   - Adduction
4. Passive range of motion of the shoulder
   - Impingement test
5. Strength testing of all major muscle groups
   - Flexor/extensor of the wrist
   - Biceps
   - Triceps
   - Supraspinatus isolation
   - Internal rotators
   - External rotators
   - Deltoid
6. Deep tendon reflexes (DTRs)
7. Peripheral pulses (check for bruits)

PALPATION

1. Supraclavicular fissure
2. Sternoclavicular joint
3. Acromioclavicular joint
4. Glenohumeral joint
5. Biceps tendon insertion
6. Muscular structures

TABLE 203-1 Tests of Shoulder Function

Test	Technique	Interpretation
Apprehension test	Abduct and externally rotate patient's arm to a position where it might easily dislocate.	Impending dislocation is signaled by noticeable look of apprehension on face of patient, with patient resisting further motion.
Drop arm test	Have patient hold affected extremity in a fully abducted position, then ask patient to slowly lower arm to side.	Rotator cuff tearing is suggested if patient's arm drops to side from a position of 90 degrees abduction.
Empty can test	Have patient hold out affected arm as if offering examiner a can of soda, then have patient turn arm to empty the contents.	Rotator cuff tendonitis is suggested if pain is produced by maneuver of "emptying the can."
Impingement test	Have patient elevate arm slowly into overhead position.	Rotator cuff tendinitis is suggested if patient experiences sharp "catches" of pain or impingement with this maneuver.
Yergason's test	Have patient fully flex elbow, then grasp flexed elbow in one hand while holding patient's wrist in other hand; to test stability of biceps tendon, externally rotate patient's arm as patient resists and, at same time, pull downward on patient's elbow.	Pain with this maneuver suggests that biceps tendon is unstable in biceps groove; no pain is experienced with a stable tendon.

pain. Active range of motion of each shoulder should be measured, including forward flexion (normal is 180 degrees), extension (normal is 70 degrees), external rotation (normal is 45 degrees), internal rotation (normal is 60 degrees), abduction (normal is 180 degrees), and adduction (normal is 180 degrees). Any clicks or crepitation suggestive of impingement should be noted. Passive range of motion should be compared with active range of motion and is particularly useful in determining whether adhesive capsulitis (frozen shoulder) is present. A person with adhesive capsulitis can generally still abduct the arm 60 degrees.

Strength testing of the individual rotator cuff muscles is then performed using resisted movements. Table 203-1 summarizes special tests of shoulder function and their associated disorders. Complete neurovascular assessment of the associated shoulder structures should also be performed documenting sensory, motor, or circulatory impairment. The spine and peripheral joints are examined for evidence of coexisting joint disease.

Evaluation of a painful shoulder is challenging because the problem is often dynamic, with pain occurring only with specific activity. It is necessary to determine if the discomfort and immobility are articular (bone) or periarticular (soft tissue structure). With bursitis or adhesive capsulitis, for example, both active and passive range of motion will be limited. Weakness on resisted movements suggests a muscle or tendon tear or neurologic compromise.[1]

DIAGNOSTICS

Diagnostic tests should be used judiciously to confirm or refine diagnoses. It is unwise to base a diagnosis on a radiologic test, as x-ray studies can be misleading or unrevealing. Radiographs and even MRIs are often negative in soft tissue problems in the young athlete[5]; this underscores the importance of a good examination.

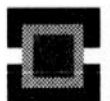

Diagnostics

Shoulder Pain

Laboratory
CBC and differential*
ESR*

Imaging
X-ray*
- Anteroposterior (AP) views
- Axillary lateral views
- Scapula Y view

MRI*
CT scan*
Ultrasound*
Arthrography*

*If indicated.

Plain x-ray films are recommended if there is a history of trauma or if arthritis or neoplastic disease is a consideration. With all significant trauma it is imperative to obtain the appropriate x-ray studies including standard anteroposterior views of the glenohumeral joint with the arm at 30 degrees external rotation, axillary lateral views, and scapula Y views that detect dislocation not seen on standard views. Occasionally, in nontraumatic presentations, calcifications from previous or chronic injuries can be seen. Spurring of the acromial process or calcium deposits in the soft tissues (seen in the tendon in calcific tendinitis) are common findings.[6] A detailed explanation of the reason for the x-ray study enables the radiologist to obtain the appropriate views.[1] X-ray findings of the cervical spine are indicated if cervical radiculopathy is suspected.

MRI or other modalities can be valuable in detecting soft tissue lesions. In older patients, however, these tests almost always reveal some "abnormality" that may have nothing to do with the presenting symptoms. Therefore these studies, which also include ultrasonography and CT scans, as well as invasive studies such as arthrography, are best ordered in consultation with a specialist, particularly when there may be a need for surgical intervention.

Laboratory studies are seldom indicated. However, CBC, erythrocyte sedimentation rate, and serologic tests for rheumatologic disorders should be performed in accordance with the history and examination findings.

DIFFERENTIAL DIAGNOSIS

The ability to correlate the history and physical examination with a functional knowledge of anatomy, an understanding of the mechanism of injury, and an ability reproduce the symptoms clinically will often diagnose the problem.[5] Shoulder disorders can be categorized as acute or chronic and as either traumatic or nontraumatic. The diagnosis of shoulder pain is simplified when there is a history of trauma. If the duration of pain is less than 2 weeks, the patient may recall an injury or fall. The difficulty comes with subacute, smoldering conditions that have an onset 6 weeks to 3 months after the incident or injury.[2]

Although instability is most common in teenagers, gradual onset of shoulder pain on the nondominant side of a middle-aged woman is more likely adhesive capsulitis. Severe acute shoulder pain with restricted movement in a laborer or athlete is likely acute calcific tendinitis.[7] Pain in the shoulder at night is rotator cuff disease until proven otherwise. Pain in the shoulder with repetitive overhead activity also suggests rotator cuff disease. Pain at rest should suggest that the problem is extrinsic to the shoulder girdle, although acute inflammatory conditions often cause night pain. Pain associated with a throwing motion may be secondary to instability. Pain in the supraclavicular area and toward the vertebral border of the scapula is often referred pain from the neck. Pain radiating down the arm, especially below the elbow, suggests a neurogenic cause.

Tendinitis

Tendinitis occurs when the tendons or surrounding tissue become inflamed, swollen, and tender. Supraspinatus tendinitis is the most common cause of shoulder pain[8] and is usually caused by degenerative changes in that tendon with advancing age. Other common causes of tendinitis include overhead or repetitive activity, a weakened rotator cuff (usually in combination with overhead activity), heavy lifting activities, and muscle strain. In rotator cuff tendinitis, abnormal repetitive stresses cause a mechanical irritation of the structures below the acromial bursa.[6] With calcific tendinitis, calcific deposits form in the rotator cuff tendon causing local mechanical irritation. Biceps tendinitis, which can result from overuse activities above the head, can lead to subacromial impingement, particularly in internal rotation. Elbow flexion against resistance usually reproduces pain located over the anterior aspect of the shoulder and upper arm.

Tendinitis often has no isolated precipitating event. Most patients complain of a deep ache in the shoulder with increasing pain on abduction and internal rotation. Determining what position or posture causes pain is diagnostic. Pain with arm elevation,

Differential Diagnosis

Shoulder Pain

Dislocation, instability, and subluxation
Adhesive capsulitis
Acute calcific tendinitis
Rotator cuff disease
Neurogenic cause
Referred pain
Malignancy
Bursitis
Tendinitis
Arthritis

Acromioclavicular joint separation
Fractures
Referred shoulder pain
- Reflex sympathetic dystrophy
- Thoracic outlet syndrome
- Cardiovascular causes
  - Pericarditis
  - Ischemia/angina
  - Dissecting aortic aneurysm

Gastrointestinal causes
- Hepatic inflammation or congestion
- Cholecystitis
- Pancreatitis

Pulmonary causes
- Pleurisy
- Pancoast's tumor

Postlaparoscopic surgery
Nerve compression/irritation

for example, is suggestive of rotator cuff tendinitis and/or subacromial bursitis. Point tenderness is often localized to the vicinity of the greater tuberosity below the acromion and along the lateral aspect of the humeral head. The reflexive shrug will be noted as the patient tries to abduct the arm. The shrug helps to reduce the pain caused by impingement on the acromion.

Generalized muscle weakness on manual muscle testing, especially with internal and external rotation, is characteristic of rotator cuff tendinitis.[6] Also the empty can test and the impingement test are useful in validating the clinical diagnosis (see Table 203-1).

Bursitis

Bursitis occurs when the bursa becomes inflamed and painful as surrounding muscles move over it. The bursa's primary function is to maintain a gliding surface between muscles and ligaments (see Chapter 188). The most common cause of bursitis is overuse syndromes. Pitching, tennis, swimming, or repetitious use of the arm at or above shoulder level can all cause subacromial bursitis.

Occasionally the calcific deposits in tendinitis may extend the inflammatory process into the subacromial bursa, producing inflammation in the wall of the subacromial bursa.

The pain is usually felt at the tip of the shoulder or along the upper third of the humerus and is referred down the deltoid muscle into the upper arm. It occurs when the arm is lifted overhead or twisted. In extreme cases pain will be present continuously and may disrupt sleep.

Rotator Cuff Tear or Rupture

Tears in the rotator cuff are more common in older adults because of degenerative changes that take place over time in tendons and lead to structural weakening that predisposes the tendon to tears, particularly after the fifth decade of life.[8] Rotator cuff disease is classified or graded to reflect progressively worsening symptomatology and functional impairment. Grade I disease of the rotator cuff, which is most common in young adults, involves acute inflammation and edema resulting from either acute trauma or repetitive overhead activity. Grade II disease, which is seen in middle-aged adults, is characterized by chronic degenerative changes without actual tear. Grade III disease, commonly observed in older adult populations, represents disruption of tendon integrity (a tear).

Excessive use of the shoulder involving repetitive stressful movement, as well as injury or repeated injuries, will produce this partial or complete rupture or disintegration of the rotator cuff. A weakened rotator cuff at the supraspinatus tendon may tear spontaneously as a result of minimal trauma, such as a fall. Tears tend not to be painful. Muscle atrophy often accompanies rotator cuff tears. Although the rotator cuff is not easily palpable, point tenderness to manual palpation is maximal just below the greater tubercle of the humerus. Incomplete ruptures produce chronic thickening of the subacromial bursa and impingement syndrome. There is little chance for spontaneous healing of a torn rotator cuff.

The patient with rotator cuff tear typically presents with complaints of shoulder pain aggravated by activity and radiating to the anterior aspect the arm. Abduction is painful and weak and tenderness may be elicited over the insertion of the greater tuberosity.[8] On examination, the patient will be unable to abduct the arm, instead producing a characteristic shoulder shrug. The drop arm test assesses the integrity of the rotator cuff and is positive with significant tears (see Table 203-1).

Shoulder Instability, Dislocation, and Subluxation

Shoulder dislocation predisposes the patient to recurrent instability. Instability results from posttraumatic capsular tear or stretch. Athletes are subject to numerous repetitive loads that can lead to symptoms of instability.[9] There are two primary types of shoulder instability: (1) traumatic, unidirectional instability and (2) atraumatic, multidirectional, bilateral, rehabilitation, inferior capsule shift. Dislocation is much more common in very young adults, with the likelihood of redislocation decreasing with advancing age. In older adults rotator cuff tears commonly occur with dislocation. A history of traumatic dislocation and medical or surgical reduction is a powerful risk factor for instability. The patient will simply complain of the shoulder "giving out." Dislocation results from trauma to the shoulder while it is hyperextended. Dislocations are often anterior and are characterized by loss of the shoulder's rounded appearance. The patient typically presents with the hands held to the side. There is prominence of the acromion, painful limitation of movement, and displacement of the humerus away from the trunk.

The apprehension test detects chronic shoulder dislocation (see Table 203-1). Yergason's test for long head of the biceps tendon stability determines whether the biceps tendon is stable in the occipital groove[10] (see Table 203-1). A palm-up hand position is used to rule out posterior dislocation.

Arthritis

Arthritis of the glenohumeral joint may be secondary to inflammatory arthritis or osteoarthritis. The distinguishing feature of shoulder arthritis is pain at rest, aggravated by movement. The patient reports a grinding sound or clicking with motion. Examination may reveal muscle wasting, crepitation, effusion, and decreased range of motion.

Although the shoulder may undergo arthritic changes from a number of causes, these changes are much better tolerated than arthritic changes occurring in the weight-bearing joints. A hot, red, swollen, and painful shoulder accompanied by fever and chills is suggestive of septic arthritis.

Shoulder Trauma

With severe shoulder trauma the differential diagnosis includes acromioclavicular separation (crepitus at and elevation at acromioclavicular joint), fractures of the clavicle or humerus, strains, sprains, and dislocation. Severe shoulder trauma not promptly responsive to conservative treatment warrants orthopedic referral.

Extrinsic Shoulder Disorders

Shoulder pain may be specific to the shoulder girdle area or may be referred from another location. Referred pain should be suspected when shoulder motion shows a painless complete arc, no specific periarticular shoulder tender point is identified, muscle strength is within normal limits, or when pain cannot be reproduced with various tests of the shoulder muscles.

Referred pain from cervical radiculopathies is common.[5] Because it is located in the thoracic dermatome area, shoulder pain can be referred from several interthoracic or abdominal organs enervated by the same nerves.

Myocardial ischemia or infarction may cause pain radiation to the left shoulder. Shoulder symptoms may also be related to diaphragmatic irritation, which shares the same root innervation (C5, C6) as the dermatome covering the shoulder's summit.

Cervical spondylosis, a herniated cervical disk, cervical trauma, or other neck problems may also cause pain radiating to the shoulder, scapula, or upper back. This pain is often felt at the superomedial angle of the scapula and may be verified by Spurling's test in which radicular pain is reproduced with head compression.[7] Sometimes a spinal fracture, in addition to causing local pain, may radiate pain to the shoulder along the course of any muscle affected by the fracture.

The shoulder may also be affected by a problem of the elbow and the distal end of the humerus, where a fracture can radiate pain proximally to the shoulder; however, this is a rather uncommon finding.[10]

Reflex sympathetic dystrophy after myocardial infarction, a cerebrovascular accident, and trauma can also cause shoulder pain. The characteristic features are persistent burning pain, diffuse tenderness, immobilization of the shoulder, and vasomotor changes in the hands. Gallbladder disease can cause scapular pain as well as right upper abdominal pain and tenderness. Pain caused by bony malignancy is usually gnawing, constant, and unrelated to movement.

MANAGEMENT

Although neither national specialty guidelines nor evidence-based practice guidelines are available as templates for approaching the management of shoulder pain, certain general principles of management apply to most presentations. Treatment includes both pharmacologic and a variety of nonpharmacologic approaches, including the triad of rest/avoidance of aggravating activities, ice packs/cold for the first few days followed by heat, and graded exercise. Other appropriate therapeutic modalities include physical therapy, nonsteroidal antiinflammatory drugs (NSAIDs) including the newer cylcooxygenase (COX)-2 inhibitors, and intraarticular corticosteroid injections. Goals of treatment center on maximizing physical comfort and preserving shoulder joint mobility and function.

When rest is prescribed for the treatment of acute shoulder pain, the patient avoids any activity that precipitates symptoms and especially the offending or "abusive" activity. Although in some situations a sling is useful, immobilization is recommended only in clinical situations where instability is apparent and never for more than 3 or 4 days. Sports and job modifications may be beneficial.[7]

Applications of ice or heat may provide relief. Ice reduces edema and bleeding and is most often recommended after trauma. Both heat and cold have been demonstrated to reduce muscle spasm and pain.[11] Ice applied topically to the affected joint for 30 minutes three or four times a day, particularly after any activity that involves use of the affected extremity, may reduce inflammation and swelling and promote comfort. Ice massage may also be of therapeutic benefit.

Restoration of normal shoulder function should begin as soon as acute pain has subsided. The overall goals of any therapeutic exercise program include maintaining or restoring full range of motion, decreasing inflammation (with ice, NSAIDs, and deep friction massage), and strengthening the rotator cuff musculature. Range-of-motion exercises including the "pendulum swing" and the "wall climb" (in which the patient "walks" his or her fingers up a wall) can be performed two or three times daily for 5 to 10 minutes and are helpful in maintaining mobility. Strengthening exercises with weight or resistance and stretching/strengthening exercises with Theraband are indicated only after the pain has subsided.

Referral to a physical therapist is recommended for a supervised exercise program. Physical rehabilitation programs should focus on restoration of functional ability as well as resolution of symptoms.[12] Adjunctive physical therapy modalities such as local heat application, electrogalvanic stimulation, ultrasound, and transverse friction massage may promote tissue extensibility and joint function in more chronic situations.

Pain-relieving medications may be indicated. The drugs of choice include NSAIDs including COX-2 inhibitors (see Table 199-1). Acetaminophen may be recommended for milder analgesia or in patients for whom NSAIDs are contraindicated. Although acetaminophen has no antiinflammatory activity, its analgesic effect is comparable to ibuprofen and naproxen with fewer side effects.[13]

Patients should be instructed to use antiinflammatory medication as prescribed, not just when pain is severe. In addition, they should be counseled about the medication's action, dosage, potential adverse effects, and drug-drug interactions. Certain NSAIDs are available over the counter and these should be discontinued if a prescription strength product is recommended.[13]

Corticosteroid injections may reduce pain and expedite functional recovery in patients with inflammatory conditions such as bursitis and tendinitis, as well as in rotator cuff impingement that does not improve with conservative therapy (see Chapter 188).

Health-promoting behaviors such as joint protection, balancing rest and exercise, and an optimistic attitude can improve outcomes as can attention to athletic and occupational considerations (e.g., workplace design, worker training, conditioning).[12]

LIFE SPAN CONSIDERATIONS

Children rarely have rotator cuff tears but commonly have shoulder joint instability (subluxations or dislocations of the glenohumeral joint). In young adults tendinitis is the most common cause of shoulder pain. Older patients rarely have problems with instability, but because the rotator cuff apparatus undergoes significant age-related changes, older patients commonly present with problems with rotator cuff and the glenohumeral joint. This results from the unique anatomy of the shoulder coupled with age-related degenerative changes.[4] Rotator cuff tears often go unrecognized or are clinically confused with degenerative tendinitis or other forms of shoulder disease in older adults.[4] Musculoskeletal disease is the leading cause of functional disability in the older population.[4]

COMPLICATIONS

The most common and worrisome complication of chronic shoulder pain is adhesive capsulitis. Adhesive capsulitis is characterized by a gradual, progressive decline in shoulder mobility often resulting from prolonged joint immobilization after a painful episode. Diffuse aching pain and limited mobility are common. Pain is related to the stretching of the restricted joint capsule. Both active and passive range of motion of the glenohumeral joint and scapula are limited. Patients may have difficulty with activities of daily living including dressing, toileting, and even feeding themselves.

INDICATIONS FOR REFERRAL/HOSPITALIZATION

A referral to an orthopedist may be indicated for more aggressive diagnostic testing, including radiographs to assess for calcifications, spurs, or arthritic changes, MRI, arthrography, ultrasonography, or electromyelography for continued muscle weakness. Arthroscopic acromioplasty may be required for debridement of bursa, subacromial decompression, repair of ligaments, and repair of tendons if a tear is present. Total shoulder replacement may be necessary for end-stage arthritic conditions of the glenohumeral joint.

Failure to respond to conservative therapy or escalating symptoms despite conservative therapy, shoulder dislocation or instability, a rotator cuff tear or rupture, severe disabling arthritis, and infection are among the definitive indications for referral. In cases where arthrocentesis or arthroscopy is indicated, referral to a rheumatologist or an orthopedist may be indicated.

PATIENT AND FAMILY EDUCATION

Patient education concerning health promotion and injury prevention is important.[14] Recovery takes time and requires a multidisciplinary approach, including patient participation. If exercise programs are not taken seriously, chronic or recurrent pain and loss of function may result. Recovery from shoulder injury and pain can be an excruciatingly slow process requiring 6 weeks to 6 months. Education regarding the healing process and the factors that affect healing including patient motivation, adherence to interventions, social support, nutrition, lifestyle behaviors, exercise, age, occupation, mental status, depression, and co-morbidities is necessary.

In addition, the importance of exercise, as well as warm-up and stretching before activities, should be stressed. Avoidance of repetitive movements and overuse should be carefully explained. For chronic conditions patients should understand that although the pain may resolve, the condition can recur. Reinforcement of the need for modification of activities, adherence to exercise regimens, ice packs, medications, and gradual resumption of activities are also necessary.

REFERENCES

1. Kern DE: Shoulder pain. In Barker LR, Burton JR, Zieve PD, editors: *Principles of ambulatory medicine*, ed 4, Baltimore, 1995, Williams & Wilkins.
2. Brunet ME, Norwood LA, Sykes TF: What to do for the painful shoulder, *Patient Care* 15:56-83, 1997.
3. Onieal ME: Problems of the shoulder, *J Am Acad Nurse Pract* 6(6): 283-285, 1994.
4. Rousseau P: Rotator cuff tears in the elderly: a brief review of two cases, *J Am Geriatr Soc* 40(6):614-617, 1992.
5. Owens S, Itamura JM: Differential diagnosis of shoulder injuries in sports, *Orthop Clin North Am* 32(3):393-398, 2001.
6. Onieal ME: Rotator cuff tendinitis, *J Am Acad Nurse Prac* 6(7): 339-340, 1994.
7. Fongemie AE, Buss DD, Rolnick SJ: Management of shoulder impingement syndrome and rotator cuff tears, *Am Fam Physician* 57(4):667-674, 1998.
8. Simon RR, Koenigsknecht SJ, editors: Fractures and rheumatology. In *Emergency orthopedics: the extremities*, ed 4, New York, 1999, McGraw-Hill.
9. Doukas WC, Speer KP: Anatomy, pathophysiology, and biomechanics of shoulder instability, *Orthop Clin North Am* 32(3):381-389, 2001.
10. Hoppenfeld S: *Examination of the spine and extremities*, London, 1976, Prentice-Hall.
11. Simon RR, Koenigsknecht SJ, editors: Soft tissue injuries, dislocations, and disorders of the shoulder and upper arm. In *Emergency orthopedics: the extremities*, ed 4, New York, 1999, McGraw-Hill.
12. Kibler WB, McMullen J, Uhl T: Shoulder rehabilitation strategies, guidelines, and practice, *Orthop Clin North Am* 32(3):527-538, 2001.
13. McCarberg BH, Herr KA: Osteoarthritis: how to manage pain and improve patient function, *Geriatrics* 56(10):14-24, 2001.
14. Boyd MD and others: *Health teaching in nursing practice: a professional model*, ed 3, Stamford, CT, 1998, Appleton & Lange.

CHAPTER 204

Sprains, Strains, and Fractures

Christine M. Wilson

DEFINITION/EPIDEMIOLOGY

Common musculoskeletal injuries include sprains, strains, dislocations, and fractures. Sprains result from a tearing of the ligaments that bind the joint as the joint is forced beyond its normal range of motion. Strains result from the overstretching or overuse of muscles. Dislocations occur when a bone is displaced at the joint so that the articulating surfaces of the bones detach. Partial displacements are called subluxations. A fracture is a break in the cortex of bone.

Fractures may be classified as closed or open. A closed (simple) fracture has no associated disruption in the continuity of the overlying skin. An open (compound) fracture has an associated disruption through the skin to the environment.

Immediate emergency department referral or physician consultation is indicated for compound fractures or any patient with neurovascular compromise of an extremity.

Strains and sprains are often cared for in private physician offices, clinics, athletic training centers, or simply at home. This makes statistical tracking of these types of injuries an impossibility.[1]

PATHOPHYSIOLOGY

Strains, sprains, and fractures are common musculoskeletal injuries. Strains are minor injuries that result when a muscle is overstretched. No actual muscle damage occurs with a muscle strain, but a sprain involves actual injury to the supporting structures of the affected joint. The degree of damage to these structures is dependent on the amount of tissue and fiber shearing and tearing that occurs.

Bone injuries can result in fractures, avulsion fractures, and dislocations. The pulling or pushing of a bone out of its normal position in the joint results in dislocation, which can be complete or incomplete.

Avulsion fractures result when a small piece of bone is chipped away, usually after a forceful injury. Stress fractures are small cracks in bone that initially may not be seen on x-ray examination. Repeat x-ray studies after 2 weeks or more may show new bone formation at the fracture site.

CLINICAL PRESENTATION

Sprains may demonstrate swelling, discoloration, and pain with movement. *Strains* also cause local pain, and, if severe, palpable swelling and/or muscle spasm. Fractures will usually present with an area of pinpoint pain. There may or may not be associated swelling, discoloration, or decreased range of motion. Dislocations involve the joint and often produce visible deformity. Patients often experience more pain with dislocations than with fractures, as the nerves, tendons, and vessels crossing the joint are disrupted. Injuries that occur as a result of crushing or compression should be evaluated immediately, as they can lead to neurovascular compromise and permanent tissue damage. It is difficult, if not impossible, to exclude a fracture without x-ray studies.

PHYSICAL EXAMINATION

In any trauma, it is essential to exclude and/or stabilize any life-threatening injuries. A good musculoskeletal examination includes an in-depth history, which should explore the mechanism of injury with a focus on the physical forces incurred by the patient. Often, this assessment is simplified by requesting the patient to use the opposite extremity to reconstruct the exact motion of the affected side during the injury.

A good history of the mechanism of injury will also provide vital information regarding the presence of a compression injury. This will permit accurate diagnosis of these injuries and allow for correct treatment and ongoing monitoring. A past medical history of arthritis, past injuries or surgery that resulted in deformity, or birth defects must be elicited.

Physical examination of the injured area includes observations of the patient favoring the affected area. Pain, swelling, discoloration, deformity, or open wounds should be noted. The joint above and below the injury should also be examined for injury. Circulatory, motor, and sensory function must be assessed. Palpation for joint laxity can be deferred until fracture is ruled out.

In an elbow injury the arm is usually flexed at the elbow with the palm toward the chest. From this position, the patient should be asked to move only the lower arm away from the body so that the hand is pointing straight ahead. If elbow pain is elicited, this is indicative of a radial head fracture.

Ankle fractures with tenderness through the mortis of the ankle can indicate an associated knee fracture. This indirect fracture of the knee is easily missed on the initial examination; therefore care should be taken to palpate the areas of the upper tibia and fibula and the knee.

When evaluating fractures, especially in adolescents or children, it is important to recall the classification method developed by Salter-Harris. A type I Salter-Harris fracture occurs when trauma causes complete epiphysis separation only, without any bone fracture.[2] At any age the diagnosis of Salter-Harris type I navicular fracture is made if the clinical examination demonstrates tenderness on palpation at the "snuffbox" (Figure 204-1).

DIAGNOSTICS

Because of the difficulty in determining the type of musculoskeletal injury based on presenting symptoms alone, radiologic examinations are often ordered. Radiologic examinations help to diagnosis fractures vs. soft tissue injury only. A

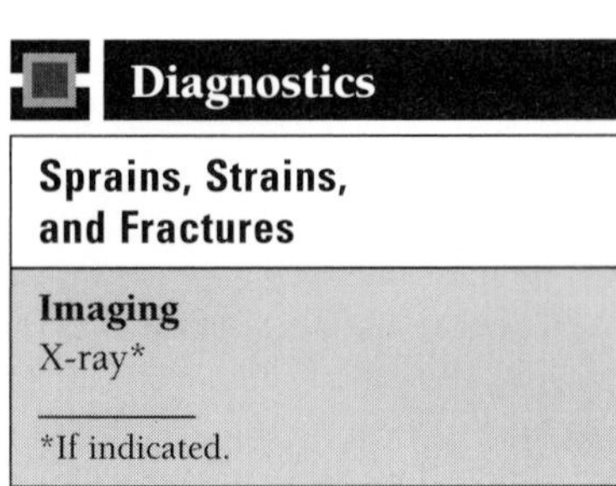

Diagnostics

Sprains, Strains, and Fractures

Imaging
X-ray*

*If indicated.

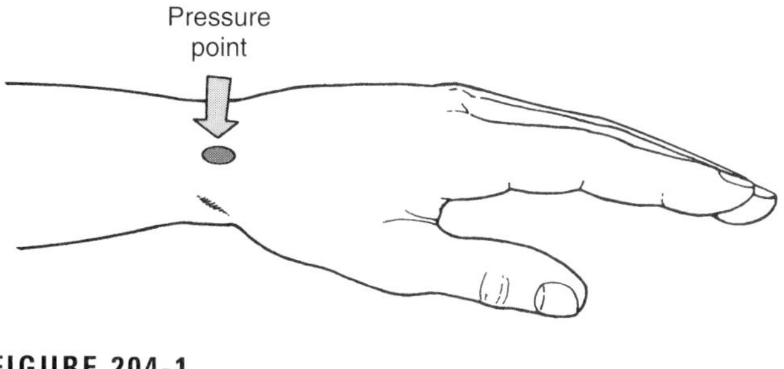

FIGURE 204-1

Palpation for Salter-Harris type I fracture at the "snuffbox" site on the wrist.

history of trauma followed by immediate signs or symptoms of pain, swelling, discoloration, and limited range of motion, and/or decreased strength are indications for x-ray studies. The ability to bear weight or the absence of swelling, however, may still require x-ray evaluation to rule out fracture.

Fractures are diagnosed when a break in the bone cortex is visible on two radiographic views. *Angulated* fractures may be either open or closed and usually refer to fractures with more than 30 degrees of angulation. A *transverse* fracture is straight across the bone. *Oblique* fractures are seen diagonally on x-ray films. *Spiral* fractures are seen as wrapping around the bone. A *greenstick* fracture is diagnosed when the bone tears as if a fresh twig were being bent in two. This is commonly seen in children, as they have a more porous cortex, which makes the bone more flexible. An *impacted* fracture occurs when both pieces of the broken bone are crushed into each other. A *comminuted* fracture is observed when the bone ends shatter with multiple fragments. *Stress* fractures are often seen in metatarsals of athletes who run on hard surfaces. The continued pounding to the bone causes it to fracture, with impaired healing resulting from repeated injury. *Jones* fracture involves a fifth metatarsal stress fracture. The fracture itself is distal to the proximal tuberosity and tends not to heal without prolonged immobilization or internal fixation. An *avulsion* or *osteochondral* fracture occurs when the ligament pulls away from the bone, bringing a bone fragment(s).

Three common clinical presentations require consideration of additional radiographic views. These are injuries to the navicular, patella, and acromioclavicular joint. Although it is possible to miss a navicular fracture with only a wrist series, the addition of an ulnar deviation view allows more complete assessment of this injury. This view is especially important in the presence of snuffbox tenderness. An injured patella may be better assessed with the sunrise view, which will clearly identify joint effusion and patella fracture. X-ray views taken of a tender acromioclavicular joint while the patient is weight bearing will confirm acromioclavicular separation and allow for grading.

DIFFERENTIAL DIAGNOSIS

Presentation of any musculoskeletal injury requires exclusion of sprains, strains, fractures, dislocations, subluxations, and ligamentous or muscle tears. A large muscle rupture may present as a convex or concave area with decreased range of motion and pain. Once traumatic injury is excluded, local and systemic causes, such as various forms of arthritis, autoimmune diseases, infection, phlebitis, or tumor, must be considered.

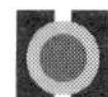 **Differential Diagnosis**

Sprains, Strains, and Fractures

Sprain	Fracture
Strain	Angulated
Dislocation	Transverse
Muscle/ligament tear	Oblique
Arthritis	Spiral
Infection	Greenstick
Phlebitis	Impacted
Tumor	Comminuted
Autoimmune disorder	Stress
	Avulsion

MANAGEMENT

Care of a fracture, strain, or sprain requires the following initial guidelines. If appropriate, blood and body fluid precautions should be followed. All jewelry must be removed from the affected limb. Irrigation with normal saline should be considered for any open wounds; then the area should be dressed and bandaged. Impaled objects must be stabilized. If a compartmental or crush injury is suspected, any restrictive dressing or clothing should be removed. Although all orthopedic injuries require assessment of neurovascular function distal to the injury, it is imperative that this function be closely monitored with a compartmental or crush injury.

Any acute orthopedic injury will respond to rest, ice, immobilization, and elevation. Extremity injuries require constant monitoring of the neurovasculature to prevent complications. If there is no joint involvement and pulses are palpable distal to the injury, the area should be splinted, immobilized, or supported as needed. If there is no palpable pulse and no joint involvement, gentle traction should be applied distally along the long axis until the pulse is palpable. The extremity should then be immobilized.

Extremity injuries involving joints should be immobilized in the presenting position. A sling and swathe can easily splint shoulder injuries. The exception to this is an anterior dislocation of the shoulder, which places the arm in abduction and requires splinting in this position. Wrapping a pillow around the joint and securing it with tape until x-ray films are obtained may comfortably splint severe ankle injuries.

Finger fractures not involving the fingertip should be splinted in the "safe" position, with the metacarpophalangeal joint in 70 degrees of flexion and the proximal interphalangeal joint in 20 degrees of flexion. This position minimizes shortening of the collateral ligaments and subsequent loss of hand function.

If radiographic findings are negative for fracture or dislocation, rest, ice, immobilization, and elevation are recommended. Minor sprains or strains may be immobilized with a simple Ace wrap. An air splint is an appropriate choice for an ankle with an inversion or eversion injury. With a knee injury, a knee immobilizer should be used to prevent compression on the plexus located in the popliteal space. If an immobilizer is unavailable, a 6-inch Ace bandage may be substituted. An nonsteroidal antiinflammatory drug is usually prescribed if it is not contraindicated. Severe injuries mandate consideration of narcotic analgesic agents. If discomfort persists for more than 10 days, an orthopedic consultation should be considered.

If the back is strained, bed rest is recommended only for the first 24 hours. This should be followed by a slow return to normal activities of daily living. Long-term bracing of back muscles will cause them to remain weak, whereas gentle reconditioning will strengthen them (see Chapter 196).

Clavicular fractures with displacement rarely result in injury to the brachial plexus and adjacent vessels. Clavicular fractures heal well, usually within 2 months. If the fracture does not involve injury to surrounding structures, it is easily managed by making the patient comfortable in a clavicular splint. Although this figure-eight bandage will not reduce a clavicular fracture, it affords great comfort for the patient.

LIFE SPAN CONSIDERATIONS

Before full maturation of the skeletal system, patients may sustain fractures as classified by Salter-Harris. Whereas a type I fracture is diagnosed by clinical examination with radiologic confirmation, types II through V are diagnosed by radiography. The most common Salter-Harris fracture is type II.

A type II fracture runs along the epiphysis with an associated triangular break in the metaphysis of the bone. Type III and type IV fractures are intraarticular. Type III fractures are uncommon and involve the joint surface as well as the epiphyseal plate and its periphery. Type IV fractures involve the joint surface, epiphysis, epiphyseal plate, and metaphysis. The prognosis for growth is poor in type IV fracture unless reduction and maintenance are flawless.[2] Type V fractures occur when a crushing trauma causes the epiphysis to compress the physis, leading to growth retardation.[2] The physis is the epiphyseal growth plate that connects the epiphysis to the rest of the bone. Trauma to this plate can cause not only a fracture, but also growth changes. If one side of the plate sustains trauma, it may stop producing cells on that side while the rest of the plate continues the growth process. The result is that the growing side enlarges while the injured side stops growing, causing the extremity to become angulated toward the stunted side. Children with angulation/physeal changes should be referred to an orthopedist. The potential for growth stoppage with physeal fractures requires 1 to 2 years of follow-up monitoring.[4] Although unusual beyond the age of 12 years, fractures of the tibia or femur may result in a growth stimulation of up to 1 cm. This could potentially lead to unequal leg length.[3]

The risk of falling and therefore fractures increases in patients over 65 years. Osteoporosis, poor physical conditioning, co-morbidities, and general frailty exacerbate this risk. Osteoporosis fractures are more common than heart disease or stroke and are a leading cause of disability and nursing home placement (see Chapter 201).

COMPLICATIONS

Complications may occur as a direct result of the injury or as a consequence of treatment provided, and they may be seen within the first hours of injury or may present weeks after trauma. Critical neurovascular structures lie close to the skeleton; thus disruption of the bone may lacerate, entrap, impale, or compress nerves and vessels at the fracture site. Finger fractures through the volar plate require splinting in extension for 6 weeks. Otherwise the injury to the extensor tendon will cause a mallet finger.

Long bone fractures of the lower extremities at any age require close monitoring. These fractures may have associated blood loss of up to 2 liters and may induce hypovolemic shock. The term *compartment* refers to an area where fascia wraps around a muscle group and its supplying arteries, veins, and nerves. Compartment syndrome may occur with any musculoskeletal injury that results in decreased vascular flow to the compartment, thereby causing muscle ischemia and necrosis. Because the fascia is inelastic, anything that increases compression, such as Ace bandages, casts, constrictive jewelry or clothing, and/or bleeding into an area, can potentiate this risk. The initial compression results in histamine release, which causes increased swelling and capillary dilation. This secondary swelling and dilation increase compression, which leads to further histamine release and more compression. The cyclic process continues, and in 2 to 4 hours irreversible muscle and nerve damage occurs. In 24 to 48 hours complete limb function is lost, and permanent deformity results. The presenting symptoms of this syndrome may include pain, paresthesias, pallor, pulselessness, and/or paralysis. Nonsurgical treatment includes stopping or decreasing activity to an asymptomatic level.[4] Cooling and elevation may slow and/or prevent this process. However, surgical intervention may be required to relieve pressure.

Volkmann's contracture is an example of compartment syndrome usually associated with a supracondylar fracture of the elbow. Many different names and descriptions are used to label compartment syndrome. It is essential that presenting signs and symptoms be identified quickly to enable successful intervention.

Acute infection resulting from an open fracture generally occurs within the first 24 to 48 hours. Gas gangrene, a rare occurrence, manifests in a contaminated open fracture approximately 72 hours after injury. Osteomyelitis, a chronic infection, presents weeks later (see Chapter 200).

After long bone, pelvic, or multiple fractures, fat embolism syndrome may occur within the first 48 to 72 hours. This is manifested by the sudden onset of respiratory distress and extreme arterial hypoxia. Pulmonary emboli are a later complication, generally occurring approximately 2 weeks after the fracture.

Delayed union refers to a fracture that is able to heal but in which the process takes longer than expected. Nonunion occurs if the fracture does not heal sufficiently to support normal limb function and pain continues. Malunion is defined as healing with a poor functional or cosmetic outcome; this generally requires surgical intervention. To protect the fracture site, a cast or brace may be used if complete union fails to occur.

Additional complications include joint stiffness, posttraumatic arthritis, implant failure, and osteochondrosis (avascular necrosis). Reflex sympathetic dystrophy should be suspected if a patient presents with prolonged, increasing pain extending beyond the anticipated period for healing along with discoloration and temperature changes of the limb.

Fracture blisters, histologically comparable to second-degree burn blisters, result from a separation of the dermis and stratified squamous resulting from edema and most commonly seen with fractures caused by severe twisting. However, they sometimes do appear with other joint or limb trauma. Fracture blisters generally emerge on parts of the body with minimal soft tissue between the skin and bone (e.g., elbow, ankle, foot, shin).[5]

INDICATIONS FOR REFERRAL/HOSPITALIZATION

Compartment syndrome requires immediate orthopedic referral. If fracture or dislocation is confirmed on x-ray examination, an orthopedist must be consulted. The orthopedist will provide instructions regarding management and/or hospitalization.

If radiographic findings are positive for fracture or dislocation, an orthopedist is usually consulted. Some primary care practices have guidelines for finger dislocation reductions. The orthopedist is consulted only if the reduction fails. Other types of dislocations, such as a shoulder, require premedication and are usually referred to emergency department physicians or orthopedists.

Physical therapy and/or occupational therapy referral should be considered in any injury not expected to resolve spontaneously in 10 days. Physical therapy may also be consulted to evaluate ambulation and teach the patient proper use of ambulatory assistive devices. Occupational therapy can be quite helpful with the appropriate splinting of hand and finger injuries and subsequent rehabilitation.

PATIENT AND FAMILY EDUCATION

In uncomplicated soft tissue injuries, elevation of the extremity should be above the level of the heart for the first 24 hours. This implies that the more distal joint should be higher than each preceding proximal joint. Ice should be applied in 20-minute intervals as often as tolerated. Instructions should include placement of a cloth between the ice and skin to prevent cold injury to the skin. Ice therapy can be continued unless muscle spasm occurs at which time a switch to moist heat is recommended.

The patient should be instructed in how to check for paresthesias, pallor, pulselessness, decreasing circulation, and/or paralysis in the extremity. Education should address the fact that pain is expected to gradually decrease and that any pain that continues, increases, or is not relieved by medication must be reported to the practitioner.

Ace bandages need to be removed every 2 to 3 hours for 15 minutes and then reapplied snugly. Ace bandages should be removed at night. If a splint or immobilizer is used, specific idiosyncrasies of that particular apparatus should be explained. If no improvement is noted in 4 or 5 days or symptoms persist beyond 10 days, reevaluation, and possibly orthopedic referral, is indicated.

Patients with casts should be even more diligent regarding elevation and neurovascular assessment. Patients should also be encouraged to wiggle their fingers or toes to prevent swelling. A cast will conduct cold. Ice contained in a plastic bag and wrapped in a thin cloth will absorb condensation and protect the cast from moisture. The cold will be conducted to the injury, which reduces swelling. Casts should be kept clean and dry. To prevent skin breakdown under or around the edges of the cast, foreign objects such as cast fragments, liquids, lotions, powders, or any device intended to relieve itching should be avoided. Instructions also need to include recommendations for weight bearing, bathing, and follow-up care.

HEALTH PROMOTION

Home and yard safety checks, especially with the older population, should be performed on a regular basis. Poor lighting or being out in the dark also accounts for many injuries. Seasonal issues including ice or wet surfaces should be addressed before accidents occur. Warm-up stretches and exercises for any sport are essential. Patients should have yearly physical examinations and ask specifically if their health and physical stature are compatible for the desired sport. Clinicians should then instruct the parents and children about specific risks. Coaches should be instructed in safe play and pediatric risks involved with their sport and then ensure that children understand and follow the rules. Training programs and instructional programs for both coaches and sports enthusiasts are essential. Safety gear should be checked for fit and worn at all times, and spotters should be used. First aid equipment/personnel should be available during any organized sport to provide immediate care of injuries. Pain needs to be acknowledged as a warning sign and activity should be stopped. The health care provider providing care to the injured patient should determine when it is safe to return to previous activity levels.

REFERENCES

1. National Center for Injury Prevention and Control: Unintentional Injury Prevention, Center for Disease Control and Prevention, NCPP. Retrieved August 12, 2002 from the World Wide Web: www.cdc.gov/ncipc/duip/duip.htm
2. Salter RB: *Textbook of disorders and injuries of the musculoskeletal system*, ed 2, Baltimore, 1983, Williams & Wilkins.
3. American Academy of Orthopaedic Surgeons: Your orthopaedic connection. About orthopaedics: growth plate fractures. Retrieved from the World Wide Web October 31, 2001: http://orthoinfo.aaos.org/fact/thr_report.cfm?Thread_ID=244&topcategory=Pediatrics.
4. Greene WB, editor: *Essentials of musculoskeletal care*, ed 2, Rosemont, Ill, 2000, American Academy of Orthopaedic Surgeons.
5. Harvey C: Compartment syndrome: when it is least expected, *Orthop Nurs* 20(3):15-23, 2001.

CHAPTER 205

Stretch Exercises

Anne LeMaitre

GENERAL GUIDELINES

Stretches should not be painful. They are most effective when muscle is maintained in a gently stretched position. Patients should be encouraged to maintain the stretch in a comfortable position, where they feel a mild stretch or tension, but no pain. Muscles respond to pain by contracting and shortening; thus stretching to the point of pain is not beneficial.

There is controversy regarding how long a stretch should be held, but it appears that holding a stretch for 15 to 30 seconds is effective. A longer (20- to 30-second) stretch allows muscles to achieve increased lengthening/flexibility, whereas a shorter duration (1 to 15 seconds) is effective in maintaining current muscle flexibility.

Stretches should be done in a relaxed position. Any stretching routine should begin with a few moments of deep breathing and relaxation. This is best done while lying supine with bent knees. The patient should focus on taking a few slow, deep, diaphragmatic breaths, then continue breathing slowly while noting any areas of increased tension and trying to release that tension. Commonly, people hold tension in their upper trapezius, facial muscles, and low back muscles.

An exercise mat should be used on a firm surface if possible. The floor generally provides a better surface than a bed or couch.

It is common to find that one leg or one side of the body is more flexible than the other side. Each side should be stretched to its comfortable tolerance, and over time the sides should become more equal.

Patients should be advised that if any stretch causes pain, they should back off and attempt to do the stretch in a more comfortable range. Often it is not the stretch that causes pain, but the technique. If a patient feels pain after stretching but cannot identify a particular stretch as an aggravant, the patient should try doing them at separate intervals during the day.

STRETCHES

Low Back Stretch (Figure 205-1)

Lie with your knees bent, feet on the mat. Bring one knee toward your chest until you feel a stretch in your low back or buttock. Use your hands to hold in a comfortably stretched position for 15 to 30 seconds. Return your foot to the mat, then repeat with the opposite leg. Perform alternately, three times on each side.

As a progression, bring one knee to your chest and keep it there while bringing the second knee to your chest, again using your hands to assist. Hold, and then lower one knee at a time. Perform three times total, trying to alternate.

Hip Flexor Stretch (Figure 205-2)

Begin as in the preceding exercise, but after bringing one knee to your chest, gently lower the opposite knee to the mat, straightening your leg. The stretch should be felt in the front of the hip of the straight leg. Hold 15 to 30 seconds. One leg at a time, return both legs to the starting position. Perform three times for each side.

Alternate method: If you do not feel a stretch in the above method, lie at the edge of the bed and bring the knee of the leg in the middle of the bed up to your chest. Lower the opposite leg off the edge of the bed, bringing your foot toward the floor until you feel a stretch. Hold as above. Perform three times on one side, then switch to the opposite side.

Lower Trunk Rotation (Figure 205-3)

Lie with your knees bent, feet on the mat. Gently rock your knees from side to side, gradually increasing how far you rock, but never forcing it. You can hold in a stretched position three times for 15 to 20 seconds, but if this is uncomfortable, just continue rocking your knees for 10 to 15 repetitions in a comfortable range.

Alternate method: Bring both knees to your chest as in the first exercise, and rock them from side to side in this position.

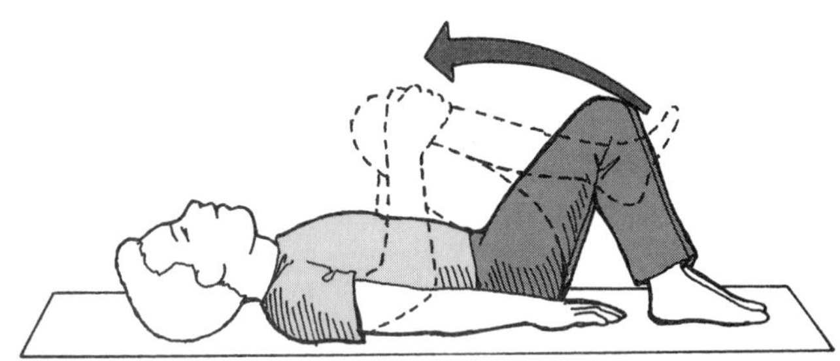

FIGURE 205-1

Low back stretch.

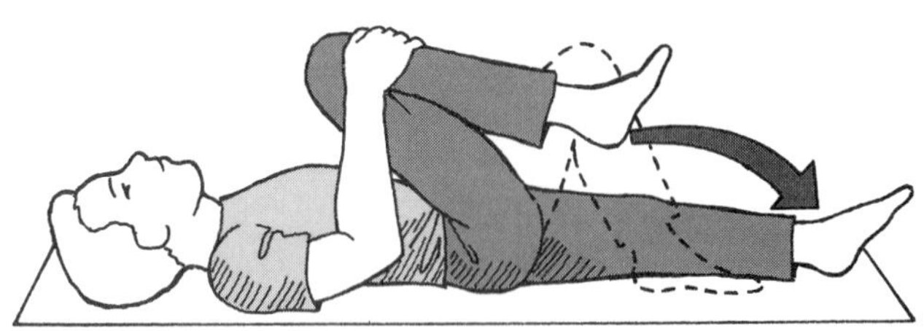

FIGURE 205-2

Hip flexor stretch.

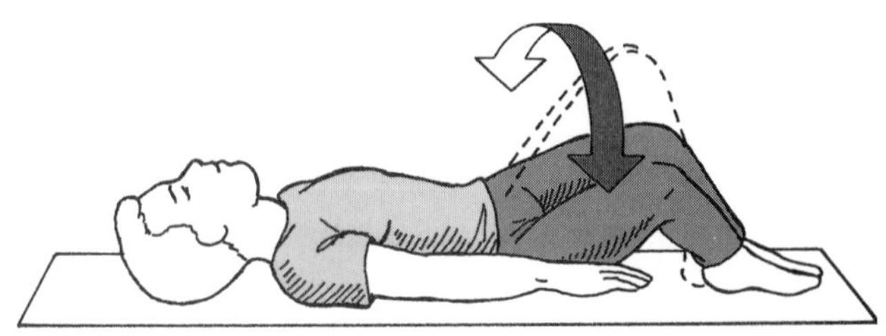

FIGURE 205-3

Lower trunk rotation.

Hamstring Stretch (Figure 205-4)

Lie with your knees bent, feet on the mat. Hook both hands behind one knee to support your thigh and straighten this leg. Keep your knee perfectly straight and raise your leg toward the ceiling until you feel a stretch in the back of your leg—it may pull from behind the knee all the way to the ischial tuberosity. Remember to hold in a gently stretched position. Perform three times on each leg. It is very common that one leg will be more flexible than the other. Stretch each as tolerated.

Mad Cat Stretch (Figure 205-5)

Gently arch your back up and down—up like an angry cat, then sagging down like a swaybacked horse. Try to move each segment of your spine. You may notice that some parts move freely, whereas other areas are stiff. Focus on increasing movement of the stiff areas.

Rocking/Bow to Mecca Stretch (Figure 205-6)

Begin rocking forward and back slowly and go a bit further each time, until you are able to sit back on your heels, with your arms outstretched in front of you, head down. Hold this position for 15 to 30 seconds. Perform three times.

Extension Stretch (Prone) (Figure 205-7)

Lie on your stomach. While keeping your stomach flat on the mat, rest on your elbows with your arms out in front of you. (Your head and shoulders should be up.) Hold 15 to 30 seconds if you feel a stretch. If not, press your hands into the mat and raise yourself so that your stomach, but not your hips, are off the mat, and hold as able (this may not be comfortable for a longer stretch).

Side Stretch (Figure 205-8)

Standing with your feet apart, raise one arm overhead, reaching for the ceiling. Hold if a stretch is felt in the side of your trunk. If not, reach your arm overhead toward the opposite side, then gently slide the opposite hand down your leg toward the knee. Stop and hold when a stretch is felt, for 15 to 30 seconds. Perform three times on each side, alternating sides.

Extension Stretch (Figure 205-9)

Stand with your feet apart, hands on hips. Slowly arch your back, raising your face to the ceiling. Gently release.

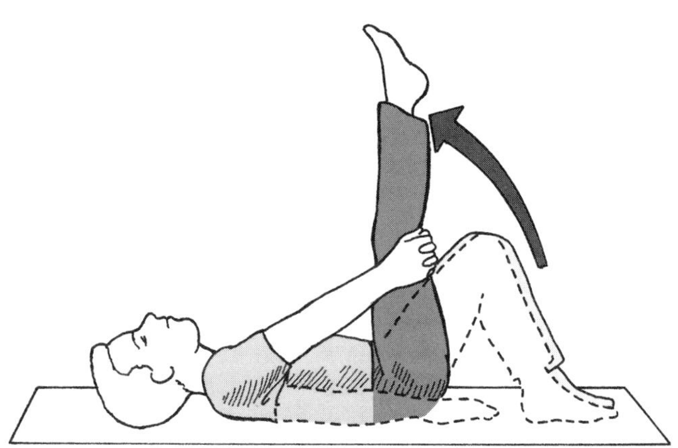

FIGURE 205-4

Hamstring stretch.

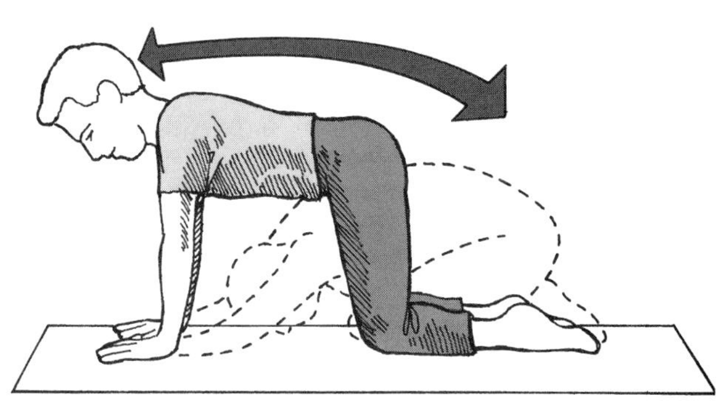

FIGURE 205-6

Rocking/bow to Mecca stretch.

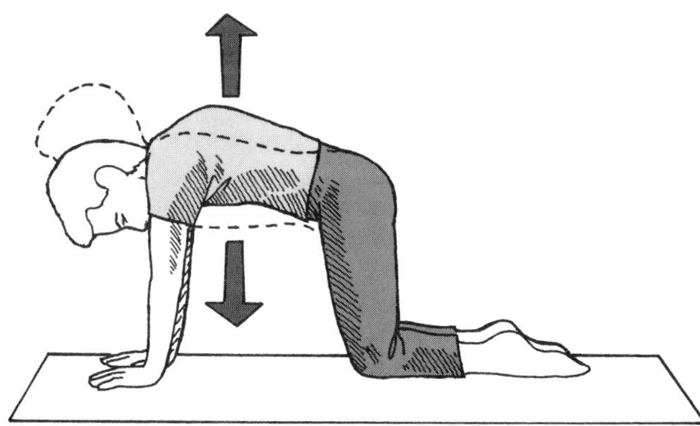

FIGURE 205-5

Mad cat stretch.

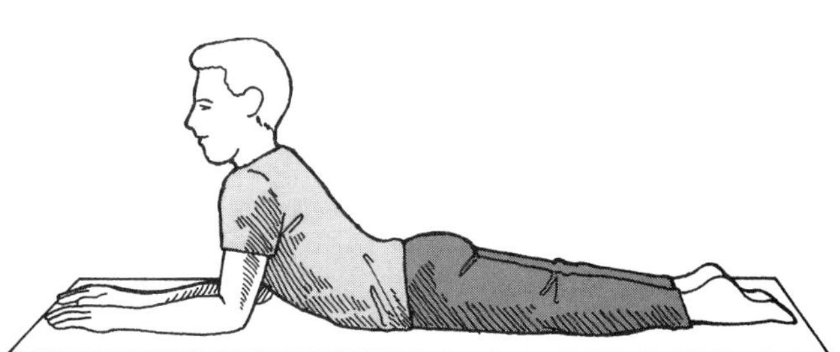

FIGURE 205-7

Extension stretch (prone).

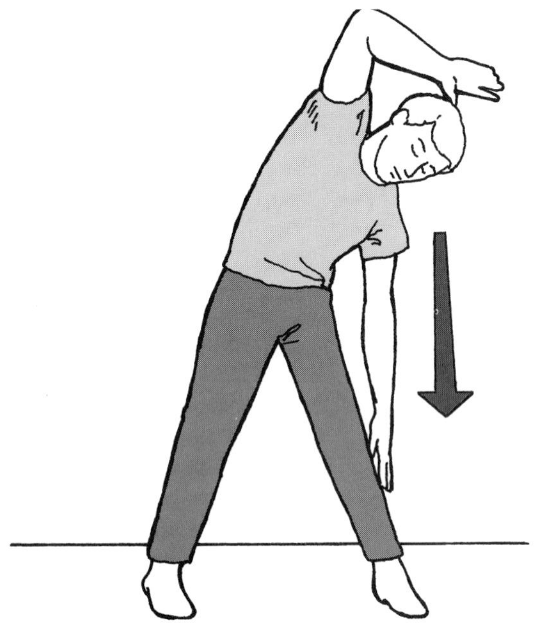

FIGURE 205-8

Side stretch.

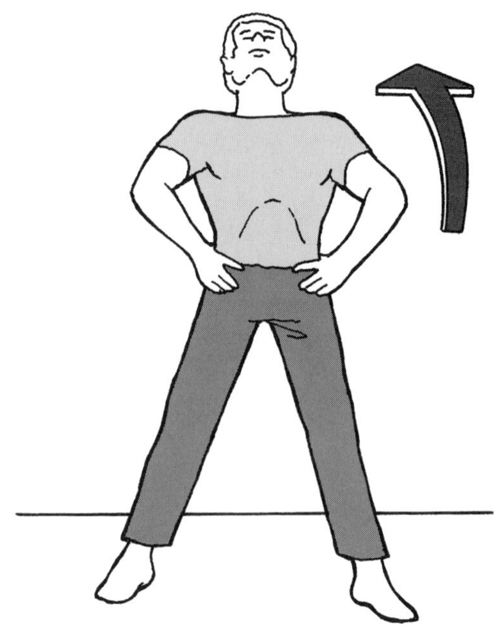

FIGURE 205-9

Extension stretch (standing).

PART 16

Evaluation and Management of Neurologic Disorders

JOANNE SANDBERG-COOK, Section Editor

CHAPTER 206

Amyotrophic Lateral Sclerosis

Noreen M. Leahy

DEFINITION/EPIDEMIOLOGY

Amyotrophic lateral sclerosis (ALS) is the most common of the progressive motor neuron diseases. New insights into the pathogenesis of ALS have led to exciting advancements in treatment regimens, making this devastating neurodegenerative disease more manageable.[1]

ALS is a progressive motor neuron disease that affects both upper motor neurons (UMNs) and lower motor neurons (LMNs) in the corticospinal and corticobulbar tracts, anterior motor horn cells, and bulbar motor nuclei. There are different forms of ALS, including sporadic, familial, and Western Pacific forms. There are also a variety of clinical variants, including progressive muscular atrophy and progressive bulbar palsy, affecting LMNs in limb and bulbar muscles, respectively. Primary lateral sclerosis and progressive pseudobulbar palsy affect UMNs in limb and bulbar muscles. Although these clinical variants may present differently early on, they all eventually affect both LMNs and UMNs.[2]

The worldwide incidence rate of ALS is 1 to 3 per 100,000 population, and the prevalence rate is between 3 and 5 per 100,000 population.[2] There appears to be a several-fold higher incidence and prevalence in the Western-specific forms (Guam, Papua New Guinea). The average age of onset is about 55 years, with a slightly increased incidence in men in the United States.[3]

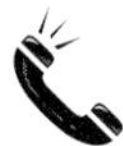

Neurology consultation is indicated for all patients with suspected ALS.

PATHOPHYSIOLOGY

The etiology of ALS remains unknown, although recent literature suggests four major hypotheses as the pathogenesis of the disease. The first describes excitotoxic stimulation as a result of accumulation of glutamate in the central nervous system. It appears that the excess glutamate is toxic to motor neurons. The second hypothesis suggests an autoimmune process with autoantibodies to the calcium channels in motor neurons. There is also a familial hypothesis that neuronal injury is secondary to altered function of superoxide dismutase and subsequent accumulation of free oxygen radicals.[4] There is growing evidence that this oxidative stress, mediated by free radicals, is important in the initiation of the disease.[5] Finally, there is a theory that deficiency in neuronal growth factors leads to degeneration of motor neurons.[4] Each of these etiologic mechanisms has a basis for specific treatment arms that are currently under investigation.

The four proposed mechanisms of etiology all lead to neuronal damage of both UMNs and LMNs. The UMNs are initially altered in the motor cortex, thereby affecting the corticospinal and corticobulbar tracts. The LMNs are affected at the anterior motor horn cells in the spinal cord and at the respective motor nuclei in the brainstem. Death of the motor neurons in the brainstem and spinal cord leads to denervation and atrophy of muscle fibers. Selectivity of the neuronal cell death completely spares sensory systems, neuronal systems controlling coordination, and components of the brain controlling cognition. ALS is also selective within the motor system, sparing ocular motility and bowel and bladder function.[3]

CLINICAL PRESENTATION AND PHYSICAL EXAMINATION

A precise documentation of the history of symptoms and a complete neurologic examination are essential. Early LMN cell death leads to an insidious onset of asymmetric weakness that is evident initially in the limbs. The initial presenting symptoms occur in the upper extremities in 40% to 60% of cases and in the lower extremities in 20% of cases. These symptoms include weakness and difficulty performing fine motor tasks. The remaining 20% to 25% of patients with ALS present with bulbar symptoms as the initial complaint.[6] These may include dysarthria, dysphagia, and drooling. LMN symptoms include muscle atrophy, hyporeflexia, fasciculations, and muscle cramps. Patients often give a history of early morning cramping while stretching in bed. One of the hallmark physical findings of this disease is fasciculations (spontaneous twitching) that tend to be of low amplitude and high frequency. If the bulbar muscles are initially involved, early symptoms include problems with chewing and swallowing and difficulty with movements of the face and tongue. UMN deterioration of the corticospinal tract leads to spasticity, hyperreflexia, and loss of dexterity. UMN involvement of the corticobulbar tract will cause dysarthria and a pseudobulbar effect. As the disease progresses, both UMN and LMN involvement becomes evident with a more symmetric distribution of the disease. Yet, even in the late stages of disease, sensation, bowel and bladder function, cognition, and ocular motility are spared.[3]

DIAGNOSTICS

The diagnosis of ALS is usually made when there are widespread UMN and LMN signs in the absence of any sensory findings. In 1994 the World Federation of Neurology presented diagnostic criteria for ALS. These include signs of LMN degeneration by clinical, electrophysiologic, or neuropathologic examination and signs of UMN degeneration by clinical examination. There also has to be a progressive spread of signs within a region or to other regions. The four regions are bulbar, cervical, thoracic, and lumbosacral. The second part of the diagnosis consists of an absence of electrophysiologic or neuroimaging evidence of other disease processes that might explain the observed clinical or electrophysiologic signs. Based on the World Federation of Neurology diagnostic criteria, the number of regions involved, and the presence and distribution of UMN and LMN signs, a degree of diagnostic certainty can be achieved.[6] At this point there are no specific biochemical or laboratory markers for ALS. Laboratory and other diagnostic studies may be necessary to exclude other disorders considered in the differential diagnosis. Routine laboratory studies,

MRI, lumbar puncture, and an electromyogram (EMG) are often ordered in consultation with the primary care physician. Other diagnostic studies may also be necessary.

DIFFERENTIAL DIAGNOSIS

Differentiating ALS from treatable neurologic disorders was always important in the past because ALS was considered an untreatable disease. Now that ALS has specific treatments, it becomes even more important to diagnose ALS early and initiate the appropriate medical therapy. Atypical features that should alert the practitioner that the patient may have a disease other than ALS include restriction of the disease to just UMNs or LMNs, involvement of neurons other than motor neurons, and EMG findings not consistent with ALS. Compression of the cervical spine, syringobulbia, multifocal motor neuropathy with conduction block, LMN axonal neuropathy, chronic lead poisoning, thyrotoxicosis, inherited enzyme disorders, benign fasciculations, poliomyelitis, and other motor neuron disorders must all be considered when evaluating a patient for possible ALS.[3]

Diagnostics

Amyotrophic Lateral Sclerosis

Laboratory	Folate
CBC and differential	Cerebrospinal fluid culture
ESR	Screening for hereditary disorders*
Serum electrolytes	
BUN	**Imaging**
Creatinine	MRI (head, foramen magnum, and cervical spine)
Serum glucose	
TSH	
Lead levels	**Other**
Calcium	EMG
Lyme titer	Lumbar puncture
Vitamin B_{12}	

*If indicated.

Differential Diagnosis

Amyotrophic Lateral Sclerosis

Benign fasciculations	Kennedy's syndrome
Cervical spine compression	Lower motor neuron axonal neuropathy
Chronic aluminum or lead poisoning	Multifocal motor neuropathy with conduction block
Drug intoxication (phenytoin or strychnine)	Syringobulbia
Familial amyotrophic lateral sclerosis	Thyrotoxicosis
Infection	Tumor
Herpes zoster	Foramen magnum
Poliomyelitis	Parasagittal tumor
Lyme disease	Vitamin deficiency/malabsorption syndrome
Tetanus	
Adult Tay-Sach's disease	

MANAGEMENT

As more is discovered regarding the mechanisms of this disease, more treatment options become available. A promising pharmacologic agent is riluzole, an antiglutamate that appears to slow progression of ALS and may improve survival in patients with early bulbar involvement.[4,7,8] The efficacy of riluzole has been evaluated in two stratified, randomized, placebo-controlled clinical studies. Riluzole significantly reduced mortality over a 21-month period in the first trial and over an 18-month period in the second trial. Early survival improved in both studies, although there was no statistical difference in mortality. The most common side effects described with riluzole are asthenia and nausea. As the dosage is increased, dizziness, diarrhea, and anorexia become more common. The most current recommendation for dosing is 50 mg every 12 hours. In addition to the aforementioned side effects, riluzole has been associated with elevations in the serum alanine aminotransferase level in a small proportion of patients. Therefore it has been recommended that liver function tests be obtained at the onset of treatment and then monthly during the first 3 months of therapy, and every 3 months thereafter.[5]

The second agent that appears to be effective in reducing motor neuron death is insulin-like growth factor–I (IGF-I), a neurotrophic growth factor.[4,9,10] IGF-I is a naturally occurring polypeptide that mediates the activity of growth hormone and has actions similar to insulin. Initial clinical trials with IGF-I suggest a reduction in mortality, along with an improvement in the quality of life. As noted with riluzole, survival curves tend to merge with those of a placebo as time increases in their respective trials.

There are many other treatments currently under investigation that may work independently or in combination with the aforementioned treatments. It is generally believed that the use of combinations of these drugs will become the standard of care in the treatment of ALS.

LIFE SPAN CONSIDERATIONS

The median duration of survival for ALS is 23 to 52 months. Most patients die from respiratory failure or infection. The two most important factors in determining survival are the patient's age and the presence or absence of bulbar symptoms at the time of diagnosis. The older the patient, the shorter the duration of survival. Similarly, patients who present with bulbar symptoms at the onset of disease have a poorer prognosis and shorter duration of survival.[6]

COMPLICATIONS

As with any chronic, terminal disease, it is important to maintain a holistic approach toward the patient. Denial and depression are common early in the disease process and are important to identify and treat to ensure the best quality of life for the patient. The patient should be evaluated for depression at every office visit. Depression is a component of the ALS disease process, and this should be explained to the patient. The treatment of choice for depression in patients with ALS is use of a selective serotonin reuptake inhibitor, although tricyclic agents can be used effectively if tolerated. It is also important to involve a multidisciplinary team early, including a social worker, dietitian, and physical, speech, occupational, and respiratory therapists.[11]

Nutritional support can be maximized with early intervention for dysphagia including referral to a speech therapist and changing the consistency of foods and fluids. Placement of a gastrostomy tube serves to maintain caloric needs and minimize the aspiration of foods and fluids. Tube feedings in these patients can be controversial, and the possible benefits as well as the risks associated with this procedure should be carefully discussed with patients.

Management of respiratory dysfunction in ALS consists of pulmonary function monitoring and the use of respiratory therapy, incentive spirometry, and positive pressure ventilation as needed. The key to delaying respiratory failure is to treat pneumonia and heart failure promptly, suction secretions appropriately, and prevent aspiration. The use of long-term assisted ventilation in ALS is controversial, although with newer ventilators on the market now, it is possible to remain ventilator dependent and still live at home.

It is important to keep these patients as functional as possible, to anticipate problems, and to provide patient awareness before problems occur. Cramping, spasticity, and pain must be treated promptly. The patient should also be vaccinated against pneumococcal infection and influenza.[12]

INDICATIONS FOR REFERRAL/HOSPITALIZATION

Because of the difficulty in diagnosis and new treatments available for ALS, it is important for all patients presenting with signs and symptoms consistent with ALS to see a neurologist. Once the diagnosis is confirmed, the role of the primary care provider becomes important. It is the role of the primary care provider to organize all of the patient's multidisciplinary care, along with identifying and treating any psychosocial issues as they present.

Impairment of respiratory function in ALS is gradual. During the year preceding death, however, the decline of respiratory function is accelerated. As previously mentioned, it is imperative to promptly treat any sign of respiratory dysfunction or any disorders that will contribute to a rapid respiratory decline. Pneumonia and heart failure should be treated in a hospital setting, especially in the latter stages of disease. Most of the hospitalizations will occur in the last year of the patient's life as respiratory function declines.

PATIENT AND FAMILY EDUCATION

ALS is a physically, mentally, and financially debilitating disease. It is important to educate patients and families about the natural history of the disease. Discussion topics must include the use of antidepressants, assistive devices, home modifications, gastrostomy tube placement, ventilatory assistance, and hospice care.

In addition, it is important that patients have the necessary physical, mental, and financial support. Forthright discussion with patients and families regarding end-of-life wishes as early as possible will benefit all involved. Patients should be encouraged to appoint a health care proxy and openly discuss end of life directives with him. Many patients will elect not to have a gastrostomy tube placed and will refuse ventilatory support. These patients should be reassured that good palliative care is available. The services of community agencies in addition to the local Visiting Nurses Association and hospice can be invaluable in supporting the patient and family.[12]

Patients and caretakers should be referred to local ALS foundations and the Internet for support and educational information.

REFERENCES

1. Miller R, Swash M: Therapeutic advances in ALS, *Neurology* 47 (suppl 4):S217, 1996.
2. Tandan R: Disorders of the upper and lower motor neurons. In Bradley WG and others, editors: *Neurology in clinical practice,* Newton, Mass, 1991, Butterworth-Heinemann.
3. Brown RH Jr: Motor neuron disease and the progressive ataxias. In Isselbacher KJ and others, editors: *Harrison's principles of internal medicine,* New York, 1994, McGraw-Hill.
4. Jerusalem F and others: ALS, *Neurology* 47(suppl 4):S218-S220, 1996.
5. Miller R, Sufit R: New approaches to the treatment of ALS, *Neurology* 48(suppl 4):S28-S32, 1997.
6. Mitsumoto H: Diagnosis and progression of ALS, *Neurology* 48 (suppl 4):S2-S8, 1997.
7. Bengimon G, Lacomblez L, Meininger V: The ALS/riluzole study group: a controlled trial of riluzole in amyotrophic lateral sclerosis, *N Engl J Med* 330:585-591, 1994.
8. Rowland LP: Riluzole for the treatment of amyotropic lateral sclerosis: too soon to tell? *N Engl J Med* 330:636-637, 1994.
9. Lewis M and others: The potential of insulin-like growth factor–I as a therapeutic for the treatment of neuromuscular disorders, *Ann NY Acad Sci* 692:201-208, 1993.
10. Gehrmann J and others: Expression of insulin-like growth factor–I and related peptides during motor neuron regeneration, *Exp Neurol* 128:202-210, 1994.
11. Gelinas DF: Patient and caregiver communications and decisions, *Neurology* 48(suppl 4):S9-S14, 1997.
12. Miller R and others: ALS standard of care consensus, *Neurology* 48(suppl 4):S33-S37, 1997.

CHAPTER 207

Bell's Palsy

Noreen M. Leahy

DEFINITION/EPIDEMIOLOGY

Bell's palsy is a term used to describe an acute, unilateral, peripheral facial palsy of unknown etiology and accounts for 60% to 75% of all cases of lower facial motor neuron paralysis.[1-3] Genetic, autoimmune, infectious, vascular, entrapment, and metabolic causes have been proposed as etiologic factors; viral causation is currently the most popular. With the use of the polymerase chain reaction technique, the herpes simplex virus genome has been isolated from the endoneurial fluid of the facial nerve.[4] Thus it may no longer be considered synonymous with "idiopathic facial paralysis."[2,4,5]

Bell's palsy is the most common cause of facial paralysis worldwide, with an incidence of about 20 per 100,000. Men and women are equally affected, although it is more common in young and middle-aged adults. There appears to be a higher prevalence in lower socioeconomic groups. Either side of the face may be affected, and the majority of patients report a recent respiratory tract infection.[2,4] Occurrence is higher in pregnant patients.[6] It is possibly more common in persons with diabetes and hypertension than in the general population.[5]

Physician consultation is indicated for patients with corneal abrasions or if the eyelid cannot close.

PATHOPHYSIOLOGY

The typical unilateral facial paralysis of Bell's palsy is assumed to be initiated by a triggering event that places physiologic stress on the body (e.g., an upper respiratory tract infection). This stressor promotes the body's protective inflammatory response with its release of acute-phase reactants. The intraneural inflammatory response results in edema of the facial nerve. If the edema is not alleviated, there is inevitable ischemia of the nerve, with resulting axonal demyelination and inevitable nerve degeneration. Varying degrees of motor control loss become obvious about 3 days after nerve demyelination. Knowledge of the topographic anatomy of the facial nerve can provide clinical clues to sites of injury.[7]

CLINICAL PRESENTATION

The typical onset is acute and progressive, with maximum paralysis attained in about half of the cases within 48 hours and in nearly all cases by day 5. Individuals may report pain behind the ipsilateral ear preceding the facial paralysis by 1 to 2 days. Typically, a smooth forehead, widened palpebral fissure, flattened nasolabial fold, and asymmetric smile are characteristic. Tearing, drooling, postauricular pain, tinnitus, and a mild hearing deficit may also be present. Complaints of altered taste (dysgeusia) and an increased sensitivity to sound (hyperacusis) may also be present, as well as a hypesthesia in one or more branches of the trigeminal nerve.[5] A complete and detailed history is essential for diagnosis, as Bell's palsy is a diagnosis of exclusion.

Other associated symptoms include a history of recent infections, especially viral illnesses such as chickenpox, mumps, mononucleosis, coxsackievirus, cytomegalovirus, human immunodeficiency virus, and influenza. The presence of chronic illnesses such as diabetes mellitus, hypertension, or hypothyroidism should be ascertained; and the patient should be queried about pregnancy, skin rashes or lesions, and insect (tick) bites. Any history of facial trauma should be carefully noted.

PHYSICAL EXAMINATION

A careful examination of the head and neck with assessment of all cranial nerves is essential. Special attention to the sensory and motor functions of the branches of the facial nerve is also necessary. Minor asymmetry of the lower face may be a normal deviation. The degree of facial weakness should be documented. Ross and colleagues[8] have developed a tool for grading the resting symmetry (compared with the normal side), the symmetry of voluntary movements, and the synkinesis (degree of involuntary muscle contraction associated with each facial expression). Clinicians may find this tool helpful in gauging the severity of neural degeneration and in establishing objective measures of recovery. A photographic record is also helpful in establishing the extent of facial muscle weakness and documenting progressive neural regeneration.

DIAGNOSTICS

Although routine laboratory tests are of little value in the diagnosis of Bell's palsy, diagnostic studies may be useful to exclude varied conditions in the differential diagnosis. If infection is suspected, a CBC and differential is indicated. A Lyme titer is useful to exclude Lyme disease. Other serologic tests to consider include TSH and blood sugar to exclude diabetes or thyroid dysfunction. If indicated, a pregnancy test should also be obtained.

Tests usually performed by an otolaryngologist or other specialist include topognostic studies (tests for tactile sensation) such as Schirmer's test (checks for tear production), acoustic reflex, and electrogustometry (salivation test). Electrophysiologic studies involve nerve excitability testing, electromyography, and electroneurography. Audiologic studies encompass pure tone audiometry and impedance tests, along with

Diagnostics

Bell's Palsy

Laboratory	Other
CBC and differential	Schirmer's test*
TSH	Acoustic reflex*
Serum glucose	Electrogustometry*
Pregnancy test (serum hCG)	EMG*
Lyme titer	Audiometry*
	ENG*
Imaging	
MRI*	

*If indicated.

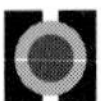

Differential Diagnosis

Bell's Palsy

Infectious conditions	Metabolic conditions
Otitis media	Pregnancy
Tuberculous mastoiditis	Diabetes
Meningitis	Hypothyroidism
Lyme disease	Trauma
Neoplastic conditions	
Leukemia	
Cholesteatoma	
Tumor	

electronystagmography. MRI and CT scans may be indicated if an intracranial tumor within the cerebellopontine angle is suspected.[7] The facial nerve in Bell's palsy may often be visualized on a gadolinium-enhanced MRI[5] and is the diagnostic choice for diagnosing cranial nerve pathology.

DIFFERENTIAL DIAGNOSIS

The list of conditions to be included in the differential diagnosis for unilateral facial paralysis is quite lengthy. Infectious, traumatic, neoplastic, immunologic, and metabolic conditions (e.g., otitis media, cholesteatoma, tumors, tuberculosis mastoiditis, meningitis, Lyme disease, leukemia, pregnancy, diabetes mellitus, and hypothyroidism) should be considered.

MANAGEMENT

Protection of the eye is the single most important goal of care for the patient with Bell's palsy. Exposure keratitis can result in blindness. The cornea should be protected with eyedrops such as methylcellulose twice a day and with an ocular lubricant at bedtime. Protective eyeglasses, moisture chambers, and upper eyelid weights are other options. If the eyelids will not close, they should be taped together, with precautions taken so that the tape does not touch the cornea. Massage of weakened facial muscles may help preserve muscle tone and provide some comfort. A splint can be used for the lower facial muscles.[5]

Drug therapy for Bell's palsy remains somewhat controversial. The use of prednisone, beginning with 60 to 80 mg/day during the first 48 hours and then tapering over the next 5 days, may be beneficial in reducing the inflammatory response and shortening the recovery period. Adour and associates[9] recommended adding a 10-day course of acyclovir (400 mg five times a day) to the regimen. Early treatment with steroids is cited as being probably effective in improving outcomes. The concomitant use of acyclovir assumes a viral (herpes simplex virus) etiology and possibly promotes more complete restoration of facial function as compared with the use of prednisone alone.[10] Surgical decompression of the facial nerve is not routinely performed.[5,10] A total of 80% of patients with Bell's palsy will recover full function spontaneously with a "watchful waiting" approach; 10% will have mild residual signs, and 10% will fail to have a return of normal facial function.[8]

LIFE SPAN CONSIDERATIONS

One fifth of cases of Bell's palsy occur during pregnancy.[6,11,12] An increase in vascular volume and pregnancy-induced hypertension may contribute to palsy of the facial nerve as a result of edema and entrapment. A viral etiology cannot be excluded. For the primary care provider giving prenatal care, it is recommended that the advice of an obstetrician be solicited and referral considered. As a rule, a prednisone taper has been shown to be helpful in resolving the inflammation if it is given early in the course of the disease. Valacyclovir may be added to the regimen at 1 g t.i.d. for 1 week. Valacyclovir is category B in pregnancy and should be used in consultation with an obstetrician.

COMPLICATIONS

Evidence of poor functional recovery can be seen in facial asymmetry as a result of muscle weakness and synkinesis. Loss of vision in the affected eye from corneal ulceration is among the worst possible outcomes. Hearing loss and permanent tinnitus are sequelae indicating damage to the auditory nerve. Physician consultation is indicated for patients with corneal abrasions or if the eyelid cannot close.

INDICATIONS FOR REFERRAL/HOSPITALIZATION

All patients with corneal abrasions or ulcerations should be referred to an ophthalmologist. Any concern for compromise of the eyesight of a patient with poor or no lid closure is also reason for referral to an ophthalmologist. For the 10% of patients who fail to recover an acceptable level of motor function, referral to a neurosurgeon or otolaryngologist for autografting of the hypoglossal nerve to the facial nerve anastomosis may provide acceptable cosmetic results.[3,13]

Generally, Bell's palsy does not require hospitalization unless there are coexisting medical or surgical problems that warrant inpatient care.

PATIENT AND FAMILY EDUCATION

Explain Bell's palsy and its usual benign clinical course. Caution the patient about corneal abrasion and instruct the patient in the use of eyedrops during the day and ocular lubricant at night. Instruct the patient in taping the eyelids closed at night, taking care to avoid the cornea. Encourage the patient to report any ocular pain, discharge, or drainage. Provide information about medications, including the name, therapeutic effects, common side effects, dosing, and any other special considerations. Encourage follow-up care for evaluation of treatment and documentation of recovery of facial function.

REFERENCES

1. Ronthal M: Bell's palsy, UpToDate. Retrieved August 2001 from the World Wide Web: www.uptodateonline.com Ver 9.3.
2. James DG: All that palsies is not Bell's, *J R Soc Med* 89:184, 1996.
3. Bauer CA, Coker NJ: Update on facial nerve disorders, *Otolaryngol Clin North Am* 29(3):445-454, 1996.
4. Murakami S and others: Bell palsy and herpes simplex virus: identification of viral DNA in endoneurial fluid and muscle, *Ann Intern Med* 124:27-30, 1996.
5. Adams RD, Victor V, Ropper AH: Diseases of the cranial nerves. In *Principles of neurology,* ed 6, New York, 1997, McGraw-Hill.
6. Billue JB: Bell's palsy: an update on idiopathic facial paralysis, *Nurse Pract* 22(8):88-105, 1997.
7. Fagan JJ, Hirsh BE: Facial nerve paralysis: initial evaluation and management, *Emerg Med* 29(10):52-70, 1997.

8. Ross BG, Fradet G, Nedzelski JM: Development of a sensitive clinical facial grading system, *Otolaryngol Head Neck Surg* 114(3):380-386, 1996.
9. Adour KK and others: Bell's palsy treatment with acyclovir and prednisone compared with prednisone alone: a double-blind, randomized, controlled trial, *Ann Otol Rhinol Laryngol* 105(5):371-378, 1996.
10. Grogan PM, Gronseth GS: Practice Parameter: steroids, acyclovir, and surgery for Bell's Palsy (an evidence-based review). Report of the Quality Standards Subcommittee of the American Academy of Neurology, *Neurology* (56):830-836, 2001.
11. Hess LW, Morrison JC, Hess DB: General medical problems during pregnancy. In DeCherney AH, Pernoll ML, editors: *Current obstetric and gynecologic diagnosis and treatment*, ed 8, Norwalk, CT, 1994, Appleton & Lange.
12. Beric A: Peripheral nerve disorders in pregnancy, *Adv Neurol* 64:179-192, 1994.
13. Seidman MD, Simpson GT, Khan MJ: Common problems of the ear. In Noble J, editor: *Textbook of primary care medicine*, St Louis, 1996, Mosby.

CHAPTER 208

Cerebrovascular Events

John Joseph Graykoski

DEFINITION/EPIDEMIOLOGY

A stroke is an interruption of blood circulation to the brain causing a neurologic deficit reflecting the area of the brain affected. Stroke can be ischemic or hemorrhagic.[1]

Ischemic stroke is most prevalent. It is occlusive in nature, which is the result of atherosclerotic disease, and progresses slowly as the affected artery becomes more occluded with plaque. Clotting in the narrowed vessel can bring about full occlusion and symptoms. Another type of ischemic stroke is the result of embolism, or the rupture of atherosclerotic plaque that travels to the brain and blocks blood flow. Atrial fibrillation can result in clot formation in the heart, which then seeds small embolic particles that travel to the brain. Lacunar strokes are seen more in older adults and in people with diabetes. They affect smaller areas of the brain by closing off arterioles.

Hemorrhagic stroke has a lower incidence than ischemic stroke but is associated with greater mortality. Subarachnoid stroke can be the result of a congenital (berry) aneurysm rupture, arteriovenous malformation, or trauma.[2] Subarachnoid stroke is a rupture of a large vessel within the protective lining of the brain. Intracerebral stroke is the rupture of a vessel within the brain itself.

Transient ischemic attacks (TIA) are small ischemic events. Neurologic deficits resolve completely within a few hours, but no more than 24 hours. A study by the University of California and Kaiser Permanente evaluated about 1700 patients presenting to the Emergency Department with TIA. Of those patients, 10% went on to have a stroke within 90 days after the event.[3] Other authors believe up to 25% of TIAs will signal impending stroke. The American Heart Association has calculated that people with TIAs have nine times the risk of a stroke.[4] These numbers reflect the growing practice of aggressive assessment and early treatment of persons presenting with TIA symptoms.

Stroke is the third leading cause of death in the United States after coronary heart disease and cancer.[5] There are approximately 600,000 cases of stroke each year, of which 100,000 are recurrences. Of all strokes, 83% were ischemic, 10% were intracerebral hemorrhage, and 7% were subarachnoid hemorrhage. More than 7.5% of ischemic strokes and nearly 38% of hemorrhagic strokes resulted in death within 30 days. Although from 1988 to 1998 the incidence of stroke fell by 15.5%, the death rate from stroke increased by 5.5%.[5]

The rate of stroke death is 58.6 per 100,000 people when all ages, sexes, and races are considered; however, it is a disease of age, with the prevalence being 404.5 per 100,000 in the over-65-year-old population. Women experience stroke at a rate 1.75 times that of men. Hispanics are twice as likely as whites to suffer a stroke. African-Americans are four times more likely to have a stroke than whites.[6]

Ischemic strokes tend to occur in older patients with other disease processes, whereas hemorrhagic strokes generally occur in healthy individuals between the ages of 40 and 60 years. Risk factors for ischemic stroke include hypertension, age, cigarette smoking, male gender, family history, race, previous stroke, carotid stenosis >80%, atrial fibrillation, congestive heart failure, mitral stenosis, prosthetic cardiac valves, myocardial infarction, and drug abuse (e.g., cocaine).[7] Other factors that may contribute to stroke are diabetes, obesity, a sedentary lifestyle, and an elevated serum cholesterol level.

Risk factors for hemorrhagic stroke include intracranial vascular anomalies, hypertension, family history, polycystic kidney disease, Ehlers-Danlos syndrome, systemic lupus erythematosus, neurofibromatosis, and tuberous sclerosis. Pregnancy, cigarette smoking, atherosclerosis, acute alcohol intoxication, and recreational drug use (e.g., cocaine) also increase the risk of hemorrhagic stroke.[8]

Stroke represents a significant burden for long-term care. Although 50% to 70% of stroke survivors regain functional independence, 15% to 30% are permanently disabled. Institutional care is required by 20% at 3 months after onset. Approximately 25% of stroke victims die within 1 year of their first stroke.[5]

Immediate emergency department referral/ physician consultation is indicated for all patients with a suspected cerebrovascular accident.

PATHOPHYSIOLOGY

Ischemic Stroke

In a thrombotic event a critical degree of atherosclerosis causes complete or relatively complete blockage of blood flow through a local area. In an embolic event a clot forms elsewhere (e.g., a fibrillating atrium), breaks off, and travels through the arterial circulation until it lodges in a vessel and blocks the flow of blood distally. The effects of arterial occlusion on brain tissue vary depending on the location of the occlusion in relation to available collateral and anastomotic channels, and on the degree and duration of the ischemia. The specific neurologic deficit relates to the location and size of the infarction or focus of ischemia. At the time of arterial occlusion, the viscosity of the blood and resistance to flow both increase, and there is sludging within the vessels. The tissue becomes pale. If the ischemia is prolonged, sludging and endothelial damage prevent normal reflow. There is cellular breakdown and swelling.[1]

Hemorrhagic Stroke

Trauma is the most common cause of subarachnoid hemorrhage.[9] Spontaneous subarachnoid hemorrhage is usually the result of rupture of an intracranial saccular aneurysm or arteriovenous malformation on the surface of the brain. A less common type of spontaneous subarachnoid hemorrhage occurs when there is bleeding within the brain tissue itself (intraparenchymal), with subsequent dissection of the hematoma through the brain and into the cerebrospinal fluid. Most of these hemorrhages are caused by hypertension, amyloid angiopathy, intraparenchymal vascular malformations, or tumors.[8]

In either embolic or hemorrhagic stroke, there is an area immediately surrounding the injury that dies within a few minutes from lack of oxygen and the failure of the oxygen-dependent adenosine triphosphate metabolic pathway. There is a broader area of injury referred to as the penumbra. In this area, the damage is more dynamic, extending over 12 to 24 hours. It is believed the release of intracellular calcium initiates the sequence of programmed cell death, or apoptosis.[10]

CLINICAL PRESENTATION

Patients with TIAs and strokes present similarly, although time is a major differentiating factor. The symptoms of cerebral ischemia are widely variable and depend on the vascular territory involved. When the carotid artery circulation is involved, symptoms reflect ischemia to the ipsilateral eye or brain. The classic visual disturbance (amaurosis fugax) is a transient, painless loss of vision, often described as a "shade" descending over the visual field.[1] Hemispheric brain ischemia usually causes weakness or numbness of the contralateral face or limbs. Language difficulties and cognitive and behavioral changes may also occur.[2] Vertebrobasilar TIAs and strokes may present with vertigo, nystagmus, diplopia, dysconjugate gaze, or deficits of cranial nerves III to XII.[2,11]

Many signs and symptoms are common to both anterior (carotid) and posterior (vertebrobasilar) circulation. These include hemiparesis, hemisensory loss, visual field defects, ataxia (difficulty with balance and coordination), dysarthria (difficulty speaking), reflex asymmetry, and Babinski's sign.[11] Headache does not usually occur in ischemic stroke but may in some cases. When present, headache is not nearly as severe as in intracerebral or subarachnoid hemorrhage, and there is no stiffness of the neck. TIAs more commonly precede ischemic stroke than hemorrhagic stroke.

In ischemic stroke there is usually a single attack, and the entire illness evolves within a few hours. However, the stroke may present in a "stuttering" fashion, with intermittent progression of neurologic deficits that extend over several hours, a day, or longer. A partial stroke may occur and even recede temporarily for several hours, after which there may be rapid progression to the full-blown stroke. The stroke may involve several parts of the body at once or only one part (e.g., a limb or one side of the face), with the other parts becoming involved in a stepwise fashion until the stroke is fully developed. The stroke may occur during sleep, with the patient remaining unaware until he or she tries to get up and discovers the paralysis.[1]

In subarachnoid hemorrhage the clinical presentation is usually heralded by the abrupt onset of a severe headache ("the worst headache of my life"), nausea and vomiting, signs of meningeal irritation, and varying degrees of neurologic dysfunction. Loss of consciousness at the time of the initial event is common but is usually short-lived. Nearly 50% of patients who present with aneurysmal subarachnoid hemorrhage give a history of atypical headaches occurring days to weeks before the definitive event.[9] These "sentinel" headaches are characteristically sudden in onset and are often associated with nausea, vomiting, and dizziness, with or without neurologic dysfunction. Some hemorrhagic events may present with seizures.

Patients with hypertensive intracerebral hemorrhage may have no consistent warning or prodromal symptoms. In the majority of cases the hemorrhage has its onset while the patient is up and active; onset during sleep is rare. The blood pressure is elevated in almost all cases. The neurologic signs and symptoms vary with the site and size of the extravasation of blood. The patient may lapse almost immediately into stupor and coma, with hemiplegia and steady deterioration to death over the next several hours. More often, the patient complains of a headache, followed within a few minutes by unilateral facial sag, slurred speech, weakness in an arm and leg, and eye deviation away from the paretic limbs. These events, occurring over a period of 5 to 30 minutes, strongly suggest intracerebral bleeding. More advanced cases are characterized by paralysis; aphasia; stupor; coma; deep, irregular respiration; dilated, fixed pupils; and, occasionally, decerebrate rigidity.[1]

PHYSICAL EXAMINATION

Findings on physical examination correspond to the location of the vascular event and associated neurologic deficit. Because TIAs are, by definition, events that last no longer than 24 hours, by the time the patient seeks medical attention all signs and symptoms may have completely resolved, leaving a normal physical examination.

DIAGNOSTICS

Diagnostic studies are necessary to determine the type of stroke and the probable etiology, as well as to detect complications. Because management is vastly different, it is important to be able to quickly differentiate ischemic stroke from hemorrhagic stroke and to exclude disorders that may occasionally present like stroke.

In the initial evaluation the most common imaging procedure performed is a head CT scan.[9] A noncontrast CT scan is better than MRI in discriminating between hemorrhagic and ischemic stroke. Patients who have atypical presentations or who have unusual findings on noncontrast CT scans ought to have a CT scan with contrast or MRI to exclude tumor. CT can miss small subcortical or cortical infarctions or lesions in the posterior fossa. Among patients with ischemic stroke, the CT scan may be normal in the first few hours but will usually show abnormalities after 12 or more hours. In hemorrhagic stroke, the head CT scan will usually be abnormal at presentation to the emergency department. If the initial CT scan shows hemorrhage, other studies (e.g., arteriogram) may be necessary to determine if an underlying vascular malformation is present.[8]

Other diagnostic studies include an ECG, chest radiograph, pulse oximetry or arterial blood gas assessment, CBC with platelets, prothrombin time, partial thromboplastin time, serum glucose, creatinine, BUN, and electrolytes. Depending on the clinical presentation, other tests may be necessary, including examination of the cerebrospinal fluid if central nervous system infection is suspected or when the clinical picture suggests subarachnoid hemorrhage but the head CT scan is negative. An electroencephalogram is indicated when the clinical picture suggests seizure. Carotid ultrasound will assess patency of the carotid arteries. Carotid arteriography or magnetic resonance angiography should be done in patients with severe carotid stenosis on ultrasound evaluation who are considered candidates for endarterectomy. A transesophageal echocardiogram[9] and Holter monitor study may be performed if the presentation is suspicious for an embolic event originating from the heart. Other laboratory tests that may be indicated include a serum cholesterol level, toxicology screening, erythrocyte sedimentation rate, hemoglobin electrophoresis, fibrinogen, serum protein electrophoresis, antiphospholipid antibody level, serologic test for syphilis, protein C level, protein S level, antithrombin III level, lupus anticoagulant, anticardiolipin antibody level, and connective tissue disease screen.

Diagnostics

Cerebrovascular Events

Initial
ECG
Pulse oximetry

Laboratory
CBC and differential
PT, PTT, international normalized ratio
Serum electrolytes
BUN
Creatinine
Serum glucose
Toxic screen*
Lipid profile
ESR
Hemoglobin electrophoresis*
Fibrinogen
Serum protein electrophoresis*
Antiphospholipid antibody*
FTA/ABS or RPR*
Protein C, protein S*
Antithrombin III*
Lupus anticoagulant*
Anticardiolipin antibody*
Connective tissue disease screening*

Imaging
CT scan of head (noncontrast)
Transesophageal echocardiogram
Chest x-ray*

Other
Carotid ultrasound
EEG*
Arteriography*
ABGs*
Lumbar puncture*
Holter or event monitoring

*If indicated.

DIFFERENTIAL DIAGNOSIS

A number of conditions may be mistaken for TIAs and stroke: migraine and migraine equivalents, simple partial or complex partial seizures, subdural hematoma, brain tumor (primary or metastatic), syncope, cardiac arrhythmia, hyperventilation, panic attack, hypoglycemia, demyelinating disease, encephalitis, suicide gestures, conversion disorders, recent cocaine or amphetamine use, transient global amnesia, systemic infection,

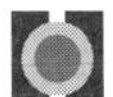

Differential Diagnosis

Cerebrovascular Events

Migraine
Seizures
Subdural/epidural hematoma
Tumor (primary, metastatic)
Syncope
Hypoglycemia
Cardiac arrhythmia
Transient global amnesia
Encephalopathy
Conversion disorder
Carpal tunnel syndrome
Hyperventilation
Panic attack
Infection (meningitis, encephalitis) or systemic infection
Drug overdose
Demyelinating disease
Nonketotic hyperosmolar coma
Postcardiac arrest ischemia

toxic/metabolic encephalopathy, and carpal tunnel syndrome, among others.[11-13]

MANAGEMENT

Initial management depends on the acuity of presentation. The patient who presents days after a probable TIA but has no current signs or symptoms of neurologic dysfunction can generally be evaluated and treated in the outpatient setting. The patient who presents acutely with neurologic signs and symptoms compatible with a TIA or stroke should be managed as a medical emergency.[12]

Initial management of suspected stroke includes assessment of the ABCs (airway, breathing, and circulation) and vital signs. The airway should be secured; oxygen should be administered by nasal cannula; a cardiac monitor, pulse oximeter, and sphygmomanometer should be attached; an IV access should be established; a physical examination should be performed; a 12-lead ECG and portable chest radiograph should be obtained; laboratory tests (as described previously) should be ordered; and an urgent noncontrast head CT scan should be obtained. If hemorrhage has occurred, a neurosurgeon should be contacted. If ischemic stroke has occurred, thrombolytic therapy should be considered if the patient meets criteria.

Careful blood pressure management is necessary in the acute ischemic stroke setting. Patients who have a stroke commonly have elevated blood pressure after the acute event. The conscious stroke patient is usually quite anxious. Often the blood pressure will fall when the patient is moved to a quieter room and allowed to rest after the initial evaluation has been completed.[7] There is evidence that an acute hypertensive response may represent a beneficial compensatory response to maintain cerebral perfusion.[14] If the brain is already ischemic, lowering the blood pressure may only exacerbate hypoperfusion and injury. Therefore except when the blood pressure is extremely high, it is best not to lower it during the first few days after an ischemic infarction. After that time, the blood pressure usually returns to the previous baseline value without additional treatment.[15] Patients with a systolic blood pressure >220 mm Hg or a diastolic blood pressure >120 mm Hg and medical conditions requiring blood pressure control may require medical intervention.

If an antihypertensive drug is necessary, labetalol is currently the drug of choice.[16] The drug is given intravenously, 20 mg, over 1 to 2 minutes. The dose may be repeated or doubled every 10 to 20 minutes, with a maximum dose of 300 mg. If no satisfactory response is obtained with labetalol, a nitroprusside infusion may be started.[16] Use of sublingual calcium antagonists should be avoided because of their rapid absorption and sometimes precipitous decline in blood pressure.[7] If antihypertensive therapy is necessary, blood pressure reduction should be gradual and gentle, and the patient should be carefully monitored. The therapy should be discontinued if there is any neurologic deterioration. In patients with subarachnoid hemorrhage, the blood pressure should be reduced to prestroke levels.

Thrombolytic Therapy

In June 1996 the U.S. Food and Drug Administration approved the use of IV recombinant tissue plasminogen activator (t-PA) for treatment of appropriately selected patients with ischemic stroke if it is administered within 3 hours from the onset of symptoms. Despite an increased incidence of bleeding complications, studies show a significant reduction in neurologic disability in patients treated with t-PA as compared with patients treated in the conventional manner.[7,17] There is no evidence that t-PA is effective after 3 hours of symptoms, and the drug has not been approved for use beyond that point. The time to treatment is the most important determinant of success in treating ischemic stroke (the sooner thrombolytic therapy is started, the better the outcome). Inclusion criteria for use of t-PA include the following: age 18 or older, clinical diagnosis of ischemic stroke, and time of onset <180 minutes before t-PA administration. The exclusion criteria list is much longer, focusing primarily on evidence of current bleeding or a risk of bleeding that is sufficient to outweigh potential benefits of t-PA treatment (see Table 32-1). Because t-PA is the only approved specific treatment for acute ischemic stroke and many patients do not fulfill the criteria for its use, the major goals of stroke management are to limit the size of the infarction, prevent and treat complications, and prevent recurrences.[17]

Surgery

Certain types of stroke may require urgent neurosurgical intervention. Neurosurgical consultation is indicated in cases of subarachnoid hemorrhage, intracerebral hemorrhage, and increased intracranial pressure causing neurologic compromise.

The patient who presents with a more remote history (days to weeks) compatible with a TIA but with no current signs or symptoms of neurologic dysfunction can be evaluated and treated in the outpatient setting (see the Diagnostics box), using the patient's history and physical examination findings to guide the testing sequence and initial treatment. Identification of the most likely cause of the TIA is vital to proper management. For example, management of the patient with severe carotid stenosis will be different from that of the patient with atrial fibrillation. Treatment for all patients with a TIA or stroke should include risk factor management.

Antiplatelet Agents

Numerous studies have demonstrated a benefit of antiplatelet agents in reducing stroke risk in patients who have had a TIA or minor stroke.[18] The relative benefit of antiplatelet therapy is remarkably constant regardless of age, gender, blood pressure, and the presence or absence of diabetes. Aspirin is the standard medical therapy used for TIAs and ischemic stroke prevention. The optimal dose remains somewhat controversial, but there is increasing evidence that lower doses are as effective as higher doses and have fewer gastrointestinal side effects. Currently prescribed regimens range from 85 to 325 mg every day.

Warfarin (Coumadin) is indicated for TIAs and stroke prevention in patients at risk for cardiac embolism. This includes patients with chronic or paroxysmal atrial fibrillation, left ventricular dysfunction with congestive heart failure, or artificial cardiac valves.

A class of antiplatelet drugs, the thienopyridines, are modestly more effective than aspirin, but the degree of additional benefit is unclear. Two representative drugs from this class include clopidogrel (Plavix) and ticlopidine (Ticlid). Ticlopidine, however, has potential side effects, which can include diarrhea, thrombotic thrombocytopenic purpura, and neutropenia. These risks require hematologic monitoring. Cost is also significantly higher.[19,20]

Carotid Endarterectomy

Carotid endarterectomy has been demonstrated to have a beneficial effect (as compared with medical therapy alone) in patients with carotid stenosis greater than 70% to 80%, but the role of endarterectomy for patients with lesser degrees of stenosis has not been clearly established.[7,18] The benefit of surgery must be weighed against potential perioperative morbidity and mortality. Carotid endarterectomy is strongly indicated in patients with a hemispheric TIA and in 70% to 99% of patients with ipsilateral carotid stenosis and should be undertaken as soon as possible in these patients because of the high risk of a full stroke.[18] Surgery for intracranial or vertebrobasilar disease has not been shown to be of any benefit.

LIFE SPAN CONSIDERATIONS

Pregnancy

Stroke during pregnancy is of course a major tragedy. Fortunately it is a rare occurrence. In a retrospective study of hospital admissions for delivery by Jaigobin and Silver, 34 strokes occurred in 50,700 patients.[21] There were 21 infarctions and 23 hemorrhages. The primary care provider can best address this through pregnancy preparation counseling for all fertile women, stressing the need for early and complete prenatal care. Close monitoring of weight, signs of proteinuria, and blood pressure changes in the gravid patient require early intervention.

Geriatric Patients

Stroke will disproportionately affect older persons. In older patients, especially those with co-morbid conditions, therapeutic interventions such as surgery or thrombolysis can be contraindicated. In these situations, comprehensive assessment of need will help determine where appropriate care can be provided. For some, sufficient capacities will remain that will enable return to home with supportive services. Others will require skilled nursing care. It is critical that the health care provider know a patient's intentions regarding end-of-life care. It is not sufficient to know whether a patient desires intubation or defibrillation in case of respiratory or cardiac arrest. Surrogate decision maker must be identified and their role defined through advance directives. More important, one should learn what a patient values in life to help guide decisions when impairments may significantly affect those aspects that bring meaning to an individual. In this way care can be tailored to the patient's wishes.

COMPLICATIONS

The main complication of a TIA is a subsequent full-blown stroke. A TIA is clearly a warning indicating the necessity for a thorough cardiovascular evaluation and appropriate management.

The complications of stroke impact virtually every organ system. Early complications of stroke include cerebral edema, increased intracranial pressure, pulmonary and urinary tract infections, sepsis, seizures, hypertension, hypotension, cardiac arrhythmias, myocardial ischemia and infarction, deep venous thrombosis, pulmonary embolism, pressure sores, depression, and extension or progression of the stroke. Later complications include permanent residual problems with mobility, activities of daily living, communication, nutrition, swallowing, behavior, continence, sexual function, limb contractures, and dementia.

A patient with an acute stroke should be admitted to the hospital, with management directed toward limiting, if possible, the amount of brain injury and preventing or ameliorating the constellation of potential complications.

Complications in the hospitalized stroke patient include pneumonia, seizures, myocardial infarction, deep venous thrombosis, pressure ulcers, hyperglycemia, hypoglycemia, depression, limb contractures, and constipation. Awareness of these potential complications and specific therapies directed toward their prevention will dramatically reduce the stroke patient's morbidity and mortality. Of particular importance is physical, occupational, and speech therapy, which should be initiated as soon as the patient is medically stable and able to participate.

INDICATIONS FOR REFERRAL/HOSPITALIZATION

All patients with a suspected acute TIA or stroke should be evaluated and managed as an emergency. Time is critical. Any patient presenting to an outpatient setting within 3 hours of symptom onset should be transported immediately to the nearest emergency department having CT and the ability to implement a thrombolytic (tPA) protocol. Clear survival benefits exist in those hospitals having dedicated stroke units.[22] A patient with a suspected TIA who presents with a more remote history and a normal current examination may be evaluated as an outpatient. Physician consultation is warranted, as the specific situation may dictate a sense of urgency similar to that of an acute TIA or stroke and warrant hospitalization for evaluation and treatment.

Even with a remote history and a current normal physical examination, hospitalization may be justified to expedite evaluation and lessen the possibility of a stroke. In certain subgroups of TIAs, including those with multiple frequent and recent ("crescendo") TIAs and those with ventricular thrombi, the early risk of stroke is particularly high.[18] The diagnostic evaluation of patients seen within 1 week of a TIA should be completed within 1 week or less. All acute strokes require hospitalization.

PATIENT AND FAMILY EDUCATION

Two elements of patient education are paramount: (1) risk factor reduction and (2) stroke symptom recognition and emergency treatment. Hypertension is the most important independent and modifiable risk factor. It is imperative that patients with hypertension be educated about their disease and the importance of medical therapy and lifestyle changes for prevention of complications such as stroke. Cigarette smoking, obesity, diabetes, a sedentary lifestyle, and hypercholesterolemia are other modifiable factors that require patient education. Despite the rapid evolution of stroke care and exciting possibilities being investigated, the most important function for the primary care provider is aggressive early identification of at-risk individuals, education for all patients, and appropriate early intervention with elevated blood pressure, glucose intolerance, obesity, smoking, and sedentary lifestyles.

The public, particularly those individuals with risk factors, must be educated about the signs and symptoms of TIAs and strokes. The term *brain attack* should be used to convey the same sense of urgency that *heart attack* carries. Factors that have been shown to be associated with delay in treatment include lack of recognition of stroke signs and symptoms, calling the primary care provider instead of the emergency medical number, living alone, onset while asleep, onset at home rather than at work, and a milder severity of stroke.[17] A study by the American Heart Association revealed that nearly two thirds of the persons surveyed could not identify even one warning sign of a stroke.[12] Patients at risk should be taught to recognize the signs and symptoms of a stroke and to call 911 as soon as symptoms occur.

Those patients who do survive suffer a wide range of physical and psychologic impairments, including motor, sensory, perceptual, cognitive, and communicative skills that may seriously interfere with adequate social interactions and the ability of the patient to engage in normal activities of daily living. The direct and indirect costs for the patient, family, and society are incalculable.

Rehabilitation services are essential to maximal stroke recovery. Intensive rehabilitation should commence within 48 hours of stabilization. The recovery stage of stroke requires significant adaptive training for the patient, family, and caregivers. The family itself will be stressed by the recovery process and will need access to counseling, peer support and other community resources.[23]

REFERENCES

1. Adams RD, Victor M: *Principles of neurology*, New York, ed 15, 1993, McGraw-Hill
2. Alper BS: Acute stroke, Dynamed. Not yet peer reviewed. Available at http://www.dynamicmedical.com.
3. 125th Annual Meeting of the American Neurological Association, Day 1: October 15, 2000. Advances in Outcomes Research, Andrew N. Wilner, MD, FACP. Retrieved November 27, 2001 from the World Wide Web: http://www.medscape.com/medscape/cno/2000/ANA/Story.cfm?story_id=1726.
4. Stroke, American Heart Association. Retrieved from the World Wide Web November 27, 2001: http://216.185.112.5/presenter.jhtml?identifier=1498.
5. 2001 Heart and Stroke Statistical Update, American Heart Association. Retrieved November 28, 2001 from the World Wide Web: http://www.americanheart.org/downloadable/heart/4838_HSSTATS2001_1.0.pdf.
6. National Vital Statistics Report, *Epidemiology* 11(1):48, 2000.
7. Gasecki AP: Stroke recurrence and prevention. Paper presented at the Neurology for Primary Care Providers Conference, San Diego, May 1997.
8. Sawin PD, Loftus CM: Diagnosis of spontaneous subarachnoid hemorrhage, *Am Fam Physician* 55(1):145-156, 1997.
9. 125th Annual Meeting of the American Neurological Association, Day 1: October 15, 2000 Technology Advances Our Understanding of Cerebrovascular Events, Rebecca Evans, MD. Retrieved November 27, 2001 from the World Wide Web.
10. XVII World Congress of Neurology, Day 1: June 17, 2001. Recent Advances in Cerebrovascular Disease, Malin Maeder-Ingvar, MD, Julien Bogousslavsky, MD. Retrieved November 28, 2001 from the World Wide Web: http://www.medscape.com/medscape/cno/2001/WCNCME/Story.cfm?story_id=2316. http://www.medscape.com/medscape/cno/2000/ANA/Story.cfm?story_id=1725.
11. Nadeua SE: Transient ischemic attacks: diagnosis and medical and surgical management, *J Fam Pract* 38(5):495-504, 1994.
12. Selman WR, Tarr R, Landis DMD: Brain attack: emergency treatment of ischemic stroke, *Am Fam Physician* 55(8):2655-2662, 1997.
13. Edmeads JG: Transient ischemic attacks: rethinking concepts in management, *Postgrad Med* 96(5):42-54, 1994.
14. Smucker WD, Disabato JA, Krishen AE: Systematic approach to diagnosis and initial management of stroke, *Am Fam Physician* 52(1):225-234, 1995.
15. Biller J: Cerebrovascular disorders in the 1990s, *Clin Geriatr Med* 7(3), 1991.
16. Koller RL, Anderson DC: Intravenous thrombolytic therapy for acute ischemic stroke: weighing the risks and benefits of tissue plasminogen activator, *Postgrad Med* 103(4):221-231, 1998.
17. Broderick JP: Practical considerations in the early treatment of ischemic stroke, *Am Fam Physician* 57(1):73-80, 1998.
18. Feinberg WM: Guidelines for the management of transient ischemic attacks: Ad Hoc Committee on Guidelines for the Management of Transient Ischemic Attacks of the Stroke Council, American Heart Association, *Heart Dis Stroke* 3(5):275-283, 1994.
19. Hankey GJ, Sudlow CLM, Dunbabin DW: Thienopyridine derivatives (ticlopidine, clopidogrel) versus aspirin for preventing stroke and other serious vascular events in high vascular risk patients (Cochrane Review). In: *The Cochrane Library*, 2, 2001. Oxford: Update Software.
20. Mohr JP and others: A comparison of warfarin and aspirin for the prevention of recurrent ischemic stroke, *N Engl J Med* 345:1444-1451,1493-1495, 2001.
21. Stroke and pregnancy, *Stroke* 31:2948, 2000. Retrieved December 10, 2001 from the World Wide Web: www.stroke.ahajournals.org/cgi/content/abstract/31/12/2948.
22. Organized Inpatient (stroke unit) Care for Stroke. Retrieved November 27, 2001 from the World Wide Web: http://www.medscape.com/Cochrane/abstracts/ab000197.html.
23. Recovery and rehabilitation. Retrieved November 27, 2001 from the World Wide Web: http://www.stroke.org/recov_rehab.cfm.

CHAPTER 209

Delirium

Karen Dick

DEFINITION/EPIDEMIOLOGY

Delirium is a serious and significant health problem for older adults and one that requires prompt recognition and treatment. Also known as acute confusional state, delirium is often the first and only indicator of underlying physical illness, such as infection, myocardial infarction, or drug toxicity in older adults. According to the DSM-IV (fourth edition of *Diagnostic and Statistical Manual of Mental Disorders*), delirium can develop from a general medical condition, substance intoxication or withdrawal, multiple etiologies, or unspecified conditions (Box 209-1).[1] It is characterized by a disturbance in attention, consciousness, and cognition. The hallmark of delirium is a clouding of consciousness, with an inability to focus, sustain, or shift attention, as well as a change in cognition, including impairment in short-term memory, disorientation, and perceptual disturbances.[1]

The incidence estimates for delirium in hospitalized medical patients range from 10% to 30% and are as high as 70% in some postoperative (orthopedic or cardiac surgery) patients.[3-8] It has been suggested that between 37% and 72% of patients who become delirious are never recognized as such and may be incorrectly labeled as having dementia, a psychiatric disorder, or unmanageable behavior.[3,9] Patients with an underlying dementia are at even greater risk for developing delirium if physically or psychologically stressed.[2]

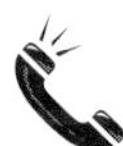

Physician consultation is indicated for patients with delirium.

BOX 209-1

DIAGNOSTIC CRITERIA FOR DELIRIUM

A. Disturbance of consciousness (i.e., reduced clarity of awareness of the environment) with reduced ability to focus, sustain, or shift attention.
B. A change in cognition (such as memory deficit, disorientation, language disturbance) or the development of a perceptual disturbance that is not better accounted for by a preexisting, established, or evolving dementia.
C. The disturbance develops over a short period of time (usually hours to days) and tends to fluctuate during the course of the day.
D. There is evidence from the history, physical examination, or laboratory findings that the disturbance is caused by the direct physiologic consequences of a general medical condition.

From American Psychiatric Association: *Diagnostic and statistical manual of mental disorders*, ed 4 (Text revision 2000), Washington, DC, 1994, The Association.

PATHOPHYSIOLOGY

There remains a lack of agreement as to the exact cause of delirium. Four mechanisms have been proposed that might explain the physiologic precipitant underlying the development of delirium[5]: (1) there is an insufficiency of cerebral metabolism as demonstrated by diffuse slowing on an electroencephalogram (EEG) in a patient with delirium, (2) a central abnormality is caused by an imbalance of central cholinergic and adrenergic metabolism, (3) there is impairment in cerebral oxidative metabolism, and (4) a stress reaction as evidenced by abnormally high circulating corticosteroids is causing the symptoms. It is likely that a combination of several physiologic, psychologic, and environmental variables, combined with the known effects of the normal aging process, triggers the acute mental status changes.

CLINICAL PRESENTATION

Delirium occurs acutely over hours to days and is characterized by fluctuations in mental status over the course of the day. This fluctuating presentation is problematic, as patients may have periods of lucidity interspersed with inattention and high distractibility, motor restlessness, speech that is difficult to follow, and perceptual disturbances that range from misinterpretations of the environment to frank visual hallucinations. Memory, particularly in relation to recent events, is often impaired, and disorientation, most commonly to time (day of the week or time of the year) or place, is usually present. Patients may also exhibit affective signs of fear, anxiety, or anger. There may be a history of a fragmented and disordered sleep-wake cycle. Symptoms may be worse in the evening and labeled "sundowning"; however, it is not clear if sundowning is a component of delirium or a separate clinical condition. Patients with a history of dementia are at greatest risk for sundowning.

Clinical subtypes of delirium have been identified and include hyperactive, hypoactive, and mixed variants.[10] The hyperactive type, manifested by agitation and restlessness, is often thought of as the typical presentation of delirium. However, the quiet, calm patient who may have the same clouding of consciousness, as well as hallucinations, is often overlooked.

Because the diagnosis of delirium is based on history, physical examination, or laboratory evidence of an underlying medical condition, careful attention to other symptomatology and conditions is necessary. In long-term care, the nursing staff can provide invaluable information as to subtle changes in behavior, appetite, or functional status that may be the warning signs of an underlying problem. Urinary tract infection and pneumonia in the frail nursing home patient often present with an altered mental status as the only indicator of an underlying problem.

Polypharmacy and biologic vulnerability for adverse effects make the older person more prone to medication-induced delirium, and a thorough review of all medications, including prescription and over-the-counter preparations, is an essential part of the assessment process.[11] Anticholinergic medications have long been implicated as a risk factor for delirium and although research results have been mixed as to the strength of the association and the relationship to severity of symptoms, these medications need to be discontinued whenever possible.[12] The patient's use of alcohol and other substances also needs to be evaluated.

It is also important to assess psychosocial and sociocultural factors to better understand the patient's baseline personality and psychologic functioning. For patients admitted to the hospital, information from family members and/or long-term care facilities can be critical in understanding premorbid behavior and function.

PHYSICAL EXAMINATION

In an attempt to identify the precipitating medical condition, a thorough review of systems, as well as a comprehensive physical examination, should be undertaken. However, this may be difficult if the patient is unable to answer questions or follow even simple commands. A detailed history from family members or other caregivers becomes critical in identifying the onset and development of symptoms, as well as in establishing that there has been a sudden change in affect, cognition, or behavior. A neurologic examination is necessary to exclude trauma and focal signs suggestive of a central nervous system disturbance (e.g., tumor, stroke, seizure).

Careful observation of the patient's gait, level of consciousness, speech, appearance, and interactions with others can be most helpful in establishing a diagnosis. Mental status testing is important to establish the degree of cognitive impairment but may have to be modified if the patient is unable to cooperate with the examination. Although it is not specific to delirium, the Folstein Mini-Mental Status Examination (MMSE) is the most commonly used evaluation tool.[13] The MMSE measures orientation, memory, attention, calculation, and language functions. Mental status examinations that were developed specifically for purposes of diagnosing delirium include the Delirium Rating Scale[14] and the Confusion Assessment Method.[15] Both are capable of assessing the complex features of delirium and of distinguishing delirium from dementia, and both are feasible for use in delirious patients.[16]

DIAGNOSTICS

It is important to note that there may be more than one contributing medical condition that leads to the development of delirium, and multiple etiologies, including substance intoxication or withdrawal, should be considered. The choice of specific diagnostic studies is guided by the history and physical examination and may include a head CT or MRI, lumbar puncture, and EEG, as well as laboratory studies. A CBC, basic metabolic profile (BMP), thyroid function test, drug levels, as well as urinalysis, culture and sensitivity should be checked. Although it is rarely done, the EEG can be helpful in confirming the diagnosis and will show a characteristic slowing of brain wave activity.[17]

DIFFERENTIAL DIAGNOSIS

DSM-IV diagnostic criteria for delirium mandate that the etiology be specified. Specific etiologies include systemic diseases, primary cerebral disease, metabolic disturbances, intoxication with exogenous substances (drugs or poisons), and withdrawal from drugs or alcohol.[5]

Diagnostics

Delirium

Laboratory
CBC and differential
ESR
Platelet count
Serum electrolytes
Serum glucose
Calcium
Magnesium
Phosphorus
BUN
Creatinine
LFTs
Vitamin B_{12}
Folate
Thiamine
Ammonia
TFTs
Blood and urine toxic screens
Medication levels
Urinalysis and culture

Imaging
Chest x-ray

Other
ECG

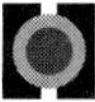

Differential Diagnosis

Delirium

Systemic Diseases
Infections: urinary tract infection, pneumonia, subacute bacterial endocarditis, meningitis
Myocardial infarction, congestive heart failure, arrhythmias, pulmonary embolus
Anemia

Primary Cerebral Disease
Cerebrovascular accident
Transient ischemic attack
Subdural hematoma
Temporal arteritis
Seizure
Head trauma

Metabolic Causes
Dehydration
Elevation or decrease in sodium, calcium, magnesium, potassium
Acid-base imbalance
Hypoxia
Hypoglycemia
Hepatic insufficiency
Renal insufficiency
Thyroid dysfunction
Vitamin deficiencies

Intoxication
Alcohol
Anticholinergics
Narcotics
Sedative-hypnotics
Antidepressants
Nonsteroidals
Heavy metal poisons

Withdrawal
Alcohol
Benzodiazepines
Sedatives and hypnotics
Narcotics

Delirium must be distinguished from other organic and psychiatric syndromes including dementia and depression. All three of these conditions have manifestations in common and can occur in the same patient at the same time; the interrelationships between them are complex. It is critical to establish the onset of symptoms, as unlike depression and dementia, the onset of delirium is acute. A psychiatric referral may be necessary to establish a diagnosis.

MANAGEMENT

Treatment of delirium is both definitive and palliative. Current practice remains empirically based without consensus for evidenced-based guidelines for diagnosis and management.[18] Definitive care is aimed at identifying and treating the precipitating causes, and palliative care is directed toward the management of such symptoms as agitation, restlessness, and hallucinations.[11] Recent studies have suggested that an interdisciplinary approach may be effective.[19-21] Generally, nonessential medications need to be tapered or discontinued. The sleep-wake cycle needs to be regulated and sensory deficits corrected. The patient should be in a setting that provides necessary medical interventions as well as close behavioral monitoring, and in an environment that maintains patient safety. Interventions such as frequent reorientation, reduced stimulation, and a calm and comforting approach can be helpful. Families can often provide a stabilizing presence and can assist with establishing a reassuring and familiar routine. Physical and chemical restraints should be avoided wherever possible.

Haloperidol and droperidol may be useful in controlling agitation and psychosis, and dosing should be guided by the patient's initial response and by frequent reassessment. Newer antipsychotics such as risperidone and olanzapine may be used in small doses for behavior management in the short term when patient and/or staff safety is compromised. Benzodiazepines are useful in the treatment of alcohol and sedative withdrawal. The goal of treatment is to promote recovery, prevent additional complications, maintain the patient's safety, and maximize function.

COMPLICATIONS

Delirium contributes to increased morbidity and mortality, longer hospital stays, functional impairment, and more permanent forms of cognitive impairment if it is not recognized and treated in a timely fashion.[4,22,23] It has been suggested that an episode of delirium may represent the unmasking of an unrecognized dementia in the setting of an acute illness. Patients who become delirious during a hospitalization have longer length of stays and higher rates of referral to skilled nursing facilities on discharge. Although it was once thought that delirium was transient in nature, there is now evidence that functional impairment may persist for up to 6 months after treatment.[24] In a prospective study of patients diagnosed with delirium during hospitalization, the 3-year mortality rate was 75% vs. 51% for control patients even when prehospital cognitive, functional, and social measures were taken into account.[25]

INDICATIONS FOR REFERRAL/HOSPITALIZATION

A diagnosis of delirium is considered a medical emergency. The need to identify, remove, or treat the underlying condition is critical to modifying the delirious state and preventing subsequent morbidities and complications. Hospitalization is an additional stressor that contributes to delirium, and decisions for treatment should be based on an evaluation of the patient's overall functional status, the ability of caregivers to provide supportive care, and, most important, the patient's safety. Patients are often admitted to the hospital with a diagnosis of mental status change as the search for the underlying cause is actively pursued.

PATIENT AND FAMILY EDUCATION

Patients who have experienced episodes of delirium report feelings of fear and anxiety and often describe vivid hallucinations. Patients and families need reassurance and explanation that the delirium is related to the medical condition and is not a sign that the patient is "crazy," is "losing his or her mind," or is becoming "senile." Patients also need an opportunity to reflect on the experience and to express their feelings.

Patients with advanced age, preexisting cognitive impairment, or severe, chronic illnesses, as well as those taking psychoactive medication, are most at risk for delirium.[11,22,23] Although many of these risk factors are not modifiable, it is important that all caregivers be able to recognize the risks and presenting signs and symptoms of delirium.

REFERENCES

1. American Psychiatric Association: *Diagnostic and statistical manual of mental disorders,* ed 4, Washington, DC, 1994, American Psychiatric Association.
2. Lipowski Z: Delirium in the elderly patient, *N Engl J Med* 320:578-582, 1989.
3. Gillick M, Serrell N, Gillick L: Adverse consequences of hospitalization in the elderly, *Soc Sci Med* 16:1033-1038, 1982.
4. Lipowski Z: Transient disorders in the elderly, *Am J Psychiatry* 140: 1426-1436, 1983.
5. Johnson J: Delirium in the elderly, *Emerg Clin North Am* 8:255-264, 1990.
6. Sadler D: Incidence, degree, and duration of postcardiotomy delirium, *Heart Lung* 10:1084-1092, 1981.
7. Smith L, Dimsdale J: Postcardiotomy delirium: conclusions after 25 years, *Am J Psychiatry* 146:452-458, 1989.
8. Williams M and others: Predictors of acute confusional states in hospitalized elderly patient, *Res Nurs Health* 8:31-40, 1985.
9. Wolanin M, Phillips L: *Confusion: prevention and care,* St Louis, 1981, Mosby.
10. Lipzin B, Levkoff S: An empirical study of delirium subtypes, *Br J Psychiatry* 161:843-845, 1992.
11. Jacobsen S: Delirium in the elderly, *Psychiatr Clin North Am* 20: 91-109, 1997.
12. Tune L: Anticholinergic effects of medication in elderly patients, *J Clin Psychiatry* 62(Suppl 21):11-14, 2001.
13. Yesavage J and others: Development and validation of a geriatric depression screening scale: a preliminary report, *J Psychiatr Res* 17(1): 37-49, 1982.
14. Trzepac P, Dew M: Further analysis of the Delirium Rating Scale, *Gen Hosp Psychiatry* 17:75-79, 1995.
15. Inouye S and others: Clarifying confusion: the confusion assessment method, *Ann Intern Med* 113:941-948, 1990.
16. Inouye S: The dilemma of delirium, *Am J Med* 97:278-288, 1994.
17. Romano J, Engel G: Delirium. I. Electroencephalographic data, *Arch Neurol Psychiatry* 51:356-377, 1944.
18. Britton A, Russel R: Multidisciplinary team interventions for delirium in patients with chronic impairment, *Cochrane Database Syst Rev,* 1(1):CD000395, 2001.

19. Rizzo J and others: Multicomponent targeted intervention to prevent delirium in hospitalized elderly patients: what is the economic value? *Med Care* 39:7, 2001.
20. Milsen K and others: A nurse-led interdisciplinary intervention program for delirium in elderly hip-fracture patients, *J Am Geriatr Soc* 49:5, 2001.
21. Inouye S: Prevention of delirium in hospitalized older patients: risk factors and targeted intervention strategies, *Ann Med* 32:257-263, 2000.
22. Levkoff S, Besdine R, Wetle T: Acute confusional states in the hospitalized elderly, *Annu Rev Gerontol Geriatr* 6:1-26, 1986.
23. Levkoff S and others: Delirium, the occurrence and persistence of symptoms among elderly hospitalized patients, *Arch Intern Med* 152:334-340, 1992.
24. Murray A and others: Acute delirium and functional decline in the hospitalized elderly patient, *J Gerontol* 48:M181-M186, 1993.
25. Curyto K and others: Survival of hospitalized elderly patients with delirium: a prospective study, *Am J Geriatr Psychiatry* 9:141-147, 2001.

CHAPTER 210

Dementia

Karen Dick

DEFINITION/EPIDEMIOLOGY

Most people enjoy a fruitful and productive period during their later years. However, for 5% to 10% of the population over age 65 and 15% to 45% of the population over age 85, these years are associated with a serious form of cognitive impairment known as dementia. It is estimated that at least 4 million people in the United States—regardless of race, creed, or socioeconomic status—are afflicted with one of these debilitating diseases. It is estimated that 14 million Americans will have dementia of the Alzheimer's type by the middle of the next century unless a cure is found.[1] Dementia is often the reason for institutionalization; the prevalence in nursing home residents is estimated to be between 60% and 80%.[2] It has long been a common belief that memory loss is an inevitable and incurable part of the aging process, making any clinical evaluation useless. However, with the recent advances in research, as evidenced by numerous clinical trials and new drug therapies, early detection, treatment, education, and support for families are critical.

The fourth edition of the *Diagnostic and Statistical Manual of Mental Disorders* (DSM-IV) defines dementia as the development of multiple cognitive deficits (including memory impairment) as a result of the direct physiologic effects of a general medical condition, the persisting effects of a substance, or multiple etiologies (e.g., the combined effects of cerebrovascular disease and Alzheimer's disease) (Boxes 210-1 to 210-3).[3] The two most common types of dementia, Alzheimer's disease and vascular dementia, account for about 80% to 90% of all dementias in older adults.[4] Other less common dementias include Lewy body, Pick's disease, Jakob-Creutzfeldt disease, and HIV dementia. Patients may also have dementia from more than one etiology; for example, Alzheimer's and vascular dementia can occur at the same time.

PATHOPHYSIOLOGY

Alzheimer's disease is characterized by amyloid plaques and neurofibrillary tangles. The number of senile plaques per microscopic field correlates with the degree of cognitive loss. Examinations of the brains of patients with Alzheimer's disease show atrophy of the cerebral cortex that is usually diffuse but may be more pronounced in the frontal, temporal, and parietal lobes.[5] The degree of atrophy does not correlate with the degree of cognitive impairment. Biochemically, there is a reduction in choline acetyltransferase, an enzyme found only in cholinergic neurons. Advances in genetic research have included the identification of ApoE, a protein involved in cholesterol transport linked to Alzheimer's disease and the identification of the beta amyloid gene on chromosome 21. Researchers continue to explore the role of inflammation and oxidative stress and their effects on neuronal health. Clinical trials are under way investigating the effects of estrogen, vitamin E, and nonsteroidal agents on the development of Alzheimer's disease.

BOX 210-1

DIAGNOSTIC CRITERIA FOR DEMENTIA OF THE ALZHEIMER'S TYPE

A. The development of multiple cognitive deficits manifested by both
   (1) memory impairment (impaired ability to learn new information or to recall previously learned information)
   (2) one (or more) of the following cognitive disturbances:
      (a) aphasia (language disturbance)
      (b) apraxia (impaired ability to carry out motor activities despite intact motor function)
      (c) agnosia (failure to recognize or identify objects despite intact sensory function)
      (d) disturbance in executive functioning (i.e., planning, organizing, sequencing, abstracting)
B. The cognitive deficits in Criteria A1 and A2 each cause significant impairment in social or occupational functioning and represent a significant decline from a previous level of functioning.
C. The course is characterized by gradual onset and continuing cognitive decline.
D. The cognitive deficits in Criteria A1 and A2 are not due to any of the following:
   (1) other central nervous system conditions that cause progressive deficits in memory and cognition (e.g., cerebrovascular disease, Parkinson's disease, Huntington's disease, subdural hematoma, normal-pressure hydrocephalus, brain tumor)
   (2) systemic conditions that are known to cause dementia (e.g., hypothyroidism, vitamin B_{12} or folic acid deficiency, niacin deficiency, hypercalcemia, neurosyphilis, HIV infection)
   (3) substance-induced conditions
E. The deficits do not occur exclusively during the course of a delirium.
F. The disturbance is not better accounted for by another Axis I disorder (e.g., Major Depressive Disorder, Schizophrenia).

From American Psychiatric Association: *Diagnostic and statistical manual of mental disorders*, ed 4 (Text revision 2000), Washington, DC, 1994, The Association.

Multiple areas of focal ischemic change characterize vascular dementia, formerly known as multiinfarct dementia. The defining lesion is the lacunar infarct. Lacunae are defined as gaps, missing areas, or holes.[6] The infarctions occur in tiny arteries deep in the brain. Patients with hypertension, diabetes, hyperlipidemia, or peripheral vascular occlusive disease are at particular risk.[2]

CLINICAL PRESENTATION

Memory loss, personality changes, language disturbances, and problems with independent activities of daily living are common presenting symptoms of dementia. A concerned family member or friend typically makes the initial presentation to a primary care provider. It may take months to years for family members to seek medical attention, as subtle changes in cognition may be overlooked or attributed to old age. Patients with dementia do not typically worry about what is wrong with them. These patients often have little understanding of the seriousness of their symptoms or of safety concerns (e.g., driving, cooking). On the other hand, patients with depression or benign forgetfulness often present to the primary care provider overly concerned about minor symptoms (e.g., forgetting a name, misplacing keys). It is an anecdotal finding in primary care that those patients worried about memory problems often have only minor problems, whereas the patients who seem unconcerned pose a major worry to providers.

Alzheimer's disease is commonly divided into three stages: early, middle, and late (Box 210-4). The initial symptom is typically short-term memory loss. The earliest stage is often accompanied by symptoms of anxiety and depression. Word finding and naming problems may emerge as symptoms progress. The second stage is characterized by a worsening of memory and language as well as judgment. Disorientation to time and place is common. There may be neuropsychiatric symptoms including paranoia, hallucinations, and delusional thinking. Urinary incontinence may be a problem. The final stage is characterized by motor rigidity, prominent neurologic abnormalities including apraxia and agnosia, severe cognitive and language impairment, and death. The average duration of the disease from diagnosis until death is 9 years.[5] Staging a patient's disease based on clinical presentation and examination can be helpful to patients and families in planning subsequent care and treatment.

BOX 210-2

DIAGNOSTIC CRITERIA FOR VASCULAR DEMENTIA

A. The development of multiple cognitive deficits manifested by both
   (1) memory impairment (impaired ability to learn new information or to recall previously learned information)
   (2) one (or more) of the following cognitive disturbances:
      (a) aphasia (language disturbance)
      (b) apraxia (impaired ability to carry out motor activities despite intact motor function)
      (c) agnosia (failure to recognize or identify objects despite intact sensory function)
      (d) disturbance in executive functioning (i.e., planning, organizing, sequencing, abstracting)
B. The cognitive deficits in Criteria A1 and A2 each cause significant impairment in social or occupational functioning and represent a significant decline from a previous level of functioning.
C. Focal neurologic signs and symptoms (e.g., exaggeration of deep tendon reflexes, extensor plantar response, pseudobulbar palsy, gait abnormalities, weakness of an extremity) or laboratory evidence indicative of cerebrovascular disease (e.g., multiple infarctions involving cortex and underlying white matter) that are judged to be etiologically related to the disturbance.
D. The deficits do not occur exclusively during the course of a delirium.

From American Psychiatric Association: *Diagnostic and Statistical Manual of Mental Disorders*, ed 4 (Text revision 2000), Washington, DC, 1994, The Association.

PHYSICAL EXAMINATION

The basic components of an evaluation for dementia include a complete physical examination (with a focus on neurologic findings, blood pressure, carotid bruits, and evidence of strokes),

BOX 210-3

DIAGNOSTIC CRITERIA FOR DEMENTIA DUE TO MULTIPLE ETIOLOGIES

A. The development of multiple cognitive deficits manifested by both
   (1) memory impairment (impaired ability to learn new information or to recall previously learned information)
   (2) one (or more) of the following cognitive disturbances:
      (a) aphasia (language disturbance)
      (b) apraxia (impaired ability to carry out motor activities despite intact motor function)
      (c) agnosia (failure to recognize or identify objects despite intact sensory function)
      (d) disturbance in executive functioning (i.e., planning, organizing, sequencing, abstracting)

B. The cognitive deficits in Criteria A1 and A2 each cause significant impairment in social or occupational functioning and represent a significant decline from a previous level of functioning.

C. There is evidence from the history, physical examination, or laboratory findings that the disturbance has more than one etiology (e.g., head trauma plus chronic alcohol use, Dementia of the Alzheimer's Type with the subsequent development of Vascular Dementia).

D. The deficits do not occur exclusively during the course of a delirium.

From American Psychiatric Association: *Diagnostic and Statistical Manual of Mental Disorders*, ed 4 (Text revision 2000), Washington, DC, 1994, The Association.

BOX 210-4

STAGES OF ALZHEIMER'S DISEASE

EARLY-STAGE DEMENTIA
Memory loss
Time and spatial disorientation
Poor judgment
Personality changes
Withdrawal or depression
Perceptual disturbances

MIDSTAGE DEMENTIA
Recent and remote memory worsens
Increased aphasia (slowed speech and understanding)
Apraxia
Hyperorality
Disorientation to place and time
Restlessness or pacing
Perseveration
Irritability
Loss of impulse control

LATE-STAGE DEMENTIA
Incontinence of urine and feces
Loss of motor skills, rigidity
Decreased appetite and dysphagia
Agnosia
Apraxia
Severely impaired communication
Possible inability to recognize family members or self in mirror
Loss of most or all self-care abilities
Severely impaired cognition
Depressed immune system

metabolic evaluation, functional status assessment, mood assessment, and mental status assessment. Many screening tools are available. The Katz Index of Activities of Daily Living, the Folstein Mini-Mental State Examination, and the Geriatric Depression Scale (short form) are helpful tools that have been used for many years and have been shown to be both valid and reliable in clinical practice.[7-9] One of the benefits of these tools is the ability to compare scores year to year to provide families with an objective description of disease progression.

DIAGNOSTICS

Because there is no single standard test for dementia and because Alzheimer's disease is a disease of exclusion, the diagnostic evaluation should determine if the patient has a reversible condition that may be contributing to or causing cognitive decline. The most important tests include thyroid-stimulating hormone, B_{12}, folate, rapid plasma reagent, and an electrolyte screen. Medications that have measurable levels, such as digoxin, carbamazepine (Tegretol), theophylline, or valproic acid (Depakote), should be measured. Alcohol or any over-the-counter medications (sleeping medications, anticholinergic cold remedies, and laxatives) should also be addressed.

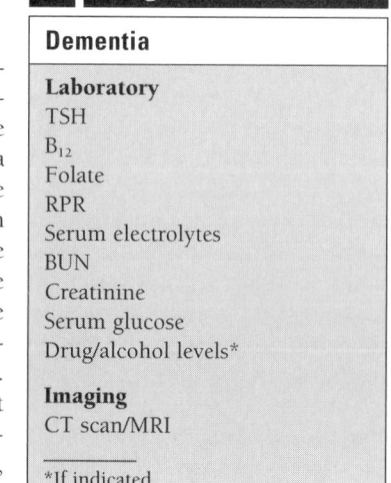

Diagnostics

Dementia

Laboratory
TSH
B_{12}
Folate
RPR
Serum electrolytes
BUN
Creatinine
Serum glucose
Drug/alcohol levels*

Imaging
CT scan/MRI

*If indicated.

Imaging studies are useful in identifying mass lesions, vascular lesions, or infections but do not confirm a diagnosis of Alzheimer's disease. Although there is lack of agreement as to the role of imaging in the workup of dementia, most geriatric specialists recommend a baseline brain imaging study (a CT scan is adequate). Neuropsychologic testing can also be useful in evaluating cognition.

DIFFERENTIAL DIAGNOSIS

Dementia has innumerable causes. The etiology of many dementias cannot yet be determined by diagnostic evaluation. Some dementia syndromes are characterized by a lack of neurologic signs (Pick's disease, Alzheimer's disease), whereas others are associated with a definitive neurologic disease such as Huntington's disease, diffuse Lewy body disease, or HIV. Delirium and depression are treatable conditions that may present with the same symptoms as dementia; however, errors on the Mini-Mental State Examination will differ. Patients with dementia have a normal level of consciousness without inattention. Patients with depression often answer questions with an "I don't know," whereas those with dementia may confabulate an answer.

Medical illnesses, drug overdoses, adverse effects of medication (especially anticholinergics or anxiolytics), sensory impairments, and nutritional deficits are all part of the differential diagnosis.

Differential Diagnosis

Dementia	
Alcoholic dementia	Depression
Medication, organic toxin, heavy metal intoxication	Vasculitis
Medical illness	Alzheimer's dementia
Liver disease	Vascular dementia
Hypothyroidism	Pick's disease
Chronic hypoglycemia	Diffuse lewy body dementia
Hypothyroidism	Huntington's disease
Adrenal insufficiency	Jakob-Creutzfeldt disease
Cushing's disease	Shy-Drager syndrome
Vitamin deficiency	Progressive supranuclear palsy
Thiamine	Parkinson's disease and other movement disorders
B_{12}	
Folic acid deficiency	
Neoplasm	
Trauma, subdural hematoma, hydrocephalus	

MANAGEMENT

Management of dementia depends on the stage of the disease. The family and community supports required are often the same for vascular dementia and Alzheimer's disease. It is important to address safety concerns, including driving competency, soon after the diagnosis is made. Laws regarding mandatory reporting of unsafe drivers vary from state to state and can be confirmed by calling the state department of motor vehicles. A kitchen safety evaluation alerts caregivers to possible problems with cooking. A health care proxy and durable power of attorney for health care can help to prevent conflicts later in the course of the disease. Encouraging families to contact the local chapter of the Alzheimer's Disease and Related Disorders Association is an important step; through this association caregivers can gain support, obtain reading material to promote understanding of the disease and behavior management, and determine the availability of respite care. There are now many web sites and online support groups that can help family members access and share information.

Because management may differ, determining which form of dementia is present is important. In addition, behavior management needs to be individualized. Certain behavioral problems are amenable to medication or to family education regarding the avoidance and management of difficult situations. Trials are under way for additional drugs that may slow progression of the disease.

Four cholinesterase inhibitor drugs are currently approved by the U.S. Food and Drug Administration. They are recommended for mild to moderate Alzheimer's disease and may be less effective as the disease process advances and fewer cholinergic neurons remain intact. These drugs include tacrine (Cognex), donepezil (Aricept), rivastigmine (Exelon), and galantamine (Reminyl). There is no evidence that these medications alter the course of the disease. For patients with vascular dementia, treatment of risk factors (e.g., hypertension, hyperglycemia, smoking, diet) may help to delay further progression. Patients with vascular dementia are often given aspirin 81 to 325 mg/day along with vitamin E 400 to 800 IU/day as prophylaxis.

COMPLICATIONS

Dementia has many complications that vary with the stages of illness. In the early stages, getting lost or having a motor vehicle accident puts patients (and others) at risk. In the middle stage, falls, incontinence, and sleep disturbances may cause further problems. Contractures, pressure ulcers, urinary tract infections, and pneumonia, all a result of immobility, are common in late and final stages of the disease. Reconditioning and nutritional deficits are also commonly seen. Patients may develop apraxia and forget how to chew and swallow. Weight loss becomes inevitable. An inability to communicate as a result of aphasia and an inability to tell caretakers about symptoms lead to further frustration and difficulty in diagnosing complications. Death is often the result of infectious complications.

Patients with end-stage dementia are eligible for referral to hospice under the Medicare Hospice benefit but must meet criteria related to bed-bound status and stage of disease. These hospice services can be provided in the home or in long-term care.

INDICATIONS FOR REFERRAL/HOSPITALIZATION

Many patients with dementia are frail, older adults with multiple medical, nursing, and social service needs. Involvement of other disciplines is helpful for patients, families, and providers. Physical therapy can optimize function by evaluating and recommending exercises or the appropriate adaptive equipment. Driving evaluations and kitchen and home safety evaluations can be performed by occupational therapists. These therapists can also recommend equipment to help with feeding. Speech therapy is necessary for swallowing or dysphagia assessments in the later stages of dementia. A neurology consultation is often helpful for patients with an unclear clinical picture. A neuropsychologist or geropsychiatrist may be able to differentiate unusual presentations of dementia, especially if depression is present.

PATIENT AND FAMILY EDUCATION

The focus of patient education is to maintain independence by emphasizing patients' strengths and allowing them to continue normal activities. A woman who is no longer able to follow a recipe may still be able to knead dough and make a loaf of her special bread with help. A grandmother unable to be left alone with her grandchild is still able to rock an infant to sleep and sing a lullaby she once heard as a child. A carpenter may no longer be able to operate electrical shop tools but may still be able to hammer and glue pieces of furniture that have been precut. Feeling robbed of self-esteem is a major detriment to function; education for families is essential. Behavioral guidance, social supports, and recognition of the difficult caregiver role will benefit both patient and caregiver and may prevent illness or injury.

Families need guidance and suggestions regarding the appropriate settings and activities for their loved ones. The decision about nursing home placement is always difficult and usually comes after community services and family support have been maximized. An acute illness or injury often precedes nursing home placement. Adult day care and group homes are appropriate in the early to early-middle stages of the disease; special care units are used during the middle stages of dementia. There is a wide variation in the philosophies, goals, and design of these units. Although many families are reluctant to enroll their relative in a program or living arrangement specifically for people with dementia, the focus of activities is at an appropriate level so that patients can participate and enjoy. The frustration of not being able to participate in activities that are too difficult is minimized. Staff members are specifically trained to handle behavioral problems in nonpharmacologic ways. Persons with late-stage dementia who are unable to participate in activities are often cared for on the general units of a nursing home.

Families also need to be able to recognize the symptoms of medical illness in a person with dementia; families should understand patients' increased susceptibility for delirium. Pneumonia without a fever or cough, a myocardial infarction without chest pain, and a urinary tract infection with no urinary symptoms are typical. A change in behavior that is noticeable only to those who know the patient well may be the only sign of illness. Families need to be given resource information about support groups, financial and legal matters, and how to tell family and friends about the diagnosis.

If caregivers are unfamiliar with resources, the Alzheimer's Disease Education and Referral Center (800-438-4380) provides information.[10] The Agency for Health Care Policy and Research has practice guidelines for practitioners and a patient and family guide for Alzheimer's disease and medical dementias.[10]

REFERENCES

1. Alzheimer's Association. Retrieved December 15, 2002, from the World Wide Web: www.alz.org
2. Beers M, Berkow R, editors: *The Merck manual of geriatrics,* ed 3, Whitehouse Station, NJ, 2000, Merck.
3. American Psychiatric Association: *Diagnostic and statistical manual of mental disorders,* ed 4, Washington, DC, 1994, American Psychiatric Association.
4. Plassman B, Breitner J: The genetics of dementia in late life, *Psychol Clin North Am* 20:59-75, 1997.
5. Kovach C: *Late-state dementia care: a basic guide,* Milwaukee, 1997, Taylor & Francis.
6. Venes D, Thomas C, editors: *Taber's cyclopedic medical dictionary,* ed 19, Philadelphia, 2001, FA Davis.
7. Katz S and others: Studies of illness in the aged: the index of ADL, *JAMA* 185:914-919, 1963.
8. Folstein M, Folstein S, McHugh P: Mini-mental state: a practical method for grading cognitive state of patients for the clinician, *J Psychiatr Res* 12:189-198, 1975.
9. Yesavage J and others: Development and validation of a geriatric depression screening scale: a preliminary report, *J Psychiatric Res* 17(1):37-49, 1982.
10. Costa P Jr and others: *Early identification of Alzheimer's diseases and related dementias. Clinical practice guideline: quick reference guide for clinicians,* AHCPR pub no 97-0703, Rockville, Md, Nov 1996, US Department of Health and Human Services, Public Health Service, Agency for Health Care Policy and Research.

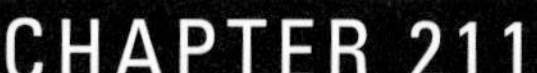

CHAPTER 211 Dizziness/Vertigo

Nancy McQueen Le

DEFINITION/EPIDEMIOLOGY

Dizziness is a common, nonspecific term used to describe a variety of subjective states with varied etiologies. Clinically it is helpful to classify dizziness into the categories of vertigo, disequilibrium, and presyncope or syncope. Differentiation of the type of dizziness experienced will dictate the direction of evaluation and treatment.

Vertigo is the illusion of movement of either one's self or the environment. This may be perceived as one's self or the environment spinning, tilting, or moving back and forth. Disequilibrium is a sense of insecurity or imbalance, an unsteadiness in walking. Although this feeling is often described as dizziness, it often occurs in the absence of abnormal head sensations.

Vertigo can be related to a peripheral or central etiology. Peripheral causes may include benign paroxysmal positional vertigo, vestibular neuronitis, acute labyrinthitis, Meniere's disease, ototoxicity, or head trauma. Central disorders include brainstem ischemia, tumors, multiple sclerosis, or a migrainous syndrome (see the Differential Diagnosis box).

A sense of wooziness or impending faint is often referred to as presyncopal light-headedness. However, light-headedness is not exclusive to a presyncopal episode and can be a feeling manifested in some states of disequilibrium or vertiginous conditions. Cardiac conditions associated with light-headedness or syncope include arrhythmias, sick sinus syndrome, mitral valve prolapse, aortic stenosis, and heart block. Dehydration, hypotension, and cough or Valsalva-related syncope are common causes of vascular-related syncope/presyncope.

It has been noted that less than half of patients complaining of dizziness actually have vertigo.[1] Hain[2] stated that even after evaluation, the largest diagnostic group is represented by dizziness of uncertain cause.

PATHOPHYSIOLOGY

Vertigo is caused by an imbalance in the vestibular system that may result from lesions in the inner ear, vestibular nerve, brainstem, or cerebellum. Less commonly, vertigo may result from lesions in the subjective sensory pathways of the thalamus or cortex, or stretch receptors in the neck.[1] Disequilibrium may result from visual impairment, bilateral or unilateral vestibular loss, proprioceptive loss, impaired cerebellar function, or involvement of motor (frontal/basal ganglia) centers. Multisensory disequilibrium describes a syndrome of impaired balance caused by some degree of combined dysfunction in the areas of vestibular, visual, and proprioceptive sensation.[3] Light-headedness or presyncope/syncope is most commonly a result of a cardiovascular problem. Etiologies include orthostatic hypotension, vasovagal episodes, hyperventilation, and decreased cardiac output. Less common causes of light-headedness include hypoglycemia and seizure activity. It is rarely a manifestation of impending stroke.

CLINICAL PRESENTATION

Dizziness is an intensely subjective sensation that may be difficult to describe. However, a thorough history will often differentiate the type of dizziness being experienced. It is helpful to start by eliciting a description of the dizziness in the patient's own words, making note of how precise or vague the details are. This description can be further guided through specific questioning and the suggestion of some varied descriptors, especially if the individual is having difficulty articulating his or her sensory experience. Further history is then directed toward defining the characteristics of the dizziness, the time course of individual episodes, the pattern of recurrences, precipitating and relieving factors, and any associated symptoms. A general medical history must be included, with special focus on neurologic and cardiovascular systems, medication history, and functional history.[1,3,4]

True vertigo is such a striking phenomenon that it is usually readily and precisely described as a clear sensation of spinning, tilting, rotating, or swaying. Associated symptoms can include nausea, vomiting, diaphoresis, disequilibrium, nystagmus, and/or blurry vision. Ear symptoms, including pain or pressure, tinnitus, or altered hearing, may be present. Disequilibrium is described as a sense of imbalance or insecurity on arising or when walking. Patients often say they are dizzy when they are not in fact vertiginous or presyncopal, but rather "off-kilter." They may have begun using a cane or "furniture walking" for unclear reasons. The sense of imbalance may be worse in the dark or may be accompanied by changes in gait characterized by a shortened step length and widened base of support.[3,4] Light-headedness is classically described as a sense of wooziness or impending faint. It is often accompanied by diaphoresis, apprehension, nausea, and, in the extreme, an actual transient "blackout" with diminished vision but with persisting vague awareness of one's surroundings.

When the description elicited is vague or ill defined, it may reflect multifactorial issues. A specific sensory experience in multisensory disequilibrium may be difficult to describe. Dizziness can also be related to psychogenic causes, such as anxiety states or agoraphobia. However, anxiety and apprehension often accompany dizziness and these complaints should not be automatically attributed to a psychogenic etiology.

PHYSICAL EXAMINATION

The physical examination in any complaint of dizziness should always include a general medical review. This information will guide a more focused examination.

The neurologic examination should include a cognitive screen. Cranial nerves are assessed with particular emphasis on visual acuity, eye movements, and nystagmus. Motor examination should include evaluation of power, muscle tone, coordination, and deep tendon reflexes. Sensory examination emphasizes basic vision and hearing assessments, as well as testing of primary sensory modalities. Gait and balance evaluation includes observation of stride, arm swing, tandem gait with eyes opened then closed, as well as Romberg's sign. A more detailed otologic evaluation includes pneumatic otoscopic examination and hearing assessment with Weber's test and the Rinne test.

Cardiovascular evaluation includes cardiac rate and rhythm, auscultation of heart sounds, carotid bruit, and blood pressure measurement. Orthostatic vital signs, both blood pressure and heart rate, should also be determined.

A neurootologic examination refers to a number of special examination procedures considered when problems related to vertigo and/or disequilibrium are suspected. These procedures specifically assess the vestibuloocular and vestibulospinal systems and help distinguish between peripheral disorders and central disorders. They include evaluation for nystagmus using Frenzel's glasses (special gogglelike glasses that remove visual fixation and magnify the eyes), position testing (Hallpike-Dix maneuver) (Box 211-1), head-fixed/body-turn maneuvers, postural sway on a foam surface, and the stepping test (marching in place with the eyes closed).[3]

DIAGNOSTICS

If a vestibular lesion is suspected, the history and examination may be augmented by vestibular laboratory testing, an audiogram, and/or neuroimaging. Vestibular laboratory testing can help differentiate peripheral from central lesions, confirm lateralization of a documented abnormality, and/or allow serial evaluation for monitoring purposes.[1,3] Laboratory studies include electronystagmography (ENG), rotational testing, and posturography.

ENG (sometimes referred to as electrooculography) is often helpful in measuring the vestibuloocular response when lesions of the vestibular system are suspected. ENG basically refers to the measurement of nystagmus via electrodes placed around the eyes. Recordings are taken under a variety of test conditions and routinely include various positions of gaze (an oculomotor test battery), caloric testing, and positional testing. Rotational testing is another means of assessing vestibular function or the vestibuloocular response. It relies on stimulation of the labyrinthine systems by having the individual sit in a computer-controlled chair that rotates in a darkened booth. Eye movements and nystagmus are recorded under a variety of rotational and gaze fixation conditions.

Posturography is a means of evaluating the vestibulospinal system through measurement of postural sway. This procedure involves the individual standing on a platform that can mechanically alter the source of proprioceptive and visual cues.

BOX 211-1

POSITIONAL NYSTAGMUS TESTING

1. The patient should first be checked for spontaneous nystagmus while seated on the examining table.
2. Next, the patient is brought quickly back to the recumbent or supine position with the head extended back 30 to 45 degrees over the end of the bed/table; and head tilted 30 to 45 degrees to one side (that is, one ear down toward the floor).
3. Repeat the above step two times, once with the head tilted to the left, then again with the head tilted to the right.
4. Observe the patient for latency, duration, direction, and fatigability or nystagmus both while positioned down and as helped to upright position.

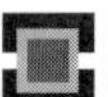

Diagnostics

Dizziness/Vertigo

Vestibular Disorders
Audiogram
CT scan or MRI/magnetic resonance angiography (with gadolinium)*
Vestibular laboratory testing*
  Electronystagmography
  Posturography

Cardiac Disorders
ECG
Holter or event monitor

Laboratory
Basic metabolic screen
  Electrolytes
  CBC and differential
  BUN/Creatinine
  Serum glucose
TSH
Vitamin B_{12}
Fluorescent treponemal antibody absorption test

*If indicated

Posturography can give valuable functional information regarding balance manifestations of lesions, whether vestibular or not, and help guide physical therapy interventions.[3,5]

Audiology evaluation, including Weber's test and the Rinne test, may have an important adjunctive role in helping establish or confirm a suspected diagnosis. Many disorders resulting in vertigo have associated hearing involvement. The presence or absence of specific hearing findings can help confirm or exclude some conditions. Most routine hearing evaluations involve a standard audiogram (a measurement of thresholds for pure-tone frequencies) and a word recognition test (the ability to repeat words presented at standardized thresholds).[1] Hearing loss is based on the etiology and defined as conductive or sensorineural.

Neuroimaging may be considered when central (brain) or structural (bony labyrinthine, internal auditory canal) lesions are amenable to visualization. Either a CT scan or MRI is appropriate, depending on what is suspected. Magnetic resonance angiography is used when vertebrobasilar insufficiency is a concern.

When multisystem disequilibrium is suspected or must be excluded, formal ophthalmology evaluation is necessary. Assessment of peripheral nerve function via EMG (electromyography) and NCV (nerve conduction velocity) in these instances can be definitive.

If cardiac issues are suspected, evaluation routinely begins with an ECG. Holter monitoring or telemetry may also be indicated if an arrhythmia is suspected. Serial orthostatic vital signs in conjunction with these studies can provide important data. An echocardiogram may be indicated to further evaluate cardiac status.

An electroencephalogram may be considered if seizure activity should be excluded. Vertigo, disequilibrium, and light-headedness are not common manifestations of seizures, and thus such testing is commonly under the guidance of a neurologist.

The choice of laboratory diagnostic studies should be guided by presentation and examination. A basic metabolic review usually includes thyroid-stimulating hormone, CBC, electrolytes, serum glucose, BUN, creatinine, vitamin B_{12}, and fluorescent treponemal antibody absorption as indicated.

DIFFERENTIAL DIAGNOSIS

Clarifying the diagnosis of dizziness begins with differentiating vertigo, disequilibrium, and light-headedness. Vertigo is a phenomenon resulting from a vast array of etiologies. Anatomically and neurologically it is helpful to start by determining whether the vertigo is caused by a peripheral or central lesion. Peripheral problems refer to problems of the inner ear or cranial nerve VIII. Peripheral lesions include vestibular neuronitis, labyrinthitis, benign positional vertigo, Meniere's disease, posttraumatic vertigo, acoustic neuroma, and ototoxic drug-induced conditions.[6] The general hallmarks of these conditions include a higher likelihood of associated nausea, a negative neurologic examination, and symptoms that are position related. Central or brain disorders usually involve the brainstem or cerebellum and include vertebrobasilar insufficiency or infarction, multiple sclerosis, posterior fossa tumor, basilar migraine, or central nervous system infection (syphilis).[6] Hallmarks of a central etiology include the presence of associated neurologic findings, and/or vertigo and nausea that are not position related.

Disequilibrium is sometimes clear from the history. In many cases the descriptions elicited are imprecise or vague yet seem to suggest balance problems rather than actual dizziness. When a description of a balance impairment in the absence of dizziness is clear, the focus turns to evaluation of multisystem impairment, in particular, vision and peripheral sensory function. Disequilibrium should be distinguished from complaints that may be based on visual complaints or related to psychogenic etiologies. Diabetes mellitus is a common etiology of a multisystem disequilibrium state. However, a number of other conditions should be considered, including cerebellar disorders, extrapyramidal system disorders, drug toxicity, and posterior fossa tumors.[6]

Light-headedness is most commonly related to cardiovascular issues. Diagnostic evaluation should exclude cardiac arrhythmia, critical aortic stenosis, vasovagal response, and orthostatic hypotension (autonomic insufficiency, volume depletion with anemia, drug-induced condition). When a psychogenic etiology is suspected, it must be considered only in the context of excluding atypical manifestations of other causes. Possible etiologies to be considered in the evaluation process include anxiety reactions, agoraphobia, hyperventilation, and depression.

MANAGEMENT

Many vestibular disorders are amenable to vestibular rehabilitation and other physical therapy interventions, with a generally limited or symptomatic role for pharmacologic agents. Some conditions respond particularly well to vestibular rehabilitation, and there are few patients who will not derive some benefit.[3] Treatments are aimed at facilitating vestibular compensation through a specific program of movements and exercises. The goal is to improve functional balance limitations, decrease dizziness, increase activity level, and improve general functional abilities.[3,5,7,8]

Medications used in treating vestibular disorders target vertigo and the associated nausea, vomiting, and anxiety.[2,7] Indications for use of these medications is dictated by the specific diagnosis. The commonly accepted vestibular suppressants are from the classes of anticholinergics (scopolamine), antihistamines

Differential Diagnosis

Dizziness/Vertigo

VESTIBULAR DISORDERS		SYNCOPE OR DISEQUILIBRIUM
Peripheral	**Central**	Cardiac arrhythmias
Benign paroxysmal positional vertigo	Vertebrobasilar insufficiency	Critical aortic stenosis
Vestibular neuronitis	Transitory ischemic attack/cerebrovascular accident	Medication effects
Bacterial labyrinthitis	Multiple sclerosis	Systemic illness
Meniere's disease	Tumor in posterior fossa	Infection
Nerve damage	Cerebellar pontine angle	Vasculitis
Ototoxic drugs	Brainstem	Endocrine (in diabetes)
Head trauma	Cerebellar	Volume depletion
Acoustic neuroma	Migraine syndrome	Valsalva
Perilymphatic fistula	Central nervous system infection	Hypotension
Physiologic	Cervical dizziness	Hypoxia
Motion sickness	Drop attacks	Severe anemia
Height vertigo		Hyperventilation
		Hypoglycemia
		Psychogenic (anxiety, depression)

(meclizine, dimenhydrinate [Dramamine], both with anticholinergic effects as well), and benzodiazepines (lorazepam [Ativan], clonazepam [Klonopin], diazepam [Valium]).[2,7]

Antiemetic medications used for the nausea associated with vestibular lesions are phenothiazines (promethazine [Phenergan], prochlorperazine [Compazine]) and antihistamines with anticholinergic properties (meclizine). Meclizine is often the drug of choice because of the vestibular suppressant and antiemetic effects, as well as the low side-effect profile.[2,7]

COMPLICATIONS

The risk of falling is greatly increased in the patient with dizziness. This is especially problematic in older patients, in whom the risk of fracture is the highest. Intractable nausea and/or vomiting associated with dizziness, although rare, can be disabling. Side effects with medications, especially anticholinergics or antihistamines, can include drowsiness, urinary retention, and confusion (especially in older patients). Benzodiazepines should be used cautiously because of the side-effect profile, as well as the potential for dependence. Other complications are related to the specific etiologies of the dizziness and may include visual disturbances, tinnitus, decreased hearing, and balance and gait disorders.

INDICATIONS FOR REFERRAL/HOSPITALIZATION

Identification of any positive neurologic signs or symptoms or the suspicion of an underlying cardiac disorder warrants prompt referral. Depending on the findings or what is suspected, immediate hospitalization or emergency department evaluation by a neurologist or cardiologist may be necessary. Acute labyrinthitis accompanied by a fever always requires urgent referral and treatment.[6] When a diagnosis remains uncertain or the response to standard treatments is suboptimal, further specialty evaluation should be pursued. If these cases involve vertigo or disequilibrium, referral to an otoneurologist or otolaryngologist is indicated for further testing, such as vestibular laboratory evaluation, or recommendations for alternate physical therapy or medication regimens. In most cases of vestibular dysfunction or disequilibrium, referral to physical therapy is recommended for a general functional evaluation or for vestibular rehabilitation. When a change is noted in a previously stable cardiac condition, prompt referral is indicated.

PATIENT AND FAMILY EDUCATION

Patient education should always include information about the diagnostic evaluation and, once a diagnosis is determined, specific information regarding the prognosis, treatment options, and complications. If an exercise program for vestibular compensation is initiated, patients should be told they may initially feel worse, but as they continue the program symptoms then subside. Specific aspects of their program should be reinforced. Other teaching emphasizes how medications can be used to relieve symptoms and the potential side effects of these agents.

The Vestibular Disorders Association is a national organization dedicated to providing information and support to people with dizziness and balance disorders. Patients can be encouraged to contact them at 503-229-7705 or online at www.vestibular.org.[8]

REFERENCES

1. Baloh RW, Honrubia V: *Clinical neurophysiology of the vestibular system*, ed 2, Philadelphia, 1990, FA Davis.
2. Hain TC: Treatment of vertigo, *Neurologist* 1(3):125-133, 1995.
3. Furman JM, Cass SP: *Balance disorders: a case study approach*, Philadelphia, 1996, FA Davis.
4. Burke M: Dizziness in the elderly, *Nurse Pract* 20(12):28-35, 1995.
5. Norre ME: Rehabilitation treatments for vertigo and related syndromes, *Crit Rev Phys Rehabil Med* 2(2):101-120, 1990.
6. Weiss HD: Dizziness. In Samuels M, editor: *Manual of neurologic therapeutics*, ed 5, Boston, 1991, Little, Brown.
7. Rascol O and others: Antivertigo medications and drug induced vertigo, *Drugs* 50(5):780-787, 1995.
8. The Vestibular Disorders Association. Retrieved September 7, 2001 and October 12, 2001 from the World Wide Web: www.vestibular.org.

CHAPTER 212

Guillain-Barré

Denise T. Bynum

DEFINITION/EPIDEMIOLOGY

Guillain-Barré (pronounced *ghee-yan bah-ray*) is an acute clinical syndrome caused by an autoimmune inflammatory destruction of the myelin sheath that covers the peripheral nerves. This destruction causes respiratory paralysis and varying degrees of rapid, progressive, and symmetric loss of motor function. Guillain-Barré syndrome (GBS) is also called polyradiculoneuritis, acute idiopathic polyneuritis, ascending paralysis, acute idiopathic polyneuritis, acute inflammatory demyelinating polyneuropathy, and acute inflammatory polyradiculopathy.

The incidence of GBS is 1 to 2 per 100,000 persons, without regard to gender, age, or race.[1,2] GBS can strike at any age but is at its highest rate in individuals 50 to 74 years old.[2] The incidence is increased in persons with Hodgkin's disease or systemic lupus erythematosus. The course is more benign in children. The mortality rate is 5%.[2] In all 20% of patients with GBS will have weakness after 1 year, 5% will have a permanent disability, and 3% may suffer a relapse of muscle weakness and tingling sensations after the initial episode.[2]

Immediate emergency department referral/ physician consultation is indicated for all patients with GBS and impending respiratory failure.

Physician consultation is indicated for all patients with suspected GBS.

PATHOPHYSIOLOGY

The cause of GBS is unclear, but it is thought to be an autoimmune disease. The macrophages and T-cells attack the myelin sheath of the peripheral and cranial nerves, causing a block in the conduction of nerve impulses. The central nervous system and sensory nerves are unaffected. GBS is occasionally triggered by surgery, pregnancy, or vaccinations. The disease may develop in hours, days, or over 3 to 4 weeks. GBS often occurs 1 to 4 weeks after a respiratory or gastrointestinal infection.[3] *Campylobacter jejuni*, an organism that causes diarrhea, is recognized as the most common organism to precede the syndrome. After this infection there may be a severe form of the disease, with increased risk of nerve deterioration, slow recovery, and longer disability. The 1976-1977 swine flu vaccines triggered an increased risk of GBS in some groups of recipients. The reason for this association has not been determined. During the 1992-1993 and the 1993-1994 flu seasons, an increased risk of approximately 1 in 1 million doses was noted when both seasons were combined. However, morbidity and mortality are greater because of influenza than because of the risk of GBS from the vaccine.[4] When GBS is preceded by a viral infection, it is postulated that the virus triggers the production of antibodies that damage the myelin sheath. This damage interferes with impulse conduction to muscle fibers.

CLINICAL PRESENTATION

It may be difficult to diagnose GBS in its earliest stages because the signs and symptoms can vary. The initial presentation of GBS is commonly weakness and/or numbness in the lower limbs that may ascend to the upper extremities; sensation impairment in a "glove and stocking" distribution; back pain; severe and persistent pain in the calves; double vision; difficulty swallowing, talking, and chewing because of the motor effects on cranial nerves; and urinary retention. Paresthesia occurs first, followed by an ascending muscle weakness and flaccid paralysis. If paralysis occurs from the head down (descending), it may occur quickly and respiratory distress occurs more often. Cognitive function and level of consciousness are not affected. Pain in the lower limbs is often the early symptom in children less than 6 years old.[5] The history should include a review of the symptom duration, medications, diet, and other medical illnesses, particularly any recent viral respiratory or gastric illness in the previous 1 to 4 weeks. The time frame from onset of symptoms to peak disability varies from hours to weeks. Most people reach the stage of greatest weakness within the first 2 weeks after symptoms appear and are at their weakest by the third week of the illness.[2] Symptoms then stabilize at this level for days, weeks or, sometimes, months. The recovery period may be a few weeks to 2 years; 80% to 90% completely recover in 1 year.[6]

PHYSICAL EXAMINATION

The first physical signs of GBS include varying degrees of progressive weakness and tingling in the legs, which eventually spread to the arms and upper body. Flaccid quadriplegia and bulbar paralysis that ascend from the extremities to the head may occur and is considered a medical emergency. Autonomic dysfunction including overreactivity or underreactivity of the sympathetic or parasympathetic nervous systems may occur, leading to disturbances of heart rate and rhythm, blood pressure, and other vasomotor disturbances. Other signs include inappropriate secretion of antidiuretic hormone, depressed or absent deep tendon reflexes, and paralysis of extraocular muscles causing ptosis. Symptoms can increase in intensity until the muscles cannot be used, leaving the patient almost totally paralyzed and unable to breathe without ventilatory assistance.

The physical examination should include vital signs, assessment of respiratory and urinary function, and a complete neurologic examination that includes the cranial nerves, deep tendon reflexes, and sensory and motor function. Sphincter disturbances are rare; therefore other diagnoses should be considered if these are present. The patellar reflexes are usually lost, with most patients being unable to walk at the peak of illness. Respiratory function can be impaired in many patients requiring mechanical ventilation.

DIAGNOSTICS

There are no specific tests to diagnose GBS; diagnosis is based mainly on the history and physical examination.[2] Diagnostic tests include CBC (there may be early leukocytosis with a shift to the

Diagnostics

Guillain-Barré
Initial
Peak flow meter
Pulse oximetry
Laboratory
CBC and differential
ESR
Serum electrolytes
BUN
Creatinine
Serum glucose
LFTs
TSH*
HIV*
Lyme titers*
Urinary porphyrin screen*
Stool for C-Diff*
ABGs*
Other
PFTs
Electromyogram
Nerve conduction velocity
Lumbar puncture

*If indicated.

left that resolves during the course of illness), erythrocyte sedimentation rate, biochemistry with electrolytes, and the following tests if differential diagnoses are suspected: thyroid-stimulating hormone, chest x-ray study, LFTs, serologic tests for HIV and Lyme disease, urinary porphyrin screen, and stool for *Clostridium difficile* toxin. Pulmonary function studies, especially of inspiratory force, should be monitored carefully and the patient placed on a ventilator at the first sign of deterioration. A referral is indicated for assessment of nerve conduction velocity (which shows marked slowing of the signals traveling along the nerve) and a spinal tap (which has a normal cell count with an increased protein concentration >400 mg/L).[2,3]

DIFFERENTIAL DIAGNOSIS

Because of the lack of objective signs, diagnosis of GBS is difficult in the early stages but is crucial to prevent death from respiratory paralysis. Patients are sometimes misdiagnosed with anxiety or hysteria. Differential diagnoses include spinal cord lesions, myasthenia gravis, poliomyelitis, acquired hypokalemia, periodic paralysis, polymyositis, botulism, acute intermittent porphyria, heavy metals, toxins, lymphoma, lung carcinoma, alcohol abuse, history of hexacarbon abuse, renal failure, hypothyroidism, AIDS, vasculitis, diphtheria, Lyme disease, diabetes, vitamin B_{12} deficiency, hereditary causes of polyneuropathy, or conditions secondary to drugs such as gold, disulfiram, phenytoin, or dapsone. Symptoms that have been noted for years suggest a hereditary cause, symptoms notes for weeks to months suggest a toxin or metabolic cause, and symptoms noted for days suggest a toxin or GBS.

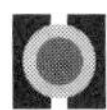

Differential Diagnosis

Guillain-Barré	
Spinal cord lesions	Polyneuropathy (hereditary, drug-induced)
Myasthenia gravis	Severe hypophosphatemia
Polio	Severe hypokalemia
Periodic paralysis	Diptheritic neuropathy
Polymyositis	Brickthorn berry intoxication
Botulism	History of hexacarbon abuse
Acute, intermittent porphyria	Lymphoma
Heavy metal poisoning	Lung cancer
Alcohol abuse	Hypothyroidism
Renal failure	Diabetes
B_{12} deficiency	
AIDS	
Vasculitis	
Lyme disease (or other tick-related paralysis)	

MANAGEMENT

There is no known cure for GBS. The goal of management is to expedite recovery, reduce disability, and prevent complications. If the clinical presentation suggests GBS, immediate hospitalization and available ventilator support are essential. Hospitalization includes IV fluids, cardiac monitoring, nutritional support, nursing care, prevention of complications, physical and occupational therapy, pain control, improved communication, relief of fear and anxiety, comfort measures, preventive skin care, and home care teaching.

Current treatment includes plasmapheresis and IV immunoglobulin therapy. Plasmapheresis reduces the severity and duration of the disease by producing a temporary reduction in circulating antibodies.[3] High-dose IV immunoglobulin therapy can lessen the immune system attack on the nerves and shorten the duration of disability. Immunoglobulin therapy is considered safer and more effective than corticosteroids.

Most patients recover from even the most severe cases of GBS, although some continue to have a certain degree of weakness. Some patients have a residual disability that requires long-term management and supervision at home. Psychologic counseling and support groups may be needed to help patients and their families adapt to the sudden paralysis and dependence on others.

COMPLICATIONS

Ventilator support plus continued monitoring for problems such as arrhythmias, infections, pneumonia, thrombus formation, autonomic dysfunction, bladder atony, gastrointestinal dysfunction, contractures, and pressure ulcers are necessary.

INDICATIONS FOR REFERRAL/HOSPITALIZATION

Because GBS is an acute inflammatory disease that can result in respiratory paralysis, it is essential that patients suspected of having this condition be evaluated by a physician. Lumbar puncture is necessary, and the majority of patients require hospitalization. A small number of patients with mild GBS can be managed as outpatients, but they require careful and frequent monitoring.

PATIENT AND FAMILY EDUCATION

At diagnosis, the patient and family should be informed of the expected course of the disease and treatment and referred to a support group. The Guillain-Barré Syndrome Foundation can be contacted at PO Box 262, Wynnewood, PA 19096, phone (610) 667-0131 or www.guillain-barre.com. The Foundation provides visits to patients by recovered persons, supplies literature, fosters research, develops local support groups, and holds an International Educational Symposia for the medical community and the general public.[7]

REFERENCES

1. Hingley A: *Campylobacter, FDA Consumer* 33(5):14-17, 1999.
2. Worsham TL: Easing the course of Guillain-Barre syndrome, *RN* 63(3):46-50, 2000.
3. Smelzer SC, Bare BG: *Brunner and Suddarth's textbook of medical-surgical nursing,* ed 9, Philadelphia, 2000, JB Lippincott.
4. Poland GA, Jacobson, RM: Vaccine safety: injecting a dose of common sense, *Mayo Clin Proc* 75(2):135-139, 2000.
5. Tang T, Noble-Jamieson C: A painful hip as a presentation of Guillain-Barre syndrome in children, *Br Med J* 322(7279):149-150, 2001.
6. Sulton LL: A multidisciplinary care approach to Guillain-Barre syndrome, *Dimens Crit Care Nurs* 20(1):16-22, 2001.
7. Guillain-Barre Syndrome Foundation International, Wynnewood, Penn. Retrieved December 16, 2002, from the World Wide Web: http://www.guillain-barre.com.

CHAPTER 213

Headache

Gretchen Van Buren

DEFINITION/EPIDEMIOLOGY

Headache is experienced by 90% to 95% of the population and is one of the 10 most common complaints in the outpatient setting.[1,2] Many people with headache are never diagnosed by a physician. Some individuals treat headaches at home, with over-the-counter (OTC) medications and home remedies such as ice packs and rest. Research has shown that even with the development of newer medications, up to 57% of patients with headaches use OTC medications, and many do not seek care for their headaches because they do not believe that satisfactory treatment is available.[3]

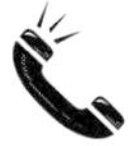

Physician consultation is indicated for patients with suspected temporal arteritis, change in mental status, nuchal rigidity, neurologic deficit, or new onset of headache.

It is essential to differentiate secondary from primary headaches because secondary headaches can be harbingers of a potentially more serious medical problem than the benign, primary headache usually seen in the office setting.[1] Secondary headaches are less common and are usually the result of an underlying disease or condition such as sinusitis, tumor, hemorrhage, temporal arteritis, or meningitis.[1,2] Once identified and treated, secondary headaches may dissipate.

Primary headaches are more common and are not symptomatic of another medical condition. These are distinct disorders that result from pathophysiologic mechanisms. Types of primary headaches include migraine with and without aura, chronic and episodic tension-type headaches, and chronic or episodic cluster headaches.[1,2]

In 1999 the estimated number of migraineurs in the United States was approximately 27 million, and the average annual indirect cost was between $5 and $17 billion.[1,4] These headaches may range in intensity from mild to severe but cause considerable distress. In general, migraine varies by age and sex, increasing in frequency to about age 40 years and declining thereafter in both men and women. Women experience migraine 3 times more often than men. Similarly, tension-type headache is seen more in women than in men, with a male-female ratio of 4:5.[5] Cluster headache, on the other hand, is more common in men than in women, with a ratio of about 7:1. Cluster attacks usually begin between the ages of 20 and 40.[6]

Clinical and research evidence has demonstrated a relationship between migraine and other disease processes, including epilepsy, major depression, and panic disorder. The neurotransmitter serotonin has been suggested as a basis for both migraine and major depression. Knowing that a co-occurrence exists helps in the treatment of each disease, as well as in providing clues to the pathophysiology of migraine.[7]

PATHOPHYSIOLOGY

There are some similarities between headache types. For migraine and tension-type headache, considerable debate has occurred over the existence of a headache continuum—there are similar features between migraine and tension-type headache. Often the headache is not a "pure" form of one or the other.[2]

The exact mechanism of a headache is still debated. Previously, headaches were thought to be caused by increased blood flow to the head, resulting in distended vessels and pressure on the nerve fibers of the brain.[1] This "vascular theory" was popular for many years until the 1930s, when Harold Wolfe identified that migraine, specifically, was due to both vascular and chemical changes within the brain.[1,8]

Many theories have since identified several neurochemicals as key elements in migraine development. Serotonin (5-hydroxytryptamine [5-HT]), a powerful vasoconstrictor, sensitizes the blood vessel walls to painful dilation. Other neurochemicals, such as dopamine and the catecholamines, may alter the excitability of the brain, as well as mediate the vasoconstriction or vasodilatation of blood vessels.[1] A polypeptide, substance P, may be responsible for propagation of pain impulses from the periphery to the central nervous system. When substance P is released, it interacts with blood vessel walls, resulting in dilation, plasma extravasation, inflammation, and pain.[8]

A similar theory postulates that central brain pathways, which may include the hypothalamus or the brainstem, are involved. Here certain chemicals are released that affect the vasodilatation, vasoconstriction, and pain associated with a migraine.[1]

In a review of the various theories, it is clear that during a headache changes occur in the vasculature of the brain, as well as in the neurochemicals found within the body. These changes are a result of a brain response to a stimuli, or "trigger." Vasodilatation and vasoconstriction subsequently cause the release of neurochemicals, which may be responsible for the headache as well as for the feelings of impending doom or fatigue that can occur before and after an attack.

CLINICAL PRESENTATION

The International Headache Society has developed criteria for various types of headache disorders. Using the criteria can be tedious and not applicable in many primary care settings, but the information may allow the practitioner to quickly differentiate the different types of primary headache conditions[9,10] (Boxes 213-1 to 213-4).

Migraine

There are two major types of migraine: migraine with aura and migraine without aura. Migraine without aura, also known as *common migraine,* is the more common of the two. In general, the patient will complain of an ipsilateral headache. The pain is described as pounding or throbbing, moderate to severe in intensity, and is aggravated by physical activity. This headache, which is episodic, will last from 4 to 72 hours and may be associated with nausea, vomiting, and photophobia/phonophobia. These patients usually retreat to a dark, quiet room until the attack is over. They often can identify a trigger that will precipitate the attacks. Triggers are an individual characteristic and may be difficult to identify because they may not always stimulate a headache. Common triggers include weather changes, foods, alcohol, altitude, delaying or skipping a meal, and hormonal changes.[1,11]

In migraine with aura, or *classic migraine,* the aura usually occurs before the onset of head pain, although sometimes it can extend into the period of headache. The classic aura, or "fortification spectrum," occurs in about 10% of patients and is described by patients as jagged lines similar to the stone fortifications found around a fort.[1,12] Visual auras can also be characterized by spots, shimmering bright lights, or areas of visual loss (scotomas). Somatosensory-type auras can also occur, with tingling or numbness of the fingers, motor disturbances such as hemiparesis or monoparesis, and cognitive disorders.[13] These visual and somatosensory disturbances usually last seconds but can last as long as 20 minutes.[1] The patient then will experience head pain and features similar to those of migraine without aura.

BOX 213-1

INTERNATIONAL HEADACHE SOCIETY CRITERIA FOR MIGRAINE WITHOUT AURA

A. At least five attacks fulfilling criteria B through D
B. Headaches lasting 4 to 72 hr (untreated or unsuccessfully treated)
C. Headache has at least two of the following characteristics:
   1. Unilateral location
   2. Pulsating quality
   3. Moderate or severe intensity (inhibits or prohibits daily activities)
   4. Aggravation by walking stairs or similar routine physical activity
D. During headache, at least one of the following symptoms:
   1. Nausea or vomiting, or both
   2. Photophobia and phonophobia
E. No evidence of related organic disease

Modified from Headache Classification Committee of the International Headache Society.

BOX 213-2

INTERNATIONAL HEADACHE SOCIETY CRITERIA FOR MIGRAINE WITH AURA

A. At least two attacks fulfilling criterion B
B. At least three of the following characteristics:
   1. One or more fully reversible aura symptoms indicating brain dysfunction
   2. At least one aura symptom develops gradually over >4 min, or two or more symptoms occur in succession
   3. No single aura symptom last >60 min
   4. Headache follows aura with a free interval of <60 min (may also begin before or simultaneously with the aura)
C. No evidence of a secondary cause

Modified from Headache Classification Committee of the International Headache Society.

BOX 213-3

INTERNATIONAL HEADACHE SOCIETY CRITERIA FOR EPISODIC TENSION-TYPE HEADACHE

A. At least 10 previous headache episodes fulfilling criteria B through D; number of days with such headache <180/yr (<15/mo)*
B. Headache lasting from 30 min to 7 days
C. At least two of the following pain characteristics:
  1. Pressing/tightening (nonpulsating) quality
  2. Mild or moderate intensity (may inhibit but does not prohibit activities)
  3. Bilateral location
  4. No aggravation by walking stairs or similar routine physical activity
D. Both of the following:
  1. Absence of nausea and vomiting (anorexia may occur)
  2. Absence of photophobia or phonophobia, or both

Modified from Headache Classification Committee of the International Headache Society.
*Chronic tension-type headache has similar criteria but occurs >15 days/mo (>180 days/yr) for >6 mo. Either condition may be associated with disorder of pericranial vessels.

BOX 213-4

INTERNATIONAL HEADACHE SOCIETY CRITERIA FOR CLUSTER HEADACHE

A. At least 5 attacks fulfilling criteria B through D
B. Severe unilateral orbital, supraorbital and/or temporal pain lasting 15 to 180 min untreated
C. Headache associated with at least one of the following signs on the side of the pain:
  1. Conjunctival injection
  2. Lacrimation
  3. Nasal congestion
  4. Rhinorrhea
  5. Forehead and facial sweating
  6. Miosis
  7. Ptosis
  8. Eyelid edema
D. Frequency of attacks: from one every other day to eight per day

Modified from Headache Classification Committee of the International Headache Society.

TABLE 213-1 Abortive Therapies for Headache

Medications	Route	Dosage	Considerations
NSAIDs			
Ibuprofen (Advil, Motrin, others)	PO	1200 mg × 1, repeat 600 mg × 2 p.r.n.	As with all NSAIDs, side effects include dyspepsia, heartburn, bleeding, and nausea or vomiting; contraindicated in patients with history of ulcer; will have better effect if taken on an empty stomach but might not be tolerated well by patient
Naproxen sodium (Anaprox DS)	PO	550 mg b.i.d. p.r.n.	
Indomethacin (Indocin)	PO or PR	25-50 mg t.i.d. p.r.n.	Indomethacin suppositories are very effective and can be used when patient complains of nausea; may need to be compounded by pharmacist
Ketorolac (Toradol)	IM	30-60 mg IM p.r.n.	Can be used as an alternative to one of the acute abortives or narcotics; should be used on a limited basis only—5-day course

Data from Solomon GD and others: Standards of care for treating headache in primary care practice, *Cleve Clin J Med 64*(7):373-383, 1996; and Schulman EA, Silberstein SD: Symptomatic and prophylactic treatment of migraine and tension-type headache, *Neurology* (2 suppl):S16-S21, 1992.
PR, Per rectum.

A prodrome can be part of a migraine.[13] Several days before the aura or start of the head pain, the person may have feelings of doom or fatigue. During this period, increased irritability, decreased energy, and food cravings are common complaints. Often this can be an early signal that a severe headache is coming and may enable the patient to use pharmacologic, as well as nonpharmacologic, modalities in the hope of aborting the attack (Table 213-1).

Tension-Type Headache

Acute tension-type headaches are described as feeling like there is a tight band around the head. Nausea and vomiting are not present, and the pain can be mild to moderate in intensity. This headache can last minutes to hours. It usually is not exacerbated by physical activity, but a common trigger is stress. Overall, the acute tension-type headache is a nagging headache that occurs fewer than 15 days per month, is present most of the day, and may start after the person wakes up. It rarely awakens the person. Chronic tension-type headache is similar in presentation to the acute type but occurs more often than 15 days per month.

Cluster Headache

The patient with cluster headache, acute or chronic, is usually awakened during the night with severe unilateral, retroorbital pain. A cluster headache will reach maximal intensity in about 15 minutes and usually lasts about 90 minutes, although some can last 3 hours.[6,14] These attacks can occur several times per

TABLE 213-1 Abortive Therapies for Headache—cont'd

Medications	Route	Dosage	Considerations
GLUCOCORTICOIDS			
Dexamethasone	PO	10-12 mg q day × 1-2 days	Should be limited to less than one treatment per month; hold NSAIDs while administering glucocorticoids; used when usual treatments have not aborted headache and it continues for several days
Prednisone	PO	Steroid taper over 7 days	
MUSCLE RELAXANTS			
Carisoprodol (Soma)	PO	350 mg ½-1 tablet PO up to q.i.d. p.r.n.	Encourage patient to start with lowest dose and increase as needed to take away tightness; this may often abort a migraine from beginning; used on headaches described as "tight" or "pressure"; used frequently with tension-type headaches; caution patient about sedation
Metaxalone (Skelaxin)	PO	400 mg 1-2 tablets t.i.d.-q.i.d. p.r.n.	
NARCOTIC ANALGESIC			
Butorphanol tartrate (Stadol)	Nasal	1 mg (1 spray in 1 nostril) followed by 1 mg in 60-90 min	Should be used only occasionally; may be diluted in half with equal part N/S to decrease side effects; can cause sedation and dysphoria; limit number of bottles per month; frequently used to abort cluster attacks
Meperidine (Demerol)	PO, IM	75-150 mg stat at headache onset; may repeat q 4-6 hr p.r.n.	Limited use only when other treatments are ineffective; overuse may contribute to rebound headaches; an antinauseant may also be needed
COMBINATION ANALGESICS			
Butalbital combination (Fioricet, Fiorinal)	PO	1-2 PO stat at headache onset; may repeat q 4 hr p.r.n.	Important to tell patient to take sufficient amount of these medications right at start of headache; adding metoclopramide to these may facilitate absorption; because of risk of rebound headache, limit to 2 days per week
ASA plus caffeine (Excedrin)	PO	1-2 PO stat at headache onset; may repeat q 4 hr p.r.n.	
OTHER			
Midrin	PO	2 caplets stat, then repeat 1 caplet q 1 hr	May cause sedation; maximum dose: 5 caplets/24 hr
Metoclopramide (Reglan, others)	PO	10 mg b.i.d. p.r.n.	May facilitate absorption of many abortives; watch for akathesia
Hydroxyzine	PO	25-mg caplets, 1-2 caplets t.i.d.-q.i.d. p.r.n. for nausea, mild pain, or sleeplessness	Very effective antinauseant; may potentiate some NSAIDs; can be used alone or in combination for mild pain
ACUTE ABORTIVES			
"Triptans"			
Sumatriptan (Imitrex)	PO	25-100 mg up to 200 mg/day p.r.n.	With all "triptans" separate all doses by at least 2 hours; common side effects are triptan sensations of flushing, tingling, chest tightness, and throat tightness that will subside after 10-20 minutes; contraindicated in presence of hypertension, coronary artery disease, myocardial infarction history, hepatic or renal dysfunction, or pregnancy; first dose of a triptan should be administered under medical supervision
	Nasal	20 mg for adults, 1 spray in 1 nostril b.i.d. p.r.n.	
	SC	6 mg SC b.i.d. p.r.n.	
Zolmitriptan (Zomig)	PO	2.5-5.0 mg b.i.d. p.r.n.; limited to three "attacks" per month; maximum dose: 10 mg/day	
Naratriptan (Amerge)	PO	2.5 mg b.i.d. p.r.n.; limited to four "attacks" per month	
Rizatriptan (Maxalt)	PO	5-10 mg; maximum dose: 30 mg/day	Available in fast-melt preparation—may be no faster than PO, but useful when nausea/vomiting present
Dihydroergotamine mesylate D.H.E. 45	SC	1 mg b.i.d. p.r.n.	Effective therapy that can last all day but can cause nausea and vomiting; should premedicate with antinauseant, such as promethazine, before administration; leg cramping is common and usually responds to dose reduction
Migranal 0.5 mg/spray	Nasal	1 spray in 1 nostril, wait 15 min, repeat q day p.r.n.	
	PR	2 mg custom suppository b.i.d. p.r.n.	
Ergotamine (Wigraine, Cafergot)	PO	1-2 tablets at headache onset; may repeat at 30-minute intervals; maximum dose: 6 mg/day	May be more effective if metoclopramide is added; can lead to ergotamine-dependency headaches; its use should be limited to 2 days per week
	PR	2-mg suppository cut into fourths; repeat one-fourth suppository q 30 min until headache abates; limit to 2 suppositories per attack	Causes severe nausea, and dose must be titrated to a subnauseating dose; premedication with an antinauseant is key to success; may not be tolerated by many patients because of severe nausea/vomiting

day. The pain is described as boring, and unlike migraineurs, these patients often cannot sit still. The severe intensity of cluster pain causes restlessness and often pacing. Patients may have thoughts of suicide.[15] Other features of cluster headache include ipsilateral injection of the conjunctiva, lacrimation, rhinorrhea, and a partial Horner's sign. For the patient with acute cluster headache, attacks will occur in groups or clusters lasting days to weeks and then subside until the next attack. There can be a period of years between attacks, and often the event will occur at the same time each year. The patient with chronic cluster headache will have the same presentation as the patient with the acute type but does not experience any remission longer than 14 days during a 12-month period. These headaches are also relatively resistant to therapy. Although it is well tolerated between attacks, alcohol often will precipitate an attack in both the patient with acute cluster headache and the patient with chronic cluster headache.[6,14,15]

PHYSICAL EXAMINATION

The history is the most important part of the evaluation. With most primary headache disorders, the diagnosis can be made on the basis of the history alone.[16] It is important that the patient characterize the headache by describing the duration, quality, and location of the pain. The presence or absence of any precipitating factors or triggers, as well as the age of onset, should be established. Associated symptoms such as nausea, vomiting, or photophobia should be explored. Can the patient be active during these headaches, or does the patient need to lie still in a dark room? How does the patient describe his or her sleep and energy? Sleep is usually labile in the person with headache, and energy may be poor. A medication profile is essential and should include medications that have been tried in the past for headache control. If OTC medications are taken, the number used per month should be identified because OTC medications are often not viewed as medications by patients. Migraine is known to be familial; therefore it is important to determine if any family member has had headaches, which might have been called "sinus headaches," "sick headaches," or headaches that were disabling. Asking about the presence or absence of any abuse is important because it has been shown that a history of abuse contributes to refractory headaches.

A targeted physical examination will confirm any information given in the history.[16] The examination in primary headache disorders is usually within normal limits. Key aspects of the physical examination should include the following:

- Funduscopic examination
- Mental status examination
- Palpation of the head, neck, and sinuses
- Evaluation of vital signs
- Palpation of the temporomandibular joint
- Examination of the cranial nerves
- Evaluation of motor and balance

Many patients with tension-type headaches and migraineurs will have tight cervical musculature. Painful biceps insertions, along with general aches and pains along the back, hips, and knees, may herald the beginning of fibromyalgia, a condition commonly seen in migraineurs. Pain and pressure on palpation of the sinuses accompanied by purulent nasal discharge may be indicative of sinusitis. The temporomandibular joints may click and pop when the mouth is opened and closed, but rarely is this the cause of a headache. Tension often is exhibited in the musculature surrounding this joint, and the subsequent bruxism may potentiate pain in this area.

Serious symptoms and findings include a headache accompanied by a stiff neck, fever, malaise, nausea or vomiting, and/or the presence of any aphasia, weakness, or poor coordination. Other danger signs include the following:

- Onset of headache after age 50
- Asymmetry of pupillary responses
- Decreased deep tendon reflexes
- Headache described as "the worst ever experienced"
- Personality change
- Onset of a new or different headache
- Onset of a headache that progressively worsens
- Presence of papilledema
- Palpable painful temporal arteries[1,16]

Further investigation and referral to a specialist or hospital would be warranted with any of these signs.

DIAGNOSTICS

The use of diagnostic studies depends on the results of the history and physical examination. Most diagnostic studies in the patient with primary headache will be unrevealing.[16] If the diagnosis is not clear or if the history or physical findings are cause for concern, diagnostic studies should be used to distinguish primary headache from a secondary condition.

Blood tests are generally not indicated, although exceptions include the use of a CBC to exclude anemia or an infectious process, erythrocyte sedimentation rate (ESR) to help exclude temporal arteritis, and thyroid function tests (TFTs) to determine thyroid dysfunction. Lyme titers or rheumatoid factors may also be indicated in some situations.

Practice guidelines recently been developed by the U.S. Headache Consortium advocate three principles for diagnostic testing: (1) testing should be avoided if it will not change the management of the patient, (2) testing is not indicated if the patient is not significantly more likely than the general public to have an abnormality, and (3) testing may make sense in a patient who is excessively concerned that he or she has a serious problem that is causing the headaches. Neuroimaging should be considered when any serious signs or symptoms are present during the physical examination but are not indicated if the patient has had these headaches for years, if there are no focal neurologic signs, and if the headache improves without the use of analgesics.

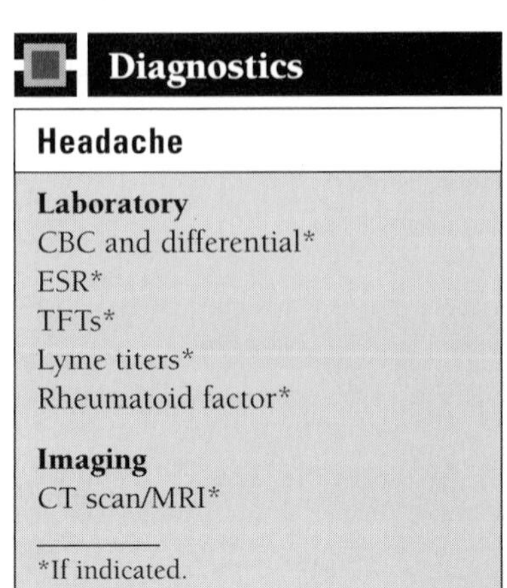

Diagnostics

Headache

Laboratory
CBC and differential*
ESR*
TFTs*
Lyme titers*
Rheumatoid factor*

Imaging
CT scan/MRI*

*If indicated.

DIFFERENTIAL DIAGNOSIS

The history and physical examination will aid in excluding potential diagnoses. The differential diagnosis includes fever, meningitis, pseudotumor cerebri, hemorrhage, rheumatologic disorders

Differential Diagnosis

Headache	
Primary Headache	Eye disorder
Migraine	Abscess
Cluster headache	Earache
Tension-type headache	
	Structural Causes
Infectious/Inflammatory Causes	Tumor
Fever	Hemorrhage
Meningitis	Aneurysm
Temporal arteritis	Subdural hematoma
Systemic lupus erythematosus	
Lyme disease	**Metabolic Causes**
Trigeminal neuralgia	Thyroid dysfunction
Rheumatoid arthritis	Pheochromocytoma
Systemic lupus erythematosus	Sleep apnea
Sinusitis	
	Other Causes
	Pseudotumor cerebri
	Posttrauma

(e.g., lupus erythematosus and rheumatoid arthritis), Lyme disease, temporal arteritis, trigeminal neuralgia, thyroid dysfunction, sleep apnea, tumor, aneurysm, and pheochromocytoma, among many others. Headache is a feature of many disease processes (see the Differential Diagnosis box).

MANAGEMENT

The U.S. Headache Consortium has developed evidence-based practice guidelines for migraine that cover both nonpharmacologic and pharmacologic modalities, with the goals of: reducing the frequency of attacks, improving the response to therapy, and restoring the patient to normal functioning. Control can be achieved after a proper diagnosis is made and proper treatment is prescribed. Currently no cure exists for primary headaches, although control is possible for most patients.[1,13,16-18]

Nonpharmacologic

Nonpharmacologic measures attempt to control the headache without medication. These methods include behavior modification, biofeedback, acupressure, and a wellness program. Behavior modification uses several methods, such as relaxation via tapes and stress management, as well as modification of daily activities. Biofeedback involves the use of instrumentation to bring under voluntary control physiologic processes of which the individual is not normally aware. For example, during a migraine attack, vasoconstriction of the periphery causes cold hands. Biofeedback training teaches migraineurs to raise hand temperature and thereby prevent an attack. The area between the thumb and the first finger (or other acupressure areas) can be depressed during a headache to offer some relief. It is thought that this pressure causes the release of endogenous endorphins and adrenocorticotropic hormones, which aborts the headache in some people.[1] A wellness program, consisting of balanced meals, regular exercise, and adequate sleep, can also be helpful in controlling headache bouts. Overall, nonpharmacologic approaches may help patients avoid triggers that might be initiating the headache.

Another important nonpharmacologic measure is having the patient keep a headache diary. The diary documents the number of headaches as well as triggers and treatment successes and failures.[18] This should be done daily by the patient because attempting to fill it in before a follow-up appointment may be less than accurate. It is important for the patient to bring the diary to office visits so information can be shared and the treatment plan can be adjusted if necessary.

Pharmacologic (Preventive)

Pharmacologic treatment can be divided into two areas: abortive and preventive. There are some clinicians who use a "stepped-care" approach when selecting treatment regimens. Here therapy would start with the least potent medication, advancing toward increased potency, and many times expense. A more sensible approach would be "stratified care," which matches the level of therapy to the intensity of the headache, regardless of potency or cost. If the attack is severe, early intervention with an appropriate therapy, such as a triptan, is in the patient's best interest.[3,9,17]

Preventive therapy is appropriate for patients if they experience more than four headaches a month, the attacks are prolonged and refractory to medicine, or the person is unable to psychologically deal with the attacks. Preventive therapy is given daily and, if successful, will decrease headache intensity and frequency. When choosing preventive treatment, the patient's history must be considered, including the presence or absence of any co-morbid conditions. For example, a connection has been shown between epilepsy and migraine; therefore anticonvulsants, such as valproic acid (Depakote) and gabapentin (Neurontin), can be used to control migraine. Diltiazem (Cardizem), a vasodilator and antihypertensive, may be selected if the patient complains of cold hands or is hypertensive. Propranolol (Inderal), which decreases the heart rate and regulates some arrhythmias, might be chosen for the patient with palpitations caused by mitral valve prolapse or panic disorders. If sleep is a problem or if chronic pain persists in the shoulders, a tricyclic antidepressant, such as amitriptyline (Elavil), may facilitate sleep and also decrease the sensation of pain.[13,19]

Both migraine and tension-type headache may result from an imbalance of neurochemicals. Adjusting these neurochemicals to a more "normal" level may decrease the number and frequency of headaches. The tricyclic antidepressants and the selective serotonin reuptake inhibitors (SSRIs), such as sertraline (Zoloft), modulate the levels of serotonin in the brain. Both the tricyclic antidepressants and the SSRIs have an extensive side effect profile. Weight gain and sexual dysfunction may not be acceptable to patients, although the starting dose for many of the medications can be very low. The SSRIs are better tolerated, but they might not be as effective for headaches as the tricyclic antidepressants.[13,19]

The mechanism of action for both beta-blockers and calcium channel blockers is not fully understood. Calcium channel blockers prevent calcium from entering the cells and therefore decrease their excitability. This may in turn prevent vascular spasm and headache. Beta-blockers affect the beta-1 receptors and inhibit the usual adrenergic responses.[19] Beyond these mechanisms, it has been theorized that they may have an effect on the serotonergic system within the brain, as well as the vascular system.

Methysergide (Sansert), a serotonin receptor antagonist, is one of the oldest and most effective agents in migraine prevention. However, serious side effects such as retroperitoneal, pulmonary, and cardiac fibrotic changes have caused it to be eliminated from first-line therapy.[19] It is often used when all other therapy has failed. It has also been found to be effective in controlling cluster attacks.

Pharmacologic (Abortive)

Abortive therapy is used to treat the intensity and duration of pain during an attack, as well as to manage associated symptoms such as nausea and vomiting. It is important to prescribe an adequate amount of medication initially. The appropriate medicine will depend on the prior response to treatment, the presence of nausea or vomiting, and the interval between headache onset and peak intensity. A patient with a severe migraine or cluster attack that peaks to full intensity within 15 minutes will most likely benefit only from parenteral therapy and not from oral medication.[13] For many patients, the pain of the headache is severe, but the associated nausea and vomiting are incapacitating. During a migraine attack, gastric emptying is slowed, causing gastric stasis. Medications that "turn the stomach back on," such as metoclopramide (Reglan), will augment the availability of the abortive therapy, enhance gastric motility, and decrease the nausea.[20]

Many of the abortive medications are powerful analgesics. When these medications, including acetaminophen, aspirin, and ibuprofen (Advil), are taken frequently, a condition called *analgesic rebound* can develop in a headache-prone individual.[20] The medications prescribed to abort a headache will essentially potentiate the headache and make it a daily condition.[1] Strict guidelines on the use of abortive medicine, as well as limitations on medication refills, need to be reviewed with the patient to prevent analgesic rebound.[1] Often refills will be limited to monthly only. Patients may be instructed to limit analgesic use to 2 days per week or less.

Simple analgesics, such as acetaminophen and aspirin, can represent first-line treatment in the management of mild to moderate headaches. Caffeine combinations (Excedrin, Anacin) can potentiate their absorption and analgesia. These medications are available without a prescription.

When simple analgesics are ineffective, combining them with a short-acting barbiturate, such as butalbital (Fioricet, Fiorinal, Esgic), may be effective. These medications should be used with caution because they can cause dependency, as well as rebound headaches if used more than 2 to 3 days per week.[1,20]

Nonsteroidal antiinflammatory drugs (NSAIDs) are helpful in treating an acute attack. Naproxen sodium (Anaprox DS, Aleve) has a longer half-life and a better safety profile than some of the other NSAIDs. Indomethacin (Indocin) is available in pill or suppository form, which is helpful for patients who experience some nausea or vomiting with their headache attacks.[13] The addition of metoclopramide to many of the NSAIDs when nausea is present will facilitate their absorption and potentiate their effect.[20]

Ergot derivatives are effective in the treatment of moderate to severe attacks that might not have responded to simple or combination analgesics. There are two forms presently in use: ergotamine tartrate (Cafergot, Wigraine) and dihydroergotamine. Ergotamine tartrate is available in both rectal and oral forms, but the rectal dose is 20 times more potent than the oral preparation.[1,13] Dosing regimens need to be reviewed with the patient and adjusted to obtain relief. Dihydroergotamine (D.H.E. 45) is available in both an injectable form and a nasal spray. The injectable form can be given via the subcutaneous or intramuscular route. The nasal form (Migranal) is easily administered and much more convenient. Because all forms of the ergots can cause nausea and vomiting, premedication with an antiemetic, such as promethazine (Phenergan) or prochlorperazine (Compazine), is necessary. Ergot derivatives may have a high potential for overuse and subsequent rebound headaches; patients need to be made aware of the risk for rebound headaches when this medication is prescribed. With the advent of the 5-HT receptor agonists, the triptans, the use of ergot derivatives is not necessarily first line, although they are very effective and less expensive.

Corticosteroids (Decadron, prednisone) are often used when the patient is unable to abort an attack and the attack continues for several days. They may be given as a one-time dose (Decadron 10 mg) or as a tapering dose (prednisone over 7 days). The side effects with the extended use of corticosteroids are serious and include aseptic necrosis of the hip and gastrointestinal bleeding; therefore frequent use is not recommended.[20]

Newer agents such as the triptans or transnasal butorphanol (TNB) (Stadol NS) have given many migraine and cluster patients relief within a short period of time. TNB is a powerful agonist-antagonist with a rapid analgesic effect.[20] Sedation is a common side effect, as is dysphoria. It should be used with caution and often is diluted before administration. Recent reports of addiction have caused TNB to be closely scrutinized; now TNB is a scheduled drug and should be prescribed with care and used with close supervision.[19,20]

The triptans target specific receptors, 5-HT, in the brain that are believed to generate headache. Relief can be almost complete, allowing a return to normal daily activities with few side effects. The triptans are arterial constrictors and should be used with great caution in the presence of known cardiac disease. There are several forms of "triptans" available: oral, transnasal, and injectable. There are slight differences between the brands of each medication; if one "triptan" is ineffective, another may prove to be effective for that patient.

Patients with cluster headache use many of the same medications and treatment regimens as do patients with migraine or tension-type headache. The cluster attack has such a rapid onset that preventing the attacks may be the key to successful treatment. Preventive therapy includes verapamil and lithium as first-line options. Verapamil is usually well tolerated and does not require the close monitoring required by lithium. Calcium channel blockers may prevent the vasospasm that occurs during a cluster attack by blocking the flow of calcium. Lithium, long used for bipolar disorder, also controls cluster headaches. Levels should be monitored, and patient education about the signs and symptoms of lithium toxicity is very important. Therapy should be slowly titrated upward. With both regimens, therapy is continued until the patient is free of any attacks for several weeks. Patients are then slowly weaned from medications. Because of the rapid onset of the cluster headache, abortive therapy needs to be in either a parenteral or a nasal form. Oxygen can be effective in as many as 75% of patients and should be delivered at a rate of 7 L/min via a nonrebreather face mask. The oxygen should be inhaled at the start of an attack. If this is effective, an oxygen tank should be readily available at all times. Both sumatriptan and butorphanol are effective treatment options for the patient with cluster headache, although overuse may be a concern in patients with chronic cluster headache.

The abortive management of tension-type headaches involves many of the same medications as used for migraine, and the same principles should be used when choosing treatments for these patients. For mild attacks NSAIDs may be helpful. Because there usually is no nausea, the use of antiemetics may not be necessary. Muscle relaxants such as metaxalone (Skelaxin) and carisoprodol (Soma), used cautiously, have been helpful with mild to moderate attacks. Triptan drugs may abort a severe tension attack as well. As with migraine, the use of these medications should be limited to 2 days a week or less to prevent rebound headaches. For many of these patients, stress may be triggering the attack, so nonpharmacologic measures are often helpful.[9]

LIFE SPAN CONSIDERATIONS

As patients age, headaches usually seem to decrease. It is uncommon for headaches to appear after the age of 50. When an older patient presents with a history of daily headache, analgesic rebound is often the cause; however, secondary processes need to be excluded.

During pregnancy the headache pattern can change. Many women will experience a decrease in headaches during the second and third trimesters, although some will see no change in the pattern. For the pregnant woman, headache control is usually limited to abortive medications only, and preventive therapy should be tapered immediately. Acetaminophen (Tylenol) and meperidine (Demerol), at dosages within normal parameters, can be safely used during pregnancy.

COMPLICATIONS

Misdiagnosis is the most serious complication. For this reason, all patients who complain of headache pain require a careful history and physical examination. Patients with positive physical findings require appropriate and timely referral. Other complications of headache include status migrainosus; dependency on narcotics, barbiturates, tranquilizers, or other agents; side effects of medication; inadequate treatment; and interruption of the activities of daily living.

INDICATIONS FOR REFERRAL/HOSPITALIZATION

Most patients with headache can be managed within the primary care setting. Indications for referral to a specialist, a headache clinic, or a neurologist include the following:

- The headache is not easily controlled by routine headache medicines, such as dihydroergotamine or sumatriptan.
- Rebound headaches or habituation limit outpatient therapy.
- Headache is new and progressively worsening.
- The patient describes it as the "worse headache of my life."
- Headache is affecting the patient's quality of life.
- Headache is accompanied by neurologic symptoms that last longer than 30 minutes or is accompanied by numbness or hemiparesis.[1,11,16]

Hospitalization of the patient with headache may be appropriate in some situations. Headaches that are resistant to treatment may be rebound headaches and require IV medication to help abort the headache. Referral to a headache specialist or neurologist for consultation may be advantageous. Consultation may be ongoing to provide frequent monitoring and adjustments. Treatment plans should include a step-by-step algorithm for patients to use when they are in the middle of an attack.

PATIENT AND FAMILY EDUCATION

Knowledge and education are important aspects of patient care. Education allows patients and their family to make choices and may enable them to regain control. During the initial examination and subsequent treatment, open communication and reassurance are necessary because many patients believe that they have a life-threatening condition. It is important they realize that their physical examination findings are normal and that the information received during the history indicates a primary headache disorder. Family members should be included in the treatment plan because headache affects both the patient and the family members.

Educational materials on headaches are widely available. Pharmaceutical companies and national groups such as the American Council for Headache Education and the National Headache Foundation have developed written information about headaches and their history, pathophysiology, treatment, and prevention. The brochures and videos are available to the public, either free of charge or at a nominal cost. Both national groups encourage headache patients and their families to join for support and information. Websites from both national groups are also available for information and support.

HEALTH PROMOTION

As reviewed in the section on management, the nonpharmacologic measures are an important part of headache treatment. This can include the modalities reviewed there but also encourages a "regular lifestyle" of going to bed at the same time, getting up at the same time, eating three meals a day, limiting alcohol and caffeine intake, and including exercise as part of one's daily routine. This wellness program may abort an attack or prevent triggers from initiating an attack. Being able to identify one's triggers through a daily diary can encourage the headache patient to modify behavior, eating habits, or lifestyle.

REFERENCES

1. Rapoport A, Sheftell F: *Headache disorders: a management guide for practitioners*, Philadelphia, 1996, WB Saunders.
2. Weiss J: Assessment and management of the client with headaches, *Nurse Pract* 18:44-57, 1993.
3. Matchar DB, McCrory DC, Gray RN: Toward evidence-based management of migraine, *JAMA* 284:2640-2641, 2000.
4. Mannix LK: Epidemiology and impact of primary headache disorders, *Med Clin North Am* 85:887-895, 2001.

5. Rasmussen BK and others: Epidemiology of headache in a general population: a prevalence study, *J Clin Epidemiol* 44):1147-1157, 1991.
6. Mathew NT: Cluster headache, *Semin Headache Manage* 1:1-12, 1996.
7. Merikangas KR: Comorbidity and migraine, *Semin Headache Manage* 1:1-2, 1996.
8. Silberstein SD: Advances in understanding the pathophysiology of headache, *Neurology* 42(suppl 2):S6-S10, 1992.
9. Ward TN: Providing relief from headache pain. Current options for acute and prophylactic therapy, *Postgrad Med* 108:121-128, 2000.
10. Headache Classification Committee of the International Headache Society: Classification & diagnostic criteria for headache disorders, cranial neuralgias, and facial pain, *Cephalalgia* 8(suppl 7):1-96, 1988.
11. Kumar KL, Mathew NT, Silberstein SD: Migraine: finding the road to relief, *Patient Care* pp 2-19, Sept 15, 1995.
12. Lance JW: Current concepts of migraine pathogenesis, *Neurology* 43(suppl 3):S11-S15, 1993.
13. Capobianco DJ, Cheshire WP, Campbell JK: An overview of the diagnosis and pharmacologic treatment of migraine, *Mayo Clin Proc* 71: 1055-1066, 1996.
14. Walling AD: Cluster headache, *Am Fam Physician* 47:1457-1463, 1993.
15. Cambell JK: Diagnosis and treatment of cluster headache, *J Pain Symptom Manage* 8:155-164, 1993.
16. Solomon GD and others: Standards of care for treating headache in primary care practice, *Cleve Clin J Med* 64:373-383, 1996.
17. Morey SS: Guidelines on migraine: part 2. General principles of drug therapy, *Am Fam Physician* 62:1915-1917, 2000.
18. Morey SS: Guidelines on migraine: part 4. General principles of preventive therapy, *Am Fam Physician* 62:2359-2360, 2000.
19. Baumel B: Migraine: a pharmacologic review with newer options and delivery modalities, *Neurology* 44:S13-S17, 1994.
20. Ward TN: Management of an acute primary headache, *Clin Neurosci* 5:50-54, 1998.

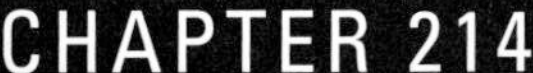

Infections of the Central Nervous System

Daniel W. O'Neill

DEFINITION/EPIDEMIOLOGY

Infections of the central nervous system (CNS) consist primarily of meningitis (inflammation of the meninges) and encephalitis (inflammation of the brain) and are caused by a variety of pathologic microorganisms. The high morbidity and mortality rates of bacterial meningitis make diagnosis and early treatment a high priority in the primary care setting. Bacterial meningitis is most common in children younger than 2 years, with a peak incidence at 3 to 8 months of age; however, it does occur throughout the life span, with a second peak incidence after 60 years of age. In the United States, the annual overall incidence rate is 3 per 100,000 persons. Despite the use of effective antimicrobial therapy, annual mortality rates remain at 5% to 20%, with up to 30% of survivors having some long-term neurologic sequelae.

Immediate emergency department referral/physician consultation is indicated for all suspected CNS infections because early treatment reduces morbidity and mortality.

PATHOPHYSIOLOGY

Encephalitis is caused primarily by enteroviruses (80% to 85% of cases) and arboviruses (transmitted via insects), with a peak incidence in the late summer months.[1] *Meningitis* is defined as either aseptic or septic, depending on the identification of bacteria on the Gram's stain or culture. Aseptic meningitis is caused mostly by enteroviruses, for which there is a good prognosis and no specific therapy. Bacterial meningitis is usually spread hematogenously from another primary source (predominantly the respiratory tract) or via contiguous spread from sinusitis, mastoiditis, or otitis media. The pathogens in meningitis are age specific. *Streptococcus pneumoniae* is the most common cause in adults. Because of the widespread overuse of oral antibiotics, there has been a dramatic rise in multidrug-resistant *S. pneumoniae:* nearly one third of isolates show penicillin resistance.[2,3] *Neisseria meningitidis* is common in adults, but *Haemophilus influenzae* has become rare since the advent of widespread immunization of infants. Older adults have a notably higher percentage of infections with gram-negative bacilli and *Listeria monocytogenes.*

Staphylococci and gram-negative bacilli are the most common causes of postoperative meningitis; staphylococci are common in patients with a cerebrospinal fluid (CSF) shunt. Risk factors for bacterial meningitis are male gender, malignancy/chemotherapy, previous basilar skull fracture or neurosurgery, sickle cell disease, complement deficiency, asplenia, alcoholism, Navajo or Eskimo descent, and exposure to a community outbreak.[4] Once the pathogen gains access to the CSF, where there is little natural host defense, there is replication and release of bacterial cell wall proteins, which stimulate cytokine release and capillary leak. This leads to the accumulation of protein and leukocytes, cerebral edema, and, ultimately, cerebral ischemia and hypoxia.

CLINICAL PRESENTATION

The onset of symptoms of CNS infection can be either acute or subacute, with progression over several days. The classic adult presentation of meningitis is fever, headache, and stiff neck (*meningismus*). Altered levels of consciousness, seizures, and hypotension predict a poor prognosis. Nausea, vomiting, and photophobia are common.[5] Older adult patients can present without fever or meningismus; they are commonly confused or even obtunded, often following an antecedent infection such as bronchitis, pneumonia, sinusitis, or urinary tract infection.[6] Encephalitis presents with signs and symptoms similar to those of meningitis but with more prevalent alterations in consciousness, focal neurologic signs, and seizures.[4]

PHYSICAL EXAMINATION

Nuchal rigidity with Kernig's and Brudzinski's signs is detectable in only 50% of cases and thus cannot be used to exclude meningitis. In older adults, nuchal rigidity has an even lower sensitivity and specificity. Kernig's sign is positive if a patient in the supine position resists passive knee extension when the hip is fully flexed on the abdomen. Brudzinski's sign is positive if a patient in the supine position actively flexes the hips when the neck is passively flexed. Purpura or petechiae are often associated with rapidly progressing meningococcemia but can be seen with other infections or can be a sign of disseminated intravascular coagulopathy. In 15% of patients, a careful neurologic examination may reveal focal deficits suggestive of brain abscess, cranial nerve inflammation, or cerebral edema. Papilledema is rarely seen; if present, it suggests venous sinus thrombosis, subdural effusion, or brain abscess.[4] Meningitis can lead to signs of increased intracranial pressure (ICP), which include depressed consciousness, sluggishly reactive or dilated pupils, ophthalmoplegia, respiratory depression, bradycardia, hypertension, posturing, hyperreflexia, and spasticity. With clinical presentation alone, it is difficult to distinguish aseptic meningitis from bacterial meningitis or encephalitis.

DIAGNOSTICS

Blood cultures (positive in 80% of patients with bacterial meningitis), CBC, and serum glucose should be obtained immediately. A lumbar puncture (LP) must be obtained in all patients with suspected meningitis or encephalitis, with the following contraindications: cardiorespiratory compromise, evidence of increased ICP, or cellulitis over the LP site. Thrombocytopenia is a relative contraindication. If there is evidence of increased ICP or focal neurologic deficits, then an immediate CT scan must be obtained before the LP. The first dose of antimicrobials should be administered before the CT scan to avoid critical delays in treatment. The CSF culture can still yield bacteria 1 to 2 hours after the first dose of antibiotics.

Diagnostics

Infections of the Central Nervous System

Laboratory
CBC and differential
Platelet count
Blood cultures
Serum glucose

Imaging
CT scan*

Other
Lumbar puncture (for CSF, protein glucose, cell count and differential, Gram's stain and culture; hold extra tubes for special studies)

*If indicated.

Opening CSF pressures should be measured, and a sample of the CSF should be sent for protein, glucose, Gram's stain, culture, and cell count with differential; extra tubes of CSF should be held for special studies, if indicated. Rapid testing of the CSF for antigens of several common pathogens is widely available but not routinely used except in cases of prior antibiotic therapy. Interpretation of CSF values is helpful in distinguishing viral from bacterial infections (Table 214-1), but it has some limitations.[7] Further testing of the CSF with viral cultures, polymerase chain reaction (PCR), specialized stains, and cultures may be indicated.

DIFFERENTIAL DIAGNOSIS

Other important viral causes of encephalitis include West Nile virus (epidemic in the United States since an outbreak in New York in 1999), herpes virus (herpes simplex virus [HSV]-1 and -2 and varicella zoster), mumps virus, lymphocytic choriomeningitis virus, and human immunodeficiency virus.[1] Nonviral causes of encephalitis and meningitis include tuberculosis (usually a more indolent course with CSF lymphocytosis and hypoglycemia), spirochetes (e.g., syphilis and Lyme disease), rickettsiae (e.g., Rocky Mountain spotted fever and typhus), protozoa (e.g., malaria), and fungal organisms, each with its own specific therapy. In patients with acquired immunodeficiency syndrome, unusual organisms such as *Toxoplasma*, *Cryptococcus*, *Histoplasma*, cytomegalovirus, *Nocardia*,

TABLE 214-1 Cerebrospinal Fluid Findings in Acute Meningitis

	Normal	Bacterial Meningitis	Viral Meningitis
Opening pressure	50-195 mm CSF	>180 mm CSF	NL or mildly increased
Cell count	<5 cells/mm^3	1000-10,000	10-1000
	(15% neutrophils)	(>80% neutrophils)	(<34% neutrophils)
Protein	15-50 mg/dl	100-500	50-100
Glucose	45-80 mg/dl	<40	NL or 20-40
CSF: Serum glucose	>0.5	<0.4	NL

NL, Normal limits.

Differential Diagnosis

Infections of the Central Nervous System

Infectious	**Noninfectious**
Herpesvirus	Carcinoma
Mumps virus	Vasculitis
Lymphocytic choriomeningitis virus	Multiple sclerosis
HIV	Intravenous immunoglobulin therapy
Tuberculosis	Drug reactions
Spirochetes	CNS hemorrhage
Rickettsiae	Postvaccination aseptic meningitis
Protozoa	
Fungal	**In Patients with AIDS**
Bacteria	Toxoplasma
West Nile virus	Cryptococcus
Lyme disease	Histoplasma
	Cytomegalovirus
	Nocardia
	Papovavirus

and papovavirus can infect the CNS. Noninfectious causes of encephalitis and meningitis are carcinoma, vasculitis, multiple sclerosis, IV immunoglobulin therapy, drug reactions (e.g., nonsteroidal antiinflammatory drugs [NSAIDs]), CNS hemorrhage, and postvaccination aseptic meningitis.[4]

MANAGEMENT

If bacterial meningitis is suspected, immediate empiric antimicrobial therapy is directed against presumptive pathogens on the basis of age and underlying health status. In most patients, a third-generation cephalosporin such as ceftriaxone (2 g every 12 hours) or cefotaxime (2 g every 6 hours) is recommended. This is supplemented with ampicillin (2 g every 4 hours) in adults older than 50 years and in those who are immunocompromised. Posttraumatic, neurosurgical, or CSF shunt patients should be started empirically on ceftazidime (2 g every 8 hours) plus vancomycin (1 to 2 g every 12 hours). If gram-positive diplococci are seen on Gram's stain or if a higher incidence of penicillin-resistant *S. pneumoniae* (>20%) is known to be present in the community, the addition of vancomycin (1 to 2 g every 12 hours) is currently recommended.[3] Other clinical factors and findings on Gram's stain and culture will direct the choice of specific antimicrobial therapy.[2,8] Adjunctive dexamethasone therapy is used in *H. influenzae* meningitis in children but is controversial for adults, unless critically ill.[8] If HSV encephalitis is suspected, IV acyclovir (10 mg/kg every 8 hours) should be initiated as well.

COMPLICATIONS

Complications of bacterial meningitis include dehydration, septic shock, hemodynamic compromise, cerebral edema, disseminated intravascular coagulopathy, myocarditis, hyponatremia, seizures, and death (still 20% in some series). Long-term sequelae are seen in 30% of survivors and consist of learning disability, hearing impairment, seizure disorder, visual and motor impairment, ataxia, hydrocephalus, or diabetes insipidus.[7] Permanent neurologic damage is seen in many cases of HSV-1, HSV-2, and Eastern equine encephalitis.

INDICATIONS FOR REFERRAL/HOSPITALIZATION

All cases of suspected meningitis or encephalitis should be immediately referred to a physician experienced in the treatment of CNS infections. All patients with suspected bacterial meningitis should be admitted to the hospital without delay for IV antimicrobial therapy, 24 hours of respiratory isolation, and close monitoring, possibly in an intensive care unit. IV fluids should be administered cautiously in the absence of hypovolemia to prevent increasing cerebral edema and hyponatremia. Consultation with specialists in infectious disease, critical care, neurology, or neurosurgery should be obtained if indicated. Neuropsychiatric testing, rehabilitation specialists, audiologists, psychiatrists, and other counselors may be needed in follow-up care.

PATIENT AND FAMILY EDUCATION

Prevention is a valuable strategy for reducing the morbidity and mortality of bacterial meningitis. The *H. influenzae* type b vaccine has proved to be very effective in lowering the attack rate in all ages; it should be strongly encouraged for infants. The 23-VALENT polysaccharide pneumococcal vaccine should be administered to eligible candidates, including all patients older than 65 years, patients who are immunocompromised, patients with chronic disease, patients without a spleen, or patients in long-term-care facilities.[6] The quadrivalent meningococcal vaccine is available for high-risk patients or travelers to endemic areas and is now recommended for adolescents entering college.[9] To control community outbreaks, chemoprophylaxis with rifampin (600 mg b.i.d. for 2 days) or ciprofloxacin (a single dose of 500 mg) is indicated for close contacts of patients with *N. meningitidis* or *H. influenzae*.

The broader implications for public health infrastructure are obvious. Effective surveillance, prevention, and control of vector-borne diseases, including West Nile virus and Eastern equine encephalitis, requires designated resources in local and state public health departments.[10] This includes public education regarding mosquito control and the prevention of mosquito and tick bites.

REFERENCES

1. Guitierrez KM, Prober CG: Encephalitis, *Postgrad Med* 103:123-143, 1998.
2. Philips EJ, Simor AE: Bacterial meningitis in children and adults, *Postgrad Med* 103:102-117, 1998.
3. Aronin SI, Quagliarelo VJ: New perspectives on pneumococcal meningitis, *Hosp Pract* 36:43-46, 49-51, 2001.
4. Tunkel AR, Scheld WM: Central nervous system infection. In Mandell GL, Bennett JE, Dolin R, editors: *Principles and practices of infectious diseases*, ed 4, Wiley Medical, 1995, New York.
5. Tunkel AR, Scheld WM: Issues in the management of bacterial meningitis, *Am Fam Physician* 56:1355-1362, 1997.
6. Miller LG, Choi C: Meningitis in older patients: how to diagnose and treat a deadly infection, *Geriatrics* 52:43-55, 1997.
7. Ashwall S: Neurologic evaluation of the patient with acute bacterial meningitis, *Neurol Clin* 13:549-573, 1995.
8. Quagliarelo VJ, Scheld WM: Treatment of bacterial meningitis, *N Engl J Med* 336:708-716, 1997.
9. Harrison LH: Preventing meningococcal infection in college students, *Clin Infect Dis* 30:648-651, 2000.
10. Guidelines for surveillance, prevention, and control of West Nile virus infection—United States, *MMWR Morb Mortal Wkly Rep* 49:25-28, 2000.

CHAPTER 215

Movement Disorders and Essential Tremor

Ann S. Bruner-Welch

Movement Disorders

DEFINITION/EPIDEMIOLOGY

There are a number of neurologic disorders that cause difficulty with movement leading to hypokinesis or hyperkinesis. Some manifest as uncontrolled, strikingly awkward muscle contractions of various parts of the body. Others present as an awkward, wide-stance gait, and still others involve exceedingly low muscle tone and inability to move various parts of the body.

These movement disorders are caused by dysfunction of the extrapyramidal system of the brain, which extends through the cerebellar and basal ganglia regions.[1,2] Movements may be physical only or may include other manifestations, such as dementia. The disorders are typically divided into categories based on one of the two affected brain regions. They may be inherited, infectious, a result of substance misuse or abuse, a result of trauma, or idiopathic.[1] They may be self-limited and resolve spontaneously, or chronic and progressive.

PATHOPHYSIOLOGY

The cerebellum is responsible for smooth, coordinated movement of the body. It influences both voluntary and involuntary motion.[1] Cerebellar dysfunction is broken down into three categories: vestibulocerebellar dysfunction (loss of flow from one movement to the next), cerebellar ataxia disorders (steadiness and gait), and cerebellar tremor (rhythmic oscillations with motion).[1] Extremity abnormalities are on the same side as the brain dysfunction. They occur whether the eyes are open or closed.[1] There is no tremor seen with the patient at rest.

The basal ganglia affects posture, muscle tone, and gracefulness. It acquires input from several parts of the body, including the cerebellum, the special sense organs, sensation, and the motor cortex. Dysfunctions of the basal ganglia affect the opposite side of the body and will be found at rest.[1] Symptoms diminish with voluntary movement.

CLINICAL PRESENTATION

The patient may complain of involuntary, awkward body movements. Symptoms can be minor to severe and include tremors, difficulty starting or stopping voluntary motion, and loss of facial muscle tone and expression. Symptoms will be worse in the presence of stress or fatigue.[1,2] Inquiry about alcohol or drug intake is necessary because alcohol can cause a severe ataxia and in other cases improve a tremor, whereas LSD can produce a parkinsonian picture. Some medications can cause tardive *dyskinesia,* a permanent change in cell receptor sites that causes slow and awkward movements. A careful medication and drug history is therefore very important and should include prescription, over-the-counter, and illicit drug use.

It is important to ascertain the age of onset, progression, what makes symptoms better or worse, the quality of movements and dysfunction, the region(s) of the body affected, the severity of disability, and timing. A family history of movement disorder should be noted.

PHYSICAL EXAMINATION

A complete neurologic examination, as well as examination of any other pertinent systems, is indicated. Subtle findings in involuntary movement may differentiate between some of the disorders. A good description of the movements, including the side of the body affected and whether the movements occur when the person is at rest or in motion, is crucial.[2-4] Depending on the disorder, deep tendon reflexes (DTRs), muscle tone, gait, and/or Romberg's sign or Babinski's reflex may be altered.[2] A Mini-Mental State Examination is also important to demonstrate any cognitive dysfunction and to monitor disease progression.[2]

Nystagmus is common with cerebellar disorders.[1] With ataxia, Romberg's test will be very difficult, if not impossible, to perform; the gait is often staggering and unsteady. Rapid, alternating movement testing reveals slow, purposeful, jerky, and uncoordinated movement. Performance of the finger-to-nose test may also jerky and overcorrected. Cerebellar (intention) tremor, like essential tremor, is a rhythmic oscillation of the finger or toe that increases as a target is approached.[1] It begins with intentional movement and is not found at rest. Cerebellar dysfunction can also affect speech, usually causing slurred, slow speech with varying amplitude, or there is a loss of the automatic movements of the body, such as the arm swing.[1,5]

With disorders of the basal ganglia, abnormal movement may be either hyperkinetic or bradykinetic, depending on which part of the basal ganglia is involved. These disorders include tremor, hemiballismus (jumping around of body parts), chorea (facial contortions and flexion/extension movements of the extremities), athetosis (twisting, wormlike movements of the face, arms, and legs, like a screwdriver), or difficult movement of the head, trunk, and extremities.[1,2] Oral motor tone can be affected, which can affect speech and ability to swallow.

DIAGNOSTICS

Diagnostic studies to consider include a head CT scan or MRI to exclude tumors or cerebellar defects. A positron emission tomography (PET) scan can help exclude parkinsonism and is being evaluated for use in the diagnosis of essential tremor.[5,6] A thyroid panel, including thyroid-stimulating hormone (TSH), is recommended to eliminate thyrotoxicosis or hyperthyroidism. An adrenal x-ray study or CT scan, or urine or blood catecholamine levels, can help exclude pheochromocytomas. This analysis should be done when the patient is symptomatic to avoid false-negative test results. Liver function tests

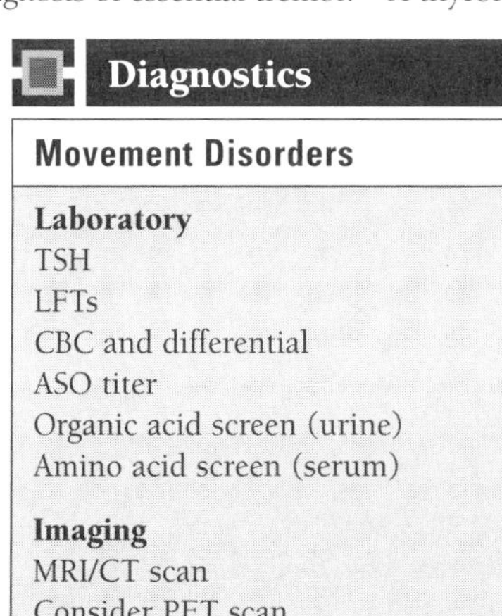

Diagnostics

Movement Disorders

Laboratory
TSH
LFTs
CBC and differential
ASO titer
Organic acid screen (urine)
Amino acid screen (serum)

Imaging
MRI/CT scan
Consider PET scan

(LFTs) will help eliminate hepatic causes for the tremor or ataxia. A CBC and antistreptolysin-O (ASO) titer can help identify infectious causes.[2,3] Serum amino acid levels and urine organic acid analysis can be used to further evaluate metabolic conditions.

DIFFERENTIAL DIAGNOSIS

The cause of movement disorders may be idiopathic or related to a number of degenerative, metabolic, or vascular disorders. Medications should always be reviewed and considered possible precipitants. Neoplasms, infection, anoxia, head trauma, brain surgery, colloid cysts, syringomyelia, and Munchausen's syndrome are also potential causes.

MANAGEMENT

Once the presence of a movement disorder has been determined, a thorough neurologic evaluation is indicated for diagnosis and treatment recommendations. Referral to a neurologist or neurosubspecialist may be indicated. In many cases treatment is directed at controlling or relieving the symptoms; there usually is no cure. For the remaining movement disorders, it is important to treat the underlying condition, such as infection, hormone imbalance, or drug withdrawal.

Disease progression and functional ability should be continually monitored.[3] Haloperidol (Haldol) and phenothiazines may be helpful for chorea and tic syndromes; clonazepam (Klonopin) may be used for myoclonus; and reserpine or haloperidol may be recommended for hemiballismus and tardive dyskinesia.[2,3]

LIFE SPAN CONSIDERATIONS

If the symptoms are severe, activities of daily living may be compromised, and a wheelchair may be necessary. Even with milder symptoms, patients may be self-conscious and experience increased anxiety, which accentuates the disorder.[2] Some patients may be able to learn compensatory strategies to alter or limit unwanted movement.[3] A physical therapist is a valuable resource for this purpose. Unfortunately, the ability to compensate may decrease as the disease progresses.[3] With some of these conditions, such as metabolic or organic acidemias, the life span can be significantly limited; some people die in childhood.

Differential Diagnosis

Movement Disorders

Degenerative Disorders
Parkinson's disease
Huntington's chorea
Supranuclear palsy
Hallervorden-Spatz disease
Olivopontocerebellar atrophies

Metabolic Disorders
Leigh's disease
Wilson's disease
Hormone deficiencies
Metabolic acidemias
Organic acidemias

Vascular Disorders
Cerebellar/basal ganglia
Bleed/infarction

Medications/Drugs
LSD-methyl-4-phenyl-1,2,3,6-tetrahydropyridine (MPTP)
Dopamine antagonists
Dopamine agonists
Tardive dyskinesia
CNS stimulants

Neoplasms
Cerebellar or basal ganglia

Other Conditions
Idiopathic infections
Anoxia
Head trauma
Syringomyelia
Munchausen's syndrome
Brain surgery
Colloid cyst

COMPLICATIONS

Some medications may cause undesired side effects. Impotence, exacerbations of asthma or emphysema, or problems with diabetic hypoglycemic control are potential concerns that should be addressed at each office visit.

The loss of facial expression is also possible.[2] Although this seems benign, facial immobility can affect nonverbal communication. Conscientious patient and family education can promote understanding of the disease process, and alternative ways of communication can be explored.

If the disease process is infectious, confinement is a consideration.

INDICATIONS FOR REFERRAL/HOSPITALIZATION

Consultation with a physician, often with a neurologist or subspecialist, is indicated for evaluation and management of the various movement disorders. Physical, occupational, and speech therapy, as well as psychiatric consultation, may be beneficial. Hospitalization is generally reserved for complications of disease rather than for the specific disease process itself.

PATIENT AND FAMILY EDUCATION

Understanding the diagnosis and prognosis is beneficial for patients and families. Facilitating the identification of resources to promote awareness of the disease process, as well as treatment options, is important. There are support and informational groups available on the Internet as well as good information in public and medical libraries.

The following are good resources for patients with movement disorders:

- Mitchel Brin, MD, Judith Balzer, MS: WEMOVE—Worldwide Education and Awareness for Movement Disorders, Mount Sinai Medical Center, 1 Gustave L. Levy Place, P.O. Box 1052, New York, NY 10029; (800) 437-MOV2 or (212) 241-8567; Fax: (212) 987-7363; website: http://www.mssm.edu/neurology/wemove/textonly.html.
- *Awakenings (Parkinson's disease):* website: http://www.parkinsonsdisease.com.
- Glaxo Neurological Center, Norton Street, Liverpool, England L3 8LR; (151) 298-2999; Fax: (151) 298-2333; website: http://www.glaxocentre.merseyside.org/. Supports people with neurologic disorders and their families.

HEALTH PROMOTION

Understanding the specific disease process can be the foundation to better health for these individuals and their families. Appropriate diet, exercise, social support, physical or occupational therapy as indicated, and assistive devices can significantly enhance quality of life.

Essential Tremor

DEFINITION/EPIDEMIOLOGY

Essential tremor is a benign, chronic neurologic condition that involves symmetric, rhythmic trembling of the upper extremities, head, and/or voice. The legs are less commonly involved.

The only clinical finding is the tremor, which may be present at rest and usually progresses over time.[4-6]

The oscillations of 4 to 12 Hz are present throughout voluntary movement and are accentuated as the hand approaches a given target.[2,5] Emotional stress will also increase the symptoms, whereas alcohol or rest will diminish them.[2,4] Known as *benign, familial, hereditary,* or *senile tremor,*[4] this is the most common of the movement disorders. Men and women are affected equally, with a mean age of onset of 45 years. The condition can begin as early as adolescence but most often begins in the sixth or seventh decade of life. An estimated 10 million people in the United States are afflicted with this condition. If more than one person in a family group has the condition, the tremor is termed *familial* or *hereditary tremor.* An autosomal dominant inheritance pattern can be identified in more than 50% of cases. If the tremor begins in old age, it is commonly termed *senile tremor.*[4-6]

PATHOPHYSIOLOGY

Although it is a neurologic disorder, little is known about the etiology of essential tremor.[4] To date, no structural defects have been identified on autopsy, and diagnostic studies are typically normal. It is believed to be caused by focal oscillatory activity within the central nervous system.[6] PET scan studies have found changes in regional blood flow in the cerebellum and inferior olivary nuclei of patients with essential tremor compared with matched control subjects.[6] It is unclear at this time if that finding is specific to essential tremor alone or is also found in other tremors. Because of the autosomal dominant inheritance, a thorough family history may prove helpful in establishing the diagnosis.[4-6] There is high variability in the rate of development of this disease.

CLINICAL PRESENTATION

For essential tremor, the patient's only complaint will be that of tremor; any additional neurologic deficits should be consideration for an alternative diagnosis.[5,6] The patient will typically complain of a tremor at rest. The tremor will become worse when the patient tries to move his or her hand and/or fingers in a purposeful manner. Furthermore, the amplitude of the tremor will increase as the patient approaches his or her desired target.[2]

The patient may have difficulty writing, eating, or performing other fine motor tasks. The head may nod ("yes" movements) or shake ("no" movements). Eyelid and facial tremor is also common.[3] The voice may quaver or shake. The tremor may be continual; however, it may also be episodic, sporadic, or intermittent.[4] Generally, the tremor will disappear during sleep. A careful history of food, coffee or caffeine, antihistamine, medication, or illicit drug intake, as well as other symptoms, will be helpful in excluding other causes for the tremor.[2]

Patients will complain that the tremor is worse during periods of increased emotional stress or when they are trying to hurry. The tremor will decrease with rest and alcohol[2]; for this reason, a careful inquiry about alcohol consumption should be elicited.

The patient will not have problems with weakness or changes in muscle tone, nor will there be problems with coordination despite the tremor. The tremor generally does not affect the lower extremities.[2]

The patient may have had the tremor for several years. It may be a disabling disease progression that has brought the patient to the primary care provider's attention. A careful history, including the age of onset, rate of progression and symmetry of the tremor, and exacerbating or alleviating factors, should be ascertained.

PHYSICAL EXAMINATION

An upper extremity tremor that cycles 6 to 10 times per second is obvious. The amplitude of this tremor will increase with voluntary movement, particularly as the patient approaches a specific target.[2] The rate of cycles per second should remain unchanged. The fingertip-to-nose test is particularly helpful in eliciting this phenomenon.[3] There may be difficulty writing or grasping small objects. Examination should include having the patient draw a circle; this is a useful marker for disease progression, as well as for monitoring treatment efficacy. The drawing should be included in the medical record. The patient's voice may quiver, and the head may shake or nod rhythmically. The eyelids and facial muscles may also twitch. All findings should be documented and updated at subsequent visits.[2,4]

Muscle tone, gait, and posture should all be normal. The lower extremities should be tremor free. The arm swing with walking should be relatively normal. DTRs should also be normal; there should be no clonus.[2] Other findings suggest an alternative diagnosis.

DIAGNOSTICS

The diagnosis is generally based on the history and examination findings. Laboratory or diagnostic testing should be considered when findings other than an isolated, generally symmetric upper extremity tremor is noted.[2]

DIFFERENTIAL DIAGNOSIS

Tremors may originate in the central nervous system, arise from metabolic abnormalities, or be induced by medication or alcohol. Central nervous system tremors may be caused by Parkinson's disease, Huntington's chorea, or Sydenham's chorea (secondary to streptococcal infections), or they may be cerebellar in nature. Metabolic tremors may be related to a thyroid abnormality, pheochromocytoma, or liver disease.

MANAGEMENT

Good Evidence for Benefit

Initially, reassurance may be all that is necessary.[2] If the tremor becomes problematic for the patient, there are a number of medication regimens that can help. Finding the medicine that is most effective but has minimal side effects may require persistent trials and evaluations. There is risk for dependence with some of the commonly prescribed medications.

The most commonly prescribed medication for this condition is propranolol (Inderal) 80 mg h.s. Symptoms should be reevaluated after 1 to 2 weeks. A number of placebo-controlled studies evaluating a number of beta-blockers clearly demonstrate their efficacy with 40% to 50% of patients experiencing relief.[6,7]

Primidone, at 50 to 350 mg at bedtime, in double-blind, placebo-controlled studies appears to be effective in reducing or eliminating tremor, especially hand tremor.[6] The dose is titrated up from 25 mg/night and increased by 50 mg each week until the tremor is controlled. Like propranolol, primidone reduces the amplitude, but not the frequency, of the tremor.

Botulinum toxin (BTX-A) has been used to effectively treat limb, vocal, palatal, and other tremors in addition to head and hand tremors. One double-blind, placebo-controlled study

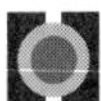

Differential Diagnosis

Essential Tremor

CNS Tremors	Medications/Drugs
Cerebellar tremor	Antihistamines
Sydenham's chorea secondary to streptococcal infections	Stimulants
Parkinsonism	Caffeine
Huntington's chorea	Alcohol withdrawal
Metabolic Tremors	Illicit drugs
Hyperthyroidism	Primary or metastatic neoplasm
Hypothyroidism	Cervical spine tumor
Pheochromocytoma	
Liver disease	

demonstrated that 75% of BTX-A–treated patients versus 27% of placebo patients reported mild to moderate benefit at 4 weeks after treatment.[6]

Other medications to consider include nadolol (Corgard) 40 mg/day, clonazepam (Klonopin) 0.5 mg t.i.d., gabapentin (Neurontin) 100 to 2400 mg/day, alprazolam (Xanax) 0.25 to 0.5 mg t.i.d., diazepam (Valium) 2 to 10 mg b.i.d. to t.i.d. increased gradually, topiramate (Topamax) 25 to 300 mg/day, nicardipine HCl (Cardene) 10 to 60 mg/day, nimodipine (Nimotop) 30 to 180 mg/day, or methazolamide (Neptazane) 50 to 100 mg b.i.d. to t.i.d.[3,6,7] These drugs have been used for many years, but limited information is available on their efficacy.

Alcohol is often listed as beneficial for tremor sufferers; however, few formal studies have been completed to demonstrate its efficacy.[4-6,8]

LIFE SPAN CONSIDERATIONS

Although essential tremor is considered a benign condition, it may have a profound effect on the patient's quality of life. The tremor may be embarrassing, particularly in younger patients. The condition may cause the patient to withdrawal socially to avoid the social implications and ramifications.[2,6,7] Careful observation for depression, alcoholism, and suicidal ideation in younger patients is very important. Antidepressants and counseling may be required to help the patient cope with the disorder.

Severe tremors can significantly interfere with activities of daily living. Basic fine motor activities can be impossible for some patients. Treatment is aimed at controlling the severity of the tremor to facilitate independence.[2,4-7]

COMPLICATIONS

Alcohol dependency is a potential complication. The patient should be advised to avoid overuse. The patient who consumes more than one glass of wine or other alcoholic preparation per day needs to be monitored closely.[3]

All of the medications used to treat the tremors have side effects, and drug-drug interactions are a concern if the patient is taking other medications. It is important to inquire about the tolerability of the medicine at all subsequent patient visits. Inquiry about sexual function and impotence is necessary because these are side effects that the patient generally will not discuss unless asked directly. Their effects on the patient's life, however, can be quite significant.

INDICATIONS FOR REFERRAL/HOSPITALIZATION

Consultation with a physician, possibly a neurologist, is warranted if the etiology is unclear. Speech therapy may be helpful if the voice tremor is severe. If conservative management fails to control severe tremors, surgical intervention is available.[4-8] Although there have been studies that evaluate the effectiveness, the patient numbers are small.[6]

Management questions or difficulty controlling the tremor with prescribed medication also warrants physician consultation.

PATIENT AND FAMILY EDUCATION

Careful education about the chronicity, progression, and prognosis of the disease is necessary. Although it is medically considered a benign condition, this disorder may have significant psychosocial implications, requiring frequent reevaluation and patient support. Patients also should understand that if the condition is hereditary, their children have a 50% chance of inheriting the same condition.[2,4]

The patient should also be advised to avoid stimulants such as caffeine, soda, or coffee. Many over-the-counter allergy and cold preparations have stimulants in them that can also accentuate the tremors.

Support groups such as the International Tremor Foundation (833 W. Washington Blvd., Chicago, IL 60607; [312] 733-1893) can be helpful..

HEALTH PROMOTION

Understanding of the disease process and support as necessary can help support the patient's health and quality of life. An appropriate diet and a good exercise program can also be beneficial. Alcohol abuse should always be a concern because consumption can limit the tremor.

REFERENCES

1. Porth C and others: *Pathophysiology: concepts of altered health states*, ed 4, Philadelphia, 1994, JB Lippincott.
2. Olson WH and others: *Symptom-oriented neurology: handbook for primary care*, ed 2, St Louis, 1994, Mosby.
3. Weiner W, Goetz C: *Neurology for the non-neurologist*, ed 3, Philadelphia, 1994, JB Lippincott.
4. Tierney L, McPhee S, Papadakis M: *Current medical diagnosis and treatment*, Norwalk, Conn, 1999, Lange Medical Publications.
5. Louis ED: Clinical practice. Essential tremor, *N Engl J Med* 345:887-891, 2001.
6. Koller WC, Deuschl G: Essential tremor, *Neurology* 54(11 suppl 4):S7, 2000.
7. Evidente VGH: Understanding essential tremor, differential diagnosis and options for treatment, *Postgrad Med* 108:138-140, 143-146, 149, 2000.
8. Rajput AH: Specificity of ethanol in essential tremor, *Ann Neurol* 40:950-951, 1996.

CHAPTER 216

Multiple Sclerosis

Nancy McQueen Le

DEFINITION/EPIDEMIOLOGY

Among the growing number of enigmatic diseases, multiple sclerosis (MS) is one of the most mysterious. The cause and cure are unknown. What *is* known is that the course of MS is predictably unpredictable and that no two people experience the disease in the same way. MS often targets individuals during their most productive years and can have a severe impact on the social, fiscal, physical, and emotional aspects of life.

MS affects up to 500,000 Americans and approximately 1.1 million persons worldwide.[1] After trauma, MS is the most common cause of disability in young adults. The onset of MS is likely to occur between 20 and 40 years of age, affecting 3 times as many females as males. Socioeconomically, MS is estimated to cost between $17,769 and $22,875 annually for each patient in the United States; for the 87,000 patients in the United Kingdom, the total is $1.2 billion per year.[2,3] In 1994, the total cost of patient care and lost wages in the United States was estimated to be $9.7 billion.[4]

The hallmark lesion in MS is called a *plaque* and was first described two centuries ago.[5] When viewed microscopically, these plaques are characterized by inflammation, destruction of myelin sheath, and eventual replacement by scar tissue. Larger plaques can be visualized with MRI. Lesions are described as demyelinating because of the loss of myelin; however, not all demyelinating lesions are caused by MS. Multiple lesions are seen in multiple locations in the central nervous system (CNS)—hence, the name *multiple sclerosis.* Table 216-1 describes the many manifestations of MS.

Clues to the etiology of MS come from the worldwide and nonrandom pattern of this disease, from the studies of structural and functional changes within the CNS, from neuroimmunologic studies, and from genetic studies, particularly studies of families and twins.[6-11] To date, no single etiologic factor has been identified.

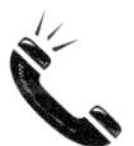

Physician consultation is indicated for all suspected cases of MS.

PATHOPHYSIOLOGY

It is theorized that MS is accompanied by, if not caused by, a disturbance in the function of the immune system. On the basis of animal models and immunopathologic studies of MS lesions, there is increasing evidence that MS results from an unknown trigger that stimulates a cell-mediated perivascular inflammatory response in genetically predisposed persons.

The sequence of these events has become better clarified. CNS-activated T lymphocytes, interacting with adhesion molecules, move into the CNS, where they presumably "see" their antigen and proliferate, and scavenger cells begin to eat away at the insulating covering on axons called *myelin.*[12] Members of the protein family called *cytokines* and *chemokines* are also recruited to the site and contribute to a series of cascading events that damage myelin-producing cells. In addition, B-lymphocyte clones produce plasma cells that secrete IgG to attack viral antigens. The antigens are myelin proteins, lipids, and molecular mimics. The response is an attack on an individual's own cells (autoimmunity). What occurs is either the result of a direct assault on myelin by an antigen or a hypersensitivity reaction that destroys myelin or the oligodendrocytes.[13]

TABLE 216-1 Manifestations of Multiple Sclerosis

	Description
Relapsing-remitting	Course punctuated with relapses (exacerbations) followed by periods of remission
Primary progressive	Accumulating disability from initial presentation onward
Secondary progressive	Accumulating disability after a period of relapsing-remitting disease
Progressive relapsing	Steadily progressive from onset, but also with acute attacks
Benign	Mild form; patient is fully functional in all neurologic systems
Malignant	Rapidly progressive course with severe disability and death
Transverse myelitis	Inflammation of spinal cord; may be single episode or harbinger of MS
Optic neuritis	Inflammation of optic nerve, often only symptom; may be first sign of MS
Devic's disease	Neuromyelitis optica transverse myelopathy and optic neuritis; considered unfinished form of MS

The oligodendrocytes (the cells that manufacture myelin) are generally not destroyed in the early stages of MS. Many oligodendrocytes appear to multiply after early attacks and even mend some of the damage, rewrapping nerve fibers with new myelin. However, they cannot keep up the replenishment for long in the presence of ongoing MS.[14] Eventually, scarred and demyelinated areas (plaque) develop.

CLINICAL PRESENTATION

Myelin acts as an insulator around axons, aiding the speed of nerve conduction while improving metabolic efficiency. Demyelination results in short circuiting, decreased conduction velocity, and even conduction block if damage is severe. The onset of symptoms of MS is often associated with a breakdown of the blood-brain barrier and a resultant loss of myelin. The venue and intensity of this process, along with its resolution and possible remyelination, determine the severity and duration of the clinical symptoms and recovery after an attack.[15] Demyelination in the cord may result in tingling, numbness, weakness, and strange sensations of tightness, banding, itching, and constriction. Imbalance or ataxia may result if the cerebellum is affected. Because MS plaques may occur in any location in the CNS, it is easy to understand why no two persons with MS have the same symptoms. Often, however, the initial presentation includes visual changes (particularly blurring or diplopia), extremity weakness, and a history of falls, or ataxia.

PHYSICAL EXAMINATION

The clinical evaluation is critical in evaluating disease status because at the present no simple laboratory or imaging technique has been validated to track the disease activity or progression of MS. The diagnosis is based on various criteria that reflect different levels of confidence. For example, a practitioner may determine that the patient has a working diagnosis of clinically definite MS, clinically probable MS, or laboratory study–supported probable MS or is at risk for MS.[16] Many patients can be diagnosed clinically on the first visit, but other situations are more difficult, especially when a patient has only transient symptoms. Diagnostic criteria include the following:

- At least two distinct episodes of neurologic significance lasting at least 24 hours and occurring at least 1 month apart
- More than one lesion at more than a single site in the CNS on neurologic examination
- Signs and symptoms that cannot be explained by another medical condition

DIAGNOSTICS

Neuroimaging may reveal demyelination and other changes that may be consistent with MS. The sensitivity of the test is very high, whereas the specificity is not. The MRI does not always correlate with the patient's clinical picture. Periods of increased MRI activity (enhanced by the use of the contrast agent gadolinium) may be associated with a deterioration of the patient's functional abilities. Less often, patients have significant clinical disease with little MRI activity. Clinically, patients who look the same (e.g., have similar disability measures) may have completely different histopathologic results and MRI activities. Through the use of serial MRI monitoring, it is now known that gadolinium enhancements may precede the clinical expression of disease activity and that the disease may be active biologically before it becomes clinically apparent.[17]

Evoked potential/evoked response (EP/ER) studies measure the electrical potential in the brain in response to stimulation of a sensory system. The time between application of the stimulus and measurement of the brain's response provides a measure of the ability of the nerves to conduct electrical impulses from one point to another. These tests are abnormal in the majority of patients with clinically definite MS. These tests also provide a measure of brain and cord *function* that complement the MRI, which provides information about brain *structure*.[18] In patients with only a single spinal cord or brain lesion, EPs may be very helpful in establishing a diagnosis of MS. Visual evoked potentials (VEPs) assess nerve conduction through the optic nerve. Brainstem auditory evoked potentials (BAEPs) and somatosensory evoked potentials (SSEPs) work similarly to assess the integrity of brain and cord pathways. VEPs are the most helpful in providing objective evidence of optic neuritis or an optic nerve lesion, even when the clinical examination is normal. VEPs tend to worsen over time.

Changes in cerebrospinal fluid (CSF) have long been used to support a clinical diagnosis of MS. A lumbar puncture may be performed if the MRI is not helpful but the clinical picture suggests MS. The most common abnormality is a selective increase in IgG. In MS, discrete bands called single oligoclonal bands may be seen with electrophoretic separation of CSF proteins. Patients must have two or more of these bands for diagnostic significance.

Further diagnostics should be guided by clinical presentation, physical examination, and consideration of the differential diagnosis.

Diagnostics

Multiple Sclerosis

Laboratory	Imaging
CSF IgG	MRI with gadolinium
Lyme titers*	
ESR*	**Other**
Antinuclear antibodies*	Evoked potential/evoked response studies
B_{12} levels	Lumbar puncture*
FTA-ABS*	

*If indicated.

DIFFERENTIAL DIAGNOSIS

Because many neurologic conditions must be considered, the differential diagnosis is extensive. CNS infections, syphilis, tumors, Lyme disease, vitamin B_{12} deficiency, and autoimmune processes such as systemic lupus erythematosus, sarcoidosis, or vasculitis should be included in the differential diagnosis.

MANAGEMENT

Co-Management with Specialists

Medical management of MS is accomplished through a true partnership with the patient, family members, and a core team of professionals, including the neurologist, primary care provider, occupational therapist, physical therapist, psychologist, and social worker. In general, the primary care provider is the primary patient advocate and coordinates the care plan, educates patients and families in all aspects of the treatment plan, initiates referrals to specialists, triages problems, identifies candidates for research

Differential Diagnosis

Multiple Sclerosis

Tumors
- Especially lymphoma or glioma of brain or spinal cord

Spinal cord compression
- Spondylosis
- Herniated disk
- Epidural tumor

Degenerative disorder
- Motor neuron disease (ALS)
- Spinocerebellar degeneration

Collagen vascular disease
- Systemic lupus erythematosus
- Polyarteritis

Neurosarcoidosis
Encephalitis
Neurosyphilis
HIV encephalopathy
Lyme disease
B_{12} deficiency
Vasculitis

protocols, monitors regular preventive services, and surveys the medication profile. The primary care provider may emphasize interventions that a patient can control rather than what is uncontrollable or unpredictable. Controllable interventions include proper exercise, rest, nutrition, stress reduction, skin care, and scrutinization of the various nonscientifically proven therapies that are available. Family issues should include parenting with disabilities, coping skills, caregiving issues, and relationship issues. Concerns about confidentiality, insurance, employment, and disability issues should also be considered.[19]

The National Multiple Sclerosis Society offers a vast array of resources for care providers, including current research, treatment and care guidelines, educational programs.[20]

Early management of multiple sclerosis begins with initiation of disease-modifying agents as indicated, and as soon as possible. Table 216-2 lists the four current immune-modulating drug therapies approved by the Food and Drug Administration (FDA) for the treatment of MS. Two are naturally occurring interferons (Betaseron and Avonex), and one is a synthetic protein (Copaxone). These three agents are approved for the treatment of relapsing-remitting MS. An antineoplastic agent (Novantrone) was approved in October 2000 for the treatment of secondary progressive and progressive relapsing MS. It is *not* approved for the treatment of primary relapsing-remitting disease. The interferons have a similar biologic activity and an adverse event profile and should not be taken during pregnancy, and patients should be monitored for depression while on treatment. The administration of Novantrone requires careful cardiac evaluation and monitoring. It also carries a lifetime accumulated dose limit due to the risk of cardiac toxicity. Of all of these agents, it carries the highest pregnancy risk warning.

Other agents that exert immunosuppressant effects include azathioprine (Imuran), methotrexate (Rheumatrex), cyclophosphamide (Cytoxan), and cladribine (Leustatin). All have been studied with varying degrees of reported efficacy.[21] In the past, corticotropin (ACTH) was used to decrease inflammation; currently, synthetic corticosteroids are more often used.[22] Their use is generally targeted for treatment of exacerbations. Short-term courses of steroids are usually well tolerated, although flushing, edema, gastrointestinal upset, insomnia, acne, euphoria, and agitation may be seen. Lithium carbonate (to modulate mood) and H_2-blockers (to prevent gastrointestinal irritation) may be given with steroids.[23]

Recent clinical trials with linomide (Roquinimex) and oral cow myelin (Myloral) in persons with secondary progressive MS have had disappointing results.[24] IV immunoglobulins (IVIGs) have shown promise in promoting spinal cord remyelination in patients with paresis from MS and visual loss from optic neuritis.[25] Other experimental therapies, including monoclonal antibodies, vaccines, bee venom therapy, plasmapheresis, and total lymphoid irradiation, have been inconclusive. Table 216-3 shows symptomatic and rehabilitative therapies that are the biggest challenge of the co-management partnership described above.

LIFE SPAN CONSIDERATIONS

In some situations, a diagnosis of MS is actually followed by relief, especially for patients who have spent years experiencing strange symptoms and have met with an indeterminable diagnosis. For others the diagnosis is difficult—the variable clinical course of MS leads to an uncertain and unpredictable future. Many persons with MS are still capable of ambulation and regular employment 20 years after diagnosis. The life span is

TABLE 216-2 Disease-Modifying Therapies for Multiple Sclerosis

	Betaseron (Interferon Beta-1b)	Avonex (Interferon Beta-1a)	Copaxone (Glatiramer Acetate)	Novantrone (Mitoxantrone)
Description	rDNA technology	rDNA technology	Synthetic mixture of four amino acids	Antineoplastic agent
Action	Antiviral/immunomodulatory	Antiviral/immunomodulatory	Immune system modifier	Immune system
Efficacy	Reduces exacerbation rate Tendency to slow disease progression	Reduces exacerbation rate Reduces rate of disability progression	Reduces exacerbation rate Trend in slowing disability progression	Reduce exacerbation rate Delay in disability progression Reduced number of treated relapses
MRI	Decrease lesion load	Changes in lesion load not statistically significant	Data unavailable	Reduced number of *new* lesions detected
Dosing	8 mIU SC q.o.d.	6 mIU IM weekly	20 mg SC daily	12 mg/m^2 IV q 3 mo Is a lifetime cumulative dose limit of 140 mg/m^2 due to cardiac toxicity
Adverse events	Flulike symptoms Injection site reaction Depression Laboratory abnormalities	Flulike symptoms Depression Laboratory abnormalities Asthenia	Immediate postinjection reaction Injection site reaction Chest pain Vasodilation	Myelosuppression Infection Sepsis Cardiac toxicity Heart failure Arrhythmias Renal failure Hyperuricemia Side effects: nausea, hair loss, menstrual disorders

TABLE 216-3 Symptomatic and Rehabilitative Therapies for Multiple Sclerosis*

Symptom	Description	Treatment Modalities
Spasticity	Very common Stiff, slow movements, spasms	PT and assistive devices Baclofen intrathecal pump implantation or, rarely, botulinum toxin (Botox) *Drug therapy:* baclofen (Lioresal), tizanidine (Zanaflex), or benzodiazepine
Fatigue	Very frequent Highly debilitating and depressing Often the reason for disability Cause unknown Aggravated by elevated temperature, reversed by cooling	OT for energy conservation techniques Cooling vest or cap Avoidance of heat *Drug therapy:* amantadine (Symmetrel), pemoline (Cylert), fluoxetine (Prozac), 4-amino-pyridine (Fampridine)
Pain	Fairly common symptom Various disagreeable sensations	Trigeminal neuralgia is common Pain from spasms relieved with antispasmodics *Drug therapy:* carbamazepine (Tegretol), phenytoin (Dilantin), gabapentin (Neurontin), or tricyclic antidepressants
Tremor	May involve hand, arm, head, eyes, or voice and be incapacitating Very difficult symptom to manage	OT can help with weighted equipment and environmental strategies *Drug therapy:* propranolol (Inderal), clonazepam (Klonopin), primidone (Mysoline), ondansetron (Zofran)
Weakness		No response to medication, but often compensated by use of adaptive equipment OT/PT evaluation for tailored exercise program
Ataxia	Incoordination and disturbance of balance and gait Worsened by spasticity, weakness, and fatigue Falls are common	Home evaluation necessary to assess safety risks
Paresthesias	Numbness, tingling, burning, coldness, revulsion when touched	No specific medications Controlled with tricyclic antidepressants
Loss of vision	Optic neuritis may be first presentation of MS Disc pallor on ophthalmoscopic examination	Generally treated with corticosteroids Regular eye examinations are a must
Dysarthria and dysphagia		Can be helped with evaluation and interventions of speech and language therapist
Paroxysms	Seizures/tonic spasms	Respond to anticonvulsants
Depression	Very common	Antidepressants plus counseling usually helpful Watch for adverse effect of medications
Bowel and bladder	Bladder fails to store or empty as evidenced by postvoid residual Bowel problem is usually constipation Fecal incontinence very distressful	Intermittent catheterization may help Medications with anticholinergic or muscle relaxant properties helpful, such as oxybutynin (Ditropan), propantheline (Pro-Banthine) Avoidance of urinary infections Surgery may be indicated for bladder or bowel when appropriate
Sexuality	Lack of interest or arousal Changes in self-esteem Problems with intimacy Impotence	
Cognition	Common complaint Memory (recall of recent events), abstract reasoning, problem solving, verbal fluency, and speed of information processing are most common deficits	Safety assessment

PT, Physical therapy; *OT,* occupational therapy.
*Note: Many medications used for MS worsen weakness and mobility.

shortened only slightly compared with that of the general population. Several factors are associated with a favorable prognosis: (1) female gender, (2) age of disease onset less than 40 years, (3) sensory symptoms without impairment in ambulation, (4) optic neuritis as an isolated first symptom, and (5) minor abnormalities of the brain MRI at the time of diagnosis.[19]

COMPLICATIONS AND INDICATIONS FOR REFERRAL/HOSPITALIZATION

The primary complications of MS are infections, usually of the urinary tract or lungs. Symptoms of infection may be underappreciated in patients with MS. Uncomplicated urinary tract infections (UTIs) may be treated in the customary fashion. Complicated UTIs require a referral for consultation and/or management. Decubiti and contractures are additional concerns and require constant monitoring.

Any infection can trigger an exacerbation of MS, which can necessitate hospitalization if functional loss is severe. Exacerbations can be discrete and easily diagnosed or more subtle and more complicated to assess. A thorough history and neurologic examination that compares current and baseline disability helps determine treatment.[26] Long-term steroid therapy contributes to bone demineralization. Bone densitometry is a useful monitor of a patient's risk for fractures or further disability. Alendronate (Fosamax) or other similar agents may be given for the prevention of osteoporosis, especially in postmenopausal women.

Many of the common symptoms of MS may become problematic enough to require specialty referrals, such as a Botox referral for spasticity, urology consult for refractory bladder problems or impotence issues, or psychiatric referral for depression.

PATIENT AND FAMILY EDUCATION

The diagnosis of MS can be devastating for patients and families. Considerable support and education about the disease process, its variability, and available therapies are essential. Careful explanation about the avoidance of precipitating triggers, including the need for rest, exercise, and a well-balanced diet, may prevent exacerbations. Community support groups may also be helpful. Research is continuous, and therefore ongoing education about new medications is particularly important. Exciting advances the understanding and treatment of MS have been made in the past decade, and the future is promising. Patients can be encouraged to contact the national Multiple Sclerosis Society ([800] FIGHTMS or http://www.nmss.org) for more information.

REFERENCES

1. Dean G: How many people in the world have multiple sclerosis? *Neuroepidemiology* 13:1-7, 1994.
2. Harvey C: *Economic costs of multiple sclerosis: how much and who pays?* New York, 1995, National Multiple Sclerosis Society.
3. Holmes J, Madgwick T, Bates D: The cost of multiple sclerosis, *Br J Med Econ* 8:181-193, 1995.
4. Andersson PB, Waubant E, Goodkin DE: How should we proceed with disease-modifying treatments for multiple sclerosis? *Lancet* 349: 586-587, 1997.
5. Holland N, Murray TJ, Reingold SC: *Multiple sclerosis: a guide for the newly diagnosed,* New York, 1996, Demos Vermande.
6. Trapp BD, Peterson J, Ransohoff RM: Axonal transection in the lesions of multiple sclerosis, *N Engl J Med* 338:278-285, 1998.
7. Correale J and others: Defective post-thymic tolerance mechanisms during the chronic progressive stage of multiple sclerosis, *Nat Med* 2:1354-1360, 1996.
8. Cook SD: *Multiple sclerosis and viruses.* Excerpts from the 4th annual meeting of America's Committee for Treatment and Research in Multiple Sclerosis, September 1997.
9. Sadovnick AD, Ebers GC: Epidemiology of multiple sclerosis: a critical overview, *Can J Neurol Sci* 20:17-29, 1993.
10. Riise T: Cluster studies in multiple sclerosis, *Neurology* 49(2 suppl 2): S27-S32, 1997.
11. Cook SD and others: Evidence for multiple sclerosis as an infectious disease, *Acta Neurol Scand Suppl* 161:34-42, 1995.
12. Lublin FD: *Excerpts from current topics in multiple sclerosis.* 49th Annual American Academy of Neurology meeting, April 1997.
13. Frozena C: Clinical snapshot: multiple sclerosis, *Am J Nurs* 97:48-49, 1997.
14. Understanding the enemy: Cedric Raine's multiple attack on multiple sclerosis, *Inside MS,* Summer 1996; 4-5.
15. Waxman SG: Demyelinating diseases: new pathological insights, new therapeutic targets (editorial), *N Engl J Med* 338:323-325, 1998.
16. Poser CM and others: New diagnostic criteria for multiple sclerosis, *Ann Neurol* 13:227-231, 1983.
17. McFarland HF and others: Using gadolinium-enhancing magnetic resonance imaging lesions to monitor activity in multiple sclerosis, *Ann Neurol* 32:758-766, 1992.
18. Bailey K and others: *Current contents in multiple sclerosis,* Monograph 4, 1996.
19. Goodkin DE, Neilley LK: *Multiple sclerosis handbook: a primer,* San Francisco, 1996, University of California Regents.
20. The National Multiple Sclerosis Society. Retrieved September 24, 2001, and October 17, 2001, from the World Wide Web: http://www.nmss.org.
21. Weinstock-Guttman B, Cohen JA: Emerging therapies for multiple sclerosis, *Neurologist* 2:342-355, 1996.
22. Goodin DS: The use of immunosuppressive agents in the treatment of multiple sclerosis: a critical review, *Neurology* 41:980-985, 1991.
23. Tselis AC: Multiple sclerosis: a pharmacotherapy update, *Formulary* 32:472-499, 1997.
24. Reingold SC: Disappointing results from five drug trials, Research Highlights, *NMSS,* Summer/Fall 1997.
25. van Engelen BGM and others: Promotion of remyelination by polyclonal immunoglobulin in Theiler's virus-induced demyelination and in multiple sclerosis, *J Neurol Neurosurg Psychiatry* 57:65-68, 1994.
26. Kurtzke JF: Rating neurologic impairment in multiple sclerosis, *Neurology* 33:1444-1452, 1983.

CHAPTER 217

Parkinson's Disease

Brenda L. Jordan

DEFINITION/EPIDEMIOLOGY

Parkinson's disease (PD) is a slowly progressing neurodegenerative disorder with an insidious onset of tremor, weakness and slowness of movement. PD is classified into four categories (see the Differential Diagnosis box). PD is the fourth most common neurodegenerative disease of patients; the age-adjusted prevalence is 1% of the population worldwide, rising from 0.6% at age 60 to 64 years to 3.5% at age 85 to 89 years. In 5% to 10% of those in whom PD develops, symptoms appear before age 40 years, with mean age of onset being 65 years. The incidence worldwide is equal in the two sexes.[1] The risk of developing PD appears to double if a first-degree relative had PD compared with people in the general population.[2,3] Although the cause of PD is unknown, research has concentrated on genetics, exogenous toxins, and endogenous toxins from cellular oxidative reactions. Those who develop PD may be affected by a combination of genetic and environmental factors, viruses, toxins, drugs containing 1-methyl-4-phenyl-1,2,3,6-tetrahydropyridine (MPTP), well water, vitamin E, and smoking.[4-6]

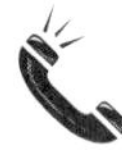

Physician consultation is recommended for patients with treatment failure or disease progression.

PATHOPHYSIOLOGY

PD develops after widespread destruction of pigmented neural cells in the zona compacta of the substantia nigra, causing the nigrostriatal tract to degenerate.[7] Consequently, the dopamine normally secreted in the caudate nucleus and putamen is no longer available. Loss of approximately 80% of the pigmented neurons in the substantia nigra, leading to a 70% to 80% depletion of striatal dopamine, is required for the appearance of clinical parkinsonism.[8] However, the large number of acetylcholine-secreting neurons that transmit excitatory signals remains active. The decreased dopaminergic activity in the striatum leads to an imbalance between dopamine and acetylcholine, and the loss of dopamine receptor sites affects the refinement of voluntary movement.[7] Thus the seven cardinal features of PD are produced: (1) tremor at rest, (2) rigidity, (3) bradykinesia, (4) hypokinesia, (5) flexed posture, (6) loss of postural reflexes, and (7) freezing phenomenon.

CLINICAL PRESENTATION

The clinical features of tremor, rigidity, and flexed posture are referred to as positive phenomena; bradykinesia, loss of postural reflexes, and freezing are negative phenomena. In general, the negative phenomena are the more disabling. Tremor at rest is recognized as the first symptom in 70% of patients with this disease.[7,8] Rest tremor, most common in the distal extremities, characteristically disappears with action but reemerges as the limbs maintain a posture. Rest tremor of the hands increases with walking and may be an early sign when others are not yet present. Tremor misdiagnosis is the most common problem for practitioners without neurology training. In general, tremors may be coarse, medium, or fine in amplitude. Most often, patients with PD exhibit a slow, coarse tremor with a rate varying from two to five oscillations per second, usually averaging four or five oscillations per second when the hand is motionless, which decreases with postural changes. There is a clear distinction from essential, or intention tremors, which appear only, or primarily, with deliberate, willed movement.[7,8]

Another classic sign is rigidity, which is an increase in muscle tone that can be elicited when one of the patient's limbs, neck, or trunk is passively moved.[7] The increased resistance to passive movement is equal in all directions and usually is manifested by a ratcheting, or cogwheeling, "give" during the movement. Rigidity of the passive limb increases when another limb is engaged in voluntary active movement.[8]

The patient with PD will often have a uniquely flexed posture involving the entire body. The head is bowed, the trunk is bent forward, the back is kyphotic, the hands are held in front of the body, and the elbows, hips, and knees are flexed. Deformities of the hands and feet may also be apparent. Lateral tilting of the trunk is common.[8]

The most common features of PD are slowness of movement (hypokinesia), loss of automatic movement (bradykinesia), and difficulty initiating movement (freezing).[7] A tendency to shuffle and a decrease in arm swing may be evident. Masked facies, a reduction in spontaneous facial expression, and decreased frequency of blinking are prevalent. The patient may tend to sit motionless or may be characterized by loss of gesturing. Speech becomes soft (hypophonia), and the voice often has a monotonous tone with lack of inflection (aprosody of speech). Some patients are not able to enunciate clearly (dysarthria) or may experience repetition of syllables (palilalia).[8]

PHYSICAL EXAMINATION

Postural reflexes can be tested by giving a sudden, firm pull on the shoulders from behind but the practitioner should be prepared to catch the patient. Rigidity, demonstrated by cogwheeling, may be tested by grasping the patient's elbow at antecubital region and slowly flexing and extending the elbow or pronating/supinating the forearm. Walking can also be marked by festination, whereby the patient walks faster and faster with short steps, trying to move the feet forward under the flexed body's center of gravity.[7,8]

The freezing phenomenon, a motor block, is a transient inability to perform active movements. It most often affects the legs but can involve eyelid opening, speaking, and writing.[7,8] The feet may appear to be glued to the ground. Because patients with PD exhibit an increased ability to perform intentional/conscious movement as opposed to automatic movement, freezing can be overcome by having patients intentionally raise their legs as if stepping over objects. Despite severe bradykinesia with marked immobility, patients with PD may rise suddenly and move normally for a short burst of motor activity (kinesia paradoxica).

DIAGNOSTICS

Diagnostic studies are usually not indicated. The earliest pathologic abnormality may be incidental Lewy bodies in the brain (a postmortem finding).[9] Diagnosis is based on the clinical presentation and physical examination. Clinical diagnostic criteria have a sensitivity of 80% and specificity of 30% compared with the "gold standard" of diagnosis at autopsy.[9] A resting tremor almost always suggests PD because it rarely is seen in other syndromes. Perhaps the most important diagnostic aid, although not an absolute confirmation, is a satisfactory response to levodopa. CT or MRI may be considered for identifying patients with lacunae in the basal ganglia because this group may respond poorly to medications.

DIFFERENTIAL DIAGNOSIS

As previously noted, the diagnosis of PD and other forms of parkinsonism is based on the response to levodopa. Bradykinesia and rigidity respond best, but lack of improvement does not exclude the diagnosis of PD. Tremor may never respond satisfactorily.

Diagnosis may be problematic in mild cases, especially if tremor is minimal or absent. For example, mild hypokinesia, or slight tremor, is commonly attributed to old age. The family history, the character of the tremor, and the lack of other neurologic signs should distinguish essential tremor from parkinsonism (see Chapter 215).

Depression, with its associated expressionless face, poorly modulated voice, and reduction in voluntary activity, can be difficult to distinguish from mild parkinsonism, especially because the two disorders may coexist. In some cases a trial of antidepressant drug therapy may be necessary.

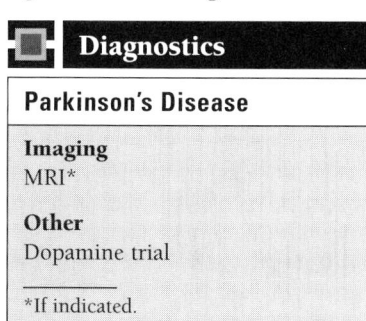

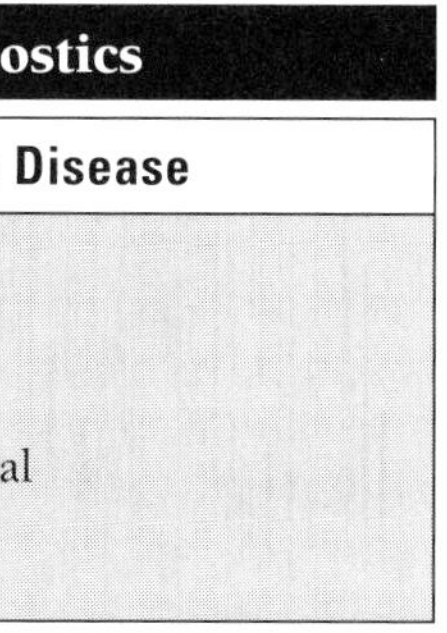
Diagnostics

Parkinson's Disease

Imaging
MRI*

Other
Dopamine trial

*If indicated.

MANAGEMENT

Judicious selection of treatment options can maximize functional gains and may even slow the progress of the disease. Treatment is individualized because each patient has a unique set of signs and symptoms, response to medications, and host of social, occupational, and emotional needs that must be considered. The goal is to maintain independence and functional ability as long as possible. Drug treatment acts in one of two ways: (1) to increase the functional ability of the underactive dopaminergic system or (2) to reduce the excessive influence of the excitatory cholinergic neurons.

Pharmacotherapy

Selegiline. Evidence exists in five randomly controlled trials (RCTs) demonstrating the benefit of selegiline in delaying the need for levodopa an average of 9 months if used for patients with early PD.[10-12] Selegiline (Eldepryl) is a monoamine oxidase-B inhibitor that delays the destruction of the nigral neurons and inhibits the metabolic breakdown of dopamine. Adverse side effects and contraindications in administering and monitoring selegiline should be noted. When given concurrently with levodopa, selegiline can increase the dopaminergic effect and contribute to dopaminergic toxicity. A maximum dose is currently considered 5 mg b.i.d.

Levodopa. Treatment is aimed at restoring the amount of dopamine reaching the basal ganglia. Unfortunately, dopamine does not cross the blood-brain barrier; thus its precursor, levodopa, must be given. Levodopa is metabolized both peripherally and centrally. The peripheral metabolism is responsible for the majority of side effects. Sinemet combines levodopa with carbidopa, which blocks peripheral metabolism, allowing much more of the levodopa to enter the brain than if it were given alone. Sinemet 25/100 contains 25 mg of carbidopa and

Differential Diagnosis

Parkinson's Disease

Idiopathic Parkinsonism
Parkinson's disease

Symptomatic Parkinsonism
Drug-induced condition: dopamine antagonists and depletors
Hemiatrophy-hemiparkinsonism
Hydrocephalus
Hypoxia
Postencephalitic infection
Parathyroid dysfunction
Manganese, carbon dioxide, 1-methyl-4-phenyl-1,2,3,6-tetrahydropyridine (MPTP) cyanide toxicity
Trauma
Tumor
Multiinfarctions

Parkinson-Plus Syndromes
Cortical-basal ganglionic degeneration
Dementia syndromes
Lytico-Bodig (Guamanian parkinsonism–dementia–amyotrophic lateral sclerosis
Multiple-system atrophy syndromes

Heredodegenerative Diseases
Hallervorden-Spatz disease
Huntington's disease
Mitochondrial cytopathies with striatal necrosis
Neuroacanthocytosis
Wilson's disease

Other Conditions
Normal aging
Essential tremor
Depression

100 mg of levodopa. The optimal dose of carbidopa is 100 to 150 mg/day, which should completely block peripheral metabolism of levodopa.

Sinemet increases therapeutic potency and avoids gastrointestinal adverse effects. Slow-release forms of carbidopa/levodopa (Sinemet CR) and benserazide/levodopa (Madopar HBS) provide a longer half-life and a lower peak plasma level of levodopa, reducing clinical fluctuations.[13,14] Once stable, the patient may be reassessed every 3 to 6 months.

After 2 to 5 years of treatment, more than 50% of patients begin to experience fluctuations in their response to levodopa. This "on-off" effect refers to the shortened duration of improvement following each drug dose, with resultant swings from intense akinesia to uncontrollable hyperactivity. Unfortunately, 75% of patients may have serious complications after 5 years of levodopa therapy. Two RCTs found no evidence that modified-release levodopa reduced motor complications or improved disease control at 5 years compared with immediate-release levodopa monotherapy in people with early PD.[13,14]

Dopamine Agonists. Evidence exists that dopamine agonist monotherapy and combination therapy reduces the incidence of irreversible motor complications of dyskinesia and fluctuations in motor response related to long-term levodopa treatment. The same systematic review and six long-term RCTs, however, found that levodopa monotherapy is slightly more effective in treating the disabling motor impairments of PD.[15] Bromocriptine (Parlodel), pergolide (Permax), ropinirole (Requip), and pramipexole (Mirapex) are dopamine agonists that can be effective adjuncts to levodopa in antiparkinsonian therapy to reduce the dosage needed for levodopa alone and to overcome some of the side effects of long-term use of levodopa.[15-18] Therefore dopamine agonists instead of levodopa in younger people with early disease is likely to be beneficial. The agonists tend to induce orthostatic hypotension when first introduced. The best starting regimen is a small dose at bedtime for the first 3 days and then a switch to daytime dosing, with a gradual increase. Bromocriptine and ropinirole may induce psychosis and confusion, whereas pramipexole induces somnolence and pergolide is more likely to induce dyskinesias.[16,17] Overall, however, all are less likely than levodopa to induce dyskinesias, which makes them useful to reduce the severity of "off" states. All dopamine agonists should be used cautiously in patients with cardiac disease.

Anticholinergics. Amantadine (Symmetrel, Symadine), an anticholinergic, may be more useful in controlling tremor and rigidity than bradykinesia but may also cause typical side effects. In older patients amantadine may cause mental changes such as depression, anxiety, or psychosis and probably should not be used in patients over the age of 70.[8] Benztropine (Cogentin) and trihexyphenidyl (Artane) also are useful anticholinergics. The potency of anticholinergics seem to decrease over time, and side effects such as blurred vision, dry mouth, bowel and bladder problems, and cognition changes limit their usefulness. Evidence of benefit of anticholinergics is unclear.

Surgery/Stereotaxic Procedures

Limited evidence exists for the benefit of pallidotomy in reducing contralateral tremor and rigidity during "off " time (periods when treatment is not working) and dyskinesia during "on" time (period when treatment is working).[19,20] There is no evidence that pallidotomy reduces the need for medical treatment.[20] Stereotaxic procedures may be effective in relieving rigidity, bradykinesia, and tremor for patients responding poorly to pharmacologic management, but evidence of benefit is unclear.[21,22]

Unilateral pallidotomy may greatly improve walking speed and precision of manual performances, but left-sided pallidotomy reduces verbal fluency.[23]

Neural Grafting. Experimental surgical implantation of adrenal medullary tissue into the nigrostriatal region, although controversial, has the advantage of being from the patient's own body. However, preliminary evidence shows high morbidity and mortality rates and improvement in the condition of the patient for only 6 months.[24] Reduction in drug doses have been possible after surgery; improved motor function, diminished "off" time, and shorter "freezing" spells have been reported.[24]

COMPLICATIONS

Especially significant is depression, which occurs in more than 50% of patients with PD and may precede motor symptoms.[8] There is debate as to whether depression is a reaction to or part of the illness. Most patients with PD exhibit behavioral changes.[25] The patient's attention span is reduced. Passivity and lack of motivation are common. Confusion, agitation, hallucinations, and mania are probably related to activation of dopamine receptors in cortical and limbic structures.[8]

The prevalence of cognitive dysfunction is estimated to be as high as 81%. However, only 15% to 20% exhibit the severe type of dementia seen in Alzheimer's disease.[26] Memory impairment is not a primary feature; rather, the patient is slow in responding to questions. Subtle signs, such as the inability to change mental set rapidly, may be present early in the disease. Concurrent task demand deficiency indicates an attentional control conflict.[8] Onset of true memory impairment soon after diagnosis of PD would suggest a dementia such as Lewy body rather than idiopathic PD.

Sensory symptoms such as pain, burning, and tingling are fairly common in the region of motor involvement.[8] However, uncomfortable sensations tend to disappear with movement. Autonomic disturbances may produce cooler skin, constipation, inadequate bladder emptying, difficulty with erection, and low blood pressure.

The freezing phenomenon is responsible for the number of hip fractures in patients with PD. Other concerns include small and slow handwriting (micrographia) and difficulty in shaving, brushing teeth, combing hair, and buttoning.[8] Bradykinesia makes rising from a deep chair, getting out of automobiles, and turning in bed difficult. Drooling saliva results from failure to swallow spontaneously. Choking and aspiration are concerns.

General side effects of overmedication with all dopamine agonists include nervousness, restlessness, and vivid nightmares, which predate hallucinations or delusions. Selegiline's adverse side effects include dizziness, confusion, hallucinations, nausea and vomiting, abdominal pain, and possible fatal reaction with concurrent meperidine or narcotic analgesic. Selegiline also is expensive.

Anticholinergics typically produce dry mouth, blurred vision, constipation, and urinary retention. Delirium is not uncommon, especially in frail older adults. Dopamine agonists tend to induce orthostatic hypotension when first introduced. Patients and their caregivers should be taught the signs and symptoms of confusion and psychosis that are to be reported to their primary care provider, as well as any changes in their overall health (e.g., cardiac changes).[8]

INDICATIONS FOR REFERRAL/HOSPITALIZATION

Collaboration with other health providers is common in the treatment of patients with PD. It is important to consult with a neurologist before committing patients to medications. Physician consultation is indicated when patients are not responding to treatment or disease is progressing. Also, if there are signs and symptoms of depression, referral to a psychiatrist should be considered. Neuropsychologic documentation of the precise nature and prevalence of the cognitive deficit has important implications in medical and psychosocial management of patients with PD.[25] Hospitalization may be considered for complications such as pneumonia, deep vein thrombosis, or pulmonary embolus. Physical therapy can improve mobility and strength, which may help to maintain independence and prevent injury. Occupational therapy can be useful; adaptive equipment can be provided to the patient and/or caregivers, and assistance can be provided to adapt the home or workplace as disability progresses.

PATIENT AND FAMILY EDUCATION

Patients should be told that levodopa is more effective when taken on an empty stomach, but this may result in nausea, particularly for the first 3 days. Some patients may report that high-protein meals tend to produce "off" states.[8] It should be explained that foods containing phenylalanine, leucine, and isoleucine, such as milk and meat, can block the absorption of levodopa from the intestine and its passage into the brain. This effect may be responsible for later diurnal response fluctuations. Side effects of dopamine agonists, including dizziness, confusion, hallucinations, or delusional thinking, should be reviewed with the patient.

Answering questions and addressing concerns honestly are part of establishing a successful practitioner-patient relationship. Reassurance and encouragement complement medication. The patient should be encouraged to contact a PD support group and a local PD information and referral center. Internet resources are also available for patients with PD. The patient may find the following resources helpful:

American Parkinson's Disease Association (APDA)
1250 Hylan Boulevard, Suite B
Staten Island, NY 10305-1946
(800) 223-2732
California: (800) 908-2732
http://www.apdaparkinson.org.

National Parkinson Foundation, Inc. (NPF)
Bob Hope Parkinson Research Center
1501 NW 9th Avenue
Miami, FL 33136-1494
(800) 327-4545
Florida: (800) 433-7022
http://www.parkinson.org.

Parkinson's Disease Foundation (PDF)
710 W. 169th Street
New York, NY 10025
(800) 457-6676
http://www.pdf.org.

Parkinson Support Groups of America
11376 Cherry Hill Road, No. 204
Beltsville, MD 20705

Informational Webstes: http://www.ninds.nih.gov; http://www.pdweb.mgh.harvard.edu.

REFERENCES

1. DeRijk MC and others: Prevalence of parkinsonism and Parkinson's disease in Europe: the Europarkinson collaborative study, *J Neurol Neurosurg Psychiatry* 62: 10-15, 1997.
2. Marder K and others: Risk of Parkinson's disease among first degree relatives: a community based study, *Neurology* 47:155-160, 1996.
3. Jaman P and others: Parkinson's disease genetics comes of age, *Br Med J* 318:1641-1642, 1999.
4. Ben-Shlomo Y: How far are we in understanding the cause of Parkinson's disease? *J Neurol Neurosurg Psychiatry* 61:4-16, 1996.
5. DeRijk M and others: Dietary antioxidants and Parkinson's disease: the Rotterdam study, *Arch Neurol* 54:762-765, 1997.
6. Tzourio C and others: Smoking and Parkinson's disease: an age-dependent risk effect? *Neurology* 49:1267-1272, 1997.
7. Tierney LM, McPhee SJ, Papadakis MA, editors: *Current medical diagnosis and treatment*, ed 35, Stamford, Conn, 1996, Appleton & Lange.
8. Tapper VJ: Pathophysiology, assessment, and treatment of Parkinson's disease, *Nurse Pract* 22:76-95, 1997.
9. Hughes AJ and others: A clinico-pathologic study of 100 cases of Parkinson's disease, *Arch Neurol* 50:140-148, 1993.
10. Lees AJ, for the Parkinson's Disease Research Group of the United Kingdom: Comparison of therapeutic effects and mortality data of levodopa and levodopa combined with selegiline in people with early, mild Parkinson's disease, *Br Med J* 311:1602-1607, 1995.
11. Przuntek and others: Seledo: a 5-year long-term trial on the effect of selegiline in early Parkinson's people treated with levodopa, *Eur J Neurol* 61:1441-1450, 1995.
12. Larson JP and others: Does selegiline modify the progression of early Parkinson's disease? Results from a five-year study, *Eur J Neurol* 6: 539-547, 1999.
13. Dupont E and others: Sustained-release Madopar HBS compared with standard release Madopar in the long-term treatment of de novo Parkinson's people, *Acta Neurol Scand* 93:14-20, 1996.
14. Block G and others for the CR First Study Group: Comparison of immediate release and controlled release carbidopa/levodopa in Parkinson's disease, *Eur Neurol* 37:23-47, 1997.
15. Ramaker C, van Hilton J: Bromocriptine/levodopa versus levodopa in early Parkinson's disease, *Parkinson Relat Disord* 5(suppl) 82, 1999.
16. Rascol O and others: A five-year study of the incidence of dyskinesia in people with early Parkinson's disease who were treated with ropinirole or levodopa, *N Engl J Med* 342:1484-1491, 2000.
17. Parkinson's Study Group: Pramipexole versus levodopa as initial treatment for Parkinson's disease, *JAMA* 284:1931-1938, 2000.
18. Rinne U: A 5-year double-blind study with cabergoline versus levodopa in the treatment of Parkinson's disease, *Parkinsonism Relat Disord* 5 (suppl):84, 1999.
19. Alkhani A, Lozano A: Pallidotomy for Parkinson's disease: a review of contemporary literature, *J Neurosurg* 94: 43-49, 2001.
20. De Bie R and others: Unilateral pallidotomy in Parkinson's disease: a randomized, single-blind, multicentre trial, *Lancet* 354: 28:1665-1669, 1999.
21. Merello M and others: Unilateral radiofrequency lesion versus electrostimulation of posteroventral pallidum: a prospective randomized comparison, *Mov Disord* 14:50-56, 1999.

22. Katayama Y and others: Double-blind evaluation of the effect of pallidal and subthalamic nucleus stimulation on daytime activity in advanced Parkinson's disease, *Parkinson Relat Disord* 7:35-40, 2000.
23. Schmand B and others: Unilateral pallidotomy in PD. A controlled study of cognitive and behavioural effects, *Neurology* 54:1058-1064, 2000.
24. Collier TJ, Springer JE: Neural graft augmentation through co-grafting, *Prog Neurobiol* 44:309-331, 1994.
25. Taylor AE, Saint-Cyr JA: The neuro psychology of Parkinson's disease, *Brain Cogn* 28:281-296, 1997.
26. Braak H and others: New aspects of pathology in Parkinson's disease with concomitant incipient Alzheimer's disease, *J Neurol Transm* 48S:1-6, 1996.

CHAPTER 218

Seizure Disorder

Karen L. Gilbert

DEFINITION/EPIDEMIOLOGY

Seizure disorder (epilepsy) is a common neurologic condition that currently affects more than 2 million people in the United States, with more than 50 cases per 100,000 people reported annually. Although the onset of seizures can occur at any age, incidence rates peak in neonates and young children, plateau, and then rise again in the older adult population. In the United States, the prevalence of seizures is approximately 5 to 10 cases per 1000 persons in the general population; the lifetime risk of developing epilepsy in one's lifetime is between 3% and 5%.[1]

Causes of seizures include genetic factors, vascular abnormalities (e.g., strokes, hemorrhages, arteriovenous malformations), significant head trauma, brain tumors, and infections such as encephalitis and meningitis. Genetic predisposition is strongest in forms of epilepsy in which the entire brain is electrically unstable. Childhood absence (petit mal) epilepsy, juvenile myoclonic epilepsy, and generalized convulsive epilepsy are syndromes with a genetic predisposition. These types account for approximately one third of all epilepsy cases, with seizures and electroencephalographic (EEG) abnormalities affecting the entire brain. The remaining types of epilepsy are related to localization, with focal electrical abnormalities usually being the result of a structural lesion. The occurrence of prolonged or complicated febrile seizures in infancy is strongly correlated with the subsequent development of temporal lobe epilepsy.[2]

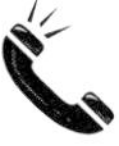

Physician consultation is indicated for suspected central nervous system lesions, status epilepticus, initiation of antiepileptic medications, treatment failures, and women with epilepsy who are contemplating pregnancy.

PATHOPHYSIOLOGY

Although the terms *epilepsy* and *seizure disorder* are often used interchangeably, they have two distinct definitions. A *seizure* can be defined as an isolated event in which a group of neurons produce excessive electrical discharges in the brain. Seizures occur when the balance between excitation and inhibition of the brain's electrical activity becomes abnormally altered in favor of excitation. Seizures can be caused by the excess production or release of an excitatory neurotransmitter, which stimulates neurons to discharge abnormally, or by a loss of inhibitory neuronal activity, which permits abnormal excitation and discharges of neurons to occur. Single seizures can be triggered by hypoxia or metabolic factors, but they do not constitute epilepsy unless they recur in a habitual and unprovoked manner. Epilepsy is characterized by recurrent seizures and is divided into syndromes on the basis of various etiologies, seizure types, associated neurologic symptoms, anatomic correlates, age, and family history. For diagnosis and treatment, it is valuable to be able to identify both the type of seizure and the epileptic syndrome.

CLASSIFICATION OF SEIZURES, EPILEPSY, AND EPILEPTIC SYNDROMES

In 1981, a commission for the International League Against Epilepsy (ILAE) developed, revised, and adopted the International Classification of Epileptic Seizures[3] (Box 218-1). The classification includes two broad categories of seizure types: partial and generalized. Partial seizures begin in a limited region of one cerebral hemisphere and show focal EEG abnormalities. Depending on the spread of electrical activity, the patient may have varying levels of consciousness. By definition, simple partial seizures are not associated with any alteration of consciousness and are usually the aura, or warning, that the patient experiences before a larger seizure. Occasionally, patients may have only simple partial sensory seizures, which makes the seizure purely subjective. If the seizure activity spreads and involves the brainstem or both hemispheres, consciousness becomes altered and the seizure is classified as complex partial. Altered consciousness and aberrations of behavior, such as automatisms, are usually associated with complex partial seizures. If such seizures spread bilaterally and involve the motor cortex, the patient may have a secondarily generalized tonic-clonic seizure.[4]

In contrast, primary generalized seizures occur when the initial electrical activity begins in both cerebral hemispheres. These seizures are usually seen with idiopathic or hereditary epilepsy. Consciousness is almost always impaired, and the seizure may be convulsive or nonconvulsive. Motor activity and EEG changes are bilateral. Nonconvulsive seizures, such as absence (petit mal) seizures, may be brief, and the patient may initially be diagnosed as a "daydreamer." The EEG characteristics of generalized spike-and-wave patterns are crucial for the proper diagnosis of these types of seizures. Convulsive seizures, such as tonic-clonic (grand mal) types, are rarely missed but can be confused with secondarily generalized tonic-clonic seizures. Being able to differentiate between these two types is helpful in prescribing the appropriate treatment, because each type may respond differently to certain antiepileptic medications. In the case of secondarily generalized seizures, it is very important to exclude an underlying structural lesion, such as a brain tumor.

To tailor treatment to the individual, it is essential that consideration be given to the seizure type as well as the epileptic syndrome to which it belongs. The International Classification of Epilepsy and Epileptic Syndromes (Box 218-2) was adopted in 1989 and allows the practitioner to categorize by seizure type, etiology, precipitating factors, age of onset, and prognosis.[5] Although epilepsy can develop at any age, certain syndromes are more age related than others. A variety of epileptic syndromes develop in early childhood. Approximately 70% of childhood epilepsies, particularly the benign partial epilepsies, remit at the time of puberty. Idiopathic, generalized epilepsy usually manifests itself by 18 years of age. After age 18, focal brain processes should be suspected. Brain tumors are a prominent cause of seizures in adults, whereas strokes are often the cause of seizures that begin late in life.[6] Symptomatic focal epilepsy syndromes account for 30% to 35% of all cases of epilepsy.[1] Seizure manifestations can be helpful in identifying which lobe of the brain is involved.[2,6,7] Table 218-1 outlines the general characteristics of partial seizures in relation to the region of seizure origin. However, it should be noted that not all seizures fit neatly into a particular syndrome. Surgical treatment is often possible if the epileptic focus is in a surgically accessible region of the brain.

CLINICAL PRESENTATION

An accurate and detailed history is important. Complicated pregnancy or childbirth, delayed childhood development, childhood diseases such as meningitis and encephalitis, significant head trauma with loss of consciousness, and a family history of epilepsy are among the significant risk factors for the

BOX 218-1

INTERNATIONAL CLASSIFICATION OF EPILEPTIC SEIZURES

I. **Partial Seizures.** Epileptic focus is in one hemisphere of the brain. Also called focal or local seizures.
   A. **Simple Partial Seizures.** Usually the aura of a complex seizure. Patient has no loss of consciousness.
      1. Motor—tonic or clonic activity of one arm or leg
      2. Sensory—such as an auditory, olfactory, visual hallucination
      3. Autonomic—such as the epigastric rising sensation
      4. Psychic—deja vu, fear, indescribable feeling
   B. **Complex Partial Seizure.** Consciousness is altered. Patient may exhibit complex behaviors.
      1. Can begin with a simple partial onset.
      2. Can begin with immediate alteration of consciousness.
   C. **Partial Seizure Evolving to Generalized.** Patient starts with a simple or complex partial seizure that evolves into a generalized tonic/clonic seizure.

II. **Generalized.** Epileptic focus is not lateralized to one hemisphere. Begins in both hemispheres of the brain simultaneously.
   A. **Nonconvulsive**
      1. Absence (petit mal)
      2. Atonic—loss of muscle tone (drop attacks)
   B. **Convulsive.** Involves motor activity.
      1. Myoclonic—abrupt muscle twitches/jerks
      2. Tonic-clonic (grand mal)—tonic, then clonic activity
      3. Tonic—involving increased muscle tone/rigidity
      4. Clonic—muscle contraction and relaxation movements

Modified from Commission on Classification and Terminology of the International League Against Epilepsy: proposal for revised clinical and electroencephalographic classification of epileptic seizures, *Epilepsia* 22(4):489-501, 1981.

development of epilepsy. New-onset seizures require the determination of any recent history of headache, illness, trauma, focal neurologic deficit, or light-headedness.

An accurate description is very important when attempting to decide whether an event was a seizure. The patient should be questioned to determine if there was a warning before the event. A gastric sensation or a feeling of déjà vu is very characteristic of temporal lobe epilepsy. A history of incontinence, injury, tongue biting, postictal confusion, lateralized weakness, or severe headache should raise suspicion of a true epileptic event. A detailed seizure history can also suggest where the seizures are originating, define seizure characteristics and frequency, and determine how the seizures are interfering with the patient's life.

PHYSICAL EXAMINATION

A general physical examination should be performed on all patients with epilepsy and should be directed toward specific disease processes and focal neurologic deficits. Skin and mucous membranes should be assessed to identify areas of injury that may be related to events that occurred while consciousness was altered. Tongue biting and cheek biting are common during tonic-clonic seizures; usually the tongue is bitten on just one side. Cardiovascular assessment is important because syncope and arrhythmias are included in the differential diagnosis of epilepsy. Postural vital signs will determine if orthostatic hypotension is a consideration. Neurologic signs such as lateralized weakness, papilledema, memory problems, or changes in reflexes can signify a structural lesion in the brain.[4,6] Most often, a patient with epilepsy will have an unremarkable physical examination.

BOX 218-2

INTERNATIONAL CLASSIFICATION OF EPILEPSY AND EPILEPTIC SYNDROMES

1. Localization related (focal, partial)
   - 1.1 Idiopathic (benign childhood epilepsy with centerotemporal spikes)
   - 1.2 Symptomatic (e.g., temporal lobe epilepsy, frontal lobe epilepsy)
   - 1.3 Cryptogenic (etiology unknown)
2. Generalized epilepsies
   - 2.1 Idiopathic (juvenile myoclonic, juvenile absence, grand mal upon awakening)
   - 2.2 Cryptogenic (Lennox-Gastaut syndrome, West syndrome)
   - 2.3 Symptomatic
3. Undetermined (neonatal types, Landau-Kleffner syndrome)
4. Special situation related (febrile seizures, metabolic seizures)

Modified from Commission on Classification and Terminology of the International League Against Epilepsy: proposal for revised clinical and electroencephalographic classification of epileptic seizures, *Epilepsia* 22(4):489-501, 1981.

DIAGNOSTICS

Clinical presentation, physical examination, and differential consideration guides diagnostic testing. A new seizure may signify a serious pathologic condition. If infection of the central nervous system (CNS) is suspected, a CBC and differential, as well as a lumbar puncture, is indicated. A chemistry profile, including calcium, is necessary to exclude hypoglycemia, electrolyte abnormalities, or renal failure. Liver function tests (LFTs) should be obtained to exclude hepatic failure. Alcohol and drug levels are necessary when indicated. MRI or CT is indicated if a tumor, trauma, or cerebrovascular accident is suspected. An electrocardiogram (ECG) should be obtained to ascertain the presence of arrhythmias or heart block.

Diagnostics

New-Onset Seizure

Laboratory
- Alcohol/drug levels*
- Serum electrolytes*
- BUN*
- Creatinine*
- Serum glucose*
- Calcium*
- CBC and differential*
- LFTs*

Imaging
- MRI/CT scan*

Other
- ECG*
- Lumbar puncture*
- EEG*

*If indicated.

TABLE 218-1 Clinical Manifestations of Complex Partial Seizures

Site	Aura	Clinical Characteristics	% of Partial Cases
Temporal	Epigastric sensation Déjà vu	Altered consciousness Oral, hand automatisms Moderate postictal confusion	75-85
Frontal	Dizziness or fear	Abrupt onset, rapid clearing Frenetic behavior Sexual automatisms Most occur during sleep	10-15
Parietal	Sensory	With or without altered consciousness Often begins with numbness, tingling, or pain	Rare
Occipital	Visual	May begin with eye twitching May include visual hallucinations May include ictal blindness	5-15

Diagnosing and classifying epilepsy and seizure types require confirmation that the patient does indeed have epileptic seizures. To appropriately treat the disorder, the practitioner must attempt to determine the cause of the epilepsy and classify it according to syndrome. A few diagnostic tests should be part of the initial evaluation.

An EEG is useful because a baseline recording of background brain waves may reveal epileptic abnormalities. Because the chance of a patient having a seizure during a routine EEG is small, ictal information may not be obtained; however, interictal epileptiform abnormalities may give localizing information and suggest epilepsy. Many patients with focal epilepsy show no focal or generalized EEG abnormalities on routine EEG. Therefore a normal EEG does not exclude a diagnosis of epilepsy. In contrast to focal epilepsy, generalized types of epilepsy often produce abnormalities of spike-and-wave activity or generalized slowing on routine EEG recordings. Interictal EEG abnormalities—either focal or generalized—are not synonymous with seizure activity, and therefore EEG abnormalities should not be the only basis for treatment.

Although neuroimaging studies can be of great value in diagnosis, the absence of structural abnormalities does not exclude a diagnosis of epilepsy. CT scans are useful for identifying large mass lesions, bleeding, subdural fluid collections, and cerebral infarcts, but they often miss more subtle changes in brain structure. MRIs provide great anatomic detail and are very useful in distinguishing small low-grade tumors, scars, and neural migration disorders from each other and from normal variants in brain structure. Except in an emergency, when the immediate availability of a CT scan is an advantage, MRIs should be the only routine imaging study in patients with epilepsy.

If a diagnosis of epilepsy cannot be made after an accurate history, EEG, or imaging study, patients should be referred to a comprehensive epilepsy center in which long-term video/EEG monitoring can be done. This type of monitoring is intended to capture an event on video with simultaneous EEG recording, and it is almost always successful in distinguishing epilepsy from nonepileptic events.

DIFFERENTIAL DIAGNOSIS

A variety of nonepileptic paroxysmal events can be confused with epileptic seizures. Psychogenic seizures, also called *nonepileptic seizures* or *pseudoseizures*, are often mistaken for epileptic seizures; if patients are treated with antiepileptic drugs, this usually makes seizure frequency increase. A careful history can help to raise the suspicion of psychogenic seizures. In such cases, seizures may be symptoms of conversion disorder and the stress of physical or sexual abuse, a part of posttraumatic stress disorder (PTSD), attention-seeking behavior, or a means of achieving secondary gain.[8] Treatment involves patient acceptance of the diagnosis of psychogenic seizures and the beginning of a comprehensive psychotherapy program.

The second most common disorder to be confused with epilepsy is syncope. Syncope presents with loss of consciousness, and convulsive syncope secondary to cerebral ischemia may mimic epileptic seizures. Syncope is often vasovagal, but cardiac causes include heart block or cardiac arrhythmia. Presyncopal symptoms such as vertigo, sensory disturbances, and tinnitus are sometimes mistaken for epileptic auras or minor seizures.

Other disorders in the differential diagnosis include tumors, cerebrovascular disease, arteriovenous malformation, trauma, CNS infection, migraines, hyperventilation syndrome, movement disorders, transient ischemic attacks, transient global amnesia, and toxic metabolic disturbances such as alcohol withdrawal seizures.[9] Occasionally, sleep deprivation may cause generalized tonic-clonic seizures. This phenomenon is not associated with a pathologic disorder.

Differential Diagnosis

Seizure Disorder

Psychogenic seizures	Toxic metabolic disturbances
Syncope	Brain tumor
Cardiac arrhythmias	Infection
Migraine	Alcoholism/drug withdrawal
Hyperventilation	Idiopathic
Movement disorders	Trauma
Transient global amnesia	Sleep deprivation
Transient ischemic attacks	Arteriovenous malformation
Cerebrovascular disease	

MANAGEMENT

The goal of management in epilepsy is to control seizures with minimal adverse effects. In more than 50% of patients with epilepsy, seizures are completely controlled with medication. An additional 20% to 30% of patients have improvement of their symptoms with medications, but they are not seizure free or may have significant side effects. The remaining 25% of seizures are medically intractable. Determination of the appropriate medical or surgical treatment is based on a variety of factors, including the patient's perception of how the seizures are interfering with life goals, economic considerations, personal support from family and friends, and the severity and complexity of the epilepsy in that patient.

Conservative

The first decision is whether to treat a patient who has had a single seizure. There has been much controversy regarding this issue because of the lack of randomized, unbiased studies. Most studies have combined multiple seizure types, which clouds interpretation of the data. In one randomized multicenter trial of 397 patients seen within 7 days of their first seizure, 36 of 204 treated patients (18%) and 75 of 193 untreated patients (38%) had a recurrent seizure within 2 years.[10] Although these results demonstrate the effectiveness of antiepileptic medication, the recurrence rate even in untreated patients is low enough that most patients with first seizures are not treated.

In a review of the literature by Beghi and others,[11] the two most consistent predictors of seizure recurrence are the presence of an abnormal EEG and an underlying etiology. In patients with an unprovoked seizure for which there was an underlying antecedent cause (e.g., a previous head injury, mental retardation, or cerebral palsy), the risk of recurrent seizures was double that of patients with an unprovoked seizure for which there was no antecedent cause. After a second seizure, the risk of recurrence increases to more than 80%.[11]

Most epilepsy specialists advocate making treatment decisions after considering the risks and benefits of the treatment for a particular patient. Elements of decision making include the

TABLE 218-2 Antiepileptic Drug Chart

Drug	Dosage Range	Side Effect Profile	Half-Life/ Peak Effect	Drug Levels	Considerations
Phenobarbital (Luminal)	60-250 mg/day PO in single or divided dose 100-300 mg IV (up to 600 mg to load)	Drowsiness, but tolerance usually develops May cause difficulties with memory and cognition May exacerbate depression in adults	*Half-life:* 96 hours +/−12 *Peak effect:* Oral: 20-60 minutes IV: 15 minutes	15-40 (levels may not stabilize for 3-4 weeks)	Do not stop abruptly May cause hyperactivity in children Used in partial and generalized seizures Effective for motor seizures
Phenytoin (Dilantin)	300-600 mg/day Loading dose: 1 g IV in divided doses	Gingival hypertrophy Mild sedation Rash, nausea, vomiting Lethargy, nystagmus, ataxia with high doses Difficulty with concentration and memory	*Half-life:* Oral: 22 hours IV: 10-15 hours *Peak effect:* 4-12 hours; 7-10 days to reach optimum levels	10-20 (levels may stay therapeutic for 7-10 days after discontinuing) Free level should be ordered if patient is also taking valproic acid	Used in partial and generalized seizures IV phenytoin and fosphenytoin are effective for treating status epilepticus
Carbamazepine (Tegretol)	600-1200 mg in divided doses	Drowsiness, dizziness, nausea/vomiting, which decrease with time Titration should be started slowly to avoid side effects Diplopia when toxic	*Half-life:* 12-17 hours *Peak effect:* 4-5 hours after regular and 3-12 hours after extended-release preparation	Normal ranges vary by laboratory: 4-12 or 8-12 Takes approximately 2 days to achieve therapeutic level	Used in partial seizures Not for absence types Should be taken with food Generics should be avoided in patients with intractable seizures
Primidone (Mysoline)	Titrated slowly by 125 mg until 250 mg t.i.d. is reached	Drowsiness, ataxia, and vertigo may occur, which usually decrease with time or dose reduction	*Half-life:* 12 hours +/−6	Levels reported as primidone and phenobarbital Primidone: 5-12 Phenobarbital: 15-40	Used in partial and generalized seizures Effective for motor seizures Should not be used by patients who are allergic to phenobarbital
Valproic acid (Depakote)	15-60 mg/kg/day Rarely exceeds 3500-4000 mg/day	Patient should be instructed on side effects of tremor and possible weight gain	*Half-life:* 6-16 hours *Peak effect:* 1-4 hours after dose	Normal range 50-100 Levels over 100 may be tolerated by some patients if well controlled	Effective in generalized seizures May increase free dilantin epoxide; free dilantin levels should be obtained if necessary
Oxcarbazepine (Trileptal)	600-2400 mg/day	Somnolence, headache, dizziness, hyponatremia	*Half-life:* 8-10 hours *Peak effect:* 4-5 hours	No established level	Similar to carbamazepine, but fewer drug interactions
Lamotrigine (Lamictal)	Without valproic acid: 300-500 mg With valproic acid: 100-150 mg Dose b.i.d.	Rash, headache, dizziness, blurred vision Blurred vision may occur more often in patients taking carbamazepine	*Half-life:* 12-27 hours (with valproic acid: 70 hours) *Peak effect:* 1.4-4.8 hours	3-14 Lamictal elimination is more rapid in patients taking hepatic enzyme-inducing AEDs	Used in partial and generalized seizures Risk of rash is higher in patients also taking valproic acid Titrated to effect, not to a certain blood level

risk to the patient according to the severity, timing, and frequency of seizures; age of seizure onset; and cognitive considerations.[12] In determining risk, it is obvious that patients with generalized tonic-clonic seizures are more at risk for injury than those with simple partial seizures. The timing of seizures is also important. Seizures that occur primarily out of sleep pose less risk. Seizures that occur only in relation to special circumstances such as alcohol consumption, sleep deprivation, or pregnancy are sometimes better treated by avoiding those factors instead of by taking antiepileptic medication. Age and cognition can be

TABLE 218-2 Antiepileptic Drug Chart—cont'd

Drug	Dosage Range	Side Effect Profile	Half-Life/ Peak Effect	Drug Levels	Considerations
Gabapentin (Neurotin)	900-3600 mg/day Titrated to 300 mg t.i.d., then increased by 300-mg increments	Somnolence, dizziness, ataxia, fatigue Side effects usually short lived Reduced interactions with other AEDs	*Half-life:* 5-9 hours *Peak effect:* 2-3 hours	Normal range 2-20 Neurontin is not appreciably metabolized, and significance of levels is uncertain	Used in partial seizures Should be taken 2 hours apart from Maalox to avoid changes in bioavailability
Topiramate (Topamax)	200-400 mg/day b.i.d. Titrated slowly at 25 mg/day/weekly increments	Somnolence, dizziness, psychomotor slowing, speech hesitancy, mood disturbances May cause weight loss Males have increased risk of kidney stones	*Half-life:* 21 hours *Peak effect:* Within 2 hours after dose	Not completely metabolized, and need for levels is uncertain	Used as an adjunct in partial seizure disorders May decrease estrogen levels in patients taking oral contraceptives Patients should increase fluid intake
Tiagabine (Gabatril)	12-32 mg Titrated by 4 mg/week	Somnolence, dizziness, headache, mild memory impairment, abdominal pain	*Half-life:* 5-13 hours *Peak effect:* 0.5-1.0 hour	Not established at this time	Used in partial seizures as an adjunctive therapy Dosage should be adjusted if hepatic disease is present
Felbamate (Felbatol)	600-3600 mg/day	Insomnia, weight loss, headache Should refer to boxed warning regarding aplastic anemia and hepatic failure	*Half-life:* 20-23 hours	Monitor concomitant drug levels Monitor CBC and LFTs frequently	Multiple drug interactions with other AEDs; drug text should be consulted for details Used in partial and generalized seizures
Levatiracetam (Keppra)	1000-3000 mg/day	Dizziness, drowsiness, asthenia, infection	*Half-life:* 6-8 hours	Not established	Use caution in patients with a history of psychosis or depression
Zonisamide (Zonegran)	100-600 mg/day	Somnolence, dizziness, anorexia, headache	*Half-life:* Alone: 63 hours With enzyme Inducers: 27-46 hours		Note: contains sulfonamides; avoid use in those with sensitivity

factors in decision making. An adolescent who has just learned to drive may be more tolerant of the side effects related to seizure control than a young adult who has just entered college.

Treatment choices vary with individual differences in etiology, seizure type, age, and psychosocial factors. Controlling seizures with a single drug should be the goal. Each drug should be titrated slowly to determine how it is tolerated, and each drug should be given a fair trial. If seizures are frequent, efficacy can be determined quickly. When changing medications, the new medication should be added to the existing regimen. When the new medication is well tolerated and an effective dose has been achieved, the first medication can be slowly reduced. If the patient's seizures remain intractable after trying several single drugs, rational combinations of medications should be tried. Drugs with different mechanisms of action and different side effect profiles usually combine well. To maintain a steady level of the drug in circulation, dosage frequency should be determined by the half-life of the drug. Table 218-2 compares the most common antiepileptic drugs (AEDs) related to dosage, peak, half-life, side effects, indications, and special considerations.

Side effects occur in approximately 30% to 40% of patients taking AEDs.[13] The side effects should be carefully monitored and the dosages adjusted to minimize the adverse effects of the medication. Rarely, an idiosyncratic reaction can occur, which can be life threatening.

Measurements of blood levels of AEDs are helpful in determining whether a therapeutic dose has been achieved. However, it is most important to follow the patient's response to treatment in relation to efficacy and side effects. With many patients, seizures are controlled with low doses and levels of medications, whereas other patients require and tolerate high levels. Some patients experience significant side effects, even when drug levels are in a normal range. In this case, it may be best to order "free" AED levels, especially if the drug is highly protein bound. Protein binding, absorption, and elimination pharmacokinetics are extremely important factors to consider in predicting side effects and drug-drug interactions. A complete list of medications, including over-the-counter preparations, should be obtained from the patient. Blood levels should be obtained at least yearly and more often if the patient is having breakthrough seizures, increased side effects, or signs of drug toxicity. In addition, CBC, electrolytes, and LFTs should be performed within 1 month of beginning a new AED.

In making a decision to discontinue AED therapy, the risk-benefit ratio should be considered. The risk for relapse is 20% to 40% in the first year of drug withdrawal.[14] Patients with the greatest risk for relapse are those with seizure disorder onset during adolescence, an abnormal EEG, an underlying neurologic condition, a definite diagnosis of primary generalized epilepsy, or a history of previous failures at discontinuing AEDs. There is insufficient evidence to establish when to withdraw AEDs in patients who are seizure free.

Surgical

Of all patients with epilepsy, 25% are refractory to medical management. Of this 25%, approximately half have focal lesions that are responsible for their seizures; these patients are good candidates for epilepsy surgery. The most common form of epilepsy surgery is a temporal lobectomy. Almost 80% of partial seizures in adults begin in the temporal lobes; a portion of one of the temporal lobes can be removed if tests consistently indicate that the seizures originate in that area. After temporal lobe surgery, success rates (complete seizure control) range from 65% to 95%.[15]

The removal of tumors, abnormal collections of blood vessels, and congenital lesions are other resective surgical options. These conditions can be found anywhere in the brain, and the best results are obtained when both the lesion and the surrounding epileptogenic brain are removed. It is often necessary to perform intracranial EEG mapping to delineate the epileptic zone and to identify cortically important areas such as the language and motor cortex, which must be avoided during surgery.

Another major type of epilepsy surgery involves dividing the corpus callosum. With this type of surgery, the nerve fibers that connect one side of the brain to the other are severed; no tissue is removed. This surgery is most helpful for secondarily generalized tonic-clonic seizures and atonic seizures. Although seizures are not completely stopped by this procedure, they are confined to one hemisphere. Impairment of consciousness, convulsive seizure activity, and falls are often eliminated or greatly reduced.

After surgery, patients remain on antiepileptic medication for several years. Patients who are seizure free for several years can consider a medication taper.

LIFE SPAN CONSIDERATIONS

Although stigma, social isolation, and depression can affect all persons with epilepsy, special concerns are recognized in specific age-groups. Many patients develop epilepsy in early adolescence. This diagnosis can have a profound effect on self-esteem and a sense of lack of control because of the unpredictability of seizures. Parental overprotection and preoccupation with the child can lead to problems within the entire family unit. Adolescents should be encouraged to take responsibility for their own care. Providing education and the forum for a trusting relationship is the initial goal for this group of patients. Factual information should be presented in a straightforward, individualized manner, and the young adult should be encouraged to be honest and open about seizure frequency and compliance issues. It is hoped that collaboration between patient and provider results in a better understanding of the importance of medication, which makes adherence to the treatment plan more likely.

In women with epilepsy there are additional concerns about contraception, fertility, and sexuality. Pregnancy, however, has unpredictable effects on seizure control. Female adolescents should be counseled about family planning and birth control options. Patients taking hepatic enzyme–inducing AEDs should be given a higher-dose oral contraceptive—one with an estrogen content of 50 μg.[16] Women with epilepsy should be encouraged to plan their pregnancies. They should also be given folate supplements in advance; some AEDs have been shown to inhibit folate action, and folate deficiency is associated with an increased risk of neural tube defects. Overall, AEDs probably double the baseline rate of birth defects. Decisions to continue or to stop taking medication during pregnancy are difficult and should be discussed with a neurologist on an individual basis. Women who continue to take AEDs during pregnancy should be enrolled in the AED pregnancy registry, which can be located through the Epilepsy Foundation of America.

Hormonal changes also have an effect on seizure control. Many women note that seizures tend to occur just before or during their menstrual cycle; this is most likely related to low progesterone levels. Progesterone has been shown to decrease neuronal excitability in animal models.[17] Little is known about the relationship of epilepsy and menopause, but one preliminary study by Harden and others[18] suggests that hormonal changes that occur during menopause may exacerbate seizures in some women, especially those using estrogen supplementation.

The onset of epilepsy in older adults has increased during the past decade. This increase is related to an increase in cerebrovascular disease and brain tumors. Special concerns for older adults include an increased risk of injury or falls during seizures, the effects of AEDs on cognition and physical abilities, and interactions between various medications. Monotherapy is most important for this population to reduce side effects and drug interactions. Dosage changes should be made slowly because older adults are more sensitive than young patients to even minor changes.

COMPLICATIONS

Complications in patients with epilepsy are usually related to seizure events. Injuries that occur during seizures include falls, burns, motor vehicle accidents, and aspiration pneumonia. Risks can be reduced by making lifestyle changes at work and during recreation. Patient advocacy helps ensure safe environments at work and school and can discourage discrimination.

Convulsive or generalized tonic-clonic status epilepticus—defined either as a continuous seizure that lasts longer than 30 minutes or as two consecutive seizures without mental clearing in between—is a medical emergency that can lead to brain damage or even death.[19] Mortality and morbidity rates are related to the etiology of status epilepticus and the time from the onset of status epilepticus until seizures are controlled. In patients with known epilepsy, one half of the hospital-reported cases of generalized convulsive status epilepticus have been associated with subtherapeutic AED levels.[20] Other causes of status epilepticus include brain infection, trauma, and stroke. Most cases of status epilepticus can be treated successfully with parenteral drug therapy, including lorazepam, phenytoin, or phenobarbital.

INDICATIONS FOR REFERRAL/HOSPITALIZATION

Physician consultation is indicated for suspected central nervous system lesions, status epilepticus, initiation of antiepileptic medications, treatment failures, and women with epilepsy who are contemplating pregnancy.

Patients with very frequent seizures or patients who meet the criteria for status epilepticus should be hospitalized for further evaluation and medication adjustment. Patients with seizures that are refractory to conventional therapy should be referred to a neurologist or epileptologist for further evaluation. If adequate seizure control is not achieved, patients should undergo presurgical and diagnostic evaluation with video EEG monitoring at a comprehensive epilepsy center. Patients who are having difficulty tolerating medications should also be referred for a neurology consultation. Patients with structural lesions should be referred promptly to a neurosurgeon for further evaluation.

PATIENT AND FAMILY EDUCATION

Epilepsy provides unique teaching opportunities because it is a chronic condition that affects all aspects of a patient's life. Patient and family education regarding safety is vital. It is imperative that patients avoid high places such as rooftops or ladders, not operate dangerous equipment that could cause cuts or crush injuries, and not swim alone. Family members should be taught simple first aid measures such as turning the patient onto his or her side and not putting objects into the mouth during a tonic-clonic seizure.

The following are other key areas for patient instruction:

- Information about the diagnosis
- Diagnostic studies
- Treatment plan
- Medication information
- Alternative or adjunctive therapies
- Safety issues/first aid for seizures
- Support services available (e.g., support groups, centers for independent living) and how to access them

HEALTH PROMOTION

Issues related to driving and other behaviors that impose a great safety risk should be discussed. Each state has varied restrictions for individuals with epilepsy who want to obtain a driver's license. Information regarding the laws of a particular state can be found by calling the state department of motor vehicles. Issues surrounding employment and psychosocial functioning should also be addressed. Resources such as vocational rehabilitation programs, clinical social workers, centers for independent living, and epilepsy support groups should be used.

Overall, moderation should be encouraged. Adequate rest, stress reduction, proper nutrition, and the avoidance of known seizure precipitants can improve seizure control.

Epilepsy is a challenging condition and requires a comprehensive approach to treatment. The goal is to treat the patient but to not make the treatment worse than the disease. Efforts in understanding the impact of epilepsy on patients will improve the ability of primary care providers to treat in an appropriate and compassionate manner.

REFERENCES

1. Shorvons S: *Handbook of epilepsy treatment,* Philadelphia, 2000, Blackwell Science, Inc.
2. French J and others: Characteristics of medial temporal lobe epilepsy. I. Results of history and physical examination, *Ann Neurol* 34:774-780, 1993.
3. Commission on Classification and Terminology of the International League Against Epilepsy: Proposal for revised clinical and electroencephalographic classification of epileptic seizures, *Epilepsia* 22:489-501, 1981.
4. Driefuss F: Classification of the epilepsies: influence on management. In Nancy Santilli, editor: *Managing seizure disorders: a handbook for health care practitioners,* Philadelphia, 1996, Lippincott-Raven.
5. Commission on Classification and Terminology of the International League Against Epilepsy: Proposal for revised classification of epilepsy and epileptic syndromes, *Epilepsia* 30:389-399, 1989.
6. Leppick I: *Contemporary diagnosis and management of the patient with epilepsy: handbooks in healthcare,* Newton, Penn, 1993, Handbooks in Health Care.
7. Williamson P: Frontal lobe seizures: problems of diagnosis and classification. In Chauvel P, Delgado-Escueta AV, editors: *Advances in neurology,* New York, 1992, Raven Press.
8. Ellis C: Considerations for individuals with developmental disabilities. In Santilli N, editor: *Managing seizure disorders: a handbook for health care practitioners,* Philadelphia, 1996, Lippincott-Raven.
9. So N, Andermann F: Differential diagnosis. In Engel J Jr, Pedley T, editors: *Epilepsy: a comprehensive textbook,* Philadelphia, 1997, Lippincott-Raven.
10. First Seizure Trial Group: Randomized clinical trial on the efficacy of antiepileptic drugs in reducing the risk of relapse after a first unprovoked tonic clonic seizure, *Neurology* 43:478-483, 1993.
11. Beghi E, Berg A, Hauser W: Treatment of single seizures. In Engel J Jr, Pedley T, editors: *Epilepsy: a comprehensive textbook,* Philadelphia, 1997, Lippincott-Raven.
12. Freeman J, Pedley T: Indications for treatment. In Engel J Jr, Pedley T, editors: *Epilepsy: a comprehensive textbook,* Philadelphia, 1997, Lippincott-Raven.
13. Santilli N: Selection and discontinuation of antiepileptic drugs. In Nancy Santilli, editor: *Managing seizure disorders: a handbook for health care practitioners,* Philadelphia, 1996, Lippincott-Raven.
14. Berg A, Shinnar S, Chadwick D: Discontinuing antiepileptic drugs. In Engel J Jr, Pedley T, editors: *Epilepsy: a comprehensive textbook,* Philadelphia, 1997, Lippincott-Raven.
15. Santilli N, Sierzant T: Surgical management of seizures. In Nancy Santilli, editor: *Managing seizure disorders: a handbook for health care practitioners,* Philadelphia, 1996, Lippincott-Raven.
16. Callahan M, Stalland N: Issues for women with epilepsy. In Nancy Santilli, editor: *Managing seizure disorders: a handbook for health care practitioners,* Philadelphia, 1996, Lippincott-Raven.
17. Morrell M: Hormones and epilepsy through the lifetime, *Epilepsia* 33(suppl 4):49-57, 1992.
18. Harden CL and others: The effect of menopause and perimenopause on the course of epilepsy, *Epilepsia* 40:1402-1407, 1999.
19. Working Group on Status Epilepticus: Treatment of status epilepticus, *JAMA* 270:854-859, 1992.
20. Ramsay E: Treatment of status epilepticus, *Epilepsia* 34(suppl 1):71-81, 1993.

CHAPTER 219

Trigeminal Neuralgia

Noreen M. Leahy

DEFINITION/EPIDEMIOLOGY

The fifth cranial nerve, the trigeminal nerve, is a large, mixed sensory and motor nerve that originates in the brainstem and travels in the cervical cord. The peripheral branches form the three sensory divisions (ophthalmic, maxillary, and mandibular), which conduct sensory impulses from the greater part of the face and head, from the cornea and conjunctiva, and from the nose and mouth. These impulses eventually terminate in the thalamus, where they are relayed to the appropriate cortical area for interpretation. The motor portion of the nerve supplies the muscles of the jaw and sphenoid areas. Rarely is the entire nerve interrupted; however, partial affection, particularly of the sensory component, is common.[1]

The most common and most elusive of the disorders that affect the sensory branches of the trigeminal nerve is trigeminal neuralgia (tic douloureux [from the French for "painful spasm"]). It has been known since ancient times, and to date there is no known cause for the majority of cases. Women are affected more often than men (3:2), and older adults more often than younger persons. The mean age of onset is 54 years for the idiopathic form and 33 years for the symptomatic form, in which an organic reason is evident.[2]

PATHOPHYSIOLOGY

Isolated or painful facial numbness may be caused by a variety of conditions, both intracranial and extracranial. Such extracranial causes may include trauma, edema, hematoma, hemorrhage, aneurysm, or neoplasm. Intracranial causes may arise from conditions affecting the eyes, ears, nose, throat, sinuses, teeth, and salivary glands. In addition, inflammatory conditions, including herpes zoster, systemic sclerosis, lupus erythematosus, multiple sclerosis, and Sjögren's syndrome, may manifest with facial pain.[3]

CLINICAL PRESENTATION

The primary feature of this disorder is recurrent paroxysms of pain in the distribution of any branch of the trigeminal nerve. The pain is usually described as burning, stabbing, sharp, penetrating, or electric shock–like and usually is on one side of the face. Males may present with unshaven faces or portions thereof. The index of suspicion for multiple sclerosis rises if the patient exhibits bilateral facial pain. The duration of each paroxysm varies from seconds to more than 15 minutes and most often involves the second and/or third branch of the trigeminal nerve.[1] Pain may recur once a month or several times per day. If the pain occurs frequently during the day, the patient may complain of unremitting facial discomfort between discrete episodes. Usually, a patient does not awaken from sleep during a paroxysm. Cold weather may dramatically increase the frequency of pain episodes.[4]

During an attack, the patient may cease talking, stop chewing, become very still, rub or pinch the face, avoid making facial expressions during conversation, grimace, or make movements of the face and jaw. Between attacks, the patient is free of symptoms except for fear of an impending attack.

PHYSICAL EXAMINATION

A characteristic feature of trigeminal neuralgia is the trigger zone: a small area of the skin or orobuccal mucosa that the patient can identify as the point that sets off an attack. Trigger points are generally in the distribution of the nerve branch experiencing the pain. Chewing, talking, facial movement, or touch may also elicit a paroxysm. Drafts or cool breezes may also precipitate symptoms.[5]

The individual may be reluctant to allow examination of the face for fear of triggering an attack. All cranial nerves should be examined in detail. The remainder of the physical examination, including the neurologic component, is normal.

DIAGNOSTICS AND DIFFERENTIAL DIAGNOSIS

The diagnosis of trigeminal neuralgia is usually made without difficulty from the history and the characteristic manner in which the patient relates the history (the patient is careful not to touch any trigger points or painful areas). However, the classic case presentation of trigeminal neuralgia may not always be encountered. Because there are innumerable causes of facial pain, prudence dictates that alternative diagnoses be investigated and that the patient be reexamined at regular intervals. The differential diagnosis should include consideration of headache, particularly migraine, acoustic neuroma, trigeminal neuroma, meningioma, aneurysms, acute polyneuropathy, chronic meningitis, and multiple sclerosis.

Results of laboratory tests are either normal or noncontributory. If alternative diagnoses are suspected, an autoimmune laboratory panel may be indicated. Magnetic resonance angiography (MRA) of the posterior fossa may be undertaken to differentiate vascular abnormalities. MRI can corroborate multiple sclerosis or mass lesions.

Diagnostics

Trigeminal Neuralgia

Imaging
Magnetic resonance tomographic angiography*
MRI*

*If indicated.

MANAGEMENT

The treatment of trigeminal neuralgia has not changed much over the past decade. Regardless of the intervention adopted, symptoms may remit spontaneously and permanently. Short-lived relief can be gained with

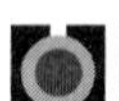

Differential Diagnosis

Trigeminal Neuralgia

Headache	Tumor
Acoustic neuroma	Dental disorders
Trigeminal neuroma	Abscess
Meningioma	Temporomandibular joint syndrome
Aneurysms	Sinusitis
Acute polyneuropathy	Migrainous neuralgia
Chronic meningitis	
Multiple sclerosis	

TABLE 219-1 Pharmacotherapy of Trigeminal Neuralgia

Generic Drug	Brand	Starting Dose	Maximum Dose	Complications
Carbamazepine	Tegretol	100-200 mg q day	200-400 mg t.i.d.	Aplastic anemia, agranylocytosis
Phenytoin	Dilantin	100-300 mg q day	300-500 mg q day	CNS effects
Gabapentin	Neurontin	100-300 mg q day	300-600 mg t.i.d.	CNS effects
Lamotrigine	Lamictal	25-50 mg q day	150-200 mg b.i.d.	Rash, Stevens-Johnson syndrome

the local administration of proparacaine into the conjunctival sac. When using anticonvulsant/antineuralgic therapy, the practitioner should titrate to the maximum therapeutic dose and avoid abrupt withdrawal (Table 219-1).

If the patient does not respond satisfactorily to the treatments provided in Table 219-1 or has relief only at a dose that causes intolerable adverse effects, combination drug therapy may be started with clonazepam (Klonopin) or a tricyclic antidepressant, such as amitriptyline (Elavil). On occasion, corticosteroids, such as methylprednisolone (Solu-Medrol), may be used. The long-acting prostaglandin E analogue misoprostol (Cytotec) has been useful in patients with trigeminal neuralgia associated with multiple sclerosis.[6]

COMPLICATIONS

Complications are usually related to management. Carbamazepine therapy may result in aplastic anemia, drowsiness, dizziness, or ataxia. Other medications also may have untoward effects. Surgical complications include facial numbness and infection, as well as the risk of any surgical procedure. Pain control may also be a significant factor, particularly if patients cannot tolerate the usually prescribed medications. In such an instance, additional management concerns may arise with weight loss, dehydration, and poor dental hygiene if chewing, liquids, and oral care are triggers.

INDICATIONS FOR REFERRAL/HOSPITALIZATION

The primary care provider is often the initial practitioner to evaluate the patient with facial pain. After a thorough history and neurologic examination, a patient presumed to have trigeminal neuralgia should be referred to a neurologist for a more comprehensive physical and imaging examination. Medical treatment may be initiated by the specialist and managed by the primary care provider. Care consists of medication initiation, observations for adverse effects, and consultation with the neurologist regarding dose adjustments and response to therapy. Referral to a neurosurgeon is indicated after medical therapies have been exhausted. Surgery is considered when medical regimens do not provide pain relief. The many procedures performed for the treatment of trigeminal neuralgia require an extensive knowledge of the brainstem and spinal anatomy and physiology, their projections, connections, and autonomic elements.[7]

Major disadvantages of radiofrequency and decompression surgery include loss of facial sensation (anesthesia dolorosa), dysesthesias, and recurrent neuralgia.[8] More traditional surgical approaches include ganglionectomy, rhizotomy, and tractotomy, in which the nerve or nerve root is ablated.

Consultation with a psychologist or psychiatrist may also be indicated, depending on the patient's adaptation skills. Multidisciplinary team meetings may be valuable in planning an approach to care. Referral to a pain center may also be an option for individuals with chronic pain.

PATIENT AND FAMILY EDUCATION

Significant education is necessary to explain the varied medication therapies, all of which are sedating. Caution about use of these medications in conjunction with use of alcohol and other medications is essential. If indicated, monitoring of laboratory tests is necessary to prevent commonly known complications of drug therapy. For patients in severe pain or those who are fearful of the next attack, it is important to consider the patient's activities of daily living, including eating, sleeping, and socializing with others. A collaborative relationship with the patient enhances a tailored, well-informed approach toward quality care.

REFERENCES

1. Adams RD, Victor M, Ropper AH: Diseases of the cranial nerves. In: *Principles of neurology,* ed 6, New York, 1997, McGraw-Hill.
2. Bowsher D: Trigeminal neuralgia: an anatomically oriented review, *Clin Anat* 10:409-415, 1997.
3. Lockerman LZ: Face and jaw pain. In Samuels MA, Faske S, editors: *Office practice of neurology,* New York, 1996, Churchill Livingstone.
4. Lechtenberg R: Trigeminal neuralgia. In Lechtenberg R, Schutta HS, editors: *Neurology practice guidelines,* New York, 1998, Marcel Dekker.
5. Adams AC: Facial pain. In: *Neurology in primary care,* Philadelphia, 2000, FA Davis.
6. Reder AT, Arnason BGW: Trigeminal neuralgia in multiple sclerosis relieved by prostaglandin-E analogue, *Neurology* 45:1097-1100, 1995.
7. Brown JA: The trigeminal complex: anatomy and physiology, *Neurosurg Clin North Am* 8:1-10, 1997.
8. Liao JJ and others: Reoperation for recurrent trigeminal neuralgia after microvascular decompression, *Surg Neurol* 47:562-568, 1997.

CHAPTER 220

Tumors of the Brain

Ann S. Bruner-Welch

DEFINITION/EPIDEMIOLOGY

A *tumor* is defined as excess tissue that develops when cells duplicate out of control somewhere in the body. The genetic "on-off" switch for replication gets stuck in the "on" position.[1,2] A tumor in the brain can be characterized as a benign or malignant expanding lesion and is either a primary tumor that originates in the brain or a secondary, metastatic tumor that originates elsewhere and travels to the brain via the blood or lymph systems. All brain tumors cause symptoms by infiltrating, expanding, and displacing healthy brain tissue.

Of all deaths from cancer, 2.4% result from tumors of the brain, with 50% of these patients dying within 1 to 3 years.[1] In the United States, approximately one third of brain tumors are primary in origin, with two thirds metastasized from other parts of the body, often the lung, breast, kidney, or gastrointestinal tract. Benign primary lesions tend to be treated more successfully than other brain tumors.

Many tumor types are identified and named for the cell of origin in the central nervous system (CNS). A meningioma originates from the meninges, an adenoma from glandular tissue, a sarcoma from CNS connective tissue, and a neuroma from neurons.[2] Tumor grading depends on cellular shape, size, and organization (Table 220-1). Staging evaluates the size and progression of tumor growth, the number of lymph nodes involved, and metastasis to other parts of the body.[3]

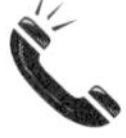

Physician consultation is indicated for all suspected brain tumors.

PATHOPHYSIOLOGY

The nervous system consists of two basic types of cells: neurons and neuroglia. Neurons carry and transmit electric impulses throughout the central and peripheral nervous systems. They are responsible for sensation, movement, the senses, and cognitive ability. New neurons are not produced after approximately 2 years of age. Therefore the incidence of tumor formation in neurons is very low.[1,2,4]

The neuroglia (nerve glue) cells are the connective tissue cells within the nervous system. There are several types of neuroglia cells, which outnumber neurons 5:1 to 10:1. Because these cells duplicate and divide throughout life, they are often the origin of primary tumors.[1,2,5]

Astrocytes are found in the gray or white matter of the brain. They twist around neurons to help form a supportive transport network, to connect neurons to blood vessels, and to help form the blood-brain barrier. Tumors in these cells are the most common and invasive of all primary brain tumors and have the poorest prognosis.[1-4,6] Oligodendrocytes also construct the semirigid support network between neurons and produce a conductive sheath around the neuronal axons and dendrites. Tumors in the oligodendrocytes are the next most common type of malignant brain tumor.[1-3] Microglia are small macrophages within the CNS. Ependymal cells are ciliated CNS epithelial cells that help circulate the cerebrospinal fluid. Neurolemmocytes (Schwann cells) are the oligodendrocytes of the peripheral nervous system (PNS). Satellite cells support ganglia in the PNS.[1-4]

CLINICAL PRESENTATION

Only generalized statements can be made about the symptoms of brain tumors.[1,4,5] These symptoms tend to be subtle and insidious in onset.[1,4,5,7] A tumor should be considered in the following specific circumstances: a stroke or seizure in a healthy gravid or postpartum patient or patients older than 20 years who have new seizures or new multiple endocrinopathies.[7] Generalized symptoms are described as follows:

- **Headache**—The most common initial symptom; typically a morning headache, sometimes rousing the patient from sleep; comes and goes, does not throb, and gradually improves during the day; worsens with exercise, coughing, or a change in body position
- **Neck pain**—Experienced by some patients
- **Seizures**—Experienced by 50% of patients
- **Mental changes**—Problems with memory, speech, communication, reasoning, or concentration; subtle or dramatic changes in interests, temperament, and affect
- **Constitutional symptoms**—Nausea, vomiting, weakness, drowsiness, loss of balance or coordination, unsteady gait, paralysis, or altered sensation
- **Vision problems**—Blurred or double vision, narrowed field of vision, crossed eyes, eye pain
- **Hearing problems**—Tinnitus, decreased hearing, earache

PHYSICAL EXAMINATION

Any areas that are pertinent to the patient's complaints should be examined because such abnormalities can aid in determining the location and extent of the tumor.[1,6] Other significant findings are elicited by careful examination of the following:

- **Eyes**—Extraocular movements (EOMs); pupils equal, round, react to light, and accommodation (PERRLA); visual fields; funduscopic examination; acuity; color
- **Ears**—Gross hearing, Weber's and Rinne's tests, audiogram as needed

TABLE 220-1 Tumor Staging

		Staging		
	Grading	T	N	M
0	Normal cell	No tumor	No nodes	No metastasis
I	Almost normal	Small tumor	A few nodes	Metastasis
II	Some changes	Moderate tumor	Many nodes	
III	Moderate changes	Large tumor		
IV	Very abnormal	Extensive tumor		

Data from Fleming ID and others: *AJCC cancer staging manual,* ed 5, Philadelphia, 1997, JB Lippincott.

T, Tumor; *N,* nodes; *M,* metastasis.

Neck—Range of motion (ROM), thyroid nodularity, palpation, nodes, suppleness
Neurologic system—Cranial nerves, deep tendon reflexes (DTRs), gait, Romberg's sign, Babinski's reflex, cerebellar testing, mental status, stereotactics, extremity sensation, motion/strength, full evaluation of focal neurologic deficits

DIAGNOSTICS

The most common diagnostic tests for brain tumors include MRI or CT.[1] Electroencephalography (EEG) may also be helpful.[4,7] If an abnormality is found, a neurooncologist may recommend a number of other studies to help define the extent of the tumor before biopsy.[1,3,4,5]

Blood tests may also be indicated, particularly if a prior tumor is being monitored. The tests look at specific hormones produced by cancers and can help to evaluate tumor progression or recurrence. A cancer specialist will indicate which antigen markers should be monitored and will clarify parameters that indicate a need for specialist evaluation.

DIFFERENTIAL DIAGNOSIS

Headaches have a variety of causes, the most common being migraines, cluster or tension headaches, and neck strain. An inquiry about trauma to exclude whiplash or a postconcussive headache is important. In addition, infectious causes, including sinusitis, otitis, herpes, meningitis, encephalitis, or abscesses, should be considered in the differential diagnosis. Other dangerous headaches include intracranial hemorrhage, stroke, trigeminal neuralgia, temporal arteritis, iritis, glaucoma, or poisoning (e.g., carbon monoxide exposure). Temporomandibular joint (TMJ) syndrome, eye strain, pseudotumor, and drug dependence and/or addiction should be considered.[4,7,8]

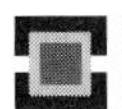
Diagnostics

Tumors of the Brain

Laboratory
Tumor markers*

Imaging
CT scan/MRI*
PET* (consult with radiologist to determine if contrast is indicated)

Other
EEG*

*If indicated.

MANAGEMENT

Physician consultation is essential if a brain or spinal cord tumor is suspected. Specific tumor treatment requires evaluation and management by the appropriate specialist. The emotional implications of a brain or spinal cord tumor diagnosis can be tremendous for the patient and family.[1,5] Tremendous support is necessary. Questions should be answered openly and honestly, and resources should be offered for questions that the primary care provider is unable to answer.

When developing a treatment plan, the provider should not only recognize the diagnosis but also consider the patient; the patient's age, life potential, desires, and physical abilities should be considered. The patient and family should be assisted with the development of the treatment plan and advanced directives if possible.

It is important that patients be safe. If a seizure or recurrent loss of consciousness is part of the clinical picture, the patient should not drive a motor vehicle. Unfortunately, this may affect the patient's mobility and ability for independent living. Offering available alternatives is helpful.

If there is evidence of increased intracranial pressure, dexamethasone (10 mg every 6 hours) should be considered. If the patient is having seizures, anticonvulsants should usually be prescribed. A 1-g loading dose of phenytoin (Dilantin) followed by 300 to 400 mg/day is recommended. If brain edema is present, a fluid shunt may be placed if the pressure continues to be a problem.[3-5,7]

If possible, both primary and metastatic tumors may be treated surgically.[3,4,7] The tumor must be in a relatively accessible area. The surgeon tries to spare normal brain or spinal cord tissue as much as possible. Radiation and, finally, chemotherapy are used as adjunctive therapies. There are also a number of alternative experiments. Clinical trials should be considered as an option.[3-5,7] (See Table 220-2 for the treatment and prognosis of primary brain tumors.)

Palliative alternatives are an essential consideration if the patient is not a candidate for the previously mentioned therapies or the therapies have failed. Hospice, for example, can be helpful in preparing and caring for the patient and family during the terminal phase of the illness.

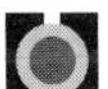
Differential Diagnosis

Tumors of the Brain

Migraine	Temporal arteritis
Cluster headache	Iritis
Tension headache	Cerebrovascular accident
Cervical tension headache	Seizure disorder
Postconcussive headache	Pseudotumor
Sinusitis	Carbon monoxide poisoning
Otitis	Herpes
Meningitis, encephalitis	Glaucoma
Abscess	TMJ syndrome
Trigeminal neuralgia	

COMPLICATIONS

Tumor growth may compress vital organs, block the flow of various fluids, and cause endocrinopathies, weakness or paralysis, and the loss of various senses. Vascular compromise, including coagulopathies, disseminated intravascular coagulopathy, cerebrovascular accidents, thrombocytopenia, intracranial hemorrhage or pressure, and thromboses, can also be problematic.[1,3,5] The mass effect from fluid accumulation or tumor growth can further damage delicate brain tissue.[1,3,5]

Tumor therapies can also cause difficulties, including immunosuppression, hair loss, weakness, fatigue, and gastrointestinal upset or bleeding. Any of the previously discussed therapies can cause neurologic or psychologic problems. Cancer metastasis or recurrence requires continual monitoring.

INDICATIONS FOR REFERRAL/HOSPITALIZATION

Neurosurgical and oncologic referral for definitive treatment is imperative, and early consultation is indicated. The development of new symptoms requires a referral to the specialist for

TABLE 220-2 Treatment and Prognosis of Primary Brain Tumors

Tumor Type	Good Evidence	Clinical Trials	Prognosis/Longevity
Astrocytoma Grade I	Surgery alone or surgery + radiation	Nitrosourea-based or biologic response modifiers	Excellent if excised
Astrocytoma Grade II or III	Surgery + radiation	Surgery if age <35 years and no enhancement on CT; chemotherapy if resistant	Good to fair "Cytoma" better than "blastoma/anaplastic"
Astrocytoma Grade IV	Surgery + radiation Surgery + radiation + chemotherapy	Radioactive polymer implant Various radiation techniques	Poor Mean survival age <65 years, 7-9 months; 11-13 months with treatment
Ependymoma: well differentiated	Surgery Surgery + radiation	Nitrosourea-based or biologic response modifiers	5-year disease free 80% if excised
Ependymoma: anaplastic or blastoma	Surgery + radiation	Chemotherapy after radiation Nitrosourea-based or biologic response modifiers if recurrent	Variable Fair to poor
Germinomas: embryonal, carcinoma, meningioma, teratoma, chorocarcinoma, craniopharyngioma	Surgery Surgery + radiation	Debulking and radiation if unresectable; chemotherapy if malignant	Better if resectable 5-year survival >85% if resected
Glioma: brainstem	Radiation	Biologic response modifiers	Poor: 44-74 weeks
Glioblastoma multiforme	Surgery + radiation + chemotherapy Surgery + radiation	Various radiation treatments Biologic response modifiers	Poor
Lymphoma: primary CNS (associated with Epstein-Barr virus)	Glucocorticoids Radiation Radiation + steroids	Chemotherapy	Poor Disease relapses within weeks 18-month survival
Lymphoma: secondary CNS (associated with B-cell lymphoma/leukemia)	Chemotherapy + radiation		Determined by the course of underlying systemic disease
Meduloblastoma	Surgery + craniospinal radiation	Debulking + radiation + chemotherapy if unresectable	>70% at 5 years <50% children survive to adulthood 50% relapse in 5 years
Meningioma	Surgery	Multiple radiation techniques	Surgery is curative if resectable
Pituitary adenoma	Surgery + radiation	Chemotherapy	Recurrence <10%
Oligodendroglioma	Surgery if <45 years and no enhancement on contrast CT Surgery + radiation	Chemotherapy + radiation after surgery if anaplastic	5 years >50% 10 years 25% Better if minimal infiltration and if surgically resectable
Schwannomas: neuroma, neurinoma neurolemmoma	Surgery Surgery + radiation	Various radiation techniques	Good

Data from CancerNet-Health Professionals: PDQ Adult Brain Tumors, National Cancer Institute National Guidelines, *Radiology* 215 Suppl:1105-1128; and Sager S, Israel M: Primary and metastatic tumors of the nervous system. In Braunwald E and others, editors: *Harrison's principles of internal medicine,* ed 15, Philadelphia, 2002, McGraw-Hill.

evaluation of specific treatments, tumor progression, or new tumor formation. In general, hospitalization is reserved for patients with severe symptoms or unstable clinical findings that cannot be safely or efficiently managed in the outpatient setting. Tumor removal may be performed in a surgical center or limited-stay hospital setting.

PATIENT AND FAMILY EDUCATION

Dietary considerations depend on tumor type, specific medications, and co-morbid illness.[5] Pharmacists and nutritionists may be helpful resources. In general, patients should be encouraged to follow a diet that is as normal and healthy as possible. A thorough understanding of the disease process is usually helpful for patients and families. Many useful books are available in public and medical center libraries, and the Internet contains an enormous amount of information and a large number of support groups.

REFERENCES

1. William J, Weiner G: *Neurology for the nonneurologist,* ed 3, Baltimore, 1994, JB Lippincott.
2. Tortora GJ: *Principles of human anatomy,* ed 6, New York, 1992, HarperCollins.

3. National Cancer Institute, CancerWeb, Adult Brain Tumor 208/01143, 1997. Retrieved August 12, 2002, from the World Wide Web: http://www.graylab.ac.uk/cancernet/101143.html.
4. Scheinburg P: *An introduction to diagnosis and management of common neurologic disorders,* ed 3, Philadelphia, 1986, Raven Press.
5. *A primer of brain tumors,* American Brain Tumor Association, 27020 River Road, Des Plaines, IL 60018; (847) 827-9910; e-mail: infoabta.org; retrieved August 12, 2002, from the World Wide Web: http://www.abta.org/booklet.htm 1997.
6. Tatter MD: WHO: the new WHO classification of tumors affecting the central nervous system, 1998. Retrieved August 12, 2002, from the World Wide Web: http://neurosurgery.mgh.harvard.edu/newwhobt.htm.
7. Cantu RC: *Neurology in primary care,* New York, 1985, Macmillan.
8. Olson WH and others: *Symptom-oriented neurology: handbook for primary care,* ed 2, St Louis, 1989, Mosby.

PART 17

Evaluation and Management of Endocrine and Metabolic Disorders

JOANNE SANDBERG-COOK, Section Editor

CHAPTER 221

Acromegaly

Suzanne Mary Rieke and Alan Ona Malabanan

DEFINITION/EPIDEMIOLOGY

Acromegaly is an insidious, chronic, debilitating disease arising from the prolonged excessive secretion of growth hormone (GH). This excess GH manifests as excessive bone and soft tissue growth. Untreated or partially treated patients with acromegaly have double the expected mortality rate of age-matched healthy subjects. The increased prevalence of hypertension and diabetes mellitus associated with acromegaly increases cardiovascular morbidity and mortality. Sleep apnea associated with acromegaly may also lead to cardiopulmonary decline. Motor vehicle accidents from daytime somnolence and sleep deprivation contribute to the overall mortality risk. Patients with acromegaly may also have an increased risk for malignancy, particularly of the colon.

Acromegaly is rare, but the diagnosis is commonly delayed or missed. Recent studies have suggested a prevalence of 40 to 60 cases per 1 million persons and an annual incidence of 3 cases per 1 million persons per year.[1] It is usually diagnosed in middle age, with a mean age at diagnosis of 40 years in men and 45 years in women. When GH excess occurs in children (before the closure of the epiphyseal plates), gigantism results.

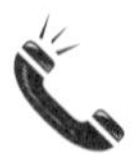

Physician consultation is indicated for all patients with suspected acromegaly.

PATHOPHYSIOLOGY

GH is secreted by cells in the anterior pituitary gland. Its secretion is regulated by the two hypothalamic hormones: growth hormone–releasing hormone (GHRH) and somatostatin (SS). GHRH stimulates both GH secretion and production, whereas SS inhibits GH secretion. GH secretion is pulsatile, with brief surges followed by long periods of inactivity. Many physiologic stimuli affect GH secretion, including stress (increased), sleep (increased), meals (increased or decreased), and aging (decreased). The variable nature of a random serum GH level limits its usefulness in diagnosing acromegaly.

Insulin-like growth factor I (IGF-I, or somatomedin C) is a GH-dependent protein produced by the liver. Its serum level is directly proportional to the 24-hour integrated serum GH level, and it is a much better indicator of GH excess than a random serum GH level. The bone and soft tissue growth in acromegaly is a direct result of the effects of GH and IGF-I. In addition, GH has several other metabolic effects, including insulin antagonism, lipolysis, and protein anabolism, resulting in glucose intolerance, decreased fat stores, and increased muscle mass.

The most common cause of GH excess is a GH-secreting pituitary adenoma. Rare (<1%) causes include GHRH-producing tumors such as hypothalamic (hamartomas), bronchial carcinoid, and pancreatic islet cell tumors. Ectopic production of GH has been described in pancreatic islet cell tumors. Acromegaly may be associated with multiple endocrine neoplasia type 1 (MEN-1); a triad of pituitary tumor, hyperparathyroidism, and pancreatic tumor; and McCune-Albright syndrome, a genetic disease associated with polyostotic fibrous dysplasia, café au lait spots, and endocrine hyperfunction.

CLINICAL PRESENTATION

Acromegaly in younger patients tends to result from more aggressive tumors and may develop relatively rapidly.[2] In older patients, it develops insidiously over many years. As mentioned previously, the diagnosis is often delayed, with most patients having symptoms for 10 to 20 years. Symptoms result from the effects of GH excess or from the pituitary mass's effect on surrounding brain structures. An evaluation of 500 patients with acromegaly revealed the following most common clinical features (in order of decreasing frequency): excessive acral growth, enlargement of facial features, soft tissue swelling, excessive sweating, headache, peripheral neuropathy, decreased energy, paresthesia, osteoarthritis, impotence, daytime somnolence, carpal tunnel syndrome, muscular weakness, depression, decreased libido, hypertrichosis, dyspnea, and galactorrhea. About half of these patients had hypertension, and 66% had abnormal glucose metabolism (either glucose intolerance or frank diabetes mellitus).[3] Visual field disturbance and amenorrhea may also be presenting complaints.

PHYSICAL EXAMINATION

The earliest and most common physical changes occur in the skin and extremities. The growth of the soft tissues produces facial puffiness, broadening of the nose, furrowing of the brow, skin thickening (bogginess) of the hands and feet, and enlargement of the tongue, uvula, and soft palate, leading to sleep apnea. Vocal cord thickening results in a deeper and coarser voice. Skin tags (acrochordon) are more common in patients with acromegaly, as are colonic polyps.

Facial bone growth leads to coarsened facial features, which are usually recognizable only when they are very severe or after review of the patient's old photographs. These changes include growth of the calvarium and mandible, producing a prominent brow, an enlarged jaw, and dental malocclusion. With growth of the jaw, there is also widening of the spaces between the teeth. Excessive rib growth produces a barrel-shaped chest. A glove and shoe size change results from bone growth in the hands and feet. Loss of lateral visual fields (bitemporal hemianopsia), papilledema, extraocular palsy, or even rhinorrhea may result from the pituitary tumor's impingement on surrounding structures.

DIAGNOSTICS

Random serum GH levels are not useful in the diagnosis of acromegaly. IGF-I, IGF-binding protein-3 (IGFBP-3), and 24-hour urine study for GH are all GH dependent and are useful as screening tests for acromegaly.[4,5] It is important that these tests be done at laboratories with age-adjusted reference ranges because GH secretion normally decreases with age. Unfortunately, normal and abnormal values for these tests may overlap.

The definitive test for acromegaly is the oral glucose tolerance test (OGTT),[5] which most clearly demonstrates pathologic GH secretion. In a normal individual, GH secretion is suppressed by an oral glucose load. This test is contraindicated in a patient with poorly controlled diabetes mellitus.

The test is conducted as follows: after an overnight fast, blood is drawn for a baseline serum glucose and GH level. Glucose 75 g is given orally. Samples for serum glucose and GH are then taken every 30 minutes for a total of 120 minutes after the oral glucose challenge. In a normal individual, GH should be suppressed to less than 2 ng/ml by radioimmunoassay (RIA) and to less than 1 ng/ml by the newer immunoradiometric assay (IRMA).[6] In a patient with acromegaly there is failure of suppression of GH after a glucose load. As newer assays become more sensitive, it is likely that these criteria will change. Results of the OGTT should always be evaluated together with the IGF-1 measurement.

After the biochemical diagnosis of acromegaly, imaging of the pituitary gland should be performed, preferably with MRI. If no pituitary tumor is seen or if generalized pituitary hyperplasia is seen, the possibility of ectopic GHRH production should be considered. A plasma GHRH determination may be helpful in this instance.

DIFFERENTIAL DIAGNOSIS

The primary differential diagnostic consideration in acromegaly is an etiologic one: What is the cause of the GH excess? A few other situations, however, should be examinted. Pseudoacromegaly is a syndrome characterized by acromegaloid features and severe insulin resistance without elevated GH or IGF-I levels. Benign familial prognathism may prompt evaluation for acromegaly, but GH and IGF-I levels are normal. Paget's disease of bone can cause bony deformities, particularly in the skull, but, again, GH and IGF-I levels should be normal. Although the OGTT is the standard test for the diagnosis of acromegaly, there are some conditions in which GH secretion fails to suppress after a glucose load. Among these are severe liver or renal disease, uncontrolled diabetes mellitus, malnutrition, anorexia nervosa, heroin addiction, and levodopa ingestion.[7]

Diagnostics

Acromegaly

Laboratory
Serum IGF-1 level
IGFBP-3
24-hour urine study for GH
Plasma GHRH*
Oral glucose tolerance test (OGTT)

Imaging
MRI

Other
Oral glucose tolerance test for GH suppression

*If indicated.

Differential Diagnosis

Acromegaly

Pseudoacromegaly	Uncontrolled diabetes
Benign familial prognathism	Malnutrition
Paget's disease	Anorexia nervosa
Severe liver disease	Heroin addiction
Severe renal disease	Levodopa ingestion

MANAGEMENT AND CO-MANAGEMENT WITH SPECIALISTS

Acromegaly should be co-managed with an endocrinologist experienced in managing acromegaly and hypopituitarism. Early diagnosis is crucial in curing this disease because the success of surgical therapy, the therapy of choice, is dependent on tumor size. Cure is defined as a reduction in IGF-1 to the age-adjusted normal range and a suppressed GH after OGTT to less than 1 ng/ml.[6] For those with small (<10 mm), well-localized pituitary tumors, the cure rate is approximately 70% to 80% at major neurosurgical centers.[6,8] The cure rate decreases to less than 50% for tumors larger than 10 mm.

For patients who are not surgical candidates and for patients with postsurgery recurrence, two alternatives exist: pituitary irradiation and medical therapy. Pituitary irradiation effects are delayed. Ten years after irradiation, 50% of patients have adequate GH suppression by old criteria (<5 ng/ml).[9] There is a high risk of hypopituitarism complicating this procedure. Medical treatment is required for patients in whom radiotherapy is ineffective.

Octreotide (an SS analogue) and bromocriptine (a dopamine agonist) are the two most commonly used medical therapies. Octreotide is given as three daily subcutaneous injections (100 to 250 μg per dose) and has produced normalization of IGF-I in 60% and GH of less than 2 ng/ml in 40% of 103 patients studied recently.[10] New long-acting formulations of SS analogues (octreotide-LAR and lantreotide) are now available and have similar efficacy with the benefit of less frequent administration (IM injection every 2 to 4 weeks).[11,12] Bromocriptine is titrated to a maximum of 20 mg/day and is given orally. It is, however, less effective than octreotide; less than 10% have normalization of IGF-1 and less than 20% have GH of less than 5 ng/ml.[9] The most common side effects are gastrointestinal for both bromocriptine (nausea and vomiting) and octreotide (diarrhea, abdominal discomfort, and gallstones). Newer agents, including a growth hormone receptor antagonist, continue to be investigated as medical treatment options.[13]

LIFE SPAN CONSIDERATIONS

When GH excess occurs in children (before the closure of the epiphyseal plates), gigantism results. Acromegaly in younger patients tends to result from more aggressive tumors and may develop relatively rapidly.[2] In older patients it develops insidiously over many years. Untreated or partially treated patients with acromegaly have double the expected mortality rate of age-matched healthy subjects. The diagnosis is often delayed, with most patients having symptoms for 10 to 20 years.

COMPLICATIONS

The complications associated with advanced acromegaly are numerous and include diabetes, hypertension, sleep apnea, osteoarthritis, peripheral neuropathies, and increased incidence of malignancy. These conditions affect quality of life and increase mortality rates. All patients need to be managed in collaboration with a physician because many of the complications may not remit after therapy of the GH excess. Complications of surgical or radiation therapy include hypopituitarism and may require consultation with an endocrinologist.

INDICATIONS FOR REFERRAL/HOSPITALIZATION

All patients suspected of having acromegaly should be referred to an endocrinologist experienced in the evaluation and treatment of acromegaly, if possible. The rarity of this condition, its increased mortality rate, and the complexity of its manifestations make this critical. Patients with evidence of pituitary tumor mass effect or hemorrhage need urgent neurosurgical referral.

Advanced acromegaly may lead to neurologic or cardiovascular complications (e.g., pituitary or myocardial infarction), requiring hospitalization. Any patient with new symptoms of headache, visual disturbance, dyspnea, or chest pain should be promptly evaluated.

PATIENT EDUCATION AND HEALTH PROMOTION

The normalization of GH and IGF-I levels is essential in the successful management of acromegaly and requires patient adherence and diligence to the prescribed medical therapy. Patients should realize that acromegaly is a chronic and progressive disease, resulting in a multitude of complications that may be avoided or delayed with prompt and appropriate therapy. Patients should be aware that the changes in physical appearance will likely not remit even with successful therapy but will likely worsen if the condition is not treated. Patients should be alerted to the symptoms of sleep apnea, diabetes mellitus, heart disease, and hypopituitarism so that appropriate evaluation and therapy may be undertaken.

REFERENCES

1. Etxabe J and others: Acromegaly: an epidemiologic study, *J Endocrinol Invest* 16:181-187, 1993.
2. Melmed S and others: Recent advances in pathogenesis, diagnosis, and management of acromegaly, *J Clin Endocrinol Metab* 80:3395-3402, 1995.
3. Ezzat S and others: Acromegaly: clinical and biochemical features in 500 patients, *Medicine* 73:233-240, 1994.
4. Grinspoon S and others: Serum insulin-like growth factor–binding protein-3 levels in the diagnosis of acromegaly, *J Clin Endocrinol Metab* 80:927-932, 1995.
5. Stoffel-Wagner B and others: A comparison of different methods for diagnosing acromegaly, *Clin Endocrinol* 46:531-537, 1997.
6. Giustina A and others: Criteria for cure of acromegaly: a consensus statement, *J Clin Endocrinol Metab* 85:526-529, 2000.
7. Wass JAH, Besser M: Tests of pituitary function. In DeGroot LJ, editor: *Endocrinology*, ed 3, Philadelphia, 1995, WB Saunders.
8. Kreutzer J and others: Surgical management of GH-secreting pituitary adenomas: an outcome study using modern remission criteria, *J Clin Endocrinol Metab* 86:4072-4077, 2001.
9. Melmed S and others: Current treatment guidelines for acromegaly, *J Clin Endocrinol Metab* 83:2646-2652, 1998.
10. Newman CB and others: Safety and efficacy of long term octreotide therapy of acromegaly: results of a multicenter trial in 103 patients: a clinical research study, *J Clin Endocrinol Metab* 80:2768-2775, 1995.
11. Colao AM and others: Long-term effects of depot long-acting somatostatin analog octreotide on hormone levels and tumor mass in acromegaly, *J Clin Endocrinol Metab* 86:2779-2786, 2001.
12. Baldelli R and others: Two-year follow-up of acromegalic patients treated with slow release lantreotide, *J Clin Endocrinol Metab* 85:4099-4103, 2000.
13. Trainer PJ and others: Treatment of acromegaly with the growth hormone-receptor antagonist pegvisomant, *N Engl J Med* 342:1171-1177, 2000.

CHAPTER 222

Adrenal Gland Disorders

Dennis M. McCullough

DEFINITION/EPIDEMIOLOGY

Adrenal gland disorders are conditions marked by inadequate or excessive amounts of glucocorticoid and mineralocorticoid hormones. These conditions can result from overproduction as a consequence of changes in the adrenal gland itself, from hypothalamic or pituitary gland dysfunction, or through the exogenous administration of corticosteroid medications. A second major hormone, aldosterone, a mineralocorticoid, is independently produced in the adrenal cortex and regulates renal and electrolyte (mineral) metabolism. Small amounts of androgens produced by the adrenal cortex also are the origin of certain clinical syndromes. Three common types of adrenal gland disorders are discussed: Addison's disease, Cushing's syndrome, and pheochromocytoma.

Addison's Disease

Historically, Addison's disease most commonly occurred as a result of bilateral destruction of the adrenal glands by tuberculosis. More recently, Addison's disease has been associated with autoimmune disturbances. Recent increases in tuberculosis worldwide may alter these patterns. Data from Great Britain suggest that the prevalence of Addison's disease is 100 per 1 million individuals, with one third of these cases being tuberculous in origin.[1]

Cushing's Syndrome

Determining the prevalence of Cushing's syndrome is complicated by pseudo-Cushing's syndrome, which is associated with both depression and obesity. Eighty percent of patients with major depression also have abnormal cortisol secretion. Thus there clearly is a spectrum of disorders associated with the overproduction of cortisol.[2] Incidental adrenal adenoma found on CT and MRI imaging suggests possible early hypercortisolism and may occur at the rate of 20 to 30 per 1 million individuals.[3]

Pheochromocytoma

A pheochromocytoma is a tumor of chromaffin cells. Ninety percent of these tumors are found in the adrenal medulla. A small percent may arise intraabdominally along the sympathetic ganglion chain, which also comprises chromaffin tissue. A malignant process occurs when the tumor spreads beyond chromaffin tissue. Pheochromocytomas are typically unilateral; however, type II bilateral involvement is common in the setting of polyglandular multiple endocrine neoplasia (MEN).

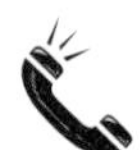

Physician consultation is indicated for patients with adrenal gland disorders.

PATHOPHYSIOLOGY

Hypothalamus-synthesized corticotropin (ACTH)-releasing hormone (CRH) regulates the secretion of ACTH, which in turn regulates the production of glucocorticoids. The glucocorticoids (cortisol) regulate the metabolic processes in the body in response to normal and abnormal both physical and psychologic. This is accomplished by altering physiologic responses that range from hepatic glucose production to inflammatory and vascular reactions.

Underproduction disorders relate to the destruction or dysfunction of some portion of the hypothalamic-pituitary-adrenal axis or to the sudden consequences of withdrawing exogenous corticosteroids after high-dose use. Autoimmune disorders currently account for most cases of Addison's disease. Because more than 90% of both adrenal glands must be destroyed or malfunctioning before clinically recognized adrenal insufficiency is present, destruction by tuberculosis, bilateral hemorrhage or vein thrombosis, medications (rifampin, ketoconazole), and rare infections (meningococcemia, AIDS, histoplasmosis) are among the very rare remaining causes. Inadequate production of cortisol in the context of severe sudden illness or trauma, particularly in chronic users of corticosteroids, is a more common manifestation.

Cushing's syndrome results from ACTH-secreting tumors of the pituitary and occasionally from other conditions, including ectopic secretion of small-cell lung carcinomas. Cortisol and ACTH levels are elevated. In rare instances, Cushing's syndrome results from primary overproduction of cortisol by the adrenal gland (low levels of serum ACTH and high levels of serum cortisol). Steroid medications systematically suppress pituitary production of ACTH, particularly when steroids are administered in high doses over long periods of time. Both short- and long-term use (>10 to 14 days) of corticosteroids are a common and appropriate part of the management of asthma, difficult dermatitis problems, various malignancies, rheumatic diseases, and a number of other acute and chronic disorders. Careful monitoring is mandatory to avoid, or to detect early, the impact on endogenous corticosteroid production.

Abnormal production of epinephrine and norepinephrine by a pheochromocytoma produces multisystem effects. Renal effects include sodium retention, increased renin secretion, and reduction of hydrostatic pressure. Cardiovascular effects involve peripheral vasoconstrictors and increased cardiac contraction. Tissue oxygen consumption and gluconeogenesis are increased.

CLINICAL PRESENTATION

Addison's disease may present suddenly, or a patient with known Addison's disease who is inadequately supplemented with corticosteroids can exhibit a sudden onset of nausea, vomiting, hypotension, and acute shock, especially during a period of severe trauma or illness. However, most presentations are chronic, with dizziness, nausea, vomiting, chronic abdominal pain, muscle cramps, hyperpigmentation, decreased libido, lethargy, weakness, weight loss, and a progressive decline of health.

Cushing's syndrome almost always presents with chronic changes; the exception is a patient who has been taking high-dose steroids over a prolonged period. Sudden weight gain, loss of menses, decreased libido, weakness, depression, insomnia, and bruising are all possible presenting symptoms.

With pheochromocytoma, there may be a family history of the disease, MEN, neurofibromatosis, or multiple neuroma syndrome. Presenting symptoms are episodic and include headache, facial flushing, diaphoresis, and palpitations. The symptomatic episodes last 15 to 30 minutes and may be precipitated by specific activities.

PHYSICAL EXAMINATION

Patients with Addison's disease appear chronically ill. They exhibit weight loss, dehydration, and increased skin pigmentation—a result of melanocyte stimulation by pituitary hormones attempting to drive the adrenal glands. Palmar creases and creases of the elbows, knees, and lips are commonly involved. Occasionally, vitiligo is reported.

Patients with Cushing's syndrome have a characteristic habitus similar to many patients with exogenous obesity. Central obesity, a "moon face" appearance caused by thickening of facial fat, the classically described "buffalo hump" dorsocervical fat pad (very common with all obesity), increased supraclavicular fat pads, hypertension, thigh muscle weakness and wasting, hirsutism, abdominal skin striae, and acne can be associated signs. Emotional lability or depression may be associated signs.

With pheochromocytoma, the physical examination is marked by a new onset of moderate to severe hypertension, with systolic pressures above 170 mm Hg. Arrhythmias or sinus tachycardia or bradycardia may be present. The course is characterized by substantial variations in blood pressure measurements.

DIAGNOSTICS

Patients with Addison's disease have an elevated serum ACTH level and suppressed levels of cortisol. Hyponatremia and hyperkalemia related to lost aldosterone production might be a serendipitous finding that suggests Addison's disease. Eosinophilia, azotemia, and hypoglycemia may be present. Adrenal antibody studies to identify autoimmune disorders should be ordered in concert with an endocrinology consultation. Chest x-ray studies and tuberculin testing are essential to exclude underlying tuberculosis.

Metabolic acidosis or decreased potassium or chloride may be present, but Cushing's syndrome is most accurately determined with measurement of the 24-hour excretion of cortisol in the urine. This excretion study is thought to be more dependable than serum ACTH and serum cortisol testing. Confirmation of the 24-hour

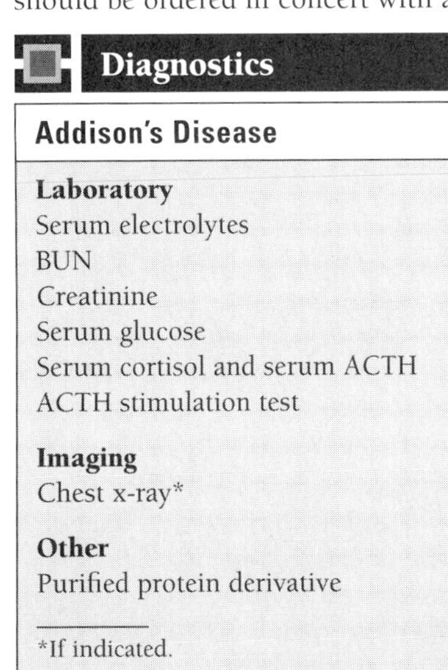
Diagnostics

Addison's Disease

Laboratory
Serum electrolytes
BUN
Creatinine
Serum glucose
Serum cortisol and serum ACTH
ACTH stimulation test

Imaging
Chest x-ray*

Other
Purified protein derivative

*If indicated.

urine cortisol elevation by two or three repeat tests is important because cortisol production can vary markedly from day to day, even in Cushing's syndrome. Pursuit of this elusive diagnosis is an appropriate aspect of a primary care practice. Suppression testing with ACTH is another laborious diagnostic process and may require careful pursuit to separate the physiology of the obese and depressed patients from that of those with true Cushing's syndrome.[4] Consultation is required for testing to separate disorders primary to the pituitary from those primary to the adrenal glands.

Elevated levels of catecholamines in a 24-hour urine collection confirm the diagnosis of pheochromocytoma. To increase accuracy, the collection must occur during a period of hypertension in association with episodes of facial flushing, diaphoresis, or palpitations. Many medications alter the accuracy of the test. For example, alcohol, amphetamines, quinidine, theophylline, tetracycline, clofibrate, and disulfiram can raise or lower catecholamine levels. Therefore a careful medication review and consultation of current test guidelines must occur. Specialist consultation concerning test results may be indicated. With abnormal test results, the presence and extent of the tumor are determined by adrenal CT scan or MRI.

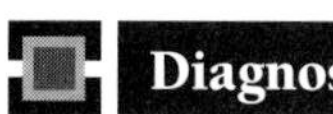

Diagnostics

Cushing's Disease

Laboratory
Creatinine
24-hour urine for cortisol
ACTH suppression test

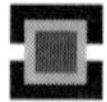

Diagnostics

Pheochromocytoma

Laboratory
24-hour urine for catecholamines, metanephrines,* and vanillylmandelic acid*

Imaging
CT scan/MRI*

*If indicated.

DIFFERENTIAL DIAGNOSIS

Both Addison's disease and Cushing's syndrome can be difficult to distinguish from normal physiology, particularly because both chronic and acute stresses have such an impact on adrenal hormone production.[5] Addisonian symptoms, when mild, can be produced by eating disorders, alcoholism, malnutrition, hyperthyroidism, diabetes, and the wasting effects of a chronic illness such as AIDS or metastatic cancer. Psychiatric symptoms, including apathy, confusion, and depression, are common with adrenal insufficiency presentations and often confound the clinical assessment. By far the most commonly seen conditions are those associated with exogenous steroid use, as well as withdrawal or inadequate steroid use in circumstances of stress. Cushing's syndrome can be confused with the presence of depression or obesity. Pheochromocytoma is most commonly confused with anxiety or labile "white coat" hypertension.

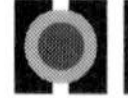

Differential Diagnosis

Adrenal Gland Disorders

Addison's Disease	**Pheochromocytoma**
Eating disorders	Essential hypertension
Alcoholism	Anxiety
Malnutrition	Intracranial neoplasm
Hyperthyroidism	Subarachnoid/intracranial hemorrhage
Diabetes	Medication withdrawal (clonidine or monoamine oxidase inhibitor)
Chronic illness	**Diencephalia epilepsy**
Psychogenic illness	
Cushing's Syndrome	
Obesity	
Depression	

MANAGEMENT

An acute adrenal crisis is best managed in the hospital, although treatment for shock with corticosteroids should begin immediately. Chronic adrenal insufficiency is generally a nonemergency and can be treated in an outpatient context with oral hydrocortisone in divided daily doses (total, 20 to 30 mg) to allow for restoration of a diurnal pattern. Individualized dosing patterns guided by patients' symptomatic responses should be carefully constructed. Mineralocorticoid replacement in Addison's syndrome is managed with fludrocortisone (dose range, 0.05 to 0.2 mg/day PO) to correct the renal disturbance and consequent hypotension. The need for replacement doses is monitored by frequent measurement of electrolytes, serum renin, serum ACTH, and judiciously timed serum cortisol levels. Careful dose adjustments can enhance a patient's sense of well-being and quality of life.

Management of Cushing's syndrome depends on the source of the hypercortisolism. Current imaging techniques have enhanced the approach to pituitary surgery and greatly aid in the search for nonadrenal sources of ACTH and adrenal sources of cortisol. In these cases, pituitary tumor resection remains the first choice for therapy. Chemotherapy treatments may be used adjunctively. Radiation therapy has a lesser role and is occasionally used for long-term management where surgery fails or is inappropriate. There are medical therapies for Cushing's syndrome, which require consultation with an endocrinologist.

The management issues for pheochromocytoma depend on an accurate diagnosis of tumor. Treatment is surgical removal of the tumor, if indicated.

COMPLICATIONS

Immediate life-threatening complications are generally confined to acute adrenal crisis. With chronic Addison's disease and Cushing's syndrome, complications are prevented by giving careful attention to the side effects of exogenous steroids and to the patient's symptoms, physiologic and emotional functioning, and metabolic status. With chronic adrenal insufficiency, complications from co-morbid conditions that result in periods of sudden adrenal inadequacy can be reduced by the availability of injectable hydrocortisone for home use. With Cushing's syndrome, osteoporosis is a common complication. In addition to monitoring for osteoporosis, patients should be observed for hypertension and diabetes. Hypertensive crisis is a potential complication of pheochromocytoma.

INDICATIONS FOR REFERRAL/HOSPITALIZATION

If acute adrenal insufficiency is suspected, immediate referral and hospitalization are required. Consultation with an endocrinologist is warranted if the diagnostic evaluation suggests either Addison's disease or Cushing's syndrome. With pheochromocytoma, referral and hospitalization are indicated for hypertensive crisis. Endocrinology and surgical evaluation for resection of the pheochromocytoma may also be indicated.

Management of an acute adrenal crisis (corticosteroid insufficiency) requires IV administration of hydrocortisone 100 mg every 6 hr for an initial 24 hours, followed by careful dose tapering. Management of hypotension, hypovolemia, and hypoglycemia is accomplished with IV administration of normal saline with 5% dextrose with careful monitoring in the hospital, often in an intensive care setting; consultation is recommended.

Patients who have been taking exogenous steroids at any time during the preceding year are at some risk for inadequate cortisol response when faced with the stress of any surgical procedure. These patients should be considered candidates for perioperative stress doses of hydrocortisone.[6] Consultation with a physician comfortable with prescribing stress steroid doses is advised. In general, for patients with known adrenal insufficiency, hydrocortisone is added to intraoperative IV fluids and infused at a rate of 5 mg/hr. During the first 24 hours after surgery, a total of 150 to 200 mg is administered. The dose is then tapered by 50% per day if the postoperative period is without complications.

PATIENT EDUCATION AND HEALTH PROMOTION

Careful explanation of Addison's disease and Cushing's syndrome and the complications of chronic exogenous steroid dependency is an important component of patient and family education. Patients with adrenal insufficiency require early assessment and medication adjustments with fever and common illnesses. In many of these situations, it is essential that hydrocortisone maintenance doses be doubled quickly. Patients and families must understand the risks of suddenly withdrawing corticosteroid medications.

Medical Alert bracelets are also vital for the recognition of emergency presentations of adrenal insufficiency. Carrying extra oral and emergency parenteral steroids is mandatory when traveling and when in remote places. The impact these diseases may have on lifestyle and reproduction should be carefully explained to the patient.

Quick access to the primary care provider should be an important goal of the provider-patient partnership. A partnership approach and attention to medication use, as well as psychologic and emotional adaptation, enables patients and families to have a reasonably full life experience.

REFERENCES

1. Willis AC, Vince FP: The prevalence of Addison's disease in Coventry, UK, *Postgrad Med J* 73:286-288, 1997.
2. Peeke PM, Chrousos GP: Hypercortisolism and obesity, *Ann NY Acad Sci* 771:665-676, 1995.
3. Ross NS: Epidemiology of Cushing's syndrome and subclinical disease, *Endocrinol Metab Clin North Am* 23:539-546, 1994.
4. Orth D: Cushing's syndrome, *N Engl J Med* 332:791-803, 1995.
5. Tsigos C, Chrousos GP: Differential diagnosis and management of Cushing's syndrome, *Annu Rev Med* 47:443-461, 1996.
6. Werbel SS, Ober KP: Acute adrenal insufficiency (review), *Endocrinol Metab Clin North Am* 22(2):303-328, 1993.

CHAPTER 223

Diabetes Mellitus

Rosemary Bill-Fleury

DEFINITION/EPIDEMIOLOGY

Diabetes mellitus (DM) is the most common metabolic disorder seen in primary care and is the leading cause of renal failure, blindness, and nontraumatic lower limb amputation. This disorder is also the third leading cause of death, a direct result of diabetes-associated complications. The new criteria increase the number of newly diagnosed diabetics to 800,000 cases per year, with more than 16 million Americans afflicted with the disease, and another 5.4 million people may have undetected diabetes. An estimated 90% to 95% of patients with diabetes have adult-onset, or type 2, diabetes; less than 10% have type 1 diabetes. These statistics may increase with the new classifications for diabetes from the International Expert Committee and the American Diabetes Association (ADA) (Box 223-1).

The prevalence of diabetes in the United States is twice as high in females as in males. Diabetes in males is more prevalent in individuals of African-American, Native-American, and Hispanic decent in comparison with white males. The chance of developing diabetes doubles with every 20% of increased body weight and decade of life.

The long-term sequelae of diabetes are the microvascular and macrovascular complications to target end organs: the eyes,

BOX 223-1

RECENT CHANGES AND CURRENT CLASSIFICATIONS OF DIABETES FROM THE INTERNATIONAL EXPERT COMMITTEE

In type 1 DM, insulin deficiency is caused by beta cell destruction, and exogenous insulin is necessary to maintain life. Ketosis prone and autoimmune in nature, type 1 DM may occur in children, young adults, or fragile older adults. Some cases have a genetic or viral basis of development.

Type 2 diabetes results from insulin resistance and/or insulin defect. It is nonketotic in nature, and individuals usually have a positive family history. Development occurs later in life secondary to obesity, sedentary lifestyle, medications, or other factors that make the individual glucose intolerant.

Secondary diabetes occurs as a result of an underlying medical condition that renders the patient glucose intolerant.

Gestational diabetes refers to glucose intolerance during pregnancy. These women are at high risk for developing type 2 (non–insulin-dependent) diabetes at a later time.

Impaired glucose tolerance refers to the intermediate stage of glucose imbalance between normal physiology and DM. This stage covers impaired fasting glucose (>110 mg/dl but <126 mg/dl) and impaired glucose tolerance (oral glucose tolerance test of >140 mg/dl and <200 mg/dl). This latter classification includes a high risk for developing diabetes and cardiovascular disease.

kidneys, heart, blood vessels, and nerves. Diabetes costs an estimated $62 million per year as a result of the long-term complications; this does not include costs associated with disability. Therefore it is evident that the key to improved lifestyle and decreased financial burden is to prevent or slow the complications of diabetes.

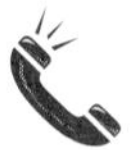

Physician consultation is indicated for patients with diabetic ketoacidosis or hyperglycemic hyperosmolar nonketotic coma, and for pregnant women with diabetes.

PATHOPHYSIOLOGY

Diabetes is characterized by glucose intolerance and hyperglycemia. The pathology of diabetes ranges from autoimmune destruction to deformities of insulin secretion, insulin action, insulin resistance, and/or basement membrane thickening. The morbidity and mortality of the disease are influenced by the glycemic control of the patient. Results from the Diabetes Control and Complications Trial and the United Kingdom Prospective Diabetes Study revealed a significant reduction in the complications of retinopathy, nephropathy, and neuropathy with glycemic control within the glycohemoglobin ranges of 6% to 7%.

Type 1 diabetes results from the destruction of the beta cells in the pancreatic islets, causing insulin deficiency. Surgery (e.g., Whipple's procedure or pancreatectomy) or autoimmune damage (e.g., various genetic or environmental insults) can also cause destruction of beta cells. Insulin deficiency impairs the uptake of glucose from intravascular to intercellular spaces, slows lipid synthesis, retards protein synthesis, and stimulates glycolysis.

In type 2 diabetes the pathology is more obscure. This disorder is identified with increased hepatic glucose production, impaired insulin secretion, and action in the peripheral tissues resulting in hyperglycemia. Fasting hyperglycemia is a result of increased hepatic glucose production from the impaired early phase of insulin secretion. Postprandial hyperglycemia is caused by the decreased uptake of glucose from the skeletal muscles. In response to the elevated blood glucose level, the insulin pathways become resistant to hormonal impulses, resulting in hyperinsulinemia. Insulin resistance by definition is the decreased sensitivity of tissue to glucose uptake. As hyperglycemia increases so does insulin resistance. The body is able to adapt and maintain homeostasis for a while, but as hyperglycemia progresses, diabetes occurs. As the degree of glucose intolerance progresses, hyperglycemia results from the insufficient insulin produced by the beta cells. Again, the body adapts for a while before diabetes occurs.

Insulin resistance is a particular problem in obese individuals. Primary insulin resistance is a defect in the target cells of insulin receptors and postreceptors, resulting in altered insulin action and sensitivity. The onset of insulin resistance can occur with hyperinsulinemia, in the fasting or fed state of the individual. The fed state is the time associated with insulin secretion from food intake to carbohydrate metabolism and synthesis of fat and protein. As insulin resistance proceeds to the peripheral levels, glucose transportation or utilization of glucose in the cell is altered. Hormones or abnormal physiologic states (e.g., puberty, pregnancy, and advanced age) cause secondary resistance. Other factors associated with the development of insulin resistance include a high-fat diet, sedentary lifestyle, smoking, and increasing weight gain. Metabolic stress, such as illness and obesity, increase the incidence of insulin resistance. An individual is considered insulin resistant when a daily intake of insulin greater than 1.5 to 2 units/kg of body weight is required.

Currently both insulin resistance and hyperinsulinemia are the focus of many research studies. In particular, researchers are concerned with the increased morbidity associated with insulin resistance, endothelial dysfunction, platelet adhesion, and cardiac disease. The full ramifications of this syndrome and its associated risk for heart disease are unclear. Weight loss, improving glucose tolerance, lipid management, and improving blood pressure may decrease the significance of this syndrome.

CLINICAL PRESENTATION

Polyuria, polydipsia, polyphagia, weight loss, and blurred vision are overt signs of diabetes. However, unexplained fatigue, paresthesia (especially in the feet), recurrent infections, and moniliasis may also signal the onset of the disorder. In type 1 diabetes the individual will be symptomatic for a short period. Then, as the glucosuria increases, nausea, vomiting, shallow breathing, hypotension, and dehydration will lead to ketosis and possibly death. Medical care is essential.

The patient with type 2 diabetes has subtle symptoms that may persist for weeks, months, or even years before detection occurs. Unfortunately, during this time vascular and neurologic complications begin to develop and progress before the diagnosis is made. Medical conditions that imply underlying diabetes include cranial nerve palsies (cranial nerve III with spared pupillary light reflex), symmetric distal polyneuropathy (stocking/glove), acanthosis nigricans, vitiligo, Dupuytren's contracture, autonomic neuropathy (characterized by tachycardia and orthostatic hypotension), increased incidence of monilial vaginitis, skin infections (furuncles and carbuncles), increased number of urinary tract infections (UTIs), and atrophic changes (hair loss, thinned skin, and decreased body temperature).

PHYSICAL EXAMINATION

The importance of the examination in the patient with diabetes is threefold: (1) to evaluate blood glucose control, as poor control leads to end-organ complications; (2) to assess for the presence or progression of end-organ damage of the eyes, heart, kidneys, nerves, and peripheral vascular system; and (3) to assess for other autoimmune disorders, such as thyroid disorders, or secondary causes for diabetes (see Box 223-1).

Annual examinations should be comprehensive. Periodic visits, every 3 months for patients with type 1 diabetes and those with type 2 diabetes with one or more complications, should be scheduled to assess end-organ involvement and glucose control. If the individual is stable and in control, visits could be every 6 months. Each examination should include height, weight, and blood pressure measurements, including comparison with age-related norms and evaluation of target end-organ involvement (Box 223-2).

DIAGNOSTICS

Diagnostic criteria for diabetes, supported by the ADA, no longer require a glucose tolerance test for definitive diagnosis. Initial diagnostic studies should include electrolytes, BUN, creatinine, serum glucose (random or fasting), lipid profile, urinalysis, and, if indicated, a thyroid-stimulating hormone study. A glycosylated hemoglobin assay indicates a percentage of glucose saturation to the hemoglobin and can be expressed with any of the A_1 fractions of the molecule: A_{1A}, A_{1B}, or A_{1C} (the largest). This test evaluates glucose control for the previous 12 weeks and is recommended every 3 months. A urine microalbumin study evaluates kidney function and should be done yearly after 5 years of diagnosis in the patient with type 1 diabetes and at the onset, and then yearly in the patient with type 2 diabetes. A 24-hour urine collection for creatinine clearance is still the "gold standard" for true evaluation of kidney function. Insulin levels and C-peptides are helpful in cases where there is concern for true diagnosis of type 1 vs. glucose intolerance. This is especially helpful when a type 1 diabetes has gone into a "honeymoon" phase.

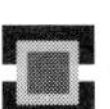

Diagnostics

Diabetes

Laboratory
Serum electrolytes
BUN
Creatinine
Serum glucose (random or fasting)
Lipid profile
Urinalysis
TSH*
Glycosylated hemoglobin*

*If indicated.

BOX 223-2

PHYSICAL EXAMINATION OF PATIENTS WITH DIABETES

Vital signs—Check blood pressure for orthostasis in blood pressure or inappropriate heart rate response (irregular, tachycardia, or bradycardia, especially with activity or position changes).
Eye—Perform funduscopic examination for bleeding, nicking, vascular changes, or retinopathy.
Oral cavity—Check for gum disease, fungal infections, or lesions.
Thyroid—Palpate for enlargement or nodules.
Neck—Auscultate for carotid bruits and evaluate for neck vein distention.
Cardiac—Auscultate heart rate for rhythm, murmurs, clicks, or extra heart sounds.
Abdomen—Assess for hepatomegaly and auscultate for abdominal bruits or aortic pulsations.
Vascular—Palpate pulses for presence and quality. Evaluate hands/fingers and feet for vibration, sensation, two-point discrimination, and proprioception.
Skin—Examine for signs of irritation, infection, redness, ulcers, lipodystrophy, and hypertrophy; give special attention to feet.
Evaluate prepubertal individuals for sexual maturation staging.

DIFFERENTIAL DIAGNOSIS

The diagnosis of diabetes has been facilitated by the recent changes in the diagnostic criteria (Box 223-3). However, secondary causes of diabetes should always be considered. These include excess of counterregulatory hormones (Cushing's syndrome, pheochromocytoma, and acromegaly), significant hypokalemia caused by glucose intolerance, hyperaldosteronism or diuretic use, and destruction to the pancreatic islet from pancreatitis (caused by alcoholism or gallbladder disease), hemochromatosis, or drug-induced islet cell injury. In addition, infection or medication may cause glucose intolerance, whereas the presence of polyuria and polydipsia may indicate DM, diabetes insipidus, or primary polydipsia.

MANAGEMENT

Insulin, an anabolic hormone produced by the beta cells of the pancreas, has a vital role in metabolism. Insulin therapy is the primary treatment for type 1 diabetes and is used in patients with type 2 diabetes with persistent hyperglycemia despite oral diabetic agents. Secretion of insulin is biphasic: prandial and basal. The prandial phase controls the initial glucose load and reuptake. The basal phase inhibits glycolysis and gluconeogenesis and maintains insulin in a steady state. Early morning hyperglycemia caused by counterregulatory hormones is controlled by basal insulin, and meal coverage is controlled by prandial insulin. Insulin therapy should pantomime this response.

The four types of insulin and three mixtures (Table 223-1) are derived synthetically from recombinant DNA (Human, Humulin). Insulin mixtures of pork or purified pork made from the pancreas of pigs are still available but no longer produced.

Differential Diagnosis

Diabetes

Cushing's syndrome	Alcoholism
Pheochromocytoma	Gallbladder disease
Acromegaly	Hemochromatosis
Diabetes insipidus	Drug-induced condition
Pancreatic disease	Infection

BOX 223-3

DIAGNOSTIC CRITERIA FOR GLUCOSE CONTROL

- Fasting plasma glucose >126 mg/dl confirmed by a repeat test
- Casual plasma glucose >200 mg/dl plus classic symptoms of diabetes
- Fasting plasma glucose >110 and <126 mg/dl = impaired glucose tolerance
- Two-hour postprandial plasma glucose >200 mg/dl after 75 g glucose load
- Two-hour postprandial glucose >140 and <200 mg/dl = impaired glucose tolerance

From American Diabetes Association (Committee Report): Report of the expert committee on the diagnosis and classification of diabetes mellitus, *Diabetes Care* 24 (Suppl 1):S5-S15, 2001.

TABLE 223-1 Insulin Types

Type	Formulation	Species	Concentration (U)	Onset	Peak	Duration	Comments
Regular	Humulin	Human	100	20-60 minutes	2-3 hours	4-8 hours	Administered intravenously, subcutaneously, and by insulin pump; mix with NPH and Lente; used for prandial glycemic control
	Human	Human	100				
Humalog	Humulin	Human	100	15-30 minutes	0.5-2 hours	3-4 hours	Administered subcutaneously; mix with NPH and Lente; used for prandial glycemic control
NovoLog	Human	Human	100	10-20 minutes	40-50 minutes	3-5 hours	Effective postprandial control—given preprandially; give SC; mix with NPH or Lente
NPH	Humulin	Human	100	1-4 hours	4-10 hours	10-16 hours	Administered subcutaneously; usually requires two injections; used for prandial glycemic control
	Human	Human	100				
	Iletin I	Pork	100	4-6 hours	8-14 hours	16-20 hours	
Lente	Humulin	Human	100	1-4 hours	4-12 hours	12-18 hours	Administered subcutaneously; longer duration than NPH; used for basal and prandial glycemic control
	Human	Human	100				
	Iletin II	Pork	100	4-6 hours	8-14 hours	16-20 hours	
Ultralente	Humulin	Human	100	6-10 hours		18-30 hours	Administered subcutaneously; used for basal glycemic control; should be used with a shorter-acting insulin for prandial glycemic control
Glargine	Human-analog			1.5 hours	Peakless	24 hours	Give SC; do not mix with any insulins; give 20% of daily dose at bedtime or one to one; if only on one shot/day, increase every four days
MIXTURES							
70/30	Humulin	Human	100				Mixture of 70% NPH + 30% regular insulin
	Human	Human	100				
50/50	Humulin	Human	100				Mixture of 50% NPH + 50% regular insulin
75/25	Humulin		100				Mixture of 75% NPH + 25% Humalog
70/30	Human		100				Mixture of 70% NPH + 30% NovoLog

There are three insulin analogues made of recombinant human insulin. Two are quick acting, lispro and aspart, and one is long acting, glargine. The two short-acting analogues are better interventions when treating postprandial blood sugars, and glargine provides true basal coverage of insulin without insulin peaks. All three analogues have demonstrated a decrease in the frequency of hypoglycemia episodes and improved glycemic control. When starting someone on insulin, synthetic insulin should be used. The advantage of using synthetic insulin over animal insulin is the decreased episodes of allergic reactions and lipoatrophy. The disadvantage of this regimen is the longer duration of animal insulin, which makes it a better choice for a single daily injection. Mixing of insulin allows a more personalized regimen for better adherence and safety. Four prepared insulin mixtures in ratios of 75/25, 70/30 Novomix, and 50/50 offer ease and safety to the individual.

Diabetes management requires a homeostatic relationship of diet, exercise/activity, illness/disease state, emotional well-being, and insulin or oral diabetic medication. Care for both type 1 and type 2 encompasses the same issues and may even require insulin. However, the role of circulating insulin differs between the two types of diabetes. Insulin therapy is used for type 1 diabetes because of insulin deficiency, whereas diet, weight loss, and exercise are appropriate initial interventions for patients with type 2 diabetes. Individuals with type 2 diabetes with persistent hyperglycemia, ketosis, pregnancy, syndrome X (see Chapter 228), or the development of complications require aggressive therapy to improve glycemic control.

TABLE 223-2 Management for Type I Diabetes

	Breakfast	Lunch	Dinner
Patients 15-18 years	$\frac{2}{3}$ to $\frac{1}{2}$ of calculated dose	Sliding scale—$\frac{1}{4}$ of calculated dose	$\frac{1}{3}$ to $\frac{1}{4}$ of calculated dose
	NPH/Lente + Humalog/NovoLog	Humalog or NovoLog	NPH/Lente + Humalog/NovoLog
	NPH/Lente + Regular	Regular	NPH/Lente + Regular
	NPH/Lente + Humalog/NovoLog		Humalog/NovoLog + NPH/Lente
	Ultralente + Humalog/NovoLog	Homalog or NovoLog	Ultralente + Humalog
			Humalog/NovoLog + Ultralente/Lantus

Start with b.i.d. insulin and then titrate upwards depending on control. Adolescents may require more insulin per day—1-1.5 units/kg or greater. Add lunchtime insulin if not able to control by AM insulin. If very active, may be able to cover with sliding scale of Humalog/NovoLog for meals and nighttime long-acting drugs such as Ultralente or Lantus. Decrease insulin dose with onset of honeymoon phase from 0.1 to 0.5 units/kg/body weight.

	Breakfast	Dinner	Bedtime
Patients 19-40 years	$\frac{2}{3}$ calculated dose	$\frac{1}{3}$ calculated dose	Ultralente/Lantus
	NPH/Lente + Humalog/ NovoLog/Regular	NPH/Lente + Humalog/ NovoLog/Regular	
	Ultralente + Humalog/ NovoLog	Ultralente + Humalog/NovoLog	
	Humalog/NovoLog	Humalog/NovoLog	

INSULIN ADJUSTMENTS

Individualized according to patient's meal plan, exercise, work/sleep hours, and lifestyle

Blood glucose monitoring is the tool regulating adjustments; testing is from one to four time per day, depending on control and financial situation

May require stationary NPH/Lente/Ultralente but adjustments in the short-acting insulin; Regular or Humalog

With episodes of early-morning hypoglycemia and/or nighttime hyperglycemia—give Humalog/NovoLog before evening meal and long-acting Ultralente or Lantus at bedtime (9-10 PM).

Modified from American Diabetes Association: *Insulin therapy of Type I diabetic: medical management,* ed 3, Alexandria, Va, 1994.

The Diabetes Control and Complications Trial (DCCT-type 1) and the United Kingdom Prospective Diabetes Study (UKPDS-type 2) both revealed the importance of glycemic control in improving outcomes by delaying or preventing vascular and neurologic ravages of the disease. Achievement of near-normal glucose levels (70 to 120 mg/dl) before meals and below 140 mg/dl 2 hours postprandially are goals for optimal glycemic control.

Type 1 Diabetes

When starting an individual on insulin, body weight, morphologic development (obese vs. muscular), age (adolescence vs. older), and activity (sedentary vs. athletic) should be considered. Physiologic insulin secretion for adults is approximately 20 to 40 units/day. The recommended starting dose for an adult is approximately 15 to 25 units of insulin in the morning before breakfast. An individual with fasting blood glucose levels above 250 mg/dl should receive an additional nighttime dose of five units before bedtime snack (preferably) or before supper should be started. The type of insulin used is dependent on the need of the patient as well as on the preference of the clinician. Glargine, a true long-acting insulin given at approximately 8 to 10 PM and lasting for 24 hours, mimics the basal rate of insulin. Therefore this may be a better choice when starting individuals on insulin. The insulin dose should be adjusted every 3 to 4 days until the fasting blood glucose level is below 120 mg/dl. The insulin should be increased by increments of 2 to 8 units in an obese individual or by 1 to 6 units in a patient with thin body frame, a frail older adult, or in a patient with frequent episodes of hypoglycemia. Use of standard insulin NPH or Lente and Ultralente also could be used to mimic both prandial and basal insulin. The dose when starting is the same but may be increased every 2 to 3 days by 2 to 4 units.

If after a few weeks the individual's glucose range is greater than 150 to 200 mg/dl at bedtime or before lunch, or if the morning insulin dose exceeds 45 units, fast-acting lispro or aspart should be added to the regimen. Regular insulin may be used as an alternative, but does not offer the immediate mealtime coverage and may be long acting enough to increase postprandial hyperglycemia and contribute to hypoglycemia before next meal if mealtime is delayed. All three insulins may be mixed with the morning and supper doses of NPH or Lente injection; however, none can be mixed with glargine. To achieve tighter control, a second or third injection of lispro/aspart could be added at lunch, and/or the evening dose of insulin could be separated into lispro/aspart insulin given before supper and NPH or Lente or glargine insulin given before the bedtime snack. Using lispro/aspart insulin before meals allows for more flexibility, better coverage of hyperglycemia (Table 223-2), and a decrease in the episodes of hypoglycemia.

Adolescent doses are calculated by weight, activity level, and needed insulin requirements to maintain optimal glycemic control (Table 223-3). Requirements for insulin increase during illness, surgery, growth spurts, and with ketoacidosis. Insulin absorption from subcutaneous tissues varies about 25% among patients. The practitioner should be aware of a possible "honeymoon" phase in the patient with newly diagnosed type 1 diabetes with recovering beta-cell function. Insulin requirements may decrease to 0.2 to 0.5 unit/kg/day during this short-term phase. The goal of the diabetes plan is to attain glycemic control with appropriate insulin doses but without symptoms of hypoglycemia or hyperglycemia.

Intensified insulin therapy encompasses multidose insulin or infusion pumps to achieve tighter glucose control. This comprehensive plan involves a close partnership with the individual with diabetes and the primary care provider or diabetic specialist. To prevent both hypoglycemia and hyperglycemia, factors such as exercise/activity, meals, mealtimes, sleep patterns, illness, and psychologic well-being must be considered when calculating insulin doses. Hypoglycemia is a serious side effect of this therapy and prevents some individuals from participating. One way of controlling day-to-day variations and preventing hypoglycemia is through home blood glucose testing. There are many different varieties of glucose monitors. The best one is the one the patient is able to use. To evaluate the range of glucose disparity between plasma and whole blood, one should test the blood using a personal glucose monitor and the laboratory at the same time. If the range is greater than 20 to 30 points another glucose monitor should be tried. Comparing different glucose monitors to each other should be avoided, as this may produce an array of results.

Individuals not appropriate for intensified insulin include (1) those with glycemic control of 70 to 120 mg/dl and without complications, (2) those with hypoglycemia unawareness, (3) those who are poorly motivated and unwilling to test their blood glucose frequently, and (4) those who have had diabetes for less than 6 months to 1 year.

Insulin adjustments are made using one type of insulin at a time. One unit of lispro insulin can decrease the blood glucose level by 50 mg/dl; regular insulin is more variable and can sometimes act like intermediate insulin. A guideline for initiating intensive insulin therapy is to take the total daily insulin dose and divide it into percentages to be taken before meals and at bedtime. For example, 35% of the total insulin dose should be taken before breakfast, 20% before lunch, 30% before supper, and 15% before bedtime. These amounts need to be fine-tuned if patients work night shifts or eat their larger meal at noontime, with a smaller meal at nighttime. When the patient is using an insulin pump, co-management with an endocrinologist is strongly recommended.

Nutrition therapy is essential in diabetic management for both type 1 and type 2 diabetes. The goal of nutrition therapy for both types is the development of the meal plan, balancing insulin with food intake and activity to achieve glycemic control. A dietitian is valuable in helping to balance medications and food intake for type 1 diabetes and is a priority for weight control and lipid management, in type 2 diabetes. Individuals with type 2 diabetes must also balance food intake (meals and snacks) with activity and the use of medications. A registered dietitian can individualize the nutrition guidelines for each individual with diabetes to attain optimal glycemic control and prevent hypoglycemia in short-term illness (Box 223-4). Lifestyle changes need special dietary adjustments with the help of a dietitian. This would include issues surrounding growth and development, pregnancy, lactation, or recovery from a severe illness.

Exercise/physical therapy has been shown to improve glycemic control. Exercise suppresses insulin and increases glucose uptake in skeletal muscle. In the individual without diabetes, counterregulatory hormones increase glucose secretion to balance glucose uptake into skeletal muscle; however, this function is lost in the individual with diabetes. Therefore to prevent

TABLE 223-3 Insulin Dosage

Life Span	Dosage
Before adolescence	0.7-0.8 units/kg/day of body weight
Adolescence	1.2-1.4 units/kg/day of body weight
Adult	0.5-1 units/kg/day of body weight
Older adult	0.5 units/kg/day of body weight
Pregnancy*	
Gestational and type 2 diabetes	30 units (2:1) NPH plus regular insulin in morning plus 5-10 units regular insulin before evening meal*
Type 1 diabetes:	
First trimester	Decrease preconception dose by 10%-20%
Second and third trimesters	0.9-1.2 units/kg of body weight over 24 hours
Postpartum and breast-feeding	0.6 units/kg of body weight

Modified from American Diabetes Association: *Medical management of pregnancy complicated by diabetes,* Alexandria, Va, 1995, The Association.

*If insulin is started before the twenty-eighth week in gestational diabetes, decrease the dose by 20%. Some may start with the nighttime injection only, then add on the daytime injection.

BOX 223-4

NUTRITION GUIDELINES FOR PATIENTS WITH DIABETES

Calories—Adequate amounts for weight control, growth and development, pregnancy and lactation

Protein—10%-20% of calories; with nephropathy, 0.8 g/kg of body weight per day

Fat—30% or less from calories with <10% calories from saturated fat; if obese or hyperlipidemic, less than 30% may be needed

Carbohydrate—Remainder of calories after protein and fat adjustments; percentage varies with individual lifestyle, activity level, and insulin level

Carbohydrate counting—Calculating dose of fast-acting insulin to correspond with amount of carbohydrate per meal; 15 g of carbohydrate equals 1 unit of regular/Humalog insulin

Cholesterol—300 mg/day; if hyperlipidemic, 200 mg/day

Fiber—20-35 g/day

Sodium—3000 mg/day; for individuals with mild to moderate hypertension, 2400 mg/day; with hypertension and nephropathy, 2000 mg/day

Alcohol—Limit to two alcoholic beverages/day (12 oz beer, 5 oz wine, or 1½ oz distilled spirits = 1 drink); ingest at meals and substitute for two fat exchanges

Data from American Diabetes Association (Committee Report): Nutrition recommendations and principles for people with diabetes mellitus, *Diabetes Care* 24 (suppl 1):S44-S47, 2001.

hypoglycemia, the individual with diabetes, especially on insulin, must balance activity with adequate food and appropriate medication. Postexercise hyperglycemia occurs in an individual with poorly controlled diabetes; this develops as a result of decreased circulating insulin and glucose uptake and increased hormonally regulated hepatic glucose. Ketosis is increased as fatty acids are broken down for energy, resulting in higher blood glucose levels and possible ketosis during exercise.

In the individual with type 2 diabetes, exercise decreases insulin resistance and increases glucose uptake. Insulin sensitivity resulting from the lag effect can last up to 48 hours. Thus medication, especially insulin, needs to be adjusted for the activity/exercise performed. Adjustment involves decreasing the insulin that is peaking at the time of exercise. In the patient with type 2 diabetes it would be optimal to decrease medication vs. increasing food consumption for the exercise regimen. Guidelines for exercise in diabetes are reviewed in Box 223-5.

Type 2 Diabetes

The mainstay of therapy for the patient with type 2 diabetes is education, diet, and exercise. However, persistent hyperglycemia and end organ compromise require pharmacologic intervention. Patients with symptomatic hyperglycemia and vascular complications require medication for immediate improvement of glycemic control. Using diet, weight loss, and exercise as treatment options entails a time frame of at least 3 to 6 months to monitor progress. If time is not an option, the use of medications must be added to the regimen of diet and exercise.

BOX 223-5

EXERCISE RECOMMENDATIONS FOR PATIENTS WITH DIABETES

TYPE 1 DIABETES

1. Eat a carbohydrate snack, 15-30 g (glass of milk, piece of fruit, half of banana) for every 30-60 minutes of low to moderate exercise.
2. Eat 25-50 g of a carbohydrate and protein snack (one half to whole sandwich [of meat] with glass of milk) for every hour of moderate to high-intensity exercise.
3. Do not exercise when blood glucose level is above 300 mg/dl or if spilling ketones.
4. Be aware of symptoms of hypoglycemia and carry readily absorbable carbohydrate.
5. Diabetics with insensitive feet should avoid running. Those with proliferative retinopathy should avoid Valsalva-like maneuvers, isometric exercises, and high-intensity strenuous exercises.
6. Individuals with hypertension should avoid heavy lifting, Valsalva-like maneuvers, and straining-type exercises.

TYPE 2 DIABETES

1. Exercise when blood glucose level is above 120 mg/dl, 1 to 3 hours after a meal.
2. Decrease insulin that is peaking at time of exercise.
3. Same as recommendations 1, 2, 4, 5, and 6 for type 1 diabetes.

The variety of oral hypoglycemic agents enables treatment individualization for improved glycemic control (Box 223-6 and Table 223-4). The sulfonylureas are the most widely used first-line oral medications for type 2 diabetes. The second-generation sulfonylureas are a better choice because of their shorter half-life and side-effect profile, particularly in older adults. Their mechanism of action affects both pancreatic and extrapancreatic tissue. Insulin production by indirect stimulation of beta cells is their primary role. Associated benefits are inhibition of glucagon release, increased insulin sensitivity and affinity to postreceptor sites by decreasing insulin resistance, and decreased hepatic insulin release. There is increased risk for drug interactions causing either hypoglycemia or hyperglycemia (Box 223-7). These drugs are not used as first-line therapy for everyone, especially a thin person with type 2 diabetes.

Biguanide (metformin), an antihyperglycemic agent, sensitizes liver, small intestine, and peripheral muscle tissue to decrease hepatic glucose production and intestinal glucose absorption. Additional benefits of metformin are enhanced glucose uptake into skeletal muscle and tissue, and improved insulin sensitivity. Studies support the effectiveness of monotherapy, with glucose ranges lowered by 25%. The advantage of using metformin as first-line therapy is the direct decrease in endogenous insulin, weight loss, and reduction in low-density lipoprotein (LDL) cholesterol, especially in the obese patient with insulin-resistant type 2 diabetes. Lactic acidosis is a potential lethal problem. Specific situations prohibiting metformin are given in Box 223-8.

The thiazolidinediones (T2Ds), pioglitazone and rosiglitazone, are antihyperglycemic medications that act in peripheral and adipose tissues and in skeletal muscle to enhance insulin sensitivity and increase glucose uptake and mobilization. Ultimately this decreases insulin resistance. Improvement of both fasting and postprandial blood glucose levels occurs over time and without stimulating insulin secretion. Both pioglitazone and rosiglitazone are indicated for use as monotherapy or in combination with insulin. However, neither is considered first-line therapy if the patient is glucose toxic because results are not fully seen for 4 to 8 weeks. Advantages to using the thiazolidinediones include the delay of beta-cell exhaustion, decrease in insulin resistance, no hypoglycemia (if used alone), and lipid improvement with triglyceride and high-density lipoprotein (HDL). Some studies have revealed a slight increase in LDL with rosiglitazone. Disadvantages of this class are weight gain, edema, and a distant association with liver disease; this was seen with troglitazone (now off the market) but not with the newer agents. However, the recommendation is to monitor liver functions every 2 months and stop the drug if serum transaminase exceeds 2.5 times the upper limit. Serum transaminase levels should then be monitored until enzymes are normal. T2Ds used with insulin may cause peripheral edema. They should be used with extreme caution in patients who are taking insulin or are at risk for congestive heart failure (CHF). They are not recommended for use in patients with class 3 or 4 CHF.

Meglitinides (repaglinide, nateglinide) are nonsulfonylurea insulin stimulators. The benefit of this class is the short and rapid release of insulin to control postprandial hyperglycemia with normal premeal glucose levels. These drugs are taken

BOX 223-6

MANAGEMENT OF TYPE 2 DIABETES MELLITUS

STEP 1

Fasting blood glucose >126 mg/dl or postprandial glucose >200 mg/dl and above ideal body weight—diet and exercise.
If within ideal body weight or no response within 3 months, go to Step 2.

STEP 2

Fasting blood glucose <140 mg/dl, glycose above 6.0

or

Postprandial above 160 mg/dl—initiate medical treatment plus Step 1; if inadequate after 3 months, go to Step 3.

Fasting blood glucose <140 mg/dl, glycose
Patient obese, dyslipidemic
Choices: metformin b.i.d. or T2Ds q.d. at low doses

Fasting blood glucose <150 mg/dl
Patient not obese or dyslipidemic
Choices: longer for diet and exercise or metformin b.i.d.

STEP 3

Combination of oral therapy; if inadequate, go to Step 4

Fasting blood glucose <140 mg/dl, glycose
Choices: acarbose 25 mg b.i.d., metformin 500 b.i.d
Actos (15-30) mg or Avandia (2-4 mg) q.d.
If not responding, add sulfonylureas or megleinides

Fasting blood glucose <150 mg/dl
Choices: metformin to maximum 100 mg b.i.d. and/or add sulfonylurea

STEP 4

Fasting blood glucose <140 mg/dl, glycose
Combination oral therapy and nighttime insulin

At evening meal, increase oral therapies to maximum

Fasting blood glucose <150 mg/dl
If fasting still high, add 10 units NPH + 2-5 units Humalog/NovoLog or Regular
If inadequate after 2-3 months, go to Step 5

STEP 5

Insulin therapy b.i.d. and orals to decrease insulin resistance

FAILED ORAL THERAPY—INSULIN THERAPY B.I.D., T.I.D., OR Q.I.D.

Stop acarbose and sulfonylureas

1. Start with Lantis or NPH 10 units at bedtime and increase to 25% of total daily formula ($\frac{1}{2}$ unit kg/day—obese; 0.5-0.7 unit/kg/day—nonobese)
2. Two injections of NPH or Lente; increase by 50% above formula ($\frac{1}{2}$-$\frac{2}{3}$ in AM and $\frac{1}{3}$-$\frac{1}{2}$ in evening)
3. Four daily injections of Humalog or NovoLog AC and Lantis, NPH, or Ultralente at bedtime. When using Lantis (galargine), start with 20% of total daily insulin dose administered at bedtime, 30% of total at breakfast, 20% at lunch, and 30% at evening meal.
4. In obese individuals with high glucose ranges, use 75/25 or 70/30 either b.i.d. in AM and at evening meal
5. Three injections of NPH or Lente + Humalog/NovoLog in AM, NovoLog or Humalog before evening meal and NPH or Lantis or Ultralente at bedtime

Data from American Diabetes Association (Position Statement): Standards of medical care for patients with diabetes mellitus, *Diabetes Care* 23(Suppl 1): S32-S34, 2000.

only before meals and should be withheld if the individual is not eating. These agents are also used in combination, especially in individuals eating a high-carbohydrate meal and in need of a boost of insulin for a shorter period. Nateglinide seems to work slightly faster than repaglinide with fewer episodes of hypoglycemia.

Alpha-glucosidase inhibitors (acarbose, miglitol) are antihyperglycemic agents that act in the small intestine by delaying the absorption of glucose from the gastrointestinal tract. The inhibition of starch and the sucrose enzymes causes lowered postprandial glucose levels. Both drugs are sufficient as monotherapy, especially with obese individuals eating a high-starch diet; however, they are more effective when used in combination with other hypoglycemic agents. Contraindications to using acarbose and miglitol include inflammatory bowel disease, colonic ulceration, obstructive bowel disease, gastroparesis, hypoglycemia unawareness, type 1 diabetes, and creatinine levels >2 mg/dl. Close monitoring of individuals with diabetes is needed for medical disorders of digestion or absorption.

Insulin may be used as first-line treatment for the patient with type 2 diabetes in the following situations: glycosylated hemoglobin >10% or glucose range >250 mg/dl, severe illness with associated complications, gestational diabetes, or in fragile older adults. However, the most common reason for use of insulin in type 2 diabetes management is secondary failure (see Table 223-4) of the oral antihyperglycemic agents. A hallmark scenario with type 2 diabetes is an elevated fasting glucose. This can be treated with a nighttime dose of 5 to 10 units of intermediate-acting

BOX 223-7

HYPOGLYCEMIA AND HYPERGLYCEMIA INDUCED BY PHARMACOKINETICS AFFECTING SULFONYLUREAS

HYPOGLYCEMIA

Displacement from albumin binding site
- Clofibrate
- Halofenate
- Salicylates
- Some sulfonamides
- Phenylbutazone, oxyphenylbutazone, and sulfinpyrazone

Prolongs half-life of sulfonylurea by interfering with metabolism
- Warfarin
- Chloramphenicol
- Monoamine oxidase inhibitors
- Sulfaphenazole
- Pyrzolone derivatives

Decreases urinary excretion of sulfonylurea
- Allpurinol
- Probenecid
- Salicylates
- Pyrazolone derivatives
- Some sulfonamides

HYPERGLYCEMIA

Shortens half-life by increasing metabolism of sulfonylurea
- Chronic alcohol use
- Rifampin

Modified from American Diabetes Association: *Physician's guide to noninsulin dependent (type 2) diabetes*, ed 3, Alexandria, Va, 1994, The Association.

insulin, NPH or Lente, or 10 units of a long-acting insulin, glargine, taken at 8 to 9 PM in addition to oral agents during the day. If control is still elusive, a daytime injection of NPH or Lente or a mixture of 75/25 or 70/30 should be initiated at a dose of 10 to 25 U every morning.

If an individual with diabetes has insulin resistance and/or early morning hyperglycemia, a combination of metformin and thiazolidinedione or the addition of a long-acting bedtime insulin should be considered. If glargine insulin is used, it should be titrated slowly every 4 days. When changing to nighttime glargine, the total daily dose of insulin should be reduced by 20%. For instance, if total insulin dose were 40 units, a starting dose of 8 units of glargine would be started at 8 to 11 PM.

Combination therapy using the previously mentioned medications along with insulin therapy allows for a more individualized regimen and affords better glycemic control without side effects and episodes of hypoglycemia. The timing of glucose testing helps with adjusting medications. Fasting and premeal testing enables an overall view of basal control. Glucose levels should be between 70 and 100 mg/dl; 1- to 2-hour postprandial testing addresses the impact of insulin secretion and beta-cell function and should be below 120 to 130 mg/dl.

Follow-up care is an integral part of diabetes management. The visits evaluate glycemic control, initiation or progression of vascular complications, and frequency and severity hypoglycemic reactions. The individual's ability to understand and manage the diabetes helps with compliance and circumventing potential problems. The frequency of visits, every 3 to 6 months, depends on diabetic control and the presence of complications. Each visit should involve evaluation of blood pressure, weight, height (check against growth chart for age), feet, and blood glucose log. Laboratory tests include a glycohemoglobin test every 3 months. A lipid profile is indicated yearly unless findings are abnormal or are being medically treated; then it is obtained every 4 to 6 months. Yearly screening should include urinary microalbumin and urinalysis, BUN, creatinine, ophthalmologic examinations, and if indicated cardiovascular evaluation. A baseline ECG is recommended after age 40 years. Exercise ECG or peripheral vascular testing should be obtained when indicated.

Pregnancy

Women with diabetes before pregnancy and pregnancy-induced diabetes (gestational diabetes) require special considerations for treatment. If diabetes is untreated or poorly treated, there is an increase in morbidity and mortality for the woman and her infant. For the woman with type 1 or type 2 diabetes, ideal glycemic control is strongly recommended before pregnancy, as well as during the pregnancy, to improve maternal and fetal outcome. The patient with gestational diabetes requires glycemic control during pregnancy. One in every 20 to 30 healthy pregnant women will develop gestational diabetes, carbohydrate intolerance, and insulin resistance. Fetal complications in untreated and poorly treated women include birth injury, macrosomia, hypoglycemia, respiratory distress syndrome, and hyperbilirubinemia. Maternal complications include an increase in cesarean section delivery, preeclampsia, postpartum hemorrhage, and an increased incidence of developing diabetes later in life.

Glucose intolerance is the result of insulin resistance during the latter half of pregnancy. Placenta and counterregulatory hormones, along with the stress of the growing fetus, increase insulin resistance. Hyperglycemia results, as beta cell reserve cannot counteract the increasing insulin resistance and the hormonal effect on blood glucose. Screening for gestational diabetes with a glucose tolerance test is not needed in women less than 25 years of age, in women of normal body weight, in women with no first-degree relative with diabetes, or in women who are not Hispanic, Native-American, Asian, or African-American. Women who require testing should have a 2- or 3-hour glucose tolerance test performed at 24 to 28 weeks' gestation. Earlier screening at 16 to 20 weeks' gestation is recommended if there is a prior history of gestational diabetes or delivery of a large-for-gestational-age infant. If the glucose tolerance test is negative, it should be repeated at the suggested time of screening (Table 223-5). The screening method is a 50-g glucose load with 1-hour plasma glucose. If the blood glucose value is ≥140 mg/dl, then the test should be repeated using either a 75- or 100-g glucose load. Glucose ranges should be as close to 80 to 120 mg/dl as possible. Table 223-6 compares laboratory values.

Management for the patient with gestational diabetes is essential. Initial treatment is an 1800- to 2200-calorie diet, as prescribed by a diabetic dietitian. Monitoring glucose values with a self-monitoring glucose monitor four times a day, including fasting and a 2-hour postprandial blood glucose reading, is also necessary. Alterations in caloric requirements are needed if the woman is obese and sedentary, or if she is very active. The key

TABLE 223-4 Oral Hypoglycemic Agents

Medication	Daily Dose Range	Actions	Comments
SULFONYLUREA-GLIPIZIDE		Stimulate insulin secretion, increase absorption of insulin, and improve glucogenesis	Side effects: hypoglycemia, weight gain; take before main meals; better for thinner patients; do not use when nursing or while pregnant
(Glucotrol)	5-40 mg		
(Glucotrol XL)	5-20 mg	Extended release—last longer	
Glyburide (Glynase)	0.75-12 mg		
(Diabeta and Micronase)	1.25-20 mg		
Glimepride (Amaryl)	1-8 mg	Great for use with bedtime insulin	
Glucovance	1.25/250-5/500	Combination of biguanide and sulfonylureas	Titrate slowly; take during meal; side effects include hypoglycemia, GI distress; same precautions as with metformin
Metaglip	5/500 dose Max: 20/2000 mg	Combination of glipazide and metformin	
MEGLITINIDES			
Repaglinide (Prandin)	0.5-4 mg bid-qid	Increase endogenous insulin postprandially; excreted in bile; short-acting; take 30 minutes before meals	Side effects include hypoglycemia, GI distress; use with caution if have renal/hepatic insufficiency
Nateglinide (Starlix)	60-120 mg	Take 30 minutes before meals	Same precautions as above
BIGUANIDES			
Metformin	500-2000 mg	Has 850 mg; decrease hepatics glucose production and increases insulin sensitivity	Take with food to decrease GI distress; do not use if have renal/hepatic insufficiency
Metformin Extended Release	500-2000 mg	Take during meals all at once	
THIAZOLIDINEDIONDES			
Rosiglitazone (Avandia)	2-8 mg	Decreases insulin resistance and increases glucose uptake	Edema; may cause anovolatory women to resume ovulation; monitor with use of OCP
Pioglitazone (Actose)	15-45 mg	Contraindicated with renal or hepatic function	Side effects may include anemia, headache, dizziness, nausea, vomiting; monitor LFTs q 2 mo for first year and regularly thereafter
Avandamet	1/500 mg-4/500 mg Max: 8/200 mg	Combination T2D/Biguanide (Avandia and Metformin)	
ALPHA GLUCOSIDASE INHIBITORS			
Acarbose (Precose)	25-300 mg	Delays carbohydrate absorption	Side effects include flatulence, diarrhea, abdominal pain
Miglitol (Glyset)	25-300 mg	Treat hypoglycemia with sucrose only	Take during meals, start slowly and titrate slowly; contraindicated with DKA, inflammatory bowel, ulcerative colitis, or bowel obstruction

Modified from Massachusetts Guidelines for Adult Diabetes Care: *Oral medications,* Massachusetts Health Promotion, June 2001, Boston.

to glycemic control is calculating appropriate carbohydrates in combination with protein and/or fat to slow glucose release. Exercise is also used to improve glycemic control. Walking or some form of nonstrenuous aerobic exercise three or four times a week for 15 to 30 minutes a day improves glycemic control. The patient is advised to start slowly, increase gradually, prevent increasing body core temperature, and stop exercising if signs of overexertion, hypothermia, fetal distress, bleeding, or uterine contractions occur. The obstetrician should be notified if symptoms of fetal distress, bleeding, or contractions develop.

Insulin therapy should be added to improve glucose control when two or more glucose readings exceed the recommended goal range (see Table 223-6). As pregnancy progresses, insulin resistance from hormonal effects can supersede even strict dietary compliance, and insulin therapy is recommended. The starting dose is approximately 20 to 30 units/day (two thirds in the morning and one third before supper) of a mixture 75/25, 70/30, or using NPH and Humalog. However, the exact amount is dependent on the insulin type and the amount needed for glycemic control. Higher doses of insulin may be necessary in the third trimester, when insulin resistance is the greatest. Adjustments in insulin doses are made in increments of 2 to 4 units every 3 days for minor elevations (120 to 140 mg/dl) or in increments of 5 to 6 units when glucose ranges are higher.

Pregnancy in the Patient with Type 1 Diabetes. Pregnancy in the patient with type 1 diabetes is considered a high-risk pregnancy that may result in life-threatening complications for both the mother (Box 223-9) and fetus (Box 223-10). Therefore it is imperative that the woman with diabetes attain ideal

BOX 223-8

METFORMIN CONTRAINDICATIONS

CONTRAINDICATIONS TO THE USE OF METFORMIN

Creatinine levels >1.5 mg/dl in men and 1.4 mg/dl in women
Hepatic dysfunction
History of alcoholism
Binge drinking

SITUATIONS REQUIRING WITHHOLDING OF METFORMIN

Acute myocardial infarction
Congestive heart failure
Use of iodine contrast
Major surgical procedures

TABLE 223-5 Screening and Diagnosis for Gestational Diabetes*

Plasma Glucose	50 g	75 g	100 g
Fasting		>95	>95 mg/dl
1 hour	<140 mg/dl	>175 mg/dl	>180 mg/dl
2 hour	<120 mg/dl	150 mg/dl	>155 mg/dl
3 hour			>140 mg/dl

Data from American Diabetes Association (Committee Report): Gestational diabetes mellitus, *Diabetes Care* 24(Suppl1):S77-S79, 2001.

*Two or more values exceeding the normal range on the 3-hour glucose tolerance test must be met for diagnosis of gestational diabetes to be made.

BOX 223-9

MATERNAL COMPLICATIONS OF DIABETES

Hyperglycemia, ketoacidosis
Pregnancy-induced hypertension
Pyelonephritis, other infections
Polyhydramnios
Preterm labor
Worsening of chronic complications
Nephropathy, neuropathy, cardiac disease

Modified from American Diabetes Association: *Medical management of pregnancy complicated by diabetes*, Alexandria, Va, 1995, The Association.

BOX 223-10

FETAL COMPLICATIONS WITH DIABETIC MOTHERS

Asphyxia
Birth injury
Cardiac hypertrophy
Congenital anomalies
Erythemia and hyperviscosity
Heart failure
Hyperbilirubinemia
Hypocalcemia
Hypoglycemia
Hypomagnesium
Increased blood volume
Intrauterine growth retardation
Macrosomia
Neurologic instability, irritation
Organomegaly
Respiratory distress
Small left colon syndrome
Stillbirth
Transient hematuria

From American Diabetes Association: *Medical management of pregnancy complicated by diabetes*, Alexandria, Va, 1995, The Association.

TABLE 223-6 Gestational Diabetes Glucose Ranges

	Premeal		2-Hour Postprandial	
	Laboratory	SMGM	Laboratory	SMGM
First trimester	≤105 mg/dl	≤100 mg/dl	≤140 mg/dl	≤120 mg/dl
Second and third trimesters	≤100 mg/dl	≤90 mg/dl	≤120 mg/dl	≤110 mg/dl

SMGM, Self-monitoring glucose monitor.

glycemic control, including a plasma glucose level of 80 to 120 mg/dl and a glycohemoglobin A_{1C} value of 6% to 7%, before pregnancy. However, if pregnancy happens first, glycemic control should be the utmost priority. There is a 1 in 10 chance of congenital anomaly in the growing fetus with poor glycemic control. For the pregnant woman with diabetes the metabolic changes that occur with the growing fetus can accelerate retinal and renal complications. Vascular complications of retinopathy, nephropathy, pregnancy-induced hypertension, and poorly controlled glycemia are strong risk factors for perinatal compromise. These individuals are at high risk and need to be monitored closely by a team of specialists, including an obstetrician, endocrinologist, nephrologist, ophthalmologist, primary care provider, dietitian, and diabetic educator.

Adjustments in insulin doses are needed for glucose control as pregnancy progresses. In the first trimester, insulin doses may be decreased because of hypoglycemia from the increase in fetal glucose transport and a loss of maternal amino acids. During the latter half of the second trimester, there is a rapid diversion to fat metabolism, resulting in higher concentrations of circulating glucose. The longer the postprandial hyperglycemia, the more glucose is transported to the fetus, thus promoting fetal growth. During this time there is also a degree of insulin resistance that occurs from the placental hormone (human placental lactogen), prolactin, and cortisol. Insulin requirements are increased during this stage and into the third trimester, then plateau around the thirty-sixth week of gestation.

Treatment changes with pregnancy. Dietary requirements, activity/exercise, glucose monitoring, and insulin requirements are adjusted for the pregnant state. Caloric requirements are increased and snacks are added, particularly during the first trimester, to prevent hypoglycemia. Multiple injections with changes in insulin type (NPH, lispro, Lente, and Ultralente) may be needed for better glycemic control. To achieve safer and improved glycemic control, home monitoring may be increased to eight times per day (fasting, before each meal, 2-hour postprandial, at bedtime, and at 2 or 3 AM). Also, reassessment for signs of retinopathy, nephropathy, and hypertension is necessary because of the metabolic changes of pregnancy. Certain oral medications are not safe during pregnancy and will have to be changed (e.g., angiotensin-converting enzyme [ACE] inhibitors).

Pregnancy in the Patient with Type 2 Diabetes. Treatment for the pregnant patient with type 2 diabetes is the same as it would be for the patient with gestational diabetes. Ideally, glycemic control should be attained before pregnancy to improve maternal and fetal outcomes. Careful monitoring of blood pressure, renal and retinal status, glycemic control, and fetal well-being by a team of specialists is necessary throughout pregnancy. Dietary and exercise guidelines and insulin requirements are the same as for gestational diabetes. If the woman is taking oral agents, these need to be discontinued and insulin started (see Table 223-3 for insulin dosing during pregnancy). Metformin (Glucophage) and the thiazolidinediones decrease insulin resistance and enhance the onset of pregnancy and can be used right up to conception. For approximately 6 months postpartum, these women may not need pharmacologic treatment. After that time, depending on weight, exercise/activity, and food intake, they may return to their prior regimen. The sulfonylureas, biguanide, ACE inhibitors, or the thiazolidinediones should not be used while breastfeeding, as these medications are transferred into breast milk.

Co-Management with Specialists

Diabetes is a progressive vascular disease requiring collaborative treatment from many specialties to prevent or slow the progression of end-organ complications. Specialists included in the co-management of individuals with diabetes throughout the life span include endocrinologists, ophthalmologists, podiatrists, cardiologists, nephrologists, obstetricians, and vascular surgeons. Consultation with an endocrinologist is required for individuals with diabetes who are receiving insulin pump therapy, for those with inadequate control (either with hyperglycemia or frequent hypoglycemia), during pregnancy, for motivational issues, and/or for the development of complications. Other referrals include routine yearly visits to an ophthalmologist for evaluation and treatment of retinopathy, cataracts, and retinal hemorrhaging, and podiatry referral for treatment of ulcers, foot deformities, foot infections, callus removal, and nail care. Once renal involvement is identified, a nephrology referral is indicated. A vascular surgeon or specialist is needed for the treatment of peripheral vascular disease, nonhealing ulcers, and/or amputation.

Other appropriate referrals include consultation with a dietitian for meal management, caloric requirements, and weight loss; an exercise physiologist or physical therapist for exercise guidelines; a social worker; and a diabetic educator.

LIFE SPAN CONSIDERATIONS

Diabetes is a progressive disease with acute and chronic phases. It encompasses all ages from newborn to older adults. With each stage of development there are issues regarding diabetes management, physical and emotional development, education and understanding, physical handicaps, nutrition, and behavioral and medical problems that will affect the diabetic treatment plan. Adolescents and older adults are at greatest risk for failure. Predictors that impede diabetic adherence to therapy include lack of practical knowledge, lack of control, vulnerability, social unacceptance, little or no family support, and fear of hypoglycemia. Other barriers include financial or occupational restraints. Integration of these issues is essential for optimal care.

Adolescents pose a particular challenge, as metabolic and biologic changes affect good blood glucose control. Early or preadolescence (12 years of age), middle adolescence (13 to 15 years of age), and late adolescence (16 to 18 years of age) impose hormonal changes that often cause relative insulin resistance as a result of changing counterregulatory hormonal responses and declining peripheral insulin action.

During adolescence, emotional and developmental issues are critical. The emotional stages of shock, denial, negotiation, anger, and acceptance can recur throughout aging. Developmental issues of individual identity, sexual identity and exploration, the drive for independence and struggles with parents and authority, and peer acceptance can impact adolescents' ability to manage their diabetes. Other concerns affecting diabetes management include athletic participation, recurrent ketoacidosis, inadequate nutrition and dieting, alcohol, drugs, and sexual activity. The primary care provider's ability to communicate and compromise without risking safety will aid the development of a trusting relationship. Education must be factual, specific, consultative vs. directive, and relevant to the adolescent's stage of development and emotional behavior. The treatment plan must be realistic and workable and agreed on by the patient and provider. Written instructions are helpful.

During young adulthood, developmental issues of career development, interpersonal relationships, self-image, health perception, and understanding of diabetes can influence glycemic control. As emotional ties to family decrease, concerns related to marriage, pregnancy and children, employment, finances, and anticipation of complications can influence diabetes management. Primary care providers must provide emotional support, educational review or expansion on previous information, and nutritional and pharmacologic reevaluation. Emphasis should be on blood glucose monitoring, appropriate physical activity, nutrition, and medical intervention to prevent hypoglycemia and maintain glycemic control.

In middle-aged and older persons, concerns about loneliness, economics, and disease progression or failing health can affect diabetic management. Financial constraints can interfere with proper food, prescribed medications, blood testing and/or insulin equipment, and medical care. Issues of weight loss, physical inactivity, failing vision or blindness, poor dexterity and/or amputation, memory impairment, hearing loss, gait disturbance or muscle weakness, sexual dysfunction, dialysis, and physical and emotional isolation can affect glycemic control. As complications develop and health begins to fail, denial, anger, hostility, and depression can threaten the emotional well-being of the older patient with diabetes and influence diabetic management. Primary care providers must provide emotional support. The maintenance of function, independence, and general well-being, as well as prevention of severe hypoglycemia and vascular compromise, should take precedence over attaining optimal glycemic control. Insulin doses at this time may need to be decreased to prevent hypoglycemia and prevent falls. In the older patient with diabetes it is essential that the patient understand and can accomplish the treatment plan. Frequent medical visits, as well as written and simplified instructions, are helpful for older adults with diabetes.

COMPLICATIONS

Psychologic Complications

The diagnosis of DM, as with any chronic illness, can be unexpected and potentially devastating. Grief is the most common reaction of an individual diagnosed with DM, and resolution is dependent on variables such as education, economics, geography, and religious and cultural adherence. The integral support of family members and friends affects the long-term acceptance of the disease progression.

Whereas 5% to 8% of the general population will experience a major depressive disorder sometime in their lifetime, there is a threefold to fourfold increase in the prevalence of depression in patients with type 1 or type 2 diabetes. Without treatment, depression in the patient with diabetes can affect glycemic control, complicating management. Careful coordination of medical therapy is necessary to avoid the unfortunate hyperglycemic side effects of most antidepressant agents.

Macrovascular Complications

Macrovascular disease in the patient with diabetes is characterized by arteriosclerosis and atherosclerosis of moderate- to large-sized arterial and venous vessel walls as well as nonatherosclerotic disease leading to vascular insufficiency, claudication, and gangrene. The vascular pathology encompasses cerebral, coronary, and peripheral circulation and is exacerbated by an "atherosclerotic environment" of hypertension, hyperlipidemia, hyperglycemia, and obesity. These diffuse atherosclerotic plaques increase the presence of tissue ischemia, thrombosis, infarction, and atheroemboli leading to tissue and organ damage. Also seen are small vessel disease and endothelial dysfunction with inappropriate vasodilatory responses.

The patient with type 2 diabetes presents a particular challenge, as many of the symptoms associated with macrovascular disease are overlooked before the onset and/or diagnosis of diabetes itself and may be present long before the development of hyperglycemia. Cerebrovascular disease, correlated with the length of time diabetes is present in the patient with type 1 diabetes and the level of glycemic control, carries a three to five times greater mortality rate than in the population without diabetes. Slurred speech, intermittent dizziness, transient loss of vision and/or paresthesia, or weakness of an arm or leg suggests a transient ischemic attack consistent with cerebral disease. In patients with type 1 diabetes these symptoms are usually discernible and easily distinguished from episodes of hypoglycemia, but in patients with type 2 diabetes the diagnosis is often less clear. Auscultation of vascular bruits over the carotid arteries and noninvasive Doppler ultrasound studies can help identify the presence and extent of cerebrovascular disease. Anticoagulant and antiplatelet medications, and/or the use of daily aspirin may help prevent a recurrence of symptoms.

Coronary artery disease (CAD) in the patient with diabetes occurs earlier and more extensively, and infarction may occur without typical symptoms. Atypical symptoms of CAD include dyspnea, fatigue, gastrointestinal complaints with exertion, periods of poor glycemic control particularly if associated with diabetic ketoacidosis, and unexplained congestive heart failure. Typical symptoms of exertional chest pain, chest tightness, and arm pain associated with activity or rest need to be evaluated for the presence of cardiovascular disease. There is a twofold to fourfold increase in patients with diabetes vs. those without diabetes. An initial or subsequent myocardial infarction is more likely to precipitate long-term complications (e.g., heart failure, arrhythmia) or death in the patient with diabetes vs. the patient without diabetes. Silent myocardial infarcts are two to three times more common in patients with diabetes. Early identification of those patients needing revascularization, either by screening or diagnostic testing (Boxes 223-11 and 223-12), is necessary to ensure aggressive medical or surgical management. Diabetic patients with known cardiac disease should be treated early with aspirin, ACE inhibition, target blood pressure control, and lipid-lowering therapy. Their medical care should be in conjunction with a cardiologist.

Dyslipidemia in patients with predominantly type 2 diabetes is characterized by hypertriglyceridemia, low HDL, and high LDL. There is a twofold to fourfold increase in risk for coronary heart disease. Patients are evaluated for fasting lipid levels, cardiovascular disease, and hypertension. Improvement of glycemic control will help to improve hypertriglyceridemia and

BOX 223-11

SCREENING/DIAGNOSTIC TESTS

- ECG
- Persantine or thallium exercise testing
- Stress echocardiogram
- SPECT sestamibi imaging
- Coronary angiography

BOX 223-12

INDICATIONS FOR CARDIOVASCULAR TESTING

- ECG persistent with ischemia
- Age >65 years with duration of type 2 diabetes >10 years
- Plans to begin vigorous exercise program
- Evaluation before renal transplantation
- Preoperative clearance for major vascular or noncardiac surgery
- Atypical cardiac symptoms
- Peripheral or carotid obstructive vascular disease
- Two or more of following risk factors in addition to diabetes:
  - Total cholesterol ≥240 mg/dl, LDL ≥160 mg/dl, or HDL <35 mg/dl
  - Blood pressure >140/90
  - Cigarette smoking
  - Positive family history or premature coronary artery disease
  - Positive micro/macroalbuminuria

From Sander GE: Diagnostic evaluation for coronary artery disease in patients with diabetes mellitus, *Cardiovascular Primer,* New Orleans, 2001, Louisiana State University School of Medicine.

may lower LDL. Thiazolidinediones may increase HDL and have some impact on LDL, but long-term data are unavailable. Nutrition therapy with a low-fat, low-cholesterol diet and aerobic exercise are first-line treatments and should be maintained in conjunction with pharmacologic intervention. Risk stratification (see Chapter 227) allows the medical practitioner to proceed in the care of the diabetic patient while decreasing the sequelae of cardiovascular disease. Optimal LDL in diabetic patients is below 100 mg/dl and optimal HDL is above 45 mg/dl. Treatment of LDL between 100 and 129 mg/dl depends on the presence of vascular disease (coronary, cerebral, and/or peripheral). Without disease the diabetic individual may be able to use nutrition therapy alone for 3 to 6 months and reserve drug therapy for LDLs >130 mg/dl (see Chapter 227). Lifestyle changes, dietary modification of lowered saturated fat and dietary cholesterol, weight loss, increased aerobic exercise, and smoking cessation must be endorsed simultaneously.

The incidence of occlusive peripheral arterial disease is four to six times higher in patients with diabetes. The pattern of lower extremity ischemia in these patients differs from that in the population without diabetes. There is a predilection for macrovascular disease, primarily in the tibial and peroneal arteries. The dorsalis pedis artery and other foot vessels are usually spared. As a direct consequence of poor peripheral circulation, infections, limb ischemia, and lower extremity ulceration are additional concerns. Early warning signs include claudication. Diagnosis by Doppler of lower extremities or by ankle-brachial index confirms the diagnosis. Treatment options include exercise, aggressive lipid and hypertension management, smoking cessation, antiplatelet medications, and the use of cilostazol.

Neuropathic Complications

Diabetic neuropathy affects up to 60% of individuals with DM and is one of the most complex and potentially catastrophic of all the diabetic complications. Although the degree and duration of hyperglycemia appear to increase the risk of nerve damage, these two factors do not reliably predict the development of neuropathy. Multiple mechanisms contribute to the pathogenesis of this diabetic complication. There are three major classes of diabetic neuropathies: peripheral or distal polyneuropathy, mononeuropathy, and diabetic autonomic neuropathy.

Peripheral polyneuropathy is the most commonly occurring neuropathic complication. Distal numbness or impaired sensation is typically symmetric and bilateral, and it can occur acutely as a complication of poor glycemic control. Initially, pain sensation and the ability to discriminate sharp stimuli are impaired, along with bilaterally absent knee or ankle jerk reflexes. Progression of sensory deficits can cause destruction of cartilage in foot joints. This destruction results in loss of normal foot architecture, leaving the foot susceptible to an arthropathy known as Charcot's joint. Charcot's joint may be difficult to distinguish from active infection with cellulitis, as both present with erythema and swelling. The presence of altered foot sensation suggests that an individual require daily foot inspection and routine podiatry visits to minimize the risk of complications.

Pain is present in about 25% of all diabetic patients with peripheral neuropathy. Nonpharmacologic treatment for painful peripheral neuropathy is aimed at avoidance of alcohol; improvement of glycemic control; use of relaxation, hypnotic, or biofeedback techniques; use of transcutaneous electrical nerve stimulation; or referral to a pain control clinic. Pharmacologic considerations include topical capsaicin, aspirin, nonsteroidal antiinflammatory drugs, and, in limited situations, narcotics. Sharp pain may respond to carbamazepine or phenytoin. Tricyclic antidepressants alone or in combination with fluphenazine, cholinergic drugs such as doxepin, and beta blockers such as phenoxybenzamine may all provide relief of symptoms when given in low doses at bedtime.

The mononeuropathies occur in large nerves or nerve roots and produce radicular symptoms. Large nerve roots in the spinal cord, chest, or abdomen, or even cranial nerves can be affected. Mononeuropathy involves both the sensory and motor neurons, producing increased or decreased sensation, weakness, and pain. The pain produced by mononeuropathies can be severe and mimic degenerative disk disease, herpes zoster, carpal tunnel syndrome, Bell's palsy, or intraabdominal conditions. Oculomotor palsy, characterized by ptosis, pain, and sparing of the pupillary reflex, occurs in patients over 50 years of age. Pain and oculomotor function improve gradually over several weeks, and full recovery usually occurs within 3 to 5 months.

Autonomic neuropathy impacts both sympathetic and parasympathetic fibers. Although any organ system may be affected, the more common effects are found in the gastrointestinal tract, genitourinary tract, and cardiovascular system. Symptoms of gastrointestinal dysfunction include esophageal motility problems and gastroparesis with impaired gastric emptying. Gastroparesis affects food absorption, affecting glycemic control. The erratic nature of gastric emptying also produces nausea and vomiting. Bowel peristaltic dysfunction is evidenced by explosive diarrhea and altered small bowel motility. These symptoms may improve with control of hyperglycemia. Gastroparesis can be addressed through dietary modifications and with the use of metoclopramide. Various modalities have been tried for controlling diarrhea including biofeedback, diphenoxylate/atropine (Lomotil), clonidine, and antibiotics.

Genitourinary complications most often consist of neurogenic bladder and sexual dysfunction. Bladder atony, characterized by a residual urine volume >150 ml, may lead to recurrent UTIs and eventual obstructive uropathy. The occurrence of more than two UTIs in 1 year indicates the need for further evaluation. Bethanechol may be helpful as a conservative measure. Sexual dysfunction in women is characterized by decreased vaginal lubrication and frequency of orgasm. Impotence can affect more than 50% of diabetic men with 10 or more years of disease. Retrograde ejaculations are also common. Psychologic, endocrine-related, medication, or alcohol-induced impotence needs to be excluded before vasodilatory substances, implantations, or vacuum devices are considered.

Cardiovascular autonomic neuropathy has two major associated syndromes: orthostatic hypotension and cardiac denervation. Orthostatic hypotension may be pronounced, with an inability to tolerate rising from a supine to an upright posture unless achieved gradually over more than 10 minutes. Cardiac denervation, characterized in later stages by a fixed heart rate in the range of 80 to 100 beats per minute, is unresponsive to stress, exercise, or tilting. These patients may suffer myocardial ischemia or infarction without pain and are at risk for cardiac arrhythmias and sudden death. They should avoid heavy exercise, aerobic exercise, and straining, and are generally not candidates for intensive insulin therapy because of the risk for hypoglycemia and potential cardiac arrhythmias.

Nephropathic Complications

Nephropathy results in end-stage renal disease (ESRD) requiring dialysis in 30% to 40% of patients with type 1 diabetes, and it is the second leading cause of death in individuals with diabetes. In all, 60% of patients with diabetes who ultimately require renal dialysis have type 2 diabetes.

Proteinuria, hypertension, edema, and renal insufficiency characterize diabetic nephropathy. Once established and without adequate medical intervention, nephropathy progresses through five stages: (1) hypertrophy and hyperfunction, (2) renal lesions, (3) incipient nephropathy, (4) clinical diabetic nephropathy, and (5) ESRD. Histologically there are three classes of renal changes: (1) glomerulosclerosis, (2) structural vascular changes, and (3) tubulointerstitial disease.

The glomerular filtration rate (GFR), usually elevated when a person is first diagnosed with diabetes, is directly related to the degree of hyperglycemia. However, it is a poor measure of renal function, as its elevation may ensue over a long "silent" period (about 15 years' duration) as histologic changes in the kidney continue. Serum creatinine, also an unreliable marker for renal disease, might not be elevated until more than 50% of function is lost and may be normal in older patients with renal damage because of decreased muscle mass.

All patients with diabetes should have a urinalysis performed and renal function assessed at least annually. Those individuals with proteinuria need closer monitoring of renal function, initiation of ACE inhibition, and screening for microalbuminuria. Microalbuminuria analysis can be performed by random spot collection, a 24-hour collection, or a timed (e.g., 4-hour or overnight) collection. Microalbuminuria is diagnostic at greater than 30 mg/24 hr excretion. Two to three positive collections in a 3- to 6-month period should exist before microalbuminuria is diagnosed. Consultation with a diabetologist or nephrologist should occur when microalbuminuria (30 to 300 mg/24 hr), overt albuminuria (>2 mg/dl), or decreased GFR (<50 ml/min) is present.

Controlling blood pressure is the single most important factor in the prevention and treatment of renal disease in the patient with diabetes. The ADA cites 120 to 130/80 mm Hg to be the normalized blood pressure goal to prevent complications of cerebral, cardiac, or other organ system functions. In patients with evidence of microvascular or macrovascular complications, a blood pressure >130/80 mm Hg should be considered abnormal. Currently, a reasonable blood pressure goal of below 130/80 mm Hg in individuals with type 2 diabetes and 120/80 mm Hg or lower in those with type 1 diabetes is the optimal goal. For individuals with systolic hypertension, blood pressure should be decreased in slow increments with careful monitoring of patient tolerance. As with all treatment options, diet, exercise, weight loss, and smoking cessation are included in treatment options. Pharmacologic intervention for blood pressure includes, in order of preference, ACE inhibitors, angiotension II inhibitors, alpha blockers, beta blockers, calcium blockers, and low-dose diuretics. Consultation with a cardiologist and/or nephrologist is recommended for patients with recalcitrant hypertension.

Additional management concerns involve reduction of the GFR by control of hyperglycemia, use of low-protein diets, and limiting the use of nephrotoxic drugs. As the creatinine increases, the use of metformin (Glucophage) may be contraindicated. Although recommended, ACE inhibitors and angiotension II inhibitors may also be nephrotoxic. In addition, monitoring the hematocrit is essential as renal failure progresses.

Microvascular Complications

Retinopathy. Annual screening for retinopathy with a dilated examination by an ophthalmologist or optometrist is recommended for all individuals with diabetes. In the 20- to 74-year age-groups, diabetic retinopathy is now the leading cause of new-onset blindness in the United States. More than 80% of patients with type 1 or type 2 diabetes will have some form of retinopathy 15 years after diagnosis. Poor glucose control, proteinuria, hyperlipidemia, and hypertension are all risk factors associated with the incidence and progression of diabetic retinopathy.

A patient presenting with initial visual blurring may have changes that result from fluid accumulation in the lens. Sorbitol, created by the conversion of glucose by aldose reductase, may be responsible. Readjusting blood glucose levels should reverse these symptoms in most patients over several weeks.

The three stages of diabetic retinopathy are characterized by individual findings and changes. Nonproliferative (or background) diabetic retinopathy (NPDR) is the earliest stage and intraretinal "dot and blot" microaneurysms can be detected. Often this form, especially in the patient with type 2 diabetes, will not progress or interfere with visual acuity. If these microaneurysms are not detected, or if the abnormal vessels leak serous fluid into macula, edema will occur with a decrease in visual acuity. Although macular edema is not detectable by monocular viewing, the presence of yellowish white, glistening, hard lipid exudates found within the retina, especially in a ring-shaped configuration, should prompt the primary care provider to suspect macular edema and refer the patient to a retinal specialist.

A diagnosis of preproliferative diabetic retinopathy (PPDR) can be made when the "dot and blot" microaneurysms become clustered, indicating nonfunctional capacity of the capillary circulation. Hypoxia is blamed for rendering the existing capillaries nonperfusing, and an angiogenic response stimulus for growth of new and abnormal blood vessels occurs. Cotton-wool spots (soft exudates), "beading" of the retinal veins, and dilated, tortuous retinal capillaries are all seen in this stage.

Proliferative diabetic retinopathy (PDR), the final and most vision-threatening stage, is characterized by increased retinal ischemia producing continued abnormal retinal vessel growth and creating neovascularization on the surface of the retina and sometimes extending into the posterior vitreous. As these new vessels bleed, a condition exacerbated by macular edema, the patient will report a new sensation of "floaters or cobwebs"

TABLE 223-7 Hypoglycemia

	Signs/Symptoms	Treatment
Mild neuroglycopenia	Hungry, weak, shaky, diaphoresis, pallor, tachycardia, paresthesia, difficulty concentrating, irritability but no changes in mental status; individual able to self-treat	15 g of simple-acting carbohydrate increases blood glucose level 40-80 mg/dl after 15 minutes Stop activity and retest in 10-15 minutes; if below 60 mg/dl, take additional 10-15 g of carbohydrate; ½ hour later, eat snack or meal consisting of one protein and one carbohydrate
Moderate neuroglycopenia	Impaired function of CNS: decreased thinking, increased emotions (anger, irritability), inability to complete tasks, some changes in mental status; individual may be able to self-treat	Take 15-30 g of simple-acting carbohydrate and then follow above instructions
Severe neuroglycopenia	Confusion, drowsiness, and progression to unconsciousness; impaired neurologic function; individual not able to self-treat	Take 30-45 g of simple-acting carbohydrate—if able to swallow—or glucagons SC if not (1 mg—adults; 0.5 mg—children <5 years; 0.25 mg—infants)

Data from Gonder-Frederick L, Cox DJ, Clarke WL: Helping patients understand and recognize hypoglycemia, *Clin Diabetes* 14:86-90, 1996.

in the eye and may experience a sudden, painless loss of vision. Retinal detachment resulting from the tractional forces of fibrous tissue can occur. This tissue, if formed on the surface of the iris and extending into the "angle" of the anterior chamber of the eye, will block the outflow of aqueous humor and increase intraocular pressure. This will manifest as severe pain, loss of vision, and development of glaucoma.

NPDR and PPDR are treated by strict adherence to blood pressure and blood glucose control and follow-up by an eye specialist. Panretinal photocoagulation using a xenon or argon laser is aimed at "spot welding" leaking microaneurysms in patients with PDR, reducing central vision loss. This is helpful in preventing further vision loss but is not beneficial in reversing already diminished visual acuity. Approximately 10% of all patients treated by photocoagulation will experience a loss of peripheral vision and night vision. Treatment of patients with mild to moderate NPDR is minimally effective. Vitrectomy, another form of treatment for severely advanced PDR, is used in patients with vitreous hemorrhage, scarring, and imminent or present retinal detachment.

Hypoglycemia. Hypoglycemia is a complication of insulin excess and results in various symptoms (Table 223-7). Neuroglycopenia occurs when the brain and central nervous system are not able to maintain normal function because of lowered glucose levels. The lowered serum glucose is classified as mild, moderate, or severe and is dependent on the symptoms of neuroglycopenia and the individual's ability to self-treat. When blood glucose levels are below 70 mg/dl (may be higher in a diabetic patient with poor control), the hypothalamus senses the decreased blood glucose and triggers the sensation of hunger. This action stimulates the nervous system to increase gastric juices and stomach contraction. The adrenal medulla secretes epinephrine and cortisol, which stimulates glycogenolysis. This slows glycogenesis (the uptake of glucose) and promotes gluconeogenesis (glucose formation from fatty and amino acids). As the blood glucose level decreases, cerebral function is altered.

Patients with diabetes have different blood glucose ranges for mild to severe hypoglycemia. A previously normal glucose range of 70 mg/dl for one individual may mean hypoglycemia for another. Therefore the individual must monitor episodes of hypoglycemia, symptoms encountered (especially unconscious episodes), and blood glucose ranges. Areas of concern in treating hypoglycemia include inadequate treatment and/or inability to recognize warning signals. Hypoglycemia unawareness is the loss of autonomic symptoms that warn the individual of the impending lowered blood glucose level. Uncontrolled diabetes or large swings in glucose ranges are risk factors for this reversible condition. Thus improvement of glycemic control will correct the process. Intensive insulin therapy and ideal blood glucose control can cause serious consequences related to hypoglycemia. Primary care providers must be aware of the influence of medications on glucose control and be wary of nighttime moderate to severe hypoglycemia, especially with neurologic impairment, and make adjustments in insulin doses and blood glucose monitoring (Box 223-13). Severe hypoglycemia left untreated can lead to death. Those at greatest risk are individuals with type 1 diabetes and older adults. Another situation affecting glycemic control is the patient who has experienced a severe hypoglycemic episode and purposefully allows the blood glucose level to remain high because of fear of a repeat hypoglycemic event. Therefore it is very important that providers and diabetic individuals collaborate on a treatment plan that is safe and comfortable.

Hyperglycemia. Ketoacidosis and hyperosmolar nonketotic acidosis are two medical emergencies of hyperglycemia that require immediate treatment and possible hospitalization.

Ketoacidosis involves profound hyperglycemia, osmotic diuresis, dehydration, and acidosis causing an increased anion gap from insulin deficiency. Symptoms associated with this process include a 12- to 24-hour history of polyuria, polydipsia, hyperventilation, and dehydration. A fruity breath, abdominal pain, nausea and vomiting, and changes in consciousness can also be present. Hospitalization can sometimes be avoided if the hyperglycemia, even with positive ketones, is treated with increased levels of insulin immediately and dehydration is prevented. Hydration is essential. Once dehydration starts, the downward spiraling process of increasing ketones, nausea and vomiting, and acidosis develops quickly. At this

BOX 223-13

DRUGS INTERFERING WITH GLYCEMIC CONTROL

INTRINSIC HYPOGLYCEMIC EFFECT

Alcohol
Salicylates
Guanethidine
Monoamine oxidase inhibitors
Beta-blockers

INTRINSIC HYPERGLYCEMIC EFFECT

Acetazolamide
Beta-blockers
Diazoxide
Diuretics (thiazides, furosemide)
Epinephrine
Estrogens
Glucagon
Glucocorticoids
Indomethacin
Interferon
Isoniazid
Nicotinic acid
Pentamidine
Phenytoin
L-Thyroxine

time, the goal of therapy includes restoring fluid and electrolyte imbalances, reversing hyperglycemia, and preventing hypoglycemia. Adequate hydration with IV fluids and replacement of potassium and insulin are the essential interventions (Figure 223-1). Once the patient is stable, the cause for ketoacidosis should be explored to prevent recurrence. Most common causes include new-onset diabetes, infection, illness or major surgery, and depression.

Prevention of ketoacidosis requires prompt dialogue between the patient and primary care provider to treat increasing hyperglycemia. Humalog insulin and an antiemetic should be available for the patient once this occurs. Sick day management guidelines (Box 223-14) can enable the individual with diabetes to actively participate in preventing ketoacidosis.

Nonketotic hyperglycemia hyperosmolar syndrome affects the patient with type 2 diabetes. Presenting symptoms include altered consciousness, shallow respiration, polydipsia, hyperglycemia, and profound dehydration. Seizures, coma, or even hemiplegia may be present. This most commonly occurs in older adults with type 2 diabetes or in newly diagnosed individuals. Diagnostic abnormalities include blood glucose ranges >600 mg/dl without ketosis or with slight ketosis, serum osmolarity >340 mOsm, increased BUN and creatinine, and mild metabolic acidosis. Precipitating causes include medications (see Box 223-13), infection, surgery or severe dialysis, excessive burns, and certain medical conditions (cerebrovascular accident, myocardial infarction, pancreatitis, gastrointestinal hemorrhage, and diabetic gangrene). Treatment includes hospitalization to reverse dehydration and hyperglycemia and to correct any electrolyte abnormalities (Figure 223-2).

BOX 223-14

SICK DAY MANAGEMENT OF PATIENTS WITH DIABETES

At time of impending illness when glucose levels are higher, ketones may be present. Some general rules:

1. Monitor blood glucose every 4 hours with symptoms of nausea, anorexia, and rising glucose levels.
2. If blood glucose level is above 275 mg/dl, test for ketones.
3. With elevated blood glucose levels, supplemental regular insulin can be given every 4 hours. Give 10% of total daily dose as supplement if blood glucose level is under 300 mg/dl. If it is above 300 mg/dl, give 20% of total daily dose as supplement. Another method is to use a sliding scale of regular insulin while sick until blood glucose levels return to previous control.
4. Maintain adequate hydration by drinking 8 ounces of calorie-free fluid hourly while awake. This can be alternated with a sodium-rich fluid, such as bouillon, consomme, or clear canned soups.
5. Continue to take diabetic medicine, even if anorexic or if nausea is present. If unable to eat, follow these guidelines: blood glucose level between 250 mg/dl and higher—drink calorie-free fluid; blood glucose between 180-250 mg/dl—drink equivalent of 15 g of carbohydrate at meal; blood glucose level less than 180 mg/dl—drink fluids with sugar or eat easily tolerated foods equivalent to meal plan.
6. Antiemetics should be prescribed for those unable to tolerate fluids by mouth, monitor closely for dehydration—may need IV fluid.

Modified from American Diabetes Association: *Medical management of insulin dependent (type 1) diabetes*, ed 3, Alexandria, Va, 1994, The Association.

Insulin Allergy

Local reactions at the injection site are the most common form of allergic reaction to insulin. Delayed hypersensitivity may also occur but remains in the area of injection. The use of synthetic or purified insulin has decreased both local and systemic reactions. Occurrence of reactions may be secondary to improper injection technique, injection of cold insulin, or the presence of preservatives. If systematic reactions do occur, the individual may require desensitization (the process of slowly reintroducing the allergic insulin at minute doses until the body no longer reacts with an allergic response). This procedure requires a series of injections of the insulin.

INDICATIONS FOR REFERRAL/HOSPITALIZATION

Guidelines based on the ADA recommendations for hospitalization include the following:

1. Acute metabolic complications: diabetic ketoacidosis (with ketonuria, blood glucose >250 mg/dl and arterial pH <7.35, and nausea and vomiting), hyperosmolar nonketotic state (with impaired mental status, dehydration, elevated plasma osmolarity, and blood glucose >400 mg/dl), and hypoglycemia with neuroglycopenia
2. Newly diagnosed diabetes in children and adolescents
3. Poor metabolic control that requires close monitoring

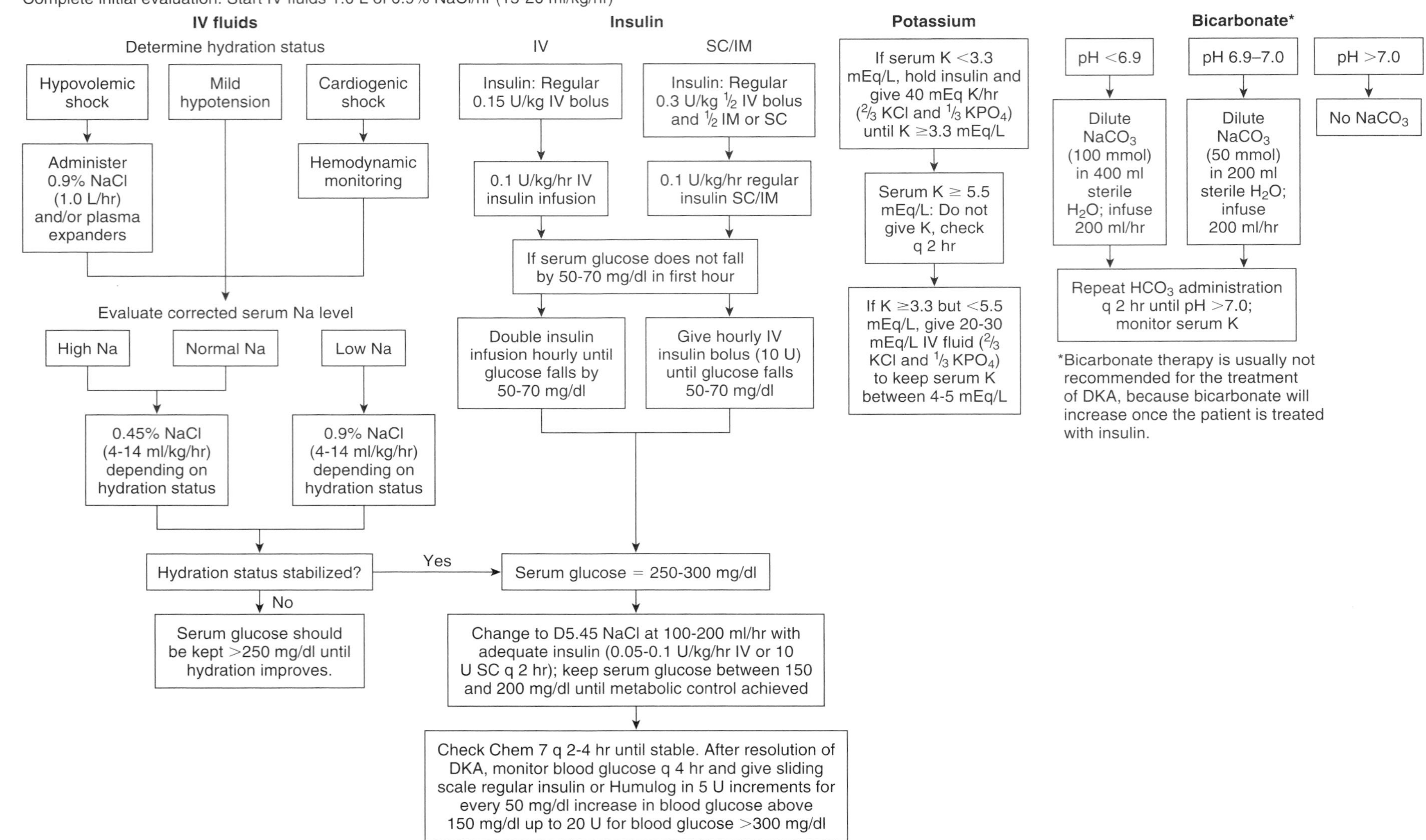

FIGURE 223-1

Management of ketoacidosis. (Data from American Diabetes Association (Position Statement): Hyperglycemic crises in patients with diabetes mellitus, *Diabetes Care* 24:S85, 2001).

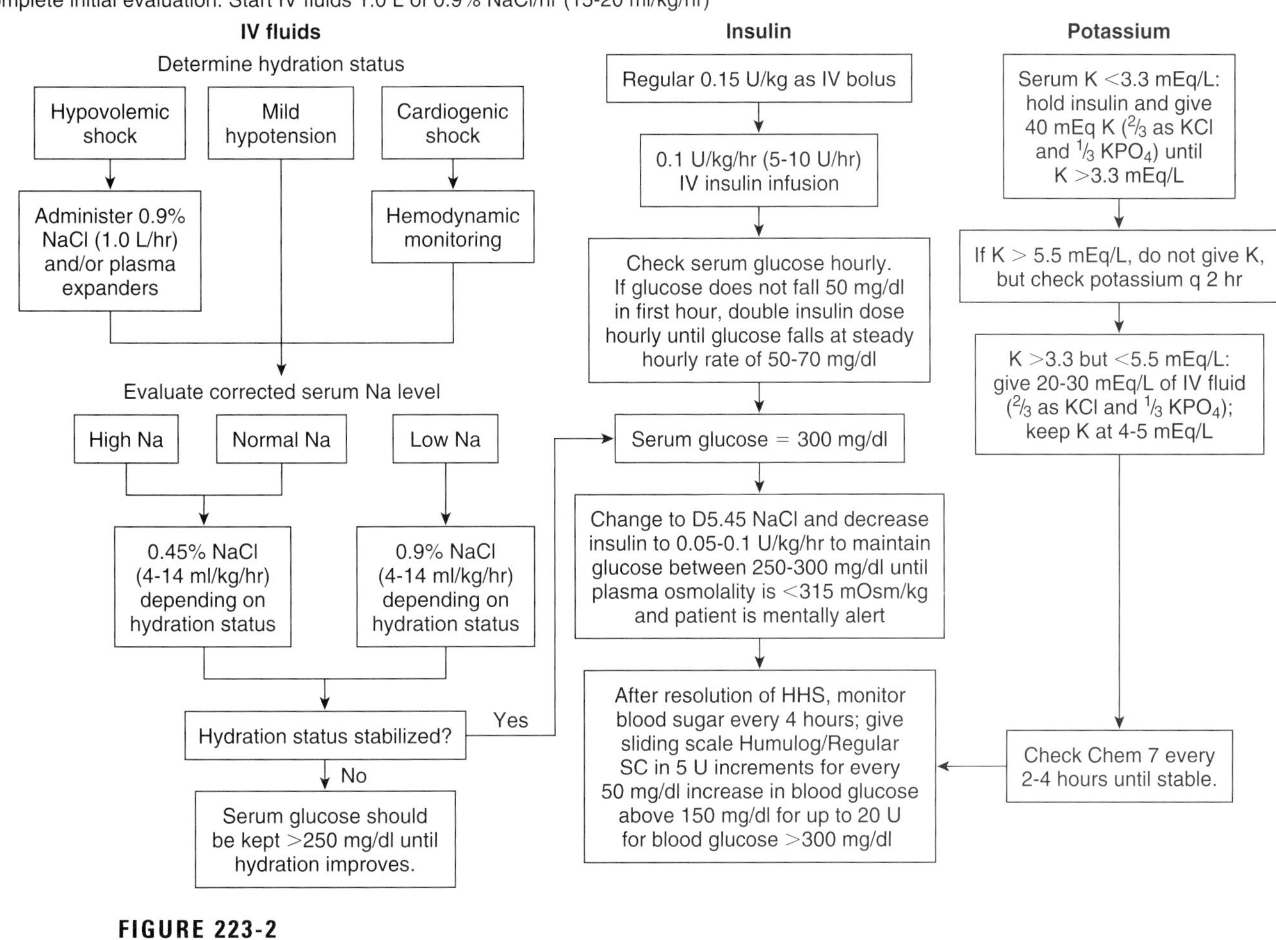

FIGURE 223-2

Hyperosmolar nonketotic syndrome. (Data from American Diabetes Association [Position Statement]: Hyperglycemic crisis in patient with diabetes mellitus, *Diabetes Care* 24:S86, 2001.)

4. Uncontrolled or newly diagnosed gestational diabetes requiring insulin
5. Institution of insulin pump or other intensive insulin therapy requiring close observation
6. Chronic vascular complications of diabetes that progress, requiring intensive treatment

Other situations requiring physician consultation include an inability to attain glucose control (either consistent hyperglycemia or hypoglycemia), pregnancy, and the development of complications.

PATIENT AND FAMILY EDUCATION

Patient education enhances glycemic control. Education is lifelong as the individual enters different life and emotional stages resulting in changes, reevaluations, and new treatment options. The length of time with the disease alters the amount of knowledge the patient may receive at a particular time. Initially, the patient with diabetes cannot process all that is needed to manage the disease. Therefore survival skills for the patient and family are devised to maintain a safe environment for managing the disease process. Diabetic educators, support groups, and diabetic classes assist the patient and family to understand diabetes management. Survival skills encompass the basic pathology of the disease, pharmacologic understanding, and recognition and treatment of hypoglycemia and hyperglycemia. In addition, education includes injection technique, home glucose monitoring, foot care, basic meal planning, and the importance of when to notify the primary care provider.

As the individual becomes accustomed to the disease, further education is needed. Areas to be reviewed are sick day management, acidosis or situations of impending emergency, the pathology of the disease and complications, adjustment of insulin guidelines, an exercise program with appropriate snacking, management during traveling, preventive care, treatment options for progressing complications of diabetes, nutrition and weight loss, use of glucagon, and options with diabetic supplies.

Diabetic education reinforced with written material and instruction improves understanding and compliance. The ADA, Department of Public Health, pharmacists, drug representatives and companies, diabetic educators, and diabetic supply resources are great sources for free written materials.

Diabetic Websites:
http://www.diabetesmonitor.com
http://www.americandiabetesassociation.com
http://www.diabetesonestop.com
http://www.aace.com

REFERENCES

1. American Diabetes Association: Clinical practice recommendations 2001, *Diabetes Care* 24(1): 512-515, 2001.
2. American Diabetes Association: *Medical management of insulin dependent (type 1) diabetes,* ed 3, Alexandria, VA, 1994, The Association.
3. American Diabetes Association: *Medical management of non–insulin dependent (type II) diabetes,* ed 3, Alexandria, VA, 1994, The Association.
4. American Diabetes Association: *Medical management of pregnancy complicated by diabetes,* ed 2, Alexandria, VA, 1995, The Association.
5. American Diabetes Association: *The fourth international workshop: conference on gestational diabetes mellitus,* Washington, DC, March 1997, The Association.
6. American Diabetes Association: Screening for diabetic retinopathy, *Diabetes Care* 24(1):S73, 2001.
7. Bakkris GL and others: Preserving renal function in adults with hypertension and diabetes: a consensus approach, *Am J Kidney Dis* 36(3):646-661, 2000.
8. Bastyr EJ and others: Therapy focused on lowering postprandial glucose, not fasting glucose, *Diabetes Care* 23(9):1236-1241, 2000.
9. Beck AT, Beamederfer A: Assessment of depression: the depression inventory in psychological measurements in psychopharmacology, *Mod Probl Pharmacopsychiatry* 7:151-169, 1974.
10. Buchanan TA: Diabetes and pregnancy: a focus on type 2 and gestational diabetes. In Olefsky JM, editor: *Current approaches to the management of type 2 diabetes,* Secaucus, NJ, 1997, Professional Postgraduate Services.
11. Caputo GM and others: Assessment and management of foot disease in patients with diabetes, *N Engl J Med* 331(13):854-860, 1994.
12. Coustan DR: Gestational diabetes mellitus. In American Diabetes Association: *Therapy for diabetes mellitus and related disorders,* Alexandria, VA, 1994, The Association.
13. Coustan DR: Gestational diabetes. In National Institutes of Health: *Diabetes in America,* ed 2, NIH Pub No 95-1468, Bethesda, MD, 1995, The Institutes.
14. DeValentine S, Fredenburg M, Loretz L: Infections of the diabetic foot, *Clin Podiatr Med Surg* 4(2):395-412, 1987.
15. Devlin JT: Exercise therapy in the management of diabetes, *Practical Diabetol* March, pp 38-44, 2001.
16. Diabetes Control Program: *Massachusetts guidelines for adult diabetes care,* Mass Department of Public Health, June 2001.
17. Dittko-Peragallo V and others: Psychosocial issues. In *A core curriculum for diabetes education,* ed 2, Chicago, 1994, American Association of Diabetes Educators.
18. The Expert Committee on the Diagnosis and Classification of Diabetes Mellitus: Report of the Expert Committee on the Diagnosis and Classification of Diabetes Mellitus, *Diabetes Care* 24(1):S5-S16, 2001.
19. Expert Panel on Detection, Evaluation, and Treatment of High Blood Cholesterol in Adults: Executive summary of the third report of the national cholesterol education program, *JAMA* 285:2486-2497, 2001.
20. Garber AJ, Gavin JR, Goldstein BJ: Understanding insulin resistance and syndrome X, *Patient Care* 30:198-211, 1996.
21. Gibbons GW: Vascular evaluation and long-term results of distal bypass surgery in patients with diabetes, *Clin Podiatr Med Surg* 12(1):129-140, 1995.
22. Giles TD, editor: *Diabetes and cardiovascular disease: a practical primer,* New Orleans, 2000, Cardiovascular Research Center.
23. Gonder-Frederick L, Cox DJ, Clarke WL: Helping patients understand and recognize hypoglycemia, *Clin Diabetes* 14(4):86-90, 1996.
24. Harris MI: Classification, diagnostic criteria, and screening for diabetes. In National Institutes of Health: *Diabetes in America,* ed 2, NIH Pub No 95-1468, Bethesda, MD, 1995, The Institutes.
25. Hirsch AT, Baum P: *Peripheral arterial disease,* Society for Vascular Medicine, May 1999, San Antonio.
26. Kahn R: Macrovascular disease. In *Medical management of insulin dependent (type 1) diabetes,* ed 2, Alexandria, VA, 1994, American Diabetes Association.
27. Kahn R: Promoting behavior change. In *Medical management of non–insulin dependent (type 2) diabetes,* Alexandria, VA, 1994, American Diabetes Association.
28. Kasden F: Teaching diabetes survival skills, *Adv Nurse Pract* 5(5): 51-54, 1997.
29. Krall LP, Beaser RS, editors: *Joslin diabetes manual,* ed 12, Philadelphia, 1996, Lea & Febiger.
30. Levin ME: Understanding your diabetic patient, *Clin Podiatr Med Surg* 4(2):315-330, 1987.
31. Levin ME: Saving the diabetic foot, *Intern Med* 90-102, 1997.
32. Lepore M and others: Pharmacokinetics and pharmacodynamics of subcutaneous injection of long acting human insulin glargine, NPH, and ultralente and continuous lispro, *Diabetes* 49:2142-2147, 2000.
33. Lipnick JA, Lee TH: Diabetic neuropathy, *Am Fam Physician* 54(8):2478-2483, 1996.
34. Luna B, Feinglos MN: Oral agents in the management of type 2 diabetes mellitus, *Am Fam Physician* 63(9):1747-1756, 2001.
35. Lustman PJ, Harper GW: Nonpsychiatric physicians' identification and treatment of depression in patients with diabetes, *Compr Psychiatry* 28(1):22-27, 1987.
36. Marcus AO: Diabetes mellitus: nephropathy and hypertension, *Clin Diabetes* 7(9), 1996.
37. Murray HJ, Boulton AJM: The pathophysiology of diabetic foot ulceration, *Clin Podiatr Med Surg* 12(1):1-17, 1995.
38. National Institutes of Health: *Diabetes in America,* ed 2, NIH Pub No 95-1468, Bethesda, MD, 1995, The Institutes.
39. Nelson JP: The vascular history and physical examination, *Clin Podiatr Med Surg* 9(1):1-17, 1992.
40. Novo Nordisk Pharmaceuticals: *Introducing Novolog, Insulin aspart,* Drug Insert, 2001.
41. O'Keefe JH and others: Improving the adverse cardiovascular prognosis of type 2 diabetes, *Mayo Clinic Proc* 74:171-180, 1999.
42. Palumbo PJ: Glycemic control, mealtime glucose excursions, and diabetic complications in type 2 diabetes, *Mayo Clinc Proc* 76:609-618, 2001.
43. Perkins AT, Morgenlander JC: Endocrinologic causes of peripheral neuropathy, *Postgrad Med* 102(3):81-106, 1997.
44. Prendergast JJ: Diabetic autonomic neuropathy, *Practical Diabetol* March, pp 7-14, 2001.
45. Professional Practice Committee and Executive Committee: Position statement: diabetic nephropathy, *Diabetes Care* 24(1): 56-57, 2001.
46. Riddle ME, Karl DM: Starting insulin for type 2 diabetes, *Postgrad Inst Med* 108(6): 3-11, 2000.
47. Rosenstock J and others: Basal insulin therapy, *Diabetes Care* 24(4):631-636, 2001.
48. Russek AS: Immediate postoperative prosthetic fitting and rehabilitation. In Haimovici H, editor: *Vascular surgery principles and techniques,* ed 3, Norwalk, CT, 1989, Appleton & Lange.
49. Scarlet JJ, Blais MR: Statistics on the diabetic foot, *J Am Podiatr Med Assoc* 79(6):306, 1989 (special communications).
50. Schulte M, Mehler PS: Slowing the progression of diabetic nephropathy, *Women's Health* 4(6):437-442, 2001.
51. Sims DS and others: Risk factors in the diabetic foot: recognition and management, *Phys Ther* 68(12):1887-1902, 1988.
52. Skyler JS: Insulin treatment. In American Diabetes Association: *Therapy for diabetes mellitus and related disorders,* Alexandria, VA, 1994, The Association.
53. Veves A, Sarnow MR: Diagnosis, classification and treatment of diabetic peripheral neuropathy, *Clin Podiatr Med Surg* 12(1):19-30, 1995.
54. Winters S, Jernigan V: Vascular disease risk markers in diabetes: monitoring and intervention, *Nurse Pract* 25(6):40-65, 2000.
55. White JR: Combination oral agent/insulin therapy in patients with type 2 diabetes mellitus, *Clin Diabetes* 15:102-111, 1997.
56. Yki-Jarvinen H, Dressler A, Ziemen M: Less nocturnal hypoglycemia and better post dinner glucose control with bedtime glargine, *Diabetes Care* 23(8):1130-1136, 2000.

CHAPTER 224

Hirsutism

Michelle E. Freshman

DEFINITION/EPIDEMIOLOGY

Hirsutism refers to excessive male pattern hair growth in women resulting from increased levels of circulating androgens. Although areas of coarse, pigmented body hair are not unusual in women, concerns regarding abundance and distribution commonly arise. Evaluation of the regions indicative of androgen excess in women helps discern physiologic from pathologic causes. When signs of virilism such as temporal balding or voice deepening accompany hirsutism, ovary and adrenal glands are more likely involved. In each individual, regardless of gender or race, the number of hair follicles is predetermined; what differs is the pigmentation, thickness, and pattern of hair as mediated by localized androgen sensitivity.[1,2]

Millions of women worldwide are affected by hirsutism. Anywhere from 5% to 10% are considered hirsute.[3,4] Coarse, pigmented hair growth on the face, breast, or lower abdomen has also been identified in 17% to 35% of women who have neither androgen excess nor polycystic ovary syndrome (PCOS) and are clinically nonhirsute.[5] Moreover, at least 25% of normal young women have such terminal hair on either their upper lip, areola, or lower abdomen.[5]

The most common underlying pathologic condition is PCOS, which affects 6% to 8%[6] of premenopausal women. In fact, 95% of women who present with progressive hirsutism have PCOS.[5] Generally less than 1% have ovarian or adrenal tumors.[7] PCOS is considered a heterogeneous syndrome. Only 40% to 60% of hirsute women have elevated levels of androgens and just as many women with PCOS may not exhibit elevated androgen levels.[8]

An important consideration for primary care providers is that 38% of women with scattered areas of alopecia, as well as 50% of patients with acne, have underlying hyperandrogenism.[9] By contrast, 5% of hirsute women have congenital adrenal hyperplasia, which may appear in later life; it a condition more prevalent in Latinas, Ashkenazi Jews, Yugoslavians, and Italians.[1]

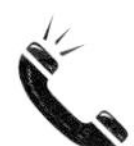

Physician consultation is indicated for all patients with suspected hirsutism.

PATHOPHYSIOLOGY

Clinical conditions of androgen excess are signaled by hirsutism and/or virilism, but may include alopecia, acne, and seborrhea. C19 steroids, androgenic compounds derived from cholesterol, are produced by the ovaries and adrenal glands. They include progesterone, 17-hydroxyprogesterone, testosterone, androstenedione, dihydrotestosterone (DHT), dehydroepiandrosterone (DHEA), estradiol, cortisol, and aldosterone.[10,11] To varying degrees, muscle, fat, and liver tissue, in addition to the ovaries and adrenals, contribute these testosterone precursors.[2] Although androgen excess manifests with abnormal laboratory values, even patients with normal or slightly elevated levels may suffer from disorders involving peripheral production and clearance or target organ sensitivity.[9] Hirsutism and virilism result from this increased testosterone activity.

Testosterone activates the skin and hair follicles via enzyme 5-alpha-reductase, which converts testosterone to the potent metabolite, DHT. This enzyme makes the difference, given similar androgen profiles, between a woman who is hirsute and one who is not. Hair expression is ultimately controlled by follicular sensitivity to 5-alpha-reductase.[7]

As early as age 6 years, children begin producing androgens. In women these levels peak around age 30 years.[7] Adrenarche is heralded by hair growth in the axillae, in the lower pubic triangle, and on the arms and lower legs. Normally, boys have more testosterone than girls, which differentiates their distribution of terminal hair.[12] Most centrally located terminal body hair responds to sex hormone production, especially the amount, duration of exposure, and "intrinsic potential of the hair," which together determine the resultant density and diameter of the hair type.[1,5]

Androgen abnormalities causing hirsutism and occasionally virilism include those found in congenital adrenal hyperplasia, acromegaly, and Cushing's syndrome. In congenital adrenal hyperplasia, any of a set of three enzyme deficiencies causes an accumulation of DHEA and androstenedione, which ultimately increases extraglandular testosterone levels. Testosterone in its various forms is ultimately excreted via urine as 17-ketosteroids. DHEA-S, the largest component, is a useful proxy for the adrenal androgen activity.[8] Finally, women with PCOS can suffer from hyperinsulinemia because of ovarian androgen production by both insulin and insulin-like growth factor receptors. The reduction of sex hormone–binding globulin in turn raises the free testosterone level.[2]

CLINICAL PRESENTATION

Inquiry into familial hair growth, a previous existence of diagnosed hirsutism, or previous treatment is an important initial screen. Constitutional or familial hirsutism is common in individuals of Mediterranean or Persian descent. Ovarian, adrenal, and menstrual function is normal in 80% of these cases, whereas 3-alpha-diol G levels relating to 5-alpha-reductase activity are increased.[8] Seasonal observations regarding hair growth resulting from neurovascular changes should be considered, as more rapid hair growth occurs in the summer months.[7]

Features of virilism, including those associated with defeminization (antiestrogenic), such as body contour changes, breast size reduction, and vaginal dryness; or masculinization, such as acne, hirsutism, oligomenorrhea, temporal balding, voice deepening, increased shoulder girth, and clitoromegaly that progresses sequentially with increasing androgen levels, should be determined.[9] Often virilism is accompanied by amenorrhea.[8] Cushingoid features, such as muscle wasting, truncal obesity, scapular fat pads, moon facies, red striae, and thin skin, are evidence of adrenocorticotropic hormone (ACTH) excess from unsuppressed androgen.

A menstrual history and menopausal status should be assessed. Any irregular or intermenstrual bleeding may indicate the presence of endometrial neoplasm. Moreover, a pregnancy history significant for hair growth may be useful in diagnosing rare conditions such as a type of ovarian tumor called a luteoma.

Use of contraceptives, anabolic steroids such as nandrolone decanoate,[13] danazol, 19-nortestosterone, or other progestins can cause hirsutism. Gonadal abnormalities are indicative of elevated androgen levels and can be ascertained by a history of abnormal sexual development. Finally, patients with PCOS or Cushing's syndrome have lipid and insulin abnormalities. Galactorrhea accompanies hyperprolactinemia and is present in 20% of patients with PCOS.[8] Dyslipidemia and hypertension are common in these populations and should be investigated further.

PHYSICAL EXAMINATION

Weight, height, and vital signs are especially pertinent given the profile of a significant proportion of patients with PCOS. Obesity is seen in patients with PCOS or Cushing's syndrome, although research in PCOS has determined that body fat varies continuously with gonadotropin abnormalities; obese and nonobese patients with PCOS do not make up distinct groups.[14] In fact, only 50% of PCOS patients are obese.[9]

An essential component of the physical examination must include an objective measurement of hair growth pattern and quantity. Regions of androgen-sensitive growth include the lip, chin, sideburns, chest, upper pubic triangle, and intergluteal area, which, when present in women, may be accompanied by seborrhea, acne, and alopecia.[15] The Ferriman-Gallwey scale is often used as an index (Table 224-1). A score of 8 or greater out of 36 is interpreted as evidence of an androgenic excess; a score greater than 15, along with other supporting evidence, is more likely correlated with neoplasms.[5] Terminal hair on the upper back, shoulders, or upper abdomen delineates virilism, as does clitoromegaly in excess of 35 mm.[2,7]

Acanthosis nigricans, the pigmented patch on the back of the neck, elbows, knuckles, knees, and intertriginous regions, is seen commonly in obese women and is indicative of insulin resistance. Although this is not a reliable sign of hyperandrogenism, it is found in 30% of hyperandrogenic women.[5,8] A

TABLE 224-1 The Ferriman-Gallwey Scale: Definition of Hair Grading at Each of 11 Sites*

Site	Grade	Definition
Upper lip	1	Few hairs at outer margin
	2	Small moustache at outer margin
	3	Moustache extending halfway from outer margin
	4	Moustache extending to midline
Chin	1	Few scattered hairs
	2	Scattered hairs with small concentrations
	3, 4	Complete cover, light and heavy
Chest	1	Circumareolar hairs
	2	With midline hair in addition
	3, 4	Fusion of these areas, with three-quarters cover
		Complete cover
Upper back	1	Few scattered hairs
	2	Rather more, still scattered
	3, 4	Complete cover, light and heavy
Lower back	1	Sacral tuft of hair
	2	Rather more, still scattered
	3	Three-quarters cover
	4	Complete cover
Upper abdomen	1	Few midline hairs
	2	Rather more, still scattered
	3, 4	Half and full cover
Lower abdomen	1	Few midline hairs
	2	Midline streak of hair
	3	Midline band of hair
	4	Inverted V-shaped growth
Arm	1	Sparse growth affecting not more than one fourth of limb cover
	2	More than this, cover still incomplete
	3, 4	Complete cover, light and heavy
Forearm	1, 2, 3, 4	Complete cover of dorsal surface, two grades of light and two grades of heavy
Thigh	1, 2, 3, 4	As for forearm
Leg	1, 2, 3, 4	As for forearm

From Mishell DR Jr, Davajan V, Lobo RA: *Infertility, contraception, and reproductive endocrinology,* ed 3, Cambridge, Mass, 1991, Blackwell Scientific Publications.
*Grade 0 at all sites indicates absence of terminal hair.

pelvic examination is performed to assess the presence of Sertoli-Leydig cysts. Cysts are palpable 85% of the time.[16]

DIAGNOSTICS

Hormonal evaluations in slow-onset, peripubertally hirsute, nonvirilized, normally menstruating patients are deferred. Diagnosis in this population relies heavily on the physical examination and evidence of virilism. In cases of hirsutism and virilization together, a preliminary investigation includes a serum testosterone level.

Testosterone levels show diurnal and menstrual phase–related fluctuation and may not truly indicate circulating levels. Therefore the ratio of the total testosterone to sex hormone–binding globulin levels may be preferred in some cases.[8] Normal levels range from 0.2 to 2.8 nmol/L. Values greater than 3.5 to 6 nmol/L prompt further investigation for tumors using pelvic or adrenal ultrasound studies.[1,15]

The DHEA-S is seen as a screen for adrenal gland production to distinguish tumors of adrenal origin.[11] An elevated DHEA-S level should be followed with an adrenal ultrasound or CT scan. An initial 24-hour urine collection for 17-ketosteroids (17-hydroxyprogesterone) and free cortisol is advised if Cushing's syndrome is suspected. A 17-hydroxyprogesterone value <200 ng/dl (6 nmol/ml) is normal, whereas a value >800 ng/dl (24 nmol/ml) indicates a 21-hydroxylase deficiency and the need for follow-up ACTH testing to determine the degree of deficiency.

A luteinizing hormone (LH)–follicle-stimulating hormone (FSH) ratio is evaluated in hirsute patients. This ratio is elevated to 2:1 or 3:1 in approximately three fourths of PCOS cases.[5,6] A glucose tolerance test and lipid profile would be valuable if dyslipidemia, insulin resistance, hyperinsulinemia, or diabetes were suspected. Galactorrhea warrants a prolactin level; increased levels are indicative of hyperprolactinemia and possible thyroid dysfunction. In these cases thyroid-stimulating hormone and FSH are also measured. The pituitary is imaged by MRI to search for a prolactinoma. The presence of a pelvic mass warrants a pelvic CT scan.

DIFFERENTIAL DIAGNOSIS

The onset of hirsutism may correspond to a variety of conditions: recent weight gain, discontinuation of oral contraceptives, initiation of progestins or steroids, and the onset of menopause or puberty. In addition, pituitary, adrenal, and ovarian tumors must be excluded. For patients with PCOS, the constellation of oligomenorrhea, acne, alopecia, and obesity is often seen in conjunction with hirsutism.[8] Finally, a subcategory of normoandrogenic hirsutism is known as idiopathic hirsutism.

A separate condition is hirsutism with concomitant virilism. Adrenal tumors (benign or malignant), enzyme deficiencies, or endocrinopathies are a consideration if virilization accompanies hirsutism. Sertoli-Leydig cell tumors can be present in patients in their twenties to forties. Hyperthecosis of the ovary usually occurs in premenopausal women. In these cases removal of the often unilaterally affected ovary returns testosterone levels to normal and reverses signs of virilism.[17] If intermenstrual or irregular bleeding is occurring in perimenopausal or premenopausal patients more than 35 years old, endometrial cancer needs to be excluded by endometrial biopsy.[1]

Hypertrichosis may be mistaken for hirsutism. Despite an abundance of fine, unpigmented hair, androgens are not involved. This type of hair growth results from conditions such as anorexia nervosa, hypothyroidism, or drug therapy such as occurs with the antihypertensive minoxidil.[7,15] Body hair is often diffusely distributed about the midline, including the face and even the forehead.[18] In familial, or constitutional hypertrichosis, genetic factors, rather than disease status, dictate the growth pattern. Unlike hirsutism, abundant familial hair growth patterns cannot be easily treated.[15] The diagnosis of hypertrichosis can be assessed by the hair type and some laboratory testing.

In the presence of elevated ACTH levels, the differential diagnosis should include Cushing's disease, glucocorticoid resistance, or anabolic steroid use. Finally, the investigation into insulin resistance conditions is warranted with hirsute patients, as hyperinsulinemia correlates inversely with sex hormone binding globulin (SHBG) concentrations, and SHBG is recognized as being inversely proportional to Ferriman-Gallwey scale scores.[15] Other considerations include congenital adrenal hyperplasia detected either in vivo or early in life, and its milder form indicated by excess cortisol precursors after an adrenal corticotropic hormone challenge. The milder case is said to affect 1:100 to 1000 in the United States and can lead to serious sinus and pulmonary illness as well as orthostatic syncope.[19]

Diagnostics

Hirsutism

Laboratory
Serum testosterone
DHEA-S
24-hour urine for 17-hydroxyprogesterone*
LSH/FSH ratio*
Prolactin*
TSH*
Glucose tolerance test*
Free cortisol*
Lipid profile*

Imaging
Pelvic ultrasound/pelvic CT scan
Abdominal ultrasound/CT scan*
MRI*

Other
ACTH stimulation test*
Dexamethasone suppression test*

*If indicated.

MANAGEMENT

Most often the causes of central hair growth are benign and can be managed effectively with a combination of medical therapy and mechanical hair removal. Because a woman's appraisal of her appearance is influenced by cosmetic, cultural,

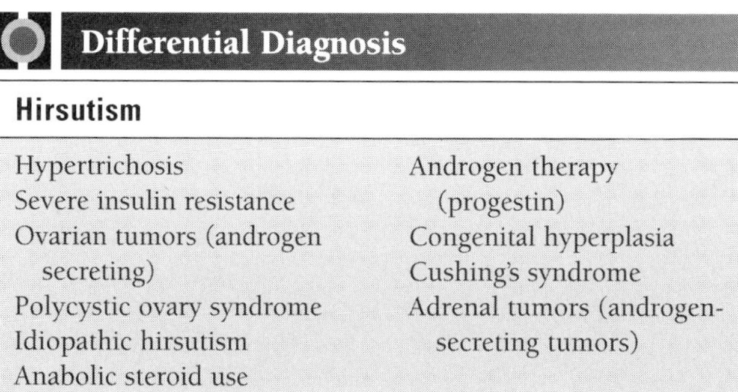
Differential Diagnosis

Hirsutism

Hypertrichosis
Severe insulin resistance
Ovarian tumors (androgen secreting)
Polycystic ovary syndrome
Idiopathic hirsutism
Anabolic steroid use
Androgen therapy (progestin)
Congenital hyperplasia
Cushing's syndrome
Adrenal tumors (androgen-secreting tumors)

and even age-determined standards,[20] in cases of normal hair growth, reassurance is essential.

Cosmetic measures are advisable in all patients who desire temporary or permanent removal of unwanted hair. Temporary methods include depilatory cream, which dissolves hair but may lead to skin irritation, allergic dermatitis, or permanent skin damage. Shaving (which may cause stubble to appear coarser and thicker) and plucking (which is uncomfortable and can stimulate hair growth, folliculitis, and scarring) can be used on small areas. Waxing removes hair at the base of the pilosebaceous unit and is more effective, although it may produce superficial burns and infection. Bleaching involves using a diluted cream preparation of hydrogen peroxide and can be effective in temporarily depigmenting hair, although in a matter of weeks, pigmented hair will return as a new growth cycle ensues.[15]

Electrolysis requires the insertion of a fine needle into the base of a hair follicle and the administration of electric current to permanently destroy the follicle. It is a popular, although costly, procedure; moreover, results vary. Caution is advised if acne, skin infection, diabetes mellitus, epilepsy, ischemic heart disease, an in situ pacemaker, or artificial joints are present. Antibiotic prophylaxis is recommended if a patient is at risk for endocardial infection or reactivation of herpes simplex.[20] Patients who choose waxing or electrolysis should be instructed to observe for possible signs of infection.

When the pattern of hair growth is hormonally caused, the goal of management is to interrupt the untoward effect of excessive testosterone on the hair follicle. Testosterone excess can be variously controlled depending on ovarian, adrenal, or peripheral tissue production (Table 224-2). A commonly accepted nonpharmacologic strategy is weight reduction.[1,5] Decreasing weight has been proved to lower insulin resistance and reduce hyperandrogenism; in fact, weight gain can worsen hirsutism.[15] Weight loss of 10% to 15% may diminish unwanted hair growth and return menses to normal.[1]

Medications are used to inhibit androgen secretion in the ovaries and adrenal glands or block testosterone and DHT. Of the varied pharmacologic options, a first-line approach includes oral estrogen/progesterone agents (oral contraceptives), which have the added benefit of treating acne and oligomenorrhea. Also, many oral medications slated for acne use diminish hirsutism.[21] Oral contraceptives inhibit LH secretion from the pituitary gland, reducing bioavailable testosterone, which decreases the stimulation of the ovarian thecal cells. 19-Nortestosterone derivatives, such as levonorgesterol, should be avoided, as they block the estrogen-mediated increase in SHBG concentration and are mildly androgenic.[15] Ultimately, the practitioner may want to stop medications after 1 to 2 years to see if any regression has been achieved and observe for return of ovulatory functioning in premenopausal women.

A second option is spironolactone, which, although better known as a potassium-sparing diuretic, serves as an antiandrogen product. It inhibits the binding of testosterone and DHT to the androgen receptor and improves the metabolic clearance of testosterone. It further limits androgen production by inhibiting cytochrome P-450 and is a popular choice for combined therapy with oral contraceptives. Side effects rarely compel patients to discontinue drug therapy; however, nausea, vomiting, abdominal discomfort, diarrhea, fatigue, mental confusion, headache, and dizziness may follow. Its mild progesterone activity has caused 80% of a sample of women taking it as sole therapy to report menstrual disturbance, especially polymenorrhea, if it is taken cyclically or continuously.[15] Of course, this method should not be used if women are already using a potassium-sparing diuretic or angiotensin II–converting enzyme inhibitors, have renal dysfunction, or are anticipating pregnancy.[8]

Popular therapy combines oral contraceptives and antiandrogens.[22] Patients who do not respond to oral contraceptives or spironolactone treatments may try one of several antiandrogen compounds, such as cyproterone acetate (CPA), finasteride, gonadotropin-releasing hormone agonist, glucocorticoids, or the antifungal ketoconazole. Of note, various CPA therapies have led to improvement in at least 70% of severely hirsute women.[20] In one study of 40 hirsute women, the efficacies spironolactone, flutamide, and finasteride at a given dose were comparable after 6 months.[23] By contrast, a randomized trial of 70 women showed that finasteride was superior to flutamide in reducing hair and impacting SHBG and DHEAS (dehydroepiandrosterone) indices.[24] Patients with accompanying insulin resistance have been started on metformin or troglitazone with improvement.[3,4,25] Eflornithine has been shown to slow hair growth by inhibiting ornithine decarboxylase at the follicle, although this is a temporary treatment.[26] Laser hair removal via ruby, Alexandrite, diode or Nd:YAG laser as well as broad band intense pulsed light therapy has been shown to produce long-lasting effects.[27] Finally, acupuncture therapy has reduced testosterone levels and body hair.[20]

TABLE 224-2 Androgen Production Inhibitors

Agent	Source of Androgen Production
Oral contraceptives	Ovarian, adrenal, peripheral
Corticosteroids	Ovarian, adrenal
Spironolactone	Ovarian, adrenal, peripheral
Cyproterone acetate	Ovarian, peripheral
Ketoconazole	Ovarian, adrenal
Progestins	Ovarian
Gonadotropin-releasing hormone agonist	Ovarian
Topical progesterone	Peripheral
5 alpha-reductase inhibitors	Peripheral

Modified from Mishell DR and others: *Infertility, contraception, and reproductive endocrinology*, ed 3, Oxford, 1991, Blackwell Scientific.

Co-management with Specialists

When an endocrinologist prescribes finasteride, flutamide, or ketoconazole for a patient, liver enzymes should be assessed regularly. Patients must not become pregnant while receiving corrective hormonal therapy. Finally, an outcome evaluation, such as reevaluating the patient with the Ferriman-Gallwey scale or reviewing the success of mechanical hair removal, is useful.

LIFE SPAN CONSIDERATIONS

Hirsutism is a sensitive issue for adolescent girls, whose peer acceptance may heavily influence their body image and resulting health behaviors. In fact, eating disorders related to PCOS are common.[15] Any menstrual cycle irregularities are of concern if they are accompanied by acne, alopecia, and hirsutism, as well as insulin resistance, as this might be a presentation of PCOS. Medication and mechanical hair removal options should be explored. Excessive hair growth can accompany pregnancy but usually disappears within 6 to 15 months postpartum.[19]

COMPLICATIONS

Failure to diagnose an adrenal or ovarian tumor that may be malignant is a serious complication of hirsutism. Surgical removal of ovarian or adrenal tumors is recommended, although postsurgical complications, such as adhesions, are possible. Diabetes and hypertension are often associated with PCOS, as well as the possibility of hyperestrogen-related cancers,[28] necessitating careful follow-up monitoring. In addition, hirsute women may be at increased risk for endometrial cancer.[1]

INDICATIONS FOR REFERRAL/HOSPITALIZATION

The evaluation of a hirsute patient is performed in consultation with a physician. Patients may be referred to an endocrinologist for androgen studies, or preliminary studies may be performed in primary care. Certainly, referral to an endocrinologist is appropriate if hirsutism is accompanied by virilism, which suggests the need for further imaging, androgen, or dexamethasone studies. There is research to support dexamethasone and triptorelin testing to differentiate between adrenal and ovarian source androgen excess.[29] An endocrinologist is also consulted for treatment failure or persistent infertility.

A nephrologist should evaluate patients with insulin resistance or renal failure. A surgical consultation is indicated for the evaluation of patients with adrenal gland or ovarian tumors.

The psychosocial effects of increasing body hair may warrant a psychiatric consultation if the hair has become a consuming concern. A mental health referral will be useful if there is reason to suspect underlying gonadal abnormality such as chromosomal mosaicism or, in rare cases, hermaphroditism. Genetic counseling, or even fetal testing, may be appropriate in some cases.

PATIENT AND FAMILY EDUCATION

Hirsute patients should be advised to avoid second-generation androgenic oral contraceptives, including norgestrel, levonorgestrel, and norethindrone, in favor of third-generation oral contraceptives.[5,15] Ethinyl estradiol 35 μg singly, or in combination with cypionate acetate 2 mg, offers good effect but must be taken for several years and is often followed by relapse of symptoms after several months of drug hiatus.[30] However, patients using third-generation oral contraceptives should be advised of the possibility of thromboembolic events. All patients taking oral contraceptives should be strictly advised to stop smoking. Use of anabolic steroids for muscle building is strongly discouraged.

Education regarding realistic expectations of cosmetic hair removal, hair loss, and hair growth suppression, as well as a reminder that even a temporary drug hiatus will likely return the patient to her previous hirsute status, is essential. It will take anywhere from 6 to 18 months to see a new "set point" in hair growth.[7]

Finally, the practitioner will need to address increased levels of anxiety and depression in women with PCOS and to provide reassurance about fears of masculinization, ridicule or social rejection, and sexual or gender identity.[15] Because pregnancy is contraindicated during therapy, pregnancy plans should be discussed in advance. Often the discontinuation of therapy will herald a return of hair growth.

HEALTH PROMOTION

Woman should be adequately counseled regarding their concerns and realistic expectations regarding future fertility and body image. For patients with PCOS, a diet high in fiber and low in refined carbohydrates is encouraged, as well as support for weight loss. Individual or group psychologic counseling can help with weight management.

REFERENCES

1. Marshburn PB, Carr BR: Hirsutism and virilization: a systematic approach to benign and potentially serious causes, *Postgrad Med* 97(1): 99-106, 1995.
2. Agarwal SK, Judd HL: What we see most, we understand least, *West J Med* 165(6):392-393, 1996.
3. Hock DL, Seifer DB: New treatments of hyperandrogenism and hirsutism, *Obstet Gynecol Clin North Am* 27(3):567-581, vi-vii, 2000.
4. Azziz R and others: Troglitazone improves ovulation and hirsutism in the polycystic ovary syndrome: a multicenter, double blind, placebo-controlled trial, *J Clin Endocrinol Metab* 86(4):1626-1632, 2001.
5. Kalve E, Klein JF: Evaluation of women with hirsutism, *Am Fam Physician* 54(1):117-124, 1996.
6. Marshall JC, Eagleston CA: Polycystic ovary syndrome: neuroendocrine aspects of polycystic ovary syndrome, *Endocrinol Metab Clin* 28(2):295-324, 1999.
7. Rittmaster RS: Hirsutism, *Lancet* 349:191-195, 1997.
8. Mishell DR and others: *Comprehensive gynecology*, ed 3, St Louis, 1997, Mosby.
9. Taylor AE: Hirsutism and androgen excess. In Carlson KJ, Eisenstat SA, editors: *Primary care of women*, St Louis, 1995, Mosby.
10. Kessel B, Liu J: Clinical and laboratory evaluation of hirsutism, *Clin Obstet Gynecol* 34(4):805-816, 1991.
11. McKenna TJ: Screening for sinister causes of hirsutism, *N Engl J Med* 331(15):1015-1016, 1994.
12. Bates GW, Cornwell CE: Iatrogenic causes of hirsutism, *Clin Obstet Gynecol* 34(4):849-851, 1991.
13. Gerritsma EJ and others: Virilization of the voice in postmenopausal women due to the anabolic steroid nandrolone decanoate (Deca-Durabolin): the effects of medication for 1 year, *Clin Otolaryngol* 19(1):79-84, 1994.
14. Taylor AE and others: Determinants of abnormal gonadotropin secretion in clinically defined women with polycystic ovary syndrome, *J Clin Endocrinol Metab* 82(7):2248-2256, 1997.
15. Conn JJ, Jacobs HS: The clinical management of hirsutism, *Eur J Endocrinol* 136:339-348, 1997.
16. Ferriman D, Gallwey JD: Clinical assessment of body hair growth in women, *J Endocrinol Metab* 21:144-147, 1961.
17. Agorastos T and others: Postmenopausal virilization due to ovarian hyperthecosis, *Arch Gynecol Obstet* 256(4):209-211, 1995.
18. Rittmaster RS: Medical treatment of androgen-dependent hirsutism, *J Clin Endocrinol Metab* 80(9):2559-2563, 1995.
19. Kroumpouzos G, Cohen LM: Dermatoses of pregnancy, *J Am Acad Dermatol* 45(1):1-19, 2001.
20. Schriock EA, Schriock ED: Treatment of hirsutism, *Clin Obstet Gynecol* 34(4):853-863, 1991.
21. Shaw JC: Antiandrogen and hormonal treatment of acne, *Dermatol Clin* 14(4):803-811, 1996.

22. Bergfeld WF: Hirsutism in women: effective therapy that is safe for long-term use. Symposium: third of four articles on troublesome skin problems, *Postgrad Med* 107(7):93-94, 99-104, 121-124, 2000.
23. Moghetti P and others: Comparison of spironolactone, flutamide, and finasteride efficacy in the treatment of hirsutism: a randomized, double blind, placebo-controlled trial, *J Clin Endocrinol Metab* 85(1): 89-94, 2000.
24. Muderris II, Bayram F, Guven M: A prospective, randomized trial comparing flutamide (250 mg/d) and finasteride (5 mg/d) in the treatment of hirsutism, *Fertil Steril* 73(5):984-987, 2000.
25. Carmina E: A risk benefit assessment of pharmacological therapies for hirsutism, *Drug Saf* 24(4):267-276, 2001.
26. Barman-Balfour JA, McClellan K: Topical eflornithine, *Am J Clin Dermatol* 2/3(197-201), 2001.
27. Lask G and others: The role of laser and intense light sources in photo-epilation: a comparative evaluation, *J Cutan Laser Ther* 1(1):3-13, 1999.
28. Marshall K: Polycystic ovary syndrome: clinical considerations, *Altern Med Rev* 6(3):272-292, 2001.
29. Bidzinska B and others: Modified dexamethasone and gonadotropin-releasing hormone agonist (Dx-GnRHa) test in the evaluation of androgen source(s) in hirsute women, *Przegl Lek* 57(7-8):393-396, 2000.
30. Kokaly W, McKenna TJ: Relapse of hirsutism following long-term successful treatment with estrogen-progestogen combination, *Clin Endocrinol* 52(3):379-382, 2000.

CHAPTER 225

Hypercalcemia and Hypocalcemia

Kathryn Blum and Kathlyn Nowak

DEFINITION/EPIDEMIOLOGY

Calcium is one of the major electrolytes necessary to maintain the human body's homeostasis and to ensure proper body functioning. Calcium ion is fundamentally important to all biologic systems.[1] If specific levels are not maintained, homeostasis is disturbed, precipitating a host of consequences, some potentially life threatening.

Hypercalcemia, a serum calcium excess, is a disorder in which the calcium level exceeds 10.5 mg/dl. Conversely, hypocalcemia is a serum calcium deficiency, with a calcium level below 8.5 mg/dl. Both disorders can be a manifestation of a serious illness such as malignancy or can be detected coincidentally by laboratory testing in a patient with no obvious illness.[2] The imbalance may have varied etiologies, may be chronic or acute, and may exhibit variable effects.

A total of 99% (1 to 2 kg) of body calcium is used to provide structural support of the bones and teeth. The remaining 1% is found in the extracellular fluid and soft tissues. Approximately 50% of plasma calcium is in the ionized, biologically active form, 10% is complexed in nonionic form, and 40% is protein bound.[1,3] It is a catalyst for muscle contraction (including cardiac), normal neuromuscular excitability, blood coagulation, exocrine and endocrine gland function, cell membrane integrity and permeability, vision, enzyme activity, and cell growth.[4]

The mechanisms regulating calcium metabolism are complex and intimately involved with those of phosphorus metabolism, both of which are regulated by parathyroid hormone (PTH), 1,25-dihydroxycholecalciferol (vitamin D_3), and calcitonin. These hormones exert their effects through feedback mechanisms on three major organ systems: the skeleton, intestinal tract, and kidneys.

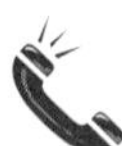

Physician consultation is indicated for patients with serum calcium levels <8.5 mg/dl or >10.5 mg/dl.

A decrease in serum calcium stimulates the production of PTH. PTH has a direct effect on calcium and phosphorus through its activity on the osteoclast, which is responsible for bone resorption. PTH also directly stimulates the kidney tubules to reabsorb calcium and excrete phosphorus, leading to a rise in serum calcium and a fall in serum phosphorus. In response to the decrease in phosphorus, vitamin D is converted by the kidneys to an active form, which is essential for intestinal absorption of calcium.[3,5] Increases in serum calcium both inhibit release of PTH and stimulate production of calcitonin from the thyroid. Calcitonin then impedes the release of calcium from the bone, resulting in decreased renal tubular absorption of calcium and decreased production of active vitamin D, thereby decreasing calcium absorption in the intestines.[3-6]

Hypercalcemia

PATHOPHYSIOLOGY

Hypercalcemia results from either increased entry or decreased loss of calcium into the circulation. Serum phosphate levels, vitamin D concentrations, and PTH are the primary determinants of both hypercalcemia and hypocalcemia. The hypercalcemia of hyperparathyroidism is directly related to the effects of increased PTH. Hypercalcemia of malignancy develops most frequently when bone resorption exceeds bone formation as a result of bony metastases. Solid tumors without metastasis and hematologic malignancies may operate via an alternative mechanism, humoral hypercalcemia of malignancy.[7,8] These tumor cells secrete PTH-related protein, which binds to PTH receptors initiating bone resorption and renal reabsorption of calcium.[8,9] Milk-alkali syndrome, a combination of hypercalcemia, metabolic alkalosis, and renal insufficiency, develops in response to the simultaneous ingestion of large amounts of calcium and absorbable alkali such as calcium carbonate.[10] Disorders involving vitamin D excess lead to increased bone resorption and intestinal absorption of calcium.

CLINICAL PRESENTATION

The severity of symptoms in hypercalcemia is directly related to the level and rate of rise of calcium. An abnormally high level may be tolerated chronically, whereas a less elevated but abrupt increase may cause significant symptoms. Clinical manifestations are associated with the depressant effect of calcium on nerve tissue excitability, as well as the contractility of cardiac, skeletal, and smooth muscle.[9]

Initial symptoms of anorexia, fatigue, malaise, lethargy, nausea, dehydration, vague abdominal pain, and constipation can be easily missed. Central nervous system symptoms include depression, impaired concentration, disorientation and confusion, memory loss, shortened attention span, inappropriate behavior, irritability, and ataxia. If they are allowed to progress, these symptoms may lead to psychosis, stupor, coma, or death. Musculoskeletal effects include muscle fatigue, hypotonia, and weakness. Decreased smooth muscle contractility of the gastrointestinal system causes anorexia, nausea, vomiting, weight loss, abdominal pain, and constipation. Decreased contractility and decreased nerve conduction of the cardiac system produce arrhythmias and increased potential for digitalis toxicity. Renal system effects include polyuria, polydipsia, and nocturia.[11,12]

PHYSICAL EXAMINATION

The physical examination is often unremarkable. Cardiovascular examination may reveal irregularity of rate and rhythm. Depression of the central nervous system is reflected in hyporeflexia, changes in sensorium, muscle weakness, tremor, lethargy, and ataxia. With severe hypercalcemia, stupor and coma may be present.

DIAGNOSTICS

The diagnosis of calcium imbalance is made by measuring the serum calcium level. Hypercalcemia is indicated if the total calcium level is greater than 10.5 mg/dl; a level less than 8.5 mg/dl is diagnostic of hypocalcemia. The level of serum calcium must be correlated with the simultaneous concentration of serum albumin. Serum calcium concentration falls by 0.8 mg/dl per 1 g/dl decrease of serum albumin. For example, with a serum calcium of 8.0 mg/dl and an albumin of 2 g/dl (2 g/dl below normal), the corrected serum calcium would be 9.6 mg/dl (2 g/dl $\times$ 0.8 = 1.6) and therefore normal.[1,4] The serum pH can be a significant factor in determining true calcium concentration; alkalosis increases the amount of calcium bound to albumin, thereby decreasing the free ionized calcium available for biologic use; the opposite occurs with an acidotic state.[1,4]

When a true calcium imbalance is confirmed, further testing should be pursued to determine the etiology. Initial testing should include measurement of intact PTH by two-sided radioimmunoassay (RIA), vitamin D metabolite levels, creatinine, amylase, magnesium, and phosphorus levels.[12,13] Measurement of PTH by RIA is most useful in distinguishing hyperparathyroidism from malignancy and in differentiating hypoparathyroidism from nonparathyroid causes.[12,13] Serum alkaline phosphatase, radiographs, and bone scans can indicate a bony origin of hypercalcemia or hypocalcemia as seen in malignancy, vitamin D excess or deficiency, osteomalacia, or Paget's disease.[12]

DIFFERENTIAL DIAGNOSIS

Hyperparathyroidism and malignancy account for the majority of all cases of hypercalcemia, with 60% attributed to primary

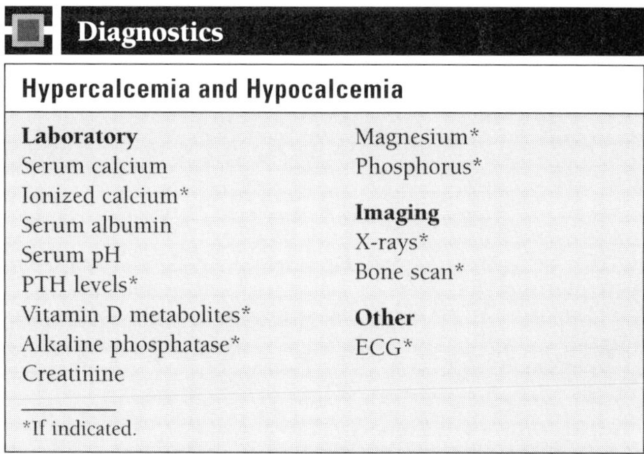

Diagnostics

Hypercalcemia and Hypocalcemia

Laboratory	Magnesium*
Serum calcium	Phosphorus*
Ionized calcium*	
Serum albumin	**Imaging**
Serum pH	X-rays*
PTH levels*	Bone scan*
Vitamin D metabolites*	**Other**
Alkaline phosphatase*	ECG*
Creatinine	

*If indicated.

Differential Diagnosis

Hypercalcemia

Hyperparathyroidism	Thiazide diuretic use
Malignancy	Addison's disease
Milk-alkali syndrome	Renal failure
Sarcoidosis	Immobilization
Granulomatous disease	Drug toxicity (lithium, theophylline)
Thyrotoxicosis	
Vitamin A or D toxicity	

hyperparathyroidism.[7,12] Milk-alkali syndrome has recently become the third leading cause of hypercalcemia.[10] The remaining causes of hypercalcemia include sarcoidosis and other granulomatous disorders, thyrotoxicosis, vitamin A and D intoxication, thiazide diuretics, Addison's disease, prolonged immobilization, theophylline or lithium toxicity, and renal failure.[5,12]

MANAGEMENT

With early recognition and rapid intervention, hypercalcemia is a reversible condition. Conversely, the mortality rate of hypercalcemia is 50% without timely intervention.[7] Treatment of hypercalcemia consists of supportive or preventive measures, emergency therapies, and treatment of the underlying disorder. Severe, symptomatic hypercalcemia requires aggressive therapy aimed at decreasing the serum calcium level by increasing renal excretion. Excretion of sodium is accompanied by excretion of calcium; thus inducing natriuresis with saline and furosemide is the emergency treatment of choice.[7,11]

Further medical therapy is specific to treatment of the underlying cause. Hyperparathyroid-induced hypercalcemia often remains silent until the onset of an acute illness or until it is detected by laboratory testing. Surgery is the treatment of choice for symptomatic patients. The asymptomatic patient risks progressive skeletal disease. Medical therapy includes estrogen/progesterone therapy, oral phosphate preparations, bisphosphonates, and loop diuretics. Despite appropriate medical management, surgery is often necessary.

Asymptomatic milk-alkali syndrome is managed primarily through withdrawal of the causative agents. This generally results in rapid correction of both hypercalcemia and metabolic alkalosis.[10] Symptomatic patients are treated with saline and furosemide to induce natriuresis and excretion of calcium.[7,11]

The primary and most effective long-term treatment of malignancy-induced hypercalcemia is antineoplastic therapy aimed at tumor eradication. Medication therapy is directed at inhibiting osteoclast activity.[12] The choice of agent depends on the urgency of treatment, renal status, bone marrow status, and hospitalized vs. nonhospitalized status of patients.[13] Four agents are available that inhibit osteoclastic activity: bisphosphonates, salmon calcitonin, plicamycin, and gallium nitrate.[14] Bisphosphonates are the drugs of choice; they are relatively nontoxic, with maximum effect occurring in 2 to 4 days. Pamidronate is currently the most widely used biphosphonate; however, zoledronic acid (Zometra), a newer agent, is proving extremely effective and longer lasting.[14,15] Calcitonin works rapidly when effective, although many patients develop tachyphylaxis within 2 to 3 days. Calcitonin in conjunction with a bisphosphonate has good efficacy.[14] Cytotoxic agents such as plicamycin and gallium nitrate should be considered as a last resort, as there is considerably greater toxicity.[12] Hydration and diuresis are a critical concurrent therapy. Medical treatment of hypercalcemia in the face of renal failure is difficult and often requires hemodialysis.

Preventive measures include moderate dietary calcium (1 g/day), adequate hydration (2 L/day), and medication scrutiny. Because immobilization perpetuates bone resorption, weight-bearing activity is critical.[16] Thiazide diuretics, lithium, vitamins A and D, and theophylline, all of which further contribute to hypercalcemia, should be discontinued. Hypercalcemia decreases cardiac responsiveness to digitalis, necessitating close regulation of this medication.

LIFE SPAN CONSIDERATIONS

The cure rate of hypercalcemia with parathyroidectomy is 90% to 98%, although subsequent therapy for hypocalcemia may be necessary. Primary hyperparathyroidism is common in older women. Confusion may occur with only a slight elevation in serum calcium and is often mistaken as a sign of aging. Fortunately, it is completely reversible with appropriate treatment.[12] Malignancy-induced hypercalcemia usually occurs late in the disease, by which time the survival rate is only 2 to 6 months. If the disease is very advanced and/or the side effects of treatment overshadow the benefits, the decision not to treat may be an appropriate choice.[13]

COMPLICATIONS

Complications of severe hypercalcemia include atonic ileus and obstipation, coma, profound muscular weakness, ataxia, pathologic fractures, renal failure, cardiac arrest, and death.

Hypocalcemia

PATHOPHYSIOLOGY

Hypocalcemia occurs with either an increased loss of calcium from the circulation (deposition in tissue, increased urinary excretion, increased binding within the circulation) or with decreased entry of calcium into the circulation (malabsorption, decreased bone resorption).[18] Hypoparathyroidism causes impaired synthesis and secretion of PTH; lack of PTH is a direct cause of hypocalcemia.[16] Pseudohypoparathyroidism is a genetic deficiency in which the PTH is adequate but there is a peripheral resistance to its effect. Malabsorption syndromes, renal failure, and liver disease interfere with the absorption of both vitamin D and calcium despite elevated levels of PTH.[16] Hyperphosphatemia deposits calcium in bone, hypermagnesemia increases peripheral resistance to PTH, and certain substances chelate calcium in the circulation, all effectively leading to hypocalcemia.[17]

CLINICAL PRESENTATION

Clinical manifestations of hypocalcemia are associated with increased excitation of nerve and muscle cells, primarily affecting the neuromuscular and cardiovascular systems.[11,16] Patients often complain of a generalized feeling of hyperirritability with restlessness, jumpiness, and sleeplessness.[6] Early symptoms of hypocalcemia include numbness and tingling, especially around the nose, lips, earlobes, and extremities. As neurologic excitability increases, irritability, depression, memory loss, psychosis, and seizure may occur. Musculoskeletal symptoms present as muscle spasm, carpopedal spasm, tetany, and laryngospasm with stridor, which can obstruct the airway, causing asphyxia.[6] Gastrointestinal symptoms include intestinal cramps and chronic malabsorption related to increased gastrointestinal motility and spasm.[16]

PHYSICAL EXAMINATION

The physical examination may reveal features of spontaneous neuromuscular irritability with hyperreflexia of deep tendons.[6,16] Chvostek's sign (contraction of the facial muscle in response to tapping the facial nerve against the bone anterior to the ear) and Trousseau's sign (carpal spasm occurring after occlusion of the brachial artery with a blood pressure cuff for 3 minutes) are usually readily elicited.[6,11] Cardiovascular examination may exhibit hypotension, impaired cardiac contractility, and bradyarrhythmias.[14] Adults suffering from chronic hypocalcemia may display coarse hair, dry and brittle nails, and scaly skin. Subcapsular cataracts can be seen with slit-lamp examination.[6,11]

DIAGNOSTICS

See Diagnostics under Hypercalcemia, p. 1019.

DIFFERENTIAL DIAGNOSIS

Chronic hypocalcemia can be ascribed to several disorders associated with an absence of PTH or with its ineffectiveness. Possible etiologies include surgery that involves the parathyroid or thyroid, idiopathic hypoparathyroidism, pseudohypoparathyroidism, vitamin D deficiency, malabsorption syndromes, severe renal or liver disease, alcoholism and poor nutritional intake, osteoblastic malignancy, pancreatitis, and hypomagnesemia or hyperphosphatemia. Clinical criteria are important in distinguishing the etiology, including the duration of illness, symptoms of associated disorders, detection of hereditary features, and a nutritional and alcohol history. Acute transient hypocalcemia can be associated with severe sepsis, burns, acute renal failure, extensive blood transfusions with citrated blood, medications, and pancreatitis.[2]

MANAGEMENT

All patients with symptomatic hypocalcemia must be treated. Severe, symptomatic hypocalcemia in the presence of tetany, arrhythmias, or seizures should be treated with IV calcium. The treatment of hypocalcemia is guided by the acuity and severity of the hypocalcemia and the associated signs and symptoms. In acute, life-threatening situations, 1 or 2 ampules of calcium gluconate are diluted in 50 to 100 ml of 5% dextrose infused over 10 to 20 minutes. With less severe symptoms, a more dilute calcium solution is infused over a longer period.[17] Serum calcium should be monitored frequently and the infusion adjusted accordingly.[3,6] Until calcium repletion has occurred, treatment of life-threatening symptoms such as hypotension and arrhythmias is refractory to medical management.[16]

Vitamin D is the cornerstone therapy for chronic hypocalcemia. Calcitriol is recommended (0.25 to 0.5 μg/day) with calcium supplementation as needed (1 to 1.5 g/day).[6] Vitamin D and calcium can be varied independently. Higher doses of vitamin D allow for more effective absorption of calcium from the intestinal tract. If intestinal absorption is inefficient, higher intakes of oral calcium permit adequate calcium assimilation. The use of thiazide diuretics with sodium restriction in hypoparathyroidism lowers urinary calcium excretion, thus allowing a lower dose of vitamin D and calcium supplementation.[2] A low serum calcium level associated with a low serum albumin level does not require replacement. Serum pH, potassium, magnesium, and phosphorus levels should be monitored and corrected if necessary. This will usually correct hypocalcemia without further intervention.

Differential Diagnosis

Hypocalcemia	
Parathyroid hormone deficiency (surgery, idiopathic hypoparathyroidism, pseudoparathyroidism, radiation)	Poor nutrition
	Malignancy
	Pancreatitis
	Hypomagnesemia
	Hyperphosphatemia
Vitamin D deficiency	Severe sepsis
Malabsorption syndromes	Burns
Renal disease	Medications
Liver disease	Extensive transfusion with citrated blood
Alcoholism	

LIFE SPAN CONSIDERATIONS

Hypocalcemia can be easily managed throughout the life span with calcium and vitamin D supplementation and monitoring of calcium levels to prevent crisis.

COMPLICATIONS

Complications of hypocalcemia are related to increased neuromuscular irritability and may precipitate laryngospasm, airway obstruction, tetany, seizures, cardiac arrhythmias, coma, or death.

Indications for Referral/Hospitalization

Treatment for both hypocalcemic crisis and hypercalcemic crisis always requires hospitalization. Immediate IV correction of the imbalance, either through replacement of calcium in hypocalcemia or through fluid replacement and diuresis in hypercalcemia, with concurrent cardiac monitoring, possible intubation, laboratory analysis, and diligent observation, is required until stabilization occurs. Referral to an endocrinologist and/or surgeon may be necessary if hyperparathyroidism is diagnosed. Malignancy-induced hypercalcemia should be managed by an oncologist.

Patient and Family Education/Health Promotion

Patient and family education should emphasize lifestyle changes, including diet, hydration, and mobility. Patients should learn to identify foods that are high in calcium and adjust their diets according to their imbalance. Maintaining mobility to promote uptake of calcium into bone should be stressed, as should the importance of adequate hydration for patients with either hypocalcemia or hypercalcemia. Patients and families should also be taught to recognize signs and symptoms of calcium imbalance. Early manifestations may be treated without hospitalization; however, if neglected, a calcium imbalance can be a truly life-threatening disorder.

REFERENCES

1. Genuth SM: Endocrine regulation of calcium and phosphate metabolism. In Berne RM and others, editors: *Physiology*, ed 4, St Louis, 1998, Mosby.
2. Potts JT: Diseases of the parathyroid gland and other hyper- and hypocalcemic disorders. In Isselbacher KJ, Braunwald E, Wilson JD, editors: *Harrison's principles of internal medicine*, ed 13, New York, 1994, McGraw-Hill.
3. Terry J: The other electrolytes—magnesium, calcium, and phosphorus, *J Intraven Nurs* 14(3):167-176, 1991.

4. Hoppe B: Taking the confusion out of calcium levels, *Nursing* 25(7):32KK-32MM, 1995.
5. Yucha CB, Toto KH: Calcium and phosphorous derangements, *Crit Care Nurs Clin North Am* 6(4):747-766, 1994.
6. Tohme JF, Bilezikian JP: Hypocalcemic emergencies, *Endocrinol Metab Clin North Am* 22(2):363-367, 1993.
7. Clayton K: Cancer-related hypercalcemia: how to spot it, how to manage it, *Am J Nurs* 97(5):42-49, 1997.
8. Rizzoli R and others: Actions of parathyroid hormone and parathyroid hormone-related protein, *J Endocrinol Invest* 15: 51, 1992.
9. Kaplan M: Hypercalcemia of malignancy: a review of advances in pathophysiology, *Oncol Nurs Forum* 21(6):1039-1048, 1994.
10. Beall DP, Scofield RH: Milk-alkali syndrome associated with calcium carbonate consumption, *Medicine* 74:89, 1995.
11. Papadakis MA: Fluid and electrolyte disorders. In Tierney LM and others, editors: *Current medical diagnosis and treatment,* ed 34, Norwalk, Conn, 1995, Appleton & Lange.
12. Mundy GR: Evaluation and treatment of hypercalcemia, *Hosp Pract* 29(6):79-84, 1994.
13. Schmitt R: Quality of life issues in lung cancer, *Chest* 103(1):515-555, 1993.
14. Bilezikian JP: Management of hypercalcemia, *J Clin Endocrinol Metab* 77:1445, 1993.
15. Majur P and others: Zolendroic acid is superior to pamidronate in treatment of hypercalcemia of malignancy: a pooled analysis of two randomized, controlled clinical trials, *J Clin Oncol* 19:558, 2001.
16. Guise TA, Mundy GR: Evaluation of hypocalcemia in children and adults, *J Clin Endocrinol Metab* 80(5):1463-1478, 1995.
17. Hobich MF: Evaluation and treatment of disorders in calcium, phosphorus, and magnesium metabolism. In Noble J, editor: *Primary care medicine,* ed 2, St Louis, 1996, Mosby.

CHAPTER 226

Hypernatremia and Hyponatremia

Terry Mahan Buttaro

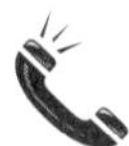

Physician consultation is indicated for serum sodium levels less than 125 mEq/L or greater than 155 mEq/L.

Hypernatremia

DEFINITION/EPIDEMIOLOGY

Hypernatremia is one of the more common electrolyte disorders in older adults. Characterized by an increase in the concentration of extracellular serum sodium and defined as a serum sodium level greater than 145 mEq/L, hypernatremia is most commonly associated with a fluid volume deficit. However, it can develop as a result of excessive sodium intake or as the result of some other diagnosis such as chronic renal disease or congestive heart failure.[1-3]

PATHOPHYSIOLOGY

Hypernatremia indicates a disruption in water homeostasis. Under normal conditions, water intake and water loss are balanced. When water loss exceeds water intake, serum osmolality rises, and thirst is stimulated. Water balance is achieved as water intake increases. Thirst receptors are stimulated when serum osmolality rises above the normal range of 290 to 295 mmol/kg. Destruction of the thirst centers in the hypothalamus as a result of neoplasm, trauma, or vascular abnormalities leads to an inadequate thirst response, and hypernatremia results. Patients who are unable to adequately express thirst, such as infants and those with a decreased sensorium, are also at risk for developing hypernatremia. Older adults are at risk because the thirst mechanism decreases with age. Frail, debilitated older adults who live alone are also at greater risk because impaired mobility may limit adequate fluid intake.[1-5]

An excess in water loss in relation to intake leads to increased serum osmolality. In response to this rise in serum osmolality, antidiuretic hormone (ADH), or vasopressin, is secreted from the posterior pituitary gland. ADH increases the permeability of the renal collecting ducts to water. As a result, water is reabsorbed in the collecting ducts, and the urine becomes more concentrated. Patients with a deficit in the production of ADH or a diminished renal response to ADH will develop hypernatremia if water losses are not corrected. Older adults are especially at risk because of the diminished renal concentrating ability that occurs with aging. Patients with diabetes insipidus develop hypernatremia when water intake is not enough to compensate for fluid loss. Also at risk for the development of hypernatremia as a result of losing large amounts of free water are patients who have osmotic diuresis because of hyperglycemia or the administration of osmotic diuretics such as mannitol.[1-6]

Hypernatremia also develops with an increase in insensible water losses. Normally, small amounts of fluids are lost from the skin, respiratory tract, and gastrointestinal tract. Conditions such as fever, tachypnea, diarrhea, vomiting, and burns increase the volume of insensible water loss. Hypernatremia results if these losses are not replaced. Patients who exercise vigorously and drink an insufficient amount of liquid and those with insufficient fluid intake in the setting of fever, vomiting, or diarrhea are at great risk for developing hypernatremia.[1-6]

Hypernatremia occurs less often as a result of excess sodium intake including rapid administration of intravenous normal saline or high solute tube feedings. The sodium excess can cause an increase in serum osmolality and expansion of extracellular volume.[1,2]

CLINICAL PRESENTATION AND PHYSICAL EXAMINATION

Patients can be asymptomatic if the hypernatremia is related to a hypothalamic lesion or complain of thirst or light-headedness. The major clinical feature of hypernatremia is a central nervous system disturbance that results from dehydration and shrinkage of brain cells. The signs and symptoms of hypernatremia are nonspecific and in general do not develop until the serum sodium level becomes greater than 150 mEq/L. Agitation, irritability, confusion, and changes in personality are early signs. Muscle twitching, spasticity, hyperreflexia, and lethargy may also be seen. Coma, seizures, and muscle weakness are later signs. Thirst is always present unless the thirst receptors are nonfunctioning. Other signs of volume depletion that may be seen include hypotension, tachycardia, and abnormal postural changes in vital signs. Weight loss, flat neck veins, and diminished skin turgor may also be seen depending on the severity of the volume loss.[1-3,6,7]

Diminished urine output is also a finding, except in patients with diabetes insipidus or osmotic diuresis as the underlying cause of the hypernatremia. Fever, flushing, and dry mucous membranes may also be present.[1-3,6,7]

Classification of the patient's fluid volume status is facilitated by evaluation of the patient's appearance, weight, and postural vital signs and careful examination of the pulmonary, cardiac, and gastrointestinal systems. Neurologic screening, including motor tone, strength, coordination, and cognitive and functional ability, is necessary to determine subtle neurologic changes.

DIAGNOSTICS

Hypernatremia is confirmed by a serum sodium level above 145 mEq/L, with serum osmolality greater than 300 mOsm/kg. Urine osmolality is increased to greater than 600 mOsm/kg except in patients taking diuretics or in those with diabetes insipidus or osmotic diuresis. Urine specific gravity is not as precise as urine osmolality but is a quick test to determine urine concentration. The urine specific gravity of patients with hypernatremia is elevated, except in the cases noted previously. Urine sodium levels can be elevated, normal, or decreased. Serum protein, hematocrit, and red blood cells will be elevated.[1-3,6,7]

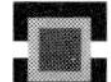

Diagnostics

Hypernatremia

Laboratory	
Serum electrolytes	Urine osmolality
CBC and differential	Urine specific gravity
Serum protein	BUN
Serum osmolality	Creatinine

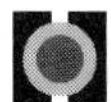

Differential Diagnosis

Hypernatremia

- Water depletion with insufficient water intake
  - Excessive sweating and increased insensible water loss
  - Diarrheal conditions
    - Viral illnesses
    - Hepatic encephalopathy with use of lactulose
  - Abnormal thirst mechanism
- Increased renal water loss with inadequate fluid intake
  - Diabetes insipidus
    - Central (pituitary) diabetes insipidus
  - Osmotic diuresis
    - Glycosuria
    - Mannitol use for diuresis
    - Chronic renal failure
  - Use of loop diuretics
- Water loss due to peritoneal dialysis
- Excessive sodium intake with inadequate water intake
  - High solute tube feedings
  - Rapid IV N/S
- Hyperactivity of the adrenal cortex

DIFFERENTIAL DIAGNOSIS

It is important that the practitioner determine the underlying cause of the sodium imbalance because treatment options vary with the etiology. The patient with hypernatremia resulting from diabetes insipidus is treated differently than the patient whose imbalance is a result of excessive diarrhea caused by the use of lactulose.

MANAGEMENT

The primary goal of treatment is the replacement of water loss and restoration of extracellular fluid volume. Oral water replacement is the safest, but replacement can be by nasogastric-gastric infusion or by IV infusion in the hospital. The replacement fluid should be a hypotonic saline solution (0.45% NaCl) or 5% dextrose in water (D_5W).[1,7] Hypernatremia of less than 24 hours' duration can be corrected over 24 hours. Patients with chronic hypernatremia should have the water deficit corrected slowly, over 24 to 48 hours, to prevent cerebral edema. Reductions of serum sodium by no more than 1 to 2 mEq/L/hr is recommended to avoid cerebral consequences. The rate of fluid administration can be calculated by dividing the water deficit by the number of hours over which the fluid is to be replaced.[1,2] Water deficit is calculated as follows:

Free water deficit = 0.6 × Body weight in kilograms × [(Plasma Na/140) − 1].

Diuretics and laxatives should be held until the deficit is corrected. The need for these medications should then be reevaluated.

The patient with hypernatremia caused by central diabetes insipidus is given vasopressin to decrease renal water losses. If the degree of hypernatremia is moderate (<155 mEq/L), 0.1 to 0.4 ml of desmopressin acetate may be given intranasally b.i.d. With more severe hypernatremia, aqueous vasopressin is given subcutaneously q 12 to 24 hours. Nephrogenesis diabetes insipidus is treated with a thiazide diuretic (usually hydrochlorothiazide, 50 mg q day) and a sodium-restricted diet (2 g/day). Serum sodium levels should be monitored closely.[1-4, 7]

LIFE SPAN CONSIDERATIONS

Hypernatremia is commonly associated with fever and dehydration and in warm environments. Patients receiving high-solute tube feedings and diuretic or laxative therapy can also be at increased risk.

COMPLICATIONS

If hypernatremia is not corrected, cerebral vascular damage occurs as a result of brain dehydration and shrinkage. Shock results if a severe volume depletion is not corrected. Patients with cardiac disease should be monitored closely for signs and symptoms of congestive heart failure, which may occur if fluid is replaced too rapidly.[1,2]

INDICATIONS FOR REFERRAL/HOSPITALIZATION

Hypernatremia may be managed on an outpatient basis if the degree of sodium imbalance is moderate and the patient is alert and able to drink sufficient amounts of fluids. Older adults living alone or those at risk for developing congestive heart failure may best be managed in an inpatient setting. Patients with severe hypernatremia (serum sodium >155 mEq/L) or severe volume depletion should be hospitalized.[1,2,7]

PATIENT AND FAMILY EDUCATION

Patients and families should understand that normally 1500 to 2000 ml of fluid should be consumed each day. Patients at risk for hypernatremia should understand the importance of maintaining proper fluid balance. Older patients in particular need to be aware of the dangers of dehydration, especially in hot weather or if fever is present. Patients who are taking diuretics or medications such as lithium and carbamazepine (Tegretol), which cause hypernatremia, need to be aware of this side effect. Patients who exercise regularly should be educated about the need for adequate fluid intake when exercising. Patients with underlying conditions that put them at risk for hypernatremia need to be educated accordingly.[1,4,6]

Hyponatremia

DEFINITION/EPIDEMIOLOGY

Hyponatremia is a common electrolyte disorder. It is a syndrome rather than a disease and has been identified with a number of varied disorders, including infections, malignancy, untoward medication effects, endocrine disorders, psychogenic polydipsia, the syndrome of inappropriate antidiuretic hormone (SIADH), AIDS, and other illnesses. These conditions seem to be related to a dysfunction in the release of ADH or renal insensitivity to the hormone. However, hyponatremia can result from any condition that leads to excess water in relation to body sodium or causes salt loss in excess of water loss.[8]

Hyponatremia is defined as a serum sodium concentration of less than 135 mEq/L and may present as an acute or a chronic condition. Acute hyponatremia customarily develops in hospitalized patients after surgery and is often associated with fluid overload. Chronic hyponatremia usually occurs outside the hospital, is acquired over a longer period, and is typically associated with less serious neurologic sequelae. It is one of the more common electrolyte disorders in older adults, but premenopausal women and children are also at risk, particularly after surgery.[9,10] Serious morbidity may occur with sodium levels less than 110 mEq/L, with mortality approaching 50% in acute hyponatremia.[9]

Hyponatremia may be classified into one of four categories by the determination of extracellular fluid volume (ECFV).[9] These include hyponatremia with hypervolemia (increased ECFV), hyponatremia with hypovolemia (decreased ECFV), hyponatremia with euvolia (normal ECFV), and pseudohyponatremia.[8,9] The first three hyponatremias are associated with decreased plasma osmolality and are considered hypotonic hyponatremias. Pseudohyponatremia has been identified with both increased and normal osmolality and may be either a hypertonic or isotonic hyponatremia.

PATHOPHYSIOLOGY

As the major extracellular cation, sodium regulates intracellular and extracellular body water and is a determinant of serum osmolality. If serum sodium levels are allowed to fall below normal limits, serum osmolality is decreased and extracellular water is permitted to seep into cells. This results in a hypotonic hyponatremia and the subsequent swelling of cerebral brain cells that causes the neurologic features associated with hyponatremia.

Normally the body responds to an excess amount of water by diuresing. Renal mechanisms and ADH control body fluid volume and the composition of body fluids. An increase in serum osmolality over the normal 275 to 295 mOsm stimulates the posterior pituitary to release ADH, which influences the distal tubules and collecting ducts in the kidneys to conserve water. As body fluid accumulates and serum osmolality becomes hypotonic, ADH is inhibited.

Hyponatremia with Increased Extracellular Volume

Hyponatremia with increased ECFV may occur with cirrhosis, congestive heart failure, nephrotic syndrome, or advanced renal failure. Hypervolemic hyponatremias are considered edematous conditions and are characterized by urine sodium less than 20 mEq/L and high urine osmolality. In renal failure, however, urine sodium may be more than 20 mEq/L. Diuretic therapy may cause the urine to have a high sodium concentration, rendering the test inaccurate.

Hyponatremia with Decreased Extracellular Volume

Hypovolemic hyponatremia consists of a sodium deficit that occurs in isolation or in addition to a water deficit. This condition can be associated with either nonrenal or renal precipitants; this is distinguished by the evaluation of the urine sodium. With renal-associated disorders (chronic renal disease, osmotic diabetic diuresis, mineralocorticoid deficiency, angiotensin-converting enzyme [ACE] inhibitors, and diuretics), urine sodium is usually greater than 20 mEq/L. In nonrenal disorders (dehydration, diarrhea, vomiting, burns, extreme exercise, diaphoresis, and third-space fluid loss), urine sodium is less than 20 mEq/L and is combined with a high urine osmolality.

Hyponatremia with Normal Extracellular Volume

SIADH is often the cause of hyponatremia associated with normal ECFV and has been identified with many conditions.[9] With SIADH, a stimulus causes an excess production of ADH, which precipitates an increase in water reabsorption, an increase in glomerular filtration rate, and a decrease in sodium reabsorption. SIADH is characterized by hypotonic hyponatremia, euvolia, increased urinary sodium (usually >20 mEq/L), a urine osmolality greater than serum osmolality, and normal renal, cardiac, hepatic, adrenal, and thyroid function. Typically, plasma urea and uric acid are within normal limits.[11]

Psychogenic polydipsia, beer potamia, and a reset osmostat have also been identified as precipitants of hypotonic hyponatremia with euvolia. Psychogenic polydipsia may be related to ACE inhibitor or lithium therapy or to a biologic or psychiatric disorder; it may also be a compensatory mechanism for medications that cause dry mouth.[9,11] Individuals with beer potamia derive the vast amount of their caloric intake from large quantities of beer, which contains relatively few solutes.[12] The reduced solute delivery to the distal tubule restricts urine production and results in hyponatremia. The reset osmostat phenomenon, or sick-cell syndrome, is found in patients with malnutrition, cancer, or other debilitating conditions. Changes in cellular metabolism cause hypothalamic osmoreceptors to reset to maintain a lowered serum osmolality.[9] The diagnosis of reset osmostat is complex. Usually BUN and creatinine are normal, but urine sodium and osmolality are variable.[9]

Euvolemic hyponatremia has also been identified in varied postoperative situations. Pain and the stress of surgery can stimulate the release of excess ADH, which may cause hyponatremia in the presence of IV hypotonic fluid replacement.[8]

Pseudohyponatremia

Pseudohyponatremia without plasma hypoosmolality has been associated with hyperproteinemia and hyperlipidemia. In these disorders, partial displacement of the sodium-containing plasma by increased numbers of lipids or proteins causes falsely lowered sodium. Both conditions are isotonic hyponatremias associated with normal plasma osmolality and are treated with correction of the hyperproteinemia or hyperlipidemia.[9]

Hyperosmolar pseudohyponatremia may be seen with conditions that elevate plasma osmolality, such as hyperglycemia, mannitol excess, and glycerol therapy. The increased serum glucose causes increased plasma osmolality, which shifts body water into the intravascular space and lowers serum sodium. Correction of plasma glucose corrects the hyponatremia.

Pseudohyponatremia may also be caused by the absorption of isotonic irrigant solutions containing glycine or sorbitol after endometrial resection or a urologic procedure.[13] The absorption of the irrigant lowers plasma sodium, but not usually plasma osmolality. Elevated serum osmolality with lowered serum sodium may occur in some cases.[11]

CLINICAL PRESENTATION AND PHYSICAL EXAMINATION

Hyponatremia should be considered in the differential diagnosis of all individuals who present with irritability, restlessness, impaired central nervous system function, history of falls, nonspecific gastrointestinal complaints, flulike symptoms, dysgeusia, unusual water-drinking behavior, or weight changes.[14] Unfortunately, the symptoms commonly associated with hyponatremia may not be apparent until the patient's sodium level has fallen below 120 mEq/L. Nonetheless, patients with even mild hyponatremia may present with headache, blurred vision, dizziness, lethargy, weakness, combativeness, extrapyramidal signs, muscle cramps, and fatigue. Stupor, seizures, psychosis, and coma are associated with sodium levels below 110 mEq/L.

DIAGNOSTICS

Determination of serum electrolytes, calcium, magnesium, phosphorus, BUN, and creatinine is essential. Calculated serum osmolality affords mathematical categorization of the hyponatremia into a hypertonic, hypotonic, or isotonic state:

$$2(\text{Na in mEq/L}) + \text{K in mEq/L} + (\text{BUN in mg/dl}/2.8) + (\text{Glucose in mg/dl}/18)$$

Uric acid, urine sodium, urine specific gravity, and urine osmolality are also useful for the classification of hyponatremia.

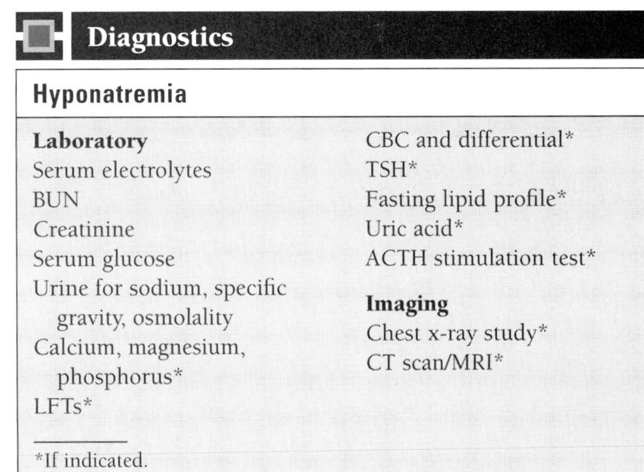

Diagnostics

Hyponatremia

Laboratory	
Serum electrolytes	CBC and differential*
BUN	TSH*
Creatinine	Fasting lipid profile*
Serum glucose	Uric acid*
Urine for sodium, specific gravity, osmolality	ACTH stimulation test*
Calcium, magnesium, phosphorus*	**Imaging**
LFTs*	Chest x-ray study*
	CT scan/MRI*

*If indicated.

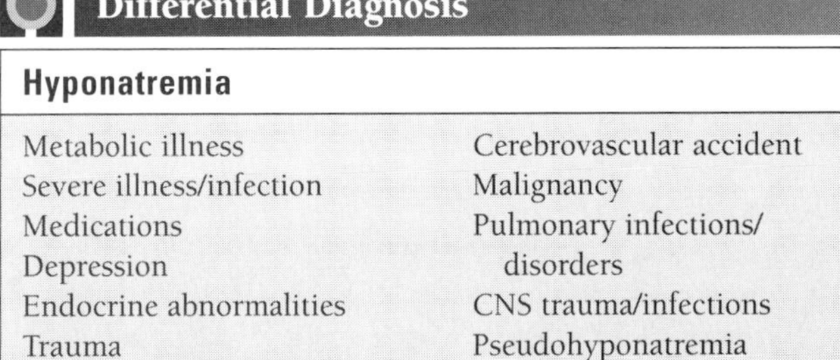

Differential Diagnosis

Hyponatremia

Metabolic illness	Cerebrovascular accident
Severe illness/infection	Malignancy
Medications	Pulmonary infections/disorders
Depression	CNS trauma/infections
Endocrine abnormalities	Pseudohyponatremia
Trauma	
Cardiovascular event	

CBC, fasting lipid profile, liver function studies, thyroid-stimulating hormone, chest x-ray studies, malignancy evaluations, definitive neurologic studies, and/or endocrine tests may be indicated to discern the underlying cause of the hyponatremia.

DIFFERENTIAL DIAGNOSIS

Metabolic disturbances, severe illness, infection, medications, depression, endocrine abnormalities, nutritional deficiencies, trauma, and cardiovascular and cerebral vascular accidents should be considered in the differential diagnosis. Additionally, fluid volume status should be determined to classify the hyponatremia.

MANAGEMENT

The volume status guides specific management decisions. Correction of the body water and sodium imbalance is the primary goal in managing hyponatremia, but correction or control of the underlying pathologic condition is also critical.

Hyponatremia with increased extracellular volume (hypervolemia) is associated with lowered serum osmolality (<280 mOsm/L), serum sodium <135 mEq/L, and increased urine osmolality. In renal failure, the urine sodium will be >20 mEq/L, but otherwise the urine sodium will be <20 mEq/L. For asymptomatic patients with serum sodium >125 mEq/L, management consists of fluid restriction (1000-1500 ml/day) and dietary sodium restriction (2-5 g/day). If the serum sodium is <125 mEq/L, the physician should be consulted and the cautious use of loop diuretics considered.

In hyponatremia with decreased extracellular volume (hypovolemia) associated with a renal disorder, serum osmolality will be <275 mOsm/L, urine sodium >20 mEq/L, and the BUN and creatinine will be increased. If diarrhea, vomiting, or dehydration is the cause of the hypovolemic hyponatremia, the serum osmolality will be <275 mEq/L, urine sodium <20 mEq/L, and the BUN and creatinine will be increased. Management consists of treating the underlying disorder, eliminating medications associated with the hyponatremia (particularly NSAIDs, thiazide diuretics, and if necessary ACE inhibitors) and, if indicated, isotonic fluid replacement to correct the fluid deficit. If the serum sodium is <125 mEq/L, consultation with the primary care physician is necessary to discuss hospitalization for IV saline.

Hyponatremia associated with euvolemia (normal extracellular volume) requires careful consideration as the underlying pathologies are considerable. In SIADH, the urine osmolality is usually >100 mOsm/L and urine sodium >20 mEq/L. BUN (<10 mg/dl) and uric acid (<4 mg/dl) are low and thyroid, renal, adrenal, and hepatic function are normal. Management consists of correcting the underlying pathology and fluid restriction. Consultation with the physician is indicated for a serum sodium <125 mEq/L to discuss hospitalization for hypertonic saline infusion or initiating demeclocycline.

Treatment of patients with psychogenic polydipsia and beer potamia consists of fluid restriction and behavioral counseling. Management of pseudohyponatremia associated with hyperglycemia consists of correcting the hyperglycemia. If an isotonic genitourinary irrigant is the cause of the hyponatremia, the irrigant should be discontinued. No treatment is necessary for hyperlipidemia or hyperproteinemia.

Co-Management with Specialists

In consultation with a physician, loop diuretics may be used with caution. Furosemide and increased oral sodium may be indicated for patients who are unable to adhere to water restriction. Furosemide is also prescribed in combination with ACE inhibitors to manage hyponatremia in severe congestive heart failure.

Demeclocycline in doses greater than 600 mg/day (300 to 600 mg PO b.i.d.) inhibits the effect of ADH on the renal tubule and has been used in the long-term management of SIADH and carbamazepine-induced hyponatremia.[13,15] Demeclocycline can increase BUN, precipitate renal toxicity, and induce fluid loss; therefore caution is advised, particularly with congestive heart failure, renal disease, or liver disease.[9] Lithium, another ADH inhibitor, has also been used for the treatment of SIADH despite its potential for precipitating psychogenic polydipsia and thyroid dysfunction.[9,15]

Urea, both oral and IV, has been successfully used to treat varied types of hyponatremia but is contraindicated in patients with gastric ulcers, renal failure, and liver disease.[16] Oral nonpeptide vasopressin antagonists may also soon be available and offer added benefit in the treatment of hyponatremia.[17]

COMPLICATIONS

Brain damage or death is the most serious complication of hyponatremia and seems to occur most often in children and premenopausal women.[13] These sequelae are associated with encephalopathy resulting from untreated hyponatremia and the untoward consequences of mistreatment.[13]

INDICATIONS FOR REFERRAL/HOSPITALIZATION

Symptoms of hyponatremia with decreased ECFV are typically those associated with hypovolemia. Treatment of the underlying disorder and isotonic fluid volume replacement in the hospital setting is indicated.[15]

Patients with acute SIADH and serum sodium less than 115 mEq/L should be hospitalized for intensive correction of both the underlying disorder and the SIADH disorder with hypertonic saline (3% NaCl), diuretics, and replacement electrolytes. To prevent central pontine myelinosis and brain damage, care must be taken to prevent hypoxia and to slowly, rather than quickly, repair the hyponatremia with hypertonic IV saline.[13,15] Hypertonic saline should not be administered more rapidly than 10 to 15 mEq/L/24 hr; urine output and serum electrolytes should be monitored hourly, and the infusion should be discontinued before the serum sodium reaches 130 mEq/L.[11]

PATIENT AND FAMILY EDUCATION

Hyponatremia and its treatment may be anxiety provoking for both patients and families. Patients and caregivers, both family and professional, need to understand the nature of the hyponatremic disorder and recognize its associated neurologic symptoms. Instructions regarding the importance of frequent weight measurements, dietary or fluid restriction, intake and output measurement, and medications (and their side effects) should be explicit and understandable. Patients and families also need to understand the importance of calling the primary care provider if the fluid restriction causes constipation or other problems. Because fluid restriction can dry oral membranes, good oral hygiene is important. Patients who are bedridden or immobile need good skin care, constant turning, and proper positioning. Frequent follow-up care with continuous evaluation of the treatment plan is imperative.

REFERENCES

1. Fried LF, Palevsky PM: Hyponatremia and hypernatremia, *Med Clin North Am* 81(3):585-609, 1997.
2. Oh MS, Carroll HJ: Disorders of sodium metabolism: hypernatremia and hyponatremia, *Crit Care Med* 20(1):94-103, 1992.
3. Brown RG: Disorders of water and sodium balance, *Postgrad Med* 93(4):227-246, 1993.
4. Bove LA: Restoring electrolyte balance: sodium and chloride, *RN* 59(11):25-29, 1996.
5. Winger JM, Hurnic T: Age-associated changes in the endocrine system, *Nurs Clin North Am* 31(4):827-844, 1996.
6. Horne MM, Heitz UE, Swearingen PL: *Fluid, electrolyte, and acid-base balance: a case study approach*, St Louis, 1991, Mosby.
7. Hobbs J: Fluid, electrolyte, and acid-base disturbances. In Mengel MB, Schwiebert LP, editors: *Ambulatory medicine: the primary care of families*, Stamford, Conn, 1996, Appleton & Lange.
8. Rutecki GW, Whittier FC: Physiologic clues to a state of disordered tonicity, *Consultant* 688-702, 1994.
9. Rousseau P: Hyponatremia among older individuals, *South Med J* 84(9):1114-1118, 1991.
10. Miller M and others: Apparent idiopathic hyponatremia in an ambulatory geriatric population, *J Am Geriatr Soc* 44(4):404-408, 1996.
11. Mulloy AL, Caruana RJ: Hyponatremic emergencies, *Med Clin North Am* 79(1):155-167, 1995.
12. Reeves WB, Andreoli TE: The posterior pituitary and water metabolism. In Wilson JD, Foster DF, editors: *William's textbook of endocrinology*, ed 8, Philadelphia, 1992, WB Saunders.
13. Fraser CL, Arieff AI: Epidemiology, pathophysiology, and management of hyponatremic encephalopathy, *Am J Med* 102(1):67-77, 1997.
14. Panayioutou H and others: Sweet taste (dysgeusia): the first symptom of hyponatremia in small cell carcinoma of the lung, *Arch Intern Med* 155(12):1325-1328, 1995.
15. Narins RG, Krishna GG: Disorders of water balance. In Stein JH and others, editors: *Internal medicine*, ed 5, St Louis, 1998, Mosby.
16. Soupart A, Decaux G: Therapeutic recommendations for management of severe hyponatremia: current concepts on pathogenesis and prevention of neurologic complications, *Clin Nephrol* 46(3):149-169, 1996.
17. Gross P, Wehrle R, Bussemaker E: Hyponatremia: pathophysiology, differential diagnosis, and new aspects of treatment, *Clin Nephrol* 46(4):273-276, 1996.

CHAPTER 227

Lipid Disorders

Philip E. Knapp

DEFINITION/EPIDEMIOLOGY

Despite significant reductions in cardiovascular disease (CVD) rates over the last three decades, CVD is still the leading cause of death in the United States, accounting for 40.6% of all deaths at a cost of over $298 billion in 2001.[1] Significant advances have been made in identifying and treating risk factors associated with CVD. As a better understanding of the process of atherosclerosis and the importance of the lipid disorders has emerged, it has become apparent that the identification and treatment of these disorders is essential if the decrease in coronary heart disease (CHD) is to continue. It is critical that these disorders are identified and evaluated, and that management plans are prescribed that match the intensity of the treatment to the level of risk for each individual.

Lipid disorders, or dyslipidemias, are generally the result of a combination of genetic and dietary factors. A serum total cholesterol level of less than 200 is considered desirable, but more than 100 million or about half of all American adults have a total cholesterol level of 200 or greater. More than 40 million, almost 20%, have total cholesterol levels of 240 or more and are clearly at increased risk for CHD.

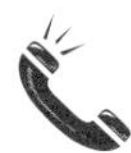

Physician consultation is recommended for all patients with lipid disorders that do not respond to treatment.

PATHOPHYSIOLOGY

Cholesterol and other lipids are normal and essential components of human cells. The liver synthesizes much of the body's cholesterol. Additional cholesterol, as well as a variety of other lipids, is absorbed from the gastrointestinal tract. Mechanisms are in place to transport them via the bloodstream to the liver where they are processed, and to the rest of the body where they are used or stored. As cholesterol and other lipids are insoluble in water, they must be combined with specialized phospholipids and proteins called apoproteins to form microscopic packages called lipoproteins, which are soluble in the plasma. Lipoproteins take the form of a lipid core containing triglycerides and cholesterol and an outer layer containing the phospholipids and the apoproteins. The apoproteins serve as ligands for the enzymes and receptors that mediate lipid metabolism.

Atherosclerosis is a pathologic process whereby cholesterol is deposited into the walls of arteries. It is influenced by a number of factors including toxins and inflammatory mediators within the bloodstream and at the level of the vessel wall. It is also influenced by the characteristics and concentrations of the various lipoproteins. These are characterized by their density and include: chylomicrons, very-low-density lipoprotein (VLDL), intermediate-density lipoprotein (IDL), low-density lipoprotein (LDL), and high-density lipoprotein (HDL).

Chylomicrons

Dietary cholesterol and triglycerides are packaged into chylomicrons within the intestine and then absorbed into the circulation. Chylomicrons serve two important physiologic functions. First, they deliver dietary fat to body tissues for energy and storage, and second, they supply dietary cholesterol to the liver, where it is either converted to bile acids or is incorporated into VLDL for transport to the rest of the body. Although not thought to be atherogenic, chylomicrons are triglyceride rich; thus a deficiency in certain enzymes and apoproteins can lead to very high serum triglyceride levels.

Very-Low-Density Lipoprotein/Intermediate-Density Lipoprotein

In the liver triglycerides and cholesterol are packaged into VLDL particles that circulate in the bloodstream. In the presence of the enzyme lipoprotein lipase, some of the triglycerides are broken down to free fatty acids, which are absorbed by the tissues. The VLDL particles are thereby made more dense and transformed into IDL. The liver will break down half of the IDL particles; the other half are transformed into LDL.

Low-Density Lipoprotein

LDL carries most of the cholesterol in the plasma and is the cause of atherogenic changes associated with the development of CHD. The principal function of LDL is to transport cholesterol to hepatic and extrahepatic cells. Although LDL particles are small, they carry approximately 70% of the circulating cholesterol in plasma. Both IDL and LDL are removed from the plasma by a single type of receptor located on the surface of many cells throughout the body—the LDL receptor. LDL's primary apoprotein is apoprotein B (Apo B), which binds to the LDL receptor during the process by which LDL is brought into the cells. One molecule of Apo B is present for each LDL particle, but the quantity of cholesterol per particle can vary considerably. The ratio of LDL cholesterol to Apo B correlates with the size of the LDL particles. Low LDL cholesterol–Apo B ratios reflect small LDL particles. It has been postulated that these smaller, denser LDL particles are more atherogenic than normal-sized LDL particles. Two theories exist on why this may be true. First, their size allows these particles to filter more easily through the arterial wall, and, second, these particles are especially vulnerable to oxidation. Small, dense LDL particles have been associated with conditions such as insulin resistance, diabetes, hypertriglyceridemia, and low HDL, all of which are independent risk factors for CHD.

It may be that measurements of apoprotein B in the blood correlate even more closely than LDL cholesterol with the risk for CHD, but this test is not available in most laboratories.[2] Elevation of a distinct form of LDL, lipoprotein (a) [Lp(a)], has been identified as an independent risk factor for the development of premature CHD in men.[3] Because there is no scientific proof that lowering Lp(a) will lower cardiovascular risk, assessment of this lipid determination at this time should be limited to research and specialized lipid clinics.

High-Density Lipoprotein

HDL has emerged as a powerful independent predictor of CHD risk. For every 1 mg/dl decrease in HDL there is a 2% to 3% increase in CHD risk. The role of HDL is twofold. First, when free cholesterol is released from cells into the plasma, it binds to HDL particles, resulting in a reverse cholesterol transport system. Cholesterol is returned to the liver, where it is excreted into bile, converted to bile acids, or reprocessed. Both the liver and intestines synthesize and secrete HDL particles. Second, HDL prevents oxidation of LDL within the arterial wall. There is an inverse relationship between VLDL remnants and small, dense LDL particles, known atherogenic factors, and HDL. Because of the inverse relationship between levels of HDL and CHD risk, low levels of HDL (<40 mg/dl) have been identified as an independent risk factor for CHD regardless of the total cholesterol. Higher HDL cholesterol has a protective effect and levels >60 mg/dl are considered to be a "negative risk factor" lowering the overall risk.

The ratio of total cholesterol to HDL cholesterol has been correlated to cardiac risk in some studies and a total cholesterol-HDL cholesterol ratio of greater than 4.5 is associated with increased cardiac risk. Use of this ratio, however, appears less useful than previously thought. Apoprotein AI (Apo AI) is the predominant lipoprotein in HDL and measurement of Apo AI in addition to the Apo B found in LDL may, in the future, allow for more accurate assessment of cardiac risk.

Increased levels of physical activity can increase HDL cholesterol levels, and this should be a target for intervention. Also, it appears that modest alcohol consumption increases HDL cholesterol and appears to reduce cardiac risk. Alcohol, however, can also increase triglycerides, and have other adverse effects. The intake of one to two alcoholic beverages per day may be beneficial in terms of overall mortality, but consumption of more alcohol than this is clearly detrimental and in many patients alcohol use can escalate. Recommending alcohol consumption to patients must be done with caution.

Triglycerides

Levels of LDL and HDL cholesterol actually represent a measurement of the amount of cholesterol contained in each kind of lipoprotein particle in the blood. Triglycerides are found in all types of lipoprotein particles. Elevations in triglycerides therefore could represent a number of different abnormalities in lipid metabolism. Nonetheless, elevated triglycerides have been identified as an independent cardiac risk factor and, when extremely elevated, can cause pancreatitis.

Role of Genetics

A person's genetic makeup plays a profound role in his lipid metabolism and the resulting risk for complications. In the well-characterized but relatively rare familial dyslipidemias single gene mutations result in a faulty apoprotein, receptor, or enzyme and a particular pattern of dyslipidemia. The most common of these is familial hypercholesterolemia, which is caused by a defect in the gene for the LDL receptor and results in very high levels of serum cholesterol sometimes above 500 mg/dl. Familial hypertriglyceridemia, familial combined hyperlipidemia, and the other familial hyperlipidemia syndromes are even rarer.

Most individuals with hyperlipidemia do not fit into one of these classic genetic syndromes. Nonetheless, more subtle genetic factors influence their lipid metabolism and predispose them to unfavorable lipid profiles, particularly when exposed to an unhealthy diet and physical inactivity.

Role of Diet and Exercise

Although genetic factors play a major role in lipid metabolism, they cannot readily be changed. Lifestyle choices can be. Dietary cholesterol and fats, especially saturated fats, have been identified as factors that contribute to deleterious lipid profiles. These dietary factors work by downregulating LDL receptors, resulting in a slowing of the breakdown of LDL particles and increased concentrations in the blood. Obesity is associated with elevated triglycerides and physical inactivity with low HDL.

Dietary cholesterol is derived only from animal products. Of the cholesterol that is consumed, 40% is absorbed, contributing to an increase in the endogenous cholesterol and raising total and LDL cholesterol levels in the plasma. It is estimated that for every 100 mg of dietary cholesterol per 1000 calories consumed per day, the serum cholesterol will increase 6 to 10 mg/dl.

There are three major types of dietary fats: saturated, monounsaturated, and polyunsaturated. Each subtype exerts different influences on lipid metabolism, with saturated fats being the most harmful. Saturated fats increase blood cholesterol levels significantly more than dietary cholesterol. Reducing saturated fats in the diet from 14% to 7% of total calories can decrease total blood cholesterol levels by close to 20 mg/dl. Within this category are a number of subtypes, based on the number of carbon bonds, not all of which adversely affect the lipid profile. Unfortunately, the major source of saturated fats in the American diet is from palmitic acid, which does increase lipid levels and is found in meats, eggs, and dairy products. Certain vegetable oils, namely tropical oils such as palm and coconut oil, are highly saturated, raise serum cholesterol significantly, and are typically found in commercially prepared cakes, muffins, cookies, and other baked goods.

Monounsaturated fats are derived from animal and plant oils. The most common source of monounsaturated fats in the American diet is from peanuts, olives, avocados, and almonds. They do not by themselves raise or lower cholesterol levels but have been shown to help preserve baseline HDL levels when substituted for other fats. Their inclusion is a major feature of the popular Mediterranean diet.

Polyunsaturated fats are considered essential fatty acids because they cannot be synthesized by the body, unlike the saturated and monounsaturated fatty acids. Polyunsaturated fats are derived from vegetable oils consisting of omega-3 fatty acids or omega-6 fatty acids found in fish products. The enthusiastic endorsement that they received in the 1980s has been dampened by recent findings. Dietary fish oils have been shown to lower total cholesterol and LDL levels while also lowering HDL levels.

There has been recent evidence for the negative effect of a particular form of unsaturated fats called trans-fatty acids.[4] These arise from vegetable oils that undergo extensive chemical processing or exposure to excess heat. The most common sources in the American diet are margarine spreads, with the stick form being more concentrated than the tub form. They are also found in commercially produced baked goods and deep-fried foods.

Despite apparent increased awareness of healthy lifestyle choices in the United States, obesity has been on the rise since 1960, and could reasonable be called an epidemic. Nearly 55% of American adults are overweight or obese.[5] Obesity causes an increase in total and LDL cholesterol by decreasing LDL receptor activity. Obesity also decreases HDL cholesterol by increasing triglyceride levels through a mechanism considered more atherogenic than the triglyceride-raising effect of a high-carbohydrate diet and/or high alcohol intake. Weighing just 20 pounds over one's ideal body weight can increase LDL cholesterol by 10 mg/dl and decrease HDL cholesterol by 3 mg/dl, resulting in a 16% increased risk for the development of CHD.

Insulin Resistance, Diabetes, and "The Metabolic Syndrome"

Adult onset or type 2 diabetes appears to stem from a combination of factors including progressive insulin resistance and inadequate insulin supply. Insulin resistance may or may not be associated with frank diabetes or even detectable high blood glucose levels. It is strongly influenced by genetic factors and is associated with abdominal obesity. Physical inactivity and a diet high in carbohydrates are major contributing factors. Insulin resistance, together with physical inactivity and obesity, often appears as part of a larger constellation of abnormalities including hypertension, high triglycerides, low HDL cholesterol, and small dense LDL particles, which are thought to be particularly atherogenic. Patients with this constellation of abnormalities, labeled as "the metabolic syndrome" or "syndrome X," have a significantly increased risk for CHD (see Chapter 228).

CLINICAL PRESENTATION

The National Cholesterol Education Project (NCEP) is an expert panel sponsored by the National Heart Lung and Blood Institute that periodically reviews the available evidence and publishes guidelines on the evaluation and treatment of lipid disorders. Their most recent report, NCEP III, reinforces earlier guidelines in the treatment of dyslipidemias, but goes further in recommending tailoring treatment goals to patients according to their overall risk for CHD.[6] Clinical evaluation should thus include a complete medical history. The clinician should attempt to elicit symptoms of occult vascular disease such as exertional angina or claudication. A detailed past medical history should be obtained with documentation of any known CHD or other atherosclerotic process such as cerebrovascular or peripheral vascular disease, as well as hypertension and diabetes. Hypothyroidism, liver disease, and renal disease can affect lipid metabolism and should be noted. Other cardiac risk factors should be documented as well, including tobacco use and a family history of early CHD.

PHYSICAL EXAMINATION

The physical examination should include accurate measurement of blood pressure, height, and weight, with determination of the body mass index. The waist-hip ratio should be measured, as it has been shown to be more specifically related to the development of CVD than weight alone. As the ratio increases from 1, so does the risk. A good general examination should be with specific attention to any signs of occult cardiac or vascular disease. In the occasional patient with very high cholesterol from a familial hyperlipidemia, one might find fatty deposits called xanthomas on tendons such as the Achilles, and on elbows, knees, and metacarpal joints, or deposits of cholesterol on the eyelids called xanthelasmas. The presence of corneal arcus, an opaque white ring about the corneal periphery, is less predictive of a lipid disorder but should trigger further evaluation if it is seen in the young adult.

DIAGNOSTICS

The NCEP III guidelines recommend lipid screening every 5 years for all adults over 20 years old (Figure 227-1). If possible this should be done with a full lipid profile obtained after 10 to 12 hours of fasting. If circumstances do not allow a fasting lipid profile, then total and HDL cholesterol only can be measured with a follow-up fasting profile for those with a total cholesterol ≥200 mg/dl or a low HDL cholesterol (<40 mg/dl).

The values in a lipid profile that are actually measured by most laboratories are total cholesterol, HDL cholesterol, and triglycerides. LDL cholesterol is then calculated from these three values according to the following equation:

$$\text{LDL cholesterol} = \text{Total cholesterol} - (\text{HDL cholesterol} + \text{Triglycerides}/5)$$

Of the three measured values only triglycerides are significantly affected by dietary intake in the 12 hours preceding the test. This in turn affects the calculated value for LDL cholesterol. If, for whatever reason, the triglyceride level is >400 mg/dl, the LDL cholesterol level cannot be accurately calculated.

Total cholesterol ≥240 mg/dl is considered high, and 200 to 239 mg/dl is considered borderline high. HDL cholesterol ≤40 mg/dl is considered low and is an independent risk factor for CHD. Triglyceride levels <150 mg/dl are considered desirable, 150 to 199 mg/dl are considered borderline high, 200 to 499 mg/dl are considered high, and triglycerides ≥500 mg/dl are considered very high. High triglycerides are also emerging as an independent risk factor for CHD, particularly when associated with low HDL.

Elevated LDL cholesterol is the lipid abnormality most closely associated with the development of CHD, and reduction in LDL

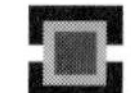 **Diagnostics**

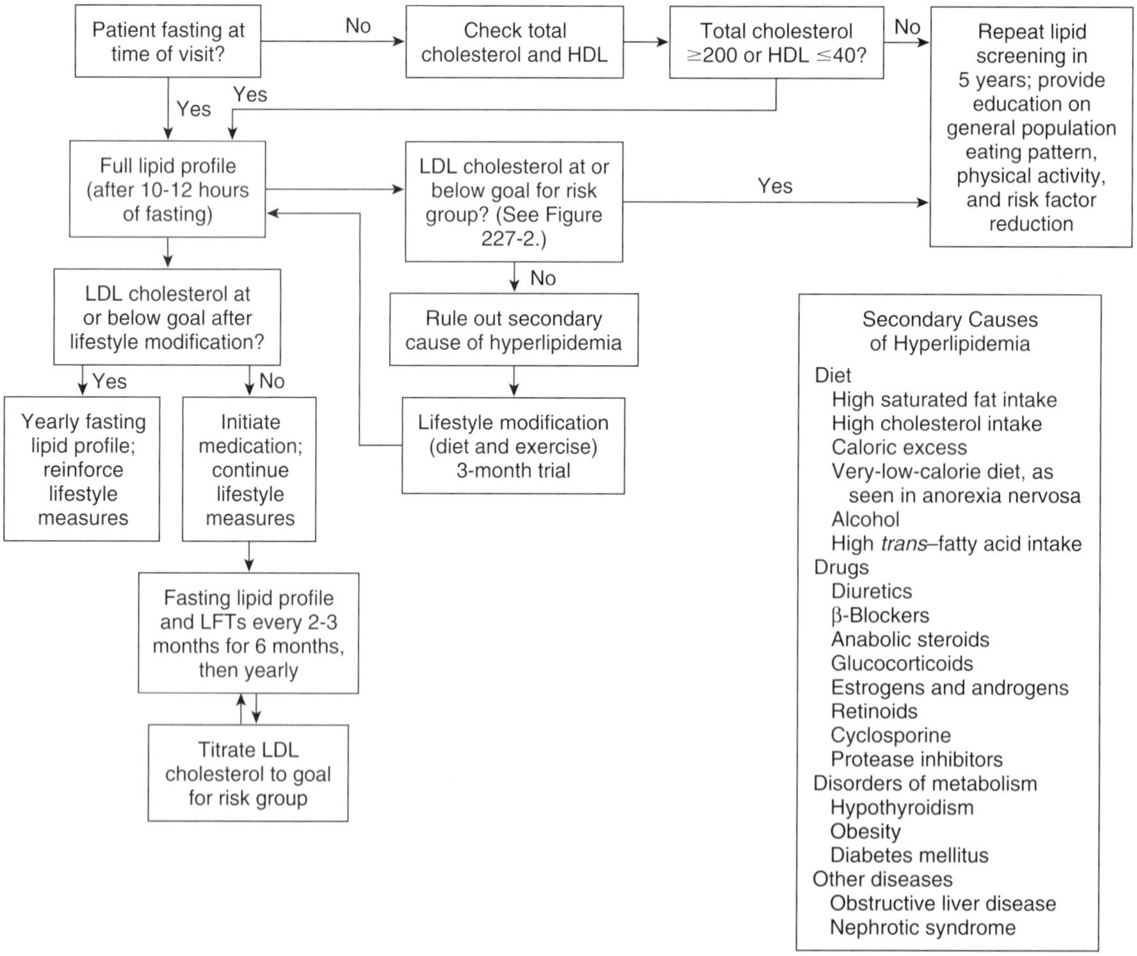

Lipid Disorders

Laboratory

Cholesterol (random total and high-density lipoprotein (HDL) every 5 years for all adults >20 years.

Lipid profile (10- to 12-hour fasting if total cholesterol is high, if borderline and two or more coronary heart disease (CHD) risk factors are present, or if HDL cholesterol is <35 mg/dl or overt CHD is present.

Patient fasting at time of visit?
No
Check total cholesterol and HDL
Total cholesterol ≥200 or HDL ≤40?
No
Repeat lipid screening in 5 years; provide education on general population eating pattern, physical activity, and risk factor reduction
Yes
Yes
Full lipid profile (after 10-12 hours of fasting)
LDL cholesterol at or below goal for risk group? (See Figure 227-2.)
Yes
No
Rule out secondary cause of hyperlipidemia
Lifestyle modification (diet and exercise) 3-month trial
LDL cholesterol at or below goal after lifestyle modification?
Yes
No
Yearly fasting lipid profile; reinforce lifestyle measures
Initiate medication; continue lifestyle measures
Fasting lipid profile and LFTs every 2-3 months for 6 months, then yearly
Titrate LDL cholesterol to goal for risk group
Secondary Causes of Hyperlipidemia
Diet
High saturated fat intake
High cholesterol intake
Caloric excess
Very-low-calorie diet, as seen in anorexia nervosa
Alcohol
High trans–fatty acid intake
Drugs
Diuretics
β-Blockers
Anabolic steroids
Glucocorticoids
Estrogens and androgens
Retinoids
Cyclosporine
Protease inhibitors
Disorders of metabolism
Hypothyroidism
Obesity
Diabetes mellitus
Other diseases
Obstructive liver disease
Nephrotic syndrome

FIGURE 227-1

Screening and treatment of hyperlipidemia should be done for all adults ≥20 years of age.

cholesterol has been clearly demonstrated to have a dramatic impact on morbidity and mortality from CHD. LDL cholesterol remains the primary target of therapy. Decisions about what level of LDL cholesterol should prompt the initiation of lifestyle modification and/or drug therapy and what the goals of therapy should be are made based on a comprehensive assessment of the individual patient's risk for CHD. The desired LDL cholesterol level for a patient therefore depends on such an individual risk assessment and is discussed in the management section.

DIFFERENTIAL DIAGNOSIS

Before embarking on therapy for a dyslipidemia, one should consider other factors that may influence lipid metabolism. Diet, as has been discussed, can have a profound effect on the lipid profile, particularly excesses in overall caloric intake, saturated fat, and dietary cholesterol. In addition, starvation states such as anorexia nervosa can cause an elevation in total serum cholesterol. Overuse of alcohol is associated with hypertriglyceridemia.

The other major causes of secondary dyslipidemia are drugs, disorders of metabolism, and certain disease states. Drugs can affect lipid metabolism in a variety of ways. Glucocorticoids and estrogens have been shown to elevate triglyceride and HDL levels, although anabolic steroids can markedly reduce HDL levels. Thiazide diuretics have been shown to raise total cholesterol, triglyceride, and LDL levels. Alpha blockers may cause increases in HDL, whereas beta blockers can decrease HDL levels and increase triglyceride levels. Angiotensin-converting enzyme inhibitors and calcium channel blockers are thought to be lipid neutral. Elevation of total cholesterol and triglyceride levels is now being reported with the use of protease inhibitors used in the treatment of HIV infection. Whether the use of these drugs over time will increase the risk for the development of CHD remains to be seen.

By far the most common metabolic disorders associated with lipid abnormalities are hypothyroidism and diabetes. Therefore a screening test for thyroid-stimulating hormone and fasting glucose should be obtained when abnormalities in the lipid profile are discovered. Stabilization to a euthyroid state should be achieved before initiation of lipid treatment. In those with diabetes, achieving adequate glycemic control will improve the lipid profile and is an integral component of therapy. Other disease states such as the nephrotic syndrome and obstructive liver disease can also cause lipid abnormalities and can be excluded by a thorough medical history, physical examination, and, if appropriate, laboratory tests including a urinalysis, BUN, creatinine and LFTs.

Differential Diagnosis

Lipid Disorders

Primary Disorders
Familial disorders

Secondary Disorders
Diet
- High saturated fat intake
- High cholesterol intake
- Caloric excess
- Very-low-calorie diet, as seen in anorexia nervosa

Alcohol
High *trans*-fatty acid intake
Drugs
- Diuretics
- Beta blockers
- Anabolic steroids
- Glucosteroids
- Estrogens and androgens
- Retinoids
- Cyclosporine
- Protease inhibitors

Disorders of metabolism
- Hypothyroidism
- Obesity
- Diabetes mellitus

Other diseases
- Obstructive liver disease
- Nephrotic syndrome

MANAGEMENT

There is clear evidence that lowering elevated LDL cholesterol will reduce the risk for new CHD events both in patients without known CHD (primary prevention), and in those with known, preexisting CHD (secondary prevention). Recent recommendations such as those in the NCEP III report and those from an expert panel at the Bethesda Conference emphasize grouping patients into more specific categories of risk for cardiac events and tailoring their management accordingly.[7]

Risk Assessment

The NCEP III recommendations group patients into three categories of risk for CHD and each group is assigned specific goals for LDL cholesterol. Those with the highest risk for CHD are treated most aggressively.

Patients in the category of highest risk generally have more than a 20% risk for an acute cardiac event in the next 10 years. This category consists of those patients with known CHD and those with a CHD "risk equivalent" or a condition that confers an equally high risk for a new cardiac event (Figure 227-2). These conditions include other known atherosclerotic diseases such as peripheral vascular disease, aortic aneurysm or cerebrovascular disease, as well as diabetes. The LDL cholesterol goal for patients in this highest risk category is ≤100 mg/dl. Patients in this group who have LDL cholesterol >130 mg/dl are almost certain to require drug therapy. Those with LDL cholesterol levels between 100 and 130 mg/dl may be adequately treated with lifestyle modification, but many advocate early initiation of drug therapy for all patients in this group with LDL cholesterol >100 mg/dl (Table 227-1).

The intermediate risk category consists of patients with two or more major risk factors for CHD other than diabetes (see Figure 227-2). Patients in this category generally have a 10-year risk for a CHD event of ≤20%. Their goal for LDL cholesterol is <130 mg/dl but decisions about when to initiate drug therapy and when to use lifestyle modification alone may require a more detailed risk assessment. Table 227-2, which is derived from data from the Framingham Heart study, quantifies patients' 10-year risk for a new CHD event according to a point scoring system based on multiple risk factors. For patients with two or more risk factors and a 10-year risk for a cardiac event between 10% and 20%, lifestyle modification and drug therapy should be considered for all patients with LDL cholesterol ≥130 mg/dl. The goal for therapy is <130 mg/dl. For those with two or more risk factors but a 10-year cardiac risk <10%, the goal remains for LDL cholesterol <130 mg/dl. Lifestyle modification should be instituted for LDL cholesterol levels above this. It is reasonable to avoid the use of cholesterol-lowering medication unless the LDL cholesterol level is ≥160 mg/dl.

The category of lowest risk for CHD consists of patients with zero or one major risk factors. They generally have a 10-year risk for a CHD event of ≤10%. Their LDL cholesterol goal is <160 mg/dl, but it is reasonable to avoid medication unless their LDL cholesterol level is ≥190 mg/dl. While patients in

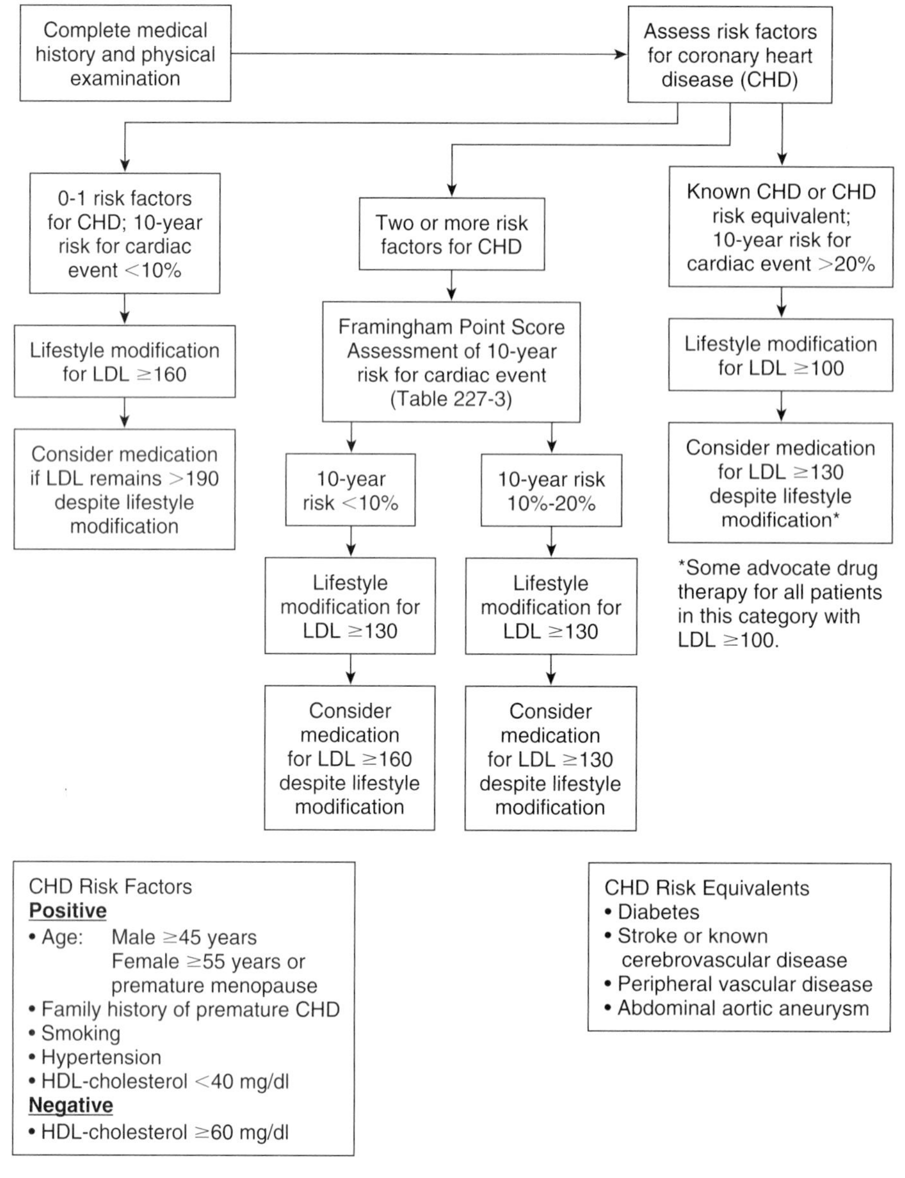

FIGURE 227-2

Risk assessment and the setting of goals for treatment in hyperlipidemia. (Data from NCEP III, *JAMA* 285: 2486-2497, 2001.)

this group have a relatively low 10-year risk for cardiac events, attention must also be paid to their risk for CHD beyond 10 years. This is more difficult to quantify and more difficult to balance against the risks and cost of long-term drug therapy. It is reasonable, however, to initiate lifestyle modification in these patients even with modest elevation of LDL cholesterol (≥130 mg/dl) to reduce their long-term risk of CHD.

Lifestyle Modification

Diet. Maximal dietary therapy will typically achieve a reduction in LDL cholesterol by 15 to 25 mg/dl, but a healthy balanced diet, exercise, and maintenance of an ideal body weight have benefits well beyond this reduction. Such benefits include a decreased tendency toward other cardiac risk factors including hypertension, insulin resistance, and diabetes.

Our understanding of the impact of diet on blood lipid levels and cardiac risk is constantly evolving. There has been some evidence that a very-low-fat diet (i.e., <10% of calories coming from fat) in conjunction with other lifestyle changes such as exercise, yoga, and meditation can reverse coronary artery disease.[8] This degree of restriction, however, is impractical for most patients. Until recently, standard dietary recommendations were to limit total dietary fat to 30% of total calories and saturated fat to 10%. Newer dietary recommendations include a slightly more liberal limit on total fat to 25% to 35% of total calories, with increased restriction of saturated fat to 7%. Saturated fats are primarily found in animal products such as meat and dairy, but also are found in certain vegetable oils such as palm and coconut.

Whenever possible, dietary fat should be the unsaturated fat found in most vegetable oils and, in particular, the monounsat-

TABLE 227-1 LDL Cholesterol Goals and Cutpoints for Therapeutic Lifestyle Changes (TLCs) and Drug Therapy in Different Risk Categories*

Risk Category	LDL Goal (mg/dL)	LDL Level at Which to Initiate Therapeutic Lifestyle Changes (mg/dL)	LDL Level at Which to Consider Drug Therapy (mg/dL)
CHD or CHD risk equivalents (10-year risk >20%)	<100	≥100	≥130 (100-129: drug optional)†
2 + Risk factors (10-year risk ≤20%)	<130	≥130	10-year risk 10%-20%: ≥130 10-year risk <10%: ≥160
0-1 Risk factor‡	<160	≥160	≥190 (160-189: LDL-lowering drug optional)

From Expert Panel on Detection, Evaluation, and Treatment of High Blood Cholesterol in Adults: Executive summary of the Third Report of the National Cholesterol Education (NCEP) Expert Panel on Detection, Evaluation, and Treatment of High Blood Cholesterol in Adults (Adult Treatment Panel III), *JAMA* 285:2486-2497, 2001.

**LDL*, low-density lipoprotein; *CHD*, coronary heart disease.

†Some authorities recommend use of LDL-lowering drugs in this category if an LDL cholesterol level of <100 mg/dL cannot be achieved by therapeutic lifestyle changes. Others prefer use of drugs that primarily modify triglycerides and HDL, e.g., nicotinic acid or fibrate. Clinical judgment also may call for deferring drug therapy in this subcategory.

‡Almost all people with 0-1 risk factor have a 10-year risk <10%; thus a 10-year risk assessment in people with 0-1 risk factor is not necessary.

urated fat found in olive oil and nuts. Evidence for this dietary strategy comes partly from study of the Mediterranean diet. Long known for their lower CHD rates, the populations of countries bordering this sea, such as Italy and Greece, typically have dietary fat intakes equal to or even higher than that of the populations of countries with high rates of CHD. Their consumption of saturated fats, however, is lower and a higher intake of monounsaturated fats, from olives and olive oil, contributes to their increased intake of fat. It is postulated that this diet helps to increase HDL and lower LDL cholesterol, thus decreasing the risk for CHD.

There is recent evidence that trans-fatty acids, which arise from excessive processing, are also atherogenic. Trans-fatty acids are found in margarine spreads, commercially produced baked goods, and deep-fried foods. These foods should be avoided when possible. Some data support the use of new "cholesterol lowering" margarine products enriched with plant sterols and stanols that inhibit the absorption of dietary cholesterol. The long-term safety of these products is currently being studied.

Actual cholesterol in the diet tends to be less detrimental to the lipid profile than saturated fats, and products labeled "low in cholesterol" often mislead patients. Nonetheless, dietary cholesterol does impact serum cholesterol and should be limited to 200 mg/day.

Replacement of fats should be from complex carbohydrates with added emphasis on increasing fiber in the diet to 20 to 30 g/day through the consumption of whole-grain breads and cereals along with fresh fruits and vegetables. Increased dietary fiber appears to have a direct effect on lowering serum cholesterol.

Fortunately, it is now required that food products in the United States are labeled with nutritional information including the amount of total fat, saturated fat, cholesterol, and dietary fiber. Despite this labeling and the increased awareness of nutrition in our society, monitoring dietary intake and adhering to dietary guidelines can be challenging for patients and for the clinicians working with them. For many, difficulties arise not only with food selection but also with portion control. Referral to a qualified nutritionist can be quite beneficial in helping patients to understand nutrition and to meet and maintain their dietary goals.

Exercise. The importance of physical activity cannot be over emphasized. It has been demonstrated in multiple studies that regular aerobic exercise increases HDL cholesterol and decreases total and LDL cholesterol and triglyceride levels. Regular aerobic exercise can also modulate and improve control of frequent coexisting risk factors such as obesity, hypertension, and insulin resistance. With exercise there is upregulation of insulin receptors on the cell membrane, thus decreasing the risk for the development of diabetes. Therefore exercise, whenever possible, should be included as in the treatment of high blood cholesterol.

All patients with known CHD embarking on a new exercise regimen should have a recent exercise tolerance test; based on the results, an appropriate exercise program can be prescribed. Consideration for exercise testing in individuals with two or more cardiovascular risk factors should be based on the clinical evaluation and the level of exercise intensity to be performed. Low to moderate expenditure, such as with moderate walking, can be safely prescribed to most asymptomatic individuals without the need or expense of an exercise test, and even low level activity can have a dramatic impact when performed regularly. When a more intensive exercise program is being considered, an exercise test should be obtained, especially for those with multiple risk factors or individuals who have been sedentary. Individuals should be encouraged to start slowly and increase their intensity and duration of exercise gradually over several weeks, with the goal of doing moderate exercise for at least 30 minutes 4 to 5 days per week.

Other Risk Factors. The presence of hyperlipidemia can be used as an opportunity to stress the importance of cessation of tobacco use. Tobacco, when combined with other risk factors,

TABLE 227-2 Point Scoring System for Coronary Heart Disease Risk

Estimate of 10-Year Risk for Men (Framingham Point Scores)

Age, yr	Points
20-34	−9
35-39	−4
40-44	0
45-49	3
50-54	6
55-59	8
60-64	10
65-69	11
70-74	12
75-79	13

Total Cholesterol, mg/dL	Points				
	Age 20-39 yr	Age 40-49 yr	Age 50-59 yr	Age 60-69 yr	Age 70-79 yr
<160	0	0	0	0	0
160-199	4	3	2	1	0
200-239	7	5	3	1	0
240-279	9	6	4	2	1
≥280	11	8	5	3	1

	Points				
	Age 20-39 yr	Age 40-49 yr	Age 50-59 yr	Age 60-69 yr	Age 70-79 yr
Nonsmoker	0	0	0	0	0
Smoker	8	5	3	1	1

HDL, mg/dL	Points
≥60	−1
50-59	0
40-49	1
<40	2

Systolic BP, mm Hg	If Untreated	If Treated
<120	0	0
120-129	0	1
130-139	1	2
140-159	1	2
≥160	2	3

Point Total	10-Year Risk, %
<0	<1
0	1
1	1
2	1
3	1
4	1
5	2
6	2
7	3
8	4
9	5
10	6
11	8
12	10
13	12
14	16
15	20
16	25
≥17	≥30

Estimate of 10-Year Risk for Women (Framingham Point Scores)

Age, yr	Points
20-34	−7
35-39	−3
40-44	0
45-49	3
50-54	6
55-59	8
60-64	10
65-69	12
70-74	14
75-79	16

Total Cholesterol, mg/dL	Points				
	Age 20-39 yr	Age 40-49 yr	Age 50-59 yr	Age 60-69 yr	Age 70-79 yr
<160	0	0	0	0	0
160-199	4	3	2	1	1
200-239	8	6	4	2	1
240-279	11	8	5	3	2
≥280	13	10	7	4	2

	Points				
	Age 20-39 yr	Age 40-49 yr	Age 50-59 yr	Age 60-69 yr	Age 70-79 yr
Nonsmoker	0	0	0	0	0
Smoker	9	7	4	2	1

HDL, mg/dL	Points
≥60	−1
50-59	0
40-49	1
<40	2

Systolic BP, mm Hg	If Untreated	If Treated
<120	0	0
120-129	1	3
130-139	2	4
140-159	3	5
≥160	4	6

Point Total	10-Year Risk, %
<9	<1
9	1
10	1
11	1
12	1
13	2
14	2
15	3
16	4
17	5
18	6
19	8
20	11
21	14
22	17
23	22
24	27
≥25	≥30

From Expert Panel on Detection, Evaluation, and Treatment of High Blood Cholesterol in Adults: Executive summary of the Third Report of the National Cholesterol Education (NCEP) Expert Panel on Detection, Evaluation, and Treatment of High Blood Cholesterol in Adults (Adult Treatment Panel III), *JAMA* 285:2486-2497, 2001.

can dramatically increase the overall risk for CHD. Hypertension and diabetes, of course, should also be well controlled.

Pharmacotherapeutic Management

Despite adherence to a prudent diet and exercise program, many will not achieve acceptable LDL levels without the addition of lipid-lowering medications. As described previously and outlined in Table 227-1, the recommendation for instituting lipid-lowering drugs and the goals of therapy should be based on the presence or absence of other risk factors. A number of medications are available for the treatment of lipid disorders. These are listed in Table 227-3 along with their expected lipid-lowering potential and side effect profiles. The general drug categories are: HMG CoA reductase inhibitors, bile acid sequestrants, nicotinic acid (niacin), fibrates, and probucol.

The most effective and best tolerated drugs for lowering LDL cholesterol are the HMG CoA reductase inhibitors or "statins." They also increase HDL cholesterol and decrease triglyceride levels. These are generally the first line agents for lipid lowering. Several large-scale, randomized, controlled trials have demonstrated dramatic reductions in morbidity and mortality from cardiac events with the use of these agents. In addition they are very safe and relatively free of side effects. There is a 1% incidence of hepatic inflammation and for this reason the liver transaminases aspartate aminotransferase and alanine aminotransferase should be checked before initiating treatment and monitored every 2 to 3 months for the first 6 months and then every 6 months thereafter. For elevations in the transaminases of 2 to 2.5 times normal during therapy, treatment should be changed and sources of co-morbid liver toxicity such as alcohol should be excluded. An even rarer potential adverse reaction to the statins is drug-induced myopathy, which can range in severity from mild myalgias to severe muscle breakdown or rhabdomyolysis with the potential for subsequent acute renal failure. Such events are extremely rare. One agent, cerivastatin or Baycol was removed from US markets in 2001 because it appeared to have a higher incidence of drug-induced myopathy, with two fatalities reported, and because several comparable and apparently safer statins are available. Patients taking HMG-CoA reductase inhibitors who complain of new muscle pain should have a creatine phosphokinase (CPK) level checked to rule out muscle breakdown. If the CPK is elevated, the drug should be discontinued and the patient should be monitored for potential renal dysfunction. In the absence of symptoms, it is not necessary to routinely monitor CPK.

Fasting lipid profiles can be checked every 2 to 3 months along with LFTs when initiating therapy. The dose of the statin can then be titrated up to that required to achieve the appropriate LDL cholesterol goal. Generally it is reasonable to do this by doubling the dose every 2 to 3 months until the maximum dose is reached or the LDL cholesterol goal is achieved.

Bile acid sequestrants (resins) such as cholestyramine have been shown to be safe and effective in lowering LDL modestly when used singularly and can further lower LDL when combined with HMG-CoA reductase inhibitors. They represent a safe alternative to statins in patients with liver disease or in those who have had an adverse reaction.

Nicotinic acid (niacin) has good LDL- and triglyceride-lowering and HDL-raising effects. It has been shown to reduce overall mortality rates in secondary prevention trials. It is widely available at reasonable cost in sustained- and immediate-release formulations. Unfortunately, its use is limited by frequent, significant, unpleasant side effects, including flushing, itching, rash, and gastrointestinal upset. In rare cases liver toxicity, hyperuricemia, and glucose intolerance have occurred. The frequency and intensity of side effects are usually dose related and can be blunted by the use of sustained-release formulations. With anticipatory guidance, gradual escalation to the mid-range doses of 2 to 3 g/day in divided doses, and pretreatment with aspirin, niacin is an effective and inexpensive option.

The fibric acids, such as gemfibrozil, are effective in lowering triglycerides and can raise HDL cholesterol. Because their effects at lowering LDL cholesterol are modest, they should be reserved for individuals with very high triglyceride levels. They may be beneficial in patients with the metabolic syndrome. Fibrates can also occasionally cause liver toxicity and require the monitoring of LFTs.

If LDL cholesterol treatment goals are not achieved with maximum doses of a single agent, then combination therapy should be considered. The addition of a bile acid sequestrant can reduce LDL cholesterol by an additional 10% and is generally safe in combination with the other classes of lipid-lowering medication. The combination of two systemic lipid-lowering drugs (e.g., niacin with a statin, or gemfibrozil with a statin) can lead to increased frequency of side effects. Collaboration with a physician or referral to a lipid specialist is recommended in these cases.

LIFE SPAN CONSIDERATIONS/SPECIFIC POPULATIONS

Younger Adults

Premenopausal women and men less than 35 years old have a relatively low short-term risk of CHD events and, as a result, there has not been clear evidence that they will benefit from pharmacologic treatment for high cholesterol. It is known, however, that atherosclerosis begins early in life and that young adults with high cholesterol are predisposed to CHD later in life. It is recommended that younger adults be screened for high cholesterol. This can be used as an opportunity for counseling regarding diet, exercise, weight control, and other risk factors such as tobacco use. Drug therapy in women less than 45 years old and men less than 35 years old should be reserved for those with LDL cholesterol levels ≥190 mg/dl despite maximal lifestyle modification, or those with other risk factors. Committing a young adult to lifelong drug therapy is a major decision and consultation with a physician is reasonable.

Middle-Aged Men

The benefits of lowering cholesterol in terms of lowering the risk for CHD had been most clearly demonstrated in men between the ages of 35 and 65 years. Men in this age-group also have particularly high prevalence of obesity, hypertension, and tobacco use. They should be targeted for aggressive lifestyle modification, lipid screening, and drug therapy when appropriate.

TABLE 227-3 Expected Lipid-Lowering Effects and Side Effects of Available Agents

Drug	Dose/Day	Total Cholesterol	LDL Cholesterol	HDL Cholesterol	Triglycerides	Side Effects	Patient Education
Niacin	2-3 g	↓10%-25%	↓20%-40%	↑15%-30%	↓45%-50%	Flushing, itching, rash, GI upset ↑Glucose, uric acid, and transaminases (TA)	Take with aspirin Avoid taking with hot fluids and ETOH Start with low dose and increase gradually over several weeks Call if prolonged nausea occurs Need to be monitored with laboratory tests
Resins	4-24 g	↓10%	↓25%	None	10% of patients will have ↑	Indigestion, bloating, gas, and constipation	Mix with uncarbonated liquid Add high-fiber foods to diet Drink plenty of fluids Start with lowest dose and advance as tolerated Need to take resins 1 hour before or 4 hours after other medication
Cholestyramine	8 g						
Colestipol	10 g						
Colesevelam	1.5-3.75 g						
Statins							
Lovastatin (Mevacor)	20-80 mg	↓15%-30%	↓20%-40%	↑5%-10%	↓10%-19%	As a class the statins are well tolerated	Take with evening meal, since most cholesterol is made in evening hours
Pravastatin (Pravachol)	10-40 mg	↓15%-30%	↓20%-30%	↑5%-10%	↓10%-15%	Increase in TA = transaminases in 1% of patients	Need to have regular laboratory measurement for efficacy and safety
Simvastatin (Zocor)	5-40 mg	↓20%-30%	↓23%-40%	↑6%-12%	↓10%-20%	Rare episode of myopathy with or without associated rhabdomyolysis	Call and report any unexplained muscle pains, tenderness, or weakness
Fluvastatin (Lescol)	20-80 mg	↓20%-30%	↓20%-32%	—	—	Infrequent GI upset, constipation, rash, headaches	Avoid grapefruit juice
Atorvastatin (Lipitor)	10-80 mg	↓27%-40%	↓36%-60%	↑7%-12%	↓17%-30%		
Gemfibrozil (Lopid)	600-1200 mg	↓6%	↓10%	↑10% (if HDL <35%, ↑25%)	↓35%	LFT abnormality Muscle aches Abdomen pain	Take 30 minutes before breakfast and dinner Need to have regular laboratory measurements of efficacy and safety

Middle-Aged Women

CHD is often perceived of as a disease more prevalent in men, but half of all CHD deaths are in women, and CHD is the leading cause of death in women over the age of 50 years. The main difference in CHD between the sexes is that the onset of CHD in women occurs on average 10 to 15 years later than in men, and rarely before menopause. Women between the ages of 45 and 75 years should be screened and treated aggressively for high cholesterol.

It is thought that the presence of estrogen in women's premenopausal years has a protective effect against the development of CHD. For this reason it was widely assumed for some time that estrogen replacement therapy (ERT) in postmenopausal women reduced morbidity and mortality from CHD, and this appeared to be confirmed in early clinical trials. In fact, ERT does appear to confer a modest reduction in LDL cholesterol and an increase in HDL cholesterol, but it also appears to increase triglycerides, which, particularly in women, have been shown to be an independent risk factor for CHD. In addition ERT is associated with an increased risk of the development of blood clots and gallbladder disease. There may also be a small increased risk of breast cancer. A recent, more comprehensive clinical trial has not shown a benefit in CHD mortality for women taking ERT, and in fact there is a possible trend towards increased mortality early in the course of treatment.[9] The benefits of ERT include protection against osteoporosis and it is effective in treating the symptoms of menopause. Decisions about initiating ERT should include a careful assessment of these factors, but it should not be advocated to reduce CHD risk or overall mortality.

The management of hyperlipidemia in middle-aged women should focus on lifestyle modification and pharmacologic therapy with lipid-lowering medication when indicated according to the standards outlined previously. Use of Table 227-2 to quantify the actual risk for the development of CHD will be helpful in directing therapy.

Older Adults

Initial studies of lipid-lowering drugs only included men younger than 65 years old; clinicians were forced to extrapolate the benefits to older adults. More recent clinical trials have included adequate numbers of men older than 65 years and women older than 75 years. The risk reduction associated with lowering LDL cholesterol by whatever means appears to persist regardless of age. Decisions regarding treatment in this group should be made on an individual basis, taking the patient's entire clinical situation into account, but lowering cholesterol whether by lifestyle modification or medication is relatively low-risk intervention.

The Metabolic Syndrome

Patients with insulin resistance, with or without frank diabetes, and the syndrome of abdominal obesity, physical inactivity, high triglycerides, and low HDL cholesterol are clearly at increased risk for CHD. It is essential in these patients to work aggressively toward increased physical activity, improvement in diet, and weight loss. Achieving good glycemic control, as always, should be a priority and may lead to improvement in the lipid profile. These patients should be targeted for aggressive treatment of LDL cholesterol even though this may not be the most prominent abnormality in their lipid profile. Whether they will also benefit from specific therapy to lower triglycerides and increase HDL cholesterol is currently under study.

COMPLICATIONS

Numerous epidemiologic, clinical, genetic, and laboratory studies support the relationship between elevated cholesterol levels and increased risk of CHD. For many years it had been thought that intervention to lower lipid levels would improve CHD outcomes, but trials of dietary modification and early lipid-lowering agents had mixed results. Then, in the 1990s, several landmark clinical trials showed dramatic benefits from lipid-lowering medication in reducing morbidity and mortality from CHD, both in patients with established CHD (secondary prevention) and those without known CHD but with risk factors (primary prevention).[10-13] These studies were limited to men between the ages of 35 and 65 years, but subsequently similar benefits have been shown for women as well, and for a broader range of ages.[14,15] The results of these studies are summarized in Table 227-4. It is thought that for a given population, a 10% reduction in the average cholesterol could produce a 30% reduction in the incidence of CHD.[16]

INDICATIONS FOR REFERRAL/HOSPITALIZATION

Treatment of lipid disorders for most individuals will not necessitate referral to a specialist. In cases where a primary genetic lipid disorder is suspected, when recommended treatment plans are not successful in achieving treatment goals, when co-morbid conditions such as liver disease limit therapy, or when combination therapy is required, referral to a lipid specialist should be considered.

PATIENT AND FAMILY EDUCATION

A patient's clear understanding of the essential role of positive lifestyle choices involving diet and exercise is the foundation for the treatment of lipid disorders. Even when drug therapy is prescribed, these lifestyle behaviors should be continued and encouraged. Studies have consistently shown that the degree of attainment of therapeutic goals is significantly influenced by lifestyle factors, and lifestyle changes can have benefits beyond their effects on the lipid profile. Lifestyle changes can involve multiple behaviors, and thus attainment should be considered a process that should and can occur over time with support and encouragement. For some, the failure to make behavior changes is not from lack of motivation but from real or perceived barriers. The focus of education should be the identification of these barriers and the development of interventions and problem-solving techniques that are meaningful and achievable for that individual. Focusing on any achievement, no matter how small, can lead to continued progress toward a healthier lifestyle. Finally, anticipatory education about the potential side effects of medication will increase the likelihood that patients will adhere to treatment plans.

HEALTH PROMOTION

Despite increasing awareness of the importance of diet, exercise, and weight control, obesity in the United States is at an all time high. Many patients, even those without hyperlipidemia,

TABLE 227-4 Summary of Recent Clinical Trials Establishing the Benefits of Lipid-Lowering Treatment

Indication	Study Title	N	Duration	Baseline LDL	Treatment	Results
Primary prevention	WOSCOPS	6595 (M)	4.9 years	>155 mg/dL	Pravastatin, 40 mg/placebo	31% reduction in coronary events 31% reduction in nonfatal MI 32% reduction in CVD deaths
	AFCAPS/TEXCAPS	6605 (M/F)	5 years	150 mg/dl ± 17 mg	Lovastatin, 20-40 mg/placebo	36% reduction in first major coronary event 33% reduction in revascularizations 35% reduction in MI (fatal and nonfatal)
Secondary prevention	4 S	4444 (M/F)	5.4 years	>190 mg/dl	Simvastatin (20-40 mg/placebo)	30% reduction in total mortality 42% reduction in cardiovascular mortality 34% reduction in major coronary events 37% reduction in CABG/PTCA
	CARE	4159 (M/F)	5 years	139 mg/dl	Pravastatin (40 mg/placebo)	24% reduction in CHD death or nonfatal MI 27% reduction in CABG/PTCA 31% reduction in stroke 46% reduction in events for women vs. 20% reduction in men
	LIPID	9014 (M/F)	6 years	Total cholesterol = 155-271 mg/dl	Pravastatin (40 mg/placebo)	24% reduction in CVD mortality 23% reduction in total mortality 29% reduction in cardiac events 23% reduction in MI 20% reduction in stroke

N, Size of study group; *WOSCOPS*, West of Scotland Coronary Prevention Study; *AFCAPS/TexCAPS*, Air Force/Texas Coronary Atherosclerosis Prevention Study; *4S*, Scandinavian Simvastatin Survival Study; *CARE*, Cholesterol and Recurrent Events; *LIPID*, Long-Term Intervention with Pravastatin in Ischemic Disease Study, *MI*, myocardial infarction; *CVD*, cardiovascular disease; *CABG*, coronary artery bypass graft; *PTCA*, percutaneous transluminal coronary angioplasty; *CHD*, coronary heart disease.

would benefit from dietary modification and increased activity. Patients with hyperlipidemia can clearly benefit from such changes.

REFERENCES

1. American Heart Association: *2001 heart and stroke statistical update*, Dallas, Texas, 2000, AHA.
2. Walldius G and others: High apolipoprotein B, Low apolipoprotein A-I, and improvement in the prediction of fatal myocardial infarction (AMORIS Study): a prospective study, *Lancet* 358:2026-2033, 2001.
3. Bostom AG and others: Elevated plasma lipoprotein (a) and coronary heart disease in men aged 55 and younger, *JAMA* 276:544-548, 1996.
4. Zock PL, Mensink RP: Dietary trans–fatty acids and serum lipoproteins in humans, *Curr Opin Lipidol* 7:34-37, 1996.
5. National Institutes of Health: *Clinical guidelines on the identification, evaluation and treatment of overweight and obesity in adults—the evidence report* , NIH Pub. No. 98-4083, Bethesda, MD, 1993.
6. Expert Panel on Detection, Evaluation, and Treatment of High Blood Cholesterol in Adults: Executive summary of the third report of the National Cholesterol Education (NCEP) Expert Panel on Detection, Evaluation, and Treatment of High Blood Cholesterol in Adults (Adult Treatment Panel III), *JAMA* 285:2486-2497, 2001.
7. Fuster V, Pearson TA, American College of Cardiology: Twenty-seventh Bethesda conference: matching the intensity of risk factor management with the hazard for coronary disease events, *J Am Coll Cardiol* 27:961-1047, 1996.
8. Ornish D and others: The Lifestyle Heart Trial, *Lancet* 336:129-133, 1990.
9. Hulley S and others: Randomized trial of estrogen plus progestin for secondary prevention of coronary heart disease in postmenopausal women. Heart and Estrogen/Progestin Replacement Study (HERS) Research Group, *JAMA* 280(7):605-613, 1998.
10. The Lipid Research Clinics Program: The lipid research clinics coronary primary prevention trial results: reduction in the incidence of coronary heart disease, *JAMA* 251(3):351-364, 1984.
11. Scandinavian Simvastatin Survival Study group: Randomized trial of cholesterol lowering in 4444 patients with coronary heart disease: the Scandinavian Simvastatin Survival Study (4S), *Lancet* 344:1383-1389, 1994.
12. Shepherd J and others: Prevention of coronary heart disease with pravastatin in men with hypercholesterolemia, *N Engl J Med* 333:1301-1307, 1995.
13. Long-Term Intervention with Pravastatin in Ischemic Disease (LIPID) Study Group: Prevention of cardiovascular events and death with pravastatin in patients with coronary heart disease and a broad range of initial cholesterol levels, *N Engl J Med* 339:1349-1357, 1998.
14. Sacks FM and others: The effect of pravastatin on coronary events after myocardial infarction in patients with average cholesterol levels, *N Engl J Med* 335(14):1001-1009, 1996.
15. Downs JR and others: Primary prevention of acute coronary events with lovastatin in men and women with average total cholesterol levels: results of AFCAPS/TexCAPS. Air Force/Texas Coronary Atherosclerosis Prevention Study, *JAMA* 279:1615-1622, 1998.
16. Cohen JD: A population based approach to cholesterol control, *Am J Med* 102(2A):23-25, 1997.

CHAPTER 228

Metabolic Syndrome X

Donna Jenell Pease

DEFINITION/EPIDEMIOLOGY

Metabolic syndrome X is a cluster of disorders that was first introduced by Reaven[1] in 1988 and is characterized by insulin resistance with hyperinsulinemia, hypertension, abdominal (central/visceral) obesity, and dyslipidemia consisting of hypertriglyceridemia, low high-density lipoprotein cholesterol (HDL-C), and increased small, dense low-density lipoprotein (LDL) particles. More recent characteristics that have been added include increased plasminogen activator inhibitor (PAI-1) levels, microalbuminuria, hyperuricemia, and microvascular angina.[2]

In 1998, the World Health Organization defined metabolic syndrome X as insulin resistance and/or glucose intolerance or diabetes mellitus together with two or more of the following components:

- Raised arterial pressure ≥160/90 mm Hg
- Raised plasma triglyceride (≥1.7 mmol or 150 mg/dl) and/or low HDL-C (<0.9 mmol, 35 mg/dl men; <1.0 mmol, 39 mg/dl women) levels
- Central obesity (waist-to-hip ratio; males >0.90; females >0.85, and/or body mass index [BMI] >30 kg/m^2)
- Microalbuminuria (urinary albumin excretion rate ≥20 μg/min or albumin/creatinine ratio ≥20 mg/g)[3]

Not all hyperinsulinemic individuals develop all of the multiple components of this syndrome, but studies have found that the greater the number of associated characteristics an individual exhibits, the more at risk is an individual of developing cardiovascular disease and/or dying.[4,5] This syndrome has also been called the *insulin resistant syndrome, cardiovascular dysmetabolic syndrome,* and *deadly quartet*.[2]

Metabolic syndrome X often occurs in the general population, mostly in individuals older than 50, and more commonly in men than in women. African Americans and Hispanics were found to be more insulin resistant than non-Hispanic whites in the Insulin Resistance and Atherosclerosis Study (IRAS).[6] It has been estimated that 25% to 35% of nonobese, normal glucose-tolerant U.S. adults have insulin resistance.[1]

It has been found that both genetic factors and environmental factors play a role in the incidence of metabolic syndrome X. Studies have found a genetic predisposition to syndrome X and the associated cardiovascular risk factors in first-degree relatives of individuals diagnosed with type 2 diabetes.[7,8] It has also been found that nonobese individuals with a family history of diabetes, hypertension, or obesity are genetically predisposed to the development of syndrome X.[9]

Various authors have speculated that there are numerous genes that may be involved in this syndrome. One such theory is the "thrifty genes" theory. These thrifty genes ensure optimal storage of surplus energy as abdominal fat during periods of fasting, but when these genes are exposed to the abundance of food in the Western diet, insulin resistance develops. Genes coding for beta$_2$ and beta$_3$ adrenergic receptors, hormone-sensitive lipase, lipoprotein lipase (LPL), skeletal muscle glycogen synthase, and regulation of insulin signaling have also been associated with features of this syndrome.[10]

An environmental factor involved with insulin resistance is the lifestyle typical of Western civilization, consisting of a high-fat diet and low levels of physical activity. High-energy intake and low-energy output have led to the increased prevalence of obesity seen today. It has been found that the adipose tissue associated with visceral/abdominal obesity contributes to insulin resistance. Studies have shown that tissue sensitivity to insulin declines by ~30% to 40% when an individual becomes >35% to 40% over ideal body weight.[11] The fat cells found in abdominal obesity are larger and are more insulin resistant. Abdominal fat is also more metabolically active, and fat lipolysis occurs more often, releasing excess free fatty acids (FFAs) that interfere with hepatic insulin clearance, thus resulting in higher levels of circulating insulin. Therefore it has been speculated that visceral obesity may be one of the leading causes of insulin resistance.[12]

PATHOPHYSIOLOGY

Insulin resistance is defined as the impaired insulin-stimulated glucose uptake by skeletal muscle, adipose tissue, or liver. The mechanisms involved in insulin resistance may consist of abnormal insulin molecules, decreased number of insulin receptors, decreased glucose transporters, and defective postreceptor activity.[2] Impairment at the receptor level is usually associated with decreased sensitivity to insulin, whereas postreceptor or cellular defects are associated with decreased responsiveness to insulin.[13] When the cells become resistant to the insulin, the body compensates by producing more insulin to overcome the resistance and to maintain normal glucose levels. Fasting hyperinsulinemia occurs in response to elevated fasting plasma glucose. This hyperinsulinemia leads to the various other abnormalities associated with syndrome X; they include hypertension, dyslipidemia, atherosclerosis, microalbuminuria, abnormalities in the fibrinolytic system, and hyperuricemia.[2]

Hypertension

It has been found that arterial blood pressure is inversely related to insulin sensitivity and directly related to fasting plasma insulin concentration. In a retrospective analysis by the European Group for the Study of Insulin Resistance (EGIR), it was found that for each 10-unit increase in insulin resistance, systolic blood pressure was 1.7 mm Hg higher and diastolic blood pressure was 2.3 mm Hg higher. This small increase is significant considering that prospective studies have found that a 2 mm Hg increase in blood pressure will produce a 17% increase in cerebrovascular disease and a 10% increase in ischemic heart disease.[14]

The hyperinsulinemia associated with insulin resistance may mediate elevated blood pressure in a number of different ways. Increases in plasma insulin concentration cause urinary sodium excretion to decline. This antinatriuretic effect of insulin has been shown to be exerted on both the proximal and distal tubules of the nephron. This renal sodium retention causes expansion of the extracellular fluid volume and leads to the hypertension associated with syndrome X.[11,15] Hyperinsulinemia can also activate the sympathetic nervous system, which leads to an increase in the plasma norepinephrine level. This may cause increased cardiac contractibility, increased heart rate, increased cardiopulmonary blood volume, and direct vasoconstriction of resistant vessels.[11,16] Because insulin is a stimulus for growth of vascular endothelial and smooth muscle cells, hyperinsulinemia may result in a thickening in arterial blood vessel walls.[12] This may lead to hypertension and may also contribute to the cardiovascular disease associated with metabolic syndrome X.

Resnick[17] speculated that there may exist an ionic basis to the hypertension and altered insulin metabolism associated with syndrome X and termed this the *ionic hypothesis*. He found that hypertension was caused by increased calcium and decreased magnesium levels and lowered arterial pH in individuals with insulin resistance.

Dyslipidemia

The lipid abnormalities found in metabolic syndrome X are elevated triglycerides, low HDL-C, and increased small, dense LDL-C particles (referred to as *pattern B*, or *atherogenic dyslipidemia*). Insulin impairs the normal suppression of FFA release from the adipose tissue. Increased FFAs released from the adipose tissue and delivered to the liver offer an efficient substrate for enhanced synthesis of triglycerides and very low-density lipoprotein (VLDL). Hyperinsulinemia results in high plasma triglyceride levels by simultaneous increasing production of VLDL and decreasing metabolism of VLDL. Furthermore, when the liver content of lipids is high, gluconeogenesis is increased, resulting in a higher production of glucose by the liver.[2] Finally, HDL-C particles are directly synthesized by the liver but are also derived from liver metabolism of VLDL remnants; therefore reduced VLDL metabolism contributes to a decrease in HDL-C.[18]

Two steps are involved in the formation of small, dense LDL particles and involve lipid transfer protein exchange. When triglyceride from VLDL is exchanged for a cholesterol ester in LDL, the VLDL becomes enriched in cholesterol ester and the LDL becomes enriched in triglyceride. If the triglyceride in LDL is hydrolyzed by LPL or hepatic lipase, a smaller, denser LDL particle will be produced. These small, dense LDL particles lead to atherosclerosis because they are able to bind to and penetrate the arterial wall and more readily undergo oxidative modification.[19] Small, dense LDL have also been linked to thicker intima-media and plaque occurrence in the femoral and carotid arteries.[20,21] These adverse effects in lipoprotein levels increase the risk of atherosclerosis, ischemic heart disease, coronary heart disease, and overall cardiovascular mortality.

Plasminogen Activator Inhibitor and Coagulation Disorders

Studies have found that levels of PAI-1 correlate significantly with insulin resistance. Elevated levels of PAI-1 reflect impaired fibrinolysis, impaired endothelial function, and increased tendency toward acute arterial thrombosis.[22] Insulin resistance also affects other coagulation factors, including platelet aggregability, platelet adhesion, levels of factor VII and factor VIII, tissue plasminogen activator (TPA), and fibrinogen.[23]

Microalbuminuria

An association between microalbuminuria and syndrome X has been found secondary to the effects of insulin on renal hemodynamics. The IRAS found that acute hyperinsulinemia causes renal vasodilatation, resulting in increased plasma flow and increased glomerular hydrostatic pressure and gradient as well as increased glomerular filtration rate. The localized elevated pressure in the glomerular vessels is involved in increased microalbumin secretion.[24,25] Microalbuminuria is a strong predictor of cardiovascular morbidity and mortality.[4]

Hyperuricemia

Increases in uric acid concentration are commonly seen in association with insulin resistance, hypertension, and dyslipidemia. Studies have found that uric acid concentration is increased in individuals with higher insulin levels, higher insulin response to glucose challenges, higher triglyceride levels, lower HDL levels, and higher blood pressure. It has been speculated that insulin resistance is correlated with a decreased urinary clearance of uric acid, suggesting a link between insulin metabolism and hyperuricemia[26,27] (Figure 228-1).

Microvascular Angina

Originally the nomenclature *syndrome X* was used by H.G. Kemp[28] in 1973 to describe microvascular angina as impaired infusion of the microvasculature of the heart occurring in the absence of macrovascular atherosclerosis. The patient with microvascular angina experiences typical anginal chest pain with a positive treadmill test but a completely normal coronary angiogram. Additional studies are ongoing to find a relationship between microvascular angina and metabolic syndrome X because recent research has found a common pathogenesis of these two disorders.[29,30]

CLINICAL PRESENTATION

Because it is difficult to accurately measure insulin resistance, the diagnosis is usually clinical based on a constellation of physical findings and laboratory characteristics. Insulin resistance can be suspected in the individual who presents with abdominal obesity, increased triglyceride, low HDL-C, and hypertension.[12]

A physical sign that is suggestive of moderate to severe insulin resistance is the hyperkeratotic condition acanthosis nigricans. This is a diffuse, hyperpigmented, velvety thickening of the cutaneous skin that is found in the neck and axillae. The onset is usually insidious, with the first visible change being darkening of the skin pigmentation so as to appear dirty. As the skin thickens, it becomes velvety, and the skin line is accentuated. Eventually the skin becomes rugose and mammillated.[31,32]

PHYSICAL EXAMINATION

The physical examination consists of accurate measurement of the blood pressure, height and weight, and BMI, or waist-to-hip ratio using the techniques described in the Diagnostics section. A patient who presents with the clinical features of metabolic syndrome X should be screened annually for hyperglycemia, glucose intolerance, and type 2 diabetes mellitus. Those presenting with the metabolic syndrome X should also be screened for the cardiovascular complications that accompany the syndrome and managed appropriately. A thorough history is also important to obtain during the assessment to determine if the patient is at risk of developing insulin resistance secondary to genetic factors or family history.[33]

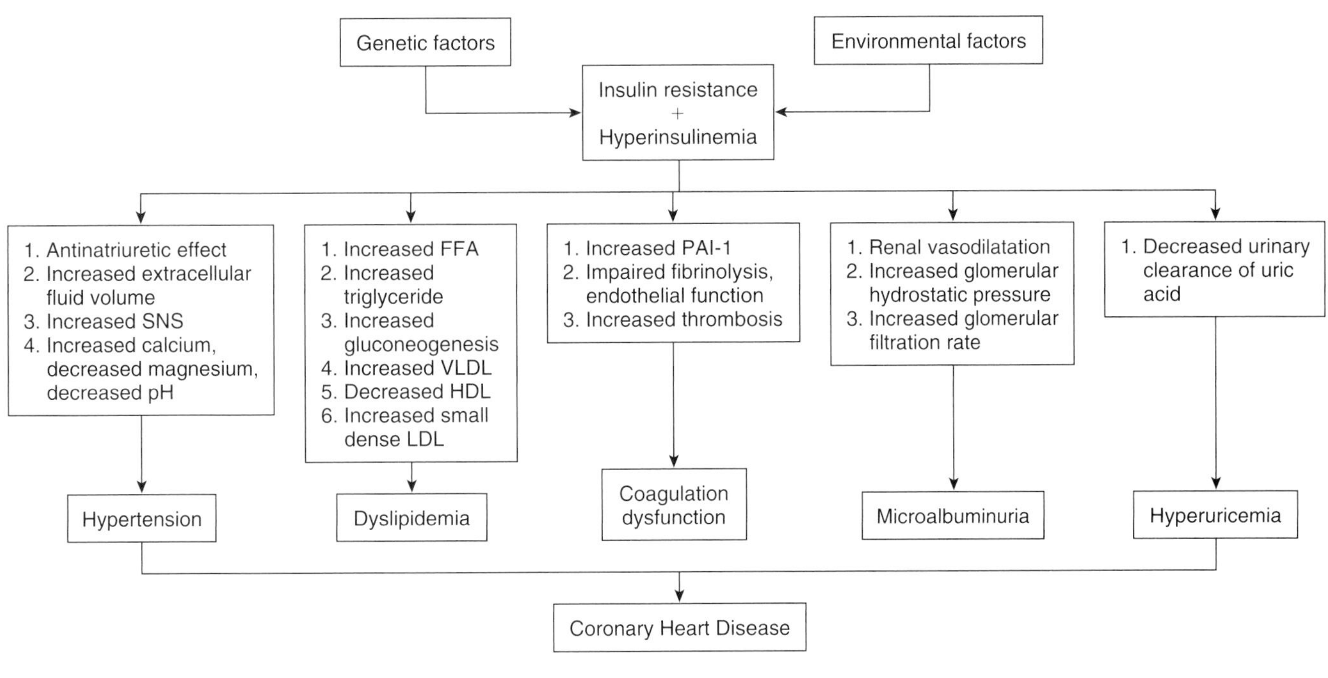

FIGURE 228-1

Role of insulin resistance and coronary heart disease. *SNS,* Sympathetic nervous system; *FFA,* free fatty acids; *VLDL,* very-low-density lipoprotein; *HDL,* high-density lipoprotein; *LDL,* low-density lipoprotein; *PAI-1,* plasminogen activator inhibitor-1.

DIAGNOSTICS

There are several techniques available for measuring insulin resistance and sensitivity; they include the euglycemic insulin clamp technique, the insulin tolerance test, the insulin suppression test, the frequently sampled intravenous glucose tolerance test, and the regional arteriovenous balance test.[34] The gold standard for determining insulin resistance is the euglycemic insulin clamp technique. This technique is usually performed in the laboratory setting. It involves infusion of exogenous insulin to maintain a constant plasma insulin level above fasting while glucose is fixed at a basal level through the infusion of glucose at varying rates. Plasma glucose levels are measured every 5 minutes, and if the glucose level falls below basal, the glucose infusion rate is increased to return plasma glucose to basal levels. The total amount of glucose infused over time is a determinant of insulin action on glucose metabolism. Insulin sensitivity is determined by the amount of glucose that has to be infused. If more glucose is infused, the individual is more sensitive to insulin. The insulin-resistant individual requires less glucose to maintain basal plasma glucose levels. This technique is complex and costly and cannot be adapted easily to the clinical setting.[35]

A more practical way of assessing insulin resistance in the clinical setting is through the measurement of the fasting plasma insulin concentration. A significant correlation has been found between fasting insulin levels and insulin action measured by the euglycemic clamp technique. A fasting serum insulin value of >10 μg/ml indicates insulin resistance.[32] High plasma insulin values with normal glucose levels are suggestive of insulin resistance. The limitation of using the fasting insulin concentration as a diagnostic tool for insulin resistance is the technique's lack of a reliable standardization of the insulin assay procedure.[35]

A variety of measures of body mass and body fat exist that measure and express different aspects of general obesity, fat distribution, patterning, and fat percentage. BMI is calculated as weight divided by height squared and measures percent of body fat or total adipose tissue. The ratio of waist and hip circumference is highly correlated with visceral adipose tissue. BMI and waist-to-hip ratio are the most routinely used anthropometric indices because they are easy to use and have a high reliability.[36]

Common laboratory tests can be used to screen for the other various features associated with metabolic syndrome X. HDL and triglyceride blood levels are measured after an 8- to 12-hour fast. Small, dense LDL can be calculated using gradient gel electrophoresis.[21] Microalbumin is measured using a random urine test. Hyperuricemia can be measured with a serum uric acid test.

DIFFERENTIAL DIAGNOSIS

Metabolic syndrome X is diagnosed based on clinical presentation, so it is important to rule out hypertension, dyslipidemia, or obesity without manifestations of insulin resistance. The differential diagnoses also include type 2 diabetes mellitus or impaired glucose tolerance (IGT), which can be excluded with laboratory testing. Other diseases characterized by insulin resistance are polycystic ovary syndrome, lipodystrophy and lipoatrophic diabetes, type A insulin resistance (insulin receptor mutations), and type B insulin resistance (anti–insulin receptor antibodies). Genetic syndromes (Down, Turner's, or muscular

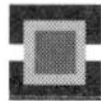 Diagnostics

Metabolic Syndrome X

Laboratory
Euglycemic insulin clamp technique
Glucose tolerance test
Fasting plasma insulin concentration
Fasting lipid profile
Urinalysis (for protein)

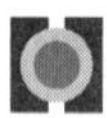 Differential Diagnosis

Metabolic Syndrome X

Diabetes Mellitus Type 2
Impaired glucose tolerance
Polycystic ovary syndrome
Lipodystrophy and lipoatrophic diabetes
Type A insulin resistance (insulin receptor mutations)
Type B insulin resistance (anti-insulin receptor antibodies)
Genetic syndromes

dystrophies), neurodegenerative disorders (Werner's syndrome and Friedreich's ataxia), and excess hormonal antagonists such as glucocorticoids, growth hormone, and catecholamines are also characterized by insulin resistance.[32,37]

MANAGEMENT

It is imperative that the different features of metabolic syndrome X be treated appropriately to prevent or lessen the risk of cardiovascular morbidity and mortality. One study found that the prevalence of coronary heart disease, myocardial infarction, and stroke as approximately threefold higher in subjects with metabolic syndrome X.[4] Methods to treat the metabolic syndrome X include both nonpharmacologic and pharmacologic measures. These management methods are divided into a three-tiered arrangement: (1) evidence exists for benefit, (2) limited evidence exists for benefit, and (3) evidence of benefit unclear.

Evidence Exists for Benefit

Nonpharmacologic treatments for insulin resistance include healthy lifestyle changes in diet and exercise. Because many individuals with the metabolic syndrome are overweight, dietary treatment should be primarily focused on weight reduction. Dietary carbohydrates with a high glycemic index increase blood glucose levels more rapidly, whereas fiber-rich low glycemic index foods are digested and absorbed more slowly and can lower triglyceride and raise HDL levels. Intake of soluble fiber has been shown to decrease postprandial glucose levels and concentrations of insulin levels. The benefits of a high-fiber diet on decreased levels of fasting plasma insulin were found in both the Coronary Artery Risk Development in Young Adults (CARDIA) Study and the Framingham Offspring Study.[38,39] Plant-based foods such as whole grains, fruits, and vegetables have also been found to decrease systolic and diastolic blood pressures and reduce the incidence of coronary heart disease.[39] A monounsaturated fatty acid diet significantly improves insulin sensitivity and the dyslipidemia associated with the metabolic syndrome X compared with a high–unsaturated fatty acid diet.[40] Dietary trials suggest that treatment of the thrombogenic disorders (elevated plasma fibrinogen and factor VIII coagulant activity levels, raised PAI-1) can be improved with a low-fat diet and a high content of foods rich in complex carbohydrates and dietary fiber.[41,42] In a recent study using female Fisher rats, it was shown that a low-fat complex-carbohydrate diet improved glucose transport, decreased hyperinsulinemia, lowered blood pressure, reduced hypertriglyceridemia, and contributed to significant weight loss.[43]

The Third Report of the Expert Panel on Detection, Evaluation, and Treatment of High Blood Cholesterol in Adults (ATP III) has identified individuals with the metabolic syndrome X as candidates for intensified therapeutic lifestyle changes and recommends that they be given the same intensive treatment as people with established heart disease. ATP III suggests a therapeutic lifestyle change diet consisting of <7% of total calories from saturated fats per day and <200 mg of cholesterol per day. ATP III also recommends consumption of foods that contain plant stanols and sterols to lower LDL and soluble fibers such as cereal grains, beans, peas, legumes, fruits, and vegetables.[44]

Exercise and physical training have been found to be beneficial in the treatment of metabolic syndrome X. Exercise improves insulin resistance by increasing glucose utilization by the muscle. Glycogen synthase activity and the number of glucose transporters translocated to the cell surface increase after exercise. Glucose disposal by the skeletal muscle and insulin sensitivity continue for many hours after completion of the exercise. This improvement in insulin sensitivity may prevent the progression of the metabolic abnormalities. The Da Qing IGT and Diabetes study found that diet and/or exercise led to significant decrease in the incidence of the development of diabetes in individuals with IGT over a 6-year period.[45] Regular aerobic training has also been shown to significantly decrease systolic and diastolic blood pressures. Physical training has been shown to decrease plasma levels of triglyceride by 15% to 30%. Exercise increases LPL activity and improves the removal of VLDL and intermediate-density lipoprotein (IDL) particles and decreases the levels of small, dense LDL associated with metabolic syndrome X. An increase in HDL may occur if exercise training is intense and prolonged. Exercise is a potent stimulus for fibrinolysis. Regular physical exercise improves fibrinolytic activity and lowers levels of PAI-1. Exercise and caloric restriction can cause weight loss and a loss of intraabdominal fat, which will decrease the insulin resistance associated with metabolic syndrome X.[46]

Recommendations for exercise in individuals with metabolic syndrome X are similar to those published by the American Diabetes Association for individuals with diabetes type 2. The American College of Sports Medicine recommend at least 20 minutes of continuous aerobic exercise performed at a minimum of 50% of VO_{2max} (maximal oxygen uptake) for 3 days a week for several weeks to improve cardiovascular fitness. It is recommended that the aerobic exercise involve the legs such as brisk walking, bicycling and swimming. The exercise session should begin with a 10 minute warm-up consisting of light aerobic activity and stretching and end with a 5-10 minute cool down period to lower the heart rate. If the individual is sedentary, a careful cardiovascular assessment may be needed prior to the initiation of an exercise program.[47]

Pharmacologic methods involve the treatment of the associated characteristics that are seen with metabolic syndrome X. Included would be antihypertensives, HMG-CoA reductase inhibitors (statins), fibric acid derivatives, aspirin therapy, possibly thiazolidinediones, and the biguanide, metformin.

The classes of antihypertensives that have been found to be effective in reducing blood pressure as well as increasing insulin sensitivity are alpha adrenergic antagonist and the angiotensin converting enzyme inhibitors. Prazosin and doxazosin have been found to increase sensitivity to insulin. Alpha adrenergic antagonists play a beneficial role in the dyslipidemia found in syndrome X. They improve lipoprotein metabolism by decreasing triglyceride and very-low-density lipoprotein concentrations and increasing HDL cholesterol. Angiotensin converting enzyme (ACE) inhibitors and angiotensin II receptor blockers (ARB) do not worsen the insulin resistance or the lipid profile and can actually prevent or retard progression of renal disease. They can also improve the microalbuminuria found in metabolic syndrome X. Calcium channel blockers are effective in lowering blood pressure and have no profound adverse effects on lipid or glucose metabolism. Beta blockers should be avoided in individuals with syndrome X since they have been found to worsen insulin resistance and decrease glucose uptake by 25-32% in studies using the euglycemic clamp technique. Beta blockers may also increase plasma triglyceride levels. Diuretics also should not be used since they can cause increased insulin resistance and worsening glucose tolerance.[11,12,15,32]

The ATP III recommends triglyceride levels <150 mg/dL, LDL levels <100 mg/dL, and HDL levels >40 mg/dL in men or >50 mg/dL in women with the metabolic syndrome X. HMG-CoA reductase inhibitors (statins) may lower LDL by 18%-55%, raise HDL by 5%-15%, and lower triglyceride by 7%-30%. If the triglyceride level is very high (>500 mg/dL), it is recommended that a fibrate or nicotinic acid be used which may decrease triglyceride levels by 20%-50%.[43] It has been found that gemfibrozil improves insulin action and flow-mediated vasodilatation as well as decreases triglyceride levels.[48]

The Hypertensive Optimal Treatment (HOT) Trial found that the daily use of aspirin has been found to be beneficial in the reduction of myocardial infarction in diabetic as well as nondiabetic individuals. Aspirin significantly reduced cardiovascular events by 15% and myocardial infarction by 36%.[49] The use of aspirin therapy in individuals with metabolic syndrome X would prove to be beneficial since these individuals are at increased risk of developing cardiovascular complications.

Limited Evidence Exists for Benefit

The Diabetes Prevention Program (DPP) is a randomized clinical trial that is currently being conducted to evaluate the safety and efficacy of interventions that may delay or prevent development of diabetes in individuals at increased risk for diabetes type 2. The interventions being examined are (1) intensive lifestyle intervention that includes at least 150 minutes of moderate-intensity exercise per week together with a healthy diet to achieve and maintain a 7% loss of body weight, or (2) metformin 850 mg b.i.d. These 2 groups are being compared with a group given standardized lifestyle recommendations and placebo b.i.d. Until the results of the DPP are available, it is reasonable for the clinician to offer non-pharmacologic interventions such as diet and exercise to promote weight loss.[50]

Recent research has demonstrated reduction in the cardiovascular risk factors with the use of the thiazolidinediones, which include rosiglitazone and pioglitazone. These drugs improve insulin resistance by sensitizing the muscle and subcutaneous cells to the effects of insulin thus lowering plasma insulin levels. The use of thiazolidinediones result in a decrease in blood pressure, improvement of dyslipidemia by lowering triglyceride levels, decreasing lipid oxidation and increasing HDL levels, improvement of fibrinolysis and endothelial function and a decrease in carotid artery intima thickness. The adverse effects include elevation of LDL, edema and weight gain. Hepatic aminotransferase levels must be monitored during the use of these drugs.[51,52]

Metformin has been shown to reduce hyperinsulinemia and insulin resistance, lower blood triglyceride levels, assist in weight reduction, and lower plasma PAI-1 levels. Metformin improves the sensitivity of cells to insulin, reduces hepatic glucose production, and increases glucose uptake in muscle and other peripheral tissues. Through these mechanisms of action, metformin has been found to reduce or prevent macrovascular complications. Serum creatinine needs to be monitored while using metformin.[12,53]

Evidence of Benefit Unclear

New studies show that the I1 imidazoline agonists, moxonidine and rilmenidine improve glucose metabolism and reduce blood pressure and microalbuminuria associated with syndrome X. Further research is currently being conducted on these new medications and their beneficial effects on the metabolic syndrome X[54,55] (Figure 228-2).

LIFE SPAN CONSIDERATIONS

Insulin resistance may occur at any age. Studies have shown that insulin resistance has been found in overweight African American children as young as 5 years old. These children also showed elevations in blood pressure and lipid levels.[56] It has also been shown that childhood obesity increases the risk for metabolic syndrome X in adulthood. This risk can be reduced if an obese child reduces his/her relative weight to become a nonobese adult. The baseline assessment of and identification of obese children can possibly lead to the prevention of adult obesity, metabolic syndrome X and cardiovascular risk.[57] Parents require education on ways to promote healthy lifestyle, proper nutrition, weight loss, and increased physical activity in young obese children. These healthy lifestyle modifications must continue through out the entire life span. The older adult may be at increased risk of developing insulin resistance secondary to increased obesity, decreases in physical activity, and changes in body mass due to muscle loss and increased adipose tissue. Older adults may need to be educated on exercise programs tailored to suit their needs or modified for the chronic illnesses that they may have. Dietary recommendations may also need to be modified to provide for the older adult's nutritional needs.[13,58]

COMPLICATIONS

As discussed earlier, the complications associated with the features of syndrome X include cardiovascular disease, atherosclerotic vascular disease, ischemic heart disease and coronary artery disease, as well as, myocardial infarction and stroke.[59,60]

Insulin resistance is the pathophysiologic hallmark of impaired glucose tolerance and diabetes type 2, and may occur decades before the clinical presentation of these diseases. As the beta cell function deteriorates and is no longer able to compensate for the insulin resistance and glucose plasma levels

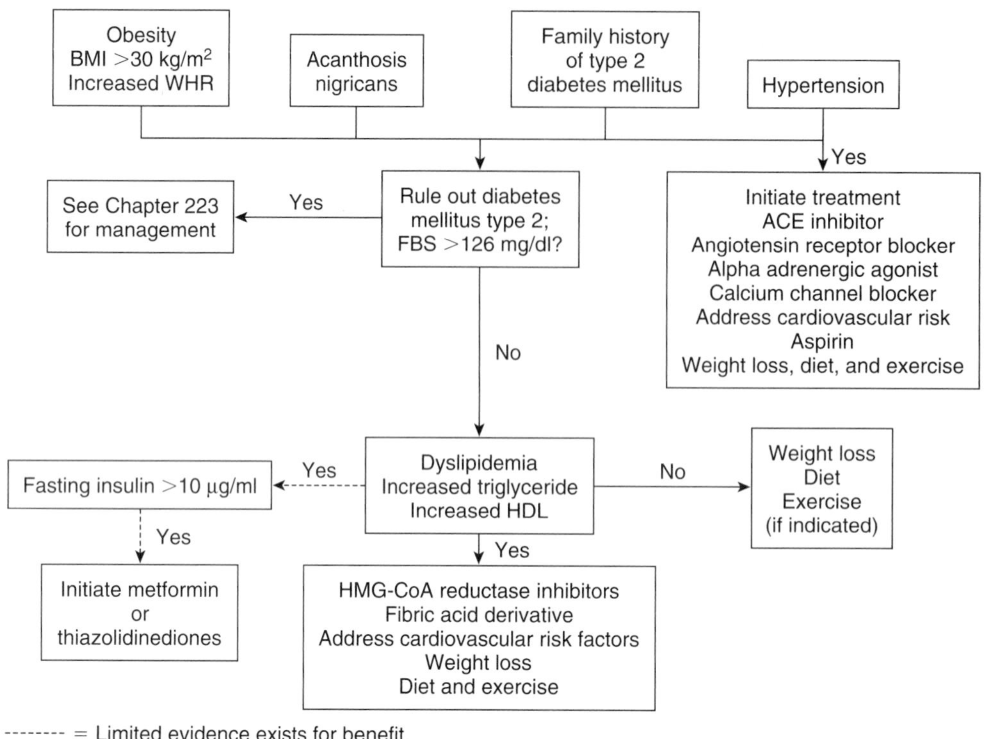

FIGURE 228-2

Algorithm for treatment of metabolic syndrome X. *BMI,* Body mass index; *WHR,* waist to hip ratio; *DM,* diabetes mellitus.

rise, a transition from insulin resistance to impaired glucose tolerance with mild increases in post-prandial glucose levels occurs and eventually results in diabetes mellitus type 2.[18]

Very high levels of triglyceride can provoke an acute episode of pancreatitis. Elevated uric acid levels may induce gout. Elevated PAI-1 may lead to clotting dysfunction and coagulation abnormalities resulting in an acute cardiovascular event such as stroke or myocardial infarction.[32]

INDICATIONS FOR REFERRAL/HOSPITALIZATION

A physician consultation is necessary when the hypertension or dyslipidemia (associated with metabolic syndrome X) is resistant to therapy. Referral to a dietitian may be beneficial to assist the individual with meal planning and weight loss. A health psychologist can provide psychologic support as well as support with realistic goal setting, stress management, and behavior modification methods. An exercise physiologist can assist in the development of a safe and effective exercise regimen.[61]

PATIENT AND FAMILY EDUCATION

Education should be focused on the pathology of the metabolic syndrome X and associated characteristics along with the complications and cardiovascular risks that accompany the syndrome. This instruction should address medication use, mechanism of action, and adverse effects. Education must be provided to the patient and the family members since meal planning and participation in a physical fitness program will benefit the patient as well as the family members involved. Family support is necessary to assist the patient with the lifestyle changes needed to decrease the risks of complications involved in the syndrome. Explaining the benefits of healthy eating and exercise can empower and motivate the patient. The discussion should involve exploring the patient's feelings towards metabolic syndrome X and the treatment regimen. The patient should be instructed on mode, frequency and intensity of exercise. Preferably, an exercise program of the patient's choice will better ensure adherence. Instructions on smoking cessation and limited use of alcohol, as well as effects on insulin resistance, triglyceride levels, and cardiovascular risks should be discussed.[12] Mutual goal setting before the initiation of treatment is necessary for the patient's success. Both written and verbal instructions must be given to patient and reinforced at each visit.

HEALTH PROMOTION

Primary health care providers are in a unique position to intervene, motivate, and influence the patient's outcome, as well as the family members, through teaching, counseling and health promotion. As discussed earlier, insulin resistance has been found in children as young as 5 years of age, therefore, it is imperative to start promoting healthy lifestyles at a very young age. Promotion of weight loss in the individual who is moderately obese can prevent the development of insulin resistance and the complications associated with the syndrome. Practitioners can assist the patient in changing harmful health behaviors through counseling on nutrition and facilitating increases in physical activity. Disease prevention and health promotion prior to the occurrence of complications associated with metabolic syndrome X is more cost-effective in terms of health care dollars as well as savings in human suffering. Through health promotion and early intervention, the occurrence of and ramifications of metabolic syndrome X can surely be decreased or possibly eliminated.

REFERENCES

1. Reaven GM: *Role of insulin resistance in human disease, Diabetes* 37: 1595-1607, 1988.
2. Timar O, Sestier F, Levy E: Metabolic syndrome X: a review, *Can J Cardiol* 16(6):779-89, 2000.
3. Alberti KGMM, Zimmet PZ: Definition, diagnosis and classification of diabetes mellitus and its complications. Part 1: diagnosis and classification of diabetes mellitus provisional report of a WHO consultation, *Diabet Med* 15(7):539-53, 1998.
4. Isomaa B, Almgren P, Tuomi T et al: Cardiovascular morbidity and mortality associated with the metabolic syndrome, *Diabetes Care* 24(4):683-9, 2001.
5. Trevisan M, Liu J, Bahsas FB et al: Syndrome X and mortality: a population-based study. Risk factor and life expectancy research group, *Am J Epidemiol* 148(10):958-66, 1998.
6. Haffner SM, D'Agostino R, Saad MF et al: Increased insulin resistance and insulin secretion in nondiabetic African-Americans and Hispanics compared with non-Hispanic whites. The insulin resistance atherosclerosis study, *Diabetes* 45: 742-8, 1996.
7. Stewart MW, Humphriss DB, Berrish TS et al: Features of syndrome X in first-degree relatives of NIDDM patients, *Diabetes Care* 18(7):1020-2, 1995.
8. Gaillard TR, Schuster DP, Bossetti BM et al: The impact of socioeconomic status on cardiovascular risk factors in African-Americans at high risk for type 2 diabetes. Implications for syndrome X, *Diabetes Care* 20(5):745-52, 1997.
9. Hunt KJ, Heiss G, Sholinsky PD et al: Familial history of metabolic disorders and the multiple metabolic syndrome: The NHLBI family heart study, *Genet Epidemiol* 19(4):395-409, 2000.
10. Groop LC: Pathogenesis of insulin resistance in type 2 diabetes. A collision between thrifty genes and an affluent environment, *Drugs* 58: S1: 11-12, 1999.
11. DeFronzo RA, Ferrannini E: Insulin resistance: A multifaceted syndrome responsible for NIDDM, obesity, hypertension, dyslipidemia and atherosclerotic cardiovascular disease, *Diabetes Care* 14(3):173-94, Mar 1991.
12. Baillie GM, Sherer JT, Weart CW: Insulin and coronary artery disease: Is syndrome X the unifying hypothesis? *Ann Pharmacother* 32: 233-47, 1998.
13. Muller DC, Elahi D, Tobin JD et al: The effect of age on insulin resistance and secretion: a review, *Semin Nephrol* 16(4):289-98, 1996.
14. Ferrannini E, Natali A, Capaldo B et al: Insulin resistance, hyperinsulinemia, and blood pressure. Role of age and obesity. European Group for the Study of Insulin Resistance (EGIR), *Hypertension* 30: 1144-9, 1997.
15. Reaven GM, Lithell H, Landsberg L: Hypertension and associated metabolic abnormalities: The role of insulin resistance and sympathoadrenal system, *N Engl J Med* 334(6):374-81, 1996.
16. Reaven GM: Pathophysiology of insulin resistance in human disease, *Physiol Rev* 75(3):473-86, 1995.
17. Resnick LM: Ionic basis of hypertension, insulin resistance, vascular disease, and related disorders. The mechanism of "Syndrome X", *Am J Hypertens* 6(4):123S-134S, 1993.
18. Granberry MC, Fonseca VA: Insulin resistance syndrome: options for treatment, *Southern Med* J 92(1):2-14, 1999.
19. Sniderman AD, Scantlebury T, Cianflone K: Hypertriglyceridemic hyperapob: the unappreciated atherogenic dyslipoproteinemia in type 2 diabetes mellitus, *Ann Int Med* 135(6):447-59, 2001.
20. Hulthe J Bokemark L, Wikstrand J et al: The metabolic syndrome, LDL particle size, and atherosclerosis: the atherosclerosis and insulin resistance (AIR) study, *Arterioscler Thromb Vasc Biol* 20(9):2140-7, 2000.
21. Reaven GM Chen YD, Jeppesen J et al: Insulin resistance and hyperinsulinemia in individuals with small, dense, low density lipoprotein particles, *J Clin Invest* 92(1):141-6, 1993.
22. Sakkinen PA, Wahl P, Cushman M et al: Clustering of procoagulation, inflammation, and fibrinolysis variables with metabolic factors in insulin resistance syndrome, *Am J Epidemiol* 152(10):897-907, 2000.
23. Vinik AI, Erbas T, Park TS et al: Platelet dysfunction in type 2 diabetes, *Diabetes Care* 24(8):1476-85, 2001.
24. Mykkanen L, Zaccaro DJ, Wagenknecht LE et al: Microalbuminuria is associated with insulin resistance in nondiabetic subjects. The insulin resistance atherosclerosis study, *Diabetes* 47: 793-800, 1998.
25. Meigs JB and others: Fasting plasma homocysteine levels in the insulin resistance syndrome: the Framingham offspring study, *Diabetes Care* 24(8):1403-10, 2001.
26. Zavaroni I and others: Changes in insulin and lipid metabolism in males with asymptomatic hyperuricemia, *J Int Med* 234: 24-30, 1993.
27. Reaven GM: Syndrome X: 6 years later, *J Int Med* 736: S13-22, 1994.
28. Kemp HG: Left ventricular function in patients with the anginal syndrome and normal coronary arteriograms, *Am J Cardiol* 32(3):375-6, 1973.
29. Botker HE and others: Myocardial insulin resistance in patients with syndrome X, *J Clin Invest* 100(8):1919-27, 1997.
30. Botker HE and others: Insulin resistance in microvascular angina (syndrome X), *Lancet* 342(8864):136-40, 1993.
31. Fitzpatrick TB: *Color atlas and synopsis of clinical dermatology*, ed 3, New York, 1997, McGraw-Hill.
32. Garvey WT, Hermayer KL: Clinical implications of the insulin resistance syndrome, *Clin Cornerstone* 1(3):13-28, 1998.
33. Minchoff LE, Grandin JA: Syndrome X: recognition and management of this metabolic disorder in primary care, *Nurse Prac* 21(6):74-86, 1996.
34. Del Prato S: Measurement of insulin resistance in vivo, *Drugs* 58 Suppl 1:3-6, 1999.
35. American Diabetes Association: Consensus development conference on insulin resistance. 5-6 November 1997, *Diabetes Care* 21(2):310-314, 1998.
36. Liese AD, Mayer-Davis EJ, Haffner SM: Development of the multiple metabolic syndrome: an epidemiologic perspective, *Epidemiol Rev* 20(2):157-72, 1998.
37. Moller DE, Flier JS: Insulin resistance: mechanisms, syndromes and implications, *N Engl J Med* 325(13):938-48, 1991.
38. Ludwig DS, Pereira MA, Kroenke CH et al: Dietary fiber, weight gain, and cardiovascular disease risk factors in young adults, *JAMA* 282: 1539-46, 1999.
39. Liu S, Manson JE: Dietary carbohydrates, physical inactivity, obesity, and the "metabolic syndrome" as predictors of coronary heart disease, *Curr Opin Lipidol* 12(4):395-404, 2001.
40. Riccardi G, Rivellese AA: Dietary treatment of the metabolic syndrome—the optimal diet, *Br J Nutr* 83 Suppl 1: S143-8, 2000.
41. Marckmann P: Dietary treatment of thrombogenic disorders related to the metabolic syndrome, *Br J Nutr* 83 Suppl 1: S121-6, 2000.
42. Jenkins DJ, Axelsen M, Kendall CW et al: Dietary fibre, lente carbohydrates and the insulin-resistant diseases, *Br J Nutr* 83 Suppl 1: S157-63, 2000.
43. Roberts CK, Vaziri ND, Liang KH et al: Reversibility of chronic experimental syndrome X by diet modification, *Hypertension* 37(5):1323-8, 2001.
44. Expert Panel on Detection, Evaluation, and Treatment of High Blood Cholesterol in Adults: Executive summary of the third report of the national cholesterol education program (NCEP) expert panel on detection, evaluation, and treatment of high blood cholesterol in adults (adult treatment panel III), *JAMA* 285(19):2486-97, 2001.
45. Pan XR, Li GW, Hu YH et al and others: Effects of diet and exercise in preventing NIDDM in people with impaired glucose tolerance: the Da Qing IGT and diabetes study, *Diabetes Care* 20(4):537-44, 1997.
46. Shahid SK, Schneider, SH: Effects of exercise on insulin resistance syndrome, *Coron Artery Dis* 11(2):103-9, 2000.

47. American College of Sports Medicine: Position stand on the recommended quantity and quality of exercise for developing and maintaining cardiorespiratory and muscular fitness in healthy adults, *Med Sci Sports Exerc* 30: 975-91, 1998.
48. Avogaro A and others: Gemfibrozil improves insulin sensitivity and flow-mediated vasodilatation in type 2 diabetic patients, *Eur J Clin Invest* 31(7):603-9, 2001.
49. Hansson L and others: Effects of intensive blood-pressure lowering and low dose aspirin on patients with hypertension: Principal results of the Hypertension Optimal Treatment (HOT) randomized trial, *Lancet* 351(9118):1755-62, 1998.
50. The Diabetes Prevention Program Research Group: The diabetes prevention program. Baseline characteristics of the randomized cohort, *Diabetes Care* 23(11):1619-29, 2000.
51. Parulkar AA and others: Nonhypoglycemic effects of thiazolidinediones, *Ann Intern Med* 134(1):61-71, 2001.
52. Sunayama S and others: Thiazolidinediones, dyslipidemia and insulin resistance syndrome, *Curr Opin Lipidol* 11(4):397-402, 2000.
53. Zimmet P, Collier G: Clinical efficacy of metformin against insulin resistance parameters. Sinking the iceberg, *Drugs* 58 Suppl. 1: 21-8, 1999.
54. Reid JL: Rilmenidine: a clinical overview, *Am J Hypertens* 13(6 Pt 2):106S-11S, 2000.
55. Prichard BN, Graham BR: I1 imidazoline agonists. General clinical pharmacology of imidazoline receptors: implications for the treatment of the elderly, *Drugs Aging* 17(2):133-59, 2000.
56. Young-Hyman D and others: Evaluation of the insulin resistance syndrome in 5- to 10-year-old overweight/obese African American children, *Diabetes Care* 24(8):1359-64, 2001.
57. Vanhala M and others: Relation between obesity from childhood to adulthood and the metabolic syndrome: population based study, *Br Med J* 317(7154):319, 1998.
58. Ferrannini E and others: Insulin action and age. European Group for the Study of Insulin Resistance (EGIR), *Diabetes* 45(7):947-53, 1996.
59. Bressler P and others: Insulin resistance and coronary artery disease, *Diabetologia* 39(11):1345-50, 1996.
60. Stout RW: Insulin and atheroma: 20-yr perspective, *Diabetes Care* 13(6):631-54, 1990.
61. Grundy SM: Hypertriglyceridemia, insulin resistance, and the metabolic syndrome, *Am J Cardiol* 83(9B):25F-29F, 1999.

CHAPTER 229

Parathyroid Gland Disorders

Suzanne Mary Rieke and Alan Ona Malabanan

DEFINITION/EPIDEMIOLOGY

The four parathyroid glands, which are located in the neck, tightly regulate serum levels of ionized calcium through the actions of parathyroid hormone (PTH). PTH is a peptide that raises serum calcium in three ways: (1) by acting directly on bone to release calcium into the extracellular fluid, (2) by acting directly on the kidney to decrease renal loss of calcium, (3) by acting indirectly on the intestinal tract, via the activation of vitamin D, to increase dietary calcium absorption. Parathyroid disorders occur through their effects on bone, kidney, serum calcium, and phosphorus.

The two major categories of parathyroid dysfunction are hyperparathyroidism (the oversecretion of PTH) and hypoparathyroidism (the undersecretion of PTH). PTH levels must be interpreted in the context of the serum calcium level. When considered in this manner, primary hyperparathyroidism can be defined as the inappropriate secretion of PTH in the setting of hypercalcemia. Secondary hyperparathyroidism is an appropriately increased secretion of PTH in the setting of low or normal serum calcium. Tertiary hyperparathyroidism is prolonged secondary hyperparathyroidism in which hypercalcemia develops; it is an initially appropriate secretion that later becomes inappropriate. Hypoparathyroidism is the inappropriately low secretion of PTH in the setting of hypocalcemia.

Automated chemistry measurements have allowed the routine detection of asymptomatic hypercalcemia, thus increasing recognition of early primary hyperparathyroidism. The estimated incidence of primary hyperparathyroidism is approximately 1:1000, with the peak incidence between the fourth and fifth decades of life. The incidence in women is higher than that in men, approximately 3:1.[1] A recent overview of cases in Rochester, Minnesota, showed a gradual unexplained decline in the incidence of hyperparathyroidism—from a peak of 129.4 per 100,000 person-years in the final 6 months of 1974 to 4.0 per 100,000 person-years in 1992.[2] With this decline, the clinical presentation of primary hyperparathyroidism has changed, with a lower incidence of severe kidney and bone disease.

Secondary hyperparathyroidism is found mainly in patients with renal insufficiency. It is usually present when the glomerular filtration rate falls below 50 ml/min.[3] Vitamin D deficiency is another important cause of secondary hyperparathyroidism, particularly in older adults and institutionalized patients.[4] Secondary hyperparathyroidism may also occur in patients being treated with glucocorticoids, which cause decreased intestinal calcium absorption.

Hypoparathyroidism is primarily a consequence of thyroid and parathyroid surgery. The incidence, which can range between 0.6% and 17%, depends on the skill of the surgeon and the type of operation.[5]

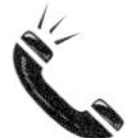

Physician consultation is indicated for all suspected cases of parathyroid disorders.

PATHOPHYSIOLOGY

In 80% to 85% of cases of primary hyperparathyroidism, excess PTH is produced by a single parathyroid adenoma. In 15% to 20% of cases, it is produced by hyperplasia of all four glands. Primary hyperparathyroidism is produced by a parathyroid carcinoma in fewer than 0.5% of cases.[1]

Excess PTH stimulates osteoclast-mediated bone degradation, releasing calcium and phosphorus into the extracellular space. As a result, prolonged exposure to excess PTH will erode bone, particularly cortical (dense) bone. Trabecular bone is relatively spared. Skeletal sites with primarily cortical bone, such as the wrist and proximal radius, are particularly at increased risk for fracture.

PTH acts on the kidney to increase calcium resorption and increase phosphorus losses. The rising serum calcium gradually exceeds the ability of the kidney to resorb the filtered calcium, thus increasing urinary calcium. Nephrocalcinosis, nephrolithiasis, and renal dysfunction may result. PTH receptors also exist on a variety of tissues, including brain, skin, and heart. The effects of PTH on these tissues are not yet well characterized.

Secondary hyperparathyroidism represents a compensation for decreased serum levels of ionized calcium. The kidney is important in calcium and phosphorus homeostasis, and renal insufficiency disturbs calcium metabolism in three ways. First, decreased phosphorus clearance and hyperphosphatemia cause a decrease in serum ionized calcium levels. Second, a decrease in renal activation of vitamin D decreases intestinal calcium absorption. Third, uremia produces PTH resistance, thus necessitating higher levels of PTH. As with primary hyperparathyroidism, excess PTH will erode bone.

Prolonged stimulation of the parathyroid glands by hypocalcemia results in hyperplasia of the glands. Occasionally this leads to autonomous parathyroid function and hypercalcemia (tertiary hyperparathyroidism).

Vitamin D deficiency results in a decrease in intestinal calcium absorption. This coupled with the daily loss of calcium in the urine and the feces leads to a net loss of calcium. To prevent overt hypocalcemia, the parathyroid glands secrete more PTH, thus releasing calcium from the bone and preserving normal serum calcium levels. Long-standing vitamin D deficiency may lead to overt hypocalcemia if calcium stores in the bone are depleted.

Hypoparathyroidism results from the destruction of the parathyroid glands, whether the result of surgery, radiation, infiltration (hemochromatosis, amyloidosis, hemosiderosis), malignancy, or autoimmune disease. As may be expected, decreased PTH affects the renal conservation of calcium, the intestinal absorption of calcium, and the degradative release of calcium from bone. Hypocalcemia results from these effects. Of note, hypomagnesemia or hypermagnesemia may decrease PTH secretion or diminish PTH action on the bone and should be considered as a potential cause of hypoparathyroidism.

CLINICAL PRESENTATION

Asymptomatic elevation of serum calcium is the most common presentation of primary hyperparathyroidism. The hypercalcemia may be masked by hypoalbuminemia. To correct for hypoalbuminemia, 0.8 mg/dl calcium should be added for every 1 g/dl below 4 g/dl albumin. Usually this hypercalcemia is accompanied by a fasting hypophosphatemia. Kidney stones are another initial presenting complaint. Some cases of primary hyperparathyroidism are found following an evaluation for osteoporosis.

Osteitis fibrosa cystica (OFC) is associated with multiple lytic bone lesions and subperiosteal bone resorption. OFC may be found in conjunction with an acute hyperparathyroid crisis in which the hypercalcemia develops quickly, causing obtundation, volume depletion, and cardiac arrhythmias. Patients with primary hyperparathyroidism may also have slightly worsened hypertension, gastrointestinal complaints, and somewhat vague symptoms of fatigue and weakness.

Hyperparathyroidism may occur as part of a familial disorder such as multiple endocrine neoplasia syndrome (MEN). MEN type I includes hyperparathyroidism, pituitary tumors, and pancreatic tumors (insulinoma, gastrinoma). MEN type IIa includes hyperparathyroidism, pheochromocytoma, and medullary thyroid carcinoma. In these disorders, the hyperparathyroidism is caused by parathyroid hyperplasia.

Secondary hyperparathyroidism is usually found with renal insufficiency and vitamin D deficiency. Patients may present with bone pain or a pathologic fracture. Risk factors for vitamin D deficiency include minimal sun exposure, minimal vitamin D dietary intake, malabsorption, prior gastric surgery, and medications that may increase the metabolism of vitamin D (e.g., rifampin and anticonvulsants). Other factors such as aging, sunscreen use, and heavily pigmented skin decrease sunlight-mediated vitamin D synthesis in the skin.

Hypoparathyroidism presents as hypocalcemia accompanied by hyperphosphatemia. The presentation can range from symptoms of perioral and digital paresthesias to life-threatening cardiac arrhythmias, seizures, and laryngospasm. The severity of presentation is dependent on the rapidity of the development of hypocalcemia. It may also depend on the presence of acidemia, which increases ionized calcium, or alkalemia, which decreases ionized calcium. Chronic hypocalcemia can produce premature cataract formation or basal ganglia calcifications, at times with a reversible Parkinson's syndrome.[6]

PHYSICAL EXAMINATION

Physical clues to primary hyperparathyroidism include band keratopathy, a white cloudiness at the border of the cornea. It may be mistaken for arcus senilis and is not specific for hypercalcemia caused by hyperparathyroidism. Occasionally, there may be bony tenderness, particularly of the sternum and tibia. Rarely, there may be a palpable neck mass that is indicative of parathyroid carcinoma.

The physical clues to hypoparathyroidism include the signs indicative of hypocalcemia. Chvostek's sign may be positive in cases of hypocalcemia. This test is performed by tapping (the point of a triangular reflex hammer or a fingertip may be used) over the facial nerve (cranial nerve VII). Contraction of the facial muscles (seen at the corner of the lip and cheek) is a positive test. Trousseau's sign may also be present in hypocalcemia. This test is performed by placing a blood pressure cuff around the biceps and inflating the cuff approximately 10 to 20 mm Hg above the systolic blood pressure. The cuff is left inflated for 3 minutes, or until a positive result is elicited. The test is positive if carpal spasm occurs (flexion at the wrist and extension of the fingers). The presence of Chvostek's and Trousseau's signs can be affected by abnormalities in acid-base balance, potassium level, and magnesium level.

DIAGNOSTICS

Laboratory testing is necessary for the diagnosis of parathyroid disease. The most useful PTH assay is the PTH immunoradiometric assay (IRMA), which allows measurement of the intact PTH molecule.

Primary hyperparathyroidism requires the assessment of PTH, serum calcium, albumin, 25-hydroxyvitamin D, and fasting phosphorus. Assessing levels of serum 1,25-dihydroxyvitamin D may be useful if medical therapy is planned. A bone mineral density assessment of a cortical bone site (e.g., radius) and a 24-hour urine collection for calcium are useful for assessing the risk for osteoporosis; renal imaging (plain film abdominal radiographs or renal ultrasound) is useful in assessing the presence of nephrolithiasis. An ECG may be useful in assessing hypercalcemic cardiotoxicity (QT shortening). Parathyroid imaging is usually not required if an experienced parathyroid surgeon is available and no prior neck surgery has been performed.

Secondary hyperparathyroidism and hypoparathyroidism require assessment of PTH, serum calcium, albumin, and fasting phosphorus. A serum 25-hydroxyvitamin D level, if less than 20 ng/ml, is useful in establishing vitamin D deficiency as the cause of the hyperparathyroidism. A serum magnesium level may also be useful in evaluating hypoparathyroidism. An ECG can reveal hypocalcemic cardiotoxicity (QT lengthening).

Diagnostics

Parathyroid Gland Disorders

HYPERPARATHYROIDISM

Laboratory
- PTH (PTH IRMA)
- Serum calcium
- Albumin
- Fasting phosphorus
- 24-hour urine calcium
- Serum 1,25-dihydroxyvitamin D*
- Serum 25-hydroxyvitamin D

Imaging
- X-rays of abdomen*
- Renal ultrasound
- Bone mineral densitometry (radius)

Other
- ECG*

HYPOPARATHYROIDISM

Laboratory
- PTH
- Serum calcium
- Albumin
- Fasting phosphorus
- Serum 1,25-dihydroxyvitamin D
- Magnesium
- Serum 25-hydroxyvitamin D

Other
- ECG*

*If indicated.

DIFFERENTIAL DIAGNOSIS

By definition, the differential diagnoses for the parathyroid diseases overlap with those of hypercalcemia and hypocalcemia (see Chapter 225). With primary hyperparathyroidism, the most important diagnosis to exclude is familial hypocalciuric hypercalcemia (FHH), an autosomal dominant trait characterized by hypercalcemia and hyperparathyroidism. With FHH, a defective calcium sensor requires higher levels of calcium to suppress PTH secretion. Patients with FHH do not have the usual sequelae of primary hyperparathyroidism and generally have a benign course. In FHH, the fractional excretion of calcium (FE_{Ca}) is generally <0.01. For patients with primary hyperparathyroidism, the FE_{Ca} is >0.013. The formula is as follows.

$$FE_{Ca} = (U_{Ca} \times P_{Cr})/(U_{Cr} \times P_{Ca})^{*}$$

Another clinical situation that produces a similar picture is lithium-related parathyroid disease. Lithium appears to raise the calcium set point through unclear mechanisms. For hypoparathyroidism, the most important diagnostic consideration is hypomagnesemia or hypermagnesemia.

MANAGEMENT

The only cure for primary hyperparathyroidism is surgery, and referral to an experienced parathyroid surgeon is important. In most instances, resection of the parathyroid adenoma or 33/4 of the 4 hyperplastic parathyroid glands corrects the hyperparathyroidism. However, the changing character of primary hyperparathyroidism, with early diagnosis and primarily asymptomatic patients, has led to an increasing role for medical therapy.

*U, Urine concentration (mg/dl) of a 24-hour specimen; P, plasma concentration (mg/dL) for calcium (Ca) and creatinine (Cr).

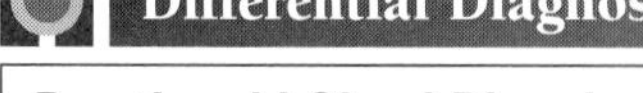

Differential Diagnosis

Parathyroid Gland Disorders

Hyperparathyroidism
- Primary hyperparathyroidism
  - Familial hyperparathyroidism
  - Familial hypocalciuric hypercalcemia
  - Lithium-related parathyroid disease
  - Adenoma
  - Radiation-induced hyperparathyroidism
  - MEN syndrome (multiple endocrine neoplasia)
  - Parathyroid carcinoma
- Secondary hyperparathyroidism
  - Chronic renal disease
  - Vitamin D deficiency
  - Thiazide-induced hypercalcemia

Hypoparathyroidism
- Idiopathic
- Iatrogenic
- Congenital
- Polyglandular autoimmune syndrome
- Metastatic cancer
- Hemochromatosis
- Amyloidosis
- Hypermagnesemia/hypomagnesemia
- Parkinson's syndrome

There is a conspicuous absence of data regarding the prediction of complications in a patient with asymptomatic primary hyperparathyroidism. A National Institutes of Health (NIH) Consensus Conference[7] issued the following guidelines favoring the choice of surgical over medical management:

- Serum calcium level >1 mg/dl above the upper limit of normal
- Substantially decreased bone mineral density (Z-score of distal radius ≤2)
- Nephrolithiasis
- Decreased renal function
- Marked hypercalciuria (>400 mg/day)
- Age <50 years

Longitudinal measurements of bone mineral density in 66 patients with asymptomatic hyperparathyroidism who were managed medically show that their bone disease did not progress at the radius and lumbar spine over 6 years of observation.[8] However, surgery in 34 patients who met the NIH criteria resulted in marked increases in bone mineral density (12.8% at the spine, 12.7% at the femoral neck, and 4% at the distal radius).[9]

Medical management of asymptomatic primary hyperparathyroidism involves maintaining adequate hydration, avoiding medications that may raise calcium (e.g., thiazide diuretics), and maintaining activity (inactivity can increase bone resorption). Dietary calcium excess and deficiency should be avoided—the former for obvious reasons and the latter because of potential increases in PTH as a result of a calcium-deficient diet. A recent study has suggested that patients with normal levels of 1,25-dihydroxyvitamin D can liberalize their calcium intake (i.e., 1000 mg of elemental calcium daily), whereas patients with elevated levels are advised to ingest less calcium daily to prevent hypercalciuria.[10]

Oral phosphorus supplementation decreases serum calcium but is limited by the risk of ectopic calcification and the potential for further raising PTH. In postmenopausal women, estrogen may decrease serum calcium but does not affect PTH levels. Bisphosphonates have not yet been shown to produce sustained decreases in serum calcium. Preliminary studies of 13 postmenopausal women with mild primary hyperparathyroidism aged 67 to 81 who were treated with alendronate for 2 years demonstrated a decrease in bone turnover markers during treatment and a statistically significant increase in body mass density at the spine (+8.6 ± 3.0%), hip (+4.8 ± 3.9%), and total body (+1.2 ± 1.4%) versus the nontreatment group. However, there was a transient decrease in serum calcium levels and statistically significant increase in serum PTH levels.[11] Calcimimetic agents that activate the calcium receptor on parathyroid cells show promise for the medical management of primary hyperparathyroidism. Their action seems to inhibit PTH release and decrease serum calcium levels.[12]

Monitoring bone mineral density and 24-hour urinary calcium annually and serum calcium semiannually is prudent. Imaging studies for occult nephrolithiasis and the assessment of creatinine clearance may be helpful.

When vitamin D deficiency and primary hyperparathyroidism coexist, repletion of vitamin D stores may be linked to increases in bone mineral density. A recent study of 229 individuals with osteoporosis found 5 subjects to have both primary hyperparathyroidism and vitamin D deficiency. After replacement of their vitamin D deficiency (50,000 IU twice a week for 5 weeks), increases in bone mineral density of 6.3% and 8.2% in the spine and hip, respectively, were seen despite persistent elevation of PTH.[13] Serum calcium levels were monitored during vitamin D therapy.

The management of secondary hyperparathyroidism depends on the cause. For renal failure, renal transplantation usually corrects the hyperparathyroidism, but it may be refractory if long-standing. Calcitriol (1,25-dihydroxycholecalciferol) and calcium therapy (to raise serum calcium and decrease serum phosphorus) is also useful in lowering PTH levels. For vitamin D deficiency, mild secondary hyperparathyroidism can be corrected with 400 to 800 IU vitamin D daily. More aggressive therapy can be undertaken with 50,000 IU vitamin D weekly for 8 weeks.

Hypoparathyroidism is difficult to treat. PTH must be given parenterally and therefore is not easily replaced. Therapy usually consists of vitamin D analogues and calcium supplements. Dairy products, which are high in phosphorus, should be avoided. Perhaps the safest medication is calcitriol, but it is also the most expensive. It is preferable to ergocalciferol (vitamin D) because it acts more quickly (days versus weeks) and has a shorter duration of action, which allows rapid titration. Hypercalciuria is the main limitation of calcitriol therapy. The absence of the PTH effect on renal conservation of calcium results in hypercalciuria as intestinal absorption of calcium increases. Calcitriol should be started at 0.25 μg PO q.d. and increased as necessary every 2 to 4 weeks to bring serum calcium into the low-normal range without producing hypercalciuria. The judicious use of thiazides may decrease urinary calcium loss and allow the normalization of serum calcium.

COMPLICATIONS

Complications may result from the parathyroid disease process or its treatment. In addition to osteoporosis and nephrolithiasis, surgery for primary hyperparathyroidism may cause hypocalcemia as a result of temporary hypoparathyroidism, vitamin D deficiency, or *hungry bone syndrome*. With hungry bone syndrome, calcium and phosphorus are rapidly incorporated into bone. This cause of hypocalcemia is more common in patients with higher serum calcium, alkaline phosphatase, or more severe bone disease.

INDICATIONS FOR REFERRAL/HOSPITALIZATION

All parathyroid disorders should be referred to a physician or an endocrinologist experienced in the treatment of parathyroid disease. If surgical therapy is indicated, a referral to an experienced parathyroid surgeon is essential.

PATIENT EDUCATION AND HEALTH PROMOTION

For patients with primary hyperparathyroidism, understanding the importance of adequate calcium and fluid intake, as well as continued monitoring of bone and calcium status, is important. Potential complications of parathyroid bone disease, such as wrist and hip fractures, should be carefully explained. For patients with secondary hyperparathyroidism, the importance of calcium and vitamin D supplementation should be stressed. For patients who undergo surgical therapy or who have hypoparathyroidism, it is essential that they recognize the symptoms of hypocalcemia and the consequences of nonadherence to therapy, including tetany, laryngospasm, cardiac arrhythmias, and seizures.

REFERENCES

1. Silverberg SJ, Bilezikian JP: Primary hyperparathyroidism: still evolving? *J Bone Miner Res* 12:856-862, 1997.
2. Wermers RA and others: The rise and fall of primary hyperparathyroidism: a population-based study in Rochester, Minnesota, 1965-1992, *Ann Intern Med* 126:433-440, 1997.
3. Bushinsky DA: Bone disease in moderate renal failure: cause, nature, and prevention. *Ann Rev Med* 48:167-176, 1997.
4. McKenna MJ: Differences in vitamin D status between countries in young adults and the elderly, *Am J Med* 93:69-77, 1992.
5. Kahky MP, Weber RS: Complications of surgery of the thyroid and parathyroid glands, *Surg Clin North Am* 73:307-321, 1993.
6. Tambyah PA, Ong BKC, Lee KO: Reversible Parkinsonism and asymptomatic hypocalcemia with basal ganglia calcification from hypoparathyroidism 26 years after thyroid surgery, *Am J Med* 94:444-445, 1993.
7. Proceedings of the NIH Consensus Development Conference on diagnosis and management of asymptomatic primary hyperparathyroidism. Bethesda, Maryland, October 29-31, 1990, *J Bone Miner Res* 6(suppl 2):S1-166, 1991.
8. Silverberg SJ and others: Longitudinal measurements of bone density and biochemical indices in untreated primary hyperparathyroidism, *J Clin Endocrinol Metab* 80:723-728, 1995.
9. Silverberg SJ and others: Increased bone mineral density after parathyroidectomy in primary hyperparathyroidism, *J Clin Endocrinol Metab* 80:720-722, 1995.
10. Locker FG, Silverberg SJ, Bilezikian JP: Optimal dietary calcium intake in primary hyperparathyroidism, *Am J Med* 102:543-550, 1997.
11. Rossini M and others: Effects of oral alendronate in elderly patients with osteoporosis and mild primary hyperparathyroidism, *J Bone Miner Res* 16:113-119, 2001.
12. Silverberg SJ and others: Short-term inhibition of parathyroid hormone secretion by a calcium-receptor agonist in patients with primary hyperparathyroidism, *N Engl J Med* 337:1506-1510, 1997.
13. Kantorovich V and others: Bone mineral density increases with vitamin D repletion in patients with coexistent vitamin D insufficiency and primary hyperparathyroidism, *J Clin Endocrinol Metab* 85:3541-3543, 2000.

CHAPTER 230

Thyroid Disorders

Jennifer C. Braimon, Naaznin Lokhandwala, and Monika Walczak

Thyroid disease in its various forms is widely prevalent in the general population. Perhaps 50% of the population has microscopic nodules; 3.5% have occult papillary carcinoma, 15% have palpable goiters, 10% have abnormal thyroid-stimulating hormone (TSH) levels, and 5% of women have overt hypothyroidism or hyperthyroidism.[1]

Hormones secreted by the thyroid gland influence a variety of metabolic processes in the body. Thyroid function is regulated by TSH, which is secreted by basophilic cells in the anterior pituitary gland in response to the secretion of thyrotropin-releasing hormone (TRH) from the hypothalamus. Control of TRH secretion is regulated in a negative-feedback fashion by the thyroid hormones. Low serum levels of thyroid hormones cause TRH release from the hypothalamus, which in turn causes TSH release from the pituitary. TSH causes increased release of thyroid hormones until a normal serum level is reached. Within the thyroid gland, thyroid function is affected by glandular organic iodine content.

The synthesis of T_4 (thyroxine) and T_3 (triiodothyronine) requires that adequate quantities of iodine enter the thyroid gland. Iodine enters from the bloodstream and is a constituent of both T_4 and T_3. These hormones are transported in the bloodstream bound to plasma proteins. The majority of T_4 is bound; only a small portion is free. However, it is free T_4 concentration in the serum that indicates thyroidal activity. Approximately 80% of serum T_3 is formed in the liver, kidney and muscle from the deiodination of T_4; the remaining 20% is secreted directly by the thyroid.[2] Alterations in the regulation of hormone secretion can have varied effects on the body (Box 230-1).

Alterations in the function of the thyroid gland may result in hypersecretion and increased metabolism (hyperthyroidism) or hyposecretion and decreased metabolism (hypothyroidism). Enlargement of the gland may also occur and take the form of localized nodules or generalized goiter. Localized nodules may be

BOX 230-1

PHYSIOLOGIC EFFECTS OF THYROID HORMONES

- Affects fetal development—secreted from 11 weeks in fetus and facilitates normal fetal growth
- Promotes basal metabolic function—regulates oxygen consumption and heat production
- Affects cardiovascular muscle contraction
- Stimulates bone resorption and, to some extent, bone formation
- Permits normal glucose metabolism, absorption, and storage
- Functions in the synthesis and breakdown of lipids
- Affects the rate of metabolism of many hormones and drugs (depends on amount of thyroid hormones)

benign or malignant, and solitary or multiple; goiters may be mild or quite extensive.

Thyroid Function Testing

Thyroid function can be evaluated in the laboratory through the use of thyroid function tests (TFTs). Thyroid structure and function can be assessed through a variety of imaging techniques and through biopsy.

TSH is the most sensitive indicator of overall thyroid function. Current techniques allow measurement of serum TSH concentrations as low as 0.01 μU/L (third-generation assay, immunometric dual-antibody [Ab] assay). This generally is the best screening test for thyroid dysfunction. Exceptions include patients with pituitary or hypothalamic (secondary or tertiary) disease and patients immediately after treatment of hypothyroidism or hyperthyroidism (when the TSH response may lag behind). In addition, various medications and nonthyroidal conditions may affect TSH levels.

TSH measurements are usually sufficient to categorize patients into one of three groups: hyperthyroid (TSH <0.3 μU/L), hypothyroid (TSH >4 μU/L), and euthyroid (TSH = 0.3 to 4 μU/L). Approximately 99% of circulating T_4 and T_3 is bound to serum proteins. It is the free, unbound T_4 that is maintained at a constant level and correlates most with the thyroid state. Free T_4 traverses cell membranes to exert its effects on body tissues. Direct measurements of free T_4 and T_3 are available but are cumbersome and technically demanding. It is usually sufficient to correct the total T_4 (TT_4) level for the concentration of thyroxine-binding globulin (TBG).

TBG determinations are inaccurate in patients with congenital absence of TBG or familial dysalbuminemic hyperthyroxinemia (FDH). Patients with FDH have aberrant albumin that binds T_4 (not T_3) with increased affinity. In FDH, laboratory tests reveal increased TT_4, normal TT_3 (total T_3), normal TSH, and normal free T_4 by equilibrium dialysis. Circumstances that increase TBG include pregnancy, acute hepatitis, inherited abnormalities, and the use of estrogen, oral contraceptives, methadone, or heroin. Decreased TBG results from acromegaly, nephrotic syndrome, cirrhosis, chronic debilitating disease, and treatment with glucocorticoids, androgens, aspirin, nonsteroidal antiinflammatory drugs (NSAIDs), and some penicillins.

If the TSH level is abnormal, T_4 and a marker for binding proteins should be obtained. The T_3U test is the resin or charcoal T_3 (radioactive T_3) uptake test; it estimates the unoccupied binding sites on TBG. The T_3U parallels the concentration of free T_4. The thyroid hormone–binding ratio (THBR) is a standard way of correcting for TBG.

$$\text{THBR} = \text{Patient's } T_3U : \text{Mean laboratory } T_3U$$

Thus the corrected T_4 (T_4 index or T_7) is calculated as follows.

$$T_4 \text{ index} = TT_4 \times \text{THBR}$$

T_3 determination is useful in diagnosis of T_3 toxicosis (normal TT_4, decreased TSH, increased TT_3) and in the diagnosis of euthyroid sick patients. With euthyroid sick syndrome, acute nonthyroidal illness, chronic disease, or caloric deprivation causes decreased peripheral conversion of T_4 to T_3 (inhibition of the type 1 deiodinase). Reverse T_3 (rT_3) is a product of T_4 degradation in the peripheral tissues. It is also secreted in insignificant amounts by the thyroid gland. Levels are elevated in states in which T_3 is decreased (i.e., patients who are euthyroid sick).

Autoantibodies to thyroglobulin (Tg) or thyroid microsomes may be found in patients with autoimmune thyroid disease. Thyroid peroxidase (TPO) is the major microsomal antigen. Anti-TPO Abs are found in patients with Hashimoto's thyroiditis and in fewer than 85% of patients with Graves' disease (autoimmune hyperthyroidism). Anti-Tg Abs are found in 20% of patients with Hashimoto's thyroiditis and fewer than 20% of patients with Graves' disease. Up to 15% of the general population have Abs to either of these antigens. Quantifying the Ab titers is not clinically useful, although some studies suggest that the severity of thyroid destruction in Hashimoto's thyroiditis is proportional to the anti-TPO titer. These tests are particularly useful in the evaluation of patients with atypical manifestations of autoimmune thyroid disease (i.e., isolated ophthalmopathy without signs of hyperthyroidism). They are also predictive of postpartum thyroiditis.[3]

Radionuclide imaging cannot be performed in patients who have recently received iodine-containing compounds (i.e., IV contrast). They may also be inaccurate (falsely low uptake) in patients who are following a high-iodine diet.

The pertechnetate scan is often used for imaging the thyroid. Pertechnetate (99m Tc04-) has the same size and charge as iodide. It is concentrated but not bound by thyroid tissues. Scans are performed 20 minutes after the administration of 99m Tc04-. Its advantages include low radiation exposure to the patient, availability, and its power of resolution (approximately 5 mm). Rarely there will be a false-positive result (i.e., "hot" or false uptake) in malignant tissues. Iodine isotopes (^{123}I, ^{125}I, and ^{131}I) are concentrated and bound by thyroid tissues. Scans are performed 4 or 24 hours after the administration of ^{123}I or ^{125}I and 48, 72, or 96 hours after the administration of ^{131}I when used to search for metastatic thyroid cancer.

Normally, the isotopes are distributed evenly throughout the thyroid gland. Each thyroid lobe is approximately 5 cm long and 2.3 cm wide. A mottled appearance is seen in Hashimoto's thyroiditis or in recently treated Graves' disease. An inhomogeneous uptake is also seen in multinodular goiters.

Nodules are classified as hot, warm, or cold according to the concentration of isotope in the nodule in comparison with the rest of the thyroid gland. Hot nodules are usually, but not always, benign. Many cold nodules (solid or cystic) are benign; however, most malignancies also appear as cold nodules. The normal radioactive iodine uptake (RAIU) is approximately 30%. Exuberant iodine supplementation is becoming more prevalent and may cause a falsely low RAIU. When ordering isotope scans, a RAIU can be ordered alone or with a scan.

Ultrasonography is used to evaluate the anatomy of the thyroid gland and to differentiate solid from cystic nodules. It is useful in detecting abnormalities >0.5 cm in diameter. It localizes the position and depth of lesions and can be used to guide fine needle aspiration (FNA). It cannot clearly assess substernal goiters because of interference from bone.

A core biopsy is used for histologic examination of thyroid tissue (i.e., the architecture is preserved) via closed-needle or open surgery. Fine needle aspiration biopsy (FNAB) obtains material for cytologic examination only. It is simple and safe but should be performed only by experienced practitioners. Initially there had been concern regarding an increased risk of cancer spreading along the needle tract from FNA, but this has not been observed. In experienced hands, FNAB is approximately 95% accurate in excluding cancer.

Goiter (Simple, Nontoxic)

DEFINITION/EPIDEMIOLOGY

Enlargement of the thyroid gland is referred to as *goiter.* It may be caused by hormonal or immunologic stimulation or may result from inflammatory, infiltrative, or metabolic conditions, including iodine deficiency or excess, neoplasia, Graves' disease, and thyroiditis.

Nontoxic (simple) goiter occurs when the thyroid gland enlarges in response to inadequate thyroid hormone production. Iodine deficiency remains the most common cause in large areas of Africa, Asia, and South America. The scarcity of iodine in the diet results in the production of TRH, which causes TSH to be secreted in large amounts. The increased TSH has two effects: (1) the retention of all available iodine by the thyroid and (2) the growth of thyroid cells. It is this latter effect that results in thyroid enlargement.

In developed countries, iodine is available in supplemented products such as table salt, fertilizers, animal feeds, and food preservatives. Therefore the most common cause of nontoxic goiter in developed countries is chronic autoimmune thyroiditis.

PATHOPHYSIOLOGY

Initially, the pathology of simple goiters demonstrates a uniformly hypertrophic, hyperplastic, and hypervascular gland. Later, fibrosis may lead to formation of multiple nodules to create a multinodular goiter. These nodules may be "hot" and concentrate iodine or "cold" and not concentrate iodine. When the nodules become autonomous, hyperthyroidism may occur, a condition known as *toxic multinodular goiter.*

Individuals with a nontoxic goiter may or may not have increased levels of TSH. When levels are normal, it is believed the gland enlarges as a response to impaired hormone synthesis by increasing thyroid mass and cellular activity. In individuals with elevated levels of TSH, the thyroid gland increases mass and activity in response to this stimulation.

CLINICAL PRESENTATION

Patients with simple goiter usually present with either diffuse or multinodular thyroid enlargement. Symptoms such as difficulty swallowing and neck pressure may be present.

Undetected and continued growth may result in the thyroid gland extending downward to a substernal location in the chest. Presentation may include symptoms that result from compression of the trachea, esophagus, and vasculature.

PHYSICAL EXAMINATION

Examination of the thyroid should begin with observation under a good examining light. The normal gland is rarely visible. It is useful to have the patient extend the neck fully to permit inspection of the gland over the trachea. It is also helpful to observe from the side to identify any enlargement between the cricoid cartilage and the suprasternal notch. Any prominence in this area should be measured with a ruler and recorded; a high likelihood of goiter exists if the prominence is >2 mm. Having the patient swallow a sip of water may enhance visualization of an enlarged gland.

Palpation may be performed either in front of or behind the patient (depending on practitioner's comfort), and the texture is noted. The texture of the thyroid can range from extremely soft to relatively firm; it may be smooth or may contain palpable nodules. Prominent glands should be measured and recorded. Thyroid size should be categorized as normal or goiter.[4] A small goiter is considered to be 1 to 2 times normal size, and a large goiter is greater than twice normal size.

The Pemberton sign is used for examination when substernal goiter is suspected. The patient is asked to elevate both arms until they touch the sides of the head. Flushing of the face, cyanosis, and respiratory distress may occur as a result of impingement of structures within the thoracic inlet.[5] Distention of neck veins may also be apparent in these patients.

DIAGNOSTICS

Laboratory studies may show low or normal free thyroxine and, most often, normal levels of TSH. Radioiodine uptake may be high, normal, or low depending on the amount of iodine in the diet and the level of TSH. Isotope scanning results depend on whether nodules are hot or cold. Thyroid ultrasound allows identification of gland size and the number and size of any nodules. If necessary for diagnosis, FNA may be performed.

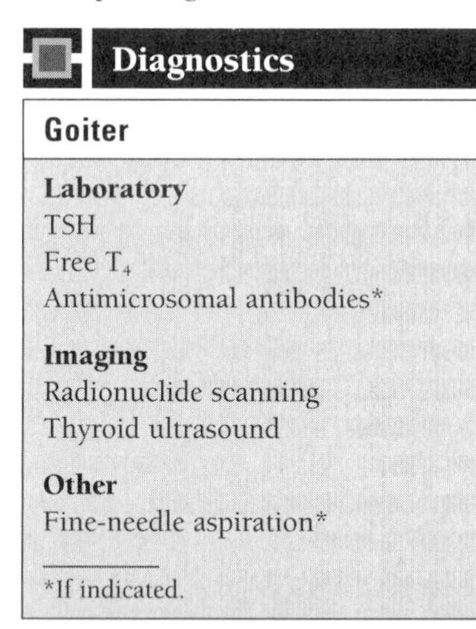

Diagnostics

Goiter

Laboratory
TSH
Free T_4
Antimicrosomal antibodies*

Imaging
Radionuclide scanning
Thyroid ultrasound

Other
Fine-needle aspiration*

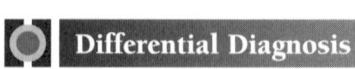

*If indicated.

DIFFERENTIAL DIAGNOSIS

Simple goiter must also be differentiated from chronic autoimmune thyroiditis and toxic multinodular goiter. A careful history of symptoms is important. Also, with chronic autoimmune thyroiditis, circulating antimicrosomal Ab levels will be elevated.

Differential Diagnosis

Goiter

Iodine deficiency of excess
Neoplasia (multinodular, malignant)
Graves' disease
Simple goiter
Thyroiditis
- Chronic autoimmune thyroiditis
- Hashimoto's thyroiditis
- Subacute thyroiditis
- Postpartum thyroiditis

Genetic goiter

MANAGEMENT

The majority of nontoxic goiters grow slowly over many years. The presence of a goiter, with no accompanying symptoms or cosmetic concerns, is not an indication for treatment. Treatment indications include venous flow obstruction, compression of the trachea or esophagus, progressive enlargement of the entire goiter or individual nodules, neck discomfort, or the presence of cosmetic concerns.[6] The treatment of nontoxic goiter may involve the use of levothyroxine to suppress glandular function, thyroidectomy, or radioiodine.

Surgical treatment, usually bilateral subtotal thyroidectomy, is the preferred treatment in otherwise healthy, young patients, especially in presence of goiters that grow substernally or continue to enlarge, causing compressive symptoms. There is little evidence that postoperative suppressive T_4 treatment prevents goiter recurrence; therefore it should not be routinely used.[6]

Levothyroxine treatment will suppress TSH, correct any hypothyroidism, and slowly reduce the size of the goiter. However, this therapy may have significant adverse effects, such as decreased bone mineral density, atrial fibrillation, and biochemical hyperthyroidism, if not monitored closely. The best candidates for this form of treatment are young patients with small diffuse goiters and a high normal TSH. Thyroxine therapy is not recommended for patients with any type of goiter or nodule and a low TSH because this therapy may cause hyperthyroidism, especially in older adults.[7,8] Some sources recommend a trial of suppressive therapy for patients with a solitary and nonfunctioning nodule, negative fine-needle aspirates, and normal or elevated TSH levels with the goal of keeping TSH at low normal levels. Such therapy may continue for 6 months to 1 year before reevaluation.

Nontoxic multinodular goiter may also be treated with radioactive iodine to reduce thyroid volume. Therapy with ^{131}I has been found to be an effective alternative with a few side effects.[9,10] This therapy is especially useful in older patients or those with cardiopulmonary disease.

COMPLICATIONS

Nontoxic goiter, even if multinodular, has few complications. Of particular concern is the potential for a multinodular goiter to develop autonomous function with ensuing hyperthyroidism. Close monitoring of TSH enables identification of this potential problem. Surgical patients with a nontoxic goiter may require special observation for airway maintenance and hormone supplementation if indicated.

INDICATIONS FOR REFERRAL/HOSPITALIZATION

Patients who have any indication for treatment of their goiter may require an endocrinology referral for discussion of an appropriate treatment and a surgical referral if thyroidectomy is selected as the treatment of choice.

PATIENT AND FAMILY EDUCATION AND HEALTH PROMOTION

It is important that patients understand the definition and cause of the nontoxic goiter. Patients need to participate in developing the plan of care and understand its rationale. Those living in inland areas or who have seafood allergies should use iodized salt. Patients should understand that nontoxic goiter is a manageable, highly livable condition that will not affect their lives in a negative way if well controlled.

Thyroid Nodules and Thyroid Cancer

DEFINITION/EPIDEMIOLOGY

A *thyroid nodule* is a palpable abnormality within an apparently normal thyroid gland. By this definition, thyroid nodules include cysts, lobules of normal thyroid tissue, and benign and malignant solid lesions. The term *nodular thyroid disease* is preferred.

With ultrasonography, approximately 50% of all single, palpable nodules are found to be in a multinodular gland. In general, nodules larger than 0.5 to 1.0 cm are palpable. Thyroid adenomas are benign neoplastic nodules within a capsule.

The prevalence of thyroid nodules depends on the method of evaluation. Palpable thyroid nodules are found in 4% to 7% of the general adult population. In a Framingham, Massachusetts, cohort, there was a 4.2% overall incidence (6.4% in women and 1.6% in men).[11] Autopsy and ultrasound studies have quoted a prevalence as high as 50%. The lifetime risk of developing a thyroid nodule is estimated to be between 5% and 10%.[12] Thyroid nodules are common, and most of them are benign. Only 3% to 5% of all thyroid nodules are malignant.

PATHOPHYSIOLOGY

Thyroid nodules may be due to adenomas, cysts, carcinomas, multinodular goiters, Hashimoto's thyroiditis, and subacute thyroiditis. Less common causes of neck lumps include the effects of prior surgery or ^{131}I, parathyroid cysts or adenomas, thyroglossal cysts, nonthyroidal lesions, and lymphomas.

Thyroid adenomas are benign, monoclonal growths. Benign thyroid tumors include embryonal, fetal, follicular, Hurthle's, and papillary adenomas. They are distinguished by their characteristic histologic appearance.[13] Malignant thyroid tumors include papillary, follicular, medullary, and anaplastic carcinomas.

CLINICAL PRESENTATION AND PHYSICAL EXAMINATION

Thyroid nodules are usually asymptomatic and are identified as a lump by patients or by practitioners during routine thyroid examinations. Recently, there have been an increasing number of thyroid nodules identified incidentally during carotid Doppler ultrasound or other neck imaging studies. Clinical features that increase the likelihood of cancer include a history of head and neck irradiation, a family history of thyroid cancer, an age $<$20 years or $>$60 years, male gender, and a history of multiple endocrine neoplasia 2 (MEN 2) or medullary thyroid cancer (MTC).[14-16] Familial thyroid tumors also occur in Cowden's disease (multiple hamartoma syndrome), Gardner's syndrome (development of multiple tumors with autosomal dominant inheritance), and familial polyposis.

An anaplastic tumor may present as an enlarging, painful mass associated with hoarseness, dysphonia, dysphagia, or dyspnea. However, patients with benign goiters may also present with compressive symptoms. Patients with anaplastic thyroid cancer may present with pathologic fractures of the spine or hip or with thoracic outlet syndrome. Patients with toxic nodules may present with symptoms of hyperthyroidism. Signs and symptoms of hyperthyroidism or hypothyroidism are usually suggestive of a benign process. However, lymphoma may develop within the thyroid gland of patients with Hashimoto's thyroiditis.

Important features noted during the physical examination include nodule size, consistency, and mobility and the presence and consistency of associated lymphadenopathy. Supraclavicular, anterior cervical, and axillary lymph nodes should be examined. Although most thyroid cancers feel firm or hard, they can be soft and fluctuant on examination. The presence of a new nodule or enlarging nodule while a patient is on thyroxine therapy is a cause for concern.

DIAGNOSTICS AND DIFFERENTIAL DIAGNOSIS

TFTs (e.g., TSH) are necessary to exclude hyperthyroidism or hypothyroidism. The routine measurement of serum calcitonin (to exclude medullary thyroid cancer) is not useful or cost effective.[17]

Historically, radionuclide imaging was the first diagnostic test used in the evaluation of solitary thyroid nodules. Although it is true that most thyroid malignancies appear as cold nodules, most cold nodules are benign. Radionuclide scanning is now used as an initial test if a hyperfunctioning nodule is suspected. It may also be useful if the results of FNA are inconclusive.

High-resolution sonography can clearly distinguish between solid and cystic components. However, ultrasonic findings correlate poorly with disease and are not believed to be useful in the routine evaluation of thyroid nodules. The major indications for use of ultrasound are as an aid to FNAB, to detect nodules too small to palpate in high-risk patients, and to map the extent of thyroid malignancy.[18]

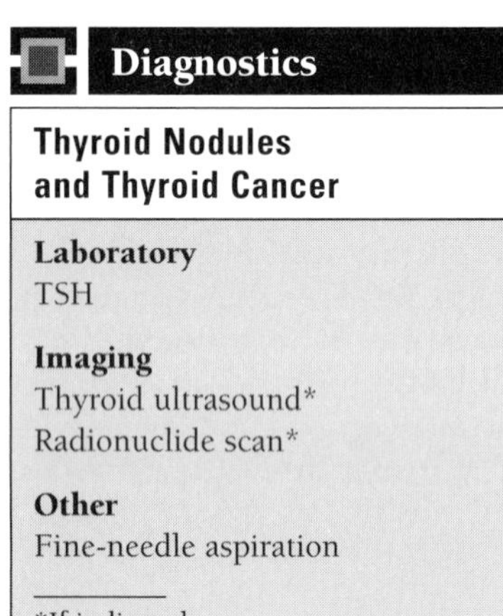

Diagnostics

Thyroid Nodules and Thyroid Cancer

Laboratory
TSH

Imaging
Thyroid ultrasound*
Radionuclide scan*

Other
Fine-needle aspiration

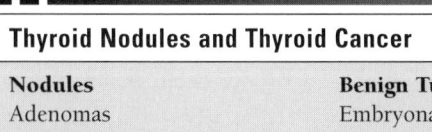

*If indicated.

Differential Diagnosis

Thyroid Nodules and Thyroid Cancer

Nodules
Adenomas
- Follicular
- Papillary
- Teratoma
- Parathyroid

Cysts
Carcinomas
Multinodular goiters
Hashimoto's thyroiditis
Subacute thyroiditis
Surgery/radiation effects
Parathyroid cysts/adenomas
Thyroglossal cysts
Nonthyroidal lesions
Lymphomas

Benign Tumors
Embryonal
Fetal
Follicular
Hürthle cell adenomas
Papillary adenomas

Malignant Carcinomas
Papillary
Follicular
Medullary
Anaplastic

FNAB is an essential diagnostic procedure for the evaluation of thyroid nodules. It is safe and technically simple but requires an experienced operator and cytopathologist. False-negative and false-positive rates are <5% with experienced users. Cytologic results are sufficient in 85% of biopsies and insufficient for diagnosis.

MANAGEMENT

The initial management of a thyroid nodule includes a complete history and physical examination. TSH levels are indicated. If there is evidence of a solitary nodule on examination, with normal TSH level, the patient should be referred to a practitioner (usually an endocrinologist) who is experienced in performing FNAB biopsies.

If the results of the cytologic tests are benign, no further evaluation is necessary. A repeat FNAB should be reserved for enlarging nodules.[19] Thyroid examinations should be performed every 6 to 12 months. T_4 suppression therapy has been shown to be somewhat effective in patients with multinodular goiters and in patients with diffuse nontoxic goiters (30% reduction in nodule size); it is less effective in the treatment of solitary nodule.[20] Because of the uncertainty of the efficacy of T_4 suppression, therapy should be individualized. Because of the untoward effects of suppression therapy on bone density, T_4 suppression is avoided in postmenopausal women unless they are taking hormone replacement therapy. A reasonable strategy is to consider the use of T_4 suppression therapy (TSH = 0.1 to 0.5 μU/ml) in men and premenopausal women. If there is shrinkage, the same dose is continued for approximately 1 year and then decreased to keep the TSH levels between 0.4 and 0.9 μU/ml. A repeat FNAB is performed if the nodules increase in size while the patient is on suppressive therapy.

If the TSH level is elevated on initial evaluation, the patient has two conditions requiring medical attention. In addition to the work-up and management of hypothyroidism, the presence of a single dominant nodule necessitates further evaluation by FNAB.

If serum TSH is suppressed, free T_4 and TT_3 values should be obtained and a radionuclide scan (^{123}I scan) performed. If the nodule is hyperfunctioning, the patient has an autonomously functioning thyroid adenoma. Patients with an adenoma who have thyrotoxicosis should be treated with radioactive iodine or surgery. Patients with subclinical thyrotoxicosis can be monitored or treated (radioactive iodine or surgery) depending on adenoma size. If the nodule is hypofunctioning on ^{123}I scan, the next step is the FNAB evaluation.

If the cytologic test results are suspicious or positive, referral to an experienced surgeon for resection is necessary. The extent of surgical resection remains controversial. For solitary lesions <1.0 cm, a lobectomy may be performed. Total thyroidectomy is indicated if there is a history of head or neck irradiation, the tumor extends beyond the thyroid capsule, or the lesion is >1.0 cm.[6] The thyroid remnant is usually ablated with ^{131}I after surgery. This eases the diagnosis and treatment of metastases. Prophylactic lymph node dissection is not generally indicated. At the time of surgery, regional lymph nodes are evaluated and removed if abnormal.

Medullary thyroid cancer and anaplastic thyroid cancers are more aggressive than well-differentiated thyroid cancers and therefore are treated differently.[21] If the cytology results are indeterminate, aspiration should be performed again. If still inconclusive, radionuclide imaging may be useful.

Patients with differentiated thyroid carcinoma are followed at 3- to 6-month intervals for 5 years after diagnosis and surgery and then at 6- to 12-month intervals if disease free. Thyroglobulin levels and whole-body scans are followed postoperatively. Serum antithyroglobulin Abs should be checked; if present, these invalidate serum thyroglobulin measurement. Patients are maintained on suppressive doses of T_4 (the goal is TSH levels of 0.2 and 0.4 μU/ml). Biannual chest x-ray examinations are necessary to exclude pulmonary metastasis in papillary carcinomas.

LIFE SPAN CONSIDERATIONS

The net mortality rate of papillary thyroid cancer is 10% to 20% over 20 to 30 years. Several factors increase the risk of death from cancer: extrathyroidal invasion (6 times the risk), metastasis (47 times), age >45 years (32 times), and size of tumor >3 cm (6 times).[22]

Various scoring systems are used to stratify patients (in terms of prognosis) with well-differentiated and medullary thyroid cancer. In the MACIS scoring system for papillary carcinoma, metastasis, age, completeness of surgery, invasion, and size are used to predict survival. The following scores are given:

- 3.0 for distant metastasis
- 3.1 for age <40 years
- 0.08 × age if >40 years
- 1.0 if surgical removal was incomplete
- 1.0 for extrathyroidal invasion
- 0.3 × size of tumor

A total score of <6.0 predicts a 99% chance for 20-year survival; 6.0 to 6.99, 89% chance; 7.0 to 7.99, 56% chance; and >8.0, 24% chance.

The Mayo Clinic scoring system for follicular carcinoma assigns 1 point to each of the following:

- Age >50 years
- Vascular invasion
- Metastatic disease at diagnosis

A total score of 0 or 1 predicts a 99% chance of 5-year survival and an 86% chance of 20-year survival. A total score of 2 or 3 predicts a 47% chance of 5-year survival and an 8% chance of 20-year survival.

The Mayo Clinic scoring system for medullary thyroid cancer predicts prognosis using the following:

- Completeness of resection
- Amyloid staining
- Local invasiveness
- Metastasis

One point is given for each of these items. A total score of 0 predicts a 100% 10-year survival rate; a score of 1 predicts a 78% survival rate; a score of 2 predicts a 26% survival rate; and a score of 3 predicts a 0% 10-year survival rate.

COMPLICATIONS

Complications of thyroid surgery include hypoparathyroidism and hoarseness from recurrent laryngeal nerve damage. Side effects of radioiodine include thyroid tenderness, dry mouth, altered taste, and nausea. Accumulative doses of >300 mCi may increase the risk of leukemia. Bone marrow suppression is seen with cumulative doses of >500 mCi. Other potential complications of radioiodine include pulmonary fibrosis and ovarian or testicular failure. Treatment doses range from 30 to 150 mCi.

INDICATIONS FOR REFERRAL/HOSPITALIZATION

Once the initial evaluation has been performed (physical examination and TSH levels), the patient is referred to a practitioner experienced in FNABs. If the cytologic test results are positive or suspicious, the patient should be referred to an experienced thyroid surgeon. After surgery the patient should be referred to thyroid specialist, who can coordinate and administer therapeutic radioactive iodine. Patients are maintained on suppressive doses of T_4.

Indications for hospitalization include respiratory compromise because of invasive tumors, as well as the administration of radioactive iodine doses above 30 mCi (requires specialized rooms).

PATIENT AND FAMILY EDUCATION AND HEALTH PROMOTION

Patients should be given instructions regarding precautions after radioactive iodine treatment or scanning. These instructions include (1) no kissing, exchanging of saliva, or sharing of food or eating utensils for 5 days; dishes should be washed in a dishwasher; (2) no close contact with infants, young children (<8 years of age), or pregnant women for 5 days; it is permissible to be in the same room; (3) no breastfeeding; (4) flushing toilets twice after urinating and washing hands thoroughly; (5) what to do if a sore throat or neck pain develops (may take acetaminophen or aspirin); and (6) notifying physician if nervousness, tremulousness, or palpitations increase.[23] Patients should be taught how to perform a self-thyroid examination.

Hyperthyroidism

DEFINITION/EPIDEMIOLOGY

Hyperthyroidism is defined as a clinical syndrome caused by the excess production or release of thyroid hormone and its clinical manifestations. Although the term *hyperthyroidism* implies that the thyroid is the source of excess thyroid hormone, *thyrotoxicosis* refers to the syndrome produced by excess thyroid hormone regardless of its source (e.g., overingestion of iodine). *Primary hyperthyroidism* is independent of TSH. TSH-dependent hyperthyroidism is called *secondary hyperthyroidism*.

TRH-dependent hyperthyroidism is referred to as tertiary hyperthyroidism. Graves' disease (autoimmune hyperthyroidism) is the most common cause of hyperthyroidism. There is a female-to-male predominance of 7:1, and it is most common in women aged 20 to 40 years. Transient hyperthyroidism (thyroiditis) needs to be excluded. Toxic multinodular goiters are usually seen in women >55 years old who have a long history of goiter. Multinodular goiters with autonomy are more susceptible to iodine-induced hyperthyroidism. Iodine sources include topical povidone-iodine (Betadine), IV contrast medium, and iodine-containing drugs. Postpartum thyroiditis (painless) occurs in approximately 5% to 9% of all pregnant women, 25% of pregnant women with type 1 diabetes, and 75% of women with high microsomal Ab titers before pregnancy.[24]

PATHOPHYSIOLOGY

Graves' disease is an autoimmune disorder in which thyroid-stimulating Ab (TSAbs) or immunoglobulins (TSIs) compete with TSH for TSH receptors on the thyroid and activate the production of cyclic adenosine monophosphate; this increases the synthesis and release of thyroid hormones. In whites, there is an increased prevalence of certain human leukocyte antigens (HLA-B8 and HLA-DR3).

Subacute thyroiditis is a postviral illness. The thyroid gland is tender, and there is evidence of multinucleated giant cells on microscopic evaluation. Silent thyroiditis (painless) is believed to be an autoimmune disorder. On microscopic examination, there is evidence of lymphocytic infiltration that may mimic Hashimoto's thyroiditis.

CLINICAL PRESENTATION AND PHYSICAL EXAMINATION

Because thyroid hormone acts on all organs, the clinical presentation is variable. The symptoms of hyperthyroidism are secondary to increased sympathetic activity and increased catabolism. Apathetic hyperthyroidism refers to patients who lack these symptoms. It is useful to describe the symptoms by organ system as shown in Table 230-1.

Lid lag may be seen with thyrotoxicosis, regardless of the origin of thyroid hormone. This symptom is caused by increased sympathetic activity. The other eye changes associated with Graves' disease are due to the action of TSIs on the connective tissue behind the eye. The NO SPECS mnemonic is used to describe the eye changes in association with Graves' disease, as follows:[24]

No signs or symptoms
Only signs, no symptoms
Soft tissue swelling
Proptosis
Extraocular muscle paresis
Corneal involvement
Sight loss (optic nerve involvement)

With subacute thyroiditis, the thyroid gland is tender, and patients often note a recent viral illness.

DIAGNOSTICS

TSH is the best screening test for primary hyperthyroidism. With primary hyperthyroidism, TSH levels will be low or undetectable. If the TSH is suppressed, a T_3U test (or any test of binding proteins) and T_4 levels should be obtained to determine the degree of hyperthyroidism. Alternatively, a free T_4 level can be obtained. TSH levels will remain suppressed for up to 3 months after treatment and therefore the free T_4 or free T_4 index must be followed. See Table 230-2 for laboratory results in different types of hyperthyroidism.

Abnormal liver function tests are common in patients with hyperthyroidism. Elevations in alkaline phosphatase, alanine aminotransferase (ALT), aspartate aminotransferase (AST), gamma glutamyltransferase (GGT), and total bilirubin levels

Diagnostics

Hyperthyroidism

Laboratory	Imaging
TSH	Radioactive iodine uptake scan*
T_4, free T_4	MRI*
Total T_3	

*If indicated.

TABLE 230-1 Signs and Symptoms of Hyperthyroidism

	Symptoms	Signs
Eyes	Dry eyes, blurry vision	See *NO SPECS* mnemonic (in text)
Neck	Diffuse goiter in patients with Graves' disease	Goiter with thyroid bruit in Graves' disease
Respiratory system	Shortness of breath	Labored respiration
Cardiac system	Palpitation, tachycardia, angina	Systolic hypertension, congestive heart failure, tachycardia, atrial fibrillation
Gastrointestinal system	Hyperphagia, hyperdefecation, weight loss, weight gain (rare), anorexia in older adults	Weight loss, weight gain (rare)
Reproductive system	Amenorrhea, menstrual irregularities, infertility	
Neuromuscular system	Proximal muscle weakness, heat intolerance, tremor	Proximal muscle weakness, hyperreflexia
Skin	Pruritus; hyperhidrosis; warm, moist palms; onycholysis (brittle nails, "Plummer's nails")	Smooth, velvety skin; warm, moist palms; onycholysis; pretibial myxedema (Graves' disease)
Skeletal system	Osteoporosis	Thyroid acropachy (Graves' disease)
Psychiatric problems	Anxiety, irritability, nervousness, sleeplessness	Visually manifest
Older adults	Anorexia, constipation, normal pulse, weight loss	

were found in a recent study in 33%, 17%, 26%, 24%, and 8% of patients, respectively.[25]

As shown in Table 230-3, a radioactive iodine uptake is useful in distinguishing Graves' disease from thyroiditis.

A scan is useful in identifying a toxic multinodular goiter or solitary nodular goiter. In patients with a diffusely enlarged gland and obvious signs of eye disease, this test is not necessary for diagnosis of Graves' disease but is needed for calculation of the radioactive iodine dose necessary if iodine ablation therapy is chosen. The erythrocyte sedimentation rate (ESR) will be increased in subacute thyroiditis. A careful review of iodine-containing medications is necessary in the evaluation of hyperthyroidism. With TSH-induced (secondary) hyperthyroidism, the TSH is inappropriately elevated in the setting of increased T_4 index. Pituitary adenomas are best visualized on MRI. With TSH adenomas, there is an increased ratio of TSH alpha subunit/TSH.

DIFFERENTIAL DIAGNOSIS

Differential diagnoses are described in the box at right. Another consideration, "hamburger thyrotoxicosis," refers to an epidemic of thyrotoxicosis in the Midwest that was eventually traced to the ingestion of hamburger meat that included the strap muscles of slaughtered cattle (including thyroid tissue). The U.S. Department of Agriculture now prohibits the use of this material.[26]

MANAGEMENT AND LIFE SPAN CONSIDERATIONS

The treatment of hyperthyroidism/thyrotoxicosis depends on the etiology of the disease and the patient's age. To simplify the discussion, the therapeutics are discussed by disease entity.

Graves' Disease

With Graves' disease, symptomatic treatment with beta blockers should be initiated to alleviate the beta adrenergic symptoms of hyperthyroidism (tremor, tachycardia). Propranolol (Inderal) can be used at doses between 10 mg and 40 mg PO every 6 hours. The dose is titrated to symptoms. Alternatively, longer-acting preparations can be used. They must be used with caution in patients with congestive heart failure and bronchospasm, and they should be avoided in pregnant women because of untoward effects on the fetus.

Medical therapy is the treatment of choice for patients younger than 20 years of age and for pregnant women. The thioamides (antithyroid drugs) include methimazole (Tapazole) and propylthiouracil (PTU). They inhibit thyroid hormone synthesis by blocking organification. In addition, PTU inhibits the peripheral conversion of T_4 to T_3. PTU is the drug of choice for pregnant women because it crosses the placenta less avidly. Thioamide therapy is described in Table 230-4 and Box 230-2.

Thioamides are generally believed to be the most effective in patients with Graves' disease and small glands. In general, they are used for 6 to 12 months and then discontinued; at that time, 30% of patients are in remission. Radioactive iodine ablation is

TABLE 230-2 Thyroid Function Tests in Hyperthyroidism

	T_3	T_4/Free T_4 Index	TSH
Graves' disease	Increase	Increase	Decrease
T_3 toxicosis	Increase	Normal	Decrease
T_4 toxicosis	Normal	Increase	Decrease
Subclinical hyperthyroidism	Normal	Normal	Decrease

TABLE 230-3 Radioactive Iodine Uptake in Different Forms of Hyperthyroidism

Decreased or Zero Radioactive Iodine Uptake	Normal or High Radioactive Iodine Uptake
Thyroiditis (subacute, painless)	Graves' disease
Iodine-induced hyperthyroidism	Toxic nodule
Exogenous etiology of hyperthyroidism	Toxic multinodular goiter
Struma ovarii	TSH-induced hyperthyroidism
Metastatic thyroid cancer postthyroidectomy	HCG-induced hyperthyroidism

HCG, Human chorionic gonadotropin.

Differential Diagnosis

Hyperthyroidism

Thyroid Disorders
- Graves' disease
- Transient hyperthyroidism
  - Subacute thyroiditis
  - Hashimoto's thyroiditis
  - Silent (lymphocytic) thyroiditis (postpartum)
- Toxic multinodular goiter
- Toxic adenoma (toxic nodular goiter)
- Exogenous (factious) hyperthyroidism
- Iodine-induced hyperthyroidism (Jod-Basedow phenomenon) (amiodarone)
- Hydatidiform mole, HCG-induced hyperthyroidism
- TSH-secreting pituitary adenoma
- Ectopic thyroxine production
  - Struma ovarii and metastatic follicular thyroid carcinoma postthyroidectomy
- Hereditary familial hyperthyroidism (activating mutation for TSH receptor)

Nonthyroid Disorders
- Anxiety
- Pheochromocytoma
- Menopause
- Pregnancy
- Metastatic carcinoma
- Cirrhosis
- Hyperparathyroidism
- Sprue
- Myasthenia gravis
- Muscular dystrophy

TABLE 230-4 Thioamide Therapy

	Propylthiouracil	Methimazole
Dosage	50-100 mg PO q 6-8 hr	5-20 mg PO q 8 hr, or 15-60 mg/day PO
Tablets	50 mg	5 mg, 10 mg
Protein binding	75%	0%
Half-life	75 minutes	4-6 hours
Placental passage	1:1	High
Breast milk concentration	Low	High
Advantages	Inhibits conversion of T_4 to T_3; safer in pregnancy	Long half-life

BOX 230-2

SIDE EFFECTS OF THIOAMIDES

- Agranulocytosis occurs in 0.2% to 0.5% of patients; usually reversible with discontinuation of medication
  Baseline CBC and differential should be obtained before initiation of treatment. Patients should be instructed to discontinue medications and call their primary care provider immediately if there are symptoms of infection (e.g., fever, pharyngitis); a CBC and differential should be obtained.
- Rash, arthralgias, myalgias (lupuslike reaction), fever (3% to 5% of patients)
- Transient, PTU-induced subclinical liver injury; need for baseline LFTs should be questioned
- Nephrotic syndrome (methimazole) (rare)
- Aplastic anemia, thrombocytopenia (rare)

generally recommended if relapse occurs. The initial clinical response may lag for 2 weeks given the increased stored thyroid hormone. TFTs are monitored every 4 to 6 weeks until the results are stable. TSH levels may remain suppressed for months, and therefore the T_4 index (or free T_4) should be followed. In pregnant women, this index should be kept at the high-normal range because of the effect of thioamides in inhibiting the fetal thyroid gland.

Radioactive iodine therapy is the treatment of choice in the United States for patients >20 years old and for those for whom thioamide therapy has failed (through noncompliance or a relapse after treatment). It is contraindicated during pregnancy and should be avoided in patients with Graves' ophthalmopathy because of the increased risk of exacerbation of eye symptoms after treatment. There is no evidence of increased incidence of long-term malignancies. Because there is a high incidence of post-treatment hypothyroidism, TFTs should be followed closely. Approximately 4 to 6 weeks after treatment, the T_4 index should be checked, and the patient should be reevaluated. If there is no evidence of hypothyroidism at that time, TSH and T_4 index should be followed monthly for 3 to 4 months and then periodically.

Surgery is recommended for pregnant women who cannot be managed with PTU or who develop side effects from it, for patients who refuse radioactive iodine and cannot tolerate thioamides, and for patients with an obstructive goiter. Complications include hypothyroidism, hypoparathyroidism, and hoarseness (recurrent laryngeal nerve damage).

Other much less commonly used medications include cholestyramine (which decreases enterohepatic circulation of thyroid hormone), organic iodides (amiodarone and ipodate, which block T_4 to T_3), lithium and iodides (which block hormone release), and glucocorticoids (which block the conversion of T_4 to T_3).

Thyroiditis

Thyroiditis may be subacute or painless or may be a result of a toxic nodule or toxic multinodular goiter. Hyperthyroid findings may result.

Subacute Thyroiditis. With subacute thyroiditis, symptomatic treatment with beta blockers can be used during the hyperthyroid phase. Different studies have shown relief of pain with the use of NSAIDs, aspirin, and glucocorticoids. Hyperthyroidism lasts for weeks to months and is followed by hypothyroidism (which lasts for months). Most patients become euthyroid, although 30% may remain hypothyroid. Recurrences are rare.

Painless (Postpartum) Thyroiditis. With painless postpartum thyroiditis, symptomatic treatment with beta blockers can be used during the hyperthyroid phase. Beta blockers are concentrated in breast milk and must be used with caution. Thyroid hormone therapy can be initiated if hypothyroid phase is severe. TFTs should be monitored closely. Although most patients become clinically euthyroid, up to 30% remain hypothyroid. This condition tends to recur with subsequent pregnancies.

Toxic Nodule. With toxic nodules, radioactive iodine ablation is the treatment of choice after beta blocker therapy. Some studies demonstrate effective therapy with alcohol ablation through repetitive percutaneous injections under ultrasound guidance. Surgical excision is another option, especially in patients with a large adenoma.

Toxic Multinodular Goiter. With toxic multinodular goiter, radioactive iodine ablation is the treatment of choice after beta blocker therapy. Other nodules may become toxic in the future and may require repeat doses of ^{131}I. Other treatment options include antithyroid drugs followed by subtotal thyroidectomy.

COMPLICATIONS

Untreated Graves' disease can lead to atrial fibrillation, congestive heart failure, angina, and osteoporosis. Thyroid storm is a rare, life-threatening form of hyperthyroidism that leads to systemic decompensation. The incidence has declined during the past few decades because of advances in medical management, but thyrotoxic crises account for approximately 1% of all hospitalizations for hyperthyroidism. Although it more commonly occurs with Graves' disease, it can be found in conjunction with other causes of hyperthyroidism.

INDICATIONS FOR REFERRAL/HOSPITALIZATION

Primary care providers can perform the initial evaluation for hyperthyroidism. Laboratory confirmation of hyperthyroidism and radioactive iodine scans should be obtained. Thioamides can be administered by practitioners who are experienced with their use. Treatment options can be discussed with patients; if radioactive iodine therapy is selected, a consultation with an endocrinologist should be obtained. An endocrinologist and an ophthalmologist should see patients with Graves' ophthalmopathy.

Patients with thyroid storm require hospitalization and should be evaluated by an endocrinologist or by a physician familiar with its treatment. Thyroid storm, or thyrotoxic crisis, requires aggressive inpatient management. The diagnosis is based on clinical findings: temperature of 38.8° to 40.5° C (102° to 105° F), profuse sweating, pulse >120 to 140 beats per minute, atrial fibrillation, restlessness, confusion, agitation, and coma. Gastrointestinal symptoms may include severe vomiting, diarrhea, and hepatomegaly with jaundice. The goals of therapy are to inhibit thyroid hormone formation and release, provide beta adrenergic blockade, provide supportive therapy, identify and treat any precipitating illness, and initiate long-term therapy to prevent further episodes of thyroid storm.

PATIENT AND FAMILY EDUCATION

Patients should understand the symptoms and treatment of hyperthyroidism and should be instructed in the "danger signs" of thyroid storm. If receiving beta blockers, they are instructed to monitor their pulse and contact their primary care physician if their pulse is <50 (or 40 if baseline heart rate is low) or >120 beats per minute.

Patients receiving thioamides should be cautioned about the rare but serious effects of agranulocytosis. They should discontinue thioamide therapy if they have signs of infection and a temperature higher than 38.3° C (101° F). Patients should be advised to call their primary care provider and have a CBC and differential blood count performed to exclude agranulocytosis. TFTs should be followed closely during pregnancy. Women with Graves' disease who have received radioactive iodine ablation in the past should be advised that TSIs could still cross the placenta. They should inform their obstetricians that they have Graves' disease so that the fetal thyroid and heart rate can be followed closely.

Hypothyroidism

DEFINITION/EPIDEMIOLOGY

Hypothyroidism is a condition resulting from the synthesis of thyroid hormone that is insufficient to meet bodily needs. It is the most common disorder of the thyroid gland. This condition usually occurs in the setting of primary hypothyroidism whereby diseases or treatments destroy thyroid tissue or prevalent conditions interfere with thyroid hormone biosynthesis. Rarely it is caused by inadequate thyroidal stimulation by TSH, which is referred to as *central* or *secondary hypothyroidism*.

If hypothyroidism is congenital or occurs during infancy or childhood, growth and development are slowed and may result in mental retardation, a condition known as *cretinism*.

In adulthood, untreated hypothyroidism results in decreased metabolic function and in the deposition of hydrophilic mucopolysaccharides in the skin and other tissues, which results in fluid and sodium retention and impairment of blood circulation and lymphatic drainage. Progressive and severe hypothyroidism with skin thickening and cardiovascular and renal manifestations is known as *myxedema*.[27]

Hypothyroidism is found in 2% of women and 0.2% of men. The prevalence increases with age, with 6% of women and 2.5% of men >60 years old having this condition. Subclinical hypothyroidism may occur in as many as 15% of persons 60 years of age or older. It has been found that, in 20% to 40% of patients, subclinical hypothyroidism progresses to overt hypothyroidism within 4 years.[28,29]

Appropriate thyroid hormone biosynthesis is dependent on dietary intake of iodides and on various geographic and environmental factors that may affect a population's ability to obtain the recommended daily allowance of iodine. In the United States, adequate dietary sources of iodine have been established to prevent iodine deficiency disorders, which may manifest as hypothyroidism or goiter. Mountainous areas such as the Himalayas and Andes or lowlands far from the ocean such as central Africa and parts of Europe are important goitrous areas in the world today.[6]

Previous irradiation for head and neck cancers may put a patient at increased risk of developing hypothyroidism. Radioactive treatment with ^{131}I therapy for hyperthyroid disorders results in hypothyroidism in most cases. Subtotal or total thyroidectomy will render a patient hypothyroid.

The most common cause of primary hypothyroidism is chronic autoimmune thyroiditis. This may take atrophic or goitrous forms. When autoimmune thyroiditis co-exists with a goiter, the condition is called Hashimoto's thyroiditis. It is believed to be a familial autoimmune condition in which the lymphocytes become sensitized to an individual's own thyroid antigens, resulting in the formation of autoantibodies. The autoantibodies react with the thyroid antigens and destroy functional tissue. This manifests itself as an increase in TSH and the presence of antithyroid Abs, including antimicrosomal Abs, anti-TPO Abs, and anti-Tg Abs. Eventually there is a drop in serum T_4 and then T_3. Younger patients most often present with goiter, whereas older patients may have more severe disease and a small (atrophic) gland.

Transient primary hypothyroidism may be encountered during the postpartum period, 2 to 6 months after delivery. This condition may be preceded by a brief period of hyperthyroidism and can result in permanent thyroid failure. Postinfectious thyroiditis may follow a similar course. A sentinel viral upper respiratory tract infection followed by an inflamed, large tender thyroid gland, and transient hyperthyroidism followed by transient or permanent hypothyroidism is the usual observed sequence of events.

Drugs with antithyroid action such as lithium, amiodarone, iodine, and radiographic contrast may cause hypothyroidism. The drug effect may be transient during the period of use or may result in permanent thyroid failure. Patients with underlying chronic autoimmune thyroiditis living in iodine-sufficient geographic areas are more susceptible to hypothyroidism when taking iodine or iodine-containing drugs.

Pituitary (or secondary) causes of hypothyroidism are not common and are usually associated with other signs of pituitary hormone insufficiency. Patients with a history of pituitary disease or tumor may be at risk for thyroid hyposecretion.

PATHOPHYSIOLOGY

There are many effects of thyroid hormone deficiency. Cardiac and metabolic consequences include impaired myocardial contractility, cardiomegaly, impaired lipid metabolism with accelerated atherosclerosis, hypertension, depressed ventilatory drive and fatigue, impaired energy utilization, and weight gain. Altered kidney and gastrointestinal performance include a reduction in glomerular filtration rate (GFR) and hyponatremia, hypomotility, and constipation respectively. Musculoskeletal effects include an increased volume of muscle and slowness of contraction leading to myopathic disorders and connective tissue thickening. This can lead to entrapment neuropathies such as carpal tunnel syndrome. In children, delayed skeletal maturation may cause growth retardation. Impaired cellular function in the brain may cause depression or psychiatric disability, and diminished erythropoiesis results in anemia.[6]

Characteristic myxedematous changes seen in untreated advanced disease are largely a result of deposition of hydrophilic mucopolysaccharides, especially hyaluronic acid, in the interstitial tissues. The hydrophilic nature of the mucopolysaccharides and increased capillary permeability to albumin create interstitial edema of heart muscle, striated muscle, and skin.

CLINICAL PRESENTATION

Presentation may range from subclinical hypothyroidism (with an asymptomatic TSH elevation) to overt myxedema (with slowed mentation and visible symptoms). The most common presenting symptom is fatigue. There may also be increased sensitivity to cold, weight gain, hoarseness, puffiness of the face and hands, heavy and irregular menstrual periods, dry skin, dry and brittle hair, depression, paresthesias, muscle aches, and constipation. A careful history will elicit the severity and duration of these symptoms. Goiter may or may not be present. Women are 5 to 7 times more likely to be affected than men, and more women present with goiter. Symptoms may be more vague and subtle in older adults and include deafness, confusion, dementia, and ataxia.

PHYSICAL EXAMINATION

The physical examination should focus on the patient's general appearance and degree of energy and animation. Any lethargy or slowness of mentation should be noted. Assessment of physical appearance includes texture, color, and general appearance of the skin. Facial expression and the texture and thickness of the hair should be noted; the patient's voice, which may be deepened, and pulse, which may be slowed, should also be assessed.

The thyroid gland may be large or small on examination and should be evaluated carefully for the presence or absence of nodules. Tenderness of the gland is suggestive of a subacute thyroiditis, whereas a nontender gland is more suggestive of chronic autoimmune thyroiditis. A rubbery, firm, symmetric goiter is characteristic of Hashimoto's thyroiditis. Deep tendon reflexes should be evaluated. Any delay in the relaxation phase, which may be most noticeable in the Achilles' tendon, should be noted. The patient's weight should be documented and compared with previous weights to determine if there has been any weight gain. Heart rate and respiratory rate should also be noted and documented.

The presence of headache or visual impairment may suggest secondary hypothyroidism, as may any other features of pituitary hormone excess or deficiencies. Postural hypotension may indicate coexistent endocrine deficiencies such as autoimmune adrenal insufficiency, as seen in Schmidt's syndrome.

DIAGNOSTICS

An ECG examination may reveal low-voltage QRS complexes and P and T waves, as well as cardiac enlargement. This may result from both dilation and pericardial effusion. Bradycardia is usually present, and diastolic blood pressure may be elevated. Respirations may be slow and shallow with advanced disease. Bowel sounds may be diminished and deep tendon reflexes slowed in the relaxation phase. Mentation may also be slowed, and the patient may appear lethargic and expressionless. Occasionally, severe depression or agitation results.

Laboratory tests reveal an elevated TSH level, which may precede symptoms or alterations in thyroid hormones. This condition is referred to as *subclinical hypothyroidism*. More advanced hypothyroidism shows low serum levels of free T_4 and a low free T_4 index. TRH testing to evaluate TSH response and therefore hypothalamic function is rarely used since the introduction of the third generation TSH. Anti-TPO Ab levels will be elevated in patients with chronic autoimmune thyroiditis. Patients often demonstrate a mild normocytic, normochromic anemia. If menstrual periods are heavy, the anemia may be microcytic. If vitamin B_{12} deficiency is present, the anemia may be macrocytic. Hypercholesterolemia may also be present.

Imaging studies are unnecessary for chronic autoimmune thyroiditis. If used, the findings may be misleading. The pattern of uptake with goitrous autoimmune thyroiditis may be variable, whereas uptake may be low with atrophic thyroiditis. An ultrasound examination may be indicated to verify the presence of a suspected nodule. FNAB may be necessary to evaluate a suspicious nodule or rapidly enlarging goiter.

DIFFERENTIAL DIAGNOSIS

Chronic autoimmune thyroiditis is differentiated from other causes of hypothyroidism by the presence of thyroid Abs. TSH levels will distinguish primary hypothyroidism from secondary causes.

Serum TBG concentrations affect serum T_4 concentrations and may mask the diagnosis of hypothyroidism. Certain drugs, such as estrogen, 5-fluorouracil, methadone, clofibrate, heroin, and tamoxifen, may increase TT_4 through increased TBG binding. Other drugs, including androgens, phenytoin, furosemide, salicylates, and corticosteroids, may decrease TT_4 by decreasing TBG binding. A normal TSH level in the presence of these findings would confirm drug effect as long as there are no symptoms of pituitary involvement.

Diagnostics

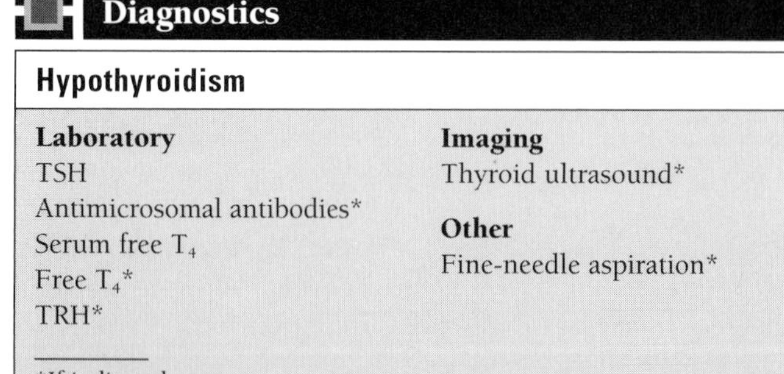

Hypothyroidism

Laboratory	Imaging
TSH	Thyroid ultrasound*
Antimicrosomal antibodies*	**Other**
Serum free T_4	Fine-needle aspiration*
Free T_4*	
TRH*	

*If indicated.

Differential Diagnosis

Hypothyroidism

Chronic autoimmune thyroiditis	Postsurgical causation
Postpartum thyroiditis	Idiopathic hypothyroidism
Radiation-induced thyroid damage	Pituitary tumor
Postinfection thyroiditis	Hypothalamic dysfunction
Medication-induced hypothyroidism (amiodarone, lithium, iodide)	Nephrotic syndrome
	Chronic nephritis
	Depression

MANAGEMENT

Hypothyroidism is treated with levothyroxine orally in amounts that return the TSH to normal levels. The desired amount is determined by the measurements of TSH and by subjective clinical criteria. The dosage necessary to achieve metabolic homeostasis is usually 1.6 μg/kg/day. Supplementation may begin with an initial dosage of 50 μg/day, with the dosage increased at 4- to 6-week intervals to 100 μg/day. In patients <30 or 40 years old with no history of other medical problems, the initial dosage of thyroxine can be 100 μg/day. Patients with ischemic heart disease or atrial fibrillation (and older patients in whom these conditions may become apparent with treatment) should start at 25 μg/day and increase by 25 μg/day every 8 weeks. An euthyroid effect is usually achieved in 4 to 6 weeks after the onset of full-dose therapy and can be adjusted, if necessary, according to TSH determinations. This daily dosage is then monitored once or twice a year to maintain a normal TSH. Estrogen administration leads to an increase in TBG levels and thus may increase thyroxine requirements in patients with hypothyroidism.[30]

Subclinical Hypothyroidism

Elevated TSH in the presence of normal thyroid hormone levels in asymptomatic patients is called *subclinical hypothyroidism* or *mild thyroid failure*. It is important to determine if the patient has goiter, a history of prior treatment for hypothyroidism, antithyroid Abs, or hypercholesterolemia. Treatment seems warranted in the presence of these conditions. Patients with subtle symptoms such as infertility, menstrual cycle irregularities, depression, and fatigue may also benefit from replacement therapy. Levothyroxine supplementation for subclinical hypothyroidism is recommended at 1.0 μg/kg/day (50 to 75 μg) and is directed toward reducing serum TSH to normal levels. Patients without any of these symptoms and with a TSH of <10 mU/ml may be monitored at yearly intervals with a TSH for progression of thyroid failure.[31]

LIFE SPAN CONSIDERATIONS

Older adults and those with known heart disease should be started at 25 μg/day of levothyroxine and increased gradually. This careful administration prevents arrhythmias, angina, and the other cardiac symptoms that may be precipitated by starting at a full daily dose. After the dose has been stabilized, annual TSH measurements are desirable. Patients should understand that supplementation is lifelong, not short term. Given the high prevalence of hypothyroidism in women >60 years of age and the presence of subtle symptoms, TSH screening is recommended in this age-group.

Patients with known hypothyroidism require close monitoring during pregnancy. A TSH should be measured during the prenatal evaluation and in every trimester thereafter. Most often thyroid hormone requirements increase during pregnancy and close monitoring will ensure appropriate levothyroxine replacement doses. Evidence has emerged that suggests intrauterine fetal development can be adversely affected in the setting of untreated hypothyroidism.[32]

Smoking has been found to impair both thyroid hormone secretion and thyroid hormone action. It may contribute to the incidence of subclinical hypothyroidism and may aggravate the clinical manifestations of overt hypothyroidism; therefore smoking cessation is advised.[33]

COMPLICATIONS

Myxedema coma, a hypothermic stuporous state that may be characterized by respiratory depression and eventually death, results from untreated hypothyroidism. It may be triggered by environmental stressors such as cold exposure or trauma and by internal stressors such as infection or medications that depress the central nervous system. These patients may require IV levothyroxine as well as glucocorticoid therapy for any coexistent adrenal insufficiency. Warming for the hypothermia, ventilation support for the respiratory depression, and treatment of any renal and electrolyte imbalances are necessary.

In patients with underlying coronary disease, angina and arrhythmias may be a complication of therapy and a cause for concern. Some patients also experience palpitations after starting levothyroxine, especially if other medications are added. This is particularly true of stimulants such as caffeine and pseudoephedrine.

Long-term, marked overtreatment with thyroxine can result in symptoms of hyperthyroidism. It can also result in bone resorption with significant decreases in bone mineral density.

INDICATIONS FOR REFERRAL/HOSPITALIZATION

Referral to a surgeon may be necessary for a large goiter that is obstructive. Referral to an endocrinologist may be necessary if there is a solitary nodule requiring biopsy or if regulation of medication is difficult. Persistent symptoms and a normal TSH level or suspicion for secondary hypothyroidism should also prompt an endocrine referral. Hospitalization may be warranted if any of the previously mentioned conditions are severe. Usually, clinical or subclinical hypothyroidism can be managed on an outpatient basis.

PATIENT AND FAMILY EDUCATION AND HEALTH PROMOTION

The most important aspect of patient education is communicating to the patient and the family that levothyroxine replacement is a permanent and necessary treatment that cannot be discontinued. Patients should be encouraged not to increase their daily dosage with out medical supervision, informed not to double the next dose if one is skipped, and advised that osteoporosis is a possible consequence of high doses. They should also understand that annual or biannual monitoring of TSH helps ensure that the medication dosage remains accurate.

Euthyroid Sick Syndrome

The *euthyroid sick syndrome* (sick euthyroidism) refers to thyroid function abnormalities in a critically ill euthyroid individual. It is characterized by hypothalamic suppression of TSH release, acute inhibition of peripheral conversion of T_4 to T_3, and an increased conversion of T_4 to rT_3. This results in low TSH levels, decreased levels of T_3 (low T_3 syndrome), and increased levels of rT_3. Euthyroid sick syndrome is seen during carbohydrate restriction, liver disease, or severe acute or chronic illness. Patients with the low free T_4 levels in addition to low T_3

TABLE 230-5 Euthyroid Sick Syndrome

	T_3	T_4	Free T_4	rT_3	TSH
Low T_3 syndrome	Decrease	Normal or increase	Normal or increase	Increase	Low
Low T_4, T_3 syndrome	Decrease	Decrease	Normal	Increase	Low

levels are severely ill and have an increased mortality rate. Total T_4 levels can be decreased even initially because of the liberation of fatty acids from ischemic or injured cells, which inhibits the binding of T_4 to TBG. A summary of laboratory tests during acute illness is provided in Table 230-5. These abnormalities resolve when the patient recovers. The TSH level rises to normal or higher than normal levels during the recovery phase; the changes are thought to be a protective adaptation to severe illness. Therapy with T_4 or T_3 has not been shown to improve outcomes and may actually worsen the situation. Given this syndrome, TFTs should not be checked in critically ill patients unless thyroid dysfunction is strongly suspected. If TFTs are checked, TSH alone does not suffice. TFTs should be interpreted in context of the current clinical scenario and time frame of illness.

Drugs and the Thyroid Gland

Pharmacologic agents may cause thyroid dysfunction or abnormalities in TFTs. The most important examples are discussed in this section.

Amiodarone is an iodine-rich pharmacologic agent used in the management of cardiac arrhythmias. It is highly lipophilic and concentrates in the thyroid gland, heart muscles, and adipose tissue. It therefore has a very long half-life, and effects on the thyroid gland can be seen up to 2 to 3 years after discontinuation of the drug. Like iodine or radiographic contrast, its effects on the thyroid gland can be variable depending on the presence of underlying autoimmune disease and the geographic iodine availability. Individuals with chronic autoimmune thyroiditis or living in iodine-sufficient areas are more likely to develop hypothyroidism when exposed to iodinated agents, whereas patients with a multinodular goiter or those residing in iodine deficient areas may be more likely to develop hyperthyroidism.[34]

Hypothyroidism is the more common thyroid disorder in patients taking amiodarone in the United States. This condition is effectively treated with LT4 replacement therapy and does not necessitate the discontinuation of amiodarone. Goals of therapy include the establishment of a high-normal TSH level and a mid- to low-normal free T_4 level.

When thyrotoxicosis develops in the setting of amiodarone, it could be caused by thyroiditis (type 1), in which the thyroid gland is inflamed, or hyperthyroidism (type 2), in which there is overactivity of the thyroid gland. Treatment ultimately depends on the nature of the disease; such cases can be diagnostically challenging and difficult to manage. Amiodarone should be discontinued. Measurement of cytokines and thyroid Abs as well as thyroid ultrasound may be helpful in differentiating these two types. Type 1 thyroiditis is treated with oral steroids, and type 2 hyperthyroidism is treated with antithyroid drugs. Ultimately, surgery may be needed in either type if thyrotoxicosis is refractory to medical intervention.

Ideally, before starting amiodarone therapy, baseline TFTs and the presence of thyroid Abs should be documented. Underlying thyroid disease and a family history of thyroid disorders should be noted; this would place the patient at increased risk of thyroid dysfunction on this drug and would alert clinicians to this possibility. TFTs should be checked at 3-month intervals after start of the medication.[34]

Interferon alpha is used in the treatment of hepatitis viruses B and C or malignant disease. Use of this agent can induce the production of thyroid Abs, resulting in hypothyroidism or thyrotoxicosis or a biphasic thyroiditis. With discontinuation of this agent, these Abs often disappear.[6]

Lithium, as used in the treatment of psychiatric conditions such as bipolar depression, can induce thyroid dysfunction. It blocks the uptake of iodine and the release of thyroid hormone and can induce chronic autoimmune thyroiditis. Clinical or subclinical hypothyroidism or a goiter in an euthyroid patient is within the spectrum of lithium-induced thyroid disease.[6]

TFT abnormalities, including a low TSH, low TT_3, and an elevated rT_3 level, are noted in patients on steroids and pressor agents. Similar abnormalities in T_3 and rT_3 are noted with amiodarone. Much like in sick euthyroid syndrome, these agents block the formation of T_3 from T_4 and most of T_4 is shunted into the formation of rT_3.

REFERENCES

1. Wang C, Crapo LM: Epidemiology of thyroid disease and implications for screening, *Endocrinol Metab Clin North Am* 26:189-219, 1997.
2. Surks MI, Ocampio E: Subclinical thyroid disease, *Am J Med* 100: 217-223, 1996.
3. DeGroot LJ and others: *The thyroid and its diseases*, New York, 1996, Churchill Livingstone.
4. Siminoski K: Does this patient have a goiter? *JAMA* 273:813-817, 1995.
5. Wallace C, Siminoski K: The Pemberton sign, *Ann Intern Med* 125: 568-569, 1996.
6. Braverman LE, Utiger RD: *Werner & Ingbar's the thyroid: a fundamental and clinical text*, ed 8, New York, 2000, Lippincott-Raven.
7. Toft A: Drug therapy: thyroxine therapy, *N Engl J Med* 331:174-180, 1994.
8. Mandel S and others: Levothyroxine therapy in patients with thyroid disease, *Ann Intern Med* 119:492-502, 1993.
9. Huysmans DA and others: Large, compressive goiters treated with radioiodine, *Ann Intern Med* 121:757-762, 1994.
10. Nygaard B and others: Radioiodine treatment of multinodular non-toxic goiter, *Br Med J* 307:828-832, 1993.
11. Vander JB, Gaston EA, Dawber TR: Significance of solitary non-toxic thyroid nodules, *N Engl J Med* 251:970, 1954.
12. Mortensen D, Woolner LB, Bennett WA: Gross and microscopic findings in clinically normal thyroid glands, *J Clin Endocrinol Metab* 15:1270, 1955.

13. Hedinger C, Williams ED, Sabin LH: The WHO histological classification of thyroid tumors: a commentary on the second edition, *Cancer* 63:908-911, 1989.
14. Belfiore A and others: High frequency of cancer in cold thyroid nodules; occurring at young age, *Acta Endocrinol* 121:197-202, 1989.
15. Belfiore A and others: Cancer risk in patients with cold thyroid nodules: relevance of iodine intake, sex, age, and multinodularity, *Am Med* 93:363-369, 1992.
16. Schneider AB and others: Radiation-induced tumors of the head and neck following childhood irradiation, *Medicine* 64:1-15, 1985.
17. Singer PA and others: Treatment guidelines for patients with thyroid nodules and well-differentiated thyroid cancer, *Arch Intern Med* 156:2165-2172, 1996.
18. Blum M, Yee J: Advances in thyroid imaging: thyroid sonography; when and how should it be used? *Thyroid Today* 3:1-13, 1977.
19. Lucas A and others: Fine-needle aspiration cytology of benign thyroid disease: value of re-aspiration, *Eur J Endocrinol* 132:677-680, 1995.
20. Ross DS: Thyroid hormone suppressive therapy of sporadic nontoxic goiter, *Thyroid* 2:263-269, 1992.
21. Heshmati H and others: Advances and controversies in the diagnosis and management of medullary thyroid carcinoma, *Am J Med* 103:60, 1997.
22. Degroot LJ, Larsen PR, Hennemann G: *The thyroid and its diseases,* New York, 1996, Churchill Livingstone.
23. Singer PA and others: Treatment guidelines for patients with hyperthyroidism and hypothyroidism, *JAMA* 273:808-812, 1995.
24. Gerstein H: Incidence of postpartum thyroid dysfunction in patients with type I diabetes mellitus, *Ann Intern Med* 118:419-423, 1993.
25. Biscoveanu M, Hasinski S: Abnormal results of liver function tests in patients with Graves' disease, *Endocrine Practice* 6:367-369, 2000.
26. Hedberg CW and others: An outbreak of thyrotoxicosis caused by the consumption of bovine thyroid gland in ground beef, *N Engl J Med* 316:993-998, 1987.
27. Hierholzer K, Finke R: Myxedema, *Kidney Int Suppl* 59:582-589, 1997.
28. Lindsay R, Toft A: Hypothyroidism, *Lancet* 349:413-417, 1997.
29. Dayan C, Daniels G: Medical progress: chronic autoimmune thyroiditis, *N Engl J Med* 335:99-107, 1996.
30. Arafah BM: Increased need for thyroxine in women with hypothyroidism during estrogen therapy, *N Engl J Med* 344:1743-1749, 2001.
31. Cooper, David S: Subclinical hypothyroidism, *N Engl J Med* 345: 260-265, 2001.
32. Haddow J and others: Maternal thyroid deficiency during pregnancy and subsequent neuropsychological development of the child, *N Engl J Med* 341:549-555, 1999.
33. Muller B and others: Impaired action of thyroid hormone associated with smoking in women with hypothyroidism, *N Engl J Med* 333:964-969, 1995.
34. Martino E and others: The effects of amiodarone on the thyroid, *Endocrine Rev* 22:240-254, 2001.

PART 18

Evaluation and Management of Hematologic Disorders

JOANNE SANDBERG-COOK, Section Editor

CHAPTER 231

Anemia

Elyse Mandell

DEFINITION/EPIDEMIOLOGY

Anemia is not a disease but rather a sign of an underlying disorder. Anemia, defined as a reduction in hematocrit or hemoglobin concentration, is not a disease but is a sign of an underlying disorder. In general, a hematocrit less than 40% or a hemoglobin concentration less than 14 g/dl for men and a hematocrit less than 37% or a hemoglobin concentration less than 12 g/dl for women suggests anemia.[1] Although certain signs and symptoms are sometimes associated with anemia, the diagnosis is often based on laboratory data alone.

PATHOPHYSIOLOGY

Erythropoiesis, the production of erythrocytes (red blood cells [RBCs]), occurs in the bone marrow of the sternum, ribs, vertebrae, pelvis, and proximal ends of the femur and humerus. Anemia results from either an underproduction of erythrocytes (also referred to as ineffective erythropoiesis) or an increased rate of their destruction. (The reader is referred to any comprehensive hematology textbook for a more detailed discussion of erythropoiesis and the pathophysiology of anemia.) Conditions or diseases that can cause hematologic disorders include dietary deficiencies, malabsorption problems, drug toxicities, metabolic disorders, blood loss (either acute or chronic), infection, malignancies, genetic disorders, and immunologic defects.[2]

CLINICAL PRESENTATION

The presentation of anemia can be quite variable, depending on the acuteness of onset and the cardiopulmonary system's ability to compensate for the anemia. If the patient is healthy and the onset of anemia is gradual, there are few signs or symptoms until the hematocrit value falls below 30%. At this point patients may begin to experience dyspnea and a mild decrease in exercise tolerance. A further reduction in hematocrit (<20% to 25%) may be associated with a markedly reduced exercise capacity, resting tachycardia, and a systolic flow murmur. Other nonspecific complaints that can accompany a moderate to severe anemia include headache, tinnitus, poor concentration, palpitations, spoon-shaped nails, brittle nails, glossitis, angular cheilitis, papillary atrophy of the tongue, poor skin turgor, anorexia, nausea, and diarrhea or constipation. Pallor of the mucous membranes of the mouth, lips, conjunctiva, nail beds, and palmar skin creases is a common sign of anemia but is of little help in judging its severity.[3]

DIAGNOSTICS

Diagnostic evaluation includes a CBC and a variety of standard tests. The reticulocyte count is the most accessible method of evaluating bone marrow production of RBCs (a direct bone marrow examination requires an invasive procedure). Reticulocytes are immature RBCs that, once released into the circulation, mature in 2 to 3 days. Normally, these cells account for less than 2% of the total RBC count.[1] Reticulocytes are larger than mature RBCs; thus conditions with increased reticulocyte counts may have slightly elevated mean corpuscular volume (MCV) and RBC size distribution width (RDW). A low reticulocyte count reflects decreased bone marrow activity (i.e., decreased RBC production). A high reticulocyte count (reticulocytosis) reflects the bone marrow's attempt to replace cells lost or prematurely destroyed. Box 231-1 identifies conditions associated with either reticulocytosis or a decreased reticulocyte count.

A hemoglobin electrophoresis allows hemoglobin chains to be separated according to differences in the charges of their subunits. It is essential for accurate diagnosis of thalassemias and hemoglobinopathies.

Other commonly used tests are related to evaluating the body's iron stores. They include serum ferritin, serum iron, total iron binding capacity (TIBC), and the percentage of transferrin saturation. These tests are essential for differentiating the etiology of a microcytic anemia.

The serum ferritin level reflects total body iron stores. It is the first laboratory value to become abnormal when iron stores are becoming depleted, even before iron deficiency anemia is reflected in RBC morphology. The serum ferritin is directly proportional to iron stores: each nanogram per milliliter of serum ferritin reflects 8 to 10 mg of stored iron.[4] Normal values are 12 to 150 μg/L for women and 10 to 345 μg/L for men.[1] Serum ferritin levels are low in iron deficiency anemia, and normal or elevated in anemia of chronic disease. Serum ferritin is also elevated in conditions unrelated to anemia such as iron overload (either transfusion-dependent or hereditary hemochromatosis), inflammatory disorders, and alcoholism.

The serum iron reflects the amount of iron bound to transferrin, a plasma carrier protein that regulates iron transport in the blood. Normal values for serum iron are 40 to 150 μg/dl for women and 40 to 160 μg/dl for men. The transferrin level is measured indirectly as the TIBC. The TIBC indicates the availability of binding sites on the protein for iron transport. Normal values for TIBC are 250 to 450 μg/dl (for both women and men).

Diagnostics

Anemias

Laboratory
CBC and differential
Peripheral smear
Reticulocyte count
Ferritin*
TIBC*
Transferrin*
Serum iron*
Stool for occult blood × 3*
Hemoglobin electrophoresis*
Folate*
B_{12}*
LFTs*
TFTs*
BUN*
Creatinine*
G6PD assay*
Erythropoietin level*
Serum hemocysteine*
Methylmalonic acid*
Coombs' direct and indirect tests*

Other
Bone marrow biopsy*

*If indicated.

The percentage of transferrin saturation can be calculated from the TIBC and the serum iron values:

$$\frac{\text{Serum iron}}{\text{TIBC}} \times 100$$

Normal values for percentage of transferrin saturation are 20% to 50%.

Most mild to moderate anemias are usually asymptomatic and are found incidentally on a routine CBC. If data from the patient's history and physical examination suggest an anemia, however, the initial laboratory tests should include a CBC with differential, reticulocyte count, and peripheral smear examination of RBC morphology. These results indicate the need for further tests.

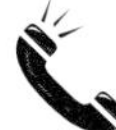

Physician consultation is recommended for hematocrit values less than 30% in patients with known coronary artery disease, and for any patient with postural vital sign changes or active bleeding. Physician consultation is also recommended for sickle cell crises, suspected aplastic anemia, or hemolytic anemia.

DIFFERENTIAL DIAGNOSIS

Anemias are generally divided into three categories based on the size of the RBCs produced by the underlying condition or disease. RBCs are normally uniform in size and shape, and alterations in their appearance can suggest a specific cause for the anemia. The degree of anisocytosis (variation in RBC size) is determined by looking at the RBC indexes on the CBC and on cell morphology seen in the peripheral smear. The RBC indexes most useful for determining variation in blood size are the MCV and the RDW. The MCV is a direct measurement averaging all of the cell sizes in the sample, and the RDW is an indirect measurement that indicates the degree of homogeneity of the sample. For example, uniformly small RBCs will have a low MCV and a normal RDW, whereas a sample with mostly small RBCs but some normal RBCs can have a low MCV, but the RDW will be increased, reflecting the heterogeneity of the sample. Based on the MCV, anemias are classified as microcytic (MCV <87 fl), normocytic (MCV of 87 to 103 fl), or macrocytic (MCV >103 fl). Variations in RBC shape (poikilocytosis) provide important diagnostic clues and in fact are often pathognomonic of underlying disease. Box 231-2 classifies commonly seen hematologic disorders according to RBC morphology.

BOX 231-1

CONDITIONS THAT CAN INFLUENCE RETICULOCYTE COUNTS

INCREASED RETICULOCYTE COUNTS

- Hemolytic anemia
  - Autoimmune hemolysis
  - RBC enzyme deficiencies
  - Traumatic or microangiopathic hemolysis
  - RBC membrane problems (hereditary spherocytosis and elliptocytosis)
- Three to 4 days following acute blood loss
- Hemoglobinopathies
- Toxin exposures
- Hypersplenism
- Following treatment of anemias
  - After adequate doses of iron to treat iron deficiency anemia
  - After adequate doses of folate or vitamin B_{12} to correct a megaloblastic anemia

DECREASED RETICULOCYTE COUNTS

- Iron deficiency anemia
- Aplastic anemia
- Untreated megaloblastic anemia
- Radiation therapy
- Marrow tumors
- Myelodysplastic syndromes

Microcytic Anemia

IRON DEFICIENCY ANEMIA

Iron deficiency anemia (IDA) is the most common type of anemia in the world and the most common nutrient deficiency. IDA predominantly affects women of reproductive age and older adults. The most common cause is chronic blood loss, especially gastrointestinal blood loss or menorrhagia.[5] Chronic gastrointestinal blood loss should be suspected as an etiology of IDA in adult men and postmenopausal women. Box 231-3 lists additional causes of iron deficiency.

Inadequate nutrition and increased requirements for iron are the principal etiologies for IDA in children and pregnant women. The prevalence of IDA during pregnancy is 3.5% to

BOX 231-2

CLASSIFICATION OF ANEMIAS BASED ON RED BLOOD CELL MORPHOLOGY

SIZE

- Microcytic (MCV <87 fl)
  - Iron deficiency
  - Thalassemia
  - Anemia of chronic disease (occasionally)
  - Sideroblastic anemia
  - Hemoglobin E disease
- Macrocytic (MCV >103 fl)
  - Megaloblastic anemia (vitamin B_{12} or folate deficiency)
- Normocytic (MCV of 87 to 103 fl)
  - Sickle cell disease
  - Anemia of chronic disease
  - Aplastic anemia
  - Hemolytic anemias

SHAPE

- Sickle
  - Sickle cell disease
- Targets
  - Thalassemias
  - Hemoglobin C, hemoglobin E
- Spherocytes
  - Hereditary spherocytosis
  - Immune hemolysis
- Elliptocytes
  - Hereditary elliptocytosis

7.4% in the first trimester and can increase to 15% to 55% in the third trimester.[6] Nutritional deficiency is more prevalent among poor women. During the past several decades, however, the frequency of nutritional IDA has decreased in women and children in the United States as a result of iron-fortified foods, iron supplementation during pregnancy, better access to health care, and support programs such as WIC (Women, Infants, and Children).[6]

Pathophysiology

Iron is an essential nutrient present in all living cells. In humans more than 70% of the total body iron content is in hemoglobin, with another 5% in myoglobin and other heme-containing enzymes.[7] The remaining 25% of iron is bound to the protein transferrin. The normal man has a total body iron content of about 4000 mg. Women have about 200 mg of total body iron, a significantly lower amount because of menstrual blood loss and lower dietary intake. The average adult normally loses approximately 1 mg of iron each day through the natural process of desquamation of cells from the skin, gastrointestinal tract, and urinary tract. The adult woman loses an additional 1 mg through normal menstruation.

The recommended daily allowance of iron is 15 mg/day in the diet of nonpregnant women and 30 mg/day for pregnant women. Most American diets consist of approximately 15 mg of elemental iron a day.[8] Dietary iron is absorbed in the duodenum of the small intestine. The amount of iron absorbed from the intestine is determined by several factors, including the iron content of the meal, the form of iron being ingested, the iron status of the individual, and the presence or absence of other substances that can enhance or inhibit iron absorption (Box 231-4).[6]

When iron requirements increase or intake declines, the small intestine increases absorption of iron to meet the increased demand. If there is no additional supply of iron to meet this increased demand, the body's iron stores begin to be depleted. At this point several hematologic parameters are affected. The ferritin levels decline as body iron stores decrease. As body iron stores are depleted, the transferrin saturation decreases, leading to a reduced supply of iron to the RBC precursors, resulting in impaired (iron-deficient) erythropoiesis. At this stage, however, an overt microcytic anemia may not yet be present. Once the iron stores are truly depleted and there is no iron available for erythropoiesis, an overt microcytic, hypochromic anemia is present, which is manifested in the CBC by a low hemoglobin concentration and decreased RBC indexes (↓MCV, ↓ mean corpuscular hemoglobin [MCH], and ↓ mean corpuscular hemoglobin concentration [MCHC]). The peripheral smear will show hypochromia, microcytosis, mild anisocytosis, and poikilocytosis. Iron studies will show a low ferritin and high TIBC.

BOX 231-3

CAUSES OF IRON DEFICIENCY

CONDITIONS LEADING TO MILD IRON DEFICIENCY*

- Inadequate diet
- Normal or heavy menses
- Blood donation
- Malabsorption
  - Partial gastrectomy
  - Malabsorption syndromes
- Increased requirements
  - Infancy and adolescence (periods of rapid growth)
  - Pregnancy
- Polycythemia vera treated with phlebotomy

CONDITIONS ASSOCIATED WITH MODERATE TO SEVERE IRON DEFICIENCY

- Chronic blood loss
  - Gastrointestinal
    - Peptic ulcer disease
    - Varices
    - Malignancy
    - Diverticulitis
  - Severe menorrhagia
- Severe malabsorption
  - Gastrectomy
  - Sprue and other malabsorption syndromes

*Usually no associated symptoms.

Clinical Presentation

Mild to moderate iron-deficient states are not associated with any clinical symptoms. Severe IDA may be asymptomatic or may be associated with signs and symptoms that are primarily those of severe anemia (i.e., nonspecific to IDA). Patients may complain of fatigue, decreased exercise tolerance, weakness, palpitations, irritability, and headaches. Complaints that are specifically related to iron store depletion include paresthesias, sore tongue, brittle nails, spoon-shaped nails (koilonychia), and pica for starch, ice, or clay.[5] In fact, a craving for ice (pagophagia) is a common symptom of women with IDA.

Physical Examination

As the severity of the anemia increases, several physical changes may become evident. The patient may demonstrate a more forceful apical pulse, tachycardia with exertion, and a systolic flow murmur. Patients may also demonstrate pallor of the conjunctiva, mucous membranes, nail beds, and palmar creases. The characteristic spooning of the nails may also be present.

BOX 231-4

FACTORS THAT INFLUENCE IRON ABSORPTION

SUBSTANCES THAT INHIBIT IRON ABSORPTION

- Soy protein
- Bran
- Dairy products
- Tea and coffee
- Calcium-rich antacids
- Vegetable sources

SUBSTANCES THAT ENHANCE IRON ABSORPTION

- Ascorbic acid (vitamin C)
- Citric acid
- Meat, poultry, and fish sources
- Other factors:
  - Low iron stores of individual
  - Low iron content of meal

Diagnostics

IDA is commonly discovered incidentally during a routine CBC. Once IDA is diagnosed, the history may reveal factors that would cause iron deficiency, such as inadequate nutrition, gastrointestinal bleeding, menorrhagia, multiple pregnancies, or a recent hemorrhage. Iron studies reveal a low serum iron level, decreased serum ferritin, increased TIBC, and decreased percent of transferrin saturation (Box 231-5). Laboratory changes occur gradually as the iron stores are depleted. The earliest laboratory change is a fall in serum ferritin, reflecting depletion of iron stores. This change is followed by a decrease in serum iron and an increase in transferrin, producing a reduction in the percentage of transferrin saturation to below 15% (this will drop below 10% as the severity progresses) and an associated increase in the TIBC. The first change in the CBC is a drop in hemoglobin. Only with increasing severity (hemoglobin <8 to 9 g/dl) do the RBCs become microcytic and hypochromic.

The underlying cause of the iron deficiency must be identified. Blood loss should be suspected until proved otherwise, especially in adult men and postmenopausal women. Older patients with suspected IDA should be thoroughly evaluated for gastrointestinal cancers.

Differential Diagnosis

Only a few diseases need to be considered in the differential diagnosis of a microcytic, hypochromic anemia. The thalassemias typically have a moderate to severe microcytosis with varying degrees of anemia but normal iron studies.

Anemia of chronic disease presents a more common diagnostic dilemma. With long-standing chronic inflammatory illnesses such as rheumatoid arthritis, the defective iron supply can result in severe microcytic, hypochromic anemia. Iron studies, especially the serum ferritin level, usually differentiate between a true IDA, anemia of chronic disease, and thalassemia (Table 231-1). Both IDA and anemia of chronic disease have low serum iron levels. The ferritin level is normal or increased in anemia of chronic disease and decreased in IDA. The TIBC is normal or low in anemia of chronic disease and increased in IDA.

Microcytosis can occur in patients with acquired (secondary to drug or toxin exposure) or inherited sideroblastic anemias. These rare conditions are characterized by the presence of ringed sideroblasts in the bone marrow and an associated inefficient erythropoiesis.[5] A bone marrow examination is necessary for diagnosis. The anemia tends to be severe (hemoglobin concentration of 6 g/dl) in the hereditary form to moderate (hemoglobin concentration of 6 to 10 g/dl) in the acquired form. Erythrocytes tend to be both normocytic and normochromic, and others will be microcytic and hypochromic. Treatment of sideroblastic anemia consists of chronic transfusions and iron chelation therapy (to prevent or treat the transfusion-dependent iron overload). Pyridoxine (vitamin B_6) therapy may sometimes partially correct the anemia in some patients, leaving them with a mild anemia that does not require chronic transfusions.

Differential Diagnosis

Microcytic Anemia

Iron deficiency anemia	Sideroblastic anemia
Thalassemia	Lead poisoning/aluminum toxicity
Anemia of chronic disease	

Management

Treatment of IDA usually begins with an oral iron preparation. The usual therapeutic dose is 60 to 120 mg of elemental iron per day in divided doses. This can be reduced to 30 mg/day once the anemia is corrected. Common side effects of iron preparations are nausea, constipation, heartburn, upper gastrointestinal discomfort, black stools, and diarrhea. Iron absorption is optimal

BOX 231-5

LABORATORY STUDIES IN IRON DEFICIENCY ANEMIA

Hemoglobin: slight decrease to marked decrease
Serum iron: decreased
TIBC: increased
Percent of transferrin saturation: decreased (<10% in severe IDA)
Serum ferritin: decreased

TABLE 231-1 Laboratory Values in Microcytic Anemias

Anemia	Hemoglobin*	MCV	MCHC	Serum Iron†	Serum Ferritin‡	TIBC§	Transferrin Saturation‖
Iron deficiency							
Early	N	N	N	N	N	N	N
Intermediate	N	N	N	↓/N	↓	High N	↓
Late	↓	↓	↓	↓	↓	↑	↓
Thalassemia minor	Low N/↓	↓	N/↓	N	N/↑	N	N
Chronic disease	Low N	N/↓	N/↓	↓	↑	↓	↑
Sideroblastic anemia	↓	↓	↓	↑	↑	N	↑

*N = 12-16 g/dl for women; 13.5-17.5 g/dl for men.
†N = 65-165 μg/dl for women; 75-175 μg/dl for men.
‡N = 12-150 μg/dl for women; 15-300 μg/dl for men.
§N = 240-450 μg/dl.
‖N = 20%-50%.

when taken 30 minutes before meals and can be reduced by as much as 40% to 50% if taken with meals. However, iron on an empty stomach can cause more side effects and can lead to discontinuation of medication. Gastrointestinal upset, the most common side effect, may be avoided by starting with a single pill per day and slowly increasing to the recommended dose.

Once an adequate dose of iron is reached, changes in the hematologic markers should be seen in just a few weeks. The hemoglobin level should begin to rise within 1 to 2 weeks. The MCV should correct within 1 to 2 months, reflecting the normalization of the erythrocyte size. Supplementation with oral iron should continue until the anemia is corrected, until the underlying cause of the deficiency is corrected, or indefinitely if the cause of the deficiency is chronic.

If the anemia is severe, if the patient has an iron malabsorption problem, or if oral iron is not tolerated, then replacement should be by parenteral iron. Patients should be referred to a hematologist for IV iron administration.

Parenteral iron is not without risk. Adverse reactions to intravenous iron are possible and include anaphylactic shock, headache, malaise, fever, generalized lymphadenopathy, phlebitis, arthralgias, and urticaria. Therefore administration of IV iron should start with a physician-supervised test dose. The patient should be carefully monitored during the test dose. If the patient tolerates this initial test dose, then the full dose can be administered.

Life Span Considerations

Iron supplementation during pregnancy is almost always required. Pregnancy places a greater demand on iron stores, especially during the last two trimesters. The daily requirement for iron can increase to 5 to 6 mg (the nonpregnant woman requires approximately 1 to 4 mg of iron per day).[6] The additional iron is needed to cover the needs of the developing fetus and placenta and to accommodate the increase in erythrocyte mass that normally occurs during the later stages of pregnancy. Diagnosing IDA during pregnancy can be difficult because of a number of phenomena that normally occur: (1) the maternal serum iron is low because of increased placental uptake, (2) the TIBC increases even in pregnant women with sufficient iron stores, and (3) the transferrin saturation declines even in nonanemic pregnant women.[6] These factors can make the serum iron, TIBC, and percent transferrin saturation inaccurate. The best indicator of IDA during pregnancy is the serum ferritin level.

Older adults with suspected IDA should be thoroughly evaluated for gastrointestinal cancers, even when their stools are negative for occult blood. Next to anemia of chronic disease, IDA is the most common cause of a microcytic anemia in older adults.[9]

Complications

Untreated IDA is especially worrisome during pregnancy. IDA may be associated with preterm delivery, low birth weight, and learning deficits. Untreated iron deficiency can lead to severe anemia and may be associated with fatigue, falls, and cardiovascular compromise.

Indications for Referral/Hospitalization

Most patients with IDA are diagnosed and treated by their primary care providers. Patients who are referred to a hematologist for any of the aforementioned reasons are generally referred back to the primary care provider once the anemia has been corrected, or at the very least, once an accurate diagnosis has been made and the patient is receiving stable iron replacement therapy.

A referral to a hematologist should be considered for the following reasons: (1) nonadherence or intolerance to oral iron replacement and persistent IDA, which will require parenteral iron therapy, and (2) persistent microcytic anemia despite iron replacement and the fact that other conditions have been excluded.

Other referrals may be required as evaluation for the cause of the iron deficiency progresses, such as referral to an internist or gastroenterologist to exclude gastrointestinal blood loss or referral to an oncologist to treat any malignancies (either gastrointestinal or gynecologic). Women of reproductive age may require referral to a gynecologist or a hematologist to evaluate severe menorrhagia (the hematology referral may be helpful to rule out von Willebrand's disease as an etiology of the menorrhagia).

Healthy patients with IDA do not require hospitalization. Patients who are unable to adequately compensate for a severe anemia may require hospitalization for cardiac or respiratory compromise that may occur.

Patient and Family Education

Patients should receive education about the use of iron supplements to ensure adequate treatment and an understanding of the prescribed regimen. Maximum absorption of iron occurs if it is ingested 30 minutes before meals. Substances that can enhance or inhibit iron absorption are listed in Box 231-4. Calcium can significantly inhibit iron absorption. Multivitamins with calcium or dairy products should be taken 1 to 2 hours after an iron supplement. Ascorbic acid may enhance absorption of iron; therefore concurrent ingestion of foods rich in vitamin C, such as orange juice, should be encouraged.[10]

There are numerous iron supplementation preparations on the market (Table 231-2), some with combinations of iron plus stool softeners, slow-release iron, or iron plus vitamin C. Patients who are intolerant of one preparation may find another for which they have fewer or no side effects. Therefore patients should be encouraged to try various preparations.

Health Promotion

Nutritional counseling is an important strategy to prevent further episodes of iron deficiency anemia and should include assessment of the patient's dietary intake. Assessment should also include the quantity and timing of iron ingestion and other substances that can interfere with iron absorption, such

TABLE 231-2 Common Iron Supplement Preparations

Preparation	Usual Dosage	Amount of Elemental Iron in Dose (mg)
Ferrous sulfate	Feosol 200 mg 1-2 q day	65
	Slow Fe 160 mg 1-2 q day	50
Ferrous gluconate	324 mg t.i.d.	36
Polysaccharide-iron complex (Niferex)	150 mg 1-2 tablets q day	150
Ferrous fumarate	150 mg 1-2 tablets q day	50

as tea, coffee, chocolate, dairy products, and high-fiber foods. Strict vegetarians who rely on vegetable sources of iron instead of animal sources should be encouraged to supplement their diets with iron-fortified vitamins or to add iron-fortified foods to their diet. Patients whose iron deficiency anemia is secondary to other conditions should be encouraged to seek appropriate medical care.

THALASSEMIA

Definition/Epidemiology

Thalassemia is a group of inherited microcytic anemias caused by abnormal hemoglobin production. Thalassemia occurs as a result of absent or insufficient production of the alpha or beta chains of normal hemoglobin. The resulting anemia depends on the type of thalassemia inherited and varies from asymptomatic to severe hemolytic anemia. All of the thalassemias produce some degree of microcytosis and hypochromia.

Thalassemia is most commonly found in people of Mediterranean, Middle Eastern, African, and Asian descent. It can be inherited concurrently with genes for the hemoglobinopathies, resulting in conditions such as sickle beta-thalassemia (Sβ-thalassemia). Thalassemia affects males and females equally.

Pathophysiology

The manifestations and severity of clinical symptoms depend on the number of chain deletions in the hemoglobin molecule.[11] Normally, adult RBCs contain predominantly hemoglobin A_1 (96% to 97% of the cell's hemoglobin) and only small amounts of hemoglobin A_2 (2.5%) and hemoglobin F (less than 1%). The thalassemia abnormalities produce changes in the normal amounts of adult hemoglobin. These quantitative changes are important in the diagnosis of thalassemia.

Inheritance of thalassemia follows an autosomal dominant pattern. Examples of this inheritance pattern can be seen in Figure 231-1.

Clinical Presentation

Patients with thalassemia are classified as having thalassemia minor, thalassemia intermedia, or thalassemia major, depending on the severity of their anemia. Throughout the world, the majority of patients have thalassemia minor. Patients with thalassemia minor generally have either little or no hematologic disease or a mild microcytic hypochromic anemia that is often mistaken for IDA.

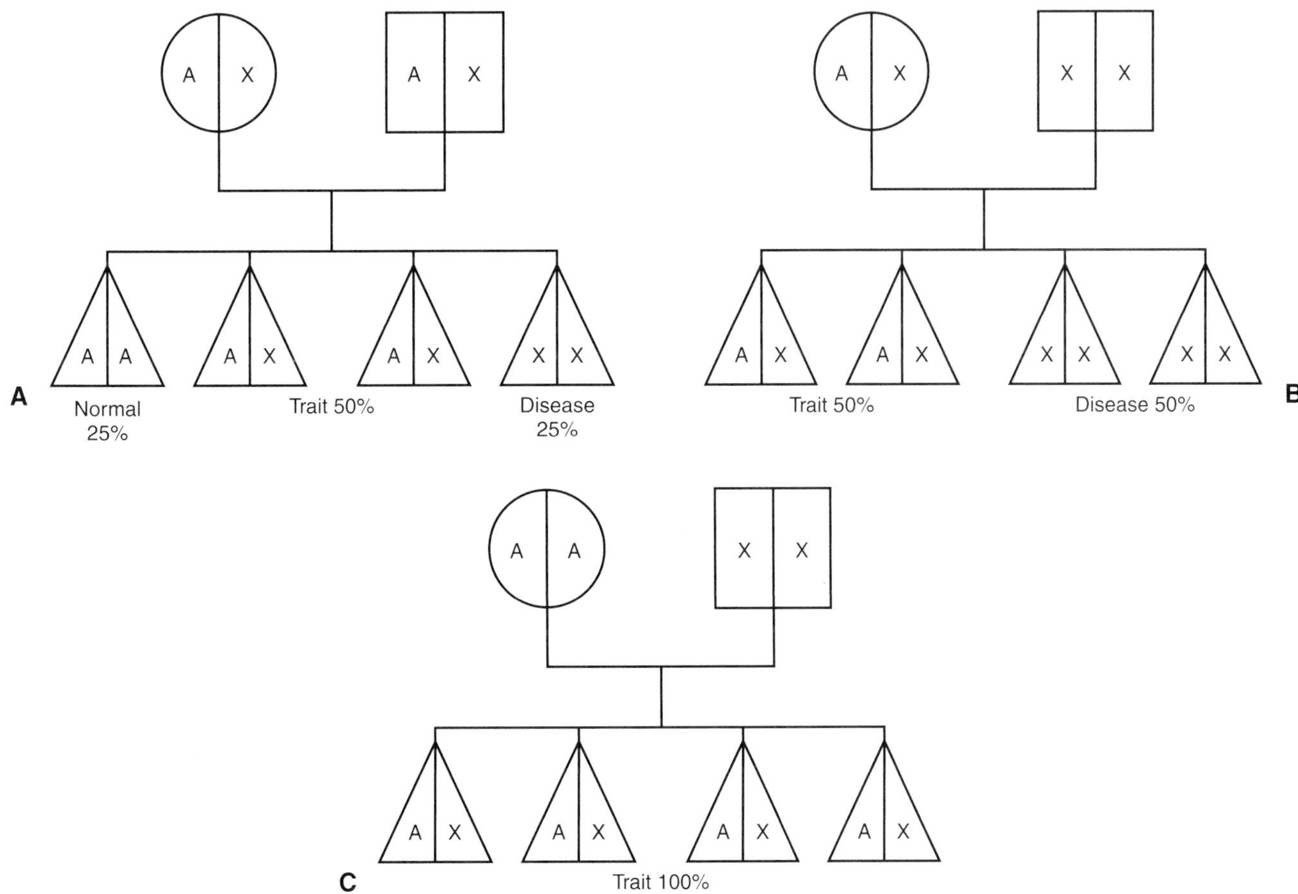

FIGURE 231-1

Inheritance patterns for autosomal genes. **A**, When both parents have a trait, offspring have a 25% chance of being normal, a 25% chance of having the disease, and a 50% chance of having the trait. **B**, When one parent has the disease and the other parent has the trait, offspring have a 50% chance of having the trait and a 50% chance of having the disease. **C**, When one parent has the disease and the other parent is normal, all offspring will have the trait. *A*, Gene for normal hemoglobin; *X*, gene for abnormal hemoglobin (S, C, E) or thalassemia.

Patients with thalassemia intermedia have a moderate microcytic and hypochromic anemia that is not transfusion dependent. Patients with thalassemia intermedia may require occasional transfusions during pregnancy or preoperatively. If patients with thalassemia intermedia begin to develop persistent clinical problems such as abnormal facies, growth retardation, or pathologic fractures, they will require regular transfusions. At this point, these patients are given the diagnosis of thalassemia major.[12]

Patients with thalassemia major (also known as Cooley's anemia) develop a severe, life-threatening anemia during their first year of life. This profound anemia is associated with developmental problems and decreased life expectancy. These patients require lifelong chronic RBC transfusions to maintain adequate hemoglobin levels.

Physical Examination

The physical examination is remarkable only in patients with thalassemia intermedia and thalassemia major. Patients can exhibit the characteristic physical changes of short stature and abnormal facies associated with cranial marrow expansion. In the United States, however, the facial abnormalities are seen primarily in patients with thalassemia intermedia, because most patients with thalassemia major are hypertransfused to normal hemoglobin levels, thus preventing the marrow expansion.[12]

Diagnostics

Patients with thalassemia intermedia or major are diagnosed during the first few years of life. The diagnosis of thalassemia minor is based on a mildly decreased hemoglobin concentration, low MCV (<80 fl), normal iron studies, and a normal hemoglobin electrophoresis with high levels of hemoglobin A_2.

Patients with thalassemia intermedia who maintain adequate hemoglobin levels without requiring transfusions exhibit signs of a mild microcytic anemia with slightly low hemoglobin and a low MCV. Patients with thalassemia major who are hypertransfused have either a low or low-normal hemoglobin level and a relatively normal MCV (because they are receiving normal blood during transfusions). Peripheral smears of both patients with thalassemia intermedia and patients with thalassemia major have typical target cells present. Patients with thalassemia major who do not receive iron chelation therapy or who are receiving subtherapeutic doses of deferoxamine (iron chelator) have iron study results that reflect their state of iron overload (very high ferritin, very low TIBC, and percent of transferrin saturation approaching 100%). Patients with thalassemia intermedia may also have similar iron studies because they can develop iron overload as a result of iron hyperabsorption rather than from transfusions.

Differential Diagnosis

In most cases the primary care provider needs to distinguish thalassemia minor from IDA. Both conditions are microcytic anemias, but results of iron studies are normal in patients with thalassemia minor. In areas with a high prevalence of immigrants from Southeast Asia, the differential diagnosis of a mild microcytic anemia must differentiate between thalassemia minor and hemoglobin E disease.

Hemoglobin E is the second most common hemoglobinopathy in the world (next to sickle cell disease). It is characterized by a mild microcytic anemia with many target cells on the peripheral smear. It closely resembles the microcytic anemia of β-thalassemia minor, but hemoglobin E is found only in people of Southeast Asian ancestry. Patients who are homozygous for hemoglobin E (EE) are clinically normal, as are patients with β-thalassemia minor. Patients can also be double heterozygotes for hemoglobin E and sickle cell disease (ES), resulting clinically in a mild sickle cell disease or combined hemoglobin E and β-thalassemia, which results in a moderate to severe transfusion-dependent anemia that will be similar to β-thalassemia major.[13] Hemoglobin E is diagnosed by hemoglobin electrophoresis.

Often, patients with thalassemia minor or hemoglobin E are given a diagnosis of IDA because of their mild microcytic anemia and are prescribed a regimen of iron replacement. Failure to correct the anemia with iron supplementation should then lead one to suspect thalassemia minor (or hemoglobin E disease if the patient is from Southeast Asia).

Management

Patients with thalassemia minor do not require medical management but should be referred for genetic counseling if family planning is an issue. Patients with thalassemia intermedia can be adequately cared for in a primary care setting, with regular attention to any changes in their anemia. Patients with thalassemia intermedia who begin to develop persistent clinical problems such as abnormal facies, growth retardation, or pathologic fractures should be referred to a hematologist to begin chronic transfusion therapy. Patients with thalassemia intermedia who hyperabsorb iron and develop iron overload require chelation therapy.

In the United States, hematologists who are familiar with the disease manage most patients with thalassemia major and intermedia. Management consists of two equally important functions: (1) regular transfusions to maintain an adequate hemoglobin level to allow for normal growth and development and (2) iron chelation therapy to prevent the complications of transfusion-dependent iron overload.

Regular transfusions of packed RBCs are the mainstay of therapy for thalassemia major. Transfusions are begun early in childhood to maintain an adequate hemoglobin level to allow for normal growth and development. Transfusions are usually necessary every 3 to 6 weeks to maintain hemoglobin levels at 9 to 10 g/dl.[14]

Chelation therapy is the standard treatment for prevention of complications from iron overload. Complications of transfusional iron overload can be profound and are the major cause of death in patients with thalassemia major who are not well chelated. Deferoxamine is a chelating agent that removes iron from tissues and allows excretion of iron in urine and stools. It is currently the only medical chelating agent available, although an oral chelator continues in clinical trials around the world. Deferoxamine must be administered parenterally, generally via a subcutaneous needle, and delivered by slow infusion over at least 8 hours to effectively remove iron. The longer the infusion period, the more effective the iron removal. Chelation therapy is usually administered 5 to 7 days a week for life. The normal subcutaneous dose is 50 to 100 mg/kg/day administered by continuous infusion during a 10- to 16-hour period. If subcutaneous administration is not tolerated, IV therapy can be attempted but requires the use of an indwelling venous catheter. The goal of chelation therapy is to reduce body iron stores and maintain a ferritin level of <1500 μg/L, which will significantly reduce the risks associated with iron overload.[15]

Bone marrow transplantation (BMT) is currently the only potential cure for thalassemia. Rund and Rachmilewitz[14] reported that more than 1000 transplantations have been done since 1982. BMT is not without serious risks. Transplant success is highest in children and in those who are well chelated, have a normal liver size and histology, and have no cardiac complications.

Other therapies (including erythropoietin, hydroxyurea, and butyrate derivatives) are currently being investigated for their potential to induce fetal hemoglobin production.[14] Increasing fetal hemoglobin production may prove especially beneficial for patients with thalassemia intermedia as a way to avoid transfusions.

Life Span Considerations

Reproductive issues are a major concern. Well-chelated and well-transfused women may be fertile. Contraception counseling should be offered to all women with thalassemia who are sexually active with male partners. There are no restrictions as to the types of contraception available to women with thalassemia.

Complications

There are many possible complications associated with both the regular transfusion regimen and the chelation therapy. However, most of the severe complications are due to iron overload.

Transfusions are usually well tolerated, but complications can occur. The development of alloantibodies can make it difficult to find suitable blood donors on a regular basis. Viral infections such as HIV and hepatitis B and C have become less of an issue, as blood products are now routinely screened for these viruses. Patients should receive hepatitis B vaccine and are periodically screened for hepatitis B antibodies, as vaccine immunity is not lifelong and may require boosters. Iron overload is the primary complication of chronic transfusions. Accumulation of excess iron leads to cirrhosis, heart failure, and endocrine problems such as diabetes mellitus, hypothyroidism, growth failure, and delayed sexual development.[14,16]

Chelation therapy can also be problematic. Chronic subcutaneous administration of deferoxamine can cause localized reactions such as scar tissue formation, itching, rash, and local irritation at the site of injection. There are also possible complications if a high dose of deferoxamine is given in the presence of low serum ferritin. These complications include toxic effects on the eye, such as cataracts, night blindness, and reduction of visual fields and acuity (these effects usually regress when deferoxamine therapy is stopped); hearing loss (high-tone deafness is irreversible despite cessation of therapy); and skeletal lesions such as pseudorickets, metaphyseal changes, and short stature (these are also irreversible complications of deferoxamine therapy).[16]

Despite the availability of iron chelation therapy, complications of iron overload are common in patients with thalassemia who are more than 10 years of age. This may be due to inadequate iron chelation early in life with resulting irreversible damage, insufficient chelation therapy, or poor compliance. Iron overload complications include endocrine, cardiac, and hepatic problems (Box 231-6). The presence of cardiac complications is an indication for continuous (24 hours a day, 7 days a week) iron chelation therapy.

Well-chelated patients with thalassemia who maintain a ferritin level <1500 μg/L do not develop the major complications of iron overload. However, many of them have growth retardation and delayed puberty. Most people with thalassemia major are unusually short and may appear younger than their age. Young women are often amenorrheic. An endocrinology consult may be indicated when the patient is nearing the age of puberty. Hormone replacement therapy, either estrogen for girls or testosterone for boys, can be initiated to hasten maturation and sexual development.

Indications for Referral/Hospitalization

Thalassemia major is a chronic lifelong disease that requires constant attention by health care providers. Ideally, hematologists or primary care providers familiar with the disease should manage these patients. Attention to issues of growth and development, compliance with transfusion and chelation therapy, reproductive issues, and assessment for the development of complications require frequent follow-up visits.

Patients with thalassemia major who are well transfused and well chelated may still experience considerable delays in puberty. These patients should be referred to a reproductive endocrinologist for possible hormone therapy.

Patients with thalassemia who receive chronic transfusion therapy and chelation therapy can lead relatively healthy and otherwise normal lives. If they are not compliant, however, the complications of iron overload will eventually lead to increasing morbidity from liver disease and, especially, cardiac disease. When patients with thalassemia major are hospitalized for any reason, they should be transfused to maintain an adequate hemoglobin concentration and maintained on IV chelation therapy.

Patient and Family Education

Patients with thalassemia major and their families assume a great deal of responsibility for their own health. Chelation therapy occurs at home, and patients must learn how to perform

BOX 231-6

COMPLICATIONS OF IRON OVERLOAD

ENDOCRINE PROBLEMS
Growth retardation
Diabetes mellitus
Hypothyroidism
Hypoparathyroidism
Disturbed pubertal development

CARDIAC PROBLEMS
Arrhythmias
Pericarditis
Cardiac failure

HEPATIC COMPLICATIONS
Cirrhosis

aseptic subcutaneous injections and use the infusion pump. Adhering to the chelation therapy schedule is essential. There are no signs and symptoms of iron overload until a fairly advanced stage; therefore it is hard for young children and especially adolescents to understand the importance of a treatment for which they see no immediate need. Adolescents will have self-image issues. Delayed puberty, the need for daily medication infusions, and frequent trips to the hospital for transfusions will constantly remind them of being different from their peers. The daily (or usually nightly) requirement for infusions can interfere with social life and complicate intimate relationships. The transfusion schedule can interfere with work or school, and most patients with thalassemia find that they require a flexible work and/or school schedule to accommodate their transfusion schedule. The availability of evening and weekend transfusions will greatly enhance the patient's well-being and adherence to the treatment schedule.

Health Promotion

Collaborating with patients and their families is important to promote patients' self-esteem and self-reliance. Patients who believe in the value of their own lives will be more likely to comply with the regular transfusion schedule and their daily chelation therapy.

Macrocytic Anemia: Megaloblastic Anemia

Definition/Epidemiology

Vitamin B_{12} and folate deficiency are the primary causes of macrocytic anemia. Both vitamins are essential for normal DNA synthesis, and tissues such as bone marrow are highly sensitive to any deficiency. Marrow precursors for all cell lines (erythroid, myeloid, and platelets) become larger than normal and are unable to complete normal growth and maturation, a condition referred to as a megaloblastic bone marrow.[7,17] The resulting ineffective erythropoiesis causes the release of macrocytic RBCs into the circulation and worsening anemia.

Folate deficiency is found in the presence of decreased dietary intake, diseases associated with malabsorption, or increased requirements such as pregnancy. Alcoholism is a common cause of folate deficiency because of alcohol's interference with folate metabolism and the usually poor dietary habits related to alcoholism. In developing countries, malabsorption syndromes such as tropical and nontropical sprue are more common etiologies.[7] Folate deficiency is also associated with neural tube defects in fetuses.

Vitamin B_{12} deficiency is most commonly caused by pernicious anemia but can also be associated with other gastrointestinal disorders. Chronic gastritis can damage parietal cells and partial or complete gastric resection results in loss of parietal cells and therefore intrinsic factor.

Pathophysiology

Dietary sources of vitamin B_{12} are found only in meat and meat by-products. When vitamin B_{12} from food reaches the small bowel, it is bound to intrinsic factor, a glycoprotein secreted by parietal cells of the stomach. The vitamin B_{12} intrinsic factor (cobalamin-IF) complex is then transported through the terminal ileum into the circulation. Vitamin B_{12} absorption cannot occur in the absence of intrinsic factor.

Once in the circulation, vitamin B_{12} is bound to the transport protein, transcobalamin II, which carries it to the liver, bone marrow, and other proliferating cells. A healthy adult receiving an adequate diet can accumulate from 1 to 10 mg of vitamin B_{12} in the liver, the major storage site.[7] Because the daily requirement of vitamin B_{12} is only 3 to 5 μg/day, most omnivorous individuals have no difficulty obtaining the necessary amounts from their diets as long as absorption is normal. Only strict vegetarians are at risk for a dietary deficiency, and it would take several years of a strict vegan diet for megaloblastosis to occur.

Pernicious anemia is the most prevalent cause of vitamin B_{12} deficiency. It is an autoimmune disease in which atrophy of the parietal cells of the stomach leads to a complete loss of intrinsic factor.[18] It often coexists with other autoimmune disorders. The onset of pernicious anemia usually occurs after age 50 years.

Dietary folate is readily available in most foods, especially green leafy vegetables; however, folate is heat labile and rapidly destroyed by prolonged cooking or food processing.[19] Body stores are limited to approximately a 3-month reserve. It is possible that a prolonged inadequate diet may not provide sufficient amounts of folate for normal DNA production, especially during pregnancy or for patients with hemolytic anemias (high rates of cell turnover). Dietary folate deficiency is relatively uncommon, as many foods, such as orange juice, are now supplemented. Folate deficiency is commonly associated with chronic alcoholism and can also be caused by the same malabsorption syndromes that lead to vitamin B_{12} deficiency (Box 231-7).

Clinical Presentation

A mild megaloblastic anemia produces few symptoms, and the CBC usually makes the diagnosis incidentally. A severe vitamin B_{12} deficiency includes signs and symptoms of marked anemia

BOX 231-7

COMMON CAUSES OF MEGALOBLASTIC ANEMIA

INADEQUATE INTAKE
Vegetarian diet devoid of animal proteins (vitamin B_{12})
Chronic alcoholism (folate)

MALABSORPTION (VITAMIN B_{12} AND FOLATE)
Lack of intrinsic factor
Gastric surgery
Inflammatory bowel disease
Sprue (tropical and nontropical)
Celiac disease
Intestinal tapeworm
Hyperthyroidism

INCREASED REQUIREMENTS (FOLATE)
Pregnancy
Hemolytic anemias

and neurologic deficits. Early neurologic symptoms include decreased vibratory sensation, loss of proprioception, and ataxia. Later involvement results in spasticity, hyperactive reflexes, and a positive Romberg's sign. These neurologic symptoms result from the formation of a demyelinating lesion of the neurons of the spinal cord and cerebral cortex.[7] Neurologic symptoms may be evident in the absence of anemia and may not resolve with correction of the deficiency. Other classic symptoms of B_{12} deficiency include a sore mouth and loss of taste.

Folate deficiency is rarely associated with any symptoms, even in the severe state. Folate deficiency is not associated with neurologic or psychiatric disorders except those caused by neural tube defects.

Physical Examination

The physical examination of a patient with severe megaloblastic anemia may reveal the classic changes associated with any severe anemia. Patients with severe vitamin B_{12} deficiency may have characteristic findings such as a smooth, red, shiny tongue and the aforementioned neurologic changes.

Diagnostics

Findings on the CBC that suggest a macrocytic anemia include low hemoglobin levels and an MCV >100. Severe anemia may also be associated with leukopenia or thrombocytopenia. In addition, the reticulocyte count will be low. The peripheral smear is also helpful in diagnosing a megaloblastic anemia. The presence of hypersegmented neutrophils and oval macrocytes are the earliest and most specific sign of a megaloblastic anemia. Serum cobalamin (vitamin B_{12}) and folate levels may help to distinguish the cause of the macrocytosis. Measuring certain metabolites of vitamin B_{12}, methylmalonic acid, and homocysteine provides additional information to help identify the cause of the anemia. The normal range of serum methylmalonic acid is 70 to 270 nm/L, and the normal serum homocysteine level ranges from 5 to 16 nm/L. Homocysteine levels are elevated in both vitamin B_{12} and folate deficiency. Methylmalonic acid levels are elevated in vitamin B_{12} deficiency and are normal in folate deficiency.

It is important to distinguish vitamin B_{12} deficiency caused by malabsorption from that caused by lack of intrinsic factor (pernicious anemia). The Schilling test has been the classic method used to verify the diagnosis of pernicious anemia but is now rarely used. Assaying for antiintrinsic factor or antiparietal cell antibodies is the currently accepted method for verifying the diagnosis of pernicious anemia. The presence of antiintrinsic factor antibodies is highly specific for pernicious anemia. However, the majority of older people found to have biochemically significant vitamin B_{12} deficiency do not have a positive Schilling test result or autoantibodies and thus do not meet the criteria for pernicious anemia.[18]

Differential Diagnosis

The differential diagnosis involves identifying whether the deficient state is due to vitamin B_{12} or folate deficiency and identifying the etiology of the vitamin deficiency itself. It is important to accurately determine the cause of the macrocytic anemia because misdiagnosis can have extremely negative consequences.

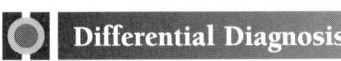

Macrocytic Anemia

Vitamin B_{12} deficiency
Folic acid deficiency
Myelodysplastic syndromes
Liver disease
Hypothyroidism
Hemolysis
Chemotherapeutic agents
Hereditary disorder
Alcoholism
Drug reaction

A vitamin B_{12} deficiency that is inappropriately treated with folic acid may result in permanent neurologic or psychiatric abnormalities.

It may also be necessary to distinguish the macrocytic anemia associated with vitamin B_{12} or folate deficiency from the macrocytosis caused by other conditions such as drug or alcohol use, liver disease, hypothyroidism, myelodysplastic syndromes, exposure to chemotherapeutic agents, or hemolysis.[20] It is also essential to consider vitamin B_{12} deficiency in the differential diagnosis of any peripheral neuropathy, dementia, or other psychiatric disorder, especially in older adults.

Management

Initial management of a macrocytic anemia depends on the severity of the anemia. Patients with life-threatening anemia may require transfusions of packed RBCs to correct the anemia. Treatment with both B_{12} and folate can be started until a definitive diagnosis is made. If the patient's cardiovascular system is unable to compensate for the degree of anemia, hospitalization may be required until the patient is stable.

Patients with asymptomatic anemia should not be treated until an accurate diagnosis is made. Treatment should then be targeted to replacement of the deficient vitamin and correction of the underlying disease, if possible. The usual treatment for vitamin B_{12} deficiency is 1000 μg of cyanocobalamin or hydroxocobalamin intramuscular injections every week for 8 weeks and then monthly for life. Reticulocytosis begins in approximately 3 days and peaks in 7 to 10 days after the initiation of vitamin replacement. The anemia should resolve over 3 to 4 weeks.

The recommended treatment of a macrocytic anemia resulting from folate deficiency is 1 mg of folic acid daily and correction of the underlying cause of the deficiency. Treatment should continue until at least a normal hemoglobin level is reached (usually in about 4 to 6 weeks) and should be continued indefinitely if the patient has an inadequate diet or if the underlying disease persists. Patients with a chronic hemolytic process, such as sickle cell disease, and pregnant patients should receive prophylactic daily supplementation of the same dose.

Patients who have had partial or total gastrectomy, ileal resection, or any other evidence of gastric atrophy or intestinal malabsorption should receive prophylactic treatment of monthly parenteral vitamin B_{12} therapy and daily folic acid supplements.

Life Span Considerations

Studies in the early 1990s by the MRC Vitamin Research Group[21] confirmed preliminary reports of an association between folate deficiency and neural tube defects. Data showed that the risk of neural tube defects is 1 to 5 per 1000 live births for the general population and approximately 10 times this amount among women with previous pregnancies involving neural tube defects. When women received supplements of folic acid before they became pregnant, the incidence of neural tube defects decreased by 72%. In 1992 the Centers for Disease Control and Prevention recommended routine supplementation before pregnancy for all women who wish to become pregnant.[22] The recommended intake is 0.4 mg/day either as a supplement or in the diet.

Annual screening for vitamin B_{12} deficiency is recommended for all older adults.[18] Screening is also recommended for patients with hematologic, neurologic, or psychiatric abnormalities suggestive of vitamin B_{12} deficiency.

Complications

The complication of undiagnosed or mistreated vitamin B_{12} deficiency is irreversible neurologic damage. Manifestations of weakness, ataxia, and poor coordination may not completely resolve with therapy, depending on the duration of the deficiency and the extent of neurologic damage. Mental status changes can range from minimal forgetfulness to severe dementia and psychosis. Patients with neurologic damage can have an almost normal blood count with normal indexes, emphasizing the need to test for vitamin B_{12} levels in patients with unexplained neurologic deficits.

Indications for Referral/Hospitalization

A primary care provider can easily manage patients who are receiving maintenance therapy of either vitamin B_{12} or folate replacement. These patients require regular visits for evaluation of therapy and monthly visits for vitamin B_{12} injections. Periodic evaluations should include a complete history and physical examination to look for the appearance or progression of any neurologic or psychiatric complications, as well as continued assessment of the underlying disease causing the vitamin deficiency. Laboratory evaluations include CBC and serum cobalamin and folate levels. A hematologist should manage patients with refractory anemia.

Patients with a severe macrocytic anemia should be referred to a hematologist for treatment. Asymptomatic patients can be treated and monitored in an outpatient setting, either by a hematologist or by the patient's primary care provider. A referral to a radiologist for administration of the Schilling test may be made in consultation with a hematologist.

As previously stated, patients with a severe, life-threatening anemia may require hospitalization for correction of the anemia. This is especially true for patients with a severe vitamin B_{12} deficiency, as they will require daily administration of parenteral vitamin B_{12} therapy to begin to correct the vitamin deficiency.

Patient and Family Education

Patients with folate deficiency secondary to an inadequate diet require nutritional counseling to learn how to properly cook and prepare foods without losing their nutritional value. Daily folic acid supplementation may be required for patients on certain drug regimens such as sulfasalazine.

Patients with megaloblastic anemia secondary to vitamin B_{12} deficiency require monthly vitamin B_{12} injections. Patients of caregivers can easily be taught this injection technique so that injections can be administered at home. Parenteral vitamin B_{12} in the absence of pernicious anemia is not effective in increasing energy in older adults.

Health Promotion

Early recognition and treatment of alcohol abuse is one preventive measure that primary care providers can take to reduce the incidence of folate deficiency anemia. Lifestyle modifications include improving dietary sources of folic acid and vitamin B_{12} and taking vitamin supplements if necessary. Primary care providers who see older patients should screen for cobalamin deficiency in cases of unexplained mental status changes and should begin therapy with vitamin B_{12} before the onset of symptoms.

Normocytic Anemia

SICKLE CELL DISEASE

Definition/Epidemiology

Sickle cell syndromes are the most common inherited hemoglobinopathies and include homozygous disease (hemoglobin SS), hemoglobin SC (also known as SC disease), Sβ-thalassemia, and a variety of other rare, abnormal hemoglobins. Patients with sickle cell disease have mild to moderate hemolytic anemia that is generally well compensated. The anemia, however, is the least serious manifestation of the disease. The hallmark of sickle cell disease is the acute vasoocclusive crisis that causes unpredictable, severe pain and organ damage.

It is known that 1 in 10 African-Americans carries the gene for sickle cell trait (AS), and about 1 in 400 is affected by SS disease. Other types of sickle cell syndromes are found in Mediterranean, Middle Eastern, and Southeast Asian populations. People with only one gene for hemoglobin S are phenotypically normal (sickle cell trait). People who inherit one gene for hemoglobin S from each parent will have SS disease. People with either hemoglobin SC or Sβ-thalassemia have inherited one gene for hemoglobin S and the other gene for either hemoglobin C or β-thalassemia. The life span of patients with SS disease is approximately 45 years; the life span is 50 to 60 years for patients with other types of sickle cell syndromes, including hemoglobin SC or Sβ-thalassemia.[23]

Pathophysiology

The hemoglobin defect occurs when valine replaces glutamic acid in the beta chain of hemoglobin, resulting in hemoglobin S.[24] Deoxygenated hemoglobin S tends to undergo irreversible polymerization, deforming the erythrocytes and giving them the pathognomonic sickle shape. The sickled cells are rigid and can be easily trapped in the microcirculation, causing obstruction, ischemia, and sometimes infarction. This process leads to the clinical consequences of severe pain and organ damage. These vasoocclusive episodes (usually referred to as "crises" or "pain crises") can occur anywhere in the body but commonly affect the joints, extremities, back, chest, abdomen, and lungs.

Clinical Presentation

Sickle cell trait has no clinical manifestations. Manifestations of sickle cell disease vary widely; some affected individuals have few painful crises and rare complications, whereas others are often hospitalized with painful crises or other complications. A study of the natural history of sickle cell disease indicated that about 5% of patients account for almost one third of hospital admissions.[25] Patients with other types of sickle cell syndromes (hemoglobin SC or Sβ-thalassemia) are reported to have milder forms of disease, although this is not always true. For example, patients with hemoglobin SC can exhibit the same range of severity as patients with SS disease.

Physical Examination

Objective manifestations of a moderate to severe hemolytic anemia include jaundice and a physiologic systolic flow murmur. Scleral icterus can range from mild to severe. The degree of scleral icterus often has no association with the severity of disease. The physiologic flow murmur secondary to anemia is often a grade I or II holosystolic murmur, which is heard best along the left sternal border. Cardiomegaly is routinely noted on the radiographs of adults with sickle cell disease and is also a compensatory manifestation of lifelong anemia.

Diagnostics

Accurate diagnosis of any sickle cell syndrome requires a hemoglobin electrophoresis. Patients with sickle cell disease have evidence of a hemolytic anemia: low hemoglobin, chronic reticulocytosis, chronic hyperbilirubinemia, and chronically elevated lactic dehydrogenase (LDH) levels. The peripheral blood smear shows mild to moderate anisocytosis and poikilocytosis with numerous sickle cells and Howell-Jolly bodies (evidence of the patient's functional asplenia). Patients with SC disease have target cells in addition to the sickle cells on their peripheral blood smears.

Unfortunately, there are no laboratory tests diagnostic of an acute painful crisis. Serial determinations of CBC during the crisis may reveal a slight increase in the anemia but give no information about the severity of the crisis.[26]

Differential Diagnosis

Most patients with sickle cell disease are diagnosed at birth. In fact, currently most states have mandatory newborn screening for sickle hemoglobin. However, it is possible for persons with very mild disease to go undiagnosed until they are in their adult years. These patients may present with a mild hemolytic anemia (low hemoglobin concentration, slight hyperbilirubinemia with elevated LDH levels, and mild reticulocytosis). A history of occasional, spontaneous painful events, usually abdominal or joint pains, should suggest a hemoglobinopathy. Accurate diagnosis requires a hemoglobin electrophoresis to differentiate among the various forms of sickle cell disease. Other possible causes of hemolytic anemia include hereditary spherocytosis, hypersplenism, autoimmune hemolysis, or a delayed hemolytic transfusion reaction.

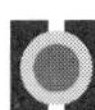

Differential Diagnosis

Normocytic Anemia

Sickle cell disorders	Hypersplenism
Sickle cell trait	Autoimmune hemolysis
Sickle cell anemia	Delayed hemocytic transfusion reaction
Sβ-Thalassemia	Aplastic anemia
Sickle cell disease	
Hereditary spherocytosis	

Management

The frequency and severity of pain crises vary tremendously among patients and even in the same patient over time. Infection, as well as physical or emotional stress, may precipitate a crisis, but the majority of crises occur spontaneously with no obvious precipitating events.[26] The sites affected in an acute crisis vary among individuals, but crises tend to recur at the same site(s) for a particular person. The quality of the pain is usually similar as well. Most patients are able to distinguish a "typical" sickle cell pain crisis from other events, such as back pain from pyelonephritis or abdominal pain resulting from cholecystitis.

Most crises are mild to moderate in severity and can be managed at home with oral analgesics (either nonsteroidal antiinflammatory drugs [NSAIDs] or oral narcotics), adequate hydration, rest, and local measures such as heat or gentle massage. Moderate to severe crises require treatment in an emergency department or a hospital-based outpatient treatment center with parenteral narcotic analgesics and hydration, as well as the same local measures described previously. Often, aggressive and early management of a crisis can prevent hospital admission. Hospitalizations for crises can last from a few days to several weeks. Patients describe a severe crisis as the most intense pain that they have ever experienced. Pain control often requires large quantities of narcotic analgesics. For many patients it is not unusual to administer 4 to 8 mg of hydromorphone as an IV bolus over 10 to 15 minutes every 30 minutes for four to six doses before achieving adequate pain relief. Many adults with sickle cell disease have learned how to manage their pain without the behavioral signs that one would expect from someone experiencing severe pain. Therefore it becomes important when evaluating a sickle cell patient in crisis to believe the patient's report and to treat the pain quickly and appropriately.

Hydroxyurea is becoming standard therapy for patients who experience three or more crises per year. Hydroxyurea induces hemoglobin F formation, which forms soluble hybrid polymers with hemoglobin S, thus reducing hemoglobin S polymer concentration and ameliorating the cellular and tissue damage related to vascular occlusion.[26] In a randomized, double-blind, placebo-controlled study of 299 patients with SS disease, hydroxyurea reduced the incidence of painful crises.[27] However, patients have varied responses to hydroxyurea. Some respond well and see a reduction in their painful crises, whereas others may see no effect or no obvious reduction in crises. Hydroxyurea is started at a dose of 15 to 20 mg/kg/day. Patients must be monitored every 2 weeks for signs of toxicity (neutrophil count $<2000/mm^3$, platelet count $<80,000/mm^3$, or hemoglobin drop of 2 g/dl) or favorable response. The dose of hydroxyurea can be increased over several months to a maximum dose of 35 mg/kg. Once stable, patients should be monitored monthly.

By definition, patients with sickle cell disease are anemic. The degree of anemia varies, but most have hematocrit concentrations that range from the high teens to the mid-20s. Patients with hemoglobin SC tend to have hematocrit values in the high 20s to mid-30s. The baseline hematocrit value tends to remain relatively stable in a given patient. Most patients are able to compensate for their level of anemia and do not require routine transfusions. In fact, transfusing patients to hematocrit concentrations in the mid-30s or higher can be dangerous, as blood viscosity increases substantially at higher hematocrit levels and the increased viscosity can worsen the tendency to sickle by slowing the RBCs' transit time through low-oxygen regions of the circulation.[28]

Like other people with hemolytic anemias, patients with sickle cell disease require daily folic acid replacement. Folate is necessary for normal erythropoiesis, and in hemolytic anemias it is rapidly consumed by the proliferating erythroid precursors. Supplemental folic acid in the amount of 1 mg/day is enough to maintain the higher rate of erythropoiesis that occurs in chronic hemolysis.

Life Span Considerations

Women with sickle cell disease can carry pregnancies to term but should be considered high risk because of the potential for obstetric complications such as spontaneous abortion, thrombophlebitis, toxemia, and pulmonary embolism after delivery. The frequency of painful crises sometimes increases during pregnancy, but the crises are treated no differently from other crises, with narcotic analgesics and hydration. Pregnancy prevention and family planning options are the same for women with sickle cell disease as they are for other women. In fact, many women experience relief from menses-related crises with the use of oral contraceptives or other hormone contraception methods.

Sickle cell disease is a chronic condition that often leads to psychosocial difficulties, as well as medical problems. Some patients experience frequent complications of their disease, making it almost impossible to participate in normal daily activities or to hold a regular job or attend school on a regular schedule. Many of these patients can benefit from rehabilitation counseling and vocational training. Often, however, many adults with sickle cell disease find that they are unable to work because of chronic pain or other multiorgan damage. These individuals are clearly disabled.

Complications

Chronic pain is a substantial problem for most adults with sickle cell disease. The severity of the pain varies greatly among patients and can change over time. Some patients can manage their chronic pain with intermittent use of mild analgesics such as NSAIDs. Most patients, however, require frequent doses of oral narcotic analgesics. Often, these patients become tolerant to narcotics, and the quantity of medication needed to control the pain can escalate over time. This physical tolerance should not be confused with psychologic addiction and drug-seeking behaviors, which are uncommon in this population.

Acute pulmonary disease has become the most common cause of death and the second most common reason for hospitalizations.[29] The term *acute chest syndrome* (ACS) is used to describe an acute pulmonary event that can be either infectious or noninfectious in its etiology. Fever, dyspnea, cough, pulmonary infiltrates, and severe chest pain usually characterize the condition. Clinically, ACS is often more severe than pneumonia in the general population, with severe hypoxia and progressive multilobar involvement despite treatment with antibiotics. Typically the patient is hospitalized for a vasoocclusive crisis and 1 to 3 days later develops respiratory distress.

The most important step in the treatment of ACS is early recognition. Potential bacterial infections should be treated with appropriate antibiotics. Single-volume exchange transfusions are the treatment of choice for ACS in patients with severe hypoxemia (Pa_{O_2} <60 mm Hg) and can have a dramatic effect on reversing the clinical course, with rapid correction of hypoxia.[30] Simple transfusions raising the hemoglobin concentration to 10 g/dl can also be beneficial in patients with mild to moderate hypoxemia.[29]

Strokes are much more common in children than in adults but can occur in the adult population.[31] Stroke in sickle cell disease is a medical emergency. The treatment of choice is an exchange transfusion followed by maintenance hypertransfusion and iron chelation therapy.[32] In 1997, the Stroke Prevention Trial showed that chronic transfusion is highly effective in reducing the risk of first stroke in children with sickle cell disease and an abnormal transcranial Doppler ultrasonography.[33] It is now recommended that children with sickle cell disease be screened by transcranial Doppler ultrasonography and started on chronic transfusion therapy if results indicate a high risk of stroke. Young patients on chronic transfusion have fewer pain episodes and a reduced risk of acute chest syndrome.[34] These same patients must be compliant with iron chelation therapy to prevent future complications from iron overload (see previously).

Priapism is defined as a persistent, painful erection of the penis and can last from several hours to several days. Priapism lasting more than 3 or 4 hours is a medical emergency, as it can cause impotence. Treatment includes hydration, analgesia, and possible transfusion (either simple or exchange). Other controversial interventions include the use of conjugated estrogens and vasodilators for nonacute cases, and surgical interventions such as aspiration and shunt placement.

There is a high risk of renal dysfunction or failure in adults with sickle cell disease. Renal failure results from sickle cell-induced damage to renal microvasculature.[35] Renal dysfunction is generally diagnosed in the third or fourth decade and eventually progresses to renal failure. Subcutaneous erythropoietin or darbapoietin to maintain appropriate hemoglobin levels is often helpful to try to prevent or reduce the need for transfusions in patients with renal insufficiency. Adults with renal failure usually require chronic transfusions and should be offered chelation therapy if necessary. Treatment of end-stage renal disease requires hemodialysis or renal transplantation.

Skin ulcerations of the lower legs are the most common cutaneous complication of sickle cell disease, causing pain and physical disfigurement. They are resistant to therapy and often exist for years (some patients report persistent ulcers for more than 10 years). In the United States, approximately 25% of patients with sickle cell disease have a history of leg ulcers.[36]

The etiology and pathogenesis of leg ulcers are not well understood. Clinical experience and epidemiology studies suggest a role for three factors: marginal blood supply to the skin of the lower extremities, local edema, and minor trauma.[36] The greatest risk factor for the development of leg ulcers is a history of previous ulcers.

The most common site of skin ulcers is over the medial or lateral malleoli; they occur less commonly over the dorsum of the foot, near the Achilles tendon. The size of the ulcers varies from a few millimeters to large, circumferential ulcers that involve the entire ankle or foot. Lesions can extend into the dermis and often into the underlying subcutaneous tissue, or even into the underlying muscle fascia. These lesions are highly susceptible to infections and other complications. Pain is the major problem and is often severe and unremitting, causing significant disability.

Treatment of existing ulcers can be difficult and frustrating, as there is no effective cure and healing is often only temporary. Zinc is important in wound healing. It is found in RBCs and is lost during hemolysis; therefore zinc deficiency is common in patients with sickle cell disease.[37] The evidence that zinc supplementation benefits the healing of ankle ulcers is controversial; however, zinc supplementation is relatively benign and therefore a reasonable addition to therapy. Other controversial treatments include chronic transfusions and skin grafting for ulcers that are resistant to more conservative therapy, but failure rates for both methods are high.

Prevention includes educating patients about the importance of preventing local trauma by wearing shoes that fit properly, using insect repellents to prevent bites, and promptly treating any minor cuts on the feet and ankles. Patients with a history of ulcers and leg edema are encouraged to wear compression stockings and to perform routine care of the skin with emollients, good local hygiene, and daily inspection for any minor traumas.

The bony skeleton is a common target of the consequences of sickling. Bone marrow necrosis, bone infarcts, avascular necrosis (AVN), and osteomyelitis are common complications. The heads of the femur and humerus are common sites for marrow infarction and necrosis. Infarcts can also occur in the spine, ribs, and sternum. Bone infarcts constitute a painful crisis and generally resolve in 1 to 2 weeks. Treatment does not differ from that of any other painful crisis and includes analgesia, hydration, and rest.

AVN commonly affects the hip and shoulder joints and is a more chronic condition than an acute bony infarct. Patients complain of severe chronic pain, limited range of motion, and pain with joint movement. Late stages are evident on plain radiographs, but MRI is much more sensitive in identifying AVN in the very early stages. Initially, NSAIDs and narcotic analgesics are the mainstay of treatment. Later stages are usually surgically corrected with core decompression and/or joint replacement.

Retinopathy is a significant problem for patients with sickle cell disease. It is more common in patients with SC disease than in those with homozygous SS disease.[38] The retinopathy resembles that seen in diabetes and is believed to be caused by ischemia to the retina. Annual ophthalmoscopy with pupillary dilation is recommended. Treatment is with laser photocoagulation.

Indications for Referral/Hospitalization

Patients with sickle cell disease can be cared for in a primary care setting. However, the chronic nature of the disease, the frequent need for acute treatment of painful crises, and the high risk for complications generally require care by specialists familiar with the disease. Many of the large urban hospitals in the United States have sickle cell centers where patients receive comprehensive care by multidisciplinary teams of physicians, nurse practitioners, physician assistants, nurses, psychologists, and social workers. These hospital-based centers allow for prompt referral to other specialists such as neurologists, cardiologists, high-risk obstetricians, and ophthalmologists.

Most of the aforementioned complications require hospitalization for treatment. Patients with moderate to severe disease also have many admissions for intractable vasoocclusive crises. These hospitalizations can last from a couple of days to several weeks.

Consultation with a social worker is recommended for issues related to school, employment, housing, and transportation.

Patient and Family Education

Patient education begins early in childhood and continues throughout life. Initially, parents are taught how to manage pain crises, to recognize signs of infection, and to administer daily medications.[39] Coping with acute and chronic pain is a lifelong issue and involves learning both pharmacologic and nonpharmacologic interventions. Educating patients on the proper use of oral analgesics and management of painful crises is important and should occur at every opportunity. Patients need to be taught to seek prompt medical attention for any complication and not wait until they can speak to their primary care provider.

The importance of preventive care must also be stressed. Routine care should include annual ophthalmologic, gynecologic, and dental examinations; periodic sickle cell clinic visits; and immunizations, including hepatitis A and B, annual influenza vaccine, pneumococcal vaccine, meningococcal vaccine, and *Haemophilus influenzae* vaccine. Patients must also be educated about the importance of maintaining folic acid replacement therapy, even if their disease is mild.

Health Promotion

Maintaining adequate hydration, regular exercise, and sufficient sleep plays a role in helping patients manage their disease. Teaching children and young adults coping skills can be beneficial and can help them manage both the acute and chronic pain associated with their disease. Annual health screenings, ophthalmologic examinations, and vaccines are recommended but easily overlooked.

Anemia of Chronic Disease

Definition/Epidemiology

Anemia of chronic disease (ACD) is usually a mild anemia associated with chronic infectious, inflammatory, malignant, and connective tissue disorders.[40] The resulting anemia can be either normocytic or microcytic. ACD is often confused with IDA when the anemia is microcytic; however, both serum iron and TIBC are low in ACD.

ACD is the most common type of anemia among hospitalized patients.[4] It can mimic or coexist with other common anemias.

Pathophysiology

The exact pathogenesis of ACD is unclear but may include several factors, one of which may be a blunted erythropoietin response to anemia. The anemia can be associated with chronic renal failure and therefore erythropoietin deficiency. Erythropoietin is a renal hormone whose normal plasma levels increase logarithmically in response to hemoglobin levels below 12 g/dl.[7] In ACD this response is lower than would be predicted by the degree of anemia.[38] Other possible mechanisms for ACD that have been suggested include a decreased RBC survival time, decreased utilization of reticuloendothelial iron for hemoglobin synthesis, and inflammatory cytokine inhibition of erythropoietin production.[4,40]

Clinical Presentation

ACD is often mild and asymptomatic. Patients generally develop symptoms that are associated with the underlying disease(s) rather than the anemia itself. Progression of anemia results in the usual symptoms of advanced anemia such as fatigue and poor activity tolerance.

Physical Examination

There are usually no changes in the physical examination associated with ACD. Any changes in the physical examination are a result of the patient's underlying disease.

Diagnostics

The CBC will usually reveal a normocytic anemia, but the anemia can occasionally be microcytic. Hematocrit levels are generally 30% to 40%. There are no distinctive changes in RBC size or shape, but if microcytosis does occur, the RDW is slightly elevated. Iron studies reveal a low serum iron level, a normal or increased ferritin level, and a normal or elevated TIBC. Bone marrow examination, if done, reveals increased bone marrow iron stores with decreased amounts of bone marrow sideroblasts. The reticulocyte count is normal.

Basically, there are no precise diagnostic criteria for ACD. ACD often coexists with IDA, but laboratory tests can be difficult to distinguish, as frequent overlap exists. The only true way to distinguish ACD from IDA is by assessment of iron stores (which are absent in IDA and normal or increased in ACD) either by bone marrow aspiration or biopsy or by evaluation of the serum ferritin levels.

Differential Diagnosis

If the clinical picture is one of a mild microcytic anemia, the differential diagnosis is between ACD and IDA. Iron studies are the most useful test to differentiate the two (see Differential Diagnosis under Iron Deficiency Anemia, p. 1069).

Management

After IDA has been excluded, a mild anemia need not be treated unless symptomatic. The standard treatment for anemia of chronic disease or renal insufficiency is recombinant human erythropoietin (rHuEPO) or darbapoetin alfa (novel erythropoiesis stimulating protein [NESP]).[41] Intermittent transfusions may be required with more severe anemias. As always, the underlying condition should be treated or optimally controlled. Treatment of the underlying disease(s) will correct the anemia.

Complications

As long as the anemia is mild, there should be no complications associated with the anemia itself. Complications of the underlying disease should be managed appropriately.

Indications for Referral/Hospitalization

Once acute reasons for the anemia have been excluded and the diagnosis of ACD confirmed, patients should be followed by the clinician who is managing the underlying medical condition. The anemia should be monitored with periodic CBCs and iron studies. Referral to a hematologist may be necessary to initiate therapy with rHuEPO or NESP or if the anemia worsens and requires other interventions.

Given that ACD is associated with chronic medical conditions, it is possible that the patient may have an acute reason for anemia, such as a drug or transfusion reaction. If there is any uncertainty about the etiology of the anemia, a referral to, or consultation with, a hematologist is appropriate.

Rarely, ACD requires hospitalization for management. Patients are sometimes hospitalized when the diagnosis is made.

Patient and Family Education

Regular visits with the primary care provider should include laboratory studies to monitor for anemia. Patients should be encouraged to contact their provider if they experience any increase in symptoms such as fatigue, decreased exercise tolerance, or shortness of breath.

Aplastic Anemia

Definition/Epidemiology

Aplastic anemia is a life-threatening condition resulting from bone marrow stem cell failure. It is characterized by a marked decrease in all hematopoietic precursors, resulting in pancytopenia.

Aplastic anemia can affect all ages and both genders. It is a rare disorder with an estimated incidence of approximately 2 to 6 cases per million people per year.[42]

Pathophysiology

Aplastic anemia is usually related to exposure to specific toxins or medications that can cause bone marrow damage. Box 231-8 includes a few of the more than 500 medications that are associated with aplastic anemia. Aplastic anemia may also be immunologic, resulting from infections or severe disease such

BOX 231-8

AGENTS ASSOCIATED WITH APLASTIC ANEMIA

TOXINS
- Radiation
- Alkylating agents
- Insecticides
- Benzene and its derivatives
- Chemotherapeutic agents

MEDICATIONS
- Antibiotics (penicillin, chloramphenicol, cephalosporins, sulfonamides)
- Antidepressants (lithium, tricyclics)
- Antiinflammatory drugs (gold salts, nonsteroidals, salicylates)
- Antimalarials
- Anticonvulsants

OTHER POSSIBLE CAUSES
- Viral: non-A, non-B hepatitis, HIV, Epstein-Barr virus
- Graft-vs.-host disease (GVHD)
- Malignancy
- Pregnancy

as liver failure; however, almost half of all cases of aplastic anemia have an unclear etiology.

Clinical Presentation

Patients may present with abnormal bleeding, infection, and anemia (from the pancytopenia). Onset is usually sudden without any other apparent illness. The history may reveal information about a recent viral infection or chronic disease, or exposure to an offending medication or toxin.

Physical Examination

The physical examination may reveal petechiae, ecchymoses, purpura, pallor of the skin and mucous membranes, and mild lymphadenopathy in the late stages. Early stages of aplastic anemia may show no significant changes on physical examination.

Diagnostics

A CBC will show pancytopenia with normocytic and normochromic RBC indexes and morphology. The reticulocyte count is also below normal, reflecting the lack of bone marrow activity. A bone marrow biopsy is essential for diagnosis and reveals a severe hypoplasia (<25% cellularity).[42]

Differential Diagnosis

Aplastic anemia is readily detected and easily distinguished from other forms of normocytic, normochromic anemias. Involvement of other cell types (myeloid, and platelets) confirms the diagnosis.

Management

Any patient presenting with suspicions of aplastic anemia should be referred to a hematologist for management. Definitive treatment is either BMT or immunosuppressive therapy.[42,43] Use of blood products to correct the anemia should be minimized to prevent alloimmunization and to reduce the risk of graft failure after BMT. The decision to transfuse a patient with aplastic anemia should be made in consultation with the hematologist who will be treating the patient.

Life Span Considerations

The treatment of choice for aplastic anemia is based on the severity of the anemia and the age of the patient. BMT is more successful in younger patients and is the treatment of choice for children and adolescents. Patients who are more than 40 years of age have a higher risk of transplant-related morbidity and mortality. Immunosuppression therapy is the treatment of choice for adults over 40 years of age.[43]

Complications

Complications of untreated aplastic anemia include sepsis and death resulting from pancytopenia. Complications of BMT include graft failure, graft-versus-host disease, and a risk of secondary malignancies. Complications of immunosuppressive therapy include relapse and death resulting from pancytopenia or evolution of aplastic anemia to myelodysplasia or leukemia.[43]

Indications for Referral/Hospitalization

All patients who are suspected of having aplastic anemia should be immediately referred to a hematologist for treatment. Patients with severe aplastic anemia require hospitalization for management of the pancytopenia and to begin treatment. Most patients who undergo BMT or immunosuppressive therapy should continue to be monitored by a hematologist or oncologist as necessary.

Patient and Family Education/Health Promotion

Aplastic anemia can be caused by exposure to toxins such as benzene and insecticides. Patients should be taught that proper handling of products such as paints and insecticides includes adequate ventilation of the work area and wearing protective clothing such as masks and gloves.

Hemolytic Anemia

Definition/Epidemiology

All of the hemolytic anemias are associated with an increased rate of RBC destruction. The clinical presentation varies according to the disease. Some patients present with chronic hemolytic states that are well compensated, and others present with acute, self-limited hemolytic episodes. The most common chronic hemolytic anemia is sickle cell disease (discussed previously). Most of the other hemolytic anemias (Box 231-9) are rare and are mentioned only briefly here.

Glucose-6-phosphate dehydrogenase (G6PD) deficiency is an inherited erythrocyte enzyme deficiency that can result in an acute hemolytic anemia. G6PD-induced hemolysis is usually precipitated either by infection or by ingestion of an oxidant drug.

The most common form of G6PD deficiency in the United States is a mild variant of the disorder that typically affects approximately 10% of African-American males.[2] In all, 20% of African-American females carry the X-linked recessive gene for G6PD deficiency. G6PD deficiency is prevalent throughout tropical and subtropical regions of the world because it provides protection against malaria infection.[44] G6PD deficiency can be also be inherited along with other hematologic disorders such as sickle cell disease.

A mild chronic hemolytic anemia can also be caused by abnormalities in erythrocyte membrane protein composition. Hereditary spherocytosis and hereditary elliptocytosis are the best examples of this abnormality.[45]

The prevalence of hereditary spherocytosis is approximately 1 in 5000 (mostly northern Europeans).[43] Hereditary elliptocytosis is also relatively common, with a prevalence of 1 in 2500 to 1 in 5000, and is observed in all racial and ethnic groups. One form of hereditary elliptocytosis is commonly

BOX 231-9

EXAMPLES OF HEMOLYTIC ANEMIAS

- Hemoglobinopathies
- Glucose-6-phosphate dehydrogenase (G6PD) deficiency
- Membrane structural defects
  - Hereditary spherocytosis
  - Hereditary elliptocytosis
- Autoimmune hemolysis
  - Warm-reacting autoimmune hemolytic anemia
  - Cold-reacting autoimmune hemolytic anemia

seen in African-Americans. Another form is common in Southeast Asia, especially Papua New Guinea.[46]

Conditions such as viral or bacterial infections, collagen vascular diseases, or lymphoproliferative disorders are associated with autoimmune hemolytic anemias.

The frequency of an autoimmune hemolytic anemia depends on the prevalence of the associated disease state in the population. Warm-reacting autoantibodies are seen in 80% to 90% of all cases of autoimmune hemolytic anemia. Idiopathic autoimmune hemolytic anemia is most commonly seen in patients older than age 50 years.[47,48]

Pathophysiology

Drugs associated with acute hemolysis in G6PD-deficient patients include aspirin and phenacetin, sulfonamides, nitrofurantoin, and primaquine. Ingestion of an offending drug can result in the denaturation of hemoglobin,[7] leading to an acute hemolytic event. Other precipitants of hemolysis include the ingestion of fava beans or mothballs, or a severe bacterial or viral infection.

The functional abnormality in hereditary spherocytosis and hereditary elliptocytosis results from defects in the structural proteins of the erythrocyte cytoskeleton, specifically, a deficiency of the protein spectrin.[45]

In the autoimmune hemolytic anemias, the patient produces autoantibodies that react with the RBCs, causing premature erythrocyte destruction. Two types of autoantibodies are produced: warm-reacting autoantibodies and cold-reacting autoantibodies. Warm-reacting antibodies are reactive with cells at 37° C, and cold-reacting antibodies are reactive at temperatures below 37° C.[49]

Clinical Presentation

Most hemolytic anemias are mild, well compensated, and associated with few signs or symptoms. If the anemia is severe, the patient presents with the usual symptoms of severe anemia such as fatigue and exercise intolerance. Patients with G6PD deficiency can present with minimal or no clinical signs. Often the first clue that a patient has the deficiency is the onset of an acute hemolytic anemia after ingestion of an oxidant drug. The hemolytic event is self-limiting and usually mild. Patients with the Mediterranean form of G6PD deficiency are at risk for more severe hemolysis.[49]

Both hereditary spherocytosis and hereditary elliptocytosis are usually characterized by a mild hemolytic anemia that is well compensated. Patients with hereditary spherocytosis, however, can have a severe hemolytic anemia, whereas patients with hereditary elliptocytosis rarely have a clinically significant hemolytic anemia. Splenomegaly, aplastic crises, pigment gallstones, and chronic leg ulcers can complicate severe hereditary spherocytosis.[45]

Most commonly, the anemia caused by autoimmune hemolysis is also mild and self-limited. Patients with a warm-reacting autoimmune hemolytic anemia can have splenomegaly and other symptoms of anemia if the hemolysis is moderate or severe. Patients also present with signs and symptoms of the underlying disease. Box 231-10 gives examples of conditions associated with warm antibody autoimmune hemolysis and conditions associated with cold antibody autoimmune hemolysis.

BOX 231-10

CONDITIONS ASSOCIATED WITH AUTOIMMUNE HEMOLYSIS

CONDITIONS ASSOCIATED WITH HEMOLYSIS DUE TO WARM AUTOANTIBODIES

- Infections
- Collagen vascular diseases
  - Systemic lupus erythematosus
  - Rheumatoid arthritis
- Lymphoproliferative disorders
  - Leukemia
  - Lymphoma
- Drugs
  - Quinidine/quinine
  - Penicillin
  - Alpha-methyldopa
- Chronic renal disease
- Idiopathic

CONDITIONS ASSOCIATED WITH HEMOLYSIS DUE TO COLD AUTOANTIBODIES

- Malignancy
- *Mycoplasma pneumoniae*
- Viral pneumonia
- Idiopathic

Physical Examination

Patients with hemolytic anemias have an essentially normal physical examination. The only remarkable evidence of hemolysis may be scleral icterus, especially in patients with chronic hemolytic anemias, such as sickle cell disease.

Diagnostics

During a mild acute hemolytic event, serologic tests show a slight decrease in hemoglobin and the RBC count, an elevated LDH level, and slight hyperbilirubinemia. Patients with chronic hemolytic anemias, even when they are well compensated, have persistent reticulocytosis.

Assays for G6PD are useful and detect most deficient patients. In some milder variants of the disease, however, the screening test may be negative for several weeks after an acute hemolytic event.

A positive family history and the presence of pathognomonic findings on the peripheral blood smear easily diagnose both hereditary spherocytosis and hereditary elliptocytosis. Patients with hereditary spherocytosis have a large number of microspherocytes on the peripheral blood smear and an elevated MCHC on the CBC. The RBCs of patients with hereditary elliptocytosis have a uniform elliptic (oval) shape.

The diagnosis of an autoimmune hemolytic anemia depends on laboratory findings of abnormal autoantibodies. Coombs' test (both direct and indirect) is used to screen for these antibodies. The direct form of Coombs' test is positive in most cases of autoimmune hemolytic anemia, transfusion reactions, and some cases of drug-induced hemolysis. The indirect form of Coombs' test is positive in cases of antibody formation from

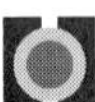

Differential Diagnosis

Hemolytic Anemia	
Sickle cell disease G6PD deficiency Hereditary disorders (hereditary spherocytosis, hereditary elliptocytosis)	Autoimmune hemolytic anemia

previous transfusions or pregnancy and in drug-induced hemolytic anemia.

Differential Diagnosis

It is important to match the clinical presentation with the possible diagnosis of a hemolytic anemia. Differential diagnoses that should be considered include whether the anemia is acute or chronic and whether the hemolysis is intravascular (such as occurs in disseminated intravascular coagulation) or extravascular (such as occurs in the hemolytic anemias previously discussed). The presence of any underlying disease will also direct the approach to the diagnosis, as many of the autoimmune disorders have predictable and expected patterns of hemolytic anemia.

Management

Management of a patient with a hemolytic anemia varies according to the individual disease state. Therefore proper management begins with an accurate diagnosis. Patients who are able to compensate for their degree of anemia generally require very little intervention. If the hemoglobin level begins to fall well below the patient's baseline, an occasional transfusion of packed RBCs may be necessary. All patients, especially if they have a chronic hemolytic anemia, require folic acid supplementation (1 mg folic acid/day) to maintain adequate erythropoiesis.

The acute, self-limited hemolysis in patients with mild G6PD deficiency rarely requires treatment. The resulting anemia is mild and resolves without intervention. Any patient presenting with an acute hemolytic event as a result of exposure to an oxidant drug should have serial CBCs measured to determine resolution of the anemia. The most important aspect of management of G6PD deficiency is ensuring the patient's awareness of the condition. All high-risk individuals should be screened, and information about what drugs and foods to avoid should be provided to all patients with the deficiency.

Patients with mild forms of hereditary spherocytosis or hereditary elliptocytosis maintain adequate hemoglobin levels and are in generally good health. Patients with severe hereditary spherocytosis may require a splenectomy to decrease the severity of the anemia.[30] These patients are also candidates for prophylactic cholecystectomy because of the high incidence of pigment gallstones (elective cholecystectomy should definitely be done if gallstones occur).

Patients with autoimmune hemolytic anemia are generally treated with some combination of corticosteroid therapy or immunosuppressive therapy, splenectomy, and transfusion with packed RBCs. The specific therapy varies according to the type and severity of the hemolytic anemia.

Life Span Considerations

Patients with G6PD deficiency, hemoglobinopathy, or a hereditary RBC membrane defect should be aware of the hereditary potential. Professional genetic counseling and screening should be offered to all patients who are considering pregnancy.

Complications

Most of the hemolytic anemias discussed here rarely cause complications, especially if the hemolysis is mild and self-limited or chronic but well compensated. Patients with more severe forms of hemolytic anemia, especially autoimmune hemolytic anemia, are at risk for acute episodes of severe hemolysis, with the associated morbidity and mortality of a severe anemia.

Indications for Referral/Hospitalization

A referral to a hematologist is prudent when an acute hemolysis does not appear to be resolving, or when the anemia is severe or does not respond to treatment. Acute hemolysis that occurs as a result of a mild form of hemolytic anemia does not require hospitalization for management. If the patient also has some other underlying condition or the anemia is severe, however, hospitalization may be required for management. As with any other type of anemia, the need for hospitalization depends on the patient's ability to compensate for the degree of anemia.

Patient and Family Education

Patients should understand the nature of their disorder well enough to be able to explain it to other health care providers. Patients with G6PD deficiency should be given a list of drugs and foods to avoid including over-the-counter products that contain aspirin or phenacetin. Patients with drug-induced hemolysis should be made aware of the types of drugs to avoid. Those with autoimmune hemolytic anemias should be made aware of the types of situations and conditions that can aggravate their anemia. All patients should be instructed to contact their primary care provider if there are any signs of increased anemia.

REFERENCES

1. Fischbach F: *A manual of laboratory and diagnostic tests*, ed 4, Philadelphia, 1992, JB Lippincott.
2. Payton RG, White PJ: Primary care of women: assessment of hematologic disorders, *J Nurse Midwifery* 40(2):120-136, 1995.
3. Shine JW: Microcytic anemia, *Am Fam Physician* 55(7):2455-2462, 1997.
4. Sears DA: Anemia of chronic disease, *Med Clin North Am* 76(3):567-579, 1992.
5. Massey AC: Microcytic anemia: differential diagnosis and management of iron deficiency anemia, *Med Clin North Am* 76(3):549-566, 1992.
6. Schwartz WJ III, Thurnau GR: Iron deficiency anemia in pregnancy, *Clin Obstet Gynecol* 38(3):443-454, 1995.
7. Hillman RS, Ault KA: Hematology. In *Hematology in Clinical practice: a guide to diagnosis and management*, New York, 1995, McGraw-Hill.
8. Wada L, King JC: Trace element nutrition during pregnancy, *Clin Obstet Gynecol* 37(3):574-586, 1994.
9. Guyatt GH and others: Diagnosis of iron-deficiency anemia in the elderly, *Am J Med* 88(3):205-209, 1990.

10. Hallberg L, Brune M, Rossander L: Iron absorption in man: ascorbic acid and dose-dependent inhibition of phytate, *Am J Clin Nutr* 49(1):140-144, 1989.
11. Lops VR, Hunter LP, Dixon LR: Anemia in pregnancy, *Am Fam Physician* 51(5):1189-1197, 1995.
12. Pearson HA: The evaluation of thalassemia intermedia. In Thalassemia intermedia: a Region I conference: proceedings from a conference on thalassemia intermedia, *Genet Res* 11(2):5-10, 1997.
13. Katsanis E and others: Hemoglobin E: a common hemoglobinopathy among children of Southeast Asian origin, *Can Med Assoc J* 137(1): 39-42, 1987.
14. Rund D, Rachmilewitz E: New trends in the treatment of beta-thalassemia, *Crit Rev Oncol Hematol* 33(2):105-118, 2000.
15. Telfer P and others: Hepatic iron concentration combined with long-term monitoring of serum ferritin to predict complications of iron overload in thalassemia major, *Br J Haematol* 110(4-II):971-977, 2000.
16. Cao A and others: 1992 *Management protocol for the treatment of thalassemia patients,* Flushing, NY, 1992, Cooley's Anemia Foundation.
17. Campbell BA: Megaloblastic anemia in pregnancy, *Clin Obstet Gynecol* 38(3):455-462, 1995.
18. Stabler S: Screening the older population for cobalamin (vitamin B_{12} deficiency), *J Am Geriatr Soc* 43(11):1290-1297, 1995.
19. Campbell NR: How safe are folic acid supplements? *Arch Intern Med* 156(15):1638-1644, 1996.
20. Savage DG and others: Etiology and diagnostic evaluation of macrocytosis, *Am J Med Sci* 319(6):343-352, 2000.
21. MRC Vitamin Research Group: Prevention of neural tube defects: results of the Medical Research Council Vitamin Study, *Lancet* 338(8760):131-137, 1991.
22. Centers for Disease Control and Prevention: Recommendations for the use of folic acid to reduce the number of cases of spina bifida and other neural tube defects, *MMWR* 41(RR-14):1-7, 1992.
23. Koshy M, Dorn L: Continuing care for adult patients with sickle cell disease, *Hematol Oncol Clin North Am* 10(6):1265-1274, 1996.
24. Vichinshy EP, Lubin BH: Sickle cell anemia and related hemoglobinopathies, *Pediatr Clin North Am* 27(2):429-447, 1980.
25. Platt OS and others: Pain in sickle cell disease: rates and risk factors, *N Engl J Med* 325:11-16, 1991.
26. Ballas SK, Mohandes N: Pathophysiology of vaso-occlusion, *Hematol Oncol Clin North Am* 10(6):1221-1240, 1996.
27. Charache S and others: Effect of hydroxyurea on the frequency of painful crisis in sickle cell anemia: investigations of the Multicenter Study of Hydroxyurea in Sickle Cell Anemia, *N Engl J Med* 332(20):1317-1322, 1995.
28. Kaul DK and others: Erythrocytes in sickle cell anemia are heterogeneous in their rheological and hemodynamic characteristics, *J Clin Invest* 72:22-31, 1983.
29. Vichinsky E, Styles L: Pulmonary complications, *Hematol Oncol Clin North Am* 10(6):1275-1288, 1996.
30. Emre U and others: Effect of transfusion in acute chest syndrome of sickle cell disease, *J Pediatr* 127(6):901-904, 1995.
31. Ohene-Frempong K: Stroke in sickle cell disease: demographic, clinical, and therapeutic considerations, *Semin Hematol* 28(3):213-219, 1991.
32. Pegelow CH and others: Risk of recurrent stroke in patients with sickle cell disease treated with erythrocyte transfusion, *J Pediatr* 126(6):896-899, 1995.
33. Adams RJ: Lessons from the Stroke Prevention Trial in Sickle Cell Anemia (STOP) study, *J Child Neurol* 15(5):344-349, 2000.
34. Miller ST and others: Impact of chronic transfusion on incidence of pain and acute chest syndrome during the Stroke Prevention Trial (STOP) in sickle-cell anemia, *J Pediatr* 139(6):785-789, 2001.
35. Wong WY, Elliot-Mills D, Powars D: Renal failure in sickle cell anemia, *Hematol Oncol Clin North Am* 10(6):1321-1331, 1996.
36. Eckman JR: Leg ulcers in sickle cell disease, *Hematol Oncol Clin North Am* 10(6):1333-1344, 1996.
37. Prasad AS, Abbasi A, Ortega J: Zinc deficiency in man: studies in sickle cell disease, *Prog Clin Biol Res* 14:211-239, 1977.
38. Clarkson JG: The ocular manifestations of sickle-cell disease: a prevalence and natural history study, *Trans Am Ophthalmol Soc* 90:481-504, 1992.
39. Gil KM and others: Daily coping practice predicts treatment effects in children with sickle cell disease, *J Pediatr Psychol* 26(3):163-173, 2001.
40. Spivak JL: The blood in systemic disorders, *Lancet* 355(9216): 1707-1712, 2000.
41. Nissenson AR: Novel erythropoiesis stimulating protein for managing the anemia of chronic kidney disease, *Am J Kidney Dis* 38(6):1390-1397, 2001.
42. Fonseca R, Tefferi A: Practical aspects in the diagnosis and management of aplastic anemia, *Am J Med Sci* 313(3):159-169, 1997.
43. Young NS, Barrett AJ: The treatment of severe acquired aplastic anemia, *Blood* 85(12):3367-3377, 1995.
44. Mehta A and others: Glucose-6-phosphate dehydrogenase deficiency, *Baillieres Best Pract Res Clin Haematol* 13(1):21-38, 2000.
45. Smedley JC, Bellingham AJ: Current problems in hematology. II: hereditary spherocytosis, *J Clin Pathol* 44(6):441-444, 1991.
46. Davies KA, Lux SE: Hereditary disorders of the red cell membrane skeleton, *Trends Genet* 5:221-227, 1989.
47. Sokok RJ, Booker DJ, Stamps R: The pathology of autoimmune hemolytic anaemia, *J Clin Pathol* 45(12):1047-1052, 1992.
48. Rosenwasser LJ, Joseph BZ: Immunohematologic diseases, *JAMA* 268(20):2940-2945, 1992.
49. Luzzatto L: Inherited haemolytic states: glucose-6-phosphate dehydrogenase deficiency, *Clin Haematol* 4(1):83-108, 1975.
50. Bolton-Maggs PH: The diagnosis and management of hereditary spherocytosis, *Baillieres Best Pract Clin Haematol* 13(3):327-342, 2000.

CHAPTER 232

Blood Coagulation Disorders

Maura Malone, Laurel McKernan,
and Leo R. Zacharski

DEFINITION/EPIDEMIOLOGY

Coagulation is the process by which blood changes from a liquid to a solid; this is a complex process involving many different initiatory and inhibitory proteins, as well as certain cells, particularly platelets. Disorders of coagulation occur for a wide variety of reasons. A quantitative deficiency or a qualitative abnormality in the coagulant or anticoagulant mechanisms may tip the balance toward either a tendency to bleed (coagulopathy) or a tendency to form clots (thrombophilia). Disorders of coagulation factors may be inherited or acquired (e.g., from illness or medications). The three most common bleeding disorders are von Willebrand's disease (vWD), hemophilia A, and hemophilia B. The gene for vWD is present in approximately 1% of the general population. Together, hemophilia A and hemophilia B occur in about 2 per 50,000 males.[1]

Determining the diagnosis required for appropriate management can be difficult, particularly with mild bleeding disorders. Patients are often referred for medical evaluation because of one of the following: a bleeding or thrombotic episode, a positive family history, or an abnormal laboratory test result found, for example, during preoperative screening. The primary care provider needs to determine, through clinical and laboratory assessment, whether these referral indicators reflect the presence of a coagulation disorder. There are many different coagulation disorders, and only the most common of these are covered in this chapter. Practical guidelines for evaluating thrombosing and bleeding disorders are discussed. Particular focus is on congenital disorders.

Extensive studies have shown that an elaborate balance exists between substances in the blood that promote clotting (called coagulation factors) and other substances that preserve blood in fluid form (called anticoagulant factors). This balance is maintained until a blood vessel is injured. The blood coagulation mechanism is designed to interpret such injuries and respond by developing a protective clot at the injury site that stops the flow of blood. Prevention of blood loss from the vasculature with injury is vital, and this process is referred to as hemostasis. The clotting mechanism is called a self-referencing system because of its ability to turn itself on and off locally to achieve a beneficial effect. It is correctly viewed as an irreducibly complex system, because a defect in any one of its many components can lead to malfunction of the entire system. The benefits of this mechanism are obvious and are taken for granted except in individuals who have a deficiency in a coagulant or anticoagulant protein, because they may bleed excessively or form pathologic clots.

The normal hemostatic response may be considered to proceed in three phases. In phase 1, blood vessels constrict, reducing blood flow from the site. In phase 2, platelets are activated by tissues, and chemicals are released almost instantaneously, resulting in the formation of a platelet plug. Phase 3 begins within seconds after platelet activation. In this phase a complex cascade, involving over a dozen protein clotting factors is triggered.[2] The end result of this cascade is the production of a powerful enzyme (thrombin) that converts fibrinogen, which is present in solution in the blood, to fibrin. Fibrin is a durable, visible mesh that seals the injured vessel (the scab). Traditionally this cascade is thought to consist of intrinsic (entirely plasma derived) and extrinsic (tissue factor initiated) pathways.[2] Abnormalities within these pathways are detected by specific tests such as the activated partial thromboplastin time (APTT) for the intrinsic pathway and the prothrombin time (PT) for the extrinsic pathway. Although the precise initiator of coagulation with injury in vivo is controversial, it is generally held that such coagulation proceeds by way of the extrinsic pathway.

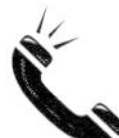

Physician consultation is recommended for patients with an international normalized ratio (INR) greater than 6.
Physician consultation is recommended for patients with a platelet count less than 100,000/mm³.

Coagulopathies

PATHOPHYSIOLOGY AND CLINICAL PRESENTATION

The manifestations of coagulopathies are determined by the type and severity of the defect. Is it a vascular disorder, platelet abnormality, or clotting factor deficiency? Is it acquired or congenital? These questions are answered through the clinical and laboratory assessment.

Patients with congenital bleeding disorders usually have a lifelong history of symptoms such as easy bruising and prolonged bleeding with cuts, surgery, or trauma. Severe deficiencies generally become evident when the affected individual becomes a toddler and is more likely to sustain minor trauma. Episodes also occur spontaneously. Milder hereditary deficiencies may go undiagnosed for years, or until significant trauma occurs or the individual undergoes surgery. In contrast, acquired disorders may become evident later in life in the absence of a past history of bleeding manifestations. New symptoms may include a recent onset of increased bruising, bleeding with trauma, nosebleeds, or a recent change in clotting test findings. These changes may be due to effects of medications or other disorders such as liver or renal disease. The type of bleeding reported may indicate which pathway is involved. Easy bruising, mucosal bleeding, and postsurgical hemorrhage are typical of a platelet disorder, whereas a history of delayed bleeding after surgery and hemorrhage into the joints and muscles are typical of a factor deficiency such as hemophilia A or B. Clinical symptoms are discussed further in the section on diagnosis. However, there are no rigid distinctions between the types of defects and their clinical manifestations.

PHYSICAL EXAMINATION

Bleeding disorders are generally diagnosed by the history and laboratory findings. The physical examination may be negative, especially with mild defects. However, a variety of findings, including bruises, petechiae, gingival bleeding, epistaxis, and hematomas, may be evident, especially in individuals with more severe defects. Some degree of bruising is very common in the general population. However, bruises that are more than just a few in number and that occur on the trunk in addition to the extremities are more significant.

DIAGNOSTICS AND DIFFERENTIAL DIAGNOSIS

The most valuable diagnostic test for a bleeding disorder is a careful, comprehensive bleeding history. The history should provide clues to the type of bleeding disorder that may be present and to laboratory tests that are indicated for further evaluation. The hemostatic response to trauma determined in the bleeding history is generally a more sensitive test of hemostatic competence than are screening laboratory tests (e.g., when evaluating a patient before surgery).[3]

There are two major elements in a bleeding history: the patient's history and the family history. The patient should be asked to describe each event in life in which a hemostatic challenge was presented. These include the response to minor cuts and scratches, surgery, dental extractions, and menstrual periods. Spontaneous bleeding may occur in the form of joint or soft tissue bleeding, epistaxis, and bruising. Bruising in the absence of trauma is more significant than bruising in response to trauma. It is particularly important to encourage the patient to quantitate the degree of bleeding. This may be done by estimating average bruise counts and location, duration of posttraumatic bleeding, duration and number of pads soaked during menstruation, and so on. Menstrual blood is normally unclotted, and the passage of clots (e.g., with urination, defecation, or pad changes) may be significant. With practice, interviewers will refine their assessment skills and assist their patients in proper interpretations because what is "normal" bleeding to one person may be "heavy" to another. Box 232-1 gives examples of interview questions for use when evaluating a patient for a bleeding disorder.

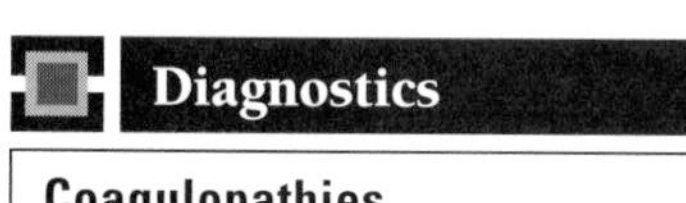

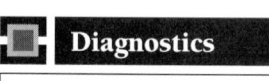

Diagnostics

Coagulopathies

Laboratory
PT, PTT
Platelet count
Bleeding time
Thrombin time
Fibrinogen levels
Peripheral smear

Differential Diagnosis

Coagulopathies

Hemophilia	HIV infection
von Willebrand's disease	Drug-induced condition
Idiopathic thrombocytopenic purpura	Connective tissue disorder
Vitamin K deficiency	Hypersplenism
Liver disease	Cushing's syndrome
Disseminated intravascular coagulation	Uremia
	Factor XI deficiency
	Marfan's syndrome

The family history is critical in assessing coagulation disorders. The genetic defect in hemophilia A and B (factor VIII and IX deficiency) is X-linked recessive and affects only males. However, the defect in families is carried by females, who are usually asymptomatic. Thus a male patient's maternal grandfather, uncles, and cousins may have bleeding that provides a clue to the diagnosis of hemophilia A or B.

Although the bleeding history is of paramount importance in the evaluation for coagulation disorders, it is not without limitations. The accuracy of information reported is largely dependent on the interviewer and his or her ability to elicit a description of previous hemostatic challenges. It is easy to miss events or receive an incomplete history. Mild bleeding disorders are difficult to identify, especially in the absence of a hemostatic challenge or in young children who may not have experienced hemostatic challenges. Spontaneous mutations are common, especially in hemophilia A and B, and consequently the family history may be negative.

While the decision as to whether to refer the patient for specialized tests is made, certain screening studies may be performed. The typical laboratory screen includes the PT, APTT, platelet count, bleeding time, thrombin time, and fibrinogen level.[3] These studies provide basic information on the integrity of the intrinsic and extrinsic pathways, as well as platelet function.

The platelet count is usually done by automated counters. Low values must be confirmed by examination of the peripheral blood smear. Common causes of a low platelet count include immune destruction, drugs, vasculitis, disseminated intravascular coagulation, and chemotherapy.

The bleeding time is a valuable screen for platelet disorders if performed by an experienced technologist. It is best done by the same individual using a standardized template method. Prolonged bleeding time generally is defined as >8 minutes. Causes of a prolonged bleeding time include thrombocytopenia (platelet count <100,000/mm^3), qualitative platelet defect, vWD, and poor (overly aggressive) technique.

PT measures the function of the extrinsic system and the common pathway. It is sensitive to abnormalities of factors VII, X, V, II, and fibrinogen.

Partial thromboplastin time (PTT) measures the function of the intrinsic system and the common pathway. It detects abnormalities of prekallikrein; high-molecular-weight kininogen; factors XII, XI, IX, VIII, X, V, and II; and fibrinogen.

A prolonged PT or APTT may be evaluated further by a test known as mixing studies, which incorporate different ratios of normal (control) and abnormal (patient) plasma. Correction of the abnormality on addition of normal plasma suggests the presence of a factor deficiency, whereas failure to correct the abnormality suggests the presence of an inhibitor, such as the lupus anticoagulant. The inhibitor acts to neutralize the added normal plasma, which then fails to correct the abnormal coagulation test. Misinterpretation of the results of mixing studies is a common cause for a request for a coagulation consultation.

If the patient has a negative bleeding history (patient and family), an underlying bleeding disorder is unlikely, and laboratory evaluation is usually not helpful. If the patient has a negative bleeding history without hemostatic challenges, such as surgery or significant trauma, and a positive family history for bleeding, screening tests may be advisable. Diagnosis may be important in planning future care, such as with trauma or elective surgery. Patients may be able to avoid unnecessary

BOX 232-1

INTERVIEW QUESTIONS FOR EVALUATING A PATIENT WITH A BLEEDING DISORDER

PATIENT HISTORY

Ecchymoses, easy and frequent bruising: How many bruises are present at a given time—6, 12, more? Are they raised or flat? Are they on the chest and trunk, or only on the limbs? Are there hematomas with injections?

Epistaxis: Are they spontaneous, or do they occur with trauma? Are they one sided or bilateral? Are they seasonal, or do they occur year-round? How many occur in a month? How long do they last, and what measures do you use to stop them? Do large clots form?

Hemostatic challenges such as injuries or lacerations? How long did the bleeding last—2 minutes, 20 minutes, longer? Did the laceration require sutures? Did the bleeding continue afterward? For how long? Have there been any fractures?

Have there been any dental extractions? Was there any excess bleeding? For how long—an hour, half a day, a day, a week?

Has there been any prior surgery? What kind? Was there any reported excess bleeding? Were any transfusions required?

Has there been any significant injury or other trauma that might challenge the coagulation mechanism?

Is the bleeding immediate, platelet-type bleeding or delayed, with deep hematomas?

Detailed menstruation history when appropriate: How long does menstruation last? How heavy is it? What is heavy? Generally, how many pads per day? Is there formation of large clots?

Has there been any recent illness? Any current medications, including over-the-counter medications (e.g., aspirin)?

Obstetric history when appropriate: Was there any bleeding during pregnancy or delivery? Was a transfusion required?

FAMILY HISTORY

Inquire about immediate family members—brothers, sisters, parents, children. Request documentation when appropriate.

Inquire about extended family on the maternal and paternal sides—grandparents, aunts and uncles, cousins.

Review a similar line of questioning as for the patient history for clinical features, surgery, trauma, transfusions, and menstrual history.

When questioning parents about their children, inquire about cephalhematomas, buccal mucosal bleeding, bleeding from the tongue or tooth extractions, bleeding with separation of the umbilical cord, bruising or hematomas with immunizations, and bruising with the onset of crawling and ambulation.

Important to note: A negative bleeding history in a young child may not rule out a bleeding disorder; rather a hemostatic challenge has not yet been encountered.

blood transfusions if a bleeding disorder is diagnosed and prophylactic treatment provided.

If the patient has a negative bleeding history and positive screening studies, extraneous factors need to be considered, such as medications (e.g., aspirin, over-the-counter cold preparations with guaifenesin), allergies (rhinitis), or illness. Circulating anticoagulants are found commonly in patients with an unexplained prolonged APTT. Occasionally the PTT may reveal the presence of a circulating anticoagulant. These may be diagnosed using mixing studies and rarely result in clinical bleeding.

If the patient has a positive bleeding history, it is essential to exclude an anatomic explanation for the bleeding. Unfortunately, routine screening tests are relatively insensitive except in the presence of severe abnormalities. Bleeding disorders that may be associated with normal screening tests include mild hemophilia, vWD, abnormal fibrinogens, and factor XIII deficiency. A positive bleeding history in a patient with normal laboratory tests suggests the need for referral to a hematologist with specialty expertise in coagulopathies.

A positive history and abnormal laboratory screening tests suggest strongly that a bleeding disorder exists, and referral to a hematologist for further evaluation is needed to determine a specific diagnosis.

Differential diagnosis of bleeding is based on the medical history, physical findings, and laboratory testing. It is important to keep in mind that the quality of coagulation test results is highly dependent on the conditions under which the samples are obtained, as well as the experience and professional quality of the coagulation laboratory. Prompt specimen processing and proper plasma storage are mandatory. Certain tests, such as platelet aggregation studies, require immediate laboratory testing using specialized equipment by highly trained and experienced technicians. Ideally, patients should be medication free for at least 2 weeks and sampled while fasting, especially when platelet aggregation tests are to be performed. It may be inadvisable to make a critical diagnosis on the basis of results obtained on plasma samples after prolonged storage or shipment to a distant laboratory. Travel by the patient to the testing laboratory for blood sampling is optimal.

MANAGEMENT AND INDICATIONS FOR REFERRAL/HOSPITALIZATION

Since 1975, hemophilia treatment centers (HTCs) have been federally funded to provide comprehensive, specialized care to person with bleeding disorders. There is evidence suggesting persons who receive care at a HTCs have a 40% lower mortality rate associated with bleeding complications.[4] Therefore, management of a patient with a known congenital bleeding disorder by a primary care provider should be conducted in conjunction with a hematologist with expertise in blood coagulation and the guidelines put forth by the Medical and Scientific Advisory Council (MASAC) and adopted by the National Hemophilia Foundation.[5] Once the patient is evaluated by a hematologist, a detailed plan of patient care should be developed that includes the MASAC guidelines for managing the patient if trauma occurs or an invasive procedure is required. A variety of plasma-derived and recombinant factor concentrates are available, and the hematologist will assist in identifying the appropriate product and dose for the patient (Table 232-1). To ensure rapid and appropriate treatment, a local supply of the appropriate replacement product should be maintained. Most patients with congenital bleeding disorders learn to recognize bleeding episodes soon after they occur and may be trained in self-administration of the clotting factor by IV administration. Surgery in the patient with a bleeding disorder should be undertaken at a facility equipped with an on-site coagulation laboratory, a full range of treatment products, and expert hematology consultation. Box 232-2 illustrates important factors to consider when assessing the type, degree, and treatment of a bleeding disorder.

Patients with a factor deficiency, such as moderate or severe hemophilia A or B, require replacement with the missing clotting protein. It is better to overestimate than to underestimate the risk of bleeding and to treat prophylactically or as soon as possible after bleeding begins. Hemostasis is more difficult to achieve once excessive bleeding has commenced. Generally speaking, any significant trauma will require replacement. Any invasive procedure, even a tooth extraction, requires pretreatment with factor concentrate. Trauma or surgery often requires many days of factor replacement accompanied by close monitoring of coagulation factor levels to ensure that hemostatic levels of the deficient clotting protein are present. Milder bleeding disorders such as mild hemophilia A and type I vWD may be corrected temporarily by administration of desmopressin acetate, either IV or by high-concentrate nasal spray. Desmopressin is a synthetic analogue of vasopressin. It is effective in releasing factor VIII and von Willebrand's factor (vWF) from endothelial cells in patients with certain mild bleeding disorders. However, reliance on desmopressin to achieve hemostasis requires prior demonstration of a rise in clotting factor levels in a previously performed trial of this drug.

BOX 232-2

ASSESSMENT OF BLEEDING EPISODE

- Type of coagulation disorder
- Degree or severity of the disorder
- Presence of co-morbidity as associated with transfusion, such as hepatitis B, hepatitis C, HIV
- Site and extent of bleeding and number of treatments
- History of response to replacement product; history of circulating inhibitors
- Replacement product: choice, dose, half-life, risks, benefits
- Are adjunct therapies (e.g., oral antifibrinolytics) required?

von Willebrand's Disease

DEFINITION/EPIDEMIOLOGY

vWD is the most common congenital bleeding disorder and occurs in approximately 1% of the general population.[6] A single gene for this disease is sufficient to cause bleeding in either males or females. vWD results from a quantitative or qualitative abnormality in vWF. vWF functions as a bridging molecule that binds to receptors exposed on the platelet surface to link them both to each other and to the area of damage on the blood vessel wall. It is important to note that vWF also serves as the carrier protein for blood coagulation factor VIII. vWF is therefore involved in both platelet and fibrin thrombus formation and typically is manifested by prolongation of both the bleeding time and the APTT. vWD can be a challenging disease to diagnose because various conditions (e.g., medications, inflammation, stress, pregnancy) can elevate vWF from abnormally low levels into the normal range, thus masking the deficiencies seen in vWD. vWD bleeding often consists of epistaxis, menorrhagia, excessive bruising, and prolonged bleeding with cuts or dental extractions and in the intraoperative or immediate postoperative period.

There are three major types of vWD. Type I vWD, the most common type, representing 70% to 80% of cases, is a quantitative deficiency of vWF.[7] Type IIA and type IIB vWD are qualitative defects in vWF, affecting about 20% to 30% of cases.[7] Type III vWD is a rare and severe homozygous form of vWD.[7] It is important to identify the correct type of vWD to prescribe correct treatment. Desmopressin acetate, which is the treatment of

TABLE 232-1 Dosing Guidelines for Factor Replacement Therapy for Patients with Hemophilia A (Factor 8 Deficiency) and Hemophilia B (Factor 9 Deficiency)

Type of Bleeding Episode		Hemophilia A: Target Factor 8 Level (%)	Hemophilia A: Factor 8 Dose (IV/kg)	Hemophilia B: Target Factor 9 Level (%)	Hemophilia B: Factor 9 Dose (IV/kg)
Minor	Mucosal bleeds (oral, nasal), skin deep lacerations, soft tissue	30-40	20	30-40	30-40
Moderate	Joint (elbow, hip, knee, ankle), muscle, soft tissue, status post trauma	40-60	20-30	50-60	50-60
Major*	CNS, head, neck, throat, eye, gastrointestinal, iliopsoas, surgical/trauma	80-100	50	80-100	75-100

*A week or more of aggressive factor replacement and close monitoring will be required.

choice for a patient with mild to moderate type I vWD, is contraindicated in type IIB vWD.[8,9] The explanation for this is beyond the scope of this text. Because of inherent variability in plasma levels of vWF, a single assay for this protein may not be sufficient for diagnosis. Furthermore, overlap exists between levels present in normal subjects and in those with mild disease. The blood type is also correlated with vWF levels. Relative ranking of vWF levels according to the blood type is as follows: AB > B > A > O. Typical screening tests for vWD include the following:

- Bleeding time—May be normal to prolonged.
- PTT—May be normal to prolonged.
- vWF antigen—Quantitative immunoassay for the amount of vWF protein present. This is typically decreased in type I disease but is low to normal in type II disease.
- vWF activity (ristocetin C activity)—Quantitative measure of the ability of vWF to clump platelets in the presence of the antibiotic ristocetin. vWF activity is decreased in type I disease and disproportionately decreased in type II disease.
- Factor VIII activity (FVIII:C)—Because vWF functions as a carrier protein for factor VIII, this test generally parallels levels of antigen unless the binding site for factor VIII on vWF is abnormal.
- Ristocetin-induced platelet aggregation (RIPA)—Special test used to distinguish between type IIa and type IIb vWD.
- vWF multimers—Test that confirms the type of vWD. vWF occurs in the plasma in multimers of various sizes. vWF multimers are clusters consisting of variable numbers of individual vWF molecules. The very large vWF multimers are biologically most active. Type II vWD is characterized by a relatively selective decrease in the larger multimers. This test is therefore helpful in distinguishing between type I and type II vWD.

Once the diagnosis is confirmed, treatment options include desmopressin and plasma-derived factor VIII concentrates that are rich in vWF.[9]

Hemophilia

DEFINITION/EPIDEMIOLOGY

Hemophilia is an X-linked recessive bleeding disorder characterized by low levels of factor VIII (hemophilia A) or factor IX (hemophilia B).[1] Such deficiencies result in defective fibrin clot formation. Minor injuries are sometimes associated with little bleeding because platelet thrombus formation is normal. However, on later breakdown of the platelet plug, bleeding may occur because of the lack of a stabilizing fibrin clot. Joint and muscle hemorrhages are common in moderate and severe hemophilia. Recurrent hemarthrosis results in hypertrophy and inflammation of the joint synovial tissue, leading to release of proteolytic enzymes that damage the articular cartilage, causing loss of joint function and long-term disability. Soft tissue hematomas may resolve with factor replacement if treated promptly; however, continued bleeding may result in compression of vital structures. Limb contractures are common, often requiring physical therapy to regain range of motion. Psoas muscle bleeding may cause vague hip pain and/or abdominal pain and are often confused with the symptoms of appendicitis or renal colic. Intracranial hemorrhage is a leading cause of death in hemophilia. A blow to the head or concussion requires immediate factor replacement. Symptomatic head trauma must be evaluated by a practitioner with expertise in neurologic injuries, including imaging studies to exclude intracranial bleeding.

Treatment of bleeding in the hemophilia patient involves prompt replacement of clotting factors or in mild hemophilia A, stimulating release of clotting factor from intracellular stores via administration of desmopressin acetate.[10] Although most patients receive treatment after bleeding is identified, preventive therapy is given before surgery or an invasive procedure. It has been shown that prophylactic infusions of clotting factor for severe hemophilia, when begun at an early age, prevents hemorrhages and associated long-term joint damage.[11] See Table 232-1 for dosing guidelines.

COMPLICATIONS

Bleeding that results from disorders of hemostasis may produce a variety of complications. For example, the chronic, recurrent joint bleeding commonly experienced by patients with hemophilia may lead to joint immobility and limb contractures. Chronic bleeding can cause anemia as well as iron deficiency. Bleeding into various organs can result in dysfunction of that organ. Such bleeding may be fatal if it occurs, for example, in the cranial cavity.

PATIENT EDUCATION AND LIFE SPAN CONSIDERATIONS

Education is an important and ongoing process. Patients should know the specific name of their bleeding disorder and be able to communicate this diagnosis to future health care providers. They should be able to recognize the signs and symptoms of their disease and know how to respond to these appropriately to ensure early and effective treatment to prevent complications. Work and leisure activities should be reviewed for practices such as contact sports that present a risk for precipitating bleeding episodes. Alcohol and medications such as aspirin and other nonsteroidal antiinflammatory drugs that aggravate bleeding tendencies should be avoided. Patients are advised to use safe medications such as acetaminophen for mild discomfort. All medications must be reviewed periodically, and new medications evaluated for their potential to increase bleeding tendencies. Wearing a medical alert bracelet or necklace is emphasized. The patient's coagulation status must be evaluated before visits to the dentist or for surgical or other invasive procedures. Genetic counseling is recommended as a component of family planning counseling.

Thrombophilia

DEFINITION/EPIDEMIOLOGY

Thrombosis is the process by which a thrombus (blood clot) forms in the living heart or vasculature. Thrombosis may occur in either the arterial or venous circulation. Thrombophilia is the state of having a condition that predisposes one to thrombosis. This term usually refers to a predisposition to venous thrombosis.

In the normal state, procoagulant enzymes trigger clot formation to ensure hemostasis after injury. These factors are balanced by inhibitory factors that maintain blood as a liquid. When this equilibrium is disturbed, hypercoagulability results. Estimates are that more than a half-million individuals in the United States experience venous thrombosis each year. Pulmonary embolism resulting in death complicates roughly 200,000 cases per year.[12] Thrombosis may occur in any vein or artery in the body, but the majority of clots form in the veins of the lower extremity.

Fortunately, medical science has produced a steady flow of new findings that have, in many cases, clarified why such clots occur and have provided effective treatment. Sometimes thrombi occur in the veins and arteries of the same patient, but usually they do not. Thrombi in arteries are commonly associated with atherosclerosis (hardening of the arteries), a condition that does not affect veins. Clots can occur in superficial veins or deep veins. Thrombi in deep veins, known as deep vein thrombosis (DVT), may be caused by defects in the blood coagulation mechanism that usually do not contribute to clotting in arteries. The following information focuses on issues surrounding the medical management of inherited thrombophilias and thrombotic events.

Our understanding of why thrombi occur has increased dramatically in recent years, along with knowledge of the mechanism of normal blood coagulation, as mentioned previously.

Knowledge of the normal, protective coagulation mechanism prompted investigators to examine substances in the blood for clues as to why thrombi develop inappropriately in veins, causing pain, tenderness, and swelling in the distal tissues. This search uncovered many different abnormalities that may either accelerate clot formation beyond control or block reactions needed to keep the blood fluid.[13] In such instances the risk of thrombosis is increased.

The precise explanation for the occurrence of venous thrombosis in a given location at a specific time is usually not apparent unless there has been an injury. Individuals with various diseases such as cancer or an inflammatory condition, or those who have been immobilized because of surgery, childbirth, injury, or even after a long trip, are more likely to develop venous thrombosis. Other risk factors include advancing age, liver disease, smoking, oral contraceptive use, pregnancy, the presence of the lupus anticoagulant, elevated homocysteine levels, and prior history of DVT. Thrombosis can also occur in otherwise healthy individuals with no obvious explanation.

PATHOPHYSIOLOGY

Virchow's triad continues to define the pathogenesis of DVT, with changes in vessel walls, blood flow, and coagulability of the blood itself contributing to risk. Abnormalities in coagulation proteins may contribute to venous thrombosis. The role of some of these (such as heparin co-factor II) is currently controversial, but others clearly predispose the patient to thrombosis and may even be quite common. For example, activated protein C-resistance (APC-R) affects about 6% of individuals of European descent. (This condition is rare in individuals of Asian or African extraction.) APC-R is due to the presence of an abnormal, or mutated, factor V molecule called factor V–Leiden (named for the city in the Netherlands where the mutation was identified).[13] The mutated factor V resists breakdown by activated protein C (one of the proteins that helps to keep blood liquid). These abnormalities are almost always inherited; they are passed from generation to generation through abnormal genes and affect both males and females. An individual with such an abnormality is said to have hereditary thrombophilia (predisposition to abnormal clot formation). An abnormality in only one of the pair of genes (heterozygote) responsible for the protein is enough to increase the risk of thrombosis. When both members of the gene pair are abnormal (homozygote), a more severe tendency toward thrombosis exists.

In addition to thrombosis risk factors well established in the literature, such as protein C, protein S, and antithrombin III deficiencies, a number of other protein defects that predispose to DVT have recently been found, including the prothrombin gene mutation and elevated factor 8 assays. However, the most prevalent hereditary defect predisposing the patient to DVT is APC-R secondary to the factor V–Leiden mutation.

A person with this defect has an eightfold increase in risk for DVT. If this person also takes oral contraceptives, the risk increases to thirty-five-fold, suggesting a synergistic interaction between the factor V–Leiden mutation and other risk factors.

CLINICAL PRESENTATION AND PHYSICAL EXAMINATION

Thrombi can form in both superficial and deep veins. Thrombi in the superficial veins present with localized tenderness at the site, redness and a feeling of warmth, and possible swelling of the affected limb. Because the vein is close to the surface, it may feel hard or ropelike when examined. The clinical features of DVT include pain, swelling, and erythema of the affected extremity. A positive Homan's sign may also be seen on dorsiflexion of the foot. Physical examination is neither sensitive nor specific for DVT, however, and further testing must be done when the condition is suspected (see Chapter 130).

DIAGNOSTICS

Ascending venography, a radiologic procedure involving injection of contrast dye into the superficial and deep veins of the leg, permits diagnosis of DVT. However, Doppler ultrasound is generally the first test performed when excluding a thrombosis event. The impedance plethysmography is also useful in diagnosis.

DIFFERENTIAL DIAGNOSIS

Abnormalities that predispose the patient to thrombosis may be acquired (e.g., in association with some other disease such as malignancy or lupus erythematosus) or hereditary (Box 232-3). Thrombophilic disorders are distinguished from one another primarily on the basis of the laboratory evaluation. The decision about which laboratory

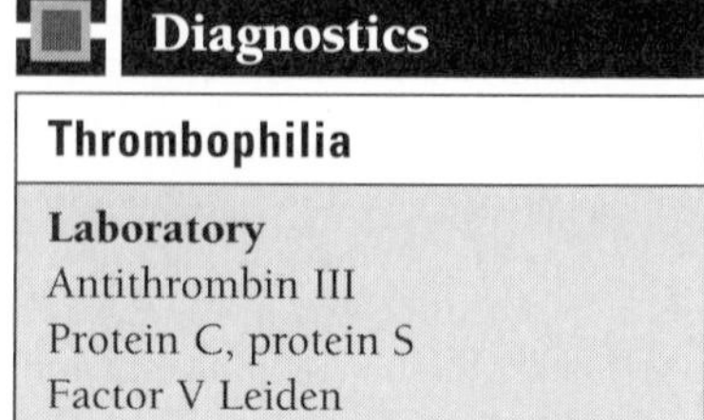

Diagnostics

Thrombophilia

Laboratory
Antithrombin III
Protein C, protein S
Factor V Leiden

tests are indicated is determined by the medical history and clinical presentation. The goal of testing is to determine whether a defect is present that may be important for planning future treatment and that may be sought in other family members who may or may not yet have had an episode of venous thrombosis.

MANAGEMENT

Management of venous thrombosis should follow the American College of Physicians Guidelines for antithrombotic therapy for prevention and treatment of thrombosis.[14] The diagnosis of hereditary thrombophilia in itself is not necessarily an indication for treatment, especially if thrombosis has not occurred. However, when venous thrombosis does occur in a patient with thrombophilia, treatment is begun immediately with anticoagulants to prevent thrombus growth and possible subsequent embolic events.

Heparin is initiated because it is immediately effective. Heparin may be given IV or subcutaneously. The dose of heparin is adjusted according to the APTT and should be aimed at 1.5 to 2.5 times the normal range for therapeutic treatment but not in excess of that, as bleeding can occur.[15]

Initial heparin therapy is typically followed by treatment with warfarin (Coumadin) 2 to 3 days later. Warfarin is given orally and is absorbed from the intestine along with other nutrients, including vitamin K. Vitamin K is required for the production of certain coagulation factors in their complete, fully active form by the liver. Warfarin competes with vitamin K so that incomplete, less active coagulation factors are produced. This takes time, usually 2 to 3 days. During this period, heparin and warfarin are given together for full protection. When the warfarin becomes effective, as measured by laboratory testing, heparin is discontinued. The patient is then maintained on warfarin as an outpatient for 3 months after a first episode of thrombus or longer for repeat episodes.

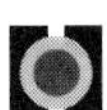

Differential Diagnosis

Thrombophilia

- Hereditary
- Disseminated intravascular coagulation
- Malignancy
- Medications (oral contraceptives)
- Autoimmune disease
- Cardiac abnormalities
  - Prosthetic valve
  - Dilated cardiomyopathy
  - Ventricular aneurysm
- Pregnancy
- Nephrotic syndrome

BOX 232-3

SOME CAUSES OF HEREDITARY THROMBOPHILIA

- Activated protein C resistance (factor V–Leiden mutation)
- Dysfibrinogenemia
- Factor XII deficiency
- Heparin cofactor II deficiency
- Histidine-rich glycoprotein deficiency
- Homocysteinuria (homocysteinemia)
- Plasminogen deficiency
- Plasminogen activator inhibitor excess
- Protein C deficiency
- Protein S deficiency
- Tissue plasminogen activator deficiency
- Mutant thrombomodulin
- Urokinase plasminogen activator deficiency
- Mutant prothrombin
- Factor VIII coagulant activity

Because warfarin and vitamin K are in competition, the effect of warfarin may be exaggerated when dietary vitamin K is inadequate. The effect of warfarin is also exaggerated where liver disease exists, and many different drugs increase or decrease warfarin's effects. Therefore it is important to identify any medications being used by the patient during anticoagulation therapy. When warfarin is stopped, the production of complete coagulation factors gradually returns over several days. The amount of warfarin required to achieve an optimal degree of therapeutic anticoagulation varies among individuals and is determined by the PT. Specific guidance on adjusting warfarin dosage according to the PT is provided in Figure 232-1. The degree of anticoagulation itself is measured on a scale referred to as the INR. Calculation of the INR is based on the PT test. However, expression of the result as the INR is preferred because it eliminates variability between laboratories and reagents used to perform the PT. The degree of warfarin anticoagulation required for maximum protection with minimum risk of bleeding depends on clinical conditions present at that time. The recommended INR range for prophylaxis to reduce the risk of recurrent thrombosis is generally between 2 and 3.[16]

Low-molecular-weight forms of heparin (LMW-H) have also recently become available for the treatment of DVT.[17] These work with antithrombin III to inhibit activated factor X to a much greater extent than it does thrombin, whereas heparin affects activated factor X and thrombin to an equivalent extent. The ability of LMW-H to block the clotting mechanism "upstream" accounts for many of the advantages of this drug. LMW-H has been shown in large, randomized clinical trials to be more effective and at least as safe as either warfarin or heparin.[17] Compared with heparin, LMW-H has a longer half-life, more consistent and complete absorption when injected subcutaneously, and fewer side effects. LMW-H is as effective when given subcutaneously as when given intravenously and usually does not require laboratory monitoring for dose determination. LMW-H tends to have superior antithrombotic properties and less risk of bleeding as compared with heparin.[18] These advantages may permit possible management of DVT without hospitalization and also safe, outpatient control of thrombosis with self-administration should warfarin fail.

An even newer treatment currently in development for DVT is a polypeptide originally isolated from the salivary gland of the medicinal leech, hirudin. This drug acts as a direct thrombin inhibitor, independent of antithrombin III. It has exceptionally high affinity and is active against both free thrombin and thrombin bound to fibrin. A number of other synthetic thrombin inhibitors are also in development. These advances and others on the horizon offer the prospect of improved care for patients with thrombophilia at reduced cost.

COMPLICATIONS

Clot formation within intact vessels compromises the vascular supply to the affected areas. With venous thrombosis the reduced flow of blood from the affected area of the body results in swelling and pain in that part. For example, a thrombus in

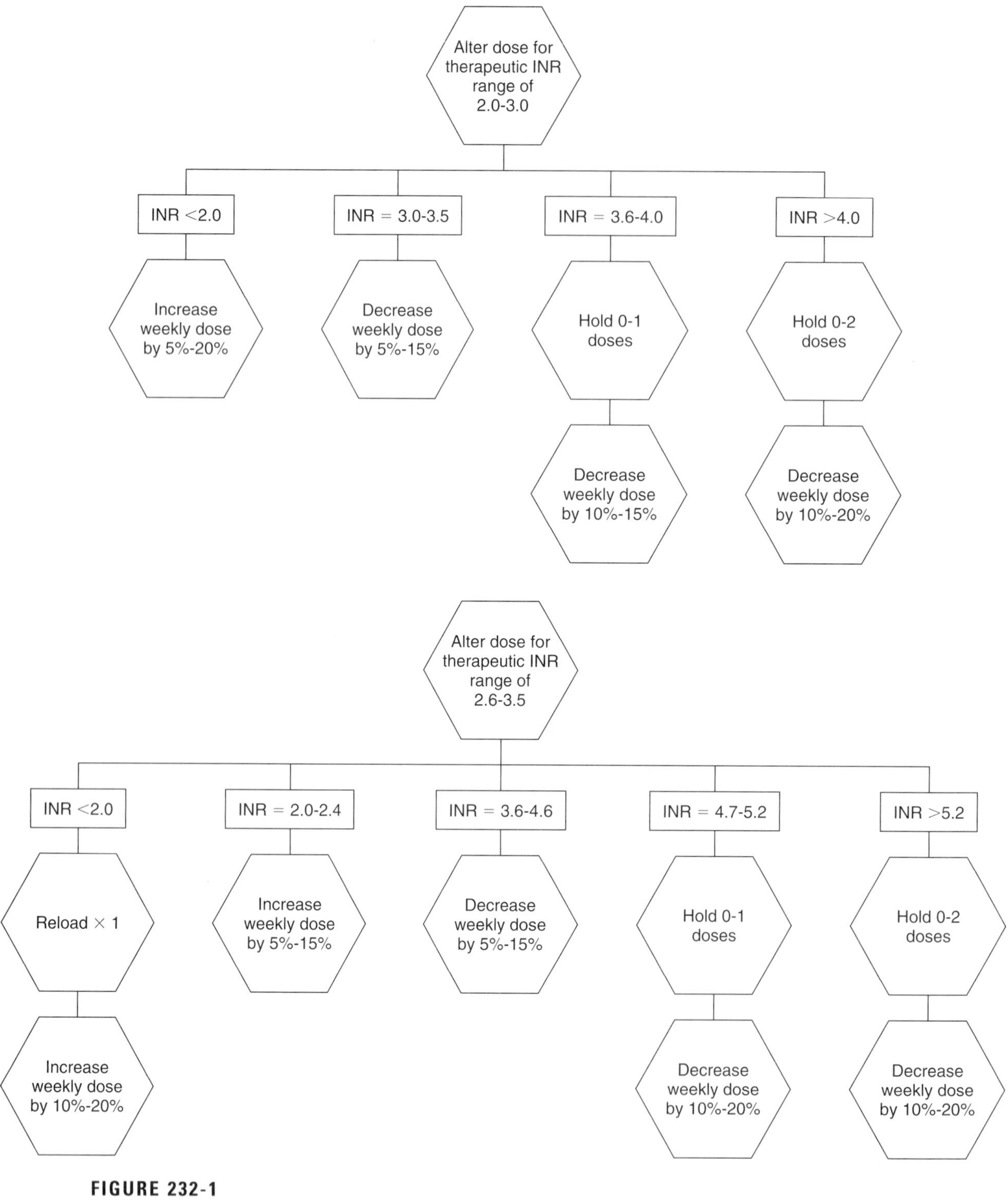

FIGURE 232-1

Warfarin dosage adjustment protocol. (From Establishing an outpatient anticoagulation clinic in a community hospital, *Am J Health Syst Pharm* 53:1154, 1996.)

the veins of the leg can result in swelling and discoloration of the foot and lower leg. When the obstruction is not relieved promptly, the swelling may become chronic and noticeable, especially after the patient has been on his or her feet for a period of time. A venous clot may extend and break off, producing an embolus that may become lodged in the small vessels of the lung (a pulmonary embolus). When such emboli are large, they can be life threatening. Clot formation in the arteries can cause complications in the organ that depends on the blood supplied by the thrombosed artery. For example, a coronary thrombosis that results in myocardial infarction can result in an arrhythmia or congestive heart failure secondary to failure of the pumping mechanism of the heart. Thrombosis of a cerebral artery can result in injury to the nervous tissue in the brain, producing changes in sensory or motor function anywhere in the body. Other examples of complications of arterial thrombosis include infarction of the kidney (renal artery thrombosis) or bowel (mesenteric artery thrombosis).

INDICATIONS FOR REFERRAL/HOSPITALIZATION

Referral to a hematologist with experience in thrombophilia should be considered for patients with a history of recurrent DVT, a family history of thrombosis, or thrombosis at an early age. Prompt investigation for a hereditary cause may result in therapeutic or preventive measures for the patient or family member.

PATIENT AND FAMILY EDUCATION AND LIFE SPAN CONSIDERATIONS

Patient education is an important component of safe and effective outpatient anticoagulation therapy. Patients need to be aware of their diagnosis and factors influencing anticoagulation treatment. Education regarding the importance of regular follow-up visits; anticoagulation dose monitoring; identifying signs of bleeding; maintaining a consistent diet; noting changes in health, diet, or medications; and avoiding hazardous activities is all part of the educational process. In addition, a regularly updated pharmacology resource should be consulted for medications that interact with warfarin, and information should be provided to patients with periodic updates.

Prolonged immobility is discouraged. There should be frequent rest breaks when the patient is immobilized, such as while driving or flying. Under such circumstances, leg stretching or walking at intervals is advisable. Patients at risk for thrombus formation need information about the signs and symptoms of clot formation and how to access appropriate care. With inherited disorders, genetic counseling is an important component of preconceptual counseling.

REFERENCES

1. Venkateswaran L and others: Mild hemophilia in children: prevalence, complications, and treatment, *J Pediatr Hematol Oncol* 20(1):32-35, 1998.
2. White II GC and others: Approach to the bleeding patient. In Colman R, editor: *Hemostasis and thrombosis: basic principles and clinical practice*, ed 3, Philadelphia, 1994, JB Lippincott.
3. Lusher J: Approach to the bleeding patient. In Nathan DG, editor: *Nathan and Oski's hematology of infancy and childhood*, ed 5, Philadelphia, 1998, WB Saunders.
4. Soucie JM and others: Mortality among males with hemophilia: relations with source of medical care, *Blood* 96(2):437-442, 2000.
5. National Hemophilia Foundation Medical and Scientific Advisory Council (MASAC): *Recommendations on the treatment of hemophilia and related bleeding disorders*, New York, 2001, National Hemophilia Foundation.
6. Sham R, Francis C: Evaluation of mild bleeding disorders and easy bruising, *Blood Rev* 8:98-104, 1994.
7. Sadler JE: A revised classification of von Willebrand disease, *Haemophilia* 3(2):11-18, 1997.
8. Mannuccio PM: Desmopressin (DDAVP) in the treatment of bleeding disorders: the first 20 years, *Blood* 9(7):2515-2521, 1997.
9. Blackwell Science Ltd: Treatment and management of Von Willebrand disease, *Haemophilia* 3(suppl 2):4-8, 1997.
10. Coyne MA, Lusher J: Guidelines for emergency care of patients with hemophilia, *Emerg Med* 4 (69):69-77, 2000.
11. Nilsson IM and others: Prophylactic treatment of severe hemophilia A and B can prevent joint disability, *Semin Hematol* 31(S2):5-9, 1994.
12. Mann KG: Thrombosis: theoretical considerations, *Am J Clin Nutr* 1657S-1664S, 1997.
13. De Stefano V, Finazzi G, Mannucci PM: Inherited thrombophilia: pathogenesis, clinical syndromes, and management, *Blood* 87(9):3531-3544, 1996.
14. Hirsh J and others: The sixth ACCP guidelines for antithrombotic therapy for prevention and treatment of thrombosis, *Am Coll Chest Phys*, Jan, pp. 15-370S, 2000.
15. Litin SC, Gastineau DA: Concise review for primary-care physicians: current concepts in anticoagulation therapy, *Mayo Clin Proc* 70: 266-272, 1995.
16. Ansell JE, Holden A, Nozzolillo E: Oral anticoagulant therapy: practical considerations, *Nurse Pract Forum* 3(2):105-113, 1992.
17. Bulle HR and others: Low molecular weight heparin in the treatment of patients with venous thrombosis, *N Engl J Med* 337(10):657-662, 1997.
18. Weitz JI: Low-molecular-weight heparins, *N Engl J Med* 337(10): 688-698, 1997.

CHAPTER 233

Leukemias

Sandra L. Creamer, Murat Anamur, Ruth M. Messer, and Sally-Ann Milne

DEFINITION/EPIDEMIOLOGY

Some of the most challenging and complex cancers to manage in the community setting are the leukemias, hematologic malignancies that affect the bone marrow and lymphatic tissue. There are two types of leukemia: acute and chronic. Acute leukemias are distinguished by an abnormal production of immature white blood cells and a rapid disease progression over approximately 6 months. Chronic leukemias display an overabundance of more mature appearing but ineffective cells. Disease progression is usually slow, over 2 to 5 years. The overproduction of leukemia cells displaces normal cells in the bone marrow and thus destroys hematopoietic performance. Depending on cell type, treatment of leukemia may be as conservative as observation or as aggressive as bone marrow transplantation. Consequences of the disease state and side effects of treatment options represent a true challenge to the primary care provider.[1]

In 2001 there were approximately 31,000 new cases of leukemia, with chronic and acute leukemia of equal incidence. There were approximately 22,000 deaths from leukemia.[2] The exact etiology of leukemia is unknown. Causes and risk factors for consideration are genetic factors and disorders, exposure to radiation, chemicals, drugs, viruses, and other bone marrow disorders and environmental factors.

Children with genetic disorders such as Down syndrome have an increased risk of developing acute leukemia. Other conditions that are associated with a high incidence of leukemia include Ellis-van Creveld syndrome, Fanconi's anemia, Kleinfelter's syndrome, Bloom syndrome, and ataxia-telangiectasia.

Exposure to ionizing radiation is the most conclusive predisposing factor associated with humans and leukemia. This became evident after World War II when a large number of Japanese survivors of the atom bomb explosion displayed an increased incidence of acute myeloid leukemia (AML) and chronic myelogenous leukemia (CML). Pioneer radiologists who were exposed to massive radiation also exhibited a high incidence of leukemia.[3]

Occupational exposure to certain chemicals increases the risk of developing leukemia. Workers exposed to benzene (a hydrocarbon used in industry and in unleaded gasoline), rubber cement, and cleaning solvents are at risk for developing leukemia. Other occupations in which workers are at risk of contracting leukemia are those that expose workers to explosives, distilleries, dyes, paints, and leather tanning. Although the relationship between leukemia and viruses remains unclear, there does appear to be a correlation between retroviruses and T-cell leukemia and hairy cell leukemia.[4]

Polycythemia vera, aplastic anemia, myelodysplastic syndromes, and other diseases of the bone marrow also appear to predispose individuals to leukemia. Environmental factors such as hair dye, cigarette smoking, and sunbathing may also increase the risk of developing leukemia.[5]

Intensive combination chemotherapy for patients with cancer has led to increased survival rates. However, these survivors must be continually evaluated for complications of the long-term cytotoxic treatment. One serious consequence is the development of a second cancer, especially myeloid leukemia. Therapy-related leukemia is generally a fatal disease. The terms *t-MDS* (treatment-related myelodysplastic syndrome) and *t-AML* (treatment-related acute myeloid leukemia) are used to describe a clinical syndrome that may imply a causal relationship, but this relationship remains to be proven.[6]

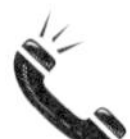

Physician consultation is indicated for all suspected cases of leukemia.

PATHOPHYSIOLOGY

Leukemia is a malignant disorder of the blood and blood-forming organs—the spleen, lymphatic system, and bone marrow. It is identified as acute or chronic depending on the onset of symptoms and the maturity of the blood cell. With acute leukemia, there is marked abnormality and uncontrolled production of the immature leukocytes. The chronic form of the disease shows an accumulation of mature-appearing cells that have lost the ability to function efficiently. The proliferation of abnormal blood cells infiltrates the bone marrow, the peripheral blood, and other organs, which causes swelling and interference with normal organ function and destroys normal hematopoiesis. All blood cell types are formed within the marrow; as leukocyte crowding persists, there is a decrease in the circulating erythrocytes and thrombocytes. This compromise leads to anemia, dyspnea, bruising, the potential for hemorrhage, and further tissue destruction.[7]

The maturation process of various blood cell lines originates from the stem cell. The stem cell line is responsible for the generation of new cells necessary to meet the body's requirements throughout a lifetime.[8] Leukemic cells are designated as either myeloid or lymphocytic according to the type of cell that predominates.

CLINICAL PRESENTATION AND PHYSICAL EXAMINATION

Acute Leukemias

The signs and symptoms of acute lymphocytic leukemia (ALL) and AML may include a viral infection with a low-grade fever, anemia with fatigue, and pallor. Initial manifestations include bleeding gums, epistaxis, ecchymosis, petechiae, and excessive bleeding after minor dental procedures, all caused by thrombocytopenia. Chloromas, the collection of blast cells in the subcutaneous tissues, may imitate a primary or metastatic carcinoma.

In general, the presenting symptoms are nonspecific. Often the primary care provider evaluates and treats a sinus, respiratory, perirectal, or urinary tract infection with poor response and may eventually discover leukemia. Because leukemia involves the lymph, spleen, and liver, diffuse lymphadenopathy and hepatosplenomegaly may be present on examination. Patients may complain of bone pain. Younger patients may experience joint pain and swelling that resembles rheumatoid arthritis; 50% of all leukemia patients have some type of ocular involvement. A funduscopic examination may reveal flame-shaped hemorrhages, which are caused by retinal leukemic infiltration; these hemorrhages are a classic sign of leukemia.[9] In AML, the skin and gums are often infiltrated with leukemic cells, and therefore an oral examination may be helpful.

Although only 2% of patients have central nervous system (CNS) involvement at the time of initial diagnosis, many may have CNS involvement at some time during the course of their leukemia. The most common signs and symptoms of leukemia that has invaded the CNS are headache, papilledema, vomiting, nuchal rigidity, and cranial nerve palsy. In AML, leukostasis occurs when the blast count exceeds 100,000 cells/mm^3, and the patient is at risk for a fatal cerebral hemorrhage.[10]

Chronic Leukemias

Patients with CML and chronic lymphocytic leukemia (CLL) are usually asymptomatic. There may be subtle changes in the WBC and differential early in the disease. A cardinal finding on physical examinations of patients with chronic leukemia is splenomegaly. The patient may complain of a mild sensation of fullness in the left upper quadrant or may have an obvious mass. Severe splenomegaly can compress surrounding organs, causing early satiety, weight loss, and peripheral leg edema related to compression of the splenic vein. As the disease progresses, other symptoms occur, such as bone pain, bleeding problems, infection, fatigue, pallor, adenopathy, fevers, and night sweats.[11]

DIAGNOSTICS AND DIFFERENTIAL DIAGNOSIS

Acute Leukemias

To confirm the diagnosis of acute leukemia, a CBC is necessary. Many patients present with anemia and thrombocytopenia, but striking abnormalities are noted in the WBC and differential. The WBC parameters vary within a wide range—from 1000 to 100,000 cells/mm^3. Most patients have counts between 5000 and 30,000 cells/mm^3.[11]

Careful examination of the blood smear is essential. The significant finding on the blood smear is an increased population of blast cells and a decrease of neutrophils and platelets. It is important to realize that as many as 10% of all patients have normal blood counts even when the marrow has been replaced by leukemic cells; therefore a bone marrow aspiration and biopsy is definitive for diagnosis. The bone marrow contents will be hypercellular, with a crowding of blast cells (60% to 90%) and a decrease in normal cellular elements. Auer rods (reddish filaments) incorporated within the blast cells confirm the diagnosis of AML.[10]

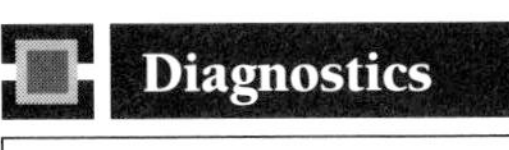

Leukemia

Laboratory
CBC and differential
Peripheral blood smear evaluation
Serum electrolytes
Uric acid
LFTs
Urinalysis

Other
Bone marrow biopsy

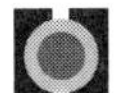

Differential Diagnosis

Leukemia

Lymphomas	Aplastic anemia
Solid tumors	Lymphoproliferative disorders
Systemic lupus erythematosus	
Megaloblastic anemia	

Biochemical studies may reveal hyperuricemia. Hyperuricemia occurs because of the high turnover rate of proliferating leukemia cells and the end-product of purine catabolism. Electrolyte disorders are common, and in acute leukemia elevated lactic dehydrogenase may occur. Therefore serum chemistries and liver function tests (LFTs) should be ordered initially. Any patient with an increased myeloblast count may be at risk for leukostasis; this condition primarily affects the lung and brain, but any organ can be involved. Lowering the blast count in a rapid fashion is necessary, usually by chemotherapy and/or leukapheresis. Therefore patients who have acute leukemia should be admitted to a tertiary center for comprehensive and aggressive management.

The differential diagnosis for ALL and AML is lymphoma, although other infiltrative processes such as solid tumors (e.g., breast cancer) must be excluded. Some patients with fever and cytopenia who have a small amount of circulating blast cells must be differentiated from reactions occurring in tuberculosis, systemic lupus erythematosus, megaloblastic anemia, and aplastic anemia. Surface antigen and serologic studies can exclude viral infections such as infectious mononucleosis. Cytogenic studies are currently being used as a diagnostic tool in determining the subtype of leukemia.[3]

Chronic Leukemias

At diagnosis, the WBC count may range from fewer than 10,000 to more than 200,000 cells/mm^3, with mature and predominantly myelocytic cells. In general, the red blood cell count is normal, but a slight degree of anemia may occur (Table 233-1). Hypereosinophilia and hyperbasophilia are common. Increased levels of uric acid in the blood and urine are also found in patients with CML. Bone marrow biopsy reveals hyperplastic myeloid cells and storage cells similar to Gaucher's cells scattered throughout the marrow. The striking biochemical abnormality in CML is the reduction or absence of leukocyte alkaline phosphatase. This, along with the positive test for Philadelphia chromosome (Ph^1), the hallmark of CML, confirms the diagnosis of CML. CML is the first cancer shown to be associated with a chromosomal abnormality.[11]

CLL is often discovered on a routine office visit when a CBC is ordered. The physical examination may be negative, but some patients have nontender adenopathy or splenomegaly. Patients may report fatigue, night sweats, occasional fever, or malaise. The majority of patients consult their primary care provider because of a painless cervical lymph node that waxes and wanes but does not disappear completely.[11]

CLL is suspected whenever an absolute lymphocytosis in the peripheral blood occurs in an adult and is sustained over

TABLE 233-1 Recommended Diagnostic Tests and Plan for the Leukemias

Tests	Acute	Chronic
CBC and differential	X	X
Chemistry profile	X	X
Uric acid	X	X
Liver profile	X	X
Urinalysis	X	X
Complete physical examination with special attention to:		
Lymph nodes		
Liver/spleen		
Oral examination		
Ophthalmic examination		
Pertinent patient history—fever, night sweats, painless lumps, fatigue, bruising, bleeding		
Refer to hematologist for:		
Bone marrow aspirate and biopsy		
Definitive diagnosis		
Treatment plan		

time. Lymphocytosis also occurs in infectious mononucleosis, pertussis, and toxoplasmosis, but in these conditions the lymphocyte count returns to normal after a few weeks.

A peripheral smear may be adequate for the diagnosis of CLL; a bone marrow biopsy will *always* reveal lymphocytosis in all cases of CLL. The lymphocyte count ranges from 10,000 to 150,000/mm^3. Because there may be a decrease in immunoglobulin levels, a serum protein electrophoresis should be performed; this test may reveal a marked decrease in levels of immunoglobulin G (IgG) and slight decreases in IgA and IgM levels. A chest x-ray study may be helpful in detecting hilar and mediastinal adenopathy.[12]

The differential diagnoses for CLL include non-Hodgkin's lymphoma, hairy cell leukemia, and a variety of other lymphoproliferative disorders.

MANAGEMENT

Acute Leukemias

Patients diagnosed with ALL and AML require aggressive chemotherapy. Treatment of AML and ALL involves induction therapy for remission and postremission therapy. The oncologist should be consulted before any medicine is prescribed for a patient who is undergoing chemotherapy for acute leukemia.

Patients with AML may also undergo a bone marrow transplant (BMT). The increasing use of both autologous and allogenic BMTs will most certainly have a profound effect on the outcome of AML. The impact of these newer approaches is under observation. Management of these patients requires a multidisciplinary approach. Expertise in transfusion management, infectious disease, care of indwelling catheters, nutrition, chemotherapy, and side effects and psychosocial counseling is required.

Approximately 50% of patients with ALL who are less than 15 years of age achieve a long-term, leukemia-free survival. Approximately 70% of all patients with AML who are less than 60 years of age achieve a complete, but short-lived, remission; only 15% remain disease free for 5 years or more. The major cause of failure to achieve remission during induction therapy is death from hemorrhage and infection.[1]

Chronic Leukemias

CML has three phases: chronic phase, accelerated phase, and terminal blast crisis phase. The chronic phase has a duration of approximately 3 years; the durations of the other phases vary. In contrast, CLL is usually a long-term disease, with reported cases lasting from 1 to 15 years.

Chronic leukemias are managed differently. Treatment consists primarily of oral antineoplastic agents in the chronic phase. In the early phase of CML, however, clinical trials report benefit with bone marrow transplant vs. alpha-interferon therapy. Discussion and referrals are extremely important and should be evaluated on a case-by-case basis. Special note should be made of imatinib (Gleevec), a drug that inhibits tyrosine kinase found in CML. This drug has shown remarkable remission-inducing activity as a single agent.[13]

In chronic leukemia there may be drug interactions, including an increased effect of anticoagulants, a decreased digoxin level, and an increased drug action of barbiturates. When in doubt, the pharmacist should be contacted to discuss any potential drug interactions. Any leukemia patient with previously diagnosed diabetes may have episodes of hyperglycemia related to corticosteroid therapy.

Patients diagnosed with leukemia who have undergone chemotherapy or perhaps a BMT are at risk for infection (bacterial, fungal, viral) and other long-term side effects of aggressive treatment. Patients with CLL are predisposed to several infectious complications that are related to the humoral immune compromise associated with the disease process, as well as to further immunosuppression from steroid therapy and cytotoxic therapy.[14] Periodic visits with the primary care provider and the hematologist/oncologist are essential for close monitoring and support.

Chemotherapy is the cornerstone of treatment for both acute and chronic leukemias. However, chemotherapy management for the leukemias varies (Box 233-1). The goal of chemotherapy is to eradicate leukemic stem cells in acute leukemia and decrease mature leukemia cells in chronic leukemia.

Chemotherapy agents have many side effects including bone marrow depression, gastrointestinal distress, nausea, vomiting, anorexia, stomatitis, diarrhea, constipation, skin rashes, alopecia, and fatigue. Specific agents have particular side effects. Daunorubicin may cause cardiotoxicity, vincristine may cause peripheral neuropathy, and asparaginase may cause elevated LFTs.

Patients who have undergone BMT need close follow-up monitoring, which usually occurs in collaboration with the tertiary center that performed the BMT. These patients are immunocompromised and intervening in a timely fashion with antibiotics and antifungal agents when indicated will improve survival and quality of life.

LIFE SPAN CONSIDERATIONS

Leukemia was once thought to be a childhood disease, but 90% of the newly diagnosed cases occur in adults. AML and CLL are the most common adult forms of the disease. ALL accounts for 80% of the childhood forms.[2]

BOX 233-1

MOST COMMONLY USED DRUGS

AML	CML	ALL	CLL
Cytosine arabinoside IV	Busulfan PO	Vincristine	Chlorambucil PO
Daunorubicin IV	Hydroxyurea PO	L-asparaginase IV	Corticosteroids PO
	Gleevec PO	Daunorubicin IV	*Advanced Stage*
	Advanced Stage	Prednisone PO	Cyclophosphamide IV
	Cytosine arabinoside IV	Methotrexate—Intrathecal	Doxorubicin IV
	Daunorubicin IV		Fludarabine IV

COMPLICATIONS

Complications of leukemia include possible sequelae from chemotherapy and BMT (e.g., secondary malignancies, infection, fertility problems). Neuropathies and cardiopathies may develop and are usually related to the aggressive treatment regimen experienced by the leukemia patient. Despite the development of more effective antibiotics, the granulocyte colony-stimulating factor, and the granulocyte-macrophage colony-stimulating factor, bacterial and fungal infections continue to be a source of morbidity and mortality in patients with prolonged neutropenia.[15] Other syndromes that are potential complications are discussed next.

Tumor Lysis Syndrome

Acute tumor lysis syndrome (ATLS) is most commonly seen in patients with AML and CML who are undergoing active treatment. ATLS occurs when a great many rapidly proliferating tumor cells are destroyed. Patients with a high WBC count, a heavy tumor burden, lymphadenopathy, and splenomegaly receiving cytotoxic chemotherapy rupture tumor cell membranes and release intracellular contents into the bloodstream.[16] ATLS is characterized by the development of acute hyperuricemia, hyperkalemia, hyperphosphatemia, and hypercalcemia, with or without acute renal failure.[16] Prevention and management of these metabolic complications require close monitoring. Renal function and chemistry values should be monitored daily. Fluid balance and electrolyte disturbances should be corrected with vigorous IV hydration and diuretics as indicated. The addition of sodium bicarbonate to maintain urinary alkalinization is recommended, as is the use of allopurinol to decrease serum uric acid levels. Monitoring of daily weights, meticulous assessment of intake and output, and observation for signs and symptoms of fluid overload are also indicated. ATLS ordinarily resolves within 4 to 7 days if adequate renal function is maintained.

Disseminated Intravascular Coagulation

Disseminated intravascular coagulation (DIC) is a hematologic disorder that occurs when there is an alteration in the blood-clotting mechanism. It may be acute or chronic and can be related to either the disease process or the treatment regimen. DIC is the most common serious hypercoagulable state that occurs in patients with cancer.[17] It is an event in which both clotting and hemorrhage exist simultaneously.

Acute leukemia, antineoplastic agents, infection, trauma, and hemolytic transfusion reactions interrupt normal body hemostasis and may initiate an episode of DIC. Spontaneous hemorrhage or the slow occult damage of multiple small clot formation within the lungs, organs of the central nervous system, or gastrointestinal tract may herald the presentation of DIC. Organ dysfunction from circulatory impairment leads to mental status changes, severe muscle pain, oliguria, and slowed gastrointestinal mobility.[16] Symptoms may range from mild chronic episodes to acute and life-threatening incidents.

Abnormal laboratory findings suggest a diagnosis of DIC. A decreased platelet count, a prolonged prothrombin and partial thromboplastin time, and a decreased fibrinogen level with an elevation of fibrin degradation products confirm the diagnosis of DIC.[18] Treatment of the underlying cause of DIC is vital. Hemorrhage is treated with replacement of fluids and blood component therapy, infection is treated with antibiotics, and cancer is treated with radiation therapy, chemotherapy, or surgery as indicated. Heparin therapy is more commonly used for the chronic DIC of malignancy associated with thrombotic, thromboembolic, or necrotizing complications. Thorough, multiple system assessments in combination with patient and family education and involvement is necessary to prevent further injury and complications associated with DIC.

Leukostasis

The predominant cell in acute leukemia is undifferentiated or immature, usually a blast cell. In leukostasis, blood sludging or stasis occurs when the blood vessels become overcrowded with these blast cells. Individuals with high WBC counts and a large tumor burden are at risk for developing leukostasis. The small, delicate pulmonary and cranial vessels are the most susceptible. If leukostasis is left untreated, rupture and hemorrhage result in ischemia and infarct. Emergent treatment includes high-dose chemotherapy or cranial radiotherapy to decrease the number of circulating blast cells. Leukapheresis (removal of white blood cells from the plasma) may also be indicated.[1]

Pancytopenia

Regardless of the treatment regimen chosen, infection, bleeding, and symptomatic anemia are the most common side effects of leukemia and its therapy. The desired effect of treatment produces severe myelosuppression. Prolonged periods of neutropenia leave the immunocompromised patient especially susceptible to infection. Until normal bone marrow function is restored, the leukemic patient lacks the normal host responses. Treatment with empiric antibiotics to prevent systemic or disseminated infection is indicated once infection is suspected. Prevention of infection must focus on providing meticulous care of any invasive treatment option and limiting unnecessary

BOX 233-2

PATIENT EDUCATION

SEPSIS/INFECTION

White blood cells are the body's defense against infection. If your white blood count is low, you are at risk for infection and should do the following:

1. Avoid crowds, malls, churches, and movie theaters.
2. Instruct sick friends and relatives to call, not visit.
3. Practice exceptionally careful personal hygiene with multiple handwashings.

Signs and symptoms of infection to report to the health care team: elevated temperature (report a fever of 37.7° C [100° F] or higher); productive cough; wound redness, swelling, or drainage; mouth sores

THROMBOCYTOPENIA

Platelets are the components of blood that play a major part in the clotting mechanism. If your platelets are low, you are at risk for increased bleeding and should do the following:

1. Use electric shavers for shaving (this includes women).
2. Apply extra caution when using any sharp objects.
3. Avoid bumps, bruises, and falls (this is not the time to rearrange furniture).
4. Avoid aspirin and aspirin-containing products.

Signs and symptoms of thrombocytopenia to report to the health care team: increased bruising, nosebleeds, bleeding gums, blood in urine or stool, increase in menstrual flow

ANEMIA

You should do the following:

1. Take frequent rest periods.
2. When moving from one position to another, do so slowly.
3. Keep warm.
4. Eat a well-balanced diet and drink plenty of fluids.

Signs and symptoms of anemia to report to the health care team: shortness of breath, ringing in the ears, fainting, pounding heart, increased heart rate, or palpitations.

MANAGEMENT OF SIDE EFFECTS OF DISEASE AND/OR TREATMENT

There is the potential for numerous side effects from your disease and/or the treatment you are receiving. The following are options for managing various side effects. If you are unable to manage these problems effectively, contact your health care team:

Fever: Take acetaminophen (Tylenol) for a temperature over 37.7° C (100° F) and call your primary care provider.

Headache: Take acetaminophen (Tylenol); if headache persists or other symptoms (e.g., visual disturbances or seizures) arise, call your health care team immediately.

Mucositis: Ask your health care team to prescribe a medication for sore mouth, and take as directed. Keep mouth clean and moist, rinsing it every 2 hours with ½ teaspoon of salt in 8 ounces of water or with a 1:3 ratio of hydrogen peroxide solution. Brush teeth gently with a soft toothbrush or an oral swab. Use only alcohol-free mouthwash. Drink plenty of liquids.

Wear dentures only for meals. Use a lip moisturizer to keep lips from becoming dry and cracked. Avoid highly spiced food, high-acid food, and very hot foods or liquids. Avoid alcohol and tobacco. See your dentist routinely.

Nausea, vomiting, and anorexia: These symptoms affect your ability to maintain a good nutritional state, which is imperative for body repair and healing. Take antinausea medications at the first sign of queasiness; do not wait until vomiting occurs. If the medication does not work, call your health care team for another type of medication; numerous antinausea medications are available. Eat small, frequent, well-balanced meals that are high in protein and calories. Have snacks. If there is a bad taste in your mouth, try chewing gum or sucking on hard candy.

Diarrhea: If you are taking laxatives, *stop.* Take an antidiarrheal preparation such as loperamide (Imodium A-D) after each *watery* stool; follow package instructions. Use the BRAT diet—bananas, rice, applesauce, and dry toast. When free of diarrhea for 24 hours, resume regular diet slowly. Avoid foods that cause diarrhea. If diarrhea persists for 24 hours despite treatment, call your health care team.

Constipation: Many pain medications cause constipation, and prevention is the best treatment. Take a natural laxative with a stool softener at bedtime. Drink at least 8 8-ounce glasses of water each day (if you have had a bone marrow transplant, you may be instructed to drink distilled water). Avoid foods that contribute to constipation. If constipation occurs, increase natural laxative with a stool softener to two or three times a day. Suppositories, enemas, and the more aggressive laxatives (e.g., milk of magnesia or magnesium citrate) may need to be added. When constipation is resolved, remove medications in reverse order, but continue the natural laxative with stool softener. If constipation persists despite treatment, contact your health care team because a more serious problem may exist.

Pain: Take pain medications as prescribed. If you are taking time-release pain medications, take them regularly to prevent pain. If you are taking pain medications only as needed, take them when the pain begins. Do not wait until pain becomes severe, because the medication will not be as effective. If taking narcotics, do not drive, operate dangerous machinery, or drink alcohol. Avoid situations that cause pain to increase. Call your health care team if the pain medication becomes ineffective or if pain changes in intensity or location.

Alopecia: Keep the head warm, because a great deal of body heat can be lost through a bare scalp. Wigs, turbans, and caps not only keep the head warm but may also help improve body image. In most cases hair will start to grow back when treatment ends. If eyelashes and eyebrows are gone, wear eye protection, especially when outdoors, to avoid injury to the eyes. Nose hair may also be lost, which may cause discomfort in cold weather; a mask may be helpful.

Fatigue: Maintain good nutrition and take a vitamin supplement. Space exercise and rest periods throughout the day. Use a time log to determine the optimum routine.

Insomnia: Avoid sleeping excessively during the day. Get some exercise daily (this may mean just walking around the house). Do not drink caffeinated beverages before bedtime. Over-the-counter diphenhydramine (Benadryl) may be effective. As a last resort, ask your health care team to consider a sleeping medication.

Depression: Review your medications; many medications and their side effects can affect emotional state. Avoid alcohol, because it can have a depressive effect. Discuss your feelings with your health care team. Join a cancer support group; if unable to do this, ask for a referral to a therapist. Eat well, exercise, and get plenty of rest.

Data from Groenwald S and others: *Cancer symptom management,* Boston, 1997, Jones & Bartlett.

invasive procedures. Education empowers patients and their families to participate in their own health practices.

Fatigue is one of the most common symptoms associated with cancer and cancer therapies. Chronic low-grade anemia, stress, and alterations in sleeping, eating, and working are known to deplete energy levels. Fatigue can be one of the most disabling complications of cancer and chemotherapy treatments, which allows feelings of hopelessness and powerlessness to occur. Supportive transfusion or erythropoietin therapies may be used. Many patients find support groups beneficial.[1]

INDICATIONS FOR REFERRAL/HOSPITALIZATION

All patients with suspected leukemia should be referred to a hematologist or oncologist for bone marrow aspiration and biopsy. Definitive diagnosis and treatment plans vary. In general, patients with acute leukemias are referred to a tertiary care center. Chronic leukemias are often managed in the community by a hematologist or oncologist. However, the primary care provider plays a major role in the co-management of the leukemias. A hematology consult is suggested before any invasive procedure such as colonoscopy, cystoscopy, or any surgery, whether minor or major.

PATIENT EDUCATION AND HEALTH PROMOTION

The educational goal for leukemia patients and their families is prevention of complications of the disease process and/or treatment, management of side effects, and access to community resources.

The major life-threatening complication of leukemia is bone marrow suppression. This may be a result of either the disease process itself or the chemotherapy instituted to treat the leukemia. The result of bone marrow suppression is a subnormal functioning of the immune system, which puts the patient at risk for sepsis, thrombocytopenia, and anemia. The health care team will notify the patient and family of laboratory results indicating that the patient is at risk.

It is the responsibility of the health care team to educate the patient and family regarding the numerous other side effects of leukemia and/or its treatment, such as fever, headache, mucositis, nausea/vomiting/anorexia, diarrhea, constipation, pain, fatigue, insomnia, and depression. Patient instructions are given in Box 233-2. After diagnosis, patients still require cancer screening tests specific for age, including mammograms, Pap smears, PSA (prostate-specific antigen), and fecal occult blood testing. Other health-promoting activities including smoking cessation, maintaining normal weight, and getting adequate exercise should be encouraged.

REFERENCES

1. Wujcik D: Leukemia. In Groenwald S and others, editors: *Cancer nursing: principles and practice*, ed 4, Boston, 1997, Jones & Bartlett.
2. American Cancer Society: *Cancer facts and figures*, Atlanta 2001, The Society.
3. Scheinberg D, Maslak P, Weiss M: Acute leukemias. In DaVita V and others, editors: *Cancer: principles and practice of oncology*, ed 6, Philadelphia, 2001, Lippincott Williams and Wilkins.
4. Linet M: Leukemias. In Harras A, editor: *Cancer rates and risks*, ed 4, Bethesda, Md, 1996, National Institutes of Health.
5. Miaskowski E: *Oncology nursing: an essential guide for patient care*, Philadelphia, 1997, WB Saunders.
6. Thirman M, Larson R: Therapy-related myeloid leukemia. *Hemat Oncol Clin North Am* 2:293-320, 1996.
7. Cotran R, Kumar V, Collins T: *Robbins pathologic basis of disease*, ed 6, Philadelphia, 1999, WB Saunders.
8. Ososki R: Leukemia. In Otto S, editor: *Oncology nursing*, St Louis, 1997, Mosby.
9. Lien-Gieschen T, McMurtry C: Orbital leukemia, *Nurse Pract* 20(1):75-77, 1996.
10. Miller K and others: Leukemia. In Osteen R, editor: *Cancer manual*, ed 9, Boston, 1996, American Cancer Society.
11. Kantarjian H, Faderl Stalpaz M: Chronic leukemia. In DeVita V and others, editors: *Cancer principles and practice of oncology*, ed 6, Philadelphia, 2001, Lippincott Williams and Wilkins.
12. Rai K, Keating M: Chronic lymphocytic leukemia. In Holland J and others, editors: *Cancer medicine*, ed 5, Hamilton, 2000, BC Decker.
13. Calabresi P, Chabner B: Chemotherapy of neoplastic diseases. In Hardman J and others, editors, *Goodman's and Gilman's the pharmacologic basis of therapeutics*, ed 10, New York, 2001, McGraw-Hill.
14. Morrison V: The infectious complications of chronic lymphocytic leukemia, *Semin Oncol* 25(1):98-106, 1998.
15. Wuest D: Transfusion and stem cell support in cancer treatment. *Hematol Oncol Clin North Am* 2:397-429, 1996.
16. Shelton BK: Oncology emergencies. In C Varriechio, editor: *A cancer sourcebook for nurses*, London, 1997, Jones & Bartlett.
17. Morris J, Holland J: Oncologic emergencies. In Holland J and others, editors: *Cancer medicine*, ed 5, 2000, Hamilton, BC Decker.
18. Arnold S and others: Paraneoplastic syndromes. In DeVita V and others, editors: *Cancer: principles and practice of oncology*, ed 6, Philadelphia, 2001, Lippincott Williams and Wilkins.

CHAPTER 234

Lymphomas

Janet H. Van Cleave

The lymphomas are a diverse group of neoplasms with varied clinical features and biologic patterns. Clonal expansion of the immune system leads to uncontrolled growth of components of the immune system composed of B, T, and/or null cells. More than 30 neoplasms of the lymphoid system are included in this group of malignancies. They can originate in any site bearing lymphoid tissue such as lymph nodes, spleen, bone marrow, and extranodal sites including the liver, gut, and rarely other viscera. This chapter addresses the malignant lymphomas, which are typically classified as either Hodgkin's lymphoma (HD) or non-Hodgkin's lymphomas (NHL). The two diseases are differentiated based on pathology and are managed differently. Therefore this chapter addresses each disease separately.

Hodgkin's Lymphoma

DEFINITION/EPIDEMIOLOGY

In the United States, it is estimated that in the year 2001 there will be 7400 new diagnoses of HD, with cases almost evenly divided between males and females. It is also estimated that there will be 1300 deaths caused by HD, again evenly divided between males and females.[1] In the United States and some industrialized European nations, there is a bimodal age-incidence occurrence. The first incidence peak is seen in people during their twenties and the second peak after age 50 years.[2] The etiology of the disease is unclear. There is no clear relationship with environmental exposures. Although no specific pathogen has been identified, it is suspected that the Epstein-Barr virus (EBV) is involved given that patients with a history of infectious mononucleosis have a threefold chance of developing HD and approximately half of all HD nodes have evidence of EBV DNA. However, there appears to be another mechanism because there is no evidence of EBV or history of mononucleosis in many patients with HD. Also, there appears to be an increased frequency of HD in patients with the AIDS, and in patients after bone marrow transplantation.[3]

CLASSIFICATION

The classification of HD has evolved over time. The older classification is the Rye classification, which associates the histopathologic subtypes to clinical behavior and prognosis. These subtypes are lymphocyte predominance, nodular sclerosis (NS), mixed cellularity (MC), and the uncommon lymphocyte depleted (LD).[2] The World Health Organization (WHO) classification proposed the categories of nodular lymphocyte predominant Hodgkin's lymphoma and classical Hodgkin's lymphoma. Classical Hodgkin's lymphoma is subdivided into NS, lymphocyte-rich classical, MC, and LD. The most common form of HD is NS, which accounts for approximately 60% of cases. The second most common histopathologic finding is MC, which occurs in 20% to 40% of presentations.[3]

PATHOPHYSIOLOGY

The primary neoplastic cell in HD is the polynucleated Reed-Sternberg cell. The majority of the lymphatic tissue of HD is composed of normal-appearing lymphocytes, plasma cells, eosinophils, neutrophils, and histiocytes existing in the varied proportion as reflected in the histologic subtypes. In HD, there is a progressive loss of cell-mediated immunity associated with the development of cutaneous anergy, lymphocytopenia, and increased susceptibility to organisms associated with depressed cell-mediated immunity and herpes zoster.[2]

CLINICAL PRESENTATION

HD generally presents as painless lymphadenopathy. Constitutional symptoms that may accompany HD include fevers, night sweats, and weight loss. The patient may also experience pruritus and pain in a lymph node region with alcohol intake. Laboratory evaluation may have nonspecific findings including a mild lymphocytosis, eosinophilia, and an elevated erythrocyte sedimentation rate (ESR).[3]

PHYSICAL EXAMINATION

Important information in the patient's history includes any constitutional symptoms of weight loss, fever, and night sweats. The history should also include information about performance status, pruritus, and alcohol tolerance.[4] The physical examination includes evaluation of the lymph node regions, size of the liver and spleen, and Waldeyer's ring inspection. Pertinent laboratory values are the complete blood count including differential and platelets, ESR, liver function tests, and renal function tests.[4,5]

DIAGNOSTICS

Staging

For more than 25 years, the four-stage clinical and pathologic Ann Arbor system has been the most widely used staging system. It yields important prognostic and treatment information (Table 234-1). In predicting survival, there are two groups within the staging system. The favorable group includes stages I, II, and IIIA, with disease-specific survival at 15 years being 96%. The less favorable group consists of stages IIIB and IV, with the disease-specific survival being 80%. Overall survival rates are 80% and 60%, respectively, for the two groups.[3]

Diagnosis

Generally, a pathologic diagnosis of HD requires an excisional biopsy of the enlarged LN. A needle aspiration or core biopsy may help document recurrent disease, but may give false-negative information because of sampling error for the initial diagnosis and is thus insufficient. A needle or surgical biopsy may be required of any extranodal sites that are suspicious for disease. Other important information can be derived from cytologic examination of effusions.[5] A staging laparotomy is performed in rare circumstances in early stage disease when supradiaphragmatic radiation therapy alone is being considered as the only method of treatment.[4] If staging laparotomy is performed, however, then a polyvalent pneumococcal vaccine should be given approximately 2 weeks before the surgery to

TABLE 234-1 ANN ARBOR STAGING SYSTEM FOR LYMPHOMA

Stage	Substage	Definition
I	I	Single node region
	IE	Single extralymphatic site or involvement by direct extension
II	II	Two or more node regions on same side of diaphragm
	IIE	Single node region plus single localized extranodal site
	IIS	Spleen
	IIES	Extralymphatic site plus spleen
III	III	Involvement on both sides of diaphragm
IV	IV	Diffuse extralymphatic involvement
A		No constitutional symptoms
B		Fevers, chills, night sweats, or weight loss

From Cheson BJ: Hodgkin's disease and the non-Hodgkin's lymphomas. In Lenhard RE, Osteen RT, Gansler T, editors: *Clinical oncology,* Atlanta, 2000, American Cancer Society.

Diagnostics

Lymphomas

Laboratory	Imaging
CBC and differential	Chest x-ray
Serum electrolytes	CT scan of chest, abdomen, pelvis, head
LFTs	Lumbar puncture
BUN	Gallium or thallium scan*
Creatinine	**Other**
Serologic evaluation for EBV	Lymph node biopsy
HIV test	Bone marrow biopsy
Toxoplasmosis titer	

*If indicated.

prevent overwhelming sepsis from encapsulated organisms.[6] Other staging diagnostics should include a chest radiograph, chest and abdominal/pelvic CT scans, and a single photon emission gallium scan. Positron emission tomography (PET) scans are being widely studied and compared with MRI and CT scans for its ability to evaluate abnormal lymph nodes.[3] A bone marrow biopsy is typically performed in patients with HD as part of initial staging.

DIFFERENTIAL DIAGNOSIS

Lymphadenopathy may be a primary or secondary sign of numerous disorders including infectious diseases, immunologic disorders, and malignant diseases[7] (see Chapter 251). Although malignant lymphadenopathy is rare in the primary care setting, malignant lymphomas should be considered when infection or an inflammatory process has been excluded.[6] A patient presenting with unexplained lymphadenopathy not related to infection or inflammation may need a biopsy to rule out malignancy.[7]

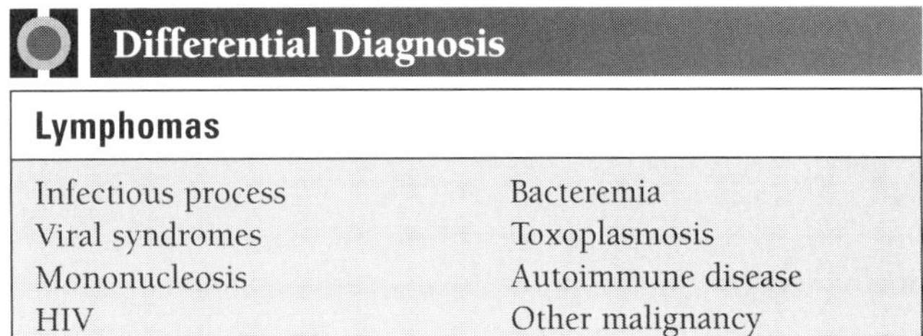

Differential Diagnosis

Lymphomas

Infectious process	Bacteremia
Viral syndromes	Toxoplasmosis
Mononucleosis	Autoimmune disease
HIV	Other malignancy

MANAGEMENT

There may be more than one treatment approach in the management of the patient with HD. The goal is to determine a course of therapy that preserves cure while minimizing long-term complications.

The course of treatment is based on the stage and prognostic factors. The adverse prognostic factors are advanced age, male gender, histologic subtype, presence of constitutional symptoms, presence of mediastinal mass, number of involved nodal regions, elevated ESR, presence of anemia, and low serum albumin.[5] The treatment for patients with early stage and favorable prognostic factor profile is generally radiation. Patients with early stage disease and an unfavorable risk profile are generally treated with both chemotherapy (typically 4 cycles) and radiation therapy. Patients in advanced stages receive an extensive course of chemotherapy (8 cycles) with or without consolidating radiation therapy.[5] A total of 80% of patients with bulky mediastinal or retroperitoneal disease who respond to therapy have a persistent radiographic abnormality that may remain longer than 1 year in half of those cases, without evidence of disease progression. Many of these patients are given additional radiation to sites of bulky disease. They should be observed closely with chest radiographs. Confirmation biopsy and therapy may be needed if the mass continues to enlarge or if disease appears outside of the radiated field. A positive PET scan may also provide evidence to differentiate residual tumor from fibrosis.[3]

Relapsing/Refractory Disease

Although HD is a relatively curable disease, 20% to 30% of patients never achieve a complete (CR) or partial remission (PR). Another 20% to 30% relapse after an initial CR. Treatment decisions with patients who have experienced relapse include review of initial therapy and duration of initial response. Patients who experience late relapses from CR or durable PR (>12 months) have a more favorable prognosis and may be treated with combination chemotherapy, with about 15% remaining in remission at 5 years. The prognosis of patients with an early relapse from CR is poor.[3] High-dose therapy with autologous bone marrow or peripheral blood stem cell support may be considered in relapsed patients.[8]

Non-Hodgkin's Lymphoma

DEFINITION/EPIDEMIOLOGY

NHLs are the fifth most common tumor type diagnosed in men and the sixth most common in women.[3] In 2001, it is estimated that there will be 56,200 new diagnoses of NHL and 26,300 deaths.[1] During the last two decades, the incidence of

NHL rose at almost 7% per year, but recently the incidence has leveled, if not decreased. The rise in occurrence was seen most strikingly in older adults and primarily in the diffuse, large B-cell histology.[3] The explanation for the rise in NHL incidence, as well as the etiology of NHL, are unknown. There is a noted increase in the frequency of aggressive NHL in patients who are on long-term immunosuppressive medicines after allogeneic BMT, as well as in patients with inherited immune defects, rheumatoid arthritis, or with HIV/AIDS. There is also an association between a variety of infectious agents and lymphomas including EBV with Burkitt's lymphoma in immunodeficient patients, human herpes virus-8 with body cavity based lymphoma, and human T-cell lymphotropic virus-1 with adult T-cell leukemia/lymphoma. Helicobacter pylori has been linked to gastric mucosa-associated lymphoid tissue (MALT) lymphomas.[5] There have also been reports of an association with environmental factors such as pesticides and agricultural chemicals, exercise, smoking, and hair dyes.[3]

Classification

There have been multiple attempts to classify lymphomas using morphology, immunophenotype, and genetic as well as clinical features to distinguish between the multiple entities that compose the non-Hodgkin's lymphomas. The earlier classifications systems, including the Working Formulation (WF) and the Revised European American Lymphoma (REAL), were recently modified by the WHO. The WF is the most commonly used classification of NHL (Table 234-2). It describes the most common lymphomas. However, it does not recognize a large variety of newly described clinicopathologic entities within the lymphomas. The REAL/WHO classification correlates the lymphoma classification with the normal lymphocyte counterpart. Therefore it is particularly applicable to uncommon lymphomas.[2]

PATHOPHYSIOLOGY

The molecular biology research of NHL has identified clues to the pathogenesis of some of these disorders. The translocation of t(14;18) is detectable at 80% to 90% of patient with follicular NHL, and the BCL2 gene has been cloned at that breakpoint. This gene overexpression prevents apoptosis, or programmed cell death. In mantle cell lymphoma, the BCL1 gene and cyclin D1 are overexpressed.[3]

CLINICAL PRESENTATION

Patients often present with signs or symptoms related to the lymphadenopathy.[3] They may also have constitutional symptoms of fevers, night sweats, and weight loss.[5]

PHYSICAL EXAMINATION

The history and physical examination can yield important information. The presence of constitutional symptoms, as described previously, can have adverse prognostic implications. Other pertinent information includes pain that can be related to sites of disease and co-morbidities such as diabetes or heart disease that may limit treatment options.[5] On physical examination there should be careful evaluation of lymph node areas, as well as the size of the liver and spleen. Other important physical examination findings may include pharyngeal involvement, thyroid mass, evidence of pleural effusion, abdominal mass, testicular mass, cutaneous lesions, and Waldeyer's ring. All of these findings may direct further investigations and therapies.

DIAGNOSTICS

Laboratory studies should include CBC, screening chemistries including glucose, calcium, albumin, lactate dehydrogenase, and beta-2 microglobulin.[5]

Staging

The initial staging evaluation provides treatment, prognostic, and clinical trial data. The Ann Arbor Staging classification is also used in NHL. There is also an International Prognostic Index that is widely used to predict outcome. It was initially developed for patients with diffuse aggressive lymphoma, but experience has shown that it applies to patients with almost all subtypes of NHL.[9]

Diagnostic Tests

An initial excisional lymph node biopsy is recommended for precise diagnosis and clarification of the histopathology. Needle biopsies may not provide enough information to distinguish between histologies of the different NHL. An aspirate or core needle biopsy may provide enough information to confirm a suspected recurrence in patients who have previously been diagnosed. The increased use of flow cytometry, cytogenetics,

TABLE 234-2 CLASSIFICATION OF NON-HODGKIN'S LYMPHOMA: THE WORKING FORMULATION

Low Grade	Intermediate Grade	High Grade
Small lymphocytic Chronic lymphocytic leukemia-type Plasmacytoid	Follicular, large cell	Immunoblastic (large cell)
Follicular, small cleaved cell	Diffuse, small cleaved cell	Lymphoblastic
Follicular, mixed (small cleaved and large cell)	Diffuse, mixed cell (small and large cell)	Small, noncleaved Burkitt Non-Burkitt
	Diffuse, large cell	

From Emmanouilides C, Casciato DA, Rosen PJ: Hodgkin and non-Hodgkin lymphoma. In Casciato DA, Lowitz BB, editors: *Manual of clinical oncology,* ed 4, Philadelphia, 2000, JB Lippincott.

and molecular genetic studies can provide information for analysis from a core needle biopsy and in some instances fine-needle biopsy when dealing with a lymphoma in the mediastinal, retroperitoneal, or other inaccessible locations.[3]

The staging workup should include CT scan of the chest/abdomen/pelvis and a gallium scan. PET scans are used more frequently, but clinical trials are needed to determine their true usefulness.[5]

DIFFERENTIAL DIAGNOSIS

See Hodgkin's Lymphoma-Differential Diagnosis.

MANAGEMENT

The current approach to the treatment of NHL is dependent on the stage and histologic subtype.

Low-Grade NHL

Low-grade histologies include small lymphocytic leukemia, follicular grades I and grade II. Only about 10% to 15% of patients with grade I or II follicular NHL initially present with stages I or II disease. These patients may be treated with local radiation therapy. Advanced stage low-grade NHL is incurable and there is no evidence that early treatment prolongs survival.[10] Because the therapies have toxicity, treatment is usually given to patients who are symptomatic. Numerous standard chemotherapies are used including single agents or combination chemotherapy involving the alkylating agents or purine analogue chemotherapy. Treatment is generally continued until a maximum response in the disease is seen. There is no clear evidence of a survival advantage in maintenance therapy.[2]

Relapsed/Refractory Disease. Patients with low-grade NHL usually relapse. Response with chemotherapy can be achieved with similar regimens, but the response is usually of shorter duration with each treatment. Patients who experience relapse can convert to a high-grade NHL, which has a poor prognosis. Early treatment of these patients may result in the possibility of disease-free survival.[3]

New Approaches. During the last few years, two new classes of drugs have influenced therapy in NHL. These drugs are the purine nucleoside analogues and monoclonal antibodies. Purine nucleoside analogues in combination with other chemotherapy drugs have resulted in impressive response rates for patients with low-grade lymphomas.[11] The first monoclonal antibody to be approved by the U.S. Food and Drug Administration for treatment of a human malignancy is rituximab. It is directed against the cells containing the CD20 receptor, which are expressed on more than 90% of B-cell lymphomas. Rituximab is generally well tolerated with the major side effects of fevers and chills. After the first infusion, most patients have no toxicity for the remainder of the treatment.[12] Monoclonal antibodies to other lymphoma antigens and monoclonal antibodies conjugated to radioisotopes are currently in clinical trials.[2]

Intermediate/High-Grade Lymphomas

Generally, patients who present with local, nonbulky disease may be treated with combination chemotherapy containing doxorubicin and radiation therapy to the site of disease. Patients with bulky disease are generally treated with cyclophosphamide, doxorubicin, vincristine, prednisone chemotherapy (CHOP). Patients may benefit from radiation therapy if the bulky disease can be encompassed in a radiation port.[2] Recent data show that the addition of rituximab to CHOP chemotherapy resulted in a significant increased rate of complete response and 2-year event-free survival in older patients with diffuse large B-cell lymphoma compared with CHOP chemotherapy alone.[13]

Within the classification of intermediate/high-grade NHL, there is a subset of less common NHL disease that may have a unique natural history and therapies. These include mantle cell lymphoma, Burkitt's/Burkitt's-like lymphoma and lymphoblastic lymphoma. Mantle cell lymphoma exhibits the worst features of lymphoma in that it is not curable and has an aggressive clinical course. Complete remission can be achieved, but the disease generally recurs with a median survival of 2.5 to 3 years.[3] Patients with mantle cell lymphoma should be considered for clinical trials.[14] Burkitt's/Burkitt's-like lymphoma and lymphoblastic lymphoma are highly aggressive, have exponential growth rate, and disseminate to the bone marrow and meninges. There has been some success in treatment of Burkitt's/Burkitt's-like lymphoma with intensive short-course chemotherapy. Lymphoblastic lymphoma may be treated similarly to lymphoblastic leukemia with dose-intensive cyclophosphamide and anthracycline and standard dose vincristine and asparaginase chemotherapy.[14]

Relapsed/Refractory Disease. Only 40% of patients treated with CHOP chemotherapy are cured. The majority of recurrences occur within 2 years. Late recurrences can demonstrate a low-grade histology, so biopsies of recurrences are necessary. The therapy of patients with relapsed/refractory disease has been investigated with some success.[15,16] Data have supported the use of high-dose chemotherapy with stem cell support in patients who are in the first or subsequent relapse and are still chemosensitive, those with primary induction failure, and those in first remission who were IPI high-intermediate/high risk categories. Patients with primary refractory disease and relapsed disease may be considered for allogeneic stem cell therapy. Clinical trials may also be offered to these patients.[14] The biologic therapies of rituximab and I131-conjugated anti-CD20 antibody (BEXXAR) have shown some clinical response.[3]

Marginal Zone Lymphomas

Marginal zone lymphomas consist of MALT NHL, monocytoid B-cell NHL, primary (nodal counterparts to MALTomas), and primary splenic lymphoma with villous lymphocytes. The MALTomas account for about 80% of the indolent NHLs of the stomach. The majority are associated with Helicobacter pylori and are highly responsive to double or triple antibiotic therapy. Splenic lymphoma is generally disseminated with peripheral blood and bone marrow involvement at diagnosis. A splenectomy can provide a prolonged clinical remission.[3]

Peripheral T-Cell NHL

Peripheral T-cell lymphoma (PTCL) consists of a diverse group of post-thymic T-cell tumors that have a mature T-cell phenotype. They make up fewer than 10% of NHL in the United States, but they generally present with advanced stage disease and constitutional symptoms, as well as a poorer prognosis in comparison with B-cell lymphoma. Classifications in this lymphoma include PTCL otherwise unspecified (generally (50% of cases), anaplastic large cell lymphoma, angioimmunoblastic T-cell lymphoma, angiocentric lymphoma, adult T-cell leukemia/lymphoma, and a few less common lymphomas. In general patients with PTCL are treated with aggressive combination chemotherapy such as CHOP. However, often they have a poor response to treatment and a high rate of relapse, with no long-term remissions.[3]

LIFE SPAN CONSIDERATIONS

Patients should be monitored carefully after treatment, and this can be coordinated with the patient's hematology/oncology physician. The necessary radiologic and laboratory studies are usually done or can be coordinated with the patient's hematologist/oncologist to ensure adequate follow-up evaluation.[17]

Under some circumstances, gonadal dysfunction can affect quality of life after treatment. Transient and sometimes permanent male sterility may occur.[6] Infertility may occur in at least 80% of women over 25 years of age who receive nitrogen mustard, vincristine, procarbazine, prednisone chemotherapy regimen. This may be reversible after up to three courses of therapy. The newer, nonalkylating agent-containing regimens have a lower risk of infertility. However, sperm banking should be considered before initiating treatment. Pregnancies occurring in patients or their partners do not appear to be associated with complications, congenital abnormalities, or spontaneous abortions.[3]

Improved treatment regimens and survival mean that many patients will return to primary care providers for care and monitoring. Advance directives should be discussed with the patient, but with the understanding that some lymphomas can be treated successfully or have an indolent course. Patients are encouraged to prepare a living will and appoint a health care proxy so that both the health care proxy and the primary care provider understand their preferences for terminal care.

COMPLICATIONS

Complications from lymphoma can occur during treatment, as a result of treatment, or from the disease itself.

During Therapy

Patients with cancer who undergo chemotherapy and radiation therapy are at risk of infection because of the immune suppression from the cancer, myelosuppression from chemotherapy, the break in skin barriers from the placement of Portacaths/central lines and/or shifts in microbial flora. The myelosuppressive effect of chemotherapy can cause neutropenia. Absolute neutropenia is defined as less than 1000 neutrophils/bands in the bloodstream and is calculated by multiplying the total number of white cells from the CBC with the total percentage of neutrophils + bands. The period of neutropenia after chemotherapy is relatively predictable, with the lowest count of neutrophils occurring approximately 10 to 14 days after chemotherapy and recovery in about 3 to 4 weeks after chemotherapy. Although fever can be a presenting sign in a patient with lymphoma, fever in a patient after chemotherapy, especially in a neutropenic patient, may be a sign of life-threatening sepsis. In addition, patients who have undergone splenectomy have a lifelong risk of overwhelming sepsis by encapsulated organisms.[18] Research shows that colony-stimulating factors (CSF) can reduce the incidence of febrile neutropenia; however, these medications can be inconvenient and expensive, and have toxicities including bone pain. Guidelines for CSF administration have been issued by the American Society of Clinical Oncology and these medications should be administered based on the recommendation of the treating hematologist/oncologist.[19]

Fatigue is a poorly understood phenomenon that affects the patient's quality of life. It can occur as a result of the treatment and/or the disease. It may be associated with anxiety/depression as well as physiologic processes related to tumor necrosis factor and interleukin-1 and other cytokines. Physiologic conditions such as anemia resulting from the chemotherapy and radiation therapy may also contribute to fatigue. A careful review of symptoms and CBC with differential is important. Current recommendations include education to relieve anxiety, activities that provide distraction, and participation in low intensity exercise.[18] Packed red blood cell transfusion should be given to patients with severe anemia. Patients with mild anemia may benefit from erythropoietin.[20]

Pain is a common complaint in cancer patients. It is experienced by one third of persons receiving treatment and two thirds who have advanced disease. A broad assessment of the symptom is important and should include location, duration, and quality, as well as the impact on the patient's life.[18] The range of strategies to relieve pain may target the etiology of the pain itself (chemotherapy and radiation therapy) and/or pharmacologic therapy using the analgesic ladder from the World Health Organization. Nonopioid and adjuvant analgesics may be used such as acetaminophen and nonsteroidal antiinflammatory drugs (NSAIDs). Potential side effects and concerns about gastrointestinal and renal toxicity may limit NSAID use. Other adjuvant analgesics may include steroids as a multipurpose therapy. Antidepressants and anticonvulsants are often used for neuropathic pain. When drug therapy does not resolve pain, consideration can be given for anesthetic, surgical, neurostimulatory, physiatric, or psychologic interventions.[21]

Posttreatment Toxicities

A serious consequence of treatment is the increased risk of a second cancer including acute myeloid leukemia (AML). The risk of secondary AML extends up to approximately 11 years posttreatment. Radiation therapy with and without chemotherapy may contribute to increased risk of solid tumors in the radiation field. Solid tumors tend to occur in the second decade posttreatment. Breast cancers in this population are often bilateral. Regular breast examination and mammography starting at an early age are recommended as part of routine posttreatment.[3]

More than two thirds of patients who undergo mantle irradiation develop thyroid disease including hypothyroidism, Graves' disease, silent thyrotoxicosis, and nodules, with a 2% risk of cancer. Mantle field irradiation also adds to the risk of cardiac toxicity.[3]

Other serious treatment complications are cardiotoxicity, which can be fatal, and pulmonary toxicity. High doses of doxorubicin can cause cardiomyopathy. Mantle-field radiotherapy can cause pericarditis, but the incidence of this complications has declined as a result of recent improvements in the delivery of radiotherapy. Mantle field radiotherapy can also cause radiation pneumonitis and chronic restrictive fibrosis. It is unclear whether radiotherapy results in the acceleration of coronary artery disease.[22] Pulmonary fibrosis or restrictive disease has also been associated with bleomycin chemotherapy.

INDICATIONS FOR REFERRAL/HOSPITALIZATION

Referrals

A patient should be referred to an hematologist/oncologist after confirming the diagnosis of malignant lymphoma. Patients with high-risk disease should be referred to a comprehensive cancer center whenever possible. These centers can often provide oncology care with access to the latest research treatments.

Patients with a diagnosis of lymphoma in remission should request that the hematologist/oncologist forward treatment records. Follow-up examinations should evaluate both the presenting sites and symptoms of the disease, as well as new symptoms or lymphadenopathy. The patient should be referred back to the hematologist/oncologist if constitutional symptoms continue or recur and if suspicious nodes are found.

There is a high prevalence of depression among cancer patients. Patients who are depressed may find psychotherapy that involves social support, coping skills, emotional expression, and cognitive restructuring helpful.[23]

Hospitalizations

The majority of treatments for lymphoma can be administered in an outpatient setting. The patient might be hospitalized for high-dose chemotherapy requiring careful monitoring of laboratory values and blood product support, as well as for episodes of febrile neutropenia.

PATIENT AND FAMILY EDUCATION

One of the most common reactions to the stress of cancer diagnosis and treatment is anxiety and depression. Education about the disease, treatment, and prognosis can help relieve anxiety. Educational and social support resources for patients include the American Cancer Society programs such as "I Can Cope,"[18] The National Cancer Institute web site, and Oncolink, an Internet resource affiliated with the University of Pennsylvania.

Nutrition education should start at diagnosis to prevent complications caused by malnutrition and weight loss often associated with treatment. Dietary counseling should address the need for calorie-, protein-rich foods.[18] Alcoholic beverages should be avoided. Given the treatment-related pulmonary and cardiac toxicity, smoking cessation should be encouraged.

REFERENCES

1. Greenlee RT and others: Cancer statistics, 2001, *CA Cancer J Clin* 51(1):15-36, 2001.
2. Casciato DA, Lowitz BB: *Manual of clinical oncology*, ed 4, Philadelphia, 2000, Lippincott.
3. Lenhard RE and others: *Clinical oncology*, Atlanta, 2001, American Cancer Society.
4. Hoppe RT and others: *NCCN Practice guidelines for Hodgkin's disease*, 2000, National Comprehensive Cancer Network.
5. Devita VT and others: *Cancer: principles & practice of oncology*, ed 6, Philadelphia, 2001, Lippincott.
6. Yarbro CH and others: *Cancer nursing*, ed 5, Boston , 2001, Jones and Bartlett.
7. Ferrer R: Lymphadenopathy: differential diagnosis and evaluation, *Am Fam Physician* 58(6):1313-1320, 1998.
8. Moskowitz CH and others: A 2-step comprehensive high-dose chemoradiotherapy second-line program for relapsed and refractory Hodgkin disease: analysis by intent to treat and development of a prognostic model, *Blood* 97(3):616-623, 2001.
9. Shipp MA and others: A predictive model for aggressive non-Hodgkin's lymphoma, *N Engl J Med* 329(14):987-994, 1993.
10. Horning SJ: Follicular lymphoma: have we made any progress? *Ann Oncol* 11(Suppl 1):S23-S27, 2000.
11. McLaughlin P and others: Fludarabine, mitoxantrone, and dexamethasone: an effective new regimen for indolent lymphoma, *J Clin Oncol* 14(4):1262-1268, 1996.
12. McLaughlin P and others: Rituximab chimeric anti-CD20 monoclonal antibody therapy for relapsed indolent lymphoma: half of patients respond to a four-dose treatment program, *J Clin Oncol* 16(8):2825-2833, 1998.
13. Coiffer and others: CHOP chemotherapy plus rituximab compared with CHOP alone in elderly patients with diffuse large-B-cell lymphoma, *N Engl J Med* 346(4):235-242, 2002.
14. Zelenetz A and others: *NCCN practice guidelines for non-Hodgkin's lymphomas*, Rockledge, Penn, 2000, National Comprehensive Cancer Network.
15. Wilson WH and others: EPOCH chemotherapy: toxicity and efficacy in relapsed and refractory non-Hodgkin's lymphoma, *J Clin Oncol* 11(8):1573-1582, 1993.
16. Rodriguez MA and others: Results of a salvage treatment program for relapsing lymphoma: MINE consolidated with ESHAP, *J Clin Oncol* 13(7):1734-1741, 1995.
17. Boyer and others: *Primary care oncology*, Philadelphia, 1999, WB Saunders.
18. Yarbro CH and others: *Cancer symptom management*, ed 2, Boston, 1999, Jones and Bartlett.
19. Ozer H and others: 2000 update of recommendations for the use of hematopoietic colony-stimulating factors: evidence-based, clinical practice guidelines, *J Clin Oncol* 18(20):3558-3585, 2000.
20. Groopman JE, Itri LM: Chemotherapy-induced anemia in adults: incidence and treatment, *J Natl Cancer Inst* 91(19):1616-1634, 1999.
21. Portenoy RK, Lesage P: Management of cancer pain, *Lancet* 353: 1695-1700, 1999.
22. Urba WJ, Longo DL: Medical progress: Hodgkin's disease, *N Engl J Med* 326(10):678-687, 1992.
23. Spiegel D: Cancer and depression, *Br J Psychiatry* 168(Suppl 30): 109-116, 1996.

CHAPTER 235

Myelodysplastic Disorders

Sandra L. Creamer and Murat Anamur

DEFINITION/EPIDEMIOLOGY

Myelodysplastic syndromes are a heterogenous group of bone marrow disorders characterized by dysplastic growth of the hematopoietic precursors and associated with hypercellular bone marrow and peripheral cytopenia. They are diseases of the stem cells. The origin and expansion of these cells are clonal, which indicates that the origin may be a single cell that evolves from a relatively benign clonal myeloid hemopathy into the frankly malignant neoplasm.

Myelodysplastic syndrome (MDS) is a relatively rare disease. The incidence increases after age 40 years to more than 20 per 100,000 septuagenarians. The median age of presentation is approximately 60 to 70 years. Males are affected about 1.5 to 2.0 times as often as females.[1] MDS is rarely hereditary, which indicates that this clonal expansion almost always is an acquired change. MDS that occurs in young patients is usually a consequence of prior damage to the stem cells from either chemotherapy or irradiation.[2]

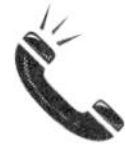

Physician consultation is indicated for all suspected cases of myelodysplastic syndrome.

PATHOPHYSIOLOGY

Research studies confirm that the marrow cells of patients with MDS are derived from a malignant clone of marrow stem cells. Because this occurs in an early stage of the maturation process, a number of hematopoietic stem cells, including white cells, red cells, and platelets, may also be derived from the malignant clone. In some cases, even lymphoid cells may be part of this abnormal clone, thus resembling leukemia.[3]

MDS has five subtypes: (1) refractory anemia, (2) refractory anemia with ringed sideroblast, (3) refractory anemia with excess blasts, (4) refractory anemia with excess blasts in transformation, and (5) chronic myelomonocytic leukemia. The best way to determine the subtype of myelodysplastic syndrome is to carefully assess the peripheral smear and the bone marrow; the number of blasts in the peripheral smear and the bone marrow will be helpful. Survival and the percentage of leukemic transformation vary depending on the MDS subtype. Refractory anemia has the best prognosis, whereas refractory anemia with excess blasts in transformation has the lowest survival rate and the highest percentage of leukemic transformation.[4]

CLINICAL PRESENTATION AND PHYSICAL EXAMINATION

The symptoms of MDS are usually the end result of cytopenia. If the anemia is the most significant sign of MDS, then the clinical signs—namely, fatigue, shortness of breath, and malaise—are related to this problem. Low platelet count may produce bleeding episodes. The immune system in patients with neutropenia is compromised; presenting symptoms may include fever and recurrent infections. Anemia occurs in more than 90% of patients and is actually the hallmark of MDS. Anemia alone may be present in only 15% of the patients, but 50% of them demonstrate signs and symptoms of thrombocytopenia or neutropenia (Box 235-1).

Chromosomal abnormalities occur in MDS. There may be a number of changes in the chromosomal structure. These nonrandom chromosome abnormalities are useful in confirming the diagnosis; however, normal cytogenetics does not exclude a diagnosis of MDS.[5]

DIAGNOSTICS

The diagnosis of MDS requires careful assessment of both a blood smear and a bone marrow specimen. The bone marrow may show a number of abnormal changes in the white blood cells, including abnormal granules, bizarre nuclear forms, and other abnormalities such as Auer rods and Pelger-Huët nuclear anomalies. The red blood cells also are significantly abnormal, showing ringed sideroblasts, megaloblastic changes, and multinuclear forms. Platelets also show abnormal changes in the bone marrow such as micromegakaryocytes, decreased ploidy, or other abnormalities. Bone marrow cellularities may be normal or increased, and myeloblasts may be seen in increased numbers.

A peripheral blood smear may show anomalies similar to those seen in the bone marrow. Red blood cells show polychromasia, tear drop formation, and fragmentation. Platelets may be large with an abnormal appearance. Neutrophils show poorly granulated, hyposegmented changes.

BOX 235-1

MYELODYSPLASTIC SYNDROME AT A GLANCE

PATHOGENESIS

Unknown.

Secondary MDS is seen after chemotherapy, irradiation, chemical exposure, BMT.

Defective maturation and uncontrolled proliferation of the malignant clone is the underlying pathogenesis for progression.

CLINICAL FINDINGS

Usually the end result of underlying cytopenia.

Fatigue, shortness of breath, bleeding, and recurrent infections may be the first sign, necessitating a CBC.

Incidental splenomegaly, lymphadenopathy, and skin changes are seen.

DIAGNOSIS

Anemia is a universal finding (80% of patients have hemoglobin less than 10 g/dl).

Leukopenia and low platelets are common.

Peripheral smear shows macrocytosis, stippling, ringed sideroblasts, hypogranulation of neutrophils, large platelets, and various other abnormalities.

DIFFERENTIAL DIAGNOSIS

Several illnesses imitate MDS and should be considered. These syndromes include vitamin B_{12} deficiency, folic acid or iron deficiency, and drug toxicity (including the effects of chemotherapy), irradiation, or alcohol-related damage. A number of toxins may also imitate changes similar to those seen in MDS. Viral infections, including the HIV virus, human parvovirus B19, and Epstein-Barr virus may create morphologic changes similar to this syndrome. Anemia of chronic disease secondary to an underlying infection, collagen vascular disease, or renal failure may also imitate MDS. Primary acute or chronic leukemia or a metastatic solid tumor with bone marrow metastasis should also be considered in the differential diagnosis. Hypersplenism, paroxysmal nocturnal hemoglobinuria, and several congenital disorders, including Down syndrome and hereditary sideroblastic anemia, may create a similar picture.[6]

MANAGEMENT

The main therapy for MDS is supportive care. This includes aggressive antibiotic coverage for major infections and supportive transfusion therapy. The use of differentiating agents, including the low-dose cytosine arabinoside and retinoic acid derivatives and 5-azacitidine, have not produced consistently good results, and routine use of these agents cannot be recommended. Corticosteroids have been used in a small number of patients; however, clear survival benefits have not be demonstrated.

Hematopoietic growth factors have also been tried. So far, there has been no clear survival benefit of using granulocyte colony-stimulating factor (G-CSF) or granulocyte-macrophage colony-stimulating factor (GM-CSF). There appears to be no significant risk of progression to acute myelogenous leukemia if G-CSF or GM-CSF is used. There does appear to be some improvement in the number of episodes of major infections, but this decrease does not translate to a major survivor benefit. There may be some benefit in the use of erythropoietin to improve the anemia, especially if the serum erythropoietin level is low; however, clinical studies now underway have yet to provide evidence indicating the use of erythropoietin injections as a standard therapy for MDS. Interleukin-3 (IL-3) has been used in early clinical studies; at this point, its exact impact remains unclear. Several trials address the use of growth factors. Because these studies are ongoing, it is difficult to recommend any particular combination of growth factors that should be used routinely in patients with MDS.

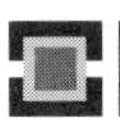

Diagnostics

Myelodysplastic Disorders

Laboratory
CBC and differential
Peripheral blood smear evaluation

Other
Bone marrow biopsy

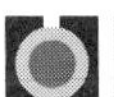

Differential Diagnosis

Myelodysplastic Disorders

Vitamin B_{12}, folic acid, or iron deficiency	Renal failure
Drug toxicity	Leukemia
Alcohol toxicity	Tumor with bone marrow metastasis
HIV	Hypersplenism
Irradiation	Paroxysmal nocturnal hemoglobinuria
Parvovirus	Down's syndrome
Epstein-Barr virus	Hereditary sideroblastic anemia
Anemia of chronic disease	
Collagen vascular disease	

Considerable progress has been demonstrated by clinical trials in understanding the biology of MDS, as well as an increasing number of new drugs currently in development. Topotecan (a topoisomerase I inhibitor) has single agent activity against MDS. Another agent, amifostine, induces responses in 30% of patients. Many studies are ongoing and an increasing body of data suggests a possible role for angiogenesis agents such as thalidomide. It is hoped that more effective therapeutic strategies will emerge.[7] Unfortunately, the use of conventional chemotherapy creates significant treatment-related deaths and cannot be recommended routinely. In future studies, however, new chemotherapy agents and the aggressive use of growth factor support may reduce the death rate; conventional chemotherapy may have a role in select groups of patients.

The only treatment that results in significant disease-free survival is bone marrow transplantation. This treatment should be reserved for patients who meet the age requirement and donor criteria of allogeneic or unrelated bone marrow transplantation. According to several studies, the younger the patient and the shorter the duration of disease before transplant, the better the overall survival rate. On the basis of these initial studies, a bone marrow transplantation should be offered to young patients with good performance status. Unfortunately, a number of patients with MDS do not meet the criteria for bone marrow transplantation; they either do not have a compatible bone marrow donor, or their performance status and age do not allow for this form of aggressive approach.[8]

COMPLICATIONS

The clinical course of MDS is inexorably progressive. Approximately 70% of patients die directly because of MDS either secondary to bone marrow failure (causing major infections or bleeding) or because of transformation to a leukemia and its complications.

Poor prognostic features include severe neutropenia, severe thrombocytopenia, and anemia. A high percentage of blasts in the bone marrow clearly indicates a poor prognosis. As far as genetic changes are concerned, single-characteristic abnormalities usually do not change the prognosis; however, multiple or complex chromosomal deletions indicate a poor prognosis. The exception to a single characteristic abnormality is monosomy,[7] which always indicates a poor prognosis; a 5q deletion has a better prognosis. MDS that develops as a sequela of chemotherapy and irradiation usually has a poor prognosis. Unfortunately, this problem is occurring more often because of the increased number of patients being treated aggressively with systemic chemotherapy, irradiation, and bone marrow transplantation. This secondary incidence of MDS currently approaches approximately 20% of cancer survivors. This certainly must be taken into consideration before the initial decision-making process regarding treatment plan.[9]

INDICATIONS FOR REFERRAL/HOSPITALIZATION

Because the definitive diagnosis of MDS requires examination of both a peripheral blood smear and a bone marrow specimen, patients are referred to a hematologist whenever this condition is suspected. Hematology should also be consulted for management of complications.

PATIENT AND FAMILY EDUCATION

The side effects and sequelae of MDS are similar to the leukemias in that bone marrow elements are altered, causing moderate to severe dysfunction. For further information, see Box 233-2.

REFERENCES

1. Lichtman M, Brennan J: Myelodysplastic disorders. In Beutler and others, editors: *William's hematology,* ed 6, New York, 2001, McGraw-Hill.
2. Beguin Y and others: Long-term follow-up of patients with acute myelogenous leukemia who received the daunorubicin, vincristine, and cytosine arabinoside regimen, *Cancer* 79(7):1351-1354, 1997.
3. Lowenthal RM, Marsen KA: Myelodysplastic syndromes, *J Hematol* 65(4):319-338, 1997.
4. Greenberg P: In Hoffman R, editor: *Hematology: basic principles and practice,* ed 2, London, 1994, Churchill-Livingstone.
5. Gilliland G: *Harvard Review: course in cancer medicine and hematology,* Boston, 1995.
6. Jacobs P: Myelodysplasia and the leukemias, *Dis Mon* 43(8):505-597, 1997.
7. Cheson BD, Valmonte CM: Clinical trials referral resource, *Oncology* 15(1):52-55, 2001.
8. Loffler H, Schmitz N, Gassman W: Intensive chemotherapy and bone marrow transplantation for myelodysplastic syndromes, *Hematol Oncol Clin North Am* 6(3):619-631, 1992.
9. Deiss A: *Non-neoplastic diseases, chemical agents, and hematologic disorders that may precede hematologic neoplasms in clinical hematology,* ed 9, Philadelphia, 1993, Lea & Febiger.

PART 19

Evaluation and Management of Rheumatic and Multisystem Disorders

JOANNE SANDBERG-COOK, Section Editor

CHAPTER 236

Common Diagnostics in Rheumatologic Disorders

Robert H. Shmerling

Diagnostic testing in patients with possible or established autoimmune disease may not be helpful or may be misleading because most of these tests have significant limitations in accuracy. Both false-positive results (abnormal findings when the patient is fine) and false-negative results (normal findings when the patient is ill) are common in autoimmune disease. Some are sensitive (usually abnormal findings when disease is present), and others are specific (usually normal findings if disease is absent), but, unfortunately, most are not both. In fact, the symptoms, findings on examination and, often, the passage of time are the most useful "tests" in patients with possible autoimmune disease. In clinical practice the most important consideration is predictive value: what does a positive or negative test result mean? Positive predictive value is the likelihood that a positive result is an indication of disease; negative predictive value is the likelihood that a disease is absent if the test result is normal. Predictive value is determined not only by the sensitivity and specificity of the test but also by the likelihood of disease, as clinically assessed, before the test is ordered. If a test is ordered when the chances of disease are low (e.g., a rheumatoid factor for a patient with low back pain), an abnormal result will often represent a clinical false-positive finding. Thus how a test is ordered by the practitioner has a direct effect on its usefulness.

These principles are crucial to interpreting test results in all fields of medicine but particularly in the rheumatic diseases, for which there is often no single result that confirms or excludes a particular illness. It is more common that these disorders are diagnosed by "the big picture," an integration of symptoms and signs, as well as test results. Often, routine tests are the most helpful, however, and occasionally, more specific (and often more expensive) testing is warranted, especially when the suspicion of rheumatic disease is moderate or high. Selective testing is recommended to avoid unnecessary expense and unhelpful, or even misleading, results. This applies also to combinations of tests, or "panels," in which more false-positive results are inevitable as the number of tests increases. It should be noted that for most tests there is no clear consensus regarding when they should be ordered.

ERYTHROCYTE SEDIMENTATION RATE

The erythrocyte sedimentation rate (ESR) is an inexpensive, widely available, and easily measured acute-phase reactant, a family of proteins that appear in the bloodstream in elevated levels during acute inflammation. As such, they are nonspecific, meaning that any cause of inflammation, including infection, tumor, or rheumatic disease, may be associated with an elevated ESR.[1] Among the rheumatic diseases the ESR is almost always elevated in giant cell (temporal) arteritis, as well as in most patients with polymyalgia rheumatica (PMR); in both of these disorders the test is monitored over time, along with symptoms and signs, to help assess disease. Among other rheumatic diseases, including systemic lupus erythematosus (SLE), rheumatoid arthritis (RA), and others, the test may be suggestive of active illness when the ESR is elevated or of improvement when the ESR is normal, but exceptions to this are common. Among nonrheumatic diseases, patients with subacute bacterial endocarditis (SBE) almost always have an elevation in ESR, but in other infectious, neoplastic, and other inflammatory states the ESR may be high or normal. The test has limited clinical use unless it has previously been proved to correlate well with clinical status, as might be true in a patient with osteomyelitis: the ESR will usually fall with treatment and may rise again if the infection relapses. Other acute-phase reactants (including ferritin, C-reactive protein, transferrin, and haptoglobin) may change in the face of inflammation as well, but these offer no clear advantage to the ESR.

RHEUMATOID FACTOR

The rheumatoid factor (RF) is an IgM antibody directed against IgG and is found in most patients with RA, as well as in several other rheumatic and nonrheumatic disorders (Box 236-1). Its usefulness is limited to patients whose chances of having RA, as estimated by the history and physical examination, are neither very low nor very high.[2] Prognostic information provided by RF testing may be more useful than its diagnostic utility because, on average, RF-positive patients with established RA will have more severe joint disease, more frequent disability, and more extraarticular disease (including nodules) compared with RF-negative patients. The higher the titer of a positive RF, the more likely it is that the patient has RA or another RF-associated illness; however, exceptions to this general rule are often encountered. High-titer RF in a patient without other findings of RA should raise the possibility of Sjögren's syndrome, SBE, or cryoglobulinemia. Because many of the "non-RA" causes of a positive RF finding (Box 236-1) are associated with arthralgia or even arthritis, there is significant potential for misdiagnosis.[3]

ANTINUCLEAR ANTIBODIES

Antinuclear antibodies (ANAs) are a heterogeneous family of possibly pathogenic autoantibodies directed against several components of cell nuclei. Almost all patients (95% to 99%) with SLE will have a positive test result; therefore a negative result is a strong argument against that diagnosis. However, up to 20% to 30% of healthy patients will have a positive test result (suggesting low specificity); a positive ANA finding certainly does not establish a diagnosis of SLE.[4] Other ANA-associated diseases include drug-induced lupus, Sjögren's syndrome, mixed connective tissue disease (MCTD), scleroderma, and RA, but for some of these, sensitivity is not high (Table 236-1). As with the RF, the higher the titer of the ANA, the more likely it is that a positive result is truly related to an ANA-associated illness such as SLE but, again, exceptions are common. The specific antigen responsible for the positive ANA, when identifiable (the specific autoantibody profile), may suggest one disease over another (see Table 236-1), but only anti-Smith (anti-Sm) and anti–double-stranded DNA (anti-dsDNA) have

BOX 236-1

DISEASES ASSOCIATED WITH A POSITIVE RHEUMATOID FACTOR

SYSTEMIC RHEUMATIC DISEASE
Rheumatoid arthritis
Sjögren's syndrome

INFECTION
Subacute bacterial endocarditis
Hepatitis virus B

LUNG DISEASE
Sarcoidosis
Asbestosis

MALIGNANCY
Leukemia
Colon cancer (case reports)

OTHER CHRONIC INFLAMMATORY DISEASE
Autoimmune hepatitis

TABLE 236-1 Rheumatic Diseases Associated with a Positive ANA Test

Disease	Comment
SLE	95%-99% of patients are ANA positive in any pattern; anti-ds-DNA and anti-Sm are highly specific but not sensitive
Drug-induced lupus	100% of patients are ANA positive; diffuse pattern, 95% of whom will have antihistone antibody specificity
Sjögren's syndrome	75% of patients are ANA positive, often in a speckled pattern as a result of anti-Ro (with or without anti-La) specificity
Scleroderma	50%-90% of patients are ANA positive, often in a high-titer speckled or nucleolar pattern
MCTD	95%-99% of patients are ANA positive, 95% of which cases are due to anti-RNP specificity
Rheumatoid arthritis	15%-30% of patients are ANA positive, usually in a diffuse pattern without presence of specific autoantibodies

SLE, Systemic lupus erythematosus; *ANA,* antinuclear antibody; *ds-DNA,* double-stranded deoxyribonucleic acid; *MCTD,* mixed connective tissue disease.

high positive predictive value for SLE. However, they are not highly sensitive because many lupus patients are negative for anti-dsDNA and anti-Sm. Routine testing for the entire autoantibody profile (antibodies to Sm, dsDNA, Ro, La, ribonucleoprotein [RNP]) for all patients being tested for ANA has low clinical usefulness.[5]

In pregnant women with or without systemic rheumatic disease, anti-Ro (also called SS-A) antibodies cross the placenta and are associated with neonatal lupus, a disease in which the newborn may manifest rash, thrombocytopenia, and heart block.[6] Consequences may be serious; therefore detection of this antibody before or during pregnancy warrants close monitoring by an obstetrician experienced in managing high-risk pregnancies.

URIC ACID

Serum uric acid (urate) is a byproduct of purine metabolism, a pathway crucial to DNA synthesis. Patients develop hyperuricemia because too little is renally excreted, too much is produced, or a combination of the two conditions. Other than obvious contributors (e.g., renal insufficiency), the underlying reason why a person underexcretes or overproduces uric acid is often unclear. Other conditions associated with elevated uric acid include diuretic use, obesity, hypertension, alcohol consumption, and myeloproliferative disorders. Although hyperuricemia generally causes no clinically evident disease, some patients develop gout or nephrolithiasis, particularly men and older women (e.g., 5 to 10 years postmenopausal). Gout is rare when the serum uric acid level is less than 5 to 6 mg/dl, but a sizeable subset of gout patients will have a high-normal level of uric acid.

Testing serum for the uric acid level in patients with definite gout is unnecessary unless treatment is planned to lower the uric acid. In addition, testing when gout is suspected, but not documented, generally yields little useful information because high-normal or high levels are so common in the general population.[7] Conversely, the finding of a low serum uric acid (e.g., less than 5 mg/dl) is a compelling argument against the diagnosis of suspected gout. For patients treated with allopurinol or probenecid to lower the uric acid level, the dosage of medications is dictated by the serum uric acid level, with a target of 5.5 mg/dl or less.

HLA-B27

The HLA-B27 immunogenetic marker is associated with spondyloarthropathies, which are present in 95% of patients with ankylosing spondylitis and in 50% to 80% of patients with the spondyloarthropathy of inflammatory bowel disease, Reiter's disease, or psoriasis. The HLA-B27 molecule may be involved in the pathogenesis of an autoimmune inflammatory response by allowing more efficient or persistent microbial tissue invasion (e.g., in Reiter's disease) through molecular mimicry between HLA-B27 and microbial antigens or by other, as-yet-unknown mechanisms. Determining a patient's HLA-B27 status has limited use, except in the case of patients with a moderate pretest probability of ankylosing spondylitis (e.g., patients with morning stiffness in the lower back that improves with exercise, especially if the stiffness is associated with oligoarthralgia, inflammatory eye disease, or radiographic changes of sacroiliitis).[8]

RADIOGRAPHY

Radiographic imaging has a high level of usefulness in suspected fracture or established, erosive RA and to document the presence and severity of osteoarthritis (especially if management would be altered by the radiographic findings, such as in the consideration of surgical intervention). However, the level of usefulness is low for the vast majority of patients with low back pain; suspected bursitis, tendinitis, cartilage or ligament injuries; or nonspecific

TABLE 236-2 Miscellaneous Diagnostic Tests and Their Indications

Diagnostic Test	Indication/Comment
Complement[9]	Suspected SLE, especially with nephritis; may correlate with disease activity
Anti-Scl-70 (topoisomerase)	Suspected diffuse scleroderma; less than 50% sensitive
Anticentromere	Suspected CREST syndrome; less than 50% sensitive
CPK	Suspected myopathy; sensitive measure of muscle injury
EMG/NCS	Suspected myopathy or neuropathy, especially if results would alter management (e.g., muscle or nerve biopsy)
Synovial fluid analysis[10]	Suspected infection or crystal disease; less compelling: to determine degree of inflammation or possible hemarthrosis
ANCA[11]	Suspected Wegener's granulomatosis, related renal vasculitides; specific types: anti-PR3 and anti-MPO
Myositis specific antibodies[12]	Suspected dermatomyositis or polymyositis; 50% sensitivity; effect on diagnosis and management unclear
Tissue biopsy	Suspected vasculitis, sarcoidosis, myositis

SLE, Systemic lupus erythematosus; *CREST,* calcinosis, Raynaud's phenomenon, esophageal dysfunction, sclerodactyly, and telangiectasia; *CPK,* Creatine phosphokinase; *EMG/NCS,* electromyogram/nerve conduction studies; *ANCA,* antineutrophilic cytoplasmic antibodies; *PR3,* proteinase 3; *MPO,* myeloperoxidase.

joint pain and early in the course of rheumatic disease, including RA. It takes 3 to 4 months for erosions characteristic of RA to be radiographically detectable. Certain circumstances warrant immediate x-ray studies; these include significant trauma, suspected bone or joint infection (although x-ray findings may be normal if disease has been present less than 10 days), and neck pain in the setting of neurologic findings or erosive RA. Normal or nonspecific radiographic findings are the rule in early RA, SLE, acute gout, and pseudogout.

MISCELLANEOUS

Other diagnostic tests are indicated in select clinical circumstances (Table 236-2).

REFERENCES

1. Sox HC, Liang MH: The erythrocyte sedimentation rate: guidelines for rational use, *Ann Intern Med* 104:515-523, 1986.
2. Shmerling RH, Delbanco TL: How useful is the rheumatoid factor? an analysis of sensitivity, specificity and predictive value, *Arch Intern Med* 152:2417-2420, 1992.
3. Shmerling RH, Delbanco TL: The rheumatoid factor: an analysis of clinical utility, *Am J Med* 91:528-534, 1991.
4. Slater CA, Davis RB, Shmerling R: Antinuclear antibody testing: a study of clinical utility, *Arch Intern Med* 156:1421-1425, 1996.
5. Homburger HA: Cascade testing for autoantibodies in connective tissue diseases, *Mayo Clin Proc* 70:183-184, 1995.
6. Buyon JP and others: Identification of mothers at risk for congenital heart block and other neonatal lupus syndromes in their children: comparison of enzyme-linked immunosorbent assay and immunoblot for measurement of anti-SS-A/Ro and anti-SS-B/La antibodies, *Arthritis Rheum* 36:1263-1273, 1993.
7. Liang MH, Fries JF: Asymptomatic hyperuricemia: the case for conservative management, *Ann Intern Med* 88:666-670, 1978.
8. Olajos A, Suranyi P: The value of HLA-B27 typing in the diagnosis of early, oligosymptomatic spondyloarthropathies, *Br J Rheumatol* 35:192, 1996.
9. Hebert LA, Cosio FG, Neff JC: Diagnostic significance of hypocomplementemia, *Kidney Int* 39:811-821, 1991.
10. Shmerling RH and others: Synovial fluid tests: what should be ordered? *JAMA* 264:1009-1014, 1990.
11. Savige J and others: International consensus statement on testing and reporting of antineutrophil cytoplasmic antibodies (ANCA), *Am J Clin Pathol* 111:507-513, 1999.
12. Love LA and others: A new approach to the classification of idiopathic inflammatory myopathy: myositis-specific autoantibodies define useful homogeneous patient groups, *Medicine* 70:360-374, 1991.

CHAPTER 237

Ankylosing Spondylitis and Related Disorders

Susan Hoch

Ankylosing Spondylitis

DEFINITION/EPIDEMIOLOGY

The seronegative spondyloarthropathies are a group of inflammatory arthritides that share many clinical, radiographic, and genetic features. The seronegative spondyloarthropathies include (1) ankylosing spondylitis, (2) reactive arthritis and Reiter's syndrome, (3) psoriatic arthritis, and (4) arthritis associated with inflammatory bowel disease (IBD). These illnesses are characterized by the presence of sacroiliitis, peripheral joint inflammation, and eye inflammation. Ankylosing spondylitis is the prototype of the seronegative spondyloarthropathies.

Ankylosing spondylitis has an estimated hospital prevalence of 0.1% to 0.2% in North America[1]; however, it is as prevalent as rheumatoid arthritis in outpatient clinic populations. Ankylosing spondylitis tends to be familial and follows the population frequency of HLA-B27. The male-female ratio, according to most studies, is between 2.5:1 and 5:1; however, some believe that the sex distribution is close to 1:1.[2] The disease usually begins in the third or fourth decade of life.

PATHOPHYSIOLOGY

A strong association with the genetically determined histocompatibility antigen HLA-B27 exists. Of note, however, is the fact that B27 by itself is neither necessary nor sufficient for development of these diseases.[3] The association with HLA-B27 is the highest in ankylosing spondylitis, where it is 95%, but only 2% to 10% of HLA-B27–positive individuals develop ankylosing spondylitis. The explanation for the link between HLA-B27 and the spondyloarthropathies remains unknown.

The pathognomonic features of ankylosing spondylitis are (1) inflammation of the bony insertions of ligaments and tendons (entheses), known as enthesitis or enthesopathy, and (2) new bone formation. The pathophysiology of this disease begins with ligamentous inflammatory granulation tissue that is gradually replaced by fibrocartilage and then ossifies.

CLINICAL PRESENTATION

Low back pain caused by sacroiliitis is the initial complaint of approximately 60% of patients. The back pain of sacroiliitis is inflammatory and can be distinguished clinically from back pain of other etiologies. It is usually insidious in onset; it is chronic, lasting for more than 3 months, with periods of exacerbation and remission. It is diffuse, poorly localized, and described as a deep ache or nagging discomfort in the lower back below the waist, in the buttocks, or in the hips. As in other types of inflammatory joint pain, the inflammatory back pain of ankylosing spondylitis worsens with bed rest and improves with exercise. Sleep disturbance is common, and patients may describe having to get up in the middle of the night to "walk off the pain." The back pain is worse in the morning and is associated with morning stiffness that is inflammatory in nature (i.e., lasts longer than 30 minutes). Patients can have intermittent sciatica occurring on alternating sides, which is pathognomonic for ankylosing spondylitis.

Spondylitis occurs in approximately 50% of patients with ankylosing spondylitis and begins in the lumbosacral spine. As the disease progresses, the upper portions of the spine are involved.

Patients may have peripheral joint involvement, and the diagnosis of ankylosing spondylitis can be made with only minimal sacroiliitis. Peripheral joint involvement is usually asymmetric, often involving large joints and is most commonly found in the lower limbs. More than 30% of patients develop chronic peripheral joint arthritis. Involvement of the hip joint can be an early manifestation in ankylosing spondylitis. Other inflammatory enthesopathic (at ligament and tendon insertions) areas of involvement peculiar to ankylosing spondylitis are the sternoclavicular joint, the costochondral joint, the Achilles tendon, and the plantar fascia. Small joints of the hands and feet are infrequently involved as opposed to rheumatoid arthritis.

Extraarticular manifestations of the disease include low-grade fever, fatigue, and weight loss. Inflammatory eye disease, usually uveitis, presents as a painful and often red eye and occurs in up to 30% of patients during the course of their disease. The inflammation is acute in onset 90% of the time, and in approximately 95% of patients the uveitis is unilateral or unilateral-alternating.[4] Cardiac involvement, most commonly aortic valve insufficiency, can be clinically silent or can dominate the clinical picture.

PHYSICAL EXAMINATION

Examination of the spine will show loss of normal lumbar lordosis. Palpable muscle spasm of the paraspinal muscles is common. Measurement of spine mobility is decreased in most patients and can be documented by (1) Schober's flexion test of the lumbosacral spine, (2) Moll's lateral flexion test of the thoracic spine, and/or (3) measurement of chest expansion.[5] Schober's flexion test measures lumbosacral flexion by having the patient stand erect and marking two points 15 cm apart in the midline—5 cm below and 10 cm above the level of the dimples of Venus. The patient is then asked to bend forward, reaching for the floor as far as possible. Normal flexion is defined as an increase in the distance between the two points of 5 cm or more in a patient under the age of 50. Moll's lateral flexion test measures lateral thoracic spine flexion by having the patient stand erect with the hands behind the head. One mark is placed in the midaxillary line at the iliac crest, and another mark is placed 20 cm above the iliac crest. The patient is asked to tilt, bending the trunk to the opposite side as far as possible, and the distance between the two marks is measured. Normal thoracic spine tilt or lateral flexion is 3 cm. Chest expansion is measured with the patient standing erect with the hands on the head. With a centimeter tape at the nipple line, the patient is asked to first maximally expire and then maximally inspire. The chest circumference should normally increase by at least 5 cm with full inspiration.

Extraarticular manifestations can produce physical findings such as the heart murmur of aortic valve insufficiency or the red, inflamed eye associated with acute iritis.

DIAGNOSTICS

Radiographic studies are the most helpful for documenting a clinical diagnosis.[6] The presence of sacroiliitis on x-ray examination definitely establishes the diagnosis of ankylosing spondylitis. Many patients will have negative findings on plain radiographs because their disease has not been sufficiently severe or long to produce radiographic changes. Magnetic resonance imaging may be able to identify sacroiliitis earlier than standard plain radiography.[7] Early sacroiliitis includes irregularity of the sacroiliac joints, with subchondral bone resorption giving a rosary-bead effect, and pseudowidening. More advanced sacroiliitis produces sclerosis, with the joint becoming indistinct and narrow over time. Complete bony fusion is seen late in the disease. Characteristic spine x-ray findings include syndesmophyte formation, which leads to bony bridging from one vertebral body to the next, producing a "bamboo" spine appearance. X-ray changes in the hip occur in up to 50% of patients and are often bilateral and symmetric with uniform joint space narrowing.

Laboratory findings can include a normochromic, normocytic anemia of chronic disease and an elevated erythrocyte sedimentation rate (ESR); however, anemia and an abnormal ESR are not necessary for the diagnosis. Rheumatoid factor and antinuclear antibodies are typically negative. HLA-B27 testing is inappropriate for screening an asymptomatic population. In the clinical setting, it should not be thought of as a routine diagnostic test, and in general because the test result does not absolutely confirm or exclude ankylosing spondylitis, it is not useful enough diagnostically to warrant its expense.[8]

DIFFERENTIAL DIAGNOSIS

For patients presenting with sacroiliitis and/or spinal disease, the principal diseases to be considered are Reiter's syndrome, psoriatic spondylitis, and spondylitis of IBD, all of which are discussed later in this chapter. In the absence of axial involvement, the most common chronic inflammatory arthritides that can be confused with ankylosing spondylitis in the 20- to 40-year age-group are (1) seronegative rheumatoid arthritis and (2) Lyme arthritis. Rheumatoid arthritis is more likely to involve the upper extremity (especially small) joints, characteristically has hand involvement, and is symmetric. Distinguishing rheumatoid arthritis from the seronegative spondyloarthropathies often requires prolonged observation of the patient. Lyme arthritis, which most commonly involves the knee, is suggested by a history of tick exposure and of erythema migrans and is established by enzyme-linked immunosorbent assay (ELISA) for *Borrelia burgdorferi* antibody, which can be confirmed by Western blot analysis.[9]

Anatomic causes of noninflammatory back pain, such as a herniated intervertebral disc, and noninflammatory arthritis of the spine, such as degenerative joint disease or disseminated idiopathic skeletal hyperostosis (DISH), produce a different pain, which is noninflammatory in nature, that is relieved by rest and aggravated by motion.

MANAGEMENT

Ankylosing spondylitis and the other seronegative spondyloarthropathies respond to first-line nonsteroidal antiinflammatory drugs (NSAIDs). The hip arthritis, sacroiliitis, and spondylitis of ankylosing spondylitis respond particularly well to the indole derivative class of NSAIDs, including indomethacin, tolmetin, and sulindac. High-dose aspirin (4 to 8 g/day) is usually not effective. Other nonsteroidal agents, particularly the ketoprofens such as ibuprofen and naproxen, are variably effective if used at high doses. The cyclooxygenase 2–specific inhibitor celecoxib appears to be equivalent to ketoprofen in short-term study and may have less gastrointestinal toxicity.[10] Second-line drugs for patients with severe or refractory ankylosing spondylitis include sulfasalazine and methotrexate; however, efficacy is predominantly in those cases with peripheral joint involvement.[11,12] New studies have provided preliminary data on the efficacy of biologic anti–tumor necrosis factor (TNF) agents, etanercept and infliximab, in spondyloarthropathies.[13]

Pain management is important to minimize spinal deformity and allow patients to exercise. Patients stoop with pain, thereby increasing the likelihood of the spine fusing in a kyphotic position.

Analgesics such as acetaminophen, muscle relaxants, and low-dose corticosteroids (5 to 7.5 mg/day) can be beneficial adjunct therapy. Patients often find the use of heat and massage helpful. Using small doses of narcotic pain relievers intermittently for short periods of time may be appropriate in selected situations. Local injections of corticosteroids can treat pain from enthesopathy. Sacroiliac joint pain may benefit from corticosteroid injection under fluoroscopic or computed tomographic guidance.

Diagnostics

Ankylosing Spondylitis and Related Disorders

Laboratory	Imaging
CBC and differential	X-ray of spine, including sacroiliac joints
ESR	X-ray of small joints of hands and feet
HLA-B27*	
Antinuclear antibody*	**Other**
C-reactive protein*	Joint fluid analysis
Uric acid*	
Elisa assay for *Borrelia burgdorferi* (Lyme)*	
Rheumatoid factor*	

*If indicated.

Differential Diagnosis

Ankylosing Spondylitis and Related Disorders

Rheumatoid arthritis	Reiter's disease
Degenerative joint disease	Psoriatic arthritis
Mechanical back pain	Spondylitis of inflammatory bowel disease
Disseminated idiopathic skeletal hyperostosis	Lyme arthritis

LIFE SPAN CONSIDERATIONS

The prognosis with ankylosing spondylitis is variable. Death from the disease itself is very unusual. Some patients have minimal aggravating symptoms that are limited to the low back and pelvis. Less commonly, patients may have progressive widespread disease with skeletal deformity and functional loss, requiring chronic medication and physical therapy. Often patients are unable to work or perform normal household tasks. Chronic medical therapy can shorten the patient's life span as a result of medication side effects. Some studies have suggested an increase in expected mortality rates over control populations, especially in individuals with higher ESRs and more inflamed peripheral joints.

Pregnancy in patients with ankylosing spondylitis does not improve symptoms, unlike what is observed in rheumatoid arthritis. The majority of women with ankylosing spondylitis have unchanged or temporarily aggravated disease activity during pregnancy. There is no effect of the disease on fertility, course of pregnancy, or delivery. However, the offspring of patients with ankylosing spondylitis are at increased risk of developing this disease.

COMPLICATIONS

Visual loss secondary to inflammatory eye disease is a major cause of disability in this disease. A variety of neurologic complications of ankylosing spondylitis can be seen in long-standing disease. These include cord compression secondary to spinal fracture or a fused spine, atlantoaxial subluxation resulting from chronic cervical involvement, cauda equina syndrome with slowly progressive sensory loss in the lumbosacral dermatomes with less frequent weakness, pain, and sphincter disturbance and tarsal tunnel syndrome caused by ankle arthritis. Cardiovascular involvement, although rare, can include ascending aortitis, aortic valve insufficiency, and conduction abnormalities. Pulmonary involvement can be seen in ankylosing spondylitis with upper lobe fibrocystic changes and chest wall restriction with restrictive lung disease. Ankylosing spondylitis is associated with bone loss and osteoporosis, particularly in the lumbar spine, placing these patients at risk for spinal fracture. Amyloid deposition is a rare complication after years of inflammatory disease and can produce nephrotic syndrome or renal failure.

INDICATIONS FOR REFERRAL/HOSPITALIZATION

Referral to a physical therapist is appropriate to promote pain relief, minimize deformity, and maintain independent function.[14] Referral to an orthopedic surgeon is indicated in the 20% to 30% of patients who develop hip arthritis that is severe enough to produce night pain, rest pain, and pain on weight bearing, impairing the ability to walk.[15] Immediate referral to an ophthalmologist is warranted for acute eye pain. Periodic ophthalmic monitoring is recommended when iritis has been a manifestation. Evaluation by a cardiologist is indicated with the presence of an aortic valve murmur. Hospitalization is rarely indicated in patients with ankylosing spondylitis. Acute catastrophic neurologic complications, congestive heart failure secondary to progressive aortic valve insufficiency, and significant gastrointestinal bleeding resulting from NSAIDs are the most likely reasons for hospitalization.

PATIENT AND FAMILY EDUCATION

Optimal management is enhanced when patients understand the chronic nature of the disease and their role in preventing disability and deformity. Patients need to learn to rest when tired and to discontinue any activity that causes joint pain to avoid disease flares. Extension exercises and regular physical activity are beneficial. Walking (shallow water) or running (deep water) in a pool are excellent exercises for increasing and maintaining trunk and neck muscle strength. Swimming is recommended because it avoids excessive stressful weight bearing. The backstroke is particularly good for stretching anterior chest muscles and strengthening posterior chest and neck extensor muscles, thereby decreasing the tendency toward kyphosis. Ongoing attention to daytime and nighttime posture minimizes deformity, and sleeping without a pillow under the head or knees is important to avoid flexion deformity.

Reactive Arthritis and Reiter's Syndrome

DEFINITION/EPIDEMIOLOGY

Reactive arthritis refers to an acute sterile inflammatory arthropathy after an infection where there is no microbial invasion of the synovium or joint space and where the prior infection is remote from the joint. Reiter's syndrome, as first described by Hans Reiter in 1916, is an example of a reactive arthritis defined by the classic triad of conjunctivitis, urethritis, and arthritis. Because as many as two thirds of patients present with an incomplete syndrome and do not fulfill all three criteria, reactive arthritis is a preferred and more general term. Reactive arthritis has been observed after both venereal and dysenteric infection and can be initiated by a number of infectious organisms. The most common infectious agents associated with reactive arthritis and Reiter's syndrome are *Salmonella, Shigella, Yersinia, Campylobacter* and *Chlamydia.*

The exact prevalence of reactive arthritis and Reiter's syndrome in the general population has not been determined but is not rare. In one study, of 260 individuals infected with *Salmonella typhimurium* during an outbreak of gastroenteritis, 19 patients (7%) developed reactive arthritis.[16] The common infection *Chlamydia trachomatis* can lead to the venereal form of Reiter's syndrome. The peak incidence of reactive arthritis and Reiter's syndrome is during the third decade of life. Postvenereal Reiter's syndrome affects men more commonly, with male/female ratios ranging from 9:1 to 5:1. The dysenteric form of Reiter's syndrome and reactive arthropathy affects males and females equally.

PATHOPHYSIOLOGY

Like ankylosing spondylitis, Reiter's syndrome has a strong association with the histocompatibility antigen HLA-B27. HLA-B27 is observed in 60% to 80% of patients with Reiter's syndrome and appears to be associated with increased disease susceptibility and severity of disease expression. As in rheumatoid arthritis, there is inflammatory synovitis with infiltration of polymorphonuclear leukocytes, lymphocytes, and plasma cells. However, unlike rheumatoid arthritis, the production of synovial pannus is rare. As in ankylosing spondylitis, there is inflammation at the insertions of ligaments and tendons (enthesopathy). Erosions, bony proliferation, and periosteal new bone formation may occur.

The relationship between the antecedent infection and the development of reactive arthritis or Reiter's syndrome is not completely understood. The HLA-B27 molecule participates in binding antigenic peptides and presenting them to $CD8^+$ T cells. That the disease does occur in patients with AIDS, who presumably lack a full complement of functional $CD4^+$ T cells, suggests a role for $CD8^+$ cells in reactive arthritis. It is of interest that most of the infectious agents associated with reactive arthritis survive and multiply within cells. Antigenic bacterial peptides derived from these intracellular organisms may then trigger reactive arthritis. The exact mechanism by which this happens is not known; one possible hypothesis is that sharing of amino acid sequence between bacterially derived peptides and self-antigens may induce autoreactivity.

CLINICAL PRESENTATION AND PHYSICAL EXAMINATION

Reactive arthritis or Reiter's syndrome can occur without documented prior infection. When there has been an antecedent infection, arthritic symptoms tend to occur 10 to 20 days later. Less than 40% of patients present with the classic triad. The eye and genitourinary tract features of the triad may take as long as 5 years to manifest. Urethritis in men may be transient and the genitourinary symptoms (cervicitis, cystitis, or mild urethritis) in women are often missed, occult, or not reported.[17] The eye inflammation presents classically as conjunctivitis, but blepharitis, keratitis, iritis, or uveitis can also be seen. The arthropathy of Reiter's syndrome is distinctive and characterized by lower extremity, asymmetric joint involvement, "sausage digits," heel pain, Achilles tendonitis, plantar fasciitis, and sacroiliitis.[18] Hip involvement is common. Approximately 50% of patients will develop sacroiliitis, and some will progress to spondylitis. Like patients with ankylosing spondylitis, they have inflammatory back pain. A classic enthesopathic (inflammation of ligament and tendon insertions) feature is dactylitis, which produces a sausage digit as a result of inflammation of the bony insertions of ligaments and tendons throughout the entire length of a digit. These sausage digits are characteristic of Reiter's syndrome and psoriatic arthritis. Enthesopathic involvement of the anterolateral ribs, pubic symphysis, and iliac crest may present with pain and/or swelling in these areas. Dermatologic manifestations include painless shallow lingual or palatal ulcerations, keratoderma blennorrhagica, and circinate balanitis. These tend to correlate with the severity of disease. Keratoderma blennorrhagica is the most common dermatologic manifestation of Reiter's syndrome, presenting as painless papulosquamous lesions on the palms or soles. The histopathology of keratoderma blennorrhagica is indistinguishable from that of pustular psoriasis. Circinate balanitis occurs in males and presents as painless, shallow ulcerative lesions on the glans of the penis that may go unnoticed.

The course of the disease is highly variable, with the initial episode often lasting 2 to 3 months. In some patients, there are recurrent acute attacks, often with disease-free intervals. About one third of patients will have sustained disease activity with a chronic course.[19] Less than 20% of patients develop chronic destructive and potentially debilitating disease.

DIAGNOSTICS

For the most part, laboratory test results are nonspecific, consistent with an inflammatory process and similar to those in ankylosing spondylitis. The ESR and C-reactive protein are elevated. There often is peripheral leukocytosis with thrombocytosis and often a mild anemia. There usually is a synovial fluid leukocytosis, often with a polymorphonuclear leukocyte predominance that is suggestive of a septic arthritis. The x-ray studies of sausage digits, Achilles tendinitis, and plantar fasciitis reveal a fluffy periosteal reaction of new bone formation. Periarticular demineralization or osteopenia is notably absent in Reiter's syndrome compared with in rheumatoid arthritis. The syndesmophytes in the vertebral spine are not as fine as in ankylosing spondylitis, are nonmarginal and denser, and may be asymmetric and skip portions of the spine.

DIFFERENTIAL DIAGNOSIS

Distinguishing between psoriatic arthritis and Reiter's syndrome can be difficult because the arthritis is similar and the skin histology is identical. Only the finding of nail pitting, characteristic of psoriatic arthritis, differentiates the two. More important, Reiter's syndrome or reactive arthritis may be misdiagnosed as seronegative rheumatoid arthritis. Reiter's syndrome can have symmetric peripheral joint involvement, but sacroiliitis is uncommon in rheumatoid arthritis. In rheumatoid arthritis, hip disease is a late sequela, and sausage digits, Achilles tendonitis, plantar fasciitis, and other presentations of enthesopathy do not occur. Dactylitis is not a feature of rheumatoid arthritis. Lyme disease presents with chronic knee arthritis and can be differentiated from Reiter's syndrome by a positive *B. burgdorferi* antibody assay.

MANAGEMENT

Reiter's syndrome responds to the same drugs as ankylosing spondylitis.[11] Sulfasalazine 2 g/day is more effective than placebo and well tolerated in patients with chronically active reactive arthritis not responsive to nonsteroidal antiinflammatory drug (NSAID) therapy.[20] Methotrexate 15 to 25 mg every week has been used with some success.[21] Patients with chlamydial infection and reactive arthritis may respond to long-term (3-month) tetracycline therapy with decreased duration of illness.[22] Reactive arthritis associated with HIV infection has been reported to improve following antiretroviral treatment with a rise in $CD4^+$ T cell count.[23]

COMPLICATIONS

The course of Reiter's syndrome is highly variable. Some patients can develop chronic, disabling arthritis and be forced to consider alternative employment options.[19]

INDICATIONS FOR REFERRAL/HOSPITALIZATION

Most patients with Reiter's syndrome can be managed by the primary care provider with initial diagnostic studies and management suggestions from a rheumatologist. In cases where the skin disease is prominent or painful, referral to a dermatologist may be helpful. A physical therapist and/or occupational therapist should be consulted for suggestions regarding exercise regimens and/or teaching regarding joint protection and energy conservation. As noted, patients with chronic, disabling arthritis may benefit from vocational counseling.

PATIENT AND FAMILY EDUCATION

Patient education should be directed toward managing the disease chronically and providing thorough familiarity with drugs and side effects. Patients receiving NSAIDs are advised to take these medications with food and should be warned of the risk of gastrointestinal bleeding associated with these medications. In cases in which gastrointestinal symptoms occur, consideration should be given to ulcer prevention with H_2 blockers and antacids. Patients who receive second-line agents such as sulfasalazine or methotrexate should be managed according to guidelines for patients with rheumatoid arthritis on these medications with regular laboratory screening.

Psoriatic Arthritis

DEFINITION/EPIDEMIOLOGY

Psoriatic arthritis is an inflammatory arthritis associated with the dermatologic condition of psoriasis. Approximately 6% of patients with mild to moderate psoriasis will develop inflammatory arthritis. Patients with severe psoriasis have a 30% to 40% incidence of joint disease, with men and women being affected equally.[24] The most common age at onset is 30 to 40 years. More extensive spinal involvement occurs in men who are positive for HLA-B27.

PATHOPHYSIOLOGY

Immune, genetic, and environmental factors influence disease expression. Some patients have elevated serum IgA and IgG levels, the presence of IgG rheumatoid factor, and even elevated immune complexes. Peripheral joint disease has been linked to HLA-B38, and axial disease to HLA-B27. Patients have been known to have flares after trauma to a joint or infection with group A streptococci. Immune mechanisms are suggested by a possible molecular similarity between streptococcal and epidermal components, which could allow T cell clones directed against streptococci to initiate the skin disease.

CLINICAL PRESENTATION AND PHYSICAL EXAMINATION

Psoriatic arthritis may occur before the onset, with, or after the onset of the skin disease.[25] Arthritis precedes the rash in 15% to 20% of patients. In these patients, nail pitting is often present before rash as an early clue to the diagnosis. The arthritis is heterogeneous, with five different clinical presentations being recognized: oligoarticular asymmetric (48%), spondyloarthropathy (24%), polyarticular symmetric (18%), distal phalangeal (8%), and arthritis mutilans (2%). Only the distal interphalangeal (DIP) joint type and arthritis mutilans type are clinically unique to psoriatic arthritis, which sets them apart from other inflammatory arthritides. Typically, patients, over time, present with overlapping forms of the disease, and most patients will eventually develop DIP involvement. As in Reiter's syndrome, sausage digits occur. Arthritis mutilans is a destructive form of arthritis in which there is significant bone erosion with decreased bone length, producing redundant skin and "opera glass" deformity. The spondylitis, when seen, is similar to that of Reiter's syndrome and can occur without sacroiliitis, be asymmetric, and skip portions of the spine.[6] Sacroiliitis in psoriatic arthritis is often asymmetric, as opposed to ankylosing spondylitis, where bilateral sacroiliac involvement is more common. Systemic involvement is limited to eye inflammation, which occurs in approximately 30% of patients. HIV infection in patients with psoriatic arthritis causes increased proliferation of the skin disease and is associated with rapidly progressive polyarticular joint involvement.

DIAGNOSTICS

Laboratory tests are mostly nonspecific, as they are in the other seronegative spondyloarthropathy. Tests for rheumatoid factor and antinuclear antibodies are negative. The ESR and C-reactive protein levels may be elevated. Hyperuricemia may result from the high-purine turnover in psoriatic skin lesions. Psoriatic synovial histology is similar to rheumatoid synovial histology, with lymphocyte and plasma cell infiltration and microvascular changes.

The radiographic changes in hands and feet are distinctive.[6] Subchondral erosions and erosions with new bone formation, called *proliferative erosions,* are seen. In late disease, radiographs of the DIP joints may show whittling and a "pencil-in-cup" appearance, which is believed to be pathognomonic of psoriatic arthritis. Osteoporosis is notably absent, and periosteal reaction can be seen along the bone shafts of sausage digits.

DIFFERENTIAL DIAGNOSIS

It is difficult to distinguish between Reiter's syndrome and psoriatic arthritis. The skin lesions of the two diseases are histologically similar. Both can present with eye disease. Nail pitting suggests psoriatic arthritis, whereas nail onycholysis can be seen in both diseases.

Polyarticular symmetric disease can present like seronegative rheumatoid arthritis, and it may be impossible to differentiate between the two. The monarticular arthritis of Lyme disease involving the knee can be differentiated from oligoarticular asymmetric psoriatic arthritis by *B. burgdorferi* antibody assay.[8] Degenerative joint disease of the DIP joints looks similar to that of psoriatic DIP joints, but psoriatic arthritis will involve morning stiffness for longer than 30 minutes, whereas degenerative joint disease will not.

MANAGEMENT

NSAIDs may be helpful in controlling the arthritis; however, many patients have continued active disease despite the use of NSAIDs and require second-line therapy. Sulfasalazine 2 to 3 g/day may provide control of joint symptoms.[26] Methotrexate 15 to 25 mg PO once a week is the drug of choice in patients with erosive joint disease and aggressive skin disease.[27] Azathioprine, gold, hydroxychloroquine (Plaquenil), retinoids, and cyclosporine have been shown to be beneficial for patients who are unresponsive to methotrexate. Anti-TNF agents, etanercept and infliximab, may offer new therapeutic options for control of psoriatic arthritis.[13,28] Oral steroids are not recommended for the treatment of psoriatic arthritis because of the flare of skin disease that may occur with withdrawal of steroid medication.

Patients with a history of alcohol ingestion who are receiving methotrexate need to be followed with percutaneous liver biopsies because the incidence of methotrexate-induced cirrhosis in patients with psoriasis who consume alcohol is significant. Patients treated with methotrexate should not drink alcohol. Patients with severe, erosive joint disease may become permanently disabled, requiring work disability and/or assistance with activities of daily living.

Suppression of the psoriatic skin disease is essential for the comfort and appearance of the patient. It may also be important in the management of the associated arthritis because flares in the skin disease may correlate with flares in the joint disease.

COMPLICATIONS

Acute iritis can lead to loss of vision. Cirrhosis of the liver can occur in patients treated with methotrexate who consume alcohol. Infection has been reported in psoriatic patients undergoing intraarticular injection, aspiration, or surgery; therefore careful preparation of the skin before surgery or arthrocentesis is necessary.

INDICATIONS FOR REFERRAL/HOSPITALIZATION

Most patients with psoriatic arthritis can be managed by the primary care provider. In cases where the joint and/or skin disease is disabling, referral to a rheumatologist and/or dermatologist for consultation may be helpful. As in other cases of inflammatory arthritis, referral to a physical therapist and/or occupational therapist for joint-protective exercise regimens, as well as teaching in joint protection and energy conservation, is very helpful. Patients disabled by joint disease may need vocational counseling.

PATIENT AND FAMILY EDUCATION

Patients should be counseled about the chronic nature of this disease. Medication regimens can be complicated and will need to be reviewed periodically. Patients taking methotrexate should understand that permanent sterility is possible and should be urged to use reliable birth control because of the possibility of birth defects. These patients should not drink alcohol. Appropriate forms of exercise may include range-of-motion and stretching exercises, as well as swimming.

Arthritis of Inflammatory Bowel Disease

DEFINITION/EPIDEMIOLOGY

The arthritis of IBD is an inflammatory arthritis associated with ulcerative colitis and Crohn's disease. Peripheral arthritis occurs in 15% to 20% of patients with IBD. Spondylitis and sacroiliitis are less common and are associated with HLA-B27 approximately 50% of the time. Approximately 16% of patients with Crohn's disease or regional enteritis will have radiographic evidence of sacroiliitis.[29] Sex distribution of ankylosing spondylitis in Crohn's disease is equal. Sacroiliac joint involvement is strongly associated with acute uveitis and occurs in 17% of patients with ulcerative colitis. In ulcerative colitis, the presence of ankylosing spondylitis has an equal sex distribution.

PATHOPHYSIOLOGY

Arthritis is one of several extraintestinal manifestations associated with ulcerative colitis and Crohn's disease. The mechanism of this association is not clearly understood; the arthritic manifestations of the disorder may be an immunologic phenomenon.

CLINICAL PRESENTATION AND PHYSICAL EXAMINATION

Two forms of arthritis occur in IBD: peripheral joint disease (a systemic manifestation of the IBD varying with bowel disease activity) and ankylosing spondylitis, which is unrelated to IBD activity. The peripheral arthritis is acute or subacute and is more common in the lower extremities than in the upper extremities. It tends to be associated with active IBD and flares when the bowel disease flares.[30]

The spondylitis seen in association with IBD is insidious and chronic and does not correlate with bowel disease activity. The joint involvement is identical to that of ankylosing spondylitis. Patients may develop inflammatory eye disease, usually uveitis, which presents as an acute, red, painful eye. This presentation is more commonly unilateral but can be bilateral.

The clinical presentation may include complaints of joint pain, back pain, or morning stiffness. Mild abdominal pain with reports of bloody or mucous stools may antedate or occur with the joint disease, indicating a direct causative relationship between the two, but joint disease can present as the first symptom.

DIAGNOSTICS

Indicators of inflammation, including ESR and C-reactive proteins, are often elevated. A mild hypochromic anemia is common. Joint fluid findings are consistent with inflammatory arthritis showing cell counts of 1500 to 50,000 cells/mm^3.

DIFFERENTIAL DIAGNOSIS

Inflammatory arthritis is seen in conjunction with gastrointestinal manifestations in a number of diseases, including vasculitis with abdominal involvement, systemic sclerosis complicated by motility dysfunction, amyloidosis, Behçet's disease, and familial Mediterranean fever.[30] This involvement is differentiated from the arthritis of IBD by the fact that the abdominal disease occurs as a complication of the disease and is not related to the cause of the arthritis.

MANAGEMENT

Sulfasalazine 2 to 3 g/day, which often controls the bowel disease, is also helpful in controlling the joint disease. Corticosteroids usually control both bowel and joint disease but are not indicated for long-term use because of drug toxicity. Azathioprine has been beneficial in patients whose disease is not controlled with sulfasalazine. NSAIDs, when tolerated, are useful for the control of joint pain. Infliximab appears to be effective and well tolerated in patients with Crohn's disease and may be steroid sparing.[31] There is no information available yet about whether the associated arthritis may respond as well.

COMPLICATIONS

Complications primarily arise with uncontrolled bowel disease. Abdominal pain and bloody diarrhea with weight loss can be severely disabling and may require hospitalization. Corticosteroid-treated patients with IBD are at risk for steroid-induced osteoporosis and should be administered appropriate calcium and vitamin D supplementation, as well as prophylactic treatment with a bisphosphonate to prevent steroid-driven bone loss.

INDICATIONS FOR REFERRAL/HOSPITALIZATION

Referral to a rheumatologist and/or a gastroenterologist may be indicated for confirmation of the diagnosis and/or treatment suggestions. Referral to a physical therapist and/or occupational therapist can be beneficial for patients dealing with severe joint disease. Dietary modifications may be helpful in controlling bowel disease, and referral to a dietitian may be useful.

PATIENT AND FAMILY EDUCATION

Patients need to understand the chronicity of this disease and the relationship between their bowel disease and their arthritis. Unlike psoriatic arthritis, there does not seem to be a correlation between the activity of the bowel and joint disease. Total colectomy may provide a cure for patients with ulcerative colitis and effect remission in the associated arthritis. This is not necessarily true for patients with Crohn's disease because the bowel inflammation can affect the remaining gastrointestinal tract even if the colon is removed. Patients need to understand their medication regimens and potential toxicities. Patients taking prednisone should be cautioned not to discontinue this medication abruptly. Dietary modifications may be crucial, and patients are often advised to adhere to a low-residue diet.

REFERENCES

1. Gran JT, Husby G: The epidemiology of ankylosing spondylitis, *Semin Arthritis Rheum* 22:319-334, 1993.
2. Calin A: The individual with ankylosing spondylitis: defining disease status and the impact of the illness, *Br J Rheumatol* 34:663-672, 1995.
3. Schumacher TM and others: HLA-B27 associated arthropathies, *Radiology* 126:289-297, 1978.
4. Tay-Kearney M and others: Clinical features and associated diseases of HLA-B27 uveitis, *Am J Ophthalmol* 121:47-56, 1996.
5. Merritt JL and others: Measurement of trunk flexibility in normal subjects: reproducibility of three clinical methods, *Mayo Clin Proc* 61: 192-197, 1986.
6. El-Khoury GY, Kathol MH, Brandser EA: Seronegative spondyloarthropathies, *Radiol Clin North Am* 34:343-357, 1996.
7. Oostveen J and others: Early detection of sacroiliitis on magnetic resonance imaging and subsequent development of sacroiliitis on plain radiography. A prospective longitudinal study, *J Rheum* 26:1953-1958, 1999.
8. Khan MA, Khan MK: Diagnostic value of HLA-B27 testing ankylosing spondylitis and Reiter's syndrome, *Ann Intern Med* 96:70-76, 1982.
9. Centers for Disease Control and Prevention: Recommendations for test performance and interpretation from the Second National Conference on Serologic Diagnosis of Lyme Disease, *MMWR* 44:590-591, 1995.
10. Dougados M and others: Efficacy of celecoxib, a cyclooxygenase 2-specific inhibitor, in the treatment of ankylosing spondylitis: a six week controlled study with comparison against placebo and against a conventional nonsteroidal anti-inflammatory drug, *Arthritis Rheum* 44:180-185, 2001.
11. Creemers MC and others: Second-line treatment in seronegative spondyloarthropathie, *Semin Arthritis Rheum* 24:71-81, 1994.
12. Toussirot E, Wendling D: Therapeutic advances in ankylosing spondylitis, *Expert Opin Invest Drugs* 10:21-29, 2001.
13. Braun J and others: New treatment options in spondyloarthropathies: increasing evidence for significant efficacy of anti-tumor necrosis factor therapy, *Curr Opin Rheum* 13:245-249, 2001.
14. Oh TH and others: Rehabilitation in the joint and connective tissue diseases. II. Inflammatory and degenerative spine diseases, *Arch Phys Med Rehabil* 76:S41-S46, 1995.
15. Sorokin R: Management of the patient with rheumatic disease going to surgery, *Med Clin North Am* 77:453-464, 1993.
16. Inman RD and others: Postdysenteric reactive arthritis. A clinical and immunogenetic study following an outbreak of salmonellosis, *Arthritis Rheum* 31:1377-1383, 1988.
17. Smith DL, Bennett RM, Regan MG: Reiter's disease in women, *Arthritis Rheum* 23:335-340, 1980.
18. Arnett FC, McLusky E, Schacter BZ: Incomplete Reiter's syndrome: discriminating features and HLA-W27 in diagnosis, *Ann Intern Med* 84: 8-12, 1975.
19. Fox R and others: The chronicity of symptoms and disability in Reiter's syndrome. An analysis of 131 consecutive patients, *Ann Intern Med* 91:190-193, 1979.
20. Clegg DO and others: Comparison of sulfasalazine and placebo in the treatment of reactive arthritis (Reiter's syndrome): a Department of Veterans Affairs Cooperative Study, *Arthritis Rheum* 39:2021-2027, 1996.
21. Lally EV, Ho G Jr: A review of methotrexate therapy in Reiter syndrome, *Semin Arthritis Rheum* 15:139-145, 1985.
22. Lauhio A and others: Double-blind, placebo-controlled study of three-month treatment with lymecycline in reactive arthritis, with special reference to Chlamydia arthritis, *Arthritis Rheum* 34:6-14, 1991.
23. McGonagle D and others: Human immunodeficiency virus associated spondyloarthropathy: pathogenic insights based on imaging findings and response to highly active antiretroviral treatment, *Ann Rheum Dis* 60:696-698, 2001.
24. Ruzicka T: Psoriatic arthritis: new types, new treatments, *Arch Dermatol* 132:215-219, 1996.
25. Smiley JD: Psoriatic arthritis, *Bull Rheum Dis* 44:1-2, 1996.
26. Clegg DO and others: Comparison of sulfasalazine and placebo in the treatment of psoriatic arthritis. A Department of Veterans Affairs Cooperative Study, *Arthritis Rheum* 39:2012-2020, 1996.
27. Cuellar ML, Espinoze LR: Methotrexate use in psoriasis and psoriatic arthritis, *Rheum Dis North Am* 23:797-809, 1997.
28. Mease PJ and others: Etanercept in the treatment of psoriatic arthritis and psoriasis: a randomized trial, *Lancet* 356:385-390, 2000.
29. Mueller CE, Seeger JF, Martel W: Ankylosing spondylitis and regional enteritis, *Radiology* 112:579-582, 1974.
30. Mielants H, Veys EM: Enteropathic arthritis. In Schumacher HR, editor: *Primer on the rheumatic diseases*, ed 10, Atlanta, 1993, Arthritis Foundation.
31. Cohen RD: Efficacy and safety of repeated infliximab infusions for Crohn's disease: 1-year clinical experience, *Inflam Bowel Dis* 7 (suppl 1): S17-S22, 2001.

CHAPTER 238

Lyme Disease

Martin Jan Bergman

DEFINITION/EPIDEMIOLOGY

Lyme disease is an infectious disease caused by the spirochete *Borrelia burgdorferi,* which is transmitted to humans by the bite of the deer tick *Ixodes dammini.* It is often accompanied by a classic rash and may involve the central nervous system (CNS), cardiac system, and musculoskeletal system. When diagnosed in a timely fashion, it is curable with conventional antibiotics, but both underdiagnosis and overdiagnosis have been a problem.

Since its first description in 1977, Lyme disease has captured the attention of the medical community and the public.[1] The investigative process involved in recognizing the disease and determining the vector and the causative agent represent a classic study in epidemiologic research. In the fall of 1975, two mothers, concerned about an unusual cluster of juvenile rheumatoid arthritis (JRA) in their communities and not satisfied with the explanations given to them by their primary care providers, notified the Connecticut Health Department and the Rheumatology Clinic at Yale University. An initial survey done by Steere, Malawista, and others revealed a cluster of 51 cases of JRA in three communities along the eastern shore of the Connecticut River. Peculiar to these cases, in addition to the "clustering" of a relatively uncommon entity, was the involvement of 12 adults with the disease, the marked seasonality of the initial presentation, and the association of the illness with an unusual rash, similar to erythema chronicum migrans. This rash was first described by a Swedish physician, Afzelius, in 1910 and was known to be associated with the bite of the sheep tick *Ixodes ricinus.* A few years later, a new member of the genius *Ixodes, I. dammini* (also called *I. scapularis),* was identified in the region where the new entity, Lyme disease (named for one of the towns, Lyme, Connecticut), was prevalent. This was followed by Burgdorfer's isolation of a spirochete, later characterized as a member of the genus *Borrelia,* from the gut of *I. dammini* and now recognized as the causative agent, *B. burgdorferi.*[2]

Much has been learned about the disease, including other manifestations, diagnostic modalities and treatments, the life cycle of the vector, and the life cycle of the organism. With this knowledge has also come much misinformation, hysteria, and exploitative behavior by the general public and less scrupulous health professionals.

Although it was best described in the late 1970s, it is obvious from studies that this disease has been around for many years. The spirochete has been isolated from the gut of a 50-year-old museum specimen, and the Europeans have known of a similar disease, Bannworth's syndrome, since the early part of the twentieth century.[3] Cases have been increasing at nearly an exponential rate since Steere's first description. The Centers for Disease Control and Prevention (CDC) report (1999 surveillance data) shows 16,273 cases being reported in 1999 in all of the United States except Montana. The majority of the cases have been found in the Northeast, Mid-Atlantic, Great Lakes, and West Coast regions, and of these a disproportionate number have been reported in New York, Connecticut, Pennsylvania, and New Jersey.[4] There is no racial or sexual predominance in this disease, but there does seem to be an association with the incidence of the disease and the encroachment of the woodlands by community development.

To understand the disease and its epidemiology, it is necessary to understand the life cycle of its primary vector, *I. dammini.*[2] New eggs hatch in the early spring, and the as-yet–uninfected larvae seek their first blood meal. The host of choice is the white-footed mouse, which is also the reservoir for the *B. burgdorferi* organism. After this meal, the now-infected ticks molt over the winter and emerge the next spring in the nymph stage. These ticks, who prefer to live in tall grasses or woods, are aggressive feeders, seeking their next blood meal from any warm-blooded, carbon dioxide–exhaling creature, including humans. It is this stage that is responsible for the vast majority of infections. After this blood meal, the tick again molts, to the adult stage, and may again seek a blood meal in the early fall and then mate, generally on the white-tailed deer, starting the cycle again. There does not appear to be any transovarial transmission of the disease; thus the newborn tick will again emerge, infection free.

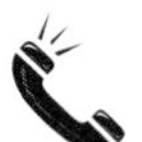

Physician consultation is recommended for patients with a positive Lyme titer or suspected Lyme disease.

PATHOPHYSIOLOGY

Because Lyme disease is a classic arthropod-borne infection, the risk of infection in hosts, such as humans, will depend on a number of factors. The infection rates of the tick vary from location to location, so that tick infection density will play a role. High-prevalence areas may have infection rates of 20% to 30% of nymphs to 50% to 65% of adult ticks, but, obviously, the host must come into contact with the tick to be bitten. The tick must then be embedded and feed long enough to transmit the disease. This is generally thought to require at least 24 hours and probably takes closer to 48 hours. This, then, affords some time for simple preventive measures, such as avoidance of grassy areas, long clothing, and tick removal, to be applied. Even when imbedded and feeding, for reasons not entirely clear and probably relating to host defenses and differences in infecting organisms, only 1% to 3% of reported tick bites ultimately cause Lyme disease.[4]

CLINICAL PRESENTATION AND PHYSICAL EXAMINATION

Once infected by *B. burgdorferi,* a patient may present in any number of ways. This is described as three, potentially overlapping stages: localized disease, early disseminated disease, and chronic disease. Any individual may present with symptoms in any of these levels of disease; they may first be seen with signs and symptoms of disseminated or late disease or may progress in a stepwise fashion from localized to early disseminated to chronic disease.

Localized Disease

Usually within 1 week to 1 month of the tick bite, the classic rash of erythema migrans (EM) will appear.[2,5] This generally occurs in the late spring and early summer and is reported in 60% to 80% of patients with Lyme disease. Usually appearing at the site of the initial bite, or the groin, axilla, or scalp, the rash is classically described as a large circular rash, at least 5 cm in diameter with central clearing (bull's eye), that expands rapidly, at a rate of about 20 cm^2/day and lasts approximately 1 to 2 weeks (Color Plates 40 and 41). This means that if there is a question as to the proper diagnosis, the rash can be measured and outlined with a marker. The patient can return to the office or clinic the next day, and at that time the rash can be remeasured and should have enlarged noticeably. This also helps to distinguish the rash from a tick bite reaction, which is an indurated erythematous lesion generally less than 3 cm in diameter (about the size of a quarter) that does not expand.[5] Most patients with EM will have some associated constitutional signs; these may include fatigue, myalgias, arthralgias, headache, conjunctivitis, lymphadenopathy, fevers, and a stiff neck. These are the symptoms that are generally described by the media as a flulike illness. Absent, however, are the sore throat, rhinorrhea, and cough that are often seen with common seasonal viral illnesses. These constitutional symptoms suggest dissemination and tend to blur the distinction between localized and disseminated disease.[5]

Not all rashes present in the classic fashion. The rash may be irregular in shape, and the central clearing does not have to be present. Central necrosis or vesicles may be noted. The rash is usually asymptomatic, but there may be warmth, tenderness, and occasional pruritus. Often these rashes are believed to be spider bites. In the northeast United States, the brown recluse spider, which is known for its bite, is essentially absent, yet the diagnosis of a brown recluse bite is often made in patients subsequently shown to have Lyme disease.[5]

Early Disseminated Disease

Early in the course, multiple skin lesions may appear, suggesting dissemination. These lesions are generally smaller than the original lesion and are not at the site of the original bite. In addition, they are more evanescent than the primary lesion and are less likely to have prominent local symptoms.

As the disease disseminates, more constitutional symptoms may be seen and more evidence of other organ system involvement may become present. These symptoms may occur anywhere from 1 week to 7 months from the original bite; typically they occur 1 to 2 months later. Nervous system dissemination occurs early in the course of the disease.[6] This may present in a peripheral form such as Bell's palsy, as any cranial neuropathy, or as a peripheral sensorimotor radiculoneuritis. Even cases of neurogenic bladders have been described. There may be subtle signs of an encephalitis manifested by changes in mood or emotional lability, or the disease may present as a frank meningitis. The severity of the headache and neck stiffness, however, is less than that of bacterial meningitis. At this time, dissemination to the heart may also occur, with the conduction system being the most commonly affected. The most common abnormality noted is a nonspecific ST-T wave change, but any conduction abnormality, including complete heart block, can occur. Fortunately, these conditions respond well to antibiotic therapy, so that when necessary, the use of a pacemaker is usually temporary. On rare occasions there may be a true myocarditis with global dysfunction, but, fortunately, this is exceedingly uncommon and usually responds to antibiotics.

The musculoskeletal system is another system that is often involved.[6] Initially, patients may notice a migratory polyarthralgia, which generally settles into a monoarticular or an oligoarticular presentation. Most commonly, the joints involved are large weight-bearing joints, with the knee being the most common site. Polyarticular involvement, although described, is very unusual and should steer the practitioner toward another diagnosis, such as rheumatoid arthritis (RA) or systemic lupus erythematosus (SLE), rather than Lyme disease. The involved joint, although markedly inflamed, is surprisingly asymptomatic, with patients complaining more of swelling than of pain. Examination of the fluid will reveal marked inflammation, and studies of the fluid for Lyme disease will be uniformly positive. Untreated, the arthropathy of Lyme disease will remit and recur, with attacks occurring approximately once or twice a year but lasting for months at a time. However, most patients respond to antibiotic therapy. Occasionally, even with adequate therapy, a patient may develop a chronic, noninfectious arthritis that will require treatment other than antibiotics.

Chronic Disease

Left untreated or unrecognized, the *Borrelia* infection will become chronic. The primary sites of chronicity are the joints, as previously discussed, and the CNS. An atrophic lesion of the skin, acrodermatitis atrophicans, has also been described, but this lesion is more common in Europe than in the United States and probably reflects differences in the infecting organisms seen in different locations.

Neuroborreliosis can manifest itself in many different ways and ranges from subtle changes of cognition to frank neuropathies. The nervous system seems to be infected relatively early in the course of the infection, often within the first month after exposure. Symptoms may start as mood changes and cognitive deficits. Abnormalities on MRI may be noted. Whether these lesions represent actual infection or "microinfarcts" is not clear. A "confusional state," suggesting an encephalitis, may develop as well. Bandlike neuropathies are not uncommon and are believed to be caused by direct invasion of the nerve by the organism, although molecular mimicry with autoimmune reactions and lymphokines has also been implicated in this presentation, as well as in the encephalopathies. In addition, the damage to the nervous system caused by the infection (or the host's immune response) can delay healing and result in some degree of residual damage and dysfunction.[7,8]

Another of the chronic manifestations of Lyme disease is fibromyalgia.[9] This chronic pain syndrome, which is associated with fatigue, malaise, sleep disturbance, and tender trigger points on examination, can be extremely disconcerting to the patient, especially given the widespread concern that the general population has with Lyme disease. Noninfectious in nature, it responds to pain control, sleep correction, and aerobic exercise but not to repeated courses of antibiotics (see Chapter 190).

DIAGNOSTICS

The diagnosis is generally straightforward but requires a high degree of clinical suspicion and appropriate use of laboratory studies. If a patient presents with an expanding, bull's-eye rash, the diagnosis is established. No further testing is necessary or indicated.[9] Testing too early in the course of the infection, before the body can produce an antibody response, can result in a false-negative finding and the impression that the rash is not caused by Lyme disease. The testing for Lyme disease, when indicated clinically and not used as a screening test, generally consists of measuring antibodies directed against the organism (an enzyme-linked immunosorbent assay [ELISA] is used) and then confirming the specificity of the testing with Western blot (WB) testing.[9] After an initial infection, the body will start to make antibodies of the IgM class. This usually begins 1 to 2 weeks after exposure and is then followed, in an additional 4 weeks, by the production of antibodies of the IgG class. Both of these antibodies may persist after treatment and do not indicate persistence of infection. Antibiotics given very early in the course of the disease can abort this antibody production and make laboratory interpretation difficult. This is one of the arguments against empiric use of antibiotics in all but established cases of Lyme disease. The initial study should always be confirmed by WB analysis because cross-reactivity with normal host flora and other disease states can lead to false-positive results and erroneous treatment regimens. In the presence of the appropriate clinical presentation and positive laboratory testing and confirmation, the diagnosis is established and therapy should be begun.

The stage of the disease must be considered when interpreting the results. For patients with a chronic manifestation, an isolated positive IgM titer without a concurrent rise in the IgG titer should raise suspicion about the validity of the study. Similarly, in a previously untreated patient with a chronic manifestation of the disease, the absence of an IgG antibody response should be considered before the initiation of a treatment regimen.

In general, the antibody production is "locally produced"; that is, the antibody will be produced in excess in the affected site. Therefore patients with CNS involvement would be expected to have antibodies not only in their blood but also in their cerebrospinal fluid (CSF). Measuring this antibody production through lumbar puncture is an essential part of the diagnosis of neuroborreliosis. In the more acute forms, a pleocytosis with lymphocytic predominance, elevated protein levels (including low levels of oligoclonal banding), and positive Lyme titers by ELISA and WB are expected. If meningitis is part of the early disseminated syndrome, these antibodies may be absent because the body has not yet had a chance to respond with antibody production. In the later stages of CNS disease, positive antibodies in either the blood or CSF are nearly universal and should always be sought. Polymerase chain reaction (PCR) studies, which measure DNA from the organism, are even more specific and are currently recommended in CSF testing as well. In patients with a chronic polyneuropathy, the CSF may be negative, but results of peripheral blood testing are nearly always positive.

Diagnostics

Lyme Disease

Laboratory
ELISA*
WB analysis*
IgM, IgG*
PCR*

Imaging
MRI*

Other
Lumbar puncture*
Synovial fluid analysis*

*If indicated.

A similar antibody response and testing regimen is recommended for Lyme arthritis; however, this time the fluid studied should be the synovial fluid. The joint fluid is highly inflammatory, and Lyme titers of both the blood and the fluid are nearly universally positive. PCR can be done to confirm the presence of the organism as well.

The role of MRI testing, which is generally nonspecific in its findings for Lyme disease, and the role of neuropsychiatric studies remain unclear. The latter may be very sensitive and specific for Lyme disease but requires a skilled evaluator and is generally not covered by most insurance plans, nor is it commonly available outside of academic centers.

New laboratory studies are being investigated that will detect the organism at an earlier stage and will be more specific for infection rather than exposure. Their availability and utility are not yet established. Polymerase chain reaction (PCR), although very specific, is technically demanding and requires that the living organism be found in the studied fluid. Unfortunately, if the small sample studied does not contain the living organism, the test will be negative, even in an established disease. The Lyme urine antigen test has given unreliable results and should not be used in the diagnosis of Lyme disease.[9]

DIFFERENTIAL DIAGNOSIS

Depending on the stage of infection, Lyme disease may be confused with a number of other diseases. Some of this confusion may be related to the myth of Lyme disease being the "great imitator," akin to syphilis. As can be seen from the previous sections, the more common presentations of Lyme disease are rather stereotypical.

During the summer months the differential diagnosis of Lyme disease always includes the far more common and benign "summer flu." Coryza, cough, and congestion will help to differentiate the viral illness from *Borrelia* infection. The EM rash may be confused for a simple cellulitis or for a spider bite. As previously noted, the local arachnid population should be considered. On the East Coast of the United States, where brown recluse spiders are usual, that diagnosis should be made reluctantly. Other arthropod-borne infections such as Rocky

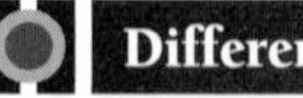

Differential Diagnosis

Lyme Disease

Influenza	Infection
Cellulitis	Tumor
Bell's palsy	Multiple sclerosis
Bacterial meningitis	Vasculitides
Reiter's disease	Depression
Gonorrheal arthropathy	Fibromyalgia
Crystalline-induced arthritis	Collagen vascular disease
Rheumatoid arthritis	

Mountain spotted fever, babesiosis, and chronic granulocytic ehrlichiosis can cause rashes and constitutional symptoms similar to those of Lyme disease and are in fact transmitted by the *I. dammini* tick.[8] Proper laboratory testing and recognition of other related symptoms and signs will help to differentiate these from Lyme disease.

In its disseminated stages, Lyme disease can be easily confused for other conditions. When a patient with any nervous system involvement is being treated, the caveat "common things happen commonly" should always be kept in mind. Thus although Lyme disease should be included in the differential diagnosis of a facial nerve palsy, even in endemic regions, the more common cause of this abnormality is still idiopathic Bell's palsy. In addition, although Lyme meningitis may be present, failure to diagnose and treat a pyogenic meningitis could have lethal complications. A lumbar puncture done at this time should show a lymphocytic or monocytic predominance if Lyme disease is the cause, distinguishing it from the polymorphonuclear reaction of a pyogenic meningitis. An elevation of the CSF protein level may be seen in both. Testing of either blood or CSF at this stage is almost uniformly positive for Lyme disease.

The arthropathy of Lyme disease is generally pauciarticular and thus can be confused with any of the other causes of oligoarthritis, such as Reiter's disease, gonorrheal infection, crystalline-induced arthritis, or even early RA. In some patients, this arthropathy has been erroneously diagnosed as a sprain or internal derangement, leading to unnecessary arthroscopic procedures. Any patient with an inflammatory arthritis, particularly of the knee, should be evaluated for Lyme disease. If the arthropathy becomes more generalized, it is less likely to be Lyme disease and more likely to be a rheumatologic illness such as RA or SLE. In the latter, rashes and neurologic involvement may confuse the presentation. Unlike Lyme disease, these conditions will not respond to antibiotics, although patients have received multiple courses of IV antibiotics for the misdiagnosis of Lyme disease.

New-onset heart block, especially in an unusual setting, such as a younger patient without a cardiac history, requires evaluation for the infection. The cardiac manifestations are otherwise relatively limited and should not be confused with other cardiac disease. Rarely, a cardiomyopathy can occur that should be excluded from the more common forms such as atherosclerotic and hypertensive cardiomyopathies.

The later manifestations of CNS involvement generally cause the most diagnostic confusion. Radicular pain may be caused by trauma or may be caused by nerve encroachment from disc disease, infections such as syphilis or herpes zoster, or tumors. Multiple levels, a seasonal onset, and bilaterality tend to favor the diagnosis of Lyme disease but are not specific findings. Headaches and memory deficits can be caused by Lyme disease, tumor, multiple sclerosis, vasculitides, collagen vascular diseases, fibromyalgia, or depression. Only a careful history, physical examination, and appropriate laboratory testing will help to differentiate these problems.

MANAGEMENT

The treatment of Lyme disease is dependent on the clinical manifestations. As with most infections, it is generally easier to eradicate the infection with less toxic or aggressive techniques, the earlier the diagnosis is made.

For most of the symptoms, except the true CNS manifestations, the treatment of choice is oral antibiotics.[3,5,10,11] In general, doxycycline 100 mg b.i.d. for 2 to 4 weeks is sufficient to treat EM rashes, myalgias and arthralgia, and mild heart block. Alternate therapies include amoxicillin 500 mg q.i.d. for 2 to 4 weeks (with or without probenecid) and cefuroxime axetil (Ceftin) 500 mg b.i.d. for 2 to 4 weeks. The arthritis is generally treated for 30 to 60 days via the oral route or for 14 to 28 days with IV antibiotics. Longer courses of antibiotics are generally reserved for later or for more severe manifestations. In children younger than 9 years old, in whom tetracyclines are to be avoided, the drugs of choice are amoxicillin 250 mg t.i.d. or 50 mg/kg/day in three divided doses or cefuroxime axetil 125 mg or 30 mg/kg b.i.d., both for 2 to 4 weeks, depending on the presentation.[10,11] What appears to be Bell's palsy, if there are absolutely no other CNS symptoms, can also be treated with the above oral regimens. However, if there is any possibility of more extensive CNS involvement, a lumbar puncture should be performed, and treatment decisions based on the results.

For all other CNS involvement or serious cardiac manifestations, or in the case of true treatment failures, the treatment of choice is a third-generation cephalosporin given intravenously.[12,13] The most common regimen is ceftriaxone 2 g/day for 3 to 4 weeks, although cefotaxime 2 g every 8 hours may also be used. In children the dosage is 75 to 100 mg/kg/day (maximum of 2 g) for ceftriaxone and 150 mg/kg/day (maximum of 6 g) in three or four[12,13] divided doses for cefotaxime. If a true cephalosporin allergy is found, treatment with chloramphenicol 50 mg/kg/day in four divided doses has been recommended, although strong consideration should be made toward rapid desensitization to a cephalosporin and treatment with that drug.

It is not uncommon for patients to develop fevers, chills, myalgias, and rashes early in the course of the antibiotic regimen. Called the Jarisch-Herxheimer reaction and also seen in treatment for syphilis, it is a response of the body to the rapid lysis of the infecting organism and should not cause the therapy to be prematurely aborted.

Treatment failures occur in approximately 10% of cases and can generally be treated intravenously. If the treatment still fails, reconsideration of the original diagnosis is necessary.[7] If the cause is fibromyalgia, treatment is rest, exercise, aerobic conditioning, and low doses of antidepressant medications to correct the sleep disturbance, and not repeated courses of antibiotics or new combinations of antibiotics.[12,13]

There are a few scenarios that are often encountered and need special mention. Even in endemic areas, only 1% to 3% of tick bites cause infection. Thus there currently is no indication for empiric treatment of a tick bite, unless the patient manifests symptoms of Lyme disease.[11] A recent study has shown a single dose of 200 mg doxycycline given within 72 hours of a known tick bite (after removal of the imbedded tick) to have some efficacy in preventing disease.[14] Treatment too early in the course of the disease can abrogate the initial antibody response, making later diagnosis difficult, and may subject the patient to a greater risk of side effects from the treatment than from the disease.

Seronegative Lyme disease (test results are negative for Lyme disease, but the patient has Lyme disease) is a rare but well-recognized entity. Generally, it occurs in a patient who took an inadequate amount or duration of antibiotic very early in the course of the disease. In this situation all other possible explanations for the symptomatology must be excluded, and fixed end points of treatment must be established before therapy is begun. Open-ended therapies of long duration have not been shown to have any efficacy and subject patients to potential serious toxicities. In addition, a previous response to an antibiotic should never be used as a criterion for making the diagnosis and continuing treatment.[13,14]

The patient who tests positive for Lyme disease on a screening test presents a different problem. In this situation the patient has clearly been exposed to the organism, but more often than not, the symptom that resulted in the testing is not caused by Lyme disease. A thorough history and physical examination should determine if there are any obvious signs of Lyme disease. If any are present, they should be treated with the appropriate regimen. If such signs are absent, a frank discussion with the patient about the risks of treatment (e.g., photosensitivity to tetracyclines, allergic reactions) versus the potential benefits of treatment is necessary to develop an appropriate treatment plan. If treatment is chosen, it should be via the oral route and for 2 to 4 weeks' duration (e.g., doxycycline 100 mg b.i.d. for 2 to 4 weeks).[8]

LYMErix, a vaccine for the prevention of Lyme disease, is no longer available commercially. However, other vaccines will be developed and approved for use in the future.

COMPLICATIONS

Although there are few complications when Lyme disease is diagnosed and treated properly, pregnancy requires special consideration.[3] Obviously, having an infection during pregnancy can be cause for great concern for any expectant parent. The spirochete has been shown to cross the placenta and infect the fetus, but, fortunately, this is a rare occurrence. In fact, studies concerned with the risk of miscarriage and congenital defects in patients with Lyme disease have not shown any increase in either compared with other pregnancies in the same region. The best approach is to treat the infected mother with amoxicillin 500 mg PO t.i.d. for 3 to 4 weeks for early localized disease and with ceftriaxone 2 g/day IV for 3 to 4 weeks for disseminated disease (tetracyclines are contraindicated in pregnancy).[15] Although no guarantees can be made, the expectant parents can in general be reassured of a normal outcome of the pregnancy.

INDICATIONS FOR REFERRAL/HOSPITALIZATION

In general, the management of early localized disease and the more common disseminated features does not require consultation with a specialist. Uncommon rashes may confound the practitioner and require consultation. Patients may require consultation with a specialist when the disease is more advanced and procedures such as a lumbar puncture or arthrocentesis are being contemplated. Because these procedures are not always welcomed by the patient, it is often best to refer the patient for a definitive procedure and evaluation, rather than potentially subjecting the patient to a procedure that may need to be repeated in the near future. In patients who have unusual manifestations such as polyarticular involvement, persistent synovitis, multiple neurologic deficits, or seronegative Lyme disease or in those for whom therapy has failed in the past, a referral to a rheumatologist, a neurologist, or an infectious disease specialist will help to secure a proper diagnosis and ensure proper therapy. It is worth repeating that even in endemic regions, other diseases such as RA, SLE, idiopathic Bell's palsy, and fibromyalgia are common entities that need to be considered, independent of Lyme disease.

Lyme disease, for the most part, is treated on an outpatient basis, requiring admission to a hospital only when the presenting feature would otherwise warrant it, independent of the cause. Thus a patient with acute meningitis or heart failure as a result of a high-degree heart block should be admitted to a hospital, but this admission would have been made regardless of the ultimate etiology of the symptom. As a rule, in patients who have not taken a cephalosporin in the past for other reasons, home IV therapy companies will require that the first dose be given in a controlled environment (e.g., a short-procedure unit or a physician's office). Antibiotic desensitization should always be done in a controlled setting, where emergency measures to treat anaphylaxis are readily available. With these exceptions, Lyme disease is easily managed in the outpatient setting.

PATIENT AND FAMILY EDUCATION

Although diagnosis and treatment are necessary in the management of this disease, the best approach to Lyme disease is avoidance of the tick bite. Patients should be instructed to wear light-colored, long-legged, and long-sleeved clothing, with socks tucked in, whenever walking through potentially endemic areas. This will make it harder for the tick to find skin to burrow into and will allow easy identification of the tick on the outside of the clothing. Insect repellents, such as DEET (diethyltoluamide), should also be considered, because these will also decrease the chance of tick bites. On returning from a wooded or grassy area, a thorough search of all body areas should be made. Any nonembedded tick can be removed and destroyed. If an embedded tick is found, it should be grasped firmly at the base of the head with a pair of tweezers and gently removed. Care should be taken to avoid crushing the embedded tick while it is still attached or removing the body of the tick while leaving the mouth parts attached. Measures such as applying petroleum jelly, oils, or lighted cigarettes to the tick to aid in removal are not effective and are potentially dangerous. The bite site should be observed for the next week for signs of induration, with any expanding rash or viral-type symptoms reported to the practitioner.

Lyme disease continues to spread as humans encroach on the wilderness, increasing the likelihood of an encounter with an infected tick. Although Lyme disease causes unwarranted anxiety and fear, with understanding of the disease process and recognition of its manifestations, the practitioner should be able to treat and cure this condition.

REFERENCES

1. Steere AC and others: Lyme arthritis: an epidemic of oligoarticular arthritis in children and adults in three Connecticut communities, *Arthritis Rheum* 20:7-17, 1977.
2. Nocton JJ, Steere AC: Lyme disease, *Adv Intern Med* 40:69-117, 1995.

3. Zemel LS: Lyme disease: a pediatric perspective, *J Rheumatol* 19 (suppl 34):1-13, 1992.
4. Lyme disease—United States, 1999, *MMWR* 50:181-185, 2001.
5. Nadelman RB, Wormser GP: Erythema migrans and early Lyme disease, *Am J Med* 98 (suppl 4A):15S-24S, 1995.
6. Steer AC and others: The overdiagnosis of Lyme disease, *JAMA* 269(14):1812-1816, 1993.
7. Sigal LH: Anxiety and persistence of Lyme disease, *Am J Med* 98 (suppl 4A):74S-83S, 1995.
8. Krause PJ and others: Concurrent Lyme disease and babesiosis, *JAMA* 275:1657-1660, 1996.
9. Steere, AC: Lyme Disease, *N Engl J Med* 345 (2): 115-125, 2001
10. Shapiro ED: Lyme disease in children, *Am J Med* 98 (suppl 4A):69S-73S, 1995.
11. Dattwyler RJ and others: Ceftriaxone compared with doxycycline for the treatment of acute disseminated Lyme disease, *N Engl J Med* 337:289-294, 1997.
12. Treatment of Lyme disease, *Med Lett* 42(1077):37-39, 2000.
13. Klempner MS and others: Two controlled trials of antibiotic treatment in patients with persistent symptoms and a history of Lyme disease, *N Engl J Med* 345:85-92, 2001.
14. Nadelman RB and others: Prophylaxis with single-dose doxycycline for the prevention of Lyme disease after an *Ixodes scapularis* tick bite, *N Engl J Med* 345:79-84, 2001.
15. Shapiro ED: Doxycycline for tick bites—not for everyone, *N Engl J Med* 345:133-134, 2001.

CHAPTER 239

Polymyalgia Rheumatica and Temporal Arteritis

Susan Hoch

DEFINITION/EPIDEMIOLOGY

Polymyalgia rheumatica (PMR) is a musculoskeletal syndrome seen in persons older than 50 years. This disorder is characterized by pain and stiffness in the neck, shoulder girdle, and pelvic girdle; an elevated erythrocyte sedimentation rate (ESR); and a dramatic, rapid response to corticosteroids. It can occur alone or in association with giant cell (temporal) arteritis (GCA). GCA is a systemic inflammatory vasculitis of large and medium-sized arteries, commonly affecting the branches of the proximal aorta that supply the neck and the extracranial structures of the head. Approximately 40% to 50% of patients with GCA have symptoms of PMR and, conversely, 15% to 20% of patients with PMR have GCA.

The average annual incidence of PMR is 52.5 per 100,000 persons 50 years of age or older.[1] It is more common in whites than in other groups, and the highest recorded incidence is in northern Europe and northern United States. Typically, patients are older than 50 years of age, and 90% are over 60 years of age. The male/female ratio is 1:2.

GCA has a prevalence of 133 per 100,000 population in people 50 years of age or older. The disease is rare before age 50, and the mean age at onset is 71 years. The incidence increases with age. It has a striking predilection for whites and is more common in females. The male/female ratio is 1:2 to 1:5. New-onset headache or visual symptoms in an older patient with or without musculoskeletal symptoms should prompt consideration of GCA. GCA is a medical emergency with the potential for the occurrence of sudden and irreversible blindness.

Physician consultation is indicated for patients with suspected polymyalgia rheumatica. Physician consultation is indicated for patients with tender temporal arteries or with suspected temporal arteritis.

PATHOPHYSIOLOGY

PMR and GCA are related disorders that seem to represent a continuum of disease. The current hypothesis is that an infectious cause or causes appear to precipitate a cellular immune response directed at the walls of specific arteries. Why these diseases specifically target individuals above the age of 50 is not known. This initial arterial insult appears to initiate a series of cellular and immunologic events with influx of interferon gamma (INF-γ) producing T-cells, macrophages, and giant cells.[2] The artery itself responds with proliferation of smooth muscle cells and the eventual production of a lumen-obstructing neointima. Molecular studies have shown differing tissue cytokine profiles in PMR and GCA that may be related to disease expression.[3] Patients with PMR symptoms seem to have higher production of interleukin-2 (IL-2), whereas higher levels of synthesis of IFN-γ, IL-1β, and platelet-derived growth factor (PDGF) seem to correlate with ischemic symptoms.[3,4] There appears to be an association between the histocompatibility antigen HLA-DR4 in both patients with PMR and GCA. In patients with large vessel (nontemporal artery) GCA, there appears to be overrepresentation of the *HLA-DRB1*0404* allele, suggesting that GCA itself is a heterogeneous entity.[5] Similarly, it is found clinically that a small proportion of patients with PMR without vascular symptoms are discovered to have arteritis on blind biopsies.

These studies suggest that heterogeneity either in the triggering agent and/or in the host's immunologic and vascular response may correlate with the variations in the clinical presentation of these syndromes.[5] GCA most commonly affects the arteries originating from the arch of the aorta. Large vessel GCA generally involves the subclavian/axillary/brachial arteries and may or may not be associated with cranial GCA. Autopsies performed on patients who died of GCA show severe involvement most commonly in the superficial temporal arteries, vertebral arteries, and ophthalmic and posterior ciliary arteries. The central retinal, carotid, subclavian, brachial, and abdominal arteries and the aorta may also be affected. Intracranial arteries are infrequently involved. The arterial lesion may be segmental or patchy with skip areas. Blindness is usually a result of occlusion of the posterior ciliary artery and, less commonly, of the central retinal artery.

CLINICAL PRESENTATION

The onset of PMR symptoms may be abrupt or subacute. Several weeks to months may elapse before the diagnosis is made. Symmetric pain and stiffness in the neck, shoulders, and hips are present, and patients report that they feel as if they have aged several decades. Difficulty in rising from a chair is reported, and gelling occurs after immobility. Morning stiffness, the time it takes for patients to reach their baseline agility and limberness, is inflammatory in nature and lasts more than 60 minutes—it often lasts as long as 2 to 3 hours. Range of motion of the hips and shoulders is usually normal, but adhesive capsulitis of the shoulder(s) with significant loss of motion (a frozen shoulder) is sometimes present. Constitutional symptoms, including fever, weight loss, lassitude, fatigue, and anorexia, are common. Muscle pain without significant muscle weakness is common. The pain is characterized by the patient as diffuse and often limits mobility. Patients will report difficulty getting in and out of a car or difficulty combing their hair. However, true muscle weakness is not usually present, although pain may limit effort in strength testing. Synovial swelling in joints such as wrists and knees has been reported but is uncommon.

GCA has varied presentations.[6] Patients may present with PMR with or without symptoms of arteritis. Headache, found in two thirds of patients, may be continuous or intermittent, can be located temporally or occipitally, and can be throbbing, aching, or sharp. A new headache in a patient over 60 years of age must raise the suspicion of GCA. A history of scalp tenderness at any time but particularly in association with headache suggests GCA. Jaw claudication (jaw pain on chewing) is pathognomonic of GCA. In addition, 20% of patients may have fever (temperature as high as 39° C [102.2° F), and 40% experience weight loss. Fatigue and anorexia occur. Approximately 15% of patients present with fever of unknown origin. Visual symptoms, including diplopia, ptosis, amaurosis fugax, and blindness, occur in 30% of patients. Fifteen percent of patients have permanent visual loss. Eye involvement is often initially unilateral and may become bilateral without treatment within 1 to 10 days. Neurologic complications occur in 31% of patients, with neuropathies occurring in 14% and strokes in 7%. Respiratory symptoms such as cough, sore throat, and hoarseness occur in 10% of patients. Tongue claudication or dysphagia secondary to ischemia of the muscles of deglutition can occur. In addition, tongue numbness, tinnitus, vertigo, and hearing loss have been reported.

PHYSICAL EXAMINATION

Most patients with PMR have normal findings on joint examination, although joint and muscle tenderness may be present. The knee and wrist may show mild swelling, usually without loss of motion. There is no muscle atrophy or true muscle weakness. When muscle strength is being tested in the upper arms, the patient is asked to abduct his or her arms to 90 degrees and resist the examiner's arms pressing downward. These patients may be unable to maintain their arms in the horizontal position because of pain elicited by the examiner's maneuver rather than because of weakness. Trigger point tenderness and pain on mild squeezing of the extremities, so characteristic of fibromyalgia, are unusual. Often it is helpful to watch people get up out of a chair and walk because the stiffness and gelling can be striking.

All patients presenting with symptoms of PMR should be examined for GCA. In normal individuals the temporal artery pulsations are easily palpable. With GCA there may be a decrease in pulsation or lack of pulsation in an involved temporal artery. The temporal, occipital, or other scalp or cervical arteries may be enlarged, erythematous, and tender. Bruits or pulse deficits may be present over the carotid, subclavian, or brachial arteries. Carotidynia may be present. Patients with visual symptoms may have funduscopic findings of disc pallor and edema, cotton-wool spots, and retinal hemorrhage progressing to optic atrophy.

DIAGNOSTICS

Most patients with PMR have an elevated erythrocyte sedimentation rate (ESR) above 40 to 50 mm/hr, and many have ESRs above 80 mm/hr. However, 7% of patients can present with ESRs below 40 mm/hr.[7] Patients presenting with PMR and low ESR appear to differ from patients with PMR and high ESR only by the occurrence of more common systemic symptoms in the high-ESR group.[7] Normochromic, normocytic anemia may be present, and liver function tests (LFTs), particularly for alkaline phosphatase, may show mild elevations. Muscle enzymes, muscle biopsy, and nerve conduction studies are normal. Rheumatoid factor (RF) and antinuclear antibody (ANA) tests are negative.

Recent MRI and shoulder ultrasonographic studies in patients with PMR have confirmed the presence of subacromial/subdeltoid bursitis in the majority of cases of PMR.[8,9] Inflammation of these bursae as well as iliopectineal bursitis and co-existent hip synovitis may account for the symptoms of diffuse shoulder and hip girdle pain and stiffness experienced by patients with PMR.[9]

Diagnostics

Polymyalgia Rheumatica

Laboratory
CBC and differential
ESR
LFTs
Creatine phosphokinase (CPK)
RF*
ANA*
TSH*
Serum protein electrophoresis*

Other
Muscle biopsy
Nerve conduction studies

*If indicated.

It has been suggested that a dramatic and rapid response to low-dose corticosteroids (15 mg/day or less) after 2 to 3 days of treatment may be an additional criteria for the diagnosis of PMR.[10] No other disease will have 100% improvement within 48 hours with steroid therapy.[11]

Like PMR, laboratory studies in GCA show evidence of inflammation. Characteristically the ESR is elevated, often above 100 mm/hr. A normochromic, normocytic anemia is commonly observed. There often is a thrombocytosis. Patients may have mildly elevated findings on LFTs, usually for alkaline phosphatase. When liver biopsies have been performed on these patients, granulomatous changes have been found, but this is not part of the usual diagnostic evaluation in this disease.

The major clinical question in establishing a diagnosis of GCA is whether to perform a temporal artery biopsy. A positive temporal artery biopsy result assuredly documents the diagnosis of GCA, yet a negative biopsy result in a setting of high clinical suspicion does not exclude this condition. This remains an area of some controversy. Biopsy results may be falsely negative because of the high incidence of skip lesions. The usefulness of performing unilateral versus bilateral temporal artery biopsy has been found to increase the diagnostic yield by only 3%.[12] Some rheumatologists believe that because of this low positive biopsy rate, biopsies should not be performed unless patients have other system involvement not explainable by GCA. In lieu of biopsy, a diagnostic trial of 40 to 60 mg of prednisone for 10 days to 2 weeks may be considered with monitoring of clinical symptoms and ESR. Others believe that the long-term commitment to high-dose corticosteroids in this older patient population is associated with significant toxicity and therefore it is useful to try to confirm who indeed has biopsy-proved temporal arteritis.

Regardless of whether a decision to perform a biopsy has been made, there should be no hesitation in beginning high-dose prednisone if there is clinical suspicion of GCA. The biopsy can be arranged in a couple of days and the pathology will not change. The consequences of delay in the institution of corticosteroids in a patient with GCA symptoms can be blindness or stroke. Based on the patient's initial clinical response, the decision to perform a biopsy can be made at a less emergent moment.

Diagnostics

Temporal Arteritis

Laboratory	Other
ESR	Temporal artery biopsy
CBC and differential	Prednisone trial
LFTs	

DIFFERENTIAL DIAGNOSIS

Rheumatoid arthritis is difficult to differentiate from PMR in older adults, particularly in the early stages, when there is little detectable synovitis and the RF is negative.[13] Continued observation or a diagnostic trial of steroids can help resolve the dilemma. Patients with little or no observable joint findings after several weeks are unlikely to have rheumatoid arthritis. Patients with symmetric synovitis of their proximal interphalangeal (PIP), metacarpophalangeal (MCP), or metatarsophalangeal (MTP) joints are not likely to have PMR. Polymyositis can present much like PMR, but patients with polymyositis have muscle weakness and may have muscle atrophy. They also have abnormal findings on muscle enzyme studies, muscle biopsies, and nerve conduction studies. Myeloma and hypothyroidism may present like PMR, but serum protein electrophoresis in myeloma and thyroid function tests in hypothyroidism will be abnormal. Fibromyalgia presents with muscle pain and tenderness, but patients will have characteristic pain on palpation of trigger points and will have a normal ESR. Degenerative joint disease (DJD) can present with neck, shoulder, and hip pain but not inflammatory morning stiffness, as in PMR. Patients with DJD have noninflammatory morning stiffness that lasts less than 30 minutes. Parkinsonism can present with muscle aching and severe stiffness but not with an elevated ESR. In addition, patients with parkinsonism may have cogwheel rigidity and tremor on examination.

Other forms of systemic vasculitis, such as Wegener's granulomatosis, hypersensitivity vasculitis, and polyarteritis nodosa, can involve the temporal arteries. Therefore all patients with symptoms of GCA who have signs or symptoms of other organ involvement require a biopsy to establish the cause of their arteritis.

Finally, the presence of any systemic inflammatory disease other than GCA is thought to exclude a diagnosis of primary PMR.

MANAGEMENT

PMR is usually curable, although relapses do occur. The duration of the disease can be as short as 6 weeks or as long as several years. It is important to keep in mind that PMR is a heterogeneous disorder with significant variation between patients in treatment duration and required dose of corticosteroids for the control of symptoms and disease process.[14] Nonetheless, many physicians treat patients with an initial dose of 10 to 15 mg prednisone for 2 to 4 weeks. The patient is monitored for control of musculoskeletal symptoms and the ESR is followed closely. With control of symptoms and ESR, tapering can begin. The

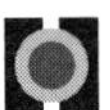

Differential Diagnosis

Polymyalgia Rheumatica

Rheumatoid arthritis
Polymyositis
Myeloma
Hypothyroidism
Fibromyalgia
Degenerative joint disease
Parkinson's disease

Differential Diagnosis

Temporal Arteritis

Wegener's granulomatosis
Hypersensitivity vasculitis
Polyarteritis nodosa

goal is to taper the dose of prednisone as quickly as possible while maintaining a normal ESR and the patient in an asymptomatic state. Again there is no single widely accepted steroid tapering protocol for PMR but many physicians will taper by no more than 1 mg every week or 2 above 10 mg prednisone and by 1 mg monthly below 10 mg. With this schedule, many patients will discontinue prednisone after slightly more than 1 year of treatment.[15]

GCA is considered a medical emergency. Treatment is begun immediately. As previously noted, in a patient with new-onset headache, temporal artery symptoms, and a suspicion of GCA, there is no reason to wait to start steroids. Corticosteroids should be initiated at a dose of 40 to 60 mg/day, the higher dose to be used where there is a stronger clinical suspicion. This high-dose steroid therapy should then be continued for 4 to 6 weeks with frequent monitoring of the patient's clinical condition and ESR. In general, there is little risk of eye complications and blindness occurring in patients with normal ESRs. The steroid dose is tapered rapidly to 20 mg/day by decrements of 2.5 to 5 mg every other week. A good rule of thumb for GCA and other forms of vasculitis, including systemic lupus erythematosus, is to taper steroids no faster than 10% of the dose per week. Steroids are then tapered slowly, as recommended for PMR. Methotrexate has shown efficacy in some studies as a steroid-sparing agent in combination with prednisone.[16] Alternate-day use of steroids is not advised. Treatment for 1 to 2 years is typical. Treatment may be necessary for as long as 5 years. Recurrences usually occur during the first 18 months after diagnosis and within 12 months of discontinuation of therapy.

Patients with both PMR and GCA should be managed to minimize the risks associated with long-term corticosteroid use in this older population. Serum potassium should be checked regularly, and potassium supplements should be prescribed if hypokalemia occurs. Serum glucose should be monitored. A baseline bone densitometry study should be performed to check for preexisting osteoporosis. Because of the risk of steroid-induced osteopenia and osteoporosis, all patients with PMR and GCA should be supplemented with 1200 mg/day of elemental calcium and 400 mg vitamin D. Treatment with estrogen, raloxiphene, or a bisphosphonate should be initiated either to prevent the development of corticosteroid-induced osteoporosis or to treat preexisting osteoporosis in a patient who is now receiving corticosteroids. Daily weight-bearing exercise should be encouraged. Patients receiving corticosteroids for either PMR or GCA should be considered immunocompromised and should receive immunization with both pneumococcal and influenza vaccines.

LIFE SPAN CONSIDERATIONS

Studies of the natural history of PMR and temporal arteritis (GCA) have not shown a reduction in survival in comparison with the general population. These are diseases of the older population exclusively. Patients are all older than 50, and most are older than 65.

COMPLICATIONS

The most significant and most common complication of PMR is GCA. Other complications often seen in patients with PMR are complications secondary to long-term corticosteroid therapy, including osteoporosis, infection, cataract formation, hypertension, hypokalemia, and glucose intolerance.

Blindness, which occurs in 15% of patients with GCA, is the most common complication of GCA. Several studies have tried to predict which patients with GCA may be at increased risk of blindness. In one recent study of 161 patients, the best predictors of irreversible blindness were the presence of amaurosis fugax and cerebrovascular accidents, suggesting that patients with other ischemic manifestations are at higher risk for ischemic visual loss.[17] Another study of a similar number of patients has suggested that thrombocytosis with a platelet count greater than 400,000/mm^3 may be a risk factor for permanent visual loss.[18] This study raises consideration of whether there is a role for antiplatelet therapy in the treatment of GCA.

There is an increased risk of aortic aneurysm and dissection in patients with GCA; this is often a late complication and may be fatal.[19] Myocardial infarction can occur. Neurologic complications include optic neuropathies, ocular motility disorders, acute auditory nerve infarction, mononeuritis multiplex, transient ischemic attack, and stroke.[20] Complications of long-term high-dose steroid use in GCA are similar to those observed in PMR but may occur more often and be more severe given the higher doses of corticosteroids and longer duration of treatment for GCA.

INDICATIONS FOR REFERRAL/HOSPITALIZATION

Physician consultation is indicated in suspected cases of PMR to assist with the differential diagnosis and determination for steroid therapy. A rheumatologist should be consulted for (1) patients who do not respond to standard steroid therapy; (2) patients with other rheumatic or neurologic disorders, making management difficult; and (3) patients with other system involvement. All patients suspected of having GCA should have physician consultation. Temporal artery biopsy is performed by an ophthalmologist, a general surgeon, or a plastic surgeon. A rheumatologist is consulted for patients with biopsy-proved GCA who do not respond to steroids.

PMR rarely warrants hospitalization unless there are life-threatening side effects of treatment, such as diabetes with blood sugar levels that are out of control or gastrointestinal bleeding. With GCA, symptoms of stroke, aortic aneurysm, or myocardial infarction would warrant hospitalization.

PATIENT AND FAMILY EDUCATION

Patients with PMR should be educated about its association with GCA. Patients should be aware of the necessity to report immediately any new headache, change in vision, scalp tenderness, difficulty chewing, or other new symptom.

Education about the dangers of corticosteroid therapy is important. The patient should be informed of the potential life-threatening risk of sudden withdrawal of corticosteroids. The patient should be instructed not to discontinue steroid therapy abruptly because doing so can cause hypoadrenalism. Obtaining a Medical Alert bracelet indicating that the patient is taking corticosteroids may be helpful. They need to be aware of common steroid side effects and the importance of contacting their primary care provider should they develop such symptoms as increased thirst, polyuria, and weight loss. Patients should be reminded to take their medication with food.

If symptoms of heartburn or nausea occur, ulcer prophylaxis with antacids and H_2 blockers is indicated. The patient should understand the risks of the development of corticosteroid-induced bone loss and the importance of behaviors such as daily weight-bearing exercise and adequate (1200 mg) calcium and (400 mg) vitamin D intake as well as the use of antiresorptive medication.

REFERENCES

1. Hunder GG: Giant cell arteritis and polymyalgia rheumatica, *Med Clin North Am* 81:195-219, 1997.
2. Weyand CM, Goronzy JJ: Pathogenic principles in giant cell arteritis, *Int J Cardiol* 75 (suppl 1):S9-S15, 2000.
3. Weyand CM and others: Disease patterns and tissue cytokine profiles in giant cell arteritis, *Arthritis Rheum* 40:19-26, 1997.
4. Weyand CM and others: Giant cell arteritis—a molecular approach to the multiple facets of the syndrome, *Ann Intern Med* 149:420-424, 1998.
5. Brack A and others: Disease pattern in cranial and large-vessel giant cell arteritis, *Arthritis Rheum* 42:311-317, 1999.
6. Hunder GG: Giant cell (temporal) arteritis, *Rheumatol Clin North Am* 16:399-409, 1990.
7. Proven A and others: Polymyalgia rheumatica with low erythrocyte sedimentation rate at diagnosis, *J Rheum* 26:1333-1337, 1999.
8. Pavlica P and others: Magnetic resonance imaging in the diagnosis of PMR, *Clin Exp Rheum* 18(4 suppl 20):S38-S39, 2000.
9. Cantini F and others: Shoulder ultrasonography in the diagnosis of polymyalgia rheumatica: a case-control study, *J Rheum* 28:1049-1055, 2001.
10. Cohen MD, Ginsburg WW: Polymyalgia rheumatica, *Rheum Dis North Am* 16:325-339, 1990.
11. Michet CJ and others: Common rheumatologic diseases in elderly patients, *Mayo Clin Proc* 70:1205-1214, 1995.
12. Boyev LR, Miller NR, Green WR: Efficacy of unilateral versus bilateral temporal artery biopsies for the diagnosis of giant cell arteritis, *Am J Ophthal* 128:211-215, 1999.
13. Hunder GG, Goronzy J, Weyland C: Is seronegative RA in the elderly the same as polymyalgia rheumatica? *Bull Rheum Dis* 43:1-3, 1994.
14. Weyand CM and others: Corticosteroid requirements in polymyalgia rheumatica, *Arch Intern Med* 159:577-584, 1999.
15. Cohen MD, Abril A: Polymyalgia rheumatica revisited, *Bull Rheum Dis* 50:1-4, 2001.
16. Jover JA and others: Combined treatment of giant-cell arteritis with methotrexate and prednisone: a randomized, double-blind, placebo-controlled trial, *Ann Intern Med* 134:106-114, 2001.
17. Gonzalez-Gay MA and others: Visual manifestations of giant cell arteritis. Trends and clinical spectrum in 161 patients, *Medicine* 79:283-292, 2000.
18. Liozon E and others: Risk factors for visual loss in giant cell (temporal) arteritis: a prospective study of 174 patients, *Am J Med* 111:211-217, 2001.
19. Evans JM, O'Fallon WM, Hunder GG: Increased incidence of aortic aneurysm and dissection in giant cell (temporal) arteritis, *Ann Intern Med* 122:502-507, 1995.
20. Caselli RJ, Hunder GG: Neurologic complications of giant cell (temporal) arteritis, *Semin Neurol* 14:349-353, 1994.

CHAPTER 240

Raynaud's Phenomenon

Bonnie L. Bermas

DEFINITION/EPIDEMIOLOGY

Raynaud's phenomenon is a vasospastic disorder that affects the blood flow to the digits. When these changes occur in isolation with a normal physical examination, the disorder is known as *primary* Raynaud's phenomenon. There are no associated autoimmune diseases, and rarely are autoantibodies present. Primary Raynaud's phenomenon characteristically occurs in women in their second to third decade of life. It is not uncommon and is thought to affect up to 10% of the population.[1] *Secondary* Raynaud's phenomenon is seen in patients who also have an autoimmune disorder such as progressive systemic sclerosis (scleroderma), systemic lupus erythematosus (SLE), or mixed connective tissue disease (MCTD). In addition to autoimmune diseases, Raynaud's phenomenon has been seen in association with migraine headaches and chest pain.[2]

Secondary Raynaud's phenomenon can also be seen as part of the CREST constellation (*c*alcinosis, *R*aynaud's phenomenon, *e*sophageal dysmotility, *s*clerodactyly, and *t*elangiectasias) and scleroderma. When Raynaud's phenomenon is seen in conjunction with scleroderma, it can portend a poor clinical outcome. Patients with SLE who have Raynaud's phenomenon often have antiphospholipid antibodies.

Secondary Raynaud's phenomenon is more severe than primary disease, and there is a greater likelihood of ulcerations and severe ischemic changes.

Physician consultation is recommended for patients with persistent pallor, coldness, tissue breakdown, and diminished pulse in the digits.

PATHOPHYSIOLOGY

In Raynaud's phenomenon, the blood vessels constrict in response to cold or stress. The resultant disturbance in circulation causes a series of color changes in the skin: white, blanched, or pale as the blood flow is reduced; blue as the affected digit loses oxygen from the decreased blood flow; and red or flushed as blood flow returns. Finally, as the attack subsides and the circulation returns to normal, usual skin color is restored. In the white or blue stages numbness, tingling, and coldness can be felt. In the red stage a feeling of warmth, burning, or swelling may be reported. Not infrequently, pain is experienced.

CLINICAL PRESENTATION

The vasospasm of Raynaud's phenomenon causes classic tricolor changes of first white (pallor), then blue (cyanosis), and then red (reperfusion hyperemia) after the vasospasm ends.[1] Episodes can be triggered by cold exposure, rapid changes in ambient temperature, or emotional stress. Attacks can occur in single or multiple digits and can spread to other digits, the other hand, or the feet. Patients can experience pain, numbness, and burning.

PHYSICAL EXAMINATION

On examination, the aforementioned classic tricolor changes can often be observed with sharp demarcation of where the spasm occurs. Submersion of the patient's hand in ice water occasionally precipitates attacks. Physical examination of the digits can reveal dilated capillary loops at the base of the nail beds. Tissue breakdown and ulcerations can also be present.

DIAGNOSTICS

The diagnosis of Raynaud's phenomenon is based on a clinical history of the classic tricolor changes. The autoantibodies anti–Scl-70 and anticentromere antibodies are useful diagnostic studies. The presence of autoantibodies and the severity of symptoms are thought to predispose patients to more systemic involvement. In particular, the presence of an anticentromere antibody is associated with the development of CREST, whereas the anti–Scl-70 antibody is more often seen in scleroderma.[3]

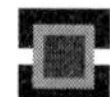

Diagnostics

Raynaud's Phenomenon

Initial
Nailfold capillary microscopy

Laboratory
Antinuclear antibody
Anti-Scl-70
Anticentomere antibody

DIFFERENTIAL DIAGNOSIS

The differential diagnosis of Raynaud's phenomenon is extensive and can be divided into several categories: occupational exposures, drug exposures, occlusive vascular disease, connective tissue disease, hematologic disorders, and others.[4] Primary Raynaud's phenomenon can be difficult to distinguish from other causes of vasospasm in the differential diagnosis. Observation of the tricolor changes is helpful.

Patients with primary Raynaud's phenomenon without the presence of autoantibodies tend to do well without medical intervention. The absence of nailfold capillaries in patients with autoantibodies improves the prognosis. CREST syndrome is a limited form of scleroderma characterized by calcinosis, Raynaud's phenomenon, esophageal dysmotility, sclerodactyly, and telangiectasias. Patients with CREST are usually spared the life-threatening organ involvement seen in scleroderma, but they are still subject to the lung disease (see Chapter 243).

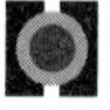

Differential Diagnosis

Raynaud's Phenomenon

Primary Disorder
Raynaud's phenomenon

Secondary Disorder
Drug-induced condition
Trauma (electric shock or repetitive injury)
Occupational injury or exposure
Connective tissue disease
- Rheumatoid arthritis
- Scleroderma
- Systemic lupus erythematosus
- Polymyositis
- Dermatomyositis

Hematologic disorders
- Polycythemia
- Cryoglobulinemia
- Waldenström's macroglobulinemia
- Cold agglutinins
- Cryofibrinogemia
- Myeloproliferative disorder

Occlusive disease/disorder
- Atherosclerosis
- Thromboembolism
- Thoracic outlet syndrome
- Buerger's disease
- Thromboangiitis obliterans
- Takayasu's arteritis

Neurologic disorder
- Cervical disk disease
- Tumor
- Cerebrovascular accident
- Poliomyelitis

Pulmonary hypertension
Reflux sympathetic dystrophy
Chilblain

MANAGEMENT

In its most benign form, Raynaud's phenomenon can be a mild inconvenience. Most patients have discomfort when Raynaud's phenomenon is triggered but have no permanent damage. Nifedipine, a calcium channel blocker, may help prevent vasospasm.[5] If vasospasms are not controlled, vasodilators such as hydralazine and prazosin can be added, provided that the blood pressure is not adversely affected. Nitropaste can be applied locally to the hands for additional relief. The most successful management is patient education.

COMPLICATIONS

In patients in whom standard medical therapy has failed and who are at risk for permanent ischemic damage, chemical ganglion sympathectomies can be tried. Alternatively, patients are hospitalized for IV administration of prostaglandin, such as prostaglandin E_1.[6] A vascular or hand surgeon can perform permanent digital sympathectomy if medical therapies fail. Unfortunately, in some patients all techniques fail and autoamputation of digits occurs.

INDICATIONS FOR REFERRAL/HOSPITALIZATION

Referral to a rheumatologist is necessary to exclude the presence of associated autoimmune disease. In severe cases, consultation with a vascular surgeon or anesthesiologist may be indicated. Patients in intractable pain or who are at risk for autoamputation of a digit or severe infection should be hospitalized under the care of a rheumatologist. A vascular surgeon should be consulted early if possible digit loss is suspected. Anesthesia can also be helpful in providing chemical ganglion sympathectomies for the relief of pain. Referral to an occupational therapist for evaluation and education can be helpful. Some patients have found biofeedback useful during attacks of Raynaud's phenomenon.

PATIENT AND FAMILY EDUCATION

Patient education is crucial, and the potentially serious nature of this disorder should be emphasized. Patients should avoid exposing their hands to the cold if at all possible. Mittens, which are preferable to gloves, should be worn as soon as the weather begins to get cool. For some patients, mittens need to be worn when grocery shopping because reaching for food items in refrigerator or freezer sections can often trigger attacks. Keeping core temperature higher by wearing hats and layering clothing may also be of benefit. Sudden temperature changes should be avoided. For many patients, emotional stress can trigger episodes, and behavioral modification and biofeedback may play a role in limiting attacks. Patients should also discontinue cigarette smoking if they are smokers. Decongestants and amphetamines should be avoided.

In some patients the protracted ischemia results in ulcerations that can become superinfected. Treatment of the infection can be difficult because local delivery of antibiotics is difficult given the impaired blood flow. Rarely, ischemia can be so profound that loss of tissue and bone stock can occur, resulting in autoamputation of digits.

REFERENCES

1. Blunt RJ, Porter JM: Raynaud's syndrome, *Semin Arthritis Rheum* 10:282-304, 1981.
2. O'Keeffe ST, Tsapatsaris NP, Beetham WP: Increased prevalence of migraine and chest pain in patients with primary Raynaud's disease, *Ann Intern Med* 116:985-989, 1992.
3. Sarkozi J and others: Significance of anticentromere antibody in idiopathic Raynaud's syndrome, *Am J Med* 83:893-898, 1987.
4. Silver R: Raynaud's phenomenon. In Stein J and others, editors: *Internal medicine*, ed 5, St Louis, 1998, Mosby.
5. Rodeheffer RJ and others: Controlled double-blind trial of nifedipine in the treatment of Raynaud's phenomenon, *N Engl J Med* 308:880-883, 1983.
6. Hauptman HW, Rudd S, Roberts WN: Reversal of the vasospastic component of lupus vasculopathy by infusion of prostaglandin E_1, *J Rheumatol* 18:1747-1752, 1991.

CHAPTER 241

Rheumatoid Arthritis

Dorothy Johnson and Francisco P. Quismorio, Jr.

DEFINITION/EPIDEMIOLOGY

Rheumatoid arthritis (RA) is an autoimmune disorder characterized by symmetric inflammatory polyarthritis and varying degrees of extraarticular involvement. A chronic fluctuating course of the disease is experienced by most patients that may result in joint destruction, deformity, disability and premature death.[1-4] Major economic and emotional disabilities can result from RA and can have a significant impact on patients' families and loved ones. More than 9 million physician visits and more than 250,000 hospitalizations occur in the United States each year because of RA.[5,6]

RA affects 1% of the adult population in the United States, with women affected 2 to 3 times more often than men. The prevalence increases with age. Despite extensive research, the etiology of RA remains unknown; however, most investigators believe that a combination of genetic, environmental, hormonal, and reproductive factors is important. RA probably occurs in a genetically susceptible person with an abnormal immune response to an undetermined antigen(s). Genetic studies have shown that RA is strongly linked to *HLA-DRB 10404* and *-DRB 10401*.[5,6]

PATHOPHYSIOLOGY

The main target of inflammation is the synovial lining of diarthrodial joints. The earliest changes in the synovial membrane are seen in the capillaries and small blood vessels. There is proliferation of the lining cells and early infiltration by T lymphocytes. Later, there is diffuse infiltration with B and T lymphocytes, macrophages, and plasma cells. The synovial membrane undergoes hyperplastic thickening with the proliferation of lining cells and fibroblasts and formation of new blood vessels. This granulation tissue called "pannus" invades the cartilage and subchondral bone and is primarily responsible for the destruction of joint structures in RA.[1-4,7]

Immune complexes in the synovial tissue activate the complement system, which then participates in the inflammatory process. Kinins, prostaglandins, and other mediators increase the permeability of blood vessels and attract leukocytes and lymphocytes into the joint. Neutrophils and macrophages ingest immune complexes and release enzymes that degrade articular cartilage and joint structures. Rheumatoid factor (RF) and possibly other autoantibodies produced locally in the synovium participate in the formation of pathogenic immune complexes.[1-4,7]

T-cells are the major infiltrating lymphocytes in the rheumatoid synovium. Many autoantigens are targeted by the immune system in RA and some autoantigens are T-cell targets. Activated T-cells proliferate, expand, and stimulate monocytes, macrophages, and synovial fibroblasts to secrete cytokines, including interleukin-1 (IL-1) and tumor necrosis factor alpha (TNF-α). Both cytokines stimulate mesenchymal cells to secrete matrix metalloproteinases that destroy cartilage and bone.

Activated T-cells stimulate B-cells to produce immunoglobulins, including RF.[1-4,7]

Venules and small blood vessels become occluded by hypertrophied endothelial cells: fibrin, platelets, and inflammatory cells. The decreased circulation along with the increased metabolic demands of hypertrophy and hyperplasia results in hypoxia and metabolic acidosis. Acidosis stimulates the release of hydrolytic enzymes from synovial cells into the surrounding tissue, causing erosion of articular cartilage as well as inflammation of ligaments and tendons.[1-4,7]

CLINICAL PRESENTATION

The onset of RA is usually insidious, occurring over a period of several weeks or months, but in 10% to 15% of patients there is an acute onset. The initial symptoms include general systemic manifestations of inflammation, weakness, weight loss, malaise, fatigue, anorexia, aching, and stiffness. Localized symptoms include painful, tender, swollen joints. Morning stiffness lasts for as long as 1 to 2 hours.[1-4,8]

The small joints of the hands, metacarpophalangeal (MCP) and proximal interphalangeal (PIP) joints, wrists and small joints of the feet, and metatarsophalangeal (MTP) joints are commonly affected initially. Joint involvement is bilateral and symmetric. The hips, knees, ankles, and shoulders may also be involved.[1-4,8]

PHYSICAL EXAMINATION

A complete medical history should be obtained in a comfortable setting. Particular attention should be paid to the location, quality, quantity, course, and alleviating factors of the patient's pain. Assessment of functional activities, activities of daily living, and instrumental activities of daily living and social support should be elicited. The patient should be evaluated for comorbid medical conditions such as hypertension, diabetes, or heart disease.[2]

Physical examination of the peripheral joints and the axial skeleton is central to the evaluation of a patient with RA. The joints should be examined in an organized manner, and report of joint pain, tenderness, degree of swelling, range of motion, and deformity should be recorded. On palpation, the inflamed joint feels warm and tender and the synovial membrane feels thickened and "boggy." The skin over the affected joint may look thin and shiny and have a ruddy color. During the joint examination the examiner should support painful or weak joints.[9]

The physical examination should include evaluation for the presence of extraarticular manifestations. Subcutaneous nodules, which are present in 20% of patients with RA, are found over pressure areas, such as the extensor surface of the elbow and other areas of trauma. Rheumatoid nodules may occasionally be found on the cardiac valves, pericardium, pleura, lung parenchyma, and spleen. Other extraarticular manifestations of RA can include signs of vasculitis (mononeuritis multiplex, skin infarcts, and ulceration), ocular signs (Sjögren's syndrome, episcleritis, and scleritis), respiratory symptoms (interstitial lung disease or pleurisy), cardiac involvement (pericarditis or valvular heart disease), and peripheral nerve entrapments.[1,2,8]

Sjögren's syndrome, seen in 0% to 30% of patients with RA, is characterized by dry eyes (keratoconjunctivitis sicca) and dry mouth (xerostomia) and is caused by immune-mediated destruction of the salivary and lacrimal glands. Felty's syndrome, an uncommon feature seen in long-standing RA, is characterized by skin ulcers, leukopenia, and increased risk for bacterial infections.[1-4,8]

DIAGNOSTICS

The diagnosis of RA is primarily based on the clinical history and physical findings. Laboratory tests, including radiographs, are used to confirm the diagnosis, exclude other conditions, and, more importantly, to predict the prognosis and develop a treatment plan for the individual patient.

Because RA can affect many organs, it is important to obtain laboratory tests at the baseline evaluation and periodically during the course of treatment. Baseline evaluation should include a CBC, acute-phase reactants, serum creatinine, hepatic panel, urinalysis, and RF. Normocytic, normochromic anemia is very common in RA. Evaluation of renal and hepatic function is necessary because many antirheumatic agents have renal and hepatic toxicity and may be contraindicated if these organs are severely impaired.

RF in RA is an IgM autoantibody that is directed against IgG antigenic determinants. Not all RA patients have a positive RF factor at the time of diagnosis, but 70% to 80% of patients will become positive during the course of disease. RA patients with high titer of RF tend to have more severe joint and extraarticular disease and worse prognosis than RF-negative patients. The titer of RF does not change rapidly with treatment, so frequent monitoring is not recommended.[1-4,8]

Acute-phase reactants are proteins that are synthesized rapidly by the liver in the presence of inflammation or tissue necrosis and include C-reactive protein (CRP), fibrinogen, complement proteins, and several other proteins. Measurement of serum concentration of CRP and erythrocyte sedimentation rate (ESR) is widely used to assess the activity of the inflammatory process in RA.[1-4,8]

Radiographs

Because the hands and feet are often involved in RA, x-ray studies of these and other affected joints establish a baseline for future evaluation of the effectiveness of treatment as well as help with the diagnosis. The radiographs of the joints and bones are often normal in early RA.[1-4,8]

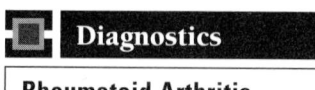

Diagnostics

Rheumatoid Arthritis

Laboratory
Erythrocyte sedimentation rate/ C-reactive protein
Rheumatoid factor
CBC and differential
BUN/creatinine
Hepatic panel (AST, ALT, and albumin)
Urinalysis
Synovial fluid analysis

Imaging
Radiography of selected involved joints

Synovial Fluid Analysis

Aspiration of an inflamed joint and examination of the synovial fluid are important to the diagnosis of RA. Normal synovial fluid is clear, viscous, and low in volume with a white cell count of <2000 cells/mm^3. In RA, the joint fluid is inflammatory with poor viscosity and a high white blood cell count of over 10,000 cells/mm^3 with a predominance of neutrophils.[1-4,8]

The American College of Rheumatology established criteria for the classification of RA that can be used as guidelines for patient diagnosis and for research classification.[8]

DIFFERENTIAL DIAGNOSIS

The differential diagnosis must consider other causes of inflammatory arthritis. Initially, systemic lupus erythematosus, psoriatic arthritis, and seronegative spondyloarthropathies (ankylosing spondylitis, reactive arthritis, enteropathic arthritis, Reiter's syndrome) may be indistinguishable from RA. Usually the presence of extraarticular manifestations of these disorders helps to establish the correct diagnosis.[1-4]

Soft tissue disorders such as fibromyalgia, a generalized pain disorder, tendonitis, bursitis, and, in older adults, polymyalgia rheumatica may confound the diagnosis of RA early in the course of the disease.

Viral infections such as human parvovirus, hepatitis viruses B and C, and HIV infection can cause symmetric polyarthritis and chronic arthralgia and should be considered in the differential diagnosis.[1-4]

MANAGEMENT

An assessment of the patient's prognosis should be made before selecting the treatment regime. Poor prognosis is suggested by early age of onset, high RF titer, elevated ESR, and swelling of more than two joints. Poor prognostic extraarticular signs are rheumatoid nodules, Sjögren's syndrome, episcleritis, scleritis, interstitial lung disease, pericardial involvement, systemic vasculitis, and Felty's syndrome.[1,2]

Nonpharmacologic Treatment

Instruction in joint protection, conservation of energy, strengthening exercises, and a range of motion program is beneficial for all RA patients. Regular participation in dynamic and aerobic conditioning exercise program improves joint symptoms, muscle strength, functional abilities, and psychologic well-being. Consultation with occupational and physical therapists for assistive and adaptive devices and education about care of joints are recommended.

Complementary and alternative therapy is of growing interest and use to RA patients. Many patients on conventional medical therapy are using acupuncture, acupressure, herbs, and other complementary modalities.[10]

Pharmacologic Therapy

Choosing a pharmacologic agent for an individual patient is based on consideration of cost, efficacy, safety, and convenience. Pharmacologic therapy often consists of a combination of nonsteroidal antiinflammatory drugs (NSAIDs), disease-modifying antirheumatic drugs (DMARDs), and/or glucocorticoids[11-13] (Table 241-1).

Nonsteroidal Antiinflammatory Drugs. The use of salicylates, NSAIDs, or selective cyclooxygenase 2 (COX-2) inhibitors to reduce joint pain and swelling and improve joint function is usually the initial drug treatment (see Table 199-1). These drugs have analgesic and antiinflammatory effects but do not alter the course of disease or prevent joint destruction. They should not be used alone as the treatment of RA.

Disease-Modifying Antirheumatic Drugs. All patients with RA are candidates for DMARD therapy. DMARDs have the potential to reduce or prevent joint damage and preserve joint integrity and function. Any RA patient taking NSAIDs with ongoing signs or symptoms of active RA such as fatigue, morning stiffness, elevated ESR, or synovitis should have DMARD therapy started promptly. Many factors influence the choice of a DMARD. Patients and their providers must select the initial DMARD based on the efficacy, ease of administration, requirements for monitoring, cost, adverse reactions, co-morbid diseases, and the prognosis of the disease. Commonly used DMARDs include methotrexate, leflunomide, hydroxychloroquine, sulfasalazine, etanercept, infliximab, and Anakinra Subcutane. Less commonly used DMARDs are gold salts, D-penicillamine, azathioprine, minocycline, and cyclosporine[11-13] (see Table 241-1).

Tumor Necrosis Factor Alpha Therapy. Biologic agents that selectively block cytokines have recently been developed for the treatment of RA. The most clinically effective anticytokine is an antagonist to TNF-α; the two medications available in the United States are etanercept and infliximab.[14]

Interleukin 1 Receptor Antagonist (IL-1Ra). IL-1 is a cytokine that has been shown to play a major role in RA synovial inflammation and joint destruction. IL-1Ra acts to block the binding of IL-1a and IL-1b to the IL-1 receptors, preventing the activation of target cells. Anakinra Subcutane, a recombinant form of IL-1Ra, has recently been approved for the treatment of RA.[15]

Glucocorticoids. Low-dose oral glucocorticoids (<10 mg prednisone daily) is highly effective in relieving symptoms in active RA. The benefits should also be weighed against adverse

Differential Diagnosis

Rheumatoid Arthritis

Fibromyalgia	Scleroderma
Osteoarthritis	Dermatomyositis polymyositis
Viral syndrome	
Soft tissue syndromes	Polymyalgia rheumatica
Spondyloarthropathies	Vasculitis
Systemic lupus erythematosus	

TABLE 241-1 DISEASE-MODIFYING ANTIRHEUMATIC DRUGS (DMARDS)

Medication	Usual Maintenance Dose
Infliximab	3 to 5 mg/kg IV every 8 weeks
Etanercept	25 mg SC 2 times a week
Anakinra Subcutane	100 mg SC once a day
Methotrexate	Oral 7.5 to 20 mg once a week SC 7.5 to 20 mg once a week
Hydroxychloroquine	200 mg twice daily
Sulfasalazine	500 to 1000 mg 2 to 3 times daily
Gold	Oral 3 mg twice daily IM 25 to 50 mg every 2 to 4 weeks

effects such as osteoporosis, hypertension, weight gain, possible hyperglycemia, cataracts, and increased skin fragility. Effectiveness of treatment should be assessed at each follow-up visit. Symptoms of inflammation indicate active disease and necessitate the need to consider changing treatment regimens. Intaarticular injection of glucocorticoids is widely used if one or two joints are actively inflamed.[1,2]

Co-Management with Specialists

The rheumatologist should provide support and consultation to the patient and his or her primary care provider. Because the level, training, and experience in the diagnosis and treatment of RA varies among primary care providers, the responsibility for diagnosis, development of a treatment plan, and monitoring of therapy should be assigned to the rheumatologist. A general maintenance plan should be developed for the patient with all health care providers participating.

LIFE SPAN CONSIDERATIONS

RA has considerable impact on quality of life. Significant work disability has been identified in patients with RA, with about one half of patients who are working at the onset of disease becoming work disabled. Direct and indirect monetary costs of RA are enormous. Pregnancy should be avoided in those RA patients taking immune-modulating medications. Patients who choose to become pregnant will experience a temporary remission is disease activity for the duration of the pregnancy. Early death has been identified in RA patients, with the life span decreased by about 10 years.[16]

COMPLICATIONS

Joint deformity with the resulting sequelae of muscle, tendon, and ligament weakening/deconditioning and joint immobilization is the most important complications. Small vessel vasculitis can cause neuropathy and skin ulcers.

Complications due to adverse reactions to medications include osteoporosis, avascular necrosis, retinal toxicity, gastrointestinal irritation and bleeding, and hepatic toxicity. Opportunistic infections may develop with the anti–TNF-α agents, systemic corticosteroids, and other immunosuppressive agents.[1-4,14]

INDICATIONS FOR REFERRAL/HOSPITALIZATION

Referral to a rheumatologist for diagnosis and treatment of RA is strongly recommended. A rheumatologist should manage medication regimens and monitor for adverse drug reactions. Referral to an orthopedic surgeon specializing in joint replacement should be considered for end-stage joint disease. Quality of life is improved and pain is relieved in most patients after joint replacement surgery. Physical and occupational therapists should be consulted for exercise programs and adaptive devices. A rheumatology nurse specialist can provide information about life style changes and community programs such as those sponsored by the Arthritis Foundation. Because most patients experience a period of grief after diagnosis, referral to a clinical psychologist or social worker should be considered. Life role adjustments will be made because of the disease, and many patients will benefit from psychologic counseling through this transition.[10,16-18]

PATIENT AND FAMILY EDUCATION

Patients should be educated about lifestyle modifications such as increased bed rest for a disease flare ups, use of adaptive aides to facilitate function, prioritizing and planning activities to accommodate fatigue, and the use of splints for painful and swollen wrists and hands. Podiatric care for foot pain should be provided, along with special shoe wear and flexible orthotic devices. Education about the need for a regular aerobic and muscle-strengthening exercise program is essential to help reduce stiffness, avoid joint contractures, and prevent osteoporosis.

Advise the patient about the benefit of warm showers in the morning as well as frequent position changes to alleviate stiffness. The use of pillows to position joints at night is contraindicated.

Education regarding medication use, restrictions, and side/adverse effects should be provided to the patient and his or her families. Warnings against stopping certain medications without notifying the provider should be stressed. Instructions should be given about dietary restrictions or recommendations as they relate to medications.[10,16-18]

Self-management programs, educational information, and exercise programs from the Arthritis Foundation are available to the patients in print form and online. Most material is available in Spanish and English.

REFERENCES

1. Harris ED Jr: Rheumatoid arthritis: pathophysiology and implications for therapy, *N Engl J Med* 322:1277-1289, 1990.
2. Klippel JH, editor: *Primer on the rheumatic diseases*, ed 11, Atlanta, 1997, Arthritis Foundation.
3. Albani S, Carson D: Rheumatoid arthritis. In Koopman WJ, editor: *Arthritis and allied conditions*, ed 13, Baltimore, 1996, Williams and Wilkins.
4. Newman S and others: *Understanding rheumatoid arthritis*, London, 1996, Routledge.
5. Silman AJ, Hochberg MC: *Epidemiology of the rheumatic diseases*, New York, 1993, Oxford University Press.
6. Allaire SL, Prashker M, Meenan R: The costs of rheumatoid arthritis, *Pharmoeconomics* 6:513-522, 1994.
7. Choy EHS, Panayi GS: Mechanisms of disease: cytokine pathways and joint inflammation in rheumatoid arthritis, *N Engl J Med* 344:907-916, 2001.
8. Arnett FC and others: The American Rheumatism Association 1987 revised criteria for the classification of rheumatoid arthritis, *Arthritis Rheum* 31:315-324, 1988.
9. Polley HF, Hunder GG: *Physical examination of the joints*, ed 2, Philadelphia, 1978, WB Saunders.
10. Affleck G and others: Appraisals of control and predictability in adapting to chronic disease, *J Personal Soc Psychol* 53:273-279, 1987
11. van der Heijde DW and others. The effectiveness of early treatment with "second-line" antirheumatic drugs: a randomized, controlled trial, *Ann Intern Med* 124:699-707, 1996.
12. Tsakonas E and others: Consequences of delayed therapy with second-line agents in rheumatoid arthritis: a 3-year follow-up on the Hydroxychloroquine in Early Rheumatoid Arthritis (HERA) study, *J Rheumatol* 27:623-629, 2000
13. Albers JM and others: Treatment strategy, disease activity, and outcome in four cohorts of patients with early rheumatoid arthritis, *Ann Rheum Dis* 60:453-458, 2001.
14. Weinblatt ME and others: A trial of etanercept, a recombinant tumor necrosis factor receptor: Fc fusion protein, in patients with rheumatoid arthritis receiving methotrexate, *N Engl J Med* 340:253-259, 1999.

15. Jiang Y and others: A multicenter, double-blind, dose-ranging, randomized, placebo-controlled study of recombinant human interleukin-1 receptor antagonist in patients with rheumatoid arthritis, *Arthritis Rheum* 43:1001-1009, 2000
16. Schiaffino KM, Revenson TA, Gibofsky A: Assessing the impact of self-efficacy beliefs of adaptation to rheumatoid arthritis, *Arthritis Care Res* 4:150-157, 1991.
17. Komatireddy GR and others: Efficacy of low resistance muscle training in patients with rheumatoid arthritis functional class II and III, *J Rheumatol* 24:1531-1539, 1997.
18. Neuberger GB and others: Effects of exercise on fatigue, aerobic fitness, and disease activity measures with rheumatoid arthritis, *Res Nurs Health* 20:195-204, 1997.

CHAPTER 242

Systemic Lupus Erythematosus

Francisco P. Quismorio and Dorothy Johnson

DEFINITION/EPIDEMIOLOGY

Systemic lupus erythematosus (SLE) is a chronic multisystemic inflammatory rheumatic disease that may cause diverse symptoms such as fatigue, joint pain, skin rashes, seizures, edema, and chest pain.[1,2] SLE has a propensity to affect women, particularly during the prime childbearing years of 15 to 35. The pathognomonic feature of SLE is the formation of autoantibodies, including antibodies to DNA. SLE can damage many organ systems, notably the joints, kidneys, lungs, and brain, and may result in severe disability and even death.

The disease is relatively uncommon, with incidence and prevalence rates that are difficult to estimate with great precision. These rates vary by geographic distribution and by demographic characteristics. Data from European and American surveys suggest that the prevalence of SLE among whites ranges from 12 to 39 per 100,000 persons.[3] The reported incidence rates of SLE in the United States also vary from 1.8 to 7.6 cases per 100,000 persons per year. SLE is up to 10 times more common in women than in men.[3] The disease is substantially more common among African-American women, among whom the prevalence may be as high as 1:250. In addition, African-American patients with SLE are more prone to experience severe damage.[4] Recent epidemiologic data suggest that the incidence of the disease may be increasing.[5]

The cause of SLE is unknown.[1,2] Its association with certain genotypes such as the *C4* null allele and various HLA haplotypes, as well as the 25% rate of concordance in identical twins, suggests that the disease is likely to be a result of an interaction between genetic makeup and one or more environmental triggers. Because certain drugs may produce SLE-like syndromes, it is speculated that certain environmental chemicals might promote the development of this autoimmune disease. An amino acid, L-canavanine, which is found in alfalfa sprouts, has been associated with the development of an SLE-like disease in macaque monkeys; this, together with reports of exacerbation in patients with established disease, suggests that dietary factors may contribute to SLE development. Other potential environmental triggers include a wide range of viruses including the Epstein-Barr virus,[6] physical trauma, and emotional stress. Differences in estrogen metabolism in women with SLE may also play a significant role in the disease.

PATHOPHYSIOLOGY

The pathophysiologic hallmark of SLE is the development of antibodies directed against components of "self" tissues, particularly structures found within cell nuclei. The first laboratory diagnostic test for the disease was described in 1948 by Hargraves and was predicated on the presence of antinuclear antibodies (ANAs) (the LE cell preparation).[1] Since then, a wide variety of autoantibodies have been described in SLE, including antibodies directed against DNA and other nuclear constituents, platelets, white blood cells, and phospholipids. The latter are a group of molecules found in cell membranes. Associated with these autoimmune phenomena is the presence of increased circulating immune complexes, which are widely deposited in the skin, basement membranes, and kidneys. These complexes are normally solubilized and cleared from the circulation by the kidneys. The reason these immune complexes fail to clear in SLE is unclear but may be related to a functional deficiency in components of the complement system resulting in failure of solubilization of immune complexes. Patients with genetic deficiencies of the early complement components C1, C2, and C4 are at an increased risk for lupus-like autoimmune disease. The reasons for autoantibody development are also unclear but may relate to defective apoptosis (programmed cell death) and failure of normal mechanisms that promote immune self-tolerance.

The deposition of immune complexes in tissues generates a local inflammatory response that may have organ-specific effects. For example, inflammation in blood vessels causes vasculitis, which may result in ischemia or infarction due to vessel occlusion. Inflammation in serosal surfaces (visceral membrane linings) may cause pleurisy or pericarditis. Immune complex deposition in the kidneys in SLE is associated with the development of glomerulonephritis.

CLINICAL PRESENTATION AND PHYSICAL EXAMINATION

SLE is a systemic inflammatory disorder characterized by relapses, remissions, and varied presentations. It can develop acutely, with obvious severe manifestations that include arthritis, nephritis, or vasculitis, or it may become apparent in an individual who has had subtle symptoms (e.g., fatigue, arthralgia, skin rashes) sporadically for many years. The facts that many of the symptoms are nonspecific (e.g., oral ulcers, arthritis) and that the ANA test is positive in approximately 5% of healthy persons lead to a tendency to overdiagnose the disorder. The American College of Rheumatology has developed and validated a set of criteria for the classification of SLE[7] (Table 242-1).

Malaise and fatigue, often profound, are common but nonspecific complaints of patients with SLE. Anorexia and weight loss may be seen in those with active disease, as may fevers, lymphadenopathy, tachycardia, and anemia.

The malar, or butterfly, rash is one of the most recognizable features of SLE, but it is observed in only 35% of patients. This is an erythematous rash on the cheeks and forehead in a sun-exposed distribution that tends to spare the nasolabial folds. Discoid rash is seen in 20% of patients with SLE. There is also a more benign form of lupus termed *discoid lupus*, in which there are no manifestations other than skin rash. Discoid lesions are thick plaques that often heal with scarring, atrophy, depigmentation, and loss of hair. Mucous membrane ulcerations are also common, occurring in the oral and nasal cavities.

Approximately one third of patients with SLE experience Raynaud's phenomenon, a syndrome characterized by episodic changes in blood flow to the extremities, accompanied by color change and often unpleasant tingling sensations (see Chapter 240). Livedo reticularis is a red mottling or lacelike appearance under the skin. Cutaneous vasculitis may manifest as erythema around the nail beds, tender skin nodules, splinter hemorrhages, or palpable purpura. Bruising or petechiae may also occur, reflecting thrombocytopenia. These manifestations are often associated with an antibody to phospholipid.

Joint pains occur in 80% to 90% of patients with SLE, and inflammatory arthritis can be objectively documented in about 50% of patients. The arthritis of SLE is nonerosive and progresses to deformity in only about 10% of patients. Osteoporosis is common in SLE as a result of a combination of steroid therapy, chronic inflammation, and inactivity. In those patients with renal insufficiency, metabolic bone disease related to vitamin D deficiency and secondary hyperparathyroidism may be a contributing factor. Inflammatory myositis is also occasionally seen in patients with SLE.

Chest pain is common in SLE and often commonly represents musculoskeletal pain. More significantly, SLE can cause serious cardiopulmonary disease, including pleurisy, pericarditis, pneumonitis, interstitial lung disease, pulmonary hemorrhage, and, occasionally, pulmonary stenosis. In addition, patients with SLE, particularly those with antiphospholipid antibodies, are hypercoagulable and at an increased risk for pulmonary embolism and resulting pulmonary hypertension. Patients with antiphospholipid antibodies are at an increased risk for valvular heart disease and Libman Sacks endocarditis and therefore are more susceptible to the development of bacterial endocarditis should they be bacteremic. SLE may also involve the myocardium, coronary arteries, and endocardium. Patients with SLE are at a greatly increased risk of the development of ischemic heart disease.[8] It has been reported that patients with SLE in the age range of 35 to 44 years have a 50-fold increased risk for myocardial infarction.[9] The full reasons for this are unclear but may relate in part to the long-term use of corticosteroids, to alterations in lipid metabolism related to changes in the endothelium, and to nephrotic syndrome; and to the sequelae of chronic inflammatory processes.[10] Hypertension is quite common in SLE, with underlying renal disease and the use of nonsteroidal antiinflammatory drugs (NSAIDs) and corticosteroids all contributing factors.

Mood change, depression, and migraine headaches are all common in SLE. SLE can also cause wide-ranging neurologic problems, the most common being cognitive dysfunction but also including psychosis, seizures, altered consciousness, stroke, and peripheral neuropathies. The effects of SLE on the brain have traditionally been attributed to inflammation in cerebral blood vessels, but recently it has been appreciated that many events may also be due to thrombosis associated with antiphospholipid antibodies.

Renal involvement is present in 25% to 50% of patients with SLE. Persistent proteinuria of more than 500 mg/day or cellular casts are observed. Glomerulonephritis occurs as a result of a deposition of immune complexes and complement components in the kidney. There is a spectrum of renal involvement ranging from mesangial disease with abnormalities of increased cellularity and deposition of immune complexes limited to the mesangium to severe diffuse proliferative glomerulonephritis with global involvement of all glomeruli. Evaluation and staging of renal disease in SLE often require a kidney biopsy, and the biopsy findings are helpful prognostically as well as in outlining further therapy. Kidney transplantation sometimes becomes necessary. Patients with SLE generally do well after

TABLE 242-1 Revised Criteria for the Classification of Systemic Lupus Erythematosus*

Criterion	Definition
1. Malar rash	Fixed erythema, flat or raised, over the malar eminences, tending to spare the nasolabial folds
2. Discoid rash	Erythematous raised patches with adherent keratotic scaling and follicular plugging; atrophic scarring may occur in older lesions
3. Photosensitivity	Skin rash as a result of unusual reaction to sunlight, by patient or physician observation
4. Oral ulcers	Oral or nasopharyngeal ulceration, usually painless, observed by a physician
5. Arthritis	Nonerosive arthritis involving two or more peripheral joints, characterized by tenderness, swelling, or effusion
6. Serositis	a. Pleuritis—convincing history of pleuritic pain or rub heard by a physician or evidence of pleural effusion *or* b. Pericarditis—documented by ECG or rub or evidence of pericardial effusion
7. Renal disorder	a. Persistent proteinuria greater than 0.5 g/day or greater than 3+ if quantitation not performed *or* b. Cellular casts—may be red cell, hemoglobin, granular, tubular, or mixed
8. Neurologic disorder	a. Seizures—in the absence of offending drugs or known metabolic derangements; e.g., uremia, ketoacidosis, or electrolyte imbalance *or* b. Psychosis—in the absence of offending drugs or known metabolic derangements; e.g., uremia, ketoacidosis, or electrolyte imbalance
9. Hematologic disorder	a. Hemolytic anemia—with reticulocytosis *or* b. Leukopenia—less than 4000/mm^3 total on two or more occasions *or* c. Lymphopenia—less than 1500/mm^3 on two or more occasions *or* d. Thrombocytopenia—less than 100,000/mm^3 in the absence of offending drugs
10. Immunologic disorder	a. Positive LE cell preparation *or* b. Anti-DNA: antibody to native DNA in abnormal titer *or* c. Anti-Sm: presence of antibody to Sm nuclear antigen *or* d. False-positive serologic test for syphilis known to be positive for at least 6 months and confirmed by *Treponema pallidum* immobilization or fluorescent treponemal antibody absorption test
11. Antinuclear antibody	An abnormal titer of antinuclear antibody by immunofluorescence or an equivalent assay at any point in time and in the absence of drugs known to be associated with "drug-induced lupus" syndrome

From Tan EM and others: The 1982 revised criteria for the classification of systemic lupus erythematosus (SLE), *Arthritis Rheum* 25:1271-1277, 1982.

*The proposed classification is based on 11 criteria. For the purpose of identifying patients in clinical studies, a person shall be said to have systemic lupus erythematosus if any four or more of the 11 criteria are present, serially or simultaneously, during any interval of observation.

transplantation because of the immunosuppression required for preventing rejection. Lupus nephritis recurs at a rate of approximately 6% in the transplanted kidney.

DIAGNOSTICS

During an exacerbation of SLE, laboratory tests reveal nonspecific evidence of systemic inflammation with an elevated erythrocyte sedimentation rate (ESR), plasma viscosity or C-reactive protein, and raised gamma globulins.[1,2] Anemia is common in SLE and may result from many factors, including iron deficiency, chronic systemic inflammation causing an anemia of chronic disease, autoimmune hemolysis with a positive Coombs antibody and, in patients with renal insufficiency, inadequate erythropoietin. Leukopenia, lymphopenia, and thrombocytopenia are also features of the disease and appear to be caused by autoantibodies. Indeed, idiopathic thrombocytopenia purpura may be the presenting manifestation of lupus. Patients with antiphospholipid antibodies are often thrombocytopenic.

A urinalysis should always be obtained both during a flare and to monitor the disease because patients who have not had previous kidney involvement can develop it de novo. BUN and creatinine should be monitored for change indicating new renal involvement or worsening renal function.

Although the ANA test is the most sensitive diagnostic test for lupus, it is not specific. The autoantibodies anti-Smith (anti-Sm) and anti–double-stranded DNA (anti-dsDNA) are more specific for the diagnosis of lupus.[7] Other autoantibodies such as anti-Ro and anti-La (also known as SSA [Sjögren's syndrome A] and SSB [Sjögren's syndrome B]) can be observed in patients with SLE and are often associated with subacute cutaneous lupus, secondary Sjögren's syndrome, and neonatal lupus. Patients with lupus often have antibodies that react with phospholipids. These autoantibodies can produce a false-positive

Diagnostics

Systemic Lupus Erythematosus

Laboratory	
Urinalysis	C-reactive proteins
CBC and differential	ANA
BUN	Anti-ds-DNA, anti-Sm
Creatinine	CH_{50}, C3, C4*
ESR	PT/PTT*
Rheumatoid factor	Lupus anticoagulant*

*If indicated.

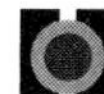

Differential Diagnosis

Systemic Lupus Erythematosus

Fibromyalgia	Polymyositis
Mixed connective tissue disease	Mixed corrective tissue disease
Rheumatoid arthritis	Drug-induced lupus
Dermatomyositis polymyositis	Multiple sclerosis
Primary Sjögren's syndrome	Drug-induced lupus
Systemic sclerosis	Psychiatric disorder

test for syphilis using the screening tests RPR or VDRL. However, the presence of syphilis can be determined in a patient with lupus by using of a more specific test for syphilis. There are several other tests that measure the presence of antibodies directed against phospholipid; these tests include assays for anticardiolipin antibodies, the so-called lupus anticoagulant test that measures a prolonged partial thromboplastin time (PTT), and the most sensitive currently available test, the diluted Russell venom viper time (DRVVT). Other autoantibodies that may be positive in patients with lupus include rheumatoid factors and antibody to ribonucleoprotein (RNP).

In contrast to other inflammatory disorders, complement levels may be reduced, indicating the deposition of immune complexes in tissues. In many patients with lupus, falls in complement levels, in particular C3, are associated with flares of nephritis. Complement can be consumed in lupus in inflammation of other tissues, including the skin. In patients with lupus, a biopsy of normal-appearing skin can show confluent immunofluorescence at the dermal-epidermal junction when stained with at least three of the following five proteins: IgG, IgM, IgA, C3, or fibrinogen (the so-called lupus band test).

DIFFERENTIAL DIAGNOSIS

SLE may be confused with a number of other disorders, particularly other autoimmune rheumatic diseases, including rheumatoid arthritis, primary Sjögren's syndrome, systemic sclerosis, mixed connective tissue disease, and polymyositis, as well as fibromyalgia, multiple sclerosis, and other conditions. Persons with fibromyalgia who happen to have a borderline positive ANA test are especially likely to be misdiagnosed as having SLE. Acute parvovirus arthropathy can mimic lupus and serologic tests can be positive.[11] Drug-induced lupus can also be caused by a number of commonly prescribed medications, including interferon alpha, quinidine, isoniazid, hydralazine, procainamide, minocycline, and others.

MANAGEMENT

Individuals diagnosed with SLE require guidance and education about the disease.[1] Avoidance of strong sunlight is often emphasized because photosensitivity and exacerbation of disease activity by sun exposure are common. Patients should be encouraged to use sunscreens with a sun protection factor (SPF) of at least 15 or sun protective clothing to avoid excessive sun exposure. In a few documented cases, exposure to unshielded fluorescent lighting has exacerbated disease activity. Modest physical exercise is considered to be helpful in maintaining cardiopulmonary fitness, avoiding obesity, and improving mood. Diet is important and often overlooked. Studies in mice with lupus-like syndromes show that diets enriched with fish oil–derived fatty acids protect mice from the development of glomerulonephritis, whereas mice fed diets enriched with lipids derived from beef tallow have an accelerated disease process.[12] Although this has not been confirmed in patients with lupus, the frequent occurrence of lipid abnormalities and the accelerated atherosclerosis in the lupus population suggest that avoidance of diets high in saturated fats is reasonable. Due to the frequent occurrence of osteoporosis in these patients, attention should be paid to ensuring adequate calcium and vitamin D in the patient's diet.

Regular health checkups with other specialties are important in the patient with lupus. Regular gynecologic care assumes an increased importance in this patient population, with recent studies showing an increased incidence of cervical dysplasia.[13] Obviously the issues regarding pregnancy and hormone replacement are complex in these patients and require communication among obstetrician/gynecologist, rheumatologist, and primary care provider. The patient with SLE will need dental consultation with attention to the need for antibiotic prophylaxis given the increased risk for infective endocarditis.[14] Where secondary Sjögren's syndrome is present, accelerated problems with caries and gingivitis are often seen. Ophthalmologic monitoring is important both to detect the appearance of dry eye caused by secondary Sjögren's syndrome and to monitor for ophthalmologic side effects of hydroxychloroquine (Plaquenil) and corticosteroids.

NSAIDs are often used for the treatment of pain, particularly joint pain, fevers, and serositis. However, careful monitoring for NSAID toxicity is suggested. Salicylate hepatitis can be seen in patients with SLE. There is an unusual syndrome of aseptic meningitis occurring after ibuprofen use that has been reported in SLE. In addition, all NSAIDs, including the newer cyclooxygenase-2 (COX-2) selective NSAIDs, have effects on the kidneys that can exacerbate hypertension, edema, and renal insufficiency in patients with SLE and renal involvement. Hydroxychloroquine is also widely used and is effective in managing the musculoskeletal, cutaneous, cognitive, and serosal aspects of the disease (Table 242-2). It has been shown to be more effective than placebo in allowing tapering of steroids and reducing flares of disease.[15]

Corticosteroids remain the mainstay of treatment for serious SLE. For discoid skin involvement, treatment with local corticosteroid cream, ointment, or injection is often helpful.

TABLE 242-2 Drugs Used in the Treatment of Systemic Lupus Erythematosus and Dosing Schedules

Drug	Dosage	Length of Treatment
Hydroxychloroquine	200 mg q day to b.i.d.	Long term
Chloroquine	250 mg q day	Long term
Prednisone (mild disease)	5-10 mg q day	Intermittent courses
Prednisone (organ-threatening disease)	20-30 mg q day	Intermittent courses
Azathioprine	75-150 mg q day	6 months to several years
Cyclophosphamide (oral)	1-4 mg/kg q day	6 months to a few years
Cyclophosphamide (IV)	0.5-1 g/m^2 monthly for 6 months	
Methotrexate (with folic acid, 1 mg q day)	7.5-15 mg q week	6 months to years

For patients with joint pain, fatigue, and more minor degrees of disease who have failed to respond to hydroxychloroquine, low-dose corticosteroids (less than 10 mg/day) may improve the quality of life. For the patient with major organ involvement (pericarditis, thrombocytopenia, autoimmune hemolytic anemia, nephritis, central nervous system lupus), corticosteroids are given in higher doses: either 40 to 60 mg/day or "pulse" therapy of 1 g methylprednisolone IV every day for 3 days. After the initial active disease begins to come under control, a variety of immunosuppressive agents have been used to control disease and allow tapering of corticosteroids (steroid sparing). The choice of immunosuppressive depends on the manifestation involved. For renal involvement, studies have shown that the combination of intravenous cyclophosphamide and prednisone is associated with better renal outcome than prednisone alone.[16] More recently mycophenolate mofetil (CellCept) has shown some short-term efficacy in lupus nephritis.[17] For patients with severe arthritis, methotrexate and, more recently, leflunomide (Arava) have been used. Azathioprine (Imuran) has shown efficacy in both renal and nonrenal lupus.

The treatment of the patient with an antiphospholipid antibody remains controversial.[18] Clearly the patient who has experienced recurrent thrombosis or a major thrombotic event such as a pulmonary embolism or stroke in the setting of SLE with an antiphospholipid antibody should be treated with anticoagulation. Studies suggest that these patients need to maintain anticoagulation in the high therapeutic range. The patient with SLE, an antiphospholipid antibody, and recurrent miscarriage should be treated with low-dose aspirin and subcutaneous heparin or low-molecular-weight heparin in future pregnancies.[19] Many rheumatologists recommend that patients with SLE who have an antiphospholipid antibody take low-dose aspirin daily even if they have not had a thrombotic event.

Patients with SLE who are at risk for osteoporosis require attention to bone health. Osteoporosis prophylaxis with calcium supplementation and vitamin D is appropriate. Measurement of bone density and implementation of osteoporosis therapy such as bisphosphonates or calcitonin may be required. Avoidance of high doses or corticosteroids and use of steroid-sparing immunosuppressives may help limit steroid-induced bone loss. Estrogens, on the other hand, should be used with caution because they may exacerbate disease activity in some patients and exacerbate thrombotic tendencies in these patients.

Optimal control of blood pressure is important because patients with SLE are at increased risk for cardiovascular disease. High blood pressure increases the risk of kidney involvement or may result from kidney involvement. Corticosteroids contribute to hypertension. Patients with Raynaud's syndrome may benefit from the use of calcium channel blockers such as nifedipine or angiotensin receptor blockers such as losartan.[20]

Many persons with SLE have difficulty maintaining employment and household work roles.[21] Use of the Americans with Disabilities Act to obtain flexible work hours, placement of filters on fluorescent lights, or other accommodations may preserve employment or enhance productivity. Methods of reducing the amount of energy expended in commuting, in doing household work, and in maintaining social activities should be explored. Women can be encouraged to adopt a manager rather than "doer" homemaker role; family counseling may help members manage family role changes necessitated by the disease.[21]

The level of social support has been linked to health status, and studies have shown that persons with rheumatic diseases with higher levels of social support have better function.[21] Telephone counseling programs have been effective in reducing feelings of depression and anxiety, as well as in improving function and providing support.[22,23] Some patients will benefit from treatment with antidepressant medications.

Influenza vaccines should be administered yearly. Consideration for the administration of pneumococcal vaccine should be given to all patients with lupus given evidence for splenic dysfunction in these patients. As mentioned previously, patients with lupus are at increased risk for infective endocarditis and therefore should receive antibiotic prophylaxis while undergoing dental, genitourinary, and other invasive procedures.[1]

LIFE SPAN CONSIDERATIONS

The prognosis for patients with SLE has improved dramatically since its first description, when the disease was universally fatal. At the present, more than 90% of patients with SLE live 10 years after the onset of symptoms, although the survival rate for those with organ-threatening disease is somewhat lower.[1,2] Certain subsets of the population appear to experience worse disease. African-Americans generally have more severe disease and a poor prognosis.[4] The reasons for this are unclear but may relate, in part, to socioeconomic factors and reduced access to health care.

Pregnancy may be problematic for both the mother and the fetus, especially for women with antiphospholipid antibodies.[1] Patients with SLE have increased fetal losses and are at increased risk for preeclampsia and premature rupture of membranes resulting in prematurity, intrauterine growth retardation, and pregnancy loss. Maternal risks include disease flares during pregnancy, exacerbation of preexistent hypertension, worsening of renal status, and pulmonary embolism. Both prednisone and methylprednisolone can be safely used in pregnancy because they are inactivated by placental enzymes and do not affect the fetus. However, pregnancy-induced diabetes or hypertension can have effects on fetal well-being. The presence of anti-Ro antibody (SSA) during pregnancy is associated with an increased risk for neonatal lupus, in particular, congenital heart block. In such patients, monitoring of fetal heart rate during the second trimester is critical. Treatment of the maternal-fetal dyad in such patients with dexamethasone (which does cross the placenta) and sometimes plasmapheresis to remove the autoantibody has been reported to reverse this syndrome. In the patient with repeated fetal loss associated with an antiphospholipid antibody, subcutaneous heparin and low-dose aspirin improve pregnancy outcome.[19]

In the patient who wishes to avoid pregnancy, birth control methods should be used by women at least during disease exacerbations, especially in those with nephritis and in those taking hydroxychloroquine, methotrexate, leflunomide, or cyclophosphamide. Both injectable Depo-Provera and progesterone-only minipills can be safely used by patients with lupus, as can barrier methods. Anecdotal experience suggests that estrogen-containing oral contraceptives may exacerbate lupus.

As young women with lupus live longer, the issue of hormone replacement at menopause becomes one of increasing concern. Current studies are pending to determine whether hormone replacement at menopause exacerbates lupus. Certainly in the patient with an anticardiolipin antibody, both estrogen and the selective estrogen receptor–modulating drug raloxifene seem to be contraindicated because of their association with hypercoagulability and venous thrombosis.

COMPLICATIONS

Fever in the patient with SLE always raises the question of whether the fever represents a flare of the underlying illness or an infectious process. Fever in these patients should be considered infectious. In particular, fever in the absence of other signs of active SLE and fever associated with leukocytosis should prompt extensive culture and search for infection. In the patient with lupus who is on corticosteroids and immunosuppressants, opportunistic organisms such as *Listeria monocytogenes, Pneumocystitis carinii, Cryptococcus neoformans,* and others should be considered. Tuberculosis remains a pathogen in these patients. Fever with digital infarcts and joint pain could represent a flare of lupus but could also be caused by infective endocarditis. In evaluating these patients, microbiologic cultures of blood, urine, cerebrospinal fluid, sputum if available, and other fluids should be done.

Previous sections have discussed some of the complications of lupus, including renal disease and renal failure, deep vein thrombosis and pulmonary embolism, stroke, coronary artery disease, and osteoporosis. Many of these complications are accelerated or worsened by corticosteroids. In particular, aseptic necrosis of bone is an unfortunate complication, and whereas it can be seen in lupus patients not treated with corticosteroids, it is much more common in the steroid-treated patient.

The use of immunosuppressives to limit corticosteroid-induced side effects is practiced by many rheumatologists. However, these agents have toxicities of their own. Of note, cyclophosphamide is associated with sustained amenorrhea and premature ovarian failure, particularly in the patient who is older than 30 years.[24]

Common causes of death from SLE are complications of infections, renal disease and its sequelae, premature atherosclerotic heart disease, thromboembolic events, central nervous system vasculitis, and suicide. It has been suggested that early death results from complications of active disease, whereas later deaths are the results of complications of therapy.

INDICATIONS FOR REFERRAL/HOSPITALIZATION

Patients with SLE should be referred at diagnosis for several reasons. Confirmation of the diagnosis of this serious illness is important because it is a life-altering disease. Even patients with relatively mild or even asymptomatic lupus require periodic assessment of disease severity and activity, an evaluation best performed by a physician familiar with lupus. Given the myriad of choices for management in this disease, rheumatologic involvement in the patient's care is important even in mild disease. In uncontrolled disease with life-threatening organ involvement and in special complications such as pregnancy and the antiphospholipid antibody syndrome, management by a rheumatologist is in the patient's best interest. Obviously other specialists, such as a dermatologist, an ophthalmologist, a high-risk obstetrician, a nephrologist, a cardiologist, an orthopedic surgeon, and a hematologist, are often consulted to manage their specific organ problems. Psychiatric or psychologic consultation may assist the patient in dealing with the lifestyle changes wrought by this illness and managing depression. An occupational therapist should design and teach methods of conserving energy and prescribe appropriate assistive technology.[25] A physical therapist should be consulted to design an appropriate exercise regimen. Nutrition counseling is indicated for those patients with obesity, diabetes, hyperlipidemia, or renal insufficiency.

PATIENT AND FAMILY EDUCATION

As with any chronic disease, patient education is essential to enable persons with SLE to skillfully self-manage the disease on a day-to-day basis. Medication management; engaging in appropriate, disease-relevant health habits; and self-monitoring activities should be encouraged. Lower socioeconomic status is associated with poorer outcome in SLE, in part because of less adherence to complex treatment regimens and self-monitoring actions, as well as a greater sense of learned helplessness.[4] These conditions can be influenced by educational programs.

The SLE Self-Help course, a group education and support program, has been developed to assist persons with disease-related self-management activities. Course evaluation has indicated improved feelings of self-worth and self-efficacy, increased enabling skills, and lowered uncertainty and depression, in addition to increased knowledge about the disease.[26] Recent changes have made the course more relevant to persons of Hispanic origin.[27] The course is available through chapters of either the Arthritis Foundation (800-283-7800) or the Lupus Foundation of America (301-670-9292; 800-558-0121; Spanish: 800-558-0231).

REFERENCES

1. Klippel JH, editor: *Primer on the rheumatic diseases,* ed 11, Atlanta, 1997, Arthritis Foundation.
2. Wallace D, Metzger A: Systemic lupus erythematosus. In Koopman WJ, editor: *Arthritis and allied conditions,* ed 13, Baltimore, 1997, Williams & Wilkins.
3. Silman AJ, Hochberg MC: *Epidemiology of the rheumatic diseases,* New York, 1993, Oxford Press.
4. Liang MH and others: Strategies for reducing excess morbidity and mortality in blacks with systemic lupus erythematosus, *Arthritis Rheum* 34:1187-1196, 1991.
5. Uramoto KM and other: Trends in the incidence and mortality of systemic lupus erythematosus 1950-1992, *Arthritis Rheum* 42:46-50, 1999.
6. James JA and others: Systemic lupus erythematosus in adults is associated with previous Epstein-Barr virus exposure, *Arthritis Rheum* 44:1122-1126, 2001.
7. Tan EM and others: The 1982 revised criteria for the classification of systemic lupus erythematosus, *Arthritis Rheum* 25:1271-1277, 1982,
8. Ward MM: Premature morbidity from cardiovascular and cerebrovascular diseases in women with systemic lupus erythematosus, *Arthritis Rheum* 42:338-346, 1999.
9. Manzi S and others: Age-specific incidence rates of myocardial infarction and angina in women with systemic lupus erythematosus: comparison with the Framingham Study, *Am J Epidemiol* 145:408-415, 1997.
10. Petri M and others: Risk factors for coronary artery disease in patients with systemic lupus erythematosus, *Am J Med* 93:513-519, 1992.
11. Trapani S, Ermini M, Falcini F: Human parvovirus B19 infection: its relationship with systemic lupus erythematosus, *Semin Arthritis Rheum* 28:319-325, 1999.
12. Prickett JD, Robinson DR, Steinberg AD: Dietary enrichment with the polyunsaturated fatty acid eicosapentaenoic acid prevents proteinuria and prolongs survival in NZB x NZW F1 mice, *J Clin Invest* 68:556-559, 1981.
13. Dhar JP and others: Abnormal cervicovaginal cytology in women with lupus: a retrospective cohort study, *Gynecol Oncol* 82:4-6, 2001.
14. Miller CS and other: Prevalence of infective endocarditis in patients with systemic lupus erythematosus, *J Am Dental Assoc* 130:387-392, 1999.
15. Anonymous: A randomized study of the effect of withdrawing hydroxychloroquine sulfate in systemic lupus erythematosus. The Canadian Hydroxychloroquine Study Group, *N Engl J Med* 324:150-154, 1991.
16. Austin HA 3rd and others: Therapy of lupus nephritis. Controlled trial of prednisone and cytotoxic drugs, *N Engl J Med* 314:614-619, 1986.
17. Chan TM and others: Efficacyof mycophenolate mofetil in patients with diffuse proliferative lupus nephritis. Hong Kong-Guangzhou Nephrology Study Group, *N Engl J Med* 343:1156-1162, 2000.
18. Ruiz-Irastorza G, Khamashta MA, Hughes GR: Antiaggregant and anticoagulant therapy in systemic lupus erythematosus and Hughes' syndrome, *Lupus* 10:241-245, 2001.
19. Cowchock FS and others: Repeated fetal losses associated with antiphospholipid antibodies: a collaborative randomized trial comparing prednisone with low dose heparin treatment, *Am J Obstet Gynecol* 166:1318-1323, 1992.
20. Dziadzio M and others: Losartan therapy for Raynaud's phenomenon and scleroderma: clinical and biochemical findings in a fifteen-week, randomized, parallel-group, controlled trial. *Arthritis Rheum* 42:2646-2655, 1999.
21. Allaire S: Employment and household work disability in women with rheumatoid arthritis, *J Appl Rehabil Couns* 23:44-51, 1992.
22. Horton R and others: Users evaluate Lupusline, a telephone peer counseling service, *Arthritis Care Res* 10:257-263, 1997.
23. Austin JS and others: Health outcome improvements in patients with systemic lupus erythematosus using two telephone counseling interventions, *Arthritis Care Res* 9:391-399, 1996.
24. Boumpas DT and others: Risk for sustained amenorrhea in patients with systemic lupus erythematosus receiving intermittent pulse cyclophosphamide therapy. *Ann Intern Med* 119:366-369, 1993.
25. Wegener ST and others, editors: *Clinical care in the rheumatic diseases,* Atlanta, 1996, American College of Rheumatology.
26. Braden CJ: Patterns of change over time in learned response to chronic illness among participants in a Systemic Lupus Erythematosus Self-Help course, *Arthritis Care Res* 4:158-167, 1991.
27. Robbins L, Allegrante JP, Paget SA: Adapting the Systemic Lupus Erythematosus Self-Help (SLESH) course for Latino SLE patients, *Arthritis Care Res* 6:97-103, 1993.

CHAPTER 243

Systemic Sclerosis (Scleroderma)

Bonnie L. Bermas

DEFINITION/EPIDEMIOLOGY

Scleroderma, or progressive systemic sclerosis (SSc), is a family of connective tissue disorders characterized by skin thickening, fibrosis, and vascular changes. These disorders can be further subclassified as progressive SSc, limited and diffuse; localized SSc; linear morphea and generalized morphea; and SSc sine SSc.[1] SSc is a relatively rare disorder affecting 1 or 2 new patients per 100,000 per year. The female/male ratio is 3:1, and the peak age of onset is in the fourth to seventh decade of life.[2] Genetics may play a role, as evidenced by familial clustering and the association of this disorder with the HLA haplotypes DR1, DR3, and DR5.[3]

The various forms of SSc, with the exception of SSc sine SSc, are unified by their skin abnormalities. In general, thickened fibrotic skin appears shiny and is smooth to the touch. On skin biopsy a decreased number of capillaries is seen, along with tissue ischemia, subintimal fibrosis, and increased collagen deposition. Both localized and systemic sclerosis have skin involvement, but only the systemic types affect the internal organs as well.[1]

PATHOPHYSIOLOGY

Fibrosis of the skin and other organs, including blood vessels, is the hallmark of SSc. The pathophysiology of SSc is a vascular lesion involving the tiny arterioles and capillaries. Endothelial abnormalities, as well as proliferation of the intima, characterize these lesions. This widespread disorder of the microvasculature eventually results in the unregulated fibrosis. When the vessels involved are present in vital organs, serious damage results. Although the etiology of the vascular lesion is poorly understood, it is believed that the immune system contributes substantially to the process. One proposed model is that a susceptible host (usually a middle-aged woman) develops illness as a response to external events (environmental toxins). These external events or stimuli remain unidentified and may be different in each individual. Early in the disease there is immune system activation, endothelial cell activation, and damage that results in fibroblast activation and end-stage pathology, including obliterative vasculopathy and fibrosis.[4]

CLINICAL PRESENTATION

SSc is a chronic multisystem disease. Initial symptoms are nonspecific and may include Raynaud's phenomenon, fatigue, and joint pain. The first specific clue to the diagnosis is skin thickening, which presents as skin puffiness of the fingers and hands.

Localized Scleroderma

There are three forms of localized SSc: (1) linear SSc, (2) morphea, and (3) generalized morphea.[5] Linear SSc preferentially affects individuals under the age of 25. The thickened skin occurs in a band or ribbonlike lesion, and the underlying subcutaneous tissues and muscle can be involved. Occasionally these lesions can cross a joint line. When this occurs, growth abnormalities and severe deformities can occur. Facial lesions can cause a scarring indentation that looks like it resulted from a knife wound—hence the name, *en coup de sabre*. Most patients with localized SSc have no internal organ involvement.

The term *morphea* refers to patches of thickened hyperpigmented or hypopigmented skin, which can occur anywhere on the body. The trunk is the most common site involved. When the patches are more widespread, the disorder is referred to as generalized morphea. The subcutaneous tissues are rarely involved.

Systemic Sclerosis

SSc is defined as more widespread skin thickening with internal organ involvement. There are three major forms. The first, limited progressive SSc, is often associated with the CREST syndrome (*c*alcinosis, *R*aynaud's phenomenon, *e*sophageal dysmotility, *s*clerodactyly, and *t*elangiectasias). Calcinosis refers to calcific deposits under the skin and is more commonly seen in the pediatric population. Raynaud's phenomenon occurs with vasospasm of the vessels that supply the digits (see Chapter 240). Subsequent tricolor changes of the fingers are seen (blue, then white, and then red). Esophageal dysmotility results from the thickening of the distal esophagus, which prevents normal peristalsis. Reflux, heartburn, and coughing are common symptoms. Sclerodactyly, or thickening of the skin of the fingers, causes loss of the normal hand architecture. Telangiectasias are venous dilations that may represent collateral vessel formation in response to ischemia. They are most commonly found on the face. The terms *limited progressive systemic sclerosis* and *CREST* are used interchangeably. The second form, diffuse SSc, is often associated with internal organ involvement, and the third form, SSc sine SSc, is an extremely rare disorder in which patients have internal organ involvement without any skin findings.[1]

Limited Systemic Sclerosis

In limited SSc, the skin thickening is limited to the hands and the face. This disorder is seen in conjunction with CREST syndrome. Patients may have some or all of the features of this syndrome. In general, patients with limited SSc have a good prognosis; approximately 10% of these patients will develop pulmonary hypertension, which can be life threatening.[6] The mortality rate in this subgroup of patients is very high.

Progressive Systemic Sclerosis

There is a more generalized skin involvement, including the proximal limbs and trunk, in progressive SSc. These patients can have extremely high morbidity and mortality rates resulting from the internal organ involvement. Patients with diffuse progressive SSc commonly develop some degree of renal disease and/or pulmonary disease. Gastrointestinal and cardiac involvement is also possible. Initially, renal disease was the major cause of complications and death, but with improved treatment, pulmonary disease is now the leading cause of death.

In *SSc sine SSc,* classic internal organ involvement such as renal and pulmonary disease occurs, but the skin is unaffected.[1]

PHYSICAL EXAMINATION

Physical examination should include a careful evaluation of the skin for evidence of skin thickening. The digits appear to have a sausage shape, and the skin is shiny and smooth. Examination of the nail beds with a capillary microscope classically shows dilated loops of some capillaries and complete loss of other vessels. The location of skin thickening should be documented (e.g., hands and face only, arms, trunk). The mouth aperture should be measured. The skin should be examined for ulcers and tissue breakdown. A careful evaluation for evidence of CREST syndrome is very important, as are blood pressure measurements.

DIAGNOSTICS

SSc is primarily a clinical diagnosis, although occasionally a skin biopsy is indicated for clarification. Baseline creatinine and pulmonary function tests (PFTs) are necessary to permit monitoring. The antinuclear antibody (ANA) test is positive in 40% to 98% of patients with SSc.[7] The anticentromere antibody and anti–Scl-70 (topoisomerase I) tests are more specific for SSc.

DIFFERENTIAL DIAGNOSIS

SSc can occasionally be confused with systemic lupus erythematosus, overlap syndrome, or mixed connective tissue disease. In general, the skin findings in SSc in conjunction with the laboratory tests are pathognomonic.

MANAGEMENT

The treatment of progressive SSc remains disappointing. Attempts to arrest disease progression have been limited, and, in general, treatment is focused toward organ specificity.

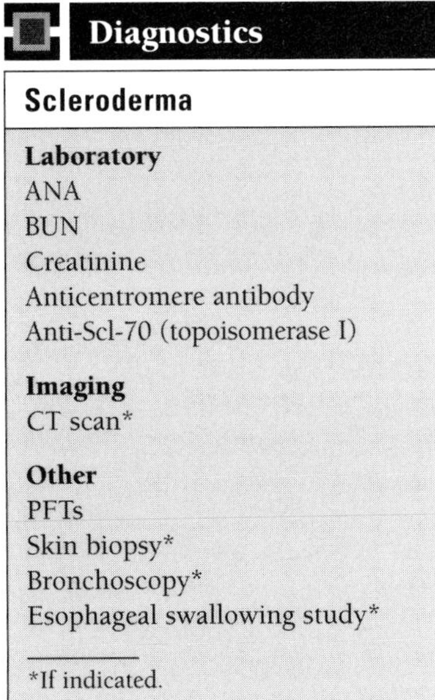

Diagnostics

Scleroderma

Laboratory
ANA
BUN
Creatinine
Anticentromere antibody
Anti-Scl-70 (topoisomerase I)

Imaging
CT scan*

Other
PFTs
Skin biopsy*
Bronchoscopy*
Esophageal swallowing study*

*If indicated.

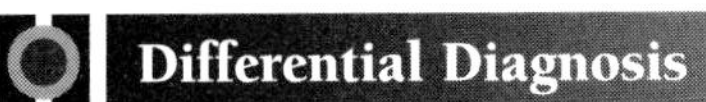

Differential Diagnosis

Scleroderma

Systemic lupus erythematosus
Mixed connective tissue disease
Localized scleroderma

One of the most widely used medications for the treatment of progressive SSc is D-penicillamine, which was first shown to have skin-thinning effects in patients treated for Wilson's disease. Unfortunately, the effectiveness of D-penicillamine has not been supported in large clinical trials.[8] Despite this, it has been used for the treatment of SSc for several decades.[9] Toxicity is high, with 47% of patients developing side effects, including bone marrow failure, proteinuria, and skin rash.[10]

Cyclophosphamide has been shown to cause some modest improvement in lung compliance but not in diffusion capacity.[11] More recently, methotrexate has been shown to cause a favorable improvement in total skin score (TSS), compared with a placebo, in a 24-week randomized double-blind trial.[12] Cyclosporine has had a modest impact on decreasing skin thickening, but no changes in pulmonary function have been shown, and the therapy could potentially exacerbate renal function.[13] There are limited data on other therapies designed to moderate inflammatory mediators such as cytokines.

The biggest strides in treatment have been made in the prevention and control of SSc renal crisis by using angiotensin-converting enzyme (ACE) inhibitors. There is a significant improvement in the survival of patients with SSc who were treated with ACE inhibitors[14]; 76% of patients treated with ACE inhibitors were alive at the end of 1 year versus 15% of those who were not treated with ACE inhibitors. However, 44% of patients with SSc treated with ACE inhibitors still require dialysis.[14]

LIFE SPAN CONSIDERATIONS

The female/male ratio of patients with SSc is 3:1, with the peak age of onset in the fourth to seventh decade of life.[2] Patients with SSc can develop life-threatening complications that shorten life. Approximately 10% of patients with CREST will develop life-threatening pulmonary hypertension[6]; the mortality rate in this subgroup of patients is very high.

Risk factors for SSc renal crisis include male sex, pregnancy, older age, and those who present with creatinine levels of greater than 3 mg/dl. SSc renal involvement is thought to be more common in African-Americans, occurs at an average age of 49 years, and occurs approximately 3 years after the onset of progressive SSc. There are other sex, age, and genetic background factors that modify disease susceptibility. The Choctaw Native Americans in Oklahoma have the highest prevalence of SSc.[4]

COMPLICATIONS

Renal Disease

Approximately half of patients with progressive SSc will have clinical evidence of renal disease, although a higher percentage of patients will have findings at blind renal biopsy. In one review of 210 patients with SSc, 94 had clinical markers of renal involvement. Seventy-six patients had proteinuria, 50 patients had hypertension, and 40 patients developed azotemia. SSc renal crisis occurred in 15 patients. On average, renal disease developed 2 to 3 years after the diagnosis of SSc was made. The urine sediment was relatively benign and acellular. On microscopic pathology, the arcuate and interlobar arteries were most commonly involved.[15] SSc renal involvement is thought to be more common in African-Americans. Early, rapid progression of skin lesions, anemia, pericardial effusion, and congestive heart failure can be precursors to renal crisis. Patients present with rapid rise in blood pressure, headaches, blurred vision, and progressive renal failure. Rarely, heart failure and seizures occur.[16] There have been case reports of patients developing SSc renal crisis after receiving doses of prednisone that were higher than 20 mg/day.[17] Other risk factors for SSc renal crisis include male sex, pregnancy, older age, and those who present with creatinine levels of greater than 3 mg/dl.

The outcome of SSc renal crisis has been vastly improved by the use of ACE inhibitors. Steen and others[14] at the University of Pittsburgh demonstrated that therapy with ACE inhibitors in 108 patients with SSc renal crisis dramatically improved the 1-year survival rate.

Pulmonary Disease

Pulmonary involvement is currently the leading cause of death in patients with both limited and diffuse forms of SSc.[18] Restrictive lung disease, decreased diffusion capacity of carbon dioxide, pulmonary fibrosis, reduced lung volumes, and pulmonary hypertension have all been described. Clinically patients may present with dyspnea and fatigue. Physical examination reveals bibasilar crackles, and there may be evidence of elevated right-sided pressures (accentuated P2, evidence of right-sided failure). Surprisingly, chest radiography may underestimate the degree of disease. High-resolution CT scans and bronchioloalveolar lavage are beneficial for making the diagnosis.

In the series of 77 patients with diffuse SSc and 88 patients with CREST syndrome reported by Steen and others, 34% of all patients had abnormal PFT findings. Patients with diffuse SSc had a decreased forced vital capacity (FVC) compared with patients with CREST, although patients with CREST tended to have lower diffusion capacities.[19] The presence of anti–Scl-70 antibodies was associated with restrictive disease. In general, patients with a restrictive pattern on PFTs had the worst prognosis, with a 5-year survival of 58%. Patients with decreased diffusing capacity of carbon dioxide or obstructive disease had a 5-year survival of 73% or 69%, respectively. There is a higher prevalence of lung cancer in patients with SSc.

Chronic reflux and aspiration may contribute to pulmonary damage by causing fibrosis and restrictive disease over time; therefore antacids and antireflux medication may be indicated.

Although patients with limited SSc and those with diffuse SSc tend to have similar incidences of pulmonary involvement, patients with limited disease (CREST) have a much higher incidence of pulmonary hypertension. It is estimated that 10% of patients with CREST will develop pulmonary hypertension.[6]

The efficacy of treatment in SSc pulmonary disease is limited. Some patients have improved after treatment with a combination of prednisone and cyclophosphamide. Conventional management of pulmonary artery hypertension includes low-flow oxygen, management of right-sided heart failure, smoking cessation, and possible anticoagulation. The calcium channel blocker nifedipine and the prostacyclin analogue epoprostenol sodium have been used with limited benefit.[20]

Gastrointestinal Disease

In patients with SSc, 75% to 90% will have involvement of the gastrointestinal tract. Esophageal dysmotility and gastrointestinal reflux are the most common findings. Gastric motility can also be impaired. Symptoms include heartburn, cough, dyspepsia, and evidence of chronic aspiration. Esophageal swallowing studies can be very useful for making the diagnosis.[21] Treatment with H_2 antagonists and protein-pump inhibitors is effective, although high-dose therapy is often necessary.

Musculoskeletal Symptoms

Arthralgias and myalgias can be the earliest symptoms of SSc. Discomfort can extend along tendons and into muscles and joints. A coarse friction rub can be heard and felt with motion of (especially) the ankle, wrist, knee, and elbow and may predict more severe disease. In late-stage disease, there are joint contractures secondary to tightened skin and reduced mobility. Muscle atrophy and weakness result from disuse and deconditioning.

Cardiac Disease

SSc can affect the heart. Symptoms can be subtle and often occur late in the course of the disease. Symptoms can include dyspnea on exertion, palpitations, and, less often, chest pain. Pericardial effusion and pericarditis have been reported. Abnormal perfusion scans may be a result of abnormalities in microcirculation and vasospasm. Interestingly, these changes can be induced by cold and prevented by nifedipine.[22]

Other complications of SSc can include depression, sexual dysfunction, and Sjögren's syndrome (dry eyes, dry mouth). Aggressive dental care and frequent use of lubricating eye drops may be necessary. Carpal tunnel syndrome can cause severe pain and may require surgical intervention.

INDICATIONS FOR REFERRAL/HOSPITALIZATION

SSc is a multisystem disease that requires a collaborative team approach. A rheumatologist with experience in this disorder should be involved in the patient's care. When appropriate, a nephrologist, pulmonologist, gastroenterologist, and cardiologist should also be consulted. These patients can have a reduced life span, with most of the deaths resulting from renal and pulmonary disease.

Patients with SSc renal crisis should be admitted to the hospital for evaluation and therapy. Declining pulmonary function or severe skin breakdown with superinfection may also necessitate hospitalization.

Patients with musculoskeletal involvement will require measures to relieve pain and prevent joint contractures. A referral to physical therapy should be made early in the course of the disease, and patients should be taught a home exercise program. Occupational therapy can be very helpful for patients with hand involvement. For patients with restricted mouth opening, good dental hygiene is essential and may require special equipment.

PATIENT AND FAMILY EDUCATION

A thorough understanding of the chronicity of the disease and an awareness of the signs and symptoms of SSc renal crisis are important for patients and families. In addition, the side effect profile of medications and any untoward effects should be understood. Careful monitoring will be necessary throughout the course of the illness and will require a partnership between the patient and the primary care provider to manage crises and maintain function.

REFERENCES

1. Subcommittee for Scleroderma Criteria of the American Rheumatism Association Diagnostic and Therapeutic Criteria Committee: Preliminary criteria for the classification of systemic sclerosis (scleroderma), *Arthritis Rheum* 23:581-590, 1980.
2. Steen VD, Medsger TA Jr: Epidemiology and natural history of systemic sclerosis, *Rheum Dis Clin North Am* 16:1-10, 1990.

3. Briggs D, Black C, Welsh K: Genetic factors in scleroderma, *Rheum Dis Clin North Am* 16:31-51, 1990.
4. White B: *Systemic sclerosis and related syndromes, epidemiology, pathology and pathogenesis in primer on the rheumatic diseases*, ed 12, Atlanta, Ga, 2001, Arthritis Foundation.
5. Falanga V: Localized scleroderma, *Med Clin North Am* 73:1143-1156, 1989.
6. Stupi AM and others: Pulmonary hypertension in the CREST syndrome variant of systemic sclerosis, *Arthritis Rheum* 28:515-524, 1986.
7. Bernstein RM, Steigerwald JC, Tan EM: Association of antinuclear and antinucleolar antibodies in progressive systemic sclerosis, *Clin Exp Immunol* 48:43-51, 1982.
8. Steen VD, Blair S, Medsger TA Jr: The toxicity of d-penicillamine in systemic sclerosis, *Ann Intern Med* 104:699-705, 1986.
9. Jayson MIV and others: Penicillamine therapy in systemic sclerosis, *Proc R Soc Med* 70 (suppl 3):82-88, 1977.
10. Clements PJ and others: High dose versus low dose D penicillamine in early, diffuse systemic sclerosis: analysis of a two year, double blind, randomized, controlled trial, *Arthritis Rheum* 42:1194-1203, 1999.
11. Silver RM and others: Cyclophosphamide and low-dose prednisolone therapy in patients with systemic sclerosis (scleroderma) with interstitial lung disease, *J Rheumatol* 20:838-844, 1993.
12. Van den Hoogen FHJ and others: Comparison of methotrexate with placebo in the treatment of systemic sclerosis: a 24-week randomized double-blind trial, followed by a 24-week observational trial, *Br J Rheumatol* 35:364-372, 1996.
13. Clements PJ and others: Cyclosporine in systemic sclerosis: results of a forty-eight week open safety study, *Arthritis Rheum* 36:75-83, 1993.
14. Steen VD and others: Outcome of renal crisis in systemic sclerosis: relation to availability of angiotensin converting enzyme (ACE) inhibitors, *Ann Intern Med* 113:352-357, 1990.
15. Cannon PJ and others: The relationship of hypertension and renal failure in scleroderma (progressive systemic sclerosis) to structural and functional abnormalities of the renal cortical circulation, *Medicine* 53:1-46, 1974.
16. Steen VD and others: Factors predicting development of renal involvement in progressive systemic sclerosis, *Am J Med* 76:779-786, 1984.
17. Steen VD, Conte C, Medsger TA Jr: Case-control study of corticosteroid use prior to scleroderma renal crisis (abstract), *Arthritis Rheum* 37 (suppl):S360, 1994.
18. Black CM: *Clinical manifestations and evaluation of scleroderma lung disease*, Wellesley, Mass, 1997, Up to Date in Medicine (serial publication: CD Rom).
19. Steen VD and others: Pulmonary involvement in systemic sclerosis scleroderma, *Arthritis Rheum* 28:759-767, 1985.
20. Black CM: *Treatment of scleroderma lung disease*, Wellesley, Mass, 1997, Up to Date in Medicine (serial publication: CD Rom).
21. Sjögren RW: Gastrointestinal features of scleroderma, *Curr Opin Rheumatol* 8:569-575, 1996.
22. Kahan A and others: Nifedipine and thallium-201 myocardial perfusion in progressive systemic sclerosis, *N Engl J Med* 314:1397-1402, 1986.

CHAPTER 244

Vasculitis

Simon M. Helfgott

DEFINITION AND EPIDEMIOLOGY

The vasculitides include a diverse group of disorders characterized by inflammation and the destruction of blood vessel walls. Clinical signs and symptoms result from the subsequent impairment of blood flow through these damaged blood vessels to the distal organ. Although specific vasculitides typically affect certain organ systems, virtually any may be involved.

The vasculitic syndromes are uncommon and data on disease incidence are imprecise. The age of onset is quite variable, ranging from infancy to old age. Drug-induced vasculitis (most commonly caused by penicillin and sulfonamides) can occur at any age. Another common disorder, giant cell arteritis, does not occur in individuals younger than 50 years of age, whereas Takayasu's arteritis is never seen in patients older than 40 years of age.

CLASSIFICATION OF VASCULITIC SYNDROMES

The systemic vasculitides can be classified according to the size of the involved vessels (Box 244-1). Small and medium-sized blood vessels are involved in polyarteritis nodosa (PAN) Churg-Strauss syndrome (CSS), and Wegener's granulomatosis (WG). Cutaneous leukocytoclastic vasculitis involves the smallest vessels in the skin. Common features of these vasculitides include prominent constitutional symptoms and a predilection for cutaneous, renal, and peripheral neurologic involvement. Differentiation of these symptoms is made on the basis of pathologic findings on biopsy. For example, giant cells may be observed in biopsies of the temporal artery in patients

BOX 244-1

THE VASCULITIDES

LARGE VESSELS
Giant cell arteritis
Takayasu's arteritis

MEDIUM-SIZED VESSELS
Polyarteritis nodosa
Kawasaki's disease

SMALL VESSELS
Wegener's granulomatosis
Microscopic polyarteritis
Henoch-Schönlein purpura
Essential cryoglobulinemic vasculitis
Cutaneous leukocytoclastic vasculitis
Drug-induced, ANCA-associated disorders
Lupus vasculitis
Behçet's disease
Drug-induced immune complex vasculitis

with giant cell arteritis. Eosinophils in large numbers are generally seen in patients with CSS.

Leukocytoclastic vasculitis typically involves the smallest blood vessels in the skin. In most cases, the skin is the only organ involved, although more widespread involvement may be observed in more severe cases. Patients present with raised, purpuric skin lesions, typically over the lower extremities (palpable purpura). They are sometimes slightly itchy; they may develop over the trunk and chest as well. The most common predisposing factor is the ingestion of a drug (known to predispose to cutaneous vasculitis) about 7 to 10 days earlier. The most common inciting drugs include antibiotics such as penicillins and sulfonamides, hydralazine, and propylthiouracil.[1]

Polyarteritis nodosa is defined as a necrotizing arteritis of medium and small arteries. Destruction of the blood vessel wall causes the development microaneurysms, which interfere with blood flow to affected organs. Patients may present with systemic complaints including weight loss and fever. Other common features include myalgias, arthralgias, palpable purpura, hypertension, and peripheral neuropathy.[1]

Wegener's granulomatosis is a vasculitis that typically involves the upper and lower airways and kidney. Involvement of the ears, nose, and throat is common. Abnormal chest radiograph may be seen with nodules, infiltrates, and cavities. Renal dysfunction resulting from a glomerulonephritis is detected by an elevated serum creatinine and a urinalysis showing red blood cells and/or red cell casts.[2]

Churg-Strauss syndrome is characterized by features of both PAN and WG. Eosinophilia and asthma characterize it. Multiorgan involvement is observed with upper and lower respiratory tract involvement, as well as kidney and peripheral nervous system inflammation.[1]

Vasculitides involving larger blood vessels include the relatively common giant cell arteritis (temporal arteritis), which is found almost exclusively in patients more than 50 years of age (see Chapter 239), and the less common Takayasu's arteritis seem primarily in women younger than 40 years of age. There is a higher incidence of Takayasu's vasculitis in women of Asian background. Patients with this vasculitis often present with signs of unequal blood pressures, arm claudication, or bruits in the neck or arms. Other presentations include cerebral vascular accident, heart failure, or ruptured aortic aneurysm. As these are all extremely unusual events in young persons, consideration should be given to Takayasu's arteritis in the appropriate clinical setting.[3]

The presentation of giant cell arteritis is varied and includes the new onset of headache, scalp tenderness, cranial pain, or jaw claudication. Fever of unknown origin is another mode of presentation. Some patients also complain of diffuse shoulder and pelvic girdle achiness (polymyalgia rheumatica). The hallmark laboratory feature of GCA is the finding of an elevated erythrocyte sedimentation rate (ESR).

Henoch-Schönlein purpura (HSP) is a form of small vessel vasculitis that may affect people of all ages, from early childhood to middle age. Typically, there is involvement of the joints (with pain and/or swelling), skin (palpable purpura), gastrointestinal tract (abdominal pain, bleeding), and kidneys (microscopic hematuria, rising serum creatinine). Although this is usually a benign disorder in children, it may be a more serious condition in adults.[1]

PATHOPHYSIOLOGY

The pathophysiology of the vasculitides is varied. The group of small to medium-sized vessel vasculitides such as WG and CSS are associated with the presence of an autoantibody, the antineutrophil cytoplasmic antibody (ANCA) in the majority of patients. Its role, if any, in the pathogenesis of the condition has not been elucidated.

Some patients with PAN are noted to have hepatitis B surface antigen. Hepatitis C may be associated with a small vessel vasculitis resulting from the deposition of cryoglobulins containing viral particles and antibody in the blood vessel wall, and subsequent destruction occurs.

Patients with a drug-induced vasculitis may have immune complex formation consisting of the foreign protein (offending drug) and its binding antibody.[4] A small percentage of patients also have a positive ANCA. Patients with either rheumatoid arthritis or systemic lupus erythematosus (SLE) may also develop a small vessel vasculitis.

CLINICAL PRESENTATION AND PHYSICAL EXAMINATION

The protean manifestations of vasculitis include systemic complaints such as fever, malaise, arthralgias, and myalgias. When present, fever rarely exceeds 38.9° C (102° F) and is not associated with chills. Depending on the organ system involved, other findings may include cough, hemoptysis, sinusitis, otitis, abdominal pain, dysesthesia, extremity weakness, and skin rash. Visual changes including monocular blindness may occur uniquely with GCA.

Perhaps the most helpful physical examination finding is the presence of palpable purpura (see Color Plate 24). These lesions are usually multiple, more often seen in distal lower extremities. They occur as a result of extravasation of red blood cells and white blood cells outside of the destroyed blood vessel wall of the small arterioles. They vary in size from a few millimeters to 1 to 2 cm in diameter. Occasionally, they are itchy. Other skin lesions including livedo reticularis, nonpalpable purpura, and cutaneous ulcers can also be seen.

A careful neurologic examination may detect findings compatible with peripheral nerve involvement (e.g., sensory dysesthesia or motor weakness). For example, wrist or foot drop may be highly suspicious for the diagnosis of a vasculitis. On the other hand, joint swelling (i.e., arthritis) is uncommon. More often, patients complain of nonspecific arthralgias and myalgias. Renal and gastrointestinal involvement usually requires a careful laboratory evaluation. Acute abdominal pain in the setting of a vasculitis may point toward either HSP or PAN. Upper respiratory signs and symptoms including sinusitis and otitis are most commonly seen in patients with WG or CSS. Cough and hemoptysis can be seen with either of these conditions, whereas asthma is unique to CSS.

DIAGNOSTICS

Establishing the diagnosis of vasculitis requires a high degree of clinical suspicion, as the multiorgan involvement can mimic many other conditions. Diagnostic studies should include a CBC (assessing for eosinophilia in CSS, thrombocytosis in WG and anemia in all), ESR, which is generally elevated, serum electrolytes, serum glucose, creatinine, BUN, and liver function

Diagnostics

Vasculitis

Laboratory	Imaging
CBC and differential	Chest x-ray study
ESR	Angiography*
Serum electrolytes	
Serum glucose	**Other**
BUN	Biopsy
Creatinine	EMG*
LFTs	
Urinalysis	
ANCA	
ANA*	

*If indicated.
ANCA, antineutrophil, cytoplasmic antibody; *ANA*, antinuclear antibody; *EMG*, electromyography.

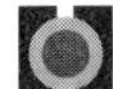

Differential Diagnosis

Vasculitis

Allergic angiitis	Cryoglobulinemia
Atheroembolic vasculitis	Inflammatory bowel disease
Serum sickness	Atheromatous embolization
Microscopic polyangiitis	Buerger's disease
Infectious endocarditis	Fibromuscular dysplasia
Viral endocarditis	Antiphospholipid antibody syndrome
Viral infections	Thrombotic thrombocytopenic purpura
Rheumatoid arthritis	Chilblain
Lupus	Atrial myxoma
Sjögren's syndrome	Ergotamine abuse
Medications (antibiotics, sulfa drugs, NSAIDs)	Pseudoxanthoma elasticum
Lymphoproliferative disorders	

NSAIDs; nonsteroidal antiinflammatory drugs.

studies. A spun, fresh, urine sediment should be carefully examined for the presence of casts and cells, which would suggest a glomerulonephritis. Recent studies confirm the utility of ANCA testing in the evaluation of vasculitis, particularly WG, CSS, and their variants. Although the majority of patients with these forms of vasculitis have a positive ANCA study, a negative test does not rule out the diagnosis. Serum cryoglobulins, hepatitis B and C serologies, and, if indicated, HIV status may also be useful tests for patients suspected of having PAN. The antinuclear antibody (ANA), rheumatoid factors, and complement levels are all of limited diagnostic value.

Tissue biopsy showing evidence of blood vessel wall necrosis and inflammation establishes the diagnosis of vasculitis. Clearly the simplest tissue to obtain is skin. Thus any patient with a suspected vasculitis should be examined carefully for skin lesions that can be biopsied.

Other useful biopsy sites include peripheral nerve when patients have symptoms suggesting nerve involvement. The sural nerve, located posterior to the lateral malleolus is a pure sensory nerve that is easily accessible for biopsy. When this procedure is performed, the adjacent gastrocnemius muscle should also be sampled to increase the diagnostic yield.

When necessary, a lung nodule can be biopsied. However, successful biopsy generally requires that the procedure be done via an open lung approach or thoracoscopy. Needle aspiration or biopsy via the bronchoscopic approach is rarely helpful.

In cases of PAN or Takayasu's arteritis, arteriography of the involved blood vessels may show characteristic angiographic changes that can establish the diagnosis.

DIFFERENTIAL DIAGNOSIS

In general, the differential diagnosis of vasculitis includes infectious diseases, such as subacute bacterial endocarditis, or bacteremia, such as meningococcemia. These are multisystem disorders that can mimic vasculitis. Similarly, cholesterol emboli syndrome may mimic vasculitis. Affected patients are older and may be using an anticoagulant medication or have undergone some vascular manipulation, such as angiography, or sustained aortic trauma days to weeks earlier. The presentation is characterized by fever, bilateral palpable purpura over the legs and feet, renal insufficiency, and eosinophilia.

Certain connective tissue diseases, such as SLE may present with features similar to vasculitis. Generally, serologic studies such as a high titer ANA or other antibodies can distinguish this condition from vasculitis. The antiphospholipid antibody syndrome is a rare disorder that may present with multiorgan dysfunction resulting from multiple thrombotic events. Patients with this syndrome have marked increases in the antiphospholipid antibodies, which target clotting factors.

MANAGEMENT

The choice of therapy depends on the severity of the involvement. For example, drug-induced vasculitis may be treated successfully simply by withholding the offending agent. Patients with systemic disease of a more serious nature generally require corticosteroids either orally or intravenously. Oral doses are generally 0.5 mg to 1.0 mg per/kg prednisone per day. For more serious disease, IV corticosteroid preparations can be given for a faster mode of onset.

If patients either have disease that is refractory to corticosteroid therapy or have developed corticosteroids-induced side effects, an additional immunosuppressant drug may be added. These drugs include cyclophosphamide, methotrexate, and azathioprine. The use of newer biologic therapy such as antitumor necrosis factor agents (e.g., infliximab or etanercept) is being evaluated in ongoing clinical studies.

COMPLICATIONS

Complications from vasculitis may often be life threatening and include neurologic events such as stroke, renal failure, pulmonary hemorrhage, or gangrene of distal extremities. The use of high-dose corticosteroids may predispose to the development of obesity, osteoporosis, hypoglycemia, infections, and osteonecrosis. The use of other immunosuppressant agents may predispose to infections as well and may also increase the risk for the development of malignancies in the long term.

INDICATIONS FOR REFERRAL/HOSPITALIZATION

All patients suspected of having a vasculitis should be referred to a rheumatologist for diagnosis and management because these conditions can be severe and life threatening.

PATIENT AND FAMILY EDUCATION

Patients diagnosed with vasculitis must understand the potentially serious nature of their condition. Although some forms of vasculitis are a limited one-time event (e.g., drug-induced or a result of HSP), others may be chronic. Mortality resulting from vasculitis has been greatly reduced thanks to earlier diagnosis and intervention with immunosuppressant therapies. Long-term survivors, however, are susceptible to complications of treatment or the disease process itself, including accelerated atherosclerosis and a higher incidence of infections resulting from immunosuppression.

Signs of worsening disease may include new rash, sensory loss, hemoptysis, hematuria, or proteinuria. A sudden headache or loss of vision should be reported immediately. Side effects of high-dose steroids, including hypertension, obesity, cataracts, skin thinning and osteoporosis, should be reviewed with both the patient and family.

Given the potentially life-threatening complications of both the diseases and treatment regimen, an open and accessible patient-provider relationship is essential.

REFERENCES

1. Jeanette JC, Falk RJ: Medical progress: small-vessel vasculitis, *N Engl J Med* 337:1512-1523, 1997.
2. Hoffman GS and others: Wegener's granulomatosis: an analysis of 158 patients, *Ann Intern Med* 116:488-98, 1992.
3. Dillon MJ, Ansell BM: Vasculitis in children and adolescents, *Rheum Dis Clin North Am* 21:1115-1136, 1995.
4. Choi HK and others: Drug-associated neutrophil cytoplasmic antibody-positive vasculitis. Prevalence among patients with high titers of antimyeloperoxidase antibodies, *Arthritis Rheum* 43:405-413, 2000.

CHAPTER 245

Barotrauma and Other Diving Injuries

Joanne Sandberg-Cook

The popularity of scuba diving has increased over the last several decades and along with it the number of patients who are at risk for injuries sustained while diving. These injuries are diverse and vary in severity from the benign to the life threatening. Many diving injuries require sophisticated medical attention emergently. These include near drowning, hypothermia, arterial gas embolism (AGE), severe decompression sickness, and poisonous bites or stings. Other diving injuries are not as serious, enabling patients to be seen by their own primary care provider or at a nearby facility.

PREDIVE PHYSICAL EXAMINATION AND DIAGNOSTICS

Because few primary care providers are trained in sports or diving medicine, it may be necessary for the diver to assess injuries on site and educate health care providers. The prediving physical examination is an opportunity for both the diver and primary care provider to be aware of potential problems. A careful history is imperative.

Diving is relatively contraindicated in any patient with a history of frequent ear infections, serous otitis, chronic sinus infections, or asthma. Tubes in the ears or chronic or intermittent aspiration suggesting an incompetent larynx are absolute contraindications, as is chronic lung disease, emphysema, and a history of spontaneous pneumothorax.[1] Known coronary artery disease, heart failure, and valvular disease or other cardiac conditions are also contraindications. Epilepsy or unstable diabetes are both contraindications to diving because of the possibility of loss of consciousness. Obesity is a hazard in that it may reflect poor physical conditioning, as well as predispose a diver to decompression sickness on the basis of nitrogen's lipid solubility.

The physical examination should reveal a normal eye, ear, nose, and throat. The tympanic membrane should be intact, and each ear should be autoinflated, using a modified Valsalva's maneuver. Normal neurologic examination findings with intact reflexes and strength are essential. The range of motion for all

Diagnostics

Barotrauma

Initial	**Imaging**
PFTs (for predive) Visual acuity (predive)	Chest x-ray (for predive, pulmonary barotraumas)
Laboratory	**Other**
CBC and differential (for predive)	ECG (for predive) Cardiac stress testing

joints should be within normal limits. Lung and heart examination findings should be completely benign without rales, wheezes, murmurs, or extra sounds. Cardiac stress testing may be recommended for divers age 45 years and older as for any other activity requiring physical exertion. Older divers are at higher risk for chronic disease and should consider annual physical evaluation for diving fitness.[2]

Recommended studies before diving include a chest x-ray film, ECG, and visual acuity testing. Pulmonary function tests, bone and joint x-rays studies, and periodic audiograms are recommended for commercial divers.[1]

PATHOPHYSIOLOGY

Most injuries sustained while diving stem directly from the differences in physical properties that exist between liquids and gases.[3] A basic understanding of the laws of physics, particularly those laws that deal with the pressure and density relative to liquids and gases, is important. During a dive the body absorbs nitrogen from the breathing gas in proportion to the surrounding pressure. Nitrogen at higher pressures can alter the electrical properties of brain function (nitrogen narcosis). Every 50 feet of depth is the equivalent of one alcoholic drink, causing many of the same impairments in judgment and coordination as alcohol intoxication.[4] If the pressure is removed too quickly, the nitrogen comes out of solution and forms bubbles in the tissue and in the bloodstream. These bubbles can cause different problems depending on where they form.[3]

Decompression sickness (DCS) is the result of bubble formation from tissue inert gas supersaturation during decompression. Risk factors for DCS include rapid ascent, deeper and longer dives, repeated dives, and failure to follow appropriate decompression procedures. Dive tables or decompression computers are used to calculate the rate of ascent based on the depth of the dive and are essential to safe diving. Following appropriate decompression procedures can reduce but not eliminate the risk of DCS.

Air embolism (AGE) occurs when a diver surfaces without exhaling or when the rate of ascent exceeds the rate at which expanding gas can exit through the tracheobronchial tree. Trapped air in the lungs expands and may rupture lung tissue, releasing gas bubbles into the circulation. These bubbles are then carried to vital organs, causing life-threatening conditions or sudden death.[1] The term *dysbarism* has been used to describe these pressure-related injuries that result in permanent tissue damage. The term *barotrauma* refers to injury of the lung, middle or inner ear, sinus, or gastrointestinal tract caused by differences in pressure. *Decompression* illness is now the preferred term when describing an injured diver who is suffering from either AGE or DCS.

CLINICAL PRESENTATION

DCS can present acutely, even while the diver is still in the water, but delayed presentation is more common. The vast majority of symptoms start within 24 hours of surfacing, although altitude exposure, including commercial air travel, can precipitate DCS after a longer time. Individual differences in physical fitness, body weight, gender, fatigue, hydration, and age may make some divers more prone to decompression sickness in spite of the use of appropriate decompression procedures.

Type I DCS can present with dull pain in limbs or joints, especially in the upper extremities.[4] Skin itching, rash, and localized swelling (lymphedema) are also common manifestations of type I DCS. Type II DCS is more severe and is characterized by neurologic or pulmonary symptoms including chest pain and cough. Nervous system involvement most often manifests as patchy numbness or paresthesias, but can also present as paralysis. Headache, dizziness (including vertigo), urinary or anal sphincter disorders (usually urinary retention), and mental status changes can also be seen. Hypovolemic shock can occur as a result of fluid shifts from intravascular to extravascular spaces.[4]

PHYSICAL EXAMINATION

A careful history of the dive is essential. Knowing where the dive took place, how deep it was, and how much time was spent at specific depths is crucial. Questions about the diver's predive condition including drug or alcohol intake should be asked. Knowledge of first aid administered at the site is helpful. Multiple systems can be affected, but the neurologic and respiratory systems in particular must be carefully assessed. Disorientation, dizziness, fatigue, and joint pain with limited ability to move are common complaints. The joint pain of limb DCS can sometimes be relieved by inflating a blood pressure cuff around the affected joint, although this is not a reliable sign. Physical findings may also include skin blotching, paralysis, weakness, ataxia, paresthesias, and paralysis. Hypotension, tachycardia, chest pain, and cough are common symptoms. Collapse with loss of consciousness may indicate hypovolemic shock.[4]

DIFFERENTIAL DIAGNOSIS

Many of the signs of DCS are identical to more common syndromes including dehydration, electrolyte imbalance, viral syndromes, and exhaustion. A CNS lesion could certainly

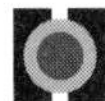

Differential Diagnosis

Barotrauma

Systemic Symptoms	**Cardiac/Pulmonary Symptoms**
Dehydration	CHF
Electrolyte imbalance	Pulmonary edema
Viral syndromes	Angina
Exhaustion	
Neurologic Symptoms	**Dermatologic Symptoms**
CNS lesions, CVA	Allergic reactions
Heat exhaustion, heat stroke	Abrasions
	Contusions
Musculoskeletal Symptoms (Limb Pain)	Envenomations
Sprains, strains, fractures	Cellulitis
Arthritis	
Herniated disk	
DVT, phlebitis	

CVA, cerebrovascular accident; *DVT*, deep venous thrombosis; *CHF*, congestive heart failure.

cause many of the neurologic symptoms discussed previously. Sprains, strains, fracture, arthritis, and herniated disk can all cause musculoskeletal pain. Congestive heart failure and pulmonary edema can cause symptoms similar to AGE. Dermatitis, allergic reactions, abrasions, contusions, or envenomations can all lead to dermatologic symptoms including cellulitis, rash, itching, or burning. Heat exhaustion or heat stroke can lead to muscle cramping or mental status changes. Deep vein thrombosis and thrombophlebitis can be a cause of limb pain but not usually joint pain.

Pulmonary Barotrauma

Pulmonary barotraumas (dysbarism) with AGE ranks second only to drowning as a cause of death in divers.[3] Trapped air in the lung expands and ruptures lung tissue, releasing air bubbles into the circulation. If a bubble lodges in the brain, stroke, seizures, paralysis, and unconsciousness can occur. Air bubbles traveling to the heart can lead to myocardial infarction or cardiac arrest. AGE can also cause minor symptoms such as numbness, tingling, or weakness of a limb. Vision and hearing losses have also been seen, all without loss of consciousness.

The pathognomonic features of air embolism include marbling of the skin of the upper body, gas emboli in the retina, and areas of pallor on the tongue, although this is rarely seen.[1] Pneumothorax can occur in conjunction with AGE or in isolation and become evident at a later time. The patient may be in respiratory distress with mild to moderate pain. Tachypnea, pallor, decreased or absent oxygen saturation, and diminished breath sounds may be noted. Mediastinal air can track cephalad into the soft tissues of the neck and cause changes in the voice.[5] A chest x-ray study usually confirms the diagnosis, although CT scan may be required.

MANAGEMENT

Medical stabilization at the nearest facility with rapid transport to the nearest recompression chamber is essential and may involve emergency care at the scene including cardiopulmonary resuscitation and intubation if indicated. Immediate treatment with inhaled 100% oxygen is highly effective in reducing symptoms while awaiting transport. The breathing of 100% oxygen reduces bubble size and enhances oxygen delivery to ischemic tissues. Injured divers are often hypovolemic and require aggressive IV hydration.

Emergency management of AGE is the same as for decompression sickness and includes on-site use of 100% inhaled oxygen therapy, medical stabilization, and transport to a recompression chamber. Patients with mild presenting symptoms, however, may experience relapse while undergoing decompression. This relapse may be on the basis of bubble interaction with blood vessel wall, causing an inflammatory response.[5] This response leads to blood vessel occlusion and cell damage, which can result in clinical deterioration or even death in spite of recompression treatments.[4] These patients are often observed in hospital and discharged with careful instructions to return if symptoms increase. Persistent problems maintaining adequate oxygen saturations may require hospitalization for chest tube placement and ongoing assessment of respiratory status.

LIFE SPAN CONSIDERATIONS

Children under the age of 12 years are usually not certified to dive, as they may lack the maturity to appreciate the inherent dangers and need for absolute adherence to the rules. Diving in pregnancy is not recommended because of risk to the fetus from the unknown effects of nitrogen diffusion across the placenta. Seniors, who are more likely to have medical problems that could affect diving, should seek initial medical clearance and annually thereafter or as health status changes.

COMPLICATIONS

Complications of decompression illness include cardiac arrest, drowning or near drowning, hypoxia, and permanent neurologic damage.[4] Initial symptoms that appear minimal can worsen over the first few hours; thus it is recommended that patients with even mild symptoms be referred to a facility with a recompression (hyperbaric) chamber and medical personnel with knowledge of diving injuries.[5]

Ear Barotrauma

Ear barotrauma was first described in 1897 and remains an important problem for both occupational and recreational divers. Again, the pathophysiology is related to an inability to equalize pressures during descent or ascent. Injuries can range from injury to the tympanic membrane (including rupture), severe middle ear damage, to inner ear labyrinthine window rupture. Symptoms associated with these problems include dizziness, tinnitus, nausea, ear pain, jaw or neck pain, and hearing difficulty.[4]

Examination of the ear canal may reveal bloody drainage and acute damage to the tympanic membrane. Inflammation of the eardrum and/or collections of fluid behind the eardrum may be seen. Nystagmus, hearing loss, and loss of balance may also be noted. The Weber's and Rinne tests may be helpful in distinguishing conductive hearing loss (caused by middle ear barotrauma) from sensorineural hearing loss (implicating either inner ear barotrauma or inner ear DCS).[1]

All patients must refrain from diving until symptoms have cleared. If symptoms are limited to the ear, referral to recompression centers is indicated only for treatment of inner ear DCS.[1] Systemic decongestants may provide symptomatic relief. Antibiotics may be necessary if purulent secretions are present. Topical antiinflammatory/antibiotic drops may be helpful in alleviating the pain of otitis externa. Occasionally, mild systemic analgesics may be needed. Most tympanic membrane ruptures heal within 4 to 5 days.

Inner ear barotrauma with vertigo and tinnitus require a period of bed rest, usually in the hospital, with medication to control vertigo and possibly sedatives to help the patient to rest comfortably.[6] Surgical exploration to repair a round window rupture may be required. Referral to an audiologist for hearing evaluation may be necessary if hearing loss is severe or persistent.

Varying degrees of hearing loss, vestibular dysfunction resulting in chronic vertigo, balance disorders, and gait disorders are the most serious complications of ear barotrauma.[7] Permanent inner ear damage can be a contraindication to further diving.

Sinus Barotrauma

Sinus barotrauma is associated with severe pain during descent. The frontal sinus is most commonly involved. Epistaxis occurs in about half of the cases.[1] Sinus barotrauma can be a problem in divers who have experienced it before and in those with a history of chronic sinus problems.

Topical and systemic nasal decongestants may provide both relief and prophylaxis for divers who are predisposed to this complication. Antibiotics may be indicated when infection is suspected. Patients who do not respond to conservative therapy should be referred to an otolaryngologist for ongoing management.[1]

Marine Animal Bites and Stings

A common source of injuries to divers is inadvertent contact with marine life. Bites and stings from sea creatures are quite common and range from the annoying to the life threatening. These injuries usually require immediate treatment, but patients who sustain multiple and/or deep wounds or serious systemic illness will require follow-up care by primary care providers. Discussion of these injuries is limited to some of the more common or toxic species found in the Western Hemisphere.

CLINICAL PRESENTATION

Although it is often not possible to identify the marine animal that caused the injury, the envenomations of the lionfish and stingray are notable for severe reactions. Symptoms, including hypotension, heart failure, respiratory distress, and death, can occur, although the number of confirmed human deaths from these encounters is much less than commonly believed.[8] Milder and delayed reactions can include regional lymphadenopathy, fever, malaise, nausea, vomiting, and delirium. The wounds inflicted are most commonly mild (erythema only) but often extremely painful. More severe encounters can result in vesicle formation, cellulitis, and necrotic breakdown. Recovery can take months, especially if the wounds are complicated by secondary infection.[3]

The sting of the sculpin, a common member of the scorpion fish family found off the coast of southern California, produces severe pain and occasionally nausea and vomiting. The venom produces protein that is rapidly broken down in the presence of heat. Treatment is immersion in water as hot as can be tolerated for 60 to 90 minutes. Once the pain is relieved, the wound should be flushed of debris and monitored for infection.[9]

The stingray can also be found in large numbers off the coast of southern California, Florida, and other warmer waters. Typically a swimmer will step on the stingray lying on the bottom in shallow water. The venom also breaks down on exposure to heat and the treatment is the same as for sculpin stings.[9]

The jellyfish envenomation is of low toxicity but is quite painful and in susceptible people, an allergic reaction can occur. First aid consists of removal of any adherent tentacles followed by a vinegar rinse. The wound is then washed with soap and water and treated with a topical hydrocortisone cream. Pain can be controlled with acetaminophen or ibuprofen.[9]

The Portuguese man-of-war, found in tropical and subtropical regions of the Pacific, as well as the northern Atlantic Gulf Stream, is infamous for its painful sting and systemic manifestations. First aid generally consists of copious flushing with either sea or fresh water, removal of visible tentacles, and applications of ice to control pain.[10]

A vinegar or acetic acid wash may help to reduce pain. Anaphylactic shock is treated with epinephrine and other supportive measures.

MANAGEMENT OF ENVENOMATIONS

Good and immediate first aid is essential to uncomplicated healing and should include immediate assessment of the patient's general status, especially if there is airway, breathing, or circulatory compromise requiring stabilization or resuscitation.[2] Gentle removal of visible spines, control of bleeding, analgesia, and transport to the nearest emergency department are recommended initial treatments.

In the emergency department, stings are managed immediately by removing tentacles and spines (if not done at the dive site) and irrigating the area. A local anesthetic should be used. Open wounds require careful and thorough irrigation and debridement of foreign bodies. Heat treatment using immersion of the affected limb into water no hotter than 114° F can be effective with specific envenomations (see previously).[7]

Wound care is then directed toward healing without secondary infection. Skin irritations and itching can be treated with warm or cool compresses and mild steroid creams. The patient's tetanus status should be ascertained and vaccine administered if longer than 10 years has elapsed since the last immunization.

INDICATIONS FOR REFERRAL/HOSPITALIZATION

All patients with DCS and pulmonary barotrauma (dysbarism) must be stabilized on site and referred to the nearest recompression (hyperbaric oxygen) chamber facility. This referral can be made more than 24 hours after a dive with treatment success. Evaluation by a sports medicine physician with specialized knowledge of diving injuries is preferred whenever possible. Patients with ear barotrauma may need to be seen and managed by an otolaryngologist, especially if they are not responding to conservative therapy. The primary care provider can manage bites and stings as long as wound healing is uncomplicated. Referral for surgical debridement may be necessary for nonhealing wounds.

PATIENT AND FAMILY EDUCATION

All divers are required to complete a standard course in diving principles and first aid. Diving certification agencies have uniform standards established by the Recreational Scuba Training Council.[4] A basic life support certification is highly recommended. Extra training in the use of oxygen in an emergency is also recommended. Divers should make every effort to avoid contact with marine life and wear protective clothing while diving. Venomous species are widespread throughout tropical, subtropical, and temperate waters and the ability to visually identify these fish is advised. Wearing appropriate gear in cold water helps to prevent hypothermia. Recreational divers are encouraged to use dive tables and computers conservatively.[1] Immunizations, especially tetanus, should be current.

The Divers Alert Network (DAN),* a nonprofit organization, provides expert medical information to the diving public and to medical providers treating diving-related injuries, promotes and supports diving research, and maintains a 24-hour emergency telephone line for diving accidents. DAN can provide medical providers with the location of the nearest recompression chamber. Primary care providers who encounter patients with possible diving-related injuries can use DAN for both emergent and nonemergent consultations and questions, especially for cases in which decompression injuries are suspected.

*DAN, The Peter B. Bennett Center, 6 West Colony Place, Durham, NC 27705; medical emergencies: (919) 684-4326; nonemergency diving questions: (919) 684-2948, Monday through Friday, 9 AM to 5 PM EST. www.diversalertnetwork.org

REFERENCES

1. Bove A, Davis JC: *Diving medicine*, Philadelphia, 1997, WB Saunders.
2. Bove AA, editor: *Medical examination of sports scuba divers*, ed 3, San Antonio, 1998, Medical Seminars Inc.
3. Mebane GV, editor: *DAN dive and travel medical guide*, Durham, NC, 1995, Diver Alert Network.
4. Pulley SA: Decompression sickness, *eMedicine Journal* 2(9) 2001.
5. Moon RE: Treatment of diving emergencies, *Crit Care Clin* 15: 429-456, 1999.
6. Paparella MM, Adams GL, Levine SC: Disease of the middle ear and mastoid. In Adams GL, Boies LR, Hilder PA, editors: *Fundamentals of otolaryngology*, ed 6, Philadelphia, 1989, WB Saunders.
7. Parell GJ, Becker GD: Inner ear barotrauma in scuba divers: a long-term follow-up after continued diving, *Arch Otolaryngol Head Neck Surg* 119(4):455-457, 1993.
8. Gallagher SA: Lionfish and stonefish, *eMedicine Journal* 2(7), 2001.
9. UCSD Healthcare: *Venomous marine animals of Southern California*. Retrieved March 30, 2002, from the World Wide Web: www.health.ucsd.edu/poison/marine.asp
10. The Portuguese man-of war, a dangerous ocean organism of Hawaii. Retrieved March 30, 2002, from the World Wide Web: www.aloha.com/~lifeguards/portue.html.

CHAPTER 246

Fatigue

Michelle E. Freshman

DEFINITION/EPIDEMIOLOGY

Fatigue is common, often presenting as an attendant rather than a primary complaint. The subjective nature of this problem compels a practitioner to rely almost entirely on the patient's perception of diminished performance. Fatigue has been cited as a chief complaint in 5% of primary care visits, accounting for more than 10 million visits a year,[1] representing 25% of the ambulatory care visits, and totaling $1 billion. Attempts to catalog the source have determined that 20% to 45% of cases are related to physical causes, and 40% to 80% are due to emotional ones.[1] One estimate of cost per patient, using the Maryland Medicare Fee Schedule from a sample of 1721 primary care physicians representing 53 managed care organizations, came to $389 (± $201); this amount was similar to that for the management of high cholesterol, but half that for low back pain at $726 (± $369).[2]

Although it is recognized that both physical and emotional components are involved, research has not yet delineated the relationship between these domains. Some define fatigue as a marked decrease in a patient's ability to exert himself or herself physically or mentally during usual activities. Others incorporate depressed affect in their definition, as well as interactions with psychologic and somatic pain.[3]

Fatigue may accompany infections or parallel a precipitous decline in health status and persist over months. In contrast to illness-related fatigue, physiologic fatigue is said to result from poor sleep hygiene, pregnancy, postpartum status, or stress.[4] Health-destructive practices such as intentional sleep deprivation, a diet of nutritionally deficient foods, a sedentary lifestyle, and excessive intake of alcohol, caffeine, or stimulant drugs also result in protracted fatigue. Physiologic fatigue is simple to remedy if the offending habits, medications, sleep disturbances, or exertional demands can be rectified.

Many medications cause fatigue. A sampling includes antipsychotics, cancer chemotherapy drugs (interferon-alfa, high-dose corticosteroids, vincristine, cisplatin), cardiac drugs (calcium channel blockers, beta blockers, diuretics), phenobarbital, carbamazepine, H_1- and H_2-receptor blockers, benzodiazepines, and sedative tricyclic antidepressants. A common source of pharmacologically induced fatigue is the chronic use of hypnotics, hypnotic withdrawal, or minor tranquilizers. Antihistamines that have anticholinergic effects can produce fatigue as a side effect.

Finally, a large population at risk for debilitating fatigue is postpartum women. Blood loss at the time of delivery coupled with sleep deprivation and the stress of caring for a newborn can contribute to profound fatigue. Postpartum "blues" occur in 50% to 85% of pregnancies. One in 1000 manifest psychosis, with a 4% mortality.[5] Although serious postpartum sequelae affect less than 10% of delivered patients, the discerning practitioner can help avert serious illness in those patients who do complain of fatigue. It is important to remember that concerned family members may be the first ones to approach the practitioner with concerns about a postpartum patient.

PATHOPHYSIOLOGY AND CLINICAL PRESENTATION

The pathophysiology of fatigue is entirely dependent on its etiology. Given the subjective nature of this complaint, a careful review of symptoms and a physical examination are required. Inquiry is first directed to sleep habits, noise, privacy, temperature discomfort, snoring, safety, difficulties with partner, and bedtime irregularity (see Chapter 16). Irregular sleeping patterns, generalized apathy, loneliness, vegetative symptoms, a change in circumstances (e.g., recent loss, a new job), anorexia, crying, hopelessness, and suicidal ideation must also be determined.

A symptom profile is constructed by assessing the effects of rest periods, such as bedtime sleep, naps, weekends, and vacation, on the perceived state of fatigue. A medication inventory of prescribed, over-the-counter, and self-prescribed drugs, including alcohol, should be elicited. Of particular concern is the use of caffeine, nicotine, amphetamines, cocaine, or central nervous system (CNS) depressants. Screening for contacts with infectious agents or vectors, including pets and other animals, may be informative if viral or bacterial symptoms are present. Pertinent family history, including a history of malignancies or recent family illnesses, should also be elicited.

Concurrent CNS illness or chronic pain produces fatigue. It is useful to know if there has been accompanying neurologic deficits such as dysphasia, tremor, gait disturbance, or dysgraphia. Fatigue often accompanies deconditioning after a prolonged illness or hospitalization. If fatigue increases during the day but is relieved by rest, rheumatologic or other organic causes are considered. Fatigue that has increased over months suggests a debilitating disease. Recurrent, irresistible attacks of daytime sleepiness—often in conjunction with a triad of cataplexy, sleep paralysis, and hypnagogic hallucinations—suggests narcolepsy.

PHYSICAL EXAMINATION

For patients with fatigue, the physical examination is an adjunct to a thorough history of the complaint. Initially, habitus, speech, cognition, balance, and gait are assessed. Measurements of postural blood pressure and pulse, with attention to pulse character, may indicate postural hypotension or cardiac arrhythmia, which can precipitate fatigue. Skin should be examined for dryness, jaundice, pallor, or lesions. Thinning hair, glossy tongue, poor skin turgor or wound healing, easy bruising, and body wasting manifest poor nutritional status. Lymphadenopathy should be noted.

A complete examination of the cardiorespiratory system should be performed with attention to the presence of respiratory rales (i.e., adventitious, irregular, or rapid breath sounds) or consolidation. Jugular venous distention, cardiac murmurs, or peripheral edema should be noted. The abdominal examination should carefully exclude ascites, bruits, organomegaly, and gastrointestinal bleeding. Neuromuscular coordination and movement, exertional strain, and joint function are included to determine if chronic disease or acute infection exists. All age- and history-appropriate cancer screenings including breast, cervical, prostate, and colon examinations are recommended.

DIAGNOSTICS

Diagnostic investigation requires persistence, as fatigue may be a manifestation of any number of organic diseases. Generally, an initial screen in cases of fatigue with a suspected physical etiology should include a stool for occult blood; CBC with differential; chemistry profile, including serum electrolytes, serum glucose, calcium, albumin, creatinine, BUN, and transaminase-aminotransferase; erythrocyte sedimentation rate; thyroid-stimulating hormone, and urinalysis. Any abnormal results require follow-up evaluation.

In addition, clinical information can be obtained from a pharyngeal culture; Monospot test; syphilis titer; and testing for hepatitis, HIV, or tuberculosis if the history and physical examination support this investigation. A chest x-ray film is ordered for suspected lung or cardiac disease. A patient with primary sleep disorder should be referred to a regional sleep disorder clinic, where a sleep study may be suggested. For patients in whom postpolio syndrome (PPS) is suspected, a nerve conduction study and an electromyogram can differentiate such cases from myasthenia gravis or other neuropathies.[7] Although myasthenia gravis may be considered a disease of older age, it can be seen in women ages 20 to 40 years of age, often triggered by an infection.[8]

DIFFERENTIAL DIAGNOSIS

The differential diagnosis for fatigue is divided into four categories: physiologic, physical, psychologic, and situational. Physiologic fatigue results from adverse external influences such as poor sleep hygiene, substance abuse, or medication side effects. Physical disorders include acute and chronic illnesses resulting from a host of systemic conditions. Some patients suffer from restless leg syndrome, which causes undetectable sleep interruption but nonrefreshing sleep as a result.[9] Any cardiac, pulmonary, hematologic, endocrine, rheumatoid, neuromuscular, skin, renal, immune, or CNS disorders may individually or

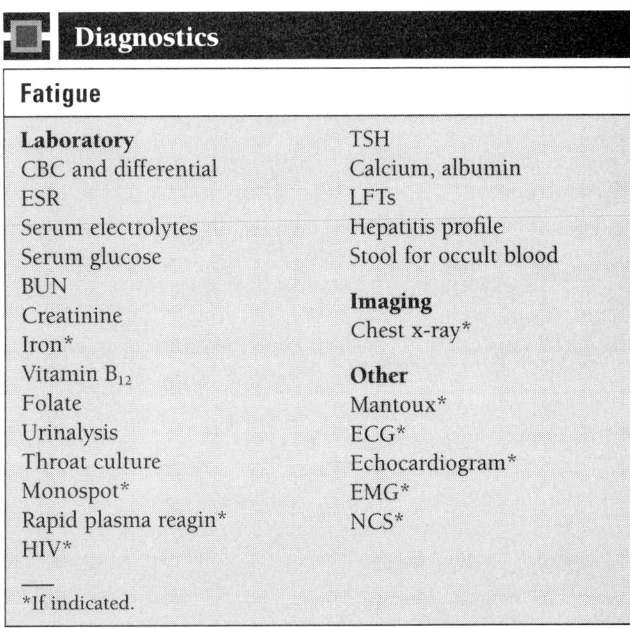

Diagnostics

Fatigue

Laboratory	TSH
CBC and differential	Calcium, albumin
ESR	LFTs
Serum electrolytes	Hepatitis profile
Serum glucose	Stool for occult blood
BUN	
Creatinine	**Imaging**
Iron*	Chest x-ray*
Vitamin B_{12}	**Other**
Folate	Mantoux*
Urinalysis	ECG*
Throat culture	Echocardiogram*
Monospot*	EMG*
Rapid plasma reagin*	NCS*
HIV*	

*If indicated.

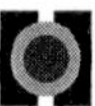

Differential Diagnosis

Fatigue

Physiologic Causes	Psychologic Causes
Poor sleep hygiene	Depression
Substance abuse	Chronic anxiety
Medication side effects	Mania, psychosis
Postpartum	Eating disorders
Health-destructive behaviors	
Physical Causes	**Situational Causes**
Anemias	Role stress
Malignancy	Unemployment
Chronic obstructive pulmonary disease	Posttraumatic stress disorder
Congestive heart failure	Grief
HIV	
Thyroid dysfunction	
Diabetes mellitus	
Acute/chronic infection	
Rheumatic disorders	
Renal insufficiency	
Postpolio syndrome	
Chronic fatigue syndrome	
Sleep apnea	
Restless leg syndrome	

collectively contribute to fatigue. Systemic disorders result from inflammation, malignancy, infection, noxious fumes, or ingested poisons.

Fatigue accompanies cardiac, pulmonary, hematologic, and metabolic disturbances. The mechanisms in most of these cases involve reduced oxygen intake, pulmonary congestion or inelasticity, or severe iron deficiency (hematocrit <20). A calorie-consuming malignancy such as pancreatic cancer is known to present with marked fatigue and few other symptoms. Morbid obesity can be a cause of fatigue, particularly in cases of sleep apnea, which may cause hemoglobin desaturation, leading to pulmonary hypertension. The decreased metabolic activity associated with hypothyroidism commonly produces sluggishness and depression, whereas hyperthyroidism in older patients can manifest as fatigue, weight loss, and disinterest. Uncontrolled diabetes mellitus causes fatigue because of significant calorie and fluid depletion. In cases of acute or chronic infection, fever and lymphadenopathy often accompany fatigue because of the long-term assault on immunologic resources. Fatigue is also associated with rheumatologic diseases but is not usually the only symptom.

Another source of chronic fatigue is the relatively prevalent phenomenon of PPS, which affects 25% to 40% of victims of poliomyelitis 30 years after the initial illness. Approximately 1.6 million people have had acute poliomyelitis in the United States.[7] It is projected that between 66% and 80% of these patients will experience some later degree of disability, usually in the form of weakness, heat or cold intolerance, or easy fatiguability.[7]

Fatigue persisting for at least 6 months and accompanied by a 50% decrease in activity level and exclusion of all other medical and psychiatric explanations warrants consideration of chronic fatigue syndrome (CFS).[4] Muscle or joint pain, headaches, sore throat, enlarged and painful nodes, and mental dullness or confusion severe enough to affect routine activity are common symptoms. Nonrestorative sleep and an extreme reaction to exertion are also reported. It is known that 4 to 10 of every 100,000 Americans older than 18 years is diagnosed with CFS. The reported ratio of women to men is 3:1, and the syndrome is seen more commonly among those in their early thirties.[3] Some sources claim that more than two thirds of patients with CFS have psychiatric disorders, most often mood, somatoform, and anxiety disorders.[4]

CFS is a diagnosis of exclusion. No definitive test exists for the syndrome. Between 20% and 60% of patients improve in 1 to 2 years, whereas others wax and wane for years.[10] Therapies that have been helpful, in addition to lifestyle adjustment, include use of antidepressants and cognitive strategies.[10] Myofascial conditions or fibromyalgia may be difficult to distinguish from CFS. Myofascial pain syndrome (see Chapter 197) involves painful, tender areas in muscles that twitch on palpation or produce an area of referred pain. This localized, short-term condition lacks systemic manifestations other than fatigue. Fibromyalgia, in contrast, has uniform trigger point associations, with fatigue and other systemic features (see Chapter 190).

Slow-onset fatigue is commonly related to psychologic distress.[11] Fatigue is often observed in depression. Research on clinically diagnosed depression has established the contribution of neurotransmitter chemistry. In addition, chronic anxiety or stress can produce neck and shoulder muscle fatigue, irregular sleeping patterns, or irritable bowel symptoms. Among the mental illnesses that tax energy reserves are anxiety, eating, or depressive disorders. Generalized anxiety produces autonomic hyperactivity, sleep disturbances, dry mouth, and bowel distress.[11]

Of note, situational factors such as increased work, school or relationship stress, unemployment, delayed effects of trauma, or bereavement provoke fatigue. CFS patients can also manifest depressive illness, although premorbid depression is not necessarily a precursor.

MANAGEMENT

The patient with fatigue requires support. The practitioner must acknowledge the fatigue as a valid complaint, worthy of further exploration. Behavioral, situational, and environmental contributions to sleep disturbance should be identified for optimal improvement. Depression should be confirmed before medication for short-term sleep management is prescribed. When generalized anxiety disorder is identified, use of benzodiazepines other than on a short-term basis is discouraged in favor of buspirone and other antidepressants such as venlafaxine.[12]

Chronic muscle fatigue and joint pain sufferers can influence the onset and toll of their illness by maintaining normal weight, avoiding exercising to the point of muscle pain, keeping body temperature warmer than air temperature (to avoid the muscle tension associated with cold), and using stress reduction, energy conservation, and time management techniques. The practitioner can empower the patient to have a sense of control over the environment by encouraging the patient to network, obtain relevant publications, and attend support groups. If endurance can be improved, a regimen of increased exercise ameliorates fatigue by improving cardiovascular functioning.[13]

If diagnosis is elusive, the patient is asked to keep a fatigue diary. Recording the time of onset, duration, severity, accompanying symptoms, relief measures, exercise, mood, diet, medications, and stressors not only helps the primary care provider, but will be helpful if future consultation is necessary.

For the subset of patients who are physically disabled by fatigue, employment considerations and alternative compensation might require a practitioner's involvement. A patient may wish to file for temporary disability, workers' compensation, job reassignment, long-term disability, or government disability funds.

LIFE SPAN CONSIDERATIONS

A patient's age and life span stressors influence the evaluation. Teenagers and newly independent young adults should be screened for deleterious health habits, given a natural tendency toward experimentation with alcohol, drugs, and irregular sleep and nutrition. Transitions and losses resulting from changes such as marriage or the death of a parent can be destabilizing. Situational depression or anxiety accompanies these developmental transitions and cause fatigue. Older patients who have nightmares or who sleepwalk may have precipitant underlying disease or may be using contributing medications.[14]

COMPLICATIONS

Complications of fatigue include daytime sleepiness, risk of injury and/or accident, poor performance, and cognitive and functional impairment.

INDICATIONS FOR REFERRAL/HOSPITALIZATION

The collaborating physician is consulted in the evaluation of the patient with fatigue. Specialist involvement is dictated by the suspected cause of the fatigue. When fatigue is long-standing, mental health referral is helpful for support. Referral is also indicated for progressive symptoms, a lack of response to therapy, or indications of life-threatening illness. It is important to consider services available to the patient with a chronic fatigue condition such as CFS or PPS, which impacts heavily on the quality of life and work. Cognitive behavior therapy has been effective with adult outpatients with CFS.[15]

Postpartum patients with fatigue are screened for anemia, thyroid disorders, and urinary tract infections. When fatigue is associated with acute depression, psychosis, cardiomyopathy, congestive heart failure or chronic obstructive pulmonary disease exacerbation, or obstructive sleep apnea resulting from morbid obesity or anatomic abnormality, patients should be referred to the appropriate specialist or acute care setting.

PATIENT AND FAMILY EDUCATION

It is important to acknowledge fatigue as a legitimate symptom of various underlying illnesses. The importance of proper nutrition, sleep, and exercise should be stressed to patients in concrete terms. This approach maximizes their health, assists them in maintaining an optimal quality of life, and provides protection against debilitating stressors and communicable illnesses. Consultation with a nutritionist, review of sleep hygiene, and an exercise tolerance test are recommended when indicated.

Alcohol, drug, tobacco and caffeine consumption has an adverse effect on restful sleep. Patients are advised to discontinue caffeine 4 to 6 hours before bed and to avoid late night snacks and stimulants such as tobacco and alcohol. Regular sleep and wake times, minimal environmental stimuli such as noise or light, regulated ambient temperature, and late afternoon or evening exertion encourage good sleep hygiene.

REFERENCES

1. Libbus MK: Women's beliefs regarding persistent fatigue, *Issues Ment Health Nurs* 17:589-600, 1996.
2. Meyer CM and others: Evaluation of common problems in primary care: effects of physician, practice, and financial characteristics, *Am J Manage Care* 6(4):457-469, 2000.
3. Gorensek MJ: Definition of fatigue and the problem of chronic fatigue, *Prim Care* 18(2):397-407, 1991.
4. Portwood MF: Chronic fatigue syndrome: a diagnosis for consideration, *Nurse Pract* 13(2):11-23, 1988.
5. Atkinson LS, Baxley EG: Postpartum fatigue, *Am Fam Physician* 50(1):113-118, 1994.
6. Friedman HH: *Problem-oriented medical diagnosis,* ed 5, Boston, 1991, Little Brown.
7. LeCompte CM: Post polio syndrome: an update for the primary health care provider, *Nurse Pract* 22(5):133-154, 1997.
8. Suarez GA: Myasthenia gravis: diagnosis and treatment, *Rev Neurol* 29(2):162-165, 1999.
9. Insomnia: assessment and management in primary care. National Heart Lung, and Blood Institute Working Group on Insomnia, *Am Fam Physician* 59(11):3029-3038, 1999.
10. Buchwald D and others: Tips on chronic fatigue syndrome, *Patient Care* 30:45-55, 1991.
11. Epstein KR: The chronically fatigued patient, *Med Clin North Am* 79(2):315-327, 1995.
12. Lydiaer RB: An overview of generalized anxiety disorder: disease state—appropriate therapy, *Clin Ther* 22(Supp A):A3-24, 2000.
13. Potempa K and others: Chronic fatigue, *Image J Nurs Sch* 18(4): 165-169, 1986.
14. Vgontzas AN: Sleep and its disorders, *Annu Rev Med* 50:387-400, 1999.
15. Price JR, Couper J: Cognitive behaviour therapy chronic fatigue syndrome in adults: Cochrane Depression, Anxiety, and Neurosis Group, *Cochrane Database Syst Rev,* Issue 2:CD001027, 2000.

CHAPTER 247

Fever

Michelle E. Freshman

DEFINITION/EPIDEMIOLOGY

A clinical encounter with a febrile patient can be one of the most challenging encounters in primary care. Such a presentation requires both skillful assessment and careful diagnostic reasoning. A temperature of 36.8° C (98.2° F), within 1° C (1.8° F), is considered normal despite the common 98.6° F attributed to Wunderlich in the 1860s who used a foot-long axillary thermometer thought to be calibrated slightly higher.[1] Generally, fever is distinguished from normal temperature variation at 37.7° C (99.9° F) or greater, which is the 99th percentile of maximum temperatures in healthy adults.[1] A low fever, 37.2° to 37.8° C (99° F to 100.4° F), may indicate viral or gastrointestinal illness; moderate, 37.8° to 40° C (100.5° F to 104° F), may reflect sinusitis or mononucleosis; and high, above 40° C, may suggest bacterial causes.[2]

Peripherally, core body temperature is thought to be best approximated by rectal temperatures, which are 0.4° C to 0.5° C (0.7° F to 1.0° F) higher than oral temperatures, which are similarly higher than axillary or tympanic measures. Although an oral temperature can be affected by variables such as digestion and hyperventilation, it is a useful proxy for the core; the axillary reading is far less reliable.[3] All individuals experience a diurnal temperature fluctuation within 1° C (1.8° F), peaking around 6 PM and falling the most during sleep. Furthermore, the basal temperature of fertile women rises just before ovulation by as much as 0.5° C (1° F).[4]

Most of the time a fever reflects a humoral response to infection, inflammation, or neoplasms. Although fevers can produce myalgias, malaise, and fatigue, some patients are unaware of fever symptoms. For example, 20% to 30% of older patients may present with low-grade elevations or below-normal temperatures despite overwhelming infection.[5]

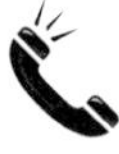

Physician consultation is recommended for patients with persistent fever unresponsive to treatment, temperature greater than 39.4° C (103° F), or fever associated with hypertension, immunocompromised status, Reye's syndrome, or mental status changes.

PATHOPHYSIOLOGY

The human body is able to maintain a consistent core temperature in the face of environmental fluctuation. When an individual develops a sustained elevated temperature, however, this suggests system deregulation in any of the three temperature control mechanisms in the body: the afferent, efferent, and neuronal control mechanisms. The afferent system is composed of thermosensors located around the mouth and fingertips, which conduct changes in heat or cold sensation to central thermosensors. This system links directly to the anterior hypothalamus. The efferent system has the capacity to generate and dissipate heat through autonomic, somatic, endocrine, and behavioral mechanisms. Finally, the neuronal system, centered in the hypothalamus, ultimately provides a negative feedback loop by way of increasing or decreasing body temperature in response to external or internal cues, including bacteria, viruses, and other pathogens.

Fever affects the body in multiple ways. A 1° C (1.8° F) increase in temperature increases the basal metabolic rate by more than 10%. Thus fever produces dehydration in the absence of increased water intake, taxes cardiac output by increasing myocardial oxygen consumption, and causes confusion, delirium, and seizures.

A fever generally produces a change in the hypothalamic set point temperature. Hyperpyrexia refers to temperatures in excess of 40° C (105° F), where the hypothalamic set point is dangerously high. This condition is seen in association with high environmental temperatures or in response to strenuous physical exercise or illness. Common clinical conditions associated with hyperpyrexia include heat cramps, heat exhaustion, and heat stroke. A body can sustain a temperature of 41° C (109° F), although this is likely to lead to brain damage, whereas a temperature in excess of 43° C (114° F) is invariably fatal. Hyperthermia, marked by an extremely high temperature and including heat stroke, severe burns, thyroid storm, and CNS lesions, results from an override of the heat-dissipating system. The set point does not change, nor are pyrogens involved. Malignant hyperthermia, seen with mottled cyanosis, is an inherited condition characterized by a febrile response to general anesthesia. It is ideally prevented by obtaining a thorough family history.

CLINICAL PRESENTATION

A complete history comprises fever symptoms and patterns, along with possible infectious agents, recent illnesses, iatrogenic medications, underlying chronic illnesses, and high-risk health behaviors. Rash, lymphadenopathy, myalgia, specific pain, hemoptysis, or a palpable mass may accompany fever. Chills with rigors are more common with bacterial infections, drug fever, or transfusions.[6] Concomitant complaints help distinguish primary sites of infection such as the tonsils, eardrums, urinary tract, or prostate, from systemic conditions. Blunt trauma or internal injury, as from ischemia, can cause inflammation and cytokine recruitment, producing fever. A review of the patient and family's immunization history, including purified protein derivative (PPD) status, past communicable diseases, and past fever and responses to fever such as seizures, is crucial. Irregularities of physiologic function including headache, rash, nausea, vomiting, and diarrhea help delineate which organ system is primarily involved.

Fever patterns may provide diagnostic clues but are thought to have limited diagnostic significance, in part as a result of antibiotic therapies.[1,7] Intermittent fevers return to normal levels at least once a day, such as occurs with malaria. Remittent fevers fall during the day but not to normal levels and can signify a systemic etiology, such as malignancy or adverse drug reaction. Sustained fevers that are consistent within a degree on a daily basis can indicate viral or bacterial infections, as well as noninfectious conditions in older individuals or the chronically ill. Relapsing fevers that come and go over several daylong or month-long cycles may reflect conditions such as typhoid or Hodgkin's disease. Hectic fevers, intermittent or remittent type with wide fluctuations, may result from pyogenic abscess or chronic tuberculosis.

PHYSICAL EXAMINATION

Although a thorough assessment of fever begins with a good history, the source of the fever may still be elusive. Signs of infection, including an injected pharynx, exanthema or vesicles, masses, areas of tenderness, and changes in mentation, should be assessed. A full skin examination (including nail beds) looking for skin tears, signs of cellulitis, rash, splinter hemorrhages, petechial or puerpural lesions, purulent wounds, or signs of dehydration is required. Sinus, nasal, ear, dental, and throat examinations are essential. Regional lymph node enlargement suggests a localized infectious process. As with any isolated lymphadenopathy, malignancy must be excluded. Heart murmurs or a rub in the setting of fever may indicate subacute endocarditis. Adventitious or irregular breath sounds may indicate pneumonia, pulmonary emboli, or pulmonary effusions. An abdominal mass, hepatosplenomegaly, guarding, or rebound tenderness indicates a probable abdominal fever source.

Calf tenderness with a palpable vascular cord is evidence of thrombophlebitis. Fever accompanied by musculoskeletal weakness may suggest drug-induced fever. Joints are evaluated for heat, erythema, swelling, and tenderness. A warm, swollen joint should be tapped to exclude infectious vs. crystal-induced arthropathies. Breast, pelvic, penile, and rectal examinations are indicated when infections or neoplasms are suspected. Neurologic signs of confusion, delirium, or focal deficits may be present in meningitis, endocarditis, brain tumor, or hemorrhage.

DIAGNOSTICS

A CBC with differential is essential. Leukocytosis with a shift to the left suggests bacterial infection, particularly when juvenile band forms, toxic granulations, or Döhle's bodies are present. Appropriate cultures such as sputum, throat, blood, or urine are obtained as indicated by the history and physical examination. A positive leukocyte esterase is indicative of pyuria and has a sensitivity of 75% to 90%.[8] Bacterial causes have demonstrable evidence in 80% of cases.[1] Targeted viral titers and antibody titers are obtained if a specific virus is suspected. Serum amylase or lipase for suspected acute pancreatitis, blood smears for malaria, thyroid studies for thyroid storm, or sedimentation rates for septic arthritis are reserved for specific inquiries.

Electrolytes can help delineate dehydration, especially in the older patient. Chest radiographs can assist in the diagnosis of pneumonias, pleural effusions, tuberculosis, sarcoidosis, or tumors. Pelvic or renal ultrasound examinations may be useful if the fever source remains elusive. A lumbar puncture is performed if meningitis is suspected. It should be noted that despite a negative PPD and chest radiograph, tuberculosis commonly presents as fever of unknown origin in its disseminated form and should be suspected in immunocompromised patients.[9]

Fevers usually resolve with little or no intervention within 2 to 3 weeks. Those fevers in excess of 38.3° C (101° F) persisting beyond 3 weeks, for which intensive investigation fails to yield a diagnosis, are considered fevers of undetermined origin and

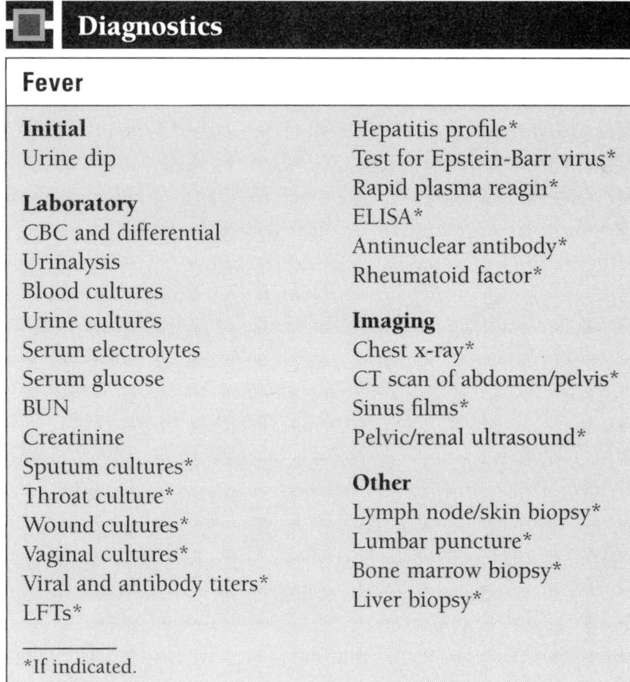

Diagnostics

Fever

Initial
Urine dip

Laboratory
CBC and differential
Urinalysis
Blood cultures
Urine cultures
Serum electrolytes
Serum glucose
BUN
Creatinine
Sputum cultures*
Throat culture*
Wound cultures*
Vaginal cultures*
Viral and antibody titers*
LFTs*
Hepatitis profile*
Test for Epstein-Barr virus*
Rapid plasma reagin*
ELISA*
Antinuclear antibody*
Rheumatoid factor*

Imaging
Chest x-ray*
CT scan of abdomen/pelvis*
Sinus films*
Pelvic/renal ultrasound*

Other
Lymph node/skin biopsy*
Lumbar puncture*
Bone marrow biopsy*
Liver biopsy*

*If indicated.

warrant hospitalization. It is rare that such a case cannot be categorized in the acute setting.[9]

DIFFERENTIAL DIAGNOSIS

Fever is best interpreted in the context of the site and signs of preexisting illness. The Differential Diagnosis box summarizes fever origins by local and systemic sources. A preliminary consideration in an otherwise well adult would be community-acquired pathogens producing upper respiratory tract infections, influenza, or pneumonia. Work, school, or home settings should be reviewed for human-, chemical-, and food-borne inoculation. Ingestion of noxious plants or prescribed, experimental, or recreational drug use may precipitate fever. In addition, contact with infected domesticated or wild animals is a concern. Cat-scratch fever, toxoplasmosis, leptospirosis, ehrlichiosis, babesiosis, brucellosis, psittacosis, rat-bite fever, and Lyme disease all originate from contact with an infected animal or insect. The tick-borne infections Rocky Mountain spotted fever, babesiosis, and ehrlichiosis are potentially fatal.

With recent foreign travel, cholera, typhoid fever, tularemia, dengue, amebiasis, plague, granulomatous infections such as tuberculosis or histoplasmosis, malaria, or various parasitic or protozoal illnesses may be acquired. Ethnic origin predisposes some to fever-producing conditions. Turks, Arabs, Armenians, and Sephardic Jews may develop familial Mediterranean fever. Sickle cell crisis is more common in Africans and their descendants (see Chapter 231).[6]

Recent surgical procedures place patients at higher risk for infections. Patients with prosthetic devices or silicone implants can develop graft-versus-host reactions or infections. Indwelling portals, including Foley catheters, percutaneous IV catheters, and peripheral lines, may be sources of infection.

A recent history of otitis media, urinary tract infection, or pneumonia may signify persistent infection. Diuretics, stool softeners, sleep medications, antiarrhythmic medications, sulfa

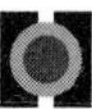

Differential Diagnosis

Fever

Infection	Factitious fever
Neoplasm	Pheochromocytoma
Drug-related fever	Anemia
Familial Mediterranean fever	Hemoglobinopathies
Inflammation	
Thyrotoxicosis	
Injury	

drugs, beta-lactamase antibiotics, thyroid medication, and often phenytoin can cause drug fever, especially after administration over multiple weeks. Corticosteroids and other immunosuppressive drugs can also cause low-grade temperature increases. Hematologic diseases such as anemias, leukemia, and lymphomas produce fevers, as can transfusion reactions. A pulmonary embolus or thrombophlebitis may be accompanied by fever. Inflammatory conditions, including thyrotoxicosis, systemic lupus erythematosus, rheumatoid arthritis, or osteomyelitis, can induce febrile states. Trauma, particularly head injury, is known to cause hyperpyrexia in some cases. Occasionally patients with mental illness or attention-seeking behaviors may fabricate the signs and symptoms of a fever; this is known as factitious fever. Finally, recent or past illicit drug use (especially IV use) or alcohol abuse, cigarette smoking, or high-risk sexual contacts suggest a host of possible conditions that should be considered in the differential diagnosis, including HIV/AIDS and oropharyngeal, lung, or hepatic malignancies.

MANAGEMENT

Most fevers are managed with antipyretic agents, cooling blankets, or excess clothing removal. Some believe that fever is a self-regulatory response that should be allowed to persist unsuppressed, with only symptomatic relief and comfort measures offered. Support for this position argues that bacterial reproduction is inhibited at higher temperatures. Judicious use of antibiotics is advised. Discomfort or suspected serious illness warrants intervention and further testing.

In treating fever, acetaminophen 325 to 650 mg q 4 hours is commonly used. Antipyretic drugs such as aspirin, acetaminophen, and nonsteroidal antiinflammatory drugs (NSAIDs) inhibit fever by blocking the formation of pyrogenic substances that elevate the hypothalamic thermostat. However, salicylates and NSAIDs are used cautiously in surgical patients to preserve platelet functioning and reduce bleeding potential.[10] Salicylates are not recommended for fever reduction in children or adolescents because of a possible risk of Reye's syndrome. Nutrition and hydration status need to be closely monitored and serial temperatures should be recorded at regular intervals. Regulating room temperature and bedding promote stabilization. A fever that is unresponsive to antibiotic therapy invites further inquiry into viral, connective tissue, immune system, or malignant etiology.

LIFE SPAN CONSIDERATIONS

There are several populations for whom continuity and coordination of care is essential because of their fragile status: nursing home patients, patients with cancer, chronically ill, homebound older adults, and IV drug users or excessive alcohol users. Malnutrition, anemia, and indwelling prostheses, appliances, or access lines also put individuals at increased risk for infection and fever when they are made vulnerable by their living situations. These patients may need ongoing supervision to monitor adherence to medications, cancer screenings, nutritional and ambulatory safety education, and continual assessment for comorbidities Infectious diseases are a major cause of fever in older adults. Common infections in this general population are pneumonias, meningitis, endocarditis, urinary tract and skin infections, and septic shock.[11] For nursing home residents, these types of infections may result in expensive and disruptive hospitalization or death. Older patients have an impaired sweating mechanism, which leads to higher risk of heat stroke.[2]

COMPLICATIONS

Complications of fever include myalgias, malaise, fatigue, rigor, sepsis, orthostatic hypotension, confusion, delirium, seizures, tachycardia, tachypnea, and shock. Older individuals have a tendency toward a lower body temperature and a diminished ability to raise the temperature in response to illness; therefore practitioners must be vigilant for subtle and persistent signs of infection.[5] Dehydration as a result of fever is a common cause of morbidity and mortality, particularly in older adults.[12] In addition, older patients admitted with pneumonia and fever >38.1° C (101° F) are twice as likely to die in the hospital as those without such as fever.[1]

INDICATIONS FOR REFERRAL/HOSPITALIZATION

Referral to a specialist is indicated if the etiology remains unknown, the patient fails to respond to treatment, or the diagnosis indicates the need for consultation. The decision to hospitalize is made if the patient is not taking fluids, is hemodynamically unstable, is hypotensive, or has persistent tachycardia or tachypnea. Hospitalization is also advised in the event of shock, sepsis, or resistant microbial infections. In the face of infective endocarditis, necrotizing fasciitis, bacterial meningitis, acute onset viral encephalitis, or other overwhelming infections that can lead to rapid deterioration, emergent care is critical.

PATIENT AND FAMILY EDUCATION

All patients should be advised to call the primary care provider for fever that is higher than 38.6° C (101.5° F) for more than 24 hours. Immunosuppressed patients, including those with AIDS and those taking chemotherapeutic drugs, should monitor their temperature daily. These patients are advised to seek care without delay if they have a temperature above 37.8° C (100° F). Other patients whose fever exceeds 41.1° C (106° F) should be treated as soon as possible with antipyretics and cooling measures while constantly monitoring rectal temperature to avoid a hypothermic response.[2]

HEALTH PROMOTION

Individuals can mitigate their risk for heat-related illnesses by attending to their fluid intake and protecting themselves from long periods of sun exposure and exertion. Adequate reserves to fight infection are created through proper nutrition, sleep, exercise, and relaxation such that fever will not render an otherwise healthy patient severely debilitated. Minimizing one's risk of infection through proper immunization and handwashing is known to be effective. Patients with underlying illness, past history of surgery, or family history of fevers do well to keep these recorded in their medical record and communicated to their care provider.

REFERENCES

1. McGee S: Temperature. In McGee S: *Evidence-based physical diagnosis*, Philadelphia, 2001, WB Saunders.
2. Schull P, editor: *Professional guide to signs and symptoms*, ed 3, Springhouse, Penn, 2001, Springhouse Corp.
3. Dinarello C, Bunn P: Fever, *Semin Oncol* 24(3):288-298, 1997.
4. McCance KL, Huether SE: *Pathophysiology: the biological basis for disease in adults and children*, ed 3, St Louis, 1998, Mosby.
5. Norman DC, Yoshikawa TT: Fever in the elderly, *Infect Dis Clin North Am* 10(1):93-99, 1996.
6. Gelfand JA, Dinarello CA: Fever and hyperthermia. In Fauci AS, editor: *Harrison's principles of internal medicine*, ed 14, New York, 1997, McGraw-Hill.
7. Cunha BA: The clinical significance of fever patterns, *Infect Dis Clin North Am* 10(1):33-44, 1996.
8. Sirinavin S: Antibiotics for treating salmonella gut infections: Cochrane Infectious Diseases Group, *Cochrane Database Syst Rev*, Issue 2, 2000.
9. Friedman HH: *Problem-oriented medical diagnosis*, ed 5, Boston, 1991, Little, Brown.
10. Litwack K: Practical points in the evaluation of postoperative fever, *J Perianesth Nurs* 12(2):100-104, 1997.
11. Jacobs LG: Infectious disease emergencies in the geriatric population, *Clin Geriatr Med* 9(3):559-575, 1993.
12. Sansevero A: Dehydration in the elderly: strategies for prevention and management, *Nurse Pract* 22(4):41-70, 1997.

CHAPTER 248

HIV Infection

Han Q. Bui

DEFINITION/EPIDEMIOLOGY

A defining characteristic of human immunodeficiency virus (HIV) infection is diversity—in presentation, in affected populations, and in complications. The challenge for the primary care provider is who to screen, at what juncture to refer, and when to suspect and investigate for deterioration.

The definition of acquired immunodeficiency syndrome (AIDS) has been refined a number of times since it was first proposed by the Centers for Disease Control and Prevention (CDC) in 1987.[1] At that time the definition included opportunistic infections, signs, and symptoms usually associated with malignant diseases, and, in women, persistent and nonresponsive cervical cancer.[2] Currently diagnostic criteria have been expanded to include laboratory confirmation for the presence of antibody to HIV and a CD4 cell count of less than 200/mm^3 (Box 248-1).[2]

Transmission of HIV occurs sexually, parenterally through either injection drug use or blood product transmission, and via mother to child prenatally or through breast milk. In the United States, men who have sex with men account for the largest number of infected individuals, followed by injecting drug users and their heterosexual partners.

In the CDC Semiannual HIV/AIDS Surveillance Report through June 2001, the cumulative number of AIDS cases reported to the CDC was 793,026, with 649,186 cases in males and 134,845 in females. Through the same reporting period, 8994 AIDS cases were in children less than 13 years old. Total deaths were 457,677, including 452,111 adults and adolescents, and 5168 children under age 15 years.

A total of 330,000 AIDS cases were reported in whites and 301,000 in African-Americans. The three states reporting the highest number of cumulative AIDS cases were New York, California, and Florida. The three leading cities were New York City, Los Angeles, and San Francisco.

According to the Joint United Nations Program on HIV/AIDS, the following trends of the worldwide epidemic (or pandemic) of HIV were evident at the end of 2001:

- Today, 40 million people are estimated to be living with HIV/AIDS. Of these, 37.2 million are adults; 17.6 million are women, and 2.7 million are children less 15 years old.
- During 2001, AIDS caused the deaths of an estimated 3 million people, including 1.1 million women and 580,000 children less than 15 years old.
- HIV is increasingly affecting women. Approximately 48%, or 17.6 million, of the 37.2 million adults living with HIV or AIDS worldwide are women.
- The overwhelming majority of people with HIV—approximately 95% of the global total—now live in the developing world.[3]

BOX 248-1

INDICATOR CONDITIONS IN CASE DEFINITION OF AIDS (ADULTS)—1997*

- Candidiasis of esophagus, trachea, bronchi, or lungs (16%)
- Cervical cancer, invasive (0.6%)
- Coccidioidomycosis, extrapulmonary (0.3%)
- Cryptococcosis, extrapulmonary (5%)
- Cryptosporidiosis with diarrhea >1 month (1.3%)
- CMV of any organ other than liver, spleen, or lymph nodes; eye (7%)
- Herpes simplex with mucocutaneous ulcer >1 month or bronchitis, pneumonitis, esophagitis (5%)
- Histoplasmosis, extrapulmonary (0.9%)
- HIV-associated dementia: Disabling cognitive and/or other dysfunction interfering with occupation or activities of daily living (5%)
- HIV-associated wasting: Involuntary weight loss >10% of baseline plus chronic diarrhea (≥2 loose stools/day ≥30 days) or chronic weakness and documented enigmatic fever ≥30 days (18%)
- Isosporiasis with diarrhea >1 month (0.1%)
- Kaposi's sarcoma in patient under 60 years (or over 60 years) (7%)
- Lymphoma, Burkitt's (0.7%), immunoblastic (2.3%), primary CNS (0.7%)
- *Mycobacterium avium*, disseminated (5%)
- *Mycobacterium tuberculosis*, pulmonary (7%), extrapulmonary (2%)
- Nocardiosis <1%
- *Pneumocystis carinii* pneumonia (38%)
- Pneumonia, recurrent bacterial (≥2 episodes in 12 months) (5%)
- Progressive multifocal leukoencephalopathy (1%)
- *Salmonella* septicemia (nontyphoid), recurrent (0.3%)
- Strongyloidosis, extraintestinal <1%
- Toxoplasmosis of internal organ (4%)

Data from Centers for Disease Control and Prevention. *HIV/AIDS Surveillance Report* 9(2):18, 1997; Website http://www.cdc.gov/hiv/stats/hivsur92.pdf.
*Indicates frequency as the AIDS-indicator condition among 42,350 reported cases in 1997.

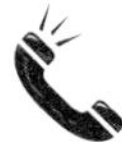

Physician consultation is recommended for patients with newly diagnosed HIV infection, a CD4 count less than 50/mm³, or suspected AIDS (diarrhea, fever, cytomegalovirus retinopathy, *Pneumocystis carinii* infection, visual changes, neurologic changes, or skin lesions).

PATHOPHYSIOLOGY

The HIV virus is a retrovirus, meaning that for replication to occur, the genomic material that is contained in the RNA must be transformed into DNA. The HIV virus commandeers the immune system's cells to achieve that goal. The HIV virus has an affinity for T lymphocytes, monocytes/macrophages, dendrite cells and, in particular, the CD4 molecule. The mechanism of viral attachment to the host cell is now recognized as involving chemokine factors, particularly CXCR4 and CCR5, which serve as co-receptors.

Approaches to preventing replication have involved blocking entry into the cell and stopping replication by inhibiting the activity of the various enzymes involved in the transformation of RNA to DNA (reverse transcriptase), integration into the host cell (integrase), and release of the immature virions and formation of mature virions (protease).

BOX 248-2

SYMPTOMATIC CONDITIONS IN HIV-1–INFECTED ADULTS AND ADOLESCENTS

- Bacillary angiomatosis
- Candidiasis, oropharyngeal (thrush)
- Candidiasis, vulvovaginal; persistent, frequent, or poorly responsive to therapy
- Cervical dysplasia (moderate or severe/cervical carcinoma in situ)
- Constitutional symptoms, such as fever (38.5° C [101.3° F]) or diarrhea lasting longer than 1 month
- Hairy leukoplakia, oral
- Herpes zoster (shingles) involving at least two distinct episodes or more than one dermatome
- Idiopathic thrombocytopenic purpura
- Listeriosis
- Pelvic inflammatory disease, particularly if complicated by tubo-ovarian abscess
- Peripheral neuropathy

Data from Centers for Disease Control and Prevention: Revised classification system for HIV infection and expanded case definition for AIDS among adolescents and adults, *MMWR* 41:1-19, 1992.

CLINICAL PRESENTATION

Patients with early HIV infection are often asymptomatic. Although 2 to 6 weeks after exposure there may be a flulike event, patients are not usually sick enough to seek medical attention. The headache, malaise, muscular aches, fever, sore throat, and other symptoms do not typically generate suspicion for the presence of HIV. As the virus becomes latent, HIV infection still will not be suspected, although transmission to others is possible during this time.

Frequent oral, pharyngeal, or vulvovaginal candidiasis or other HIV-related conditions may be presenting signs of HIV infection and signal the need for testing (Box 248-2).[2] Other illnesses are considered AIDS indicators and also suggest the need for diagnostic evaluation.

Once the diagnosis of HIV is established, the initial assessment is designed to (1) identify risky behaviors that could lead to further spread of HIV or compromise the health of the individual, (2) identify cues in the history or physical examination that may indicate evidence of advancing HIV disease or AIDS, and (3) determine future needs for follow-up care and health teaching.[4] The initial visit provides the opportunity to establish rapport, as well as to perform an in-depth health assessment.[5]

BOX 248-3

ASPECTS OF THE HIV-SPECIFIC HISTORY

SOCIAL HISTORY

Sexual activities

Sex with men, women, or both
Preferred sexual activities
Absolutely safe behavior: abstinence or mutually monogamous with a noninfected partner
Very safe behavior: noninsertive sexual practices
Probably safe behavior: insertive sexual practices with the use of condoms and spermicide
Risky behavior: everything else
Use of condoms (both male and female), including application, removal, use of lubricants, and difference in condom efficacy
Engaging in sex with multiple partners
Use of mood-affecting drugs before or during sexual activities
Whether HIV disease has been diagnosed in anyone with whom the patient has had sex

Needle Exposure

Use of drugs via IV route; sharing of needles, syringes, and other drug paraphernalia
Other needle-exposure activities, such as tattoos, acupuncture, treatment by unskilled individuals or "folk doctors," or sharing of prescribed drugs between friends
Whether HIV disease has been diagnosed in anyone with whom patient has shared needles

Occupational History

Current employment status
Patient's occupation and responsibilities in relation to risk potential for HIV exposure
Whether patient has experienced any exposures
What type of health care follow-up the patient has pursued since exposure
Patient's knowledge level regarding signs and symptoms of seroconversion and need for follow-up

Travel

Within past 10 years
Sexual activities when traveling in areas where the number of AIDS cases is high, such as New York, California, New Jersey, Texas, Florida, or countries such as Haiti or Zaire
Treatment for illnesses or accidents while traveling
Immigration history and potential exposures in country of origin

FAMILY HISTORY

Including medical and mental health problems, including but not limited to substance use in the home or by other family members, tuberculosis, and HIV infection

MEDICATION HISTORY

Current or previous use of medication that may suppress the immune system, such as steroids; current treatment for chemical dependence if applicable

NUTRITION AND USE OF MOOD-AFFECTING AGENTS

Nutrition history (see Box 248-4)
Use of mood-affecting drugs, such as alcohol, marijuana, cocaine, crack, LSD, quaaludes, amphetamines, barbiturates, tranquilizers, amyl or butyl nitrate (called "poppers"), heroin, "crystal meth," or "ecstasy"
Route of administration: oral, inhalation (including sniffing, snorting, and smoking), IV, or subcutaneous ("skin popping")
Any current or previous treatment for substance abuse

MEDICAL HISTORY

Usual source and patterns of seeking health care
HIV testing in the past: has it ever been recommended, where was it done, and what were the results; does the patient have documentation
Major diseases, including but not limited to tuberculosis; hepatitis A, B, or C; mononucleosis; hemophilia and receiving treatment with clotting replacements such as factor VIII; cancer; and tuberculosis
Treatment for psychiatric/emotional disorders
Transfusion donor or recipient
Date of last chest x-ray and tuberculin test and results

CHILDHOOD ILLNESSES

Including but not limited to varicella and immunization history, including measles, mumps, rubella (MMR); last tetanus booster; hepatitis A or B vaccination; Pneumovax, influenza, bacillus Calmette-Guérin (BCG), as well as anergy panel testing

SEXUALLY TRANSMITTED DISEASES

Including but not limited to syphilis, gonorrhea, amebiasis, herpes simplex (oralis or genitalis), *Giardia lamblia* enteritis, chlamydia, condylomas, trichomoniasis, and pelvic inflammatory disease (PID)

GYNECOLOGIC HISTORY

Menstrual history
Pregnancy history, including abortions
Methods of birth control
Last Papanicolaou (Pap) test and results

Specific aspects of the baseline history pertinent to HIV infection are presented in Box 248-3.

PHYSICAL EXAMINATION

The goals of the physical examination are screening for active problems, establishing disease stage, and documenting baseline:

Vital signs: Baseline vital signs (weight, blood pressure, pulse rate, temperature, respiratory rate, oxygen saturation)
Eyes: Baseline extraocular movement, pupil size, reactivity, retinal examination, visual acuity, and visual fields
Ears: Hearing, intact tympanic membrane (potential for invasion), healthy canal
Oropharynx: Pigmented lesions; exudate; missing, tender, or decaying teeth; gum inflammation or tenderness; appearance of pharyngeal lymphoid tissue; oral candidiasis; hairy leukoplakia
Pulmonary, Cardiac: As for any primary care examination

Abdominal: Organomegaly, masses, focal tenderness
Genitalia: Condylomata, ulcers, abnormalities beneath foreskin, discharge, testicular lesions or atrophy
Pelvic: Vaginal discharge, inflammation, cervical lesions, masses, tenderness, Pap smear, sexually transmission disease (STD) cultures if appropriate
Rectal: Condylomata, ulcers, mass lesions, tenderness, prostate tenderness, Pap smear, STD cultures if appropriate
Skin: Fungal infections (periungual, feet, groin, axilla), edema, pigmented lesions (Kaposi's sarcoma), nodules, condylomata,
Lymph nodes: Enlargement (document size), asymmetric or focal enlargement, tenderness
Neurologic: Careful baseline examination
Mental status: Careful baseline examination

DIAGNOSTICS

In the United States and other affluent nations, definitive diagnosis is dependent on laboratory confirmation of the presence of antibody to HIV-1, usually by enzyme-linked immunosorbent (ELISA) testing and Western blot confirmation. The sensitivity of the ELISA test, the purpose of which is not to miss HIV-positive individuals, is balanced by the specificity of the Western blot test. It is prudent with any new patient, even those identified as being HIV-positive, to repeat the ELISA and Western blot tests. An exception to this repeat approach is a patient with documented viral load testing.

New patients whose serostatus is unknown or questionable should be counseled about the distinctions of anonymous vs. confidential testing. Concerns about inadvertent disclosures or the reactions of insurance companies may result in a desire for anonymous testing.

Baseline laboratory studies are essential to (1) determine the need for antiretroviral therapy, (2) identify existing problems, and (3) guide the selection of medications that may affect preexisting conditions such as liver or kidney disease. A listing of laboratory studies commonly ordered with initial evaluation is given in Table 248-1.[6-11]

HIV activity can be monitored by measuring viral load, which is also referred to as viral burden. By measuring the amount of HIV RNA in plasma, the amount of HIV activity that is taking place in the body can be more accurately quantified, thus enabling appropriate patient treatment (Table 248-2). RNA is the substance that programs reproduction. HIV RNA viral load tests (1) measure the amount of HIV RNA in plasma, (2) quantify HIV activity, (3) determine prognosis, (4) indicate the need for antiretroviral treatment, (5) evaluate the efficacy of prescribed antiretroviral therapy, and (6) identify treatment failure. In the HIV-positive patient three tests used to measure viral load include (1) quantitative reverse transcription polymerase chain reaction (RT-PCR), (2) branched-chain DNA (bDNA), and (3) nucleic acid sequence-based amplification.

Test results are reported in the number of viral copies per milliliter. Fewer than 10,000 copies/ml indicate a low risk for advancing disease. Test results that show 10,000 to 100,000 copies/ml indicate a medium risk for advancing disease, and more than 100,000 copies/ml indicate a high risk for advancing disease. Testing is usually performed as part of the initial evaluation, when CD4 cell counts indicate a clinical problem, and 3 to 4 weeks after starting or changing antiretroviral therapy. Illnesses such as influenza, herpes, or pneumonia can cause a temporary increase in viral load. Because immunizations such as influenza or tetanus can also cause a temporary increase, testing should not be performed in the presence of any of these situations.

Diagnostics

HIV Infection

Laboratory
ELISA (if positive, Western blot)
CBC and differential
CD4 and T-cell count
Others (see Table 248-1)

The current classification system for HIV-1 infection/AIDS in adults and adolescents was implemented in January 1993.[2] Three major changes occurred with the 1993 revision: (1) instead of identifying clinical categories, CD4 T lymphocyte counts were emphasized; (2) a CD4 T-cell count of less than 200/mm^3 ("14% of total lymphocytes") was added to the AIDS case surveillance definition; and (3) three new AIDS-indicator diseases were added—pulmonary tuberculosis, recurrent pneumonia, and invasive cervical cancer. The 1993 revised classification system is presented in Table 248-3.[2]

Patients infected with HIV-1 should be classified on the basis of existing guidelines for the medical management of HIV-1. The *lowest* accurate, but not necessarily the most recent, CD4 T-lymphocyte count should be used for classification purposes.

The three CD4 T-lymphocyte categories are defined as follows: category 1, 500 cells/mm^3; category 2, 200 to 499 cells/mm^3; and category 3, $<$200 cells/mm^3. These categories correspond to CD4 T-lymphocyte counts per microliter of blood and guide clinical and therapeutic actions in the management of adolescents and adults with HIV-1. In addition, patients are placed in clinical categories—clinical category A, B, or C—to guide management strategies.

Clinical category A includes adults or adolescents who exhibit asymptomatic infection, persistent generalized lymphadenopathy, or acute (primary) HIV-1 infection with accompanying illness or a history of acute HIV-1 infection. Many practitioners recommend antiretroviral therapy to treat patients classified as category A.

Clinical category B consists of adolescents or adults who have symptomatic conditions that are not included among the conditions listed in clinical category C and that meet at least one of the following criteria: (1) are attributed to HIV-1 infections or are indicative of a defect in cell-mediated immunity, and (2) are considered by physicians to have a clinical course or to require management that is complicated by HIV-1 infection. For classification purposes, category B conditions take precedence over those in category A. For example, a patient should be classified in clinical category B if he or she was previously treated for oral or persistent vaginal candidiasis but is now free of symptoms and has not developed a category C disease.

Category C includes the clinical conditions listed in the AIDS surveillance case definition. For classification purposes, a patient remains in category C once a category C condition has occurred. Being familiar with the specific AIDS indicator diseases is essential not only for understanding the clinical needs of the patient but also for determining eligibility for entitlements such as Social Security and Medicare.

TABLE 248-1 Initial Laboratory Studies for the HIV-Infected Person

Tests	Comments
CD4+ T-cell count/ percentage and CD4 +/ CD8+ ratio	Quantifies immunologic status of an individual. CD4+ T-cell counts less than 200/mm^3 indicate an increased risk for developing AIDS-indicator diseases. Absolute numbers may vary significantly from test to test; the percentage is considered a more stable numeric value. Treatment decisions should be based on serial counts rather than on a single test result.
HIV RNA viral load test	Quantifies HIV activity in an infected individual. Counts >100,000 copies/ml are associated with a high risk for developing an AIDS-indicator disease. Should not be performed if acute illness (e.g., bacterial pneumonia, tuberculosis, herpes simplex infection) is present or if patient has recently received an immunization, because these events can cause increases in serum plasma HIV RNA lasting 2-4 weeks. Treatment decisions should be based on serial counts rather than on a single test result.
CBC and differential	Complications often seen in HIV disease include erythropenia, anemia, low platelet counts and thrombocytopenia, and leukopenia.
Multichannel chemistry panel	Abnormal findings seen in HIV disease: Alanine aminotransferase, serum glutamic pyruvic transaminase (ALT, SGPT)—Increased with hepatitis, alcohol abuse, heart or liver injury, and several of the drugs used to treat HIV and related conditions. Albumin—Low levels are seen in infection (e.g., hepatitis), malignancy, and malnutrition. Used to monitor overall nutritional status and monitor outcomes of nutritional interventions. Alkaline phosphatase—Increased in liver disease (e.g., biliary obstruction associated with cytomegalovirus disease), as well as an indicator of drug toxicity. Aspartate aminotransferase, serum glutamic oxaloacetic transaminase (AST, SGOT)—Abnormal findings are usually associated with alcohol abuse, liver disease, and drug toxicity. Bilirubin—Increased in liver disease, drug toxicity causing cholestasis, and hemolytic disorders. Elevation in the absence of other abnormal liver function tests may be a normal variant. Blood urea nitrogen (BUN)—Increased in kidney disease and toxicity to drugs. Decreased in low-protein diets. Cholesterol (total)—Commonly decreased in HIV disease. Increased in liver and kidney disease and in familial hyperlipoproteinemias. Creatinine—Increased in kidney disease. Decreased in debilitative states or decreased muscle mass. Gamma-glutamyltransferase (GGT, γ-GT)—Increased in liver disease and recent alcohol intake. Protein (total)—Increased with elevated levels of immunoglobulins seen in infection (e.g., hepatitis, HIV), liver disease, and some malignancies. Triglycerides—Increased with HIV disease progression and may result from drug therapy. High levels may indicate predisposition to pancreatitis.
Urinalysis	May reflect renal, metabolic, or nutritional disease.
Tuberculin skin test (Mantoux test) with or without anergy panel testing	HIV-infected individuals are vulnerable to tuberculosis, especially in congregate living settings such as prisons, hospitals, residences, and shelters. All PPD-negative HIV-infected individuals should be tested annually. Because of a lack of standardization of reagents and inconsistent test results, routine anergy panel testing, along with the tuberculin test, is no longer recommended.
Chest x-ray examination	Repeated for signs and symptoms of pulmonary disease and for patients newly identified as having a positive PPD result.
Pregnancy test	Performed if the menstrual history, symptoms, and physical examination indicate the likelihood of pregnancy.
Papanicolaou (Pap) test	For abnormal or uninterpretable results, a colposcopy should be considered.
Venereal Disease Research Laboratory (VDRL) test or rapid plasma reagin (RPR) screening test	High rates of coinfection in HIV populations; false-negative and false-positive results, although rare, do occur; patients with negative results who are sexually active should be tested yearly; patients with positive test results should have fluorescent treponema antibody absorption (FTA-ABS) test performed for confirmation; sexual partners should be evaluated.
Gonorrhea culture	All women (even if free of symptoms) should be screened; all men with symptoms should be tested; evaluations should include possibility of pharyngeal and/or rectal infection; sexual partners should be evaluated.
Chlamydia culture	All women (even if free of symptoms) should be screened; all men with symptoms should be tested; sexual partners should be evaluated.
Hepatitis A panel	Prevalence is high in sexually active men who have sex with men, injecting and noninjecting illegal drug users, and persons who have clotting factor disorders; for these individuals who test negative, HAV vaccination is recommended.
Hepatitis B panel	Prevalence of past exposure is high in most HIV-infected populations in the Untied States; if result is negative and patient is at continued risk of having HBV infection, vaccination is recommended.
Hepatitis C panel	Especially indicated for IV drug users and patients with abnormal liver function tests.
Toxoplasmosis serologic test	Repeat testing may be considered for seronegative patients when CD4+ T-cell count is less than 100/mm^3 and patients are unable to tolerate trimethoprim/sulfamethoxazole.
Cytomegalovirus tests	May be performed initially for baseline data on previous exposure and/or current disease.
Varicella serologic test	May be considered for baseline data in patients who cannot provide a history of chickenpox or shingles.
Glucose-6-phosphate dehydrogenase level (G6PD)	Inherited deficiency seen in men, and some women, of African-American, Asian, or Mediterranean descent. Deficiency predisposes patient to hemolytic anemia when exposed to drugs such as dapsone, primaquine, and sometimes sulfonamides.

TABLE 248-2 Indications for Plasma HIV RNA Testing

Clinical Indication	Information Provided	Clinical Importance
Syndrome consistent with acute, primary HIV infection	Establishes a diagnosis when HIV antibody test is negative or indeterminate	Diagnosis of HIV disease
Initial evaluation of newly diagnosed HIV infection	Baseline viral load, also referred to as the set point	Used to make a decision whether or not to start antiretroviral therapy
Every 3-4 months in patients not on therapy	Detects changes in viral activity	Used to make a decision whether or not to start antiretroviral therapy
4 to 8 weeks after starting antiretroviral therapy	Initial assessment of the efficacy of the prescribed therapy	Provides information as to whether or not the prescribed therapy should be continued or changed
3 to 4 months after starting antiretroviral therapy	To determine the maximum effects of antiretroviral therapy	Provides information as to whether or not the prescribed therapy should be continued or changed
Every 3-4 months while on antiretroviral therapy	To monitor the durability of antiretroviral therapy effect	Provides information as to whether or not the prescribed therapy should be continued or changed
A clinical event occurs (e.g., an infection) or a decline in CD4+ T cells	To determine if there is a correlation with the clinical event or decline in CD4+ T cells with the viral load	Provides information as to whether or not the prescribed therapy should be continued or changed

From US Department of Health and Human Services, Public Health Service: *Guidelines for the use of antiretroviral agents in HIV-infected adults and adolescents*, Rockville, Md, 1997, US Department of Health and Human Services.

NOTES:

1. Viral load testing should not be performed during an acute illness (e.g., bacterial pneumonia, tuberculosis, HSV infection, PCP) or near the time immunizations are administered, since these types of situations can cause increases in the plasma HIV RNA for 2-4 weeks.
2. When changes are noted in either HIV RNA or CD4+ T-cell test results, they should be verified with a repeat test before starting or making any changes in therapy.
3. The HIV RNA should be measured by using the same assay method and the same laboratory to prevent intralaboratory or intramethod variations in test results.
4. When plasma HIV RNA testing identifies HIV infection, the definitive diagnosis should be confirmed by ELISA and Western blot testing (performed 1-2 weeks after the initial indeterminate test).

TABLE 248-3 1993 Revised Classification System for HIV Infection and Expanded AIDS Surveillance Case Definition for Adolescents and Adults

	Clinical Categories*		
CD4 + T-Cell Categories	A. Asymptomatic, Acute (Primary) HIV or PGL	B. Symptomatic, Not A or C Conditions	C. AIDS-Indicator Conditions†
1. ≥500/mm³	A1	B1	C1
2. 200-499/mm³	A2	B2	C2
3. <200/mm³ AIDS-indicator T-cell count	A3	B3	C3

Modified from Centers for Disease Control and Prevention: Revised classification system for HIV infection and expanded case definition for AIDS among adolescents and adults, *MMWR* 41:1-19, 1992.

*Shaded areas are AIDS-defining categories.

†See Box 248-1.

DIFFERENTIAL DIAGNOSIS

In the absence of confirming data indicating antibodies to HIV, other causes of immune dysfunction must be considered. Immune dysfunction can be primary, as noted in idiopathic failure of normal immune function, or secondary, as a consequence of clinical disease (e.g., malignancies, immunosuppressive agents, malnutrition, chromosomal abnormalities, hypercatabolism of immunoglobulin, hereditary metabolic defects, or congenital or surgical asplenia) (Table 248-4).

Idiopathic CD4 T-lymphocytopenia (ICL) resembles HIV but occurs rarely. ICL is diagnosed in the presence of low CD4 T-cell counts (<300/mm³, or <20% of total lymphocytes) without laboratory evidence of HIV infection or other cause.[12]

MANAGEMENT

The primary goal of care for an HIV-positive patient is to prevent complications associated with the HIV illness trajectory. Clinical monitoring, health promotion education, immunizations for disease prevention, and primary prophylaxis of AIDS-indicator diseases are essential.

Monitoring is achieved by continual assessment of the patient's clinical status. The CD4 T-cell count is used as the surrogate marker indicating the degree of immune functioning and, along with viral load testing, is used to guide decisions regarding the institution of antiretroviral therapy and primary prophylaxis to prevent common opportunistic infections. Based on accumulated AIDS surveillance data, the probability of developing

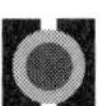

Differential Diagnosis

HIV Infection

Malignancy	Hereditary metabolic defects
Immunosuppressive agents	Congenital or surgical asplenia
Malnutrition	Idiopathic CD4 T-lymphocytopenia
Chromosomal abnormalities	
Hypercatabolism of immunoglobulin	

TABLE 248-4 Secondary Causes of Immune Dysfunction*

Dysfunction	Cause
Infectious diseases	HIV infection X-linked lymphoproliferative syndrome
Malignancy	Thymoma Lymphoma Hodgkin's disease Leukemia
Immunosuppressive agents	Radiation therapy Steroids Cytotoxic drugs Chemotherapy
Malnutrition	—
Chromosomal abnormalities	Bloom's syndrome Fanconi's anemia Down's syndrome
Hypercatabolism of immunoglobulin	Familial hypercatabolism of immunoglobulin Myotonic dystrophy Intestinal lymphangiectasia
Hereditary metabolic defects	Transcobalamin II deficiency Zinc deficiency Biotin-dependent carboxylase deficiency
Other	Congenital or surgical asplenia

*Table compiled by Susan Cross-Skinner, MSN, RNCS.

P. carinii pneumonia is significantly increased when the CD4 T-cell count falls below 200/mm^3, and the probability of developing disease from *Mycobacterium avium-intracellulare* is increased with a CD4 T-cell count less than 50/mm^3. The primary prophylaxis of AIDS-indicator diseases is outlined in Table 248-5.

Although high viral loads are generally correlated with low counts, and low levels are correlated with high CD4 T-cell counts, the correlation is inconsistent.[13] Therefore CD4 T-cell counts are not reliable substitutes for viral load tests when attempting to determine the degree of HIV disease activity or evaluate the efficacy of treatment. The recommended schedule for HIV RNA testing is given in Table 248-2.

Immunizations for disease prevention are carefully monitored, as HIV-infected patients cannot receive some vaccines (Table 248-6).[9,10,14-17] Patients with HIV disease can and should be immunized against preventable infectious diseases, including influenza and pneumococcal pneumonia. HIV-positive persons caring for children receiving oral polio vaccine should avoid contact for 3 weeks after immunization.

Antiretroviral therapy should be offered to (1) all patients with acute HIV syndrome, (2) those within 6 months of HIV seroconversion, and (3) all patients who are symptomatic from HIV infection. For asymptomatic patients, treatment should be offered to individuals with fewer than 350 CD4 T-cells/mm^3 or plasma HIV RNA levels exceeding 30,000 copies/ml (bDNA assay) or 55,000 copies/ml (RT-PCR assay) (Table 248-7).[18]

The choice of antiretroviral therapy is one of the most critical decisions made in the care of patients with HIV. This critical decision is made in conjunction with an HIV specialist and is tailored to the individual patient. Preservation of future treatment options and identification of an alternative therapy if the first choice fails are significant factors in the decision-making process. Antiretroviral drug selection is made from the currently available drugs listed in Table 248-8.[19]

At this time, the preferred recommendation for an initial drug combination as of this writing is based on the guideline from The HIV/AIDS Treatment Information Service, which is outlined in Table 248-9.[19]

LIFE SPAN CONSIDERATIONS

There were 135,000 cases of AIDS reported in women through June 2001. A total of 300 to 400 children are born with HIV each year in the United States. Without antiretroviral drugs during pregnancy, mother-to-child transmission has ranged from 16% to 25% in North America and Europe. The Institute of Medicine, American Academy of Pediatrics, and American College of Gynecology have recommended universal HIV testing and patient notification as a routine component of prenatal care. Maternal-infant transmission of HIV can occur antepartum, intrapartum, or postpartum with breastfeeding: 25% to 40% of vertical transmissions occurs in utero, 65% to 70% occurs intrapartum. Breastfeeding carries an additional 14% risk with established HIV infection and 29% risk with primary HIV infection. Women with HIV infection in the United States should not breastfeed.

There is correlation between high maternal viral load and transmission rate. Transmission is observed at every viral load level including undetectable levels. There is no HIV RNA threshold below which there is no risk of transmission. Zidovudine (ZDV) (Retrovir) has been shown to decrease transmission regardless of HIV RNA levels. Infected pregnant women should have ZDV added to their antiretroviral regimens regardless of HIV RNA levels and CD4 count. Treated women have a 66% percent risk reduction of vertical transmission.

Regarding modes of delivery, women whose viral loads are greater than 1000 should be counseled regarding the potential benefit of scheduled cesarean section to reduce the risk of perinatal HIV transmission. Current data do not demonstrate a benefit of C/S in reducing HIV transmission after labor or rupture of membranes has occurred.

Newborns of women with HIV infection should be started on a 6-week course of prophylactic ZDV. A baseline CBC with

TABLE 248-5 Primary Prophylaxis of AIDS-Indicator Disease

Pathogen	Indication	First Choice	Alternatives
STRONGLY RECOMMENDED AS STANDARD OF CARE			
Pneumocystis carinii	CD4+ count <200/μl or oropharyngeal candidiasis or unexplained fever ≥2 weeks	Trimethoprim/sulfamethoxazole (TMP/SMZ)	Dapsone, or dapsone *plus* pyrimethamine *plus* leucovorin, or aerosolized pentamadine, via Respirgard 11 nebulizer
Mycobacterium tuberculosis			
Isoniazid-sensitive	PPD or tuberculin skin test reaction ≥5 mm *or* prior positive PPD result without treatment *or* contact with case of tuberculosis	Isoniazid *plus* pyridoxine × 9 months	Rifampin
Isoniazid-resistant	Same; high probability of exposure to isoniazid-resistant tuberculosis	Rifampin *plus* pyrazinamide × 2 months	Rifabutin
Multidrug (isoniazid and rifampin)-resistant	Same; high probability of exposure to multidrug-resistant tuberculosis	Choice of drugs requires consultation with public health authorities	None
Toxoplasma gondii	IgG antibody to *Toxoplasma* and CD4+ count <100/mm³	TMP/SMZ	Dapsone *plus* pyrimethamine *plus* leucovorin
Mycobacterium avium-intracellulare complex	CD4+ count <50/mm³	Clarithromycin or azithromycin	Rifabutin; azithromycin *plus* rifabutin
Streptococcus pneumoniae	All patients	Pneumococcal vaccine (CD4+ ≥200 μl)	None
Varicella zoster virus (VZV)	Significant exposure to chickenpox or shingles for patients who have no history of either condition or, if available, negative antibody to VZV	Varicella zoster immune globulin (VZIG), ideally within 48 hours	Acyclovir
GENERALLY RECOMMENDED			
S. Pneumoniae	All patients	Pneumovax IMX1	None
Hepatitis B virus	All susceptible (anti-HBc-negative) patients	Engerix B or Recombivax HB	None
Influenza virus	All patients (annually, before influenza season)	Whole or split virus	Rimantadine or amantadine
NOT RECOMMENDED FOR MOST PATIENTS; INDICATED FOR USE ONLY IN UNUSUAL CIRCUMSTANCES			
Candida species	CD4+ count <50/μl	Fluconazole	
Bacteria	Neutropenia	Granulocyte colony-stimulating factor (GCSF) or granulocyte-macrophage colony-stimulating factor (GMCSF)	
Cryptococcus neoformans	CD4+ count <50/μl	Fluconazole	Itraconazole
Histoplasma capsulatum	CD4+ count <100/μl endemic geographic area	Itraconazole	None
Cytomegalovirus (CMV)	CD4+ count <50/μl and CMV antibody positivity	Oral ganciclovir	None
Coccidioidomycosis	CD4+ count <200	Fluconazole	None

differential should be obtained in the newborn before starting ZDV. *P. carinii* pneumonia prophylaxis should be started at age 6 weeks until HIV is ruled out or until 1 year of age.[20]

COMPLICATIONS

Complications associated with HIV infection include opportunistic infection, nutritional deficiencies, and multisystem abnormalities that affect virtually all body systems. The devastating extent of HIV infection can be appreciated by reviewing the list of opportunistic infections in Box 248-1 and the list of HIV-related complications categorized by body system in Table 248-10.[21,22] Close monitoring of clinical status is imperative in all HIV-positive patients to prevent complications. Complications can be categorized as they occur in early, intermediate, and late or advanced stages of HIV infection.

Common complications in early disease (CD4 cell count >500/mm³) affect the lymphatic and integumentary systems. Lymphadenopathy is common, as are dermatologic conditions such as seborrhea, psoriasis, folliculitis, disseminated scabies, and aphthous ulcerations.

Intermediate-stage HIV (CD4 counts of 200 to 499/mm³) conveys increased risk for opportunistic infections; skin conditions and oral lesions may intensify, and bacterial respiratory infections (sinusitis, pneumonia, bronchitis) occur more frequently. Arthralgias, myalgias, headache, diarrhea, fever, herpes simplex, and fatigue are common. Shingles and candidiasis

TABLE 248-6 Immunizations for HIV-Infected Adults*

Immunization	Comments
Haemophilus influenzae B (Hib) vaccine	Should be considered.
Hepatitis A vaccine	Should be screened first for past infection. Although not specifically recommended for HIV-infected individuals, hepatitis A vaccine is recommended for sexually active men who have sex with men, injecting and noninjecting drug users, and persons with clotting factor disorders.
Hepatitis B vaccine	Should be screened first for past infection. Should be offered to sexually active men who have sex with men, commercial sex workers, injecting drug users, heterosexual men and women with STDs or different sex partners, and household or sexual contacts of HbsAg carriers.
Immune globulin	Recommended to prevent measles or hepatitis A following exposure.
Influenza vaccine	Recommended annually. Usually produces protective antibodies in HIV-infected persons with minimal manifestations of HIV disease and high CD4+ T-cell counts. Alternatives for influenza prophylaxis include rimantadine or amantadine.
Measles-mumps-rubella (MMR) vaccine	Although live-virus or live-bacteria vaccines should not be administered to HIV-infected individuals, MMR is considered safe and is recommended when indicated.
Pneumococcal vaccine	Recommended at 6-year intervals.
Varicella-zoster immune globulin (VZIG)	Indicated for severely immunocompromised persons after significant exposure to chickenpox or herpes zoster. An alternative to VZIG is a 3-week course of oral acyclovir.
Other vaccines	Vaccines containing killed or inactivated antigens such as diphtheria-tetanus-pertussis vaccine, enhanced inactivated polio vaccine, meningococcal vaccine, rabies vaccine, cholera vaccine, plague vaccine, and anthrax vaccine may be used for the same indications as for persons with a healthy immune system. Yellow fever vaccine, oral polio vaccine, and bacillus Calmette-Guérin (BCG) are contraindicated. Inactivated (parenteral) typhoid vaccine or typhoid (Vi) polysaccharide vaccine should be used in place of live oral typhoid (Ty21a) vaccine.

*Any vaccine may produce a transient elevation in the HIV RNA level of an HIV-infected person.

TABLE 248-7 Indications to Initiate Antiretroviral Therapy

Clinical Category	CD4 Cell Count	Plasma HIV RNA	Recommendation
Symptomatic (AIDS or severe symptoms)	Any value	Any value	
Asymptomatic AIDS	Any value	Any value	
Asymptomatic AIDS	CD4 cell count 200 to 350 cells/mm^3	Any value	Treatment should usually be offered; controversy exists for patients with viral load <20,000 cells/ml due to low probability of AIDS-defining diagnosis within 3 years.
Asymptomatic AIDS	CD4 cell count >350/mm^3	>30,000 (bDNA) or >55,000 (RT-PCR)	Some experts would treat, since viral load at this threshold predicts a 3-year risk of AIDS in 30% despite high baseline CD4 cell count. Some would defer therapy and monitor CD4 cell count.
Asymptomatic AIDS	CD4 cell count >350/mm^3	<30,000 (bDNA) or <55,000 (RT-PCR)	Many experts would defer therapy and observe, recognizing that the 3-year risk of developing AIDS in untreated patients is <15%

Data from HIV/AIDS Treatment Information Service http://www.hivatis.org/guidelines/adult/Aug13_01/text/index.html.

are not unusual. Renal insufficiency and proteinuria may be present.[23]

The risk of developing a typical HIV-associated condition increases markedly once CD4 cell counts drop below 200/mm^3. Opportunistic infections and malignancies are common at this late stage and include *P. carinii* infection, toxoplasmosis, encephalitis, cryptosporidiosis, tuberculosis, B-cell lymphoma, Kaposi's sarcoma (a malignant, raised purple lesion), and esophageal candidiasis.[23] Neurologic conditions observed during this late stage include neuritis, cranial nerve palsies, retinopathy, and peripheral neuropathies.[23] Cervical or rectal cancers, hematologic abnormalities, and endocrine disturbances are also common complications.

Advanced disease is characterized by CD4 cell counts of <50/mm^3. Development of coexisting opportunistic infections with relapse after initially successful treatment is typical. The

TABLE 248-8 Antiretroviral Drugs Approved by the Food and Drug Administration for HIV

Brand Names	Generic Names	Firm Name	Approval Date
COMBINATION NUCLEOSIDE REVERSE TRANSCRIPTASE INHIBITORS (NRTIs)			
Trizivir	abacavir, zidovudine, lamivudine	Glaxo Wellcome	14 November 00
Combivir	zidovudine, lamivudine	Glaxo Wellcome	26 September 97
Trizivir	abacavir, zidovudine, and lamivudine	Glaxo Wellcome	14 November 00
SINGLE NUCLEOSIDE REVERSE TRANSCRIPTASE INHIBITORS (NRTIs)			
Epivir, 3TC	lamivudine	Glaxo Wellcome	November 95
HIVID, ddC	zalcitabine	Hoffmann-La Roche	19 June 92
Retrovir, AZT	zidovudine	Glaxo Wellcome	19 March 87
Videx, ddI	didanosine	Bristol Myers-Squibb	09 October 91
Zerit, d4T	stavudine	Bristol Myers-Squibb	24 June 94
Ziagen	abacavir	Glaxo Wellcome	17 December 98
NUCLEOTIDE REVERSE TRANSCRIPTASE INHIBITORS (NRTIs)			
Viread	tenofovir	Gilead Sciences, Inc.	26 October 01
PROTEIN INHIBITORS (PIS)			
Agenerase	amprenavir	Glaxo Wellcome	15 April 99
Crixivan	indinavir	Merck & Co., Inc.	13 March 96
Fortovase	saquinavir	Hoffmann-La Roche	07 November 97
Invirase	saquinavir	Hoffmann-La Roche	06 December 95
Kaletra	lopinavir, ritonavir	Abbott Laboratories	15 September 00
Norvir	ritonavir	Abbott Laboratories	01 March 96
Viracept	nelfinavir	Agouron Pharmaceuticals	14 March 97
NONNUCLEOSIDE REVERSE TRANSCRIPTASE INHIBITORS (NNRTIs)			
Rescriptor	delavirdine	Pharmacia & Upjohn	04 April 97
Sustiva	efavirenz	DuPont Pharmaceuticals	17 September 98
Viramune	nevirapine	Boehringer Ingelheim Pharmaceuticals, Inc.	21 June 96

Data from FDA website: http://www.fda.gov/oashi/aids/virals.html.

TABLE 248-9 Initial Regimen from DHHS Guidelines (One from Column A and one from Column B)

	Column A	Column B
PREFERRED NNRTIs+ NRTIs or PIs + NRTIs	Sustiva	d4T + 3TC AZT + ddI AZT + 3TC d4T + ddI ddI + 3TC
	Crixivan Viracept Norvir + Invirase Norvir + Crixivan Norvir + Kaletra	d4T + 3TC AZT + ddI AZT + 3TC d4T + ddI ddI + 3TC
ALTERNATIVE 3 NRTIs or PI + NRTIs or NNRTIs + NRTIs	Ziagen	AZT + ddC
	Rescriptor Viramune	AZT + ddC
	Agerenase Norvir Fortovase Viracept + Fortovase	AZT + ddC

Data from Guidelines for the Use of Antiretroviral Agents in HIV-Infected Adults and Adolescents. Retrieved August 13, 2001, from the World Wide Web: http://www.hivatis.org/guidelines/adult/Aug13_01/text/index.html.

PI, Protease inhibitor; *NNRTI*, nonnucleoside reverse transcriptase inhibitor; *NRTI*, nucleotide reverse transcriptase inhibitors.

TABLE 248-10 HIV-Related Complications

Organ/System	Condition
Central nervous system	Aseptic meningitis, cranial neuropathy, cognitive impairment, peripheral sensory neuropathy (PSN)
Eyes	Uveitis
Cardiovascular system	Cardiomyopathy, myocarditis, vaculitis
Pulmonary system	Lymphocytic or nonspecific interstitial pneumonitis
Hematologic system	Anemia, granulocytopenia, thrombocytopenia
Gastrointestinal system	Enteropathy, malabsorption, pancreatitis
Renal system	Glomerulosclerosis, glomerulonephritis, nephritic syndrome, uremia
Musculoskeletal system	Reiter's syndrome, psoriatic arthritis, arthritis, arthralgia
Integumentary system	Xerosis, seborrheic dermatitis, psoriasis, atopic dermatitis
Gynecologic system	Cervicitis
Endocrine system	Adrenalitis, thyroiditis, lipid metabolism dysfunction, gonadal (male) dysfunction

Data from Ungvarski PJ: Co-morbidities of HIV/AIDS. In Holzemer WL, Portillo CJ, editors: *HIV/AIDS nursing care summit proceedings,* Washington, DC, 1994, American Academy of Nursing; and Ungvarski PJ and others: Adolescents and adults: HIV disease care management. In Ungvarski PJ, Flaskerud JH, editors: *HIV/AIDS: a guide to primary care management,* Philadelphia, 1999, WB Saunders.

possibility of *M. avium-intracellulare* complex, cytomegalovirus retinitis, aspergillosis, and progressive multifocal leukoencephalopathy (PML) must be entertained. In particular, disorders of the brain may be noted. HIV dementia and PML produce a progressive decline in mental and motor function. However, HIV dementia may improve with antiretroviral therapy. HIV wasting syndrome, an unexplained weight loss of more than 10 pounds, also frequently occurs in advanced disease.

As newer therapies to treat HIV infection have been introduced, additional complications have been noted. Metabolic complications, including new-onset diabetes, elevated triglyceride levels, and abnormal fat distribution have been noted.[24] These complications have been observed, especially in patients taking protease inhibitors (PIs).[24]

Because new-onset diabetes has developed in patients receiving PI therapy, it is prudent to obtain and monitor serum glucose levels before and during PI therapy. Patients with a family history of type 2 diabetes may be more likely to develop this complication.[22] Management of new-onset diabetes includes diet modification and exercise alone or in combination with oral hypoglycemic agents. For patients with preexisting diabetes, traditional management approaches are still indicated but require closer monitoring, because PI therapy may cause hypoglycemia. In both situations the patient's weight should be monitored carefully and nutritional counseling should be a priority, as many patients progressively lose weight in conjunction with the development of diabetes.

Extremely high triglyceride levels (>1000 mg/dl) have also resulted from PI therapy.[22] However, hypertriglyceridemia has also been associated with HIV disease progression. Serum cholesterol and triglyceride levels should be monitored both before and during PI therapy. A history of coronary artery disease, smoking, or obesity should be considered when including PI therapy as part of a combination drug regimen.

Abnormal fat distribution has also been reported in association with PI therapy. A loss of subcutaneous fat in the extremities and face, along with increased adipose tissue in the abdomen, posterior neck, and upper back, may be noted.[24] Although liposuction and surgical excision have been tried, recurrences have been reported. Hyperglycemia, blood lipid abnormalities, and abnormal fat distribution increase the risk of cardiovascular complications.

INDICATIONS FOR REFERRAL/HOSPITALIZATION

HIV-positive patients can be well cared for in primary care but require careful, frequent monitoring of both the patient and viral load. Multiple guidelines and resources are available, and all primary care providers should be familiar with the diagnosis and management of HIV infection. A collaborative relationship with an HIV specialist benefits both the patient and provider.

Routine illness associated with normal CD4 cell counts does not require specialist evaluation or hospitalization. However, specific findings and decreased CD4 cell counts may indicate the need for referral to the appropriate specialist or hospitalization for treatment of complications. Signs and symptoms guide specific evaluation. For example, visual changes require ophthalmologic evaluation. Depression may require psychiatric consultation, whereas neurologic changes may indicate the need for neuropsychiatric evaluation.

Because HIV is a chronic illness with potentially devastating social and financial implications, these aspects of the illness must be anticipated and addressed. A social service referral, vocational counseling, and support groups may all be beneficial.

PATIENT AND FAMILY EDUCATION

The diagnosis of HIV infection is devastating. Patients need support through the diagnostic process and treatment to enable them to cope with this chronic and potentially life-threatening illness. Individual physical, emotional, social, and spiritual resources should be continually assessed so that support networks can be established. Substance use needs to be addressed. The use of illicit substances does not automatically eliminate a patient from consideration for antiretroviral therapy.

It is crucial that patients be provided information about HIV testing, prevention of transmission, prevention of opportunistic infection, available treatments, and antiretroviral therapy. In particular, the antiretroviral therapy regimen is complex, and troublesome side effects should be explained. General health maintenance issues encompass recommendations for stress management, exercise, sexual practices, food safety, water safety, skin and mouth care, household cleaning, pet care, smoking cessation, medication use, travel, and frequency of health care visits (Table 248-11).[4] Nutritional information is

TABLE 248-11 Topical Outline for Health Teaching for the HIV-Positive Person

Topic	Purpose
Stress management	Reduce HIV illness-related psychologic distress
Exercise	Maintain lean muscle mass
Sexual practices	Prevent transmission of HIV and acquisition of an STD
Procreation	Provide complete and accurate information for patient to make an informed choice about getting pregnant
Nutrition	Focus on a high-protein, high-calorie, low-fat diet with vitamin supplements
Food safety	Prevent foodborne infection
Water safety	Prevent waterborne infection
Skin care	Prevent secondary skin infections and skin breakdown
Hair care	Minimize hair loss seen in HIV infection
Mouth care	Decrease potential for secondary infection
Handwashing	Decrease potential for secondary infection
Household cleaning	Decrease potential for secondary infection and transmission of pathogens to other household members
Pet care	Decrease potential for secondary infection
Alcohol drinking	May have negative effect on CD4+ T-cell count and disease progression
Smoking	Decrease risk for recurrent sinus and lung infections, oral lesions, and periodontal disease
Drug use	Prevent bloodborne disease transmission
Travel	Decrease potential for secondary infection
Health care follow-up	Decrease potential for complications of HIV disease

Data from Ungvarski PJ, Schmidt J: Nursing management of the adult client. In Flaskerud JH, Ungvarski PJ, editors: *HIV/AIDS: a guide to nursing care*, ed 3, Philadelphia, 1998, WB Saunders.

BOX 248-4

QUICK NUTRITION SCREEN

Question	*Yes*	*No*
1. Without wanting to, I have lost 10 pounds or more in the last 6 months.		
2. I have problems eating because of my current health status.		
3. I eat less than three times a day.		
4. I eat meat or other proteins like beef, poultry, peanut butter, dried beans, etc., less than three times a day.		
5. I eat bread, cereals, rice, pasta, etc., less than four times a day.		
6. I eat fruits or vegetables or drink juice less than four times a day.		
7. I drink/eat milk products like milk, cheese, yogurt, etc., less than three times a day.		
8. I have three or more drinks of beer, liquor, or wine almost every day.		
9. I don't always have enough money to buy the food I need.		
10. I don't have any place to cook or to keep my foods cold.		
11. I don't take any vitamin or mineral supplements.		
12. I often have one or more of the following *(circle all that apply):* diarrhea, nausea, heartburn, bloating, vomiting, no/poor appetite, feel too tired, pain.		
13. When I take my medicines, I get *(circle all that apply)* diarrhea, nausea, heartburn, bloating, vomiting, no/poor appetite, feel too tired.		
14. I smoke cigarettes, cigars, or chew tobacco every day.		
15. I often don't feel like eating, food shopping, or cooking.		
16. I have problems when I eat or drink milk products (like getting cramps, or bloating).		
17. I have a problem when I eat high-fat or greasy foods (like a stomachache, pain in my belly, or diarrhea).		
18. I have tooth, swallowing, or mouth problems.		
19. I have to watch what I eat because of certain health problems like *(circle all that apply)* diabetes, high blood pressure, kidney		
or liver problems.		
20. I am pregnant or breastfeeding.		

From US Department of Health and Human Resources, Public Health Service: *Guidelines for the use of antiretroviral agents in HIV-infected adults and adolescents,* Rockville Md, 1997, The Department.

critically needed by all HIV-infected patients, as weight loss and decreases in lean muscle mass occur in the course of the disease. Early identification and correction of nutritional deficiencies can maintain lean muscle mass, thus prolonging survival.[25]

A quick nutrition screen that identifies potential nutritional problems is provided in Box 248-4.[26]

Other critical topics that should be explored include disclosure, financial, and legal issues, because children and spouses may be involved. It is important to address naming a durable power of attorney, advance directives (including naming a health care proxy), and identifying potential guardian issues before difficulties arise.

The challenge and opportunity of care for HIV-infected patients and their families are not only providing the clinical care, which is profound, but also caring for a patient who is part of a complex social system. Primary care providers can accept the challenge inherent in HIV/AIDS care and use the opportunity to engage in health promotion for all individuals infected and affected by HIV. Furthermore, primary care providers can use this opportunity to empower patients to advocate for their own needs—physical, psychologic, social, and spiritual.

REFERENCES

1. Revision of the CDC surveillance case definition for acquired immunodeficiency syndrome. Council of State and Territorial Epidemiologists; AIDS Program, Center for Infectious Diseases, *MMWR Morb Mortal Wkly Rep* 36(Suppl 1):1S-15S, 1987.
2. Centers for Disease Control and Prevention: *HIV/AIDS Surveillance Report* 9(2):18, 1997. www.cdc.gov/hiv/stats/hivsur92.pdf.
3. Center for Disease Control and Prevention: US HIV and AIDS cases reported through June 13(1), 2001. Retrieved February 21, 2003, from the World Wide Web: http://www.cdc.gov/hiv/stats/hasr1301.htm
4. Ungvarski PJ, Schmidt J: Nursing management of the adult client. In Flaskerud JH, Ungvarski PJ, editors: *HIV/AIDS: a guide to nursing care,* ed 3, Philadelphia, 1998, WB Saunders.
5. Carmichael CG, Carmichael JK, Fischl MA: *HIV-AIDS primary care handbook,* Norwalk, Conn, 1995, Appleton & Lange.
6. AIDS Institute, Medical CARE Criteria Committee: HIV medical evaluation and preventative care. In *Protocols for the medical care of HIV infection,* ed 7, Albany, NY, 1995, New York State Department of Health.
7. Bartlett JG, Gallant JE: *Medical management of HIV infection,* 2001-2002 ed, Baltimore, 2002, The Johns Hopkins University Division of Infectious Diseases and AIDS Service. Website: http://www.hopkins-aids.edu/publications/book/book_toc.html
8. Centers for Disease Control and Prevention: Prevention of hepatitis A through active or passive immunization: recommendations of the Advisory Committee on Immunization Practices, *MMWR Morbid Mortal Wkly Rep* 45(RR-15):1-30, 1996.
9. Centers for Disease Control and Prevention: Preventative therapy for HIV-infected persons: revised recommendations, *MMWR Morbid Mortal Wkly Rep* 46(RR-15):1-13, 1996.
10. Centers for Disease Control and Prevention: 1997 USPHS/IDSA guidelines for the prevention of opportunistic infections in persons infected with human immunodeficiency virus, *MMWR Morbid Mortal Wkly Rep* 46(RR-12):1-46, 1997.
11. Cornelson B: HIV primary care evaluation and management. In Fanning MM, editor: *HIV infection: a clinical approach,* ed 2, Philadelphia, 1997, WB Saunders.
12. Fauci AS: CD4+ T-lymphocytopenia without HIV infection: no lights, no camera, just facts, *N Engl J Med* 328(6):429-431, 1993.
13. Mellors JW and others: Prognosis in HIV-1 infection predicted by the quantity of virus in plasma, *Science* 272(5265):1167-1170, 1996.
14. Centers for Disease Control and Prevention: Update on Adult Immunization Practices Advisory Committee (ACIP), *MMWR Morbid Mortal Wkly Rep* 40(RR-12):1-94, 1991.

15. Centers for Disease Control and Prevention: Recommendations of the Advisory Committee on Immunization Practices (ACIP): use of vaccines and immune globulins in persons with altered immunocompetence, *MMWR Mortal Wkly Rep* 42(RR-4):1-18, 1993.
16. Centers for Disease Control and Prevention: Prevention and control of influenza: recommendations of the Committee on Immunization Practices (ACIP), *MMWR Morbid Mortal Wkly Rep* 46(RR-9):1-25, 1997.
17. Centers for Disease Control and Prevention: Prevention of pneumococcal disease: recommendations of the Committee on Immunization Practices (ACIP), *MMWR Morbid Mortal Wkly Rep* 46(RR-8):1-24, 1997.
18. U.S. Food and Drug Administration: Antiretroviral drugs approved by FDA for HIV. Retrieved November 7, 2001from the World Wide Web: http://www.fda.gov/oashi/aids/virals.html.
19. HIV/AIDS Treatment Information Service: Guidelines for the Use of Antiretroviral Agents in HIV-infected adults and adolescents. Retrieved August 13, 2001 from the World Wide Web: http://www.hivatis.org/guidelines/adult/Aug13_01/text/index.html
20. The National Pediatric & Family HIV Resource Center: HIV infection and pregnancy: managing mother and baby. Retrieved March 2002 from the World Wide Web: http://www.pedhivaids.org/preventing/
21. Ungvarski PJ: Co-morbidities of HIV/AIDS. In Holzemer WL, Portillo CJ, editors: *HIV/AIDS nursing care summit proceedings*, Washington, DC, 1994, American Academy of Nursing.
22. Ungvarski PJ and others: Adolescents and adults: HIV disease care management. In Ungvarski PJ, Flaskerud JH, editors: *HIV/AIDS: a guide to primary care management*, ed 4, Philadelphia, 1999, WB Saunders.
23. Saag MS: Clinical spectrum of human immunodeficiency virus diseases. In Devita VT and others, editors: *AIDS: etiology, diagnosis, treatment and prevention*, ed 4, Philadelphia, 1997, Lippincott-Raven.
24. Galli M and others: Incidence of adipose tissue alterations in first-line antiretroviral therapy: The LipoICONa study, *Arch Inter Med* 162(22):2621-2628.
25. Kotler DP and others: Magnitude of body-cell-mass depletion and timing of death from wasting in AIDS, *Am J Clin Nutr* 50(3):444-447, 1998.
26. US Department of Health and Human Services, Public Health Service, Health Resources Administration: *Health care and HIV: nutrition guide for providers and clients*, Rockville, Md, 1996, The Department.

CHAPTER 249

Immunodeficiency

Susan Cross-Skinner

DEFINITION/EPIDEMIOLOGY

An estimated 1 in every 500 people in the United States is born with an immune system defect.[1,2] Many more acquire impairments later in life that can have serious health implications. Isolated immunoglobulin (Ig)A deficiency and common variable immunodeficiency syndrome are the common immunodeficiencies among people of European descent. Isolated IgA occurs in approximately 1 in 500 to 700 individuals. Other primary immunodeficiency disorders are relatively rare and have a frequency of approximately 1 in 10,000 individuals.[3,4]

Disorders of the immune system may be categorized as primary defects or secondary to an underlying disorder. The World Health Organization has identified and classified more than 50 primary immunodeficiency disorders.[5] Primary immunodeficiency disorders are a result of abnormalities in the development and maturation of cells of the immune system. Patients who have genetic mutations impairing B- or T-lymphocyte function have one of three major clinical presentations: a deficiency of antibody production, a deficiency of cellular immunity, or deficiencies of both.[6]

Primary immunodeficiencies are characterized by susceptibility to devastating bacterial, fungal, and viral infections. Secondary characteristics include increased frequency of autoimmune diseases and malignancies of the lymph system, reticular system, and gastrointestinal tract. Many severe forms of primary immunodeficiencies are diagnosed in the first 6 years of life[3]; however, immunodeficiencies may become apparent at any age. Early diagnosis, appropriate management of infections, effective prophylactic therapy, and treatment options such as exogenous Ig and bone marrow transplantation have improved outcomes for patients with primary immunodeficiency disorders over the last decade (Table 249-1).

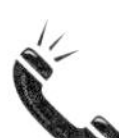

Physician consultation is indicated for all patients with suspected immunodeficiency disorders.

PATHOPHYSIOLOGY

The primary immunodeficiency disorders are a result of abnormal development and maturation of immune system cells (cell differentiation) with resultant defects in humoral and cell-mediated immunity. Defects in differentiation can cause immature development of lymphocytes, defects in antibody production or release, or impaired T-cell or phagocyte function. In addition, deficiencies of complement components or functions have been associated with an increased incidence of infections.[1]

Primary immunodeficiencies are congenital and are classified according to the mode of inheritance and whether the defect involves T-cells, B-cells, or both T- and B-cells. Many primary

TABLE 249-1 Selected Primary Immunodeficiency Disorders

Disorder	Functional Immune Deficiency	Inheritance Pattern	Therapy
B-CELL DISORDERS			
X-linked agammaglobulinemia	Antibody Pre–B-cell maturation	XL	Antibiotics Immunoglobulin
Common variable hypogammaglobulinemia	Antibody Cell-mediated immunity B-cell maturation	AR	Antibiotics Immunoglobulin
Transient hypogammaglobulinemia of infancy	None: immunogloblins low, but antibodies present Usually resolves by 16-30 months	Unknown	Antibiotics Immunoglobulins
Selective IgA deficiency	IgA B-cell maturation	XL AR?	Antibiotics Immunoglobulins in rare cases
IgG subclass deficiency	IgG and IgA Chromosomal deletion	AR	
T-CELL DEFICIENCIES			
DiGeorge's syndrome	T-cell deficiency Faulty embryonic development of third and fourth pharyngeal pouches: hypoplasia or aplasia of thymus gland		Transplantation of fetal thymic tissue Calcium and vitamin D Bone marrow transplantation
Chronic mucocutaneous candidiasis	T-cell deficiency No T-cell receptor for *Candida* antigens		Antifungal agents
COMBINED B- AND T-CELL DISORDERS			
Severe combined immunodeficiency syndrome (SCID)	Antibody B- and T-cell maturation Adenosine deaminase (ADA) deficiency	XL AR	Bone marrow transplantation Irradiated erythrocytes to replace ADA Gene therapy
Wiskott-Aldrich syndrome	IgM T-cell function decreases as disease progresses	XL	Antibiotics Bone marrow transplantation
Ataxia-telangiectasia	IgA Variable T-cell deficiency	AR	Antibiotics Bone marrow transplantation
PHAGOCYTE DISORDERS			
Chronic granulomatous disease (CGD)	Neutrophil function	XL	Antibiotics Interferon-gamma

immunodeficiencies are inherited with an X-linked or autosomal recessive pattern. Until the last decade, little was understood about the fundamental problems underlying these conditions. As a result of advances in human molecular genetics, the abnormal genes have been identified in a growing number of defects. Within the last 8 years, the molecular basis of five X-linked immunodeficiency disorders have been discovered. These include X-linked agammaglobulin, X-linked immunodeficiency with hyperimmune globulin M, Wiskott-Aldrich syndrome, and X-linked severe combined immunodeficiency (SCID).[7] Some autosomal recessive genetic defects have also been identified.[7]

Secondary immunodeficiencies are acquired or associated with some underlying disorder and are not caused by intrinsic abnormalities in the development and function of the immune system. HIV infection and malnutrition are the two most common causes of secondary immunodeficiency. Other causes include malignancy, immunosuppressive agents, and systemic inflammatory diseases such as rheumatoid arthritis and systemic lupus erythematosus.[8] Secondary immunodeficiencies must be considered in the differential diagnosis of patients with multiple or recurrent infections.

CLINICAL PRESENTATION

A patient with an incompetent immune system presents with a pattern of recurrent bacterial or viral infections that are difficult to manage despite standard recommended antibacterial and antiviral therapy. Infections can be caused by a variety of pathogens, including normal flora, common environmental organisms, and unusual or opportunistic agents. There is often a slow recovery or poor response to treatment. Signs and symptoms associated with primary immunodeficiency disorders include chronic diarrhea, eczema, hepatosplenomegaly, autoimmune diseases, and failure to thrive in infants and children.

The type of infection at presentation can often provide clues to the nature of the immunologic defect. Patients with a defect in humoral immunity (antibody production) may present with recurrent or chronic sinopulmonary infections, meningitis, or bacteremia. Pathogens commonly involved include *Haemophilus influenzae, Streptococcus pneumoniae,* and staphylococci.[2] Children presenting with persistent lymphadenitis or recurrent abscesses caused by low-virulence, gram-negative organisms, such as *Escherichia coli, Serratia* sp., or *Klebsiella* sp., may have an abnormality in phagocyte function. Recurrent skin infections with catalase-positive *Staphylococcus aureus* and recurrent gingivitis are also characteristic of a phagocyte defect.[8] The occurrence of *H. influenzae* meningitis in an older child or adult warrants consideration of a defect in humoral immunity. Chronic otitis media occurs frequently in adult patients with low levels of immunoglobulins and is a significant finding because of its rarity in immunocompetent adults. The intestinal parasite *Giardia lamblia* is often the cause of diarrhea in patients with impaired immunity. Multiple episodes of chickenpox and measles may occur with impaired humoral immunity as a result of impaired antibody production and the absence of long-lasting immunity.[2]

Individuals with a defect in cell-mediated immunity are susceptible to viral, fungal, and other opportunistic infections. Infections with herpes simplex, varicella zoster, and cytomegalovirus are common and tend to be more severe than expected, with increased risk of dissemination. Patients with T-cell defects are at high risk for developing pneumonia caused by the protozoan *Pneumocystis carinii*. Mucocutaneous infections resulting from *Candida albicans* are common and often difficult to manage. T-cell deficiency is often accompanied by abnormalities in antibody responses. Consequently, individuals with T-cell defects are also at risk for overwhelming bacterial infections.[1-3,9]

PHYSICAL EXAMINATION

A careful history and physical examination usually provide evidence to identify the nature of the immune system defect. However, a normal examination does not exclude an underlying immunodeficiency. The history should include a detailed description of infections, including age of onset, site(s), patterns of recurrence, response to treatment, and pathogens if known. More severe immunodeficiency disorders such as SCID, characterized by defects in both B- and T-cells, can present with life-threatening infections in the first few months of life.[8] The patient's immunization history and response to immunizations should be assessed. A history of normal response to smallpox vaccination or contact dermatitis resulting from poison ivy suggests an intact cellular immunity.[2] Associated symptoms such as eczema, diarrhea, or arthritis should be noted. Risk factors for HIV infection should be assessed. A history of weight loss, enlarged lymph nodes, night sweats, fever, ecchymosis, pruritus, or epistaxis should be obtained. The medical history should identify childhood illnesses, recurrent infections, autoimmune diseases, cancer, and a history of splenectomy. A complete medication history should be obtained. A family history of unexplained death from infection may be significant.[8]

A complete physical examination should be performed with the goal of identifying the site and source of infection. HIV infection and malignancy should be excluded. Lymphadenopathy, petechiae, weight loss, gingivostomatitis, dental erosions, signs of sinusitis, tympanic membrane scarring, absence of tonsillar tissue and lymph nodes, hepatosplenomegaly, pruritus, rashes, and chronic diarrhea are associated findings that are consistent with primary and secondary immunodeficiency disorders.[8] A neurologic examination should be included. Progressive ataxia in a young child could be the first sign of ataxia-telangiectasia before immunodeficiency becomes apparent.[10]

DIAGNOSTICS

When an immunodeficiency disorder is suspected, initial diagnostic studies should include laboratory tests that are broadly informative, reliable, readily available, and cost-effective. Efforts should be made to identify pathogens through appropriate cultures and serology. Initial evaluation by the primary care provider should include a CBC with differential, erythrocyte sedimentation rate (ESR), serology, cultures, antigen detection for HIV, and a quantitative Ig panel.[1-3,8,9] If the ESR is normal, chronic bacterial infection is unlikely. If the absolute neutrophil count is normal, congenital and acquired neutropenias are excluded. If the absolute lymphocyte count is normal, the patient is not likely to have a T-cell defect. A normal platelet count excludes Wiskott-Aldrich syndrome. Howell-Jolly bodies on red blood cells are significant for congenital asplenia.[9] A quantitative Ig panel evaluates B-cell function. Low or absent levels of specific immunoglobulins warrant further evaluation. The most cost-effective test for evaluating T-cell function is delayed hypersensitivity skin testing, which can be used for adults and children more than 6 years old. Commonly used extracts include those for *C. albicans,* mumps, *Trichophyton* organisms, and tuberculosis. If findings are positive, virtually all primary T-cell defects are excluded.[2,9]

Killing defects of phagocytic cells should be suspected if the patient has recurrent staphylococcal, gram-negative bacterial, or fungal infections. A nitroblue tetrazolium test is used to screen for this disorder, A CH_{50} assay should be ordered to screen for complement defects. This assay measures the integrity of the entire complement pathway.[8,9]

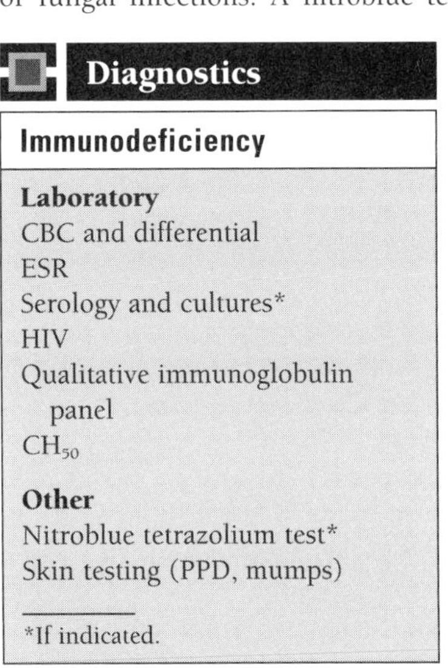
Diagnostics

Immunodeficiency

Laboratory
CBC and differential
ESR
Serology and cultures*
HIV
Qualitative immunoglobulin panel
CH_{50}

Other
Nitroblue tetrazolium test*
Skin testing (PPD, mumps)

*If indicated.

If the results of these screening tests are abnormal, or if the clinical presentation suggests an immunologic defect when the screening tests are normal, the patient should be referred to a specialist in the field of immunology, who will perform more specific and definitive immunologic studies.

Differential Diagnosis

Immunodeficiency

Primary
- Congenital

Secondary
- Infectious diseases
- Malignancies
- Immunosuppressive agents
- Malnutrition
- Hereditary metabolic defects
- Chromosomal abnormalities

DIFFERENTIAL DIAGNOSIS

The differential diagnosis should include primary and secondary causes of immune dysfunction. Both B- and T-cell deficiencies can occur in association with secondary immunodeficiencies. Categories of secondary immunodeficiencies include infectious diseases, specifically HIV/AIDS; malignancies; immunosuppressive agents; malnutrition; hereditary metabolic defects; and chromosomal abnormalities (see Table 248-4).[2,3]

MANAGEMENT

There are two goals of treatment when providing care for a patient with a primary immunodeficiency: (1) minimize the occurrence and impact of infections on the overall health of the individual, and (2) replace the defective component of the immune system by passive transfer or transplantation when possible.[1] Prompt and vigorous use of antibiotics to eradicate and prevent bacterial and fungal infections is crucial to minimize the impact of infection. The principles of antibiotic therapy are not different from those used with other patients; however, an index of suspicion for bacterial and fungal infection should remain high in this population. Prophylactic antibiotic therapy may be used for recurrent or recalcitrant infections. Prophylactic antibiotics are recommended for children and adults with significant T-cell defects because of the risk for pneumocystis pneumonia. Trimethoprim-sulfamethoxazole is commonly prescribed.[8] Replacement or correction of the defective immune component is specific to the disorder and may be accomplished by administration of exogenous immunoglobulins; administration of cytokines such as interleukin-2, granulocyte-macrophage colony-stimulating factor (GM-CSF), or interferon-gamma; or bone marrow transplantation.[1-3,9,11]

Appropriate use of antibiotics and regular administration of Ig replacement therapy have been shown to be effective as either primary or supportive therapy for agammaglobulinemia, X-linked immunodeficiency, Wiskott-Aldrich syndrome, and all forms of SCID. The most common form of replacement therapy is IV immunoglobulin (IVIG).[12,13] IVIG preparations consist primarily of IgG antibodies with small amounts of other classes of antibodies. IVIG therapy is indicated in the case of severe impairment of antibody-forming capacity in the setting of recurrent or severe infections. Replacement therapy with IVIG is contraindicated in patients with selective IgA deficiency or common variable immunodeficiency where there is no detectable IgA because of the risk of anaphylactic reaction.[12,13]

The usual administration schedule for IVIG is 300 to 400 mg/kg each month.[12,13] Because of the differences in half-life of IVIG in individual patients and the fact that individual IVIG lots vary in antibody concentration, serum IgG levels should be measured before each infusion, and the dose of IVIG adjusted accordingly. Trough serum IgG concentrations 4 weeks after treatment should be maintained at 400 to 500 mg/dl. Infusion intervals may be shortened or lengthened, depending on the trough IgG concentration and the patient's clinical condition. Potential side effects include diaphoresis, tachycardia, flank pain, nausea, vomiting, and hypotension within the first 30 minutes of the infusion. Chills, fever, headache, myalgia, and fatigue may occur at the end of the infusion and continue for several hours. HIV is inactivated by the ethanol used in preparation of the immune serum globulin and IVIG. These preparations are also free of hepatitis antigen.[2,14] Infusion of fresh plasma, 10 to 20 ml/kg at intervals of 3 to 4 weeks, can also be used as antibody replacement therapy. This regimen has the advantage of replacing IgM and IgA, as well as IgG, but should be used only in rare cases when IgM antibodies are needed to control extremely resistant infections because of the risk of transmitting hepatitis and other viruses.[2]

Most immunodeficiencies involving severe abnormalities of T-cell function are treated with stem cell transplantation under the care of a specialist. Stem cell transplantation can be effective in restoring immune competence in patients diagnosed with such immunodeficiencies as SCID, DiGeorge syndrome, leukocyte adhesion deficiency, and Wiskott-Aldrich syndrome.[13] Patients with DiGeorge syndrome are also treated with the thymic hormone thymosin or with transplantation of fetal thymic tissue with the goal of T-cell function restoration.[1-3,9,14] Patients with abnormalities in T-cell function should be assessed for fungal, parasitic, and opportunistic infections and treated aggressively with careful follow-up care.

Cytokines are also useful treatment modalities for specific immunodeficiencies. Interferon-gamma therapy is used to treat patients with chronic granulomatous disease. GM-CSF is used to stimulate white blood cell proliferation in the presence of neutropenia.[1]

Patients with T-cell deficiencies should receive only blood products that are leukocyte poor, irradiated, and virus free to avoid graft-versus-host disease and cytomegalovirus infection.[8] Patients with adenosine deaminase–related SCID should receive irradiated erythrocytes as an element of treatment.

Genetic engineering and gene therapy are promising and important treatment tools for a variety of genetic defects of the immune system. Gene therapy has been successful in the treatment of X-linked SCID and is being studied for the treatment of adenosine deaminase deficiency, leukocyte adhesion deficiency, Wiskott-Aldrich syndrome, and other disorders.[7,15,16]

LIFE SPAN CONSIDERATIONS

A patient diagnosed with a primary immunodeficiency syndrome lives with a chronic, often fatal disease that requires diligent care, careful follow-up evaluation, and monitoring over the entire life span. Infants diagnosed with severe immunodeficiency syndromes often die of overwhelming infection early in life. However, approximately two thirds of immunodeficient patients live to adulthood.[2] Many patients can be effectively cared for in primary care; however, some patients require specialty care and monitoring over their life span. Patients should be monitored closely for malignancies and autoimmune diseases. The majority of malignancies are seen in patients with ataxia telangiectasia, Wiskott-Aldrich syndrome, and common variable immunodeficiency.[14] Bone marrow transplant recipients should be monitored for complications of initial treatment and potential late side effects of treatment. Family members of the affected individual also require specialized care. Relatives of patients with Ig deficiencies should be screened for immune defects, genetic defects, autoimmune disorders, and malignancies.[3,9,15] Mothers of male infants diagnosed with an X-linked disorder and both parents of children diagnosed with a disorder known to have an autosomal recessive inheritance pattern should be referred for genetic testing and counseling. Intrauterine diagnosis of some primary immunodeficiencies is possible.[9,15]

A patient diagnosed with an immunodeficiency disorder often has a shortened life span. Death may occur from infection or complications of disease or treatment. Use of community or mental health resources to provide support for the patient and family is an important component of care.

COMPLICATIONS

Complications associated with immunodeficiency include recurrent bacterial, viral, or fungal infection; malignancy, especially of the lymph and reticular system; and autoimmune diseases such as rheumatoid arthritis, lupus erythematosus, multiple sclerosis, or systemic sclerosis. Primary immunodeficiency is often associated with chronic diarrhea, eczema, or failure to thrive. Zoster infections are commonly recurrent and are at high risk for dissemination.

INDICATIONS FOR REFERRAL/HOSPITALIZATION

Patients should be referred to an immunologist when the diagnosis of immunodeficiency disorder is suspected. Once the definitive diagnosis is made and a plan of care is developed by the specialist, the patient can be cared for in a collaborative fashion. Infections can be diagnosed and managed by the primary care provider. Patients requiring specialized therapy such as Ig replacement therapy or transplantation with bone marrow or stem cells should receive this care under the supervision of the immunologist or a hematologist. Relatives of affected individuals should be referred for genetic testing and counseling as appropriate.

Diligent follow-up care of patients with primary immunodeficiency is necessary for effective management of infections and minimization of the sequelae of chronic infection (e.g., bronchiectasis). Patients should be closely monitored for the development of autoimmune diseases and malignancy. It is necessary for the primary care provider to communicate with the specialist to establish a plan of care that is comprehensive and ensures careful, coordinated follow-up care.

PATIENT AND FAMILY EDUCATION/HEALTH PROMOTION

Patients with primary immunodeficiency disorders should understand the importance of avoiding contact with individuals with known contagious diseases, and they should be able to identify and report signs and symptoms of infection. It is essential that these patients seek care at the first sign of infection. Good personal hygiene, proper nutrition, and adaptation of health behaviors such as regular exercise and stress management should be recommended to promote good health and support immune function.

Immunocompromised patients should have current childhood, adolescent, and adult vaccinations as recommended by the U.S. Public Health Advisory Committee on Immunization Practices.[17] Live attenuated vaccines, such as oral polio, varicella, and bacille Calmette-Guérin (BCG), should not be given to children with suspected or diagnosed antibody or T-cell deficiencies because of the risk of vaccine-induced infection. Inactivated polio vaccine should be given to household members to prevent transmission of the virus by shedding of the attenuated virus in stool. MMR, varicella, and BCG can be given to family members.[8] In addition, immunocompromised adults should receive the 23-valent pneumococcal vaccine, with revaccination every 5 years, plus yearly influenza vaccine. *H. influenzae* vaccine is recommended for asplenic patients and immunocompromised patients.[17] A vaccine for *S. aureus* is currently being studied in Phase III clinical trials and is being recommended for patients at high risk, patients with eczema, and patients with neutrophil dysfunction.[18]

REFERENCES

1. Hyde RM: *Immunology,* ed 3, Philadelphia, 1995, Williams & Wilkins.
2. Fauci AS and others: *Harrison's principles of internal medicine,* vol 2, ed 14, New York, 1994, McGraw-Hill.
3. Hoffman R and others: *Hematology: principles and practice,* ed 2, New York, 1995, Churchill Livingstone.
4. Stiehm ER, editor: *Immunologic disorders in infants and children,* Philadelphia, 1996, WB Saunders.
5. Rosen FS, Cooper MD, Wedgwood RJP: The primary immunodeficiencies, *N Engl J Med* 333(7):431-440, 1995.
6. Austen KF, Frank MM, Atkinson JP, editors: *Samter's immunologic diseases,* vol 1, ed 6, Philadelphia, 2001, Lippincott Williams and Wilkins.
7. Buckley RH and others: Human severe combined immunodeficiency: genetic phenotypic, and functional diversity in one hundred eight infants, *J Pediatr* 130:378-387, 1997.
8. Woroniecka M, Ballow M: Office evaluation of children with recurrent infection, *Pediatr Clin North Am* 47(6):1211-1224, 2000.
9. Buckley RH: Immunodeficiency diseases, *JAMA* 268(20):2797-2806, 1992.
10. Regueiro JR and others: Ataxia telangiectasia: a primary immunodeficiency revisited, *Immunol Allergy Clin North Am* 20:177-206, 2000.
11. Horwitz ME: Stem cell transplantation for inherited immunodeficiency disorders, *Pediatr Clin North Am* 47(6):1371-1382, 2000.
12. Oates JA, Wood AJJ: The use of intravenous immune globulin in immunodeficiency diseases, *N Engl J Med* 325(2):110-117, 1991.
13. Schwartz SA: Intravenous immunoglobulin treatment of immunodeficiency disorders, *Pediatr Clin North Am* 47(6):1355-1369, 2000.
14. Filipovich AH and others: The immunodeficiency cancer registry: a research resource, *Am J Pediatr Hematol Oncol* 9(2):183-184, 1987.
15. Condotti F: The potential for therapy of immune disorders with gene therapy, *Pediatr Clin North Am* 47(6):1389-1405, 2000.
16. Salima HBA and others: Sustained correction of X-lined severe combined immunodeficiency by EX-VIVO gene therapy, *N Engl J Med* 346(16):1185-1192, 2002.
17. Update on immunization recommendations, *J Am Acad Nurse Pract* 2(2):32-38, 1998.
18. Gordon A: Vaccines and vaccination, *N Engl J Med* 345(14):1042-1052, 2001.

CHAPTER 250

Infectious Mononucleosis

Patricia Polgar Bailey

DEFINITION/EPIDEMIOLOGY

Infectious mononucleosis is an acute, self-limited, generally benign illness that occurs in both children and adults after primary infection with Epstein-Barr virus (EBV), cytomegalovirus (CMV), and other infectious agents. The classic manifestation of this syndrome includes fever, pharyngitis, and lymphadenopathy, although atypical presentations also occur. This syndrome was first described in the 1880s; however, the term *infectious mononucleosis* was not used until the 1920s. The link between EBV and infectious mononucleosis was not discovered until the late 1960s.[1]

In this chapter, the term *Epstein-Barr virus-associated infectious mononucleosis* (EBV-IM) is used to refer to infectious mononucleosis caused by acute EBV infection. The term *non-Epstein-Barr virus-associated infectious mononucleosis* (non-EBV-IM) is used to refer to the clinical syndrome of infectious mononucleosis that is caused by an agent other than EBV. The term *infectious mononucleosis* is used to refer to the triad of fever, pharyngitis, and lymphadenopathy regardless of the infectious agent. This chapter deals primarily with the presentation, evaluation, and management of EBV-IM, the most common type of acute infectious mononucleosis, which is seen in 20% to 70% of adolescents and young adults.[2]

The peak rate of EBV-IM occurs between the ages of 15 and 19 years in industrialized countries, and the annual incidence in this age-group is 345 to 671 cases per 100,000. In persons 35 years or older, the annual incidence of EBV-IM decreases dramatically to 2 to 4 cases per 100,000. The incidence of EBV-IM is 30 times higher in whites than in African-Americans. No gender differences have been noted. Interestingly, more than 90% of adults worldwide have serologic evidence of prior EBV infection, which indicates that a significant number of EBV infections are atypical or without clinical manifestations. The chance of developing infectious mononucleosis after EBV infection appears to increase from childhood to young adulthood; it is estimated that less than 10% of children develop infectious mononucleosis post-EBV exposure, but up to 20% to 70% of adolescents have a chance of developing EBV-IM after acute EBV infection.[2]

PATHOPHYSIOLOGY

Infectious mononucleosis can be caused by a variety of infectious agents other than EBV, including CMV, herpes virus 6, HIV, adenovirus, hepatitis A virus, influenza A and B viruses, and rubella virus. In addition, infectious mononucleosis is also associated with some neoplasms. Transmission of infectious mononucleosis varies depending on the specific causative infectious agent. Transmission of EBV-IM occurs through exposure to oropharyngeal secretions, although blood products have also been reported as a source of transmission. EBV is a relatively fragile DNA herpes virus that cannot survive for long outside the host. The virus initially infects the oral epithelial cells and then spreads to the B-lymphocytes, which then circulate through the reticuloendothelial system, causing a significant but time-limited immunologic response. Many of the signs and symptoms associated with the clinic presentation of EBV-IM are the result of this immunologic response. The incubation time of EBV-IM is usually between 30 and 50 days. Acute EBV infection stimulates the production of antibodies against EBV antigens, which remain present lifelong.[1]

CLINICAL PRESENTATION

The classic triad of symptoms of acute infectious mononucleosis include fever, pharyngitis, and lymphadenopathy. However, infectious mononucleosis often manifests atypically, making diagnosis difficult. Pharyngitis is usually diffuse, with exudates present in approximately 30% of cases. Lymphadenopathy usually affects the anterior and posterior cervical chain and may also be diffuse. Temperatures may be as high as 40° C (104° F) and may last as long as 2 weeks. Symptoms that may precede, as well as persist throughout, the acute phase of illness include malaise, anorexia, and fatigue. Symptoms of EBV-IM usually peak approximately 7 days after onset and become less pronounced during the next 1 to 3 weeks. Based on reports, splenic enlargement occurs in 40% to 100% of cases, although studies that have included ultrasonography as part of the evaluation suggest that splenomegaly may be more common than not.[1]

Less common signs and symptoms of EBV-IM include upper airway compromise, abdominal pain, rash, hepatomegaly, jaundice, and eyelid edema. The rash, which occurs in approximately 5% to 10% of individuals, may be macular, urticarial, petechial, and erythema multiforme.[1,3]

PHYSICAL EXAMINATION

The physical examination may reveal an ill- or non-ill-appearing individual depending on degree of fever, associated signs and symptoms, and length of time since onset of symptoms. The classic clinical manifestation of fever, pharyngitis, and lymphadenopathy raise suspicion for EBV-IM. The anterior and posterior cervical chains should be assessed for lymphadenopathy, which may be diffuse. An abdominal examination identifies splenomegaly and hepatomegaly, which are complications of EBV-IM, especially in older adults. Rash and jaundice should be noted as they are associated with EBV-IM in some cases.

DIAGNOSTICS

The most useful laboratory test is the serologic test for heterophil antibodies, as these may be demonstrable at the onset of illness or may appear later in the course of the illness. The accuracy of the test varies depending on the specific kit and reagent used, with the sensitivity and specificity ranging from 63% to 84% and 84% to 100%, respectively. The likelihood of positive heterophil antibodies in response to acute infection increases in direct response to the length of time since onset of symptoms. In addition, individuals more than 4 years of age are more likely to have positive antibodies in response to acute illness.[1]

False-positive heterophil antibody results, albeit rare, have also been associated with lymphoma, viral hepatitis, and autoimmune disease. In addition, 10% to 43% of individuals with acute infectious mononucleosis may have titers that are lower than the range associated with positive infection.[1,3,4]

If the heterophil antibody test is negative, but EBV-IM is still highly suspect, then further testing may be helpful. Blood tests for viral capsid antigen (VCA) immunoglobulin (Ig)G, and IgM and for EBV nuclear antigens (EBNA) can be obtained, as they also indicate acute infection. VCA IgG and IgM generally become positive within 1 to 2 weeks of infection, but VCA IgM becomes undetectable after 6 months. EBNA IgG becomes detectable 6 to 12 weeks after infection and can also be useful in making a diagnosis.[1]

DIFFERENTIAL DIAGNOSIS

The triad of fever, pharyngitis, and lymphadenopathy are associated with a number of diagnoses in addition to acute infectious mononucleosis. If symptoms have been present for only a few days, group A beta-hemolytic streptococcal pharyngitis or a viral upper respiratory infection should be considered. It is important to remember, however, that individuals with a positive streptococcus culture may also have acute infectious mononucleosis. Individuals with a negative throat culture for group A beta-hemolytic streptococcus and symptoms that persist for more than a week are highly suspect for acute infectious mononucleosis.

MANAGEMENT

Treatment of uncomplicated EBV-IM is primarily supportive. Nonsteroidal antiinflammatory drugs or acetaminophen can be used for fever reduction. Aspirin should be avoided, as it has been associated with Reye's syndrome in a few cases of acute EBV.[5] Bed rest may be helpful during the acute phase of the illness depending on the degree of fatigue. Individuals with splenomegaly should be encouraged to refrain from strenuous physical activity for 3 to 4 weeks to avoid the risk of splenic rupture before resolution of the splenomegaly. Studies have shown that neither corticosteroids nor acyclovir reduced the severity of individual symptoms or the duration of symptoms. Therefore current management guidelines do not include the use of either of these agents in the treatment of acute uncomplicated EBV-IM, although corticosteroids may be useful in the treatment of several complications associated with EBV-IM. Most patients with EBV-IM recover spontaneously in approximately 2 to 4 weeks.[1]

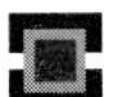

Diagnostics

Infectious Mononucleosis

Heterophile antibody	CBC and differential*
Viral capsid antigen (VCA) IgG and IgM*	Liver function tests*
EBV nuclear antigen (EBNA)*	Abdominal ultrasonography*

*If indicated.

Differential Diagnosis

Infectious Mononucleosis

Infectious Causes
- Bartonellosis (cat-scratch disease)
- Corneybacterium diphtheriae
- Cytomegalovirus
- Epstein-Barr virus
- Hepatitis A and B viruses
- HIV
- Human herpesvirus 6
- Lyme disease
- Malaria
- Meningococcemia
- Rubella
- *Salmonella* bacteremia
- *Streptococcus* pharyngitis
- Syphilis
- Toxoplasmosis
- Trichinosis
- Tuberculosis

Noninfectious Causes
- Juvenile rheumatoid arthritis
- Kawasaki syndrome
- Lymphoma
- Sarcoidosis
- Systemic lupus erythematosus

Drugs
- Dapsone
- Phenytoin
- Sulfonamides

LIFE SPAN CONSIDERATIONS

Older individuals are at risk for misdiagnosis of EBV-IM because the disease is relatively uncommon in older adults, occurring in only 3% to 10% of those 40 years of age or older. In addition, older adults with acute infectious mononucleosis often present differently; fever is present in more than 90% of individuals, but pharyngitis and lymphadenopathy are seen in less than 50% of patients.[2] The risk of EBV-associated liver disease is more common in older adults, however, and hepatitis, cholestasis, and hepatomegaly are seen in substantial numbers of older adults with EBV-IM as well. Jaundice is seen in more than 20% of older individuals.[2] Similarly, the risk of EBV-IM-associated hepatic failure, as well as other complications, increases with age. Nonetheless, the prognosis for EBV-IM is good even in older individuals.

COMPLICATIONS

The most common complications of EBV-IM, albeit rare, include upper airway obstruction, hepatomegaly, splenomegaly, and splenic rupture. In 1% to 2% of cases, EBV-IM has been associated with neurologic complications including cranial nerve palsies, Guillain-Barré syndrome, encephalitis, and peripheral neuropathies. In rare, cases EBV-IM has been associated with fatal cases of conduction abnormalities and myocarditis. Various ophthalmologic problems have been associated with EBV-IM including keratitis, uveitis, retinopathy, and periorbital cellulitis. Complications of EBV-IM can also result in a variety of renal pathologies including nephritic syndrome, hemolytic uremic syndrome, and renal failure. Hematologic complications include aplastic anemia, thrombocytopenia, and acute monoarthritis.[1,5]

The association between EBV-IM and chronic fatigue has been controversial for some time. Transient fatigue is part of acute infectious mononucleosis; however, the evidence for EBV-associated chronic fatigue is questionable. In fact, the Centers for Disease Control and Prevention does not consider workup for EBV infection to be useful in the evaluation of individuals suffering from chronic fatigue. Several studies have found that psychiatric morbidity and distress are associated with delayed recovery or development of chronic fatigue syndrome, although it has been difficult to confirm these findings.[6]

INDICATIONS FOR REFERRAL/HOSPITALIZATION

Infectious mononucleosis caused by EBV is generally a self-limiting disease of young adults. However, mild liver enzyme abnormalities are not uncommon and hepatitis is a rare but well-recognized complication of EBV infection that generally resolves spontaneously. Infectious mononucleosis is rarely seen in older adults; however, the potential for complications appears to increase in the older population, and several cases of severe cholestatic jaundice associated with infectious mononucleosis have been reported in this age-group. Abdominal imaging should be obtained in such cases to rule out a malignant extrahepatic biliary obstruction, and acute EBV infection should be considered in patients presenting with cholestasis. Because this complication is rare, it is generally not established until more common causes have been eliminated and serology consistent with EBV infection has been obtained.[7]

PATIENT AND FAMILY EDUCATION

Education about the nature of the illness and prognosis is important. Acute infectious mononucleosis has been referred to colloquially as the "kissing disease," and it is important to communicate that transmission through oropharyngeal secretions occurs in a variety of ways other than kissing. Changes in routines and schedules during the first few of weeks should be encouraged to allow for sufficient rest. The fact that acute infectious mononucleosis is usually an uncomplicated self-limiting illness is reassuring, especially during the first few weeks when the manifestations are most pronounced. However, education about the possible complications is important so that proper treatment can be initiated should any complications occur.

REFERENCES

1. Godshall SE, Kirschner JT: Infectious mononucleosis: complexities of a common syndrome, *Postgrad Med* 107(7):175-186, 2000.
2. Auwaerter PG: Infectious mononucleosis, *JAMA* 281(5):454-459, 1999.
3. Schooley RT: Epstein-Barr virus (infectious mononucleosis). In Mandell GL and others, editors: *Mandell, Douglas, and Bennett's principles and practice of infectious diseases,* ed 4, New York, 1995, Churchill Livingstone.
4. White PD and others: Incidence, risk and prognosis of acute and chronic fatigue syndromes and psychiatric disorders after glandular fever, *Br J Psychiatry* 173:475-481, 1998.
5. Bailey RE: Diagnosis and treatment of infectious mononucleosis, *Am Fam Physician* 49(4):879-888, 1994.
6. Buchwald DS and others: Acute infectious mononucleosis: characteristic of patients who report failure to recover, *Am J Med* 109:531-537, 2000.
7. Tahan V and others: Infectious mononucleosis presenting with severe cholestatic liver disease in the elderly, *J Clin Gastroenterol* 33(1):88-89, 2001.

CHAPTER 251

Lymphadenopathy

Michelle E. Freshman

DEFINITION/EPIDEMIOLOGY

Lymphadenopathy refers to nontender lymph nodes that have enlarged or changed in consistency. Lymphadenitis is defined as tender, warm, red nodes; suppurative lymphadenitis includes fluctuance. In 56% of physical examinations, there are incidental but palpable nodes.[1] Lymph nodes vary in size between 0.5 and 2.5 cm in diameter.[2] These enlargements are often related to inflammation or infection in younger patients but become more suspicious in older patients. Neck masses in patients between 15 and 35 years of age are most often associated with an infection such as mononucleosis. Congenital disorders and neoplasms may also cause neck masses in this age-group. With the exception of thyroid disease, 90% of neck masses in patients over 50 years of age are malignant.[3] The "rule of 80s" refers to patients over 40 years of age who regularly smoke or drink alcohol who present with a neck mass: 80% of all nonthyroid neck masses are neoplastic, 80% of those are malignant, 80% of those are metastatic, and 80% of those arise from primary sites above the clavicle.[4]

PATHOPHYSIOLOGY

The lymph nodes are integral to the lymphatic drainage system and provide filtration of foreign substances through the action of lymphocytes, monocytes, and macrophages. They are located in clusters around the lymphatic veins, where excess interstitial fluid is accumulated, processed, and later returned to hematologic circulation. More than 1000 lymph nodes exist in the body, with one third of these located in the head and neck. Only a small number of lymph nodes are normally palpable.[3]

Because development of the lymphatic system is linked to venous development, the lymphatic ducts run along venous tracks.[3] Lymph fluid ultimately reaches one of two large ducts in the thorax: the right lymphatic duct or the thoracic duct. The right lymphatic duct drains lymph from the right upper body—mediastinum, lungs, and esophagus—into the right supraclavicular vein; the thoracic duct drains lymph from the rest of the body, including the abdominal cavity, into the left supraclavicular vein.

Lymph nodes filter foreign substances and protein byproducts from the bloodstream and swell in response to viral or bacterial antigens. This swelling is caused by the proliferation of monocytes (the precursors to macrophages) or B- and T-lymphocytes. Along with the lymph nodes, other lymphoid organ tissues—including the tonsils, spleen and, sometimes, the liver—may enlarge. Splenomegaly associated with lymphadenopathy may reflect lymphocytosis generated by infection, macrophage proliferation, or a tumor. Generalized lymphadenopathy may indicate malignancy or systemic disease. The lymph system can be infiltrated by malignant cells and other cells not normally present in the nodes.

CLINICAL PRESENTATION

Because lymphadenopathy is often related to infection or inflammation in patients less than 50 years old, a thorough symptom analysis including infectious contacts or exposures (e.g., deer ticks, bird droppings, cat feces) may suggest a nonmalignant condition.[5] Foreign travel or travel to endemic infectious areas of the United States requires investigation. Questions regarding occupational exposure to livestock, asbestos, or silicone are also useful. Patients should be asked about any previous abdominal, thoracic, breast, head and neck, pelvic, or lower extremity surgeries; silicon implant products or prostheses; cancer diagnosis or family history; irradiation; and chemotherapy.

A review of systems should include all areas of the skin for irregular or nonhealing lesions. A history of scalp pruritus (e.g., seborrheic dermatitis, scabies infection), conjunctivitis, eye pain, photophobia, visual complaints, unilateral ear pain, difficulty hearing, nose or throat pain or discharge, odynophagia, impaired swallowing, acidic food intolerance, voice changes or persistent hoarseness, mastoid swelling or pain, dental maladies, denture malocclusion, facial paralysis, and muscular strain of the head or neck should be obtained from the patient.

The patient's breastfeeding history may indicate mastitis. Gastrointestinal symptoms suggestive of malabsorption, complaints of diarrhea or constipation, or back pain with relief in the fetal position can be associated with abdominal or inguinal lymphadenopathy.[6] Any signs of external or internal bleeding, such as hemoptysis, hematuria, melena, or menorrhagia, should be pursued to exclude malignancy. New medications and long-term prescriptions are worth reviewing for potential drug hypersensitivities. Phenytoin and typhoid vaccination can result in generalized lymphadenopathy.[2] Inquiry into the incidence and frequency of blood transfusions, sexually transmitted diseases, cigarette smoking, and illegal drug or alcohol abuse is also necessary. Tobacco and alcohol used together increases the risk of head and neck cancer greatly.[4] Iodine deficiency is a risk factor for thyroid cancer.[4]

Essential to the diagnosis is the duration and extent of the lymph node enlargement. It is also important to establish unilateral or bilateral involvement, tenderness, and other symptoms.

PHYSICAL EXAMINATION

The history and location of the lymphadenopathy guide the physical examination. Careful assessment for generalized lymphadenopathy is essential.

Differentiating between normally palpable cervical, axillary, and inguinal lymph nodes and enlarged nodes can be subtle. Smaller nodes greater than 1.5 cm and larger nodes in excess of 3 cm are considered abnormal.[2] The node should be characterized by degree of fluctuance, firmness, matted or shoddy quality, mobility or immobility, and tenderness or nontenderness. Unilateral or bilateral involvement, hard and fixed position, and symmetry or asymmetry may indicate malignancy (Box 251-1). Skin quality, accompanying or overlying vessels, and visible pulsations or bruits should be assessed.[3] A swollen node that is warm, tender, and rapidly enlarging may represent lymphadenitis and is suggestive of an infection at the drainage terminal. Lymphedema is an interruption and blockage in drainage and may result from a variety of causes. Primary lymphedema refers to congenital malformations; secondary refers to traumatic injury resulting from cancer obstruction, radiation, recurrent infection, or surgery.

Evaluation of the cervical nodes requires full muscle relaxation and midline positioning. Both anterior and posterior cervical nodes can indicate carcinomas of the head or neck. The presence of posterior cervical adenopathy more often suggests an infectious etiology.[6] A supraclavicular node can be elicited by a Valsalva maneuver in thin individuals.[6] Axillary nodes are terminal lymph drains for the upper extremities and can become enlarged as a result of breast malignancies or cellulitis of the hand or arm. Observed in both abducted and adducted positions, most axillary adenopathy is benign.[6] However, a woman of any age with a positive axillary node requires a mammography to exclude breast cancer. Liver and spleen examinations are essential.

Inguinal or retroperitoneal nodes may be difficult to palpate unless they are grossly enlarged; however, pain or a feeling of fullness may be present.[7] Unilateral or bilateral presentation is an important consideration, because the former is more often malignant. Bilateral presentation is also less common, except in syphilis.[6] Men can present with unilateral malignant lymphedema of the leg in cases of disseminated prostate cancer; it is termed lymphoma in women usually over 40 years of age with a characteristic postsurgical, radiation, or infection history.[8]

DIAGNOSTICS

A peripheral blood smear may be one of the most beneficial initial screens for lymphadenopathy.[1,6] Routine diagnostics to exclude infectious diseases may be indicated and include CBC with differential, a throat culture, a heterophil antibody or Monospot screen, an enzyme-linked immunosorbent assay/Western blot and rapid plasma reagin (RPR), a Venereal Disease Research Laboratory test, or a fluorescent treponemal antibody absorption test for secondary stage syphilis, especially in presentation with palmar rash. If indicated, Lyme disease titers should be obtained. Other cultures and screening tests should not be ordered unless the history or physical examination suggests specific etiologies. Liver function tests are important in the presence of hepatomegaly; renal disease or metastasis would be suggested by abnormal urinalysis, BUN, creatinine. Thyroid studies are warranted in suspected cases of thyroiditis, goiter, or carcinoma, for which a serum calcitonin might provide further confirmatory evidence.

BOX 251-1

LYMPHADENOPATHY: IMPORTANT FINDINGS ON PHYSICAL EXAMINATION

Nonneoplastic—Enlarged, flat, relatively soft
Neoplastic—Enlarged, irregular, and rubbery hard
Infectious—Enlarged, with a variable degree of hardness (may be fluctuant), tenderness, erythema, heat, and pain
Other factors—Presence or absence or hepatosplenomegaly; anatomic location and extent of lymphadenopathy

From Hess CE: Approach to patients with lymphadenopathy and splenomegaly. In Thorup OA Jr, editor: *Leavell and Thorup's fundamentals of clinical hematology*, Philadelphia, 1987, WB Saunders.

A chest radiograph for hilar adenopathy differentiates tuberculosis, sarcoidosis, and other infectious diseases from malignancy. Ultrasound (to avoid administering iodine contrast to thyroid lesions), CT, and positive technetium scans are reserved for soft tissue masses. A bone scan is ordered to confirm metastasis. Firm, immobile, nontender nodes greater than 1 cm are an indication for biopsy, whether by fine needle aspiration or open excision, as is slowly progressive lymphadenopathy in a patient who lacks other symptoms.[6] Typing and clinical staging of lymphomas require a specialist (see Chapter 234).

DIFFERENTIAL DIAGNOSIS

Lymphadenopathy may be related to an acute infectious process, a long-standing illness, malignancy, endocrine disorders, drug sensitivity, or other conditions. Drugs specifically known to produce lymphadenopathy include diphenylhydantoin, hydralazine, para-aminosalicylic acid, and allopurinol. Illnesses associated with lymphadenopathy include HIV/AIDS, syphilis, chancroid, Hodgkin's lymphoma, leukemia, and perhaps systemic lupus erythematosus, rheumatoid arthritis, and chronic fatigue syndrome. Most infectious processes that coincide with lymphadenopathy last fewer than 2 weeks. Mononucleosis classically presents with lymphadenopathy, pharyngitis, and fever. Parasitic toxoplasmosis from contact with cat feces, varicella, brucellosis, histoplasmosis, fungal coccidioidomycosis, and CMV are other infectious considerations. Hyperthyroidism, lipid storage diseases, sarcoidosis, and amyloidosis should also be included in the differential diagnosis.

Head and neck area lymphadenopathy coupled with a history of smoking and/or alcohol should raise a high index of suspicion for cancer if accompanied by hoarseness, hemoptysis, otalgia or hearing loss, facial nerve deficits, nasal obstruction or bleeding, throat pain or difficulty swallowing, or nonhealing ulcers.[4]

Inguinal lymphadenopathy may be confused with a hernia, vessel malformations, lipomas, or ectopic endometrial, testicular, or splenic tissue.[6] Cat-scratch disease, lymphogranuloma venereum, or herpesvirus can present with a unilateral, tender, and enlarged inguinal node. An asymptomatic unilateral enlargement suggests a malignant neoplasm or lymphoma.[6] A supraclavicular node enlargement or an asymptomatic, generalized lymphadenopathy pose the greatest risk for malignancy.[3,6] Fever, weight loss (10% in 6 months), night sweats, and pruritus occur in approximately 30% cases of Hodgkin's lymphoma and 10% of cases of non–Hodgkin's lymphoma.[9] Hodgkin's disease is particularly prevalent in young adults, but, if treated early, has excellent long-term survival rates.[10] Cervical mycobacterial lymphadenitis or scrofula, an extrapulmonary form of tuberculosis, accounts for 5% of head and neck lymphadenopathy and should be of particular concern in immunocompromised or AIDS patients.[11] Pain is often associated with infection or rapidly growing nodes within their capsule, although hemorrhage resulting from tissue death in a cancerous node also causes pain.[1]

Diagnostics

Lymphadenopathy

Laboratory	
Peripheral blood smear	Urinalysis*
CBC and differential	BUN, creatinine*
Heterophil antibody (monospot)*	TSH*
HIV*	**Imaging**
RPR or VDRL*	Chest x-ray*
Throat culture*	CT scan*
LFTs*	Ultrasound*
Epstein-Barr virus*	Bone scan*
Cytomegalovirus*	**Other**
Toxoplasmosis*	Purified protein derivative*
Lyme titer*	Lymph node biopsy*

*If indicated.

MANAGEMENT

Symptomatic relief of viral infections and appropriate antibiotic therapy for bacterial, mycobacterial, fungal, rickettsial, and chlamydial infections is indicated. Abscesses and other deep structure infections are treated in the hospital and may require surgery for drainage. Congenital or benign growths can be surgically removed. Evidence of malignancy requires a referral to the appropriate specialist. Patients with lymphadenopathy of unclear etiology also require physician consultation.

Co-Management with Specialists

It is imperative that patients with malignancies have continued primary care services to monitor for physical and psychosocial complications. It is also important that patients receive drug level monitoring, counseling, and weight management during chemotherapy. Patients and family should receive support for psychologic distress that may result from functional loss, hair loss, and other cosmetic change. Advance directives are often most comfortably discussed with primary care providers and communicated to the consultant. End-of-life care may be best managed at home with the help of the family and community volunteers and hospice services.

LIFE SPAN CONSIDERATIONS

With lymphadenopathy, an age greater than 50 years is correlated with an increased likelihood of malignancy.[3] As patients age, some lose muscular mass in the neck. As a result, some structures, including the hyoid bone, carotid bulbs, and thyroid, may become more pronounced or appear asymmetric and be mistaken for abnormalities.[4] Older adults can develop immunoblastic lymphadenopathy with a host of symptoms including combined autoimmune hemolytic anemia, polyclonal gammopathy, hepatosplenomegaly, and rash.[7] Older patients diagnosed with life-threatening infections or malignancies may decline treatment, especially if they suffer from other chronic diseases; they should be supported through these difficult decisions.

COMPLICATIONS

Given the variety of structures in the head and neck, a single enlarged node or a group of nodes might be mistaken for benign or congenital growths. Unfortunately, if an oropharyngeal or laryngeal cancer is missed, local metastasis may result. Untreated

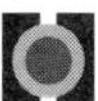

Differential Diagnosis

Lymphadenopathy

Disorder	*Associated Findings*
Mononucleosis-type syndromes	Fatigue, malaise, fever, atypical lymphocytosis
Epstein-Barr virus*	Splenomegaly in 50% of patients
Toxoplasmosis*	80% to 90% of patients are asymptomatic
Cytomegalovirus*	Often mild symptoms: patients may have hepatitis
Initial stages of HIV infection*	"Flu-like" illness, rash
Cat-scratch disease	Fever in one third of patients; cervical or axillary nodes
Pharyntitis due to group A streptococcus, gonococcus	Fever, pharyngeal exudates, cervical nodes
Tuberculosis lymphadenitis*	Painless, matted cervical nodes
Secondary syphilis*	Rash
Hepatitis B*	Fever, nausea, vomiting, icterus
Lymphogranuloma venereum	Tender, matted inguinal nodes
Chancroid	Painful ulcer, painful inguinal nodes
Lupus erythematosus*	Arthritis, rash, serositis, renal, neurologic, hematologic disorders
Rheumatoid arthritis	Arthritis
Lymphoma*	Fever, night sweats, weight loss in 20%-30% of patients
Leukemia*	Blood dyscrasias
Serum sickness*	Fever, malaise, arthralgia, urticaria, exposure to antisera or medications
Sarcoidosis	Hilar nodes, skin lesions, dyspnea
Kawasaki disease*	Fever, conjunctivitis, rash, mucous membrane lesions
Less Common Causes of Lymphadenopathy	
Lyme disease*	Rash, arthritis
Measles*	Fever, conjunctivitis, rash, cough
Rubella*	Rash
Tularemia	Fever, ulcer at inoculation site
Brucellosis*	Fever, sweats, malaise
Plague	Febrile, acutely ill with cluster of tender nodes
Typhoid fever*	Fever, chills, headache, abdominal complaints
Still's disease*	Fever, rash, arthritis
Dermatomyositis*	Proximal weakness, skin changes
Amyloidosis*	Fatigue, weight loss

Modified from Ferrer R: Lymphadenopathy: differential diagnosis and evaluation, *Am Fam Physician* 58(6):1318, 1998.
*Causes of generalized lymphadenopathy

or inadequately treated group A beta-hemolytic streptococcus may lead to rheumatic heart disease and glomerulonephritis and therefore warrants sufficient testing. A negative rapid strep test should be followed with a throat culture, and possibly the antistreptolysin-O titer to identify chronic carriers.[12] Tonsillar capsule abscesses can follow chronic or recurrent infections.[12] Infection can travel along the carotid sheath to the chest; therefore a CT scan might be required to determine surgical strategy.[12] Complications related to prescribed drugs, especially antibiotics and chemotherapeutic agents, are common.

INDICATIONS FOR REFERRAL/HOSPITALIZATION

Patients with unusual infectious diseases (e.g., those resulting from foreign travel or communicable illnesses), cases of rare animal or environmental exposure, chronic inflammatory diseases such as systemic lupus erythematosus, or a diagnosis of malignancy should be referred to the appropriate specialist. The crucial decision point for primary care providers is *when* to biopsy a node for a definitive diagnosis. A referral to an otolaryngologist or general surgeon might precede a visit to the oncologist. Immunosuppressed patients with AIDS, malignancy, or other illnesses may require hospitalization for intensive nutritional, antiinfective, and chemotherapeutic support.

PATIENT AND FAMILY EDUCATION

Patients with lymphadenopathy need reassurance that most cases are benign and require only watchful waiting. Nodes that persist for more than 4 weeks require further investigation. Ongoing cancer screening for early cancer detection significantly increases the odds for survival.

HEALTH PROMOTION

Because many diseases involving lymph node enlargement in otherwise healthy adults are sexually transmitted, patients should be well informed of their health risks for genital and oral contagion. Frank discussion with patients, as well as support of communication and condom use between partners, is critical. Cancer prevention strategies include eliminating all forms of tobacco, reducing alcohol consumption to less than three drinks a day, and protecting skin from ultraviolet radiation and occupational hazards. Health behaviors that fortify the immune system such as proper nutrition, sleep, exercise, emotional support, and stress management promote health and assist recovery. Patients are often able to find educational and social support in local or state chapters of national disease foundations.

REFERENCES

1. Pangalis GA and others: Clinical approach to lymphadenopathy, *Semin Oncol* 20(6):570-582, 1993.
2. *Lymphadenopathy. Professional guide to signs and symptoms,* ed 3, Springhouse, Pa, 2001, Springhouse Corporation.
3. Olsen KD: Evaluation of masses in the neck, *Prim Care* 17(2):415-435, 1990.
4. Prisco MK: Evaluating neck masses, *Nurse Pract* 25(4):30-32, 35-36, 38, 2000.
5. Shaffer S: Benign lymphoproliferative disorders, *Semin Oncol Nurs* 12(1):29-37, 1996.
6. Segal GH, Clough JD, Tubbs RR: Autoimmune and iatrogenic causes of lymphadenopathy, *Semin Oncol* 20(6):611-626, 1993.
7. Dowd TR, Stewart FM: Primary care approach to lymphadenopathy, *Nurs Pract* 19(12):36-44, 1994.
8. McGee S: *Evidence-based physical diagnosis,* Philadelphia, 2001, WB Saunders.
9. Erikson JM: Update on Hodgkin's disease, *Nurs Pract* 19(11):63-68, 1994.
10. Morrison C, Gordon S, Yeo TP: Hodgkin's disease in primary care, *Nurse Pract* 25(7):44, 47-50, 2000.
11. Weber AL, Siciliano A: CT and MR imaging evaluation of neck infections with clinical correlations, *Radiol Clin North Am* 38(5):941-968, 2000.
12. Richardson MA: Otolaryngology for the internist, *Med Clin North Am* 83(1):75-83, 1999.

CHAPTER 252

Weight Loss

Michelle E. Freshman

DEFINITION/EPIDEMIOLOGY

The average American is able to maintain his or her body weight within a range of 0.5 to 1.0 kg annually.[1] Although not all weight loss is ominous, a loss in excess of 5% body weight in 6 months or 10% within 1 year typically warrants further investigation.[1-3] Among older adults in particular, involuntary weight loss may result from a broad spectrum of physiologic and/or psychosocial factors. Within the nursing home population, the Omnibus Budget Reconciliation Act of 1987 established strict criteria for unintentional weight loss: 5% decrease in actual body weight in 30 days or 10% in 6 months.[4] Such a threshold has been shown to be independently and highly predictive of mortality and associated with increased morbidity.[2-4] Although annual prevalence and incidence within this subgroup have not been well established,[3,5] 2-year mortality rate among a group of 91 older adults was reported to be 25% among those initially hospitalized with an unexplained weight loss.[2,5] Moreover, 20% of 850 patients treated in England from a pool of 1611 surveyed demonstrated malnutrition on admission.[6]

PATHOPHYSIOLOGY

Protein-energy malnutrition occurs when the supply of proteins and/or calories is inadequate to maintain weight. In most industrial societies a combination of the conditions *marasmus*-insufficient calories and *kwashiorkor*-protein deficiency often occurs as evidenced by changes in body composition, systemic weakness, and laboratory abnormalities.[7] Unintentional weight loss can be categorized by one of the following: decreased calorie intake, decreased calorie absorption, and insufficient calorie intake to meet increased metabolic demands. Functional anorexia may be due to disinterest, obstacles to mastication, a depressed sense of taste and smell, delayed gastric emptying time, or pain with elimination. Decreased calorie absorption results from malabsorption, vomiting, diarrhea, and urinary frequency. Increased metabolism occurs with hyperactivity, hyperthyroidism, and tumor growth. Regardless of the cause, the pathway by which weight loss occurs has not yet been fully explained.[2] There is a pathophysiologic connection between weight loss and infection through the diminished capacity of cell-mediated and humoral immune systems to mount an adequate response; other humoral system secretions in the setting of illness produce anorexia.[2]

CLINICAL PRESENTATION

Patients are often unaware of weight changes and, in the absence of consistent health records, may only recollect the observations of others or demonstrate unconsciously cinched-in clothing as evidence of weight loss. A record of the quantity, quality, and regularity of intake assists in the investigation. A diet history is of utmost importance. Situational stress or anxiety can explain unintentional weight loss. Changes in mood, affect, or coping can point to a psychogenic origin.[8]

An inquiry into food affordability, availability, preparation, safety, and social isolation is essential. An older patient with early dementia may have trouble sequencing the steps necessary to procure and prepare food.

Recent adoption of proscribed food practices, such as veganism or religious fasting, coupled with inadequate education can lead to unintentional weight loss. For those who report polyphagia or polydipsia and appear to have lost weight, a set of endocrine disorders should be included in the differential diagnosis including hyperthyroidism, diabetes mellitus, diabetes insipidus, and adrenal insufficiency. Symptoms associated with decreased intake such as fever, night sweats, dyspnea, and/or mental status changes suggest underlying infection, malignancy, or possible neurologic impairment.

Swallowing difficulties may cause a patient to alter the types or amounts of food eaten. Common reasons for decreased appetite include dysgeusia, pain with chewing, heartburn, and gastric pain before or after eating or associated with eating fatty or acidic foods. Disturbances such as nausea, vomiting, abdominal bloating, flatulence, constipation, and diarrhea affect intake. Milk products associated with these latter complaints might signal lactose malabsorption. Bloody stool can indicate hemorrhoid, inflammatory bowel disease, or malignancy. Fatty, odorous stool can point to gallbladder disease or malabsorption syndromes. Individuals may also try to prevent diarrhea by avoiding food.[5] A history of chronic diarrhea, whether secondary to bacterial or parasitic exposure or as a result of underlying illness or recent hospitalization, should be elicited.

Premorbid health conditions can tax a patient's reserves to a degree that interferes with adequate nutrition and hydration. Fatigue, shortness of breath, or impaired mobility may make the duration of a meal exhausting, causing the patient to eat less. Older adults experience a diminished thirst drive, as well as taste and smell.[9] Obtaining a smoking, alcohol, and drug history is essential; patients who abuse alcohol may drink rather than eat or have vitamin deficiencies that cause anorexia. A history of behaviors that put people at risk for disease, including HIV, should be elicited. Immunocompromised states can exist along with wasting syndrome. Surgical repair or resection of the intestine can cause bowel torsion and constipation to the point of anorexia.

A review of medications, especially if there is evidence of polypharmacy, is necessary. Drugs that affect taste and smell include digoxin, theophylline, and angiotensin-converting enzyme inhibitors. Many other medications, including antiviral agents and macrolide antibiotics, as well as antineoplastic medications, can cause anorexia.[8] Anticholinergics produce dry mouth and, along with narcotics, potassium, iron, nonsteroidal antiinflammatory drugs, and calcium channel agonists, promote constipation.[3,4] Psychotropic drugs can disturb eating behaviors.[4] Excessive use of diuretics or laxatives should also be explored; amphetamine use, digitalis, and thyroid medication can all cause anorexia.

PHYSICAL EXAMINATION

General appearance, habitus, affect, speech, cognition, and recall provide basic information. Weight loss can be determined if a previsit weight is available and should be calculated as a percentage change from baseline. Weight charts are not as useful in patients over 75 years of age. Vital signs indicate orthostasis or arrhythmias, suggestive of underlying cardiac disease and disability. Dyspnea, arrhythmias, diminished breath sounds, wheezing, and ankle edema suggest cardiopulmonary problems that may interfere with appetite or energy demands. Functional limitations are usually evident with minimal exertion.[5]

Pallor, jaundice or rash, skin texture and turgor, hair consistency and distribution, and poor wound healing should be noted. Hyperpigmentation of the joints, waist, mouth, and palmar creases is associated with adrenal insufficiency.[10] Serial skinfold measurement may be helpful to determine the percentage of body fat. Muscle wasting at the temples and intercostal spaces, which is more commonly seen in older adults, should be assessed in context. Exophthalmos typifies hyperthyroidism. An oropharyngeal examination looking for glossitis, ulcers, exudates, masses, ill-fitting or odorous dentures, tooth or gum decay, and missing teeth should be carefully performed. The temporomandibular joint should be palpated and gently extended to assess pain or crepitation. Lymphadenopathy, neck masses, and a diminished swallow reflex may warrant further studies. Thyroid enlargement requires further testing for thyroid dysfunction.

Breast examination is important given the increasing incidence of cancers associated with aging. An abdominal examination that is positive for acute rigidity, masses, hepatomegaly, midepigastric tenderness, or ascites may indicate problems of digestion or absorption. A pelvic examination with cervical screening should be included, if indicated. Rectal ulcers, lesions, hemorrhoids, swollen prostate or nodule, or painful defecation resulting from underlying disease process may be seen on examination.

DIAGNOSTICS

A thyroid-stimulating hormone to exclude hyperthyroidism is especially warranted among women over 40 years of age and generally in those over 70 years of age who have signs of tachycardia and fatigue[11] (see Chapter 230). An abnormal CBC with differential is helpful in determining the presence of infection or malignancy. A positive screen for anemia should be followed by evaluation of serum iron, ferritin, B_{12}, and folate levels. A chemistry

Diagnostics

Weight Loss

Laboratory
TSH
CBC and differential
Calcium
Serum electrolytes
Alkaline phosphatase
Serum glucose
LFTs
Cholesterol
BUN
Creatinine
Serum albumin
Iron, B_{12}, folate, ferritin*
Urinalysis
Stool for occult blood
Stool for ova and parasites*
Stool for fecal fat*
Stool for culture*

Imaging
Ultrasound (abdominal, pelvic, renal)*

Other
Endoscopy*
Barium swallow*
Echocardiogram

*If indicated.

profile, including calcium, potassium, alkaline phosphatase, liver function studies, serum electrolytes, serum glucose, serum albumin, BUN, and creatinine, would suggest nutritional deficiencies or other underlying diseases. The combination of low serum albumin and high alkaline phosphatase in a retrospective inpatient analysis was 17% sensitive but 87% specific for neoplasia.[1] A urinalysis can reveal infection or unmask diabetes or uremia associated with early anorexia.[2] A chest x-ray study is helpful if pulmonary pathology is suspected. Age- and history-appropriate cancer screenings should be incorporated. Glucose tolerance testing is appropriate for suspected diabetes.

Although a stool evaluation for occult blood is indicated, testing for ova and parasites, culture, or fat content is based on clinical presentation and physical signs. If the patient's history suggests a possible esophageal stricture or gastric or duodenal ulcer, an upper and lower endoscopy and/or barium swallow is appropriate. Pelvic, renal, and abdominal ultrasounds; echocardiography; and lung studies should be reserved to confirm suspected abdominal, renal, gynecologic, cardiac, or pulmonary causes of weight loss. Sigmoidoscopy or colonoscopy is appropriate for high suspicion of intestinal disease. Because judicious testing has been shown to elucidate about 75% of the cases of weight loss among older adults, a straightforward approach is best guided by physical examination and history.[5] Finally, a low score on the Mini Mental State Examination for cognitive functioning (<24) should raise the question of dementia; a positive depression inventory should lead a provider to further explore situational or psychologic diagnoses.

DIFFERENTIAL DIAGNOSIS

From a summary of seven studies, it can be concluded that the three most common diagnoses associated with weight loss are

Differential Diagnosis

Weight Loss

Decreased Caloric Intake	Decreased Caloric Absorption
Malignancies	Uncontrolled diabetes mellitus
Gastrointestinal/bowel distress	Renal disease
Depression/anxiety/stress/hypomania	Small bowel disease
Anorexia nervosa/bulimia	AIDS wasting syndrome
Poor nutrition	Post–gastrectomy surgery
Alcoholism	Alcoholism/liver disease
Congestive heart failure	Repeated vomiting or diarrhea from illness/chemotherapy
Chronic respiratory disease	Gallbladder disease
HIV/AIDS/infectious diseases	Open skin wounds
Poor dentition	**Increased Metabolic Demands**
Decreased smell/taste	Hyperthyroidism
Functional obstacles to eating	Malignancies
Decreased access to food	Fever
Dementia	Mania
Social isolation	Chronic respiratory disease
Drug side effects	Cocaine abuse

cancer, gastrointestinal disorders, and psychiatric problems.[3] Yet weight loss is a hallmark of many systemic diseases such as cardiac, respiratory, or bowel disease; diabetes; hyperthyroidism; and a host of psychiatric illnesses including schizophrenia and mania. In fact, the psychiatric component is said to be significant: 25% of older adults seen in outpatient settings have been found to have any of a constellation of depressive symptoms; 10% of those surveyed had major depressive disorders.[5] Because depression factors heavily into weight loss, these statistics are significant. Furthermore, 25% of patients diagnosed with Alzheimer's disease are thought to be both depressed and demented; all eventually suffer from decreased thirst and appetite.[5] Despite the clinical visit, upwards of 25% of cases may defy diagnosis and therefore follow-up evaluation is critical in this population, as most cases are rarely occult.[1,2] One interesting rubric is worth noting. The difference between a patient's actual loss and perceived loss has been used to predict the nature of the cause: an underestimation of greater than 0.5 kg is correlated with organic disease with a sensitivity of 40% and a specificity of 92%; and overestimation of greater than 0.5 kg is predictive of inorganic disease with a sensitivity of 70% and a specificity of 81%.[7]

MANAGEMENT

The primary goals are to provide adequate energy, protein, and micronutrients, as well as treat the underlying disease. Medications can either reverse nausea and/or increase appetite, such as the progestogens megestrol acetate and dronabinol, and the corticosteroid prednisone. Megestrol acetate has been seen to improve geriatric appetite, enjoyment of life, and well-being, increasing weight after 3 months.[12] Young patients with anorexia from AIDS wasting syndrome can be given cyproheptadine, a serotonin antagonist, but this medication should be avoided in older patients.[3] Anabolic steroids might be used with cancer cachexia syndrome.[13] Antidepressants should be chosen carefully because some selective serotonin reuptake inhibitors are known to decrease appetite. With severe wasting or when oral feeding is not safe or desirable, enteral tube feedings or parenteral feedings can supplement or supplant oral feedings.

LIFE SPAN CONSIDERATIONS

As older adults experience the physiologic changes that uniquely predispose them to weight loss, it is important to monitor weight and nutrition before weight loss occurs. Body mass peaks in men during their forties and in women during their fifties; in subsequent years, shifts in fat stores and fat atrophy occur.[2] Smell and taste sensations also change, which diminishes the pleasurable experience of eating. Because older age brings limitations in abilities, a thorough evaluation of functional independence and safety may clarify meal-related problems. Weight loss that is related to a disease process, acute illness, or depression may be difficult to recover, particularly in older adults,[3] so optimal management requires a team effort. This is particularly true in institutionalized settings where contributing factors such as eating dependency or illness can be assessed more globally. Anticipating malnutrition and weight loss during acute episodes is likely to be crucial to the care of the vulnerable patient, because catching up on depleted stores is difficult.[14]

INDICATIONS FOR REFERRAL/HOSPITALIZATION

If available, the services of a dietitian or nutritionist are invaluable. Occupational, physical, and speech therapists can help patients with functional or swallowing problems. Medical specialists, including oncologists, neurologists, and psychologists, should be consulted when necessary.

Any patient with severe anorexia, a weight loss in excess of 35% of ideal body weight, hypokalemia, hypotension, or prerenal azotemia related to dehydration requires immediate hospitalization to prevent sudden death.[15] Patients with wasting syndromes, including cancer, HIV/AIDS, or failure to thrive, may require hospitalization for gastric tube placement and feedings or parenteral nutrition. An unchecked decline in weight and functional status can result in a spiraling decline in health with potentially dire consequences.

COMPLICATIONS

Complications include severe malnutrition, weakness, loss of muscle mass, orthostatic hypotension, falls, immobility, and skin breakdown. Immunocompromised patients and older adults are at special risk for weight loss. Because the course of a debilitative process and recovery is compounded by weight loss, patients who are at risk require nutritional evaluation and support whether in hospital or home settings.

PATIENT AND FAMILY EDUCATION

Teaching patients simple nutritional concepts and encouraging them to keep a food diary may be helpful. Suggestions for increasing meal attractiveness include flavor enhancement through polyunsaturated butters, oils, dressings, jellies, and creamers; increased fiber; and increased fluid content. Zinc deficiency can lead to dysgeusia, so adding a multivitamin along with protein-rich snacks and nutritional supplements may significantly improve appetite and intake.[2,5] Facilitating food procurement with prepackaged meals or home-delivered foods can make a difference. Increasing activity, social engagement, and a sense of functional capability in the face of dysfunction or physical limitation also improves quality of life. Appetite may also be improved with a simplified regimen that reduces the number of medications taken, eliminating those that might be contributing to the problem. Because weight loss can be a late sign of renal or cardiac disease, it important to encourage patients to seek medical advice to maximize their quality of life.[10]

HEALTH PROMOTION

Primary prevention of weight loss includes promoting activities that support safe access to food, medical, and dental services, as well as socialization for those at social or financial risk of decreased intake. For those who already suffer from underlying illness, vigilance against communicable disease, receiving scheduled Pneumovax and flu vaccines, managing sleeping requirements by preventing overexertion or poor sleep hygiene, and making adjustments in diet for tastes and preferences help safeguard nutritional status. Managing side effects such as constipation, nausea/vomiting, and gas; focusing on the favorite meal of the day; and choosing easy-to-prepare foods with adequate flavorings are important strategies to optimize the experience.

REFERENCES

1. Wise GR, Craig D: Evaluation of involuntary weight loss: where do you start? *Postgrad Med* 95(4):143-150, 1994.
2. Reife CM: Significance of involuntary weight loss, *Med Clin North Am* 79(2):299-313, 1995.
3. Wallace JI, Schwartz RS: Involuntary weight loss in elderly outpatients: recognition, etiologies, and treatment, *Clin Geriatr Med* 13(4):717-735, 1997.
4. Fabiny AR, Kiel DP: Assessing and treating weight loss in nursing home residents, *Clin Geriatr Med* 13(4):737-751, 1997.
5. Robbins LJ: Evaluation of weight loss in the elderly, *Geriatrics* 44(4):31-37, 1989.
6. Edington J and others: Prevalence of malnutrition on admission to four hospitals in England. The malnutrition prevalence group, *Clin Nutr* 19(3):191-195, 2000.
7. McGee S: *Evidence-based physical diagnosis*, Philadelphia, 2001, WB Saunders.
8. Williams B, Waters D, Parker K: Evaluation and treatment of weight loss in adults with HIV disease, *Am Fam Physician* 60(3):843-854, 1999.
9. Lipschitz DA: Screening for nutritional status in the elderly, *Prim Care* 21(1):55-67,1994.
10. Holmes HN, editor: *Professional guide to signs and symptoms*, ed 3, Springhouse, Penn, 2001, Springhouse Corp.
11. Kennedy JW, Caro JF: The ABCs of managing hyperthyroidism in the older patient, *Geriatrics* 51(5):22-32, 1996.
12. Yeh SS and others: Improvement in quality of life measures and stimulation of weight gain after treatment with megestrol acetate oral suspension in geriatric cachexia: results of a double-blind, placebo-controlled study, *J Am Geriatr Soc* 48(5):485-492, 2000.
13. Puccio M, Nathanson L: The cancer cachexia syndrome, *Semin Oncol* 24(3):277-287, 1997.
14. Moriguti JC and others: Involuntary weight loss in elderly individuals: assessment and treatment, *Sao Paulo Med J* 119(2):72-77, 2001.
15. Waldrop R: Anorexia nervosa, eMedicine (May 21, 2001). Retrieved January 6, 2002, from the World Wide Web: http://www.emedicine.com.

PART 20

Evaluation and Management of Oncologic Disorders

JOANN TRYBULSKI, Section Editor

CHAPTER 253

Collaborative Management of the Oncology Patient

Jane Williams and Marcia L. Patterson

Optimal cancer care depends on careful planning across multidisciplinary care settings to reduce the risk of fragmentation and ensure a continuum of care. Many patients belong to managed care insurance plans requiring primary care providers (PCP) to serve as gatekeepers. A 1995 study found that the majority of oncology patients regard their oncologist as their PCP and are opposed to having a managed-care gatekeeper.[1] However, it is important that the PCP be viewed as a valuable member of the cancer-care team, not as a resented formality. Therefore it is necessary that all providers have a basic understanding of cancer-specific risk factors, presenting signs and symptoms, diagnostic tools, treatment options, prognosis, psychosocial issues, and available support systems.

Approximately three fourths of all cancer risks are elements that individuals can control themselves. These include dietary habits, the use of tobacco products or alcohol, sun exposure, physical activity, and risky sexual behaviors. Emphasizing healthy lifestyle practices is a principal component of primary care, not only for cancer prevention but also for overall disease prevention.

The American Cancer Society (ACS) offers cancer-specific guidelines for screening asymptomatic patients, and evidence-based screening guidelines can be obtained from the National Cancer Institute.[2,3] The PCP needs to be involved in quality screening activities, which include (but are not limited to) the following comprehensive examinations: breast, gynecologic (women), genitourinary (men), colorectal, skin, and oral head and neck. Screening tests should be performed according to age-appropriate recommended guidelines and need to include mammography, cervical smears, fecal occult blood test, prostate-specific antigen test, and flexible sigmoidoscopy or colonoscopy. The PCP will most likely detect cancer and will provide the first source of information regarding diagnosis and possible treatment options before referring the patient to the oncologist or cancer center.

New information about genetic testing is widely available. Although only 5% to 10% of cancers are hereditary, providers must be diligent in obtaining accurate family histories to establish the possibility of a hereditary cancer syndrome. If this possibility does exist, the patient should be informed about the potential personal risk for cancer and about available surveillance and management strategies, including self-examinations, screening examinations, diagnostic tests, and cancer prevention strategies.[4] Patients at high risk for certain cancers may need additional screening. For example, women suspected of being at risk for inheriting a mutation in the BRCA-1 (breast and ovarian) gene need to continue monthly breast self-examinations, increase clinical breast examinations to annually if between ages 20 and 40 years (some authorities even recommend every 6 months), and have annual mammograms beginning at least 10 years earlier than the youngest age of diagnosis in a relative. In addition, an annual CA_{125} and transvaginal ultrasound screening for ovarian cancer is advised. Other high-risk guidelines can be obtained from the ACS.[2] If indicated, a referral to a National Cancer Institute–designated comprehensive cancer center that offers genetic testing and counseling is appropriate.

After a diagnosis of cancer, a timely referral for treatment increases the opportunity for optimal outcomes. In many cases these outcomes include improved rates of cure, longer survival rates, and improved quality of life. The Consensus Statement of the American Federation of Clinical Oncologic Societies states that "cancer care requires that the patient has access to a multidisciplinary team of cancer providers across the full continuum of care and coordination of services, including prevention, early detection, staging evaluation, initial and subsequent treatment, palliative care, supportive therapies, long-term follow-up, rehabilitation, psychosocial services, and hospice."[5] It also states that PCPs who lack the experience and skills to provide necessary and appropriate care be encouraged to refer patients for specialty care.[5] With shortened hospital stays, management of cancer patients has moved from the hospital to the home. In such cases, collaboration with the oncology team in managing symptoms and monitoring for complications becomes essential.

Caring for the cancer patient can place inordinate burdens on family and friends. Assessing caregiver readiness and availability to care for the patient is imperative. The primary care giver must be aware of the established support systems and the availability of additional community resources such as breast cancer support groups, the United Ostomy Association, I Can Cope, Candlelighters, and Can Care. The local ACS chapter is another excellent resource. Successful home care also depends on such factors as cultural beliefs, role delineation, and existing interpersonal conflicts. Additionally, personal values surrounding narcotic analgesic use and beliefs about death and dying should be explored.

The PCP is an essential patient resource between appointments with the oncologist, especially if the oncologist is in another city, or if the PCP is monitoring the patient for management of other chronic conditions. If the PCP is not receiving reports and updates from the oncologist, he or she should contact the oncologist and request to receive all vital information that will affect patient outcomes. This information includes current disease status, patient condition and prognosis, current and recent treatment, and future treatment plans. This approach allows the PCP to adequately monitor various symptoms, accurately answer patient questions regarding treatment side effects, and reinforce information given by the oncologist.

Communication must clearly define areas of responsibility between the PCP and oncologist, and should be *task oriented.*[6] For example, if the PCP agrees to monitor laboratory values for neutropenia, anemia, thrombocytopenia, kidney function, and liver function, he or she must be aware of critical laboratory parameters that require management by the oncology team or referral to a specialist. Additionally, the PCP can reinforce to the patient those signs and symptoms such as fever, mental status change, increasing pain, persistent vomiting, and so on that indicate the need for urgent evaluation. Establishment of a collaborative relationship between the oncology team and the PCP ensures safe and continuous care, minimizes potential complications, and promotes patient and provider confidence.

Health care reform has redirected patient care. Both patients with cancer and cancer survivors are especially vulnerable to the risk of fragmentation of care when migrating from specialist to generalist or from hospital to home care. Consistent personnel who know the patient's situation are the key components for successful delivery of health care. It is the responsibility of the patient and all members of the multidisciplinary health care team to identify needs and form a collaborative plan so that outcomes of care can be maximized.

REFERENCES

1. Blum D, Glajchen M, Calder K: Access to specialty care for oncology patients: the case for designating the oncologist as gatekeeper, *Proc Annu Meet Am Soc Clin Oncol* 14:A1673, 1995.
2. American Cancer Society: Cancer specific prevention and early detection. Retrieved March 3, 2003, from the World Wide Web: http://www.cancer.org/docroot/PED/ped_0.asp.
3. National Cancer Institutes: Cancer specific early detection. Retrieved March 3, 2003, from the World Wide Web: http://www.nci.nih.gov/cancer_information/.
4. American Cancer Society: *Cancer and genetics: answering your patients' questions*, Huntington, NY, 1997, PRR.
5. Consensus Statement of the American Federation of Clinical Oncologic Societies: *Oncol Nurs Forum* 25(1), 1998.
6. Buckman R: Communication in palliative care: a practical guide. In Doyle D, Hank G, MacDonald N, editors: *Oxford textbook of palliative medicine*, ed 2, Oxford, 1998, Oxford University Press.

CHAPTER 254

Basic Principles of Oncology Treatment

Karen Borden and Debra Toran

Treatment of any cancer is multifaceted and involves a multidisciplinary team that includes physician specialists, nurses, pharmacists, social workers, and other health care professionals. Primary care providers must act as patient advocates and must play a central role in coordinating the effort among all involved disciplines.

The oldest treatment for cancer is surgery. The early 1800s marked the modern era of elective surgery for visceral tumors in frontier America.[1] Approximately 55% of all patients with cancer are now treated with surgical intervention.[2] Surgery is effectively used for cancer prevention, definitive treatment, rehabilitation, and palliation. Using combinations of surgery, chemotherapy, radiotherapy, biotherapy, and genetic therapy, disease-free intervals have been significantly lengthened and survival benefits have been recognized. Radiation and chemotherapy, historically relegated to palliative roles, have become adjuncts for local disease and are even curative for some early-stage cancers.[3]

The first approach to any cancer treatment is determined by tumor type. One major role of surgery is to obtain tissue for an accurate histologic diagnosis.[1] After a histologic diagnosis has been established, the patient is staged. Staging is based on specific criteria and differs according to the tumor type. In the earliest stages of the disease, the tumor is localized and a cure is possible through local or regional therapy. If the tumor stage is higher, the cancer is no longer localized and the chance of curing the patient diminishes. Once the tumor type and stage are determined, the treatment plan is created. This plan considers the risk-benefit ratio of various options, the overall physical condition of the patient, the patient's consent, the availability of treatment facilities, and any financial restrictions.

RADIOTHERAPY (RADIATION THERAPY)

Radiotherapy may be the sole treatment for cancer but is often combined with surgery or chemotherapy and biologic therapy. Although treatment techniques and equipment may vary, the important principles of radiotherapy form a basis on which a course of treatment is chosen and designed for each patient.[3] The goals of radiotherapy may be to cure, control, or palliate.

Radiation therapy has become more effective with the development of high-energy linear accelerators and technical improvements in delivery.[3] Various types of equipment and beams are used in radiotherapy. Equipment can be categorized according to use: (1) external radiation, or teletherapy (radiation from a source at a distance from the body), or (2) brachytherapy (radiation from a source placed within the body or a body cavity).

Teletherapy produces x-rays of varying energies (orthovoltage or megavoltage). The higher the voltage, the greater the depth of penetration of the x-ray beam. Disadvantages of teletherapy include poor depth of penetration, severe skin reactions resulting from high doses at the skin level, and bone necrosis (bone absorbs more radiation than soft tissue). Megavoltage equipment has distinct advantages over an orthovoltage beam. Megavoltage equipment provides deeper penetration, more uniform absorption of radiation, and greater skin sparing. Equipment used in megavoltage therapy includes the Van de Graaff machine, cobalt and cesium units, and betatron and linear accelerators.[4] The dose of radiation is determined by the radiosensitivity of the tumor. The Gray system international unit is the accepted term for radiation dosages: 1 Gray (Gy) equals 100 rads (radiation absorbed doses); 1 cGy equals 1 rad.[5]

Historically, radium and radon have provided the source of removable interstitial and intracavitary radiation; radon has been used primarily for permanent implants. Marie Curie, who discovered radium, recognized its importance early and endorsed the medical use of radium isotopes. These now have been largely replaced by synthetic isotopes.[3]

Brachytherapy involves placement of these sources of radioactive material within or near a tumor and is the treatment of choice for a variety of malignancies. It is often combined with teletherapy and may be used preoperatively or postoperatively. Radioactive isotopes for brachytherapy application are contained in a variety of forms such as wires, ribbons, tubes, needles, grains, seeds, or capsules. The source is selected by the radiotherapist according to the site to be treated, size of the lesion, and whether the implant is temporary or permanent. Brachytherapy is given at either a low-dose rate or a high-dose rate, which produces the same effect in a shorter time period.[4]

It is usually assumed that DNA is the critical target for the effects of radiotherapy. A cell damaged by radiation loses its reproductive integrity but may divide at least once before its offspring are reproductively sterile. Some delay in division is usually produced, even in cells that are not damaged lethally.[3] Other factors that affect the biologic response to radiotherapy include oxygen effect (well-oxygenated tumors have a greater response), linear energy transfer (the rate at which energy is lost from different types of radiations while traveling through matter), relative biologic effectiveness, and fractionation.[3]

After the patient has been evaluated and a decision to use external beam therapy has been made, a simulation is performed. Simulation localizes the tumor and defines the volume to be treated. The field of treatment is determined by tattooing the area to be irradiated. Special immobilization devices, such as custom casts or molds, may be used.[4]

For patients not receiving whole-body irradiation, certain treatment-related side effects may develop. Predictable side effects of irradiation for a particular tumor type often occur. Factors that predict side effects include the following: the exact body tissue treated, the daily dose and total dosage given, the particular method of radiation delivery, and individual factors (e.g., the patient's age and genetic makeup). Many symptoms do not develop until 10 to 14 days into treatment, and some do not subside until 2 or more weeks after treatments have ended.[3] Common side effects include fatigue, anorexia, mucositis, xerostomia, radiation caries, esophagitis, dysphagia, nausea, vomiting, diarrhea, tenesmus, cystitis, urethritis, alopecia, skin reactions, and bone marrow depression.[5]

In the future, radiation oncology will be characterized by continuous improvement of treatment techniques and increased application of multimodal therapy. Radiotherapy has come a long way since its beginning in the 1800s. The future holds promise for advances in cancer treatment, with radiotherapy playing a major role in primary treatment and in combined modality approaches.

The responsibility of the primary care provider is to monitor for complications and collaborate with oncologists or radiotherapists. For the treatment phase of radiotherapy, the provider should monitor vital signs, prepare the patient's gastrointestinal tract to reduce inflammation, and provide physical and emotional support. After treatment is completed, the management of subsequent local reactions is crucial.

CHEMOTHERAPY

The word *chemotherapy* was introduced by Paul Ehrlich in the early 1900s.[6] Chemotherapeutic agents have traditionally been classified by their mechanism of action, chemical structure, or biologic source. Alkylating agents were the first modern chemotherapeutic agents and were a product of the secret weapons programs in the two world wars. After an explosion in Italy, physicians noticed that many of the soldiers exposed to the resultant gases died from atrophy of the lymph glands and bone marrow suppression.[5] After this discovery, a similar chemical called nitrogen mustard was given to patients with metastatic lymphomas; this resulted in transient but promising antitumor responses (Table 254-1).[7]

During the last 5 years molecular analysis of the DNA of both normal and neoplastic cells has defined the mechanisms by which chemotherapy causes cell death. Understanding how chemotherapy works and how genetic change can result in resistance to therapy has enabled new types of treatment. These therapies combine molecular, genetic, and biologic strategies to increase the sensitivity of abnormal cells to treatment and to protect the normal tissues of the body from therapy-induced side effects.[6] Discovery of these new strategies could change the way therapy is delivered over the next few years and improve treatment outcomes, especially in patients with cancers that are resistant to standard therapy.

Administering and monitoring chemotherapy requires an understanding of the principles of carcinogenesis and cellular kinetics.[7] Carcinogenesis is the process by which one or more normal cells undergo genetic changes, leading to malignant transformation. The direct exposure of DNA to a carcinogen may lead to irreversible genetic damage that allows this malignant transformation. The cell cycle is a sequence of steps through which both normal and abnormal cells grow and reproduce.[8] This process involves five phases: M, the period of cell division; G_1, the postmitotic period (in the proliferative cycle); G_0, the postmitotic period (temporarily out of the proliferative cycle); S, the period of DNA synthesis; and G_2, the premitotic period (RNA and protein synthesis). These cell-cycle kinetics are altered when a cell becomes malignant. Chemotherapy agents can be classified according to the phase of the cell cycle in which they are active (Box 254-1).

Chemotherapy is used as an induction treatment for advanced disease, as an addition to local methods of treatment,

TABLE 254-1 Common Oncology Medications

Drugs	Uses
PLATINUM COMPLEXES	
Carboplatin and cisplatin	Ovarian cancer; endometrial, head and neck, lung, testicular, breast cancers; relapsed acute leukemia; non-Hodgkin's lymphoma; testicular, ovarian, bladder, uterine, cervical, lung, head and neck sarcoma
NITROGEN MUSTARDS	
Chlorambucil, cyclophosphamide, estramustine, ifosfamide, mechlorethamine, and melphalan	CLL; HD; NHL; ovarian cancer; choriocarcinoma; lymphosarcoma
AZIRIDINE	
Thiotepa	Ovarian, breast, superficial bladder cancer; HD; CML; CLL; bronchogenic carcinoma; malignant effusions (intracavitary); BMT for refractory leukemia, lymphoma
ALKYL SULFONATE	
Busulfan	CML; BMT
NITROSOUREAS	
Carmustine, lomustine, and streptozocin	Brain and refractory brain cancer; multiple myeloma; HD; NHL; melanoma; BMT; GI carcinomas; NSCLC; pancreatic islet-cell carcinoma; carcinoid colon; hepatoma
NONCLASSIC ALKYLATORS	
Dacarbazine, procarbazine, altretamine	Malignant melanoma; HD; sarcoma; neuroblastoma; NHL; brain, lung, ovarian, breast, cervical cancer
ANTIMETABOLITES	
Methotrexate, fludarabine, mercaptopurine, thioguanine, cladribine, pentostatin, cytarabine, floxuridine, fluorouracil, gemcitabine	Breast, head, neck, GI, lung cancer; ALL; CNS leukemia; Burkitt's lymphoma; CLL; CML; AML; multiple myeloma; hairy-cell leukemia; NHL; lymphoma; pancreatic, renal cell, prostate, ovarian cancer
Hydrea (substituted urea)	CML; ALL; ovarian, head and neck cancer; melanoma; essential thrombosis; polycythemia
NATURAL PRODUCTS	
Bleomycin, dactinomycin, daunorubicin, doxorubicin, idarubicin, mitoxantrone, mitomycin, etoposide, teniposide, docetaxel, paclitaxel, vinblastine, vincristine, vinorelbine, irinotecan, topotecan	Skin, bladder, breast, ovarian, testicular, vulvar, penile, thyroid, gastric, colorectal, uterine, cervical, pancreatic, and renal cancers; reticulum cell sarcoma; HD; squamous cell cancer of head and neck; Wilm's tumor; Ewing's sarcoma; AML; ALL; NHL; SCLC; CML; NSCLC; melanoma; rhabdomyosarcoma
Asparaginase (enzyme)	ALL; CML; AML

ALL, acute lymphocytic leukemia; *AML,* acute myelogenous leukemia; *BMT,* Bone marrow transplant; *CLL,* chronic lymphocytic leukemia; *CML,* chronic myelogenous leukemia; *HD,* Hodgkin's disease; *NHL,* non-Hodgkin's lymphoma; *NSCLC,* non–small-cell lung cancer; *SCLC,* small-cell lung cancer.

or as the primary treatment for patients with localized cancer. Chemotherapy agents may also be directly instilled into tumor sanctuaries (e.g., the brain or meninges) or perfused into specific regions of the body most affected by the cancer.[6]

Among patients receiving chemotherapy, there is a wide patient diversity in both therapeutic response and unacceptable toxicity observed. This variability can be attributed to differences in patient characteristics, the chemotherapeutic agents given, and the type of tumor being treated.[8] Patient factors include toxicity response, organ dysfunction, previous treatments, and age. The occurrence and severity of toxicity are widely variable among patients and often require a dose reduction or a treatment delay.

Chemotherapy can be given with a curative goal by using primary or adjuvant therapy. Primary chemotherapy is used when no other modality is available. Neoadjuvant chemotherapy is given before alternative treatments (e.g., surgery) in patients who present with primarily local disease.[9] Adjuvant chemotherapy is given systemically after surgical resection of the primary tumor, with the goal being to improve the potential for cure. Administering a combination of clinically effective antitumor drugs is the standard chemotherapeutic approach for most malignancies. This technique provides a maximal cell kill for resistant cells, reduces the development of resistant cell lines, and minimizes toxicity.[6]

Administration of chemotherapy may be assigned to the primary care provider when an oncologist is not available. It is critical that the provider be aware of the hazards of extravasation associated with certain IV agents, including doxorubicin, vincristine, vinblastine, dactinomycin, mitomycin, carmustine,

BOX 254-1

CELL-CYCLE ACTIVITY

S-PHASE AGENTS
Antimetabolites
- Cytarabine
- Doxorubicin
- Fludarabine
- Gemcitabine
- Hydroxyurea
- Mercaptopurine
- Methotrexate
- Prednisone
- Procarbazine
- Thioguanine

CELL-CYCLE-PHASE–NONSPECIFIC AGENTS
Alkylating agents
Antibiotics
Nitrosoureas
Miscellaneous

M-PHASE AGENTS
Vinca alkaloids
- Vinblastine
- Vincristine
- Vinorelbine

Podophyllotoxins
- Etoposide
- Teniposide

Taxanes
- Docetaxel
- Paclitaxel

G_2-PHASE AGENTS
Bleomycin

G_1-PHASE AGENTS
Asparaginase
Corticosteroids

daunorubicin, idarubicin, teniposide, and nitrogen mustard.[7] Unfamiliar agents must be checked for potential effects of extravasation by calling a pharmacist or reading the drug label. The best treatment for extravasation is prevention. Proper central venous access is essential.

It is important that the provider differentiate among toxic chemotherapeutic reactions and distinguish these reactions from complications related to the tumor itself. Myelosuppression is the most common and the most lethal dose-limiting side effect of chemotherapy. It is critical that patients with neutropenia be referred to an oncologist or an emergency department. Other common adverse effects of cancer and its therapy include fatigue, anorexia, diarrhea, constipation, nausea/vomiting, cardiotoxicity, neurotoxicity, pulmonary toxicity, hepatotoxicity, hemorrhagic cystitis, nephrotoxicity, and gonadal toxicity.[6]

Treatment of cancer has progressed from early experiments with mustard gas derivatives to the current abundance of drugs at the oncologist's disposal. These drugs include growth factors such as erythropoietin and colony-stimulating factors, which prevent specific chemotherapy side effects. Research efforts continue to focus on improving quality of life through evaluation of new drug therapies and reevaluation of existing treatments. Biologic therapies such as interferon and interleukin-2 are also being investigated for their ability to control tumor growth and generation and to restore, augment, or modulate their ability to fight cancer. Antibody-based immunotherapies, otherwise known as monoclonal antibodies, have been found to be effective both alone and in combination with other therapies for the treatment of cancer. Although many of the monoclonal antibodies are still under clinical investigation, they offer a safe and specific new approach to treating cancer cells and sparing normal tissue.[9,10] Gene therapy is an attempt to alter patients' genetic material to fight or prevent disease. Future research endeavors include combining chemotherapy, biologic therapy, and gene therapy to achieve optimal patient outcomes.

Primary care providers have diverse responsibilities to patients receiving chemotherapy. Understanding the different tumor types and chemotherapeutic agents and their toxicities is essential when caring for these patients. Direct communication and collaboration between the oncologist and primary care provider is necessary for the recognition of subtle but potentially life-threatening changes in the patient's condition. Given the research that is currently under way to improve effective therapies and to prevent and manage their side effects, there is great reason for optimism.

REFERENCES

1. Rosenberg S: Principles of cancer management in surgical oncology. In DeVita VT, Hellman S, Rosenberg SA, editors: *Cancer: principles and practice of oncology,* ed 5, Philadelphia, 1997, JB Lippincott.
2. Younger J: Principles of radiation therapy. In Goroll AH, May LA, Mulley AG, editors: *Primary care medicine,* ed 4, Philadelphia, 2000, JB Lippincott.
3. Hellman S: Principles of cancer management in radiation therapy. In DeVita VT, Hellman S, Rosenberg SA, editors: *Cancer: principles and practice of oncology,* ed 5, Philadelphia, 1997, JB Lippincott.
4. Iwamato RR: Radiation therapy. In Varricchio C and others, editors: *A cancer sourcebook for nurses,* ed 7, Atlanta, 1997, American Cancer Society.
5. Bucholtz JD: Radiation. In Gross J, Johnson BJ, editors: *Handbook for oncology nursing,* ed 3, Boston, 1998, Jones & Bartlett.
6. Hubbard SM, Gakassi A: Chemotherapy. In Gross J, Johnson BL, editors: *Handbook of oncology nursing,* ed 3, Boston, 1998, Jones & Bartlett.
7. DeVita V: Principles of cancer management in chemotherapy. In DeVita VT, Hellmans S, Rosenberg SA, editors: *Cancer: principles and practice of oncology,* ed 5, Philadelphia, 1997, JB Lippincott.
8. Page R, Rhodes V, Pazdur R: Cancer chemotherapy. In Pazdur R and others, editors: *Cancer management: a multidisciplinary approach,* ed 5, New York, 2001, PRR.
9. Chabner B, Longo D: *Cancer chemotherapy and biotherapy: principles and practice,* ed 3, Philadelphia, 2001, Lippincott Williams and Wilkins.
10. Yarbro C and others: *Cancer nursing: principles and practice,* ed 5, Boston, 2000, Jones & Bartlett.

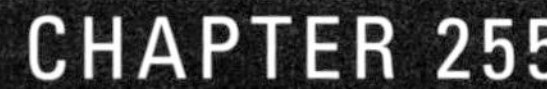

CHAPTER 255

Detection of Tumor of Unknown Origin

Renato Lenzi

DEFINITION/EPIDEMIOLOGY

Unknown primary carcinoma (UPC) is defined as the presence of documented metastatic cancer in the absence of an identifiable primary tumor site. Because identification of the primary site forms the basis for predicting expected behavior and assigning the appropriate therapy of malignant diseases, the absence of a primary site poses a major challenge. In patients with UPC, the reason the primary site cannot be diagnosed remains unknown. Investigators have speculated that the tumor either remains below the limits of clinical or radiographic detection or regresses spontaneously.

Of the large population of patients referred to a cancer center, approximately 1% have metastases from an unknown primary site.[1] Higher prevalence rates of 3% to 15% have been reported but probably reflect differences in referral patterns, demographics, and the extent of the evaluation performed. Patients with UPC are heterogeneous in their clinical presentation and have widely varying clinical courses. As a group, these patients have a historically poor median survival of 11 months. Except for a slight preponderance of male patients, the demographics (age and ethnicity) generally mirror those of the general cancer patient population.[1]

PATHOPHYSIOLOGY

Findings of chromosome 1 deletion, translocations, and gene amplification in UPC suggest that these tumors may rapidly progress to reach the ability to metastasize. It has been speculated that specific genetic changes of UPC may support metastatic but not local growth. Although UPC would be expected to have a high rate of *p53* mutations because of the metastatic potential and clinical aggressiveness, the measured frequency of *p53* mutations is low (26%).[2] This suggests that *p53* mutations may not have a major role in tumor progression. Furthermore, there appear to be no differences in microvessel density between metastases from unknown primary sites and those from primary tumors originating in the colon or breast.[3]

CLINICAL PRESENTATION

The clinical presentations of patients with UPC vary widely, which probably reflects the heterogeneous nature of the underlying malignancies. Subgroups of patients with similar clinical presentations have been identified as having disease that is responsive to therapy and/or has longer survival times. These favorable subsets include (1) women with peritoneal carcinomatosis, (2) women with metastatic adenocarcinoma or carcinoma confined to the axillary nodes, (3) patients with inguinal node metastases of squamous cell carcinoma histology, (4) patients with squamous cell carcinoma confined to lymph nodes in the high or mid neck, and (5) patients with neuroendocrine involvement. Moreover, it has been shown that patients presenting with lymph node involvement have longer median survival times than patients presenting with lung, liver, or bone metastases.[1]

TABLE 255-1 Tumor Histology of 1109 Patients with Unknown Primary Carcinoma

Histology	Patients	% of Total
Adenocarcinoma	646	58.3
Well differentiated	14	
Moderately differentiated	45	
Poorly differentiated	220	
Mucinous	46	
No descriptor/other	321	
Carcinoma	317	28.6
Poorly differentiated	161	
Undifferentiated	21	
Large cell	9	
Small cell	14	
No descriptor/other	112	
Squamous	68	6.1
Neuroendocrine	48	4.3
Adenosquamous	7	0.6
Pathology not available for review/other	23	2.1

Data from Abbruzzese JL, Abbruzzese MC, Lenzi R: Unpublished data, M. D. Anderson Cancer Center, Houston, Tex.

The tumor histology of 1109 consecutive UPC patients is portrayed in Table 255-1. Glandular differentiation sufficient to permit a diagnosis of adenocarcinoma was identified in approximately 60% of patients with UPC. Nearly 30% of patients were diagnosed with carcinoma, and more than half of these had evidence of poorly differentiated or undifferentiated carcinoma. Squamous cell carcinoma and neuroendocrine carcinoma together accounted for 10% of patients and were associated with more favorable median survival times. Patients with carcinoma also have a longer median survival time (12 months) than patients with adenocarcinoma (9 months), but their survival advantage is not as pronounced as that of patients with squamous cell carcinoma (24 months) and neuroendocrine carcinoma (33 months).

PHYSICAL EXAMINATION

The initial evaluation should focus on signs and symptoms that could identify the primary site (e.g., blood in stool, persistent cough) and should include an inquiry regarding the family history of cancer. The physical examination should include a skin evaluation of the skin; a careful breast and pelvic examination (for women); and a testicular, rectal, and prostate examination (for men). Areas with lymph nodes should be examined for adenopathy.

DIAGNOSTICS

A limited and focused evaluation that includes a pathologic review, careful physical examination, CBC, chemistry survey (SMA-12 or SMA-20), chest radiography, and a CT scan of the abdomen and pelvis in all patients, prostate-specific antigen levels in men, and a mammography in women has been shown to be effective in identifying the majority of treatable primary malignancies.[4] Additional studies are performed only as needed to pursue abnormalities that are revealed during the initial evaluation. This strategy identified a primary malignancy in 20% (179 patients) of a consecutive group of 879 patients referred with suspected UPC.[4]

A pathologic examination is the most important step in determining the primary site or identifying a unique histologic subset that is amenable to therapy.[4] Good communication between the primary care provider and pathologist is needed to determine whether the use of more sophisticated techniques (e.g., histochemical and immunohistochemical staining, electron microscopy, or molecular studies) will contribute to the evaluation of a particular patient. Such special studies are not recommended in every case but are extremely useful in patients diagnosed with undifferentiated carcinoma or poorly differentiated carcinoma after a review of hematoxylin and eosin–stained slides.[5,6]

DIFFERENTIAL DIAGNOSIS

At the beginning of the diagnostic evaluation, it is very important to ascertain whether the patient has a neoplastic process. A small but significant percentage of the patients referred with a diagnosis of metastatic carcinoma of unknown primary are found on further evaluation not to have cancer.

In the majority of cases the diagnosis is made on the basis of radiographic studies, and the initial evaluation does not include a biopsy. For example, a patient with osteoporosis and compression fractures of single or multiple vertebral bodies may be initially diagnosed with metastatic bone lesions. Clarification of the diagnosis is usually accomplished with a biopsy of the suspected metastatic site. However, caution needs to be used in the planning of invasive diagnostic modalities because complications can result from the diagnostic procedure itself. For example, a liver biopsy may produce adverse results if performed to diagnose a liver lesion that is actually a hemangioma. In such cases the diagnosis can be made with a high rate of confidence by the use of noninvasive testing such as an MRI or a tagged red cell scan. Lesions that appear to be metastatic may indeed represent the primary cancer. For example, multiple liver lesions thought to be metastatic from an unknown site may represent a primary multifocal hepatocellular carcinoma. Sometimes the primary tumor displays an unusual pattern of tumor growth, and more sophisticated imaging studies such as an indium-111–octreotide scan are necessary.[7]

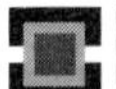

Diagnostics

Tumor of Unknown Origin

Pathology
Review of biopsy material
- Morphology
- Immunohistochemistry*
- Molecular and chromosomal studies*

Repeat biopsy*

Laboratory
CBC and differential
Complete chemistry profile
Prostate-specific antigen (PSA) for men
Beta-hCG and alpha-fetoprotein†

Imaging
Chest x-ray
CT scan of abdomen/pelvis
Mammogram for women

*If indicated.
†If extragonadal germ cell syndrome is suspected.

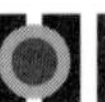

Differential Diagnosis

Tumor of Unknown Origin

Clinicopathologic subgroups with favorable prognosis
Extragonadal germ cell syndrome
Women with peritoneal carcinomatosis
Women with isolated axillary node involvement
Squamous cell carcinoma in inguinal nodes
Squamous cell carcinoma in high or midneck nodes
Poorly differentiated neuroendocrine carcinoma

MANAGEMENT

The treatment of patients in whom the primary site or a unique histologic subtype (e.g., melanoma, lymphoma, sarcoma) has been identified should follow disease-specific guidelines. The treatment of patients presenting with features matching one of the favorable subsets is as follows.

Male gender, an age less than 50 years, and rapidly growing and poorly differentiated carcinomas involving predominantly midline structures (mediastinum, retroperitoneum) are typical features of the extragonadal germ cell syndrome. A careful pathologic review will identify the true germ cell histologies; molecular studies of chromosome 12 may be extremely helpful in establishing the diagnosis.[8] These patients should be treated aggressively with the chemotherapy regimens used for testicular cancer. Patients with poorly differentiated carcinomas without histologic evidence of germ cell features are much less responsive to therapy but should be given a trial of platinum-based chemotherapy.[9]

Women presenting with isolated peritoneal carcinomatosis have a survival advantage compared with all women with UPC and should be treated according to the guidelines established for therapy of advanced (stage III) ovarian carcinoma. Although in some patients the underlying primary malignancies may be gastrointestinal in nature, the lack of effective treatment for gastrointestinal malignancies justifies tailoring the initial chemotherapy regimen to a possible ovarian primary. Cytoreductive surgery followed by cisplatin-based combination chemotherapy produces favorable survival in approximately 10% to 20% of these patients.

In women, the most common cause of carcinomas confined to the axillary nodes is occult breast cancer. Biopsy material should be analyzed for estrogen and progesterone receptors. These patients should be treated similarly to patients with a breast primary tumor of a corresponding stage.[7] Overall, the survival rate appears to be similar to that of patients with breast cancer. Inguinal node metastases of unknown origin with squamous cell carcinoma histology (a rare clinical presentation) require careful inspection of the skin; endoscopic evaluation of the anal canal, rectum, and distal genitourinary tract; and a gynecologic examination in women. Patients in whom the primary tumor cannot be identified and who do not have additional sites of disease should undergo lymph node dissection of the affected area. Local radiotherapy is often administered after surgery.

Squamous cell carcinoma is found in more than 70% of patients with involved nodes high in the neck or in the mid neck. The most common occult primary sites include the nasopharynx, tonsil, base of the tongue, and hypopharynx. The first step is to perform fine-needle aspiration of an involved node, which often has a high diagnostic yield. If squamous cell carcinoma is diagnosed, the patient should undergo CT studies of the neck and a thorough ear, nose, and throat evaluation that consists of direct laryngoscopy with random biopsy samples from the tonsil, nasopharynx, and base of the tongue. If no primary tumor is found, the patient should undergo neck dissection followed by radiotherapy. Patients with extensive adenopathy are often treated with platinum-based chemotherapy. The exact role of chemotherapy and the best sequencing of the modalities in these patients are unclear. The overall 5-year survival rate is 30% to 50%, depending on the extent of the disease at diagnosis.[10]

Poorly differentiated neuroendocrine carcinoma is a clinicopathologic entity that is recognized for its responsiveness to therapy. Morphologically, these tumors are very poorly differentiated. Histochemical stains are usually positive for chromogranin, synaptophysin, or nonspecific enolase (NSE). These patients often present with diffuse hepatic or bone metastases. Neuroendocrine carcinomas do not have the indolent histologic or clinical features of typical carcinoid tumors, islet cell tumors, or paragangliomas, for which observation is often appropriate; they are often responsive to cisplatin-based chemotherapy.[11]

The majority of patients with UPC do not fit into one of the previously described subsets. Palliative chemotherapy, with either investigational or standard agents, should be considered in patients with good performance status.[12,13] A combination of carboplatin and paclitaxel is the standard regimen for these patients, resulting in an overall response rate of approximately 38%. Best results have been observed in patients with nodal/pleural disease and in women with peritoneal carcinomatosis. Patients with multiorgan involvement or bone or liver metastases have a lower rate of response of approximately 15% and a shorter median survival.[14] In a study of patients treated with carboplatin, paclitaxel, and etoposide, a 3-year survival rate of 14% was observed.[15]

Co-Management with Specialists

The delivery of care to patients with UPC often requires a multidisciplinary team to provide adequate integration and planning of multimodality care. This care involves specialists in medical oncology, radiotherapy, surgery, and pain and symptom management.

LIFE SPAN CONSIDERATIONS

The median survival for patients with UPC is relatively short (11 months). Consideration should be given to prompt identification of patients in the more treatable subsets. This can usually be accomplished if the limited and focused evaluation previously described is used; the goal is timely administration of therapy without the undue delay of prolonged and unproductive testing.

COMPLICATIONS

As with other patients with metastatic cancer, patients with UPC are at risk for a broad spectrum of complications. Complications directly related to the disease process include spinal cord compression from metastatic disease, hypercalcemia of malignancy, ureteral and biliary obstruction, development of pleural and pericardial effusions, and ascites. Complications related to treatment include chemotherapy-induced alopecia, nausea, vomiting, diarrhea, and mucositis, as well as febrile neutropenia, anemia, and thrombocytopenia, which often require the transfusion of blood products. Narcotic analgesics are often necessary for pain control and may cause respiratory depression, hallucinations, somnolence, nausea, vomiting, and severe constipation. Radiation treatment may cause fatigue and, depending on the anatomic area being treated, hair loss, esophagitis with dysphagia, gastritis, diarrhea, rectal pain/burning, and cystitis with dysuria. Clinically significant anxiety and depression are often observed in these patients.

INDICATIONS FOR REFERRAL/HOSPITALIZATION

Diagnostic evaluation and therapeutic decisions for patients with UPC are complex and require referral to a physician who specializes in the treatment of cancer patients. Hospitalization may be required for adequate management of symptoms and complications related to either the disease process (e.g., spinal cord compression, bleeding, hypercalcemia, intractable pain) or treatment side effects (e.g., intractable nausea and vomiting, febrile neutropenia, thrombocytopenia with bleeding). Hospitalization may also be required for the administration of chemotherapy or for procedures such as surgical stabilization of metastatic bone lesions or excision of limited metastatic disease.

PATIENT AND FAMILY EDUCATION

A diagnosis of UPC is a major challenge for patients and families. The lack of knowledge of the primary tumor results in diagnostic and therapeutic uncertainties and can generate anxiety in the primary care provider and patient.[4] It is important to emphasize that although the primary site is not known, there are guidelines to help choose the most effective treatment for each patient. Patients need education regarding the side effects of chemotherapy and radiotherapy and need to be taught to recognize the complications that require immediate medical attention. It is also important to educate patients in the appropriate use of pain medications. Finally, it is often necessary to educate and communicate with these patients on emotionally charged topics such as "do not resuscitate" status and the shift from chemotherapy to supportive care only. Training staff in dealing with these difficult aspects of patient communication will increase their confidence in dealing with these issues and has been shown to contribute to improved patient adjustment.[16]

REFERENCES

1. Abbruzzese JL and others: Unknown primary carcinoma: natural history and prognostic factors in 657 consecutive patients, *J Clin Oncol* 12:1272-1280, 1994.
2. Bar-Eli M and others: p53 gene mutation spectrum in human unknown primary tumors, *Anticancer Res* 13(5A):1619-1623, 1993.

3. Hillen HF and others: Microvessel density in unknown primary tumors, *Int J Cancer* 74:81-85, 1997.
4. Abbruzzese JL and others: Analysis of a diagnostic strategy for patients with suspected tumors of unknown origin, *J Clin Oncol* 13:2094-2103, 1995.
5. Abbruzzese JL, Raber MN: Unknown primary carcinoma. In Abeloff MD and others, editors: *Clinical oncology*, New York, 1995, Churchill Livingstone.
6. Hainsworth JD and others: Poorly differentiated carcinoma of unknown primary site: clinical usefulness of immunoperoxidase staining, *J Clin Oncol* 9:1931-1938, 1991.
7. Lenzi R and others: Detection of primary breast cancer presenting as metastatic carcinoma of unknown primary origin by ^{111}In-pentetreotide scan, *Ann Oncol* 9:213-216, 1998.
8. Motzer RJ and others: Molecular and cytogenetic studies in the diagnosis of patients with poorly differentiated carcinomas of unknown primary site, *J Clin Oncol* 13:274-282, 1995.
9. Lenzi R and others: Poorly differentiated carcinoma and poorly differentiated adenocarcinoma of unknown origin: favorable subsets of patients with unknown primary carcinoma? *J Clin Oncol* 15:2056-2066, 1997.
10. Buzaid AC, Abbruzzese MC, Abbruzzese JL: Carcinoma of unknown primary site. In Greene HL, Johnson WP, Lemcke D, editors: *Decision making in medicine: an algorithmic approach*, St Louis, 1998, Mosby.
11. Hainsworth JD, Johnson DH, Greco FA: Poorly differentiated neuroendocrine carcinoma of unknown primary site: a newly recognized clinicopathologic entity, *Ann Intern Med* 109:364-371, 1988.
12. Lenzi R and others: Phase II study of cisplatin, 5FU and folinic acid in patients with tumors of unknown primary origin, *Eur J Cancer* 29A:1634, 1993.
13. Hainsworth JD and others: Carcinoma of unknown primary site: treatment with 1-hour paclitaxel, carboplatin, and extended-schedule etoposide, *J Clin Oncol* 15:2385-2393, 1997.
14. Briasoulis E and others: Carboplatin plus paclitaxel in unknown primary carcinoma: a phase II Hellenic Cooperative Oncology Group study, *J Clin Oncol* 18:3101-3107, 2000.
15. Greco FA and others: Carcinoma of unknown primary site, *Cancer* 89:2655-2660, 2000.
16. Baile WF and others: Improving physician-patient communication in cancer care: outcome of a workshop for oncologists, *J Cancer Educ* 12:166-173, 1997.

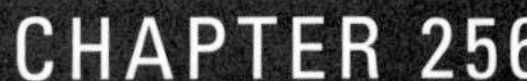

CHAPTER 256

Gastrointestinal Symptoms in the Oncology Patient

Jane Williams and Marcia L. Patterson

DEFINITION/EPIDEMIOLOGY

Cancer patients can experience numerous disorders of the digestive system. These disorders can be related to the treatment (e.g., chemotherapy, radiation, surgery) or the disease (e.g., neoplasm, infection, functional, obstruction, motility alterations, or malabsorption). The prevention of complications and early detection of lower-grade toxicity permit fewer and more easily managed sequelae. This chapter focuses on the most common problematic symptoms, which include nausea and vomiting, constipation and diarrhea, anorexia, and the oral manifestations of mucositis, xerostomia, and dysphagia.

PATHOPHYSIOLOGY

The secretory and absorptive abilities of the gastrointestinal (GI) tract facilitate the essential functions of digestion and nutrient uptake. The other essential function is to maintain a barrier between the host and potentially harmful pathogens in the lumen. The mucosal epithelium has a very rapid turnover—every 24 to 72 hours. It is believed that this rapid restitution of functioning cells may both reduce the risk of malignancy and create the environment for neoplastic disorders, which are common in the GI tract.[1]

Nausea is described as an unpleasant, wavelike sensation that is experienced in the back of the throat, the epigastrium, or both and may or may not culminate in vomiting.[1] *Vomiting* is defined as the forceful expulsion of the contents of the stomach, duodenum, or jejunum through the oral cavity.[1] The most common causes of nausea and vomiting (N&V) are emetogenic chemotherapy drugs and radiotherapy to the GI tract, liver, or brain. Other possible causes include other medications (e.g., opioids, antimicrobials, or bronchodilators), intestinal obstructions, fluid and electrolyte imbalances, constipation, tumor invasion of the GI tract or liver, and brain metastatis.[1,2] The mechanisms of nausea are believed to be controlled by alterations of the parasympathetic autonomic nervous system. Vomiting results from (1) the stimulation of a complex reflex that is coordinated by the vomiting center (VC), which is located in the medulla, and (2) by afferent stimulation of the chemoreceptor trigger zone (CTZ), which is also located in the medulla.[2]

Constipation may be described as stool that is infrequent, dry, hard, and difficult to pass, or there may be a feeling of incomplete evacuation.[3] It is important to consider the patient's perception of well-being and usual pattern of evacuation rather than a standard norm. The most common constipating chemotherapy agents are the vinca alkaloids, which result in autonomic nerve dysfunction and can lead to decreased peristalsis and paralytic ileus.[3,4] Chemotherapy-induced N&V may also contribute to constipation through decreased oral intake. Cancer patients may also be prone to constipation from the use of narcotic agents, aluminum antacids, anticonvulsants, anticholinergic drugs, antispasmodics, diuretics, tricyclic antidepressants, antiinflammatory drugs, and muscle relaxants. Primary or metastatic tumors of the bowel may result in extraluminal compression on the intestine itself, which blocks the passage of stool, or in interference with the colon's neural innervation. This can also be seen with pelvic cancer, malignant ascites, paraneoplastic syndromes, spinal cord compression, hypercalcemia, organ failure, or debility with advanced disease. Fatigue and immobility may also be a contributing factor.[3,4]

Diarrhea can be described as an increase in stool volume and in water content of the feces, or as three or more bowel movements per day.[1] The most common cause of cancer-related diarrhea is abdominal irradiation and chemotherapy agents such as 5-fluorouracil, methotrexate, actinomycin D, cytarabine (ara-C), or doxorubicin. These treatments result in the destruction of the actively dividing epithelial cells of the bowel, which leads to mucosal atrophy and shortened, denuded villae. The bowel lining becomes slick, the contents move through more rapidly, and the resorption of fluids is decreased. Patients who are immunosuppressed are more susceptible to infectious organisms such as *Clostridium difficile*, which causes excessive mucosal secretion of fluid and electrolytes by the bowel mucosa.

Anorexia is characterized by a decrease in appetite and food intake. The resulting weight loss may lead to cachexia, a syndrome of progressive wasting that may be irreversible and fatal. Interferences of physiologic, psychologic, and social stimuli can decrease food intake and nutritional status. Appetite suppression results from the secretion of cytokines that act as anorexigenic agents. Physiologic factors include N&V, taste alterations, constipation, dysphagia, odynophagia, fatigue, infection, and stomatitis. Psychologic factors include anxiety and depression. Social factors include the inability to eat, personal or cultural preferences, or the loss of the patient's usual eating companions when hospitalized. Medical causes can be related to tumors, bowel obstruction, fever, metabolic disorders (hepatic and renal dysfunction), and ectopic hormone production by tumors. Head and neck surgery may affect the ability to eat normally because of altered facial architecture. Radiotherapy can lead to glossitis, stomatitis, esophagitis, and altered taste. In addition to chemotherapy agents, antibiotics, antifungal agents, and pain medications may produce a loss of appetite.

All mucous membranes are at risk for the effects of systemic chemotherapy, but the most common sites for mucositis are the oral cavity and the esophagus. The most common mucosatoxic agents are 5-fluorouricil, methotrexate, bleomycin, doxorubicin, actinomycin D, vinblastine, docetaxel, etoposide, mitoxantron, cytarabine, daunorubicin, vindesine, and floxuridine.[5] With irradiation, tissues that are in the treatment field will be predisposed to mucositis as a result of mitotic death of the basal cells in the epithelium.[6] The risk of developing mucositis is not the same for all patients and is not the same for each drug regimen. The mucosa may become dry, inflamed, ulcerated, and painful. Pain is the major clinical problem and may render the patient unable to practice adequate oral hygiene, eat properly, or communicate.

Xerostomia is a decrease in the quantity and quality of saliva, resulting in thick, ropy saliva that interferes with nutrition, taste, and speech. It is a direct result of radiotherapy to the head and neck region, which destroys the taste buds and the cells responsible for the secretion of saliva. Xerostomia may be of long duration (months to years). Dental caries can result from xerostomia and the alteration of bacterial flora in the mouth. Symptoms suggestive of oropharyngeal dysphagia include difficulty in initiating a swallow, regurgitation of liquid through the nose, aspiration with swallowing, and an inability to propel a bolus of food into the esophagus. Patients with esophageal dysphagia complain of retrosternal fullness after swallowing and the feeling that food is stuck in the esophagus.

CLINICAL PRESENTATION

A complete assessment that includes documentation of alterations in sleep patterns and the evolution of change in constitutional symptoms, such as weight loss (>10 pounds over 4 weeks), fever, anorexia, or alteration in bowel habits, is important. A thorough history of associated GI symptoms, patterns and relationships to intake of food, and treatment history should be elicited. An assessment of factors that exacerbate or relieve symptoms; the quality, region or location, severity (scale), and timing or duration of symptoms; and any change in pattern or character of pain (or symptom), which might denote progression of disease, is also necessary.

PHYSICAL EXAMINATION

The oral cavity should be inspected for integrity of mucosa, ulcerations, the presence of thrush or exudate, erythema, and gingivitis. Using a gloved finger and tongue depressor ensure thorough examination of the oral mucosa and oropharynx. The abdomen should be inspected, auscultated, and palpated. Inspection is done first and may detect striae, distention, and contour abnormalities. Jaundice can be detected by inspecting the skin and conjunctivae. Auscultation of bowel sounds in all quadrants is done next, with palpation and percussion performed last. Rebound tenderness, vomiting, visible peristalsis, and altered bowel sounds are indicative of obstruction. Paralytic obstruction is characterized by absent bowel sounds, whereas hyperactive high-pitched bowel sounds can indicate mechanical obstruction. Palpation can detect presence of masses, hepatosplenomegaly, inguinal lymphadenopathy, and asymmetry of contour. Ascites can be detected by testing for shifting dullness of the abdomen. Digital rectal examinations are avoided if the patient is neutropenic or thrombocytopenic.

DIAGNOSTICS

Laboratory data serve to confirm or exclude a diagnosis and warn of potential complications in a cancer patient with altered GI function. For example, a chemistry profile consisting of electrolytes, BUN, and creatinine determines the presence of fluid and electrolyte imbalances that can result from prolonged vomiting, diarrhea, and anorexia. Kidney function can deteriorate rapidly in a dehydrated patient who has received nephrotoxic chemotherapy. Additional laboratory levels that are helpful include magnesium and phosphorous. These can drop precipitously in a patient with altered GI function, especially after receiving chemotherapeutics (e.g., cisplatin and ifosfamide) that affect their excretion. Ileus can be caused by hypomagnesemia, hypophosphatemia, hypokalemia, or hypercalcemia. A CBC can detect neutropenia, thrombocytopenia, and anemia, all of which can be related to GI symptomatology. A urinalysis is indicated if urinary tract infection is a suspected cause of the N&V. Serum albumin, particularly prealbumin, can be useful in assessing nutritional status. Liver enzymes, sometimes referred to as liver function tests, may be ordered if serious hepatic dysfunction is suspected as a source of GI symptoms.

The tests mentioned are basic panels that are generally ordered in cancer patients with GI symptoms. Additional tests are indicated based on the differential diagnoses for that particular patient. For example, a stool test for occult blood (three sequential specimens) should be ordered if GI bleeding is suspected, and a stool test for *C. difficile* is indicated for relentless diarrhea, particularly in a patient who has received broad-spectrum antibiotics. A KUB radiograph (kidneys, ureters, and bladder) is helpful in diagnosing intestinal obstruction and ileus.

DIFFERENTIAL DIAGNOSIS

It is important to recognize other conditions with presentations similar to cancer-related GI symptoms. Gastroenteritis, hepatitis, pancreatitis, cholecystitis, peptic ulcer disease, ileus, uremia, urinary tract infection, hypercalcemia, and psychogenic or anticipatory vomiting should be considered when evaluating the patient with GI complaints. Other possibilities include anorexia nervosa, irritable bowel syndrome, increased intracranial pressure, vestibular disorders, and acute myocardial infarction. Pregnancy is a possibility that must be considered in sexually active women of child-bearing age. Knowing the details of the symptom's onset, along with the patient's past medical history, risk factors for other diseases, and side effects of current treatment, is essential in identifying the most likely cause of the GI symptoms.

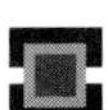

Diagnostics

Gastrointestinal Symptoms in the Oncology Patient

Laboratory
CBC and differential
Serum electrolytes
BUN
Creatinine
Serum glucose
Serum calcium*
Serum magnesium*
Serum phosphorus*
Serum HCG*
LFTs*
Serum albumin and total protein*
Stool for occult blood/*C. difficile**
Urinalysis*

Imaging
KUB*

*If indicated.

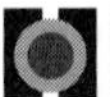

Differential Diagnosis

Gastrointestinal Symptoms in the Oncology Patient

Irritable bowel	Constipation
Gastroenteritis	Pregnancy
Hepatitis	Increased intracranial pressure
Pancreatitis	Vestibular disorder
Peptic ulcer disease	Acute myocardial infarction
Ileus	Anorexia nervosa
Uremia	Psychogenic vomiting
Urinary tract infection	

MANAGEMENT

Nausea and Vomiting

Effective antiemetic regimen interrupt the stimulation of the VC. No one antiemetic controls all types of N&V for all patients. There are important patient-related factors that affect control of N&V, including gender, age, and alcohol intake. N&V are not as well controlled in females as in males, particularly if the females are young (<30 years of age) or menstruating.[2] Individuals with a high alcohol intake (>5 drinks/day) have better control of vomiting than those with low or no alcohol intake.[2] Delayed N&V is not as well managed as acute N&V. Patients with a history of motion sickness or a propensity for N&V (pregnancy, migraine headaches) may be more prone to delayed or anticipatory N&V.[2]

Combination chemotherapy may be classified as low, moderate, or severe emetic potential (Box 256-1). Evidence-based studies support the administration of serotonin (5-HT_3) inhibitor antagonists such as ondansetron for chemotherapeutics with high-emetic potential.[7] Serotonin inhibitors have been found to be more effective in preventing acute N&V rather than delayed or anticipatory N&V. Clinical evidence does not demonstrate any difference in efficacy among the different 5-HT_3 antagonist agents.[7]

Evidence has also shown that combinations of antiemetic agents are significantly more effective than single agents.[7] For example, combinations of a steroid and a 5-HT_3 antagonist provides the best control of N&V in patients with high-dose cisplatin regimens.[2,7]

Several other classes of agents are less effective and may have more side effects because they are less selective than 5-HT_3 antagonists. Metoclopramide also acts as a serotonin receptor

BOX 256-1

COMBINATION ANTIEMETIC REGIMENS

LOW EMETIC POTENTIAL*
Dexamethasone 10 to 20 mg IV 30 minutes before chemotherapy

MODERATE EMETIC POTENTIAL*
5-HT_3 antagonist IV 30 minutes before chemotherapy
or Dexamethasone 10 to 20 mg IV 30 minutes before chemotherapy

SEVERE EMETIC POTENTIAL*
5-HT_3 antagonist IV plus dexamethasone 10 to 20 mg IV 30 minutes before chemotherapy

BREAKTHROUGH NAUSEA AND VOMITING
Metoclopramide 2 mg/kg IV plus diphenhydramine 50 mg IV every 3 to 4 hours as needed

DELAYED NAUSEA AND VOMITING (BEGINS MORE THAN 24 HOURS AFTER CHEMOTHERAPY)
Metoclopramide 20 to 30 mg PO q.i.d. plus dexamethasone 4 to 8 mg PO b.i.d. for 2 days

Data from M.D. Anderson Cancer Center, Houston, TX; and Gralla RJ and others: Recommendations for the use of antiemetics: evidence-based, clinical practice guidelines, *J Clin Oncol* 17:2971-2994, 1999.
*Emetic potential is dependent on chemotherapy agent, dose, and schedule.

antagonist and, when combined with dexamethasone, is especially beneficial in delayed N&V. Phenothiazines (prochlorperazine) and butyrophenones (haloperidol and droperidol) block dopamine receptors in the CTZ and inhibit the VC by blocking autonomic afferent impulses via the vagus nerve. However, they induce more extrapyramidal symptoms in patients under 30 years of age. Benzodiazepines such as lorazepam and antihistamines such as diphenhydramine are useful adjuncts for their antianxiety effect and prevention of the extrapyramidal reactions associated with some antiemetics, although they are not recommended for single-agent use. Cannabinoids, both inhaled (marijuana) and oral (marinol), have been found to have some antiemetic activity but significantly less than other agents.[7]

Some patients can learn to interrupt the association of N&V with chemotherapy through the use of behavioral interventions; progressive muscle relaxation, hypnosis, imagery, biofeedback, or distraction may be valuable. Any adverse sounds or smells that stimulate the VC should be minimized in the environment. Patients who experience sustained episodes of N&V may be encouraged to avoid eating their "favorite foods" to possibly avoid food aversions after treatment subsides.

Constipation

The management of constipation should first include the prevention and elimination of precipitating factors. Once constipation occurs, bowel management includes increasing fluid intake to 2 quarts of fluid per day. Regular exercise should be encouraged for all patients. Physical therapy can be consulted for coordination of an exercise regimen for bed-bound patients and those with physical limitations. Fiber intake should be increased by consuming more fruits (including figs, dates, prunes), vegetables, and whole grains. Two to four ounces of prune juice or a hot liquid before a large meal may be helpful.[4] The patient should be given privacy for defecation; the use of a bedpan should be avoided if at all possible. Patients receiving narcotics should also receive a senna derivation and a stool softener.[4] If the constipation continues, use of osmotic laxatives is encouraged. Rectal agents should be avoided in cancer patients who are at risk for thrombocytopenia or leukopenia. If a patient is immunocompromised, there should be no manipulation of the anus because this can lead to fissures or abscesses, which are portals of entry for infection.[1]

Diarrhea

The management of diarrhea may begin with dietary interventions such as low-fiber, high-calorie, and high-protein meals. Identification and avoidance of aggravating foods, such as milk products or high-fat foods, are helpful.[8] Pharmacologic measures may also be used. Anticholinergic drugs such as diphenozylate plus atropine, and loperamide reduce gastric secretions and decrease intestinal peristalsis. Opiate drugs bind to receptors on the smooth muscle of the bowel, slowing intestinal motility and increasing fluid absorption. Octreotide acetate, which is reserved for patients with excessive diarrhea, inhibits the release of intestinal hormones (including serotonin and gastrin), prolongs intestinal transit time, and increases intestinal water and electrolyte transport.[3] Topical agents containing hydrocortisone or dibucaine are useful for perianal irritation. Glucocorticoid retention enemas are often used for radiation-induced proctitis.[6] Stool cultures should be obtained to exclude infectious agents such as *C. difficile*, which is commonly reported in patients receiving chemotherapy. Antidiarrheal medications should be avoided in patients with GI infections.

Anorexia

Anorexia can be managed through education, behavioral changes, and pharmacologic methods. Consultation with a nutritionist can be valuable for exploring high-calorie options, food supplements, appetizing recipes, and visually appealing presentations. Increased physical activity and smaller, more frequent meals may also be helpful. Simple maneuvers such as having a family member share a meal, serving a favorite wine or beer, or using special table settings may be helpful. Several pharmacologic agents have been helpful in managing anorexia. The most common is megestrol acetate, which may inhibit tumor necrosis factor and increase weight gain. Other agents include metoclopramide, which increases gastric emptying and is useful for patients with early satiety or delayed gastric emptying; cannabinoids, which appear to increase appetite and control N&V; and dexamethasone, which stimulates appetite and induces a sense of well-being.[8] Patients who continue to have significant anorexia or weight loss may require formal nutritional support, such as enteral or parenteral feeding.

Oral Hygiene/Stomatitis

The systematic performance of oral hygiene may be of greater value in preventing or reducing stomatitis than the actual agents used. Therefore it is important to develop with the patient a plan for oral care that includes daily plaque removal and mouth rinses at least after meals and at bedtime. Soft toothbrushes and dental floss should be used regularly unless there is danger of mucosal injury or there is evidence of thrombocytopenia. In that instance, foam brushes can be used. Mouth rinses should be nonirritating and nondrying and include normal saline, sodium bicarbonate, or diluted hydrogen peroxide. Hydrogen peroxide should be avoided when new granulation surfaces are visible in the mouth.[9] Evidence has shown that sucking on ice chips or popsicles may reduce the severity of mucositis.[10,11] The lips should be lubricated often to keep them moist and comfortable. Topical formulations that are available to relieve the pain and inflammation of stomatitis are numerous and should be individualized for each patient. Camp-Sorrell[3] has several excellent tables for oral care and the prevention of complications. An example of a good universal solution is a combination of Maalox or Kaolin-Pectin, viscous lidocaine, and diphenhydramine. In general, patients should avoid all tobacco products, alcohol, and foods that cause irritation, such as hot, spicy, or coarse-textured foods.[5]

Xerostomia/Saliva Problems

The thick, ropy saliva of xerostomia makes eating difficult and unpleasant. Oral care before meals may help to freshen the mouth. Increasing fluids during meals will help to moisten food and aids in swallowing. Patients should be encouraged to eat soft foods that are moistened with milk or gravy and to avoid dry, spicy, and acidic foods. The use of humidified air may help prevent mucous membranes from drying and cracking. Lubricating agents such as saliva substitutes are expensive and may or may not be useful. Some authorities have suggested swishing liquid corn oil or vegetable oil in the mouth. Papain and amylase will dissolve and break up thick saliva in some patients. Papain is found naturally in papaya and meat tenderizers. Amylase is found in papaya but can sting the mouth.

COMPLICATIONS

Complications of GI symptoms are varied and depend on the severity or grade of toxicity. For example, significant stomatitis in the presence of neutropenia can be life threatening and requires aggressive antibiotic management. Severe GI toxicities can create friable, edematous, and ulcerative mucosal insults, resulting in anorexia, malabsorption, malnutrition, dehydration, and intractable pain. Mechanical or paralytic obstruction of the bowel is serious and difficult to diagnose early in its presentation; any suspicion of this complication should be promptly referred to a GI specialist.

INDICATIONS FOR REFERRAL/HOSPITALIZATION

Certain symptoms may indicate a complication and therefore require a referral to the oncologist, with possible hospitalization. These symptoms include acute or refractory N&V, acute or refractory pain, acute anemia, dysphagia, dehydration, orthostatic hypotension, intractable diarrhea or constipation, refractory metabolic disorders, a mass noted on examination or on the radiologic image, or a weight loss of 4.5 kg (10 pounds) in 4 weeks.

PATIENT AND FAMILY EDUCATION

Patients and families need to understand the importance of notifying the primary care provider if GI symptoms occur. Written instructions, as well as verbal discussion of treatments for nausea, vomiting, diarrhea, constipation, and oral hygiene, will assist patients in controlling problematic symptoms. A list of symptoms that indicate a need to call the primary care provider should also be available to the patient and family. Prompt recognition and reporting of gastrointestinal symptoms, particularly when accompanied by fever, chills, or signs of dehydration, may help to avoid serious sequelae.

REFERENCES

1. National Cancer Institute: Other complications/side effects; PDQ supportive care/screening. Retrieved August 12, 2002, from the World Wide Web: http://www.cancernet.nci.nih.gov.
2. Gralla RJ, Pisters KM, Kris MG: Chemotherapy-induced nausea and vomiting. In Pazdur R and others, editors: *Cancer management: a multidisciplinary approach*, ed 4, New York, 2000, PRR.
3. Camp-Sorrell D: Chemotherapy: toxicity management. In Groenwald SL and others, editors: *Cancer nursing: principles and practice*, ed 5, Boston, 2000, Jones & Bartlett.
4. Bisanz A: Managing bowel elimination problems in patients with cancer, *Oncol Nurs Forum* 24:679-686, 1997.
5. Kostler WJ and others: Oral mucositis complicating chemotherapy and/or radiotherapy: options for prevention and treatment, *CA Cancer J Clin* 51:290-315, 2001.
6. Nicolaou N: Prevention and management of radiation toxicity. In Pazdur R and others, editors: *Cancer management: a multidisciplinary approach*, ed 4, New York, 2000, PRR.
7. Gralla RJ and others: Recommendations for the use of antiemetics: evidence-based, clinical practice guidelines, *J Clin Oncol* 17:2971-2994, 1999.
8. Wadler S and others: Recommended guidelines for the treatment of chemotherapy-induced diarrhea, *J Clin Oncol* 16:3169-3178, 1998.
9. Grant MM, Rivera LM: Anorexia, cachexia, and dysphagia: the symptom experience, *Semin Oncol Nurs* 11:266-271, 1995.
10. Rocke LK and others: A randomized clinical trial of two different durations of oral cryotherapy for prevention of 5-fluorouracil-related stomatitis, *Cancer* 72(9): 2234-2238, 1993.
11. Edelman MJ and others: Phase I trial of edatrexate plus carboplatin in advanced solid tumors: amelioration of dose-limiting mucositis by ice chip cryotherapy, *Invest New Drugs* 16:69-75, 1998.

CHAPTER 257

Management of Cancer Pain

Annabel D. Edwards

DEFINITION/EPIDEMIOLOGY

Fear of pain and suffering is a common experience for most patients who are diagnosed with cancer. Unfortunately, despite advances in the science of pain and improvements in the global consciousness about the problem of pain, it remains an *undertreated* problem.[1,2] Health care providers are faced with several barriers in their efforts to effectively manage pain.[3] Knowledge deficits exist because of a lack of academic attention to pain mechanisms and treatment in most medical, nursing, and pharmacy curricula. Attitudes about pain and misconceptions about related issues—particularly treatment with opioids—and difficulties in dealing with the subjective nature of pain contribute to the reluctance to aggressively use the necessary tools to manage pain. Fears of addiction and dependence are major factors in undertreatment despite considerable evidence that the development of these problems is rare even with the prolonged use of opioids. Impediments also include the monitoring and regulatory controls applied to opioid use, particularly in states that require triplicate prescriptions.[4]

The International Association for the Study of Pain defines pain as "an unpleasant sensory and emotional experience associated with actual or potential tissue damage, or described in terms of such damage." The association goes on to say that pain is always subjective. This means that the patient's self-report of pain is the only true indicator of its presence and severity. The impact of pain is also unique to the individual. The most practical definition is that "pain is whatever the experiencing person says it is, existing whenever he says it does."[5]

PATHOPHYSIOLOGY

The key to treating pain effectively is to identify the underlying cause(s) wherever possible. Pain can be nociceptive or neuropathic in nature or a combination of both. Factors such as inflammation and myofascial pain may contribute to the overall pain problem.[6]

Nociceptive pain is the most common mechanism and is a function of the normal nervous system. Nociceptors are the receptors that respond to noxious stimuli and transmit a message through the peripheral nerves, to the spinal cord, and then up to the cerebral cortex, where the message is interpreted. Some motor responses are initiated (e.g., withdrawal of an extremity from a heat source) from the spinal cord, whereas others are initiated by higher brain centers. Nociceptive pain may also be classified as somatic (i.e., arising from soft tissue and musculoskeletal structures) or visceral (i.e., arising from the internal organs). Nociceptive pain is characteristically described as "dull," "sharp," "aching," or "heavy," although other adjectives might be used. There are fewer pain fibers in the viscera as well as a convergence of visceral and cutaneous afferent fibers at the dorsal horn of the spinal cord, which accounts for the fact that visceral pain may be referred to other areas. Many cancer pain syndromes demonstrate classic referral patterns. For example, pain associated with cancer of the pancreas is very often experienced as back pain. Neuropathic pain does not rely on the activation of the nociceptors. It develops as a result of injury to the peripheral nerves, spinal cord, or brain tissue. Nerves are injured or damaged by being cut, crushed, compressed, stretched, burned, frozen, or exposed to toxic agents such as chemotherapy drugs or viruses. The result of the injury is a cascade of events that create both anatomic and neurochemical changes in the neurons. A severed peripheral nerve may send out tendrils as it tries to regrow, but the tendrils may tangle together to form a neuroma, which can be painful under light pressure. An imbalance in the number of sodium channels along the axon may occur as the nerve tries to repair itself, allowing for ectopic impulses to be generated. Common examples of neuropathic pain syndromes include postherpetic neuralgia, phantom pain, and peripheral neuropathy. Neuropathic pain is characteristically described as "burning." Other common descriptors include "tingling," "shocking," or "jolting." Neuropathic pain often has a delayed onset from the time of the precipitating injury. Over that time, the perception of normally mild and nonpainful stimuli (e.g., touch) can change to being exquisitely sensitive or painful (allodynia). Neuropathic pain may also be accompanied by sympathetic dysfunction. An injured nerve may develop an electrical or a chemical interaction with sympathetic nerve fibers, providing continuous stimuli to peripheral nerves.[7]

Many pain syndromes are accompanied by inflammation that either contributes to or is the primary underlying mechanism of the pain. The inflammatory response includes the release of prostaglandins and leukotrienes that sensitize peripheral nerves to painful stimuli. Associated swelling causes pressure on the nerves or other sensitive structures. With bone metastases, inflammation may account for much of the pain.

CLINICAL PRESENTATION

Pain associated with cancer has many presentations. It may evolve slowly from an awareness of "discomfort" with increasing intensity, or it may be acute and severe in onset. Because it is possible for pain to be experienced before a tumor is clinically detectable, caution should be exercised even in patients for whom no evidence of disease can be found—and especially in patients who have a history of cancer and have been free of disease for some time.

A thorough history includes identification of the pattern, characteristics, severity, and impact of the pain. There are many instruments, such as the Brief Pain Inventory, that can be used to conduct a comprehensive pain assessment.[8] The *PQRST* mnemonic is a simple and practical tool to guide pain assessment (Box 257-1).

The severity of pain cannot be measured by any direct or physiologic means. Patient report is the only valid means of establishing the degree or intensity of the pain. The most convenient method, and one that most patients can use, is to ask for a rating on a 0-to-10 scale, where 0 indicates no pain and 10 indicates the worst possible pain. Other scales can be used if preferred by the patient. Several versions of a "faces scale" that show a range of happy to sad/hurting faces accompanied by a numerical scale are available. These scales are useful for children (ages 3 and up) or for patients with communication difficulties (e.g., a language barrier or an inability to speak). It is important to use one scale consistently with the individual so that you have a sense of the change in status or impact of your interventions over time.

To interpret the ratings given by patients, it must be remembered that these are *subjective* measures and therefore have no "normal values." In general, ratings of 1 to 4 are considered to be mild pain, 5 to 6 are described as moderate, and 7 or greater as severe.[9] Because there is considerable individual variation in the way patients use these scales, comparison among patients should be avoided except for aggregate analysis for research and quality assurance purposes.

PHYSICAL EXAMINATION

Patients can experience significant pain without appearing to be suffering. Coping abilities vary widely among individuals. With persistent pain, physiologic and psychosocial adaptations usually occur; signs, including elevated pulse, blood pressure, and even behaviors such as grimacing, may not be seen. The physical examination should be focused initially on the painful area(s) to identify any lesions, inflammation, vascular changes, edema, or pain on palpation. Sensory changes in the affected part or new areas should also be carefully assessed because such changes often herald new disease or injury from other sources, such as chemotherapy. Changes in motor capacity, joint range of motion, and muscle strength should also be observed. The patient needs to be observed ambulating, wherever possible, to determine the impact of pain on movement and functional ability. If the patient complains of back pain, there should be a high suspicion that impending cord compression is possible. One test is to apply firm compression over the spinous processes to determine if pain is elicited; if it is, further work-up is indicated.

BOX 257-1

PQRST PAIN ASSESSMENT GUIDE

P—PATTERN
Location
Timing (e.g., constant, intermittent, at night)
Onset and duration

Q—QUALITIES
Characteristics (e.g., sharp, burning)

R—RESPONSE/REACTION
What activities make it better or worse
Response to heat, cold, etc.
Psychosocial responses/ impact on quality of life

S—SEVERITY
Intensity of pain (e.g., 0-10 scale)

T—TREATMENTS
What drugs have been used (current and past)
Other treatments, interventions
What has worked, what has not worked

DIAGNOSTICS

There is no specific imaging or laboratory technique with which to directly study pain. The diagnostic evaluation should be guided by the location and nature of the pain and by an understanding of the natural history of the underlying disease. Relevant x-ray studies and scans should be reviewed and repeated periodically. CT scans may be indicated to identify masses that involve the vital organs or lymphadenopathy. Plain films and a bone scan should be obtained if bone metastases are suspected. The bone scan is a sensitive test that can show disease before it is visible on the x-ray film; however, it is not as specific and may be positive for other inflammatory processes. Plain films may be negative until 30% to 50% of the cortical bone has been destroyed. An MRI is usually necessary to evaluate for nerve root or epidural cord compression. Epidural cord compression is an oncologic emergency, and the patient may present with a complaint of back pain *without* any signs of neurologic impairment. Patients with a history of tumors that tend to metastasize to the bone (especially breast, lung, and prostate) should undergo an MRI promptly to exclude cord impingement. With cord compression, the earliest possible intervention (e.g., steroids, surgery, radiotherapy) is critical to preserve neurologic function.[10,11]

DIFFERENTIAL DIAGNOSIS

Pain is a significant problem for the majority of cancer patients at some point during the course of their disease. Although pain can occur at any time and can be related to tumor involvement or tumor treatment, the incidence and severity of pain increase as the disease progresses. Common treatment-related cancer pain syndromes include those associated with surgery, chemotherapy, radiotherapy, and biologic therapy.[12,13] Surgical patients may, for example, experience postmastectomy, postthoracotomy, or phantom pain. Some chemotherapy agents, such as the vinca alkaloids and cisplatin, can cause peripheral neuropathies; extravasational agents can cause significant tissue and

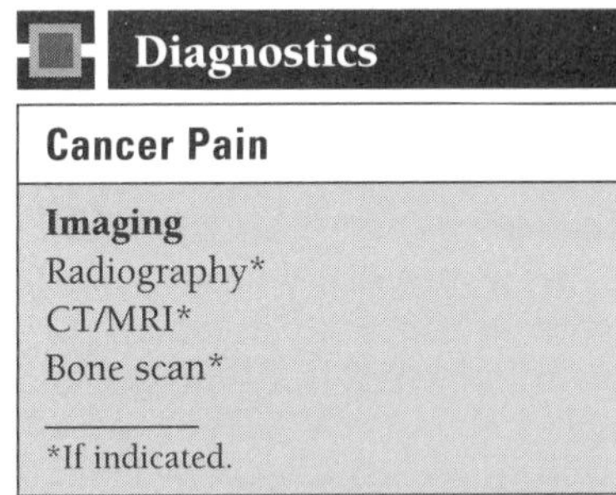

Diagnostics

Cancer Pain

Imaging
Radiography*
CT/MRI*
Bone scan*

*If indicated.

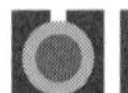

Differential Diagnosis

Cancer Pain

Tumor-related pain	Treatment-related pain
Peripheral neuropathies	Chemotherapy
Cervical, brachial, and lumbosacral	Radiotherapy
Acute and postherpetic neuralgia	Biologic therapy
Mucositis	Postsurgical
	Bone metastasis
	Epidural cord compression
	Preexisting chronic pain
	Abdominal obstruction
	Nonmalignant pain

nerve damage. Radiation effects can be early (e.g., mucositis) or late (e.g., brachial plexopathy or osteoradionecrosis). Biologic agents such as interferon can cause peripheral neuropathy and joint pain, both of which can be transient or chronic.

Tumor-related pain can result from the compression of pain-sensitive structures by a mass (e.g., epidural cord compression), or it can be related to direct infiltration, especially of the nervous and musculoskeletal systems. Pain resulting from bone metastasis is one of the most severe and disabling types of pain. Patients may also experience pain that is unrelated to the tumor or its treatment. Many patients have preexisting chronic pain problems (e.g., low back pain, migraine, diabetic neuropathy). These syndromes must be assessed and included in the treatment plan.

Other causes of pain must always be considered. Herpes zoster in either the acute or chronic stage can cause sharp, burning, or aching pain and follows a dermatomal distribution. Obstruction, constipation, ileus, peptic ulcer disease, gallbladder disease, pancreatitis, and appendicitis are examples of diseases and conditions that can cause abdominal pain. Mucositis may cause severely painful lesions of the oral mucosa.

MANAGEMENT

Effective pain management, particularly for the patient with advanced cancer, requires a comprehensive approach that often involves the use of multiple modalities. Opioids (the preferred term for narcotic analgesics) are the mainstay of pain management.[14,15] However, adjuvant pharmacologic management and surgical, anesthetic, and nonpharmacologic interventions play an important role in care. Figure 257-1 presents a broad overview and decision-making algorithm for pain management of the patient with cancer. Adjuvant drugs to enhance pain control (e.g., the tricyclic antidepressants and anticonvulsant drugs for neuropathic pain or those targeted to manage side effects) are appropriate at any stage, if indicated.

Unfortunately, opioids are among the most underused and misunderstood category of drugs. To use opioids effectively, it is important to distinguish between key terms that are often misapplied in practice: *addiction, dependence,* and *tolerance.* The phenomenon known as *pseudoaddiction* must also be recognized.

Addiction is chiefly a psychologic and behavioral problem in which controlled substances are used for reasons other than pain. For someone who is addicted, obtaining and taking drugs become the primary focus of existence, and drug use is continued despite the risks (social and physical) involved. Illegitimate drug use resulting in addiction is destructive in nature. In contrast, legitimate use of opiates for pain relief can improve the overall ability of the body to fight off and cope with disease and significantly improve the patient's quality of life and ability to function and carry out normal life activities, limited only by the disease and related disability. It is very rare for a patient being treated for pain to become addicted.

Dependence is not synonymous with or diagnostic of addiction. Dependence is a physiologic process resulting from adaptation to the presence of a drug. Its only clinical significance is the potential for a withdrawal syndrome (e.g., vomiting, diarrhea, cramping, and diaphoresis). The avoidance of withdrawal may promote drug-seeking behaviors, but this has no clinical significance to the patient with pain as long as the dose is properly tapered when no longer needed to relieve the pain.

Patients are often reluctant to take opioids in the early stages of cancer for fear that they may become "immune" to them—that is, the drug will not work when it is "really needed." It may be that patients confuse tolerance with "immunity." Tolerance is a phenomenon whereby a higher dose of a drug is required over time to maintain the same therapeutic effect. The possible development of tolerance is sometimes of great concern to health care providers who worry about the amount of medications that they give to a patient. Fortunately, tolerance is much less of a problem than once thought; to the extent it does occur, it can be overcome by upward dose titration. Experience with cancer patients has shown that patients with stable pain may stay on the same dose for years without decreasing efficacy.[16] When dose escalation (especially a rapid increase) is required, progression of disease is the most common reason for the change.[13,16] Opioid medications do not have a ceiling dose and so can be continually titrated based on need.

Pseudoaddiction is a recently recognized phenomenon. Many patients who have been labeled as "difficult" and "drug seeking" are in fact simply being undertreated for their pain.[17] Factors contributing to the development of pseudoaddiction include the administration of opioids at intervals greater than their expected duration of action or doses that are too low or of insufficient potency for the type of pain experienced. Patients who have endured unrelieved pain may become more aggressive in seeking relief and may increase their dose; as a consequence, they may call frequently and earlier than expected for more medication. Although these actions may serve as warning signs to alert the practitioner to abuse, the adequacy of treatment must be assessed thoroughly before a judgment can be made.

Opioids are classified as pure agonists, mixed agonist-antagonists, or partial agonists (Box 257-2). The pure agonists can be relied on to produce effective analgesia and, except for meperidine, can be titrated to pain relief without having a ceiling effect. Meperidine (Demerol) is not recommended for sustained or high-dose use. The metabolite normeperidine often causes central nervous system excitability (delirium, tremors, seizures, and even death), and the potential is enhanced in older persons and in patients with renal insufficiency or hepatic impairment.[15,18]

The mixed agonist-antagonist opioids produce analgesia but can also reverse analgesia. These drugs are also associated with a fairly high incidence of psychotomimetic side effects and, like meperidine, are not recommended for long-term use. The most serious consequence arises when agonist-antagonists are given to a patient who has been taking a pure agonist opioid. In this situation, the agonist-antagonist acts as an antagonist by displacing the agonist from the opiate receptors, which precipitates withdrawal and reverses analgesia. Withdrawal and exacerbation of pain not only impair quality of life but also pose considerable risk to critically ill and debilitated patients. For this reason, the injudicious use of naloxone, a pure opioid antagonist, is also to be avoided because respiratory depression is rare in the opioid-tolerant patient. In rare cases, the rapid infusion of naloxone can even lead to severe pulmonary edema.[19,20] The action of partial agonists is not well understood and, in general, has limited usefulness in the treatment of cancer pain.

The key principle for effective pain control with opioids is to titrate the dose to achieve the desired outcome.[14,15] Considerable variability in dosage exists from one patient to another. Some opioids (e.g., morphine and hydromorphone) are classified as "strong," and others (e.g., codeine and hydrocodone) are classified as "weak." However, these opioids are actually capable of producing equally effective analgesia if given in sufficient doses. The "weak" opioids are usually combined with aspirin or acetaminophen, and dosing is limited by the potential for renal and hepatic toxicity associated with the nonopioid drug.

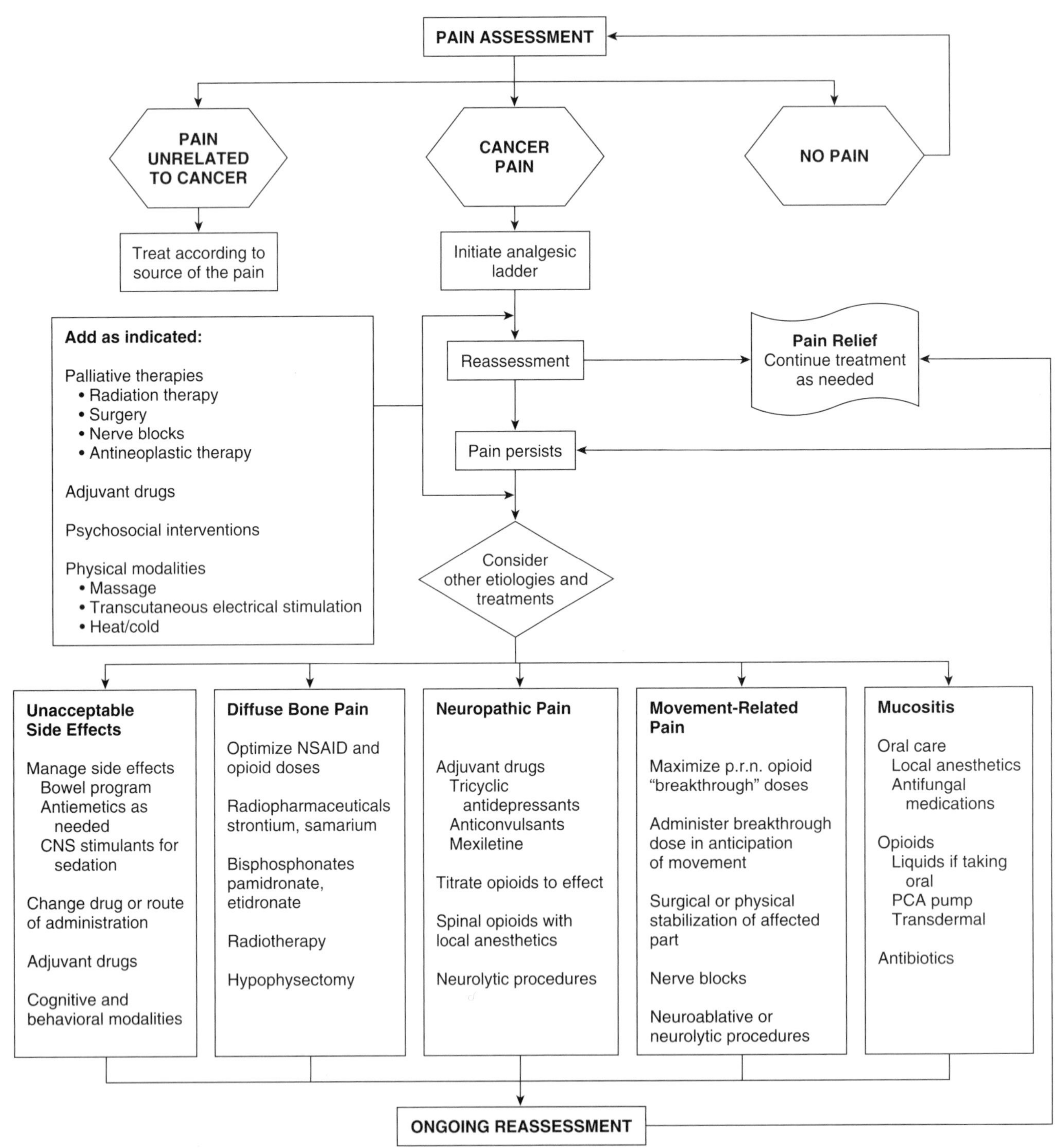

FIGURE 257-1

Cancer pain management and flow chart. (From Department of Health and Human Services, Public Health Service, Agency for Health Care Policy and Research, Rockville, Md, 1994, The Department.)

Table 257-1 demonstrates the relative equianalgesic doses for some of the commonly used opioids. Morphine is used for comparison because it is the most widely used opioid and more is known about its pharmacokinetics, but any of the agonist opioids can be used. Using the table, one drug or route can be changed to another. For example, a dose of hydromorphone requires only 1.5 mg to produce approximately the same analgesia as 10 mg of morphine. The table also shows the ratio of each drug required for oral (including rectal or feeding tube administration) use compared with parenteral (systemic) use. An orally administered drug can be equally potent to a parenterally administered one *if* the dose is adjusted to compensate for biotransformation.[14] Opioids administered via the gastrointestinal tract are subject to a first-pass effect, whereby a portion of the drug is metabolized to nonanalgesic substances as it is routed through the hepatic circulation before being circulated systemically. If a patient is receiving adequate analgesia from 10 mg of morphine sulfate given parenterally, it takes 30 mg to achieve the *same* effect if given orally because approximately 20 mg is metabolized before reaching the systemic circulation. The parenteral-to-oral ratio varies from drug to drug. It must be remembered that these equianalgesic comparisons are only guides—the relationship between the drugs is not absolute. In addition, the longer that a patient is taking an opioid, the less accurate are these relationships due to what is called *cross-tolerance*. In fact, it is often the case that when changing from one opioid to another in a patient who has been using opioids over time, the amount of the new opioid being used might need to be anywhere from 10% to 50% of the amount the chart recommends.

The oral route of administration is the route of choice in most situations because of simplicity and cost-effectiveness.[14,15] However, opioids are extremely versatile drugs and can be given via numerous routes. The choice of route and drug depends on a variety of patient factors, including: (1) the nature and stability of the pain, (2) the functional status of the gastrointestinal tract, (3) patient/caregiver abilities to manage the regimen (e.g., cognitive function, psychomotor skills), (4) side effects, (5) dosage forms/availability, and (6) cost. More invasive routes of administration, such as parenteral, epidural,

BOX 257-2

OPIOID CLASSIFICATIONS

PURE AGONISTS

Codeine (Tylenol #3 or #4*)
Fentanyl (Sublimaze, Duragesic)
Hydrocodone (Vicodin,* Lortab*)
Hydromorphone (Dilaudid)
Levorphanol (Levo-Dromoran)
Meperidine (Demerol)
Methadone (Dolophine)
Morphine (MSIR, Roxanol, MS Contin,† Oramorph,† Kadian†)
Oxycodone (Percocet,* Percodan,‡ Roxicodone, Oxycontin†)
Propoxyphene (Darvon, Darvocet*)

AGONIST-ANTAGONISTS

Butorphanol (Stadol)
Nalbuphine (Nubain)
Pentazocine (Talwin)

PARTIAL AGONISTS

Buprenorphine (Buprenex)
Dezocine (Dalgan)

*Combination containing acetaminophen.
†Sustained or controlled-release delivery system.
‡Combination containing aspirin.

TABLE 257-1 Analgesic Equivalence Conversion Guide

Drug	Parenteral Dose (mg)	Oral Dose (mg)	Parenteral-to-Oral Ratio	Duration of Action[a] (hours)
Morphine	10	30	3[b]	3-4
Oramorph, MS Contin	—	30	—	8-12
Kadian	—	30	—	24
Methadone[c]	10	20	2	4-8
Hydromorphone	1.5	7.5	5	3-4
Fentanyl[d]	100 μg	—	—	1
Meperidine[e]	75	300	4	3-6
Levorphanol[c]	2	4	2	6-8
Codeine	130	200	1.5	3-4
Oxycodone	—	15	—	3-4
Oxycontin	—	10	—	12
Hydrocodone	—	30[f]	—	3-4
Propoxyphene[e]	—	100	—	3-6

[a]Lower figure represents expected duration for parenteral administration.
[b]Conversion factor for chronic dosing; single doses may require 6:1 factor.
[c]Long half-life; observe for drug accumulation and side effects after 2-5 days.
[d]Intravenous or transdermal delivery.
[e]Not recommended for long-term or high-dose use because of toxic metabolites (normeperidine, norpropoxyphene).
[f]Equivalence data not substantiated. Clinical experience suggests use as mild, initial-use opioid.

and intrathecal, increase the risk for complications (e.g., infection), are usually more costly, and should be reserved for carefully selected patients.

Opioids should be administered on a schedule that is based on their expected duration of action. "As needed" (p.r.n.) dosing leads to greater peaks and valleys in analgesic blood levels between doses, especially if patients wait until the pain is severe before requesting medication. The administration of medications on a p.r.n. basis is most appropriate for isolated moments of incident pain as the only treatment or as supplemental dosing for acute exacerbations ("breakthrough pain"), over and above scheduled long-acting medication.[14,15]

Rapid dose titration is needed for severe, uncontrolled pain or in response to interventions such as surgery. Short-term use of parenteral administration may be required. In such situations, use of the patient-controlled analgesia (PCA) pump is ideal. The on-demand patient-administered dose used on a p.r.n. basis with or without a continuous (basal) infusion allows for individualized dosing and sustained analgesia. As a way to better understand the use of long-acting opioids in combination with short-acting opioids, a patient with insulin-dependent diabetes serves as an example of the principle.[20] Typically, a long-acting form of insulin serves as the baseline. However, blood glucose levels are not steady: they respond to a host of influences. Regular insulin is given to treat episodic hyperglycemia. Pain is also a dynamic state influenced by a host of factors. Controlled-release drugs, continuous infusions, and transdermal delivery systems can be used to provide sustained analgesia, much like long-acting insulin.[21,22] Regular, short-acting opioids can be used to treat the breakthrough pain associated with activity, treatments, or other factors. It can also be used as a preventive approach to pain control. When an event or activity (e.g., walking) is known to provoke pain, the p.r.n. dose should be taken about 30 to 45 minutes in advance of that activity whenever possible.

COMPLICATIONS

Vigilant management is critical to the success of pain therapy and is needed to avoid the complications associated with pain therapy. Side effects are among the most common reasons cited for opioid failure and premature abandonment of therapy.[23] A patient who experiences nausea, sedation, or clouded thinking has often been improperly labeled as being "allergic" to opioids. Fortunately, a true allergy to opioids is rare. Some side effects, particularly nausea and sedation, are usually transient and improve once tolerance develops. Tolerance to another side effect of opioids, respiratory depression, develops quite rapidly and is rare after a few days of drug exposure. Most patients develop a tolerance to the emetic and sedating effects over several days. Sedation is most likely to be related to sleep deprivation, which is to be expected in patients who have experienced unrelieved pain. Daytime sedation usually abates once pain control is achieved and sleep is restored. Instead of sacrificing pain control if sedation persists, sedation can be treated by increasing caffeine intake or adding a stimulant such as methylphenidate (Ritalin) or dexamphetamine (Dexedrine).

Nausea and/or vomiting can be managed with antiemetics on a scheduled basis initially and then p.r.n. once the opioid dose is stabilized. Often, nausea is directly related to decreased bowel function and resolves when the constipation is corrected. Unfortunately, patients do not develop a tolerance to the constipating effects of opioids, and it is a rare patient who does not need an aggressive bowel management program. For patients who have not had a bowel movement in more than 3 to 5 days, it is essential that a serious effort be made to restore bowel function. Proper hydration and a diet with foods rich in fiber are important. Regular use of stool softeners with senna is often adequate to maintain a reasonable bowel regimen. If not, more aggressive therapies such as Miralax, lactulose, Dulcolax suppositories, or citrate of magnesia can be used. There are also preprepared enemas that can be purchased. In a very refractory situation, laxatives and enemas may need to be repeated every 6 hours.[24] Once a reasonable regimen has been restored, a prophylactic regimen should be initiated using a combination of a senna laxative and stool softener (Senekot-S) titrated to maintain a normal, comfortable bowel movement at least every other day. If, at any time, there is concern that an ileus is pres-ent, the patient needs to be medically evaluated, which might mean having an abdominal x-ray study.

Less common opioid side effects include urinary retention and myoclonus. Urinary retention is often transient and can be temporarily relieved with straight catheterization or by changing to another opioid. Myoclonus, the intermittent muscle jerking that occurs especially during sleep, is usually seen at higher opioid doses and is of no consequence unless it disrupts sleep or is significant enough to increase pain. If myoclonus is bothersome, a low dose of a muscle relaxant such as diazepam (2 mg t.i.d.) or clonazepam (Klonopin, 1 mg every h.s.) is usually effective. If myoclonus persists, the opioid may need to be changed.

Other complications of pain management include an increased risk of gastrointestinal bleeding with the use of nonsteroidal antiinflammatory drugs (NSAIDs) or corticosteroids.

INDICATIONS FOR REFERRAL/HOSPITALIZATION

A pain specialist should be consulted if efforts to titrate the dose to desired effect and manage the related side effects are not successful. If a pain specialist is not available, a local hospice organization is an excellent resource. Consultation is essential whenever a more invasive route of administration or other interventions are indicated. It should be remembered that some pain problems are relatively easily managed through the use of simple procedures performed in a pain center (e.g., epidural steroid injections, trigger point injections, celiac plexus block). Multidisciplinary pain specialty teams are being established to combine the expertise of such diverse fields as neurology, anesthesia, neurosurgery, nursing, psychology, and physical medicine.

PATIENT AND FAMILY EDUCATION

Patient education regarding the management of side effects is essential to ensuring good pain management. Patients should be encouraged to anticipate that side effects will improve with adaptation and that they can be treated without sacrificing pain relief. Patients and families should also be encouraged to discuss with the primary care provider their concerns about pain management, including the fear of pain, the fear of addiction, and possible misconceptions about the management of cancer pain. This approach will involve patients in the care plan and promote pain control.

REFERENCES

1. Marks RM, Sachar EJ: Undertreatment of medical inpatients with narcotic analgesics, *Ann Intern Med* 78:73-181, 1973.
2. Melzack R: The tragedy of needless pain, *Sci Am* 262:27-33, 1990.
3. Hill CS, Fields WS, Thorpe DM: A call to action to improve relief of cancer pain. In Hill CS, Fields WS, editors: *Drug treatment of cancer pain in a drug-oriented society: advances in pain research and therapy,* New York, 1989, Raven Press.
4. Hill CS: A review and commentary on the negative influence of licensing and disciplinary boards and drug enforcement agencies on pain treatment with opioid analgesics, *J Pharm Care Pain Symp Control* 1:33, 1993.
5. McCaffery M, Pasero A: *Pain: clinical manual,* ed 2, St Louis, 1999, Mosby.
6. Payne R: Pathophysiology of cancer pain. In Foley KM, Bonica JJ, Ventafridda V, editors: *Advances in pain research and therapy,* vol 16, New York, 1990, Raven Press.
7. Fields HL: *Pain,* New York, 1987, McGraw-Hill.
8. Daut RL, Cleeland CS, Flanery RC: Development of the Wisconsin Brief Pain Questionnaire to assess pain in cancer and other diseases, *Pain* 17:197-210, 1983.
9. Serlin RC and others: When is cancer pain mild, moderate or severe? Grading pain severity by its interference with function, *Pain* 61:277-284, 1995.
10. Fisher G, Mayer DK, Struthers C: Bone metastases, part I: pathophysiology, *Clin J Oncol Nurs* 1:29-35, 1997.
11. Weinstein SM: Management of spinal neoplasm and its complications. In Berger A, Portenoy RK, Weissman DE, editors: *Principles and practices of supportive oncology,* Philadelphia, 1998, Lippincott-Raven.
12. Foley KM: The treatment of cancer pain, *N Engl J Med* 313:84-95, 1985.
13. Cherny JI, Portenoy RK: The management of cancer pain, *CA Cancer J Clin* 44:262-303, 1994.
14. Hill CS: Oral opioid analgesics. In Patt RB, editor: *Cancer pain,* Philadelphia, 1993, JB Lippincott.
15. Jacox A, Carr DB, Payne R: *Management of cancer pain: clinical practice guideline no 9,* AHCPR publication No. 94-0592, Rockville, Md, 1994, Agency for Health Care Policy and Research, US Department of Health and Human Services, Public Health Service.
16. Foley KM: Changing concepts of tolerance to opioids: what the cancer patient has taught us. In Chapman CR, Foley KM, editors: *Current and emerging issues in cancer pain: research and practice,* New York, 1993, Raven Press.
17. Weissman DE, Haddox JD: Opioid pseudoaddiction: an iatrogenic syndrome, *Pain* 35:363-366, 1989.
18. Kaiko RF and others: Central nervous system excitatory effects of meperidine in cancer patients, *Ann Neurol* 13:180-185, 1983.
19. Schwartz JA, Koenigsberg MD: Naloxone-induced pulmonary edema, *Ann Emerg Med* 16:1294-1296, 1987.
20. Thorpe DM: The insulin-dependent diabetic as a model for pain management, *Dimens Oncol Nurs* 4:36-38, 1990.
21. Portenoy RK: Continuous infusion of opioid drugs in the treatment of cancer pain: guidelines for use, *J Pain Sympt Manage* 1:223-228, 1986.
22. Payne R: Transdermal fentanyl: suggested recommendations for clinical use, *J Pain Sympt Manage* 7:40-44, 1992.
23. Texas Cancer Council Workgroup on Pain Control in Cancer Patients, Hill CS, editor: *Guidelines for treatment of cancer pain,* ed 2, Austin, 1997, The Council.
24. Bisanz A: Managing bowel elimination problems in patients with cancer, *Oncol Nurs Forum* 24:679-686, 1997.

CHAPTER 258

Oncology Complications and Paraneoplastic Syndromes

Jane Williams

An oncologic emergency is an acute, potentially life-threatening event that is directly or indirectly related to cancer or its treatment. If left unrecognized and untreated, significant morbidity or death may result. An oncologic emergency may also occur in an individual not previously diagnosed with cancer. Because cancer manifests itself in various ways, it must be considered part of the differential diagnosis of many complex medical events. In addition, because the nature of these entities is emergent and requires treatment of the underlying cancer, all of these syndromes require urgent referral to an oncologist.

Common structural emergencies consist of superior vena cava syndrome (SVCS) and spinal cord compression. Metabolic emergencies include hypercalcemia, syndrome of inappropriate antidiuretic syndrome, and tumor lysis syndrome. Other oncologic emergencies not discussed in this chapter include sepsis and disseminated intravascular coagulation.

Immediate emergency department referral/physician consultation is indicated for patients with angioedema, dyspnea, stridor, papilledema, seizures, and other signs of superior vena cava syndrome.
Immediate emergency department referral/physician consultation is indicated for back pain accompanied by focal weakness, ataxia, or bowel/bladder dysfunction.
Immediate emergency department referral/physician consultation is indicated for patients with serum calcium level of >12.0 mg/dl.
Immediate emergency department referral/physician consultation is indicated for patients with tumor lysis syndrome.
Immediate emergency department referral/physician consultation is indicated for patients with serum sodium level of <125 mEq/L.

Superior Vena Cava Syndrome

DEFINITION/EPIDEMIOLOGY

SVCS occurs when blood flow through the superior vena cava (SVC) is obstructed. Lung cancer is responsible in approximately 70% of SVCS cases.

PATHOPHYSIOLOGY

Any pathologic process that invades the lymphatics or structures of the superior mediastinum can encroach on the thin-walled, compliant SVC and cause obstruction of venous return to the heart. SVCS may result from external compression, direct invasion, or thrombosis of the SVC. The most common cause of SVC obstruction is malignancy, usually lung cancer, lymphoma, or breast cancer.[1] The most common nonmalignant cause of SVCS is thrombosis of the SVC associated with indwelling central venous catheters.[2]

CLINICAL PRESENTATION AND PHYSICAL EXAMINATION

SVCS is usually insidious in onset. The severity of presentation depends on the underlying cause, rapidity of obstruction, concurrent thrombosis, location of obstruction, and adequacy of collateral circulation. Swelling of the face, neck, chest, or upper extremities; dyspnea; erythema; cough; or orthopnea are classic presenting complaints.[2] Other symptoms include headache, dizziness, visual disturbances, hoarseness, chest pain, and dysphagia.[2] Physical findings include venous distention in the upper body, facial edema, plethora, cyanosis, arm and hand edema, telangiectasias of the chest and upper back, tachypnea, hoarseness, and stridor.[1,2] Neurologic abnormalities resulting from increased intracranial pressure include papilledema, agitation, lethargy, confusion, seizures, and coma.

DIAGNOSTICS

A chest x-ray examination commonly reflects a superior mediastinal mass or widening, a hilar mass, adenopathy, and pleural effusion. An MRI or a CT scan of the chest is indicated to localize the level of SVC obstruction and identify the presence of intrinsic or extrinsic obstruction, superimposed thrombosis, collateral circulation, mediastinal adenopathy, masses, and other sites of unrecognized disease in the chest. Because the underlying pathology in many patients with new-onset SVCS is not identified, other diagnostic evaluations (biopsies) are almost always required before the definitive therapy can be administered.

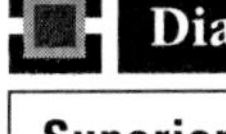

Diagnostics

Superior Vena Cava Syndrome

Imaging
Chest x-ray
CT scan/MRI

Other
Biopsy

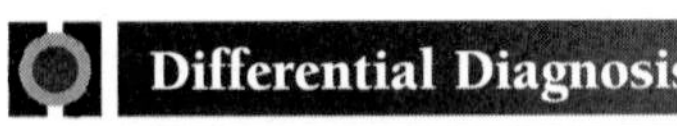

Superior Vena Cava Syndrome

Idiopathic mediastinal fibrosis
Tuberculosis
Histoplasmosis
Goiter
Aortic aneurysm
Thrombosis
Constrictive pericarditis

DIFFERENTIAL DIAGNOSIS

With SVCS, idiopathic mediastinal fibrosis, tuberculosis, histoplasmosis, and aneurysm of the aortic arch are among the differential diagnoses.[1] Other diagnoses to consider are constrictive pericarditis and thrombosis from indwelling catheters or pacemaker leads.

MANAGEMENT AND COMPLICATIONS

Treatment is directed at the underlying cause. If a neoplasm is found, mediastinal irradiation is often the primary treatment.[1-3] Temporary measures to alleviate discomfort include bed rest with elevation of the upper body, supplemental oxygen, and limited IV fluids.[3] Venipuncture and IV lines should not be placed in the upper extremities. There may be temporary symptomatic improvement with diuretic therapy, but dehydration may increase the risk for thrombosis and exacerbate the SVCS.[1-3] The use of short-term corticosteroids to reduce the inflammation and edema associated with the tumor is controversial; however, corticosteroids and bronchodilators are indicated if stridor or airway compromise is present.[2] Intubation or an emergency tracheostomy may be necessary. Patients with central nervous system (CNS) signs require high doses of dexamethasone to relieve increased intracranial pressure.[1] If the SVCS is a result of thrombosis, thrombolytic agents (urokinase or streptokinase) are effective if initiated within 7 days of symptom onset.[2] Other less commonly used treatments include balloon angioplasty, caval stenting, and surgical bypass.[2] If left untreated, patients will develop marked venous distention, laryngeal edema, stridor, increased intracranial pressure, sagittal sinus thrombosis, and cerebral edema.

INDICATIONS FOR REFERRAL/HOSPITALIZATION AND PATIENT AND FAMILY EDUCATION

See Indications for Referral/Hospitalization and Patient and Family Education under Syndrome of Inappropriate Diuretic Hormone, p. 1212.

Spinal Cord Compression

DEFINITION/EPIDEMIOLOGY

Epidural spinal cord compression (SCC) occurs in approximately 5% of patients with cancer, with the majority of cord compressions in adults arising from metastatic breast, lung, or prostate cancer. Other cancers that cause spinal cord metastases include lymphoma, melanoma, renal cancer, sarcoma, and myeloma.[4,5]

PATHOPHYSIOLOGY

SCC usually results when metastasis from a vertebral body extends into the epidural space or when a vertebral body collapses, resulting in a compression fracture. Direct extension of a paraspinous tumor through a vertebral foramen will also compress the spinal cord.[4] The compression of the spinal cord impairs blood flow, resulting in spinal cord edema, ischemia, and infarction.

CLINICAL PRESENTATION AND PHYSICAL EXAMINATION

The signs and symptoms of SCC depend on the area of spinal cord involved. The thoracic spine is involved most often (70%), followed by the lumbosacral (20%) and cervical (10%) vetebrae.[2] In 70% to 95% of patients, the presenting symptom is a constant, dull, aching back pain that is often worse when the patient is supine (opposite of the usual finding with a herniated disc).[4] The pain, which antedates the diagnosis of SCC by days to many months, is exacerbated by movement, sneezing, straining, or neck flexion.[4,5] Weakness, especially of the lower extremities, is the second most common symptom. It may be preceded or accompanied by sensory loss or paresthesia that ascends to the level of compression.[2] The loss of proprioception produces ataxia. Autonomic dysfunction such as urinary frequency, urgency, urinary retention, constipation, and sexual impotence are late manifestations and are associated with a poor prognosis.[4,5] Physical findings may include tenderness to palpation of the involved vertebrae, hyperactive deep tendon reflexes, and an extensor plantar response.[2]

DIAGNOSTICS

MRI is the preferred diagnostic test for SCC. A CT scan or myelography is reserved for patients who cannot undergo an MRI (e.g., patients who have cardiac pacemakers or are claustrophobic).[4] Patients with cancer who present with a new complaint of back pain should undergo an evaluation for SCC.

DIFFERENTIAL DIAGNOSIS

Other clinical situations may mimic SCC by causing motor or sensory deficits of the neck or upper and lower back or by causing pain. These situations include thoracic outlet syndromes, osteoarthritis of the spine, periarthritis of the shoulder, a herniated disk, sacroiliitis, facet joint degenerative arthritis, spinal stenosis, irritation of the sciatic nerve, compression fractures from osteoporosis, epidural abscess, ankylosing spondylitis, leaking aortic aneurysm, and renal stones.

MANAGEMENT

Clear indications of SCC in the cancer patient (e.g., focal weakness, ataxia, bowel or bladder dysfunction accompanied by back pain) demand an emergent evaluation and a referral. Immediate therapy includes the use of steroids (dexamethasone is the most commonly used). The optimum loading dose and maintenance dose are controversial. An IV loading dose of 10 to 100 mg is given followed by 4 to 24 mg every 6 hours. After 2 days, therapy is switched to 4 to 8 mg oral dexamethasone every 6 hours. Steroid doses are tapered every 4 days.[4] If neurologic decline results from dose reduction, the dose is maintained at effective levels during definitive treatment.

The decision to proceed with surgery, radiotherapy, or chemotherapy is based on the type of cancer. Radiotherapy alone is the definitive treatment for most patients.[4] Surgical decompression is indicated in the following situations: the histopathology of the cancer is unknown, neurologic deterioration develops during or after radiotherapy, the cancer is radiation resistant, a pathologic fracture causes compression by bone, or the spine is unstable.[2,4] Chemotherapy can be used for chemosensitive tumors (e.g., small cell lung cancer, lymphoma) and is usually used in adjunct to radiotherapy.[2,4]

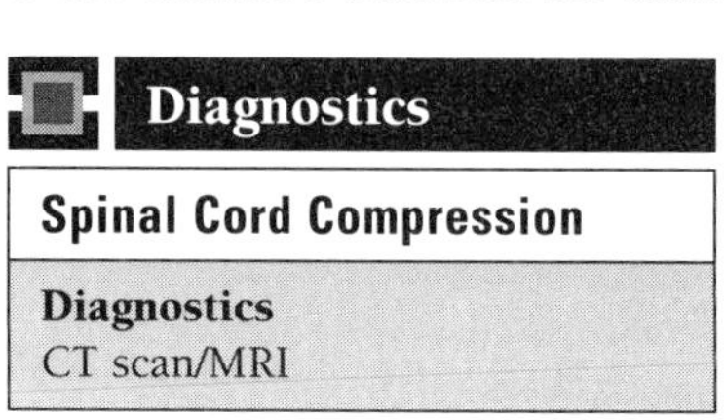

Diagnostics

Spinal Cord Compression

Diagnostics
CT scan/MRI

Differential Diagnosis

Spinal Cord Compression	
Thoracic outlet syndrome	Spinal stenosis
Osteoarthritis	Sciatic nerve irritation
Periarthritis of shoulder	Epidural abscess
Sacroiliitis	Leaking aortic aneurysm
Herniated disk	Renal stones
Facet joint degenerative arthritis	Ankylosing spondylitis
	Compression fractures

COMPLICATIONS

If left untreated or undiagnosed, SCC can result in paraplegia, quadriplegia, or loss of bowel or bladder function. In most patients, motor function and sphincter control cannot be regained once they have been lost. Neurologic deficits are more likely to reverse with a gradual rather than a rapid compression.[4,5]

INDICATIONS FOR REFERRAL/HOSPITALIZATION AND PATIENT AND FAMILY EDUCATION

See Indications for Referral/Hospitalization and Patient and Family Education under Syndrome of Inappropriate Diuretic Hormone, p. 1212.

Hypercalcemia

DEFINITION/EPIDEMIOLOGY

The most common metabolic emergency in patients with cancer is hypercalcemia, which develops when the rate of calcium mobilization from bone exceeds the renal threshold for calcium excretion. The serum calcium level is >11.0 mg/dl. The most common malignancies associated with hypercalcemia are cancers of the breast, lung, kidney, head/neck, esophagus, thyroid, and prostate; lymphomas; and multiple myeloma.[2,6]

PATHOPHYSIOLOGY

The mechanisms involved in hypercalcemia of malignancies were thought to be related primarily to bone resorption resulting from metastatic bone lesions. Although bone metastasis results in hypercalcemia, recent evidence suggests that certain tumors secrete a variety of hormonal factors that stimulate osteoclast activity, resulting in the release of calcium from the bone. Several of these humoral factors are parathyroid hormone–related protein, osteoclast-activating factors, transforming growth factors, hematopoietic colony-stimulating factors, prostaglandins (E series), and 1,25-dihydroxyvitamin D.[2,6] Other phenomena that can contribute to and worsen hypercalcemia are immobility, dehydration, and renal insufficiency.[6,7]

CLINICAL PRESENTATION AND PHYSICAL EXAMINATION

Most patients with hypercalcemia present with nonspecific symptoms of fatigue, anorexia, nausea/vomiting, polyuria, polydipsia, and constipation.[6,8,9] The neurologic symptoms begin with vague muscle weakness, lethargy, apathy, and hyporeflexia and then progress to stupor and coma.[6,8,9] Ventricular extrasystoles and idioventricular rhythms can occur, especially in the presence of digoxin.

DIAGNOSTICS

With hypercalcemia, serum calcium level is elevated and serum phosphorus level is often low. Because calcium binds to albumin, total calcium measurements can be greatly affected by changes in albumin concentrations. Hypoproteinemia is often seen in cancer patients; therefore the measurement of total serum calcium may understate the severity of the disorder. It is useful to obtain an initial measurement of ionized serum calcium; alternatively, total serum calcium can be adjusted for the level of serum protein using the following equation.

$$\text{Corrected calcium (mg/dl)} = \text{Measured calcium (mg/dl)} - [\text{Albumin (g/dl)} + 4]$$

Other changes include a shortened QT interval on the ECG.[6]

DIFFERENTIAL DIAGNOSIS

Other than neoplasia, causes of hypercalcemia to consider include primary or secondary hyperparathyroidism, acromegaly, adrenal insufficiency, sarcoidosis or other granulomatous disorders, Paget's disease of bone, hypophosphatasia, familial hypocalciuric hypercalcemia, and renal failure. Other causes are immobilization, complications of renal transplantation, medication-induced hypercalcemia (thiazide diuretics, lithium), excessive intake of vitamin D or A, and the milk-alkali syndrome (secondary to calcium ingestion for osteoporosis prevention).[6,7]

MANAGEMENT

Oral or parenteral rehydration is recommended as initial therapy for all patients with hypercalcemia. IV normal saline is generally preferred for hospitalized patients, with infusion rates of 250 to 500 ml/hr used in the initial hours.[2] Strict attention to adequate urine output and fluid balance is critical. Furosemide is used primarily to prevent hypervolemia after euvolemia has been achieved with saline infusion. If renal function is normal, 20 to 40 mg furosemide IV may be initiated after volume expansion is achieved, with subsequent doses given if the urine output is less than 150 to 200 ml/hr.[2]

Hospitalization is recommended for patients with a serum calcium level of 12.0 mg/dl or greater (3.0 mmol/L) or for patients who have symptoms other than mild fatigue and constipation. For moderate to severe hypercalcemia (total calcium, ≥12.0 mg/dl), saline hydration alone does not generally reduce the serum calcium, and antiresorptive drug therapy should be instituted within the first 24 hours. Third-generation bisphosphonates (pamidronate or zoledronic acid), calcitonin, or gallium nitrate is recommended.[2,4,6,8]

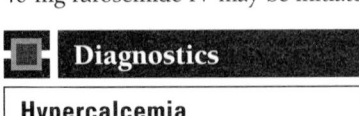

Diagnostics

Hypercalcemia

Laboratory
Serum calcium
Serum phosphorus
Serum albumin
Total protein
Ionized serum calcium

Other
ECG

Differential Diagnosis

Hypercalcemia

Primary or secondary hyperparathyroidism	Renal failure or transplantation
Acromegaly	Medication-induced hypercalcemia
Adrenal insufficiency	Excessive vitamin D or A ingestion
Sarcoidosis	Immobilization
Granulomatous disease	Milk-alkali syndrome
Paget's disease of the bone	
Hypophosphatasia	
Familial hypocalciuric hypercalcemia	

COMPLICATIONS

Without treatment, symptoms progress to profound alterations in mental status, psychotic behavior, seizures, coma, and, ultimately, death. Prolonged hypercalcemia eventually causes permanent renal tubular abnormalities with renal tubular acidosis, glucosuria, aminoaciduria, and hyperphosphaturia. Sudden death from cardiac arrhythmias may occur when serum calcium rises acutely.[6,7]

INDICATIONS FOR REFERRAL/HOSPITALIZATION AND PATIENT AND FAMILY EDUCATION

See Indications for Referral/Hospitalization and Patient and Family Education under Syndrome of Inappropriate Diuretic Hormone, p. 1212.

Tumor Lysis Syndrome/Hyperuricemia

DEFINITION/EPIDEMIOLOGY

Tumor lysis syndrome (TLS) is a metabolic imbalance that occurs with the rapid killing and lysis of neoplastic cells and the subsequent release of large quantities of intracellular potassium, phosphorus, and nucleic acids into the bloodstream.[6] Patients with acute leukemia, high-grade lymphoma, and, to a lesser degree, solid tumors (e.g., breast cancer, small-cell lung cancer, squamous cell carcinoma of the head and neck, hepatoblastoma, multiple myeloma) and myeloproliferative disorders are at high risk for the development of this syndrome.[5,6]

PATHOPHYSIOLOGY

The metabolic consequences of cell death include the catabolism of nucleic acid purines by xanthine oxidase to produce uric acid. High levels of uric acid crystallize in the distal tubule of the nephron, with resultant acute obstructive uropathy and renal failure. The massive release of other intracellular products, such as potassium and phosphorus, may lead to life-threatening concentrations. This syndrome is characterized by hyperuricemia, uric acid nephropathy, hyperkalemia, hyperphosphatemia, and hypocalcemia.[5,6]

CLINICAL PRESENTATION AND PHYSICAL EXAMINATION

Although urate nephropathy/TLS is sometimes reported at the time of the initial cancer diagnosis, most cases develop within 1 to 2 days of the initiation of cytotoxic treatment. Patients develop rapidly progressive oliguria with signs of uremia. Edema, fluid overload, hypertension, congestive heart failure, and seizures may result. Acute hyperkalemia and hypocalcemia may result in cardiac arrhythmias, syncope, and sudden death. Hypocalcemia may cause mild muscle cramps, tetany, and seizures. Hyperphosphatemia may aggravate renal failure. Acidosis and anuria may ensue.

DIAGNOSTICS

Serum electrolytes, uric acid, phosphorus, calcium, and creatinine should be checked several times per day for 3 to 4 days after the initiation of cytotoxic therapy. If hyperkalemia or hypocalcemia develops, an ECG should be evaluated and the possible cardiac arrhythmia monitored.

DIFFERENTIAL DIAGNOSIS

Gout is the most common cause of hyperuricemia. Other causes of uremia include primary hyperuricemia from specific enzyme defects (Lesch-Nyhan syndrome, glycogen storage disease) and decreased renal clearance of uric acid secondary to intrinsic kidney disease.[5,6]

MANAGEMENT AND COMPLICATIONS

Treatment is aimed at prevention by identifying patients at risk. Prophylactic measures include the initiation of allopurinol 300 to 600 mg/day starting 1 to 2 days before therapy and continuing until there is no evidence of TLS; vigorous hydration with approximately 3000 ml/day; and diuresis with urinary pH of at least 7.0 before cytotoxic therapy is begun. The urine may be alkalinized by adding 100 mEq sodium bicarbonate to each liter of IV fluid.[5,6] Hyperkalemia can be managed with an oral sodium-potassium exchange resin (sodium polystyrene sulfonate [Kayexalate] 15 g PO every 6 hours) or combined with insulin glucose therapy. Hyperphosphatemia can be controlled with the ingestion of aluminum hydroxide antacid. The hypocalcemia usually responds to the correction of hyperphosphatemia. Calcium replacement is usually not indicated because of the risk of producing acute nephrocalcinosis and increased renal failure by the precipitation of calcium phosphate in the kidney. Any of the previously mentioned imbalances may be severe enough to require temporary hemodialysis.[5,6]

INDICATIONS FOR REFERRAL/HOSPITALIZATION AND PATIENT AND FAMILY EDUCATION

See Indications for Referral/Hospitalization and Patient and Family Education under Syndrome of Inappropriate Diuretic Hormone, p. 1212.

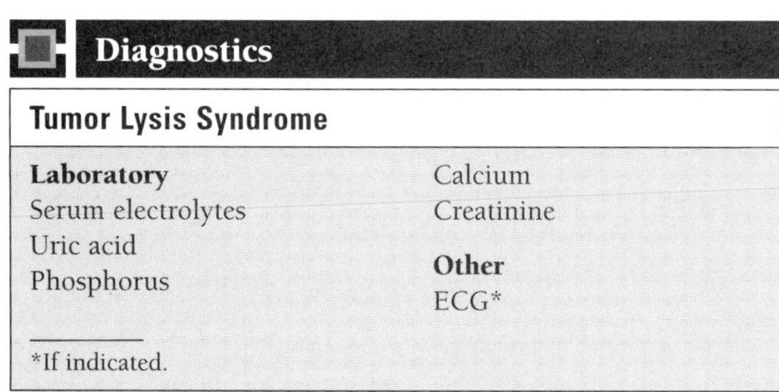

Diagnostics

Tumor Lysis Syndrome

Laboratory	Calcium
Serum electrolytes	Creatinine
Uric acid	**Other**
Phosphorus	ECG*

*If indicated.

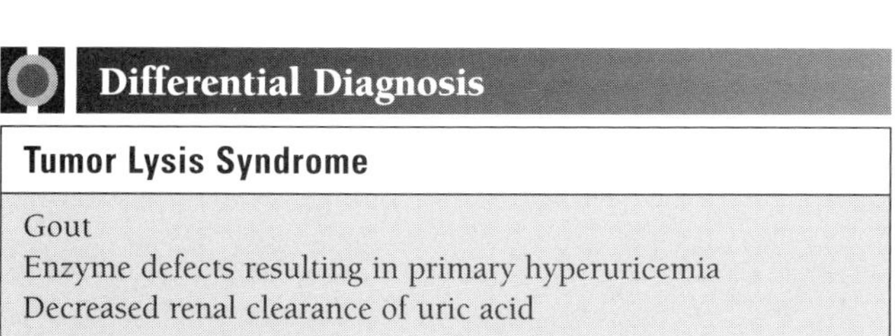

Differential Diagnosis

Tumor Lysis Syndrome

Gout
Enzyme defects resulting in primary hyperuricemia
Decreased renal clearance of uric acid

Syndrome of Inappropriate Antidiuretic Hormone

DEFINITION/EPIDEMIOLOGY

Syndrome of inappropriate antidiuretic hormone (SIADH) is a paraneoplastic syndrome that develops when excessive amounts of ADH are present, causing excessive water retention. Ectopic ADH secretion has been noted in small-cell lung cancer and in primary tumors with metastatic lesions to the brain and lung.[2,5]

PATHOPHYSIOLOGY

SIADH is characterized by excessive urinary loss of sodium and excessive retention of water by the renal tubules, as well as by reduced levels of serum sodium and serum osmolality. Because the normal regulation of ADH release occurs from both the CNS and the chest via baroreceptors, any disorders affecting the CNS (structural, metabolic, psychiatric, or pharmacologic) or the lungs may cause SIADH.[7] With excessive ADH secretion, excessive water is reabsorbed in the collecting ducts, and a dilutional hyponatremia occurs.

CLINICAL PRESENTATION AND PHYSICAL EXAMINATION

With mild hyponatremia, early manifestations include thirst, anorexia, mild nausea and vomiting, weight gain without edema, muscle cramps, headache, and mild lethargy.[5,7] Patients become more symptomatic as hyponatremia develops rapidly or as sodium levels fall below 115 mg/dl. Signs and symptoms include hyporeflexia, confusion, oliguria, seizures, and coma.[5,7]

DIAGNOSTICS

With SIADH, the serum sodium level is less than 135 mEq/L, serum osmolality is less than 280 mOsm/kg, urinary sodium is greater than 20 mEq/L, and urine osmolarity is greater than 500 mOsm/kg.[2] Serum and urine electrolytes, osmolality, and creatinine should be measured. Thyroid and adrenal dysfunction may also need to be excluded.[7] A chest x-ray and CT scan may be ordered to evaluate pulmonary or neurologic disorders that may cause excessive ADH production.

Diagnostics

Syndrome of Inappropriate Antidiuretic Hormone

Laboratory
Serum electrolytes
Serum osmolality
Urine sodium
Urine osmolality
BUN
Creatinine
TSH*

Imaging
Chest x-ray*
CT scan*

*If indicated.

DIFFERENTIAL DIAGNOSIS

The differential diagnosis of hyponatremia includes liver disease, congestive heart failure, renal failure, hypothyroidism, adrenal insufficiency, psychogenic polydipsia, and idiosyncratic drug reaction (thiazide diuretics, angiotensin-converting

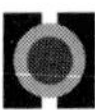

Differential Diagnosis

Syndrome of Inappropriate Antidiuretic Hormone

Small-cell cancer of the lung	Pseudohyponatremia
Metastatic cancer to brain or lungs	Hypothyroidism
Liver disease	Polydipsia
Congestive heart failure	Reset osmostat
Renal failure	Beer potamia
Adrenal insufficiency	CNS infection
Medication-induced hyponatremia	CNS trauma (stroke, hemorrhage)
	Pulmonary infection (tuberculosis)

enzyme inhibitors). Other causes include CNS infection (meningitis, abscess), CNS trauma (hemorrhage, stroke), and pulmonary infections (tuberculosis).[2,7]

MANAGEMENT AND COMPLICATIONS

Treatment of mild to moderate SIADH (serum sodium level of 120 to 134 mEq) with minimal symptoms consists of limiting fluid intake to 500 to 1000 ml/24 hr. If SIADH is refractory or if patients can be managed on an outpatient basis, demeclocycline (600 to 1200 mg/day in divided doses) may be used.[2] Patients with significant neurologic impairments (coma, seizures) require hospitalization for treatment with 3% saline by slow infusion at a rate sufficient to increase the serum sodium level by 0.5 to 1.0 mEq/L/hr.[7] Untreated SIADH or too rapid an increase in serum sodium may result in severe neurologic impairment or death[2] (see Chapter 226).

INDICATIONS FOR REFERRAL/HOSPITALIZATION

All of the complications discussed in this chapter are considered emergencies. Patients will usually require hospitalization and are often sent to an emergency medical center. Because most of these complications are related to progression of the cancer, patients must be referred to the oncologist for further management.

PATIENT AND FAMILY EDUCATION

In any emergency, patients and their families are frightened, but they also want honest explanations regarding their situation. The patient should be told possible causes for the symptoms being experienced and the possible plan of action, and they should be reassured that the oncologist is being notified immediately. Once treatment is initiated, the patient will benefit from reinforcement from the primary care provider regarding instructions for medications, activities, and further warning signs that need to be reported.

REFERENCES

1. Yahalom J: Superior vena cava syndrome. In DeVita VT, Hellman S, Rosenberg SA, editors: *Cancer: principles and practice of oncology,* Philadelphia, 2001, Lippincott-Raven.
2. Escalante CP and others: Oncologic emergencies and paraneoplastic syndromes. In Pazdur R and others, editors: *Cancer management: a multidisciplinary Approach,* New York, 2000, PRR.
3. Tierny LM, Messina LM: Blood vessels and lymphatics. In Tierney LM, McPhee SJ, Papaakis MA, editors: *Current medical diagnosis and treatment,* Norwalk, Conn, 1998, Appleton & Lange.
4. Fuller BG, Heiss J, Oldfield EH: Spinal cord compression. In DeVita VT, Hellman S, Rosenberg SA, editors: *Cancer: principles and practice of oncology,* Philadelphia, 2001, Lippincott-Raven.
5. Rugo HS: Cancer. In Tierney LM, McPhee SJ, Papaakis MA, editors: *Current medical diagnosis and treatment,* Norwalk, Conn, 1998, Appleton & Lange.
6. Warrell R: Metabolic emergencies. In DeVita VT, Hellman S, Rosenberg SA, editors: *Cancer: principles and practice of oncology,* Philadelphia, 2001, Lippincott-Raven.
7. Okuda T, Kurokawa K, Papaakis MA: Fluid and electrolyte disorders. In Tierney LM, McPhee SJ, Papaakis MA, editors: *Current medical diagnosis and treatment,* Norwalk, Conn, 1998, Appleton & Lange.
8. Kaye TB: Hypercalcemia: how to pinpoint the cause and customize treatment, *Postgrad Med* 97:153-160, 1995.
9. Edelson GW, Kleerekoper M: Hypercalcemic crisis, *Med Clin North Am* 79:79-92, 1995.

PART 21

Evaluation and Management of Mental Health Disorders

TERRY MAHAN BUTTARO, Section Editor

CHAPTER 259

Alcohol Abuse

Joseph Rampulla

DEFINITION/EPIDEMIOLOGY

Alcoholism is a term used to describe recurrent maladaptive drinking that is difficult to control and results in adverse consequences. Alcoholism generally refers to long-term problematic alcohol consumption, whereas more specific terms (e.g., *alcohol intoxication, alcohol withdrawal*) are best used to describe an acute condition. Alcohol abuse, or "problem drinking," refers to a pattern of intermittent maladaptive alcohol consumption that includes continued drinking despite knowledge of specific medical consequences; drinking despite medical recommendations to stop; drinking while driving, working, or operating hazardous equipment; and the experience of recurrent problems such as arrests, work impairment, a failure to meet financial obligations, and alcohol-related family problems. Alcohol has a ubiquitous and normative presence in human society; as a result, problems with alcohol use are found among all ethnic, economic, and gender groups.

Alcohol abuse usually includes episodes of binge drinking, which is defined by the Substance Abuse and Mental Health Services Administration (SAMHSA) as drinking five or more drinks on at least one occasion in a 30-day period.[1] A drink is usually considered to be 12 ounces of beer, 5 ounces of table wine, or 1.5 ounces of distilled spirits. Alcohol abuse is generally considered a less severe condition than dependence, but binge drinkers probably contribute to more highway fatalities than dependent alcoholics.[2] Alcohol dependence develops when repetitive heavy drinking causes cellular adaptive changes; the individual then requires a baseline level of alcohol to maintain homeostasis. The development of alcoholism is multifactorial, and there is little question that the risk for developing alcoholism runs in families.

In 2000 it was estimated that 104 million persons (46.6% of the United States population) 12 years of age or older had used alcohol in the past month, with approximately 46 million engaging in binge drinking.[3] Reported alcohol use among teenagers has remained stable 1990 through 1999, with minor upward trends in the early 1990s and a slight decline in later years.[4] Alcohol-related motor vehicle deaths have steadily declined in this time period from 8.9 to 5.8 per 100,000.[5]

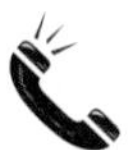

Physician consultation is indicated for delirium tremens, withdrawal symptoms, and psychotic behavior.

PATHOPHYSIOLOGY

Ethyl alcohol is a low-molecular-weight alcohol that primarily acts as a central nervous system sedative; this effect is thought to be related primarily to its effects on the gamma-aminobutyric acid (GABA) system and possibly to alterations in cellular membrane fluidity. The perceived stimulant effect of alcohol may be caused by depressant effects on the cerebral cortex, resulting in disinhibition and excitement. It is likely that alcohol somehow affects all neurotransmitter-receptor complexes, including opiate-mediated dopamine levels in the brain reward center and *N*-methyl-D-aspartate (NMDA) glutaminergic receptors.[6] Serotonin neurotransmission dysfunction appears to contribute to early-onset alcoholism.[7]

Alcohol is absorbed from the stomach and small intestine; the presence of food delays absorption. Infinitely miscible in water, alcohol distributes to all bodily tissues in concentrations roughly proportional to their water content. Alcohol is metabolized in the liver by two principal pathways: (1) alcohol dehydrogenase (ADH) catalyzes degradation of alcohol to acetaldehyde, which is then metabolized by aldehyde dehydrogenase (ALDH); and (2) the liver's microsomal ethanol oxidizing system (MEOS) increases in activity with chronic exposure to alcohol. Both of these pathways reduce a co-factor, nicotinamide-adenine dinucleotide (NAD), to NADH. Excess NADH produces a wide range of metabolic derangements, including fatty liver, hypertriglyceridemia, and hypoglycemia.[8]

In the absence of liver failure, the hepatic metabolism of alcohol and several other drugs is somewhat increased in chronic alcoholics. It takes 1 hour for most individuals to oxidize 7.5 to 10 ml of alcohol, with the excess accumulating and causing toxicity. The effects of alcohol toxicity are roughly related to both the blood alcohol concentration (BAC) and the tolerance of the individual. BAC is influenced by the amount and rate of ingestion and absorption, body weight, and rate of metabolism. Women generally achieve a higher BAC per drink than men, possibly because of their smaller body water compartment and lesser gastric ADH activity.[8] BAC can be estimated by measuring the amount in saliva or expired air. A level of 0.10% (100 mg/dl) is generally considered the BAC that results in clinical intoxication. Taking individual differences into account, a BAC of 50 mg/dl causes mild tranquilization; a BAC of 50 to 150 mg/dl causes impairment in coordination, speech, judgment, and concentration. BACs above 150 mg/dl cause delirium or stupor. Levels of consciousness decline at 300 to 400 mg/dl, which leads to unconsciousness and, with increasing levels, respiratory depression, cardiovascular collapse, and death. Partial tolerance develops and is associated with cross-tolerance to other drugs that affect the GABA system, such as benzodiazepines and barbiturates. Tolerance develops in several ways: (1) intracellular adaptation; (2) metabolically, in which the liver metabolizes alcohol more rapidly, and (3) behaviorally, in which a person changes his or her lifestyle to accommodate dependence. In patients who are alcohol dependent, an abstinence syndrome develops when alcohol levels decline.[9]

Alcohol Withdrawal (Abstinence)

Withdrawal from alcohol produces a range of manifestations, from mild emotional symptoms to life-threatening autonomic instability. Because withdrawal syndrome develops when the BAC falls below the level to which the individual has adapted, highly tolerant individuals may experience withdrawal even with a substantial level of alcohol in their system. Concommitant misuse of other substances complicates the presentation of patients in withdrawal (see Chapter 268). Within a few hours after the last drink, anxiety, headache, nausea, hypervigilance, tachycardia, and mild tremors develop. Diaphoresis, photophobia, hyperreflexia, a more rapid pulse, elevated blood pressure, more pronounced tremors, and auditory, visual, and/or tactile hallucinations constitute manifestations of more severe withdrawal. Some form of hallucination is common and they persist in a small number of patients long after withdrawal. Grand mal seizures, which are usually self-limited and short-lived, may occur during the first week of withdrawal and typically 12 to 48 hours after the last drink. With uncomplicated alcohol withdrawal, temperature does not usually rise to greater than 38.1° C (100.5° F). Major withdrawal can be dangerous because it may herald the development of delirium tremens, may aggravate a serious co-morbid condition such as coronary artery disease and cerebral vascular disease, or may provoke status epilepticus.

Delirium tremens (DTs) are a severe withdrawal syndrome characterized by deterioration of mental status and instability of the autonomic nervous system. DTs usually develop within 24 to 72 hours of the last drink. The development of disorientation, confusion, frank hallucinations, and elevated temperature in the setting of alcohol withdrawal should be considered an urgent situation. The mortality rate for DTs has been declining in recent years with better recognition and more aggressive treatment.[9]

CLINICAL PRESENTATION

The earliest manifestations of alcoholism are psychosocial, including behavioral and emotional instability, family and marital dysfunction, and difficulties with work, school, and the law. Alcoholism affects those around the patient. The first indicator of a problem is often a secondary report from the patient's spouse, child, or employer. A history of arrests for driving while intoxicated, disorderly behavior, or assault are highly suggestive of alcoholism. Patients with alcoholism and/or other substance use disorders are likely to benefit from early intervention, which makes screening appropriate in the primary care setting.

As a screening tool, the *CAGE* questions regarding *C*oncern about drinking, *A*ggravating others by drinking, *G*uilt about drinking, and taking an "*E*ye-opener" drink in the morning can be woven into standard history taking (Box 259-1).[10] These questions should be asked if the patient reports drinking or drug use when asked about medications or lifestyle. The CAGE questions were derived from the 24-question Michigan Alcoholism Screening Test (MAST). Two or more positive answers suggest an alcohol use disorder, but like any structured questionnaire this should be interpreted contextually. A patient who answers "yes" to one question but is grossly tremulous is more likely to have a problem than a patient who scores a 4 but drinks only twice a year. Answers of "yes" to any question should be pursued by follow-up questions. Asking the two questions "Have you, in the last year, drunk or used more drugs than you meant to?" and "Have you felt that you wanted or needed to cut down on your drinking or drug use in the past year?" may be as effective as CAGE with the advantage of screening for both alcohol and drug concerns.[11]

Health problems that suggest the presence of alcoholism include emotional difficulties, poor nutrition, trauma, seizures, unexplained tachycardia, refractory hypertension, dyspepsia, liver disease, pancreatitis, and peripheral neuropathy (see the Complications section).

BOX 259-1

CAGE QUESTIONNAIRE

"Have you ever felt you ought to	Cut down on your drinking?"
"Have people	Annoyed you by criticizing your drinking?"
"Have you ever felt bad or	Guilty about your drinking?
"Have you ever had an	Eye-opener drink first thing in the morning?

From Ewing J: Detecting alcoholism: the CAGE questionnaire, *JAMA* 252:1905-1907, 1984.

PHYSICAL EXAMINATION

There often are no abnormal physical findings unless the patient is intoxicated, is in withdrawal, or indulges in chronic heavy alcohol use. The patient's general mental status and vital signs should be noted. Postural blood pressure and pulse changes may indicate gastrointestinal bleeding. The smell of alcohol strongly suggests alcohol dependence, because even the heaviest drinkers will not drink before a primary care appointment. The head should be observed for signs of recent or old trauma, facial flushing, and rhinophyma. Facial puffiness in the morning often follows a drinking binge. Unusual bruises, abrasions, and burns should raise the suspicion of an alcohol problem. Older drinkers, especially older patients who have recently been prescribed medications that interact with alcohol, are prone to falls. Ataxia characterized by a wide or stepping gait may result from secondary cerebellar deterioration. Early peripheral neuropathy is suggested by diminished lower extremity touch and/or temperature sensations.

DIAGNOSTICS

Several laboratory values are altered by excessive alcohol use. No laboratory test demonstrates better screening properties than the CAGE questions. Mean corpuscular volume (MCV) is elevated from impaired folate utilization and probably from direct bone marrow toxicity. It may not return to normal for months, even with folate substitution. Affected liver enzymes include gamma-glutamyltransferase (GGT), aspartate aminotransferase (AST), alanine aminotransferase (ALT), and alkaline phosphatase (AP). All liver enzyme levels are nonspecific when interpreted in isolation. The GGT returns to normal after approximately 3 weeks of abstinence and is useful for tracking abstinence. In contrast to chronic viral hepatitis, alcohol causes the AST level to rise in excess of the ALT level. Carbohydrate-deficient transferrin (CDT) levels are elevated in male patients who have been drinking heavily for 1 week or longer and may be useful as an indicator of the severity of drinking.[12]

DIFFERENTIAL DIAGNOSIS

Because alcoholism affects every body system, the physical symptoms and findings may indicate numerous pathologies. Hypertension, hyperlipidemia, cardiac arrhythmias, cardiac myopathy, liver disease, peptic ulcer disease, pancreatitis, or injury may be the first physical indication of this disorder.

Psychologic disorders that may be associated with alcoholism include anxiety, depression, and social isolation, and dysfunction. Other forms of substance abuse should also be considered in the differential diagnosis. Alcohol and nicotine are the earliest and most enduring substances of abuse that persons with major mental illness use for self-medication.

MANAGEMENT

When alcoholism is suspected, a follow-up appointment should be scheduled to further explore the issue. This discussion is usually better accepted when addressed within the context of the patient's overall health and quality of life. Patients may be susceptible to using other substances, and this should be kept in mind. Clinician's concerns about drinking and the evidence that supports these concerns should be shared and reinforced. It is helpful if a spouse or significant other is willing to accompany the patient to the appointment, although patients often reject this suggestion in the beginning. A brief intervention by a primary care provider and advice to cut down on drinking may ultimately be the most effective interventions for reducing drinking problems. The approach should be empathetic, nonaccusatory, and concerned. In brief, primary care providers should (1) provide feedback on their impression of the problem (including historical and physical evidence about alcoholism and its severity), (2) inform the patient about safe consumption limits while offering recommendations about changing and sources of help, (3) assess the patient's readiness to change and to negotiate goals and strategies, and (4) arrange a follow-up visit.[13] Brief interventions for heavy-drinking college students have been associated with reduction in drinking and adverse consequences, although it is not clear how much improvement is due to the intervention and how much is due to the normal maturation of the students.[14]

In a formal intervention, the important people in a patient's life (e.g., spouse, work supervisor, and primary care provider) meet together to confront the patient, express concern, and help the patient recognize the need for treatment. This type of intervention should be conducted with an experienced consultant; it should be rehearsed, with the logistics of referral worked out in advance.

Alcoholics Anonymous (AA) is the prototype community self-help group and for decades has provided millions of people with a foundation for alcoholism recovery. The focus and tone of individual meetings can differ, and patients may need to attend several before finding a meeting in which they feel comfortable. In summary, the 12 steps of recovery (12-Step program) in AA ask that participants begin to acknowledge that they have a problem, that there is a spiritual dimension to life beyond their control, that personal relationships should be healed, and that recovering persons should use experiences and insight to help other alcoholics. These principles are the same at all AA meetings, and the only requirement for attendance is a desire to stop using alcohol or mind-altering drugs. The advantage of the recommendation to attend "90 meetings in 90 days" is that it helps patients to get into a routine of AA attendance, begin to understand that their problems are shared by others, and begin to establish a relationship with a member that has achieved successful sobriety. Some patients engage better with cognitive behavior–oriented groups such as Rational Recovery; others benefit from church attendance. In-depth, insight-oriented psychotherapeutic approaches have not been shown to be helpful in assisting with early recovery, but they may be helpful for patients who have established long-term sobriety.

Family members often experience more distress than the patient. Most counseling centers have services for family members, including Al-Anon meetings. Al-Anon and its affiliate Ala-Teen provide group support to family members. The major goals for family members of alcoholics are to understand that they are not to blame for the patient's alcoholism, to recognize the role that the patient's alcoholism plays in family functioning, and to limit enabling behaviors.

Pharmacologic adjuncts include medications to prevent major withdrawal, drugs to reduce craving, antidepressants (usually selective serotonin reuptake inhibitors) for persistent dysthymia or coexisting depression, and/or disulfiram (Antabuse) as aversive therapy. Patients should also receive thiamine, multivitamin, and folic acid supplementation. Selective serotonin reuptake inhibitors may be helpful for mood stability and reduced alcohol consumption, particularly if there is coexisting depression.[15]

Benzodiazepines have consistently been shown to be the safest and most effective drugs to assist with alcohol detoxification. Outpatient detoxification is labor intensive and requires the patient to have good involved social support and the clinician to have ready inpatient backup. If outpatient detoxification is preferred and attempted, one good general guideline for detoxification begins with 50 to 100 mg of chlordiazepoxide and then 25 to 50 mg every 4 to 6 hours p.r.n. The patient returns the next day and then receives 25 mg once or twice a day p.r.n.[16] The patient should be referred for inpatient detoxification if the patient resumes drinking or has worsening withdrawal symptoms while following this regimen. Higher doses are generally

Diagnostics

Alcohol Abuse

Laboratory	Creatinine*
Blood alcohol*	Total protein*
LFTs*	Albumin*
Amylase*	Calcium*
Lipid profile*	Phosphorus*
PT/PTT*	Magnesium*
CBC and differential*	Carbohydrate-deficient transferrin*
BUN*	

*If indicated.

Differential Diagnosis

Alcohol Abuse

Hypertension	Seizure disorder
Hyperlipidemia	Endocrine disorder
Cardiac arrhythmias	Depression
Cardiac myopathy	Anxiety
Liver disease	Bipolar disorder
Peptic ulcer disease	Substance abuse
Pancreatitis	

used when patients are admitted for inpatient detoxification. Inpatient detoxification consists of usually brief (approximately 1 week) admission to a facility, during which the patient is monitored and given medication to prevent major withdrawal. Initially, sufficient medication is given to produce mild sedation, and this is tapered over several days. Patients attend AA meetings and group and individual counseling while plans for aftercare are developed.

Naltrexone is an opioid antagonist that appears to reduce the desire to drink and supports abstinence at a dosage of 50 mg/day.[17] Because it is mildly hepatotoxic, liver function test results should be evaluated before treatment and at 1, 3, and 6 months. A recent study questions the effectiveness of naltrexone. No difference was found between those patients receiving counseling and naltrexone and those receiving counseling and placebo interventions.[18]

Acamprosate is a novel anticraving medication that is widely used in Europe, although it is not yet approved in the United States. It appears to reduce the activity of hyperactive glutaminergic neurons and to stimulate GABA transmission.[15] Patients treated with acamprosate have shown a greater rate of treatment completion, abstinence, and/or reduced drinking days with minimal side effects.[19]

Some practitioners begin aversive treatment with disulfiram (Antabuse) after the first couple of days of verifiable abstinence. Disulfiram interferes with the metabolism of acetaldehyde, causing headache, flushing, nausea, vomiting, and, sometimes, chest pain. It is used as an adjunct to counseling and may help patients to resist temptation while in the early stages of recovery.[16] It is generally contraindicated in patients who are not currently engaged in counseling and in patients who have neurologic impairment, cardiovascular disease, and a history of past drinking while taking disulfiram. Patients need to be warned explicitly about the nature of the reaction and warned to avoid any alcohol-containing products. Patients should know to come to the emergency department if a reaction occurs.

COMPLICATIONS

The earliest physical complications are usually related to trauma or poisoning. Drinking is a factor in almost half of all motor vehicle fatalities, half of all violent deaths, and approximately one third of all suicides. One fourth of all motor vehicle–related deaths among children younger than 15 years of age involves alcohol.[20] Trauma accompanies alcoholism so often that a history of two or more major injuries after 18 years of age is strongly suggestive of alcoholism.[16] Also, alcoholism greatly increases the risk of becoming homeless. Overall quality of life is perceived as very poor by alcoholics and appears to improve with reduction in drinking or abstinence.[21] Older alcohol abusers are more likely to develop long-term impairments in ability to work and in their ability to function independently at home.[22]

Nutritional and Metabolic

Drinking causes nutritional deficiencies in two primary ways. As a source of energy, alcohol may be consumed in preference to food, leading to deficiencies of macronutrients. Alcohol hinders the absorption of any vitamin that is absorbed in the small intestine, most notably thiamine (B_1), folic acid, pyridoxine (B_6), niacin, and vitamin A. Pancreatitis, chronic gastritis, and liver disease are common co-morbid conditions that impair the absorption and use of nutrients. Alcohol ketosis results from starvation after a period of heavy drinking that has caused vomiting and an inability to hold down food or fluids. This condition resolves with the administration of IV glucose solutions, but thiamine must be administered first to prevent toxic cerebral accumulation of glucose in the brain. Chronic alcohol ingestion suppresses the production and function of the white blood cells, which results in increased susceptibility to tuberculosis, pneumonia, and skin infections.[23] Hyperuricemia, blood sugar dysregulation, and hypogonadism are caused by excess NADH.[8]

Neurologic

Alcohol and its metabolite acetaldehyde are direct neurotoxins whose effects are compounded by associated nutritional deficiencies. The entire picture of the effects of alcohol on the brain are not clear. Although brain atrophy appears to be more common among older drinkers than among abstainers, the reverse is true for white matter defects.[24] "Moderate" alcohol consumption has even been linked with a lower risk of both Alzheimer's disease and vascular dementia.[25]

Familiar syndromes that are clearly related to excessive alcohol use include Wernicke's encephalopathy, Korsakoff's psychosis, hepatic encephalopathy, convulsive disorders, and neuropathy.[26] Wernicke-Korsakoff syndrome is the frequent coexistence of Wernicke's encephalopathy and Korsakoff's psychosis. Wernicke's encephalopathy is an acute neurologic syndrome that is characterized by confusion, ocular palsies (nystagmus, paralysis of the external ocular muscles), and ataxia. The primary cause is thiamine deficiency, and the acute syndrome can be treated with IV thiamine. Treatment must be initiated quickly, because the damage can become irreversible. Korsakoff's psychosis is an amnesic syndrome that often appears after episodes of Wernicke's encephalopathy or DTs. It is characterized by impaired memory, with the preservation of most other neurologic functions. Recent memory and the ability to encode new information are the most evident deficits. Confabulation is common but not universal. Wernicke-Korsakoff syndrome can improve over time with alcohol abstinence, vitamin supplementation, and compensatory cognitive strategies. A more generalized dementia from the direct toxic effects of alcohol and its metabolites generally improves after 3 weeks of abstinence.

Hepatic encephalopathy is the deterioration of mental status in patients with cirrhosis and may result from portal-systemic shunting of venous blood and a subsequent failure to detoxify several toxins, most notably ammonia and GABA. Precipitants include drinking binges, central nervous system depressants, and physiologic stressors such as gastrointestinal bleeding and infections. It begins with inattention, reversal of the sleep-wake cycle, and asterixis, and it may progress to delirium and coma. Treatment is abstinence and administration of a cathartic disaccharide. The most common alcohol-related cause of generalized seizures is alcohol withdrawal. Individuals with alcoholism are also prone to other seizure foci as a result of head trauma and metabolic derangements. Peripheral neuropathy is characterized by limb paresthesias, diminished sensation, and sometimes shooting neuropathic pains. This may progress to permanent motor weakness and chronic pain. Manifestations of peripheral neuropathy are often complicated by coexisting alcoholic cerebellar degeneration.[9,26]

Cardiovascular

There are several cardiovascular consequences of alcoholism, possibly the most serious of which is dilated cardiomyopathy. Acetaldehyde is directly toxic to the myocardium. This is often aggravated by a coexisting thiamine deficiency (beriberi). Orthopnea is usually the first symptom, and an enlarged heart is noted on chest films. The "holiday heart" syndrome, in which the patient experiences runs of tachyarrhythmias, including atrial fibrillation, is probably an antecedent of cardiomyopathy.[9] Excessive alcohol use causes 5% to 20% of hypertension in the United States and usually improves with abstinence. Drinking three or more standard drinks per day doubles the risk of hypertension that is resistant to therapy.[27] Binge drinking appears to cause wider swings in blood pressure than steady alcohol consumption, and this is thought to contribute to increase susceptibility to "Monday morning heart attacks."[28] On the other hand, numerous studies repeatedly demonstrate the cardioprotective effects of low to moderate alcohol use, thought to possibly be due to beneficial effects on lipid profiles and reduced platelet aggregation.[27]

Gastrointestinal

Alcoholism contributes to four major esophageal disorders. Alcohol decreases lower esophageal pressure, contributing to reflux esophagitis; frequent vomiting can result in mucosal tears of the lower esophagus (Mallory-Weiss syndrome); portal hypertension causes esophageal varices; and, when used with nicotine, alcohol increases the incidence of esophageal adenocarcinoma.[29] Erosive gastritis is probably a result of the direct toxic effects of alcohol on the mucosa as well as increased susceptibility to *Helicobacter pylori* infections. Alcoholism is the major cause of chronic pancreatitis, which can result in a chronic pain syndrome and pancreatic insufficiency with diabetes often unresponsive to oral agents. Acute exacerbations of pancreatitis can be life threatening from necrosis and acute respiratory distress syndrome. Heavy prolonged alcohol use is associated with the progression of colon adenomas to high-risk adenomas or colorectal cancer.[30]

There are three major pathologic forms of alcoholic liver disease—fatty liver, alcoholic hepatitis, and cirrhosis—all of which may exist simultaneously. Excess NADH contributes to the deposition of hepatic fat and an enlarged liver that usually improves with abstinence. Alcoholic hepatitis results from an acute inflammatory response to alcohol and its metabolites. Patients may present with right upper quadrant pain, icterus, and AST increased in comparison to ALT. Cirrhosis and fibrotic derangement of liver acini may be subclinical and insidious or may first be noted with the onset of an acute complication, such as ruptured esophageal varices. Coagulopathies develop as a consequence of impaired clotting factor synthesis. Edema develops as a consequence of depressed albumin synthesis.

Fetal Alcohol Syndrome

Pregnancy is perhaps the most important contraindication to alcohol use; a safe level of drinking during pregnancy has not been defined. The major manifestations of fetal alcohol syndrome (FAS) are intellectual impairment and developmental delays, growth retardation, and characteristically abnormal facial features (short palpebral fissures, flattening of the midface, and a thin upper lip). More subtle behavioral and learning difficulties are termed *fetal alcohol effect,* but these cannot be diagnosed before the child reaches school age.

INDICATIONS FOR REFERRAL/HOSPITALIZATION

Inpatient treatment should be considered for patients with a history of severe withdrawal, who are drinking all day long, who are medically ill, or who are abusing other substances. Patients with repeated seizures, severe intoxication, or mental status changes that are not obviously attributable to intoxication, recent head trauma, fevers, postural hypotension or tachycardia, shortness of breath, chest pain, severe abdominal pain, severe vomiting, or diarrhea often need to be seen in the emergency department for stabilization and consideration for hospitalization. Pregnant women who are alcohol dependent should be referred for inpatient detoxification; this needs to be coordinated with the patient's obstetric team and often involves making arrangements for child care, and it should be done in conjunction with a treatment program that has experience with the treatment of pregnant women. If a patient does not yet have prenatal care, such care should be arranged urgently.

PATIENT AND FAMILY EDUCATION

Careful explanation about the dangers associated with alcohol should be reviewed with the patient, and treatment options should be explored. The importance of safety considerations for patients and others should be stressed. Encouragement and support are essential to enable the patient to make the necessary lifestyle changes to attain sobriety. Patients will often ask about or allude to the idea of resuming alcohol use in a controlled manner. This may be possible for some patients and life-threatening for others. Studies on returning to controlled drinking conflict. It is probably best to advise continued abstinence in patients who have had health or repeated social problems related to their drinking.

The following are resources for patients with alcoholism:

Al-Anon Family Group Headquarters, Inc.
1600 Corporate Landing Parkway
Virginia Beach, VA 23454
(757) 563-1600; (757) 563-1655
Website: http://www.al-anon.org/helppro.html

Alcoholics Anonymous
PO Box 459
Grand Central Station
New York, NY 10163
(212) 870-3400
Website: http://www.alcoholics-anonymous.org/index.html (general); http://www.alcoholics-anonymous.org/pro/engpro.html_(information for professionals)

Rational Recovery
Rational Recovery Systems, Inc.,
PO Box 800
Lotus, CA 95651
(530) 621-4374 or (530) 621-2667, weekdays 8 AM to 4 PM
Fax: (530) 622-4296
Website: http://www.rational.org/recovery/

REFERENCES

1. Substance Abuse and Mental Health Services Administration (SAMHSA): *National household survey on drug abuse: population estimates, 1996,* DHHS publication No. (SMA) 97-3137, Washington, DC, 1997, US Department of Health and Human Services.
2. Duncan DF: Chronic binge drinking and drunk driving, *Psychol Rep* 80:681-682, 1997.
3. Substance Abuse and Mental Health Services Administration (SAMHSA): *2000 National household survey on drug abuse,* Washington, DC, The Administration. Retrieved August 12, 2002, from the World Wide Web: http://www.samhsa.gov/oas/NHSDA/2kNHSDA.
4. Johnston LD, O'Malley PM, Bachman JG: *The monitoring the future survey results on adolescent drug use: review of key findings* (NIH Publication No. 02-5105), Bethesda, Md, 2001, National Institute of Drug Abuse.
5. Centers for Disease Control and Prevention: National drunk and drugged driving prevention month—December 2000, *MMWR Morb Mortal Wkly Rep* 49:1073, 2000.
6. Tsai G, Gastfriend DR, Coyle JT: The glutamatergic basis of human alcoholism, *Am J Psychiatr* 152:332-340, 1995.
7. Heinz A and others: Serotonergic dysfunction, negative mood states, and response to alcohol, *Alcohol Clin Exp Res* 25:487-495, 2001.
8. Lieber CS: Medical disorders of alcoholism, *N Engl J Med* 333:1058-1065, 1995.
9. MacDonald J, Twardon EM, Shaffer HJ: Alcohol. In Friedman LS and others, editors: *Source book of substance abuse and addiction,* Baltimore, 1996, Williams & Wilkins.
10. Ewing J: Detecting alcoholism: the CAGE questionnaire, *JAMA* 252:1905-1907, 1984.
11. Brown RL and others: A two-item conjoint screen for alcohol and other drug problems, *J Am Board Fam Pract* 14:95-106, 2001.
12. Gronhoek M, Henriksen JH, Becker U: Carbohydrate-deficient transferrin: a valid marker of alcoholism in population studies: results from the Copenhagen City Heart Study, *Alcohol Clin Exp Res* 19:457-461, 1995.
13. Samet JH, Rollnick S, Barnes H: Beyond CAGE: a brief clinical approach after detection of substance abuse, *Arch Intern Med* 156:2287-2293, 1996.
14. Baer JS and others: Brief intervention for heavy-drinking college students: 4 year follow-up and natural history, *Am J Public Health* 91: 1310-1316, 2001.
15. Gastfriend DR, Elman I, Solhkha R: Pharmacotherapy of substance abuse and dependence, *Psychiatr Clin North Am* 5:211-229, 1998.
16. Clark WD: Alcohol problems. In Noble J and others, editors: *Textbook of primary care medicine,* ed 2, St Louis, 1996, Mosby.
17. Volpicelli JR and others: Naltrexone in the treatment of alcohol dependence, *Arch Gen Psychiatr* 49:876-880, 1992.
18. Krystal JH and others: Naltrexone in the treatment of alcohol dependence, *N Engl J Med* 345:1734-1739, 2001.
19. Mason BJ: Treatment of alcohol-dependent outpatients with acamprosate: a clinical review, *J Clin Psychiatr* 62 (suppl 20):42-48, 2001.
20. Centers for Disease Control and Prevention: Alcohol-related traffic fatalities involving children: United States, 1985-1996, *MMWR Morb Mortal Wkly Rep* 46:1129-1133, 1998.
21. Foster JH and others: Quality of life in alcohol-dependent subjects—a review, *Qual Life Res* 8:255-261, 1999.
22. Osterman J, Sloan FA: Effects of alcohol consumption on disability among the near elderly: a longitudinal analysis, *Milbank Q* 79:487-515, iii, 2001.
23. Schuckit MA: Alcohol and alcoholism. In Wilson JD and others, editors: *Harrison's principles of internal medicine,* New York, 1991, McGraw-Hill.
24. Mukamal K and others: Alcohol consumption and subclinical findings on magnetic resonance imaging of the brain in older adults: the cardiovascular health study, *Stroke* 32:1939-1946, 2001.
25. Ruitenberg A and others: Alcohol consumption and risk of dementia: the Rotterdam Study, *Lancet* 359:281-286, 2002.
26. Levesque CA, Sabin TD: Dementing illnesses. In Noble J and others, editors: *Textbook of primary care medicine,* ed 2, St Louis, 1996, Mosby.
27. Cushman WC: Alcohol consumption and hypertension, *J Clin Hypertens* 3:166-172, 2001.
28. Marques-Vidal P and others: Different alcohol drinking and blood pressure relationships in France and Northern Ireland: the PRIME study, *Hypertension* 38:1361-1366, 2001.
29. Burakoff R: Esophagus. In Noble J and others, editors: *Textbook of primary care medicine,* ed 2, St Louis, 1996, Mosby.
30. Bardou M and others: Excessive alcohol consumption favours high risk polyp or colorectal cancer occurrence among patients with adenomas: a case control study, *Gut* 50:38-42, 2002.

CHAPTER 260

Anxiety Disorders

Willadene Walker Schmucker

DEFINITION/EPIDEMIOLOGY

Anxiety is normally a helpful emotion that rouses the individual to action and alerts the individual to danger. Everyone has anxiety; it is common to feel anxiety before a "first date," when beginning a new job, or before an examination. In general, anxiety is a state of tension that occurs in the body as a warning to keep the body safe and out of danger. An anxiety disorder, on the other hand, often disrupts daily life. Individuals with anxiety disorders feel anxious most of the time and without apparent reason. The anxious feelings can be so uncomfortable that an individual may stop everyday activities of daily living to avoid the discomfort or may have immobilizing bouts of anxiety. Many people misunderstand anxiety disorders and think individuals should be able to overcome their symptoms through sheer willpower.[1]

Anxiety is commonly defined as an unpleasant and overriding mental tension that has no apparent identifiable cause and is accompanied by physical distress and disruption in activities of daily living. Uhde and Nemiah[2] provide a more formal definition of anxiety: a pathologic state characterized by a feeling of dread and accompanied by somatic signs indicative of a hyperactive autonomic nervous system, differentiated from fear, which has a known cause. Anxiety is considered a disorder when it becomes a problem in daily life. There are several anxiety disorders: generalized anxiety disorder (GAD), simple phobias, panic disorder (sometimes accompanied by agoraphobia), posttraumatic stress disorder (PTSD), obsessive-compulsive disorder (OCD), social phobias (general social phobia and performance anxiety), and atypical anxiety.[3]

According to research sponsored by the National Institute of Mental Health (NIMH), anxiety disorders are the most common mental illnesses in the United States, some of the most commonly underdiagnosed disorders, and the most successfully treated disorders after diagnosis. More than 23 million Americans have one or more of the identified anxiety disorders, and each year billions of dollars are lost in the workplace as a result.[4] In addition, with undiagnosed anxiety disorders, an undetermined amount of the health care dollar is spent on additional medical testing to exclude a medical condition. As a group, anxiety disorders afflict nearly 9% of Americans during any 6-month period.[5]

Symptoms of anxiety disorders can be so severe that sufferers are almost totally disabled—too terrified to leave their homes, to enter the elevator that takes them to their offices, or to shop for food. NIMH research shows that anxiety disorders (1) have an age of onset from late childhood to adulthood, (2) affect a higher ratio of females to males as a group across several of the individual disorders, and (3) have a family link to prevalence, with an 80% to 90% concordance in monozygotic twins for GAD.[3] Many people have a single anxiety disorder, but it is not unusual for an anxiety disorder to be accompanied by another illness, such as depression, an eating disorder, alcoholism, drug abuse, or other anxiety disorder. In these cases, the other illnesses also need to be treated.[6] According to NIMH sources, "anxiety disorders are real, identifiable brain diseases. Current research suggests that anxiety disorders arise from a combination of genetic vulnerability with an environmental 'second hit.' In addition, we are beginning to understand the specific circuits in the brain that are malfunctioning in PTSD, OCD, and perhaps panic disorder. Through this research we will be able to develop new and better therapies."[4]

Immediate psychiatric evaluation is required for all patients with suicidal/homicidal ideation.

PATHOPHYSIOLOGY

Congress designated the 1990s as the Decade of the Brain, and a massive effort is under way to overcome the major mental disorders. The NIMH supports sizable and multifaceted research programs on anxiety disorders and their causes, diagnosis, treatment, and prevention. This research involves studies of anxiety disorders in human subjects and investigations of the biologic basis for anxiety and related phenomena in animals. A large database of information regarding the pathophysiology of anxiety disorders has been derived from these investigations. For example, in positron emission tomography (PET) studies of OCD, a decreased metabolism has been demonstrated in the orbital gyrus, caudate nuclei, and cingulate gyrus; with panic, an increased PET blood flow has been demonstrated in the right parahippocampus; in anxiety, this increase in blood flow is demonstrated in the frontal lobe.[7] Using classification criteria from the fourth edition of the *Diagnostic and Statistical Manual of Mental Disorders (DSM-IV)*, studies have shown that mitral valve prolapse is present in 50% of the subjects identified with panic disorder.[2]

Probably no single situation or condition causes anxiety disorders. Instead, physical and environmental triggers may combine to create a particular anxiety illness. More recent studies have indicated that biochemical imbalances may be the source. Scientists speculate that all thoughts and feelings result from complex electrochemical interactions in the central nervous system. Moreover, some studies indicate that infusions of certain biochemicals can cause a panic attack in some individuals. According to this theory, the treatment of anxiety should correct these biochemical imbalances.[5]

Other theories from the psychologic field of study have been used to define the cause of anxiety disorders. Psychoanalytic theory attributes anxiety to unconscious impulses that threaten to burst into consciousness and produce anxiety. According to this theory, defense mechanisms are used to ward off anxiety. Learning theory attributes the cause of anxiety to frustration or stress. Norepinephrine, serotonin, and dopamine regulate mood, movement, and blood pressure, and they stimulate and initiate postsynaptic impulse conduction. Debate exists as to the exact imbalance that leads to an anxiety disorder. Excess levels of serotonin or norepinephrine characterize anxiety, but there is disagreement regarding whether the problem reflects excess production, blockage, or impaired uptake of these neurotransmitters. Another explanation of anxiety disorders relates to the hypothesis that some individuals have an overly sensitive response system.

The treatment of chemical imbalances underlies the treatment of all anxiety disorders. Because the biologic function of "anxiety" is a useful and protective natural function of the body, the elimination of "anxiety" is not possible or desired. However, *control* of the noxious symptoms of an anxiety disorder is desired and necessary to prevent the long-term adverse effects on the body of the almost constant hyperproduction of certain neurochemicals. It is hypothesized that noradrenergic, gamma-aminobutyric acid (GABA)ergic, and serotonergic neuronal systems in the frontal lobe and limbic system are the areas from which the pathophysiology of anxiety disorders arise.[2]

CLINICAL PRESENTATION

One of the most striking aspects of anxiety disorders are the similar statements that patients voice during the initial interview (Box 260-1). It is essential that the primary care provider pay close attention to the words patients use to describe their feelings. Key words to note include *tense, uptight, on edge, hassled, nervous, dread, jumpy, jittery, edgy, vulnerable, worried,* and *anxious.* Individuals with panic disorder often believe they are going to die during a panic attack and often convince others of this fact; they are in such distress that, to all outward evaluation, it seems they are indeed going to die. A rapidly worsening medical condition, substance-induced anxiety, and a psychologic response to stressors associated with a medical condition should be excluded. Anxiety should be considered to be a potential diagnosis in the presentation of physical symptoms such as shortness of breath, nervousness, gastrointestinal upset, palpitations, fatigue, muscle aches, tension, and sleep disorders.[8] It is easy to overlook biologic inheritance, but genes influence health and behavior from birth to death. In an initial interview, investigation of family members with similar symptoms is an important consideration.

BOX 260-1

COMMON STATEMENTS VOICED DURING INITIAL INTERVIEW

- I have butterflies in my stomach.
- There is a lump in my throat.
- I think I'm going crazy.
- I don't go out anymore.
- I know something bad is going to happen.
- I feel a black cloud over my head.
- My mind just goes blank.
- I know this isn't rational, but I can't seem to shake this feeling of doom.
- I have been feeling "on edge" a lot lately.
- I know something awful is wrong with me.
- I can feel my heart beating in my chest.
- I can't breathe.
- I'm going to die.
- I'm so easily fatigued/irritable/restless.
- I have had a lot of "worries" lately.
- I have been under a lot of stress.
- I shake all the time.
- My hands sweat.
- I have to go to the bathroom so much.

PHYSICAL EXAMINATION

Anxiety disorders emerge from a malfunction of neurobiologic substances that alert individuals to danger.[8] A complete physical examination is necessary to exclude any underlying physical condition. The physical complaints related to an anxiety disorder include dizziness, light-headedness, diarrhea, frequent urination and urgency, tachycardia, shortness of breath, tingling in the extremities, tremors, hyperreflexes, gastrointestinal distress, palpitations, hypertension, syncope, muscle tightness, sweating, nausea, and vomiting. However, individuals may not "fit" the expected profile for the symptoms observed. Young, healthy-appearing individuals present with shortness of breath, heart palpitations, a fear of dying, and other symptoms. Older patients also experience anxiety symptoms, but because they "fit" the expected profile for many disease processes, the diagnosis of anxiety is often overlooked.

DIAGNOSTICS

Diagnostic tests should be guided by the history and physical examination. ECG and baseline laboratory studies are also indicated. In addition, many tests are available as an initial screen for anxiety disorders. Standardized instruments include the Zung Anxiety Self-Assessment Scale and the Hamilton Anxiety and Depression Scales. Although these tests are easily administered and scored, they do not replace a formal evaluation but rather serve as a database. It is essential to remember that individuals may be physically ill and have an anxiety disorder. Individuals under stress from medical conditions may also experience nonpathologic anxiety.

According to Valente,[8] diagnosing untreated anxiety disorders may be challenging. Patients complain of diverse somatic symptoms during brief primary care visits. The DSM-IV diagnostic criteria have shortcomings—mild symptoms may be overlooked because symptoms of physical illness and anxiety overlap (Box 260-2). Serious sequelae of anxiety disorders include suicide risk, alcohol/chemical dependency, sexual dysfunction, and vulnerability to physical illness.[8] Screening for anxiety disorders is necessary because a large and growing percentage of anxious individuals are now treated in primary care settings.

Diagnostics

Anxiety Disorders

Laboratory
TSH*
CBC and differential*
Serum electrolytes*
BUN*
Creatinine*
Serum glucose*

*If indicated.

DIFFERENTIAL DIAGNOSIS

Hyperthyroidism, hypoglycemia, hyperglycemia, pheochromocytoma, cardiac conditions, vestibular dysfunctions, hyperparathyroidism, temporal lobe epilepsy, and other organic conditions should be considered in the differential diagnosis. Alcohol and

BOX 260-2

DIAGNOSTIC CRITERIA FOR GENERALIZED ANXIETY DISORDER

A. Excessive anxiety and worry (apprehensive expectation) occurring more days than not for at least 6 months about a number of events or activities (such as work or school performance).

B. The person finds it difficult to control the worry.

C. The anxiety and worry are associated with three (or more) of the following six symptoms (with at least some symptoms present for more days than not for the past 6 months).
Note: Only one item is required in children.
(1) restlessness or feeling keyed up or on edge
(2) being easily fatigued
(3) difficulty concentrating or mind going blank
(4) irritability
(5) muscle tension
(6) sleep disturbance (difficulty falling or staying asleep, or restless, unsatisfying sleep)

D. The focus of anxiety and worry is not confined to features of an Axis I disorder, e.g., the anxiety or worry is not about having a Panic Attack (as in panic Disorder), being embarrassed in public (as in Social Phobia), being contaminated (as in Obsessive-Compulsive Disorder), being away from home or close relatives (as in Separation Anxiety Disorder), gaining weight (as in Anorexia Nervosa), having multiple physical complaints (as in Somatization Disorder), or having a serious illness (as in Hypochondriasis), and the anxiety and worry do not occur exclusively during Posttraumatic Stress Disorder.

E. The anxiety, worry, or physical symptoms cause clinically significant distress or impairment in social, occupational, or other important areas of functioning.

F. The disturbance is not due to the direct physiologic effects of a substance (e.g., a drug of abuse, a medication) or a general medical condition (e.g., hyperthyroidism) and does not occur exclusively during a Mood Disorder, a Psychotic Disorder, or a Pervasive Developmental Disorder.

From American Psychiatric Association: *Diagnostic and statistical manual of mental disorders*, ed 4 (Text revision 2000), Washington DC, 1994, The Association.

drug dependencies, factitious disorders, malingering, adjustment reactions, borderline personality disorders, dementia, delirium, psychoses, schizophrenia, depression, somatization disorders, dysthymia, and other psychiatric illnesses must be considered.

Co-morbid conditions and mixed disorders often occur with the anxiety disorders; there is a complicated two-way interaction between anxiety disorders and co-morbid medical disorders. Although anxiety can mimic or exacerbate various medical conditions, it can also be the result or expression of those same disorders. Approximately 25% of medical patients complaining of anxiety have an underlying physical pathology at the root of their complaint.[9] Anxiety may actually be an early reaction to the onset of major medical problems and may be caused by underlying cardiopulmonary, endocrine, gastrointestinal, neurologic, metabolic,

 **Differential Diagnosis**

Anxiety Disorders

Medical Disorders	Psychiatric Disorders
Cardiac conditions	Acute situational anxiety
Central nervous system disorders	Adjustment reaction
Hyperglycemia/hypoglycemia	Alcohol and drug dependencies
Hyperparathyroidism	Borderline personality disorder
Hyperthyroidism	Delirium
Medications	Dementia
Nutritional problems	Depression
Pheochromocytoma	Dysthymia
Respiratory disorders	Factitious disorder
Stimulants (e.g., caffeine)	Generalized anxiety disorder
Temporal lobe epilepsy	Malingering
Vestibular dysfunctions	Panic disorder
	Phobias
	Posttraumatic stress disorder
	Psychosis
	Schizophrenia
	Somatization disorder

and drug-related causes. Factors that increase the likelihood of underlying illness include an onset of anxiety symptoms after 35 years of age, a lack of a personal or family history of anxiety disorders, the absence of significant stressors or emotional traumas, and a poor response to standard antianxiety medications.[10]

MANAGEMENT

Treatment that has shown to be most effective for the anxiety disorders combines education, brief counseling, self-management techniques, and medications.[8] Education includes an explanation of the biologic etiology of anxiety, a provision of written information, an explanation of available treatments, an emphasis on the effectiveness of treatments, strategies for coping, and relaxation.[11] Anxiety disorders respond effectively when there is an understanding of individual symptoms and an ability to identify cues and learn self-management techniques. Progressive relaxation, routine noncompetitive exercise, music, and medication help reduce anxiety.[12]

Studies demonstrate a synergistic effect of multiple treatment approaches.[13] The pharmacologic treatment of anxiety has increased with the advent of more specific drug therapies. Nine classes of drugs may be used to treat anxiety. Barbiturates (which are seldom used because of their potential for toxicity, interaction, and abuse), glycerol derivatives, benzodiazepines, antihistamines, tricyclic antidepressants, selective serotonin reuptake antidepressants, antipsychotics, azaperone, and beta blockers are commonly used as treatments for primary anxiety disorders. Benzodiazepines should be used with psychotherapy and stress management; however, they create an addictive tolerance over time and become ineffective for long-term management. The treatment of anxiety disorders often involves the short-term use of benzodiazepines to reduce symptoms until other medications become effective. If used, they should be tapered slowly after a limited period of use. Medication management alone provides some symptom relief, but the prognosis improves if self-management strategies are included.[8]

Selective serotonin reuptake inhibitors (SSRIs) are helpful with virtually all anxiety disorders, with the initial starting doses and final effective dose varying by disorder. Any of the SSRIs—citalopram (Celexa), paroxetine (Paxil), fluoxetine (Prozac), sertraline (Zoloft), or venlafaxine (Effexor)—can be effective; however, patients must understand there is a 3- to 5-week initial period before the medication becomes fully effective. Benzodiazepines should be used sparingly and for short periods until the SSRIs become effective. Buspirone (BuSpar) is a good choice as an initial medication for patients without depressive symptoms. The recommended beginning dose of BuSpar is 5 to 10 mg b.i.d. Patients with anxiety disorders often "overreact" to medications, so medications should be started slowly. Beginning doses of the SSRIs are 10 mg for Celexa, 5 to 10 mg for Paxil, 10 mg for Prozac, 25 mg for Zoloft, and 37.5 mg for Effexor. Doses are titrated according to the side effect profile and at 1- to 2-week intervals. Side effects for the SSRIs include gastrointestinal distress, dry mouth, and sexual dysfunction. Drug-drug interactions need to be assessed before medications are prescribed. OCD can be treated effectively with SSRIs, and several medications, including clomipramine (Anafranil) and fluvoxamine (Luvox), are specific to symptoms of OCD. Tricyclic antidepressants are also sometimes useful, but the side effect profile and the potential for lethal overdose make these medications a less likely choice. If patients continue to experience symptoms after a fair trial on medication, a referral is recommended; this dual-treatment approach has been shown to be most effective. Recent research also demonstrates the importance of ethnicity in psychopharmacologic management of depression and anxiety disorders, with sometimes profound implications for efficacy and safety. Because different ethnic groups respond differently to therapy, primary care providers are advised to use ethnically sensitive approaches to assessment and treatment.[13]

Education regarding the adverse effects that caffeine, alcohol, and over-the-counter and prescribed stimulants have on anxiety is useful. Patients often do not wish to reduce their use of these chemicals, but education about the biologic effects may encourage them to do so.

Coordination of health care services with individuals who have anxiety disorders may prove difficult. Clearly, the "health care provider" shopping performed by patients with anxiety disorders leads to frustration of both the provider and the patient. Often heard are the following phrases: "No one can tell me what is wrong," "I have been everywhere but I can't get any relief," and "I am so worried about my health." The coordination of the primary health care provider and mental health care provider is essential to provide successful treatment.[14]

One difficulty reported in several studies is the accurate diagnosis of anxiety disorders.[15] *DSM-IV*, the standard for mental health care providers, is cumbersome and difficult to use by primary care providers. To simplify the task of primary care providers, the American Psychiatric Association published a primary care version of the *DSM-IV* in 1995. This version, the *DSM-IV-PC* (primary care) groups psychiatric disorders by their presenting symptoms.[15] The use of this manual to provide accurate diagnosis and treatment of anxiety disorders will substantially improve outcomes.[16]

LIFE SPAN CONSIDERATIONS

Anxiety disorders occur across the life span and are associated with distressing physical symptoms and a tendency to worry about health issues. These symptoms often bring patients to primary care providers, who may be frustrated by seemingly unexplained somatic complaints. Extensive studies document that parental anxiety disorders are a potent risk for child psychiatric disorders and behavioral problems. Although some of this risk is attributable to shared genetic vulnerability, it is likely that parenting by an ill mother also contributes substantially to the development of such disorders. In one study of children whose mothers had anxiety disorders, as many as 80% had emotional disturbances.[17]

The family members of patients with anxiety disorders may also be affected. Different psychosocial factors are likely to have an impact on anxiety disorders at different stages of the life span. Anxiety impairs quality of life; when the underlying disorder is treated, quality of life improves. Bereavement and loss, childbearing, the postpartum period, life changes (e.g., retirement), and the loss of health and independence in older adults all are times for the potential emergence of anxiety disorders. Primary care providers are likely to see these patients and should be aware of this potential. Older patients have a potential risk for falls and are vulnerable to cognitive impairments, memory impairments, and disorientation from the medications used to treat their anxiety.

COMPLICATIONS

Only one in four patients with an anxiety disorder is correctly diagnosed and treated. Undiagnosed anxiety disorders have a negative impact on many aspects of life—they interfere with and diminish a patient's quality of life. Anxiety disorders increase health concerns and the use of medical services, including urgent care costs and visits. Beyond the direct cost of frequent and often unnecessary visits, undiagnosed anxiety disorders adversely affect social and occupational functioning, causing frequent work absences and the loss of untold hours of productivity. Serious complications of untreated anxiety include alcohol and chemical dependency, suicide risk, sexual dysfunction, and an increased vulnerability to physical illness.[18]

INDICATIONS FOR REFERRAL/HOSPITALIZATION

Meredith and others[19] demonstrated that primary care providers often do not detect anxiety disorders and that the outcome of detection and referral of patients with anxiety disorders significantly increases a positive health outcome. Referral to a mental health practitioner should be considered when an anxiety disorder is diagnosed and the initial treatment has not been successful. Although primary care providers can treat anxiety disorders, studies have shown improved outcomes with specialized mental health care.[20]

Individuals with anxiety disorders are often hospitalized to exclude co-morbid medical conditions. Medical causes must be excluded when an individual presents in acute distress with complaints of cardiovascular symptoms such as palpitations, sweating, and chest pain. Anxiety disorders often accompany stroke and diseases of the cardiovascular, endocrine, neurologic, metabolic, and respiratory systems. The co-morbid medical condition often indicates a need for hospitalization, but treatment of the anxiety disorder often shortens the hospitalization and increases positive outcomes.[13]

Patients with suicidal ideation require careful psychiatric evaluation and potential hospitalization. A mental health evaluation is recommended when a patient's thought processes are significantly impaired or when psychosis is present (see Chapter 266). Evaluation of dementia, delirium, and psychosis also requires referral to a mental health care provider.

PATIENT AND FAMILY EDUCATION

The educational component of the treatment of anxiety disorders is the core to treatment success and positive outcome; this fact cannot be overemphasized. The ability of the individual to develop positive coping strategies depends on the education of both the individual and family members.[17]

Many techniques exist to facilitate the education of patients with anxiety disorders. Some of these techniques include positive self-talk, imagery, a daily mood log, realistic goals, exercise, relaxation exercises, behavioral therapy, family therapy, insight-oriented psychotherapy, hypnosis, supportive therapy, cognitive therapy, brief psychotherapy, and systematic desensitization.

Because of the nature of the disease process, patients with anxiety disorders are particularly difficult to educate at times. The motor and visceral effects of anxiety also have effects on thinking, perception, and learning. This fact needs to be considered in the education of both patients and their families. Anxiety tends to produce confusion and distort perception, not only of time and space but also of people and the meaning of events. These distortions can interfere with learning by lowering concentration, reducing recall, and impairing the ability to relate one item to another (association).[3] The provision of written information is often necessary to overcome the difficulties these patients experience.

Education should include the fact that anxiety disorders can be treated effectively. To reduce anxiety, patients must learn and practice difficult skills. Consistent and reliable support, coaching, and the belief that "you can do it" from significant others is helpful.[8] Investigating a patient's preferred learning style is an important consideration. Patients gradually learn strategies for coping with anxiety if provided with the support and instructional material necessary to accomplish their goal. Educational audiotapes, videos, books, how-to manuals, relaxation, breathing exercises, self-talk instruction, nonnegative thinking guidance, and distraction techniques are useful teaching methods. Just informing an individual on "how to fix the problem," "get control," or "set your mind to it" is not effective. Short-term psychotherapy is very useful and effective in helping individuals understand anxiety, identify cues, and learn self-management techniques. Research shows that individual and family education is an integral part of the treatment package for anxiety disorders and that treatment outcomes are significantly improved with the use of a combined treatment strategy. Studies have also shown a synergistic effect of proven psychosocial treatments and proven drug treatments.[13] The following brochures, which provide more detailed information on various anxiety disorders and related topics, are available by from the NIMH*:

Understanding Panic Disorder (NIH publication No. 93-3482)
Obsessive-Compulsive Disorder (NIH publication No. 94-3755)
Medications (DHHS publication No. [ADM] 92-1509)

HEALTH PROMOTION

Anxiety is a part of our everyday life; all the generally accepted positive lifestyle behaviors promote the management of anxiety: sufficient rest, a healthy and balanced diet, regular exercise, routine medical check-ups, and following a routine. A family history of relatives with anxiety disorders increases the individual's risk for the development of an anxiety disorder. Education is the key to early intervention.

Anxiety often refers to the feeling or emotion of fear when the cause of the emotion is sometimes obscure; the events of September 11, 2001, have brought to the forefront identifiable fears. People during this time of terrorism are not unclear about the source of their fear. They know exactly what they are afraid of and it is not an irrational anxiety. The key to limiting the growth of anxiety disorders due to a steady state of heightened fear is education.[21] The way to promote health and deal with rational fears is through the use of reason and logic.

*Room 7C-02, 5600 Fishers Lane, Rockville, Md 20857.

REFERENCES

1. Top sites for anxiety. Retrieved August 12, 2002, from the World Wide Web: www.anxiety.org.
2. Uhde TW, Nemiah JC: Panic and generalized anxiety disorders. In Kaplan HI, Sadock BJ, *Comprehensive textbook of psychiatry*, ed 5, Baltimore, 1989, Williams & Wilkins.
3. National Anxiety Foundation: What are anxiety disorders? Retrieved August 12, 2002, from the World Wide Web: www.lexington-online.com/naf.whatare.html.
4. U.S. Department of Health and Human Services, National Institutes of Health: Health information. Retrieved August 12, 2002, from the World Wide Web: www.nih.gov/health/.
5. American Psychiatric Association—Public Information: Anxiety disorders. Retrieved August 12, 2002, from the World Wide Web: www.psych.org/public_info/anxiety_day.cfm.
6. U.S. Department of Health and Human Services, National Institutes of Health. Retrieved August 12, 2002, from the World Wide Web: www.nimh.nih.gov/.
7. Lucey JV and others: Brain blood flow in anxiety disorders, *Br J Psychiatr* 171:346-350, 1997.
8. Valente S: Diagnosis and treatment of panic disorder and generalized anxiety in primary care, *Nurse Pract* 21:26-38, 1996
9. Sherborne CD and others: Comorbid anxiety disorder and the functioning and well-being of chronically ill patients of general medical providers, *Arch Gen Psychiatry* 53:889-895, 1996.
10. Rosenbaum JF, Pollack MH: Anxiety. In Cassem NH, editor: *Massachusetts General Hospital handbook of general hospital psychiatry*, ed 3, St Louis, 1991, Mosby.
11. Wise MG, Griffies WS: A combined treatment approach to anxiety in the medically ill, *J Clin Psychiatr* 56 (suppl 2):14-19, 1995.
12. Leaman TL: Generalized anxiety disorder: an evolving concept, *Anx Profil* 1:4-5, 1993.
13. Barlow DH, Lehman CL: Advances in the psychosocial treatment of anxiety disorders, *Arch Gen Psychiatry* 53:727-735, 1996.
14. Eisenberg L: Treating depression and anxiety in primary care: closing the gap between knowledge and practice, *N Engl J Med* 326:1080-1085, 1992.
15. Retrieved August 12, 2002, from the World Wide Web: www.ama-assn.org/sci-pubs/journals/archive/jama/vol_275/no_24/mn6113.htm.
16. Selected health psychology research findings. Retrieved August 12, 2002, from the World Wide Web: www.healthpsych.com/research.html.

17. Shear MK, Mammen O: Anxiety disorders in primary care: a life-span perspective, *Bull Menninger Clin* 612:A37-A53, 1997.
18. Gorman JM, Papp LA: Drug treatment strategies for GAD, *Anx Profil* 1:6-8, 1993.
19. Meredith LS and others: Treatment typically provided for comorbid anxiety disorders, *Arch Fam Med* 6:231-237, 1997.
20. Jonas BS, Franks P, Ingram DD: Are symptoms of anxiety and depression risk factors for hypertension? *Arch Fam Med* 6:244-256, 1997.
21. National Anxiety Foundation. Retrieved August 12, 2002, from the World Wide Web: http://lexington-on-line.com/naf.html.

CHAPTER 261

Bipolar Disorder

Claire J. Barrett

DEFINITION/EPIDEMIOLOGY

People experience a wide range of moods throughout their lifetimes, and often from one day to the next. This is an expected part of living and usually is not problematic. However, some people experience mood disorders that are more extreme fluctuations of their baseline mood. These fluctuations affect thoughts, feelings, physical health, behavior, and social functioning. Bipolar disorder is a mood disorder characterized by a vacillation between depressed (low) and manic (elevated) mood states.

Symptoms of the disorder may vary over time within the same patient or may remain similar across episodes. These symptoms also vary across a population afflicted with the disease. Because bipolar disorder is characterized by mood cycles, the clinical presentation may vary widely from a manic to a depressed episode. There are medications to treat the symptoms, and therefore early recognition of the disorder can aid in recovery. If left untreated, symptoms may become quite severe. Because episodes are often recurrent, it is important to have a treatment plan and it is important for the patient and the practitioner to maintain open communication.

Bipolar disorder is most thoroughly explained in the fourth edition of the *Diagnostic and Statistical Manual of Mental Disorders (DSM-IV)*. The clinical presentation is characterized by one or more manic or mixed episodes during a patient's lifetime. The patient has often also had a major depressive episode, but such an episode is not necessary for diagnosis.[1]

Approximately 1% of the population experiences a bipolar I disorder over the course of lifetime. The prevalence for bipolar II disorder is probably significantly higher because it is underdiagnosed. The lifetime prevalence for a major depressive disorder is approximately 15%, but this proportion may approach 25% in women.[2] In contrast to major depression, bipolar disorder affects men and women equally. However, gender may play a role in the timing of bipolar episodes.[2] Men are more likely to have a manic episode first, whereas women are more likely to have an initial depressive episode.[1] Women may also experience an onset of symptoms during the postpartum period, and women who have the disorder are at increased risk for experiencing additional episodes postpartum.[1] The premenstrual period may also be associated with the exacerbation of symptoms.[1]

In a study across several countries, bipolar disorder rates are notably consistent, whereas major depression rates vary widely.[3] Although the differential incidence of the disorder by racial or ethnic group has not been reported, mood disorders and schizophrenia have been underdiagnosed and overdiagnosed in patients whose cultures or races differ from that of their health care providers.[2] This may be related both to stereotypes and assumptions about races or ethnic groups and to the way in which people of different cultural, ethnic, or racial groups describe their symptoms.

The age of onset for a bipolar disorder can fall within a wide range but is generally between 15 and 30 years. Newly diagnosed mania rarely occurs in children or in adults over the age of 65 years. The initial episodes may be depressive; approximately 10% to 15% of adolescents with major depressive episodes are diagnosed with bipolar disorder later in life.[2]

There seems to be a genetic link among mood disorders, with the risk increasing with increases in the proportion of genes shared with an afflicted person.[4] This link is supported by a concordance rate for monozygotic twins that is approximately 3 times that noted in dizygotic twins.[4,5] In an National Institute of Mental Health–Yale University study, affective disorders occurred much more frequently in first-degree relatives of patients with affective disorders than in relatives of patients in a control group.[5] Despite the evidence supporting a genetic link, a specific mode of genetic transmission has not yet been found.[4]

Immediate psychiatric evaluation is required for all patients with suicidal/homicidal ideation. Approximately 25% of individuals with bipolar disorder will attempt suicide.[6]

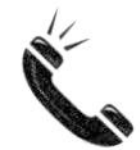

Physician consultation is indicated for patients with psychosis or violent behavior.

PATHOPHYSIOLOGY

Bipolar disorder is a biologic illness; however, its specific cause is still unknown. Reports from neuroimaging studies suggest that the thalamus, hypothalamus, amygdala, caudate, prefrontal cortex, and cerebellum may be involved in pathophysiology.[7] The neurotransmitters serotonin, norepinephrine, dopamine, and acetylcholine and second-messenger pathways have also been implicated.[8] In many patients, dysregulation of the hypothalamic-pituitary-adrenal axis and of circadian rhythms has been identified.[4] The search for gene carriers has been the subject of much study, but no single gene has been identified.[9,10] It is probable that there is a complex interaction between genetic and environmental factors.

CLINICAL PRESENTATION

Observation of the patient's behaviors and attention to the patient's description of symptoms are valuable for diagnosis. The clinical presentation of bipolar disorder varies depending on whether the presenting episode is manic or depressive. Subtypes of bipolar disorder include bipolar I disorder, in which the disorder presents for the first time with a manic episode and almost always has depressions as well. In bipolar II disorder, hypomania rather than mania occurs. Bipolar II disorder is more difficult to diagnose because hypomania may not be seen as problematic but the person is seen as happy or energetic, especially if he or she able to avoid serious consequences. The person then may present only during depressive episodes, thus jeopardizing effective treatment.

A working knowledge of the common symptoms enables appropriate questions to be directed toward the patient during any stage of illness. Manic states involve heightened mood, sexuality, and impulsivity. Increased energy results in a decreased need for sleep, faster speech, and physical activity. Although mania is often thought to be a grouping of exaggerated positive characteristics, certain stages of mania are quite painful to the patient. Increased irritability, paranoia, and suspicion may also be evident.[11]

Mania can begin as hypomania, a state most easily described as a less severe manic phase and one in which the patient's mood might be euphoric and self-confident. Thinking may be affected at times, because thoughts move quickly. However, the patient may enjoy this feeling because it allows for increased productivity, creativity, and energy.[11]

The progression from hypomania to a full-blown manic episode is gradual, but the actual time involved varies from person to person and episode to episode. During acute mania, cognition and perception often become psychotic; delusions or hallucinations may be experienced. Because thinking is so quick and tangential, patients are often very distractible. When speaking, cognitive symptoms become obvious to others in the form of loose associations between ideas and, at times, the flight of ideas from one topic to another. Behavior can be bizarre and inappropriate and may seem disorganized.[11]

Patients with bipolar disorder can become violent and destructive or, more specifically, homicidal or suicidal. Although the beginning stage of mania is usually pleasurable, the later stages can be frightening and, finally, painful. By the height of the mania, the patient is in great pain but is usually apathetic.[12] During all stages of mania; it is crucial that a patient's risk of harm to self or others be assessed.

Depressive episodes are on the opposite end of the mood spectrum and have a very different presentation from that of mania. Although speech, movement, and thoughts are increased and quicker in mania, depression tends to decrease pleasure and to slow speech, thoughts, energy, and sexuality. Mood is negative and pessimistic, and the patient can be irritable, paranoid, and angry.[11]

Depression can be simple or psychotic. Simple depression usually includes morbid preoccupations and, frequently, suicidal thoughts. Sleeping and eating patterns are often altered and are characterized by decreased appetite and difficulty in getting to sleep or staying asleep.[11] As with mania, psychotic depression may also include mood-congruent hallucinations and delusions. Mixed episodes are those in which symptoms of mania and depression occur at the same time.

The course of an individual's illness may be influenced by very high rates of co-morbid alcohol or substance abuse. Almost two thirds of patients with the disorder will meet the diagnostic criteria for an addictive disorder over their lifetime.

PHYSICAL EXAMINATION

The physical examination may reveal symptoms indicative of bipolar disorder, but the time frame and controlled setting limit the range of observable symptoms. The provider's office does not allow for observation of the patients as they function in their own environment, where many of the previously described symptoms could be observed. In addition, patients in an acute state of mania or depression are much less likely than a healthy individual to keep a scheduled appointment. Symptoms of mania or depression likely to be observed during a physical examination are rapid, slowed, or incoherent speech; changes in weight; irritability; grandiosity; distractibility; and overt psychosis.

DIAGNOSTICS

The commonly accepted method of diagnosing bipolar disorder is the use of *DSM-IV* criteria. Although the criteria for diagnosis are listed in the following paragraphs, the *DSM-IV* itself should be consulted for the most comprehensive information. An understanding of the criteria for a manic or major depressive episode, as well as the criteria for several disorders important in the differential diagnosis, is imperative for the diagnosis of a bipolar I disorder. The essential feature of a bipolar I disorder is a clinical course that includes one or more manic or mixed episodes. Often the patient has had one or more episodes of major depression; however, such an episode is not necessary for diagnosis.[1] Mood problems resulting from the use of substances, medical conditions, or other diagnoses are not to be counted toward diagnosis.[1]

A major depressive episode is manifested by feeling sad, blue, or "down in the dumps" or by losing interest in normally enjoyable activities and by having at least four of the following:

- Insomnia or hypersomnia
- Significant weight loss or gain
- Impaired concentration, indecisiveness
- Psychomotor agitation or retardation
- Loss of energy, fatigue
- Feelings of worthlessness or guilt
- Thoughts of suicide or death

The feelings must be present daily or almost daily for at least 2 weeks.

In addition to meeting the preceding symptom criteria, these symptoms must not meet criteria for a mixed episode, and they must cause clinically significant distress or difficulties in important areas of functioning (i.e., social, occupational). In addition, symptoms must not be a result of the direct effects of a substance or medical condition, and they may not be better explained by bereavement[2] (see Chapter 264 for more information on depression).

To meet the criteria for a manic episode, defined as a period of abnormally and persistently elevated, expansive, or irritable mood,[1] the mood must last at least 1 week unless hospitalization is necessary sooner. Three to four of the following must be manifested in a significant manner and persistent:

- Inflated self-esteem or grandiosity
- Decreased need for sleep
- More talkative than usual or pressure to keep talking
- Flight of ideas, racing thoughts
- Distractibility
- Increased goal-directed activity or psychomotor agitation
- Excessive involvement in pleasurable activities, which might result in painful consequences

Diagnostics

Bipolar Disorder	
Laboratory	Chemistry panels
TSH*	Urine toxicology*
CBC and differential	

*If indicated.

These symptoms must not be part of a mixed episode. The mood disturbance must also be severe enough to result in impaired occupational, social, or relationship functioning; to necessitate hospitalization to prevent harm; or to include psychotic features. Again, the symptoms must not be better explained by the physiologic effects of a substance or medical condition.[1]

DIFFERENTIAL DIAGNOSIS

The diagnosis of a psychiatric illness differs from that of a physical illness because there are no laboratory tests from which to draw conclusive diagnoses. Diagnosis and treatment are based on the patient's report of symptoms, observation, and the elimination of other diagnoses. This emphasizes the importance of obtaining a thorough history. When possible, family interviews can be helpful in providing a more objective description of recent events. Schizophrenia, schizoaffective disorder, posttraumatic stress disorder, abuse of alcohol, cocaine, or amphetamines, and personality disorders can mimic or coexist with bipolar disorder.[13,14] In the primary care setting, clinicians see patients with medical illnesses with symptoms that resemble manic episodes, including thyrotoxicosis, partial complex seizures, systemic lupus erythematosus, cerebrovascular accident, HIV, tertiary syphilis, and steroid-induced mood symptoms.[13,15] For this reason, evaluation should include physical examination with particular focus on neurologic and endocrine systems, observation for signs of alcohol or other substances, and laboratory testing that includes thyroid function tests, CBC, chemistry panels, and urine toxicology for possible substance abuse. Patients previously treated for depression with medication or electroconvulsive therapy may exhibit signs of mania; in such cases, a diagnosis should not be based on these symptoms.[1]

Bipolar I disorder is distinguished from other mood disorders by matching the criteria for diagnosis with the patient's symptoms. It is distinguished from major depressive disorder by the presence of only one manic or mixed episode in the patient's lifetime. It is less easily distinguished from bipolar II disorder, in which the only difference is the presence of one or more manic or mixed episodes (bipolar I) as opposed to hypomanic episodes (bipolar II). Cyclothymic disorders also share similar criteria with bipolar I disorder and are differentiated by the duration and nature of symptoms. With cyclothymic disorder, the hypomanic and depressive symptoms are present but do not meet the criteria for manic episodes or major depressive episodes.[1]

MANAGEMENT

During the acute phase of the illness, the focus should be on management of the presenting symptoms and on securing the

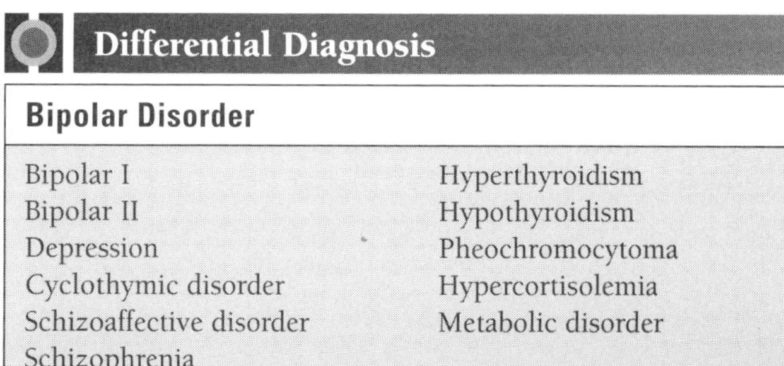
Differential Diagnosis

Bipolar Disorder	
Bipolar I	Hyperthyroidism
Bipolar II	Hypothyroidism
Depression	Pheochromocytoma
Cyclothymic disorder	Hypercortisolemia
Schizoaffective disorder	Metabolic disorder
Schizophrenia	

safety of the person. The person in this phase may be suicidal, psychotic, or displaying such poor judgment that they pose an imminent risk to self. Hospitalization may be necessary until the severity of symptoms abates. The continuation phase can last weeks to months. The goal is to reach full remission of symptoms and to restore the patient to full functioning. The maintenance phase aims to maintain remission and should last at least 1 year after resolutions of symptoms. Lifetime maintenance is recommended for patients who have had three or more manic episodes.

The major components of treatment include psychopharmacology, psychotherapy, and education. Psychotherapy is indicated to facilitate the resolution of issues that may contribute to or be exacerbated by the symptoms. Co-morbid substance abuse and personality disorders seem to predict poorer outcomes for patients with bipolar disorder, and therapy may be helpful in managing these conditions.[16] Family therapy can enable the patient and significant others to work through problems resulting from or contributing to the disorder. Support groups, such as the National Alliance for the Mentally Ill and the Depressive and Manic-Depressive Association, allow individuals and significant others to receive support from peers who understand.

A psychiatrist or practitioner skilled in the use of psychiatric medications should manage all medications used to treat bipolar disorder. A psychiatric evaluation is standard before beginning treatment, and system functions should be monitored throughout the course of treatment. Because toxic and therapeutic levels of lithium are often close, serum levels should be carefully monitored.

Medications commonly used during a manic episode to reduce symptoms include lithium carbonate, a mood stabilizer, anticonvulsants, antipsychotics, and benzodiazepines. Lithium, divalproex sodium, and carbamazepine are mood stabilizers and the drugs of choice. The choice of a mood stabilizer is often based on previous history, side effect profiles, and any coexisting medical illness. For example, lithium is contraindicated in patients with severe renal disease, and valproate is contraindicated in patients with hepatic impairment. For patients who do not respond to a single mood stabilizer, combinations of mood stabilizers are being used, particularly lithium and valproate.[17] Anticonvulsants may be more effective than lithium in patients with mixed mania and depression.[6] In addition, patients with rapid cycling are less likely to respond to lithium than to valproate or carbamazepine.[6]

Antipsychotics may be used as adjunctive therapy in the manic phase. The use of typical antipsychotics (e.g., haloperidol) may be associated with extrapyramidal symptoms and tardive dyskinesia. The atypical antipsychotics such as olanzapine or risperidone may not cause the preceding side effects but are associated with weight gain, glucose intolerance, and hyperlipidemia. Clozapine may be especially useful for patients with refractory bipolar illness but is associated with the risk of agranulocytosis.

Hypomania may be a precursor of either a manic or a depressive episode. It is often characterized by a decrease in sleep time. Addressing this symptom with a benzodiazepine, a higher dose of mood stabilizer, or a low dose of a stabilizing antipsychotic may end the hypomanic state.[18] However, the potential for benzodiazepine abuse plus the already high rates of substance abuse among individuals with bipolar disorder limits their use outside the acute setting.

Additional anticonvulsants such as lamotrigine, gabapentin, and topiramate have shown promise but are not yet part of the standard treatment of bipolar disorder. Electroconvulsive therapy remains a reliable and effective treatment for manic episodes nonresponsive to psychopharmacology.

Treatment of the depressed phase of bipolar disorder has not been extensively studied and is controversial. In many cases, a mood stabilizer alone, usually lithium, may be useful. When additional medications are needed, either a selective serotonin reuptake inhibitor or bupropion is less likely to precipitate a rapid switch to mania than is a tricyclic antidepressant or a monoamine oxidase inhibitor. Unlike treatment of an episode of unipolar depression, antidepressant treatment of the depressed phase of bipolar disorder should be limited to the acute episode. Antidepressants should not be used without the concomitant administration of a mood stabilizer.

LIFE SPAN CONSIDERATIONS

As patients with bipolar disorder age, it may be beneficial to consult a geriatric psychiatrist or similarly trained professional. With increasing age and without treatment, the interval between mood episodes decreases and the duration of the episodes increases.[19] The ongoing use of powerful medications may require the monitoring of various body systems for adverse effects or decreased tolerance.

COMPLICATIONS

The complications of bipolar disorder are primarily psychosocial. Recurrences of symptoms often result in the stigma associated with inappropriate behavior. Relationships and employment are jeopardized by behaviors that are perceived as harmful or hurtful to the patient and others. Diminished financial status and credit are often the result of excessive spending and disregard for repayment during manic episodes.

Harm to self or others is the most severe consequence of bipolar disorder. Patients should be regularly monitored for mood changes that may indicate an impending acute episode. Because alcoholism is often a secondary complication associated with the disorder, the risks and results of alcoholism must also be considered if present. Careful exploration of suicidal or homicidal ideation is ongoing. It is important that the provider determine the level of impulsivity and judgment, as well as consider whether impairment may result in unreported feelings. Although importance should be placed on the patient's perceptions, these accounts may not be indicative of the actual level of danger because objectivity is obscured during an episode. In these cases, collateral informants, clinical judgment about impulsivity, knowledge of a history of dangerous or violent behavior, and knowledge of the patient's ability to convey risk accurately are infinitely valuable pieces of information.

INDICATIONS FOR REFERRAL/HOSPITALIZATION

Treatment for bipolar disorder is best administered by a psychiatrist or psychiatric nurse practitioner. Hospitalization on a psychiatric unit may be necessary if the mood disorder presents a danger to the patient or others or results in grave disability of the patient to provide for his or her basic needs. Mania may precipitate anger and violence at the threat of intervention. Anger, delusions, and hallucinations may result in homicidality or suicidality. In depressed patients, an inability to care for self and a failure to thrive may warrant hospitalization. Certainly, suicide is also a risk during a major depressive episode. To ensure patient safety, it is important that medication management and control of the disorder occur in a secure setting, where the patient will not be allowed to harm himself or herself or others.

PATIENT AND FAMILY EDUCATION

Of all patients with bipolar disorder, 85% to 95% will have a recurrence.[5] Therefore it is important to educate the patient and family about the signs and symptoms of an impending episode of depression or mania. Because the early stages of mania can be quite pleasant, likely progression of the disorder to more unpleasant stages should be discussed. Encouraging continuity with medications through education about risks and benefits can prove helpful in the quest to maintain stable mood. As always, efforts to minimize side effects maximize patient involvement in treatment and to address patient concerns are valuable. It is very important to encourage the patient to become as informed about the illness as possible. There are many published biographies and self-help books and informative sites on the Internet that can serve as valuable resources.

Education of family and friends can increase support for the patient. By teaching significant others about the disorder and risk associated with the refusal of treatment options, everyone can share in noticing the warning signs and creating plans with the patient to manage symptoms and increase safety.

REFERENCES

1. American Psychiatric Association: *Diagnostic and statistical manual of mental disorders*, ed 4, Washington, DC, 1994, The Association.
2. Kaplan HI, Sadock BJ, Grebb JA: *Kaplan and Sadock's synopsis of psychiatry*, ed 7, Baltimore, 1994, Williams & Wilkins.
3. Weissman MM and others: Cross-national epidemiology of major depression and bipolar disorder, *JAMA* 276:293-299, 1996.
4. Tsuang MT, Faraone SV, Green R: Genetic epidemiology of mood disorders. In Papolos DF, Lachman HM, editors: *Genetic studies in affective disorders*, New York, 1994, John Wiley & Sons.
5. Charney EA, Weissman MM: Epidemiology of depressive and manic syndromes. In Georgotas A, Cancro R, editors: *Depression and mania*, New York, 1988, Elsevier.
6. Keck PE Jr, McElroy SL, Arnold L: Bipolar disorder, *Med Clin North Am* 85:645-661, 2001.
7. Calabrese JR and others: A double-blind placebo-controlled study of lamotrigine monotherapy in outpatients with bipolar I depression, *J Clin Psychiatr* 60:79-88, 1999.
8. Potash JB, DePaulo JR: Searching high and low: a review of the genetics of bipolar disorder, *Bipolar Disord* 2:8, 2000.
9. Craddock N, Jones I: Molecular genetics of bipolar disorder, *Br J Psychiatr* 178:S128, 2001.
10. Goodwin F, Jamison KR: *Manic depressive illness*, New York, 1990, Oxford University Press.
11. Schad-Somers SP: *On mood swings*, New York, 1990, Plenum Press.
12. Sachs G: Approach to the patient with elevated, expansive, or irritable mood. In Stern TA, Herman JB, Slavin PL, editors: *The MGH guide to psychiatry in primary care*, New York, 1998, McGraw-Hill.
13. Blazer D: Mood disorders. In Kaplan HI, Sadock BJ, editors: *Comprehensive textbook of psychiatry*, ed 5, Baltimore, 1995, Williams and Wilkins.
14. Hilty DM, Brady KT, Hales RE: A review of bipolar disorder among adults, *Psychiatr Serv* 50:201-213, 1999.
15. Jefferson JW: Lithium. In Goodnick PA, editor: *Predictors of treatment response in mood disorders*, Washington, DC, 1996, American Psychiatric Press.
16. Freeman MP, Stoll AL: Mood-stabilizer combination: a review of safety and efficacy, *Am J Psychiatry* 155:12-21, 1998.
17. Glick ID and others: Psychopharmacologic treatment strategies for depression, bipolar disorder, and schizophrenia, *Ann Intern Med* 134:47, 2001.
18. Krauthammer C, Klerman GL: Secondary mania: manic syndromes associated with antecedent physical illness or drugs, *Arch Gen Psychiatry* 30:74-79, 1978.
19. Winokur G and others: Alcoholism in manic-depressive (bipolar) illness, and the primary-secondary distinction, *Am J Psychiatry* 152:365-372, 1995.

CHAPTER 262

Depressive Disorders

Nancy S. Mahan

DEFINITION/EPIDEMIOLOGY

Although approximately 10 million Americans (20% of the population) suffer from depression, only one third of them seek treatment. Of this one third, most seek treatment in a primary care setting. In primary care, patients often present with vague somatic complaints that have no known medical etiology. Such complaints may mask an underlying and potentially severe depressive disorder. Depression goes largely undetected for many patients given the lack of attunement to such concerns by many primary care practitioners. Additionally, because of the brief amount of time that practitioners can spend talking with and getting to know their patients given health care reimbursement protocols, accurate diagnosis of major depressive disorder can easily be missed except in patients with extreme symptoms.

Although people often refer to feeling depressed, it is important to note that depressive disorders differ from the experiences that everyone occasionally has of feeling down for a week or two. It is normal for children, adolescents, adults, and older adults to have ranges of emotional experience and expression that involve a case of the blues or to experience times of sadness, grief, irritability, and/or melancholy. In general, these experiences pass with time and support and do not require medical or psychiatric care. When these experiences become more acute in severity or more chronic in nature, treatment is needed. To determine appropriate interventions and treatments, it is imperative to discern the differences between these types of experiences.

Depressive disorders are illnesses that affect mood and result in a range of feelings and symptoms including anhedonia; feelings of helplessness, hopelessness, worthlessness, and guilt; sleep disruption; changes in appetite; irritability; impairment in occupational and interpersonal functioning; feelings of personal failure; rejection sensitivity; a propensity to interpret events, thoughts, and affect states from a negative perspective; difficulty with concentration; decreased energy and fatigue; psychomotor disturbances; and recurrent thoughts of or a preoccupation with death and/or suicide. In some instances, psychotic distortions in thoughts, perceptions, and/or beliefs emerge as hallucinations or delusions. Depressive illnesses render enormous suffering for patients and families and commonly result in the erosion of hope, the promise for a future, faith, and overall quality of life. In the most acute stages, a patient may be at significant risk of suicide; 10% to 15% of individuals diagnosed with major depressive disorder successfully complete suicide.[1]

Both nature and nurture play a strong role in the etiology of depressive disorders. Although there is a significant genetic component that predisposes individuals to develop a major depressive disorder, several environmental factors also put a person at risk. These factors include gender (women are two to three times more likely than men to develop the disorder), a history of traumatic events, premature parental loss, personality (specifically introversion), negligent or abusive parenting, no or few social supports, and the occurrence of recent stressful events.

Several types of depressive disorders and current research suggest that the etiology of depressive disorders may vary significantly depending on the neurologic pathogenesis of a particular syndrome or symptom cluster. Initially, episodes of depression are commonly precipitated by stressful life events (e.g., death of a loved one, divorce). However, for individuals who go on to experience persistent episodes, the psychosocial precipitants appear to play a decreasing, if not irrelevant, role. The differing types of depressive disorders include major depressive disorder (MDD), dysthymic disorder, substance-induced depressive disorder, seasonal affective disorder, postpartum depression, psychotic depression, bipolar disorder, and atypical depression.

Major Depressive Disorder

It is estimated that approximately 1 out of 10 people treated in a primary care setting have MDD.[1] As defined by the fourth edition of the *Diagnostic and Statistical Manual of Mental Disorders Text Revision* (DSM-IV-TR), episodes of MDD can be single or recurrent. More than 50% of people who have a single episode go on to have a recurrent episode.[2] If left untreated, each episode can last as long as 2 years in one third of all patients, resulting in significant impairment in psychosocial functioning and quality of life. According to Kessler and others,[3] there is a very high lifetime co-morbidity of MDD with anxiety disorders (58%). There is also a high co-morbidity with substance abuse disorders (38.6%).[3] The high co-morbidity of MDD with anxiety and substance abuse disorders generally results in more serious impairment in functioning and an increased severity and persistence of symptoms. Individuals in whom anxiety and/or substance abuse disorders complicate a depressive illness are more depressed and are depressed longer. The diagnostic criteria for MDD are listed in Box 262-1.

The recurrence of depressive episodes is likely if an individual has had only a partial recovery. The more episodes experienced, the more likely an individual will have depressive episodes in the future. If a person has had three episodes, the likelihood of experiencing another episode is 90%.[2]

Further aggravating the debilitating symptoms that occur with MDD is the worry about suicide. Approximately 1 out of 10 people with MDD die as a result of suicide. Suicide associated with MDD is significantly higher among adolescents and among persons with associated substance abuse, panic, and/or psychotic disorders. However, depression is usually highly treatable, with most people enjoying full or partial recovery. Approximately one fourth of individuals with depression do not experience full recovery between episodes. This is most common for people who have what is called a double depression, in which an episode of MDD occurs after (at minimum) a 2-year period of dysthymic disorder.

There is a much higher incidence of depression among women (twice as high for adolescent girls and women as compared with adolescent boys and men).[2] This difference may be related to hormonal differences and social conditioning.

BOX 262-1

CRITERIA FOR MAJOR DEPRESSIVE DISORDER

A. Five (or more) of the following symptoms have been present during the same 2-week period and represent a change from previous functioning; at least one of the symptoms is either (1) depressed mood or (2) loss of interest or pleasure.

Note: Do not include symptoms that are clearly due to general medical condition, or mood-incongruent delusions or hallucinations.

(1) depressed mood most of the day, nearly every day, as indicated by either subjective report (e.g., feels sad or empty) or observation made by others (e.g., appears tearful) **Note:** In children and in adolescents, can be irritable mood

(2) markedly diminished interest or pleasure in all, or almost all, activities most of the day, nearly every day (as indicated by either subjective report or observations made by others)

(3) significant weight loss when not dieting or weight gain (e.g., a change of more than 5% of body weight in a month), or decrease or increase in appetite early every day. **Note:** In children, considerable failure to make expected weight gains

(4) insomnia or hypersomnia nearly every day

(5) psychomotor agitation or retardation nearly every day (observable by others, not merely subjective feelings of restlessness or being slowed down)

(6) fatigue or loss of energy nearly every day

(7) feelings of worthlessness or excessive or inappropriate guilt (which may be delusional) nearly every day (not merely self-reproach or guilt about being sick)

(8) diminished ability to think or concentrate, or indecisiveness, nearly every day (either by subjective account or as observed by others)

(9) recurrent thoughts of death (not just fear of dying), recurrent suicidal ideation without a specific plan, or a suicide attempt or a specific plan for committing suicide

B. The symptoms do not meet the criteria for a Mixed Episode.

C. The symptoms cause clinically significant distress or impairment in social, occupational, or other important areas of functioning.

D. The symptoms are not due to the direct physiologic effects of a substance (e.g., a drug of abuse, a medication) or a general medical condition (e.g., hypothyroidism).

E. The symptoms are not better accounted for by Bereavement, i.e., after the loss of a loved one, the symptoms persist longer than two months or are characterized by marked functional impairment, morbid preoccupation with worthlessness, suicidal ideation, psychotic symptoms, or psychomotor retardation.

From American Psychiatric Association: *Diagnostic and statistical manual of mental disorders,* ed 4 (Text revision 2000), Washington DC, 1994, The Association.

Women commonly experience aggression/frustration against the self, whereas men learn to direct it outwardly. In addition, women may be more comfortable than men in seeking help regarding depressive symptoms.

Dysthymic Disorder

A diagnosis of dysthymic disorder can be made when the onset of depressive symptoms is less discreet, when the symptom picture is less acute, and when the experience has been more chronic in nature (Box 262-2). The duration of these more chronic symptoms must be in excess of 2 years (1 year in children). In general, patients who suffer from dysthymia do not require hospitalization because their symptoms are less acute. Although patients respond to pharmacotherapy, talk psychotherapy is often needed to assist in coping with the more chronic assaults to self-esteem and the feelings of hopelessness and inadequacy. Such persistently chronic feelings of worthlessness can put patients at risk for suicide and substance abuse.

Substance-Induced Depressive Disorder

A diagnosis of substance abuse-induced depression should be given whenever depressive symptoms (either a depressed or elevated, irritable mood) emerge as a result of the use of illegal drugs, medications, or toxins. Depressive symptoms may emerge as a result of the physiologic effect of, or withdrawal from, the drug or toxin. This information must be obtained through the patient history or by reviewing laboratory results. As opposed to a diagnosis of substance intoxication or withdrawal, a diagnosis of substance abuse-induced depression should occur when symptoms exceed what is usually seen with intoxication and withdrawal syndromes or when symptoms are severe enough to warrant independent evaluation and treatment. A list of mood-altering medications is provided in Box 262-3.

Seasonal Affective Disorder

Some individuals experience episodes of MDD that emerge in the fall and last through the winter and cannot be attributed to other biologic or psychosocial stressors. The higher the latitude, the more prevalent the incidence of these seasonal depressions. In addition to more traditional treatment with therapy and medications, exposure to intense light has been shown to be effective in ameliorating symptoms.

Postpartum Depression

When the onset of depression occurs within 4 weeks after the birth of an infant, the condition is called postpartum depression. The overall symptoms are similar to MDD, but in addition the mother often has psychotic symptoms that involve delusional thoughts about her infant and potentially her other children. Postpartum depression occurs in up to 1 in 500 births and in its most severe forms can be dangerous for the infant, because it can result in infanticide.[2] The mother is often

BOX 262-2

DIAGNOSTIC CRITERIA FOR DYSTHYMIC DISORDER

A. Depressed mood for most of the day, for more days than not, as indicated either by subjective account or observation by others, for at least 2 years. **Note:** In children and adolescents, mood can be irritable and duration must be at least 1 year.

B. Presence, while depressed, of two (or more) of the following:
   (1) poor appetite or overeating
   (2) insomnia or hypersomnia
   (3) low energy or fatigue
   (4) low self-esteem
   (5) poor concentration or difficulty making decisions
   (6) feelings of hopelessness

C. During the 2-year period (1 year for children or adolescents) of the disturbance, the person has never been without symptoms in Criteria A and B for more than 2 months at a time.

D. No Major Depressive Episode has been present during the first 2 years of the disturbance (1 year for children and adolescents); i.e., the disturbance is not better accounted for by chronic Major Depressive Disorder, or Major Depressive Disorder, in Partial Remission.
   Note: There may have been a previous Major Depressive Episode provided there was a full remission (no significant signs or symptoms for 2 months) before development of the Dysthymic Disorder. In addition, after the initial 2 years (1 year in children or adolescents) of Dysthmic Disorder, there may be superimposed episodes of Major Depressive Disorder, in which case both diagnoses may be given when the criteria are met for a Major Depressive Episode.

E. There has never been a Manic Episode, a Mixed Episode, or a Hypomanic Episode, and criteria have never been met for Cyclothymic Disorder.

F. The disturbance does not occur exclusively during the course of a chronic Psychotic Disorder, such as Schizophrenia or Delusional Disorder.

G. The symptoms are not due to the direct physiologic effects of a substance (e.g., a drug abuse, a medication) or a general medical condition (e.g., hypothyroidism).

H. The symptoms cause clinically significant distress or impairment in social, occupational, or other important areas of functioning.

Specify if:
   Early Onset: if onset is before age 21 years
   Late Onset: if onset is age 21 years or older
Specify (for most recent 2 years of Dysthymic Disorder):
   With Atypical Features

From American Psychiatric Association: *Diagnostic and statistical manual of mental disorders,* ed 4 (Text revision 2000), Washington DC, 1994. The Association.

very anxious, labile, and panicky; is prone to uncontrollable crying; and, in addition to treatment, needs significant emotional support and assistance with the infant (and any other children). Separation from the infant may be necessary despite the disruptions this can cause in the development of normal attachment. The mother may need to cease breastfeeding if pharmacologic interventions are initiated.

Psychotic Depression

With psychotic depression, a patient exhibits all the signs and symptoms of MDD, as well as psychotic symptoms that are not related to the presence of another psychotic disorder such as schizophrenia. Psychotic symptoms may include delusions and/or hallucinations. Psychotic depression is associated with a high incidence of suicide and commonly warrants inpatient care until the patient is stabilized. Pharmacologic treatment should include antidepressant and antipsychotic medications.

Bipolar Disorder

Bipolar disorder is characterized by episodes of mania and depression, or extreme highs and lows (see Chapter 261). Psychotic features may or may not be present during manic episodes.

Atypical Depression

Atypical depression is characterized by atypical features. For example, a patient sleeps excessively as opposed to experiencing insomnia, eats excessively rather than demonstrates disinterest in eating, or describes more persistent feelings of irritability and anxiety as opposed to melancholia.

All patients with suicidal/homicidal ideation require immediate psychiatric evaluation.

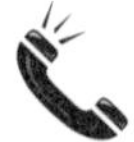

Physician consultation is indicated for patients who do not respond to the treatment plan.

PATHOPHYSIOLOGY

To date, the most convincing research in the pathophysiology of depressive disorders suggests deficiencies in serotonergic neurotransmission (Box 262-4).

BOX 262-3

MEDICATIONS NOTED TO ALTER MOOD

MEDICATIONS ASSOCIATED WITH INTOXICATION
Alcohol
Amphetamine and related substances
Anxiolytics
Cocaine
Hallucinogens
Hypnotics
Inhalants
Opioids
Phencyclidine/related substances
Sedatives

MEDICATIONS ASSOCIATED WITH WITHDRAWAL
Alcohol
Amphetamines and related substances
Anxiolytics
Cocaine
Hypnotics
Sedatives

OTHER MEDICATIONS NOTED TO EVOKE MOOD SYMPTOMS
Analgesics
Anesthetics
Anticholinergics
Anticonvulsants
Antihypertensives
Antiparkinsonian medications
Antiulcer medications
Oral contraceptives
Psychotropic medications
Muscle relaxants
Steroids
Sulfonamides

Data from American Psychiatric Association: *Diagnostic and statistical manual of mental disorders*, ed 4 (Text revision 2000), Washington DC, 1994, The Association.

BOX 262-4

DATA SUPPORTING SEROTONIN DYSFUNCTION IN MAJOR DEPRESSION

1. There are decreased concentrations of brain serotonin and cerebrospinal fluid 5-HIAA in many depressed patients.
2. Most antidepressant agents have been shown to increase the efficacy of central serotonin neurotransmission.
3. A reduction in both central and peripheral 5-HT reuptake sites has been found in depressed subjects.
4. Neuroendocrine challenges have demonstrated that the postsynaptic serotonin-mediated stimulation of prolactin is blunted in patients who are depressed.

Modified from Stoudemire A: *Clinical psychiatry for medical students*, ed 2, Philadelphia, 1994, Lippincott-Raven.

CLINICAL PRESENTATION

Disability, loss of health, aging and its accompanying losses, economic stresses secondary to health problems, chronic pain, and a range of other somatic complaints that may be a reaction to the illness can complicate or mask an underlying depressive disorder. A careful, complete history, including exploration of the following questions, is needed to determine the presence of a depressive disorder. An affirmative response to one or several of these inquiries may suggest the presence of a depressive syndrome:

- Is there a family history of affective disorders or addictive disorders?
- Does the patient have a previous history of depression?
- Does the patient have a history of suicide attempts or a family history of suicide attempts?
- Has the patient endured a recent loss?
- Does the patient have difficulty falling or staying asleep? Does the patient sleep too much?
- Does the patient feel helpless, hopeless, worthless, or excessively guilty?
- Does the patient experience anhedonia?
- Is the patient excessively irritable?
- Has the patient had a significant unintentional weight loss or gain?
- Have the patient's feelings and behaviors resulted in disruptions in family, relational, or occupational functioning?
- Does the patient describe an overwhelming sense of impending doom?
- Is there evidence of psychomotor retardation or psychomotor agitation?
- Does the patient have thoughts or plans for suicide?
- If the patient is a child or adolescent, has there been a significant change in his or her behavior (e.g., an affable child becomes socially isolated)?

PHYSICAL EXAMINATION

A thorough history and examination are necessary to identify the substances or general medical conditions responsible for the symptoms. The physical examination may be negative, but weight gain or loss, confusion, or psychomotor agitation may be present.

DIAGNOSTICS

It is necessary to exclude a physiologic cause for the patient's symptoms. There are no current diagnostic or laboratory tests that provide definitive information regarding the presence or absence of a depressive disorder.

Potential medical conditions should be excluded before beginning treatment for depression; however, several assessment scales are useful in determining the presence of symptoms that may suggest evidence of a depressive disorder. Commonly used instruments include the Center for Epidemiological Studies Depression Scale, the Beck Depression Inventory, the Zung Self-Rating Scale, and the Hamilton Rating Scale for Depression. The first three are completed by the patient and rely on self-report. The Hamilton scale is interviewer rated.

DIFFERENTIAL DIAGNOSIS

Multiple medical disorders present with depressive symptoms, including immunologic disorders (e.g., lupus, HIV-related illnesses, and multiple sclerosis), terminal illnesses, myocardial infarction, substance abuse disorders, infectious diseases (e.g., tuberculosis and postviral fatigue syndrome), and neurologic conditions (e.g., Parkinson's disease, seizures, dementias). If there are psychotic symptoms not related to an underlying psychotic disorder, it is important to exclude brain tumors and thyroid problems. In addition, certain medications cause iatrogenic depressive symptoms.

MANAGEMENT

Major depressive disorder can be treated in the primary care arena, primarily through the use of pharmacotherapy. Many patients, however, benefit from specialized treatment by psychiatrically trained professionals, as they can augment medications with a range of psychosocial treatments that serve to better enhance outcomes. Some patients do not consider treatment by a psychiatrist or other mental health professional because of the stigma that continues to pervade behavioral health disorders and their treatments. Principal considerations for referral to a specialist are the severity of the patient's condition, the existence of coexistent psychiatric disorders, the patient's network of familial and personal supports, and the patient's likely adherence to a treatment plan. Although adherence to treatment is an issue in most medical illnesses, a trusting relationship with the practitioner directly influences patients' adherence specific to major depressive disorder. Remission may take time, and often patients must tolerate side effects of the medications that interfere with adherence. Many primary care practitioners do not always have the time to develop and maintain the frequency of contact that many patients require to get better. Additionally, given the potential for suicide and the chronicity of depressive disorders for a large portion of patients, ongoing consultation or referral to a psychiatric specialist is often indicated.

Depressive disorders are generally responsive to adequate treatments; most patients get better, enjoy premorbid activities, and resume their previous level of functioning. A significant number of patients get better with aggressive treatment but never fully recover or return to their previous level of functioning. A small percentage of patients are unresponsive to existing treatments. Risk factors for patients who appear to be resistant to treatment include failure to adhere to the prescribed treatment plan, presence of one or more coexisting psychiatric or medical illnesses, or underlying psychodynamic issues that interfere with a patient's capacity to see and feel worthy or psychologically healthy (or where secondary gains or reinforcement of the sick role is more compelling than wellness). In some situations, the patient may have a more rapid cycling bipolar illness that can appear as MDD but is responsive to different treatment interventions.

Because depressive disorders are associated with high lethality, the first task of assessment is to evaluate the patient's potential risk for self-harm and to ensure patient safety. Treatment can be initiated once safety is established (depending on acuity of the symptoms and potential for suicide, inpatient care may be warranted). The most effective treatment for depressive disorders is a combination of antidepressant medication and psychosocial interventions.

It is common for patients with depressive disorders to receive inadequate pharmacologic treatment, especially in the primary care arena. However, antidepressant medications have shown enormous efficacy in the treatment and amelioration of depressive disorders.

The American Psychiatric Association (APA) has developed practice guidelines for the treatment of major depressive disorder that are specific to differing phases of the illness: acute (0 to 16 weeks), continuation (16 to 18 weeks), and maintenance (18+ weeks). In the acute phase, an antidepressant (selective serotonin reuptake inhibitor [SSRI]) should be initiated and the patient should be closely monitored. Medications should be introduced slowly to minimize side effects. Tricyclic antidepressants and SSRIs are appropriate antidepressants prescribed by primary care providers. Both types of medications are equally efficacious, but the side effect profile of SSRIs is generally less problematic for patients. Monoamine oxidase inhibitors, the earliest medications used to treat depressive disorders, are used rarely in contemporary practice because of their extensive interactions with medications and foods. They should generally be prescribed when other medication classes have been ineffective and only to those patients who can follow adherence guidelines carefully.

In general, it takes approximately 4 to 6 weeks to yield a significant reduction or remission of symptoms. Patients who have a favorable response to medications should be encouraged to continue taking these medications for at least 4 months after a positive response. Commonly prescribed antidepressants are described in Table 262-1; antidepressants are often chosen by their side effect profile.

If there is only partial or no remission in symptoms, either the medication dosage should be increased or another antidepressant should be tried. The APA's practice guideline indicates that when another medication is tried, it should first be from the same class. If two medication trials from the same class are unsuccessful, then a medication from another class should be tried. Similarly, other classes can be tried if results are not favorable. If there continues to be no response, adjunctive treatment with a medication that will potentiate the SSRI, such as lithium, may be tried. When medications are not effective and the depressive symptoms are severe, electroconvulsive therapy (ECT) should be considered.

ECT involves passing an electrical current through the brain to induce a series of generalized seizures. Current research is inconclusive with regard to how ECT actually works, but it is hypothesized that these seizures render changes in

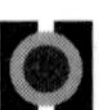

Differential Diagnosis

Depressive Disorder	
Immunologic disorder	Neurologic condition
Terminal illness	Adrenal dysfunction
Myocardial infarction	Thyroid dysfunction
Substance abuse disorders	Tumor
Infectious disease	Medication-induced depression
Postviral fatigue syndrome	

TABLE 262-1 Commonly Used Antidepressant Medications

Generic Name	Starting Dose* (mg/day)	Usual Dose (mg/day)
TRICYCLICS AND TETRACYCLICS		
Tertiary Amine Tricyclics		
Amitriptyline	25-50	100-300
Clomipramine	25	100-250
Doxepin	25-50	100-300
Imipramine	25-50	100-300
Trimipramine	25-50	100-300
Secondary Amine Tricyclics		
Desipramine†	25-50	100-300
Nortriptyline†	25	50-200
Protriptyline	10	15-60
Tetracyclics		
Amoxapine	50	100-400
Maprotiline	50	100-225
SELECTIVE SEROTONIN REUPTAKE INHIBITORS†		
Citalopram	20	20-60‡
Fluoxetine	20	20-60‡
Fluvoxamine	50	50-300‡
Paroxetine	20	20-60‡
Sertraline	50	50-200‡
DOPAMINE-NOREPINEPHRINE REUPTAKE INHIBITORS		
Bupropion†	150	300
Bupropion, sustained release	150	300
SEROTONIN-NOREPINEPHRINE REUPTAKE INHIBITORS		
Venlafaxine†	37.5	75-225
Venlafaxine, extended release	37.5	75-225
SEROTONIN MODULATORS		
Nefazodone	50	150-300
Trazodone	50	75-300
NOREPINEPHRINE-SEROTONIN MODULATOR		
Mirtazapine	15	15-45
MONOAMINE OXIDASE INHIBITORS (MAOI)		
Irreversible, Nonselective		
Phenelzine	15	15-90
Tranylcypromine	10	30-60
Reversible MAOI-A		
Moclobemide	150	300-600
Selective noradrenaline reuptake inhibitor		
Reboxetine	§	§

From the American Psychiatric Association: *American Psychiatric Association practice guideline for the treatment of patients with major depressive disorder,* ed 2, Washington, DC, 2000, American Psychiatric Publishing.

*Lower starting doses are recommended for older patients and for patients with panic disorder, significant anxiety or hepatic disease, and general co-morbidity.

†These medications are likely to be optimal medications in terms of the patient's acceptance of side effects, safety, and quantity and quality of clinical trial data.

‡Dose varies with diagnosis; see text for specific guidelines.

§FDA approval is anticipated. When available, consult manufacturer's package insert or the Physician's Desk Reference for recommended starting and usual doses.

neurotransmitter receptors. Changes in these receptors are similar to those seen in patients who have been on long-term pharmacotherapy with antidepressants.

Current research suggests that ECT is one of the safest treatments for MDD and psychotic depression. It works quickly (one of its prime benefits) and has often proven useful for patients who are unresponsive to lengthy trials of varied antidepressant medications. Because ECT causes short-term, temporary confusion and memory loss, it is often conducted while the patient is hospitalized. It also renders minor structural changes in the brain; the long-term implications of such changes are unknown. For many with MDD or psychotic depression, ECT is lifesaving. The temporary problems of memory loss and confusion pale in terms of the exigencies of suffering with acute depressive symptoms and the resulting loss of quality of life or risk as a result of suicide.

Also during the acute phase, psychosocial treatments added to the pharmacologic regimen serve to enhance outcomes. Current research supports the effectiveness of cognitive behavioral therapy for most patients with depressive disorders. Other therapies that can be helpful include behavioral, interpersonal, or psychodynamic therapies. Because of the stress of depressive disorders on the family, marital and/or family therapy may also be helpful. In the acute phase of the disorder, once there is partial remission of symptoms, patients with suicidal ideation may often be at more risk. This increased risk occurs because the person has more energy to act on their suicidal thoughts and plans. This risk must be closely monitored by the practitioner, and the patient should be hospitalized, as needed, in a secure setting to ensure patient safety.

Practice guidelines for the continuation phase of treatment have been determined based on whether this is the first or a recurring episode of depression. For patients who have experienced their first episode, and who evidence remission of depressive symptoms, medication should be slowly decreased. The patient should be monitored carefully for evidence of recurring symptoms. Patients with two or more episodes of MDD should be considered for long-term maintenance therapy at the dose that alleviated their symptoms.

As with the acute phase, in the continuation phase of treatment, psychotherapies that augment pharmacologic interventions should be continued to effectively monitor patients and provide them with education and support that enables them to pick up on early detection of recurring symptoms and improve their overall functioning. Cognitive therapy examines and works to change negative thought patterns that are common to patients with depressive disorders. These negative thought patterns (e.g., all-or-nothing thinking, catastrophic thinking, negative self-image, negative interpretation of events and experiences, a negative anticipation of the future) reinforce depressive affects. With training and practice, these disordered thoughts can be altered by stopping such thoughts and replacing them with more positive or neutral thoughts. Other types of psychotherapies (e.g., interpersonal, psychodynamic, existentialist, self-psychology, relational, and family) work to decrease the patient's isolation, improve self-understanding and esteem, and work toward making changes that improve quality of life.

In the maintenance phase of treatment, the patient who has had more than two episodes of major depressive disorder should continue taking medications, but does not require such intensive monitoring by the practitioner. Adjunctive therapies may continue to enhance long-term outcome in that they assist the patient in maintaining adherence to the treatment plan and because they enable the patient to develop an understanding of the factors that led to their depression. Although there are strong biologic underpinnings to depressive illnesses, there are a variety of lifestyle factors that make one more vulnerable to depressive disorders, and often the patient must make his or her peace with life circumstances or make changes in the service of improved well-being and mental health. Such changes can be facilitated by participation in behavioral therapies.

Regardless of the phase of treatment, when more than one practitioner is involved, communication between providers can be essential in managing the patient's symptoms, adherence, and relapses. Communication protocols should be negotiated up front with the patient and whenever possible include the patient as an active partner in the treatment planning and review.

LIFE SPAN CONSIDERATIONS

Although depressive disorders can emerge at any point in a patient's life span, recurring episodes are more the norm than the exception. Thus it is important that practitioners, patients, and family members recognize the chronic nature of depressive disorders for most patients.

As previously noted, various life events can precipitate a first episode of depressive illness such as a significant loss, development of a serious medical condition, or birth of a child as with postpartum depression. However, subsequent recurring episodes are not strongly correlated with precipitating conditions or events.

People from all age-groups (including toddlers) can experience serious depressive disorders. Depending on age, different symptom clusters are apparent. In children, irritability is a far more prominent symptom than sadness. Depressed children are often more socially withdrawn and have more somatic complaints, especially headaches and stomachaches. Although children may not understand the meaning or consequences of death, the risk for suicide exists even with young children, particularly if there has been a suicide by a family member or friend. One of the most predictive risk factors for children who commit suicide is the presence of a problem that they believe is completely unsolvable. Although some children can describe their feelings and share their thoughts, this ability depends on the child's developmental level (and personality); assessment of depression must rely more heavily on observations of behavior. Episodes of depression cause significant disruptions in a child's capacity to successfully maneuver through the normal stages of development and as a result may render developmental arrest and further precipitate a variety of psychosocial challenges.

Depression in adolescents is difficult to assess and, unfortunately, is often not diagnosed or treated accurately. It is twice as common in females as in males. Irritable mood is common, and sadness is not necessarily a requisite symptom. Suicide is the second leading cause of death among adolescents, and such suicides often erupt in clusters in communities as a result of the phenomenon of contagion.

Older adults may not complain outwardly about depressive symptoms but may instead describe a range of somatic complaints. Depression in older adults is often characterized by a prominence of cognitive symptoms such as memory loss, confusion, disorientation, and distractibility. Other prominent symptoms include the presence of somatic or persecutory delusions, agitation, and irritability. Depression has a poorer prognosis in older adults (with a higher relapse rate, a higher incidence of suicide, and a lower remission of symptoms), and some research suggests that this is particularly evident for older adults experiencing a psychotic depression. The differential diagnosis can be difficult with geriatric patients because of the frequent co-morbidity of serious medical conditions that may mimic or include depressive symptoms. Assessment of depression can be further complicated by the normative experiences involved in coping with loss, social isolation, and/or grief, all of which can be experienced more often by adults in later life. ECT may be indicated for older adults who do not respond to psychopharmacologic treatment.

COMPLICATIONS

The most serious complication of depressive disorders is the high risk for suicide. The risk is quite high for adolescents, older adults, and patients who suffer from concomitant substance abuse, psychosis, and/or anxiety disorders. Suicide is most prevalent at the beginning or end of a depressive episode.[1] Research indicates that 80% of people who kill themselves shared their intentions with others before their successful suicide.[1] Although there are no guaranteed methods for predicting suicide, there are ways to assess increased risk, and there are several assessment scales such as the Beck Suicidal Ideation Scale and the Risk Estimator Scale for Suicide. Given the high correlation of helplessness with suicidality, the Beck Helplessness Scale is also a useful assessment scale. Although assessment scales differ, they generally review a combination of demographic and psychologic factors that statistically indicate that the patient may be at risk. Some of the primary risk factors include the following:

- The presence of another psychiatric disorder, specifically a substance abuse disorder, anxiety (particularly panic disorder), or a psychotic disorder
- A history of successful suicide(s) by a family member or friend
- A history of previous attempts
- The presence of a specific plan (the risk increases significantly if the patient also has the means to carry out this plan)
- The presence of command hallucinations or delusional depression
- Recent loss
- Serious medical illness
- Gender (men complete more suicides because they use more lethal means, such as guns and hanging; women make more suicide attempts and have a higher tendency to use methods involving drug overdose, cutting, and gas)
- Age (older adults have the highest incidence)
- Race (whites have a higher incidence of suicide than nonwhites)
- An experience of helplessness, guilt, shame, desperation, or humiliation (these experiences are highly correlated with suicide)[4]

INDICATIONS FOR REFERRAL/HOSPITALIZATION

Concern regarding a patient's potential for self-harm mandates immediate consultation with another colleague or physician. If a patient has a significant prior medical history of depression, or if the depressive symptoms are unresponsive to pharmacologic and psychosocial interventions, it is recommended that additional consultation be secured. For situations in which the patient has other complicating medical problems, a pharmacologic consultation should be secured to maximize treatment effectiveness. Indications for hospitalization or referral include the following:

- Suicidality
- Inability to care for oneself
- Initiation of ECT
- Evaluation and treatment with psychotherapy and/or cognitive therapy
- Education and support for family members
- Treatment of children, adolescents, and older adults

PATIENT AND FAMILY EDUCATION

It is important that patients and families receive education regarding the physiology of mood disorders and the symptoms identified with depression. A thorough understanding of the chronicity of depression, prognosis, importance of treatment, and medication side effects is essential. A collaborative patient-provider relationship and frequent monitoring (two to three times weekly) until the patient is stable provide support for the patient and permit early identification of risk factors for treatment failure and suicide.

HEALTH PROMOTION

Given the widespread incidence of depressive illnesses in the general public, education and routine screening as part of the physical examination should be implemented by all primary care practitioners. Such proactive practice will increase the detection of depressive disorders and, over time, will minimize the stigma associated with depression and other psychiatric conditions and their treatment. Simultaneously, such education and early detection will enable patients to receive requisite treatment and reduce their often considerable suffering. Many clinics and hospitals additionally participate in National Depression Screening Day activities at local schools, religious institutions, shopping malls, and community centers. National Depression Screening Day takes place in early to mid October of every year and is part of the National Institute of Mental Health's Mental Illness Awareness Month.

REFERENCES

1. Kaplan H, Sadock B: *Synopsis of psychiatry: behavioral sciences/clinical psychiatry*, ed 8, Baltimore, 1998, Williams & Wilkins.
2. American Psychiatric Association: *Diagnostic and statistical manual of mental disorders*, ed 4, Text Revision, Washington, DC, 1994, The Association.
3. Kessler RC and others: Comorbidity of DSM III-R major depressive disorder in the general population: results from the US National Comorbidity Survey, *Br J Psychiatry* 168(Suppl 30):17-38, 1996.
4. Hales RE, Yudofsky SC, Talbott JA, editors: *The American Psychiatric Press textbook of psychiatry*, ed 2, Washington, DC, 1994, American Psychiatric Press.

CHAPTER 263

Eating Disorders*

Barbara E. Wolfe, Eran D. Metzger, and David C. Jimerson

DEFINITION/EPIDEMIOLOGY

Anorexia nervosa and bulimia nervosa are psychiatric disorders characterized by excessive concern with body shape and weight. Impaired psychosocial functioning often accompanies these disorders, and serious medical consequences may arise as a result of the behavioral manifestations of the illness. Diagnostic criteria and clinical characteristics are reviewed in detail later.

Eating disorders occur in approximately 2% to 3% of female adolescents and young adults.[1-3] Typically bulimia nervosa is more common than anorexia, although the reverse may be true in some cultures.[4] Women are 10 times more likely than men to be affected by an eating disorder. White women tend to report greater disturbances in eating, as well as body dissatisfaction, compared with minority groups, although ethnic differences appear to diminish when formal clinical disorders are examined.[5] Age of onset is typically during adolescence and young adulthood. The course of the illness is quite variable and is often influenced by medical complications and psychiatric co-morbidity. For patients with anorexia nervosa, crude mortality rates are approximately 5% with fatalities associated with co-morbid psychopathology and a history of bingeing and purging behavior.[6]

PATHOPHYSIOLOGY

Psychologic and environmental factors are likely to influence the development of an eating disorder. Recent research has been directed at understanding potential biologic influences, including variations in neurochemicals involved in the modulation of eating behavior. Laboratory studies have shown that stimulation of carbohydrate intake may result from increased activity of norepinephrine and neuropeptide Y in the hypothalamus. Serotonin and cholecystokinin suppress food intake and increase satiety. Dopamine and opiates influence food cravings and the food reward system. Studies in laboratory animals suggest that leptin decreases food intake while also increasing the use of energy.

Initial studies have demonstrated abnormalities in several of these neurochemical systems in patients with active symptoms of anorexia nervosa and bulimia nervosa. However, little is known regarding which of these alterations may be a consequence of the illness itself. Investigations suggest that, although some abnormalities return to normal with the remission of symptoms, certain changes (e.g., in the serotonin system) may be more persistent.

CLINICAL PRESENTATION

Patients with anorexia nervosa typically exhibit denial regarding the potential seriousness of their reduced weight state. Despite life-threatening cachexia, these patients maintain a need to lose

*Supported in part by a USPHS grant (K07 MH00965) from the National Institute of Mental Health.

weight, often reflecting distortions in body image. Many patients with anorexia nervosa have other coexisting psychiatric disorders.[7] Depression is common, with depressive symptoms often remitting after weight restoration. An estimated 25% to 50% of patients with anorexia nervosa have a lifetime history of an anxiety disorder, including obsessive-compulsive disorder, panic disorder, social phobia, or generalized anxiety disorder. Up to one third of patients with anorexia nervosa, particularly those with the binge-eating/purging type, have a co-morbid alcohol or substance abuse/dependence disorder.

Patients with bulimia nervosa characteristically present with feelings of shame and embarrassment regarding their symptoms. Efforts to maintain the secrecy of the disorder are often accompanied by social withdrawal and a denial of illness. Psychiatric co-morbidity is common.[7] As many as half of the patients with bulimia nervosa have a lifetime history of major depression. Alcohol and substance abuse/dependence disorders are also common, perhaps reflecting increased impulsivity in this patient group. Approximately one third of patients with bulimia nervosa have a lifetime history of an anxiety disorder, which generally includes social phobia, obsessive-compulsive disorder, or generalized anxiety disorder.

Other conditions that may be evident on presentation include personality disorders and trauma history. Dependent, avoidant, obsessive-compulsive, and borderline are the most commonly occurring personality disorders in patients with eating disorders.[7] Borderline personality disorder appears to more frequent in bulimia nervosa than in anorexia nervosa, perhaps contributing to impulse dysregulation and self-destructive behavior at times observed in this patient group. Sexual trauma in patients with eating disorders has been widely reported in the literature, although a causal relationship between an eating disorder and trauma history remains to be elucidated.

PHYSICAL EXAMINATION

A comprehensive psychiatric history, medical history, and physical examination are customarily recommended for the initial assessment of a patient with an eating disorder. The initial appearance of a patient with anorexia nervosa may be deceptive if the primary care provider is under the assumption that all such patients appear outwardly cachectic. Loose-fitting or baggy clothes are common attire for patients with this disorder and often disguise weight loss. Body weight for a female adolescent with anorexia nervosa is typically below a body mass index of approximately 18 kg/m^2. Vital sign abnormalities include depression of core body temperature and bradycardia (e.g., pulse in the range of 40 to 60 beats per minute). However, heart rate may manifest tachycardia in the event of dehydration, or tachyarrhythmia secondary to ipecac-induced cardiomyopathy. Blood pressure is generally low, and postural changes in heart rate and blood pressure typically exceed the normal range.

Dry skin and decreased turgor indicate dehydration, and temporal wasting may be apparent. Thinning hair, a sign of malnutrition, is often noted. Lanugo, a covering of dry, downy hair, may be observed over the neck, cheeks, forearms, and legs. The skin may adopt a yellow hue as a result of hypercarotenemia. Examination of the mouth often reveals poor dentition related to self-induced vomiting. These dental changes are most commonly observed on the interior aspects of the molars, which exhibit a subtle loss of luster and mild discoloration where the gastric acid has eroded the enamel. Skin abrasion or scarring over the carpal-metacarpal joints (Russell's sign) is additional evidence of a history of self-induced vomiting.

Examination of the chest and abdomen reveals protruding ribs and a dramatically reduced abdominal girth, with protrusion of the iliac crests. Cardiac auscultation often uncovers abnormalities in heart rhythm. A neurologic examination may show motor weakness that accompanies muscle wasting. Hypothyroidism secondary to malnutrition may result in a characteristic latency in deep tendon reflexes.

Unlike patients with anorexia nervosa, patients with bulimia do not typically present with the physical signs of severe cachexia, but laboratory studies may reveal evidence of malnutrition related to abnormal dietary patterns. Physical signs of self-induced vomiting (dental erosion, Russell's sign) may be apparent in patients who use this method of purging. Patients who binge and self-induce vomiting may also have enlarged salivary glands, particularly the parotid glands. Preliminary research suggests a correlation between salivary gland enlargement and elevated serum amylase.[8] Rarely, binge eating and self-induced vomiting can result in severe medical complications such as esophagitis, esophageal tears, or gastric perforation.

DIAGNOSTICS

The fourth edition of the *Diagnostic and Statistical Manual of Mental Disorders* (DSM-IV-TR) published specific criteria defining anorexia nervosa and bulimia nervosa (Boxes 263-1 and 263-2).[9] Individuals who do not meet formal criteria for anorexia nervosa or bulimia nervosa may fall under the diagnostic category of Eating Disorder Not Otherwise Specified. This latter diagnostic category currently includes the DSM-IV provisional diagnosis (in need of further study) identified as Binge Eating Disorder, which characterizes individuals who experience regular binge eating but do not engage in routine compensatory behaviors to prevent weight gain.

DIFFERENTIAL DIAGNOSIS

Alternative medical and psychiatric diagnoses should be considered during the initial evaluation, particularly when the clinical presentation is atypical. Such characteristics include an unusual age of onset or an absence of symptoms related to a preoccupation with body weight and shape. Medical illnesses that may mimic some aspects of anorexia nervosa include peptic ulcer disease,

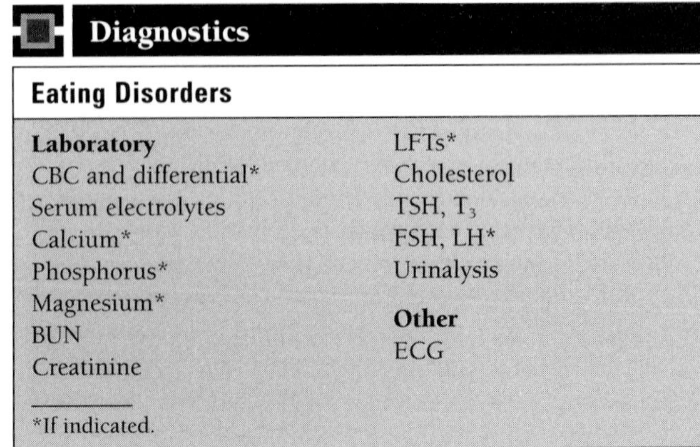

Diagnostics

Eating Disorders

Laboratory	LFTs*
CBC and differential*	Cholesterol
Serum electrolytes	TSH, T_3
Calcium*	FSH, LH*
Phosphorus*	Urinalysis
Magnesium*	**Other**
BUN	ECG
Creatinine	

*If indicated.

hyperthyroidism, primary or secondary adrenocortical insufficiency, AIDS, and cancer. A voracious appetite is associated with the rarely occurring Kleine-Levin syndrome. A change in body weight and eating patterns can accompany psychiatric conditions such as drug abuse (e.g., alcohol, cocaine, and other stimulants), major depression, and schizophrenia. A preoccupation with body shape, without the additional eating disorder diagnostic characteristics, raises the possibility of body dysmorphic disorder.

COMPLICATIONS

Clinical laboratory abnormalities are often encountered in patients with eating disorders, particularly when malnutrition is marked and purging behaviors are frequent. For nonhospitalized, normal-weight individuals, initial laboratory tests often include a CBC, electrolytes, BUN and creatinine levels, and urinalysis.[10] In the presence of severe symptoms or poor nutritional states, LFTs and the measurement of serum calcium, magnesium, and phosphorous may be indicated.[10] An initial ECG may be particularly valuable in the presence of severely low body weight, significant malnutrition, or a history of regular abuse of syrup of ipecac. Levels of serum follicle-stimulating hormone (FSH) and luteinizing hormone (LH) are sometimes included as part of an evaluation of amenorrhea for individuals at normal weight. Serum estradiol levels and the measurement of bone mineral density (e.g., dual energy x-ray absorptiometry) provide indices of bone loss and the risk for fracture, and may be indicated for individuals with prolonged low-weight states.

The hematologic profile associated with anorexia nervosa reflects nutrition-related anemia and may also reveal leukopenia and thrombocytopenia. Mineral and electrolyte abnormalities can include decreased chloride, calcium, magnesium, and phosphate. BUN levels may be increased as a result of dehydration or decreased in association with muscle wasting. Malnutrition may result in elevated serum levels of hepatic enzymes and cholesterol.

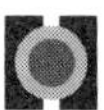

Differential Diagnosis

Eating Disorders

Medical	Psychiatric
AIDS	Body dysmorphic disorder
Cancer	Drug abuse
Hyperthyroidism	Major depression
Kleine-Levin syndrome	Schizophrenia
Peptic ulcer disease	
Primary/secondary adrenocortical insufficiency	

BOX 263-1

DIAGNOSTIC CRITERIA FOR ANOREXIA NERVOSA

A. Refusal to maintain body weight at or above a minimally normal weight for age and height (e.g., weight loss leading to maintenance of body weight less than 85% of that expected; or failure to make expected weight gain during period of growth, leading to body weight less than 85% of that expected).

B. Intense fear of gaining weight or becoming fat, even though underweight.

C. Disturbance in the way in which one's body weight or shape is experienced, undue influence of body weight or shape on self-evaluation, or denial of the seriousness of the current low body weight.

D. In postmenarcheal females, amenorrhea, i.e., the absence of at least three consecutive menstrual cycles. (A woman is considered to have amenorrhea if her periods occur only following hormone, e.g., estrogen, administration.)

Specify type:

Restricting Type: during the current episode of Anorexia Nervosa, the person has not regularly engaged in binge-eating or purging behavior (i.e., self-induced vomiting or the misuse of laxatives, diuretics, or enemas)

Binge-Eating/Purging Type: during the current episode of Anorexia Nervosa, the person has regularly engaged in binge-eating or purging behavior (i.e., self-induced vomiting or the misuse of laxatives, diuretics, or enemas)

From American Psychiatric Association: *Diagnostic and statistical manual of mental disorders*, ed 4 (Text revision 2000), Washington DC, 1994, The Association.

BOX 263-2

DIAGNOSTIC CRITERIA FOR BULIMIA NERVOSA

A. Recurrent episodes of binge eating. An episode of binge eating is characterized by both of the following:
(1) eating, in a discrete period of time (e.g., within any 2-hour period) an amount of food that is definitely larger than most people would eat during a similar period of time and under similar circumstances
(2) a sense of lack of control over eating during the episode (e.g., a feeling that one cannot stop eating or control what or how much one is eating)

B. Recurrent inappropriate compensatory behavior in order to prevent weight gain, such as self-induced vomiting; misuse of laxatives, diuretics, enemas, or other medications; fasting; or excessive exercise.

C. The binge eating and inappropriate compensatory behaviors both occur, on average, at least twice a week for 3 months.

D. Self-evaluation is unduly influenced by body shape and weight.

E. The disturbance does not occur exclusively during episodes of Anorexia Nervosa.

Specify type:

Purging Type: during the current episode of Bulimia Nervosa, the person has regularly engaged in self-induced vomiting or the misuse of laxatives, diuretics, or enemas

Nonpurging Type: during the current episode of Bulimia Nervosa, the person has used other inappropriate compensatory behaviors, such as fasting or excessive exercise, but has not regularly engaged in self-induced vomiting or the misuse of laxatives, diuretics, or enemas

From American Psychiatric Association: *Diagnostic and statistical manual of mental disorders*, ed 4 (Text revision 2000), Washington DC, 1994, The Association.

Commonly observed endocrine alterations include elevations in serum cortisol and growth hormone levels. A history of secondary amenorrhea is characteristically associated with decreased levels of FSH, LH, estrogen, and progesterone. Although levels of TSH are often normal, a malnutrition-related sick euthyroid syndrome is associated with reduced concentrations of serum triiodothyronine (T_3).

In general, patients with bulimia nervosa in whom malnutrition is less marked have fewer abnormalities on routine laboratory tests.[10] Anemia is common, particularly among patients who are strict vegetarians. In patients with frequent self-induced vomiting, electrolyte measurements may reveal increased concentrations of serum bicarbonate, which suggests metabolic alkalosis. Less commonly, laxative abuse may contribute to decreased serum bicarbonate levels. Self-induced vomiting, laxative abuse, and diuretic abuse may result in hypokalemia, hypochloremia, and hypomagnesemia. Severe hypokalemia, with an increased risk for life-threatening arrhythmia, can occur in patients with bulimia nervosa but is a relatively uncommon finding in outpatients. Repeated use of syrup of ipecac to induce vomiting may increase the risk for cardiomyopathy resulting from emetine toxicity.

ECG disturbances occur in both anorexia nervosa and bulimia nervosa. In anorexia nervosa, severe malnutrition is commonly associated with bradycardia. Abnormalities in heart rhythm, including prolonged QT intervals, may rarely be associated with sudden death. As previously noted, hypokalemia may be observed in both disorders, contributing to prolonged ventricular repolarization as reflected in QT prolongation or "U" waves.

MANAGEMENT

Successful medical management of patients with eating disorders involves ongoing thorough assessment, planning, intervention, and evaluation. It is dependent on communication and collaborative efforts with other health care professionals who are involved in the care or treatment of the patient. Communication with the patient is crucial to establishing the critically needed therapeutic alliance.

For patients with anorexia nervosa, medical stability and restoration of body weight to the point of resumption of normal bodily function (e.g., restoration of menses) are a primary concern. The monitoring of body weight provides an index of nutritional changes, with frequency of assessment based on the patient's weight status. For the adolescent patient, ongoing monitoring of developmental growth is important and includes regular measurement of body height and weight. Weight gain is achieved based on the patient's ability to increase caloric intake. Caloric intake may initially start in the range of 1000 to 1600 kcal/day, with a progressive increase to allow for body weight restoration and maintenance.[10] Refeeding during a significantly low-weight malnourished state requires careful assessment of vital signs, electrolytes, and signs and symptoms of fluid overload. Excessive or rapid refeeding has been associated with seizures, cardiac arrhythmias, delirium, and in rare instances congestive heart failure.[11] Vitamin, mineral, and food supplements may be necessary during the initial weight gain phase.

Periodic monitoring of serum electrolytes should be considered in cases of anorexia nervosa or bulimia nervosa, and particularly for individuals with frequent purging behaviors who are at increased risk for hypokalemia.[12] A finding of hypokalemia should be followed up with an ECG, with attention given to possible cardiac conduction and rhythm disturbances.

The potential role of psychotropic medications in the initial management of an eating disorder is evaluated in the context of presenting symptoms and co-morbid conditions. In general, medications are not a first-line treatment for anorexia nervosa unless co-morbid conditions such as major depression, severe anxiety disorder, or psychosis necessitate such intervention.[10] There is little evidence that psychotropic medications contribute to weight gain in anorexia nervosa, although preliminary data suggest that antidepressant medications of the serotonin selective reuptake inhibitor (SSRI) class (e.g., fluoxetine) may help to prevent relapse after weight restoration.[13]

Outpatient psychotherapy is often effective for bulimia nervosa and is advantageous as an initial treatment modality for many patients. Medications may be part of an initial treatment plan for patients with bulimia nervosa, particularly as placebo-controlled trials have shown that administration of an antidepressant agent may contribute to a diminished frequency of binge-eating and purging behaviors, even in the absence of current depression. Medications also may be particularly beneficial for patients who show a limited response to an initial period of psychotherapy or manifest a co-morbid condition. The SSRIs have received particular attention, in part because of their relatively favorable side effect profile.[14] Tricyclic antidepressants are an alternative for patients who are refractory to SSRIs, although these medications may require more frequent monitoring of blood pressure and cardiac functioning. Use of tricyclic antidepressant agents necessitates extreme caution with patients at risk for suicide attempt. Monoamine oxidase inhibitors are generally avoided, given that adherence to the required low-tyramine diet may prove difficult for a patient with an eating disorder.

Management of eating disorders is ideally conducted by a multidisciplinary team and often includes a primary care provider, dietitian, and individual psychotherapist. Consultation with an endocrinologist may be particularly helpful in assessing the cause of amenorrhea during the initial evaluative phase. Referral for a dental examination is indicated for patients engaged in self-induced vomiting. A psychiatric clinician can make important contributions to the assessment and treatment planning phases, as well as provide individual or group psychotherapy and a referral to appropriate support groups. A family therapist may also play an important role, particularly in the treatment of children and adolescents. The psychiatric clinician or a consultant psychopharmacologist often manages psychotropic medication intervention.

LIFE SPAN CONSIDERATIONS

Although the age of onset of eating disorders typically occurs during adolescence or young adulthood, the illness can be present and recur during other life phases. Relapse is likely to happen during periods of increased stress. Patients with bulimia nervosa are most vulnerable to relapse during the first 6 months after psychiatric treatment for the disorder.[15] Eating disorders are often chronic conditions; although symptoms of bulimia nervosa are responsive to treatment, complete abstinence from binge eating may be a difficult goal in short-term treatment.[16] Certain metabolic sequelae of an eating disorder, such as decreased bone mineral density, may have residual consequences later in life.

INDICATIONS FOR REFERRAL/HOSPITALIZATION

Weight loss and medical complications may become severe enough to warrant hospitalization. Significant electrolyte disturbances, for example, can require inpatient cardiac monitoring. Severe malnutrition may result in transient cognitive impairment to the extent that the patient is incapable of making a valid decision about care; in such instances, involuntary hospitalization may be necessary to ensure safety. Hospitalization is also indicated in the presence of significant co-morbid psychiatric conditions such as depression with suicidal ideation.

Although uncommon, enteral and parenteral alimentation may be considered during hospitalization when a severely malnourished patient is medically compromised and unable to comply with less invasive measures. These modes of refeeding can be accompanied by serious medical risks and may require intensive medical monitoring for potential problems. A refusal of life-sustaining care may require legal petitioning for a medical guardian.

Hospitalization provides patients with an opportunity to discontinue potentially harmful forms of purging while receiving intensive psychologic and medical support. Laxatives, diuretics, and diet pills can usually be discontinued rapidly, with symptomatic treatment of the resultant constipation or edema. Medical-psychiatric inpatient units often have specific, behaviorally oriented protocols for working with patients with eating disorders. Partial hospital programs provide an alternative to inpatient hospitalizations for symptomatic patients who can be treated in a less restrictive setting.

PATIENT AND FAMILY EDUCATION

Education about the disorder, medical consequences, nutritional needs, and treatment options is important for patients and families. Information regarding specific interventions (e.g., medication treatment) is necessary not only for informed consent but also for enhancing adherence to the treatment regimen. For younger patients, it is often important to educate family members about the etiology, course of illness, prognosis, and treatment of the disorder. Attention to these needs helps to build the alliance required for treatment adherence and longitudinal medical monitoring.

HEALTH PROMOTION

Risk factors are not fully understood, and it is unlikely that there will prove to be a single cause for eating disorders; however, there are several identifiable "at risk" groups for whom primary prevention may be important. Adolescence, for example, is a time of developmental body change, weight gain, challenge to self-esteem, peer pressure, and increased external influences related to body image. Teens may be particularly vulnerable to media messages that portray an unrealistic waif-like figure as the "ideal" body shape. In an era where more than one third of the U.S. adult population is overweight, dieting behavior is rampant. Dieting behavior is thought to be a potential risk factor for an eating disorder because it often precedes the onset of illness. Individuals participating in activities such as ballet, gymnastics, wrestling, or crew may be prone to pressures related to minimizing body weight. Thus they may be vulnerable to the use of compensatory behaviors to prevent weight gain. Although all of these groups may be at risk, it is clear that no single stressor provides a comprehensive explanation for the development of an eating disorder. Thus the context in which a set of risk factors operates is likely to be important for expression of the disorder in the person who may, for example, be biologically or genetically vulnerable.

Although in their infancy, primary prevention strategies are currently being tested in the research community. Although there seems to be little argument about the potential value of primary prevention, there is less agreement with regard to the content of such programs. Some critics fear that educational components focused on compensatory behaviors used to prevent weight gain, for example, have the potential for introducing unhealthy behaviors to vulnerable individuals who may have not otherwise known about them. Programs that focus on positive eating habits, nutritional values, positive-self-esteem, and coping strategies seem likely to be beneficial, although the long-term effectiveness in preventing an eating disorder remains unknown.

REFERENCES

1. Garfinkel PE and others: Bulimia nervosa in a Canadian community sample: prevalence and comparison of subgroups, *Am J Psychiatry* 152(7):1052-1058, 1995.
2. Walters EE, Kendler KS: Anorexia nervosa and anorexic-like syndromes in a population-based female twin sample, *Am J Psychiatry* 152(1):64-71, 1995.
3. Lewinsohn PM, Striegel-Moore RH, Seeley JR: Epidemiology and natural course of eating disorders in young women from adolescence to young adulthood, *J Am Acad Child Adolesc Psychiatry* 39(10):1284-1292, 2000.
4. Nakamura K and others: Prevalence of anorexia nervosa and bulimia nervosa in a geographically defined area in Japan, *Int J Eat Disord* 28(2):173-180, 2000.
5. Wildes JE, Emery RE: The roles of ethnicity and culture in the development of eating disturbances and body dissatisfaction: a meta-analytic review, *Clin Psychol Rev* 21(4):521-551, 2001.
6. Herzog DB and others: Mortality in eating disorders: a descriptive study, *Int J Eat Disord* 28(1):20-26, 2000.
7. Braun DL, Sunday SR, Halmi KA: Psychiatric comorbidity in patients with eating disorders, *Psychol Med* 24(4):859-867, 1994.
8. Metzger ED and others: Salivary gland enlargement and elevated serum amylase in bulimia nervosa, *Biol Psychiatry* 45(11):1520-1522, 1999.
9. American Psychiatric Association: *Diagnostic and statistical manual of mental disorders*, ed 4, Washington DC, 1994, The Association.
10. American Psychiatric Association: Practice guideline for the treatment of patients with eating disorders (revision), *Am J Psychiatry* 157(1 Suppl):1-39, 2000.
11. Kohn MR, Golden NH, Shenker IR: Cardiac arrest and delirium: presentations of the refeeding syndrome in severely malnourished adolescents with anorexia nervosa, *J Adolesc Health* 22:239-243, 1998.
12. Wolfe BE and others: Laboratory screening for electrolyte abnormalities and anemia in bulimia nervosa: a controlled study, *Int J Eat Disord* 30(3):288-293, 2001.
13. Kaye WH and others: Double-blind placebo-controlled administration of fluoxetine in restricting- and restricting-purging type anorexia nervosa, *Biol Psychiatry* 49(7):644-652, 2001.
14. Jimerson DC and others: Medications in the treatment of eating disorders, *Psychiatr Clin North Am* 19(4):739-754, 1996.
15. Olmsted MP, Kaplan AS, Rockert W: Rate and prediction of relapse in bulimia nervosa, *Am J Psychiatry* 151(5):738-743, 1994.
16. Fairburn CG and others: The natural course of bulimia nervosa and binge eating disorder in young women, *Arch Gen Psychiatry* 57(7):659-665, 2000.

CHAPTER 264

Grief

Alice Bolton

DEFINITION/EPIDEMIOLOGY

Grief is a normal response to loss. It is dynamic, pervasive, highly individualized, and found in all age-groups.[1] It is estimated that 10 million people in the United States are grieving each year.[2]

Grieving usually occurs after a person experiences the death of a loved one—a family member, spouse, child, close friend, or pet. A grief response can also occur in response to other losses, such as a job or career loss, loss of physical health or abilities, divorce, financial loss, or the diminishing health of a spouse or loved one.

Many health care providers are uncomfortable with death and loss, which is reflected in their attitudes toward the bereaved. Avoidance is common. To prevent such responses, providers must be aware of their own feelings about death and loss. Clichéd responses should be avoided, and the loss should be acknowledged. Most people prefer a sincere word or gesture. Books and continuing education seminars are helpful in achieving a comfort level that permits discussion about death and grief.

Immediate psychiatric evaluation is required for all patients with suicidal/homicidal ideation.

CLINICAL PRESENTATION

The length of the grief process varies. Estimates of 2 months to 2 years have been given. Individuals experience stages of grief: denial, anger, bargaining, depression, and acceptance.[3] The process is ongoing, does not follow a rigid order or time frame, and may fluctuate between or even skip stages. The stages of grief are not necessarily all obvious; they may be repeated many times and are often not completed before moving on to another stage.

PHYSICAL EXAMINATION

Physical complaints, which are often vague, are common during the grieving period. Office visits to the primary care provider may become more frequent.[4] Sleep and appetite disturbances are reported. Sad faces, crying, and anxiety are seen.

DIAGNOSTICS

Although there are no definitive laboratory tests to diagnose grief, there has been research on the response of the immune system.[5] At this time, research findings are not sufficiently significant to enable a diagnosis of grief by laboratory testing. The physical symptoms of patients must be taken seriously, with disorders such as diabetes, anemia, hypothyroidism, hyperthyroidism, gastrointestinal, or cardiac abnormalities excluded as indicated.

DIFFERENTIAL DIAGNOSIS

Horowitz and others[6] have proposed diagnostic criteria for complicated grief. These criteria include a loss that occurred at least 14 months ago; the experience of severe emotional symptoms related to memories and yearnings of the lost relationship that interfere with daily functioning during the previous month; isolating; avoiding contact with circumstances or situations that remind the person of the deceased; loss of interest in social, recreational, or work activities to a degree that it becomes problematic; severe disruption in sleep patterns; and feelings of being alone or empty.[6]

Complicated grief and major depression are considered when diagnosing a grief reaction. A major depressive disorder is characterized by a change from a previous level of functioning during a 2-week period, with either a depressed mood or a loss of pleasure or interest in almost all activities. Symptoms associated with this disorder are prevalent all or most of the day. These include weight loss or gain not related to dieting, increased or decreased appetite every day, sleep disturbance every day, low energy or fatigue every day, psychomotor retardation or agitation, diminished concentration, inability to make decisions, excessive guilt or feelings of worthlessness, or a suicide ideation, intent, plan, or attempt. These symptoms may not result from a substance use disorder or medical condition and may significantly interfere with the patient's ability to function. The fourth edition of the *Diagnostic and Statistical Manual of Mental Disorders* (DSM-IV-TR) differentiates these symptoms from bereavement by setting a time frame of 2 months for the bereavement period. If the symptoms of normal grief persist and remain severe after this period, a major depressive episode is considered as a diagnosis.[7]

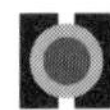

Differential Diagnosis

Grief

Grief
May be present up to 2 months after loss
Guilt related to the deceased
Thoughts of death related to the deceased
Intact self-esteem
Short-lived functional impairment
No hallucinations; may "hear" voice of deceased or "see" image of deceased

Complicated Grief
Occurs up to 14 months after bereavement for 1 month
Feelings of being alone or empty
Present and problematic functional impairment
Isolation
Avoidance of situations reminiscent of the deceased

Major Depression
Severe and persistent after bereavement, lasting 2 weeks or more
Thoughts of death
Feelings of worthlessness
Prolonged and marked functional impairment
Possible auditory or visual hallucinations unrelated to the deceased

Normal bereavement is similar to complicated grief and major depression and may include feelings of sadness, insomnia, poor appetite, and weight loss.

MANAGEMENT

Treatment considerations for an uncomplicated grief reaction include bereavement support groups, books, empathetic responses from health care providers, and short-term medications for symptom relief.[8] Support group information should be available for the patient. The primary care provider should be knowledgeable about the group and its affiliations and leadership.

Medication is the final consideration in treatment of the grief response. The primary concern should be to allow the process to unfold and progress toward resolution. However, there are occasions when short-term symptom relief is indicated. Benzodiazepines (clonazepam, lorazepam, and alprazolam) prescribed in small doses for infrequent use may be helpful for the anxiety and insomnia associated with grief.[9] Current research is inconclusive regarding the benefits of benzodiazapine use during bereavement.[10] There is a risk for addiction when prescribing such medications, and therefore they should not be prescribed for patients with any type of substance abuse history. Patients must be monitored for signs of abuse, particularly tolerance. Taking more of the drug to achieve the desired effect is a clear indication of trouble. Limiting the number of tablets dispensed is an effective way to monitor use and prevent abuse. Clonazepam or lorazepam 0.5 mg b.i.d. or t.i.d. is usually more than adequate to provide relief of anxiety and insomnia. No more than 15 to 20 tablets need be dispensed weekly. Benzodiazepines are used with extreme caution in older adults because there is a great risk for falls and mental confusion in this age-group.[10] Follow-up office visits at frequent intervals (every 2 weeks) provide an opportunity to assess the patient's progress, identify any complications, and provide emotional support.

Antidepressants may be indicated for some patients during the grief process.[11] Those who have not responded to short-term use of antianxiety agents (2 weeks) may benefit from a selective serotonin reuptake inhibitor (SSRI) or tricyclic agent. Although the SSRIs (fluoxetine, sertraline, paroxetine, citalopram) usually produce a maximum antidepressant benefit in 2 to 5 weeks, many patients report a decrease in anxiety within a week or even days of therapy. Although some drug interactions have been reported, SSRIs have proven to be relatively safe. The side effect profile is usually benign when therapy is initiated with a low dose—half the recommended starting dose. Older patients most often respond favorably to one fourth of the recommended starting dose. Sedation and some anxiolytic effect can be achieved using tricyclic antidepressants (nortriptyline, doxepin) and nefazodone and trazodone. Limited evidence exists for use of bupropion sustained release for bereavement.[12]

A bedtime dose of trazodone, nefazodone, mirtazapine (atypical antidepressants), or a tricyclic agent can provide immediate insomnia relief; the antidepressant effect occurs in approximately 3 to 6 weeks. The tricyclics have a greater potential for adverse interactions yet can be safely prescribed if used with caution. Prescribing tricyclics for older adults is usually not advised because of the anticholinergic effects.[10] Awareness of potential drug-drug interactions is needed before prescribing any agent.

LIFE SPAN CONSIDERATIONS

Grieving occurs in all age-groups. Children may fear abandonment or the loss of others they love, as well as guilt or responsibility for the loss.[13] They may begin to have behavioral problems at home or school. Evidence exists that the loss of a parent in childhood is linked to psychosocial problems in adults when the family relationship is poor.[14]

COMPLICATIONS

Adverse effects related to grief are major depression, complicated grief, physical illness, and suicide. A thorough history, including a brief psychosocial assessment, is needed to screen the at-risk population. It is helpful to ask questions related to living arrangements, availability of transportation, friends, socialization, and diet. Inquiries about feelings of sadness or depression, thoughts of suicide, and coping skills are necessary. Illness resulting from accidents is common in the bereavement period. Stress-related illness and substance abuse are common during the first year of grieving.

Complicated grief is a risk for older adults, for individuals who lose a spouse or child, for individuals in poor health, and for those with severe coexisting and preexisting stressors.[15,16] Individuals who have had dependent relationships, have lacked social support, or have had ambivalent relationships are also at risk for complicated grief.[17,18]

A major depressive episode is an additional risk. A depression screening tool is helpful to diagnose major depression, and many are available at no cost from pharmaceutical companies. The primary care provider may choose to prescribe an SSRI to treat the depression. Individual and/or group therapy is a beneficial adjunct to medication. Assessment for suicide risk is necessary at each visit. Office appointments should be scheduled at frequent intervals to assess the patient's response to medication and risk factors.

Patients are often treated by several health care providers, all of whom may prescribe medications and other interventions. For the patient's safety and to avoid duplication and drug interactions, it is essential that all providers be aware of these treatments and medications.

INDICATIONS FOR REFERRAL/HOSPITALIZATION

Major depression and complicated grief can be time consuming to treat in the primary care setting. Often patients present with somatic symptoms that require frequent clinic visits, assessments, and testing. Anxiety may be a component of the depression. Patients may not be able to clearly express their concerns, and they may require more time than the routine visit allows. Antidepressant medications may take from 2 to 5 weeks to reach a beneficial effect, and dose titrations or a trial of an alternative antidepressant may delay the treatment progress.

A referral to psychiatric care may be threatening to a patient because of the bias of mental illness in today's society. Psychiatric care is often associated with incapacitation or insanity. Immediate psychiatric intervention is indicated for suicidal thoughts, intent, and attempts; for patients who have not responded to one or two trials of antidepressants; for patients who require more time than the practitioner has available; and for patients whom the practitioner is not comfortable treating.

The patient can be prepared for referral if the psychiatric intervention is not an emergency. Approaches that are empathetic and honest are best. Presenting depression as a treatable, biologic disorder similar to other medical conditions is helpful to the patient's understanding.

Immediate hospitalization is indicated when patients pose a threat to themselves or others. Primary care providers must be aware of the mental health act in their practice locale and take appropriate action. All states have provisions for involuntary placement for evaluation in mental health emergencies.

Some primary care providers refer patients with uncomplicated grief reactions to mental health services. Advanced practice registered nurse practitioners in mental health, licensed clinical social workers, mental health counselors, and psychologists can assess, diagnose, and treat mental health disorders. In many states, advanced practice registered nurse practitioners prescribe medications and provide psychotherapy.

Many people are not covered by prescription plans, and for these people the cost of medications may be prohibitive. Many pharmaceutical companies make medications available through indigent drug programs. The indigent patient program can be initiated by calling the specific drug company. In addition, psychotherapy is not a covered service with many insurance plans, and many patients are unable to pay out-of-pocket. Local mental health clinics may provide some therapy. Other providers may offer services on a sliding scale.

PATIENT AND FAMILY EDUCATION

Grieving is a normal process in response to loss. An awareness of the predisposing factors to complicated grief may aid in its prevention. The maintenance of mental, physical, and religious health is reported as a positive indicator of successful grieving.[19]

Emotional support is essential as a patient progresses through the grieving process. It is helpful for the patient to know that the feelings associated with grieving are natural and that the intensity of these feelings will wax and wane as the process continues.

Weight loss is not uncommon during this period. Patients report having no appetite. Nutrition education stressing the necessity to eat balanced meals is indicated. Patients are often unaware of the importance of nutrition to emotional health. A liquid dietary supplement may be suggested if there is the potential for a nutritional deficit. These supplements may be substituted for one or two meals or used as additional nutrition.

Some patients find support and comfort in their faith. Others may reject their religious ties, blaming God for their loss. Assurance that this is often part of the process is important.

Maintaining a routine is an essential component of a healthy lifestyle. Patients should be encouraged to have a regular bedtime and waking time each day. Scheduling activities outside the home is also important. Maintaining social contacts is essential, but patients should also know that quiet time alone is acceptable. Exercise in some form is beneficial and need not be strenuous.

Medication education is important. Patients should understand the side effects, risks, purposes, and use of the medications prescribed. A list of concurrent medications should also be reviewed for potential drug interactions or duplication. This approach offers an opportunity to assess a patient's knowledge of the medication and health status and also provides an opportunity for teaching. Education about the use of as-needed medications should also be reviewed, because patients often do not understand this concept. Specific instructions are needed rather than a blanket "when, if, or as you need it" statement. Although many patients report they would never abuse medication or become addicted, abuse and dependence can occur without initial intent. Therefore it is important that patients receive education about the risk for dependence with certain medications. The primary care provider continually assesses and educates patients about medication use.

Most people do not consider alcohol to be a drug. The potential for drug and alcohol interaction should be assessed as medications are reviewed. Often a primary care provider does not ask about alcohol consumption, or patients may minimize their intake. Teaching about the depressant effects of alcohol is especially needed in this population.

It is often helpful to include the family in grief education to stress the nature of the grief response, in particular the universality and individuality of the phenomenon and the fact that it is a process. Expectations of family and friends can help or hinder the grieving progress. Education is the key to better understanding—the resolution of grief depends on it.

For further assistance, patients can be referred to the Grief Recovery Institute at (800) 445-4808. AARP offers grief and loss programs, aarp.org/grief programs.

REFERENCES

1. Cowles KV, Rodgers BL: The concept of grief: a foundation for nursing research and practice, *Res Nurs Health* 14(2):119-127, 1991.
2. Sullivan MD: Maintaining good morale in old age, *West J Med* 167(4):276-284, 1997.
3. Kubler-Ross E, Wessler S, Avioli LV: On death and dying, *JAMA* 221(2):174-179, 1972.
4. Fenner P, Manchershaw A: A group approach to overcome loss: a model for a bereavement service in general practice, *Prof Nurse* 8(10):680-684, 1993.
5. Lindstrom TC: Immunity and somatic health in bereavement: a prospective study of 39 Norwegian widows, *Omega* 35(12): 1997.
6. Horowitz M and others: Self-regard: a new measure, *Am J Psychiatry* 153(3):382-385, 1996.
7. American Psychiatric Association: *Diagnostic and statistical manual of mental disorders*, ed 4 Text Revision, Washington, DC, 2000, The Association.
8. Shear MK and others: Traumatic grief treatment, a pilot study, *Am J Psychiatry* 158(9):1506-1508, 2001.
9. Anderson EG: Grief recovery: helping those who've had to say goodbye, *Geriatrics* 52(9):103-104, 1997.
10. Warner J, Metcalfe C, King M: Evaluating the use of benzodiazapines following recent bereavement, *Br J Psychiatry* 178(1):36-41, 2001.
11. Guze B, Richeimer S, Szuba MP: *The psychiatric drug handbook*, St Louis, 1992, Mosby.
12. Zizook S and others: Buprion sustained release for bereavement: results of an open trial, *Clin Psychiatry* 62(4):227-230, 2001.
13. Stuber M, Mesrkhai VH: What do we tell children? Understanding childhood grief, *West J Med* 174(3):187-191, 2001.
14. Luecken LJ: Attachment and loss experiences during childhood are associated with hostility, depression, and social support, *J Psychosom Res* 49(1):85-91, 2000.
15. Pasternak RE and others: The posttreatment illness course of depression in bereaved elders: high relapse/recurrence rates, *Am J Geriatr Psychiatry* 5(1):54-59, 1997.

16. Prigerson HG and others: The inventory of complicated grief: a scale to measure certain maladaptive symptoms of loss, *Psychiatry Res* 59 (1-2):65-79, 1995.
17. Zisook S, Shuchter SR: Uncomplicated bereavement, *J Clin Psychiatry* 54(10):365-372, 1993.
18. Jacobs S: *Pathological grief*, Washington, DC, 1993, American Psychiatric Press.
19. Levin JS: Religion and health: is there an association, is it valid, is it causal? *Soc Sci Med* 38(11):1475-1482, 1994.

CHAPTER 265

Posttraumatic Stress Disorder

Nancy S. Mahan

DEFINITION/EPIDEMIOLOGY

Posttraumatic stress disorder (PTSD) is a psychiatric disorder characterized by a wide range of symptoms that have developed in response to a significant and overwhelming stressful incident or from chronic exposure to intolerable stressful conditions (see Box 265-2). The individual experiences the stressful incident or incidents as a life-or-death threat to his or her safety and personal integrity. He or she has often witnessed death or extremely horrendous conditions in which the life or integrity of others is threatened or actually occurs.

Initially conceptualized in response to symptoms experienced by military personnel during World War I who were exposed to gruesome situations in combat, and further developed in subsequent wars, the diagnosis of PTSD has expanded to include anyone who evidences serious impairment in psychologic, occupational, and interpersonal functioning as a result of exposure to traumatic events that are considered beyond the scope of normative life experiences. Examples of such traumatic experiences include those endured by survivors of the Holocaust or resettlement/re-education camps, prisoners of war and other hostage situations, survivors of terrorist attacks, adults and children who have been raped or who have been persistently sexually abused or battered, people involved in severe accidents (e.g., motor vehicle accident in which the driver witnesses his/her children dying), and those who have experienced other natural disasters such as earthquakes, tornadoes, volcano eruptions, or floods.

Although included in the Anxiety Disorders section of the fourth edition of the *Diagnostic and Statistical Manual of Mental Disorders Text Revision* (DSM-IV-TR), there is also strong support to consider PTSD a dissociative disorder, given the high prevalence of dissociative symptoms that are observed and believed by many survivors of trauma. For many people beleaguered with PTSD, the trinity of coexisting anxiety, depressive, and dissociative symptoms is a common feature of their nights and days. Fortunately, a resurgence of research over the last two decades regarding PTSD has furthered our understanding of this complex disorder and simultaneously enhanced the overall effectiveness of treatment and interventions that serve to ameliorate symptoms and salvage one's once distressed soul. The DSM-IV-TR cites that:

The person's response to the event must involve intense fear, helplessness, or horror (or in children, the response must involve disorganized or agitated behavior) . . . The characteristic symptoms resulting from the exposure to the extreme trauma include persistent reexperiencing of the traumatic event, persistent avoidance of stimuli associated with the trauma and numbing of general responsiveness . . . and persistent symptoms of increased arousal . . . The full symptom picture must be present for more than 1 month, . . . and the disturbance must cause significant distress or impairment in social, occupational, or other important areas of functioning.[1]

Not everyone exposed to extreme traumatic incident[s] develops PTSD. Some people are more resilient than others to such stressors, whereas others evidence considerable vulnerability. Factors that influence the short- and long-term development of this disorder are listed in Box 265-1.

Immediate psychiatric consultation is indicated for patients with suicidal or homicidal ideation.

PATHOPHYSIOLOGY

Research suggests that exposure to trauma alters the normal functioning of brain chemistry at both the time of exposure and later when the person experiences other stresses that may replicate the traumatic experience. The part of the brain that is primarily involved in one's response to fear, other emotions, and behavior is the limbic system: particularly the amygdala and the hippocampus. The amygdala registers hyperarousal, which diminishes the functioning of the hippocampus. As reviewed in van der Kolk and others, "the amygdala is most clearly implicated in the evaluation of the emotional meaning of incoming stimuli...[it is] thought to integrate internal representations of the external world in the form of memory images with emotional experiences associated with those memories."[2] The hippocampus is responsible for the development and operation of declarative memory and when impaired (by the hyperarousal of the amygdala) is unable to function optimally, interfering with the person's memory encoding and retention and his or her ability to infer a narrative cognition regarding what events have occurred.

Several neuroendocrine abnormalities are present in PTSD and current evidence suggests that any or several of the following systems are involved: catecholamines, corticosteroids, serotonin, and endogenous opioids. Catecholamines, specifically, norepinephrine and epinephrine, are chronically increased in persons with PTSD. Similarly, the number of glucocorticoid receptors are also altered, generally reflecting a lowered cortisol level in persons with a history of exposure to trauma. Research supports that cortisol response appears to be blunted in people with a previous traumatic exposure.[2] Research demonstrates that animals that are shocked with no means of escape evidence less serotonin in the central nervous system, which is why many of the selective serotonin reuptake inhibitors (SSRIs), a class of antidepressant medications, have efficacy in the pharmacologic treatment of PTSD. Lowered levels of serotonin have "repeatedly been correlated with impulsivity and aggression."[2]

Endogenous opioids play an important role in the way in which an organism initially experiences a traumatic event (or events) and how they are later triggered with stimuli that somehow mimics or resembles early traumatic exposure. Release of these endogenous opioids is responsible for the development of stress-induced analgesia, which serves to decrease pain and panic. This mechanism is initially an adaptive protection for an organism, although when overused often has maladaptive consequences for a person. Opioid release also interferes with how memories are processed, stored, and recalled. This dissociative process, common to people who suffer with PTSD, can serve to protect the individual exposed to overwhelming stimulation or fear, but also impairs memory and integration of the experience into a meaningful or narrative understanding of the event[s]. Secretion of endogenous hormones similarly interferes with normal brain processing. As discussed by van der Kolk and others:[2]

> Physiologic arousal in general can trigger trauma related memories; conversely, trauma-related memories precipitate generalized physiologic arousal. It is likely that the frequent reliving of a traumatic event in flashbacks or nightmares causes a re-release of stress hormones, which further kindle

BOX 265-1

FACTORS INFLUENCING THE DEVELOPMENT OF POSTTRAUMATIC STRESS DISORDER

- The person's developmental level at the time of exposure to the traumatic event[s]: the younger the person the more likely the person will not have other life experience to buffer the experience or the cognitive capacities to put the event[s] into an understandable context. For example, severe sexual and/or physical abuse of young children fundamentally interferes with their development of a stable sense of self and the capacity for affect regulation. Because such trauma commonly occurs at the hands of primary caregivers or a known, formerly trusted adult, such experiences compromise a child's ability to develop stable attachments that are requisite for identity formation, future interpersonal and relational competence, and the realization of developmental tasks that unfold in a normative manner.
- The length of exposure: people are less likely to develop long-term symptoms after one incident of exposure to a traumatic event as compared with persistent exposure
- One's temperament and personality, along with previous life experience[s] that may serve to either buffer or potentiate symptom development
- The availability of help immediately after the incident and after early development of symptoms can minimize the development or severity of symptoms of clinical PTSD
- Family history of psychiatric illness that predisposes a person toward more vulnerability
- One's proximity to the traumatic exposure
- Evidence of dissociation at the time of the exposure—as indicated by van der Kolk and others, "dissociation at the moment of the trauma appears to be the single most important predictor for the establishment of PTSD"[2]
- The severity of the traumatic event
- The nature of the traumatic event (i.e., whether it occurred at the hands of others, such as in war or in child abuse, or whether it occurred as a result of natural disasters)

> the strength of the memory trace. Such a positive feedback loop could cause subclinical PTSD to escalate into clinical PTSD (Pittman et al, 1993) in which the memories appear so strong and powerful that Pittman and Orr (1990) have called them "the black hole" in the mental life of the PTSD patient. They attract all associations to themselves, and sap current life of its significance.[2]

Additionally, trauma-related memories often surface in fragments or in sensory or emotional memories, leading many specialists in the trauma field to propose that the body remembers what the mind cannot bear. The inability to articulate a narrative of the traumatic event is one of the characteristics of the brain's inability to recall with clarity exactly what happened under symptoms of extreme stress.

CLINICAL PRESENTATION

The patient presents with symptoms, such as anxiety or depression, that on inquiry are associated with a history of exposure to extreme stressful event[s] beyond the scope of normal human suffering, and that place the individual at such a substantive level of stress that the mind cannot tolerate it. Although initially PTSD was considered to be a rare phenomenon, recent research suggests that it may have widespread prevalence given the large number of people who have witnessed or experienced combat, violent death, extreme battery, or sexual assault, making it one of the more prevalent of psychiatric disorders, second only to depression. When the trauma occurs to a very young child, it is unlikely that the child will be able to articulate in words what occurred. Instead, what one observes behaviorally may be suggestive of trauma, through reenactment of terrorized, terrorizing, or sexualized activity in play; increased nightmares; regression to earlier developmental behaviors; and increased somatization.

In addition to the signs and symptoms described in Table 265-1, patients may also show evidence of the following:

- Presence of a range of dissociative symptoms that are determined by the severity and persistence of the trauma. Some people describe milder symptoms as "spacing out" or "numbing out." More severe symptoms involve the development of alters (multiple personalities) as is evident in dissociative identity disorder
- Acute symptoms of depression, which may include suicidality
- Feelings of numbness, depersonalization (the feeling as if one is detached from himself/herself and observing himself/herself from a distance), derealization (feeling unreal), and detachment from relationships and situations

TABLE 265-1 Management of Posttraumatic Stress Disorder

Signs or Symptoms	Pharmacologic Interventions	Therapeutic and Behavioral Interventions
For depression	Antidepressants, particularly those SSRIs that have sedative effects enabling the patient to sleep better and simultaneously reduce anxiety	Secure psychotherapy that provides monitoring, support, treatment, and hope. Cognitive treatment for thoughts associated with the depressed affect has been found to be useful when combined with pharmacologic interventions. Depressed individuals often evidence catastrophic or all-or-nothing thought patterns that can be relearned through identification, restatement, and practice.
For suicidality	Antidepressant medications should be initiated and continued	For chronic suicidality, identification of increased risk (i.e., increased risk factors include the presence of a plan, the means to enact this plan, the presence of command hallucinations, use of substances, having more energy after an acute depressive episode, etc) must be continually assessed. When a patient is acutely suicidal, the patient should be hospitalized in a locked setting to ensure safety.
For acute episodes of psychotic symptoms	Use antipsychotic medications	Educate the person about psychotic symptoms occasionally associated with acute stress reactions. Ensure safety, assess orientation, provide as-needed monitoring and aggressive treatment aimed at ameliorating symptoms.
For dissociative episodes	No medications have demonstrated efficacy	Assist the person is getting grounded and out of the dissociative episode. A variety of interventions can be helpful in bringing the person back to the present. Techniques such as having the person hold ice packs on face and neck (providing the traumatic exposure did not involve cold sensations), having the person open eyes and attempt to give words to the experience, and holding tightly onto a small object to regain composure have been found to be useful anecdotally.
For autonomic hyperactivity	Antiadrenergics such as clonidine, guanfacine, or propranolol	Relaxation exercises such as diaphragmatic breathing can assist the patient with shortness of breath and help with overall discomfort.
For persistent reexperiencing of intrusive sensations	MAOIs, tricyclics, SSRIs	Grounding techniques such as those mentioned previously can bring the person back to the present and reestablish safety.

SSRI, Selective serotonin reuptake inhibitor; *MAOIs,* monoamine oxidase inhibitors.

- Somatization (this is particularly evident when the exposure to the traumatic incident[s] has [have] occurred in childhood and symptoms usually include stomachaches or headaches)
- Problems with concentration, generally resulting from overwhelming anxiety or depression
- Overreliance on substances or activities to ameliorate painful symptoms such as flashbacks, irritability, rage, and nightmares
- Chronic affective dysregulation
- Loss of a sense of self-agency
- Self-mutilation is often seen in people with severe histories of childhood abuse. Self-injury differs from suicide attempts (although one can accidentally kill oneself in an act intended for self-harm). As adhered by Herman, "self injury is intended not to kill but rather to relieve unbearable emotional pain and many survivors regard it, paradoxically, as a form of self preservation."[3]

PHYSICAL EXAMINATION

It is generally not common for patients presenting in a primary or acute care setting to disclose their personal history specific to traumatic exposure. Often, people do not consider such experience as relevant to their overall health status, or think to share it with their caretakers. It is helpful when taking a history as part of a physical examination to inquire nonjudgmentally about the patient's previous recollection of any exposure to traumatic events, in much the same manner that one takes a drug and alcohol or a sexual history. Similarly, it is important to note that often the person may not have any recollection of the traumatic event because of repression or amnesia that characteristically can cloud such overwhelming experiences. In the case of exposure to certain traumatic stimuli, the person may not remember the event[s] or may remember only fragments of the event[s].

For all patients, it is imperative to first establish a relationship that honors safety. This is particularly true for a person with PTSD, who may be triggered by intrusive procedures that occur as part of the routine physical examination. It can be helpful to tell patients what you are going to do and the reason why you are proceeding with specific interventions. One way to assist patients in remaining grounded is to ensure them that they can request that you stop or further explain any procedure, and that they are welcome to have a supportive person with them through most procedures and examinations, should they find this helpful.

DIAGNOSTICS

Currently laboratory tests to diagnose PTSD are not available; however, a variety of scales are used in assessment for PTSD in research and increasingly in some clinical settings (Box 265-2.) Van der Kolk advocates for the use of a battery of different such scales to optimize sensitivity and specificity of differing symptom presentations. Some of these scales include the PTSD Symptom Scale Interview (PSS-I), the PTSD Symptom Scale Self-Report (PSS-S), the Structured Interview for DSM III R (SCID), the Structured Interview for PTSD (SI-PTSD), the PTSD Interview, the Clinician Administered PTSD Scale (CAPS), the PTSD Checklist, and the Modified PTSD Symptom Scale Self-Report (MPSS-S).[2]

DIFFERENTIAL DIAGNOSIS

Although the symptom picture may appear similar to those characterized by acute anxiety disorder, major depression, brief psychotic disorder, psychotic disorders, obsessive compulsive disorder, or other medical illnesses in which acute anxiety, depression, and/or psychosis emerge, the patient's history of exposure to severely traumatic incident[s] is the definitive feature for a diagnosis of PTSD. Although adjustment disorder emerges as a result of an identifiable stressor, it is not characterized by extreme stress such as that experienced by someone feeling the fear or likelihood of death or witnessing such severe traumatic events that are considered unbearable. Acute stress disorder can present with similar sequelae of symptoms; however, symptoms always occur within 4 weeks of exposure to the traumatic event[s] and are resolved within 4 weeks of the initial presentation of symptoms.

MANAGEMENT

Given that PTSD affects a person biologically, psychologically, interpersonally, and spiritually, a multimodal approach to treatment generally renders effective results. In cases of severe symptomatology, the person should be treated by a psychiatric clinician who has demonstrated expertise in working with people with PTSD and their families (see Table 265-1).

LIFE SPAN CONSIDERATIONS

As previously noted, the age that the patient is first exposed to the traumatic incident[s] has implications for how he or she comes to understand the trauma and its meaning in his or her life. Younger children have less life experience with which they can buffer the painful impacts of traumatic exposure. They also have less cognitive capacity to understand and think through the event[s], their resulting distressing symptoms, and their consequences for their overall functioning and well-being.

People can reexperience traumatic symptoms long after exposure, which can make this a particularly confusing and challenging disorder for patient to understand and address. For example, a woman may not have had any significant difficulties after her personal experience of sexual victimization, but may experience acute symptoms when her daughter approaches the age at which she, herself, was traumatized.

COMPLICATIONS

Acute exacerbations of PTSD and chronic PTSD symptoms can render significant impairment in personal, occupational, and interpersonal functioning. The erosion of hope that is commonly evident with persistent symptoms and the high co-morbidity of depression, anxiety disorders (particularly panic disorder and phobias), and substance abuse disorders affect individuals' overall health status biologically, psychologically, and spiritually. Avoidance of situations and places in which the traumatic memories or

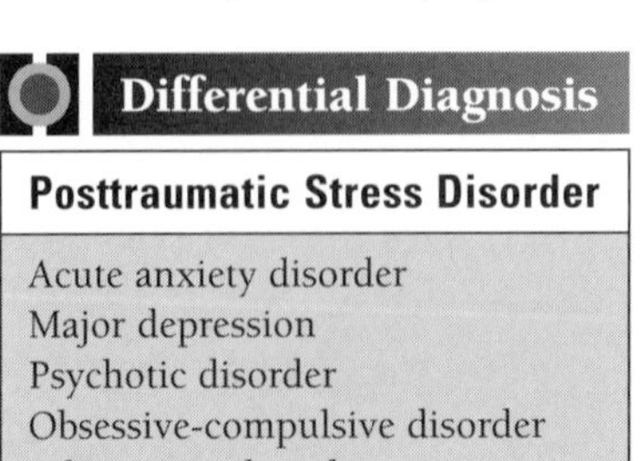
Differential Diagnosis

Posttraumatic Stress Disorder

Acute anxiety disorder
Major depression
Psychotic disorder
Obsessive-compulsive disorder
Adjustment disorder
Acute stress disorder

BOX 265-2

DIAGNOSTIC CRITERIA FOR POSTTRAUMATIC STRESS DISORDER

A. The person has been exposed to a traumatic event in which both of the following were present:
   (1) the person experienced, witnessed, or was confronted with an event or events that involved actual or threatened death or serious injury, or a threat to the physical integrity of self or others
   (2) the person's response involved intense fear, helplessness, or horror. Note: In children this may be expressed instead by disorganized or agitated behavior

B. The traumatic event is persistently experienced in one (or more) of the following ways:
   (1) recurrent and intrusive distressing recollections of the event, including images, thoughts, or perceptions. Note: In young children, repetitive play may occur in which themes or aspects of the trauma are expressed
   (2) recurring distressing dreams of the event. Note: In children, there may be frightening dreams without recognizable content
   (3) acting or feeling as if the traumatic event were recurring (includes a sense of reliving the experience, illusions, hallucinations, and dissociative flashback episodes, including those that occur on awakening or when intoxicated). Note: In young children, trauma-specific reenactment may occur
   (4) intense psychologic distress at exposure to internal or external cues that symbolize or resemble an aspect of the traumatic event
   (5) physiologic reactivity on exposure to internal or external cues that symbolize or resemble an aspect of the traumatic event

C. Persistent avoidance of stimuli associated with the trauma and numbing of general responsiveness (not present before the trauma), as indicated by three (or more) of the following:
   (1) efforts to avoid thoughts, feelings, or conversations associated with the trauma
   (2) efforts to avoid activities, places, or people that arouse recollections of the trauma
   (3) inability to recall an important aspect of the trauma
   (4) markedly diminished interest or participation in significant activities
   (5) feeling of detachment or estrangement from others
   (6) restricted range of affect (e.g., unable to have loving feelings)
   (7) sense of a foreshortened future (e.g., does not expect to have a career, marriage, children, or a normal life span)

D. Persistent symptoms of increased arousal (not present before the trauma), as indicated by two (or more) of the following:
   (1) difficulty falling or staying asleep
   (2) irritability or outbursts of anger
   (3) difficulty concentrating
   (4) hypervigilance
   (5) exaggerated startle response

E. Duration of the disturbance (symptoms in criteria B, C, and D) is more than 1 month.

F. The disturbance causes clinically significant distress or impairment in social, occupational, or other important areas of functioning.

Specify if:
   Acute: if duration of symptoms is less than 3 months
   Chronic: if duration of symptoms is 3 months or more

Specify if:
   With delayed onset: if onset of symptoms is at least 6 months after the stressor

From the American Psychiatric Association: *Diagnostic and statistical manual of mental disorders,* ed 4 (Text revision 2000), Washington DC, 1994, The Association.

symptoms are reexperienced results in constricted capacities to live more fully. In acute phases, symptoms of PTSD can render a person at risk for harm to himself or herself or others. Management of the symptoms must be aggressive to provide requisite safety for the patient and others.

INDICATIONS FOR REFERRAL/HOSPITALIZATION

Patients with a primary disorder of PTSD should be referred to a psychiatrist or psychiatric clinician who has the skills and expertise in PTSD to maximize the patient's successful treatment. Hospitalization is indicated in the following situations:

- Acute anxiety that is nonresponsive to pharmacologic interventions
- Acute depression with suicidal or homicidal features
- Homicidal ideation (with intention to hurt or kill a specific person or persons)
- Inability for the patient to care for himself or herself
- Dissociative episodes in which the patient cannot account for time that has elapsed or in which the patient's sense of self presents as disorganized and fragmented, or in which multiple personalities emerge

PATIENT AND FAMILY EDUCATION

It is important to explain to patients and families basic information about the physiology of PTSD, and the signs and symptoms that are identified with PTSD. Thorough understanding of PTSD, its prognosis, the importance of treatment, and medication side effects is essential. With adequate information and support, providers and patients can develop an individualized treatment plan to assist the patient through exacerbations of the disorder. Frequent monitoring (two to three times a week) until stable and a collaborative patient-provider relationship provide support for the patient and permit early identification of risk factors for treatment failure and the potential of self-harm or harm toward others.

HEALTH PROMOTION

There is evidence that people with a preexisting psychiatric illness may be more likely to develop PTSD when exposed to traumatic events; thus, it is important for patients with other disorders to receive ongoing treatment for them. There is also evidence that early intervention after a traumatic event is beneficial in reducing the likelihood that a person will develop PTSD or reduce the severity of the symptoms. As a result, many public health programs and school systems have now implemented Critical Stress Incident Debriefing programs after a traumatic incident occurs to minimize the long-term impact of a stressful event or events on a person or community.

REFERENCES

1. American Psychiatric Association: *Diagnostic and statistical manual of mental disorders*, ed 4, Text Revision, Washington, DC , 2000, The Association.
2. van der Kolk BA and others, editors: *Traumatic stress—the overwhelming experience on mind, body, and society*, New York, 1996, The Guilford Press.
3. Herman J: *Trauma and recovery*, New York, 1992, Basic Books.

CHAPTER 266

Psychotic Disorders

Cindy D. Campbell

DEFINITION/EPIDEMIOLOGY

Psychosis in itself is not a diagnosis but rather a presenting set of symptoms.[1] It may be a diagnostic symptom of a number of psychiatric disorders, or it may indicate an underlying metabolic or neurologic illness or a toxic reaction to a medication. The fourth edition of the *Diagnostic and Statistical Manual of Mental Disorders Text Revision* (DSM-IV-TR) defined psychosis as an impairment in reality testing that can include such symptoms as hallucinations and delusions.[2] Hallucinations may be auditory, visual, tactile, somatic, olfactory, or gustatory in nature.[2] Hallucinations need to be differentiated from illusions, which have as their basis some external stimuli that is then misinterpreted. A delusion is any persistent belief with no factual basis. Types of delusions include paranoid delusions, ideas of reference, thought insertion, and thought broadcasting.

Psychosis can be a symptom of a number of underlying conditions such as schizophrenia and dementia. It is estimated that the incidence of schizophrenia is between 0.7 and 1.4 per 10,000 individuals per year.[3] This rate is consistent across cultures and geographic locations.[2] Schizophrenia can be seen in children, adolescents, adults, and older individuals. It is estimated that between 2% and 4% of individuals over 65 years old have a diagnosis of Alzheimer's-type dementia.[2] In older adults, psychosis often occurs in association with a diagnosis of dementia.

Immediate psychiatric evaluation is required for all patients with suicidal/homicidal ideation.

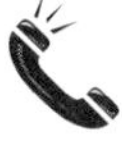

Physician consultation is indicated for increased psychotic behavior or for the development of tardive dyskinesia.

PATHOPHYSIOLOGY

Research to identify the etiology of schizophrenia is ongoing. The most promising theory is the biologically based neurotransmitter and receptor site theory.[4] This theory involves a number of transmitter systems—dopamine, serotonin, and gamma-aminobutyric acid—all of which appear to play a role. No single neurotransmitter system is ultimately responsible for schizophrenia. Schizophrenia is likely to be a complex combination of neurotransmitter availability, receptor sensitivity, and other mediating neural pathways. It is believed that either an alteration in neurotransmitters or a genetic vulnerability is inherited. The combination of genetics and life stressors leads to schizophrenia.[4]

Alzheimer's-type dementia is the most common type of dementia. Some families experience higher rates of Alzheimer's disease than others; therefore there is believed to be some genetic component.[5] Other theories include disorders of the neurotransmitters, an infectious process, or exposure to toxins.[5]

CLINICAL PRESENTATION

Psychosis may present in a variety of ways. A patient may be actively psychotic and obviously hallucinating; this is evident if the patient is responding to unseen stimuli by talking out loud when nobody else is present. However, often the presentation is not so obvious. Patients experiencing a schizophrenic decompensation are quite reluctant to discuss their unusual thought processes. The more obvious thought disturbances are paranoid delusions, ideas of reference, thought insertion, and thought broadcasting. A paranoid delusion may include the belief that one is being monitored electronically by unknown persons. An individual who believes that a conversation on the radio or a newspaper article pertains specifically to himself or herself is said to be experiencing ideas of reference. Thought insertion is the belief that thoughts are being placed inside one's head. Thought broadcasting is the belief that one's thoughts are being broadcasted to the world at large.

A psychosis may appear as speech disorganization, behavior disorganization, or catatonia. These conditions are more likely to be found in children.[6] Disorganized speech may be evidenced by an inability to complete a train of thought or by speaking words in no comprehensible order. Disorganized behavior is observed as an inability to complete any goal-directed activity such as activities of daily living. Catatonia is an extreme lack of reaction to outside stimuli; the individual may stare into space for hours, completely unresponsive to any verbal or physical stimuli. A less obvious sign of psychosis is thought blocking, which is evidenced by lengthy pauses between words and frequent losses of trains of thought. Thought blocking may be so severe that the individual forgets the question before formulating a response.

Psychosis related to dementia often presents itself as aggressive behavior accompanied by paranoia and delusions. Current estimates project that somewhere between 30% and 73% of individuals with Alzheimer's disease experience psychotic symptoms.[7,8] Individuals with Alzheimer's disease may suddenly fail to recognize their spouse and, believing there is a stranger in the home, may become combative. Such experiences may exacerbate paranoia and delusional thinking.

PHYSICAL EXAMINATION

A comprehensive physical examination is essential to exclude an underlying medical cause of psychosis. It is important that the primary care provider not make an immediate psychiatric diagnosis in a patient previously undiagnosed with a psychiatric disorder. A thorough medical evaluation is also indicated, even in patients with a known psychiatric history. Psychosis may hamper communication about serious medical illness.

DIAGNOSTICS

Numerous conditions may cause psychosis. It is necessary to first establish the origin of psychotic symptoms, which will dictate treatment. To determine if a medical or psychiatric diagnosis is appropriate, certain laboratory tests are necessary, including CBC, BUN, glucose, creatinine, electrolytes, LFTs, and urine toxic screen.[9] Results of these tests help the provider reach an appropriate diagnosis. The DSM-IV-TR also has specific criteria by which to define schizophrenia and brief psychotic disorder (Boxes 266-1 and 266-2).

A mental status examination is also essential to establish the patient's orientation and ability to perform executive functioning and to obtain a general overview of the patient's cognitive impairment. This information aids in determining a differential diagnosis. Neuropsychologic testing is another valuable

Diagnostics

Psychotic Disorders

Laboratory
CBC and differential
BUN
Creatinine
Serum glucose
Serum electrolytes
LFTs
Urine for toxic screen

Imaging
CT scan*

*If indicated.

BOX 266-1

DIAGNOSTIC CRITERIA FOR BRIEF PSYCHOTIC DISORDER

A. Presence of one (or more) of the following symptoms:
(1) delusions
(2) hallucinations
(3) disorganized speech (e.g., frequent derailment or incoherence)
(4) grossly disorganized or catatonic behavior

Note: Do not include a symptom if it is a culturally sanctioned response pattern.

B. Duration of an episode of the disturbance is at least 1 day but less than 1 month, with eventual full return to premorbid level of functioning.

C. The disturbance is not better accounted for by a Mood Disorder With Psychotic Features, Schizoaffective Disorder, or Schizophrenia and is not due to the direct physiologic effects of a substance (e.g., a drug of abuse, a medication) or a general medical condition.

Specify if:

With Marked Stressor(s): (brief reactive psychosis): if symptoms occur shortly after and apparently in response to events that, singly or together, would be markedly stressful to almost anyone in similar circumstances in the person's culture

Without Marked Stressor(s): if psychotic symptoms do *not* occur shortly after, or are not apparently in response to events that, singly or together, would be markedly stressful to almost anyone in similar circumstances in the person's culture

With Postpartum Onset: if onset within 4 weeks postpartum

From American Psychiatric Association: *Diagnostic and statistical manual of mental disorders*, ed 4 (Text revision 2000), Washington DC, 1994, The Association.

BOX 266-2

DIAGNOSTIC CRITERIA FOR SCHIZOPHRENIA

A. *Characteristic symptoms:* Two (or more) of the following, each present for a significant portion of time during a 1-month period (or less if successfully treated):
   (1) delusions
   (2) hallucinations
   (3) disorganized speech (e.g., frequent derailment or incoherence)
   (4) grossly disorganized or catatonic behavior
   (5) negative symptoms, i.e., affective flattening, alogia, or avolition

   Note: Only one Criterion A symptom is required if delusions are bizarre or hallucinations consist of a voice keeping up a running commentary on the person's behavior or thoughts, or two or more voices conversing with each other.

B. *Social/occupational dysfunction:* For a significant portion of the time since the onset of the disturbance, one or more major areas of functioning such as work, interpersonal relations, or self-care are markedly below the level achieved prior to the onset (or when the onset is in childhood or adolescence, failure to achieve expected level of interpersonal, academic, or occupational achievement).

C. *Duration:* Continuous signs of the disturbance persist for at least 6 months. This 6-month period must include at least 1 month of symptoms (or less if successfully treated) that meet Criterion A (i.e., active-phase symptoms) and may include periods of prodromal or residual symptoms. During these prodromal or residual periods, the signs of the disturbance may be manifested by only negative symptoms or two or more symptoms listed in Criterion A present in an attenuated form (e.g., odd beliefs, unusual perceptual experiences).

D. *Schizoaffective and Mood Disorder exclusion:* Schizoaffective Disorder and Mood Disorder With Psychotic Features have been ruled out because either (1) no Major Depressive, Manic, or Mixed Episodes have occurred concurrently with the active-phase symptoms; or (2) if mood episodes have occurred during active-phase symptoms, their total duration has been brief relative to the duration of the active and residual periods.

E. *Substance/general medical condition exclusion:* The disturbance is not due to the direct physiologic effects of a substance (e.g., a drug of abuse, a medication) or a general medical condition.

F. *Relationship to a Pervasive Developmental Disorder:* If there is a history of Autistic Disorder or another Pervasive Developmental Disorder, the additional diagnosis of Schizophrenia is made only if prominent delusions or hallucinations are also present for at least a month (or less if successfully treated).

Classification of longitudinal course (can be applied only after at least 1 year has elapsed since the initial onset of active-phase symptoms):

Episodic With Interepisode Residual Symptoms (episodes are defined by the reemergence of prominent psychotic symptoms); *also specify if:* **With Prominent Negative Symptoms**

Continuous (prominent psychotic symptoms are present throughout the period of observation); *also specify if:* **With Prominent Negative Symptoms**

Single Episode In Partial Remission; *also specify if:* **With Prominent Negative Symptoms**

Single Episode In Full Remission

Other or Unspecified Pattern

From American Psychiatric Association: *Diagnostic and statistical manual of mental disorders,* ed 4 (Text revision 2000), Washington DC, 1994, The Association.

tool for establishing an accurate psychiatric diagnosis. Testing consists of a battery of written and verbal tests administered by a qualified licensed practitioner, who administers the tests and interprets the results.

No specific diagnostic tests are indicative of schizophrenia or dementia. Research to determine the role certain structural abnormalities play in the development and treatment of schizophrenia continues. Depending on the situation, a CT scan may be used to determine the presence of structural abnormalities. A CT scan is required if neurologic indicators are present, if the patient is experiencing a psychosis of sudden onset, or if the patient is experiencing a psychosis for the first time.[9] MRI, positron emission topography, and single proton emission CT scans indicate that enlarged ventricles, decreased temporal and hippocampus size, increased basal ganglia, and abnormal glucose utilization in the prefrontal cortex are consistently found in patients with schizophrenia when examined as a group.[2] Autopsies have shown that the brains of patients with Alzheimer's disease contain neurofibrillary tangles and protein-based neuritic plaques. This differs from other dementias and normal aging, as the plaques and tangles are present in greater numbers and locations in individuals with Alzheimer's disease.[5]

DIFFERENTIAL DIAGNOSIS

Numerous conditions may be responsible for psychosis. Medical diagnoses to be considered in the differential diagnosis include metabolic disorders (e.g., hypoglycemia, hypothyroidism, hyperthyroidism, porphyria), nutritional deficiencies, neurologic disorders (e.g., brain lesion, encephalitis, Parkinson's disease, Huntington's chorea, cerebrovascular accident, seizure disorder), exposure to heavy metals, and medication toxicity (e.g., digitalis, theophylline, steroids, antiparkinsonian medications).[9] Psychiatric diagnoses to be considered include schizophrenia, major depression with psychotic features, bipolar disorder, substance abuse and/or withdrawal (alcohol, benzodiazepines, LSD [lysergic acid diethylamide], PCP [phencyclidine hydrochloride], stimulants, cocaine, marijuana), and medication toxicity (anticholinergics). In older adults it is necessary to consider dementia

Differential Diagnosis

Psychotic Disorders

Heavy metal exposure	Neurologic disorder
Medication/substance toxicity	Brain lesion
Antiparkinsonian	Cerebrovascular accident
Digitalis	Encephalitis
Steroids	Huntington's chorea
Theophylline	Parkinsons' disease
Anticholinergics	Seizure disorder
Substance abuse	Nutritional deficiencies
Metabolic disorder	Psychiatric disorders
Hypoglycemia	Bipolar disorder
Hypothyroidism	Dementia
Hyperthyroidism	Major depression
Porphyria	Schizophrenia

(Alzheimer's dementia, vascular dementia, or dementia resulting from a specific medical condition such as HIV, Parkinson's disease, and others). In children it is necessary to exclude pervasive developmental disorders.[10,11]

MANAGEMENT

The treatment of choice for psychosis is the use of antipsychotic medications, which are also known as neuroleptics or major tranquilizers. These medications are divided into high-potency, low-potency, and atypical antipsychotic medications and should be prescribed and monitored by a psychiatric provider. The low-potency antipsychotic drugs (chlorpromazine [Thorazine], thioridazine [Mellaril], and mesoridazine [Serentil]) are highly sedating and are associated with increased anticholinergic side effects such as weight gain, constipation, blurred vision, urinary retention, and dry mouth. These medications are particularly useful for patients experiencing agitation or sleeplessness in association with psychotic symptoms. They also have a lower potential for causing extrapyramidal side effects (EPSs). At present, thioridazine (Mellaril) is used only when all other attempts at stabilization have been exhausted because of the potential for cardiac QTc prolongation.

The high-potency antipsychotics (haloperidol [Haldol], thiothixene [Navane], fluphenazine [Prolixin], perphenazine [Trilafon], molindone [Moban], Orap, trifluoperazine [Stelazine], loxapine [Loxitane]) tend to be less sedating but have an increased tendency to cause EPSs. The atypical antipsychotic drugs (clozapine [Clozaril], risperidone [Risperdal], olanzapine [Zyprexa], quetiapine [Seroquel], ziprasidone [Geodon]) are reported to have decreased tendency to cause EPSs and may have a decreased tendency to cause tardive dyskinesia (TD). However, these medications are too new for this to be established with certainty. Serlect and Zeldox did not gain approval by the U.S. Food and Drug Administration (FDA). All antipsychotic medications have the potential to cause TD. They also have the potential to lower the seizure threshold and therefore should be used with caution in patients with seizure disorder.[11,12]

Supportive psychotherapy for both the patient and family is equally important. It is well known that the impact of schizophrenia can be greatly reduced with early aggressive intervention.[4] Other treatment options necessary at various times during the course of the disease include case management and vocational rehabilitation. As with any major disorder, patient and family education and the use of community resources are essential. Respite care is also a useful intervention for families experiencing caregiver stress.

Co-Management with Specialists

A psychiatric health care provider treats most patients with psychosis. Therefore treatment with the primary care provider and any other specialty providers must be closely coordinated. Antipsychotic medications should never be discontinued abruptly and, ideally, dosages should never be decreased without serious consideration by the patient, family, and the psychiatric health care provider. Although a patient may appear to be completely free of psychosis, this is usually a result of the antipsychotic medication. Because each psychotic episode incurs a risk that the patient may not return to the previous level of functioning, lowering or discontinuing antipsychotic medications is a serious decision.

Accurate medication records are necessary because of interactions and potentiation of medications and because many medications can exacerbate psychosis. Although the use of the medication in question may be necessary, collaboration with the psychiatric health care provider can allow for an adjustment in the antipsychotic medications.

LIFE SPAN CONSIDERATIONS

The use of antipsychotic medications in children and adolescents has not yet been approved by the FDA. Nevertheless, in many cases it is necessary to use these medications for patients less than 18 years of age who are experiencing psychotic symptoms. Consideration should be given to the age and weight of the child, and consent must be obtained from both the child and the custodial parents or legal guardian.[13] As always, the dose should be started low and slowly titrated up to the minimum effective dose. Atypical antipsychotic medications should be selected for use in children. These medications may have a decreased incidence of TD, but the incidence of TD increases with length of time on the medication. When making the initial assessment of children, it is necessary to obtain information from parents, siblings, and teachers.[6,11]

It is always necessary to determine pregnancy before initiating antipsychotic medications in females of childbearing age. In certain extenuating circumstances it may be necessary to use antipsychotic medications during pregnancy. In such cases, the benefits must clearly outweigh the risks. A thorough discussion of the potential side effects must be discussed, and a referral to a neonatologist is recommended.

Antipsychotic medications should be used with care in older adults. A much lower dose of medication is often required because of the decreased ability to metabolize it.[14] Older adults may be taking a multitude of medications, and drug interactions must be carefully assessed. The risk for falls, lowered blood pressure, and orthostatic changes with these medications is a primary concern, as dizziness can result in falls and fractures.[15] The anticholinergic side effects of the antipsychotic medications may increase confusion in this population. Risperidone (Risperdal), a newer atypical antipsychotic medication, has recently been suggested as the antipsychotic of choice in older adults because of its decreased incidence of side effects.[16] However, the cost of a newer agent is often prohibitive in this population.

COMPLICATIONS

All antipsychotic medications have the potential to cause uncomfortable side effects, which often cause patients to stop taking their medications. EPSs include dystonia, tremors, akathisia (an intolerable restlessness and need to pace), and a shuffling gait. Medications available to combat these unpleasant side effects include benztropine (Cogentin) and trihexyphenidyl (Artane). However these medications have their own side effects, which can include increased psychosis and anticholinergic effects. Amantadine (Symmetrel) is also used for gait disturbances and muscle stiffness. Other treatment options for antipsychotic side effects include the beta blocker propranolol (Inderal) for tremors and akathisia and benzodiazepines for akathisia. Inderal may worsen postural hypotension, and benzodiazepines should be avoided if possible because of their potential for both addiction and increased risk for falls in older adults.

The most frightening side effect of the antipsychotic medications is TD. It is a sometimes irreversible condition characterized by involuntary muscle movements of the mouth, jaw, and tongue. The incidence of TD is estimated to be between 3% and 5% per year.[2] There is no known treatment, but clonazepam (Klonopin) may ease the symptoms. If symptoms of TD develop, the antipsychotic medication must be tapered immediately to discontinuation if at all possible. Of the patients who are able to be kept off of antipsychotic medications, approximately one third experience resolution of TD within 3 months, and approximately 50% within 18 months.[2] The decision regarding whether or not a patient can remain free of antipsychotic medications is best decided between the patient and the specialty psychiatric health care provider.

The atypical antipsychotic clozapine (Clozaril) has the potential to cause life-threatening agranulocytosis. Consequently, one of the requirements is that all patients taking this medication have their white blood cell (WBC) count monitored weekly. This may change to biweekly after 6 months of normal results. The medication is dispensed from the pharmacy after confirmation of an acceptable WBC count.

Neuroleptic malignant syndrome (NMS) is the most serious complication of antipsychotic administration and is potentially fatal. Although the clinical presentation of NMS may vary, it is usually associated with an elevated temperature and muscle rigidity. In addition, at least two of the following must be present: diaphoresis, dysphagia, tremor, incontinence, mutism, tachycardia, labile blood pressure, leukocytosis, elevated creatine phosphokinase, and a change in level of consciousness.[2] NMS usually occurs within the first 3 months of initiating the medication but can occur at any time, even after the patient has been maintained on a medication for months.[2]

Weight gain, hyperlipidemia, hyperglycemia, and diabetes mellitus are emerging as health risks of antipsychotic therapy.[17] Hyperprolactinemia is a less common occurrence.

Psychosis has many complications. In patients with schizophrenia, psychosis may progressively worsen over time, resulting in decreased functional ability, particularly if medications are not taken consistently. Each exacerbation of the illness has the potential to last longer and be more severe. It is possible that the patient may never return to the previous level of functioning.

Whether a result of schizophrenia or dementia, treatment-resistant psychosis may result in the need for a series of medication trials, which can be frustrating for both the patient and the caregivers. Care must be taken to provide a safe environment during this process. Patients with psychosis may also have a potential for violence. This potential must be carefully and continually assessed, because patients may feel threatened by the environment as a result of the hallucinations.

INDICATIONS FOR REFERRAL/HOSPITALIZATION

Psychosis is often only a symptom of a severe brain disorder and therefore needs to be managed by a psychiatric health care provider. Any patient experiencing psychosis needs to have the benefit of a full psychiatric evaluation to ensure proper diagnosis and treatment. Psychosis in children or adolescents should be managed by a psychiatric health care provider, preferably one with a specialty in child and adolescent psychiatry.

Hospitalization is often necessary during an acute exacerbation of a psychotic illness. This determination is best made by a psychiatric health care professional. However, any health care provider who believes a patient to be in imminent danger of harming either himself or herself or someone else should immediately initiate procedures for a psychiatric consultation.

PATIENT AND FAMILY EDUCATION

Patients and their families must be educated about psychosis and the available treatments so that they may make informed health care decisions. The side effects of medications are often frightening to both patients and families. A thorough discussion of the potential side effects and a plan to manage them can greatly alleviate the concerns of patients and families when deciding whether to use an antipsychotic medication. They must also be informed that psychosis is a biochemical illness with extreme psychosocial ramifications that respond to chemical intervention. As with any serious illness, patients must understand that, even if they are feeling better, medications need to be continued.

HEALTH PROMOTION

Hyperglycemia, hyperlipidemia, and weight gain can be managed with a combination of diet and exercise. It must be acknowledged, however, that many of the symptoms of a psychotic disorder include low motivation and indifference to personal appearance and hygiene. Consequently expectations must be kept realistic and achievable and should be highly individualized.

REFERENCES

1. Preston J, Johnson J: *Clinical psychopharmacology made ridiculously simple*, ed 3, Miami, 1997, MedMaster.
2. American Psychiatric Association: *Diagnostic and statistical manual of mental disorders*, ed 4, Text Revision, Washington, DC, 2000, The Association.
3. Hafner H, van der Heiden W: Epidemiology of schizophrenia, *Can J Psychiatry* 42(2):139-151, 1997.
4. Munich R: Contemporary treatment of schizophrenia, *Bull Menninger Clin* 61:189-220, 1997.
5. Tariot P: Neurobiology and treatment of dementia. In Salzman C, editor: *Clinical geriatric psychopharmacology*, ed 2, Baltimore, 1992, Williams & Wilkins.

6. Volkmar F: Childhood and adolescent psychosis: a review of the past 10 years, *J Am Acad Child Adolesc Psychiatry* 35:843-851, 1996.
7. Lacro J, Jeste D: Geriatric psychosis, *Psychiatr Q* 68:247-259, 1997.
8. Wilson R and others: Hallucinations, delusions, and cognitive decline, *J Neurol Neurosurg Psychiatry* 69:172-177, 2000.
9. Hyman S: *Manual of psychiatric emergencies,* ed 2, Boston, 1988, Little, Brown.
10. Gartner J, Weintraub S, Carlson G: Childhood-onset psychosis: evolution and comorbidity, *Am J Psychiatry* 154:256-261, 1997.
11. Dulcan M, Martini D: *Concise guide to child and adolescent psychiatry,* ed 2,Washington DC, 1999, American Psychiatric Press.
12. Green W: *Child and adolescent psychopharmacology,* ed 2, New York, 1995, Williams & Wilkins.
13. McClellan J, Werry J: Practice parameters for the assessment and treatment of children and adolescents with schizophrenia, *J Am Acad Child Adolesc Psychiatry* 33(5):616-635, 1994.
14. Salzman C: *Psychiatric medications for older adults: the concise guide,* New York, 2001, The Guilford Press.
15. Lamy P, Salzman C, Nevis-Olesen J: Drug prescribing patterns, risks, and compliance guidelines. In Salzman C, editor: *Clinical geriatric psychopharmacology,* ed 2, Baltimore, 1992, Williams & Wilkins.
16. Zayas E, Grossberg G: The treatment of psychosis in late life, *J Clin Psychiatry* 59(suppl 1):5-10, 1998.
17. Sussman N: Review of atypical antipsychotics and weight gain, *J Clin Psychiatry* 62 (suppl 23):5-12, 2001.

CHAPTER 267

Somatization Disorder

Alice Bolton, Cindy D. Campbell, and Willadene Walker Schmucker

DEFINITION/EPIDEMIOLOGY

Somatization disorder is one of the somatoform disorders. This disorder generally develops before 30 years of age and is characterized by frequent, varied, and long-lasting somatic complaints that have no basis in physical dysfunction. Individuals with a somatization disorder do not accept the psychologic basis of their problems and insist on obtaining medical help. They are viewed by health care providers as frustrating or irritating because they do not get better and keep coming back. Somatization disorder represents a significant cost to the health care system.

There are six types of somatoform disorders: (1) body dysmorphic disorder, (2) conversion disorder, (3) hypochondriasis, (4) somatization disorder, (5) somatoform pain disorder, and (6) undifferentiated somatoform disorder.[1] The essential feature of these disorders is the presence of a physical or somatic complaint in the absence of any demonstrable organic findings or any known physiologic mechanisms that can account for the complaint or explain the findings. There is also the presumption of associated psychologic factors or unconscious conflicts to account for the syndrome.[2]

Previously known as Briquet's syndrome, somatization disorder differs in specific criteria from the other somatoform disorders. With a somatization disorder, complaints are not limited to one organ system and are not caused by any medical disorder. To meet the criteria for classification as a somatization disorder, the patient must have experienced symptoms before 30 years of age and must have at least four pain symptoms, two gastrointestinal symptoms, one sexual symptom, and one pseudoneurologic symptom.[1] These unexplained symptoms are not intentionally feigned or produced.[1] The severity of somatization disorder is assessed from a total count of any of the following: complaints, the search for medical treatment, the use of medication, or lifestyle adjustments for different symptoms.[3]

The onset of a somatization disorder usually occurs in adolescence or early adulthood. It occurs predominantly in women (1% to 2% of the female population) and tends to be associated with sociopathy and alcoholism in male relatives.[4] In research conducted by Faravelli and others,[5] all somatoform disorders were much more common in women, with somatization, conversion, and body dysmorphic disorders found only among females in their inquiry. Kroenke and others[6] report that the diagnosis of a somatization disorder involves lifetime symptoms, with more than one fourth of all health care provider visits attributable to somatoform disorders.[6] All somatoform disorders seem to be more common in less-educated, lower socioeconomic groups and in those of low occupational status. Studies have shown a concordance rate of 29% in monozygotic twins and 10% in dizygotic twins.[7] Cultural factors may influence the gender ratio for somatization disorder. This particular somatoform disorder occurs only rarely in men in the United States; a higher frequency is reported in Greek and Puerto Rican men.[1]

Immediate psychiatric evaluation is required for all patients with suicidal/homicidal ideation.

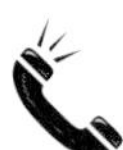

Physician consultation is indicated for patients who do not respond to the treatment plan for somatization disorder.

PATHOPHYSIOLOGY

Somatization is one of the oldest of all known psychologic diagnoses. The first reference to this type of phenomenon appeared in Egyptian documents in approximately 1900 BC; it was also commented on by the Greeks. In its modern form, it was first defined in 1859 by Briquet, a French physician who identified patients with medical symptoms but no demonstrable medical disease.[6,8] The cause of somatization disorder is unknown. Rossi[9] has suggested that patients with this disorder have no conscious control over their somatization because it is tied to neuropsychophysiologic state–dependent memory, but they do have control over whether they embellish their symptoms and disabilities.

The suspected etiology of somatization disorder lies in the mind-body connection. One body of research reports an interrelated link between psychosocial and genetic factors, including identification with a parent who models the sick role, suppression or repression of anger toward others and turning this anger inward toward self, a punitive personality organization with a strong superego, and low self-esteem. There seems to be a genetic link, with a 10% to 20% incidence of mothers and/or sisters of patients also being afflicted.[7] Some studies have suggested a neuropsychologic basis for somatization disorder. These investigations propose that patients with this disorder have characteristic attentional and cognitive impairments that result in a faulty perception and assessment of somatosensory input. Impairments include excessive distractibility, an inability to habituate to repetitive stimuli, and partial and circumstantial associations. Cultural and ethnic factors are important to note because they influence the patient's self-report of symptoms.[10]

CLINICAL PRESENTATION

Patients with somatization disorder often have "seen every health care provider in town." The nature of the disorder is chronic and lifelong, generally beginning in adolescence and lasting through the life cycle if left untreated. Individuals often present with complex and inconsistent medical histories. Laboratory tests are generally not significantly abnormal, and reported symptoms may be the result of a faulty assessment of somatosensory input by the individual.

There are 35 symptoms reviewed to indicate a diagnosis of somatization disorder. To receive this diagnosis, the patient must display 13 or more of these 35 symptoms, and these symptoms must lack an acceptable medical explanation. If the physical examination reveals no acceptable medical explanation, the following 7 symptoms are recommended as an initial screen for somatization disorder: (1) pain in extremities, (2) shortness of breath, (3) amnesia, (4) burning sensation in sexual organs or rectum (other than during intercourse), (5) difficulty swallowing, (6) vomiting, and (7) painful menstruation.[9] Patients with somatization disorder report a belief that they have "always been sickly" and that "nobody has been able to help me." Somatization disorder has a fluctuating course, and afflicted individuals are rarely asymptomatic. It is unusual for them to go for more than 1 year without some medical attention. These individuals describe their symptoms in vivid, colorful, exaggerated, emotional, and dramatic terms. Instead of the simple "I can't swallow," an individual with somatization disorder would likely say, "I can't swallow, it's as if I have someone's hands around my throat, squeezing their fingers deeply into my neck." These individuals often dress in an exhibitionistic manner and are sometimes seductive. They usually describe significant distress and interpersonal problems and often report marital, occupational, and social problems. When describing their histories they are often vague, imprecise, inconsistent, and disorganized. Suicide threats are common, but actual suicides are rare.[7]

PHYSICAL EXAMINATION

Somatoform disorders are a diagnostic challenge because the symptoms encountered are nonspecific and can overlap with a multitude of medical conditions. Caution is always necessary so that underlying and potentially treatable mental and general medical disorders are not overlooked.[6] A thorough physical examination is necessary, even in patients with a psychiatric history. As is always the case, it is important that the primary care provider not be swayed by a suspicion of a psychiatric diagnosis in patients previously undiagnosed with a psychiatric disorder. Although the provider may be tempted to forgo the physical examination in a patient previously diagnosed with a somatoform disorder, these individuals can also develop serious medical illnesses.

DIAGNOSTICS

Given the array of potential symptoms, an appropriate clinical investigation is indicated. The fourth edition of the *Diagnostic and Statistical Manual of Mental Disorders (DSM-IV)* has specific criteria for defining a somatization disorder (Box 267-1). The initial diagnostic tests should be guided by the history and physical examination. However, characteristically there is a lack of findings on diagnostic studies.[1] Health care providers treating this condition often find themselves walking a fine line between an appropriate clinical investigation and an exhaustive but nonproductive battery of testing.[11] Neuropsychologic testing is a valuable tool in establishing an accurate psychiatric diagnosis. This procedure consists of a battery of written and verbal tests administered by a licensed individual who is qualified to administer and interpret the results.

DIFFERENTIAL DIAGNOSIS

Symptom presentation may be indicative of numerous medical conditions. Three clues may indicate the presence of somatization disorder: (1) the physical complaints often involve multiple organ systems; (2) the symptoms have appeared early (before age 30), appear to be chronic, and lack physical findings or structural abnormalities; and (3) there is an absence of diagnostic abnormalities that are characteristic of the indicated

BOX 267-1

DIAGNOSTIC CRITERIA FOR SOMATIZATION DISORDER

A. A history of many physical complaints beginning before age 30 years that occur over a period of several years and result in treatment being sought or significant impairment in social, occupational, or other important areas of functioning.

B. Each of the following criteria must have been met, with individual symptoms occurring at any time during the course of the disturbance:

(1) *Four pain symptoms:* a history of pain related to at least four different sites or functions (e.g., head, abdomen, back, joints, extremities, chest, rectum, during menstruation, during sexual intercourse, or during urination)

(2) *Two gastrointestinal symptoms:* a history of at least two gastrointestinal symptoms other than pain (e.g., nausea, bloating, vomiting other than during pregnancy, diarrhea, or intolerance of several different foods)

(3) *One sexual symptom:* a history of at least one sexual or reproductive symptom other than pain (e.g., sexual indifference, erectile or ejaculatory dysfunction, irregular menses, excessive menstrual bleeding, vomiting throughout pregnancy)

(4) *One pseudoneurologic symptom:* a history of at least one symptom or deficit suggesting a neurologic condition not limited to pain (conversion symptoms such as impaired coordination or balance, paralysis or localized weakness, difficulty swallowing or lump in throat, aphonia, urinary retention, hallucinations, loss of touch or pain sensation, double vision, blindness, deafness, seizures; dissociative symptoms such as amnesia; or loss of consciousness other than fainting)

C. Either (1) or (2)

(1) After appropriate investigation, each of the symptoms in Criterion B cannot be fully explained by a known general medical condition or the direct effects of a substance (e.g., a drug of abuse, a medication)

(2) When there is a related general medical condition, the physical complaints or resulting social or occupational impairment are in excess of what would be expected from the history, physical examination, or laboratory findings

D. The symptoms are not intentionally produced or feigned (as in factitious disorder or malingering).

From American Psychiatric Association: *Diagnostic and statistical manual of mental disorders*, ed 4 (Text revision 2000), Washington, DC, 2000, American Psychiatric Association, p. 490.

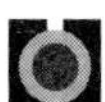

Differential Diagnosis

Somatization Disorder

Medical Disorders	Psychiatric Disorders
Hyperparathyroidism	Factitious disorder
Systemic lupus erythematosus	Generalized anxiety disorder
Multiple sclerosis	Malingering
Porphyria	Mood disorders
	Panic disorder
	Posttraumatic stress disorder
	Schizophrenia

medical condition.[1] Many medical conditions also present as vague somatic symptoms and must excluded in the differential diagnosis. These include hyperparathyroidism, porphyria, multiple sclerosis, and lupus.[1] It is essential to remember that such presentations in an older patient are most likely indicative of a medical condition.[1]

A number of psychiatric disorders must also be considered; these include schizophrenia, panic disorder, generalized anxiety disorder, mood disorders, posttraumatic stress disorder, factitious disorder, and malingering.[1,11,12]

MANAGEMENT

It is helpful to view the development of somatization disorder as an unhealthy coping skill.[13] Because any number of symptoms may be present, it is important to focus on symptom relief. If the patient is experiencing a high level of anxiety or significant depressive symptoms, a selective serotonin reuptake inhibitor (SSRI) antidepressant may be helpful. It is essential that the patient be involved in some type of therapy, the goal of which is to develop healthier methods of coping. Cognitive behavioral therapy is also useful and can assist with the reduction of somatization by not reinforcing this behavior.[12] Group therapy in combination with regular consultation with a primary care provider can also be helpful in treating somatoform disorders. There also may be additional medical or psychiatric illnesses that require appropriate treatment.

Because these patients often seek health care from many providers, it is of utmost importance to obtain a thorough history, including current medications and treatments. Queries about past and current interventions to seek symptom relief may help the provider to discover a duplication of treatment interventions or dangerous drug interactions. Communication among all health care providers is necessary. Records from previous and current providers may be required.

When narcotic analgesics or other controlled substances are considered in treatment, precautions must be taken to avoid dependence or addiction.

LIFE SPAN CONSIDERATIONS

By definition, symptoms of somatoform disorder begin before age 30. Woman are diagnosed more often with the disorder in the United States, whereas men of Puerto Rican or Greek descent are diagnosed more often.

Life span considerations involve quality of life for the individual and family as well as monetary concerns.

COMPLICATIONS

Complications associated with any somatoform disorder include unnecessary medical treatment and operations, financial distress, impairment in work and social activities, family discord, iatrogenic effects from multiuse and overuse of medical interventions, substance-related disorders, and suicide.[1,14] Treatment is often sought from several providers, which places the patient at risk for dangerous interactions from treatment combinations. Each operation or hospitalization adds health risks. Time is lost from work, which often creates job insecurity. Families suffer from loss of the patient's interaction, loss of parental guidance, or loss of spousal support. The risk for dependence on narcotic analgesics is great. Depression and suicide risk increase as the condition progresses.

INDICATIONS FOR REFERRAL/HOSPITALIZATION

Somatoform disorders present a challenge in primary care. Because the condition is not readily recognized, considerations for referral are not definitively identified. The primary care provider might consider the following as guidelines for referral: the patient's medical and surgical history, the frequency and nature of primary care and specialist office visits, and response to interventions. A psychosocial assessment may provide clues to the causative nature of the disorder. Childhood abuse has been correlated with the development of somatoform disorders.[15] A mental health referral is made after the provider has excluded any physical reason for the patient's symptoms.

With the advent of managed care, hospitalizations for somatoform disorder have been limited. Outpatient evaluations are more prevalent. Patients with a somatoform disorder and a co-morbid personality disorder may be at risk for suicide. For the patient's safety, any indication of suicide risk requires an immediate referral to a psychiatric health care provider. All states have provisions for emergency inpatient evaluation for patients who pose a danger to themselves or others. Providers should be familiar with the mental health act in their practice locale.

PATIENT EDUCATION

Many patients are prescribed medications for symptom relief. Education about the side effects, risks, purposes, and use of medications is stressed. A review of medications and an assessment of the effectiveness of the intervention are made at each office visit. Patients are advised to write down their questions and concerns before the visit; such communication may provide clues to a diagnosis.

Although often seen in primary care, somatization is not often treated in this setting. Nevertheless, the primary care provider often continues to be the medical provider. The challenge to the provider is to distinguish somatic symptoms from those with an actual biologic origin. The provider has the opportunity to assess and educate the patient about treatment. Educating the patient about the importance of continuing mental health treatment is essential. A decrease in the use of health care has been associated with patients' ability to distinguish between mental health issues and physical symptoms.[14]

HEALTH PROMOTION

Health promotion is difficult to define in this diagnosis. The nature of the disorder is to displace emotional responses with magnified physical symptomology. Those persons identified at risk for developing the disorder should receive psychotherapy and other supportive interventions early in life. Those persons diagnosed would benefit from ongoing treatment focusing on developing and maintaining effective coping skills and on developing and maintaining a healthy lifestyle: regular exercise, appropriate diet, routine physical examination, adequate rest, and maintaining a routine.

REFERENCES

1. American Psychiatric Association: *Diagnostic and statistical manual of mental disorders*, ed 4, Text Revision, Washington, DC, 2000, The Association.
2. Barsky AJ, Borus JF: Somatization and medicalization in the era of managed care, *JAMA* 27:1931-1934, 1995.
3. Servan-Schreiber D, Tabas G, Kolb R: Somatizing patients: part II. Practical management, *Am Fam Physician* 61:1423-1428, 1431-1432, 2000. Retrieved August 12, 2002, from the World Wide Web: www.aafp.org/afp/20000215/1073.html.
4. Berkow R: Somatoform disorders. In Beers MH, Berkow R, editors: *The Merck manual of diagnosis and therapy*, ed 17, Whitehouse Station, NJ, 2002, Merck & Co, Inc. Retrieved August 12, 2002, from the World Wide Web: www.merck.com/pubs/mmanual/section15/chapter186/186b.htm.
5. Faravelli C and others: Epidemiology of somatoform disorders: a community survey in Florence, *J Affect Disord* 20:135-141, 1996.
6. Kroenke K and others: Multisomatoform disorder, *Arch Gen Psychiatry* 54:352-358, 1997.
7. Kaplan H, Sadock B: *Synopsis of psychiatry, behavioral sciences, clinical psychiatry*, ed 6, Baltimore, 1991, Williams & Wilkins.
8. Bruns D: *The problem of somatizaton*, Greeley, Colo, 1998, Health Psychology and Rehabilitation. Retrieved August 12, 2002, from the World Wide Web: www.healthpsych.com/somatization.html.
9. Rossi E, Cheek D: *Mind-body therapy: methods of ideodynamic healing in hypnosis*, Baltimore, 1988, WW Norton.
10. Noyes R and others: A family study of hypochondriasis, *J Nerv Ment Dis* 185:223-232, 1997.
11. Peveler R, Kilkenny L, Kinmouth A: Medically unexplained physical symptoms in primary care: a comparison of self-report screening questionnaires and clinical opinion, *J Psychosom Res* 42:245-252, 1997.
12. Gooch J, Wolcott R, Speed J: Behavioral management of conversion disorder in children, *Arch Phys Med Rehabil* 78:264-268, 1997.
13. Badura A and others: Dissociation, somatization, substance abuse, and coping in women with chronic pelvic pain, *Obstet Gynecol* 90:405-410, 1997.
14. Morse D, Suchman A, Frankel R: The meaning of symptoms in 10 women with somatization disorder and a history of childhood abuse, *Arch Fam Med* 6:468-476, 1997.
15. Farley M, Keaney J: Physical symptoms, somatization, and dissociation in women survivors of childhood sexual assault, *Women Health* 25:33-45, 1997.

CHAPTER 268

Substance Abuse

Joseph Rampulla

DEFINITION/EPIDEMIOLOGY

Patients afflicted with addiction have health, emotional, family, social, legal, and spiritual troubles that are vexing to the patient, the family, and the primary care provider. The HIV epidemic, the cocaine surge of the 1980s, the heroin surge of the 1990s, the advent of designer drugs, and the recognition of other morbidity and mortality associated with substance abuse has increasingly brought this problem to the attention of primary care providers. Patients with an addiction usually incur higher medical costs than patients with other chronic conditions.[1]

Although serious substance abuse disorders are rarely permanently reversed by a single treatment episode, formal treatment and brief counseling by a primary care provider reduce substance abuse and its hazards over time. Alcohol and nicotine are the most widely abused substances in the United States, resulting in the greatest burden of substance use–related suffering, meriting discussion in separate chapters. Nicotine dependence is discussed in Chapter 21, and Chapter 259 is devoted to alcohol abuse. In 2000, 14 million U.S. adults, representing 6.3% of the population, were estimated to be current users of illicit drugs, and 86.9 million were estimated to have used illicit drugs in their lifetime.[2] More than 50% of American youth are estimated to have tried an illicit drug by grade 12.[3]

The term *addiction* refers to a syndrome in which there is overriding concern with the use and acquisition of a drug, despite the negative consequences. Addiction involves drug obsession, self-dose escalation, and health, family, emotional, and economic deterioration. Addiction also usually implies a degree of tolerance and physiologic dependence. The term *abuse* usually refers to a problematic pattern of substance use that is not necessarily associated with a defined withdrawal syndrome. Not all patients who develop a physiologic dependence are "addicted." Physiologic dependence inevitably develops with the therapeutic use of several medications, such as opiates that are appropriately prescribed for chronic pain and corticosteroids that are prescribed for refractory inflammatory conditions. Although these patients may experience abstinence syndromes, they usually do not display addictive behaviors and should not be diagnosed with a substance use disorder on this basis alone.

The term *abstinence* can refer to the stereotyped adverse physiologic or psychologic syndromes of drug withdrawal; this term is often used interchangeably with the term *withdrawal*. An individual who is abstinent is drug free, whereas an individual in recovery is in the long-term process of attending to the spiritual, physical, and psychosocial needs that have been affected by addiction. *Withdrawal* refers to the process of removing the drug of dependence from the body, whereas *detoxification* generally refers to the process of administrating tapering doses of the same or cross-tolerant drugs to assist with withdrawal.

Tolerance refers to the need to increase the amount of drug to achieve the same effects. Because individuals who are tolerant have adapted to a certain level of drug use, they can experience both intoxication and abstinence at the same time. *Relapse* is the return to problematic drug use after a significant period of abstinence; it may involve a different drug than the patient's original drug of choice. A common example of this is the abstinent opioid addict who develops alcoholism.

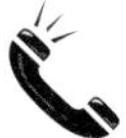

Psychiatric consultation is indicated for patients with suicidal/homicidal ideation.

PATHOPHYSIOLOGY

Addictive disorders are chronic relapsing conditions. The etiology of addictive disorders is probably the result of interactions among genetic and temperament susceptibility, psychosocial factors, and drug availability. Major hazards include overdose; withdrawal; violence and unintentional injuries; pregnancy and neonatal complications; social, economic, and family dysfunction; and the complications of injection drug use (IDU). Drugs can be conveniently, although not precisely, classified as central nervous system (CNS) depressants, opioids, stimulants, psychotomimetics and hallucinogens, inhalants, nicotine, and anabolic steroids.

On a neurobiologic level, addiction appears to be driven by activation of the dopaminergic neurons in the ventral tegmental area–nucleus accumbens (VTA-NA) of the brain in complex interaction with endogenous opioids (endorphins), gamma-aminobutyric acid (GABA), serotonin channels, acetylcholine, and adrenergic systems.[4] Drugs act at various sites to stimulate brain reward, thereby reinforcing repeated use. Long-term alterations in brain reward pathways may explained persistent heightened vulnerability to drug effects and continued dependence long after the clinical physical dependence has resolved. Such alterations may in part explain the chronic relapsing nature of addiction.

Major Drugs of Abuse

Drugs from one class can be used to enhance the desired or attenuate the undesired effects of drugs from another class. Understanding the features of these drug classes should be tempered by the knowledge that addicted patients usually take drugs from more than one category at a time.

Central Nervous System Sedatives. The major CNS sedatives are alcohol, barbiturates, benzodiazepines, and other compounds that are similar to either barbiturates or benzodiazepines. GABA is the major inhibitory neurotransmitter that lowers cell excitability, and sedatives generally depress brain activity by augmenting the GABA systems. Mild manifestations of sedative intoxication include tranquilization, fine lateral nystagmus, and slightly decreased alertness. Moderate intoxication is manifested as ataxia, slurred speech, coarse nystagmus, and sedation. An overdose of these substances produces somnolence, staggering, and marked dysarthria; this can progress to coma, respiratory depression, and death. The major hazards of sedative abuse include a dangerous abstinence syndrome, unintentional injuries, and overdose. Alcohol alters CNS membrane fluidity and interacts with GABA receptors, producing sedative effects (see Chapter 259). Although the perinatal effects of alcohol are well known, such research regarding other sedatives is sparse.

Barbiturates, which are derivatives of barbituric acid, both enhance and mimic the effect of GABA, thus depressing all brain activity. They are classified by their onset and duration of action, although their wide distribution in body fat and muscle compartments makes the relationship between serum concentration and action variable. Their prescribed use for sedation has largely been replaced by benzodiazepines, but phenobarbital is still useful for epilepsy and butabarbital combinations are effective for headaches. Barbiturates have a much narrower therapeutic index than do benzodiazepines. Chronic use may cause slowed learning, impaired memory, sleep disturbances, and emotional lability. The short-acting (e.g., pentobarbital) and intermediate-acting (e.g., amobarbital) barbiturates are most often abused. Long-acting barbiturates (e.g., phenobarbital) are not considered intoxicating, but individuals with addiction often take them in high doses with alcohol, producing dangerous impairment and toxicity. The chronic metabolism of barbiturates induces hepatic enzymes that can speed the metabolism of other sedatives, phenytoin, and warfarin. Because tolerance to barbiturates is incomplete, chronic users are still vulnerable to overdose. The drugs methaqualone (Quaalude), methyprylon, and glutethimide are synthetic compounds that are similar in toxicity and effect to barbiturates.

Benzodiazepines, formerly referred to as minor tranquilizers, facilitate the action of GABA at specific sites. They are often prescribed for relief of anxiety, insomnia, or muscle spasm or tension; for acute management of agitation; and for acute treatment of convulsions. Cross-tolerance and a wide therapeutic index make benzodiazepines good agents to assist with alcohol detoxification. In general, benzodiazepines are effective and have a wide margin of safety; however, their misuse is widespread among addicts. Their abuse potential seems to be associated with speed of onset and potency, with rapidly acting drugs (e.g., diazepam, clonazepam, and alprazolam) having the greatest potential for abuse and slower-acting compounds (e.g., oxazepam and prazepam) having the least. The high potency of clonazepam and alprazolam, with 1 mg roughly equivalent to 10 mg of diazepam, appears to contribute to their abuse potential and street value.[5] All benzodiazepines are metabolized to inactive compounds in the liver. Longer-acting benzodiazepines first require hepatic oxidation, which produces active drug metabolites. Flunitrazepam (Rohypnol) is a high-potency and short-acting benzodiazepine that has been implicated in acquaintance rape. It is prescribed for insomnia in many countries and is smuggled into the United States for illicit use. Zolpidem (Ambien) and Zaleplon (Sonata) are newer short-acting synthetic hypnotics that are similar in action to the benzodiazepines.

Gamma-hydroxybutyrate (GHB) is an emerging sedative of abuse that is a synthetic formulation of a normally occurring neurotransmitter. It induces anesthesia, petit mal seizures, and probably dependence. It is often synthesized in home laboratories; several deaths have been attributed to the ingestion of home GHB recipes that include lye. Emergency department reports of overdose and other GHB-related medical emergencies have risen sharply in recent years. These estimates are imprecise because GHB is short-acting and difficult to detect with laboratory tests.[6]

The severity of withdrawal from sedatives is generally proportional to the level and duration of use, with barbiturates and rapidly acting, high-potency benzodiazepines producing the most severe syndromes. Restlessness, anxiety, and mild tremors usually develop approximately 12 to 24 hours after discontinuation of a short-acting drug. The onset may be delayed for several days if the primary drug is long acting. Chronic liver dysfunction may increase drug storage and thereby delay the manifestations of withdrawal. Escalating symptoms, increased tremors, dissociative and perceptual symptoms, increased pulse and blood pressure, and hyperreflexia develop. At this point the patient becomes prone to convulsions, even if properly treated. If left untreated, withdrawal can progress to an acute psychosis that resembles delirium tremens. Patients experiencing high-dose sedative withdrawal need to be treated on an inpatient basis with a long-acting sedative like phenobarbital. Patients may be given a challenge dose of pentobarbital to estimate their habit and to guide dosing.[5]

Low-dose sedative withdrawal is a different phenomenon that is primarily characterized by waxing and waning anxiety, insomnia, irritability, and mild tremors. These individuals may or may not be addicted per se but may instead be physiologically dependent on therapeutic benzodiazepine regimens. Tapering of the benzodiazepine dose may take as long as 6 months. Patients usually benefit from additional psychosocial support and must be cautioned that they may experience a recurrence of the original symptoms for which they were initially prescribed the medication.

Opioids. Opioids produce their effects by interacting with endogenous opioid receptors throughout the CNS and intestines. Morphine is the prototypical opioid, with heroin (diacetylmorphine) the form most often seriously abused. There has been an increasing trend in new heroin use since 1992, although this trend appears to be leveling off. In 2000 approximately 2.8 million Americans report using heroin at some time in their lives.[7] Heroin is illegal in the United States and is sold on the streets as a white or brown powder; it is usually diluted with sugar, talc, baking soda, aspirin, or quinine. It is sometimes mixed with scopolamine, strychnine, or other poisons. Heroin may be insufflated (snorted), smoked, or dissolved and injected. Most heroin users eventually turn to IV use and rarely return to other routes.[8] Synthetic opioids include methadone, propoxyphene, meperidine, and fentanyl. Tramadol (Ultram) is a newer synthetic with both mu and kappa opioid activity. Overuse can provoke convulsions, but so far reports of abuse have been low.[9]

There has been an emerging problem with the illicit use of the sustained-release formulation of the prescription analgesic oxycodone. The sustained-release coating is easily bypassed by crushing the pill, making high-potency drug available for rapid effects. Tablets are reported to sell on the street for $0.50 to $1.00 per milligram.[10] Popular because of its excellent analgesic efficacy, the manufacturer is currently working on new formulations that would be less susceptible to abuse.

Opioids are useful for relief of pain and suffering, for cough suppression, and for their antidiarrheal effects. With a few individual differences, most opioids display similar pharmacologic actions and vary mostly in kinetics. Although chronic administration inevitably produces some degree of physiologic dependence, susceptibility to the development of addiction varies among individuals. Addiction, overdose, and premature labor are the most serious complications directly caused by opiates, with most other complications caused by IV drug use and hazardous lifestyles. The long-term mortality rate for heroin addicts may be 50 to 100 times that of the general population.[11] The use of home-synthesized meperidine and fentanyl analogues is associated with disastrous toxicity.

Aloofness, calmness, and mild sedation characterize opioid intoxication. A warm flush and sudden sensation of pleasure accompany injection, sometimes with mild nausea and vomiting. Individuals experience vague itching and characteristically scratch their nose. Opioid intoxication usually produces drowsiness and slowed movement but with less mental slowing than that caused by sedatives. Pupils constrict and respiratory rate and bowel motility decrease, effects that persist even if the individual has a high level of tolerance. Blood pressure and pulse are mildly decreased.

Stupor that progresses to coma, markedly slow and shallow respirations, and pulmonary edema characterize opioid overdose. Meperidine overdose and/or cerebral anoxia may produce dilated pupils; meperidine or propoxyphene overdose may produce seizures. Acute frothy pulmonary edema and eosinophilia are the prominent features of a hypersensitivity type of overdose. Naloxone, an intravenously administered pure opioid antagonist, reverses the stupor, usually precipitating an opioid abstinence syndrome. It is short acting, and the patient should be observed for at least 24 hours, especially if overdose with a long-acting opioid is suspected. A legion of other toxic, neurologic and metabolic causes should be sought when a patient who is stuporous does not respond to naloxone.

A stereotypic abstinence syndrome develops as blood levels of opiates decline. The timing of this syndrome varies with the duration of the drug's effect—withdrawal from long-acting opiates begins later and lasts longer. Severity is proportional to the size and duration of the habit. The syndrome starts with overwhelming fatigue and is followed by restlessness, pupillary dilation, temperature intolerance, general aches/arthromyalgias, increased respiratory rate and yawning, runny eyes and nose, piloerection, sweating, and hyperactive bowels. Nausea, vomiting, and an elevated blood pressure and pulse may occur. Vital signs may reveal little about withdrawal severity, with respiratory rate being the most affected by opioid withdrawal. The most reliable physical signs are pupillary dilation and constantly hyperactive bowel sounds. The patient is unable to sleep despite the administration of sedatives. Objectively, the syndrome resembles an acute episode of influenza that is accompanied by parasympathetic hyperactivity and intense drug craving. The syndrome can precipitate premature labor but otherwise is not dangerous. It is now recognized that protracted, low-level symptoms may persist for months or years.

Pharmacologic treatment of abstinence may include tapering doses of the long-acting opioid methadone, the alpha-2 adrenergic antihypertensive clonidine, or the mixed opioid agonist-antagonist drug buprenorphine. Clonidine attenuates some abstinence symptoms and, in combination with other medication for myalgias, abdominal cramps, and insomnia, can help to withdraw patients from opioids. When abstinence is established, patients can begin taking naltrexone, an antagonist that blocks the effect of opioids and assists some highly motivated addicts to maintain drug abstinence. Patients should be cautioned that naltrexone will block the effects of opioid analgesics, and liver function tests (LFTs) should be monitored.

Methadone detoxification may be prescribed only through specially licensed drug treatment programs or for patients who are acutely hospitalized for a coexistent medical condition. Methadone maintenance involves the administration of high oral doses of methadone to substitute for and to block the effect of illicit opioids. Although patients remain physiologically dependent, these programs have repeatedly demonstrated effectiveness in reducing illicit opioid use and the harm associated with opioid addiction. Methadone maintenance is the treatment of choice for heroin addicts who are pregnant. Their neonates are born physically dependent but can be safely withdrawn in the nursery. Methadone maintenance programs should also provide counseling, case management, and other support services. Higher dosage (80 to 100 mg/day) appear to be more effective than lower doses.[12] Remaining on methadone for 1 year or longer is associated with better overall outcomes in terms of alcohol use, illicit drug use, and criminal involvement.[13] *levo*-Acetyl-alpha-methadol (LAAM) is a longer-acting synthetic opiate that may be given three times per week and has recently been approved for use by several clinics that already dispense methadone.

Federal approval of the use of buprenorphine for detoxification and maintenance is pending. It is already widely used in inpatient detoxification programs, and studies have so far indicated that it is nearly as effective as methadone in helping to achieve abstinence from illicit opioids.[14]

Central Nervous System Stimulants. CNS stimulants comprise a wide array of drugs that increase alertness, cause excitation, and sometimes cause euphoria. Stimulant drugs include cocaine, amphetamines, and methylphenidate, as well as several amphetamine-like psychotomimetic compounds. Use of stimulants in the United States appears to have declined or leveled off in recent years.[15]

Major stimulants are often used in combination with opioids or sedatives. Mild stimulant intoxication is manifest by increased alertness, hyperactivity, anorexia, blood pressure, and pulse elevation. Intoxication is manifest by euphoric excitement, hyperstimulation, and grandiosity. Chronic stimulant users develop nervousness, irritability, insomnia and, often, paranoia. Depression, hypersomnia, lethargy, poor concentration, and drug craving characterize stimulant withdrawal.

Cocaine hydrochloride has the properties of a CNS and peripheral nervous system stimulant and local anesthetic. The major methods of cocaine use involve sniffing, injecting, or vaporization (smoking "crack"). Cocaine enhances the effects of dopamine, serotonin, and norepinephrine by elevating synaptic levels. MRI changes have been noted with both cocaine administration and during drug-free episodes of cocaine craving.[16]

Restlessness, agitation, paranoia, and panic characterize acute toxicity. Blood pressure and pulse increase, and pupils dilate. Overdose can produce cardiac arrhythmias, including ventricular fibrillation and seizures. Vasospasm can cause myocardial, cerebral, or hepatic infarction, even in users with normal arteries.

This also contributes to the premature separation of membranes when used during pregnancy. Different routes of administration account for different intoxication effects. The onset is within minutes when inhaled nasally and within seconds when injected or smoked. The duration of effect is brief, and the withdrawal syndrome appears quickly; this reinforces use and leads to frequent administration and the accumulation of metabolites. Alcohol and cocaine together form cocaethylene, a compound that appears to intensify cocaine's euphoric effects and possibly increases the risk for sudden death. The need for frequent multiple injections of cocaine probably increases the risk of acquiring HIV infection compared with other IV drugs of abuse. Prostitution often accompanies crack cocaine addiction, which makes cocaine smoking an independent risk factor for sexually transmitted disease. The prenatal effects of cocaine use have not been as drastic as originally feared. Cocaine-exposed infants and young children display delayed motor development and impaired ability to regulate attention.[17]

Amphetamine and amphetamine-like stimulants have effects that are qualitatively similar to those of cocaine, but their effects are more prolonged. The two most commonly abused forms of these substances are methamphetamine, which is synthesized in home laboratories, and methylphenidate, which is diverted from pharmaceutical supplies. The methods of methamphetamine use involve the oral route, sniffing, smoking, and injection. Tolerance develops rapidly, and users become sensitized and seizure prone. Chronic heavy use causes a paranoid psychosis that is difficult to manage, and it may cause long-term degeneration of dopaminergic neurons. IV amphetamine use is associated with the development of vasculitis. Inadvertent subcutaneous injections of methylphenidate produce deep purulent abscesses.

Adolescent use of 3,4-methylene dioxymethamphetamine (MDMA), also known as "ecstasy," has increased in recent years.[18] MDMA has a chemical structure similar to both amphetamines and mescaline and produces both stimulant and hallucinogenic effects. MDMA stimulates the release of serotonin, producing a feeling of empathy and closeness and an enhanced sense of pleasure, confidence, and endurance, with effects lasting several minutes to hours. Psychologic effects include confusion, depression, sleep problems, and anxiety that may persist for weeks. Physical effects include muscle tension, involuntary teeth-clenching, blurred vision, faintness, elevated blood pressure and pulse, and altered control of body temperature. The drug, which allows users to dance for extended periods of time, is usually used in hot crowded nightclubs, increasing the risk for hyperthermia, dehydration, and heart or kidney failure.[19] The drug appears to cause long-lasting serotonin neuron loss and memory damage.[20]

Stimulant users who have persistent depression may benefit from antidepressant therapy, but no medication has been demonstrated to effectively treat stimulant withdrawal or drug craving. Sedation is often necessary during acute toxicity, and medications are often needed for detoxification from a coexisting dependence on sedatives and/or opioids.

Psychotomimetics and Hallucinogens. Psychotomimetics and hallucinogens are an informal category of drugs that alter perceptions and/or mimic psychotic or dissociative states. Included in this category are cannabinoids, lysergic acid diethylamide (LSD) and similarly acting hallucinogens, and phencyclidine (PCP). As with stimulant drugs, no medication has been demonstrated to effectively treat hallucinogen withdrawal or drug craving. Sedation is often needed during episodes of acute toxicity.

Cannabinoids, in the form of marijuana, are the active ingredients in the leaves or resin of the *Cannabis sativa* hemp plant; they are either smoked or taken orally. Marijuana is the most commonly abused illicit substance. Intoxication produces a mildly dissociated and dreamy mental state, an elevated pulse, dilated pupils, an increased appetite, and a characteristic odor. In high doses it may produce hallucinations and, idiosyncratically, paranoia. Marijuana use is greatest in adolescence and young adulthood, and possibly hinders emotional development and initiative. Heavy users appear to be prone to a mild abstinence syndrome that consists of nervousness, restlessness, and an appetite and sleep disturbance.

PCP and the related compound ketamine are dissociative anesthetics whose action closely mimics schizophrenia. PCP is most commonly smoked but can be absorbed via any route. Toxicity is dose dependent, with individuals varying markedly in their responses. Mild toxicity includes giddiness, elation, expansiveness, and mild dissociative states. Highly toxic individuals display disorientation, a bizarre affect, rotary nystagmus, ataxia, tachycardia, and a dissociative lack of concern with pain or the external world. These individuals are prone to self-mutilation and are difficult to contain despite sedation. Deaths from overdose are caused by hypertensive crisis, respiratory arrest, and status epilepticus.

The true hallucinogenic drugs are ergots (LSD), phenylalkylamines (mescaline), indolealkylamines (psilocybin), and the amphetamine-like drug MDMA (ecstasy). As with cannabis, young people are the main users of hallucinogens. LSD is the prototype and appears to produce its action by serotonin inhibition and dopamine stimulation. It is highly potent, and its effects are noted with oral ingestions of tiny fractions of a gram.

Tolerance to hallucinogens develops rapidly, sometimes after a single dose. Giddiness, visual and other sensory distortions, marked dissociation, widely dilated pupils, and peripheral vasoconstriction characterize intoxication. Patients may develop acute panic or psychosis. The effects last 8 to 12 hours; some patients report recurrent manifestations months to years later.

Inhalants. The term *inhalant* describes an informal grouping of differing substances that are used by inhaling their vapors. Solvents (e.g., acetone, benzene, toluene), nitrous oxide gas, and volatile nitrites (e.g., amyl nitrite, butyl nitrite) are members of this group. Solvent inhalation produces a rapid onset of sedative-like intoxication, including dizziness, drowsiness, slurred speech, and ataxia. Chronic complications include cerebral atrophy, peripheral neuropathy, toxic hepatitis, and bone marrow toxicity, as well as the complications associated with lead poisoning and other impurities. Nitrous oxide is usually obtained from medical or laboratory supplies or from commercial aerosol sprays. It displaces CNS oxygen rapidly after inhalation, causing an acute euphoric state followed by a brief period of sedation; the major hazard is anoxia. The effect of the volatile nitrites is short-lived flushing, dizziness, euphoria, and hypotension. Chronic use can lead to methemoglobinemia, which is evidenced by cyanosis that does not respond to oxygen administration.

Anabolic Steroids. Anabolic steroids are synthetic derivatives of testosterone that are used to enhance athletic performance and build lean muscle mass. They are usually smuggled from outside the United States and sold surreptitiously in gymnasiums. Internet user groups have been a recent supply source. Injection is the most common route of use, which makes the user susceptible to the hazards of unsterile injections. Toxicity is characterized by aggression, irritability, impulsiveness, and elation. Users also have disturbed hormonal cycles, acne, hair loss, excessive muscle growth, testicular atrophy or clitoral hypertrophy, breast enlargement or atrophy, liver toxicity, and elevated low-density lipoprotein. A common pattern of use is "cycling," which involves taking these drugs for weeks and then stopping them for short periods. Lethargy, restlessness, insomnia, and anorexia often occur with abstinence.

Injection Drug Use. IDU violates the first line of defense of the body, leaving the user vulnerable to infection, chemical impurities, and immediate drug toxicity. This method of use is obviously a greater hazard when injection equipment is shared. The Centers for Disease Control and Prevention reports that in 1999, 25% of HIV infections in adults were acquired by injecting drugs.[21] HIV-1 has been found to remain viable in used syringes for as long as 6 weeks.[22] Immunologic abnormalities include hypergammaglobulinemia, which may be related to repeated intravenous introduction of impurities or hepatitis C. Chronic rheumatologic conditions are a consequence, as sometimes are false-positive serologic tests for syphilis. Neurologic complications include brain abscesses from endocarditis, cerebral anoxia, and transverse myelitis. Lung granulomas and abscesses can result from particles and pathogens that filter through the pulmonary circulation. Endocarditis may result from bacteria and fungi that settle in the endocardium. In the United States, IDU is the major means of transmission for hepatitis viruses B and C and has been linked to serious outbreaks of hepatitis D. Most injection drug users have serologic evidence of remote hepatitis virus B exposure. Renal disease may be the result of immune complex deposition, endocarditis, or nephrotoxic impurities. Vertebral osteomyelitis from hematologic seeding of the cancellous bone is the most common serious musculoskeletal condition associated with IDU. Cellulitis, subcutaneous abscesses, and fascial abscesses are a common result of injection infiltration outside of the vein. Phlebitis is common, particularly when irritating drugs are injected. Poor venous access complicates the care of these patients, particularly when the management of comorbid conditions calls for frequent laboratory testing. This is a major disincentive for addicts to seek health care. Needle exchange and other "harm reduction" methods have been used with some success and much controversy to reduce the public and individual health hazards of IDU.

CLINICAL PRESENTATION AND PHYSICAL EXAMINATION

Patients may have no history of a recognized addictive disorder, may be actively addicted, may be in early recovery, or may have a history of addiction and be well established in recovery. As a screening tool, the *CAGE* questions regarding *C*oncern about drinking, *A*ggravating others by drinking, *G*uilt about drinking, and taking an "*E*ye-opener" drink in the morning can be adapted to include other drugs[23] (see Box 259-1).These questions can be woven into a standard history and should be asked if patients report drinking or drug use when asked about medications or lifestyle. Poor compliance and requests for disability testimony by an otherwise healthy patient should raise concerns about the presence of substance abuse. Behavioral problems appear first, and early manifestations of addiction are rarely apparent with routine examination. The time of the last substance use can be asked when reviewing medications, and the temporal relationship between substance use and symptoms should be considered.

Addiction-related causes of fever are endocarditis, acute retroviral syndrome and HIV-associated infections, anticholinergic ingestion, and sedative withdrawal. Withdrawal from opioids will cause chills and sweats that are not accompanied by fever. A simultaneously elevated pulse and blood pressure often results from sedative withdrawal or stimulant toxicity. Weight may fluctuate because of an irregular diet, wasting infections, or chronic liver disease. Generalized edema may be due to liver failure from chronic hepatitis, kidney failure from glomerulopathies, or heart failure from valvular insufficiency or cardiomyopathy. Overwhelming lethargy and fatigue accompany withdrawal from stimulants and very early opioid withdrawal. Varying degrees of lethargy are seen with coexisting vegetative depressions, chronic hepatitis, and kidney failure. Headaches commonly accompany alcohol and cocaine withdrawal. Sudden headaches may be related to cocaine-induced venospasms. Many addicts have a history of head trauma or brain abscess; therefore it is helpful if cranial nerve deficits are noted in initial examinations. Visual changes may be caused by retinal emboli from IDU or from several complications of HIV infection. Sedatives may cause diplopia. The sclerae should be examined for icterus. Opioid withdrawal or cannabis, stimulant, or hallucinogen intoxications dilate the pupils, and the use of opioids causes pupils to constrict. Sedative and alcohol intoxication causes nystagmus. Rotary nystagmus is a unique feature of PCP intoxication. Nasal heroin or cocaine use causes mucosal inflammation. Perforation of the nasal septum is caused by mucosal vasoconstriction and subsequent tissue ischemia with cocaine use. Inhalation of hot crack vapors can cause flaming pharyngitis and tonsillar swelling. Apart from well-known HIV-related adenopathy, IV drug users often have swollen lymph nodes in response to local injections. The cervical spine is a possible focus of osteomyelitis.

Due to hypersensitivity, nasal heroin use causes a bronchitis that resembles severe asthma. The bronchitis tends to get worse with each subsequent exposure and is difficult to control with steroids and bronchodilators if the patient continues to inhale heroin. Cocaine may make the heart hyperdynamic through its adrenergic effects, or it may slow myocardial impulses through its anesthetic effects. Ischemic chest pain can result from vasospasm that damages the intima and predisposes the patient to subsequent coronary artery disease. A variety of cocaine-induced arrhythmias can cause sudden death. Patients with endocarditis are usually febrile, with a new or changed murmur, petechiae, and possible signs of metastatic infections. A wide pulse pressure may represent secondary aortic regurgitation. The strain of acute sedative withdrawal may precipitate a serious cardiac event in a patient with preexisting cardiac disease.

Evidence of ascites should be determined in a patient with increasing abdominal girth. Mild tenderness in the right upper quadrant may be the only clinical manifestation of chronic hepatitis. The visceral pain and hyperactive bowel sounds from opioid withdrawal can be severe enough to mimic an acute abdominal emergency. Bleeding in the stool may be from alcohol-induced gastritis, liver congestion, coagulopathies, or hemorrhoids from opioid-related constipation.

The usual desperate life of a patient with addiction leaves little time and energy for concern regarding regular Papanicolaou (Pap) tests and breast, testicular, rectal, and prostate examinations. In addition to neglecting these health maintenance examinations, addicts often exchange sex for drugs, adding to the concern about sexually transmitted diseases. Many addicts also have a history of sexual trauma and avoid genital examinations, which they can find quite frightening. The possibility of pregnancy is a consideration with all fertile female patients.

Vertebral tenderness raises the question of osteomyelitis or epidural abscess. Swollen and tender joints suggest septic arthritis from injected pathogens, gonorrhea, or syphilis. Arthromyalgias may be a prominent feature of opioid withdrawal. Arthromyalgias may also commonly accompany polyarteritis syndromes, which are associated with IV amphetamine abuse and with hepatitis C. Localized muscle hypertrophy and calcification from repeated needle manipulation ("drug abuser's elbow") may present as a worrisome mass.

Getting to know patients over time is the most useful way for the primary care provider to understand the neurologic and psychiatric conditions. Intoxication with alcohol or sedatives causes incoordination. Broad-based gaits are associated with alcohol-induced cerebellar degeneration. Intention tremors are the conspicuous physical sign of sedative withdrawal. Compression and trauma are the most common causes of mononeuropathy. Neuropathy of the ulnar or radial nerves sometimes follows prolonged periods of unconsciousness and results from compression of the nerves against the bony prominences. Peripheral manifestations of alcoholism and/or thiamine deficiency include proximally progressing decreased peripheral sensation and deep tendon reflexes. Symmetric hyperreflexia suggests stimulant drug toxicity or sedative withdrawal, whereas sedative toxicity causes reflexes to be sluggish. Seizure disorders are complicated by multiple drug use, head trauma, and past cerebral anoxia. Stimulant toxicity and withdrawal from sedatives or alcohol are the most common causes of drug-related convulsions. Substance abuse is the most common precipitant of psychiatric symptoms.

Edema of the hands without coexisting ankle or facial edema is usually a result of damaged veins. Needle marks from cocaine injection are usually multiple and recent, whereas those from heroin use are more deliberately tracked along large veins. Venous insufficiency and attendant complications are common, especially in older addicts. Injection of irritating substances causes chemical phlebitis with varying degrees of severity. Palmar erythema suggests chronic liver disease. Patients often have scars from cigarette burns or wrist cutting.

DIAGNOSTICS

The use of laboratory tests should be individualized and based on the clinical presentation. Toxicology testing is essential in evaluating many emergency situations. Drug screening may be useful in monitoring patients in treatment programs or receiving prescriptions for controlled substances, but it may give little information about addiction per se because screening tests reflect use during a fairly narrow period of time. Commercially prepared urine enzyme immune assays are the most commonly used drug screening tests, giving a positive or negative test for several classes but not all drugs of abuse. Drugs concentrate in the urine, making urine tests generally better for screening purposes than serum tests. Chromatography tests are necessary for specific serum levels of specific substances. Because psychiatric symptoms are so often caused or influenced by substance use, toxicology tests may be most useful in evaluating refractory psychiatric symptoms

Anemia and thrombocytopenia are often due to liver disease or HIV infection. Liver function abnormalities are often due to viral hepatitis or alcoholism. Hepatitis and syphilis serologic screening should be conducted at some time. Patients should be counseled and offered HIV testing in the office or given information about anonymous HIV test sites. Urine or blood human chorionic gonadotropin (hCG) testing for pregnancy is often indicated in guiding the pace, intensity, and nature of treatment plans. Baseline renal function tests are useful in detecting glomerular nephropathies associated with IV drug use. Baseline thyroid function tests are useful because sedatives and stimulants can mimic hypothyroidism or hyperthyroidism, respectively, whereas their abstinence syndromes cause the reverse effects. Patients usually need frequently neglected routine health maintenance screening tests such as PAP smears and lipid levels.

MANAGEMENT

Conveying a hopeful attitude is important. There is no way to predict when a single episodic encounter may the time that the patient makes substantial progress. Because substance use disorders are often chronic conditions that progress slowly over time, primary care providers address a patient's substance abuse problems, monitor progress, and provide regular supportive counseling. This provides the patient with a stable relationship during which harm reduction and keeping up with health maintenance can pay off in long-term benefits.

The primary care brief intervention format of (1) providing feedback of relevant data, (2) emphasizing patient responsibility and self-efficacy, (3) advising about recommended change, (4) providing a menu of helpful options, and (4) taking an empathetic approach is helpful whether or not the patient enters a formal treatment program. Patients should be counseled about risk-reduction strategies such as not sharing needles, using condoms, and not driving while using. The provider should be familiar with local treatment, consultation, and case management services and have a handy referral list.

Although several studies suggest that an inpatient detoxification is unlikely to affect the long-term course of addiction, it may be needed to stabilize the patient and facilitate entry into more long-term treatment. Other treatment often is impossible without detoxification first. Individual motivated patients sometimes significantly reduce drug use after a brief detoxification without other services.[24]

Common formal treatment programs include outpatient methadone maintenance, long-term residential treatment programs, outpatient drug-free programs, and short-term inpatient rehabilitation programs. Some patients find regular acupuncture to be an effective treatment for detoxification and craving. Most outpatient substance abuse counseling is based on cognitive-behavioral and/or 12-Step models (see Chapter 259). Patients in longer-term recovery often benefit from insight-oriented therapy. Intensive outpatient/partial hospitalization programs for less-stable patients are designed to provide a daily therapeutic milieu while having the advantage of allowing patients to stay at home or even participating in the evening while attending work during the day. Long-term residential programs offer a drug-free therapeutic living environment that is staffed by counselors and usually other recovering addicts. The optimal duration of involvement in long-term residential treatment appears to be 6 months.[25] These programs are especially helpful in supporting the recovery of addicts who are homeless and reintegrating them into society. Residential programs for these patients usually require a more lengthy stay. Adolescent programs should include strong peer and family components.

The primary care provider may become a collaborative part of the treatment team and/or continue to treat the patient's medical conditions, encourage continuing participation in the program, and schedule follow-up visits after treatment termination to monitor progress and help prevent relapse. How to judiciously prescribe controlled substances is one of the major difficulties providers face in caring for these patients. Drug-seeking patients may feign symptoms and request medications for longer periods of time than their medical conditions dictate. Medications that can be abused may reinitiate craving and addiction in patients who have achieved drug abstinence, whereas inadequately treated pain, depression, or anxiety may also be a trigger for relapse. Recognizing that symptom relief is a legitimate goal of care, the guidelines of the Drug Enforcement Agency (DEA) ask providers to consider the following when controlled substances are indicated: the severity of the patient's symptoms and ability to tolerate them, the patient's reliability in taking medications, and the addiction liability of the medication. The DEA also recognizes that patients have a corresponding obligation to comply with the prescriber's instructions.[26]

Opiates, barbiturates, and stimulants are Schedule II drugs and have the highest potential for abuse. In general, prescribing opiates to treat opiate withdrawal is restricted to methadone programs and acute medical situations such as hospital admission. Schedule III and IV medications are considered by the DEA to have a lower potential for abuse. Prescriptions of controlled substances should be written only for recognized indications and for limited amounts, and they are usually recommended for finite time periods. The number of doses to be dispensed should be written out both in longhand and numerically to discourage alteration. It is good practice to consult with addiction and/or pain specialists when prescribing controlled substances to patients with addiction. Pharmacologic treatment includes prescribing detoxification regimens and/or naltrexone to block alcohol craving and the effects of opioids. Antidepressant medications (usually selective serotonin reuptake inhibitors) may be useful for dysthymic states that persist after detoxification. The antidepressant trazodone is a useful adjunctive medication for persistent insomnia. It has a low potential for overdose and addiction, but its efficacy varies. When used to assist with sleep, a low dose is taken approximately 30 to 40 minutes before going to bed.

COMPLICATIONS

There are a myriad of complications of drug abuse, and they affect patients and families socially, psychologically, legally, and physically. Every body system can be affected, placing the patient at risk for cardiac arrhythmias, infections, injuries, seizures, coma, and liver, heart, or kidney failure.

INDICATIONS FOR REFERRAL/HOSPITALIZATION

Referral to an inpatient or outpatient addiction program should always be discussed with actively addicted patients. Referral to the emergency department should be considered for patients with unexplained fevers, delirium, overdose, severe sedative withdrawal, vital sign instability, severe headaches, chest pain, acute shortness of breath, acute abdominal pain and gastrointestinal bleeding, or active suicidality. These patients often need to be stabilized and considered for hospitalization. Hospitalized substance abusers are notoriously difficult patients who are often unwelcome and sometimes undertreated for discomfort. In addition to assisting with the medical aspects of care, collaboration with the inpatient team helps humanize the patient and helps the hospital staff recognize and work with problematic behaviors. Patients on methadone should be kept on their usual dosage and receive normal or slightly higher doses of pain medication as indicated by their medical conditions.

Emergency department/physician consultation should be considered for patients with unexplained fevers, delirium, overdose, severe sedative withdrawal, vital sign instability, severe headaches, chest pain, acute shortness of breath, acute abdominal pain and gastrointestinal bleeding, or active suicidality.

Medical clearance is often requested of the primary care provider before admission to a detoxification or rehabilitation program. A brief history and physical examination are necessary to identify and stabilize acute health problems. It is helpful to know what resources are available at the program for which the patient is being cleared, because the program may or may not have medical support or medication on site. It should be clear to both the patient and the program that "medically clear" does not mean that the patient does not have outstanding health problems that need future attention; it is simply an assessment that the patient is stable enough to enter a program.

PATIENT AND FAMILY EDUCATION

Both patients and families need to understand that resources are available to help with addiction. As with the patient, a feeling of hopefulness should be conveyed to significant others. The importance of recognizing symptoms of infections and other complications, plus the need to seek treatment when necessary, should be emphasized. The disease, treatment, nutritional counseling, and side effects of prescribed medications should be carefully explained. Frequent follow-up is important both for health promotion and to help patients and families cope with the devastating effects of substance abuse.

The following are sources of information for patients with substance abuse problems:

Center for Substance Abuse Prevention (CSAP)
5600 Fishers Lane, Rockwall II Building, 9th floor
Rockville, MD 20857
(301) 443-0365
Website: http://www.samhsa.gov/centers/csap

Center for Substance Abuse Treatment (CSAT)
5600 Fishers Lane, Rockwall II Building, Suite 618
Rockville, MD 20857
(301) 443-5052
Website: www.samhsa.gov/centers/csat
Hotline: (800) 662-HELP; for information and treatment resources

Directory of state alcohol and drug abuse agencies:
Website: http://www.treatment.org_states

Hazelden
CO.3, PO Box 11
Center City, MN 55012-0011
(800) 257-7810
Website: http://www.hazelden.org/index.dbm

SAMHSA, Office of Applied Studies
5600 Fishers Lane
Rockville, MD 20857
(301) 443-6239; (301) 443-4795 (general information about SAMHSA)
Website: http://www.drugabusestatistics.samhsa.gov
SAMHSA distributes a National Directory of Drug Abuse and Alcoholism Treatment and Prevention Programs (1-800-729-6686).

Treatment Improvement Protocols (TIPs) are provided as a service of the Substance Abuse and Mental Health Service Administration's Center for Substance Abuse Treatment (CSAT). TIPs can be obtained through:

The National Clearinghouse for Alcohol and Drug Information (NCADI)
PO Box 2345
Rockville, MD 20852
(301) 468-2600; (800) 729-6686
Website: http://www.samhsa.gov/centers/clearinghouse

REFERENCES

1. Garnick DW and others: Do individuals with substance abuse diagnoses incur higher charges than individuals with other chronic conditions? *J Subst Abuse Treat* 14:457-465, 1997.
2. Substance Abuse and Mental Health Services Administration (SAMHSA): *2000 National household survey on drug abuse,* Washington, DC, The Administration. Retrieved August 12, 2002, from the World Wide Web: www.samhsa.gov/oas/NHSDA/2kNHSDA.
3. Johnston LD, O'Malley PM, Bachman JG: *Demographic subgroup trends for various licit and illicit drugs, 1975-2000* (Monitoring the Future Occasional Paper No. 53), Ann Arbor, MI, 2001, Institute for Social Research. Retrieved August 12, 2002, from the World Wide Web: www.monitoringthefuture.org.
4. Hyman SE: Why does the brain prefer opium to broccoli? *Harvard Rev Psychiatry* 2:43-46, 1994.
5. Wesson DR, Center for Substance Abuse Treatment: *Detoxification from alcohol and other drugs,* Rockville, Md, 1995, DHHS publication No. (SMA) 95-3046, Treatment Improvement Protocol (TIP) Series, No. 19, US Department of Health and Human Services.
6. National Institute of Drug Abuse: Conference highlights increasing GHB abuse, *NIDA Notes* 16(2), May 2001.
7. Substance Abuse and Mental Health Services Administration (SAMHSA): *2000 National household survey on drug abuse,* Washington, DC, The Administration. Retrieved August 12, 2002, from the World Wide Web: http://www.samhsa.gov/oas/NHSDA/2kNHSDA.
8. Strang J and others: How constant is an individual's route of heroin administration? data from treatment and non-treatment samples, *Drug Alcohol Depend* 46:115-118, 1997.
9. Cicero TJ and others: A postmarketing surveillance program to monitor Ultram (tramadol hydrochloride) abuse in the United States, *Drug Alcohol Depend* 57:7-22, 1999.
10. US Department of Justice: *Drugs and chemicals of concern: Oxycodone,* Washington, DC, August 2001, The Department. Retrieved August 12, 2002, from the World Wide Web: http://www.deadiversion.usdoj.gov/drugs_concern/oxycodone/summary.htm.
11. Hser YI and others: A 33-year follow-up of narcotic addicts, *Arch Gen Psychiatry* 58:503-508, 2001.
12. Strain EC and others: Moderate vs high-dose methadone in the treatment of opioid dependence: a randomized control trial, *JAMA* 281:1000-1005, 1999.
13. Simpson DD, Joe GW, Rowan-Szal GA: Drug abuse treatment retention and process effects on follow-up outcomes, *Drug Alcohol Depend* 48:227-235.
14. Barnett PG, Rodgers JH, Bloch DA: A meta-analysis comparing buprenorphine to methadone for treatment of opioid dependence, *Addiction* 96:683-690, 2001.
15. Substance Abuse and Mental Health Services Administration (SAMHSA): *2000 National household survey on drug abuse,* Washington, DC, The Administration. Retrieved August 12, 2002, from the World Wide Web: http://www.samhsa.gov/oas/NHSDA/2kNHSDA.
16. Breiter HC and others: Acute effects of cocaine on human brain activity and emotion, *Neuron* 19:591-611, 1997.
17. Smeriglio VL, Wilcox HC: Prenatal drug exposure and child outcome, *Clin Perinatol* 26:1-16, 1999.
18. Bolla KI, McCann UD, Ricaurte GA: Memory impairment in abstinent MDMA ("ecstasy") users, *Neurology* 51:1532-1537, 1998.
19. Centers for Disease Control and Prevention: *HIV prevention strategic plan through 2005.* Retrieved November 17, 2001, from the World Wide Web: www.cdc.gov/hiv/pubs/prev-strat-plan.pdf.
20. Heimer R, Abdal N: Viability of HIV-1 in syringes: implications for interventions among injection drug users, *AIDS Reader* 10:410-417, 2000.
21. Ewing J: Detecting alcoholism: the CAGE questionnaire, *JAMA* 252:1905-1907, 1984.
22. Chutuape MA and others: Detoxification beneficial as a stand-alone treatment, *DATA* 20:1-6, 2001.
23. McCusker J and others: The effects of planned duration of residential drug abuse treatment on recovery and HIV risk behavior, *Am J Public Health* 87:1637-1644, 1997.
24. Severinghaus J, Kinney J: Medical management. In Kinney J, editor: *Clinical manual of substance abuse,* ed 2, St Louis, 1996, Mosby.
25. Johnston LD, O'Malley PM, Bachman JG: *Demographic subgroup trends for various licit and illicit drugs, 1975-2000* (Monitoring the Future Occasional Paper No. 53), Ann Arbor, MI, 2001, Institute for Social Research. Retrieved August 12, 2002, from the World Wide Web: http://monitoringthefuture.org/.
26. Johnston LD, O'Malley PM, Bachman JG: *Demographic subgroup trends for various licit and illicit drugs, 1975-2000* (Monitoring the Future Occasional Paper No. 53), Ann Arbor, MI: Institute for Social Research. Retrieved August 12, 2002, from the World Wide Web: http://monitoringthefuture.org.

INDEX

A

Page numbers followed by *f* indicate figures; *b* indicates boxes, and *t* indicates tables

B

E

F

G

H

O

P

ISBN 0-323-02032-1